A Dictionary Of Medical Science Containing A Concise Explanation Of The Various Subjects And Terms Of Physiology, Pathology, Hygiene, Therapeutics, Pharmacology, Obstetrics, Medical Jurisprudence, &C., With The French And Other Synonymes; Notices Of Climate, And Of Celebrated Mineral Waters; Formulæ For Various Officinal, Empirical, And Dietetic Preparations, Etc (Volume 5)

Robley Dunglison

Alpha Editions

This Edition Published in 2020

ISBN: 9789354300905

Design and Setting By
Alpha Editions
www.alphaedis.com
Email – info@alphaedis.com

As per information held with us this book is in Public Domain.
This book is a reproduction of an important historical work. Alpha Editions
uses the best technology to reproduce historical work in the same manner
it was first published to preserve its original nature. Any marks or number
seen are left intentionally to preserve its true form.

Entered, according to the Act of Congress, in the year 1851, by

BLANCHARD AND LEA,

in the Office of the Clerk of the District Court of the United States, in and for the Eastern District of Pennsylvania.

Printed by T. K. & P. G. Collins.

TO

ROBERT M. PATTERSON, M.D.

EX-PRESIDENT OF THE AMERICAN PHILOSOPHICAL SOCIETY, ETC. ETC.

ONCE HIS COLLEAGUE IN THE UNIVERSITY OF VIRGINIA,

ALWAYS HIS FRIEND,

This Work is Dedicated,

WITH UNCHANGED AND UNCHANGEABLE SENTIMENTS, BY

THE AUTHOR.

PREFACE TO THE EIGHTH EDITION.

In issuing a new edition of his Dictionary the Author has, again, the pleasure to express his acknowledgments for the reception it has met with from the profession. The last two editions comprised about nine thousand subjects and terms not contained in the edition immediately preceding, many of which had been introduced into medical terminology in consequence of the progress of the science, and others had escaped him in the previous revisions.

That the author has not suffered his exertions to diminish, in the preparation of the present edition, is sufficiently manifested by the fact, that he has added about *four thousand terms*, which are not to be found in the last. These additions have necessarily required a great amount of labour, which has been cheerfully bestowed, however, in order that the work might be rendered still more worthy of the vast favour which it has experienced. It has been the anxious desire of the author to make it a satisfactory and desirable—if not indispensable—lexicon, in which the student may search without disappointment for every term that has been legitimated in the nomenclature of the science; and the present very carefully revised, greatly enlarged, and accurately printed edition cannot fail to be more extensively useful, and to offer stronger claims to the attention of the practitioner and student, than any of its predecessors.

ROBLEY DUNGLISON.

PHILADELPHIA, 18 GIRARD STREET.

EXTRACT FROM THE

PREFACE TO THE SECOND EDITION.

THE present undertaking was suggested by the frequent complaints, made by the author's pupils, that they were unable to meet with information on numerous topics of professional inquiry,—especially of recent introduction,—in the medical dictionaries accessible to them. It may, indeed, be correctly affirmed, that we have no dictionary of medical subjects and terms which can be looked upon as adapted to the state of the science. In proof of this, the author need but remark, that he has found occasion to add several thousand medical terms, which are not to be met with in the only medical lexicon at this time in circulation in the country.

The author's object has not been to make a mere lexicon or dictionary of terms, but to afford, under each, a condensed view of its various medical relations, and thus to render the work an epitome of the existing condition of medical science. In its preparation, he has freely availed himself of the English, French, and German works of the same nature, and has endeavoured to add every subject and term of recent introduction, which has fallen under his notice; yet, with all his care, it will doubtless be found that subjects have been omitted. The numerous additions, however, which he has made, and his strong desire to be useful, "by removing rubbish and clearing obstructions from the paths through which learning and genius press forward to conquest and glory," will, he trusts, extenuate these and other objections that might be urged against the work; especially when the toil, which every compiler of a dictionary must endure, is taken into consideration; a toil which has been so forcibly depicted by the great English Lexicographer, as well as by the distinguished SCALIGER:

"Si quelqu'un a commis quelque crime odieux,
S'il a tué son père, ou blasphémé les Dieux,
Qu'il fasse un Lexicon: s'il est supplice au monde
Qui le punisse mieux, je veux que l'on me tonde."

EXPLANATION.

If the simple synonymy of any term be needed, a mere reference to the term may be sufficient; but if farther information be desired, it may be obtained under the term referred to. For example, the French word *Tronc* is said to be synonymous with *Trunk*. This may be sufficient for the inquirer: should it not, the requisite information may be found by turning to *Trunk*.

ABBREVIATIONS ARBITRARILY EMPLOYED.

Arab.	Arabic.	Nat. Ord.	Natural Order.
Ch.	Chaussier.	P.	Portuguese.
D.	Dutch.	Ph. D.	Pharmacopœia of Dublin.
Da.	Danish.	Ph. E.	" Edinburgh.
E.	English.	Ph. L.	" London.
F.	French.	Ph. P.	" Paris.
F. *or* Fah.	Fahrenheit.	Ph. U. S.	" of the United States of America.
Fam.	Family.		
G.	German.		
Heb.	Hebrew.	R.	Réaumur.
I.	Italian.	S.	Spanish.
Ir.	Irish.	S. g.	Specific Gravity.
L.	Latin.	Sax.	Anglo-Saxon.
Linn.	Linnæus.	Sex. Syst.	Sexual System.
		Sw.	Swedish.

A NEW DICTIONARY
OF
MEDICAL SCIENCE.

A.

A

A, before a consonant; *An* before a vowel, *a, av,* have, in the compound medical terms, a privative or debasing signification, like that of the particles *in, im, un, ir,* in English. Thus: *Stheni'a* means strength;—*Astheni'a,* want of strength;—*Anæmia,* want of blood, &c. Occasionally, in compound words, they have an intensive meaning.

AACHEN, Aix-la-Chapelle.

A, or $\overline{\text{aa}}$. See Abbreviation.

AARZHIL, MINERAL WATERS OF. A. is in the canton of Berne in Switzerland. The chief spring contains chlorides of calcium and sodium, sulphates of lime and soda, oxyd of iron, and sulphohydric acid gas.

AASMUS, Anhelatio.

ABACH, MINERAL WATERS OF. A hydrosulphuretted saline spring, not far from Ratisbon or Regentsberg in Bavaria.

ABAISSEMENT, Depression: see Cataract—*a. de la Matrice*, Prolapsus uteri.

ABAISSEUR DE L'AILE DU NEZ, Depressor alæ nasi—*a. de l'angle des lèvres*, Depressor anguli oris—*a. de la lèvre inférieure*, Depressor labii inferioris—*a. de la machoire inférieure*, Digastricus—*a. de l'œil*, Rectus inferior oculi.

ABALIENATIO MENTIS, Insanity.

ABALIENA'TUS. *Corrup'tus,* Corrupted; from *ab,* and *alienus,* 'different.' *Membra abaliena'ta.* Limbs dead or benumbed. — Celsus, Scribonius Largus.

ABANGA. Name given by the inhabitants of St. Thomas to the fruit of a palm tree, the seeds of which they consider very useful in diseases of the chest, in the dose of three or four, two or three times a day.

ABAPTIST'A. *Abaptiston* or *Abaptis'tum,* from *a,* privative, and βαπτιζειν, 'to plunge.' A term applied to the old trepan, the conical shape of which prevented it from plunging suddenly into the cavity of the cranium.

ABAPTISTON, Abaptista.

ABAPTISTUM, Abaptista.

ABAREMO-TEMO. A Brazilian tree, which grows in the mountains, and appears to be a mimosa. Piso relates that the decoction of its bark, which is bitter and astringent, was applied in that country, to ulcers of a bad character.

ABARNAHAS, Magnesia.

ABARTICULATIO, Diarthrosis and Synarthrosis.

ABATARDISSEMENT, Degeneration.

ABATTEMENT, Prostration.

ABATTIS, Giblets.

ABBREVIATION

ABBECOURT, MINERAL WATERS OF. A chalybeate spring, six leagues from Paris, and one from Poissy. It was once much frequented, but is now abandoned.

ABBEVILLE, MINERAL WATERS OF. An acidulous chalybeate at Abbeville, in the department of Somme, France.

ABBREVIA'TION, *Abbrevia'tio, Brachyn'sis, Brachys'mos, Abbreviatu'ra.* (F.) *Abréviation,* from *brevis,* 'short.' Abbreviations are chiefly used in medicinal formulæ. They are by no means as frequently employed now as of old, when every article had its appropriate symbol. The chief abbreviations now adopted are the following:

℞. *Recipe,* Take.

A. $\overline{\text{aa}}$, ANA, (ανα) *utriusque,* of each.

ABDOM. *Abdomen.*

ABS. FEBR. *Absente febre,* In the absence of fever.

AD. or ADD. *Adde* or *addatur.*

AD LIB. *Ad libitum,* At pleasure.

ADMOV. *Admoveatur,* Let it be applied.

ALTERN. HOR. *Alternis horis,* Every other hour.

ALV. ADSTRICT. *Alvo adstrictâ,* The bowels being confined.

AQ. *Aqua,* Water.

AQ. COMM. *Aqua communis,* Common water.

AQ. FONT. *Aqua fontis,* Spring water.

AQ. BULL. *Aqua bulliens,* Boiling water.

AQ. FERV. *Aqua fervens,* Hot water.

AQ. MARIN. *Aqua marina,* Sea water.

B. A. *Balneum arenæ,* A sand-bath.

BALS. *Balsamum,* Balsam.

BB. BBDS. *Barbadensis,* Barbadoes.

BIB. *Bibe,* Drink.

BIS IND. *Bis indies,* Twice daily.

B. M. *Balneum mariæ,* A salt water bath.

BOL. *Bolus.*

BULL. *Bulliat,* Let it boil.

BUT. *Butyrum,* Butter.

B. V. *Balneum vaporis,* A vapour-bath.

CÆRUL. *Cæruleus,* Blue.

CAP. *Capiat,* Let him take.

C. C. *Cornu cervi,* Hartshorn.

C. C. U. *Cornu cervi ustum,* Burnt hartshorn.

C. M. *Cras mane,* To-morrow morning.

C. N. *Cras nocte,* To-morrow night.

C. V. *Cras vespere,* To-morrow evening.

COCHL. *Cochleare,* A spoonful.

COCHL. AMPL. *Cochleare amplum,* A large spoonful.

COCHL. INF. *Cochleare infantum,* A child's spoonful.

COCHL. MOD. or MED. *Cochleare modicum* or *medium,* A dessert-spoonful.

COCHL. PARV. *Cochleare parvum*, A tea-spoonful.
COL. *Cola*, and *Colaturæ*, Strain, and to the strained.
COMP. *Compositus*, Compound.
CONF. *Confectio*, Confection.
CONS. *Conserva*, Conserve.
CONT. *Continuetur*, Let it be continued.
COQ. *Coque*, Boil.
CORT. *Cortex*, Bark.
CRAST. *Crastinus*, For to-morrow.
CUJ. *Cujus*, Of which.
CUJUSL. *Cujuslibet*, Of any.
CYATH. *Cyathus*, A glassful.
CYATH. THEÆ, A cup of tea.
D. *Dosis*, A dose.
D. et S. *Detur et signetur*, (placed at the end of a prescription.)
D. D. *Detur ad*, Let it be given in or to.
D. D. VITR. *Detur ad vitrum*, Let it be given in a glass.
DEAUR. PIL. *Deaurentur pilulæ*, Let the pills be gilded.
DEB. SPISS. *Debita spissitudo*, A due consistence.
DEC. *Decanta*, Pour off.
DECUB. *Decubitus*, Lying down, going to bed.
DE D. IN D. *De die in diem*, From day to day.
DEJ. ALV. *Dejectiones alvi*, Alvine evacuations.
DEP. *Depuratus*, Purified.
DET. *Detur*, Let it be given.
DIEB. ALTERN. *Diebus alternis*, Every other day.
DIEB. TERT. *Diebus tertiis*, Every third day.
DIG. *Digeratur*, Let it be digested.
DIL. *Dilutus*, Dilute.
DIM. *Dimidius*, One-half.
DIST. *Distilla*, Distil.
DIV. *Divide*, Divide.
DONEC ALV. SOLUT. FUER. *Donec alvus soluta fuerit*, Until the bowels are opened.
DRACH. *Drachma*, A drachm.
EJUSD. *Ejusdem*, Of the same.
ENEM. *Enema*, A clyster.
EXHIB. *Exhibeatur*, Let it be exhibited.
EXT. SUPER ALUT. *Extende super alutam*, Spread upon leather.
F. *Fiat*, Let it be made.
F. PIL. *Fiat pilula*, Make into a pill.
F. VENÆS. or F. VS. *Fiat venæsectio*, Let bleeding be performed.
FEB. DUR. *Febre durante*, The fever continuing.
FEM. INTERN. *Femoribus internis*, To the inside of the thighs.
FIST. ARMAT. *Fistula armata*, A bag and pipe, a clyster pipe and bladder fitted for use.
FL. *Fluidus*, and *Flores*, Fluid, and Flowers.
FRUST. *Frustillatim*, In small pieces.
GEL. QUAVIS, *Gelatinâ quâvis*, In any kind of jelly.
G. G. G. *Gummi guttæ Gambiæ*, Gamboge.
GR. *Granum*, A grain.
GTT. *Gutta*, A drop.
GTT. or GUTT. QUIBUSD. *Guttis quibusdam*, With some drops.
GUM. *Gummi*, Gum.
GUTTAT. *Guttatim*, By drops.
HOR. DECUB. *Horâ decubitûs*, At bed-time.
HOR. INTERM. *Horis intermediis*, At intermediate hours.
H. S. *Horâ somni*, At bed-time.
INF. *Infunde*, Infuse.
IND. *Indies*, Daily.
INJ. ENEM. *Injiciatur enema*, Let a clyster be given.
IN PULM. *In pulmento*, In gruel.
JUL. *Julepus*, A julep.
LAT. DOL. *Lateri dolenti*, To the pained side.
LB. and LIB. *Libra*, A pound weight.
LBS. LLB, *Libræ*, Pounds.

LIQ. *Liquor*.
M. *Misce*, Mix.
MAC. *Macera*, Macerate.
MAN. *Manipulus*, A handful.
MAN. PRIM. *Manê primo*, Early in the morning.
MIC. PAN. *Mica panis*, Crumb of bread.
MIN. *Minimum*, The 60th part of a drachm by measure.
MITT. *Mitte*, Send.
MITT. SANG. *Mittatur sanguis*, Let blood be drawn.
MOD. PRÆSCRIPT. *Modo præscripto*, In the manner directed.
MOR. SOL. *More solito*, In the usual manner.
MUC. *Mucilago*, Mucilage.
N. M. *Nux moschata*, Nutmeg.
O. *Octarius*, A pint.
OL. *Oleum*, Oil.
OL. LINI, S. I. *Oleum lini sine igne*, Cold-drawn linseed oil.
OMN. BID. *Omni biduo*, Every two days.
OMN. BIH. *Omni bihorio*, Every two hours.
OMN. HOR. *Omni horâ*, Every hour.
OMN. MAN. *Omni mane*, Every morning.
OMN. NOCTE, Every night.
OMN. QUADR. HOR. *Omni quadrante horæ*, Every quarter of an hour.
O. O. O. *Oleum olivæ optimum*, Best olive oil.
OV. *Ovum*, An egg.
OX. *Oxymel*.
OZ. *Uncia*, An ounce.
P. *Pondere*, By weight.
P. and PUG. *Pugillus*, A pugil.
P. Æ. *Partes æquales*, Equal parts.
PART. VIC. *Partitis vicibus*, In divided doses.
PERACT. OP. EMET. *Peractâ operatione emetici*, The operation of the emetic being over.
PIL. *Pilula*, A pill.
POST SING. SED. LIQ. *Post singulas sedes liquidas*, After every liquid evacuation.
POT. *Potio*, A potion.
P. P. *Pulvis patrum*, Jesuits' bark.
P. RAT. ÆTAT. *Pro ratione ætatis*, According to the age.
P. R. N. *Pro re natâ*, As occasion may be.
PULV. *Pulvis*, A powder.
Q. P. *Quantum placeat*, As much as may please.
Q. S. *Quantum sufficiat*, As much as is sufficient.
QUOR. *Quorum*, Of which.
Q. V. *Quantum volueris*, As much as you wish.
RAD. *Radix*, Root.
RAS. *Rasuræ*, Shavings.
RECT. *Rectificatus*, Rectified.
RED. or REDIG. IN PULV. *Redactus in pulverem*, or *Redigatur in Pulverem*, Powdered, or Let it be powdered.
REG. UMBIL. *Regio umbilici*, The umbilical region.
REPET. *Repetatur*, Let it be repeated.
S. A. *Secundum artem*, According to art.
SEM. *Semen*, Seed.
SEMI-DR. *Semi-drachma*, Half a drachm.
SEMI-H. *Semi-hora*, Half an hour.
SERV. *Serva*, Keep, preserve.
SESQUIH. *Sesquihora*, An hour and a half.
SESUNC. *Sesuncia*, An ounce and a half.
SI NON VAL. *Si non valeat*, If it does not answer.
SI OP. SIT. *Si opus sit*, If there be need.
SI VIR. PERM. *Si vires permittant*, If the strength will permit.
SOLV. *Solve*, Dissolve.
SP. and SPIR. *Spiritus*, Spirit.
Ss. *Semi*, One half.
ST. *Stet*, Let it stand.
SUB FIN. COCT. *Sub finem coctionis*, Towards the end of the boiling.
SUM. *Sumat*, Let him take; also, *Summitates*, The tops.

S. V. *Spiritus vini*, Spirit of wine.
S. V. R. *Spiritus vini rectificatus*, Rectified spirit of wine.
S. V. T. *Spiritus vini tenuior*, Proof spirit of wine.
SYR. *Syrupus*, Syrup.
TEMP. DEXT. *Tempori dextro*, To the right temple.
T. O. *Tinctura opii*, Tincture of opium.
TR., TRA. and TINCT. *Tinctura*, Tincture.
TRIT. *Tritura*, Triturate.
V. O. S. or VIT. OV. SOL. *Vitello ovi solutus*, Dissolved in the yolk of an egg.
VS. *Venæsectio*, Venesection.
Z. Z. Anciently *myrrh*: now *zinziber* or ginger.
℔, *Libra*, A pound.
℥, *Uncia*, An ounce.
ℨ, *Drachma*, A drachm.
℈, *Scrupulum*, A scruple.
℞, *Minimum*, A minim.
ss, *Semissis*, or half; iss, one and a half.
j, one; ij, two; iij, three; iv, four, &c.
The same system is not always followed in abbreviating. The subjoined will exhibit the usual mode:
℞
Infus. Colomb.   f ℥iss
Tinct. Gent. c.   f ℨi
Syr. Cort. Aurant.   f ℨss
Tinct. caps.   gtt. xl. M.
Capt. coch. ij. p. r. n.
This, written at length, is as follows:
Recipe
Infusi Colombæ sesqui-fluidunciam.
Tinctura Gentianæ Compositæ fluidrachmam.
Syrupi Corticis Aurantiorum semi-fluidrachmam.
Tincturæ Capsici guttas quadraginta.
Misce.
Capiat cochlearia duo pro re natâ.
ABCÈS, Abscess—*a. Aigu*, see Abscess—*a. Chaud*, see Abscess—*a. Chronique*, see Abscess—*a. Par congestion*, see Abscess—*a. Diathésique*, see Abscess—*a. Froid*, see Abscess—*a. Métastatique*, see Abscess—*a. Scrofuleux*, see Abscess—*a. Soudain*, see Abscess.
ABDO'MEN, from *abdere*, 'to conceal;'—*Etron, Hypogas'trion, Hypoca'lium, Epis'chion, Lap'ara, Hypochoi'lion, Gaster, Hypou'trion, Nedys, Abdu'men, Venter, Venter imus, Venter in'fimus, Alvus, U'terus, The belly*, (F.) *Ventre, V. inférieur, Bas ventre*. The largest of the three splanchnic cavities, bounded, above, by the diaphragm; below, by the pelvis; behind, by the lumbar vertebræ; and at the sides and fore part, by muscular expansions. It is distinguished into three anterior regions, from above to below; viz. the epigastric, umbilical, and hypogastric, each of which is itself divided into three others, one middle, and two lateral: thus, the *epigastric region* comprises the *epigastrium* and *hypochondria;* the *umbilical*, the *umbilicus* and *flanks* or *lumbar regions;* and the *hypogastric*, the *hypogastrium* and *iliac regions*. None of these regions has its limits well defined. The chief viscera contained in the cavity of the abdomen, *Cœ'lia, Cavum Abdom'inis*, are the stomach, intestines, liver, spleen, pancreas, kidneys, &c. It is lined by the peritoneum.
ABDOMEN, PENDULOUS, Physconia.

ABDOM'INAL, *Abdomina'lis, Ventra'lis*, Ventral. That which belongs to the Abdomen, as *abdominal muscles, abdominal viscera*, &c.

ABDOMINIS EXPLORATIO, Abdominoscopia.

ABDOMINISCOP'IA, *Gastroscop'ia*. A hybrid word, from *Abdomen*, 'the lower belly,' and σκοπεω, 'I view;' Laparoscop'ia, Abdom'inis Explora'tio. Examination of the lower belly as a means of diagnosis. See Auscultation.

ABDUCENS LABIORUM, Levator anguli oris.
ABDUCENTES, Motor oculi externus.
ABDUCTEUR DE L'ŒIL, Rectus externus oculi—*a. de l'oreille*, Abductor auris—*a. du gros orteil*, Abductor pollicis pedis—*a. du petit orteil*, Abductor minimi digiti pedis—*a. court du pouce*, Abductor pollicis brevis—*a. long du pouce*, Abductor longus pollicis.

ABDUC'TION, *Abduc'tio*, from *abducere*, to separate, (*ab* and *ducere*, 'to lead.') The movement which separates a limb or other part from the axis of the body.
The word has also been used synonymously with *Abrup'tio, Apag'ma, Apoclas'ma*, a fracture near the articular extremity of a bone, with separation of the fragments.

ABDUC'TOR, same etymon. (F.) *Abducteur*. A muscle which moves certain parts by separating them from the axis of the body.

ABDUCTOR AURICULARIS, Abductor auris—*a.* Indicis pedis, Prior indicis pedis, Posterior indicis pedis—*a.* Medii digiti pedis, Prior medii digiti pedis—*a.* Minimi digiti, Flexor parvus minimi digiti—*a.* Minimi digiti, Prior minimi digiti—*a.* Oculi, Rectus externus oculi—*a.* Pollicis manûs, and *a.* Brevis alter, Abductor pollicis brevis.

ABDUCTOR AURIS, *Abductor auricula'ris.* (F.) *Abducteur de l'oreille.* A portion of the *posterior auris*, whose existence is not constant, which passes from the mastoid process to the concha.

ABDUCTOR IN'DICIS, *Semi-interos'seus in'dicis.* A muscle which arises from the os trapezium and metacarpal bone of the thumb, and is inserted into the first bone of the forefinger. Its use is to bring the forefinger towards the thumb.

ABDUCTOR MIN'IMI DIG"ITI, *Carpo-phalan'geus min'imi digiti, Carpo-phalangien du petit doigt, Exten'sor ter'tii interno'dii minimi digiti*—(Douglas.) *Hypoth'enar minor metacarpeus*. See Flexor parvus. It originates fleshy from the os pisiforme, and from the annular ligament near it; and is inserted, tendinous, into the inner side of the base of the first bone of the little finger. *Use*, to draw the little finger from the rest.

ABDUCTOR MINIMI DIGITI PEDIS, *Calco-subphalangeus minimi digiti, Calcaneo-phalangien du petit orteil, Parath'enar major*—(By Winslow, the muscle is divided into two portions,—*Parathenar major* and *metatarseus*.) *Calcaneosous-phalangien du petit orteil*—(Ch.) (F.) *Abducteur du petit orteil*. This muscle forms the outer margin of the sole of the foot, and is immediately beneath the plantar aponeurosis. It arises, tendinous and fleshy, from the outer side of the protuberance of the os calcis, and from the root of the metatarsal bone of the little toe, and is inserted into the outer part of the root of the first bone of the little toe. *Use*, to draw the little toe outwards.

ABDUCTOR POL'LICIS BREVIS, *Abductor Pollicis Manûs, Scapho-carpo-super-phalangeus Pollicis, Sus-phalangien du pouce, A. pollicis manus* and *A. brevis alter*—(Albinus.) (F.) *Abductor court du pouce, Carpo-sus-phalangien du pouce*—(Ch.) A short, flat, triangular muscle, which arises from the anterior surface of the os scaphoides and the annular ligament of the carpus, and terminates at the outside of the upper extremity of the first phalanx of the thumb. A particular portion, on the inner side of this muscle, is called, by Albinus, *Abductor brevis alter*.

ABDUCTOR LONGUS POLLICIS, *A. l. P. Manûs, Extensor ossis metacarpi pollicis manûs, Extensor primi internodii*—(Douglas,) *Extensor primus Pollicis, Cubito-radi-sus-métacarpien du pouce*,

Cubito-sus-métacarpien du pouce,—(Ch.) (F.) *Abducteur long du pouce.* A long, thin muscle, arising from the posterior surface of the ulna, radius; and interosseous ligament, and inserted at the outer side of the upper extremity of the first metacarpal bone.

ABDUCTOR POLLICIS PEDIS, *Calco-sub-phalangeus Pol'licis.* (F.) *Abducteur du gros orteil.* This muscle arises, fleshy, from the anterior and inner part of the protuberance of the os calcis, and tendinous from the same bone where it joins with the os naviculare. It is inserted, tendinous, into the internal os sesamoideum and root of the first bone of the great toe. *Use*, to pull the great toe from the rest.

The name *Abductor* has been given also to all those interosseous muscles of the hand and foot, which perform the motion of abduction on the fingers or toes, and to muscles which execute the same function on other parts of the body.

ABDUMEN, Abdomen.

ABEBÆ'OS, from *a*, neg. and βέβαιος, 'firm,' *Infir'mus, Deb'ilis.* Weak, infirm, unsteady.

ABEILLE, Bee.

ABELMELUCH. One of the names of the Ricinus, according to some authors.—Prosper Alpinus says that a tree, which grows about Mecca, is so called. Its seeds, which are black and oblong, are said to be a most violent cathartic.

ABELMOSCHUS, Hibiscus abelmoschus—a. Moschatus, Hibiscus abelmoschus.

ABELMUSK, Hibiscus abelmoschus.

ABENSBERG, MINERAL WATERS OF. A. is a city of Bavaria, where there is a cold, sulphureous spring.

ABERRATIO, Aberration—a. Lactis, Galactoplania—a. Mensium, Menstruation, vicarious—a. Menstruorum, Menstruation, vicarious.

ABERRA'TION, *Aberra'tio*, from *aberrare*, (*ab* and *errare*,) 'to stray,' 'to wander from.' This word has several meanings.

1. The passage of a fluid of the living body into an order of vessels not destined for it. In this sense it is synonymous with the *Error Loci* of Boerhaave.

2. The flow of a fluid towards an organ different from that to which it is ordinarily directed; as in cases of vicarious hemorrhage. *Aberrations of sense* or *judgment* are certain errors in the perceptions, or certain derangements of the intellectual faculties.

The word is used in optics to designate the dispersion of the rays of light in passing through a lens.

ABERRATION, CHROMATIC, Aberration of Refrangibility.

ABERRATION OF REFRANGIBIL'ITY, *Chromat'ic aberra'tion*, exists, when, as in a common lens, the rays that pass near the circumference of the lens are decomposed, so that a coloured image is observed. This aberration in the human eye is corrected by the iris, which does not permit the rays to fall near the circumference of the lens, and also by the crystalline lens itself, which, owing to its structure, serves the purposes of an achromatic glass.

ABERRATION, SPHERICAL, Aberration of sphericity.

ABERRATION OF SPHERIC''ITY or *spher'ical aberra'tion* takes place, when the rays, as in a common lens, which pass through the centre of the lens, and those which pass near the circumference, are unequally refracted, so that they do not meet at a common focus.

This aberration of sphericity in the human eye is corrected by the iris.

ABESSI, Realgar.

ABEVACUA'TIO, *Apoceno'sis*, from *ab*, and *evacuare*, 'to empty.' An evacuation. A partial or imperfect evacuation. By some it is applied to an immoderate evacuation.—Kraus.

ABHAL. A fruit well known in India, and obtained from a species of cypress. It passes for an emmenagogue.

ABIES, Pinus picea—a. Balsamea, Pinus balsamea.

ABIES BALSAMIFERA, Pinus balsamea—a. Canadensis, Pinus Canadensis—a. Excelsa, see Pinus abies—a. Gallica, Pinus picea—a. Larix, Pinus larix—a. Pectinata, Pinus picea—a. Picea, Pinus picea—a. Rubra, Pinus rubra.

ABIGA, Teucrium Chamæpitys.

ABIOSIS, Death.

ABIOTOS, Conium maculatum.

ABIRRITA'TION. *Abirrita'tio*, from *ab*, privative, and *irritatio*, 'irritation.' This word strictly means absence or defect of irritation. The disciples of Broussais used it to indicate a pathological condition, opposite to that of irritation. It may be considered as synonymous with debility, asthenia, &c.

ABLACTATIO, Weaning.

ABLASTES, Sterile.

ABLATIO, Extirpation.

ABLEPH'ARUS, from *a*, privative, and βλέφαρον, 'eyelid.' One who has no eyelids.

ABLEPSIA, Cæcitas.

ABLUENTIA, Detergents.

ABLU'TION, *Ablu'tio, Aponip'sis, Cataclys'mus*, from *abluere*, (*ab* and *luere*,) 'to wash.' A name given to legal ceremonies in which the body is subjected to particular affusions. Ablution (especially of the extremities) with cold or tepid water is employed, therapeutically, to reduce febrile heat. Also, the washing by which medicines are separated from the extraneous matters mixed with them.

ABNORMAL, Abnormous.

ABNORMITY, Anomalia.

ABNOR'MOUS, *Abnor'mal*, (F.) *Anormal*, from *ab*, 'from,' and *norma*, 'rule.' Not conformable to rule; irregular.

ABOLI''TION, *Aboli''tio*, destruction or suppression, from *ab* and *luere* (?) 'to wash.' A word, often employed, especially by the French, to express the complete suspension of any symptom or function. *Abolition of the sight*, e. g. is the complete loss of sight.

ABOMA'SUS, *Aboma'sum, Enys'tron, Rennet.* The lowermost or fourth stomach of ruminating animals.

ABOMINATIO, Disgust.

ABONDANCE, Plethora.

ABORSIO, Abortion.

ABORSUS, Abortion.

ABORTICIDIUM, Fœticide.

ABORTIF, Abortive.

ABORTIFACIENS, Abortive.

ABORTION, *Abor'tus, Abor'sus, Abor'sio, Dysto'cia aborti'va, Omoto'cia, Paracye'sis abortus, Amblo'sis, Amblo'ma, Amblos'mus, Ec'bolē, Embryotoc'ia, Diaph'thora, Ectro'sis, Examblo'ma, Examblo'sis, Ectros'mos, Apopalle'sis, Apopal'sis, Apaph'thora, Phthora, Convul'sio u'teri, Deperdi'tio.* (F.) *Avortement, Blessure,* Miscarriage, from *ab* and *oriri*, 'to rise,' applied to that which has arisen out of season. The expulsion of the fœtus before the seventh month of utero-gestation, or before it is *viable*. The causes of this accident are referrible either to the mother, and particularly to the uterus; or to the fœtus and its dependencies. The causes, in the mother, may be: —extreme nervous susceptibility, great debility, plethora; faulty conformation, &c.; and it is frequently induced immediately by intense mental emotion, violent exercise, &c. The causes seated in the fœtus are its death, rupture of the membranes, &c. It most frequently occurs between the 8th and 12th weeks of gestation. The symptoms of abortion are:—uterine hemorrhage with or without flakes of decidua, with intermitting pain. When abortion has once taken place, it is extremely apt to recur in subsequent pregnancies about the same period. Some writers have called abortion, when it occurs prior to three months, *Effluxion*. The treatment must vary according to the constitution of the patient and the causes giving rise to it. In all cases, the horizontal posture and perfect quietude are indispensable.

ABORTION is likewise applied to the product of an untimely birth,—*Abor'tus, Abor'sus, Apoble'ma, Apob'olè, Ecblo'ma, Amblothrid'ion, Ectro'ma, Fruc'tus immatu'rus,* Abortment. (F.) *Avorton, Avortin.*

TO ABORT, *Abori'ri.* To miscarry. (F.) *Avorter.*

ABOR'TIVE, *Aborti'vus, Ecbol'ius, Amblo'ticus, Amblothrid'ium, Ambol'icus, Phthor'ius, Apophthor'ius, Ectrot'icus, Abortifa'ciens, Acyte'rius, Expel'lens, Phthiroc'tonus, Phthoroc'tonus, Ecbol'icus, Contrac'tor u'teri, Accelera'tor Partûs, Parturient, Parturifa'cient, Ecbolic.* (F.) *Abortif.* A medicine to which is attributed the property of causing abortion. There is probably no direct agent of the kind.

ABORTMENT, Abortion.

ABORTUS, Abortion.

AROUCHEMENT, Anastomosis.

ABOULAZA, a tree of Madagascar, used, according to Flacourt, in the practice of the country, in diseases of the heart.

ABOUTISSEMENT, Suppuration.

ABRABAX, *Abrasax, Abraxas.* A mystic term, expressing the number 365, to which the Cabalists attributed miraculous properties.

ABRACADA'BRA: the name of a Syrian Idol, according to Selden. This word, when pronounced and repeated in a certain form and a certain number of times, was supposed to have the power of curing fevers and preventing many diseases. It was figured on amulets and worn suspended around the neck.

אברכדברא
אברכדבר
אברכדב
אברכד
אברכ
אבר
אב
א

ABRACALAN, A cabalistic term to which the Jews attributed the same virtue as to the word ABRACADABRA.

ABRASAX, Abrabax.

ABRA'SION, *Abra'sio, Aposyr'ma, Apoxys'mus,* from *abradere,* (*ab* and *radere,*) 'to rasp.' A superficial excoriation, with loss of substance, under the form of small *shreds,* in the mucous membrane of the intestines,—(F.) *Raclures des Boyaux.* Also, an ulceration of the skin, possessing similar characters. According to Vicq d'Azyr, the word has been used for the absorption of the molecules composing the various organs.

ABRATHAN, Artemisia abrotanum.

ABRAXAS, Abrabax.

ABRÉVIATION, Abbreviation.

ABRICOT, Prunus Armeniaca.

ABROSIA, Abstinence.

ABROTANUM, Artemisia abrotanum—a.

Cathsum, Artemisia abrotanum—a. Mas, Artemisia abrotanum.

ABROTONI'TES, (οινος, 'wine,' understood.) Wine impregnated with Artemisia Abrotanum or Southernwood.

ABROTONUM, Artemisia Abrotanum.

ABRUPTIO, Abduction.

ABRUS PRECATO'RIUS, *Liq'uorice Bush, Red Bean, Love pea.* A small ornamental shrub, found from Florida to Brazil, as well as in Egypt and the West Indies; *Nat. Ord.* Leguminosæ. *Sex. Syst.* Monadelphia enneandria; having beautiful scarlet seeds with a black spot. The roots and leaves are sweet mucilaginous demulcents. The seeds of the American kind are considered to be purgative and poisonous.

ABSCESS, from *abscedo,* (*abs,* and *cedere,*) 'I depart,' or 'separate from.' *Absces'sus, Absces'sio, Aphiste'sis, Aposte'ma, Ecpye'ma, Ecpye'sis, Reces'sus, Impos'thume.* (F.) *Abcès, Dépôt.* A collection of pus in a cavity, the result of a morbid process. See Pyogenia, and Suppuration.

The French have various distinctive terms for Abscesses.

ABCÈS CHAUD, AIGU, SOUDAIN, is one which follows violent inflammation.

ABCÈS FROID, CHRONIQUE, SCROFULEUX, one which is the result of chronic or scrofulous inflammation.

ABCÈS PAR CONGESTION, A. *diathésique,* a symptomatic abscess; one which occurs in a part at a distance from the inflammation by which it is occasioned: e. g. a *lumbar abscess;* in which the inflammation may be in the lumbar vertebræ, whilst the pus exhibits itself at the groin.

ABSCESS, METASTAT'IC, *Absces'sus metastat'icus,* (F.) *Abcès métastatique;* A. *consécutif,* an abscess, which forms suddenly, and sometimes without any precursory signs of inflammation, in a part of the body remote from one in a state of suppuration, and without presenting a sufficient reason for its development in the place which it occupies. It is a consequence of phlebitis.

ABSCESS, PERFORATING OF THE LUNG, see Lung, perforating abscess of the—a. PSOAS, Lumbar abscess—a. Retropharyngeal, see Retropharyngeal.

ABSCESSUS CAPITIS SANGUINEUS NEONATORUM, Cephalæmatoma—a. Cerebri, Encephalopyosis—a. Gangræanescens, Anthrax—a. Gangrænosus, Anthrax—a. Lacteus, Mastodynia apostematosa—a. Lumborum, Lumbar abscess—a. Mammæ, Mastodynia apostematosa—a. Metastaticus, Abscess, metastatic—a. Nucleatus, Furunculus—a. Oculi, Hypopyon—a. Pectoris, Empyema—a. Pulmonum, Pneumapostema—a. Renalis, Nephrapostasis—a. Spirituosus, Aneurism—a. Thoracis, Empyema—a. Urinosus, Urapostema.

ABSCISSIO PRÆPUTII, Circumcision.

ABSCIS'SION, *Abscis'io, Abscis'sio,* from *abscidere* or *abscindere,* 'to cut off,' *Apoc'opè, Apothrau'sis, Diac'opè.* Excision or extirpation of a part, especially of a soft part.—Fabricius Hildanus.

Fracture or injury of soft parts, with loss of substance.—Hippocrates.

Diminution, or loss of voice.—Celsus.

Sudden and premature termination of a disease.—Galen.

ABSCONSIO, Sinus.

ABSENCE DU BRUIT RESPIRATOIRE, see Murmur, respiratory.

ABSINTHI'TES, αψινθιτης, *Apsinthi'tes,* Wine impregnated with Absinthium or Wormwood.—Dioscorides.

ABSINTHIUM, (Ph. U. S.,) Artemisia absinthium—a. Marinum, Artemisia maritima—a. Maritimum, Artemisia maritima—a. Ponticum, Artemisia pontica—a. Romanum, Artemisia pontica—a. Santonicum, Artemisia santonica—a. Vulgare, Artemisia absinthium.

ABSORBANT, Absorbent.

ABSOR'BENT, *Absor'bens*, from *absorbere*, (*ab* and *sorbere*,) 'to drink, to suck up.' (F.) *Absorbant*. That which absorbs.

ABSORBENT SYSTEM is the collection of vessels, *Vasa absorben'tia seu resorben'tia*, and glands, which concur in the exercise of absorption.

A medicine used for absorbing acidity in the stomach and bowels, as magnesia, chalk, &c. *Insertens, Resor'bens, Sat'urans*.

Also, any substance, such as cobweb, sponge, &c., which, when applied to a bleeding surface, retains the blood, and forms with it a solid and adhesive compound, which arrests the hemorrhage.

ABSORPTIO, Absorption—a. Sanguinis, Hæmorrhophesis.

ABSORP'TION, *Resorp'tio, Inhala'tio, Imbibi"tio, Absorp'tio, Anar'rhophē, Anarrophe'sis, Catapino'sis, Rhoëbdo'sis, Catarrhophe'sis, Catar'rhophē;* same etymon. The function of absorbent vessels, by virtue of which they take up substances from without or within the body. Two great divisions have been made of this function. 1. *External absorption*, or the *absorption of composition*, which obtains from without the organs the materials intended for their composition; and, 2. *Internal absorption*, or the *absorption of decomposition*, which takes up from the organs the materials that have to be replaced by the exhalants.

By *external absorption* is meant not only that which takes place at the external surface of the body, but also that of the mucous membranes of the digestive and respiratory passages. Hence, again, the division of external absorption into *cutaneous—resorp'tio cuta'nea seu cutis, inhala'tio cutis,—intestinal or digestive*, and *pulmonary or respiratory*.

Internal absorption is also subdivided into, 1. *Molecular* or *interstitial, nutritive, organic*, or *decomposing*, which takes up from each organ the materials that constitute it, so that the decomposition is always in equilibrio with the deposition. 2. The *absorption of recrementitial secreted fluids*, such as the fluid of serous membranes, synovia, &c. As these are constantly exhaled on surfaces which have no external outlet, they would augment indefinitely, if absorption did not remove them in the same proportion as that in which they are deposited. 3. The *absorption of a part of the excrementitial fluids*, as they pass over the excretory passages.

Absorption does not effect the decomposition of the body immediately. It merely prepares the fluid which has to be eliminated by the secretory organs.

The great agents of external absorption are the veins and chyliferous vessels; of internal absorption, probably the lymphatics. In the chyliferous vessels and lymphatics the fluid is always found to possess the same general properties. In them, therefore, an action of elaboration or selection must have taken place. The veins, on the other hand, seem to exert no selection. Any fluid, possessing the necessary tenuity, passes through the coats of the vessel readily by imbibition, and proceeds along with the torrent of the circulation. Watery fluids in this manner enter the blood when they are taken into the stomach. Substances that require digestion, on the other hand, must pass through the chyliferous vessels and thoracic duct.

ABSORPTION OF COMPOSITION, see Absorption—a. Cutaneous, see Absorption—a. of Decomposition, see Absorption—a. Digestive, see Absorption—a. External, see Absorption—a. of Excrementitial Secreted Fluids, see Absorption—a. Internal, see Absorption—a. Intestinal, see Absorption—a. Interstitial, see Absorption—a. Molecular, see Absorption—a. Nutritive, see Absorption—a. Organic, see Absorption—a. Pulmonary, see Absorption—a. of Recrementitial Secreted Fluids, see Absorption—a. Respiratory, see Absorption.

ABSTÈME, Abstemious.

ABSTE'MIOUS, *Abste'mius, Aoi'nos*, from *abs*, 'without,' and *temetum*, 'wine.' (F.) *Abstème*. Used by the ancient writers, as well as by the French, in the sense only of its roots; one who abstains from wine or fermented liquors in general.

ABSTERGENTIA, Detergents.
ABSTERSIVA, Detergents.
ABSTERSORIA, Detergents.

AB'STINENCE, *Abstinen'tia*, from *abs*, 'from,' and *tenere*, 'to hold,' *Abros'ia, Asit'ia, Liman'chia, Limocton'ia*, Fasting. Privation, usually voluntary, as when we speak of *abstinence from pleasure, abstinence from drink*, &c. It is more particularly used to signify voluntary privation of certain articles of food. Fasting is a useful remedial agent in certain diseases, particularly in those of an inflammatory character.

ABSUS, a kind of cassia—*C. Absus*—which grows in Egypt and in India, the seeds of which, pulverized and mixed with powdered sugar have been employed, in form of a dry collyrium, in the endemic ophthalmia of Egypt.

ABU'LIA; from *a*, 'privative,' and $βουλη$, 'will.' Loss of the will, or of volition.

ABU'LICUS; same etymon. One who has lost the power of will or of volition.

ABUS DE SOI-MÊME, Masturbation.

ABUTA, Pareira brava.

ABU'TILON CORDA'TUM, *Sida abutilon*, Yellow mallow. An indigenous plant, common from Canada to Mexico, which resembles common mallow in its medical virtues, being mucilaginous and demulcent.

ABVACUA'TIO, an excessive or colliquative evacuation of any kind.

ACACIA, (Ph. U. S.) Acaciæ gummi—a. Catechu, Catechu—a. False, Robinia pseudo-acacia—a. Germanica, see Prunus spinosa—a. Giraffæ, see Accaciæ gummi—a. Horrida, see Acaciæ gummi—a. Indica, Tamarindus—a. Nilotica, see Acaciæ gummi—a. Nostras, see Prunus spinosa—a. Senegal, see Acaciæ gummi—a. Vera, see Acaciæ gummi—a. Zeylonica, Hæmatoxylon Campechianum.

ACACIÆ GUMMI, *Aca'cia*, from *ακη*, 'a point,' so called in consequence of its spines, *G. Aca'ciæ Arab'icæ, G. Arab'icum, G. Acanth'inum, G. Leucum, G. Theba'icum, G. Serapio'nis, G. Lamac, G. Senega*, or *Seneca*, (see Senegal, gum,) *Gum Ar'abic*. (F.) *Gomme Arabique*. The gum of the *Aca'cia* seu *Mimo'sa Nilot'ica, Aca'cia vera, Spina Ægyptiaca*, of Upper Egypt, *Nat. Ord.* Mimoseæ. *Sex. Syst.* Polygamia Monœcia. It is in irregular pieces, colourless or of a pale yellow colour, hard, brittle, of a shining fracture, transparent, soluble in water, and insoluble in alcohol, s. g. 1·4317.

It is mucilaginous; but is rarely used, except in pharmacy. Sometimes it is administered alone as a demulcent.

Acacia Horrida and *A. Giraffæ*, of South Africa, yield a good gum.

ACAJOU, Anacardium occidentale.

ACAJUBA OFFICINALIS, Anacardium occidentale.

ACAL'YPHA VIRGIN'ICA, *Three-seeded mer'cury.* Order, Euphorbiaceæ, indigenous, flowering in August, is said to have expectorant and diuretic properties.

ACAM'ATUS, from *a*, priv., and *καμνω*, 'I labour.' This word has been sometimes used for a good constitution of the body. According to Galen, it means that position in which a limb is intermediate between flexion and extension; a position which may be long maintained without fatigue.

ACAMPSIA, Contractura.

ACANOS, Onopordium acanthium.

ACANOS SPINA, Onopordium acanthium.

ACANTHA, Vertebral column. Also, Spinous process of a vertebra.

ACANTHAB'OLUS, *Acan'thulus, Volsel'la,* from *ακανθα,* 'a spine,' and *βαλλω,* 'I cast out.' A kind of forceps for removing extraneous substances from wounds.—Paulus of Ægina, Fabricius ab Aquapendente, Scultetus, &c.

ACANTHALZUCA, Echinops.

ACANTHE FAUSSE, Heracleum spondylium.

ACANTHIUM, Onopordium acanthium.

ACANTHULUS, Acanthabolos.

ACANTHUS MOLLIS, same etymon as Acacia, *Melamphyl'lum, Branca ursi'na seu vera, Brankur'sine, Bear's Breech.* (F.) *Pied d'ours.* This plant is mucilaginous like Althæa, and is used as a demulcent.

ACAPATLI, Piper longum.

ACAR'DIA, from *a*, priv., and *καρδια,* 'the heart.' The state of a fœtus without a heart.

ACARDIOTROPHIA, Heart, atrophy of the.

AC'ARICIDE, from *acarus,* and *cædere,* 'to kill.' A destroyer of acari, — as of the acarus scabies.

ACARICOBA. The Brazilian name for *Hydrocot'ylē umbella'tum,* used by the Indians as an aromatic, alexipharmic, and emetic.

ACARON, Myrica gale.

ACARP'Æ, from *a,* 'privative,' and *καρπος,* 'fruit.' A division of the family of cutaneous diseases by Fuchs, in which there is no "fruit," (Germ. *Frucht,*) or production from the cutaneous surface — tubercles, vesicles or pustules. Lentigo, Chloasma, Argyria, and Pityriasis belong to it.

AC'ARUS, from *a,* privative, and *καρης,* 'divisible.' A minute insect, one species of which has been noticed by several observers, in the itch. The *Acarus Scabiei,* see Psora.

ACARUS CIRO, see Psora — a. Comedonum, Acarus Folliculorum.

AC'ARUS CROS'SEL. An insect supposed by Mr. Crosse, of England, to have been developed in a solution of silicate of potassa when submitted to slow galvanic action, for the purpose of obtaining crystals of silex. It did not, however, prove to be a new formation.

ACARUS FOLLICULO'RUM, *Entozo'on Folliculo'rum, A. Oomedo'num, De'modex folliculo'rum, Simo'nea folliculo'rum, Steatozo'on folliculo'rum, Macrogas'ter plat'ypus.* An articulated animalcule, discovered in the sebaceous substance of the cutaneous follicles. According to Professor Owen, it belongs to the Arachnida.

ACARUS SCABIEI, Acarus, see Psora.

ACATALEP'SIA, from *a,* privative, and *καταλαμβανω,* 'I comprehend.' Uncertainty in diagnosis. Its opposite is Catalepsia.—Galen.

ACĀTAP'OSIS, from *a* privative, and *καταποσις,* 'deglutition.' Incapacity of swallowing. Vogel has given this name to difficulty of deglutition.

ACATASTAT'IC, *Acatastat'icus,* from *a,* priv., and *καθιστημι,* 'to determine.' An epithet given to fevers, &c., when irregular in their periods or symptoms.—Hippocrates.

ACATHAR'SIA, from *a,* priv., and *καθαιρζω,* 'I purge;' *Sordes,* Impurities. Omission of a purgative.—Foësius.

ACATSJAVAL'LI, a Malabar plant, which is astringent and aromatic. A bath of it is used in that country in cases of hemicrania. It is supposed to be the *Cassytha filiformis* of Linnæus.

ACAWERIA, Ophioxylum serpentinum.

ACCABLEMENT, Torpor.

ACCÉLÉRATEUR, Accelerator urinæ.

ACCELERATOR PARTUS, Abortive.

ACCELERA'TOR URI'NÆ, *Bulbo-caverno'sus, Bulbo-urétral —* (Ch.) *Ejacula'tor Semi'nis, Bulbosyndesmo-caverneux.* (F.) *Accélérateur,* from *ad* and *celer,* 'quick.' A muscle of the penis, which arises, fleshy, from the sphincter ani and membranous part of the urethra, and tendinous from the crus and beginning of the corpus cavernosum penis. In its course it forms a thin, fleshy layer, the inferior fibres of which run more transversely than the superior, which descend in an oblique direction; the muscles of both sides completely enclosing the bulb of the urethra. It is inserted into its fellow by a tendinous line running longitudinally on the middle of the bulb. Its use is to propel the urine or semen forwards.

ACCENT, *Sonus vocis,* from *ad* and *canere, cantum,* to sing. Inflection or modification of the voice, which consists in raising or dropping it on certain syllables.

The accent exhibits various alterations in disease.

ACCÈS, Paroxysm.

ACCES'SION. *Acces'sio,* from *accedo,* (*ad* and *cedere,*) 'I approach.' The invasion, approach, or commencement of a disease.

ACCESSOIRE, Accessory—*a.* du *long Fléchisseur commun des orteils:* see Flexor longus digitorum pedis profundus perforans (accessorius)—*a. de l'Obturateur interne,* Ischio-trochanterianus —*a. du pied d'Hippocampe:* see Cornu ammonis —*a. du Sacro-lombaire:* see Sacro-lumbalis.

ACCESSORIUS FLEXOR LONGUS DIGITORUM PEDIS; see Flexor longus digitorum pedis profundus perforans (accessorius)—a. Pedis hippocampi;—see Cornu ammonis.

AC'CESSORY, *Accesso'rius,* (F.) *Accessoire, Annexe,* same etymon. A consequence or dependence on any thing; as *accessory ligament, muscle, nerve,* &c.

ACCESSORY OF THE PAROT'ID is a name given by Haller to a small gland, which accompanies the parotid duct, and is commonly a mere prolongation of the parotid itself. See Parotid.

ACCESSORY SCIENCES TO MEDICINE are those which do not relate directly to the science of man in a state of health or disease; as physics, chemistry, &c.

ACCESSORY OF THE PAR VAGUM, Spinal nerve. The term *accessory* is also given to several muscles.

ACCESSUS, Coition.

ACCIDENS, Symptoms—*a. Consecutifs,* Consecutive phenomena.

AC'CIDENT, *Ac'cidens,* from *accidere,* (*ad* and *cadere,*) 'to happen.' A casualty; an unforeseen event. The French use the term in nearly the same sense as *symptom.* It means also an unexpected symptom.

ACCIDEN'TAL, *Adventi''tious.* That which happens unexpectedly.

The French give the name *Tissus accidentels,* to those adventitious textures, that are the result of a morbid process.

ACCIP'ITER, *Hi'erax,* 'ιεραξ, 'the hawk,' from *accipere* (*ad* and *capio,*) 'to take.' *Menec'ratis Accip'iter.* (F.) *Épervier.* A bandage applied over the nose, so called from its likeness to the claw of a hawk.

ACCLI'MATED, *Clima'ti assue'tus,* (from *ad* and *clima.*) A word of recent introduction from the French, which means 'accustomed to a climate.'

ACCLIMATEMENT, Acclimation.

AC'CLIMATION, *Seas'oning.* (F.) *Acclimatement.* The act of becoming acclimated, or accustomed to a climate.

The constitution of a person, who goes to live in another and a very different climate, usually experiences changes, which are frequently of an unfavourable character, and the study of which is of considerable importance in medicine.

ACCOM'PANIMENT, *Adjun'ction.* (F.) *Accompagnement,* (*compagnon,* 'an associate.') That which is joined to any thing.

Accompaniment to the cataract is a whitish, viscid substance, which sometimes surrounds the opake crystalline, and remains after the operation for cataract, causing a secondary cataract.

ACCOUCHÉE, Puerpera.

ACCOUCHEMENT, Parturition—*a.* Laborious, Dystocia—*a. Contre nature,* see Presentation, preternatural—*a. Laborieux,* Laborious labour.

ACCOUCHEUR, (F.) *Adju'tor Partus, Obstet'ricans, Obstetri"cius, Maieu'ter, Maieu'tes.* He who practises the art of midwifery. *A physician-Accoucheur, a Surgeon-Accoucheur, a Man-midwife,* &c.

ACCOUCHEUSE, Midwife.

ACCOUPLEMENT, Coition.

ACCOUTUMANCE, Habit.

ACCRE'TION, *Accre'tio,* from *ad,* 'to,' and *crescere,* 'to increase." Augmentation; also, increase by juxtaposition.

ACCROISSEMENT, Increase.

ACCUSATIO, Indication.

ACE'DIA, *Incu'ria,* from *a,* privative, and *κηδος,* 'care.' Want of care, neglect. Also, fatigue.—Hippocrates.

ACELLA, Axilla.

ACENINOSUS, Curative.

ACEOGNOSIA, Pharmacognosia.

ACEOLOGIA, Materia Medica.

ACEPHALIA, see Acephalous.

ACEPH'ALOBRACHUS, from *a,* privative, *κεφαλη,* 'head,' and *βραχιων,* 'arm.' A fœtus without head or arms.

ACEPHALOCHI'RUS, from *a,* privative, *κεφαλη,* 'head,' and *χειρ,* 'hand.' A fœtus without head or hands.

ACEPH'ALOCYST, *Acephalocys'tis,* from *a,* privative, *κεφαλη,* 'head,' and *κυστις,* 'bladder.' A hydatiform vesicle, without head or visible organs, ranked amongst the Entozoa, although possessed of few animated characteristics. In no organ of the body are acephalocysts so frequently found as in the liver. Generally it is the 'multiple acephalocyst,' *A. socia'lis* seu *prolif'era,* which is met with. At times, however, it is the 'solitary acephalocyst,' *A. eremi'ta* seu *ster'ilis.*

The *acephalocystis endog"ena* has a firm coat, and is composed of different layers, which have numbers of smaller hydatids within them, and are thrown off from the interior of the parent cyst. This species has hence been termed *endogena,* to distinguish it from the *A. exog"ena* of ruminant animals, in which the young vesicles are developed from the exterior of the parent vesicle.—See Hydatid.

ACEPHALOGAS'TER, *Athoracoceph'alus,* from *a* privative, *κεφαλη,* 'head,' and *γαστηρ,* 'the belly.' A name given to monsters devoid of head, chest, and abdomen; or to those which have an abdomen, but no chest or head.

ACEPHALOS'TOMA, from *a* privative, *κεφαλη,* 'head,' and *στομα,* 'mouth.' An acephalous fœtus, at the upper part of which there is an opening resembling a mouth.

ACEPHALOTHO'RUS, from *a* privative, *κεφαλη,* 'head,' and *θωραξ,* 'chest,' *Apectoceph'alus.* A monster devoid of head or chest.

ACEPH'ALOUS, from *a* privative, and *κεφαλη,* 'head.' A monster born devoid of head. The condition is called *Acepha'lia.*

ACER, Acrid.

ACER PALMIFOLIUM, A. Saccharinum.

ACER SACCHARI'NUM, *A. palmifo'lium.* Maple, Sugar Maple. (F.) *Érable.* This tree contains a large amount of sweet sap, whence a considerable quantity of sugar may be extracted. When purified, this sugar can scarcely be distinguished from that obtained from the cane.—See Saccharum.

ACERA'TES LONGIFO'LIA, *Long-leaved green Milkweed; Order,* Asclepiadaceæ; indigenous, flowering in June and July; has the properties of the order. See Asclepias.

ACERATO'SIS, from *a* privative, and *κερας,* 'horn.' Defective development of the corneous tissue.

ACERB', *Acer'bus, Stryphnos,* from *acer,* 'sharp.' A savour, or taste, compounded of the acid, bitter, and astringent; such as is met with in unripe fruits, &c.

ACER'CUS, from *a* privative, and *κερκος,* 'a tail.' A monster devoid of tail.—Gurlt.

ACE'RIDES, *Acero'des,* from *a* privative, and *κηρος,* 'wax.' Plasters devoid of wax.—Galen.

ACERODES, Acerides.

ACERO'SUS, *Achyro'des, Pithyri'nus,* from *αχυρον,* 'chaff.' *Furfura'ceous.* An epithet used by Hippocrates, for the coarsest bread, made of flour not separated from the chaff.—Foësius.

ACERVULUS CEREBRI. See Pineal Gland —*a.* Glandulus Pinealis, see Pineal Gland.

ACES'CENCY, *Acescen'tia,* from *acescere,* 'to grow sour,' (*ακις,* 'a point,' *acer,* 'sharp.') A disposition to acidity. The humourists believed that the animal humours are susceptible of this change.

ACESIA, Cure.

ACESIS, Curation, Cure, Medicament.

ACESMA, Medicament.

ACESMIUS, Curable.

ACESMUS, Cure.

ACESODYNES, Anodyne.

ACESOPHORUS, Curative.

ACESTER, Physician.

ACESTIS, Medicament.

ACESTOR, Physician.

ACESTORIA, Medicine.

ACESTORIS, Midwife.

ACESTOS, Curable.

ACESTRA, Needle.

ACESTRIA, Midwife.

ACESTRIS, Midwife.

ACESTRUM, Medicament.

ACETA MEDICATA, Acetica.

ACETABULA UTERINA, Cotyledons.

ACETAB'ULUM, from *acetum,* 'vinegar,' because it resembles the old vinegar vessel, *oxybaph'ion.* A measure capable of containing the eighth part of a modern pint. Athenæus. Galen. See Cotyloid. According to Castelli, the lobes or cotyledons of the placentæ of ruminating animals have been so called.

ACETABULUM, Cotyle, Cotyloid—*a.* Humeri, see Glenoid—*a.* Marinum, Umbilicus marinus.

ACETA'RIA, same etymon. A salad or pickle.

ACETAS, Acetate.

AC"ETATE, *Ace'tas.* A salt formed by the union of the acetic acid with an alkaline, earthy, or metallic base. The acetates chiefly used in medicine are the acetates of ammonia, lead, potash, and zinc.

ACE'TICA, *Ace'ta Medica'ta.* (F.) *Vinaigres Médicinaux.* Pharmaceutical preparations of vinegar.

ACE'TICUM AC"IDUM, *Acidum Ace'ticum for'tius, A. A. fortè, A. Ace'ticum purum, Ace'tum radica'lè, Oxos, Ace'tic Acid, Strong Ace'tous Acid, Acidum Aceto'sum fortè, Rad'ical Vin'egar, Spir'itus Ven'eris (when made from verdigris,) Spirit of Verdigris.* Concentrated acetic acid, prepared by decomposing an acetate and receiving the acetic acid by distillation, has a very pungent and grateful odour, and an acid and acrid taste. Its s. g. is about 1.046, and it is very volatile.

It is stimulant, rubefacient, and escharotic, and is applied to the nostrils in syncope, asphyxia, headache, &c. It destroys warts.

An *Aromatic Spirit of Vinegar, Ac"idum Ace'ticum Camphora'tum, A. aceto'sum camphora'tum,* is formed of this *strong acid,* ʒvj, *Camphor,* ʒss, *Ol. Caryoph.* gtt. xv.

A strong Acetic Acid was ordered by the London pharmacopœia prepared from wood. It was called *Vinegar of wood, Improved distilled Vinegar, Pyrolig'neous Acid, Ace'tum Ligno'rum,* and its strength was such, that 87 gr. of crystallized subcarbonate of soda should saturate 100 grains of the acid.

Ac"idum Ace'ticum Dilu'tum, A. A. ten'uè, Ace'tum destilla'tum, Acidum ace'ticum, Acidum aceto'sum destilla'tum, Acidum ace'ticum debil'ius, Distil'led vin'egar, (F.) *Acide Acétique faible, Vinaigre distillé,* is prepared by distilling vinegar, until seven-eighths have passed over. An *Acidum aceticum dilutum, Diluted acetic acid,* is made by mixing half a pint of the strong acetic acid with five pints of distilled water.—Ph. U. S. Its properties are like those of vinegar.

ACETIQUE, MARTIALE, Ferri Acetas.

AC"ETUNE, from *acetum,* 'vinegar.' *Spir'itus pyro-ace'ticus ligno'sus, Pyro-ace'tic spirit, Pyroace'tic, Ether, Mesit'ic Al'cohol, Bihydrate of Mesit'ylene;* erroneously called *Naphtha* and *Wood Naphtha.* A limpid, colourless liquid, having a peculiarly penetrating and slightly empyreumatic odour. Its density in the liquid state, is almost the same as that of alcohol, 0.7921. Its taste is disagreeable, and analogous to that of peppermint. It is miscible in all proportions with water, alcohol, and ether. It may be prepared by distilling a mixture of two parts of crystallized acetate of lead and one part of quicklime in a salt-glaze jar (gray-beard,) the lower part of the jar being coated with fire-clay; and a bent glass tube, half an inch in diameter, adapted to the mouth by a cork, so as to form a distillatory apparatus. The jar is supported on the mouth of a small furnace, by which the lower part only is heated to redness, and the vapours are conducted into a Liebig's condenser. The product is repeatedly redistilled from quicklime, until its boiling point is constant at 132°.

It has been brought forward as a remedy in phthisis pulmonalis; but evidently with unfounded pretensions. It is an excitant, and may be serviceable in chronic bronchitis. The dose is ten to forty drops three times a day, diluted with water.

ACETOSA ALPINA, Rumex alpinus—a. Nostras, Rumex acetosa—a. Pratensis, Rumex acetosa—a. Romana, Rumex scutatus—a. Rotundifolia, Rumex scutatus—a. Scutata, Rumex scutatus—a. Vulgaris, Rumex acetosa.

ACETOSELLA, Oxalis acetosella.

ACE'TUM, *ὄξυς, Οξυς, Ace'tum Vini, A. Britan'nicum, Common Vinegar, Acidum aceto'sum, A'legar, Ace'tum Cerevis'iæ,* (F.) *Vinaigre;* from *ακις,* 'a point,' *acer,* 'sharp.' A liquor obtained by the acetous fermentation. Vinegar has a pungent odour, and a pleasant acid taste. One fluid ounce of the Acetum of the United States Pharmacopœia is saturated by about 35 grains of crystallized bicarbonate of soda. It is refrigerant in fevers; antiseptic, and anti-narcotic; and externally is stimulant and discutient.

Vinegar Whey is made by stirring a small wineglassful of vinegar, sweetened with a dessert spoonful of *sugar,* in a pint of *milk ;* boiling for fifteen minutes, and straining. Like tamarind whey it is an agreeable drink in febrile affections.

ACE'TUM AROMAT'ICUM, *Acidum Ace'ticum Aromat'icum, Ace'tum Theriaca'lè, A. quatuor furum, Thieves' Vinegar, Vinegar of the four Thieves, Marseilles Vinegar,* (F.) *Vinaigre Aromatique, V. des quatre voleurs,* (*Rorismarin. cacum. sicc., Fol. Salviæ* sing. ʒj. *Lavand. flor. sicc.* ʒiv. *Caryoph. cont.* ʒss. *Acid. Acet.* Oij. Macerate 7 days, and filter.—Ph. E.) Odour, pungent and aromatic. Used as a perfume.

ACETUM BRITANNICUM, Acetum.

ACE'TUM CANTHAR'IDIS, *Vinegar of Cantharides,* (*Cantharid.* in pulv. ʒiij. *Acid. acet.* f ʒv., *Acid. pyrolign.* f ʒxv : *Euphorb.* in pulv. crass. ʒss. Mix the acids; add the powders; macerate for seven days; strain; express strongly, and filter the liquor.—Ph. E. The London College macerates *cantharid.* ʒij in *acid. acet.* Oj. for eight days; expresses and strains.) It is used as a prompt vesicant.

ACE'TUM COL'CHICI, *Vinegar of meadow saffron.* (*Colchic. rad. contus.* ʒij ; *Acid. acetic. dilut.* seu *Acet. destillat.* Oij ; Ph. U. S. 1851. It may also be made by displacement.) It is used as a diuretic, and also in gout. Dose f ʒss. to ʒiss.

ACETUM DESTILLATUM ; see Aceticum acidum —a. Lignorum : see Aceticum acidum—a. Mulsum dulce, Oxyglycus—a. Opii, Guttæ Nigræ—a. Quatuor furum, Acetum Aromaticum—a. Radicale, Aceticum Acidum—a. Rosatum Oxyrrhodinon.

ACETUM SCILLÆ, *Acidum Ace'ticum Scillit'icum. Vinegar of Squills,* (F.) *Vinaigre scillitique,* (*Scillæ* contus. ʒiv ; *Acet. destillat.* Oij ; Ph. U. S. It may also be made by displacement.) Diuretic, expectorant, and emetic. Dose f ʒss to ʒij as a diuretic and expectorant.

ACETUM THERIACALE, Acetum aromaticum.

ACEYTE DE SAL. A remedy for bronchocele used in S. America. Roulin found it to contain a portion of iodine.

ACHACANA. A species of cactus, in the province of Potosi in Peru. Its root is thick and fleshy, and of a conical shape. It is a good edible, and is sold in the markets of the country.

ACHANACA. A plant of the kingdom of Mely in Africa. It is used by the natives as an antisyphilitic.

ACHAOVAN, a species of Egyptian chamomile.—Prosper Alpinus.

ACHAOVAN-ABIAT. The Egyptian name of *Cineraria maritima,* used in female diseases.

ACHAR, Atchar.

ACHE, Apium graveolens—a. *des Montagnes,* Ligusticum levisticum.

ACHEI'LIA, *Achi'lia,* from *a,* priv., and χειλος, 'lip.' A malformation, consisting in a deficiency of a lip or lips.

ACHEI'LUS, *Achi'lus,* same etymon. One who is without lips.

ACHEIR, *Achir, De'manus,* from *a,* privative, and χιρ, 'hand.' One devoid of hands.—Galen.

ACHEI'RIA, *Achi'ria:* same etymon. The state of being devoid of hands.

ACHEROIS, Populus.

ACHIA, *Achiar.* A name given in India to the pickled shoots of the bamboo.

ACHIA, Atchar.

ACHIAR, Achia.

ACHIC'OLUM, *Achit'olus, Hidrote'rion, Suda'rium, Fornix, Tholus, Sudato'rium.* The sweating-room in the ancient bagnios.

ACHILIA, Acheilia.

ACHILLE'A AGE'RATUM, *A. Visco'sa, Balsami'ta fœmin'ea, Eupato'rium* MES'UES, *Age'ratum, Cos'tus horto'rum minor, Maudlin, Maudlin Tansey;* (F.) *Achillée Visqueuse; Nat. Ord.* Compositæ; *Sub. Ord.* Anthemideæ; *Sex. Syst.* Syngenesia Polygamia superflua,—has the same properties as tansey, bitter and aromatic, and is used in like affections.

ACHILLE'A ATRA'TA, *Herba Gen'ipi veri,* (F.) *Achillée Noire,* has similar virtues.

ACHILLE'A MILLEFO'LIUM, *Achille'a Myriophyl'lon, Chrysoc'oma, Millefo'lium, Chiliophyl'lon, Lumbus Ven'eris, Common Yarrow or Milfoil.* (F.) *Millefeuille.* The leaves and flowers have an aromatic smell, and a rough, bitterish, somewhat pungent taste. They have been used in dyspepsia, flatulence, &c. An extract of the plant, made with proof spirit, has been called *Achilleï'num;* and is used by the Italians in intermittent fever.

ACHILLE'A PTAR'MICA, *Pseudo-py'rethrum, Py'rethrum sylves'trē, Draco sylves'tris, Tarchon sylvestris, Sternutamento'ria, Dracun'culus Praten'sis, Sneeze-wort, Bastard Pel'litory, Ptar'mica.* (F.) *Herbe à éternuer.* The roots and flowers have a hot, biting taste, approaching that of pyrethrum. Their principal use is as a masticatory and sialogogue.

ACHILLEA VISCOSA, A. Ageratum.

ACHILLÉE NOIRE, Achillea atrata—*a. Visqueuse,* Achillea ageratum.

ACHILLEINUM, see Achillea Millefolium.

ACHILLE'IS. A beautiful species of barley, mentioned by Theophrastus and Galen, called after Achilles, a labourer. The decoction was used in fevers and jaundice.—Hippocrates.

ACHIL'LIS TENDO, *Funis* HIPPOC'RATIS, *Corda seu Chorda* HIPPOC'RATIS, *Corda magna, Nervus latus,* (F.) *Tendon d'Achille.* The strong tendon of the gastrocnemii muscles above the heel: so called, because it was the only vulnerable part of ACHILLES, or because of its strength. See Tendon.

ACHILUS, Acheilus.

ACHIMBASSI. An archiater or chief of physicians. A name given, at Grand Cairo, to a magistrate who licenses physicians.

ACHIR, Acheir.

ACHIRIA, Acheiria.

ACHITOLUS, Achicolum.

ACHLYS, Caligo.

ACHMELLA, Spilanthus acmella.

ACHNE. Lint. See Linteum. Also, small mucous flocculi seen in front of the cornea.—Hippocrates.

ACHOL'IA, from *a,* privative, and χολη, 'bile.' Deficiency or want of bile.

ACH'OLUS: same etymon. One deficient in bile.

ACHOR, Porrigo larvalis.

ACHO'RES. A term often employed by the ancients to designate both *crusta lac'tea,* and small superficial ulcerations on the skin of the face and head. See Porrigo Larvalis.

ACHORES CAPITIS, Porrigo scutulata.

ACHORION SCHÖNLEINI. See Porrigo favosa.

ACHORIS'TUS, from *a,* priv., and χωριζω, 'I separate.' Any sign which necessarily accompanies a state of health or disease.

ACHOUROU. The Caraib name for a species of myrtle used in dropsy.

ACHRAS AUSTRALIS, Sapota—*a.* Sapota, Sapota—*a.* Zapota, Sapota.

ACHROI, *Achromatis'ti, Achro'mati, Achro'mi,* from *a,* privative, and χρωμα, 'colour.' Pale individuals.—Hippocrates. It is nearly synonymous with λειφαιμοι, *leipha'mia,* persons without colour; bloodless.

ACHROMASIA, Decoloration.

ACHROMATI, Achroi.

ACHROMAT'IC, *Achromat'icus;* same etymon. A lens, so constructed as to correct the aberration of refrangibility of common lenses, is so termed. The *Crystalline* is an achromatic lens.

ACHROMATISTI, Achroi.

ACHROMATOPSIA, *Chromatopseudop'sia, Chromatometablep'sia, Dyschromatop'sia, Parachro'ma, Parora'sis, Visus de'color, Colour blindness, Idiop'tcy, Dal'tonism,* from *a,* privative, χρωμα, 'colour,' and οντομαι, 'I see.' Incapability of distinguishing colours; a defect situate in the cerebral part of the visual organ. Persons so circumstanced have been termed by Mr. Whewell, *Idiopts.* See Acyanoblepsia and Anerythropsia.

ACHROMI, Achroi.

ACHYLO'SIS, from *a,* privative, and χυλος, 'juice, chyle.' Defective chylosis or formation of chyle.

ACHYMO'SIS, from *a,* privative, and χυμος, 'juice, chyme.' Defective chymification.

ACHYRODES, Acerosus.

ACHYRON, Furfur.

A'CIA, from ακις, a point. A word used by Celsus, which has puzzled commentators,—some believing it to have meant a needle; others the thread; and others, again, the kind of suture. *"Acia mollis, non nimis torta."*—Celsus, Galen. (Chifflet thinks it meant the thread.—Antwerp, 1638.)

ACID, *Ac"idus, Oxys.* (F.) *Acide, aigre,* from *ακις,* 'a point;' sharp; sour; especially as applied to odorous or sapid substances. The French also use the term *aigre,* when referring to the voice, in the sense of sharp and shrill:—*as une voix aigre, vox aspera.*

ACID, ACETIC, Aceticum acidum — *a.* Acetic, dilute, see Aceticum acidum.

ACID, ACETOUS, STRONG, Aceticum acidum — *a.* Aerial, Carbonic acid — *a.* Antimonious, Antimonium diaphoreticum—*a.* Arsenious, Arsenicum album—*a.* Auric, see Gold—*a.* Azotic, Nitric acid—*a.* Benzoic, Benjamin, flowers of—*a.* Boric, Boracic acid—*a.* Calcareous, Carbonic acid —*a.* Carbonaceous, Carbonic acid—*a.* Carbonous, Oxalic acid—*a.* Chromic, see Chromic acid—*a.* Citric, Citric acid—*a.* Cyanhydric, Hydrocyanic acid—*a.* Cyanhydric, Hydrocyanic acid—*a.* Gastric, Gastric juice.

ACID, GALLIC, *Ac"idum Gall'icum.* (F.) *Acide Gallique.* This acid is found in most of the astringent plants that contain tannic acid of the kind obtained from galls. It is in delicate silky needles, usually somewhat yellowish, inodorous, and of a harsh, somewhat astringent taste. It dissolves in one hundred parts of cold and three parts of boiling water. It is very soluble in alcohol, and but slightly so in ether.

It has been highly extolled in internal hemorrhage, especially from the urinary organs and uterus. Dose from ten to twenty grains.

The last Pharmacopœia of the United States (1851) directs it to be made by exposing a thin paste of *powdered galls* and *distilled water* for a month, adding the water from time to time to preserve the consistence; expressing the paste; boiling the residue in distilled water; filtering through animal charcoal, and crystallizing.

ACID, HIPPU'RIC, Ac''idum Hippu'ricum, Uroben'zoic acid. An acid found in the urine of graminivorous animals. It is contained in human urine, especially after benzoic acid has been taken. See Hippuria.

ACID, HYDRIOD'IC, Ac''idum Hydriod'icum. This acid is made by mixing solutions of iodide of potassium and tartaric acid; filtering the liquor to separate the bitartrate of potassa, and adding water to make the resulting hydriodic acid of definite strength.

It has been used in the same cases as the preparations of iodine in general, but is rarely employed.

ACID, HYDROCHLORONITRIC, Nitro-muriatic acid—a. Hydrocyanic, Hydrocyanic acid—a. Hydrocyanic, dilute, see Hydrocyanic acid—a. Hydrosulphuric, Hydrogen, sulphuretted—a. Hydrothionic, Hydrogen, sulphuretted—a. Igasuric: see Jatropha curcas.

ACID, IODIC, Ac''idum Iod'icum, (F.) Acide Iodique. This is obtained by boiling iodine with nitric acid; or by decomposing iodate of baryta by dilute sulphuric acid. It is a white, transparent solid, slightly deliquescent, and very soluble in water. It has been given with sulphate of quinia in hoarseness, scrofula, incipient phthisis, chronic inflammation, syphilis, &c. Dose three to six grains, or more.

ACID OF LEMONS, Citric acid—a. Lithic, Uric acid—a. Dephlogisticated marine, Chlorine—a. Mephitic, Carbonic acid—a. of Milk, Lactic acid—a. Muriatic, see Muriaticum acidum—a. Muriatic, dilute, see Muriaticum acidum—a. Nitric, see Nitric acid—a. Nitric, dilute, see Nitric Acid—a. Nitro-hydrochloric, Nitro-muriatic acid—a. Nitro-Muriatic, see Nitro-Muriatic Acid—a. Nitrous, dephlogisticated, Nitric acid—a. Oxyseptonic, Nitric acid—a. Polygalic: see Polygala senega—a. Prussic, Hydrocyanic acid—a. Pyroligneous: see Aceticum acidum—a. Pyrolignic, Pyroligneous acid—a. of Sorrel, Oxalic acid—a. of Sugar, Oxalic acid—a. Sulphuric, see Sulphuric acid—a. Tannic, Tannin—a. Uric, Uric acid—a. Urobenzoic, A. Hippuric—a. Urous, Uric oxide—a. Urylic, Uric acid—a. Chromique, Chromic acid.

ACIDE ACÉTIQUE FAIBLE, see Aceticum acidum—a. Boracique, Boracic acid—a. Chromique, Chromic acid—a. Gallique, Acid, gallic—a. Hydrocyanique, Hydrocyanic acid—a. Hydrosulfurique, Hydrogen, sulphuretted—a. Iodique, Acid, iodic—a. Lactique, Lactic acid—a. Nitrique, Nitric acid—a. Phosphorique, Phosphoric acid—a. Prussique, Hydrocyanic acid—a. Sulfureux, Sulphurous acid—a. Sulfurique, Sulphuric acid—a. Sulfurique delayé, Sulphuricum acidum dilutum—a. Tannique, Tannin.

ACIDITATIO, Acidities.

ACID'ITIES, Aco'res, Acidita'tio, Ac''idum morbo'sum, Ac''idum prima'rum via'rum, Oxytes, Sordes ac''idæ. (F.) Aigreurs. Sourness of the stomach, the result of indigestion, indicated by acid eructations, &c. The affection is very common in children, and must be obviated by absorbents, as magnesia, chalk, &c., and by regulated diet.

ACIDOLOG''IA, from $\alpha\kappa\iota\varsigma$, 'a point, a sharp instrument,' and $\lambda o\gamma o\varsigma$, 'a description.' A description of surgical instruments.

ACIDOM'ETER, (F.) Acidomètre, Pèse-acide, from acid, and $\mu\epsilon\tau\rho o\nu$, measure. A hydrometer for determining the density of acids.

AC''IDS, Ac''ida, Aco'res, are liquid, solid, or gaseous bodies, possessed of a sour, more or less caustic taste, and the principal character of which is the capability of saturating, wholly or in part, the alkaline properties of bases.

Acids, in general, are refrigerent and antiseptic. Their particular uses are pointed out under the individual articles.

To ACID'ULATE. (F.) Aiguiser, Aciduler. To render acidulous, or slightly acid.

ACID'ULOUS, Acid'ulus, Oxo'des, Oxoï'des. (F.) Acidule, Aigrelet. Substances are so called which possess a sourish taste, as tamarinds, cream of tartar, &c.

ACIDULOUS FRUITS. Oranges, gooseberries, &c.

ACIDULOUS WATERS, Aquæ Acidulæ. Mineral waters containing carbonic acid gas sufficient to render them sourish. See Waters, mineral.

ACIDULOUS WATER, SIMPLE, Aqua Ac''idi Carbon'ici, (Ph. U. S.) Aqua a'eris fixi, Aqua acid'ula simplex, Liquor seu Aqua Sodæ efferves'cens, Aqua Carbona'tis Sodæ acid'ula, Soda water, Mineral water, (F.) Eau Acidule simple, is water impregnated with fixed air.

Water, so impregnated, is cooling, and slightly stimulating. It is used beneficially in dyspepsia, and in cases of vomiting, &c.

ACIDUM ACETICUM, Aceticum acidum—a. Aceticum aromaticum, Acetum aromaticum—a. Aceticum camphoratum: see Aceticum acidum—a. Aceticum dilutum: see Aceticum Acidum—a. Aceticum empyreumaticum, Pyroligneous acid—a. Aceticum Scilliticum, Acetum scillæ—a. Acetosellæ, Oxalic acid—a. Acetosum, Acetum—a. Allantoicum, Allantoic acid—a. Amnicum, Amniotic acid—a. Arsenicosum, Arsenious acid—a. Arsenicosum, (Ph. U. S.) Arsenious acid—a. Azoticum, Nitric Acid—a. Benzoicum, Benjamin, Flowers of—a. Boracicum, Boracic acid—a. Borussicum, Hydrocyanic acid—a. Carbonicum, Carbonic acid—a. Citricum, Citric acid—a. Gallicum, Acid, gallic—a. Hydriodicum, Acid hydriodic—a. Hydrocarbonicum, Oxalic acid—a. Hydrochloricum, Muriaticum acidum—a. Hydrocyanicum, Hydrocyanic acid—a. Hydrocyanicum dilutum, see Hydrocyanic Acid—a. Hydrothionicum liquidum, see Hydrosulphuretted water—a. Iodicum, Acid, iodic—a. Jatrophicum, see Jatropha curcas—a. Lacticum, Lactic acid—a. Ligneum, Pyroligneous acid—a. Ligni pyro-oleosum, Pyroligneous acid—a. Lithicum, Uric acid—a. Marinum concentratum, Muriaticum acidum—a. Morbosum, Acidities—a. Muriaticum, Muriaticum acidum—a. Muriaticum dilutum, Muriatic acid—a. Muriaticum nitroso-oxygenatum, Nitro-muriatic acid—a. Nitri, Nitric acid—a. Nitricum, Nitric acid—a. Nitricum dilutum, Nitric acid—a. Nitro-Muriaticum, Nitro-muriatic acid—a. Oxalinum, Oxalic acid—a. Phosphoricum, Phosphoric acid—a. Primarum viarum, Acidities—a. Prussicum, Hydrocyanic acid—a. Pyro-aceticum, Pyroligneous acid—a. Pyrolignosum, Pyroligneous acid—a. Pyroxylicum, Pyroligneous acid—a. Quercitannicum, Tannin—a. Sacchari, Oxalic acid—a. Saccharinum, Oxalic acid—a. Salis, Muriaticum acidum—a. Salis culinaris, Muriaticum acidum—a. Salis marini, Muriaticum acidum—a. Septicum, Nitric acid—a. Succinicum, Succinic acid—a. Sulphuricum, Sulphuric acid—a. Sulphuricum alcoolisatum, Elixir acidum Halleri—a. Sulphuricum aromaticum, Sulphuric acid, aromatic—a. Sulphuricum dilutum, Sulphuric acid, diluted—a. Sulphuris volatile, Sulphurous acid—a. Sulphurosicum, Sulphurous acid—a. Tannicum, Tannin—a. Tartari essentiale, Tartaric acid—a. Tartaricum, Tartaric acid—a. Tartarosum, Tartaric acid—a. Uricum, Uric acid—a. Urolithicum, Uric acid—a. Vitriolicum, Sulphuric acid—a. Vitriolicum aromaticum, Sulphuricum acidum aromaticum—a. Vitriolicum alcohole aromaticum, Sulphuricum acidum aromaticum—a. Vitriolicum vinosum, Elixir acidum Halleri—a. Zooticum, Hydrocyanic acid—a. Zootinicum, Hydrocyanic acid.

ACIDURGIA, Surgery (operative.)
ACIER, Chalybs.

ACIES, Chalybs—a. Digitorum manus, Phalanges of the fingers—a. Diurna, Hemeralopia.

ACINE'SIA, *Acine'sis, Akine'sia, Immobil'itas, Quies, Requies, Requie'tio, Esych'ia, Erem'ia*, from *a*, privative, and κινησις, motion,' κινεω, 'I move.' Rest. Immobility. Also, the interval between the systole and diastole of the heart—*Parasys'tolē.*

Under the term *Acineses*, Remberg includes the paralytic neuroses, or those that are characterized by defect of motive power.

ACINI OF MALPIGHI, Corpora Malpighiana.

ACINIFORMIS (TUNICA) Choroid, Uvea.

AC"INUS, *Ac"inus glandulo'sus*, from *ac"inus*, 'a grape-stone.' A *glandiform corpuscle* or *granulation*, in which secretion was supposed to take place, and the excretory radicle to arise. Acini are the *glob'uli arteria'rum ter'mini* of Nichols. The term *ac"ini glandulo'si* has also been given to glands, which, like the pancreas, are arranged as it were in clusters. See Lobule.

ACIPENSER, see Ichthyocolla.

ACIURGIA, Surgery, (operative.)

ACLEITROCARDIA, Cyanopathy.

ACMAS'TICUS, from ακμη, 'the top,' and σαω, 'I remain.' A fever which preserves an equal degree of intensity throughout its course. It is also called *Homot'onos*. The Greeks gave it the name of *Epacmas'ticos*, and *Syn'ochos*, when it went on increasing,—and *Paracmas'ticos*, when it decreased.—Galen.

ACMÉ, *Vigor, Cor'yphē, Culmina'tio, Status, Fastig"ium.* The period of a disease at which the symptoms are most violent. *Archē*, Αρχη, is 'the commencement;' *anab'asis, αναβασις*, 'the period of increase;' and *acmē, ακμη*, 'the height.'

ACMELLA, Spilanthus acmella—a. Mauritiana, Spilanthus acmella.

ACMON, Incus.

ACNÉ, *Acna, Ion'thus varus, Varus, Psydra'cia Acne, Stone Pock, Whelk, Bubucle*, (F.) *Dartre pustuleuse disséminée.* A small pimple or tubercle on the face.—Gorræus. Foësius thinks the word ought to be *Acme;* and, according to Cassius, it is, at all events, derived from ακμη, 'vigour;' the disease affecting those in the vigour of life, especially.

Willan and Bateman have adopted the term in their Nosology of cutaneous diseases, and placed it in the Order, TUBERCULA. Acne, with them, is an eruption of distinct, hard, inflamed tubercles, sometimes continuing for a considerable length of time, and sometimes suppurating slowly and partially. They usually appear on the forehead, temples and chin, and are common to both sexes; but the most severe forms are seen in young men. They require but little management, and consist of four varieties; *Acne indura'ta, A. simplex*, (*Haploäcnē,*) *A. puncta'ta* (*Ion'thus varus puncta'tus, Punctæ muco'sæ, Comedo'nes* or *Maggot Pimple,*) and *A. rosa'cea.*—See Gutta Rosea.

ACNE ROSACEA, Gutta rosea—a. of the Throat, Pharyngitis, follicular.

ACNES'TIS, from *a*, privative, and κναειν, 'to scratch.' The part of the spine which extends, in quadrupeds, from between the shoulders to the loins. According to Pollux, the middle of the loins. The vertebral column.

ACNESTOS, Cneorum tricoccum.

ACOÉ, Audition, Ear.

ACOE'LIOS, from *a*, privative, and κοιλια, 'belly.' Devoid of belly. One who is so emaciated as to appear to have no belly.—Galen.

ACOËMETER, Acoumeter.
ACOËMETRUM, Acoumeter.
ACOËNOSI, Aconusi.
ACOËSIS, Audition.
ACOGNOSIA, Pharmacognosia.
ACOLASIA, Intemperance.
ACOLOGY, Materia Medica.
ACONE, Mortar.

ACONIT À GRANDS FLEURS, Aconitum cammarum—a. *Salutaire*, Aconitum anthora.

ACONITA, see Aconitum napellus.

ACONITE, Aconitum—a. Folia, see Aconitum —a. Radix, see Aconitum.

ACONITI FOLIA, see Aconitum — a. Radix, see Aconitum.

ACONITIA, see Aconitum napellus.
ACONITIN, see Aconitum napellus.
ACONITINE, see Aconitum napellus.
ACONITIUM, see Aconitum napellus.

ACONI'TUM, from *Ac'onē*, a place in Bithynia, where it is common. *Cynoc'tonon, Pardalian'ches, Pardalian'chum, Canici'da, Ac'onite, Wolfsbane, Monkshood. Nat. Ord.* Ranunculaceæ. *Sex. Syst.* Polyandria Trigynia.

ACONITUM, Aconite, in the Pharmacopœia of the United States, 1842, is the leaves of Aconitum napellus, and A. paniculatum. In the last edition, 1851, *Aconiti folia* is the officinal name for the leaves; *Aconiti radix* for that of the root.

ACONI'TUM AN'THORA, *Aconi'tum Salutif'erum,* seu *nemoro'sum* seu *Candol'lei* seu *Jacquini* seu *eul'ophum* seu *anthoroïdeum, An'thora vulga'ris, An'thora, Antith'ora, Sal'utary Monkshood, Wholesome Wolfsbane, Yellow helmet flower.* (F.) *Aconit salutaire.* The root of this variety, as of all the rest, is poisonous. It is used as a cathartic and anthelmintic. Dose ƺss to ƺj.

ACONITUM ANTHOROIDEUM, A. anthora.

ACONI'TUM CAM'MARUM, *A. panicula'tum, A. macran'thum, A. Kusnezo'vii*, (F.) *Aconit à grands fleurs*, resembles Aconitum Napellus in properties.

ACONITUM CANDOLLEI, A. anthora—a. Eulophum, A. anthora—a. Jacquini, A. anthora—a. Kusnezovii, A. cammarum—a. Macranthum, A. cammarum.

ACONI'TUM NAPEL'LUS, *Napel'lus verus, Aconi'tum, Common Monkshead* or *Wolfsbane, A. Neomonta'num.* (F.) *Chaperon de Moine.* The leaves are narcotic, sudorific, and deobstruent (?) They have been used in chronic rheumatism, scrofula, scirrhus, paralysis, amaurosis, &c. The active principle is called *Aconit'ia, Aconiti'na, Aconi'ta, Aconit'ium* or *Aconitine.* A form for its preparation is contained in the Ph. U. S. (1851.) It is made by treating an *alcoholic extract of the root* with *dilute sulphuric acid;* precipitating by *solution of ammonia;* dissolving the precipitate in *dilute sulphuric acid;* treating with *animal charcoal;* again precipitating with *solution of ammonia;* washing with water, and drying. It requires 150 parts of cold and 50 of boiling water to dissolve it, but is readily dissolved by alcohol and ether. It neutralizes the acids, and forms with them uncrystallizable salts. It has been used internally, and especially applied externally, in neuralgic cases, iatraleptically and endermically. Dose of Aconitum, gr. j. to gr. iij.

ACONITUM NEMOROSUM, A. anthora—a. Neomontanum, A. napellus—a. Paniculatum, A. cammarum—a. Racemosum, Actæa spicata—a. Salutiferum, A. anthora.

ACONU'SI, *Acoën'osi, Acoën'osi*, from ακοη, 'audition,' and νουσος, 'disease.' *Morbi au'rium et audi'tūs.* Diseases of the ears and audition.

ACOÖNOSI, Aconusi.

AC'OPIS. Same etymon as the next. Pliny

gives this name to a precious stone, which was boiled in oil and used against weariness.

AC'OPON, from *a*, privative, and κοπος, 'weariness.' A remedy against weariness—Foësius, Gorræus, &c. *Ac'opum*,—Celsus, Pliny. See Anagyris.

ACOPRIA, Constipation.

ACOPROSIS, Constipation.

ACOR BENZOÏNUS, Benjamin—a. Boracicus, Boracic acid—a. Succineus, Succinic acid—a. Sulphuris, Sulphuric acid—a. Tartaricus, Tartaric acid.

ACORE BÂTARD, Iris pseudacorus—a. *Faux*, Iris pseudacorus—a. *Odorant*, Acorus calamus.

ACORES, Acids, and Acidities.

ACOR'IA, from *a*, privative, and κορεω, 'I satiate.' An inordinate or canine appetite.—Hippocrates.

ACORI'TES. A wine made of Acorus.—Dioscorides.

ACOR'MUS, from *a*, privative, and κορμος, 'trunk.' A monster devoid of a trunk.—Gurlt.

ACORN, JUPITER'S, Fagus castanea—a. Oily, Guilandina moringa—a. Sardinian, Fagus castanea.

ACORNS. See Quercus alba.

ACORUS ADULTERINUS, Iris pseudacorus.

Ac'ORUS CAL'AMUS. *A. Verus, Cal'amus Aromat'icus, C. Odora'tus, Cal'amus vulga'ris, Typha Aromat'ica, Acorus Brazilien'sis, Clava Rugo'sa, Sweetflag* or *Ac'orus, Flagroot, Sweet cane, Myrtle Flag, Sweet grass, Sweet root, Sweet rush*. (F.) *Jonc roseau* ou *Canne aromatique, Acore odorant. Nat. Ord.* Aroideæ; Acoraceæ. (Lindley.) *Sex. Syst.* Hexandria Monogynia. The rhizoma—*Cal'amus* (Ph. U. S.)—is stomachic and carminative, but is rarely used. It is regarded as a good adjuvant to bark in quinia and intermittents.

Ac'ORUS PALUSTRIS, Iris pseudacorus—a. Vulgaris, Iris pseudacorus.

ACOS, Medicament.

ACOS'MIA, from *a*, privative, and κοσμος, 'order, ornament,' Disorder, irregularity in the critical days, according to Galen, who uses the word κοσμος for regularity in those days. Others, and particularly Pollux, call bald persons ακοσμοι, because they are deprived of one of their most beautiful ornaments.

ACOUM'ETER, *Acouŏm'eter, Acoëm'eter, Acoëm'etrum, Acu'meter, Acusim'eter*, (F.) *Acoumètre*, from ακουω, 'I hear,' and μετρον, 'measure.' An instrument designed by M. Itard for measuring the degree of hearing.

ACOUMÈTRE, Acoumeter.

ACOUOPHO'NIA, *Copho'nia;* from ακουω, 'I hear,' and φωνη, 'voice,' "*Aus'cultatory Percus'sion*." A mode of auscultation, in which the observer places his ear on the chest, and analyzes the sound produced by percussion.—Donné.

ACOUS'MA, an imaginary noise. Depraved sense of hearing.

ACOUS'TIC, *Acus'ticus*. That which belongs to the ear; as *Acoustic nerve, Acoustic trumpet*.

ACOUSTIC MEDICINE is one used in diseased audition.

ACOUS'TICS, *Acus'tica*. (F.) *Acoustique*. The part of physics which treats of the theory of sounds. It is also called *Phonics*.

ACOUSTIQUE, Acoustics.

ACQUA BINELLI, Aqua Binellii—a. Brocchieri, Aqua Brocchierii—a. Monterossi, Aqua Binellii—a. di Napoli, Liquor arsenicalis—a. della Toffana, Liquor arsenicalis.

ACQUETTA, Liquor Arsenicalis.

ACQUI, MINERAL WATERS OF. These thermal sulphureous springs are in Piémont. Their temperature is 167° Fahr., and they contain sulphohydric acid and chloride of sodium.

ACQUIRED DISEASES, *Morbi acquisi'ti, M. adventi'tii, M. epicte'ti. Adventitious diseases*. (F.) *Maladies acquises*. Diseases which occur after birth, and which are not dependent upon hereditary predisposition.

ACRAI'PALA, from *a*, privative, and κραιπαλη, 'drunkenness.' Remedies against the effects of a debauch.—Gorræus.

ACRA'LEA, from ακρος, 'extremity.' The extreme parts of the body, as the head, hands, feet, nose, ears, &c.—Hippocrates and Galen. See Acrea.

ACRA'NIA, from *a*, privative, and κρανιον, 'the cranium.' Want of cranium, wholly or in part.

ACRA'SIA, from *a*, privative, or 'bad,' and κρασις, 'mixture.' Intemperance. Excess of any kind.—Hippocrates.

It has been employed to denote debility, synonymously with *Acratia;* but this may have been a typographical inaccuracy.

ACRATI'A, from *a*, privative, and κρατος, 'strength.' Impotence; weakness, fainting.

ACRATIS'MA, from *a*, privative, and κεραννυμι, 'to mix.' A breakfast, consisting of bread steeped in wine, not mixed with water.—Galen, Athenæus.

ACRATOM'ELI, from ακρατον, 'pure wine,' and μελι, 'honey.' Wine mixed with honey.

ACRATOPE'GÆ, *Akratope'gæ*, from *a*, privative, and κρατος, 'strength,' and πηγη, 'a spring.' Mineral waters having no marked chemical qualities.

ACRATOPOS'IA, from *Acratum*, and ποσις, 'drink.' The drinking of pure or unmixed wine.

A'CRATUM, ακρατον, from *a*, privative, and κρατος, 'strength.' Unmixed wine,—*Acratum vinum, Vinum merum*.

ACRATURE'SIS, from *Acratia*, 'weakness,' and ουρον, 'urine.' Inability to void the urine from paralysis of the bladder.

ACRE. The extremity or tip of the nose.

A'CREA, *Acrotéria*, from ακρος, 'the summit.' The extreme parts of the body, as the feet, hands, ears, &c.

Also the extreme parts of animals that are used as food. *Acrocolia*.

ACRID, from ακρος, 'a point or summit,' or from ακις, 'a point,' *Acer*. An epithet for substances which occasion a disagreeable sense of irritation or of constriction at the top of the throat.

Acrid heat, (F.) *Chaleur âcre*, is one that causes a hot tingling sensation at the extremities of the fingers.

ACRID POISON, See Poison.

ACRIDS, in Pathology, are certain imaginary substances, supposed by the humourists to exist in the humours, and to cause various diseases. See Acrimony.

ACRIDOPH'AGI, from ακρις, 'a locust,' and φαγω, 'I eat.' *Locust-eaters*. Acridophagous tribes are said to exist in Africa.—Strabo.

AC'RIMONY, *Acu'itas, Acrimo'nia*, from *acer*, 'acrid,' ακις, 'a point.' Acrimony of the humours. An imaginary acrid change of the blood, lymph, &c., which, by the humourists, was conceived to cause many diseases.

ACRIN'IA, from *a*, privative, and κρινω, 'I separate.' A diminution in the quantity, or a total suspension, of the secretions.

ACRIS, a sharp bony prominence. Also, the locust.

ACRI'SIA, *Acri'sis*, from *a*, privative, and κρισις, 'judgment.' A condition of disease, in which no judgment can be formed; or in which an unfavourable opinion must be given.—Hipp and Galen.

ACRISIS, Acrisia.

ACRIT'ICAL, *Ac'ritos,* from *a,* privative, and *κρισις,* 'judgment.' That which takes place without any crisis, or which does not foretell a crisis; as *a critical symptom, abscess,* &c.

ACRITOS, Acritical.

ACRIVIOLA, Tropæolum majus.

ACROAMA, Audition.

ACROASIS, Audition.

ACROBYS'TIA, *Acropos'thia,* from ακρος, 'top,' and βυω, 'I cover.' The extremity of the prepuce.—Hippocrates. Rufus.

ACROCHEIR', *Acrochir', Acrocheir'on,* from ακρος, 'extremity,' and χειρ, 'the hand.' The forearm and hand. Gorræus. Also, the hand.

ACROCHOR'DON, from ακρος, 'extremity,' and χορδη, 'a string.' A tumour which hangs by a pedicle. A kind of hard wart, *Verru'ca pensi'lis.*—Aëtius, Celsus.

ACROCHORIS'MUS, from ακρος, 'extremity,' and χορευω, 'I dance.' A kind of dance, with the ancients, in which the arms and legs were violently agitated.

ACROCOLIA, Acrea.

ACROCOLIUM, Acromion.

ACROD'RYA, from ακρος, 'extremity,' and δρυς, 'a tree.' Autumnal fruits, as nuts, apples, &c.

ACRODYN'IA, *Erythe'ma acrod'ynum, E. acrodyn'ia,* (F.) *Acrodynie,* from ακρος, 'extremity,' and οδυνη, 'pain.' A painful affection of the wrists and ankles especially, which appeared in Paris as an epidemic, in 1828 and 1829. It was supposed by some to be rheumatic, by others to be owing to spinal irritation.

ACROLENION, Olecranon.

ACROMASTIUM, Nipple.

ACROMIA, Acromion.

ACRO'MIAL, *Acromia'lis.* Relating to the Acromion.

ACROMIAL AR'TERY, *External Scap'ular, A. Arte'ria Thorac''ica humera'lis, Artère troisième des Thoraciques,*—(Ch.) *A. Thoracique humérale,* arises from the anterior part of the axillary artery, opposite the upper edge of the pectoralis minor. It divides into two branches: one, *superior;* the other, *inferior,*—the branches of which are distributed to the subclavius, serratus major anticus, first intercostal, deltoid, and pectoralis major muscles, as well as to the shoulder joint, &c. They anastomose with the superior scapular, thoracic, and circumflex arteries.

ACROMIAL NERVES, *Nervi acromia'les.* Branches of the fourth cervical nerve, which are distributed to the acromial region.

ACROMIAL VEIN has the same arrangement as the artery.

ACRO'MIO-CORACOI'DEUS. Belonging to the acromion and coracoid process.

The triangular ligament between the acromion and coracoid process of the scapula is so called.

ACRO'MION, *Acro'mium, Acro'mia, Acro'mis,* from ακρος, 'the top,' and ομος, 'the shoulder.' *Os Acro'mii, Hu'merus summus, Armus summus, Mucro hu'meri, Rostrum porci'num, Caput Scap'ulæ, Acroco'lium.* The process which terminates the spine of the scapula, and is articulated with the clavicle.

ACROMIS, Acromion.

ACROMPHALIUM, Acromphalon.

ACROM'PHALON, *Acrompha'lium,* from ακρος, 'the top,' and ομφαλος, 'the navel.' The extremity of the umbilical cord, which remains attached to the fœtus after birth.

ACROMYLE, Patella.

ACEU-NARCOTIC, See Poison.

A'CRONYX, from ακρος, 'the summit,' and ονυξ, 'the nail.' Growing in of the nail.

ACROPARAL'YSIS, from ακρος, 'extremity,' and παραλυσις, 'palsy;' *Paral'ysis extremita'tum,* Palsy of the extremities. Fuchs.

ACROPOSTHIA, Acrobystia.

ACROPSI'LON, from ακρος, 'extremity,' and ψιλος, 'naked.' The extremity of the glans penis.

ACRORIA, Vertex.

ACRORRHEU'MA, *Rheumatis'mus extremita'tum,* from ακρος, 'extremity,' and ρευμα, 'defluxion rheumatism.' Rheumatism of the extremities.

ACROS, ακρος, 'extremity, top.' The strength of the Athletæ, and of diseases; the prominences of bones: the extremities of the fingers, &c. See Acrocheir, Acromion, &c.

ACROTERIA, Acrea. See Extremity.

ACROTERIASIS, Acroteriasmus.

ACROTERIAS'MUS, *Acroteri'asis,* from ακροτηρια, 'the extremities;' hence ακρωτηριαζειν, 'to mutilate.' Amputation of the extremities.

ACROTHYM'ION, from ακρος, 'top,' and θυμος, 'thyme.' A kind of conical, rugous, bloody wart, compared by Celsus to the flower of thyme.

ACROT'ICA, from ακρος, 'summit.' Diseases affecting the excernent functions of the external surface of the body.

Pravity of the fluids or emunctories that open on the external surface; without fever or other internal affection as a necessary accompaniment. The 3d order of the class *Eccrit'ica* of Good.

ACROTISMUS, Asphyxia.

ACT, *Actus,* from *actum,* past participle of *agere,* 'to do,' 'a thing done.' The effective exercise of a power or faculty. The action of an agent. *Acte* is used by the French, to signify the public discussion, which occurs in supporting a thesis:—thus, *soutenir un Acte aux Écoles de Médecine,* is, 'to defend a Thesis in the Schools of Medicine.'

ACTÆ'A CIMICIF'UGA, *A. racemo'sa.*

ACTÆ'A RACEMO'SA, *A. Cimicif'uga, Cimicif'uga,* (Ph. U. S.) *C. racemo'sa, Macro'trys racemo'sa, Bot'rophis Serpenta'ria* (?) *Serpenta'ria nigra,* Black snakeroot, Richweed, Cohosh, Squaw root, Rattleweed, Black Cohosh. (F.) *Actée à grappes, Serpentaire noire.* Nat. Ord. Ranunculaceæ. Sex. Syst. Polyandria Pentagynia. A common plant in the United States. The root is astringent; and, according to Barton, has been successfully used, in the form of decoction, as a gargle in putrid sore throat. A decoction of the root cures the itch. It is acro-narcotic, and has been used in rheumatism, acute and chronic; chorea, &c.

ACTÆ'A SPICA'TA, *Christophoria'na spica'ta, Aconi'tum racemo'sum, Baneberry, Herb Chris'topher.* (F.) *Herbe St. Christophe.* A perennial herbaceous European plant, the root of which resembles that of the black hellebore. The root is cathartic, and sometimes emetic, and in overdoses may produce dangerous consequences.

Actæ'a America'na, of which there are two varieties, *A. alba* and *A. rubra,*—*white and red cohosh,* is indigenous in the United States. It has the same properties as *A. spicata.*

ACTE, Sambucus.

ACTÉ, Act.

ACTÉE à GRAPPES, Actæa racemosa.

ACTIF, Active.

ACTIO, Action, Function.

AC'TION, *Ac'tio, Opera'tio, Energi'a, Praxis:* from *agere, actum,* 'to act.' Mode in which one object influences another.

The *animal actions* are those that occur in the animal body: the *vital,* those that are essential to life: the *physiological,* those of a healthy character: the *pathological,* or *morbific,* those that occur in disease, &c. The ancients divided the *physiological actions* into *vital, animal, natural, sexual, particular, general,* &c. See Function.

ACTIONES NATURALES, see Function.
ACTIVE, same etymon. *Dras'ticus, Acti'vus, Sthen'icus, Hypersthen'icus.* (F.) *Actif.* This adjective is used, in *Pathology*, to convey the idea of superabundant energy or strength. *Active symptoms, e. g.* are those of excitement. In *Therapeutics,* it signifies *energetic:*—as, an *active treatment.* The French use the expression *Médecine agissante,* in contradistinction to *Médecine expectante.* In Physiology, *active* has a similar signification, many of the functions being divided into active and passive.
ACTON. A village near London, at which there is a purgative mineral spring, like that at Epsom.
AC'TUAL. Same etymon as *active.* That which acts immediately. A term usually restricted to the red-hot iron, or to heat in any form; in contradistinction to the *potential* or *virtual*, which is applied to caustics or escharotics.
ACTUA'RIUS. Originally a title of dignity given to the Byzantine physicians.
ACTUS PARTURITIONIS, Parturition.
ACUITAS, Acrimony.
ACULEUS LIGNEUS, Splinter.
ACUMETER, Acoumeter.
A'CUPUNCTURE, *Acupunctu'ra,* from *acus,* 'a needle,' and *punctura,* 'a puncture.' A surgical operation, much in use amongst the Chinese and Japanese, which consists in puncturing parts with a very fine needle. It has been employed, of late years, in obstinate rheumatic affections, &c., and apparently with success. Acupuncture is likewise a mode of infanticide in some countries; the needle being forced into the brain through the fontanelles, or into the spinal marrow, &c.
ACURGIA, Surgery (operative.)
ACUS, Needle—a. Capitata, Pin—a. Invaginata, see Needle—a. Ophthalmica, see Needle—a. Paracentica, Trocar—a. Paracentetica, Trocar—a. Triquetra vulgaris, Trocar—a. Veneris, Eryngium campestre.
ACUSIMETER, Acoumeter.
ACUSIS, Audition.
ACUSTICA, Acoustics.
ACUSTICUS, Auditory.
ACUTE, *Acu'tus, Oxys,* ὀξύς, (*acis,* 'a point.') (F.) *Aigu.* A disease which, with a certain degree of severity, has a rapid progress, and short duration, is said to be "acute."—*Oxynose'ma, Oxyn'osos, Oxynu'sos.*
Diseases were formerly subdivided into *Morbi acutis'simi,* very acute, or those which last only three or four days: *M. subacutis'simi,* which continue seven days: and *M. subacu'ti,* or those which last from twenty to forty days.
The antithesis to *acute* is chronic. *Acute,* when applied to pain, sound, cries, &c., means *sharp.*
ACUTENACULUM, Porte-aiguille.
ACYANOBLEP'SIA, from *a,* privative, κυανος, 'blue,' and βλέπω, 'I see.' Defective vision, which consists in incapability of distinguishing blue.—Göthe. See Achromatopsia.
ACYESIS, Sterilitas.
ACYRUS, Arnica montana.
ACYTERIUS, Abortive.
ADACA. The *Sphæran'thus In'dicus,* a Malabar plant, which is acrid and aromatic.
ADAC'RYA, from *a,* privative, and δακρυω, 'I weep.' Defective secretion of tears.
ADÆMONIA, Anxiety.
ADAKO'DIEN. A Malabar plant of the family Apocyneæ, used in that country in diseases of the eyes.
AD'ALI, *Lip'pia.* A Malabar plant, which the Orientals regard as an antidote to the bite of the *naja.*

ADAMANTINE SUBSTANCE, Enamel of the teeth.
ADAMAS, Diamond.
ADAMI'TA, *Adami'tum.* A very hard, white calculus.—Paracelsus.
The first word has been used for stone in the bladder: the second for lithiasis or the calculous condition.
ADAM'S APPLE, Pomum Adami.
ADANSONIA DIGITATA, Baobab.
ADAPTER, from *ad* and *apto,* 'I fit.' A tube employed in pharmaceutical operations for lengthening the neck of a retort; or in cases where the opening of the receiver is not large enough to admit the beak of the retort.
ADAR'CE, *Adar'cion, Adar'cis* A concretion found about the reeds and grass in the marshy regions of Galatia, and hiding them, as it were: hence the name, from *a,* privative, and δερκω, 'I see.' It was formerly in repute for cleansing the skin from freckles, &c.
ADARIGO, Orpiment.
ADARNECH, Orpiment.
ADARTICULATIO, Arthrodia.
AD CUTEM ABDOM'INIS (ARTERIA.) The *superficial artery of the abdomen,*—a branch of the crural or femoral, which arises at the lower part of Poupart's ligament and ascends towards the umbilicus, being distributed to the integuments.
ADDAD. A Numidian plant; bitter and poisonous.
ADDEPHAG"IA, *Adephag"ia,* from ἀδὴν, 'much,' and φαγειν, 'to eat.' *Voraciousness.* Galen and Hoffman have given this name to voracious appetite in children affected with worms. Sauvages refers it to Bulimia. Also, the goddess of gluttony.
ADDER'S TONGUE, Ophioglossum vulgatum.
ADDITAMEN'TUM. A term once used synonymously with *Epiphysis.* It is now restricted to the prolongation of two cranial sutures, the lamboidal and squamous.
ADDITAMENTUM COLI, Appendix vermiformis cæci—a. Necatum, Olecranon—a. ad Sacrolumbalem, see Sacro-lumbalis—a. Uncatum ulnæ, Olecranon—a. Ulnæ, Radius.
ADDUCENS OCULI, Rectus internus oculi.
ADDUCTEUR DE L'ŒIL, Rectus internus oculi—a. du Gros orteil, Adductor pollicis pedis—a. Premier ou moyen, Adductor longus femoris—a. du Pouce, Adductor pollicis manûs—a. Second ou petit, Adductor brevis—a. Troisième ou grand, Adductor magnus.
ADDUC'TION, *Adduc'tio,* from *ad,* 'to,' and *ducere,* 'to draw.' *Parago'ge.* The action by which parts are drawn towards the axis of the body.
The muscles which execute this function are called *Adduc'tors.*
ADDUCTOR MEDII DIGITI PEDIS, Posterior medii digiti pedis—a. Oculi, Rectus internus oculi.
ADDUC'TOR METACAR'PI MIN'IMI DIG"ITI, *Metacar'peus, Car'po-metacar'peus min'imi dig"iti,* is situate between the adductor and flexor, next to the metacarpal bone. It arises, fleshy, from the unciform process of the os unciforme, and from the contiguous part of the annular ligament of the wrist, and is inserted, tendinous and fleshy, into the fore-part of the metacarpal bone of the little finger, from its base to its head.
ADDUC'TOR POL'LICIS MANÛS, *A. Pol'licis, A. ad min'imum dig"itum, Metacar'po-phalan'geus pol'licis*—(Ch.) (F.) *Adducteur du pouce.* A muscle which arises, fleshy, from almost the whole length of the metacarpal bone of the middle finger, and is inserted into the inner part of the root of the first bone of the thumb.

ADDUC'TOR POL'LICIS PEDIS, *Antith'enar, Metatar'so-subphalan'geus pollicis.*—(Ch.) *Tarsometatarsi-phalangien du pouce.* (F.) *Adducteur du gros orteil.* Arises by a long, thin tendon, from the under part of the os calcis, from the os cuboides, os cuneiforme externum, and from the root of the metatarsal bone of the second toe. It is divided into two fleshy portions, and is inserted into the external sesamoid bone, and root of the metatarsal bone of the great toe.

Bichat has given the general name, *Adductors,* to those of the interosseous muscles of the hand or foot, which perform the action of adduction.

ADDUCTOR TERTII DIGITI PEDIS, Prior tertii digiti pedis.

ADDUCTORS OF THE THIGH. These are three in number, which have, by some anatomists, been united into one muscle—the *Triceps Adduc'tor Fem'oris.*

1. *Adduc'tor longus fem'oris, Adduc'tor fem'oris primus, Triceps minor, Pu'bio-femora'lis*—(Ch.) (F.) *Premier ou moyen adducteur.* Arises by a strong tendon from the upper and fore part of the os pubis and ligament of the symphysis, at the inner side of the pectinalis. It runs downwards and outwards, and is inserted by a broad, flat tendon, into the middle of the linea aspera.

2. *Adduc'tor brevis, A. fem'oris secun'dus, Triceps secun'dus, Sub-pubio-femora'lis* — (Ch.) (F.) *Second* ou *petit Adducteur.* Arises tendinous from the os pubis, at the side of its symphysis, below and behind the last muscle. It runs obliquely outwards, and is inserted by a short, flat tendon into the inner and upper part of the linea aspera, from a little below the trochanter minor to the beginning of the insertion of the adductor longus.

3. *Adduc'tor magnus, Adduc'tor fem'oris tertius et quartus, Triceps magnus, Is'chio-femora'lis*—(Ch.) (F.) *Troisième* ou *grand adducteur,* is much larger than either of the others. It arises from the ramus of the pubis, from that of the ischium, and from the tuber ischii, and is inserted into the whole length of the linea aspera. Near the lower part of the linea aspera it is pierced by a kind of oblique, fibrous canal, through which the crural artery and vein pass.

ADEC. The inner man.—Paracelsus.

ADECTA, Sedatives.

ADELIPARIA, Polysarcia.

ADELODAGAM. A bitter Malabar plant, used in asthma, catarrh, and gout.

ADELPHIA, see Adelphixia.

ADELPHIX'IA, *Adelphixis;* from *αδελφος,* 'brother.' Consanguinity of parts in health or disease. *Frater'nitas, Fratra'tio.* Hippocrates used the word *Adel'phia,* for diseases that resemble each other.

ADELPHIXIS, Sympathy.

ADEMONIA, Depression, Nostalgia.

ADEMOSYNE, Depression, Nostalgia.

ADEN, *αδην,* 'a gland;' hence *Adenalgia, Adeniform, &c.*—see Gland.

ADENAL'GIA, *Adenodyn'ia,* from *αδην,* 'a gland,' and *αλγος,* 'pain.' Glandular pain.

ADENECTOP'IA, from *αδην,* 'a gland,' and *εκτοπος,* 'removed from its place.' Dislocation of a gland.

ADENEMPHRAX'IS, from *αδην,* 'a gland,' and *εμφραξις,* 'obstruction.' Glandular obstruction.

ADEN'IFORM, *Adeniform'is, Adenol'des, Adenoid,* from *Aden,* 'a gland,' and *Forma,* 'form or resemblance.' *Glan'diform,* or resembling a gland.

ADÉNITE LYMPHATIQUE, Lymphadenitis.

ADENI'TIS, from *αδην,* 'a gland,' and *itis,* a termination denoting inflammation. *Phlegma'sia adeno'sa* seu *glandulo'sa.* Glandular inflammation.

ADENITIS LYMPHATICA, Lymphadenitis.

ADENI'TIS MESENTER'ICA, *Mesenter'ic Ganglioni'tis.* Inflammation of the mesenteric glands.

ADENITIS PALPEBRARUM CONTAGIOSA, see Ophthalmia.

ADENOCHIRAPSOLOG"IA, from *αδην,* 'a gland,' *χειρ,* 'the hand,' *απτω,* 'I lay hold of,' and *λογος,* 'a description.' The doctrine of curing scrofula or the king's evil by the royal touch.

ADENOCHON'DRIUS, from *αδην,* 'a gland,' and *χονδρος,* 'a cartilage.' Relating to gland and cartilage, — for example, *Arthrophy'ma adenochon'drium,* a tumefaction of the glands and cartilages of joints.

ADENODYNIA, Adenalgia.

ADENOG'RAPHY, *Adenogra'phia,* from *αδην,* 'a gland,' and *γραφω,* 'I describe.' That part of anatomy which describes the glands.

ADENOID, Adeniform.

ADENOIDES, Adeniform.

ADENOL'OGY, *Adenolog"ia,* from *αδην,* 'a gland,' and *λογος,* 'a description.' A treatise on the glands.

ADENOMALA'CIA, from *αδην,* 'a gland,' and *μαλακια,* 'softening.' Mollescence or softening of a gland.

ADENO-MENINGEAL, see Fever, adeno-meningeal.

ADENONCOSIS, Adenophyma.

ADE'NO-PHARYN'GEUS, from *αδην,* 'a gland,' and *φαρυγξ,* 'the pharynx.' Some fleshy fibres, which pass from the constrictor pharyngis inferior to the thyroid gland, have received this name. Their existence is not constant.

ADE'NO-PHARYNGI'TIS. Same etymon. Inflammation of the tonsils and pharynx.

ADENOPHTHALMIA, Ophthalmia tarsi.

ADENOPHY'MA, *Adenon'cus, Adenonco'sis,* from *αδην,* 'a gland,' and *φυμα,* 'a swelling.' Swelling of a gland, or glandiform ganglion. (F.) *Glandage.* *Adenophyma* is used by some to signify a soft glandular swelling;—*Adenoncus,* one of a harder character.—Kraus.

ADENOPHYMA INGUINALIS. Bubo.

ADENOSCIR'RHUS, *Adenosclero'sis,* from *αδην,* 'a gland,' and *σκιρρος,* 'induration.' Scirrhous induration of a gland.

ADENOSCLEROSIS, Adenoscirrhus.

ADENOSIS SCROPHULOSA, Scrofula.

ADENO'SUS, (*Absces'sus.*) A hard, glandular abscess, which suppurates slowly.—M. A. Severinus.

ADENOT'OMY, *Adenotom'ia,* from *αδην,* 'a gland,' and *τεμνω,* 'I cut.' Dissection of the glands.

ADEPHAGIA, Addephagia, Boulimia.

ADEPS, *Adeps Suillus, Oxyn'gium, Pingue'do.* Pig's flare. The fat of the hog. In the Ph. U. S. the prepared fat of *Sus scrofa,* free from saline matter.

ADEPS ANSERI'NUS, *Adeps an'seris* or *Goose grease,* (F.) *Graisse d'Oie,* is emollient. It has been used as an emetic.

ADEPS CANTHARIDIBUS MEDICATUS, Unguentum lyttæ medicatum—a. Cortice Daphnes gnidii medicatus, Unguentum epispasticum de Daphne gnidio—a. Humanus, Liquamumia—a. Hydrargyro medicatus, Unguentum Hydrargyri—a. ex Hydrargyro mitius dictum cinereum, Unguentum oxidi hydrargyri cinereum—a. Hydrargyri muriate oxygenato medicatus, Unguentum muriatis hydrargyri oxygenati medicatum—a. Hydrargyri nitrate medicatus, Unguentum hydrargyri nitratis —a. Hydrargyri oxido rubro et plumbi aceta me-

diatus, Unguentum ophthalmicum—a. Lauro medicatus, Unguentum laurinum—a. Ovilli, Sevum—a. Papavere, hyoscyamo, et belladonnâ medicatus, Unguentum populeum—a. Sulfure et ammoniso muriate medicatus, Unguentum sulphuratum ad scabiem—a. Sulfure et carbonate potassæ medicatus, Unguentum sulphuratum alcalinum ad scabiem—a. Tartaro stibii medicatus, Unguentum antimonii tartarizati—a. Oxido zinci medicatus, Unguentum oxidi zinci impuri.

ADEPS PRÆPARA'TUS, *Hog's lard, Barrow's grease, Lard, Ax'unge, Axun'gia, Adeps suil'lus præpara'tus, A. præpara'tus, Axun'gia porci'na,* (F.) *Graisse de Porc, Saindoux,* is prepared by melting pig's flare, and straining it. This is called *rendering* the lard. Lard is emollient, but is chiefly used for forming ointments and plasters.

ADEPT, Alchymist.

ADEP'TA MEDICI'NA. Medicine, which treated of diseases contracted by celestial operations, or communicated from heaven.

ADEPTA PHILOSOPHIA, Alchymy.

ADFLATUS, Afflatus.

ADHÆRENTIA, Adherence.

ADHÆSIO, Adherence.

ADHATO'DA, *Justic"ia adhato'da.* The *Malabar Nut Tree.* (F.) *Noyer de Ceylon.* Used in India for expelling the dead foetus in abortion. The word is said to convey this meaning in the Ceylonese.

ADHE'RENCE, *Adhe'sion, Adhæren'tia, Concre'tio, Atre'sia, Pros'physis, Proscolle'sis, Adhæ'sio,* from *adhærere,* (*ad* and *hærere,*) 'to stick to.' These words are usually employed synonymously. The French often use *adherence* for the state of union, and *adhesion* for the act of adhering.

ADHESION, Adherence.

ADHE'SIVE INFLAMMA'TION is that inflammation which terminates by an adhesion between inflamed and separated surfaces, and which was, at one time, supposed to be necessary for such adhesion.

Adhe'sive is also an epithet for certain plasters which stick closely to the skin.

ADIANTHUM, Adiantum.

ADIANTUM, A. pedatum.

ADIANTUM ÆTHIOP'ICUM. A South African plant, *Nat. Ord.* Filices, an infusion of which is sometimes used as an emollient in coughs, and in diseases of the chest.

ADIANTUM ALBUM, Asplenium ruta muraria—a. Aureum, Polytrichum.

ADIAN'TUM CAPIL'LUS VEN'ERIS, *A. Coriandrifo'lium* seu *Nigrum, Capil'lus Ven'eris,* from *a,* privative, and *διαινω,* 'to grow wet,' from the leaves not being easily moistened. *Maiden hair.* (F.) *Capillaire de Montpellier.* A European plant, of feeble, aromatic and demulcent properties. It is used for forming the *Sirop de Capillaire* or *Capillaire.*

ADIANTUM CORIANDRIFOLIUM, A. Capillus Veneris.

ADIANTUM NIGRUM, A. Capillus Veneris.

ADIAN'TUM PEDA'TUM, *A. Canaden'sē* seu *Patens, Adiantum, Capil'lus Ven'eris Canaden'sis, Herba Ven'eris, Filix Ven'eris, Canada Maidenhair, American Maidenhair, Rockfern, Sweetfern,* (F.) *Capillaire du Canada,* has the same properties. *Capillaire* was once made from this. See Adiantum.

ADIANTUM RUBRUM, Asplenium trichomanoides.

ADIAPHORO'SIS, *Adiaphore'sis,* from *a,* privative, *δια,* 'through,' and *φορος,* 'a pore.' Defect or suppression of perspiration, *Adiapneus'tia.*

ADIAPH'OROUS, *Adiaph'orus, Indiff'erens,*

Neutral. A medicine which will neither do harm nor good.

ADIAPNEUSTIA, Adiaphorosis.

ADIARRHŒ'A, from *a,* privative, and *διαρρειν,* 'to flow.' Retention of any excretion.—Hippocrates.

ADICE, Urtica.

ADIPATUS, Fatty.

ADIPEUX, Adipose.

ADIPOCERA, *Adipocire*—a. Cetosa, Cetaceum.

ADIPOCIRE, Adipoce'ra, from *adeps,* 'fat,' and *cera,* 'wax.' The base of biliary calculi, called also *Chol'esterine.* Also, a sort of soap, formed from animal matter under certain circumstances. (F.) *Gras des Cadavres, Gras des Cimetières.* The human body, when it has been for some weeks in water, assumes this appearance; and it has been a subject of legal inquiry, what length of time is necessary to produce it. This must, of course, depend upon various circumstances, as climate, season, &c.

ADIPOCIRE DE BALEINE, Cetaceum.

AD'IPOSE, *Ad'ipous, Adipo'sus,* from *adeps,* 'fat.' (F.) *Adipeux.* That which relates to fat—as *Adipose membrane, A. vessels,* &c. See Fatty.

AD'IPOSE SARCO'MA of ABERNE'THY, *Emphy'ma sarco'ma adipo'sum,* is suetty throughout, and enclosed in a thin capsule of condensed areolar substance, connected by means of minute vessels. It is chiefly found on the fore and back parts of the trunk. See Sarcoma.

ADIPOSIS. See Polysarcia.

ADIPO'SIS HEPAT'ICA, *Pimelo'sis hepat'ica, Fatty liver, Fatty degeneration of the liver,* (F.) *Dégénérescence graisseuse du Foie.* Fatty disease of the liver.

ADIPOSUS, Fatty.

ADIPOUS, Fatty.

ADIP'SIA, *Dipso'sis expers.* Absence of thirst.

ADIP'SON, *Adip'sum,* from *a,* privative, and *διψα,* 'thirst.' Any substance which relieves thirst. Applied to a decoction of barley to which oxymel was added.—Hippocrates.

ADIPSOS, Glycyrrhiza.

AD'ITUS, 'an entrance,' 'an approach;' from *adere, aditum,* 'to go to.' *Pros'odos.* The entrance to a canal or duct, as *Aditus ad Aquæductum Fallopii.*

ADITUS AD INFUNDIBULUM, Vulva.

ADIULIS'TOS, from *a,* privative, and *διυλιζω,* 'I strain.' Unstrained wine for pharmaceutical purposes.—Gorræus.

ADJUNCTUM, Accompaniment.

ADJUTOR PARTUS, Accoucheur.

AD'JUVANT, *Ad'juvans,* from *adjuvare,* 'to aid.' A medicine, introduced into a prescription to aid the operation of the principal ingredient or basis. Also, whatever assists in the removal or prevention of disease.

ADNASCENTIA, Prosphysis.

ADNATA (TUNICA,) Conjunctiva.

ADNÉE (MEMBRANE,) Conjunctiva.

ADOLES'CENCE, *Adolescen'tia, Juven'tus, Ætas bona, Youth;* from *adolescere* (*ad* and *olescere*) 'to grow.' (F.) *Jeunesse.* The period between puberty and that at which the body acquires its full development; being, in man, between the 14th and 25th years; and, in woman, between the 12th and 21st.

ADOLES'CENS, *Ju'venis, Hebe'tes, hebe'ter, Hebe'tor.* A youth. A young man in the period of adolescence.

ADO'LIA. A Malabar plant, whose leaves, put in oil, form a liniment, used in facilitating labour.

ADOR, Zea mays.

ADORION, Daucus carota.

ADOUCISSANT, Demulcent.

AD PONDUS OM'NIUM. The weight of the whole. In a prescription it means, that any particular ingredient shall equal in weight the whole of the others.

ADRAGANT, Tragacantha.

ADRA RIZA, Aristolochia clematitis.

ADROBO'LON, from αδρος, 'great,' and βωλος, 'mass.' The bdellium of India, which is in larger pieces than that of Arabia.

ADROS, αδρος, 'plump and full.' Applied to the habit of body, and also to the pulse.—Hippocrates.

ADSARIA PALA, Dolichos pruriens.

ADSPIRATIO, Aspiration, Inspiration.

ADSTANS, Prostate.

ADSTITES GLANDULOSI, Prostate.

ADSTRICTIO Astriction, Constipation.

ADSTRICTORIA, Astringents.

ADSTRINGENTIA, Astringents.

ADULAS'SO. The *Justitia bivalvis*. A small shrub, used in India as a local application in gout.

ADULT, see Adult age.

ADULT AGE, *Andri'a*, from *adolescere*, 'to grow to,' (*ad* and *olere, olitum*, 'to grow.') *Viril'ity*. The age succeeding adolescence, and preceding old age. In the civil law, an adult is one, who, if a boy, has attained the age of fourteen years; and, if a girl, of twelve. In the common law, one of full age. *Adult, Adul'tus*, is also used for one in the adult age.

ADULTERATIO, Falsification.

ADULTUS, see Adult age.

ADUNCATIO UNGUIUM, Onychogryphosis.

ADURENS, Caustic,

ADURION, Rhus coriaria.

ADUST, *Adus'tus*, from *adurere*, (*ad* and *urere*,) 'to burn.' The blood and fluids were formerly said to be adust, when there was much heat in the constitution and but little serum in the blood.

ADUSTIO, Adustion, Burn.

ADUS'TION, *Adus'tio*. State of the body described under Adust. In surgery, it signifies *cauterization*.

ADVENTITIOUS DISEASES, Acquired diseases.

ADVENTITIUS, Accidental.

ADYNA'MIA, *Impoten'tia*; from *a*, privative, and δυναμις, 'strength,' *Adyna'sia, Adyna'tia*. Considerable debility of the vital powers; as in typhus fever. Some Nosologists have a class of diseases under the name *Adynamiæ, Ec'lyses, Morbi asthen'ici*.

ADYNAMIA VIRILIS, Impotence.

ADYNAM'IC, *Adynam'icus, Hypodynam'ic, Hypodynam'icus*; same etymon. Appertaining to debility of the vital powers.

ADYNASIA, Adynamia.

ADYNATIA, Adynamia.

ADYNATOCOMIUM, Hospital.

ADYNATODOCHIUM, Hospital.

ADYNATOS, Sickly.

ÆDŒA, Genital Organs.

ÆDŒ'AGRA, from αιδοια, 'genital organs,' and αγρα, 'seizure.' Gout in the genitals.

ÆDŒAG'RAPHY, *Ædœagraph'ia*, from αιδοια, 'organs of generation,' and γραφω, 'I describe.' A description of the organs of generation.

ÆDŒAL'OGY, *Ædœalog''ia*, from αιδοια, 'the pudendum,' and λογος, 'a description.' A treatise on the organs of generation.

ÆDŒAT'OMY, *Ædœatom'ia, Ædœotom'ia, Ædœot'omia, Ædœot'omy*, from αιδοια, 'the pudendum,' and τεμνω, 'I cut.' Dissection of the parts of generation.

ÆDŒI'TIS, *Ædœoti'tis, Medel'tis*; from αιδοια, 'genital organs,' and *itis*, denoting inflammation. Inflammation of the genital organs.

ÆDŒOBLENORRHŒA, Leucorrhœa.

ÆDŒODYN'IA, from αιδοια, 'genital organs,' and οδυνη, 'pain.' Pain in the genitals. Pudendagra.

ÆDŒOGARGALUS, Masturbation, Nymphomania.

ÆDŒOGARGARISMUS, Masturbation, Nymphomania.

ÆDŒOMANIA, Nymphomania.

ÆDŒON, Inguen.

ÆDŒOPSOPHESIS, Ædœopsophia.

ÆDŒOPSOPH'IA, *Ædœopsophe'sis*, from αιδοια, 'the pudendum,' and ψοφειν, 'to make a noise.' Emission of wind by the urethra in man, by the vagina in woman.—Sauvages and Sagar.

ÆDŒOPSOPHIA UTERINA, Physometra.

ÆDŒOTITIS, Ædœitis—æ. Gangrænosa, Colpocace—æ. Gangrænosa puellarum, Colpocace infantilis—æ. Gangrænosa puerperarum, Colpocace puerperarum.

ÆDŒOTOME, Ædœatomy.

ÆDŒOTOMIA, Ædœatomy.

ÆDŒOTOMY, Ædœatomy.

ÆDOPTOSIS, Hysteroptosis—æ. Uteri, Prolapsus uteri—æ. Uteri inversa, Uterus, inversion of the—æ. Uteri retroversa, Retroversio uteri—æ. Vaginæ, Prolapsus V.—æ. Vesicæ, Exocyste.

ÆEIG'LUCES, *Aeig'luces*, from αει, 'always,' and γλυκυς, 'sweet.' A kind of sweet wine or must.—Gorræus.

ÆGAGROPI'LA, *Ægagropi''lus*, from αιγαγρος, 'the rock goat,' and πιλος, 'hair,' *Bézoar d'Allemagne, Pila Dama'rum* seu *Rupicapra'rum*. A ball composed of hairs, found in the stomach of the goat: once used medicinally.—Bezoar.

ÆGEIROS, Populus.

ÆGER, Sick.

Æ'GIAS, *Ægis, Æglia, Æ'gides*, from αιξ, 'the goat;' why, is not known. (F.) *Aige* or *Aigle*. There is obscurity regarding the precise meaning of this word. It was used to designate an ulcer, or speck on the transparent cornea.—Hippocrates. Maître Jean uses it for a calcareous deposit between the conjunctiva and sclerotica.

ÆGIDES, Ægias.

Æ'GILOPS, *An'chilops, An'kylops*, from αιξ, 'goat,' and ωψ, 'the eye.' An ulcer at the greater angle of the eye, which sometimes does not penetrate to the lachrymal sac, but at others does, and constitutes fistula lachrymalis.—Galen, Celsus, Oribasius, Aëtius, Paulus of Ægina, &c.

ÆGI'RINON. An ointment of which the fruit or flower of the poplar was an ingredient; from αιγειρος, 'the black poplar.'

ÆGLIA, Ægias.

ÆGOCERAS, Trigonella fœnum.

ÆGOLETHRON, Ranunculus flammula.

ÆGONYCHON, Lithospermum officinale.

ÆGOPHONIA. Egophony.

ÆGOPHONICUS, Egophonic.

ÆGOPODIUM PODAGRARIA, Ligusticum podagraria.

ÆGRIPPA, Agrippa.

ÆGRITUDO, Disease—æ. Ventriculi, Vomiting.

ÆGROTATIO, Disease.

ÆGROTUS, Sick.

ÆGYP'TIA. An epithet for several medicines, mentioned by Galen, Paulus of Ægina, and Myrepsus.

ÆGYP'TIA MOSCHATA, Hibiscus abelmoschus.

ÆGYP'TIA STYPTE'RIA, Αιγυπτια στυπτηρια, *Egyptian alum*. Recommended by Hippocr.

ÆGYP'TIA UL'CERA; *Egyptian ulcers*. Ulcers of the fauces and tonsils, described by Aretæus, as common in Egypt and Syria.

ÆGYPTIACUM, Ægyp'tion, Mende'sion, Mel Ægyptiacum, Phar'macum Ægyptiacum. A preparation of vinegar, honey, and verdigris, scarcely used now, except by veterinary surgeons as a detergent. See Linimentum Æruginis.

ÆGYPTION, Ægyptiacum.

ÆGYPTIUM MEDICAMENTUM AD AURES, Pharmacum ad aures.

ÆGYPTIUS PESSUS: Ægyptian pessary. A pessary, composed of honey, turpentine, butter, oil of lily or of rose, saffron, each one part; with sometimes a small quantity of verdigris.

AEICHRYSON, Sedum.

ÆIPATHEIA, see Continent (Disease.)

AEIPATHIA, see Continent (Disease.)

ÆMOPTOICA PASSIO, Hæmoptysis.

ÆNEA, Catheter.

ÆOLECTHYMA, Variola.

ÆOLLION, Varicella.

ÆOLLIUM, Varicella.

ÆON, αιων. The entire age of a man from birth till death.—Hippocrates, Galen. Also, the spinal marrow. See Medulla Spinalis.

ÆONESIS, Fomentation.

ÆONION, Sedum.

ÆO'RA, from αιωρεω, 'I suspend.' Gestation, swinging.—Aëtius, Celsus, &c.

ÆQUALIS, Equal.

ÆQUA'TOR OC'ULI. The line formed by the union of the upper and under eyelid, when they are closed. It is below the middle of the globe.

ÆQUIVOCUS, Equivocal.

AËR, Air.

AËRATION OF THE BLOOD, Hæmatosis.

AËRATUS, Carbonated.

AÉRÉ, Carbonated.

ÆREOLUM, Æreolus, Chalcus. The sixth part of an obolus by weight, consequently about 2 grains.

Æ'RESIS, αιρεσις, 'the removal of any thing.' A suffix denoting a removal or separation, as Aphærěsis, Diærěsis, &c.

AËRGIA, Torpor.

AËRIF'EROUS, Aërifer, (F.) Aérifère, from aer, 'air,' and ferre, 'to carry.' An epithet for tubes which convey air, as the larynx, trachea, and bronchia.

AËRIFLUX'US. The discharge of gas, and the fetid emanations from the sick. Flatulence.—Sauvages.

AËRODIAPH'THORA, from ανρ, 'air,' and διαφθορα, 'corruption.' A corrupt state of the air.

AËRO-ENTERECTASIA, Tympanites.

AËROL'OGY; Aërolog"ia, Aërolog"icè, from ανρ, 'air,' and λογος, 'a description.' That part of physics which treats of the air, its qualities, uses, and action on the animal economy.

AËR'OMANCY, Aëromanti'a, from ανρ, 'air,' and μαντυα, 'divination." An art in judicial astrology, which consists in the foretelling, by means of the air, or substances found in the atmosphere.

AËROMELI, Fraxinus ornus.

AËROPÉRITONIE, see Tympanites.

AËROPHOB'IA, from ανρ, 'air,' and φοβος, 'fear.' Dread of the air. This symptom often accompanies hydrophobia, and sometimes hysteria and other affections.

AËROPHOB'ICUS, Aëroph'obus; same etymon. One affected with aerophobia.

AËROPHOBUS, Aerophobicus.

AËROPHTHORA, Aerodiaphthora.

AËROPLEURIE, Pneumothorax.

AËROSIS, Pneumatosis, Tympanites.

AËROTHORAX, Pneumothorax.

ÆRUCA, Cupri subacetas.

ÆRU'GINOUS, Æerugino'sus, Io'des, from Ærugo, 'verdigris.' (F.) Érugineux. Resembling verdigris in colour; as the bile when discharged at times from the stomach.

ÆRU'GO, ιος, from æs, 'copper.' The rust of any metal, properly of brass. See Cupri Subacetas.

Ærugo Ferri, Ferri subcarbonas—æ. Plumbi, Plumbi subcarbonas.

ÆS, Cuprum.

ÆSCHOS, αισχος. Deformity of the body generally, or of some part.—Hippocrates.

ÆS'CULUS HIPPOCAS'TANUM, from esca, 'food,' [?] Casta'nea equi'na, Pavi'na, Horsechestnut, Buck-eye. (F.) Marronier d'Inde. Nat. Ord. Hippocastaneæ. Sex. Syst. Heptandria Monogynia. The bark has been advised as a substitute for cinchona. Both bark and fruit are astringent. Externally, it has been employed, like cinchona, in gangrene.

ÆSECAVUM, Brass.

ÆSTATES, Ephelides.

ÆSTHE'MA, αισθημα, gen. αισθηματος, 'a sensation, a perception.' See Sensation and Sensibility. In the plural, æsthe'mata, the apparatuses of the senses.

ÆSTHEMATOL'OGY, Æsthematolog"ia; from αισθημα, and λογος, 'a description.' The doctrine of, or a treatise on, the senses, or on the apparatus of the senses.

ÆSTHEMATONU'SI, Æsthematorganonu'si, from αισθημα, and νουσοι, 'diseases.' Diseases affecting sensation.

ÆSTHEMATORGANONUSI, Æsthematonusi.

ÆSTHE'SIS, Aisthe'sis, from αισθανομαι, 'I feel.' The faculty of being affected by a sensation. Perception. Sensibility, as well as the senses themselves. See Sense.

ÆSTHETERION, Sensorium.

ÆSTHET'ICA, from αισθανομαι, 'I feel.' Diseases affecting the sensations. Dulness, depravation or abolition of one or more of the external organs of sense. The 2d order, class Neurotica, of Good. Also, agents that affect sensation.—Pereira.

ÆSTIVUS, Estival.

ÆSTUARIUM, Stove.

ÆSTUATIO, Ardor, Ebullition, Fermentation.

ÆSTUS, Ardor.

Æstus Volat'icus. Sudden heat, scorching or flushing of the face.—Vogel.

ÆTAS, Age—æ. Bona, Adolescence—æ. Decrepita, Decrepitude—æ. Mala, Senectus—æ. Provecta, Senectus—æ. Senilis, Senectus.

ÆTHER, Ether, from αιθηρ, 'air,' or from αιθω, 'I burn.' Liquor æthe'reus. A volatile liquor obtained by distillation from a mixture of alcohol and a concentrated acid. See Æther sulphuricus, and Ether.

Æther Chloricus, Chloroform; Ether, chloric.

Æther Hydrocyan'icus, Æther Prus'sicus, Hydrocyan'ic Ether, Hydrocya'nate of Eth'erine, Cyan'uret of Eth'ule, (F.) Éther Hydrocyanique, has been advised in hooping-cough, and where the hydrocyanic acid is indicated. Dose, 6 drops.

Æther Lignosus, Acetone.

Æther Martialis, Tinctura seu Alcohol sulfurico-æthereus ferri.

Æther Muriat'icus, Muriat'ic or Chlorohydric Ether, Mu'riate of Etherine, Chloride of Ethyle. This ether, on account of its volatility, can only be kept in cool places. It has the properties of the other ethers, and when used, is generally mixed with an equal bulk of alcohol. It has been employed as an anæsthetic. A Chlorinated Chlorohydric Ether, (F.) Éther Chlorhydrique chloré, formed by the action of Chlorine on Chlorohydric Ether, has been introduced into practice as a local anæsthetic.

Æther Nitricus Alcoolisatus, Spiritus ætheris nitrici—æ. Pyro-aceticus, Acetone.

Æther Sulphu'ricus, *Æ. Vitriol'icus, Naphtha Vitrioli, Sul'phuric Ether.* Ether prepared from *sulphuric ether* and *alcohol.*

Rectified Ether, Æther rectifica'tus, prepared by distilling 12 oz. from a mixture of *sulphuric ether*, f℥xiv, *fused potass,* ℥ss. and *distilled water,* f℥ij, is a limpid, colourless, very inflammable, volatile liquor; of a penetrating and fragrant odour, and hot pungent taste. Its s. g. is 0.732.

Æther Sulphuricus, Sulphuric Ether of the Pharmacopœia of the United States (1842), *Æther* of that of 1851, is formed from *alcohol*, Oiv; *sulphuric acid,* Oj; *potassa,* ʒvj; *distilled water*, f℥iij; distilling and redistilling according to the process there laid down. The specific gravity of this ether is 0.750.

It is a diffusible stimulant, narcotic and antispasmodic, and is externally refrigerant. Dose, gtt. xxx to f℥iss. When ether is inhaled, it is found to be a valuable anæsthetic agent: and is employed with advantage in spasmodic affections, and in surgical operations. See Anæsthetic.

The Parisian Codex has an *Æther ace'ticus,* an *Æther muria'ticus* seu *hydrochlor'icus,* an *Æther ni'tricus* seu *nitro'sus*, and an *Æther phosphora'tus.* They all possess similar virtues. See Anæsthetic.

Æther Sulphuricus Acidus, Elixir acidum Halleri— æ. Sulphuricus cum alcohole, Spiritus ætheris sulphurici—æ. Sulphuricus cum alcohole aromaticus, Spiritus ætheris aromaticus.

Æther Terebinthina'tus, *Terebinth'inated ether,* made by mixing gradually two pounds of *alcohol*, and half a pound of *spirit of turpentine*, with two pounds of *concentrated nitric acid*, and distilling one-half the mixture with a gentle heat. Employed externally and internally in biliary calculi, rheumatism, &c. Dose 20 to 40 drops, in honey or yolk of egg.

Æthereа Herba, Eryngium maritimum.

Æthe'real, *Ethe'real, Ethe'reous, Æthe'reus,* (F.) *Éthérée.* An ethereal tincture, (F.) *Teinture éthérée*, is one formed by the action of sulphuric ether, at the ordinary temperature, on medicinal substances. An ethereal oil is a volatile oil. See Olea Volatilia.

Ætherizatio, Etherization.

Ætherizatus, Etherized.

Æthe'reo-Oleo'sa (Remedia), from *Ætheroleum*, 'a volatile oil.' Remedies, whose properties are dependent upon the volatile oil they contain.

Ætherolea, Olea volatilia.

Æthiop'icus Lapis, Ethiopian stone. A stone formerly supposed to be possessed of considerable virtue.—Oribasius.

Æthiopifica'tio, *Æthiopopoï'sis, Æthiopis'mus, Æthiopio'sis*, from *Æthiops*, and *facere*, 'to make.' The mummy-like colouring of the skin, induced at times by the use of mercurial ointment: and seen in bodies poisoned by arsenic.

Æthiopiosis, Æthiopificatio.

Æthiopis, Salvia sclarea.

Æthiopismus, Æthiopificatio.

Æthiopopoesis, Æthiopificatio.

Æ'thiops, from αιθω, 'I burn,' and ωψ, 'countenance.' A black or burnt countenance. The ancients gave this name to certain oxides and sulphurets of metals, which were of a black colour.

Æthiops Albus, Albino— æ. Alcalisatus, Hydrargyrum cum cretâ — æ. Animal, see Choroid.

Æthiops Martia'lis. *Ferri Deutox'ydum nigrum.* The black deutoxide of iron: once in repute as a tonic.

Æthiops Mineralis, Hydrargyri sulphuretum nigrum—æ. Narcoticus, Hydrargyri sulphuretum nigrum—æ. per se, Hydrargyri oxydum cinereum —æ. Saccharatus, Hydrargyrum saccharatum— æ. Vegetabilis, see Fucus vesiculosus.

Æthol'ices, from αιθω, 'I burn.' Fiery pustules on the skin. Some have considered them to have been *boils*.

Æthusa Ammi, Sison ammi.

Æthu'sa Cyna'pium, *Fool's Parsley*, (F.) *Faux Persil, Petite Ciguë. Family,* Umbelliferæ. *Sex. Syst.* Pentandria Digynia. A poisonous plant, which has been mistaken for true parsley, producing nausea, vomiting, headache, giddiness, sopor, and at times, fatal results. It resembles conium in its action.

Æthu'sa Meum, *Meum, M. Athaman'ticum,* seu *Anethifo'lium, Athaman'ta Meum, Ligus'ticum Capilla'ceum* seu *Meum, Ses'eli Meum, Meu, Spignel, Baldmoney.* (F.) *Éthuse, Méum.* The root has been advised as carminative, stomachic, &c.

Ætiol'ogy, *Ætiolog''ia, Etiol'ogy, Aitiolog''ia*, from αιτια, 'cause,' and λογος, 'a discourse.' The doctrine of the causes of disease.

Æti'tes, from ατος, 'an eagle.' *Eagle-stone, Pierre d'Aigle, Hydrate de tritoxide de fer.* This stone was formerly supposed to facilitate delivery, if bound on the thigh; and to prevent abortion, if bound on the arm. It was also called *Lapis Collymus.*

Ætoi Phlebes, Temporal veins.

Ætolion, Cnidia grana.

AFFADISSEMENT, (F.) from *fade*, 'insipid.' That condition of the digestive function in which the appetite is diminished, the sense of taste blunted, and the action of the stomach enfeebled; a state usually accompanied by general languor.

AFFAIBLISSEMENT, Asthenia.

AFFAIRES, Menses.

AFFAISSEMENT, Collapsus.

AFFECTIO, Affection—a. Arthritica Cordis, Cardiagra—a. Hypochondriaca, Hypochondriasis—a. Hysterica, Hysteria—a. Sarmatica, Plica—a. Tympanitica, Tympanites.

Affec'tion, *Affec'tio*, from *afficio* or *affectare* (*ad* and *facere*,) 'to move or influence.' Any mode in which the mind or body is affected or modified.

AFFECTION TYPHOÏDE, see Typhus—a. *Vaporeuse,* Hypochondriasis.

AFFECTIONES ANIMI, Affections of the mind.

Affections of the Mind, *Affec'tus* seu *Passio'nes* seu *Affectio'nes* seu *Conquassatio'nes* seu *Confusio'nes* seu *Turbatio'nes* seu *Perturbatio'nes an'imi*, (F.) *Affections de l'âme* include not only the different passions, as love, hatred, jealousy, &c., but every condition of the mind that is accompanied by an agreeable or disagreeable feeling, as pleasure, fear, sorrow, &c.

In Pathology, *Affection, Pathos, Pathe'ma*, is synonymous with disease: thus we speak of a *pulmonary affection,* a *calculous affection,* &c.

AFFECTIONS DE L'ÂME. Affections of the mind.

Affec'tive. That which affects, touches, &c. Gall gives the term *affective faculties* (F.) *Facultés affectives,* to functions dependent upon the organization of the brain, comprising the sentiments, affections, &c.

Affectus, Passion—a. Faucium pestilens, Cyanche maligna—a. Hyderodes, Hydrops—a. Spasmodico-convulsivus labiorum, Neuralgia faciei.

Af'ferent, *Af'ferens, Centrip'etal, Esod'ic*, from *affero*, (*ad* and *fero,* 'to carry,') 'I bring.' Conveying inwards, as from the periphery to the centre. The vessels which convey the lymph to the lymphatic glands, are called *afferent.* Also,

AFFION 53 AGGLUTINANT

nerves that convey impressions towards the nervous centres—*nervi sntobænon'tes.*
AF'FION, *Of'fium, O'pium.* The Bantamese thus designate an electuary of which opium is the basis, and which they use as an excitant.
AFFLA'TUS, *Adfla'tus, Epipnoi'a,* from *ad,* 'to,' and *flare* 'to blow.' Any air that strikes the body and produces disease.
AF'FLUENCE, *Af'flux,* from *affluere,* (*ad* and *fluerc,* 'to flow,') 'to flow to.' A flow or determination of humours, and particularly of blood, towards any part.
AFFLUXUS, Fluxion.
AFFUSIO, Affusion—a. Frigida, see Affusion—a. Orbicularis, Placenta.
AFFU'SION, *Affu'sio, Pros'chysis, Epich'ysis,* from *ad,* 'to,' and *fundere, fusum,* 'to pour.' The action of pouring a liquid on any body. *Affusions,* Rhyptolu'siæ, cold and warm, are used in different diseases. The *cold affusion, Affu'sio* seu *Perfu'sio frig"ida,* is said to have been beneficial in cutting short typhus fever and scarlatina, if used during the first days. It consists in placing the patient in a tub, and pouring cold water over him; then wiping him dry, and putting him to bed. The only precaution necessary, is, to use it in the state of greatest heat and exacerbation; not when chilliness, or topical inflammation, is present.
AFIUM, Opium.
AFTER-BIRTH, Secundines.
AFTER-PAINS, see Pains, labour.
AGACEMENT, (F.) from ακαζειν, 'to sharpen.' The setting on edge.
AGACEMENT DES DENTS. A disagreeable sensation experienced when acids are placed in contact with the teeth. *Tooth edge.* Setting the teeth on edge.
AGACEMENT DES NERFS. A slight irritation of the system, and particularly of the organs of sense and locomotion, corresponding nearly to the English *Fidgets.*
AGALACTATIO, Agalactia.
AGALAC'TIA, *Agalax'ia, Agalac'tio, Agalacta'tio, Defec'tus lac'tis, Oligoga'lia, Oligogalac'-tia,* from *a,* privative, and γαλα, 'milk.' Absence of milk in the mammæ.
AGALAXIA, Agalactia.
AGAL'LOCHUM, from αγαλλομαι, 'to become splendid,' *Calambac, Calambouk, Lig'num Agal'-lochi veri, Lig'num Al'oës, L. Aspal'athi, Xylo-aloës, Aloes wood.* A resinous and very aromatic wood of the East Indies, from *Excæca'ria Agal'-locha, Oynometra Agal'lochum, Aloëx'ylon Agal'-lochum.* Used in making pastils, &c. — Dioscorides, Oribasius, Paulus.
AGAMOUS, see Cryptogamous.
AG'ARIC, *Agar'icum.* A genus of plants in the Linnæan system, some of which are edible, others poisonous. It was so called from Agaria, a region of Sarmatia.—Dioscorides. Among the edible varieties of the Boletus, the following are the chief. 1. The *Agar'icus edu'lis* seu *Arven'sis* seu *Sylvat'icus* seu *Campes'tris,* (F.) *Agaric comestible et champignon de couche.* 2. The *Agar'icus odora'tus,* (F.) *Mousseron.* The most common poisonous varieties are the *Agar'icus neca'tor,* (F.) *Agaric meurtrier:* and 2. The *Agaricus acris,* (F.) *Agaric âcre;* besides the *Auranite,* a sub-genus, which includes several species. One of the most delicate is the *Agaricus Aurantiacus,* but care must be taken not to confound it with the *A. Pseudo-aurantiacus,* which is very poisonous. The A. aurantiacus is called, in French, *Oronge.* See Poisons, Table of.
AGARIC, see Boletus igniarius—a. Blanc, Boletus laricis—a. de Chêne, Boletus igniarius—a. Female, Boletus igniarius—a. of the Oak, Boletus igniarius—a. Odorant, Dædalea suaveolens—a. White, Boletus laricis.
AGARICUM, Boletus igniarius.
AGARICUS, Boletus igniarius—a. Albus, Boletus laricis—a. Arvensis, see Agaric—a. Aurantiacus, Amanitæ, Bolites—a. Auriculæforma, Peziza auricula—a. Campestris, see Agaric—a. Chirurgorum, Boletus igniarius—a. Igniarius, Boletus igniarius—a. Laricis, Boletus laricis—a. Pseudo-aurantiacus, Amanitæ—a. Quercûs, Boletus igniarius—a. Sylvaticus, see Agaric.
AGASYLLIS GALBANUM, Bubon galbanum.
AGATHIS DAMARRA, Pinus damarra.
AGATHOSMA CRENATUM, Diosma crenata.
AGATHOTES CHIRAYITA, Gentiana chirayita.
AGA'VE AMERICA'NA, A. *Ramo'sa, American Agave, American aloe, Maguey,* from αγαυος, 'admirable.' *Nat. Ord.* Bromeliaceæ. *Sex. Syst.* Hexandria Monogynia. This plant has been considered diuretic and antisyphilitic. The favourite drink of the Mexicans—*Pulque*—is the fermented juice of this plant.
AGAVE RAMOSA, A. Americana.
AGAVE VIRGIN'ICA, *Rattlesnake's master:*—grows in the Southern States. The root is very bitter. It has been used in tincture as a carminative in colic; and as a remedy for bites of serpents.
AGE, 'ηλικια, *Heli'kia, Ætas;* — Of uncertain etymon. Period of life. Time that has elapsed since birth, &c. Five ages are often designated in the life of man. 1. First infancy (*Infan'tia;*) 2. Second infancy (*Pueri"tia;*) 3. Adolescence (*Adolescen'tia:*) 4. The adult age (*Viril'itas:*) 5. Old age (*Senec'tus.*)
AGENEIOS, Imberbis.
AGEN'ESIS, from *a,* privative, and γενεσις, 'generation.' Imperfect development of any part of the body; as *cerebral agenesis,* i. e. imperfect development of the brain in the fœtus.
AGENNESIA, Impotence, Sterilitas.
AGENNESIS, Impotence.
AGENOSO'MUS; from *a,* privative, γεννau, 'I generate,' and σωμα, 'body.' A malformation in which the fissure and eventration are chiefly in the lower part of the abdomen; the urinary or sexual apparatus absent or very rudimentary.
AGENT, *Agens,* from *agere,* 'to act.' Any power which produces, or tends to produce an effect on the human body. Morbific agents, (F.) *Agens morbifiques,* are the causes of disease;—therapeutical agents, (F.) *Agens thérapeutiques,* the means of treating it.
AGER NATURÆ, Uterus.
AGERA'SIA, *Insenescen'tia,* from *a,* privative, and γηρας, 'old age.' A vigorous and green old age.
AGERATUM, Achilleæ ageratum.
AGE'RATUS LAPIS. A stone used by cobblers to polish shoes. It was formerly esteemed discutient and astringent. — Galen, Oribasius, Paulus.
AGES, Palm.
AGEUSIA, Ageustia.
AGEUS'TIA, *Agheus'tia, Ageu'sia, Apogeus'-tia, Apogeu'sis, Dysæsthe'sia gustato'ria, Parageu'sis,* from *a,* priv., and γευσις, 'taste.' Diminution or loss of taste, *Anæsthe'sia linguæ.* Sauvages, Cullen.
AGGLOM'ERATE, *Agglomera'tus,* from *agglomerare* (*ad* and *glomerare,* 'to wind up yarn in a ball,') 'to collect together.' Applied to tumours or glands in aggregation.
AGGLU'TINANT, *Agglu'tinans, Collet'icus, Glu'tinans,* from *gluten,* 'glue' (F.) *Agglutinand, Agglutinatif, Glutinatif.* Remedies were for-

merly so called, which were considered capable of uniting divided parts.—Paulus.

Plasters are called *agglutinants*, (F.) *agglutinatifs*, which adhere strongly to the skin. Certain bandages are likewise so termed. (F.) *Bandelettes agglutinatives*.

TO AGGLU'TINATE. The French use the word *agglutiner*, in the sense of 'to reunite;' as *agglutiner les lèvres d'une plaie*, 'to reunite the lips of a wound.'

AGGLUTINATIF, Agglutinant.
AGGLUTINATIO, Coition.
AGGLUTINA'TION, *Colle'sis, Epicolle'sis, Proscolle'sis, Glutina'tio*, from *agglutinare*, 'to glue together.' The first degree of adhesion. Also, the action of agglutinants.
AGGLUTINER, To agglutinate.
AG'GREGATE, *Aggrega'tus*, from *aggregare*, (*ad* and *gregare*,) 'to flock together,' 'to assemble together.' Glands are called *aggregate* which are in clusters. See Peyeri Glandulæ. *Aggregate pills*, (F.) *Pilules agrégatives*, signified, formerly, those which were believed to contain the properties of a considerable number of medicines, and to be able to supply their place.
AGHEUSTIA, Ageustia.
AGHOUL, Agul.
AGIAHA'LID or AGIHA'LID or AGRAHA'LID. An Egyptian and Ethiopian shrub, similar to *Ximenia*. The Ethiopians use it as a vermifuge. The fruit is purgative.
AGIHALID, Agiahalid.
AGISSANT, Active.
AGITATION, *Agita'tio, Done'sis;* from *agere*, 'to act.' Constant and fatiguing motion of the body, *Tyrbē, Tyrba'sia, In'quies*,—or distressing mental inquietude,—*An'imi Agita'tio*.
AGITATORIUS, Convul'sive.
AGLOS'SIA, from *a*, privative, and γλωσσα, 'the tongue.' A malformation, which consists in the want of a tongue.
AGLOSSOS'TOMA, from *Aglossia*, and στομα, 'mouth.' A mouth without a tongue.
AGLOSSOSTOMOG'RAPHY, *Aglossostomogra'phia*, from *a*, priv., γλωσσα, 'the tongue,' στομα, 'the mouth,' and γραφω, 'I describe.' Description of a mouth without a tongue.—Roland (of Saumur).
AGLUTI'TION, *Agluti'tio*, from *a*, priv., and *glutire*, 'to swallow.' A hybrid term, designating impossibility of swallowing.—Linnæus.
AGMA, Fracture.
AGMATOLOG''IA, from *αγμα*, fracture, and λογος, 'a description.' The doctrine of fractures. A treatise on fractures.
AGME, Fracture.
AGMINA DIGITORUM MANUS, Phalanges of the fingers.—a. Membrana, Amnios.
AGMINATED GLANDS, Peyer's glands.
AGNA'THIA, from *a*, priv., and γναθος, 'jaw.' A malformation, which consists in the want of the jaw, especially of the lower.
AGNINA MEMBRANA, Amnios.
AGNOI'A, *Agnœ'a* from *a*, priv., and γινωσκω, 'I know.' State of a patient who does not recognise individuals.—Hippocrates, Galen, Foësius.
AGNUS CASTUS, Vitex.
AGO'GE, αγωγη. The order or condition of a disease.—Hippoc., Galen. Likewise the state of the air.—Hippoc., Galen, Gorræus, Foësius.
AGOGUE, αγωγος, a leader,' from αγω, 'I lead or expel.' Hence *Cholagogue*, an expeller of bile: *Hydragogue*, &c.
AGOMPHI'ASIS, *Agompho'sis*, from *a*, privative, and γομφοω, 'I nail.' Looseness of the teeth.—Gorræus. See Gomphiasis.
AGOMPHOSIS, Agomphiasis.
AGON, Agony.

AGONE, Hyoscyamus.
AGONIA, Sterilitas.
AGONISMA, Agony.
AGONISMUS, Agony.
AGONIS'TICA, from αγων, 'a combat.' The part of ancient gymnastics, which had reference to the combats of the Athletæ.

Also, very cold water, given internally, to calm febrile heat.—Paulus of Ægina.
AGONIZANS, Psychorages.
AGONOS, Sterile.
AG'ONY, *Agon'ia, Agon, Agonis'ma, Agonis'mus, Mochthus, Mogus, Psychorag''ia, Psychorrhag''ia, Angor*, from αγων, 'a combat.' The last struggle of life.—Galen, Gorræus, &c. The agony, which is of longer or shorter duration, is characterized by great change in the features, gradual abolition of sensation and motion, loss of voice, dryness or lividity of the tongue and lips, rattling in the throat, small and intermittent pulse, and coldness of the extremities. This state is not present in those who die suddenly. See Facies Hippocratica.
AGOS'TUS, from αγω, 'I lead.' The fore arm from the elbow to the fingers. Also, the palm of the hand.—Gorræus. See Palm.
AGRA, αγρα, from αγρεω, 'I seize hold of.' A seizure, as *Odontagra*, a tooth seizure, toothache; *Chiragra, Podagra*, &c.
AGRAFE DE VALENTIN. A kind of forceps with parallel branches, employed by Valentin in the operation for hare lip, to effect the approximation of the edges of the wound.
AGRAHALID, Agiahalid.
AGRÉGATIVES PILULES. See Aggregate.
AGRIA, Herpes exedens.
AGRIAMPELOS, Bryonia alba.
AGRICOCCIMELEA, Prunus Spinosa.
AGRIFOLIUM, Ilex aquifolium.
AGRIMONIA, Agrimony—a. Eupatoria, Agrimony—a. Odorata, Agrimony—a. Officinalis, Agrimony.
AG'RIMONY, *Agrimo'nia, A. Eupato'ria seu odora'ta seu officina'lis, Caf'al, Lap'pula hepat'ica, Cockle-bur, Stickwort*. (F.) *Aigremoine*. *Nat. Ord.* Rosaceæ. *Sex. Syst.* Icosandria Digynia. A mild astringent and stomachic. Dose, in powder, from ʒj to ʒj.
AGRIMONY, HEMP, Eupatorium cannabinum.
AGRIOCASTANUM, Bunium bulbocastanum, Lycoperdon tuber.
AGRIOCINARA, Sempervivum tectorum.
AGRIORIGANUM, Origanum majorana.
AGRIOSELINUM, Smyrnum olusatrum.
AGRIOTHYM'IA, from αγριος, 'ferocious,' and θυμος, 'disposition.' Ferocious insanity.—Sauvages.
AGRIPALMA GALLIS, Leonurus cardiaca.
AGRIP'PA, *Ægrip'pa*, from *æger partus*, 'difficult birth:' or perhaps from αγρα, 'taking, or seizure,' and πους, 'the foot.' This term has been given to those born by the feet. It is pretended that the family of Agrippa obtained their name from this circumstance. Parturition, where the feet present, is called *Agrippæ partus, Agrippi'nus partus*.
AGRIPPINUS PARTUS, see Agrippa.
AGRO DI CEDRO, see Citrus medica.
AGROPYRUM LÆVISSIMUM, Triticum repens.
AGROSTIS, Bryonia alba.
AGRUNA, Prunus spinosa.
AGRYPNIA, Insomnia.
AGRYPNOCOMA, Coma vigil.
AGRYPNO'DES, from αγρυπνος, 'sleepless.' Characterized by sleeplessness, as *Febris Agrypnodes*, a fever accompanied with sleeplessness.

AGRYPNOTICUS, Anthypnotic.
AGRYP'NUS, αγρυπνος. Sleepless; vigilant.
AGUA DE VERUGA, see Verugas.
AGUARDIENTE, Brandy. See also Spirit.
—*a. de Italia*, see Spirit.
A'GUE, from Gothic, *agis*, 'trembling.' (?) Intermittent fever.
AGUE AND FEVER, Intermittent fever.
AGUE CAKE, *Placen'ta febri'lis, Physco'nia sple'nicum, P. splenica, Splenis Tumor;* (F.) *Gâteau fébrile*. A visceral obstruction—generally in the spleen—which follows agues, and is distinctly felt by external examination. To a greater or less degree, it is not uncommon.
AGUE, DEAD, see Fever, masked. Ague drop, tasteless, Liquor arsenicalis—a. Dumb, see Fever, masked—a. Free, Laurus sassafras—a. Leaping, see Leaping ague—a. Quartan, Quartan—a. Tertian, Tertian fever—a. Weed, Eupatorium perfoliatum.
AGUL, *Aghoul, Alha'gi*, the *Hedisa'rum* seu *Hedysa'rum alhagi*. A thorny shrub of Persia and Mesopotamia, which affords manna. The leaves are purgative.
AGY'ION, from *a*, priv., and *γυιον*, 'limb.' Mutilated or wanting limbs.—Hippocr. Weak, feeble.—Galen.
AGYR'IAS, from *αγυρις*, 'a collection.' Opacity of the crystalline.—Aëtius, Paré.
AGYRTA, from *αγυρις*, 'a crowd.' Formerly, a stroller who pretended to supernatural powers. Subsequently, a quack or illiterate pretender. See Charlatan.
AGYRTIA, Charlatanry.
AHO'RA, from *a*, privative, and *ωρα*, 'youth.' Tardy development of the organs:—the opposite to *Hyperho'ra*.
AHOUAI, Thevetia ahouai.
AHUSAL, Orpiment.
AHYPNIA, Insomnia.
AIDE, (F.) *Ad'jutor min'ister*. An assistant to a surgeon in his operations.
AIDOROMANIA, Nymphomania.
AIERSA, Iris Germanica.
AIGE, Ægias.
AIGLE, MINERAL WATERS OF. Near the city of this name, in Normandy, is the chalybeate spring of Saint Xantin, much used in the 16th and 17th centuries.
AIGLE, Ægias.
AIGRE, Acidulous—*a. Voix*. See Acid.
AIGRELET, Acidulous.
AIGRETTE, see Typha latifolia.
AIGREMOINE, Agrimony.
AIGREURS, Acidities.
AIGU, Acute.
AIGUILLE, Needle—*a. à Acupuncture*, see Needle—*a. à Appareil*, see Needle—*a. à Bec de Lièvre*, see Needle—*a. à Cataracte*, see Needle—*a. de Deschamps*, see Needle—*a. Engainée*, see Needle—*a. à Fistule*, see Needle—*a. à. Gaine*, see Needle—*a. à Ligature*, see Needle—*a. à Manche*, see Needle—*a. à Séton*, see Needle—*a. à Suture*, see Needle.
AIGUILLON, (F.) *Spina Helmon'tii*. A term used since the time of Van Helmont to designate the proximate cause of inflammation. According to him, an inflamed part is in the same condition as if an *aiguillon* or thorn were thrust into it.
AIGUISER, to Acidulate.
AIL, Allium.
AILE, Ala, *Aileron*.
AILERON, (F.) *Extre'ma Ala* seu *Pin'nula*, diminutive of (F.) *Aile*, a wing. The extremity of the wing of a bird, to which the great feathers are attached.

AILERONS DE LA MATRICE. Three folds at the base of the broad ligaments of the uterus, which are occupied by the ovary and its ligament, the Fallopian tube, and the round ligament.
AIMA, 'αιμα, see Hæma.
AIMANT, Magnet.
AIMATERA, Hepatirrhœa.
AIMORRHŒA, Hæmorrhagia.
AIMORRHOIS, Hæmorrhois.
AINE, Inguen.
AIPATHIA, Continent disease.
AIPI, Jatropha manihot.
AIPIMA COXERA, Jatropha manihot.
AIPIPOCA, Jatropha manihot.
AIR, *Aër, Pneuma*, from *αω*, 'I breathe.' Common Air, Atmospheric air (F.) *Air atmosphérique*, is an invisible, transparent, inodorous, insipid, ponderable, compressible, and elastic fluid, which, under the form of the atmosphere, surrounds the earth to the height of 15 or 16 leagues.
Air is essentially composed of two gases, oxygen and nitrogen, in the proportion of 20 of the former to 80 of the latter. Oxygen is the vital portion, but the nitrogen is necessary to dilute it. Air also contains a small portion of carbonic acid gas, and has always floating in it aqueous vapour, different terrestrial emanations, &c. Its effects upon the human body vary according to its greater or less density, temperature, moisture, &c.; hence, change of air is found extremely serviceable in the prevention and cure of certain morbid conditions. See Climate and Respiration.
AIR ACIDE VITRIOLIQUE, Sulphurous acid—*a. Alcalin*, Ammonia—*a. Atmosphérique*, Air.
AIR BLADDER, *Swim-bladder, Swimming bladder*; (F.) *Vessie natatoire*. An abdominal organ in many fishes, sometimes communicating by means of a duct with the alimentary canal, at others, not, which is considered by some to belong to the respiratory system. Its contents are the elements of atmospheric air, but in different proportions; and its chief and general function appears to be to regulate the specific gravity of the fish.
AIR CELLS OF THE LUNGS, Bronchial cells; see Cellule—a. Chamber, Folliculus aeris—a. Dephlogisticated, Oxygen—a. Empyreal, Oxygen—*a. du Feu*, Oxygen—a. Factitious, Carbonic acid—a. Fixed, Carbonic acid—*a. Gaté*, Azote—a. Inflammable, Hydrogen, Hydrogen carburetted.
AIR PASSAGES, (F.) *Voies aériennes, V. aérifères*. The larynx, trachea, bronchia, &c.
AIR, PURE, Oxygen—a. Solid, of Hales, Carbonic acid—*a. Vicié*, Azote—a. Vital, Oxygen.
AIRAIN, Bell-metal, Brass.
AIRE, Areola.
AIRELLE ANGULEUSE, Vaccinium myrtillus—*a. Ponctuée*, Vaccinium vitis idæa.
AIRIGNE, Hook.
AIRTHREY, MINERAL WATERS OF. Airthrey is situate about two miles north of Stirling, Scotland. The waters are saline cathartics; containing chloride of sodium, chloride of calcium, sulphate of zinc, and chloride of magnesium.
AISSELLE, Axilla.
AISTHESIS, Æsthesis.
AITHOMO'MA, from *αιθος*, 'black.' A black condition of all the humours of the eye. A. Paré.
AITIA, Cause.
AITIOLOGY, Ætiologia.
AITION, Cause.

AIX-LA-CHAPELLE, MINERAL WATERS OF. Called by the Germans, Aachen. A thermal, sulphureous, mineral water, which contains, in 1000 grammes, 28.54 cubic inches of sulphohydric acid gas, 18.05 cubic inches of carbonic acid gas, 0.1304 grammes of carbonate of lime, 0.0440 grammes of carbonate of magnesia, 0.5444 grammes of carbonate of soda, 2.3697 grammes of chloride of sodium, 0.2637 of sulphate of soda, and 0.0705 of silica. The temperature is 134° Fahrenheit.

The *factitious water of Aix-la-Chapelle, A'qua Aquisgranen'sis*, (F.) *Eau d'Aix-la-Chapelle*, is made by adding *pure water* f℥xvijss, *to hydrosulphuretted water* f℥iv., *carbonate of soda* gr. xx, *chloride of sodium* gr. ix.—Ph. P.

There are thermal sulphureous springs at Aix in Savoy (98°), and some thermal springs at Aix in Provence (91°).

AIZOON, Sempervivum tectorum.

A'JUGA, A. *pyramida'lis, Consol'ida me'dia, Bu'gula, B. pyramida'lis, Teu'crium pyramida'lē, Upright Bugloss, Middle Consound.* (F.) *Bugle pyramidale.* This plant is subastringent and bitter.

AJUGA CHAMÆPITYS, Teucrium chamæpitys.

AJUGA REPTANS, Bu'gula, B. reptans, Common Bugle, (F.) *Bugle rampante*, has similar properties.

AKATALIS, Juniperus communis.
AKATERA, Juniperus communis.
AKINESIA, Acinesia.
AKOLOGY. Matéria Medica.
AKRATOPEGÆ, Acratopegæ.

ALA, *Pinna, Pteryx*, 'a wing.' (F.) *Aile*. A term often used by anatomists for parts which project like a wing from the median line; as the *Alæ nasi, Alæ of the uterus,* &c. See Axilla and Pavilion of the Ear. Also, Pterygium.

ALA EXTREMA, see Aileron.

ALABAS'TER, *Alabas'trum.* (F.) *Albâtre, Alabastri'tes.* A variety of compact gypsum; of which an ointment was once made;—the *unguen'tum alabastri'num;* used as a discutient. Alabaster likewise entered into several dentifrices.

ALABASTRITES, Alabaster.

ALÆ INTERNÆ MINORES CLITORIDIS, Nymphæ—a. Majores, Labia pudendi—a. Minores, Nymphæ—a. Muliebres minores, Nymphæ—a. Nasi, see Nasus—a. Pudendi Muliebris, Labia pudendi—a. Pulmonum, see Pulmo—a. of the Uterus, see Ala—a. Vespertilionis, see Uterus.

ALAITER, from (F.) *lait*, 'milk.' To suckle.
ALALIA, Mutitas.
ALAMBIC, Alembic.

ALANFU'TA. A name given by the Arabians to a vein, situate between the chin and lower lip, which they were in the habit of opening in cases of fœtor of the breath.—Avicenna.

ALAQUE'CA. The Hindoostanee name of a stone, found in small, polished fragments, which is considered efficacious in arresting hemorrhage when applied externally. It is a sulphuret of iron.

ALARES MUSCULI, Pterygoid muscles.

ALA'RES VENÆ. The superficial veins at the fold of the arm.

ALA'RIA OSSA. The wing-like processes of the sphenoid bone.

ALA'RIS, *Ala'tus, Aliform'is;* from *ala,* 'a wing.' Wing-shaped; winged.

ALATERNUS, COMMON, Rhamnus alaternus—a. Latifolius, Rhamnus alaternus.

ALA'TUS. *Pterygo'des, Homo ala'tus.* One whose scapulæ project backwards like wings.

ALBAD'ARAN. The sesamoid bone of the metatarso-phalangal joint of the great toe. The Rabbis and Magicians attributed extraordinary virtues to it.—Arabians.

ALBAGIAZI, Sacrum.
ALBAMENTUM, Albumen ovi.

ALBAN, SAINT, MINERAL WATERS OF. A French acidulous chalybeate, in the department of the Loire.

ALBARAS ALBA, Lepra alphoides—a. Nigra, Lepra nigricans.
ALBARÆS, Lepra alphoides.
ALBAROS, Lepra alphoides.
ALBÂTRE, Alabaster.
ALBEDO UNGUIUM, see Nail.
ALBIN D'ŒUF, Albumen ovi.
ALBINISM, see Albino.
ALBINISMUS, see Albino.

ALBI'NO 'White.' *Leucæ'thiops, Æthiops albus, Dondo,* from *albus,* 'white.' (F.) *Blafard, Nègre-blanc.* A spanish word applied to individuals of the human race who have the skin and hair white; the iris very pale, bordering on red; and the eyes so sensible, that they cannot bear the light of day. This condition, which has been called *Leucæthio'pia, Alpho'sis Æthiop'ica, Albinoïs'mus, Albinis'mus, Al'binism, Leucopathi'a,* is seen more frequently in the Negro. Both sexes are exposed to it. It does not seem to be true, that there are tribes of Albinos in the interior of Africa.

ALBINOISMUS, see Albino.
ALBOR OVI, Albumen ovi.

AL'BORA. A kind of itch or complicated leprosy.—Paracelsus.

ALBOT, Crucible.
ALBOTIM, Terebinthina.

ALBUGIN'EA, *Tu'nica albugin'ea, A. Testis, Perites'tis, Dura mater testis, Membra'na capsula'ris testis.* (F.) *Albuginée, Tunique albuginée.* A strong, fibrous, and resisting membrane, which immediately envelopes the testicle, and has, at its upper part, an enlargement, called corpus Highmorianum. From its inner surface it sends off a number of flat, filiform prolongations or septa, between which are contained the seminiferous vessels. Externally it is covered by the tunica vaginalis testis.

ALBUGINÉE, Albuginea, Albugineous.

ALBUGIN'EOUS, *Albugin'eus,* 'white,' from *albus,* (F.) *Albuginée.* A term applied to textures, humours, &c., which are perfectly white.

ALBUGIN'EOUS FIBRE, (F.) *Fibre albuginée.* A name given by Chaussier to what he considers one of the four elementary fibres.

The albugineous fibre is linear, cylindrical, tenacious, elastic, but little extensible, and of a shining, satiny appearance. It forms fasciæ or fasciculi, which constitute the tendons, articular ligaments, and aponeuroses; hence the name *Albugineous membranes,* given by Chaussier to the fibrous membranes.

Gauthier considered, that the rete mucosum consists of four layers, to two of which he gives the names *membra'na albugin'ea profun'da* and *membra'na albugin'ea superficia'lis,* respectively.

ALBUGINI'TIS, (F.) *Albuginite.* A term employed by some authors for inflammation of the albugineous tissue. Thus, gout and rheumatism are regarded as species of the genus albuginitis.

ALBUGO OCULORUM, Leucoma—a. Ovi, Albumen ovi.

ALBULA, Leucoma.

ALBUM CANIS, Album græcum—a. Ceti, Cetaceum.

ALBUM GRÆCUM, *Oynoc'oprus, Spo'dium Græco'rum, Album Canis, Stercus Cani'num Album.* The white dung of the dog. It consists almost wholly of *phosphate of lime*, from the bones used as food. It was formerly applied as a discutient to the inside of the throat in quinsies, but is now justly banished from practice.

ALBUM NIGRUM. The excrement of the mouse.
ALBUM OCULI, see Sclerotic.
ALBUM RHAZIS. A white ointment made of cerusse and lard, prescribed by the Arabian physician Rhazes.

ALBU'MEN, *Leuco'ma, Ooni'nē, Ozemun*, from *albus*, 'white.' (F.) *Albumine*. An immediate principle of animals and vegetables, which constitutes the chief part of the white of egg. It is found in the serum, chyle, synovia, serous fluids, &c. There is not much difference in chemical composition between animal and vegetable albumen, fibrin and casein: fibrin alone appears, however, to be possessed of plastic properties. Also, the white of the eye. See Sclerotic.

ALBU'MEN OVI, *Albu'mor, Albu'go Ovi, Albor Ovi, Can'didum Ovi, Albu'men, Olare'ta, Ovi albus liquor, Albumen'tum, Lac avis* or *white of egg*, (F.) *Blanc d'œuf*, (Old F.) *Albin d'œuf*, is used in pharmacy for suspending oils, &c., in water. See Ovum.

ALBUMINE, Albumen.
ALBUMINU'RIA. A hybrid term from '*Albumen*,' and ουρον, 'the urine.' A condition of the urine in which it contains albumen, the presence of which is indicated by its coagulation on the application of adequate heat.

ALBUMINURORRHÉE, Kidney, Bright's disease of the.

ALBUMOR, Albumen ovi.
AL'CAEST, *Al'cahest, Al'chaest*, perhaps from (G.) all, 'all,' and geist, 'spirit.' A word invented by Paracelsus to designate a liquor, which, according to him, was capable of removing every kind of swelling.

The same word was used by Van Helmont for a fancied universal solvent, capable of reducing every body to its elements.

ALCAEST OF GLAUBER is a thick liquor obtained by detonating nitrate of potassa on hot coals, which transforms it into subcarbonate of potassa.

ALCAEST OF RESPOUR is a mixture of potassa and oxyd of zinc.

ALCAHEST, Alcaest.
ALCAHOL, Alcohol.
ALCALES'CENCE, *Alkales'cence, Alcalescen'tia*. The condition in which a fluid becomes alkaline.

ALCALESCENCE OF THE HUMOURS was an old notion of the humourists. It can only occur during the putrid fermentation of animal matters, which contain azote, and produce ammonia.

ALCALIN'ITY is the quality of being alcaline.

AL'CALI or *Alca'li, Al'kali*, from *al* (Arab.,) 'the,' and *kali*, the name of the *Salso'la Soda*, a plant which contains a large quantity of one of the principal alkalis—*soda*. The alkalis are substances soluble in water, possessing generally a urinous, acrid, and caustic taste, turning the syrup of violets green, and restoring to blue infusion of litmus, which has been reddened by acids; reddening the yellow of turmeric, and having the greatest tendency to unite with acids, whose character they modify, and form salts with them. In medicine we understand by this term *Potassa, Soda*, or *Ammonia*.

ALCALI, CAUSTIC, *Al'kali Caus'ticum*. A pure alkali. One deprived of its carbonic acid.

ALCALIS, FIXED, Soda and potassa; VOLATILE ALCALI, Ammonia.

ALCALI AMMONIACUM ACETATUM, Liquor ammoniæ acetatis—a. Ammoniacum fluidum, Liquor ammoniæ—a. Fixum tartarizatum, Potassæ tartras—a. Minerale sulphuricum, Soda, sulphate of—a. Tartari aceto saturatum, Potassæ acetas—a. Vegetabile salito dephlogisticatum, Potassæ murias hyperoxygenatus—a. Vegetabile tartarizatum, Potassæ tartras—a. Vegetabile vitriolatum, Potassæ sulphas—a. Volatile acetatum, Liquor ammoniæ acetatis—a. Volatile aeratum, Ammoniæ carbonas—a. Volatile ex sale ammoniaco, Ammoniæ carbonas.

ALCALIGENE, Azote.
ALCALINITY. See Alkalescence.
ALCANA, Anchusa officinalis.
ALCANNA MAJOR LATIFOLIA DENTATA, Prinos—a. Orientalis, Lawsonia inermis—a. Spuria, Anchusa tinctoria—a. Vera, Lawsonia inermis.

ALCEA, Hibiscus abelmoschus—a. Ægyptiaca, Hibiscus abelmoschus—a. Indica, Hibiscus abelmoschus.

ALCE'A RO'SEA, *Common hollyhock*. Emollient, like Althæa.

ALCHACHENGE, Physalis.
ALCHACHIL, Rosmarinus.
ALCHAEST, Alcahest.
ALCHEMIL'LA, said to have been celebrated with the Alchemists [?] *A. vulga'ris, Common Ladies' Mantle, Pes Leo'nis, Leontopo'dium*, (F.) *Pied de Lion*. Formerly in great repute as an astringent in hemorrhage.

ALCHEMY, Alchymy.
ALCHITRAM, see Pinus Sylvestris.
ALCHITURA, see Pinus Sylvestris.
ALCHOOL, Alcohol.
ALCHORNEA LATIFOLIA, see Alcornoque.
AL'CHYMY, *Al'chemy, Alchemi'a, Alchimi'a, Adep'ta Philosoph'ia*, from *al*, an Arabic particle, signifying 'superiority, excellence,' and *Ohimia*, 'Chymistry.' This word was formerly synonymous with Chymistry; but, from the 7th century, it has been applied to the mysterious art of endeavouring to discover a universal remedy, and a mode of transmuting the baser metals into gold: an operation to which they gave the name *Opus magnum*, and *Philosopher's stone*.

Alchymy has also been called *Scien'tia vel Philosoph'ia Hermet'ica*, from an idea that Hermes or Mercury was its inventor.

Harris has well defined this chimerical art: '*Ars sine arte, cujus principium est mentiri, medium laborare, et finis mendicare.*'

AL'CHYMIST, *Flatua'rius, Adept'*. One pretending to alchymy.

ALCOCALUM, Cynara scolymus.
AL'COHOL, *Al'cahol, Alchool, Alkol, Alcol, Al'cool, Al'kool*. An Arabic word, formerly used for an impalpable powder, and signifying 'very subtile, much divided.' At the present day it is applied to highly rectified spirit of wine:—see *Spiritus rectificatus* or rectified spirit, distilled from dried subcarbonate of potassa. In the Ph. U. S. Alcohol is rectified spirit of the specific gravity 0.835.

Alcohol is an inflammable liquor, lighter than water, of a warm, acrid taste, colourless, transparent, and of a pungent, aromatic smell. It is the product of the distillation of vinous liquors; is miscible with water in all proportions, and is the direct solvent of resins, balsams, &c. Various other vegetable principles are soluble in it, and hence it is used, in different states of concentration, in the preparation of *elixirs, tinctures, essences,* &c.

Alcohol acts on the animal body as a powerful stimulus: as such, in a dilute form, it is used in the prevention and cure of disease. Its habitual and inordinate use is the cause of many serious affections, of a chronic character especially, as visceral obstructions, dropsy, &c.

ALCOHOL ÆTHEREUS FERRATUS, A. Sulfurico-æthereus ferri—a. cum Aloe perfoliatâ, Tinctura aloes—a. Ammoniæ et guaiaci, Tinctura guaiaci ammoniata—a. Ammoniatum, Spiritus ammoniæ—a. Ammoniatum aromaticum, Spiritus ammoniæ aromaticus—a. Ammoniatum fœtidum, Spiritus ammoniæ fœtidus—a. Amylicum, Oil, Fusel—a. cum Aromatibus sulphuricatus, Sulphuricum acidum aromaticum—a. cum Aromatibus compositus, Tinctura cinnamomi composita—a. Castoriatum, Tinctura castorei—a. cum Crotone cascarillâ, Tinctura cascarillæ—a. Dilutum, Spiritus tenuior—a. Ferratus, Tinctura ferri muriatis—a. cum Sulphate ferri tartarisatus, see Ferrum tartarisatum—a. cum Guaiaco officinale ammoniatus, Tinctura guaiaci ammoniata—a. Iodii, Tinctura Iodinæ—a. cum Opio, Tinctura opii—a. Sulphuricatum, Elixir acidum Halleri—a. Sulphuricum, Elixir acidum Halleri—a. Sulphuris, Carbonis sulphuretum—a. Vini, Spiritus rectificatus.

ALCOHOL'IC, *Alcohol'icus,Spirituo'sus,Spir'-ituous.* Relating to or containing alcohol—as an *alcoholic* drink or remedy.

ALCOL, Alcohol.

ALCOLÆ, Aphthæ.

ALCOOL, Alcohol—a. *Camphré,* Spiritus camphoræ.

ALCOOLAT, Tincture.

ALCOOLATUM, Tincture—a. Antiscorbuticum, Tinctura de Cochleariis—a. Carminativum Sylvii, Tinctura de Cochleariis—a. de Croco compositum, Tinctura de Croco composita.

ALCOOLISER (F.) Formerly, 'to reduce into an impalpable powder.' No longer used.

ALCOOLOMETER, Areometer.

ALCORNOQUE (F.) *Cortex Alcornoco.* The bark of *Alchor'nea latifo'lia,* of Jamaica, which has been considered capable of curing phthisis. It is bitter, tonic, and slightly astringent. Dose of the powder ℈i to ʒss.

AL'CYON, *Hal'cyon.* A swallow of Cochin China, whose nest is gelatinous and very nutritious. It has been proposed in medicine as analeptic and aphrodisiac.

ALCYO'NIUM, *Bastard sponge.* The ashes were formerly employed as dentrifices: they were believed proper for favouring the growth of the hair and beard, and were used in Alopecia.

ALDABARAN, Albadaran.

ALDEHYDE, see Anæsthetic.

ALDER, AMERICAN, Alnus serratula—a. Black, Prinos, Rhamnus frangula—a. European, Alnus glutinosa.

ALE, Cerevisia.

ALEACAS, Glycyrrhiza.

ALECOST, Tanacetum balsamita.

ALECTO'RIUS LAPIS, *Alecto'ria;* from αλεκτωρ, 'a cock.' The name of a stone, supposed to exist in the stomach of the cock, or, according to others, in that of the capon, four years old. Many marvellous properties were formerly attributed to it, which are as groundless as its existence. There are no stones in the stomach, except what have been swallowed.

ALEGAR, Acetum.

ALEHOOF, Glechoma hederacea.

ALEIMMA, Liniment.

ALEIPHA, Liniment.

ALEIPTE'RIUM, from αλειφω, 'I anoint.' The place in the ancient gymnasium where the combatants anointed themselves.

ALEIP'TRON. Same etymon. A box for containing ointments.

ALEMA, Farina.

ALEM'BIC (*Arab.*) *Moorshead, Capitel'lum, Capit'ulum, Am'bicus,* (F.) *Alambic.* A utensil made of glass, metal, or earthen ware, adapted for distillation. A *still.* It consists of a *body* or *cucurbit,* (F.) *cucurbite, chaudière,* to which is attached a *head* or *capital,* (F.) *chapiteau,* and out of this a *beak* descends laterally to be inserted into the *receiver, worm, condenser,* or *refrigerator,* (F.) *serpentin, réfrigérant,* as the case may be.

ALEM'BROTH (*Salt.*) *Sal Alembroth.* The alchymists designated by this name, and by those of *Sal sapien'tiæ, Sal artis, Sal vitæ* and *S. Scien'tiæ,* the product resulting from the sublimation of a mixture of corrosive sublimate and sal ammoniac. It is stimulant, but not employed.

ALÈSE, (F.) *Alèze, Lin'teum,* from αλεξω, 'I preserve.' A *guard.* A cloth arranged in several folds, and placed upon a bed, so as to *guard* it from the lochial or other discharges.

ALETON, Farina.

ALETRIS, A. farinosa.

AL'ETRIS, *A. Farino'sa, Stargrass, Starwort, Blazing star, Aloe-root, Bitter grass, Black root, Unicorn root, Ague root, Ague grass, Devil's bit, Mealy starwort,* (F.) *Alétris Meunier, Nat. Ord.* Asphodeleæ. *Sex. Syst.* Hexandria Monogynia. This plant is an intense and permanent bitter, and is used as a tonic and stomachic. It is common in the United States.

ALEURON, Farina.

ALEUROTESIS, see Cribration.

ALEXANDERS, Smyrnium olusatrum.

ALEXANDRI ANTIDOTUS AUREA. See Alexandrine.

ALEXAN'DRINE, *Emplas'trum Alexan'dri.* A garlic plaster, invented by Alexander, contemporary of Mesuë. Other ancient preparations were called 'Alexandrine;' as the *Alexan'dri antid'otus au'rea,* used in apoplexy ; the *Collyr'ium siccum Alexandri'num,* or *'Collyrium of King Alexander,'* mentioned by Aëtius.

ALEXICACUM, Amuletum, Alexipharmic.

ALEXIPHAR'MIC, *Alexiphar'macus, Antiphar'macus, Alexica'cus, Caco-alexite'ria, Lexiphar'macus,* (F.) *Alexipharmaque,* from αλεξειν, 'to repel,' and φαρμακον, 'poison.' A term formerly used for medicines which were considered proper for expelling from the body various morbific principles, or for preventing the bad effects of poisons taken inwardly.

ALEXIPYRETICUS, Febrifuge.

ALEXIR, Elixir.

ALEXITE'RIA, *Cacalexite'ria,* from αλεξασθαι, 'to assist.' Originally, *alexiterium* was used synonymously with remedy. In more modern times it has been applied to a class of medicines, that counteract poisons placed in contact with the exterior of the body, in contradistinction to alexipharmic.

ALEXITERIUM CHLORICUM, see Disinfection—a. Nitricum, see Disinfection.

ALÈZE, Alèse.

ALFUSA, Tutia.

ALGA MARINA, Pila marina.

ALGALIE, Catheter.

AL'GAROTH, *Al'garot, Algaro'thi Pulvis, Pulvis Angel'icus, Ox'idum seu Submu'rias Stib'ii præcipitan'do para'tum, Antimo'nii Ox'ydum, Ox'idum antimo'nii Nitro-muriat'icum, Ox'idum Stib'ii Ac'ido Muriat'ico oxygena'to para'tum, Mercu'rius Vitæ, Mercu'rius Mortis, Flowers of Antimony,* (F.) *Oxyde d'Antimoine,* so called from Victor Algarothi, a Veronese physician. The *sub-muriate of protoxide of antimony,* separated from the muriate of antimony by washing away some of its acid. It was formerly much used as an emetic, purgative, and diaphoretic.

ALGE'DON, from αλγος, 'pain.' Violent pain about the neck of the bladder, occasionally occurring in gonorrhœa.—Cockburn.

ALGEDON, Pain.
ALGEMA, Pain.
ALGESIS, Pain.
ALGETICUS, see Algos.
AL'GIDUS, from *algor*, 'cold.' That which is accompanied by coldness.
AL'GIDA FEBRIS, F. *horrif'ica*, F. *hor'rida*, F. *quer'quera*, F. *erymo'des*, Bry'cetus, Bry'chetus. (F.) *Fièvre algide*, *Algid Fever*. A pernicious intermittent, accompanied by icy coldness, which is often fatal in the second or third paroxysm.
ALGOR, Rigor.
ALGOS, αλγος, 'pain.' See Pain. Hence, *Alget'icus*, 'painful,' as *Epilep'sia alget'ica*. The suffix *algia* has the same signification, — as in *Cephalalgia, Pleuralgia, Neuralgia*, &c.
ALGOSPAS'MUS, from αλγος, 'pain,' and σπασμος, 'spasm.' Painful spasm or cramp of the muscles.
ALHAGI, Agul.
ALHANDAL, see Cucumis colocynthis.
ALHASEF, Sudamina.
ALIBILIS, Nutritious.
AL'ICA, *Hal'ica, Farina'rium, Chondrus*, from *alere*, 'to nourish.' A grain from which the ancients made their tisanes; supposed, by some, to have been the *Triticum spelta*. At times, it seems to have meant the tisane itself.
AL'ICES, from αλιζω, 'I sprinkle.' Spots which precede the eruption of small pox.
ALIENATIO, Anomalia—a. Mentis, Insanity.
ALIENATION, MENTAL, Insanity.
ALIENUS, Delirious.
ALIFORMES MUSCULI, Pterygoid muscles.
ALIFORMIS, Alaris, Pterygoid.
ALIGULUS, Confection.
ALIMA, Aliment.
ALIMELLÆ, Parotid.
AL'IMENT, *Alimen'tum, Al'ima, Harma'lia, Nutri'men, Nu'triens, Sustentac'ulum, Ciba'rium, Broma, Oomis'tě, Cibus, Esca, Nutri'tus, Nutrimen'tum, Sitos, Trophē*. (F.) *Aliment, Nourriture*, from *alere*, 'to nourish.' Food. Any substance which, if introduced into the system, is capable of nourishing it and repairing its losses.

The study of aliments forms one of the most important branches of hygiene. They are confined to the organized kingdom,—the mineral affording none.

As regards the immediate principles which predominate in their composition, they have been classed, but imperfectly, as follows:—

TABLE OF ALIMENTS.

1. *Feculaceous.*	Wheat, barley, oats, rye, rice, Indian corn, potato, sago, peas, beans, &c.
2. *Mucilaginous.*	Carrot, salsify, beet, turnip, asparagus, cabbage, lettuce, artichoke, melon, &c.
3. *Saccharine.*	Sugar, fig, date, raisin, apricot, &c.
4. *Acidulous.*	Orange, currant, gooseberry, cherry, peach, strawberry, raspberry, mulberry, prune, pear, apple, sorrel, &c.
5. *Oleaginous and Fatty.*	Cocoa, olive, sweet almond, nut, walnut, animal fat, oil, butter, &c.
6. *Caseous.*	Different kinds of milk, cheese.
7. *Gelatinous.*	Tendon, aponeurosis, true skin, cellular texture; very young animals.
8. *Albuminous.*	Brain, nerve, eggs, &c.
9. *Fibrinous.*	Flesh and blood.

Dr. Prout has four great classes—the *aqueous, saccharine, oleaginous*, and *albuminous*: — Dr. Pereira twelve;—the *aqueous, mucilaginous* or *gummy, saccharine, amylaceous, ligneous, pectinaceous, acidulous, alcoholic, oily* or *fatty, proteinaceous, gelatinous*, and *saline*.

Liebig divides them into two classes:—the NITROGENIZED OF PLASTIC ELEMENTS OF NUTRITION, in which he comprises *vegetable fibrin, vegetable albumen, vegetable casein, flesh* and *blood*; and the NON-NITROGENIZED ELEMENTS OF RESPIRATION, in which he comprises, *fat, starch, gum, cane sugar, grape sugar, sugar of milk, pectin, bassorin, wine, beer* and *spirits*. The former alone, in his view, are inservient to the nutrition of organized tissue: the latter are burnt in respiration, and furnish heat.

The following simple arrangement is, perhaps, as little objectionable as any:

1. *Nitrogenized Aliments*, (*Albuminous*, of Prout.)	Fibrinous (Glutinous') Albuminous. Caseinous.
2. *Non-nitrogenized Aliments*,	Amylaceous. Saccharine. Oleaginous.

The second division might be still farther simplified, inasmuch as amylaceous aliments are convertible into sugar during the digestive process; and, from both, oleaginous matter may be formed.

ALIMENTARY TUBE, Canal, alimentary.
ALIMENTATION, *Alimenta'tio*. The act of nourishing.
ALIMENTUM, Aliment, Pabulum.
ALIMOS, Glycyrrhiza.
ALINDE'SIS, from αλινδομαι, 'to be turned about.' A species of exercise, which consisted in rolling in the dust, after having been anointed with oil.—Hippocrates.
ALIPÆ'NOS, *Alipæ'num, Alipan'tos*, from α priv., and λιπαινω, 'to be fat.' An epithet formerly given to every external remedy, devoid of fat or moisture; such as powders.—Galen.
ALIPANTOS, Alipænos.
ALIP'TA, *Alip'tes*, αλιπτης, 'I anoint.' He who anointed the Athletæ after bathing. The place where this was done was called *Alipte'rium*.
ALIPTERIUM, see Alipta.
ALIP'TICA, same etymon. The part of ancient medicine, which treated of inunction, as a means of preserving health.
ALISIER BIANC, Cratægus aria.
ALISMA, A. plantago, Arnica montana—a. Grammifolia, A plantago—a. Lanceola'ta, A. plantago.
ALIS'MA PLANTA'GO, *Alisma, A. lanceola'ta* seu *graminifo'lia, Planta'go aquat'ica, Water Plantain*, (F.) *Plantain d'Eau. Nat. Ord*. Alismaceæ. *Sex. Syst*. Hexandria Polygynia. The fresh root is acrid, and the dried leaves will vesicate. The leaves have been proposed as substitutes for Uva Ursi.
ALITURA, Nutrition.
AL'IPALE, *O'leum Galli'næ*. An ancient pharmaceutical name for pullets' fat.
ALKALESCENCE, Alcalescence.
ALKALI, see Alcali—a. Ammoniacum causticum, Ammonia—a. Ammoniacum spirituosum, Spiritus ammoniæ—a. Minerale nitratum, Soda; nitrate of—a. Minerale phosphoratum, Soda, phosphate of—a. Minerale salinum, Soda, muriate of—a. Vegetable, Potash—a. Vegetabile cum aceto, Potassæ acetas—a. Vegetabile fixum causticum, Potassa fusa—a. Volatile, Ammonia—a Volatile causticum, Ammonia—a. Volatile, concrete, Ammoniæ carbonas—a. Volatile nitratum, Ammoniæ nitras—a. Volatile tartarizatum, Ammoniæ tartras—a. Volatile vitriolatum, Ammoniæ sulphas.
ALKANET, BASTARD, Lithospermum officinale—a. Dyer's, Anchusa tinctoria—a. Garden, Anchusa officinalis—a. Officinal, Anchusa officinalis.
ALKAR, Medicament.

ALKEKENGI, Physalis.

ALKER'MES, *Confec'tio Alker'mes, Alcher'mes*. A celebrated electuary, composed of a multitude of substances. It was so called from the grains of kermes contained in it. It was used as a stimulant. Also, kermes.

ALKERVA, see Ricinus communis.

ALKITRAN, Cedria.

ALKOL, Alcohol.

ALKOOL, Alcohol.

ALLA, Cerevisia.

ALLAITEMENT, Lactation.

ALLAMAN'DA, *A. Cathar'tica seu grandiflo'ra, Ore'lia grandiflo'ra, Gal'aripe, Echi'nus scandens, Apoc"ynum scandens*. A shrub, native of Guiana, the infusion of whose leaves is said by Linnæus to be useful in Colica Pictonum.

ALLANTODES, Allantois.

ALLAN'TOIC ACID, *Ac"idum allanto'icum*. A peculiar acid, found in the liquor of the allantois of the cow.

ALLANTOIDES, Allantois.

ALLAN'TOIS, *Allantoï'des, Allanto'des, Membra'na urina'ria, .M seu Tunica Farcimina'lis, M. Intestina'lis*, the *Allantoid Vesicle*, from αλλος, 'a sausage,' and ειδος, 'shape.' A sort of elongated bladder, between the chorion and amnion of the fœtus, which is thrown out from the caudal extremity of the embryo, and communicates with the bladder by the urachus. It is very apparent in quadrupeds, but not in the human species. As the allantois is developed, its walls become very vascular, and contain the ramifications of what become the umbilical artery and vein, which, by the elongation of the allantois, are brought through the villi of the chorion, into indirect communication with the vessels of the mother.

ALLANTOTOX'ICUM, from αλλας, 'a sausage,' and τοξικον, 'a poison.' Sausage poison (G.) Wurstgift. The Germans have given this name to a poison developed in sausages formed of blood and liver.

ALLELUIA, Oxalis acetosella.

ALLE'VIATOR: from *ad*, 'to,' and *levare*, 'to raise.' A soother. An instrument for raising invalids, invented by Mr. Jenks, of Rhode Island. It consists of two upright posts, about six feet high, each supported by a pedestal; of two horizontal bars at the top, rather longer than a common bedstead; of a windlass of the same length, placed six inches below the upper bar; of a cogwheel and handle; of linen belts from six to twelve inches wide; of straps secured at one end of the windlass; and at the other having hooks attached to corresponding eyes in the linen belts, and of a head-piece made of netting. The patient lying on his mattress, the surgeon passes the linen belts beneath his body, attaching them to the hooks on the ends of the straps, and adjusting the whole at the proper distance and length, so as to balance the body exactly, and then raises it from the mattress by turning the handle of the windlass. To lower the patient again, and replace him on the mattress, the windlass must be reversed.

ALLGOOD, Chenopodium bonus Henricus.

ALLHEAL, Heracleum spondylium.

ALLIA'CEOUS, *allia'ceus*, from *allium*, 'garlic.' Belonging to garlic, as *alliaceous* odour.

ALLIAIRE, Alliaria.

ALLIA'RIA, from *allium*, its smell resembling garlic. *A. cfficina'lis, Erys'imum allia'ria seu cordifo'lium, Sisymbrium allia'ria, Jack-in-the-hedge, stinking hedge Mustard, Hedge Garlic, Sauce-alone, Hes'peris allia'ria*, (F.) *Alliaire*. This plant has been sometimes given in humid asthma and dyspnœa. It is reputed to be diaphoretic, diuretic, and antiscorbutic.

The Parisian Codex has a compound syrup of alliaria, *Sirop d'érysimum composé*, which is used in hoarseness.

ALLIGATURA, Fascia, Ligature.

ALLIOTICUS, Alterative.

AL'LIUM, from *oleo*, 'I smell.' *A. sati'vum, Theriaca rustico'rum, Ampelop'rasum, Scor'odon, Scordon, Garlic*, (F.) *Ail*. *Nat. Ord.* Asphodeleæ. *Sex. Syst.* Hexandria Monogynia. A native of Sicily, but cultivated for use. The *bulbs* or *cloves, Ag'lithes*, have a strong, offensive, and penetrating odour, and a sweetish, biting, and caustic taste. *Internally*, garlic is stimulant, diuretic, expectorant, emmenagogue (?), diaphoretic, and anthelmintic. *Externally*, it is rubefacient, maturative, and repellent.

Dose, one to six cloves, swallowed whole, or from f ℨss to f ℨij. of the juice.

Taylor's Remedy for Deafness, a nostrum, appears to consist of garlic, infused in *oil of almonds*, and coloured by *alkanet root*.

ALLIUM ASCALONICUM, Échalotte.

AL'LIUM CEPA, *Cepa vulga'ris, Common Onion, Cepul'la, Orom'myon*, (F.) *Oignon*. Acrid and stimulating, and possessing very little nutriment. Onions have been used as stimulants, diuretics, and anthelmintics. The boiled or roasted onion, as a cataplasm, is emollient and maturating. The fresh root is rubefacient. The expressed juice is sometimes used in otalgia and in rheumatism.

ALLIUM GALLICUM, Portulaca.—a. Plantagineum, A. Victoriale.

AL'LIUM PORRUM, *Porrum, P. sati'vum, Prasum*, the *Leek* or *Porret* ; (F.) *Poireau, Porreau*. It possesses the same property as the onion.

The virtues of the genus *Allium* depend upon an acrid principle, soluble in water, alcohol, acids, and alkalies.

ALLIUM REDOLENS, Teucrium scordium.

AL'LIUM VICTORIA'LE, *A. plantagin'eum, Cepa victoria'lis, Victoria'lis longa*. The root, which, when dried, loses its alliaceous smell and taste, is said to be efficacious in allaying the abdominal spasms of pregnant women (?).

ALLOCHET'IA, *Allotriochet'ia*, from αλλος, 'another,' and χεζειν, 'to go to stool.' The discharge of extraneous matters from the bowels. The discharge of fæces by an abnormous opening.

ALLOCHOOS, Delirious.

ALLOCHROMA'SIA, from αλλος, 'another,' and χρωμα, 'colour.' A change of colour.

ALLŒOPATHIA, Allopathy.

ALLŒOPATHIC, Allopathic.

ALLŒOSIS, Alteration.

ALLŒOTICUS, Alterative.

ALLOIOSIS, Alteration.

ALLOIOTICUS, Alterative.

ALLONGEMENT, Elongation.

ALLOPATH, Allopathist.

ALLOPATHES, Allopathic.

ALLOPATH'IC, *Allopath'icus, Allœopath'ic, Allœopath'icus, Allop'athes, Heteropath'ic*, from αλλος, 'another,' and παθος, 'affection.' Relating to the ordinary method of medical practice, in contradistinction to the homœopathic.

ALLOP'ATHIST, *Al'lopath*, same etymon. One who follows allopathy.

ALLOP'ATHY, *Allopathi'a, Allœopathia, Hypenantio'sis, Hypenantio'ma, Cura'tio contrario'rum per contra'ria*, same etymon. The opposite to homœopathy. The ordinary medical practice.

ALLOPHASIS, Delirium.

ALLOTRIOCHETIA, Allochetia.

ALLOTRIODON'TIA, from αλλοτριος, 'foreign,' and οδους, 'a tooth.' Transplantation of teeth.

ALLOTRIOEC'CRISIS, from αλλοτριος, 'foreign,' and εκκρισις,' 'separation.' The separation of extraneous matters from the body in disease.

ALLOTRIOGEUSTIA, Parageustia.

ALLOTRIOPHAGIA, Malacia.

ALLOTRIOTEX'IS, from αλλοτριος, 'foreign,' and τεξις, 'parturition.' The bringing forth of an abnormous fœtus.

ALLOTRIU'RIA, from αλλοτριος, 'foreign,' and ουρον, 'urine.' Admixture of foreign matters with the urine.

AL'LOTROPISM; from αλλος, 'another,' and τροπος, 'a turn or change.' A term recently introduced into chemistry; the object of which is to express the property possessed by certain simple bodies, of assuming different qualities on being subjected to certain modes of treatment. Carbon, for example, furnishes three forms — plumbago, charcoal, and diamond.

ALLSPICE, see Myrtus pimenta — a. Bush, Laurus Benzoin — a. Carolina, Calycanthus — a. Wild, Laurus Benzoin.

ALLUCINATIO, Hallucination.

ALLURE, Influenza.

ALMA, Water.

ALMARIAB, see Plumbi oxydum semivitreum.

ALMEZERION, Cneorum tricoccum.

ALMOND, Amygdala.

ALMOND BLOOM. A liquid cosmetic, formed of Brazil dust ℥j, water Oiij; boil and strain; and add isinglass ℥vj, grana sylvestria ℥ij, or cochineal ℥ij, alum ℥j, borax ℥iij; boil again, and strain through a fine cloth.

ALMOND CAKE, see Amygdala — a. of the Ear, Tonsil — a. Earth, Arachis hypogæa — a. Paste, see Amygdala — a. Powder, see Amygdala — a. of the Throat, Tonsil.

ALNUS, A. glutiḟosa — a. Communis, A. glutinosa.

ALNUS GLUTINO'SA, Alnus, A commu'nis, Bet'ula glutino'sa seu emargina'ta, Europe'an Alder. A tree which grows in Europe, in moist places. The bark and leaves are astringent and bitter; and hence are employed in intermittents, and as a tonic and astringent.

ALNUS SERRAT'ULA, American Alder, has similar properties.

ALNUS NIGRA, Rhamnus frangula.

ALOCHI'A, from a, privative, and λοχεια, 'lochia.' Absence of the lochial discharge.

ALOËDA'RIUM. A compound medicine, containing aloes. — Gorræus.

ALOE, Aloes.

ALOE ROOT, Aletris farinosa.

AL'OËS, Al'oë, Fel Natu'ræ. The inspissated juice of the Aloe. Nat. Ord. Asphodeleæ. Sex. Syst. Hexandria Monogynia.

ALOES BARBADENSIS, A. hepatica — a. Bombay, A. hepatica — a. des Barbades, A. hepatica.

ALOES CABALLI'NA, A. Guinien'sis, Horse-aloes. Used chiefly for horses. It is collected in Spain and Portugal, and is very coarse.

ALOES EN CALÉBASSES, A. hepatica.

ALOES, CAPE, Shining Aloes; a cheap and excellent form of aloes, collected at the Cape of Good Hope, from Aloe ferox, A. Africana, A. spicata, and other species.

ALOES, EAST INDIA, A. Succotorina — a. Guiniensis, A. Caballina.

ALOES HEPAT'ICA, A. vulga'ris, A. Barbaden'sis, Hepat'ic aloes, Bombay aloes, Barba'does aloes, A. vulga'ris extrac'tum, (F.) Aloes en calébasses, A. des Barbades. This species has a very disagreeable odour, and an intensely bitter and nauseous taste. Properties the same as the last.

ALOES, HORSE, A. Caballina — a. Lucida, A. Succotorina — a. Socotrine, A. Succotorina — a. Spicata extractum, A. Succotorina.

ALOES SUCCOTORI'NA, Soc'otrine aloes, Turkey aloes, East India aloes, Aloës lu'cida, A. Zoctori'nia, A. spica'ta extrac'tum, An'ima Aloës, is the best species. Its odour is not unpleasant; taste very bitter, and slightly aromatic; colour reddish-brown, with a shade of purple; mass hard, friable; fracture conchoidal and glossy; soluble in dilute alcohol. Powder of a bright cinnamon-yellow colour. It is cathartic, warm, and stimulating; emmenagogue, anthelmintic, and stomachic. As a cathartic, it affects the rectum chiefly. Dose, as a cathartic, gr. v. to ℈j. in pill.

ALOES, TURKEY, A. Succotorina — a. Vulgaris, A. hepaticus. — a. Wood, Agallochum — a. Zoctorinia, A. Succotorina.

ALOËT'IC, Aloët'icus. A preparation which contains aloes.

ALOEXYLON, Agallochum.

ALOGOTROPH'IA, from αλογος, 'disproportionate,' and τροφη, 'nutrition.' Irregular nutrition. Used particularly to designate the irregular manner in which the nutrition of bones is effected in rickety individuals.

ALOPECES, Psoæ.

ALOPE'CIA, from αλωπηξ, 'a fox;' (this animal being said to be subject to the affection.) Capillo'rum deflu'vium, Athrix depi'lis, Phalacro'tis, Depila'tio, Tricho'sis Athrix, Gangræ'na Alope'cia, Atrich'ia, Deflu'vium seu Lapsus Pilo'rum, Lipsotrich'ia, Vulpis morbus, Baldness. Falling off of the hair; loss of the hair. When this is confined to the crown of the head, it is called calvities, although the terms are often used synonymously.

ALOPECIA AREATA, Porrigo decalvans — a. Circumscripta, Porrigo decalvans — a. Partialis, Porrigo decalvans.

ALOUCHE, Cratægus aria.

ALOUCH'I. The name of a gum procured from the canella alba tree.

ALOUCHIER, Cratægus aria.

ALPAM. A shrub which grows on the coast of Malabar. Certain parts of this, infused in oil, form an antipsoric ointment. The juice of the leaves, mixed with that of calamus, is employed against the bites of serpents.

ALPHENIC, Saccharum candidum.

ALPHITEDON, see Fracture.

ALPH'ITON, αλφιτον, Polen'ta, Fari'na. Any kind of meal. Toasted barley-meal. — Hippocrates. Polenta means also a food composed of Indian meal, cheese, &c. See Farina.

ALPHON'SIN, Alphon'sinum. A kind of bullet forceps, similar to a Porte-crayon, so called from the inventor, Alphonso Ferri, of Naples. — Scultetus.

ALPHOS, Lepra alphoides.

ALPHOSIS ÆTHIOPICA, see Albino.

ALPINIA CARDAMOMUM, Amomum cardamomum — a. Galanga, Maranta galanga.

ALPISTE, Phalaris Canadiensis.

ALSANDERS, Smyrnium olusatrum.

ALSI'NE ME'DIA, A. avicula'rum seu vulga'ris, from αλσος, 'a grove,' because growing abundantly in the woods. Morsus Galli'næ, Holos'teum Alsi'në, Stella'ria me'dia, Mouse-ear, Chickweed, (F.) Mouron des Oiseaux, Morgoline. This plant, if boiled tender, may be eaten like spinach, and forms an excellent emollient poultice. It was formerly regarded as a vulnerary and detergent.

ALTAFOR, Camphor.

ALTER SEXUS, Sex, female.

ALTERANS, Alterative.

ALTÉRANT, Alterative.

ALTERA'TION, Altera'tio, from alter, 'other,' Alloio'sis, Allœo'sis. This word is used in France to express a morbid change which supervenes in the expression of the countenance (*altération de la face,*) or in the structure of an organ (*altération organique,*) or in the nature of fluids excreted (*altération de l'urine, des larmes, du lait, &c.*)

Altération is also used in an entirely different sense, to express intense thirst in disease. In this case its etymology is different. It comes from *haléter*, and was formerly written *halétération.*

AL'TERATIVE, *Al'terans, Alloiot'icus, Allæot'icus, Alliot'icus, Immu'tans.* An agent considered to be capable of producing a salutary change in a disease, but without exciting any sensible evacuation. As medicine improves, this uncertain class of remedies becomes, of necessity, diminished in number. See Eutrophie.

(F.) *Altérant.* The French term likewise means, that which causes thirst,—*Siticulo'sus, Dipset'icus,* as *altérer* means both to change, and to cause thirst. *S'altérer* is to experience a change for the worse,—*corrum'pi.*)

ALTERCANGENON, Hyoscyamus.
ALTERCUM, Hyoscyamus.
ALTHÆ'A, from αλθειν, 'to heal;' *A. officina'lis, Malvavis'cum, Aristalthæ'a, Hibis'cus, Ibis'chus, Ibis'cha mismal'va, Bismal'va, Marsh mallow.* (F.) *Guimauve.* Nat. Ord. Malvaceæ. *Sex. Syst.* Monadelphia Polyandria. The leaves, *Althæ'æ fo'lia,* and root, *Althæ'æ radix,* contain much mucilage. They are emollient and demulcent, and are employed wherever medicines, possessing such properties, are required. In the Ph. U. S., Althæa is the root of Althæa officinalis.

ALTHANAIHA, Orpiment.
ALTHEUS, Physician.
ALTHEXIS, Curation.
ALTHOS, Medicament.
ALTILIBAT, Terebinthina.
ALU'DEL, *Alu'tel, Vitrum sublimato'rium.* A hollow sphere of stone, glass, or earthen ware, with a short neck projecting at each end, by means of which one glass might be set upon the other. The uppermost had no aperture at the top. Aludels were formerly used in the sublimation of various substances.

A'LULA; diminutive of *ala,* 'a wing.' A little wing.

ALUM, Symphytum—a. Cataplasm, Coagulum aluminosum—a. Egyptian, Ægyptia stypteria.

ALUM, ROCHE, *Alu'men de Rochi,* (F.) *Alun de Roche.* So called from Roccha in Syria, where there was a manufactory of it. It is in pieces of the size of an almond, covered with a reddish efflorescence.

Common Roche Alum, A. Rochi Gallis. Fragments of common alum, moistened and shaken with prepared bole. It is white when broken.

ALUM, SOLUTION OF, COMPOUND, Liq. aluminis compos.

ALUM ROOT, Geranium maculatum, Heuchera cortusa.

ALU'MEN, (an Arabic term, *alum,*) *Alum, Hypersul'phas alu'minæ et Potas'sæ, Potas'sæ alu'mino-sulphas, Sul'phas Aluminæ Acid'ulus cum Potas'sâ, Sulphas Alu'minæ, Sul'phas Kal'ico-alumin'icum, Sulphas alumina'ris, Supersul'phas alu'minæ et potas'sæ, Argil'la sulphu'rica alcalisa'ta, A. vitriola'ta, Stypte'ria, Supersul'phas Argil'læ alcalisa'tum, Argilla Kalisulphurica.* (F.) *Alun.*

ALUMEN CATINUM, Potash of commerce — a. Fixum, see Potash — a. Kinosatum, Pulvis sulphatis aluminæ compositus.

ALU'MEN COMMU'NE, *Common alum, English alum, Rock alum, Alumen facti"tium, A. crystal'linum, A. ru'peum,* (F.) *Alun d'Angleterre,* is the variety usually employed. It is in octahedral crystals, but generally in large, white, semitransparent masses; has a sweetish, styptic taste; effloresces in the air, and is soluble in 16 parts of water at 60°. It is tonic and astringent, and as such is used internally and externally. Dose, gr. v. to xv.

ALU'MEN EXSICCA'TUM, *Alu'men ustum, A. calcina'tum, Sulphas alu'minæ fusus, Argil'la sulphu'rica usta,* Burnt alum, dried alum. (F.) *Alun calciné,* (*Alum* melted in an earthen vessel until ebullition ceases.) Escharotic.

ALU'MEN ROMA'NUM, *Roman alum, A. Ru'tilum, A. Rubrum.* (F.) *Alun de Rome.* In crystals, which are of a pale red when broken, and covered with a reddish efflorescence.

ALUMINA, ACETATE OF, *Aluminæ Acetas*—a. Depurata, Argilla pura—a. Pura, Argilla pura—a. Sulphate of, Aluminæ Sulphas.

ALU'MINÆ ACE'TAS, *Argil'læ Ace'tas, Ac''etate of Alu'mina.* A deliquescent salt, obtained by the addition of *acetate of lead* to *sulphate of alumina and potassa.* It possesses the same properties as the sulphate of alumina.

ALU'MINÆ ET POTASSÆ HYPERSULPHAS, *Alumen*—a. et Potassæ supersulphas, Alumen—a. Sulphas, Alumen.

ALU'MINÆ SULPHAS, *Argillæ Sulphas, Sulphate of Alu'mina.* Simple sulphate of alumina may be made by the direct combination of *alumina* and *sulphuric acid,* and contains 30 per cent. of the former, to 70 per cent. of the latter. It is a deliquescent salt; and is an excellent antiseptic and detergent to ulcers. It is chiefly used to preserve dead bodies — a strong solution being injected into the arteries.

ALUMINÆ SULPHAS ACIDULUS CUM POTASSÂ, *Alumen*—a. Sulphas fusus, Alumen exsiccatum.

ALUMINE FACTICE, Argilla pura.
ALUN, Alumen.
ALUNSEL, Gutta.
ALUS, Symphytum.
ALUSIA, Hallucination—a. Hypochondriasis Hypochondriasis.
ALUTEL, Aludel.
ALVAQUILLA, Psoralea glandulosa.
ALVARAS NIGRA, Ichthyosis.
ALVEARIUM, Auditory canal, external.
ALVE'OLAR, *Alveola'ris,* from *alveus,* 'a cavity.' (F.) *Alvéolaire.* That which relates to the alveoli.

ALVE'OLAR ARCHES, (F.) *Arcades alvéolaires,* are formed by the margins or borders of the two jaws, which are hollowed by the Alveoli.

ALVE'OLAR ARTERY, *Supra-maxillary A., Artère sus-maxillaire* of Chaussier, arises from the internal maxillary, descends behind the tuberosity of the upper jaw, and gives branches to the upper molar teeth, gums, periosteum, membrane of the maxillary sinus, and buccinator muscle.

ALVEOLAR BORDER, *Limbus alveola'ris.* The part of the jaws, that is hollowed by the alveoli.

ALVE'OLAR MEMBRANES are very fine membranes, situate between the teeth and alveoli, and formed by a portion of the sac or follicle which enclosed the tooth before it pierced the gum. By some this membrane has been called the *alveolodental periosteum.*

ALVE'OLAR VEIN. This has a similar distribution with the artery.

ALVÉOLE, Alveolus.
ALVEOLI DENTIS, see Alveolus.
ALVÉOLO-LABIAL, Buccinator.
ALVE'OLUS, same etymon. *Bo'trion, Bo'thrion, Odontoboth'rium, Odontophat'nē, Frena, Mortariolum, Hol'micos, Præscpiolum, Phatnē, Phat'nion, Præsepium, Patnē, Pathnē.* (F.) *Alvéole.* The alveoli are the *sockets of the teeth,*

ALVEUS 63 AMBON

Alve'oli dentis, Ma'nia seu *Caver'næ den'tium,* into which they are, as it were, driven. Their size and shape are determined by the teeth which they receive, and they are pierced at the apex by small holes, which give passage to the dental vessels and nerves.

ALVEUS, Auge — a. Ampullosus, Receptaculum chyli — a. Ampullescens, Thoracic duct — a. Communis: see Semicircular canals — a. Utriculosus: see Semicircular canals.

ALVI EXCRETIO, Defecation — a. Fluxus aquosus, Diarrhœa — a. Laxitas, Diarrhœa — a. Profluvium, Diarrhœa.

ALVIDUCUS, Laxative.

ALVINE, *Alvi'nus,* from *alvus,* 'the abdomen.' That which relates to the lower belly, as *alvine dejections, alvine flux, alvine obstructions,* &c.

ALVUM EVACUANS, Cathartic.

ALVUS, Abdomen, Uterus—a. Adstricta, Constipation—a. Cita, Diarrhœa—a. Dura, Constipatio—a. Renum, Pelvis of the kidney — a. Tarda, Constipation—a. Viridis, Dejection.

ALYCE, Anxiety.

AL'YPON, from *a,* priv., and λυπη, 'pain.' An acrid, purging plant, described by Matthiolus. By some it has been supposed to be the *Globula'ria alypum* of botanists.

ALYSIS, Anxiety.

ALYSMUS, Anxiety.

ALYSSUM PLINII, Galium Mollugo.

ALYSSUS, Antihydrophobic.

AL'ZILAT. In some of the Arabian writers, a weight of three grains.—Ruland and Johnson.

AMABILE, Lacuna Labii Superioris.

AMADOU, Boletus igniarius.

AMADOUVIER, Boletus igniarius.

AMAIGRISSEMENT, Emaciation.

AMANDES, see Amygdala.

AMANI'TÆ, from *a,* privative, and μανια, 'madness:' i. e. 'not poisonous.' A name given, by the Greeks and Romans, to the edible *champignons. Amanita* forms, at the present day, a genus, some of which are edible, others poisonous. Amongst others, it contains the *Agaricus aurantiacus* and *A. pseudo-aurantiacus.*

AMARA DULCIS, Solanum dulcamara.

AMARACI'NUM. An ancient and esteemed plaster, containing several aromatics, the marjoram, *αμαρακος,* in particular.

AMARACUS, Origanum majorana—a. Tomentosus, Origanum dictamnus.

AMARITIES, Bitterness.

AMARITUDO, Bitterness.

AMAROR, Bitterness.

AMARUCACHU, Polyanthes tuberosa.

AMA'RUS, *Picros,* 'bitter.' (F.) *Amèr.* The bitter principle of vegetables is the great natural tonic, and hence *bitters,* as they are termed collectively, belong to the class of tonics. Several are used in medicine; the chief are, gentian, quassia, cinchona, calumba, dog-wood, &c.

AMASE'SIS, *Amasee'sis,* from *a,* privative, and μασησις, 'mastication.' Mastication when impeded or impracticable.

AMATORIUM, Lacuna labii superioris.

AMATORII, Oblique muscles of the eye.

AMATORIUM VENEFICIUM, Philter.

AMATORIUS MUSCULUS, Obliquus superior oculi.

AMAURO'SIS, *Obfusca'tio, Offusca'tio,* from *αμαυρος,* 'obscure.' *Drop serene, Gutta sere'na, Cataract'a nigra, Paropsis amauro'sis, Immobil'itas pupil'læ, Suffu'sio nigra, Black cat'aract.* (F.) *Goutte-sereine, Cataracte noire, Anopticonervie* (Piorry.) Diminution, or complete loss of sight, without any perceptible alteration in the organization of the eye; generally, perhaps, owing to loss of power of the optic nerve or retina. Counter-irritants are the most successful remedial agents, although the disease is always very difficult of removal, and generally totally incurable.

AMAUROSIS DIMIDIATA, Hemiopia—a. Imperfecta, Hypo-amaurosis.

AMAUROT'IC, *Amaurot'icus;* same etymon. Affected with amaurosis.

AMAUROTIC CAT'S EYE, *Galeamauro'sis.* A name given by Beer to an amaurotic affection, accompanied by a remarkable change of colour in the pupil, which presents, apparently in the fundus of the eye, a lighter tint, yellowish or brownish yellow, instead of its natural clear black.

AMA'ZIA, from *a,* privative, and μαζος, 'breast.' A monstrosity, in which there is absence of one or both breasts.

AMBARUM, Ambergris — a. Cineritium, Ambergris.

AMBE, from αμβαινω, 'I ascend;' *Ambi.* A superficial eminence on a bone. Also, an old surgical machine for reducing dislocations of the shoulder; the invention of which is ascribed to Hippocrates. It is no longer used. — Hippocrates, Scultetus. See Crista.

AMBER, Succinum — a. Liquid: see Liquidamber styraciflua.

AM'BERGRIS, *Ambra gri'sea, Ambor, Ambar, Ambra cinera'cea, A. ambrosiaca, Ambarum, Suc'cinum cine'reum, S. gri'seum, Am'barum cineri''tium.* A concrete substance, of the consistence of wax, cineritious colour, studded with yellow and blackish spots, and exhaling a very pleasant odour. It seems highly probable that ambergris is formed in the intestines of the whale, and voided with its excrements. Like all aromatic substances, ambergris is slightly antispasmodic and excitant; but it is oftener employed as a perfume than as a medicine.

AMBIA. A liquid, yellow bitumen, the smell and virtues of which are similar to those of the resin tacamahaca. It is obtained from a spring in India.

AMBICUS, Alembic.

AMBIDEX'TER, *Amphidex'ius,* from *ambo,* 'both,' and *dexter,* 'right.' One who uses *both* hands with equal facility. Celsus says the surgeon ought to be '*non minus sinistrâ quam dextrâ promptus.*' One of the aphorisms of Hippocrates says, that a woman is never ambidexter. This is a mistake.

AMBILÆVUS, Ampharisteros.

AMBITUS GENITALIS MULIEBRIS, Vestibulum.

AMBLOMA, Abortion.

AMBLOSIS, Abortion.

AMBLOSMUS, Abortion.

AMBLOTHRIDION, see Abortion.

AMBLOTHRIDIUM, Abortive.

AMBLOTICUS, Abortive.

AMBLUS, *αμβλυς,* 'obscure.' Hence, AMBLYAPH'IA, from *αμβλυς,* 'obscure,' and *'αφη,* 'feeling.' Dulness of the sense of touch.

AMBLYOGMOS, Amblyopia.

AMBLYO'PIA, from *αμβλυς,* 'obscure,' and *ωψ,* 'the eye.' *Ambly'osmos, Amblyog'mos, Amplio'pia* (so called by some, according to Castelli, *ob ignorantiam Græcæ linguæ,*) *Hebetu'do visûs, Feebleness of sight,* (F.) *Vue faible.* First degree of Amaurosis.—Hippocrates.

AMBLYOPIA CREPUSCULARIS, Hemeralopia—a. Dissitorum, Myopia—a. Meridiana, Nyctalopia—a. Proximorum, Presbytia.

AMBLYOSMOS, Amblyopia.

AMBOLICUS, Abortive.

AMBON, *αμβων,* 'the raised rim of a shield or dish,' from *αμβαινω,* 'I ascend.' The fibro-cartilaginous rings or *bourrelets*, which surround the articular cavities, as the glenoid cavity of the scapula, the acetabulum, &c., have been so called —Galen. See Crista.

AMBOR, Ambergris.

AMBRA, Succinum—a. Ambrosiaca, Ambergris—a. Cineracea, Ambergris.

AMBRAGRISEA, Ambergris.

AMBRE BLANC, Succinum (album) — a. Jaune, Succinum.

AMBRETTE, Hibiscus abelmoschus.

AMBRO'SIA, from *a,* privative, and βροτος, 'mortal.' Food which makes immortal, or the food of immortals. The food of the gods — Homer. See also, Chenopodium botrys.

AMBROSIA ELATIOR, see A. Trifida.

AMBRO'SIA MARIT'IMA. A plant which grows on the shores of the Levant, and has a pleasant, bitter and aromatic taste. It is given in infusion, as a tonic and antispasmodic.

AMBRO'SIA TRIF'IDA, *Horseweed, Richweed, Horsemint, Horsecane, Bitterweed, Great Ragweed, Wild Hemp.* This indigenous plant is found in low grounds and along streams, from Canada to Georgia, and west to Louisiana and Arkansas. It is an annual, and flowers in August and September. An infusion has been recommended locally in mercurial salivation.

Ambrosia Elatior, Ragweed, is said by Dr. R. E. Griffith to have much more developed sensible properties.

AMBROSIE DU MEXIQUE, Chenopodium ambrosioides.

AMBULANCE, (F.) from *ambulare,* 'to walk.' A military hospital attached to an army, and moving along with it. Also called *Hôpital ambulant.*

AMBULATIO, Walking.

AM'BULATORY, *Am'bulans, Ambulati'vus, Am'bulative,* (F.) *Ambulant.* A morbid affection is said to be 'ambulatory,' (F.) *ambulante,* when it skips from one part to another; as *Erisypèles ambulants,* &c. When blisters are applied successively on different parts of the body, they are called *Vésicatoires ambulants.*

AMBULEIA, Cichorium intybus.

AM'BULI. The Brachmanic name for an Indian aquatic herb, which appears to belong to the family *Lysimachiæ.* The whole plant has a sweet smell. Its decoction has a very bitter taste, and is an excellent febrifuge. It is also taken in milk in cases of vertigo.

AM'BULO FLATULEN'TUS ET FURIO'SUS, *Flatus furio'sus, Vare'ni.* Painful, mobile, and periodical tumours affecting different parts, which were once considered as the effect of very subtile vapours—Michaelis. Their nature is by no means clear.

AMBUSTIO, Burn.

AMBUTUA, Pareira brava.

AMBUYA-EMBO. A very beautiful, creeping aristolochia of Brazil, the decoction of which is exhibited successfully in obstructions. It is also used in fumigation and in baths as a tonic.

AME, Anima.

AMELI. A Malabar shrub, belonging to a genus unknown. The decoction of its leaves is said to relieve colic. Its roots, boiled in oil, are used to repel tumours.

AMELIA, Apathy.

AMENIA, Amenorrhœa, Emmenagogues.

AMENOMA'NIA. A hybrid word, formed from the Latin *amœnus,* 'agreeable,' and μανια, 'mania.' A gay form of insanity.

AMENORRHŒ'A, *Parame'nia obstructio'nis, Menocryph'ia, Menosta'sia, Apophrax'is, Arrhœ'a, Defec'tus seu Reman'sio seu Cessa'tio men'sium,* *Menstrua'tio impedi'ta, Ischome'nia, Ame'nia,* from *a,* privative, μην, 'a month,' and ρεω, 'I flow.' *Suppression of the menses,* (F.) *Suppression du flux menstruel.* This suppression is most commonly symptomatic, and hence the chief attention must be paid to the cause. Usually, there is an atonic state of the system generally, and hence chalybeates and other tonics are advisable.

Two great varieties of Amenorrhœa are commonly reckoned. 1. *A. Emansio'nis, Eman'sio men'sium, Menis'chesis, Menos'chesis, Menstrua'tio retenta, Men'sium reten'tio, Retention of the menses,* when the mensés do not appear at the usual age: and, 2. *Suppres'sio Men'sium, Suppres'sio Menstruatio'nis, Amenorrhœ'a Suppressio'nis, Interrup'tio menstruatio'nis, Menstrua'tio suppressa,* in which the catamenia are obstructed in their regular periods of recurrence. See Emansio Mensium, and Menses.

AMENORRHŒA DIFFICILIS, Dysmenorrhœa—a. Emansionis, see Amenorrhœa—a. Hymenica, see Hymenicus — a. Partialis, Dysmenorrhœa — a. Suppressionis, see Amenorrhœa.

AMENTIA, Dementia: see, also, Fatuitas, and Idiotism—a. Senilis, Dementia of the aged.

AMER, Amarus.

AMERICAN, see Homo.

AMERICANUM TUBEROSUM, Solanum tuberosum.

AMERTUME, Bitterness.

AM'ETHYST, *Amethys'tus,* from *a,* privative, and μεθυω, 'I am drunk.' A precious stone, to which the ancients attributed the property of preventing drunkenness. It was also used as an anti-diarrhœic and absorbent — Pliny, Albertus Magnus.

AMETH'YSUM, *Amethys'tum, (remedium,)* Same etymon as the last. A remedy for drunkenness.

AMETRIA, Intemperance. Also, absence of the uterus; from *a,* privative, and μητρα, 'the uterus.'

AMICULUM, Amnios.

AMIDON, IODURE D', Starch, Iodide of.

AMIDUM, Amylum.

AMINÆA, Anime.

AMINÆ'UM VINUM, *Aminæ'an wine,* highly esteemed as a stomachic. Virgil distinguishes it from the Falernian.—Pliny, Macrobius, &c.

AMMA, Truss.

AMMI, *Ammi majus* seu *cicutæfo'lium* seu *vulga'ré* seu *Bolberi, Am'mios murica'ta, A'pium ammi, Bishop's weed.* The seeds of this plant are aromatic and pungent. They are said to be carminative and diuretic, and are tonic and stomachic.

AMMI BOLBERI, Ammi — a. *des Boutiques,* see Sison ammi—a. Cicutæfolium, Ammi—a. Verum, see Sison ammi —a. Vulgare, Ammi.

AMMION, Hydrargyri sulphuretum rubrum.

AMMIOS MURICATA, Ammi.

AMMISMUS, Psammismus.

AMMOCHO'SIA, *Ammocho'sis,* from αμμος, 'sand,' and χεω, 'I pour.' *Arena'tio.* Putting the human body in hot sand, for the cure of disease.

AMMO'NIA, *Ammo'nia* or *Ammoni'acal gas, Volatile al'kali, Al'cali ammoni'acum caus'ticum, A. volat'ilè caus'ticum, Ammo'nia caus'tica, A. pura, Ammoni'acum, A. caus'ticum, Gas ammoniaca'lè, Mephi'tis urino'sa,* (F.) *Ammoniaque, Air alcalin, Gaz ammoniacal.* An alcali, so called, because obtained principally by decomposing *sal ammoniac (muriate of ammonia)* by lime. This gas is colourless, transparent, elastic, of a pungent, characteristic odour, and an acrid urinous taste. It turns the syrup of violets green, and its specific gravity is 0·596. When inhaled, largely diluted with common air, it is a powerful irritant. When unmixed, it instantly induces suffocation.

AMMONIA, ACETATE OF, SOLUTION OF, Liquor ammoniæ acetatis—a. Arseniate of, Arseniate of ammonia—a. Benzoate of, Ammoniæ benzoas—a. Caustica liquida, Liquor ammoniæ—a. Chlorohydrate of, Ammoniæ murias—a. Citrate of, Ammoniæ citras—a. Hydriodate of, Ammonium, iodide of—a. Hydrochlorate of, Ammoniæ murias—a. Hydrosulphuret of, Ammoniæ sulphuretum—a. Iodide of, see Iodine—a. Liniment of, strong, Linimentum ammoniæ fortius—a. Liquid, Liquor Ammoniæ—a. Muriatica, Ammoniæ murias—a. Nitrate, Ammoniæ nitras—a. Phosphate of, Ammoniæ phosphas—a. Præparata, Ammoniæ carbonas—a. Pura liquida, Liquor ammoniæ—a. Solution of, Liquor ammoniæ—a. Solution of, stronger, Liquor ammoniæ fortior—a. Tartrate of, Ammoniæ tartras.

AMMO'NIAC, GUM, *Ammoni'acum*, (Ph. U. S.) *Gum'mi Ammoni'acum*, *Armoni'acum*, *Matorium*, (F.) *Ammoniac*, *Gomme ammoniaque*, so called from Ammonia in Lybia, whence it is brought. A gum-resin, the concrete juice of *Dore'ma ammoni'acum*, of Persia: a species of a genus allied to Ferula. It is in irregular, dry masses and tears, yellow externally, whitish within. Its odour is peculiar, and not ungrateful: taste nauseous, sweet, and bitter. It forms a white emulsion with water: is soluble in vinegar; partially so in alcohol, ether, and solutions of the alcalies.

Gum ammoniacum is expectorant, deobstruent(?) antispasmodic, discutient, and resolvent. It is chiefly used, however, in the first capacity, and in the formation of certain plasters.

Two varieties are met with in the market, *Guttæ ammoni'aci*, the best; and *Lapis ammoni'aci*, the more impure.

AMMONIACÆ NITRAS, Ammoniæ nitras—a. Sulphas, Ammoniæ sulphas.

AMMONIACUM, Ammonia, Ammoniac Gum—a. Succinatum, Spiritus ammoniæ fœtidus—a. Volatile mite, Ammoniæ carbonas.

AMMONIÆ ACETAS, Liquor ammoniæ acetatis—a. Arsenias, Arseniate of Ammonia.

AMMO'NIÆ BEN'ZOAS, *Ben'zoate of Ammonia*. A salt formed by the union of benzoic acid and ammonia, which has been prescribed for the removal of gouty depositions of urate of soda in the joints. It is regarded as a good diuretic.

AMMONIÆ CAR'BONAS, *A. Subcar'bonas*, *A. Sesquicar'bonas*, *Salt of bones*, *Sal Os'eium*, *Salt of wood-soot*, *Sal Fulig"inis*, *Salt of urine*, *Volatile Sal Ammoniac*, *Baker's salt*, *Al'cali volat'ilĕ aëra'tum*, *A. volat'ilĕ ammoniaca'lĕ*, *A. volat'ilĕ ex sale ammoni'aco*, *Ammoni'acum volat"ilĕ mitĕ*, *Ammo'nium carbon'icum*, *A. subcarbo'neum*, *Carbonas ammo'niæ alkali'nus* seu *incomple'tus* seu *superammoni'acus*, *Hypocar'bonas ammo'niæ*, *Flores salis ammoni'aci*, *Sal cornu cervi volat'ilĕ*, *Sal volat'ilis salis ammoni'aci*, *Concrete volatile alkali*, *Carbonate* or *Subcarbonate of ammonia*, *Ammo'nia præpara'ta*, *Sal volat'ilĕ*, *Smelling salt*, (F.) *Carbonate d'ammoniaque*, *Sel volatil d'Angleterre*, (Ammon. muriat. ℔j; Cretæ ℔iss. Sublime — Ph. U. S.) A white, striated, crystalline mass; odour and taste pungent and ammoniacal: soluble in two parts of water: insoluble in alcohol: effloresces in the air. It is stimulant, antacid, diaphoretic, and antispasmodic. Dose, gr. v. to xv.

Carbonate of ammonia is at times used to form effervescing draughts. One scruple saturates six fluidrachms of lemon-juice, twenty-six grains of crystallized tartaric acid, and twenty-six grains of crystallized citric acid.

AMMONIÆ CITRAS, *Citrate of Ammo'nia*. Made by saturating lemon or lime juice, or a solution of citric acid, with carbonate of ammonia. Dose, f ʒss.

It may be made extemporaneously, and taken in an effervescing state. Seventeen grains of citric acid or half a fluidounce of lemon-juice will be sufficient for thirteen grains of carbonate of ammonia.

AMMONIÆ CUPRO-SULPHAS, Cuprum ammoniatum.

AMMONIÆ ET FERRI MURIAS, Ferrum ammoniatum—a. Ferro-citras, Ferri ammonio-citras—a. Hydriodas, Ammonium, iodide of—a. Hydrosulphuretum, Liquor fumans Boylii—a. Hypocarbonas, Ammoniæ Carbonas.

AMMO'NIÆ MU'RIAS, *Mu'riate of Ammo'nia*, *Hydrochlo'rate of Ammo'nia*, *Chlorohydrate of Ammo'nia*, *Sal Ammoni'acum*, *Sal Ammo'niac*, *Sal Ammoni'acus*, *Ammo'nia Muriat'ica*, *Ammo'nium Muria'tum*, *Hydrochlo'ras Ammo'niæ*, *Sal Armoni'acum*, *Salmiac*, *Fuli'go Al'ba Philosopho'rum*, *Misadir*, (F.) *Muriate d'Ammoniaque*. A saline concrete, formed by the combination of muriatic acid with ammonia. In Egypt it is manufactured in large quantities by subliming the soot formed by burning camel's dung — 26 pounds of the soot yielding 6 pounds. It is also prepared, in great quantities, by adding sulphuric acid to the volatile alkali obtained from soot, bones, &c., mixing this with common salt, and subliming.

Muriate of ammonia is inodorous, but has an acrid, pungent, bitterish, and urinous taste. Three parts of cold water dissolve one. Soluble also in 4·5 parts of alcohol. It is aperient and diuretic, but seldom used internally. Externally, it is employed, producing cold during its solution, in inflammations, &c.

AMMO'NIÆ NITRAS, *Nitrate of Ammonia*, *Al'kali volat'ilĕ nitra'tum*, *Sal ammoni'acus nitro'sus*, *Ammo'nia nitra'ta*, *Nitras ammoni'acæ*, *Nitrum flammans*, (F.) *Nitrate d'Ammoniaque*. A salt composed of nitric acid and ammonia. It is diuretic and deobstruent.(?) Externally, it is discutient and sialogogue.

AMMO'NIÆ PHOSPHAS, *Phosphate of Ammo'nia*, (F.) *Phosphate d'Ammoniaque*. This salt has been recommended as an excitant, diaphoretic, and discutient. More recently, it has been proposed as a new remedy for gout and rheumatism, as a solvent for uric acid calculus, and for, diseases, acute and chronic, connected directly with the lithic acid diathesis.

AMMONIÆ SESQUICARBONAS, A. carbonas.

AMMONIÆ SULPHAS, *Sulphate of Ammo'nia*, *Sulphas ammoni'acæ*, *Ammo'nium sulphu'ricum*, *Al'kali volat'ilĕ vitriola'tum*, *Sal Ammoni'acum secre'tum* GLAUBERI, *Sal secre'tus* GLAUBERI, *Vitriolum ammoniaca'lĕ*, (F.) *Sulphate d'Ammoniaque*. Formed by adding sulphuric acid either to sal ammoniac or to ammoniacal liquor. Its properties are like those of the muriate of ammonia.

AMMO'NIÆ SULPHURE'TUM, *Sul'phuret of Ammo'nia*, *Hydrosul'phuret of Ammo'nia*, *Ammo'nium Sul'hydra'tum*, *Hydrosul'phas Ammonia*, *Spir'itus* BEGUI'NI, *Sp. fumans* BEGUI'NI, *Sul'phure'tum ammoni'acæ*, *Sp. salis ammoni'aci sulphura'tus*, *Liquor ammo'nii hydrothi'odis*, *Hydrosulphure'tum Ammo'nicum*, *Hydrarg. ammoniaca'lĕ aquo'sum*, *Hydrog"eno-sulphure'tum ammoni'acæ liq'uidum*, *Spir'itus sul'phuris volat'ilis*, *Hepar sulphuris volat'ilĕ*, BOYLE'S or BEGUINE'S *fuming spirit*, (F.) *Hydrosulphate sulfurĕ d'Am-*

moniaque, Liqueur fumante de BOYLE, *Sulfure hydrogéné d'Ammoniaque, Hydrosulfure d'Ammoniaque.* Odour very fetid; taste nauseous and styptic; colour dark yellowish green. It is reputed to be sedative, nauseating, emetic, disoxygenizing, (?) and has been given in diabetes and diseases of increased excitement. Dose, gtt. viij. to gtt. xx.

AMMO'NIÆ TARTRAS, *Al'kali volat'ilē tartarisa'tum, Sal Ammoni'acum tarta'reum, Tar'tarus ammo'niæ, Tartrate of Ammo'nia,* (F.) *Tartrate d'Ammoniaque.* A salt composed of tartaric acid and ammonia. It is diaphoretic and diuretic; but not much used.

AMMONIAQUE, Ammonia—*a. Arséniaté d',* Arseniate of ammonia—*a. Hydrosulfure d',* Ammoniæ sulphuretum—*a. Hydrosulfate sulfuré d',* Ammoniæ sulphuretum—*a. Liquide,* Liquor ammoniæ—*a. Phosphate d',* Ammoniæ phosphas—*a. Sulfure hydrogéné d',* Ammoniæ sulphuretum.

AMMONII IODIDUM, Ammonium, iodide of.

AMMONII IODURETUM, Ammonium, iodide of.

AMMONIO-CUPRICUS SUBSULPHAS, Cuprum ammoniatum.

AMMO'NION, from αμμος, 'sand.' An ancient collyrium of great virtues in many diseases of the eye, and which was said to remove sand from that organ.

AMMONIUM ARSENICICUM, Arseniate of ammonia—a. Carbonicum, Ammoniæ carbonas—a. Hydroiodicum, Ammonium, iodide of—a. Iodatum, Ammonium, iodide of.

AMMO'NIUM, I'ODIDE OF, *Iod'idum seu Iodure'tum ammonii, Ammonium Ioda'tum seu Hydroiod'icum, Hydri'odas ammo'niæ, Hydri'odate of ammo'nia.* This salt is formed by saturating liquid hydriodic acid with caustic ammonia, and evaporating the solution. It is applied in the form of ointment (ʒj *ad adipis* ʒj) in lepra, psoriasis, &c.

AMMONIUM MURIATICUM MARTIATUM SEU MARTIALE, Ferrum ammoniatum—a. Muriatum, Ammoniæ murias—a. Subcarboneum, Ammoniæ carbonas—a. Sulfhydratum, Ammoniæ sulphuretum—a. Sulphuricum, Ammoniæ sulphas.

AMNA ALCALIZATA, Water, mineral, saline.

AMNEMOSYNE, Amnesia.

AMNE'SIA, *Amnest'ia, Amnemos'ynē,* from *a,* privative, and μνησις, 'memory.' *Moria imbec''ilis amne'sia, Obliv'io, Recollectio'nis jactu'ra, Dysæsthe'sia inter'na, Debil'itas memo'riæ, Memo'ria dele'ta,* (F.) *Perte de Mémoire,* 'loss of memory.' By some Nosologists, amnesia constitutes a genus of diseases. By most, it is considered only as a symptom, which may occur in many diseases.

AMNESTIA, Amnesia.

AMNI TIS, Amnitis.

AMNIOCLEP'SIS, from *Amnios,* and κλεπτω, 'I steal or take away clandestinely.' Premature escape of the liquor amnii.

AMNIORRHŒ'A, from *amnios,* and ρεω, 'I flow.' A premature discharge of the liquor amnii.

AM'NIOS, *Am'nion, Am'nium, Hym'nium, Charta virgin'ea, Armatu'ra, Agni'na membra'na, Pellu'cida membra'na, Galea, Scepar'num, Indu'sium, Amic'ulum, Membra'na fœtum invol'vens.* The innermost of the enveloping membranes of the fœtus:—so called because first observed in the sheep, (?) αμνος, 'a sheep.' It is thin, transparent, perspirable, and possesses many delicate, colourless vessels, which have not been injected. It is generally considered to be produced by a fold of the external layer of the germinal membrane, rising up, and gradually enveloping the embryo. Its external surface is feebly united to the cnorion by areolar and vascular filaments. Its inner surface is polished, and is in contact with the body of the fœtus and the liquor amnii.

AMNIOT'IC ACID, *Ac''idum am'nicum vel amniot'icum.* A peculiar acid, found by Vauquelin and Buniva in the liquor amnii of the cow.

AMNI'TIS, *Amnit'tis,* from *Amnion* and *itis,* inflammation. Inflammation of the Amnion.

AMŒNOMA'NIA, from *amœnus,* 'agreeable,' and *mania.* A form of mania in which the hallucinations are of an agreeable character.

AMOME FAUX, Sison amomum.

AMO'MUM CARDAMO'MUM, *A. repens* seu *racemo'sum, A. verum, Alpin'ia cardamo'mum, Caro'pi, Mato'nia Cardamo'mum, Eletta'ria Cardamo'mum, Cardamo'mum Minus, Lesser* or *officinal Car'damom,* (F.) *Cardamome de la Côte de Malabar, Cardamome.* The seeds of this East India plant have an agreeable, aromatic odour, and a pungent, grateful taste. They are carminative and stomachic: but are chiefly used to give warmth to other remedies. The fruit is called *Amomis.* Dose, gr. v. to ℈j.

AMOMUM CURCUMA, Curcuma longa.

AMOMUM GALANGA, Maranta G.

AMOMUM GRANUM PARADI'SI, *Cardamo'mum majus, Meleguet'ta, Maniguet'ta, Cardamo'mum pipera'tum, A. max'imum,* (F.) *Graines de Paradis.* Greater cardamom seeds resemble the last in properties. They are extremely hot, and not much used.

AMOMUM HIRSUTUM, Costus—a. Montanum, see Cassumuniar—a. Pimenta: see Myrtus pimenta—a. Repens, A. cardamomum—a. Sylvestre, see Cassumuniar—a. Zedoaria, Kæmpferia rotunda—a. Zerumbet, see Cassumuniar.

AMOMUM ZIN'GIBER, *Zin'giber officina'lē, Zin'giber album, Z. nigrum, Z. commu'nē, Zin'ziber, Ginger,* (F.) *Gingembre.* The *white* and *black ginger, Zin'ziber fuscum* et *album,* are the rhizoma of the same plant, *Zin'giber officina'lē,* the difference depending upon the mode of preparing them.

The odour of ginger is aromatic; taste warm, aromatic, and acrid. It yields its virtues to alcohol, and in a great degree to water. It is carminative, stimulant, and sialogogue.

Preserved Ginger, Zingib'eris Radix Condi'ta, Radix Zingib'eris condi'ta ex Indiâ alla'ta, is a condiment which possesses all the virtues of ginger.

Ginger-Beer Powders may be formed of *white sugar,* ʒj. and ℈ij. *ginger,* gr. v. *subcarbonate of soda,* gr. xxxvj in each *blue* paper: *acid of tartar,* ℈iss in each *white* paper,—for half a pint of water.

Oxley's Concentrated Essence of Jamaica Ginger is a solution of *ginger* in *rectified spirit.*

AMOR, Love.

AMORGE, Amurca.

AMORPHUS, Anhistous, Anideus.

AMOSTEUS, Osteocolla.

AMOUR, Love—*a. Physique,* Appetite, venereal.

AMOUREUX (muscle.) Obliquus superior oculi.

AMPAC, *Amp'acus.* An East India tree, the leaves of which have a strong odour, and are used in baths as detergents. A very odoriferous resin is obtained from it.

AMPAR, Succinum.

AMPELOCARPUS, Galium aparine.

AMPELOPRASUM, Allium.

AMPELOP'SIS QUINQUEFO'LIA, *Virgin'ian Creeper, American Ivy, Fiveleaved Ivy, Woody Climber.* An indigenous climbing plant. *Family,* Vitaceæ; which flowers in July. It has been advised as an expectorant.

AMPELOS, Vitis vinifera—a. Agria, Bryonia

alba—a. Idæa, Vaccinium Vitis Idæa—a. Oinophoros, Vitis vinifera.

AMPHAMPHOTERODIOPSIA, Diplopia.

AMPHARIS'TEROS, *Ambilæ'vus*, 'awkward;' from αμφι, and αριστερος, 'the left.' Opposed to ambidexter.

AMPHEMERINOS, Quotidian.

AMPHEMERUS, Quotidian.

AMPHI, αμφι, 'both, around, on all sides.' Hence, a prefix in many of the following terms.

AMPHIAM, Opium.

AMPHIARTHRO'SIS, from αμφι, 'both,' and αρθρωσις, 'articulation.' A mixed articulation, in which the corresponding surfaces of bones are united in an intimate manner by an intermediate body, which allows, however, of some slight motion. Such is the junction of the bodies of the vertebræ by means of the intervertebral cartilages. This articulation has also been called *Diarthrose de Continuité*. The motion it permits is but slight.

AMPHIBLESTRODITIS, Retinitis.

AMPHIBLESTROIDES, Reticular.

AMPHIBLESTROMALA'CIA, from *amphiblestroï'des* (membrana) the retina, and μαλακια, 'softening.' Mollescence or softening of the retina.

AMPHIBRAN'CHIA, from αμφι, 'around,' and βραγχια, 'the throat.' *Amphibron'chia*. The tonsils and neighbouring parts.—Hippocrates.

AMPHICAUSTIS, Vulva.

AMPHID'EUM, from αμφι, 'around,' and δεω, 'I bind.' The outermost margin of the cervix uteri; the *Labium uteri*.

AMPHIDEXIUS, Ambidexter.

AMPHIDIARTHRO'SIS, from αμφι, 'about,' and διαρθρωσις, 'a moveable joint.' A name given by Winslow to the temporo-maxillary articulation, because, according to that anatomist, it partakes both of ginglymus and arthrodia.

AMPHIESMA CORDIS, Pericardium.

AMPHIMERINA, Pertussis—a. Hectica, Hectic fever.

AMPHIMERINOS, Quotidian.

AMPHION, Maslach.

AMPHIPLEX, Perinæum.

AMPHIPNEUMA, Dyspnœa.

AMPHISMELA, Knife, double-edged.

AMPHISMILE, Knife, double-edged.

AMPHISPHAL'SIS, *Circumac'tio*, *Circumduc'tio*, from αμφι, 'around,' and σφαλλω, 'I wander.' The movement of circumduction used in reducing luxations.—Hippocrates.

AMPHODIPLOPIA, see Diplopia.

AM'PHORA, per syncop. for αμφιφορευς, from αμφι, 'on both sides,' and φερω, 'I bear :' because it had two handles. A liquid measure among the ancients, containing above seven gallons. Also called *Quadrant'al*, *Cera'mium*, *Ceram'nium*, *Cadus*.

AMPHORIC RESPIRATION, see Cavernous Respiration.

AMPHOTERODIPLOPIA, see Diplopia.

AMPHRODIPLOPIA, Diplopia.

AMPLEXATIO, Coition.

AMPLEXUS, Coition.

AMPLIFICATIO, Platynosis.

AMPLIOPIA, Amblyopia.

AMPOSIS, Anaposis.

AMPOULES, Essera.

AMPUL'LA, (L.) 'A bottle.' A membranous bag, shaped like a leathern bottle. See *Cavitas Elliptica*. In pharmacy, a receiver.

AMPULLA CHYLIFERA SEU CHYLI, Receptaculum chyli.

AMPULLÆ, Phlyctænæ.

AMPUTATION, *Amputa'tio*, from *amputare*, (am, 'around,' and *putare*,) 'to cut off.' *Apot'-*omē, *Apotom'ia*. The operation of separating, by means of a cutting instrument, a limb or a part of a limb, or a projecting part, as the mamma, penis, &c., from the rest of the body. In the case of a tumour, the term *excision*, *removal*, or *extirpation*,(F.) *Resection*, is more commonly used.

AMPUTATION, CIRCULAR, is that in which the integuments and muscles are divided circularly.

AMPUTATION, FLAP, (F.) *A. à lambeaux*, is when one or two flaps are left so as to cover the stump, when the limb has been removed.

AMPUTATION, JOINT, *Exarticula'tio*, (F.) *A. dans l'article* ou *dans la contiguité des membres*, is when the limb is removed at an articulation.

Each amputation requires a different process, which is described in works on operative surgery.

AMPUTATION, SPONTANEOUS, See Spontaneous.

AMULET, Amuletum.

AMULETTE, Amuletum.

AMULE'TUM, from *amoliri*, 'to remove.' An *Amulet*, *Periam'ma*, *Apotropæ'um*, *Periap'ton*, *Phylacte'rion*, *Apoteles'ma*, *Exarte'ma*, *Alexica'cum*, *Præservati'vum*, *Probasca'nium*, *Probascan'tium*, (F.) *Amulette*. Any image or substance worn about the person for the purpose of preventing disease or danger.

AMUR'CA, *Amur'ga*, αμοργη. The marc or grounds remaining after olives have been crushed and deprived of their oil. It has been used as an application to ulcers.

AMURGA, Amurca.

AMUSA, Musa Paradisiaca.

A'MYCE, *Amycha*, *Amy'xis*. Excoriation, Scarification.

AMYCHA, Amyce.

AMYC'TICA, from αμυσσω, 'I lacerate,' Medicines which stimulate and vellicate the skin.—Cælius Aurelianus.

AMYDRIASIS, Mydriasis.

AMYEL'IA, from *a*, privative, and μυελος, 'marrow.' A monstrous formation, in which there is an absence of spinal marrow.

AMYG'DALA, same etymon as Amyctica; because there seem to be fissures in the shell. The *Almond*, of which there are two kinds; *Amyg'dalæ ama'ræ* and *A. dulces*, (F.) *Amandes amères*, and *A. douces*, obtained from two varieties of *Amyg'dalus communis* or *A. sati'va*, a native of Barbary. *Nat. Ord.* Amygdaleæ. *Sex. Syst.* Icosandria Monogynia.

The taste of *Amygdala dulcis* is soft and sweet; that of *A. amara*, bitter. Both yield, by expression, a sweet, bland oil. The bitter almond contains Prussic acid. They are chiefly used for forming emulsions.

AMYG'DALÆ PASTA, *Almond Paste*, a cosmetic for softening the skin and preventing chaps, is made of *bitter almonds*, blanched, ℥iv, *white of one egg; rose water*, and *rectified spirit*, equal parts, or as much as is sufficient.

AMYG'DALÆ PLACEN'TA, *Almond Cake*, is the cake left after the expression of the oil. The ground Almond Cake, Almond Powder, *Fari'na Amygdala'rum*, is used instead of soap for washing the hands.

AMYGDALA, Tonsil. Also, a lobule or prominence of the cerebellum, so called from its resemblance to an enlarged tonsil. This and its fellow of the opposite side form the lateral boundaries of the anterior extremity of the *valley*, and are in great part covered by the medulla oblongata. The Amygdalæ are seated on either side of the uvula, in the fourth ventricle.

AMYGDALATUM, Emulsio Amygdalæ.

AMYGDALE, Tonsil.

AMYG'DALIN, *Amygdali'num*, *Amygdali'na*, *Amyg'daline*. A principle contained in bitter almonds, which is prepared by pressing the bruised almonds between heated plates to separate the fat oil; boiling the residue in alcohol; evaporating, and treating with ether, which precipitates the amygdaline in a crystalline powder. A weak solution of it, under the influence of a small quantity of *emulsin* or *synaptase*, which constitutes the larger portion of the pulp of almonds, yields at once oil of bitter almonds and hydrocyanic acid.

AMYGDALITIS, Cynanche tonsillaris.
AMYGDALUS, see Amygdala.
AMYGDALUS COMMUNIS, see Amygdala.
AMYG'DALUS PER'SICA, *Per'sica vulga'ris*. The *common peach-tree*, (F.) *Pêcher*. The leaves and flowers have been considered laxative. They are bitter and aromatic, and have been given in hæmaturia, nephritis, &c. The fruit is one of the pleasant and wholesome summer fruits, when ripe. The kernels, *Amyg'dalæ Per'sicæ*, as well as the flowers, contain prussic acid.

Peach Brandy is distilled from the fruit, and is much used in the United States.

AMYGMOS, Scarification.
AMYLA'CEA (*remedia*), from *amylum*, 'starch.' Remedies whose chief medicinal constituent is starch.
AMYLEON, Amylum.
AMYLI IODIDUM, Starch, iodide of — a. Ioduretum, Starch, iodide of.
A'MYLUM, *A'midum, Fec'ula, Amyl'eon, Amyl'ion*, from *a*, priv., and μυλη, 'a mill,' because made without a mill. *Starch*, (F.) *Amidon, Amylon, Starch of Wheat, Fari'na, Trit'ici fari'na, Amylum triti''ceum seu Trit'ici, Fec'ula Amyla'cea*, is inodorous and insipid, white and friable. It is insoluble in cold water and alcohol, but forms with boiling water a strong, semi-transparent jelly. It is demulcent, and is used as an emollient glyster, and as the vehicle for opium, when given *per anum*. Starch is met with abundantly in all the cereal grains, in the stalks of many of the palms, in some lichens, and in many tuberous roots, particularly in the bulbs of the orchis.

AMYLUM AMERICANUM, see Arrow root — a. Cannaceum, *Tous-les-mois* — a. Iodatum, Starch, iodide of — a. Manihoticum, see Jatropha manihot — a. Marantaceum, Arrow-root — a. Palmaceum, Sago — a. Querneum, Racahout.

A'MYON, from *a*, priv., and μυον, 'a muscle,' *Emuscula'tus*. Without muscle. Applied to the limbs, when so extenuated that the muscles cannot be distinguished.

AMYOSIS, Synezizis.
AMYRIS COMMIPHORA, see Bdellium.
AM'YRIS ELEMIF'ERA, (F.) *Balsamier Élémifère*. *Nat. Ord.* Terebinthaceæ. *Sex. Syst.* Octandria Monogynia. The plant whence it has been supposed GUM ELE'MI is obtained. This gum or resin is brought from the Spanish East and West Indies. *Brazilian Elemi*, according to Dr. Royle, is produced by *Icica Icicariba*; *Mexican Elemi*, by *Ela'phrium elemiferum*; and *Manilla Elemi*, by *Cana'rium commu'nè*. It is softish, transparent, of a pale whitish colour, inclining a little to green, and of a strong, though not unpleasant smell. It is only used in ointments and plasters, and is a digestive.

AMYRIS GILEADENSIS, see A. opobalsamum.
AM'YRIS OPOBAL'SAMUM, (F.) *Balsamier de la Meoque, Bal'sem, Bal'samum*. The plant from which is obtained the BALSAM OF MECCA, *Bal'samum genui'num antiquo'rum, Balsamela'on, Ægyptiacum Bal'samum, Bal'samum Asiat'icum, B. Juda'icum, B. Syriacum, B. e Meccâ, Cocobal'samum, B. Alpi'ni, Oleum Bal'sami, Opobal'samum, Xylobal'samum, Balsam or Balm of Gilead*, (F.) *Baume Blanc, B. de Constantinople blanc, B. de Galaad, B. du Grand Caire, B. Vrai, Térébinthine de Giléad, T. d'Égypte, T. du Grand Kaire, T. de Judée*. A resinous juice obtained by making incisions into *Amyris opobal'samum* and *A. Gileaden'sis* of Linnæus, *Balsamaden'dron Gileaden'sè* of Kunth. The juice of the fruit is called *Carpobal'samum*; that of the wood and branches *Xylobal'samum*. It has the general properties of the milder Terebinthinates.

AMYRIS TOMENTOSUM, Fagara octandra.
AMYRON, Carthamus Tinctorius.
A'MYUS, from *a*, privative, and μυς, 'a mouse, a muscle.' Weak or poor in muscle.
AMYX'IA, from *a*, privative, and μυξα, 'mucus.' Deficiency of mucus.
AMYXIS, Amyce, Scarification.
ANA, *ana*, a word which signifies 'of each.' It is used in prescriptions as well as ā and āā, its abbreviations. As a prefix to words, it means 'in,' 'through,' 'upwards,' 'above,' in opposition to *cata*; also 'repetition,' like the English *re*. Hence,—

ANAB'ASIS, from αναβαινω, 'I ascend.' The first period of a disease, or that of increase.— Galen. See Augmentation.
ANABEXIS, Expectoration.
ANABLEP'SIS, from *ανα*, 'again,' and βλεπω, 'I see.' Restoration to sight.
ANABOLÆ'ON, *Anabole'us*, from αναβαλλω, 'I cast up.' An ointment for extracting darts or other extraneous bodies.
ANAB'OLE, from *ανα*, 'upwards,' and βαλλω, 'I cast.' *Anago'gē, Anaph'ora, Anacine'ma, Anacine'sis*. An evacuation upwards. An act by which certain matters are ejected by the mouth. In common acceptation it includes, *exspuition, expectoration, regurgitation*, and *vomiting*.

ANABROCHIS'MUS, *Anabron'chismus*, from *ανα*, 'with,' and βροχος, 'a running knot.' An operation for removing the eye-lashes, for example, when they irritate the eye, by means of a hair knotted around them—Hippocrates, Galen, Celsus, &c.

ANABRONCHISMUS, Anabrochismus.
ABABROSIS, Corrosion, Erosion.
ANACAMPSEROS, Sedum telephium.
ANACAR'DIUM OCCIDENTA'LE, *Acajuba occidenta'lis, Cassu'vium pomif'erum, Cashew* (W. Indies.) (F.) *Ac'ajou*. *Nat. Ord.* Terebinthaceæ. *Sex. Syst.* Enneandria Monogynia. The *Oil of the Cashew Nut, O'leum Anacar'dii,* (F.) *Huile d'Acajou*, is an active caustic, and used as such in the countries where it grows, especially for destroying warts, &c.

ANACARDIUM ORIENTALE, Avicennia tomentosa.
ANACATHAR'SIS, from *ανα*, 'upwards,' and καθαιρειν, 'to purge.' Purgation upwards. Expectoration. See, also, Repurgatio.
ANACATHARSIS CATARRHALIS SIMPLEX, Catarrh.
ANACATHARTICUS, Expectorant.
ANACESTOS, Incurable.
ANACHREMPSIS, Exspuition.
ANACHRON, Soda.
ANACINEMA, Anabole, Exspuition.
ANACINESIS, Anabole, Exspuition.
ANACLASIS, Repercussion.
ANACLINTE'RIUM, *Anaclin'trum, Recubito'rium*, from ανακλινω, 'I recline.' A long chair or seat, so formed that the person can rest in a reclining posture.
ANACLINTRUM, Anaclinterium.
ANACOLLE'MA, from *ανα*, 'together,' and κολλαω, 'I glue.' A healing medicine.
ANACOLLEMATA, Frontal bandages.

ANACOLUP'PA. A creeping plant of Malabar, the juice of which, mixed with powdered pepper, passes in India as a cure for epilepsy, and as the only remedy for the bite of the naja. It is supposed to be *Zapa'nia nodiflo'ra.*
ANACOLUTHIE, Incoherence.
ANACOMIDE, Restauratio.
ANACONCHYLIASMUS, Gargarism.
ANACONCHYLISMUS, Gargarism.
ANACTESIS, Restauratio.
ANACTIRION, Artemisia.
ANACYCLEON, Charlatan.
ANACYCLUS OFFICINARUM, see Anthemis Pyrethrum—a. Pyrethrum, Anthemis pyrethrum.
ANADESMUS, Fascia.
ANADIPLO'SIS, from ava, 'again,' and διπλοω, 'I double.' *Epanadiplo'sis, Epanalep'sis, Reduplica'tio.* The redoubling which occurs in a paroxysm of an intermittent, when its type is double.—Galen, Alexander of Tralles.
ANADORA, Ecdora.
ANAD'OSIS, from αναδιδωμι, 'I distribute.' Purgation upwards, as by vomiting. Congestion of blood towards the upper parts of the body. *Anadosis* seems also to have occasionally meant chylification, whilst *diadosis* meant capillary nutrition,—Hippocrates, Galen.
ANAD'ROME, from ava, 'upwards,' and δρεμω, 'I run.' The transport of a humour or pain from a lower to an upper part.—Hippocr. Also, the globus hystericus.
ANÆDŒ'US, from αν, privative, and αιδοια, 'organs of generation.' A monster devoid of sexual organs.
ANÆMATOPOIE'SIS, from α, αν, privative, 'αιμα, 'blood,' and ποιεω, 'I make.' Impeded or obstructed hæmatosis.
ANÆMATO'SIS, *Anhæmato'sis,* from α, αν, privative, and 'αιμα, 'blood.' Defective hæmatosis or preparation of the blood. Anæmia.
ANÆ'MIA, *Exæ'mia, Anæ'masis, Anhæ'mia, Anhæmato'sis, Polyanhæ'mia, Anæmo'sis, Oligæ'mia, Oligohæ'mia, Hypæ'mia, Hydroæ'mia, Hydræ'mia, Anæ'mia,* (F.) *Anémie, Polyanhémie, Hydrohémie, Exsanguinity, Bloodlessness:* from α, priv., and 'αιμα, 'blood.' Privation of blood; — the opposite to plethora. It is characterised by every sign of debility. Also, diminished quantity of fluids in the capillary vessels:—the opposite to *Hyperæmia.*—The essential character of the blood in anæmia is diminution in the ratio of red corpuscles.
ANÆ'MIC, *Anem'ic, Anæ'micus;* same etymon. Appertaining to Anæmia,—as an "*anæmic* person;" "*anæmic* urine."
ANÆMOCH'ROÜS, from α, αν, privative, 'αιμα, 'blood,' and χροα, 'colour.' Devoid of colour, pale.
ANÆMOSIS, Anæmia.
ANÆMOT'ROPHY, *Anæmotroph'ia:* from αν, privative, 'αιμα, 'blood,' and τροφη, 'nourishment.' A deficiency of sanguineous nourishment. —Prout.
ANÆMYDRIA, Anhydræmia.
ANÆSTHE'SIA, *Anæsthe'sis, Insensibil'itas, Analge'sia, Parap'sis expers,* (F.) *Anesthésie:* from α, privative, and αισθανομαι, 'I feel.' Privation of sensation, and especially of that of touch, according to some. It may be general or partial, and is almost always symptomatic.
ANÆSTHESIA LINGUÆ, Ageustia—a. Olfactoria, Anosmia.
ANÆSTHESIS, Anæsthesia.
ANÆSTHET'IC, *Anesthet'ic, Anæsthet'icus, Anesthérique;* same etymon. as *Anæsthesia.* Relating to privation of feeling, as an "*anæsthetic agent;*" one that prevents feeling, as chloroform inhaled during a surgical operation. Different agents have been used as anæsthetics,—sulphuric ether, chloroform, chloric ether, compound ether, chlorohydric and nitric ethers, bisulphuret of carbon, chloride of olefiant gas, benzin, aldehyde, light coal-tar naphtha, &c.; but the first four are alone employed as agents.
ANÆSTHETIZA'TION, (F.) *Anesthétisation;* same etymon. The condition of the nervous system induced by anæsthetics.
ANÆSTHISIA, Insensibility.
ANAGAL'LIS, from ava, and γαλα, 'milk,' from its power of coagulating milk. *A. arven'sis, A. Phænic''ea, Red Pim'pernel, Scarlet Pimpernel.* Nat. Ord. Primulaceæ. *Sex. Syst.* Pentandria Monogynia. (F.) *Mouron rouge.* A common European plant; a reputed antispasmodic and stomachic.
Another species—*Anagal'lis cæru'lea* is a mere variety of the above.
ANAGALLIS AQUATICA, Veronica Beccabunga.
ANAGARGALICTON, Gargarism.
ANAGARGARISMUS, Gargarism.
ANAGARGARISTON, Gargarism.
ANAGLYPHE, Calamus scriptorius.
ANAGOGE, Anabole, Rejection.
ANAGRAPHE, Prescription.
ANAG'YRIS, *Anag'yrus, Ac'opon, Anag'yris fœ'tida, Stinking Bean Trefoil.* Native of Italy. The leaves are powerfully purgative. The juice is said to be diuretic, and the seeds emetic.—Dioscorides, Paulus.
ANAGYRUS, Anagyris.
ANAL, *Ana'lis.* That which refers to the anus;—as *Anal region,* &c.
ANAL'DIA, (F.) *Analdie;* from α, privative, and αλδειν, 'to grow.' Defective nutrition.
ANALEMSIA, Analepsia.
ANALENTIA, Analepsia.
ANALEP'SIA, *Analep'sis, Analen'tia, Analem'sia,* from ava, 'fresh,' and λαμβανειν, 'to take.' Restoration to strength after disease.—Galen. A kind of sympathetic epilepsy, originating from gastric disorder. See Epilepsy.
Also, the support given to a fractured extremity;—*Appen'sio.*—Hippocrates.
ANALEPSIS, Convalescence, Restauratio.
ANALEP'TICA, *Anapsyc'tica, Psychot'ica, Refecti'ʋa, Reficien'tia, Analep'tics,* same etymon. Restorative medicines or food; such as are adapted to recruit the strength during convalescence:—as sago, salep, tapioca, jelly, &c.
ANALEPTIC PILLS, JAMES'S, consist of *James's Powder, Gum Ammoniacum,* and *Pills of Aloës* and *Myrrh,* equal parts, with *Tincture of Castor,* sufficient to form a mass.
ANALGE'SIA, *Anal'gia,* from α, priv., and αλγος, 'pain.' Absence of pain both in health and disease. See Anæsthesia.
ANALGIA, Analgesia.
AN'ALOGUE, *Anal'ogus;* from ava, 'again,' and λογος, 'a description.' A part in one organised being which has the same function as another part in another organised being.
ANALOGOUS TISSUES, see Tissues.
ANALOSIS, Atrophy.
ANALTESIS, Restauratio.
ANALTHES, Incurable.
ANAMIRTA COCCULUS, Menispermum cocculus—a. Paniculata, Menispermum cocculus.
ANAMNES'TIC, *Anamnes'ticum,* from ava, 'again,' and μναομαι, 'I remember.' A medicine for improving the memory. See, also, Commemorative.
ANANAS, Bromelia ananas—a. Aculeata, Bromelia ananas—a. Americana, Bromelia pinguin —a. Ovata, Bromelia ananas — Wild, broad leaved, Bromelia pinguin.

ANANAZIP'TA. A word formerly scrawled on amulets to charm away disease.

ANANDRI'A, from *a, av*, privative, and *avηρ*, 'a man.' Want of manliness. Impotence in the male. The state and act of emasculation.

ANANEO'SIS, *Renova'tio*; from *ava*, 'again,' and *νεος*, 'new.' Renovation or renewal,—as of the blood by the chyliferous vessels and lymphatics.

ANAPETI'A, *Expan'sio mea'tuum*, from *ava*, and *πεταω*, 'I dilate.' A state opposite to the closure of vessels—Galen.

ANAPHALANTI'ASIS, *Anaphalanto'ma*, from *αναφαλαντιας*, 'bald.' Loss of the hair of the eyebrows. Also, baldness in general.

ANAPHALANTOMA, Anaphalantiasis.

ANAPHE, Anaphia.

ANAPH'IA, *Anhaph'ia, An'aphè*, from *a, av*, priv., and '*αφη*, 'touch.' Diminution or privation of the sense of touch.

ANAPHLASMUS, Masturbation.

ANAPHONE'SIS, from *ava*, 'high,' and *φωνη*, 'voice.' Exercise of the voice: vociferation:—the act of crying out. *Vocifera'tio, Clamor*.

ANAPHORA, Anabole.

ANAPHRODIS'IA, from *a*, priv., and *Αφροδιτη*, 'Venus,' *Defec'tus Ven'eris*. Absence of the venereal appetite. Sometimes used for *Impotence* and *Sterility*.

ANAPHRODISIAC, Antaphrodisiac.

ANAPHROMELI, Mel despumatum.

ANAP'LASIS, *Anaplasmus*, from *αναπλασσω*, 'I restore.' *Confirma'tio, Reposi''tio*. Restoration. Union or consolidation of a fractured bone—Hippocrates.

ANAPLASMATIC, Anaplastic.

ANAPLASMUS, Anaplasis.

ANAPLAS'TIC, *Anaplas'ticus;* same etymon. An epithet applied to the art of restoring lost parts, or the normal shape—as '*Anaplastic Surgery*.' See Morioplastice. Also an agent, that increases the amount of plastic matter—fibrin—in the blood; *Anaplasmat'ic*.

ANAPLERO'SIS, from *αναπληροω*, 'I fill up.' Repletion. That part of surgical therapeutics whose object is to supply parts that are wanting. Also, *Apposition* or *Prosthesis*.

ANAPLEROTICUS, Incarnans.

ANAPLEU'SIS, *Fluctua'tio, Innata'tio*, from *αναπλειν*, 'to swim above.' The looseness or shaking of an exfoliated bone; or of a carious or other tooth, &c.—Hippocrates, Paulus.

ANAPLOSIS, Growth.

ANAPNEUSIS, Respiration.

ANAPNOE, Respiration.

ANAPNOENU'SI; from *Anapnoē*, 'respiration,' and *νουσος*, 'disease.' Diseases of the respiratory organs.

ANAPNOMETER, Spirometer.

ANAPODISIS UTERI, Retroversio Uteri.

ANAPODISMUS UTERI, Retroversio Uteri.

ANAPODOPHYLLUM CANADENSE, Podophyllum peltatum.

ANAP'OSIS, *Am'posis*, from *ava*, 'again,' and *ποσις*, 'drink.' A recession of humours from the circumference to the centre of the body—Hippocrates.

ANAPSE, Auante.

ANAPSIA, Cæcitas.

ANAPSYCTICA, Analeptica.

ANAPTYSIS, Expectoration.

ANAPTYXIS, Growth.

ANARCOTINA, Narcotine.

ANARRHEGNU'MINA, from *αναρρηγνυμι*, 'I break out again.' Fractures are so called when they become disunited; as well as ulcers when they break out afresh.

ANARRHI'NON, from *ava*, 'upwards,' and *ριν*, 'the nose.' That which returns by the nose—Gorræus.

According to others, that which issues by the skin; from *ava*, and *ρινος*, 'the skin.'

ANARRHINUM, Sternutatory.

ANARRHOE, Anarrhœa.

ANARRHŒ'A, *Anar'rhoē, Anarrho'pia, Anas'tasis*, from *ava*, 'upwards,' and *ρεω*, 'I flow.' Afflux of fluid towards the upper part of the body.

ANARRHOPHE, Absorption.

ANARRHOPHENU'SI; from *anarrhophe*, 'absorption,' and *νουσος*, 'disease.' Diseases of the absorbents.

ANARRHOPHESIS, Absorption.

ANARRHOPIA, Anarrhœa.

ANAR'THRUS, from *av*, priv., and *αρθρον*, 'a joint.' Without a joint. One who is so fat that his joints are scarcely perceptible—Hipp.

ANASAR'CA, from *ava*, 'through,' and *σαρξ*, 'the flesh.' *Anasarch'a, Catasar'ca, Aqua intercus seu inter cutem, Hyposar'ca, Hydrops cellula'ris totius cor'poris, H. Anasar'ca, H. inter'cus seu subcuta'neus seu cellulo'sus seu cuta'neus seu telæ cellulo'sæ, Katasar'ca, Episarcid'ium, Hy'deros, Hydaton'cus, Hyderon'cus, Hydron'cus, Hydrosar'ca, Hydroder'ma, Hydrop'isis vera, Sar'cites, Polylym'phia, Hyposarcid'ius, Leucophlegma'tia, General dropsy, Dropsy of the cellular membrane*, (F.) *Anasarque*. Commonly, it begins to manifest itself by swelling around the ankles; and is characterized by tumefaction of the limbs and of the soft parts covering the abdomen, thorax, and even the face, with paleness and dryness of the skin, and pitting when any of these (especially the ankles) are pressed upon. Like dropsy in general, Anasarca may be *active* or *passive;* and its treatment must be regulated by the rules that are applicable to general dropsy. At times, the symptoms are of an acute character, and the effusion sudden, constituting *Dermatoch'ysis, Hydrops Anasar'ca acu'tus, Œde'ma cal'idum, Œ. acu'tum, Œ. febri'lē* of some. See Hydrops.

ANASARCA HYSTERICUM, Anathymiasis — a. Pulmonum, Hydropneumonia, Œdema of the Lungs—a. Serosa, Phlegmatia dolens.

ANASARCHA, Anasarca.

ANASARQUE, Anasarca.

ANASISMUS, Concussion.

ANASPADIA, see Anaspadiæus.

ANASPA'DIAS, *Epispa'dias*, from *ava*, 'upwards,' and *σπαω*, 'I draw.' One whose urethra opens on the upper surface of the penis.

ANASPADISIS, see Anaspadiæus.

ANASPADISMUS, see Anaspadiæus.

ANAS'PASIS, *Anaspasm'us*, from *ανασπαω*, 'I contract.' *Retrac'tio*. Contraction, especially of the bowels. The condition is called *Anaspa'dia, Anaspad'isis*, and *Anaspadis'mus*—Hippocrates.

ANASPASMUS, Anaspasis.

ANASSA, Bromelia ananas.

ANASTALTICA, Styptics.

ANASTASIS, Anarrhœa. Also, restoration from sickness. Convalescence.

ANASTŒCHEIO'SIS, from *ava*, 'again,' and *στοιχειον*, 'element.' *Reëlementa'tio*. Resolution of a body or its parts into their elements—Galen.

ANASTOMO'SIS, from *ava*, 'with,' and *στομα*, 'a mouth.' *Inoscula'tio seu Reu'nio vaso'rum, Exanastomo'sis, Concur'sus*, (F.) *Abouchement*. Communication between two vessels. By considering the nerves to be channels, in which a nervous fluid circulates, their communication likewise has been called *Anastomosis*. By means of anastomoses, if the course of a fluid be arrested in one vessel, it can proceed along others.

ANASTOMOSIS ANEURISMATICA, Telangiectasia—a. Jacobson's;—see Petrosal ganglion.

ANASTOMOT'ICS, *Anastomot'ica.* Same etymon. Certain medicines were formerly so called, which were believed to be capable of opening the mouths of vessels:—as aperients, diuretics, &c.

ANASTOMOT'ICUS MAGNUS, (RAMUS,) (F.) *Artère collatérale interne, A. collatérale du coude,* is a branch of the brachial artery which comes off a little above the elbow, and bestows branches to the brachialis internus, to the under edge of the triceps, and to the muscles, ligaments, &c., about the elbow joint. See, also, Articular arteries of the knee.

ANASTROPHE UTERI, Inversio uteri.

ANATASIS, Extension.

ANATHYMIAMA, Anathymiasis.

ANATHYMI'ASIS, *Anathymi'ama,* from ανα, 'upwards,' and θυμα, 'fumigation.' (*Œde'ma fugax, Œde'ma spas'ticum, Œde'ma hyster'icum, Anasar'ca hyster'icum.* An uncertain and transient swelling or inflation, said to have been observed at times in nervous and hysterical persons. It also means Exhalation, Fumigation, and Hypochondriasis.

ANATOLE UNGUIUM, see Nail.

ANATOME, Anatomy—a. Animata, Physiology.

ANATOMIA, Anatomy—a. Animalis, Zootomy—a. Comparata, Zootomy—a. Comparativa, Zootomy—a. Viva, Physiology.

ANATOMIE, Anatomy—*a. Chirurgicale,* see Anatomy—*a. des Régions,* see Anatomy.

ANAT'OMIST, *Anatom'icus.* One who occupies himself with anatomy. One versed in Anatomy.

ANAT'OMY, *Anat'omē, Anatom'ia, Prosec'tio,* from ανα, and τεμνειν, 'to cut,' (F.) *Anatomie.* The word *Anatomy* properly signifies *dissection;* but it has been appropriated to the study and knowledge of the number, shape, situation, structure, and connexion,—in a word, of all the apparent properties of organised bodies. Anatomy is the science of organisation. Some have given the term a still more extended acceptation, applying it to every mechanical decomposition, even of inorganic bodies. Thus, *Crystallography* has been termed the *Anatomy* of crystallized minerals. Anatomy has also been called *Morphol'ogy, Somatol'ogy, Somatot'omy, Organol'ogy,* &c. It assumes different names according as the study is confined to one organized being, or to a species or class of beings. Thus, *Androt'omy,* or *Anthropot'omy,* or *Anthropog'raphy,* or *Anthroposomatol'ogy,* is the Anatomy of man:—*Zoötomy,* that of the other species of the animal kingdom: and *Vet'erinary Anat'omy* is the anatomy of domestic animals: but when the word is used abstractly, it means *human Anatomy,* and particularly the study of the organs in a physiological or healthy state. *Physiological Anatomy* is occasionally used to signify the kind of anatomy which investigates structure with a special view to function. The Anatomy of the diseased human body is called *Patholog''ical* or *Morbid Anatomy,* and when applied to Medical Jurisprudence, *Foren'sic Anatomy.* Several of the organs possessing a similarity of structure, and being formed of the same tissues, they have been grouped into Systems or Genera of Organs; and the study of, or acquaintance with, such systems, has been called *General Anat'omy, Histol'ogy,* or *Morphot'omy,* whilst the study of each organ in particular has been termed *Descriptive Anatomy. Histology* is, however, more frequently applied to the *Anatomy of the Tissues,* which is called, also, *Tex'tural* and *Microscopic Anatomy.* Descriptive Anatomy has been divided into *Skeletol'ogy* which comprises *Osteol'-ogy,* and *Syndesmol'ogy;* and into *Sarcol'ogy,* which is subdivided into *Myol'ogy, Neurol'ogy, Angiol'ogy, Adenol'ogy, Splanchnol'ogy,* and *Dermol'ogy. Sur'gical Anat'omy, Medico-Chiurgical Anatomy, Topograph'ical Anat'omy, Re'gionale Anat'omy,* (F.) *Anatomie Chiurgicale, A. des Régions,* is the particular and relative study of the bones, muscles, nerves, vessels, &c., with which it is indispensable to be acquainted before performing operations. *Compar'ative Anat'omy* is the comparative study of each organ, with a view to an acquaintance with the modifications of its structure in different animals or in the different classes of animals. *Transcendent'al* or *Philosoph'ical Anatomy* inquires into the mode, plan, or model upon which the animal frame or organs are formed; and *Artifi'cial Anat'omy* is the art of modelling and representing in wax or other substance, the different organs or different parts of the human body, in the sound or diseased state. *Phytot'omy* is the anatomy of vegetables, and *Picto'rial Anatomy,* anatomy artistically illustrated.

ANATOMY, ARTIFICIAL, see Anatomy—a. Comparative, see Anatomy, Zootomy—a. Descriptive, see Anatomy—a. Forensic, see Anatomy—a. General, see Anatomy—a. Human, see Anatomy—a. of Man, see Anatomy—a. Medico-chirurgical, see Anatomy—a. Microscopic, see Anatomy—a. Morbid, see Anatomy—a. Pathological, see Anatomy—a. Philosophical, see Anatomy—a. Physiological, see Anatomy—a. Pictorial, see Anatomy—a. Practical, see Dissection—a. Regional, see Anatomy—a. Surgical, see Anatomy—a. Textural, see Anatomy—a. Topographical, see Anatomy—a. Transcendental, see Anatomy—a. Veterinary, see Anatomy.

ANATON, Soda.

ANATREPSIS, Restauratio.

ANATRESIS, Perforation, Trepanning.

ANATRIBE, Friction.

ANATRIPSIS, Friction.

ANATRIPSOL'OGY, *Anatripsolog''ia, Anatriptolog''ia,* from ανατριψις, 'friction,' and λογος, 'a discourse.' A treatise on friction as a remedy.

ANATRIPTOLOGIA, Anatripsology.

ANATRON, Natrum, Soda.

ANAT'ROPE, from ανα, 'upwards,' and τρεπω, 'I turn.' Subversion. A turning or subversion or inverted action of the stomach, characterized by nausea, vomiting, &c.—Galen. We still speak of the stomach turning against any thing.

ANAUDIA, Catalepsy, Mutitas.

ANAXYRIS, Rumex acetosa.

ANAZESIS, Ebullition.

ANAZOTURIA, see Urine.

ANCHA, Haunch.

ANCHILOPS, Ægilops.

ANCHORALIS PROCESSUS, Coracoid.

ANCHUSA ANGUSTIFOLIA, A. Officinalis—a. Incarnata, A. Officinalis—a. Lycopsoides, A. Officinalis.

ANCHU'SA OFFICINALIS, *A. Angustifo'lia* seu *Incarna'ta* seu *Lycopsol'des, Alca'na, Lingua Bovis, Buglos'sum sylves'trē, Offic''inal* or *Garden Al'kanet* or *Bugloss; Nat. Ord.* Boragineæ. *Sex. Syst.* Pentandria Monogynia. (F.) *Buglose.* A native of Great Britain. The herb was formerly esteemed as a cordial in melancholia and hypochondriasis; but it is now rarely used. It is also called *Buglos'sa, Buglos'sum angustifo'lium majus, B. vulga'rē majus, B. sati'vum.*

ANCHU'SA TINCTO'RIA, *Alcan'na spu'ria, Dyer's Bugloss, Anc'bium, Buglos'sum Tincto'rum, Lithosper'mum villo'sum, Dyer's Al'kanet,* (F.) *Orcanette.* A European plant. The medical

properties are equivocal. It is used to give a beautiful red colour to ointments.
ANCHYLOSIS, Ankylosis.
ANCISTRON, Hamulus.
ANCOLIE, Aquilegia vulgaris.
ANCON, Elbow, Olecranon.
ANCONAD, see Anconal Aspect.
ANCONAGRA, Pechyagra.
ANCO'NAL; from *αγκων*, 'the elbow.' Relating, or appertaining to, the elbow or the olecranon.
ANCONAL ASPECT. An aspect towards the side on which the ancon or elbow is situated. — Barclay. *Anco'nad* is used by the same writer adverbially, to signify 'towards the anconal aspect.'
ANCONÉ, Anconeus.
ANCONE'US, from *αγκων*, 'the elbow.' A term once applied to every muscle attached to the olecranon. Winslow distinguished four:—the *great, external, internal,* and *small;* the first three being portions of the same muscle, the *triceps brachialis.* The last has, alone, retained the name. It is the *Ancone'us minor* of Winslow, the *Ancone'us vel Cubita'lis* RIOLA'NI of Douglas, the *Epicondylo-Cubita'lis* of Chaussier, the *Brevis Cu'biti,* (F.) *Anconé*, and is situate at the upper and back part of the fore-arm. It arises from the external condyle of the os humeri, and is inserted into the posterior edge of the upper third of the ulna. Its use is to aid in the extension of the fore-arm.
ANCONEUS EXTERNUS, see Triceps extensor cubiti — a. Internus, see Triceps extensor cubiti — a. Major, see Triceps extensor cubiti.
ANCTE'RES. *Fibulæ* or *Olaspe,* by which the lips of wounds were formerly kept together. —Celsus, Galen.
ANCTERIASMUS, Infibulation.
ANCU'BITUS, *Petrifac'tio.* An affection of the eye, in which there is a sensation as if sand were irritating the organ.
ANCUNNUEN'TÆ. A name formerly given to menstruating females.
ANCUS, *Ankus,* from *αγκων*, 'the elbow.' One who cannot extend his arms completely.
Also, the deformity resulting from a luxation of the humerus or fore-arm. — Hippocrates.
ANCYLE, Ankylosis.
ANCYLOBLEPHARON, Ankyloblepharon.
ANCYLODERE, Torticollis.
ANCYLODERIS, Torticollis.
ANCYLODONTIA, Ankylodontia.
ANCYLOGLOSSIA, Ankyloglossia.
ANCYLOMELE, Ankylomele.
ANCYLOMERISMUS, Ankylomerismus.
ANCYLOSIS, Ankylosis.
ANCYLOTOMUS, Ankylotomus.
ANCYRA, Hook.
ANCYROID CAVITY, Digital cavity.
ANCYROIDES PROCESSUS, Coracoid.
ANDA. A tree of Brazil;—*Anda Gome'sii, Joanne'sia princeps. Nat. Ord.* Euphorbiaceæ. *Sex. Syst.* Monœcia Monadelphia. An oil is obtained from the seeds by pressure, 50 to 60 drops of which act as a cathartic. The fruit is an oval nut, containing two seeds. These have the taste of the chestnut; but are strongly cathartic, and even emetic. The shell is astringent, and is used as such in diarrhœa, &c.
ANDELY, MINERAL WATERS OF. Andely is in France, near Gysore, and eight leagues from Rouen. The water is cold, and a weak chalybeate. It is used in chlorosis and abdominal obstruction.
ANDERSON'S PILLS, Pilulæ Aloes et Jalapæ.
ANDIRA IBAI, Geoffræa Vermifuga—a. Inermis, Geoffræa inermis—a. Racemosa, Geoffræa inermis—a. Surinamensis, Geoffræa Surinamensis.
ANDRACHAHARA, Sempervivum tectorum.

ANDRACHNE, Arbutus unedo, Portulaca.
ANDRANATOM'IA, *Andranat'omē, Androtom'ia, Androt'omē, Anthropot'omy,* from *ανηρ,* genitive *ανδρος,* 'a man,' and *τεμνειν,* 'to cut.' The anatomy of man.
ANDRI'A. Adult age. Manhood.
ANDRI'A MU'LIER, *Mulier Hermaphrodit'ica.* A female hermaphrodite.
ANDROGEN'IA, from *ανηρ,* 'man,' and *γενεσις,* 'generation.' The procreation of males. — Hippocrates.
ANDROG'YNUS, from *ανηρ,* 'a man,' and *γυνη,* 'a woman.' A hermaphrodite. An effeminate person. — Hippocrates.
ANDROLEPSIA, Conception.
ANDROMANIA, Nymphomania.
ANDROM'EDA ARBO'REA, *Sorrel Tree, Sour Tree, Sour Wood, Elk Tree, Elk Wood, Sorrel Wood, Sour Leaf,* (F.) *Andromédier.* A small indigenous tree; *Nat. Ord.* Ericeæ, *Sex. Syst.* Decandria Monogynia; found in the Alleghany Mountains and the hills and valleys diverging from them, as far as the southern limits of Georgia and Alabama; but seldom north of Virginia. The leaves are refrigerant and astringent, and have been used to make a kind of lemonade, which has been given in fevers.
ANDROM'EDA MARIA'NA, *Broad-leaved Moorwort.* A decoction of this American plant is said to have been successfully employed as a wash, in a disagreeable affection,—not uncommon amongst the slaves in the southern parts of the United States,—called the *Toe Itch,* and *Ground Itch.*—Barton.
ANDROPOGON BICORNIS, Juncus odoratus —a. Citratus, Juncus odoratus—a. Citriodorus, Juncus odoratus, Nardus Indica—a. Nardus, Calamus Alexandrinus, Nardus Indica — a. Schœnanthus, Juncus odoratus.
ANDROSACE, Umbilicus marinus — a. Matthioli, Umbilicus marinus.
ANDROSÆMUM, Hypericum perforatum.
ANDROTOMY, Andranatomia.
ANDRUM. An East India word, latinized by Kæmpfer, signifying a kind of elephantiasis of the scrotum, endemic in southern Asia.
ANÉANTISSEMENT (F.), *Vir'ium extinc'tio.* This word is often employed hyperbolically, by patients in France, to signify excessive fatigue, debility or syncope.
ANEBIUM, Anchusa tinctoria.
ANEBUS, Impuber.
ANECPYE'TUS, from *εν,* for *ανευ,* 'without,' and *πυεω,* 'I promote suppuration.' That which does not suppurate, or is not likely to suppurate.
ANEGER'TICA, from *ανεγειρω,* 'I awaken.' The art of resuscitating the apparently dead.
ANEILE'MA, *Aneile'sis,* from *ανειλεσθαι,* 'to be rolled upwards.' Applied particularly to the motion of air in the intestines and the tormina accompanying it. — Hippocrates.
ANEILESIS, Aneilema.
ANEMIA, Anæmia.
ANEMO'NE. The *Wind Flower:* from *ανεμος,* 'the wind,' because it does not open its flowers until blown upon by the wind.
ANÉMONE DES BOIS, Anemone nemorosa.
ANEMONE COLLINA, A. Pulsatilla—a. Hepatica, Hepatica triloba—a. Intermedia, A. Pulsatilla.
ANEMO'NE NEMORO'SA, *Ranun'culus albus seu nemoro'sus, Wood anem'ony,* (F.) *Anémone des bois.* The herb and flowers are poisonous, acrid, and corrosive. They have been used as rubefacients.
ANEMO'NE PRATEN'SIS, *A. Sylves'tris, Pulsatil'la ni'gricans seu praten'sis.* This plant has si-

milar properties with the last. It is also called *Meadow Anemony*, (F.) *Pulsatille noire, P. des prés.*

ANEMO'NE PULSATILL'LA, *A. Colli'na* seu *Interme'dia* seu *Praten'sis* seu *Rubra, Pulsatil'la vulga'ris, Herba ventis, Nola culina'ria, Pasque flower*, (F.) *Coquelourde*, possesses like properties.

ANEMONE RUBRA, A. Pratensis—a. Rue-leaved, Thalictrum anemonoides—a. Sylvestris, A. Pratensis.

ANEMONY, Anemone hepatica—a. Meadow, Anemone pratensis—a. Wood, Anemone nemorosa.

ANEMOS, Wind.

ANENCEPHALIA, see Anencephalus.

ANENCÉPHALOTROPHIE, from *αν*, privative; *εγκεφαλος*, 'the encephalon,' and *τροφη*, 'nourishment.' Atrophy of the encephalon.

ANENCEPH'ALUS, from *a*, privative, and *εγκεφαλος*, 'brain.' A monster devoid of brain. —Bonetus. G. St. Hilaire. Also one that has a part only of the brain;—*Paraceph'alus*. The condition has been called *Anencephal'ia*. A weak, silly person.—Hippocrates.

ANENERGESIA, Debility.

ANENERGIA, Debility.

ANENTERONERVIA, Colic.

ANEPISCHESIS, Incontinentia.

ANEPITHYM'IA, from *α*, priv., and *επιθυμια*, 'desire.' Many nosologists have used this word for a loss of the appetites, as of those of hunger, thirst, venery, &c.

ANEPITHYMIA CHLOROSIS, Chlorosis.

ANER. *ανηρ*, genitive *ανορος*. A man.

ANERETHIS'IA, *Inirritabil'itas*, from *a*, priv., and *ερεθισις*, 'irritability.' Defect of irritability. —Swediaur.

ANERYTHROP'SIA, from *αν*, priv., *ερυθρος*, 'red,' and *οψις*, 'vision.' Defective vision, which consists in an incapability of distinguishing red.

ANESIS, Remission.

ANESTHÉSIE, Anæsthesia.

ANESTHÉSIE EXTATIQUE. The aggregate of phenomena of impaired feeling produced especially by the manipulations of the animal magnetizer.—Andral.

ANESTHETIC, Anæsthetic.

ANESTHÉSIQUE, Anæsthetic.

ANESTHETIZATION, Anæsthetization.

ANESON, Anethum.

ANESUM, Pimpinella anisum.

ANET, Anethum.

ANETH, Anethum graveolens.

ANE'THUM, *Ane'son, Ane'ton, Ane'thum Fœnic'ulum* seu *Sege'tum* seu *Piperi'tum, Fœnic'ulum, F. Officinale, F. vulga'ré, F. Dulcé, Ligus'ticum fœnic'ulum, Fan'culum, Fennel* or *Finckle, Mar'-athrum, Anet, Sweet Fennel*, (F.) *Fenouil* ou *Anis doux. Nat. Ord.* Umbelliferæ. *Sex. Syst.* Pentandria Digynia. The seeds *Fœnic'ulum*, (Ph. U. S.) have an aromatic odour, and warm, sweetish taste. They are carminative. The oil — *Oleum Fœnic'uli* — is officinal in the Ph.U. S. The root is said to be pectoral and diuretic.

ANETHUM FŒNICULUM, Anethum.

ANE'THUM GRAVEOLENS, *Anethum, Pastina'ca Anethum* seu *Graveolens, Fer'ula Graveolens, A. horten'sé, Dill*, (F.) *Aneth, Fenouil puant.* A native of the south of Europe. The seeds are stimulant and carminative. Dose, gr. xv to ʒj.

Oleum Ane'thi, Oil of Dill, (F.) *Huile d'Aneth*, possesses the carminative properties of the plant.

ANETHUM PASTINACA, Pastinaca Sativa—a. Piperitum, Anethum—a. Segetum, Anethum.

ANETICUS, Anodyne.

ANETON, Anethum.

ANETUS, Intermittent fever—a. Quartanus, Quartan—a. Quotidianus, Quotidian—a. Tertianus, Tertian fever.

ANEURAL'GICON, from *α*, privative, *νευρον*, 'nerve;' and *αλγος*, 'pain.' A name given by Dr. C. T. Downing to an instrument used by him to allay pain in nerves. It is a kind of fumigating apparatus, in which dried narcotic and other herbs are burnt, the heated vapour being directed to any part of the body.

AN'EURISM, *Aneurys'ma, Aneurys'mus, Aneuris'ma, Cedma*, from *ανευρυνειν*, 'to dilate or distend.' *Dilata'tio Arteria'rum, Ecta'sia, Embory'sma, Exangi'a aneuris'ma, Arterieurys'ma, Artereurys'ma, Hæmatoce'lē arterio'sa, Absces'sus spirituo'sus, Arterieo'tasis*, (F.) *Anévrysme, Aneurisme*. Properly, Aneurism signifies a tumour, produced by the dilatation of an artery; but it has been extended to various lesions of arteries, as well as to dilatations of the heart.

There are various kinds of aneurism. The following are the chief.

I. When the blood, which forms the tumour, is enclosed within the dilated coats of the artery. This is the TRUE ANEURISM, *Aneurys'ma verum, Hernia Arteria'rum*, (F.) *Anévrysme vrai.*

II. When the blood has escaped from the opened artery, it is called SPURIOUS or FALSE ANEURISM, *Aneuris'ma spu'rium, Ruptu'ra Arte'riæ, Arteriorrhex'is, Arteriodial'ysis, Ecchymo'ma arterio'sum*, (F.) *Anévrysme faux.* The latter is divided into three varieties.

1. *Diffused False Aneurism*, (F.) *Anévrysme faux, primitif, diffus, noncirconscrit* ou *par infiltration*, which occurs immediately after the division or rupture of an artery, and consists of an extravasation of blood into the areolar texture of the part.

2. *Circumscribed False Aneurism*, (F.) *Anévrysme, faux consécutif, circonscrit* ou *par épanchement, enkysté* ou *sacciforme, tumeur hémorrhagiale circonscrite*, in which the blood issues from the vessel some time after the receipt of the wound, and forms itself a sac in the neighbouring areolar membrane.

3. *An'eurism by Anastomo'sis*, or *Var'icose An'eurism, Phlebarteriodial'ysis, Aneurys'ma veno'-so-arterio'sum, A. varico'sum*, (F.) *Anévrysme par anastomose* ou *variqueux, A. par érosion, A. de* POTT, *A. des plus petites artères*, which arises from the simultaneous wounding of an artery and vein;—the arterial blood passing into the vein, and producing a varicose state of it.

III. MIXED ANEURISM, (F.) *Anévrysme mixte*, is that which arises from the dilatation of one or two of the coats, with division or rupture of the other. Some authors have made two varieties of this.

1. *Mixed external Aneurism*, where the internal and middle coats are ruptured, and the areolar is dilated.

2. *Mixed internal Aneurism*, in which the internal coat is dilated, and protrudes, like a hernial sac, through the ruptured middle and outer coats. This variety has been called *Aneurys'ma Her'niam Arte'riæ sistens.*

Aneurisms have been likewise termed *traumat'ic* and *sponta'neous*, according as they may have been caused by a wound, or have originated spontaneously. They have also been divided into *internal* and *external*.

The *internal aneurisms* are situate in the great splanchnic cavities, and occur in the heart and great vessels of the chest, abdomen, &c. Their diagnosis is difficult, and they are often inaccessible to surgical treatment.

The *external aneurisms* are situate at the exte-

rior of the head, neck, and limbs, and are distinctly pulsatory.

Aneurisms, especially the internal, may be combated by a debilitant treatment, on the plan of Valsalva, which consists in repeated bloodletting, with food enough merely to support life. In external aneurism, the artery can be obliterated. This is usually done by applying a ligature above the aneurismal tumour.

ANEURISM, DISSECTING, is one in which, owing to rupture of the inner and middle coats of an artery, the blood makes itself a channel between these coats and the outer coat.

In many cases, the lesion appears to consist in a separation of the laminæ of the middle coat, between which the blood forms itself a channel.

ANEURISMS OF THE HEART, *Cardion'chi, Cardieurys'ma*, (F.) *Anévrysmes du cœur*, have been divided into *active* and *passive*. The former can scarcely be esteemed aneurisms, as they most commonly consist of increased thickness of the parietes of the heart, which diminishes its cavity instead of increasing it. The term *Hypertrophy of the heart*, better indicates their character. *Passive aneurism, Oardiec'tasis*, on the contrary, is attended with extenuation of the parietes of the organ, and enlargement of the cavities. The physical signs of *dilatation of the heart* are the following:—The action of the heart is not visible, and no impulse is conveyed to the hand. On percussion, there is a loss of resonance over a larger surface than usual, but the dulness is much less intense than that which accompanies hypertrophy. On auscultation, the action of the heart is only slightly felt, and communicates at once the impression of its diminished power. The impulse is feebler than usual. Both sounds are widely transmitted over the thorax, and are not much fainter at a distance from their point of origin.

Partial or *true aneurism of the heart—Cardiec'tasis partia'lis, Aneurys'ma consecuti'vum cordis*, is sometimes seen,—rarely, however.

The name *Aneurism of the Valves of the heart* has been given to pouch-like projections of the valves into the auricles.

ANEURISM BY ANASTOMOSIS, see Aneurism—a. Brasdor's operation for, see Brasdor—a. External, see Aneurism—a. False, see Aneurism—a. False, circumscribed, see Aneurism—a. False, diffused, see Aneurism—a. Internal, see Aneurism—a. Mixed, see Aneurism—a. Mixed, external, see Aneurism—a. Mixed, internal, see Aneurism—a. Spontaneous, see Aneurism—a. Spurious, see Aneurism—a. Traumatic, see Aneurism—a. True, see Aneurism—a. Valsalva's method of treating, see Aneurism—a. Varicose, see Aneurism.

ANEURISMA, Aneurism.

ANEURIS'MAL, *Aneurys'mal, Aneurismat'ic, Aneurysmat'ious, Aneurisma'lis*. That which belongs to Aneurism.

ANEURISMAL SAC or CYST, (F.) *Sac ou Kyste anévrysmal*, is a sort of pouch, formed by the dilatation of the coats of an artery, in which the blood, forming the aneurismal tumour, is contained.

ANEURISMATIC, Aneurismal.
ANEURYSM, Aneurism.
ANEURYSMA, Aneurism—a. Cordis activum, Heart, hypertrophy of the—a. Herniam arteriæ sistens, see Aneurism—a. Spurium, see Aneurism—a. Varicosum, see Aneurism—a. Venoso-arteriosum, see Aneurism—a. Verum, see Aneurism.
ANEURYSME, Aneurism.
ANEURYSMUS, Aneurism, Dilatation.
ANÉVRYSME, Aneurism — a. de l'Aorte, Aorteurysma—a. *Circonscrit*, see Aneurism—a. *de Pott*, see Aneurism—a. *des Plus petites artères*, see Aneurism—a. *Diffus*, see Aneurism—a. *Enkysté*, see Aneurism—a. *Faux*, see Aneurism—a. *Faux consécutif*, see Aneurism—a. *Mixte*, see Aneurism—a. *par Anastomose*, see Aneurism—a. *par Épanchement*, see Aneurism—a. *par Érosion*, see Aneurism—a. *par Infiltration*, see Aneurism a. *Primitif*, see Aneurism—a. *Sacciforme*, see Aneurism—a. *Variqueux*, see Aneurism—a. *Vrai*, see Aneurism.

ANFION, Maslach.

ANFRACTUOSITÉS CÉRÉBRALES, Anfractuosities, cerebral—a. *Ethmoïdales*, see Anfractuosity.

ANFRACTUOS'ITY, *Anfrac'tus, Gyrus*, from *am*, 'around,' and *frangere, fractum*, 'to break.' A groove or furrow. Used in anatomy to signify sinuous depressions or *sulci*, of greater or less depth, like those which separate the convolutions of the brain from each other. These

ANFRACTUOSITIES, CEREBRAL, *Anfrac'tus Cer'ebri, Gyri Cer'ebri, Intestin'ula Cer'ebri*, (F.) *Anfractuosités Cérébrales*, are always narrow, and deeper at the upper surface of the brain than at its base; and are lined by a prolongation of the pia mater.

The Ethmoid Cells are, sometimes, called *Anfractuosités ethmoïdales*.

ANFRACTUS, Anfractuosity—a. Cerebri, Anfractuosities (cerebral.)

ANGECTASIA, Angiectasis.
ANGEIAL, Vascular.
ANGEIECTASIA, Angiectasis.
ANGEIECTASIS, Angiectasis.
ANGEIECTOMA, Angiectasis.
ANGEIOG'RAPHY, *Angiog'raphy, Angeiograph'ia*, from αγγειον, 'a vessel,' and γραφη, 'a description.' The anatomy of the vessels.

ANGEIOHYDROG'RAPHY, *Angiohydrog'raphy, Angeiondrog'raphy, Angeiohydrogra'phia, Hydrangiograph'ia*, from αγγειον, 'a vessel,' 'υδωρ, 'water,' and γραφω, 'I describe.' A treatise on the lymphatics.

ANGEIOHYDROT'OMY, *Angiohydrot'omy, Angeiondrot'omy, Angeiohydrotom'ia, Hydrangiotom'ia*, from αγγειον, 'a vessel,' 'υδωρ, 'water,' and τεμνω, 'to cut.' Dissection of the lymphatics.

ANGEIOLEUCI'TIS, *Angioleuci'tis, Lymphangei'tis, Lymphangi'tis, Lymphangioi'tis, Hydrangei'tis, Lymphi'tis, Lymphati'tis, Inflamma'tio vaso'rum lymphatico'rum*, from αγγειον, 'a vessel,' λευκος, 'white,' and *itis*, inflammation. (F.) *Inflammation des vaisseaux lymphatiques* ou *des tissus blancs*. Inflammation of the lymphatics: lymphatic or scrofulous inflammation.

ANGEIOL'OGY, *Angiol'ogy, Angeiolog''ia*, from αγγειον, 'a vessel,' and λογος, 'a discourse.' A discourse on the vessels. The anatomy of the vessels. It includes *Arteriol'ogy, Phlebol'ogy*, and *Angeiohydrol'ogy*.

ANGEIOMALA'CIA, *Angiomala'cia*; from αγγειον, 'a vessel,' and μαλακια, 'softening.' Mollescence or softening of vessels.

ANGEIOMYCES, Hæmatodes fungus.
ANGEION, Vessel.
ANGEIONDROGRAPHY, Angeiohydrography.
ANGEIONDROTOMY, Angeiohydrotomy.
ANGEIONOSUS, Angeiopathia.
ANGEIONUSUS, Angeiopathia.
ANGEIOPATHI'A, *Angiopathi'a, Angeion'osus, Angeionu'sus, Angio'sis*, from αγγειον, 'a vessel,' and παθος, 'a disease.' Disease of the vessels.

ANGEIOPLEROSIS, Plethora.
ANGEIOPYRA, Synocha.
ANGEIORRHAGIA, Hæmorrhagia activa.
ANGEIORRHŒ'A, (F.) *Angeiorrhée*; from

αγγειον, 'a vessel,' and ρεω, 'I flow.' Passive hemorrhage.
ANGEIOSIS, Angiosis.
ANGEIOSTEGNOSIS, Angiemphraxis.
ANGEIOSTENOSIS, Angiemphraxis.
ANGEIOSTEO'SIS, *Angiosto'sis*, from αγγειον, 'a vessel,' and οστεωσις, 'ossification.' Ossification of vessels.
ANGEIOSTROPHE, see Torsion.
ANGEIOTELECTASIA, Telangiectasia.
ANGEIOT'OMY, *Angiot'omy*, *Angeioton'ia*, from αγγειον, 'a vessel,' and τεμνειν, 'to cut.' Dissection of vessels.
ANGEI'TIS, *Angii'tis*, *Angioi'tis*, *Inflamma'tio vaso'rum*, (F.) *Angéite*. Inflammation of vessels in general.
ANGELIC ROOT, Angelica lucida.
ANGEL'ICA, *Angel'ica Archangel'ica* seu *Hispa'na* seu *Sati'va*, *Archangel'ica officina'lis*, *Garden Angelica*, (F.) *Angélique*, *Racine de Saint Esprit*. So called from its supposed angelic virtues. *Nat. Ord.* Umbelliferæ. *Sex. Syst.* Pentandria Digynia. Native of Lapland. The roots, stalk, leaves, and seed, are aromatic and carminative. A sweetmeat is made of the root, which is agreeable.
ANGELICA ARCHANGELICA, Angelica.
ANGEL'ICA ATROPURPU'REA, *Angelica* (Ph. U. S.) *Masterwort*. An indigenous species, growing over the whole United States, and admitted into the secondary list of the Pharmacopœia of the United States. Virtues, same as those of the Angelica of Europe.
ANGELICA LEVISTICUM, Ligusticum levisticum.
ANGELICA LU'CIDA, *Angelic root*, *Bellyache root*, *Nendo*, *White root*, an indigenous plant, the root of which is bitterish, subacrid, fragrant, aromatic, stomachic, and tonic.
ANGELICA OFFICINALIS, Imperatoria—a. Paludapifolia, Ligusticum levisticum—a. Sativa, Angelica, A. sylvestris.
ANGEL'ICA SYLVES'TRIS, *A. sati'va*, *Seli'num Sylves'trě* seu *Angel'ica* seu *Pubes'cens*, *Imperato'ria Sylves'tres* seu *Angelica*, *Wild Angel'ica*, (F.) *Angélique sauvage*. Possesses similar properties to the last, but in an inferior degree. The seeds, powdered and put into the hair, are used to destroy lice.
ANGELICA SYLVESTRIS, Ligusticum podagraria —a. Tree, Aralia spinosa.
ANGELI'NÆ CORTEX. The bark of a Grenada tree, which has been recommended as anthelmintic and cathartic.
ANGÉLIQUE, Angelica—a. *Sauvage*, Angelica sylvestris.
ANGELOCACOS, Myrobalanus.
ANGEMPHRAXIS, Angiemphraxis.
ANGIDIECTASIA, Trichangiectasia.
ANGIDIOSPONGUS, Hæmatodes fungus.
ANGIECTASIA VENOSA, Varix
ANGIEC'TASIS, *Angiecta'sia*, *Angecta'sia*, *Angieurys'ma*, *Angeiecto'ma*, from αγγειον, 'a vessel,' and εκτασις, 'dilatation.' Any dilatation of vessels.—Gräfe and Alibert. *Telangiectasia*.
ANGIEMPHRAX'IS, *Angemphrax'is*, *Angiosteno'sis*, *Angeiostegno'sis*, from αγγειον, 'a vessel,' and εμφραξις, 'obstruction.' Obstruction of vessels.
ANGIEURYSMA, Angiectasis.
ANGIITE, Inflammation, Angeitis.
ANGIITIS, Angeitis.
ANGI'NA, *Febris Angino'sa*, *Isthmi'tis*, *Quinsy* or *Sore Throat*; from *angere*, 'to suffocate.' Inflammation of the supra-diaphragmatic portion of the alimentary canal, and of the air passages. The Latin writers applied the term to every disease in which deglutition or respiration, separately or united, was affected, provided that such affection was above the stomach and lungs.— Boerhaave speaks of the angina of the moribund, which is nothing more than the dysphagia or difficult deglutition preceding death. See Cynanche.

ANGINA APHTHOSA, Aphthæ—a. Arnosa, Œdema of the glottis—a. Bronchialis, Bronchitis—a. Canina, Cynanche trachealis—a. Cordis, Angina pectoris—a. cum Tumore, Cynanche tonsillaris— a. Epidemica, Cynanche maligna—a. Epiglottidea, Epiglottitis—a. Erysipelatosa, Erythrarche —a. Exudatoria, Cynanche trachealis—a. Externa, Cynanche parotidæa—a. Faucium, Isthmitis—a. Faucium Maligna, Cynanche maligna—a. Felliculosa of the pharynx, Pharyngitis follicular—a. Gangrænosa, Cynanche maligna—a. Humida, Cynanche trachealis—a. Inflammatoria, Cynanche, Cynanche trachealis—a. Laryngea, Laryngitis —a. Laryngea Œdematosa, Œdema of the glottis—a. Linguaria, Glossitis—a. Maligna, Angina pellicularis, Cynanche maligna, Pharyngitis, diphtheritic—a. Maxillaris, Cynanche parotidæa —a. Membranacea, Cynanche trachealis—a. Mitis, Isthmitis.
ANGI'NA NASA'LIS, *Nasi'tis posti'ca*. An inflammation of the posterior portion of the Schneiderian membrane lining the nose. Also, Coryza.
ANGI'NA ŒDEMATO'SA, (F.) *Angine œdémateuse*, *Œdème de la Glotte*. An œdematous swelling of the glottis: the effect of chronic cynanche laryngea. See Œdema of the Glottis.
ANGINA PALATINA, Hyperoitis—a. Paralytica, Pharyngoplegia—a. Parotidæa Externa, Cynanche parotidæa.
ANGI'NA PEC'TORIS, *A. cordis*, *Sternal'gia*, *Asthma spas'tico-arthrit'icum incon'stans*, *Asthma diaphragmat'icum*, *Arthri'tis diaphragmatica*, *Orthopnæ'a cardi'aca*, *Sternodyn'ia syncop'tica et pal'pitans*, *S. syncopa'lis*, *Cardiog'mus cordis sinis'tri*, *Astheni'a pectora'lis*, *Angor pec'toris*, *Stenocar'dia*, *Diaphragmat'ic gout*. *Asthma convulsi'vum*, *Asthma arthrit'icum*, *Cardioneural'gia*, *Nearal'gia brachiothorac'ica*, *Hyperæsthe'sia plexus cardi'aci*, *A. dolorif'icum*, *Syn'copē angino'sa* seu *angens*, *Cardiod'ynē spasmod'ica intermit'tens*, *Pnigopho'bia*, *Prunel'la*, *Suspir'ium cardi'acum*, *Pneumonal'gia*, *Suffocative Breastpang*, (F.) *Angine de Poitrine*, *Névrose du Cœur*. A disease, the precise pathology of which is not known. The principal symptoms are, violent pain about the sternum, extending towards the arms; anxiety, dyspnœa, and sense of suffocation. It is an affection of great danger, and is often connected with ossification, or other morbid condition of the heart. It appears to be neuropathic, and has been termed *Neuralgia of the Heart*. Some, however, employ this last term for an acutely painful intermittent affection of the heart, which seems to differ from angina pectoris more in regard to the small number of parts which are drawn into morbid consent with the affected cardiac nerves, than in regard either to its nature or appropriate treatment. The most powerful stimulating and narcotic antispasmodics are required during the paroxysm.
ANGI'NA PELLICULA'RIS, *A. malig'na*, *Diptheri'tis of the throat*. A name given to those inflammations about the throat, in which exudations or false membranes are thrown out, during the phlogosis of the mucous membranes. *Aphthæ*, *Tracheitis*, when accompanied with the membraniform exudation, are, with some, examples of diphtheritic inflammation.
ANGINA PERNICIOSA, Cynanche trachealis—a. Pestilentialis, Pharyngitis, diphtheritio—a. Polyposa, Cynanche trachealis—a. Polyposa seu membranacea, Cynanche trachealis—a. Pseudo-membranosa, Pharyngitis, diphtheritic—a. Pulposa,

rior of the head, neck, and limbs, and are distinctly pulsatory.

Aneurisms, especially the internal, may be combated by a debilitant treatment, on the plan of Valsalva, which consists in repeated bloodletting, with food enough merely to support life. In external aneurism, the artery can be obliterated. This is usually done by applying a ligature above the aneurismal tumour.

ANEURISM, DISSECTING, is one in which, owing to rupture of the inner and middle coats of an artery, the blood makes itself a channel between these coats and the outer coat.

In many cases, the lesion appears to consist in a separation of the laminæ of the middle coat, between which the blood forms itself a channel.

ANEURISMS OF THE HEART, *Cardion'chi, Cardieurys'ma,* (F.) *Anévrysmes du cœur,* have been divided into *active* and *passive.* The former can scarcely be esteemed aneurisms, as they most commonly consist of increased thickness of the parietes of the heart, which diminishes its cavity instead of increasing it. The term *Hypertrophy of the heart,* better indicates their character. *Passive aneurism, Cardiec'tasis,* on the contrary, is attended with extenuation of the parietes of the organ, and enlargement of the cavities. The physical signs of *dilatation of the heart* are the following:—The action of the heart is not visible, and no impulse is conveyed to the hand. On percussion, there is a loss of resonance over a larger surface than usual, but the dulness is much less intense than that which accompanies hypertrophy. On auscultation, the action of the heart is only slightly felt, and communicates at once the impression of its diminished power. The impulse is feebler than usual. Both sounds are widely transmitted over the thorax, and are not much fainter at a distance from their point of origin.

Partial or *true aneurism of the heart—Cardiec'tasis partia'lis, Aneurys'ma consecuti'vum cordis,* is sometimes seen,—rarely, however.

The name *Aneurism of the Valves of the heart* has been given to pouch-like projections of the valves into the auricles.

ANEURISM BY ANASTOMOSIS, see Aneurism—a. Brasdor's operation for, see Brasdor—a. External, see Aneurism—a. False, see Aneurism—a. False, circumscribed, see Aneurism—a. False, diffused, see Aneurism—a. Internal, see Aneurism—a. Mixed, see Aneurism—a. Mixed, external, see Aneurism—a. Mixed, internal, see Aneurism—a. Spontaneous, see Aneurism—a. Spurious, see Aneurism—a. Traumatic, see Aneurism—a. True, see Aneurism—a. Valsalva's method of treating, see Aneurism—a. Varicose, see Aneurism.

ANEURISMA, Aneurism.

ANEURIS'MAL, *Aneurys'mal, Aneurismat'ic, Aneurysmat'icus, Aneurisma'lis.* That which belongs to Aneurism.

ANEURISMAL SAC or CYST, (F.) *Sac* ou *Kyste anévrysmal,* is a sort of pouch, formed by the dilatation of the coats of an artery, in which the blood, forming the aneurismal tumour, is contained.

ANEURISMATIC, Aneurismal.

ANEURYSM, Aneurism.

ANEURYSMA, Aneurism—a. Cordis activum, Heart, hypertrophy of the—a. Herniam arteriæ sistens, see Aneurism—a. Spurium, see Aneurism—a. Varicosum, see Aneurism—a. Venoso-arteriosum, see Aneurism—a. Verum, see Aneurism.

ANÉURYSME, Aneurism.

ANEURYSMUS, Aneurism, Dilatation.

ANÉVRYSME, Aneurism—a. *de l'Aorte,* Aorteurysma—a. *Circonscrit,* see Aneurism—a. *de Pott,* see Aneurism—a. *des Plus petites artères,* see Aneurism—a. *Diffus,* see Aneurism—a. *Enkysté,* see Aneurism—a. *Faux,* see Aneurism—a. *Faux consécutif,* see Aneurism—a. *Mixte,* see Aneurism—a. *par Anastomose,* see Aneurism—a. *par Épanchement,* see Aneurism—a. *par Érosion,* see Aneurism—a. *par Infiltration,* see Aneurism a. *Primitif,* see Aneurism—a. *Sacciforme,* see Aneurism—a. *Variqueux,* see Aneurism—a. *Vrai,* see Aneurism.

ANFION, Maslach.

ANFRACTUOSITÉS CÉRÉBRALES, Anfractuosities, cerebral—a. *Ethmoïdales,* see Anfractuosity.

ANFRACTUOS'ITY, *Anfrac'tus, Gyrus,* from *am,* 'around,' and *frangere, fractum,* 'to break.' A groove or furrow. Used in anatomy to signify sinuous depressions or *sulci,* of greater or less depth, like those which separate the convolutions of the brain from each other. These

ANFRACTUOSITIES, CEREBRAL, *Anfrac'tus Cer'ebri, Gyri Cer'ebri, Intestin'ula Cer'ebri,* (F.) *Anfractuosités Cérébrales,* are always narrow, and deeper at the upper surface of the brain than at its base; and are lined by a prolongation of the pia mater.

The Ethmoid Cells are, sometimes, called *Anfractuosités ethmoïdales.*

ANFRACTUS, Anfractuosity—a. Cerebri, Anfractuosities (cerebral.)

ANGECTASIA, Angiectasis.

ANGEIAL, Vascular.

ANGEIECTASIA, Angiectasis.

ANGEIECTASIS, Angiectasis.

ANGEIECTOMA, Angiectasis.

ANGEIOG'RAPHY, *Angiog'raphy, Angeiograph'ia,* from αγγειον, 'a vessel,' and γραφη, 'a description.' The anatomy of the vessels.

ANGEIOHYDROG'RAPHY, *Angiohydrog'raphy, Angeiondrog'raphy, Angeiohydrogra'phia, Hydrangiograph'ia,* from αγγειον, 'a vessel,' ὑδωρ, 'water,' and γραφω, 'I describe.' A treatise on the lymphatics.

ANGEIOHYDROT'OMY, *Angiohydrot'omy, Angeiondrot'omy, Angeiohydrotom'ia, Hydrangiotom'ia,* from αγγειον, 'a vessel,' ὑδωρ, 'water,' and τεμειν, 'to cut.' Dissection of the lymphatics.

ANGEIOLEUCI'TIS, *Angioleuci'tis, Lymphangei'tis, Lymphangi'tis, Lymphangoi'tis, Hydrangei'tis, Lymphi'tis, Lymphati'tis, Inflamma'tio vaso'rum lymphatico'rum,* from αγγειον, 'a vessel,' λευκος, 'white,' and *itis,* inflammation. (F.) *Inflammation des vaisseaux lymphatiques* ou *des tissus blancs.* Inflammation of the lymphatics: lymphatic or scrofulous inflammation.

ANGEIOL'OGY, *Angiol'ogy, Angeiolog''ia,* from αγγειον, 'a vessel,' and λογος, 'a discourse.' A discourse on the vessels. The anatomy of the vessels. It includes *Arteriol'ogy, Phlebol'ogy,* and *Angeiohydrol'ogy.*

ANGEIOMALA'CIA, *Angiomala'cia ;* from αγγειον, 'a vessel,' and μαλακια, 'softening.' Mollescence or softening of vessels.

ANGEIOMYCES, Hæmatodes fungus.

ANGEION, Vessel.

ANGEIONDROGRAPHY, Angeiohydrography.

ANGEIONDROTOMY, Angeiohydrotomy.

ANGEIONOSUS, Angeiopathia.

ANGEIONUSUS, Angeiopathia.

ANGEIOPATHI'A, *Angiopathi'a, Angeion'osus, Angeionu'sus, Angio'sis,* from αγγειον, 'a vessel,' and παθος, 'a disease.' Disease of the vessels.

ANGEIOPLEROSIS, Plethora.

ANGEIOPYRA, Synocha.

ANGEIORRHAGIA, Hæmorrhagia activa.

ANGEIORRHŒ'A, (F.) *Angeiorrhée ;* from

αγγειον, 'a vessel,' and ρεω, 'I flow.' Passive hemorrhage.

ANGEIOSIS, Angiosis.
ANGEIOSTEGNOSIS, Angiemphraxis.
ANGEIOSTENOSIS, Angiemphraxis.
ANGEIOSTEO'SIS, *Angiosto'sis*, from αγγειον, 'a vessel,' and οστεωσις, 'ossification.' Ossification of vessels.
ANGEIOSTROPHE, see Torsion.
ANGEIOTELECTASIA, Telangiectasia.
ANGEIOT'OMY, *Angiot'omy*, *Angeiotom'ia*, from αγγειον, 'a vessel,' and τεμνειν, 'to cut.' Dissection of vessels.
ANGEI'TIS, *Angii'tis*, *Angioi'tis*, *Inflamma'tio vaso'rum*, (F.) *Angéite*. Inflammation of vessels in general.
ANGELIC ROOT, Angelica lucida.
ANGEL'ICA, *Angel'ica Archangel'ica* seu *Hispa'na* seu *Sati'va*, *Archangel'ica officina'lis*, *Garden Angelica*, (F.) *Angélique, Racine de Saint Esprit*. So called from its supposed angelic virtues. *Nat. Ord.* Umbelliferæ. *Sex. Syst.* Pentandria Digynia. Native of Lapland. The roots, stalk, leaves, and seed, are aromatic and carminative. A sweetmeat is made of the root, which is agreeable.
ANGELICA ARCHANGELICA, Angelica.
ANGEL'ICA ATROPURPU'REA, *Angelica* (Ph. U. S.) *Masterwort*. An indigenous species, growing over the whole United States, and admitted into the secondary list of the Pharmacopœia of the United States. Virtues, same as those of the Angelica of Europe.
ANGELICA LEVISTICUM, Ligusticum levisticum.
ANGELICA LU'CIDA, *Angelic root*, *Bellyache root*, *Nendo*, *White root*, an indigenous plant, the root of which is bitterish, subacrid, fragrant, aromatic, stomachic, and tonic.
ANGELICA OFFICINALIS, Imperatoria—a. Paludapifolia, Ligusticum levisticum—a. Sativa, Angelica, A. sylvestris.
ANGEL'ICA SYLVES'TRIS, *A. sati'va*, *Seli'num Sylves'tré* seu *Angel'ica* seu *Pubes'cens*, *Imperato'ria Sylves'tres* seu *Angelica*, *Wild Angel'ica*, (F.) *Angélique sauvage*. Possesses similar properties to the last, but in an inferior degree. The seeds, powdered and put into the hair, are used to destroy lice.
ANGELICA SYLVESTRIS, Ligusticum podagraria —a. Tree, Aralia spinosa.
ANGELI'NÆ CORTEX. The bark of a Grenada tree, which has been recommended as anthelmintic and cathartic.
ANGÉLIQUE, Angelica—a. *Sauvage*, Angelica sylvestris.
ANGELOCACOS, Myrobalanus.
ANGEMPHRAXIS, Angiemphraxis.
ANGIDIECTASIA, Trichangiectasia.
ANGIDIOSPONGUS, Hæmatodes fungus.
ANGIECTASIA VENOSA, Varix
ANGIEC'TASIS, *Angeiecta'sia*, *Angecta'sia*, *Angieurys'ma*, *Angeiecto'ma*, from αγγειον, 'a vessel,' and εκτασις, 'dilatation.' Any dilatation of vessels.—Gräfe and Alibert. *Telangiectasia*.
ANGIEMPHRAX'IS, *Angemphrax'is*, *Angeiosteno'sis*, *Angeiostegno'sis*, from αγγειον, 'a vessel,' and εμφραξις, 'obstruction.' Obstruction of vessels.
ANGIEURYSMA, Angiectasis.
ANGIITE, Inflammation, Angeitis.
ANGIITIS, Angeitis.
ANGI'NA, *Febris Angino'sa*, *Isthmi'tis*, *Quinsy* or *Sore Throat*; from *angere*, 'to suffocate.' Inflammation of the supra-diaphragmatic portion of the alimentary canal, and of the air passages. The Latin writers applied the term to every disease in which deglutition or respiration, separately or united, was affected, provided that such

affection was above the stomach and lungs.— Boerhaave speaks of the angina of the moribund, which is nothing more than the dysphagia or difficult deglutition preceding death. See Cynanche.

ANGINA APHTHOSA, Aphthæ—a. Aquosa, Œdema of the glottis—a. Bronchialis, Bronchitis—a. Canina, Cynanche trachealis—a. Cordis, Angina pectoris—a. cum Tumore, Cynanche tonsillaris—a. Epidemica, Cynanche maligna—a. Epiglottidea, Epiglottitis—a. Erysipelatosa, Erythranche a. Exudatoria, Cynanche trachealis—a. Externa, Cynanche parotidæa—a. Faucium, Isthmitis—a. Faucium Maligna, Cynanche maligna—a. Folliculosa of the pharynx, Pharyngitis, follicular—a. Gangrænosa, Cynanche maligna—a. Humida, Cynanche trachealis—a. Inflammatoria, Cynanche, Cynanche trachealis—a. Laryngea, Laryngitis—a. Laryngea Œdematosa, Œdema of the glottis—a. Linguaria, Glossitis—a. Maligna, Angina pellicularis, Cynanche maligna, Pharyngitis, diphtheritic—a. Maxillaris, Cynanche parotidæa —a. Membranacea, Cynanche trachealis—a. Mitis, Isthmitis.

ANGI'NA NASA'LIS, *Nasi'tis posti'ca*. An inflammation of the posterior portion of the Schneiderian membrane lining the nose. Also, Coryza.

ANGI'NA ŒDEMATO'SA, (F.) *Angine œdémateuse*, *Œdème de la Glotte*. An œdematous swelling of the glottis; the effect of chronic cynanche laryngea. See Œdema of the Glottis.

ANGINA PALATINA, Hyperoitis—a. Paralytica, Pharyngoplegia—a. Parotidæa Externa, Cynanche parotidæa.

ANGI'NA PEC'TORIS, *A. cordis*, *Sternal'gia*, *Asthma spas'tico-arthrit'icum incon'stans*, *Asthma diaphragmat'icum*, *Arthri'tis diaphragmatica*, *Orthopnœ'a cardi'aca*, *Sternodyn'ia syncop'tica et pal'pitans*, *S. syncopa'lis*, *Cardiog'mus cordis sinis'tri*, *Astheni'a pectora'lis*, *Angor pec'toris*, *Stenocar'dia*, *Diaphragmat'ic gout*. *Asthma convulsi'vum*, *Asthma arthrit'icum*, *Cardioneural'gia*, *Nearul'gia brachiothorac''ica*, *Hyperæsthe'sia plexus cardi'aci*, *A. dolorif'icum*, *Syn'copé angino'sa* seu *angens*, *Cardiod'ynē spasmod'ica intermit'tens*, *Pnigopho'bia*, *Prunel'la*, *Suspir'ium cardi'acum*, *Pneumonal'gia*, *Suff'ocative Breastpang*, (F.) *Angine de Poitrine*, *Névrose du Cœur*. A disease, the precise pathology of which is not known. The principal symptoms are, violent pain about the sternum, extending towards the arms; anxiety, dyspnœa, and sense of suffocation. It is an affection of great danger, and is often connected with ossification, or other morbid condition of the heart. It appears to be neuropathic, and has been termed *Neuralgia of the Heart*. Some, however, employ this last term for an acutely painful intermittent affection of the heart, which seems to differ from angina pectoris more in regard to the small number of parts which are drawn into morbid consent with the affected cardiac nerves, than in regard either to its nature or appropriate treatment. The most powerful stimulating and narcotic antispasmodics are required during the paroxysm.

ANGI'NA PELLICULA'RIS, *A. malig'na*, *Diphtheri'tis of the throat*. A name given to those inflammations about the throat, in which exudations or false membranes are thrown out, during the phlogosis of the mucous membranes. *Aphthæ*, *Tracheitis*, when accompanied with the membraniform exudation, are, with some, examples of diphtheritic inflammation.

ANGINA PERNICIOSA, Cynanche trachealis—a. Pestilentialis, Pharyngitis, diphtheritic—a. Polyposa, Cynanche trachealis—a. Polyposa seu membranacea, Cynanche trachealis—a. Pseudo-membranosa, Pharyngitis, diphtheritic—a. Pulposa.

rior of the head, neck, and limbs, and are distinctly pulsatory.

Aneurisms, especially the internal, may be combated by a debilitant treatment, on the plan of Valsalva, which consists in repeated bloodletting, with food enough merely to support life. In external aneurism, the artery can be obliterated. This is usually done by applying a ligature above the aneurismal tumour.

ANEURISM, DISSECTING, is one in which, owing to rupture of the inner and middle coats of an artery, the blood makes itself a channel between these coats and the outer coat.

In many cases, the lesion appears to consist in a separation of the laminæ of the middle coat, between which the blood forms itself a channel.

ANEURISMS OF THE HEART, *Cardion'chi, Cardieurys'ma,* (F.) *Anévrysmes du cœur,* have been divided into *active* and *passive.* The former can scarcely be esteemed aneurisms, as they most commonly consist of increased thickness of the parietes of the heart, which diminishes its cavity instead of increasing it. The term *Hypertrophy of the heart,* better indicates their character. *Passive aneurism, Cardiec'tasis,* on the contrary, is attended with extenuation of the parietes of the organ, and enlargement of the cavities. The physical signs of *dilatation of the heart* are the following:—The action of the heart is not visible, and no impulse is conveyed to the hand. On percussion, there is a loss of resonance over a larger surface than usual, but the dulness is much less intense than that which accompanies hypertrophy. On auscultation, the action of the heart is only slightly felt, and communicates at once the impression of its diminished power. The impulse is feebler than usual. Both sounds are widely transmitted over the thorax, and are not much fainter at a distance from their point of origin.

Partial or *true aneurism of the heart*—*Cardiec'tasis partia'lis, Aneurys'ma consecuti'vum cordis,* is sometimes seen,—rarely, however.

The name *Aneurism of the Valves of the heart* has been given to pouch-like projections of the valves into the auricles.

ANEURISM BY ANASTOMOSIS, see Aneurism—a. Brasdor's operation for, see Brasdor—a. External, see Aneurism—a. False, see Aneurism—a. False, circumscribed, see Aneurism—a. False, diffused, see Aneurism—a. Internal, see Aneurism—a. Mixed, see Aneurism—a. Mixed, external, see Aneurism—a. Mixed, internal, see Aneurism—a. Spontaneous, see Aneurism—a. Spurious, see Aneurism—a. Traumatic, see Aneurism—a. True, see Aneurism—a. Valsalva's method of treating, see Aneurism—a. Varicose, see Aneurism.

ANEURISMA, Aneurism.

ANEURIS'MAL, *Aneurys'mal, Aneurismat'ic, Aneurysmat'icus, Aneurisma'lis.* That which belongs to Aneurism.

ANEURISMAL SAC or CYST, (F.) *Sac ou Kyste anévrysmal,* is a sort of pouch, formed by the dilatation of the coats of an artery, in which the blood, forming the aneurismal tumour, is contained.

ANEURISMATIC, Aneurismal.

ANEURYSM, Aneurism.

ANEURYSMA, Aneurism—a. Cordis activum, Heart, hypertrophy of the—a. Herniam arteriæ sistens, see Aneurism—a. Spurium, see Aneurism—a. Varicosum, see Aneurism—a. Venoso-arteriosum, see Aneurism—a. Verum, see Aneurism.

ANEURYSME, Aneurism.

ANEURYSMUS, Aneurism, Dilatation.

ANÉVRYSME, Aneurism—a. *de l'Aorte, Aorteurysma*—a. *Circonscrit,* see Aneurism—a. *de Pott,* see Aneurism—a. *des Plus petites artères,* see Aneurism—a. *Diffus,* see Aneurism—a. *Enkysté,* see Aneurism—a. *Faux,* see Aneurism—a. *Faux consécutif,* see Aneurism—a. *Mixte,* see Aneurism—a. *par Anastomose,* see Aneurism—a. *par Épanchement,* see Aneurism—a. *par Érosion,* see Aneurism—a. *par Infiltration,* see Aneurism a. *Primitif,* see Aneurism—a. *Sacciforme,* see Aneurism—a. *Variqueux,* see Aneurism—a. *Vrai,* see Aneurism.

ANFION, Maslach.

ANFRACTUOSITÉS CÉRÉBRALES, Anfractuosities, cerebral—a. *Ethmoïdales,* see Anfractuosity.

ANFRACTUOS'ITY, *Anfrac'tus, Gyrus,* from *am,* 'around,' and *frangere, fractum,* 'to break.' A groove or furrow. Used in anatomy to signify sinuous depressions or *sulci,* of greater or less depth, like those which separate the convolutions of the brain from each other. These

ANFRACTUOSITIES, CEREBRAL, *Anfrac'tus Cer'ebri, Gyri Cer'ebri, Intestin'ula Cer'ebri,* (F.) *Anfractuosités Cérébrales,* are always narrow, and deeper at the upper surface of the brain than at its base; and are lined by a prolongation of the pia mater.

The Ethmoid Cells are, sometimes, called *Anfractuosités ethmoïdales.*

ANFRACTUS, Anfractuosity—a. Cerebri, Anfractuosities (cerebral.)

ANGECTASIA, Angiectasis.

ANGEIAL, Vascular.

ANGEIECTASIA, Angiectasis.

ANGEIECTASIS, Angiectasis.

ANGEIECTOMA, Angiectasis.

ANGEIOG'RAPHY, *Angiog'raphy, Angeiograph'ia,* from αγγειον, 'a vessel,' and γραφη, 'a description.' The anatomy of the vessels.

ANGEIOHYDROG'RAPHY, *Angiohydrog'raphy, Angeiondrog'raphy, Angeiohydrogra'phia, Hydrangiograph'ia,* from αγγειον, 'a vessel,' ὑδωρ, 'water,' and γραφω, 'I describe.' A treatise on the lymphatics.

ANGEIOHYDROT'OMY, *Angiohydrot'omy, Angeiondrot'omy, Angeiohydrotom'ia, Hydrangiotom'ia,* from αγγειον, 'a vessel,' ὑδωρ, 'water,' and τεμνειν, 'to cut.' Dissection of the lymphatics.

ANGEIOLEUCI'TIS, *Angioleuci'tis, Lymphangei'tis, Lymphangi'tis, Lymphangioi'tis, Hydrangei'tis, Lymphi'tis, Lymphati'tis, Inflamma'tio vaso'rum lymphatico'rum,* from αγγειον, 'a vessel,' λευκος, 'white,' and *itis,* inflammation. (F.) *Inflammation des vaisseaux lymphatiques ou des tissus blancs.* Inflammation of the lymphatics: lymphatic or scrofulous inflammation.

ANGEIOL'OGY, *Angiol'ogy, Angeiolog"ia,* from αγγειον, 'a vessel,' and λογος, 'a discourse.' A discourse on the vessels. The anatomy of the vessels. It includes *Arteriol'ogy, Phlebol'ogy,* and *Angeiohydrol'ogy.*

ANGEIOMALA'CIA, *Angiomala'cia;* from αγγειον, 'a vessel,' and μαλακια, 'softening.' Mollescence or softening of vessels.

ANGEIOMYCES, Hæmatodes fungus.

ANGEION, Vessel.

ANGEIONDROGRAPHY, Angeiohydrography.

ANGEIONDROTOMY, Angeiohydrotomy.

ANGEIONOSUS, Angeiopathia.

ANGEIONUSUS, Angeiopathia.

ANGEIOPATHI'A, *Angiopathi'a, Angeion'osus, Angeionu'sus, Angio'sis,* from αγγειον, 'a vessel,' and παθος, 'a disease.' Disease of the vessels.

ANGEIOPLEROSIS, Plethora.

ANGEIOPYRA, Synocha.

ANGEIORRHAGIA, Hæmorrhagia activa.

ANGEIORRHŒ'A, (F.) *Angeiorrhée;* from

αγγειον, 'a vessel,' and ρεω, 'I flow.' Passive hemorrhage.
ANGEIOSIS, Angiosis.
ANGEIOSTEGNOSIS, Angiemphraxis.
ANGEIOSTENOSIS, Angiemphraxis.
ANGEIOSTEO'SIS, *Angiosto'sis*, from αγγειον, 'a vessel,' and οστεωσις, 'ossification.' Ossification of vessels.
ANGEIOSTROPHE, see Torsion.
ANGEIOTELECTASIA, Telangiectasia.
ANGEIOT'OMY, *Angiot'omy, Angeiotom'ia*, from αγγειον, 'a vessel,' and τεμνειν, 'to cut.' Dissection of vessels.
ANGEI'TIS, *Angii'tis, Angioi'tis, Inflamma'tio vaso'rum*, (F.) *Angéite*. Inflammation of vessels in general.
ANGELIC ROOT, Angelica lucida.
ANGEL'ICA, *Angel'ica Archangel'ica* seu *Hispa'na* seu *Sati'va, Archangel'ica officina'lis, Garden Angelica*, (F.) *Angélique, Racine de Saint Esprit*. So called from its supposed angelic virtues. *Nat. Ord.* Umbelliferæ. *Sex. Syst.* Pentandria Digynia. Native of Lapland. The roots, stalk, leaves, and seed, are aromatic and carminative. A sweetmeat is made of the root, which is agreeable.
ANGELICA ARCHANGELICA, Angelica.
ANGEL'ICA ATROPURPU'REA, *Angelica* (Ph. U. S.) *Masterwort*. An indigenous species, growing over the whole United States, and admitted into the secondary list of the Pharmacopœia of the United States. Virtues, same as those of the Angelica of Europe.
ANGELICA LEVISTICUM, Ligusticum levisticum.
ANGELICA LU'CIDA, *Angelic root, Bellyache root, Nendo, White root*, an indigenous plant, the root of which is bitterish, subacrid, fragrant, aromatic, stomachic, and tonic.
ANGELICA OFFICINALIS, Imperatoria—a. Paludapifolia, Ligusticum levisticum—a. Sativa, Angelica, A. sylvestris.
ANGEL'ICA SYLVES'TRIS, *A. sati'va, Seli'num Sylves'tre* seu *Angel'ica* seu *Pubes'cens, Impera'toria Sylves'tres* seu *Angelica, Wild Angel'ica*, (F.) *Angélique sauvage*. Possesses similar properties to the last, but in an inferior degree. The seeds, powdered and put into the hair, are used to destroy lice.
ANGELICA SYLVESTRIS, Ligusticum podagraria —a. Tree, Aralia spinosa.
ANGELI'NÆ CORTEX. The bark of a Grenada tree, which has been recommended as anthelmintic and cathartic.
ANGÉLIQUE, Angelica—a. *Sauvage*, Angelica sylvestris.
ANGELOCACOS, Myrobalanus.
ANGEMPHRAXIS, Angiemphraxis.
ANGIDIECTASIA, Trichangiectasia.
ANGIDIOSPONGUS, Hæmatodes fungus.
ANGIECTASIA VENOSA, Varix
ANGIEC'TASIS, *Angeiecta'sia, Angecta'sia, Angieurys'ma, Angeiecto'ma*, from αγγειον, 'a vessel,' and εκτασις, 'dilatation.' Any dilatation of vessels.—Gräfe and Alibert. *Telangiectasia*.
ANGIEMPHRAX'IS, *Angemphrax'is, Angeiosteno'sis, Angeiostegno'sis*, from αγγειον, 'a vessel,' and εμφραξις, 'obstruction.' Obstruction of vessels.
ANGIEURYSMA, Angiectasis.
ANGIITE, Inflammation, Angeitis.
ANGIITIS, Angeitis.
ANGI'NA, *Febris Angino'sa, Isthmi'tis, Quinsy* or *Sore Throat;* from *angere*, 'to suffocate.' Inflammation of the supra-diaphragmatic portion of the alimentary canal, and of the air passages. The Latin writers applied the term to every disease in which deglutition or respiration, separately or united, was affected, provided that such affection was above the stomach and lungs.—Boerhaave speaks of the angina of the moribund, which is nothing more than the dysphagia or difficult deglutition preceding death. See Cynanche.

ANGINA APHTHOSA, Aphthæ—a. Aquosa, Œdema of the glottis—a. Bronchialis, Bronchitis—a. Canina, Cynanche trachealis—a. Cordis, Angina pectoris—a. cum Tumore, Cynanche tonsillaris—a. Epidemica, Cynanche maligna—a. Epiglottidea, Epiglottitis—a. Erysipelatosa, Erythranche a. Exudatoria, Cynanche trachealis—a. Externa, Cynanche parotidæa—a. Faucium, Isthmitis—a. Faucium Maligna, Cynanche maligna—a. Folliculosa of the pharynx, Pharyngitis, follicular—a. Gangrænosa, Cynanche maligna—a. Humida, Cynanche trachealis—a. Inflammatoria, Cynanche, Cynanche trachealis—a. Laryngea, Laryngitis—a. Laryngea Œdematosa, Œdema of the glottis—a. Linguaria, Glossitis—a. Maligna, Angina pellicularis, Cynanche maligna, Pharyngitis, diphtheritic—a. Maxillaris, Cynanche parotidæa —a. Membranacea, Cynanche trachealis—a. Mitis, Isthmitis.

ANGI'NA NASA'LIS, *Nasi'tis posti'ca*. An inflammation of the posterior portion of the Schneiderian membrane lining the nose. Also, Coryza.
ANGI'NA ŒDEMATO'SA, (F.) *Angine œdémateuse, Œdème de la Glotte*. An œdematous swelling of the glottis; the effect of chronic cynanche laryngea. See Œdema of the Glottis.
ANGINA PALATINA, Hyperoitis—a. Paralytica, Pharyngoplegia—a. Parotidæa Externa, Cynanche parotidæa.
ANGI'NA PEC'TORIS, *A. cordis, Sternal'gia, Asthma spas'tico-arthrit'icum incon'stans, Asthma diaphragmat'icum, Arthri'tis diaphragmatica, Orthopnœ'a cardi'aca, Sternodyn'ia syncop'tica et pal'pitans, S. syncopa'lis, Cardiog'mus cordis sinis'tri, Astheni'a pectora'lis, Angor pec'toris, Stenocar'dia, Diaphragmat'ic gout. Asthma convulsi'vum, Asthma arthrit'icum, Cardioneural'gia, Nearul'gia brachiothorac''ica, Hyperæsthe'sia plexus cardi'aci, A. dolorif'icum, Syn'copè angino'sa* seu *angene, Cardiod'ynè spasmod'ica intermit'tens, Pnigopho'bia, Prunel'la, Suspir'ium cardi'acum, Pneumonal'gia, Suff'ocative Breastpang*, (F.) *Angine de Poitrine, Névrose du Cœur*. A disease, the precise pathology of which is not known. The principal symptoms are, violent pain about the sternum, extending towards the arms; anxiety, dyspnœa, and sense of suffocation. It is an affection of great danger, and is often connected with ossification, or other morbid condition of the heart. It appears to be neuropathic, and has been termed *Neuralgia of the Heart*. Some, however, employ this last term for an acutely painful intermittent affection of the heart, which seems to differ from angina pectoris more in regard to the small number of parts which are drawn into morbid consent with the affected cardiac nerves, than in regard either to its nature or appropriate treatment. The most powerful stimulating and narcotic antispasmodics are required during the paroxysm.
ANGI'NA PELLICULA'RIS, *A. malig'na, Diptheri'tis of the throat*. A name given to those inflammations about the throat, in which exudations or false membranes are thrown out, during the phlogosis of the mucous membranes. *Aphthæ, Tracheitis*, when accompanied with the membraniform exudation, are, with some, examples of diphtheritic inflammation.
ANGINA PERNICIOSA, Cynanche trachealis—a. Pestilentialis, Pharyngitis, diphtheritic—a. Polyposa, Cynanche trachealis—a. Polyposa seu membranacea, Cynanche trachealis—a. Pseudo-membranosa, Pharyngitis, diphtheritic—a. Pulposa.

Cynanche trachealis—a. Sanguinea, Cynanche tonsillaris.

ANGINA SICCA, (F.) *Angine sèche*, is a chronic inflammation of the pharynx, with a distressing sense of dryness and heat, in chronic diseases of the stomach and lungs. See Pædanchone.

ANGINA SIMPLEX, Isthmitis.

ANGINA SQUIRRO'SA, (F.) *Angine squirreuse*, consists in difficulty of deglutition, caused by scirrhous disorganization of the pharynx or œsophagus, or by enlarged tonsils.

ANGINA STRANGULATORIA, Cynanche trachealis—a. Strepitosa, Cynanche trachealis—a. Suffocatoria, Cynanche trachealis—a. Synochalis, Cynanche tonsillaris—a. Thyreoidea, Thyreoitis—a. Tonsillaris, Cynanche tonsillaris—a. Trachealis, Cynanche trachealis—a. Ulcerosa, Cynanche maligna—a. Uvularis, Staphylœdema, Uvulitis—a. Vera et Legitima, Cynanche tonsillaris.

ANGINE GUTTURALE, Cynanche tonsillaris—*a. Laryngée*, Laryngitis—*a. Laryngée et trachéale*, Cynanche trachealis—*a. Laryngée œdémateuse*, Œdema of the glottis—*a. Œsophagienne*, Œsophagitis—*a. Pharyngée*, Cynanche parotidæa—*a. de Poitrine*, Angina pectoris—*a. Sèche*, Angina sicca—*a. Simple*, Isthmitis—*a. Squirreuse*, Angina Squirrosa—*a. Tonsillaire*, Cynanche tonsillaris.

ANGINEUX, Anginosa.

ANGINO'SA, (F.) *Angineux*. That which is accompanied with angina; as *Scarlati'na angino'sa*.

ANGIOCARDI'TIS, from αγγειον, 'a vessel,' and *carditis*, 'inflammation of the heart.' Inflammation of the heart and great vessels.

ANGIOGRAPHY, Angeiography.

ANGIOHÉMIE, Hyperæmia.

ANGIOHYDROGRAPHY, Angeiohydrography.

ANGIOHYDROTOMY, Angeiohydrotomy.

ANGIOITIS, Angeitis.

ANGIOLEUCITIS, Angeioleucitis.

ANGIOLOGY, Angeiology.

ANGIOMALACIA, Angeiomalacia.

ANGIOMYCES, Hæmatodes fungus.

ANGIONOSUS, Angeiopathia.

ANGIONUSUS, Angeiopathia.

ANGIOPATHIA, Angeiopathia.

ANGIOPLEROSIS, Plethora.

ANGIOPYRA, Synocha.

ANGIO'SIS, from αγγειον, 'a vessel.' *Angeio'sis, Angeiopathi'a*. Under this term Alibert includes overy disease of the blood vessels.

ANGIOSTEGNOSIS, Angiemphraxis.

ANGIOSTENOSIS, Angiemphraxis.

ANGIOSTOSIS, Angeiostosis.

ANGIOSTROPHE, See Torsion.

ANGIOTELECTASIA, Telangiectasia.

ANGIOTEN'IC, *Angeioten'ic, Angioten'icus* seu *Angeioten'icus*, from αγγειον, 'a vessel,' and τεινειν, 'to extend.' An epithet given to inflammatory fever, owing to its action seeming to be chiefly exerted on the vascular system.

ANGIOTOMY, Angeiotomy.

ANGLE, *An'gulus*, from αγκυλος, 'a hook.' The space between two lines which meet in a point.

ANGLE, FA'CIAL, pointed out by Camper, is formed by the union of two lines, one of which is drawn from the most prominent part of the forehead to the alveolar edge of the upper jaw, opposite the incisor teeth — the *facial line* — and the other from the meatus auditorius externus to the same point of the jaw. According to the size of the angle it has been attempted to appreciate the respective proportions of the cranium and face, and, to a certain extent, the degree of intelligence of individuals and of animals. In the white varieties of the species, this angle is generally 80°; in the negro not more than 70°, and sometimes only 65°. As we descend the scale of animals, the angle becomes less and less; until, in fishes, it nearly or entirely disappears. Animals which have the snout long, and facial angle small, such as the snipe, crane, stork, &c., are proverbially foolish, at least they are so esteemed; whilst intelligence is ascribed to those in which the angle is more largely developed, as the elephant and the owl. In these last animals, however, the large facial angle is caused by the size of the frontal sinuses:—so that this mode of appreciating the size of the brain is very inexact, and cannot be depended upon.

The following is a table of the angle in man and certain animals:

FACIAL ANGLES.

Man	from 68° to 88° and more.
Sapajou	65
Orang-Utang	56 to 58
Guenon	57
Mandrill	30 to 42
Coati	28
Pole-cat	31
Pug-dog	35
Mastiff	41
Hare	30
Ram	30
Horse	23

ANGLE, OCCIPITAL, OF DAUBENTON, is formed by a line drawn from the posterior margin of the foramen magnum to the inferior margin of the orbit, and another drawn from the top of the head to the space between the occipital condyles. In man, these condyles, as well as the foramen magnum, are so situate, that a line drawn perpendicular to them would be a continuation of the spine; but in animals they are placed more or less obliquely; and the perpendicular is necessarily thrown farther forward, and the angle rendered more acute.

ANGLE, OPTIC, (F.) *Angle optique*, is the angle formed by two lines, which shave the extremities of an object, and meet at the centre of the pupil.

ANGOISSE, Angor.

ANGOLAM. A very tall Malabar tree, which possesses vermifuge properties.

AN'GONE, *Præfoca'tio Fau'cium* seu *Uteri'na* seu *Matri'cis, Strangula'tio uteri'na, Suffoca'tic uteri'na* seu *hyster'ica, Globus hyster'icus, Orthopnœ'a hyster'ica, Dyspha'gia globo'sa, D. hyster'ica, Nervous Quinsy*. A feeling of strangulation, with dread of suffocation. It is common in hysterical females, and is accompanied with a sensation as if a ball arose from the abdomen to the throat.

ANGOR, *Anguish*, (F.) *Angoisse*. Extreme anxiety, accompanied with painful constriction at the epigastrium, and often with palpitation and oppression. It is frequently an unfavourable symptom.

ANGOR, Agony, Orthopnœa—a. Faucium, Isthmitis—a. Pectoris, Angina pectoris.

ANGOS, Bubo, Uterus, Vessel.

ANGOURION, Cucumis sativus.

ANGUIS, Serpent.

ANGUISH, Angor.

ANGUISH, FEBRILE, *Angor Febri'lis*. The combination of weariness, pain, anxiety, and weakness affecting the head and neck, which is so generally observed at the commencement of fever.

ANGULAIRE DE L'OMOPLATE, Levator scapulæ.

AN'GULAR, *Angula'ris*, from *angulus*, 'an angle,' (F.) *Angulaire*. That which relates to an angle.

ANGULAR ARTERY AND VEIN. A name given,

1. to the termination of the facial artery and vein, because they pass by the greater angle of the eye; and, 2. to the facial artery and vein themselves, because they pass under the angle of the jaw. See Facial.

ANGULAR NERVE is a filament furnished by the inferior maxillary, which passes near the greater angle of the eye.

ANGULAR PROCESSES of the frontal bone are seated near the angles of the eyes. See Orbitar.

ANGULARIS, Levator scapulæ.

ANGULI-SCAPULO-HUMÉRAL, Teres major.

ANGULUS OCULARIS, Canthus.

ANGURIA, Cucurbita citrullus.

ANGUSTATIO, Arctatio—a. Cordis, Systole—a. Intestini recti vel ani, Stricture of the rectum.

ANGUS'TIA, *Angusta'tio*, *Stenocho'ria*. Anxiety, narrowness, strait, constriction.

ANGUSTIA ABDOMINALIS, Pelvis, (Brim)—a. Perinæalis, Pelvis, (Outlet.)

ANGUSTURA, Cusparia febrifuga—a. False, Brucea antidysenterica, and Strychnos nux vomica—a. Spuria, Brucea antidysenterica, and Strychnos.

ANGUSTURE, FAUSSE, Brucea antidysenterica—*a. Ferrugineuse*, Brucea antidysenterica—*a. Vraie*, Cusparia febrifuga.

ANHÆMATOSIA, Asphyxia, Anæmia.

ANHÆMIA, Anæmia.

ANHAPHIA, Anaphia.

ANHELA'TIO, from *anhelo*, 'I pant.' *Anhel'itus*, *Aas'mus*, Panting, *Anhelation*, (F.) *Essoufflement*. Short and rapid breathing. See Dyspnœa.

Anhelatio is sometimes employed synonymously with asthma.

ANHELITUS, Breath.

ANHIS'TOUS, from *a*, *av*, privative, and '*ιστος*, 'organic texture,' '*Anorganic*.' *Amor'phus*. The tunica decidua uteri is termed by Velpeau the *anhistous membrane*.

ANHUIBA, Laurus sassafras.

ANHYDRÆ'MIA, *Anæmyd'ria*, from *av*, privative, *υδωρ*, 'water,' and '*αιμα*, 'blood.' A condition of the blood in which there is a diminution in the quantity of the serum.

ANICE'TON, *Anice'tum*, *Mesia'mum*, from *a*, privative, and *νικη*, 'victory,' 'invincible.' A plaster much extolled by the ancients in cases of achores. It was formed of litharge, cerussæ, thus, alum, turpentine, white pepper, and oil.

ANI'DEUS, from *av*, privative, and *ειδος*, 'shape.' *Amorphus*. A monster devoid of shape.—J. G. St. Hilaire.

ANIDRO'SIS, from *a*, privative, and '*ιδρως*, 'sweat.' *Sudo'ris nul'litas* vel *priva'tio*. Absence of sweat. Deficiency of perspiration.—Hippocrates.

ANILEMA, Borborygmus, Tormina.

ANILESIS, Borborygmus, Tormina.

ANILITAS, see Dementia.

AN'IMA, *An'imus*, *Mens*, *Psyché*. The mind, breath, &c., from *ανεμος*, 'wind or breath.' (F.) *Âme*. The principle of the intellectual and moral manifestations. Also, the principle of life:—the life of plants being termed *An'ima vegetati'va*, (F.) *Âme végétative*; that of man, *An'ima sensiti'va*, (F.) *Âme sensitive*.

The *Anima* of Stahl, *An'ima Stahlia'na*, was a fancied intelligent principle, which he supposed to preside over the phenomena of life,—like the *Archæus* of Van Helmont.

Under the term *Anima mundi*, the ancient philosophers meant a universal Spirit, which they supposed spread over every part of the universe.

The precise seat of the mind in the brain has given rise to many speculations. The point is unsettled.

With the ancient chemists, *Anima* meant the active principle of a drug separated by some chemical management.

ANIMA ALOES: see Aloes, Succotorina—a. Articulorum, Hermodactylus—a. Hepatis, Ferri sulphas—a. Pulmonum, Crocus—a. Rhei, Infusum rhei—a. Stahliana, see Anima—a. Vegetativa, Plastic force.

AN'IMAL, *Zoön*. A name given to every animated being. The greater part of animals have the power of locomotion; some can merely execute partial movements, such as contraction and dilatation. In other respects it is often a matter of difficulty to determine what is an animal characteristic. The study of animals is called *Zoöl'ogy*.

AN'IMAL, (adjective,) *Anima'lis*. That which concerns, or belongs to, an animal.

ANIMAL HEAT, *Calor anima'lis*, *C. nati'vus*, *Cal'idum anima'lē*, *C. inna'tum*, *Biolych'nion*, *Flam'mula vita'lis*, *Therma em'phytum*, *Thermum em'phytum*, *Ignis anima'lis* seu *natura'lis* seu *vita'lis*, (F.) *Chaleur animale*, is the caloric constantly formed by the body of a living animal, by virtue of which it preserves nearly the same temperature, whatever may be that of the medium in which it is placed. This formation seems to take place over the whole of the body, and to be connected with the action of nutrition.

The following are the natural temperatures of certain animals; that of man being 98° or 100°.

ANIMALS.	Temperatures.
Arctic Fox	107
Arctic Wolf	105
Squirrel	
Hare	104
Whale	
Arctomys citillus, *zizil*—in summer	103
Do. when torpid,	80 to 84
Goat,	103
Bat, in summer,	102
Musk,	
Marmota bobac,—*Bobac*,	101 or 102
House mouse,	101
Arctomys marmota, *marmot*,—in summer,	101 or 102
Do. when torpid	43
Rabbit,	100 to 104
Polar Bear,	100
Dog,	
Cat,	
Swine,	100 to 103
Sheep,	
Ox,	
Guinea-pig,	100 to 102
Arctomys glis,	99
Shrew,	98
Young wolf,	96
Fringilla arctica, *Arctic finch*,	111
Rubecola, *redbreast*,	
Fringilla linaria, *lesser red poll*,	110 or 111
Falco palumbarius, *goshawk*,	
Caprimulgus Europeus, European goat-sucker,	100
Emberiza nivalis, *snow-bunting*,	109 to 110
Falco lanarius, *lanner*,	
Fringilla carduelis, *goldfinch*,	
Corvus corax, *raven*,	109
Turdus, *thrush*, (of Ceylon,)	
Tetrao perdix, *partridge*,	
Anas clypeata, *shoveler*,	
Tringa pugnax, *ruffe*,	
Scolopax, limosa, *lesser godwit*,	
Tetrao tetrix, *grouse*,	108
Fringilla brumalis, *winterfinch*,	
Loxia pyrrhula,	
Falco nisus, *sparrowhawk*,	
Vultur barbatus,	
Anser pulchricollis,	
Colymbus auritus, *dusky grebe*,	107
Tringa vanellus, *lapwing*, wounded,	
Tetrao lagopus, *ptarmigan*,	
Fringilla domestica, *house sparrow*,	107 to 111

ANIMALS.	Temperature.
Strix passerina, *little owl*,	
Hæmatopus ostralegus, *sea-pie*,	
Anas penelope, *widgeon*,	106
Anas strepera, *gadwall*,	
Pelecanus carbo,	
Falco ossifragus, *sea-eagle*,	
Fulica atra, *coot*,	105
Anas acuta, *pintail-duck*,	
Falco milvus, *kite*, (wounded,)	
Merops apiaster, *bee-eater*,	104
Goose,	
Hen,	
Dove,	103 to 107
Duck,	
Ardea stellaris,	
Falco albicollis,	103
Picus major,	
Cossus ligniperda,	89 to 91
Shark,	83
Torpedo marmorata,	74

ANIMAL KINGDOM, (F.) *Règne Animal*, comprises all animated beings.

ANIMAL LAYER, see *Tache embryonnaire*.

ANIMAL MAGNETISM, see Magnetism, animal.

ANIMALCULA SEMINALIA, Spermatozoa—a. Spermatica, Spermatozoa.

ANIMAL'CULE, *Animal'culum;* diminutive of *animal.* A small animal. An animal well seen only by means of the microscope.

ANIMALCULES, SEMINAL, Spermatozoa—a. Spermatic, Spermatozoa.

ANIMAL'CULIST, *An'imalist.* One who attempts to explain different physiological or pathological phenomena by means of animalcules.

ANIMALCULUM, Animalcule.

ANIMALIST, Animalculist.

ANIMAL'ITY, *Animal'itas.* Qualities which distinguish that which is animated. That which constitutes the animal.

ANIMALIZA'TION, *Animalisa'tio.* The transformation of the nutritive parts of food into the living substance of the body to be nourished.

To AN'IMATE, *Anima're.* To unite the living principle with an organized body. The French use it in the sense of,—to excite or render active; as, *animer un vésicatoire:* to excite a blister to suppurate.

ANIMATIO FŒTUS, see Quickening.

ANIMA'TION, *Zoö'sis, Anima'tio*, from *anima,* 'the soul or mind.' The act of animating. The state of being enlivened.

ANIMATION, SUSPENDED, Asphyxia.

AN'IME, *Gum an'imé, Amina'a, Can'camy, Gummi an'imé, Can'camum.* A resin obtained from the trunk of *Hymen'æa cour'baril.* It has been given as a cephalic and uterine. It is not used. The plant is also called *Cour'baril.*

ANIMÉ, (F.) An epithet applied to the countenance, when florid, in health or disease.

ANIMELLÆ, Parotid.

ANIMI CASUS SUBITUS, Syncope—a. Deliquium, Syncope—a. Pathemata, Passions.

AN'IMIST, from *anima,* 'the soul.' One who, following the example of Stahl, refers all the phenomena of the animal economy to the soul. The soul, according to Stahl, is the immediate and intelligent agent of every movement, and of every material change in the body. Stahl therefore concluded, that disease is nothing more than a disturbance or disorder in the government of the economy, or an effort by which the soul, attentive to every morbific cause, endeavours to expel whatever may be deranging the habitual order of health. See Stahlianism.

ANIMUS, Anima, Breath.

ANIS, Pimpinella anisum—a. *Aigre,* Cuminum Cyminum—a. *de la Chine,* Illicium anisatum—a. *Doux,* Anethum—a. *Étoilé,* Illicium anisatum.

ANISA'TUM, from *Anisum,* 'Anise.' A sort of medicated wine, formerly prepared with honey, wine of Ascalon, and aniseed.

ANISCALPTOR, Latissimus dorsi.

ANISCHURIA, Enuresis.

ANISE, Pimpinella anisum—a. Star, Illicium anisatum, I. Floridanum—a. Tree, Florida, Illicium Floridanum—a. Tree, yellow-flowered, Illicium anisatum.

ANISEED, see Pimpinella anisum.

ANISI SEMINA, see Pimpinella anisum.

ANISO'DUS LU'RIDUS, *Nican'dra anom'ala, Phy'salis stramo'nium, Whittle'ya stramo'nifolia.* A plant of Nepal, possessed of narcotic properties, and resembling belladonna and tobacco. It dilates the pupil, and is used in diseases of the eye like belladonna. It is given in alcoholic tincture (dried leaves ʒj. to alcohol f℥viij). Dose, 20 drops internally in the 24 hours.

ANISOPHYLLUM IPECACUANHA, Euphorbia Ipecacuanha.

ANISOS'THENES, *Inæqua'li rob'ore pollens.* That which is unequal in strength: from *α,* priv., *ισος,* 'equal,' and *σθενος,* 'strength.' An epithet applied particularly to the muscular contractility which, in the sick, is sometimes augmented in certain muscles only,—in the flexors, for example.

ANISOT'ACHYS, from *α,* priv., *ισος,* 'equal,' and *ταχυς,* 'quick.' An epithet for the pulse, when quick and unequal—Gorræus.

ANISUM, Pimpinella anisum—a. Africanum frutescens, Bubon Galbanum—a. Fruticosum galbaniferum, Bubon galbanum—a. Officinale, Pimpinella anisum—a. Sinense, Illicium anisatum—a. Stellatum, Illicium anisatum—a. Vulgare, Pimpinella anisum.

ANKLE, Astragalus, Malleolus.

ANKUS, Ancus.

ANKYLOBLEPH'ARON, *Ancylobleph'aron, Palpebra'rum coal'itus,* from *αγκυλη,* 'contraction,' and *βλεφαρον,* 'eyelid.' A preternatural union between the free edges of the eyelids. Likewise called *Symbleph'aron, Symblepharo'sis,* and *Pros'physis.*

Also, union between the eyelids and globe of the eye.—Aëtius.

ANKYLODON'TIA, from *αγκυλος,* 'crooked,' and *οδους,* 'a tooth.' An irregular position of the teeth in the jaws.

ANKYLOGLOS'SIA, *Ancyloglos'sia, Concre'tio linguæ,* from *αγκυλος,* 'crooked,' or 'contracted,' and *γλωσσα,* 'the tongue.' Impeded motion of the tongue in consequence of adhesion between its margins and the gums; or in consequence of the shortness of the frænum: the latter affection constituting *Tongue-tie, Olopho'nia lin'guæ frœna'ta.* It merely requires the frænum to be divided with a pair of scissors.

ANKYLOGLOSSOT'OMUM, from *ankyloglossia,* 'tongue-tie,' and *τομη,* 'incision.' An instrument used in the operation for tongue-tie.

ANKYLOME'LE, *Ancylome'lē,* from *αγκυλος,* 'crooked,' and *μηλη,* 'a probe.' A curved probe. —Galen.

ANKYLOMERIS'MUS, *Ancylomeris'mus,* from *αγκυλη,* 'a contraction, and *μερος,* 'a part.' Morbid adhesion between parts.

ANKYLOPS, Ægilops.

ANKYLO'SIS, *Ancylo'sis, Anchylo'sis, An'cylē, Stiff Joint,* from *αγκυλος,* 'crooked.' An affection, in which there is great difficulty or even impossibility of moving a diarthrodial articulation. It is so called, because the limb commonly remains in a constant state of flexion. Anchylosis is said to be *complete* or *true,* when there is an intimate adhesion between the synovial surfaces, with union of the articular extremities of the bones. In the *incomplete* or *false* anchylosis, there is obscure motion, but the fibrous parts around the joint are more or less stiff and thickened. In the treatment of this last state, the joint must be gently and gradually exercised; and oily, relaxing applications be assiduously employed.

ANKYLOSIS SPURIA, Rigiditas articulorum.

ANKYLOT'OMUS, *Ancylot'omus*, from αγκυλος, 'crooked,' and τεμνειν, 'to cut.' Any kind of curved knife.—Paulus. An instrument for dividing the frænum linguæ.—Scultetus.

ANNEAU, Ring—a. *Crural*, Crural canal—a. *Diaphragmatique*, Diaphragmatic ring—a. *Fémoral*, Crural canal—a. *Inguinal*, Inguinal ring—a. *Ombilical*, Umbilical ring.

ANNEXE, Accessory, Appendix.

ANNI CRITICI, Climacterici (anni)—a. *Decretorii*, Climacterici (anni)—a. *Fatales*, Climacterici (anni)—a. *Genethliaci*, Climacterici (anni) a. *Gradarii*, Climacterici (anni)—a. *Hebdomadici*, Climacterici (anni)—a. *Heroici*, Climacterici (anni)—a. *Natalitii*, Climacterici (anni)—a. *Scalares*, Climacterici (anni)—a. *Scansiles*, Climacterici (anni).

ANNOTA'TIO, *Episema'sia*. Under this term some have included the preludes to an attack of intermittent fever—as yawning, stretching, somnolency, chilliness, &c.

ANNOTTO, see Terra Orleana.

AN'NUAL DISEASES, *Morbi an'nui*, *M. anniversa'rii*, (F.) *Maladies annuelles*. A name given, by some, to diseases which recur every year about the same period. *Febris annua*, (F.) *Fièvre annuelle*, is a term used for a fancied intermittent of this type.

ANNUENS, Rectus capitis internus minor.

ANNUIT"IO, *Nodding*, from *ad*, 'to,' and *nutus*, 'a nod.' A gesture denoting assent in most countries. Also, the state of somnolency, when the individual is in the erect or sitting posture, with the head unsupported, in which the power of volition over the extensor muscles of the head is lost, and the head drops forward.

AN'NULAR, *Annula'ris*, *Cricoï'des*, (*annus*, 'a circle.') Any thing relating to a ring, or which has the shape or fulfils the functions of a ring; from *annulus*, 'a ring,' itself.

ANNULAR FINGER, *Ring Finger*, *Dig"itus annula'ris*, *Param'esos*. The fourth finger, so called from the wedding ring being worn thereon.

ANNULAR GANGLION, see Ciliary ligament.

ANNULAR LIG'AMENT, *Transverse ligament*, *Cru'cial ligament*. A strong ligamentous band, which arches across the ring of the atlas, from a rough tubercle upon the inner surface of one articular process, to a similar tubercle on the other. It serves to retain the odontoid process of the axis in connexion with the anterior arch of the atlas.

AN'NULAR LIG'AMENT OF THE RA'DIUS, is a very strong fibro-cartilaginous band, which forms, with the lesser sigmoid cavity of the cubitus, a kind of ring, in which the head of the radius turns with facility.

AN'NULAR LIG'AMENTS OF THE CARPUS, *Armil'læ manus membrano'sæ*, are two in number. The one, *anterior*, is a broad, fibrous, quadrilateral band, extending transversely before the carpus, and forming the gutter, made by the wrist, into a canal. It is attached, externally, to the trapezium and scaphoïdes; and internally to the os pisiforme and process of the unciforme. It keeps the tendons of the flexor muscles, median nerve, &c., applied against the carpus.

The *posterior* ligament is situate transversely behind the joint of the hand, and covers the sheaths of the tendons, which pass to the back of the hand. Its fibres are white and shining, and are attached, externally, to the inferior and outer part of the radius; internally to the ulna and os pisiforme.

AN'NULAR LIG'AMENTS OF THE TARSUS are two in number. The *anterior* is quadrilateral, and extends transversely above the instep. It is attached to the superior depression of the os calcis, and to the malleolus internus. It embraces the tendons of the extensor muscles of the toes, the *tibialis anticus*, and *peroneus anticus*. The *internal* is broader than the last. It descends from the malleolus internus to the posterior and inner part of the os calcis, with which it forms a kind of canal, enclosing the sheaths of the tendons of the *tibialis posticus*, *o flexor longus digitorum pedis*, and *F. longus pollicis pedis*, as well as the plantar vessels and nerves.

ANNULAR VEIN, *Vena annula'ris*, is situate between the annular finger and the little finger. Aëtius recommends it to be opened in diseases of the spleen.

ANNULARIS, Cricoid: see Digitus—a. *Ani*, Sphincter ani.

ANNULI CARTILAGINEI, see Tracheæ—a. *Cartilaginosi Tracheæ*, see Tracheæ.

ANNULI-TENDINO-PHALANGIENS, Lumbricales manus.

ANNULUS, Dactylius, Vulva—a. *Abdominis*, Inguinal ring—a. *Albidus*, see Ciliary (body)— a. *Cellulosus*, Ciliary ligament—a. *Ciliaris*, Ciliary ligament—a. *Fossæ ovalis*: see Ovalis fossa —a. *Gangliformis*, see Ciliary (body)—a. *Repens*, Herpes circinatus—a. *Umbilicalis*, Umbilical ring —a. *Ventriculi*, Pylorus—a. *Vieussenii*, see Ovalis fossa.

ANO, *ανω*. A prefix denoting 'above, up.'

ANOCHI'LUS, from *ανω*, 'above,' and χειλος, 'lip.' The upper lip. Also, one who has a large upper lip.

ANOCŒLIA, Stomach.

ANO'DIA, from *αν*, priv., and *ωδη*, 'song.' An unconnected or dissonant mode of speech.

ANOD'IC, *Anod'icus*, from *ανω*, 'above, up,' and '*οδος*, 'a way.' Tending upwards. An epithet applied by Dr. Marshall Hall to an ascending course of nervous action.

ANODIN, Anodyne.

ANODIN'IA, from *a*, *αν*, privative, and *ωδις*, 'a labour pain.' Absence of labour pains.

ANODMIA, Anosmia.

ANODUS, Edentulus.

AN'ODYNE, *Anod'ynus*, *Antod'ynus*, *Antid'ynous* (improperly,) *Paregor'icus*, *Anet'icus*, *Antal'gicus*, *Acesod'ynes*, (F.) *Anodin* ou *Anodyn*, from *a*, *αν*, privative, and *οδυνη*, 'pain.' Anodynes are those medicines which relieve pain, or cause it to cease; as opium, belladonna, &c. They act by blunting the sensibility of the encephalon, so that it does not appreciate the morbid sensation.

ANODYN'IA, *Indolen'tia*. Cessation or absence of pain. Vogel has given this name to a genus of diseases, characterized by a cessation of pain, and the exasperation of other symptoms; as we see in gangrene.

ANODYNUM MINERALE, Potassæ nitras sulphatis paucillo mixtus.

ANŒ'A, *Anoia*, from *a*, privative, and *νους*, 'mind.' Delirium, imbecility. See Dementia and Idiotism.

ANOESIA, Dementia.

ANOESIA ADSTRICTA, Melancholy.

ANOIA, Anœa.

ANOMAL, Anomalous.

ANOMALES, Anomalous.

ANOMA'LIA, from *αν*, privative, and *ομαλος*, 'regular.' *Abnor'mitas*, *Aliena'tio*. Anomaly, abnormity, irregularity. In Pathology, anomaly means something unusual in the symptoms proper to a disease, or in the morbid appearances presented by it.

ANOMALIA NERVORUM, Nervous diathesis.

ANOMALOTROPHIES, from αν, privative, ομαλος, 'regular,' and τροφη, 'nourishment.' A class of diseases, which consist in modifications in the nutrition of organs.—Gendrin.

ANOM'ALOUS, *Anom'alus, Anom'ales;* the same etymon. Irregular; contrary to rule. (F.) *Anomal.* In Medicine, a disease is called anomalous, in whose symptoms or progress there is something unusual. Affections are also called anomalous, which cannot be referred to any known species.

ANOMALOUS, Irregular.

ANOMMATUS, Anophthalmus.

ANOMOCEPH'ALUS, from α, priv., νομος, 'rule,' and κεφαλη, 'head.' One whose head is deformed.—Geoffroi Saint-Hilaire.

ANOM'PHALUS, from αν, priv., and ομφαλος, 'the navel.' One devoid of navel. Many writers have endeavoured to show that Adam and Eve must have been ανομφαλοι, as they could not have had umbilical vessels.

ANO'NA TRIPET'ALA. A tree of the *family* Anoneæ or Anonaceæ; *Sex. Syst.* Polyandria polygynia, from fifteen to twenty feet high, native of South America, which bears a delicious fruit called *Chirimoya*. Both the fruit and flowers emit a fine fragrance, which, when the tree is covered with blossom, is almost overpowering—Tschudi.

ANONIS, Ononis.

ANONYME, Innominatum.

ANON'YMOUS, *Anon'ymus, Innomina'tus,* (F.) *Anonyme,* from αν, privative, and ονομα, 'name.' That which has no name.

The word has been applied to many parts of the body:— to the *Anonymous bone* or *Os innominatum:*—the *Anonymous foramen* or *Foramen innominatum,* &c.

ANOPHRESIA, Anosmia.

ANOPHTHAL'MUS, *Anom'matus,* from αν, privative, and οφθαλμος, 'an eye.' A monster devoid of eyes.

ANOPS'IA, from αν, priv., and ωψ, 'the eye.' A case of monstrosity in which the eye and orbit are wanting.

ANOPTICONERVIE, Amaurosis.

ANOR'CHIDES, from αν, priv., and ορχις, 'a testicle.' They who are without testicles.—Fortunatus Fidelis.

ANOREX'IA, from αν, priv., and ορεξις, 'appetite. *Inappeten'tia, Limo'sis expers,* (F.) *Perte d'appetit.* Absence of appetite, without loathing. Anorexia or want of appetite is symptomatic of most diseases. Also, Indigestion, Dyspepsia.

ANOREXIA EXHAUSTO'RUM, Frigidity of the stomach—a. Mirabilis, Fasting.

ANORGANIC, see Anhistous, and Inorganic.

ANORMAL, Abnormous.

ANOS'IA, from α, priv., and νοσος, 'disease.' Health. Freedom from disease.

ANOS'MIA, from α, privative, and οσμη, 'odour.' Loss of smell. Diminution of the sense of smell. Called, also, *Anosphre'sia, Anosphra'sia, Anophre'sia, Parosmia, Anod'mia, Anosmo'sia, Olfactús amis'sio, O. defic''iens, Dysœsthe'sia olfacto'ria, Anœsthe'sia olfacto'ria, Odora'tus deper'di:us,* (F.) *Perte de l'Odorat.*

ANOSMOSIA, Anosmia.

ANOSPHRASIA, Anosmia.

ANOSPHRESIA, Anosmia.

ANSE (F.), *Ansa* (L.), signifies, properly, the handle of certain vessels, usually of an arched form. By analogy, it has been applied to that which is curved in the form of such handle. Thus, the French speak of *Anse intestinale* to signify a portion of intestine, supported by its mesentery, and describing a curved line:— also, of *Anse nerveuse, Anse anastomotique,* &c.

Anse de fil is used, in Surgery, to designate a thread, curved in the form of an *Anse.*

ANSERINA, Potentilla anserina.

ANSÉRINE, Chenopodium ambrosioides—a. *Anthelmintique,* Chenopodium anthelminticum—a. *Bon Henri,* Chenopodium Bonus Henricus—a. *Botrys,* Chenopodium Botrys—a. *Fétide,* Chenopodium vulvaria—a. *Vermifuge,* Chenopodium anthelminticum.

ANTAC''IDS, *Anti-acids, Antiac''ida, Inverten'tia,* from *anti,* 'against,' and *acida,* 'acids.' Remedies which obviate acidity in the stomach. They are chemical agents, and act by neutralizing the acid. Those chiefly used are ammonia, calcis carbonas, calx, magnesia, magnesiæ carbonas, potassa, potassæ bicarbonas, p. carbonas, sodæ bicarbonas, and s. carbonas. They are, of course, only palliatives, removing that which exists, not preventing the formation of more.

ANTAG'ONISM, *Antagonis'mus, Antis'tasis,* from αντι, 'against,' and αγωνιζειν, 'to act.' Action in an opposite direction. It applies to the action of muscles that act in a contrary direction to others. In estimating the force of the muscles, this antagonism must be attended to.

ANTAG'ONIST, *Antagonis'ta.* A muscle whose action produces an effect contrary to that of another muscle. Every muscle has its antagonist, because there is no motion in one direction without a capability of it in another.

ANTALGICUS, Anodyne.

ANTAPHRODIS'IAC, *Antaphrodit'ic, Antaphrodisiacus, Anaphrodisiacus, Anaphrodisiac, Anterot'icus,* from αντι, 'against,' and αφροδισιακος, 'aphrodisiac.' A substance capable of blunting the venereal appetite.

ANTAPHRODITIC, Antaphrodisiac.

ANTAPOD'OSIS, from ανταποδιδωμι, 'I return in exchange.' The succession and return of the febrile periods.—Hippocrates.

ANTAPOPLECTICUS, Antiapoplectic.

ANTARTHRITIC, Antiarthritic.

ANTASTHENICUS, Tonic.

ANTASTHMATICUS, Antiasthmatic.

ANTATROPH'IC, *Antatroph'icus, Antat'rophus, Antiatroph'icus,* from αντι, 'against,' and ατροφια, 'atrophy.' A remedy opposed to atrophy or consumption.

ANTEBRACHIAL, see Antibrachial.

ANTECENDEN'TIA. The precursory or warning symptoms of a disease.

ANTELA'BIA, *Prochei'la,* from *ante,* 'before,' and *labia,* 'the lips.' The extremity of the lips.

ANTELOPE, Antilopus.

ANTEMBALLOMENUM, Succedaneum.

ANTEM'BASIS, from αντι, and εμβαινω, 'I enter.' *Mu'tuus ingres'sus.* The mutual reception of bones.—Galen.

ANTEMETIC, Antiemetic.

ANTENDEIXIS, Counter-indication.

ANTENDIXIS, Counter-indication.

ANTENEAS'MUS, from αντι, 'against,' and νεαν, 'audacious.' One furious against himself. Mania, in which the patient attempts his own life.—Zacchias.

ANTENNA'RIA DIOI'CA, *Gnapha'lium Dioi'cum, Hispid'ula, Pes cati, Elichry'sum monta'num, Diœ'cious Everlast'ing, Oatsfoot,* (F.) *Pied de chat.* A common European plant, which has been advised in hemorrhage, diarrhœa, &c.

ANTEPHIALTIC, Antiephialtic.

ANTEPILEPTIC, Antiepileptic.

ANTEPONENS, Anticipating.

ANTEREI'SIS, from αντι, 'against,' and ερειδω, 'I support.' The resistance—the solidity—of bones.—Hippocrates.

ANTÉRIEUR DU MARTEAU, Laxator tympani—a. *de l'Oreille*, Anterior auris.

ANTE'RIOR, *Anti'cus*, from *ante*, 'before.' Situate before. Great confusion has prevailed with anatomists in the use of the terms *before*, *behind*, &c. Generally, the word *anterior* is applied to parts situate before the median line, the body being in the erect posture, with the face and palms of the hands turned forwards; and the feet applied longitudinally together.

ANTE'RIOR AU'RIS (*Muscle*,) *Auricula'ris ante'rior*, *At'trahens auric'ulam* (F.) *Auriculaire antérieur*, *Antérieur de l'oreille*, *Zygomato-oriculaire*. A small muscle, passing from the posterior part of the zygoma to the helix. *Use*, to draw the ear forwards and upwards.

ANTERIOR MALLEI, Laxator tympani.

ANTEROTICUS, Antaphrodisiac.

ANTEUPHORBIUM, Cacalia anteuphorbium.

ANTEVER'SION, *Antever'sio*, *Antrover'sio*, from *ante*, 'before,' and *vertere*, *versum*, 'to turn.' Displacement of the uterus, in which the fundus is turned towards the pubes, whilst its orifice is towards the sacrum. It may be caused by extraordinary size of the pelvis, pressure of the viscera on the uterus, &c.; and is recognised by examination *per vaginam*. See Retroversio uteri.

ANTHÆMOPTY'ICUS, *Antihæmoptyicus*, from αντι, 'against,' and *hæmoptysis*, 'spitting of blood.' Against spitting of blood. A remedy for spitting of blood — *antihæmoptyicum* (*remedium*.)

ANTHÆMORRHAGICUS, Antihemorrhagic.

ANTHECTICUS, Antihectic.

ANTHELIT'RAGUS, (F.) *Anthélitragien*. One of the proper muscles of the pavilion of the ear.

ANT'HELIX, *Anti-helix*, from αντι, 'before,' and 'ελιξ, 'the helix.' An eminence on the cartilage of the ear, in front of the helix, and extending from the concha to the groove of the helix, where it bifurcates.

ANTHELMIN'TIC, *Anthelmin'ticus*, *Antiscol'icus*, *Anthelmin'thicus*, *Antiscolet'icus*, *Helmin'thicus*, *Helminthago'gus*, *Antivermino'sus*, *Vermif'ugus*, *Ver'mifuge*, from αντι, 'against,' and 'ελμινς, 'a worm.' A remedy which destroys or expels worms, or prevents their formation and development. The chief anthelmintics are, Chenopodium, Mucu'na, Oleum animale Dippelii, Oleum Terebinthinæ, Sodii Chloridum, Spigelia, and Pulvis Stanni. See Worms.

ANTHEMA ERUPTIO, Exanthem.

AN'THEMIS COT'ULA, from ανθω, 'I flower.' *A. fœt'ida*, *Cot'ula*, *C. fœ'tida*, *Cota*, *Cynan'themis*, *Chamæme'lum fœ'tidum*, *An'themis Noveboracen'sis*, *Chamomil'la spu'ria seu fœ'tida*, *Mayflower*, *Mayweed*, *Stinking Chamomile*, *Wild Cham'omile*, *Dog's fennel*, *Dilly*, *Dilweed*, *Fieldweed*, *Pissweed*. *Nat. Ord.* Compositæ Corymbiferæ. *Sex. Syst.* Syngenesia Superflua. (F.) *Maroute*, *Camomille fétide*, *Camomille puante*. This plant has a very disagreeable smell: and the leaves have a strong, acrid, bitterish taste. It is reputed to have been useful in hysterical affections.

ANTHEMIS FŒTIDA, A. cotula.

AN'THEMIS NO'BILIS, *A. odora'ta*, *Chamæme'lum*, *Chamæme'lum No'bilē*, *Chamomil'la Roma'na*, *Euan'themon*, *An'themis*, *Chamæme'lum odora'tum*, *Leucan'themum*, *Matrica'ria*, (F.) *Camomille Romaine*. The leaves and flowers — *Anthemis*, Ph. U. S.—have a strong smell, and bitter, nauseous taste. The flowers are chiefly used. They possess tonic and stomachic properties, and are much given as a pleasant and cheap bitter. A simple infusion is taken to produce, or to assist vomiting. Externally, they are often used in fomentations.

The *O'leum Anthem'idis* possesses the aromatic properties of the plant, but not the bitter and tonic. Consequently, the '*Chamomile Drops*,' as sold by the druggists, must be devoid of the latter qualities. They are made by adding *Ol. anthem.* f℥j. to *Sp. vini rectif.* Oj.

ANTHEMIS NOVEBORACENSIS, A. Cotula.

ANTHEMIS ODORATA, A. cotula.

AN'THEMIS PY'RETHRUM, *Py'rethrum*, *Anacyc'lus pyrethrum*, *Pyrethrum verum*, *Buphthal'mum Cre'ticum*, *Denta'ria*, *Herba saliva'ris*, *Pes Alexandri'nus*, *Spanish Chamomile*, *Pellitory of Spain*. (F.) *Pyrèthre*, *Racine salivaire*, *Pied d'Alexandre*. The root is hot and acrid, its acrimony residing in a resinous principle. It is never used except as a masticatory in toothache, rheumatism of the face, paralysis of the tongue, &c. It acts as a powerful sialogogue.

The Pellitory of the shops in Germany is said to be derived from *Anacyc'lus officina'rum*; a plant cultivated in Thuringia for medicinal purposes.

AN'THEMIS TINCTO'RIA, *Buphthal'mi Herba*, *Dyer's Chamomile*, a European plant, has a bitter and astringent taste, and has been regarded stomachic and vulnerary. (F.) *Camomille des Teinturiers*, *Œil de Bœuf*.

ANTHEMIS VULGARIS, Matricaria Chamomilla.

ANTHE'RA, from ανθηρος, 'florid,' so called from its florid colour. A remedy compounded of several substances, myrrh, sandarac, alum, saffron, &c. It was used under the form of liniment, collyrium, electuary, and powder.—Celsus, Galen.

ANTHEREON, Mentum.

ANTHORA, Aconitum anthora — a. Vulgaris, Aconitum anthora.

ANTHORIS'MA, from αντι, 'against,' and ορισμα, 'boundary.' *Tumor diffu'sus*. A tumor without any defined margin.

ANTHOS: see Rosmarinus — a. Sylvestris, Ledum sylvestre.

ANTHRA'CIA, from ανθραξ, 'coal.' *Carbun'cular Exan'them*. An eruption of tumours, imperfectly suppurating, with indurated edges, and, for the most part, a sordid and sanious core. A genus in the order *Exanthematica*, class *Hæmatica* of Good, and including Plague and Yaws.

ANTHRACIA, Anthracosis — a. Pestis, Plague — a. Rubula, Frambœsia.

ANTHRACION, see Anthrax.

AN'THRACOID, *Anthraco'des*, from ανθραξ, 'coal,' and ειδος, 'resemblance.' (F.) *Charbonneux*. As black as coal. Accompanied by or resembling anthrax.

ANTHRACOMA, Anthrax.

ANTHRACONECROSIS, see Sphacelus.

ANTHRACOPHLYCTIS, see Anthrax.

ANTHRACOSIA, Anthrax.

ANTHRACO'SIS, *Anthra'cia*, *Carbo Palpebra'rum*, from ανθραξ, 'a coal.' A species of carbuncle, which attacks the eyelids and globe of the eye.— Paulus of Ægina. Also, a carbuncle of any kind. It has been used for the "black lung of coal miners," which is induced by carbonaceous accumulation in the lungs. *Pseudo-melanot'ic formation*, (Carswell). When ulceration results from this cause, *black phthisis*, (F.) *Phthisie avec Mélanose*, exists. See Melanosis.

ANTHRACOSIS PULMONUM, see Melanosis.

ANTHRACOTYPHUS, Plague.

ANTHRAKOK'ALI, *Lithanthrakok'ali*, from ανθραξ, 'coal,' and *kali*, 'potassa.' An article introduced as a remedy in cutaneous diseases. It is formed by dissolving carbonate of potassa in 10 or 12 parts of boiling wa'er and adding as much slacked lime as will separate the potassa. The filtered liquor is placed on the fire in an iron vessel, and suffered to evaporate, until neither froth nor effervescence occurs, and the liquid presents a smooth surface like oil. To this, levigated coal is added in the proportion of 160 grammes to 192 grammes of potassa. The mixture is stirred, and removed from the fire, and the stirring is continued, until a black homogeneous powder results. A *sulphuretted anthrakokali* is made by mixing accurately 16 grammes of sulphur with the coal, and dissolving the mixture in the potassa as directed above. The dose of the simple and sulphuretted preparations is about two grains three times a day.

ANTHRAX, ανθραξ, 'a coal,' *Antrax, Carbo, Rubi'nus verus, Codesel'la, Erythe'ma gangræno'sum, Grantris'tum, Pruna, Per'sicus Ignis, Pyra, Granatris'tum, Phyma Anthrax, Erythema anthrax, Carbun'culus, Anthraco'sia, Anthraco'ma, Absces'sus gangræne'cens, A. gangræno'sus, Furun'culus malig'nus, F. gangræno'sus, Carbuncle,* (F.) *Charbon.* An inflammation, essentially gangrenous, of the cellular membrane and skin, which may arise from an internal or external cause. In the latter case it is called *Anthra'cion, Vesic'ula gangrænes'cens, Anthracophlyc'tis, Pustule maligne; Bouton d'Alep, Feu Persique, (Persian fire), Malvat, Bouton malin, Puce maligne,* and is characterized at the outset by a vesication or bleb filled with a sero-sanguinolent fluid, under which a small induration is formed, surrounded by an areolar inflammation, which becomes gangrenous. It has been thought by some to be induced altogether by contact with the matter of the carbuncle of animals, or of the exuviæ of the bodies of such as had died of the disease, but it is now known to arise primarily in the human subject. This form of carbuncle has received different names, many of them from the places where it has prevailed;— *Carbun'culus contagio'sus* seu *Gal'licus* seu *Hunga'ricus* seu *Polon'icus* seu *Septentriona'lis, Morbus pustulo'sus Fin'sicus, Pus'tula gangrænosa* seu *Liv'ida Estho'nia, Pemphigus Hungar'icus.*

Anthrax is a malignant boil, and its treatment is similar to that which is required in case of gangrene attacking a part.

ANTHRAX PULMONUM, Necropneumonia.

ANTHRISCUS CEREFOLIUM, Scandix cerefo'lium — a. Humilis, Chærophyllum Sylvestre — a. Procerus, Chærophyllum Sylvestre.

ANTHROPE, Cutis.

ANTHROPIAT'RICA (MEDICINA,) from ανθρωπος, 'man,' and ιατρος, 'a physician.' Medicine applied to man in contradistinction to animals.

ANTHROPOCHEMIA, Chymistry (human).

ANTHROPOCHYMY, Chymistry, (human).

ANTHROPOGEN'IA, *Anthropogen'esis, Anthropog"eny,* from ανθρωπος, 'man,' and γενεσις, 'generation.' The knowlege, or study, or phenomena of human generation.

ANTHROPOG'RAPHY, *Anthropograph'ia,* from ανθρωπος, 'man,' and γραφη, 'a description.' Anthropology. A description of the human body.

ANTHROPOL'ITHUS, from ανθρωπος, 'man,' and λιθος, 'a stone.' The petrifaction of the human body or of any of its parts. Morbid concretions in the human body.

ANTHROPOL'OGY, *Anthropolog"ia,* from ανθρωπος, 'man,' and λογος, 'a discourse.' A treatise on man. By some, this word is used for the science of the structure and functions of the human body. Frequently, it is employed synonymously with *Natural History* and *Physiology of man.*

ANTHROPOMAGNETISMUS, Magnetism, animal.

ANTHRO'POMANCY, *Anthropomanti'a,* from ανθρωπος, 'a man,' and μαντεια, 'divination.' Divination by inspecting the entrails of a dead man.

ANTHROPOM'ETRY, from ανθρωπος, 'a man,' and μετρον, 'measure.' Measurement of the dimensions of the different parts of the human body.

ANTHROPOMORPHUS, Atropa mandragora.

ANTHROPOPH'AGUS, (F.) *Anthropophage,* from ανθρωπος, 'a man,' and φαγω, 'I eat.' A name given to one who eats his own species.

ANTHROPOPH'AGY, *Anthropopha'gia,* same etymon. The custom of eating human flesh. A disease in which there is great desire to eat it.

ANTHROPOS, Homo.

ANTHROPOSCOPIA, Physiognomy.

ANTHROPOTOMY, Andranatomia.

ANTHUS, Flos.

ANTHYPNOT'IC, *Anthypnot'icus, Antihypnot'ic, Agrypnot'ic,* from αντι, 'against,' and 'υπνωτικος, 'stupefying.' A remedy for stupor.

ANTHYPOCHON'DRIAC, *Anthypochondri'acus,* from αντι, 'against,' and 'υποχονδριακος, 'hypochondriac.' A remedy for hypochondriasis.

ANTHYSTER'IC, *Antihyster'ic, Antihyster'icus,* from αντι, 'against,' and 'υστερα, 'the uterus.' A remedy for hysteria.

ANTI, αντι, as a prefix, in composition, generally means 'opposition.'

ANTIADES, Tonsils.

ANTIADITIS, Cynanche tonsillaris.

ANTIADON'CUS, from αντιαδες, 'the tonsils,' and ογκος, 'tumour.' A swelling of the tonsils. — Swediaur. *Anti'ager* has a similar meaning.

ANTIADONCUS INFLAMMATORIUS, Cynanche tonsillaris.

ANTIAPOPLEC'TIC, *Antiapoplec'ticus, Antapoplec'ticus, Apoplec'ticus,* from αντι, 'against,' and αποπληξια, 'apoplexy.' A remedy for apoplexy.

ANTIARIS TOXICARIA, see Upas.

ANTIARTHRIT'IC, *Antarthrit'ic, Antiarthrit'icus, Antipodag'ric,* from αντι, 'against,' and αρθριτις, 'the gout,' (F.) *Antigoutteux.* A remedy for gout.

ANTIASTHEN'IC, *Antiasthen'icus,* from αντι, 'against,' and ασθενεια, 'debility.' A remedy for debility.

ANTIASTHMAT'IC, *Antiasthmat'icus, Antasthmat'icus,* from αντι, 'against,' and ασθμα, 'asthma.' A remedy for asthma.

ANTIATROPHICUS, Anatrophic.

ANTIBALLOMENUM, Succedaneum.

ANTIBDELLA, Antlia sanguisuga.

ANTIBRA'CHIAL, *Antibrachia'lis.* That which concerns the fore-arm. — Bichat. J. Cloquet suggests that the word should be written *antebrachial,* from *ante,* 'before,' and *brachium,* 'the arm:'— as *antebrachial region, antebrachial aponeurosis,* &c.

ANTEBRA'CHIAL APONEURO'SIS, (F.) *Aponévrose antébrachiale,* is a portion of the aponeurotic sheath which envelops the whole of the upper limb. It arises from the brachial aponeurosis, from a fibrous expansion of the tendon of the biceps muscle, from the epicondyle, epitrochlea, and, behind, from the tendon of the triceps brachialis. Within, it is inserted into the cubitus, &c.; and, below, is confounded with the two annular ligaments of the carpus. It is covered by the skin, by veins, lymphatics, and by filaments of superficial nerves; it covers the muscles of the fore-arm, adheres to them, and sends between them several fibrous septa, which serve them for points of insertion.

ANTIBRACHIUM, Fore-arm.

ANTIBRO'MIC, *Antibro'micus*, from αντι, 'against,' and βρωμος, 'fœtor.' A *Deo'doriser*. An agent that destroys offensive odours — as chloride of zinc, simple sulphate of alumina, &c.

ANTICACHEC'TIC, *Anticachec'ticus*, Anticacochym'ic, from αντι, 'against,' and καχεξια, 'cachexy.' A remedy against cachexy.

ANTICACOCHYMIC, Anticachectic.

ANTICAN'CEROUS, *Anticancero'sus*, *Anticancro'sus*, *Anticarcinom'atous*, *Antiscir'rhous*, from αντι, 'against,' and καρκινωμα, 'cancer,' carcinoma. Opposed to cancer.

ANTICANCROSUS, Anticancerous.

ANTICARCINOMATOUS, Anticancerous.

ANTICARDIUM, *Fossette du cœur*, Scrobiculus cordis.

ANTICATAR'RHAL, *Anticatarrha'lis*, *Anticatarrholcus*, from αντι, 'against,' and καταρρος, 'catarrh.' A remedy for catarrh.

ANTICAUSOD'IC, *Anticausot'ic*, *Anticausod'icus*, from αντι, 'against,' and καυσος, 'a burning fever.' A remedy for *causus* or inflammatory fever.

AMTICAUSOTIC, Anticausodic.

ANTICHEIR, Pollex, see Digitus.

ANTICHŒRADICUS, Antiscrofulous.

ANTICHOLERICA, Sophora heptaphylla.

ANTIC"IPATING, *Antic"ipans*, *Antepo'nens*, *Prolept'icus*. A periodical phenomenon, recurring at progressively shorter intervals. An anticipating intermittent is one in which the intervals between the paroxysms become progressively less.

ANTICNEMIUM, Shin.

ANTICŒUR, Scrobiculus cordis.

ANTICOL'IC, *Anticol'icus*, from αντι, 'against,' and κωλικος, 'the colic.' That which is opposed to colic.

ANTICOMMA, *Contre-coup*.

ANTICOPE, *Contre-coup*.

ANTICRUSIS, *Contre-coup*.

ANTICRUSMA, *Contre-coup*.

ANTICUS, Anterior.

ANTIDARTREUX, Antiherpetic.

ANTIDEIXIS, Counter-indication.

ANTIDIARRHŒ'IC, *Antidiarrhœ'icus*. A remedy for diarrhœa. Opposed to diarrhœa.

ANTID'INIC, *Antidin'icus*, *Din'icus*, from αντι, 'against,' and δινος, 'vertigo.' Opposed to vertigo.

AN'TIDOTAL, *Antidota'lis*, same etymon as *antidote*. Relating to an antidote; possessed of the powers of an antidote.

ANTIDOTA'RIUM, from αντιδοτον, 'an antidote.' A dispensatory. A pharmacopœia or formulary.

AN'TIDOTE, *Antid'otum*, from αντι, 'against,' and διδωμι, 'I give.' Originally this word signified an *internal remedy*. It is now used synonymously with *counter-poison*, *Antiphar'macum*, and signifies any remedy capable of combating the effect of poisons.

A List of Substances reputed as Antidotes.

1. METALS.
Iron Filings.
Zinc Filings.

2. ACIDS.
Tannic Acid.
Acetic or Citric Acid.

3. SALTS.
Alkaline or Earthy Sulphates.
Chloride of Sodium.
Hypochlorite of Soda or of Lime.

4. ALKALINES.
Ammonia.
Carbonates of Ammonia.
Carbonates of Soda.
Magnesia.
Carbonate of Magnesia.
Lime Water.

Chalk.
Soap.

5. SULPHURETS.
Sulphuretted Hydrogen, dissolved in water.
Sulphuret of Potassium.

6. HALOIDS.
Chlorine.

7. METALLIC OXIDES.
Hydrated Sesqui-oxide of Iron.
Mixed Oxides of Iron.

8. ORGANIC SUBSTANCES.
Albuminous Substances, (Albumen, Casein, and Gluten.)
Starch.
Oil.
Animal Charcoal.

ANTIDOTUM HERACLIDIS, Enneapharmacos — a. Mithridatium, Mithridate.

ANTIDYNAMICA, Debilitants.

ANTIDYNOUS, Anodyne.

ANTIDYSENTER'IC, *Antidysenter'icus*, from αντι, 'against,' δυς, 'with difficulty,' and εντερον, 'intestine.' Opposed to dysentery.

ANTIEMET'IC, *Antemet'ic*, *Antiemet'icus*, from αντι, 'against,' and εμετικος, 'emetic.' A remedy for vomiting.

ANTIEPHIAL'TIC or ANTEPHIAL'TIC, *Antiephial'ticus*, from αντι, 'against,' and εφιαλτες, 'nightmare.' A remedy for nightmare.

ANTIEPILEP'TIC or ANTEPILEP'TIC, *Antiepilep'ticus*, from αντι, 'against,' and επιληψια, 'epilepsy.' A remedy for epilepsy.

ANTIFEBRILIS, Febrifuge.

ANTIGALAC'TIC, *Antigalac'ticus*, *Antilac'teus*, from αντι, 'against,' and γαλα, 'milk.' (F.) *Antilaiteux*. Opposed to the secretion of milk, or to diseases caused by the milk.

ANTIG'ONI COLLYR'IUM NIGRUM, *Black collyrium* of ANTIG'ONUS. It was composed of cadmia, antimony, pepper, verdigris, gum Arabic, and water.

ANTIGUA, see West Indies.

ANTIHÆMOPTYICUS, Anthæmoptyicus.

ANTIHEC'TIC, *Antithec'ticus*. *Anthec'ticus*, from αντι, 'against,' and 'εξις, 'habit of body.' The *Antihec'ticum* POTE'RII is the white oxyd of antimony; also called *Diaphoret'icum Jovia'lē*.

ANTIHELIX, Anthelix.

ANTIHELMINTICUS, Anthelmintic.

ANTIHEMORRHAG"IC, *Antihæmorrhag"icus*, *Anthæmorrhag"icus*; from αντι, 'against,' and 'αιμορραγια, 'hemorrhage.' That which is against hemorrhage; an antihemorrhagic remedy.

ANTIHEMORRHOID'AL, *Antihæmorrholda'lis*, from αντι, 'against,' and 'αιμορροιδες, 'hemorrhoids.' A remedy for hemorrhoids.

ANTIHERPET'IC, *Antiherpet'icus*, from αντι, 'against,' and 'ερπις, 'herpes.' (F.) *Antidartreux*. A remedy for herpes.

ANTIHYDROPHOB'IC, *Antihydrophob'icus*, *Antylis'sus*, *Alys'sus*, from αντι, 'against,' 'υδωρ, 'water,' and φοβος, 'dread.' A remedy for hydrophobia.

ANTIHYDROP'IC, *Antihydrop'icus*, *Hydrop'icus*, from αντι, 'against,' and 'υδρωψ, 'dropsy.' A remedy for dropsy.

ANTIHYPNOTIC, Anthypnotic.

ANTIHYSTERIC, Antihysteric.

ANTI-ICTERIC, *Anti-icter'icus*, *Icter'icus*, from αντι, 'against,' and ικτερος, 'jaundice.' A remedy for jaundice.

ANTI-IMPETIGENES, SOLOMON'S, see Liquor Hydrargyri oxymuriatis.

ANTILABIUM, Prolabium.

ANTILACTEUS, Antigalactic.

ANTILAITEUX, Antigalactic.

ANTILEP'SIS, *Apprehen'sio*, ● from αντιλαμβανω, 'I take hold of.' The mode of attaching a bandage over a diseased part, by fixing it upon the sound parts. — Hippocrates. The mode of securing bandages, &c., from slipping. Treatment by revulsion or derivation.

ANTILETHAR'GIC, *Antilethar'gicus*, from αντι, 'against,' and ληθαργικος, 'affected with lethargy.' A remedy for lethargy.

ANTILITH'ICS, *Antilith'ica*, *Lith'ica*, from αντι, 'against,' and λιθος, 'a stone.' A substance that prevents the formation of calculi in the urinary organs.

The chief antilithics — according as the calculi are lithic acid or phosphatic — are alkalies or acids; with revellents, especially change of air; tonics, as diosma crenata, (?) and uva ursi. (?)

ANTILLY, MINERAL WATERS OF. A

celebrated French medicinal spring, near Méaux, in France. The waters have not been analysed; but astonishing and chimerical effects have been ascribed to them.

ANTILOBIUM. Antitragus, Tragus.

ANTILOI'MIC, *Antiloi'micus, Antilœ'mic, Antipestilentia'lis,* from αντι, 'against,' and λοιμος, 'the plague.' A remedy for the plague.

ANTIL'OPUS. The *An'telope.* (F.) *Gazelle.* An African animal, whose hoofs and horns were formerly given in hysteric and epileptic cases.

ANTILYSSUS, Antihydrophobic.

ANTIMEL'ANCHOLIC, *Antimelanchol'icus,* from αντι, 'against,' and μελαγχολια, 'melancholy.' A remedy for melancholy.

ANTIMEPHIT'IC, *Antimephit'icus,* from αντι, 'against,' and *mephitic.* A remedy against mephitic or deleterious gases.

ANTIMOINE, Antimonium—*a. Beurre d',* Antimonium muriatum—*a. Chlorure d',* Antimonium muriatum—*a. Oxide d',* Algaroth—*a. Oxide blanc d',* Antimonium diaphoreticum—*a. Soufre doré d',* Antimonii sulphuretum præcipitatum—*a. Sulfure d',* Antimonium—*a. Sulfuré, hydrosulphure rouge d',* Antimonii sulphuretum rubrum—*a. Verre d',* Antimonii vitrum.

ANTIMO'NIAL, *Antimonia'lis, Stibia'lis,* from *antimonium,* 'antimony.' A composition into which antimony enters. A preparation of antimony.

ANTIMO'NIAL POWDER, *Pulvis antimonia'lis, Ox'idum antimo'nii cum phos'phatĕ calcis, Phosphas calcis stibia'tus, P. Cal'cicum stibia'tum, Pulvis Jame'sii, Pulvis stibia'tus, Pulvis de phos'phatĕ calcis et stib'ii compos'itus,* Factitious JAMES'S *Powder,* SCHWANBERG'S *Fever Powder,* CHENEVIX'S *Antimonial Powder,* (F.) *Poudre antimoniale composée* ou *de* JAMES. A peroxide of antimony combined with phosphate of lime. (*Take of common sulphuret of antimony,* ℔j; *hartshorn shavings,* ℔ij. Roast in an iron pot, until they form a gray powder. Put this into a long pot, with a small hole in the cover. Keep it in a red heat for two hours, and grind to a fine powder.) This preparation has long been esteemed as a febrifuge: but it is extremely uncertain in its action. The ordinary dose is 6 or 8 grains.

ANTIMONIALE CAUSTICUM, Antimonium muriatum.

ANTIMONIATUM SULPHUR, Antimonii sulphuretum præcipitatum—*a.* Tartar, Antimonium tartarizatum.

ANTIMONII (BUTYRUM,) Antimonium muriatum—*a.* Calx, Antimonium diaphoreticum—*a.* Cerussa, Antimonium diaphoreticum—*a.* et Potassæ tartras, Antimonium tartarizatum—*a.* Murias, Antimonium muriatum—*a.* Oleum, Antimonium muriatum—*a.* Oxydulum hydrosulphuratum aurantiacum, Antimonii sulphuretum præcipitatum—*a.* Oxydum, Algaroth—*a.* Oxydum auratum, Antimonii sulphuratum præcipitatum—*a.* Oxidum nitro-muriaticum, Algaroth—*a.* Oxydum cum sulphure vitrifactum, Antimonii vitrum—*a.* Oxydum sulphuretum vitrifactum, Antimonii vitrum—*a.* Oxysulphuretum, A. sulphuretum præcipitatum—*a.* Potassio-tartras, Antimonium tartarizatum—*a.* Regulus medicinalis, Antimonium medicinale—*a.* Sal, Antimonium tartarizatum—*a.* Sulphur auratum, Antimonii sulphuretum præcipitatum—*a.* Sulphur præcipitatum, Antimonii sulphuretum præcipitatum—*a.* Sulphuretum, Antimonium—*a.* Tartras, Antimonium tartarizatum—*a.* Tartras et Potassæ, Antimonium tartarizatum—*a.* Vitrum hyacinthinum, Antimonii vitrum.

ANTIMO'NII SULPHURE'TUM PRECIPITA'TUM, *Sulphur antimonia'tum, Hydrosulphure'tum stibio'sum cum sul'phurĕ, Oxo'des stib'ii sulphura'tum, Oxyd'ulum antimo'nii hydrosulphura'tum auranti'acum, Ox'ydum aura'tum antimo'nii, Sulphure'tum stib'ii oxydula'ti, Hydro-sulfure'tum lu'teum ox'ydi stib'ii sulfura'ti, Sulphur antimo'nii præcipita'tum, Sulphur aura'tum antimo'nii, Golden Sulphur of Antimony.*

Antimo'nii Sulphure'tum Præcipitatum, A. Oxysulphuretum, (F.) *Soufre doré d'Antimoine,* of the London Pharmacopœia, is nearly the same as the old *Kermes Mineral.* It is a powder of an orange colour, of a metallic, styptic taste. It is emetic, diaphoretic, and cathartic, according to the dose; and has been chiefly used in chronic rheumatism, and in cutaneous affections. Dose, gr. j. to gr. iv.

Antimonii Sulphuretum Præcipitatum of the United States Pharmacopœia, is made by boiling together *Sulphuret of Antimony,* in fine powder, *Solution of Potassa,* and *distilled water;* straining the liquor while hot, and dropping into it *Diluted Sulphuric Acid* so long as it produces a precipitate.

ANTIMO'NII SULPHURE'TUM RUBRUM, *Red Sul'phuret of An'timony, Hydrosulfure'tum stib'ii rubrum, Sub-hydrosul'fas stib'ii, Hydro-sulphure'tum rubrum stib'ii sulphura'ti, Pulvis Carthusiano'rum, Kermes mineral,* (F.) *Hydrosulfure rouge d'Antimoine sulfuré, Vermillon de Provence.* Properties the same as the last. Dose, gr. j. to gr. iv.

ANTIMO'NII VITRUM, *Glass of Antimony, Antimo'nii ox'ydum sulphure'tum vitrifac'tum, Ox'ydum stib'ii semivit'reum, Antimo'nium vitrifac'tum, Ox'idum antimo'nii cum sul'phure vitrifac'tum, Vitrum stib'ii, Antimo'nii vitrum hyacin'thinum, Oxyd'ulum stib'ii vitrea'tum,* (F.) *Verre d'Antimoine.* (Formed by roasting powdered common antimony in a shallow vessel, over a gentle fire, till it is of a whitish gray colour, and emits no fumes in a red heat; then melting it, on a quick fire, into a clean, brownish-red glass.) It has been used for preparing the tartarized antimony and antimonial wine.

ANTIMONIOUS ACID, Antimonium diaphoreticum.

ANTIMO'NIUM, from αντι, 'against,' and μονος, 'alone;' *i. e.* not found alone: or according to others, from αντι, 'against,' and *moine,* 'a monk;' because, it is asserted, certain monks suffered much from it. *Stibi, Stib'ium, Reg'ulus Antimo'nii, Minera'lium, Gynæce'um, Magne'sia Satur'ni, Marcasi'ta plum'bea, Platyophthal'mon, Stim'mi, Aurum lepro'sum, Antimo'nium crudum, Antimo'nii sulphure'tum, Sulphure'tum stib'ii nigrum, Common Antimony, Sulphuret of Antimony,* (F.) *Antimoine, Sulfure d'Antimoine.* Sulphuret of antimony is the ore from which all the preparations of antimony are formed. In Pharmacy, it is the native sesquisulphuret of antimony, purified by fusion. When prepared for medical use, by trituration and levigation, it forms a powder of a black, or bluish gray colour, which is insoluble. It is slightly diaphoretic and alterative, and has been used in chronic rheumatism, cutaneous diseases, &c.

ANTIMONIUM ALBUM, Bismuth.

ANTIMO'NIUM CALCINATUM, Antimonium diaphoreticum.

ANTIMO'NIUM DIAPHORET'ICUM, *Diaphoret'ic Antimony, Antimo'nious Acid, Min'eral Bez'oard, Antimo'nium Calcina'tum, Mineral Diaphoret'ic, Matière perlée de* KERKRING, *Peroxide of Antimony, Calx Antimo'nii, Antimo'nium diaphoret'icum lotum, Cerus'sa Antimo'nii, Calx Antimo'nii elo'ta, Oxo'des stib'ii album, Ox'idum stibio'sum, Deutoxide of An'timony, Ox'idum stib'ii album median'tĕ nitro confectum, Potassa biantimo'nias,* (F.) *Oxide blanc d'Antimoine préparé par le moyen du nitre.* (*Common antimony,* ℔j; *purified nitre*, ℔iij.—Throw it by spoonfuls into a red-hot crucible; powder and wash. The flowers that stick to the side of the crucible must be carefully separated, otherwise they render it emetic.) Dose, gr. x. to xxx.

ANTIMONIUM EMETICUM, A. tartarizatum.
ANTIMO'NIUM MEDICINA'LE, *Reg'ulus Antimo'nii Medicina'lis, Medicinal Reg'ulus of Antimony.* (*Antimon. sulphur.* ℥v. *Potass. subcarb.* ℥i. *Sodii chlorid.* ℥iv. Powder, mix, and melt. When cold, separate the scoriæ at top, powder the mass, and wash it well.) It is conceived to be more active than common antimony.

ANTIMO'NIUM MURIA'TUM, *Antimo'nii Mu'rias, Chlor'uret of An'timony, Chlorure'tum stib'ii, Spuma viridis draco'num, Deuto-murias stib'ii sublima'tus, Butter of Antimony, Muriate of Antimony, Chloride of Antimony, Buty'rum Antimo'nii, O'leum Antimo'nii, Buty'rum stib'ii, Caus'ticum antimonia'lē, Antimonium sali'tum,* (F.) *Chlorure d'Antimoine, Beurre d'Antimoine.* (Common antimony and corrosive sublimate, of each equal parts: grind together, and distil in a wide-necked retort, and let the butyraceous matter that comes over, run, in a moist place, to a liquid oil.) A caustic, but not much used as such. Sometimes taken as poison.

ANTIMONIUM SALITUM, Antimonium muriatum.
ANTIMO'NIUM TARTARIZA'TUM, *Tartris Antimo'nii, Tartar Antimonia'tum, Sal Antimo'nii, Tartrae Potas'sæ stibio'sus* seu *stibia'lis, Tartris lixiv'iæ stibia'tus, Deuto-tartras potas'sæ et stib'ii, Tar'tarus emet'icus, Tar'tarum emet'icum, Tartras antimo'nii, Tartras Antimo'nii et Potassæ, Antimo'nii et Potassa Tartras* (Ph. U. S.), *Antimo'nii potas'sio-tartras, Antimo'nium emet'icum, Tar'tarized An'timony, Tartrate of An'timony and potas'sa, Potassio-tartrate of Antimony, Emet'ic Tartar, Tartar Emetic,* (F.) *Tartre stibié, Tartre Émétique, Émétique;* in some parts of the United States, vulgarly and improperly called *Tartar:* (Made by digesting *sulphuret of antimony* in a mixture of *nitric* and *muriatic acids* with the aid of heat; filtering the liquor, and pouring it into *water:* freeing the precipitate from acid, by washing and drying it; adding this powder to *bitartrate of potassa* in boiling *distilled water;* boiling for an hour, and after filtering the liquor while hot, setting it aside to crystallize.—Ph. U. S.) Tartarized antimony is emetic, sometimes cathartic and diaphoretic. Externally, it is rubefacient. Dose, as an emetic, gr. j. to gr. iv. in solution: as a diaphoretic, gr. one-sixteenth to gr. one-quarter.

The empirical preparation, called NORRIS'S DROPS, consist of a solution of *tartarized antimony* in *rectified spirit*, disguised by the addition of some vegetable colouring matter.

ANTIMONIUM VITRIFACTUM, Antimonii vitrum.
ANTIMONY, BUTTER OF, Antimonium muriatum—a. Chloride of, Antimonium muriatum—a. Chloruret of, Antimonium muriatum—a. Deutoxide of, Antimonium diaphoreticum—a. Flowers of, Algaroth—a. Glass of, Antimonii vitrum—a. Golden sulphur of, Antimonii sulphuretum præcipitatum—a. Medicinal, regulus of, Antimonium medicinale—a. Muriate of, Antimonium muriatum—a. Peroxide of, Antimonium diaphoreticum —a. Potassio-tartrate of, Antimonium tartarizatum—a. Submuriate of, Protoxide of, Algaroth—a. Sulphuret of, red, Antimonii sulphuretum rubrum—a. Tartarized, Antimonium tartarizatum —a. Vegetable, Eupatorium perfoliatum.

ANTIMONY AND POTASSA, TARTRATE OF, Antimonium tartarizatum.

ANTINEPHRIT'IC, *Antinephret'ic, Antinephret'icus,* from *αντι,* 'against,' and *νεφριτις,* 'nephritis.' A remedy for inflammation of the kidney.

ANTINEUROPATHIC, Nervine.
ANTINEUROTIC, Nervine.
ANTINIAD, see Antinial.
ANTIN'IAL, from *αντι,* 'against,' and *ινιον,* 'the ridge of the occiput.' An epithet for an aspect towards the side opposite to the *inion,* or ridge of the occiput.—Barclay. *Antiniad* is used adverbially by the same writer, to signify 'towards the antinial aspect.'

ANTI'OCHI HI'ERA. A preparation extolled by the ancients in melancholy, hydrophobia, epilepsy, &c. It was formed of germander, agaric, pulp of colocynth, Arabian stœchas, opoponax, sagapenum, parsley, aristolochia, white pepper, cinnamon, lavender, myrrh, honey, &c.

ANTIOCHI THERIACA. A theriac employed by Antiochus against every kind of poison. It was composed of thyme, opoponax, millet, trefoil, fennel, aniseed, nigella sativa, &c.

ANTIODONTAL'GIC, *Antodontal'gic, Antodontal'gicus, Odontal'gic, Odont'ic, Antiodontal'gicus,* from *αντι,* 'against,' and *οδονταλγια,* 'toothache.' A remedy for toothache.

ANTIORGAS'TIC, *Antiorgas'ticus,* from *αντι,* 'against,' and *οργαω,* 'I desire vehemently.' A remedy for orgasm or erethism, and for irritation in general.

ANTIPARALYT'IC, *Antiparalyt'icus,* from *αντι,* 'against,' and *παραλυσις,* 'palsy.' Opposed to palsy.

ANTIPARASIT'IC, *Antiparasit'icus, Antiphtheiriacus, Phthi'rius, Parasit'icide;* from *αντι,* 'against,' and *παρασιτος,* 'a parasite.' An agent that destroys parasites, as the different vermin that infest the body. The chief antiparasitics are *Cocculus, Staphisagria, Veratrum album,* and certain of the mercurial preparations.

ANTIPARASTATI'TIS, from *αντι,* 'opposite,' and *παραστατης,* 'the epididymis;' also, 'the prostate,' and *itis,* denoting inflammation. Inflammation of Cowper's glands.

ANTIPATHI'A, from *αντι,* 'against,' and *παθος,* 'passion, affection.' Aversion. A natural repugnance to any person or thing.

ANTIPATH'IC, *Antipath'icus,* (F.) *Antipathique.* Belonging to antipathy. Opposite, contrary,—as *humeurs antipathiques;* humours opposed to each other. Also, palliative.

ANTIP'ATRI THERIACA, *Theriac of* ANTIP'ATER. A farrago of more than 40 articles: used as an antidote against the bites of serpents.

ANTIPERIOD'IC, *Antiperiod'icus, Antityp'icus,* from *αντι,* 'against,' and *περιοδος,* 'period.' A remedy which possesses the power of arresting morbid periodical movements;—e. g. the sulphate of quinia in intermittents.

ANTIPERISTAL'TIC, *Antiperistal'ticus, Antivermic'ular,* from *αντι,* 'against,' and *περιστελλω,* 'I contract.' An inverted action of the intestinal tube.

ANTIPERIS'TASIS, from *αντι,* 'against,' and *περιστασις,* 'reunion, aggregation.' A union of opposite circumstances: the action of two contrary qualities, one of which augments the force of the other. The peripateticians asserted, that it is by Antiperistasis, that fire is hotter in winter than in summer. Theophrastus attributes the cause, which renders man more vigorous, and makes him digest more readily in winter, to the augmentation of heat caused by Antiperistasis.

ANTIPER'NIUS, from *αντι,* 'against,' and *Pernio,* 'a chilblain.' A remedy against chilblains;—as *Unguen'tum antiper'nium,* an ointment for chilblains.

ANTIPERTUSSIS, see Zinci sulphas.
ANTIPESTILENTIALIS, Antiloimic.
ANTIPHARMACUS, Alexipharmic.
ANTIPHLOGIS'TIC, *Antiphlogis'ticus,* from

αντι, 'against,' and φλεγω, 'I burn.' Opposed to inflammation;—as *Antiphlogistic remedies, A. regimen,* &c.

ANTIPHTHEIRIACA, *Antiphthiriaca,* from αντι, 'against,' and φθειριαω, 'I am lousy.' A remedy used to destroy lice.

ANTIPHTHIS'ICAL, *Antiphthis'icus,* from αντι, 'against,' and φθισις, 'consumption.' Opposed to phthisis.

ANTIPHYSICA, Carminatives.

ANTIPHYS'ICAL, *Antiphys'icus,* from αντι, 'against,' and φυσω, 'I blow.' An expeller of wind: a carminative.

It has also been used for any thing preternatural; here, the derivation is from αντι, 'against,' and φυσις, 'nature.' The French sometimes say, *'Un goût antiphysique,' 'an* unnatural taste.'

ANTIPLAS'TIC, *Antiplas'ticus, Plastilyt'ic, Plastilyt'icus,* from αντι, 'against,' and πλαστικος, 'formative.' Antiformative. An agent that diminishes the quantity of plastic matter—fibrin—in the blood.

ANTIPLEURIT'IC, *Antipleuret'icus, Antipleuret'ic,* from αντι, 'against,' and πλευριτις, 'pleurisy.' Opposed to pleurisy.

ANTIPNEUMON'IC, *Antipneumon'icus,* from αντι, 'against,' and πνευμονια, 'disease or inflammation of the lungs.' A remedy for disease or inflammation of the lungs.

ANTIPODAGRIC, Antiarthritic.

ANTIPRAX'IS, from αντι, 'against,' and πρασσω, 'I act.' A contrary state of different parts in the same patient: e. g. an increase of heat in one organ, and diminution in another.

ANTIPSOR'IC, *Antipso'ricus, Antisca'bious,* from αντι, 'against,' and ψωρα, 'the itch.' (F.) *Antigaleux.* Opposed to the itch.

ANTIPUTRID, Antiseptic.

ANTIPY'IC, *Antipy'icus,* from αντι, 'against,' and πυον, 'pus.' Opposed to suppuration.

ANTIPYRETIC, Febrifuge.

ANTIPYROT'IC, *Antipyrot'icus,* from αντι, 'against,' and πυρ, 'fire.' Opposed to burns or to pyrosis.

ANTIQUARTANA'RIUM, *Antiquar'tium.* A remedy formerly used against quartan fever.

ANTIQUUS, Chronic.

ANTIRHACHIT'IC, *Antirhachit'icus,* from αντι, 'against,' and *rachitis.* Opposed to rachitis, or rickets.

ANTIRHEUMAT'IC, *Antirrheumat'icus;* from αντι, 'against,' and ρευμα, 'rheumatism.' A remedy for rheumatism.

ANTIRHINUM ACUTANGULUM, A. Linaria—a. Auriculatum, A. Elatine.

ANTIRHI'NUM ELATI'NE, *A. auricula'tum, E. hasta'ta, Elati'ně, Lina'ria elati'ně, Cymbala'ria elati'ně, Fluellen* or *Female Speedwell,* was formerly used against scurvy and old ulcerations.

ANTIRHI'NUM HEDERACEUM, A. Linaria—a. Hederæfolium, A. Linaria.

ANTIRHI'NUM LINA'RIA, *A. hedera'ceum seu hederæfo'lium seu acutan'gulum, Lina'ria, L. vulga'ris seu cymbala'ria, Elati'ně cymbala'ria, Cymbala'ria mura'lis, Osy'ris, Urina'ria, Common Toad Flax,* (F.) *Linaire.* The leaves have a bitterish taste. They are reputed to be diuretic and cathartic. An ointment made from them has been extolled in hemorrhoids.

ANTISCABIOUS, Antipsoric.

ANTISCIRRHOUS, Anticancerous.

ANTISCOLETICUS, Anthelmintic.

ANTISCOLICUS, Anthelmintic.

ANTISCORBU'TIC, *Antiscorbu'ticus,* from αντι, 'against,' and *scorbutus,* 'the scurvy.' Opposed to scurvy.

ANTISCROF'ULOUS, *Antiscroph'ulous, Antiscrofulo'sus, Antistrumo'sus, Antichærad'icus.* Opposed to scrofula.

ANTISEP'TIC, *Antisep'ticus, Antipu'trid,* from αντι, 'against,' and σηπτος, 'putrid.' *Antiputredino'sus.* Opposed to putrefaction. The chief antiseptics, internally or externally employed, are *Acidum Muriaticum, Acidum Nitricum, Acidum Sulphuricum, Aluminæ sulphas, Carbo Ligni, Calx Chlorinata, Chlorinum, Cinchona* and its active principles, *Creasote, Dauci Radix, Fermentum Cerevisia, Soda Chlorinata,* and *Zinci Chloridum.*

ANTISIAL'AGOGUE, *Antisialago'gus, Antisi'alus,* from αντι, 'against,' and σιαλον, 'saliva.' A remedy against ptyalism.

ANTISPASIS, Derivation, Revulsion.

ANTISPASMOD'IC, *Antispasmod'icus, Antispas'ticus,* from αντι, 'against,' and σπαω, 'I contract.' Opposed to spasm. The whole operation of antispasmodics is probably revulsive. The following are the chief reputed antispasmodics. *Æther Sulphuricus, Asafœtida, Castoreum, Dracontium, Moschus, Oleum Animale Dippelii,* and *Valeriana*—with the mental antispasmodics, abstraction, powerful emotions, fear, &c. Of direct antispasmodics, we have no example.

ANTISPASTICUS, Antispasmodic, Derivative.

ANTISTASIS, Antagonism.

ANTISTERIG'MA, from αντι, 'against,' and στηρυγμα, 'a support.' A fulcrum, support, crutch.—Hippocrates.

ANTISTER'NUM, from αντι, 'against,' and στερνον, 'the sternum.' The back.—Rufus.

ANTISTRUMOUS, Antiscrofulous.

ANTISYPHILIT'IC, *Antisyphilit'icus,* from αντι, 'against,' and *syphilis,* 'the venereal disease.' Opposed to the venereal disease.

ANTITASIS, Counter-extension.

ANTITHENAR, Opponens pollicis, Adductor pollicis pedis.

ANTITHERMA, Refrigerants.

ANTITHORA, Aconitum anthora.

ANTITRAG'ICUS, *Antitra'geus,* (F.) *Muscle de l'Antitragus, M. antitragien.*—(Ch.) Belonging to the antitragus. A small muscle is so called, the existence of which is not constant. It occupies the space between the antitragus and anthelix.

ANTITRAGIEN, Antitragicus.

ANTIT'RAGUS, from αντι, 'opposite to,' and τραγος, 'the tragus,' *Antilo'bium, Oblo'bium.* A conical eminence on the pavilion of the ear, opposite the tragus.

ANTITYP'IA, from αντι, 'against,' and τυπτω, 'I strike.' Resistance. Hardness. Repercussion.

ANTITYPICUS, Antiperiodic.

ANTIVENE'REAL, *Antivene'reus,* from αντι, 'against,' and *Venus,* 'Venus.' The same as Antisyphilitic. Formerly it was used synonymously with Antaphrodisiac.

ANTIVERMICULAR, Antiperistaltic.

ANTIVERMINOSUS, Anthelmintic.

ANT'LIA or ANTLI'A, from αντλειν, 'to pump out.' A syringe; a pump. Hence, *Antlia lac'tea, Lactisu'gium,* a breast-pump; and *Antlia sanguisu'ga, Antibdella, Hiru'do artificia'lis,* the exhausting syringe used in cupping.

ANTLIA GASTRICA, Stomach-pump.

ANTODONTALGIC. Antiodontalgic.

ANTODYNUS, Anodyne.

ANTRAX, Anthrax.

ANTRE, Antrum — a. *d'Hyghmore,* Antrum of Highmore.

ANTROVERSIO, Anteversio.

ANTRUM, 'A cavern,' *Cavern'a, Bar'athrum,* (F.) *Antre.* A name given to certain cavities in bones, the entrance to which is smaller than the bottom.

ANTRUM AURIS, Tympanum — a. Buccinosum,

Cochlea, Labyrinth — a. Dentale, see Tooth — a. Pylori, see Stomach.

ANTRUM OF HIGHMORE, *Antrum Highmoria'num, Antrum Genæ, Antrum maxilla'ré* vel *maxil'læ superio'ris, Genyan'trum, Max'illary Sinus, Sinus Genæ pituita'rius*, (F.) *Antre d'Hyghmore, Sinus Maxillaire.* A deep cavity in the substance of the superior maxillary bone communicating with the middle meatus of the nose. It is lined by a prolongation of the Schneiderian membrane.

ANULUS, *Fossette.*

ANURESIS, Ischuria.

ANURIA, Ischuria.

ANUS, 'a circle,' *Podex, Potex, Mol'yne, Molyn'ie, Dactyl'ios, Oath'edra, Oyr'ceon, Cys'earos, Oysthos, Aph'edra, Aph'edron, Hedra, Proctos, Archos, Sedes, Culus, Cu'leon.* The circular opening situate at the inferior extremity of the rectum, by which the excrement is expelled. The *fundament.* The *scat.* The *body.* The *seat*, (F.) *Siége.*

ANUS also signifies the anterior orifice of the *Aqueduct of* Sylvius. By some, this *Anus*, called also, *Fora'men commu'né poste'rius*, has been supposed to form a communication between the back part of the third ventricle and the lateral ventricles. It is closed up, however, by the tela choroides, and also by the fornix, which is intimately connected with this. The foramen is situate between the commissura mollis of the optic thalami and the pineal gland.

ANUS, ARTIFICIAL. An opening made artificially, to supply the natural anus. The term is often used to include preternatural anus.

ANUS, CONTRACTED, (F.) *Anus rétréci.* A state of the anus when, from some cause, it is constricted.

ANUS, IMPERFORATE. A malformation, in which there is no natural anus. See Atresia ani adnata.

ANUS, PRETERNAT'URAL, (F.) *Anus contre nature, A. anormal.* An accidental opening which gives issue to the whole or to a part of the fæces. It may be owing to a wound, or, which is most common, to gangrene attacking the intestine in a hernial sac.

This term is also employed, as well as *Anus devié, devious anus,* to the case where the anus, instead of being in its natural situation, is in some neighbouring cavity, as the bladder, vagina, &c.

ANXI'ETY, *Anxi'etas, Anxi'etude, Adæmo'nia, Dyspho'ria anxi'etas, Alys'mus, Al'ycé, Al'ysis, Asé,* from *angere,* Gr. *αγχειν,* 'to strangle, to suffocate.' A state of restlessness and agitation, with general indisposition, and a distressing sense of oppression at the epigastrium. *Inquietude, anxiety,* and *anguish,* represent degrees of the same condition.

ANYPNIA, Insomnia.

AOCHLE'SIA, from *a,* priv., and *οχλος,* 'disturbance.' Tranquillity. Calmness.

AOR'TA, *Arte'ria magna, A. crassa, A. max'ima, Hæmal Axis,* of Owen. (F.) *Aorte.* This name was given by Aristotle to the chief artery of the body. It may have been derived from *αορτεομαι,* 'I am suspended,' as it seems to be suspended from the heart; or from *αηρ,* 'air,' and *τηρεω,* 'I keep,' because it was supposed to contain air. It is probable that Hippocrates meant by *αορται* the bronchia and their ramifications. The aorta is the common trunk of the arteries of the body. It arises from the left ventricle of the heart, about opposite to the fifth dorsal vertebra, passes upwards *(ascending Aorta,)* forms the *great arch of the Aorta,* and descends along the left of the spine *(descending Aorta,)* until it reaches the middle of the fourth or fifth lumbar vertebra, where it bifurcates, to give origin to the common iliacs. The aorta is sometimes divided into the *Thoracic* or *pectoral,* and the *Abdominal.* For the arteries which arise from it, &c., see Artery.

AORTEURYS'MA, from *αορτη,* 'the aorta,' and *ευρυς,* 'dilated.' Aneurism of the Aorta, (F.) *Anévrysme de l'Aorte, Aortiectasie.* By carefully auscultating over the dorsal vertebræ, a bellows' sound, with a deep and not always perceptible impulse, may be detected.

AOR'TIC, *Aor'ticus.* Relating to the Aorta. The *Aortic ventricle,* (F.) *Ventricle Aortique,* is the left ventricle. The *Aortic valves* are the sigmoid valves at the origin of the Aorta, &c.

AORTIEOTASIE, Aorteurysma.

AORTI'TIS, *Inflamma'tio Aor'tæ,* from *Aorta,* and *itis,* denoting inflammation. Inflammation of the aorta.

AORTRA, *Aortron.* A lobe of the lungs.—Hippocrates.

AO'TUS, from *a,* privative, and *ους,* 'an ear.' A monster devoid of ears.—Gurlt.

APAG'MA, *Apoclas'ma, Apocecaulis'menon,* from *απο,* 'from,' and *αγω,* 'I remove.' Separation, abduction. Separation of a fractured bone.—Galenus, Foësius.

APAGOGE, Defecation, Inductio.

APALACHINE, Ilex vomitoria — *a. à Feuilles de Prunier,* Prinos—a. Gallis, Ilex vomitoria.

APAL'LAGE, *Apallax'is,* from *αναλαττω,* 'I change.' Mutation, change. It is generally taken in a good sense, and means the change from disease to health.—Hippocrates.

APALLAXIS, Apallage.

APALOT'ICA, from *απαλοτης,* 'softness, tenderness.' Fortuitous lesions or deformities affecting the soft parts. The first order in the class *Tychica,* of Good.

APANTHESIS, Apanthismus.

APANTHIS'MUS, *Apanthe'sis,* from *απο,* 'from,' and *ανθεω,* 'I flower.' The obliteration of parts previously inservient to useful purposes, as of the ductus venosus and ductus arteriosus, which are essential to fœtal existence, but are subsequently unnecessary. See, also, Stuprum.

APANTHRO'PIA, from *απο,* 'from,' and *ανθρωπος,* 'man.' Detestation of man; desire for solitude.—Hippocrates. One of the symptoms of hypochondriasis.

APAPHRISMOS, Despumation.

APARACH'YTUM VINUM, from *a,* priv., and *παραχυω,* 'I pour over.' The purest wine: that which has not been mixed with sea-water.—Galen.

APARINE, Galium aparine—a. Hispida, Galium aparine.

APARTHROSIS, Diarthrosis.

AP'ATHY, *Apathi'a, Ameli'a,* from *a,* privative, and *παθος,* 'affection.' (F.) *Apathie.* Accidental suspension of the moral feelings. It takes place in very severe diseases, particularly in malignant fevers.

APECHE'MA, from *απο,* 'from,' and *ηχος,* 'sound.' Properly the action of reflecting sound. In medicine, it is synonymous with the Latin *Contrafissura,* a counter-fissure, a counter-blow.—Gorræus, Celsus.

APECTOCEPHALUS, Acephalothorus.

APEL'LA, *Appel'la, Leipoder'mos, Recuti'tus,* from *a,* priv., and *pellis,* 'skin.' One whose prepuce does not cover the glans.—Galenus, Linnæus, Vogel. Retraction or smallness of any other soft appendage.—Sagar. One who is circumcised.

APEPSIA, Dyspepsia.

APE'RIENT, *Ape'riens, Aperiti'vus,* from *aperire, (ad* and *pario,)* 'to open.' *Res'erans.* A laxative. (F.) *Apéritif.* A medicine which gently opens the bowels. The term had formerly a much more extensive signification, and, like *Catalyt'icum*, was given to a substance supposed to have the power of opening any of the passages, and even the blood-vessels.

APERIS'TATON, *Aperis'tatum*, from *a*, privative, and περιστημι, 'I surround.' An epithet for an ulcer not dangerous nor considerable, nor surrounded by inflammation.

APÉRITIF, Aperient.

APERITIVUS, Aperient.

APERTOR OCULI, Levator palpebræ superioris.

APERTO'RIUM, from *aperio*, 'I open.' An instrument for dilating the os uteri during labour.

APERTURA, Mouth — a. Anterior ventriculi tertii cerebri, Vulva (cerebri) — a. Pelvis superior, see Pelvis.

APEUTHYSMENOS, Rectum.

APEX, *Mucro*. The point or extremity of a part: — as the apex of the tongue, nose, &c.

APEX LINGUÆ, Proglossis.

APHÆRESIS, Apheresis, Extirpation.

APHALANGI'ASIS, from *a*, 'intensive,' and φαλαγξ, 'phalanx.' The fourth stage of Oriental leprosy, which is recognised chiefly by a gangrenous condition of the fingers.

APHASSOM'ENOS, from αφασσω, 'I touch, I feel.' The touching of the parts of generation of the female as a means of diagnosis. — Hippocrates. See Esaphe.

APHEDRA, Anus.

APHEDRIA, Menses.

APHEDRON, Anus.

APHELI'A, αφελης, 'simple.' Simplicity. The simple manners of the sect of Methodists in teaching and practising medicine.

APHELX'IA, from αφελκω, 'I abstract.' Voluntary inactivity of the whole or the greater part of the external senses to the impressions of surrounding objects, during wakefulness. *Revery*, (F.) *Rêverie*. Dr. Good has introduced this into his Nosology, as well as *Aphelx'ia socors* or *absence of mind* — A. *inten'ta* or *abstraction of mind*: and A. *otio'sa*, *Stu'dium ina'nē*, *brown study* or *listless musing*.

APHEPSEMA, Decoction.

APHEPSIS, Decoction.

APHE'RESIS, *Aphæ'resis*, from αφαιρεω, 'I take away.' An operation by which any part of the body is separated from the other. Hippocrates, according to Foësius, uses the expression *Aphæ'resis San'guinis* for excessive hemorrhage; and Sennertus, to express the condition of an animal deprived both of the faculties of the mind and of the mind itself.

APH'ESIS, from αφιημι, 'I relax.' A remission. This word expresses sometimes the diminution or cessation of a disease; at others, languor and debility of the lower extremities. See Languor, and Remission.

APHILAN'THROPY, *Aphilanthro'pia*, from *a*, privative, φιλεω, 'I love,' and ανθρωπος, 'a man.' Dislike to man. Love of solitude. Vogel has given this name to the first degree of melancholy.

APHISTĒSIS, Abscess.

APHODEUMA, Excrement.

APHODUS, Excrement.

APHONETUS, Aphonus.

APHO'NIA, *Liga'tio linguæ*, *Loque'la abol'ita*, *Defec'tus loque'læ*, *Dyspho'nia*, (of some,) *Aph'ony*, (F.) *Aphonie*, *Perte de la Voix*, from *a*, privative, and φωνη, 'voice.' Privation of voice, or of the sounds that ought to be produced in the glottis. When aphonia forms part of catarrh or of 'cold,' it is commonly of but little consequence; but when produced by causes acting on the nervous system, as by some powerful emotion, or without any appreciable lesion of the vocal apparatus, (*Laryngo-paralysis*,) it frequently resists all remedies.

APHONIA, Catalepsy — a. Surdorum, Mutitas Surdorum.

APHONICUS, Aphonus.

APHO'NUS, *Apho'nicus*, *Apho'netus*; same etymon. Relating to aphonia.

APHONY, Aphonia.

APHORIA, Sterilitas.

APHORICUS, Sterile.

APHORUS, Sterile.

APHOR'ME, αφορμη, 'occasion.' The external and manifest cause of any thing. The occasional cause of a disease. — Hippocrates.

APHRO'DES, 'frothy,' from αφρος, 'foam,' and ειδος, 'resemblance.' Applied to the blood and the excrements. — Hippocrates.

APHRODISIA, Coition, Puberty.

APHRODIS'IAC, *Aphrodisiacus*, from Αφροδιτη, 'Venus.' (F.) *Aphrodisiaque*. Medicine or food believed to be capable of exciting to the pleasures of love; as ginger, cantharides, &c. They are generally stimulants.

APHRODISIACUS, Venereal.

APHRODISIASMUS, Coition.

APHRODISIOG'RAPHY, from Αφροδιτη, 'Venus,' and γραφω, 'I describe.' Etymologically, this term means a description of the pleasures of love, but it has been placed at the head of a work describing the venereal disease.

APHROG'ALA, from αφρος, 'foam,' and γαλα, 'milk.' *Lac spumo'sum*. A name formerly given to milk rendered frothy by agitation.

APHRONIA, Apoplexy.

APHRONITRUM, Natrum, Soda.

APHROSYNE, Delirium, Insanity.

APHTHÆ, *Aphta*, *Apthæ*, from αττω, 'I inflame.' *Thrush* or *sore mouth*, *Aphtha lactu'cimen*, A. *Infan'tum*, *Lactu'cimen*, *Lactucim'ina*, *Al'colæ*, *Lactu'mina*, *Em'phlysis aphtha*, *Ulcera serpen'tia oris*, *Pus'tula oris*, *Febris aphtho'sa*, *Angi'na aphtho'sa*, *Vesic'ulæ gingiva'rum*, *Stomati'tis exsudati'va*, *S. vesiculo'sa infan'tum*, *Stomap'yra*, *S. aphtha*, *Prunel'la*, *White Thrush*, *Milk Thrush*. Aphthæ consist of roundish, pearl-coloured vesicles, confined to the lips, mouth, and intestinal canal, and generally terminating in curd-like sloughs. In France, the Aphthæ of children, *Aphthes des Enfans*, is called *Muguet*, *Millet*, *Blanchet*, *Catarrhe buccal* and *Stomatite crémeuse pultacée*, *Pultaceous inflammation of the Mouth*; and generally receives two divisions — the *mild* or *discreet*, (F.) *Muguet bénin* ou *discret*, and the *malignant*, (F.) *Muguet malin* ou *confluent*, the *Black Thrush*. Common Thrush is a disease of no consequence, requiring merely the use of absorbent laxatives. The malignant variety, which is rare, is of a more serious character, and is accompanied with typhoid symptoms, — *Typhus aphthoïdeus*.

APHTHÆ ADULTORUM, Stomatitis, aphthous — a. Præputii, Herpes præputii — a. Serpentes, Cancer aquaticus.

APHTHE GANGRÉNEUX, Cancer aquaticus.

APHTHES DES ENFANS, Aphthæ.

APHTHEUX, Aphthous.

APHTHO'DES, *Aphthoïdes*, *Aphthoïdeus*, from *aphthæ*, and ειδος, 'resemblance.' Aphthous-like. Resembling aphthæ.

APH'THOUS, *Aphtho'sus*, (F.) *Aphtheux*. Belonging to aphthæ; complicated with aphthæ; as *Aphthous Fever*.

APIASTRUM, Melissa.

APICES CRURUM MEDULLÆ OBLONGATÆ, Corpora striata — a. Digitorum, Pupulæ.

APILEPSIA, Apoplexy.

APIONTA, see Excretion.

APIOS, Pyrus communis.
APIS, Bee.
API'TES, from απιον, 'a pear.' Perry.—Gorræus.
APIUM, A. graveolens—a. Ammi, Ammi—a. Anisum, Pimpinella anisum—a. Carvi, Carum.
APIUM GRAVEOLENS, *Apium Paluda'pium, Beli'num, Ses'eli graveolens, Sium graveolens, S. a'pium, Smallage,* (F.) *Ache. Nat. Ord.* Umbelliferæ. *Sex. Syst.* Pentandria Digynia. The plants, roots, and seeds are aperient and carminative. *Selery* is a variety of this.
APIUM HORTENSE, A. graveolens—a. Montanum, Athamanta aureoselinum—a. Paludapium, A. Graveolens—a. Petræum, Bubon Macedonicum.
APIUM PETROSELI'NUM, *Apium Horten'se* seu *vulga'ri, Eleoseli'num* (?), *Grielum, Petroseli'num, Common Parsley,* (F.) *Persil.* The root—*Petroselinum,* (Ph. U. S.)—and seeds are diuretic and aperient.
APIUM SIUM, Sium nodiflorum—a. Vulgare, A. graveolens.
APLAS'TIC, *Aplas'ticus,* from *a,* privative, and πλασσω, 'I form.' That which is not capable of forming; that which does not serve to form, or is not organisable.
APLASTIC ELEMENT; one which is unsusceptible of any further amount of organization.—Gerber.
APLESTIA, Ingluvies, Intemperance.
APLEU'ROS, from *a,* privative, and πλευρος, 'a rib.' One without ribs.—Hippocrates, Galen.
APLOT'OMY, *Aplotom'ia,* from απλοος, 'simple,' and τεμνω, 'I cut.' A simple incision.
APNEUSTIA, Apnœa, Asphyxia.
APNŒ'A, from *a,* privative, and πνεω, 'I respire.' *Asphyx'ia, Apneus'tia.* Absence of respiration, *Respira'tio abol'ita,* or insensible respiration. Also, Orthopnœa.
APNŒA INFANTUM, Asthma Thymicum.
APNŒASPHYXIA, Asphyxia.
APNUS, απνους, same etymon. One devoid of respiration. An epithet applied by authors to cases in which the respiration is so small and slow, that it seems suspended.—Castelli. It is probable, however, that the word was always applied to the patient, not to the disease.
APO, απο, a prefix denoting 'from, of, off, out,' Hence—
APOBAMMA, Embamma.
APOBAINON, Eventus.
APOBESOMENON, Eventus.
APOBIOSIS, Death.
APOBLEMA, Abortion.
APOBOLE, Abortion.
APOBRASMA, Furfur.
APOCAPNISMUS, Fumigation.
APOCATASTASIS, Considentia, Restauratio.
APOCATHARSIS, Catharsis.
APOCATHARTICUS, Cathartic.
APOCECAULISMENON, Apagma.
APOCENO'SIS, *Aposceno'sis,* from απο, 'out,' and κενωσις, 'evacuation.' A partial evacuation, according to some, in opposition to Cenosis, which signifies a general evacuation.—Cullen and Swediaur apply it to morbid fluxes.
APOCENOSIS, Abevacuatio—a. Diabetes mellitus, Diabetes—a. Ptyalismus mellitus, see Salivation—a. Vomitus pyrosis, Pyrosis.
APOCHOREON, Excrement.
APOCHREMMA, Sputum.
APOCHREMPSIS, Exspuition.
APOCH'YMA, from αποχεω, 'I pour out.' A sort of tar, obtained from old ships, which is impregnated with chloride of sodium. It was used as a discutient of tumours.— Aëtius, Paulus, Gorræus.

APOCIN GOBE-MOUCHE, Apocynum androsæmifolium.
APOCLASMA, Abduction, Apagma.
APOCLEISIS, Asitia, Disgust.
APOC'OPE, from απο, and κοπτω, 'to cut.' Abscission. A wound with loss of substance. Fracture with loss of part of a bone. Amputation.
APOCOPUS, Castratus.
APOCRISIS, Contagion, Excrement, Secretion.
APOCROUS'TIC, *Apocrous'tica* seu *Apocrus'tica,* (remed'ia,) from απο, 'out,' and κρουω, 'I push.' An astringent and repellent.—Galenus.
APOCRUSTICA, Apocroustic.
APOCYESIS, Parturition.
APOC"YNUM ANDROSÆMIFO'LIUM, from απο, and κυων, 'a dog,' because esteemed, of old, to be fatal to dogs. *Dog's Bane, Bitter Dog's Bane, Milkweed, Bitterroot, Honeybloom, Catchfly, Flytrap, Ip'ecac,* (F.) *Apocin gobe-mouche, A. amer. Nat. Ord.* Apocyneæ. *Sex. Syst.* Pentandria Digynic. The root of this plant is found from Canada to Carolina. Thirty grains evacuate the stomach as effectually as two-thirds of the amount of Ipecacuanha, by which name it is known in various parts of the eastern states. It is in the secondary list of the Pharmacopœia of the United States.
APOC"YNUM CANNAB'INUM, *Indian Hemp.* This American plant possesses emetic, cathartic, diaphoretic and diuretic properties, and has been strongly recommended in dropsy. It has been given in decoction,— ℨij of the root boiled in three pints of water to two. A wine-glassful for a dose.
APOCYNUM NOVÆ ANGLIÆ HIRSUTUM, Asclepias tuberosa—a. Orange, Asclepias tuberosa—a. Scandens, Allamanda.
APODACRYT'ICUS, *Delachrymati'vus,* from απο, 'from,' and δακρυω, 'I weep.' A substance, supposed to occasion a flow of the tears, and then to arrest them.—Columella, Pliny, Galenus.
APODEMIALGIA, Nostalgia.
APOD'IA, from *a,* privative, and πους, 'a foot.' Want of feet; hence *Apous* or *Apus,* one who has no feet.
APODYTE'RIUM, *Coniste'rium, Spoliato'rium, Spolia'rium,* from αποδυω, 'I strip off.' The ante-room, where the bathers stripped themselves in the ancient gymnasia.
APOGALACTISMUS, Weaning.
APOGALACTOS, Exuber.
APOGEUSIS, Ageustia.
APOGEUSTIA, Ageustia.
APOGLAUCOSIS, Glaucosis.
APOGON, Imberbis.
APOG'ONUM, from απο, and γινομαι, 'I exist.' A living fœtus in utero.—Hippocrates.
APOLEPISIS, Desquamation.
APOLEPISMUS, Desquamation.
APOLEP'SIS, *Apolep'sia, Apolip'sis,* from απολαμβανω, 'I retain.' Retention, suppression.—Hippocrates. Asphyxia.
APOLEX'IS, from απολεγω, 'I cease.' Old age, decrepitude.
APOLINO'SIS, from απο, and λινον, 'a flaxen thread.' The mode of operating for fistula in ano, by means of a thread of *Homolinon* or *Linum crudum.*—Hippocrates, Paulus.
APOLIPSIS, Apolepsis.
APOLLINARIS ALTERCUM, Hyoscyamus.
APOLUTICA, Cicatrisantia.
APOLYS'IA, *Apol'ysis,* from απολυω, 'I loosen.' Solution. Relaxation. Debility of the limbs or looseness of bandages.—Erotian. Expulsion of the fœtus and its dependencies. Termination of a disease.—Hippocrates, Galen.

APOMATHE'MA, *Apomathe'sis*, from ἀπό, and μανθάνω, 'I learn.' Forgetfulness of things taught.—Hippocrates.

APOM'ELI, from ἀπό, 'of,' and μέλι, 'honey.' An oxymel or decoction made of honey.—Galen, Aëtius, Paulus, &c.

APOMEXIS, Munctio.

APOMYLE'NAS, from ἀπομυλλαίνω, 'I make a wry mouth.' One who pushes his lips forwards, pressing them against each other. Occasionally a symptom of nervous fever.—Galen, Erotian.

APOMYTHO'SIS, from ἀπομύσσω, 'I snore.' A disease in which there is stertor.—Sauvages, Sagar.

APOMYXIA, Nasal mucus.

APONEUROG'RAPHY, *Aponeurogra'phia*, from ἀπονεύρωσις, an 'aponeurosis,' and γραφή, 'a description.' A description of the Aponeuroses.

APONEUROL'OGY, *Aponeurolog''ia*, from ἀπονεύρωσις, 'an aponeurosis.' and λόγος, 'a discourse.' *Aponeurosiol'ogy.* The anatomy of the aponeuroses.

APONEUROSIOLOGY, Aponeurology.

APONEURO'SIS, *Aponevro'sis*, from ἀπό, 'from,' and νεῦρον, 'a nerve.' *Pronerva'tio*, *Denerva'tio*, *Enerva'tio*, *Expan'sio nervo'sa*, (F.) *Aponeurose, Aponévrose.* The ancients called every white part νεῦρον, and regarded the Aponeurosis as a nervous expansion. The Aponeuroses are white, shining membranes, very resisting, and composed of fibres interlaced. Some are continuous with the muscular fibres, and differ only from tendons by their flat form. They are called *Aponeuroses of insertion*, (F.) *Aponévroses d'insertion*, when they are at the extremities of muscles, and attach them to the bone;—*Aponeuroses of intersection*, (F.) *Aponévroses d'intersection*, if they interrupt the continuity of the muscle, and are continuous on both sides with muscular fibres. Others surround the muscle, and prevent its displacement: they are called *enveloping Aponeuroses*, (F.) *Aponévroses d'enveloppe.*

APONEUROSIS, Fascia—a. Crural, Fascia lata—a. Femoral, Fascia lata—a. Iliac, Fascia iliaca.

APONEUROSI'TIS, from *aponeurosis*, and *itis*, 'denoting inflammation.' Inflammation of an aponeurosis.

APONEUROT'IC, *Aponeurot'icus.* What relates to Aponeuroses:—thus, we say *Aponeurotic expansion, Aponeurotic muscle*, &c.

APONEUROT'OMY, *Aponeurotom'ia*, from ἀπονεύρωσις, 'aponeurosis,' and τέμνω, 'I cut.' Anatomy of aponeuroses.

Aponeurotomy has, also, been proposed for the division, (*débridement*) of filaments, &c., in aponeurotic openings, and for the section of fasciæ.

APONÉVROSE PÉDIEUSE, see Pedal Aponeurosis—*a. Superficielle de l'Abdomen et de la Cuisse*, Fascia superficialis.

APONEVROSIS, Aponeurosis.

APON'IA, from *a*, privative, and πόνος, 'pain.' Freedom from pain.

APONIPSIS, Ablution.

APOPALLE'SIS, *Apopal'sis*, from ἀποπάλλω, 'I throw off.' Expulsion. Protrusion.—Hippocrates. Also, Abortion.

APOPATE'MA, *Apop'athos, Apop'atus.* The excrement, and the place where it is deposited.—Dioscorides, Erotian.

APOPEDASIS, Luxation.

APOPHLEGMATISANS PER NARES, Errhine—a. per Os, Sialogogue.

APOPHLEGMATISAN'TIA, *Apophlegmatison'ta, Apophlegmatis'mi*, from ἀπό, 'out,' and φλέγμα, 'phlegm.' Medicines which facilitate the upward expulsion of mucus from the mucous membrane of the digestive or air passages; as gargles, masticatories, &c.

APOPHLEG'MATISM, *Apophlegmatis'mus.* The action of Apophlegmatisantia.—Galen.

APOPHLEGMATISMI, Apophlegmatisantia.

APOPH'RADES, from ἀπόφρας, 'unlucky.' An epithet applied to unlucky days, (*dies nefandi.*) Days on which a favourable change is not expected to occur in a disease.—A. Laurentius.

APOPHRAXIS, Amenorrhœa.

APOPHTHAR'MA, *Apoph'thora*, from ἀπό, and φθείρω, 'I corrupt.' Abortion, as well as a medicine to procure abortion.

APOPHTHORA, Abortion.

APOPHTHORIUS, Abortive.

APOPHY'ADES, from ἀπό, 'from,' and φύω, 'I spring.' The ramifications of veins and arteries.—Hippocrates.

APOPHYSE BASILAIRE, Basilary process—*a. Engainante* ou *vaginale*, Vaginal process—*a. Pyramidale*, see Temporal Bone—*a. Pétrée*, see Temporal Bone.

APOPHYSES ÉPINEUSES, Spinous processes of the vertebræ.

APOPH'YSIS, from ἀπό, 'from,' and φύω, 'I rise,' *Ec'physis, Proces'sus, Appendix, A process of a bone, Prominen'tia ossis contin'ua.* When the apophysis is yet separated from the body of the bone by intervening cartilage, it is called *Epiph'ysis*. The apophyses or processes are, at times, distinguished by epithets, expressive of their form: as *A. styloid, A. coracoid*, &c. Others are not preceded by the word apophysis; as *Trochanter, Tuberosity*, &c.

APOPH'YSIS OF INGRAS'SIAS is a term applied to the lesser ala of the sphenoid bone.

APOPHYSIS OF RAU, *Grêle apophyse du Marteau*: see Malleus.

APOPHYSIS ZYGOMATICA, Zygomatic process.

APOPIES'MA, from ἀποπιέζω, 'I compress.' Hippocrates uses the term to signify a fancied expression or forcing out of humours by the application of bandages in wounds and fractures.

APOPLANESIS, Error loci.

APOPLEC'TIC, *Apoplec'ticus*. Referring to Apoplexy. This word has various significations. It is applied, 1. To individuals labouring under apoplexy: 2. To remedies proper for combating apoplexy: 3. To the constitution, temperament, or make, *Architectu'ra apoplec'tica, Hab'itus apoplec'ticus*, which predisposes to it, and, 4. To the symptoms which characterize apoplexy; as *Apoplectic sleep, A. stroke, A. stertor*, &c. The jugular veins have also, by some, been called *Apoplectic veins, Venæ apoplec'ticæ.*

APOPLECTICUS, Antiapoplectic, Apoplectic.

APOPLECTIC CELL. A cavity remaining in the encephalon, after the effusion of blood and its subsequent absorption.

APOPLEXIA, Apoplexy—a. Catalepsia, Catalepsia—a. Cerebralis, see Apoplexy—a. Cerebri, see Apoplexy—a. Cordis, Hæmocardiorrhagia—a. Hydrocephalica, Hydrocephalus internus—a. Hepatica, Hepatorrhagia — a. Medullaris, Apoplexia myelitica—a. Meningæa, Apoplexy, meningeal.

APOPLEXIA MYELIT'ICA; *A. Medulla'ris, A. Spina'lis, A. Rachia'lis, Hæmor'rhachia, Myelorrhag''ia, Myelapoplex'ia*, (F.) *Apoplexie de la Moëlle épinière, Hémorrhagie de la Moëlle épinière, Hémato-myélie, Hémo-myélorrhagie, Hématorrhachis*. Hemorrhage into the spinal marrow.

APOPLEXIA NERVOSA, Apoplexy, nervous—a. Nervosa traumatica, Concussion of the brain—a. Pituitosa, see Apoplexy—a. Pulmonalis, see Hæmoptysis — a. Pulmonum, see Hæmoptysis — a.

Renalis, Apoplexy, renal — a. Rachialis, A. myelitica — a. Sanguinea, see Apoplexy — a. Serosa, see Apoplexy — a. Simplex, Apoplexy, nervous — a. Spasmodica, Apoplexy, nervous — a. Spinalis, Apoplexia myelitica. — a. Temulenta, see Temulentia.

APOPLEXIE CAPILLAIRE, Mollities cerebri — a. Cérébrale, Apoplexy, Hémorrhagie cérébrale.

APOPLEXIE FOUDROYANTE, 'Thundering Apoplexy.' A form of apoplexy, which is intense and rapidly fatal.

APOPLEXIE MENINGÉE, Apoplexy, meningeal — a. De la Moëlle Épinière, Apoplexy, spinal.

AP'OPLEXY, *Apoplex'ia*, from ατοπληττειν, 'to strike with violence.' At the present day, the term apoplexy is employed by many writers to signify *interstitial hemorrhage*, (F.) *Hémorrhagie interstitielle*, or every effusion of blood, which occurs suddenly into the substance of an organ or tissue. Hence, we speak of cerebral apoplexy, pulmonary apoplexy, &c. &c. Formerly it was always — and still is by many — used in a restricted sense, to signify, in other words, the train of phenomena, which characterize cerebral apoplexy. This disease, *Hæmorrha'gia Cer'ebri, Aphro'nia, Carus Apoplex'ia, Coma Apoplex'ia, Apoplex'ia cer'ebri sanguin'ea, A. cerebra'lis, Encephalorrhag"ia, San'guinis ictus, Hæmatenceph'alum, Pulpex'ia, Sidera'tio, Apileps'ia, Morbus atton'itus, Gutta, Theople'gia, Theoplex'ia*, (F.) *Apoplexie, A. cérébrale, Hématoëncephalie, Coup de sang*, is characterized by diminution, or loss of sensation and mental manifestation; by the cessation, more or less complete, of motion; and by a comatose state, — circulation and respiration continuing. It generally consists in pressure upon the brain; either from turgescence of vessels, or from extravasation of blood: hence the terms *Hæmenceph'alus, Hémorrhagie cérébrale*, and *Hémoëncephalorrhagie*, applied to it by some. The general prognosis is unfavourable; especially when it occurs after the age of 35. When Apoplexy is accompanied with a hard, full pulse, and flushed countenance, it is called *Apoplexia sanguin'ea, Cataph'ora coma;* when with a feeble pulse and pale countenance, and evidences of serous effusion, *Apoplex'ia sero'sa, A. pituito'sa, Serous Apoplexy, Cataph'ora hydrocephal'ica, Encephaloch'ysis seni'lis, Hydroceph'alus acu'tus senum, Hydroëncephalorrhée*, (Piorry), *Hydropisie cérébrale suraigüé, Hydrorrhagie.*

In *Nervous Apoplexy, Apoplex'ia nervo'sa seu spasmod'ica, A. simplex, Simple apoplexy*, no lesion whatever may be perceptible on dissection, although the patient may have died under all the phenomena that are characteristic of apoplexy.

APOPLEXY OF THE HEART, Hæmocardiorrhagia.

APOPLEXY, MENINGE'AL, *Apoplex'ia meningæ'a*, (F.) *Apoplexie méningée, Hémorrhagie méningée.* Hemorrhage from the meninges of the brain or spinal marrow, generally into the great cavity of the arachnoid.

APOPLEXY, NERVOUS, see Apoplexy — a. Pulmonary, see Hæmoptysis — a. Simple, A. Nervous.

APOPLEXY, RENAL, *Apoplex'ia rena'lis.* A condition of the kidney, characterized by knotty, irregular, tuberculated eminences, some of a deep black colour. Effusion of blood into the substance of the kidney.

APOPLEXY, SEROUS, see Apoplexy — a. Spinal, Apoplexia myelitica.

APOPNEUSIS, Exhalatio.
APOPNIXIS, Suffocation.
APOPNOE, Exspiratio.
APOPNŒA, Exspiratio.
APOPSYCHIA, Syncope.
APOPTO'SIS, from αποπιπτω, 'I fall down.' A relaxation of bandages. — Erotian.
APORRHOE, Aporrhœa.
APORRHŒ'A, *Apor'rhoë, Apor'rhysis, Deflu'vium*, from αποῤῥεω, 'I flow from.' An emanation, effluvium, contagion. — Moschion. A falling off of the hair, according to some.
APORRHYSIS, Aporrhœa.
APOSCEM'MA, *Aposcep'sis*, from αποσκηπτω. 'I lie down, I direct myself towards.' Afflux of fluids towards a part. Metastasis. The first word has been applied to the excrements. — Hippocrates, Galen.
APOSCENOSIS, Apocenosis.
APOSCEPARNIS'MUS, *Deascia'tio*, from απο and σκεπαρνον, 'a hatchet.' Wound of the cranium, by a cutting instrument, in which a piece of the bone has been cut out, as with a hatchet. — Gorræus.
APOSCEPSIS, Aposcemma.
APOS'CHASIS, *Aposchas'mus*, from ατοσχαζω, 'I scarify.' *Scarifica'tion.* A slight superficial incision in the skin. Also, blood-letting. — Hippocrates.
APOS'IA, *Sitis defec'tus*, from α, privative, and ποσις, 'drink.' Want of thirst, absence of desire for liquids.
APOSI'TIA, from απο, 'from,' and σιτος, 'food.' Aversion for food. — Galen. See Disgust.
APOSIT'IC, *Aposit'icus;* the same etymology. Any substance which destroys the appetite, or suspends hunger.
APOSPAS'MA, from αποσπαω, 'I tear or lacerate.' (F.) *Arrachement.* A solution of continuity, especially of a ligament; *Rhegma ligamenta'rē, Lacera'tio ligamenta'ria.*
APOSPHACEL'ISIS, *Aposphacelis'mus*, from απο, and σφακελος, 'mortification.' Gangrene in wounds and fractures, owing to the bandages being too tight. — Hippocrates.
APOSPHINX'IS, αποσφιγξις, constriction, compression. The action of a tight bandage. — Hippocrates.
APOSPONGIS'MUS, the act of sponging for any purpose. — Gorræus.
APOSTALAG'MA, *Apostag'ma*, from απο, 'from,' and σταλαζω, 'I drop.' The ancient name for the saccharine liquor which flows from grapes when not yet pressed.
APOS'TASIS, from απο, and ιστημι, 'I stop.' The ancients had different significations for this word. It was most commonly used for an abscess. The separation of a fragment of bone by fracture. Removal of disease by some excretion, &c.
APOSTAX'IS, from αποσταζω, 'I distil from.' *Staxis.* The defluxion of any humour, as of blood from the nose. — Hippocrates.
APOSTE'MA, from απο, 'from,' and ιστημι, 'I settle,' or from αφιστημι, 'I recede from.' This word is used by the ancients somewhat vaguely. It meant an affection in which parts, previously in contact, are separated from each other by a fluid collected between them. The moderns regard it as synonymous with *Abscess.* Some, even of the moderns, have applied it to any watery tumour, and even to tumours in general.

APOSTEMA CEREBRI, Encephalopyosis — a. Empyema, Empyema — a. Parulis, Parulis — a. Phalangum, *Fourche* — a. Psoaticum, Lumbar abscess.
APOSTERIG'MA, from αποστηριζω, 'I support.' Any thing that supports a diseased part, as a cushion, a pillow, &c. — Galen. A deep-seated and inveterate disease of the intestines. — Hippocrates.

APOS'THIA, *Leipoder'mia*, from *a* privative, and τοσθια, 'prepuce.' Want of prepuce.

APOSTOLO'RUM UNGUENT'UM, *Dodecaphar'macum, Ointment of the Apostles.* So called, because as many solid ingredients entered into its composition as there were apostles. It contained several resins and gum-resins, yellow wax, oil, vinegar, verdigris, &c., and was formerly employed as a vulnerary.

APOS'TROPHE, from απο, and στρεφω, 'I turn.' An aversion or disgust for food.—Paulus. Also, the direction of humours towards other parts.

APOSYRMA, Abrasion, Desquamation.

APOTELES'MA, from απο, and τελεσμα, 'completion.' The result or termination of a disease. See, also, Amuletum.

APOTHANASIA, see Death.

APOTHE'CA, *Pharmace'um, Pharmacopo'lium*, from απο, and τιθημι, 'to place.' Any place where things are kept, and therefore 'a shop,' and particularly a wine cellar. A place or vessel wherein medicines are kept. See Pharmacopolium.

APOTHECARIES' HALL. The Hall of the Corporation or Society of Apothecaries of London, where medicines are prepared and sold under their direction, &c. This Company obtained a charter of incorporation in the 15th year of James the First. No general practitioner can establish himself in England or Wales, without having obtained a license from the Court of Examiners of the Company.

APOTH'ECARY, *Apotheca'rius, Dispensa'tor, Pharmacopo'la, Pigmenta'rius, Pharmacopoe'us, Pharma'ceus, Pharmaceu'ta, Rhizot'omus, Myropo'les, Myropo'lus, Pharmacter, Pharmacurgicus, Pharmacur'gus, Pharmaceu'tist*, same derivation, (F.) *Apothicaire, Pharmacien, Pharmacopole*. In every country except Great Britain, it means one who sells drugs, makes up prescriptions, &c. In addition to these offices, which, indeed, they rarely exercise, except in the case of their own patients, the Apothecaries in England form a privileged class of practitioners—a kind of sub-physician.

APOTHERAPEI'A, *Apotherapi'a, Apotherapeu'sis*, from αποθεραπευω, (απο and θεραπευω,) 'I cure.' A perfect cure.—Hippoc. In the ancient Gymnastics, it meant the last part of the exercises:—the friction, inunction, and bathing, for the purpose of obviating fatigue, or curing disease.—Galen, Gorræus.

APOTHERAPEUSIS, Apotherapeia.

APOTHER'MUM, from απο, and θερμη, 'heat.' A pickle made of mustard, oil, and vinegar.—Galen.

APOTH'ESIS, from αποτιθημι, 'I replace.' The position proper to be given to a fractured limb, after reduction.

APOTHICAIRE, Apothecary.

APOTHICAIRERIE, (F.) from αποθηκη, 'a warehouse, shop.' The same as Apotheca; also, a gallipot.

APOTHLIM'MA, from απο, and θλιβω, 'I press from.' Anciently, the dregs, and sometimes the expressed juice, *Succus expres'sus*, of plants.—Gorræus.

APOTHRAU'SIS, from αποθραυω, 'I break.' Fracture of a bone, with spicula remaining. Extraction of a spiculum of bone.—Gorræus. Also, Abscission.

APOTILMOS, Evulsion.

APOT'OKOS, from απο, and τικτω, 'I bring forth.' An abortive fœtus.—Hippocrates.

APOTOME, Amputation.

APOTOMIA, Amputation.

APOTROPÆUM, Amuletum.

APOTROPE, Aversion. Also, deviation—as of a limb—*Parat'ropē*.

APOXYSMUS, Abrasion.
APOZEM, Decoction.
APOZESIS, Decoction.

APPARA'TUS, *Parasceu'ē*, from *ad* and *parare*, 'to prepare.' This word signifies a collection of instruments, &c., for any operation whatever. (F.) *Appareil*.

In surgery, it means the methodical arrangement of all the instruments and objects necessary for an operation or dressing. By extension, the French give the name *Appareil, Caisse chirur'gica*, to the case or drawers in which the apparatus is arranged.

Apparatus has likewise been applied to the different modes of operating for the stone.—See Lithotomy.

In *Physiology*, Apparatus (*Appareil*) is applied to a collection of organs, all of which work towards the same end. *A system of organs* comprehends all those formed of a similar texture. An *apparatus* often comprehends organs of very different nature. In the *former*, there is analogy of structure; in the *latter*, analogy of function.

APPARATUS ALTUS, see Lithotomy.

APPARATUS IMMOV'ABLE, (F.) *Appareil immobile, Immovable Bandage, Permanent Bandage*. An apparatus for fractures, which is generally formed by wetting the bandages in some substance, as starch or dextrin, which becomes solid, and retains the parts *in situ*.

APPARATUS LATERALIS, see Lithotomy — a. Major, see Lithotomy—a. Minor, see Lithotomy.

APPAREIL, Apparatus, *Boîtier* — a. *Grand*, see Lithotomy—a. *Haut*, see Lithotomy—a. *Immobile*, Apparatus, immovable—a. *Lateralisé*, see Lithotomy — a. *Petit*, see Lithotomy — a. *Pigmental*, Pigmental apparatus.

APPAREILS DE FORMATION, (F.) Gall admits, in the brain, two kinds of fibres; the one, divergent, proceeding from the cerebral peduncles to the convolutions, and constituting what he calls *appareils de formation :* the other, convergent, and proceeding from the convolutions to the centre of the organ, constituting what he calls *appareils de réunion*. The *first*, as a whole, form the organs of the mental faculties : the *latter* are commissures, which unite parts of the organ that are double and in pairs.

APPAUVRI, Impoverished.

APPENDICE, Appendix—a. *Cœcal*, Appendix vermiformis cæci—*a. Digital*, Appendix vermiformis cæci — a. *Sous-sternale*, Xiphoid cartilage — a. *Sus-sphenoïdale du cerveau*, Pituitary gland—*a. Xiphoïde*, Xiphoid cartilage.

APPENDICES COLI ADIPOSÆ, Appendiculæ epiploicæ—*Épiploïques*, Appendiculæ epiploicæ.

APPENDICULA CEREBRI, Pituitary gland — a. Vermiformis cæci, see Appendix — a. Epiploica, Epiploic appendage.

APPENDIC'ULÆ PINGUEDINO'SÆ, *Epiploic appendages, Appendic'ulæ Epiplo'icæ, Appen'dices coli adipo'sæ, Omen'tula,* (F.) *Appendices Epiploïques*. Prolongations of the peritoneum beyond the surface of the great intestine, which are analogous in texture and arrangement to omenta.

APPEN'DIX, *Epiph'ysis*, from *appendere*, (*ad* and *pendere*, 'to hang,') 'to hang from.' Any part that adheres to an organ or is continuous with it:—seeming as if added to it. *An appendage;* an apophysis, (F.) *Appendice, Annexe*.

APPENDIX AURICULÆ, see Auricles of the Heart.

APPENDIX CEREBRI, Pituitary gland — a. ad Cerebrum, Cerebellum—a. Cutanea Septi Narium, Statica Septi Narium—a. to the Epididymis, Vasculum aberrans—a. Ventriculi, Duodenum.

APPENDIX VERMIFOR'MIS, *Appendic'ula Ver-*

miför'mis Cæ'ci, Tubus Vermicula'ris Cæci, Ec'-phyas, Additamen'tum Coli, Appen'dix Cæ'ci, (F.) *Appendice vermiforme, A. cæcal* ou *digital.* A vermicular process, the size of a goose-quill, which hangs from the intestine cæcum. Its functions are unknown.

APPENSIO, see Analeptia.

AP'PETENCE, *Appeten'tia,* from *appetere,* (*ad* and *petere,*) 'to desire.' An ardent, passionate desire for any object.

APPETIT, PERTE D', Anorexia.

AP'PETITE, *Appeti'tus, Appeten'tia, Appeti''-tia,* (*ad* and *petere,*) 'to seek,' *Cupi'do, Orex'is, Ormè:* same etymology as the last. An internal sensation, which warns us of the necessity of exerting certain functions, especially those of digestion and generation. In the latter case it is called *venereal appetite,* (F.) *Appetit vénérien:* in the former, simply *appetite,* (F.) *Appetit* ou *Appetition.* If the desire for food, occasioned by a real want, be carried to a certain extent, it is called *hunger,* when solid food is concerned; *thirst,* when liquid. Appetite and hunger ought not, however, to be employed synonymously: they are different degrees of the same want. Hunger is an imperious desire: it cannot be provoked, like the appetite. It is always allayed by eating: but not so the appetite; for, at times, it may be excited in this manner. They are very generally, however, used synonymously.

APPETITE, MORBID, Limosis.

AP'PETITE, VENE'REAL, Venereal desire, (F.) *Le génésique, Amour physique.* The instinctive feeling that attracts the sexes towards each other to effect the work of reproduction.

APPETITUS CANINUS, Boulimia—a. Deficiens, Dysorexia.

APPLE, ADAM'S, Pomum Adami—a. Bitter, Cucumis colocynthis—a. Curassoa, Aurantium curassaventium—a. Eye, see Melon—a. May, Podophyllum peltatum—a. Root, Euphorbia corollata.

APPLE TEA, *Apple water.* Slice two large, not over-ripe *apples,* and pour over a pint of boiling *water.* After an hour, pour off the fluid, and, if necessary, sweeten with sugar.

APPLE TREE, Pyrus malus.

APPLICA'TA, from *applicare,* (*ad* and *plicare,* 'to fold,') 'to apply.' A word, unnecessarily introduced into medical language, to express the objects which are applied immediately to the surface of the body, as clothes, cosmetics, baths, &c.—Hallé.

APPLICA'TION, *Applica'tio,* (same etymon,) in a moral signification, is synonymous with Attention. Also, the act of applying one thing to another; as the application of an apparatus, of a bandage, blister, &c.

APPREHEN'SIO, from *ad* and *prehendere,* 'to take.' This word is employed in various senses. It means catalepsy or catoche.—Paul Zacchias. A kind of bandage for securing any part. Also, a therapeutical indication.

APPROCHE, Coition.

APPROXIMA'TION, *Approxima'tio,* from *ad* and *proximus,* 'nearest.' Ettmuller gave this name to a pretended method of curing disease, by making it pass from man into some animal or vegetable, by the aid of immediate contact.

APRAC'TA, from *a,* priv., and *πρασσω,* 'I act.' Without action. An epithet for the parts of generation, when unfit for copulation or generation.

APRICATIO, Insolation.

APRICOT, Prunus Armeniaca.

APROCTUS, see Atretus.

APROSO'PIA, *Triocephal'ia,* from *a,* priv., and *προσωπον,* 'the face.' A malformation, which consists in the face being deficient.

APROSOPUS, Microprosopus.

APSINTHIA'TUM, from *αψινθιον,* 'wormwood.' A sort of drink made of wormwood.—Aëtius.

APSINTHITES, Absinthites.

APSYCHIA, Syncope.

APSYXIA, Syncope.

APTHÆ, Aphthæ.

APTYS'TOS, from *a,* priv., and *πτυω,* 'I spit.' Devoid of expectoration. An epithet given to certain pleurisies, in which there is no expectoration.—Hippocrates.

APUS, see Apodia.

APY'ETOS, from *a,* priv., and *πυον,* 'pus.' An external affection, which does not end in suppuration.

APYIQUE, Apyos.

AP'YOS, from *a,* priv., and *πυον,* 'pus,' (F.) *Apyique.* That which does not afford pus.

APYRECTIC, Apyretic.

APYRENOMELE, Apyromele.

APYRET'IC, *Apyret'icus, Apyree'tic, Apyrec'-ticus, Apyr'etus,* from *a,* priv., and *πυρ,* 'fire, fever.' Without fever. This epithet is given to days in which there is no paroxysm of a disease, as in the ease of an intermittent, as well as to some local affections which do not induce fever. Urticaria is sometimes called an *apyretic exanthem.*

APYREX'IA. The same etymology. Absence of fever; *Dialem'ma, Dialeip'sis, Dialip'sis, Tempus intercala're, Interval'lum, Intermis'sio.* Apyrexia is the condition of an intermittent fever between the paroxysms: the duration of the apyrexia, consequently, depends on the type of the intermittent. Occasionally, the term has been applied to the cessation of the febrile condition in acute diseases.

APYROME'LE, *Apyrenome'le,* from *a,* priv., *πυρην,* 'a nut,' and *μηλη,* 'a sound.' A sound or probe, without a button or nut. It is the *Melo'tis, Specil'lum auricula'rium* or *Auricular sound* of Galen.

AQUA, Urine, Water—a. Acidi carbonici, Acidulous water—a. Acidula hydrosulphurata, Naples water (factitious)—a. Aeris fixi, Acidulous water (simple)—a. Alkalina oxymuriatica, *Eau de Javelle*—a. Aluminis compositus, Liquor, a. c.—a. Aluminosa Bateana, Liq. aluminis compositus—a. Ammoniæ, Liquor ammoniæ—a. Acetatis ammoniæ, Liquor ammoniæ acetatis—a. Ammoniæ carbonatis, Liquor ammoniæ subcarbonatis—a. Ammoniæ caustica, Liquor ammoniæ—a. Amnii, Liquor Amnii.

AQUA AMYGDALA'RUM CONCENTRA'TA, (F.) *Eau d'Amandes amères, Water of bitter almonds.* Made by bruising well two pounds of *bitter almonds;* adding, whilst triturating, ten pounds of *spring water,* and four pounds of *alcohol;* letting the mixture rest in a well-closed vessel, and then distilling two pounds. Used instead of the Aqua Laurocerasi, and the Hydrocyanic acid.

An *Aqua amyg'dalæ ama'ræ,* Bitter Almond water, has been introduced into the last edition of the Ph. U. S., 1851, (*Ol. amygdal. amar.* ℈xvj.; *Magnes. Carbon.* ℥j.; *Aquæ* Oij.)

AQUA ANISI FORTIS, Spiritus anisi—a. Aquisgranensis, see Aix-la-Chapelle—a. Auditoria, Cotunnius, Liquor of—a. Aurantii, see Citrus aurantium—a. Azotica oxygenata, Aqua nitrogenii protoxydi—a. Balsamica arterialis, Aqua Binellii—a. Bareginensis, Baréges water—a. Barytæ Muriatis, see Baryta, muriate of—a. Bellilucana, Balaruc waters—a. Benedicta, Liquor calcis—a. Benedicta composita, Liquor calcis compositus—a. Benedicta Rulandi, Vinum antimonii tartarizati.

AQUA BINE'LLII, *Acqua Binelli. A. Monteroesi,*

Aqua Balsam'ica arteria'lis, (F.) *Eau de Binelli*, *Eau de Monterossi*. A celebrated Italian hæmostatic, invented by one Binelli. Its composition is unknown, but its virtues have been ascribed to creasote; although there is reason for believing it to possess no more activity than cold water.

AQUA BROCCHIE'RII, *Acqua Brocchieri*, *Brocchieri water*, (F.) *Eau de Brocchieri*, *Eau styptique de Brocchieri*. A supposed styptic, which made much noise at Paris at one time. It is devoid of efficacy. Dr. Paris found nothing in it but water perfumed by some vegetable essence.

AQUA BORVONENSIS, Bourbonne-les-Bains, mineral waters of—a. Bristoliensis, Bristol water—a. Calcariæ ustæ, Liquor calcis—a. Calcis, Liquor calcis—a. Calcis composita, Liquor calcis compositus—a. Camphoræ, Mistura camphoræ—a. Camphorata, Bates's, see Cupri sulphas—a. Carbonatis sodæ acidula, Acidulous water, simple—a. Catapultarum, *Arquebusade, eau d'*—a. Chlorini, see Chlorine.

AQUA CINNAMO'MI, *Cinnamon Water*. Distilled water of Cinnamon Bark. Prepared also in the following manner. *Ol. Cinnam.* f ʒss; *Magnes. Carbon.* ʒj; *Aq. destillat.* Oij. Rub the oil and carbonate of magnesia; add the water gradually, and filter. (Ph. U. S.)

AQUA CINNAMOMI FORTIS, Spiritus Cinnamomi—a. Colcestrensis, Colchester, mineral waters of.

AQUA COLORA'TA, 'coloured water.' A name given to a prescription in which simple coloured water is contained. Used in hospital cases, more especially, where a *placebo* is demanded.

AQUA CUPRI AMMONIATA, Liquor c. a.—a. Cupri vitriolati composita, Liquor cupri sulphatis composita—a. inter Cutem, Anasarca—a. Destillata, Water, distilled—a. Florum aurantii, see Citrus aurantium—a. Fluviatilis, Water, river.

AQUA FŒNIC'ULI, *Fennel water*. The distilled water of fennel seed. It may be prepared also like the aqua cinnamomi.

AQUA FONTANA, Water, spring—a. Fortis, Nitric acid—a. Hepatica, Hydrosulphuretted water—a. Hordeata, Decoctum hordei—a. Imbrium, Water, rain—a. Intercus, Anasarca—a. Inter Cutem, Anasarca—a. Juniperi composita, Spiritus juniperi compositus—a. Kali, Liquor potassæ subcarbonatis—a. Kali caustici, Liquor potassæ—a. Kali præparati, Liquor potassæ subcarbonatis—a. Kali puri, Liquor potassæ—a. Kali subcarbonatis, Liquor potassæ subcarbonatis—a. Labyrinthi, Cotunnius, liquor of—a. Lactis, Serum lactis—a. ex Lacu, Water, lake—a. Lithargyri acetati composita, Liquor plumbi subacetatis dilutus—a. Luciæ, Spiritus ammoniæ succinatus—a. Marina, Water, sea—a. Medicata, Water, mineral.

AQUA MENTHÆ PIPERI'TÆ, *Peppermint Water*. The distilled water of peppermint. It may be prepared like the aqua cinnamomi.

AQUA MENTHÆ PIPERITIDIS SPIRITUOSA, Spiritus menthæ piperitæ—a. Menthæ viridis, Spearmint water; see Aquæ menthæ piperitæ—a. Menthæ vulgaris spirituosa, Spiritus menthæ viridis—a. Mineralis, Water, mineral—a. Mirabilis, Spiritus pimentæ—a. Mulsa, Hydromeli—a. Natri Oxmyuriatici, Liquor sodæ chlorinatæ—a. Neapolitana, Naples water, (factitious)—a. Nephritica, Spiritus myristica.

AQUA NITROGEN'II PROTOX'YDI, *Protox'ide of Ni'trogen Water*, *Aqua asot'ica oxygena'ta*, *Searle's patent oxyg"enous aërated water*. A patent solution of protoxide of nitrogen, said to contain five times its own bulk of gas. It has been recommended as a nervine, and excitant in nervous conditions, dyspepsia, &c. It has also been used in cholera, and to counteract the evil consequences of drunkenness. The dose is f ʒvj, or ʒviij, two or three times a day; or, in dyspepsia, as a beverage between meals.

AQUA NIVATA, Water, snow—a. Nucis moschatæ, Spiritus myristicæ—a. Ophthalmica, Liquor zinci sulphatis cum camphorâ—a. Paludosa, Water, marsh—a. Pedum, Urine—a. Pericardii, see Pericardium—a. Picea, see Pinus sylvestris—a. Picis, see Pinus sylvestris—a. Pluvialis, Water, rain—a. Potassæ, Liquor potassæ—a. Pulegii spirituosa, Spiritus pulegii—a. Putealis, Water, well—a. ex Puteo, Water, well—a. Rabelli, Elixir acidum Halleri—a. Raphani composita, Spiritus armoraciæ compositus—a. Regia, Nitromuriatic acid.

AQUA ROSÆ, *Rose Water*, *Rhodostag'ma*, (*Ros. centifol.* ℔viij: *Aquæ* cong. ij. M. Distil a gallon—Ph. U. S.)

AQUA SALUBRIS, Water, mineral—a. Sapphrina, Liquor cupri ammoniata—a. Saturni, Liquor plumbi subacetatis dilutus—a. Sclopetaria, *Arquebusade eau d'*—a. Seminum anisi composita, Spiritus anisi—a. Seminum carui fortis, Spiritus carui—a. Sodæ effervescens, Acidulous water, simple—a. Soteria, Water, mineral—a. Stygia, Nitro-muriatic acid—a. Styptica, Liquor cupri sulphatis composita—a. Sulphurata simplex, Hydrosulphuretted water—a. Sulphureti ammoniæ, Liquor fumans Boylii—a. Thediana, *Arquebusade eau d'*—a. Theriacalis Bezoardica, Chylostagma diaphoreticum Mindereri—a. Tofana, Liquor arsenicalis—a. Tosti panis, Toast water—a. Traumatica Thedenii, *Arquebusade eau d'*—a. Vegeto-mineralis, Liquor plumbi subacetatis dilutus—a. Viciensis, Vichy water—a. Vitriolica camphorata, Liquor zinci sulphatis cum camphorâ—a. Vitriolica cærulea, Solutio sulphatis cupri composita—a. Vulneraria, *Arquebusade eau d'*—a. Zinci vitriolati cum camphorâ, Liquor zinci sulphatis cum camphorâ.

AQUÆ ACIDULÆ, Acidulous waters—a. Badiguæ, Bath, Mineral waters of—a. Badizæ, Bath, Mineral waters of—a. Bathoniæ, Bath, Mineral waters of—a. Buxtonienses, Buxton, Mineral waters of—a. Cantuarienses, Canterbury, waters of—a. Chalybeatæ, Waters, mineral, chalybeate.

AQUÆ DESTILLA'TÆ, *Distilled Waters*, *Hydrola'ta*, (F.) *Hydrolats*. These are made by putting vegetable substances, as roses, mint, pennyroyal, &c., into a still with water, and drawing off as much as is found to possess the aromatic properties of the plant. To every gallon of the distilled water, 5 oz. of spirit should be added to preserve it. The *simple distilled waters* are sometimes called *Aquæ stillatit"iæ sim'plices*: the *spirituous*, *Aquæ stillatit"iæ spirituo'sæ*, but more commonly *Spir'itus*.

AQUÆ MARTIALES, Waters, mineral, chalybeate—a. Metus, Hydrophobia—a. Minerales acidulæ, Waters, mineral, gaseous—a. Minerales ferruginosæ, Waters, mineral, chalybeate—a. Minerales sulphureæ, Waters, mineral, sulphureous—a. Stillatitiæ, Aquæ destillatæ—a. Solis, Bath, mineral waters of.

AQUÆDUC'TUS, *Aq'ueduct*, from *aqua* 'water,' and *ducere, ductum,* 'to lead.' (F.) *Aqueduc*. Properly, a canal for conducting water from one place to another. Anatomists have used it to designate certain canals.

AQUÆDUCTUS CEREBRI, Infundibulum of the brain—a. Cotunnii, Aquæductus vestibuli.

AQUÆDUC'TUS COCH'LEÆ, (F.) *Aqueduc du Limaçon;*—a very narrow canal, which proceeds from the tympanic scala of the cochlea to the posterior edge of the *pars petrosa*.

AQUÆDUC'TUS FALLO'PII, *Canal spiroïde de l'os temporal* of Chaussier, (F.) *Aqueduc de Falope.* A canal in the pars petrosa of the temporal bone, which extends from the meatus auditorius internus to the foramen stylo-mastoideum, and gives passage to the facial nerve. The opening into this aqueduct is called *Hia'tus Fallo'pii.*

AQUÆDUC'TUS SYL'VII, *Cana'lis eminen'tiæ quadrigem'inæ,* (F.) *Aqueduc de Sylvius, Iter ad quartum ventric'ulum, Cana'lis me'dius, Canal intermédiare des ventricules* of Chaussier. A canal forming a communication between the third and fourth ventricles of the brain.

AQUÆDUC'TUS VESTIB'ULI, *Aquæductus Cotun'nii, Canal of Cotun'nius,* (F.) *Aqueduc du vestibule* ou *Aqueduc de Cotugno.* This begins in the vestibule, near the common orifice of the two semicircular canals, and opens at the posterior surface of the *pars petrosa.*

AQUALIC'ULUS, from *aqualis,* 'a water-pot.' That part of the abdomen which extends from the umbilicus to the pubes. See Hypogastrium. It has also been applied to the stomach or intestinal canal.

AQUAS'TER. A word used, by Paracelsus, to express the visions or hallucinations of patients.

AQUEDUC, Aqueduct—*a. de Cotugno*—Aquæductus vestibuli—*a. de Fallope,* Aquæductus Fallopii—*a. du Limaçon,* Aquæductus cochleæ—*a. de Sylvius,* Aquæductus Sylvii—*a. du Vestibule,* Aquæductus vestibuli.

AQUEDUCT, Aquæductus.

A'QUEOUS, *A'queus, Aquo'sus, Hydato'des. Hydro'des,* from *aqua,* 'water,' (F.) *Aqueux,* Watery. The absorbents or lymphatics are sometimes called, in France, *Conduits* ou *Canaux aqueux.*

AQUEOUS HUMOUR OF THE EYE, *Humor aquo'sus, Albugin'eous humour, Oöei'des, Oo'des, Hydatoï'des, Hydato'des, Ova'tus* seu *Orifor'mis humor,* (F.) *Humeur aqueuse.* The limpid fluid which fills the two chambers of the eye, from the cornea to the crystalline, and which is, consequently, in contact with the two surfaces of the iris. Quantity, 5 or 6 grains: s. g. 1.0003. It contains albumen, chloride of sodium, and phosphate of lime in small quantity; and is enveloped in a fine membrane:—*the membrane of the aqueous humour, Tunica propria* seu *Vagi'na humo'ris a'quei* seu *Membra'na Demuria'na* seu *Descemet'ii, Membrane of Demours* or *of Descemet;* although these last terms are by some appropriated to a third layer of the cornea.

AQUEUS, Aqueous.

AQUIDUCA. Hydragogues.

AQUIFOLIUM, Ilex aquifolium—*a.* Foliis deciduis, Prinos.

AQUILA, Hydrargyri submurias, Sulphur. The alchymists used this word for sublimed sal ammoniac, precipitated mercury, arsenic, sulphur, and the philosopher's stone. See Hydrargyri Submurias, and Sulphur.

AQ'UILA CŒLEST'IS; a sort of panacea, of which mercury was a constituent.

AQ'UILA LACH'RYMÆ; a liquor prepared from several ingredients, especially from calomel.

AQ'UILA PHILOSOPHO'RUM. The alchymists, whose terms were always mysterious, called mercury thus, when reduced to its original form.

AQ'UILA VEN'ERIS; an ancient preparation, made by subliming verdigris and sal ammoniac.

AQUILÆ VENÆ, Temporal veins.

AQUILE'GIA, *A. vulga'ris, A. sylves'tris* seu *Alpi'na, Common Columbine* or *Columbine,* (F.) *Ancolie.* The seeds, herb, and flowers were formerly used in jaundice and cutaneous diseases. They are still retained in many of the Pharmacopœias of continental Europe.

AQUILEGIA ALPINA, Aquilegia.

AQUILEGIA CANADENSIS, *Wild Columbine,* is indigenous, and flowers in April and June. The seeds are said to be tonic.

AQUILEGIA SYLVESTRIS, Aquilegia—*a.* Vulgaris, Aquilegia.

AQUO-CAPSULITIS, Aquo-membranitis.

AQUO-MEMBRANI'TIS, *Keratoïri'tis, Aquocapsuli'tis.* Inflammation of the anterior chamber of the eye. A badly compounded term, denoting inflammation of the capsule or membrane of the aqueous humour.

AQUULA, Ceratocele, Hydatid, Hydroa—a. Acustica, Cotunnius, liquor of.

AQUULA seu AQUA MORGAGNII. The minute portion of water which escapes when an opening is made into the capsule of the crystalline.

ARA PARVA, a small altar;—a kind of bandage invented by Sostratus, which represents the corners of an altar.—Galen.

AR'ABE; a wound, a blow.—Erotian.

ARAB'ICA ANTID'OTUS HEPAT'ICA, *Ar'abic Hepat'ic An'tidote.* A powder composed of myrrh, costus, white pepper, &c. It was administered in new wine.

ARAB'ICUS LAPIS. A sort of white marble, analogous to alabaster, found in Arabia. It was regarded as absorbent and desiccative, and was employed in hemorrhoids.

ARABIS BARBAREA, Erysimum barbarea.

AR'ABIS MALAG'MA. An antiscrofulous medicine, composed of myrrh, olibanum, wax sal ammoniac, iron pyrites, &c.—Celsus.

AR'ABS, MEDICINE OF THE. The Arabians kept the torch of medical science illuminated during a dark period of the middle ages. Before the year of the Hegira, they had schools of medicine; but these were most flourishing during the 10th, 11th, and 12th centuries. The chief additions made by them to medical science were in the departments of pharmacy and in the description of diseases. Their principal writers were Avicenna, Serapion, Averrhoes, Hali Abbas, Moses Maimonides, Avenzoar, Rhazes, Albucasis, &c.

ARACACHA, Conium moschatum.

ARACHIS AFRICANA, A. hypogea—a. Americana, A. Hypogea.

AR'ACHIS HYPOGE'A, *A. America'na, A. Africa'na, Arachni'da hypogea, Ground nut, Pea nut, Earth almond,* (S.) *Mane;* erroneously called *Pistachio nut,* in the South; *Pindars* of the West Indies. Cultivated in the Southern States. The seeds are oily, and are eaten. A kind of inferior chocolate may be made of them.

ARACH'NE, αραχνη, 'a spider,' 'a cobweb.' Hence—

ARACHNIDA HYPOGEA, Arachis hypogea.

ARACHNI'TIS, *Arachnoïdi'tis, Arachnodei'tis, Inflammation of the Arachnoid.* A variety of phrenitis.

ARACHNODEITIS, Arachnitis.

ARACHNOID CANAL, see Canal, arachnoid.

ARACHNOID OF THE EYE. The lining membrane of a cavity, supposed by some to exist between the sclerotic and choroid.

ARACH'NOID MEMBRANE, *Meninx Me'dia, Arachnoïdeus, Arachno'des,* from αραχνη, 'a cobweb,' and ειδος, 'form, resemblance;' *Tu'nica ara'nea, Arachno'des, T. crystal'lina, Menin'gion.* A name given to several membranes, which, by their extreme thinness, resemble spider-webs. — Celsus and Galen called thus the membrane of the vitreous humour,—the *tunica hyaloidea.* The moderns use it now for one of the membranes of the brain, situate between the dura mater and pia mater. It is a serous membrane, and composed of two layers; the *external* being confounded, in the greater part of its extent, with the dura mater, and, like it, lining the interior of the cranium and spinal canal; the *other* being extended over the brain, from which it is separated by the pia mater, without passing into the sinuosities between the convolutions, and penetrating into the interior of the brain by an opening at its posterior part under the corpus callosum. It forms a part of the investing sheath of the nerves, as they pass from the encephalic cavities. Its chief uses seem to be;—to envelop, and, in some measure, protect the brain, and to secrete a fluid for the purpose of keeping it in a state best adapted for the proper performance of its functions.

ARACHNOIDITIS, Arachnitis.

ARACK′, *Arrack;* (East Indian.) A spirituous liquor made in India in various ways, often from rice, sometimes from sugar fermented along with the juice of the cocoa nut; frequently from toddy, the juice which flows from the cocoa-nut tree by incision, and from other substances. It is a strong, heating spirit.

ARACK, MOCK, is made by adding ℈ij of *Benzoic acid* to *a quart of rum.* The celebrated Vauxhall punch is made with such arack.

ARACOUCHINI, Icica aracouchini.

ARACUS AROMATICUS, Vanilla.

AR′ADOS, from αραδω, 'I am turbulent.' The agitation excited in the stomach by the coction of aliments of different nature.—Hippocrates. Likewise, the motion produced by cathartics.

ARÆOMA, Interstice.

ARÆOMETER, Areometer.

ARÆOT′ICA, from αραιοω, 'I rarefy.' Medicines supposed to have the quality of rarefying the humours. See Rarefaciens.

ARAKI, see Spirit.

ARALIA CANADENSIS, Panax quinquefolium.

ARA′LIA HIS′PIDA, *Dwarf Elder*, is said to be diuretic, and has been recommended, in decoction, in dropsy.

ARA′LIA NUDICAU′LIS, *Nardus America′nus, Small Spikenard, Wild Liq′uorice, Sweet root, False Sarsaparil′la,* (F.) *Petit nard.* This American plant is said to be a mild stimulant and diaphoretic, and has been recommended as a substitute for sarsaparilla. It is used, also as a tonic. It is in the secondary list of the Pharmacopœia of the United States.

ARA′LIA RACEMO′SA, *American Spikenard,* has the same properties as A. Nudicaulis.

ARA′LIA SPINO′SA, *Angel′ica Tree, Prickly Ash, Toothach Tree, Spikenard Tree, Prickly Elder, Shotbush, Pigeon Tree.* Its properties are not clear. The berries, and a tincture of them, have been employed, it is said, successfully in *toothach.* A spirituous infusion has also been used in colic.

ARANEA, Araneæ Tela — a. Tarentula, see Tarentula.

ARA′NEÆ TELA, *Ara′nea, Ara′neum, Cobweb,* (F.) *Toile d'Araignée.* Formerly, this substance was much employed, and supposed to possess extraordinary virtues, especially when applied to the wrists. It has been recently used again in intermittents. The spider itself, softened into a plaster and applied to the forehead and temples, is said by Dioscorides to prevent ague. Cobweb is a mechanical styptic, and is so applied, at times.

ARANEO′SA URI′NA. A term applied to the urine when loaded with filaments, like cobwebs.

ARANEO′SUS (PULSUS); a term employed to express extreme weakness of pulse; when the movements resemble those of a delicate net raised by the wind.

ARANEUM, Araneæ Tela.

ARA′NEUM ULCUS, *Astakil′los*. A name given by Paracelsus to a malignant, gangrenous ulcer, extending from the feet to the legs.

ARARA, Myrobalanus citrina.

ARASCON, Nymphomania, Satyriasis.

ARATRUM, Vomer.

ARAUCARIA DOMBEYI, Dombeya excelsa.

ARBOR BENIVI, Benjamin—a. Indica, Laurus cassia—a. Maris, Coral—a. Thurifera—Juniperus Lycia—a. Uteri Vivificans, Palmæ uteri plicatæ.

ARBOR VITÆ, (F,) *Arbre de vie.* A name given to an arborescent appearance, observed on cutting the cerebellum longitudinally; and which results from the particular arrangement of the white substance with the cineritious. Also, the Thuya occidentalis.

ARBOR VITÆ UTERINUS, Palmæ uteri plicatæ.

ARBOR VITÆ OF THE UTERUS, Palmæ uteri plicatæ.

AR′BORES. A morbid alteration of the skin, which precedes its ulceration. Ruland.

ARBOUSIER, Arbutus unedo.

ARBRE DE VIE, Arbor Vitæ.

ARBUSCULA GUMMIFERA BRAZILIENSIS, Hypericum bacciferum.

ARBUTUS, A. Unedo—a. Trailing, A. Uva ursi, Epigæa repens.

AR′BUTUS UVA URSI, *Arctostaph′ylos Uva ursi, Maira′nia uva ursi. Nat. Ord.* Ericeæ. *Sex. Syst.* Decandria Monogynia. (F.) *Busserolle* ou *Raisin d'Oura.* The leaves—(*Uva Ursi,* Ph. U. S.)—of this plant are tonic and astringent, and have been employed, chiefly, in diseases of the urinary organs. Dose of the powder from gr. xv. to ʒss. The English names are *Trailing Ar′butus, Bear's Whortleberry* or *Bearberry, Mountain-box, Redberry, Upland Cranberry, Foxberry, Checkerberry.*

AR′BUTUS UNE′DO, *Ar′butus, Andrach′nē, Une′-do, Une′do papyra′cea,* κομαρος, (F.) *Arbousier.* A decoction of the leaves is astringent, and has been used in diarrhœa.

ARC, *Arch, Arcus.* Any part of the body resembling an arch in form; as the *Arch of the colon,* (F.) *Arc du colon,*—the transverse portion of that intestine:—*Arch of the Aorta, Arcus aor′-tæ.* (F.) *Crosse de l'Aorte,* &c., the turn which the aorta takes in the thorax.

ARCA ARCANORUM, Hydrargyrum—a. Cordis, Pericardium.

ARCADE ANASTOMOTIQUE, Arch, anastomotic—*a. Crurale,* Crural arch—*a. Inguinale,* Crural arch—*a. Orbitaire,* Orbitar arch—*a. Pubienne,* Pubic arch—*a. Zygomatique,* Zygomatic arch.

ARCADES DENTAIRES, Dental arches—*a. Palmaires,* Palmar arches.

ARCADI-TEMPORO-MAXILLAIRE, Temporalis.

ARCÆ′US or ARCŒ′US, BALSAM OF, (F.) *Baume d'Arcæus.* A kind of soft ointment used in sores, contusions, &c. It is made by melting two parts of mutton suet, one part of hog's lard, turpentine and rosin, each one part and a half: straining and agitating till cold.

ARCANSON, Colophonia.

ARCA′NUM, from *arca,* 'a chest.' A secret, a *nostrum,* a *quack* or *empir′ical med′icine,* (F.) *Arcane.* A remedy whose composition is kept secret; but which is reputed to possess great efficacy.

ARCANUM CORALLINUM, Hydrargyri nitrico-oxydum — a. Duplicatum, Potassæ sulphas — a. Tartari, Potassæ acetas.

ARCEAU, Arculus, Cradle.

ARCEUTHOS, Juniperus communis.

ARCH, ANASTOMOT'IC, (F.) *Arcade Anastomotique*, is the union of two vessels, which anastomose by describing a curved line. The vessels of the mesentery anastomose in this manner.

ARCH OF THE AORTA, see Aorta—a. Crural, see Crural arch — a. Femoral, see Crural arch — a. Gluteal, see Gluteal aponeurosis—a. Hæmal, see Hæmal arch—a. Inguinal, see Crural arch—a. Orbital, see Orbitar arch—a. of the Palate, see Palate bone—a. of the Pubis, see Pubic arch—a. Subpubic, see Subpubic arch—a. Superciliary, see Superciliary arches—a. Zygomatic, see Zygomatic arch.

ARCHES OF THE PALATE. These are two in number on each side of the throat, one of which is termed *anterior*, the other *posterior*.

The *anterior arch* arises from the middle of the velum palati, at the side of the uvula, and is fixed to the edge of the base of the tongue.

The *posterior* arch has its origin, likewise, from the side of the uvula, and passes downwards to be inserted into the side of the pharynx. The anterior arch contains the circumflexus palati, and forms the isthmus faucium. The posterior arch has, within it, the levator palati, and between the arches are the tonsils.

ARCHÆ'US, *Archæ'us*, from αρχη, 'commencement,' (F.) *Archée*. A word invented by Basil Valentine, and afterwards adopted by Paracelsus and Van Helmont. The latter used it for the internal principle of our motions and actions. This archæus, according to Van Helmont, is an immaterial principle, existing in the seed prior to fecundation, and presiding over the development of the body, and over all organic phenomena. Besides this chief archæus, whose seat Van Helmont placed in the upper orifice of the stomach, he admitted several of a subordinate character, which had to execute its orders; one, for instance, in each organ, to preside over its functions; each of them being subject to anger, caprice, terror, and every human failing.

ARCHANGEL, NEW, MINERAL SPRINGS. About twenty miles to the north of New Archangel, Sitka Island, on the N. W. coast of North America, are some thermal sulphureous waters, the temperature of one of which is upwards of 153° of Fahr. They are much celebrated.—Sir Geo. Simpson.

ARCHANGELICA, Lamium album.

ARCHANGELICA OFFICINALIS, Angelica.

ARCHE, αρχη, *Init'ium, Princip'ium, Primor'dium, Ori'go, Inva'sio*. The first attack of a disease.

ARCHECPTOMA, Proctocele.

ARCHÉE, Archæus.

ARCHELL, CANARY, Lichen roccella.

ARCHELOG"IA, from αρχη, 'beginning,' and λογος, 'a discourse.' A treatise on fundamental principles;—of medicine, for example.

ARCHEN'DA. A powder of the leaves of the *ligustrum*, used by the Ægyptians after bathing, to obviate the unpleasant odour of the feet.— Prosper Alpinus.

ARCHIA'TER, *Archia'trus, Protomed'icus, Protia'tros*, from αρχη, 'authority,' and ιατρος, 'physician.' The original signification of this word is a matter of dispute. Some consider, with Mercurialis, that it meant physician to a prince, king, emperor, &c.: others, with C. Hoffman, apply it to every physician who, by his situation, is raised above his colleagues. The former opinion seems to have prevailed,—*Archiatre des Rois de France* being applied to the chief physician to the kings of France.

ARCHIG"ENI MORBI. Acute diseases; because they hold the first rank: from αρχη, 'beginning,' and γινομαι, 'I am.'

ARCHIMAGIA, Chymistry.

ARCHINGEAY, MINERAL WATERS OF. Archingeay is situate in France, three leagues from St. Jean d'Angely. The waters are prised in all diseases. They seem to contain carbonate of lime, a little chloride of sodium, carbonate of iron, and some bitumen.

ARCHITECTURA APOPLECTICA, Apoplectic make.

ARCHITIS, Proctitis, Rectitis.

ARCHOCELE, Proctocele.

ARCHOPTOMA, Proctocele.

ARCHOPTOSIS, Proctocele.

ARCHORRHA'GIA, from αρχος, 'the anus,' and ῥεω, 'I flow.' *Archorrhœ'a*. Hemorrhage from the anus.

ARCHORRHŒA, Archorrhagia.

ARCHOS, Arcus, Rectum.

ARCHOSTEGNOMA, Stricture of the Rectum.

ARCHOSTEGNOSIS, Stricture of the Rectum.

ARCHOSTENOSIS, Stricture of the Rectum.

ARCHOSYRINX, Fistula in ano.

AR'CIFORM, *Arcifor'mis*, from *arx, arcis*, 'a top or ridge,' and *forma*, 'shape.' An epithet given to certain fibres, *Fibræ arciform'es*, of the anterior pyramids of the medulla oblongata, which take a curved course around the inferior extremity of each corpus olivare and ascend towards the cerebellum.

ARCTA'TIO, *Arctitu'do*, from *areto*, 'I make narrow;' *Angusta'tio, Coareta'tio*. Contraction, (F.) *Rétrécissement*, of a natural opening or of a canal, and especially of the vulva, of the orifice of the uterus, or of the intestinal canal. Constipation, (see Stegnosis.) Reunion by suture or infibulation. — Scribonius Largus, Paul Zacchias, &c.

ARC'TITUDO, Arctatio.

ARCTIUM, A. lappa—a. Bardana, A. lappa.

ARCTIUM LAPPA. The root and seed of the *Clit'bur, Barda'na, Arctium, A. barda'na seu majus seu minus seu tomento'sum, l'laphis, Lappa glabra, Lappa major, L. persona'ta, Persola'ta, Persolla'ta, Persolu'ta, Burdock*, (F.) *Bardane, Glouteron*. *Nat. Ord.* Compositæ. *Sex. Syst.* Syngenesia æqualis. Root diuretic: seed cathartic. It has been used in decoction in diseases of the skin and in syphilis.

ARCTIUM MAJUS, A. lappa—a. Minus, A. lappa —a. Tomentosum, A. lappa.

ARC'TOPUS ECHINA'TUS. A South African plant, *Nat. Ord.* Umbelliferæ, which is demulcent and diuretic, somewhat approaching sarsaparilla. The decoction of the root is employed in syphilis, lepra, and chronic cutaneous affections of all kinds.

ARCTOSTAPHYLOS UVA URSI, Arbutus uva ursi.

ARCTU'RA, from *areto*, 'I straighten.' The effects of a nail grown into the flesh, *Arctu'ra unguis*.—See Onychogryphosis.

ARCTURA UNGUIUM. The growing in or inversion of the nails. See Onychogryphosis.

ARCUA'TIO, *Concava'tio*. An anterior gibbosity or projection of the sternum.

ARCUEIL, MINERAL WATERS OF. Arcueil is about one league south of Paris. The water contains carbonic acid, carbonate of lime, sulphate of lime, chloride of sodium, and some deliquescent salts.

A celebrated society held its meetings at this village, of which Berthollet, Humboldt, La Place, &c., were members.

ARCULA CORDIS, Pericardium.

ARCULÆ. The Orbitar Fossæ: κοιλιδες. — Rufus of Ephesus.

ARC'ULUS, diminutive of *arcus*, 'an arch.' A small arch; a cradle, (F.) *Arceau, Archet*. A semicircular box or basket used for preventing the bed-clothes from coming in contact with injured or diseased parts. An ordinance of the Grand Duke of Tuscany forbade mothers to sleep with an infant near them, unless it was put under a solid cradle.

ARCUS MEDULLARIS, Fornix—a. Senilis, Gerotoxon—a. Subpubicus, Subpubic arch—a. Superciliaris, Superciliary arches—a. Unguium, see Nail—a. Zygomaticus, Zygomatic arch.

ARDALOS, Excrement.
ARDAS, Excrement.
ARDENT, *Ardens*, from *ardere*, 'to burn.'
ARDENT FEVER, (F.) *Fièvre ardente*. The *Causus*, *Synocha*, or inflammatory fever.
ARDENT or INFLAMED EYES, (F.) *Yeux ardens*. The eyes are so called when injected red.
ARDENT URINE, (F.) *Urine ardente*. Urine of a deep red.
ARDESIA HIBERNICA, Hibernicus lapis.
ARDEUR, Ardor—a. du *Cœur*, Cardialgia—a. *d'Estomac*, Ardor ventriculi, Pyrosis—a. de la *Fièvre*, Ardor Febrilis—a. *d'Urine*, Ardor Urinæ.
AR'DOR, (F.) *Ardeur*. Heat. A feeling of burning, of violent heat; *Æstus*, *Æstua'tio*, *Cau-so'ma*.
ARDOR FEBRI'LIS, (F.) *Ardeur de la Fièvre*. The hot period of fever.
ARDOR STOMACHI, Pyrosis.
ARDOR URI'NÆ, (F.) *Ardeur d'Urine*. A scalding sensation occasioned by the urine in passing over the inflamed mucous membrane of the urethra, or over the neck of the bladder.
ARDOR VENEREUS, Heat.
ARDOR VENTRIC'ULI, *Ebullit'io Stom'achi*, (F.) *Ardeur d'Estomac*. Heartburn. See Cardialgia and Pyrosis.
A'REA, 'a void place,' 'an open surface.' A Latin word used by some authors to designate a variety of Alopecia, in which the hair changes colour, but does not fall off; also, Porrigo decalvans.
AREA GERMINATIVA, *Tache embryonnaire*.
AREA PELLU'CIDA. An elliptical depression in the ovum, filled with a pellucid fluid, in the centre of which is the germ.
AREA VASCULO'SA, see Circulus venosus.
ARE'CA. The fruit—*Are'ca* nut, *Betel* nut—of *Are'ca Cat'echu*, A. *Faufel*, *Caun'ga*; Nat. Ord. Palmæ; Sex. Syst. Monœcia Monadelphia; (F.) *Arec*, is astringent and tonic, and enters into the composition of the *Betel*, the great masticatory of the Orientals.
ARE'CA CATECHU, see Areca.
ARECA FAUFEL, see Areca.
AREFAC'TION, *Arefac'tio*, *Xeran'sis*, ξηρανσις, from *arefacere*, 'to make dry,' (*arere*, 'to dry,' and *facere*, 'to make.') The process of drying substances, prior to pulverization.
ARENA, see Gravel.
ARENAMEN, Bole Armenian.
ARENA'TIO, *Chosis*, Sand or Earth Bath; from *arena*, 'sand;' *Saburra'tio*. The application of hot sand to the body. *Pedilu'via* of sand were formerly used in Ascites.
ARENO'SA URI'NA, *Sandy Urine*. Urine when it deposits a sandy sediment.
ARENO'SUS, Sabulous. Also, one who passes sandy urine.
ARENULA, see Gravel.
ARE'OLA. A diminutive of *Area*, (F.) *Aire*. Anatomists understand by *Areola*, the interstices between the fibres composing organs; or those existing between laminæ, or between vessels which interlace with each other.
Areola is, also, applied to the coloured circle *Halo*, *Haloes*, which surrounds the nipple, *Are'-ola papilla'ris*, and which becomes much darker during pregnancy; as well as to the circle surrounding certain vesicles, pustules, &c., as the pustules of the small-pox, the vaccine vesicle, &c. Chaussier, in such cases, recommends the word *Aure'ola*, (F.) *Auréole*.

AREOLA PAPILLARIS, see Areola.
AREOLA, TUBERCLES OF THE, see Mamma.
ARE'OLAR, *Areola'ris*. Appertaining to an areola.
AREOLAR EXHALATIONS are those recrementitial secretions, which are effected within the organs of sense, or in parenchymatous structures,—as the aqueous, crystalline and vitreous humours, &c.
AREOLAR TISSUE, Cellular Tissue.
AREOM'ETER, *Arœom'eter*, *Gravim'eter*, *Alcoölom'eter*, *Aërostat'ic Balance*, from αραιος, 'light,' and μετρον, 'measure:' i. e. '*measure of lightness*.' An instrument, so called, because first employed to take the specific gravity of fluids lighter than water. The *Areometer of Baumé*, which is the most used in Pharmacy, particularly in France, consists of a tube of glass, largely expanded towards its inferior extremity, and terminating, below, by a small ball, containing mercury or lead, which serves it as a balance, so that it may remain upright in the fluid. This tube is furnished with a graduated scale. If the fluid into which the Areometer is plunged be heavier than water, the instrument rises: if lighter, it sinks. There are various Areometers, as those of the Dutch, of Fahrenheit, Nicholson, &c. The Areometer is also called *Hydrom'eter*, (F.) *Aréomètre*, *Pèse-liqueur*.

There are some hydrometers which have a general application for determining the specific gravities of liquids,—as Fahrenheit's, Nicholson's, Guyton de Morveau's, and the common glass hydrometers, including Baumé's, Cartier's, Twaddle's, Zanetti's, and the specific gravity beads; others intended for special application,—as for estimating the comparative strength of spirits; the comparative densities of syrups, oils, &c.,—as Guy Lussac's, Sikes's and Dicat's hydrometers, and the saccharometer, urinometer, and elæometer.

SCALE OF BAUMÉ'S AREOMETER WITH CORRESPONDING SPECIFIC GRAVITIES.

1. *Ascending Scale for light liquids.*

Scale of Baumé.	Specific Gravities.	Substances.
	700	Pure hydrocyanic acid.—*Gay Lussac.*
66	715	Very pure sulphuric ether.
60	742	The same concentrated.
50	782	
48	792	Equal parts of alcohol and ether.
42	819	Very pure alcohol for phamaceutical purposes.
40	827	
36	847	Pure alcohol. Naphtha.
33	863	Alcohol of commerce.
32	868	Essential oil of turpentine.
30	878	
26	900	Hydrocyanic acid of Scheele and pure hydrocyanic acid, mixed with an equal portion of water. (*Robiquet.*)
25	906	Acetic ether.
23	915	
Id.	Id.	Nitric ether.
23	923	Muriatic ether. Liquid ammonia. Olive oil.
Id.	Id.	
20	935	Brandy.
18	948	
13	960	Burgundy wine.
12	986	
11	993	Bordeaux wine.
10	1000	Distilled water.

2. *Descending Scale for heavy liquids.*

Scale of Baumé.	Specific Gravities.	Substances.
0	1000	Common distilled water.
1	1007 / 1009	Distilled vinegar.
2	1014	Common vinegar.
3 / 4	1032	Cow's milk.
10	1075 / 1091	Concentrated acetic acid.
12		
20	1161	
21	1180 / 1210	Liquid hydrochloric acid.
25		
30	1261	Boiling syrup.
35	1321	Cold syrup.
		Common nitric acid.
40	1384 / 1398	Concentrated nitric acid.
41		
45	1454	
Id.	Id.	Phosphoric acid for medical use.
50	1532	
60	1714	
66	1847	Very concentrated sulphuric acid.
70	1946	Very concentrated phosphoric acid.

ARES. A term invented by Paracelsus to designate the principle on which depends the form of mercury, sulphur, and salt. These the alchymists regarded as the three bodies that give birth to every other.

AR'ETE, *αρετη*, 'virtue.' Mental or corporeal vigour.—Hippocrates.

ARETHU'SA, *A. bulbo'sa*; indigenous. Order, Orchideæ. The bruised bulbs are used in toothach; and as cataplasms to tumours.

A'REUS. A pessary mentioned by Paulus of Ægina.

ARGEL, Cynanchum oleæfolium.

AR'GEMA, *Ar'gemon*, *Ar'gemus*, from *αργος*, 'white.' *Fos'sula*, (F.) *Encavure*. A white spot or ulceration of the eye.—Hippocrates. See Leucoma.

ARGEM'ONE, MEXICA'NA, *Thorn Poppy, Prickly Poppy, Yellow Thistle*. A native of Mexico, but naturalized in most parts of the world. *Nat. Ord.* Papaveraceæ. *Sex. Syst.* Polyandria Monogynia. The juice resembles gamboge, and has been used as a hydragogue. The seeds are employed in the West Indies as a substitute for ipecacuanha. They are also used as a cathartic.

ARGENSON, MINERAL WATERS OF. A chalybeate situate at Argenson in Dauphiny: used in cases of obstruction, jaundice, &c.

ARGENT, Argentum—a. *Chlorure d', æce* Argentum—a. *Cyanure d'*, see Argentum—a. et *d'Ammoniaque, chlorure d'*, see Argentum—a. *Iodure d'*, see Argentum—a. *Oxide d'*, see Argentum.

ARGENTERIA, Potentilla anserina.

ARGENTI CHLORIDUM, see Argentum—a. et Ammoniæ chloridum, see Argentum—a. et Ammoniæ chloruretum, see Argentum—a. Cyanidum, see Argentum—a. Cyanuretum, see Argentum—a. Iodidum, see Argentum—a. Ioduretum, see Argentum.

ARGEN'TI NITRAS, *Argen'tum Nitra'tum, Sal argen'ti*, *Argentum Nit'ricum*, (F.) *Nitrate d'Argent, Azotate d'Argent, Nitrate of Silver.* This preparation is sometimes kept in crystals, the *Nitras Argen'ti in crystal'los concre'tus, Nitrate d'Argent crystallisé* of the Codex of Paris, *Luna potab'ilis, Crystalli Lunæ, Argen'tum nit'ricum crystallisa'tum. Nitras argenti crystal'linus, Nitrum luna'ré, Hydrago'gum* BOY'LEI. Generally, however, it is in the fused state: and it is this which is admitted into most Pharmacopœias, and which, besides the name *Nitras Argenti*, is called *Ni'tras argen'ti fusus, Caus'ticum luna'ré, Lapis* *inferna'lis, Argen'tum nit'ricum fu*—— *and* —— *caustic,* (F.) *Nitrate d'argent fondu, Pierre infernale.*

In the Pharmacopœia of the United States, it is directed to be prepared as follows:—Take of *silver*, in small pieces, ℥j.; *nitric acid*, f℥vij., *distilled water*, f℥ij. Mix the acid with the water, and dissolve the silver in the mixture in a sand bath; then crystallize, or gradually increase the heat, so that the resulting salt may be dried. Melt this in a crucible over a gentle fire, and continue the heat until ebullition ceases; then immediately pour it into suitable moulds.

The *virtues* of nitrate of silver are tonic, and escharotic. It is given in chorea, epilepsy, &c.; locally, it is used in various cases as an escharotic. Dose, gr. 1-8 to gr. 1-4 in pill, three times a day.

When silver is combined with iodine, it is said to have the same effect as the nitrate, and not to produce the slate colour of the surface, which is apt to follow the protracted use of the latter.

ARGENTI OXIDUM, see Argentum.

ARGENTILLA VULGARIS, Potentilla anserina.

AR'GENTINE, *Argento'sus*, same etymon as the next. Pertaining to silver; as an 'argentine solution,' or solution of a salt of silver.

ARGENTINE, Potentilla anserina.

ARGEN'TUM, *Ar'gyrus*, from *αργυς*, 'white,' *Silver, Luna, Dia'na,* (F.) *Argent.* A solid metal of a shining white appearance; insipid; inodorous; highly sonorous; malleable and ductile; somewhat hard; crystallizable in triangular pyramids; fusible a little above a red heat; and volatizable; s. g. 10.4. Not used in medicine, unless in some places for silvering pills. SILVER LEAF, *Argen'tum folia'tum*, is the state in which it is used for this purpose.

ARGENTUM DIVI'SUM, *metallic silver*, in very fine powder, has been recommended internally in syphilis.

The CHLORIDE (*Argen'ti chlo'ridum, Argen'tum muriat'icum, A. chlora'tum, A. sali'tum. Chlorure'tum Argen'ti, Chlor'uret* or *Mu'riate of Silver,* (F.) *Chlorure d'Argent ;*) the CYANURET; the IODIDE (*Argen'ti Io'didum, Argen'tum Ioda'tum, Iodure'tum Argen'ti, Iod'uret of Silver,* (F.) *Iodure d'Argent ;*) the OXIDE (*Argen'ti ox'idum, Argen'tum oxyda'tum,* (F.) *Oxide d'Argent,* and the CHLORIDE of AMMONIA and SILVER (*Argen'ti et Ammo'niæ chlo'ridum, Argen'tum muriat'icum ammonia'tum, Chlorure'tum Argen'ti et Ammo'niæ, Chlo'ruret of Silver and Ammonia, Ammonio-chloride of Silver,* (F.) *Chlorure d'Argent et d'Ammoniaque,* have been used in syphilis. At first, these different preparations were administered iatraleptically on the gums; the chloride, the cyanide and the iodide in the dose of 1-12th of a grain; the chloride of silver and ammonia in the dose of 1-14th of a grain, and the oxide of silver and divided silver in the dose of 1-8th and 1-4th of a grain. M. Serre, of Montpellier, who made many trials with them, soon found that these doses were too small; he therefore raised that of the chloride to 1-10th, and of the iodide to 1-8th of a grain, without any inconvenience resulting. The dose of the other preparations was likewise increased in a similar ratio. M. Serre extols the preparations of silver—used internally as well as iatraleptically—as antisyphilitics, but they are not to be depended upon.

The *Oyanuret* or *Cyanide of Silver, Argen'ti Oyanure'tum, A. Cyan'idum, Argen'tum cyanogena'tum,* (F.) *Oyanure d'argent,* is thus directed to be prepared in the Ph. U. S. (1842.) *Argent. Nit.* ℥xv. *Acid Hydrocyan., Aq. destillat.* āā Oj. Having dissolved the nitrate of silver in the water, add the hydrocyanic acid, and mix them.

Wash the precipitate with distilled water and dry it. In the last edition of the Pharmacopœia, (1851,) it is directed to be prepared as follows:—*Nitrate of Silver*, dissolved in *distilled water*, is put into a tubulated glass receiver; *Ferocyanuret of Potassium*, dissolved in *distilled water*, is put into a tubulated retort, previously adapted to the receiver. *Dilute Sulphuric Acid* is added to the solution in the retort; and, by means of a sand-bath and a moderate heat, distillation is carried on until the liquid that passes over no longer produces a precipitate in the receiver. The precipitate is then washed with distilled water, and dried.

The Oxide of Silver, *Argen'ti Ox'idum*, has been introduced into the last edition of the Ph. U. S. (1851.) It is made by precipitating a solution of the *Nitrate of Silver* by *solution of Potassa*, drying the precipitate.

ARGENTUM CHLORATUM, see Argentum — a. Cyanogenatum, see Argentum — a. Fugitivum, Hydrargyrum — a. Fusum, Hydrargyrum — a. Iodatum, see Argentum — a. Liquidum, Hydrargyrum — a. Mobile, Hydrargyrum — a. Muristicum, see Argentum — a. Muriaticum Ammoniatum, see Argentum — a. Oxydatum, see Argentum — a. Salitum, see Argentum — a. Vivum, Hydrargyrum.

ARGIL, PURE, Argilla pura.

ARGILE OCHREUSE PÂLE, Bolus Alba.

ARGILLA BOLUS FLAVA, Terra Lemnia — a. Bolus rubra, Bole Armenian — a. Ferruginea rubra, Bole Armenian — a. Kalisulphurica, Alumen — a. Palida, Bolus alba.

ARGILLA PURA, *Terra Alu'minis*, *T. bola'ris*, seu *argilla'cea pura*, *Alu'mina depura'ta*, pure Argil or Alumina, (F.) *Alumine factice*. This substance, which is prepared by drying alum and exposing it, for twenty or twenty-five minutes, to a red heat, until the sulphuric acid is driven off, has been recommended in indigestion as antacid, as well as in vomiting and diarrhœa accompanied with acidity. The dose to a very young child is from ʒss to ʒj; to older children from ʒj to ʒij.

ARGILLA SULPHURICA ALCALISATA, Alumen — a. Sulphurica usta, Alumen exsiccatum — a. Supersulphas alcalisatum, Alumen — a. Vitriolata, Alumen.

ARGILLÆ ACETAS, Aluminæ acetas — a. Sulphas, Aluminæ sulphas.

ARGOL, RED, Potassæ supertartras impurus — a. White, Potassæ supertartras impurus.

ARGUMENTUM INTEGRITATIS, Hymen.

ARGY'RIA, from αργυρος, 'silver.' The discoloration of the skin occasioned by the internal use of nitrate of silver.

ARGYROCHÆTA, Matricaria.

ARGYROPH'ORA, from αργυρος, 'silver,' and φερω, 'I bear.' A name given, by Myrepsus, to an antidote which he regarded as extremely precious.

ARGYROTROPHEMA, *Blancmanger*.

ARGYRUS, Argentum.

ARHEUMAT'IC, *Arheumat'icus*, from *a*, privative, and ρευμα, 'fluxion or rheumatism.' One without fluxion or rheumatism.

ARIA, Cratægus aria.

ARICI'NA, *Cus'conin*, *Cusco-Cincho'nia*, so called from Arica in South America, the place where it is shipped. An alkali found in Cusco Bark, which is very similar in many of its properties to Cinchonia. Cusco was the ancient residence of the Incas.

ARIC'YMON, from αρι, an intensive particle, and κυειν, 'to conceive.' A name given to a female who conceives readily.—Hippocrates.

ARIDE'NA. A Latin word employed to designate the leanness of any part. — Ettmuller, Sauvages.

ARID'ITY, *Arid'itas*. (F.) *Aridité*, from *arere*, 'to dry.' The French use the word *Aridité* to express the dryness of any organ, and particularly of the skin and tongue, when such dryness is so great as to render the organ rough to the touch. *Aridité* also means the lanuginous appearance of the hair in some diseases in which they seem covered with dust.

ARIDU'RA. Wasting or emaciation of the whole or of any part of the body; Marasmus, Atrophy.

ARIDURA CORDIS, Heart, atrophy of the — a. Hepatis, Hepatrophia.

ARIKA, see Spirit.

ARISTALTHÆA, Althæa.

ARISTOLOCHI'A, from αριστος, 'very good,' and λοχεια, 'parturition;' so called, because the different varieties were supposed to aid parturition. Birthwort, (F.) *Aristoloche*. Several varieties were once in use.

ARISTOLOCHIA CAVA, Fumaria bulbosa.

ARISTOLOCHI'A CLEMATI'TIS, *Aristolochi'a Vulga'ris* seu *Ore'tica*, *Adra Riza*, *Aristolochi'a ten'uis*, (F.) *Aristoloche ordinaire*, *Upright Birthwort*. The root has been considered stimulant and emmenagogue, and as such has been used in amenorrhœa, chlorosis, and cachexia.

ARISTOLOCHIA CRETICA, A. Clematitis — a. Fabacea, Fumaria bulbosa.

ARISTOLOCHI'A LONGA, and A. ROTUN'DA, (F.) *Aristoloche longue et ronde*, Long and Round *Birthwort*. Virtues the same as the preceding.

ARISTOLOCHI'A PISTOLOCHI'A, *Pistolochi'a Aristolochi'a*, *Polyrrhi'za*. This variety has an aromatic odour, and an acrid and bitter taste. (F.) *Aristoloche crénelée*.

ARISTOLOCHI'A SERPENTA'RIA, *Serpenta'ria*, *Vipera'ria*, *Viperi'na Virginia'na*, *Colubri'na Virginia'na*, *Contrayer'va Virginia'na*, *S. Virginia'na*, (F.) *Serpentaire et Aristoloche serpentaire de Virginie*, *Colurine de Virginie*, *Virginia Snakeroot*, *Snakeroot Birthwort*, *Snakeweed*, *Snagrel*. Virtues — tonic, stimulant; and, as such, employed in debility, intermittents, &c.

ARISTOLOCHIA TENUIS, A. Clematitis — a. Trifida, A. Trilobata.

ARISTOLOCHI'A TRILOBA'TA, *A. trif'ida*, (F.) *Aristoloche trilobée*. A plant of Surinam and Jamaica; possessing the general virtues of the Aristolochiæ. The other varieties of Aristolochia have similar properties.

ARISTOLOCHI'A VULGARIS ROTUNDA, Fumaria bulbosa.

ARISTOLOCH'IC, *Aristoloch'icus*. Same etymology. An old term for remedies supposed to have the property of promoting the flow of the lochia.—Hippocrates, Theophrastus, Dioscorides, &c.

ARIS'TON MAGNUM, and ARISTON PARVUM. These names were formerly given to pharmaceutical preparations, used in phthisis, tormina, and fever.—Avicenna.

ARISTOPHANEI'ON. A sort of emollient plaster, prepared with four pounds of pitch, two of apochyma, one of wax, an ounce of opoponax, and half a pint of vinegar. — Gorræus. Not used.

ARKANSAS, MINERAL WATERS OF. About 5 miles from the Washita river, and about a quarter of a degree north of the Louisiana line, there are about 70 of those springs. They are thermal, varying from 138° to 150° Fahrenheit, and are employed in rheumatism, cutaneous affections, &c.

ARLADA, Realgar.

ARLES, MINERAL WATERS OF. Thermal sulphureous springs in the department of Pyrénées Orientales, France. Their temperature is 103° to 145° of Fahr., and they contain sulphohydric acid.

ARM, Brachium.

ARMA, Penis—a. Ventris, Penis.

ARMAMENTARIUM, Arsenal—a. Chirurgicum, see Arsenal.

ARMATORY UNGUENT, Hoplochrysma.

ARMATURA, Amnios.

ARMÉ, from *αρω*, 'I adapt.' Any physiological or mechanical junction or union of parts.—Hesychius. A suture, as of the cranium.—Galen.

ARMENIACA EPIROTICA, Prunus Armeniaca — a. Malus, Apricot. See Prunus — a. Vulgaris, Prunus Armeniaca.

ARMENIAN STONE, Melochites.

ARMENITES, Melochites.

ARMILLÆ MANUS MEMBRANOSÆ, Annular ligaments of the carpus.

ARMOISE BLANCHE, Artemisia rupestris —a. *Commune*, Artemisia vulgaris—a. *Estragon*, Artemisia dracunculus—a. *Ordinaire*, Artemisia vulgaris.

ARMONIACUM, Ammoniac, gum.

ARMORA'CIA. In the Pharmacopœia of the United States, the fresh root of Cochlearia armoracia.

ARMORACIA RUSTICANA, Cochlearia armoracia —a. Sativa, Cochlearia armoracia.

ARMOUR, Condom.

ARMURE DES JAMBES, see Cornu ammonis.

ARMUS, Humerus—a. Summus, Acromion.

AR'NICA MONTA'NA. Derivation uncertain. Arnica, Leopard's Bane, Doron'icum Ger*man'icum* seu *Oppositifo'lium*, D. *Ar'nica*, *Alis'na*, *Ac''yrus*, *Diuret'ica*, Arnica *Plauen'sis*, *Panace'a lapso'rum*, *Ptar'mica monta'na*, *Caltha* seu *Calen'dula Alpi'na*, (F.) *Arnique*, *Bétoine des Montagnes*, *Tabac des Vosges*, *Tabac ou Bétoine des Savoyards*, *Doronic d'Allemagne*. *Sex. Syst.* Syngenesia Polygamia superflua. *Nat. Ord.* Synantheræ. The plant and flower are considered, or have been considered, narcotic, stimulant, emmenagogue, &c.; and, as such, have been given in amaurosis, paralysis, all nervous affections, rheumatism, gout, chlorosis, &c. Dose, gr. v to x, in powder. In large doses, it is deleterious.

ARNICA SPURIA, Inula dysenterica—a. Suedensis, Inula dysenterica.

ARNOGLOSSUM, Plantago.

ARNOTT'S DILATOR, see Dilator, Arnott's.

ARO'MA, *Ar'tyma*, 'perfume :' (*αρι*, 'very,' and *οσμη* or *οδμη*, 'odour.') *Spir'itus Rector*, (F.) *Arome*. The odorous part of plants. An emanation—frequently imponderable, from bodies—which acts on the organ of smell, and varies with the body exhaling it.

AROMAT'IC, *Aromat'icus*, (F.) *Aromate*. Any odoriferous substance obtained from the vegetable kingdom which contains much volatile oil, or a light and expansible resin. Aromatics are used in perfumes, in seasoning, and embalming. In medicine they are employed as stimulants. Ginger, cinnamon, cardamoms, mint, &c., belong to this class.

AROMATOPO'LA, from *αρωμα*, 'an odour,' and *πωλεω*, 'I sell.' An apothecary or druggist. One who sells spices.

ARON, Arum.

AROPH. A barbarous word, which had various significations with the ancients. Paracelsus employed it to designate a lithonthriptic remedy. The mandragora, according to some. Also, a mixture of bread, saffron and wine.—Van Helmont.

AROPH PARACELSI, Ferrum ammoniatum.

ARQUEBUSADE EAU D', *Aqua traumat'ica Thede'nii*, *Aqua Thedia'na*, *Aqua sclopeta'ria*, *Aqua vulnera'ria*, *Aqua catapulta'rum*, *Mistu'ra vulnera'ria ac''ida*. A sort of vulnerary water, distilled from a farrago of aromatic plants. Rosemary ℔iss, millefoil, thyme, each ℔ss. Proof spirit 2 gallons—distil a gallon. This is one form.

ARRABON, Arraphon.

ARRACHEMENT, (F.) from *arracher*, 'to tear out,' *Apospas'ma*, *Abrup'tio*, *Avul'sio*. Act of separating a part of the body by tearing it from the bonds connecting it with others. Evulsion. Laceration.

Arrachement is applied to certain operations, as to the *extraction of a tooth*, the *extirpation of a polypus*, &c.

ARRACK, Arack. See Spirit.

AR'RAPHON, *Ar'rabon*, from *a*, priv., and *ραφη*, 'a suture,'—'without suture.' A term applied to the cranium when it presents no sutures.

ARRECTIO, Erection.

ARREPTIO, Insanity.

ARRESTA BOVIS, Ononis spinosa.

ARRÊT D'HILDAN, Remora Hildani.

ARRÊTE BŒUF, Ononis spinosa.

ARRHŒ'A, from *a*, privative, and *ρεω*, 'I flow,' The suppression of any flux. Amenorrhœa.

ARRHOSTEMA, Disease.

ARRHOSTENIA, Disease.

ARRHOSTIA, Disease, Infirmity.

ARRHYTHMUS, Cacorrhythmus.

ARRIBA, Geoffræa vermifuga.

ARRIÈRE-BOUCHE, Pharynx — a. - *Dent*, see Dentition—a.-*Faix*, Secundines.

ARRIÈRE-GOUT, (F.) 'after taste.' The taste left by certain bodies in the mouth for some time after they have been swallowed, owing perhaps to the papillæ of the mouth having imbibed the savoury substance.

ARRIÈRES NARINES, Nares, posterior.

ARROCHE, Atriplex hortensis — a. *Puant*, Chenopodium vulvaria.

ARROSEMENT, Aspersion.

ARROWHEAD, Sagittaria variabilis.

ARROW LEAF, Sagittaria variabilis.

ARROW POISON. This differs with different tribes of Indians. By some, the poison capsicum, and infusions of a strong kind of tobacco, and of euphorbiaceæ are mixed together, with the poisonous emmet, and the teeth of the formidable serpent, called by the Peruvian Indians *Miuamaru* or *Jergon*,—*Lachesis picta* of Tschudi.

ARROW ROOT, *Fec'ula Maran'tæ*, *Am'ylum maranta'ceum*, A. *America'num*. The fecula of the rhizoma of *Maran'ta Arundina'cea*, which, like all feculæ, is emollient and nutritive, when prepared with water, milk, &c.

Dr. Carson has shown, that *Florida arrow-root* is derived from *Za'mia integrifo'lia* or *Z. pu'mila*, *Sugar pine ; Bermuda arrow root* being obtained from Maranta arundinacea. Florida arrow root, as well as the farina, is known in the Southern States under the name *Coonti* or *Coontie*.

According to Dr. Ainslie, an excellent kind of arrow root is prepared in Travancore from the root of *Curcuma angustifolia*.

Arrow root mucilage is made by rubbing *arrow root powder* with a little *cold water*, in a basin, by means of the back of a spoon, until it is completely mixed with the water; then pouring *boiling water* over it, stirring assiduously until a soft, gelatinous, tenacious mucilage is formed; and, lastly, boiling for five minutes. A tablespoonful of arrow root powder is sufficient to make a pint of mucilage. It may be moderately sweetened; and wine or lemon juice may be added.

With milk also it forms a bland and nutritious article of diet.

ARROW ROOT, BRAZILIAN. The fecula of Jatropha Manihot.

ARROW ROOT, COMMON, see Solanum tuberosum.

ARROW ROOT, EAST INDIAN. The fecula of the tubers of Curcuma angustifolia or narrow-leaved Turmeric.

ARROW ROOT, ENGLISH, Arrow root, common.

ARROW WOOD, Euonymus, Viburnum dendatum.

ARS CABALISTICA, Cabal—a. Chymiatrica, Chymiatria—a. Clysmatica nova, Infusion of medicines—a. Coquinaria, Culinary art—a. Cosmetica, Cosmetics—a. Culinaria, Culinary art—a. Empirica, Empiricism—a. Hermetica, Chymistry—a. Homœopathica, Homœopathy—a. Hydriatrica, Hydrosudotherapeia—a. Infusoria, Infusion of medicines—a. Machaonia, Medicina—a. Majorum, Chymistry—a. Medica, Medicina—a. Obstetricia, Obstetrics—a. Sanandi, Art, healing—a. Separatoria, Chymistry—a. Spagirica, Chymistry—a. Veterinaria, Veterinary Art—a. Zoiatrica, Veterinary Art.

ARSALTOS, Asphaltum.

ARSATUM, Nymphomania.

ARSENAL, (F.) *Chirapothe'ca, Armamenta'rium, A. chirur'gicum.* A collection of surgical instruments. A work containing a description of surgical instruments.

ARSEN'IATE, *Arsen'ias.* A salt formed by a combination of arsenic acid with a salifiable base.

ARSENIATE OF AMMONIA, *Arsen'ias Ammo'niæ, Ammo'nium Arsenic'icum,* (F.) *Arséniate d'Ammoniaque.* This preparation is highly extolled in cutaneous diseases. A grain of the salt may be dissolved in an ounce of distilled water, and 20 to 25 drops be commenced with as a dose.

ARSENIATE OF IRON, *Arsen'ias Ferri, Ferrum Arsenia'tum, F. Arsen'icum oxydula'tum,* (F.) *Arséniate de Fer.* This preparation has been applied externally to cancerous ulcers. An ointment may be made of ℨss of the arseniate, ℨij of the phosphate of iron, and ℨvj of spermaceti ointment. The arseniate has also been given internally in cancerous affections, in the dose of one-sixteenth of a grain.

ARSENIATE OF PROTOX'IDE OF POTAS'SIUM, *Proto-arsen'iate of Potas'sium, Arsen'iate of Potassa, Arsen'ias Potassæ, Arsenias Kali.* Properties the same as those of arsenious acid.

ARSENIATE OF QUINIA, Quiniæ Arsenias.

AR'SENIC, *Arsen'icum.* A solid metal; of a steel-gray colour; granular texture; very brittle; volatilizing before melting; very combustible and acidifiable. It is not dangerous of itself, and only becomes so by virtue of the facility with which it absorbs oxygen.

ARSENIC BLANC, Arsenicum album.

ARSENIC, IODIDE OF, *Arsen'ici Io'didum seu Teriod'idum, A. Iodure'tum, Arsen'icum Ioda'tum;* formed by the combination of *arsenious acid* and *iodine.* This preparation, applied externally, has been highly extolled in various cutaneous affections. An ointment may be made of three grains of iodide to ℨj of lard. It has also been given internally in the dose of a tenth of a grain in similar affections.

ARSENIC, OXIDE OF, Arsenicum album—a. Oxide of, White, Arsenicum album—a. White, Arsenicum album.

ARSENIC AND MERCURY, IODIDE OF, *Hydrar'gyri et Arsen'ici Io'didum, Double I'odide of Mer'cury and Ar'senic, Iodo-arsenite of Mer'cury.* A compound, which has been proposed as more efficacious than either the iodide of arsenic or the iodide of mercury. It is made by triturating 6.08 grains of metallic *arsenic;* 14.82 grains of *mercury;* 49 of *iodine,* with a fluidrachm of *alcohol,* until the mass has become dry, and from being deep brown has become pale red. Eight ounces of *distilled water* are poured on, and, after trituration for a few moments, the whole is transferred to a flask; half a drachm of *hydriodic acid,* prepared by the acidification of two grains of iodine, is added, and the mixture is boiled for a few moments. When the solution is cold, make the mixture up to f℥viij with distilled water. This is called by Mr. Donovan, the proposer, *Liquor Arsen'ici et Hydrar'gyri Io'didi,* each drachm of which by measure consists of water ℨj, arsenious acid gr. 1-8th; peroxide of mercury gr. 1-4th, iodine converted into hydriodic acid gr. 3-4ths. In the last edition of the *Ph. U. S.* it is directed to be made of *Arsenici Iodidum* and *Hydrargyri Iodidum rubrum,* each gr. xxxv; and *Aqua destillata* Oss; dissolving by rubbing, heating to the boiling point, and filtering.

The dose of *Donovan's Solution,* is from ♏xv to f℥ss two or three times a day.

It has been used successfully in inveterate cutaneous diseases.

ARSEN'ICAL PASTE, (F.) *Pâte Arsénicale.* This application to cancers is formed of 70 parts of *cinnabar,* 22 of *dragon's blood,* and 8 of *arsenious acid;* made into a paste with saliva, when about to be applied.

ARSENICI IODIDUM, Arsenic, Iodide of—a. Ioduretum, Arsenic, Iodide of—a. Teriodidum, Arsenic, iodide of.

ARSENICISM'US, *Intoxica'tio Arsenica'lis.* Poisoning by arsenic.

ARSEN'ICUM ALBUM; *White Ar'senic, Oxide of Ar'senic, Ratsbane, Arsen'ici ox'ydum album, Calx Arsen'ici alba, Ac''idum Arsenico'sum, A. Arsenio'sum* (Ph. U. S.), *Arsen'ious acid, White oxide of arsenic,* (F.) *Arsenic blanc.* An acid which is met with in commerce, in compact, white, heavy, fragile, masses; of a vitreous aspect, opake, and covered with a white dust; of an acrid and nauseous taste; without smell when cold; volatilizable by heat, and exhaling the odour of garlic: soluble in water, alcohol and oil; crystallizable in regular octahedrons. It is this that is meant by the name arsenic, as commonly used.

ARSEN'ICUM ALBUM SUBLIMA'TUM, *Sublimed Oxide of Arsenic,* is the one employed in medicine. It is tonic and escharotic, and is the most virulent of mineral poisons. It is used in intermittents, periodical headachs, neuroses, &c. Dose, gr. one-tenth to one-eighth in pill. See Poisons, *Table of.*

ARSENICUM IODATUM, Arsenic, Iodide of—a. Rubrum Factitium, Realgar.

ARSENIS POTASSÆ, Arsenite of protoxide of potassium—a. Potassæ aquosus, Liquor arsenicalis—a. Potassæ liquidus, Liquor arsenicalis.

AR'SENITE, *Ar'senis.* A salt, formed by a combination of the arsenious acid with a salifiable base.

AR'SENITE OF PROTOX'IDE OF POTAS'SIUM, *Proto-ar'senite of Potas'sium, Ar'senite of Potassa, Ar'senis Potassæ.* An uncrystallizable and colourless salt, which forms the basis of the liquor arsenicalis, which see.

ARSENITE OF QUINIA, Quiniæ arsenis.

ARSE-SMART, Persicaria—a. Biting, Polygonum hydropiper.

ART, HEALING, *Ars Sanan'di, Medici'na.* The appropriate application of the precepts of the best physicians, and of the results of experience to the treatment of disease.

ART, VETERINARY, Veterinary art.

AR'TABE, *αρταβη*. Name of a measure for dry substances, in use with the ancients, equal at times, to 5 modii: at others, to 3; and at others, again, to 7.—Galen.

ARTANTHE ELONGATA, see Matico.

AR'TELSHEIM, MINERAL WATERS OF. These German waters have been much recommended in hysteria, gout, palsy, &c. Their physical or chemical properties have not been described.

ARTEMIS'IA, *Anacti'rion*. Called after a queen of the name, who first employed it; or from *Αρτεμις*, 'Diana;' because it was formerly used in diseases of women, over whom she presided. The Gauls called it *Bricumum*.

ARTEMIS'IA ABROT'ANUM, *Abrot'anum, Abrot'onum, Abrot'anum Catheum, Abrot'anum mas, Abrathan, South'ernwood, Oldman*, (F.) *Aurone, Aurone mâle, Aurone des jardins, Garderobe, Citronelle*. Supposed to be possessed of stimulant properties.

Oil of Southernwood, O'leum Abrot'ani, (F.) *Huile d'Aurone*, possesses the aromatic properties of the plant.

ARTEMIS'IA ABSIN'THIUM, *Absin'thium, Absin'thium vulga'rē, Apsin'thium, Barypi'cron, Common Wormwood*, (F.) *Absinthe*. Properties:—tonic and anthelmintic. The *Oil of Wormwood, O'leum Absin'thii*, (F.) *Huile d'Absinthe*, contains the aromatic virtues of the plant.

ARTEMISIA AFRA, a South African species, is tonic, antispasmodic and anthelmintic; and has been used in debility of the stomach, visceral obstructions, jaundice and hypochondriasis. It is taken in infusion, decoction and tincture. A strong infusion is used by the Cape Colonists as a collyrium in weakness of the eyes; and the pounded leaves and stalks are employed as discutients in œdema and sugillations.

ARTEMISIA ALBA, A. Santonica—a. Balsamita, A. Pontica.

ARTEMISIA BIEN'NIS, *Biennial Wormwood*; indigenous.

ARTEMISIA BOTRYS, Chenopodium ambrosioides.

ARTEMIS'IA CAMPES'TRIS, *Field Southernwood*, (F.) *Aurone des Champs*. This possesses the same properties as *A. Abrot'anum*.

ARTEMISIA CHENOPODIUM, Chenopodium botrys.

ARTEMISIA CHINEN'SIS, *A. In'dica, A. Moxa*. From this the Chinese form their moxas.

ARTEMISIA CONTRA, A. Santonica.

ARTEMISIA DRACUN'CULUS, *Tar'agon*, (F.) *Armoise estragon*. Virtues:—the same as the last.

ARTEMIS'IA GLACIA'LIS, *Silky Wormwood*;

ARTEMISIA INDICA, Artemisia Chinensis, A. Santonica;

ARTEMISIA LEPTOPHYLLA, A. Pontica;

ARTEMISIA MARIT'IMA, *Absin'thium Marit'num seu Marit'imum, Sea Wormwood, Maritime Southernwood*;

ARTEMISIA MOXA, A. Chinensis; and

ARTEMIS'IA PON'TICA, *A. Roma'na seu Tenuifo'lia seu Balsami'ta seu Leptophyl'la, Absinthium Pon'ticum seu Roma'num, Roman Wormwood, Lesser Wormwood*, possess like virtues;—as well as

ARTEMISIA ROMANA, A. Pontica;

ARTEMISIA RUBRA, A. Santonica; and

ARTEMIS'IA RUPES'TRIS, *Creeping Wormwood, Gen'ipi album*, (F.) *Armoise blanc, Génipi blanc*. This variety has aromatic virtues, and is used in intermittents, and in amenorrhœa.

ARTEMIS'IA SANTON'ICA, *Santon'icum, Arte-mis'ia contra, Semen contra Vermes, Semen contra, S. Zedoa'riæ, Oanni Herba, Chamæcedris, Chamæcyparis'sus, Semen Cinæ, Hagiosper'mum, Sanc'tum Semen, Absin'thium Santon'icum, Sementi'na, Xantoli'na, Scheba Ar'abum, Artemis'ia Juda'ica, Sina seu Cina Levan'tica, Wormseed, Tartarian Southernwood*, (F.) *Barbotine*. Virtues:—anthelmintic and stimulant. Dose, gr. x. to ʒj in powder.

ARTEMISIA TENUIFOLIA, A. Pontica.

ARTEMIS'IA VULGA'RIS, *Artemis'ia rubra et alba, Oin'gulum Sancti Joan'nis, Mater Herba'rum, Berenisecum, Bubasteor'dium, Canapa'cia, Mugwort*, (F.) *Armoise ordinaire, A. Commune, Herbe de Saint Jean*. This, as well as some other varieties, possesses the general tonic virtues of the Artemisiæ. Artemisia vulgaris has been highly extolled by the Germans in cases of epilepsy. Dose of the powder, in the 24 hours, from ʒss to ʒj.

ARTÈRE, Artery—a. *Brachial*, Brachial artery—a. *Brachio-céphalique*, Innominata arteria—a. *Bronchique*, Bronchial artery—a. *Ciliaire*, Ciliary artery—a. *Clitorienne*: see Clitoris—a. *Cæcale*: see Colic arteries—a. *Collatérale du coude*, Anastomoticus magnus ramus—a *Collatérale externe*, Arteria profunda humeri—a. *Collatérale interne*, Anastomoticus magnus ramus—a. *Coronaire des lèvres*, Labial artery—a. *Coronaire Stomachique*, Coronary artery—a. *Crurale*, Crural artery—a. *Deuxième des thoraciques*, Arteria thoracica externa inferior—a. *Épineuse*, Meningeal artery, middle—a. *Fémoro-poplitée*, Ischiatic artery—a. *Fessière*, Gluteal artery—a. *Gastrique droite*, petite, Pyloric artery—a. *Gutturo-maxillaire*, Maxillary artery, internal—a. *Honteuse externe*, Pudic, external, artery—a. *Honteuse interne*, Pudic, internal, artery—a. *Humérale profonde*, Arteria profunda humeri—a. *Iliaque primitive*, Iliac artery—a. *Innominée*, Innominata arteria—a. *Irienne*, Ciliary artery—a. *Ischio-penienne*: see Pudic, internal, artery—a. *Médiane antérieure*, Spinal artery, anterior—a. *Médiane postérieure du rachis*, Spinal artery, posterior—a. *Méningée moyenne*, Meningeal artery, middle—a. *Mentonnière*, Mental foramen—a. *Mesocéphalique*, Basilary artery—a. *Mésocolique*: see Colic artery—a. *Musculaire du bras*, Arteria profunda humeri—a. *Musculaire du bras, grande*: see Collateral arteries of the arm—a. *Musculaire grande de la cuisse*, Arteria profunda femoris—a. *Opisthogastrique*, Cœliac artery—a. *Orbitaire*, Ophthalmic artery—a. *de l'Oraire*, Spermatic artery—a. *Pelvi-crurale*, Crural artery—a. *Pelvi-crurale*, Iliac artery—a. *Pelvienne*, Hypogastric artery—a. *Première des thoraciques*, Arteria thoracica externa superior—a. *Radio-carpienne transversale palmaire*, Radio-carpal artery—a. *Scrotale*, Pudic, external, artery—a. *Sous-clavière*, Subclavian artery—a. *Sous-pubio-fémorale*, Obturator artery—a. *Sous-pubienne*, Pudic, internal, artery—a. *Sous-sternal*, Mammary, internal—a. *Sphéno-épineuse*, Meningeal artery, middle—a. *Stomogastrique*, Coronary artery—a. *Sus-carpienne*: see *Sus-carpien*—a. *Sus-maxillaire*, Alveolar artery—a. *Sus-maxillaire*, Buccal artery—a. *Sus-métatarsienne*, Metatarsal artery—a. *Sus-pubienne*, Epigastric artery—a. *Testiculaire*, Spermatic artery—a. *Thoracique humérale*, Acromial artery—a. *Trachélocervical*: see Cerebral arteries—a. *Trochantérienne*, Circumflex artery of the thigh—a. *Troisième des thoraciques*, Acromial artery—a. *Tympanique*, Auditory artery, external—a. *Urétale*: see Ciliary artery—a. *Vulvaire*, Pudic, external, artery.

ARTERIA, Artery—a. Ad Cutem Abdominis, see Ad Cutem abdominis, (arteria)—a. Anonyma,

Innominata artery—a. Aspera, Trachea—a. Cerebralis, Carotid, internal—a. Cervicalis, Basilary artery—a. Coronaria dextra, Pyloric artery—a. Crassa, Aorta—a. Externa cubiti, Radial artery—a. Dorsalis metacarpi, Metacarpal artery—a. Duræ matris media maxima, Meningeal artery, middle—a. Encephalica, Carotid, internal—a. Gastrica superior, Coronary artery—a. Ilio-colica: see Colic arteries—a. Iliaca interna, Hypogastric artery—a. Iliaca posterior, Hypogastric artery—a. Magna, Aorta—a. Magna pollicis, Princeps pollicis—a. Malleolaris externa: see Tibial arteries—a. Malleolaris interna: see Tibial arteries—a. Mammaria externa, A. Thoracica externa, inferior—a. Maxima, Aorta—a. Media anastomotica: see Colic arteries—a. Meningæa media, Meningeal artery, middle—a. Muscularis femoris, A. Profunda femoris—a. Pharyngea suprema, Pterygoid artery—a. Profunda cerebri: see Cerebral arteries—a. Pudenda communis, Pudic, internal, artery—a. Pudica, Pudic, internal, artery—a. Ramulus ductus Pterygoidei, Pterygoid artery—a. Spheno-spinosa, Meningeal artery, middle—a. Spinalis, A. Profunda humeri—a. Sternalis, Mammary, internal—a. Supra-orbitalis, Frontal artery—a. Sylviana: see Cerebral arteries—a. Thoracica axillaris vel alaris, Scapular artery, inferior—a Thoracica humeralis, Acromial artery—a. Transversalis colli: see Cerebral arteries—a. Transversalis humeri, Scapular artery, superior—a. Ulnaris, Cubital artery—a. Uterina hypogastrica, Uterine artery—a Vasta posterior, A. Profunda femoris.

ARTE'RIAC, *Arteri'acus*. A medicine prescribed in diseases of the windpipe. Also arterial.

ARTE'RIÆ ADIPO'SÆ. The arteries which secrete the fat about the kidneys are sometimes so called. They are ramifications of the capsular, diaphragmatic, renal, and spermatic arteries.

ARTERIÆ APOPLECTICÆ, Carotids—a. Capitales, Carotids—a. Ciliares, Ciliary arteries—a. Corporis callosi cerebri, Mesolobar arteries—a. Jugulares, Carotids—a. Lethargicæ, Carotids—a. Mesolobicæ, Mesolobar arteries—a. Præparantes, Spermatic arteries—a. Somniferæ, Carotids—a. Soporales, Carotids—a. Soporariæ, Carotids—a. Venosæ, Pulmonary veins.

ARTE'RIAL, *Arteri'acus, Arterio'sus*. Belonging to arteries.

ARTERIAL BLOOD, (F.) *Sang artériel*. Red blood is so called because contained in the arteries. The pulmonary veins, however, also contain red blood: hence the name *arterial veins*, (F.) *Veines artérielles*, applied to them.

ARTE'RIAL DUCT, *Cana'lis arterio'sus, Ductus arterio'sus, D. Botal'lii*, (F.) *Canal artériel, C. Pulmo-aortique*, is the portion of the pulmonary artery which terminates in the aorta in the fœtus. When this duct is obliterated after birth, it is called *Arte'rial Lig'ament*, (F.) *Ligament artériel*.

ARTERIAL SYSTEM includes all the arteries, from their origin in the heart to their termination in the organs. See Vascular System.

ARTERIALIZATION OF THE BLOOD, Hæmatosis.

ARTÉRIARCTIE,, from αρτηρια, 'artery,' and αρκτο, 'I straiten.' Contraction of an artery.

ARTERIECTASIS, Aneurism.

ARTERIECTOP'IA, from αρτηρια, 'artery,' and εκτοπος, 'out of place.' Dislocation of an artery.

ARTERIEURYSMA, Aneurism.

ARTERIITIS, Arteritis.

ARTERIODIALYSIS, see Aneurism.

ARTERIOG'RAPHY, *Arteriogra'phia*: from αρτηρια, 'artery,' and γραφη, 'a description.' A description of the arteries.

ARTERIOLA. A small artery.

ARTERIOL'OGY, *Arteriolog'ia*; from αρτηρια, 'artery,' and λογος, 'a discourse.' A treatise on the arteries.

ARTE'RIO-PITU'ITOUS. An epithet applied to vessels which creep along the interior of the nostrils.—Ruysch.

ARTERIORRHEXIS, see Aneurism.

ARTERIOS'ITAS, from *Arteria*, 'an artery.' A condition of the blood in which it preserves in the veins the arterial character.—The opposite to Venositas.

ARTERIOSITAS SANGUINIS, Prædominium sanguinis arteriosi.

ARTÉRIOSTEIE, from αρτηρια, 'artery,' and οστεον, 'a bone.' Ossification of an artery.—Piorry.

ARTERIOT'OMY, *Arteriotom'ia*, from αρτηρια, 'an artery,' and τεμνω, 'I cut.' This word has been used for the dissection of arteries. Most commonly, however, it means a surgical operation, which consists in opening an artery, to draw blood from it. Arteriotomy is chiefly used in inflammatory affections of the head, when the blood is generally obtained from the temporal artery. See Blood-letting.

ARTERI'TIS, *Arteri'tis, Infiamma'tio Arteria'rum*, (F.) *Artérite, Inflammation des artères;* from αρτηρια, 'an artery,' and *itis*, a termination denoting inflammation. Inflammation of an artery. Inflammation of the inner coat of an artery is termed *Endo-arteri'tis*, or *Endonarteri'tis;* of the outer, *Exo-arteri'tis* or *Exarteri'tis*.

AR'TERY, *Arte'ria*, (F.) *Artère*, from αηρ, 'air,' and τηρειν, 'to preserve,' *quasi*, 'receptacle of air,' because the ancients believed that it contained air. They, at first, gave the name *Artery* to the trachea, αρτηρια τραχεια, because it is filled with air; and afterwards they used the same term for the arteries, properly so called, probably because they commonly found them empty in the dead body. We find, also, φλεβες to designate the arteries, called by the Latins *Venæ mican'tes pulsat'iles*. Arteries, with the moderns, signify the order of vessels, which arise from the two ventricles of the heart, and have valves only at their origin. They are cylindrical, firm, and elastic canals; of a yellowish white colour; little dilatable; easily lacerable; and formed, 1. Of an external, laminated or areolar membrane, of a dense and close character. 2. Of a middle coat composed of fibres, which does not, however, contract on the application of the galvanic stimulus; and 3. Of an inner coat, which is thin, diaphanous, reddish, and polished.

The use of the arteries is to carry the blood from the heart to the various parts of the system. It will be obvious, however, that they cannot all convey *arterial* blood. The pulmonary artery, for example, is destined to convey the *venous* blood to the lungs, there to be converted into *arterial;* whilst the pulmonary veins convey *arterial* blood back to the heart.

TABLE OF THE PRINCIPAL ARTERIES OF THE BODY.

All the other arteries take their rise from the Pulmonary Artery, or the Aorta: and the names generally indicate the parts to which they are distributed.

I. ARTERIA PULMONALIS.

The Pulmonary Artery arises from the right ventricle, and soon divides into a right and left branch, one of which is distributed to each lung.

II. ARTERIA AORTA.

The Aorta arises from the left ventricle. It is the common trunk of the arteries of the body, and may be divided into five portions.

a. *Arteries furnished by the Aorta at its origin.*
  1. A. Cardiaca or coronaria anterior.
  2. A. Cardiaca or coronaria posterior.

b. *Arteries furnished by the Aorta at its arch.*

The arch of the Aorta gives off, to the left, two considerable trunks—the *Arteria carotidea primitiva*, and *A. subclavia;* and, to the right, a single trunk, which is larger—the *A. innominata*, or *Brachio-cephalica*, which divides into the *primitive carotid* and *subclavian*.

A. ARTERIA CARO-TIDEA PRIMITIVA. { Divides into A. Carotidea externa, A. Carotidea interna.

a. A. Carotidea externa. { Furnishes, 1. *A. Thyroidea superior.*
2. *A. lingualis*, which gives off the A. dorsalis linguæ and A. sublingualis.
3. *A. facialis* vel *A. Maxillaris externa*, which furnishes the A. palatina inferior, the A. submentalis, and A. coronaria superior and inferior.
4. *A. occipitalis*, which gives off the A. mastoidea posterior.
5. *A. auricularis posterior*, which gives off A. stylo-mastoidea.
6. *A. pharyngea inferior*.

The external carotid ultimately divides into the temporal artery and internal maxillary.

1. *A. Temporalis.* { Furnishes *A. transversalis faciei*, *A. auricularis anterior*, and *A. temporalis media*.

2. *A. Maxillaris interna.* { Furnishes 13 branches, viz. *A. meningea media*, *A. dentaris inferior*, *A. temporalis profunda posterior*, *A. masseterina*, *A. pterygoidea*, *A. buccalis*, *A. temporalis profunda anterior*, *A. alveolaris ; A. suborbitaris, A. vidiana, A. pterygopalatina* or *pharyngea superior*, *A. palatina superior*, and *A. sphenopalatina*.

b. A. Carotidea interna. { Furnishes, 1. *A. ophthalmica*, which gives off A. lachrymalis, A. centralis retinæ, A. supraorbitaria vel superciliaris, A. ciliares posteriores, A. ciliares longæ, A. muscularis superior et inferior, A. ethmoidalis posterior et anterior, A. palpebralis superior et inferior, A. nasalis, and A. frontalis. 2. *A. communicans, Willisii.* 3. *A. choroidea.* 4. *A. cerebralis anterior.* 5. *A. cerebralis media.*

B. ARTERIA SUBCLAVIA. { Furnishes, 1. *A. vertebralis*, which gives off A. spinalis anterior et posterior, A. cerebellosa inferior, and forms—by uniting itself with that of the opposite side—the A. basilaris, divided into A. cerebellosa superior and A. cerebralis posterior. 2. *A. thyroidea inferior*, which gives off A. cervicalis ascendens. 3. *A. mammaria interna*, which gives off the A. mediastina anterior and A. diaphragmatica superior. 4. *A. intercostalis superior.* 5. *A. cervicalis transversa.* 6. *A. scapularis superior.* 7. *A. cervicalis posterior* vel *profunda*. Farther on, the subclavian artery continues its progress under the name *A. axillaris*.

A. Axillaris. { Furnishes, 1. *A. acromialis.* 2. *A. thoracica superior.* 3. *A. thoracica inferior* vel *longa* vel *mammaria externa.* 4. *A. scapularis inferior* vel *communis.* 5. *A. circumflexa posterior.* 6. *A. circumflexa anterior.* Farther on, the axillary artery continues under the name *A. brachialis*.

A. Brachialis. { Furnishes *A. humeralis profunda* vel *collateralis externa.* 2. *A. collateralis interna.* It afterwards divides into the *radial* and *cubital* arteries.

1. *A. Radialis.* { Gives off *A. recurrens radialis*, *A. dorsalis carpi*, *A. dorsalis metacarpi*, *A. dorsalis pollicis*, and terminates in forming the *Arcus palmaris profundus*.

2. *A. Cubitalis.* { Gives off *A. recurrens cubitalis anterior* and *posterior : A. interossea anterior* and *posterior*. which latter furnishes *A. recurrens radialis posterior*. It terminates in forming the *superficial palmar arch*, which gives off *A. Collaterales digitorum*.

c. *Arteries given off by the Aorta in the Thorax.*

These arteries are, { 1. *A. Bronchica, dextra et sinistra.*
2. *A. œsophagea* (to the number of four, five, or six.)
3. *A mediastina posteriores.*
4. *A. intercostales inferiores* vel *aorticæ* (to the number of eight, nine, or ten.)

d. *Arteries furnished by the Aorta in the Abdomen.*

These branches are, { 1. The *A. diaphragmatica* vel *phrenica dextra et sinistra.*

2. *A. Cœliaca.* { Which divides into three branches, 1. *A. coronaria ventriculi.* 2. *A. Hepatica*, which gives off A. pylorica, A. gastro-epiploica dextra and A. cystica ; and, lastly, the *A. splenica*, which gives off A. gastro-epiploica sinistra and Vasa brevia.

3. *A. Mesenterica superior* { Which gives off at its concavity the *A. colica dextra superior, media et inferior*, and at its convex part from 15 to 20 Rami intestinales.

4. *A. Mesenterica inferior.* { Which gives off *A. colica superior media*, and *inferior*, and divides into A. hæmorrhoidales superiores.

5. The *A. Capsulares mediæ* (to the number of two on each side.)
6. *A. Renales* vel *Emulgentes.*
7. *A. Spermaticæ.*
8. *A. Lumbares* (to the number of four or five on each side.)

e. *Arteries resulting from the Bifurcation of the Aorta.*

The Aorta, a little above its Bifurcation, gives off the *A. sacra media*, and divides into *A. iliaca primitiva*.

A. Iliaca primitiva. { Divides into *A. Iliaca interna* and *A. Iliaca externa*.

a. A. Iliaca interna. { Furnishes, 1. *A. ilio-lumbaris.* 2. *A. sacra lateralis.* 3. *A. glutea* vel *iliaca posterior*. 4. *A. umbilicalis.* 5. *A. vesicalis.* 6. *A. obturatoria.* 7. *A. hæmorrhoidea media.* 8 *A. uterina.* 9. *A. vaginalis.* 10. *A. ischiatica.* 11. *A. pudenda interna*, which gives off the *A. hæmorrhoidales inferiores*, *A, of the septum, A. transversa perinæi, A. corporis cavernosi*, and *A. dorsalis penis*.

b. A. Iliaca externa. { Furnishes, 1. *A. epigastrica.* 2. *A. iliaca anterior* vel *circumflexa ilii*, and is continued afterwards under the name of *Crural Artery*.

A. Cruralis. { Furnishes; 1. *A. subcutanea abdominalis.* 2. *A. pudenda superficialis* and *profunda.* 3. *A. muscularis superficialis.* 4. *A. muscularis profunda*, which gives off the A. circumflexa externa and interna, and the three Perforantes, distinguished into superior, middle, and inferior. Farther on, the crural artery continues under the name *A. Poplitæa*.

A. Poplitæa. { Furnishes, 1. *A. Articulares superiores, interna, media, et externa.* 2. *A. Gemellæ.* 3. *A. Articulares inferiores, interna et externa.* 4. *A. tibialis antica*, which, at the foot, takes the name, *A. dorsalis tarsi*, and gives off the tarsal and metatarsal arteries. In the leg, the popliteal artery divides into the peroneal and posterior tibial.

1. *A. Peronæa.* { Divides into *A. peronea antica* and *A. peronæa postica*.

2. *A. Tibialis postica.* { Divides into *A. plantaris interna* and *A. plantaris externa.* The latter, by anastomosing with the *A. dorsalis tarsi*, forms the plantar arch, whence arise *Rami superiores* vel *perforantes postici*, *A. Inferiores postici et antici*, which give off Rami perforantes antici.

ARTERY, ANGULAR, Facial artery—a. Articular, Circumflex artery—a. Brachiocephalic, Innominata arteria—a. Central of the retina, Central artery of the retina—a. Central of Zinn, Central artery of the retina—a. Cephalic, Carotid—a. Cerebral posterior, Vertebral—a. Cervico-scapular, see Cervical arteries—a. Coronary of the lips, Labial artery—a. Crotaphite, Temporal artery—a. Fibular, Peroneal artery—a. Gastric inferior,

Gastro-epiploic artery — a. Gastro-hepatic, see Gastro-epiploic artery — a. Genital, Pudic (internal) artery — a. Guttural inferior, Thyroideal A. inferior — a. Guttural superior, Thyroideal A. superior — a. Humeral, Brachial artery — a. Iliac posterior, Gluteal artery — a. Iliaco-muscular, Ileo-lumbar artery — a. Labial, Facial artery — a. Laryngeal superior, Thyroideal artery, superior — a. Maxillary internal, Facial artery — a. Median of the sacrum, Sacral artery, anterior — a. Nasal, lateral, large, Spheno-palatine artery — a. Palatolabial, Facial artery — a. Pericephalic, Carotid (external) — a. Pharyngeal, superior, Pterygopalatine artery — a. Phrenic, Diaphragmatic artery — a. Posterior of the brain, see Cerebral arteries — a. External scapular, Acromial artery — a. Spinal, Meningeal artery, middle — a. Subclavian right, Innominata arteria — a. Subscapular, Scapular artery, inferior — a. Superficial of the abdomen, Ad cutem abdominis (arteria) — a. Supramaxillary, Alveolar artery — a. Suprarenal, Capsular artery — a. Thoracic, internal, Mammary internal — a. Urethro-bulbar, Transverse perineal artery — a. Vesico-prostatic, Vesical artery — a. Vidian, Pterygoid artery.

ARTETIS'CUS; from *artus*, 'a limb.' One who has lost a limb.

ARTEURYSMA, Aneurism.

ARTHANI'TA, from *apros*, 'bread;' the *Cyclamen* or *Sowbread*. It was formerly made into ointment, *Unguen'tum Arthani'tæ*, with many other substances, and was employed as a purgative, being rubbed on the abdomen.

ARTHANITA CYCLAMEN, Cyclamen.

ARTHETICA, Teucrium chamæpitys.

ARTHRAGRA, Gout — a. Anomala, Gout, anomalous — a. Genuina, Gout, regular — a. Legitima, Gout, regular — a. Normalis, Gout, regular — a. Vera, Gout, regular.

ARTHRALGIA, Arthrodynia, Gout. See Lead rheumatism.

ARTHRELCO'SIS, from *apθρov*, 'a joint,' and *ἑλκωσις*, 'ulceration.' Ulceration of a joint.

ARTHREMBOLE'SIS, same etymon as the next. The reduction of a fracture or luxation.

ARTHREM'BOLUS, from *apθρov*, 'a joint,' *εν*, 'in,' and *βαλλω*, 'I cast.' An ancient instrument used in the reduction of dislocations.

ANTHRETICA, Teucrium chamæpitys.

ARTHRIT'IC, *Arthrit'icus*, from *apθρov*, 'a joint.' (F.) *Arthritique, Goutteux*. That which relates to gout or arthritis, as *arthritic symptoms*, &c.

ARTHRITICUS VERUS, Gout.

ARTHRITIF'UGUM; from *arthritis*, 'gout,' and *fugare*, 'to drive away.' A remedy that drives away gout. Heyden terms cold water, internally, the *arthritif'ugum magnum*.

ARTHRITIS, Gout, Arthrophlogosis, Arthrosia — a. Aberrans, Gout (wandering) — a. Acuta, Gout (regular) — a. Arthrodynia, Rheumatism, chronic — a. Asthenica, Gout (atonic) — a. Atonic, Gout (atonic) — a. Diaphragmatica, Angina Pectoris — a. Erratica, Gout (wandering) — a. Hydrarthros, Hydrarthrus — a. Inflammatoria, Gout (regular) — a. Juvenilis, see Rheumatism, acute — a. Maxillaris, Siagonagra — a. Nodosa, Gout (with nodosities) — a. Planetica, Gout (wandering) — a. Podagra, Gout — a. Rheumatica, see Rheumatism, acute — a. Rheumatismus, Rheumatism, acute — a. Retrograda, Gout (retrograde).

. ARTHROC'ACE, from *apθρov*, 'a joint,' and *κακος*, 'bad.' Disease of the joints; and especially caries of the articular surfaces. Spina ventosa.

ARTHROCACE COXARUM, Coxarum morbus.

ARTHROCACOLOG"IA, from *arthrocacia* — according to Rust, a chronic disease of the joints; and *λογος*, 'a description.' The doctrine of chronic diseases of the joints.

ARTHROCARCINO'MA, from *apθρov*, 'a joint,' and *καρκινωμα*, 'cancer.' Cancer of the joints.

ARTHROCHONDRI'TIS, from *apθρov*, 'a joint,' *χονδρος*, 'a cartilage,' and *itis*, denoting inflammation. Inflammation of the cartilages and joints.

ARTHRO'DIA, from *apθρov*, 'a joint.' *Adarticula'tio*. A moveable joint, formed by the head of a bone applied to the surface of a shallow socket, so that it can execute movements in every direction. *Arthro'dium* is 'a small joint;' diminutive of Arthrodia.

ARTHRODYN'IA, *Arthronal'gia, Arthral'gia*, from *apθρov*, 'articulation,' and *οδυνη*, 'pain.' Articular pain. Pain in the joints. See Rheumatism, chronic.

ARTHRODYNIA PODAGRICA, Gout.

ARTHROL'OGY, *Arthrolog"ia*, from *apθρov*, 'a joint,' and *λογος*, 'a description.' A description of the joints. The anatomy of the joints.

ARTHROM'BOLE, from *apθρov*, and *βαλλω*, 'I cast.' Coaptation, reduction. Reduction of a luxated or fractured bone.

ARTHROMENINGITIS, Meningarthrocace.

ARTHRON, 'a joint.' The ancients used the word *Arthron*, for the articulation of bones with motion, in opposition to *Symphysis*, or articulation without motion.

ANTHRONALGIA, Arthrodynia.

ARTHRON'CUS, *Arthrophy'ma*; from *apθρov*, 'a joint,' and *ογκος*, 'a swelling.' Tumefaction of a joint.

ARTHRONEMPYESIS, Arthropyosis.

ARTHROPHLOGO'SIS, from *apθρov*, 'a joint,' and *φλεγω*, 'I burn;' *Arthri'tis, Ostarthro'sis*. Inflammation of the joints.

ARTHROPHYMA ADENOCHONDRIUM, see Adenochondrius.

ARTHROPYO'SIS, *Arthronempye'sis*, from *apθρov*, 'a joint,' and *πυον*, 'pus.' Suppuration or abscess of the joints.

ARTHRO-RHEUMATISMUS, Rheumatism (acute.)

ARTHRO'SIA, from *apθρow*, 'I articulate.' *Arthritis*, (of some.) Inflammation, mostly confined to the joints; severely painful; occasionally extending to the surrounding muscles. A genus of diseases in the Nosology of Good, including *Rheumatism, Gout, Articular inflammation, Jointache*, &c.

ARTHROSIA ACUTA, Rheumatism, acute — a. Chronica, Rheumatism, chronic — a. Lumborum, Lumbago — a. Podagra, Gout — a. Podagra complicata, Gout (retrograde) — a. Podagra larvata, Gout (atonic) — a. Podagra regularis, Gout (regular.)

ARTHROSIS, Articulation.

ARTHROSPON'GUS, from *apθρov*, 'a joint,' and *σπογγος*, 'a sponge.' A white, fungous tumour of the joints.

ARTHROTRAU'MA, from *apθρov*, 'a joint,' and *τραυμα*, 'a wound.' A wound of a joint.

AR'TIA. According to some, this word is synonymous with *αρτηρια*; others use it synonymously with *Trachea*.

ARTIOHAUT, Cynara scolymus.

ARTICHOKE, Cynara scolymus.

ARTICLE, Articulation.

ARTICOCALUS, Cynara scolymus.

ARTIC'ULAR, *Articula'ris*: from *artus*, 'a joint;' *articulus*, 'a small joint.' That which relates to the articulations; — as the *articular capsules*, &c.

ARTICULAR ARTERIES OF THE ARM, Circumflex arteries of the arm.

ARTIC'ULAR AR'TERIES OF THE KNEE arise from the popliteal artery, and surround the tibio-femoral articulation. Although of a small size, they are important, as they furnish blood to the lower extremity after the operation for popliteal aneurism. They are distinguished into *superior* and *inferior*. The *superior articular arteries, popliteal articular arteries*, are commonly three in number; one of which is *internal*, another *external*, and another *middle*, the *az'ygous artic'-ular*. The first, *Ramus anastomot'icus magnus*, anastomoses by one branch with the external circumflex; and by another with the external superior articular. The *second* anastomoses with the external circumflex, the superior internal articular, and the inferior external articular; and the *third* is distributed within the joint. The *inferior articular arteries* are two in number: an *internal* and *external*. The former anastomoses with the internal superior articular and the external inferior articular. The latter anastomoses with the recurrent branch of the anterior tibial, and the external superior articular. To each articular artery there is an *articular nerve*.

ARTIC'ULAR FACETTES' are the contiguous surfaces, by means of which the bones are articulated.

ARTICULAR PROCESSES, see Vertebræ.

ARTIC'ULAR VEINS of the knee follow the same course as the arteries.

ARTICULATIO, Articulation—a. Artificialis, Pseudarthrosis—a. Notha, Pseudarthrosis.

ARTICULA'TION, *Joint, Articula'tio, Arthro'sis, Assarthro'sis, Artic'ulus, Junctu'ra, Cola, Conjunc'tio, Nodus, Commissu'ra, Compa'ges, Syntax'is, Har'mus, Vertic'ula, Vertic'ulus, Vertic'ulum*, (F.) *Articulation, Article*. Same etymon. The union of bones with each other, as well as the kind of union.

TABLE OF ARTICULATIONS.

Articulations are generally divided into *Diarthroses* or moveable articulations, and *Synarthroses* or immoveable.

Diarthroses. { 1. Amphiarthrosis.
2. Diarthrosis, orbicular vague. { Enarthrosis. Arthrodia.
3. Alternative or Ginglymus, which admits of varieties.

Synarthroses. { 1. Suture.
2. Harmony.
3. Gomphosis.
4. Schindylesis.

The articulations are subject to a number of diseases, which are generally somewhat severe. These may be physical, as wounds, sprains, luxations, &c.; or they may be organic, as ankylosis, extraneous bodies, caries, rheumatism, gout, hydrarthroses, arthropyosis, &c.

ARTICULATION means also the combination of letters which constitute words. See Voice.

ARTICULATION, FALSE, *Pseudarthro'sis, Artic'ulus falsus*, (F.) *A. fausse, A. accidentelle, A. contre nature, A. anormale*. A false joint, formed between fragments of bone, that have remained ununited; or between a luxated bone and the surrounding parts.

ARTICULATION EN CHARNIÈRE, Ginglymus—*a. de la Hanche*, Coxo-femoral articulation.

ARTICULI DIGITORUM MANUS, Phalanges of the fingers—a. Digitorum pedis, Phalanges of the toes.

ARTICULO MORTIS, see Psychorages—a. Spinalis, Semispinalis colli.

ARTIFI"IAL, *Artificia'lis*, (F.) *Artificiel*; from *ars, artis*, 'art,' and *facere*, 'to make.' That which is formed by art.

ARTIFICIAL EYES are usually made of enamel, and represent a sort of hollow hemisphere, which is applied beneath the eyelids, when the eye is lost.

ARTIFICIAL TEETH are made of ivory, porcelain, &c.

PIÈCES D'ANATOMIE ARTIFICIELLES, are preparations of anatomy, modelled in wax, plaster, paper, &c.

ARTISCOCCUS LÆVIS, Cynara scolymus.

ARTIS'CUS, from ἄρτος, 'bread.' See Trochiscus. A troch of the shape of a small loaf. Also, and especially, a troch made of vipers.

ARTOCAR'PUS. The *Bread-fruit Tree*, (F.) *Jaquier*. A Polynesian tree, so called because the fruit, which is milky, and juicy, supplies the place of bread to the inhabitants. It grows to the height of 40 feet.

ARTOCARPUS INTEGRIFOLIA, Caoutchouc.

ARTOC'REAS, from ἄρτος, 'bread,' and κρέας, 'flesh.' A kind of nourishing food made of various aliments boiled together.—Galen.

ARTOG'ALA, from ἄρτος, 'bread,' and γάλα, 'milk.' An alimentary preparation of bread and milk. A poultice.

ARTOM'ELI, from ἄρτος, 'bread,' and μέλι, 'honey.' A cataplasm of bread and honey.—Galen.

ARTUS, Membrum.

ARTYMA, Aroma, Condiment.

ARUM, A. maculatum, and A. triphyllum—a. Americanum betæ foliis, Dracontium fœtidum.

ARUM DRACUN'CULUS, *Dracun'culus polyphyl'lus, Colubri'na Dracon'tia, Erva de Sancta Maria, Gig'arus serpenta'ria, Arum polyphyl'lum, Serpenta'ria Gallo'rum*. Family, Aroideæ. Sex. Syst. Monœcia Polyandria. The roots and leaves are very acrimonious. The plant resembles the A. *macula'tum* in its properties.

ARUM ESCULEN'TUM, *Cala'dium esculen'tum, Taro, Kalo*. The foliage and roots possess acrid qualities, which are dissipated by baking or boiling; in which form it is used as food by the people of Madeira, the Polynesians, &c.

ARUM MACULA'TUM, *Aron, Arum* (of the older writers), *A. vulga'rë, Cuckoo Pint, Barba Aaro'nis, Serpenta'ria minor, Zin'giber German'icum, Sacerdo'tis penis, Wake Robin, Priest's pintle*, (F.) *Gouet, Pied de Veau*. The fresh root is stimulant internally. Dose, ℨj. of the dried root. Externally, it is very acrid. From the root of this Arum a starch is prepared, which is called *Portland Island Sago, Gersa serpenta'riæ, Cerus'sa serpenta'riæ, Fec'ula ari macula'ti*.

ARUM, THREE-LEAVED, Arum triphyllum.

ARUM, TRIPHYL'LUM, *Three-leaved arum*, (F.) *Pied de Veau triphylle, Indian Turnip, Dragon Root, Dragon Turnip, Pepper Turnip*. This plant grows all over the United States, and is received into the Pharmacopœia under the title *Arum*. The recent root, or Cormus—Arum, (Ph. U. S.)—is very acrimonious, and has been employed in asthma, croup, and hooping-cough. Boiled in lard, it has been used in tinea capitis, and in milk in consumption.

ARUM VIRGINICUM, Peltandra Virginica—a. Vulgare, A. maculatum.

ARUMARI, Caramata.

ARUNDO BAMBOS, Bamboo—a. Brachii major, Ulna—a. Brachii minor, Radius—a. Indica, Sagittarium alexipharmacum—a. Major, Tibia—a. Minor, Fibula—a. Saccharifera, see Saccharum.

ARVA, Ava.

ARVUM, Vulva—a. Naturæ, Uterus.

ARY-ARYTENOIDÆUS, Arytenoidæus—a. Epiglotticus, Arytæno-epiglotticus.

ARYTÆ'NA, ἀρύταινα, 'a ladle.' Hence,

ARYTÆ'NO-EPIGLOT'TICUS, *Arytæ'noepiglottidæ'us, Ary-epiglot'ticus.* That which belongs to the arytenoid cartilages and epiglottis. Winslow gives this name to small, fleshy fasciculi, which are attached, at one extremity, to the arytenoid cartilages, and, by the other, to the free edge of the epiglottis. These fibres do not always exist. They form part of the arytenoid muscle of modern anatomists.

AR'YTENOID, *Arytænoï'des, Arytenoïdæ'us,* from αρυταινα, 'a ladle,' and ειδος, 'shape.' Ladle-shaped.

ARYTENOID CAR'TILAGES, *Cartilag"ines arytenoï'des, C. guttura'les, C. Gutturi'næ, C. gutturifor'mes. C. triq'uetræ, Guttur'nia,* are two cartilages of the larynx, situate posteriorly above the cricoid, which, by approximation, diminish the aperture of the glottis. Their upper extremities or cornua are turned towards each other, and are now and then found loose, in the form of appendices, which are considered, by some, as distinct cartilages, and termed *cuneiform* or *tuberculated Cartilages* or *Cornic'ula Laryn'gis.*

ARYTENOID GLANDS, *Gland'ulæ Arytenoïdæ'æ,* are small, glandular, whitish bodies, situate anterior to the A. cartilages. They pour out a mucous fluid to lubricate the larynx.

ARYTENOIDÆ'US, (F.) *Arytenoïdien.* A small muscle, which passes from one arytenoid cartilage to the other, by its contraction brings them together, and diminishes the aperture of the glottis. Winslow divided the muscle into three portions;—the *Arytenoïdæ'us transver'sus,* or *Ary-arytenoïdæ'us,* and two *Arytenoïdæ'i obli'qui.*

ARYTH'M, *Aryth'mus,* from *a*, privative, and ρυθμος, 'rhythm,' 'measure.' Irregular. This word is applied chiefly to the pulse.

ASA, Asafœtida. See Assa.

ASAFŒ'TIDA, *Assafœ'tida, Assafet'ida, Stercus diab'oli, Cibus Deo'rum, Asa, Devil's dung, Food of the Gods.* A gum-resin — the concrete juice of *Fer'ula Assafœ'tida, Narthex Assafœ'tida. Order,* Umbelliferæ. It is in small masses of a whitish, reddish, and violet hue, adhering together. Taste bitter and subacrid: smell insupportably alliaceous. The Asiatics use it regularly as a condiment.

Its medical properties are antispasmodic, stimulant, and anthelmintic. Dose, gr. v to xx, in pill.

ASAGRÆA OFFICINALIS, see Veratrina.

AS'APES, 'crude,' *Asep'ton.* A term applied to the sputa, or to other matters evacuated, which do not give signs of coction.

ASAPH'ATUM, from *a*, privative, and σαφης, 'clear.' This term has been applied to collections in the sebaceous follicles of the skin, which may be pressed out like little worms, with a black head. See Acne.

ASAPHI'A, from *a*, privative, and σαφης, 'clear.' *Dyspho'nia immodula'ta palati'na, Parapho'nia guttura'lis; P. palati'na.* Defective articulation, dependent upon diseased palate.— Hippocrates, Vogel.

ASARABACCA, Asarum — a. Broad-leaved, Asarum Canadense.

ASAR'CON, from *a*, privative, and σαρξ, 'flesh.' Devoid of flesh. Aristotle uses the term for the head when it is but little fleshy, compared with the chest and abdomen.

ASARET, Asarum — a. *du Canada,* Asarum Canadense.

ASARI'TES, from ασαρον, 'the asarum.' A diuretic wine, of which asarum was an ingredient. —Dioscorides.

AS'ARUM, from *a*, privative, and σαιρειν, 'to adorn:' because not admitted into the ancient coronal wreaths; *As'arum Europæ'um, A. officina'lë, Nardus Monta'na, Nardus Rust'ica, As'arum,* (F.) *Asaret ou Cabaret, Oreille d'homme, Oreillette, Girard-Roussin, Nard Sauvage. Fam.* Aroideæ. *Sex. Syst.* Dodecandria Monogynia. The plant, used in medicine, is the *As'arum Europæ'um, Asarabac'ca,* and of this the leaves. They are emetic, cathartic, and errhine, but are hardly ever employed, except for the last purpose.

ASARUM CANADEN'SE, *A. Carolinia'num, Canada Snakeroot, Wild Ginger, Colt's Foot, Broad-leaf Asarabacca, Indian Ginger, Heart Snakeroot,* (F.) *Asaret du Canada.* The root *As'arum,* (Ph. U. S.) is used as a substitute for ginger, and is said to act as a warm stimulant and diaphoretic.

ASARUM CAROLINIANUM, A. Canadense — a. Europæum, see Asarum — a. Hypocistis, Cytinus hypocistis — a. Officinale, see Asarum.

ASBESTOS SCALL, see Eczema of the hairy scalp.

ASCAIN, MINERAL WATERS OF. Ascain is a village, situate about a league from St. Jean-de-Luz, in France. The water is a cold chalybeate.

ASCARDAMYC'TES, from *a*, privative, and σκαρδαμυττω, 'I twinkle the eyes.' One who stares with fixed eyes, without moving the eyelids. — Hippocrates.

ASCARICIDA ANTHELMINTICA, Vernonia anthelmintica.

ASCARIDE LOMBRICOÏDE, Ascaris lumbricoides—a. *Vermiculaire,* Ascaris vermicularis.

AS'CARIS, pl. ASCAR'IDES, from ασκαριζω, 'I leap.' A genus of intestinal worms, characterized by a long, cylindrical body, extenuated at the extremities; and having a mouth furnished with three tubercles, from which a very short tube is sometimes seen issuing. Formerly, there were reckoned two varieties of the Ascaris—the *As'caris lumbricoï'des, Lumbri'cus, L. teres hom'inis, Scolex, As'caris gigas hom'inis,* (F.) *Lombricoïde, Ascaride lombricoïde, Lombric, L. Teres,* or long round worm; and the *As'caris Vermicula'ris* — the Ascaris proper — the *thread worm* or *maw worm.* The former is alone included under the genus, at present — a new genus having been formed of the *A. vermicularis,* under the name Oxyuris. It is the *Oxyu'ris vermicula'ris,* (F.) *Ascaride, A. vermiculaire, Oxyure vermiculaire.*

A new species of entozoa has been found by Dr. Bellingham, the *As'caris ala'ta.*

ASCARIS ALATA, see Ascaris — a. Gigas hominis, see Ascaris—a. Lumbricoides, see Ascaris —a. Trichuria, Trichocephalus—a. Vermicularis, see Ascaris.

AS'CELES, *As'keles, Carens cru'ribus,* from *a*, privative, and σκελος, 'a leg.' One who has no legs.

ASCELLA, Axilla.

ASCEN'DENS, from *ascendere,* (ad and *scandere,*) 'to ascend.' (F.) *Ascendant.* Parts are thus called, which are supposed to arise in a region lower than that where they terminate. Thus, *Aorta ascendens* is the aorta from its origin to the arch : *Vena cava ascendens,* the large vein which carries the blood from the inferior parts to the heart: *Obliquus ascendens (muscle,)* the lesser oblique muscle of the abdomen, &c.

ASCEN'SUS MORBI. The period of increase of a disease.

ASCESIS, Exercise.

ASCHIL, Scilla.

ASCHISTODAC'TYLUS, *Syndac'tylus:* from *a*, privative, σχιστος, 'cleft;' and δακτυλος, 'a finger.' A monster whose fingers are not separated from one another.—Gurlt.

AS'CIA, *Axinê,* 'an axe,' *Scepar'nos, Dol'abra, Fas'cia spira'lis.* Name of a bandage mentioned by Hippocrates and Galen, and figured by Scultetus, in the shape of an axe or hatchet.—Galen. See Doloire.

ASCILLA, Axilla.

ASCI'TES, from ασκος, 'a bottle:'— *Aski'tes, Hydroce'lē Peritonœ'i, Hydrops Abdom'inis, H. Ascites, Hydrogas'ter, Hydroperitone'um, Hydrocœ'lia, Hydre'trum, Ascli'tes, Œlioch'ysis, Dropsy of the lower belly, Dropsy of the Peritone'um,* (F.) *Ascite, Hydro-péritonie, Hydropisie du Bas-ventre.* A collection of serous fluid in the abdomen. Ascites proper is dropsy of the peritoneum; and is characterized by increased size of the abdomen, by fluctuation and the general signs of dropsy. It is rarely a primary disease; but is always dangerous, and but little susceptible of cure. Most generally, it is owing to obstructed circulation in some of the viscera, or to excitement of the vessels of the abdominal organs. The treatment is essentially the same as that of other dropsies. Paracentesis, when had recourse to, can only be regarded as a palliative.

Dropsy of the peritoneum may also be saccated or in cysts, and occasionally the fluid accumulates exterior to the peritoneum, *Hydrepigas'trium.* When in cysts it is termed *Hydrocys'tis, Hydrops abdom'inis sacca'tus, H. cys'ticus* and *Asci'tes sacca'tus.*

ASCITES HEPATO-CYSTICUS, Turgescentia vesiculæ felleæ—a. Ovarii, Hydrops ovarii—a. Purulentas, Pyocœlia—a. Saccatus, see Ascites, Hydroærion, and Hydrops ovarii.

ASCLEPI'ADÆ, *Asclepi'ades;* from Ασκληπιος, 'Æsculapius.' The *priest physicians*, who served in the ancient temples of Æsculapius, and who took their name from being his descendants.

ASCLÉPIADE, Asclepias vincetoxicum.

ASCLEPIAS ALBA, A. vincetoxicum—a. Apocynum, A. Syriaca.

ASCLE'PIAS ASTHMAT'ICA, *Cynan'chum Ipecacuan'ha,* (F.) *Ipecacuanha blanc de l'Ile de France.* A creeping plant of the Isle of France, regarded as a specific in asthma.

ASCLEPIAS CRISPA, Gomphocarpus crispus.

ASCLEPIAS CURASSAV'ICA, *Bastard Ipecacuanha, Redhead, Bloodweed.* The leaves are emetic in the dose of one or two scruples. It is the *Ipecacuanha blanc* of St. Domingo.

ASCLEPIAS DECUM'BENS; the root. Escharotic, cathartic, sudorific, diuretic.

ASCLEPIAS, FLESH-COLOURED, A. Incarnata.

ASCLEPIAS GIGANTE'A. The milky juice is very caustic. It is used in Malabar against herpes; and, mixed with oil, in gout. See Mudar.

ASCLE'PIAS INCARNA'TA, *Flesh-coloured asclepias.* The root of this plant, which grows in all parts of the United States, has the same virtues as A. Syriaca.

ASCLEPIAS OBOVATA, A. Syriaca.

ASCLEPIAS PROC"ERA (?) *Beidelossar; Beidelsar.* An Egyptian plant, the leaves of which are made into a plaster, and applied to indolent tumours. The milky juice is caustic, and is used as such.

ASCLEPIAS PSEUDOSARSA, Hemidesmus Indicus—a. Pubescens, A. Syriaca.

ASCLEPIAS SYRIACA, *A. pubes'cens, A. apoc"ynum, A. obova'tu seu tomento'sa, Common Silkweed, Milk Weed,* (F.) *Herbe à la houette.* The cortical part of the root has been given, in powder, in asthmatic and pulmonic affections in general, and, it is said, with success.

ASCLE'PIAS SULLIVAN'TII, *Smooth Milkweed, Silkweed:* indigenous, possesses the same virtues as the next.

ASCLEPIAS TOMENTOSA, A. Syriaca.

ASCLE'PIAS TUBERO'SA, *Butterfly Weed, Pleurisy Root, Flux Root, Wind Root, White Root, Orange Swallow Root, Silk Weed, Canada Root, Orange Apoc"ynum, Tuberous Rooted Swal'low Wort. Nat. Ord.* Asclepiadeæ. *Sex. Syst.* Pentandria Digynia. Said to have been first recommended by the Asclepiades. In Virginia and the Carolinas, the root of this plant has been long celebrated as a remedy in pneumonic affections. It is sudorific, and the powder acts as a mild purgative. Its chief powers are said to be expectorant, diaphoretic, and febrifuge. It is occasionally given to relieve pains of the stomach from flatulency and indigestion.

ASCLEPIAS VINCETOX'ICUM, *A. Alba, Cynan'chum Vincetox'icum, Vincetox'icum, V. Officina'lē, Hirundina'ria, Apoc"ynum Novæ An'gliæ hirsutum,* &c., *Swallow- Wort, White Swallow-Wort,* (F.) *Asclépiade, Dompte-venin.*

The root is said to be stimulant, diuretic, and emmenagogue, but is hardly ever used.

ASCLEPIASMUS, Hæmorrhois.

ASCLITES, Ascites.

ASCO'MA, from ασκος, 'a bottle.' The eminence of the pubes at the period of puberty in females.—Rufus of Ephesus.

ASE, Anxiety.

ASELLI, Onisci aselli.

ASELLUS, Oniscus.

ASE'MA CRISIS, κρισις ασημα, from α, privative, and σημα, 'a sign.' A crisis occurring unexpectedly and without the ordinary precursory signs.

ASEPTON, Asapes.

ASH, BITTER, Quassia—a. Blue, Fraxinus quadrangulata—a. Mountain, Sorbus acuparia—a. Prickly, Aralia spinosa, Xanthoxylum clava Herculis—a. Prickly, shrubby, Xanthoxylum fraxineum—a. Stinking, Ptelea trifoliata—a. Tree, Fraxinus excelsior—a. White, Fraxinus Americana.

ASIT"IA, from α, privative, and σιτος, 'food.' Abstinence from food. Want of appetite,—*Fastid'ium cibo'rum, Apoclei'sis.*

ASIUS LAPIS, Assius Lapis.

ASJAGAN, *As'jogam.* An Indian tree, the juice of whose leaves, mixed with powdered cumin seeds, is employed in India in colic.

ASJOGAM, Asjagan.

ASKELES, Asceles.

ASKITES, Ascites.

ASO'DES, *Asso'des,* from αση, 'disgust,' 'satiety.' A fever accompanied with anxiety and nausea; *Fe'bris aso'des* vel *azo'des.*

ASPALASO'MUS, from ασπαλαξ, 'a mole,' and σωμα, 'body.' A genus of monsters in which there is imperfect development of the eyes.—I. G. St. Hilaire. Also, a malformation, in which the fissure and eventration extend chiefly upon the lower part of the abdomen; the urinary apparatus, genitals and rectum opening externally by three distinct orifices.—Vogel.

ASPALTUM, Asphaltum.

ASPARAGINE, see Asparagus.

ASPAR'AGUS, *Aspar'agus officina'lis, Common Asparagus, Spar'agus, Sper'agus, Sparrow Grass, Grass. Nat. Ord.* Asphodeleæ. *Sex. Syst.* Hexandria Monogynia. *Aspar'agi officina'lis Tu'rio'nes,* (F.) *Asperge.* The fresh roots are diuretic, perhaps owing to the immediate crystallizable principle, Asparagine. The young shoots are a well known and esteemed vegetable diet. They communicate a peculiar odour to the urine. A syrup made of the young shoots and an extract of the roots has been recommended as a sedative in heart affections.

ASPA'SIA. A ball of wood soaked in an infusion of galls, and used by females for constringing the vagina.

ASPEN, AMERICAN, Populus tremuloides—a. European, Populus tremula.

ASPERA ARTERIA, Trachea.
ASPERGE, Asparagus.
ASPERITAS ARTERIÆ ASPERÆ, Raucedo.
ASPÉRITÉ DES PAUPIÈRES, Trachoma.
ASPER'ITY, *Asper'itas*, roughness. Asperities are inequalities on the surfaces of bones, which often serve for the insertion of fibrous organs.
ASPERMATIA, Aspermatismus.
ASPERMATIS'MUS, *Asper'mia, Asperma'tia*, from *a*, privative, and σπερμα, 'sperm.' Reflux of sperm from the urethra into the bladder, during the venereal orgasm.
ASPERMIA, Aspermatismus.
ASPERSIO, Catapasma, Fomentation.
ASPER'SION, *Asper'sio*, from *aspergere* (ad and *spargere*.) 'to sprinkle,' (F.) *Arrosement*. Act of sprinkling or pouring a liquid *guttatim* over a wound, ulcer, &c.
ASPERULA, Galium aparine.
ASPER'ULA ODORA'TA, *Ga'lium odora'tum, Matrisyl'va, Hepat'ica stella'ta*, (F.) *Aspérule odorante* ou *Muguet des bois, Hépatique étoilée*. Fam. Rubiaceæ. *Sex. Syst.* Tetrandria Monogynia. *Sweet-scented Wood-roof*. Said to be diuretic, deobstruent, tonic, and vulnerary.
ASPÉRULE ODORANTE, Asperula odorata.
ASPHALTI'TES, *Nephri'tes, Nephri'tis, Prima Vertebra lumba'ria*, same etymon as asphaltum. A name given by some to the last lumbar vertebra.—Gorræus.
ASPHAL'TUM, *Nep'ta, Arsal'tos, Asphal'tum*, from ασφαλιζειν, 'to strengthen.' With the Greeks, this word signified any kind of bitumen. It is now restricted chiefly to the BITU'MEN OF JUDÆ'A, *B. Juda'icum, A. sol'idum, Jews' Pitch, Karabē* of Sodom, (F.) *Asphalte*. It is solid, friable, vitreous, black, shining, inflammable, and of a fetid smell. An oil is obtained from it by distillation. It enters into the composition of certain ointments and plasters.
It is collected on the surface of the water of the Dead Sea or Lake Asphaltites, in Judæa.
ASPHARINE, Galium aparine.
ASPHOD'ELUS, *A. Ramo'sus, A. Albus, A. Maris, Has'tula Regis*, (F.) *Lis asphodèle*. The bulbs of this southern European plant have an acrimony which they lose in boiling water. They contain a fecula with which bread has been made, and have been considered diuretic. They have been used as a succedaneum for the squill.
ASPHYX'IA, from *a*, priv., and σφυξις, 'pulse,' *Defec'tus Pulsūs, Acrotis'mus, Sidera'tio, Sydera'tio*. For a long time, Asphyxia was confined to the sense of 'suspension of circulation or Syncope.' It now generally means *suspended animation*, produced by the nonconversion of the venous blood of the lungs into arterial *Apnœ'a, Apneus'tia, Apnœasphyx'ia, Anhæmato'sia, Ec'lysis pneumo-cardi'aca*. Owing to the supply of air being cut off, the unchanged venous blood of the pulmonary artery passes into the minute radicles of the pulmonary veins, but their peculiar excitability requiring arterial blood to excite them, stagnation takes place in the pulmonary radicle, and death occurs chiefly from this cause, — not owing to venous blood being distributed through the system, and 'poisoning' it, as was the idea of Bichat. *Onrus asphyx'ia, Mors appa'rens, Mors putati'va, Pseudothan'atos, Apparent death*, (F.) *Mort apparente*, is characterized by suspension of respiration, of the cerebral functions, &c. Several varieties of Asphyxia have been designated.

1. ASPHYX'IA OF THE NEW-BORN, *A. neonato'rum*. This is often dependent upon the feeble condition of the infant, not permitting respiration to be established.

2. ASPHY'IA BY NOXIOUS INHALA'TION or inhalation of gases, some of which cause death by producing a spasmodic closure of the glottis: others by the want of oxygen, and others are positively deleterious or poisonous.

3. ASPHYX'IA BY STRANGULA'TION or *Suffoca'tion*; produced by mechanical impediment to respiration, as in strangulation.

4. ASPHYX'IA BY SUBMER'SION, *A. by drowning, A. Immerso'rum*, as occurs in the drowned, who perish in consequence of the medium in which they are plunged, being unfit for respiration. See Submersion.

Mr. Chevalier has used the term *Asphyx'ia Idiopath'ica*, for fatal syncope owing to relaxation of the heart. See Suffocation.
ASPHYX'IA IMMERSORUM, A. by submersion—a. Local:—see Gangrene—a. Neonatorum, A. of the new-born—a. Pestilenta:—see Cholera—a. Pestilential:—see Cholera.

ASPHYX'IAL. Relating to asphyxia—as '*asphyxial* phenomena.'
ASPHYXIE DES PARTIES, Gangrene—a. *Lente des nouveau-nés*, Induration of the cellular tissue.
ASPHYX'IED, *Asphyxiated*, same etymon. In a state of asphyxia.
ASPIC, Aspis; also, Lavendula.
ASPIDISCOS, Sphincter ani externus.
ASPID'IUM ATHAMAN'TICUM. A South African fern, *Nat. Ord.* Filices, which is possessed of anthelmintic properties. Its caudex, in the form of powder, infusion, or electuary, has been found excellent in helminthiasis, and especially in tapeworm.
ASPIDIUM CORIACEUM, Calagualæ radix—a. Depastum, Polypodium filix mas—a. Discolor, see Calagualæ radix—a. Erosum, Polypodium filix mas—a. Filix fœmina, Asplenium filix fœmina—a. Ferrugineum, see Calagualæ radix—a. Filix mas, Polypodium filix mas.
ASPIRATIO, Inspiration.
ASPIRA'TION, *Adspira'tio, Aspira'tio*, from *aspirare* (ad and *spirare*) 'to breathe.' The French sometimes use the term synonymously with inspiration. It also means the act of attracting or sucking like a pump. Imbibition. Also, the pronunciation of a vowel with a full breath.
ASPIS, ασπις. A name given by the ancients to a venomous serpent—the *Ægyptian viper* of Lacépède, (F.) *Aspic*. Its bite is very dangerous, and it is supposed to have been the reptile which Cleopatra used for her destruction.
ASPLE'NIUM, from *a*, priv., and σπλην, 'the spleen.' *Spleenwort, Miltwaste*.
ASPLENIUM AUREUM, A. ceterach.
ASPLE'NIUM CET'ERACH, *A. au'reum seu latifo'lium, Gymnogram'mē ceterach, Doradil'la, Blechnum squamo'sum, Scolopen'dria, Athyr'ion, Cet'erach officina'rum seu canarien'sis, Grammi'tes cet'erach seu au'rea, Gynop'teris ceterach, Vitta'ria ceterach*, (F.) *Doradille*. Supposed to be subastringent and mucilaginous, and has been recommended as a pectoral. It has also been given in calculous cases.
ASPLE'NIUM FILIX FŒ'MINA, *Polypo'dium filix fœmina, P. mollē seu denta'tum seu inci'sum seu trif'idum, Aspidium filix fœmina, Athyr'ium filix fœmina seu mollē seu ova'tum seu trif'idum, Pteris palus'tris, Female fern, Spleenwort*, (F.) *Fougère femelle*. The root of this plant resembles that of the male fern, and is said to possess similar anthelmintic virtues. The name *female fern* is also given to *Pteris aquilina*.

ASPLENIUM LATIFOLIUM, A. ceterach — a. Murale, A. ruta — a. Obtusum, A. ruta muraria.
ASPLE'NIUM RUTA MURA'RIA, *A. mura'lē seu obtu'sum, Paronych'ia, Phylli'tis ruta mura'ria, Scolopen'drium ruta mura'ria, Wallrue, White Maidenhair, Tentwort, Adian'tum album, Ruta mura'ria, Sal'via Vitæ,* (F.) *Rue des murailles, Sauve-vie.* Used in the same cases as the last.
ASPLE'NIUM SCOLOPEN'DRIUM, *Scolopendrium officina'rum* seu *lingua* seu *phylli'tis* seu *vulga'rē, Scolopen'dra, Scolopen'dria, Hart's Tongue, Spleenwort, Phylli'tis, Lingua cervi'na Blechnum lignifo'lium,* (F.) *Scolopendre, Langue de cerf.* Properties like the last.
ASPLE'NIUM TRICHOMANOI'DES, *A. Trichom'anes, Phylli'tis rotundifo'lia, Calyphyl'lum, Trichom'anes, T. crena'ta, Adian'tum rubrum, Common Maidenhair, Polyt'richum commu'nē,* (F.) *Polytric.* Properties like the last.
ASPREDO, Trachoma — a. Miliacea, Miliary fever.
ASPRÊLE, Hippuris vulgaris.
ASSACOU, Hura Brasiliensis.
ASSA DOUX, Benjamin — a. Dulcis, Benjamin — a. Odorata, Benjamin.
ASSABA. A Guinea shrub, whose leaves are considered capable of dispersing buboes.
ASSAFETIDA, Asafœtida.
ASSAFŒTIDA, Asafœtida.
ASSAIERET. A compound of bitter, stomachic, and purgative medicines in the form of pill. — Avicenna.
ASSAISONNEMENT, Condiment.
ASSAKUR, Saccharum.
ASSALA, see Myristica moschata.
ASSARTHROSIS, Articulation.
ASSA'TIO, *Opte'sis* The boiling of food or medicines in their own juice, without the addition of any liquid. Various kinds of cooking by heat. — Galen.
ASSELLA, Axilla.
AS'SERAC, *Assis.* A preparation of opium or of some narcotic, used by the Turks as an excitant.
ASSERCULUM, Splint.
ASSERVATION, Conservation.
ASSES' MILK, see Milk, asses.
ASSES' MILK, ARTIFICIAL, see Milk, asses.
AS'SIDENS, from *ad,* 'to,' and *sedere,* 'to be seated.' That which accompanies or is concomitant. An epithet applied to the accessory symptoms, *Assiden'tia signa,* and general phenomena of disease.
ASSIDENTIA SIGNA, see Assidens.
ASSIMILA'TION, *Assimila'tio, Simila'tio, Appropria'tio, Exomoio'sis, Homoio'sis, Threpsis, Threp'ticē:* from *assimilare,* (*ad,* and *similare,*) 'to render similar.' The act by which living bodies appropriate and transform into their own substance matters with which they may be placed in contact.
ASSIS, Asserac.
AS'SIUS LAPIS, *A'sius Lapis.* A sort of stone or earth found near the town of Assa in the Troad, which had the property of destroying proud flesh.
ASSODES, Asodes.
ASSOUPISSEMENT, Somnolency.
ASSOURON, see Myrtus Pimenta.
ASSUETUDO, Habit.
ASSULA, Splint.
ASSULTUS, Attack.
ASSUMPTIO, Prehension.
ASTACI FLUVIATILIS CONCREMENTA, Cancrorum chelæ.
ASTACUS FLUVIATILIS, Crab.
ASTAKILLOS, Araneum ulcus.
ASTARZOF. An ointment, composed of li-

tharge, frog's spawn, &c. Also, camphor, dissolved in rose water. — Paracelsus.
ASTASIA, Dysphoria.
ASTER ATTICUS, Bubonium.
ASTER CORDIFOLIUS, *Heart-leaved Aster,* A. Puniceus, *Rough-stemmed Aster,* and other indigenous species, *Order* Compositæ, possess aromatic properties.
ASTER DYSENTERICUS, Inula dysenterica — a. Heart-leaved, A. cordifolius — a. Helenium, Inula Helenium — a. Inguinalis, Eryngium campestre — a. Officinalis, Inula helenium.
ASTER, ROUGH-STEMMED, A. Puniceus — a. Undulatus, Inula dysenterica.
ASTE'RIA GEMMA, *Aste'rius, Astroi'tes, As'trios, Astrob'olus.* The ancients attributed imaginary virtues to this stone, — that of dispersing *Nævi Materni,* for example.
ASTERIAS LUTEA, Gentiana lutea.
ASTEROCEPHALUS SUCCISA, Scabiosa succisa.
ASTHENES, Infirm.
ASTHENI'A, *Vis imminu'ta,* from *a,* priv., and σθενος, 'force,' 'strength.' Want of strength, debility. (F.) *Affaiblissement.* Infirmity. A word used in this sense by Galen, and employed, especially by Brown, to designate debility of the whole economy, or diminution of the vital forces. He distinguished it into *direct* and *indirect:* the former proceeding from diminution of stimuli; the latter from exhaustion of incitability by the abuse of stimuli.
ASTHENIA DEGLUTITIONIS, Pharyngoplegia — a. Pectoralis, Angina Pectoris.
ASTHENICOPYRA, Fever, adynamic.
ASTHENICOPYRETUS, Fever, adynamic.
ASTHENO'PIA, *Debil'itas visûs,* (F.) *Affaiblissement de la Vue,* from *a,* priv., σθενος, 'strength,' and ωψ, 'the eye.' Weakness of sight; *Weak-sightedness.*
ASTHENOPYRA, Fever, adynamic, Typhus.
ASTHENOPYRETUS, Fever, adynamic.
ASTHMA, from ασθμα, 'laborious breathing;' from αω, 'I respire.' *A. spas'ticum adulto'rum, A. Senio'rum, A. Convulsi'vum, A. spas'ticum intermit'tens, Dyspnœ'a et orthopnœ'a convulsi'va, Malum Cadu'cum pulmo'num, Broken-windedness, Nervous asthma,* (F.) *Asthme, A. nerveux.* Difficulty of breathing, recurring at intervals, accompanied with a wheezing sound and sense of constriction in the chest; cough and expectoration. Asthma is a chronic disease, and not curable with facility. Excitant and narcotic antispasmodics are required.
There are no pathognomonic physical signs of asthma. In some cases, the respiration is universally puerile during the attack. In the spasmodic form, the respiratory murmur is very feeble or absent during the fit; and in all forms percussion elicits a clear pulmonary sound. The disease generally consists in some source of irritation, and occasionally, perhaps, in paralysis of the pneumogastric nerves, *Bronchoparaly'sis, Paraly'sis nervi vagi in parte thorac''ica,* more frequently of the former — all the phenomena indicating constriction of the smaller bronchial ramifications. The treatment is one that relieves spasmodic action — narcotics, counter-irritants, change of air, &c.
ASTHMA ACU'TUM, of Millar, *A. spas'ticum infan'tum, Cynan'chē Trachea'lis spasmod'ica,* (F.) *Asthme aigu.* Probably, spasmodic croup. (?) See Asthma Thymicum.
ASTHMA AERIUM, Pneumothorax — a. Aërium ab Emphysemate Pulmonum, Emphysema of the Lungs — a. Arthriticum, Angina Pectoris.
ASTHMA, CARDIAC. Dyspnœa dependent upon disease of the heart.

ASTHMA CONVULSIVUM, Angina pectoris — a. Diaphragmaticum, Angina Pectoris — a. Doloriﬁcum, Angina pectoris — a. Emphysematicum, Pneumothorax.

ASTHMA, GRINDERS', *Grinders' Rot*. The aggregate of functional phenomena, induced by the inhalation of particles thrown off during the operation of grinding metallic instruments, &c. The structural changes induced are enlargement of the bronchial tubes, expansion of the pulmonary tissue, and phthisis.

ASTHMA GYPSEUM, A. pulverulentum — a. Hay, Fever, hay.

ASTHMA HU'MIDUM, *Humid, Common*, or *Spitting asthma*, is when the disease is accompanied with expectoration. It is also called *A. humora'lē, A. flatulen'tum, A. pneumon'icum, Blennotho'rax chron'icus*, &c.

ASTHMA INFANTUM, Cynanche trachealis — a. Infantum Spasmodicum, A. Thymicum — a. Koppian, A. Thymicum — a. Laryngeum Infantum, A. Thymicum — a. Montanum, A. pulverulentum — a. Nervous, Asthma — a. Nocturnum, Incubus.

ASTHMA PULVERULEN'TUM, *A. gyp'seum, A. monta'num*. The variety of asthma to which millers, bakers, grinders and others are subject.

ASTHMA SICCUM, so called when the paroxysm is sudden, violent, and of short duration; cough slight, and expectoration scanty; spasmodic constriction.

ASTHMA SPASTICO-ARTHRITICUM INCONSTANS, Angina pectoris — a. Spasticum Infantum, A. Thymicum.

ASTHMA THY'MICUM, *A. T. Kop'pii, A. spas'ticum infan'tum, A. infan'tum spasmo'dicum, Thymasth'ma, Cynan'chē trachea'lis spasmod'ica, Spasmus glot'tidis, Asthma larynge'um infan'tum, A. intermit'tens infan'tum, A. Dentien'tium, A. period'icum acu'tum, Koppian Asthma, Thymic Asthma, Laryngis'mus strid'ulus, Laryngo-spasmus, Apnœ'a infan'tum, Spasm of the larynx, Spasm of the glottis, Croup-like inspiration of infants, Child-crowing, Spasmodic croup, Pseudocroup, Spu'rious croup, Cer'ebral croup, Suf'focating nervous catarrh*, (F.) *Laryngite striduleuse, Faux Croup, Pseudo-croup nerveux, Spasme de la Glotte et du Thorax*. A disease of infants, characterized by suspension of respiration at intervals; great difficulty of breathing, especially on waking, swallowing, or crying; ending often in a fit of suffocation, with convulsions. The pathology of the disease has been supposed to consist in an enlargement of the thymus gland, or of the glands of the neck pressing on the pneumogastric nerves. (?) The ear, on auscultation, at a distance from the chest, detects an incomplete, acute, hissing inspiration, or rather cry; whilst the expiration and voice are croupal, both at the accession and termination of the paroxysm. The heart's action has been observed to be distinct and feeble.

These symptoms are often accompanied by rigidity of the fingers and toes; the thumb being frequently drawn forcibly into the palm of the clenched hand, whence the name *Carpo-pedal spasm*, applied, at times, to the disease.

ASTHMA TYPICUM. Asthma characterized by periodicity.

ASTHMA UTERI, Hysteria — a. Weed, Lobelia inflata.

ASTHMAT'IC, *Asthmat'icus, Pnoeolyt'icus*, Affected with asthma. Relating to asthma.

ASTHME AIGU, Asthma acutum — a. *Nerveux*, Asthma.

AS'TOMUS, from *a*, privative, and στομα, 'a mouth.' One without a mouth. Pliny speaks of a people in India without mouths, who live *anhelatu et odore!*

ASTRAGALE COL D', Collum astragali.

ASTRAGALOIDES SYPHILITICA, Astragalus exscapus.

ASTRAG'ALUS, *Talus*, the Ankle, *Qua'trio, Quar'tio, Quater'nio, Diab'ebos, Peza, Cavic'ula, Cavil'la, Tetro'ros, As'trion, Os Bullist'æ*, from αστραγαλος, 'a die,' which it has been considered to resemble. (?) A short bone situate at the superior and middle part of the tarsus, where it is articulated with the tibia. It is the *ankle bone, sling bone*, or *first bone of the foot*. The anterior surface is convex, and has a well-marked prominence, supported by a kind of neck, and hence has been called the *head of the astragalus*. The astragalus is developed by two points of ossification.

ASTRAG'ALUS EXS'CAPUS, *Astragaloï'des syphilit'ica, Stemless Milk-vetch*, (F.) *Astragale à gousses velus. Nat. Ord.* Leguminosæ. *Sex. Syst.* Diadelphia Decandria. The root is said to have cured confirmed syphilis.

ASTRAG'ALUS TRAGACANTHUS, see Tragacanth.

ASTRAG'ALUS VERUS, *Spina hirci, Astrag'alus aculea'tus, Goat's thorn, Milk-vetch*. The plant which affords *Gum Trag'acanth*. See Tragacantha.

ASTRANTIA, Imperatoria — a. Diapensia, Sanicula.

AS'TRAPE, *Corusca'tio, Fulgur, Fulmen, Lightning*. Galen reckons it amongst the remote causes of epilepsy.

ASTRIC'TION, *Astric'tio, Stypsis, Adstric'tio, Constric'tio*, from *astringere*, (ad and *stringere*,) 'to constringe.' Action of an astringent substance on the animal economy.

ASTRICTORIA, Astringents.

ASTRINGENT ROOT, Comptonia asplenifolia.

ASTRINGENTS, *Astringen'tia, Adstricto'ria, Adstringen'tia, Stryphna, Catastal'tica, Constringen'tia, Contrahen'tia, Stegno'tica, Syncrit'ica, Astricto'ria*. Same etymon. Medicines which have the property of constringing the organic textures. External astringents are called *Styptics*.

The following are the chief astringents: Acidum Sulphuricum, A. Tannicum, Alumen, Argenti Nitras, Catechu, Creasoton, Cupri Sulphas, Tinct. Ferri Chloridi, Liquor Ferri, Nitratis, Ferri Sulphas, Gallæ, Hæmatoxylon, Kino, Krameria, Liquor Calcis, Plumbi Acetas, Quercus Alba, Quercus Tinctoria, Zinci Sulphas,

ASTRION, Astragalus.

ASTRIOS, Asteria gemma.

ASTROBLES, from αστρον, 'a star,' and βαλλω, 'I strike.' One struck by the stars (*sidera'tus*.) One who is in a state of sideration — in an apoplectic state. — Gorræus.

ASTROBOLIS'MUS, *Heli'asis, Helio'sis; same etymology. Sidera'tion* or action of the stars on a person. Apoplexy. — Theophrastus, Gorræus.

ASTROBOLOS, Asteria gemma.

ASTROITIS, Asteria gemma.

ASTROL'OGY, *Astrolog''ia*, from αστρον, 'a star,' and λογος, 'a discourse.' The art of divining by inspecting the stars. This was formerly considered to be a part of medicine; and was called *Judicial Astrology*, to distinguish it from astronomy.

ASTRON'OMY, *Astronom'ia*, from αστρον, 'a star,' and νομος, 'a law,' 'rule.' A science which makes known the heavenly phenomena, and the laws that govern them. Hippocrates places this and astrology amongst the necessary studies of a physician.

ASTRUTHIUM, Imperatoria.

ASTYPHIA, Impotence.

ASTYSIA, Impotence.
ASUAR, Myrobalanus Indica.
ASULCI, Lapis lazuli.
ASYNODIA, Impotence.
ATACTOS, Erratic.
ATARACTAPOIE'SIA, *Ataractopœ'sia*, from *a*, privative, *ταρακτος*, 'troubled,' and *ποιειν*, 'to make.' Intrepidity, firmness; a quality of which, according to Hippocrates, the physician ought to be possessed in the highest degree.
ATARAX'IA, from *a*, privative, and *ταραξις*, 'trouble,' 'emotion.' Moral tranquillity, peace of mind.
AT'AVISM, from *atavus*, 'an old grandsire or ancestor, indefinitely.' The case in which an anomaly or disease, existing in a family, is lost in one generation and reappears in the following.
ATAX'IA, from *a*, privative, and *ταξις*, 'order.' Disorder, irregularity. Hippocrates employs the word in its most extensive acceptation. Galen applies it, especially, to irregularity of pulse; and Sydenham speaks of *Ataxia Spirituum* for disorder of the nervous system. Ataxia, now, usually means the state of disorder that characterizes nervous fevers, and the nervous condition.
ATAXIA SPIRITUUM, Nervous diathesis. See Ataxia.
ATAX'IC. *Atax'icus*; same etymon. Having the characters of ataxia.
ATCHAR, *A'chia, Achar*. A condiment used in India. It is formed of green fruits of various kinds, — garlic, ginger, mustard, and pimento, pickled in vinegar.
ATECNIA, Sterilitas.
ATELEC'TASIS, from *ατελης*, 'imperfect, defective,' and *εκτασις*, 'dilatation.' Imperfect expansion or dilatation; as in
ATELEC'TASIS PULMO'NUM, *Pneumonatelec'tasis, Pneumatelec'tasis*. Imperfect expansion of the lungs at birth, from *ατελης*, 'imperfect,' and *εκτασις*, 'dilatation.' Giving rise to *Cyano'sis pulmona'lis*.
AT'ELES, *ατελης*, 'imperfect, defective.'—Hence,
ATELOCHEI'LIA, from *ατελης*, 'imperfect,' and *χειλος*, 'lip.' A malformation which consists in an imperfect development of the lip.
ATELOËNCEPHAL'IA, from *ατελης*, 'imperfect,' and *εγκεφαλον*, 'the encephalon.' State of imperfect development of the brain.—Andral.
ATELOGLOS'SIA, from *ατελης*, 'imperfect,' and *γλωσσα*, 'tongue.' A malformation which consists in an imperfect development of the tongue.
ATELOGNA'THIA, from *ατελης*, 'imperfect,' and *γναθος*, 'the jaw.' A malformation which consists in an imperfect development of the jaw.
ATELOMYEL'IA, from *ατελης*, 'imperfect,' and *μυελος*, 'marrow.' State of imperfect development of the spinal marrow.—Béclard.
ATELOPROSO'PIA, from *ατελης*, 'imperfect,' and *προσωπον*, 'the face.' A malformation which consists in imperfect development of the face.
ATELORACHIDIA, Hydrorachis.
ATELOSTOM'IA, from *ατελης*, 'imperfect,' and *στομα*, 'mouth.' One whose mouth is imperfectly developed.
ATER SUCCUS, Atrabilis.
ATHAMAN'TA, from Athamas, a place in Thessaly. A genus of plants.
ATHAMANTA ANNUA, A. Cretensis.
ATHAMAN'TA AUREOSELI'NUM, *Oreoseli'num, O. legit'imum* seu *nigrum, Seli'num oreoseli'num, Peuced'anum oreoseli'num, Apium monta'num, Black Mountain Parsley*, (F.) *Persil de Montagne*. The plant, seed and roots, are aromatic. It has been considered attenuant, aperient, deob-

struent, and lithontriptic. The distilled oil has been used in toothach.
ATHAMAN'TA CRETEN'SIS seu CRETI'CA, *A. an'nua, Libano'tis annua* seu *Creten'sis* seu *hirsu'ta, Daucus Oreticus; D. Candia'nus, Myrrhis an'nua, Candy Carrot*. The seeds of this plant are acrid and aromatic. They have been used as carminatives and diuretics.
ATHAMANTA MACEDONICA, Bubon Macedonicum—a. Meum, Æthusa meum.
ATHANASIA, Tanacetum.
ATHANA'SIA, from *a*, privative, and *θανατος*, 'death.' An antidote for diseases of the liver, jaundice, gravel, &c. It consisted of saffron, cinnamon, lavender, cassia, myrrh, juncus odoratus, honey, &c., and was esteemed to be sudorific.
ATHARA, Athera.
ATHELAS'MUS, from *a*, privative, and *θηλη*, 'a breast or nipple.' Impracticability of giving suck; from want of nipple or otherwise.
ATHELXIS, Sucking.
ATHE'NA. Name of a plaster, recommended by Asclepiades, and composed of oxide of copper, sublimed oxide of zinc, sal ammoniac, verdigris, gall nuts, and a variety of resinous and other ingredients.—Oribasius, Aëtius, and P. Æginets.
ATHENIO'NIS CATAPO'TIUM. A pill, composed of myrrh, pepper, castor, and opium; used to allay coughing.—Celsus.
ATHE'RA, *Atha'ra*, from *αθηρ*, 'an ear of corn.' A kind of pap for children: also, a kind of liniment.—Dioscorides, Pliny.
ATHERAPEUTUS, Incurable.
ATHERO'MA, from *αθηρα*, 'pap or pulp,' *Emphy'ma encys'tis athero'ma, Mollus'cum, Pulta'tio*. A tumour formed by a cyst containing matter like pap or *Bouillie*.
ATHEROM'ATOUS, *Atheromato'des*. Having the nature of Atheroma.
ATHLE'TA, from *αθλος*, 'combat.' Athletæ were men who exercised themselves in combat at the public festivals.—Vitruvius.
ATHLET'IC, *Athlet'icus;* concerning *Athletæ*. Strong in muscular powers.—Foësius.
ATHORACOCEPHALUS. Acephalogaster.
ATHRIX, *At'richus;* from *a*, privative, and *θριξ, τριχος*, 'hair.' Bald. One who has lost his hair.
ATHRIX DEPILIS, Alopecia.
ATHYM'IA, *An'imi defec'tus et anxi'etas, An'imi demis'sio, Tristit''ia, Mæror, Lypē*, from *a*, priv., and *θυμος*, 'heart,' 'courage.' Despondency. The prostration of spirits often observable in the sick.—Hippocrates. Melancholy.—Swediaur. See Panophobia.
ATHYMIA PLEONECTICA, see Pleonectica.
ATHYRION, Asplenium ceterach.
ATHYRIUM FILIX FŒMINA, Asplenium filix fœmina—a. Filix mas, Polypodium filix mas —a. Molle, Asplenium filix fœmina—a. Ovatum, Asplenium filix fœmina—a. Trifidum, *Asplenium filix fœmina*.
ATLANTAD, see Atlantal.
ATLAN'TAL; same etymon as *Atlas*. Relating or appertaining to the atlas.
ATLANTAL ASPECT. An aspect towards the region where the atlas is situated.—Barclay. *Atlantad* is used by the same writer to signify 'towards the atlantal aspect.'
ATLANTAL EXTREMITIES. The upper limbs.
ATLANTION, Atlas.
ATLAS, *Atlan'tion*, from *ατλαω*, 'I sustain.' The *first cervical ver'tebra;* so called, from its supporting the whole weight of the head, as Atlas is said to have supported the globe on his shoulders. Chaussier calls it *Atloid*. This ver-

tebra in no respect resembles the others. It is a kind of irregular ring, into which, anteriorly, the *processus dentatus* of the second vertebra is received. Posteriorly, it gives passage to the medulla spinalis.

ATLOID'O-AXOID, (F.) *Atloïdo-axoïdien*. Relating to both the Atlas and the Axis or Vertebra Dentata.

ATLOIDO-AXOID ARTICULATION. The articulation between the first two cervical vertebræ.

ATLOIDO-AXOID LIG'AMENTS. These are two in number; one *anterior* and another *posterior*, passing between the two vertebræ.

ATLOID'O-OCCIP'ITAL. Relating to the atlas and occiput. The *Atloïdo-occip'ital Articula'tion* is formed by the condyles of the occipital bone and the superior articular surfaces of the Atlas. The *Atloïdo-occipital* muscle is the Rectus capitis posticus minor.

ATLOÏDO-SOUS-MASTOÏDIEN, Obliquus superior oculi—a. *Sous-occipitale*, Rectus capitis lateralis.

ATMIATRI'A, *Atmidiat'ricē*, from ατμος, 'vapour,' and ιατρεια, 'treatment.' Treatment of diseases by fumigation.

ATMIDIATRICE, Atmiatria.

ATMISTERION, Vaporarium.

ATMOS, Breath.

AT'MOSPHERE, *Atmosphæ'ra*, from ατμος, 'vapour,' and σφαιρα, 'a sphere:'—as it were, *Sphere of vapours*. The atmosphere is a spherical mass of air, surrounding the earth in every part; the height of which is estimated at 15 or 16 leagues. It presses on the surface of the earth, and this pressure has, necessarily, sensible effects on organized bodies. The surface of the human body being reckoned at 15 square feet, it is computed that a pressure of 33,000 pounds or more exists under ordinary circumstances; and this pressure cannot be increased or diminished materially, without modifying the circulation and all the functions.

ATMOSPHERIZATION, Hæmatosis.

ATOCIA, Sterilitis.

ATOL'MIA, from *a*, priv., and τολμα, 'confidence.' Want of confidence; discouragement. A state of mind, unfavourable to health, and injurious in disease. It is the antithesis of *Eutol'mia*.

ATONIA, Atony—a. Ventriculi, Gasterasthenia.

AT'ONY, *Aton'ia*, *Infir'mitas et Remis'sio vi'rium*, *Languor*, *Lax'itas*, from *a*, priv., and τονος, 'tone,' 'force.' Want of tone. Weakness of every organ, and particularly of those that are contractile. Violent gastritis has been described by Scribonius Largus under a similar name, *Aτονον*, *At'onon*.

ATRABIL'IARY, *Atrabil'ious*, *Atrabilia'ris*, *Atrabilio'sus*, from *ater*, 'black,' and *bilis*, 'bile.' An epithet given by the ancients to the melancholic and hypochondriac, because they believed the Atrabilis to predominate in such.

ATRABILIARY CAPSULES, ARTERIES and VEINS. The renal capsules, arteries and veins; the formation of Atrabilis having been attributed to them.

ATRABI'LIS, same etymon, *Ater succus*, *Black Bile* or *melancholy*. According to the ancients, a thick, black, acrid humour, secreted, in the opinion of some, by the pancreas; in that of others, by the supra-renal capsules. Hippocrates, Galen, Aëtius, and others, ascribe great influence to the Atrabilis in the production of hypochondriasis, melancholy, and mania. There is really no such humour. It was an imaginary creation.—Arretæus, Rufus of Ephesus, &c.

ATRACHELOCEPH'ALUS, from *a*, priv., τραχηλος, 'neck,' and κεφαλη, 'head.' A monster whose neck is partially or wholly deficient.

ATRACHE'LUS. Same etymon. One who is very short-necked.—Galen.

ATRAC'TYLIS GUMMIF'ERA, *Car'duus pi'neus*, *Ixinē*, *Gummy-rooted Atractylis*, *Pine Thistle*. The root, when wounded, yields a milky, viscid juice, which concretes into tenacious masses, and is said to be chewed with the same views as mastich.

ATRAGENE, Clematis vitalba.

ATRAMEN'TUM, *A. Suto'rium*, Ink, *Calcan'thon*, (F.) *Encre*. It has been advised as an astringent, and as an external application in herpetic affections.

ATRAMENTUM SUTORIUM, Ferri sulphas.

ATRESIA, Adherence, Imperforation. See Monster.

ATRE'SIA ANI ADNA'TA, *Anus Imperfora'tus*, *Imperfora'tio ani*, (F.) *Imperforation de l'anus*. Congenital imperforation of the intestinal canal.

ATRETISMUS, Imperforation.

ATRETOCEPH'ALUS, from ατρητος, 'imperforate,' and κεφαλη, 'head.' A monster, in which some of the natural apertures of the head are wanting.—Gurlt.

ATRETOCOR'MUS, from ατρητος, 'imperforate,' and κορμος, 'trunk.' A monster in which the natural apertures of the trunk are wanting.—Gurlt.

ATRE'TUS, from *a*, priv., and τραω, 'I perforate.' *Imperfora'tus*, *Imper'forate*. One whose anus, or parts of generation, are imperforate, (*aproc'tus*).

AT'RICES. Small tumours, which appear occasionally around the anus. Some commentators consider the word to be synonymous with condylomata.—Forestus.

ATRICHIA, Alopecia.

ATRICHUS, Athrix.

AT'RICI. Small sinuses in the vicinity of the anus, not penetrating the rectum.

ATRIPLEX FŒTIDA, Chenopodium vulvaria.

ATRIPLEX HORTEN'SIS, *A. Sati'va*, (F.) *Arroche*, *Bonne Dame*. The herb and seed of this plant have been exhibited as antiscorbutics.

At'riplex al'imus, *A. Portulacoï'des*, and *A. Pat'ula*, are used as pickles, and have similar properties.

AT'RIPLEX MEXICANA, Chenopodium ambrosioides—a. Odorata, Chenopodium botrys—a. Olida, Chenopodium vulvaria.

ATRIUM CORDIS DEXTER, Sinus dexter cordis—a. Cordis sinistrum, Sinus pulmonalis—a. Vaginæ, Vestibulum.

AT'ROPA, from Ατροπος, 'immutable,' 'the goddess of destiny;' so called from its fatal effects.

ATROPA BELLADON'NA, *Belladon'na*, *B. baccif'era seu trichot'oma*, *Deadly Nightshade*, *Sola'num letha'lē*, *Sola'num mani'acum*, *S. Furio'sum*, *Sola'num melanocer'asus*, (F.) *Belladone*, *Morelle furieuse*, *Belle Dame*. Nat. Ord. Solaneæ. Sex. Syst. Tetrandria Monogynia. The leaves—Belladonna (Ph. U. S.) are powerfully narcotic, and also diaphoretic, and diuretic. They are occasionally used where narcotics are indicated. Sprinkling the powdered leaves over cancerous sores has been found to allay the pain; and the leaves form a good poultice. Dose, gr. ½ to gr. j of the powdered leaves.

ATROPA MANDRAG'ORA, *Mandrag'ora*, *M. verna'lis seu officina'lis seu acau'lis*, *Circa'a*, *Anthropomorph'us*, *Malum terres'trē*, *Mandrake*. The boiled root has been used in the form of poultice in indolent swellings.

ATROPHIA, Atrophy, Tabes — a. Ablactatorum, Brash, weaning — a. Cerebri, Phrenatrophia — a. Cordis, Heart, atrophy of the — a. Glandularis, Tabes mesenterica — a. Hepatis, Hepatatrophia — a. Infantum, Pædatrophia, Tabes mesenterica — a. Intestinorum, Enteratrophia.

ATROPHIA LACTAN'TIUM, *Tabes nutri'cum seu lac'tea.* The atrophy of nursing women.

ATROPHIA LIENIS, Splenatrophia — a. Mesenterica, Tabes mesenterica — a. Testiculi, Orchidatrophia.

ATROPHIE, Atrophy — *a. Mésentérique,* Tabes mesenterica.

ATROPHIED, see Atrophy.

AT'ROPHY, *Maras'mus Atro'phia, Atro'phia Maras'mus, Ma'cies, Contabescen'tia, Tabes, Marco'res, Analo'sis,* from *a,* a privative, and τροφη, 'nourishment.' (F.) *Atrophie, Dessèchement.* Progressive and morbid diminution in the bulk of the whole body or of a part. Atrophy is generally symptomatic. Any tissue or organ thus affected is said to be *atrophied.*

ATROPHY OF THE HEART, see Heart, atrophy of the.

AT'ROPINE, *Atropi'na, Atro'pia, Atro'pium, Atropi'num,* (F.) *Atropine.* The active principle of *Atropa Belladonna,* separated by Brandes, by a process similar to that for procuring morphia.

ATTACHE, Insertion.

ATTACK, *Insul'tus, Assul'tus, Irrep'tio, Inva'sio, Eis'bolè, Lepsis,* (F.) *Attaque.* A sudden attack, invasion or onset of a disease. A seizure.

ATTAGAS, Attagen.

AT'TAGEN, *At'tagas,* the *Fran'colin.* Celebrated with the ancients both as food and medicine. — Martial, Aristophanes.

ATTANCOURT, MINERAL WATERS OF. A mineral water in France, at Attancourt, in Champagne; about three leagues north of Joinville. The water is a chalybeate, and contains sulphate of lime. In large doses it is purgative.

ATTAQUE, Attack — *a. des Nerfs,* Nervous attack.

ATTELLE, Splint.

ATTENÖTING, MINERAL WATERS OF, in Bavaria. The water contains carbonic acid, carbonates of lime and soda, sulphates of lime and magnesia, chloride of sodium, iron, and alum. It is much used in skin diseases, fistula, old ulcers, calculi, and hemorrhoids.

ATTEN'UANTS, *Attenuan'tia, Leptun'tica,* (F.) *Leptontiques,* from *tenuis,* 'thin.' Medicines which augment the fluidity of the humours.

ATTENUA'TION, *Attenua'tio;* same etymon. Thinness, emaciation. A term used by the homœopathists in the sense of dilution or division of remedies into infinitesimal doses.

ATTIRANT, Attrahent.

AT'TITUDE, *Situs Cor'poris.* Low Latin, *aptitudo;* from Latin *aptare,* 'to fit.' Situation, position of the body. The attitudes are the different postures which man is capable of assuming. In *General Pathology,* the attitude will often enable the physician to pronounce at once upon the character of a disease, or it will aid him materially in his judgment. In St. Vitus's dance, in fractures, luxations, &c., it is the great index. It will also indicate the degree of nervous or cerebral power; hence the sinking down in bed is an evidence of great cerebral debility in fever. The position of a patient during an operation is also an interesting subject of attention to the surgeon.

ATTOL'LENS AUREM, *Attol'lens Auric'ulæ, Leva'tor Auris, Supe'rior Auris, Attol'lens Auric'ulam, Auricula'ris supe'rior,* (F.) *Auriculaire supérieur, Temporo-auriculaire.* A muscle of the ear, which arises, thin, broad, and tendinous, from the tendon of the occipito-frontalis, and is inserted into the upper part of the ear, opposite to the anti-helix. It raises the ear.

ATTOLLENS OCULI, Rectus superior oculi — a. Oculum, Rectus superior oculi.

ATTOUCHEMENT, Masturbation.

ATTRACTION OF AGGREGATION, Cohesion, force of.

ATTRACTIVUM, see Magnet.

ATTRACTIVUS, Attrahent.

ATTRACTORIUS, Attrahent.

ATTRAHENS AURICULAM, Anterior auris.

AT'TRAHENT, *At'trahens, Attracti'vus, Attracto'rius,* from *ad,* 'to,' and *traho,* 'I draw.' (F.) *Attractif, Attirant.* Remedies are so called, which attract fluids to the parts to which they are applied, as blisters, rubefacients, &c.

ATTRAPE-LOURDAUT, (F.) A bistoury invented by a French surgeon, called Biennaise, and used in the operation for hernia. See Bistouri caché.

ATTRITA, Chafing.

ATTRITIO, Attrition, Chafing.

ATTRIT"ION, *Attrit"io, Ecthlim'ma,* from *ad,* and *terere,* 'to bruise.' Friction or bruising. Chafing. — Galen. Also, a kind of cardialgia. — Sennertus. Likewise, a violent contusion.

ATTRITUS, Chafing.

ATYP'IC, *Atyp'icus, At'ypos,* from *a,* privative, and *τυπος,* 'type.' That which has no type. Irregular. Chiefly applied to an irregular intermittent. — *Febris atypica.*

ATYPOS, Erratic.

AUANSIS, Drying.

AUAN'TÈ, *Anap'sè,* from αυανσις, 'desiccation.' Hippocrates gave this name to a disease, the principal symptom of which was emaciation. Atrophy.

AUBE-VIGNE, Clematis vitalba.

AUBÉPINE, Mespilus oxyacantha.

AUBERGINE, Solanum Melongena.

AUBIFOIN, Cyanus segetum.

AUCHEN, Collum.

AUCHENORRHEUMA, Torticollis.

AUCHE'TICUS, from αυχην, 'the neck.' One affected with stiff neck or torticollis.

AUDE, Voice.

AUDINAC, MINERAL WATERS OF. Audinac is situate in the department of Arriège, France. The water contains a small quantity of sulphohydric acid, carbonic acid, sulphates of lime and magnesia, carbonates of lime and iron, and a bituminous substance. Temp. 67° Fahr. It is much used in chronic rheumatism, herpes, scrofulous diseases, &c.

AUDIT"ION, from *audire,* 'to hear;' *Audit"io, Audi"tus, A'coè, Acro'ama, Acro'asis, Acoë'sis, Acu'sis.* Hearing. The act of hearing, The sensation arising from an impression made on the auditory nerves by the vibrations of the air, produced by a sonorous body. The physiology of Audition is obscure. It probably takes place: — 1. By the vibrations being communicated from the membrana tympani along the chain of small bones to the membrane of the foramen ovale. 2. By means of the air in the cavity of the tympanum, the membrane of the foramen rotundum is agitated. 3. The transmission may be made by means of the bony parietes. In these three ways the vibrations produced by a sonorous body may reach the auditory nerve. Audition may be *active* or *passive;* hence the difference between *listening* and simply *hearing*

AU'DITORY, *Audito'rius, Auditi'vus, Acus'ticus.* That which relates to audition.

AUDITORY ARTERIES AND VEINS, are vessels which enter the auditory canals, and are, like them, distinguished into *internal* and *external*. The *external auditory artery, A. Tympanique*—(Ch.) is given off by the styloid, a branch of the external carotid: the *internal* is a branch of the basilary artery, which accompanies the auditory nerve, and is distributed to it. The *Auditory Veins* empty into the internal and external jugulars.

AUDITORY CANAL, EXTERNAL, *Mea'tus audito'rius exter'nus, Alvea'rium, Scapha, Scaphus,* (F.) *Conduit auditif externe, Conduit auriculaire,* commences at the bottom of the concha, at the *Fora'men auditi'vum exter'num,* passes inwards, forwards, and a little downwards, and terminates at the membrana tympani. It is partly cartilaginous, partly osseous, and partly fibrous.

AUDITORY CANAL. INTERNAL, *Mea'tus audito'rius inter'nus, Porus* seu *Sinus acus'ticus, Cyar,* (F.) *Conduit auditif interne, C. labyrinthique,* is situate in the posterior surface of the pars petrosa of the temporal bone. From the *Fora'men auditi'vum inter'num,* where it commences, it passes forwards and outwards, and terminates by a kind of *cul-de-sac, mac'ula cribro'sa,* perforated by many holes, one of which is the orifice of the Aquæductus Fallopii; and the others communicate with the labyrinth.

AUDITORY NERVE, *Nerf labyrinthique*—(Ch.) is the *Portio Mollis* of the, seventh pair. It arises from the corpus restiforme, from the floor of the fourth ventricle, and by means of white striæ, from the sides of the calamus scriptorius. As it leaves the encephalon, it forms a flattened cord, and proceeds with the facial nerve through the foramen auditivum internum, and as far as the bottom of the meatus, where it separates from the facial, and divides into two branches, one going to the cochlea, the *cochlear;* the other to the vestibule and semi-circular canals, the *vestibular.*

AUGE, *Al'veus.* Some of the older anatomists gave this name to a reservoir, into which liquids flow in an interrupted manner, so that it is alternately full and empty. Such are the ventricles and auricles of the heart.

AUGMENTA'TION, from *augere,* 'to increase;' *Augmen'tum, Incremen'tum, Anab'asis, Auc'tio, Auxis, Progres'sio, Progres'sus, Auxe'sis.* The stage of a disease in which the symptoms go on increasing.

AULISCUS, Canula. See Fistula.

AULOS, Canula, Fistula. See Vagina, and Foramen.

AUMALE, MINERAL WATERS OF. Aumale is a town of Upper Normandy, in the country of Caux. Several springs of ferruginous mineral waters are found there, whose odour is penetrating, and taste rough and astringent. They are tonic, and employed in debility of the viscera, &c.

AUNE NOIRE, Rhamnus frangula.

AUNÉE, Inula helenium — *a. Dysentérique,* Inula dysenterica.

AURA, *Pnoë.* A vapour or emanation from any body, surrounding it like an atmosphere. Van Helmont regarded the vital principle as a gas and volatile spirit, which he called *Aura vitalis.*

In *Pathology,* Aura means the sensation of a light vapour, which, in some diseases, appears to set out from the trunk or limbs; and to rise towards the head. This feeling has been found to precede attacks of epilepsy and hysteria, and hence it has been called *Aura Epilep'tica,* and *A. hyste-'ica.*

AURA SAN'GUINIS. The odour exhaled by blood newly drawn. See Gaz Sanguinis.

AURA SEM'INIS, *A. semina'lis, Spir'itus geni-ta'lis:*—A volatile principle fancied to exist in the sperm, and regarded by some as the fecundating agent. Such is not the case.

AURA VITALIS, Vital principle.

AURAL MEDICINE AND SURGERY. Otiatria.

AURANCUM, see Ovum.

AURANITE, see Agaric.

AURAN'TIA CURASSAVEN'TIA, *Curasso'a apples or oranges.* Immature oranges, checked, by accident, in their growth. They are a grateful, aromatic bitter, devoid of acidity. Infused in wine or brandy they make a good stomachic. They are also used for *issue peas.*

AURANTIA CURASSAVICA, see Citrus aurantium — a. Poma, see Citrus aurantium.

AURANTII CORTEX, see Citrus aurantium.

AURANTIUM, Citrus aurantium.

AURELIANA CANADENSIS, Panax quinquefolium.

AUREOLA, Areola.

AURI CHLORETUM CUM CHLORETO NATRII, see Gold—a. Chloridum, Gold, murias of—a. Chloretum, Gold, muriate of—a. Cyanidum, see Gold—a. Cyanuretum, see Gold—a. Iodidum, see Gold — a. Ioduretum, see Gold — a. et Natri chloruretum, see Gold—a. Murias, Gold, muriate of—a. Nitro-murias, see Gold — a. Oxidum, see Gold—a. Terchloridum, see Gold—a. Tercyanidum, see Gold — a. Teroxidum, see Gold.

AURICHALCUM, Brass.

AURICLE, *Auric'ula,* (F.) *Auricule, Oricule.* Diminutive of *auris,* an ear. The auricle of the ear. See Pavilion.

AURICLES OF THE HEART, *Cavita'tes innomina'tæ,* (F.) *Oreillettes,* are two cavities; one right, the other left, each communicating with the ventricle of its side. These two cavities receive the blood from every part of the body. Into the *right* auricle, the two venæ cavæ and coronary vein open: into the *left,* the four pulmonary veins. Chaussier calls the former the *Sinus of the Venæ Cavæ:*—the latter, the *Sinus of the Pulmonary Veins.* The foliated or dog's ear portion of each auricle is called *Appen'dix auric'ulæ.* See Sinus.

AURICULA JUDÆ, Peziza auricula—a. Muris, Hieracium Pilosella—a. Muris major, Hieracium murorum.

AURICULAIRE, see Digitus—*a. Postérieur,* Retrahens auris—*a. Supérieur,* Attollens aurem.

AURIC'ULAR, *Auricula'ris, Oric'ular,* from *auricula,* 'the ear.' That which belongs to the ear, especially to the external ear.

AURIC'ULAR AR'TERIES AND VEINS, *Oriculaires*—(Ch.), are divided into *anterior* and *posterior.* The *anterior* are of indeterminate number. They arise from the temporal artery, and are distributed to the meatus auditorius externus, and to the pavilion of the ear. The *posterior* auricular is given off by the external carotid, from which it separates in the substance of the parotid gland. When it reaches the inferior part of the pavilion of the ear it bifurcates; one of its branches being distributed to the inner surface of the pavilion, the other passing over the mastoid process, and being distributed to the temporal and posterior auris muscles, &c. Before its bifurcation it gives off the *stylo-mastoid artery.* The *Anterior and Posterior Auricular Veins* open into the temporal and external jugular.

AURICULAR FINGER, (F.) *Doigt auriculaire,* is the little finger, so called because, owing to its size, it can be more readily introduced into the meatus auditorius.

AURICULAR NERVES are several. 1. The *auricular branch, Zygomato-auricular,* is one of the ascending branches of the cervical plexus.

It ramifies and spreads over the two surfaces of the pavilion. 2. The *auricular* or *superficial temporal*, *Temporal-cutaneous*—(Ch.) is given off from the inferior maxillary. It ascends between the condyle of the jaw and the meatus auditorius externus, sends numerous filaments to the meatus and pavilion, and divides into two twigs, which accompany the branches of the temporal artery, and are distributed to the integuments of the head. There is also a *posterior auricular* furnished by the facial.

AURICULARIA SAMBUCI, Peziza auricula.
AURICULARIS ANTERIOR, Anterior auris —a. Superior, Attollens aurem.
AURICULE, Auricle, Pavilion of the ear.
AURIC'ULO-VENTRIC'ULAR, *Auric'ulo-ventricula'ris*. That which belongs to the auricles and ventricles of the heart. The communications between the auricles and ventricles are so called. The *Tricuspid* and *Mitral Valves* are auriculo-ventricular valves.
AURI'GA. A species of bandage for the ribs, described by Galen. See, also, Liver.
AURIGO, Icterus—a. Neophytorum, Icterus Infantum.
AURIPIGMENTUM, Orpiment—a. Rubrum, Realgar.
AURIS, Ear.
AURISCALPIUM, Earpick.
AURISCOP'IUM, *Au'riscope*, from *auris*, 'the ear,' and σκοπεω, 'I view.' An instrument for exploring the ear.
AURIST, *Otia'ter*, *Otia'trus*, Ear-doctor, Ear-surgeon; from *auris*, 'the ear.' One who occupies himself chiefly with the diseases of the ear and their treatment.
AURIUM FLUCTUATIO, Bombus—a. Marmorata, Cerumen—a. Sibilus, Bombus—a. Sonitus, Bombus—a. Sordes, Cerumen—a. Susurrus, Bombus.
AURONE, Artemisia abrotanum—*a. des Champs*, Artemisia campestris—*a. des Jardins*, Artemisia abrotanum—*a. Mâle*, Artemisia abrotanum.
AURUGO, Icterus.
AURUM, Gold—a. Chloratum, Gold, muriate of—a. Chloratum natronatum, see Gold—a. Foliatum, Gold leaf—a. in Libellis, Gold leaf—a. Leprosum, Antimonium—a. Limatum, see Gold —a. Muriaticum, see Gold—a. Muriaticum natronatum, see Gold.
AURUM MUSI'VUM, *Aurum Mosa'icum*, *Sulph'uret of Tin*, *Deutosulphuret* or *Persulphuret of tin*. (*Quicksilver, tin, sulphur, sal ammoniac*, āā, equal parts. The tin being first melted, the quicksilver is poured into it, and then the whole are ground together, and sublimed in a boltheud. The aurum musivum lies at the bottom.) It is used in some empirical preparations.
AURUM OXYDATUM, see Gold—a. Oxydulatum muriaticum, Gold, muriate of—a. Nitro-muriaticum, see Gold—a. Salitum, Gold, muriate of.
AUS'CULTATE, TO; from *auscultare*, 'to listen.' To practise auscultation. 'To *auscult*' is at times used with the same signification.
AUSCULTA'TION, *Ausculta'tio*, *Echos'copê*, act of listening. Buisson has used it synonymously with *listening*. Laënnec introduced *auscultation* to appreciate the different sounds which can be heard in the chest, and in the diagnosis of diseases of the heart, lungs, &c. This may be done by the aid of an instrument called a *stethoscope*, one extremity of which is applied to the ear, the other to the chest of the patient. This mode of examination is called *Mediate Auscultation*, (F.) *Auscultation médiate*,—the application of the ear to the chest being *immediate auscultation*.

The act of exploring the chest is called *Stethoscop'ia*, and *Thoracoscop'ia*; of the abdomen, *Abdominoscop'ia*.
AUSCUL'TATORY, *Auscultato'rius*; *Auscul'tory*, *Auscul'tic*, (with some.) Belonging or having relation to auscultation.
AUSCULTATORY PERCUSSION, see Acouophonia.
AUSTERE', *Auste'rus*. Substances which produce a high degree of acerb impression on the organs of taste.
AUSTRUCHE, Imperatoria.
AUTALGIA DOLOROSA, Neuralgia, facial, Pleurodynia—a. Pruriginosa, Itching—a. Vertigo, Vertigo.
AUTARCI'A, from αυτος, 'himself,' and αρκεω, 'I am satisfied.' Moral tranquillity.—Galen.
AUTEMES'IA, from αυτος, 'self,' and εμεσις, 'vomiting.' Spontaneous or idiopathic vomiting. —Alibert.
AUTEMPRESMUS, Combustion, human.
AUTHE'MERON. A medicine which cures on the day of its exhibition; from αυτος, 'the same,' and 'ημερα,' 'day.'
AUTHYGIANSIS, Vis medicatrix naturæ.
AUTOCHIR, *Autochi'rus*, *Suici'da*, from αυτος, 'himself,' and χειρ, 'hand.' One who has committed suicide. A self-murderer or suicide.
AUTOCHIRIA, Suicide.
AUTOCINE'SIS, *Motus volunta'rius*, from αυτος, 'self,' and κινησις, 'motion.' Voluntary motion.
AUTOC'RASY, *Autocrati'a*, *Autocrato'ria*, from αυτος, 'himself,' and κρατος, 'strength.' Independent force. Action of the vital principle, or of the instinctive powers towards the preservation of the individual. See Vis Medicatrix Naturæ. Also, the vital principle.
AUTOCRATIA, Autocrasy, Vis Medicatrix naturæ.
AUTOCRATORIA, Autocrasy—a. Physiatrice, Vis medicatrix naturæ.
AUTOCTONIA, Suicide.
AUTOG"ENOUS; from αυτος, 'self,' and γινναω, 'I generate.' A term applied by Mr. Owen to parts or elements that are usually developed from distinct and independent centres; as in the case of the different parts or elements that form a vertebra.
AUTOGONIA, Generation, equivocal.
AUTOLITHOT'OMUS, from αυτος, 'himself,' λιθος, 'a stone,' and τεμνειν, 'to cut.' One who operates upon himself for the stone.
AUTOMAT'IC, *Automat'icus*, *Autom'atus*, from αυτοματος, 'spontaneous.' That which acts of itself. Those movements are called *automatic*, which the patient executes without any object; apparently without volition being exercised:—involuntary motions, *motus automat'ici seu autom'ati seu involunta'rii*.
AUTOMNAL, Autumnal.
AUTONOM'IA, *Vis medicatrix naturæ*. The word *Autonomia* is occasionally employed by the French and Germans for the peculiar mechanism of an organized body. Thus, although individuals of the same species may differ in outward conformation, their mechanism or instinctive laws, (*Autonomia*,) may be the same.
AUTONYCTOBATIA, Somnambulism.
AUTOPEP'SIA, from αυτος, 'self,' and πεπτω, 'I concoct.' Self-digestion,—as of the stomach after death.
AUTOPHIA, Autopsia.
AUTOPHO'NIA, (F.) *Retentissement autophonique*, from αυτος, 'self,' and φωνη, 'voice.' An auscultatory sign pointed out by M. Hourmann, which consists in noting the character of the observer's own voice, while he speaks with his head placed close to the patient's chest. The voice, is

is alleged, will be modified by the condition of the subjacent organs. The resonance, thus heard, he terms *retentissement autophonique*. This diagnostic agency Dr. R. G. Latham proposes to term *heautophon'ice*.

AUTOPHONIA, Suicide.

AUTOPHOSPHORUS, Phosphorus.

AUTOPLAS'TIC, *Autoplas'ticus;* from αυτος, 'self,' and πλαστικος, 'formative.' Relating to autoplasty or plastic surgery.

AUTOPLASTICE, Morioplastice.

AUTOPLASTY, Morioplastice.

AUTOP'SIA, *Au'topsy;* from αυτος, 'himself,' and οψις, 'vision.' *Autoph'ia, Autoscop'ia.* Inspection; examination by one's self; self-inspection. Often improperly used for the following:

AUTOP'SIA CADAVER'ICA, (F.) *Autopsie ou Ouverture cadavérique.* Attentive examination after death,—*Examination post mortem, Sectio Cadaveris, Dissection, Nec'roscopy, Nec'ropsy, Necroscop'ia, Necrop'sia, Necrop'sis,*—practised for the purpose of investigating the causes and seat of an affection of which a person may have died, &c.

AUTOP'SIA CADAVER'ICA LEGA'LIS, *Sec'tio cadav'eris legalis, Obduc'tio,* is the examination after death for medico-legal purposes.

AUTOPYROS, Syncomistos.

AUTOSCOPIA, Autopsia.

AU'TOSITE, from αυτος, 'self,' and σιτος, 'nourishment.' A single monster, capable of deriving nourishment from its own proper organs, in contradistinction to *Omphalosite.*

AUTOTHERAPIA, Vis medicatrix naturæ.

AUTUMN, *Autum'nus, Phthiropo'ron,* (F.) *Automne.* One of the seasons of the year, between the 28d of September and the 21st of December. In all climates, the Autumn or Fall is liable to disease; a combination of local and atmospheric causes being then present, favourable to its production.

AUTUM'NAL; *Autumna'lis,* (F.) *Automnal.* Relating to Autumn; as *Autumnal Fruits, Autumnal Fevers,* &c.

AUTUMNAL FEVER, generally assumes a bilious aspect. Those of the intermittent kind are much more obstinate than when they appear in the spring.

AUXESIS, Augmentation, Increase.

AUXIL'IARY, *Auxilia'ris,* from *auxilium,* 'aid.' (F.) *Auxiliaire.* That which assists, or from which assistance is obtained.

AUXILIARY MEDICINE is one which assists the principal medicine or basis. It is synonymous with Adjuvant.

AUXILIARY MUSCLES are those which concur in the same movement. Some anatomists have applied the term to several ligaments, as well as to the fleshy fibres, which hang from the *sacrospinalis* muscle.

AUXILIUM, Juvans, Medicament.

AUXIS, Augmentation, Increase.

AVA, *Arva, Kava.* An intoxicating narcotic drink, made by chewing the Piper methisticum. It is much used by the Polynesians.

AVAILLES, WATERS OF. A small village in France, 13 leagues S. S. E. of Poitiers, at which there is a cold saline chalybeate. It contains chlorides of sodium and calcium, sulphate and subcarbonate of soda, iron, &c.

AVANT-BOUCHE, (F.) *Os anti'cum.* This name has been applied by some to the *mouth,* properly so called—in contradistinction to the *Arrière bouche* or *Pharynx.*

AVANT-BRAS, Fore-arm.

AVANT-CŒUR, Scrobiculus cordis.

AVANT-GOUT, (F.) *Prægusta'tio;* a foretaste; prægustation.

AVANT-MAIN, (F.) *Adver'sa Manus.* The inside of the hand, when extended.

AVANT-PIED, (F.) The most advanced part of the foot.

AVANT-POIGNET, (F.) The anterior part of the wrist.

AVELINE, Corylus avellana (nut).

AVELLANA, Corylus avellana—a. Cathartica, Jatropha curcas.

AVE'NA, *Oats, Bromos.* The seeds of *Ave'na sati'va. Nat. Ord.* Gramineæ. *Sex. Syst.* Triandria Digynia. (F.) *Avoine.* Oats are used as food for man, in some parts, particularly in the North of England and Scotland. When deprived of the husks they form *Groats.* Reduced to meal, —*Arenæ Fari'na, Oatmeal*— they are applied as cataplasms to promote suppuration. The dry meal is sprinkled over erysipelatous parts.

Oatmeal gruel, Water gruel, is prepared as follows:— Take of oatmeal ℥ij; *soft water* Oiss. Rub the meal in a basin, with the back of a spoon, in a moderate quantity of the water, pouring off the fluid after the grosser particles have subsided, but whilst the milkiness continues; and repeat the operation until no more milkiness is communicated to the water. Put the washings in a pan, after having stirred them well, in order to suspend any fecula, which may have subsided; and boil until a soft, thick, mucilage is formed.

It is a good demulcent, and is used also as a vehicle for clysters.

AVENA EXCORTICATA, Groats.

AVENÆ FARINA, see Avena.

AVENHEIM, MINERAL WATERS OF. Avenheim is three leagues from Strasburg: near it is an aperient mineral water.

AVENNES, MINERAL WATERS OF. Avennes is a village in the department of Hérault in France: near it is a saline spring, the temperature of which rises to 84° Fahrenheit.

AVENS, COMMON, Geum urbanum — a. Water, Geum rivale — a. White, Geum Virginianum.

AVERICH, Sulphur.

AVERRHO'A BILIM'BI, *Bilim'bi, Bilimbing teres.* An Indian tree, which has a fruit that is too acid to be eaten alone. It is used as a condiment, and in the form of syrup as a refrigerant.

AVERRHO'A CARAM'BOLA, called after Averrhoës; *Malum Coën'sē, Prunum stella'tum, Tam'ara, Conga, Caram'bolo.* An Indian tree, whose fruits are agreeably acid. The bark, bruised, is employed as a cataplasm, and its fruit is used as a refrigerant in bilious fever and dysentery.

AVER'SION, *Aver'sio, Apot'ropē;* from *avertere,* (a and *vertere*) 'to turn from.' Extreme repugnance for any thing whatever.

AVERSION, (F.) also means, in therapeutics, the action of medicines which turn the afflux of fluids from one organ, and direct them to others; being synonymous with *counter-irritation,* or rather *revulsion* or *derivation.*

AVERTIN, (F.) A disease of the mind, which, according to Lavoisien, renders the patient obstinate and furious.

AVEUGLE, Cæcus.

AVEUGLEMENT, Cæcitas — a. *de Jour,* Nyctalopia—a. *de Nuit,* Hemeralopia.

AVICEN'NIA TOMENTO'SA, *A. Africa'na seu resinif'era seu nit'ida, Bon'tia ger'minans,* called after Avicenna. The plant which affords the *Malac'ca Bean* or *Anacar'dium Orienta'lē* of the Pharmacopœias, *Semecar'pus Anacar'dium.* The oil drawn from the bark of the fruit is a corrosive, and active vesicatory, but it is not used.

AVICULA CIPRIA, Pastil—a. Margaritifera, see Pearl.

AVOIN, Avena.
AVORTEMENT, Abortion.
AVORTER, to Abort.
AVORTIN, Abortion.
AVORTON, Abortion.
AVULSIO, Arrachement.
AVULSION, Evulsion.
AX, MINERAL WATERS OF. Ax is a small town in the department of Arriège, France; where there are several sulphurous springs, the temperature of which varies from 77° to 162° of Fahrenheit.
AXE, Axis—*a. de l'Œil*, Axis of the eye.
AX'EA COMMISSU'RA, *Trochoï'des*. A pivot-joint. See Trochoid.
AXIL'LA, *Ala, Ascel'la, Assel'la, Ascil'la, Acel'la, Cordis emuncto'rium, Malē, Hypo'mia, Fo'vea axilla'ris, Mas'chalē, Mas'chalis*, (F.) *Aisselle*. The cavity beneath the junction of the arm with the shoulder; the *armpit;* (F.) *Creux de l'Aisselle*. It is bounded, anteriorly, by a portion of the pectoralis major; posteriorly, by the latissimus dorsi. It is covered with hair, contains much areolar membrane, lymphatic ganglions, important vessels and nerves, and numerous sebaceous follicles, furnishing an odorous secretion. In consequence of such secretion, the ancients called it *emuncto'rium cordis*.
AX'ILLARY, *Maschaliæ'us*, (F.) *Axillaire*, from *axilla*, 'the armpit.' Belonging to the armpit.
AXILLARY ARTERY, *Arte'ria axilla'ris;* a continuation of the subclavian, extending from the passage of the latter between the scaleni muscles as far as the insertion of the pectoralis major, when it takes the name of *Brachial*.
AXILLARY GLANDS are lymphatic glands seated in the armpit; into which the lymphatic glands of the upper extremity open.
AXILLARY NERVE, *Scap'ulo-hu'meral* (CH.), *Nerf circonflexe. Artic'ular nerve;* arises from the posterior part of the brachial plexus, particularly from the last two cervical pairs and the first dorsal. It is chiefly distributed to the posterior margin of the deltoid.
AXILLARY VEIN, *Vena Axilla'ris, Vena Subala'ris*. This vein corresponds with the artery; anterior to which it is situate. It is a continuation of the *brachial veins;* and, at its termination, assumes the name *Subclavian*.
AXINE, Ascia.
AXIRNACII. An Arabic word, used by Albucasis to designate a fatty tumour of the upper eyelid, observed particularly in children.
AXIS, *Axon*, (F.) *Axe*. A right line which passes through the centre of a body.
AXIS, CEREBRO-SPINAL, see Encephalon—a. of the Cochlea, Modiolus—a. Cylinder of Nerve, see Nerve fibre—a. Cœliac, Cœliac artery.
AXIS OF THE EYE, (F.) *Axe de l'œil*, called also, *Vis'ual Axis* and *Optic Axis*, is a right line, which falls perpendicularly on the eye, and passes through the centre of the pupil.
AXIS, HÆMAL, Aorta—a. Neural, see Encephalon.
AXIS, is also the second vertebra of the neck, *Axon, Epistroph'eus, Epis'trophus, Maschalister:* the *Ver'tebra Denta'ta*, (F.) *Essieu*. So called, because it forms a kind of axis on which the head moves. Chaussier calls it *Axoïde*, from αξων, 'axis,' and ειδος, 'shape.'
AXOIDE, Axis—*a. Occipitale*, Rectus capitis posticus major.
AXOID'O-ATLOID'EUS. What refers to both the axis and atlas, as *Axoido-atloidean* articulation.
The lesions of the Axoido-atloidean, are, 1. Fracture of the *Proces'sus Denta'tus*. 2. Rupture of the odontoid ligament, and consequently passage and pressure of the process behind the transverse ligament: and, 3. The simultaneous rupture of the odontoid and transverse ligaments. These different accidents are fatal.
AXOIDO-ATLOIDIEN, Oblicuus inferior capitis.
AXON, Axis.
AXUNGE, Adeps præparata.
AXUNGIA, Pinguedo—a. Gadi, Oleum Jecoris Aselli—a. de Mumiâ, Marrow—a. Articularis, Synovia—a. Piscina Marina, Oleum Jecoris Aselli —a. Porcina, Adeps præparata.
AYPNIA, Insomnia.
AZARNET, Orpiment.
AZARUM, Asarum.
AZEDARACH, Melia Azedarach.
AZEDARACHA AMŒNA, Melia Azedarach.
AZOODYNA'MIA, from *a*, priv., ζωη, 'life,' and δυναμις, 'strength.' Privation or diminution of the vital powers.
AZO'RES, CLIMATE OF. The Azores or Western Islands are said to afford one of the best examples of a mild, humid, equable climate to be met with in the northern hemisphere. It is slightly colder and moister than that of Madeira, but even more equable. Sir James Clark thinks, that a change from the Azores to Madeira, and thence to Teneriffe—one of the Canaries—would prove more beneficial to the phthisical valetudinarian than a residence during the whole winter in any one of those islands.
AZOTATE D'ARGENT, Argenti nitras.
A'ZOTE, *Azo'tum*, from *a*, priv., and ζωη, 'life.' *Ni'trogen, Al'caligene, Gas azo'ticum, Nitrogen'ium*, (F.) *Azote, Nitrogène, Air gaté, Air vicié*, is a gas which is unfit for respiration. It is not positively deleterious, but proves fatal, owing to the want of oxygen. It is one of the constituents of atmospheric air, and a distinguishing principle of animals. Vegetables have it not generally diffused, whilst it is met with in most animal substances. It has been variously called, *phlogistic air, vitiated air, &c.;* has been looked upon as sedative, and recommended to be respired, when properly diluted, in diseases of the chest.
AZOTE, PROTOXIDE OF, Nitrogen, gaseous oxide of.
AZOTED, Nitrogenized.
AZOTENÈSES, from *azote*, and νοσος, 'disease.' Diseases fancied to be occasioned by the predominance of azote in the body.—Baumes.
AZOTIZED, Nitrogenized.
AZOTURIA, see Urine.
AZUR, Coral, Small.
AZU'RIUM. A compound of two parts of mercury, one-third of sulphur, and one-fourth of sal ammoniac.—Albertus Magnus.
AZ'YGES, *Az'ygos, Az'ygous, sine pari*, from *a*, priv., and ζυγος, 'equal.' Unequal. The *sphenoid bone*, because it has no fellow. Also, a process, *Proces'sus Az'yges, Rostrum sphenoïda'lē*, projecting from under the middle, and forepart of this bone.
AZYGOS GANGLION, see Trisplanchnic Nerve.
AZYGOUS ARTICULAR ARTERY, see Articular arteries of the skull.
AZYGOUS MUSCLE, *Azygos U'vulæ*, is the small muscle which occupies the substance of the uvula. —Morgagni. The name is, however, inappropriate, as there are two distinct fasciculi, placed along-side each other, forming the *Pal'ato-staphyli'ni, Staphyli'ni* or *Epistaphyli'ni* muscles, *Staphyli'ni me'dii* of Winslow.
AZYGOUS VEIN, *Vena Azygos, Veine Prélombo-*

thoracique—(Ch.), *Vena sine pari, Vena pari carens*, (F.) *Veine sans Paire.* This vein was so called by Galen. It forms a communication between the *V. cava inferior* and *V. cava superior*, permitting the blood to pass freely between the two. It rises from the vena cava inferior, or from one of the lumbar or renal veins, passes through the diaphragm, ascends along the spine to the right of the aorta and thoracic duct, and opens into the V. cava superior, where it penetrates the pericardium. On the left side, the SEMI-AZ'YGOS, *Left bron'chial* or *left superior intercos'tal vein, Vena demi-azygos, V. hemi-az'yga, Veine petite prélombo-thoracique*—(Ch.) presents, in miniature, nearly the same arrangement.

AZYMIA HUMORUM, Crudity of the humours.

AZ'YMUS, from *a*, priv., and ζυμη, 'leaven.' Asymous bread is unfermented, unleavened bread.—Galen.

B.

BABEURRE, Buttermilk.
BABILLEMENT, Loquacity.
BABUZICARIUS, Incubus.
BAC'ARIS, *Back'aris.* A name given by the ancients to an ointment, described by Galen under the name *Ointment of Lydia*. It was sometimes employed in diseases of the womb.—Hippocrates.

BACCÆ BERMUDENSES, Sapindus saponaria—b. seu Grana actes, see Sambucus ebulus—b. Jujubæ, Jujube—b. Myrtillorum, see Vaccinium myrtillus—b. Norlandicæ, Rubus arcticus—b. Piperis Glabri, see Piper Cubeba—b. Piscatoriæ, see Menispermum cocculus—b. Zizyphi, see Jujube.

BACCAR, *Bac'caris, Bac'charis*. An herb used by the ancients in their garlands, to destroy enchantment. Perhaps, the *Digitalis purpurea*. Some authors have erroneously thought it to be the *Asarum*.

BACCHARIS, Baccar.
BACCHI'A, from *Bacchus*, 'wine.' A name applied to the red or pimpled face of the drunkard. See Gutta rosea.

BACCHICA, Hedera helix.
BACHARIS, Bacaris.
BACHELOR'S BUTTONS, see Strychnos nux vomica.
BACHER'S TONIC PILLS, Pilulæ ex Helleboro et Myrrhâ.
BACILE, Crithmum maritimum.
BACIL'LUM, *Bacillus, Bac'ulus, Bac'culus:* 'a stick.' This name has been applied to a kind of troch, composed of expectorants, and having the shape of a stick. Also, a suppository. *Bacillum* was used by the ancient chemists for several instruments of iron.

BACK-ACH ROOT, Liatris.
BACKSTROKE OF THE HEART, Impulse, diastolic.
BACOVE, Musa sapientum.
BACTYRILOBIUM FISTULA, Cassia fistula.
BACULUS, Bacillum.
BADEN, MINERAL WATERS OF. Baden is a town six miles from Vienna. Here are 12 springs, containing carbonates of lime and magnesia; sulphates of lime, and magnesia, and soda; and chlorides of sodium and aluminum. The water is used in diseases of the skin, rheumatism, &c. There are two other towns of the same name; one in Suabia, and the other in Switzerland, about 12 miles from Zürich, where are mineral springs. The waters of the last two are thermal sulphureous.

BADEN-BADEN, MINERAL WATERS OF. Celebrated thermal springs, situate about a league from the high road to Basle and Frankfort. Their temperature varies from 130° to 154° Fahrenheit.

BADER, Bather.
BADIAGA. A kind of sponge, sold in Russia, the powder of which is said to take away the livid marks from blows and bruises in a few hours. Its nature is not understood.

BADIANE, Illicium anisatum.
BADISIS, Walking.
BADUKKA, Capparis badukka.
BAG, DUSTING, see Dusting-bag.
BAGEDIA, Pound.
BAGNÈRES-ADOUR, MINERAL WATERS OF. Bagnères-Adour is a small town in the department of *Hautes Pyrénées*, having a great number of mineral springs; some, cold chalybeates; others, thermal salines; but the greatest part sulphureous and warm.

BAGNÈRES DU LUCHON is a small town in the department of *Haute Garonne*, on the frontiers of Spain. It has been for a long time famous for its numerous sulphureous springs, the temperature of which is from 69° to 148° of Fahrenheit.

BAGNIGGE WELLS. A saline mineral spring in London, resembling the Epsom.
BAGNIO, Baignoire.
BAGNOLES, MINERAL WATERS OF. Bagnoles is a village in the department of Orne. The water resembles that of *Bagnères de Luchon*.

BAGNOLS, MINERAL WATERS OF. Bagnols is a village, two leagues from Mende, in the department of Lozère. The waters are hydrosulphurous and thermal: 109° Fahrenheit.

BAGOAS, Castratus.
BAGUENAUDIER, Colutea arborescens.
BAHA'MA ISLANDS, CLIMATE OF. The climate of the Bahamas is not considered to be well adapted for consumptive patients, on account of the rapid alternations of temperature, and the prevalence of winds, often of a dry, cold character. Still, the phthisical valetudinarians from most portions of the United States might derive advantage from a residence there during the winter months. The accommodations are not, however, good, or numerous.

BAHEL, *Colum'nea longifo'lia*. A labiated plant of Malabar, whose leaves, bruised, are applied as cataplasms to suppurating tumours.

BAHEL SCHULLI, Genista spinosa Indica.
BAIGNEUR, Bather.
BAIGNOIRE (F.), *Baptiste'rium*, a *Bathing tub, Bagnio, So'lium, Pisci'na*. The vessel or place in which bathing is performed. *Baignoire oculaire*, an *eye-bath*,—a small vessel for bathing the eyes.

BAILLEMENT, Yawning.
BAILLON, Speculum oris.
BAIN, Bath—b. *Chaud*, Bath, hot—b. *Électrique*, Bath, electric, see Electricity—b. *Entier*, Bath, general—b. *de Fauteuil*, Bath, hip—b. *Frais*, Bath, tepid—b. *Froid*, Bath, cold—b. *Marie*, Bath, water—b. *Médicinal*, Bath, medicated—b. *de Pied*, Bath, foot, Pediluvium—b. *de Sable*, Bath, sand—b. *de Siège*, Bath, hip—b. *Tempéré*, Bath, tepid, B. Temperate—b. *de Tête*,

BAINS, MINERAL WATERS OF. These are situate at Plombières, department of the Vosges. They are said to be saline and thermal by some; others deny them any medical properties.

BALAMPULLI, Tamarindus.
BALANCE, AREOSTATIC, Areometer.
BAL'ANCEMENT, *Compensa'tion*, from (F.) *balance*, 'a balance,' itself from *bis*, 'twice,' and *lanx*, 'a dish.' A law of teratogeny, as maintained by Geoffroy St. Hilaire, by which exuberance of nutrition in one organ is supposed to involve, to a greater or less extent, the total or partial atrophy of some other,—and conversely.

BALANDA, Fagus Sylvatica.
BALANEUM, Bath.
BALANISMUS, Suppository.
BALANITIS, Gonorrhœa spuria.
BALANOBLENNORRHŒA, Gonorrhœa spuria.
BALANOCASTANUM, Bunium Bulbocastanum.
BALANORRHŒA, Gonorrhœa spuria.
BA'LANUS, βαλανος, 'glans,' 'an acorn.' The glans penis. Hence, *Balanoblennorrhœ'a*, Blennorrhœa of the glans; and *Balani'tis*, Inflammation of the glans. Suppositories and pessaries were called *Bal'ani*.

BALANOS PHŒNICOS, Date.
BALANUS, Glans, Suppository—b. Myrepsica, Guilandina moringa.
BALARUC, MINERAL WATERS OF. Baluc is a town in the department of Hérault, in France. The waters are saline and thermal. They contain carbonic acid, carbonate of lime, carbonate of magnesia, chlorides of sodium, calcium, and magnesium, sulphate of lime, and a little iron. They are considered tonic, and are largely used. Their temperature is about 118° Fahrenheit.

BALARUC WATER, FACTIT"IOUS, (F.) *Eau de Balaruc; Aqua Belliluca'na* is made of *simple acidulous water* (containing twice its bulk of carbonic acid) f℥xxss; *chloride of sodium*, ℨiss; *chloride of calcium*, gr. xviij; *chloride of magnesium*, gr. lvi; *carbonate of magnesia*, gr. j.
BALATRO, Bambalio.
BALAUSTINE FLOWERS, see Punica granatum.
BALBIS, βαλβις, 'a foundation.' Any oblong cavity.—Galen. Hippocrates, in his treatise on the joints, gives the name *Balbito'des* to the olecranon cavity of the humerus.
BALBUS, (F.) *Bègue*. One habitually affected with stammering. A stammerer.
BALBU'TIES, *Psellis'mus, Psel'lotes, Blœ'sitas, Baryglos'sia, Dysla'lia, Mogila'lia, Ischopho'nia, Battaris'mus, Bamba'lia, Hœsita'tio, Loque'la blœ'sa*, (F.) *Balbutiement, Bégaiement*. Stammering, St. Vitus's Dance of the Voice. Also, vicious and incomplete pronunciation, in which almost all the consonants are replaced by the letters B and L; *Traulis'mus*.
BALCHUS, Bdellium.
BALD, Athrix.
BALDMONEY, Æthusa meum.
BALDNESS, Alopecia, Calvities—b. Limited, Porrigo decalvans—b. Partial, Porrigo decalvans.
BALENAS, Leviathan penis.
BALIMBAGO, Hibiscus populeus.
BALINEATOR, Bather.
BALINEUM, Bath.
BALL. Pila.
BALLISMUS, Chorea.
BALLISTA, Astragalus.
BALLON, Receiver.
BALLONNEMENT, Tympanites.
BALLOTA FŒTIDA, *B. vulga'ris* seu *nigra*,

Marru'bium nigrum, Black Horehound, Stinking H., (F.) *Marrube noir*. This plant is esteemed to be antispasmodic, resolvent, and detersive. (?)
BALLOTA LANA'TA, *Leonu'rus lana'tus*. A plant of the *Nat. Family*, Labiatæ, *Sex. Syst.* Didynamia Gymnospermia, which grows in Siberia. The whole plant, with the exception of the root, has been recommended in dropsy, and in rheumatism and gout, as a diuretic. It is usually given in decoction (℥ss to ℨj to f℥viij of water.)

BALLOTTEMENT, (F.) *Agita'tion, Succus'sion, Mouvement de Ballottement, Repercus'sion*, means the motion impressed on the fœtus in utero, by alternately pressing the uterus by means of the index finger of one hand introduced into the vagina; the other hand being applied on the abdomen. It is one of the least equivocal signs of pregnancy.

BALLSTON SPA. This village is situate in Saratoga County, New York. The spring Sans Souci belongs to the class of Acidulous Chalybeates. It contains iodide of sodium. There is also a sulphur spring.

BALM, Melissa—b. Apple, Momordica balsamina—b. Bastard, Melitis Melissophyllum—b. of Gilead, Solomon's, see Tinctura cardamomi—b. of Gilead, Poplar, Populus candicans—b. of Gilead tree, Dracocephalum Canariense—b. Indian, Trillium latifolium—b. Mountain, Monarda coccinea—b. Red, Monarda coccinea—b. Stinking, Hedeoma.

BALMONY, Chelone glabra.
BALNEA CŒNOSA, *Boue des eaux*.
BALNEARIUM, Hypocaustum.
BALNEARIUS, Bather.
BALNEATOR, Bather.
BALNEOG'RAPHY, *Balneograph'ia*, from βαλανειον, 'a bath,' and γραφη, 'a description.' A description of baths.
BALNEOL'OGY, *Balneolog"ia*, from βαλανειον, 'a bath,' and λογος, 'a description.' A treatise on baths.
BALNEOTHERAPI'A, from βαλανειον, 'a bath,' and θεραπεια, 'treatment.' Treatment of disease by baths.
BALNEUM, Bath—b. Acidum, Bath, acid—b. Alkalinum, Bath, alkaline—b. Animale, Bath, animal—b. Antipsoricum, Bath, antipsoric—b. Anti-syphiliticum, Bath, antisyphilitic—b. Arenæ, Bath, sand—b. Gelatinosum, Bath, gelatinous—b. Mariæ, Bath, water—b. Medicatum, Bath, medicated—b. Sulphuris, Bath, sulphur.

BALSAM, *Bal'samum, Bol'eson, Bel'eson*, (F.) *Baume*. This name is given to natural vegetable substances, concrete or liquid, but very odorous, bitter, and piquant: composed of resin, benzoic acid, and sometimes of an essential oil; — which allow benzoic acid to be disengaged by the action of heat; readily dissolved in volatile oil, alcohol, and ether; and, when treated with alkalies, afford a soluble benzoate, and throw down resin. We know of only five balsams:—those of Peru, and Tolu, Benzoin, *solid* Styrax or Storax, and *liquid* Styrax. (See those different words.) There are, however, many pharmaceutical preparations and resinous substances, possessed of a balsamic smell, to which the name *balsam* has been given; but they differ essentially in composition and properties: hence the distinction of balsams into *natural* and *artificial*. The *natural balsams* include the five before mentioned; the *artificial* the remainder.

BALSAM, ACOUS'TIC, *Bal'samum Acous'ticum*, (F.) *Baume acoustique*. A mixture of fixed and essential oils, sulphur, and tinctures of fetid gums. Used in cases of atonic deafness, dropped into the ear. The *acoustic balsam* of Dr. Hugh

Bath, head—*b. Tiède*, Bath, tepid—*b. Très froid*, Bath, cold—*b. de Vapeur*, Bath, vapour. Smith is made by mixing three drachms of ox-gall with one drachm of *balsam of Peru*.

BALSAM, AMERICAN. see Myroxylon Peruiferum — b. Anodyne, Bates's Linimentum saponis et opii.

BALSAM, APOPLEC'TIC, *Bal'samum, Apoplec'ticum*, (F.) *Baume apoplectique*. A medicine composed of several *balsams* properly so called, resins, and volatile oils. It is of a stiff consistence, is worn in ivory boxes about the person, and is smelled at in headachs, &c.

BALSAM APPLE, Momordica balsamina.

BALSAM OF ARCŒ'US, *Bal'samum Arcœi, Unguen'tum El'emi*, (F.) *Baume d'Arcœus*. A soft ointment; sometimes employed in wounds, ulcers, &c. It is made by melting, with a gentle heat, two parts of mutton suet, one of lard, one and a half of turpentine, and as much resin.

BALSAM, CANADA, see Pinus balsamea—b. Canary, Dracocephalum Canariense—b. Capivi, Copaiba.

BALSAM OF CARPA'THIA, *Bal'samum Carpath'icum*, (F.) *Baume de Carpathie*. The resin of the *Pinus Cembra*, a tree, which grows in Switzerland, Libya, and the Krapac mountains in Hungary.

BALSAM, CHALYB'EATE, *Bal'samum Chalybeu'tum*, (F.) *Baume d'acier ou d'aiguilles*. A mixture of nitrate of iron, alcohol, and oil, prepared by dissolving needles in nitric acid. It was formerly employed in frictions in pains of the joints.

BALSAM, COMMANDER'S, Tinctura benzoini composita—b. for Cuts, Tinctura benzoini composita.

BALSAM, CORDIAL, OF SENNER'TUS, *Bal'samum Cordia'lē Senner'ti*, (F.) *Baume cordiale de Sennert*. A stimulant medicine, composed of the essential oils of citron, cloves, and cinnamon, of musk, and ambergris. Dose, 6 to 15 drops.

BALSAM OF FIERABRAS. A celebrated Spanish vulnerary balsam, mentioned by Cervantes; the composition of which was oil, rosemary, salt and wine. (?)

BALSAM, SPIR'ITUOUS, OF FIORAVENTI, *Bal'samum Fioraven'ti spirituo'sum*, (F.) *Baume de Fioraventi spiritueux*. Different products of the distillation of resinous and balsamic substances, and of a number of aromatic substances, previously macerated in alcohol, have been thus called. The *Spirituous Balsam of Fioraventi*, the only one now used in friction, in chronic rheumatism, is the first product of the distillation from a sand-bath. It is entirely alcoholic. The *Oily Balsam of Fioraventi* is obtained by removing the residue, and distilling it in an iron vessel, at a white heat. It has the appearance of a citrine-coloured oil. The *Black Balsam of Fioraventi* is the black oil, obtained when the temperature is sufficient to carbonize the substances in the cucurbit.

BALSAM OF FIR, see Pinus balsamea.

BALSAM OF FOURCROY or of LABORDE, (F.) *Baume de Fourcroy ou de Laborde*. A kind of liniment composed of aromatic plants, balsams, resins, aloes, turpentine, theriac, and olive oil. Used in chaps of the skin and nipples.

BALSAM, FRIAR'S, Tinctura benzoini composita.

BALSAM OF GENEVIÈVE, (F.) *Baume de Geneviève*. An ointment composed of wax, turpentine, oil, red saunders, and camphor. Used in contused wounds, gangrene, &c.

BALSAM OF HONEY (HILL'S.) A tincture made of *tolu, honey* (ā ā ℔j) and *spirit*, (a gallon.) A pectoral, used in coughs. The committee of the New York College of Pharmacy recommend the following formula:—(*Gum. Benzoin*. ℥v, *Bals. Tolut*. ℥j, *Mellis* ℥viij, *Alcohol*. Oiij—digest for 10 days and filter.) See Mel.

BALSAM OF HOREHOUND (FORD'S.) A tincture of *horehound, liquorice-root, camphor, opium, benzoin, dried squills, oil of aniseed*, and *honey*. It has the same properties as the above. See Marrubium.

BALSAM, HUNGARIAN, see Pinus mughos.

BALSAM, HYPNOT'IC, *Bal'samum Hypnot'icum*, (F.) *Baume Hypnotique*. A preparation of which opium, hyoscyamus, camphor, and some other sedative substances form the basis. It is used externally in friction, to provoke sleep.

BALSAM, HYSTER'IC, *Bal'samum Hyster'icum*, (F.) *Baume Hystérique*. A preparation made of opium, aloes, asafœtida, castor, distilled oils of rue, amber, &c. It is held to the nose, applied to the navel, or rubbed on the hypogastrium in hysterical cases.

BALSAM, INDIAN, see Myroxylon peruiferum.

BALSAM OF LEICTOURE of CONDOM or VINCEGUERRE, *Bal'samum Lectoren'sē*. A strongly stimulant and aromatic mixture of camphor, saffron, musk, and ambergris, dissolved in essential oils. The ancients burnt it for the purpose of purifying the air of a chamber, when infected with a disagreeable odour.

BALSAM OF LIFE OF HOFF'MAN, *Bal'samum Vitæ Hoffman'ni*, (F.) *Baume de Vie d'Hoffman*. A tincture, composed of essential oils and ambergris, employed internally and externally as a stimulant. A mixture of essential oils without alcohol constitutes the *Saxon Balsam, Bal'samum apoplec'ticum, B. aromat'icum, B. cephal'icum, B. Saxon'icum, B. nervi'num, B. SCHERZERI, B. Stomach'icum*. Employed in friction as a stimulant.

BALSAM OF LIFE, Decoctum aloes compositum —b. of Life, Turlington's, see Tinctura benzoini composita.

BALSAM OF LOCATEL'LI OF LUCATEL'LI, *Bal'samum Lucatel'li*, (F.) *Baume de Lucatel*. A sort of ointment, composed of wax, oil, turpentine, sherry, and balsam of Peru, coloured with red saunders. It was once administered in pulmonary consumption.

BALSAM OF MECCA, see Amyris opobalsamum — b. Mexican, see Myroxylon Peruiferum — b. Natural, see Myroxylon peruiferum.

BALSAM, GREEN, OF METZ, *Bal'samum Vir'idē Metcn'sium, Bal'samum Vir'idē*, (F.) *Baume vert de Metz, Baume de Feuillet, Huile verte, O'leum ox'ydi cupri vir'idē*. This is composed of several fixed oils, holding, in solution, subcarbonate of copper, sulphate of zinc, turpentine, aloes, and the essential oils of cloves and juniper. It is green and caustic, and is employed to hasten the cicatrization of atonic ulcers,

BALSAM, NEPHRIT'IC, OF FULLER, *Bal'samum Nephret'icum Fulleri*. A liquid medicine, composed of oils, resins, and balsams, which have experienced an incipient state of carbonization from concentrated sulphuric acid. It was given in the dose of 15 to 30 drops in certain affections of the kidneys.

BALSAM, NERVOUS, *Bal'samum Nervi'num*, (F.) *Baume nervin ou nerval*. A kind of ointment, composed of fatty bodies, volatile oils, balsam of Peru, camphor, &c. It is employed in friction in cases of sprains and rheumatic pains.

BALSAM, PARALYT'IC, OF MYNSICHT. A sort of liniment or soft mixture of the essential oils of different aromatic plants, oils of turpentine and amber.—Lémery.

BALSAM OF PAREI'RA BRAVA, *Bal'samum Parei'ræ bravæ*. A soft mixture of balsam, resin, muriate of ammonia, and powder of the root of *Pareira brava*. It is given internally, to excite the urinary secretion.

BALSAM, PERUVIAN, see Myroxylon Peruiferum — b. of Peru, red, see Toluifera balsamum — b. of Peru, white, see Myroxylon Peruiferum.

BALSAM OF RACKASI'RA or of RAKASI'RI. This substance is of a yellowish-brown colour; semitransparent; fragile, when dry, but softening by heat; adhering to the teeth, when chewed. It has a smell similar to that of the Balsam of Tolu, and is slightly bitter. It is brought from India in gourd shells, and has been employed in diseases of the urinary and genital organs, especially in gonorrhœa.

BALSAM, RIGA. Prepared from the shoots of the Scotch Fir, macerated in spirit of wine. *Internally,* stimulant and diuretic; *externally,* a vulnerary. See Pinus Cembra.

BALSAM OF SATURN, *Bal'samum Satur'ni*. A solution of acetate of lead in spirit of turpentine, concentrated by evaporation; to which camphor has been added. This balsam was applied to hasten the cicatrization of wounds.

BALSAM OF THE SAMAR'ITAN, (F.) *Baume du Samaritain*. A sort of liniment, prepared by boiling together, at a gentle heat, equal parts of wine and oil. It is said to have been the ointment used by the Samaritan of the Gospel to cure a patient covered with ulcers.

BALSAM, SAXON, Balsam of Life of Hoffmann.

BALSAM OF SULPHUR, *Bal'samum Sul'phuris,* (F.) *Baume de Soufre*. A solution of sulphur in oil.—*B. sulph. anisa'tum,* (F.) *B. de Soufre anisé*. A solution of sulphur in essential oil of aniseed; given as a carminative.—*B. Sulph. succina'tum,* (F.) *B. de Soufre succiné*. A solution of sulphur in oil of amber. — *B. Sulphuris terebinthina'tum, Common Dutch Drops,* (F.) *B. de soufre térébinthiné*. A solution of sulphur in essential oil of turpentine, administered as a diuretic.—The *Balsam of Sulphur of* RULAND is a solution of sulphur in linseed oil or nut oil.

BALSAM OF SYM'PATHY, *Balsamum Sympath'icum,* (F.) *Baume de Sympathie*. A balsam, used in the days when sympathetic influence was strongly believed in. It was composed of the raspings of a human skull, blood, and human fat, and was applied to the instrument which had inflicted the wound.

BALSAM, THIBAUT'S. A tincture of myrrh, aloes, dragon's blood, flowers of St. John's wort, and Chio turpentine. *Internally,* diuretic; *externally,* vulnerary.

BALSAM OF TOLU, see Toluifera Balsamum.

BALSAM, TRANQUIL, *Bal'samum tranquil'lum seu tranquil'lans,* (F.) *B. tranquille*. A liquid medicine employed, externally, in the shape of friction: it is prepared by macerating and boiling, in olive oil, narcotic and poisonous plants,—belladonna, mandragora, hyoscyamus, &c.—and afterwards infusing, in the filtered decoction, different aromatic plants. It was employed as an anodyne.

BALSAM, TURKEY, Dracocephalum Canariense.

BALSAM OF TUR'PENTINE, *Dutch Drops, Bal'samum Terebin'thinæ*. Obtained by distilling oil of turpentine in a glass retort, until a red balsam is left. It possesses the properties of the turpentines.

BALSAM, VERVAIN'S, Tinctura Benzoini composita.

BALSAM, VUL'NERARY, OF MINDERE'RUS, *Bal'samum vulnera'rium Mindere'ri,* (F.) *B. vulnéraire de* MINDERER. A kind of liniment, composed of turpentine, resin elemi, oil of St. John's wort, and wax. Employed in friction, and as a dressing to wounds.

BALSAM WEED, Impatiens fulva — b. Wound, Tinctura Benzoini composita.

BALSAMADENDRON GILEADENSE, Amyris Gileadensis — b. Myrrha, see Myrrha.

BALSAMARIA INOPHYLLUM, see Fagara octandra.

BALSAMELÆON, Myroxylon Peruiferum.

BALSAM'IC, *Balsam'icus,* from βαλσαμον, 'balsam.' Possessing the qualities of balsams. *Balsamic odour:* — a sweet, faint, and slightly nauseous smell. *Balsamic substance:* — one resembling the balsams in property.

BALSAMIER ÉLÉMIFÈRE, Amyris elemifera — *b. de la Mecque*, Amyris opobalsamum.

BALSAMINA, Momordica balsamina.

BALSAMINE, Momordica balsamina.

BALSAMITA FŒMINEA, Achillea ageratum — b. Major, Tanacetum balsamita — b. Mas, Tanacetum balsamita.

BALSAM'ITA SUAV'EOLENS, *B. odora'ta, B. maris, Mentha Saracen'ica, M. Roma'na. Fam.* Compositæ Corymbiferæ. *Sex. Syst.* Syngenesia Polygamia superflua. A plant, common in the south of France, and cultivated in the gardens; where it bears the names *Menthecoq, Grand baume, Baume des Jardins*. Its smell is strong and aromatic, and taste hot. It is used for the same purposes as tansey, i. e. as a stimulant, vermifuge, &c.

BALSAMITA SUAVEOLENS, Tanacetum balsamita—b. Vulgaris, Tanacetum balsamita.

BALSAMO-SACCHARUM, Elæo-Saccharum.

BALSAMUM, see Balsam, Amyris opobalsamum—b. Ægyptiacum, see Amyris opobalsamum b. Album, see Myroxylon Peruiferum—b. Alpini, Dracocephalum Canariense—b. Alpini, see Amyris opobalsamum — b. Anodynum, Linimentum saponis et opii — b. Apoplecticum, Balsam of life of Hoffmann — b. Aromaticum, Balsam of life of Hoffmann — b. Asiaticum, see Amyris opobalsamum — b. Braziliense, Copaiba — b. Calaba, see Fagara octandra — b. Canadense, see Pinus balsamea — b. Catholicum, Tinctura benzoini composita — b. Cephalicum, Balsam of life of Hoffmann—b. Copaibæ, Copaiba—b. Genuinum antiquorum, see Amyris opobalsamum — b. Hyperici simplex, see Hypericum perforatum — b. Judaicum, see Amyris opobalsamum — b. Libani, see Pinus cembra—b. Mariæ, see Fagara octandra— b. e Meccâ, see Amyris opobalsamum — b. Mercuriale, Unguentum hydrargyri nitratis—b. Nervinum, Balsam of life of Hoffmann — b. Opodeldoc, Linimentum saponis camphoratum—b. Ophthalmicum rubrum, Unguentum hydrargyri nitrico-oxydi—b. Persicum, Tinctura benzoini composita—b. Peruanum, see Myroxylon Peruiferum b. Saturninum, Unguentum plumbi superacetatis — b. Scherzeri, Balsam of life of Hoffmann — b. Stomachicum, Balsam of life of Hoffmann — b. Styracis, Styrax—b. Styracis benzoini, Benjamin b. Succini, see Succinum — b. Sulphuris Barbadense, Petroleum sulphuratum — b. Sulphuris simplex, Oleum sulphuratum — b. Syriacum, see Amyris opobalsamum — b. Tolutanum, see Toluifera balsamum — b. Tranquillans seu Tranquillum, Balsam, tranquil—b. Traumaticum, Tinctura benzoini composita — b. Universale, Unguentum plumbi superacetatis — b. Viride, Balsam, green, of Metz; see Fagara octandra.

BALSAMUS PALUSTRIS, Mentha aquatica.

BALSEM, Amyris opobalsamum.

BAMBA, Bamboo.

BAMBALIA, Balbuties.

BAMBA'LIO, *Bam'balo, Bala'tro,* from βαμβαινω, 'I speak inarticulately.' One who stammers or lisps, or utters inarticulate sounds. According to KRAUSE, one who speaks as if he had pap in his mouth, or as if the tongue were paralyzed.

BAMBOO, (F.) *Bambou, Bambu. Fam.* Gramineæ. *Sex. Syst.* Hexandria Monogynia. The young shoots of *Bambos arundina'cea, Arun'do bambos, Bambu'sa arundina'cea,* and of *Bambos verticilla'ta,* contain a saccharine pith, of which the people of both the Indies are very fond. They are sometimes made into a pickle.

BAMBOS ARUNDINACEA, Bamboo — b. Verticillata, Bamboo.

BAMBUSA ARUNDINACEA, Bamboo.

BAMIX MOSCHATA, Hibiscus abelmoschus.

BAMMA, from βαπτω, 'I plunge,' 'a paint; a dye.' Anciently, liquids were so called, in which certain bodies were plunged, to moisten or soften them. In the case of tea, for instance, into which bread is dipped, the tea would be the *bamma*.

BANANA, Musa sapientum.

BANANIER, Musa sapientum.

BANAUSIA, Charlatanry.

BANC D'HIPPOCRATE, Bathron.

BANCAL, (F.) One who has deformed legs. It includes the *valgus*, *compernis*, and *varus*, which see.

BANCROCHE, (F.) A vulgar epithet for a rickety individual.

BAND, PRIMITIVE, see Nerve Fibre.

BAN'DAGE, *Desma, Syndes'mus, Hypodes'mis, Hypodesma, Hypodes'mus,* (the last three signify properly an under bandage.) A *binder,* from Sax. bindan, 'to bind.' This word, with the French, is generally used to express the methodical application of rollers, compresses, &c., *Ban'daging, Syn'desis,* to fix an apparatus upon any part,—corresponding to the words *deliga'tio, fascia'tio, fascia'rum applica'tio, epid'esis.* With us the noun is usually applied to the result of the application, or to the bandage itself;—a sense in which the French employ the word *Bande*. Bandages are *simple* or *compound*. The simple bandage is *equal*, if the turns are applied circularly above each other; *unequal*, if the turns are not accurately applied upon each other. If each turn of the bandage be only covered one-third, it forms the *doloire* of the French; if the edges touch only slightly, it is the *moussé;* if the turns are very oblique and separated, it is the *spiral* or *creeping*, (F.) *rampant;* if folded upon each other, it is termed the *reversed*, (F.) *renversé*. By uniting various kinds of bandaging, we have the *compound;* and these compound bandages have received various names expressive of their figure, or of the parts to which they are applied, as *capistrum, spica*, &c. Bandages are divided, also, as regards their uses, into *uniting, dividing, retaining, expelling, compressing*, &c.

BANDAGE or **ROLLER,** *Fas'cia, Tæ'nia, Epides'mos, Vin'culum,* the *Bande* of the French, is derived from (G.) binden, 'to bind.' It may be made of linen, flannel, or other stuff capable of offering a certain resistance. The two extremities of a bandage are called *tails,* (F.) *chefs,* and the rolled part is termed its *head*, (F.) *globe*. If rolled at both extremities, it is called a *double-headed roller* or *bandage,* (F.) *Bande à deux globes*.

BANDAGE, BODY, *Manti'lă,* (F.) *Bandage de Corps,* is used for fixing dressings, &c., to the trunk. It is formed of a towel, napkin, or some large compress, folded three or four times; the extremities of which are fastened by pins. This is again fixed by means of the *scapulary bandage,* which is nothing more than an ordinary bandage, stitched to the anterior and middle part of the napkin, passing over the clavicles and behind the head, to be attached to the back part of the napkin.

BANDAGE, COMPRESSING, or **ROLLER,** *Fascia compressi'va* seu *convolu'ta,* (F.) *Bandage compressive* ou *roulé*, is the simple *roller* with one head; and is employed in cases of ulcers, varices, &c., of the limbs. Whenever this roller is applied to the lower part of the limbs, it is carried upwards by the *doloire* and *reversed* methods above described.

BANDAGE DIVISIF, Dividing bandage — *b. en Doloire, Doloire*.

BANDAGE, EIGHTEEN-TAILED, *Fas'cia octod'ecim capit'ibus,* (F.) *Bandage à dix huit chefs.* This bandage is made of a longitudinal portion of a common roller; and with a sufficient number of transverse pieces or tails, to cover as much of the part as is requisite. It is a very useful bandage, inasmuch as it can be undone without disturbing the part.

BANDAGE, GALEN'S, *B. for the Poor, Fas'cia Gale'ni* seu *Pau'perum,* (F.) *Bandage de Galien* ou *des Pauvres, Ga'lea,* is a kind of *cucullus* or hood, (F.) *Couvrechef*, divided into three parts on each side; of which GALEN has given a description. See Cancer, Galeni.

BANDAGE, HERNIAL, see TRUSS — b. Immovable, Apparatus, immovable.

BANDAGE, INGUINAL, *Fas'cia inguina'lis*. A bandage for keeping dressings applied to the groin. It consists of a cincture, to which is attached a triangular compress, adapted for covering the groin. To the lower extremity of this, one or two bandages are attached, which pass under the thigh, and are fixed to the posterior part of the cincture. This bandage may be either simple or double.

Other bandages will be found described under their various names.

BANDAGE, PERMANENT, Apparatus, immovable — b. of the Poor, see Cancer Galeni; and Bandage, Galen's.

BANDAGE OF SEPARATE STRIPS, or B. OF SCULTE'TUS, *Fas'cia fasci'olis separa'tim dispos'itis* seu *Sculte'ti,* (F.) *Bandage à bandelettes séparées* ou *de Scultet*. This is formed of linen strips, each capable of surrounding once and a half the part to which they have to be applied, and placed upon each other, so as to cover successively one-third of their width. It is used chiefly for fractures, requiring frequent dressing.

BANDAGE, UNDER, Hypodesmis—b. *Unissant,* Uniting bandage.

BANDAGING, see Bandage—b. Doctrine of, Desmaturgia.

BAN'DAGIST. One whose business it is to make bandages, and especially those for hernia.

BANDE, Bandage. The word *Bande,* in anatomy, is used by the French for various narrow, flat, and elongated expansions. *Bande d'Héliodore*, is a kind of bandage for supporting the mammæ.

BANDEAU, (F.) A kind of simple bandage, which consists of a piece of cloth, folded four times, and applied round the head. There is also the *Bandeau* ou *Mouchoir en triangle* or *triangular bandage*, a kind of couvrechef, made of a square piece of cloth, or of a handkerchief, folded diagonally, and applied round the head.

BANDELETTE, (F.) Diminutive of *Bande, Fasciola, Tæniola, Vitta;* a narrow bandage, strip, or fillet. Also Tænia semicircularis.

BANDELETTES AGGLUTINATIVES, small strips, covered with a glutinous plaster. *Vittæ agglutinan'tes*. See Agglutinant.

BANDELETTES DECOUPÉES, are strips of linen, notched on one edge, and covered, on one side, with ointment. They are applied to wounds to prevent the lint from sticking, and the laceration of the cicatrix.

BANDELETTE SEMICIRCULAIRE, Tænia semicircularis—b. *des Cornes d'ammon,* Corpus fimbriatum—b. *des Éminences pyriformes,* Tænia semicircularis—b. *de l'Hippocampe,* Corpora fimbriata.

BANDURA, Nepentha destillatoria.
BANDY-LEGGED, Cnemoscoliosis.
BANEBERRY, Actæa spicata.
BANGUE, *Bhang, Bangi* or *Beng, Sedhee, Subjee.* Adanson believes this to be the *Nepenthes* of the ancients. The largest leaves and capsules without the stalks of *Can'nabis In'dica,* (F.) *Chanvre Indien, Indian hemp,* probably identical with *C. sativa. Family,* Urticeæ. *Sex. Syst.* Diœcia Pentandria. The leaves and flowers of Cannabis are narcotic and astringent. They are chewed and smoked. The seeds, mixed with opium, areca, and sugar, produce a kind of intoxication, and are used for this purpose by the people of India. An alcoholic extract of the plant, *Churrus,* has been used in India, and since then in Europe and in this country as a narcotic, and anti-convulsive, in the dose of from half a grain to ten or more. It requires, however, great caution in its administration. The pure resin—*Cannabine*—is active in the dose of two-thirds of a grain.
The dried plant, which has flowered, and from which the resin has not been removed, called *Gunjah* or *Ganjah, Haschisch, Haschich, Hachisch* or *Chaschisch,* of the Arabs, consists of the tops and tender parts only of the plant, collected immediately after inflorescence, and simply dried.
BANICA, Pastinaca sativa.
BANILAS, Vanilla.
BANILLA, Vanilla.
BANILLOES, Vanilla.
BANISTE'RIA ANGULO'SA. This plant, in Brazil and the Antilles, passes for a powerful sudorific, and an antidote to the poison of serpents.
BANKSIA ABYSSINICA, Hagenia Abyssinica—b. Speciosa, Costus.
BANNIÈRES, MINERAL WATERS OF. Bannières is a village in Quercy, diocess of Cahors, France. The waters are probably chalybeate. They are celebrated in amenorrhœa, cachexia, jaundice, &c.
BA'OBAB, *Adanso'nia digita'ta,* of Africa; *Nat. Ord.* Bombaceæ; one of the largest productions of the vegetable kingdom. Its fruit is called, in the country, *Pain de singe.* The pulp is sourish, and agreeable to eat: and a refreshing drink is made from it, which is used in fevers. Prospero Alpini and Dr. L. Frank think that the *Terra Lemnia* was prepared, in Egypt, from the pulp. All the parts of the Baobab abound in mucilage. The bark has been given as a substitute for cinchona.
BAPTISIA LEUCANTHA, see Sophora tinctoria—b. Tinctoria, Sophora tinctoria.
BAPTISTERIUM, *Baignoire.*
BARAQUETTE, (F.) A name given by Rasous, physician at Nismes in France, to a catarrhal epidemy, which occurred there in 1761. See Influenza.
BARATHRON, Juniperus sabina.
BARATHRUM, Antrum.
BARBA, Beard—b. Aaronis, Arum maculatum—b. Capræ, Spiræa ulmaria—b. Hirci, Tragopogon—b. Jovis, Sempervivum tectorum.
BARBADOES, see West Indies—b. Leg, see Elephantiasis.
BARBAREA, Erysimum Barbarea—b. Stricta, Erysimum Barbarea.
BARBAROS'SÆ PIL'ULÆ, *Barbaros'sa's Pills.* An ancient composition of quicksilver, rhubarb, diagridium, musk, &c. It was the first internal mercurial medicine, which obtained any real credit.
BARBE, Beard—*b. de Bouc,* Tragopogon.
BARBEAU, Cyanus segetum.

BARBER-CHIRUR'GEONS. A Corporation of London, instituted by king Edward IV. The barbers were separated from the surgeons, by 18 Geo. II., c. 15; and the latter were erected into a *Royal College of Surgeons* at the commencement of the present century.
BARBERS, ARMY, see Bathers.
BARBERIE, MINERAL WATERS OF. These mineral waters are half a league from Nantes. They contain carbonic acid, chlorides of magnesium and sodium, sulphate of magnesia, carbonates of magnesia, lime, and iron. They are used as chalybeates.
BARBERRY, Oxycantha Galeni—b. American, see Oxycantha Galeni.
BARBIERS. A variety of paralysis chiefly prevalent in India; and by many considered to be the same as Beriberi. Beriberi is commonly an acute disease. Barbiers is generally chronic.
BARBITIUM, Beard.
BAR-BONE, Pubis, os.
BARBOTINE, Artemisia Santonica.
BARBULA CAPRINA, Spiræa ulmaria.
BARCLAY'S ANTIBILIOUS PILLS, Pilulæ antibiliosæ.
BARDADIA, Pound.
BARDANA, Arctium lappa—b. Minor, Xanthium.
BARDANE PETITE, Xanthium.
BARÉGES, MINERAL WATERS OF. Baréges is a village in the department of Hautes Pyrénées, near which are several springs. They are sulphureous and thermal, the heat varying from 85° to 112° Fahrenheit. They contain chlorides of magnesium and sodium, sulphates of magnesia and lime, carbonate of lime, sulphur, &c. These springs have long enjoyed a high reputation, and are daily advised in cutaneous and scrofulous affections, &c.
FACTITIOUS BARÉGES WATER, *Aqua Bareginen'sis,* (F.) *Eau de Baréges,* is made by adding, *hydrosulphuretted water,* f ʒiv, to *pure water,* f ʒxvijss, *carbonate of soda,* gr. xvj, *chloride of sodium,* gr. ss. Bottle closely.
BARGADA, Convolvulus pes capriæ.
BARGOU. An alimentary preparation formed of ground oats, boiled to a proper consistence with water.
BARIGLIA, Soda.
BARII CHLORIDUM, Baryta, muriate of—b. Iodidum, Baryta, hydriodate of.
BARILLA, Soda—b. Alicant, Soda—b. Carthagena, Soda—b. Turkey, Soda.
BARILLOR, Soda.
BARIUM, *Ba'ryum, Baryt'ium, Pluto'nium,* from βαρυς, 'heavy.' The metallic base of baryta, so called from the great density of its compounds.
BARIUM, CHLORIDE OF, Baryta, muriate of—*b. Chlorure de,* Baryta, muriate of—b. Iodide of, Baryta, hydriodate of—b. Protoxide of, Baryta.
BARK, Cinchona—b. Bitter, Pinckneya pubens—b. Calisaya, Cinchonæ cordifoliæ cortex—b. Caribæan, Cinchonæ Caribææ cortex—b. Carthagena, see Cinchona—b. Crown, Cinchonæ lancifoliæ cortex—b. Elk, Magnolia glauca—b. Essential salt of, see Cinchona—b. Florida, Pinckneya pubens—b. Georgia, Pinckneya pubens—b. Gray, see Cinchona—b. Huanuco, see Cinchona—b. Indian, Magnolia glauca—b. Jesuit's, Cinchona—b. Loxa, Cinchonæ lancifoliæ cortex—b. Pale, Cinchonæ lancifoliæ cortex—b. Maracaybo, see Cinchona—b. Peruvian, Cinchona—b. Pitaya, Cinchonæ Caribææ cortex—b. Red, Cinchonæ oblongifoliæ cortex—b. Saint Lucia, Cinchonæ Caribææ cortex—b. Santa Martha, see Cinchona—b. Silver, see Cinchona—b. Yellow, Cinchonæ cordifoliæ cortex.

BARLERIA BUXIFOLIA, Cara schulli.
BARLEY, PEARL, see Hordeum—b. Scotch, Hordeum—b. Water, Decoctum hordei.
BARM, Yest.
BARNET, MINERAL WATERS OF. Barnet is not far from London. The water is of a purging quality, like that of Epsom, and about half the strength.
BAROMACROM'ETER, *Pædobaromacrom'eter, Pædom'eter*, from βαρος, 'weight,' μακρος, 'long,' and μετρον, 'measure.' An instrument invented by Stein to indicate the length and weight of a new-born infant.
BAROM'ETER, *Baroscop'ium, Ba'roscope*, from βαρος, 'weight,' and μετρον, 'measure.' (F.) *Baromètre.* An instrument which measures the weight of the air. A certain degree of density in this medium is necessary for health. When we ascend high mountains great inconvenience is experienced, owing to the diminished density. Changes of this character are indicated by the Barometer or weather-glass.
BA'ROS, βαρος, 'heaviness.' Employed by the Greek physicians to designate the feeling of lassitude and heaviness observable in many diseases. —Hippocrates, Galen.
BAROSCOPE, Barometer.
BAROSMA CRENATA, Diosma crenata.
BAROTES SALITUS, Baryta, muriate of.
BARRAS, see Pinus sylvestris.
BARRE, MINERAL WATERS OF. Barre is a small town, six leagues from Strasburg. The waters are thermal, and contain much iron, calcareous salt, &c. They are diuretic and tonic.
BARRE (F.) *Barrure, Vara*, 'a bar.' A projection or prolongation of the symphysis pubis: —a deformity rendering delivery difficult.
BARRÉE (F.) A term applied, in France, to a female whose pelvis has the deformity described under Barre.
BARRÉES, (DENTS.) The molar teeth, when the roots are spread or tortuous, so that they cannot be extracted without being broken; or without a portion of the alveolar arch being removed.
BARREL OF THE EAR, Tympanum.
BARRENNESS, Sterilitas.
BARROS, Terra Portugallica.
BARRURE, Barre.
BARTON'S FRACTURE, see Fracture of the Radius, Barton's.
BARYCOCCALON, Datura stramonium.
BARYCOITA, Barycoia.
BARYECOI'A, *Barycoi'ta, Bradyecoi'a, Paracu'sia obtu'sa, Disecoi'a, Dysecœ'a, Audi'tus diffic'ilis, Obaudi'tio, Obaudi'tus, A. gravis, A. imminu'tus, Hypocopho'sis, Hypokyro'sis*, (F.) *Dureté d'Oreille*, from βαρυς, 'heavy,' and ακοη, 'hearing.' Hardness of hearing, incomplete deafness. See Cophosis, and Deafness.
BARYGLOSSIA, Balbuties, Baryphonia.
BARYI HYDRAS IODATI, Baryta, hydriodate of.
BARYLALIA, Baryphonia.
BARYOD'YNE, from βαρυς, 'heavy,' and οδυνη, 'pain.' A dull, heavy pain.
BARYPHO'NIA, *Baryglos'sia, Baryla'lia, Loque'la impedi'ta*, from βαρυς, 'heavy,' and φωνη, 'voice.' Difficulty of voice or speech.
BARYPICRON, Artemisia abrotanum.
BARYSOMATIA, Polysarcia adiposa.
BARYSOMATICA, Polysarcia adiposa.
BARY'TA, from βαρυς, 'heavy,' *Terra ponderos'a, Bary'tes, Protox'ide of Ba'rium, Heavy Earth, Ponderous Earth*, (F.) *Baryte, Barite, Terre pesante.* This earth and its soluble salts are all highly corrosive poisons. It is never employed in medicine in the pure state. When externally applied, it is caustic, like potassa and soda.
BARY'TA, CARBONATE OF, *Barytæ Car'bonas*, (F.) *Carbonate de Baryte*, is only used officinally to obtain the muriate.
BARYTA, HYDRI'ODATE OF, *Barytæ Hydriodas, Baryta Hydriod'ica, Hydras Baryi Ioda'ti*, (in the dry state,—*Iodide of Barium, Barii Iod'idum, B. Ioda'tum*,) has been given in scrofulous and similar morbid conditions. It may be administered internally in the dose of one eighth of a grain three or four times a day, and be applied externally to scrofulous swellings, in the form of ointment, (gr. iv to ℥j of lard.)
BARYTA HYDRIODICA, Baryta, hydriodate of.
BARYTA, MU'RIATE OR HYDROCHLORATE OF, *Bary'tæ mu'rias, Chlo'ride of Ba'rium, Ba'rii Chlo'ridum* (Ph. U. S.), *Chlo'ruret of Ba'rium, Terra pondero'sa sali'ta seu muria'ta, Sal muriat'icum barot'icum, Baro'tes sali'tus*. (F.) *Chlorure de barium*, is the combination chiefly used. The Muriate of Baryta may be formed as follows: *Baryt. Carbon.* in frustulis, ℔j, *Acid. Muriat.* f℥xij, *Aquæ*, Oiij. Mix the acid with the water, and gradually add the Carbonate of Baryta. Toward the close of the effervescence, apply a gentle heat, and, when the action has ceased, filter the liquor, and boil it down so that crystals may form as it cools. Ph. U. S.
It is given in the form of the *Solu'tio Muria'tis Barytæ, Liquor Barii Chlo'ridi*, Ph. U. S., *Aqua barytæ muria'tis*, (F.) *Solution de Muriate de Baryte*, (*Muriate of Baryta*, one part; *distilled water*, three parts,) and is employed in scrofulous cases, worms, and cutaneous diseases. Externally, to fungous ulcers and to specks on the cornea.
BARYTÆ CARBONAS, Baryta (Carbonate)—b. Hydriodas, Baryta, hydriodate of—b. Murias, Baryta, muriate of.
BARYTE, Baryta—*b. Carbonate de*, Barytæ carbonate of.
BARYTHMIA, Melancholy.
BARYTIUM, Barium.
BARYUM, see Barium.
BAS-FOND, see Urinary Bladder.
BAS-LASSÉ, Stocking, laced.
BAS VENTRE, Abdomen.
BASAAL. The name of an Indian tree, the decoction of whose leaves, in water, with ginger, is used as a gargle in diseases of the fauces. The kernels of the fruit are vermifuge.
BASANASTRA'GALA, from βασανος, 'torture,' and αστραγαλος, 'the astragalus.' Pain in the ankle joint; gout in the foot.
BASANIS'MOS, from βασανιζειν, 'to explore.' 'A touch-stone.' Investigation or examination' —Hippocrates, Galen.
BASE, *Basis*, from βαινω, 'I proceed,' 'I rest,' 'I support myself.' That which serves as a foundation or support. That which enters, as a principal matter, into a mixture or combination. In anatomy, it is employed in the former sense, as *Base of the Cranium, Base of the Brain—Basis seu Parimen'tum cere'bri; Base of a process, &c., Base of the heart—Basis vel coro'na cordis.* In the art of prescribing, *Basis* is the chief substance which enters into a compound formula.
BASEMENT MEMBRANE, see Membrane, basement.
BASIATIO, Coition.
BASIATOR, Orbicularis oris.
BASIL, BUSH, Ocymum caryophyllatum—b. Citron, Ocymum basilicum — b. Common, Ocymum basilicum—b. Small, Ocymum caryophyllatum—b. Wild, Chenopodium vulgare—b. Wild,

Cunila mariana — b. Wild, Pycnanthemum incanum.

BASILAD, see Basilar Aspect.

BAS'ILAR, *Basila'ris, Bas'ilary*, (F.) *Basilaire.* That which belongs to the base, from βασις, 'base.' This name has been given to several parts, which seem to serve as basis to others. The sacrum and sphenoid have been hence so called.

BASILAR ARTERY, *A. basila'ris, A. cervica'lis,* (F.) *Artère ou Tronc basilaire, A. mesocéphalique* (Ch.) The union of the two vertebral arteries. It ascends along the middle groove on the inferior surface of the tuber, and is supported, beneath by the *Fossa basilaris.* It terminates in the posterior cerebral arteries.

BASILAR ASPECT, An aspect towards the base of the head.—Barclay. *Basilad* is used adverbially by the same writer to signify 'towards the basilar aspect.'

BASILAR FOSSA, (F.) *Gouttière ou Fosse basilaire,* is the upper surface of the basilary process, —so called because it is channeled like a *Fossa* or *Gutter.* The *Tuber annulare* rests upon it.

BASILAR PROCESS, *Proces'sus basila'ris ossis occip'itis, P. cuneifor'mis ossis occip'itis,* (F.) *Apophyse Basilaire, Prolongement sous-occipital, Cu'neiform Process,* is the bony projection, formed by the inferior angle of the os occipitis, which is articulated with the sphenoid.

BASILAR SINUS, Sinus transversus.

BASILAR SURFACE, (F.) *Surface basilaire,* is the inferior surface of the process. It is covered by the mucous membrane of the pharynx.

BASILAR VERTEBRA. The last vertebra of the loins.

BASIL'IC, *Basil'icus,* from βασιλικος, 'royal.' This name was given, by the ancients, to parts which they conceived to play an important part in the animal economy.

BASILIC VEIN, *Vena basil'ica, V. cu'biti inte'rior,* (F.) *Veine Basilique, Veine cubitale cutanée* of Chaussier. This vein is one of those on which the operation of blood-letting is performed. It is situate at the internal part of the fold of the elbow, in front of the humeral artery, and is formed by the *anterior* and *posterior cubital veins,* and by the *median basilic.* It terminates, in the arm-pit, in the axillary vein. The ancients thought, that the basilic of the right arm had some connexion with the liver, and hence they called it *hepatic.* The vein of the left arm, for a similar reason, they called *splenic.* The *Median Basilic Vein,* (F.) *Veine médiane basilique,* is one of the branches of the preceding vein. It joins the median cephalic at an acute angle, or rather by a transverse branch, and receives some branches of the deep radial and cubital veins, and a considerable subcutaneous vein —the *common median.*

BASILIC COMMUN, Ocymum basilicum—b. *Sauvage, grand,* Chenopodium vulgare.

BASIL'ICON, *Basil'icum.* 'Royal,' or of great virtue. An ointment, composed of yellow wax, black pitch, and resin, of each one part, olive oil, four parts. Hence it was called *Unguen'tum Tetraphar'macum,* (τετραφαρμακα, 'four drugs.')—Celsus. Scribonius Largus.

BASILICON, *Basilicum,* of the Parisian Codex, is the *Onguent de Poix et de Cire.* In most Pharmacopœias, it is represented by the *Unguen'tum* or *Cera'tum Resi'næ.* It is used as a stimulating ointment. See Ceratum Resinæ, and Unguentum Resinæ Nigræ.

BASILICUM, Basilicon, Ocymum Basilicum — b. Citratum, Ocymum basilicum — b. Majus, Ocymum basilicum.

BASILISCUS, Syphilis.

BASIO-CERATO-CHONDRO-GLOSSUS, Hyoglossus.

BASIO-CER'ATO-GLOSSUS, from βασις, 'base,' κερας, 'cornu,' and γλωσσα, 'tongue.' A name given to a part of the hyoglossus, which is inserted into the cornu of the os hyoides and base of the tongue.

BASIOCES'TRUM, from βασις, 'the base,' and κεστρα, 'a dart.' An instrument for opening the head of the fœtus in utero, invented by Mesler, a German.

BA'SIO-GLOS'SUS, *Hypseloglos'sus, Hyobasioglossus, Ypseloglos'sus,* from βασις, 'base,' and γλωσσα, 'the tongue.' A name formerly given to the portion of the hyoglossus which is inserted into the base of the os hyoides.—Riolan, Thomas Bartholine. See Lingual Muscle.

BASIO PHARYNGÆ'US, from βασις, 'base,' and φαρυγξ, 'the pharynx.' A name given to some fibres of the constrictor pharyngis medius. —Winslow.

BASIS, see Prescription—b. Cerebri, Base of the Brain—b. Cordis, Radix cordis—b. Corporis, Sole.

BASSI-COL'ICA. Name of a medicine composed of aromatics and honey. — Scribonius Largus.

BASSIA BUTYRACEA, see Spirit, (Arrack.)

BASSIN, Pelvis—b. *Oculaire,* Scaphium oculare.

BASSINER, to foment.

BASSINET, Pelvis of the kidney, Ranunculus bulbosus.

BAS'SORA, GUM. A gum, obtained from a plant unknown, which came originally from the neighbourhood of Bassora, on the Gulf of Persia, whence its name. It is in irregularly shaped pieces, white or yellow, and intermediate in its transparency between gum Arabic and gum tragacanth. Only a small portion is soluble in water. The insoluble portion is a peculiar principle, called *Bassorin.* It is not used in medicine; but bassorin enters into the composition of several substances.

BASSORIN, see Bassora gum.
BASSWOOD, Tilia.
BATA, Musa Paradisiaca.
BATABAS, Solanum tuberosum.

BATA'TAS. The inhabitants of Peru gave this appellation to several tuberous roots, especially to *Convolvulus Batatas* or *Sweet Potato.* Our word, Potato, comes from this.

BATEMAN'S PECTORAL DROPS, see Pectoral Drops, Bateman's.

BATERION, Bathron.

BATES'S ANODYNE BALSAM, Linimentum saponis et opii.

BATH, Anglo-Saxon, baÐ, *Bal'neum, Balane'um, Baline'um, Loutron,* (F.) *Bain.* Immersion, or stay, for a longer or shorter duration, of the whole or a part of the body, in some medium, as water. Act of plunging into a liquid, sand, or other substance, in which it is the custom to bathe, *Plunge Bath.* Also, the vessel in which the water is put for bathing. Also, a public or private establishment for bathing.

In *Pharmacy,* a vessel, placed over a fire, and filled with any substance, into which another vessel is placed, containing matters for digestion, evaporation, or distillation.

BATH, ACID, *Bal'neum ac"idum* (*Acid. muriat.* ℔ij; *Aquæ,* cong. lxvi. One half, one third, or one fourth the quantity of acid is more frequently employed.)

BATH, ACID, SCOTT'S, see Scott's Acid Bath.

BATH, AIR, HOT, see Bath, hot—b. Air, warm, see Bath, hot.

BATH, AL'KALINE, *Bal'neum alkali'num.* This

may be made of half a pound or a pound of *pearlash* or of *carbonate of soda*, to sixty-six gallons of water.

BATH, AN'IMAL, *Balneum Anima'lĕ*, consists in wrapping an animal recently killed, or its skin, around the body, or some part of it.

BATH, ANTIPSOR'IC, *Bal'neum antipso'ricum*. Recommended in cases of itch and other cutaneous diseases. (*Potass. sulphuret.* ℥iv, *Aquæ cong.* lx.)

BATH, ANTISYPHILIT'IC, *Bal'neum antisyphilit'icum, Mercu'rial bath*. Made by dissolving from two drachms to an ounce of the corrosive chloride of mercury in sixty gallons of water.

BATH, ARM, *Brachilu'vium*. A bath for the arm.

BATH, COLD, see Bath, hot—b. Cool, see Bath, hot.

BATH, DRY, is one made of ashes, salt, sand, &c. The ancients used these frequently for therapeutical purposes.

BATH, EARTH, Arenatio.

BATH, ELEC'TRIC, (F.) *Bain électrique*, consists in placing the person upon an insulated stool, communicating, by a metallic wire, with the principal conductor of the electrical machine in action. The Electric Bath produces general excitement of all the functions, and especially of the circulation and secretions.

BATH, FOOT, *Pedilu'vium*, (F.) *Bain de Pied*, a bath for the feet.

BATH, GELAT'INOUS, *Bal'neum gelatino'sum*. Made by dissolving two pounds of *gelatin* in a gallon of *water*.

BATH, GENERAL, (F.) *Bain Entier*, is one in which the whole body is plunged, except the head; in contradistinction to the *partial bath*, *Merobalane'um, Merobal'neum*.

BATH, HALF, *Semicu'pium, Excathis'ma, Inces'sio, Inces'sus*, is one adapted for half the body. One, for receiving only the hips or extremities, is also so called.

The *Sitz-bath*, (G.) Sitzbad, of the hydropathists is a tub of cold water, in which the patient sits for a variable period.

BATH, HAND, *Manulu'vium*, (F.) *Bain de Main* ou *Manuluve*, is a bath for the hands.

BATH, HEAD, *Oapitilu'vium*, (F.) *Bain de Tête* ou *Capitiluve*, a bath for the head.

BATH, HIP, *Coxælu'vium*, (F.) *Bain de Fauteuil, Bain de Siége*, is one in which the lower part of the trunk and upper part of the thighs are immersed.

BATH, HOT, *Balneum Cal'idum, Zestolu'sia*, (F.) *Bain chaud*, is a bath, the temperature of which is 98° and upwards; the WARM BATH from 92° to 98°; the TEPID BATH, (F.) *Bain Tiède, Balneum tep'idum*, from 85° to 92°; the TEMPERATE BATH, (F.) *Bain tempéré*, from 75° to 85°; the COOL BATH, (F.) *Bain frais*, from 60° to 75°; the COLD BATH, *Balneum frig'idum, Frigida'rium*, (F.) *Bain froid, Bain trés froid*, (of some,) from 30° to 60°; and the VAPOUR BATH, *Balneum vapo'ris*, (F.) *Bain de Vapeur, Étuve Humide*, from 100° to 130°, and upwards. See Vaporarium. A WARM AIR BATH, or HOT AIR BATH, consists of air the temperature of which is raised.

BATH, MED'ICATED, *Balneum Medica'tum*, (F.) *Bain médicinal*, is a bath, formed of decoctions or infusions of vegetable substances, or of any ingredient, introduced into the water for therapeutical purposes.

BATH, MERCURIAL, Bath, antisyphilitic — b. Nitro-muriatic acid, Scott's acid bath.

BATH, PLUNGE, see Bath.

BATH, SAND, *Balneum Are'næ*, (F.) *Bain de Sable*, consists of a vessel filled with sand, and placed over the fire. Into this vessel, the one is put which contains the substance to be evaporated. See Psammismus.

BATH, SEA WATER, *Balneum Mar'iæ*, (F.) *Bain Marie*, consists of a vessel filled with boiling sea water, or salt water, in which the vessel is placed, that contains the substance to be evaporated. *Bain Marie* is, however, at the present day often employed for any form of water bath.

BATH, SHOWER, *Implu'vium*, is one in which the water is made to fall like a shower on the body. See Douche.

BATH, SITZ, see Bath, half.

BATH, STEAM, may be formed by introducing steam into a properly closed vessel in place of water, as in the water bath.

BATH, SUCCES'SION, *Transition bath*. A term applied to the rapid succession or transition from a cold to a warm or hot bath, or conversely.—Bell.

BATH, SULPHUR, *Bal'neum Sulph'uris*. A bath much used in psora, and other chronic cutaneous affections. It may be composed of two ounces of diluted sulphuric acid, and eight ounces of sulphuret of potassium added to each bath.

BATH, TAN. An astringent bath, prepared, at times, by boiling two or three handfuls of ground oak-bark,—such as is used by tanners—in two or three quarts of water, for half an hour, and then adding the decoction to the water of the bath.

BATH, TEMPERATE, see Bath, hot—b. Tepid, see Bath, hot.

BATH, TRANSITION, Bath, succession.

BATH, VAPOUR, see Bath, hot, and Vaporarium—b. Warm, see Bath, hot.

Bathing is much employed in the treatment of disease. The cold bath, especially the cold sea bath, is a sedative and indirect tonic: the warm bath a relaxant; and the hot bath a stimulant.

The regular use of the bath is extremely conducive to health; but if too much indulged in, it is apt to produce injurious effects.

BATH, MINERAL WATERS OF, *Aquæ Batho'niæ vel Bad'izæ, Aquæ Solis, Aquæ Bad'iguæ*. Celebrated thermal springs at Bath, in England. They contain but little impregnation, and are chiefly indebted to their temperature, from 112° to 117° Fahrenheit, for their utility. The main ingredients are sulphate of lime, chloride of sodium, sulphate of soda, carbonate of lime, protoxide of iron, free carbonic acid and azote.

These waters are employed in the most heterogeneous cases; and are serviceable where the simple thermal springs are indicated, as in rheumatism, paralysis, &c.

BA'THER, same etymon; *Balnea'rius, Balinea'tor, Balnea'tor*, (F.) *Baigneur*. One who bathes. Anciently, the name was given to those that administered baths to the diseased,—the *Étuvistes* of the French. At the present day, in remote districts in Germany, the country people call their medical practitioners Bäder, or 'bathmen,' and Feldscheeren, or 'army barbers.'

BATHMIS, *Bathmus*, 'base, support.' The cavity of a bone, which receives the eminence of another; and especially the two *Fossettes* at the inferior extremity of the humerus into which the processes of the ulna are received, during the flexion and extension of the fore-arm.

BATHRON, *Bathrum Hippoc'ratis, Scamnum Hippoc'ratis, Bate'rion*, 'a step, a ladder.' (F.) *Banc d' Hippocrate*. An instrument, used for the extension of a limb, in cases of fracture or luxation. The description of it is found in Galen, Oribasius, and Scultetus, with a figure.

BATHRUM HIPPOCRATIS, Bathron.

BATIA, Retort.

BATISSE, MINERAL WATERS OF. Batisse is three leagues from Clermont, in France. The water is tepid, and contains subcarbonate and sulphate of soda, sulphates of lime and iron, muriate of magnesia, and carbonate of lime.

BATOS, Rubus Idæus.

BATRACHUS, Ranula.

BATTALISM'US, *Battaris'mus*, from βαρτα-ξυν, 'to stammer.' Balbuties. Stammering with incapacity to pronounce the R.

BATT'ALUS, *Bat'tarus*, same etymon. A stammerer, a stutterer.

BATTARISMUS, Battalismus.

BATTARUS, Battalus.

BATTATA VIRGINIANA, Solanum tuberosum.

BATTEMENS DOUBLES, see *Bruit du Cœur fœtal.*

BATTEMENT, Pulsation.

BAUDRICOURT, MINERAL WATERS OF. Baudricourt is a town of France, two leagues and a half from Mirecourt. The waters are sulphureous.

BAUDRUCHES, Condom.

BAUHIN, VALVE OF, *Valve of* TUL'PIUS, *V. of* FALLO'PIUS, *V. of* VARO'LIUS, *Il'eo-cœcal Valve, Ileo-colic Valve, Val'vula Ilei, Val'vula Coli, V. Cœci, Oper'culum Ilei, Sphincter Ilei*. This name is given to the valve situate transversely at the place where the ileum opens into the cœcum, and which Bauhin says he discovered at Paris, in 1759. It had, however, been previously described by several anatomists; as by Vidus Vidius, Postius, &c.

BAUME, Balsam—*b. d'Acier*, Balsam, chalybeate—*b. Aromatique*, Balsam, aromatic—*b. d'Aiguilles*, Balsam, chalybeate—*b. Apoplectique*, Balsam, apoplectic—*b. d'Arcœus*, Arcœus, balsam of; see, also, Balsam of Arcœus—*b. d'Arcéus*, Unguentum elemi compositum—*b. Benjoin*, Benjamin *b. Blanc*, see Amyris Opobalsamum—*b. du Brésil*, Copaiba—*b. de Canada*, see Pinus balsamea—*b. de Cannelle*, Laurus cinnamomum—*b. de Carpathie*, Balsam of Carpathia—*b. de Carthagène*, see Toluifera balsamum—*b. de Constantinople blanc*, see Amyris opobalsamum—*b. de Copahu*, Copaiba —*b. Cordiale de Sennerte*, Balsam, cordial, of Sennertus — *b. d'Eau à feuilles ridées*, Mentha crispa—*b. de Feuillet*, Balsam, green, of Metz— *b. de Fioraventi spiritueuse*, Balsam, spirituous, of Fioraventi —*b. de Fourcroy* ou *de Laborde*, Balsam of Fourcroy or Laborde—*b. de Galaad*, see Amyris opobalsamum—*b. de Geneviève*, Balsam of Geneviève—*b. Grand*, Tanacetum balsamita—*b. du Grand Caire*, see Amyris opobalsamum — *b. Hypnotique*, Balsam, Hypnotic—*b. Hystérique*, Balsam, hysteric—*b. des Jardins*, Mentha viridis—*b. de Lucatel*, Balsam, Lucatelli's—*b. Nervin*, Balsam, nervous—*b. de Perou*, see Myroxylon Peruiferum—*b. du Samaritain*, Balsam of the Samaritan—*b. Saxon*, Balsam, Saxon—*b. de Soufre*, Balsam of sulfur—*b. de Sympathie*, Balsam of sympathy—*b. Tranquille*, Balsam, tranquil—*b. de Tolu*, see Toluifera balsamum—*b. de Vanille*, Vanilla—*b. Vert*, see Fagara octandra—*b. Vert de Metz*, Balsam, green, of Metz—*b. de Vie d'Hoffmann*, Balsam of Life, of Hoffmann—*b. de Vie de Lelièvre*, Tinctura aloes composita — *b. Vrai*, see Amyris opobalsamum — *b. Vulneraire de Minderer*, Balsam, vulnerary, of Mindererus.

BAURAC, (*Arab.*) Nitre, or salt in general. From this word comes Borax.

BAURIN, MINERAL WATERS OF. Baurin is a village four leagues from Roye, department of Somme. The waters are strongly chalybeate.

BAVE, (F.) *Sali'va ex ore fluens, Spuma, Humor Sali'vus*. Frothy, thick, viscid saliva, issuing from the mouth. This *drivelling* or *slavering*, we see in children, old people, &c. The term is, also, applied to the frothy liquid, which flows from the mouth of rabid animals. Sauvages uses it synonymously with salivation.

BAY, CASTOR, Magnolia glauca — b. Rose, Rhododendron chrysanthemum — b. Rose, American, Rhododendron maximum—b. Sweet, Laurus — b. White, Magnolia glauca and M. macrophylla.

BDALSIS, Sucking.

BDELLA, Hirudo.

BDEL'LIUM. *Myrrha imperfec'ta, Bolchon, Madeleon, Balchus*. A gum-resin, brought from the Levant and India, and supposed to be obtained from a species of *Amyris*, little known. It is solid, brittle, of a deep brown colour, of an acrid and bitter taste, and sweet odour. It was much vaunted by the ancients, but is now little employed. Two different gum-resins have been in the shops distinguished by the names *Indian* and *African bdellium*. Dr. Royle was informed that the former was obtained from *Am'yris Commiph'ora*, growing in India and Madagascar. The latter is said to be from *Heudelo'tia Africa'na*, which grows in Senegal.

BDELLOM'ETER, from βδέλλα, 'a leech,' and μετρον, 'measure.' An instrument, proposed as a substitute for the leech; inasmuch as we can tell the quantity of blood obtained by it, whilst we cannot by the leech. It consists of a cupping-glass, to which a scarificator and exhausting syringe are attached.

BDELLUS, Fart.

BDELYGMIA, Fart.

BDELYGMUS, Fart.

BDESMA, Flatulence.

BDOLUS, Fart.

BEAD TREE, Melia Azedarach.

BEAN, CARTHAGENA, Habilla de Carthagena — b. Egyptian, Nymphæa nelumbo — b. French, Phaseolus vulgaris — b. Garden, common, Vicia faba—b. Indian, Catalpa—b. Kidney, Phaseolus vulgaris — b. Malacca, Avicennia tomentosa — b. Pontic, Nymphæa nelumbo — b. Red, Abrus precatorius — b. Sacred, Nelumbium luteum — b. St. Ignatius's, Ignatia amara—b. Trefoil tree, see Cytisine.

BEAN TREE, WHITE, Cratægus aria.

BEARBERRY, Arbutus uva ursi.

BEARD, *Barba, Pogon, Genei'on, Barbi'tium*, (F.) *Barbe*. The hair which covers a part of the cheeks, the lips, and chin of the male sex, at the age of puberty.

BEAR'S BREECH, Acanthus mollis—b. Foot, Helleborus fœtidus — b. Fright, Heptallon graveolens—b. Whortleberry, Arbutus uva ursi.

BEARWEED, Veratrum viride.

BEASTINGS, Colostrum.

BEATING OF THE HEART, see Heart.

BEAUGENCY, MINERAL WATERS OF. Beaugency is a quarter of a league from Orleans. The waters contain subcarbonate of soda, iron, magnesia, and lime. They are tonic and aperient.

BEAUMONT ROOT, Gillenia trifoliata.

BEAUVAIS, MINERAL WATERS OF. These waters are chalybeate. Beauvais is in Picardie, France.

BEAVER, Castor fiber — b. Wood, Magnolia glauca—b. Tree, Magnolia macrophylla.

BEBEERIA, see Bebeeru.

BEBEERINE, see Bebeeru.

BEBEERU, *Sipeeri*. A tree of British Guiana, which yields two alkalies—*Bebeeria, Beberi'na, Bebee'ria,* and *Sipeerine;* and in its properties resembles the Cinchona. It has been referred to *Nectan'dra Rodiei*. The timber of the tree is known to ship-builders by the name *green* heart. The *Sulphate of Bebeeria* has been employed in intermittents. *Warburg's Fever Drops, Tinctu'ra antifebri'lis Warburgi*, an empirical antiperiodic preparation, have by some been considered to be a tincture of the seeds of the Bebeeru, but this is questionable.

BEC, (F.) *Rostrum*, Beak. This name has been applied to various parts.

BEC CORACOÏDIEN, (F.) *Cor'acoid beak*, is the end of the coracoid process.

BEC DE CUILLER, *Ham'ulus*. An instrument used for the extraction of balls. It consists of an iron rod, 7 or 8 inches long, having at one extremity a small cavity, into which the ball is received to be drawn outwards. See Cochleariformis.

BEC DE GRUE MUSQUÉ, Geranium Moschatum—*b. de Grue Robertin*, Geranium Robertianum—*b. de Lièvre*, Harelip.

BEC DE LA PLUME À ÉCRIRE, (F.) *Beak of the Calamus Scripto'rius*, is a small cavity at the superior part of the medulla oblongata, which forms part of the 4th ventricle.

BEC (LE,) MINERAL WATERS OF. Bec is six leagues from Rouen, in Normandy. The water is strongly chalybeate.

BECCABUNGA, Veronica Beccabunga.

BECHÆSTHE'SIS, from βηξ, 'cough,' and αισθησις, 'sensation.' The excitement or desire to cough.

BECHIA, Tussis.

BECHIAS, Tussis.

BE'CHICS, *Be'chica, Becha, Bec'chica, Be'chita*, from βηξ, 'cough,' (F.) *Béchiques*. Medicines adapted for allaying cough.

BECHITA, Bechic.

BECHIUM, Tussilago.

BECHORTHOPNŒA, Pertussis.

BECUIBA, Ibicuiba.

BED'EGAR, *Bedeguar, Bedeguard, Spon'gia Cynos'bati, Fungus Rosa'rum, F. Cynos'bati*, (F.) *Pomme mousseuse, Éponge d'eglantier*. An excrescence, which makes its appearance on different species of wild roses, and which is produced by the puncture of a small insect,—*Cynips Rosæ*. It was formerly employed as a lithontriptic and vermifuge, but is not now used. It was slightly astringent.

BEDFORD, MINERAL WATERS OF. Bedford is a village, situate on the great Western Turnpike road from Philadelphia to Pittsburg, a few miles east of the chief elevation of the Alleghany mountains. There are various springs, saline, chalybeate and sulphureous.—The most celebrated contains carbonic acid, sulphate of magnesia, chlorides of sodium and calcium, and carbonate of iron.

BEDSTRAW, Galium verum — b. Ladies, greater, Galium mollugo, Galium verum — b. Rough, Galium asprellum — b. Ladies, rough, Galium asprellum.

BEE, Sax. beo. *Apis, A. mellif'ica seu domest'ica, Meli'sa, Melitta*, (F.) *Abeille*. This insect was formerly exhibited, when dried and powdered, as a diuretic.

BEE IN THE BONNET, see Insanity.

BEEBREAD, Propolis.

BEECH, Fagus sylvatica—b. Drop, Orobanche Virginiana — b. Drops, false, Hypopitys lanuginosa — b. Albany, Pterospora Andromedea — b. Mast, see Fagus sylvatica.

BEEF ESSENCE, see Beef tea.

BEEF TEA, *Jus bovi'num*. An infusion of beef, much used in debilitating maladies, and in convalescence. It may be made as follows: Take two pounds and a half of *lean beef*; cut it in small pieces into three parts of *water* in an earthen pipkin; let this simmer, but never boil, until the liquor is consumed to a pint and a half: then strain carefully. It ought to be entirely free from fat or grease.—Dr. E. J. Seymour.

Essence of beef—as it has been called—may be made by putting a pound of good beef, freed from fat, and cut into small pieces, into a porter-bottle, corking lightly. The bottle must be put into boiling water, and kept there until the water has been boiling at least half an hour. As the boiling goes on, the cork may be inserted a little more tightly, to retain the contents of the bottle. The juices of the beef are thus separated, and constitute the 'essence,' which may be seasoned to the taste. It contains much nutriment.

BEEN, Centaurea behen.

BEER, Cerevisia— b. Black, see Falltranck— b. Pipsissewa, see Pyrola umbellata.

BEET, Beta.

BÉGAIEMENT, Balbuties.

BEGMA,—according to some, *Bregma*,—from βηοσειν or βρησσειν, 'to expectorate after coughing.' Coughing; also, the sputum or expectorated matter.—Hippocrates.

BEGO'NIA. The *Begonia grandiflo'ra* and *B. tomento'sa* have astringent roots, which are used in Peru in cases of hemorrhage, scurvy, low fevers, &c.

BÈGUE, Balbus.

BEHEN ABIAD, Centaurea behen — b. Album, Centaurea behen — b. Officinarum, Cucubalus behen — b. Rouge, Statice limonium — b. Vulgaris, Cucubalus behen.

BEHMEN ACKMAR, Statice limonium.

BEIAHALALEN, Sempervivum tectorum.

BEIDELSAR, Asclepias procera.

BEJUIO, Habilla de Carthagena.

BELA-AYE or BE-LAHE. A tonic and astringent bark of a Madagascar tree. Du-petit-Thouars and Sonnerat think it may be substituted for the Simarouba.

BELADAMBOC. A species of convolvulus of the Malabar coast, which contains an acrid milky juice. From this a liniment is formed with oil and ginger, which is used against the bites of rabid animals.

BE-LAHE, Bela-aye.

BELA-MODAGAM. A kind of *Scævola* of the Malabar coast, the leaves of which are considered diuretic and emmenagogue.

BELANDRE, (F.) A litter, surrounded with curtains, in which patients are sometimes carried to hospitals.

BELCHING, Eructation.

BELEMNOID, Belenoid.

BELEMNOIDES PROCESSUS, Styloid processes.

BEL'ENOID, BEL'ONOID, BEL'EMNOID or BEL'OID, *Belenoï'des* or *Belemnoï'des Proces'sus*, from βελος, 'an arrow,' and ειδος, 'shape.' This name has been given to styloid processes in general—*Processus belenoï'des*.

BÉLESME, see Bellesme.

BELESON, Balsam, Mussænda frondosa.

BELILLA, Mussænda frondosa.

BELINUM, Apium Graveolens.

BELI OCULUS, Belloculus.

BELL, CANTERBURY, Campanula trachelium.

BELLADONE, Atropa belladonna.

BELLADON'NA, in the Pharmacopœia of the United States, is the officinal name of the leaves of Atropa Belladonna.

BELLADONNA BACCIFERA, Atropa belladonna— b. Trichotoma, Atropa belladonna.

BELLE DAME, Atropa belladonna.

BELLEGU, Myrobalanus.

BELLEREGI, Myrobalanus.

BELLESME, MINERAL WATERS OF.

B**ellesme** is about three leagues from Montagne in France. The waters are chalybeate.

BELLEY, MINERAL WATERS OF. The waters at Belley, department of Ain, in France, are saline aperients.

BELLIDOIDES, Chrysanthemum leucanthemum.

BELLIS, *Bellus* ('pretty,') *B. peren'nis* seu *minor* seu *horten'sis, Sym'phytum min'imum, Bruisewort, Common Daisy,* (F.) *Paquerette vivace, petite Marguerite.* The leaves and flowers are rather acrid. They were, at one time, considered to cure different species of wounds. See Osmitopsis asteriscoides.

BELLIS HORTENSIS, Bellis—b. Major, Chrysanthemum leucanthemum — b. Minor, Bellis — b. Perennis, Bellis — b. Pratensis, Chrysanthemum leucanthemum.

BELL METAL, *Cal'cocos,* (F.) *Airain, Métal des cloches.* An alloy of copper, zinc, tin, and a small quantity of antimony, used for making bells. The mortars of the apothecary are often formed of this material. They require to be kept clean, to avoid the formation of verdigris.

BELLOC'ULUS, *Beli Oc'ulus.* A kind of gem, which the Assyrians considered efficacious in the cure of many diseases. They imagined that the figure of an eye could be seen in it, and hence its name, *Bel's Eye.*

BELLON, Colic, metallic.

BELLOTAS, see Ilex major.

BELLOWS' SOUND, *Bruit de soufflet*—b. s. Encephalic, see Bruit de soufflet.

BELLOWS' SOUND, FUNIC, a single murmur of the bellows kind, synchronous with the first sound of the heart; heard by some observers, and referred by them to diminished calibre of the umbilical arteries, either by pressure or stretching of the funis, or both.

BELLOWS' SOUND, PLACENTAL, *Bruit placentaire.*

BELLWORT, SMALLER, Uvularia perfoliata.

BELLY, *Venter;* from Ir. bolg, 'the belly, a bag or pouch.' At the present day, the abdomen. Formerly, all the splanchnic cavities were called *bellies;* — the *lower belly, venter in'fimus,* being the abdomen; the *middle belly, venter me'dius,* the thorax; and the *upper belly, venter supre'mus,* the head. Also, the womb. See Venter.

BELLY-ACH, Colica — b. Dry, Colic, metallic—b. Root, Angelica lucida.

BELLY-BAND, Belt, Russian.

BELLY, POT, Physconia.

BELMUSCHUS, Hibiscus abelmoschus.

BELNILEG, Myrobalanus.

BELOID, Belenoid.

BELOIDES PROCESSUS, Styloid processes.

BELONE, Needle.

BELONODES, Styloid.

BELONOID, Belenoid.

BEL'S EYE, Belloculus.

BELT, RUSSIAN, *Ventra'lě,*—vulgarly, *Bellyband,* — *Abdominal supporter.* A broad bandage applied to the abdomen, so as to support, and make methodical pressure upon it. Different forms have been termed *obstetric binders, uteroabdominal supporters, &c.*

BELUL'CUM, from βελος, 'a dart,' and 'ελκω, 'I draw out.' An instrument used for extracting darts or arrows. Many instruments of this kind have been noticed by surgeons.—Ambrose Paré, Fabricius ab Aquapendente.

BELZOE, Benjamin.

BELZOIM, Benjamin.

BELZOINUM, Benjamin.

BEN, Guilandina moringa—b. of Judæa, Benjamin—b. Nut, Guilandina moringa.

BENATH, Pustule.

BENEDICTA SYLVESTRIS, Geum rivale.

BENEDICTUM LAXATIVUM, Confectio sennæ.

BÉNÉFICE DE LA NATURE, Beneficium naturæ—*b. de Ventre,* see Beneficium naturæ.

BENEFIC"IUM NATU'RÆ, (F.) *Bénéfice de la nature.* This term is used by the French pathologists, for cases, in which diseases have got well without medical treatment. With them, *Bénéfice de nature,* or *B. de ventre,* is synonymous also with *Alvi Proflu'vium;*—a spontaneous diarrhœa, often acting favourably either in the prevention or cure of disease.

BENEL, Croton racemosum.

BENEOLENS, from *bene,* 'well,' and *olere,* 'to smell.' *Euo'des, Suaveolens.* A sweet-scented medicine, as gums, &c.

BENG, Bangue.

BENGALE INDORUM, Cassumuniar.

BENGAL ROOT, Cassumuniar.

BENGI, Hyoscyamus.

BENIGN', *Benig'nus, Eueth'es,* (F.) *Bénin, Bénigne.* Diseases of a mild character are so called: as well as medicines whose action is not violent, as a *Benign Fever, Febris benig'na im-pu'tris, &c.*

BÉNIN, Benign.

BEN'JAMIN, *Ben'zoin, Benzo'inum* (Ph. U. S.), *Benzo'inum verum, Benzo'inum, Assa odora'ta, Benjui, Benjuin, Assa dulcis, Ben'jaoy, Benjo'-inum, Belzoë, Belzoim, Ben'zoë, Sty'racis Benzo'-ini Bal'samum, Liquor Cyreni'acus, Croton Benzoë, Ben of Judæ'a, Acor Benzo'inus, Sal Ac"idum* seu *essentia'lě* seu *volat'ilě Benzoës,* (F.) *Benjoin, Baume Benjoin, Assa doux.* A resinous, dry, brittle substance, obtained from *Styrax Benzoin, Arbor Benivi, Laurus Benzoin,* of Sumatra. The odour is extremely fragrant, and taste slightly aromatic. It is principally used for the preparation of the acid which it contains. It is also employed in some vulnerary tinctures, and as an expectorant. Benzoic Acid, *Ac"idum Benzo'icum,* is obtained from it by sublimation. The purest Benjamin is in *amygdaloid masses:* hence called (F.) *Benjoin amygdaloïde.*

BEN'JAMIN, FLOWERS OF, *Ben'zoic Acid, Ac"-idum Benzo'icum, Flores Benzoës, Flores Benzo'-ini, Ac"idum Benzo'icum per sublimatio'nem,* (F.) *Acide Benzoïque.* This acid exists in all the balsams, but chiefly in Benzoin, from which it is obtained by sublimation. It is in vanilla, canella, the urine of infants, and of herbivorous animals. Its odour is aromatic and fragrant; taste hot, slightly acidulous, and agreeable. The crystals consist of white, satiny flakes, slightly ductile. It is probably stimulant; and has been used, as such, in chronic catarrh; but it has little efficacy.

BENJAOY, Benjamin.

BENJOINUM, Benjamin.

BENJUI, Benjamin.

BEN MOENJA. A Malabar tree. An alexipharmic decoction is made of its roots, in the country, which is much praised in cases of malignant fever. Its bark, boiled with *Calamus aromaticus* and salt, forms a decoction used in bites of poisonous serpents.

BENNE, Sesamum orientale.

BENNET, HERB, Geum urbanum, and G. Virginianum.

BENOÎTE, Geum urbanum — *b. Aquatique,* Geum rivale — *b. des Ruisseaux,* Geum rivale — *b. de Virginie,* Geum Virginianum.

BENZIN, see Anæsthetic.

BENZOATE OF AMMONIA, Ammoniæ benzoas.

BENZOE, Benjamin.

BENZOENIL, Vanilla.

BENZOIN, Benjamin—b. Odoriferum Laurus Benzoin.

BERBERINE, see Oxycantha Galeni.
BERBERIS, Oxycantha Galeni—b. Canadensis, see Oxycantha Galeni.
BERCE, Heracleum spondylium.
BERENDAROS, Ocymum basilicum.
BERENICE, Succinum.
BERENICIUM, Potassæ nitras.
BERENISECUM, Artemisia vulgaris.
BERGAMOTE, *Bergamot'ta*, (F.) *Bergamotte*. A small orange, of a very agreeble taste; and peculiar odour. From its bark an oil, *Oleum Berga'mii*, (Ph. U. S.) is obtained, which is much employed as a perfume, and sometimes in medicine.
BER'IBERI, *Beribe'ria, Syn'clonus Beribe'ria, Indosyn'clonus, Paral'ysis Ber'iberi*, from *beri* in the Singhalese language, which signifies 'weakness;' therefore, beriberi, 'great weakness.' This word is also said to be Hindusthanee, and to mean a *sheep*.— Bontius. Beriberi is an Indian disease, little known in Europe. It consists in debility and tremors of the limbs,—sometimes, indeed, of the whole body; with painful numbness of the affected parts, &c.:—the patient walking doubled; and imitating the movements of sheep! Some authors have esteemed it rheumatic; others, paralytic; others, to be a kind of chorea. It is, almost always, incurable; is rarely fatal; and is treated by exercise, stimulant friction, sudorifics, &c. It is sometimes called *Bar'biers*, but this would seem to be a different disease.
BERICOCCE, Prunus armeniaca.
BERLE NODIFLORE, Sium.
BERLUE, Metamorphopsia.
BERMU'DAS, CLIMATE OF. Pulmonary invalids are occasionally sent to Bermuda, but the principal objection to a winter residence there, is the prevalence of strong winds; especially of the dry, sharp, and cold north-west winds, during the winter and spring. Still, it affords a good winter retreat for the phthisical, from any part of the United States, provided due care be selected in choosing a suitable locality. The neighbourhood of Hamilton has been strongly recommended with this view.
BERNARD THE HERMIT, Cancellus.
BERRIES, INDIAN, see Menispermum cocculus—b. Turkey, yellow, see Piper cubeba.
BERS. A sort of electuary, composed of pepper, seed of the white hyoscyamus, opium, euphorbium, saffron, &c. The Egyptians used it as an excitant.—Prospero Alpini.
BERU, MINERAL WATERS OF. Beru is in Champagne, France. The waters are slightly chalybeate.
BERULA, Sium nodiflorum—b. Angustifolia, Sium nodiflorum.
BESASA, Ruta.
BESICLES, Spectacles.
BESOIN, Want—*b. de Respirer*, see Want—*b. de la Vie*, Necessary of life. .
BESSANEM. A word used by Avicenna, for redness of the skin, limbs, and face, produced by the action of cold.
BESSON, } See Gemellus.
BESSONNE,
BETA. The *Beet, Sic'ula*, (F.) *Bette, Betterave*. Family, Chenopodeæ. *Sex. Syst.* Pentandria Digynia. A genus of plants, of which the following are the chief varieties.
BETA HY'BRIDA, *Root of Scarcity*. Root red, outside; white, within. Very nutritive; yields sugar.
BETA VULGA'RIS ALBA, *White Beet*. The root yields sugar, and the leaves are eaten as a substitute for spinach.

BETA VULGA'RIS RUBRA, *Red Beet*. Root red and nutritive; yields a small quantity of sugar.
BETEL, *Piper Betel*. A species of pepper, cultivated in several parts of India. The East Indians are in the habit of chewing the leaves with lime and areca; and they give the name *Betel* to this preparation. It is used in all the equatorial countries of Asia. Betel is said to be tonic and astringent. It is also called *Bette, Bètre, Betle*. See Areca.
BETHROOT, Trillium latifolium—b. Broadleaf, Trillium latifolium.
BÉTISE, Dementia.
BÉTOINE, Betonica officinalis—*b. des Montagnes*, Arnica Montana—*b. des Savoyards*, Arnica montana.
BÉTON, Colostrum.
BETONICA AQUATICA, Scrophularia aquatica.
BETON'ICA OFFICINA'LIS, *Cestron, Beton'ica purpu'rea, Veton'ica Cordi*, &c., *Bet'ony, Wood Betony, Psychot'rophum, Veroni'ca purpu'rea*, (F.) *Bétoine*. Family, Labiatæ. *Sex. Syst.* Didynamia Gymnospermia. Betony was in much esteem amongst the ancients, who employed the flowers and leaves, in decoction, in gout, sciatica, cephalalgia, &c. It was so called, according to Pliny, from being in great repute among the Vettones, or Bettones, an ancient people of Spain. Antonius Musa is said to have written a volume in praise of it; recommending it in no less than 47 different diseases. It has, however, little or no virtue. The leaves are said to be aperient, and the root emetic.
BETONICA PAULI, Veronica.
BETONY, Betonica officinalis—b. Paul's, Lycopus sinuatus, Lycopus Virginicus — b. Water, Scrophularia aquatica—b. Wood, Betonica officinalis.
BÊTRE, Betel.
BETTE, Beta.
BETTERAVE, Beta.
BET'ULA ALBA. The *Birch*, (F.) *Bouleau commun*. The young leaves are slightly odorous, astringent, and bitter. They are applied to wounds and ulcers. They have been regarded as antiscorbutic and anthelmintic. The tree furnishes a saccharine juice, which is considered antiscorbutic and diuretic.
BETULA EMARGINATA, Alnus glutinosa—b. Glutinosa, Alnus glutinosa.
BETULA LENTA, *Sweet Birch, Black Birch, Cherry Birch, Mountain Mahogany*, is an American species, the bark and leaves of which have the smell and taste of Gaultheria procumbens. An infusion is sometimes made of them, and used as an excitant and diaphoretic. The volatile oil is nearly if not wholly identical with that of Gaultheria.
BEURRE, Butter—*b. de Bambouc*, Butter of bambouc—*b. de Cacao*, Butter of cacao—*b. de Coco*, Butter of cocoa—*b. Végétale*, Persea gatissima.
BEUVRIGNY, MINERAL WATERS OF. Beuvrigny is in the vicinity of Bayeux in Normandy. The water is chalybeate.
BÉVUE, Diplopia.
BEX, Tussis—b. Convulsiva, Pertussis—b. Humida, Expectoration—b. Theriodes, Pertussis.
BEXIS, Tussis.
BEXU'GO. Under this name, a purgative root was formerly introduced into Europe from Peru. It is supposed to have been the root of a Hippocratea.
BEZ'OAR, *Bez'aar, Bez'chard, Pa'zahar*, from Persian Pa, 'against,' and *zahar*, poison. *Lapis Besoar'dicus, Cal'culus Bez'oar, Enterol'ithus Be-*

soar'dus, Bezoard. A calculous concretion, found in the stomach, intestines, and bladder of animals. Wonderful virtues were formerly attributed to these Bezoars. There were two great varieties: the *Bez'oar orienta'lĕ, An'imal Bezoar'ticum orienta'lĕ,* formed in the fourth stomach of the gazelle of India (*Gazel'la In'dica,* or rather *Antil'opĕ cervica'pra :*) and the *Bez'oar occidenta'lĕ, Animal Bezoar'ticum occidenta'lĕ,* found in the fourth stomach of the *wild goat* or *chamois* of Peru. These substances were esteemed to be powerful alexipharmics; but the former was the more valued. It was believed that no poison, and no eruptive, pestilential, or putrid disease, could resist its influence. As so many virtues were ascribed to it, other animal concretions were substituted for it; and factitious Bezoards were made of crabs' eyes and claws, bruised and mixed with musk, ambergris, &c.

Bez'oar Bovi'num, (F.) *Bézoard de Bœuf, Bezoard of the beef.* A concretion formed in the fourth stomach of beeves; also, a biliary calculus found in the gall-bladder.

Bez'oar of the Deer, *B. of the Lach'rymal Fossa of the Deer, Deer's Tears.* A moist, highly odorous, fatty matter, found below the anterior canthus of the orbit of the red deer—*Cervus el'ephas.* It has been used, like castor, as an antispasmodic, in the dose of from 5 to 15 grains, two or three times a day.

Bezoar Equinum, Bezoar of the horse — b. Hystricis, Bezoar of the Indian porcupine.

Bez'oard of Cayman. This was once much prized. It is now unknown.

BÉZOARD D'ALLEMAGNE, Ægagropila.

Bez'oard of the Chamois, and B. of the Horse, *Bezoar equi'num, Hippol'ithus,* &c., exhibit their origin in the name.

Bez'oard of the Indian Por'cupine. *Bez'oar Hys'tricis, Lapis Porci'nus, Lapis Malucen'cis, Petro del Porco,* (F.) *Bézoard de Porc-Épic,* was formerly the dearest of all the Bezoards, and was sold at an enormous price in Spain and Portugal.

Bez'oard Mineral, Antimonium diaphoreticum—b. Vegetable, see Calappite.

BEZOAR'DIC, *Bezoar'dicus,* (F.) *Bézoardique;* concerning the bezoard. Bezoardic medicines are those supposed to possess the same properties with the bezoard; as antidotes, alexiteria, alexipharmics, cordials.

BEZOARDICA RADIX, Dorstenia contrayerva.

BEZOAR'DICUM SATUR'NI. A pharmaceutical preparation, regarded by the ancients as antihysteric. It was formed of protoxide of lead, butter of antimony, and nitric acid.

Bezoar'dicum Huma'num. Urinary calculi were formerly employed under this name as powerful alexipharmics.

Bezoar'dicum Jovia'le. A sort of greenish powder, used as a diaphoretic, and formed of antimony, tin, mercury, and nitric acid.

Bezoar'dicum Luna're. A medicine formerly regarded as a specific in epilepsy, convulsions, megrim, &c. It was prepared of nitrate of silver, and butter of antimony.

Bezoar'dicum Martia'le. A tonic medicine, used by the ancients in diarrhœa. It was prepared from the tritoxide of iron and butter of antimony.

Bezoar'dicum Mercuria'le. A medicine, formerly vaunted as an antisyphilitic, and prepared from the mild chloride of mercury, butter of antimony, and nitric acid.

Bezoar'dicum Minera'le; the deutoxide of antimony; so called because its properties were supposed to resemble those of animal bezoard.

Bezoar'dicum Sola're. A diaphoretic medicine, prepared of gold filings, nitric acid, and butter of antimony.

Bezoar'dicum Ven'eris. A pharmaceutical preparation, formerly employed in lepra, diseases of the brain, &c.; which was made from filings of copper, butter of antimony, and nitric acid.

BHANG, Bangue.

BI, as a prefix to words, has the same signification as Di.

BIAIOTHANATI, Biothanati.

BIBITORIUS, Rectus internus oculi.

BIBLIOG'RAPHY, MED'ICAL, from $\beta\iota\beta\lambda o\varsigma$, 'a book,' and $\gamma\rho\alpha\phi\omega$, 'I describe.' Skill in the knowledge of medical books. The most distinguished medical biographers have been: J. A. Van der Linden, Amstelod. 1662, octavo, (L.) M. Lipenius, Francf. ad Mœn. 1679, fol. (L.) G. A. Mercklein, Norimb. 1686, (L.) J. J. Manget, Genev. 1695 to 1731, (L.) Tarin (anatomical,) Paris, 1753, (F.) A. von Haller, Zürich, 1774, &c.. (L.) Vigiliis von Creutzenfeld (surgical,) Vindob. 1781, (L.) C. G. Kühn, Lips. 1794, (L.) C. L. Schweickard (anat., phys., and legal medicine,) Stuttgard, 1796 to 1800, (L.) G. G. Ploucquet, Tubing. 1808 to 1814, (L.) C. F. Burdach, Gotha, 1810 to 1821, (G.) J. S. Ersch, (since 1750,) Leips. 1822, (G.) Th. Ch. Fr. Enslin, (of Germany, since 1750,) Berlin, 1826, (G.) J. B. Montfalcon, Paris, 1827, (F.) J. Forbes, M. D., F. R. S., London, 1835. A. C. P. Callisen, Copenhagen, 1845, (G.) E. Morwitz, Leipzig, 1849, (G.)

BICAUDALIS, Retrahens auris.

BICAUDA'TUS, *Cauda'tus,* 'double-tailed.' A monster having two tails.

BICEPHA'LIUM, *Dicepha'lium.* A hybrid word, from *bi* and $\kappa\epsilon\phi\alpha\lambda\eta$, 'head.' Sauvages applies this epithet to a very large sarcoma on the head, which seems to form a double head.

BICEPHALUS, Dicephalus.

BICEPS, from *bis*, 'twice,' and *caput*, 'head.' That which has two heads. This name has been particularly given to two muscles; one belonging to the arm, the other to the thigh.

Biceps Exter'nus Mus'culus. The long portion of the *Triceps Brachia'lis.*—Douglas.

Biceps Flexor Cruris, *Biceps Cruris, Biceps,* (F.) *Biceps Crural, Biceps Fem'oris, Is'chio-fem'oro-péronier*—(Ch.) A muscle on the posterior part of the thigh; one head arising from the tuberosity of the ischium, and the other from a great part of the linea aspera. It is inserted into the top of the fibula. It serves to bend the leg on the thigh.

Biceps Flexor Cu'biti, *Biceps Bra'chii, Cor'aco-radia'lis, Biceps, Biceps manûs, Biceps inter'nus, Biceps inter'nus hu'meri,* (F.) *Scapulo-radial,* (Ch.)—*Biceps Brachial.* A muscle, situate at the anterior and internal part of the arm; extending from the edge of the glenoid cavity and from the top of the coracoid process to the tuberosity of the radius. It bends the fore-arm upon the arm.

BICHE DE MER, Sea Slug. A molluscous animal, belonging to the genus Holothuria, which is caught amongst the islands of the Feejee group, New Guinea, &c., and when prepared finds a ready sale in China, where it is used as an ingredient in rich soups.

BICHET, Terra Orleana.

BICHICH'IÆ. Pectoral medicines, composed of liquorice juice, sugar, blanched almonds, &c.— Rhazes.

BICHIOS, Dracunculus.

BICHO, Dracunculus—b. di Culo, Proctocace.

BICHOS. A Portuguese name for the worms

that penetrates the toes of people in the Indies; and which are destroyed by the oil of the cashew nut.

BICIP'ITAL, from *biceps* (*bis* and *caput*) 'two-headed.' Relating to the biceps.

BICIP'ITAL GROOVE, (F.) *Coulisse* ou *Gouttière bicipitale, Coulisse humérale,* (CH.,) is a longitudinal groove, situate between the tuberosities of the os humeri, which lodges the long head of the biceps.

BICIP'ITAL TU'BERCLE, *Bicipital tuberos'ity,* (F.) *Tubérosité bicipitale;*—a prominence near the upper extremity of the radius, to which the tendon of the biceps is attached.

BICORNE RUDE, Ditrachyceros.

BICUS'PID, *Bicuspida'tus*, from *bis*, 'twice,' and *cuspis*, 'a spear.' That which has two points or tubercles.

BICUS'PID TEETH, *Dentes Bicuspida'ti*, (F.) *Dents bicuspidées,* the small molares. See Molar.

BIDENS ACMELLA, Spilanthus acmella.

BIDET, (F.) *Bidet;* pronounced *beeday*. A small horse formerly allowed to each trooper for carrying his baggage. Hence, perhaps, applied to a chamber bathing apparatus, which has to be bestridden. It is a useful arrangement, in case of hemorrhoids, prolapsus ani, affections of the sexual organs, &c.

BIECHO, Bische.

BIÈRE, Cerevisia.

BIESTINGS, Colustrum.

BIFÉMORO-CALCANIEN, Gastrocnemii.

BI'FURCATION, *Bifurca'tio,* from *bis*, 'twice,' and *furca*, 'a fork.' Division of a trunk into two branches; as the *bifurcation of the trachea, aorta,* &c.

BIGASTER, Digastricus.

BIG BLOOM, Magnolia macrophylla.

BIGEMINAL BODIES, Quadrigemina tubercula.

BIGGAR. A disease of Bengal, remarkable for the intensity and danger of the cerebral symptoms.—Twining.

BIG-LEAF, Magnolia macrophylla.

BIGLES, see Strabismus.

BIGNONIA CATALPA, Catalpa—b. Radicans, Tecoma radicans.

BIGNO'NIA IN'DICA. The leaves are employed in India, as emollients, to ulcers.

BIJON, see Pinus sylvestris.

BILAZAY, MINERAL WATERS OF. Bilazay is a town in France, two leagues from Thouar, department of Deux Sèvres, near which is a thermal sulphureous spring. Temperature about 77° Fahrenheit.

BILBERRY, Vaccinium myrtillus — b. Red, Vaccinium vitis idæa.

BILE, *Bilis, Fel, Chol'os, Cholē, Choler,* (F.) *Bile, Fiel.* A yellow, greenish, viscid, bitter, nauseous fluid, secreted by the liver. It is distinguished into *hepatic* and *cystic;* according as it flows immediately into the duodenum from the liver or from the gall-bladder. It contains, according to Muratori, water; a peculiar fatty matter; colouring matter, (*Cholepyr'rhin* or *Bili-phæ'in;*) cholesterin, combined with soda; picromel or *bilin;* extract of flesh, mucus; soda, phosphate of soda; phosphate of lime, and chloride of sodium.

The use of the bile is to remove from the body superfluous hydro-carbon; and it is probably insorvient to useful purposes in digestion.

BILE, Furunculus — b. Black, Atrabilis — b. *de Bœuf*, see Bile — b. *Repandue*, Icterus.

BILE OF THE BEAR, *Gall of the Bear, Fel Ursi,* was thought to be anti-epileptic; and that of the *Eel, Fel anguil'læ,* to facilitate labour.

BILE OF THE OX, *Gall of the Ox, Ox Gall, Fel Tauri, Fel Bovis, F. Bovi'num,* (F.) *Bile de Bœuf,* was once reputed cosmetic and detergent, antiotalgic and emmenagogue; as well as to possess the power of facilitating labour. It has also been given as a bitter stomachic and anthelmintic; and as a tonic and laxative, in cases of deficiency of the biliary secretion.

BIL'IARY, *Bilia'ris, Bilia'rius, Fel'leus.* That which relates to bile.

BIL'IARY APPARA'TUS, *B. organs, B. passages.* The collection of parts that concur in the secretion and excretion of bile: — viz. the liver, pori biliarii or tubuli biliferi; hepatic, cystic, and choledoch ducts, and gall-bladder.

BIL'IARY CONCRE'TIONS are concretions found in some parts of the biliary apparatus.

BILIARY DUCTS, Pori biliarii.

BILIEUX, Bilious.

BILIMBI, Averrhoa bilimbi.

BILIMBING TERES, Averrhoa bilimbi.

BILIN, Picromel.

BIL'IOUS, *Bilio'sus, Chol'icus, Chol'ius, Fellin'eus, Epich'olos, Picroch'olos, Fel'leus.* (F.) *Bilieux.* That which relates to bile, contains bile, or is produced by bile. An epithet given to certain constitutions and diseases, which are believed to be the effect of superabundance of the biliary secretion: as *Bilious temperament, B. symptoms, B. fever.*

BILIPHÆIN, see Bile.

BILIS FLUXIO, Cholera morbus.

BILITICUS, Cholagogue.

BILIVERD'IN, from *bilis*, 'bile,' and *viridis*, 'green.' On adding an acid to a solution of the yellow colouring matter of bile, a precipitate of green flocculi takes place, which possesses all the properties of chlorophyll, or the green colouring matter of leaves. This is the *biliverdin* of Berzelius.

BILOCULAR, see Unilocular.

BILUMBI BITING-BING, Malus Indica.

BI'MANUS, from *bis* and *manus*, 'a hand.' One that has two hands. A term applied only to man, because he is the sole mammiferous animal that possesses two perfect hands.

BINDER, Bandage.

BINDERS, OBSTETRIC, see Belt, Russian.

BINDWEED, Polygonum aviculare — b. Fiddle-leaved, Convolvulus panduratus — b. Great, Convolvulus sepium — b. Lavender-leaved, Convolvulus Cantabrica—b. Sea, Convolvulus soldanella—b. Virginian, Convolvulus panduratus.

BINKOHUMBA, Phyllanthus urinaria.

BINOC'ULAR, *Binocula'ris:* same etymon as the next. Relating to or affecting both eyes—as '*binocular vision*'—vision with both eyes; or from impressions made upon both retinæ, which are amalgamated into *single vision.*

BINOC'ULUS, *Bin'ocle, Diophthal'mica Fas'cia, Oc'ulis duplex,* from *bis*, 'twice,' and *oculus,* 'an eye.' (F.) *Œil double.* A bandage applied over both eyes. It was, also, formerly called *Diophthal'mus.*

BIN'SICA. Disorder of the mind. According to VAN HELMONT, an atrophy of the organ of imagination.

BIOCHYMIA, Chymistry, vital.

BIOD, Vis vitalis.

BIODYNAM'ICS, *Biodynam'ica, Biodynam'icē, Biosoph'ia,* from βιος, 'life,' and δυναμις, 'power,' 'force.' The doctrine of the vital activity, or forces.

BIOGAMIA, Magnetism, animal.

BIOLOGY, Physiology.

BIOLYCHNION, *Biolych'nium,* from βιος, 'life,' and λυχνιον, 'a lamp.' Innate heat, vital heat, animal heat. *Lych'nium, Lychnid'ium, Thermum em'phytum, Flamma seu Flum'mula vita'lis* seu *cordis.* Also, a secret preparation of which BEGUIN and BURGRAVE make mention.

BIOLYSIS, see Biolytic.

BIOLYT'IC, *Biolyt'icus;* from βιος, 'life,' and λυσις, 'solution.' Relating to the destruction of life. A '*biolytic* agent' is one that causes *biol'ysis,* or destruction of life.—Schultz.

BIOMAGNETISMUS, Magnetism, animal.

BIONOMY, Physiology.

BIOPHÆNOMENOLOGIA, Physiology.

BIOS, βιος. Life. Also, what is necessary for the preservation of life.

BIOSOPHIA, Biodynamics.

BIOSTATICS, Statistics, medical.

BIOTE, Life.

BIOTHAN'ATI, *Biaiothan'ati,* from βιος, 'life,' and θανατος, 'death.' Those who die of a violent death very suddenly, or as if there was no space between life and death.

BIOTIC, Vital.

BIOTICS, Physiology.

BIOTOMIA, Vivisection.

BIPARIETAL SUTURE, Sagittal suture.

BIPIN'NA, from *bis,* 'twice,' and *pinna,* 'a wing-feather.' A term used by the ancients for a diminutive penis, not exceeding in size two quills.

BIR, Thorax.

BIRA, Cerevisia.

BIRCH, Betula alba—b. Black, Betula lenta—b. Cherry, Betula lenta—b. Sweet, Betula lenta.

BIRDS' NEST, Hypopitys lanuginosa.

BIRTH, CROSS, Presentation, preternatural b. Live, see Born alive—b. Plural, see Multiparous.

BIRTHWORT, Aristolochia—b. Snakeroot, Aristolochia serpentaria.

BISCHE, *Biecho.* A malignant kind of dysentery, which often prevails in the island of Trinidad.

BISCUIT, *Biscoc'tus, bis,* 'twice,' and *coctus,* 'baked,' (F.) *bis* and *cuit,* 'twice baked.' A kind of dry, hard bread, or cake, which is variously made; and, when without eggs or butter, is easy of digestion. It was formerly called *Di'pyri'tes,* and *Di'pyros.*

BISCUIT, MEAT. An alimentary preparation, proposed by Mr. G. Borden, Jr., of Texas, which consists in combining the matters extracted from meat by boiling with flour, so as to form biscuits; which keep well, and are of course nutritive.

BISERMAS, Salvia sclarea.

BISFERIENS, Dicrotus.

BISHOP'S WEED, Ammi.

BISLINGUA, Ruscus hypoglossum.

BISMALVA, Althæa.

BISMUTH, *Antimo'nium album, Chalcitas, Luna imperfec'ta, Stannum glacia'lë* seu *cinereum, Bismu'thum, Wismu'thum. Reg'ulus of Bis'muth, Marcasi'ta, Tin glass,* (F.) *Étain gris, É. de Glace.* A metal, in spicular plates, of a yellowish-white colour; s. gr. 9.822; fusible at 400° Fahrenheit, and volatilizable at a high temperature. It is used only in the preparation of the subnitrate.

BISMUTH, OXYD OF, Bismuth, Subnitrate of—b. Regulus of, Bismuth.

BISMUTH, SUBNI'TRATE OF, *Bismu'thi subni'tras, Marcasi'ta alba, Plumbum cine'reum, Magiste'rium Marcasi'tæ* seu *Bismuthi, Bismu'thum Nit'ricum, B. Subnit'ricum, Nitras Subbismu'thicum, Nitras Bismuthi, Calx Vismu'thi, Bismu'thum oxydula'tum album, Oxyd of Bismuth, Mag"istery of Bismuth, Pearl White, Spanish White.* (F.) *Sousnitrate de bismuth, Oxide blanc de B., Blanc de fard, Blanc de perle.* (*Bismuth.* in frustulis, ℥j. Acid nitric. f℥ij. Aq. destill. q. s. Mix a fluid ounce of distilled water with the nitric acid, and dissolve the bismuth in the mixture. When the solution is complete, pour the clear liquor into three pints of distilled water, and set the mixture by, that the powder may subside. Lastly, having poured off the supernatant fluid, wash the subnitrate of bismuth with distilled water, wrap it in bibulous paper, and dry with a gentle heat. Ph. U. S.) It is considered to be tonic and antispasmodic, and has been chiefly used in gastrodynia.

BISMUTH, VALE'RIANATE OF, *Bismu'thi valeri'anas, Bismu'thum valerian'icum.* Prepared by mixing a neutral solution of *oxide of bismuth* in *nitric acid,* with *valerianate of soda;* washing, and drying the precipitate. Used in gastrodynia, chronic gastralgia, neuralgia, and chronic palpitation, as a nervine. Dose, ½ a grain to 2 grains, three or four times a day, in pill.

BISMUTHI NITRAS, Bismuth, Subnitrate of—b. Valerianas, Bismuth, valerianate of.

BISMUTHUM, Bismuth — b. Nitricum, Bismuth, subnitrate of — b. Oxydulatum album, Bismuth, subnitrate of—b. Subnitricum, Bismuth, subnitrate of — b. Valerianicum, Bismuth, valerianate of.

BISPIRUS, Dipnoos.

BISSUM, Hydrangea arborescens.

BISSUS. The silky filaments which fix the *Pinna Mari'na* to the rocks. In Italy and Corsica, clothes are made of these, which are considered to favour perspiration, and are recommended to be worn next the skin in rheumatism, gout, &c. See Byssus.

BISTORT, OFFICINAL, Pylygonum bistorta—b. Virginian, Polygonum virginianum.

BISTORTA, Polygonum bistorta.

BISTORTIER, (F.) A name given by the *Pharmacien* to a long wooden pestle used for reducing soft substances to powder, and in the preparation of electuaries.

BISTOURI, (F.) *Pistorien'sis gla'dius, Scalpel'lus, Scal'peum, Bistoury.* A small cutting-knife, used in surgery,—so called, according to Huet, from the town of Pistori, which was formerly celebrated for the manufacture of those instruments. A bistoury has the form of a small knife, and is composed of a blade and handle. The blade, which is most commonly movable in the handle, may be fixed by a button, spring, &c. When fixed in the handle, the bistoury is called by the French, *B. à lame fixe* ou *dormante.*

The chief bistouries are:—1. The STRAIGHT B. (F.) *B. droit,* in which the blade and cutting edge are straight, the point being fine, round, or square. 2. The CONVEX B. (F.) *B. convexe;* the blade of which is convex at the cutting edge, concave at the back. 3. The CONCAVE B. (F.) *B. concave;* the blade of which is concave at its edge, and convex at the back. 4. BLUNT-POINTED B. (F.) *B. boutonné;* the blade of which has a button at its extremity. 5. The BLUNT OR PROBE-POINTED BISTOURY OF POTT; concave at its cutting edge, and its point blunt; so that it can be carried on the palmar surface of the index finger, to divide the stricture, in strangulated hernia. Sir Astley Cooper has recommended a useful modification of this, to avoid wounding the intestine, should it come in contact with the edge of the knife. His Bistoury has an edge of not more than eight lines in length, situate about five lines from the point. 6. BISTOURI À LA LIME, (F.) is a straight bistoury; the blade fixed in the handle, the extremity with a button, and the edge made with a file. It is chiefly used for dilating parts. 7. BISTOURI ROYAL, (F.) A Bistoury used in operating upon Louis XIV., for fistula in ano. 8. BISTOURI GASTRIQUE, (F.) A complicated instrument, invented by Morand, for dilating wounds of the abdomen. 9. BISTOURI CACHÉ, *B. herniaire*, ou *Attrape-lourdaud de Biennaise, Forceps decepto'ria*. A curved bistouri, the blade of which is placed in a canula, whence it issues on pressing a spring.

The word *Bistouri* is used by the French, at times, where we would employ knife.

BIT NOBEN, *Salt of Bitu'men, Padnoon, Soucherloon, Khala mimuc*. A white, saline substance, which is a Hindoo preparation of great antiquity, and has been supposed to be the *Sal asphalti'tes and Sal Sodome'nus* of the ancients. It is used by the Hindoo in the prevention or cure of almost all diseases.

BITHNIMAL'CA, *Gas'teranax*. Two unmeaning words, used by Dolæus, to designate an active principle supposed to have its seat in the stomach, and to preside over chymification, &c.

BITIOS DE KIS, Proctocace.

BITTER, Amarus — b. Bark, Pinckneya pubens — b. Bloom, Chironia angularis — b. Holy, Hiera picra — b. Redberry, Cornus Florida — b. Root, Apocynum androsæmifolium, Gentiana Catesbæi, Menyanthes verna — b. Sweet nightshade, Solanum Dulcamara — b. Sweet vine, Solanum Dulcamara.

BIT'TERNESS, *Amaritu'do, Amarit'ies, Amaror, Pi'cria*, (F.) *Amertume*. A particular taste, which belongs to many substances. In some diseases there is a sense of bitterness felt in the mouth.

BITTERS, COLUMBO, Tinctura Calumbæ — b. Spirit, Tinctura gentianæ composita—b. Wine, Vinum gentianæ compositum.

BITTERSWEET, Solanum dulcamara.

BITTERWEED, Ambrosia trifida.

BITTERWOOD TREE, Quassia.

BITTOS. A disease, in which the chief symptom is an acute pain in the anus.—Chomel.

BITUMEN, GLUTINOUS, Pissasphaltum — b. Judaicum, Asphaltum — b. of Judæa, Asphaltum—b. Petroleum, Petrolæum—b. Malta, Pissasphaltum — b. Salt of, Bitnoben — b. Solidum, Asphaltum.

BIVENTER, Digastricus — b. Cervicis, Complexus musculus — b. Maxillæ, Digastricus.

BIVENTRAL LOBE OF THE CEREBELLUM, see Lobe, biventral.

BIXA AMERICANA, see Terra Orleana — b. Orleana, see Terra Orleana — b. Orellana, see Terra Orleana.

BLABE, Wound.

BLACCIÆ, Rubeola.

BLACIA, Debility.

BLACKBERRY, AMERICAN, see Rubus fruticosus — b. High or standing, see Rubus fruticosus.

BLACK DOSE, see Infusum Sennæ compositum.

BLACK DRAUGHT, see Infusum Sennæ compositum.

BLACK DROP, Guttæ nigræ.

BLACK LION. A term given to a sloughing syphilitic ulcer, under which the British soldiers suffered greatly in Portugal.

BLACK ROOT, Aletris farinosa, Leptandria purpurea.

BLACKWATER, Pyrosis.

BLADDER, GALL, see Gall Bladder—b. Irritable, Cysterethismus — b. Swim, Air bladder — b. Urinary, see Urinary Bladder.

BLADUM, *Blé*.

BLÆSITAS, *Blæsa lingua*. Some authors have used this word as synonymous with stammering. See Balbuties. Sauvages understands by it a defect in pronunciation, which consists in substituting soft consonants for those that are hard; as the z for s, the D for T, the s for G and J, &c. Also, Lisping, *Traulis'mus, Trau'lotes*, (F.) *Blésite, Blé (parler)*.

BLÆSOPODES, see Kyllosis.

BLÆSOPUS, see Kyllosis.

BLÆSUS. A distortion; especially the outward distortion of the legs. Also, a stammerer.

BLAFARD, (F.) *Pal'lidus, Pallid'ulus*. This epithet is sometimes given to the skin, when pale and dull; but, most frequently, to the flesh of a wound, when it has lost its colour, and become white. The word is, also, sometimes used synonymously with Albino.

BLANO DE BALEINE, Cetaceum — b. de Fard, Bismuth, subnitrate of—b. de *l'Œil*, Scleroticº—b. *d'Œuf*, Albumen ovi—b. *de Perle*, Bismuth, subnitrate of.

BLANC-MANGER, (F.) *Cibus albus, Leucopha'gium, Leucoph'agum, Argyrotrophe'ma*. An animal jelly, so called on account of its colour, combined with an emulsion of sweet almonds, to which sugar has been added, and some aromatic. It is sometimes prescribed as a nutriment in convalescence and chronic diseases.

BLANC-RAISIN, Blanc Rhazis.

BLANC RHAZIS, *Blanc-raisin*. An ointment composed of cerussa, white wax, and olive oil.

BLANCA, Plumbi subcarbonas.

BLANCH, TO, from (F.) *blanchir*, 'to whiten, to bleach.' To whiten by depriving of the outer rind; as 'to *blanch* almonds;' i. e. to peel them.

BLANCHET, (F.) A blanket. A term given, by the French Pharmaciens, to the woollen strainer through which they filter syrup and other thick fluids. See, also, Aphthæ.

BLANCHING, Etiolation.

BLANCNON ORIBASII, Polypodium filix mas.

BLAS. An unmeaning term, invented by Van Helmont to designate a kind of movement in the body; at times, local,—at others, under extraneous influence. Thus, he speaks of the *Blas meteoros* of the heavenly bodies, and the *Blas huma'num*, that which operates in man.

BLAS ALTERATIVUM, Plastic force.

BLASÉ, (F.) An epithet given to one whom the abuse of enjoyment has prevented from any longer deriving satisfaction or pleasure from it.

BLASTE'MA, *Blaste'sis*, from βλαστανω, 'I bud.' A germ. The sense of this word, which is often used by Hippocrates, is obscure. Castelli thinks it means the eruption of some morbific principle at the surface of the body. Also, the matrix or general formative element of tissues.

BLAS'TEMAL, *Blastema'lis*. Relating or appertaining to a blastema, — as 'blastemal formations,' those that are formed from a blastema.

BLASTODERMA, see Molecule.

BLATTA BYZAN'TIA, *Unguis odora'tus*, (F.) *Blatte de Bysance*. This name seems, formerly, to have been given to a marine production from some of the Conchylia. It had an agreeable smell, a reddish tint, and the shape of a nail. It was prescribed in epilepsy, hysteria, and hepatic obstructions. Rondelet affirms that it was the production of the shell-fish *murex* or *purpura*; and that the name *Blatta* is derived from the Greek βλαττος, 'purple.'

BLAVELLE, Centaurea cyanus.

BLAVÉOLE, Centaurea cyanus.

BLAVEROLLE, Centaurea cyanus.

BLAZING-STAR, Chamælirium luteum, Liatris.

BLÉ, *Bladum*. This word answers, in France,

to the word *Corn* in England; i. e. any kind of grain employed for making bread. Wheat being most commonly used for this purpose, *Blé* is sometimes restricted to this. *Blé méteil* is a mixture of wheat and rye.

BLÉ CORNU, Ergot—*b. d'Espagne*, Zea mays—*b. d'Italie*, Zea Mays—*b. Métteil*, see *Blé*—*b. Noir*, Polygonum fagopyrum—*b. de Turquie*, Zea mays.

BLÉ (PARLER,) Blæsitas.
BLEABERRY, Vaccinium myrtillus.
BLEACHING LIQUID, *Eau de javelle*.
BLEAR-EYE, Lippitudo.
BLEB, Bulla.
BLECHNON, Polypodium filix mas.
BLECHNUM LIGNIFOLIUM, Asplenium Scolopendrium—b. Squamosum, Asplenium ceterach.
BLECHROPYRA, see Blechros.
BLECHROPYRUS, Typhus mitior.
BLECHROS, βληχρος, 'weak, feeble, slow.' An epithet applied to different affections, and particularly to fevers. Hence *Blechrop'yra*, 'a slow fever:' *Blechrosphyg'mia*, 'a slow pulse.'
BLECHROSPHYGMIA, see Blechros.
BLED. Corn.
BLEEDING, Bloodletting, Hæmorrhagia.
BLEEDING FROM THE NOSE, Epistaxis—b. Heart, Cypripedium luteum.
BLÊME, (F.) This word has nearly the same signification as *Blafard*. Generally, however, it includes, also, emaciation of the countenance.
BLENNA, Mucus—b. Narium, Nasal mucus.
BLENNADENI'TIS, from βλεννα, 'mucus,' αδην, 'a gland,' and *itis*, denoting inflammation. Inflammation of mucous follicles.
BLENNELYT'RIA, from βλεννα, 'mucus,' and ελυτρον, 'a sheath.' A discharge of mucus from the vagina. Leucorrhœa.—Alibert.
BLENNEM'ESIS. *Blennoëm'esis, Vom'itus pituito'sus*, from βλεννα, 'mucus,' and εμεσις, 'vomiting.' Vomiting of mucus.
BLENNENTERIA, Dysentery.
BLENNISTH'MIA, from βλεννα, 'mucus,' and ισθμος, 'the gullet.' Increased flow of mucus from the pharynx and larynx.—Alibert.
BLENNOCHEZIA, Diarrhœa, mucous.
BLENNOCYSTIDES, Bursæ mucosæ.
BLENNODES, Muciform.
BLENNOËMESIS, Blennemesis.
BLENNOG''ENOUS, *Blennog''enus, Mucif'ic, Mucif'icus*, from βλεννα, 'mucus,' and γενναω, 'I form.' Forming or generating mucus. Breschet and Roussel de Vauzème describe an apparatus of this kind for the secretion of the mucous matter that constitutes the cuticle, composed of a glandular parenchyma or organ of secretion situate in the substance of the true skin, and of excretory ducts, which issue from the organ, and deposite the mucous matter between the papillæ.
BLENNOIDES, Muciform.
BLENNOIDEUS, Muciform.
BLENNOPHTHALMIA, Ophthalmia, (purulent.)
BLENNOP'TYSIS, from βλεννα, and πτυω, 'I spit.' Expectoration of mucus. Catarrh.
BLENNOPYRA, *Blennopy'ria*, from βλεννα, and πυρ, 'fire.' Alibert has classed, under this head, various fevers with mucous complications; as *Mesenteric fever, Adeno-meningeal fever*, &c.
BLENNORRHAGIA, Gonorrhœa—b. Genitalium, Leucorrhœa—b. Notha, Gonorrhœa spuria—b. Spuria, Gonorrhœa spuria.
BLENNORRHAGIC EPIDIDYMITIS, Hernia humoralis.

BLENNORRHAGIE FAUSSE, Gonorrhœa spuria—*b. du Gland*, Gonorrhœa spuria.
BLENNORRHINIA, Coryza.
BLENNORRHŒ'A, *Blennorrhoë, Blennorrhag''ia, Phlegmorrhœ'a, Phlegmorrhag''ia*, from βλεννα, 'mucus,' and ρεω, 'I flow.' Inordinate secretion and discharge of mucus. Also, Gonorrhœa.
BLENNORRHŒA CHRONICA, (gleet,) see Gonorrhœa—b. Genitalium, Leucorrhœa—b. Luodes, Gonorrhœa impura—b. Nasalis, Coryza—b. Oculi, see Ophthalmia—b. Oculi gonorrhoica, see Ophthalmia—b. Oculi neonatorum, see Ophthalmia—b. Oculi purulenta, see Ophthalmia—b. Urethralis, Gonorrhœa, Cystorrhœa—b. Ventriculi, Gastrorrhœa—b. Vesicæ, Cystorrhœa.
BLENNO'SES, from βλεννα, 'mucus.' Affections of the mucous membranes.—Alibert.
BLENNOTHORAX, Catarrh, Peripneumonia notha—b. Chronicus, Asthma humidum.
BLENNOTORRHŒA, Otirrhœa.
BLENNURETHRIA, Gonorrhœa.
BLENNURIA, Cystorrhœa.
BLEPHARADENITIS, Ophthalmia Tarsi.
BLEPHARANTHRACO'SIS, *Blephari'tis gangræno'sa, Carbuncula'tio Oc'uli*. Gangrenous inflammation of the eyelids.
BLEPHARELOSIS, Entropion.
BLEPHARIDES, Cilia.
BLEPHARIDOPLASTICE, Blepharoplastice.
BLEPHARISMUS, Nictation.
BLEPHARITIS, Ophthalmia tarsi—b. Gangrænosa, Blepharanthracosis.
BLEPHAROBLENNORRHŒA, Ophthalmia, purulent—b. Neonatorum, see Ophthalmia (purulenta infantum.)
BLEPH'ARO-CONJUNCTIVI'TIS, *Blepharosyndesmi'tis*, from βλεφαρον, 'an eyelid,' and *conjunctiva*. Ophthalmia affecting the conjunctiva and eyelids.
BLEPHARODYSCHRŒ'A, from βλεφαρον, the 'eyelid,' δυς, 'with difficulty,' and χροα, 'colour.' Discoloration of the eyelid. Nævus of the eyelid.—Von Ammon.
BLEPHARŒDEMA AQUOSUM, Hydroblepharon.
BLEPHARON, Palpebra—b. Atoniaton, Blepharoptosis.
BLEPHARONCO'SIS, *Blepharon'cus, Blepharophy'ma, Palpebra'rum Tumor*, from βλεφαρον, 'eyelid,' and ογκος, 'tumour.' A tumour of the eyelid.
BLEPHARONCUS, Blepharoncosis.
BLEPHAROPTHALMIA, Ophthalmia tarsi—b. Neonatorum, see Ophthalmia—b. Purulenta, Blepharopyorrhœa.
BLEPHAROPHTHALMITIS GLANDULOSA, Ophthalmia, purulent, of infants.
BLEPHAROPHYMA, Blepharoncosis.
BLEPHAROPLAS'TICE, *Blepharidoplas'tice, Insit''io Cilio'rum*, from βλεφαρον, 'the eyelid,' and πλαστικος, 'forming,' 'formative.' The formation of a new eyelid.
BLEPHAROPLEGIA, Blepharoptosis.
BLEPHAROPTO'SIS, *Blepharople'gia, Casus pal'pebræ superio'ris, Delap'sus pal'pebræ, Prolap'sus pal'pebræ, Propto'sis pal'pebræ, Pto'sis pal'pebræ, Atoniaton blepharon*, from βλεφαρον, 'the eyelid,' and πτωσις, 'fall.' A falling down of the upper eyelid over the eye, caused by a paralysis of the *Levator palpebræ superioris* muscle. This paralysis is an unfavourable symptom, as it is generally connected with a state of the brain favouring apoplexy or palsy.
BLEPHAROPTOSIS ECTROPIUM, Ectropium—b. Entropion, Entropion.

BLEPHAROPYORRHŒ'A, *Blepharophthal'mia purulen'ta, Pyorrhœ'a pal'pebræ,* from βλεφαρον, 'eyelid;' πυον, 'pus,' and ρεω, 'I flow.' Secretion of pus from the eyelids.

BLEPHARO-PYORRHŒA NEONATORUM, see Ophthalmia (purulenta infantum.)

BLEPHARORRHŒ'A, from βλεφαρον, 'eyelid,' and ρεω, 'I flow.' A discharge of mucus from the eyelids.

BLEPHAROSPAS'MUS, from βλεφαρον, 'eyelid,' and σπασμος, 'spasm.' A spasmodic action of the orbicularis palpebrarum muscle.

BLEPHAROSYNDESMITIS, Blepharoconjunctivitis.

BLEPHAROTIS, Ophthalmia tarsi—b. Glandularis contagiosa, see Ophthalmia.

BLEPHAROTITIS, Ophthalmia tarsi.

BLEPHAROTOSIS, Ectropium.

BLEPHAROXYS'TUM, *Blepharoxys'trum,* from βλεφαρον, 'eyelid,' and ξυω, 'I scrape.' An instrument used, by the ancients, for removing callosities, which made their appearance in the affection called, by the Greeks, τραχωμα.—Paulus of Ægina, Gorræus.

BLEPHIL'IA HIRSU'TA, *Ohio Horsemint, Hairy Horsemint;* an indigenous plant of the Mint family, Labiatæ, which has the aromatic properties of the Mints.

BLÉSITÉ, Blæsitas.

BLESSURE, Abortion, Wound.

BLESTRIS'MUS. Restlessness of the sick.—Hippocrates.

BLETA. A word, used by Paracelsus for white or milky urine, arising from diseased kidneys. *Blota alba* has the same meaning.

BLEU DE PRUSSE, Prussian blue.

BLEVILLE, MINERAL WATERS OF. Bleville is a village about two miles from Havre. The waters are acidulous chalybeate.

BLIGHT IN THE EYE, Ophthalmia, catarrhal.

BLINDNESS, Cæcitas—b. Colour, Achromatopsia.

BLISTER, *Vesicato'rium, Emplas'trum Vesicato'rium, Emplas'trum Lyttæ, Epispas'ticum, Blister plaster,* from *vesica,* 'a bladder,' (F.) *Vésicatoire, Vésicant.* Any substance which, when applied to the skin, irritates it, and occasions a serous secretion, raising the epidermis, and inducing a vesicle. Various articles produce this effect, as cantharides, mustard, garou, euphorbium, garlic, ammonia, &c. Blisters are used as counter-irritants. By exciting a disease artificially on the surface, we can often remove another which may be at the time existing internally. A *perpetual blister* is one that is kept open for a longer or a shorter time by means of appropriate dressings.

BLISTER or *vesication* also means the vesicle produced by vesicatories.

BLISTER, MAG"ISTRAL, (F.) *Vésicatoire magistral.* A prompt means of producing vesication recommended by M. Valleix. It is prepared as follows:—Take powdered cantharides and wheatflower, of each equal parts; vinegar, a sufficient quantity to form a soft paste.

BLISTER BEETLE, Cantharis.

BLISTER FLY, Cantharis.

BLISTER PLASTER, Blister.

BLISTERWEED, Ranunculus acris.

BLISTERING FLY, Cantharis—b. Paper, see Sparadrapum vesicatorium—b. Tissue, Sparadrapum vesicatorium.

BLITUM AMERICANUM, Phytolacca decandra.

BLOOD, Anglo-Saxon, bloð, from bleðan, 'to bleed.' *Sanguis, Cruor, Lapis anima'lis, Hæma,* 'αιμα, (F.) *Sang.* An animal fluid formed chiefly from the chyle; acquiring important properties during respiration; entering every organ through the circulation; distributing the nutritive principles to every texture, and the source of every secretion. The blood is white in the molluscous and inferior animals, which have been, hence, called *white-blooded,* to distinguish them from the *red-blooded,* which class includes the mammalia, birds, reptiles, and fishes. Human blood is composed of water, albumen, fibrin, an animal colouring substance, a little fatty matter—*hæmatelæ'um,* and different salts; as chlorides of potassium and sodium, phosphate of lime, subcarbonate of soda, lime, magnesia, oxide of iron, and lactate of soda, united with an animal matter. *Arterial blood* is of a florid red colour, strong smell, temp. 100°; s. g. 1.049. *Venous blood* is of a brownish red: temp. 98°; s. g. 1.051. The difference in colour has given occasion to the first being called *red blood;* the latter, *black.* The former, which is distributed from the heart, is nearly the same through its whole extent: the latter is the remains of the arterial blood after the different elements have been taken from it in nutrition, and probably differs in composition. It likewise contains different substances absorbed. Venous blood, taken from a vessel and left to itself, becomes solid, and separates into two distinct parts, —the *serum* or watery, supernatant fluid; and the *cruor, coag'ulum, crassamen'tum, hepar seu placen'ta san'guinis, placen'ta cruo'ris, in'sula, thrombus,* or *clot.* The serum is chiefly water, holding albumen in solution and the salts of the blood. The clot contains the fibrin, colouring matter — *hæmatosin,* a little serum, and a small quantity of salts. M. Le Canu found the blood to be composed—in 1000 parts—of water, 785.590; albumen, 69.415; fibrin, 3.565; colouring matter, 119.626; crystallizable fatty matter, 4.300; oily matter, 2.270; extractive matter soluble in alcohol and water, 1.920; albumen combined with soda, 2.010; chlorides of sodium and potassium; alkaline phosphates, sulphates, and subcarbonates, 7.304; subcarbonate of lime and magnesia, phosphate of lime, magnesia and iron, peroxide of iron, 1.414; loss, 2.586. The four principal components of the blood are fibrin, albumen, corpuscles, and saline matter. In the *circulating blood* they are thus combined—

Fibrin,
Albumen, } In solution forming *Liquor Sanguinis.*
Salts,

Red Corpuscles—suspended in the Liquor Sanguinis.

In *coagulated blood* they are thus combined:

Fibrin, } Forming the *crassamentum* or
Red Corpuscles, } clot.
Albumen, } Remaining in solution, forming
Salts, } *serum.*

The following table exhibits the computations of different physiologists regarding the weight of the circulating fluid—arterial and venous.

	lbs
Harvey, Lister, Moulins,	8
Abildguard, Blumenbach, Lobb, Lower,	10
Sprengel	............10 to 15
Günther	............15 to 20
Blake	............16½ to 18½
Müller and Burdach	20
Wagner	............20 to 25
Quesnai	27
F. Hoffmann	28
Haller	............28 to 30
Young	40
Hamberger	80
Keill	100

The proportion of arterial blood to venous is about 4 to 9.

Much attention has been paid to the varying condition of the blood in disease. The average proportion of each of the organic elements in 1000 parts of healthy blood is as follows, according to Le Canu, and MM. Andral and Gavarret:—fibrin, 3; red corpuscles, 127; solid matter of the serum, 80; water, 790.

Dried human blood was, at one time, considered to be anti-epileptic; that of the goat, dried, *Sanguis hirci sicca'tus,* sudorific and antipleuretic.

BLOOD, ARTERIAL, see Blood — b. Black, see Blood—b. Black, Vascular system of, see Vascular—b. Casein, Globulin—b. Corpuscles, Globules of the blood—b. Disease, Hæmatonosos—b. Disks, Globules of the blood—b. Dried, see Blood—b. Loss of, Hæmorrhagia—b. Red, see Blood—b. Red, system of, see Vascular — b. Spitting of, Hæmoptysis — b. Venous, see Blood — b. Vomiting of, Hæmatemesis—b. White, Lymph.

BLOODING, Bloodletting.

BLOODLESSNESS, Anæmia.

BLOOD-LETTING, *Missio* seu *Detrac'tio San'guinis, Hæmax'is, Cataschas'mus, Blooding, Bleeding,* (F.) *Saignée, Émission sanguine.* A discharge of a certain quantity of blood produced by art: an operation which consists in making an opening into a vessel to draw blood from it. When practised on an artery, it is called *Arteriot'omy;* on a vein, *Phlebot'omy, Venæsec'tio, Venesec'tion;* and on the capillary vessels, *local* or *capillary,* in contradistinction to the former, which is termed *general.* Blood-letting is used both during the existence of a disease, as in inflammation, and in the way of prophylaxis. It is employed to fulfil various indications. 1. To diminish the actual mass of blood;—when it is termed, by the French pathologists, *Saignée évacuative.* In such case, fluids ought not to be allowed too freely afterwards. 2. To diminish the turgescence in any particular organ—((F.) *Saignée révulsive, Revulsive bloodletting or bleeding, Venæsec'tio revulso'ria,* when performed far from the part affected; and *Saignée dérivative,* when near.) 3. To diminish the consistence of the blood, (F.) *Saignée spoliative.* The immediate effects of blood-letting are: diminution of the mass of blood and of heat; retardation of the pulse, and sometimes syncope. Blood-letting from the veins —*phlebotomy,* is practised on the subcutaneous veins of the neck, the face, the fore-arm, and the leg; sometimes on those of the hand or foot. The necessary apparatus consists of a bandage or riband, a compress of rag, and a lancet or phleam.

The veins selected for the operation, are, 1. *In the fold of the arm,* five;—the cephalic, basilic, the two median, and the anterior cubital. 2. *In the hand,* the cephalic and salvatella. 3. *In the foot,* the great and little saphena. 4. *In the neck,* the external jugular. 5. *In the forehead,* the frontal. 6. *In the mouth,* the ranine. The operation of phlebotomy in the limbs is performed by tying a circular bandage round the limb, in order that the subcutaneous veins may become turgid by the course of the blood being obstructed: the bandage not being so tight, however, as to compress the arteries of the limb. A puncture is made into the vein, and the desired quantity allowed to flow. The ligature is now removed, and a compress and retaining bandage applied. *Capillary* or *local blood-letting* is practised on the skin or mucous membranes, by means of leeches, the lancet, or cupping.

BLOODLETTING, CAPILLARY, see Bloodletting—b. Derivative, see Bloodletting— b. Evacuative, see Bloodletting—b. General, see Bloodletting—b. Local, see Bloodletting — b. Revulsive, see Bloodletting—b. Spoliative, see Bloodletting.

BLOODLIKE, Sanguine.

BLOODROOT, Sanguinaria Canadensis.

BLOODSHOT, Hyperæmic.

BLOODSTONE, Hæmatites.

BLOOD VESICLE, Globule of the blood.

BLOOD VESSEL, (F.) *Vaisseau sanguin.* vessel destined to contain and convey blood.

BLOOD VESSEL, BREAKING, BURSTING, RUPTURING OF A. Hæmorrhagia.

BLOODWEED, Asclepias curassavica.

BLOODWORT, Sanguinaria Canadensis.

BLOODY, *Sanguin'eus, Cruen'tus, Sanguin'eous,* (F.) *Sanguin.* Having the character of blood. Relating to blood. See Sanguine.

BLOOM, HONEY, Apocynum androsæmifolium.

BLOTA ALBA, Bleta.

BLOW, *Ictus, Plegè,* (F.) *Coup.* Effect produced by one body striking another. The impression made by any body which strikes us, or against which we strike;—a common cause of wounds, contusions, fractures, &c.

BLOWING SOUND, *Bruit de Souffle.*

BLUE-BELLS, Gentiana catesbæi.

BLUE-BERRY, Caulophyllum thalictroides, Lantana.

BLUE BOTTLE, Centaurea cyanus, Cyanus segetum.

BLUE STONE, Cupri sulphas.

BLUET DES MOISSONS, Cyanus segetum.

BLUSH, see Flush.

BLUSH, CUTANEOUS, see Efflorescence.

BOA, *Boia.* An eruption of red, ichorous pimples.—Pliny. See, also, Hidroa and Sudamina.

BOA UPAS, Upas.

BOÆ, Syphilis.

BOBERRI, Curcuma longa.

BOCHIUM, Bronchocele.

BOCIUM, Bronchocele.

BOCKLET, MINERAL WATERS OF. The springs of Bocklet, in Bavaria, are acidulous chalybeates.

BODY, *Corpus, Soma,* (F.) *Corps;* from (Teutonic) *boden,* the 'fundus or bottom.' (?) The human body is the collection of organs which compose the frame. At times, however, body is used synonymously with *trunk.* We say, also, *body of the femur, of the sphenoid,* &c., to designate the shaft or middle portion of those bones; *body of the uterus,* &c. Also, the rectum.

BODY, COMING DOWN OF THE, Proctocele.

BODY-SNATCHER, Resurrectionist.

BOE, Cry.

BOELLI, Intestines.

BOETHEMA, Medicament.

BOG-BEAN, Menyanthes trifoliata.

BOHON UPAS, Upas.

BOIA, Boa.

BOIL, Furunculus—b. Gum, Parulis—b. Malignant, see Furunculus—b. Wasp's nest, see Furunculus.

BOIS DE CAMPÈCHE, Hæmatoxylum Campechianum—*b. de Chypre,* Rhodium lignum—*b. de Couleuvre,* see Strychnos—*b. de Marais,* Cephalanthus occidentalis—*b. de Plomb,* Dirca palustris — *b. Puant,* Prunus padus — *b. de Rose,* Rhodium lignum—*b. de Sappan,* Cæsalpinia sappan—*b. Sudorifique,* Wood, sudorific.

BOISSE, MINERAL WATERS OF. These waters are situate about half a league from Fontenay-le-Compte, in France. They are purgative, and seem to contain carbonate and sulphate of lime and chloride of sodium.

BOISSON, Drink.

BOÎTE, (F.) A *box* or *case*, *Capsa*, *Pyxis*. An apparatus for the reception of any matters which it may be desirable to preserve. In *Surgery* and *Anatomy Boîtes à dissection, B. à amputation, B. à trépan, B. à cataracte*, &c., mean the cases containing these various instruments. *Boîte du Crane* is the bony case which receives the brain. *Boîte* is, also, the portion of the stem of the trephine which receives the pyramid or centre-pin. *Boîte de Petit* is a machine, invented by M. Petit, to retain the fractured portions of bone in apposition, when the leg has been fractured in a complicated manner. *Boîte* is, also, a kind of case put before an artificial anus to receive the fæces, which are continually being discharged. The vulgar, in France, give the name *Boîte* to various articulations,—*B. de genou, B. de la hanche; "knee-joint, hip-joint."*

BOÎTEMENT, Claudication.

BOÎTIER, (F.) *Appareil, Cap'sula unguenta'ria, Capsa'rium. A Dressing-case.* A box, containing salves and different apparatus, used more particularly by the dressers in hospitals.

BOL, Bolus—*b. d'Arménie,* Bole, Armenian—*b. Blanc,* Bolus alba.

BOLA, Myrrha.

BOLCHON, Bdellium.

BOLE, *Bolus*, (F.) *Bol, Terre bolaire*, meant, with the older writers, argillaceous earth, used as an absorbent and alexipharmic. The various boles had different forms given to them, and were stamped, as in the following:

BOLE ARME'NIAN, *Bole Arme'niac, B. Ar'menic, Argil'la ferrugin'ea rubra, A. Bolus rubra, Sinapi'sis, Arena'men, Bolus Orienta'lis, Bolus Armeniaca, B. Arme'nia, B. rubra,* (F.) *Bol d'Arménie.* A red, clayey earth, found not only in Armenia, but in several countries of Europe,—in Tuscany, Silesia, France, &c. It was once esteemed a tonic and astringent, and was applied as a styptic. It is now, scarcely, if ever, used. It consists of argil, mixed with lime and iron.

BOLESIS, Coral.

BOLESON, Balsam.

BOLET ODORANT, Dædalea suaveolens.

BOLETUS AGARICUS, B. Laricis—b. Albus, Boletus laricis—b. Discoideus, Dædalea suaveolens.

BOLE'TUS ESCULEN'TUS, (F.) *Morelle.* An eatable mushroom, found in the woods in Europe, and much admired by *Gastronomes.* It was formerly esteemed to be aphrodisiac.

BOLETUS FULVUS, B. igniarius—b. Hippocrepis, B. igniarius.

BOLE'TUS IGNIA'RIUS. The systematic name for the *Ag'aric, Agar'icus, Agar'icum* of the Pharmacopœias, *Agar'icus Chirurgo'rum, Agar'icus Querctis* seu *ignia'rius, Polyp'orus ignia'rius, Is'ca, Bole'tus ungula'tus* seu *fulvus* seu *hippocrepis* seu *obtu'sus,* Spunk, *Am'adou,* Punk, *Fungus Ignia'rius, Fungus Querci'nus, Agaric of the Oak, Touchwood, Touchwood Boletus, Female Agaric, Tinder,* (F) *Agaric de chêne, Amadouvier.* It was formerly much used by surgeons as a styptic.

BOLE'TUS LAR'ICIS, *B. Larici'nus, Fun'gus Lar'icis, Polyp'orus officina'lis, Agar'icus albus* seu *Lar'icis, Polyp'orus officina'lis, A. Albus op'timus, B. purgans, B. albus, B. agar'icus, B. officina'lis, White Agaric,* (F.) *Agaric blanc.* On the continent of Europe it has been given as a cathartic and emetic, as well as to moderate the sweats in phthisis.—De Haen. Externally, styptic.

BOLETUS OBTUSUS, B. igniarius—b. Officinalis, B. laricis—b. Purgans, Boletus laricis—b. Salicis, Dædalea suaveolens—b. Suaveolens, Dædalea suaveolens—b. Touchwood, Boletus igniarius.

BOLI MARTIS, Ferrum tartarisatum.

BOLISMOS, Boulimia,

BOLI'TES. The mushroom; perhaps the *Agar'icus Aurantiacus.*—Pliny, Martial, Seutonius, Galen. It was so called, in consequence of its shape,—from *Bolus.*

BOLUS, βωλος, a morsel, a mouthful, a bole, (F.) *Bol.* A pharmaceutical preparation, having a pilular shape, but larger; capable, however, of being swallowed as a pill.

BOLUS ALBA, *Terra Sigilla'ta, Argil'la pallid'ior:* called *sigilla'ta,* from being commonly made into small cakes or flat masses, and stamped or *sealed* with certain impressions. (F.) *Bol blanc, Terre Sigillée, Argile ochreuse pâle.* It was used like *Bole Armenian,* and was brought from Etruria. See Terra.

BOLUS, ALIMEN'TARY, *Bolus Alimenta'rius.* The bole formed by the food, after it has undergone mastication and insalivation in the mouth; and been collected upon the tongue prior to deglutition.

BOLUS ORIENTA'LIS. A kind of bolar earth, only distinguished from Bole Armenian in being brought from Constantinople. See Bole, Armenian.

BOLUS RUBRA, Bole, Armenian.

BOMA'REA SALSIL'LA. The inhabitants of Chili use this plant as a sudorific. It is given in infusion in cutaneous diseases.

BOMBAX, Gossypium.

BOMBEMENT, Bombus.

BOMBUS, *Au'rium fluctua'tio, A. Sib'ilus, A. Son'itus, A. Susur'rus,* (F.) *Bombement.* A kind of ringing or buzzing in the ears;—characterized, according to SAUVAGES, by the perception of blows or beating repeated at certain intervals. Also, Borborygmus. See Flatulence, and Tinnitus Aurium.

BOMBYX MORI, see Sericum.

BON, Coffea Arabica.

· BONA. Phaseolus vulgaris.

BONANNIA OFFICINALIS, Sinapis alba.

BONA FEVER, see Fever, Bona.

BONDUE, Gymnocladus Canadensis.

BONE, *Os, Os'teon, Os'teum,* (F.) *Os,* Saxon, ban. The bones are the solid and hard parts, which form the basis of the bodies of animals of the superior classes; and the union of which constitutes the *skeleton.* The human body has, at the adult age, 208 bones, without including the 32 teeth, the ossa Wormiana, and the sesamoid bones. Anatomists divide them, from their shape, into 1. *Long bones*, which form part of the limbs, and represent columns for supporting the weight of the body, or levers of different kinds for the muscles to act upon. 2. *Flat bones*, which form the parietes of splanchnic cavities; and, 3. *Short bones*, met with in parts of the body where solidity and some mobility are necessary. Bones are formed of two different textures; *spongy* and *compact.* They afford, on analysis, much phosphate and carbonate of lime, a little phosphate of magnesia, phosphate of ammonia, oxides of iron and manganese, some traces of alumina and silica, gelatin, fat, and water. The uses of the bones are mentioned under each bone. They give shape to the body, contain and defend the viscera, and act as levers to the muscles.

TABLE OF THE BONES.

BONES OF THE HEAD.	Bones of the Cranium or Skull.	Frontal	1
		Parietal	2
		Occipital	1
		Temporal	2
		Ethmoid	1
		Sphenoid	1
	Bones of the Face.	Superior Maxillary	2
		Jugal or Cheek	2
		Nasal	2
		Lachrymal	2
		Palatine	2
		Inferior Spongy	2
		Vomer	1
		Inferior Maxillary	1
	Dentes or Teeth.	Incisores	8
		Cuspidati	4
		Molares	20
	Bone of the Tongue.	Hyoid	1
	Bones of the Ear.	Malleus	2
		Incus	2
		Orbiculare	2
		Stapes	2
BONES OF THE TRUNK.	Vertebræ.	Cervical	7
		Dorsal	12
		Lumbar	5
	Sacrum		1
	Os Coccygis		1
	The Thorax.	Sternum	1
		Ribs	24
	The Pelvis.	Innominatum	2
BONES OF THE UPPER EXTREMITY.	The Shoulder.	Clavicle	2
		Scapula	2
	The Arm.	Humerus	2
	Fore-arm.	Ulna	2
		Radius	2
	The Hand. Carpus or Wrist.	Naviculare	2
		Lunare	2
		Cuneiforme	2
		Orbiculare	2
		Trapezium	2
		Trapezoides	2
		Magnum	2
		Unciforme	2
		Metacarpus	10
		Phalanges	28
BONES OF THE LOWER EXTREMITY.	The Thigh.	Femur	2
	The Leg.	Patella	2
		Tibia	2
		Fibula	2
	The Foot. Tarsus or Instep.	Calcis Os	2
		Astragalus	2
		Cuboides	2
		Naviculare	2
		Cuneiforme	6
		Metatarsus	10
		Phalanges	28

Total, 240

BONE-ACH, Osteocopus — b. Back, Vertebral column — b. Bar, Pubis, os — b. Blade, Scapula — b. Boat-like, Os scaphoides — b. Breast, Sternum — b. Crupper, Coccyx.

BONE FEVER, see Inflammation.

BONE, HAUNCH, Ilion — b. Interparietal, Interparietal bone — b. Rump, Coccyx — b. Share, Pubis — b. Splinter, Fibula.

BONE NIPPERS, *Osteul'cum, Tenac'ula*, from *teneo*, 'I hold.' (F.) *Tenaille incisive.* An instrument used for cutting off splinters and cartilages. It is a kind of forceps, the handles of which are strong, and the edges, which touch each other, cutting.

BONEBINDER, Osteocolla.

BONE-DOCTOR, *Renoueur.*

BONESET, Eupatorium perfoliatum — b. Upland, Eupatorium sessilifolium.

BONE-SETTER, *Renoueur.*

BONES, BRITTLENESS OF THE, Fragilitas ossium — b. Friability of the, Fragilitas ossium — b. Salt of, Ammoniæ carbonas — b. Softening of the, Mollities ossium.

BONIFACIA, Ruscus hypoglossum.

BONNE DAME, Atriplex hortensis.

BONNES, MINERAL WATERS OF. Bonnes is a village six leagues from Pau, in the department *Basses Pyrénées*, France. Here are several thermal springs. They were celebrated as early as the time of Francis I., under the name *Eaux d'Arquebusade*. They contain chlorides of sodium and magnesium, sulphates of magnesia and lime, sulphur, and silica. The temperature is from 78° to 98° Fahrenheit.

The *factitious* EAU DE BONNES is made of *Hydrosulphuretted water*, f℥iv; *pure water*, Oj. and f℥ss; *chloride of sodium*, gr. xxx; *sulphate of magnesia*, gr. i.

BONNET, Reticulum.

BONNET A DEUX GLOBES, *Bonnet d'Hippocrate.*

BONNET D'HIPPOCRATE, *Cap of Hippoc'rates, Mitra Hippocrat'ica, Fas'cia capita'lis, Pi'leus Hippocrat'icus.* A kind of bandage, the invention of which is ascribed to Hippocrates. It consists of a double-headed roller, passed over the head so as to envelop it like a cap. The French, also, name it, *Bonnet à deux globes, Capeline de la tête.*

BONNYCLABBER, *Clabber*, from Irish, *baine*, 'milk,' and *clabar*, 'mire.' In Ireland, sour buttermilk. In this country, the thick part of sour milk.

BONPLANDIA ANGUSTURA, Cusparia febrifuga — b. Trifoliata, Cusparia febrifuga.

BONTIA GERMINANS, Avicennia tomentosa.

BONUS GENIUS, Peucedanum — b. Henricus, Chenopodium bonus Henricus.

BONY, Osseous.

BOON UPAS, Upas.

BOONA, Phaseolus vulgaris.

BOOTIA VULGARIS, Saponaria.

BOOTIKIN. A glove with a partition for the thumb, but no separate ones for the fingers — like an infant's glove — made of oiled silk. — Dr. E. J. Seymour. Horace Walpole speaks in raptures of the benefit he derived from bootikins in gout.

BORAC''IC ACID, *Ac''idum Borac''icum, Sal sedati'vus* HOMBER'GI, *Boric Acid,* (F.) *Acide boracique.* An acid obtained from borax, which was once looked upon as sedative. It was also called *Acor Borac''icus, Sal vitrioli narcot'icum, Sal volat'ile Bora'cis,* and *Flores Bora'cis.*

BORAGE, Borago officinalis.

BORA'GO OFFICINA'LIS, *Buglos'sum verum, Bug. latifo'lium, Borra'go, Corra'go.* Borago hortensis, Borage, (F.) *Bourrache.* Nat. Ord. Boragineæ. *Sex. Syst.* Pentandria Monogynia. The leaves and flowers have been considered aperient.

BORAS SUPERSODICUS, Borax.

BORATHRON, Juniperus Sabina.

BORAX, *Boras Sodæ, Sodæ Bibo'ras, Subboras Sodæ, Boras supersat'urus sodæ, Soda Boraxa'ta, Chrysocol'la, Capis'trum auri, Subborate of protox'ide of So'dium, Subprotobo'rate of Sodium, Boras Sodæ alcales'cens seu alcali'num, Boras superso'dicus, Borax Ven'etus, Subbo'ras Na'tricum, Borax'trion, Nitrum facti''tium, &c. Subbo'rate* or *Biborate of Soda, Borate of Soda,* (F.) *Borate* ou *Sous-borate de Soude, Borate suraturé de soude.* It is found in an impure state in Thibet and Persia. It is inodorous; taste cool, and somewhat alkaline; soluble in 12 parts of water. Borax is seldom used except as a lotion in aphthæ.

BORATE OF MERCURY has been recommended as an antisyphilitic.

BORAXTRION, Borax.

BORBON'IA RUSCIFO'LIA. A small South African shrub, used in asthma and hydrothorax. In decoction, it is given as a diuretic. — Pappe.

BORBORUS, Fimus.

BORBORYG'MUS, from βορβορυζω, 'I make a dull noise.' *Murmur* seu *Bombus* seu *Motus Intestino'rum, Anile'ma, Anile'sis, Cælopsoph'ia, Intona'tio intestina'lis, Murmur ventris* seu *intestina'lis, Borborygm,* (F.) *Gargouillement, Grouillement d'Entrailles.* The noise made by flatus in the intestines. This happens often in health, especially in nervous individuals.

BORD, (F.) *Margo, Edge, Margin.* Anatomists have so named the boundaries of an organ. Thus, the bones, muscles, &c., have *bords* as well as bodies. The 'free edge,' *bord libre,* is one not connected with any part; the 'adhering edge,' *bord adhérent,* one that is connected; and the *bord articulaire,* or 'articular margin, or edge,' that which is joined to another bone.

BORD OILIAIRE, Ciliary margin.

BORDEAUX, MINERAL WATERS OF. Near this great city, in the south-west of France, is a saline, chalybeate spring. It contains oxide of iron, carbonate and sulphate of lime, chlorides of sodium and calcium, subcarbonate of soda, and sulphate of magnesia.

BORE, Boron.

BORGNE, (F.) *Cocles, Unoc'ulus, Luscus, Luscio'sus.* One who has only one eye, or sees only with one. The word has been used, figuratively, for *blind,* in surgery and anatomy. See Cæcus.

BORIUM, Boron.

BORKHAUSENIA'CAVA, Fumaria bulbosa.

BORN; past particle of *bear,* (F.) *né.* Brought forth from the womb.

BORN ALIVE. It has been decided by English judges, that 'to be born alive,' means that acts of life must have been manifested after the whole body has been extruded; and that respiration *in transitu* is not evidence that a child was born alive. It must be 'wholly born alive;' hence respiration may be a sign of *life,* but not of *live birth.*

BORON, *Bo'rium, Borum.* (F.) *Bore.* A simple substance, the basis of boracic acid; obtained, by heating potassium with boracic acid, as a dark olive-coloured powder, devoid of taste and smell. Heated in the air or in oxygen, it is converted into boracic acid.

BOR'OSAIL, *Zael.* Æthiopian names for a disease, very common there, which attacks the organs of generation, and appears to have considerable analogy with syphilis.

BORRAGO, Borago officinalis.

BORRI, Curcuma longa.

BORRIBERRI, Curcuma longa.

BORSE, MINERAL WATERS OF. Borse is a village in Béarn. The waters are chalybeate.

BORUM, Boron.

BOSA. An Ægyptian name for a mass, made of the meal of darnel, hemp-seed, and water. It is inebriating.—Prospero Alpini.

BOSCHESJESMANSTHEE, Methys oophyllum glaucum.

BOSOM, see Mamma.

BOSSA, Plague token.

BOSSE, Hump, Protuberance — *b. Nasale,* Nasal protuberance.

BOSWELLIA SERRATA, see Juniperus lycia.

BOTAL FORA'MEN, *Fora'men Bota'li* seu *Botal'lii;* the *Fora'men ova'lis,* (F.) *Trou de Botal, Trou ovale.* A large opening which exists in the fœtus in the partition between the two auricles of the heart; and by means of which the blood passes from one to the other. Its discovery is generally attributed to Leonard Botallus, Botal, or Botalli, who wrote in 1562. It was spoken of, however, by Vesalius, and even by Galen.

BOTANE, Herb.

BOTANICAL DOCTOR, Herb-doctor.

BOTANIQUE MÉDICALE, Botany, medical.

BOT'ANY, MED'ICAL, *Botan'ica Med'ica, Medici'na Botan'ica, Phytolog"ia med'ica;* from βοravη, 'an herb,' (F.) *Botanique Médicale.* The knowledge of the properties, characters, &c., of those vegetables which are used in medicine.

BOTAR'GO, (F.) *Botargue.* A preparation made in Italy and the south of France, with the eggs and blood of the *Mugilceph'alus* or *Mullet ;* strongly salted, after it has become putrescent. It is used as a condiment.

BOTARGUE, Botargo.

BOTHOR. An Arabic term for abscess in the nares. It means, also, a tumour in general; especially those which are without solution of continuity.

BOTHRIOCEPH'ALUS, *Botrioceph'alus latus, Bothrioceph'alum, Botrioceph'alus,* from βοθριον, 'a small pit,' and κεφαλη, 'head,' *Tæ'nia lata, T. vulga'ris, Lumbri'cus latus, Plate'a, T. os'culis lateral'ibus gem'inis, T. grisea, T. membrana'cea, T. tenel'la, T. denta'ta, T. huma'na iner'mis, Hal'ysis membrana'cea, T. prima, T. os'culis lateral'ibus solita'riis, T. aceph'ala, T. osculis superficial'ibus, T. à anneaux courts, T. non armé, Ver solitaire, Broad Tape worm.* Common in Switzerland, Russia, and some parts of France. It inhabits the intestines of man, and extends to an enormous length. A broken specimen has been obtained 60 yards long.—Goëze.

BOTH'RION, *Both'rium,* from βοθρος, 'a pit, cavity,' &c. An *alveolus* or small fossa. A small deep ulcer on the cornea.—Galen, Paulus of Ægina. See *Fossette.*

BOTHRIUM, Bothrion, *Fossette.*

BOTHROS, Fovea.

BOTIN, Terebinthina.

BOTIUM, Bronchocele.

BOTOTHINUM. An obscure term, used by Paracelsus to denote the most striking symptom of a disease:—the *Flos morbi.*

BOTOU, Pareira brava.

BOTRIOCEPHALUS, Bothriocephalus.

BOTRION, Alveolus.

BOTROPHIS SERPENTARIA, Actæa racemosa.

BOTRYS, Chenopodium botrys, see Vitis vinifera — *b.* Ambroisioides, Chenopodium ambrosioides—*b.* Americana, Chenopodium ambrosioides — *b.* Anthelminticum, Chenopodium anthelminticum—*b.* Mexicana, Chenopodium ambrosioides.

BOTTINE, (F.) A thin *boot* or *buskin, O'crea le'vior.* An instrument, which resembles a small boot, furnished with springs, straps, buckles, &c., and used to obviate distortions of the lower extremities in children.

BOTTLE-NOSE, Gutta rosea.

BOTTLE-STOOP. In Pharmacy, an arrangement for giving the proper inclination to a bottle containing a powder, so as to admit of the contents being readily removed by the knife, in dispensing medicines. It consists of a block of wood with a groove in the upper surface, to receive the bottle in an oblique position.

BOUBALIOS, Momordica elaterium, Vulva.

BOUBON, Bubo.

BOUCAGE MAJEUR, Pimpinella magna—*b. Mineur,* Pimpinella saxifraga — *b. Petit,* Pimpinella saxifraga.

BOUCHE, Mouth.

BOUCLEMENT, Infibulation.

BOUES DES EAUX, (F.) *Boues Minérales, Bal'nea Cœno'sa.* The mud or swamp, formed near mineral springs, impregnated with the substances contained in such springs, and consequently possessing similar properties. The *Boues* are applied generally and topically, in France, at the springs of St. Amand, Bagnères de Luchon,

Bagnols, Baréges; in the United States, at the White Sulphur in Virginia, &c.
BOUES MINÉRALES, Boues des eaux.
BOUFFE, (F.) The small eminence, formed by the junction of the two lips.—*Dulaurens.*
BOUFFISSURE, Puffiness.
BOUGIE, (F.) A wax candle: *Candel'ula, Cande'la, C. ce'rea, Cande'la medica'ta, Ce'reum medica'tum, Cereolus Chirurgo'rum, Dæ'dion, Specil'lum ce'reum, Virga ce'rea, Cereolus.* A flexible cylinder, variable in size, to be introduced into the urethra, œsophagus, rectum, &c., for the purpose of dilating these canals, when contracted. A *Simple Bougie* is composed of solid and insoluble substances; as plaster, elastic gum, catgut, &c. It acts of course only mechanically.
BOUGIE, MED'ICATED, (F.) *B. Médicamenteuse,* has the addition of some escharotic or other substance to destroy the obstacle; as in the *Caustic Bougie,* which has a small portion of *Lunar Caustic* or *Common Caustic* inserted in its extremity. Ducamp has recommended a Bougie, which swells out near its extremity, for the better dilating of the urethra. This he calls *B. à ventre.* The *metallic Bougie,* invented by Smyth, is a composition of metal, allowing of great flexibility; and a *hollow Bougie* is one, with a channel running through it, to be used in the same manner as the catheter, or otherwise.
BOUILLIE (F.), *Pultic'ula,* Pap, from (F.) *bouillir,* ' to boil.' Flour, beaten and boiled with milk. It is a common food for infants.
BOUILLON, (F.) from *bouillir,* ' to boil,' *Jus, Sorbit'io.* A liquid food, made by boiling the flesh of animals in water. The osmazome, gelatin, and soluble salts dissolve; the fat melts, and the albumen coagulates. Bouillon is nourishing, owing to the gelatin and osmazome. The *Jus de Viande* is a very concentrated Bouillon, prepared of beef, mutton, veal, &c.
BOUILLON, in common language, in France, means a round fleshy excrescence, sometimes seen in the centre of a venereal ulcer.
BOUILLON BLANC, Verbascum nigrum.
BOUILLONS MÉDICINAUX ou *PHARMACEUTIQUES, Medicinal* or *Pharmaceutic Bouillons,* contain infusions or decoctions of medicinal herbs. The *Bouillon aux herbes* is generally composed of *sorrel* or *beet.*
BOUILLON d'OS, (F.) *Bouillon from bones,* is obtained by treating bones with muriatic acid, in order to dissolve the earthy parts. The gelatin, which remains, is then boiled with a little meat and vegetables.—D'Arcet. Bouillon, however, can be easily obtained from the bones of roast meat by simple coction.
BOUILLONNEMENT, Ebullition.
BOUIS, Buxus.
BOULE D'ACIER, Ferrum tartarizatum—*b. de Mars,* Ferrum tartarizatum—*b. de Molsheim,* Ferrum tartarizatum—*b. de Nancy,* Ferrum tartarizatum.
BOULEAU COMMUN, Betula alba.
BOULESIS, Voluntas.
BOULIM'IA, *Bulim'ia, Bulim'ius, Bu'limus, Bou'limos, Bulimi'asis, Bolismos, Eclim'ia, Fames cani'na, Appeti'tus caninus, Appeten'tia cani'na, Adepha'gia, Cynorex'ia, Orex'is cyno'des, Bupi'na, Bupei'na, Phagæ'na, Phagedæ'na, Fames Bovi'na, F. Lupi'na,* from βους, ' an ox,' and λιμος, 'hunger;' or from βς, augmentative particle, and λιμος, 'hunger,' (F.) *Boulimie, Faim canine, F. dévorante, Polyphagie.* An almost insatiable hunger. A *canine appetite.* It is sometimes seen in hysteria and pregnancy; rarely under other circumstances.
BOULIMIE, Boulimia.

BOULOGNE, MINERAL WATERS OF. Boulogne is in the department of Pas-de-Calais, France. The waters are chalybeate.
BOUQUET ANATOMIQUE DE RIOLAN, (F.) from *bouquet,* a collection of flowers or other substances tied together. A name given, by some anatomists, to the collection of ligaments and muscles, inserted into the styloid process of the temporal bone.
BOUQUET FEVER, Dengue.
BOURBILLON, see Furunculus (core.)
BOURBON-LANCY, MINERAL WATERS OF. Bourbon-Lancy is a small village in the department of Saône-et-Loire, France; where there are thermal saline springs, containing carbonic acid, chloride of sodium, and sulphate of soda, chloride of calcium, carbonate of lime, iron, and silica. Their heat is from 106° to 135° Fahrenheit.
BOURBON L'ARCHAMBAUT, MINERAL WATERS OF. This town is in the department of Allier, six leagues west from Moulins, and has been long celebrated for its thermal chalybeate waters. They contain sulphohydric acid, sulphate of soda, magnesia, and lime, carbonate of iron, and silica. Their temperature varies between 136° and 145° Fahrenheit.
BOURBONNE-LES-BAINS, MINERAL WATERS OF. These springs are seven leagues from Langres, department of Haute-Marne, France. They are thermal and saline, and have been long celebrated. Temperature from 106° to 133° Fahrenheit. The *Factitious water,* (F.) *Eau de Bourbonne-les-Bains, Aqua Borvonen'sis,* is composed of *water,* containing twice its bulk of *carbonic acid,* f℥xxss; *chloride of sodium,* f℥j, *chloride of calcium,* gr. x, &c.
BOURBOULE, MINERAL WATERS OF. A village near Mount d'Or, where there are two thermal saline springs.
BOURDAINE, Rhamnus frangula.
BOURDONNEMENT, Tinnitus aurium.
BOURDONNET, Pulvil'lus, P. e linamen'tis confec'tus, P. rotun'dus, Dossil. A term in French surgery for charpie rolled into a small mass of an olive shape, which is used for plugging wounds, absorbing the discharge, and preventing the union of their edges. In cases of deep and penetrating wounds, as of the abdomen or chest, a thread is attached to them by which they may be readily withdrawn, and be prevented from passing altogether into those cavities.
BOURGÈNE, Rhamnus frangula.
BOURGEON, Granulation, Papula—*b. Charnu,* Granulation.
BOURGEONS, Gutta rosea.
BOURRACHE, Borago officinalis.
BOURRELET (F.), A Pad, a *Border.* A fibro-cartilaginous border, which surrounds certain articular cavities, such as the glenoid cavity of the scapula and the acetabulum; by which the depth of those cavities is augmented.
BOURRELET ROULÉ, Cornu ammonis.
BOURSE à BERGER, Thlaspibursa—*b. à Pasteur,* Thlaspibursa.
BOURSES, (LES,) Scrotum.
BOURSOUFLURE, Puffiness.
BOUTON, Papula—*b. d'Alep,* see Anthrax—*b. Malin,* see Anthrax—*b. d'Or,* Ranunculus acris.
BOUTONNIÈRE (F.), *Fissu'ra, Incis'io.* A small incision made into the urethra to extract a calculus from the canal, when it is too large to be discharged.
Also, a small incision or puncture, made in the peritoneum, or above the pubis, to penetrate the bladder in certain cases of retention of urine.

BOVACHEVO, Datura sanguinea.
BOVILLÆ, Rubeola.
BOVISTA, Lycoperdon.
BOWEL, Intestine.
BOWLEGGED, see Cnemoscoliosis.
BOWMAN'S ROOT, Euphorbia corollata, Gillenia trifoliata, Leptandria purpurea.
BOXBERRY, Gaultheria.
BOX, MOUNTAIN, Arbutus uva ursi.
BOX TREE, Buxus, Cornus Florida.
BOXWOOD, Cornus Florida.
BOYAU, Intestine.
BRABYLON, Prunum Damascenum.
BRACHERIOLUM, Truss.
BRACHERIUM, Truss.
BRACHIA COPULATIVA, see Peduncles of the Cerebellum.
BRACHIA PONTIS, see Peduncles of the Cerebellum.
BRACHIÆUS, Brachial — b. Internus, Brachialis anterior.
BRA'CHIAL, *Brachia'lis*, *Brachiæ'us*, from *Brachium*, 'the arm.' What belongs to the arm.
BRACHIAL APONEURO'SIS. An aponeurosis, formed particularly by expansions of the tendons of the latissimus dorsi, pectoralis major, and deltoides muscles, and which completely envelops the muscles of the arm.
BRACHIAL ARTERY, *Arte'ria brachia'lis*, *Hu'meral Artery*, (F.) *Artère ou Tronc brachial*. The artery, which extends from the axilla to the bend of the elbow; where it divides into *A. cubitalis* and *A. radialis*. It passes along the internal edge of the biceps, behind the median nerve and between the accompanying veins. Under the name *Brachial Artery*, M. Chaussier includes the subclavian, axillary, and humeral, the last being the *brachial proper*.
BRACHIAL MUSCLE, ANTERIOR, *Mus'culus Brachia'lis Ante'rior*, *Brachia'lis internus*, *B. anti'cus*, *Brachiæ'us*, *Brachiæ'us internus*, (F.) *Muscle brachial interne*, *Huméro-cubital*—(Ch.) This muscle is situate at the anterior and inferior part of the arm, and before the elbow-joint. It arises, fleshy, from the middle of the os humeri, and is inserted into the coronoid process of the ulna. *Use*. To bend the fore-arm.
BRACHIAL PLEXUS, *Plexus Brachia'lis*, is a nervous plexus, formed by the interlacing of the anterior branches of the last four cervical pairs and the first dorsal. It is deeply seated in the hollow of the axilla, and extends as far as the inferior and lateral part of the neck. It gives off the *thoracic* nerves, *supra* and *infra scapular*, and the *brachial* (which are six in number), the *axillary*, *cutaneous*, *musculo-cutaneous*, *radial*, *cubital*, and *median*.
BRACHIAL VEINS are two in number, and accompany the artery, frequently anastomosing with each other: they terminate in the axillary. Under the term *Brachial Vein*, Chaussier includes the humeral, axillary, and subclavian.
BRACHIALE, Carpus.
BRACHIAL'GIA, *Neural'gia Brachia'lis*, from βραχιον, 'the arm,' and αλγος, 'pain.' Pain in the arm, neuralgia of the arm.
BRACHIALIS, Brachial—b. Anticus, Brachial muscle—b. Externus, see Triceps extensor cubiti—b. Internus, Brachial muscle.
BRACHIERIUM, Truss.
BRACHILE, Truss.
BRACHILUVIUM, Bath, arm.
BRACHIO-CEPHALIC ARTERY, Innominata arteria—b. Veins, Innominatæ venæ.
BRA'CHIO-CU'BITAL, *Brachio-cubita'lis*. That which belongs both to the arm and cubitus. This name has been given to the internal lateral ligament of the elbow-joint; because it is attached to the os brachii or os humeri and to the cubitus or ulna.
BRACHIOCYLLO'SIS, from βραχιων, 'the arm,' and κυλλωσις, 'the act of making crooked.' Curvature of the arm inwards.' Paralysis or loss of power from curvature of the arm.
BRACHION, Brachium.
BRACHION'CUS, from βραχιων, 'the arm,' and ογκος, 'a swelling.' A tumour of the arm.
BRA'CHIO-RA'DIAL, *Brachio-radia'lis*. That which belongs to the brachium and radius. This name has been applied to the external lateral ligament of the elbow-joint, because it is attached to the humerus and to the radius. See Supinator radii longus.
BRACHIORRHEU'MA, *Rheumatis'mus bra'chii*, from βραχιων, 'the arm,' and ρευμα, 'defluxion, rheumatism.' Rheumatism of the arm.
BRACHIROLUM, Truss.
BRA'CHIUM, *Bra'chion*, *Lacer'tus*, (F.) *Bras*, the arm. The arm from the shoulder to the wrist, or the part between the shoulder and elbow. See Humeri, Os.
BRA'CHIUM ANTE'RIUS. A rounded process, which passes from the anterior pair of the corpora quadrigemina (*nates*) obliquely outwards into the thalamus opticus.
BRACHIUM MOVENS QUARTUS, Latissimus dorsi.
BRA'CHIUM POSTE'RIUS. A rounded process, which passes from the posterior pair of the quadrigemina (*testes*) obliquely outwards into the optic thalamus.
BRACHUNA, Nymphomania, Satyriasis.
BRACHYAU'CHEN, from βραχυς, 'short,' and αυχην, 'neck.' One who has a short neck.
BRACHYCEPH'ALÆ, (Gentes) 'short heads,' from βραχυς, 'short,' and κεφαλη, 'head.' In the classification of Retzius, those nations of men whose cerebral lobes do not completely cover the cerebellum—as the Sclavonians, Fins, Persians, Turks, Tartars, &c.
BRACHYCHRON'IUS, from βραχυς, 'short,' and χρονος, 'time.' That which continues but a short time. A term applied to diseases which are of short duration.—Galen.
BRACHYGNA'THUS, from βραχυς, 'short,' and γναθος, 'the under jaw.' A monster with too short an under jaw.—Gurlt.
BRACHYNSIS, Abbreviation.
BRACHYPNŒA, Dyspnœa.
BRACHYP'OTI, from βραχυς, 'short,' and ποτης, 'drinker.' They who drink little, or who drink rarely. Hippoc., Galen, Foësius.
BRACHYRHYN'CHUS; from βραχυς, 'short,' and ρυγχος, 'snout.' A monster with too short a nose.
BRACHYSMOS, Abbreviation.
BRACING, Corroborant.
BRACKEN, Pteris aquilina.
BRADYÆSTHE'SIA, from βραδυς, 'difficult,' and αισθησις, 'sensation.' Impaired sensation.
BRADYBOLISMUS, Bradyspermatismus.
BRADYECOIA, Deafness.
BRADYLOG'IA, *Dysla'lia*; from βραδυς, 'difficult, and λογος, 'a discourse.' Difficulty of speech.
BRADYMASE'SIS, *Bradymasse'sis*, improperly *Bradymaste'sis*, *Manduca'tio diffic'ilis*, from βραδυς, 'difficult,' and μασησις, 'mastication.' Difficult mastication. See Dysmasesis.
BRADYMASTESIS, Bradymasesis.
BRADYPEP'SIA, *Tarda cibo'rum concoc'tio*, from βραδυς, 'slow,' and πεπτω, 'I digest.' Slow digestion.—Galen. See Dyspepsia.
BRADYSPERMATIS'MUS, *Bradybolis'mus*, *Ejacula'tio sem'inis imped'ita*, *Dyspermatis'mus*, from βραδυς, 'slow,' and σπερμα, 'sperm.' A slow emission of sperm.
BRADYSU'RIA, *Tenes'mus vesi'cæ*, (F.) Té-

seems vésical, from βραδυς, 'difficult,' and ουρειν, 'to pass the urine.' Painful evacuation of the urine, with perpetual desire to void it. Dysuria.
BRADYTOCIA, Dystocia.
BRAG'GET, *Braggart, Bragwort.* A name formerly applied to a tisan of honey and water. See Hydromeli.
BRAI, LIQUIDE, see Pinus sylvestris — b. Sec, Colophonia.
BRAIN, Cerebrum—b. Fag, see Nervous diathesis—b. Little, Cerebellum—b. Pan, Cranium.
BRAINE, MINERAL WATERS OF. Braine is a small village, three leagues from Soissons, France, which has purgative waters similar to those of Passy.
BRAKE, COMMON, Pteris Aquilina—b. Rock, Polypodium vulgare, Polypodium incanum — b. Root, Polypodium vulgare.
BRAMBLE, AMERICAN HAIRY, see Rubus fruticosus—b. Common, Rubus fruticosus.
BRAN, Furfur.
BRANC-URSINE BÂTARDE, Heracleum spondylium.
BRANCA GERMANICA, Heracleum spondylium—b. Ursina, Acanthus mollis—b. Vera, Acanthus mollis.
BRANCH, from (F.) *Branche,* originally, probably, from βραχιων, 'an arm,'(?) because branches of trees, &c., go off like arms. A term applied, generally, to the principal division of an artery or nerve. The word is commonly used synonymously with *Ramus;* but often, with the French, *Branche* signifies the great division;—*Rameau,* Lat. *Ramus,* the division of the branches; and *Ramuscules,* Lat. *Ramusculi,* the divisions of these last.
The French, also, speak of the *branches* of the pubis for the *Rami* of that bone, *branches* of the Ischium for the rami of the ischium, &c.
BRANCHES DE LA MOËLLE ALLONGÉE (PETITES) Corpora restiformia.
BRANCHI, *Branchæ.* Swellings of the tonsils, or parotid, according to some;—of the thyroid gland, according to others.
BRAN'CHIA, (Gr.) βραγχια. The gills or respiratory organs of fishes, corresponding to the lungs of terrestrial animals.
BRANCHUS, βραγχος, *Rauce'do.* A catarrhal affection of the mucous membrane of the fauces, trachea, &c.—Galen. Hoarseness.
BRANCI, Cynanche tonsillaris.
BRANCIA, Vitrum.
BRANDY, (G.) Branntwein, Dutch, Brandwijn, 'burnt wine.' *Vinum adus'tum seu crema'tum, Aqua Vitæ,* (F.) *Eau de vie,* (S.) *Aguardiente.* The first liquid product obtained by distilling wine. It is composed of water, alcohol, and an aromatic oily matter, which gives it its flavour. Brandy is a powerful and diffusible stimulant, and as such is used in medicine. It has been also called *Liquor Aquile'gius.* See Spirit.
BRANDY, APPLE, see Pyrus malus — b. Egg, see Ovum.
BRANKS, Cynanche parotidæa.
BRANKURSINE Acanthus mollis.
BRANNTWEIN, Brandy.
BRAS. See Oryza.
BRAS, Brachium—*b. du Cervelet,* Corpora restiformia.
BRASDOR'S OPERATION FOR ANEURISM. An operation by ligature, proposed by Brasdor, which consists in the application of the ligature on the distal side of the tumour.
BRASÉGUR, MINERAL WATERS OF. Braségur is a place in the diocess of Rhodez, where there are cathartic waters.

BRASENIA, B. Hydropeltis.
BRASE'NIA HYDROPEL'TIS, *Brase'nia, B. pelta'ta, Hydropel'tis purpu'rea, Gelat'ina aquat'ica, Frogleaf, Little Water Lily, Water Jelly, Water shield, Deerfood.* An indigenous plant, *Nat. Ord.* Ranunculaceæ, *Sex. Syst.* Polyandria Polygynia, flourishing from Kentucky to Carolina and Florida; and covering the surface of ponds, marshes, &c. The fresh leaves are mucilaginous, and have been used in pulmonary complaints, dysentery, &c., like Cetraria.
BRASENIA PELTATA, B. Hydropeltis.
BRASH, WATER, Pyrosis.
BRASH, WEANING, *Atroph'ia Ablactato'rum.* A severe form of diarrhœa, which supervenes at times on weaning. The *Maladie de Cruveilhier* appears to be a similar affection.
BRASILETTO, see Cæsalpinia.
BRASIUM, Malt.
BRASMOS, Fermentation.
BRASS, Sax. bpar, *Welsh,* prês. *Aurichal'cum, Orichal'cum, Æsecavum, Chrysochal'cos,* (F.) *Airain.* A yellow metal, formed by mixing copper with calamine. The same general remarks apply to it as to copper. See Cuprum.
BRAS'SICA, *Crambē, Bras'sica olera'cea: B. capita'ta seu cuma'na* of the old Romans. The Cabbage, (F.) *Chou potager. Family,* Cruciferæ. *Sex. Syst.* Tetradynamia Siliquosa. Cato wrote a book on its virtues. It is a vegetable by no means easy of digestion when boiled; when raw, it appears to be more digestible. When forming a solid globular mass, like a head, it is the *B. Capita'ta,* (F.) *Chou-Cabus, Chou Pommé.*
BRASSICA CANINA, Mercurialis perennis — b. capitata, Brassica—b. Cumana, Brassica.
BRAS'SICA ERU'CA, *B. his'pida, Eru'ca, E. fœ'tida seu sati'va, Sina'pis eru'ca, Sisym'brium erucas'trum, Garden Rocket, Roman Rocket,* &c., (F.) *Chou Roquette, Roquette.* This was considered by the Romans an aphrodisiac, — Columella. The seeds were ordinarily used.
BRAS'SICA FLOR'IDA, — *Bras'sica Pompeia'na* of the ancients—the *Cauliflower, Caulis Flor'ida,* (F.) *Chou-fleur,* is a more tender and digestible variety.
The Broc'coli, *B. Sabel'lica* of the Romans, *B. Ital'ica,* belongs to this variety.
BRASSICA HISPIDA, B. eruca — b. Italica, B. Florida— b. Marina, Convolvulus soldanella.
BRAS'SICA NAPUS, *Napus Sylvestris, Bunias, Rape,* (F.) *Navette.* The seed yields a quantity of oil.
BRASSICA NIGRA, Sinapis nigra—b. Oblonga, B. rapa—b. Oleracea, Brassica—b. Pompeiana, B. Florida.
BRAS'SICA RAPA, *Rapa rotun'da seu oblon'ga, Rapum majus, Rapa napus, Sina'pis tubero'sa, Turnip,* (F.) *Chou navet, Navet, Rave.* The turnip is liable to the same objection (but to a less extent) as the cabbage.
BRASSICA SABELLICA, B. Florida.
BRATHU, Juniperus sabina.
BRATHYS, Juniperus sabina.
BRAYER, Truss.
BRAYERA ANTHELMINTICA, Hagenia Abyssinica.
BRAZIL WOOD, Cæsalpinia echinata.
BREAD, see Triticum.
BREAD. GLUTEN. Bread made of wheat dough deprived of the chief portion of its starch by washing. Bread, made of gluten only, cannot be eaten, on account of its hardness and toughness; hence one fifth of the normal quantity of starch is allowed to remain, and in this form the

bread is said to be tolerably light, eatable, and moderately agreeable.

BREAD, HOUSEHOLD, Syncomistos.
BREAD-FRUIT TREE, Artocarpus.
BREAST, Thorax, Mamma—b. Abscess of the, Mastodynia apostematosa.
BREAST-GLASS, *Milk-glass.* A glass applied to the nipple to receive the milk when secreted copiously by the mamma.
BREAST, IRRITABLE, Neuralgia Mammæ.
BREAST-PANG, SUFFOCATIVE, Angina pectoris.
BREAST-PUMP, Antlia Lactea.
BREATH, *Sax.* b*r*æ*t*e, *Hal'itus, Anhel'itus, An'imus, Spir'itus, At'mos,* (F.) *Haleine.* The air expelled from the chest at each expiration. It requires to be studied in the diagnosis of thoracic diseases especially. See Respiration.
BREATH, OFFENS'IVE; *Fœtor Oris, Catostomatosphre'sia, Hal'itus oris fœ'tidus, Ozē.* An offensive condition, which is usually dependent upon carious teeth, or some faulty state of the secretions of the air passages. The internal use of the chlorides may be advantageous.
BREATH, SATURNINE, see Saturnine—b. Short, Dyspnœa.
BREATHING AIR, see Respiration.
BREATHING, DIFFICULTY OF, Dyspnœa.
BRECHET, (F.) The *Brisket.* This name is given in some parts of France to the *cartilago ensiformis,* and sometimes to the sternum itself.
BRECHMA, Bregma.
BRECHMUS, Bregma.
BRÉDISSURE, (F.) *Trismus Capistra'tus.* Incapacity of opening the mouth, in consequence of preternatural adhesion between the internal part of the cheek and gums; often occasioned by the abuse of mercury.
BREDOUILLEMENT, (F.) *Tituban'tia.* A precipitate and indistinct mode of utterance, in which a part only of the words is pronounced, and several of the syllables viciously changed. This defect is analogous to stuttering, but differs from it in being dependent on too great rapidity of speech; whilst stuttering is characterized by continual hesitation, and frequent repetition of the same syllables.
BREED, Race.
BREEDING, Generation, Pregnant.
BREEDING, CROSS. The act of raising or breeding from different stocks or families.
BREEDING-IN-AND-IN. The act of raising or breeding from the same stock or family.
BREGMA, *Brechma, Brechmus,* from βρεχειν, 'to sprinkle;' *Fontanel'la, Sin'ciput.* The top of the head was thus called, because it was believed to be humid in infants; and, according to some, because it was conceived to correspond to the most humid part of the brain.
BREGMATODYMIA, see Cephalodymia.
BRENNING, Burning.
BREPHOCTONON, Conyza squarrosa.
BREPHOTROPHE'UM, *Ecthelobrephotrophe'um,* from βρεφος, 'a new-born child,' and τρεφειν, 'to nourish.' A foundling hospital.
BRÉSILLET, Cæsalpinia sappan.
BRE'VIA VASA, *Short Vessels.* This name has been given to several branches of the splenic arteries and veins, which are distributed to the great *cul-de-sac* of the stomach.
BREVIS CUBITI, see Anconeus.
BRICK, (F.) *Brique.* Hot bricks are sometimes need to apply heat to a part, as to the abdomen in colic, or after the operation for popliteal aneurism; or, reduced to very fine powder, and mixed with fat, as an application to herpetic and psoric affections.
BRICKS, *Fornaces Testæ* or *Tiles* were formerly bruised in vinegar, and the liquid was used as a specific in cutaneous affections. They entered, also, into a cerate used for scrofulous humours, &c. To the *Terra Forna'cum,* or *Brick earth,* the same virtues were assigned.
BRICUMUM, Artemisia.
BRIDE (F.), A bridle. *Fræ'nulum, Retinac'ulum.* This term is given, in the plural, to membranous filaments, which are found within abscesses or deep-seated wounds, and which prevent the exit of pus. The term is, also, applied to preternatural adhesions, which occur in cicatrices of the skin, in the urethra, or in inflamed serous or synovial membranes.
BRIER, WILD, Rosa canina.
BRIGHT'S DISEASE OF THE KIDNEY, see Kidney, Bright's disease of the.
BRIGHTON, CLIMATE OF. The air of this fashionable watering place, on the south coast of England, is dry, elastic, and bracing. According to Sir James Clark, its climate appears to the greatest advantage in the autumn and early part of the winter; when it is somewhat milder and more steady than that of Hastings. Accordingly, it is adapted for all cases in which a dry and mild air at this season of the year proves beneficial. In the spring months, owing to the prevalence of, and its exposure to, north-east winds, the climate is cold, harsh, and exciting to the delicate. It is well adapted for convalescents, and for all who require a dry and bracing sea air.
BRIMSTONE, Sulphur.
BRINE, Muria.
BRINTON ROOT, Leptandria purpurea.
BRION, Corallina.
BRIQUE, Brick.
BRIQUEBEC, MINERAL WATERS OF. This town is three leagues from Cherbourg, in France. The water contains chloride of iron.
BRISE-PIERRE ARTICULÉ, (F.) An instrument invented by Jacobson for crushing the stone in the bladder.
BRISTOL HOT WELL, *Bristolien'sis Aqua.* Bristol is about thirteen miles from Bath, in England. The water is an almost pure thermal; slightly acidulated. It contains chlorides of magnesium and sodium, sulphate of soda, sulphate of lime, carbonate of lime, carbonic acid, oxygen and azote. Temperature, 74° Fah. The Hot Well has been long celebrated. Its action is like that of thermal waters in general. The climate of Bristol is mild, and hence the water has been celebrated for the cure of incipient pulmonary consumption. See Clifton.
BRIZOCERAS, Ergot.
BROAD, *Sax.* b*r*ǣ*d, Latus,* (F.) *Large.* Any body is so termed whose transverse extent is considerable compared with its length. The *Broad Bones,* such as the frontal, parietal, occipital, iliac, aid in forming the parietes of splanchnic cavities. *Broad Muscles* generally occupy the parietes of cavities, and especially those of the chest and abdomen. The epithet has also been applied to other parts—as to the *broad ligaments* of the womb, &c.
BROCCOLI, Brassica sabellica.
BROCHOS, βροχος, *Laqueus.* A bandage.
BROCH'THUS, βρογχος, *Gula.* The throat. Also, a kind of small drinking vessel.—Hipp.
BROCHUS, βροχος. This name has been given to one who has a very prominent upper lip. According to others, it means one whose teeth project in front of the mouth.
BRO'DIUM. A synonym of *Jus* or *Jus'culum.* Broth, or the liquor in which any thing is boiled. *Bro'dium salis*—a decoction of salt.
BROIEMENT, see Cataract, Laceration.

BROKEN DOSES, see Doses, broken.
BROKEN-WINDEDNESS, Asthma.
BROMA, Aliment, Bromine.
BROMATO‑CCRISIS, Lientery.
BROMATOG'RAPHY, *Bromatograph'ia, Bromog'raphy, Bromograph'ia*, from βρωμα, 'food,' and γραφη, 'a description.' A description of aliments.
BROMATOL'OGY, *Bromatolog''ia, Sitiol'ogy*, from βρωμα, 'food,' and λογος, 'a discourse.' A treatise on food.
BROME, Bromine.
BROMEGRASS, Bromus ciliatus — b. Soft, Bromus ciliatus.
BROME'LIA ANA'NAS, called after Olaus Bromel, a Swede. *Car'duus Brasilia'nus, Ana'nas ova'ta seu aculea'ta, Anas'sa, Capa-Isiak'ka, Ana'nas* or *Pine Apple*. A West India tree, which produces the most delicious of fruits.
BROME'LIA PINGUIN, *Ana'nas America'na, Pinguin, Broad-leaved wild Ana'nas*, &c. The West India plant, which affords the *Pinguin* fruit. The fruit is refrigerant, and the juice, when ripe, very austere. It is used to acidulate punch. A wine is made from the Pinguin, which is very intoxicating, and has a good flavour.
BROMIC, *Bro'micus*: same etymon as Bromine. Containing bromine.
BROMIDE OF IRON, see Bromine — b. of Mercury, see Bromine — b. of Potassium, see Bromine.
BROMIDRO'SIS, from βρωμος, 'stench,' and 'ιδρως, 'sweat.' Offensive sweat.
BROMINE, *Bro'minum, Bromin'ium, Broma, Bromin'eum, Bro'mium, Bro'mina, Bromum, Mu'rina, Muride, Brome*. A simple body, of a very volatile nature, and highly offensive and suffocating odour, whence its name, from βρωμος, 'a stench.' It is met with chiefly in sea-water, and in many animal and vegetable bodies that live therein. It has likewise been found in many mineral waters of this and other countries. In its chemical relations, it may be placed between chlorine and iodine. With oxygen it forms an acid,—the *Bromic*, and with hydrogen another— the *Hydrobromic*.
PURE BROMINE, BROMIDE OF IRON, (dose, gr. į or ij,) and BROMIDE OF POTASSIUM, have been used medicinally, and chiefly in scrofulosis,— internally, as well as applied externally. Bromine may be dissolved in forty parts of distilled water, and six drops be commenced with as a dose. BROMIDES OF MERCURY (*Hydrar'gyri Bro'mida*) have been given in syphilis. The *protobromide* and the *bibromide* are analogous in composition and medicinal properties to the corresponding iodides of mercury.
BROMIUM, Bromine.
BROMOGRAPHY, Bromatography.
BROMOS, βρωμος. One of the cerealia, supposed, by some, to be oats. See Avena.
BROMOSUS, Fetid.
BROMUM, Bromine.
BROMUS CILIA'TUS, *B. purgans, Brome grass*; indigenous: *Order*, Gramineæ; is said to be emetic, and anthelmintic (?), cathartic and diuretic. It purges cattle.
BROMUS GLABER, Triticum repens.
BROMUS MOLLIS, *Soft Brome Grass*. The seeds are said to cause giddiness in man; and to be fatal to poultry.
BROMUS PURGANS, B. ciliatus.
BROMUS TEMULENTUS, Lolium temulentum.
BRONCHES, Bronchia — *b. Ganglions lymphatiques des*, Bronchial glands.
BRONCHI, Bronchia.
BRON'CHIA, *Bron'chiæ, Bronchi*, from βροyχος, 'the throat.' The Latins used the term *Bronchus*, for the whole of the trachea; whilst they called its ramifications *Bronchia. Bronchia, Bronchiæ*, and *Bronchi*, (F.) *Bronches*, now mean the two tubes, with their ramifications, which arise from the bifurcation of the trachea, and carry air into the lungs,—*Can'nulæ pulmo'num*.
BRONCHIA, DILATATION OF THE, *Dilated Bronchia*. The physical signs of this condition are the following:—*Percussion* usually clear, but not unfrequently less so than natural, although very seldom quite dull. *Auscultation* detects coarse mucous or gurgling rhonchi, increased by the cough, combined with, or replaced by, bronchial or cavernous respiration, which is often effected as if by a sudden puff or whiff. The resonance of the voice is increased, but it seldom amounts to perfect pectoriloquy. The most common situations for dilated bronchia are the scapular, mammary, or lateral regions. They are almost always confined to one side.
BRONCHIA, OBLITERATION OR COMPRESSION OF THE. The inspiratory murmur on auscultation is weaker or wholly suppressed over a limited portion of the chest; the expiration is generally more distinct and prolonged: all the other conditions are natural.
BRONCHIÆ, see Bronchia.
BRON'CHIAL, *Bronchic, Bronchia'lis, Bron'chicus*. That which relates to the bronchia.
BRONCHIAL ARTERIES, (F.) *Artères Bronchiques*. These are generally two in number, one going to each lung. They arise from the thoracic aorta, and accompany the bronchia in all their ramifications.
BRONCHIAL CELLS, (F.) *Cellules bronchiques*. The *Air-cells*; the terminations of the bronchia.
BRONCHIAL COUGH, (F.) *Toux bronchique, T. tubaire*. This generally accompanies bronchial respiration. They both indicate obstruction to the entrance of air into the air-cells.
BRONCHIAL GLANDS, *Glan'dulæ Vesalia'næ, Glands of Vesa'lius*, (F.) *Glandes bronchiques* ou *Ganglions lymphatiques des bronches*, are numerous glands of an ovoid shape; of a reddish hue in the infant, and subsequently brown and black, seated in the course of the bronchia. Their functions are unknown. The bronchial glands may be presumed to be affected by scrofulosis, when, in addition to the existence of tumours in the neck, percussion gives a dull sound under the upper and central part of the sternum, whilst there is no appreciable lesion of the lungs.
BRONCHIAL NERVES, (F.) *Nerfs bronchiques*, are furnished by the two pulmonary plexuses.
BRONCHIAL PHTHISIS, see Phthisis bronchial— b. Respiration, see Murmur, respiratory.
BRONCHIAL VEINS arise from the last divisions of the arteries of the same name, and pass, on the right side, into the vena azygos; on the left, into the superior intercostal.
BRONCHIC, Bronchial.
BRONCHIEC'TASIS, *Dilata'tio bronchio'rum*, from βροyχος, 'a bronchus,' and εκτασις, 'dilatation.' Dilatation of one or more bronchial tubes.
BRONCHIITIS, Bronchitis.
BRON'CHIOLE, *Bronchiolum, Bronchiolus*; diminutive of *Bronchium* or *Bronchus*. A minute bronchial tube.
BRONCHIOSTENO'SIS. from βροyχος, 'a bronchus,' and στενωσις, 'contraction.' Contraction or narrowness of the bronchi.
BRONCHITE CONVULSIVE, Pertussis.
BRONCHI'TIS, *Bronchii'tis, Inflamma'tio bronchio'rum, Catar'rhus Pulmo'num, C. bronchio'rum, Pleuri'tis hu'mida, P. bronchia'lis, Bronchoe'tasis, Pul'monary Catarrh, Angi'na bronchialis*, (F.) *Inflammation des Bronches*. Inflammation of the lining membrane of the

bronchial tubes. This is always more or less present in cases of pulmonary catarrh; and is accompanied by cough, mucous expectoration, dyspnœa, and more or less uneasiness in breathing. The *acute* form is accompanied with all the signs of internal inflammation, and requires the employment of antiphlogistics followed by revulsives. The *chronic* form, *Tussis seni'lis, Catar'rhus seni'lis, Rheuma catarrha'lē, Peripneumo'nia notha, Bronchorrhœ'a acu'ta, Winter cough, Chronic Catarrh*, may be confounded with phthisis; from which it must be distinguished mainly by the absence of hectic fever and of the physical signs that are characteristic of the latter, as well as by the nature of the expectoration, which is generally mucous, although at times muco-purulent. When the expectoration is little or none, the bronchitis is said to be dry, dry catarrh, (F.) *Catarrhe Sec.*

When bronchitis affects the smaller tubes, it is termed *capil'lary bronchi'tis, bronchi'tis capilla'ris, bronchoc'acē infanti'lis* (?), and is often fatal to children. *Vesic'ular bronchitis* is the term proposed by MM. Rilliet and Barthez for the *vesicular pneumonia* of children.

BRONCHITIS, Catarrh—b. Asthenica, Peripneumonia notha—b. Capillary, see Bronchitis—b. Convulsiva, Pertussis—b. Membranacea, Polypus bronchialis—b. Plastic, Polypus bronchialis—b. Pseudomembranous, Polypus bronchialis—b. Summer, Fever, hay—b. Vesicular, see Bronchitis.

BRONCHIUS, Sterno-thyroideus.
BRONCHLEMMITIS, Polypus bronchialis.
BRONCHOCACE, Peripneumonia notha—b. Infantilis, see Bronchitis.
BRONCHO-CATARRHUS, Catarrh.
BRONCHOCE'LĒ, from βρογχος, 'a bronchus,' and κηλη, 'tumour.' An inaccurate name for the affection which is called, also, *Bo'chium, Botium, Hernia gut'turis, Guttur tu'midum seu globo'sum, Trachelophy'ma, Hernia guttura'lis, Thyroce'lē, Thyreoce'lē, Tracheoce'lē, Thyremphrax'is, Thyreophrax'ia, Thyreon'cus, Thyron'cus, Deiron'cus, Deron'cus, Thyrophrax'ia, Gossum, Go'tium, Exechebron'chus, Gongro'na, Struma, Glans, Bo'cium, Her'nia bronchia'lis, Tracheloce'lē, Tuber gutturo'sum, Gutte'ria*, &c., the Derbyshire neck, Swelled neck, Wen, *Goître*, &c., (F.) *Goître, Goître, Hypertrophie du Corps Thyroïde, Grosse Gorge, Gros Cou.* This is no rupture, but consists of an enlargement of the thyroid gland. It is common at the base of lofty mountains in every part of the world; and has been supposed to be owing to the drinking of snow-water, but it occurs where there is no snow. The tumour is sometimes very extensive. Iodine has great power over it, and will generally occasion its absorption, when the case has not been of such duration as to have ended in a cartilaginous condition.

BRONCHOCEPHALITIS, Pertussis.
BRONCHOPARALYSIS, Asthma.
BRONCHOPHONY, Resonance.
BRONCHOPLAS'TIC, *Bronchoplas'ticus*, from βρογχος, 'a bronchus,' and πλασσω, 'I form.' An epithet given to the operation for closing fistulæ in the trachea.

BRONCHOPNEUMO'NIA, from βρογχος, 'a bronchus,' and *Pneumonia*. Inflammation of the bronchia and lungs.

BRONCHORRHŒ'A, (F.) *Bronchorrhée, Catarrhe pituiteux, Phlegmorrhagie pulmonaire, Flux bronchique*, from βρογχος, 'bronchus,' and ῥεω. 'I flow.' An increased secretion of mucous from the air passages, accompanied or not by inflammation:—a gleet, as it were, of the pulmonary mucous membrane.

BRONCHORRHŒA ACUTA, Bronchitis (chronic.)
BRONCHOSTASIS, Bronchitis.
BRONCHOTOME, *Bronchot'omus*, from βρογχος, and τεμνειν, 'to cut.' A kind of lancet, with a blunt and rounded point, mounted on a handle, and fitted to a canula, which passes in along with it, and is allowed to remain in the opening made in the trachea.

BRONCHOT'OMY, *Bronchotom'ia*, (F.) *Bronchotomie*. Same etymology. A surgical operation, which consists in making an opening either into the trachea, (*Tracheot'omy:*) into the larynx, (*Laryngot'omy:*) or into both, (*Tracheo-laryngot'omy*,) to extract foreign bodies or to permit the passage of air to the lungs. These different parts are divided transversely or vertically, according to circumstances.

BRONCHUS, see Bronchia. Trachea.
BROOKLIME, Veronica beccabunga.
BROOM, Sophora tinctoria, Spartium scoparium—b. Butcher's, Ruscus—b. Clover, Sophora tinctoria—b. Indigo, Sophora tinctoria—b. Rape, of Virginia, Orobanche Virginiana—b. Spanish, Spartium junceum—b. Yellow, Sophora tinctoria.

BROSSADIÈRE, MINERAL WATERS OF. Brossardière is a chateau in Bas-Poitou, France. The waters contain carbonates of iron and lime, chloride of sodium, and sulphate of lime. They are aperient.

BROSSE, Brush.
BROTH, CHICKEN, see Chicken Broth.
BROTH, VEGETABLE. Take two *potatoes*, a *carrot*, and an *onion*, all cut fine; boil in a quart of *water* for an hour, adding more water from time to time, so as to keep the original quantity; flavour with *salt*, and a small quantity of *potherbs;* strain. A little mushroom catchup improves the flavour.

BROUILLARD, Caligo.
BROUS'SAIST. One who is a believer in, and professor of, the physiological and pathological opinions of Broussais. The system itself was called BROUSSAISM, or the *Physiological Doctrine.*

BROW, Front—b. Ague, Neuralgia frontalis.
BROWN RED, Colcothar.
BROWN'IAN, *Browno'nian, Bruno'nian.* Relating to the system or opinions of John Brown.
BROWNISM, *Bru'nonism, Bruno'nianism.* The doctrines of Brown.
BROWNIST, *Browno'nian, Bruno'nian.* A follower of the system of Brown.
BRU'CEA ANTI-DYSENTER'ICA. Called after Bruce, the Abyssinian traveller. *B. ferrugin'ea, Angustu'ra spu'ria*, (F.) *Fausse Angusture, A. Ferrugineuse.* The systematic name of the plant whence was obtained—it was supposed—*false Angustura* or false *Cusparia Bark.* It is really the bark of Strychnos nux vomica.
BRUCIA, Brucine.
BRUCINE, *Bru'cia, Bruci'na, Bruci'num, Bru'cium, Pseudangusturi'num, Cancirami'num, Vom'icine.* An organic, salifiable base, discovered in the false angustura—*Brucea anti-dysenter'ica*, and obtained from *Strychnos nux vom'ica.* It is of a pearly white; crystallizes in oblique prisms with a parallelogrammatic base; is very bitter, slightly acrid and styptic, and soluble in water, but more so in alcohol. Brucia is a less active poison than strychnia. It resembles it, however, and may be used as a substitute for it and for the extract of nux vomica. Dose, half a grain.

BRUCKENAU, MINERAL WATERS OF. These springs are in Bavaria, and contain carbonic acid and iron.

BRUCOURT, MINERAL WATERS OF. Brucourt is three leagues and a half from Caen, in Normandy. The waters contain carbonic acid, chloride of sodium, and sulphate of soda, much sulphate of lime, &c.

BRUISE, Contusion.

BRUISE ROOT, Stylophorum diphyllum.

BRUISEWORT, Bellis saponaria.

BRUISSEMENT, (F.) Frem'itus. This word has much the same signification as Bourdonnement, as well as Bruit.

BRUIT, (F.) 'Sound.' A French term, applied to various sounds heard on percussion and auscultation, viz.

BRUIT DE CRAQUEMENT, B. de Tiraillement, Bruit de cuir neuf, 'sound of crackling, or bursting, or of new leather.' A sound produced by the friction of the pericardium, when dried and roughened by inflammation.

BRUIT DU CŒUR FŒTAL, Battemens doubles; Double bruit du Cœur du Fœtus. The pulsations of the fœtal heart heard in auscultation in the latter half of utero-gestation.

BRUIT DE CUIR NEUF, Bruit de craquement.

BRUIT DE DIABLE, Ronflement du Diable, Bruit de souffle à double courant, 'noise of the diable or humming-top.' Venous hum. A high degree of Bruit de soufflet, heard on auscultating the arteries or veins—probably the latter—of the neck in chlorosis. It denotes an impoverished state of the blood.

BRUIT DOUBLE DU CŒUR DU FŒTUS, Bruit du Cœur fœtal—b. de Frôlement, see Frôlement.

BRUIT DE FROISSEMENT PULMONAIRE, see Froissement pulmonaire.

BRUIT DE FRÔLEMENT PÉRICARDIQUE, see Frôlement pericardique.

BRUIT DE FROTTEMENT ASCENDANT ET DESCENDANT, 'Sound of friction of ascent and descent.' Sounds produced by the rubbing of the lung against the parietes of the chest, as it rises and falls during inspiration and expiration. They are distinctly heard in pleuritis, when the pleura has become roughened by the disease. Friction sounds, Rubbing sounds, To-and-fro sounds are also heard in pericarditis and peritonitis.

BRUIT HUMORIQUE, B. Hydropneumatique. The sound afforded on percussion when organs are filled with liquid and air.

BRUIT HYDROPNEUMATIQUE, Bruit humorique.

BRUIT DE MOUCHE (F.), 'fly sound.' A sound analogous to the Bruit de diable—so called from its likeness to the buzzing of a fly:—heard on auscultating the neck in chlorotic cases.

BRUIT MUSCULAIRE. The sound accompanying the first sound of the heart, referred by some to muscular contraction. Called, also, Bruit rotatoire, in consequence of its having been thought to resemble the rumbling of distant wheels.

BRUIT MUSICAL, Sifflement modulé.

BRUIT DE PARCHEMIN. 'Parchment tone.' A sound as if produced by two sheets of parchment applied to each other. It is said to be produced by thickening and rigidity of the valves of the heart.

BRUIT PLACENTAIRE, B. de soufflet placentaire, B. utérin, Souffle utérin, Souffle placentaire, Placental bellows' sound, Utero-placen'tal murmur, U'terine murmur. The bellows' sound heard on auscultating over the site of the placenta in a pregnant female. It does not appear to be owing to the placental vessels: but to the uterine tumour pressing upon the large vessels of the mother.

BRUIT DE POT FÉLÉ; 'Sound of a cracked vessel.' This sound is heard on percussion, when a cavern in the lungs is filled with air, and has a narrow outlet.

BRUIT DE RACLEMENT, 'Sound of scraping.' A sound produced by the scraping of hard, solid membranes, as the pericardium, against each other.

BRUIT DE RÂPE, 'Sound of a rasp.' A sound heard during the contraction of either the auricles or ventricles. It is constant; and the contraction of the cavity is more prolonged than natural, and emits a hard, rough, and—as it were—stifled sound.

It indicates contraction of the valvular orifices by cartilaginous deposits, or ossification, and is better heard near the apex of the heart, if the auriculo-ventricular valves be concerned,—near the base if the semilunar valves be the seat of the disease.

BRUIT ROTATOIRE, Bruit musculaire.

BRUIT DE SCIE, or 'saw-sound,' and BRUIT DE LIME À BOIS, or 'file-sound,' resemble the Bruit de Râpe.

BRUIT DE SOUFFLE À DOUBLE COURANT, Bruit de Diable.

BRUIT DE SOUFFLET, Bruit de Souffle, 'bellows' sound,' 'blowing sound.' A sound like that of a bellows, heard occasionally by the ear applied to the chest during the contraction of the ventricles, auricles, or large arteries. It coexists with affections of the heart, but is heard, also, without any disease in that organ,—whenever, indeed, an artery is compressed. An Encephalic bellows' sound, has been described by Drs. Fisher and Whitney. It is heard on applying the ear to the occiput or to the top of the head; and is considered to indicate turgescence of vessels, or inflammation. When such turgescence exists, the vessels are compressed, and the compression gives rise to the sound in question.

BRUIT DE SOUFFLET PLACENTAIRE, Bruit placentaire—b. de Tiraillement, Bruit de craquement.

BRUIT DE TAFFETAS. 'Sound of Taffeta.' 'Sarcenet sound.' A respiratory sound, so named, by M. Grisolle, from its resembling the sound caused by the tearing of a piece of taffeta; and which he considers to indicate hepatization of the lung, limited to the surface, in pneumonia.

BRUIT TYMPANIQUE, 'Tympanic sound.' The clear sound afforded by percussing the stomach and intestines when containing air.

BRUIT UTÉRIN, B. placentaire.

BRULURE, Burn.

BRUNELLE, Prunella.

BRUNNER'S GLANDS, Brunneri Glan'dulæ, Glandulæ solita'riæ, Solitary glands, Solitary follicles, Second pan'creas. Compound muciparous follicles, seated between the mucous and muscular coats of the stomach, along the two curvatures of that organ, and in the duodenum; so called from their discovery having been generally attributed to Brunner. The solitary intestinal follicles are often known, at the present day, as the glands of Brunner, although Brunner restricted the latter term to the glands of the duodenum.

BRUNONIAN, Brownian.

BRUNONIANISM, Brownism.

BRUNUS, Erysipelas.

BRUSCUS, Ruscus.

BRUSH, Scop'ula, (F.) Brosse. A well known instrument, used in medicine chiefly for the following purposes. 1. To clean the teeth. 2. To remove the saw-dust which adheres to the teeth of the trephine, during the operation of trephining. 3. To rub the surface of the body, for the purpose of exciting the skin, and favouring transpiration. Westring, a Swedish physician, has recommended metallic brushes for the purpose of conveying galvanism to a part. These brushes consist of a plate of ebony fitted to another of gold, in which threads of the same metal are fixed;—the brush being connected with one of the poles of the galvanic pile.

BRUSH, STOMACH, Excutia ventriculi.
BRUTA, Juniperus sabina.
BRU'TIA. A sort of thick pitch, obtained from Brutia, in Italy. From *Pix Brutia* was obtained the *O'leum Pici'num*.
BRUTIA, Instinct.
BRUTINO, Terebinthina.
BRUXANELL. A Malabar tree, the bark and leaves of which have a strong smell, and are astringent. On the coast of Malabar, its juice, mixed with butter, is applied to boils. Its bark is esteemed to be diuretic, and its roots anti-arthritic.

BRUYÈRE VULGAIRE, Erica vulgaris.
BRUYÈRES, MINERAL WATERS OF. Bruyères is a small village, 7½ leagues from Luneville. The waters are aciduous and chalybeate.
BRYCETOS, see Algidus.
BRYCHETHMOS, Rugitus.
BRYCHETOS, see Algidus.
BRYGMA, *Brygmus, Trisis, Prisis, Prismus, Odontopri'sis, Stridor Den'tium*, (F.) *Grincement des Dents*. Grinding of the teeth. A common symptom, in children, of gastric or other derangement, but often present when there is no reason to suspect any.
BRYO'NIA AFRICA'NA. A South African remedy, common amongst the Hottentots, which, in the form of decoction, acts simultaneously as an emetic, cathartic, and diuretic. It is used by the natives in cutaneous diseases, dropsy, and syphilis. The tincture is a powerful emetic and cathartic.—Thunberg.
BRYO'NIA ALBA; *White Bry'ony, Vitis alba sylves'tris, Agros'tis, Agriam'pelos, Am'pelos a'gria, Archeos'tris, Echetro'sis, Bryo'nia as'pera, Cedros'tis, Chelido'nium, Labrus'ca, Melo'thrum, Ophrostaph'ylon, Psilo'thrum, Bryonia Dioi'ca*. Nat. Ord. Cucurbitaceæ. Sex. Syst. Monœcia Monadelphia. (F.) *Couleuvrée, Vigne vierge, V. blanche*. The root is large and succulent, and has an acrid, bitter, and disagreeable taste. It is a drastic cathartic. Externally, it has been applied, in form of cataplasm, in gout. When repeatedly washed, a good starch is obtained from it. The active principle has been separated from it, and called *Bry'onine*.
BRYONIA MECHOACANNA NIGRICANS, Convolvulus jalapa—b. Peruviana, Convolvulus jalapa.
BRYONINE, see Bryonia alba.
BRYONY, WILD, Sycios angulatus.
BRYTIA, Marc of grapes.
BRYTON, Cerevisia.
BU, βου, abbreviation of βους, 'an ox;' in composition expresses, 'excess, greatness.' Hence *Bulimus, Buphthal'mia*, &c.
BUBASTECORDIUM, Artemisia vulgaris.
BUBE, Pustule.
BUBO, βουβων, *Pano'chia, Panus inguina'lis, Adenophy'ma inguina'lis, Bubonopa'nus, Bubonon'cus, Bubon'cus, Oambu'ca, Angus, Boubon, Codoce'lle, Codoscel'la*, (F.) *Bubon, Poulain*. In the works of Hippocrates and Galen, this word sometimes signifies the groin—*Inguen;* at others, the inguinal glands; and at others, again, swelling or inflammation of these parts. The moderns apply the term to an inflammatory tumour seated in the groin or axilla, and they generally distinguish, 1. *Simple* or *Sympathetic Bubo*, which is independent of any virus in the economy. 2. *Venereal Bubo*, (F.) *Bubon vénérien*, which is occasioned by the venereal virus. 3. *Pestilential Bubo*, or *B. symptomatic of the Plague*. The last two have by some been called *malignant Bubo*, (F.) *Bubon malin*.

Primary Bubo, (F.) *Bubon primitif*, shows itself with the first symptoms of syphilis: the *consecutive* not till afterwards.
BUBON, Bubo, Inguen—b. Gummiferum, see Ammoniac gum.

BUBON D'EMBLÉE, (F.) An enlargement and suppuration of one or more of the inguinal glands, not preceded by any other of the more common forms of venereal disease, nor by any other syphilitic symptom.

BUBON GAL'BANUM. The systematic name of a plant which has been supposed to afford galbanum; *Meto'pion, Mato'rium*. The plant is also called *Fer'ula Africa'na, Oreoseli'num Africa'num, Ani'sum frutico'sum galbanif'erum, Ani'sum Africa'num frutes'cens, Seli'num Galbanum, Agasyll'is gal'banum, The long-leaved* or *lovage-leaved Gal'banum*. Nat. Ord. Umbelliferæ. The plant can scarcely, however, be considered to be determined. Galbanum is the gummi-resinous juice. Its odour is fetid, and taste bitter and acrid: the agglutinated tears are of a white colour, on a ground of reddish-brown. It forms an emulsion, when triturated with water, and is soluble in proof spirits of wine, and vinegar: s. g. 1.212. It has been given as an antispasmodic, and expectorant, in pill or emulsion. Dose, from gr. 10 to 60. Externally, it is applied as a cataplasm.

Bubon galbanum is a South African plant; and is reputed to be an excellent diuretic, under the name of *Wild Celery*. A decoction of the leaves is given in dropsy and gravel. According to Pappe, the resinous matter, which exudes from the stem, differs in appearance, smell, and in every respect, from Gummi Galbanum.

BUBON MACEDON'ICUM, *Athaman'ta Macedon'ica, Petroseli'num Macedon'icum, A'pium petræ'um, Petra'pium*, (F.) *Persil de Macédoine, Macedo'nian Parsley*. Its properties are similar to those of common parsley, but weaker and less grateful. The seeds are an ingredient in the celebrated compounds, Mithridate and Theriac.

BUBONA, Nipple.
BUBONALGIA, from βουβων, 'the groin,' and αλγος, 'pain.' Pain in the groin.
BUBONCUS, Bubo.
BUBO'NIUM, *Aster At'ticus, Golden Starwort*. A plant anciently supposed to be efficacious in diseases of the groin, from βουβων, 'the groin.'
BUBONOCE'LE, from βουβων, 'the groin,' and κηλη, 'tumour,' 'rupture.' *Her'nia inguina'lis*, (F.) *Hernie inguinale, In'guinal Hernia*, or *Rupture of the Groin*. Some surgeons have confined this term to hernia when limited to the groin, and have called the same affection, when it has descended to the scrotum, *Oscheoce'lē*, or *Scrotal Hernia*. The rupture passes through the abdominal ring: and, in consequence of the greater size of the opening in the male, it is more frequent in the male sex.
BUBONONCUS, Bubo.
BUBONOPANUS, Bubo.
BUBONOREX'IS, from βουβων, 'the groin,' and ρηξις, 'a rupture.' A name given to bubonocele when accompanied with a division of the peritoneum, or when, in other words, it is devoid of a sac.
BUBON'ULUS, *Bubon'culus*. A diminutive of *Bubo*. A painful swelling of the lymphatics of the penis, extending along the dorsum of that organ to the groin. It is an occasional accompaniment of gonorrhœa.

BUBUKLE. A word used by Shakspeare for a red pimple on the nose.

BUBUNCULUS, Bubonulus.

BUCAROS, Terra Portugallica.

BUCCA, *Gnathos.* The mouth. The cheek and hollow of the cheek. Also, the vulva.

BUCCAC'RATON, from *Bucca,* and κραω, 'I mix.' A morsel of bread sopped in wine, which served of old for a breakfast.—Linden.

BUCCAL, *Bucca'lis,* from *Bucca,* 'the mouth,' or rather 'the cheek.' That which concerns the mouth, and especially the cheek.

BUCCAL ARTERY, *A. Sus-maxillaire,* (Ch.) arises from the internal maxillary or from some of its branches, as the *Temporalis profunda antica,* or the *Alveolar.* It distributes its branches to the buccinator muscle, and to the buccal membrane.

BUCCAL GLANDS, *Molar Glands.* Mucous follicles, seated in the buccal membrane, opposite the molar teeth. They secrete a viscid humour, which mixes with the saliva, and lubricates the mouth.

BUCCAL MEMBRANE, (F.) *Membrane Buccale.* The mucous membrane, which lines the interior of the mouth.

BUCCAL NERVE, or *Buccina'tor Nerve, Buccolabial*—(Ch.,) is given off by the inferior maxillary. It sends its branches to the cheek, and especially to the buccinator muscle.

BUCCAL VEIN follows the artery.

BUC'CEA, *Buccel'la.* The fleshy excrescence of nasal polypus, so called because it was believed to proceed from the mouth.—Paracelsus. Also, a mouthful.

BUCCELA'TON, *Buccela'tus.* A loaf-shaped cathartic medicine; made chiefly of scammony. —Aëtius, Paulus of Ægina.

BUCCELLA'TIO. A mode of arresting hemorrhage, by applying a pledget of lint to the bleeding vessel.—Avicenna, Fallopius.

BUCCINA, Turbinated bones.

BUCCINA'TOR, from *buccinare,* 'to sound the trumpet.' The *Buccina'tor Muscle, Retrac'tor An'guli Oris, Bucco-Alvéolo-maxillaire, Alréolo-labial* — (Ch.,) *Manso'rius,* is situate in the substance of the cheeks. It extends between the posterior portions of the alveolar arches of the two jaws and the commissure of the lips, which it draws backward. It assists in mastication, by pushing the food back towards the teeth; and, if the cheeks be distended by air, its contraction forces it out.

BUCCO. One who is blub-cheeked, or widemouthed.

BUCCO-ALVÉOLO-MAXILLAIRE, Buccinator.

BUCCO-LABIAL NERVE, Buccal nerve.

BUCCO-PHARYNGE'AL, *Bucco-Pharynge'us,* (F.) *Bucco-Pharyngien.* Belonging to the mouth and pharynx. The *Bucco-pharynge'al Aponeuro'sis* or *Intermax'illary Lig'ament,* extends from the internal ala of the pterygoid process to the posterior part of the lower alveolar arch, and affords attachment, anteriorly, to the buccinator, and, posteriorly, to the constrictor pharyngis superior.

BUC'CULA, from *Bucca,* 'the mouth.' A small mouth. The fleshy part beneath the chin. —Bartholine.

BUCERAS, Trigonella foenum — b. Foenum Græcum, Trigonella foenum Græcum.

BUCHU, Diosma crenata—b. Leaves, Diosma crenata.

BUCKBEAN, Menyanthes trifoliata—b. American, Menyanthes verna.

BUCKBERRY, Vaccinium stamineum.

BUCKET FEVER, Dengue.

BUCKEYE, Æsculus hippocastanum.

BUCKHO, Diosma crenata.

BUCKTHORN, PURGING, Rhamnus.

BUCKWHEAT, Polygonum fagopyrum — b. Plant, eastern, Polygonum divaricatum.

BUCNEMIA, see Elephantiasis — b. Tropica, see Elephantiasis.

BUCTON, Hymen.

BUFF, INFLAMMATORY, Corium phlogisticum.

BUFFY COAT, Corium phlogisticum.

BUG, (BED,) Cimex.

BUGANTIA, Chilblain.

BUG'GERY, *Sod'omy, Sodom'ia, Co'itus Sodomit'icus,* (I.) *Bugarone.* Said to have been introduced by the Bulgarians. A carnal copulation against nature, as of a man or woman with any animal; or of a man with a man, or a man unnaturally with a woman. The unnatural crime.

BUGLE, Prunella— b. Common, Ajuga reptans—b. Pyramidale, Ajuga—b. Rampante, Ajuga reptans — b. Water, Lycopus Virginicus — b. Weed, Lycopus.

BUGLOSE, Anchusa officinalis.

BUGLOSS, DYER'S, Anchusa tinctoria—b. Garden, Anchusa officinalis—b. Upright, Ajuga.

BUGLOSSA, Anchusa officinalis.

BUGLOSSUM ANGUSTIFOLIUM MAJUS, Anchusa officinalis—b. Latifolium, Borago officinalis — b. Sativum, Anchusa officinalis — b. Sylvestris, Anchusa officinalis — b. Tinctorum, Anchusa tinctoria — b. Verum, Boracic acid — b. Vulgare majus, Anchusa officinalis.

BUGRANDE ÉPINEUSE, Ononis spinosa.

BUGRANE, Ononis spinosa—*b. des Champs,* Ononis arvensis.

BUGULA, Ajuga—b. Chamæpitys, Teucrium chamæpitys — b. Pyramidalis, Ajuga — b. Reptans, Ajuga reptans.

BUIS, Buxus.

BUISARD, MINERAL WATERS OF. Buisard is two leagues from Chateau-Thierry, in France. The water contains chloride of calcium and carbonate of lime.

BULB, *Bulbus,* (F.) *Bulbe.* A name, given by anatomists to different parts which resemble, in shape, certain bulbous roots. The *Bulb of the Aorta* is the great sinus of the Aorta. *Bulb of a Tooth;* the vascular and nervous papilla contained in the cavity of a tooth. The *Bulb* or *Root of the Hair* is the part whence the hair originates. The *Bulb of the Urethra* is the dilated portion formed by the commencement of the *Corpus spongiosum* towards the root of the penis. We say, also, *Bulb,* for *Globe, of the eye.*

BULB OF THE EYE, see Eye—b. of the Female, Bulbus vestibuli — b. Rachidian, see Medulla oblongata.

BULBE, Bulb—*b. du Vagin,* Bulbus vestibuli —*b. de la Voûte à trois Piliers,* Mamillary tubercles.

BULBI FORNICIS, Mamillary tubercles—b. Priorum Crurum Fornicis, Mamillary tubercles.

BULBOCASTANEUM, Bunium bulbocastanum.

BULBO-CAVERNOSUS, Accelerator urinæ— *b. Syndesmo-caverneux,* Accelerator urinæ — *b. Uréthral,* Accelerator urinæ.

BULBOCODIUM, Narcissus pseudonarcissus.

BULBONACH, Lunaria rediviva.

BULBUS, Bulb.

BULBUS ESCULEN'TUS. The *Es'culent Bulb:* a particular kind, so denominated by the ancients. It is supposed to have been the *Cepa Ascalon'ica.*—Dioscorides, Celsus, Pliny, &c.

BULBUS GLANDULOSUS, Proventriculus — b. Oculi, see Eye — b. Olfactorius, see Olfactory Nerves — b. Pili, see Hair — b. Rachidicus, see Medulla oblongata—b. Vaginæ, B. vestibuli.

BULBUS VESTIB'ULI, *B. Vagi'næ, Plexus retiform'is, Crura clitor'idis inter'na, Bulb or Semibulb of the Female,* (F.) *Bulbe du Vagin.* A closepacked plexus of intricately anastomosing veins, inclosed in a fibrous investment, — being an immediate continuation and extension of the *pars intermedia,* and occupying the space between the beginning or vestibule of the vagina and the rami of the pubic arch. It is regarded by Louth, Taylor, Morgagni and Kobelt as the analogue of the male bulb.

BULBUS VOMITO'RIUS. A plant, said by Dioscorides to be emetic and diuretic. It is the *Musk-grape flower,* according to Ray,—the *Hyacinthus Muscari.*

BULESIS, Voluntas.

BULGA, Vulva.

BULIMIA, Boulimia.

BU'LITHOS, from βους, 'an ox,' and λιθος, 'a stone.' A bezoar or stone, found in the kidneys, gall-bladder, or urinary bladder of an ox or cow.

BULLA, (F.) *Bulle.* A *Bleb.* A portion of the cuticle, detached from the skin by the interposition of a transparent, watery fluid. It forms the 4th order in Willan's and Bateman's arrangement of cutaneous diseases, and includes erysipelas, pemphigus, and pompholyx. By some, Bulla has been used synonymously with *Pemphigus.* See, also, Hydatid.

BULLACE PLUM, Prunus invitia.

BULLÆ ROTUNDÆ CERVICIS UTERI, Nabothi glandulæ.

BULL-FISTS, Lycoperdon.

BUMELLIA, Fraxinus excelsior.

BUNA, Coffea Arabica.

BUNDURH, Corylus avellana.

BUNIAS, Brassica napus.

BU'NIOID, *Bunioi'des, Na'piform;* from βουνιον, 'a turnip,' and ειδος, 'resemblance.' An epithet for a form of cancer, bearing some resemblance to a turnip.

BUNION, Bunyon.

BUNI'TES VINUM. A wine, made by infusing the *Bunium* in must. It is stomachic, but scarcely ever used.

BUNIUM, Carvi, Carum.

BU'NIUM BULBOCAS'TANUM, βουνιον, so called, it has been supposed, from growing on hills, from βουνος, 'a hill.' *Balanocas'tanum, Bu'nium minus, Sium bulbocastanum, Scandex bulbocastanum, Carum bulbocastanum.* The systematic name of a plant, whose root is called *Pig-nut, Agriocas'tanum, Nu'cula terres'tris, Bulbocas'tanum majus et minus, Earth-nut, Hawknut, Kipper-nut,* (F.) *Terre-noix.* The root is tuberous, and is eaten raw or roasted. It has been supposed to be of use in strangury. It is not employed in medicine.

BUNNIAN, Bunyon.

BUN'YON, *Bun'ion, Bun'nian,* from βουνος, 'an eminence.' (?) An enlargement and inflammation of the bursa mucosa at the inside of the ball of the great toe.

BUOPHTHALMIA, Buphthalmia.

BUPEINA, Boulimia.

BUPHTHALMI HERBA, Anthemis tinctoria.

BUPHTHAL'MIA, *Buophthal'mia, Buphthal'mos, Elephantom'ma,* from βους, 'an ox,' and οφθαλμος, 'an eye.' *Ox-eye.* Under this name, the generality of authors have designated the first stage of nydrophthalmia. Others, with Sabatier, mean, by it, turgescence of the vitreous humour, which, by pushing the iris forwards, forms around the crystalline a sort of border

BUPHTHALMUM CRETICUM, Anthemis Pyrethrum — b. Majus, Chrysanthemum leucanthemum.

BUPHTHALMUS, Hydrophthalmia, Sempervivum tectorum.

BUPINA, Boulimia.

BUPLEUROIDES, Bupleurum rotundifolium.

BUPLEU'RUM ROTUNDIFO'LIUM, *Bupleu'ron, Bupleuroï'des,* from βου, augmentative, and πλευρον, 'side,' (F.) *Buplèvre, Percefeuille, Round-leaved Hare's Ear, Thorowwax.* The herb and seeds are slightly aromatic. It was formerly celebrated for curing ruptures, being made into a cataplasm with wine and oatmeal.

BUPLÈVRE, Bupleurum rotundifolium.

BURAC. Borax. Also, any kind of salt. (Arabic.)

BURDOCK, Arctium lappa — b. Lesser, Xanthium— b. Prairie, Silphium terebinthaceum.

BURIAL ALIVE, Zoothapsis.

BURIS, Hernia, accompanied by scirrhous tumefaction; or, perhaps, a scirrhous tumour only.—Avicenna.

BURN. Sax. bernan or bȳrnan, 'to burn or bren.' *Us'tio, Ambus'tio, Adus'tio, Tresis Causis, Erythe'ma Ambus'tio, Causis, Encau'sis, Pyricaus'tum, Combustu'ra, Catacau'ma, Combus'tio,* (F.) *Brûlure.* An injury produced by the action of too great heat on the body. Burns are of greater or less extent, from the simple irritation of the integument to the complete destruction of the part. The consequences are more or less severe, according to the extent of injury, and the part affected. Burns of the abdomen, when apparently doing well, are sometimes followed by fatal results. Their treatment varies,—at times, the antiphlogistic being required; at others, one more stimulating.

BURNEA, see Pinus Sylvestris.

BURNET, CANADA, Sanguisorba Canadensis.

BURNETT'S DISINFECTING LIQUID. A solution of chloride of zinc, first used by Sir William Burnett for preserving timber, canvass, &c., from dry rot, mildew, &c., and afterwards as an antibromic and antiseptic, especially in the case of dead bodies.

BURNING, *Brenning.* A disease mentioned by old historians, from which authors have unsuccessfully endeavoured to demonstrate the antiquity of syphilis.—Parr.

BURNING OF THE FEET, see Feet, burning of the.

BURNT HOLES. A variety of rupia, popularly known in Ireland under this name; and not unfrequent there amongst the ill-fed children of the poor.

BUR-REED, GREAT, Sparganium ramosum.

BURRHII SPIR'ITUS MATRICA'LIS. The *Spirit of Burrhus for diseases of the Womb.* It is prepared by digesting, in alcohol, equal parts of myrrh, olibanum, and mastic. Boerhaave frequently prescribed it.

BURSA CORDIS, Pericardium — b. Pastoris, Thlaspi bursa—b. Testium, Scrotum—b. Virilis, Scrotum.

BURSÆ MUCO'SÆ, *Bursæ muco'sæ vesicula'res, Bursæ seu Cap'sulæ synovia'les, Blennocys'tides, Sacci muco'si, Vesi'cæ unguino'sæ ten'dinum, Vagi'næ Synovia'les, Synovial Crypts or Follicles,* (F.) *Bourses Synoviales.* Small membranous sacs, situate about the joints, particularly about the large ones of the upper and lower extremities, and, for the most part, lying under the tendons. They are naturally filled with an oily kind of fluid, the use of which is to lubricate surfaces over which the tendons play. In consequence of bruises or sprains, this fluid sometimes collects to a great extent. The bursæ are, generally, either of a roundish or oval form, and they have been arranged under two classes, the *spherical* and the *vaginal*.

BURSÆ SYNOVIALES, Bursæ mucosæ.

BURSAL, *Bursa'lis*. Relating or appertaining to bursæ,—as a '*bureal* tumour.'

BURSALIS, Obturator internus.

BURSERA ACUMINATA, B. gummifera.

BURSE'RA GUMMIF'ERA, *B. acumina'ta, Terebinth'us gummifera, Jamaica Bark Tree.* A resin exudes from this tree, which, as met with in the shops, is solid externally; softish internally; of a vitreous fracture; transparent; of a pale yellow colour; turpentine smell, and sweet, perfumed taste. It has been used like balsams and turpentines in general, and is called, by the French, *Cachibou, Chibou*, and *Resine de Gomart.*

BURST, Hernia, Hernial.

BURSTEN, see Hernial.

BURSULA, Scrotum.

BURTHISTLE, Xanthium.

BURWEED, Xanthium.

BURWORT, Ranunculus acris.

BUSSANG, MINERAL WATERS OF. Bussang is a village in the department of Vosges, France. The waters are acidulous chalybeates.

BUSSEROLLE, Arbutus uva ursi.

BUS'SII SPIR'ITUS BEZOAR'TICUS, *Bezoar'dic Spirit of Bussius.* A preparation, regarded as sudorific, diuretic, and antispasmodic; obtained by distilling subcarbonate and muriate of ammonia, amber, oil of cedar or juniper, &c.

BUTE, ISLAND OF, CLIMATE OF. This island is in the Frith of Clyde, about 18 miles below Greenock. The climate is mild and equable, but rather moist; and, as a winter residence, it holds out advantages for those only that appear to demand such a condition of the atmosphere. The climate resembles, in character, that of the S. W. of England and France, and the Channel islands; although its temperature is lower.

BU'TEA FRONDO'SA, *Erythri'na monosper'ma, Rudolph'ia frondo'sa,* see Kino. A tree, common in Bengal, and in the mountainous parts of India; *Nat. Ord.* Leguminosæ; from which *gum butea* flows. Dr. Pereira found this gum to be identified with a specimen marked *gummi rubrum astringens*—the *gomme astringente de Gambie* of M. Guibourt. By some, this gum has been confounded with kino.

BUTIGA, Gutta rosea.

BUTOMON, Iris pseudacorus.

BUTTER, from βουτυρον; itself from βους, 'ox,' and τυρος, 'any thing coagulated.' *Buty'rum, Pice'rion,* (F.) *Beurre.* A sort of concrete oil, obtained from the cream that forms on the surface of the milk furnished by the females of the mammalia; especially by the cow and the goat. Fresh butter is very nutritious, whilst the rancid is irritating. The ancient chemists gave the name *Butter* to many of the metallic chlorides. It has also been applied to vegetable substances, which resemble, in some respects, the butter obtained from milk.

BUTTER OF BAMBOUC or BAMBUC, (F.) *Beurre de Bambouc* ou *Bambuk.* A vegetable oil obtained from a species of almond, and used in Senegal in neuralgic and rheumatismal pains.

BUTTER OF CA'CAO, *Oil of Ca'cao, Oleum Cacao epissa'tum, O. Theobro'mæ Cacao expres'sum,* (F.) *Beurre de Cacao, Huile de Cacao.* A fat substance, of a sweet and agreeable taste, obtained from the *Theobroma* cacao, or chocolate nut.

BUTTER OF COCOA, (F.) *Buerre de Coco.* A fatty, concrete substance, which separates from the milk of the cocoa nut. It is sweet and agreeable.

BUTTERBUR, Tussilago petasites.

BUTTERCUPS, Ranunculus acris.

BUTTERFLY-WEED, Asclepias tuberosa.

BUTTERMILK, (F.) *Bab, urre, Lait de Beurre.* The thin, sour milk, separated from the cream by churning. It contains caseum and a little butter. It is a refreshing drink when newly made.

BUTTERWORT, Pinguicola vulgaris.

BUTTOCK-HUMP, Steatopyga.

BUTTONBUSH, Cephalanthus occidentalis.

BUTTONWOOD SHRUB, Cephalanthus occidentalis.

BUTUA, Pareira brava.

BUTYRUM, Butter — b. Amygdalarum dulcium, Confection (almond)—b. Saturni, Unguentum plumbi superacetatis— b. Zinci, Zinci chloridum.

BUVEUR, Rectus internus oculi.

BUXTON, MINERAL WATERS OF, *Buxtonien'ses Aquæ.* Buxton is a village in Derbyshire. The springs are thermal, and about 82° Fahrenheit. They contain sulphate of soda, chloride of calcium, chloride of sodium, chloride of magnesium, carbonate of lime, carbonic acid, and azote. They are used in cases in which thermal springs, in general, are recommended. They contain little or no mineral impregnation.

BUXUS, *Buxus sempervi'rens.* The *Box-tree,* (F.) *Buis* ou *Bouis.* The leaves are bitter and aromatic, and, as such, have been used in medicine, in cases of worms, dyspepsia, &c., in the form of decoction. They are sometimes, also, added to beer. The seed was anciently called *Carthe'gon.*

BYNE, Malt.

BY'RETHRUM. A sort of cap or *Couvrechef*, filled with cephalic substances.—Forestus.

BYRSA, βυρσα. A leather skin to spread plasters upon.

BYRSODEP'SICON. A tan stuff, with which CÆLIUS AURELIANUS sprinkled wool, which he applied in certain cases to the umbilical region: from βυρσα, 'leather,' and δεψω, 'I tan.'

BYRSODEPSICUM PRINCIPIUM, Tannin.

BYSAU'CHEN, from βυω, 'I stop up,' and αυχην, 'the neck.' A morbid stiffness of the neck. One with a short neck,—*Simotrache'lus.*

BYSSOS, Vulva.

BYSSUS, *Byssum.* The ancients gave this name to several vegetable substances, which were used for the fabrication of stuffs prized for their fineness, colour, and rarity of material. It is now chiefly applied to the filaments, by the aid of which the acephalous mollusca attach their shells to the rocks. Byssus was formerly also applied to the *female pudendum.*

BYTHOS, βυθος, 'depth.' An epithet used by Hippocrates for the fundus of the stomach.

C.

C. This letter in the chemical alphabet signifies nitre. It is also sometimes used in prescriptions for calx.

CAA-AP'IA, *Dorste'nia Brazilien'sis* seu *cordifo'lia* seu *placentoi'des* seu *vitel'la*. The root, according to Piso, is employed as emetic and anti-diarrhœic.

CAA-ATAY'A. A plant of Brazil, supposed to be a species of gratiola. It is very bitter, and considered to be one of the best indigenous cathartics.

CAACICA, Euphorbia capitata.

CAA-GHIYU'YO, *Frutex bac'cifer Brazilien'sis.* A shrub of Brazil, whose leaves, in powder, are considered detersive.

CAAOPIA, Hypericum bacciferum.

CAAPEBA, Pareira brava.

CAAPONGA, Crithmum maritimum.

CAAROBA. A Brazilian tree, whose leaves, in decoction, promote perspiration. See Ceratonia.

CABAL, *Cab'ala, Cabal'la, Cal'bala, Caba'lia, Kab'ala, Gaballa.* This word is from the Hebrew, and signifies knowledge transmitted by tradition. Paracelsus and several authors of the 16th and 17th centuries have spoken much of this species of magic, which they distinguished into *Judaic* or *theologian*, and *Hermetic* or *medicinal;* the latter being, according to them, the art of knowing the most occult properties of bodies by an immediate communication with spirits,—the knowledge being thus acquired by inspiration, and incapable of inducing error. It was also called *Ars cabalis'tica*, 'cabalistic art.'

CABAL'HAU. A plant of Mexico, according to Dalechamps, which passes for an antidote to white hellebore, and yet is used for poisoning arrows. It is unknown to botanists.

CAB'ALIST, *Cabalis'ta.* One instructed in the Cabal.

CABALLATION, Cynoglossum.

CABARET, Asarum.

CABBAGE, Brassica—c. Cow, Nymphæa odorata—c. Irish, Dracontium fœtidum—c. Skunk, Dracontium fœtidum—c. Swamp, Dracontium fœtidum—c. Water, Nymphæa odorata—c. Tree, Geoffræa inermis—c. Bark tree, Geoffræa inermis.

CABBAGIUM, Geoffræa inermis.

CABUREIBA, Myroxylon Peruiferum.

CABUREICIBA, see Myroxylon Peruiferum.

CACÆ'MIA, *Cachæ'mia*, from κακος, 'bad,' and 'αιμα, 'blood.' A faulty or morbid condition of the blood.

CACÆSTHE'SIS, *Cacæsthe'sis, Cacoæsthe'sis*, from κακος, 'bad,' and αισθησις, 'feeling.' Morbid sensation. Morbid general feeling. Indisposition.

CACAFERRI. Ferri subcarbonas.

CAC'AGOGUE, *Cacago'gus*, from κακκη, 'excrement,' and αγειν, 'to expel.' An ointment, composed of alum and honey; which, when applied to the anus, produced an evacuation.—Paulus of Ægina.

CACALEXITERIA, Alexiteria.

CACA'LIA ANTEUPHOR'BIUM, *Anteuphor'bium.* A plant, which Dodoens and others considered to be capable of tempering the caustic properties of euphorbium. It is also called *Klein'ia*.

Many varieties of the Cacalia are used, in different countries, chiefly as condiments.

CA'CAO, *Ca'coa, Caca'vi, Quahoil, Cacava'ta.* The cocoa or chocolate nut; fruit of *Theobro'ma Cacao, Co'coa Cacavif'era, Ca'cao minor* seu *sati'va, Cacao theobro'ma; Family, Malvaceæ. Sex. Syst.* Polydelphia Pentandria.

CACATION, Defecation.

CACATORIA, Diarrhœa.

CAC'ATORY, *Cacato'rius*, from *cacare*, 'to go to stool.' *Febris cacato'ria;* a kind of intermittent fever, accompanied by copious alvine evacuations.—Sylvius.

CACAVATA, Cacao.

CACAVI, Cacao, Jatropha manihot.

CACCE, Excrement.

CACCION'DE. A sort of pill, chiefly formed of catechu, recommended by Baglivi in dysentery.

CACEPHEBOTE'SIA, from κακος, 'bad,' and εφιβοτης, 'puberty.' Morbid puberty. Disease occurring at the period of puberty.

CACHANG-PARANG. A sort of bean of Sumatra, mentioned by Marsden, whose seeds are given in pleurisy. Jussieu considers it to be the *Mimo'sa scandens*.

CACHEC'TIC, *Cachec'tes, Cachec'ticus*, same etymon as *Cachexia*. One attacked with cachexia. Belonging to cachexia. *Cachec'tica remed'ia* are remedies against cachexia.

CACHEN-LAGUEN, Chironia Chilensis.

CACHEX'IA, from κακος, 'bad,' and 'εξις, 'habit.' *Status cachec'ticus, Cachexy, Dysthe'sis*, (F.) *Cachexie*. A condition in which the body is evidently depraved. A bad habit of body, chiefly the result of scorbutic, cancerous, or venereal diseases when in their last stage. Hence we hear of a *Scorbutic Cachexia, Cancerous Cachexia*, &c. Sauvages and Cullen have included under this head a number of diseases—consumptions, dropsies, &c. Cachexia has been sometimes confounded with diathesis. *Cachexia Icter'ica* is jaundice or icterus itself, or a disposition thereto. Fluor albus is sometimes called *Cachexia Uterina*.

CACHEXIA AFRICANA, Chthonophagia—c. Calculosa, Lithia—c. Cancerous, see Cancer—c. Chlorotic, Chlorosis—c. Dysthetica, Dyscrasia—c. Icterica, Icterus—c. Lymphatica farciminosa, see Equinia.

CACHEXIA LONDINEN'SIS. The paleness and other evidences of impaired health presented by the inhabitants of London. A similar cachexia is seen in those of other crowded cities.

CACHEXIA, MARSH, (F.) *Cachexie paludéenne*. The state of cachexy observed in malarious districts.

CACHEXIA SATURNINE, Saturnismus.

CACHEXIA, SCORBUTIC, see Purpura — c. Scrophulosa, Scrofula.

CACHEXIA SPLE'NICA. The state of scorbutic cachexia, which often accompanies diseases, especially enlargement of the spleen, *Splenal'gia Bengalen'sis*, in India.

CACHEXIA VENEREA, Syphilis—c. Venous, Venosity—c. Virginum, Chlorosis.

CACHEXIE, Cachexia — c. *Paludéenne*, Cachexia, marsh.

CACHEXY, Cachexia.

CACHIBOU, see Bursera gummifera.

CACHINLAGUA, Chironia chilensis.

CACHINNA'TIO, from *cachinno*, 'I laugh aloud.' A tendency to immoderate laughter, as in some hysterical and maniacal affections.

CACHIRI. A fermented liquor made, in Cayenne, from a decoction of the rasped root of the manioc. It resembles perry.

CACHLEX. A small stone or pebble, found

on the sea shore. One of these, when heated in the fire, and cooled in whey, communicates an astringency to the liquid, so that it was anciently esteemed to be useful in dysentery.—Galen.

CACHOS. An oriental fruit, apparently of a Solanum, which is esteemed lithontriptic.

CACHOU, Catechu.

CACHRYS LIBANO'TIS. An umbelliferous plant which grows in Africa and the South of Europe. It is aromatic and astringent. Its seeds are extremely acrid.

CACHRYS MARITIMA, Crithmum maritimum.

CACHUN'DE. An Indian troch or pastile composed of amber, mastic, musk, cinnamon, aloes, rhubarb, galanga, pearls, rubies, emeralds, garnets, &c. It is regarded by the people of India as an antidote, stomachic and antispasmodic.

CACO, κακο, properly only an abbreviation of κακος. In composition it means something defective; as in the following words.

CACOÆSTHESIS. Cacæsthesis.

CACO-ALEXITERIA, Alexipharmic.

CACOCHO'LIA, from κακος, 'bad,' and χολη, 'bile.' Diseases induced by a depraved condition of the bile.

CAC'OCHROI, *Cac'ochri*, from κακος, 'bad,' and χροα, 'colour.' Diseases in which the complexion is morbidly changed in colour.

CACOCHYL'IA, from κακος, 'bad,' and χυλος, 'chyle.' Depraved chylification.

CACOCHYM'IA, *Kakochym'ia*, *Corrup'tio Humo'rum*, from κακος, 'bad,' and χυμος, 'juice,' 'humour.' *Cacoch'ymy*. Depravation of the humours.

CACOCHYMIA PLUMBEA, Lead poisoning — c. Scorbutica, see Purpura — c. Scrophulosa, Scrofula — c. Venerea, Syphilis.

CACOCH'YMUS, *Cacochym'icus*. One attacked with cacochymia. Belonging to cacochymia.

CACOCNE'MUS, *Cacocne'micus*, *Malis suris prædi'tus*; from κακος, 'bad,' and κνημη, 'the leg.' One who has bad legs.

CACOCORE'MA, from κακος, 'bad,' and κορεω, 'I purge, or cleanse.' A medicine which purges off the vitiated humours.

CACODÆ'MON, from κακος, 'bad,' and δαιμων, 'a spirit.' An evil spirit, to which were ascribed many disorders. The nightmare.

CACO'DES, from κακος, 'bad,' and οζειν, 'to smell,'—*malè olens*. Having a bad smell; *Caco'dia*, *Cacos'mia*.

CACODIA, see Cacodes.

CACOËTHES, *Cacoeth'icus*, from κακος, 'bad,' and ἐθος, 'disposition, habit,' &c. Of a bad or vitiated character, as *ulcus cacoë'thes*, an ulcer of a malignant character.

CACOËTHICUS, Cacoethes.

CACOGALAC'TIA, *Cacoga'lia*, from κακος, 'bad,' and γαλα, gen. γαλακτος, 'milk.' A bad condition of the milk.

CACOGALAC'TICA, same etymon as the last. One who suffers from a bad condition of the milk.

CACOGALIA, Cacogalactia.

CACOGEN'ESIS, from κακος, 'bad,' and γενεσις, 'generation.' A morbid formation.

CACOMORPHIA, Deformation.

CACOMORPHOSIS, Deformation.

CACOPATHI'A, *Pas'sio Mala*, from κακος, 'bad,' and παθος, 'affection.' A distressed state of mind.—Hippocrates.

CACOPHO'NIA, from κακος, 'bad,' and φωνη, 'voice,' *vitia'ta vox*. A dissonant condition of voice.

CACOPLAS'TIC, *Cacoplas'ticus*, *Dysplasmat'ic*; from κακος, 'bad,' and πλασσω, 'I form.' Susceptible of only a low degree of organization, as the indurations resulting from low or chronic inflammation, fibro-cartilage, cirrhosis, &c.

CACOPRA'GIA, *Cacoprax'is*, from κακος, 'bad,' and πραττω, 'I perform.' Depraved condition of the organic functions.

CACOPRAXIS, Cacopragia.

CACORRHACHI'TIS, from κακος, 'bad,' and ῥαχις, 'the spine.' *Cacor'rhachis*, *Cacorhachis*, *Cacorhachi'tis*, *Spondylal'gia*. Deformity of the spine. Disease of the spine. Spontaneous luxation of the vertebræ and ribs dependent upon internal causes.

CACORRHYTH'MUS, *Arrhyth'mus*, from κακος, 'bad,' and ῥυθμος, 'rhythm,' 'order.' Irregular.

CACO'SIS. *Mala disposit"io*, (F.) *Vice*. A bad condition of body.—Hippocrates. A diseased condition in general.

CACOSIT'IA, from κακος, 'bad,' and σιτιον, 'aliment.' Disgust or aversion for food — *Fastid'ium cibo'rum*.

CACOSMIA, see Cacodes.

CACOSOMI'UM, from κακος, 'bad,' and σωμα, 'the body.' An hospital for leprosy, and incurable affections in general.

CACOSPERMA'SIA, *Cacosperma'tia*, *Cacosper'mia*, from κακος, 'bad,' and σπερμα, 'sperm.' A bad condition of the sperm.

CACOSPHYX'IA, from κακος, 'bad,' and σφυξις, 'pulse.'—*Vitio'sus pul'sus*. Bad state of pulse.—Galen.

CACOSPLANCH'NIA, from κακος, 'bad,' and σπλαγχνον, 'a viscus.' Indigestion. The emaciation dependent upon imperfect digestion.— Siebenhaar.

CACOSTOM'ACHUS, from κακος, 'bad,' and στομαχος, 'the stomach.' What disagrees with the stomach. Indigestible.—Gorræus.

CACOSTOMATOSPHRESIA, Breath, offensive.

CACOS'TOMUS, from κακος, 'bad,' and στομα, 'a mouth.' Having a bad mouth.

CACOTHYM'IA, *Vit'ium An'imi*, from κακος, 'bad,' and θυμος, 'mind,' 'disposition.' A vitious state of mind.—Linden.

CACOTRIBULUS, Centaurea calcitrapa.

CACOTRICH'IA, from κακος, 'bad,' and θριξ, τριχος, 'hair.' Disease of the hair.

CACOTROPH'IA, from κακος, 'bad,' and τροφη, 'nutrition.'—*Vitio'sa nutrit"io*;—disordered nutrition.—Galen.

CACOU, Cagot, Catechu.

CACOU'CIA COCCIN'EA, *Coucin'ea*, *Cocin'ea*, *Schousbæ'a coccin'ea*, *Tikimma*. A perennial twining shrub of South America, the plant of which, as well as the fruit, is possessed of emeto-cathartic properties.

CACTIER, Cactus opuntia.

CACTUS OPUN'TIA, *Opun'tia*. The *Indian Fig*, (F.) *Cactier*, *Raquette*, *Figuier d'Inde*. This plant grows in South America, Spain, Italy, &c. Its fruit, which has the shape of the fig, is of a sweetish taste, and colours the urine red when eaten. Its leaves are considered refrigerant.

The fruits of different species of cactus are called *Tunas*.

CADA'BA, *Stroe'mia*. A genus of the family Capparideæ, natives of India and Arabia. The young shoots of the *Cada'ba farino'sa* are considered to be an antidote against venomous bites.

CADA'VER, *Ptoma*, *Necron*. A *dead body*; a subject; a carcass, (F.) *Cadavre*. The word has been supposed to come from *cado*, 'I fall;' and by some to be a contraction from *caro data vermibus*, 'flesh given to the worms.' (?)

CADAV'EROUS, *Cadav'eric*, *Cadavero'sus*, *Necro'des*, (F.) *Cadaréreux*. Belonging to the dead body; as *cadaverous smell*. The *Cadav'erous* or *Hippocrat'ic face* (see Face,) is an unfavourable sign in disease, and generally denotes a fatal termination.

CADAV'EROUS or CADAV'ERIC HYPERÆ'MIA. The hypostatic hyperæmia observed in depending parts of the dead body.

CADDY INSECT, see Ectozoa.

CADE, Juniperus oxycedrus.

CADEJI-INDI, Malabathrum.

CADEL-AVANACU, Croton tiglium.

CADIA. An Egyptian, leguminous plant. The Arabs attribute to its fresh leaves the power of relieving colic.

CADIVA INSANIA, Epilepsy.

CADMIA, Calamina, Tutia.

CADMI'I SULPHAS, *Cadmi'um sulphu'ricum, Sulphas Cadmi'cus, Meli'ni Sulphas, Klapro'thii Sulphas, Klapro'thium Sulphu'ricum, Melinum Sulphu'ricum, Sulphate of Cadmium.* Used in spots on the cornea, and in chronic torpid inflammation of the conjunctiva, in the quantity of half a grain to a grain to the ounce of water.

CADMIUM SULPHURICUM, Cadmii Sulphas.

CADTCHU, Catechu.

CADUCA HUNTERI, Decidua — c. Passio. Epilepsy.

CADU'CITY, *Imbecil'litas, Debil'itas, Cadu'citas,* from *cadere,* 'to fall.' The French use the word *Caducité* for the portion of human life which is comprised generally between 70 and 80 years. The age which precedes decrepitude. It is so termed in consequence of the limbs not usually possessing sufficient strength to support the body. The precise age must of course vary in individuals.

CADUQUE, Decidua membrana—*c. Réfléchie,* see Decidua membrana—*c. Vraie,* Decidua membrana.

CADURCUS, Vulva.

CADUS, καδος. A Greek measure equal to ten gallons English.—Pliny. Amphora.

CÆCA, FORAM'INA (ANTERIUS ET POSTERIUS) are situate at the fore and back parts of the tuber annulare of the brain, and at the extremities of the depression made by the vertebral artery. The former is placed between the nerves of the third; and the latter between those of the sixth pair.

CÆCÆ HÆMORRHOI'DES, *Blind Piles,* (F.) *Hémorrhoides aveugles,* are those unaccompanied by any discharge.

CÆCAL, *Cæca'lis.* Belonging to the cæcum, from *cæcus,* 'blind, hidden.' The *Cæcal arteries and veins* are the branches of the *Arteriæ et venæ colicæ dextræ inferiores,* distributed to the cæcum.

CÆCATRIX, Cicatrix.

CÆ'CITAS, *Cæ'citas, Cæcitu'do, Ablep'sia, Obcæca'tio, Occæca'tio, Anap'sia, Ty'phlotes, Typhlo'sis, Blindness,* (F.) *Aveuglement, Cécité, Perte de la vue.* Cæcitas may be dependent upon many different diseases, — as upon amaurosis, specks, hypopyon, cataract, glaucoma, ophthalmia, atrophy of the eye, &c.

CÆCITAS CREPUSCULARIS, Hemeralopia — c. Diurna, Nyctalopia — c. Nocturna, Hemeralopia.

CÆCITUDO, Cæcitas.

CÆCUM, *Cæcum, Intesti'num cæcum, Monom'achon, Monom'acum, Monoco'lon, Monocu'lum, Typhlo'teron monoco'lon, Typhlot'erum, Typhlo-en'terum, Init''ium intesti'ni crassi, Saccus Intestini crassi seu Coli, Cæcum Caput coli, Caput coli, Prima cella coli, Init''ium extu'berans coli,* from *cæcus,* 'blind.' The *Blind Gut,* so called from its being perforated at one end only. That portion of the intestinal canal which is seated between the termination of the ileum and commencement of the colon; and which fills, almost wholly, the right iliac fossa; where the peritoneum retains it immovably. Its length is about three or four fingers' breadth. The *Ileo-cæcal valve* or *Valve of* Bauhin shuts off all communication between it and the ileum; and the *Appendix vermiformis cæci* is attached to it.

CÆCUM FORA'MEN of the frontal bone is a small cavity at the inferior extremity of the internal coronal crest or crista. — *Fronto-ethmoidal foramen,* (F.) *Trou aveugle* ou *borgne.* Morgagni has given the same name to the small cavity in the middle of the upper surface of the tongue, near its base; the sides of which are furnished with mucous follicles—*Lacune de la langue*—(Ch.)

CÆCUM, PHLEGMONOUS TUMOUR OF THE, Typhlo-enteritis.

CÆCUS. 'Blind.' One deprived of sight, *Typhlops,* (F.) *Aveugle, Borgne.* In anatomy, it is used to designate certain holes or cavities, which end in a *cul-de-sac;* or have only one opening.

Blind Ducts of the Ure'thra, (F.) *Conduits aveugles de l'urèthre,* are the *Mucous Lacu'næ of the Ure'thra.*

CÆLA-DOLO, Torenia Asiatica.

CÆMENTUM, Lute.

CÆRULEUM BEROLINENSE, Prussian blue—c. Borussicum, Prussian blue.

CÆRULOSIS NEONATORUM, Cyanopathy.

CÆSALPI'NIA, *Cæsalpi'nia sappan, Sappan* or *Sampfen wood,* (F.) *Brésillet, Bois de Sappan.* A small Siamese tree, the wood of which is used in decoction, in cases of contusion.

Brazil wood, Pernambuco or *Fernambuco wood,* formerly used as an astringent, is the wood of CÆSALPIN'IA ECHINA'TA. This is the proper Brazil wood; but another variety in commerce is the *Brasiletto,* from *Cæsalpinia Brasiliensis,* and *C. crista,* which grow in the West Indies.

The *Nicaragua* or *Peach-wood* is analogous to this, and is said to be derived from a species of Cæsalpinia.

The kernel of CÆSALPIN'IA BONDUCELL'A, the seed of which is called in India *Kutkuleja* and *Kutoo Kurunja,* is given as a febrifuge tonic. Dose, ten grains.

CÆSA'REAN SEC'TION, *Cæsa'rean opera'tion, Tomotoc'ia, Cæsa'rea sectio, Partus cæsa'reus, Opera'tio cæsa'rea, Metrotom'ia,* (F.) *Opération Césarienne,* from *cædere,* 'to cut.' An incision made through the parietes of the abdomen and uterus to extract the foetus. In this manner, Julius Cæsar is said to have been extracted.—Pliny. It is also called *Hysterotom'ia, Hysterotomotoc'ia, Gastrometrotom'ia, Gasterhysterot'omy, Gastrometrot'omè, Gastrohysterot'omy,* (F.) *Opération Césarienne.* An incision has been made into the uterus through the vagina, constituting the *Vaginal Cæsarean Section, Gastrelytrotom'ia, Gastrocolpotom'ia, Laparacolpotom'ia, Laparoëlytrotom'ia,* (F.) *Opération césarienne vaginale.* The Cæsarean section may be required when the mother dies before delivery;— when there is some invincible obstacle to delivery from the faulty conformation of the pelvis; or when the child has passed into the abdominal cavity in consequence of rupture of the uterus.

CÆSARIES, Capillus.

CÆSIUS, Glaucoma.

CÆ'SONES, *Cæ'sares.* Children brought into the world by the Cæsarean operation.

CÆSU'LIÆ. They who have gray eyes.

CÆSURA, Cut.

CÆTCHU, Catechu.

CAF, Camphor.

CAFAL, Agrimony.

CAFAR, Camphor.

CAFÉ, Coffee.

CAFÉ À LA SULTANE. This name has been given to an infusion or decoction of the ground *coques* or pericarps which surround the coffee.

CAFÉ CITRIN. The aqueous infusion of unroasted coffee, so called on account of its yellowish tint.

CAFEYER, Coffea Arabica.

CAFFA, Camphor.

CAFIER, Coffea Arabica.

CAFUR, Camphor.

CAGAS'TRUM. The principal or germ of diseases which are communicable.—Paracelsus.

CAGNEUX, Cagot. See Kyllosis.

CAGOSANGA, Ipecacuanha.

CAGOTS, (F.) A name given to deformed and miserable beings, met with in the Pyrenees, Bern, and Upper Gascony, in France, where they are also called *Capots.* In other districts they are called *Gézits, Gézitains, Orétins, Gahets, Capons, Coliberts, Cacous, Cagneux,* &c. See *Crétin.* The word *Cagot* is supposed to be an abbreviation of *Canis Gothus.* 'Dog of a Goth.'

CAGUE-SANGUE, *Caquesangue.*

CAHINCÆ RADIX, Caincæ radix.

CAI'EPUT OIL, *Cajeput oil, Kyaput'ty, Cajupu'ti O'leum.* The volatile oil of the leaves of *Melaleu'ca Cajapu'ti,* a native of the Moluccas. The oil has a strong, fragrant smell, like camphor; taste pungent and aromatic. It is stimulant, and useful where the essential oils in general are employed. It has also been called *Oil of Witneben,* from the person who first distilled it.

CAILLE. Tetrao coturnix.

CAILLEAU, Lantana.

CAILLÉ, Curds.

CAILLELAIT BLANC, Galium mollugo—c. *Vraie,* Galium verum.

CAILLOT, Coagulum.

CAINANÆ RADIX, Caincæ radix.

CAÏN'CÆ RADIX, *Radix Chiococ'cæ, R. Cainc'næ* seu *Caninanæ* seu *Cahincæ* seu *Kahincæ* seu *Serpenta'riæ Brazilien'sis, Cainca Root.* The bark of the roots of *Chiococc'a anguif'uga, Ch. densifo'lia,* and, perhaps, *Ch. racemo'sa,* a plant of the *Family* Rubiaceæ. *Sex. Syst.* Pentandria Monogynia, of Linnæus. It is bitter, tonic, and diuretic, but has not been long introduced. Dose of the powder, from ᴆj to ᴆss.

Dr. John H. Griscom, of New York, considers there is a remarkable analogy between the Caincæ and the *Apocynum cannabinum.*

CAINITO, Chrysophyllum Cainito.

CAIPA SCHORA. A cucurbitaceous Malabar plant, the fruit of which has a pyriform shape. The juice is drunk in that country for the purpose of arresting hiccough. The fruit, when unripe, is emetic.

CAISSE, Case—c. *du Tambour,* Tympanum.

CAITCHU, Catechu.

CAJAN, Phaseolus creticus.

CAJUPUTI, Cajeput.

CAKES, WORM, STORY'S. These were composed of *calomel* and *jaсap,* made into cakes, and coloured with *cinnabar.*

CALABASH TREE, NARROW-LEAVED, Crescentia Cujete.

CALADIUM ESCULENTUM, Arum esculentum.

CALAF, *Salix Ægyptiaca.* A large-leaved Egyptian willow, called, also, *Ban.* The distilled water of the flowers, called *Macahalef,* passes, in that country, for an excellent antaphrodisiac. It is also used as an antiloimic, antiseptic, and cordial.

CALAGUALA, see Calagualæ radix.

CALAGERI, Vernonia anthelmintica.

CALAGIRAH, Vernonia anthelmintica.

CALAGUA'LÆ RADIX, *Calague'læ Radix.* The root of *Polypo'dium Calagua'la* seu *adiantifor'mĕ* seu *coria'ceum* seu *ammifo'lium* seu *argen'teum* seu *pol'itum, Aspid'ium coria'ceum* seu *ferrugin'eum* seu *dis'color, Tecta'ria calahuala* seu *ferrugin'ea, Calaguala, Calahuala.* It has been exhibited in Italy in dropsy, pleurisy, contusions, abscesses, &c. Its properties are not, however, clear.

CALAHUALA, see Calagualæ radix.

CALAMANDRINA, Teucrium chamædrys.

CALAMBAC, Agallochum.

CALAMBOUK, Agallochum.

CALAME'DON, from καλαμος, 'a reed.' This word has had various significations. Some have used it for an oblique fracture of a bone; the fractured portions having the shape of the nib of a pen. Others have used it for a longitudinal fracture; and others, again, for one that is comminuted.

CALAMI'NA, *Cal'amine,* from *calamus,* 'a reed,' so called from its reed-like appearance. *Cadmi'a, Cathmir, Cadmi'a lapido'sa aëro'sa, Cadmi'a Fos'silis, Lapis Aëro'sus, Calim'ia, Lapis Calamina'ris, Calamina'ris, Car'bonas Zinci impu'rus,* (F.) *Pierre calaminaire.* Native impure carbonate of zinc. Calamine is chiefly used for pharmaceutical purposes in the form of the CALAMINA PRÆPARA'TA, *Lapis Calamina'ris præpara'tus, Car'bonas zinci impu'rus præpara'tus, Zinci car'bonas præpara'tus, Prepared Calamine;* —Calamine reduced to an impalpable powder by roasting and levigation. In this state it is sprinkled or dusted on excoriated parts, or to prevent excoriation, &c.

CALAMINARIS, Calamina.

CALAMINT, Melissa Calamintha — c. Field, Melissa nepeta — c. Mountain, Melissa grandiflora — c. Spotted, Melissa nepeta.

CALAMINTA HUMILIOR, Glecoma hederacea.

CALAMINTHA, Melissa C.—c. Anglica, Melissa nepeta—c. Erecta Virginiana, Cunila Mariana — c. Hederacea, Glechoma hederacea — c. Magno flore, Melissa grandiflora — c. Montana, Melissa grandiflora—c. Nepeta, Melissa nepeta—c. Parviflora, Melissa nepeta — c. Pulegii odore, Melissa nepeta—c. Trichotoma, Melissa nepeta.

CAL'AMUS, καλαμος, 'the reed.' In the Pharmacopœia of the U. S. the rhizoma of acorus calamus.

CALAMUS ALEXANDRI'NUS. Celsus has thus called a medicine, which was long confounded with *Calamus Aromaticus.* It is not a root, however, but the stalk of a plant of India and Egypt, probably the *Andropo'gon Nardus.* It entered into the theriaca, and has been regarded as antihysteric and emmenagogue; — *Calamus aromaticus verus.*

CALAMUS AROMATICUS, Acorus calamus — c. Aromaticus verus, Calamus Alexandrinus — c. Draco, C. rotang — c. Indicus, see Saccharum — c. Odoratus, Acorus calamus, Juncus odoratus.

CALAMUS ROTANG, *C. Draco.* The systematic name of a plant, whence *Dragon's Blood, Sanguis Draco'nis, Cinnab'aris Græco'rum, Draconthæ'ma,* (F.) *Sang-Dragon,* is procured. It is the red, resinous juice, obtained, in India, from wounding the bark of the *Calamus Rotang.* It has been used as an astringent in hemorrhages, &c.; but is now rarely employed.

CALAMUS SCRIPTO'RIUS, *Anag'lyphè,* 'a writing pen,' (F.) *Fossette angulaire du quatrième ventricule.* A small, angular cavity, situate at the superior extremity of the medulla, in the fourth ventricle of the brain, which has been, by some supposed to resemble a pen.

CALAMUS VULGARIS, Acorus calamus.

CALAPPITE. Rumphius has given this name to calculous concretions, found in the interior of certain cocoa nuts. The cocoa tree itself the Malays call *Calappa*. These stones are, likewise, termed *Vegetable Bezoards*. The Malays attribute potent virtues to them, and wear them as amulets.

CALASAYA, Cinchonæ cordifoliæ cortex.

CALBALA, Cabal.

CALBIA'NUM. The name of a plaster in Myrepsus, the composition of which we know not.

CALCADINUM, Ferri sulphas.

CALCAIRE, Calcareous.

CALCA'NEAL, *Calca'neus*, from *calx*, 'the heel.' Having relation to the calcaneum, as '*calcaneal* arteries.'

CALCANÉO-PHALANGIEN DU PETIT ORTEIL, Abductor minimi digiti pedis—c. *Phalanginien commun*, Extensor brevis digitorum pedis—c. *Sous-phalangettien commun*, Flexor brevis digitorum pedis—c. *Sous-Phalanginien commun*, Flexor brevis digitorum pedis—c. *Sousphalangien du petit orteil*, see Abductor minimi digiti pedis—c. *Sus-phalangettien commun*, Extensor brevis digitorum pedis.

CALCA'NEUM, from *calx*, 'the heel.' *Calca'neus, Calcar, Cal'cia, Ichnus, Os Calcis, Pterna, Pter'nium*. The largest of the tarsal bones: that which forms the heel. It is situate at the posterior and inferior part of the foot; is articulated above and a little anteriorly with the astragalus; anteriorly, also, with the os cuboides. Its posterior surface,—called *Heel, Talus, Calx*, (F.) *Talon*,—gives attachment to the tendo-achillis: the lower has, posteriorly, two tuberosities, to which the superficial muscles of the sole of the foot are attached. The *small Apoph'ysis or lateral Apophysis of the Calca'neum*, (F.) *Petit Apophyse ou Apophyse latérale du Calcanéum*, is a projection at the upper surface of this bone, on which is formed the posterior portion of the cavity that receives the astragalus. The *great Apoph'ysis, anterior Apoph'ysis of the Calca'neum*, is the projection which corresponds, on one side, with the cuboides; and on the other forms the anterior part of the facette which receives the astragalus.

CALCANTHON, Atramentum.

CALCAR, Calcaneum, Ergot—c. Avis, Hippocampus minor.

CALCA'REOUS, *Calca'reus, Calca'rius;* from *calx*, 'lime.' (F.) *Calcaire*. Containing lime:— as *calcareous concretions, O. depositions*, &c.

CALCAREUS CARBONAS, Creta.

CALCARIA CHLORATA, Calcis chloridum—c. Chlorica, Calcis chloridum—c. Phosphorica, see Cornu cervi—c. Pura, Calx—c. Pura liquida, Liquor calcis.

CALCARIÆ CHLORUM, Calcis chloridum.

CALCATOR, Ferri sulphas.

CALCATREPPOLA, Centaurea calcitrapa.

CALCE'NA, CALCE'NON, CALCENO'NIA, CALCINO'NIA. Words employed by Paracelsus to designate the concretions of tartrate of lime which form in the human body.

CALCENOS, Calcetus.

CALCEOLA'RIA, from *calceolus*, 'a small slipper;' *Slipperwort*.

CALCEOLA'RIA PRIMATA is used in Peru as a laxative.

CALCEOLA'RIA TRIF'IDA is esteemed to be febrifuge.

CALCE'TUS, *Calceno'nius, Calce'nos*. That which abounds in tartrate of lime. An adjective used by Paracelsus in speaking of the blood; *Sanguis calce'tus*. Hence came the expression *Calcined blood, Sang calciné*.

CALCEUM EQUINUM, Tussilago.

CALCHOIDEA, (OS.) Cuneiform bone.

CALCIA, Calcaneum.

CALCIGEROUS CELL, see Tooth.

CALCIG'RADUS, *Pternob'ates*, from *calx*, πτερνα, 'the heel,' and βαινω, 'I walk.' One who walks on his heels.—Hippocrates.

CALCII CHLORURETUM, Calcis murias—c. Oxychloruretum, Calcis chloridum—c. Oxydum, Calx viva—c. Protochloruretum, Calcis chloridum.

CALCINA'TION, *Calcina'tio, Calci'non, Concrema'tio*, from *calx*, 'lime.' The act of submitting to a strong heat any infusible mineral substance, which we are desirous of depriving either of its water, or of any other volatilizable substance, that enters into its composition; or which we wish to combine with oxygen. *Alum* is calcined to get rid of its water of crystallization;— *chalk*, to reduce it to the state of pure lime, by driving off the carbonic acid; and *certain metals* are subjected to this operation to oxidize them.

CALCINATUM MAJUS POTERII, Hydrargyrum præcipitatum.

CALCINONIA, Calcena.

CALCIS BICHLORURETUM, Calcis chloridum—c. Carbonas, Creta—c. Carbonas durus, Creta, Marmor—c. Carbonas friabilis, Creta.

CALCIS CAR'BONAS PRÆCIPITA'TUS, *Precip'itated Car'bonate of Lime, Precipitated Chalk*. This preparation, introduced into the last edition of the Pharmacopœia of the United States, is prepared as follows: *Liq. Calcii Chlorid*. Ovss; *Sodæ Carbonat*. ℔vj; *Aquæ destillat*. q. s. Dissolve the carbonate of soda in six parts of distilled water; heat this and the solution of chloride of calcium, separately, to the boiling point, and mix. Wash the precipitate repeatedly with distilled water, and dry on bibulous paper. It has the same properties as creta præparata, and is preferred to it in certain cases,—for example, as an ingredient in tooth powders, owing to its freedom from gritty particles.

CALCIS CHLO'RIDUM; *Chlo'ride of Lime, Chlo'ruret of Lime, Hypochlo'rite of Lime, Chlorite of Lime, Oxymu'riate of Lime, Calx chlorina'ta*, (Ph. U.S.) *Protoxichlor'uret of Calcium, Calca'ria chlora'ta, Chlorum Calca'riæ, Chloretum Calca'riæ, Calcaria Chlo'rica, Oxychlorure'tum Calcii, Protochlorure'tum Calcii, Chlorure'tum Oxidi Calcii, Bichlorure'tum Calcis, Oxymu'rias Calcis, Calcis Hypochlo'ris, Calx oxymuriat'ica, Bleaching Powder, Tennant's Powder*, (F.) *Protoxichlorure de Calcium, Chlorure de Chaux, Oxichlorure de Chaux, Chlorure d'Oxide de Calcium, Bichlorure de Chaux, Oximuriate de Chaux, Muriate suroxigéné ou Oxigéné de Chaux, Poudre de Blanchement, P. de Tennant*. A compound resulting from the action of chlorine on hydrate of lime. Chloride of lime is a most valuable disinfecting agent, (see Disinfection,) when dissolved in the proportion of one pound to six gallons of water. It has likewise been employed both internally and externally in various diseases, as in scrofula, fœtor oris, foul ulcers, &c. &c.

CALCIS HEPAR, Calcis sulphuretum—c. Hydras, see Calx—c. Hypochloris, Calcis chloridum.

CALCIS MU'RIAS; *Muriate of Lime, Calx sali'ta, Calcii Chlorure'tum seu Chlo'ridum, Chloride of calcium*, (F.) *Chlorure de calcium, Muriate ou Hydrochlorate de Chaux*. This salt has been given, in solution, as a tonic, stimulant, &c., in scrofulous tumours, glandular obstructions, general debility, &c. A *Solu'tio Muria'tis Calcis, Liquor Calcis Muria'tis, Solution of Muriate of Lime, Liquid Shell*, may be formed of *Muriate of Lime* ℥j. dissolved in *distilled water* f℥ij. The LIQUOR CALCII CHLORIDI or *Solution of Chlo-*

ride of Calcium, of the Pharmacopœia of the United States, is prepared as follows: — *Marble*, in fragments, ℥ix, *Muriatic acid*, Oj; *Distilled water*, a sufficient quantity. Mix the acid with a half pint of the water, and gradually add the marble. Towards the close of the effervescence apply a gentle heat, and, when the action has ceased, pour off the clear liquor and evaporate to dryness. Dissolve the residuum in its weight and a half of distilled water, and filter. Dose, from gtt. xxx to fℨj, in a cupful of water.

CALCIS OXYMURIAS, Calcis chloridum.

CALCIS SULPHURE'TUM; *Hepar Calcis, Sul'-phuret of Lime*, (F.) *Proto-hydrosulfate de Calcium, Hydrosulfate de chaux*. Principally used in solution, as a bath, in itch and other cutaneous affections.

CALCITEA, Ferri sulphas.

CALCITEOSA, Plumbi oxydum semivitreum.

CALCITHOS, Cupri subacetas.

CALCITRAPA, Centaurea Calcitrapa, Delphinium consolida — c. Hippophæstum, Centaurea calcitrapa — c. Stellata, Centaurea calcitrapa.

CALCIUM, CHLORIDE OF, Calcis murias — c. *Chlorure de*, Calcis murias — c. *Chlorure d'oxide de*, Calcis chloridum — c. *Protohydrosulfate de*, Calcis sulphuretum — c. *Protoxichlorure de*, Calcis chloridum — c. Protoxichloruret of, Calcis chloridum — c. Protoxide of, Calx.

CALCO-SUBPHALANGEUS MINIMI DIGITI, Abductor minimi digiti pedis — c. Subphalangeus pollicis, Abductor pollicis pedis.

CALCOCOS, Bell-metal.

CALCOIDEA, (ossicula,) Cuneiform bones.

CALCOTAR, Ferri sulphas.

CALCUL, Calculus.

CALCULEUX, Calculous.

CALCULI, see Calculus — c. Articular, see Calculi Arthritic; and Concretions, articular.

CALCULI, ALTERNATING, see Calculi, urinary.

CALCULI, ARTHRIT'IC, *Tophi, Tuber'cula arthrit'ica, Chalk-stones, Nodes*, (F.) *Pierres crayeuses, Calculs arthritiques, Nœuds*. Concretions, which form in the ligaments, and within the capsules of the joints, in persons affected with gout. They are composed of uric acid, soda, and a little animal matter; very rarely, urate of lime and chloride of sodium are met with. Similar calculi are found in other parts besides the joints.

CAL'CULI, BIL'IARY, *Cal'culi bilio'si* seu *fell'ei* seu *bilia'rii, Bil'iary Concretions, Gall-stones, Cholel'ithus, Cholel'ithus*, (F.) *Calculs biliaires, Pierres au fiel*. Some of these contain all the materials of the bile, and seem to be nothing more than that secretion thickened. Several contain *Picromel*; and the greater part are composed of from 88 to 94 parts of *Cholesterin*, and of from 6 to 12 of the yellow matter of the bile. Biliary calculi are most frequently found in the gall-bladder: at other times, in the substance of the liver, in the branches of the *Ductus hepaticus*, or in the *Ductus Communis Choledochus*. The first are called *Cystic;* the second *Hepatic;* and the last, sometimes, *Hepatocystic*. The causes which give rise to them are very obscure. Often they occasion no uneasiness, and at other times the symptoms may be confounded with those of hepatitis. At times, they are rejected by the mouth, or by the bowels, along with a considerable quantity of bile, which had accumulated behind them; at other times they occasion violent abdominal inflammation, abscesses, and biliary fistulæ, rupture of the gall-bladder, and fatal effusion into the peritoneum. The passage of a gall-stone is extremely painful; yet the pulse is not at first affected. Antiphlogistics, when there is inflammatory action, and strong doses of opium, to allay the pain and spasm, with the warm bath, are the chief remedies. Solvents are not to be depended upon. They cannot reach the calculi.

CALCULI, BONE EARTH, see Calculi, urinary — c. Compound, see Calculi, urinary — c. Cystic, see Calculi, urinary.

CAL'CULI, OF THE EARS, (F.) *Calculs de l'Oreille*. Hard, light, and inflammable concretions, which occur in the *meatus auditorius externus*, and are merely indurated cerumen. They are a frequent cause of deafness. They can be easily seen, and may be extracted by appropriate forceps, after having been detached by injections of soap and water.

CALCULI FELLEI, Calculi, biliary — c. Fusible, see Calculi, urinary.

CAL'CULI, LACH'RYMAL, (F.) *Calculs lacrymaux*. Concretions sometimes, but rarely, form in the lachrymal passages, where they occasion abscesses and fistulæ, which do not heal until they are extracted. No analysis has been made of them.

CALCULI, LITHIC, see Calculi, urinary.

CAL'CULI OF THE MAMMÆ, (F.) *Calculs des Mamelles*. Haller gives a case of a concretion, of a yellowish-white colour, which had the shape of one of the excretory ducts of the mammary gland, having been extracted from an abscess seated in that organ.

CALCULI, MULBERRY, see Calculi, urinary.

CAL'CULI OF THE PAN'CREAS, (F. *Calculs du Pancréas*. These are but little known. Analogy has induced a belief that they resemble the salivary. Some have supposed that certain transparent calculi, rejected by vomiting, or passed in the evacuations, have proceeded from the pancreas, but there seems to be no reason for this belief.

CAL'CULI OF THE PINEAL GLAND, (F.) *Calculs de la Glande Pinéale*. These have been frequently met with. No symptom announces their presence during life. They are composed of phosphate of lime.

CAL'CULI OF THE PROSTATE, *Prostat'ic cal'culi*. These are not very rare. They have generally the same composition as the preceding. They usually present the symptoms common to every tumefaction of the prostate, and sometimes those of calculi in the bladder.

CAL'CULI PUL'MONARY, (F.) *Calculs pulmonaires*. These concretions are very frequently met with in the dead body, without seeming to have produced unpleasant symptoms during life. At other times, they are accompanied with all the symptoms of phthisis, *Phthisie calculeuse*, of Bayle. At times they are expectorated without the supervention of any unpleasant symptom. They are usually formed of carbonate of lime and animal matter.

CAL'CULI, SAL'IVARY, *Cal'culi saliva'les, Sialol'ithi*, (F.) *Calculs salivaires*. Concretions, usually formed of phosphate of lime and animal matter, which are developed in the substance of the salivary glands or in their excretory ducts. In the first case, they may be mistaken for a simple swelling of the gland; in the second, they may generally be detected by the touch. They may be extracted by incision in the interior of the mouth. The calculus developed in the sublingual ducts has been called *Cal'culus sublingua'lis* and *Ran'ula lapide'a*.

CAL'CULI, SPERMAT'IC, (F.) *Calculs spermatiques*. These have been sometimes found in the vesiculæ seminales after death. They cannot be detected during life. No analysis has been made of them.

CAL'CULI OF THE STOMACH AND INTES'TINES, *Enterol'ithus, E. Cal'culus, Coprol'ithus, Concre-*

tio'nes alvi'næ, (F.) *Calculs de l'estomac, C. intestinaux, Pierres stercorales, Concrétions intestinales*. Calculi of the stomach are rare, and have almost always been carried thither by the antiperistaltic action of the intestines. The symptoms occasioned by them are those of chronic gastritis. It has been imagined that the continued use of absorbent powders, as magnesia, will give occasion to them.

Intestinal concretions, (F.) *Calculs intestinaux*, are not uncommon in animals (see BEZOARD:) but they are rare in man. The causes which give rise to them are little known: sometimes a biliary calculus affords them a nucleus. Their composition varies. They are light, hard, very fetid, and not inflammable. They are formed, ordinarily, between the valvulæ of the small intestines, or in the cells of the large, and sometimes in old herniæ. Whilst they do not obstruct the passage of the alimentary mass, they produce no unpleasant symptoms. At times, the movable tumour which they form may be felt through the parietes of the abdomen. They are generally evacuated *per anum*.

CAL'CULI OF THE TONSILS. Calculous concretions, which sometimes form in the tonsils. (F.) *Calculs des Amygdales*. They are easily recognised by the sight and touch: sometimes they are discharged by spitting, either alone or with the pus of an abscess occasioned by their presence. They have not been analyzed.

CALCULI, TRIPLE, see Calculi, urinary—c. Uric, see Calculi, urinary.

CAL'CULI, U'RINARY, *Urol'ithi*, (F.) *Calculs urinaires, Pierres urinaires*. Concretions which form from the crystallizable substances in the urine, and which are met with not only in the whole course of the urinary passages, but in fistulous openings wherever the urine stagnates naturally or accidentally. Their causes are but little known. They are more common at the two extremities of life than at the middle, and more so in some countries and districts than in others. At times, a clot of blood, a portion of mucus, &c., form the nucleus. The symptoms and treatment vary according to the seat of the calculus. There is no such thing probably as a medical solvent, See Urinary Calculi.

Modern chymists have demonstrated the existence of several components of urinary calculi, viz., *Lithic Acid, Phosphate of Lime, Ammoniaco-Magnesian Phosphate, Oxalate of Lime, Cystic Oxide*, and *Xanthic Oxide*, with an animal cementing ingredient. The varieties of calculi, produced by the combination or intermixture of these ingredients, are thus represented by Dr. Paris.

A TABULAR VIEW OF DIFFERENT SPECIES OF URINARY CALCULI.

SPECIES OF CALCULI.	EXTERNAL CHARACTERS.	CHYMICAL COMPOSITION.	REMARKS.
1. LITHIC OR URIC.	FORM, a flattened oval. S. G. generally exceeds 1,500. *Colour*, brownish or fawn-like. *Surface*, smooth. *Texture*, laminated.	It consists principally of *Lithic Acid*. When treated with nitric acid, a beautiful pink substance results. This calculus is slightly soluble in water, abundantly so in the pure alkalies.	It is the prevailing species; but the surface sometimes occurs finely tuberculated. It frequently constitutes the *nuclei* of the other species.
2. MULBERRY.	*Colour*, dark brown. *Texture*, harder than that of the other species. S. G. from 1.428 to 1.976. *Surface*, studded with tubercles.	It is *oxalate of lime*, and is decomposed in the flame of a spirit lamp swelling out into a white efflorescence, which is *quick-lime*.	This species includes some varieties, which are remarkably smooth and pale-coloured, resembling *hempseed*.
3. BONE EARTH	*Colour*, pale brown or gray; *surface*, smooth and polished; *structure*, regularly laminated; the laminæ easily separating into concrete crusts.	Principally *phosphate of lime*. It is soluble in muriatic acid.	
4. TRIPLE.	*Colour*, generally brilliant white. *Surface*, uneven, studded with shining crystals, less compact than the preceding species. Between its laminæ small cells occur, filled with sparkling particles.	It is an *ammoniaco-magnesian phosphate*, generally mixed with phosphate of lime. Pure alkalies decompose it, extracting its ammonia.	This species attains a larger size than any of the others.
5. FUSIBLE.	*Colour*, grayish white.	A compound of the two foregoing species.	It is very fusible, melting into a vitreous globule.
6. CYSTIC.	Very like the triple calculus, but it is unstratified and more compact and homogenous.	It consists of *cystic oxide*. Under the blowpipe it yields a peculiarly fetid odour. It is soluble in acids, and in alkalies, even if they are fully saturated with carbonic acid.	It is a rare species.
7. ALTERNATING.	Its section exhibits different concentric laminæ.	Compounded of several species, alternating with each other.	
8. COMPOUND.	No characteristic form.	The ingredients are separable only by chymical analysis.	

1. *Renal Calculi*, (F.) *Calculs rénaux*. These have almost always a very irregular shape: at times, there is no indication of their presence: at others, they occasion attacks of pain in the kidneys, sometimes accompanied with bloody or turbid urine. Often, they cause inflammation of the kidneys, with all its unpleasant results. They are generally formed of uric acid, animal matter, and oxalate of lime, with, sometimes, phosphates. The treatment will have to vary, according to the absence or presence of inflammatory signs,—relieving the irritation by opiates. A surgical operation can rarely be applicable.

2. *Calculi of the Ureters*, (F.) *Calculs des Urétères*. These come from the kidneys, and do not produce unpleasant effects, unless they are so large as to obstruct the course of the urine, and to occasion distention of the whole of the ureters above them; or unless their surface is so rough as to irritate the mucous membrane, and occasion pain, hemorrhage, abscesses, &c. The

pain, during the passage, is sometimes very violent, extending to the testicle of the same side in the male; and occasioning a numbness of the thigh in both sexes. The treatment consists in general or local blood-letting, warm bath, and opiates.

3. *Calculi, Vesical; Stone in the Bladder,* Lith'ia Vesica'lis, Lithi'asis cys'tica, Lithi'asis vesica'lis, Cysto-lithi'asis, Dysu'ria calculo'sa, D. irrita'ta, Cal'culus vesi'cæ, (F.) Culculs vésicaux. These are the most common. Sometimes, they proceed from the kidneys: most commonly, they are formed in the bladder itself. Sense of weight in the perinæum, and sometimes of a body rolling when the patient changes his position; pain or itching at the extremity of the glans in men; frequent desire to pass the urine; sudden stoppage to its flow; and bloody urine—are the chief signs which induce a suspicion of their existence. We cannot, however, be certain of this without sounding the patient. Sometimes, when of a small size, they are expelled: most commonly, they remain in the bladder, the disorganization of which they occasion, unless removed by a surgical operation.

4. *Calculi Ure'thral.* They almost always proceed from the bladder. The obstruction, which they cause to the passage of the urine, the hard tumour, and the noise occasioned when struck by a sound, indicate their presence. They are removed by incision.

5. *Calculi of Fis'tulous passages.* These arise when there is some fistulous opening into the urethra. They can be readily recognised, and may generally be extracted with facility. (F.) *Calculs placés hors des voies urinaires.* See Urinary Calculi.

CAL'CULI OF THE U'TERUS, (F.) *Calculs de l'Utérus.* These are very rare. The signs, which indicate them during life, are those of chronic engorgement of the uterus. Their existence, consequently, cannot be proved till after death.

CALCULIFRAGUS, Lithontriptic.

CAL'CULOUS, (F.) *Calculeux, Graveleux.* That which relates to calculi, especially to those of the bladder.

CALCULS BILIAIRES, Calculi, biliary— *c. de l'Estomac,* Calculi of the stomach—*c. de la Glande Pinéale,* Calculi of the pineal gland—*c. Intestinaux,* Calculi of the stomach and intestines —*c. Lacrymaux,* Calculi, lachrymal—*c. des Mamelles,* Calculi of the mammæ —*c. de l'Oreille,* Calculi in the ears —*c. du Pancréas,* Calculi of the Pancreas—*c. Placés hors des voies urinaires,* Calculi of fistulous passages —*c. Pulmonaires,* Calculi, pulmonary—*c. Rénaux,* Calculi, renal— *c. Salivaires,* Calculi, salivary—*c. Spermatiques,* Calculi, spermatic—*c. Urinaires,* Calculi, urinary — *c. des Urétères,* Calculi of the ureters —*c. de l'Utérus,* Calculi of the uterus—*c. Vésicaux,* Calculi, vesical.

CAL'CULUS, *Lapis, Lithos,* λίθος. A diminutive of *calx,* a lime-stone. (F.) *Calcul, Pierre.* Calculi are concretions, which may form in every part of the animal body, but are most frequently found in the organs that act as reservoirs, and in the excretory canals. They are met with in the tonsils, joints, biliary ducts, digestive passages, lachrymal ducts, mammæ, pancreas, pineal gland, prostate, lungs, salivary, spermatic and urinary passages, and in the uterus. The causes which give rise to them are obscure.

Those that occur in reservoirs or ducts are supposed to be owing to the deposition of the substances, which compose them, from the fluid as it passes along the duct; and those which occur in the substance of an organ are regarded as the product of some chronic irritation. Their general effect is to irritate, as extraneous bodies, the parts with which they are in contact; and to produce retention of the fluid, whence they have been formed. The symptoms differ, according to the sensibility of the organ and the importance of the particular secretion whose discharge they impede. Their *solution* is generally impracticable: spontaneous expulsion or extraction is the only way of getting rid of them.

CALCULUS BEZOAR, Bezoard — c. Dentalis, Odontolithus — c. Encysted, *Calcul chatonné*—c. Sublingualis, see Calculi, salivary — c. Vesicæ, Calculus, vesical.

CALDAS, WATERS OF. Caldas is a small town, ten leagues from Lisbon, where are mineral springs, containing carbonic and hydrosulphuric acid gases, carbonates and muriates of lime and magnesia, sulphates of soda and lime, sulphuret of iron, silica, and alumina. They are much used in atonic gout. They are thermal. Temperature 93° Fahrenheit.

CALDE'RIÆ ITAL'ICÆ. Warm baths in the neighbourhood of Ferrara, in Italy, much employed in dysuria.

CALEBASSES, Cucurbita lagenaria.

CALEFA'CIENTS, *Calefacien'tia, Therman'tica,* from *calidus,* 'warm,' and *facio,* 'I make.' (F.) *Échouffants.* Substances which excite a degree of warmth in the part to which they are applied, as mustard, pepper, &c. They belong to the class of stimulants.

CALEFACTIO, *Échauffement.*
CALENDULA ALPINA, Arnica montana.
CALEN'DULA ARVEN'SIS, *Caltha Arven'sis seu officina'lis, Wild Mar'igold,* (F.) *Souci des Champs.* This is, sometimes, preferred to the last. Its juice has been given, in the dose of from f℥j to f℥iv, in jaundice and cachexia.
CALEN'DULA OFFICINA'LIS, *C. Sati'va, Chrysan'themum, Sponsa solis, Caltha vulga'ris; Verruca'ria, Single Mar'igold, Garden Mar'igold,* (F.) *Souci, S. ordinaire.* Family, Synanthereæ, Syngenesia necessaria, Linn. So called from flowering every *calend.* The flowers and leaves have been exhibited as aperients, diaphoretics, &c., and have been highly extolled in cancer.

CALENDULÆ MARTIALES, Ferrum ammoniatum.

CALENTU'RA, from *calere,* 'to be warm.' The word, in Spanish, signifies fever. A species of furious delirium to which sailors are subject in the torrid zone:—a kind of phrenitis, the attack of which comes on suddenly after a broiling day, and seems to be characterized by a desire in the patient to throw himself into the sea. It is only a variety of phrenitis.

CALENTURA CONTINUA, Synocha.
CALENTU'RAS; *Palo de Calentu'ras.* Pomet and Leméry say, that these words are sometimes applied to cinchona. Camelli says, they mean, also, a tree of the Philippine Isles, the wood of which is bitter and febrifuge.

CALF OF THE LEG, Sura.
CALICE, Calix.
CALICES RÉNALES, see Calix.
CALICO BUSH, Kalmia latifolia.
CALIDARIUM, see Stove.
CALIDUM ANIMALE, Animal heat— c. Innatum, Animal heat.
CALIGATIO, Dazzling.
CALI'GO. 'A mist.' *Achlys,* (F.) *Brouillard.* An obscurity of vision, dependent upon a speck on the cornea: also, the speck itself; *Caligo cor'neæ, Mac'ula corneæ, M. semipellu'cida, Phtharma caligo, C. à nephel'io, Hebetu'do visûs, C. à Leuco'wata, Neb'ula, Opake cornea, Web-eye,* (F.)

11

Nouage de la Cornée, Taye, Obscurcissement de la vue.

CALIGO LENTIS, Cataract — c. Pupillæ, Synesisis — c. Synizesis, Synezisis — c. Tenebrarum, Hemeralopia.

CALIHACHA CANELLA, Laurus cassia.

CALIX, *Calyx, Infundib'ulum,* from καλιξ, 'a cup.' (F.) *Calice, Entonnoir.* Anatomists have given this name to small membranous canals, which surround the papillæ of the kidney, and open into its pelvis, whither they convey the urine:—*Cal'ices rena'les, Cylind'ri membrana'cei Renum, Fis'tulæ ure'terum renum, Canales membra'nei Renum, Tu'buli pelvis renum.* Their number varies from 6 to 12 in each kidney.

CALIX VOMITORIA, Goblet, emetic.

CALLEUX, Callous.

CALLIBLEPH'ARUM, from καλλος, 'beauty,' and βλιψαρον, 'eyelid.' A remedy for beautifying the eyelids.

CALLICANTHUS, Calycanthus.

CALLICOCCA IPECACUANHA, Ipecacuanha.

CALLICREAS, Pancreas.

CALLIOMARCHUS, Tussilago.

CALLIPÆ'DIA, from καλλος, 'beauty,' and παις, παιδος, 'a child.' The art of begetting beautiful children. This was the title of a poem by Claude Quillet, in 1655; "*Callipædia sive de pulchræ prolis habendæ ratione.*" The author absurdly supposes, that the beauty of children is affected by the sensations which the mother experiences during her pregnancy.

CALLIPERS OF BAUDELOCQUE, see Pelximeter.

CALLIPESTRIA, Cosmetics.

CALLIPHYLLUM, Asplenium trichomanoides.

CALLIP'YGOS, from καλλος, 'beauty,' and πυγη, 'buttocks.' A cognomen of Venus, owing to her beautiful nates.

CAL'LITRIS ECKLO'NI. A South African tree, *Nat. Ord.* Coniferæ, from the branches and cones of which a gum exudes, that resembles Gum Sandarac. This is successfully used in the form of fumigations in gout, rheumatism, œdematous swellings, &c.

CALLITRIS CUPRESSOÏDES, a common shrub in the neighbourhood of Cape Town, exudes a similar substance.

CALLOSITAS, Induration — c. Palpebrarum, Scleriasis—c. Vesicæ, Cystauxe.

CALLOS'ITY, *Callos'itas, Scyros, Tylē, Tylus, Tylo'ma, Tylo'sis, Dermatosclero'sis, Dermatotylo'ma, Dermatotylo'sis, Dermatot'ylus, Porus, Ecphy'ma Callus.* Hardness, induration, and thickness of the skin, which assumes a horny consistence, in places where it is exposed to constant pressure. (F.) *Durillon.* Also the induration, which is observed in old wounds, old ulcers, fistulous passages, &c.

CALLOUS, *Callo'sus, Ochtho'des,* from *callus,* 'hardness.' (F.) *Calleux.* That which is hard or indurated. A *Callous Ulcer* is one whose edges are thick and indurated.

CALLUM PEDIS, Instep.

CALLUNA ERICA, Erica vulgaris — c. Vulgaris, Erica vulgaris.

CALLUS, *Calus, Callum, Osteot'ylus,* (F.) *Cal.* The bony matter, thrown out between the fractured extremities of a bone, which acts as a cement, and as a new bony formation. The words are, likewise, used occasionally in the same sense as Callosity.

CALLUS, PROVISIONAL. When the shaft of a long bone has been broken through, and the extremities have been brought in exact juxtaposition, the new matter, first ossified, is that which occupies the central portion of the deposit, and thus connects the medullary cavities of the broken ends, forming a kind of plug, which enters each. This was termed by M. Dupuytren the provisional Callus.

CALMANTS, Sedatives.

CALME, (F.) The interval that separates the paroxysms of an acute or chronic disease. When the type is intermittent, the word *intermission* is used.

CALOMBA, Calumba.

CALOMEL, Hydrargyri submurias.

CALOMEL STOOLS. A term applied to the green, spinach-like, evacuations occasioned by the internal use of the mild chloride of mercury.

CALOMELANOS TORQUETI, Hydrargyri submurias.

CALOMELANOS TURQUETI. A name given by Riverius to purgative pills, prepared with calomel, sulphur, and resin of jalap.—Dictionaries.

CALOMELAS, Hydrargyri submurias.

CALO'NIA, καλωνια. An epithet formerly given to myrrh.—Hippocrates. See Myrrha.

CALOPHYLLUM INOPHYLLUM, see Fagara octandra.

CALOR, Heat — c. Animalis, Animal heat — c. Nativus, Animal heat.

CALORICITÉ, (F.) *Caloric"itas.* The faculty possessed by living bodies of generating a sufficient quantity of caloric to enable them to resist atmospheric cold, and to preserve, at all times and in every part, a temperature nearly equal. See Animal Heat.

CALORIFA'CIENT, *Calorif'iant, Califa'ciens, Calorifi'ans:* from *calor,* 'heat,' and *facere,* 'to make.' Having the power of producing heat. Relating to the power of producing heat.

CALORIFICA'TION, *Calorifica'tio,* from *calor,* 'heat,' and *fieri,* 'to be made.' The function of producing animal heat.

CALORINÈSES, from *calor,* 'heat.' The name under which M. Baumes proposes to arrange all diseases, characterized by a sensible change in the quantity of animal heat. The *Calorinèses* form the first class of his Nosology.

CALOTROPIS GIGANTEA, Mudar — c. Mudarii, Mudar.

CALOTTE, (F.) *Pile'olum.* Anatomists sometimes give the name, *Calotte aponévrotique,* to the aponeurosis of the occipito-frontalis muscle, which covers it externally; and that of *Calotte du crane* to the *scull-cap.*

Calotte is also applied to an adhesive plaster, with which the head of a person labouring under tinea capitis is sometimes covered, after the hair has been shaved off. This plaster is pulled suddenly and violently off, in order to remove the bulbs of the hair. It means, also, a sort of coif made of boiled leather, worn by those who have undergone the operation of trepanning, &c.

CALOTTE D'ASSURANCE, Condom.

CALTHA ALPINA, Arnica montana — c. Arvensis, Calendula arvensis—c. Officinalis. Calendula arvensis — c. Vulgaris, Calendula officinalis.

CALTROPS, see Trapa natans.

CALUM'BA, *Colom'bo, Calom'ba, Colom'ba,* (Ph. U. S.;) *Columbo, Radix Columbæ,* (F.) *Calumbe* ou *Columbe.* The root of *Menisper'mum palma'tum, Coc'culus palma'tus,* indigenous in India and Africa. Its odour is slightly aromatic; taste unpleasantly bitter. It is tonic and antiseptic. Dose, gr. 10 to ʒj in powder.

CALUMBA, AMERICAN, *Frase'ra Walteri, F. Carolinien'sis, F. Officina'lis, Sweer'tia difform'is, Sw. Frase'ra, American or Marietta Columbo, Indian Lettuce, Yellow Gentian, Golden Seal, Meadow pride, Pyr'amid,* is used in the same cases as the true Calumba.

CALUS, Callus.
CALVA, Cranium.
CALVA, *Calva'ria.* The cranium; the upper part especially; the skull-cap;—the *Vault of the Cranium, Cam'era.*
CALVARIA, Cranium.
CALVA'TA FERRAMEN'TA. Surgical instruments, which have a head or button.
CALVER'S PHYSIC, Leptandra Virginica.
CALVIT"IES, *Calvit"ium, Phal'acra, l'hala-cro'sis, Glabrit"ies, Ophi'asis, Depila'tio Cap'-itis, Phalacro'ma, Madaro'sis, Lipsotrich'ia, Baldness,* &c., from *calvus,* 'bald,' (F.) *Chauveté.* Absence of hair, particularly at the top of, and behind, the head. *Calvit"ies palpebra'rum,*—loss of the eye-lashes.
CALX, Lime, *Ca'rium Terræ, Protox'ide of Cal'cium, Calca'ria pura,* (F.) *Chaux.* The lime, employed in pharmacy, should be recently prepared by calcination. When water is sprinkled over caustic lime, we have *slaked lime, hydrate of lime,*—the *Calcis Hydras* of the London pharmacopœia.
CALX, see Calcaneum — c. Chlorinata, Calcis chloridum—c. Cum kali puro, Potassa cum calce —c. Salita, Calcis murias—c. Bismuthi, Bismuth, subnitrate of.
CALX E TESTIS ; lime prepared from shells. It has probably no medicinal advantages over that prepared from marble.
CALX OXYMURIATICA, Calcis chloridum.
CALX VIVA, *Ox'idum Cal'cii, Calx recens, Fumans nix, Calx usta, Calx et Calx vira, Lime or Quicklime,* (F.) *Chaux vive.* The external operation of calx viva is escharotic, but it is rarely used. Lime is a good disinfecting agent. It is employed internally in the form of Liquor Calcis.
CALYCANTH'US, *C.Flor'idus, Callican'thus,*(?) *Caroli'na Allspice, Sweet-scented shrub, Sweet shrub.* An indigenous plant; *Order,* Calycanthaceæ; with purplish flowers, of strong, agreeable odour, which appear from March to June. The root is possessed of emetic properties.
CALYPTRANTHES CORYOPHYLLATA, Myrtus caryophyllata.
CALYSTEGIA SEPIUM, Convolvulus sepium —c. Soldanella, Convolvulus soldanella.
CALYX, Calix.
CAMARA, Calva.
CAMAREZ, MINERAL WATERS OF. Camarez is a small canton near Sylvanès, in the department of Aveyron, France, where there are acidulous chalybeates.
CAMARO'SIS, *Camaro'ma,* from καμαρα, 'a vault;' *Camera'tio, Testudina'tio Cra'nii.* A species of fracture of the skull, in which the fragments are placed so as to form a vault, with its base resting on the dura mater. — Galen, Paulus of Ægina.
CAMBING. A tree of the Molucca Islands, from the bark of which a kind of gum-resin exudes, which has been highly extolled in dysentery. It appears to have some resemblance to the simarouba.—Rumphius.
CAMBIUM, '*Exchange.*' A name formerly given to a fancied nutritive juice, which was supposed to originate in the blood, to repair the losses of every organ, and produce their increase. —Sennertus.
CAMBO, MINERAL WATERS OF. A village in the department of Basses Pyrénées, France, where there are two mineral springs; the one an acidulous chalybeate, the other sulphureous. Temperature, 62° to 69° Fahrenheit.
CAMBODIA, Cambogia.
CAMBO'GIA, from Cambodia, in the East Indies, where it is obtained. Hence, likewise, its names *Cambo'dia, Cambo'gium, Gambo'gia, Gam-bo'gium, Gambu'gium.* It is called, also, *Gutta, Gutta gamba, Gummi Gutta, Catagau'na, Cattagau'ma, Chrysopus, Laxati'vus Ind'icus, Gummi Bo'gia. G. gaman'dræ, G. de Goa, G. de Jemu, Chitta jemoco, Gutta Gaman'dræ, Gummi ad Pod'-agram, Camboge or Gamboge,* &c., (F.) *Gomme Gutte. Ord.* Guttiferæ. A yellow juice obtained from *Hebradendron Cambogioï'des,* and other plants of the natural family Guttiferæ, but it is not known from which of them the officinal camboge is obtained. It is inodorous, of an orange yellow colour; opake and brittle; fracture, glassy; is a drastic cathartic, emetic and anthelmintic; and is used in visceral obstructions and dropsy, and wherever powerful hydragogue cathartics are required. Dose from gr. ij to vi, in powder, united with calomel, squill, &c.
CAMBOGIA GUTTA, Garcinia cambogia.
CAMBU'CA, *Cambuc'ca membra'ta.* Buboes and venereal ulcers, seated in the groin or near the genital organs.—Paracelsus. See Bubo.
CAMELÉE, Cneorum tricoccum.
CAMERA, Chamber, Fornix, Vault—c. Cordis, Pericardium — c. Oculi, Chamber of the eye.
CAMERATIO, Camarosis.
CAMFOROSMA, Camphorosma.
CAMINGA, Canella alba.
CAMISIA FŒTUS, Chorion.
CAMISOLE, Waistcoat, strait.
CAMMARUS, Crab.
CAMOMILLE FÉTIDE, Anthemis cotula — *c. Puante,* Anthemis cotula—*c. Romaine,* Anthemis nobilis—*c. des Teinturiers,* Anthemis tinctoria — *c. Vulgaire,* Matricaria chamomilla.
CAMOSIERS, WATERS OF. Camosiers is a canton, two leagues from Marseilles, where are two springs containing carbonate of lime, sulphur, chloride of sodium, &c. They are purgative, and used in skin complaints.
CAMOTES, Convolvulus batatas.
CAMPAGNE, MINERAL WATERS OF. Campagne is in the department of Aude, France. The waters contain sulphate and chlorohydrate of magnesia. Temperature, 80° Fahrenheit.
CAMPAN'ULA. Diminutive of *Campana.* A bell.
CAMPANULA TRACHE'LIUM, *Canterbury Bell* or *Throatwort,* was formerly used, in decoction, in relaxation of the fauces. It is, also, called *Cervica'ria.*
CAMPE, Flexion.
CAMPHIRE, Camphor.
CAMPHOR, from Arab. *Ca'phur* or *Kam'phur, Cam'phora, Caphura, Caffa, Caf, Cafur, Caphora, Altafor, Camphire, Camphor,* (F.) *Camphre.* A concrete substance, prepared, by distillation, from *Laurus Camphora, Per'sea Cam'fora,* an indigenous tree of the East Indies. *Order,* Laurineæ. Its odour is strong and fragrant: it is volatile, not easily pulverizable; texture crystalline. Soluble in alcohol, ether, oils, vinegar, and slightly so in water. Its properties are narcotic, diaphoretic, and sedative. Dose, gr. v. to ℈j. Dissolved in oil or alcohol, it is applied externally in rheumatic pains, bruises, sprains, &c.
CAMPHOR WATER, Mistura Camphoræ.
CAMPHORA'CEOUS, *Camphora'ceus.* Relating to or containing camphor;—as a '*camphoraceous* smell or remedy.'
CAMPHORATA HIRSUTA et C. MONSPELIENSIUM, Camphorosma Monspeliaca.
CAMPH'ORATED, *Camphora'tus,* (F.) *Camphré.* Relating to camphor; containing camphor; as a *camphorated smell,* a *camphorated draught.*
CAMPHOROS'MA MONSPELIACA, *C. Pe-ren'nis,* from *Camphor,* and οσμη, 'odour.' *Sela'go, Camphora'ta hirsu'ta* seu *Monspeli-en'sium, Hairy*

Camphoros'ma, (F.) *Camphrée de Montpellier.* Family, Atriplicese. Sex. Syst. Tetrandria Monogynia. This plant, as its name imports, has an odour of camphor. It is regarded as diuretic, diaphoretic, cephalic, antispasmodic, &c. It is also called *Chamæpeu'cé* and *Stinking Ground Pine.*

CAMPHOROSMA PERENNIS, C. Monspeliaca.
CAMPHRE, Camphor.
CAMPHRÉ, Camphorated.
CAMPHRE DE MONTPELLIER, Camphorosma Monspeliaca.

CAMPOMANE'SIA LINEATIFO'LIA. A tree, twenty to thirty feet high, which grows in Peru, and whose fruit—*palillo*, of a bright yellow colour, and as large as a moderate-sized apple—has an exceedingly agreeable scent, and is one of the ingredients in making the perfumed water called *mistura*.—Tschudi.

CAMPSIS, *Flex'io, Curva'tio, Inflex'io.* Bone or cartilage, forcibly bent from its proper shape, without breaking.—Good.

CAMPSIS DEPRESSIO, Depression.

CAMPYLOR'RHACHIS; from καμπυλος, 'crooked,' and ραχις, 'spine.' A monster whose spine is crooked.—Gurlt.

CAMPYLORRHI'NUS; from καμπυλος, 'crooked,' and ριν, 'nose.' A monster whose nose is crooked.—Gurlt.

CAMPYLOTIS, Cataclasis.
CAMPYLUM, Cataclasis.
CAMUS, (F.) *Simus, Resi'mus, Simo, Silo, Silus.* One who has a short, stumpy nose. The French speak of *Nez camus,* 'short nose.'

CANADA BURNET, Sanguisorba canadensis.

CANAL, *Cana'lis, Ductus, Mea'tus, Porus, Och'etos,* (F.) *Conduit.* A channel for affording passage to liquids, or solids, or to certain organs.

CANAL, ALIMEN'TARY, C. *Diges'tive, Cana'lis ciba'rius* vel *digesti'vus, Ductus ciba'rius, Tubus alimenta'ris* seu *intestino'rum, Diges'tive Tube, Aliment'ary Duct* or *Tube.* The canal extending from the mouth to the anus.

CANAL, ARACH'NOID, *Cana'lis Bichat'ii, Canal of Bichat.* A canal formed by the extension of the arachnoid over the transverse and longitudinal fissures of the brain, which surrounds the vena magna Galeni. The orifice of the canal has been termed the Foramen of Bichat.

CANAL ARTÉRIEL, Arterial duct — c. *de Bartholin,* Ductus Bartholinus — c. *of Bichat,* Canal, arachnoid—c. *Bullular,* of Petit, *Godronné canal* — c. *Carotidien,* Carotid canal — c. *Cholédoque,* Choledoch duct—c. *Ciliary,* Ciliary canal —c. *of Cotunnius,* Aquæductus vestibuli — c. *of Fontana,* Ciliary canal—c. *Goudronné, Godronné canal—c. Hépatique,* Hepatic duct.

CANAL, HY'ALOID. A cylindrical passage, described by M. J. Cloquet as formed by the reflection of the hyaloid membrane into the interior of the vitreous body around the nutritious artery of the lens. M. Cruveilhier has never been able to see it.

CANAL, INCI'SIVE, see Palatine canals—c. Infraorbitar, Suborbitar canal—c. *Inflexe de l'os temporal,* Carotid canal—c. *Intermédiare des ventricules,* Aquæductus Sylvii.

CANAL INTES'TINAL. *Cana'lis* seu *Ductus intestina'lis.* The portion of the digestive canal formed by the intestines.

CANAL OF JACOBSON, Canal, tympanic.

CANAL, MED'ULLARY. The cylindrical cavity in the body or shaft of a long bone, which contains the marrow.

CANAL, NASAL, Lachrymal canal.

CANAL OF NUCK. A cylindrical sheath formed around the round ligaments of the uterus by a prolongation of the peritoneum into the inguinal canal.

CANAL DE PETIT, *Godronné canal* — c. *Pulmo-aortique,* Arterial duct — c. Rachidian, Vertebral canal.

CANAL OF SCHLEMM. A minute circular canal, discovered by Professor Schlemm, of Berlin. It is situate at the point of union of the cornea and sclerotica.

CANAL, SPINAL, Vertebral canal — c. *Spiroïde de l'os temporal,* Aquæductus Fallopii—c. *de Stenon,* Ductus salivalis superior — c. *Thoracique,* Thoracic duct — c. *Veineux,* Canal, venous — c. Vulvo-uterine, Vagina — c. *de Warthon,* Ductus salivalis inferior.

CANAL, TYM'PANIC, *Cana'lis tympan'icus, Canal of Ja'cobson.* A canal which opens on the lower surface of the petrous portion of the temporal bone, between the carotid canal and the groove for the internal jugular vein. It contains Jacobson's nerve.

CANAL, VENOUS, *Cana'lis* seu *Ductus veno'sus,* (F.) *Canal veineux.* A canal, which exists only in the fœtus. It extends from the bifurcation of the umbilical vein to the vena cava inferior, into which it opens below the diaphragm. At times, it ends in one of the infra-hepatic veins. It pours into the cava a part of the blood, which passes from the placenta by the umbilical vein. After birth, it becomes a fibro-cellular cord.

CANAL OF WIRSUNG, see Pancreas.

CANA'LES BRESCHETI. Canals in the diploë for the passage of veins; so called after M. Breschet.

CANALES CIRCULARES, Semicircular canals—c. Cochleæ, Scalæ of the cochlea—c. Lachrymales, Lachrymal ducts—c. Membranei renum, see Calix —c. Tubæformes, Semicircular canals.

CANALICULATED, Grooved.
CANALICULATUS, *Cannélé,* Grooved.
CANALICULÉ, Grooved.

CANALICULI HAVERSIANI, Canals, nutritive — c. Lachrymales, Lachrymal ducts — c. Limacum, Lachrymal ducts — c. Semiculares, Semicircular canals—c. Vasculosi, Canals, nutritive—c. of Bone, see Lacunæ of Bone.

CANALIC'ULUS, diminutive of *canalis,* 'a channel.' A small channel. See Lacunæ of Bone.

CANALIS, Meatus— c. Arteriosus, Arterial duct—c. Bichatii, Canal, arachnoid—c. Canaliculatus, Gorget—c. Caroticus, Carotid canal—c. Deferens, Deferens, vas — c. Eminentiæ quadrigeminæ, Aquæductus Sylvii—c. Intestinorum, Intestinal tube—c. Lachrymalis, Lachrymal or nasal duct—c. Medius, Aquæductus Sylvii—c. Medullæ Spinalis, see Vertebral column—c. Nerveus fistulosus renum, Ureter—c. Orbitæ nasalis, Lachrymal or nasal duct — c. Scalarum communis, Infundibulum of the cochlea—c. Semicircularis horizontalis, see Semicircular Canals — c. Semicircularis verticalis posterior, see Semicircular Canals — c. Semicircularis verticalis superior, see Semicircular canals—c. Tympanicus, Canal, tympanic—c. Urinarius, Urethra—c. Vidianus, Pterygoid canal.

CANALS OF HAVERS, Canals, nutritive of bones—c. Haversian, Canals, nutritive, of bones.

CANALS, NUTRITIVE, *Canals for the nutrition of bones, Ductus nutrit'ii, Canalic'uli vasculo'si* seu *Haveresia'ni, Haver'sian Canals, Canals of Havers,* (F.) *Canaux nourriciers* ou *du Nutrition des os, Conduits nourriciers* ou *nutriciers.* The canals through which the vessels pass to the bones. They are lined by a very fine lamina of compact texture, or are formed in the texture itself. There is, generally, one large nutritious canal in a long bone, situate towards its middle.

CANAPACIA, Artemisia vulgaris.

CANARIES, CLIMATE OF. The climate of the Canaries greatly resembles that of Madeira. That of the latter, however, is more equable, and the accommodation for invalids much superior.

CANARIUM COMMUNE, see *Amyris elemifera*.

CANARY-SEED, *Phalaris Canariensis*.

CANAUX AQUEUX, see Aqueous—*c. Demicirculaires*, Semicircular canals—*c. Éjaculateurs*, Ejaculatory ducts—*c. Nourriciers*, Canals, nutritive—*c. de Nutrition des os*, Canals, nutritive.

CANAUX DE TRANSMISSION. According to Bichat, the bony canals intended to give passage to vessels and nerves going to parts more or less distant: as the *Cana'lis Carot'icus*, &c.

CANAUX VEINEUX, *Venous Canals*. The canals situate in the diploë, which convey venous blood.

CAN'CAMUM. A mixture of several gums and resins, exported from Africa, where it is used to deterge wounds. Dioscorides calls, by the name καγκαμον, the tears from an Arabian tree, which are similar to myrrh, and of a disagreeable taste. He advises it in numerous diseases. This name is given, also, to the Anime.

CANCAMY, Anime.

CAN'CELLATED, *Cancella'tus*, (F.) *Cancellé*; from *Cancelli*, 'lattice-work.' Formed of cancelli, as the 'cancellated structure of bone.'

CANCEL'LI, 'Lattice-work.' The *Cellular* or *Spongy Texture of Bones*, (F.) *Tissu celluleux*; consisting of numerous cells, communicating with each other. They contain a fatty matter, analogous to marrow. This texture is met with, principally, at the extremities of long bones; and some of the short bones consist almost wholly of it. It allows of the expansion of the extremities of bones, without adding to their weight; and deadens concussions.

CANCEL'LUS, from *cancer*, 'a crab.' A species of crayfish, called the *Wrong Heir*, and *Bernard the Hermit*: which is said to cure rheumatism, if rubbed on the part.

CANCER, 'a crab.' *Car'cinos*, *Lupus cancro'sus*. A disease, so called either on account of the hideous appearance which the ulcerated cancer presents, or on account of the great veins which surround it, and which the ancients compared to the claws of the crab: called also *Carcino'ma*. It consists of a scirrhous, livid tumour, intersected by firm, whitish, divergent bands; and occurs chiefly in the secernent glands. The pains are acute and lancinating, and often extend to other parts. The tumour, ultimately, terminates in a fetid and ichorous ulcer,—*Ulcus cancro'sum*. It is distinguished, according to its stages, into *occult* and *open*; the former being the scirrhous, the latter the ulcerated condition. At times, there is a simple destruction or erosion of the organs, at others, an *encephaloid* or *cerebriform*, and, at others, again, a *colloid* degeneration.

For its production, it requires a peculiar diathesis, or cachexia. The following table, from Dr. Walshe, exhibits the characters of the three species of carcinoma:

The use of irritants in cancerous affections is strongly to be deprecated. When the disease is so situate that excision can be practised, the sooner it is removed the better.

Encephaloid.	*Scirrhus.*	*Colloid.*
Resembles lobulated cerebral matter.	Resembles rind of bacon traversed by cellulo-fibrous septa.	Has the appearance of particles of jelly inlaid in a regular alveolar bed.
Is commonly opake from its earliest formation.	Has a semi-transparent glossiness.	The contained matter is strikingly transparent.
Is of a dead white colour.	Has a clear whitish or bluish yellow tint.	Greenish yellow is its predominant hue.
Contains a multitude of minute vessels.	Is comparatively ill-supplied with vessels.	Its vessels have not been sufficiently examined as yet.
Is less hard and dense than scirrhus.	Is exceedingly firm and dense.	The jelly-like *matter* is exceedingly soft; a colloid *mass* is, however, firm and resisting.
Is frequently found in the veins issuing from the diseased mass.	Has not been distinctly detected in this situation.	The pultaceous variety has been detected in the veins.
The predominant microscopical elements are globular, not always distinctly cellular, and caudate corpuscula.	The main microscopical constituents are juxtaposed nuclear cells; caudate corpuscular do not exist in it.	Is composed of shells in a state of *emboîtement*.
Occasionally attains an enormous bulk.	Rarely acquires larger dimensions than an orange.	Observes a mean in this respect.
Has been observed in almost every tissue of the body.	Its seat, as ascertained by observation, is somewhat more limited.	Has so far been seen in a limited number of parts only.
Very commonly co-exists in several parts or organs of the same subject.	Is not unusually solitary.	Has rarely been met with in more than one organ.
Is remarkable for its occasional vast rapidity of growth.	Ordinarily grows slowly.	Grows with a medium degree of rapidity.
Is frequently the seat of interstitial hemorrhage and deposition of black or bistre-coloured matter.	Is comparatively rarely the seat of these changes.	
When softened into a pulp, appears as a dead white or pink opake matter of creamy consistence.	Resembles, when softened, a yellowish brown semitransparent gelatinous matter.	Undergoes no visible change of the kind.
Subcutaneous tumours are slow to contract adhesion with the skin.	Scirrhus thus situate usually becomes adherent.	
Ulcerated encephaloid is frequently the seat of hemorrhage, followed by rapid fungous development.	Scirrhous ulcers much less frequently give rise to hemorrhage; and fungous growths (provided they retain the scirrhous character) are now more slowly and less abundantly developed.	
The progress of the disease after ulceration is commonly very rapid.	There is not such a remarkable change in the rate of progress of the disease after ulceration has set in.	
It is the most common form under which secondary cancer exhibits itself.		
Is the species of cancer most frequently observed in young subjects.	Is much less common before puberty.	Has so far been observed in adults only.

CANCER ALVEOLARIS, Colloid.

CANCER AQUAT'ICUS, *Gan'grenous stomati'tis, Cancrum Oris, Gangrænop'sis, Canker of the mouth, Gangrenous sore mouth, Sloughing Phagedæ'na of the mouth, Water Canker:* called, also, *Aphthæ serpen'tes, Gangræ'na Oris, Noma, Nomē, Nomus, Pseudocarcino'ma la'bii, Stomac'acē gangræno'sa, Cheiloc'acē, Uloc'acē, Uli'tis sep'tica, Cheilomala'cia, Scorbu'tus Oris, Stomatomala'cia pu'trida, Stomatosep'sis, Stomatonecro'sis, Carbun'culus labio'rum et gena'rum,* (F.) *Cancer aquatique, Stomatite gangréneuse, S. Charbonneuse, Gangrène de la Bouche, Sphacèle de la Bouche, Féyarite, Aphthe gangréneux.* Certain sloughing or gangrenous ulcers of the mouth,—so called, perhaps, because they are often accompanied with an afflux of saliva. The disease is not uncommon in children's asylums, and demands the same treatment as hospital gangrene;—the employment of caustics, and internal and external antiseptics.

CANCER AQUATIQUE, Cancer aquaticus, Stomacace—*c. Aréolaire,* Colloid—*c. Astacus,* see Cancrorum chelæ—*c. Black,* Melanosis—*c. Caminariorum, Cancer, chimney-sweepers'*—*c. Cellular, Encephaloid*—*c. Cérébriforme,* see Encephaloid.

CANCER, CHIMNEY-SWEEPERS', *Sootwart, Cancer mundito'rum, Cancer purgato'ris infumic'uli, Cancer scu carcino'ma scroti, Cancer caminario'rum, Oscheocarcino'ma, Oschocarcino'ma,* (F.) *Cancer des Ramoneurs.* This affection begins with a superficial, painful, irregular ulcer with hard and elevated edges occupying the lower part of the scrotum. Extirpation of the diseased part is the only means of effecting a cure.

CANCER, DAVIDSON'S REMEDY FOR, see Conium maculatum—*c. du Foie, Hépatosarcomie*—*c. Fibrous,* Scirrhus.

CANCER GALE'NI, (F.) *Cancer de Galien.* A bandage for the head, to which Galen gave the name *cancer*, from its eight heads resembling, rudely, the claws of the crab. It is now supplied by the bandage with six *chefs* or heads, which is called the *Bandage of Galen* or *B. of the Poor.*

CANCER DE GALIEN, Cancer Galeni—*c. Gelatiniform,* Colloid—*c. Gelatinous,* Colloid—*c. Hard,* Scirrhus—*c. Intestinorum,* Enteropathia cancerosa—*c. des Intestins,* Enteropathia cancerosa—*c. of the Lung,* Phthisis, cancerous—*c. Lupus,* Lupus—*c. Medullaris,* Encephaloid—*c. Melæneus,* Melanosis—*c. Mélane,* Melanosis—*c. Melanodes,* Cancer, melanotic.

CANCER, MELANOT'IC, *Cancer melano'des, Carcino'ma melano'des.* A combination of cancer and melanosis.

CANCER MOLLIS, see Encephaloid—*c. Mou,* Encephaloid—*c. Munditorum,* Cancer, chimney-sweepers'—*c. Oculi,* Scirrhophthalmus—*c. Oris,* Stomacace—*c. Ossis,* Spina ventosa—*c. Pharyngis et œsophagi,* Læmoscirrhus—*c. Purgatoris infumiculi,* Cancer, chimney-sweepers'—*c. Soirrhosus,* Scirrhus — *c. Scroti,* Cancer, chimney-sweepers'—*c. Soft,* Hæmatodes fungus—*c. of the Stomach,* Gastrostenosis cardiaca et pylorica—*c. Uteri,* Metro-carcinoma.

CANCÉREUX, Cancerous.

CANCER ROOT, Orobanche Virginiana, Phytolacca decandra.

CANCEROMA, Carcinoma.

CAN'CEROUS, *Cancro'sus, Carcino'sus,* (F.) *Cancéreux.* Relating to cancer; as *Cancerous ulcer, Cancerous diathesis,* &c.

CANCHALAGUA, Chironia Chilensis.

CANCRENA, Gangrene.

CAN'CROID, *Cancro'des, Cancroï'des, Carci-* *no'des, Carcinoïdes, Cancroï'deus,* from *cancer* and *ειδος,* 'form.' That which assumes a cancerous appearance. Cancroid is a name given to certain cutaneous cancers by Alibert: called also *Cheloid* or *Keloid* (χελυς, 'a tortoise,' and *ειδος,* 'likeness,') from their presenting a flattish raised patch of integument, resembling the shell of a tortoise.

CANCROMA, Carcinoma.

CANCRO'RUM CHELÆ, *Oc'uli vel Lap'ides Cancro'rum, Lapil'li cancro'rum, Concremen'ta As'taci fluviat'ilis, Crab's stones* or *eyes,* (F.) *Yeux d'écrevisse.* Concretions found, particularly, in the *Cancer As'tacus* or Cray-fish. They consist of carbonate and phosphate of lime, and possess antacid virtues, but not more than chalk.

CANCROSUS, Cancerous, *Chancreuse.*

CANCRUM ORIS, Cancer Aquaticus, Stomacace.

CANDELA, *Bougie* — *c. Fumalis,* Pastil — *c. Medicata, Bougie* — *c. Regia,* Verbascum nigrum.

CANDELARIA, Verbascum nigrum.

CANDI, *Candum, Canthum, Can'tion:* 'white, bleached, purified.' Purified and crystallized sugar. See Saccharum.

CANDIDUM OVI, Albumen ovi.

CANDYTUFT, BITTER, Iberis amara.

CANEFLOWER, PURPLE, Echinacea purpurea.

CANE, SUGAR, see Saccharum — *c. Sweet,* Acorus calamus.

CANELÉ, Grooved.

CANELLA, see Canella alba.

CANEL'LA ALBA, diminutive of *Canna,* 'a reed,' so called because its bark is rolled up like a reed. *Cortex Wintera'nus spu'rius, Canella Cuba'na, C. Wintera'nia, Cinnamo'mum album, Cortex Antiscorbu'ticus, C. Aromat'icus, Costus cortico'sus, Camin'ga, Canella* of Linnæus, and of Ph. U. S., *Canella Bark, Canella,* (F.) *Canelle ou Canelle blanche, Fausse Écorce de Winter, Écorce Cariocostine. Fam.* Magnoliaceæ. *Sex. Syst.* Dodecandria Monogynia. This bark is a pungent aromatic. Its virtues are partly extracted by water; entirely by alcohol. It is a stimulant, and is added to bitters and cathartics.

CANELLA CARYOPHYLLATA, Myrtus caryophyllata—*c. Cubana,* C. alba, Laurus cassia—*c. Malabarica et Javensis,* Laurus cassia.

CANELLIFERA MALABARICA, Laurus cassia.

CANEPIN, (F.) A fine lamb's skin or goat's skin, used for trying the quality of lancets.

CANICACEOUS, Furfuraceous.

CAN'ICÆ. Meal, in which there is much bran. Also, coarse bread; or bread in which there is much bran—*Panis Canica'ceus.*

CANICIDA, Aconitum.

CANIC'ULA; the *Dogstar,* from *canis,* 'a dog;' Σειριος, Sirius, (F.) *Canicule.* This star, which gives its name to the *Dogdays, Dies canicula'res,* because they commence when the sun rises with it, was formerly believed to exert a powerful influence on the animal economy. The Dog-days occur at a period of the year when there is generally great and oppressive heat, and therefore—it has been conceived—a greater liability to disease.

CANIF, Knife.

CANIN, Canine.

CANINANÆ RADIX, Caincæ radix.

CANINE, *Cani'nus, Cyn'icus, κυνικος,* from *canis,* 'a dog.' (F.) *Canin.* That which has a resemblance to the structure, &c., of a dog.

CANINE FOSSA, *Fossa Cani'na, Infra-orbitar* or *Suborbitar fossa,* (F.) *Fosse Canine.* A small depression on the superior maxillary bone, above the *dens caninus*, which gives attachment to the *caninus* or levator anguli oris muscle.

CANINE LAUGH, *Sardon'ic laugh, Risus Cani'nus* seu *Sardon'icus* seu *Sardo'nius, R. de Sardo'nia, R. involunta'rius, R. spas'ticus, Tortu'ra Oris, Distor'sio Oris, Gelas'mus, Sardi'asis, Sardoni'asis, Trismus Sardon'icus* seu *cyn'icus, Spasmus musculorum faciei* seu *cyn'icus, Prosopospasmus*, (F.) *Ris canin, R. Sardonique, R. Sardonien, R. moqueur.* A sort of laugh, the facial expression of which is produced particularly by the spasmodic contraction of the *Caninus* muscle. Probably, this expression, as well as *Cynic Spasm, Spasmus caninus* seu *cyn'icus, Convul'sio cani'na, Trismus cyn'icus*, may have originated in the resemblance of the affection to certain movements in the upper lip of the dog. The *Risus Sardon'icus* is said to have been so called from similar symptoms having been induced by a kind of Ranunculus that grows in Sardinia.

CANINE TEETH, *Dentes Cani'ni, Cynodon'tes, D. Lania'rii, D. angula'res, cuspida'ti, columella'res, ocula'res, morden'tes, Eye Teeth,* (F.) *Dents canines, laniaires, angulaires, oculaires, œillères* ou *conoïdes.* The teeth between the lateral incisors and small molares, of each jaw;—so named because they resemble the teeth of the dog.

CANINUS, Levator anguli oris — c. Sentis, Rosa canina — c. Spasmus, see Canine Laugh.

CANIRAM, Strychnos nux vomica.

CANIRAMINUM, Brucine.

CANIRUBUS, Rosa canina.

CANIS INTERFECTOR, Veratrum sababilla —c. Ponticus, Castor fiber.

CANIT"IES, from *canus*, 'white.' *Whiteness* or *grayness of the hair*, and especially of that of the head. (F.) *Canitie.* When occurring in consequence of old age, it is not a disease. Sometimes, it happens suddenly, and apparently in consequence of severe mental emotion. The causes, however, are not clear. See Poliosis.

CANKER, Stomacace — c. of the Mouth, Cancer aquaticus — c. Water, Cancer aquaticus.

CANNA, see Tous-les-Mois, Cassia fistula, Trachea — c. Brachii, Ulna — c. Domestica cruris, Tibia — c. Fistula, Cassia fistula — c. Indica, Sagittarium alexipharmacum — c. Major, Tibia — c. Minor, Fibula, Radius — c. Solutiva, Cassia fistula.

CANNABIN, Bangue.

CANNAB'INA, from *κανναβις*, 'hemp.' Remedies composed of Cannabis Indica.—Pereira.

CANNABINA AQUATICA, Eupatorium cannabinum.

CANNABIS INDICA, Bangue. See, also, Churrus, and Gunjah.

CAN'NABIS SATI'VA, (F.) *Chanvre, Chambrie.* The seed of this—*Hempseed, Sem'ina Can'nabis*, (F.) *Chènevis*, is oily and mucilaginous. The decoction is sometimes used in gonorrhœa.

CANNACORUS RADICE CROCEA, Curcuma longa.

CANNAMELLE, see Saccharum.

CANNE AROMATIQUE, Acorus calamus— c. *Congo, Costus* — c. *de Rivière, Costus* — c. *à Sucre*, see Saccharum.

CANNEBERGE, Vaccinium oxycoccos — c. *Ponctuée*, Vaccinium vitis idæa.

CANNELÉ ou *CANELÉ*, (F.) from *canalis*, 'a canal:' *Sulca'tus, Stria'tus, Canalicula'tus.* Having a canal or groove — as *Muscle cannelé* (Lieutaud,) the Gemini; *Corps cannelés* ou *striés*, the Corpora striata; *Sonde cannelée*, a grooved sound, &c. See Grooved.

CANNELLE, Laurus cinnamomum — c. *Blanche*, Canella alba — c. *de la Chine*, Laurus cassia — c. *de Coromandel*, Laurus cassia — c. *Fausse*, Laurus cassia — c. *Giroflée*, Myrtus cary-ophyllata — c. *des Indes*, Laurus cassia — c. *de Java*, Laurus cassia — c. *de Malabar*, Laurus cassia — c. *Matte*, Laurus cassia — c. *Officinale*, Laurus cinnamomum — c. *Poirée*, see Wintera aromatica.

CANNULA, Canula.

CANNULÆ PULMONUM, Bronchia.

CANOPUM, see Sambucus.

CANOR STETHOSCOPICUS, *Tintement métallique.*

CANTABRICA, Convolvulus Cantabrica.

CANTABRUNO, Furfur.

CANTARELLUS, Meloe proscarabæus.

CANTATIO, Charm.

CANTERBURY, WATERS OF, *Aquæ Cantuarien'ses.* The waters of Canterbury in Kent, England, are impregnated with iron, sulphur, and carbonic acid.

CANTERIUM, Cantherius.

CANTHARIDE TACHETÉE, Lytta vittata.

CANTHARIDINE, see Cantharis.

CAN'THARIS, from *κανθαρος*, 'a *scarabæus;' Musca Hispan'ica, Mel'oë vesicato'rius, Cantharis vesicato'ria, Lytta vesicato'ria, Blistering Fly, Blisterfly, Blisterbeetle, Spanish Fly, Fly,* (F.) *Cantharides, Mouches, M. d'Espagne.* This fly is much employed in medicine. It is the most common vesicatory. Given internally, and even when absorbed from the skin, it affects the urinary organs, exciting strangury. This may be prevented, in cases of blisters, by interposing between the blistering plaster and skin a piece of tissue paper. Diluents relieve the strangury. Dose, half a grain to one grain. If kept dry, the flies will retain their activity for many years. Their active principle, *Can'tharidin, Cantharidi'na*, has been separated from them.

CANTHARIS VITTATA, Lytta vittata.

CANTHE'RIUS, *Cante'rium.* The cross-piece of wood in the apparatus used by Hippocrates for reducing luxations of the humerus.

CANTHI'TIS. Inflammation of the canthus of the eye.

CANTHOPLAS'TICE, from *κανθος*, 'the angle of the eye,' and *πλαστικος*, 'formative.' The formation, by plastic operation, of the angle of the eye.

CANTHUM, Candi.

CANTHUS, *Epican'this, An'gulus ocula'ris, Fons lachryma'rum.* The corner or angle of the eye. The *greater canthus* is the *inner angle, Hircus, Hir'quus, Rhanter;* the *lesser canthus*, the *outer angle, Paro'pia, Pega.*

CANTIA'NUS PULVIS. A cordial powder, known under the name '*Countess of Kent's powder*,' composed of coral, amber, crab's eyes, prepared pearls, &c. It was given in cancer.

CANTION, Candi.

CAN'ULA, *Can'nula, Au'liscus, Aulos.* Diminutive of *Canna*, 'a reed;' *Tu'bulus*, (F.) *Canule* ou *Cannule.* A small tube of gold, silver, platinum, iron, lead, wood, elastic gum, or gutta percha, used for various purposes in surgery.

CA'OUTCHOUC. The Indian name for *Indian Rubber, Elas'tic Gum, Gum Elastic, Gummi elas'ticum, Cauchuc, Resi'na elas'tica* seu *Cayennen'sis, Cayenne Resin, Cautchuc.* A substance formed from the milky juice of *Hæ'vea* seu *Herea Guianen'sis, Jat'ropha elas'tica* seu *Sipho'nia Cahuchu, S. elas'tica, Ficus Indica*, and *Artocar'pus integrifo'lia*:—South American trees. It is insoluble in water and alcohol; but boiling water softens and swells it. It is soluble in the essential oils and in ether, when it may be blown into bladders. It is used in the fabrication of catheters, bougies, pessaries, &c.

CAP, PITCH, see Depilatory.

CAPA-ISIAKKA: Bromelia ananas.

CAPBERN, WATERS OF. Capbern is in

the department Hautes-Pyrénées, France. The waters contain sulphates and carbonates of lime and magnesia, and chloride of magnesium. Temperature, 75° Fahrenheit. They are purgative.

CAPELET, Myrtus caryophyllata.

CAPELI'NA, *Capelli'na*, (F.) *Capeline;* A Woman's Hat, in French; *Capis'trum*, from *caput*, 'head.' A sort of bandage, which, in shape, resembles a riding-hood. There are several kinds of *Capelines.* 1. That of the head, *C. de la tête, Fas'cia capita'lis.* See *Bonnet d'Hippocrate. C. of the clavicle*, employed in fractures of the acromion, clavicle and spine of the scapula. *C. of an amputated limb*—the bandage applied round the stump.

CAPELLINA, Capelina.
CAPER BUSH, Capparis spinosa.
CAPER PLANT, Euphorbia lathyris.
CAPERS, see Capparis spinosa.
CAPETUS, Imperforation.
CAPHORA, Camphor.
CAPHURA, Camphor.

CAPILLAIRE, Capillary, see Adiantum capillus veneris — *c. du Canada*, Adiantum pedatum — *c. de Montpellier*, Adiantum capillus veneris.

CAPILLAMEN'TUM, from *Capillus*, 'a hair,' *Capillit''ium, Tricho'ma, Trichoma'tion.* Any villous or hairy covering. Also, a small fibre or fibril.

CAP'ILLARY, *Capilla'ris, Capilla'ceus*, from *capillus*, 'a hair.' (F.) *Capillaire.* Hair-like; small.

CAP'ILLARY VESSELS, *Vasa capilla'ria*, (F.) *Vaisseaux capillaires*, are the extreme radicles of the arteries and veins, which together constitute the *capillary, intermediate,* or *peripheral vascular system,*—the *metha'mata* or *methæmatous* blood channels of Dr. Marshall Hall. They possess an action distinct from that of the heart.

CAPILLATIO, Trichismus.
CAPILLATUS, Impuber.
CAPILLITIUM, Capillamentum, Entropion, Scalp.
CAPILLORUM DEFLUVIUM, Alopecia.

CAPIL'LUS, quasi *Capitis Pilus, Coma, Chætē, Crinis, Pilus, Thrix, Cæsa'ries,* (F.) *Cheveu.* This term is generally applied to the hair of the head, *Pili seu Honor cap'itis,* the characters of which vary, according to races, individuals, &c. Hairs arise in the areolar membrane, where the bulb is placed, and are composed of two parts—*one*, external, tubular, and transparent, of an epidermoid character; the *other*, internal and *sui generis*, which communicates to them their colour. The hair is insensible, and grows from the root.

CAPILLUS VENERIS, Adiantum capillus veneris —c. V. Canadensis, Adiantum pedatum.

CAPIPLE'NIUM, *Capitiple'nium*, from *caput*, 'the head,' and *plenum*, 'full.' A word, employed with different significations. A variety of catarrh. —Schneider. A heaviness or disorder in the head common at Rome, like the καρηβαρια, *Carebaria*, of the Greeks.—Baglivi.

CAPISTRATIO, Phimosis.
CAPISTRUM, Capeline, Chevestre, Trismus—c. Auri, Borax.

CAPIS'TRUM, *Phimos, Cemos*, κημος, 'a halter.' This name has been given to several bandages for the head.—See Capeline, Chevestre.

CAPITALIA REMEDIA, Cephalic remedies.
CAPITALIS, Cephalic.
CAPITELLUM, Alembic, see Caput.
CAPITEUX, Heady.
CAPITILU'VIUM, from *caput*, 'the head,' and *lavare*, 'to wash.' A bath for the head.

CAPITIPLENIUM, Capiplenium.
CAPITIPURGIA, Caput purgia.
CAPITITRAHA, from *caput*, 'the head,' and *trahere*, 'to draw.' Instruments which, like the forceps, draw down the head of the fœtus when impacted in the pelvis.

CAPITO'NES, from *caput*, 'the head.' *Macroceph'ali, Proceph'ali.* Fœtuses whose heads are so large as to render labour difficult.

CAPITULUM, Alembic, Condyle, see Caput—c. Costæ, see Costa — c. Laryngis, Corniculum laryngis — c. Martis, Eryngium campestre — c. Santorini, Corniculum laryngis.

CAPITULUVIUM, Bath, (head.)
CAPNISMOS, Fumigation.
CAPNITIS, Tutia.
CAPNOIDES CAVA, Fumaria bulbosa.
CAPNORCHIS, Fumaria bulbosa.
CAPNOS, Fumaria.
CAPON, Cagot.

CAPON SPRINGS. A pleasant summer retreat, situated in a gorge of the North Mountain, in Hampshire co., Va., 23 miles W. of Winchester The waters in the vicinity are sulphurous and chalybeate; — those at the springs alkaline and diuretic.

CAPOT, Cagot.

CAP'PARIS SPINO'SA, *Cap'paris, Cappar, Ca'pria, Prickly Caper Bush,* (F.) *Câprier. Family,* Capparideæ. *Sex. Syst.* Polyandria Monogynia. The bark of the root, and the buds, have been esteemed astringent and diuretic. The buds are a well known pickle.—*Capers*, (F.) *Câpres.*

CAPPARIS BADUC'CA, *Baduk'ka.* A species of caper, cultivated in India on account of the beauty of its flowers. The Orientals make a liniment with its juice, with which they rub pained parts. The flowers are purgative.

CAPPONE, WATERS OF. At Cappone, in the isle of Ischia, are waters containing carbonate of soda, chloride of sodium and carbonate of lime. Temp. 100° Fah.

CAPREOLA'RIS, from *capreolus*, 'a tendril.' *Cissoides, Elicoides,* (F.) *Capréolaire.* Twisted.

CAPREOLA'RIA VASA. Some have called thus the spermatic arteries and veins, on account of their numerous contortions.

CAPREOLUS, Helix.
CAPRES, see Capparis spinosa.
CAPRIA, Capparis spinosa.
CAPRICORNUS, Plumbum.
CAPRIER, Capparis spinosa.
CAPRIFOLIA, Lonicera periclymenum.
CAPRIFOLIUM DISTINCTUM, Lonicera periclymenum—c. Periclymenum, Lonicera periclymenum — c. Sylvaticum, Lonicera periclymenum.

CAPRILOQUIUM, Egophony.
CAPRIZANS PULSUS, see Pulse, caprizant.
CAPSA, *Boîte*, Capsule, Case—c. Cordis, Pericardium.

CAPSARIUM, *Boîtier.*
CAPSELLA BURSA PASTORIS, Thlaspi bursa.

CAPSICUM, see Capsicum annuum.

CAP'SICUM AN'NUUM, from καπτω, 'I bite.' The systematic name of the plant whence *Cayenne Pepper* is obtained, — *Piper In'dicum seu Hispan'icum, Sola'num urens, Siliquas'trum Plin'ii, Piper Brazilia'num, Piper Guineen'sē, Piper Calecu'ticum, Piper Tur'cicum, C. Hispan'icum, Piper Lusitan'icum, Cayenne Pepper, Guin'ea Pepper,* (F.) *Piment, Poivre d'Inde, Poivre de Guinée, Corail des Jardins.* The pungent, aromatic properties of *Baccæ Capsici, Capsicum Berries, Capsicum* (Ph. U. S.), are yielded to ether, alcohol, and water. They are highly stimulant and rube-

facient, and are used as a condiment. Their active principle is called *Capsicin*.
CAPSICUM HISPANICUM, Capsicum annuum.
CAPSIQUE, Capsicum annuum.
CAPSITIS, see Phacitis.
CAPSULA, *Boîtier* — c. Articularis, Capsular ligament — c. Cordis, Pericardium — c. Dentis, Dental follicle — c. Lentis, see Crystalline — c. Nervorum, Neurilemma.
CAPSULÆ SEMINALES, Vesiculæ S. — c. Synoviales, Bursæ mucosæ.
CAPSULAIRE, Capsular.
CAP'SULAR, *Capsula'ris,* (F.) *Capsulaire.* Relating to a capsula or capsule.
CAPSULAR ARTERIES, *Suprare'nal Arteries and Veins.* Vessels belonging to the suprarenal capsules. They are divided into superior, middle, and inferior. The first proceed from the inferior phrenic, the second from the aorta, and the third from the renal artery. The corresponding veins enter the phrenic, vena cava, and renal.
CAPSULAR LIG'AMENT, *Ligamen'tum capsula'rē, Cap'sula articula'ris, Artic'ular capsule, Fibrous capsule,* (F.) *Ligament capsulaire, Capsule articulaire, Capsule fibreux,* &c. Membranous, fibrous, and elastic bags or capsules, of a whitish consistence, thick, and resisting, which surround joints.
CAPSULE, *Cap'sula, Capsa,* a box, or case, (F.) *Capsule.* This name has been given, by anatomists, to parts bearing no analogy to each other.
CAPSULE, CELLULAR, OF THE EYE, see Eye.
CAPSULE, FIBROUS, Capsular ligament.
CAPSULE, GELAT'INOUS, *Cap'sula gelat'ina, Capsule of gelatin.* A modern invention by which copaiba and other disagreeable oils can be enveloped in gelatin so as to conceal their taste.
CAPSULE OF GLISSON, *Cap'sula GLISSO'NII, C. commu'nis* GLISSO'NII, *Vagi'na Portæ, V.* GLISSO'NII. A sort of membrane, described by Glisson, which is nothing more than dense areolar membrane surrounding the vena porta and its ramifications in the liver.
CAPSULE OF THE HEART, *Cap'sula cordis.* The pericardium.
CAPSULE, OCULAR, see Eye.
CAPSULE, RENAL, *Suprare'nal* or *Atrabil'iary C., Renal Gland, Glan'dula suprarena'lis, Cap'sula rena'lis, suprarena'lis vel atrabilia'ris, Ren succenturia'tus, Nephrid'ium,* (F.) *Capsule surrénale* ou *atrabiliaire.* A flat, triangular body, which covers the upper part of the kidney, as with a helmet. A hollow cavity in the interior contains a brown, reddish or yellowish fluid. The renal capsules were long supposed to be the secretory organs of the fancied atrabilis. They are much larger in the fœtus than in the adult. They are probably concerned in lymphosis.
CAPSULE, SEM'INAL, *Cap'sula semina'lis.* BARTHOLINE thus designates the extremity of the vas deferens, which is sensibly dilated in the vicinity of the vesiculæ seminales. Some anatomists apply this name to the vesiculæ themselves.
CAPSULE, SYNO'VIAL, *Capsula Synovia'lis.* A membranous bag, surrounding the movable articulations and canals, which gives passage to tendons. Synovial capsules exhale, from their articular surface, a fluid, whose function is to favour the motions of parts upon each other. See Bursa mucosa, and Synovia.
CAPSULE SURRÉNALE ou *ATRABILIARE,* Capsule, renal.
CAPSULITIS, see Phacitis.
CAPUCHON, Trapezius.
CAPUCINE, Tropæolum majus.
CAPULIES, Prunus capulin.

CAPULUS, Scrotum.
CAPUT, 'the head.' Also, the top of a bone or other part, (F.) *Tête.* The head of small bones is sometimes termed *capit'ulum, capitell'um, cephalid'ium, ceph'alis, cephal'ium.* Also, the glans penis.
CAPUT ASPERÆ ARTERIÆ, Larynx — c. Coli, Cæcum — c. Gallinaceum, see Gallinaginis caput — c. Gallinaginis, see Gallinaginis caput — c. Genitale, Glans — c. Lubricum, Penis — c. Monachi, Leontodon Taraxacum — c. Obstipum, Torticollis — c. Penis, Glans.
CAPUT PUR'GIA, *Capitipur'gia.* Remedies, which the ancients regarded as proper for purging the head: — *errhines, sternutatories, apophlegmatisantia,* &c. Prosper Alpinus makes the *caput purgia* to be the same as errhines; and the *apophlegmatismi* the same as the masticatories of the moderns.
CAPUT SCAPULÆ, Acromion.
CAPUT SUCCEDA'NEUM. A term sometimes used for the tumefied scalp, which first presents in certain cases of labour.
CAPUT TESTIS, Epididymis.
CAQUE-SANGUE, Caque-sangue. Old French words which signify *Bloody evacuations,* (F.) *Déjections sanguinolentes.* They come from *cacare,* 'to go to stool,' and *sanguis,* 'blood.' Under this term was comprehended every affection, in which blood is discharged from the bowels.
CARA SCHULLI, *Frutex In'dicus spino'sus, Barle'ria buxifo'lia.* A Malabar plant, which, when applied externally, is maturative and resolvent. The decoction of its root is used, in the country, in ischuria.
CARABAC'CIUM. An aromatic wood of India, of a yellowish colour, and a smell like that of the clove. Its decoction and infusion are given as stomachics and antiscorbutics.
CAR'ABUS. A genus of coleopterous insects. Two species, the *chrysoceph'alus* and *ferrugin'eus,* have been recommended for the toothach. They must be pressed between the fingers, and then rubbed on the gum and tooth affected.
CARACTÈRE, Character, Symbol.
CARAGNA, Caranna.
CARAMATA, *Arumari.* A tree in the inland parts of Pomeroon. It furnishes a febrifuge bark, which Dr. Hancock says may be used in typhoid and remittent fevers where cinchona is either useless or pernicious.
CARAMBOLO, Averrhoa carambola.
CARAN'NA, *Caragna, Tacamahaca, Caragna, Caran'næ Gummi, G. Brel'isis, Gum Caran'na,* (F.) *Caragne, Gomme Caragne* ou *Carane.* A gum-resinous substance, which flows from a large tree in New Spain, and is obtained from South America in impure masses. It preserves its softness for a long time, has an aromatic smell, and a slightly acrid and bitter taste. It was formerly used as a vulnerary and in plasters.
CARAWAY, Carum.
CARBASA, Linteum.
CARBASUS, Linteum.
CARBO, *Carbo Ligni, Charcoal,* (F.) *Charbon.* Fresh Charcoal is antiseptic. It is used to improve the digestive organs in cases of worms, dyspepsia, &c.; as a cataplasm to gangrenous and fetid ulcers, tinea, &c., and forms a good tooth-powder. Dose, gr. x to ʒj. Also, Anthrax.
CARBO ANIMA'LIS, *Carbo carnis, Animal charcoal,* (F.) *Charbon animal.* In the Pharmacopœia of the United States, it is directed to be prepared from bones. It is given in the same cases as *Carbo Ligni,* and has been extolled in cancer. Dose, gr. ss. to gr. iij.
The Pharmacopœia of the United States con

tains a formula for the preparation of CARBO ANIMA'LIS PURIFICA'TUS, *Purified animal charcoal* (*Carbon. animal.* ℔j; *Acid muriat., Aquæ* ää f℥xij.) Pour the muriatic acid, previously mixed with the water, gradually upon the charcoal, and digest with a gentle heat for two days, occasionally stirring the mixture. Having allowed the undissolved portion to subside, pour off the supernatant liquor, wash the charcoal frequently with water until it is entirely free from acid, and lastly dry it.

CARBO FOS'SILIS, *Lithanthrax*, Stone coal.

CARBO HUMA'NUM. The human excrement.—Paracelsus.

CARBO LIGNI, Carbo—c. Mineralis, Graphites—c. Palpebrarum, Anthracosis—c. Spongiæ, Spongia usta.

CARBON, SESQUI-IODIDE OF, Carbonis sesqui-iodidum—c. Bisulphuret of, Carbonis sulphuretum—c. Sulphuret of, Carbonis sulphuretum c. Terchloride of, Chloroform.

CAR'BONAS or CARBO'NAS. A *carbonate*. (F.) *Carbonate*. A salt, formed by the combination of carbonic acid with a salifiable base.

CARBONAS NATRICUM, Sodæ carbonas.

CARBONATE D'AMMONIAQUE, Ammoniæ carbonas.

CAR'BONATED, *Carbona'tus, Aëra'tus*, (F.) *Carboné, Aéré*. That which is impregnated with carbonic acid.

CARBONÉ, Carbonated.

CARBONEUM CHLORATUM, Chloroform.

CARBON'IC ACID, *Ac"idum Carbon'icum, Solid Air of Hales, Factitious Air, Fixed Air, Carbona'ceous Acid, Calca'reous Acid, Aërial Acid, Mephit'ic Acid, Spir'itus letha'lis*, (F.) *Acide Carbonique*. This gas, which neither supports respiration nor combustion, is not often used in medicine. It is the main agent in effervescent draughts, fermenting poultices, &c. It is often found occupying the lower parts of mines—when it is called the *choke damp*—caverns, tombs, wells, brewers' vats, &c., and not unfrequently has been the cause of death. Lime thrown into such places soon absorbs the acid.

CARBO'NIS SESQUI-IOD'IDUM, *C. Sesqui-Iodure'tum, Sesqui-I'odide* or *Sesqui-Iod'uret of Carbon*. This is made by mixing concentrated alcoholic solutions of iodine and potassa, until the former loses its colour; a solution is obtained from which water throws down a yellow precipitate—the sesqui-iodide of carbon. It has been used in enlarged glands and in some cutaneous affections, applied externally, (ʒss to ʒvj of cerate.)

CARBO'NIS SULPHURE'TUM, *Sulphure'tum Carbo'nii, Sul'fidum Carbo'nii, Carbo'nium Sulphura'tum, Al'cohol Sul'phuris, Bisulphure'tum Carbo'nii, Sulphuret of Carbon, Bisulphuret of Carbon, Carburet of Sulphur*, (F.) *Sulfure de Carbon*. This transparent, colourless fluid, which has a very penetrating, disagreeable odour, and a taste which is cooling at first, but afterwards acrid and somewhat aromatic, is a diffusible excitant. It is diaphoretic, diuretic, and has been said to have proved emmenagogue. It is also used in nervous diseases as an antispasmodic. Dose, one drop to four, repeated frequently.

It is used externally, where a cooling influence has to be rapidly exerted, and has been inhaled as an anæsthetic.

CARBONIUM SULPHURATUM, Carbonis sulphuretum.

CARBUNCLE, Anthrax—c. Fungous, Terminthus—c. of the Tongue, Glossanthrax—c. Berry, Terminthus.

CARBUNCLED FACE. Gutta rosea.

CARBUNCULAR EXANTHEM, Anthracia.

CARBUNCULATIO OCULI, Blepharanthracosis.

CARBUNCULUS, Anthrax—c. Anginosus, Cynanche maligna—c. Contagiosus, see Anthrax—c. Gallicus, see Anthrax—c. Hungaricus, see Anthrax—c. Labiorum et genarum, Cancer aquaticus—c. Polonicus, see Anthrax—c. Pulmonum, Necropneumonia—c. Septentrionalis, see Anthrax.

CARBUN'CULUS RUBI'NUS. A red, shining, and transparent stone, from the Isle of Ceylon; formerly employed in medicine as a preservative against several poisons, the plague, &c.

CARBUNCULUS ULCUSCULOSUS, Cynanche maligna.

CAR'CAROS, from καρκαιρω, 'I resound,' 'I tremble.' A fever, in which the patient has a general tremor, accompanied with an unceasing noise in the ears.

CARCINODES, Cancroid, *Chancreuse*.

CARCINOIDES, Cancroid.

CARCINO'MA, *Cancero'ma, Cancro'ma*, from καρκινος, 'a crab.' Some authors have thus called indolent tumours different from cancer; others, incipient cancer; and others, again, the species of cancer in which the affected structure assumes the appearance of cerebral substance; but the majority of authors use Carcinoma in the same sense as Cancer.

CARCINOMA ALVEOLARE, Colloid—c. Fibrosum, Scirrhus—c. Hæmatodes, Hæmatodes fungus—c. Intestinorum, Enteropathia cancerosa—c. Linguæ, Glossocarcinoma—c. of the Liver, Hepatoscirrhus—c. Medullare, Encephaloid—c. Melanodes, Cancer, melanotic—c. Melanoticum, Melanosis—c. Simplex, Scirrhus—c. Spongiosum, Encephaloid, Hæmatodes fungus—c. Scroti, Cancer, chimney-sweepers'—c. Uteri, Metrocarcinoma, Metroscirrhus—c. Ventriculi, Gastroscirrhus; see Gastrostenosis cardiaca et pylorica.

CARCINOM'ATOUS. Relating to Cancer.

CARCINOME MOU ET SPONGIEUX, Encephaloid—*c. Sanglant*, Encephaloid, Hæmatodes fungus.

CARCINOS, Cancer.

CARCINO'SES, (G.) Karsinosen, from καρκινος, 'a crab.' A family of diseases, according to the classification of Fuchs; which embraces the different forms of Cancer.

CARCINOSUS, Cancerous.

CARCINUS SPONGIOSUS, Encephaloid.

CARDAMANTICA, Cardamine pratensis, Lepidium Iberis.

CARDAMINDUM MAJUS, Tropæolum majus.

CARDAMINE FONTANA, Sisymbrium nasturtium—c. Nasturtium, Sisymbrium nasturtium.

CARDAMI'NE PRATEN'SIS, *Cardami'ne, Cardaman'tica, Nastur'tium Aquat'icum, Car'damon, Culi flos, Ibe'ris soph'ia, Nastur'tium praten'së, Ladies-smock, Cuckoo-flower, Common Bitter Cress*, (F.) *Cresson élégant, Cresson des près, Passerage sauvage*. Ord. Cruciferæ. The flowers have been considered useful as antispasmodics, in the dose of ʒj to ʒij. They are probably inert.

CARDAMOM, LESSER, Amomum cardamomum.

CARDAMOME, Amomum cardamomum—*c. de la Côte de Malabar*, Amomum cardamomum.

CARDAMOMUM MAJUS, Amomum grana paradisi—c. Minus, Amomum cardamomum—c. Piperatum, Amomum grana paradisi—c. Wild, Fagarastrum Capense.

CARDAMON, Cardamine pratensis.

CARDAMUM MAJUS, Tropæolum majus.

CARDÈRE, Dipsacus sylvestris—*c. Cultivé*, Dipsacus fullonum.

CARDIA, καρδια, 'the heart.' *Stom'achus*,

Orific"ium sinis'trum seu Ingres'sus supe'rior ventric'uli. The superior or œsophageal orifice of the stomach, — *Orific"ium ventric'uli sinis'trum.* Also, the Heart.

CAR'DIAC, *Cardi'acus,* from καρδια, 'the heart;' or the upper orifice of the stomach. (F.) *Cardiaque.* Relating to the heart or to the upper orifice of the stomach. A cordial.

CARDIAC AR'TERIES, *Cor'onary arteries,* (F.) *Artères cardiaques* ou *coronaires,* are two in number. They arise from the aorta, a little above the free edge of the sigmoid valves, and are distributed on both surfaces of the heart.

CAR'DIAC GAN'GLION, *Gan'glion cardi'acum,* situated beneath the arch of the aorta to the right side of the ligament of the ductus arteriosus. It receives the superior cardiac nerves of opposite sides of the neck, and a branch from the pneumogastric, and gives off numerous branches to the cardiac plexuses.

CARDIAC NERVES, (F.) *Nerfs cardiaques.* These are commonly three on each side; a *superior, middle* and *inferior,* which are furnished by corresponding cervical ganglia. Commonly, there are but two on the left side; the upper and middle, which draw their origin from the last two cervical ganglia. Scarpa calls the *superior—Cardi'acus superficia'lis;* the *middle—C. profun'dus* seu *C. magnus;* and the *inferior—C. parvus* seu *minor.* There are, besides, *Cardiac fil'aments,* (F.) *Filets cardiaques,* furnished by the par vagum or pneumo-gastric nerve, which become confounded with the above.

CARDIAC PLEXUS, *Plexus cardi'acus.* There are three cardiac plexuses. 1. The *great cardiac plexus* is situated upon the bifurcation of the trachea. It is formed by the convergence of the middle and inferior cardiac nerves; and by branches from the pneumogastric, descendens noni, and first thoracic ganglion. 2. The *anterior cardiac plexus* is situated in front of the ascending aorta near its origin. It is formed by filaments from the superior cardiac nerves; from the cardiac ganglion; and from the great cardiac plexus. Filaments from this plexus accompany the left coronary artery, and form the *anterior coronary plexus.* 3. The *posterior cardiac plexus* is seated upon the posterior part of the ascending aorta near its origin. It is formed by numerous branches from the great cardiac plexus. It divides into two sets of branches, which together constitute the *posterior coronary plexus.*

CARDIAC VEINS, *Coronary veins,* (F.) *Veines Cardiaques,* are commonly four in number; two anterior and two posterior. They open into the right auricle by one orifice, which is furnished with a valve, and is called, by Portal, *Sinus coronaire du Cœur.*

CARDIACA CRISPA, Leonurus cardiaca — c. Passio, Cardialgia — c. Trilobata, Leonurus cardiaca — c. Vulgaris, Leonurus cardiaca.

CARDIACUS, Cordial, Stomachal.

CARDIAGMUS, Cardialgia.

CARDI'AGRA, *Affec'tio arthrit'ica cordis;* from καρδια, 'the heart,' and αγρα, 'seizure.' Gout of the heart.

CARDIAG'RAPHY, *Cardiagra'phia,* from καρδια, 'the heart,' and γραφη, 'a description.' An anatomical description of the heart.

CARDIAL'GIA, *Cardi'aca Passio, Col'ica Ventric'uli, Spasmus Ventric'uli, Perodyn'ia, Cordo'lium, Cardilæ'a, Dyspepsodyn'ia, Dyspepsiodyn'ia, Dyspeptodyn'ia, Peratodyn'ia, Cardiod'ynē, Gastral'gia, Gasteral'gia, Gastrocol'ia, Gastrod'ynē, Pas'sio Cardi'aca, Stomachal'gia, Stomacal'gia, Gastrodyn'ia, Cardi'acus Morbus, Cardiog'mus, Cardialgy;* from καρδια, 'the cardiac orifice of the stomach,' and αλγος, 'pain.' *Pain of the stomach,* (F.) *Douleur de l'Estomac, D. névralgique de l'Estomac.* Also, *Heartburn,* (F.) *Cardialgie, Ardeur d'Estomac, A. du Cœur.* Impaired appetite, with gnawing or burning pain in the stomach or epigastrium,— *Morsus* vel *ardor ventric'uli, Morsus stom'achi, Soda, Limo'sis cardial'gia mordens, Rosio Stom'achi* seu *Ventric'uli:* — a symptom of dyspepsia.

CARDIALGIA INFLAMMATORIA, Gastritis — c. Sputatoria, Pyrosis.

CARDIALOG"IA, from καρδια, 'the heart,' and λογος, 'a discourse.' A treatise on the heart.

CARDIANASTROPHE, Ectopia cordis.

CARDIARCTIE, Heart, concentric hypertrophy of the.

CARDIA'RIUS; same etymology. A name given to a worm, said to have been found in the heart or pericardium.

CARDIATOM'IA, from καρδια, 'the heart,' and τεμνειν, 'to cut.' Dissection of the heart.

CARDIATROPHIA, Heart, atrophy of the.

CARDIAUXE, Heart, hypertrophy of the.

CARDIECTASIS, see Aneurism of the heart — c. Partialis, Aneurism of the heart.

CARDIELCOSIS; from καρδια, 'the heart,' and 'ελκος, 'an ulcer.' Ulceration of the heart.

CARDIETHMOLIPOSIS, Steatosis cordis.

CARDIEURYSMA, Aneurism of the heart.

CARDILÆA, Cardialgia.

CARDIM'ELECH, from καρδια, 'the heart,' and מלך, *Melek,* (Hebr.,) 'a governor.' A suppositious active principle seated in the heart, and governing the vital functions.—Dolæus.

CARDINAL FLOWER, Lobelia cardinalis — c. Blue, Lobelia syphilitica.

CARDINAL PLANT, Lobelia cardinalis.

CARDINAMENTUM, Ginglymus, Gomphosis.

CARDIOBOTANUM, Centaurea benedicta.

CARDIOCE'LE, from καρδια, 'the heart,' and κηλη, 'rupture.' Hernia of the heart, especially into the abdominal cavity.

CARDIOCLASIE, Cardiorrhexis.

CARDIOD'YNE, *Cardiodyn'ia;* from καρδια, 'the heart, the stomach,' and οδυνη, 'pain.' Pain in the heart. Also, Cardialgia.

CARDIODYNE SPASMODICA INTERMITTENS, Angina pectoris.

CARDIOG'MUS. Hippocrates employed this word synonymously with cardialgia. In the time of Galen it was used, by some writers, for certain pulsations of the heart, analogous to palpitations. Sauvages understood by *Cardiogmus* an aneurism of the heart or great vessels, when still obscure. Also, Angina pectoris.

CARDIOGMUS CORDIS SINISTRI, Angina pectoris.

CARDIOMALA'CIA, *Malaco'sis* seu *Mala'cia* seu *Malax'is* seu *Mollit"ies Cordis,* (F.) *Ramollissement du Cœur,* from καρδια, 'the heart,' and μαλακια, 'softness.' Softening of the heart, caused by inflammation of the organ, or a consequence of some lesion of the function of nutrition.

CARDIOMYOLIPOSIS, Steatosis cordis.

CARDIONCHI, see Aneurism.

CARDIONEURALGIA, Angina pectoris.

CARDIOPALMUS, Cardiotromus.

CARDIOPERICARDITIS, see Pericarditis.

CARDIORRHEU'MA, *Rheumatis'mus cordis;* from καρδια, 'the heart,' and ρευμα, 'defluxion, rheumatism.' Rheumatism of the heart.

CARDIORRHEX'IS, *Cardioclasie,* (Piorry,) *Ruptu'ra cordis,* (F.) *Rupture du Cœur,* from καρδια, 'the heart,' and ρηξις, 'laceration.' Laceration of the heart.

CARDIOSCLÉROSIE, (Piorry) from καρδια, 'the heart,' and σκληρος, 'hard.' (F.) *Endurcissement du Cœur.* Induration of the heart.

CARDIOSTENO'SIS, *Stenocar'dia,* from καρ-

δια, 'the heart,' and στενωσις, 'contraction.' Contraction of the openings of the heart.

CARDIOTRAU'MA, from καρδια, 'the heart,' and τραυμα, 'a wound.' A wound of the heart.

CARDIOT'ROMUS, *Palpita'tio Cordis trep'idans, Cardiopal'mus, Trepida'tio Cordis,* from καρδια, 'the heart,' and τρομος, 'tremor.' Rapid and feeble palpitation, or fluttering of the heart.

CARDIOT'ROTUS, from καρδια, 'the heart,' and τιτρωσκω, 'I wound.' One affected with a wound of the heart.—Galen.

CARDIPERICARDITIS, see Pericarditis.

CARDITE, Carditis.

CARDI'TIS, from καρδια, 'the heart, and the termination *itis.* Inflammation of the fleshy substance of the heart. *Empres'ma Cardi'tis, Inflamma'tio Cordis, Inflamma'tio Cardi'tis, Cauma Cardi'tis, Myocardi'tis, Cardi'tis Muscula'ris,* (F.) *Inflammation du Cœur, Cardite.* The symptoms of this affection are by no means clear. They are often confounded with those of pericarditis, or inflammation of the membrane investing the heart. Carditis, indeed, with many, includes both the inflammation of the investing membrane and that of the heart itself. See Pericarditis, and Endocarditis.

CARDITIS EXTERNA, Pericarditis—c. Interna, Endocarditis—c. Muscularis, Carditis—c. Membranosa, Pericarditis—c. Polyposa, Polypi of the heart—c. Serosa, Pericarditis.

CARDO, Ginglymus.

CARDOPATIUM, Carlina acaulis.

CARDUUS ALTILIS, Cynara scolymus—c. Benedictus, Centaurea benedicta—c. Brazilianus, Bromelia ananas—c. Domesticus capite majori, Cynara scolymus—c. Hemorrhoidalis, Cirsium arvense.

CAR'DUUS MARIA'NUS, *Car'duus Ma'riæ, Sil'ybum, S. Maria'num seu macula'tum, Carthamus macula'tus, Cir'sium macula'tum, Car'duus lac'teus, Spina alba, Common Milk Thistle,* or *Ladies' Thistle,* (F.) *Chardon-Marie.* The herb is a bitter tonic. The seeds are oleaginous. It is not used.

CARDUUS PINEUS, Atractylis gummifera—c. Sativus, Carthamus tinctorius—c. Sativus nonspinosus, Cynara scolymus—c. Solstitialis, Centaurea calcitrapa—c. Stellatus, Centaurea calcitrapa—c. Tomentosus, Onopordium acanthium—c. Veneris, Dipsacus fullonum.

CAREBARESIS, Carebaria.

CAREBA'RIA or CAREBARI'A, *Carebare'sis,* from καρη, 'the head,' and βαρος, 'weight.' *Scordine'ma, Cereba'ria, Scordinis'mus, Cardine'ma.* Heaviness of the head.—Hippocrates, Galen.

CARE'NA, *Kare'na.* The twenty-fourth part of a drop.—Ruland and Johnson.

CAREUM, Carum.

CAREX ARENARIA, Sarsaparilla Germanica.

CARIACOU. A beverage, used in Cayenne, and formed of a mixture of cassava, potato, and sugar fermented.

CARICA, Ficus carica.

CAR'ICA PAPA'YA, *Papaw tree,* (F.) *Papayer. Ord.* Artocarpeæ. A native of America, India, and Africa. The fruit has somewhat of the flavour of the pumpkin, and is eaten like it. The milky juice of the plant and the seed and root have been regarded as anthelmintic.

CAR'ICUM. Said to have been named after its inventor Caricus. *Car'ycum.* A detergent application to ulcers; composed of black hellebore, sandarach, copper, lead, sulphur, orpiment, cantharides, and oil of cedar.—Hippocrates.

CARIE, Caries—*c. des Dents,* Dental gangrene.

CARIÉ, Carious.

CA'RIES, *Nigrit'ies Os'sium.* An *ulceration of bone,—Necrosis* being death of a bone. It resembles the gangrene of soft parts. Hence it has been termed *Caries gangræno'sa, Gangræ'na Ca'ries, G. Os'sium, Tere'do, Arro'sio, Euros,* (F.) *Carie.* It is recognised by the swelling of the bone which precedes and accompanies it; by the abscesses it occasions; the fistulæ which form; the sanious character, peculiar odour and quantity of the suppuration, and by the evidence afforded by probing. The most common causes of caries are blows;—the action of some virus, and morbid diathesis. When dependent on any virus in the system, *this* must be combated by appropriate remedies. When entirely local, it must be converted, where practicable, into a state of necrosis or death of the affected part. For this end stimulants, the actual cautery, &c., are applied.

CARIES, DENTIUM, Dental gangrene—c. Pudendorum, see Chancre—c. of the Vertebræ, Vertebral disease—c. Vertebrarum, Vertebral disease.

CARIEUX, Carious.

CARIM CURINI, Justitia ecbolium.

CARI'NA, 'a ship's keel.' The vertebral column, especially of the fœtus. Also, the breastbone bent inwards. Hence, *Pectus carina'tum:* —the chest affected with such deformity.

CA'RIOUS, *Cario'sus, Euro'des,* (F.) *Carié, Carieux.* Affected with caries.

CARIUM TERRÆ, Calx.

CARIVE, Myrtus pimenta.

CARIVILLANDI, Smilax sarsaparilla.

CARLINA, 'Carline Thistle.'

CARLI'NA ACAUL'IS, *C. chamæ'leon, Chamæ'leon album, Cardopa'tium,* (F.) *Carline sans tige,* which grows in the Pyrenees, and on the mountains of Switzerland, Italy, &c., has been recommended as a tonic, emmenagogue, and sudorific.

CARLINA CHAMÆLEON, C. acaulis.

CARLINE SANS TIGE, Carlina acaulis.

CARLO SANCTO RADIX. '*St. Charles's Root*': found in Mechoachan, in America. The bark is aromatic, bitter and acrid. It is considered to be sudorific, and to strengthen the gums and stomach.

CARLSBAD, MINERAL WATERS OF. Carlsbad is a town in Bohemia, 24 miles from Egra, celebrated for its hot baths. The water contains about 47 parts in the 100 of purging salts. It is a thermal saline; temperature 121° to 167° Fahrenheit. The constituents are—carbonic acid, sulphate of soda, carbonate of soda, and chloride of sodium.

CARMANTINE, Justitia pectoralis—c. *Pectorale,* Justitia pectoralis.

CARMEN, 'a verse.' An amulet. A charm, which, of old, often consisted of a verse. See Charm.

CARMINANTIA, Carminatives.

CARMINATIVA, Carminatives.

CARMIN'ATIVES, *Carminan'tia seu Carminati'va,* from *carmen,* 'a verse,' or 'charm,' *Antiphys'ica, Physago'ga, Xan'tica,* (F.) *Carminatifs.* Remedies which allay pain, 'like a charm,' (?) by causing the expulsion of flatus from the alimentary canal. They are generally of the class of aromatics.

The FOUR GREATER CARMINATIVE HOT SEEDS, *Quat'uor sem'ina cal'ida majo'ra carminati'va,* were, of old, anise, carui, cummin, and fennel.

The FOUR LESSER CARMINATIVE HOT SEEDS, *Quat'uor sem'ina cal'ida mino'ra,* were bishop's weed, stone parsley, smallage, and wild carrot.

CARMOT. A name given, by the alchymists, to the matter which they believed to constitute the Philosopher's stone.

CARNABADIA, Carum, (seed.)

CARNABADIUM, Cuminum cyminum.

CARNATIO, Syssarcosis.

CARNATION, Dianthus caryophyllus.

CARNELIAN, Cornelian.
CARNEOLUS, Cornelian.
CAR'NEOUS, *Car'neous, Carno'sus, Sarco'des, Incarna'tus,* from *caro,* 'flesh.' (F.) *Charnu.* Consisting of flesh, or resembling flesh.

CARNEOUS COLUMNS, *Fleshy Columns, Colum'næ Carneæ,* of the heart, (F.) *Colonnes charnues,* are muscular projections, situate in the cavities of the heart. They are called, also, *Mus'culi Papilla'res.*

CARNEOUS FIBRES, *Fleshy Fibres, Mus'cular Fibres,* (F.) *Fibres charnues* ou *musculaires,* are fibres belonging to a muscle.

CARNEUM MARSUPIUM, Ischio-trochanterianus.

CARNIC'ULA. Diminutive of *caro,* 'flesh.' The gum,—Gingiva.—Fallopius.

CARNIFICA'TIO, Carnification — c. Pulmonum, Hepatisation of the lungs.

CARNIFICA'TION, *Carnifica'tio,* from *caro,* 'flesh,' and *fieri,* 'to become.' *Transformation into flesh.* A morbid state of certain organs, in which the tissue acquires a consistence like that of fleshy or muscular parts. It is sometimes observed in hard parts, the texture becoming softened, as in *Osteo-sarcoma.* When it occurs in the lungs, they present a texture like that of liver. Such is the condition of the fœtal lung.

CARNIFOR'MIS ABSCES'SUS. An abscess, which ordinarily occurs in the neighbourhood of the articulations, and whose orifice is hard, the sides thick and callous.—M. A. Severinus.

CARNIV'OROUS, *Carniv'orus, Sarcoph'agus, Creatoph'agus, Oreoph'agus,* (F.) *Carnivore,* from *caro,* 'flesh,' and *voro,* 'I eat.' That which eats flesh. Any substance which destroys excrescences in wounds, ulcers, &c.

CARNOSA CUTIS, Panniculus carnosus.

CARNOS'ITAS, (F.) *Carnosité,* from *caro,* 'flesh.' A fleshy excrescence.

CARNOS'ITIES OF THE URE'THRA, *Car'uncles in the Ure'thra,* (F.) *Carnosités* ou *Caroncules de l'urètre.* Small fleshy excrescences or fungous growths, which were, at one time, presumed to exist in the male urethra, whenever retention of urine followed gonorrhœa.

M. Cullérier uses the term *Carnosité vénérienne* for a cutaneous, cellular, and membranous tumour, dependent upon the syphilitic virus. See, also, Polysarcia.

CARNOSUS, Carneous.

CARO, Flesh—c. Accessoria, see Flexor longus digitorum pedis profundus perforans, (accessorius)—c. Excrescens, Excrescence—c. Fungosa, Fungosity—c. Glandulosa, Epiglottic gland—c. Luxurians, Fungosity—c. Orbicularis, Placenta—c. Parenchymatica, Parenchyma—c. Quadrata, Palmaris brevis—c. Quadratus Sylvii, see Flexor longus digitorum pedis profundus perforans, (accessorius)—c. Viscerum, Parenchyma.

CAROB TREE, Ceratonia siliqua.
CAROBA ALNABATI, Ceratonium siliqua.
CARODES, Carotic.
CAROLI, see Chancre.

CAROLI'NA, NORTH, MINERAL WATERS OF. In the counties of Warren, Montgomery, Rockingham, Lincoln, Buncomb, and Rowan, there are mineral springs. They belong generally to the sulphureous or acidulous saline.

CAROLINA, SOUTH, MINERAL WATERS OF. They are numerous. Pacolet Springs, on the west bank of Pacolet River, contain sulphur and iron. Many, with similar properties, but not held in estimation, are scattered about the State.

CARONCULE, Caruncle—c. *Lachrymale,* Caruncle.

CARONCULES MYRTIFORMES, *Caruncule myrtiformes — c. de l'Urètre,* Carnosities of the urethra.

CAROPI, Amomum cardamomum.
CAROSIS, Somnolency.
CAROTA, see Daucus carota.

CAROT'IC, *Carot'icus, Carot'id, Carot'idus, Caro'des, Com'atose,* from καρος, 'stupor.' (F.) *Carotique.* Relating to stupor or *carus*—as a *carotic state,*—or to the carotids.

CAROTIC ARTERIES, Carotids—c. Ganglion, see Carotid Nerve—c. Nerve, Carotid nerve—c. Plexus, see Carotid Nerve.

CAROTICA, Narcotics.
CAROTICUS, Carotic.
CAROTID, Carotic.

CAROT'IDS, *Carot'ides, Carot'icæ, Carotideæ, Capita'les, Jugula'res, Sopora'les, Sopora'riæ, Soporif'eræ, Somnif'eræ, Apoplec'ticæ, Lethar'gicæ (Arte'riæ),* the *Carot'id Ar'teries, Cephal'ic Arteries,* (F.) *Artères Carotides;* from καρος, 'stupor.' The great arteries of the neck, which carry blood to the head. They are divided into, 1. *Primitive* or *common;* the left of which arises from the aorta, and the right from a trunk, common to it and the subclavian. 2. *External* or *pericephal'ic,* branch of the primitive, which extends from the last to the neck of the condyle of the lower jaw; and, 3. *Internal, Arte'ria cerebra'lis* vel *encephal'ica,* another branch of the primitive, which, arising at the same place as the external, enters the cranium, and terminates on a level with the fissure of Sylvius, dividing into several branches.

CAROTID or CAROTIC CANAL, *Cana'lis Carot'icus, Canal inflexe de l'os temporal*—(Ch.), *Canal carotidien,* is a canal in the temporal bone, through which the carotid artery and several nervous filaments pass.

CAROTID or CAROTIC FORAMINA, *Foram'ina Carot'ica,* (F.) *Trous carotidiens,* are distinguished into *internal* and *external.* They are the foramina at each extremity of the *Canalis Caroticus.*

CAROTID GANGLION, see Carotid nerve.

CAROTID NERVE, *Carotic nerve, Nervus carot'icus.* A branch from the superior cervical ganglion of the great sympathetic, which ascends by the side of the internal carotid. It divides into two portions, which enter the carotid canal, and, by their communication with each other and the petrosal branch of the vidian, form the *carotid plexus.* They also frequently form a small gangliform swelling on the under part of the artery —the *carotic* or *carotid* or *cavernous ganglion, ganglion of Laumonier.*

CAROTID PLEXUS, see Carotid nerve.
CAROTTE, Daucus carota.
CAROUA, Carum, (seed.)
CAROUBIER, Ceratonium siliqua.
CAROUGE, see Ceratonium siliqua.
CARPASA, Carbasa.

CARPA'SIUM, *Car'pasum,* and *Carpe'sium.* Dioscorides, Pliny, Galen, &c., have given these names, and that of *Carpasos,* to a plant, which cannot now be determined, and whose juice, called *Opocar'pason,* οποκαρπασον, passed for a violent, narcotic poison, and was confounded with myrrh.

CARPATHICUM, see Pinus cembra.
CARPE, Carpus.
CARPENTARIA, Achillea millefolium.
CARPESIUM, Carpasium.

CARPHO'DES, *Carphoides,* from καρφος, 'flocculus,' and ειδος, 'resemblance.' Flocculent, stringy; — as *mucus carphodes,* flocculent or stringy mucus.

CARPHOLOG"IA, *Tilmus, Carpolog"ia, Crocidis'mus, Crocydis'mus, Flocco'rum vena'tio, Floccile'gium, Tricholog"ia, Crocidix'is, Floccila'tion, Floccita'tion,* from καρφος, '*floc'culus,*' and λεγω, 'I collect,' or 'pluck.' (F.) *Carphologie.* Action of gathering flocculi. A delirious picking of the bed-clothes, as if to seek some substance, or to pull the flocculi from them. It denotes great cerebral irritability and debility, and is an unfavourable sign in fevers, &c.

CARPHOS, Trigonella fœnum.

CARPIA, Linteum.

CARPIÆUS, Palmaris brevis.

CAR'PIAL, *Car'pian, Carpia'nus, Carpia'lis*, (F.) *Carpien*. Belonging to the Carpus.

CAR'PIAL LIG'AMENTS, (F.) *Ligaments Carpiens*, are, 1. The fibrous fasciæ, which unite the bones of the carpus; and, 2. The annular ligaments, anterior and posterior.

CARPIAN, Carpial.

CARPIEN, Carpial.

CARPISMUS, Carpus.

CARPOBALSAMUM, see Amyris opobalsamum.

CARPOLOGIA, Carphologia—c. Spasmodica, Subsultus tendinum.

CARPO-METACARPEUS MINIMI DIGITI, Adductor metacarpi minimi digiti—c. *Métacarpien du petit doigt*, Opponens minimi digiti—c. *Métacarpien du pouce*, Opponens pollicis — c. Phalangeus minimi digiti, Abductor minimi digiti —c. *Phalangien du petit doigt*, Abductor minimi digiti—c. *Phalangien du petit doigt*, Flexor parvus minimi digiti—c. *Phalangien du pouce*, Flexor brevis pollicis manus—c. *Sus-phalangien du pouce*, Abductor pollicis brevis.

CARPO-PEDAL, from *carpus*, 'the wrist,' and *pes, pedis*, 'the foot.' Relating to the wrist and foot.

CARPO-PEDAL SPASM, *Cer'ebral spasmod'ic croup*. A spasmodic affection of the chest and larynx in young children, accompanied by general or partial convulsions. The disease commonly occurs between the third and ninth month, and is characterized by excessive dyspnœa, accompanied by a loud croupy noise on inspiration; the thumbs being locked, and the hands and feet rigidly bent for a longer or shorter period. The seat of the disease is evidently in the cerebrospinal axis, primarily or secondarily: generally, perhaps, it is owing to erethism seated elsewhere, but communicated to the cerebro-spinal centre, and reflected to the respiratory and other muscles concerned. It seems to be connected with dental irritation, and consequently, in the treatment, where such is the case, the gums should be freely divided; after which, cathartics and revulsives, with the use of narcotics and appropriate diet, will generally remove the affection; for although extremely alarming, it is often not attended with great danger. See Asthma thymicum.

CARPOS, Fruit.

CARPOT'ICA, from καρπος, 'fruit.' Diseases affecting impregnation. Irregularity, difficulty or danger produced by parturition:—the 3d order, class *Genetica*, of Good.

CARPUS, *Carpis'mus, Brachia'lē, Rasce'ta, Raste'ta, Rascha, Rase'ta, Raset'ta*, the *wrist*. (F.) *Carpe, Poignet*. The part between the forearm and hand. Eight bones compose it, (in two rows.) In the superior row there are, from without to within — the *Scaphoïdes* or *navicula'rē, Luna'rē* or *semiluna'rē, Cuneifor'mē*, and *Orbicu-lu'rē* or *pisifor'mē*. In the lower row—*Trape'-sium, Trapezoïdes, Magnum*, and *Uncifor'mē*.

CARRAGEEN MOSS, Fucus crispus.

CARRÉ DE LA CUISSE, Quadratus femoris - -c. *des Lombes*, Quadratus lumborum — c. *du Menton*, Depressor lubii inferioris — c. *du Pied*, Extensor brevis digitorum pedis.

CARREAU, Tabes mesenterica.

CARRÉE, see Flexor longus digitorum pedis profundus perforans, (accessorius.)

CARRELET, (F.) *Acus triangula'ris*. A straight needle, two or three inches long, the point of which is triangular; and which the ancients used in different operations. Also, a wooden, triangular frame for fixing a cloth through which different pharmaceutical preparations are passed.

CARROT, CANDY, Athamanta cretensis—c. Deadly, Thapsia—c. Plant, Daucus carota.

CARTHAMUS MACULATUS, Carduus marianus.

CAR'THAMUS TINCTO'RIUS, *Am'yron, Cnicus, Crocus German'icus, Crocus Saracen'icus, Car'thamum officina'rum, Car'duus sati'vus, Safra'num, Saffron-flower, Safflower, Bastard Saffron, Dyer's Saffron*, (F.) *Carthame, Safran bâtard, Carthame des Teinturiers*. Family, Cynarocephaleæ. *Sex. Syst.* Syngenesia Polygamia æqualis. The seeds are aromatic, cathartic, and diuretic; yet to the parroquet they are an article of food; hence their name, *Graines de Parroquet*. The flowers, *Car'thamus*, (Ph. U. S.) are employed as a cosmetic, and are a reputed diaphoretic. [?]

CARTHEGON, see Buxus.

CAR'TILAGE, *Chondros, Car'tilago*, (F.) *Cartilage*. A solid part of the animal body, of a medium consistence between bone and ligament, which in the fœtus is a substitute for bone, but in the adult exists only in the joints, at the extremities of the ribs, &c. Cartilages are of a whitish colour, flexible, compressible, and very elastic, and some of them apparently inorganic. They are composed, according to J. Davy, of .44 albumen, .55 water, and .01 phosphate of lime.

CARTILAGE ANONYME, Cricoid, (cartilage)—c. Epiglottic, Epiglottis—c. *Mucroné*, Xiphoid Cartilage—c. Supra-arytenoid, Corniculum laryngis—c. Tarsal, see Tarsus.

CARTILAGES, ARTICULAR, *Obdu'cent Car'tilages*, invest bony surfaces, which are in contact; hence they are called *investing* or *incrusting cartilages*, (F.) *Cartilages de revêtement ou d'encroûtement*.

CARTILAGES, INTERARTICULAR, are such as are situate within the joints, as in the knee joint.

CARTILAGES OF OSSIFICA'TION are such as, in the progress of ossification, have to form an integrant part of bones; as those of the long bones in the new-born infant. They are termed *temporary*; the others being *permanent*. All the cartilages, with the exception of the articular, are surrounded by a membrane analogous to the periosteum, called *Perichon'drium*.

CARTILAGES OF THE RIBS are, in some respects, only prolongations of the ribs. Those of the nose, of the meatus auditorius, and Eustachian tube, present a similar arrangement. Other cartilages resemble a union of fibrous and cartilaginous textures; hence their name *Fibro-cartilages*.

CARTILAGES, SEMILUNAR, see Semilunar — c. Sigmoid, Semilunar cartilages.

CARTILAGINES GUTTURALES, Arytenoid cartilages—c. Semilunares, Semilunar cartilages—c. Sigmoideæ, Semilunar cartilages.

CARTILAGINIS ARYTENOIDÆÆ CAPITULUM, Corniculum laryngis.

CARTILAG"INOUS, *Cartilagin'eus, Cartilagino'sus, Chondro'des, Chondroï'des*, (F.) *Cartilagineux*. Belonging to, or resembling cartilage.

CARTILAGINOUS, TISSUE, see Tissue.

CARTILAGO, Cartilage — c. Clypealis, Thyroid cartilage — c. Ensiformis, Xiphoid cartilage — c. Guttalis, Arytenoid cartilage — c. Innominata, Cricoid—c. Mucronata, Xiphoid cartilage— c. Peltalis, Thyroid cartilage, Xiphoid cartilage — c. Scutiformis, Thyroid cartilage — c. Uvifer, Uvula—c. Xiphoides, Xiphoid cartilage.

CARUM, from Caria, a province of Asia. A'pium carvi, Bu'nium carvi, Ligus'ticum carvi, See'eli carvi seu carum, Sium carvi, Ca'reum, Carum car'vi, Carvi, Cumi'num praten'sē, Carus, Car'uon, the Car'away, (F.) Carvi, Cumin des prés. Family, Umbelliferæ. Sex. Syst. Pentandria Digynia. The seeds, Carnaba'dia, Car'oua, are carminative. Dose, gr. x to ʒij, swallowed whole or bruised. The oil, Oleum Car'ui, (F.) Huile de carvi, has the properties of the seeds. Dose, gtt. ij to vj.

CARUM BULBOCASTANUM, Bunium bulbocastanum.

CAR'UNCLE, Carun'cula, diminutive of caro, 'flesh.' A small portion of flesh, Sar'cium, Sarcid'ium. A fleshy excrescence,—Ecphy'ma carun'cula, (F.) Caroncule.

CARUNCLE, Carnositas.

CARUNCLES IN THE URETHRA, Carnosities.

CARUN'CULA LACHRYMA'LIS, (F.) Caroncule lacrymale. A small, reddish, follicular body, situate at the inner angle of the eye. It secretes a gummy substance.

CARUNCULÆ CUTICULARES, Nymphæ.

CARUNCULÆ MAMILLA'RES. The extremities of the lactiferous tubes in the nipples. The olfactory nerves have been so called by some.

CARUNCULÆ MYRTIFOR'MES, O. Vagina'les, Glan'dulæ myrtifor'mes, (F.) Caroncules myrtiformes. Small, reddish tubercles, more or less firm, of variable form, and uncertain number, situate near the orifice of the vagina, and formed by the mucous membrane. They are regarded as the remains of the hymen.

CARUNCULÆ PAPILLARES, Papillæ of the kidney.

CARUN'CULOUS, Carun'cular. Relating to caruncles or carnosities.

CARUON, Carum.

CARUS. κάρος, Sopor caro'ticus, Profound sleep. The last degree of coma, with complete insensibility, which no stimulus can remove, even for a few instants. Sopor, Coma, Lethargia, and Carus, are four degrees of the same condition.

CARUS APOPLEXIA, Apoplexy — c. Asphyxia, Asphyxia—c. Catalepsia, Catalepsy—c. Ecstasis, Ecstasis—c. Hydrocephalus, Hydrocephalus internus—c. ab Insolatione, Coup de soleil—c. Lethargus, Lethargy—c. Lethargus cataphora, Somnolency — c. Lethargus vigil, Coma vigil — c. Paralysis, Paralysis — c. Paralysis paraplegia, Paraplegia—c. Veternus, Lethargy.

CARVI, Carum.

CARYA, Juglans regia — c. Basilica, Juglans regia.

CARYEDON CATAGMA, see Fracture.

CARYOCOST'INUS, Caryocostinum. An electuary prepared of the costus and other aromatic substances, &c. It was cathartic. See Confectio scammoniæ.

CARYON PONTICON, Corylus avellana (nut.)

CARYOPHYLLA, Geum urbanum.

CARYOPHYLLATA AQUATICA, Geum rivale—c. Nutans, Geum rivale—c. Urbana, Geum urbanum—c. Vulgaris, Geum urbanum.

CARYOPHYLLUM RUBRUM, Dianthus caryophyllus.

CARYOPHYLLUS AMERICANUS, see Myrtus pimenta—c. Aromaticus, Eugenia caryophyllata — c. Hortensis, Dianthus caryophyllus — c. Pimenta, Myrtus Pimenta — c. Vulgaris, Geum urbanum.

CARYO'TI. The best kind of dates.—Galen.

CAS RARES (F.), Rare cases. This term is used, by the French, for pathological facts, which vary from what is usual. See a celebrated article under this head in the Dictionnaire des Sciences Médicales, Vol. IV.

CASAMUM, Cyclamen.

CASAMUNAR, Cassumuniar.

CAS'CARA, CASCARIL'LA. Spanish words, which signify bark and little bark, under which appellations the bark (Cinchona) is known in Peru. They are now applied to the bark of Croton cascarilla. The bark-gatherers are called Cascarilleros.

CASCARILLA, Croton cascarilla.

CASCARILLEROS, see Cascara.

CASCHEU, Catechu.

CASE, Capsa, Theca, (F.) Caisse. This name is given to boxes for the preservation of instruments, or of medicines necessary in hospital or other service. We say, e. g. — A case of amputating, or of trepanning instruments.

CASE, Casus, from cadere, casum, 'to fall.' The condition of a patient; — as a case of fever, &c. (F.) Observation. Also, the history of a disease.

CASEARIUS, Cheesy.

CA'SEIN, Caseine, Ca'seum, Galactine, Caseous matter; from caseus, 'cheese.' The only nitrogenized constituent of milk. It is identical in composition with the chief constituents of blood,—fibrin and albumen, all being compounds of protein. A similar principle exists in the vegetable, Vegetable Casein or Legu'min, Veg''etable Gluten. It is chiefly found in leguminous seeds —peas, beans, lentils. Like vegetable albumen, Casein is soluble in water; and the solution is not coagulable by heat.

CASEIN, BLOOD, Globulin.

CASEOSUS, Cheesy.

CASEOUS MATTER, Casein.

CASEUM, Casein.

CASEUS, Cheese—c. Equinus, Hippace.

CASEUX, Cheesy.

CASHEW, Anacardium occidentale.

CASHOO. An aromatic drug of Hindoostan, said to possess pectoral virtues.

CASHOW, Catechu.

CASIA, Laurus cassia.

CASMINA, Cassumuniar.

CASMONAR, Cassumuniar.

CASSA, Thorax.

CASSADA ROOT, Jatropha manihot.

CASSAVA ROOT, Jatropha manihot.

CASSE AROMATIQUE, Laurus cassia — c. en Bâtons, Cassia fistula—c. en Bois, Laurus cassia — c. des Boutiques, Cassia fistula — c. Séné, Cassia senna.

CASSE-LUNETTES, Cyanus segetum, Euphrasia officinalis.

CASSEENA, Ilex vomitoria.

CASSENOLES, see Quercus infectoria.

CASSIA, Laurus cassia — c. Absus, Absus — c. Acutifolia, C. senna — c. Ægyptian, C. senna — c. Alexandrina, C. fistula — c. Bonplandiana, C. fistula.

CASSIA CHAMÆCRIS'TA, Prairie senna, Partridge Pea, Wild Senna. An indigenous plant, Fam. Leguminosæ, which flowers in August. It resembles Cassia Marilandica in properties.

CASSIA CINNAMOMEA, Laurus cassia — c. Caryophyllata, Myrtus caryophyllata — c. Canella, Laurus cassia — c. Egyptian, Cassia senna — c. Excelsa, C. fistula.

CAS'SIA FIS'TULA, Cas'sia nigra, Cassia fistula'ris, C. Alexandri'na seu excel'sa seu Bonplandia'na, Canna, Canna soluti'va, Canna fistula, Cathartocar'pus, Bactyrilo'bium fis'tula, Purging Cassia, (F.) Casse Canéficier, Casse en Bâtons, Casse des Boutiques. The pulp of Cassia Fistula or Cathartocar'pus Fistula; Fam. Leguminosæ; Sex. Syst. Decandria Monogynia, Pulpa Cas'siæ, Cassiæ Aramen'tum, Cassiæ Fistulæ

Pulpa, (Ph. U. S.), which is obtained in long pods, is black, bright, and shining; sweet, slightly acid, and inodorous. It is laxative in the dose of ʒiv to ʒj.

CASSIA LANCEOLATA, C. senna — c. Lignea, Laurus cassia — c. Lignea Malabarica, Laurus cassia.

CASSIA MARILAN'DICA, *Senna America'na, American Senna, Wild Senna, Locust plant*, (F,) *Séné d'Amérique*. The leaves of this plant are similar, in virtue, to those of cassia senna. They are, however, much inferior in strength.

CASSIA NIGRA, C. fistula — c. Officinalis, C. senna — c. Orientalis, C. senna — c. Purging, Cassia fistula.

CASSIA SENNA, *C. lanceola'ta seu acutifo'lia seu orienta'lis seu officina'lis*. The name of the plant which affords senna. It is yielded, however, by several species of the genus cassia. The leaves of senna, *Sennæ Folia, Senna Alexandri'na, Senna Ital'ica, Sena, Senna* or *Ægyptian Cassia*, (F.) *Séné, Casse Séné*, have a faint smell, and bitterish taste. The active part, by some called *Cathartin*, is extracted by alcohol and water. Their activity is injured by boiling water. They are a hydragogue cathartic, and apt to gripe. Dose of the powder, Ɖj to ʒj. Infusion is the best form.

The varieties of senna, in commerce, are *Tinnivelly Senna, Bombay* or *Common India Senna, Alexandrian Senna, Tripoli Senna*, and *Aleppo Senna*.

CASSIÆ ARAMENTUM, see Cassia fistula — c. Fistulæ pulpa, see Cassia fistula — c. Flores, see Laurus cinnamomum.

CASSIALA, Hyssopus.

CASSIDA GALERICULATA, Scutellaria galericulata.

CASSIDE BLEUE, Scutellaria galericulata.

CASSINA, Ilex vomitoria.

CASSINE CAROLINIANA, Ilex paraguensis — c. Evergreen, Ilex vomitoria — c. Peragua, Ilex paraguensis.

CASSIS, Ribes nigrum.

CASSITEROS, Tin.

CASSUMU'NIAR, *Cassamu'nar, Casmonar, Zerumbet, Casmina, Ri'sagon, Ben'galā Indo'rum, Rengal Root*, (F.) *Racine de Bengale*. A root, obtained from the East Indies, in irregular slices of various forms; some cut transversely, others longitudinally. It is an aromatic bitter, and is consequently tonic and stimulant. It was once considered a panacea, and has been referred to *Zingiber Cassumuniar, Z. Clifford'ia* seu *purpureum, Amo'mum monta'num*, and to *Zingiber Zerumbet, Z. spurium, Amo'mum Zerumbet* seu *sylves'tre*.

CASSUVIUM POMIFERUM, Anacardium occidentale.

CAS'SYTA FILIFORM'IS. A South African plant, *Nat. Ord*. Laurineæ, which is employed by the Cape colonists as a wash in scald head, and as an antiparasitic.

CAST, Caste.

CASTALIA SPECIOSA, Nymphæa alba.

CASTANEA, Fagus castanea, see also Fagus castanea pumila — c. Equina, Æsculus Hippocastanum — c. Pumila, Fagus castanea pumila.

CASTE, *Cast*, from (P.) *Casta*, 'race or lineage.' A name given, by the Portuguese in India, to classes of society, divided according to occupations, which have remained distinct from the earliest times. Hence a separate and fixed order or class. See Half-caste.

CASTELLAMARE DI STABIA, WATERS OF. Castellamare di Stabia is a town in Naples, in the Principato Citra, 15 miles S. S. E. of Naples. There are two springs, the one sulphureous, the other chalybeate.

CASTELLETTO ADONO, WATERS OF. These waters, situate near Acqui, in Italy, are sulphureous.

CASTERA-VIVENT, WATERS OF. Castera-Vivent is a small village in the department of Gers, near which is a cold acidulous chalybeate, and another which is sulphureous and thermal. Temp. 84° Fahrenheit.

CASTIGANS, Corrigent.

CASTIGLIO'NIA LOBA'TA, *Piñoncillo tree*. A tree, which is cultivated in some parts of Peru, and grows wild in abundance. Its beautiful fruit, when roasted, has an agreeable flavour. When an incision is made into the stem, a clear bright liquid flows out, which, after some time, becomes black and horny-like. It is a very powerful caustic.

CASTJOE, Catechu.

CASTLE-LEOD, WATERS OF. A sulphureous spring in Ross-shire, Scotland, celebrated for the cure of cutaneous and other diseases.

CASTOR BAY, Magnolia glauca.

CASTOR FIBER, *Fiber, Canis Pon'ticus*, the *Beaver*. (F.) *Castor*. It furnishes the Castor. Rondelet recommends slippers made of its skin in gout. Its blood, urine, bile, and fat, were formerly used in medicine.

CASTOR OIL PLANT, Ricinus communis.

CASTO'REUM, *Casto'rium, Castor, Castoreum Ros'sicum et Canaden'sē*, from καστωρ, 'the beaver,' quasi γαστωρ, from γαστηρ, 'the belly,' because of the size of its belly. (?) A peculiar matter found in bags, near the rectum of the beaver, *Castor fiber*. Its odour is strong, unpleasant, and peculiar; taste bitter, subacrid; and colour orange brown. It is antispasmodic, and often employed. Dose, gr. x to Ɖj.

CASTORINA, from *Castoreum*, 'castor.' Medicines containing castor.

CASTRANGULA, Scrophularia aquatica.

CASTRAT, Castratus.

CASTRA'TION, *Castra'tio, Ec'tomē, Ectom'ia, Evira'tio, Excastra'tio, Eteticula'tio, Extirpa'tio testiculo'rum, Detesta'tio, Exsec'tio viril'ium, Eunuchis'mus, Orchotom'ia, Orcheot'omy, Orchidot'omy*, (F.) *Châtrure*. The operation of removing the testicles. Sometimes the term is employed for the operation when performed on one testicle; hence the division into *complete* and *incomplete castration*. Castration renders the individual incapable of reproduction.

CASTRATO, Castratus.

CASTRA'TUS, (I.) *Castra'to, Ectom'ius, Emascula'tus, Evira'tus, Exsec'tus, Desec'tus, Extesticula'tus, Ex maribus, Intestab'ilis, Intesta'tus, Spado, Apoc'opus, Bago'as*, from *castrare*, 'to castrate.' (F.) *Castrat, Châtré*. One deprived of testicles. This privation has a great influence on the development of puberty. It is adopted to procure a clearer and sharper voice; and in the East, the guardians of the Harem, for the sake of security, are converted into *Castra'ti* or *Eu'nuchs*, ευνουχοι. *Eunuchs* have generally both testes and penis removed.

CASUS, Prolapsus, Symptom — c. Palpebræ superioris, Blepharoptosis — c. Uvulæ, Staphyloedema.

CAT TAIL, Typha latifolia.

CATA, Κατα, 'downwards,' 'after,' applied to time: at times, it gives additional force to the radical word. A common prefix, as in —

CATAB'ASIS, from καταβαινω, 'I descend.' An expulsion of humours downwards. Also, a descent, *Descen'sus, Descen'sio*, — as of the testicles, *Descen'sus testiculo'rum*.

CATABLE'MA, καταβλημα, (κατα and βαλλειν,)

'any thing let fall, as a curtain,' *Epible'ma, Perible'ma.* The outermost bandage which secures the rest.

CATABYTHISMOMA'NIA, from καταβυθισμος, 'submersion,' and μανια, 'mania.' Insanity, with a propensity to suicide by drowning.

CATACASMUS, Cupping, Scarification.

CATACAUMA, Burn.

CATACAUSIS, Combustion, human—c. Ebriosa, Combustion, human.

CATACERAS'TICUS, from κατακεραννυμι, 'I temper,' 'I correct.' The same as *Epicerasticus.* A medicine capable of blunting the acrimony of humours.

CATACHASMOS, Scarification.

CATACHRISIS, Inunction.

CATACHRISTON, Liniment.

CATACH'YSIS, *Effu'sio, Perfu'sio,* from καταχεω, 'I pour upon.' Affusion with cold water.—Hippocrates. Decantation.

CATAC'LASIS, from κατακλαζω, 'I break to pieces.' *Cam'pylum, Campylo'tis.* Distortion, or spasmodic fixation of the eyes; spasmodic occlusion of the eyelids; also, fracture of a bone.—Hippocrates, Vogel.

CATACLEIS'; from κατα, 'beneath,' and κλεις, 'the clavicle;' 'a lock or fastening,' κατακλεια, (κατα and κλειω), I lock up. This term has been applied to many parts, as to the first rib, the acromion, the joining of the sternum with the ribs, &c.

CATACLEI'SIS, same etymon. A locking up. The act of locking up. Morbid union of the eyelids.

CATACLYS'MUS, *Cataclys'ma, Cata'clysis,* from κατακλυζειν, 'to submerge, inundate.' A *Clyster.* Hippocr. Others mean, by the term, a shower-bath, or copious affusion of water; *Cataone'sis.* Ablution, Douche.

CATÆONESIS, Catantlema, Cataclysmus.

CATAGAUNA, Cambogia.

CATAGMA, Fracture—c. Fissura, Fissure, see Contrafissura—c. Fractura, Fracture.

CATAGMAT'ICS, *Catagmat'ica remed'ia,* from καταγμα, 'fracture.' Remedies supposed to be capable of occasioning the formation of callus.

CATAGOGLOS'SUM, from καταγειν, 'to draw down,' and γλωσσα, 'the tongue.' An instrument for pressing down the tongue, See Glossocatochus.

CATAGRAPHOLOGIA, Pharmacocatagraphologia.

CATALEN'TIA. Epilepsy, or some disease resembling it.—Paracelsus.

CATALEPSIA SPURIA, Ecstasis.

CAT'ALEPSY, *Catalep'sia, Catalep'sis, Cat'oche, Cat'ochus, Cat'ocha Gale'ni, Morbus atton'itus Celsi, Hyste'ria catalep'tica, Congela'tio, Deten'tio, Encatalep'sis, Aphonia*—(Hippcr.,) *Anau'dia*— (Antigenes,) *Apprehen'sio, Contempla'tio, Stupor vig''ilans, Prehen'sio, Carus Catalep'sia, Oppres'sio, Comprehen'sio*—(Cœl. Aurelian,) *Compren'sio, Apoplex'ia Catalep'sia,* from καταλαμβανω, 'I seize hold of.' *Trance* (?) (F.) *Catalepsie.* A disease in which there is sudden suspension of the action of the senses and of volition; the limbs and trunk preserving the different positions given to them. It is a rare affection, but is seen, at times, as a form of hysteria. Some of the Greek writers have used the word in its true acceptation of a *seizure, surprise,* &c.

CATALEPTIC, *Catalep'ticus,* same etymon. Relating to catalepsy. Affected with catalepsy.

CATALEP'TIC METHOD, *Meth'odus Catalep'tica.* The administration of external agents when internal agents are inapplicable.

CATALOT'IC, *Catalot'icus,* from καταλοω, 'to break or grind down.' A remedy which removes unseemly cicatrices.

CATAL'PA, *C. Arbo'rea, Bigno'nia Catal'pa, Catal'pa Cordifo'lia, C. Arbores'cens seu Bignoniol'des* seu *Syringæfolia, Cataw'ba tree, Indian Bean.* A decoction of the pods of the Catalpa, an American tree, of the *Nat. Fam.* Bignoniaceæ, Didynamia Angiospermia, has been recommended in chronic nervous asthma.

CATALPA ARBOREA, Catalpa—c. Bignonioides, Catalpa—c. Cordifolia, Catalpa—c. Syringæfolia, Catalpa.

CATAL'YSIS, Paralysis, from κατα, and λυω, 'I dissolve or decompose.' *The action of presence* in producing decomposition; as when a body which possesses what has been termed *catalytic force* resolves other bodies into new compounds by mere contact or presence, without itself experiencing any modification.

CATALYTIC FORCE, see Catalysis.

CATAMENIA, Menses—c. Alba, Leucorrhœa.

CATAME'NIAL, *Catamenia'lis, Men'strual, Men'struus, Men'struous,* (F.) *Menstruel,* from κατα, and μην, 'a mouth.' Appertaining or relating to the catamenia.

CATAMENIORUM FLUXUS IMMODICUS, Menorrhagia.

CATANANCE, Cichorium intybus.

CATANGELOS, Ruscus.

CATANTLE'MA, *Catantle'sis,* from κατα, 'upon,' and αντλαω, 'I pour.' *Cateone'sis* and *Oatæone'sis.* Ablution with warm water. A fomentation.—Moschion, Marcellus Empiricus.

CATAPAS'MA, from καταπασσω, 'I sprinkle.' *Catapas'tum, Consper'sio. Epipas'ton, Pasma, Sympas'ma, Empas'ma, Diapas'ma, Xer'ion, Asper'sio, Epispas'tum, Pulvis asperso'rius.* A compound medicine, in the form of powder, employed by the ancients to sprinkle on ulcers, absorb perspiration, &c.—Paulus of Ægina.

CATAPH'ORA, 'a fall,' from καταφερω, 'I throw down.' A state resembling sleep, with privation of feeling and voice. Somnolency. According to others, Cataphora is simply a profound sleep, which it is difficult to rouse from—in this sense being synonymous with Sopor.

CATAPHORA COMA, see Apoplexy — c. Hydrocephalica, see Apoplexy — c. Cymini, Theriaca Londinensis—c. Magnetica, Somnambulism, magnetic.

CATAPHRAC'TA, *Cataphrac'tes,* a *Cuirass,* from καταφρασσω, 'I fortify.' A name given by Galen to a bandage applied round the thorax and shoulders. It was also called *Quadri'ga.*

CATAPIESIS, Depression.

CATAPINOSIS, Absorption.

CATAP'LASIS, from κατακλασσω, 'to besmear.' The act of besmearing or overlaying with plaster.

CAT'APLASM, *Cataplas'ma, Epiplas'ma. Bæos, Poultice, Pultice,* from κατακλασσειν, (κατα and κλασσειν, 'to form or mould,') 'to besmear.' (F.) *Cataplasme.* A medicine applied externally, under the form of a thick pap. Cataplasms are formed of various ingredients, and for different objects. They may be *anodyne, emollient, tonic, antiseptic, irritating,* &c. A simple poultice acts only by virtue of its warmth and moisture. Mealy, fatty substances, leaves of plants, certain fruits, crumb of bread, &c., are the most common bases. The chief poultices which have been officinal are the following:— *Anodyne* — c. Cicutæ, c. Digitalis. *Antiseptic*—c. Carbonis, c. Dauci, c. Fermenti, c. Acetosæ, c. Cumini. *Emollient*—c. Lini, c. Panis, c. Mali maturi. *Irritating*—c. Sinapis, c. Sodii chloridi, c. Quercûs Marini. *Tonic* and *Astringent*—c. Alum, c. Goulard, c. of Roses.

The Parisian Codex has some other medinal

cataplasms. 1. *Cataplas'ma anod'ynum*, made of poppy and hyoscyamus. 2. *Cataplas'ma emolliens*, made of meal and pulps. 3. *Cataplas'ma ad suppuratio'nem promoven'dam*, of pulps and basilicon. 4. *Cataplas'ma rubefa'ciens* vel *antipleurit'icum*, formed of pepper and vinegar.

The only cataplasms, the preparation of which it is important to describe, are some of the following: CATAPLASM, ALUM, Coagulum Aluminosum.— c. of Beer grounds, see Cataplasma Fermenti.— c. Carrot, Cataplasma Dauci.—c. Charcoal, Cataplasma carbonis ligni.

CATAPLASMA BYNES, see C. Fermenti.

CATAPLAS'MA CARBO'NIS LIGNI, *Charcoal Cataplasm* or *poultice*. Made by adding powdered charcoal to a common cataplasm. Used as an antiseptic to foul ulcers, &c.

CATAPLAS'MA DAUCI, *Carrot Cataplasm* or *poultice*. Made by boiling the root of the Carrot until it is soft enough to form a poultice. Used in fetid ulcers.

CATAPLAS'MA FÆCULÆ CEREVISIÆ, see C. Fermenti.

CATAPLAS'MA FERMENT'I, *C. efferves'cens, Yeast Cataplasm* or *Poultice*, (F.) *Cataplasme de Levure*. (Take of meal ℔j, yeast, ℔ss. Expose to a gentle heat.) It is antiseptic, and a good application to bruises. A *Cataplasm of Beer Grounds*, *Cataplasma Fæ'culæ Cerevis'iæ*, C. Bynes, is used in the same cases.

CATAPLAS'MA SINA'PIS, *C. Sina'peos, Sin'apism, Mustard Cataplasm* or *Poultice*, (F.) *Cataplasme de Moutard* ou *Sinapisme*. (*Mustard* and *Linseed meal* or *meal* āā equal parts. *Warm vinegar* or *water*, q. s.) A rubefacient and stimulant applied to the soles of the feet in coma, low typhus, &c., as well as to the pained part in rheumatism, &c.

CATAPLEX'IS, *Stupor*, from κατα, and πλησσω, 'I strike.' The act of striking with amazement. Appearance of astonishment as exhibited by the eyes in particular. See Hæmodia.

CATAPOSIS, Deglutition.

CATAPOTION, Pilula.

CATAPSYX'IS, from καταψυχω, 'I refrigerate'; *Peripsyx'is*. Considerable coldness of the body, without *rigor* and *horripilatio*.—Galen, *Perfric'tio*. Coldness in the extreme parts of the limbs.—Hippocrates.

CATAPTO'SIS, *Deciden'tia*, a *fall*. This word, at times, expresses the fall of a patient, attacked with epilepsy, or apoplexy; at others, the sudden *resolution* of a paralytic limb.

CATAPULTA VIRILIS, Penis.

CATAPUTIA MINOR, Euphorbia lathyris, Ricinus communis.

CAT'ARACT, *Catarac'ta, Catarrhac'ta, Suffu'sio Oc'uli, S. Lentis crystall'inæ, Phtharma cataract'ta, Cali'go lentis, Gutta opa'ca, Hypoc'hyma, Hopoc'hysis, Hopoph'ysis, Phacoscoto'ma, Paropsis catarac'ta, Glauco'ma Woulhou'si*, from καταρασσειν (κατα and ρασσειν), 'to tumble down.' A deprivation of sight, which comes on, as if a veil fell before the eyes. Cataract consists in opacity of the crystalline lens or its capsule, which prevents the passage of the rays of light, and precludes vision. The causes are obscure. *Diagnosis*.—The patient is blind, the pupil seems closed by an opake body, of variable colour, but commonly whitish:—the pupil contracting and dilating. Cataracts have been divided, by some, into *spurious* and *genuine*. The *former*, where the obstacle to vision is between the capsule of the lens and the uvea: the *latter*, where it is in the lens or capsule. A *lenticular cataract* is where the affection is seated in the lens;—a *capsular* or *membranous*, in the capsule. The *capsular* is divided again, by Beer, into the *anterior*, *posterior*, and *complete capsular cataract*. When the capsule is rendered opake, in consequence of an injury, which cuts or ruptures any part of it, it thickens, becomes leathery, and has been called *Catarac'ta arida siliquo'sa*. *Catarac'ta Morgagnia'na lactea* vel *purifor'mis*, is the *milky* variety, in which the crystalline is transformed into a liquid similar to milk, (F.) *Cataracte laiteuse*; or, as generally defined, in which there is opacity of the fluid situate between the lens and its capsule. The *cap'sulo-lentic'ular* affects both lens and capsule, and Beer conceives the liquor Morgagni, in an altered state, may contribute to it. Cataracts are also called *hard*, *soft*, (*Phacomala'cia*,) *stony*, (F. *pierreuse*,) *milky* or *cheesy*, (*laiteuse* ou *caséuse, Galactocatarac'ta, Catarac'ta lactic'olor*,) according to their density:—white, pearly, yellow, brown, gray, green, black, (F.) *blanche, perlée, jaune, brune, grise, verte, noire*, according to their colour:—*fixed* or *vacillating*, —*catarac'ta capsulo-lenticula'ris fixa* vel *trem'ula*, (F.) *fixe* ou *branlante*, according as they are fixed or movable behind the pupil. They are likewise called *Catarac'tæ marmora'ciæ, fenestra'tæ, stella'tæ, puncta'tæ, dimidia'tæ*, &c., according to the appearances they present.

They may also be *simple*, or *complicated* with adhesion, amaurosis, specks, &c.; and *primary* or *primitive*, when *opake* before the operation;—*secondary*, when the opacity is the result of the operation.

The following classification of cataracts is by M. Desmarres:

CLASS I. *True Cataracts.*

a. Lenticular Cataracts.	Hard.	Green. Black. Osseous. Stony or chalky. Striated,etiolated, barred, dehiscent, with three branches, &c.
	Soft.	Disseminated, or dotted. Congenital. Traumatic. Glaucomatous. Morgagnian, or interstitial.
	Liquid.	Cystic, purulent, fetid.
	Other varieties, soft, hard, or liquid.	Shaking, or floating. Luxated.
b. Capsular Cataracts.	Anterior. Posterior.	Pyramidal or vegetant. Arid siliquose.
c. Capsulo-ventricular Cataracts.	All the varieties of lenticular and capsular cataracts.	
d. Secondary Cataracts.	Lenticular. Capsular. Capsulo-lenticular.	

CLASS II. *False Cataracts.*

Fibrinous.
Purulent.
Sanguineous.
Pigmentous.

Cataract is commonly a disease of elderly individuals, although, not unfrequently, *congen'ital*. It forms slowly; objects are at first seen as through a mist: light bodies appear to fly before the eyes, and it is not until after months or years that the sight is wholly lost. No means will obviate the evil except an operation, which consists in removing the obstacle to the passage of the light to the retina. Four chief methods are employed for this purpose. 1. *Couching* or *Depression*, *Hyalonix'is*, *Hyalonyx'is*, (F.) *Abaissement, Déplacement de la Cataracte*. This consists in passing a cataract needle through the sclerotica and subjacent membranes, a little above the transverse diameter of the eye; and at about two lines' distance from the circumference of the transparent cornea, until the point arrives in the posterior chamber of the eye. With this the crystalline is depressed to the outer and lower part of the globe of the eye, where it is left. 2. *By absorption*,—by the French termed *broiement*, or *bruising*. This is performed in the same manner as the former; except that, instead of turning the crystalline from the axis of the visual rays, it is divided by the cutting edge of the needle, and its fragments are scattered in the humours of the eye, where they are absorbed. 3. *By extraction*, which consists in opening, with a particular kind of knife, the transparent cornea and the anterior portion of the capsule of the crystalline; and causing the lens to issue through the aperture. Each of the processes has its advantages and disadvantages, and all are used by surgeons. 4. Some, again, pass a cataract needle through the transparent cornea and pupil to the crystalline, and depress or cause its absorption. This is called Keratonyxis, which see.

CATARACT, BLACK, Amaurosis — c. Capsular, see Cataract — c. Capsulo-lenticular, see Cataract — c. Central, Centradiaphanes — c. Cheesy, see Cataract — c. Congenital, see Cataract — c. Complicated, see Cataract — c. Fixed, see Cataract — c. Genuine, see Cataract — c. Hard, see Cataract — c. Lenticular, see Cataract — c. Membranous, see Cataract — c. Milky, see Cataract — c. Opake, see Cataract — c. Primary, see Cataract — c. Primitive, see Cataract — c. Secondary, see Cataract — c. Simple, see Cataract — c. Soft, see Cataract — c. Spurious, see Cataract — c. Stony, see Cataract — c. Vacillating, see Cataract.

CATARACTA, Cataract — c. Arida siliquosa, see Cataract — c. Capsulo-lenticularis, see Cataract — c. Centralis, Centradiaphanes — c. Dimidiata, see Cataract — c. Fenestrata, see Cataract — c. Glauca, Glaucoma — c. Lacticolor, see Cataract — c. Liquida, Hygrocataracta — c. Marmoracea, see Cataract — c. Morgagniana, see Cataract — c. Nigra, Amaurosis — c. Punctata, see Cataract — c. Stellata, see Cataract.

CATARACTE, ABAISSEMENT DE LA, see Cataract — *c. Blanche*, see Cataract — *c. Branlante*, see Cataract — *c. Brune*, see Cataract — *c. Caséuse*, see Cataract — *c. Déplacement de la*, see Cataract — *c. Fixe*, see Cataract — *c. Grise*, see Cataract — *c. Jaune*, see Cataract — *c. Laiteuse*, see Cataract — *c. Noire*, Amaurosis, see Cataract — *c. Perleé*, see Cataract — *c. Pierreuse*, see Cataract — *c. Verte*, see Cataract.

CATARACTÉ, (F.) *Catarac'tus, Catarac'tâ vitia'tus*. One affected with cataract. The French use this term, both for the eye affected with cataract and the patient himself.

CATARIA, see Nepeta — c. Vulgaris, Nepeta.

CATARRH', *Catar'rhus, Catar'rhopus, Catarrheu'ma, Rheuma, Deflux'io, Catastag'ma, Phlegmatorrhag''ia, Phlegmatorrhœ'a*, from κατα, 'downwards,' and ρεω, 'I flow.' A discharge of fluid from a mucous membrane. The ancients considered catarrh as a simple flux, and not as an inflammation. Generally it partakes of this character, however. *Catarrh* is, with us, usually restricted to inflammation of the mucous membrane of the air-passages: the French extend it to that of all mucous membranes; (F.) *Flux muqueux, Fluxion catarrhale*.

Catarrh, in the English sense, *Broncho-catar'-rhus, Pul'monary Catarrh, Lung fever*, (vulgarly,) *Rheuma Pec'toris, Destilla'tio Pec'toris, Catar'rhus Pec'toris, C. Pulmo'num, C. Pulmona'lis, C. Bronchia'lis, Blennop'tysis, Tus'sis catarrha'lis, simplex, Grave'do* (of many), *Febris Catarrha'lis, Blennotho'rax, Bronchi'tis, Catar'rhus à Fri'gorē*, (F.) *Catarrhe pulmonaire, Fièvre Catarrhale, Rhume de Poitrine*, a *Cold*, is a superficial inflammation of the mucous follicles of the trachea and bronchi. It is commonly an affection of but little consequence, but apt to relapse and become chronic. It is characterized by cough, thirst, lassitude, fever, watery eyes, with increased secretion of mucus from the air-passages. The antiphlogistic regimen and time usually remove it. — Sometimes, the inflammation of the bronchial tubes is so great as to prove fatal.

CATARRH, ACUTE, OF THE UTERUS, see Metritis — c. Chronic, Bronchitis, (chronic) — c. Dry, see Bronchitis — c. Pulmonary, Bronchitis, Catarrh — c. Rose, Fever, hay — c. Suffocating nervous, Asthma, Thymicum — c. Summer, Fever, hay.

CATARRH', EPIDEM'IC, *Catar'rhus epidem'icus, C. à conta'gio, Rheuma epidem'icum*. Catarrh prevailing owing to some particular *Constitutio aëris*, and affecting a whole country, — *Influenza*.

CATARRHACTA, Cataract.

CATAR'RHAL, *Catarrha'lis, Catarrho'icus, Catarrhoït'icus, Catarrhoët'icus*. Relating to catarrh, — as *Catarrhal Fever*.

CATARRHE AIGUË DE L'UTÉRUS, see Metritis — *c. Buccal*, Aphthæ, — *c. Convulsive*, Bronchitis — *c. Gastrique*, Gastritis — *c. Guttural*, Cynanche tonsillaris — *c. Intestinal*, Diarrhœa — *c. Laryngien*, Laryngitis — *c. Nasal*, Coryza — *c. Oculaire*, Ophthalmia — *c. de l'Oreille*, Otirrhœa — *c. Pharyngien*, Cynanche parotidea — *c. Pituiteux*, Bronchorrhœa — *c. Pulmonaire*, Catarrh — *c. Sec*; see Bronchitis — *c. Stomacal*, Gastrorrhœa — *c. Utérin*, Leucorrhœa — *c. Vesical*, Cystorrhœa.

CATARRHEC'TICA, from καταρρηγνυμι, 'I break down.' Remedies considered proper for evacuating; — as diuretics, cathartics, &c. Hippocrates.

CATARRHEUMA, Catarrh.

CATARRHEUX (F.) *Catarrho'sus*. One subject to catarrh; affected with catarrh.

CATARRHEX'IA, *Catarrhex'is*; same etymon as *Catarrhectica*. The action of Catarrhectica. Also, effusion; evacuation of the bowels.

CATARRHEXIS, Catarrhexia, Excrement — c. Vera, Hæmatochezia.

CATARRHŒA, Rheumatism.

CATARRHOET'ICUS, from καταρρεω, 'I flow from.' An epithet for disease produced by a discharge of phlegm; catarrhal.

CATAR'RHOPA PHY'MATA, from καταρροπος, καταρροπης, 'sloping downwards.' Tubercles tending downwards, or with their apices downwards.

CATARRHOPHE, Absorption.

CATARRHOPHESIS, Absorption.

CATARRHO'PIA, *Catar'rhysis*, from κατα 'downwards,' and ροπη, 'inclination.' An afflux of fluids towards the inferior parts, and especially towards the viscera of the abdomen. The Greek word αναρροπια expresses an opposite phenomenon, or a tendency towards the upper parts.

CATARRHOPUS, Catarrh.

CATARRHOS'CHESIS, from καταρρος, 'catarrh,' and σχεσις, 'suppression.' The suppression of a mucous discharge.

CATARRHUS, Defluxion, Tussis — c. Æstivus, fever, hay — c. Bellinsulanus, Cynanche parotidæa — c. Bronchialis, Catarrh — c. Bronchiorum, Bronchitis — c. à Contagio, Influenza — c. Epidemicus, Influenza, Catarrh, epidemic—c. Genitalium, Leucorrhœa—c. Gonorrhœa, Gonorrhœa—c. Intestinalis, Diarrhœa—c. Laryngeus, Laryngo-catarrhus—c. ad Nares, Coryza—c. Nasalis, Coryza—c. Pulmonalis, Catarrh—c. Pulmonum, Bronchitis, Catarrh—c. Senilis, Bronchitis, (chronic)—c. Suffocativus Barbadensis, C. trachealis—c. Trachealis, Laryngo-catarrhus—c. Urethræ, Gonnorrhœa pura—c. Urethralis, Gonorrhœa—c. Vesicæ, Cystorrhœa.

CATARRHYSIS, Catarrhopia, Defluxion.
CATARTISIS, Catartismus.
CATARTIS'MUS, *Catar'tisis*, from καταρτιζειν, 'to repair, replace.' The coaptation of a luxated or fractured bone, or hernia.
CATASARCA, Anasarca.
CATASCEUE, Structure.
CATASCHASMUS, Bloodletting, Scarification.
CATASTAGMUS, Catarrh, Coryza.
CATASTALAGMUS, Coryza, Distillation.
CATASTALTICA, Hæmatostatica, Sedatives.
CATAS'TASIS, from καθιστημι, 'I establish.' The constitution, state, condition, &c., of anything.—Hippocrates. Also the reduction of a bone. See Constitution, and Habit of Body.
CATAT'ASIS, from κατατεινω, 'I extend'. Extension. The extension and reduction of a fractured limb.—Hippocrates.
CATATHLIPSIS, Oppression.
CATAWBA TREE, Catalpa.
CATAXIS, Fracture.
CATCH FLY, Apocynum androsæmifolium, Silene Virginica.
CATCHUP, Ketchup.
CAT'ECHU. The extract of various parts of the *Aca'cia Cat'echu*, *Mimo'sa Cat'echu*, *Caæt'chu*, an oriental tree. The drug is also called *Terra Japon'ica*, *Extrac'tum Catechu*, *Japan Earth*, *Cascheu*, *Cadtchu*, *Cashow*, *Caitchu*, *Castjoe*, *Cacau*, *Cate*, *Kaath*, *Cuti*, *Cutch*, *Coïra*, *Succus Japon'icus*, (F.) *Cachou*. It is a powerful astringent, and is used in diarrhœa, intestinal hemorrhage, &c. Dose, gr. xv to ʒss, in powder.
CATECHU, SQUARE, see Nauclea gambir.
CATEIAD'ION, from κατα, and ϊα, 'a blade of grass.' A long instrument thrust into the nostrils to excite hemorrhage in headach.—Arctæus.
CATENÆ MUSCULUS, Tibialis anticus.
CATEONESIS, Catantlema.
CATGUT, Galega Virginiana.
CATHÆ'RESIS, καθαιρεσις, 'subtraction, diminution.' Extenuation or exhaustion, owing to forced exercise.—Hippocrates. The action of catheretics.
CATHÆRETICUS, Catheretic.
CATHARETICUS, Cathartic.
CATHARISMOS, Depuration.
CATHAR'MA, *Purgament'um*. The matter evacuated by a purgative, or by spontaneous purging: also, a cathartic.
CATHAR'MUS, Same etymon; a purgation.—Hippocrates. Also, the cure of a disease by magic, &c.
CATHAR'SIS, from καθαιρειν, (καθ' and αιρειν, 'to take away,') 'to purge.' *Purga'tio*, *Apocathar'sis*, *Copropho'ria*, *Coprophore'sis*. A natural or artificial *purgation* of any passage;—mouth, anus, vagina, &c.
CATHAR'TIC, *Cathar'ticus*, *Cathare'ticus*, *Cathor'ma*, *Coprocrit'icum*, *Coprago'gum*, *Lustramen'tum*, *Purgans medicament'um*, *Trichili'um*, *Dejecto'rium Remed'ium*, *Eccathar'ticus*, *Hypacticus*, *Hopochoret'icus*, *Alvum evac'uans*, *Hypel'atos*, *Lapac'ticus*, *Apocathar'ticus*. Same etymon. (F.) *Cathartique*. A medicine which, when taken internally, increases the number of alvine evacuations. Some substances act upon the upper part of the intestinal canal, as *calomel* and *colocynth*; others, on the lower part, as *aloes*; and some on the whole extent, as *saline* purgatives. Hence a choice may be necessary. Cathartics are divided into purgatives and laxatives. The following is a list of the chief cathartics:

Aloe, Cassia Marilandica, Colocynthis, Elaterium, Gamboga, Hydrargyri Chloridum mite, Hydrargyri Oxydum nigrum, Hydrarg. cum Magnesiâ, Jalapa, Juglans, Magnesia. Magnesiæ Carbonas, Magnesiæ Sulphas, Manna, Mannita, Oleum Euphorbiæ Lathyridis, Oleum Ricini, Oleum Tiglii, Podophyllum, Potassæ Acetas, Potassæ Bisulphas, Potassæ Sulphas, Potassæ Bitartras, Potassæ Tartras, Rheum, Scammonium, Senna, Sinapis, Sodæ et Potassæ Tartras, Sodæ Phosphas, Sodæ Sulphas, Sodi Chloridum, Sulphur, Veratria, Aquæ Minerales Sulphureæ et Salinæ, Enemata, Suppositoria.

CATHARTIN, see Cassia Senna, and Convolvulus jalapa.
CATHARTIQUE, Cathartic.
CATHARTOCARPUS, Cassia fistula.
CATHEDRA, Anus.
CATHEMERINUS, Quotidian.
CATHEMERUS, Quotidian.
CATHERET'IC, *Cathæret'icus*, *Ectylot'icus*, *Sarcoph'agus*, from καθαιρειν, 'to eat,' 'destroy.' Substances applied to warts, exuberant granulations, &c., to eat them down. Mild caustics.
CATH'ETER, from καθιημι (καθ', and ιημι, 'to send,') 'I explore.' *Æne'a*, *Al'galie*, *Cathete'ris*, *Demissor*, *Immis'sor*. A hollow tube, introduced by surgeons into the urinary bladder, for the purpose of drawing off the urine. Catheters are made of silver or elastic gum. See Bougie. The French generally use the word *catheter* for the solid *sound* or *staff*; and *algalie* and *sonde* for the hollow instrument.
CATHETER, NASAL. An instrument, invented by M. Gensoul, of Lyons, for catheterizing the ductus ad nasum. It is hook-shaped; the extremity, bent at a right angle, is about an inch in length, suited to the distance of the lower orifice of the duct from the nostril, and likewise to the length and form of the duct, with a slight spiral turn.
CATHETERIS, Catheter.
CATHETERISIS, Catheterismus.
CATHETERIS'MUS, *Cathete'risis*, *Catheterisa'tio*, *Cath'eterism*, *Catheteriza'tion*, *Immis'sio Cathete'ris*, same etymon. The introduction of a catheter or sound into the bladder or Eustachian tube. Also probing a wound. Melosis.
CATHETERIZATION, Catheterismus.
CATH'ETERIZE. To perform the operation of catheterism;—in other words, to introduce the catheter, to probe or sound a cavity.
CATHID'RYSIS, from καθιδρυω, 'I place together.' Reduction of a part to its natural situation.
CATHMIA, Plumbi oxydum semi-vitreum.
CATHMIR, Calamina.
CATHOD'IC, *Cathod'icus*; from καθ', 'downwards,' and ὁδος, 'a way.' An epithet applied by Dr. Marshall Hall to a downward course of nervous action.
CATH'OLIC HUMOURS, (F.) *Humeurs Catholiques*, are the fluids spread over the whole body.
CATHOLICON, Panacea.
CATHOL'ICON DUPLEX. An ancient purging electuary, chiefly composed of cassia, tamarinds, rhubarb, senna, &c.
CATHOLICUM, Panacea.
CATIL'LIA. A weight of nine ounces.
CATILLUS, Cup.
CATINUS FUSORIUS, Crucible.

CATLING, Knife, double-edged.

CATO, κατω, 'below,' 'beneath.' This word, in the writings of Hippocrates, is often used for the abdomen, especially the intestines. When he advises a remedy κατω, he means a purgative; when ανω, 'above or upwards,' an emetic. As a prefix, *Cato* means 'beneath,' as in

CATOCATHARTIC, *Catocathar'ticus*, from κατω, 'downwards,' and καθαιρω, 'I purge.' A medicine which purges downwards. One that produces alvine evacuations. The antithesis to *Anacathartic*.

CATOCHA GALENI, Catalepsy.

CAT'OCHE, *Cat'ocheis, Cat'ochus*, from κατεχω, 'I retain,' 'I hold fast.' This word has, by some, been used synonymously with Catalepsy; by others, with Coma vigil; by others, with Tetanus.

CATOCHUS, Catoche, Ecstasis—c. Cervinus, Tetanus—c. Holotonicus, Tetanus—c. Infantum, Induration of the cellular tissue.

CATOMIS'MOS, from κατω, 'beneath,' and ωμος, 'shoulder;' *Subhumera'tio*. A mode with the ancients of reducing luxation of the humerus by raising the body by the arm.—Paulus of Ægina.

CATOPTER, Speculum.

CATOP'TRIC EXAMINATION OF THE EYE. When a lighted candle is held before the eye, the pupil of which has been dilated by belladonna, three images of it are seen—two erect, and one inverted:—the former owing to reflection from the cornea and anterior surface of the crystalline; the latter owing to reflection from the posterior layer of the crystalline. This mode of examining the eye has been proposed as a means of diagnosis between cataract and amaurosis. In the latter, all the images are seen.

CATOPTROMANCY, from κατοπτρον, (κατα, and οπτομαι,) 'a mirror,' and μαντεια, 'divination.' A kind of divination by means of a mirror.

CATOPTRON, Speculum.

CATORCHI'TES. A kind of sour wine, prepared with the orchis and black grape, or dried figs. It was formerly employed as a diuretic and emmenagogue.—Dioscorides. Called, also, *Syci'tes*.—Galen.

CATORETICUS, Purgative.

CATOTERICUS, Purgative.

CATO'TICA, from κατω, 'beneath.' Diseases infecting internal surfaces. Pravity of the fluids or emunctories, that open on the internal surfaces of organs. The second order in the class *Eccritica* of Good.

CATOX'YS, *Peracu'tus*, from κατα, 'an intensive,' and οξυς, 'acute.' Highly acute; as *Morbus Catoxys, M. Peracu'tus*, a very acute disease.

CAT'S EYE, AMAUROTIC, see Amaurotic.

CAT'SFOOT, Antennaria dioica.

CATTAGAUMA, Cambogia.

CATTITEROS, Tin.

CATULOTICA, Cicatrisantia.

CATU-TRIPALI, Piper longum.

CAUCALIS CAROTA, Daucus carota—c. Sanicula, Sanicula.

CAUCALOIDES, Patella.

CAUCASIAN, see Homo.

CAUCHEMAR, Incubus.

CAUCHEVIEILLE, Incubus.

CAUCHUC, Caoutchouc.

CAUDA, Coccyx, Penis.

CAUDA EQUI'NA. The spinal marrow, at its termination, about the second lumbar vertebra, gives off a considerable number of nerves, which, when unravelled, resemble a horse's tail,—hence the name; (F.) *Queue de Cheval, Q. de la Moëlle Épinière*. See Medulla Spinalis.

CAUDA SALAX, Penis.

CAUDAL, *Caudate, Cauda'lis, Cauda'tus;* from *cauda*, 'a tail.' Relating or appertaining to a tail. Having a tail or tail-like appendage:— as '*caudal* or *caudate* corpuscles'—corpuscles having a tail-like appendage, as in cancerous growths.

CAUDATE, Caudal.

CAUDATIO, Clitorism.

CAUDATUS, Bicaudatus.

CAUDIEZ, MINERAL WATERS OF. Caudies is a small town, nine leagues from Perpignan, in France, where there is a thermal spring, containing a little sulphate of soda and iron.

CAUDLE: (F.) *Chaudeau, chaud*, 'warm or hot.' A nourishing gruel given to women during the childbed state. The following is a form for it: Into a pint of fine gruel, not thick, put, whilst it is boiling hot, the yolk of an egg beaten with sugar, and mixed with a large spoonful of cold water, a glass of wine, and nutmeg. Mix the whole well together. Brandy is sometimes substituted for the wine, and lemon peel or capillaire added. It is also sometimes made of gruel and beer, with sugar and nutmeg.

CAUL, from (L.) *caula*, 'a fold,' *Pilus, Pile'olus, Ga'lea, Vitta,* (F.) *Coeffe, Coiffe*—(*Etre né coeffé*—'to be born with a caul.') The English name for the omentum. When a child is born with the membranes over the face, it is said to have been '*born with a caul.*' In the catalogue of superstitions, this is one of the favourable omens. The caul itself is supposed to confer privileges upon the possessor; hence the membranes are dried, and sometimes sold for a high price. See Epiploon.

CAULE'DON, *Cicye'don*, from καυλος, 'a stalk.' A transverse fracture.

CAU'LIFLOWER, (G.) Kohl, 'cabbage,' and *flower* [?], Brassica Florida.

CAULIFLOWER EXCRES'CENCE, *Excrescen'tia Syphilit'ica*, (F.) *Ohoufleur*. A syphilitic excrescence, which appears about the origin of the mucous membranes, chiefly about the anus and vulva, and which resembles, in appearance, the head of the cauliflower.

CAULIS, Penis—c. Florida, Brassica Florida.

CAULOPHYL'LUM THALICTROI'DES, *Leon'tice thalictroi'des, Blueberry Cohosh, Cohosh, Cohush, Blueberry, Papoose Root, Squaw Root, Blue Ginseng, Yellow Ginseng,* a plant of the *Family* Berberideæ; *Sex. Syst.* Hexandria Monogynia, which grows all over the United States, flowering in May and June. The infusion of the root is much used by the Indians in various diseases. To it are ascribed emmenagogue and diaphoretic virtues.

CAULOPLE'GIA, from καυλος, 'the male organ,' and πληγη, 'a wound,' or 'stroke.' An injury or paralysis of the male organ.

CAULORRHAGIA, Stimatosis—c. Ejaculatoria, Spermato-cystidorrhagia—c. Stillatitia, Urethrorrhagia.

CAULORRHŒA BENIGNA, Gonorrhœa pura.

CAULUS, Penis.

CAUMA, καυμα, 'a burnt part,' from καιω, 'I burn.' Great heat of the body or atmosphere. Synocha, Empresma.

CAUMA BRONCHITIS, Cynanche trachealis—c. Carditis, Carditis—c. Enteritis, Enteritis—c. Gastritis, Gastritis—c. Hæmorrhagicum, Hæmorrhagia activa—c. Hepatitis, Hepatitis—c. Ophthalmitis, Ophthalmia—c. Peritonitis, Peritonitis—c. Phrenitis, Phrenitis—c. Pleuritis, Pleuritis—c. Podagricum, Gout—c. Rheumatismus, Rheumatism, acute.

CAUMATO'DES, *Causmate'rus*, from καυμα, 'fire-heat.' Burning hot. *Febris caumato'des, F. causo'des.* Inflammatory fever. Synocha.

CAUNGA, Areca.

CAUSA CONJUNCTA, Cause, proximate—c. Continens, Cause, proximate.

CAUSÆ ABDITÆ, Causes, predisponent or remote—c. Actuales, Causes, occasional—c. Præincipientes, Causes, procatarctic—c. Proëgumenæ, Causes, predisponent.

CAUSE, *Cau'sa, Ai'tia, Ai'tion.* An act which precedes another, and seems to be a necessary condition for the occurrence of the latter. The causes of disease are generally extremely obscure; although they, sometimes, are evident enough. The *predisponent* and *occasional* causes are the only two, on which any stress can be laid; but as authors have divided them differently, a short explanation is necessary.

CAUSE, AC'CESSORY, (F.) *Cause Accessoire.* One which has only a secondary influence in the production of disease.

CAUSES, ACCIDENT'AL, *Common Causes,* (F.) *Causes Accidentelles,* are those which act only in certain given conditions; and which do not always produce the same disease. Cold, e. g., may be the accidental cause of pneumonia, rheumatism, &c.

CAUSES CACHÉES, C. occult—c. Common, C. accidental—c. Exciting, C. Occasional—c. Essential, C. Specific—c. *Déterminantes,* C. Specific —c. *Éloignées,* C. Predisponent.

CAUSES, EXTERN'AL, (F.) *Causes externes,* are such as act externally to the individual; as air, cold, &c.

CAUSES FORMELLES, (F.) are such as determine the form or kind of disease. They differ from the *Causes matérielles,* which are common to a set of diseases; as, to the neuroses, phlegmasiæ, &c.

CAUSES, HIDDEN, C. Occult.

CAUSES, INTERN'AL, (F.) *Causes Internes,* are those which arise within the body;—as mental emotions, &c.

CAUSES, MECHAN'ICAL, (F.) *Causes mécaniques,* are those which act mechanically, as pressure upon the windpipe in inducing suffocation.

CAUSES, NEG'ATIVE, (F.) *Causes négatives,* comprise all those things, the privation of which may derange the functions;—as abstinence too long continued. They are opposed to *positive causes,* which, of themselves, directly induce disease;—as the use of indigestible food, spirituous drinks, &c.

CAUSES, OBSCURE, C. Occult.

CAUSES, OCCA'SIONAL, *Exci'ting Causes, Causæ actua'les,* (F.) *Causes occasionelles,* are those which immediately produce disease. The occasional causes have been divided into the *cognizable* and *non-cognizable.*—C. J. B. Williams.

	I. *Cognizable Agents.*
	1. Mechanical.
	2. Chemical.
	3. Ingesta.
	4. Bodily exertion.
	5. Mental emotion.
EXCITING	6. Excessive evacuation.
CAUSES	7. Suppressed or defective evacuation.
OF	8. Defective cleanliness, ventilation and draining.
DISEASE.	9. Temperature and changes.
	II. *Non-Cognizable Agents.*
	1. Endemic.
	2. Epidemic. } Poisons.
	3. Infectious.

CAUSES, OCCULT', *Hidden causes, Obscure causes,* (F.) *Causes occultes* ou *cachées* ou *obscures.* Any causes with which we are unacquainted; also, certain inappreciable characters of the atmosphere, which give rise to epidemics.

CAUSES, PHYS'ICAL, (F.) *Causes Physiques,*—those which act by virtue of their physical properties; as form, hardness, &c. All vulnerating bodies belong to this class.

CAUSES, PHYSIOLOG''ICAL, (F.) *Causes Physiologiques,* those which act only on living matter; —narcotics, for example.

CAUSES, PREDISPO'NENT, *Remote causes, Causæ proëgu'menæ, Causæ ab'ditæ, Causæ remo'tæ;* (F.) *Causes prédisponantes, Causes éloignées,*—those which render the body liable to disease. They may be *general,* affecting a number of people, or *particular,* affecting only one person.

CAUSES, PRIN'CIPAL, (E.) *Causes principales* —those which exert the chief influence on the production of disease, as distinguished from the *accessory causes.*

CAUSES, PROCATARC'TIC, *Causæ procatarc'ticæ, Causæ præincipien'tes,* from προκαταρκτικος, 'the origin or beginning of a thing,' (καταρχω, 'I begin,' and προ, 'before.') These words have been used with different significations. Some have employed them synonymously with *predisponent* or *remote causes;* others with *occasional* or *exciting causes.*

CAUSE PROCHAINE, C. proximate.

CAUSE, PROX'IMATE, *Causa prox'ima vel con'tinens* vel *conjunc'ta,* (F.) *Cause continente* ou *prochaine,* may be the disease itself. Superabundance of blood, e. g., is the proximate cause of plethora.

CAUSES, Remote, C. predisponent.

CAUSES, SPECIF'IC, *Essen'tial causes,* &c., (F.) *Causes spécifiques, C. essentielles, C. déterminantes;* those which always produce a determinate disease; special contagion, for example.

CAUSIS, Burn, Ebullition, Fermentation, Incendium, Ustion.

CAUSOMA, Inflammation.

CAUS'TIC, *Caus'ticus, Cauteret'icus, Diæret'icus, Ero'dens, Adu'rens, Urens, Pyrot'icus,* from καιω, 'I burn.' (F.) *Caustique.* Bodies, which have the property of causticity; and which consequently, burn or disorganize animal substances. The word is also used substantively. The most active are called *Escharot'ics.* Caustics are also termed 'corrosives.'

CAUSTIC BEARER, *Porte-pierre.*

CAUSTICA ADUSTIO, Cauterization.

CAUSTIC''ITY, *Caustic''itas,* from καυστικος, 'that which burns,' (καιω, 'I burn.) The impression which caustic bodies make on the organ of taste; or, more commonly, the property which distinguishes those bodies.

CAUSTICOPHORUM, *Porte-pierre.*

CAUSTICUM ÆTHIOP'ICUM, *Unguen'tum Melan'icum caus'ticum.* A sort of paste, made by rubbing powdered *saffron* with concentrated *sulphuric acid,* recommended by Velpeau as a caustic in cases of gangrenous and carcinomatous ulcers. The acid is the caustic: the saffron, the constituent merely.

CAUSTICUM ALKALINUM, Potassa fusa—c. Americanum, Veratrum sabadilla—c. Antimoniale, Antimonium muriatum.

CAUSTICUM COMMU'NE, *Poten'tial Cautery, Common Caustic, Caute'rium potentia'lè, Lapis sep'ticus, Caus'ticum commu'nè mit'ius.* This consists of *quicklime* and *black soap,* of each equal parts.

CAUSTICUM COMMUNE, Potassa fusa—c. Commune acerrimum, Potassa fusa—c. Commune fortius, Potassa cum calce—c. Lunare, Argenti nitras —c. Potentiale, Potassa fusa—c. Salinum, Potassa fusa—c. Viennense fusum Filhos, see Powder, Vienna.

CAUSTIQUE, Caustic.
CAUSTIQUE FILHOS, see Powder, Vienna.
CAUSTIQUE DE VIENNE, Powder, Vienna.

CAUSUS, from καιω, 'I burn.' A highly ardent fever; *Deu'rens.* Pinel regards it as a complication of bilious and inflammatory fever; Broussais, as an intense gastritis, accompanied with bilious symptoms. See Synocha.

CAUSUS, ENDEMIAL, OF THE WEST INDIES, Fever, Yellow — c. Tropicus endemicus, Fever, Yellow.

CAUTER, Cauterium.

CAUTÈRE, Cauterium, Fonticulus — *c. Inhérent*, Inherent cautery.

CAUTERETICUS, Caustic.

CAUTERETS, MINERAL WATERS OF. Cauterets is a *bourg* seven leagues from Baréges *(Hautes-Pyrénées,)* France. The waters are hydrosulphurous and thermal—temperature 123° F. They are used in the same cases as the Baréges water.

CAUTERIASMUS, Cauterization.

CAUTE'RIUM, *Cauterium actua'lĕ, Cauter, Cau'tery, Inusto'rium, Rupto'rium, Ignis actua'lis,* from καιω, 'I burn.' (F.) *Cautère, Feu actuel.* A substance, used for 'firing,' burning or disorganizing the parts to which it is applied. Cauteries were divided by the ancients into *actual* and *potential.* The word is now restricted to the red-hot iron; or to positive burning. It was, formerly, much used for preventing hemorrhage from divided arteries; and also with the same views as a blister. The term *Poten'tial Cautery, Caute'rium potentia'lĕ, Ignis potentia'lis,* (F.) *Feu potentiel,* was generally applied to the *causticum commune,* but it is now used synonymously with caustic in general. *Cautère* also means an issue.

CAUTERIUM ACTUALE, Cauterium.

CAUTERIZA'TION, *Cauterisa'tio, Cauterias'mus, Exus'tio, Inus'tio, Caus'tica Adus'tio.* Firing. The effect of a cautery. The French, amongst whom cauterization is much used, distinguished five kinds: 1. *Cautérisation Inhérente,* which consists in applying the actual cautery freely, and with a certain degree of force, so as to disorganize deeply. 2. *Cautérisation transcurrente,* which consists in passing the edge of the *Cautère cultellaire,* or the point of the *Cautère conique* lightly, so as not to disorganize deeply. 3. *Cautérisation par pointes,* which consists in applying on the skin, here and there, the hot point of the conical cautery, with sufficient force to cauterize the whole thickness of the skin. 4. *Cautérisation lente,* slow cauterization, by means of the moxa. 5. *Cautérisation objective,* which consists in holding the cautery at some distance from the part to be acted upon by it.

CAU'TERIZE; *Caustico adurere;* (F.) *Cautériser.* To apply the cautery. To burn with a cautery.

CAUTERY, Cauterium — c. Potential, Causticum commune.

CAVA, Vulva.

CAVA VENA, *Vena hepati'tes.* The hollow or deep-seated vein. (F.) *Veine cave.* A name given to the two great veins of the body, which meet at the right auricle of the heart. The *vena cava supe'rior, thorac"ica* vel *descen'dens,* is formed by the union of the subclavians; and receives successively, before its termination at the upper part of the right auricle, the *inferior thyroid, right internal mammary, superior diaphragmatic, azygos,* &c. The *vena cava infe'rior, abdomina'lis* vel *ascen'dens,* arises from the union of the two *primary iliacs,* opposite the fourth or fifth lumbar vertebra, receives the *middle sacral, lumbar, right spermatic, hepatic,* and *inferior diaphragmatics,* and opens at the posterior and inferior part of the right auricle.

CAVATIO, Cavity.

CAVEA, Cavity—c. Narium, Nares.

CAVER'NA, *Antrum.* 'A cavern.' This term has been used for the female organs of generation. See Cavity, and Vulva.

CAVERNA NARIUM, Nares.

CAVERNÆ DENTIUM, Alveoli dentium—c. Frontis, Frontal Sinuses.

CAVERNEUX, Cavernous.

CAV'ERNOUS, *Caverno'sus,* (F.) *Caverneux.* Filled with small cavities or caverns,—as a sponge.

CAVERNOUS BODIES, *Cor'pora Caverno'sa* of the penis, *Cor'pora nervo'sa, C. Ner'veo-spongio'sa Penis,* (F.) *Corps Caverneux.* The corpus cavernosum is a kind of cylindrical sac, composed of cells; separated, through its whole extent, by a vertical, incomplete septum, *Septum pectinifor'mĕ,* and forming nearly two-thirds of the penis. The *corpus cavernosum,* on each side, arises from the ascending portion of the ischium, and terminates obtusely behind the glans. The arteries of the corpora cavernosa come from the internal pudic. See Helicine Arteries. Nerves are found on the surface of the outer membrane, but they do not appear to penetrate the substance, and the smooth muscular fibre has been traced into the fibrous parietes of the cells, as in the case of all erectile tissues.

J. Müller's researches have led him to infer, that both in man and the horse, the nerves of the corpora cavernosa are made up of branches proceeding from the organic as well as the animal system, whilst the nerves of animal life alone provide the nerves of sensation of the penis.

CAVERNOUS BODIES, *Corpora Cavernosa of the Clit'oris,* are two hollow crura, forming the clitoris.

CAVERNOUS BODY OF THE VAGI'NA, *Corpus Caverno'sum Vagi'næ, Plexus retiform'is,* is a substance composed of blood-vessels and cells, similar to those of the penis and clitoris, which covers the outer extremity of the vagina, on each side. It serves to contract the entrance to the vagina during coition.

CAVERNOUS GANGLION, see Carotid or Carotic Nerve.

CAVERNOUS RESPIRA'TION, (F.) When a cavity exists in the lungs, and one or more ramifications of the bronchia terminate in it, a loud tubal noise is emitted, provided the cavity be not filled with fluid, which is called *cavernous respiration.* In this condition, the cough is *cavernous* likewise, (F.) *Toux Caverneuse.* When the capacity of the cavern is very great, the sound of the respiration is like that produced by blowing into a decanter, with the mouth at a little distance from the neck. This kind of cavernous respiration has been called *amphoric,* from *amphora,* 'a flask;' (F.) *Respiration amphorique, Souffle amphorique, S. métallique.*

The *Veiled Puff,* (F.) *Souffle voilé,* is a modification of the cavernous respiration, in which, according to Laënnec, "a sort of movable veil interposed between the excavation and the ear" seems to be agitated to and fro. It is a sign which is not attended to.

CAVERNOUS SINUS, *Sinus Caverno'sus, Sinus polymor'phus* seu *Receptac'ulum, S. sphenoidalis, Receptac'ulum sellæ equi'næ lat'eribus appos'itum,* (F.) *Sinus caverneux.* The *Cav'ernous Si'nuses* are venous cavities of the dura mater, filled with a multitude of reddish, soft filaments, intersecting each other; and, as it were, reticulated. They commence behind the inner part of the sphenoid fissure, pass backwards on the sides of the fossa pituitaria, and terminate by opening into a cavity, common to the superior and inferior petrosal sinuses. They receive some meningeal veins, the ophthalmic veins, &c. The anterior extremity of each cavernous sinus has been named the *ophthal'mic sinus.*

CAVERNOUS TEXTURE or TISSUE, (F.) *Tissu caverneux.* The spongy substance which forms the greater part of the penis and clitoris. It seems to consist of a very complicated lace-work of arteries and veins; and, probably, of nervous filaments, with small fibrous plates, which form by their decussation numerous cells communicating with each other. This spongy texture produces erection, by dilating and swelling on the influx of blood; and probably, also, by virtue of some property inherent in it.

CAVIALE, Caviare.

CAVIARE', *Caviar, Caviale, Kaviac.* A culinary preparation, much used by certain people, and made on the shores of the Black and Caspian Seas, from the roe of the sturgeon, mixed with salt and other condiments.

CAVIC'ULA, *Cavil'la,* from *cavus,* 'hollow.' The ankle or space between the malleoli. Some have given this name to the os cuneiforme. See Astragalus.

CAVICULÆ PEDIS NODUS, Tarsus.

CAVILLA, Astragalus, Cavicula.

CAVITAS ANTROSA AURIS, Tympanum—c. Buccinata, Cochlea—c. Cochleata, Cochlea.

CAVITAS DIGITATA VENTRICULI LATERALIS, Cornu posterius ventriculi lateralis.

CAV'ITAS ELLIP'TICA, *Ampul'la, Sinus ampulla'ceus.* A dilatation at one end of the semicircular canals of the ear.

CAVITAS HUMERI GLENOIDES, see Glenoid—c. Narium, Nares—c. Oculi, Orbit—c. Oris, Mouth—c. Pulpæ, see Tooth.

CAVITATES CEREBRI, Ventricles of the brain—c. Duræ matris, Sinuses of the dura mater—c. Innominatæ, Auricles of the heart—c. Interscapulares, see Interscapularis.

CAVITÉ, Cavity—*c. Dentaire,* Dental cavity—*c. des Épiploons,* see Peritonæum—*c. du Tympan,* Tympanum.

CAV'ITY, *Cav'itas, Cavum, Cœ'lotes, Cœlon, Ca'vea, Caver'na, Cava'tio,* (F.) *Cavité.* Every thing hollow, as the cranium, mouth, nasal fossæ, &c.

CAVITIES, SPLANCHNIC, (F.) *Cavités splanchniques,* are those which contain the viscera. They are three in number;—the cranium, chest, and abdomen. The cavities of bones, connected with joints or otherwise, are described under their particular denominations.

CAVUM, Cavity—c. Abdominis, see Abdomen.

CAVUM CRA'NII, *Venter Supre'mus.* The cavity formed by the proper bones of the cranium.

CAVUM DENTIS, see Tooth — c. Narium, Nares—c. Oris, Mouth—c. Tympani, Tympanum.

CAYAN, Phaseolus Creticus.

CAZABI, Jatropha manihot.

CEANOTHOS, Cirsium arvense.

CEANOTHUS AMERICANUS, Celastrus—c. Trinervis, Celastrus.

CEAR, Heart.

CEASMA, Fissure.

CEBI GALLI'NÆ. The liver of the fowl, bruised.—Castelli.

CEBIP'ARA. A large Brazilian tree, whose bitter and astringent bark is used in making antirheumatic baths and fomentations

CECES, see Quercus alba.

CÉCITÉ, Cæcitas.

CEDAR, RED, Juniperus Virginiana.

CEDEIA, Embalming.

CEDMA, Aneurism, Varix.

CED'MATA, κεδματα. Rheumatic pains of the joints, especially of the hips, groin, or genital organs. A form of gout or rheumatism.

CEDRAT, Citrus medica.

CEDRELE'UM, from κεδρος, 'the cedar,' and ελαιον, 'oil.' The oil of cedar.—Pliny.

CE'DRIA, *Ce'drium, Ce'drinum, Cedri lach'ryma, Alkitran.* The oil or resin which flows from the cedar of Lebanon. It was supposed to possess great virtues. — Hippocrates, Foësius, Scribonius Largus, Dioscorides. It has been supposed to be the same as the pyroligneous acid. See Pinus Sylvestris.

CE'DRINUM VINUM, *Cedar Wine.* A wine prepared by steeping half a pound of bruised cedar berries in six French pints of sweet wine. It is diuretic and subastringent.

CEDRI'TES, from κεδρος, 'the cedar.' A wine prepared from the resin of cedar and sweet wine. It was formerly employed as a vermifuge, &c.

CEDRIUM, Cedria.

CEDROMELA, see Citrus medica.

CEDRON, see Simaba cedron.

CEDRONELLA, Melissa—c. Triphylla, Dracocephalum canariense.

CEDROS, Juniperus lycia.

CEDROSTIS, Bryonia alba.

CEDRUS BACCIFERA, Juniperus sabina—c. Mahogani, Sweetenia mahogani.

CEINTURE, Cingulum, Herpes zoster.

CEINTURE BLANCHE DE LA CHOROÏDE, Ciliary ligament.

CEINTURE DARTREUSE, Herpes zoster—*c. de Hildane,* Cingulum Hildani—*c. de Vif Argent,* Cingulum mercuriale.

CELANDINE, Impatiens—c. Common, Chelidonium majus—c. Lesser, Ranunculus ficaria—c. Poppy, Stylophorum diphyllum.

CELAS'TRUS, *Celas'tus, Ceano'thus America'nus* seu *triner'vis, New Jersey Tea, Red Root.* Used by the American Indians, in the same manner as lobelia, for the cure of syphilis. It is slightly bitter and somewhat astringent. A strong infusion of the dried leaves and seeds has been recommended in aphthæ, and as a gargle in scarlatina.

CELASTRUS SCANDENS, *Climbing Stafftree.* A climbing American shrub, the bark of which is said to possess emetic, diaphoretic, and narcotic properties.

CELATION, (F.) *Concealment,* from *celare,* 'to conceal.' A word used by French medicolegal writers for cases where there has been concealment of pregnancy or delivery.

CELE, κηλη, 'a tumour, protrusion, or rupture;' a very common suffix, as in hydrocele, bubonocele, &c. See Hernia.

CEL'ERY, (F.) *Céleri.* The English name for a variety of *Apium graveolens.*

CELERY, WILD, Bubon galbanum.

CELETA, see Hernial.

CELIA, Cerevisia.

CÉLIAQUE, Cœliac.

CELIS, κηλις, 'a spot, a stain.' A *macula,* or spot on the skin.

CELL, *Cella.* A small cavity. The same signification as cellule. Also, a vesicle composed of a membranous *cell-wall,* with, usually, liquid contents. The whole organized body may be regarded as a congeries of cells having different endowments, each set being concerned in special acts, connected with absorption, nutrition, and secretion, wherever an action of selection or elaboration has to be effected. These cells are generally termed *primary, elementary,* or *primordial.* When they give rise to other cells, they are, at times, termed *parent* or *mother cells;* the resulting cells being termed *daughter cells.*

CELL, APOPLECTIC, see Apoplectic cell — c. Bronchic, Cellule, bronchic — c. Calcigerous, see Tooth — c. Daughter, see Cell — c. Elementary, see Cell.

CELL, EPIDER'MIC or EPITHE'LIAL. The cells or corpuscles that cover the free membranous surfaces of the body, and which form the epidermis and epithelium, are termed '*epidermic* or *epithelial cells.*' They are developed from germs furnished by the subjacent membrane.

CELL, EPITHELIAL, Cell, epidermic — c. Fat, see Fatty vesicles — c. Germ, Cytoblast — c. Germinal, see Cytoblast — c. Nucleated, see Cytoblast.

CELL LIFE. The life which is possessed by the separate cells that form the tissues, and by which the nutrition of the tissues is presumed to be effected.

CELL, MOTHER, see Cell — c. Parent, see Cell.

CELL, PIGMENT. Pigment cells are mingled with the epidermic cells, and are most manifest in the coloured races. They are best seen on the inner surface of the choroid of the eye, where they form the *pigmentum nigrum*.

CELL, PRIMARY, see Cell — c. Primordial, see Cell.

CELL WALL, see Cell.

CELLA TURCICA, Sella Turcica.

CELLULA, Cellule.

CELLULÆ, see Colon — c. Medullares, see Medullary membrane — c. Pulmonales, Cellules bronchic, see Pulmo — c. Bronchicæ, see Cellule.

CEL'LULAR, *Cellula'ris, Cellulo'sus*, (F.) *Cellulaire*. Composed of cells or cellules, from *cella* or *cellula*, 'a cell.'

CEL'LULAR MEM'BRANE, *Membra'na cellulo'sa, M. Cellula'ris, — M. adipo'sa, M. pinguedino'sa*, of some, *Pannic'ulus adipo'sus*, — Membrane formed of cellular tissue, (F.) *Membrane cellulaire*. Generally used for the tissue itself.

CEL'LULAR SYSTEM. The whole of the cellular tissue of the human body.

CELLULAR TISSUE, *Tela cellula'ris, T. cellulo'sa, T. Hippoc'ratis cribro'sa, Ethmyphē, reticula'ted, filamentous, laminated, crib'riform, porous, are'olar*, and *mucous Tissue, Retic'ular* or *cellular substance, Contex'tus cellulo'sus*, (F.) *Tissu cellulaire, réticulé, lamineux, cribleux, poreux, aréolaire, muqueux*, &c., is the most common of all the organic tissues. It contains irregular *areolæ* between the fibres, as well as serum, fat, and the adipous tissue. Of the fibres, some are of the *yellow* elastic kind; but the greater part are of the *white* fibrous tissue, and they frequently present the form of broad flat bands, in which no distinct fibrous arrangement is perceptible. See Fibrous.

The cellular tissue or texture unites every part of the body, determines its shape, and by its elasticity and contractility, and by the fluid which it contains in its cells, facilitates the motion of parts on each other.

Cellular tissue has been divided by anatomists into the external, general or common cellular tissue — *textus cellula'ris interme'dius* seu *laxus*, which does not penetrate the organs, — the cellular texture which forms the envelopes of organs —*textus cellula'ris strictus*, and that which penetrates into the organs, accompanying and enveloping all their parts, — the *textus cellula'ris stipa'tus*, constituting the basis of all the organs. It has likewise been termed *Textus organ'icus* seu *parenchyma'lis*.

CELLULAR TISSUE OF BONES, see Cancelli.

CEL'LULE, *Cel'lula*, diminutive of *cella*, 'a cavity.' A small cavity. (F.) *Cellule*. Cellules are the small cavities between the laminæ of the cellular tissue, corpora cavernosa, &c.

CELLULES or CELLS, BRONCHIC, *Cel'lulæ Bron'chicæ* seu *Pulmona'les, Pori pulmo'num, Vesic'ulæ pulmonales*. The air-cells of the lungs. See Pulmo.

CELLULES BRONCHIQUES, Bronchial cells.

CELLULITIS VENENATA, see Wound.

CEL'LULOSE, same etymon as *Cellules*. The substance which is left after the action upon any kind of vegetable tissue of such solvents as are fitted to dissolve out the matter deposited in its cavities and interstices. It has been affirmed, that the tunicated or ascidian mollusca have, in their integuments, a considerable quantity of it.

CELLULOSUS, Cellular.

CELOLOG"IA, from κηλη, 'rupture,' and λογος, 'a discourse.' The doctrine of hernia. A treatise on hernia.

CELOSO'MUS, from κηλη, 'a rupture,' and σωμα, 'body.' A monster in which the trunk is malformed, and eventration or displacement of the viscera exists.

CELOTES, see Hernial.

CELOTOM'IA, *Kelotom'ia, Celot'omy*, from κηλη, 'a rupture,' and τεμνειν, 'to cut.' An operation, formerly employed for the radical cure of inguinal hernia; which consisted, principally, in passing a ligature round the hernial sac and spermatic vessels. It necessarily occasioned atrophy and loss of the testicle; and did not secure the patient against the return of the disease. The intestines were, of course, not included in the ligature. Also, the operation for hernia in general. — *Herniot'omy*.

CELOT'OMUS, same etymon. *Herniot'omus*. A knife used in the operation for hernia. Adjectively, it means relating to celotomy, like *Celotom'icus*.

CELSA. A term, used by Paracelsus for a cutaneous disease, dependent, according to him, on a false or heterogeneous spirit or vapour, concealed under the integuments, and endeavouring to escape. Perhaps the disease was *Urticaria*.

CELSUS, METHOD OF, see Lithotomy.

CELTIS OCCIDENTA'LIS, *Sugarberry, Hackberry*. Order, Ulmaceæ: indigenous, flowering in May. The bark is said to be anodyne and cooling; the berries are sweet and astringent. It has been used in dysentery.

CEMBRO NUTS, see Pinus cembra.

CEMENT. A glutinous substance introduced into a carious tooth to prevent the access of air or other extraneous matters. The following is an example: (℞. *Sandarac*. ʒij; *Mastich*. ʒi; *Succin*. gr. x. *Æther*. ʒj; Dissolve with the aid of heat.) *Ostermaier's Cement for the teeth* is prepared of finely powdered *caustic lime*, thirteen parts; anhydrous *phosphoric acid*, twelve parts. When introduced into a carious tooth, it becomes solid in about two minutes.

CEMENTERIUM, Crucible.

CEMENTUM, see Tooth.

CENANGIA, Ceneangia.

CENCHRON, Panicum miliaceum.

CENDRÉ, Cineritious.

CENDRE DU LEVANT, Soda.

CENDRES GRAVÉLÉES, see Potash — *e. de Sarment*, see Potash.

CENEANGI'A, *Cenangi'a*, from κενος, 'empty,' and αγγειον, 'a vessel.' Inanition. Empty state of vessels. — Galen.

CENEMBATE'SIS, from κενος, 'empty,' and εμβαινω, 'I enter.' Paracentesis. Also, the act of probing a wound or cavity; *Melo'sis*.

CENEONES, Flanks.

CENIGDAM, Ceniplam.

CENIGOTAM, Ceniplam.

CENIPLAM, *Cenigdam, Cenigotam, Cenipa-*

tam. The name of an instrument anciently used for opening the head in epilepsy.—*Paracelsus.*

CENIPOTAM, Ceniplam.

CENO′SIS, from κενος, 'empty.' *Ine′sis, Inethmos.* Evacuation. It is sometimes employed synonymously with inanition, and opposed to repletion,—*Exinanit′′io.*

CENOT′ICA, from κενωσις, 'evacuation.' Diseases affecting the fluids. Morbid discharges or excess, deficiency or irregularity of such as are natural. The first order, class *Genetica,* of Good; also, Drastics.

CENTAU′REA BEHEN, *Serrat′ula behen, Behen abiad, Behen album, Been,* White Behen. *Ord.* Gentianeæ. Astringent.

CENTAU′REA BENEDIC′TA, *Car′duus benedic′tus, Cnicus sylves′tris, Cnicus benedic′tus, Cardiobot′anum, Blessed* or *Holy Thistle,* (F.) *Chardon bénit. Fam.* Cynarocephaleæ. *Sex. Syst.* Syngenesia Polygamia frustranea. A strong decoction of the herb is emetic:—a strong infusion, diaphoretic (?); a light infusion, tonic and stomachic. Dose, gr. xv to ʒj of the powder.

CENTAU′REA CALCITRA′PA, *Calcitra′pa, Calcatrep′pola, Car′duus solstitia′lis, Carduus stella′tus, Ja′cea ramosis′sima, Cacotrib′ulus, Calcitrap′pa stella′ta* seu *hippophæstum, Stella′ta rupi′na, Centau′rea stella′ta, Common Star-Thistle, Star-Knapweed,* (F.) *Centaurée étoilée, Chardon etoilé, Chaussetrappe, Pignerole.* It is possessed of tonic properties, and has been given in intermittents, dyspepsia, &c. It is not much used.

CENTAU′REA CENTAU′RIUM, *Rhapon′ticum vulga′ré, Centaurium magnum, Centaurium majus, Greater Cen′taury, Centaurium officina′lě,* (F.) *Centaurée grande.* It is a bitter; and was formerly used as a tonic, especially the root.

CENTAU′REA CY′ANUS, *Cy′anus, Blue bottle, Corn-flower,* (F.) *Blavelle, Blavéole, Blavérolle.* The flowers were once much used as a cordial, tonic, &c. They are now forgotten.

CENTAUREA STELLATA, Centaurea calcitrapa.

CENTAURÉE ÉTOILÉE, Centaurea calcitrapa—*c. Grande,* Centaurea centaurium—*c. Petite,* Chironia centaurium.

CENTAUREUM, Chironia centaurium.

CENTAURIS, Chironia centaurium.

CENTAURIUM MAGNUM, Centaurea centaurium—*c.* Minus vulgare, Chironia centaurium —*c.* Officinale, Centaurea centaurium—*c.* Parvum, Chironia centaurium.

CENTAURY, AMERICAN, Chironia angularis—*c.* Greater, Centaurea centaurium—*c.* Lesser, Chironia centaurium.

CENTESIS, Paracentesis, Puncture.

CENTIGRAMME, (F.) from *centum,* 'a hundred,' and γραμμα, 'gramme,' *Centigram′ma.* The hundredth part of a gramme. A centigramme is equal to about the fifth part of a French grain, gr. .1543, Troy.

CENTILITRE, Centili′tra, from *centum,* 'a hundred,' and λιτρα, 'litre.' An ancient Greek measure for liquids:—the hundredth part of a litre—equal to nearly 2.7053 fluidrachms.

CENTIMÈTRE, Centim′eter; the hundredth part of a metre—equal to about four lines. .3937 English inch.

CENTIMORBIA, Lysimachia nummularia.

CENTINERVIA, Plantago.

CENTINODE, Polygonum aviculare.

CENTINODIA, Polygonum aviculare.

CENTO VIRGINALIS, Hymen.

CENTRAD, see Central aspect.

CENTRADIAPH′ANES, *Catarac′ta centra′lis,* from κεντρον, 'centre,' *a,* privative, and διαφανης, 'transparent.' Cataract owing to obscurity of the central portion of the crystalline.

CENTRAL, *Centra′lis,* from *centrum,* 'the centre.' Relating or appertaining to the centre.

CENTRAL AR′TERY OF THE RET′INA, *Arte′ria Centra′lis Ret′inæ, Central Artery of Zinn.* This artery is given off from the arteria ophthalmica, and penetrates the optic nerve a little behind the ball of the eye; running in the axis of the nerve, and spreading out into many small branches upon the inside of the retina. When the nerve is cut across near the eye, the orifice of the divided artery is observable. This was formerly called *Porus Op′ticus.*

CENTRAL ASPECT. An aspect towards the centre of an organ.—Barclay. Centrad is used by the same writer adverbially, to signify 'towards the central aspect.'

CENTRE OF ACTION. The viscus in which the whole or a great part of any function is executed, and to which several other organs contribute. Thus, the vital activity seems to be wholly centred in the stomach, during chymification; in the duodenum, during chylification. In like manner, the uterus becomes a centre of action during gestation.

CENTRE, EPIGAS′TRIC. The ganglions and nervous plexuses, formed by the great sympathetic and pneumogastric nerves, in the epigastrium, around the cœliac artery; where the impressions received from various parts of the body seem to be centred.

CENTRE OF FLUX′ION. The part towards which fluids are particularly attracted. An irritated organ is said to be a centre of fluxion.

CENTRES, NERVOUS, (F.) *Centres nerveux.* The organs, whence the nerves originate; as the brain and spinal marrow.

CENTRE, OPTIC, see Optic centre.

CENTRE, OVAL, *Centrum Ova′lě, C. O. Vieussé′nii, Tegumen′tum ventriculo′rum cer′ebri.* When the two hemispheres of the brain are sliced away, till on a level with the corpus callosum, the medullary part in each is of an oval shape: hence called *centrum ovalě minus,* (F.) *centre medullaire hémiphéral.* The two centres of the opposite sides, together with the corpus callosum, form the *centrum ovalě of Vieus′sens.* Vieussens supposed all the medullary fibres to issue from that point, and that it was the *great dispensatory of the animal spirits.*

CENTRE, PHRENIC, *Ten′dinous Centre of the Di′aphragm, Centrum Phren′icum, C. Ner′veum* or *C. Tendino′sum* seu *tendin′eum,* (F.) *Centre phrénique* ou *C. tendineux du Diaphragme.* The central aponeurosis or *cordiform tendon* of the diaphragm.

CENTRE OF SYMPATHET′IC IRRADIA′TIONS, (F.) *Centre d'irradiations sympathiques.* Any organ which excites, sympathetically, the action of other organs, more or less distant from it; and with which it seems to have no immediate communication.—Marjolin.

CENTRE, TENDINOUS, OF THE DIAPHRAGM, Centre, phrenic.

CENTROMYRINE, Ruscus.

CENTRUM, see Vertebræ—*c.* Commune, Solar plexus—*c.* Nerveum, Centre, phrenic—*c.* Opticum, Optic centre—*c.* Ovale, Centre, oval—*c.* Ovale minus, see Centre, oval—*c.* Ovale of Vieussens, Centre, oval—*c.* Semicirculare geminum, Tænia semicircularis—*c.* Tendinosum, Centre, phrenic.

CENTRUM VITA′LE, *Nodus* seu *Fons vita′lis,* (F.) *Nœud vital.* A term applied, at times, to the medulla oblongata: at others, to the medulla oblongata, and the medulla spinalis as far as the second cervical nerve of the spinal marrow, in any part of which a wound would seem to be instantly fatal. It is the nervous centre of respiration and deglutition.

CENTRY, Chironia angularis.

CENTUM CAPITA, Eryngium campestre.

CENTUMNODIA, Polygonum aviculare.

CEPA ASCALONICA, Bulbus esculentus, Echalotte — c. Victorialis, Allium victoriale — c. Vulgaris, Allium cepa.

CEPÆA, Veronica beccabunga.

CEPHAËLIS IPECACUANHA, Ipecacuanha.

CEPHALÆ'A, *Headach*, (F.) *Céphalée*, from κεφαλη, 'head.' Some use the term synonymously with cephalalgia; others, for a periodical headach; others, again, for a more violent headach than cephalalgia implies; and others for a chronic headach. The last was its ancient signification.

Cephalæ'a spasmod'ica, Cephalal'gia spasmod'ica, C. Nauseo'sa, Sick-headach, is characterized by partial, spasmodic pain; often shifting from one part of the head to another: chiefly commencing in the morning, with sickness and faintness. It is extremely apt to recur, notwithstanding every care.

CEPHALÆA ARTHRITICA, Cephalagra — c. Hemicrania, Hemicrania — c. Nauseosa, C. Spasmodica — c. Pulsatilis, Crotaphe.

CEPHALÆMATO'MA, from κεφαλη, 'head,' and 'αιμα, 'blood;' *Cephalæmato'ma neonato'rum, Ecchymo'ma cap'itis, E. capitis recens nato'rum, Thrombus neonato'rum, Absces'sus cap'itis sanguin'eus neonatorum, Tumor cap'itis sanguin'eus neonato'rum, Cephalophy'ma, Craniohæmaton'cus*. A sanguineous tumour, sometimes developed between the pericranium and the bones of the head of new-born children. Similar tumours are met with occasionally above other bones, and at all periods of existence.

CEPHALÆMATOMA NEONATORUM, Cephalæmatoma.

CEPHALÆ'MIA, *Hyperæ'mia cer'ebri, H. Cap'itis, Encephaloæ'mia*, (F.) *Hyperémie ou Congestion du cerveau, Encéphalohémie, H. cérébrale, Congestion cérébrale*. Accumulation of blood in the vessels of the brain.

CEPHALAGO'GUS, *Cephaloduc'tor, Capitiduc'tor*, from κεφαλη, 'head,' and αγωγος, 'a leader, a driver.' An instrument used for drawing down the fœtal head.

CEPH'ALAGRA, from κεφαλη, 'the head,' and αγρα, 'seizure.' *Cephalæ'a arthrit'ica, Meningi'tis arthrit'ica*. Gout in the head.

CEPHALAGRA'PHIA, from κεφαλη, 'the head,' and γραφη, 'a description.' An anatomical description of the head.

CEPHALAL'GIA, *Cephalopo'nia, Cephalodyn'ia, Encephalodyn'ia, Homonopa'gia*, from κεφαλη, 'the head,' and αλγος, 'pain;' *Encephalal'gia, Dolor Cap'itis, D. cephal'icus, Soda, Pain in the head; Headach*, (F.) *Ce'phalalgie, Mal à tête*. Every kind of headach, whether symptomatic or idiopathic, is a cephalalgia. It is ordinarily symptomatic, and has to be treated accordingly.

CEPHALALGIA CONTAGIOSA, Influenza — c. Inflammatoria, Phrenitis.

CEPHALALGIA PERIOD'ICA, *Febris intermit'tens cephal'ica larva'ta, Intermittent headach*. Headach which returns periodically; properly, perhaps, a form of neuralgia.

CEPHALALGIA PULSATILIS, Crotaphe — c. Spasmodica, see Cephalæa.

CEPHALALOG"IA, from κεφαλη, 'the head,' and λογος, 'a discourse.' An anatomical dissertation on the head.

CÉPHALANTHE D'AMÉRIQUE, Cephalanthus occidentalis.

CEPHALAN'THUS OCCIDENTA'LIS, *Buttonwood shrub, Buttonbush, White Ball, Little Snowball, Swampwood, Pond Dogwood, Globeflower*, (F.) *Céphalanthe d'Amérique, Bois de Marais*. An ornamental shrub, *Nat. Ord.* Rubiaceæ; *Sex. Syst.* Tetrandria Monogynia, which grows all over the United States, near streams and ponds, and flowers in July and August. The bark of the root has been used as an antiperiodic tonic.

CEPHALARTICA, Cephalic remedies.

CEPHALATOM'IA, *Cephalotom'ia*, from κεφαλη, 'the head,' and τεμνειν, 'to cut.' Anatomy, or dissection, or opening of the head.

CEPHALE, Head.

CEPHALIC, *Cephal'icus, Capita'lis*, from κεφαλη, 'the head.' (F.) *Céphalique*. Relating to the head.

CEPHAL'IC REM'EDIES, *Cephal'ica vel Capita'lia remed'ia*, are remedies capable of relieving affections of the head, especially headach: — *Cephalar'tica*.

CEPHAL'IC VEIN, *Vena Cephal'ica, Vena Cap'itis*, (F.) *Veine céphalique, Veine radiale cutanée* of Chaussier. The great superficial vein at the outer part of the arm and fore-arm. It begins on the back of the hand, by a number of radicles, which unite into a single trunk, called the *Cephalic of the Thumb, Cephal'ica Pol'licis*, (F.) *Veine céphalique du pouce*. It ascends along the anterior and outer part of the fore-arm, where it forms the *superficial radial*. At the fold of the elbow it receives the *median cephalic*, ascends along the outer edge of the biceps, and opens into the axillary vein. The name *Cephalic* was given to it by the ancients, because they thought it had some connexion with the head, and that blood-letting ought to be performed on it, in head affections.

Chaussier calls the internal jugular, *Veine céphalique*, and the primary or common carotid, *Artère céphalique*.

CEPHALIDIUM, see Caput.

CEPHALI'NE. The base or root of the tongue. —Gorræus.

CEPHALIS, see Caput.

CEPHALITIS, Phrenitis.

CEPHALIUM, see Caput.

CEPHALODUCTOR, Cephalagogus.

CEPHALODYM'IA, *Encephalodym'ia;* from κεφαλη, 'head,' and δυω, 'I enter into.' A class of double monstrosities, in which the heads are united. It is divided into two genera, *Frontodym'ia* and *Bregmatodym'ia;* in the former the union being between the ossa frontis; in the latter between the bregmata. — Cruveilhier.

CEPHALODYNIA, Cephalalgia.

CEPHALŒDEMA, Hydrocephalus.

CEPHALOID, Encephaloid.

CEPHALOMA, Encephaloid.

CEPHALO-MENINGITIS, Meningo-cephalitis.

CEPHALOM'ETER, from κεφαλη, 'the head,' and μετρον, 'measure.' An instrument for measuring the different dimensions of the fœtal head, during the process of accouchement. A kind of forceps.

CEPHALON'OSUS, from κεφαλη, 'the head,' and νοσος, 'disease.' This term has been applied to the *Febris Hungar'ica*, in which the head was much affected. See Fever, Hungaric. Others have so called any cerebral disease or fever.

CEPHALOPAGES, Symphyocephalus.

CEPH'ALO-PHARYNGÆ'US, from κεφαλη, 'the head,' and φαρυγξ, 'the pharynx:' belonging to the head and pharynx. Winslow has given this name to the portion of the *constrictor pharyngis superior*, which is attached, above, to the inferior surface of the basilary process of the os occipitis. The *Ceph'alo-pharynge'al Aponeuro'-*

sis is a thin, fibrous membrane, which is attached to the basilary process, and gives insertion to the fibres of the *constrictor superior pharyngis*.

CEPHALOPHYMA, Cephalæmatoma.

CEPHALOPONIA, Cephalalgia.

CEPHALO-RACHIDIAN, Cephalo-spinal.

CEPHALOSOMATODYM'IA, *Encephalosomatodym'ia*; from κεφαλη, 'head,' σωμα, 'body,' and δυω, 'I enter into.' A double monstrosity, in which the union is between the heads and the trunks. Of this there are varieties:—for example, *Infra-maxillosternodym'ia*, where the union is with the inferior maxillary bones and sterna; and *Prosoposternodym'ia*, between the faces and sterna.—Cruveilhier.

CEPHALO-SPINAL, *Cephalo-spina'lis*, *Ceph'alo-rachid'ian*, *Cer'ebro-spinal*, *Cranio-spinal*. A hybrid term, from κεφαλη, 'head,' and *spina*, 'spine.' Belonging to the head and spine.

CEPH'ALO-SPINAL FLUID, *Cephalo-rachid'ian fluid*, *Cerebro-spinal fluid*, *Flu'idum cer'ebrospina'lê*, *Subarachnoidean fluid*, is an exhaled fluid, which is found beneath the arachnoid, wherever pia mater exists in connexion with the brain and spinal cord. It seems to have a protecting office, and to keep up a certain degree of pressure on the organ,—at least in the spinal canal.

CEPHALOTHORACOSTERU'MENUS, from κεφαλη, 'head,' θωραξ, 'the chest,' and στερειν, 'to rob.' A monster without head or chest.

CEPHALOTOMIA, Eccephalosis.

CÉPHALOTRIBE, (F.) An instrument invented by Baudelocque, the nephew, for crushing the head of the fœtus in utero; from κεφαλη, 'the head,' and τριβω, 'I bruise.' It consists of a strong forceps, the blades of which are solid: 16 lines broad, and 3 thick. The handles are perforated at their extremity to receive a screw with three threads, the direction of which is very oblique, so as to allow great rapidity of rotation, and the screw is moved by a winch 6 inches long, to increase the force of the pressure. The bones of the head are easily crushed by it.

CEPHALOTRIP'SY, *Cephalotrip'sis*; same etymon as *Cephalotribe*. The operation of crushing the head of the fœtus in utero.

CEPHALOTRYPESIS, Trepanning.

CEPHALOXIA, Torticollis.

CEPULLA, Allium cepa.

CER, Heart.

CERA FLAVA et CERA ALBA, *Ceros*, Yellow and White Wax, (F.) *Cire Jaune* et *Blanche*. An animal substance prepared by the bee, and by some plants, as the *Ceroxylon* and *Myri'ca cerif'era*. Its colour is yellow, and smell like that of honey, but both are lost by bleaching. It is demulcent and emollient; is sometimes given in the form of emulsion, in diarrhœa and dysentery, but is chiefly used in cerates and ointments.

CERÆ'Æ, from κερας, 'a horn,' κεραιαι. The Cornua of the uterus.—Rufus of Ephesus.

CERAMICÈ, *Cerami'tis*, from κεραμος, 'potter's earth.' A sort of earth used as a cataplasm in peripneumony.—Hippocrates.

CERAMIUM, Amphora — c. Helminthochortus, Corallina Corsicana.

CERAMNIUM, Amphora.

CERAMURIA, see Urine.

CERANTHEMUS, Propolis.

CERAS, κερας, 'genitive,' κερατος, 'horn,' *Cornu*; also, the Cornea. Hence, *Ceratectomia*, *Ceratocele*, &c.

CERASION, see Prunus cerasus.

CERAS'MA, from κεραννυμι, 'to mix:' something mixed. A mixture of hot and cold water. *Metaceras'ma*.—Gorræus.

CERASUM, see Prunus cerasus.

CERASUS ACIDA, Prunus cerasus — c. Avium, Prunus avinum, P. nigra—c. Dulcis, Prunus nigra—c. Hortensis, Prunus cerasus—c. Laurocerasus, Prunus laurocerasus—c. Padus, Prunus padus — c. Racemosus sylvestris, Prunus padus —c. Rubra, Prunus cerasus—c. Serotina, Prunus Virginiana — c. Virginiana, Prunus Virginiana — c. Vulgaris, Prunus cerasus.

CÉRAT BLANC ou *DE GALIEN*, Ceratum Galeni — *c. de Blanc de Baleine*, Ceratum cetacei — *c. de Goulard*, Ceratum plumbi — *c. pour les Lèvres*, Cerate for the lips — *c. de Plomb composé*, Ceratum plumbi compositum — *c. de Savon*, Ceratum Saponis—*c. de Suracétate de plomb*, Ceratum plumbi superacetatis.

CE'RATE, *Cera'tum*, from κηρας, Lat. *cera*, 'wax,' *Cerela'um*, *Cero'ma*, *Cero'nium*, *Cero'tum*, *Ceratomalag'ma*, (F.) *Cérat*. A composition of wax, oil, or lard, without other ingredients.

CERATE, *Simple Cerate*, *Cera'tum*, *Cera'tum simplex*. (F.) *Cérat Simple*. (*White wax*, ℥iv, *Lard*, ℥viij.) It is applied as an emollient to excoriations, &c.

CERATE, BELLEVILLE'S, see Unguentum Hydrargyri nitrico-oxydi.

CERATE OF CAL'AMINE, *Cera'tum Calami'næ*, *C. Calamin. præpar.*, *C. Carbona'tis zinci impu'ri*, *C. Zinci Carbona'tis*, *Cera'tum lap'idis Calamina'ris*, *Cera'tum epulot'icum*, Cerate of Carbonate of Zinc, Turner's Cerate, Healing Salve, (F.) *Cérat de Pierre Calaminaire*, *C. de Calamine*, *Calamin.*, *Ceræ flavæ*, ā ā ℥iij, *adipis*, ℔j. Melt the wax and lard together, and, on cooling, add the carbonate of zinc and stir till cool.—Ph. U. S.)

CERATE OF CANTHAR'IDES, *Cera'tum Canthar'idis*, *Blister Ointment*, *Ointment of Spanish Flies*, *Unguen'tum ad vesicato'ria*, *Unguen'tum Pul'veris Mel'oës vesicato'rii*, *Ung. epispas'ticum fortius*, *Cera'tum Lyttæ*, (F.) *Cérat de Cantharides*. (*Spermaceti cerate* ℥vj, *Cantharides in powder*, ℥j. The cerate being softened by heat, stir in the flies.) This cerate of the European Pharmacopœias is used to keep blisters, issues, &c., open. See Unguentum Lyttæ. For the Cerate of Spanish flies of the U. S. Pharmacopœia, see Emplastrum Lyttæ.

CERATE, GOULARD'S, Ceratum Plumbi compositum.

CERATE, KIRKLAND'S NEUTRAL. (*Diachyl.* ℥viij, *olive oil* ℥iv, *prepared chalk* ℥iv: when nearly cool, add *Acet. dest.* ℥iv, *plumb. superacet.* ℥iij.) A cooling emollient.

CERATE OR POMA'TUM FOR THE LIPS, *Cera'tum labia'lê rubrum*, *Pomma'tum ad labia demulcen'da*.—Ph. P. (F.) *Cérat ou Pommade pour les lèvres*, (*Wax* 9 *parts*; *oil* 16 *parts*; — *coloured with alkanet*.)

CERATE, LEAD, COMPOUND, Ceratum plumbi compositum.

CERATE, MARSHALL'S. (*Palm oil* ℥vi. *calomel* ℥j, *sugar of lead* ℥ss, *ointment of nitrate of mercury* ℥ij.)

CERATE, RESIN, COMPOUND, Ceratum Resinæ compositum — c. Savine, Ceratum sabinæ — c. Soap, Ceratum saponis— c. Spermaceti, Ceratum cetacei — c. of Superacetate or sugar of lead, Ceratum plumbi superacetatis — c. Turner's, Cerate of calamine — c. of Carbonate of zinc, Cerate of calamine.

CERATECTOM'IA, from κερας, 'the cornea,' and εκτομος, 'cut out.' An incision through the cornea. See Ceratotomia.

CERATIA, Ceratonium siliqua.

CERATI'ASIS, from κερας, 'horn.' A morbid condition characterized by corneous growths.

CERATION, Siliqua.

CERATI'TIS, *Kerati'tis*, from κερας, 'the cornea,' and *itis*, 'inflammation.' Inflammation of the cornea, *Cerati'tis, Ceratodei'tis, Ceratomeningi'tis, Cornei'tis, Inflamma'tio cor'neæ.*

CERATIUM, Ceratonium siliqua.

CER'ATO, in composition, in the names of muscles, is used for the cornua of the os hyoides; —as Cerato-glossus.

CERATOCE'LE, *Aquula, Uva'tio, Prominen'tia Cor'ncæ, Hernia Cor'neæ, Ceratodeoce'lē,* from κερας, 'horn,' and κηλη, 'tumour.' A protrusion of the transparent cornea, or rather of the membrane of the aqueous humour through an opening in the cornea.

CERATODEÏTIS, Ceratitis.

CERATODEOCELE, Ceratocele.

CERATODEONYXIS, Ceratonyxis.

CERATODES MEMBRANA, Cornea.

CERATOGLOS'SUS, *Keratoglos'sus,* from κερας, 'horn,' and γλωσσα, 'the tongue.' A muscle, extending from the great cornu of the os hyoides to the base of the tongue. It is a part of the hyoglossus.

CERATOIDES, Cornea.

CERATOLEUCOMA, Leucoma.

CERATO'MA, *Cerato'sis,* from κερας, 'horn.' A horny growth, or horny formation.

CERATO-MALAGMA, Cerate.

CERATO-MENINGITIS, Ceratitis.

CERATO-MENINX, Cornea.

CERATO'NIA SIL'IQUA. The *Carob Tree, Cera'tium, Cera'tia, Sil'iqua dulcis, Caro'ba Al-nabati, Sweetpod,* (F.) *Caroubier (Fruit, Ca-rouge.)* This—the fruit of the *Ceratonia siliqua*—is mucilaginous, and employed in decoction, where mucilages are indicated.

CERATONYX'IS, *Keratonyx'is, Ceratodeo-nyx'is,* from κερας, 'the cornea,' and νυσσω, 'I puncture.' An operation by which the crystalline is depressed by means of a needle introduced into the eye through the cornea. Some divide the crystalline into fragments with the needle, and leave them to the action of the absorbents. The operation is as old as the 17th century.

CER'ATO-PHARYNGE'US, *Ker'ato-Pharynge'us,* from κερας, 'horn,' and φαρυγξ, 'the pharynx.' The *great and small Cer'ato-pharynge'i* are small fleshy bundles, forming part of the *Hyopharyngeus* of Winslow.

CERATOPLAS'TICE, from κερας, 'the cornea,' and πλαστικος, 'forming, formative.' The operation for the formation of an artificial cornea. It has not been practised on man.

CERATORRHEX'IS, *Ruptu'ra cor'neæ,* from κερας, 'the cornea,' and ρηξις, 'rupture.' Rupture of the cornea.

CERATOSIS, Ceratoma.

CER'ATO-STAPHYLI'NUS, *Ker'ato-staphyli'nus,* from κερας, 'horn,' and σταφυλη, 'the uvula.' Some fleshy fibres of the *Thyro-Staphylinus* of Winslow.

CERATOTOM'IA, *Ceratectom'ia,* from κερας, 'cornea,' and τεμνειν, 'to cut.' *Section of the transparent cornea.* This incision is used in the operation for cataract, to give exit to pus effused in the eye, in case of hypopyon, &c.

CERATOT'OMUS, *Keratot'omus, Kerat'omus,* from κερας, 'cornea,' and τεμνειν, 'to cut.' A name given by Wenzel to his knife for dividing the transparent cornea, in the operation for cataract. Many modifications of the instrument have been made since Wenzel's time. See Knife, cataract.

CERATUM, Cerate—c. Album, Ceratum cetacei, Ceratum Galeni—c. de Althææ, Unguentum de Althææ—c. Calaminæ, Cerate of Calamine—c. Cantharidis, Cerate of Cantharides, Emplastrum Lyttæ—c. de Cerussā, Unguentum plumbi subcarbonatis.

CERA'TUM CETA'CEI, *Cera'tum spermaceti, Ce-ra'tum album, C. Ceti, Unguen'tum adipoce'ræ ceto'rum, Liniment'um album, Emplas'trum Sperm'-atis Ceti, Spermaceti Cerate,* (F.) *Cérat de blanc de baleine.* (*Spermaceti* ℨj, *white wax* ℨiij, *olive oil* f℥vi. Ph. U. S.) A good emollient to ulcers, &c.

CERATUM CETI, Ceratum cetacei — c. Cicutæ, Ceratum conii — c. Citrinum, Ceratum resinæ.

CERA'TUM CONI'I, *Cera'tum Cicu'tæ.* (*Ung. conii* ℔j, *cetacei* ℨij, *ceræ albæ* ℨiij.) A formula in Bartholomew's Hospital: occasionally applied to cancerous, scrofulous sores, &c.

CERATUM EPULOTICUM, Corate of calamine.

CERA'TUM GALE'NI, *Cera'tum album, C. refrig''-erans Gale'ni, Unguen'tum cera'tum, U. amygdali'num, U. simplex, Emplas'trum ad fontic'ulos, O'leo-cera'tum aquā subac'tum, Cold Cream,* (F.) *Cérat blanc ou de GALIEN.* (*White wax* 4 *parts; oil of sweet almonds* 16 *parts;* add, when melted, *water or rose-water* 12 *parts.* Ph. P.) A mild application to chaps, &c.

CERATUM LABIALE RUBRUM, Cerate for the lips — c. Lapidis calaminaris, Corate of calamine — c. Lithargyri acetati compositum, Ceratum plumbi compositum — c. Lyttæ, Cerate of cantharides—c. Mercuriale, Unguentum hydrargyri —c. Picatum, Pisselæum.

CERATUM PLUMBI COMPOS'ITUM, *Cera'tum Lithar'gyri Aceta'ti Compos'itum, Goulard's Ointment, Cera'tum subaceta'ti plumbi medica'tum, C. Plumbi Subaceta'tis* (Ph. U. S.), *Cera'tum Satur'ni, Compound Lead Cerate, Goulard's Cerate,* (F.) *Cérat de Goulard, C. de Plomb composé.* (*Liq. plumb. subacet.* ℨiiss; *ceræ flavæ,* ℨiv; *ol. oliv.* ℨix; *camphoræ,* ℨss. Ph. U. S.) Its virtues are the same as the next.

CERATUM PLUMBI SUPERACETA'TIS, *Unguen'tum Cerus'sæ Aceta'tæ, Cerate of Superacetate or Sugar of Lead, Cera'tum Plumbi Aceta'tis, Unguentum Acetatis Plumbi,* (F.) *Cérat de suracétate de Plomb.* (*Acetate of lead,* ℨij; *white wax,* ℨij; *olive oil,* ℔ss.) Cooling and astringent.

CERATUM REFRIGERANS GALENI, Ceratum Galeni.

CERATUM RESI'NÆ, *C. Resi'næ flavæ, C. cit'rinum, Unguen'tum basil'icon flavum, Ung. Resi'næ flavæ, Ung. Resino'sum, Resin Cerate or Ointment, Yellow Basil'icon, Basil'icon Ointment.* (*Resin. flav.* ℨv; *Ceræ flav.* ℨij; *Adipis,* ℨviij; Ph. U. S.) A stimulating application to old ulcers, &c. Digestive.

DR. SMELLOME'S *Ointment for the Eyes* consists of finely powdered *verdigris,* ℨss, rubbed with oil, and then mixed with an ounce of *ceratum resinæ.*

CERATUM RESI'NÆ COMPOS'ITUM, *Compound Resin Cerate,* (*Resin., Sevi, Ceræ flavæ,* āā ℔j; *Terebinth.* ℔ss; *Ol. Lini,* Oss. Melt together, strain through linen, and stir till cool. Ph. U. S.)

CERATUM SABI'NÆ, *Unguentum Sabinæ, Savine Cerate,* (F.) *Cérat de Sabine.* (*Savine,* in powder, ℨij; *Resin Cerate,* ℔j. Ph. U. S.) Irritative, 'drawing.' Used in the same cases as the cerate of cantharides.

CERATUM SAPO'NIS, *Soap Cerate,* (F.) *Cérat de Savon.* (*Liq. Plumb. subacetat.,* Oij; *Sapon.* ℨvj; *Ceræ albæ,* ℨx; *Ol. olivæ,* Oj. Boil the solution of subacetate of lead with the soap over a slow fire, to the consistence of honey, then transfer to a water-bath, and evaporate until all the moisture is dissipated; lastly, add the wax, previously melted with the oil, and mix.—Ph. U. S.) It is applied in cases of sprains or fractures.

CERATUM SATURNI, Ceratum Plumbi compositum—c. Simplex, Cerate simple—c. Spermaceti, Ceratum cetacei — c. Subacetati plumbi medicatum, Ceratum plumbi compositum—c. Tetrapharmacum, Pisselæum.

CERATUM ZINCI CARBONATIS, *Cerate of Carbonate of Zinc.* (*Zinci carbonat. præparat.* ℨij; *Ung. simpl.* ℨx. Ph. U. S.) Used in the same cases as the Ceratum Calaminæ.

CERAU'NION, from κεραυνος, 'thunder,' 'a thunderbolt.' *Lapis fulmin'eus.* A kind of stone, which was believed to be formed during thunder; and to be possessed of the power of inducing sleep, and numerous other prophylactic virtues. It was rubbed on the knee, breast, &c., in swellings of those parts.

CERBERUS TRICEPS, Pulvis cornachini.

CERCA'RIA. A genus of agastric, infusory animalcules, one of the most curious of which inhabits the tartar of the teeth. The spermatozoa are presumed by some to belong to this genus.

CERCHNASMUS, Cerchnus.

CERCHNOMA, Cerchnus.

CERCHNUS, *Cerchnas'mus, Cerchnum, Cerchno'ma,* from κεχρνω, 'I render hoarse.' A rough voice produced by hoarseness. See Rattle.

CER'CIS, κερκις. A sort of pestle for reducing substances to powder. Also, the radius or small bone of the arm. See Pilum, and Radius.

CERCLE, Circulus—*c. de la Choroïde,* Ciliary ligament—*c. Ciliare,* Ciliary ligament.

CERCO'SIS, from κερκος, 'a tail.' *Men'tula mulie'bris,* the *Clit'oris.* Some authors have employed the word synonymously with nymphomania and elongation of the clitoris; and with *Polypus Uteri,* the *Sarco'ma Cerco'sis* of Sauvages.

CERCOSIS CLITORIDIS, Clitorism — c. Externa, Clitorism.

CEREA, Cerumen.

CEREA'LIA, from CERES, 'goddess of corn.' (F.) *Céréales (Plantes.)* The cerealia are gramineous plants, the seed of which serve for the nourishment of man:—as wheat, barley, rye, &c. At times, the same term is applied to some of the leguminous plants.

CEREBARIA, Carebaria.

CEREBEL'LA URI'NA. Urine of a whitish appearance, of the colour of the brain or cerebellum, from which Paracelsus thought he could distinguish diseases of that organ.

CEREBELLI'TIS, badly formed from *cerebellum,* and *itis,* denoting inflammation. *Parencephali'tis, Inflamma'tio cerebel'li.* Inflammation of the cerebellum: a variety of phrenitis or encephalitis.

CEREBEL'LOUS, *Cerebello'sus,* from *cerebellum,* 'the little brain.' (F.) *Cérébelleux.* Chaussier has given this epithet to the vessels of the cerebellum. These are three in number; two of which are *inferior:* the larger, *inferior cerebelli,* which arises from the posterior cerebral or vertebral; and the smaller, whose existence is not constant, from the meso-cephalic or basilary: —the third, called *A. cérébelleuse supérieure (superior cerebelli,)* is also a branch of the basilary.

CEREBEL'LOUS AP'OPLEXY, *Apoplex'ia cerebello'sa:* apoplexy of the cerebellum.

CEREBEL'LUM, diminutive of *Cerebrum; C. parvum, Appen'dix ad cer'ebrum, Cer'ebrum poste'rius, Encra'nion, Encra'nis, Epencra'nis, Parencephʼalis, Parencephʼalus, Encephalʼium, Encephʼalis opisʼthius, Micrencephaʼlium, Micrencephʼalum, Little brain,* (F.) *Cervelet.* A portion of the medullary mass, contained in the cavity of the cranium. It fills the lower occipital fossæ below the tentorium, and embraces the tuber annulare and medulla. It is composed, like the brain, of vesicular and tubular substance, arranged in laminæ, as it were; so that, when a section is made of it, it has an arborescent appearance, called *Arbor vitæ.* The cerebellum is divided into two *lobes* or *hemispheres* or *lateral masses,* and each lobe is again subdivided into *Montic'uli* or *Lobules.* In the cerebellum are to be observed the *crura cerebelli,* the *fourth ventricle,* the *valvula magna cerebri,* the *processus vermiculares,* superior and inferior, &c.

CER'EBRAL, *Cerebra'lis,* (F.) *Cérébral,* from *cerebrum,* 'the brain.' Belonging to the brain: similar to brain.

CEREBRAL APOPHYSIS, Pineal gland.

CEREBRAL AR'TERIES are three on each side: — the *anterior* or *artery of the corpus callosum,* and the *middle, arte'ria Sylvia'na,* are furnished by the internal carotid:—the *posterior* or *posterior and inferior artery of the brain, A. profunda cerebri,* arises from the vertebral. Chaussier calls these arteries *lobaires,* because they correspond with the anterior, middle, and posterior lobes, whilst he calls the trunks, whence they originate, *cerebral.*

CEREBRAL NERVES are those which arise within the cranium, all of which, perhaps, with the exception of the olfactory, originate from the medulla oblongata. See Nerves.

In *Pathology,* an affection is called *cerebral,* which specially occupies the brain. *Fièvre cérébrale, Cerebral fever,* is a variety in which the head is much affected.

CEREBRIFORM Encephaloid.

CEREBROPATHY, see Nervous diathesis.

CEREBRO-MALACIA, Mollities cerebri.

CEREBRO-SPINAL, Cephalo-spinal. A *cerebro-spinal* or *cerebro-spinant* is a neurotic, which exercises a special influence over one or more functions of the brain and spinal cord, and their respective nerves.—Pereira.

CEREBRO-SPINAL AXIS, see Encephalon.

CEREBRO-SPINANT, Cerebro-spinal.

CER'EBRUM or CERE'BRUM. The brain. (F.) *Cerveau, Cervelle.* This term is sometimes applied to the whole of the contents of the cranium: at others, to the upper portion;—the posterior and inferior being called cerebellum. The brain, properly so called, extends from the os frontis to the superior occipital fossæ. Anteriorly, it rests on the orbitar vaults: behind this, on the middle fossæ of the base of the cranium; and, posteriorly, on the *tentorium cerebello superextensum.* The *upper surface* is divided by a deep median cleft (*Scissure interlobaire,* — Ch.) into two halves, called *hemispheres,* which are united at the base by the *corpus callosum.* At its surface are numerous *convolutions.* The *inferior surface* exhibits, from before to behind, three *lobes,* distinguished into *anterior, middle,* and *posterior.* The middle is separated from the anterior by the *fissure of* SYLVIUS; and from the posterior, by a shallow furrow which corresponds to the upper portion of the *pars petrosa. Internally,* the brain has, on the median line, the *corpus callosum, septum lucidum, fornix, pineal gland,* and *third ventricle:*—and laterally, the *lateral ventricles,* in which are the *corpora striata, optic thalami,* &c. It is contained in a triple envelope, (see Meninges.) Its texture is pulpy, and varies according to age. Two substances may be distinguished in it—the *white, medullary, tubular* or *fibrous — medullʼa cerʼebri,* and the *cortical, cineritious, vesicular,* or *gray.* The former is white; and occupies all the interior and base of the brain. The latter is grayish and softer. It is situate particularly at the surface of the organ.

The brain receives several arterial vessels, furnished by the internal carotid and vertebral. Its veins end in the sinuses. It is the material organ of the mental and moral manifestations. According to Gall, each part is the special seat of one of those faculties, and the brain and cerebellum, inclusive, are called by him '*the nervous system of the mental faculties.*' See Craniology.

The substance of the nervous system—*Neurine* has been analyzed by Vauquelin, and found to contain water, 80.00; white fatty matter, 4.53; red fatty matter, called *cerebrine*, 0.70; osmasome, 1.12; albumen, 7.00; phosphorus, 1.50; sulphur, acid phosphates of potassa, lime, and magnesia, 5.15.

CEREBRUM ABDOMINALE, Solar plexus—c. Elongatum, Medulla oblongata—c. Parvum, Cerebellum—c. Posterius, Cerebellum.

CEREFOLIUM, Scandix cerefolium—c. Hispanicum, Chærophyllum odoratum—c. Sylvestre, Chærophyllum sylvestre.

CERELÆUM, Cerate.

CEREOLUS, *Bougie.*

CERERISIA, Cerevisia.

CEREUM MEDICATUM, *Bougie.*

CEREUS, *Bougie.*

CEREVIS'IA, quasi *Cereris'ia, Cervis'ia, Oe'lia, Zythus, Zythum, Liquor Cer'eris, Vinum hordea'ceum, Bira, Bryton, βρυτον, Barley wine,* from Ceres, 'corn;' whence it is made. Ale (*Alla,*) *Beer, Porter,* (F.) *Bière, Cervoise.* These fluids are drunk by the inhabitants of many countries habitually, and in Great Britain and Germany more than in others. They are nourishing, but not very easy of digestion. The old dispensatories contain numerous medicated ales, which are no longer in use.

CEREVISIA NIGRA, see Falltranck.

CERFEUIL, Scandix cerefolium—*c. Musqué,* Chærophyllum odoratum—*c. Sauvage,* Chærophyllum sylvestre.

CERION, Favus, Porrigo favosa.

CÉRISIER, Prunus cerasus—*c. à Grappes,* Prunus padus—*c. de Virginie,* Prunus Virginiana.

CERNIN, SAINT, WATERS OF. St. C. is a parish in the diocess of St. Flour, Upper Auvergne, France. The water is a chalybeate. It is called *Eau du Cambon.*

CERNOS, Capistrum.

CEROE'NĒ, *Cerou'nē,* or *Cirouĕ'nē, Ceroĕ'num,* from κηρος, 'wax,' and οινος, 'wine.' A plaster composed of *yellow wax, mutton suet, pitch, Burgundy pitch, bole Armeniac, thus* and *wine.* It was used as a strengthening plaster. Sometimes it contained neither wax nor wine.

CEROMA, Cerate.

CEROMANTI'A, from κηρος, 'wax,' and μαντεια, 'divination.' The art of foretelling the future, from the figures which melted wax assumes, when suffered to drop on the surface of water.

CERONIUM, Cerate.

CEROPIS'SUS, from κηρος, 'wax,' and πισσα, 'pitch.' A depilatory plaster, composed of pitch and wax.

CEROS, Cera.

CEROSTROSIS, Hystriciasis.

CEROTUM, Cerate.

CEROXYLON, see Cera flava et alba.

CERUA, Ricinis communis.

CERU'MEN, from *cera,* 'wax.' *Ceru'men Au'rium, Ce'rea, Aurium Sordes, Sordic'ulæ au'rium, Marmora'ta Au'rium, Cypselē, Ceru'minous Humour, Ear-wax, Cyp'selis, Fu'gilē,* (F.) *Cire des Oreilles.* A name given to the unctuous humour, similar to wax in its physical properties, which is met with in the *meatus auditorius externus.* It is secreted by glands, situate beneath the skin lining the meatus. It lubricates the meatus, preserves the suppleness of the lining membrane, prevents the introduction of bodies floating in the atmosphere, and by its bitterness and unctuousness prevents insects from penetrating.

CERU'MINOUS, *Cerumino'sus,* (F.) *Cérumineux.* Relating to cerumen.

CERUMINOUS GLANDS, *Ceru'minous Follicles,* (F.) *Glands cérumineuses* ou *Follicules cérumineuses.* Glands or follicles which secrete the cerumen.

CERUSSA ACETATA, Plumbi superacetas—c. Alba Hispanica, Plumbi subcarbonas—c. Alba Norica, Plumbi subcarbonas—c. Psymmithron, Plumbi subcarbonas—c. Serpentaria, see Arum maculatum.

CERUSSE, Plumbi subcarbonas.

CERUS'SEA URI'NA. A term used by Paracelsus for the urine, when of a colour like cerusse.

CERVARIA ALBA, Laserpitium latifolium.

CERVEAU, Cerebrum.

CERVELET, Cerebellum.

CERVELLE, Cerebrum.

CERVI ELAPHI CORNU, Cornu cervi, see Cervus.

CER'VICAL, *Cervica'lis,* from *cervix,* 'the back of the neck.' *Trache'lian.* Every thing which concerns the neck, especially the back part.

CERVICAL AR'TERIES are three in number: 1. The *ascending, anterior,* or *superficial,* a branch of the inferior thyroid, distributed to the scaleni muscles and integuments. 2. The *transverse* (*Cervico-scapulaire*—Ch.), a branch of the axillary artery, or of the subclavian: distributed to the *levator scapulæ, trapezius,* &c. 3. The *posterior* or *profound, A. transversa'lis colli, Trachélo-cervicale*—(Ch.) a branch of the subclavian, distributed to the deep-seated muscles on the anterior and posterior parts of the neck. See, also, Princeps Cervicis (arteria.)

CERVICAL GAN'GLIONS. The three ganglions of the great sympathetic. The *cervical glands* or lymphatic glands of the neck are, also, so called. See Trisplanchnic nerve.

CERVICAL LIG'AMENTS. These are two in number. 1. The *anterior,* extending from the basilary process of the occipital bone to the anterior part of the first cervical vertebra. 2. The *posterior* or *supraspi'nous, Ligamen'tum Nu'chæ,* which extends from the outer occipital protuberance to the spinous process of the seventh cervical vertebra. In animals with large heads it is very strong.

CERVICAL NERVES are eight in number on each side, and form the *eight cervical pairs,* which are the first given off from the spinal marrow.

CERVICAL PLEXUS, *Plexus Trachélo-sousçutané* (Ch.) The nervous net-work formed by the anterior branches of the first three cervical nerves, above the posterior scalenus muscle, and at the outer side of the pneumogastric nerve, carotid artery, and jugular vein.

CERVICAL REGION, ANTERIOR, DEEP, *Prœver'tebral region.* The region of the neck, occupied by three pairs of muscles placed immediately in front of the cervical and three superior dorsal vertebræ:—viz. the rectus capitis anticus major, the rectus capitis anticus minor, and longus colli; —hence termed *prevertebral muscles.*

CERVICAL VEINS have nearly the same distribution as the arteries.

CERVICAL VER'TEBRÆ. The first seven vertebræ of the spine.

CERVICALIS DESCENDENS, see Hypoglossus and Sacro-lumbalis.

CERVICARIA, Campanula trachelium.

CERVICI-DORSO-SCAPULAIRE, Rhomboideus—*c. Dorso-costal,* Serratus posticus superior—*c. Dorso-mastoïdien et dorso-trachélien,* Splenius—*c. Mastoïdien,* Splenius.

CER'VICO-FA'CIAL, *Cervi'co-facia'lis.* Belonging to the neck and face.

CERVICO-FACIAL NERVE, *Nervus cervico-facialis.* A branch of the facial nerve, distributed to the neck and face.

CERVISIA, Cerevisia.

CERVISPINA, Rhamnus.

CERVIX, *Collum.* The neck. A neck.

CERVIX OBSTIPA, Torticollis—c. Uteri, Collum uteri.

CERVOISE, Cerevisia.

CERVUS, *Cerva.* The horn of the *Cervus El'aphus,* called *Cornu, Cervi El'aphi Cornu, Cornu Cervi'num, Hartshorn,* (F.) *Corne de cerf,* contains 27 parts of gelatin to the 100. A jelly made from the shavings is emollient and nutritive.

The *Stag's Pizzle, Pria'pus Cervi,* was once considered to be aphrodisiac. Dose, ʒj to ʒij, in powder.

CERVUS ALCES. The *Elk,* (F.) *Élan.* The *hoof* of this animal was anciently used as an antiepileptic. The animal, it was asserted, was subject to attacks of epilepsy, and always cured them by putting its hoof into the ear. The hoof was also worn as an amulet.

Cornu Ustum, Burnt Hartshorn, has been used as an antacid, but it consists of 57 parts of *phosphate,* and only one of *carbonate* of lime. It is, therefore, not of much use.

CÉSARIENNE OPÉRATION, Cæsarean section.

CESSATIO MENSIUM, Amenorrhœa.

CESTRI'TES. A wine prepared from betony, (κεστρον, 'betony.')

CESTRON, Betonica officinalis.

CETA'CEUM, from κητος, 'a whale.' *Album Ceti, Adipoce'ra ceto'sa, Steari'num ceta'ceum, Spermacet'i,* (F.) *Blanc de Baleine, Cétine, Adipocire de Baleine.* An inodorous, insipid, white, crystallized, friable, unctuous substance, obtained from the brain of the *Physe'ter Macroceph'alus* or *Spermaceti Whale,* and other varieties of whale. S. g. .9433: melts at 112°. It is demulcent and emollient, and has been given in coughs and dysentery, but is mostly used in ointments. Dose, ʒss to ʒiss, rubbed up with sugar or egg.

CETERACH OFFICINARUM, Asplenium ceterach.

CÉTINE, Cetaceum.

CETRARIA ISLANDICA, Lichen islandicus.

CETRARIN, see Lichen islandicus.

CETRARIUM, see Lichen islandicus.

CEVADILLA HISPANORUM, Veratrum sabadilla.

CÉVADILLE, Veratrum sabadilla.

CHAA, Thea.

CHÆREFOLIUM, Scandix cerefolium.

CHÆROPHYL'LUM, from χαιρω, 'I rejoice,' and φυλλον, 'a leaf.' Scandix cerefolium.

CHÆROPHYLLUM CEREFOLIUM, Scandix cerefolium — c. Angulatum, Ch.sylvestre.

CHÆROPHYL'LUM ODORA'TUM, *Scandix Odora'ta, Myrrhis Odora'ta seu Major, Cicuta'ria odora'ta, Cerefo'lium Hispan'icum, Sweet Cic"ely,* (F.) *Cerfeuil musquée ou d'Espagne,* has the smell of aniseed, and is cultivated on account of its aromatic properties.

CHÆROPHYL'LUM MONOGYNUM, Ch. sylvestre—c. Sativum, Scandix.

CHÆROPHYL'LUM SYLVES'TRE, *Cicuta'ria, Chærophyl'lum tem'ulum seu monog'ynum seu angula'tum seu verticella'tum, Anthris'cus hu'milis seu proc"erus, Cerefo'lium Sylves'trE, Bastard Hemlock, Wild Chervil* or *Cow-weed,* (F.) *Cerfeuil sauvage, Persil d'Âne,* is a slightly fetid aromatic, but is not used.

CHÆROPHYLLUM TEMULUM, Chærophyllum sylvestre—c. Verticillatum, Ch. sylvestre.

CHÆTE, Capillus.

CHAFING, *Erythe'ma Intertri'go, Intertri'go, Paratrim'ma, Paratrip'sis, Diatrim'ma, Attri'ta, Attrit"io,* from *èchauffer,* 'to heat.' Fret. Erosions of the skin; *Attri'tus,* (F.) *Échauffemens, Écorchures.* The red excoriations which occur in consequence of the friction of parts, or between the folds of the skin, especially in fat or neglected children. Washing with cold water and dusting with hair-powder is the best preventive. When occurring between the nates and in the region of the perinæum, from long walking,—*Intertri'go pod'icis, Proctal'gia intertrigino'sa,*—it is vulgarly designated by the French *Entrefesson.*

CHAIR, Flesh.

CHAIR, OBSTETRIC, Labour chair.

CHAISE PERCÉE, Lasanum.

CHALASIS, Relaxation.

CHALASMUS, Relaxation.

CHALAS'TICUS, from χαλαω, 'I relax.' A medicine proper for removing rigidity of the fibres.—Galen. An emollient or relaxant.

CHAL'AZA, *Chala'zion, Chalazium, Chalazo'sis, Poro'sis, Grando, Tophus, Hail,* (F.) *Grêle, Gravelle.* A hard, round, transparent tumour, developed in different parts of the body, more especially in the substance of the eyelids.—Also, the Cicatricula of the egg. Generally, however, in the language of ovologists, the *chalazæ* or *poles* are, in the egg of the bird, the more dense internal layer of the albumen, which adheres to the yolk, and is continued, in the form of two spirally twisted bands, towards the extremities of the egg. The twisting is considered to be produced by the revolving motion of the egg in its descent through the oviduct.

CHALAZÆ, see Chalaza.

CHALCANTHUM, Ferri sulphas — c. Album Zinci sulphas.

CHALCEDONIUS, Cornelian.

CHALCITAS, Bismuth.

CHALCITES, Colcothar.

CHALCOIDEUM, (os), Cuneiform bone.

CHALCOS, Cuprum, Æreolum.

CHALCUS, Æreolum.

CHALEUR, Heat—c. Acre, see Acrid—c. *Animale,* Animal heat, see Heat—c. *des Animaux,* see Heat.

CHALEURS DU FOIE, Heat.

CHALINI, see Lip.

CHAL'INOPLASTY, *Chalinoplas'tice*; from χαλινος, 'frænum,' 'a bridle,' and πλασσω, 'I form.' The operation for forming a new frænum.

CHALK, Creta — c. Red, Rubrica febrilis — c. Stones, Calculi, arthritic.

CHALYB'EATE, *Chalybea'tus, Ferrugin'eus, Ferrugino'sus, Ferra'tus, Martia'lis, Ferru'ginous, Mar'tial,* (F.) *Ferrugineux*; from *chalybs,* 'iron or steel.' Of, or belonging to iron; containing iron. Any medicine into which iron enters, as chalybeate mixture, pills, waters, &c. See Waters, Mineral.

CHALYBIS RUBIGO, Ferri subcarbonas.

CHALYBS, from *Chalybes*; a people of Pontus, who dug iron out of the earth; *A'cies, Steel.* The *Proto-carburet of iron,* (F.) *Acier.* As a medicine, steel does not differ from iron.

CHALYBS TARTARIZATUS, Ferrum tartarizatum.

CHAMA, Cheme.

CHAMÆACTE, Sambucus ebulus.

CHAMÆBATOS, Fragaria.

CHAMÆCEDRIS. Artemisia santonica.

CHAMÆCISSUS, Glechoma hederacea.

CHAMÆCLEMA, Glechoma hederacea — c. Hederacea, Glechoma hederacea.

CHAMÆCYPARISSUS, Artemisia santonica.

CHAMÆDROPS, Teucrium chamædrys.

CHAMÆDRYI'TES. A wine, in which the *Teu'crium Chamædrys* has been infused.

CHAMÆDRYS, Rubus chamæmorus, Teucrium Ch.—c. Incana maritima, Teucrium marum—c. Marum, Teucrium marum—c. Minor repens, Teucrium Ch.—c. Palustris, Teucrium scordium—c. Scordium, Teucrium scordium—c. Vulgaris, Teucrium Ch.

CHAMÆGEIRON, Tussilago.
CHAMÆLÆAGNUS, Myrica gale.
CHAMÆLAÏTES. A wine impregnated with *Chamælea, Daphne Alpi'na.*
CHAMÆLEA, Cneorum tricoccum.
CHAMÆLEON ALBUM, Carlina acaulis.
CHAMÆLEUCE, Tussilago.
CHAMÆLINUM, Linum catharticum.
CHAMÆLIR'IUM LU'TEUM, *Vera'trum lu'teum, Helo'nias lu'tea, H. Dioi'ca, Devil's Bit, Blazing star;* indigenous; *Order,* Melanthaceæ; flowering in June; is acrid. An infusion of the root has been given as an anthelmintic; a tincture, as a tonic.
CHAMÆMELUM, Anthemis nobilis — c. Fœtidum, Anthemis cotula — c. Nobile, Anthemis nobilis — c. Odoratum, Anthemis nobilis — c. Vulgare, Matricaria chamomilla.
CHAMÆMORUS, Teucrium chamæpitys, Rubus chamæmorus — c. Norwegica, Rubus chamæmorus.
CHAMÆPEUCE, Camphorosma Monspeliaca.
CHAMÆPITUI'NUM VINUM. A wine, in which the leaves of the *Chamæ'pitys, Teu'crium Chamæ'pitys,* have been infused.
CHAMÆPITYS, Teucrium chamæpitys — c. Anthyllus, Teucrium iva — c. Moschata, Teucrium iva.
CHAMÆPLION, Erysimum.
CHAMÆRAPH'ANUM, from χαμαι, 'on the ground,' and ραφανος, 'the radish.' So Paulus of Ægina calls the upper part of the root of the *Apium.*
CHAMÆ'ROPS SERRAT'ULA, *Saw Palmetto.* A farina is prepared from the roots of this plant, which is used by the Indians, in Florida, as diet.
CHAMBAR, Magnesia.
CHAMBER, *Cam'era,* (F.) *Chambre.* A term used in speaking of the eye, in which there are two chambers, *Came'ræ oc'uli:* — an *anterior* and a *posterior;* (F.) *Chambre antérieure et postérieure.* The *anterior* is the space between the cornea and the anterior part of the iris :—the *posterior,* the space between the iris and anterior surface of the crystalline. They are filled with the aqueous humour, and communicate by the opening in the pupil.
CHAM'BERLAIN'S RESTOR'ATIVE PILLS. This nostrum, recommended in scrofula, and all impurities of the blood, has been analyzed by Dr. Paris, and found to consist of *cinnabar, sulphur, sulphate of lime,* and a little vegetable matter. Each pill weighs 3 grains.
CHAMBRE, Chamber.
CHAMBRIE, Cannabis sativa.
CHAMELEA, Daphne Alpina.
CHAMOMILE, DOGS', Matricaria chamomilla — c. Dyers', Anthemis tinctoria — c. German, Matricaria chamomilla — c. Spanish, Anthemis pyrethrum — c. Stinking, Anthemis cotula — c. Wild, Anthemis cotula, Matricaria glabrata.
CHAMOMILLA FŒTIDA, Anthemis cotula — c. Nostras, Matricaria chamomilla — c. Romana, Anthemis nobilis — c. Spuria, Anthemis cotula.
CHAMPACA, Michelia champaca.
CHAMPIGNON, Fungus — c. *de l'Appareil des Fractures,* Clavaria — c. *de Couche,* see Agaric — c. *de Malte,* Cynomorion coccineum.
CHANCELAGUA, Canchalagua.
CHANCRE, (F.) *Ulcus cancro'sum, Ulcus'culum cancro'sum.* A sore, which arises from the direct application of the venereal virus; hence it is almost always seated, in men, on the penis. The French use the word *Chancre,* in popular language, for cancerous ulcers, the malignant aphthæ of children, &c. Formerly, the terms *Car'oli* and *Ca'ries pudendo'rum* were used for venereal pustules or sores on the parts of generation.

CHANCRE LARVÉ. A concealed chancre, such as has been supposed by M. Ricord to give occasion to gonorrhœa virulenta.

CHANCREUX, *Chancreuse,* (F.) *Cancro'sus, Carcino'des.* Having the nature of chancre, or of cancer.

Bouton Chancreux. A small tumour of a cancerous nature, which makes its appearance on the face — most frequently on the upper lip — *Noli me tangere.*

CHANT DES ARTÈRES *Sifflement modulé.*

CHANVRE, Cannabis sativa — c. *Indien,* Bangue.

CHAOMANTI'A. The alchymists meant, by this word, the art of predicting the future from observation of the air. The word *Chaos* was used by Paracelsus for the air; (μαντεια, 'divination.')

CHAOSDA, Plague.

CHAPERON DE MOINE, Aconitum napellus.

CHAPITEAU, Alembic.

CHAPPEDONADE, Chappetonade.

CHAPPETONADE, *Chappedonade,* (F.), *Vom'itus rabio'sus.* Vomiting accompanied by furious delirium, attacking strangers in hot countries.

CHAR'ACTER, χαρακτηρ, 'A mark or impression.' (F.) *Caractère.* In Pathology it is used synonymously with stamp or appearance. We say, "A disease is of an unfavourable character," "The prevailing epidemic has a bilious character," &c. In *Mental Philosophy* it means — that which distinguishes one individual from another, as regards his understanding and passions. See Symbol.

CHARA'DRIUS. Ælian thus calls a bird, which was reputed to cure jaundice. The word now means the plover.

CITARANTIA, Momordica elaterium.

CHARBON, Anthrax carbo.

CHARBONNEUX, Anthracoid.

CHARCOAL, Carbo — c. Animal, Carbo animalis.

CHARDON AUX ÂNES, Onopordium acanthium — c. *Bénit,* Centaurea benedicta — c. *à Bonnetier,* Dipsacus fullonum — c. *Étoilé,* Centaurea calcitrapa — c. *à Foulon,* Dipsacus fullonum — c. *Hémorrhoïdal,* Cirsium arvense — c. *Marie,* Carduus Marianus — c. *Roland,* Eryngium campestre.

CHAR'LATAN, from Ital. *ciarlare,* 'to talk much;' *Circula'tor, Circumfora'neus, Periodeu'tes, Pseudomed'icus, Agyr'ta, Anacyc'leon,* A *Quack,* an *Empirical Pretender,* an *Emp'iric.* Originally, one who went from place to place to sell a medicine, to which he attributed marvellous properties. By extension — any individual, who endeavours to deceive the public by passing himself off as more skilful than he really is. According to Ménage, the word comes from *circulatanus,* a corruption of *circulator.*

CHAR'LATANRY, *Agyr'tia, Banau'sia,* the conduct or action of a charlatan. (F.) *Charlatanerie, Charlatanisme, Quackery, Empiricism.*

CHARLOCK, Sinapis arvensis.

CHARM, Lat. *Carmen,* 'a verse,' because charms often consisted of verses, whence comes the Italian, *Ciarma,* (F.) *Charme,* with the same signification. *Canta'tio, Incantamen'tum.* A trick, a spell, an enchantment. A sort of magic, or superstitious practice, consisting of words, characters, &c., by which it was believed, that individuals might be struck with sickness or death, or be restored to health.

The following are specimens of old charms — *verses charms:*

For stanching Blood, (Pepys.)
Sanguis mane in te
Sicut Christus fuit in se;
Sanguis mane in tuâ venâ
Sicut Christus in suâ poenâ;
Sanguis mane fixus,
Sicut Christus quando fuit crucifixus.

For Cramp, (Pepys.)
Cramp be thou faintless,
As our lady was sinless,
When she bare Jesus.

For the Foot when asleep, (Coleridge.)
Foot! foot! foot! is fast asleep!
Thumb! thumb! thumb! in spittle we steep;
Crosses three we make to ease us,
Two for the thieves, and one for Christ Jesus.

The same charm served for cramp in the leg, with this substitution:

The devil is tying a knot in my leg!
Mark, Luke, and John, unloose it, I beg!—
Crosses three, &c.

For a Burn, (Pepys.)
There came three angels out of the East;
The one brought fire, the other brought frost.
Out fire; in frost.
In the name of the Father and Son and Holy Ghost.
Amen.

CHARNIÈRE, Ginglymus.
CHARNU, Carneous.
CHARPIE, Linteum—c. *Brute*, see Linteum
—c. *Rapée*, see Linteum.
CHARTA ANTIARTHRITICA, Gout paper
—c. Antirheumatica, Gout paper—c. Vesicatoria,
see Sparadrapum Vesicatorium — c. Virgines,
Amnios.
CHARTRE, Tabes mesenterica.
CHAS, (F.) *Acûs fora'men*. The *eye of a needle*. Sometimes, this opening is near the point of the instrument, as in the ligature needle.
CHASCHISCH, see Bangue.
CHASME, Yawning.
CHASPE, Variola.
CHASSE (F.), *Manu'brium*. A kind of handle composed of two movable laminæ of horn, shell, or ivory, united only at the extremity, which holds the blade of the instrument,—as in the common bleeding lancet.
CHASSIE (F.), *Lema, Lippa, Glama, Glemē, Gra'mia, Lemos'itas;* the *gum of the eye*. A sebaceous humour, secreted mainly by the follicles of Meibomius, which sometimes glues the eyelids together.
CHASSIEUX (F.) *Lippus;* covered with *Chassie*—as *Paupières chassieuses*.
CHASTE TREE, Vitex.
CHÂTAIGNE, see Fagus castanea—c. *d'Eau*, Trapa natans.
CHÂTAIGNIER COMMUN, Fagus castanea
—c. *Nain*, Fagus castanea pumila.
CHATEAU-LANDON, WATERS OF. A town three leagues from Nemours, in France. The waters contain alum and iron.
CHATEAU-SALINS, WATERS OF; a town in the department of La-Meurthe, France. The waters contain carbonate of lime, sulphates of lime and magnesia, and chlorides of magnesium and sodium.
CHATELDON, MINERAL WATERS OF. Chateldon is in the department of Puy-de-Dôme, France. The waters contain carbonic acid and iron.
CHATEL-GUYON, MINERAL WATERS OF. A village in France, in the department Puy-de-Dôme, near which there are five thermal acidulous springs. Temperature, 86° Fahrenheit.
CHATON (F.), 'a husk.' In pathology, it means a *funda* or cavity formed by the irregular or *hour-glass contraction* of the uterus, in which the placenta is often retained or *enchatonné* after the birth of the child. It is detected by passing the fingers along the cord as far as the part which is contracted, when the placenta will not be discoverable.

The treatment consists in relaxing by a large dose of an opiate, then passing the fingers along the cord, and gradually dilating the opening through which it passes, until it permits the hand to go through. The placenta must then be grasped and gently withdrawn.

CHATON, Vaginal process.
CHATONNÉ, CALCUL, (F.) *Calculus incarcera'tus, Eucys'ted Cal'culus, Calcul enkysté*. A urinary calculus, adherent to the inner surface of the bladder, so that it is immovable, and cannot pass to the different parts of that organ. This happens when calculi form in some natural or accidental cavity of the bladder; or when the organ, by ulceration, gives rise to fungi, which surround the calculus; or when it is lodged in the orifice of the ureter or urethra.
CHATONNÉ, PLACENTA, (F.) The placenta when retained as above described. See *Chaton*.
CHATONNEMENT, (F.) *Incarcera'tio, Chatonnement du placenta, Enkystement*.—Hour-glass contraction of the uterus. See *Chaton*.
CHATOUILLEMENT, (F.) This word sometimes means the action of *tickling* or titillation (*Titilla'tio*,) and, at others, the sensation which gives rise to the action (*Pruri'tus*,) Itching.
CHÂTRÉ, Castratus.
CHÂTRURE, Castration.
CHAUDEAU, Caudle.
CHAUDEBOURG, MINERAL WATERS OF. C. is three quarters of a league from Thionville, in France. The waters contain iron, sulphate of lime, sulphate of magnesia, and carbonate of lime.
CHAUDEPISSE, Gonorrhœa impura—c. *Cordée*, Gonorrhœa cordata—c. *Tombée dans les Bourses*, Hernia humoralis.
CHAUDES-AIGUËS, MINERAL WATERS OF. A small town in the department of Cantal, France, where there is a number of saline springs containing carbonic acid, carbonate of soda, and chloride of sodium. Temp. 190° Fahrenheit.
CHAUDIÈRE, see Alembic.
CHAUFFOIR (F.), *Linteum Calefacto'rium*. According to the *Académie*, a warmed cloth, used either for the purpose of warming a patient, or to apply to a female recently delivered.
CHAUSSE, (F.) *Chausse d'Hippocrate, Manche d'Hippocrate, Man'ica Hippoc'ratis, Man'ica, Hippocrates' Sleeve*. A conical bag, made of flannel, for straining liquids.
CHAUSSE-TRAPPE, Centaurea calcitrapa.
CHAUVETÉ, Calvities.
CHAUX, Calx—c. *Bichlorure de*, Calcis chloridum—c. *Chlorure de*, Calcis chloridum—c. *Hydrochlorate de*, Calcis murias—c. *Hydrosulfate de*, Calcis sulphuretum—c. *Muriate de*, Calcis murias—c. *Muriate oxigéné de*, Calcis chloridum—c. *Muriate suroxigéné de*, Calcis chloridum—c. *Oxichlorure de*, Calcis chloridum—c. *Oximuriate de*, Calcis chloridum—c. *Vive*, Calx viva.
CHECKER-BERRY, Arbutus uva ursi.
CHEEK, Gena.
CHEESE, Sax. cere, (L.) *Ca'seus, Tyros, Pectē*, (F.) *Fromage*. An aliment, prepared from the caseous and oleaginous parts of milk. Fresh cheeses owe their chief medical properties to the immediate principle, essentially cheesy, to which the name *ca'seum* or *ca'sein* has been applied. Those, which have been recently salted, are digested with comparative facility. The flavour

of cheese is owing to an ammoniacal caseate. On the whole, cheese itself is not easy of digestion, although it may stimulate the stomach to greater exertion, and thus aid in the digestion of other substances.

CHEESE RENNET, Galium verum.

CHEE'SY, *Casea'rius, Caseo'sus, Tyro'des,* (F.) *Caseux* ou *Caséeux.* Having the nature of cheese.

CHEF, Bandage (tail.)

CHEGOE, *Chique.*

CHEGRE, *Chique.*

CHEILI'TIS, *Chili'tis,* from χειλος, 'a lip.' Inflammation of the lip. See Chilon.

CHEILOC'ACE, from χειλος, 'a lip,' and κακος, 'evil.' *Labrisul'cium.* A disease, characterized, it is said, by swelling, induration, and slight redness of the lips without inflammation; reputed, but without any authority, to be common in England and Scotland, amongst children. Also, the thickness of the upper lip of scrofulous children. See Stomacace, and Cancer aquaticus.

CHEILOCARCINO'MA, from χειλος, 'a lip,' and καρκινωμα, 'a cancer.' Cancer of the lip.

CHEILOMALACIA, Cancer aquaticus, Stomacace.

CHEILON, Chilon.

CHEILON'CUS, *Cheilophy'ma,* from χειλος, 'lip,' and ογκος, 'swelling.' A swelling of the lip.

CHEILOPHYMA, Cheiloncus.

CHEILOPLAS'TICE, *Chiloplas'tice,* from χειλος, 'lip,' and πλαστικις, 'forming.' The operation for an artificial lip.

CHEILOS, Lip.

CHEIMA, Cold.

CHEIMETLON, Chilblain.

CHEIMIA, Rigor.

CHEIR, Manus.

CHEIRAN'THUS CHEIRI, from χειρ, 'the hand,' and ανθος, 'flower.' The systematic name of the *Common Yellow Wall Flower, Vi'ola lu'tea, Leucoïum lu'teum, Keyri, Cheiri,* (F.) *Géroflée* ou *Violier jaune.* The flowers have been esteemed nervine, narcotic, and deobstruent.

CHEIRAP'SIA. The action of rubbing or scratching, from χειρ, 'the hand,' and απτω, 'I touch.' A troublesome symptom in the itch.

CHEIRIATER, Surgeon.

CHEIRIS'MA, *Cheiris'mus.* The act of touching:—handling. Any manual operation.

CHEIRIXIS, Surgery.

CHEIRONOM'IA, *Chironom'ia,* from χειρονομεω, 'I exercise with the hands.' An exercise, referred to by Hippocrates, which consisted in using the hands, as in our exercise of the dumb-bells.

CHEIROPLETHES, Fasciculus.

CHEIROSIS, Subactio.

CHELA, *Chelē.* This word has several significations. *Chela,* a forked probe used for extracting polypi from the nose. *Chelæ* — chaps, or cracks on the feet, organs of generation, &c. *Chelæ* likewise means claws, especially those of the crab. See Cancrorum Chelæ.

CHELÆ PALPEBRARUM, see Tarsus.

CHELAPA, Convolvulus jalapa.

CHELE, Chela.

CHÉLIDOINE GRANDE, Chelidonium majus—c. *Petite,* Ranunculus ficaria.

CHELIDON, χελιδων, the hollow at the bend of the arm; *Hirundo.*

CHELIDONIA ROTUNDIFOLIA MINOR, Ranunculus ficaria.

CHELIDONIUM, Bryonia alba—c. Hæmatodes, Ch. majus.

CHELIDO'NIUM MAJUS, *Ch. hæmato'des,* from χελιδων, 'a swallow,' because its flowering coincides with the appearance of the swallow. *Papa'ver Cornicula'tum, P. lu'teum, Common Cel'andine, Tetterwort,* (F.) *Chélidoine grande, L'Éclaire.* Family, Papaveraceæ. *Sex. Syst.* Polyandria Monogynia. The root and recent plant have been considered aperient and diuretic. Externally, the juice has been employed in some cutaneous diseases.

CHELIDONIUM MINUS, Ranunculus ficaria.

CHELIDO'NIUS LAPIS. A name given to stones, which, it was pretended, existed in the stomach of young swallows. They were formerly believed capable of curing epilepsy.

CHELOID, Cancroid.

CHELO'NE, χελωνη, 'a tortoise.' An instrument for extending a limb; so called, because in its slow motions, it resembled a tortoise.—Oribasius. See Testudo.

CHELO'NE GLABRA, *Common Snake head, Turtle head, Turtle bloom, Shellflower, Balmony.* An indigenous plant, *Sex. Syst.* Didynamia angiospermia; blossoming from July to November. The leaves are bitter and tonic; without any aromatic smell, and with very little astringency.

CHELO'NIA MYDAS, *The Green Turtle.* This species of turtle abounds on the coast of Florida. It is the one so prized by the epicure.

CHELO'NION, *Chelo'nium,* from χελωνη, 'a tortoise,' from its resembling in shape the shell of that animal. The upper, gibbous part of the back.—Gorræus. The scapula.

CHELONOPH'AGI, from χελωνη, 'the tortoise,' and φαγω, 'I eat.' An ancient name for certain tribes, who dwelt on the coasts of the Red Sea, and who lived only on tortoises. — Pliny, Diodorus of Sicily.

CHEL'SEA PEN'SIONER. An empirical remedy for rheumatism and gout, sold under this name. (*Gum guaiac,* ℨj; *powdered rhubarb,* ℨij; *cream of tartar,* ℨj; *flowers of sulphur,* ℨj; *one nutmeg,* finely powdered: made into an electuary with a pound of *clarified honey.*) Dose, two spoonfuls.

CHEL'TENHAM, MINERAL WATERS OF. C. is a town in Gloucestershire, England, nine miles from Gloucester, and 94 W. of London. Its water is one of the most celebrated natural purgatives in England. It is a saline, acidulous chalybeate, and is much frequented. Its main constituents are chloride of sodium, sulphate of soda, sulphate of magnesia, carbonic acid and carbonate of iron.

CHELTENHAM SALTS. These are sometimes made from the waters; at others, factitiously. The following is a formula: *Sodii chlorid., magnes. sulphat., sodæ sulph.,* āā lbj: dissolve, filter, evaporate to dryness; then add *Ferri sulph.,* ℨss.

CHELTENHAM WATER, ARTIFICIAL, may be made of *Epsom salt,* gr. xij; *iron filings,* gr. j; *Glauber's salt,* ℨvj; *water,* 4 gallons; impregnated with the gas from *marble powder* and *sulphuric acid,* āā ℨij.

CHELYS, Thorax.

CHELYS'CION, from χελυς, 'the chest.' A short, dry cough.—Galen, Hippocrates, Foësius.

CHEME, *Chama, Che'ramis.* An ancient measure, equivalent to about two teaspoonfuls.

CHEMEUTICE, Chymistry.

CHEMIA, Chymistry.

CHEMIATER, Chymiater.

CHEMIATRIA, Chymiatria.

CHEMICO-HISTOLOGY, see Chymico-histology.

CHEMICUS, Chymical, Chymist.

CHEMIST, Chymist.

CHEMISTRY, Chymistry.

CHEMO'SIS, from χημη, 'an aperture,' or from χυμος, 'a humour.' A name given to ophthalmia, when the conjunctiva, surrounding the cornea, forms a high ring, making the cornea seem, as it were, at the bottom of a well. By some, it is used synonymously with *ophthalmia membranarum.* See Ophthalmia.

CHEMOTICE, Chymistry.
CHEMOTICUS, Chymical.
CHENAY, MINERAL WATERS OF. Chenay is a town in France, two leagues from Rheims. The waters are chalybeate.

CHÊNE, Quercus alba—c. *Marin*, Fucus vesiculosus—c. *Petit*, Teucrium chamædrys—c. *Vert*, Ilex aquifolium.

CHÊNEVIS, see Cannabis sativa.

CHENOBOSCON, Potentilla anserina.

CHENOC'OPRUS, from χην, 'a goose,' and κοπρος, 'dung.' The *dung of the goose* is so designated in some old Pharmacopœias. It was formerly employed as a febrifuge and diuretic.

CHENOPODIUM AMBROSIACUM, Ch. ambrosioïdes.

Chenopo'dium Ambrosioï'des, *Ch. suffructico'sum*, from χην, 'a goose,' and πους, 'a foot;' *Botrys Mexica'na*, *At'riplex Mexica'na*, *Chenopo'dium ambrosiacum* seu *Mexica'num*, *Botrys*, *Ambrosioï'des Mexica'na*, *Botrys America'na*, *Artemis'ia Botrys*, *Mexico Tea*, *Spanish Tea*, (F.) *Ansérine*, *Thé du Mexique*, *Ambrosie du Mexique*. The infusion was once drunk as tea. It has been given in paralytic cases; and in the United States is said to be used as an anthelmintic indiscriminately with Ch. anthelminticum.

Chenopo'dium Anthelmin'ticum, *Chenopo'dium*, *Botrys anthelmin'tica*, *Wormseed*, *Wormgoosefoot*, *Wormseed goosefoot*, *Jerusalem Oak* of America, *Goosefoot*, *Stinkweed*, (F.) *Ansérine anthelmintique*, *A. vermifuge*. This plant grows plentifully in the United States. The fruit—*Chenopodium*, (Ph. U. S.)—is much used in cases of worms. Dose of the powder, from a teaspoonful to a tablespoonful or more. The oil, *O'leum Chenopo'dii*, (Ph. U. S.), from 8 to 10 drops, is more frequently exhibited. It is as much used in America as the *Semen Santon'ici* is in England.

Chenopo'dium Bonus Henri'cus, *Chrysolach'anum*, *Mercuria'lis*, *Bonus Henri'cus*, *Tota bona*, *Lap'athum unctuo'sum*, *Chenopo'dium*, *Ch. sagitta'tum*, *Pes anseri'nus*, *English Mercury*, *Allgood*, *Angular-leaved goosefoot*, (F.) *Ansérine Bon Henri*, *Épinard sauvage*. The leaves are emollient, and have been applied to ulcers, &c. It has also been considered refrigerant and eccoprotic.

Chenopo'dium Botrys, *Botrys*, *Botrys vulga'ris*, *Ambro'sia*, *Artemis'ia Chenopo'dium*, *At'riplex odora'ta*, *At'riplex suav'eolens*; the *Jerusalem Oak*, (Eng.) (F.) *Ansérine Botrys*, possesses anthelmintic properties, and was once given in diseases of the chest, palsy, &c. It is useless.

Chenopodium Fœtidum, Chenopodium vulvaria—c. Olidum, Ch. vulvaria.

Chenopodium Quinoa, *Quinua*. A nutritious, wholesome, and agreeable article of food with the Peruvians. The leaves, before the plant attains maturity, are eaten as spinach: but the seeds are most generally used as food, boiled in milk or broth, and sometimes cooked with cheese and Spanish pepper.

Chenopodium Sagittatum, Ch. Bonus Henricus—c. Suffructicosum, Ch. ambrosioïdes.

Chenopodium Vulva'ria, *At'riplex fœ'tida*, *At'riplex ol'ida*, *Vulva'ria*, *Garos'mum*, *Raphex*, *Chenopo'dium Fœ'tidum* seu *ol'idum*, *Stinking Orach* or *Goosefoot*, (F.) *Vulvaire*, *Arroche puant*, *Ansérine fétide*. The fetid smell has occasioned it to be used as an antispasmodic and nervine.

CHEOPINA, Cheopine.
CHEQUERBERRY, Gaultheria.
CHERAMIS, Cheme.
CHERBACHEM, Veratrum album.
CHERBAS, Lettuce.

CHERMES, Kermes.
CHERNIBIUM, Urinal.
CHERRY, BIRD, Prunus padus — c. Tree, red, Prunus cerasus — c. Tree, black, Prunus avium — c. Tree, wild, Prunus Virginiana — c. Water, Kirschwasser — c. Wild cluster, Prunus padus— c. Winter, Physalis.
CHERSÆ, Fæces.
CHERVIL, Scandix cerefolium—c. Wild, Chærophyllum sylvestre.
CHESIS, from χιζειν, 'to go to stool.' A more frequent desire to evacuate the bowels.
CHEST, Thorax.
CHEST-EXPLORATOR, see Explorator, chest.
CHESTNUT TREE, Fagus castanea.
CHEVAUCHEMENT, (F.) *Os'sium superposit'io vel equita'tio, Parallax'is, Parallag'ma*. The riding of one bone over another after fracture, giving rise to shortening of the limb. See Riding of Bones.
CHEVELURE, Scalp.
CHEVESTRE, *Chevêtre*, *Capis'trum*, from *caput*, 'the head.' A bandage, applied round the head in cases of fracture or luxation of the lower jaw. According to the mode in which it is made, it is called *simple*, *double*, *oblique*, &c.
CHEVEU, Capillus.
CHEVILLE DU PIED, Malleolus.
CHÈVRE-FEUILLE, Lonicera periclymenum.
CHEYLETUS SCABIEI, see Psora.
CHEZANAN'CE, from χιζω, 'I go to stool,' and αναγκη, 'necessity.' An ointment composed of honey and alum, and rubbed on the anus to occasion evacuation.—Paulus of Ægina.
CHIA, *Chia terra*, from *Chios*, an island where it was found. A kind of white earth, formerly used for burns.—Galen.
CHI'ACUM COLLYR'IUM. A collyrium consisting of several drugs and Chian wine.—Paulus of Ægina.
CHIADUS, Furunculus.
CHIAS'MUS, *Chias'ma*, *Chiasm*, from χιαζω, to form like the letter χ. The crucial union of parts,—as the *optic commissure* or *chiasm* of the optic nerves,—*Chias'mus* seu *Chias'ma nervo'rum optico'rum*.
CHIASTER, Kiaster.
CHIAS'TOS. Same etymon. A bandage so called because it resembles the letter χ.—Oribasius.
CHIBOU, see Bursera gummifera.
CHICHA. A drink made in Peru with Indian meal dried in the sun, and fermented with water. Its taste is that of bad cider. It is also made from rice, peas, barley, &c.
CHICKEN-BREASTED, see Lordosis.
CHICKEN-BROTH. When chicken-tea is boiled down one-half, with the addition of a little *parsley* or *celery*, and the *yolk* of an egg previously beaten up in two ounces of soft water, it forms a soup much relished by the convalescent.
CHICKEN-PEPPER, Ranunculus abortivus.
CHICKENPOX, Varicella.
CHICKEN-TEA, *Chicken-water*. This may be prepared as follows: Take a small chicken, freed from the skin and fat between the muscles; and, having divided it longitudinally, remove the lungs, liver, and every thing adhering to the back and side-bones: cut the whole—bones and muscles—into very thin slices; put into a pan with a sufficient quantity of boiling water; cover the pan; and simmer with a slow fire for two hours. Put the pan upon the stove for half an hour, and strain through a sieve.
Used where the lightest animal diet is indicated.
CHICKEN-WATER, Chicken-tea.

CHICKWEED, Alsine media.
CHICORÉE DES JARDINS, Cichorium endivia—c. Sauvage, Cichorium intybus.
CHIENDENT, Triticum repens.
CHIGGO, Chique.
CHIGGRE, Chique.
CHIGOE, Chique.
CHIL'BLAIN, Per'nio, Bugan'tia, Erythe'ma Per'nio, Erythe'ma à Fri'goré, Cheimet'lon, Chimet'lum, Chimon, Malce, from chill, 'cold,' and blain, 'a pustule.' (F.) Engelure. An erythematous inflammation of the feet,—hands, &c., occasioned by cold. It is very common in youth—not so in the adult or in advanced age. It is apt to degenerate into painful, indolent ulcerations, called Kibes. Chilblains are prevented by accustoming the parts to exposure; and are treated by stimulant, terebinthinate and balsamic washes, ointments, and liniments.
CHILD-BEARING, Parturition.
CHILD-BED, Parturient.
CHILD-BED FEVER, Puerperal fever.
CHILD-BIRTH, Parturition.
CHILD-CROWING, Asthma thymicum.
CHILDHOOD, Infancy.
CHILD-MURDER, Infanticide.
CHILDREN'S BANE, Cicuta maculata.
CHILL, see Lima.
CHILI, MINERAL WATERS OF. The most celebrated mineral springs of Chili, in South America, are those of Peldehues and Cauquenes. The former are not far from St. Jago. They consist of two springs, one thermal, the other cold. The hot spring is clear, inodorous, and contains soda and carbonic acid. The cold spring contains iron and sulphate of soda. Cauquenes is much resorted to by invalids during the summer. Mineral waters are very common in Chili.
CHILIOGRAMMA, Kilogramme.
CHILIOPHYLLON, Achillea millefolium.
CHILITES, Cheilitis.
CHILL, Rigor.
CHI'LON, Chei'lon, Cheili'tis, from χειλος, 'a lip.' Inflammation of the lips.—Vogel. One who has a thick lip; Labeo, Labes.
CHILOPLASTICE, Cheiloplastice.
CHIMAPHILA, Pyrola umbellata.
CHIMETLUM, Chilblain.
CHIMIA, Chymistry.
CHIMIATER, Chymiater.
CHIMIATRIA, Chymiatria.
CHIMIE, Chymistry.
CHIMISTE, Chymist.
CHIMON, Chilblain, Cold.
CHINA, Cinchona, Smilax china—c. American or West India, Smilax pseudo-china—c. Occidentalis, Smilax pseudo-china—c. Orientalis, Smilax china—c. Ponderosa, Smilax china—c. Root, Smilax china—c. Spuria nodosa, Smilax pseudo-china—c. Vera, Smilax china.
CHINCAPIN, Fagus castanea pumila—c. Water, Nelumbium luteum.
CHINCHE, Cimex.
CHINCHINA, Cinchona.
CHINCHUNCHULLI, Ionidium marcucci.
CHINCOUGH, Pertussis.
CHINESE, MEDICINE OF THE, Medici'na Sin'ica. Medicine has been long, but most imperfectly, practised by the Chinese. From their therapeutics we have obtained the old operations of acupuncture and moxibustion.
CHING'S WORM LOZENGES, see Worm Lozenges, Ching's.
CHININUM, Quinine. See Chinium.
CHINIO'IDINE, Chino'ïdine, Chinoïdi'na, Quinoïdine; from China, 'Cinchona.' A substance presumed to be an alkaloid by Sertürner, who separated it from cinchona. It has been sup-posed to be a mixture of quinia, cinchonia, and a peculiar resinous matter, but according to Liebig it is simply the alkaloid quinia in an amorphous state.
CHINIUM ACETICUM, Quiniæ acetas — c. Arsenicosum, Quiniæ arsenias—c. Citricum, Quiniæ citras—c. Ferrocyanogenatum, Quiniæ Ferrocyanas — c. Hydrochloricum, Quiniæ, murias — c. Hydroiodicum, Quiniæ hydriodas — c. Lacticum, Quiniæ lactas—c. Muriaticum, Quiniæ murias—c. Nitricum, Quiniæ nitras—c. Phosphoricum, Quiniæ phosphas—c. Salitum, Quiniæ murias—c. Sulphuricum, Quiniæ sulphas—c. Tannicum, Quiniæ et Cinchoniæ tannas—c. Valerianicum, Quiniæ valerianas.
CHINNEYWEED, Lichen roccella.
CHINOLEINUM, Leukoleinum.
CHINQUAPIN, Fagus castanea pumila.
CHINWHELK, Sycosis.
CHIOCOCCÆ RADIX, Caincæ radix.
CHIOLI, Furunculus.
CHION, Snow.
CHIQUE, (F.) Puce pénétrante, Pulex Pen'-etrans, Tick, Chiggre, Chig'oe, Chiggo, Chegre, Cheg'oë, Jigger. A small insect in America and the Antilles, which gets under the epidermis, and excites great irritation.
CHIR, Manus.
CHIRAETA, Gentiana chirayta.
CHI'RAGRA, from χειρ, 'hand,' and αγρα, 'a seizure.' Gout in the hand.
CHIRAPOTHECA, Arsenal.
CHIRAPSIA, Friction.
CHIRARTHRI'TIS, from χειρ, 'hand,' αρθρον, 'joint,' and itis, denoting inflammation. Inflammation of the joints of the hand.
CHIRAYITA, Gentiana chirayta.
CHIRAYTA, Gentiana chirayta.
CHIRETTA, Gentiana chirayta.
CHIRHEUMA, Chirrheuma.
CHIRIATER, Surgeon.
CHIRIATRIA, Surgery.
CHIRIMOYA, Anona tripetala.
CHIRISIS, Surgery.
CHIRISMUS, Surgery.
CHIRIXIS, Surgery.
CHIROCYRTO'SIS, from χειρ, 'the hand,' and κυρτωσις, 'crookedness.' Crookedness of the hand.
CHI'ROMANCY, Chiromanti'a, Vaticin'ium chiroman'ticum, Palm'istry, from χειρ, 'the hand,' and μαντεια, 'divination.' (F.) Chiromancie. Art of divining by inspection of the hand.
CHIRONAX, Surgeon.
CHIRO'NIA, (from Chiron, Χειρων, the Centaur, who is said to have discovered its use.) A genus of plants. Fam. Gentianeæ.
CHIRO'NIA ANGULA'RIS, Amer'ican Cen'taury, Rosepink, Wild Suc'cory, Bitterbloom, Centry, Sabba'tia, S. Angula'ris. Every part of this plant is a pure and strong bitter, which property is communicated alike to alcohol and water. It is used as a tonic and stomachic.
CHIRO'NIA CENTAU'RIUM, Centau'rium minus seu vulga'ré, Centau'rium parvum, Gentia'na centau'rium seu Gerar'di, Centau'rium minus, Erythræ'a Centau'rium, Hippocentaurea centau'rium, Centau'reum, Centau'ris, Smaller Cent'aury, Lesser Centaury, (F.) Centaurée petite. The tops of the lesser Centaury, Centau'rii Cacu'mina, are aromatic and tonic, and are sometimes employed as such.
CHIRO'NIA CHILEN'SIS, Gentia'na Cachenlahuen, Cachen-laguen, Chachinlagua, Chancelagua, Erythræ'a Chilensis, Gentia'na Peruvia'na. A very bitter plant, indigenous in Chili. It possesses the virtues of the Chironeæ. Given in infusion—(℥j, to water Oj.)

CHIRONI'UM, from χειρον, 'bad, malignant.' An ulcer difficult of cure :—of a swollen, hard, and callous nature.—Galen. Some have supposed the word to come from Chiron, the Centaur, who was unable to cure such ulcers.

CHIRONOMIA, Cheironomia.

CHIROP'ODIST, (F.) *Pédicure.* One who treats diseases of the hands and feet, or rather whose profession it is to remove corns and bunyons; from χειρ, 'the hand,' and πους, 'the foot.'

CHIRORRHEUMA, Chirrheuma.

CHIROSIS, Subactio.

CHIROSTROPHO'SIS, from χειρ, 'the hand,' and στροφειν, 'to turn.' Distortion of the hand.

CHIROTHE'CA, from χειρ, 'the hand,' and θηκη, 'a sheath.' A bandage for the hand. A kind of bandage in which the fingers and hand are enveloped in spiral turns. When the whole hand and fingers are covered, it is called the *double* or *complete Chirotheca, Ch. comple'ta, Vinctu'ra omnibus dig''itis;* and when only a finger is covered, the *half* or *incomplete, Ch. incomple'ta, Vinctu'ra pro uno diy''ito.* See *Gantelet.*

CHIROTRI'BIA, from χειρ, 'the hand,' and τριβω, 'I rub.' Friction with the hand. According to others, dexterity in an art.—Hippocrates, Galen.

CHIRRHEU'MA, *Chirorrheu'ma, Rheumatis'mus manûs,* from χειρ, 'the hand,' and ρευμα, 'flux.' Rheumatism of the hand.

CHIRURGEON, Surgeon.

CHIRURGI PHYSICI, see Surgeon.

CHIRURGIA, Surgery—c. Anaplastica, Morioplastice—c. Curtorum, Morioplastice—c. Infusoria, Infusion of medicines—c. Transfusoria, Transfusion.

CHIRURGICUS, Surgical.

CHIRURGIE, Surgery—*c. Militaire,* Surgery, military.

CHIRURGIEN, Surgeon—*c. Consultant,* Consulting Surgeon—*c. Hernieux,* see Hernial.

CHIRURGIQUE, Surgical.

CHIRURGUS, Surgeon.

CHIST. An Arabic word which signifies the sixth part. The sixth part of the *Congius* or gallon.

CHITON, Tunic.

CHITONISCUS, Indusium.

CHITTICK'S NOSTRUM, see Nostrum.

CHIUM VINUM. From *Chios,* the island where it was produced; *Chian wine;* used by the physicians of antiquity in cases of defluxions and ophthalmiæ.—Scribonius Largus.

CHLI'AROS, χλιαρος, 'tepid.' A name given to slight fevers, in which the heat is not great.—Galen.

CHLIAS'MA, χλιασμα, same etymon. A tepid and moist fomentation.—Hippocrates.

CHLOAS'MA, *Pityri'asis versic'olor, Mac'ula hepat'ica, Pannus hepat'icus, Hepat'izon, Phazè, Pha'cea, Phacus,* (F.) *Taches hépatiques, Chaleurs du foie, Éphélide scorbutique, Liverspot,* from χλοος, 'a greenish-yellow colour.' A cutaneous affection, characterized by one or more broad, irregular-shaped patches, of a yellow or yellowish-brown colour, occurring most frequently on the front of the neck, breast, abdomen, and groins. The patches do not generally rise above the surface. There is usually some degree of itching.

The causes are not very evident. Sulphur externally—in any and every form—generally removes it speedily. Should there be difficulty, the external use of the remedy in baths or fumigations may succeed.

CHLORA, Chlorine.

CHLORAS KALICUS DEPURATUS, Potassæ murias hyperoxygenatus.

CHLORASMA, Chlorosis.

CHLORE, Chlorine—*c. Liquide,* see Chlorine.

CHLORETUM CALCARIÆ, Calcis chloridum.

CHLORIASIS, Chlorosis.

CHLORIC ETHER, CONCENTRATED, see Ether, chloric—c. Ether, Strong, see Ether, chloric.

CHLORINE, from χλωρος, 'green.' *Chlo'rinum, Chlorin'ium, Chlora, Oxymuriat'ic Acid Gas, Oxygenated Muriatic Acid Gas, Dephlogisticated Marine Acid, Hal'ogene, Mu'rigene, Chlorum,* (F.) *Chlore.* So far as we know, this is an elementary substance. It is a greenish, yellow gas, of a strong suffocating smell, and disagreeable taste; incapable of maintaining combustion and respiration, and very soluble in water. One of its characteristics is, that of destroying, almost immediately, all vegetable and animal colours. It is employed in fumigations as a powerful disinfecting agent. A very dilute solution, *Aqua seu Liquor Chlo'rini,* (F.) *Chlore liquide,* has been administered internally, in certain cases of diarrhœa and chronic dysentery. Immersion of the hands and arms in it has often removed itch and other cutaneous affections. It has also been inhaled in a dilute state in the early stage of phthisis, but it is of doubtful efficacy, and is better adapted for chronic bronchitis.

CHLORINE, BISULPHURET OF, Sulphur, chloride of.

CHLO'ROFORM, *Chloroform'um, Carbo'neum chlora'tum, Superchlo'ridum formyl'icum, Perchloride* and *Terchloride of Formyl,* called also, but not correctly, *Terchloride of Carbon,* and *Chloric ether, Æther chlo'ricus,* (F.) *Chloroforme,* so called on account of the connexion of chlorine with formic acid, is a colourless, oleaginous liquid, of a sweetish ethereal odour, hot, aromatic, and peculiar taste. The specific gravity of that of the Ph. U. S. is 1.49. It may be obtained by distilling from a mixture of chlorinated lime and alcohol,—rectifying the product by redistillation, first from a great excess of chlorinated lime, and afterwards from strong sulphuric acid. It has been used with advantage in asthma, and in diseases in which a grateful soothing agent is required. Dose, fʒss to fʒj, diluted with water. It has likewise been prescribed with great success as an anæsthetic agent in spasmodic diseases; and to obtund sensibility in surgical operations and in parturition,—especially in the way of inhalation; but its use requires caution. See Anæsthetic.

CHLOROFORM, TINCTURE OF, Ether, chloric.

CHLOROFORMIZA'TION, *Chloroformisa'tio.* The aggregate of anæsthetic phenomena occasioned by the inhalation of chloroform.

CHLOROPHYLLE, Fecula, green.

CHLORO'SIS, from χλωρος, 'green,' *Pal'lidus Morbus, Fædus Vir'ginum color, Pal'lidus color virgin'eus, Pallidus morbus, Pallor vir'ginum, Icterit''ia alba, Ic'terus albus, Leucopathi'a, Morbus virgin'eus, Morbus Parthen'ius, Fædi colo'res, Dyspep'sia chloro'sis, Febris amato'ria, Cachexia vir'ginum, Febris vir'ginum, Febris alba, Anepithym'ia chloro'sis, Chloras'ma, Chloros'ma, Chlori'asis, Citto'sis, Green-sickness,* (F.) *Chlorose, Pâles-couleurs.* A disease which affects young females, more particularly those who have not menstruated. It is characterized by a pale, lurid complexion, languor, listlessness, depraved appetite and digestion, palpitation, &c. The disease generally goes off on the occurrence of the menstrual flux; but sometimes it is long before this is established, and, at times, the catamenia are in much larger quantity than usual. To this last form M. Trousseau has given the name *chlorose hémorrhagique.*

The blood of chlorosis is generally thin, light-coloured, and deficient in red corpuscles; and the clot is in less proportion to the serum than in health. On auscultation, a bellows' sound has been almost invariably detected over the heart, and a continuous blowing sound in the larger arteries, (especially the carotids and subclavians,) re-enforced by each systole of the ventricle, and resembling the buzzing of a humming-top, the cooing of doves, the whistling of air through a key-hole, &c., (see *Bruit*.) Very similar sounds are heard in the arteries after copious hemorrhage: they seem, therefore, to coincide with enfeebled circulation.

Tonics — as iron — are usually required in the treatment, — the disease most commonly occurring in those in whom there is considerable torpor of the system.

CHLOROSIS ÆTHIOPUM, Chthonophagia — c. Amatoria, Hectic fever — c. Gigantea, see Polysarcia.

CHLOROSMA, Chlorosis.

CHLOROT'IC, *Chlorot'icus*, (F.) *Chlorotique*. Affected with chlorosis, or pertaining to chlorosis; — as *chlorotic female, chlorotic symptoms*, &c.

CHLORUM, Chlorine.

CHLORURE DE CARBON, Chloroform — *c. d'Or*, Gold, Muriate of.

CHLORURETUM OXIDI CALCII, Calcis chloridum.

CHOA, Chu.

CHOA'CUM EMPLAS'TRUM NIGRUM. A black plaster, mentioned by Celsus, and composed of equal parts of litharge and resin. The litharge was first boiled in oil.

CHOAK, Cynanche trachealis — c. Wolf, Lycanche.

CHOANA, Pelvis — c. Cerebri, Infundibulum of the brain.

CHOANE, Infundibulum.

CHOANORRHAGIA, Epistaxis.

CHOAVA, Coffea Arabica.

CHOCOLATA, Chocolate — c. cum Osmazomâ, see Osmazome.

CHOC'OLATE, *Chocola'tum, Chocola'ta, Succola'ta, Succocolla'ta*. Dr. Alston says, that this word is compounded from two East Indian words: — *chooo*, 'sound,' and *atte*, 'water,' because of the noise made in its preparation. An alimentary paste prepared from the kernels of *Theobro'ma cacao* or *Cacao*, with sugar, and often aromatics. (See Cacao.) The chocolate thus simply prepared — as it is met with, indeed, in commerce — is called in France *Chocolat de santé*. It is not very easy of digestion.

The *chocolat à la vanille* contains three ounces of *vanilla* and two of *cinnamon* to twenty pounds of *common chocolate*. The addition of the aromatic renders it somewhat more digestible. Chocolates may likewise be medicated.

CHOCOLATE, OSMAZOME, see Osmazome.

CHOCOLATE ROOT, Geum Virginianum.

CHOCUS, Chu.

CHŒNICIS, Trepan.

CHŒNION, Cord.

CHŒNOS, Cord.

CHŒRAS, Scrofula.

CHOIROS, Vulva.

CHOKE DAMP, Carbonic acid.

CHOLA, Chole.

CHOLÆ'MIA; from χολη, 'bile,' and 'αιμα, 'blood.' A morbid state, in which bile exists in the blood. Jaundice.

CHOLAGO, Cholas.

CHOL'AGOGUE, *Cholago'gus, Chole'gos, Fellid'ucus, Bilit'icus*, from χολη, 'bile,' and αγω, 'I expel.' The ancients gave this name to cathartics, which were reputed to cause the flow of bile.

CHOLANSIS, Cholosis.

CHOLAS, χολας, plur. χολαδες. The epigastric region. *Chola'go*. The intestines.—Homer.

CHOLASMA, Cholosis.

CHOLÈ, *Cholus, Chola*, 'bile,' in composition. Hence:

CHOLEC'CHYSIS, *Cholen'chysis*; from χολη, 'bile,' and εγχυσις, 'effusion.' Effusion of bile.

CHOLECYST, Gall-bladder.

CHOLECYSTEURYS'MA, from χολη, 'bile,' κυστις, 'bladder,' and ευρυσμα, 'dilatation.' Dilatation of the gall-bladder.

CHOLECYSTI'TIS, *Inflamma'tio Vesi'cæ fell'ea, I. cyst'idis fell'ea, Cysti'tis fel'lea, Hepati'sis cyst'ica*, from χολη, 'bile,' and κυστις, 'bladder.' (F.) *Inflammation de la Vésicule du Fiel, Cholécystite*. Inflammation of the gall-bladder.

CHOL'EDOCH, *Choled'ochus*; from χολη, 'bile,' and δεχος, 'containing or receiving.' The *Ductus choledochus* seu *hep'ato-cyst'icus, Ductus communis choledochus*, (F.) *Conduit ou Canal Cholédoque*, is the duct formed by the union of the hepatic and cystic ducts, which pours the hepatic and cystic bile into the duodenum.

CHOLEDOCI'TIS, from *choledochus*, and *itis*; a suffix denoting inflammation. Inflammation of the choledoch duct.

CHOLEDOG'RAPHY, *choledogra'phia, Cholegraph'ia, Cholograph'ia*, from χολη, 'bile,' and γραφειν, 'to describe.' A description of what relates to the bile and biliary organs.

CHOLEDOL'OGY, *Choledolog"ia, Cholelog"ia, Chololog"ia*, from χολη, 'bile,' and λογος, 'a discourse.' A treatise on the bile and biliary organs.

CHOLEGOS, Cholagogue.

CHOLEGRAPHIA, Choledography.

CHOLEHÆMIA, Icterus.

CHOLEIA, Claudication.

CHOLELITHIA, Cysthepatolithiasis — c. Icterus, Icterus.

CHOLELITHIASIS, Cysthepatolithiasis.

CHOLELITHUS, Calculi, biliary.

CHOLELOGIA, Choledology.

CHOLEMES'IA, *Cholem'esis*, from χολη, 'bile,' and εμεσις, 'vomiting.' Vomiting of bile.

CHOLENCHYSIS, Cholecchysis.

CHOLEPYRA, Fever, bilious.

CHOLEPYRETUS, Fever, bilious.

CHOLEPYRRHIN, see Bile.

CHOLER, Bile. Anger was supposed to be produced by a superabundance of bile; hence the term *Choler* for anger.

CHOL'ERA, *Chol'era-morbus, Cholera nostras, Cholera vulga'ris, Sporad'ic Chol'era, Cholerrha'gia, Pas'sio choler'ica, Fellif'lua passio, Morbus fellif'luus, Hol'era, Bilis flux'io*, (F.) *Choladrée lymphatique, Hydrocholadrée, Choléra-morbus sporadique, Ch. Europe'en, Trousse-galant*, from χολη, 'bile,' and ρεω, 'I flow.' According to others, from χολαδες, 'intestines,' or from χελρα, 'the gutter of a house to carry off the rain.' The higher degrees have been called *Centroganglii'tis*, and *Myelι ganglii'tis*. A disease characterized by anxiety, gripings, spasms in the legs and arms, and by vomiting and purging (generally bilious:) vomiting and purging are, indeed, the essential symptoms. The disease is most common in hot climates, — and in temperate climates, during summer. In India, *Spasmod'ic chol'era, Asiat'ic cholera, Malig'nant ch., In'dian ch., Epidem'ic ch., Pestilen'tial ch., Asphyx'ia pestilen'ta, Pestilen'tial asphyx'ia, Chol'eric Pest'-ilence, Eastern ch., Orien'tal ch., Cholera orienta'lis, Ch. In'dica, Ch. Epidem'ica, Typhus Bengalen'sis, Chol'ero-typhus, Ganglioni'tis peripher'-ica et medulla'ris, Hymenoganglii'tis, Pantoganglii'tis, Cholerrhæ'a lymphat'ica, Psorenter'ia*;

CHORIONITIS. Induration of the Cellular tissue.

CHOROID, *Choroi'deus, Choroi'des, Chorioi'des, Chorio'des,* from χοριον, 'the chorion,' and ειδος, 'shape,' 'resemblance.' Several parts are so called, which resemble the chorion, in the multitude of their vessels.

CHOROID MUSCLE, Ciliary muscle.

CHOROI'DEA seu CHORIOI'DEA TU'NICA, *Ch. Membra'na,* or simply *the Choroid, Tu'nica vasculo'sa Oc'uli, T. œiniform'is seu rhagoi'des,* (F.) *Membrane choroïde, Choroïde.* A thin membrane, of a very dark colour, which lines the sclerotica, internally. The part behind the iris is called *Uvea.* It is situate between the sclerotica and retina, has an opening, posteriorly, for the passage of the optic nerve; and terminates, anteriorly, at the great circumference of the iris, where it is continuous with the ciliary processes. According to Ruysch, the choroid consists of two layers, to the innermost of which his son gave the name *Tu'nica Ruyschia'na, Membra'na Ruyschia'na,* (F.) *Membrane Ruyschienne.* The internal surface of the membrane is covered with a dark pigment, consisting of several layers of pigment cells, called *Pigmen'tum nigrum, Stratum pigmen'ti, Ophthalmochroï'tes, Æthiops animal,* (F.) *Enduit choroïdien.* Its use seems to be, to absorb the rays of light after they have traversed the retina.

CHOROI'DES PLEXUS, *Plexus choroï'deus seu reticula'ris, Vermes cer'ebri, Choroid Plexus.* Two membranous and vascular duplicatures of the pia mater, situate in the lateral ventricles. They are fixed to the *Tela choroïdea* by one edge, and are loose and floating at the other.

CHOROIDEA TELA, (F.) *Toile choroïdienne.* A kind of vasculo-membranous prolongation of the pia mater, which lines the lower surface of the fornix united with the corpus callosum. It is stretched above the third ventricle, and covers the posterior commissure and corpora quadrigemina. Anteriorly, the tela choroïdea is continuous with the plexus choroides.

CHOROIDEÆ VENÆ, *Venæ Gale'ni,* (F.) *Veines choroïdiennes.* Two veins, that creep along the tela choroïdea; into which almost all those of the lateral ventricles, of the upper part of the cerebellum, of the pineal gland, and the corpora quadrigemina open. The Venæ Galeni open into the *sinus quartus* or *fourth sinus.*

CHOROÏDE, CEINTURE BLANCHE DE LA, Ciliary ligament—*c. Commissure de la,* Ciliary ligament.

CHOROÏDITIS, Choriodeitis.

CHOROÏ'DO-RETINI'TIS. Inflammation of the choroid and retina.

CHOROMANIA, Chorea.

CHOSES CONTRE NATURE, Res contra naturam—*c. Naturelles,* Res naturales—*c. non Naturelles,* Res non naturales.

CHOSIS, Arenatio.

CHOU CABUS, Brassica capitata—*c. Croûte, Sauer Kraut*—*c. Fleur,* Brassica Florida—*Cauliflower excrescence*—*c. Marin,* Convolvulus soldanella—*c. Navet,* Brassica rapa—*c. Pommé,* Brassica capitata—*c. Potager,* Brassica—*c. Roquette,* Brassica eruca.

CHREMMA, Sputum.

CHREMPSIS, Exspuition.

CHRISIS, from χριω, 'I anoint.' The action of anointing. Inunction.

CHRISMA, same etymon. The act of anointing. The salve or liniment used. Prurigo.

CHRISTI MANUS. Troches prepared from refined sugar boiled in rose-water with or without prepared pearls.

CHRISTOPHER HERB, Actæa spicata.

CHRISTOPHORIANA SPICATA, Actæa spicata.

CHRISTOS, χριστος, from χριω, 'I anoint.' Any medicine applied under the form of liniment or ointment.

CHROA, *Chræa, Chroma.* Colour in general. The surface of the body. The skin.

CHRŒAS, Scrofula.

CHROMA, Chroa.

CHROMATOG"ENOUS, from χρωμα, 'colour,' and γενναω, 'I make.'

CHROMATOG"ENOUS APPARA'TUS. A particular apparatus for producing the colouring matter of the skin, composed of a glandular or secreting parenchyma, situate a little below the papillæ, and presenting special excretory ducts, which pour out the colouring matter on the surface of the true skin.—Breschet.

CHROMATOMETABLEPSIA, Achromatopsia.

CHROMATOPHO'BIA, from χρωμα, 'colour,' and φοβος, 'dread.' Morbid sensibility to certain colours.

CHROMATOPSEUDOPSIA, Achromatopsia.

CHROMATOPSIA, Chromopsia.

CHROMIC ACID, *Ac"idum Chro'micum,* (F.) *Acide chromique.* Obtained by crystallization from a mixture of *bichromate of potassa,* and *oil of vitriol.* It has been used as an escharotic in external hemorrhoids.

CHROMIDRO'SIS, from χρωμα, 'colour,' and ιδρως, 'sweat.' Abnormal coloration of the perspiratory secretion.

CHROMOP'SIA, *Chromop'ia, Chromatop'sia, Chrotop'sia, Chrup'sia, Crop'sia, Visus colora'tus, Suffu'sio colo'rans,* from χρωμα, 'colour,' and οψις, 'vision.' A state of vision in which a coloured impression is made on the retina. Said to be occasionally observed in jaundice.

CHRONAGUNEA, Menstruation.

CHRONIC, *Chron'icus, Chro'nius, Polychro'nius, Invetera'tus, Anti'quus, Denæ'us,* from χρονος, 'time.' Of long duration.

CHRONIC DISEASES, *Morbi chron'ici, Macronos'iæ, Macro'siæ,* (F.) *Maladies Chroniques,* are those whose duration is long, or whose symptoms proceed slowly. The antithesis to *chronic* is *acute.*

CHRONO, from χρονος, 'time.' A prefix to terms denoting inflammation of a part, to show that such inflammation is chronic.—Piorry.

CHRONO-HÉPATITE, Hepatitis, chronic.

CHRONO-NÉPHRITE, Nephritis (chronic.)

CHRONO-THERMAL, from χρονος, 'time,' and θερμη, 'heat.' Relating to time and temperature. An epithet given to a fanciful 'system' by Dr. Samuel Dickson, which maintains, that there can be no increase or diminution of temperature without motion; no motion without time; that motion consists in attraction and repulsion; that attraction and repulsion are peculiar to electric action; and hence, that medicines must change the motions of the system, and be electrical in their operation.

CHROTOPSIA, Chromopsia.

CHRUPSIA, Chromopsia.

CHRYSALEA, Nitro-muriatic acid.

CHRYSANTHEMUM, Calendula officinalis.

CHRYSAN'THEMUM LEUCAN'THEMUM, from χρυσος, 'gold,' and ανθος, 'a flower.' The Ox-eye daisy, *Daisy, Whiteweed, Goldens, Maudlinwort, Bellis major seu praten'sis, Buphthal'mum majus, Leucan'themum vulga'rē, Matrica'ria Leucanth'emum, Bellidioi'des, Consol'ida media, Oc'ulus Bovis,* (F.) *Chrysanthème, Chrysène, Grand Marguerite des prés.* The flowers and herb are slightly acrid; and were once used in pulmonary diseases.

CHRYSANTHEMUM PARTHENIUM, Matricaria parthenium.

CHRYSE, from χρυσος, 'gold.' The name of a yellow plaster, described by Paulus of Ægina, and composed of thus, alum, lead, colophony, resin, oil, and orpiment, boiled in vinegar.

CHRYSENE, Chrysanthemum leucanthemum.

CHRYSITIS, see Plumbi oxidum semivitreum.

CHRYSOBALANUS GALENI, see Myristica moschata.

CHRYSOCALIS, Matricaria.

CHRYSOCHALCOS, Brass.

CHRYSOCOLLA, Borax.

CHRYSOCOMA, Millefolium.

CHRYSOLACHANUM, Chenopodium bonus Henricus.

CHRYSOL'ITHUS, Chrys'olite, from χρυσος, 'gold,' and λιθος, 'stone.' A precious stone, of a golden colour, regarded by the ancients as cardiac, cephalic, &c.

CHRYSOMELIA, see Citrus aurantium.

CHRYSOPHYL'LUM CAINI'TO, from χρυσος 'gold,' and φυλλον, 'a leaf.' Cainito, Siderox'ylon, Broad-leaved Star-apple. A tree of the Antilles, which produces one of the best fruits of the country. There are several varieties of it.

CHRYSOPHYLLUM GLYCIPHLÆUM, Monesia.

CHRYSOPUS, Cambogia.

CHRYSOS, Gold.

CHRYSOSPERMUM, Sempervivum tectorum.

CHRYZA FIBRAUREA, Coptis.

CHTHONOPHA'GIA, Cachex'ia Africa'na, Mala'cia Africano'rum, Pica Africano'rum, Leucophlegma'tia Æthio'pum, Chloro'sis Æthiopum, Dirt-eating, (F.) Mal d'Estomac, from χθων, 'earth,' and φαγω, 'I eat.' A disorder of the nutritive functions observed amongst the negroes of the South and of the West Indies, in which there is an irresistible desire to eat earth. It is accompanied by most of the signs of chlorosis.

CHU, Choa or Chus, χυς, Chocus. A liquid measure amongst the Greeks, answering to the Congius of the Romans, and containing six sextarii, or twelve Attic cotylæ, or nine pints.—Galen.

CHURRUS, see Bangue.

CHUTE, Prolapsus—c. du Fondement, Proctocele—c. de la Matrice, Procidentia uteri—c. des Oufs, see Parturition—c. du Rectum, Proctocele.

CHYLAIRE, Chylous.

CHYLAR, Chylous.

CHYLARION, Chyle.

CHYLE, Chylus, Succus nutrit"ius, from χυω, 'I flow.' The word, in Hippocrates, means Tisane or Decoction of Barley, Chyla'rion, χυλαριον. Galen first used it in its present sense;—i. e. for a nutritive fluid, extracted by intestinal absorption, from food which has been subjected to the action of the digestive organs. It is of a whitish appearance; is separated from the chyme in the duodenum, and the rest of the small intestines, and is absorbed by the chyliferous vessels, which arise at the mucous surface of the intestine. Along these it passes through the mesenteric glands to the thoracic duct, and is finally poured into the left subclavian. It is composed, like the blood, of a coagulable part and of serum. Chyle corpuscles or globules, exist in it, the average size of which is about 1-4600th of an inch. See Chyme.

CHYLE CORPUSCLES, see Chyle.

CHYLEUX, Chylous.

CHYLIF'EROUS, Chy'lifer, Chylif'erus, Chyloph'orus; from chylus, 'chyle,' and ferre, 'to carry.' Chyle-bearing.

CHYLIF'EROUS VESSELS, Vasa Chylif'era seu Chylos'era, Viæ chylif'eræ, Venæ lacteæ, Vasa lactea. The Lacteals. (F.) Vaisseaux chylifères, V. Lactés. Vessels which convey the chyle from the intestines to the thoracic duct.

CHYLIFICA'TION, Chylifica'tio, Chylo'sis, Chylopoie'sis, Præpara'tio chyli, from chylus, 'chyle,' and facere, 'to make.' Formation of chyle by the digestive processes.

CHYLINE, Cyclamen.

CHYLISMA, Succus expressus.

CHYLIS'MUS, from χυλος, 'juice.' The act of expressing the juice of vegetables, &c.

CHYLOCYSTIS, Receptaculum chyli.

CHYLODES, Chylous.

CHYLODIABETES, Chyluria.

CHYLODIARRHŒA, Cœliac flux.

CHYLODOCHIUM, Receptaculum chyli.

CHYLOG'RAPHY, from χυλος, 'chyle,' and γραφη, 'a description.' A description of the anatomy, &c., of the chyliferous vessels.

CHYLOPOIESIS, Chylification.

CHYLOPOIET'IC, Chylopoiet'icus, Chylopoi'sus, from χυλος, 'chyle,' and ποιεω, 'I make.' Relating to or connected with the formation of chyle. Chiefly applied to the organs immediately concerned in it; as the stomach, intestines, omenta, and mesentery. Assistant Chylopoietic:—applied to viscera which aid in the formation of chyle, as the liver and pancreas.

CHYLORRHŒA, Cœliac flux—c. Pectoris, Chylothorax—c. Renalis, Chyluria—c. Urinalis, Chyluria.

CHYLOSIS, Chylification.

CHYLOSTAG'MA DIAPHORET'ICUM MINDERE'RI. A compound prepared by distilling the theriac of Andromachus, the mithridate of Damocrates, and other alexipharmics, &c. It is nearly the same preparation as the Aqua Theriaca'lis Bezoar'dica.

CHYLOTHO'RAX, Pleurorrhœ'a chylo'sa, Chylorrhœ'a Pec'toris, Hydrotho'rax chylo'sus; from χυλος, 'chyle,' and θωραξ, 'the chest.'— Effusion of chyle into the chest, owing to the rupture of a chyliferous vessel.

CHYLOUS, Chylar, Chylo'sus vel Chyla'ris, Chylo'des, (F.) Chyleux, Chylaire. Relating to the chyle; or having some analogy to that fluid.

CHYLU'RIA, Diabe'tes lac'tea, D. Chylo'sus, Chylodiabe'tes, Galactu'ria, Fluxus cœliacus per Renes, Pyu'ria lac'tea, P. Chylo'sa, Cœliaca urina'lis, C. rena'lis Chylorrhœ'a urina'lis, Ch. rena'lis, from χυλος, 'chyle,' and ουρον, 'urine.' (F.) Diabète chyleux. A discharge of milky urine, without any apparent lesion of the kidneys or bladder.

CHYLUS, Chyle, Decoction, Succus.

CHYME, Chymus, χυμος, 'juice,' from χυω, 'I flow.' The pulp, formed by the food, mixed with the supra-diaphragmatic and gastric secretions, after it has been for some time in the stomach. In this it continues until it reaches the biliary and pancreatic ducts, which open into the duodenum; where the conversion into chyle occurs, which is absorbed by the chyliferous vessels,— the excrementitious portion of the food traversing the large intestine to be evacuated per anum. Castelli asserts, that Chyme and Chyle were used in an inverse sense by the ancients, from that accepted at present.

CHYMI, Humours.

CHYMIA, Chymistry—c. Organica, Chymistry, organic—c. Pharmaceutica, see Chymistry.

CHYMIA'TER, Chimia'ter, Chemia'ter, from χυμεια or χημεια, 'chymistry,' and ιατρος, 'a physician,' Iatro-chym'icus. A chemical physician.

CHYMIATRI'A, Chymiatri'a, Chemiatri'a, Iatro-chemi'a, Medici'na spagir'ica, Ars Chymiat'rica, from χυμεια or χημεια, 'chymistry,' and ιατρεια, 'cure.' The art of curing by chemical means.

CHYM'ICAL, Chem'ical, Chem'icus, Chemo'ticus. A medicine formed by the aid of chymistry, in contradistinction to Galenical.

CHYM'ICO-HISTOL'OGY, *Chym'ico-histolog''-ia, Chem'ico-histol'ogy.* The doctrine of the organic chemistry and morphology of tissues.

CHYMICOPHANTA, Chymist.

CHYMICUS, Chymical, Chymist.

CHYMIE, Chymistry.

CHYMIFICA'TION, *Chymifica'tio, Chymo'sis,* from χυμος, 'juice,' and *facere,* 'to make.' Formation of chyme.

CHYM'IST, *Chem'ist, Chem'icus, Chymicophan'ta, Chym'icus,* (F.) *Chimiste* ou *Chymiste.* One acquainted with chymistry. In Great Britain it has, also, the signification of "one who sells chemicals."

CHYMISTE, Chymist.

CHYM'ISTRY, *Chem'istry, Chemi'a, Chymi'a, Chimi'a, Chemeu'ticĕ, Chemot'icĕ, Philosoph'ia per ignem, Spagy'ria, Pyrotech'nia, Pyrosoph'ia, Ars hermet'ica, Archima'gia, Ars mago'rum, Ars separato'ria, Ars spagir'ica;* from χυμος, 'juice,' or from Arab, *chema,* 'a secret.' (F.) *Chimie* ou *Chymie.* A branch of the natural sciences, whose object is to investigate the nature and properties of bodies, simple and compound, inorganic and organized; and to study the force or power, by virtue of which every combination is effected. It investigates the action between the integrant molecules or atoms of bodies.

Organic Chemistry, Chymi'a organ'ica, Organochemi'a, is the chymistry of organized substances,—animal and vegetable.

Animal Chym'istry, Zoöch'emy or *Zoöch'ymy, Zoochemi'a,* is the chymistry of substances afforded by the dead or living animal body. This branch of chymistry has been farther subdivided into *physiological,* when it considers the changes produced in organized bodies in health, *pathological,* when it regards those produced by organic or other diseases. *Anthropochymy, Anthropochemi'a,* is the chymistry of the human body. Chymistry is called *Therapeu'tical* or *Pharmaceu'tical, Pharmaco-chymi'a, Chymi'a pharmaceu'tica,* when it is engaged in the analysis of simple medicines; in improving the prescribing and preparing of chemical and Galenical medicines; in the means of preparing them, and detecting adulterations, &c. *Hygiĕn'ic Chym'istry* is that which is applied to the means of rendering habitations healthy, of analyzing the air we breathe, preventing the occurrence of disease, pointing out healthy aliments, and appreciating the influence of professions, &c. on the health of man. All these different subdivisions, with vegetable chymistry, are, at times, included under the head of *Medical Chym'istry, Phytochymistry;* at others, the term comprehends only the *Animal, Vegetable* and *Pharmaceutical* subdivisions.

Vital Chemistry, Biochymi'a, is that which is executed under the influence of vitality.

A knowlege of chymistry is of great importance to the physician. Many of the functions are of a chemical nature: many diseases require a chemical mode of treatment; and, without an acquaintance with it, two or more substances might be given in combination, which, by forming a chemical union, might give rise to other compounds, possessing very different virtues from the components taken singly, and thus the prescriber be disappointed in the results.

CHYMISTRY, ANIMAL, see Chymistry—c. Hygienic, see Chymistry—c. Medical, see Chymistry—c. Organic, see Chymistry—c. Pharmaceutic, see Chymistry—c. Therapeutical, see Chymistry—c. Vegetable, see Chymistry—c. Vital, see Chymistry.

CHYMOCHEZIA, Cœliac flux.

CHYMOPLANIA, (G.) Chymoplanien, Dyschymosen, from χυμος, 'juice,' and πλανη, 'wandering.' A transposition of secretions:—a family of diseases in the classification of Fuchs, which includes icterus, uroplania, menoplania and galactoplania.

CHYMORRHŒA, Cœliac flux, Lientery.

CHYMOSIN, Pepsin.

CHYMOSIS, Chymification.

CHYMOZEMIA, Hypercrinia.

CHYTLEN, RADIX. A cylindrical root, bitter and inodorous, brought from China. It is held by the Chinese to be stomachic. — Murray.

CHYT'LON, χυτλον, from χεω, 'I pour out.' A liquid formerly used for rubbing the body after bathing.

CIBARIUM, Aliment.

CIBA'RIUS PANIS, 'Coarse bread.' Bread made of second flour. — Celsus.

CIBA'TIO. *Trophē.* The taking of food. In Pharmacy, it is the same as Incorporation.

CIBUS, Aliment—c. Albus, *Blancmanger*—c. Deorum, Asafœtida.

CICATRICE, Cicatrix.

CICATRICES OVARIORUM, Stigmata ovariorum.

CICATRIC'ULA. Diminutive of *Cicatrix.* A *small cica'trix, Stigma.* The term is, also, applied to a small white spot, called the tread, *chal'asa, chala'zium,* observable at the surface of a fecundated egg. See Molecule.

CICATRISAN'TIA, *Epulot'ica, Synulot'ica, Apulot'ica, Catulot'ica, Ulot'ica.* Remedies formerly considered to be capable of producing cicatrization.

CICA'TRIX, *Cæca'trix, Ulē, Oulē,* from *cæcare,* 'to conceal,' because it conceals the wound. (F.) *Cicatrice.* The union of parts, which have been divided. A *scar* or formation, of a reddish colour, afterwards whitish, and of variable thickness, which takes place at the surface of wounds or ulcers after their cure. A cicatrix may vary much in shape, consistence, and thickness. The cicatrix of a bone is called Callus. A *vic''ious cica'trix,* (F.) *Cicatrice vicieuse,* is one which interferes with the action of the parts on which it occurs. The *scars* after small-pox, are called *Pits* or *Pockmarks,* (F.) *Coutures par la petite vérole.*

CICATRIX VARIOLÆ, Pockmark.

CICATRIZA'TION, *Cicatrisa'tio, Epulo'sis, Synulo'sis.* The process by which a cicatrix is formed. Every tissue, except the nails, epidermis, hair, and enamel is, probably, capable of cicatrization.

CICELY, SWEET, Chærophyllum odoratum, Osmorrhiza longistylis, Scandix odorata.

CICER ARIETI'NUM. The *Cicer* plant, *Erebin'thus,* (F.) *Cicérole, Pois Chiche.* The seeds are ground into flour, and used as bread in some countries.

CICER LENS, Ervum lens.

CI'CERA TAR'TARI. Small pills of turpentine and cream of tartar—of the size of a vetch or *cicer.*

CICERBITA, Sonchus oleraceus.

CICÉROLE, Cicer arietinum.

CICHO'RIUM ENDIV'IA. The systematic name of the *Endive, Endiv'ia, Endi'va, In'tubum, In'tybum (Antiq.), Scariola, In'tybus horten'sis,* (F.) *Chicorée des Jardins, Scariole. Family,* Cichoraceæ. *Sex. Syst.* Syngenesia Polygamia æqualis. It is a common pot herb, and is eaten as salad.

CICHO'RIUM IN'TYBUS, *Seris, Seriola, In'tubum errat'icum.* The systematic name of the *Wild Suc'cory, Wild Cich'ory, Cich'ory, Wild Endive, Ambulei'a, Heliotro'pion, Catanan'cē, Cicho'reum,* (F.) *Chicorée sauvage.* It is bitter, and was once used as a tonic. The root, roasted and ground, is often used instead of, or mixed with, coffee.

CHICORY, WILD, Cichorium intybus.
CICI, Ricinis communis.
CICINDE'LA, *Lam'pyris, Noctil'uca, Nited'ula.* The *Glow-worm.* (F.) *Ver luisant.* This insect was once thought to be anodyne and lithontriptic.
CICIS, see Quercus infectoria.
CIGON'GIUS; an ancient measure, containing 12 pints.
CICUTA, Conium maculatum.
CICU'TA AQUAT'ICA, *Cicu'ta viro'sa, Cicuta'ria aquat'ica, Corian'drum cicu'ta,* Water Hemlock, Cowbane, (F.) *Ciguë aquatique* ou *vireuse.* Family, Umbelliferæ. *Sex. Syst.* Pentandria Digynia. A violent poison, often eaten by mistake for *Wild Smallage, Apium Graveolens.* It produces tremors, vertigo, burning at the stomach, and all the symptoms occasioned by the *Narcotico-acrid* class of poisons.

CICU'TA MACULA'TA, (F.) *Ciguë d'Amérique,* American water hemlock, American Hemlock, Snakeweed, Death of man, Water parsley, Poison root, Wild Hemlock, Children's bane, is analogous in botanical character and medical properties to the European species. See Conium Maculatum.

CICUTA MAJOR, Conium maculatum—c. Major fœtida, Conium maculatum—c. Stoerkii, Conium maculatum—c. Terrestris, Conium maculatum—c. Virosa, Cicuta aquatica—c. Vulgaris, Conium maculatum.

CICUTARIA, Chærophyllum sylvestre—c. Aquatica, Cicuta aquatica, Phellandrium aquaticum—c. Odorata, Chærophyllum odoratum.

CIDER, *Poma'ceum,* (F.) *Cidre.* This word is said to have been formerly written *sidre,* and to have come from *Sic'era,* σικερα, which signifies any kind of fermented liquor other than wine. It is made from the juice of apples, and, when good, is a wholesome drink.

CIDRE, Cider.

CIGNUS; an ancient measure, which contained about two drachms.

CIGUË AQUATIQUE, Cicuta aquatica—*c. d'Amérique,* Cicuta maculata—*c. d'Eau,* Phellandrium aquaticum—*c. Grande,* Conium maculatum—*c. Ordinaire,* Conium maculatum—*c. Petite,* Æthusa cynapium—*c. Vireuse,* Cicuta aquatica.

CIL'IA, *Blephar'ides, Pili palpebra'rum.* The *eyelashes.* The hairs on the eyelids. (F.) *Cils.* Their use seems to be, to prevent the entrance into the eye of light bodies flying in the atmosphere; and to diminish, in certain cases, the intensity of light. Also, the tarsi. Also, a peculiar sort of moving organs, resembling small hairs, *vi'bratory* or *vi'bratile cil'ia, Cil'ia vibrato'ria,* (F.) *Cils vibratils,* which are visible with the microscope in many animals. These organs are found on parts of the body, which are habitually in contact with water, or other more or less fluid matters, and produce motion in these fluids, impelling them along the surface of the parts. Cilia have been found to exist in all vertebrated animals except fishes, having been discovered on the respiratory and uterine mucous membranes of mammalia, birds, and reptiles.

The terms *"vibratory motion"* and *"ciliary motion"* have been used to express the phenomena exhibited by the moving cilia; and it is probable, that this motion is concerned in the progression of fluids along the membranes. As yet, the motion has been observed only in the direction of the outlets of canals.

CILIAIRE, Ciliary.

CIL'IARY, *Cilia'ris,* (F.) *Ciliaire.* Relating to the eyelashes, or to *cilia.* This epithet has, also, been applied to different parts, which enter into the structure of the eye; from the resemblance between some of them *(the ciliary processes)* and the eyelashes.

CILIARY AR'TERIES, *Arte'riæ cilia'res,* (F.) *Artères ciliaires.* These are furnished by the ophthalmic artery. They are distinguished into 1. Short or *posterior (Art. uvéales*—Chauss.) 30 or 40 in number, which are distributed to the ciliary processes. 2. *Long,* (*Art. Iriennes* of Chauss.,) two in number, which, by the anastomoses of their branches, form two arterial circles at the anterior surface of the iris: and, 3. The *anterior, Arte'riæ cilia'res anterio'res* of Haller, the number of which is variable. These pierce the sclerotic a few lines from its union with the cornea; and are principally distributed to the iris.

CILIARY BODY, *Corpus Cilia'rë, Nexus Stamin'eus Oc'uli, Coro'na Cilia'ris, Ciliary Disc,* (F.) *Corps ciliaire.* A ring of the choroid surrounding the crystalline in the manner of a crown; placed behind the iris and the ciliary circle. It resembles the disk of a radiated flower, and is formed by the union of the ciliary processes. See Ciliary Muscle.

CILIARY CANAL, *Canal of Fonta'na.* A small, extremely narrow circular space, formed between the ciliary circle, the cornea, and the sclerotica. It can be filled with injection, and it is not certain that it is not the cavity of a blood-vessel.

CILIARY CIRCLE, Ciliary ligament — c. Disc, Ciliary body—c. Ganglion, Ophthalmic ganglion.

CILIARY LIG'AMENT, *C. Circle* or *Ring, Ligamen'tum* seu *Instertit"ium cilia'rë, L. l'ridis, Plexus cilia'ris, An'nulus* seu *Cir'culus* seu *Or'bic'ulus cilia'ris, A. cellulo'sus, Com'missure of the Uvea, Commissure de la Choroïde,*—(Ch.,) (F.) *Ligament* ou *Cercle ciliaire, Cercle de la Choroïde, Ceinture blanche de la Choroïde.* A species of greyish ring, of a pulpy consistence, situate between the choroid, iris, and sclerotica. The internal surface of the choroid is uniform, until it approaches within ten lines and a-half of the edge of the cornea; here a dentated line is observed, termed *ora serra'ta.* The outer surface presents the *an'nulus al'bidus* seu *gangliform'is,* the anterior edge of which unites to the inner surface of the sclerotica and constitutes the *ciliary ligament.*

CIL'IARY MARGIN OT TARSAL MARGIN of the eyelids; (F.) *Bord ciliaire.* The edge in which the cilia or eyelashes are situate.

CILIARY MOTION, see Cilia.

CILIARY MUSCLE, *Mus'culus cilia'ris.* The part of the orbicularis palpebrarum in the vicinity of the ciliary margin. Also, the greyish, semi-transparent structure behind the ciliary ligament and covering the outside of the ciliary body. By its contraction the ciliary processes, and with them the lens, must be drawn towards the cornea. It appears to be the same muscle as the *Tensor choroïdeæ* or *choroid muscle* of some anatomists.

CILIARY NERVES (*Nerfs Iriens,*—Chauss.) (F.) *Nerfs ciliaires.* These are 12 to 16 in number. They arise from the nasal nerve, and particularly from the anterior part of the ophthalmic ganglion; and unite in two fasciculi, which pass around the optic nerve, and pierce the sclerotica near the entrance of that nerve into the eye. They are lost in the ciliary ligament.

CILIARY PLEXUS, C. Ligament.

CILIARY PROC"ESSES, *Proces'sus cilia'res, Rad'ii* seu *Striæ cilia'res, Rayons sous-iriens*—(Ch.,) (F.) *Procès ciliaires.* Triangular folds, sixty or eighty in number, placed at the side of each other, and radiating, so as to resemble the disk of a radiated flower. They are lodged in depressions at the anterior part of the vitreous humour. The uses of these processes are not known.

CILIARY RING, Ciliary ligament.

CILIARY STRIÆ are numerous, pale, radiated striæ in the posterior portion of the *Corpus ciliare*, but so covered by the *Pigmentum nigrum* as not to be distinctly seen till the paint is removed. The ciliary processes are formed by these striæ.

CILIARY VEINS, (F.) *Veines ciliaires*, follow nearly the same course as the arteries. In the choroid they are so tortuous, that they have received the name *Vasa vortico'sa*. They open into the ophthalmic vein.

CILIARY ZONE, *Zona seu Zo'nula Cilia'ris, Membran'ula Coro'næ Cilia'ris*. Under the corpus ciliare, the capsule of the vitreous humour sends off an external lamina, which accompanies the retina, and is inserted, with it, into the forepart of the capsule of the lens, a little before its anterior edge. This is the *Zonula ciliaris, Zonula Zin'nii* or *Zonula of Zinn, Coro'na Cilia'ris, Orbic'ulus Cilia'ris*. It is of a striated appearance and circular form, and assists in fixing the lens to the vitreous humour.

CIL'IATED, *Cilia'tus;* from *cilia*. Provided with cilia—as "*ciliated* epithelium," the epithelium to which vibratory cilia are attached.

CILLEMENT, Nictation.

CILLO. A name given by some authors to those whose upper eyelid is perpetually tremulous;—a trembling, which in some cases is called *Life's blood*. "To have life's blood in the eye," in other words, is to have this affection. Vogel calls it *Cillo'sis*.

CILLOSIS, Cillo.

CILS, Cilia—c. Vibratila, see Cilia.

CIMEX, Κορις, *Cimex lectula'rius*. The Wall or House or Bed Bug or *Chinche*. (F.) *Punaise*. Six or seven of these, given internally, are said to have prevented ague! There is scarcely any thing which is sufficiently disgusting, that has not been exhibited for this purpose, and with more or less success. The bug has also been esteemed emmenagogue.

CIMICIFUGA, Actæa racemosa.

CIMO'LIA PURPURES'CENS, *Terra Saponaʼria, Terra Fullon'ica, Fuller's Earth*. A compact, bolar earth, employed in the arts. Used at times as a cooling application to inflamed nipples, &c.

CIMO'LIA TERRA, *Cimo'lia alba, Smectis, Smectris, Cimo'lus;* from Κιμωλος, an island in the Cretan Sea, where it is procured. It was formerly used as an astringent, &c.—Scribonius Largus, Pliny. Probably, the same as the last.

CINA CINA, Cinchona—c. Levantica, Artemisia Santonica.

CINABARIS, Hydrargyri sulphuretum rubrum.

CINABARIUM, Hydrargyri sulphuretum rubrum.

CIN'ABRA, *Grasus*. The smell of a he-goat. A rank smell, like that of the armpit, *Hircus ala'rum*.

CINÆDIA, Masturbation.

CINARA HORTENSIS, Cynara scolymus—c. Scolymus, Cynara Scolymus.

CINCHO'NA. So called from the Spanish Viceroy's lady, the Countess de Cinchon, who was cured of fever by it at Lima, about 1638. Called also *Cortex seu Pulvis Jesuit'icus, Jesuit's Bark* or *Powder, Cortex Patrum*, because it was introduced into Europe by the Jesuits; and also *Pulvis Comitis'sæ* or the *Countess's Powder*, and *Cardinal del Lugo's Powder, Cortex Cardina'lis de Lugo*, because he introduced it at Rome. It is the pharmacopœial name of several kinds of barks from various species of Cinchona, from the western coast of South America. *Nat. Order*, Cinchonaceæ. *Sex. Syst.* Pentandria Monogynia. Called, also, *Cortex, Bark, Peruvian Bark, English Remedy, Cortex China, Cortex Chinæ Regius, China, Chincki'na, Palos de Calentura, Kina Kina, (Bark of Barks,) Kinki'na, Cina Cina, Quina Quina, Quinqui'na, Magnum Dei donum*, (F.) *Quinquina*.

CINCHO'NÆ CARIBÆ'Æ CORTEX, from *Exostem'ma Caribæ'um, Caribæ'an Bark; Saint Lucia Bark*, (F.) *Écorce de Saint Lucie, Quinquina Piton*, from *Exoste'ma floribund'um;* and the *Pitaya Bark, Quinquina bi'color*, from an exostemma (?) or from strychnos pseudoquina (?), are useful substitutes for the cinchona of Peru. These are the most important spurious barks. They contain neither quinia nor cinchonia.

CINCHONÆ CORDIFO'LIÆ CORTEX, *Cortex flavus, Cinchonæ officina'lis cortex flavus, Yellow Bark, Calisay'a Bark*, (F.) *Quinquina jaune ou jaune royal, Calasaya*. Odour aromatic; taste strong, bitter, astringent. Not rolled; often without the epidermis, which is very thick and inert; light, friable; fracture fibrous. Active principle *Quinia*.

CINCHONÆ LANCIFO'LIÆ CORTEX, *Cortex Peruvia'nus, Cortex pal'lidus, Cinchonæ officina'lis cortex commu'nis, Cinchona pallida, Pale Bark, Loxa Bark, Crown Bark*, (F.) *Quinquina gris de Loxa, Quinquina Orange*. Its odour is aromatic; taste pleasant, bitter, and astringent. The pieces are rolled in double or single quills. Epidermis brown, cracked; fracture resinous. Internally of a cinnamon colour. Its active principle is *Cinchonia*.

CINCHONÆ OBLONGIFO'LIÆ CORTEX, *Cortex ruber, Cinchonæ officina'lis cortex ruber, Red Bark*, (F.) *Quinquina rouge*. Odour and taste the same as the pale, but more intense: in large flat pieces, solid, heavy, dry; fracture short and smooth; of a deep brownish-red colour. Although this variety of bark is assigned to the Cinchona oblongifolia by some, it would seem, that nothing is certainly known as to its source. Active principles, *Cinchonia* and *Quinia*.

The last three are the only officinal varieties in the Pharmacopœia of the United States. There are many other varieties, however, which are genuine cinchona barks, and yet have not been considered worthy of an officinal position. The Edinburgh Pharmacopœia admits, indeed, *Cinchona cinerea, Grey bark, Silver bark* or *Huanuco bark*, which is obtained around Huanuco in Peru, and belongs to the class of pale barks. Amongst the genuine but inferior barks are those brought from the northern Atlantic ports of South America, which, in commerce, are variously called *Carthagena, Maracaybo* and *Santa Martha barks*.

All these barks are bitter, astringent, tonic, and eminently febrifuge. The yellow bark has been thought equal to any of the others, but the red contains more active principle. The discovery of their active principles is one of the most important gifts of modern chymistry. Still, in pernicious intermittents, the bark, in substance, is often demanded. It is employed in every disease in which there is deficient tone, but in cases where the stomach is much debilitated, the powder had better be avoided in consequence of the woody fibre, which might disagree. Externally, it is used in enemata, gargles, &c., and in gangrenous ulcerations. When it excites nausea, an aromatic may be added to it; if purging, opium; if costiveness, rhubarb, &c. Dose, ʒss to ʒj or more.

ESSENTIAL SALT OF BARK, as it is called, is an extract, prepared by macerating the bruised substance of bark in cold water, and submitting the infusion to a very slow evaporation.

CINCHONA OFFICINALIS (CORTEX FLAVUS,) Cinchonæ cordifoliæ cortex—c. Pallida, Cinchonæ lancifoliæ cortex—c. of Virginia, Magnolia glauca.

CINCHONIA, Cinchonine — c. Tannate of, Quinæ et cinchoniæ tannas.

CINCH'ONINE, *Cinchoni'na, Cinchonin, Cincho'nia*. The active principle of *Cincho'na lancifo'lia*. An organic, crystalline alkali; of a white colour, and bitter, slightly astringent taste; very soluble in alcohol and ether, but almost insoluble in water.

Sulphate of Cinchonia, which is formed directly from cinchonia, is soluble in water and alcohol. The action of the sulphate of cinchonia is similar to that of the sulphate of quinia; but it is less energetic, and consequently requires to be given in a larger dose.

CINCHONINE, TARTRATE OF, see Quinine, tartrate of.

CINCHONISM, Quininism.

CINCIN'NULUS. A little lock or curl of hair.

CINCIN'NUS. A curled or frizzled lock. The hair on the temples.

CINC'LICIS, *Cinclis'mus*, 'agitation; rapid and frequent motion.' The movement of the thorax in dyspnœa.—Hippocrates. It has been used, also, synonymously with nictation.

CINCLISMUS, Cinclisis.

CINEFACTIO, Incineration.

CINE'MA, *Cine'sis*, from κινεω, 'I move.' Motion.

CINERARIA MARITIMA, Achaovan, Abiat.

CINERES CLAVELLATI, see Potash — c. Gravellati, see Potash — c. Russici, Potash of commerce.

CINEREUS, Cineritious.

CINERIT"IOUS, *Ciner'eus*, from *cineres*, 'ashes;' (F.) *Cendré*. Of the colour of ashes. The *cortical substance* of the brain, and the vesicular neurine in general, have been so called. See Cortex Cerebri, and Neurine.

CINESIS, Cinema, Motion.

CINETH'MICS, from κινεω, 'I move.' The science of movements in general.

CINETIC, Motory.

CINET'ICA. Same etymon. Diseases affecting the muscles, and characterized by irregular action of the muscles or muscular fibres, commonly denominated *Spasm*. The 3d order in the class *Neurotica* of Good. Also, agents that affect the voluntary or involuntary motions.—Pereira.

CINETUS, Diaphragm.

CINGULARIA, Lycopodium.

CIN'GULUM, *Zone*, from *cingo*, 'I bind.' (F.) *Ceinture*. A cincture. A girdle. The part of the body, situate below the ribs, to which the girdle is applied. The *waist*.

CIN'GULUM HILDA'NI, *Zo'nula Hilda'ni*, (F.) *Ceinture de Hildane*. A leathern girdle formerly used for the reduction of luxations and fractures of the extremities.

CIN'GULUM MERCURIA'LE, *C. Sapien'tiæ, C. Stultit"iæ*. A woollen girdle, containing mercurial ointment. It was used as an antisyphilitic, and in diseases of the skin. (F.) *Ceinture de vif argent*.

CINGULUM SANCTI JOANNIS, Artemisia vulgaris.

CINIS FÆCUM, see Potash—c. Infectorius, see Potash.

CINNABARIS, Hydrargyri sulphuretum rubrum — c. Græcorum, see Calamus rotang.

CINNAMOMUM, Laurus cinnamomum — c. Album, Canella alba—c. Aromaticum, see Laurus cinnamomum—c. Culilawan, Laurus Culilawan—c. Indicum, Laurus cassia—c. Magellanicum, Wintera aromaticon—c. Malabaricum, Laurus cassia — c. Zeylanicum, Laurus cinnamomum.

CINNAMON, see Laurus cinnamomum — c. Malabar, Laurus cassia—c. Wild, Laurus cassia.

CINON'OSI, from κινεω, 'I move,' and νοσος, 'a disease.' Diseases of motion.

CINOPLANE'SIS, from κινεω, 'I move,' and πλανησις, 'a wandering about.' Irregularity of motion.

CINQUEFOIL, Potentilla reptans—c. Marsh, Comarum palustre — c. Norway, Potentilla Norvegica.

CINZILLA, Herpes zoster.

CION, Uvula.

CI'ONIS. The *U'vula*. Also, tumefaction, or elongation of the uvula; *Staphylodial'ysis*.

CIONI'TIS, from κιονις, 'the uvula,' and *itis*, 'inflammation.' Inflammation of the uvula, *Uvuli'tis*.

CIONORRHAPHIA, Staphyloraphy.

CIOT'OMY, *Ciotom'ia, Cionot'omy, Cionotom'ia*, from κιων, 'the uvula,' and τομη, 'incision.' Excision of the uvula when too long.

CIPIPA, see Jatropha manihot.

CIRCÆA, Atropa mandragora, Circæa Lutetiana.

CIRCÆ'A LUTETIA'NA, *Circæ'a, Paris'ian Circæ'a*, from Circe, the enchantress; *Enchant'ers' Nightshade*, (F.) *Herbe de Saint Étienne, Herbe aux Sorciers*. This plant, common in the vicinity of Paris, was formerly considered to be resolvent and vulnerary. It was also supposed to possess wonderful magical and enchanting properties.

CIRCINUS, Herpes zoster.

CIRCLE, Circulus — c. Ciliary, Ciliary ligament — c. of Willis, see Circulus.

CIRCOCELE, Cirsocele.

CIRCONCISION, Circumcision.

CIRCONFLEXE, Circumflexus.

CIRCONSCRIT, Circumscribed.

CIRCONVOLUTION, Convolution.

CIRCUIT, *Circu'itus;* in pathological language, generally means 'period,' 'course.'

CIRCUITUS, Period, Circuit.

CIR'CULAR, *Circula'ris*, from *circulus*, 'a circle.' (F.) *Circulaire*. Having the form of a circle; as *Circular Amputation*, &c.

The French use the expression "*Une circulaire*," for a *turn* of a bandage around any part.

CIRCULAR SINUS of Ridley, Sinus coronarius.

CIRCULA'TION, *Circula'tio, Cyclophor'ia, Periodus san'guinis*, from *circulus*, 'a circle;' or rather, from *circum*, 'around,' and *ferre, latum*, 'to carry.' (F.) *Circulation*. Physiologists give this name to the motion of the blood through the different vessels of the body—*sanguimotion;*—to that function, by which the blood, setting out from the left ventricle of the heart, is distributed to every part of the body by the arteries; — proceeds into the veins, returns to the heart, enters the right auricle, and passes into the corresponding ventricle, which sends it into the pulmonary artery to be distributed to the lungs, whence it issues by the pulmonary veins, and passes into the left auricle. From this it is sent into the left ventricle, and is again distributed by means of the arteries.

CIRCULA'TION, CAP'ILLARY, *C. des Parenchymes*, is that which takes place in the capillary vessels; and is, in some measure, independent of the action of the heart. See Capillary Vessels.

CIRCULATION, PULMON'IC or LESSER, is the circle from the right to the left side of the heart by the lungs. — The GREATER or SYSTEMAT'IC or SYSTEM'IC, is that through the rest of the system.

CIRCULATOR, Charlatan.

CIR'CULATORY, *Circulato'rius;* same etymon as circulation. Relating to the circulation as of the blood;—*sanguimo'tory*.

CIR'CULUS. A circle or ring, *Cyclus*, or

rios, (F.) *Cercle*. Any part of the body which is round or annular, as *Cir'culus Oc'uli*—the globe, bulk, or orb of the eye.—Hippocr., Galen. It is, also, applied to objects, which by no means form a circle,—as to the *Circle of Willis*, *Cir'culus arterio'sus Willis'ii*, which is an *anastomotic circle* at the base of the brain, formed by the anterior and the posterior cerebral arteries and the communicating arteries of Willis.

CIRCULUS ARTERIO'SUS I'RIDIS. The artery which runs round the iris, and forms a circle.

CIRCULUS ARTERIOSUS WILLISII, Circle of Willis, see Circulus — c. Ciliaris, Ciliary ligament — c. Membranosus, Hymen.

CIRCULUS QUAD'RUPLEX; a kind of bandage used by the ancients.

CIRCULUS TONSILLA'RIS. A plexus formed by the tonsillitic branches of the glosso-pharyngeal nerve around the base of the tonsil.

CIRCULUS VENO'SUS, *Figu'ra veno'sa, Vena seu Sinus termina'lis*. The venous circle in the embryo, which bounds the *Area Vasculosa* or *Vascular Area*.

CIRCUMAGENTES, Oblique muscles of the eye.

CIRCUMCAULALIS MEMBRANA, Conjunctiva.

CIRCUMCISIO, Circumcision — c. Fœminarum, see Circumcision.

CIRCUMCIS'ION, *Circumcis'io, Posthet'omy, Præcis'io* seu *Abscis'io Præpu'tii, Circumciru'ra, Circumsec'tio, Perit'omē*, from *circum*, 'around,' and *cadere*, 'to cut.' (F.) *Circoncision*. An ancient operation, performed by some nations as a religious ceremony. It consists in removing circularly a portion of the prepuce of infants;—a custom, which was probably suggested with a view to cleanliness. In cases of extraordinary length of prepuce, or when affected with disease, the operation is sometimes undertaken by surgeons. A similar operation is performed, amongst the Ægyptians, Arabians, and Persians, on the female, *Circumcis'io fœmina'rum*, by removing a portion of the nymphæ, and at times the clitoris.

CIRCUMCISURA, Circumcision.

CIRCUMDUCTIO, Perisphalsis.

CIRCUMDUCTIONIS OPIFEX, Obliquus superior oculi.

CIRCUMFLEX, *Circumflex'us*, from *circum*, 'around,' and *flexus*, 'bent.' (F.) *Circonflexe*. Curved circularly. A name given to several organs.

CIRCUMFLEX or ARTIC'ULAR AR'TERIES of the arm are distinguished into *anterior* and *posterior*. They arise from the axillary, and are distributed around the shoulder.

CIRCUMFLEX ARTERIES OF THE THIGH are distinguished into *external* and *internal*,—A. Soustrochantériennes—Ch. They are given off from the *Profunda*, and surround the head of the thigh bone.

CIRCUMFLEX MUSCLE, *Circumflexus Mus'culus, Tensor Pala'ti, Peristaphyli'nus exter'nus* vel *inferior, C'rcumflex'us Pala'ti Mollis, Spheno-salpingo-staphyli'nus* seu *Staphyli'nus exter'nus, Mus'culus tubæ novæ, Pala'to-salpingeus, Pter'ygo-staphyli'nus, Petro-salpin'go-staphyli'nus, Spheno-pter'ygo-palati'nus, Salpingo-staphyli'nus*, (F.) *Palato-salpingien*. A muscle, which arises from the spinous process of the sphenoid bone, and is inserted into the *velum pendulum palati*. Its use is to stretch the velum.

CIRCUMFLEX NERVE. This arises from the brachial plexus by a common trunk with the musculo-spiral nerve. It divides into numerous branches, which are distributed to the deltoid.

CIRCUMFLEX VEINS follow the arteries.

CIRCUMFORANEUS, Charlatan.

CIRCUMFU'SA. Hallé has thus designated the first class of subjects that belong to Hygiene —as atmosphere, climate, residence, &c.; in short, every thing which acts constantly on man externally and generally.

CIRCUMGYRATIO, Vertigo.

CIRCUMLIGATURA, Paraphimosis.

CIRCUMLIT"IO, from *circumlino*, 'I anoint all over.' *Perich'risis, Perichris'ton*. A term formerly used for liniments, but especially for those applied to the eyelids.

CIRCUMOSSALE, Periosteum.

CIR'CUMSCRIBED, *Circumscrip'tus*, (F.) *Circonscrit*. A term applied, in pathology, to tumours, which are distinct at their base from the surrounding parts.

CIRCUMSECTIO, Circumcision.

CIRCUMVALLATÆ PAPILLÆ, see Papillæ of the Tongue.

CIRE JAUNE ET BLANCHE, Cera flava et alba—c. *des Oreilles*, Cerumen.

CIRIOS, Circulus.

CIRON, Acarus, Psora.

CIRRHAGRA, Plica — c. Polonorum, Plica.

CIRRHON'OSUS; from κιρρος, 'yellow,' and νοσος, 'disease.' A disease of the fœtus, in which there is a yellow coloration of the serous membranes.—Siebenhaar.

CIRRHOSE DU FOIE, Cirrhosis.

CIRRHO'SIS, *Cirrhono'sis, Kirrhono'sis*, from κιρρος, 'yellow.' A yellow colouring matter, sometimes secreted in the tissues, owing to a morbid process. Also, called *Cirrho'sis* or *Kirrho'sis*.

CIRRHO'SIS HEP'ATIS, see Hepatatrophia. *Gran'ulated, gran'ular, mam'millated, tuber'culated*, and *hob-nailed liver*, (F.) *Cirrhose du Foie*. It appears to be dependent upon repletion of the terminal extremities of the biliary ducts with bile, along with atrophy of the intervening parenchyma. Hence the liver is smaller in size, or atrophied.

CIRRHOSIS HEPATIS, see Cirrhosis.

CIRRHOSIS OF THE LUNG, *Cirrho'sis pulmo'num*. Dr. Corrigan has described a condition of the lung under this name, the general character of which he considers to be a tendency to consolidation or contraction of the pulmonary tissue, with dilatation of the bronchial tubes.

CIRRHOSIS PULMONUM, C. of the Lung.

CIR'SIUM ARVEN'SE, *Car'duus hemorrhoida'lis, Ceano'thos*, (F.) *Chardon hémorrhoïdal*. A common plant, used in France in the form of cataplasm in hemorrhoids; and worn as an amulet.

CIRSIUM MACULATUM, Carduus marianus.

CIRSOCE'LE, *Circoce'lē, Cirsos'cheum*, from κιρσος, 'varix,' and κηλη, 'hernia;' *Var'icose Her'nia*. The greater part of authors have employed the term synonymously with *Varicocele*. Pott gives it a different signification. *Varicocele*, he calls the tumour formed by the veins of the scrotum; *Circocele, Funic'ulus varico'sus*, the varicose dilatation of the spermatic veins. The scrotum feels as if it contained earthworms. It is commonly an affection of no consequence, demanding merely the use of a suspensory bandage.

CIRSOI'DES, *Cirso'des*, from κιρσος, 'varix,' and ειδος, 'resemblance.' Varicose, or resembling a varix. Rufus of Ephesus, according to James, applies this term to the upper part of the brain, as well as to the spermatic vessels.

CIRSOM'PHALUS, from κιρσος, 'varix,' and ομφαλος, 'navel.' Varicose dilatation of the veins surrounding the navel. The term has, likewise, been applied to the aneurismal dilatation of the arteries of that region; called also, *Varicompha'alus*, (F.) *Hargne anévrysmale, Aneurismal Hernia*.

CIRSOPHTHAL'MIA, *Cirsophthal'mus, Telangiecta'sia oculi*, from κιρσος, 'varix,' and οφθαλμος, 'the eye;' *Var'icose ophthal'mia, Ophthalmia varico'sa, Varicos'itas conjuncti'væ*. A high degree of ophthalmia, in which the vessels of the conjunctiva are considerably injected.

CIRSOSCHEUM, Cirsocele.

CIRSOT'OMY, *Cirsotom'ia*, from κιρσος, 'a varix,' and τομη, 'an incision.' Any operation for the removal of varices by incision.

CIRSUS, Varix.

CIRSYDROSCHEOCE'LE, from κιρσος, 'varix,' υδωρ, 'water,' οσχεον, the 'scrotum.' Varicocele with water in the scrotum.

CISEAUX, Scissors.

CISSA, Malacia.

CISSAMPELOS, Pareira brava.

CISSAM'PELOS CAPEN'SIS, *Nat. Ord.* Menispermaceæ, grows in almost every mountainous part of the Cape of Good Hope. The root is used as an emetic and cathartic by the Boers.

CISSARUS, Cistus Creticus.

CISSI'NUM, from κισσος, 'ivy.' Name of a plaster of ivy, used in wounds of the nerves or tendons.—Paulus of Ægina.

CISSOIDES, Capreolaris.

CISSOS, Hedera helix.

CISTERN, LUMBAR, Receptaculum chyli.

CISTER'NA, from κιστη, (L.) *Cista*, 'a chest.' (F.) *Citerne*. This term has been applied to various parts of the body, which serve as reservoirs for different fluids. The fourth ventricle of the brain has been so called.—Arantius.

CISTERNA CHYLI, Receptaculum chyli.

CISTHORUS, Cistus Creticus.

CISTOCELE, Cystocele.

CISTUS CANADENSIS, Helianthemum Canadensis.

CISTUS CRE'TICUS, *C. salvifo'lius* seu *tau'ricus, Cis'thorus, Cis'sarus, Dorycin'ium, Gum Cistus. Sex. Syst.* Polyandria Monogynia. The systematic name of the plant whence the *Labda'num, Labda'men* or *Lada'num, Gum'mi Labda'num*, is obtained. *Lada'num* is a gum-resinous substance, of a very agreeable smell, found in the shops in great masses. Its colour is blackish-green; taste, warm and bitter. It is but little used now. Formerly, it was a component of warm plasters, and was prescribed internally as a stomachic. Ladanum is also obtained from *Cistus ladanif'erus*, and *C. laurifo'lius*.

CISTUS, GUM, Cistus Creticus—c. Salvifolius, C. Creticus—c. Tauricus, C. Creticus.

CITERNE LOMBAIRE, Receptaculum chyli.

CITHARUS, Thorax.

CITRAGO, Melissa.

CITRARIA, Melissa.

CITRAS CHINICUS, Quiniæ citras.

CITREA MALUS, see Citrus medica.

CITREOLUS, Cucumis sativus.

CITRIC ACID, *Acidum cit'ricum, Acid of Lemons, Ac"idum Limo'num*, (F.) *Acide citrique*. This acid is found in the lemon, orange, &c. It is in rhomboidal prisms, which slightly effloresce on exposure to the air. It dissolves in a twelfth part of its weight in boiling water, and has an extremely acid but agreeable taste. It is employed in medicine as antiseptic, refrigerant and diuretic. Rubbed up with sugar and with a little of the essence of lemon, it forms the *dry Lemonade*, (F.) *Limonade sèche*.

CITRINE OINTMENT, Unguentum hydrargyri nitratis.

CITRON, see Citrus medica—c. Tree, see Citrus medica.

CITRONELLE, Artemisia abrotanum, Melissa.

CITRUL, SICILIAN, Cucurbita citrullus.

CITRULLUS, Cucurbita citrullus.

CITRULLUS AMA'RUS. An African plant, *Nat. Ord.* Cucurbitaceæ, called by the Boers *Bitterappel* or *Wild Watermelon*, the pulp of which, like that of colocynth, is a drastic cathartic.

CITRULLUS COLOCYNTHIS, Cucumis colocynthis.

CITRUS, see Citrus medica—c. Acida, see Lime.

CITRUS AURAN'TIUM. The systematic name of the Orange Tree, *Auran'tium, A. Hispalen'sē, Malus Auran'tia Major, Malus Auran'tia, Auran'tium vulga'rē, Malus Auran'tia vulga'ris, Ci'trus vulga'ris. Nat. Ord.* Aurantiaceæ. *Sex. Syst.* Polyadelphia Icosandria. The fruit are called *Mala Au'rea, Chrysome'lia, Neran'tia, Martia'na Poma, Poma Auran'tia, Auran'tia Curassav'ica, Poma Chinen'sia, Oranges*. The *Flowers of the Orange, Flores Naphæ*, are highly odoriferous, and used as a perfume. On distillation, they yield a small quantity of essential oil—*O'leum Auran'tii, Oleum* vel *Essen'tia Nero'li*,—with spirit and water, the *Aqua Florum Auran'tii, Aqua aurantii, Orange-flower water*. They were once used in convulsive and epileptic cases. The leaves, *Fo'lia Auran'tii*, have a bitterish taste, and furnish an essential oil. They have been used for the same purposes as the flowers. The yellow rind of the fruit, *Cortex Auran'tii, Orange Peel*, is an aromatic bitter, and is used in dyspepsia, and where that class of remedies is required. The *Juice, Succus Auran'tii, Orange juice*, is a grateful acid, and used as a beverage in febrile and scorbutic affections.

CITRUS BERGAMIA, Citrus mella rosa—c. Limetta, see Citrus mella rosa.

CITRUS MED'ICA, *C. Limo'num*. The systematic name of the *Lemon Tree*. The *Lemon, Limo'num malum, Limo'num Bacca, Malus Med'ica, Malus Limo'nia Ac"ida, Cit'rea Malus, Citrus*, (F.) *Citron, Cédrat*, has a fragrant odour, depending upon the essential oil, *O'leum Limo'nis*, of the rind. The outer rind, *Cortex Limo'num, Lemon Peel, Zest, Flave'do Corticum Citri*, is used in the same cases as the *Cortex Auran'tii*.

The *juice, Succus Limo'nis*, (F.) *Suc du Limon, Suc de Citron*, is sharp, but gratefully acid, the acidity depending upon the citric acid it contains, and is given as a refrigerant beverage in febrile affections. In doses of half an ounce to an ounce, three times a day, it has appeared to exert a markedly sedative influence on the circulation, and has been given, apparently with benefit, in acute rheumatism and rheumatic gout. Alone, or combined with wine, it is prescribed in scurvy, putrid sore throat, &c. Its general properties are refrigerant and antiseptic. Sweetened and diluted, it forms *Lemonade*. *Artificial lemonjuice* is made by dissolving an ounce of citric acid in fourteen fluidounces of water; adding a few drops of essence of lemon.

Lemonpeel tea, or *water*, is made by paring the rind of one *lemon*, previously rubbed with half an ounce of *sugar*: the peelings and sugar are then put into a jar, and a quart of boiling *water* is poured over them. When cold, the fluid must be poured off, and a tablespoonful of lemon juice be added.

It is an agreeable drink in fevers.

Cit'ron Tree is likewise considered to belong to the same species—*Cit'rus Med'ica*. Its fruit is called *cedrome'la*. It is larger and less succulent than the lemon. *Citron juice*, when sweetened with sugar, is called by the Italians *Agro di Cedro*.

CITRUS MELLA ROSA of De Lamarck, another

variety of *Citrus Medica*, affords the Bergamote, as also do *Citrus Limet'ta* and *C. Berga'mia*.

CITRUS VULGARIS, Citrus aurantium.

CITTA, Malacia.

CITTARA, MINERAL WATERS OF. These springs are in the Isle of Ischia, near the sea. They contain carbonate and sulphate of lime, and chloride of sodium. Their temperature is 100° Fahrenheit.

CITTOS, Hedera helix.

CITTOSIS, Chlorosis, Malacia.

CIVETTA, *Zib'ethum, Civ'et*, (F.) *Civette*. An unctuous perfume, of a very penetrating odour, obtained from different mammalia of the *Viver'ra* kind, particularly from *Viver'ra civet'ta*. It is contained in a fold of the skin, situate between the anus and the organs of generation.

CLABBER, Bonnyclabber.

CLABBERGRASS, Galium verum.

CLADES GLANDULARIA, Plague.

CLADISCOS, Ramusculus.

CLADONIA ISLANDICA, Lichen islandicus.

CLADO'NIA RANGIFER'RINA. The ancients regarded this European plant as pectoral and stomachic. It enters into the composition of the *Poudre de Chypre*.

CLADOS, Ramus.

CLADRAS'TIS TINCTO'RIA, *Virgil'ia, Yellow Ash, Fustic Tree, Yellow Locust*. An indigenous tree, which flourishes from Kentucky to Alabama. The bark of the tree and the roots are cathartic.

CLAIRET, Claret.

CLAIRVOYANCE (F.), 'Clear-seeing.' A clearness of sight, said to be communicated by animal magnetism, which not only enables the *magnetized* persons to see in the dark, through stone walls, &c., but even to observe prospects, whilst he may fancy he is flying in the air, which he has never seen previously. It need hardly be said, that the possession of such powers is fabulous.

CLAMMY WEED, Polanisea graveolens.

CLAMOR, Cry.

CLANGOR, Oxyphonia.

CLAP, Gonorrhœa impura.

CLAPIER (F.), A clapper, *Latib'ulum*, from κλεπτειν, 'to conceal.' A purulent *foyer* of disease; concealed in the flesh or under the skin. See Sinus.

CLAPWORT, Orobanche Americana.

CLAQUEMENT, Odontosynerismus.

CLAR'ET, (*Vin clair* [?]), *Clare'tum, Vin de Bordeaux*, (F.) *Clairet*. A pleasant French wine, which may be used whenever wine is required. Also, a wine impregnated with spice and sugar, called likewise *Vinum Hippocrat'icum* seu *Medica'tum, Potus Hippocrat'icus, Hip'pocrae, Hyp'-pocras*. Schröder speaks of a *Clare'tum al'terans*, and a *C. purgans*.

CLARETA, Albumen ovi.

CLARETUM, Claret.

CLARIFICA'TION, *Clarifica'tio, Depura'tion*, from *clarus*, 'clear,' and *facio*, 'I make.' A pharmaceutical operation, which consists in separating from a liquid every insoluble substance, held in suspension by it, that affects its transparency. *Decanting* and *filtering* are the operations necessary for this purpose.

CLARY, COMMON, Salvia sclarea.

CLASIS, Fracture.

CLASMA, Fracture.

CLASS, *Clas'sis*, (F.) *Classe*. An assemblage of a certain number of objects. In *Natural History* and in *Medicine*, a group of objects or individuals having one or more common characters. The classes are divided into *orders*, the orders into *genera*, the *genera* into *species*, and these last into *varieties*.

CLASSIFICA'TION, *Classifica'tio*, from *classis*, 'a class,' and *facio*, 'I make.' The formation of classes. A methodical distribution of any objects whatever into classes, orders, genera, species, and varieties. See Nosography, and Nosology.

CLASSY, MINERAL WATERS OF. Classy is near Laon in Picardy, France. The waters are chalybeate.

CLAUDICATIO, Claudication — c. Anatica, Vacillatio.

CLAUDICA'TION, *Claudica'tio*, from *claudicare*, 'to be lame.' The act of halting or limping. *Lameness, Clau'ditas, Cholo'sis, Cholei'a, Cholo'ma*, (F.) *Claudication, Boitement*. This condition does not constitute any special disease, but is produced by different causes or affections. It may be the result of the shortening or elongation of one of the lower limbs, of ankylosis of the joints, palsy of the muscles, pain, &c.

CLAUDITAS, Claudication.

CLAUSTRUM GUTTURIS, Isthmus of the fauces — c. Palati, Velum pendulum palati — c. Virginitatis, Hymen.

CLAUSU'RA, from *claudere*, 'to shut.' An imperforation of any canal or cavity.

CLAUSU'RA UTERI. Preternatural imperforation of the uterus.

CLAVA MYOSA, Acorus calamus.

CLAVALIER À FEUILLES DE FRÊNE, Xanthoxylum clava Herculis.

CLAVA'RIA CORALLOÏ'DES, *Coralloides Fungus, Coralwort*. Said to be corroborant and astringent. A kind of clavaria, called (F.) *Digital blanc, Digital humain, Champignon de l'appareil des fractures*, formed of digitations, grouped together, and two or three inches in length, is said to have been often found, formerly at the *Hôtel Dieu* of Paris, on the splints of white wood used in the treatment of fractures, in autumn.—H. Cloquet.

CLAVATIO, Gomphosis.

CLAVEAU, Murr.

CLAVELÉE, Murr.

CLAVES CALVARIÆ, Wormiana Ossa.

CLAV'ICLE, *Clavic'ula, Clavis, Clavic'ulus, Lig'ula, Fur'cula, Os Jug'uli, Jug'ulum, Cleis, Clei'dion*, from *clavis*, 'a key,' (F.) *Clavicule*. The *collar-bone*. The clavicle is shaped like the letter S, and is placed transversely at the upper part of the thorax. It is articulated, at one extremity, with the sternum; at the other with the acromion process of the scapula. It gives attachment, *above*, to the *Sterno-cleido mastoideus*; *below*, to the *Subclavius*; *before*, to the *Pectoralis major* and *Deltoides*; and *behind*, to the *Trapezius*. It serves as a point of support for the muscles of the arm, and protects the vessels and nerves passing to that extremity.

The fibres, connecting the lamellæ or plates of bones, have also been called *Clavic'uli* or *Nails*.

CLAVIC'ULAR, *Clavicula'ris*; same etymon. Relating to the clavicle or collar-bone.

CLAVICULAR NERVES, *Nervi clavicula'res*. Branches of the fourth cervical nerve, which are distributed to the clavicular region.

CLAVICULE, Clavicle.

CLAVICULI, see Clavicle.

CLAVIS, Clavicle, Key—c. Anglica, Key.

CLAVUS. A nail. *Helos, Gomphos*, (F.) *Clou*. This word is employed in medicine in various senses. It means, 1. A *Corn*, from its resemblance to the head of a nail. 2. Certain condylomatous excrescences of the uterus. 3. A callous tumour, which forms on the white of the eye, and resembles a nail, the *Clavus Oc'uli*, (F.) *Clou de l'œil*. This last, by some, is considered to be synonymous with staphyloma; by others, with staphyloma of the cornea. Also, the penis.

CLAVUS HYSTER'ICUS, *Monopa'gia, Monope'-gia*, (F.) *Clou hystérique*. An acute pain, confined to a small point of the head, described by the sick as resembling that which would be produced by a nail driven into the head. It has been particularly noticed in hysterical females;—hence its name. It is called *Ovum hyster'icum*, when the pain occupies a greater extent.

CLAVUS SECALINUS, Ergot—c. Secalis, Ergot—c. Siliginis, Ergot.

CLEANSINGS, Lochia.

CLEARSEEING, *Clairvoyance*.

CLEARWEED, Pilea pumila.

CLEAVAGE; from Anglo-Saxon cleoꝼan, 'to split.' The natural line of separation exhibited by certain substances, as minerals, when subjected to mechanical force. The term has been applied to the separation of muscles into longitudinal and circular striæ, when mechanical violence is used.

CLEAVERS, Galium aparine.

CLEAVERS' BEES, Galium aparine.

CLEAVEWORT, Galium verum.

CLEF DU CRANE, Wormianum os — *c. de Garengeot*, Key—*c. à Noix*, see Key—*c. à Pivot*, see Key—*c. à Pompe*, see Key.

CLEFT, Rima, see Monster — c. Palate, see Harelip.

CLEIDAGRA, Cleisagra.

CLEIDION, Clavicle.

CLEIDO-COSTAL, Costo-clavicular.

CLEI'DO-MASTOÏ'DEUS. Albinus thus designates the posterior portion of the sterno-cleido-mastoideus, which he considers a separate muscle. It has been corrupted into *clino-mastoïdeus*.

CLEIS, Clavicle, Key.

CLEIS'AGRA, *Cleid'agra*, from κλεις, 'the clavicle,' and αγρα, 'a seizure.' Gout in the clavicle.—A. Paré.

CLEMATIS DAPHNOIDES MAJOR, Vinca minor—c. Corymbosa, C. erecta.

CLEM'ATIS ERECT'A, *C. recta seu flam'mula seu corymbo'sa, Clemati'tis erec'ta, Flam'mula Jovis, Upright Virgin's Bower*, (F.) *Clématite droite*. *Family*, Ranunculaceæ. *Sex. Syst.* Polyandria Polygynia. The leaves contain an acrid principle. They have been esteemed anti-venereal; and, in the form of powder, have been used as an escharotic.

CLEMATIS FLAMMULA, C. erecta—c. Recta, C. erecta—c. Sepium, c. Vitalba.

CLEMATIS VITAL'BA, *C. se'pium seu sylves'tris, Vital'ba, Vior'na, Atra'gene, Trav'eller's Joy, Common Virgin's Bower*, (F.) *Clématite, Herbe aux gueux, Aubevigne*. It has been used in the same cases as the former. In infusion it has been applied in cases of itch.

The leaves of CLEMATIS CRISPA—C. FLAMMULA, *sweet-scented Virgin's bower*—C. VIRGIN'ICA, *common Virgin's bower*—and C. VIORNA, *Leather-flower*, have similar properties.

CLÉMATITE, Clematis vitalba—*c. Droite*, Clematis recta.

CLEMATITIS ERECTA, Clematis erecta.

CLEO'NIS COLLYR'IUM. A collyrium described by Celsus, composed of equal parts of Samian earth, myrrh, and thus, mixed with white of egg.

CLEONIS GLUTEN. An astringent formula of myrrh, frankincense, and white of egg.

CLEP'SYDRA, from κλεπτω, 'I conceal,' and 'υδωρ, 'water.' An instrument contrived by Paracelsus to convey fumigation to the uterus.

CLEPTOMANIA, Kleptomania.

CLEVES, MINERAL WATERS OF. This spring is a quarter of a league from Cleves, in Westphalia. It contains carbonate and sulphate of iron.

CLIFFORT'IA ILICIFO'LIA. *Nat. Ord.* Rosaceæ. A common South African plant, used by the Boers as an emollient expectorant in catarrh.

CLIFTON, CLIMATE OF. The vicinity of Clifton and of Bristol, England, appears to be the mildest and driest climate in the west of England; and, consequently, the best winter residence, in that part of the country, for invalids. It is, also, a favourable summer climate, and is surrounded by numerous places of agreeable resort, suited for those who may pass the season there.

For the mineral waters of Clifton, see Bristol Hot Well.

CLIGNEMENT, Nictation, Scardamygmus.

CLIGNOTEMENT, Nictation.

CLIMA, Climate.

CLIMAC'TERIC, *Climacter'icus, Climater'icus*, from κλιμακτηρ, 'a step.' (F.) *Climactérique* ou *Climatérique*. A word, which properly signifies 'by degrees.' It has been applied to certain times of life, regarded to be critical.

At present, the word *Climacteric* is chiefly applied to certain periods of life, at which great changes occur, independently of any numerical estimate of years. Such are the period of puberty in both sexes: that of the cessation of the menses in women, &c.

CLIMACTERIC YEARS, *Anni Climacter'ici*, are, according to some, all those in the life of man, which are multiples of the number 7, *Septen'niads*. Others have applied the term to years, resulting from the multiplication of 7 by an odd number. Some have admitted only three *climacterics*; others, again, have extended them to multiples of 9. Most, however, have considered the 63d year as the *Grand Climacteric*; — 63 being the product of the multiplication of 7 by 9, and all have thought that the period of three, seven, or nine, which they respectively adopted, was necessary to the entire renewal of the body; so that there was, at these times, in the economy, none of the parts of which it had previously consisted. The climacteric years have also been culled, *(Anni) hebdomad'ici, scala'res, grada'rii, scan'siles, genethliaci, natalit''ii, fata'les, crit'ici, decreto'rii, hero'ici*, &c. All the notions on the subject are essentially allied to the doctrine of numbers of Pythagoras.

CLIMATE, *Clima, Inclina'tio cœli*, (F.) *Climat*, Gr. κλιμα, 'a region.' In geography, the word *climate* is applied to a space on the terrestrial globe, comprised between two circles parallel to the equator, and arbitrarily measured according to the length of the days. In a hygienic point of view, we understand by *climate*, since Hippocrates, a country or region, which may differ from another in respect to season, qualities of the soil, heat of atmosphere, &c. Climate, indeed, embraces, in a general manner, all the physical circumstances belonging to each region, — circumstances which exert considerable influence on living beings. The dark complexion of the inhabitants of the torrid zone is easily distinguishable from the paleness of those of the frigid, — so are the diseases. They are all modified, more or less, by climate or locality. Hot climates predispose to abdominal complications in febrile affections; cold climates to thoracic, &c.

One of the most important considerations with regard to climates is their comparative fitness for the residence of invalids, and especially of those who are liable to, or suffering under catarrhal or consumptive affections. The great object, in such cases, is to select a climate which will admit of regular and daily exercise in the open air, so that the invalid may derive every advantage which this form of revulsion is capable of effecting. To an inhabitant of the northern and middle portions of the United States — and the same applies to Great Britain, France, and the northern parts of the old world — a more southern climate alone affords these advantages in an eminent degree. During the summer months, there are few, if any, diseases, which require a milder climate than that of the United States, or of the milder districts of Europe. The temperature of the winter months is, consequently, the most important object of attention. Equability of temperature is essential, inasmuch as all sudden changes interfere with the great desideratum — exercise in the open air. In the whole continent of North America the changes are very sudden and extensive. It is not uncommon for the range to be 40°, between two successive days. So far, therefore, as this applies, the American climate is not well adapted to the invalid. In the southern portions, however, of the Union, this objection is counterbalanced by many advantages.

The following tables exhibit the mean temperature of the year, and of the different seasons — with the mean temperature of the warmest and coldest months at different places in America, Europe, Africa, &c., as deduced from the excellent paper of Von Humboldt on Isothermal Lines, the Meteorological Registers kept by the surgeons of the United States army, the work of Sir James Clark on Climate, &c.

Certain of the tables show the mean monthly temperature, maximum, minimum and range, as well as the greatest daily, and mean daily range during the corresponding months — but of different years — at some of the prominent retreats for the valetudinarian in Great Britain, on the continent of Europe, and in the African islands. It is proper, however, to remark, that in no situations, except in those to which an asterisk is affixed, was the register thermometer used. In the others, the observations were made during the *day* only, and consequently the numbers given are far below the real range throughout the twenty four hours. The places are ranged in the order of their mean temperature.

TABLE OF MAXIMUM, MINIMUM, AND RANGE OF TEMPERATURE.

PLACES.	DECEMBER.			JANUARY.			FEBRUARY.			MARCH.			APRIL.		
	Max.	Min.	Range	Max.	Min.	Range	Max.	Min.	Range	Max.	Min.	Range	Max.	Min.	Range
Sidmouth*	54	25	29	47	21	26	52	27	25	56	26	30	60	31	29
Penzance*	56	34	22	54	28	26	55	33	22	59	34	25	62	36	26
Pau	56	25	31	56	21	35	60	35	25	65	35	30	71	43	28
Montpellier	57	32	25	53	27	26	55	30	25	58	35	23	64	41	23
Nice	59	40	19	58	27	31	58	37	21	65	41	24	69	46	23
Rome	60	31	29	58	29	29	60	33	27	65	37	28	74	44	30
Naples	61	34	27	58	29	29	60	31	29	69	38	31	78	43	35
Madeira	68	52	16	69	50	19	68	51	17	69	51	18	72	55	17

TABLE OF MEAN TEMPERATURE.

PLACES.	DECEMBER.	JANUARY.	FEBRUARY.	MARCH.	APRIL.
Sidmouth	43.00	36.30	42.00	45.00	51.00
Penzance	46.50	43.00	44.50	46.50	48.50
Pau	41.53	38.89	44.96	46.80	55.79
Montpellier	46.00	42.00	45.00	47.00	53.00
Nice	48.60	45.85	49.00	51.45	57.00
Rome	49.62	47.65	49.45	52.05	56.40
Naples	50.50	46.50	48.50	52.00	57.00
Madeira	60.50	59.50	58.50	61.06	62.50

TABLE OF DAILY RANGE OF TEMPERATURE.

PLACES.	DECEMBER.		JANUARY.		FEBRUARY.		MARCH.		APRIL.	
	Mean daily range.	Greatest daily range.	Mean daily range.	Greatest daily range.	Mean daily range.	Greatest daily range.	Mean daily range.	Greatest daily range.	Mean daily range.	Greatest daily range.
Sidmouth		13		13		12		12		13
Penzance	3		4		6		8		9	
Pau	7	13	7	16	9	16	9	17	8	18
Montpellier	9		8		9		14		14	
Nice	6	14	8	16	9	18	9	17	11	18
Rome	9	15	11	16	10	18	12	19	13	20
Naples	9	13	9	14	11	19	11	18	14	20
Madeira*	11	14	11	17	9	13	10	14	9	13

1. AMERICA, &c.

Places.	Latitude.	Mean temperature of several years.	Mean temperature of different seasons.				Mean temperature of	
			Winter.	Spring.	Summer.	Autumn.	Warmest month.	Coldest month.
Nain..............	57°.08'	26°.42'	0°.60	23°.60	48°.38	33°.44	51°.80	11°.20
Fort Brady, Mich....	46 .39	41 .37	14 .09	37 .89	61 .83	43 .94	62 .87	12 .65
Quebec, L. C........	46. 47	41 .74	14 .18	38 .04	68 .00	46 .04	73 .40	13 .81
Eastport, Me........	44 .54	42 .44	23 .44	38 .58	60 .54	45 .43	63 .52	20 .91
Fort Howard, Mich..	44 .40	44 .50	20 .82	41 .40	68 .70	45 .18	73 .67	17 .95
Fort Crawford, Miss..	43 .03	45 .52	23 .76	43 .09	69 .78	46 .74	71 .34	20 .14
Cambridge, Mass.....	42 .21	50 .36	33 .98	47 .66	70 .70	49 .82	72 .86	29 .84
Council Bluffs, Miss..	41 .25	50 .82	27 .38	46 .38	72 .84	48 .60	75 .92	27 .19
Newport, R. I........	41 .30	51 .02	38 .82	46 .87	68 .70	53 .83	71 .46	32 .14
Philadelphia........	39 .56	53 .42	32 .18	51 .44	73 .94	56 .48	77 .00	32 .72
New York	40 .40	53 .78	29 .84	51 .26	79 .16	54 .50	80 .78	25 .34
Cincinnati	39 .06	53 .78	32 .90	54 .14	72 .86	54 .86	74 .30	30 .20
Monticello, Va.......	37 .58	55 .40	37 .67	54 .67	73 .33	56 .50	75 .00	36 .00
Washington, D. C....	38 .53	55 .56*	36 .80	53 .83	75 .90	56 .59	79 .13	34 .66
Smithville, N. C.....	34 .00	58 .88	53 .44	64 .76	80 .46	68 .15	82 .93	50 .69
Charleston, S. C.....	32 .47	60 .18	51 .09	66 .73	80 .89	67 .55	82 .81	49 .43
Natchez, Miss.......	31 .34	64 .76	48 .56	65 .48	79 .16	66 .02	79 .70	46 .94
Pensacola, Flor......	30 .28	68 .77†	55 .13	69 .67	82 .57	69 .05	83 .55	53 .80
St. Augustine, do....	29 .48	72 .23	59 .29	71 .47	82 .73	75 .15	83 .94	56 .60
Tampa Bay, do....	27 .57	72 .37	61 .24	72 .93	80 .14	75 .26	80 .72	58 .70
Vera Cruz..........	19 .11	77 .72	71 .96	77 .90	81 .50	78 .62	81 .86	71 .06
Havana	23 .10	78 .08	71 .24	78 .98	83 .30	78 .98	83 .84	69 .98
Bahamas	26 .40 to 27 .5	78 .3*	71.	77.	83.	80.	90.	64.
Barbadoes	13 .10	79 .3	76 .7	19.	81.	80.		
Cumana	10 .27	81 .86	80 .24	83 .66	82 .04	80 .24	84 .38	79 .16

St. Louis, Missouri, Lat. 38° 46'. Mean temp. 55° .86. New Harmony. Lat. 38° 11'. Mean temp. 56° .74. New Orleans, Lat. 30°. Mean temp. 69° .01. Baton Rouge, Lat. 30° .26'. Mean temp. 68° .07. Jamaica, coast, Mean temp. 80° .6.

2. EUROPE, AFRICA, &c.

Places.	Latitude.	Mean temperature of several years.	Mean temperature of different seasons.				Mean temperature of	
			Winter.	Spring.	Summer.	Autumn.	Warmest month.	Coldest month.
Geneva.............	48°.12'	49°.28'	34°.70	47°.66	64°.94	50°.00	66°.56	34°.16
Gosport	48 .1	50 .24*	40 .44	47 .63	62 .00	50 .88		
Newport, Isle of Wight	50 .40	51 .00	40 .31	49 .00	63 .09	51 .63		
Sidmouth..........		52 .10	40 .43	50 .66	63 .83	53 .50		
Penzance...........	52 .11	51 .80	44 .03	49 .63	60 .70	53 .36		
Undercliff		51 .11	42 .14	29 .26	60 .28	52 .76		
Hastings	50 .52	57 .00	40 .11	45 .77	60 .45	51 .00		
Bute	55 .42	48 .25	39 .62	46 .66	58 .02	48 .59		
Cove of Cork.......	51 .54	51 .58	43 .90	49 .43	61 .26	51 .73		
Jersey..............	49 .13	53 .06	43 .82	50 .97	62 .84	54 .63		
Paris...............	48 .50	51 .08	38 .66	49 .28	64 .58	51 .44	65 .30	36 .14
Pau................	43 .7	54 .95	41 .79	54 .96	67 .41	55 .64		
Sienna	43 .24	55 .60	40 .50	54 .10	70 .80	57 .10		
Nantes.............	47 .13	55 .62†	42 .23	53 .10	70 .73	56 .41	70 .52	39 .02
Bordeaux..........	44 .50	56 .48	42 .08	56 .46	70 .88	56 .30	73 .04	41 .00
Montpellier	43 .36	57 .60	44 .20	53 .33	71 .30	61 .30		
Avignon............		58 .20	42 .60	57 .13	74 .66	59 .00		
Florence	43 .46	59 .00	44 .30	56 .00	74 .00	60 .70		
Nice	43 .42	59 .48	47 .82	56 .23	72 .26	61 .63		
Marseilles	43 .17	59 .50‡	45 .50	57 .56	72 .50	60 .08		
Toulon	43 .07	59 .90	43 .30	53 .70	74 .30	59 .00		
Leghorn...........	43 .33	60 .00§	46 .30	57 .60	74 .10	62 .00		
Genoa..............	44 .25	60 .37	44 .57	58 .60	74 .03	62 .94		
Pisa	43 .43	60 .60	46 .03	57 .20	75 .15	62 .80		
Rome	41 .53	60 .40	45 .86	57 .74	75 .20	62 .78	77 .00	42 .26
Naples	40 .54	61 .40	48 .50	58 .50	70 .83	64 .50		
St. Michaels, Azores..	37 .47	62 .40	57 .83	61 .17	68 .33	62 .33		
Cadiz	36 .32	62 .88	52 .90	59 .53	70 .43	65 .35		
Madeira, Funchal....	32 .37	64 .56	59 .50	62 .20	69 .83	67 .23		
Algiers.............	36 .48	69 .98	61 .52	65 .66	80 .24	72 .50	82 .76	60 .08
Canaries, Santa Cruz.	28 .28	70 .94	64 .65	68 .87	76 .68	74 .17		
Cairo..............	30 .02	72 .32	58 .46	73 .58	85 .10	71 .42	85 .82	56 .12

London, Lat. 51° .30'. Mean temp. 50° .36. Environs of London, Mean temp. 48° .81. Perpignan, Mean temp. 59° .54. Lyons, Mean temp. 55° .76. Nismes. Mean temp. 60° .26.

In the United States, the most favourable region for the phthisical invalid is that of Florida,—especially of Pensacola. St. Augustine is frequently chosen, but it is liable to north-east storms, which interfere with the out-door movements of the valetudinarian, and are the source of much discomfort. Still, great benefit has often been derived from it as a winter retreat. Of the Atlantic Isles, Madeira appears to be best adapted for the consumptive, and those affected with chronic bronchitis. In Italy, Rome, and Pisa,—and in England, Torquay and Undercliff, are to be preferred. Chronic rheumatism and gout are benefited by a warm climate, which, again, is unfavourable to those who are predisposed to cerebral diseases, especially to such as are characterized by debility and mobility of the nervous system—as paralysis, epilepsy, mania, &c. Hypochondriasis and dyspepsia require rather change of climate and travelling exercise than a sojourn in any one. (See the Author's Human Health, Philad. 1844.)

For the mortality of different countries and cities, see Mortality.

CLIMATERIC, Climacteric.

CLIMATIC, *Climat'icus*. Belonging to, or dependent upon climate.

CLIMATIC DISEASES, *Morbi climat'ici*, are such as are caused by climate.

CLIMBER, WOODY, Ampelopsis quinquefolia.

CLINE, κλινη, 'a bed.' Hence:
CLINIATER, Clinical physician.
CLINIATRIA, Clinical medicine.
CLINIATRUS, Clinical physician.
CLINIC, see Clinique.
CLINICA, Clinical medicine.
CLIN'ICAL, *Clin'icus*, (F.) *Clinique*, from κλινη, 'a bed.' Relating to a bed.

CLINICAL LECTURE, (F.) *Leçon Clinique.* One given at the bed-side, or on a particular case or cases.

CLINICAL MED'ICINE, *Cliniatri'a, Clin'ica, Clin'icè*, (F.) *Médecine clinique.* That which is occupied with the investigation of diseases at the bed-side, or individually.

CLINICAL PHYSICIAN, *Clinia'ter, Clinia'trus.* One who teaches clinical medicine.

CLINICE, Clinical medicine.
CLINICUM, *Clinique.*
CLINIQUE (F.), Clinical. *Clinique, Clin'icum*, is also used substantively, for *École Clinique* or *Clinical School:* a school in which medicine is taught by examining diseases on the patients themselves. Thus, the French say,—La *Clinique* de la Charité: "The *Clinical School* of the Hospital *La Charité.*" The term has been introduced into this country, and anglicised *Clinic.*

CLINODES, Clinoid.
CLINOID, *Clinoï'des, Olino'des, Clinoï'deus*, from κλινη, 'a bed,' and ειδος, 'form.' Resembling a bed.

CLINOID PROC"ESSES, (F.) *Apophyses clinoïdes*, are four processes at the upper surface of the sphenoid bone, which have been compared to the posts of a bed. On them the pituitary gland rests. They are divided into *anterior* and *posterior.* Each of the anterior terminates in a point called *Transverse Spinous Process.*

CLINOÏDEUS, Clinoid.
CLINOPODIA, Thymus mastichina.
CLINOPODIUM ARVENSE, C. vulgare—c. Majus, C. vulgare.

CLINOPO'DIUM VULGA'RE, from κλινη, 'a bed,' and πους, 'foot,' so called from the shape of its flowers, *Clinopodium arven'sè* seu *majus*, *Oc'ymum sylvestrè, Thymus sylvat'icus, Wild Basil*, (F.) *Grand Basilic sauvage.* A European plant, which was formerly considered to be an antidote to the bites of venomous animals, to facilitate labour, relieve strangury, stop diarrhœa, &c.

CLIQUETIS, Crepitation.

CLISEOM'ETER, *Clisiom'eter*, from κλισις, 'inclination,' and μετρον, 'a measure.' An instrument, intended to measure the degree of inclination of the pelvis and to determine the relation between the axis of the pelvis and that of the body.—Osiander, Stein.

CLITBUR, Arctium lappa.

CLITORICARCINO'MA, from κλιτορις, 'clitoris,' and καρκινωμα, 'cancer.' Cancer of the clitoris.

CLITORIDES INFERIORES LATI ET PLANI MUSCULI, Constrictores cunni.

CLIT'ORIS, from κλητωρ, 'a servant who invites guests.' (?) *Dulce'do Amor'is, Venus, Myrton, Murton, Murtum, Œstrum, Penis mulie'bris* seu *fœmineus, Men'tula mulie'bris, Membrum mulie'brè, Superla'bia, Cerco'sis, Hypoder'mis, Nympha, Nymphè, Epider'rhis, Libi'dinis Sedes, Tunic'ula, Orista.* A small, round organ, situate at the upper part of the vulva, and separated by a small space from the anterior commissure of the labia. Its base is surrounded by a slight fold, similar to the prepuce; and it is, internally, of the same structure as the *corpora cavernosa penis.* The artery of the clitoris, (F.) *A. Clitorienne*, is a branch of the internal pudic. The *vein* communicates with the internal pudic, and the *nerve* with the pudic.

CLIT'ORISM, *Clitoris'mus.* A word, invented to express the abuse made of the clitoris. Also, an unusually large clitoris, *Cerco'sis extern'a* seu *Clitor'idis, Cauda'tio.*

CLITORI'TIS, *Clitoriti'tis*, from κλιτορις, 'clitoris,' and *itis*, 'denoting inflammation.' Inflammation of the clitoris.

CLITORITITIS, Clitoritis.

CLITORIUM, Vulva.

CLOA'CA, (F.) *Cloaque*, from κλυζω, 'I wash.' The pouch at the extremity of the intestinal canal, in which the solid and liquid excretions are commingled in birds, fish and reptiles. In the male, it gives exit to the excrements, sperm and urine: in the female, to the eggs, fæcal matters, and urine.

CLOANX, Orpiment.

CLOAQUE, Cloaca.

CLOCHE, (F.) A popular expression in France for a blister or other vesicle.

CLOISON, Septum — c. *des Fosses nasales*, Septum narium — c. *Transparente*, Septum lucidum.

CLONIC, *Clon'icus*, from κλονος, 'agitation,' 'motion.' (F.) *Clonique.* Irregular convulsive motions. Convulsion with alternate relaxation; in contradistinction to *tonic*, which signifies a constant rigidity ;—*Clonus, Clon'ici partia'les.*

CLONIC SPASM, see Spasm.

CLONICI UNIVERSALES, Synclonus.

CLONIQUE, Clonic.

CLONIS, Sacrum.

CLONISM, *Clonis'mus ;* same etymon. Clonic spasm.—Baumes.

CLONO'DES, from κλονος, 'agitation,' and ειδος, 'resemblance.' Convulsive. Galen applies this term to the pulse, when convulsive, as it were, and unequal. He compares the sensation it communicates to the finger to that produced by a bundle of sticks or rods in vibration.

CLONOS EPILEPSIA, Epilepsy — c. Hydrophobia, Hydrophobia.

CLONUS, Synclonus — c. Nictitatio, Nictation —c. Palpitatio, Palpitation—c. Pandiculatio, Pandiculation—c. Pandiculatio maxillarum, Yawning

—c. Singultus, Singultus—c. Sternutatio, Sneezing—c. Subsultus, Subsultus tendinum.
CLOPEMANIA, Kleptomania.
CLOPORTES ORDINAIRES, Onisci aselli.
CLOSE-STOOL, Lasanum.
CLOT, Coagulum—c. of Blood, see Blood.
CLOTBUR, Xanthium.
CLOTHING, Vestitus.
CLOTTY, *Grumo'sus*, (F.) *Grumeleux*. Composed of clots.
CLOU, Clavus, Furunculus—*c. Hystérique*, Clavus hystericus—*c. de l'Œil*, Clavus oculi.
CLOUDBERRIES, Rubus chamæmorus.
CLOUDBERRY TREE, Rubus chamæmorus.
CLOVE, see Eugenia caryophyllata—c. Bark, see Myrtus caryophyllata—c. Pink, Dianthus caryophyllus—c. July flower, Dianthus caryophyllus.
CLUBFEET, Kyllosis.
CLUBMOSS, Lycopodium—c. Common, Lycopodium complanatum—c. Fir, Lycopodium selago—c. Upright, Lycopodium selago.
CLUNES, Nates.
CLUNE'SIA, from *Clunes*, 'the nates.' *Proctal'gia, Procti'tis*. An inflammation of the buttocks.—Vogel.
CLUNIS, Sacrum.
CLUPEA THRYSSA. The *Yellow-billed Sprat;* a very poisonous fish of the West Indies.
CLUTIA ELUTERIA, Croton cascarilla.
CLYDON, Flatulence.
CLYPEALIS (Cartilago.) Thyroid cartilage.
CLYSANTLIUM, Syringe, Clyster.
CLYSIS, *Clysmus*. Same etymon as clyster. The application of a clyster. Washing out by means of a clyster.
CLYSMA, Clysis, Clyster, Enema—c. Tonicum, Enema fœtidum.
CLYSMA'TION, same etymon as clyster. A diminutive of clysma. A small clyster.
CLYSMUS, Clysis, Enema.
CLYSOIRE, (F.) An apparatus for administering enemata, consisting of a long funnel-shaped tube of elastic gum, furnished with a pipe at the apex.
CLYSOPOMPE, Syringe, Clyster.
CLYSTER, *Clyste'rium, Clysma, Enclys'ma, Clysmus, En'ema, Lavamen'tum*, from κλυζειν, 'to wash.' (F.) *Clystère, Larement, Remède*. A liquid, thrown into the large intestines by means of a syringe, or bladder and pipe properly prepared, &c.; the nozzle of the syringe or pipe being introduced into the anus. See Enema.
CLYSTER, ANODYNE, Enema anodynum—c. Common, Enema commune—c. Domestic, Enema commune—c. Fetid, Enema fœtidum—c. Pipe, Elasma—c. Purging, Enema catharticum—c. Starch and opium, Enema anodynum—c. Tobacco, Enema tabaci—c. Turpentine, Enema terebinthinæ—c. Uterinus, Sparallium.
CLYSTÈRE, Enema.
CNEME, Leg, Tibia.
CNEMODACTYLÆUS, Extensor communis digitorum pedis.
CNEMOLORDO'SIS, from κνημη, 'the leg,' and λορδωσις, 'the state of being bent forward.' Bending of the leg forward.
CNEMOSCOLIO'SIS, from κνημη, 'leg,' and σκολιωσις, 'bending,' especially sideways. Bending of the leg sideways. The state of being bowlegged, or bandy-legged.
CNEORON, Daphne gnidium.
CNEORUM TRICOC'CUM, *Almere'rion, Ac-nes'tos, Chamæle'a, Widow-wail, Spurge-Olive*, (F.) *Camelée*. This plant, a native of Southern Europe, contains a very irritating, acrid principle. The ancients employed its leaves as a powerful purgative. It is now sometimes used for deterging ulcers.
CNESIS, *Cnesmos, Cnismos*. A painful itching.—Galen.
CNESMA, Itching.
CNESMOS, Cnesis, Itching, Prurigo.
CNICELÆ'UM, from κνικος, 'carthamus,' and ελαιον, 'oil.' Oil of carthamus.—Dioscorides.
CNICUS, Carthamus tinctorius—c. Sylvestris, Centaurea benedicta.
CNIDELÆ'ON, *Cnidelæ'um*, from κνιδεις, 'cnidia,' and ελαιον, 'oil.' Oil made from the grana cnidia or mezereon berries.—Dioscorides.
CNID'IA GRANA. *Cnidii Cocci, Coccognid'ia, Æto'lion, Coccum*. The berries of the Daphne gnidium.—Foësius.
CNIDIUM SILAUS, Peucedanum silaus—c. Tenuifolium, Sison ammi.
CNIDO'SIS. A pungent itching, compared to that produced by the *Urtica urens* or *Nettle*. (κνιδη.)—Hippoc. Urticaria; urticatio.
CNIP'OTES, *Pruri'tus*. Itching. The dry ophthalmia, *Xerophthal'mia*.
CNISMOREGMIA, Pyrosis.
CNISMOS, Cnesmos.
CNISSA, see Nidorous.
CNISSOREG'MIA, from κνισσα, 'the smell of burnt fat,' and οργω, 'I put forth;' *Ructus nidoro'sus*. A nidorous eructation, as of rotten eggs.
CNYMA, κνυμα. A slight itching. Also, a puncture or vellication.—Galen.
COACUM, Phytolacca decandra.
COAGMENTATIO, Gomphosis.
COAGULABLE LYMPH, Fibrin, Liquor sanguinis.
COAG'ULANTS, *Coagulan'tia*, from *coagulare*,—itself from *co* and *agere*, 'to act together.' Remedies, or poisons, supposed to possess the power of coagulating the blood, or to give consistency to animal fluids. The word and the absurd notions connected with it are equally abandoned.
COAGULA'TION, *Coagula'tio, Thrombo'sis*. The conversion of a liquid into a more or less soft and tremulous mass. Many animal and vegetable fluids are capable of coagulation.
COAG'ULUM, *Grumus*, (F.) *Caillot, Grumeau*, ('a small clot.') A soft mass formed in a coagulable liquid. The *Clot of the Blood* is particularly so called—the *Cruor, Insula, Placen'ta, Hepar San'guinis, Crassamen'tum, Sanguis concre'tus;*—the red mass, composed of fibrin, serum, and colouring matter, which separates when the blood is left to itself. See Blood. The word is also applied, in pathology, to the sanguineous concretions, which form in different natural and accidental cavities; and which, when they occur at the mouth of a divided artery, sometimes suspend the flow of blood. This is, indeed, one of the means by which hemorrhage is arrested.
COAG'ULUM ALU'MINIS, *Coag'ulum Alumino'-sum, Cataplas'ma alu'minis, Alum curd* or *cataplasm*. This is made by beating the white of egg with a little alum, until a coagulum is formed. It is applied in cases of ophthalmia, where an astringent is necessary.
COALES'CENCE, *Coalescen'tia, Coalit"io par'tium*, from *coalescere*, 'to run together,' (from *cum*, 'with,' and *alere*, 'to nourish,) *Sym'physis, Pros'physis*. The adhesion or union of parts previously separated, as in case of wounds and preternatural adhesions or malformations. See Monster.
COALITIO PARTIUM, Coalescence.
COALIT"ION, *Coalit"io*. The same etymon as coalescence. It has been used in the same cases; as well as to express the action of several

parts of the frame, which have the same nutrition.

COALITUS, Symphysis.

COALTER'NÆ FEBRES. A name given to two intermittents, which attack a person at the same time, but whose paroxysms are distinct: so that the attack of one supervenes when the other has ceased. The term *Double Intermittent* expresses the same meaning.

COAPTA'TION, *Coapta'tio*, from *cum*, 'with,' and *aptare*, 'to adjust,' 'adapt;' *Parago'gē*. The act of adapting the two extremities of a fractured bone to each other; or of restoring a luxated bone to its place. Coaptation must be effected gently. Usually, extension and counter-extension are, in the first place, necessary.

COARTICULATIO, Diarthrosis, Synarthrosis.

COARCTATIO, Arctatio, Coarctation, Stricture — c. Ventriculi, Stricture of the Stomach.

COARCTA'TION, *Coarcta'tio*, from *coarctare*, 'to straiten.' Stricture. Avicenna speaks of *Coarctation of the Pulse*.

COAT, BUFFY, Corium phlogisticum.

COBALT, PROTOXIDE OF, Smalt.

COBHAM, MINERAL WATERS OF. Cobham is seven miles from Kingston, in Surrey, England. The waters are weak saline purgatives.

COBRA DI CAPELLO, Crotalus horridus.

COBWEB, Araneæ tela.

COCASH, Erigeron Philadelphicum.

COCCA'RIUM. A very small pill.

COCCI GRANUM, Kermes—c. Orientales, see Menispermum cocculus.

COCCIGIO-CUTANÉ SPHINCTER, Sphincter ani externus.

COCCINELLA, Coccus cacti.

COCCINEL'LA SEPTEMPUNCTA'TA, *Lady-bird, Lady-cow, Lady-bug*. This insect, bruised upon an aching tooth, has long been regarded as antiodontalgic.

COC'CION, κοκκιον. A weight, mentioned by Myrepsus; the same as the siliqua.

COCCIONELLA, Coccus cacti.

COCCOBALSAMUM, see Amyris opobalsamum.

COCCOGNIDIA, Cnidia grana.

COCCOLOBA UVIFERA, see Kino.

COCCONES, see Punica granatum.

COCCULÆ OFFICINARUM, see Menispermum cocculus.

COCCULUS CRISPUS, Menispermum tuberculatum—c. Indi aromatica, see Myrtus pimenta—c. Indicus, see Menispermum cocculus—c. Palmatus, Columba—c. Suberosus, Menispermum cocculus.

COCCUM, Cnidia grana, Kermes—c. Baphicum, Kermes—c. Infectorium, Kermes—c. Scarlatinum, Kermes—c. Tinctorum, Kermes.

COCCUS, Coccus cacti—c. Americanus, Coccus cacti.

Coccus CACTI. The systematic name of the *Coch'ineal Insect, Coccinel'la, Cochinil'la, Coccionel'la, Coccinil'la, Ficus In'diæ grana, Coccus Polon'icus, Scarabæ'olus hemisphæ'ricus, Cochinelif'era cochinil'la, Coccus America'nus, Coccus In'dicus Tincto'rius, Cochinelle, Coccus ;* the *Coch'ineal Animal,* (F.) *Cochenille, Graine d'Écarlate.* The cochineal insects have a faint, heavy odour; their taste is acrid, bitterish, and astringent : colour blackish-red externally,—purple-red within. They are used chiefly for giving a red colour to tinctures, &c. They were, at one time, esteemed astringent, stimulant, diuretic, and anodyne.

Coccus ILICIS, Kermes—c. Indicus tinctorius, Coccus cacti—c. Indicus, see Menispermum cocculus—c. Polonicus, Coccus cacti.

COCCYCEPH'ALUS, *Coccy'go-ceph'alus*, from *coccyx* and *κεφαλη*, 'the head.' A monster whose head has the shape of the os coccygis.

COCCYGEAL, Coccygeus—c. Nerve, see Sacral Nerves.

COCCYGE'US, *Coccyge'al*, from κοκκυξ, because it is inserted into the coccyx; *Ischio-Coccygeus*, (F.) *Ischio-coccygien*. Belonging both to the ischium and coccyx. The muscle *Ischio-coccygeus, Leva'tor Coccy'gis, Triangula'ris Coccy'gis.* It arises from the spinous process of the ischium, and is inserted into the extremity of the sacrum; and into nearly the whole length of the os coccygis laterally. It retains the coccyx in place, and prevents it from being forced backwards during the evacuation of the fæces.

COCCYGIO-ANAL, Sphincter ani externus.

COCCYGIO-CUTANÉ SPHINCTER, Sphincter ani externus.

COCCYGOCEPHALUS, Coccycephalus.

COCCYMELEA, Prunus domestica.

COCCYX, 'a cuckoo,' whose bill it is said to resemble; *Os Coccy'gis, Cauda, Ossis sacri acu'men, Os Al'agas, Rump Bone, Crupper Bone, Cu'culus, Uropyg'ion, Spon'dylis, Spondyl'ium.* An assemblage of small bones, attached to the lower part of the sacrum; the curvature of which it prolongs, and of which it seems to be an appendage. Generally, it consists of four bones. Behind the base of the coccyx are two small tubercular eminences. These are called *Cornua of the Coccyx*.

COCHEMAR, Incubus.

COCHENILLE, Coccus cacti.

COCHERIA, Cochia.

COCHIA, *Cocchia, Coche'ria,* from *κοκκος*, 'berry,' 'seed,' or from *κεχυω*, 'to flow profusely.' An ancient name for several officinal purgative pills; thus called, either because they produced copious evacuations, or were shaped like a seed.

COCHIN LEG, see Elephantiasis.

COCHINEAL, Coccus cacti.

COCHINELIFERA COCHINILLA, Coccus cacti.

COCHINILLA, Coccus cacti.

COCH'LEA. A *Snail's shell*, (F.) *Limaçon, Coquille.* Anatomists have given this name to the most anterior of the three cavities which constitute the labyrinth of the ear, the *Pelvis Au'rium, Concha auris inter'na, Cav'itas cochlea'ta, C. buccina'ta, Antrum buccino'sum, Concha Labyrin'thi, Troch'lea labyrinth'i:* — and that of *Scalæ of the Cochlea,* (F.) *Rampes du limaçon,* to two spiral cavities in the interior of the cochlea. One of these scalæ terminates at the *Fenes'tra rotun'da,* and is called *Scala tympani:* the other opens at the anterior and inferior part of the vestibule : it is called *Scala vestib'uli.*

COCHLEA, SCALÆ OF THE, see Cochlea.

COCHLEAR, Cochleare—c. Auriculare, Earpick—c. Nerve, see Auditory Nerve.

COCHLEA'RE, *Ooch'lear, Cochlea'rium,* from *cochlea;* its bowl resembling a shell. A *spoonful,* (F.) *Cuillerée;* abbreviated in prescriptions usually to *coch.* See Abbreviation. Also, a scoop.

COCHLEA'RE MAGNUM, a tablespoonful; *C. Me'dium,* a dessert or pap-spoonful; and *C. Min'imum,* a teaspoonful.

COCHLEA'RIA, from *cochleare,* 'a spoon,' so called from its resemblance. *C. officinalis.*

COCHLEA'RIA ARMORA'CIA, *Raph'anus rustica'nus, Armora'cia, A. sati'va, A. rustica'na, Raph'anus mari'nus, Raph'anus sylves'tris, Raph'anus magna, Horseradish.* Family, Cruciferæ. *Sex. Syst.* Tetradynamia Siliculosa. (F.) *Raifort sauvage, Oran, Cran de Bretagne.* The root of horseradish is frequently used at table; and has long been in the Materia Medica. It is stimulant and diuretic. Externally it is rubefacient.

COCHLEA'RIA CORON'OPUS, *Coron'opus, Coron'opus Ruel'lii* seu *depres'sus* seu *vulga'ris, Lepid'ium squama'tum, Senebie'ra coron'opus, Wild Scurvy Grass, Swine's Cress,* (F.) *Corne de Cerf.* This European plant is considered to be diuretic and antiscorbutic. The term *Coron'opus* was given, by the ancients, to various plants.

COCHLEA'RIA HORTENSIS, Cochlearia officinalis.

COCHLEA'RIA OFFICINA'LIS, *Cochlearia, C. horten'sis* seu *pyrena'ica* seu *vulga'ris, Lemon Scurvy Grass, Common Scurvy Grass,* (F.) *Cranson, Herbe aux cuillers.* It has been considered a powerful antiscorbutic. It is sometimes eaten in salad.

COCHLEA'RIA PYRENA'ICA, C. officinalis — c. Vulgaris, C. officinalis.

COCHLEARIFOR'MIS, from *cochleare,* 'a spoon,' and *forma,* 'shape;' (F.) *Bec de Cuiller.*

COCHLEARIFORMIS PROCES'SUS, *Cochlear'iform process.* A small, very thin plate, which separates the bony portion of the Eustachian tube from the canal for the passage of the tensor tympani.

COCHLEA'RIS. A gelatinous looking tissue, seen on opening the cochlea, by which the membranous zone is connected, at its outer or convex margin, with the outer wall. It is supposed by Todd and Bowman to be muscular; and to have a preservative office, being placed to defend the cochlear nerves from undue vibrations of sound, in a way analogous to that in which the iris protects the retina from excessive light.

COCHLEARIUM, Cochleare.

COCHO'NE, κοχωνη. The junction of the ischium, near the seat or breech.—Foësius. The breech proper, from the hip-bones to the anus. The perinæum. The coccyx.

COCIL'IO. A weight of eleven ounces.

COCKLE-BUR, Agrimony.

COCKLES, INDIAN, see Menispermum cocculus.

COCKMINT, Tanacetum balsamita.

COCKUP HAT, Stillingia.

COCLES, *Borgne.*

COCO, Cocos nucifera.

COCO OF THE MALDIVES, *Cocos de Maldi'vâ.* The fruit of a palm, called *Lodoïce'a* by Commerson. It was formerly termed, in the shops, *Nux Med'ica,* and enjoyed great reputation.

COCOA, Cacao.

COCOA CACAVIFERA, Cacao.

COCOBAY, Mal de San Lazaro.

COCOS BUTYRA'CEA. The name of the plant which affords the *palm oil, O'leum pal'mæ,* obtained chiefly from the fruit, by bruising and mixing the kernels with water, without the aid of heat, by which the oil is separated and rises to the surface. It is of the consistence of an ointment, with little taste, and a strong, though not disagreeable, smell. It is applied to sprains, &c.; but has no advantages over other oils. It has been called, also, *O'leum Palmæ seba'ceum, O. Ax'um nucum cocos butyra'ceæ* and *Mackaw fat.* It is procured likewise from the *Ela'is Gwineen'sis,* and *Ela'is Occidenta'lis,* two species of palms.

COCOS NUCIF'ERA, *Palma cocos,* (F.) *Cocotier. Order,* Palmæ. The systematic name of the plant whose fruit is the cocoa nut. (F.) *Coco.* It is an agreeable kernel, but not easy of digestion. *Emulsions, orgeat,* &c., are made from it. The *juice* of the cocoa, when fermented, forms wine, and arrack is distilled from it.

COCOTE, Influenza.

COCOTIER, Cocos nucifera.

COCTIO, Coction, Digestion—c. Ciborum, Digestion—c. Morbi, Coction.

COC'TION, *Coc'tio, Pepsis, Pepan'sis, Pepas'mos, Sympep'sis, Concoc'tion,* from *coquere,* 'to boil.' This word has been employed in various senses. 1. With the ancients, *coction* meant the particular kind of alteration which the food experiences in the digestive organs, particularly in the stomach. It meant a preparation from its *crude* state. 2. It expressed the *maturation* or change, which the humeral pathologists believed morbific matter experiences before elimination. It was considered, that coction, *Coc'tio morbi,* was produced during the violence of the disease; and hence this was called the *Period of Coction.* See Humorism.

COD, or CODS, Scrotum.

COD-OIL, Oleum jecoris aselli.

COD-LIVER OIL, Oleum jecoris aselli.

CODAGAPALA BARK, Nerium antidysentericum.

CODE, Codex.

CODEIA, Codeine.

COD'EINE, *Codei'a, Codei'num, Papaveri'num,* from κωδια, 'a poppy head.' An alkaloid, discovered, by Robiquet, in opium, in 1832. It is soluble in water, alcohol and ether, and unites readily with acids. As a hypnotic, Magendie thinks one grain of codeia equal to half a grain of morphia. The muriate of codeia appears to be stronger than the pure codeia.

CODESELLA, Anthrax.

CODEX. A collection of laws. (F.) *Code.* By extension, a collection of approved medical formulæ, with the processes necessary for forming the compounds referred to in it. The Parisian Pharmacopœia is styled *Codex medicamenta'rius.*

CODEX MEDICAMENTARIUS, Formulary, see Codex.

CODIA, Papaver (capsule.)

CODOCELE, Bubo.

CODOSCELLA, Bubo.

CŒCAL, Cæcal.

CŒCITAS, Cæcitas.

CŒCUM, Cæcum.

COEFFE, Caul.

CŒ'LIA, κοιλια, κοιλη, 'a hollow place.' This word generally meant a cavity in the body:—the abdomen, in particular. It has also been used for the alimentary canal, &c.: — ανω κοιλια, 'the stomach,' κατω κοιλια, 'the abdomen.' Also, an alvine evacuation; excrement.

CŒ'LIAC, *Cœliacus, Gastrocœ'liacus, Gastrocœ'licus,* (F.) *Cœliaque* ou *Céliaque,* from κοιλια, 'the cavity of the abdomen.' Relating to the cavity of the abdomen.

CŒLIAC ARTERY, *A. Cœ'liaca, Cœliac axis, A. opistogastrique,* Ch., *A. Cœliaque, Tronc cœliaque, Trépied de la cœliaque,* is situate above the pancreas, and behind the upper part of the stomach. It arises from the anterior part of the abdominal aorta, where it passes between the pillars of the diaphragm, and soon divides into the *coronaria ventriculi, hepatic,* and *splenic* arteries.

CŒLIAC FLUX, *Cœliac Passion, Cœliaca chylo'sa, Diarrhœ'a chylo'sa, D. chymo'sa, Fluxus chylo'sus* seu *cœliacus, Passio cœliaca, P. Ventriculo'sa, Chymoche'sia, Fluor albus intestino'rum, Chylorrhœ'a, Chymorrhœ'a, Cœliaca lac'tea, Morbus cœliacus, Chylodiarrhœ'a, Galactodiarrhœ'a, Sedes lactescen'tes, Gastrorrhœ'a,* (F.) *Flux cœliaque.* A species of diarrhœa, in which the food is discharged by the bowels in an undigested condition. By some, defined to be diarrhœa attended with discharges of chyle or chyme. It is, in general, symptomatic of tubercular disease of the mesenteric glands. See Lientery.

CŒLIAC PASSION, Cœliac flux.

CŒLIAC PLEXUS, *Solar Plexus, Plexus mesenter'ii pro'prius et max'imus,* P. *ganglifor'mis semiluna'ris,* (F.) *Plexus médian ou opistogastrique,* (Ch.,) Pl. *Cœliao ou solaire, Ganglion de* VIEUSSENS, is formed of numerous nervous filaments, which proceed from the semilunar ganglia of the great sympathetic. It is strengthened by several branches of the right and left pneumogastric nerves; is seated around the trunk of the cœliac artery, behind the stomach, and furnishes the secondary plexuses — the *diaphragmatic, coronary of the stomach, splenic* and *hepatic,* which accompany the arteries of the same name.

CŒLIACA, from κοιλιακος, 'cœliac.' Diseases of the digestive organs; the 1st class in Good's *Nosology.* It comprises two orders, *Enterica* and *Splanchnica.* Also, medicines that act on the digestive organs.—Pereira.

CŒLIACA CHYLOSA, Cœliac flux — c. Lactea, Cœliac flux — c. Renalis, Chyluria — c. Urinalis, Chyluria.

CŒLIÆ'MIA, *Hyperæ'mia abdom'inis, Conges'tio abdomina'lis,* from κοιλια, 'the abdomen,' and 'αιμα, 'blood.' Hyperæmia or congestion of the blood-vessels of the abdomen.

CŒLIAGRA, *Gastri'tis* seu *Enteri'tis* seu *Col'ica* seu *Diarrhœ'a arthrit'ica.* Gout of the abdomen.

CŒLIALGIA, Tormina.

CŒLIAQUE, TRÉPIED DE LA, Cœliac artery.

CŒLIOCELE, see Hernia, hypogastric.

CŒLIOCHYSIS, Ascites.

CŒLIOCYESIS, Pregnancy, abdominal.

CŒLIODYNIA, Colic.

CŒLIOLYSIA, Diarrhœa.

CŒLION'CUS, *Cœliophy'ma,* from κοιλια, 'the abdomen,' and ογκος, 'a tumour.' A tumour of the abdomen.

CŒLIOPHYMA, Cœlioncus.

CŒLIOPHY'MATA, *Tuber'cula peritonæ'i,* from κοιλια, 'the cavity of the abdomen,' and φυμα, 'a hard tumour.' Tubercles of the peritoneum.

CŒLIOPSOPHIA, Borborygmus.

CŒLIOPYO'SIS, from κοιλια, 'the abdomen,' and πυωσις, 'suppuration.' Suppuration in the abdomen or its parietes.

CŒLIORRHŒA, Diarrhœa.

CŒLIORRHEU'MA, *Rheumatis'mus abdom'inis,* from κοιλια, 'the abdomen,' and ρευμα, 'defluxion, rheumatism.' Rheumatism of the muscles of the abdomen.

CŒLIOSPAS'MUS, from κοιλια, 'abdomen,' and σπασμος, 'spasm.' Spasm or cramp of the abdomen.

CŒLO'MA, from κοιλος, 'hollow.' A round ulcer of the cornea, broader and deeper than that described under the name *Bothrion.*

CŒLON, Cavity.

CŒLOPHTHAL'MUS, from κοιλος, 'hollow,' and οφθαλμος, 'eye.' One who is hollow-eyed.

CŒLOSTOM'IA, from κοιλος, 'hollow,' and στομα, 'mouth.' A defect in speaking, when the voice seems as if it came from a cavern;—that is, obscure, and as if at a distance.

CŒLOS'TOMUS, same etymon. One who has a hollow voice.

CŒLOTES, Cavity.

CŒNÆSTHE'SIS, from κοινος, 'common,' and αισθησις, 'feeling.' *Conæsthe'sis.* Common feeling. Some German writers mean, by this, a sixth sense. It is the feeling of self-existence or individuality, and is manifested by the sense of buoyancy or depression, which we experience without any known cause;—by involuntary shuddering, feeling of chill or glow, &c.

CŒNOLOGIA, Consultation.

CŒ'NOTES, κοινοτης, 'commonness,' from κοινος, 'common.' The physicians of the methodic sect asserted that all diseases arise from *relaxation, stricture,* or a mixture of both. These were called *Cœnotes:* or what diseases have in common.

COETUS, Coition.

CŒUR, Heart.

COF'FEA ARAB'ICA, *C. vulga'ris, Jas'minum Arab'icum,* (F.) *Caftier,* and *Cafeyer.* Family, Rubiaceæ. *Sex. Syst.* Pentandria Monogynia. The plant which affords coffee, *Choava, Bon, Buna,* (F.) *Café.* Originally from Yemen.

The infusion of coffee is an agreeable and wholesome article of diet. It is, to a certain extent, a tonic, and is employed as such in convalescence, especially from fevers, &c. In cases of poisoning by opium, and in old asthmas, its use has been extolled. For this purpose the *Moka* is the best. It ought to be newly torrefied, but not too much burnt; should be strong, and drunk soon after grinding. *Factitious Coffees* have been, from time to time, recommended, but they are infinitely inferior to the genuine. Various *substitutes* have been proposed; *wheat, barley, hollyberries, acorns, sunflower seeds, beechmast, peas, beans, succory-root, seeds of gooseberries* and *currants* left in making wine, and washed, —*sliced turnips,* &c. These have been roasted, with the addition of a little butter or oil: but they have not the aroma of coffee. The best substitute is said to be the seeds of the *Yellow water flag, Gladiolus luteus* or *Iris pseudacorus.*

Hunt's Œconomical Breakfast Powder consisted of rye, roasted with a little butter.

COFFEE-TREE, Gymnocladus Canadensis.

COFFEE, WILD, Triosteum.

COGNITIO PHYSIOLOGICA, Physiology.

COHABITATIO, Coition.

COHABITA'TION, *Cohabita'tio,* from *cum,* 'with,' and *habitare,* 'to dwell.' The act of dwelling together. In legal medicine, it means the consummation of marriage.—*Copulation.*

COHE'SION, *Cohæsio,* from *cum,* 'with,' and *hærere,* 'to stick.' *Vis cohæsio'nis, Vis adhæsio'nis, Vis attractio'nis,* Force of *cohe'sion, Attraction of cohesion,* A. *of aggrega'tion,* is that force in the particles of matter, whereby they are connected in such a way as to resist any attempt towards their removal or separation. This force has to be attended to, in the management of disease. Emollients, rubbed into a part, act by diminishing the cohesion.

COHIBENS, Epischeticus.

COHOBA'TION, *Cohoba'tio, Coho'bium, Co'hob, Co'hoph.* Distillation of a liquid — already distilled—on the same substances. When this is repeated three or four times, it is called *Recohoba'tion.*

COHOL. Synonym of Alcohol. Also, a dry collyrium.—Avicenna.

COHOSH, Actæa racemosa, Caulophyllum thalictroïdes — c. Black, Actæa racemosa — c. Blueberry, Caulophyllum thalictroïdes.

COHUSH, Caulophyllum thalictroïdes.

COIFFE, Caul.

COIGN, see Pyrus cydonia.

COIGNASSIER, Pyrus cydonia.

COÏNCIDEN'TIA. Some authors have translated, by this term, the word *parempto'sis,* used by Galen to designate the occlusion of the foramen opticum by a humour, proceeding from the base of the brain, and occasioning blindness.— Castelli.

COIN'DICANT, *Coin'dicans,* from *con,* 'with,' and *indico,* 'I indicate.'

COIN'DICANT SIGNS are those which furnish the same indications; or which confirm the indication afforded by another sign:—*συνενδεικνυμενα.*

COIRA, Catechu.

COIRAS, Scrofula.

COIT, Coition.

COIT"ION, *Oo'itus, Co'etus,* from *coëo,* (con, and *eo,* 'to go,') 'to go together.' *Copula'tion, Copula'tio, Cop'ula Carna'lis, Aphrodi'sia, Aphrodisiasm'us, Epip'locē, Acces'sus, Basia'tio, Amplexa'tio, Amplex'us, Conven'tus, Complex'io, Conju'gium, Agglutina'tio, Lagne'a, Lagneu'ma, Lagnei'a, Mixis, Permis'tio, Permix'tio, Syndyas'mus, Synu'sia, Concu'bitus, Congres'sus, Cohabita'tio, Venus, Res Vene'rea, Concu'bitus vene'reus, Prœ'lium, Duell'um vene'reum, Noctur'na bella, Concil'ia corpora'lia, Homil'ia, Ven'ery, Sexual intercourse,* (F.) *Coit, Approche, Accouplement.* The carnal union of the sexes.

COITUS, Coition—c. Difficilis, Dyssynodus—c. Sodomiticus, Buggery.

COL, Collum—c. *de la Matrice,* Collum uteri—c. *Utérin,* Collum uteri.

COLA, Articulation.

COLATIO, see Colatura.

COLATO'RIUM, *Hylister,* from *colare,* 'to strain.' A strainer of any kind. (F.) *Couloir.* A term by which the ancient physicians described every canal or conduit through which the excrementitious humours of the body are evacuated. Ulcers, fistulæ, setons, caustics, &c., have been called *artificial* or *accidental Colatoria,* because they were considered to be passages by which the animal economy is freed from some morbific matter.

COLATUM, see Colatura.

COLATU'RA, from *colare,* 'to strain.' *Cola'tum,* (F.) *Colature.* A filtered or strained liquor. It likewise means straining a liquid, — *Cola'tio, Diy'lisis, Diylis'mus, Hy'lisis, Hylis'mus.*

COL'CHESTER, MINERAL WATERS OF. *Aqua Colcestren'sis.* The waters of Colchester are of the bitter purging kind, similar to those of Epsom.

COLCHICIA, see Colchicum autumnale.

COL'CHICUM AUTUMNA'LE, from the country Colchis. *Meadow Saffron, Col'chicum, Coum,* (F.) *Colchique, Tue-chien, Mort aux chiens, Safran des prés, Safran bâtard.* Family, Colchicaceæ. *Class,* Hexandria. *Order,* Monogynia. The bulb or root (*Bulbus* vel *Radix* vel *Cormus,*) and the seeds are the parts used in medicine. The taste is acrid, excoriating the mouth; but the acrimony is lost by drying. It is narcotic, diuretic, and cathartic; and has been given in dropsy, gout, and rheumatism. Dose, from gr. j to vj of the fresh bulb. It is supposed to be the active ingredient of the *Eau médicinale d'Husson.* The active principle is called *Colchic"ia.* The Colchicum, in an over-dose, is an acro-narcotic poison.

Dr. Wilson's Tincture for the Gout is said to be merely an infusion of Colchicum, or *Col'chicin.*

COLCHICUM ZEYLANICUM, Kæmpferia rotunda.

COLCHIQUE, Colchicum autumnale.

COL'COTHAR, *Col'cothar Vitrioli, Henri'cus rubens, Chalci'tis, Brown red, Rouge, Crocus, Oxidum Ferri rubrum, Tritox'ydum Ferri, Sulphas Ferri calcina'tum, Ferrum vitriola'tum ustum, Terra vitrioli dulcis, Crocus martis vitriolatus* seu *adstrin'gens,* (F.) *Rouge d'Angleterre, Safran de Mars astringent.* The red oxide of iron, obtained by calcining sulphate of iron to redness, with or without the contact of air. It possesses the general properties of the preparations of iron, and has been applied to stanch blood, &c.

COLD, *Frigus, Psychos,* (F.)·*Froid.* The sensation produced by the abstraction of caloric from our organs,—*Cheima, Chimon.* See Heat. Three degrees of cold are generally distinguished in disease. 1. The simple feeling of cold (*Algor*), 2. *Chilliness* (*Horror*), and 3. *Shivering* (*Rigor*). Cold is employed in medicine, chiefly, as a refrigerant and sedative.

COLD IN THE EYE, Ophthalmia, catarrhal — c. in the Head, Coryza.

COLEITIS, Colposis.

COLEOCELE, see Hernia.

COLŒDEMA, Elytrœdema.

COLEOPTOSIS, Prolapsus vaginæ.

COLEORRHEX'IS, from χολεος, 'a vagina or sheath,' and ρηξις, 'rupture.' Laceration or rupture of the vagina.

COLEOSITIS, Leucorrhœa.

COLEOSTEGNO'SIS, *Colpostegno'sis, Colpostenochor'ia, Colposynize'sis,* from χολεος, 'a vagina or sheath,' and στεγνωσις, 'constriction.' Narrowness of the vagina, natural or acquired.

COLÈRE, Rage.

COLES, Penis.

COLEUS, Vagina.

COLIBERT, Cagot.

COLIC, *Co'licus,* from κωλον, 'the colon.' (F.) *Colique.* Relating to the colon.

COLIC ARTERIES, *Arte'riæ colicæ,* (F.) *Artères Coliques,* are six in number, three of which, given off by the *superior mesenteric,* are called *Colicæ dextræ;* and three, proceeding from the inferior mesenteric, *Colicæ sinis'træ.* All proceed towards the colon, passing between the two laminæ of the peritoneum, which form the mesocolon, where they ramify and anastomose with each other. The first, *Colica dextra, Ramus col'ica dexter,* is called *C. dextra superior,* (*Méso-colique,*— Ch.) The second, *C. dextra media, Colica media, Ramus colicus medius, Arteria media anastomot'ica,* (*C. droite,* Ch.,) and the third, *C. dextra infe'rior* or *Ileo-colica,* (*A. cæcale,*— Ch.) Of the three *Colicæ sinistræ,* the first or *superior* is called, by Chaussier, *Colica magna sinis'tra;* the second or *media* is not distinguished from the preceding, as they often arise from a common trunk; and the third is called by Chaussier *Colica parva sinis'tra.* To these arteries as many veins correspond, which open into the great and little mesenteric.

COLIC LOBE OF THE LIVER is the great lobe of that organ.

COLIC, *Co'lica Passio, Colica, Bellyache, Col'icē, Colicodyn'ia, Cœliodyn'ia, Dolo'res intestino'rum, Dolor co'licus, Dysenteronerv'ia, Anenteroner'via, Enteral'gia, Gripes, Mulligrubs.* In its etymological acceptation, Colic signifies an affection or pain in the colon. But it is employed in a more extensive signification. It includes every acute pain of the abdomen, aggravated at intervals. The word has often, however, epithets affixed to it, which render it more or less precise. See Tormina.

COLIC, CRAPULENT, Colica crapulosa—c. Devonshire, Colic, metallic— c. Horn, Priapismus — c. Lead, Colic, metallic — c. Madrid, Colica Madridensis — c. Menstrual, Colica menstrualis — c. Metallica, Colica metallica — c. Painters', Colic, metallic — c. Plumbers', Colic, metallic — c. of Poitou, Colic, metallic — c. of Prostitutes, Colica scortorum — c. Saturnine, Colic, metallic — c. of Surinam, Colic, metallic—c. Uterine, Colica uterina—c. Weed, Dicentra Canadensis—c. Worm, Colica verminosa.

COLICA ACCIDENTALIS, Colica crapulosa —c. Acuta, Enteritis—c. Arthritica, Cœliagra.

CO'LICA BILIO'SA, *Bil'ious Colic,* (F.) *Colique Bilieuse.* Colic, occasioned by an accumulation of bile in the intestines or in its own passages.

The *treatment* required resembles that proper for the next variety.

COLICA CALLO'SA. Colic attended with sense of stricture in some parts of the intestinal canal; often of flatulency and pain; the flatulency gradually passing off by the stricture; the bowels tardy; and at length discharging small liquid stools.

COLICA CONVULSI'VA, *C. Spasmod'ica, C. pitui-to'sa, C. nervo'sa, C. idiopath'ica, Enterospasm'us.* Colic, not the symptom of any other affection. It is characterized by griping pain in the bowels, chiefly about the navel, with vomiting and costiveness,—the pain increasing at intervals. The indications are to clear the intestines, and allay spasm. Calomel and opium—castor oil and opium—emollient and cathartic enemata, with fomentations, wet or dry, to the abdomen, usually succeed.

COLICA CRAPULO'SA, *C. accidenta'lis, C. helluo'num, Crap'ulent colic, Surfeit, Colic from overeating,* (F.) *Colique d'Indigestion.* A colic, arising from eating indigestible aliments, or digestible aliments in too great abundance. The remedy is obvious.

COLICA DAMNONIORUM, Colic, metallic—c. Febricosa, Colica inflammatoria—c. Figulorum, Colica metallica.

COLICA FLATULEN'TA, *Infla'tio, Gastrodyn'ia flatulen'ta, Physospas'mus, Pneumato'sis enter'-ica,* (F.) *Colique flatulente, C. flatueuse, C. venteuse.* Colic, arising from an accumulation of air in the intestines. It is very common in infants, and may be relieved by aromatics, especially when combined with antacids — for example, oil of aniseed with magnesia.

COLICA HELLUONUM, Colica crapulosa.

COLICA HEMORRHOIDA'LIS, *Hemorrhoid'al Colic,* (F.) *Colique hémorrhoïdale.* A kind of colic, supposed to precede hemorrhoids or to supervene on their suppression.

COLICA HEPAT'ICA, *Hepatal'gia, Hepatalgia Calculo'sa, Hepat'ic colic,* (F.) *Colique hépatique.* Pain in the region of the liver, chiefly about the gall-bladder, occasioned by the passing of a biliary calculus through the cystic and choledoch ducts.

COLICA IDIOPATHICA, Colica convulsiva — c. Ileus, Ileus.

COLICA INFLAMMATO'RIA, *C. Phlogis'tica, C. plethor'ica, C. febrico'sa, C. pulsat'ilis, Inflam'-matory colic.* The same as enteritis.

COLICA LAPPONICA, see Seta equina—c. Lochialis, Dyslochia—c. Madridensis, Colic of Madrid —c. Nervosa, Colica convulsiva, Colic, metallic—c. Phlogistica, Colica inflammatoria.

COLICA MADRIDEN'SIS, *Colic of Madrid, Madrid Colic.* A species of colic, endemic in several provinces of Spain, whose nature is not clear. Its symptoms resemble those occasioned by lead.

COLICA MENSTRUA'LIS, *Men'strual Colic,* (F.) *Colique menstruelle.* Colic, which precedes or accompanies the menstrual evacuation, or which is owing to the suppression of that evacuation.

COLICA METAL'LICA, *Metal'lic Colic, Painters' Colic, Colica Pic'tonum, Colic of Poitou, Colica Saturni'na, C. Figulo'rum, Colic of Surinam', Bellon, Dev'onshire Colic, Dry Bellyache, Saturnine Colic, Lead Colic, Plumbers' Colic, Rachial'-gia Pic'tonum, R. Pictavien'sium, Morbus Metal'-licus, Colicople'gia, Colica Rachial'gia, Rachial'-gia, Colica Damnonio'rum, C. Plumbario'rum, Paral'ysis rachialgia, Colica nervo'sa, Colica Picto'rum, Palmus Plumba'rius,* (F.) *Dysentéronervis Saturnina, Colique de Poitou, Colique végétale* (?), *Colique des peintres, Colique de plomb, C. métallique, C. Saturnine, C. des barbouilleurs.* Under this head is generally described the colic produced by lead, as well as the other colics mentioned in the synonymy; and they certainly resemble each other greatly, although some of them are more like bilious colic. There is not much to distinguish this variety of colic from others. The same violent pain about the navel is present, with retraction of the abdomen towards the spine. It is apt also to occasion palsy. The only difference of treatment is in the necessity for employing more opium along with the purgative. The paralytic sequelæ must be treated by change of air, rubbing the spine, exercise, &c. Treating the disease upon general principles is infinitely more philosophical, and more successful than the empirical management at *La Charité,* Paris, which it is unnecessary to detail.

COLICA NEPHRET'ICA, *Nephret'ic Colic,* (F.) *Colique Néphrétique.* Acute pains, which accompany nephritis, and especially calculous nephritis, or the passage of a calculus into the ureter.

COLICA PICTONUM, Colic, metallic — c. Pictorum, Colic, metallic—c. Pituitosa, Colica convulsiva — c. Plethorica, Colica inflammatoria — c. Plumbariorum, Colic, metallic — c. Pulsatilis, Colic, inflammatory — c. Rachialgia, Colic, metallic—c. Saturnina, Colica metallica.

COLICA SCORTO'RUM, *Colic of Pros'titutes.* A form of colic, said by Dr. Martin Hassing, of Copenhagen, to have been frequently observed by him amongst that unfortunate class of beings. It may well be doubted whether any special affection of the kind appertains to them.

COLICA SPASMODICA, Colica convulsiva, Ileus.

COLICA STERCO'REA, *Colica Stipa'ta, Stercora'-ceous Colic,* (F.) *Colique stercorale.* A species of colic, ascribed to the retention of fæcal matters in the intestines. The retention is itself, however, an effect, that may be caused in the same manner as the colic pains themselves.

COLICA STIPATA, Colica stercorea.

COLICA UTERI'NA, *Hys'tero-col'ica, Uterine Colic,* (F.) *Colique utérine.* Pain seated in the uterus, sometimes called *Hysteral'gia.*

COLICA VENTRICULI, Cardialgia.

COLICA VERMINO'SA, *Helminthocol'ica, Worm Colic,* (F.) *Colique vermineuse.* Abdominal pain, occasioned by the presence of worms in the intestines.

COLICODYNIA, Colica.

COLICOPLEGIA, Colic, metallic.

COLIMAÇON, Limax.

COLIQUE, Colic—c. *des Barbouilleurs,* Colica metallica—c. *Hépatique,* Colica hepatica—c. *d'Indigestion,* Colica crapulosa—c. *Métallique,* Colica metallica — c. *de Miserere,* Ileus — c. *de Miséricorde,* Ileus — c. *des Peintres,* Colica metallica—c. *de Plomb,* Colica metallica—c. *de Poitou,* Colica metallica—c. *Saturnine,* Colica metallica—c. *Venteuse,* Colica flatulenta — c. *Végétale,* Colica metallica.

COLIQUES, Pains, (after.)

COLI'TIS, from κωλον, 'the colon, and *itis,* denoting inflammation; *Coloni'tis, Enteri'tis co'-lica,* (F.) *Inflammation du colon.* Inflammation of the peritoneal or mucous membrane of the colon. The former is termed *Serocoli'tis,* and *Exocoli'tis;* the latter, *Endocoolitis* and *Dysentery.*

COLIX, Trochiscus.

COLLA PISCIUM, Ichthyocolla.

COLLAPSE, Collapsus.

COLLAP'SUS, *Collapse, Conciden'tia;* from *col,* or *cum,* 'with,' and *labor, lapsus,* 'to fall.' (F.) *Affaissement.* A complete prostration of strength, either at the commencement or in the progress of a disease.

COLLAR-BONE, Clavicle.

COLLARD, Dracontium foetidum — c. Cow,

Dracontium fœtidum — c. Polecat, Dracontium fœtidum.

COLLARIUM SALINUM, Haloderæum.

COLLAT'ERAL, *Collatera'lis*, from *cum*, 'with,' and *latus*, 'side.' That which accompanies or proceeds by the side of another.

COLLAT'ERAL AR'TERIES OF THE ARM, *Arte'riæ Collatera'les Bra'chii*, (F.) *Artères collatérales du bras.* They are given off by the brachial, and are distinguished into, 1. The *collateral—superior or external* (*Grandes musculaires du bras*—Ch.) which arise from the inner part of the brachial, and extend as far as the inferior and external part of the arm. 2. The *collateral — inferior or internal* (*Collatérales du Coude*—Ch.) which arise from the brachial, near the elbow-joint, and descend towards the upper part of the fore-arm.

The vessels which pass to the fingers and toes are also called *collateral.*

Speaking generally, *collateral branches* are those which follow nearly the same course as the vessel whence they emanate.

COLLATERALIS, Ischio-cavernosus.

COLLE-CHAIR, Sarcocolla.

COLLE DE POISSON, Ichthyocolla.

COLLEC'TION, *Collec'tio*, from *colligere*, 'to gather.' This word is often united to the epithet *purulent, serous*, &c., to express a *gathering* of pus, serum, &c.

COLLESIS, Agglutination.

COLLETICUS, Agglutinant.

COLLEY'S DEPILATORY, see Depilatory.

COLLIC"LÆ. 'Drains to collect and convey away water.' See *GOUTTIÈRE.* Union of the ducts passing from the puncta lachrymalia, *Collic"iæ puncto'rum lacryma'lium.*

COLLICULI NERVI ETHMOIDALIS, Corpora striata — c. Nervorum opticorum, Thalami nervorum opticorum—c. Vaginæ, Nymphæ.

COLLICULUS CAVEÆ POSTERIORIS VENTRICULORUM LATERALIUM, Hippocampus minor.

COLLIER (F.), *A collar.* A name given to certain eruptions which surround the neck like a collar.

COLLIGAMEN, Ligament.

COLLIGATIO, Syndesmosis.

COLLINSO'NIA, *C. Canaden'sis, C. decussa'ta, Horseweed, Horsebalm, Richweed, Richleaf, Heal-all, Stoneroot, Knotroot, Knotweed.* This indigenous plant is possessed of diuretic properties, which seem to reside in a volatile oil. Infusion is the best form of administration. The leaves in domestic practice are applied to wounds and bruises.

COLLINSONIA DECUSSATA, C. Canadensis.

COLLIQUAMEN'TUM, from *colliqueo*, (con and *liquere*,) 'I melt.' The first rudiments of an embryo.—Harvey.

COLLIQUA'TION, *Colliqua'tio, Eliqua'tio, Syntex'is, Ectex'is, Solu'tion, Dissolu'tion.* The ancients meant, by this term, the progressive diminution of the solid parts, with copious excretion of liquids by one or more passages. They thought, that all the solids melted; and that the liquids, and particularly the blood, lost a portion of their density.

COLLIQ'UATIVE, *Colliquati'vus, Colliques'-cens*, from *colliquescere*, 'to grow liquid.' (F.) *Colliquatif.* An epithet given to various discharges, which produce rapid exhaustion. Hence we say, *Colliquative sweats, Colliquative diarrhœa*, &c.

COLLIQUESCENS, Colliquative.

COLLISIO, Contusion.

COLLIX, Trochiscus.

COLLODES, Glutinous.

COLLO'DION, *Collo'dium, Ethe'real Solu'tion of Gun-cotton, Magnard's Adhesive Liquid;* from κολλα, 'glue.' A solution obtained by dissolving gun-cotton, (F.) *Fulmicoton*, in a mixture of rectified ether and alcohol, in the proportion of about 16 parts of the former to 1 of the latter. When applied to a part, the ether evaporates, and the solid adhesive material is left, which contracts. Hence it is used in cases of wounds, to keep their edges together. It forms, also, a coating, and has been applied in abrasions, and in cases of burns. In various chronic cutaneous diseases, it has been applied with advantage; and has been employed to give a coating to pills, which it deprives of their taste, without interfering with their action.

Collodion is in the last edition of the Ph. U. S. (1851.)

COLLODION, CANTHAR'IDAL, *Collo'dium vesi'cans seu cantharida'le.* Prepared by exhausting, by displacement, a pound of coarsely powdered *cantharides* with a pound of *sulphuric ether*, and three ounces of *acetic ether.* In two ounces of this saturated solution of cantharides, twenty-five grains of *gun-cotton* are dissolved. By painting the surface with a little of this solution, vesication is produced, as with the plaster of cantharides.

COLLODIUM, Collodion—c. Cantharidale, Collodion, cantharidal—c. Vesicans, Collodion, cantharidal.

COLLOID, *Colloï'des*, from κολλα, 'glue,' and ειδος, 'resemblance;' *Cancer alveola'ris, Carcino'ma alveola'rē*, (F.) *Cancer alvéolaire, c. Gélatiniforme, Gelatinous cancer.* An epithet applied to a product of morbid secretion, resembling glue, or particles of jelly inlaid in a regular alveolar bed. The three species of cancer or carcinoma are,—*Encephaloid, Scirrhus*, and *Colloid.* See Cancer.

COLLO'MA, from κολλα, 'glue.' A name proposed by Dr. Walshe for the gelatiniform matter, which is of common occurrence in cysts. It is transparent, amorphous, and devoid of vessels and nerves.

COLLONO'MA, from κελλα, 'glue.' A peculiar gelatinous tumour, consisting of a remarkably soft gelatiniform tissue, which trembles on being touched.—J. Müller.

COLLOSTRUM, Colostrum.

COLLOURION, Collyrium.

COLLUM, *Cervix, Trache'los, Auchen*, (F.) *Col, Cou.* The part of the body situate between the head and chest. Also, a part of an organ resembling the neck, as in the following cases.

COLLUM ASTRAG'ALI, *Cervix Astrag'ali, Neck of the Astragalus*, (F.) *Col de l'astragale.* A depression, which separates the anterior extremity of the astragalus from its body.

COLLUM COSTA'RUM, *Cervix Costa'rum, Neck of the Ribs*, (F.) *Col des Côtes.* The narrow part of the ribs, between the head and tubercle.

COLLUM DEN'TIUM, *Cervix Dentium, Neck of the Teeth*, (F.) *Col ou Collet des Dents.* The part of the teeth between the corona and fang, which is embraced by the gum.

COLLUM FEM'ORIS, *Cervix Fem'oris, Neck of the Thigh-bone*, (F.) *Col du Fémur.* The long narrow, and oblique portion of the os femoris, which separates the head from the two trochanters.

COLLUM FIB'ULÆ, *Cervix Fib'ulæ, Neck of the Fibula*, (F.) *Col du Péroné.* A slight narrowness seated below the head or upper extremity of the fibula.

COLLUM HU'MERI, *Cervix Hu'meri, Neck of the Hu'merus.* A circular, depressed portion, which separates the head of the os humeri from its two tuberosities. Some surgeons place the neck below the tuberosities, no precise line of demarcation indicating its extent.

COLLUM MANDIB'ULÆ vel MAXIL'LÆ INFERIO'-RIS, *Cervix Mandib'ulæ* seu *Maxillæ Inferio'ris, Neck of the lower jaw*, (F.) *Col de l'os maxillaire inférieure*. A depression observable on each side of the lower jaw, immediately below the condyles.

COLLUM OBSTIPUM, Torticollis.

COLLUM OSSIS MAGNI vel CAPITA'TI, *Cervix ossis magni* vel *Capita'ti, Neck of the Os Magnum*, (F.) *Col du grand Os*. A circular depression beneath the head of this bone of the carpus.

COLLUM RA'DII, *Cervix Radii, Neck of the Radius*, (F.) *Col du Radius*. A narrow portion of the radius, which supports the head of the bone.

COLLUM SCAP'ULÆ, *Cervix Scap'ulæ, Neck of the Scap'ula*, (F.) *Col de l'Omoplate*. A narrow portion, observable below the glenoid cavity of the scapula, which seems to separate it, as it were, from the rest of the bone.

COLLUM U'TERI, *Cervix U'teri, Jug'ulum Uteri, Neck of the Uterus*, (F.) *Col de la Matrice, Col utérin*. A narrow, cylindrical, and flattened portion of the uterus, which terminates it inferiorly, and opens into the vagina by the *Os Uteri* or *Os Tincæ*. This neck is perceptible on examination *per vaginam*, until near the end of utero-gestation. As the uterus enlarges, however, it becomes shorter and wider, so that a manifest difference exists between its condition at seven and nine months.

COLLUM VESI'CÆ, *Cervix Vesi'cæ, Neck of the Bladder*, (F.) *Col de la Vessie*. The anterior part of the base of the bladder, which resembles the neck of a bottle, and is continuous with the urethra.

COLLURIUM, Collyrium.
COLLUTIO, Gargarism.
COLLUTO'RIUM, from *colluere*, 'to wash out.' A mouth-wash.
COLLUTORIUM ADSTRINGENS, Mel boracis.
COLLU'VIES, from *colluo*, 'I cleanse.' Filth, excrement. Discharge from an old ulcer.
COLLUVIES GASTRICA, *Embarras gastrique*.
COLLYR'IUM, *Collu'rium, Collu'rion*, from κωλυω, 'I check,' and ρεω, 'I flow,' or from κολλα, 'glue,' and ουρα, 'tail;' (F.) *Collyre*. The ancients designated, by this term, a solid medicine, of a long, cylindrical shape; proper to be introduced into the vagina, anus, or nostrils. They are said to have given it this name because it was shaped like a *Rat's Tail*, and because there entered into its composition powders and glutinous matters.—Celsus, Oribasius, Scribonius Largus. At the present day, Collyrium means an application to the eye. Some are *pulverulent* and *dry, Ophthalmempas'ma, Collyr'ium siccum*, but the greatest part are *liquid, Hygrocollyr'ia;* and receive different epithets, as *astringent, emollient,* &c. The term is now little more than synonymous with *Eye-water*. Collyria are generally extemporaneous formulæ.

COLLYRIUM SICCUM, see Collyrium—c. Siccum Alexandrinum, see Alexandrine.

COLOBO'MA, κολοβωμα, 'any thing truncated or shortened.' A mutilated or maimed organ.

COLOBO'MA IRIDIS, *Irido-coloboma*. A congenital peculiarity of the iris, consisting in a fissure of its lower portion, and a consequent prolongation of the iris to the margin of the cornea.

COLOBO'SIS, κολοβωσις. The act of curtailing or mutilating; mutilation.

COLOCHOLO'SIS, from κωλον, 'the colon,' and χολη, 'bile.' Bilious dysentery, *Dysenter'ia bilio'sa*.

COLOCYNTH, Cucumis colocynthis.

COLOMBINE, COMMON, Aquilegia vulgaris.
COLOMBA, Calumba.
COLON, *C. Cæcum, Monen'terum, Colum, Intesti'num majus, I. cellula'tum, I. crassum et plenum, I. grandé, I. laxum*. That portion of the large intestines which extends from the cæcum to the rectum. It is said to have been so called from κοιλον, 'hollow,' or from κωλυω, 'I arrest,' because the excrements are arrested, for a considerable time, in its sacs,—*cel'lulæ*. The colon is usually divided into four portions. 1. The *right lumbar* or *ascending, Colon dextrum*, situate in the right lumbar region, and commencing at the cæcum. 2. *Transverse colon, Colon transver'sum, transverse arch of the colon*, the portion of the colon which crosses from the right to the left side, at the upper part of the abdomen. 3. The *left lumbar* or *descending colon, Colon sinis'trum*, extending from the left part of the transverse arch, opposite the outer portion of the left kidney, to the corresponding iliac fossa. 4. The *Iliac colon* or *Sigmoid flexure of the colon*, (F.) *Colon iliaque* ou *S. du colon*, the portion of the intestine which makes a double curvature in the left iliac fossa, and ends in the rectum.

The muscular fibres, as in the cæcum, are in three flat stripes, *Tæ'niæ* seu *Fas'ciæ Ligamen-to'sæ*.

COLON, *Membrum*—c. Inflammation of the, Colitis.

COLON, TORPOR OF THE. A disease in which the muscular coat of the colon acts with deficient energy; giving occasion to distention of the intestine, which, by pressing upon the other organs, may interfere so much with their functions, as to lead to distressing gastric, cardiac and other disorders.

COLONITIS, Colitis, Dysentery.
COLONNE, *Columna*—c. *Vertébrale*, Vertebral column.
COLONNES CHARNUES, Carneæ columnæ—c. *Charnues du Cœur*, Columnæ carneæ.
COLOPHANE, Colophonia.
COLOPHANY, Colophonia.
COLOPHO'NIA, so called from Colophon, a city of Ionia; *Phrycté, Fricta, Pix Græca, Resi'na nigra, Colophany, Colophony, Black Rosin, Pitch, Brown Rosin*, (F.) *Colophone, Colophane, Arcanson, Brai sec*. The black resin, which remains in the retort, after the distillation, by means of a strong fire, of common turpentine. It is used like the turpentines in general, and in some pharmaceutical preparations.
COLOPHONY, Colophonia.
COLOQUINTE, Cucumus colocynthis.
COLOQUINTIDA, Cucumus colocynthis.
COLOR VIRGINEUS PALLIDUS, Chlorosis—c. *Virginum fœdus*, Chlorosis.
COLORECTITIS, Dysentery.
COLOSTRA, Colostrum.
COLOSTRATIO, Colostration.
COLOSTRA'TION, *Colostra'tio*. Disease in new-born children, attributable to the colostrum.
COLOS'TRUM, *Culos'tra, Collostrum, Colus'trum, Troph'alis, Protog'ala, Neog'ala, Primum Puer'peræ lac, Pytia, Pyetia*, (*Biestings* or *Beastings* in the cow, &c.,) from κολον, 'food,' (?) (F.) *Béton*. The first milk after accouchement. It contains more serum and butter, and less casein than common milk, and seems to possess an evacuant property, which renders it fit to aid in the expulsion of the meconium. *Colostrum* formerly meant an emulsion prepared of turpentine and yolk of egg.

COLOUR-BLINDNESS, Achromatopsia.
COLOURS, ACCIDENT'AL, *Op'posite colours, Complemen'tary* and *Harmon'ic colours*. If the eye has been for some time regarding a particu-

lar colour, the retina becomes insensible to this colour; and if, afterwards, it be turned to a sheet of white paper, the paper will not seem to be white, but will be of the colour that arises from the union of all the rays of the solar spectrum, except the one to which the retina has become insensible. Thus, if the eye be directed for some time to a *red* wafer, the sheet of paper will seem to be of a *bluish-green*, in a circular spot of the same dimensions as the wafer. This bluish-green image is called an *oc'ular spectrum*, because it is impressed upon the eye and may be retained for a short time; and the colour *bluish-green*, is said to be the *accidental colour* of the red. If this experiment be made with wafers of different colours, other accidental colours will be observed, varying with the colour of the wafer employed, as in the following table:—

Colour of the Water.	Accidental colour, or colour of the ocular spectrum.
Red	Bluish green
Orange	Blue.
Yellow	Indigo.
Green	Violet with a little red.
Blue	Orange red.
Indigo	Orange yellow.
Violet	Yellow-green.
Black	White.
White	Black.

If all the colours of the spectrum be ranged in a circle, in the proportions they hold in the spectrum itself, the accidental colour of any particular colour will be found directly opposite. Hence, the two colours have been termed *opposite colours*. It will follow from what has been said, that if the primary colour, or that to which the eye has been first directed, be added to the accidental colour, the result must be the same impression as that produced by the union of all the rays of the spectrum — *white* light. The accidental colour, in other words, is what the primitive colour requires to make it white light. The primitive and accidental colours are, therefore, *complements* of each other; and hence accidental colours have also been called *complementary colours*. They have likewise been termed *harmonic*, because the primitive and its accidental colour *harmonize* with each other in painting.

COLPAL'GIA, from κολπος, 'vagina,' and αλγος, 'pain.' Pain in the vagina.

COLPATRE'SIA, *Elytratre'sia*, from κολπος, 'vagina,' and ατρητος, 'without opening.' Imperforation of the vagina.

COLPEMPHRAX'IS, from κολπος, 'vagina,' and εμφραξις, 'obstruction.' Obstruction of the vagina by foreign bodies.

COLPEURYNTER, Speculum vaginæ.

COLPITIS, Colposis.

COLPOC'ACE, *Ædœoti'tis gangræno'sa, Gangræ'na genita'lium et vagi'næ*. Putrescency or gangrene of the vagina and labia.

COLPOPACE INFANTI'LIS, *Ædœoti'tis gangræno'sa puella'rum, Noma pudendo'rum*. Gangrene or putrescency of the vagina and genitals in young children.

COLPOCACE PUERPERA'RUM, *Ædœoti'tis Gangræno'sa puerpera'rum, Tocodomycodori'tis malig'na vagina'lis* (Ritgen). Sloughing of the vagina and genitals in puerperal women.

COLPOCELE, Elytrocele.

COLPOCYSTOTOM'IA, from κολπος, 'vagina,' κυστις, 'bladder,' and τομη, 'incision.' *Sectio vagi'no-vesica'lis*. Lithotomy through the vagina.

COLPODESMORRAPH'IA, from κολπος, 'vagina,' δεσμος, 'ligament,' and ραφη, 'suture.' The removal of a part of the mucous membrane of the vagina for the radical cure of prolapsus vaginæ et uteri.

COLPŒDEMA, Elytrœdema.

COLPOPTOSIS, Prolapsus vaginæ.

COLPORRHA'GIA, *Elytrorrha'gia*, from κολπος, 'vagina,' and ρηγνυμι, 'I break forth.' Discharge of blood from the vagina.

COLPORRHAPHY, Elytrorrhaphy.

COLPORRHEX'IS, *Ruptu'ra vagi'næ*; from κολπος, 'vagina,' and ρηξις, 'rupture.' Rupture of the vagina. Also, colporrhagia.

COLPORRHŒA, Leucorrhœa.

COLPOS, Sinus, Vagina.

COLPO'SIS. Inflammation of the vagina. Synonymous with *Elytroï'tis, Elytri'tis, Coleï'tis, Colpi'tis*. See Leucorrhœa.

COLPOSTEGNO'SIS, *Coleostegno'sis*, from κολπος, 'vagina,' and στεγνοω, 'I close.' Atresia, or obliteration of the vagina.

COLPOSTENOCHORIA, Coleostegnosis.

COLPOSYNIZESIS, Coleostegnosis.

COLPOT'OMY, *Colpotom'ia*, from κολπος, 'vagina,' and τομη, 'incision.' An incision of the vagina in parturition.

COLT'S FOOT, Asarum Canadense, Tussilago.

COL'UBER BERUS. The systematic name of the viper, *Vi'pera*, (F.) *Couleuvre, Vipère*. A poisonous reptile—the poison lying in small sacs near its teeth. The flesh is innocent, and has been often taken in scrofula, and in cutaneous disorders in general, but it is inefficacious.

COLUBRINA, Polygonum bistorta — c. Dracontia, Arum dracunculus — c. Lusitanica, Euphorbia capitata — c. Virginiana, Aristolochia serpentaria.

COLUM, Colon.

COLUMBINE, Aquilegia vulgaris — c. Wild, Aquilegia Canadensis.

COLUMBO, Calumba — c. American, see Calumba — c. Marietta, see Calumba.

COLUMELLA, Pillar, Uvula.

COLUM'NA, *Column*, (F.) *Colonne*. Anatomists use this word for parts which resemble a column or pillar; hence for the penis.

COLUMNA ADSTANS INGUINIBUS, Penis — c. Dorsi, Vertebral column.

COLUM'NA NASI. The cartilaginous part of the septum of the nostrils. See Nares.

COLUMNA ORIS, Uvula — c. Spinalis, Vertebral column — c. Virginitatis, Hymen — c. Foraminis ovalis, see Ovalis fossa — c. Valvulæ Vieussenii, see Valvula Vieussenii — c. Vertebralis, Vertebral column.

COLUM'NÆ CAR'NEÆ, *Colum'næ Cordis, Lacer'ti* vel *Lacer'tuli* vel *Funes* vel *Fascic'uli ter'etes Cordis, Trabes* seu *Trabec'ulæ Cordis*, (F.) *Colonnes charnues du cœur*. Small, fleshy columns, which project, more or less, into the auricles and ventricles of the heart, whose use appears to be to prevent too great dilatation of those cavities. A few of these *columnæ* — see *Musculi papilla'res* — are attached by one extremity to the walls of the heart, and, by the other, give insertion to chordæ tendineæ.

COLUMNÆ CARNEÆ of the Rectum, see Rectum — c. Papillares, see Columnæ Carneæ.

COLUMNEA LONGIFOLIA, Babel.

COLUMNS, MEDIAN, POSTERIOR OF THE MEDULLA OBLONGATA, Funiculi graciles — c. of Morgagni or of the Rectum, see Rectum — c. of the Spinal Marrow, see Vertebral Nerves.

COLUS JOVIS, Salvia sclarea.

COLUSTRUM, Colostrum.

COLU'TEA, *C. Arbores'cens, C. hirsu'ta, Senna German'ica, Bladder Senna*, (F.) *Baguenaudier, Faux Séné. Fam.* Leguminosæ. *Sex. Syst.* Diadelphia Decandria. The leaves are slightly purgative, and are often mixed with those of the cassia senna.

COLUVRINE DE VIRGINIE, Aristolochia serpentaria.

COLYM'BADES, *Pickled Olives*. These, when bruised and applied to a burnt part, were supposed to be able to prevent vesication.—Dioscorides.

COLYMBIFERA MINOR, Mentha crispa.

COMA, *Semisom'nis, Semisopi'tus, Semisopo'rus, Subeth*, (Arab.) A profound state of sleep, from which it is extremely difficult to rouse the individual. It is a symptom which occurs in many diseases. Two varieties are distinguished, 1. *Coma vigil, Coma agrypno'des, Perrigil'ium, Vigil'iæ nim'iæ, Typho'nia, Veter'nus, Veternos'itas, Agrypnoco'ma, Carus lethar'gus vigil. Typhoma'nia*, which is accompanied with delirium. The patient has his eyes closed, but opens them when called; and closes them again immediately. This state is accompanied with considerable restlessness. 2. *Coma Somnolen'tum, C. Comato'des;* —in which the patient speaks when roused, but remains silent and immovable in the intervals. Coma is a deeper sleep than *sopor*, but less so than *lethargy* and *carus*.

COMA, Capillus — c. Agrypnodes, see Coma — c. Apoplexia, Apoplexy — c. Cæsarea, Plica — c. Comatodes, see Coma—c. Somnolentum, Somnolency, see Coma — c. Vigil, see Coma.

COMACON, Myristica moschata.

COMAN'DRA UMBELLA'TA, *Bastard Toadflax;* indigenous; *Order*, Santalaceæ: flowering in May and June; has been used in fevers by some of the Indian tribes.

COMAROS, Arbutus unedo.

COMA'RUM PALUS'TRE, *Potentil'la palus'tris, Marsh Cinquefoil*. An indigenous plant, *Family*, Rosaceæ, which flowers in June. It is possessed of astringent virtues.

CO'MATA, from κωμα. Diseases characterized by diminution of the powers of voluntary motion, with sleep or impaired state of the senses.—Cullen.

COMATEUX, Comatose.

COMATODES, Comatose.

COM'ATOSE, *Comato'des, Carot'icus, Caro'des*, (F.) *Comateux*. Relating to or resembling coma: —as *comatose sleep, comatose fever*, &c.

COMBUSTIBILITY, PRETERNATURAL, Combustion, human.

COMBUSTIO, Burn — c. Spontanea, Combustion, human.

COMBUS'TION, HUMAN, *Sponta'neous Combus'tion* or *Preternat'ural Combustibil'ity, Catacau'sis, Tachencau'sis, Incen'dium sponta'neum, Combus'tio sponta'nea, Autempreem'us, Catacau'sis ebrio'sa*, (F.) *Combustion humaine, C. spontanée*. These terms have been applied to the extraordinary phenomenon of a rapid destruction of the human body, by being reduced to ashes either spontaneously or by the contact of an ignited substance. It is said to have occurred in the aged, and in those that were fat and hard drinkers. In such, Dr. Traill has found a considerable quantity of oil in the serum of the blood. Vioq d'Azyı, Lair, and Dupuytren think it necessary, that the body should be placed in contact with an ignited substance. Le Cat, Kopp, and Marc are of opinion that this is not necessary. The former appears to be the more probable view.

COMBUSTURA, Burn.

COMEDONES, see Acne.

COMES ARCHIATRORUM, see Exarchiater.

COMESTIBLE, (F.) *Edu'lis*, from *comedere*, 'to eat.' *Eatable*, (F.) *Édule*. Esculent. When this word is used substantively, in French as in English, it means solid food.

COMEZ. Half a drop.—Ruland.

COMFREY, Symphytum—c. Spotted, Pulmonaria.

COMISTE, Aliment.

COMMANDUCATIO, Mastication.

COMMEM'ORATIVE, *Commemorati'vus*, from *commemorare*, (*con* and *memor*,) 'to cause to remember.' That which recalls, or rather which is recalled.

COMMEMORATIVE SIGNS, (F.) *Signes commemoratifs*, are those, deduced from circumstances which have gone before; or rather, according to others, those which point out the preceding condition of the patient. They are also called *Anamnes'tic signs*.

COMMENSUM, Symmetry.

COMMERCIUM, Sympathy.

COMMI, Gummi.

COM'MINUTED, *Comminu'tus*, from *comminuere*, (*con* and *minuo*,) 'to break to pieces.' (F.) *Comminutif*. A *comminuted fracture* is one in which the bone is broken into a number of pieces.

COMMINU'TION, *Comminu'tio, Thrypsis, Leio'sis*. Same etymon. Fracture of a bone into a number of pieces.

COMMISSURA, Articulation.

COMMISSURA ANTERIOR CEREBRI, Commissure, anterior, of the Brain.

COMMISSU'RA BREVIS. A lobule or prominence of the inferior vermiform process of the cerebellum, situate in the incisura posterior, below the horizontal fissure.

COMMISSURA LABIORUM, Prostomia—c. Magna cerebri, Corpus callosum—c. Nervea, Syndesmosis—c. Ossium carnea, Syssarcosis.

COMMISSURA POSTERIOR CEREBRI, Commissure, posterior, of the Brain.

COMMISSURA SIMPLEX. A small lobule or prominence of the superior vermiform process, near the incisura posterior of the cerebellum.

COMMISSU'RAL; same etymon as commissure. Of or belonging to a commissure.

COM'MISSURE, *Commissu'ra, Compa'ges, Compagina'tio, Sym'physis, Sym'bolè;* from *committo*, (*con* and *mitto*,) 'I join together.' A point of union between two parts: thus, the commissures of the eyelids, lips, &c., are the angles, which they form at the place of union. See Fibres, converging.

COM'MISSURE, ANTE'RIOR, OF THE BRAIN, *Commissu'ra ante'rior cer'ebri*, (F.) *Commissure antérieure du cerveau*. A small medullary fasciculus, situate transversely at the anterior part of the third ventricle, and uniting the two hemispheres.

COMMISSURE, GREAT, OF THE BRAIN, *Commissu'ra Magna Cer'ebri*, (F.) *Grande commissure du cerveau*, which unites the two hemispheres for some extent, is the *Corpus callo'sum*.

COMMISSURE, MIDDLE, OF THE BRAIN. A layer of gray substance uniting the thalami optici.

COMMISSURE, OBLIQUE OR INTERCEREBRAL, see Valvula Vieussenii — c. Optic, see Chiasmus.

COMMISSURE, POSTERIOR, OF THE BRAIN, *Commissu'ra poste'rior cer'ebri*. A medullary band, situate at the posterior part of the third or middle ventricle.

COMMISSURE OF THE UVEA, Ciliary ligament.

COMMISSURE DE LA CHOROIDE, Ciliary ligament.

COMMO'SIS, from κομμοω, 'I adorn.' The art of concealing natural deformities, as by painting the face. See, also, Propolis.

COMMO'TICE, in the older writers, meant the art of communicating factitious beauty to a person. Painting the face; *Comopor'ia*.

COMMOTIO, Motion, Concussion—c. Cerebri Concussion of the brain.

COMMOTION, Concussion — *c. du Cerveau*, Concussion of the brain.

COMMU'NICANS, from *communis*, 'common.' *Conjun'gens*. That which communicates or establishes a communication. Communicant. There are two *Arteriæ Communican'tes*, both within the cranium;—the one *anterior*, very short, and extending transversely from one anterior cerebral artery to the other,—the other *posterior*, called also *Communicans Willis'ii*, which passes from the internal carotid to the posterior cerebral artery. It is a branch of the basilary.

COMMUNICANS NONI. A long slender nervous branch, formed by filaments from the first, second and third cervical nerves, which descends upon the outer side of the internal jugular vein, and forms a loop with the descendens noni over the sheath of the carotids.

COMMUNICANS PERONEI, see Communicans poplitei.

COMMUNICANS POPLITE'I, *C. tibia'lis* (*nervus.*) A large nerve, which arises from the popliteal; and, at a variable distance below the articulation of the knee, receives the *communicans peronei* from the peroneal nerve,—the two forming the *external saphenous nerve*.

COMMUNICANS TIBIALIS, Communicans poplitei.

COMPACT, *Compac'tus*, from *con* and *pangere*, 'to strike, to fix.' Solid, close. (F.) *Compacte*. The term *Compact Tissue* is given to the hardest and closest parts of bone.

COMPAGES, Articulation, Commissure — c. Ossium per Lineam Simplicem, Harmony — c. Vertebrarum, Vertebral column.

COMPAGINATIO, Commissure.

COMPAS D'ÉPAISSEUR, see Pelvimeter.

COMPASSIO, Sympathy.

COMPEBA, Piper cubeba.

COMPENSATION, *Balancement*.

COMPEPER, Piper cubeba.

COMPER'NIS; from *con*, and *perna*, 'a gammon of bacon with the leg on.' One who has his knees turned inwards. A case of distortion of the legs.

COMPETENTIA MEMBRORUM OMNIUM, Symmetry.

COMPLAINT, Disease.

COMPLAINT, FAMILY, see Hereditary.

COMPLEMENTAL AIR, see Respiration.

COMPLEMENTARY AIR, see Respiration.

COMPLETIO, Plethora.

COMPLEX, *Complex'us*, from *con*, 'with,' and *plectere*, 'to twist.' Embracing several distinct things. Chaussier uses this term, in his anatomical descriptions, for *complicated*.

COMPLEXIO, Coition, Complexio, Confusio, Temperament.

COMPLEXION, *Complex'io*. This is often employed, in English, for the colour of the face, as "He has a *good complexion*,"—a "*sallow complexion*," &c. It formerly had a more extensive signification, and still has in France. It signifies the aggregate of physical characters presented by any individual, considered with respect to his external arrangement or condition. It means more than *constitution*, for which it is used synonymously in many cases; and differs from *temperament*, which is less the external condition of the body than the state or disposition of the organs in health.—H. Cloquet.

COMPLEXUS, Complex.

COMPLEXUS MINOR, *Mastoïdeus latera'lis, Trachè'lo-mastoïdeus,* (F.) *Trachélo-mastoïdien, Muscle petit Complexus*. It arises from the transverse processes of the last four cervical vertebræ, and is inserted into the mastoid process.

COMPLEXUS MUS'CULUS, *Biven'ter Cervi'cis, Complexus Major, Dorso-trachélon-occipital, Tra-*

chélo-occipital (Ch.), (F.) *Muscle grand complexus*. A muscle, situate at the hind part of the neck, where it extends from the interval that separates the two prominent ridges on the posterior surface of the os occipitis to the transverse and articular processes of the last six cervical vertebræ, as well as to those of the first five dorsal. It serves to straighten, incline, and turn the head.

COMPLICA'TION, *Complica'tio*, from *con*, 'with,' and *plicare*, 'to fold.' In medicine, it means the presence of several diseases, *morbi complica'ti seu perplex'i*, or of several adventitious circumstances foreign to the primary disease.

COMPOSIT"ION, *Composit'io*, from *componere*, (*con* and *ponere*, 'to place;' 'to place together.' *Syn'thesis*. The act of composing or compounding,—of medicines for example; *Iamatosyntax'is*. Also, the Compound, *Compos'itum*, or thing compounded. Likewise, a *combination*.

COMPOSITUM, Compound.

COMPOUND. Same etymology; to mix medicines. To mingle different ingredients into one whole. Used adjectively, *compound* signifies the result of the union of several medicinal agents, as "a *compound* medicine."

COMPREHENSIO, Catalepsy.

COMPRENSIO, Catalepsy.

COM'PRESS, *Compres'sa, Splenium, Speniola, Splenis'cus, Pla'gula, Penicil'lum, Penic'ulum*, from *comprimere*, (*con*, and *premere*, 'to press,') 'to press together.' (F.) *Compresse*. Folded pieces of lint or rag, so contrived as, by the aid of a bandage, to make due pressure upon any part. According to their shape, direction, and use, compresses have been called *long* ((F.) *longuettes*,) *square* (*carrées*,) *triangular, prismatic, graduated* (*graduées*,) *split* (*fendues*,) *fenêtrées, criblées, croix de Malte, oblique, circular, dividing* (*divisives*,) *uniting* (*unisantes*,) *cribriform*, &c.

The Umschlag or compress of the hydropathists is a cloth, well wetted with cold water, applied to the surface near the supposed seat of disease, securely covered with a dry cloth, and changed as often as it becomes dry. It is sometimes covered with a layer of oiled silk, to prevent evaporation.

COMPRESSEUR DE DUPUYTREN, Compressor of Dupuytren — *c. du Nez*, Compressor nasi — *c. de la Prostate*, Compressor prostatæ.

COMPRESSIO, Compression, Thlipsis.

COMPRES'SION, *Compressio, Enerei'sis*. Same etymology. Pressure; methodical compression. An agent frequently had recourse to in surgery. We *compress* a limb, affected with *œdema, varices, hydrops articuli, callous ulcer*, &c. The abdomen is *compressed* after delivery, after *paracentesis abdominis*, &c. The compression is produced by means of the roller, laced stocking, &c., according to the part, and to the particular case. *Moderate pressure* aids the contractility of parts, and excites the action of the absorbents; so that large tumours at times disappear after it has been used for some time. A greater degree of pressure occasions, still more, the emaciation of the part, but it is apt to impede the circulation. *Pressure* is often used to stop or moderate the flow of blood in cases of aneurism or wounds of arteries and veins. In such cases, the compression may be *immediate*, when applied upon the artery itself, or it may be *mediate*, when applied through the integuments and soft parts. The French use the term *Compression immédiate latérale* for that which is exerted perpendicularly to the axis of a vessel, so as to flatten its sides. It is practised with the finger, forceps, tourniquet, compresses, &c.

COMPRES'SION OF THE BRAIN. This may arise either from coagula of blood, a soft tumour, a bony excrescence, a depressed portion of the skull, or the presence of some foreign body. The effects vary, according as the compression takes place *suddenly* or *gradually*. When *suddenly*, the symptoms are of the comatose or apoplectic character. When *gradually*, mania, convulsions, &c., are more likely to occur. Compression, arising from a depressed portion of skull, requires the use of the trephine.

COMPRES'SIVE, *Compressi'vus*. That which compresses. A *compressive bandage* is one that compresses the parts to which it is applied.

COMPRES'SOR or COMPRESSO'RIUM OF DUPUYTREN, (F.) *Compresseur de Dupuytren.* An instrument for compressing the femoral artery, invented by Dupuytren. It is constructed on the same principles as the tourniquet of J. L. Petit, from which it only differs in this respect;—that, instead of being maintained in its place by a strap, which always compresses more or less the circumference of the limb, the two pads are placed at the extremities of a semicircle of steel, which, by passing from one to the other without touching the parts, limits the pressure to two opposite points of the thigh, and permits the collateral circulation to go on.

COMPRESSOR NARIS, *Renæ'us, Nasa'lis, Transversa'lis Nasi, Myrtiform'is, Dilatato'res ala'rum nasi, Constric'tor Nasi, C. Na'rium, C. Naris, Triangula'ris Nasi,* (F.) *Maxillo-narinal, Sus-maxillo-nasal,* — (Ch.,) *Compresseur du nez, Transversal du nez.* A muscle, situate at the sides of the nose; flat and triangular. It arises from the inner part of the fossa canina, and passes to the dorsum of the nose; where it is confounded with that of the opposite side.

COMPRESSOR or CONSTRICTOR OF NUCK. An instrument for compressing the urethra, to obviate incontinence of urine. It consists of a girdle of iron, which surrounds the pelvis, to which is fixed a plate of the same metal, that compresses the urethra *in perinæo.*

COMPRESSOR PROS'TATÆ, *Prostat'icus supe'rior, Pubio-prostat'icus, Sub-pubio-prostat'icus,* (F.) *Compresseur de la prostate.* A muscle, admitted by ALBINUS, which is formed of the anterior fibres of the *Levator ani*, that embrace the prostate. It is the *Prostat'icus supe'rior* of WINSLOW.

COMPRES'SOR URE'THRÆ. A muscle consisting of two portions—one of which is *transverse* in its direction, and, in consequence of its having been particularly described by Mr. Guthrie, has been called *Guthrie's muscle*. It arises from the ramus of the ischium, and passes inwards to embrace the membranous urethra. The other portion is *perpendicular*, descending from the pubis and passing down to be inserted into the transverse portion of the muscle. This portion has been considered by many to be only the anterior fibres of the levator ani; and having been described by Mr. Wilson, it has been called *Wilson's muscle.*

COMPRESSOR VENÆ DORSA'LIS PENIS. A small muscle, distinctly seen in animals, less distinctly in man, which arises from the ramus of the pubis, and ascending in a direction forwards is inserted above the vena dorsalis, joining with its fellow of the opposite side on the mesial line. Its use is supposed to compress the vein in erection. It is sometimes called the *muscle of Houston*, after Dr. Houston of Dublin.

COMPRESSORIUM, Compressor.

COMPTO'NIA ASPLENIFO'LIA, *Liquidam'-bar peregri'na, L. asplenifo'lia, Myoica asplenifo'lia, Sweet Fern, Shrubby Sweet Fern, Sweet bush, Fern bush, Fern gale, Spleenwort bush, Meadow fern, Astringent root.* An indigenous shrubby plant, which grows in sandy or stony woods from New England to Virginia. It possesses tonic and astringent properties, and is used as a domestic remedy in diarrhœa, &c., in the form of decoction.

COMPUNCTIO, Paracentesis, Puncturing.
CONÆSTHESIS, Cœnæsthesis.
CONARIUM, Pineal gland.
CONATUS, Effort.
CONCARNATIO, Syssarcosis.

CONCASSER, (F.), from *conquassare*, (*con*, and *quassare*, 'to shake much,') 'to break to pieces;' 'to comminute.' To reduce roots, woods, &c. into small fragments, in order that their active principles may be more readily separated from them.

CONCAU'SA, *Concaus'sa, Synæ'tion.* A cause which co-operates with another, in the production of disease.

CONCAVITAS CONCHULARIS CEREBRI, Infundibulum of the brain.
CONCAVUM PEDIS, Sole.

CONCENTRAN'TIA, from *con* and *centrum*, 'a centre.' A name once given to absorbents of acids.

CONCENTRA'TION. *Concentra'tio.* A word sometimes used, in medical theories, to express an afflux of fluids, or a convergence of sensibility or of vital force, towards an organ. It is applied, also, to the pulsation of arteries, when not easily felt under the finger.

POULS CONCENTRÉ, (F.) A term applied by the French to a pulse of the above character.

CONCEPTACULA SEMINARIA, Vesiculæ seminariæ.
CONCEPTACULUM, Uterus, Vessel.
CONCEPTIO, Conception — c. Vitiosa, Pregnancy. extra-uterine.

CONCEPTION, *Concep'tio, Concep'tus, Cye'sis, Syllep'sis, Androlep'sia*, from *concipio*, (*con* and *capio*,) 'I conceive.' The impregnation of the ovum by the positive contact of the male sperm, whence results a new being. The whole subject of conception is most mysterious. It seems to occur as follows. During the sexual union, the male sperm passes along the uterus and Fallopian tubes: the fimbriated extremities of the latter seize hold of the ovarium; and the sperm in this manner comes in contact with a maturated ovum, and impregnates it. The fecundated ovum remains some time in the ovarium, but at length bursts its covering, is laid hold of by the fimbriated extremity of the Fallopian tube, and passes along the tube into the cavity of the uterus, where it remains for the full period of utero-gestation. Some are of opinion, that the ovum is not impregnated until it has entered the Fallopian tubes, or uterus.

CONCEP'TION, FALSE, *Falsus Concep'tus, Spu'rium germen,* (F.) *Fausse conception, Faux germe.* An irregular, preternatural conception, the result of which is a mole or some similar production, instead of a properly organized fœtus. See Mole.

CONCEP'TUS. The first rudiments of the fœtus, after conception. Also, conception.
CONCEPTUS FALSUS, Conception, false.

CONCHA, *Conchus*. A liquid measure, amongst the Athenians, equal to half an ounce. Anatomists apply this term to several hollow parts of the body;—as the *Concha of the Ear*,—*Concha Auris, Concha Auric'ulæ*; (F.) *Conque*,—the hollow part of the cartilage of the external ear. It has, also, been applied to the genital organs of the female; to the patella, &c.

CONCHA, Patella, Turbinated bone (middle,) Vulva — c. Auris interna, Cochlea — c. Cerebri, Infundibulum of the brain—c. Genu, Patella—c. Inferior, Turbinated bone, (inferior) — c. Labyrinthi, Cochlea — c. Morgagniana, Turbinated bone, (superior) — c. Narium superior, Turbinated bone, (superior).

CONCHÆ NARIUM, Turbinated bones.

CONCHA'RUM ANTIFEBRI'LE. A febrifuge and sudorific preparation in Bates's *Pharmacopœia.* It was composed of vinegar, musselshells, and water of *Carduus benedictus.*

CONCHO-HELIX. A small, fleshy, fasciculus, attached to the concha of the ear and helix. It is also called the *small muscle of the helix.*

CONCHUS, *Concha.* The cranium. In the plural, it means the orbitar cavities.—Castelli.

CONCHUS OCULI, Orbit.

CONCHYLIA, Turbinated bones.

CONCIDENTIA, Collapse.

CONCILIA CORPORALIA, Coitus.

CONCIL'IUM. A milky plant, referred to by Pliny as aphrodisiac and antiphthisical. Adanson considers it to be a *Campanula.*

CONCOC'TED, *Concoc'tus, Matura'tus, Pepei'rus;* from *con* and *coquere,* 'to boil.' Brought to maturity; ripe; concocted; digested.

CONCOCTIO, Coction—c. Tarda, Dyspepsia.

CONCOCTION, Coction.

CONCOMBRE ORDINAIRE, Cucumis sativus—c. *Sauvage,* Momordica elaterium.

CONCOMITANS, Concomitant.

CONCOM'ITANT, *Concom'itans,* from *con* and *comitare,* (itself from *comire, — cum* and *ire,*) 'to go with.' That which accompanies. A symptom which accompanies others.

CONCREMATIO, Calcination.

CONCREMENTA ZOOHYLICA, see Zoohylica.

CONCREMENTUM, Concretion.

CONCRETIO, Adherence, Concretion — c. Palpebrarum cum bulbo oculi, Symblepharosis.

CONCRE'TION, *Concre'tio, Concremen'tum,* from *concrescere,* (*con* and *crescere,*) 'to condense, thicken, become solid:' *Pexis, Sympex'is, πηξις, συμπηξις.* The act of becoming thick or solid. It was once used synonymously with adhesion or growing together, — as, *"concretion of the toes."* Most commonly, it is applied to extraneous and inorganic bodies, of a solid character, met with in different textures, after certain chronic inflammations; or which make their appearance in the joints or in the reservoirs for excrementitial fluids. *Concretion* is, therefore, frequently synonymous with *Calculus,* and is then rendered, in Latin, by the word *Concrementum.* But *Concretion* has a more extensive signification than *Calculus;* thus, accidental ossifications or deposits of phosphate of lime in certain organs, and especially in the liver and lungs, are properly called *osseous concretions.* They could not well be called *osseous calculi.*

CONCRETION, FIBRINOUS, SANGUINEOUS, POLYPIFORM, or POLYPUS, OF THE HEART, see Polypus—c. Intestinalis, Calculus of the Stomach and Intestines.

CONCRETIONES ALVINÆ, Calculi of the stomach and intestines.

CONCUBITUS, Coition—c. Venereus, Coition.

CONCUR'SUS, from *concurrere,* (*con,* and *currere, cursum,* 'to run,') 'to meet together,' *Syn'dromē.* The congeries or collection of symptoms, which constitute and distinguish a particular disease.

CONCUS'SION, *Commo'tion,* from *concutio,* (*con* and *quatere,* 'to shake,') 'I shake together.' *Concus'sio, Thlasma Concus'sio, Commo'tio, Anasis'mus, Tinagmus,* (F.) *Commotion.* In *Surgery,* it is used for the agitation often communicated to one organ by a fall upon another; as to the brain from a fall on the breech, &c.

In all severe injuries; in sudden encephalic hemorrhage, and in overwhelming emotions, a *concussion* or *shock* is felt to a greater or less extent in the nervous system, which requires the careful attention of the physician.

CONCUSSION OF THE BRAIN, *Commo'tio Cer'ebri, Apoplex'ia nervo'sa traumat'ica, Encephalosis'mus,* (F.) *Commotion du Cerveau,* sometimes gives rise to alarming symptoms, even to abolition of the functions of the brain, yet without any sensible organic disease. Slight concussion of the brain, called *stunning,* consists in vertigo, tinnitus aurium, loss of memory, and stupefaction; all these being temporary. When more severe, there is instant loss of sensation and volition, vomiting, the patient being as if in a sound sleep, but there is no stertorous breathing. Pulse variable, generally more rapid and feeble than in compression; extremities cold. Little can be done here, till reaction has occurred: after this, the case must be treated according to general principles, — by bleeding, blisters, cold applied to the head, &c. After severe concussion, a patient, although apparently well, is not safe till some time after the accident.

CONDENSAN'TIA, from *con* and *densus,* 'dense;' *Incrassan'tia.* Medicines esteemed proper for inspissating the humours.

CONDENSATIO, Condensation, Stegnosis.

CONDENSA'TION, *Condensa'tio, Inspissa'tio.* Increase in density of the blood and other liquids, or of the solids, which enter into the composition of the human body.

CONDENSER, see Alembic.

CONDEN'SER, LIEBIG'S. A distillatory arrangement, invented by Liebig, in which the tube conveying the vapour is made to pass through another tube, the calibre of which is such as to leave a space between the two, through which a stream of water may be made to run.

CON'DIMENT. *Condimen'tum, Ar'tyma, Hedys'ma, Conditu'ra,* from *condire,* 'to season.' (F.) *Assaisonnement.* Some substances are called, at times, *aliments,* and at others, *condiments,* according as they constitute the basis or the accessory to any dish: such are cream, butter, mushrooms, olives, &c. Others are always *condiments,* as they are only used to improve the savour of food, and contain but little nutritive matter. Such are pepper, salt, cinnamon, &c. Almost all condiments are possessed of stimulant properties.

CONDIT, Confection.

CONDI'TUM, same etymon. A pharmaceutical compound of wine, honey, and some aromatics, especially pepper. Also, a confection.

CONDITURA CADAVERUM, Embalming.

CONDOM, *Armour,* (F.) *Baudruche, Redingote Anglaise, Gant des Dames, Calotte d'assurance.* The intestinum cæcum of a sheep, soaked for some hours in water, turned inside out, macerated again in weak, alkaline ley, — changed every twelve hours, and scraped carefully to abstract the mucous membrane, leaving the peritoneal and muscular coats exposed to the vapour of burning brimstone, and afterwards washed with soap and water. It is then blown up, dried, cut to the length of seven or eight inches, and bordered at the open end with a riband. It is drawn over the penis prior to coition, to prevent venereal infection and pregnancy.

CONDUCTIO, Tonic spasm, Convulsion.

CONDUCTION, VIBRATIONS OF, see Sound.

CONDUC'TOR, *Direc'tor, Itinera'rium,* (F.) *Conducteur;* from *con,* 'with,' and *ducere,* 'to lead.' That which conducts. The *Conductor* was an instrument, formerly used in the high operation for the stone, for directing the forceps into the bladder.

CONDUIT, Canal — c. *Auditif externe,* Auditory canal, external—*c. Auditif interne*, Auditory canal, internal — *c. Auriculaire*, Auditory canal, external—*c. Cholédoque*, Choledoch duct—*c. Déférent*, Deferens—*c. d'Eustache*, Eustachian tube —*c. Gutturale de l'oreille*, Eustachian tube—*c. Labyrinthique*, Auditory canal, internal — *c. Ptérygoïdien*, Pterygoid canal—*c. Sousorbitaire*, Suborbitar canal — *c. Spermatique*, Deferens (vas)—*c. Thoracique*, Thoracic duct—*c. Vidien*, Pterygoid canal.

CONDUITS ADIPEUX, Fatty canals — *c. Aqueux*, see Aqueous — *c. Aveugles de l'urèthre*, see Cæcous—*c. Dentaires*, Dental canals—*c. Éjaculateurs*, Ejaculatory ducts—*c. Lacrymaux*, Lachrymal ducts—*c. Lactifères*, Lactiferous vessels —*c. Nourriciers*, Canals, nutritive—*c. Nutriciers*, Canals, nutritive.

CONDYLARTHRO'SIS, from κονδυλος, 'a condyle,' and αρθρον, 'a joint.' Articulation by condyles. An elongated head or condyle, received into an elliptical cavity.

CON'DYLE, *Con'dyla*, *Con'dylus*, *Capit'ulum*, from κονδυλος, 'a knot, eminence.' An articular eminence, round in one direction, flat in the other. A kind of process, met with more particularly in the ginglymoid joints;—such as the condyles of the occipital, inferior maxillary bone, &c. Some anatomists have applied the term, however, to eminences that are not articular,—as to the lateral tuberosities at the inferior extremity of the *os humeri*, and even to certain depressions, — as to the concave articular surfaces at the upper extremity of the tibia. Chaussier calls the transverse root of the zygomatic process *Condyle of the temporal bone*.

CONDYLI DIGITORUM MANUS, Phalanges of the fingers.

CONDYLIEN, see Condyloid Foramina.
CONDYLIUS, Condyloid.

CON'DYLOID, *Condyloï'deus*, *Condylo'des*, *Condyl'ius*, from κονδυλος, a ' condyle,' and ειδος, 'shape.' Having the shape of a condyle.

CONDYLOID FORAM'INA, *Foram'ina Condyloidea*, (F.) *Trous condyloïdiens*, *Fosses condyloïdiénnes*. These are distinguished into *anterior* and *posterior*. They are four in number, seated in the occipital bone;—two anterior, and two posterior to the *condyles* or *condyloid processes* of the same bone, and to depressions, which are called *Fossæ Condyloideæ*.

As the word *Condyloïdien* means—'that which has the shape of a condyle,' — it has been judiciously proposed by some French anatomists that *condylien* should be used in preference, in the case of the foramina and fossæ.

CONDYLOÏDIEN, see Condyloid Foramina.

CONDYLO'MA, *Condylo'sis*, *Con'dylus*, *Verru'ca carno'sa*, from κονδυλος, 'a knot,' 'an eminence.' A soft, fleshy excrescence, of an indolent character, which appears near the orifice of the genital organs and rectum, and occasionally on the fingers and toes. It is a consequence of the syphilitic virus. Such tumours are also called *Dermophy'mata vene'rea*.

CONDYLOSIS, Condyloma.
CONDYLUS, Condyloma.
CONESSI CORTEX, Nerium antidysentericum.

CONFEC'TIO, *Confec'tion*, from *conficio*, (*con*, and *facere*, 'to make,') 'I make up.' *Alig'ulus*, (F.) *Confiture*, *Condit*. In general it means any thing made up or preserved with sugar. In the late London Pharmacopœias, it includes the articles before called electuaries and conserves. *Confec'tio* or *Confec'tum* also means *Confectionary*.

CONFECTIO ALKERMES, Alkermes.
CONFECTIO AMYGDALA'RUM, *Almond Confection*, *Almond Paste*, *Pasta re'gia*, *P. Amygdali'na*, *Pasta Emulsi'va*, *Buty'rum Amygdala'rum Dul'cium*, (F.) *Confection d'Amandes*. (*Sweet almonds*, ℥j; *gum acacia*, ℥j; *white sugar*, ℥iv. Blanch the almonds, and beat into a paste.) A good mode of keeping almonds in a state fit for making emulsions.

CONFECTIO ARCHIG"ENI, *C. Pauli'na*. (*Castor, long pepper, black pepper, storax, galbanum, costus, opium*, of each ℥ss; *saffron*, ℥ij; *syrup of wormwood*, ℥ij.) It was much recommended as a stimulant in nervous affections.

CONFECTIO AROMAT'ICA, *Electua'rium Aromat'icum*, *C. Cardi'aca*, *C. Raleigha'na*, *Aromatic Confection*, *Sir Walter Raleigh's Cordial*. The following is the Ph. U. S. formula. (*Pulv. aromat.* ℥vss; *croci*, in pulv. ℥ss; *syrup. aurant.* ℥vj; *Mel despumat.* ℥ij. Rub the aromatic powder with the saffron; then add the syrup and honey, and beat together until thoroughly mixed.) Dose, ℈j to ℈j.

CONFECTIO AURANTIO'RUM, *C. Auran'tii Cor'ticis*, (Ph. U. S.), *Conser'va Cor'ticum Aurantio'rum*, *C. Cor'ticis Exterio'ris Aurantii Hispalen'sis*, *C. Flaved'inis Corticum Aurantiorum Hispalen'sium*, *Conser'va Aurantii*, *C. Citri Aurantii*, *Confection of the Orange*, *Conserve of Orange Peel*. (*Yellow part of the peel of the orange*, ℔j; *rectified sugar*, ℔iij; beat into a conserve.) It is stomachic, and an agreeable vehicle, corrigent, and adjuvant for other remedies. Dose, ℥ss.

CONFECTIO CARDIACA, Confectio aromatica.

CONFECTIO CAS'SIÆ, *Electua'rium Cassiæ Fis'tulæ*, *E. Cassiæ*, *E. e Cassiâ*, *E. laxati'vum*, *Conserva Cassiæ*, *Electuarium Cassiæ tamarinda'tum seu leniti'vum*, *Electua'rium e Cassiâ*, *Diacas'sia cum Mannâ*, *Cassia Confection*. (*Cassia pulp*, ℔ss; *manna*, ℥ij; *tamarind pulp*, ℥j; *syrup of roses*, ℔ss. Bruise the manna, dissolve by heat, mix the pulp, and evaporate.) It is gently laxative. Dose, ℥ss.

CONFECTIO DAMOCRATIS, Mithridate.

CONFECTIO HAMEC,—so called from an Arabian physician, — was composed of the bark of the *yellow myrobalans, black myrobalans, violets, pulp of colocynth, polypodium of the oak, leaves of wormwood, thyme, aniseed, fennel, red roses, pulps of prunes, raisins, sugar, honey, senna, rhubarb*, &c. It was used as a purgative in glysters.

CONFECTIO HYACIN'THI, *Hy'acinth Confection*, *Electua'rium seu Confec'tio de Croco emenda'ta olim dicta de hyacin'this*, (Ph. P.) A tonic and slightly astringent confection, composed, according to Baumé, of *terra sigillata, crab's stones, cinnamon, leaves of the dittany of Crete, myrrh, saffron, syrup of lemon, camphor, Narbonne honey, oil of lemon*, &c.: and formerly the hyacinth was added, whence its name.

CONFECTIO O'PII, *Electua'rium Opia'tum*, *Confectio Opia'ta*, *Philo'nium Londinen'se*, *Theriaca Edinen'sis*, *Philo'nium Roma'num*, *Electua'rium Theba'icum*. *Opium Confection*, (*Opium*, in powder, ℈vss; *Pulv. aromat.* ℥vj; *Mel despumat.* ℥xiv; mix thoroughly. One grain of opium in 36:—Ph. U. S.) It is narcotic and stimulant. Dose, gr. x to ℈j.

CONFECTIO PAULINA, Confectio Archigeni — *c. ex Capitibus papaveris*, Diacodium.

CONFECTIO PIP'ERIS NIGRI, *Ward's Paste for Fis'tula*. (*Black pepper, elecampane root*, each ℔j; *fennel seed*, ℔iij; *white sugar*, ℔j.) Dose, size of a nutmeg, three or four times a day.

CONFECTIO RALEIGHANA, Confectio aromatica.

CONFECTIO ROSÆ CANI'NÆ, *Conser'va Rosæ Cani'næ*, *Conserva Cynos'bati*, *C. Cynor'rhodi*, *Rob Cynos'batos*, *Confection* or *Conserve of Dog Rose*. (*Pulp of dog rose*, ℔j; *sugar*, ℥xx. Incorporate. Ph. L.) It is chiefly used as a vehicle for other remedies.

CONFECTIO ROSÆ, *C. Rosæ Gal'lica, Conser'va Rosæ Gal'licæ, Conserva Rosæ, C. Florum Rosa'rum Rubra'rum, C. Florum Rosæ Rubræ, Rhodosac'charum, Sac'charum Rosa'ceum, C. Rosæ Rubræ, Confection of the Red Rose*. (Red roses, in powder, ℥iv; *Sugar,* in powder, ℥xxx; *Clarified honey,* ℥vj; *Rose water,* f℥viij. Rub the roses with the rose water at a boiling heat; then add gradually the sugar and honey, and beat until thoroughly mixed.— Ph. U. S.) It is astringent, and chiefly used as a vehicle for other remedies.

CONFECTIO RUTÆ, *Confection of Rue*. (Rue leaves dried, carraway seeds, bay berries, of each ℥iss; sagapenum, ℥iv; black pepper, ℥ij; honey, ℥xvj; Mix.) It is given in clysters, as an antispasmodic and carminative.

CONFECTIO DE SAN'TALIS, *Confection of the Sanders,* (F.) *Confection de Sandaux*. (Sandal wood, red coral, bole armeniac, terra sigillata, kermes berries, tormentil root, dittany, saffron, myrtle, red roses, calcined hartshorn, and cloves.) It was formerly used as an astringent.

CONFECTIO SCAMMO'NIÆ, *Electua'rium Scammo'nii, Electuarium e Scammo'nio, Caryocostinum, Confection of Scam'mony*. (Powdered scammony, ℥iss; bruised cloves, powdered ginger, āā ℥vj; oil of carraway, ℥ss; syrup of roses, q. s.) A stimulating cathartic. Dose, ℈ss to ʒj.

CONFECTIO SENNÆ, *Electua'rium Cassiæ Sennæ, E. Sennæ cum Pulpis, E. Sennæ compos'itum, Benedic'tum Laxati'vum, Electuarium ape'riens, E. cathol'icum commu'ne, E. diapru'num, E. cocoprot'icum, E. Sennæ, E. e Sennâ, E. leniti'vum, Confection of Senna,* &c. (Senna leaves, ℥viij; figs, ℔j; tamarind pulp, cassia pulp, pulp of French prunes, each ℔ss; coriander seed, ℥lv; liquorice root, ℥iij; sugar, ℔iiss; water, Oiv. Rub the senna and coriander together: separate 10 ounces of the powder with a sieve; boil the residue with the figs and liquorice root in the water to one-half; press out the liquor and strain. Evaporate the liquor by means of a water bath to a pint and a half; add the sugar, and form a syrup. Rub the pulps with the syrup, gradually added; throw in the sifted powder, and beat till thoroughly mixed.—Ph. U. S.) It is a laxative, and is used in habitual constipation, and in constipation during pregnancy. Dose, ℈ss to ℥ss.

CONFECTIO DE THURE, *Frank'incense Confection,* (F.) *Confection d'Encens*. A compound of coriander seeds, nutmeg, thus, liquorice, mastich, cubebs, prepared hartshorn, conserve of red roses, sugar, &c.

CONFECTION, Confectio—*c. d'Amandes,* Confection, almond—*c. d'Encens,* Confectio de Thure—*c.* Frankincense, Confectio de Thure—*c.* of the Orange, Confectio aurantiorum—*c.* of the Red rose, Confectio rosæ Gallicæ—*c.* of Rue, Confectio rutæ—*c. de Sandaux,* Confectio de santalis—*c.* of the Sanders, Confectio de santalis.

CONFECTUM, Confection.

CONFERVA HELMINTHOCORTOS, Corallina Corsicana.

CONFER'VA RIVA'LIS. This species of *River Weed* has been recommended in cases of spasmodic asthma, phthisis, &c.

CONFIRMANTIA, Tonics.

CONFIRMED, Consummatus.

CONFITURE, Confection.

CONFLUENT, *Con'fluens,* from *con,* and *fluere,* 'to flow.' An epithet for certain exanthematous affections, in which the pimples, pustules, &c., run together. It is particularly applied to small-pox, so circumstanced. Some authors have called scarlatina or scarlet fever *Confluent Measles, Morbil'li Confluen'tes*.

CONFLUENT DES SINUS, Torcular Herophili.

CONFLUEN'TIA, *Confœdera'tio;* same etymon as Confluent. A term, employed by Paracelsus to express the concordance between a disease and its remedies.

CONFLUXIO, Sympathy.

CONFŒDERATIO, Confluentia.

CONFORMATIO, Conformation, Structure.

CONFORMA'TION, *Conforma'tio, Diap'lasis, Diaplas'mus, Structure,* from *conformare,* (*con,* and *formare,* 'to form,') 'to arrange,' 'dispose.' The natural disposition or arrangement of the body.

Faulty conformation, (F.) *Vice de conformation,* is vice of original formation; existing, of course, from birth. In French surgery, *Conformation* is used synonymously with *Coaptation,* and both it, *Diaplasis* and *Anaplasis* mean, also, restoration to the original form—as in fractures, &c.

CONFORTANTIA, Tonics.

CONFORTATIVA, Tonics.

CONFORTER (F.), *Confirma'rē, Conforta'rē, Corrobora'rē*. To make stronger — to give energy. *Conforter l'estomac,* 'to strengthen the stomach.'

CONFRICA'TION, *Confrica'tio,* from *confricare,* (*con,* and *fricare,*) 'to rub.' The action of reducing a friable substance to powder, by rubbing it between the fingers; and of expressing the juice of a plant with the hand.

CONFRICA'TRIX, from *con,* 'with,' and *fricare,* 'to rub.' A female who practises masturbation.

CONFU'SÆ FEBRES. Intermittents, whose paroxysms are irregular and confused.—Bellini.

CONFU'SIO, from *confundo,* (*con* and *fundere,* 'to pour,') 'I mix together;' *Syn'chisis*. A disease of the eye, which consists in the mixture of the humours.— Galen. In modern times, Synchysis has been applied to a morbid state of the vitreous body, in which it is reduced to a diffluent condition. It has, also, been used synonymously with *Complexio*.

CONFUSIONES ANIMI, Affections of the mind.

CONGEE DISCHARGES, Rice-water discharges.

CONGELANTIA, Congelativa.

CONGELATIO, Catalepsy.

CONGELA'TION, *Congela'tio, Conglacia'tio, Gela'tio,* from *congelo,* (*con* and *gelare,*) 'I congeal,' 'I freeze.' The action of congealing, of passing to the solid state by the abstraction of heat; as *congelation of water, mercury,* &c. The term had once other acceptations. 1. It was synonymous with *concretion*. 2. With *coagulation,* in which sense it is still occasionally employed. 3. The ancients called all diseases, produced by cold, *congelations,* as well as those in which there was a kind of stupor or torpor—particularly catalepsy. Also, Frostbite.

CONGELATI'VA MEDICAMEN'TA, *Conglutinan'tia, Congelan'tia*. Medicines, considered capable of uniting or consolidating wounds, &c.

CON'GENER, *Congen'erous,* from *con,* 'with,' and *genus,* 'kind.' (F.) *Congénère*. Of the same kind or species. Resembling each other in some manner. When applied to muscles, it means, that they concur in the same action; in opposition to the word *antagonist,* or that which acts in an opposite direction.

In France *Congénères* is applied to those who join in the dissection of the same subject.

CONGENIALIS, Congenital.

CONGENITÆ NOTÆ, Nævus.

CONGEN'ITAL, *Con'genite, Congenita'lis, Congen'itus, Syngen'icus,* from *con,* 'with,' and *gen-*

tus, 'begotten.' (F.) *Congénial* ou *Congénital*. Diseases which infants have at birth: hence, *Congenital affections* are those that depend on faulty conformation; as *congenital hernia*, *congenital cataract*, &c. See Connate.

CONGESTED, Hyperæmic.

CONGESTIO, Congestion — c. Abdominalis, Cœliæmia — c. Pectoris, Stethæmia — c. Pulmonum, Stethæmia — c. Sanguinis, Congestion.

CONGES'TION, *Conges'tio*, *Rhopē*, from *congerere*, 'to amass, 'accumulate,' &c. *Symph'ora*, *Hæmatepago'gē*, *Hæmatosymphore'sis*, *Hæmatosynago'gē*, *Hæmorme'sis*, *Symphore'ma*, *Symphore'sis*, *Synathrois'mus*, *Synathroe'sis*, *Sanguinis Congestio*, *Engorgement*. Accumulation of blood — *hyperæmia* — in an organ. It is an important symptom in febrile and other disorders. It may arise either from an extraordinary flow of blood by the arteries, or from a difficulty in the return of blood to the heart by the veins. More often, perhaps, it is owing to the latter cause, and is termed *venous congestion*, *stasis* or *stagnation* — being not unusually attended with symptoms of oppression and collapse.

CONGESTION OF THE ABDOMEN, Cœliæmia — c. of the Brain, Stethæmia — c. *Cérébrale*, Cephalohæmia — c. *du Cerveau*, Encephalohæmia — c. of the Lungs, Stethæmia — c. *des Poumons*, Stethæmia — c. *Sanguine rachidienne*, Hypermyelohæmia.

CONGESTIVE FEVER, see Fever, congestive.

CONGLACIATIO, Congelation.

CONGLO'BATE, *Congloba'tus*, from *conglobare*, (*con*, and *globus*, 'a ball,') 'to collect,' 'to gather into a ball.' (F.) *Conglobé*.

CONGLOBATE GLAND, *Glan'dula congloba'ta*, *Glandula Muco'sa*, *Hydraden*, *Globate gland*, *Lymphat'ic gan'glion*, (F.) *Glande Conglobée*, *Ganglion lymphatique*. A round body, formed of lymphatic vessels, connected together by cellular structure, but having neither a cavity nor excretory duct. The mesenteric, inguinal and axillary glands are of this class.

CONGLOBÉ, Conglobate.

CONGLOM'ERATE, *Couglomera'tus*, from *con*, and *glomerare*, 'to gather in a heap.' *Glom'erate*, *Glomera'tus*, (F.) *Conglomérē*. Heaped together.

CONGLOM'ERATE GLANDS, *Glan'dulæ conglomera'tæ*, *Glan'dulæ vasculo'sæ*, are those whose lobules are united under the same membrane; as the liver, kidney, testicle, &c.

CONGLOMERATIO INTESTINORUM, Epiploce intestinalis.

CONGLUTINANTIA, Congelativa.

CONGRÈS, (F.) *Congress*, *Congres'sus*, from *congredi*, *congressus*, (*con*, and *gradi*, 'to go,') 'to go together.' This term, which has often been used synonymously with *Coition*, means, also, the ocular proof, formerly ordered by judicial authority, in the presence of surgeons and matrons, to test the impotence or capabilities of parties; — a most unsatisfactory and indecent exhibition. It was forbidden by the Parliament of Paris in the year 1667.

CONGRESSUS, Coition.

CONI VASCULO'SI. Conical bundles, formed by the vasa efferentia of the testis; having their base towards the epididymis, into the tube of which they enter.

CONIA, κονια. A wine, prepared by fermenting the must of the grape on tar previously washed in sea-water. — Orfila. See, also, Lixivium.

CONIASIS, Incrustation.

CONIOSTOSIS, Pulverization.

CONIS, Pulvis.

CONISTERIUM, Apodyterium.

CONI'UM, *C. macula'tum*, *Corian'drum macula'tum*, *Cicuta major* seu *macula'ta* seu *Stoerkii*, *Ahi'otes*, *Cicuta terres'tris*, *Cicuta major fœ'tida*, *C. vulga'ris*, Common Hemlock, Hemlock, Poison parsley, Spotted parsley, (F.) *Ciguë ordinaire*, *C. grande*. *Nat. Ord.* Umbelliferæ. *Sex. Syst.* Pentandria Digynia. The leaves and seeds are narcotic and poisonous in an over-dose. Light destroys the virtues of the leaves; and, therefore, the powder should be kept in opaque bottles, well corked. It has been used as a palliative in cancer and other painful affections; but is not equal to opium.. Externally, it has been applied in fomentation to cancerous and scrofulous ulcers. Dose, gr. ij to x.

Da'vidson's Remedy for Cancer is said to consist of *powdered hemlock* and *arsenious acid*.

CONIUM MOSCHA'TUM, *Aracacha*. A very agreeable and nutritive kind of tuberous vegetable, in flavour not unlike celery, which grows on the coast of Peru, but is more abundant on the projecting ridges of the Cordilleras, and on the eastern declivity of the Andes. It is cooked by being either simply boiled in water, or made into a kind of soup. — Tschudi.

CONJONCTIVE, Conjunctiva.

CONJONCTIVITE, see Ophthalmia — c. *Blennorrhagique*, see Ophthalmia.

CONJUGAISON, Conjugation.

CONJUGA'TION, *Conjuga'tio*, from *conjugare*, (*con*, and *jugum*, 'a yoke,') 'to yoke together.' (F.) *Conjugaison*. Assemblage, union, — *Conjugium*.

CONJUGATIO'NIS FORAM'INA, (F.) *Trous de conjugaison*. The apertures at the sides of the spine, formed by the union of the notches of the vertebræ. They give passage to the nerves of the spinal marrow, and to the vessels which enter or issue from the vertebral canal.

CONJUGIUM, Coition, Conjugation.

CONJUNC'TI (MORBI), from *conjungere*, (*con* and *jungere*,) 'to join together.' Diseases joined together. Authors have distinguished two kinds of these: one, in which the diseases go on simultaneously — *morbi connex'i*; the other, in which they succeed each other — *morbi consequen'tes*.

CONJUNCTIO, Articulation.

CONJUNCTIVA, CUTICULAR, Xerophthalmia — c. Granular, Trachoma.

CONJUNCTI'VA MEMBRA'NA, *Circumcaula'lis*, *Epipeph'ycos*, *Tu'nica agna'ta*, *Tu'nica adna'ta*, *T. conjuncti'va*, *Tunda oc'uli*, (F.) *Conjonctive*, *Membrane adnée*. A mucous membrane, so called because it unites the globe of the eye with the eyelids. It covers the anterior surface of the eye, the inner surface of the eyelids, and the *caruncula lachrymalis*. It possesses great general sensibility, communicated to it by the fifth pair.

CONJUNCTIVITIS, Ophthalmia — c. Ægyptiaca, Ophthalmia, purulent — c. Blennorrhagica, see Ophthalmia — c. Catarrhalis, Ophthalmia, catarrhal — c. Gonorrhoica, see Ophthalmia — c. Puro-mucosa catarrhalis, Ophthalmia, catarrhal — c. Puro-mucosa contagiosa vel Ægyptiaca, Ophthalmia, purulent.

CONJUNGENS, Communicans.

CONNATE, from *con* and *natus*, 'born with.'

CONNATE DISEASES, (F.) *Maladies connées*, *Morbi conna'ti*, are such as an individual is born with: — *connate* having the same signification as *congenital*. A difference has been made by some, however; those diseases or conditions which are dependent upon original conformation, being called *congenital*; — whilst the diseases or affections that may have supervened during gestation or delivery, are termed *connate*.

CONNEC'TICUT, MINERAL WATERS OF. There is a mineral spring at Stafford, in this state, twenty-four miles from Hartford, which has obtained more celebrity than any one in New England. Its principal ingredients are iron and carbonic acid. It, consequently, belongs to the class of acidulous chalybeates. There are other springs in the state, of which, however, little that is accurate is known.

CONNERVATIO, Syndesmosis.

CONNEXIO OSSIUM CARNOSA, Syssarcosis—c. Cartilaginea, Synchondrosis—c. Ligamentosa, Syndesmosis.

CONNUTRI'TUS, *Syn'trophos*, from *con*, 'with,' and *nutrior*, 'I am nourished.' A disease is so called which has grown up, as it were, with an individual, or has been connate with him. —Hippocrates, Galen.

CONOID, *Conoï'deus, Conoï'des*, from κωνος, 'a cone,' and ειδος, 'shape.' (F.) *Conoïde*. Resembling a cone.

CONOID LIG'AMENT. A ligament, passing from the coracoid process to the scapula, and forming part of the *coraco-clavicular* ligament of some anatomists.

CONOIDAL SUBSTANCE OF THE KIDNEY, see Kidney.

CONOIDES CORPUS, Pineal gland.

CONOPHTHALMIA, Staphyloma corneæ.

CONQUASSANT, (F.) *Conquassans*, from *con*, 'with,' 'together,' and *quassare*, 'to shake.' *Douleurs conquassantes* are the pains of parturition, at the time of their greatest intensity, when the head is engaged in the pelvis.

CONQUASSA'TION, *Conquassa'tio, Quassa'tio, Quassatu'ra*. Same etymon. A pharmaceutical operation, which consists in dividing, with a pestle, fresh vegetables, fruits, &c. See Confrication.

CONQUASSATIONES ANIMI, Affections of the mind.

CONQUE, Concha.

CON'SCIOUSNESS, DOUBLE. A somnambulistic condition, in which the individual leads, as it were, two lives, recollecting in each condition what occurred in previous conditions of the same character, but knowing nothing of the occurrences of the other. See Duality of the Mind.

CONSEC'UTIVE, *Consecuti'vus*, from *con*, 'with,' and *sequor*, 'to follow.'

CONSECUTIVE PHENOM'ENA OR SYMPTOMS, (F.) *Phénomènes ou accidens consécutifs*, are such as appear after the cessation of a disease, or, according to others, during its decline; but without having any direct connexion with it.

CONSENSUAL, see Instinctive.

CONSENSUS, Consent of parts, Sympathy.

CONSEN'SUS OCULO'RUM. The intimate association between the two eyes, as exemplified in their consentaneous action in health, and often in disease.

CONSENT OF PARTS, *Consen'sus, Consen'sus par'tium, Sympathi'a*, from *con*, and *sentire*, 'to feel;' (F.) *Consentement des Parties*. That relation of different parts of the body with each other which is more commonly denominated sympathy.

CONSENTEMENT DES PARTIES, Consent of parts.

CONSERVA'TION, *Conserva'tio, Phylax'is*, from *conservare*, (*con*, and *servare*,) 'to preserve;' (F.) *Conservation, Asservation*. The art of preserving any object of pharmacy, any remedial agent, &c., from decay.

CONSER'VA, *Conserve*. Same etymon. A pharmaceutical preparation, composed of a vegetable substance and a sufficient quantity of sugar. The London and American pharmacopœias prefer the term CONFECTION.

CONSERVA ABSIN'THII, *C. absin'thii marit'imi, Conserve of Wormwood*. (*Leaves* ℔j, *sugar* ℔iij.) It has been employed as a tonic, stomachic, and vermifuge.

CONSERVA ANGEL'ICÆ, (Ph. P.) *Conserve d'Angélique, C. of Angel'ica*. (*Pulp of root 250 parts; white sugar*, boiled in a decoction of the root, and reduced to the consistence of a solid electuary, 1000 parts.) It is tonic, aromatic, and stomachic.

CONSERVA DE A'PIO GRAVEOLEN'TE (Ph. P.), *Conserve d'Ache, Conserve of Smallage*. Prepared like the preceding. Reputed to have the same properties.

CONSERVA ARI, *Conserve of Arum*. (*Fresh root* ℔ss, *sugar* ℔iss.) Esteemed to be diuretic and stimulant.

CONSERVA AURANTII, Confectio aurantiorum— c. Cassiæ, Confectio cassiæ — c. Citri aurantii, Confectio aurantiorum.

CONSERVA COCHLEA'RIÆ HORTEN'SIS, *Conserve of Lemon Scurvy Grass*. (*Leaves* ℔j, *sugar* ℔iij.) Reputed to be stimulant and antiscorbutic.

CONSERVA CORTICIS EXTERIORIS AURANTII HISPALENSIS, Confectio aurantiorum — c. Corticum aurantiorum, Confectio aurantiorum — c. Florum rosarum rubrarum, Confectio rosæ Gallicæ — c. Cynosbati, Confectio rosæ caninæ — c. Cynorrhodi, Confectio rosæ caninæ — c. Flavedinis corticis aurantiorum Hispalensium, Confectio aurantiorum.

CONSERVA LU'JULÆ, *C. Folio'rum lu'julæ, Conserve of Woodsorrel*. (*Leaves* ℔j, *sugar* ℔iij.) Gratefully acid and refrigerant.

CONSERVA MENTHÆ, *C. Menthæ folio'rum, C. Menthæ sati'væ, Conserve of Mint*. (*Leaves* ℔j, *sugar* ℔iij.) Stomachic in nausea and vomiting.

CONSERVA PRUNI SYLVES'TRIS, *Pulpa pruno'rum sylves'trium condi'ta, C. Prunæ sylvestris, Conserve of Sloes*, (*Pulp* 1 part, *sugar* 3 parts.) Possessed of astringent properties.

CONSERVA ROSÆ, Confectio rosæ Gallicæ — c. Rosæ caninæ, Confectio rosæ caninæ — c. Rosæ Gallicæ, Confectio rosæ Gallicæ.

CONSERVA SCILLÆ, *Conserve of Squill*. (*Fresh squills* ℥j, *sugar* ℥x.) Possesses the diuretic and other virtues of the squill.

CONSERVE, Conserva, see Confectio — c. *d'Ache*, Conserva de apio graveolente — c. of Aloes, Conserva pruni sylvestris — c. of Lemon scurvy grass, Conserva cochleariæ hortensis — c. of Mint, Conserva menthæ — c. of Orange, Confectio aurantiorum — c. of Roses (red), Confectio rosæ gallicæ — c. of Smallage, Conserva de apio graveolente — c. of Woodsorrel, Conserva lujulæ — c. of Wormwood, Conserva absinthii.

CONSERVES, Spectacles.

CONSIDEN'TIA. This word has two acceptations. 1. It is synonymous with *Apocatastasis*; and, 2. It signifies contraction of any cavity or canal:—See Synezisis.

CONSISTEN'TIA. A Latin term employed in two senses. 1. When joined to the word *Morbi* or *Ætatis*, it expresses the acme of a disease, or the age at which the constitution has acquired its full strength. 2. By *Consisten'tia humo'ris* is meant the density of a humour.

CONSOLIDA MAJOR, Symphytum — c. Media, Ajuga, Chrysanthemum leucanthemum — c. Minor, Prunella — c. Regalis, Delphinium consolida — c. Rubra, Tormentil — c. Saracenica, Solidago virgaurea.

CONSOLIDAN'TIA, *Consolidati'va Medicamen'ta*, from *con*, and *solidus*, solid. Substances, formerly given for the purpose of consolidating wounds, or strengthening cicatrices.

CONSOLIDATIVA, Consolidantia.

CONSOMMÉ, Consumma'tum, Zomos. Soup, strongly charged with gelatin, and consequently very nutritious, although not proportionally easy of digestion.

CONSOMPTION, Consumption.

CONSONANCE, see Sound.

CON'SONANT, *Con'sonans*, from *consono*, 'to sound together,' (*con*, 'with,' and *sono*, 'to sound,') because it is generally believed that a consonant cannot be properly expressed, except when conjoined with a vowel. Physiologically, a breath, or a sound produced in the larynx, which suffers more or less interruption in its passage through the vocal tube.

CONSORTIUM, Sympathy.

CONSOUDE, GRANDE, Symphytum.

CONSOUND, MIDDLE, Ajuga.

CONSPERSIO, Catapasma.

CONSPICILLA, Spectacles.

CONSPIRATIO, Sympathy.

CONSTELLA'TUM UNGUEN'TUM. An ointment composed of cleansed earthworms! dried and pulverized; and of the fat of the bear or wild boar. It was formerly employed in toothach, and to hasten the cicatrization of wounds.

CONSTERNATIO, Stupor.

CON'STIPATED, *Constipa'tus*. (F.) *Constipé*. Affected with constipation. Costive.

CONSTIPATIO, Constipation, Stegnosis.

CONSTIPA'TION, *Constipa'tio*, from *constipare*, (*con* and *stipare*,) 'to cram close.' *Obstipa'tio, Adstric'tio, Arcta'tio, Obstipa'tio* seu *Reten'tio* *alvi'na, Ischocoi'lia, Alvus adstric'ta, A. Tarda, A. Dura, Obstruc'tio* seu *Suppres'sio alvi, O. Ductus alimenta'rii, O. intestina'lis, Torpor intestino'rum, Stypsis, Constipa'tio alvi, Copros'tasis, Acop'ria, Acopro'sis, Coproëpis'chesis, Ischocop'ria, Dyscoi'lia*, (F.) *Échauffement, Ventre resserré, Cost'iveness, Fæcal Reten'tion, Alvine obstruction.* A state of the bowels, in which the evacuations do not take place as frequently as usual; or are inordinately hard, and expelled with difficulty. It may be owing either to diminished action of the muscular coat of the intestines, or to diminished secretion from the mucous membrane, or to both. Cathartics will usually remove it; after which its exciting and predisponent causes must be inquired into and obviated to render the cure permanent.

CONSPIPATUS, Constipated.

CONSTIPÉ, Constipated.

CONSTITUENS, Vehicle, see Prescription.

CONSTITUTIO, Constitution, Habit of body — c. Aeris, Constitution of the atmosphere — c. Epidemica, Constitution, epidemic — c. Nervosa, Nervous diathesis.

CONSTITUTION, *Constitu'tio, Catas'tasis, Statue*, from *con*, and *statuere*, from *stare*, 'to stand.' A collection of several parts, forming a whole. In medicine, *Constitution* means the state of all the organs of the human body considered in regard to their special and relative arrangement, order, or activity. A *good constitution* is one in which every organ is well developed, and endowed with due energy, so that all perform their functions with equal facility. Any want of equilibrium in their development and energy forms a difference in the constitution. We say that a man is of a *good* or *robust*, a *delicate* or *weak constitution*, when he is commonly healthy, or commonly labouring under, or unusually susceptible of, disease.

CONSTITU'TION OF THE AT'MOSPHERE, *Constitu'tio A'ëris*, (F.) *Constitution Atmosphérique*. The condition of the atmosphere, as regards dryness and humidity, temperature, heaviness, direction of the winds, &c., considered as respects its influence on the animal economy.

CONSTITUTION, EPIDEM'IC, *Constitu'tio epidem'ica, Med'ical Constitution*, (F.) *Constitution médicale, C. épidémique*. The aggregate of meteorological conditions, so far as they are appreciable, during which diseases prevail epidemically.

CONSTITU'TIONAL, (F.) *Constitutionnel*. Belonging to the constitution of an individual; to his manner of being; as *constitutional phthisis, c. gout*, &c. By some, this epithet has been given to diseases, produced by the constitution of the atmosphere; but this acceptation is not common.

CONSTRICTEURS DE LA VULVE, Constrictores cunni — *c. du Vagin*, Constrictores cunni.

CONSTRICTIO, Astriction, Systole.

CONSTRICTIVA, Styptics.

CONSTRIC'TOR, from *constringere*, (*con*, and *stringere*,) 'to bind.' (F.) *Constricteur*. That which binds in a circular direction. A sphincter. Different muscles are so called.

CONSTRICTOR ANI, Sphincter ani externus — c. of Nuck, Compressor of Nuck.

CONSTRICTORES ALARUM NASI, Depressor alæ nasi.

CONSTRICTO'RES CUNNI, *C. Vagi'næ* seu *Vulvæ, Clitor'idis inferio'res lati et plani mus'culi, Sphincter Vagi'næ*, (F.) *Constricteurs du vagin, C. de la Vulve*. Small muscles, which originate beneath the clitoris, descend along the sides of the vagina, and terminate by becoming confounded with the *transversus perinæi* and *external sphincter ani* muscles. Their use is to contract the entrance of the vagina.

CONSTRICTORES ISTHMI FAUCIUM, Glossostaphylinus.

CONSTRICTO'RES LARYN'GIS. Lieutaud describes, under the name *Grand constricteur du Larynx*, the muscle *Crico-arytenoîdeus latera'lis* with the *Thyro-arytenoideus*.

CONSTRICTO'RES NASI, Compressor naris.

CONSTRICTOR ŒSOPH'AGI, *Constrictor of the Œsoph'agus*, (F.) *Constricteur de l'Œsophage, Muscle œsophagien*. A fasciculus of fleshy, circular fibres, at the upper part of the œsophagus.

CONSTRICTORES ORIS, Orbicularis oris — c. Palpebrarum, Orbicularis palpebrarum.

CONSTRICTO'RES PHARYN'GIS, *Constrictors of the Pharynx, Sphincter Gulæ*. Muscular expansions which assist in forming the parietes of the pharynx. Three of these are generally admitted. 1. The *Constric'tor Pharyn'gis infe'rior, Crico-Pharyngeus* and *Thyro-pharyngeus*, (F.) *Crico-thyro-pharyngien*. It is broad, very thin, quadrilateral, seated superficially, extending from the thyroid and cricoid cartilages as far as the middle of the pharynx, and uniting, on the median line, with that of the opposite side. 2. The *Constrictor Pharyngis Me'dius, Hyo-pharyngeus* and *Chondro-pharyngeus, Syndes'mo-pharyngeus*, (F.) *Hyoglosso-basi-pharyngien*, occupies the middle part of the pharynx. It is triangular, and attached, anteriorly, to the great and little cornu of the os hyoides; to the stylohyoid ligament; and terminates, posteriorly, by joining its fellow of the opposite side. 3. The *Constrictor Pharyngis supe'rior, Ceph'alo-pharyngeus, Glosso-pharyngeus, Mylo-pharyngeus, Pter'ygo-pharyngeus*, (F.) *Pterygo-syndesmo-staphili-pharyngien*, is quadrilateral, and extends from the internal ala of the pterygoid process, from the inter-maxillary ligament, from the internal oblique line of the jaw, and from the base of the tongue to the posterior part of the pharynx.

The constrictors of the pharynx contract it. They can likewise approximate the ends to each other. Chaussier considers those and the *stylopharyngeus* as but one muscle, and includes all under this last name.

CONSTRICTORES VAGINÆ, C. cunni — c. Vulvæ, C. cunni.

CONSTRINGENTIA, Astringents, Styptics.

CONSUETUDO, Habit — c. Menstrua, Menses.

CONSULTA'TION, *Consulta'tio, Delibera'tio, Cœnolog"ia, Conten'tio, Symbolen'sis,* from *consulere, consultum,* 'to hold council.' This word has several acceptations. In English, it means, almost always, the meeting of two or more practitioners, to deliberate on any particular case of disease. In France, it signifies the written result of such deliberations, as well as the opinion of a physician, given to a patient, who consults him, either personally or by writing.

CONSULT'ING PHYSIC"IAN or SURGEON, (F.) *Médecin* ou *Chirurgien consultant.* One who consults with the attending practitioner, regarding any case of disease. Some physicians, surgeons, and accoucheurs confine themselves to consulting practice.

CONSUMMATUM, *Consommé.*

CONSUMMA'TUS, from *con, cum,* 'with,' and *summus,* 'the whole.' Confirmed; established; developed,—as *Phthisis consumma'ta,* 'confirmed consumption.'

CONSUMP'TION, from *consumere,* (*con* and *sumere,*) 'to waste away;' *Consump'tio, Consum'tio, Syntex'is,* (F.) *Consomption.* Progressive emaciation or wasting away. This condition precedes death in the greater part of chronic diseases, and particularly in *phthisis pulmonalis:* on this account it is, that phthisis has received the name *consumption.*—See Phthisis. *Fièvre de Consomption, Consumptive fever,* is the same as *Hectic fever.*

CONSUMPTION OF THE BOWELS, Enterophthisis—c. Pulmonary, Phthisis pulmonalis.

CONSUMPTI'VA. Same etymology. Caustics, used for the destruction of fungi. *Burnt alum, lunar caustic,* &c., were formerly so called.

CONSUMTIO, Consumption.

CONTABESCEN'TIA, from *contabescere,* (*con* and *tabescere,*) 'to grow lean.' Consumption, marasmus, atrophy, &c.

CONTACT, *Contac'tus,* from *con* and *tangere,* 'to touch.' The state of two bodies that touch each other. In the theory of contagious diseases, we distinguish *immediate* or *direct contact,* as when we touch a patient labouring under one of those diseases; and *mediate* or *indirect contact,* when we touch, not the patient himself, but objects that have touched or emanated from him. The air is, most commonly, the medium by which this last kind of contact is effected.

CONTA'GION, *Conta'gio, Conta'ges, Conta'gium, Aporrhœ'a, Apoc'rysis.* Same etymon. The transmission of a disease from one person to another by direct or indirect contact. The term has, also, been applied, by some, to the action of miasmata arising from dead animal or vegetable matter, bogs, fens, &c., but in this sense it is now abandoned. Contagious diseases are produced either by a virus, capable of causing them by inoculation, as in small-pox, cow-pox, hydrophobia, syphilis, &c., or by miasmata, proceeding from a sick individual, as in plague, typhus gravior, and in measles and scarlatina. Scrofula, phthisis pulmonalis, and cancer, have, by some, been esteemed contagious, but apparently without foundation. Physicians are, indeed, by no means unanimous in deciding what diseases are contagious, and what not. The contagion of plague and typhus, especially of the latter, is denied by many. It seems probable, that a disease may be contagious under certain circumstances and not under others. A case of common fever, arising from *common causes,* as from cold, if the patient be kept in a close, foul situation, may be converted into a disease, capable of producing emanations, which may excite a similar disease in those exposed to them. *Contagion* and *infection* are generally esteemed synonymous. Frequently, however, the former is applied to diseases not produced by contact; as measles, scarlet fever, &c., whilst *infection* is used for those that require positive contact; as itch, syphilis, &c., and conversely. Diseases, which cannot be produced in any other way than by contagion, are said to have their origin in *specific contagion;* as small-pox, cow-pox, measles, hydrophobia, syphilis, &c. Those which are produced by contagion, and yet are supposed to be sometimes owing to other causes, are said to arise from *common contagion;* as typhus, cynanche parotidæa, &c.

CONTA'GIONIST. One who believes in the contagious character of a particular disease,—as of yellow fever.

CONTA'GIOUS, *Contagio'sus.* Capable of being transmitted by mediate or immediate contact; —as a *contagious disease, contagious fever, contagious effluvia,* &c.

CONTAGIUM, Contagion, Miasm.

CONTEMPLABILES DIES, Critical days.

CONTEMPLATIF, (F.) *Contemplati'vus,* (*con* and *templum.*) Appertaining to contemplation. The predominant idea of the melancholic — of the monomaniac — is sometimes called *contemplative.*

CONTEMPLATIO, Catalepsy.

CONTEMPLATIVUS, *Contemplatif.*

CONTENSIO, Tension.

CONTENTIO, Consultation.

CONTEX'TURE, *Contextu'ra, Contex'tus,* from *con* and *texere,* (quasi *tegsere,* from *tegere,* 'to cover,') 'to weave,' 'to make a web.' Arrangement of parts; — texture. A name given, metaphorically, to the structure of organized bodies; as *the contexture of muscles, fibres,* &c. See Tissue, and Texture.

CONTIGUITY, DIARTHROSIS OF, see Continuity.

CON'TINENCE, *Continen'tia,* from *continere,* (*con* and *tenere,* 'to hold or keep,') 'to contain oneself;' 'to restrain.' Restraint. Abstinence from, or moderation in, the pleasures of physical love.

CONTINENS, Continent.

CON'TINENT, *Continens.* Restrained. This word is synonymous, also, with *Continued;* (F.) *Continu.*

CONTINENT CAUSE, *Causa conjunc'ta,* is a cause, real or presumed, which, having given rise to a disease, continues to act during the whole of its duration. It may be considered synonymous with proximate cause. A *continent fever, Febris continens,* is one which preserves during its whole course, the same degree of intensity, without any remission or sensible exacerbation. A disease which continues uninterruptedly, has been also called *Æipathei'a, Aeipathei'a* or *Aipathi'a.*

CONTINENTIA, Continence.

CONTIN'UED FEVER, *Febris contin'ua, F. con'tinens, F. anabat'ica, F. assid'ua.* A fever which presents no interruption in its course. Continued fevers form a division in the class *Pyrexiæ* of Cullen, and include three genera,—*Synocha, Synochus,* and *Typhus.* It is proper to remark, that some of the older writers make a distinction between the continual fever, συνεχης, *febris continua,* and the *synochus* or *febris continens.* Thus, Rhases states that the synochus or *continens* is a fever, which consists of one paroxysm from beginning to end; whilst the *continua* is allied to intermittents.

CONTINU'ITY, *Continu'itas.* An adhesion of two things between each other, so that they cannot be separated without fracture or laceration.

CONTINUITY, DIARTHRO'SES OF, (F.) *Diarthroses de Continuité,* are movable joints, in which the bones are continuous, but do not touch immediately, there being between them a ligamentous substance, whose flexibility permits motion. The vertebral articulations are examples of this. DIARTHROSES OF CONTIGU'ITY, *Diarthroses de Contiguité*, on the other hand, are movable articulations, in which the bones are not continuous, but touch by surfaces covered with a cartilaginous layer, which is always moistened by synovia.

CONTINUITY, SOLUTION OF, *Solu'tio contin'ui*, is any division of parts, previously continuous. Wounds and fractures are *solutions of continuity*. The word *Continuity* is opposed to *Contiguity:* the latter meaning the condition of two things which are near each other, or touch without uniting. There is *contiguity* between the head of the humerus and the glenoid cavity of the scapula, but not *continuity*.

CONTONDANT, Contunding.

CONTORSIO, Contorsion—c. Columnæ vertebralis, Rhachiostrophosis.

CONTOR'SION, *Contor'tio*, from *contorqueo*, (*con* and *torquere*, 'to wring,') 'I twist about.' Violent movement of a part, accompanied with a kind of torsion; as *contortion of the face*.

CONTRAAPERTU'RA, from *contra*, 'against,' and *aperio*, 'I open.' A *counter-opening; Contra-incis'io, Incis'io prio'ri oppo'sita*, (F.) *Contre-ouverture*. An incision, made in the most depending part of a wound or abscess, when the first opening is not situate in a manner favourable for the discharge of the pus.

CONTRAEXTENSIO, Counter-extension.

CONTRAC'TILE, *Contrac'tilis*, from *contrahere*, (*con* and *trahere*,) 'to draw together.' Capable of contracting. The fibre of muscles is *contractile*.

CONTRACTILITÉ, Contractility—*c. par défaut d'Extension*, Elasticity — *c. de Tissu*, Elasticity.

CONTRACTIL'ITY, *Contractil'itas:* same etymon; (F.) *Contractilité*. That vital property, which gives, to certain parts, the power of contracting. The muscles of locomotion are endowed with a power of *voluntary contractility*, or one dependent immediately on the action of the brain: — the muscles of the viscera of digestion, and other internal organs, enjoy an *involuntary contractility*. *Contractility* and *irritability* are frequently used synonymously to signify the property possessed by any tissue of *contracting* on the application of an appropriate stimulus.

CONTRACTILITY, Irritability.

CONTRACTIO CORDIS, Systole.

CONTRAC'TION, *Contrac'tio*. Same etymon; *Sys'tolĕ*. Action of contracting. When we speak of the *contraction of a muscle*, we mean the phenomenon it exhibits during the time it is in action.

CONTRACTOR UTERI, Abortive.

CONTRACTU'RA. Same etymon. *Acamp'sia, Enta'sia articula'ris, Rigor ar'tuum, Muscular Stiff-joint*. A state of permanent rigidity and progressive atrophy of the flexor muscles, which prevents the motions of extension beyond a certain limit. The affected muscles form hard cords beneath the skin. On dissection, they are found converted into tendinous fibres, the fleshy fibres having almost disappeared, when the disease has been of any duration. It succeeds, frequently, other diseases, particularly rheumatism, neuralgia, convulsions, syphilis, colica pictonum, &c. The warm bath, vapour bath, or thermal waters, oleaginous embrocations, mechanical extension of the limbs, &c., are the chief means of treatment.

CONTRAFISSU'RA, from *contra*, 'against,' and *findo, fissum*, 'I cleave;' *Repercu'sio, Reson'itus, Cutag'ma Fissura contraja'cens, Apeche'ma, Anticom'ma, Antic'opĕ, Anticru'sis, Anticrusma, Infortu'nium, Counterstroke*, (F.) *Contre-coup, Contre-fente, Contre-fracture*. A fracture, contusion, or injury, produced, by a blow, in a part distant from that which is struck. Five species of *contrafissura* or *contre-coups* may occur in the skull. 1. When the internal table yields and fractures. 2. When the bone breaks in any other part than the one struck. 3. When a bone, which has been struck, remains uninjured, and its neighbour is fractured. 4. When the bone is fractured in a place diametrically opposite to that struck, as in fractures at the base of the cranium, from a fall on the vertex; and lastly, when the violence of the blow produces a separation of the neighbouring or distant sutures. These fractures of the skull are also called *Fractures par résonnance*.

CONTRAHENTIA, Astringents, Styptics.

CONTRAÏNCISIO, Contra-apertura.

CONTRAÏNDICATIO, Counter-indication.

CONTRAÏRRITATIO, Counter-irritation.

CONTRALUNA'RIS, from *contra*, 'against,' and *luna*, 'the moon.' An epithet for a woman who conceives during the menstrual discharge.— Dietrich.

CONTRASTIMULANS, Contro-stimulants.

CONTRAYERVA, Dorstenia contrayerva—c. Balls, Pulvis contrayervæ compositus—c. Lisbon, Dorstenia contrayerva — c. Mexican, Psoralea pentaphylla—c. Nova, Psoralea pentaphylla—c. Virginiana, Aristolochia serpentaria.

CONTRECOUP, Contra-fissura.

CONTREÉXTENSION, Counter-extension.

CONTREFENTE, Contra-fissura.

CONTREFRACTURE, Contra-fissura.

CONTREÏNDICATION, Counter-indication.

CONTREOUVERTURE, Contra-apertura.

CONTREXEVILLE, MINERAL WATERS OF. Contrexeville is a town in France in the department of Vosges, four leagues from Neufchâteau. The waters contain carbonate of iron, chloride of calcium, and carbonate of lime, chloride of sodium, a bituminous substance, and free carbonic acid. They are frequented by those labouring under cutaneous, scrofulous, and calculous affections.

CONTRIT''IO, *Syntrim'ma, Syntrip'sis, Tritu'ra, Tritus, Trit''io, Tripsis*, from *contero*, 'I bruise or make small:' *Comminu'tion, Trituration*.

CONTROSTIM'ULANT, *Contrastim'ulans, Hyposthen'ic*, from *contra*, 'against,' and *stimulus*, 'that which excites.' A substance that possesses a particular, debilitating property, acting upon the excitability in a manner opposite to stimulus. A name given to therapeutical agents, which, according to the Italian theory of *Contro-stimulus*, are endowed with the property of diminishing excitement by a specific action. These agents are by no means clearly defined.

CONTROSTIMULUS. Same etymon. The name given by Rasori, about thirty years ago, to a new medical doctrine, of which he was the originator—*La nuova Dottrina Medica Italiana*. It is founded on the contro-stimulant property attributed to a certain number of medicines. In this doctrine, as in that of Brown, under the name *excitability*, a fundamental principle of physiology is admitted, by virtue of which living beings are endowed with an aptitude for feeling the action of external agents or exciting influences, and of reacting on these influences. When this excitability is too great, there is excess of stimulus or *Hypersthenia'a:* when too little, there is deficiency or *Hyposthenia'a*. Diseases, *general* and *local*, are divided into three great classes, or into, 1. *Hypersthenic;* 2. *Hyposthenic;* 3. *Irritative*. The contro-stimulant physicians admit only two classes of medicines — *stimulants* and *contro-stimulants*.

CONTUND'ING, *Contu'sing, Contun'dens*, from *contundere*, (*con* and *tundere*,) 'to bruise.' (F.) *Contondant.* That which causes contusions. An epithet given to round, blunt, vulnerating projectiles, which bruise or lacerate parts without cutting them.
CONTUS, Contused.
CONTUS, Penis.
CONTU'SED. Same etymon. (F.) *Contus.* Affected with contusion. Thus we say — a *contused wound.*
CONTU'SION, *Contu'sio*, a *Bruise, Collis'io, Phlasma, Thlasis, Thlas'ma, Th. contu'sio, Rhegê, Rhegma, Rhegmus, Famex, Famis, Famix,* (F.) *Meurtrissure.* Same etymon. An injury or lesion —arising from the impulse of a body with a blunt surface—which presents no loss of substance, and no apparent wound. If the skin be divided, the injury takes the name of *contused wound.* The differences of contusions, as to extent, are of course infinite. When slight, the blood stagnates in the capillaries of the skin, or is effused into the subcutaneous areolar tissue. Time and cold applications remove it. When the texture of the parts has been lacerated, there is effusion of blood, with more or less torpor in the part. Cooling applications, general or topical bleeding, emollients, poultices, &c., are here necessary, according to circumstances. In the severest kinds of contusion, all the soft and solid parts, except the skin, are bruised, and, at times, reduced to a kind of pap. When the disorganization is to this extent, there is no hope except in amputation. A deep contusion of the soft parts has been called *Sarcoth'lasis,* and *Sarcothlas'ma.*
CONUS ARTERIO'SUS, *Infundib'ulum of the heart.* The portion of the right ventricle from which the pulmonary artery proceeds, forms a prominence on the right side of the anterior furrow of the heart, and is prolonged towards the left, becoming narrower at the same time, so as to form a funnel-shaped projection, which extends a little beyond the base of the ventricles. This is the *Conus arteriosus.*
CONUS VASCULOSUS, see Coni Vasculosi.
CONVALES'CENCE, *Convalescen'tia, Analep'sis, Anas'tasis, Reconvalescen'tia,* from *convalescere,* (*con* and *valescere*) 'to grow well.' *Exanas'trophê.* Recovery of health after disease. The time which elapses between the termination of a disease and complete restoration of strength.
CONVALLARIA ANGULOSA, C. polygonatum.
CONVALLA'RIA MAIA'LIS, from *convallis*, 'a valley,'—from its abounding in valleys. *Lil'ium Convall'ium, Convalla'ria, C. mappi, Maian'themum, Lily of the Valley, May Lily,* (F.) *Muguet, Muguet de Mai.* The recent flowers are reputed to be aromatic, cephalic, errhine, and cathartic. They are not used.
CONVALLARIA MAPPI, C. Maialis.
CONVALLA'RIA MULTIFLO'RA, *Polygon'atum multiflo'rum,* which grows in this country and in Europe, has analogous properties.
CONVALLA'RIA POLYGON'ATUM. The systematic name of *Solomon's Seal, Convalla'ria angulo'sa, Polygon'atum uniflo'rum seu ancepe seu vulga'rê, Sigil'lum Salomo'nis, Polygon'atum.* The root was once used as an astringent and tonic. It is, also, a reputed cosmetic.
CONVENTUS, Coition.
CONVER'SION, *Conver'sio,* from *con* and *vertere,* 'to turn.' Change from one state into another.
CONVERSION OF DISEASES, (F.) *Conversion des maladies,* is the change or transformation of one disease into another.
CONVOLU'TION, *Convolu'tio,* from *convolvere,* (*con* and *volvere*) 'to entwine;' *Epipha'rion,*

Gyrus, Helig'mus, (F.) *Circonvolution.* The rolling of any thing upon itself.
CONVOLU'TIONS, CER'EBRAL, *Gyri seu Plicatu'ræ seu Spiræ seu Proces'sus enteroï'dei Cer'ebri,* are the round, undulating, tortuous projections observed at the surface of the brain. In them Gall's organs, of course, terminate.
CONVOLU'TION, INTER'NAL, *C. of the Corpus Callo'sum, Convolution d'Ourlet* (Foville). A cerebral convolution of great extent, the principal portion of which is found on the inner surface of each hemisphere above the corpus callosum. In front it bends downwards and backwards to the fissure of Sylvius, and behind it extends to the middle lobe and forms the hippocampus major.
CONVOLU'TIONS, INTES'TINAL, are the turns made by the intestines in the abdomen.
CONVOLU'TION, SUPRA-OR'BITAR. A convolution of the brain, which exists on the inferior surface of the anterior lobe, and rests upon the roof of the orbit.
CONVOLVULUS, Intussusceptio, Ileus.
CONVOL'VULUS BATA'TAS. Same etymon. *C. In'dicus, Camotes; the Sweet Potato, Spanish Potato.* This is the only esculent root of the genus Convolvulus. It is much eaten in the United States.
CONVOL'VULUS CANTAB'RICA, *Cantab'rica, Lavender-leaved Bindweed,* has been considered anthelmintic and actively cathartic.
CONVOLVULUS INDICUS, C. Batatas.
CONVOL'VULUS JALA'PA. A systematic name of the Jalap plant, properly *Ipomœ'a Jalapa seu macrorhi'sa. Jala'pium, Jalo'pa, Mechoaca'na nigra, Jalappa, Jalapa, Jalap Root, Gialappa, Xalappa, Bryo'nia Mechoacan'a ni'gricans, Bryo'nia Peruvia'na, Chela'pa, Rhabar'barum Nigrum, Gelappium,* (F.) *Jalap,* is procured from South America. Its odour is nauseous; taste sweetish and slightly pungent. It is solid, hard, heavy, brittle; fracture resinous; internally, light gray; externally, covered with a deep brown, wrinkled bark. Its operation is cathartic, the resinous part griping violently. Dose, 10 gr. to ʒss. A drop or two of any essential oil may prevent it from griping. An active principle has been separated from Jalap, to which the names *Jalapin* and *Cathartin* have been given.
CONVOLVULUS MAJOR ALBUS, Convolvulus sepium—c. Maritimus, Convolvulus soldanella.
CONVOL'VULUS MECHOACAN, *Mechoaca'na Radix, Jalappa alba, Rhabar'barum album, Mechoacan,* (F.) *Rhabarbe blanche.* A Mexican convolvulus, the root of which possesses aperient properties, and was once extensively used instead of jalap.
CONVOLVULUS MEGALORHIZUS, C. Panduratus.
CONVOL'VULUS PANDURA'TUS, *C. Megalorhi'sus, Pseudo-mechoaca'na, Fiddle-leaved Bindweed, Hog Potato, Virginian Bindweed, Wild Pota'to, Mech'ameck, M. Bindweed, Wild Jalap, Man in the ground, Wild Rhubarb, Wild Potato-Vine, Kassau'der, Kassa'der, Kussauder,* (F.) *Liseron Mechamec.* In Virginia, and some other parts of the United States, the root of this plant has been much recommended in cases of gravel. It is used either in powder or decoction.
CONVOLVULUS PERENNIS, Humulus lupulus.
CONVOLVULUS PES CA'PREÆ, *Bargada.* A plant used in India as a cataplasm in arthritic cases.
CONVOLVULUS REPENS, C. sepium.
CONVOLVULUS SCAMMO'NEA seu SCAMMO'NIA, *C. Syriacus.* The systematic name of the *Scam'mony Plant.* A Syrian and Mexican plant; the concrete gummi-resinous juice of which, *Scammo'nia, Scammonia Gummi Resi'na, Scammonium, S. Syriacum, Diagryd'ium, Dacrydion, Scamme-*

ny, *Mahmoudy*, (F.) *Scammonée d'Alep*, comes to us in blackish-gray fragments, becoming whitish-yellow when touched with wet fingers. It is a drastic, hydragogue cathartic. Dose, gr. iij to gr. xv, triturated with sugar.

CONVOLVULUS, SEA, Convolvulus Soldanella.

CONVOL'VULUS SE'PIUM, *Convolvulus major albus* seu *repens* seu *Tugurio'rum, Calyste'gia se'pium, Great Bindweed,* (F.) *Liseron des Haies: Grand Liseron.* The juice of this plant is violently purgative, and is given in dropsical affections.

CONVOL'VULUS SOLDANEL'LA. The systematic name of the *Sea Convolvulus, Bras'sica Mari'na, Calyste'gia Soldanella, Sea Bindweed, Convol'vulus Marit'imus, Soldanel'la,* (F.) *Chou Marin.* The leaves of this plant are said to be drastic cathartic; but they are not much, if at all, used.

CONVOLVULUS SYRIACUS, Convolvulus scammonia—c. Tugurlorum, C. sepium.

CONVOL'VULUS TURPE'THUM, *Turpe'thum.* The systematic name of the *Turbith* plant. (F.) *Racine de Turbith.* The cortical part of the root of this species of convolvulus is brought from the East Indies. It is a cathartic, but not used.

CONVULSIBILITAS, see Subsultus tendinum.

CONVULSIF, Convulsive.

CONVULSIO, Convulsion—c. Canina, see Canine laugh.

CONVUL'SIO CEREA'LIS, *Convulsio ab Ustilag'inĕ, Ergotis'mus spasmod'icus, Myrmeci'asis, Rapha'nia, Myrmecias'mus, Convul'sio Solonien'sis, Myrmecis'mus, Myrmeco'sis, Cereal Convulsion,* (F.) *Convulsion céréale, Ergotisme convulsif, Convulsion de Sologne.* A singular disorder of the convulsive kind, attended with a peculiar tingling and formication in the arms and legs; hence called by the Germans Kriebelkrankheit. It is said to be endemic in some parts of Germany, and to arise often from the use of spoiled corn.

CONVULSIO HABITUALIS, Chorea—c. Indica, Tetanus—c. Raphania, Raphania—c. Soloniensis, C. cerealis, Ergotism—c. Tonica, Tonic spasm—c. Uteri, Abortion.

CONVUL'SION, *Spasmus, Convul'sio,* from *convallere,* (con and *vellere,*) ' to tear,' ' to pull together;' *Conduc'tio, Hieran'osis, Disten'tio nervo'rum, Spasmus clon'icus, Convul'sio clon'ica, Eclamp'sia, Syspa'sia Convul'sio, Hyperspasm'ia, Clonic Spasm.* This word has several acceptations. It means any violent perversion of the animal movements. The word *Convul'sions* generally, however, signifies alternate contractions, violent and involuntary, of muscles, which habitually contract only under the influence of the will. This alternate contraction, when slight, is called *tremor;* when strong and permanent, *tetanus, trismus, &c. Spasms, Cramp, Risus Sardonicus,* and *St. Vitus's Dance* are *convulsions.*

CONVULSION, SALAAM', *Eclamp'sia nutans.* A name given to a singular kind of convulsion in children, in which there is a peculiar bobbing of the head forward.—Sir Charles Clarke.

CONVULSION DE SOLOGNE, Convulsio cerealis.

CONVULSIONNAIRE, (F.) A name given, during the last century, to individuals who had, or affected to have, convulsions, produced by religious impulses.

CONVULSIONS OF CHILDREN, Eclampsia —c. *des Enfans,* Eclampsia—c. *des Femmes enceintes et en couches,* Eclampsia gravidarum et parturientium—c. Puerperal, Eclampsia gravidarum et parturientium. See Mania, dancing.

CONVUL'SIVE, *Convulsi'vus, Spasmo'des, Agitato'rius,* (F.) *Convulsif.* That which is accompanied by, or is analogous to, convulsions, as *convulsive cough, convulsive disease.*

CONYZA, Inula dysenterica—c. Coma aurea, Solidago Virgaurea—c. Major, C. squarrosa—c. Media, Inula dysenterica.

CONY'ZA SQUARRO'SA, *C. Major, Brephoc'tonon, In'ula squarro'sa, Great Fleabane* or *Spikenard,* (F.) *Herbe aux mouches.* A European plant, whose strong and disagreeable odour was formerly considered to be destructive to flies, fleas, &c. Its infusion in wine was once used as an emmenagogue and anti-icteric; and in vinegar as an anti-epileptic.

COOKERY, Culinary art.

COOLWEED, Pilea pumila.

COONTIE or COONTI, see Arrowroot.

COÖPERCULUM OCULI, Palpebra.

COÖPERTORIUM, Thyroid cartilage.

COÖSTRUM. The middle part of the diaphragm.—Ruland.

COPAHU, Copaiba.

COPA'IBA. The resinous juice of *Copaif'era officina'lis* seu *Jacquini, Copaiva officina'lis,* and other species of Copaifera; *Family,* Leguminosæ. *Sex. Syst.* Decandria Monogynia. It is the *Copaiferæ officina'lis Resi'na, Bal'samum Copaibæ, B. Brasilien'sĕ, B. de Copaibâ, B. Capi'vi, Balsam of Copaiba* or *Copaiva,* (vulgarly pronounced *capee'vy,*) (F.) *Copahu, Baume de Copahu, B. du Brésil, Térébinthe de Copahu.* Its odour is peculiar, but not unpleasant; taste pungent, bitter; consistence, syrupy; colour yellowish, and transparent. It is soluble in alcohol, ether, and the expressed oils. S. g. 0.950. Its properties are stimulant and diuretic; in large doses it is purgative. It acts on the lining membrane of the urethra, and on mucous membranes in general. It is given in gonorrhœa, gleet, leucorrhœa, &c., in the dose of gtt. x to ʒj, twice or thrice a day. Should symptoms of urticaria or diarrhœa arise, the dose is too large, and must be diminished. It can be inspissated by means of magnesia so as to be made into pills, and a plan has been devised for enveloping it in gelatin, so that its taste is entirely concealed. See Capsules, gelatinous.

COPAIFERA JACQUINI, see Copaiba—c. Officinalis, see Copaiba.

COPAIVA OFFICINALIS, see Copaiba.

COPAL', *Copale, Resina Copal, Gummi copalli'num.* A resinous substance brought from the East Indies, South America, and the western coast of Africa, which flows spontaneously from *Elæocar'pus Copalif'era* or *Vate'ria Ind'ica,* and probably from different species of *Hymæa'a.* It is a stimulant. like all the resins, and, dissolved in rectified spirit of wine, has been used in cases of spongy gums and looseness of the teeth; but it is now only employed in varnishes.

COPE, Cut.

COPHOMA, Cophosis.

COPHONIA, Acouophonia.

COPHO'SIS, *Copho'ma, Coph'otes, Sur'ditas, Paracu'sis, Dysæsthe'sia audito'ria;* from κωφος, ' deaf.' (F.) *Surdité.* Diminution or loss of hearing. Cullen uses the word synonymously with *Dysecœa,* and Pinel with *Paracou'sia* or *Parac'oä.* According to Sauvages, *Cophosis* differs from both,—from *Dysecœa,* because in it the sonorous rays cannot reach the labyrinth; and from *Paracousia,* which consists in a confused state of hearing.

Cophosis seems, usually, to be synonymous with deafness.—*Paracou'sis Sur'ditas.*

COPHOTES, Cophosis.

COPOS, *Lassitu'do, Fatiga'tio, Las'situde, Fatigue.* A state of body in which most of the animal functions are exerted with less promptitude and vigour than common. The ancients admitted three species: 1. That arising from plethora, *Lassitu'do tensi'va, tono'des*; 2. From plethora and increased heat combined, *Lassitu'do phlegmono'sa, æstuo'sa, phlegmono'des*; and, 3. Owing to a morbid condition of the humours, *Lassitu'do ulcero'sa, helco'des.*

COPPER, Cuprum—c. Ammoniated, Cuprum ammoniatum—c. Ammonio-sulphate of, Cuprum ammoniatum—c. Subacetate of, Cupri subacetas—c. Sulphate of, Cupri sulphas—c. Ammoniacal sulphate of, Cuprum ammoniatum.

COPPERAS, Ferri sulphas—c. White, Zinci sulphas.

COPPER-NOSE, Gutta rosea.

COPRACRASIA, Scoracrasia.

COPRACRATIA, Scoracrasia.

COPRAGO'GUM, from κοπρος, 'fæces,' and αγω, 'I bring away.' *Stercus è primis viis edu'cens.* A cathartic. The name of a laxative electuary, mentioned by Ruland.

COPRECCRITICUS, Coprocriticus.

COPREM'ESIS, *Copriěm'esis, Vom'itus fæculen'tus* seu *ster'coris*: same etymon as the next. Vomiting of fæces.

COPREM'ETUS, *Coproěm'etus, Copriěm'etus, Merdiv'omus,* from κοπρος, 'excrement,' and εμεω, 'I vomit.' One who vomits fæces.—Hippocrates.

COPRIEMESIS, Copremesis.

COPRIEMETUS, Copremetus.

COPROCRIT'ICUS, *Coprecerit'icus,* from κοπρος, 'excrement,' and κρινω, 'I separate.' A mild cathartic; an eccoprotic.

COPROEMETUS, Copremetus.

COPROEPISCHESIS, Constipation.

COPROLITHUS, see Calculi of the stomach and intestines.

COPROPHORESIS, Catharsis.

COPROPHORIA, Catharsis.

COPRORRHŒA, Diarrhœa.

COPROS, Excrement.

COPROSCLEROMA, Coprosclerosis.

COPROSCLERO'SIS, from κοπρος, 'excrement,' and σκληροω, 'I harden.' Induration of fæcal matters; *Coprosclero'ma.*

COPROSTASIS, Constipation.

COPTE, *Copton,* from κοπτω, 'I beat or pound.' A sort of cake, composed of vegetable substances, which the ancients administered internally, and applied to the epigastric region in the form of cataplasm.

COPTIS, *Coptis trifo'lia, Nigel'la, Helleb'orus trifo'lius, Fibra au'rea, Chryza fibrau'rea, Anemo'nē Grönlan'dica, Gold thread, Mouth root.* The root of this—*Coptis,* (Ph. U. S.)—is much used in Massachusetts, in aphthous and other ulcerations of the mouth, as a local application. It is a pure bitter, and can be used, wherever such is indicated.

COPTIS TEETA, *Mishme Teeta,* (Upper Assam), *Honglane,* (Chinese). The root of this plant is considered to be a powerful tonic and stomachic.

COPTON, Copte.

COPULA, Ligament—c. Carnalis, Coition—c. Cartilaginea, see Synchondrosis—c. Magna cerebri, Corpus callosum.

COPULATION, Coition.

COPYO'PIA, *Kopyo'pia,* (F.) *Lassitude oculaire,* from κοπος, 'fatigue,' and ωψ, 'the eye.' Fatigue of vision. Weakness of sight. Inability of the eye to sustain continued exertion.

COQ, Phasianus Gallus.

COQUE DU LEVANT, see Menispermum cocculus—c. d'Œuf, see Ovum—c. Levant, see Menispermum cocculus.

COQUELICOT, Papaver rhœas.

COQUELOURDE, Anemone pulsatilla.

COQUELUCHE, Influenza, Pertussis.

COQUEN'TIA MEDICAMENT'A, from *coquere,* 'to digest.' Medicines which were formerly believed to be proper for favouring the coction or digestion of food.

COQUERET, Physalis.

COQUETTE, Influenza.

COQUILLE, Cochlea—c. d'Œuf, see Ovum.

COR, A corn. Also, Heart.

COR BOVINUM, Heart, hypertrophy of the.

CORACOBRACHIÆUS, Coracobrachialis.

COR'ACO-BRA'CHIAL, *Cor'aco Brachia'lis.* Belonging both to the coracoid process and arm.

CORACO-BRACHIALIS (Muscle), *Coracobrachiæ'us, Coraco-huméral*—(Ch.), *Perfora'tus* CASSE'RII, *Perforatus,* is situate at the inner and upper part of the arm. It arises from the coracoid process of the scapula, and is inserted at the middle part of the inner side of the humerus. It carries the arm forwards and inwards, raising the humerus a little. It can, also, by acting inversely, depress the shoulder.

CORACO-CLAVIC'ULAR, *Coraco-clavicula'ris.* Belonging to the coracoid process and clavicle.

CORACO CLAVICULAR LIGAMENT,—called, also, *Omo-clavicular,*—serves to unite the clavicle to the coracoid process. It is very irregular, and formed of two fasciculi, which the greater part of anatomists have described as particular ligaments, under the names *Conoid* and *Trapezoid.*

CORACODES, Coracoid.

CORACO-HUMERALIS, Coraco-brachialis—c. Hyoideus, Omohyoideus—c. Radialis, Biceps flexor cubiti.

COR'ACOID, *Coracoī'deus, Coracoī'des, Coraco'des, C. Proces'us, Cornicula'ris Processus, Crow's-beak-like Process, Proces'sus anchora'lis, rostriform'is, ancyroī'des,* from κοραξ, 'a crow,' and ειδος, 'resemblance.' (F.) *Coracoīde.* Resembling the beak of a crow. A name given by Galen, (and still retained,) to the short, thick process, situate at the anterior part of the upper margin of the scapula; which has some resemblance to the beak of a crow. This process gives attachment to the *Coraco-clavic'ular* and *Coraco-acro'mial* ligaments, and to the *Coraco-brachia'lis, Pectora'lis minor,* and *Biceps* muscles.

CORACOID LIG'AMENT, *Ligamen'tum coracoī'deum,* (F.) *L. Coracoīdien.* This name is given to the small fibrous fasciculus, which converts the notch, at the superior margin of the scapula, into a foramen.

CORAIL, Coral—c. *des Jardins,* Capsicum annuum.

CORAL, *Coral'lium, Coral'lus, Arbor Maris, Azur, Bolesis,* from κορεω, 'I adorn,' and 'αλς, 'the sea.' (F.) *Corail.* One of the most beautiful productions of the deep. It is fixed to submarine rocks, in the form of a shrub; and is of a bright red colour. It is the habitation of a multitude of animals, of the Zoophyta order, and is formed of a calcareous substance, secreted by the animals themselves. It is in very hard, concentric layers; covered, externally, by a species of porous bark, full of cellules, each of which contains one of these animals. Linnæus calls the red coral, *Isis nob'ilis,* and M. de Lamarck, *Coral'lium rubrum.* It is much fished for on the coasts of Barbary and Sicily. Coral was formerly esteemed tonic, absorbent, astringent, &c.; but analysis has shown, that it contains only carbonate of lime and a little gelatin.—Dioscorides, Pliny, Oribasius, the *Geoponica,* &c. The *Corallium album* is a hard, white, calcareous brittle substance, the nidus of the *Madrep'ora ocula'ta.* It has been given as an absorbent.

CORALLI'NA. Diminutive of *Corallium:* *Muscus marit'imus, Corallina officinæ'lis, Brion,*

Corallina alba, Sea Cor'alline, White Worm-weed. The production of an animal, which belongs to the genus *Pol'ypi*, and which is found in all the seas of Europe;—particularly in the Mediterranean. It has the appearance of a plant, is homogeneous, an inch or two in height, of a white, reddish, or greenish colour, salt taste, and marine smell. It contains gelatin, albumen, chloride of sodium, phosphate, carbonate and sulphate of lime, carbonate of magnesia, silica, oxide of iron, and a colouring principle. It was once much used as a vermifuge; but is not now employed. Dose, ʒss to ʒj, in powder.

CORALLINA CORSICA'NA, *C. rubra, Helminthochorton, Helminthochort'um, Elminthochorton, Muscus helminthochortos, Melithochorton, Muscus coralli'nus seu Mari'nus seu Cor'sicus, Confer'va Helminthochortos, Sphærococcus helminthochortos, Gigarti'na helminthochorton, Coralli'na melitochorton, Lemithochorton, Fucus Helminthochorton, Cera'mium helminthochort'us, Corsican Worm-weed,* (F.) *Coralline de Corse, Mousse de Corse.* It is a mixture of several marine plants and zoophytes, as the *fucus, ceramium, ulva, coralline, confervæ,* &c., and has gained great reputation for destroying all kinds of intestinal worms, when given in strong decoction. The Geneva Pharmacopœia directs an officinal syrup — the *Sirop de Coralline.*

CORALLINE DE CORSE, Corallina Corsicana.

CORALLOIDES FUNGUS, Clavaria coralloides.

CORALWORT, Clavaria coralloides.

CORD, *Funis, Funic'ulus, Chœnos, Chœ'nion,* χοινος, χοινιον, from the Latin *Chorda,* which is itself derived from χορδη, 'intestine;' and, afterwards, was applied to musical cords or strings, made of the intestines of animals. See Chorda.

CORD, UMBILICAL, Funiculus umbilicalis.

CORDS. VOCAL, *Cords of Ferrein, Chordæ vocales, Ch. Ferre'nii.* A name given to the ligaments of the glottis, which Ferrein compared to stretched cords, and to which he attributed the production of voice. See Thyreo-arytenoid Ligament.

CORDA, Chorda — c. Hippocratis, Achillis tendo — c. Magna, Achillis tendo — c. Spinalis, Medulla spinalis.

CORDE DU TAMBOUR, Chorda tympani —c. *du Tympan,* Chorda tympani.

CORDÉE, Chordee.

CORDIA AFRICANA, Sebestina—c. Domestica, Sebestina—c. Myxa, Sebestina—c. Obliqua, Sebestina—c. Sebestina, Sebestina—c. Smooth-leaved, Sebestina.

COR'DIAL, *Cordia'lis, Cardi'acus,* from *cor, cordis,* 'the heart.' A tonic or excitant medicine, judged to be proper for exciting the heart. A warm stomachic.

CORDIAL, GODFREY'S, see Godfrey's Cordial—c. Nervous, Brodum's, see Tinctura gentianæ composita — c. Sir Walter Raleigh's, Confectio aromatica — c. Warner's, see Tinctura rhei et sennæ.

CORDIFORM TENDON OF THE DIAPHRAGM, Centre, phrenic.

CORDINE'MA, from καρα, 'the head,' and δινεω, 'I move about.' Headach, accompanied with vertigo. See Carebaria.

CORDIS EMUNCTORIUM, Axilla.

CORDOLIUM, Cardialgia.

CORDON (F.), *Funic'ulus,* diminutive of *funis,* 'a cord.' A term applied to many parts, which resemble a small cord.

CORDON NERVEUX, Ramus Nervo'sus. A principal division of a nerve, or the nervous trunk itself.

CORDON OMBILICALE, Funiculus umbili- calis—c. *Spermatique,* Spermatic chord—c. *Testiculaire,* Spermatic chord.

CORDONS SUS-PUBIENS, Round ligaments of the uterus—c. *Vasculaires,* Round ligaments of the uterus.

CORE, Pupil, see Furunculus.

CORECTOMIA, Coretomia.

CORECTOP'IA, from κορη, 'the pupil,' εκ, 'out of,' and τοπος, 'place.' Displacement of the pupil. A condition of the iris in which one segment is larger than the other; so that the pupil is not in the centre.—Von Ammon.

COREDIALYSIS, Coretomia.

CORE'MATA, from κορεω, 'I cleanse.' Remedies proper for cleansing the skin. — Paulus of Ægina.

COREMETAMORPHOSIS, Dyscoria.

COREMORPHO'MA, same etymon as the next. A morbid change in the shape of the pupil.

COREMORPHO'SIS, *Conforma'tio pupill'æ artificia'lis;* from κορη, 'the pupil,' and μορφωσις, 'formation.' The operation for artificial pupil. See Coretomia.

COREON'CION, *Coron'cion, Coreon'cium,* from κορη, 'the pupil,' and ογκινον, 'a hook.' An instrument, used for the formation of artificial pupil by Langenbeck. It is hooked at its extremity. A *double-hooked forceps,* used by Von Gräfe, is similarly named.

COREOP'SIS TRICHOSPER'MA, *Tickweed sunflower, Tickseed sunflower.* An indigenous plant, of the Composite *Family,* with large golden-yellow rays, which flowers in September. It is said to have been used as an alterative.

CORETODIALYSIS, Coretomia.

CORETOMEDIALYSIS, Coretodialysis.

CORETOM'IA, from κορη, 'the pupil,' and τεμνειν, 'to cut.' *Corotom'ia, Coretotom'ia, Iridotom'ia, Corectom'ia, Coretonectom'ia, Iridectom'ia, Iridectomedial'ysis, Iridectomodial'ysis, Coredial'ysis, Corodial'ysis, Coretodial'ysis, Coretomedial'ysis, Iridodial'ysis.* Various operations for the formation of artificial pupil are so termed. The last five signify the separation or tearing asunder of the iris from the ciliary ligament; the preceding five the incision of the iris, *with* loss of substance; and the remainder signify a simple incision of the iris, *without* loss of substance. When a portion of the iris is left strangulated in the wound, it is termed *Iridenclei'sis, Iridencleis'mus,* and *Iridotenclei'sis.*

CORETONECTOMIA, Coretomia.

CORETOTOMIA, Coretomia.

CORIANDER, Coriandrum sativum.

CORIANDRUM CICUTA, Cicuta virosa — c. Maculatum, Conium maculatum.

CORIAN'DRUM SATI'VUM, *Corian'der, Corian'non,* (F.) *Coriandre.* Family, Umbelliferæ. *Sex. Syst.* Petandria Digynia. The systematic name of the *Corian'drum* of the pharmacopœias; *Corian'non.* The seeds of the coriander have an aromatic odour, and grateful, pungent taste. They are carminative; but are chiefly used to cover the taste of other medicines.

CORIANNON, Coriandrum sativum.

CORIGEEN, Fucus crispus.

CORIITIS, Cytitis.

CORINTHIACÆ, see Vitis corinthiaca.

CORION, Corium, Hypericum perforatum.

CORIS, Cimex—c. Monspeliensis, Symphytum Petræum.

CO'RIUM, *Chrion,* (F.) *Cuir.* The skin of animals is so called, especially when tanned. The *cutis vera,* or the thickest part of the human skin.

CORIUM PHLOGIS'TICUM, *Crusta pleuret'ica, C. inflammato'ria, C. phlogis'tica, Inflam'matory Crust* or *Buff, Buffy Coat,* (F.) *Couenne, C. Pleurétique, C. Inflammatoire.* The grayish crust or buff, varying in thickness, observed on blood drawn from a vein during the existence of violent inflammation, pregnancy, &c. It is particularly manifest in pleurisy, and hence one of its names. For its production, it appears to be requisite, that there should be an increase in the proportion of the fibrinous element of the blood over that of the red corpuscles, with increased aggregation of those corpuscles. Under such circumstances, the buffy coat assumes a concave appearance on its upper surface, and the blood is, therefore, said to be *cupped.*

The buff is generally believed to consist of fibrin; but, according to the researches of Mulder, it is composed of a binoxide of protein, which is insoluble in boiling water, and a tritoxide which is soluble. These oxides are comprehended by him under the name *oxyprotein.*

When the blood presents the above appearance, it is said to be *buffy.*

CORK, Suber.

CORMIER, Sorbus domestica.

CORMUS. In botany, when the stem of a plant, without creeping or rooting, is distended under ground, retaining a round or oval form, it is so called. The Cormus is vulgarly termed a root,—*radix.*

CORN, (Saxon *corn,*) (G.) Kern. In England, this word means the *Cerealia,* or those seeds, which grow in ears, not in pods. In the United States, *Corn* always means *Indian Corn.* Its English sense corresponds to the French *Blé* or *Bled.*

CORN, *Clavus, Clavus Pedis, Ecphy'ma Clavus, Gemur'sa,* (F.) *Cor, Ognon,* from *cornu,* a 'horn.' A small, hard, corneous tumour, which forms upon the foot, generally on the toes; and is commonly produced on the most projecting parts, by the pressure of too tight shoes. A part of the corn is raised above the skin, and forms a round tumour, like the head of a nail: the other portion, which serves as its base, is buried more or less deeply in the integuments, and occasionally extends as far as the tendons and periosteum. Corns may, sometimes, be removed, by immersing the feet in warm water, but commonly they return. They can, likewise, be destroyed by the knife or caustic, or by paring them down and pulling them out by the roots; but these operations are not always as simple as they seem. In the way of palliation, they must be constantly pared; and, for the purpose of preventing pressure, any soft plaster, spread upon linen or leather, may be applied, with a hole in the centre to receive the corn; and layer after layer of plaster be added, until they attain the level of the corn. When very irritable, the lunar caustic, rubbed over the surface, will generally diminish irritability surprisingly, and in a mode not easy of explanation.

CORN, Zea mays—c. Guinea, Panicum Italicum—c. Indian, Zea mays—c. Wild, Matricaria chamomilla—c. Flag, Gladiolus vulgaris—c. Flower, Centaurea cyanus—c. Salad, Valeriana dentata—c. Squirrel, Dicentra Canadensis.

CORNALINE, Cornelian.

CORNE, Cornu—c. *d'Ammon,* Cornu ammonis c. *de Bélier,* Cornu ammonis—c. *de Cerf,* Cervus, Cornu cervi, Cochlearia coronopus — c. *de Chamois,* Cornu rupicapræ—c. *de la Peau,* Cornu.

CORNÉ, Corneous.

COR'NEA, *Cornea transpa'rens, C. pellu'cida, C. lu'cida, Ceras, Sclerot'ica ceratoï'des, Ceratoï'des* seu *Cerato'des membra'na, Ceratome'ninx, Membra'na cornea;* from *cornu,* 'horn.' The *transparent cornea.* (F.) *Cornée.* One of the coats of the eye, so called because it has some resemblance to horn. It is termed *transparent* to distinguish it from the *opake* — *Cornea opa'ca* or *Sclerotic.* It is convex, anteriorly; concave, posteriorly; forming nearly one-fifth of the anterior part of the eye, and representing a segment of a sphere about seven lines and a half, or in. 0.625 in diameter. It seems to be constituted of laminæ in superposition, but of the precise number anatomists are not agreed. Henle assigns it four; the third, a very solid cartilaginous lamella, being called *Membrane de Demours* or *M. de Descemet.* Messrs. Todd and Bowman assign it five layers.

CORNEA, CONICAL, Staphyloma of the cornea—c. Opake, Caligo—c. Opaca, Sclerotic—c. Sugarloaf, Staphyloma of the cornea.

CORNÉE, Cornea.

CORNEITIS, Ceratitis.

CORNEL, AMERICAN RED-ROD, Cornus sericea — c. Large-flowered, Cornus Florida — c. Panicled, Cornus paniculata.

CORNE'LIAN, *Carne'lian, Chalcedo'nius, Carne'olus, Lapis Carne'olus, Corne'lus, Corne'olus, Lapis Sard'ius,* (F.) *Cornaline.* A precious, semitransparent stone, found in Sardinia. The ancients ascribed to it a number of absurd properties.

CORNELUS, Cornelian.

CORNEOLUS, Cornelian.

COR'NEOUS, *Cor'neus,* (F.) *Corné.* Having the nature or appearance of horn.

CORNEOUS TISSUE is that which forms the nails. The *corneous membrane* is the *cornea.*

CORNES DE LIMAÇON (F.), *Snail's Horns.* A name given by Anel to the lachrymal puncta and ducts.

CORNES DE LA MATRICE, Cornua uteri —c. *de la Peau,* Horny excrescences.

CORNESTA, Retort.

CORNET ACOUSTIQUE, Ear-trumpet — c. *Moyen,* Turbinated bone, middle—c. *de Morgagni,* Turbinated bone, superior.

CORNETS DE BERTIN, Sphenoidal cornua —c. *Sphénoïdaux,* Sphenoidal cornua.

CORNICHON, see Cucumis sativus.

CORNICULARIS PROCESSUS, Coracoid process.

CORNIC'ULUM, diminutive of *cornu,* 'a horn.' 'a little horn.' A species of cupping instrument, shaped like a trumpet, having a hole at the top for sucking the air out, to diminish the pressure in its interior.—Scultetus, Hildanus.

CORNICULUM LARYN'GIS, *Capit'ulum Santori'ni* seu *Laryn'gis, Supra-arytenoid Car'tilage, Capit'ulum Cartilag''inis arytenoïdeæ.* A small, very movable, cartilaginous tubercle, found on the arytenoid cartilages.

CORNIER, Cornus Florida.

CORNIFICATION, *Racornissement.*

CORNINE, see Cornus Florida.

CORNOUILLER, Cornus Florida — c. *à Feuilles arrondies,* Cornus circinata—c. *à Grandes fleurs,* Cornus Florida—c. *Soyeux,* Cornus sericea.

CORNU, *Ceras, Corn,* Horn. (F.) *Corne.* A conical, hard, epidermeous projection, which grows on the heads of certain animals, serving them as a weapon of offence and defence. Anatomists have given this name to parts of the human body, which have nearly the same shape as the horns of animals.

CORNU. A horny excrescence; a corneous wart. which occasionally forms on the skin, and requires the use of the knife; (F.) *Corne de la Peau.*—See Corn. Also, Cornu Cervi.—See Cervus. Also, a Retort.

CORNU ACUSTICUM, Ear-trumpet.

CORNU AMMO'NIS, *Cornu Arie'tis, Hippocam'pus major, Pes hippocam'pi major, Pes hippopot'ami major, Protuberan'tia cylind'rica, Vermis Bomby''inus, Proces'sus cer'ebri latera'lis,* (F.) *Corne d'Ammon, Corne de Bélier, Grande Hippocampe,*

Pied de cheval marin, Protubérance cylindroïde (Ch.), *Bourrelet roulé.* A broad, considerable eminence, curved on itself, and situate at the posterior part of the lateral ventricle. Its surface presents two or three tubercles separated from each other by shallow grooves.

The *Accesso'rius Pedis Hippocamp'i*, (F.) *Accessoire du pied d'hippocampe*, is a prominence, usually formed by the base of the inferior cornu of the lateral ventricle of the brain. It is merely a fold of the hemisphere, and was by Malacarne called *Cuissart* ou *Armure des Jambes.*

CORNU ANTERIUS seu ANTI'CUM VENTRIC'ULI LATERA'LIS; *Anterior Cornu of the Lat'eral Ven'tricle.* The portion of the lateral ventricle of the brain, which is lodged in the middle of the lobe, and forms the commencement of that cavity.

CORNU CERVI, *Cornu, Cornu Cervi'num, Cervi El'aphi Cornu, Hartshorn,* (F.) *Corne de cerf.* The horns of various species of the stag. They contain about 27 per cent. of gelatin. The *Shavings, Raspatu'ra* seu *Ras'ura Cornu Cervi, C. C. raspa'tum,* boiled in water, have, consequently, been esteemed emollient and nutritive.

Hartshorn Jelly may be made as follows:— Hartshorn shavings, ℥vj; boil in *water* Oiv to Oij; strain, and add, whilst hot, of *lemon-juice*, two tablespoonfuls; *white sugar*, ℥vj; and *Sherry wine*, two glasses.

A good nutriment for the sick, where wine is not improper.

When burnt, the shavings constitute the *Cornu cervi calcina'tum, Cornu ustum, Phosphas Calcis, Calca'ria phosphor'ica,* (F.) *Corne de cerf calcinée,* which consists of 57.5 per cent. of phosphate of lime. It has been used as an antacid, but is wholly inert, as its composition would indicate. It contains only 1 per cent. of carbonate of lime.

Hartshorn was once supposed to possess a bezoardic power.

CORNU CERVINUM, Cervus, Plantago coronopus—c. Ethmoidal, Turbinated bone, middle.

CORNU DESCEN'DENS VENTRIC'ULI LATERA'LIS, *Dig"ital Cav'ity, Descending* or *inferior cornu of the lateral ventricle.* The termination of the lateral ventricle in the middle lobe of the brain, behind the fissure of Sylvius.

CORNU, MIDDLE, Turbinated bone, middle.

CORNU POSTE'RIUS seu POSTI'CUM VENTRIC'ULI LATERA'LIS, *Cav'itas digita'ta, Posterior Cornu of the Lateral Ventricle.* The triangular prolongation of the lateral ventricle of the brain into the substance of the occipital lobe.

CORNU RUPICA'PRÆ, (F.) *Corne de Chamois.* The horn of the chamois. It has the same properties as the *Cornu Cervi.*

CORNUA, Turbinated bones.

CORNUA CARTILAG"INIS THYROÏDEÆ. Eminences on the thyroid cartilage, distinguished into *great* or *superior*, which are articulated with the great cornu of the os hyoides;— and into *small* or *inferior*, united with the cricoid cartilage.

CORNUA COCCY'GIS, *Cornua of the Coccyx.* Two small, tubercular eminences at the base of the coccyx, which are articulated with those of the sacrum.

CORNUA CUTANEA, Horny excrescences.

CORNUA HYOÏDEI OSSIS, *Radi'ces ossis hyoï'dei, Cornua of the Hyoid Bone.* Four fragments of the os hyoides, situate above the body of the bone, and distinguished into the *small* or *superior*, and the *great* or *lateral*.

CORNUA LACHRYMALIA, Lachrymal ducts — c. Limacum, Lachrymal ducts, see Lachrymal puncta.

CORNUA SACRA'LIA, *Cornua of the Sacrum.* Two tubercles, situate at the posterior and inferior surface of the sacrum, which are sometimes united.

CORNUA, STYLOID, see Hyoides, os.

CORNUA U'TERI, *Cornua of the U'terus, Ceræa, κεραιαι, Plec'tanæ,* (F.) *Cornes de la Matrice.* The angles of the uterus, where the Fallopian tubes arise. Sometimes applied to the Fallopian tubes themselves.

CORNUE, Retort.
CORNUE TUBULÉE, see Retort.
CORNUMUSA, Retort.
CORNUS AMOMUS, C. sericea—c. Blue berried, C. Sericea.

CORNUS CIRCINA'TA, *Round-leaved Dogwood,* (F.) *Cornouiller à feuilles arrondies.* The bark of this variety has been used for similar purposes with the next.

CORNUS FLOR'IDA, *Dogwood, Dogtree, Boxtree, Bitter Redberry, Large-flowered Cornel, Male Great-flowered Dogwood, Florida Dogwood, Virginia Dogwood, Boxwood (New England),* (F.) *Cornouiller, Cornier, C. à grandes fleurs.* The bark of this beautiful tree, which grows everywhere in the United States, has been long employed as a substitute for cinchona. Dose, from ℨss to ℨj. Its active principle has been separated from it, and received the name of *Cornine.*

CORNUS FOEMINA, C. sericea — c. Mas odorata, Laurus sassafras.

CORNUS PANICULA'TA, *Pan'icled Cornel,* indigenous, has been used as a substitute for Cornus Florida.

CORNUS RUBIGINOSA, C. sericea—c. Sanguinea, Sebestina, C. sericea.

CORNUS SERI"CEA, *Cornus amo'mus, C. fœ'mina, C. rubigino'sa, C. Sanguin'ea, Swamp Dogwood, Red Willow, Rose Willow, New England Dogwood, Female Dogwood, Silky-leaved Dowood, American Red-rod Cornel, Blueberried Dogwood, Blueberried Cornus,* (F.) *Cornouiller soyeux.* The bark, it is said, has been found little inferior to *Cinchona Pallida* in intermittents.—Barton.

CORNUTA, Retort.
CORODIALYSIS, Coretomia.
CORONA, Crown — c. Ciliaris, Ciliary body — c. Dentis, Crown of a tooth — c. Glandis, Crown of the glans—c. Posterior ulnæ, Olecranon.

CORO'NA RA'DIANS, *Radiating Crown of Reil.* Fasciculi of white fibres radiate in all directions from every part of the surface of the optic thalamus, excepting its inner side, which is free and corresponds to the third ventricle; the anterior of these fibres pass directly forwards, the middle fibres outwards, and the posterior backwards, forming the *coro'na ra'dians.*

CORONA REGIA, Trifolium melilotus—c. Ulnæ, Olecranon—c. Veneris, Crown of Venus.

CORONÆ CILIARIS MEMBRANULA, Ciliary zone—c. Palpebrarum, see Tarsus.

CORONAD, see Coronal Aspect.

CORO'NAL, *Corona'lis, Corona'rius.* Relating to the *crown;* from *corona,* 'a crown.' A name formerly given to the frontal bone, because on it partly reposes the crown of kings.

CORONAL ASPECT. An aspect towards the plane of the *corona* or crown of the head. *Coronad* is used adverbially to signify 'towards the coronal aspect.'—Barclay.

CORONAL SUTURE, *Sutu'ra corona'lis, S. Fronto-parieta'lis, Puppis Sutu'ra, S. Arcua'lis.* The suture of the head, which extends from one temporal bone to the other, over the *crown* of the head, and unites the parietal bones with the frontal. The *Suture Coronale* of the French anatomists is the suture which unites the two halves of the os frontis at the early period of life. It is a prolongation of the sagittal.

CORONALE, MINERAL WATERS OF. These waters are found near Lucca, in Italy. They received their name from an erroneous notion, that they are particularly adapted for curing diseases of the os frontis. Their temperature is 95° Fahrenheit. They contain free carbonic acid, sulphates of lime and magnesia, chlorides of sodium and magnesium, &c., and some iron.

CORONARIUS, Coronal.

COR'ONARY, *Corona'rius*, (F.) *Coronaire*, from *corona*, 'a crown.' Resembling a crown.

COR'ONARY AR'TERY OF THE STOMACH, *Arte'ria Corona'ria Ventric'uli*, *A. Gas'trica supe'rior*, (F.) *Artère coronaire stomachique*, *A. Stomogastrique* (Ch.), is one of the branches of the cœliac, which passes towards the superior orifice of the stomach, extends along its lesser curvature, and ends by anastomosing with the pyloric branch of the hepatic. This artery furnishes branches to the inferior part of the œsophagus, the cardiac orifice, the great *cul-de-sac*, the middle part of the stomach, the lesser omentum, and anastomoses with the other arteries of those organs.

CORONARY LIGAMENT of the liver is a reflection of the peritoneum, which surrounds the posterior margin of the liver. The same term is likewise applied to ligaments which unite the radius and ulna.

CORONARY PLEXUS OF THE HEART. The *anterior* and *posterior coronary plexuses* of the heart are derived from the anterior and posterior cardiac plexuses. See Cardiac Plexus.

CORONARY PLEXUS OF THE STOMACH. This plexus of nerves is given off from the upper part of the solar plexus.

CORONARY SINUS OF THE HEART, Sinus, coronary, venous — c. Sinus of Ridley, Sinus coronarius.

CORONARY VEIN OF THE STOMACH, *Vena Corona'ria Ventric'uli*, accompanies the artery, and terminates in the vena porta. Sömmering, and some other anatomists, call all the four arteries of the stomach *Corona'riæ Stomach'icæ*.

CORONCION, Coreoncion.

CORO'NE, from κορώνη, 'a crow.' The coronoid process of the lower jaw.

COR'ONOID, *Coronoï'des*, from κορώνη, 'a crow,' and ειδος, 'shape,' 'resemblance.' Resembling the beak of a crow. This name has been given to two *processes*. One, situate at the anterior and superior part of the ramus of the os maxillare inferius, and affording attachment to the temporal muscle: the other, called, also, *sharp process*, situate at the superior part of the ulna, anterior to the great sigmoid fossa, and forming a part of the hinge of the elbow-joint.

CORONOPODIUM, Plantago coronopus.

CORONOPUS, Cochlearia coronopus — c. Depressus, Cochlearia coronopus — c. Ruellii, Cochlearia coronopus — c. Vulgaris, Cochlearia coronopus.

COROTOMIA, Coretomia.

CORPORA ALBICANTIA, Mammillary tubercles — c. Arantii, Noduli Arantii, Tubercula A. — c. Bigemina, Quadrigemina corpora — c. Candicantia, Albicantia corpora, Mammillary tubercles — c. Cavernosa, Cavernous bodies — c. Fibrosa, *Corps Fibreux*.

COR'PORA FIMBRIA'TA, *Tænia Hippocam'pi*, *Fimbriated* or *fringed bodies*, (F.) *Corps Frangés*, *C. Bordés*, *Bandelettes des Cornes d'Ammon*, *Bandelette de l'Hippocampe*. The thin, flattened, and very delicate band, situate along the concave edge of the cornu ammonis, which is a continuation of the posterior crura of the fornix.

CORPORA GENICULA'TA, (F.) *Corps Géniculés*, *C. génouillés*. Eminences situate at the lower and outer part of the optic thalami. Each optic tract commences at the *corp'us genicula'tum exter'num*. The *corpus genicula'tum intern'um* is merely a tubercle inserted into the bend or knee, formed by the corpus geniculatum externum.

CORPORA GLOBOSA CERVICIS UTERI, Nabothi glandulæ — c. Lutea, see Corpus luteum.

COR'PORA MALPIGHIA'NA, *Malpig'hian Bodies*, *Ac"ini*, *Cor'puscles* or *Glomerules of Malpig'hi*. Scattered through the plexus formed by the blood-vessels and uriniferous tubes in the kidney, a number of small dark points may be seen with the naked eye, which received their name from Malpighi, their describer. Each of these, under the microscope, is found to consist of a convoluted mass of blood-vessels, which constitutes the true *glandule*, *corpuscle* or *glomerule of Malpighi*. It was at one time supposed that the tubuli uriniferi originate in them; but this does not appear to be the case. Their use is not positively known, but as they have been traced by Mr. Bowman into the commencement of the urinary tubes, in which they lie uncovered, it has been supposed that their office may be to separate the watery portions of the blood to be mixed with the proper urinous matter.

CORPORA MAMMILLARIA, Mammillary tubercles — c. Nervio-spongiosa Penis, Corpora cavernosa — c. Nervosa, Corpora cavernosa.

CORPORA OLIVA'RIA, *C. ova'ta*, *Eminen'tiæ Oliva'res* seu *ova'les latera'les*, *Oli'væ*, *Prominen'tiæ Semiöva'les Medullæ Oblonga'tæ*, (*Éminences latérales*, Ch.) Oblong, whitish eminences, situate at the occipital surface of the medulla oblongata, exterior to the corpora pyramidalia.

CORPORA OVATA, Corpora olivaria — c. Pisiformia, Mammillary tubercles.

CORPORA PYRAMIDA'LIA, *Eminen'tiæ pyramida'les* seu *media'næ inter'næ*, *Pyra'mides*, (F.) *Corps pyramidaux*, *Pyramides antérieures* (Gall), *Éminences pyramidales* (Ch.) Two small medullary eminences, placed alongside each other, at the occipital surface of the medulla oblongata, between the corpora olivaria. These bodies have also been called *Corpora Pyramidalia anti'ca*, to distinguish them from the *C. olivaria*, which have been called *Corpora Pyramidalia latera'lia*.

CORPORA PYRAMIDALIA POSTERIORA, Corpora restiformia — c. Quadrigemina, Q. corpora.

CORPORA RESTIFOR'MIA, *Crura medul'læ oblonga'tæ*, *Pedun'culi medullæ oblonga'tæ*, *Corpora pyramidalia posterio'ra*, *Proces'sus à cerebell'o ad medull'am oblonga'tam*, *Pos'terior pyramids*, *Ped'uncles of the medul'la oblonga'ta*, *Inferior peduncles of the cerebellum*, (F.) *Corps restiformes*, *Cuisses postérieures*, *Pyramides postérieures*, *Racines*, *Bras* ou *Jambes du cervelet*, *Pétites branches de la moëlle allongée*, *Pédoncules du cervelet*. Two medullary projections, oblong, and of a whitish appearance, which proceed from each side of the upper extremity of the medulla oblongata, and contribute to the formation of the cerebellum.

CORPORA STRIA'TA, *Grand ganglion supérieur du cerveau* (Gall), *Couches des nerfs ethmoïdaux*, *Corps cannelés*, *Eminen'tiæ Lenticula'res*, *Collic'uli Nervi Ethmoïda'lis*, *Ap'ices Crurum medul'læ oblonga'tæ*, *Gan'glion cer'ebri ante'rius*, *Anterior cerebral ganglion*, (F.) *Corps striés*. Pyriform eminences of a slightly brownish-gray colour, which form part of the floor of the lateral ventricles of the brain. When cut, a mixture of gray and white substance is seen, arranged alternately, to which they owe their name. The tract of fibres that ascends from the anterior pyramids passes chiefly into them. Willis considered that the soul resided there.

CORPORA STRIATA SUPERNA POSTERIORA, Thalami nervorum opticorum — c. Wolffiana, see Corpus Wolffianum.

CORPS, Body—c. Bordés, Corpora fimbriata—c. Calleux, Corpus callosum—c. Cannelés, Corpora striata—c. Caverneux, Corpora cavernosa—c. Cendré, Corpus dentatum—c. Ciliaire, Corpus dentatum—c. Dentelé, Corpus dentatum—c. Étranger, Extraneous body—c. Festonné, Corpus dentatum.

CORPS FIBREUX, *Corpora Fibro'sa.* Bayle has given this name to adventitious fibrous productions of a round form, more or less adherent, and sometimes having a pedicle, which form in certain parts of the body, particularly in the substance of the uterus.

CORPS FRANGÉS, Corpora fimbriata—c. Géniculés, Corpora geniculata—c. Godronné, Fascia dentata—c. Hyaloïde, Corpus vitreum—c. d'Hygmore ou d'Highmore, Corpus Highmori—c. Jaune, Corpus luteum—c. Muqueux, Corpus mucosum—c. Organisés, Organized bodies—c. Pampiniforme, Corpus pampiniforme—c. Pyramidaux, Corpora pyramidalia—c. Restiformes, Corpora restiformia—c. Rhomboïde, Corpus dentatum—c. Striés, Corpora striata—c. Thyroïde, Thyroid gland—c. Variciforme, Epididymis—c. Variqueux, Corpus pampiniforme, Epididymis—c. Vitré, Corpus vitreum.

CORP'ULENT, *Corpulen'tus, Obe'sus, Crassus, Fat, Fleshy.* Having an unusual development of fat or flesh in proportion to the frame of the body.

CORPULEN'TIA, *Cor'pulence,* from *corpus,* 'the body,' and *lentus,* 'thick,' is synonymous with Obesity and Polysarcia.

CORPULENTIA CARNOSA, Torositas.

CORPUS, *Soma,* A Body. Any object which strikes one or more of our senses. Gases, liquids, metals, vegetables, animals, are so many bodies. Natural bodies have been divided into *animal, vegetable,* and *mineral;* or into *inorganic,* including the mineral kingdom; and *organized,* including the animal and vegetable. The chief differences between organized and inorganic bodies consists in the former having an *origin by generation, growth by nutrition,* and *termination by death:* the latter a *fortuitous origin, external growth,* and a *termination by chemical or mechanical force.*

Many parts of the frame have, also, been distinguished by this name, as *Corpus Callosum, C. Mucosum,* &c. See Body.

CORPUS ADENIFORME, Prostate—c. Adenoides, Prostate—c. Adiposum, Pinguedo—c. Alienum, Extraneous—c. Annulare, Pons varolii.

CORPUS CALLO'SUM, *Commissu'ra Magna cer'ebri, Trabs Medulla'ris* seu *Cer'ebri, Trabec'ula* seu *Cop'ula magna cer'ebri,* (F.) *Corps Calleux, Voûte médullaire, Plafond des ventricules du cerveau, Mésolobe* (Ch.) A white, medullary band, perceived on separating the two hemispheres of the brain, which it connects with each other. La Peyronie regarded it as the seat of the soul. On it are seen longitudinal and transverse fibres—*Striæ longitudina'les Lancis'ii,* and *Striæ transver'sæ Willis'ii.* The anterior portion, which bends downwards, is termed *genu;* the posterior flexure, *sple'nium.* The fibres, which curve backwards into the posterior lobes from the posterior border of the corpus callosum, have been termed *Forceps;* those which pass directly outwards into the middle lobes from the same point, *Tape'tum;* and those which curve forwards and inwards from the anterior border to the anterior lobes, *forceps anterior.*

CORPUS CILIARE, CHiary Body, Corpus dentatum, see Ciliary—c. Cinereum, Corpus dentatum—c. Conoïdes, Pineal gland—c. Crystalloïdes, Crystalline.

CORPUS DENTA'TUM, *C. Denticula'tum, C. Cilia'rē,* (F.) *Corps dentelé, Corps festonné.* A central, oval nucleus, of cineritious substance, met with in the cerebellum; the circumference of which exhibits a number of indentations, surrounded by medullary substance.—Vicq d'Azyr. It is seen by dividing the cerebellum vertically into two equal parts.—The same body has been called *Corps cendré* ou *ciliaire* ou *rhomboïde, Corpus Cine'reum, C. Rhomboïdeum* seu *Rhomboïdalē, Ganglion du cervelet, Noyau central des Pédoncules du cervelet, Nucleus dentatus* seu *fimbria'tus* seu *centra'lis* seu *rhomboïda'lis, Substan'tia rhomboïdea, Gan'glion cilia'rē, Gan'glion cerebelli.* The term *Corpus denta'tum, Nu'cleus oli'væ,* is also given to the ganglion of the corpus olivare, which, like that of the cerebellum, is a yellowish-gray dentated capsule, open behind, and containing medullary matter, from which a fasciculus of fibres proceeds upwards to the corpora quadrigemina and thalami optici.

CORPUS DENTICULATUM, c. Dentatum—c. Discoïdes, Crystalline—c. Externum, Extraneous body—c. Extraneum, Extraneous body—c. Geniculatum, see Corpora Geniculata—c. Glandiforme, Prostate—c. Glandosum, Prostate—c. Glandulosum, Prostate.

CORPUS GLANDULO'SUM MULIE'RUM, *Gland'ulæ Pros'tatæ mulis'rum.* A vascular, spongy eminence, which surrounds the orifice of the urethra, and projects at its under part.

CORPUS HIGHMO'RI, *C. Highmoria'num, Mediasti'num testis, Mea'tus semina'rius,* (F.) *Corps d'Hygmore* ou *d'Highmore, Sinus des Vaisseaux séminifères,* (Ch.) An oblong eminence, along the superior edge of the testicle, which seems formed of a reflection of the tunica albuginea, through which the principal trunks of the seminiferous vessels pass before they reach the epididymis.

CORPUS INCOMPREHENSIBLE, Thymus.

CORPUS LU'TEUM, (F.) *Corps jaune.* A small yellowish body, perceived in the ovarium, and left after the rupture of one of the vesicles. It was, for a long time, considered an evidence of previous impregnation; but it is now maintained that *Corpora lutea* may be met with in unquestionable virgins; although the corpora lutea of virgins have been generally regarded to differ materially, in size and character, from those of impregnation, which have been called *true corpora lutea,* in contradistinction to the other, which have been called *false corpora lutea.*

CORPUS MUCO'SUM, *C. reticula'rē, Retē muco'sum, Mucus* seu *Retē* seu *Stratum Malpig'hii, Retic'ulum cuta'neum* seu *muco'sum, Mesoderm'um, Mucous web,* (F.) *Corps muqueux.* The second layer of the skin has been so called. It is situate between the *cutis vera* and *cuticle,* and gives colour to the body. In the white varieties of our species it is colourless; in the negro, black. By some anatomists the existence of such a layer, distinct from the epidermis, is denied.

CORPUS OKENSE, Corpus Wolffianum.

CORPUS PAMPINIFOR'ME, *C. Varico'sum,* from *pampinus,* 'a tendril.' *Cor'pus pyramida'lē, Hedera'ceus plexus, Plexus pampiniform'is, Plexus vasculo'sus funic'uli spermatici pampiniformis,* (F.) *Corps pampiniforme, C. Variqueux.* The plexus or retiform arrangement of the spermatic arteries and veins in the cavity of the abdomen, anterior to the psoas muscle.

CORPUS PAPILLARE, *Textus Papilla'ris, Corpus reticula'rē.* The nervous and vascular papillæ situate beneath the epidermis, called by Breschet *Neurothelic apparatus.*

CORPUS PHACOIDES, Crystalline—c. Pituitare, Pituitary gland—c. Psalloides, Lyra—c. Pyramidale, Corpus pampiniforme—c. Reticulare, Corpus mucosum, Corpus Papillare—c. Rhomboïdale,

Corpus dentatum—c. Rhomboideum, Corpus dentatum—c. Thymiamum, Thymus—c. Thymicum, Thymus — c. Thyreoideum, Thyroid gland — c. Turbinatum, Pineal gland—c. Varicosum, Corpus pampiniforme, Spermatic chord — c. Varicosum testis, Epididymis.

CORPUS SPONGIO'SUM URE'THRÆ, *Substan'tia spongio'sa ure'thræ*. This substance arises before the prostate gland, surrounds the urethra, and forms the bulb. It then proceeds to the end of the corpora cavernosa, and terminates in the glans penis, which it forms. Kobelt describes, in the female, as the analogue to the corpus spongiosum of the male, a venous plexus, which, as it lies between the glans clitoridis, and the part that corresponds, in the male, to the bulb of the urethra, he terms *pars interme'dia*.

CORPUS VIT'REUM, *Humor Vitreus, H. Hyaloï'des* seu *hyal'inus, Glacia'lis humor, Vitreous humor*, (F.) *Corps vitré, C. hyaloïde, Humeur hyaloïde*. The transparent mass, of a gelatinous consistence, which fills the eye, behind the crystalline. It is contained in cells, formed by the *tunica hyaloidea*.

CORPUS WOLLFIA'NUM, *Corpus Oken'ii, Wolffian body*. At a very early period of fœtal formation, bodies are perceptible, which were first described by Wolff, as existing in the fowl, and in the mammalia by Oken. According to Müller, they disappear in man very early, so that but slight remains of them are perceptible after the 9th or 10th week of pregnancy. They cover the region of the kidneys and renal capsules, which are formed afterwards; and they are presumed to be the organs of urinary secretion during the first periods of fœtal existence.

CORPUSCLES, BLOOD, Globules of the blood —c. Bone, see Lacunæ of Bone—c. Caudate, see Caudate — c. Chyle, see Chyle.

CORPUSCLES, EXUDA'TION. The organizable nuclei contained in fibrinous fluids, which are the origin of the new tissues formed from such fluids

CORPUSCLES, GANGLION, see Neurine — c. Glandiform, Acinus — c. Lymph, see Lymph — c. of Malpighi, Corpora Malpighiana — c. Mucous, see Mucus — c. Osseous, see Lacunæ of bone.

CORPUSCLES, PACIN'IAN, so called from Filippo Pacini, an Italian physician, who, it is generally conceived, first noticed them in 1830. They appear, however, to have been depicted in 1741 by Lehmann, from a preparation by A. Vater, who called them *Papillæ* and *P. nerveæ*. Hence, it has been proposed by J. C. Strahl (1848) to call them *Vaterian corpuscles* or *Corpuscles of Vater* (Vater'sche Körperchen.) Small bodies connected with the cutaneous nerves of the palm and sole. They have also been found sparingly and inconstantly in nerves at the wrist and elbow; in the upper arm, fore-arm, and thigh, and intercostal nerve, the sacral plexus, solar plexus and the plexuses adjacent to it. In each corpuscle there is the termination of a nervous filament. Their uses are not known.

CORPUSCLES OF PURKINJE, see Canaliculus—c. Pus, see Pus—c. Pyoid, see Pus—c. Splenic, see Spleen—c. of Vater, C. Pacinian—c. White granulated, see Globulin.

CORPUSCULA ARANTII, Tubercula A.— c. Glandularum similia intestinorum, Peyeri glandulæ — c. Globosa cervicis uteri, Nabothi glandulæ — c. Ossium, see Lacunæ of bone.

CORPUSCULUM ARANTII, see Sigmoid valves — c. Sesamoideum, see Sigmoid valves.

CORRAGO, Borago officinalis.

CORRE, *Corsè*, from κειρω, 'I shave.' (?) The temples or the part of the jaws, which it is usual to shave.—Gorræus.

CORRECTIF, Corrigent.

CORRECTION, *Correc'tio*, from *corrigere*, (*con*, and *regere*, 'to rule or order,') 'to correct.' The act of correcting medicines; that is, of diminishing their energy or obviating unpleasant effects, by mixing them with substances which mitigate their operation.

CORRECTORIUS, Corrigens.

CORRELATION, see Synergy.

CORRIGEEN MOSS, Fucus crispus.

COR'RIGENT, *Cor'rigens, Correcto'rius, Castigans, Infrin'gens, Emen'dans*: same etymon. (F.) *Correctif*. That which corrects. A corrigent, in a pharmaceutical formula, is a substance added to a medicine to mollify or modify its action. In the following formula, the aloes, if not corrected, might induce tormina. The *Oleum Menthæ* is added as a corrigent.

R Aloes ʒj
 Olei Menthæ gtt. v
 Syrup q. s. *ut fiant Pilulæ* xvj

CORRIG"IA. A leathern strap. By extension, the term has been applied to the tendons and ligaments.

CORROB'ORANT, *Corrob'orans, Rob'orans, Muscula'ris, Restau'rans, Restor'ative, Bracing*, from *corroborare*, (*con*, and *robur*, 'strength,') 'to strengthen.' (F.) *Corroborant, Corroboratif, Fortifiant*. Any substance which strengthens and gives tone. Wine, for example, is a corroborant. See Tonic.

CORROBORANTIA, Tonics.

CORROBORATIF, Corroborant.

CORRODANT, Corrosive.

CORRODENS, Corrosive.

CORROSIF, Corrosive.

CORRO'SION, *Corro'sio, Diabro'sis, Anabro'sis, Ero'sio*, from *con*, and *rodere, rosum*, 'to gnaw.' The action or effect of corrosive substances.

CORRO'SIVE, *Corro'dens, Diabrot'icus, Corrosi'vus*, same etymon. (F.) *Corrosif, Corrodant*. Corrosives are substances, which, when placed in contact with living parts, gradually disorganize them. *Caustic alkalies, Mineral acids, Corrosive sublimate*, are *corrosives*. They act either *directly*, by chemically destroying the part,—or *indirectly*, by causing inflammation and gangrene.

CORROSIVE POISON, see Poison.

CORRUGATIO, Corrugation — c. Cutis, Wrinkle.

CORRUGA'TION, *Corruga'tio, Synæ'rema*, from *con*, and *ruga*, 'a wrinkle.' Wrinkling, Frowning, (F.) *Froncement :* the contraction of the *Corrugato'res Supercil'ii* muscles. Corrugation of the skin is often owing to the application of styptic medicines : it is rendered by them unequal and rugous.

CORRUGATOR COITERII, Corrugator supercilii.

CORRUGA'TOR SUPERCIL'II, from *corrugare*, 'to wrinkle;' same etymon. *Mus'culus supercil'ii, Supercilia'ris, Mus'culus fronta'lis verus* seu *Corruga'tor Coite'rii*, (F.) *Cutanéo-sourcilier, Muscle Sourcilier* ou *Surcilier, M. Fronto-Sourcilier*. A muscle situate in the eyebrows. It is attached, by its inner extremity, to the superciliary ridge, and is confounded, externally, with the occipito-frontalis and orbicularis palpebrarum. It carries the eyebrow inwards, and wrinkles the skin of the forehead.

CORRUP'TION, *Corrup'tio, Phthora, Diaph'-thora*, from *corrumpere, corruptum*, (*con*, and *rumpere*, 'to break,) 'to destroy.' Act of corrupting. State of being corrupted. Reaction of the particles of a body upon each other. It is probable that something like corruption may take place even in the living body.

CORSE, Corre.
CORSET, from (F.) *corps,* 'the body.' *Stethodesm'ium, Stethodesm'is, Stethodesm'us, Tu'nica Thora'cis, Thorax, Pectora'lā.* An article of dress, which closely embraces the trunk, and is much used by females in civilized countries. When corsets or stays are worn very tight, many serious evils result from the unnatural compression.

Different bandages, more or less complicated, which embrace the greater part of the trunk, are likewise so called.

CORSET DE BRASDOR. The name of a bandage invented by one Brasdor, to keep *in situ* the fragments of a fractured clavicle.

CORTALON, Senecio.

CORTEX, *Phloios, Phloos, Phlous, Lemma, Bark,* (F.) *Écorce.* This word has often been applied exclusively to Cinchona: thus, we say *Bark—the cortex* or *bark κατ' ἐξοχην.* It means, also, any bark.

CORTEX ADSTRING"ENS BRASILIEN'SIS. An astringent bark introduced from Brazil into Germany in the year 1828. It is said to be obtained from *Mimosa cochleacarpa seu virgina'lis.* It has been used with advantage in all cases in which astringent barks in general are indicated. Dose of the powder ʒj to ʒss.

CORTEX ALCOMOCO, *Alcomoque*—c. Anisi stellati, see Illicium anisatum—c. Antiscorbuticus, Canella alba—c. Aromaticus, Canella alba—c. Aurantii, see Citrus aurantium—c. Canellæ Malabaricæ, Laurus cassia—c. Cardinalis del Lugo, Cinchona—c. Caryophyllatus, see Myrtus caryophyllata—c. Caryophylloides, Laurus culilawan.

CORTEX CER'EBRI. The *Cor'tical, Cinerit"ious, Vesic'ular* or *Gray substance of the Brain.* The gray portion observed at the exterior of the cerebrum and cerebellum; so called because it forms a kind of bark to the medullary substance. Gall considers, that this substance forms the nerves; and therefore calls it *Substance matrice des Nerfs.*

The name *cortical* is likewise given to the external substance of the kidneys, because it is of a deeper colour than the inner part of the organ, and forms a kind of envelope to it.

CORTEX CHACARILLÆ, Croton Cascarilla—c. Chinæ, Cinchona—o. Chinæ regius, Cinchona—c. Crassior, Laurus cassia—c. Culilaban, see Laurus Culilawan—c. Culilawan, Laurus Culilawan—c. Eleutheriæ, Croton cascarilla—c. Flavus, Cinchonæ cordifoliæ cortex—c. Lavola, see Illicium anisatum—c. Magellanicus, see Wintera aromatica.

CORTEX OVI, *Cortical membrane.* This membrane, so called by Boer and Granville, is usually regarded as a uterine production, and designated *Decid'ua reflex'a.* They consider it to surround the ovule, when it descends into the uterus, and to enclose the shaggy chorion. It is absorbed during the first months of utero-gestation, so as to expose the next membrane to the contact of the decidua, with which a connexion takes place at the part where the placenta is to be formed. In that part, Boer and Granville consider, that the Cortex Ovi is never altogether obliterated, but only made thinner, and in process of time is converted into a mere pellicle or envelope, which not only serves to divide the filiform vessels of the chorion into groups or cotyledons, in order to form the placenta, but also covers those cotyledons. This Dr. Granville calls *membra'na pro'pria.* See Decidua membrana.

CORTEX PALLIDUS, Cinchonæ lancifoliæ cortex --c. Patrum, Cinchona—c. Peruvianus, Cinchona ʌ. Profluvii, Nerium antidysentericum—c. Ruber, Cinchonæ oblongifoliæ cortex — c. Striata dentium, Enamel of the teeth — c. Thuris, Croton cascarilla—c. Winteranus, see Wintera aromaticum—c. Winteranus spurius, Canella alba.

COR'TICAL, *Cortica'lis;* from *cortex,* 'bark.' Belonging to bark.

CORTICAL MATTER OF THE BRAIN, Cortex Cerebri—c. Membrane, Cortex Ovi—c. Substance of the Kidney, see Kidney—c. Substance of the Teeth, see Tooth.

CORTUSA AMERICANA, Heuchera cortusa.

CORU. An Indian tree, the bark of whose root furnishes a milky juice, which is employed in diarrhœa and dysentery. It is also called *Coru Canar'ica.*

CORUSCATIO, Astrape.

CORVISARTIA HELENIUM, Inula helenium.

CORYBAN'TIASM, *Corybantias'mus, Corybantis'mus,* from Κορυβας, one of the Corybantes. A name formerly given to a kind of phrensy, in which the sick were tormented by fantastic visions, and perpetual want of sleep.

CORYDALIS BULBOSA, Fumaria bulbosa—c. Cava, Fumaria bulbosa—c. Tuberosa, Fumaria bulbosa.

COR'YLUS AVELLA'NA, *Bundurk, Cor'ylus, Avella'na, The Hazel-nut Tree,* (F.) *Coudrier, Noisetier; Family,* Amentaceæ; *Sex. Syst.* Monœcia Polyandria. The nut,—*Filbert,* (F.) *Aveline; Hazel-nut,* (F.) *Noisette,*—of this tree, is much eaten in many countries. Like all nuts, it is by no means easy of digestion. It is the *Nux avella'na, καρυον Ποντικον,* of the ancients.

COR'YLUS ROSTRA'TA, *Beaked Hazel.* An indigenous shrub, *Nat. Ord.* Amentaceæ; *Sub-order,* Cupuliferæ: *Sex. Syst.* Monœcia Polyandria; the nut of which is surrounded by a coriaceous and scaly involucre, terminating in a tube covered with short and thick bristles. These bristles have been given as an anthelmintic in the same cases and doses as mucuna.

CORYMBETRA, Hedera helix.

CORYNE, Penis.

CORYPHE, Acme, Vertex—c. Cordis, see Mucro.

CORY'ZA, *Grave'do, Rhini'tis, Catastag'mos, Catastalag'mos, Stillicid'ium Na'rium, Phlegmatorrhag''ia, Blennorrhœ'a nasa'lis, Blennorrhin'ia, Des'tillatio, Catar'rhus ad Nares, C. nasa'lis, Rhinocatar'rhus, Angi'na nasa'lis:* vulgarly, '*running at the nose,*' '*a cold in the head:*' in French, *Rhume de cerveau, Catarrhe nasal, Enchifrènement;* in Old English, *Pose* or *Mur;* whence *Murren* and *Murrain;* from κορυς, or καρα, 'the head,' and ζεω, 'I boil.' Inflammation, attended with increased discharge, of the Schneiderian membrane lining the nose, and the sinuses communicating with it. The affection generally subsides without any medical treatment.

Chronic Coryza is termed, also, *Ozæ'na be sig'na.*

CORYZA ENTONICA, Ozæna—c. Maligna, Ozæna—c. Ozænosa, Ozæna—c. Purulenta, Ozæna—c. Scarlatinosa, Rhinocace—c. Ulcerosa, Ozæna—c. Virulenta, Ozæna.

COSCINISMUS, Cribration.

COSCINOI, see Cribration.

COSMESIS, Cosmetics.

COSMET'ICA, *Ars cosmet'ica, Callipis'tria, Cosme'sis,* (F.) *Cosmétique,* from κοσμειν, 'to adorn,' 'to embellish.' The art of improving the beauty. *Cosmetic, Stilbo'ma,* is, also, used for the different means employed for that purpose; as the compounds into which enter the oxides of lead, bismuth, mercury, arsenic, &c. All these, however, injure the skin, and often give rise to unpleasant cutaneous affections. Frequent ablution with cold water and bathing are the best cosmetics. Essences, soaps, and all the preparations intended for the toilet, fall, also, under this head.

COSMET'ICS, *Are cosmet'ica, Callipis'tria, Cosme'sis,* (F.) *Cosmétique,* from κοσμειν, 'to

COSMÉTIQUE, Cosmetics.

COSMETOL'OGY, *Cosmetolog"ia*, from κοσμειν, 'to adorn;' and λογος, 'a discourse.' A treatise on the dress, and cleanliness of the body.

COSMOS, from κοσμος, 'the world,' 'order,' &c. The order which was supposed to preside over critical days. Hippocrates and others have termed κοσμοι, 'bracelets,' employed, not only as ornaments (κοσμειν, 'to adorn,') but as therapeutical agents.

COSSA, Haunch.

COSSUM. A malignant ulcer of the nose, often of a syphilitic character.—Paracelsus.

COSSUS, *Cossis*. A sort of white, short, thick worm or larve, found in trees, logs of wood, &c., and used by the Romans as a great article of *gourmandise*. They were, also, applied to ulcers.— Pliny. The term has, likewise, been given to small vermiform pimples on the face—Acne— which arise from inflammation of the sebaceous follicles.

COSTA, *Pleura, Pleurum, Pleuro'ma*. A *Rib*, from *custodire*, 'to guard,' 'defend:' (F.) *Côte*. The ribs are 24 in number;—12 on each side. They are irregular, long, bony curves: slightly flattened, and situate obliquely at the sides of the chest. The intervals between them are called *Intercos'tal spaces*, (F.) *Espaces intercostaux*, and they are numbered *first, second, third*, &c., reckoning from above to below. They have been distinguished into *Costæ veræ, Pleurapoph'yses* of Owen, *True ribs*, (F.) *Vraies Côtes, Côtes sternales, Côtes vertébro-sternales* (Ch.,) and into *Costæ spu'riæ, Mendo'sæ Costæ, Nothæ Costæ, False ribs, Côtes asternales* (Ch.,), *Fausses Côtes*. The true or *sternal ribs*, as they have also been called, are the first 7; which are articulated at one extremity to the spine, and at the other, by means of their cartilages, *hæmapophyses* of Owen, to the sternum. The *false ribs* are the remaining 5: the uppermost three being united, by means of their cartilages, to the cartilage of the last true rib. The others are free at their external extremity, and, hence, have been called *Floating ribs, Côtes flottantes*. The vertebral extremity of each rib is slightly expanded. It is called the head of the rib—*Capit'ulum Costæ*: the space between this and the *tubercle* is the *collum* or *neck*. Anterior to the tubercle is the *angle*. The *angle* is the part where the bone bends to form the lateral part of the thorax.

COSTÆ CAPITULUM, see Costa—c. Mendosæ, see Costa—c. Spuriæ, see Costa—c. Veræ, see Costa.

COSTAL, *Costa'lis*, from *costa*, 'a rib.' Appertaining or relating to a rib—as '*costal* cartilage.'

COSTIVE, Constipated.

COSTIVENESS, Constipation.

COSTMARY, Tanacetum balsamita.

COSTO-ABDOMINAL, Obliquus externus abdominis—c. *Basi-scapulaire*, Serratus magnus— s. *Claviculaire*, Subclavian muscle.

COSTO-CLAVIC'ULAR, *Costo-Clavicula'ris*. Belonging to the ribs and clavicle.

COSTO-CLAVIC'ULAR LIG'AMENT, *Cleidocostal Ligament*, is a fibrous, flattened fascia, which extends, obliquely, from the cartilage of the first rib to the inferior surface of the clavicle.

COSTO-CORACOÏDIEN, Pectoralis minor —c. *Scapulaire*, Serratus magnus.

COSTO-STERNAL, *Costo-Sterna'lis*. Relating to the ribs and sternum. The articulation of the sternum with the anterior extremity of the first seven ribs.

COSTO-TRACHELIA'NUS. Relating to the ribs and to the *trachelian* or transverse processes of the neck. Under the name *Costo-trache'lian*, Chaussier designates the *anterior* and *posterior scaleni*.

COSTO-TRANSVERSA'RIUS. Relating to the ribs, and to the transverse processes.—Bichat gave this name to the articulation of the tuberosities of the ribs with the transverse processes of the spine.

COSTO-VER'TEBRAL, *Costo-vertebra'lis*. Belonging to the ribs and vertebræ.—Bichat gave this name to the articulation of the head of the ribs with the vertebræ, and to the ligaments connected with it.

COSTO-XIPHOID, *Costo-xiphoï'deus*. The name of a ligament, which unites the cartilage of the seventh rib to the xiphoid or ensiform cartilage.

COSTUS. The ancients seem to have given this name to several plants. One has borne the appellation, since the time of Dioscorides,—the *Costus Arab'icus, Costus In'dicus, C. specio'sus seu ama'rus, dulcis, orienta'lis, Amo'mum hirsu'tum, Helle'nia grandiflo'ra, Bank'sia specio'sa, Tsia'na*, (F.) *Canne Congo, Canne de Rivière*: Family, Amomeæ, *Sex. Syst.* Monandria Monogynia; the root of which is aromatic, and has been considered tonic, carminative, diuretic, emmenagogue, &c. The virtues of the ancient costus are highly extolled.—Theophrastus, Dioscorides, Pliny, Galen.

COSTUS AMARUS, &c., Costus—c. Arabicus, Costus—c. Corticosus, Canella alba—c. Hortorum, Tanacetum balsamita—c. Hortorum minor, Achillea ageratum—c. Indicus, Costus—c. Nigra, Cynara scolymus—c. Speciosus, Costus.

COSTYLE, Cotyle.

COTA, Anthemis cotula.

COTARO'NIUM; an obscure term, used by Paracelsus for a universal solvent: such a thing as does not exist.

CÔTE, Costa.

CÔTES, COL DES, Collum costarum—c. *Asternales*, see Costa—c. *Fausses*, see Costa—c. *Flottantes*, see Costa—c. *Sternales*, see Costa—c. *Vertébrosternales*, see Costa—c. *Vraies*, see Costa.

COTIGNAC, (pron. *cotinniac.*) A kind of conserve or preserve, prepared from quinces not entirely ripe, and sugar. It is esteemed stomachic and astringent.

COTON, Gossypium.

COTONIA, Pyrus cydonia.

COTTON, Gossypium.

COTULA, Anthemis cotula—c. Fœtida, Anthemis cotula.

COTULA MULTIF'IDA. A South African plant, which is used by the Hottentots in rheumatism, scalds and cutaneous diseases.

COTUN'NIUS, LIQUOR OF, *Liq'uor Cotun'nii, L. of Cotug'no, Aquula acus'tica, Aqua auditória, Per'ilymph*, (F.) *Lymphe de Cotugno*. A transparent, slightly viscid fluid, which fills all the cavities of the internal ear, and of which Cotugno made mention. It is also called *Aqua Labyrinth'i.*

COTURNIX, Tetrao coturnix.

COT'YLE, *Cot'yla, Cotyle'don, Cos'tylē*; the same as *Acetab'ulum*. A hollow cavity in a bone, which receives the head of another bone: particularly 'the *cotyloid* cavity.' Κοτυλη signified a drinking cup, and, indeed, any thing hollow, as the hollow of the hand.—Athenæus.

COTYLEDON, Cotyle—c. Marina, Umbilicus marinus.

COTYLE'DON ORBICULA'TA. A plant of South Africa, *Nat. Ord.* Crassulaceæ. The fresh juice is used in epilepsy; and Dr. Pappe speaks well of it. The leaves form a good application to hard corns. *Crass'ula arbores'cens* has the same properties.

COTYLE'DON UMBILI'CUS, *C. U. Vene'ris, Navelwort, Venus's Navelwort*, (F.) *Nombril de Vénus*. A plant of the *Family*, Crassulaceæ, which grows in Europe on old walls and rocks. The leaves are emollient and applied externally to piles, inflamed parts, &c. Internally, the juice has been given in epilepsy. The flowers have been used in calculous cases, and in dropsy.

COTYLE'DONS, (κοτυληδών, 'the hollow of a cup,') *Acetab'ula uteri'na*. The lobes which, by their union, form the placenta.

COT'YLOID, *Cotyloï'des, Cotyloï'deus, Cotylo'des*, from κοτυλη, 'a drinking cup,' and ειδος, 'form.' Resembling the ancient κοτυλη. The name of a hemispherical cavity, situate in the os innominatum, which receives the head of the os femoris;—*Fossa cotyloïdea, Sinus Coxæ, Acetab'ulum, Pyxis.*

COT'YLOID LIG'AMENT, *Ligamen'tum Cotyloïdeum*, (F.) *Ligament cotyloïdien*, is a very thick, fibro-cartilaginous ring, surrounding the cotyloid cavity, the depth of which it increases.

COU, Collum — *c. du Pied*, Instep — *c. Gros*, Bronchocele.

COUCH GRASS, *Triticum repens.*

COUCHE, *Couches*, (F.), from *coucher*, 'to lie down.' This word is used, 1. For *parturition, accouchement* or *delivery* (*puerpe'rium, parturi"tio;*) hence, *une couche heureuse*, 'a happy delivery;' *une fausse couche*, 'a premature delivery:' and, 2. For the time during which a female remains in bed on account of delivery, — *Tempus puerpe'rii*, the *child-bed state*. The *Lochia* have been termed *Suites de couches*. *Couche* also means a layer, bed or thalamus, as,

COUCHE CELLULEUSE, Membrana granulosa.
COUCHER, Decubitus.

COUCHES DES NERFS ETHMOÏDAUX, Corpora striata — *c. des Nerfs oculaires*, Thalami nervorum opticorum — *c. des Nerfs optiques*, Thalami nervorum opticorum — *c. Optiques*, Thalami nervorum opticorum.

COUCHING, see Cataract.
COUCINEA COCCINEA, Cacoucia coccinea.
COUDE, Elbow.
COUDE-PIED, Instep.
COUDÉE, Cubitus.
COUDRIER, Corylus avellana.

COUENNE, (F.), *Cutis suil'la*. A term given to various parts of the human skin, which are prominent, hard, brownish, and often covered with rough hairs, so as to form patches not very unlike the skin of the hog. It is a malformation, occurring during intra-uterine existence, and remaining for life. See also, Nævus, and Corium phlogisticum.

COUENNE INFLAMMATOIRE, Corium phlogisticum — *c. Pleurétique*, Corium phlogisticum.

COUGH, *Tussis* — c. Bronchial, C. tubal — c. Root, Trillium latifolium.

COUGH, TUBAL, *Bron'chial cough, Tussis bron'chica*, (F.) *Toux tubaire, T. bronchique*. Cough is so termed, when the succussion communicated by it to the parietes of the chest is very energetic, and a sensation is experienced by the ear as if a column of air was traversing with much noise, strength, and rapidity, tubes with solid walls.

COUGH, WINTER, Bronchitis, (chronic.)
COUGHING, Tussis.
COULER, To strain.
COULEUVRE, Coluber berus.
COULEUVRÉE, Bryonia alba.

COULISSE, (F.) 'A groove, a gutter.' Anatomists designate, by this name, every deep groove or channel in a bone, in which a tendon plays;— such as the *Coulisse Bicipitale* or *Bicipital Groove* of the Humerus.

COULISSE BICIPITALE, Bicipital groove—

c. Humérale, Bicipital groove.
COULOIR, Colatorium.
COUM, Colchicum autumnale.

COUN'TENANCE, *Vultus, Voltus, Visage*, (F.) *Figure, Visage:* from *cum*, 'with,' and *teneo*, 'I hold.' The form of the face. The system of the features.

COUNTER-EXTEN'SION, *Contra-exten'sio, Antit'asis*, (F.) *Contre-extension*, from *contra-extendere*, 'to extend in a contrary direction.' It consists in retaining firmly and immovably the upper part of a limb, whilst extension is practised on the lower, in cases of fracture or luxation.

COUNTER-INDICA'TION, *Contra-indica'tio, Antendeix'is, Antendix'is, Antideixis*. An indication contrary to another. (F.) *Contre-indication*. Any circumstance, which acts as an obstacle to the employment of such therapeutical means as seem to be indicated by other circumstances.

COUNTER-IRRITANT, see Counter-irritation — c. Granville's, (Lotion,) Granville's Counter-irritant.

COUNTER-IRRITA'TION, *Contra-irrita'tio* An irritation, excited in a part of the body, with the view of relieving one existing in another part. The remedies used for this purpose are called *Counter-irritants*, and form a most valuable class of remedial agents. See Derivation.

COUNTERSTROKE, Contrafissura.
COUNTING, METHOD OF, Method, numerical.

COUP, Blow—*c. de Feu*, Wound, gunshot.

COUP DE MAÎTRE ou TOUR DE MAÎTRE, (F.) A masterly stroke or performance. Applied to a mode of introducing the sound or catheter into the bladder, which consists in first passing it with its convexity towards the abdomen of the patient, and giving it a half turn towards the right groin, when its extremity has reached the root of the penis under the symphysis pubis. There is no advantage in this mode of introduction.

COUP DE SANG, (F.) A common term, used by some physicians in France, to designate the loss of sensation and motion, which results from hemorrhage in the brain, or from simple congestion in the vessels of that organ. See Apoplexy. Some authors have comprehended, under the same denomination, different hemorrhages, which occur in the areolar texture of the face, lungs, skin, &c.

COUP DE SOLEIL, (F.) *Siri'asis, Seiri'asis, Siriasis Ægyptiaca, Ictus solis, Ictus sola'ris, Insola'tio, Encephali'tis insolatio'nis, Phreni'tis calentu'ra, Stroke of the sun, Ægyptian Starstroke* or *Sunstroke*. Any affection produced by the action of the sun on some region of the body;—head, hands, arms, &c. A very common effect of exposing the naked head to the sun is inflammation of the brain or its meninges, which Sauvages calls *Carus ab Insolatio'ne, Morbus solstitia'lis.*

COUPE-BRIDE, Kiotome.
COUPEROSE, Gutta rosea.
COUPURE, Cut, Wound (incised.)
COURANTE, Diarrhœa.

COURAP. A distemper, very common in India, in which there is a perpetual itching of the surface, and eruption. It is of an herpetic character, and appears chiefly on the axilla, groins, breast, and face.

COURBARIL, see Anime.

COURBATURE, (F.) *Acer'ba lassitu'do, Violent lassitude, Fatigue*. An indisposition, characterized by a sensation, as if the limbs were bruised; general feeling of debility, extreme lassitude; and, sometimes, slight fever. It appears immediately after severe exercise, but sometimes not till the next day. Rest removes it.

COURBURE, Curvature.
COURGE, Cucurbita pepo.

COURMI or CURMI, κουρμι, κυρμι. A fermented liquor, made from barley. A kind of ale or beer.—Dioscorides.

COURO-MOELLI. An Indian tree, the bark of which is said to be anti-venomous.

COURON'DI, *Couron'do*. An evergreen tree of India, the juice of which, mixed with warm whey, is said to cure dysentery.—Ray.

COURONNE CILIAIRE, *Godronné canal* — *c. du Dent*, Crown of a tooth—*c. du Gland*, Crown of the glans—*c. du Trépan*, Crown of the trepan —*c. de Vénus*, Crown of Venus.

COURONNE RAYONNANTE (F.) A term given by Reil to the fan-shaped terminations of the crura cerebri in the brain.

COURONNEMENT (F.), *Coro'na*. A vulgar expression, sometimes used to designate the circular ring, which the os uteri forms around the head of the child at a certain period of accouchement:—the head seeming to be surrounded, as it were, by a crown. The head is then said to be *au couronnement*.

COURS DE VENTRE, Diarrhœa.
COURSE, Running.
COURSES, Menses.
COURT, Short.
COURTE HALEINE, Dyspnœa.
COUSIN, Culex.
COUSSINET, Pad.
COUTEAU, Knife — *c. à Amputation*, Knife, amputation—*c. à Cataracte*, Knife, cataract—*c. Courbe*, Knife, crooked — *c. à Crochet*, Knife, crotchet—*c. Désarticulateur*, Knife, double-edged —*c. Droit*, Knife, amputation—*c. de Feu*, Cultellaire — *c. Interosseux*, Knife, double-edged — *c. Lenticulaire*, Knife, lenticular — *c. Lithotome* — Knife, lithotomy — *c. en Serpette*, Knife *en serpette*—*c. Symphysien*, see Symphyseotomy—*c. à Deux tranchans*, Knife, double-edged.

COUTOU'BEA ALBA, *Ex'acum spica'tum, Pi'erium spica'tum*. A plant of Guiana, which is very bitter, and is considered, in the country, to be emmenagogue, anthelmintic, and antidyspeptic.

COUTURES PAR LA PETITE VÉROLE, see Cicatrix.

COUTURIER, Sartorius.
COUVERCLE, see Crucible.
COUVRECHEF (F.), *Cucul'lus, Fascia'tio cuculla'ta, Scepaster'ium, Scepas'trum*. A bandage, applied to the head for retaining certain dressings, &c. *in situ*. The French surgeons distinguish two kinds. 1. The *Grand Couvrechef* ou *Servette en carré* (*Cucul'lus major*,) which is formed of a napkin or large square compress: and, 2. The *Petit Couvrechef* ou *Mouchoir en triangle* (*Cucul'lus minor*,) formed of a napkin or other square compress, folded from one angle to the other diagonally opposite to it.

COUVRECHEF, see Bandage, Galen's.
COVE, CLIMATE OF. On the northern side of Cork Harbour, in Ireland, is the Island of Cove. The town of Cove is on the southern acclivity of a hill running from east to west. It is, consequently, sheltered from the north winds, and receives the full force of the sun. It is one of the mildest climates in Great Britain, and corresponds in its influence on disease with the south-west of England. It is well adapted as a winter retreat for the phthisical.

COVOLAM, *Cratæ'va Marmelos*. The bark of this tree is tonic: the unripe fruit is astringent: but, when ripe, is delicious.

COWBANE, Cicuta aquatica.
COWBERRY, Vaccinium vitis idæa.
COWHAGE, Dolichos pruriens.
COWITCH, Dolichos pruriens.
COWPARSNEP, Heracleum lanatum.

COWPER'S GLANDS, *Ac'cessory glands*, (F.) *Glandes accessoires, G. de Cowper, Prostates inférieures* ou *Petites prostates*. Two small ovoid groups of mucous, reddish follicles, situate behind the bulb of the urethra, before the prostate, the excretory ducts of which open into the bulbous portion of the urethra. They are also called *Glan'dulæ anterpros'tatæ*, and *G. pros'tatæ inferi'ores*.

COWPER'S GLANDS IN THE FEMALE, *Glands of Duverney, Glands of Bartholinus, Pros'tata mulie'bris* seu *Bartholi'ni*, are situate at each side of the entrance of the vagina, beneath the skin covering the posterior or inferior part of the labia. They are rounded, but elongated, flat, and bean-shaped; their long diameter varying from five to ten lines; their transverse, from two and a half to four and a quarter; and their thickness from two and a quarter to three lines. Like Cowper's glands in the male, they are not invariably present. The secretion from them is a thick, tenacious, grayish-white fluid, which is emitted in great quantity during sexual intercourse; and is probably the fluid, supposed, of old, to be the female sperm.

COWPOX, Vaccina—*c*. Inoculation, Vaccination — *c*. Itch, see Itch, cowpox — *c*. Vesicle, see Vaccination.

COWRAP, Impetigo.
COWSLIP, Primula veris—*c*. Jerusalem, Pulmonaria.
COWWEED, Chærophyllum sylvestre.
COXA, Haunch.
COXÆLUVIUM, Bath, hip.
COXAGRA, Neuralgia femoro-poplitæa.
COXAL'GIA, *Merocoxal'gia, Osphyal'gia, Osphyalge'ma*. A word of hybrid origin, from *coxa*, 'hip,' and αλγος, 'pain.' Pain in the hip. A sign of rheumatic or other inflammation—*Coxi'tis*, or of some disease about the hip-joint. See Neuralgia femoro-poplitæa, and Coxarum morbus.

COXARTHRITIS, Coxitis.
COXARTHROCACE, Coxarum morbus.
COXA'RUM MORBUS, *Oxen'dicus* seu *Coxa'rius morbus, Arthroc'acë coxa'rum, Coxarthroc'acë, Osphyarthroc'acë, Coxal'gia* (of some), *Hip disease*. A scrofulous caries, and often spontaneous luxation of the head of the os femoris, occasioning permanent shortening of the limb, and not unfrequently hectic and death.

COXEN'DIX, Haunch. This word has been used synonymously with ischium; and anatomists have also applied it to the ilia, *Ossa Coxen'dicis*.

COXI'TIS, *Coxarthri'tis*, a hybrid term, from *Coxa*, 'the hip,' and *itis*, denoting inflammation. Inflammation of the hip-joint.

COXO-FEM'ORAL, *Coxo-femora'lis*. Belonging to the coxal bone or ileum, and to the os femoris. *Ilio-femoral* has the same signification.

COXO-FEM'ORAL ARTICULA'TION, *Il'io-Femoral A.*, (F.) *Articulation de la Hanche*, the *Hip joint*. The head of the femur and the articular cavity are covered by a *diarthrodial cartilage* and *synovial capsule*; and by a very *strong capsular* or *articular ligament* attached to the circumference of the cotyloid cavity, and to the neck of the femur. There is, also, a *round* or *interarticular ligament*, passing from the inferior notch of the cotyloid cavity to the rough depression at the top of the caput femoris; and a *cotyloid ligament*,— a sort of thick, cartilaginous ring, situate on the edge of the cotyloid cavity, and converting the inferior notch into a foramen. These are the great means of union in this extensive articulation.

CRAB, *As'tacus fluviat'ilis, Cancer, Gam'marus, Gam'barus, Cam'marus*, (F.) *Crabbe, Ècrevisse, Escrevice*. A shell-fish much used as an article of diet. Like other shell-fish it is apt to disagree, and excite urticaria, &c.

CRABE, Crabyaws.

CRABLOUSE; a species of *Pedic'ulus*, *P. Pubis*, which infests the pudendum and axilla. (F.) *Morpion*. It is easily destroyed by the white precipitate of mercury, or by mercurial ointment.

CRABS' EYES, Cancrorum chelæ—c. Stones, Cancrorum chelæ.

CRABYAWS, (F.) *Crabe*. A name in the West Indies for a kind of ulcer on the soles of the feet, with edges so hard, that they are difficult to cut.

CRACHAT, Sputum.

CRACHEMENT, Excreation—c. *de Pus*, Vomica, Phthisis pulmonalis—c. *de Sang*, Hæmoptysis.

CRACHOTEMENT (F.), from *cracher*, 'to spit.' The frequent spitting of a small quantity of saliva.

CRACKLING OF LEATHER, see *Craquement de cuir*.

CRACOW GROATS, Semolina.

CRADLE, Sax. *cnabel*, *Ar'culus*, *Solen*, (F.) *Arceau* ou *Archet*. A semicircle of thin wood, or strips of wood, used for preventing the contact of the bed-clothes in wounds, fractures, &c. An ordinance of the Grand Duke of Tuscany forbade mothers and nurses to sleep with a child near them, unless it was placed under a solid cradle of this kind, in order that no accident might arise from *overlaying*.

CRÆ'PALE, from κραιπαλη, *Crap'ula*, 'drunkenness, surfeit.' A derangement of the functions of the brain, &c., produced by wine or any other fermented liquor.—Galen.

CRAIE, Creta.

CRAMA, κραμα, from κεραω, 'I mix.' A mixture of any kind. Dilute wine.

CRAMBE, Cabbage.

CRAM'BION, from κραμβη, 'cabbage.' A decoction of cabbage.—Hippocrates.

CRAMP, from (G.) krampfen, 'to contract.' *Crampus*, *Enta'sia systrem'ma*, *Tet'anus dolorif'icus*, *Myospas'mus*, *Spasmus muscula'ris*, *Myal'gia*, *Rhegē*, *Rhegma*, *Rhegmus*. A sudden, involuntary, and highly painful contraction of a muscle or muscles. It is most frequently experienced in the lower extremities, and is a common symptom of certain affections:—as of *Colica Pictonum* and *Cholera Morbus*. Friction and compression of the limb, by means of a ligature applied round it above the muscles affected, will usually remove the spasm.

CRAMP, SCRIVENERS', Cramp, Writers'.

CRAMP OF THE STOMACH, (F.) *Crampe de l'Estomac*. A sudden, violent, and most painful affection of the stomach, with sense of constriction in the epigastrium. It seems to be the effect of the spasmodic contraction of the muscular coat of the stomach, and requires the use of the most powerful stimulants and antispasmodics, of which opium is the best.

CRAMP, WRITERS', *Graphospasm'us*, *Mogigraph'ia*, (F.) *Crampe des Écrivains*, *Scriv'eners' Cramp*, *Stam'mering of the Fingers*. A condition of the fingers, in which they are unable to hold the pen, or in which one or more of the muscles of the fingers are irregularly and irresistibly contracted.

CRAMPE DES ÉCRIVAINS, Cramp, Writers'.

CRAMPE DE L'ESTOMAC, Cramp of the stomach.

CRAN DE BRETAGNE, Cochlearia armoracia.

CRANBERRY, Vaccinium oxycoccos — c. American, Common, see Vaccinium oxycoccos — c. Upland, Arbutus uva ursi.

CRANE, Cranium — c. *Humain*, Cranium humanum.

CRANE'S BILL, Geranium—c. Spotted, Geranium maculatum — c. Stinking, Geranium Robertianum.

CRANIOCELE, Encephalocele.

CRANIOHÆMATONCUS, Cephalæmatoma.

CRANIOL'OGY, *Cranios'copy*, *Craniolog"ia*, *Phrenol'ogy*, *Cranioscop'ia*, *C. Gallia'na*, *Encephaloscop'ia*, *Doctri'na Gallia'na*. Words, introduced, since Gall, into medical language. The first two terms are respectively derived from κρανιον, 'cranium,' λογος, 'a discourse,' and σκοπειν, 'to examine.' They signify a description, or simply an examination of the different parts of the external surface of the cranium, in order to deduce from thence a knowledge of the different intellectual and moral dispositions. Strictly speaking, it is by *Cranioscopy* that we acquire a knowledge of *Craniology*, *Organology* or *Cranology*, as it has been variously termed. These words are generally, however, used in the same sense. The cranium being moulded to the brain, there are as many prominences on the bone, as there are projections at the surface of the brain. According to Gall, each projection, which he calls an *organ*, is the seat of a particular intellectual or moral faculty, and all persons endowed with the same faculty, have, at the same part of the brain, a prominence, which is indicated, externally, by a bump or projection in the bony case. The *System* of Gall is made to comprise 27 prominences, which answer to 27 faculties. The following Table exhibits these supposed organs, and their seat.

CEREBRAL ORGANS AND THEIR SEAT, ACCORDING TO GALL.

1. *Instinct of generation, of reproduction; amativeness; instinct of propagation; venereal instinct.* (German.) Zeugungstrieb, Fortpflanzungstrieb, Geschlechtstrieb.	Seated in the cerebellum. It is manifested at the surface of the cranium by two round protuberances, one on each side of the nape of the neck.
2. *Love of progeny; philoprogenitiveness.* (G.) Jungenliebe, Kinderliebe.	Indicated at the external occipital protuberance.
3. *Attachment, friendship.* (G.) Freundschaftsinn.	About the middle of the posterior margin of the parietal bone, anterior to the last.
4. *Instinct of defending self and property; love of strife and combat; combativeness; courage.* (G.) Muth, Raufsinn, Zanksinn.	Seated a little above the ears, in front of the last, and towards the mastoid angle of the parietal bone.
5. *Carnivorous instinct; inclination to murder; destructiveness; cruelty.* (G.) Wurgsinn, Mordsinn.	Greatly developed in all the carnivorous animals; forms a prominence at the posterior and superior part of the squamous surface of the temporal bone, above the mastoid process.

6. *Cunning; finesse; address; secretiveness.*
(G.) List, Schlauheit, Klugheit.
7. *Desire of property; provident instinct; cupidity; inclination to robbery; acquisitiveness.*
(G.) Eigenthumssinn, Hang zu stehlen, Einsammlungssinn, Diebsinn.
8. *Pride; haughtiness; love of authority; elevation.*
(G.) Stolz, Hochmuth, Hohensinn, Herrschsucht.
9, *Vanity; ambition; love of glory.*
(G.) Eitelkeit, Ruhmsucht, Ehrgeiz.
10. *Circumspection; foresight.*
(G.) Behutsamkeit, Vorsicht, Vorsichtigheit.
11. *Memory of things; memory of facts; sense of things; educability; perfectibility; docility.*
(G.) Sachedächtniss, Erziehungsfähigkeit, Sachsinn.
12. *Sense of locality; sense of the relation of space; memory of places.*
(G.) Ortsinn, Raumsinn.
13. *Memory of persons; sense of persons.*
(G.) Personensinn.
14. *Sense of words; sense of names; verbal memory.*
(G.) Wordgedächtniss, Namensinn.
15. *Sense of spoken language; talent of philology; study of languages.*
(G.) Sprachforschungssinn, Wortsinn, Sprachsinn.
16. *Sense of the relations of colour; talent of painting.*
(G.) Farbensinn.
17. *Sense of the relations of tones; musical talent.*
(G.) Tonsinn.
18. *Sense of the relations of numbers; mathematics.*
(G.) Zahlensinn.
19. *Sense of mechanics; sense of construction; talent of architecture; industry.*
(G.) Kunstsinn, Bausinn.
20. *Comparative sagacity.*
(G.) Vergleichender Scharfsinn.
21. *Metaphysical penetration; depth of mind.*
(G.) Metaphysischer Tiefsinn.
22. *Wit.*
(G.) Witz.
23. *Poetical talent.*
(G.) Dichtergeist.
24. *Goodness; benevolence; mildness; compassion; sensibility; moral sense; conscience; bonhommie.*
(G.) Gutmüthigkeit, Mitleiden, moralischer Sinn, Gewissen.
25. *Imitation; mimicry.*
(G.) Nachahmungssinn.
26. *God and religion; theosophy.*
(G.) Theosophisches Sinn.
27. *Firmness; constancy; perseverance; obstinacy.*
(G.) Stetigkeit, Festersinn.

The first nineteen of these, according to Gall, are common to man and animals; the remaining eight, man possesses exclusively. They are, consequently, the attributes of humanity.

ORGANS ACCORDING TO SPURZHEIM.
1. Amativeness.—2. Philoprogenitiveness.—3. Inhabitiveness.—4. Adhesiveness or Attachment.—5. Combativeness.—6. Destructiveness.—

Above the meatus auditorius externus, upon the sphenoidal angle of the parietal bone.

Anterior to that of cunning, of which it seems to be a prolongation, and above that of mechanics, with which it contributes to widen the cranium, by the projection which they form at the side of the frontal bone.

Behind the top of the head, at the extremity of the sagittal suture, and on the parietal bone.

Situate at the side of the last, near the posterior internal angle of the parietal bone.

Corresponds to the parietal protuberance.

Situate at the root of the nose, between the two eyebrows, and a little above them.

Answers to the frontal sinus, and is indicated externally by two prominences at the inner edge of the eyebrows, near the root of the nose, and outside of the organ of memory of things.

At the inner angle of the orbit.

Situate at the posterior part of the base of the two anterior lobes of the brain, on the frontal part of the bottom of the orbit, so as to make the eye prominent.

Also at the top of the orbit, between the preceding and that of the knowledge of colour.

The middle part of the eyebrows, encroaching a little on the forehead.

A little above and to one side of the last; above the outer third of the orbitar arch.

On the outside of the organ of the sense of the relation of colour, and below the last.

A round protuberance at the lateral base of the frontal bone, towards the temple, and behind the organs of music and numbers.

At the middle and anterior part of the frontal bone, above that of the memory of things.

In part confounded with the preceding. Indicated at the outer side of the last by a protuberance, which gives to the forehead a peculiar hemispherical shape.

At the lateral and outer part of the last; and giving greater width to the frontal prominence.

On the outer side of the last; divided into two halves by the coronal suture.

Indicated by an oblong prominence above the organ of comparative sagacity; almost at the frontal suture.

At the outer side of the last.

At the top of the frontal bone and at the superior angles of the parietal bone.

The top of the head; at the anterior and most elevated part of the parietal bone.

7. Constructiveness.—8. Acquisitiveness.—9. Secretiveness.—10. Self-esteem.—11. Love of Approbation.—12. Cautiousness.—13. Benevolence.—14. Veneration.—15. Firmness.—16. Conscientiousness or Justice.—17. Hope.—18. Marvellousness.—19. Wit.—20. Ideality.—21. Imitation.—22. Individuality.—23. Form.—24. Size.—25. Weight and Resistance.—26. Colour.—27. Locality.—28. Numeration.—29. Order.—30. Eventu-

ality.—31. Time.—32. Melody or Tune.—33. Language.—34. Comparison.—35. Causality.

A fundamental principle with the *Craniologists* or *Phrenologists* is,—that the brain does not act as a single organ, but that it consists of a plurality of organs: but, were we able to admit this, the assignment of the seat of different faculties could not but be considered premature.

CRANIOM'ETRY, *Craniomet'ria;* from κρανιον, 'the cranium,' and μετρον, 'measure.' Measurement of the skull.

CRANIOPATHI'A; from κρανιον, 'the cranium,' and παθος, 'disease.' Disease of the cranium.

CRANIOSCOPY, Craniology.

CRANIO-SPINAL, Cephalo-spinal.

CRANIO'TABES; from *cranium*, 'the skull,' and *tabes*, 'wasting.' A softening of the bones of the cranium, and a consequent thinness of those bones,—as the occiput, (*soft occiput*,)—which are much exposed to pressure. It is a variety of rickets.—Elsässer.

CRANIOT'OMY, *Craniotom'ia;* from κρανιον, 'the cranium,' and τομη, 'incision.' The operation of opening the head in parturition.

CRANIOTOMY FORCEPS. An instrument, resembling the lithotomy forceps, for laying hold of and breaking down the bones of the head, in parturition.

CRANIUM, *Cra'nion, Cranum, Calva'ria, Sca'phion, Conchus, Calva, Olla cap'itis, Theca cer'ebri, Brain-pan,* the skull; from κρανος, 'a helmet,' or from κρανιον, 'head.' (F.) *Crane.* The collection of bones which form the case for lodging the brain and its membranes, as well as their vessels, and some of the nerves. These bones are eight in number—the *frontal, occipital,* two *parietal,* two *temporal,* the *sphenoid,* and *ethmoid.* Besides these, there might be considered, as belonging to the cranium, the cornua sphenoidalia, the bones of the ear, and the ossa Wormiana. Dr. Prichard has characterized the primitive forms of the skull according to the width of the *Bregma,* or space between the parietal bones: 1. The *Stenobregmate,* (στενος, 'narrow,') or Ethiopian variety. 2. The *Mesobregmate,* (μεσος, 'middle,') or Caucasian variety; and 3. The *Platybregmate,* (πλατυς, 'broad,') or Mongolian variety.

CRANIUM HUMA'NUM, *Human Cra'nium,* (F.) *Crane humain.* This was anciently much used in prescriptions, and was considered anti-epileptic, alexipharmic, antiloimic, &c.

CRANOMANCY, *Cranomanti'a,* from κρανον, 'the head,' and μαντεια, 'divination.' (F.) *Cranomancie.* The art of divining—from the inspection of the head or cranium—the moral dispositions and inclinations of individuals.

CRANSON, Cochlearia officinalis.

CRANSSAC, MINERAL WATERS OF. Cranssac is a village in the department of Aveyron, six leagues from Rhodez, which possesses acidulous chalybeate springs, that have been known for a long time.

CRANTER, from κραινειν, 'to finish,' 'render perfect.' The *Dens Sapien'tiæ* has been so called.

CRANUM, Cranium.

CRAPULA, Cræpula.

CRAQUEMENT DE CUIR, (F.) 'Crackling of leather.' A sound like the crackling of new leather, sometimes heard on examining the heart with the stethoscope. It has been supposed to be symptomatic of pericarditis.

CRAQUEMENT PULMONAIRE, (F.) 'Pulmonary crackling.' This *bruit* or sound consists in a succession of small cracklings, heard during inspiration, and almost always at the top of the lung. It is heard at the commencement of phthisis.

CRASIS; from κεραννυμι, 'I mix.' A mixture of the constituents of a fluid; as the *crasis of the blood, humours,* &c. The word has also been employed in a more extensive signification, as synonymous with *Constitution, Temperament,* &c.

CRASPEDON, Staphylœdema.

CRASSAMEN'TUM, from *crassus,* 'thick.' The thick part or deposit of any fluid. It is particularly applied to the clot of the blood.

CRASSAMENTUM SANGUINIS, see Blood.

CRASSE, (F.) Dirt or impurity. A sort of layer or *enduit,* which covers the skin, where cleanliness is not attended to; and which is sometimes the result of the cutaneous exhalation; at others, of extraneous matter adhering to the surface of the body.

CRASSE'NA. A term by which Paracelsus designated the saline, putrescent, and corrosive principles, which, he thought, gave rise to ulcers and tumours of different kinds.

CRASSULA, Sedum telephium — c. Arborescens, see Cotyledon orbiculata—c. Portulacacea, c. Tetragona.

CRAS'SULA TETRAGO'NA. A South African succulent plant, which is somewhat astringent. Boiled in milk it is used in diarrhœa. *Crassula portulacacea* is said to be used in similar cases.

CRASSUS, Corpulent.

CRATÆ'GUS A'RIA, from κρατος, 'strength,' owing to the hardness of the wood. *Mes'pilus, M. A'ria, Aria seu Sorbus, S. Aria seu Alpi'na, White Bean Tree,* (F.) *Alisier blanc, Alouche, Alouchier.* The fruit, which is of the size of a small pear, is slightly astringent, and somewhat agreeable to the taste. It has been employed in diarrhœa.

CRATÆVA MARMELOS, Covolam.

CRATERAU'CHEN, from κρατερος, 'strong,' and αυχην, 'neck.' One with a strong neck: as well as a strong neck itself.

CRATEVÆSIUM, Sisymbrium nasturtium.

CRATOS, Force.

CRAUTE, MINERAL WATERS OF. Craute is a village five leagues from Autun, in France, where are mineral springs, containing sulphohydrate of magnesia, chloride of sodium, chloride of lime, sulphate of lime, and carbonate of magnesia.

CRAVATE SUISSE (F.) A band of the longitudinal or superficial layer of the muscular fibres of the stomach, along the lesser curvature of the organ, the shape of which it assists in preserving;— so called, on account of a fancied resemblance to a Swiss cravat.

CRAYEUX, Cretaceous.

CRAYON NOIR, Graphites.

CRAZINESS, Insanity.

CRAZY, Insane.

CREA, Shin.

CREAM, *Oremor,* (F.) *Crème.* A thick, unctuous matter, of a yellowish-white colour, and sweet, agreeable taste, which rises to the surface of milk, if kept at rest. It is composed of butter, serum, and casein.

Crème is a name given in France to *bouillies* prepared with farina of different kinds; as the *Cream of Rice,* (F.) *Crème de Riz, C. of Barley,* (F.) *C. d'Orge,* &c.

CREAM, COLD, Ceratum Galeni, Unguentum Aquæ rosæ—c. of Tartar, Potassæ supertartras.

CRE'ASOTE, *Cre'osote, Creaso'tum, Kre'asote, Oreaso'ton, Creazo'ton;* from κρεας, 'flesh,' and σωτηρ, 'a preserver.' A substance discovered not long ago by Reichenbach. It is obtained from tar, by distillation, and appears to be the active antiseptic and medicinal agent in tar-water and crude pyroligneous acid. It is a colourless transparent fluid, of a penetrating and disagreeable odour, and is freely soluble in alcohol and acetic acid. Its taste is bitter. S. g. 1.037. It coagulates albumen, whence its hæmostatic power. It is a most powerful antiseptic; and has been largely administered in hemorrhages both internally and externally. As an external application, it has been used in burns, ulcers, especially those of a sloughing character, chronic cutaneous affections, and has been applied to tapeworm when protruded, &c. Internally, it has been administered in phthisis, vomiting, diabetes mellitus, nervous diseases, chronic glanders, &c. The dose internally is one or two drops. Externally, it is sometimes applied pure; at others, diluted, and commonly with water, (f℥ss to f℥vj;) or in the form of ointment, (f℥ss to ℥j of cerate.)

CRE'ATINE, *Cre'atin*, *Creati'na*, *Kre'atine*, from κρεας, 'flesh.' A nitrogenized crystallizable neutral substance, obtained by the agency of water and heat in making broths and soups. It does not combine either with acids or alkalies.

By the action of strong acids, creatine is converted into *Creatinine* or *Kreatinine*, a substance which has a strong alkaline reaction, and forms crystallizable salts with acids. It preëxists to a small extent in the juice of flesh; and is found in conjunction with creatine in urine.

CREATININE, see Creatine.

CREATOPHAGUS, Carnivorous.

CREAZOTON, Creasote.

CREEPER, TRUMPET, Tecoma radicans—c. Virginia, Ampelopsis quinquefolia, Tecoma radicans.

CREMASON, Pyrosis.

CREMAS'TER, *Suspendic'ulum*, *Eleva'tor Testic'uli*, *Mus'culus Testis*, *M. Testicon'dus*. That which suspends; from κρεμαω, 'I suspend.' The Greeks designated, by this term, the spermatic chord, or all the parts by which the testicle is, as it were, suspended; but, since Vesalius, it has received its present limited meaning. The cremaster is a very thin, muscular fascia—sometimes hardly perceptible—which detaches itself from the internal oblique muscle; passes through the abdominal ring, and vanishes around the tunica vaginalis; serving to draw up the testicle, and to move it slightly. It has been, also, called *Tunica Erythroï'des* and *Suspenso'rium Testis*.

CREMAS'TERIC, *Cremaster'icus*, same etymon as '*Cremaster*. Appertaining or relating to the cremaster,—as '*cremasteric* artery,'—a branch of the epigastric.

CRÈME, Cream—c. *de Soufre*, Sulphur præcipitatum—c. *de Tartre*, Potassæ supertartras.

CREMER. The common name for a disease frequent in Hungary, which is produced by excess in eating and drinking.—Chomel.

CREMNOI, plural of κρημνος, 'a steep bank.' The lips of an ulcer. The *Labia puden'di*.—Hippocrates, Foësius. Hence:

CREMNON'CUS, from κρημνος, 'the labia pudendi,' and ογκος, 'a tumour.' A swelling of the labia pudendi.

CREMOR, Cream—c. Tartari, Potassæ supertartras—c. Urinæ, see Urine.

CRENA, *Crenatu'ra*, *Dentic'ulus*, (F.) *Crénelure*. In the plural, the small teeth or projections in the bones of the cranium, by means of which an accurate junction is formed at the sutures. *Crénelure* has also been used in *surgery*, for the gutter or groove in certain instruments, which is generally intended to secure the passage of cutting instruments; the groove, for example, of a director.

CRENATURA, Crena.

CRÉNELURE, Crena.

CRE'OLE, (S.) *Criollo*; from (S.) *criar*, 'to create or foster.' A native of America, or of the West Indies, born of parents who have emigrated from the Old World, or from Africa. Hence there may be white as well as black creoles.—Tschudi.

CREOPHAGUS, Carnivorous.

CREPALIA TEMULENTA, Lolium temulentum.

CREPANELLA, Plumbago Europæa.

CREPA'TIO, *Crepa'tura*, from *crepare*, 'to make a noise.' The action of bursting any seed by ebullition. *Coque ad crepatu'ram*, 'Boil till it bursts.'

CREPATURA, Hernia.

CREPIDINES PALPEBRARUM, see Tarsus.

CREP'ITANT, *Crep'itating*, *Crep'itans*; same etymon. Crackling.

Râle Crépitant Sec à Grosses Bulles, 'dry crackling noise with formation of large bubbles,' is heard in pulmonary emphysema, when the distention becomes greater and greater, and is followed by rupture of the vesicles. The air forcing itself a passage in the interlobular areolar tissue, gives rise to this *Râle* during inspiration.

Râle Crépitant Sec of Laënnec, *R. vésiculaire*. The *crepitant rattle*, heard, during respiration, in severe pneumonia and in œdema of the lung; so termed on account of the analogy between the sound and that occasioned by pressing a healthy lung between the fingers. It resembles the sound produced by rubbing slowly and firmly between the finger and thumb a lock of hair near the ear. The *Rhonchus crepitans redux*, (F.) *Râle crépitant redux*, is the sound heard in respiration coexistent with the resolution of pneumonia. It indicates the return of the cells to the pervious condition.

CREPITA'TION, *Crep'itus*, from *crepitare*, 'to make a noise.' *Crackling*. Crepitation or *crepitus*, (F.) *Cliquetis*, has been used, in *Surgery*, to designate the noise occasioned by the friction of fractured bones, when the surgeon moves them in certain directions. When it cannot be heard at a distance, it may be detected by the immediate application of the ear, or by the use of the stethoscope. *Crepitus* or *crackling* is, likewise, met with in cases of gangrene, when air is effused into the areolar membrane—provided the part be carefully examined with the fingers. The same term is used for the cracking of the joints in health or disease.

CREPITUS, Crepitation, Fart—c. Lupi, Lycoperdon.

CRESCENTIA, Growth.

CRESCEN'TIA CUJE'TE; called after Crescentio, an Italian writer on agriculture; *Cujete*, *Narrow-leaved Calabash Tree*. The pulp of the fruit of this West India plant is acidulous. It is used in diarrhœa and headach; and, in syrup, for diseases of the chest.

CRESCENTIÆ, Waxing kernels.

CRESERA, see Cribration.

CRESPINUS, Oxycantha Galeni.

CRESS, BITTER, COMMON, Cardamine pratensis—c. Garden, Lepidium sativum—c. Indian, Tropæolum majus—c. Penny,Thlaspi—c. Swines', Cochlearia coronopus—c. Water, Sisymbrium nasturtium—c. Water, marsh, Nasturtium palustre.

CRESSES, DOCK, Lapsana—c. Sciatica, Lepidium Iberis.

CRESSI, Sisymbrium nasturtium.

CRESSON ALÉNOIS, Lepidium sativum — c. *Élégant*, Cardamine pratensis—c. *de Fontaine*, Sisymbrium nasturtium — c. *des Indes*, Tropæolum majus — c. *des Jardins*, Lepidium sativum—c. *du Mexique*, Tropæolum majus — c. *de Para*, Spilanthus oleraceus — c. *des Prés*, Cardamine pratensis.

CREST, Crista — c. of the Ilium, see Crista of the Ilium—c. of the Pubis, see Crista of the Pubis—c. of the Tibia, see Crista of the Tibia—c. of the Urethra, see Crista urethralis.

CRETA, *Car'bonas calcis friab'ilis, Car'bonas calca'reus, Glisomar'go, Melia Terra, Chalk, Car- bonate of Lime,* (F.) *Craie.* Native friable carbonate of lime.

CRETA PREPARA'TA, *Car'bonas Calcis præpara'tus, Prepared Chalk.* (Prepared by levigation.) Used externally, as an absorbent; internally, as an antacid. Dose, gr. x to ʒj or more.

CRETA'CEOUS, *Creta'ceus,* (F.) *Crayeux,* from *creta,* 'chalk.' Containing, or relating to, or having the characters of, chalk; as 'cretaceous mixture, cretaceous tubercles.'

CRÊTE, Crista—*c. de Coq,* Crista galli—*c. de l'Ethmoïde,* Crista galli — *c. Uréthrale,* Gallinaginis caput.

CRÊTES DE COQ, see Crista.

CRÉTIN. One affected with cretinism. The word is said to come from *Chrétien,* "Christian," because the Crétin, being in a state of idiocy, is incapable of committing any sin (?) See Cagot.

CRET'INISM, *Cretinis'mus, Cret'inage, Cyrto'sis Cretinis'mus, Kretinis'mus, Micrenceph'alon.* An epidemic affection in the low, deep, narrow situations of the Valais; in the valley of Aost, Maurienne, a part of Switzerland, the Pyrenees, Tyrol, &c. It is a state of idiocy, commonly accompanied by an enormous goître, and is often hereditary. The unfortunate crétin is little better than the animals around him. He rarely attains an advanced age. Like idiocy, cretinism has been divided into *complete* and *incomplete.*

CREUSET, Crucible.

CREUX DE L'AISSELLE, see Axilla.

CREUX DE L'ESTOMAC, *Fossette du cœur.*

CREUX DE LA MAIN, Palm.

CREUZNACH, MINERAL WATERS OF. The springs of Creuznach are in Germany. They contain iodine, bromine, and the chlorides of sodium and calcium.

CREUZOT, MINERAL WATERS OF. C. is a mountain to the north-east of Mount Cenis. Near it is a saline chalybeate spring.

CREVASSE, (F.) *Rima,* from *crever,* 'to break or crack.' A *crack,* a *cleft.* The words *crevasse, gerçure, fissure,* and *rhagade* are often used synonymously for small longitudinal cracks or chaps of a more or less painful character. Sometimes, *crevasse* is employed to designate the solutions of continuity or ruptures, which supervene in distended parts, in the urinary passages, uterus, &c.: it is then synonymous with rupture.

CRI, Cry.

CRIBLÉ, Cribratus.

CRIBRA, see Cribration.

CRIBRA'TION, *Cribra'tio, Coscinis'mus,* from *cribrare,* 'to sift.' *Sifting.* A pharmaceutical operation, which consists in separating the finer parts of drugs from the coarser. *Sieves. Drumsieves* are used for this purpose. These were formerly called *Cribra; Cos'cinoi.* A sieve for separating the bran from meal was termed *Cre'sera, Aleurote'sis, Cribrum Pollina'rium.*

CRIBRA'TUS, *Cribro'sus,* from *cribrum,* 'a sieve.' (F.) *Criblé.* Having holes like a sieve. *Lame criblée, Crib'riform plate,* is the horizontal lamina of the ethmoid bone—so called because it is perforated like a sieve. Through the perforations the olfactory nerves pass.

La'mina Cribro'sa of Albinus; *Crib'riform lamel'la* — a circular spot, perforated with small holes, seen when the optic nerve is regarded from the inside, after removing the retina and choroid. From these holes the medullary matter may be expressed.

CRIB'RIFORM, *Cribrifor'mis,* from *cribrum,* 'a sieve,' and *forma,* 'form.' The ethmoid bone was formerly so called:—*Os Cribrifor'mĕ.*

CRIBRIFORM COMPRESS. A square piece of linen pierced with a number of holes. This is spread with cerate and applied to a suppurating surface, the holes being intended for the escape of the pus.

CRIBRIFORM FASCIA, see Fascia, cribriform—*c.* Lamella, see Cribratus—*c.* Plate of the Ethmoid, see Cribratus.

CRIBROSUS, Cribratus.

CRIBRUM POLLINARIUM, see Cribration.

CRICARYTENODES, Crico-arytenoid.

CRICELLA'SIA, *Cricila'sia,* from κρικος, 'a circle,' and ελαυνω, 'I drive.' An exercise with the ancients, which appears to have been the same as the childish play of rolling the hoop.

CRICK IN THE NECK. A painful rheumatic affection of the muscles of the neck, which causes the person to hold his head to one side in a characteristic manner.

CRICO-ARYT'ENOID, *Crico-arytenoïdeus, Cricaryteno'des.* Relating to the cricoid and arytenoid cartilages.

CRICO-ARYT'ENOID MUSCLE, *Crico-arytenoïdeus latera'lis, Crico-latéro-aryténoïdien.* A muscle which proceeds from the lateral part of the superior edge of the cricoid cartilage to the outer and anterior part of the base of the arytenoid cartilage. It carries the arytenoid cartilage outward and forwards.

CRICO-ARYT'ENOID, POSTE'RIOR; *Crico-arytenoïdeus posti'cus, Crico-créti-aryténoïdien, Dilatateur postérieur du Larynx.* A small, triangular muscle, seated at the back part of the larynx. It extends from the prominent line, at the middle of the posterior surface of the cricoid cartilage, to the outer and posterior part of the base of the arytenoid cartilage.

CRICO-ARYTENOIDEUS SUPE'RIOR, of Winslow, forms part of the *Arytenoïdeus* of modern anatomists.

CRICO-CRÉTI-ARYTÉNOÏDIEN, Cricoarytenoid, posterior — *c. Latéro-aryténoïdien,* Crico-arytenoid.

CRICO-PHARYNGEAL, *Crico-Pharyngeus.* Belonging to the cricoid cartilage and pharynx.

CRICO-PHARYNGEUS muscle, of Winslow, is a fleshy bundle, which forms part of the *Constrictor Pharyngis inferior.* He calls the other part *Thyro-pharynge'us,* and proposes to call the whole *Thyro-crico-pharyngeus.*

CRICO-THYREOIDES, Crico-Thyroidean.

CRICO-THYROIDEAN, *Crico-thyroid, Crico-thyreo'des, Crico-thyreoï'des, Crico-thyreoïdeus.* Belonging to the cricoid and thyroid cartilages.

CRICO-THYROID MEMBRANE is of a fibrous nature, and extends from the upper edge of the cricoid cartilage to the inferior edge of the thyroid.

CRICO-THYROID MUSCLE, *Crico-thyroïdeus,* (F.) *Dilatateur antérieur du larynx,* is a small fleshy bundle, of a triangular shape, at the anterior and inferior part of the larynx. It extends from the outer surface of the cricoid cartilage to the lateral parts of the inferior margin of the thyroid cartilage; and its use is, to approximate, anteriorly, the corresponding margins of the cricoid and thyroid cartilages; and thus to stretch the ligaments of the glottis, which it contracts by separating the thyroid cartilage from the arytenoid.

CRICO-THYRO-PHARYNGIEN, Constrictor pharyngis.

CRICOID, *Cricoï'deus, Cricoï'des, Cricoï'des, Annula'ris, Cymbala'ris,* from κρικος, 'a ring,' and ειδος, 'form.' Having the form of a ring. A name given to one of the cartilages of the larynx, *Cartila'go innomina'ta,* (F.) *Cartilage anonyme,* which is situate at its lower part, between the thyroid and first ring of the trachea. It is much higher behind than before.

CRICOIDES, Annular, Cricoid.
CRICOS, Ring.
CRIMNO'DES, *Crimnoï'des*, from κριμνον, 'coarse meal,' and ειδος, 'resemblance.' Resembling meal.
CRIMNO'DES URI'NA. Urine that deposits a sediment like meal.
CRIMNON, Farina.
CRINA'LE, from *crinis*, 'hair.' An instrument formerly used to compress in cases of fistula lachrymalis. It has its name from the circumstance of its having at one end a small cushion stuffed with hair.—Scultetus.
CRINA'TUM. A species of fumigation, used by Paulus of Ægina. The roots of lilies entered into the process; hence its name,—from κρινον, 'the lily.'
CRINES, Hair.
CRINIS, Capillus.
CRINOM'YRON, from κρινον, 'the lily,' and μυρον, 'ointment.' *Unguen'tum lilia'ceum*, U. *Ægyp'tium album*, U. *Susi'num*. An ointment, composed of lilies and some aromatic plants.—Gorræus.
CRINON, Lilium candidum.
CRIOLLO, Creole.
CRIOMYX'OS. In antiquity, one who had much mucus flowing from his nasal fossæ, like the ram; from κριος, 'a ram,' and μυξα, 'mucus.'
CRISIS, *Diac'risis*, *Dijudica'tio*, 'decision;' from κρινω, 'I decide.' This word has been used in various acceptations. Some mean by *crisis of a disease*, when it augments or diminishes considerably, becomes transformed into another, or ceases entirely. Some have used the word to signify only the favourable changes which supervene in disease; others, for the change going on in the acme or violence of the disease. Others, again, have given this name only to a rapid and favourable change, joined to some copious evacuation or eruption; whilst others have applied the term to the symptoms that accompany such change, and not to the change itself;—thus including, under the same denomination, the *critical* phenomena and the *crisis*.
CRISPA'TION, *Crispatu'ra*, from *crispare*, 'to wrinkle.' A contraction or spasmodic constriction, which supervenes in certain parts, either spontaneously or by the influence of some morbific cause or therapeutical agent. The capillary vessels of a wound are, by the French, termed *crispés*, when, immediately, after an operation, the blood does not flow from them. The skin is said to be *crispée*, when contracted, and the bulbs of the hair become more prominent. *Crispation* of the nerves is a slight convulsive motion of external or internal parts, much less than that which occurs in convulsion.
CRISTA, *Ambé*, *Ambon*. A crest. (F.) *Crête*. A name given to several bony projections; also, to the clitoris.
The word *Crêtes* (F.), *Cristæ*, is also used, in France, for fimbriated excrescences, which form at the anus, and near the genital organs; and are commonly owing to the syphilitic virus. *Crêtes de Coq* are syphilitic excroscences, resembling, in form, the crest of the cock.
CRISTA GALLI; two Latin words, signifying the *comb of a cock*, (F.) *Crête de l'ethmoïde*, *C. de Coq*. A flat, triangular process, rising above the cribriform plate of the ethmoid bone, and resembling a cock's comb. It gives attachment to the anterior part of the falx cerebri.
CRISTA OR CREST OF THE IL'IUM, is the superior margin of the ilium :—the *Crista or Crest of the Tib'ia*, the anterior edge, the shin; and the *Crista or Crest of the Pubis*, the posterior sharp edge on the upper surface of the bone. Winslow calls the nymphæ *Cristæ of the clit'oris*; and Chaussier, the veru montanum, *Crista Urethra'lis, Crest of the Urethra*.
CRISTA INTERNA, Frontal spine—c. Tibiæ, Shin—c. Urethralis, Gallinaginis caput.
CRISTA VESTIB'ULI, *Eminen'tia pyramida'lis*. A crest which divides the vestibule of the ear into two fossæ,— one inferior and hemispherical, called *Fo'vea hemisphæ'rica*; the other superior and semi-elliptical, *Fovea ellip'tica seu semiellip'tica*. Morgagni has described a third groovelike fossa, *Reces'sus seu Fo'vea sulciform'is*, situate at the mouth of the common orifice of the two superior semicircular canals.
CRISTÆ CLITORIDIS, Nymphæ.
CRISTALLIN, Crystalline.
CRISTALLINE, Mesembryanthemum crystallinum.
CRITHE, Hordeolum, Hordeum, Penis.
CRITHIDION, Hordeolum.
CRITHMUM MARIT'IMUM, *Crithmum, Cachrys marit'ima, Fœnic'ulum mari'num, Samphire*, (F.) *Passe-pierre, Perce-pierre, Fenouil marin, Bacile*. Family, Umbelliferæ. Sex. Syst. Pontandria Digynia. A plant which grows on the sea-coasts, has a spicy, aromatic flavour, and is used, pickled, as a condiment.
The *Caaponga* of Brasil is a kind of crithmum.
CRIT'ICAL, *Crit'icus*. Belonging to a crisis.
CRITICAL DAYS, *Dies crit'ici, D. judicato'rii, D. Decreto'rii, D. Prin'cipes, D. Radica'les, D. Contemplab'iles, D. Internun'cii*, (F.) *Jours critiques*, are those on which a crisis, it is imagined, is most likely to happen. According to Hippocrates and Galen, the greatest number of fevers terminate favourably on the 7th day, and many on the 14th;—these two days being the most propitious. Next to these come, in order of efficiency, the 9th, 11th, 20th or 21st, 17th, 5th, 4th, 3d, 18th, 27th, and 28th. The sixth day was called by Galen, the *Tyrant*, τυραννος, because the crises that happened then were generally unfavourable. After this, the most unfavourable were the 8th, 10th, 12th, 16th, and 19th. The 13th was a sort of neutral day; the crises which happened on it being neither favourable nor unfavourable. Days were, also, divided into *Intercalary*, on which the crises happened less frequently, and were less complete than on the *critical* or *indicatory*;—and into *vacant* and *nondecretory*, on which a crisis hardly ever occurred. According to this division, they were enumerated as follows:

Critical days .... 7th, 14th, 20th, 27th, 34th, 40th, 60th, &c.
Indicatory days ..... 4th, 11th, 17th, 24th, &c.
Intercalary days .... 3d, 5th, 6th, 9th, &c.
Non-decretory days.. 2d, 8th, 10th, 12th, 13th, &c.

Fortunate crises were considered to be indicated by favourable signs appearing three days before.
CRITICAL PERIOD, see Menses.
CROCHET, Crotchet.
CROCIDISMUS, Carphologia.
CROCIDIXIS, Carphologia.
CRO'CINUM, from κροκος, 'saffron.' Made with saffron; coloured with saffron.
CROCO'DES, from κροκος, 'saffron,' and ειδος, 'resemblance.' Certain troches into which saffron entered as an ingredient.—Paulus of Ægina.
CROCODI'LEA, *Stercus Lacer'tæ*. The excrements of the crocodile, which the Arabists extolled as a remedy for cutaneous diseases, and which was long used as a cosmetic.
CROCODILIUM, Echinops.
CROCOMAG'MA, from κροκος, 'saffron,' and μαγμα, 'a kneaded or squeezed mass.' A kind

of troch, composed of saffron and spices.—Galen, Dioscorides, Paulus of Ægina, Scribonius Largus.

CROCUS, *C. sati'vus* seu *officina'lis* seu *Austriacus, Medici'na Tristit'iæ, Panace'a vegetab'ilis, Zaffran, An'ima Pulmo'num, C. Orienta'lis, Jovis flos, Saffron*, (F.) *Safran*. Order, Irideæ. The stigmata are the parts used in medicine. They are brought from the East. The odour is aromatic, and the taste aromatic, pungent, and bitter:—the colour deep orange red. Its virtues are yielded to alcohol, wine, vinegar and water. Its operation has been considered stimulant, exhilarating and diaphoretic. It is not much used.

Cake Saffron is sometimes met with. It consists of one part of saffron and nine of marigold, made into a cake with oil, and pressed.

CROCUS, Colcothar — c. Antimonii, Oxydum stibii sulphuratum — c. Austriacus, Crocus — c. Germanicus, Carthamus tinctorius — c. Indicus, Curcuma longa — c. Martis adstringens, Colcothar — c. Martis aperiens, Ferri subcarbonas — c. Martis vitriolatus, Colcothar — c. Metallorum, Oxydum stibii sulphuratum — c. Officinalis, Crocus — c. Orientalis, Crocus — c. Saracenicus, Carthamus tinctorius — c. Sativus, Crocus.

CROCYDISMUS, Carphologia.

CROISÉ, (F.) *Crossed*. An epithet given to paralysis, when it attacks the arm of one side and the leg of another.

CROISSANCE, Growth.

CROISSANCES, Waxing kernels.

CROISSANTS, Waxing kernels.

CROIX DE MALTE, *Sple'nium Crucia'tum, Maltese Cross, Cross of Malta*. A compress, having the form of the Maltese cross. It is made of a piece of square linen, folded in four, and divided with scissors from each angle to a small distance from the centre. It is used especially after amputation of the fingers, penis, and limbs.

When the compress is cut in two of its angles only, it is called the *Half Maltese Cross,—Demicroix de Malte*.

CROMMYON, Allium cepa.

CROMMYOXYREG'MIA, from κρομμυον, 'an onion,' οξυς, 'acid,' and ρηγνυμι, 'to break out.' Sour, fetid eructations, exhaling a smell similar to that of onions.

CROPALE, Nerium antidysentericum.

CROPSIA, Chromopsia.

CROSS, MALTESE, *Croix de Malte*.

CROSSE DE L'AORTE, Arch of the aorta.

CROSSES PALMAIRES, Palmar arches.

CROSSWORT, Eupatorium perfoliatum, Lysimachia quadrifolia.

CROTALOPHORUS, Crotalus horridus.

CROT'ALUS HOR'RIDUS, *Crotaloph'orus*. The *Rattlesnake, Cobra di Capello*, (F.) *Crotale*. A venomous reptile of North America. Its poison is virulent. It is so called from the rattle in its tail, (κροταλον, 'a rattle,' 'a small bell.')

CROT'APHE, *Crota'phium*, from κροταφος, 'temple.' *Cephalal'gia Pulsat'ilis, Cephalæ'a Pulsat'ilis, Sphygmoceph'alus*. A pulsatory pain, chiefly in the temples, with drumming in the ears.

CROTAPHITE ARTERIES, Temporal arteries.

CROTAPHITES, Temporal muscle.

CROTAPHIUM, Crotaphe.

CROTAPHUS, Temple, Temporal bone.

CROTCHET, *Hamus*. A small hook or crook. (F.) *Crochet*. An obstetrical instrument, whose name indicates its shape, and which is used in the extraction of the fœtus, when it becomes necessary to destroy it to expedite delivery. Crotchets are differently formed; some are sharp, others blunt; some contained in a sheath, others naked.

CROTON BENZOÉ, Benjamin.

CROTON CASCARIL'LA, *Cortex Eleuthe'ria, Croton Eleuthe'ria* seu *Elute'ria, Clu'tia Elute'ria, Thus Judæo'rum, Chacaril'læ cortex, Cascaril'la, Eleute'ria, Gascaril'la*. Order, Euphorbiaceæ. *Sex. Syst.* Monœcia Monadelphia. (F.) *Quinquina aromatique, Cascarille*. The bark of *Croton Cascarilla* of the Bahamas, *Cortex Thuris*, has a slightly aromatic odour, and bitterish, aromatic taste. The smoke has the odour of musk. The active parts are an essential oil and bitter extractive. They are completely extracted by proof spirit. It is tonic and stomachic. Dose, gr. xv to ʒss or more, in powder.

CROTON ELEUTHERIA, Croton cascarilla — c. Jamalyota, C. tiglium — c. Lacciferum, see Lacca — c. Oil, Croton tiglium.

CROTON RACEMO'SUM, *Beenel*. A small Malabar tree, whose aromatic root, boiled in oil of sesame, is employed, by the orientals, as a liniment in headach and rheumatism.

CROTON TIG'LIUM, *c. Jamalyo'ta, Cadel-Avanaeu*. A Ceylonese plant, every part of which is endowed with medicinal power. The *root* is a drastic cathartic: the wood, *Lignum Pava'næ, Pavana wood*, and the *seed*, have like virtues. The seeds have been long known under the names, *Grana Moluc'cæ, Til'ii Grana*, and *Grana Tig'lii* seu *Tig'lia*. From these seeds the *Croton Oil, O'leum Tig'lii*, is expressed. It is of a pale, brownish-yellow colour, and hot, biting taste; and is a most powerful drastic cathartic. Dose, from half a drop to three drops, made into pills with crumb of bread. It is also applied externally as a rubefacient, 3 to 5 drops being rubbed on the part; or one part of the oil and three parts of olive oil may be added together, and a little of this be rubbed on.

CROTO'NE, κροτωνη. A fungus, which grows on trees, and is produced by an insect, from κροτων, 'a tick.' By extension, applied to a fungous tumour developed on the periosteum.

CROUP, Cynanche trachealis — c. Bronchial, Polypus bronchialis — c. Cerebral, Asthma thymicum — c. Cerebral spasmodic, Carpo-pedal spasm — c. Chronic, Polypus bronchialis — c. Faux, Asthma thymicum, see Cynanche trachealis.

CROUP, HYSTER'IC. A spasmodic affection of the laryngeal muscles by no means unfrequent in hysterical females,— the paroxysm consisting in a long protracted, loud and convulsive cough, followed at times by crowing respiration, and by dyspnœa so great as to threaten suffocation. The treatment is that advised for hysteria.

CROUP, PSEUDO, Asthma thymicum — c. Pseudo-nerveux, Asthma thymicum — c. Spasmodic, see Asthma thymicum, and Cynanche trachealis — c. Spurious, Asthma thymicum.

CROUPE, see Croupion.

CROUPION (F.) *Uropyg'ium, Orrus, Orrhos*, the *Rump*. The region of the coccyx. The *Crupper*, (F.) *Croupe*.

CROUP-LIKE INSPIRATION OF INFANTS, Asthma thymicum.

CROÛTE, Crusta — c. *De lait*, Porrigo larvalis — c. *Laiteuse*, Porrigo larvalis.

CROÛTEUX, *Crustacé*.

CROWFOOT, Geranium maculatum — c. Bristly, Ranunculus Pennsylvanicus — c. Bulbous-rooted, Ranunculus bulbosus — c. Marsh, Ranunculus sceleratus — c. Meadow, Ranunculus acris — c. Small-flowered, Ranunculus abortivus — c. Water, smaller, Ranunculus flammula.

CROWN, *Coro'na, Steph'ane*. In anatomy, this name is given to parts of a circular form, which surmount other portions of the same body. Thus, the *Crown of a Tooth, Coro'na Dentis*, (F.) *Couronne du Dent*, is the portion of the tooth which projects above the gum.

CROWN OF THE GLANS, *Coro'na* seu *Tor'ulus glandis*, (F.) *Couronne du gland*, is the round, almost circular, ring, which circumscribes the base of the glans.

CROWN OF THE TREPAN, *Modi'olus*, (F.) *Couronne du Trépan*, is a species of saw, in form of a crown, or rather of a portion of a cylinder, having grooves on its external surface, and teeth at its lower extremity; the other being fitted to the handle of the trepan.

CROWN OF VENUS, *Coro'na Ven'eris, Gutta Rosa'cea Syphilit'ica*, (F.) *Couronne de Vénus*. Red, rosy pustules, dry or moist, on the face; but particularly on the forehead and temples, owing to constitutional syphilis.

CROWSBEAK-LIKE PROCESS, Coracoid process.

CRU'CIAL, from *crux, crucis*, 'a cross.' *Crucia'lis, Crucia'tus*. Having the shape of a cross. Appertaining to a cross.

CRUCIAL BANDAGE, T Bandage.

CRUCIAL INCIS'ION, *Incisu'ra crucia'lis*, (F.) *Incisio cruciale*. An incision made in the form of a cross. Often employed for exposing the cranium, for the purpose of applying the trepan.

CRUCIAL LIGAMENT OF THE ATLAS, Annular ligament of the Atlas.

CRUCIAL LIG'AMENTS, (F.) *Ligaments croisés*, L. *cruciformes*. Two strong ligaments within the knee-joint. The *anterior* passes obliquely from a depression anterior to the spine of the tibia to the posterior and inner part of the external condyle of the femur: — the *other*, the *posterior*, extends from the posterior part of the spine of the tibia to the anterior and outer part of the internal condyle.

CRUCIA'TI DOLO'RES, Excruciating pains.

CRU'CIBLE, from *crux, crucis*, 'a cross:' so called — it has been supposed — from being made in the shape of a cross, or from having a cross impressed upon it: *Crucib'ulum, Cati'nus fuso'rius, Tigil'lum, Albot, Cemente'rium*, (F.) *Creuset*. A vessel of earth, silver, platinum, gold, black-lead, &c., for receiving substances, which have to be exposed to a strong heat. It is sometimes covered with a *top* or *lid*. (F.) *Couvercle*.

CRU'CIFORM, from *crux, crucis*, 'a cross,' and *forma*, 'shape;' *Cruciform'is, Cross-shaped*. A name given to the ligaments which close the articulations of the phalanges; and likewise to the *crucial* ligaments.

CRUDE, *Crudus, Omus*: Raw, unripe, not concocted.

CRUDITAS MORBI, see Crudity—c. Ventriculi, see Crudity.

CRU'DITY, *Cru'ditas, Om'otes, Status Crudita'tis*, from *crudus*, 'crude,' 'unprepared,' *Incoctus. Rawness, Crudeness*. This has received several acceptations. 1. It expresses the quality of certain aliments, which have not experienced the action of fire. 2. The condition of matters in the digestive tube, which have not undergone the digestive changes,—*cru'ditas ventrio'uli*; and, 3. In the language of the Humorists, it means the condition of the morbific matter in a sick individual, *cru'ditas morbi*, when it has not yet been prepared or concocted by the action of the organs,— *Asym'ia humo'rum*.

The word is used in the plural, *Cru'dities*, synonymously with *crude matters*. (F.) *Matières crues*. It is applied to those, when contained in the stomach and intestines.

CRUELS, Scrofula.

CRUENTA EXSPUITIO, Hæmoptysis.

CRUES (*Matières*,) see Crudity.

CRUME'NA VESI'CÆ. The cavity of the urinary bladder.

CRUOR. The signification of this word is very vague. It has been used to designate blood in general, venous blood, extravasated or coagulated blood, and the colouring matter.

CRUOR SANGUINIS, see Blood.

CRUORIN, Hæmatin.

CRUPPER, *Croupion*—c. Bone, Coccyx.

CRUPSIA, Metamorphopsia.

C R U R A. The plural of *Crus*, 'a leg. (F.) *Cuisse*. Applied to some parts of the body, from their resemblance to legs or roots; as the *Crura cerebri, Crura cerebelli*, &c.

CRURA ANTERIORA MEDULLÆ OBLONGATÆ, Peduncles of the brain — c. Cerebelli ad Corpora Quadrigemina, see Peduncles of the cerebellum— c. Cerebelli ad Pontem, see Peduncles of the cerebellum — c. Clitoridis interna, Bulbus vestibuli— c. Medullæ oblongatæ, Corpora restiformia, Thalami nervorum opticorum, see Peduncles of the cerebellum—c. Posteriora medullæ oblongatæ, Peduncles of the cerebellum.

CRURÆUS, Cruralis.

CRURAL, *Crura'lis*, from *crus*, 'the thigh, and lower limb.' What belongs to the thigh or lower limb.

CRURAL ARCH, *In'guinal Arch, Fem'oral Arch*, (F.) *Arcade crurale, A. inguinale* (Ch.), POUPART'S *Lig'ament, L. of Fallo'pius*. This arch is formed by the internal portion of the inferior edge of the aponeurosis of the obliquus externus muscle, which is attached, at one end, to the pubis; at the other, to the anterior and superior spinous process of the ilium. At its posterior and inner part, the aponeurosis, forming the arch, sends off a falciform reflection, which is attached along the crest of the pubis, and is known under the name of GIMBERNAT'S *Ligament*. Beneath this arch, the vessels, nerves, and muscles make their exit from the pelvis to the thigh.

CRURAL ARTERY, *Fem'oral Artery*, (F.) *Artère crurale, A. Pelvi-crurale*,—(Ch.,) is the continuation of the external iliac. It extends from the crural arch to the aperture in the triceps, or to the ham. Chaussier applies the name *Artère crurale* to the trunk, which extends from the primitive or common iliac to the tibial arteries; embracing, of course, the external iliac, femoral, and popliteal.

CRURAL CANAL, *Crural Ring, Fem'oral canal* or *ring*. M. Jules Cloquet has described this canal with minuteness, and given it the name *Anneau crural, Anneau fémoral*. It is nearly an inch long, triangular, more spacious above than below, and shorter and broader in the female than in the male. Its upper orifice is bounded, anteriorly, by the crural arch; posteriorly, by the crista of the pubis; on the outer side by the psoas and iliacus muscles, covered by the iliac aponeurosis, and, at the inner, by Gimbernat's ligament. This orifice is covered by the peritoneum, and, according to M. Cloquet, is closed by a more or less resisting septum, which he has named *Septum crurale, Crural septum*. In its course, the crural canal has its anterior parietes formed by the superficial expansion of the fascia lata: the posterior by the pectineus, covered by the deep-seated expansion of the fascia; and more externally by the psoas and iliacus muscles, covered by an expansion of the *fascia iliaca*. Its inferior orifice is formed by the foramen of the fascia lata, which gives passage to the vena saphæna. It is at the upper orifice of this canal, that *Femoral* or *Crural Hernia, Hernie inguinale* of Chaussier, occurs; which would be more common, were it not for the fibrous cellular septum there situate.

CRURAL NERVE proceeds from the lumbar plexus, and is situate at the outer side of the psoas muscle and crural artery. After it has passed under the crural arch, it divides into cutaneous and muscular branches. One of the branches, which is larger than the rest, is called the *Saphœ'na nerve.* It gives off filaments to the integuments of the knee, to the inner part of the leg, and to the dorsal surface of the foot. The remainder of the branches of the *crural* are distributed to the anterior and inner part of the thigh. The *Ac'cessory of the Crural Nerve* is a term given to the 4th and 5th pairs of lumbar nerves.

CRURAL PLEXUS of Chaussier is the union of the anterior branches of the last four pairs of lumbar nerves, and the first four sacral; forming the *lumbar* and *sacral* plexuses of most anatomists.

CRURAL RING, Crural canal—c. Septum, see Crural canal.

CRURAL VEIN, *Fem'oral Vein,* has the same arrangement as the artery. It receives only one great branch, the saphæna.

CRURAL, Triceps cruris.

CRURA'LIS, *Cruræ'us.* A part of the *Triceps crural* of the French, or of the *Trifémororotulien* of Chaussier. The cruralis is situate at the anterior, outer, and inner part of the thigh. It arises, fleshy, from between the two trochanters, adheres firmly to most of the fore part of the os femoris, and is inserted, tendinous, into the upper part of the patella, behind the rectus. Its use is to assist the vasti and rectus in the extension of the leg. Under *Muscle Triceps Crural,* the French describe the cruralis and the two vasti. Some small muscular slips, sometimes found under the crurœus muscle, and inserted into the capsular ligament of the knee-joint, have been called *Sub-cruræ'i.*

CRURIS RADIUS, Fibula.

CRUS, Leg, Thigh.

CRUST, Eschar.

CRUSTA. A crust or scab. (F.) *Croûte.* An assemblage of small flakes, formed by the drying up of a fluid secreted by the skin.

The lining membrane of the stomach and intestines has been called *Crusta villo'sa.*

CRUSTA ADAMANTINA DENTIUM, Enamel of the teeth.

CRUSTA GENU EQUI'NÆ, *Hippogonyol'epus, Sweat or Knee Scab, Mock or Encircled Hoof Knees, Hangers, Corium phlogistoma, Gutta Claws, Night Eyes, Horse Crust.* This morbid secretion from the horse has been advised in cases of epilepsy. It is used in the form of powder, (gr. ij to gr. xx;) and of tincture.

CRUSTA INFLAMMATORIA, Corium phlogisticum — c. Lactea, Porrigo larvalis, P. lupinosa — c. Membranacea, Peristroma—c. Petrosa, see Tooth c. Phlogistica, Corium phlogisticum — c. Pleuretica, Corium phlogisticum—c. Pruriginosa, Gutta rosea—c. Serpiginosa, Gutta rosea—c. Vermicularis, Peristroma—c. Villosa linguæ, see Tongue —c. Villosa ventriculi, see Stomach.

CRUSTACÉ, (F.) Alibert has substituted this word, in his Nosology, for *croûteux,* 'crusty.' Having crusts or scabs; as *Dartre crustacée.*

CRUS'TULA. A small shell or scab. An ecchymosis of the conjunctiva.

CRUSTUMI'NATUM. A rob, prepared from the *Pyra Crustumi'na* or *Crustumeri'na,* (so called from Crustuminum, a town in Italy, where they grew,) boiled with honey or in rain-water.— Aëtius.

CRUX CERVI. An ancient appellation for the bone in the heart of the stag. It was once considered useful in diseases of the heart.

CRY, *Clamor, Boë,* (F.) *Cri.* The sound of the unarticulated voice. The native voice, which the idiot and deaf possess equally with the man of genius and hearing. The cry of the new-born child has been called *Vagi'tus,* (F.) *Vagissement.* We say, "*A cry of joy, of pleasure, of pain,*" &c., according to the expression which it may convey to the hearer.

CRYMO'DES, from κρυμος, 'cold.' A continued fever, *Febris crymo'des,* in which the internal parts feel hot, and the external cold; and which was attributed to an erysipelatous inflammation of the lungs.—Aëtius, Gorræus.

CRYMODYN'IA, from κρυμος, 'cold,' and οδυνη, 'pain.' Chronic rheumatism, and all its modifications.—Baumes.

CRYMO'SIS, from κρυμος, 'cold.' Diseases caused by the action of cold.—Baumes.

CRYPSOR'CHIS, from κρυπτω, 'I conceal,' and ορχις, 'a testicle.' *Cryptor'chis, Testicon'dus.* One in whom the testes have not descended into the scrotum. The state is called, *Cryptorchidis'mus, Parorchid'ium.*

CRYPTA, from κρυπτος, 'concealed.' *Follic'ulose gland, Lacu'na, Follic'ulus,* (F.) *Crypte, Follicule.* A *crypt* or *follicle* is a small, roundish, hollow body, situate in the substance of the skin or mucous membranes, and constantly pouring the fluid which it secretes on their surfaces.

The use of the cryptal or follicular secretion, is to keep the parts on which it is poured supple and moist, and to preserve them from the action of irritating bodies with which they have to come in contact.

The little rounded appearances at the ends of the small arteries, in the cortical substance of the kidney, are also called *Cryptæ.*

CRYPTÆ SEBACEÆ, Sebaceous glands.

CRYPTE, Crypta.

CRYPTOCEPH'ALUS, from κρυπτος, 'concealed,' and κεφαλη, 'head.' A monster whose head is excessively small, and does not appear externally.—G. St. Hilaire.

CRYPTOCOCCUS, Fermentum, Torula cerevisiæ.

CRYPTODID'YMUS, *Fœtus in fœtu.* A monstrosity, in which one fœtus is found contained in another.

CRYPTOG'AMOUS, *Cryptogam'ic, Cryptogam'icus;* from κρυπτος, 'concealed,' and γαμος, 'marriage.' An epithet applied by botanists to plants whose organs of fructification are concealed or not manifest. *Ag'amous* plants are those whose sexual organs are not known.

CRYPTOPY'IC, *Cryptopy'icus,* from κρυπτω, 'I conceal,' and πυον, 'pus.' A state of disease, kept up by an occult abscess.

CRYPTOPYICUS, Cryptopyic.

CRYPTORCHIDISMUS, see Crypsorchis.

CRYPTORCHIS, Crypsorchis.

CRYPTS OF LIEBERKÜHN, see Intestine —c. Synovial, Bursæ mucosæ.

CRYSTAL, MINERAL, Potassæ nitras fusus sulphatis paucillo mixtus.

CRYSTAL'LI. Vesicles filled with a watery fluid. They are also called *crystal'linæ.* Probably the pemphigus of modern writers.

CRYSTALLI LUNÆ, Argenti nitras.

CRYSTALLIN, Crystalline.

CRYSTAL'LINA, from κρυσταλλος, 'crystal.' A vesicle or phlyctæna, filled with serum, and appearing on the prepuce or in the vicinity of the anus, surrounded by a reddish extravasated areola. It may be syphilitic or not. See Crystalli.

CRYSTALLINA TUNICA, Arachnoid membrane.

CRYS'TALLINE, *Crystal'linus.* Having the appearance of crystal.

CRYS'TALLINE, *Crys'talline humour, C. Lens, Crys'talline body, Crystal'linus, Lens crystal'lina, Lens crystalloï'des* vel *Corpus Crystal'linum, C Discoï'des, C. Crystalloï'des, C. Phacoï'des, Humor crystal'linus, H. glacia'lis, Phacé, Phacos Phacus, Gemma Oculi,* (F.) *Cristallin* ou *Crystal* lin, *Humeur crystalline, Corps crystallin, Lentille crystalline.* A lenticular, transparent body, situate between the vitreous and aqueous humours of the eye, at the union of the anterior third with the two posterior thirds of the organ. It is composed of a soft exterior substance; and an interior, forming a solid nucleus, in which a number of elliptical layers is perceptible. It is contained in a *capsule,* called *Tu'nica ara'nea* vel *crystal'lina, Cap'sula lentis,* and receives, at its posterior surface, a small branch of the central artery of the retina, which is always readily distinguishable in the fœtus, prior to the seventh month of utero-gestation.

The use of the crystalline is to refract the rays of light, and to serve as an achromatic glass: for which its laminæ or layers, increasing in refractive power from the circumference to the centre, admirably adapt it.

CRYSTALLINO-CAPSULITIS, see Phacitis.
CRYSTALLION, Plantago psyllium.
CRYSTALLITIS, Phacitis.
CRYS'TALLOID, *Crystalloï'des,* from κρυσταλ- λος, 'crystal,' and ειδος, 'form,' 'resemblance.' Resembling crystal or the crystalline. The *capsule* or *membrane of the crystalline.* Also, the crystalline itself.
CRYSTALLUS MINERALIS, Potassæ nitras fusus sulphatis paucillo mixtus.
CRYTHE, Hordeolum.
CTEDON, Fibre.
CTEIS, Pubes.
CTESIPHON'TIS MALAG'MA. A plaster employed and described by Celsus.
CUBA, see Havana.
CUBAL SINI, Piper cubeba.
CUBATIO, Decubitus.
CUBEBA, Piper Cubeba.
CUBIFORMIS, Cuboid.
CUBIT, Ulna—c. Top of the, Olecranon.
CU'BITAL, *Cubita'lis, Ulnar, Ulna'ris.* Connected with or relating to the *cubitus,* or to the inner and posterior part of the forearm.

CUBITAL ARTERY, *Arte'ria cubita'lis, A. ulna'ris,* arises from the humeral a little below the bend of the elbow; proceeds along the anterior and inner part of the forearm; passes anterior to the ligamentum annulare of the carpus, and goes to form, in the palm of the hand, the superficial palmar arch. Besides the numerous muscular branches, which it gives off in its course, it sends posteriorly the common trunk of the *interosseous arteries,* and internally, the two *cubital recurrents, anterior* and *posterior,*—articular branches, which anastomose on the inside of the elbow with the divisions of the humeral artery.

CUBITAL MUSCLES are two in number. 1. The *Cubita'lis ante'rior, C. inter'nus, Flexor carpi ulna'ris, Ulna'ris inter'nus, Epitrochli-cubito-carpien, Cubito-carpien* — (Ch.), is a long muscle, situate at the anterior and inner part of the forearm. It arises from the inner condyle of the os humeri, at the inner side of the olecranon, and from the posterior edge of the ulna, and is inserted by a tendon into the os pisiforme. Its use is to bend the hand on the forearm, by directing it slightly inwards. 2. The *Cubitalis poste'rior* seu *exter'nus, Exten'sor Carpi ulna'ris, Ulna'ris exter'nus, Cubite'us exter'nus, Cubito-sus-métacarpien*—(Ch.), is situate at the posterior part of the forearm. It arises from the external condyle of the os humeri, and is inserted into the superior extremity of the fifth bone of the metacarpus. Its use is to extend the hand, inclining it a little inwards.

CUBITAL NERVE, *Ulnar nerve, Cubito-digital*—(Ch.), is furnished by the last two or three nerves of the brachial plexus, and is distributed to the inner and anterior side of the forearm; to the inner part of the palm and of the back of the hand, and to the last two or three fingers.

CUBITAL VEINS, DEEP-SEATED, and the *Recurrent cubital veins,* accompany the corresponding arteries. The superficial cubital veins belong to the basilic. Chaussier calls them *cuta'neous cubital.*

CUBITALE (OS), Cuneiform bone.
CUBITALIS RIOLANI, see Anconeus.
CUBITEUS EXTERNUS, see Cubital muscles.
CUBITO-CARPIEN, see Cubital muscles—*c. Cutané (nerf),* Cutaneous nerve — *c. Phalangettien commun,* Flexor profundus perforans — *c. Radi-sus-métacarpien du pouce,* Abductor longus pollicis—*c. Radial,* Pronator radii quadratus.
CUBITO-SUPRAPALMA'RIS. Belonging to the cubitus and to the supra-palmar or dorsal surface of the hand. Chaussier gives this name: 1. To a small artery, which is given off by the cubital or ulnar, a little above the wrist. 2. To a vein, which accompanies this artery.

CUBITO-SUS-MÉTACARPIEN, see Cubital muscles—*c. Sus-métacarpien du pouce,* Abductor longus pollicis — *c. Sus-Phalangettien de l'index,* Extensor proprius indicis — *c. Sus-phalangettien du pouce,* E. longus pollicis — *c. Sus-phalangien du pouce,* E. pollicis brevis.

CU'BITUS, κυβιτον, *Cy'biton.* The *Elbow.* Also, one of the bones of the forearm. See Ulna, and Forearm.

CUBITUS, (F.) *Coudée,* the ancient name of a measure 18 inches long.
CUBITUS SUPINUS, see Decubitus.
CU'BOID, *Cuboï'des, Cuboï'deus, Cubo'des, Cubifor'mis, Cyboï'des, Cyrtoï'des, Grandino'sum Os, Tes'sara, Tesseræ os, Os va'rium,* from κυβος, 'a cube,' and ειδος, 'form.' Having the form of a cube. This name was given, by Galen, to one of the bones of the tarsus, and is still retained. It is situate at the anterior and outer part of the tarsus; and is articulated, *behind,* with the calcaneum; *before,* with the last two metatarsal bones, and *within,* with the third os cuneiforme, and sometimes with the scaphoides. Its inferior surface has an oblique groove for the tendon of the *peroneus longus.*

CUCKOO FLOWER, Cardamine pratensis.
CUCKOW BREAD, Oxalis acetosella.
CUCKOW PINT, Arum maculatum.
CUCU'BALUS BEHEN, *Behen officina'rum* seu *vulga'ris, Sile'nè infla'ta* seu *crassifo'lia* seu *Tho'rei, Visca'go behen.* This plant was once considered alexipharmic and cordial. It is the *Spatling Poppy.*
CUCULLARIS, Trapezius.
CUCULA'TUM MAJUS. A barbarous term, used by Ruland, for brandy and spirit of wine.
CUCULLATA, Sanicula.
CUCULLUS, *Couvrechef,* Cucupha, Infundibulum of the cochlea.
CUCULUS, Coccyx, Pertussis.
CUCUMBER, Cucumis sativus — c. Indian, Medeola Virginica—c. Squirting or wild, Momordica elaterium—c. Star, one-seeded, Sycios angulatus—c. Tree, Magnolia acuminata.
CUCUMER, Cucumis sativus.
CUCUMIS, Penis — c. Agrestis, Momordica elaterium.
CU'CUMIS COLOCYN'THIS, *Citrul'lus Colocynthis.* Officinal names of the *Colocynth* or *Bitter Apple, Colocyn'thin, Coloquint'ida, Alhan'dal* (Arab.), *Bitter Gourd, Bitter Cucumber,* (F.) *Coloquinte.* Family, Cucurbitaceæ. *Sex. Syst.* Monœcia Monadelphia. A Turkey and Cape of Good Hope plant. The spongy part or medulla of the fruit, *Colocyn'thidis Pulpa, Cucu'meris Colocyn'thidis Pulpa,* has a bitter, nauseous, and acrime-

nious taste, and is a strong cathartic, acting chiefly on the upper part of the intestines. It is scarcely ever used, except in combination.

CUCUMIS MELO. The sytematic name of the *Melon Plant, Melo, Common Melon,* (F.) *Melon.* The fruit is an agreeable article of diet, but not very digestible, unless when ripe. The seeds possess mucilaginous properties.

CUCUMIS SATI'VUS. The systematic name of the *Cu'cumber plant, Cucumis, Angou'rion, Citre'olus, Cu'cumer* or *Cur'vimer,* from its curved shape. (F.) *Concombre ordinaire.* The cucumber is used, when young, as a pickle, when it is called a *Gherkin,* (F.) *Cornichon.* It is not a fruit easy of digestion. The seeds are mucilaginous.

CUCUMIS SYLVESTRIS, Momordica elaterium.

CU'CUPHA, *Cu'cullus, Pi'leus, Sac'culus cephal'icus.* A sort of coif or cap, with a double bottom, between which is enclosed a mixture of aromatic powders, having cotton for an excipient. It was formerly used as a powerful cephalic.

CUCUR'BITA, *à curvitate,* owing to its shape. A gourd. See Cupping-glass.

CUCURBITA ANGURIA, C. citrullus.

CUCUR'BITA CITRUL'LUS, *C. Angu'ria* seu *pinnatif'ida.* The systematic name of the *Watermelon plant; Citrul'lus, Angu'ria, Tetrangu'ria, Sicilian Citrul, Water-melon.* Family, Cucurbitaceæ; *Sex. Syst.* Monœcia Monadelphia. (F.) *Melon d'eau, Pastèque.* The juice of the fruit is very abundant, whence its name. The *Watermelon* is extremely refreshing and agreeable, when made cool, and is eaten like the common melon. It is very much used in the United States.

CUCURBITA LEUCANTHA, C. lagenaria.

CUCUR'BITA PEPO, *Pepo.* The systematic name of the *Common Pompion, Oucur'bita.* The seeds of this plant, as well as those of *Cucur'bita lagena'ria, Bottle-gourd,* contain a large proportion of oil, capable of forming emulsions; but they are not used.

Both the fruit of CUCUR'BITA LAGENA'RIA, *C. leucan'tha, Pepo lagena'rius,* (F.) *Calebasses,* and that of CUCUR'BITA PEPO, *Pepo vulga'ris,* (F.) *Potiron, Courge,* are eaten.

CUCURBITA PINNATIFIDA, C. citrullus.

CUCURBITAIN, Cucurbitinus.

CUCURBITATIO, Cupping.

CUCURBITE, see Alembic.

CUCURBITI'NUS, (F.) *Oucurbitain.* This name was formerly given to the *Tænia solium,* because composed of rings which resemble the seeds of the *gourd,*—*cucurbita.* The ancients believed, that the rings, which are sometimes discharged, were so many separate worms. See Tænia.

CUCURBITULA, Cupping-glass.

CUCURBITULÆ CRUENTÆ, Cupping with the scarificator—c. cum Ferro, Cupping with the scarificator—c. Siccæ, Cupping, dry.

CUDWEED, Gnaphalium margaritaceum.

CUILLERÉE, Cochleare.

CUIR, Corium.

CUISSART. A wooden leg. See Cornu ammonis.

CUISSE, Thigh, Crus — *c. Postérieure du cervelet,* Corpus restiforme.

CUISSON, (F.) A smarting, burning pain.

CUIVRE, Cuprum — *c. Ammoniacal,* Cuprum ammoniatum — *c. et Ammoniaque sulfate de,* Cuprum ammoniatum — *c. Limailles de,* see Cuprum — *c. Sous-acétate de,* Cupri subacetas — *c. Sulfate de,* Cupri sulphas.

CUIVREUX, (F.) *Copper-coloured,* (F.) *Teint cuivreux.* A copper-coloured complexion, such as is observed in cancerous affections. Syphilitic ulcers of the throat, &c., are often copper-coloured.

CUJETE, Crescentia cujete.

CULBIC"IO. A Latin word, employed by old writers as synonymous with ardor urinæ and gonorrhœa.

CULBUTE, (F.) 'A tumble head-over-heels.' A movement which the fœtus has been supposed to execute at the end of the 7th month of utero-gestation; and by means of which, it was presumed, the head presented towards the orifice of the uterus; a change of situation, which is impracticable in ordinary circumstances.

CULCITA SALINA, Halotyle.

CULEON, Anus.

CU'LEUS. A measure containing 20 barrels, or 40 urns, equal to 180 gallons.—Pliny, Gorræus.

CULEX, (F.) *Cousin.* A genus of insects, unhappily too well known in almost every part of the world, on account of their bites, which give rise to painful, local inflammation. The *gnats* and *musquitoes* belong to this genus.

CULI FLOS, Cardamine pratensis.

CULILAWAN, see Laurus culilawan.

CU'LINARY ART, from *culina,* 'a kitchen.' Cookery, *Res culina'ria, Res coqua'ria, Ars culina'ria, A. coquina'ria, Magei'ricê.* The art of preparing meats for the table. In judging of the dietetic properties of various kinds of aliment, the culinary process to which they have been subjected will always have to be considered. Many of the writers on the culinary art have been physicians.

CULLITLAWAN, see Laurus culilawan.

CULMINATIO, Acme.

CULTELLAIRE, (F.) from *cultellus,* a 'little knife.' *Le cautère cultellaire,* known also under the name *Couteau de feu, Fire-knife,* is used for what the French term the *Cautère transcurrente.* (See Cauterization.) It is shaped like a small hatchet.

CULTELLUS, Culter, Knife—c. Anceps, Knife, double-edged—c. Uncus, Knife, crotchet.

CULTER, *Cultel'lus,* from *colo, cultum,* 'I cultivate.' A *coulter,* a *knife, scalpel, machæ'ra, machæ'rion, machæ'ris.* Also, the third lobe of the liver, so called from some fancied resemblance. —Theophilus Protospatarius.

CULTER CURVUS, Knife, crooked—c. Falcatus, Knife, crooked—c. Lenticularis, Knife, lenticular —c. Rectus, Knife, amputation—c. Tonsorius, Razor.

CULTRIV'OROUS, *Cultriv'orus,* from *culter,* 'a knife,' and *vorare,* 'to devour.' Individuals, who have seemed to swallow knives with impunity, have been so called;—*Knife-eaters.*

CULUS, Anus.

CULVER'S ROOT, Leptandra purpurea.

CUMAMUS, Piper cubeba.

CUMIN, Cuminum cyminum — *c. des Prés,* Carum.

CUMI'NUM CYMI'NUM. The systematic name of the *Cummin plant, Cumi'num minu'tum* seu *Roma'num, Cymi'num, Cumi'num, Carnaba'dium.* Family, Umbelliferæ. *Sex. Syst.* Pentandria Digynia. (F.) *Cumin, Anis aigre.* The seeds of cummin, which is a native of Egypt, have a warm, bitterish, disagreeble taste. Water extracts their odour, and spirit takes up both odour and taste. They are not used, except in a plaster, which bears their name. When drunk in wine, the ancients believed they produced paleness; hence, Horace called cummin *exsangue;* and Juvenal, *pallens.*—Dioscorides, Pliny.

CUMINUM MINUTUM, C. cyminum — c. Nigrum, Nigella — c. Pratense, Carum — c. Romanum, C. cyminum.

CUMMIN, Cuminum cyminum.

CU'MULUS, 'a heap or pile.' A rounded prominence, in the centre of the proligerous disk, in which there is a small opake cavity that contains the ovum. See *Tache embryonnaire.*

CUMULUS, GERMINAL, *Tache embryonnaire*—c. Germinativus, *Tache embryonnaire* — c. Proligerus, *Tache embryonnaire.*

CUNEA'LIS SUTU'RA. The suture formed between the great and little alæ of the sphenoid bone and the os frontis.—Blasius.

CUNÉEN (F.), *Cunea'nus.* Relating to the cuneiform bones.

Articulations Cunéennes; — the joints between the cuneiform bones, as well as between them and other parts.

Ligaments Cunéennes; — the ligaments which hold the cuneiform bones together.

CU'NEIFORM, *Cuneifor'mis, Sphenoi'des,* from *cuneus,* 'a wedge,' and *forma,* 'shape.' *Wedge-shaped.* This name has been given to several bones. 1. To the sphenoid. 2. To a bone of the carpus, situate between the os lunare and os orbiculare. It is, also, called *Os Pyramida'lĕ, Os Triq'uetrum,* and *Os Cubita'lĕ.* 3. To the basilary process of the occipital bone: and, 4. To three of the bones of the tarsus, which are distinguished, according to *situation,* reckoning from within outwards, into *first, second,* and *third,* —or *internal, middle,* and *external:* and according to *size,* reckoning in the same order, into *great, small,* and *middle-sized.* The posterior surface of these bones is united to the anterior face of the scaphoides; the anterior surface with the corresponding metatarsal bones; and, in addition, the external surface of the third is articulated, behind, with the cuboides. They are also called *Chalcoi̇dea* or *Chalcoi̇dea ossic'ula.*

CUNEIFORM CARTILAGES OF THE LARYNX are two small cylinders of fibro-cartilage, about seven lines in length, and enlarged at each extremity. By the base, the cartilage is attached to the middle of the external surface of the arytenoid; and its upper extremity forms a prominence on the border of the aryteno-epiglottidean fold of membrane. They are sometimes wanting.

CU'NEO-CU'BOID, *Cuneo-cuboideus.* Belonging to the cuneiform bones and cuboides.

CUNEO-CUBOID ARTICULA'TION is formed by the third cuneiform bone and cuboides. It is furnished with a synovial capsule, and two *cuneocuboid ligaments:* — a *dorsal* and a *plantar.*

CU'NEO-SCA'PHOID, *Cuneo-scaphoi'des.* Belonging to the cuneiform bones and scaphoid.

CUNEO-SCAPHOID ARTICULA'TION is formed by the posterior surfaces of the three ossa cuneiformia, and the anterior surface of the scaphoid. It is furnished with a synovial capsule and ligaments, some of which are *dorsal,* others *plantar.*

CUNILA, Satureia capitata.— c. Bubula, Origanum.

CUNI'LA MARIA'NA, *Saturei'a organoi'des, Calamin'tha grec'ta Virginia'na, Ditt'any, American Dit'tany, Mountain Dittany, Mint-leaved Cunila, Maryland Cunila, Stonemint, Wild Basil, Sweet Horsemint,* (F.) *Cunile d'Amérique,* A small indigenous herb, growing on dry, shady hills, from New England to Georgia, and flowering in June and July. Its medical properties are dependent upon essential oil, like the mints.

CUNILA, MARYLAND, Cunila mariana—c. Mint-leaved, C. mariana—c. Muscula, Inula dysenterica — c. Pulegioides, Hedeoma pulegioides — c. Sativa, Satureia hortensis.

CUNILAGO, Inula dysenterica.

CUNILE D'AMÉRIQUE, Cunila mariana.

CUNNUS, Vulva.

CUP, *Scutel'la, Catil'lus, Patel'la, Excip'ula,* (F.) *Palette, Poëlette, Poïlette, Vase à saigner.* A small vessel of a determinate size, for receiving the blood during venesection. It generally contains about four ounces. A bleeding of two cups is, consequently, one of eight ounces.

CUPIDITAS, Voluntas — c. Desedendi, Voluntas desedendi.

CUPIDO, Appetite. Also, Cupid, the god of love, in ancient mythology;—*Deus copulatio'nis.*

CUPOLA, see Infundibulum of the cochlea.

CUPPED, see Corium phlogisticum.

CUPPING, *Catacasm'us,* from (F.) *couper,* 'to cut;' or to draw blood in vessels resembling *cups; Applica'tio cucurbita'rum seu cucurbitula'rum, Cucurbita'tio.* A species of blood-letting, performed by a *scarificator,* and glass, called a cupping-glass, *Cucurbit'ula, Cucurb'ita, Sic'ua,* (F.) *Ventouse.* The lancets are placed in such a manner in the scarificator, that, when it is applied upon the affected part, the whole are, by means of a spring, pushed suddenly into it. After scarification, the cupping-glass, which has been previously exhausted by heat, or by an exhausting syringe, is applied. The pressure of the air within the glass being thus diminished, the necessary quantity of blood may be drawn. See Bdellometer. *Dry cupping, Cucurbit'ula sicca,* is the application of the glasses, without previous scarification. (F.) *Ventouses sèches.* It is used to prevent the activity of absorption from any wounded part; occasionally, to excite suppuration in indolent abscesses; and to remove the pus when an abscess is opened. *Cupping,* taken without any epithet, means the abstraction of blood by means of the scarificator and cups:— (F.) *Ventouses scarifiées,* (L.) *Cucurbitula cruentæ, C. cum Ferro.* The verb 'to cup,' signifies to draw blood by cupping.

CUP-PLANT, Silphium perfoliatum.

CUPRESSUS, C. sempervirens—c. Arbor vitæ, Thuya occidentalis.

CUPRESS'US SEMPERVI'RENS, *C. pyramida'lis.* The systematic name of the *Cupres'sus, Cyparis'sus, Cypress,* (F.) *Cyprès.* The berries, leaves, and wood, have been considered astringent and useful in intermittents. The whole plant abounds with a bitter, aromatic, and terebinthinate fluid.

CUPRI AMMONIO-SULPHAS, Cuprum ammoniatum—c. et Ammoniæ sulphas, Cuprum ammoniatum—c. Diäcetas, C. subacetas.

CUPRI LIMATU'RA, *Filings of Copper,* (F.) *Limailles de Cuivre,* have been used in hydrophobia. It has been remarked under *Cuprum,* that they are inert.

CUPRI RUBIGO, Cupri subacetas.

CUPRI SUBACE'TAS, *C. Diace'tas, Æru'go, Ver'digris, Hispan'icum vir'idĕ, Prasi'num viridĕ, Cupri Rubi'go, Crystals of Venus, Vir'idĕ Æ'ris. Æru'ca, Cal'cithos, Subac''etate of Copper,* (F.) *Sous-acétate de Cuivre, Vert-de-gris, Crystaux de Vénus, Verdet.* Impure subacetate of copper. This, as usually met with, is in masses, difficult to break; not deliquescent; foliaceous; of a fine bluish-green colour, and salt taste. It is tonic, emetic, escharotic, and detergent; but scarcely ever employed internally. Chiefly used in detergent ointments. Dose, as a tonic, under ½ gr.: emetic, from gr. j to gr. ij. Powdered verdigris appears to be the active ingredient in *Smellome's Eye-salve,* which may be imitated by rubbing half a drachm of finely powdered verdigris with a little oil, and then mixing it with an ounce of yellow basilicon.

An ointment composed of one drachm of finely powdered verdigris, with an ounce of lard or spermaceti ointment, is used in psoriasis, tetter, &c.

CUPRI SULPHAS, *Vitriolum Cupri, Vitriolum Ven'eris, V. Cyp'rium, V. Cyp'rinum, V. Cæru'-*

iewn, V. *Roma'num, Cuprum Vitriola'tum, Lapis Caru'leus, Sulphate of Copper, Blue Stone, Blue Vitriol, Roman Vitriol, Mortooth*, (F.) *Sulfate de Cuivre*, is in rhomboidal, rich, blue, semi-transparent, efflorescing crystals. The taste is harsh, styptic, and corrosive. It is soluble in four parts of water at 60°, and is tonic, emetic, astringent, and escharotic. As a tonic, it has been used in epilepsy, intermittents, &c. Dose, as a tonic, gr. ¼ to gr. ij, in pill; as an emetic, gr. ij to x, in water. A very weak solution is sometimes used in ophthalmia and in gleet; and it forms the basis of BATES's *Aqua camphora'ta*, which has been recommended, diluted with sixteen parts of water, in the purulent ophthalmia of children.

CUPRI SULPHAS AMMONIACALIS, Cuprum ammoniatum—c. Vitriolum, Cupri sulphas.

CUPRUM, *Chalcos, Æs, Venus* of the Alchymists: *Copper, Cyp'rium, Vir'idē monta'num*, (F.) *Cuivre*. Its odour is peculiar and sensible when rubbed; taste disagreeable and metallic; colour red-yellow. S. g. 7.87; ductile; very malleable; less hard than iron; easily oxidised. In its metallic state, it exerts no action on the system. When swallowed, it undergoes no deleterious change. Copper cannot be dissolved whilst tin is in the mixture, and hence the utility of tinning copper vessels. Copper culinary vessels are harmless under ordinary cleanliness, provided the substances be not suffered to remain in them till cold. The salts of copper are very deleterious.

CUPRUM AMMONIA'TUM, *C. Ammoniaca'lē, C. Ammoni'acum, C. ammoni'aco-sulphu'ricum, Ammonia'ted Copper, Ammoni'acal Sulphate of Copper, Ammoniure'tum Cupri, Sal anti-epilep'ticus of* WEISSMAN, *Sulfas Cupri ammoniaca'lis, S. ammoni'aca cupra'tus, Sub-sulfas Ammo'nio-cu'pricus, Sulfas Cupri et Ammo'niæ, Deuto-Sulfas Cupri et Ammo'nia, Cupri Ammo'nio-sulphas, Ammo'nia Cupro-sulphas, Ammo'nio-sulphate of Copper*, (F.) *Sulfate de cuivre et d'ammoniaque, Cuivre ammoniacal.* (*Cupri Sulph.* ʒss; *Ammon. Carb.* ʒvj. Rub in a glass mortar till effervescence ceases. Wrap the ammoniated copper in bibulous paper, and dry with a gentle heat. Keep in a well-stopped glass bottle.—Ph. U. S.) A crystalline powder of a rich violet colour, and hot, styptic taste. By exposure to air, it becomes partly converted into carbonate of copper. It is tonic and astringent, and has been chiefly employed in epilepsy and other obstinate spasmodic diseases. Dose, gr. ¼ gradually increased to gr. iv, in pill.

CUPRUM VITRIOLATUM, Cupri sulphas.

CU'PULAR, *Cupula'ris*, (F.) *Cupulaire;* from *cupula*, 'a small cup.' Of or belonging to a cupula.

CUPULAR CAU'TERY, *Cautère cupulaire*, is an iron in the shape of a cupula, formerly used to cauterize the skin of the cranium in certain diseases, as epilepsy, chronic headach, &c.

CURA, *Cura'tio, Merim'na, Merim'nē.* Attention to, or treatment or cure of, a disease. Keuchen defines *Cura*, 'medicine,' and *Curator*, 'the physician.' Curatio, also, sometimes means purification; as, *Adeps suilla curata.*—Scribonius Largus.

CURA AVENA'CEA. A decoction of oats and succory roots, in which a little nitre and sugar are dissolved. Used as a refrigerant.

CURA DERVATIVA, Derivation—c. Fumigatoria, Thymiatechny.

CURA MAGNA. 'Great cure.' A term employed, at times, for a method of treatment preferable to all others. Thus ptyalism has, by many, been considered the "*cura magna*" for syphilis.

CURA MEDIANA, Transfusion—c. Palliativa, see Palliative—c. Radicalis, see Palliative—c. Revulsoria, see Derivation.

CU'RABLE, *Sanab'ilis, Aces'tos, Aces'mius, Ide'imos*, (F.) *Guérissable.* That which is susceptible of cure. An epithet applied to both patients and diseases.

CURARE, *Wourali, Woorara, Wowrari, Wooraru, Wurali, Urari, Urali, Ourary, Voorara.* A very energetic vegetable poison, employed by the South American Indians to poison their arrows. It is said to be obtained from the bark of a species of convolvulus, called *Vejuco de Mavacure*, but is referred by Martius to *Strychnos Guianen'sis*, and by Dr. Schomburg to *S. toxica'na.*

CURA'TIO, *Mede'la, Sana'tio, A'cesis, Althex'is, Althax'is, Therapei'a, Iasis, Curation,* The aggregate of means employed for the cure of disease. See Therapeutics.

CURATIO, Cura, Cure—c. Contrariorum per Contraria, Allopathy—c. Morbi per Inediam, Limotherapeia.

CU'RATIVE, *San'ative, Healing, Acesopho'rus, Acesino'rus.* Relating to the cure of a disease. *Curative Indications* are those which point out the treatment to be employed. *Curative Treatment,* that employed in the cure of disease, in opposition to *preservative* or *prophylactic treatment.* We say, also, *Curative Process, Curative Means,* &c.

CURATOR INFIRMORUM, *Infirmier.*

CURCULIO, Penis.

CURCUMA ANGUSTIFOLIA, see Arrowroot—c. Aromatica, Kæmpferia rotunda.

CURCUMA LONGA, *Cur'cuma, Amo'mum Cur'cuma, Borri, Bor'riberri, Cober'ri,* (Hindoostan,) *Crocus In'dicus, Terra Mer'ita, Cannac'orus radi'cē cro'ceo; Family, Amomeæ; Sex. Syst.* Monandria Monogynia; *Mayel'la, Kua Kaha, Cyp'erus In'dicus,* κυκυρος *Ινδικος* of Dioscorides (?), *Turmeric,* (F.) *Racine de Safran, Safran des Indes, Souchet des Indes.* Turmeric root—the rhizoma of curcuma longa—is brought from the East Indies; but is possessed of very little, if any, medicinal efficacy. It is one of the ingredients in *Curry Powder.*

CURCUMA ZEDOARIA, see Kæmpferia rotunda—c. Zerumbet, see Kæmpferia rotunda.

CURD, ALUM, Coagulum aluminosum.

CURDS, *Curds of Milk,* (F.) *Caillé, Lait caillé.* The coagulated part of milk.

CURE; from *cura,* 'care.' *Aces'ia, A'cesis, Aces'mus, Cura'tio, C. felix, Sana'tio, San'itas,* (F.) *Guérison.* A restoration to health; also, a remedy; a restorative.

CURE-ALL, Geum Virginianum, Œnothera biennis.

CUREDENT, Dentiscalpium.

CURE DU RAISIN, Grape-cure.

CURE-LANGUE, (F.) *Lingua scalpium, Tongue-scraper.* An instrument of ivory, tortoise-shell, &c., shaped like a knife or rasp, for removing the mucous coating which covers the tongue after sleep, &c.

CURE-OREILLE, Ear-pick.

CURETTE, Scoop.

CURMI, Courmi.

CURRANT, BLACK, Ribes nigrum—c. Red, Ribes rubrum.

CURRANTS, see Vitis Corinthiaca.

CURRY or CURRIE POWDER. A condiment, formed of various spices, and eaten with rice, particularly in India. The following is one of the forms of its preparation: *Sem. coriand.* ʒxviij, *pip. nigr.* ʒij, *cayen.* ʒj, *rad. curcumæ, sem. cumini,* āā ʒiij, *sem. fænugr.* ʒiv : mix.

CURSUMA HÆMORRHOIDALIS HERBA, Ranunculus ficaria.

CURSUS, Running—c. Matricis, Leucorrhœa c. Menstruus, Menses.

CURVAMEN, Curvature.

CURVATEUR DU COCCYX, Curvator Coccygis.

CURVATIO, Campsis.

CURVA'TOR COCCY'GIS, (F.) *Ourvateur du Coccyx*. Sömmering gives this name to a small bundle of fleshy fibres, which descends on the middle of the coccyx, uniting on each side with the ischio-coccygei muscles. It is a part of those muscles.

CUR'VATURE, *Ourvatu'ra, Ourva'men, Flexu'ra, Gnamp'sis,* from *curvus,* 'crooked;' *Cyrto'ma,* (F.) *Courbure.* The condition of a line or surface, which approximates more or less to the form of an arc; as the curvatures of the spine, duodenum, stomach, &c. Accidental curvatures of bones are the effect of rickets, or *Mollities ossium.* The Greeks called the curvature of the spine, 'υβος, σκολιος, and λορδος, according as the deviation was backwards, laterally, or forwards.

CURVE OF CARUS, see Pelvis.

CURVED LINES, (F.) *Courbes Lignes.* Two crooked lines or projections on the posterior surface of the occipital bone. They are distinguished into *superior* and *inferior.* Some lines on the os innominatum are also so called.

CURVIMER, Cucumis sativus.

CUSCO-CINCHONIA, Aricina.

CUSCUTA, C. Europæa.

CUSCUTA CHLOROCARPA, see C. Glomerata.

CUSCU'TA EPITH'YMUM, *C. minor.* The systematic name of the *Dodder of Thyme. Epith'ymum, Epith'ymum Cuscu'ta seu Cre'ticum.* A parasitical plant, possessed of a strong, disagreeable smell, and a pungent taste, very durable in the mouth. It was once used as a cathartic in melancholia.

CUSCUTA EUROPÆ'A seu *major* seu *vulga'ris* seu *tetran'dra* seu *filiform'is, Cuscu'ta, Epith'ymum officina'rum,* was conceived to possess similar properties.

CUSCUTA FILIFORMIS, C. Europæa.

CUS'CUTA GLOMERA'TA, and CUSCUTA CHLOROCARPA, *Dodder, Amer'ican Dodder,* indigenous plants, are bitterish, subastringent, tonic, and anti-periodic.

CUSCUTA MAJOR, C. Europæa—c. Minor, C. Epithymum—c. Tetrandra, C. Europæa—c. Vulgaris, C. Europæa.

CUSPARIA BARK, see C. Febrifuge—c. Bark, False, Brucea antidysenterica, and Strychnos nux vomica.

CUSPA'RIA FEBRIF'UGA, *Bonplan'dia trifo'lia'ta* seu *angustu'ra, Angustu'ra, Galipæ'a febrifuga.* Order, Rutaceæ. The South American tree, which furnishes the *Cuspa'ria* or *Angustura Bark,* (F.) *Angusture vraie, Quinquina faux de Virginie.* According to Dr. Hancock, however, the Angustura bark is derived from *Galipæ'a officinalis, Sex. Syst.* Decandria Monogynia, *Nat. Ord.* Diosmeæ; and this view has been adopted in the Pharmacopœia of the United States. Its odour is peculiar; taste intensely bitter and slightly aromatic; pieces thin; externally, gray and wrinkled; internally, yellowish-fawn; fracture, short and resinous. It yields its virtues to water and to proof spirit. It is tonic, stimulant, and aromatic. Dose, gr. v to xx or more, in powder.

CUSPIS. A spear. This name has been given to the glans penis.—Rolfink. It meant, also, a kind of bandage.

CUSTODIA VIRGINITATIS, Hymen.

CUSTOS, Vulva.

CUT, from (F.) *couteau,* 'a knife,' or from West Gothic, *kota,* 'to cut;' or from κεττω, 'I cut.' *Cæsu'ra, Tomē, Incis'io, Vulnus simplex, Tresis vulnus simplex, Copē,* (F.) *Coupure.* A common expression for the division or solution of continuity made by a sharp instrument.

CUTAM'BULUS, from *cutis,* 'skin,' and *ambulo,* 'I walk.' 'Walking in the skin.' An epithet given to certain parasitical animals, which creep under the skin; such as the Guinea-worm; and to certain pains felt between the skin and flesh, as it were.

CUTANEAL, Cutaneous.

CUTANÉO-SOURCILIER, Corrugator supercilii.

CUTA'NEOUS, *Cuta'neal, Cuta'neus,* (F.) *Cutané,* from *cutis,* 'the skin.' Belonging to the skin.

CUTANEOUS DISEASES, *Eruptions, Epiphy'mata,* are the numerous affections of a morbid character to which the skin is liable,—*Dermatopathi'a, Dermato'ses.*

Chronic cutaneous diseases may be thus classified:

1. Exanthematous	Urticaria. Roseola. Erythema.
2. Vesicular	Pemphigus. Rupia. Herpes. Eczema.
3. Pustular	Impetigo. Ecthyma. Scabies. (?)
4. Papular	Lichen. Strophulus. Prurigo.
5. Squamous	Lepra. Psoriasis. Pityriasis.
6. Folliculous	Acne. Sycosis. Ichthyosis. Trichosis. Favus.

CUTANEOUS EXHALATION AND ABSORPTION are those which take place from the skin.

CUTANEOUS, MIDDLE POSTERIOR, see Sciatic nerve, lesser.

CUTANEOUS NERVES, *Cutaneal Nerves,* so called, of the upper extremity, are two in number. They are given off from the brachial plexus. The *internal cutaneous, Cubito-cutané,* (Ch.,) descends along the inner part of the arm, and divides above the elbow into two branches; the outermost of which follows the outer edge of the biceps, and spreads over the anterior and inner part of the forearm; and the innermost accompanies the basilic vein, passing to the corresponding side of the hand and little finger. The *external cutaneous, Radio-cutané* (Ch.,) *Mus'culo-Cuta'neus, Per'forans CASSE'RII,* passes outwards, perforates the coraco-brachialis; descends along the anterior and outer part of the arm; passes as far as the middle fold of the elbow under the median cephalic; and descends along the anterior and outer edge of the forearm. At some distance above the wrist, it divides into two branches; an *outer,* which is distributed on the back of the hand, the thumb and index finger; and an *inner,* which descends on the muscles of the thumb into the palm of the hand, and divides into fine filaments, which may be traced to the fingers.

Cutaneous nerves, Middle cutaneous, two in number, are branches of the crural or femoral nerve. They are distributed to the integument of the middle and lower part of the thigh and of the knee.

Nervus Cutaneus Minor, Lesser internal cutaneous nerve, Nerve of Wrisberg, takes its origin from the axillary plexus, but is more particularly connected with the ulnar nerve. It soon separates from the ulnar, running afterwards between it and the inner side of the arm. A little below the axilla it divides into two branches, which are distributed to the arm.

Chaussier calls the *cephalic* and *basilic veins* the *Radial* and *Cubital Cutaneous.*

CUTCH, Catechu.
CUTI, Catechu.
CUTICULA, Epidermis.
CUTIO, Oniscus.
CUTIS, *Pellis, Pella, Co'rium, Derma, Deris, Anthro'pē, Anthro'pen, Skin,* (F.) *Peau.* A dense, resisting membrane, of a flexible and extensible nature, which forms the general envelope of the body; and is continuous with the mucous membranes, through the different natural apertures. It is generally considered to be formed of three distinct layers — the *epidermis, rete* or more properly *corpus mucosum,* and *corium.* Some anatomists, however, separate it into several others. Its outer surface is covered by a number of small eminences, called papillæ, which are generally regarded as essentially nervous and vascular. The skin is our medium of communication with external bodies. It protects the subjacent parts; is the seat of touch, and through it are exhaled the watery parts of the blood, which are not needed in the nutrition of the body. The state of the skin, as regards heat and dryness, affords useful information in pathological investigations. Its colour, too, requires attention: the paleness of disease is as characteristic as the rosy complexion of health. The colour of the skin varies according to the age, sex, &c. As a general rule, it is finer in the female and child than in the male and adult. In old age it becomes light-coloured, thin, and dry. It likewise varies according to the races, &c.

CUTIS ANSERINA, Horrida cutis — c. Carnosa, Panniculus carnosus — c. Extima, Epidermis — c. Linguæ, see Tongue — c. Suilla, Couenne — c. Summa, Epidermis — c. Tensa Chronica, Induration of the cellular tissue — c. Ultima, Epidermis.

CUTITIS, Cytitis, Erysipelatous inflammation.
CUTTING ON THE GRIPE, see Lithotomy.
CUTTLE FISH, Sepia.
CUTTUBUTH, *Cutubuth, Leucomo'ria, Melanchol'ia errabund'a.* The Arabian physicians gave this name to a species of melancholy, accompanied with so much agitation, that the patients cannot remain tranquil for the space of an hour.

CUURDO CANELLA, Laurus cinnamomum.
CYANODERMIA, Cyanopathy.
CYAN'OGEN, (F.) *Cyanogène;* from κυανος, 'blue,' and γεννάω, 'I generate.' So called from its being an ingredient in Prussian blue. It forms, with oxygen, the cyanic and other acids; with hydrogen, the hydrocyanic acid.

CYANOP'ATHY, *Cyanopathi'a, Cyano'sis, C. cardi'aca, Cyanoder'mia, Acleitro-cardia* (Piorry), *Hæmato-cyano'sis, Kyano'sis, Morbus cæru'leus, Cærulo'sis neonato'rum,* from κυανος, 'blue,' and παθος, 'affection.' (F.) *Cyanose, Maladie bleu, Ictère bleu.* A disease in which the surface of the body is coloured blue. It is often symptomatic, and commonly depends on a direct communication between the cavities of the right and left side of the heart. Such communication does not, however, always occasion the *blue disease,* but it is generally thought that the disease never exists without this state of parts; or without some obstacle to the circulation in the right side of the heart. The blueness does not seem to be owing to the admixture of black and red blood. A child affected with blueness is said to be *cyanosed,* (F.) *Cyanosé.*

CYANOSE, Cyanosis.
CYANOSE, see Cyanosis.
CYANOSIS, Cyanopathy — c. Pulmonalis, Atelectásis pulmonum.

CYANURETUM FERRO-ZINCICUM, Zinci ferro-hydrocyanas.

CYANUS, Centaurea cyanus — c. Ægyptiacus, Nymphæa nelumbo.

CY'ANUS SEG"ETUM, *Bluebottle,* (F.) *Bluet des Moissons, Barbeau, Aubifoin, Casse-Lunettes.* The flowers of this European plant, when distilled with water, have been used in ophthalmia.

CYAR, κυαρ. 'The eye of a needle,' 'a small hole.' The *Meatus audito'rius internus.* See Auditory canal, (internal.)

CYATHIS'CUS, diminutive of κυαθος, 'a bowl.' The concave part of a sound, made like a small spoon, as in the case of the ear-pick.

CY'ATHUS, 'a bowl.' A measure, both of the liquid and dry kind, equal to about an ounce and a half, or to the tenth part of a pint. According to Pliny and Galen, about 10 drachms.

CYATHUS CEREBRI, Infundibulum of the brain.
CYBE, Head.
CYBITON, Cubitus.
CYBOIDES, Cuboid.
CYCAS CIRCINALIS, see Sago — c. Revoluta, see Sago.

CYC'EON, from κυκαω, 'I mix together.' The ancient name of a medicine of the consistence of pap, composed of wine, water, honey, flour, barley meal, and cheese. — Hippocrates.

CYC'LAMEN EUROPÆ'UM, *Arthani'ta, A. cyc'lamen, Cyclam'inus, Cyssan'themon, Cyocophyl'lon, Panis porci'nus, Cas'amum, Ckyli'nā,* 'sow-bread.' *Fam.* Primulaceæ. *Sex. Syst.* Pentandria Monogynia. (F.) *Pain du Porceau.* The fresh root is said to be acrid, bitter, drastic, and anthelmintic. Dose, ʒj. For external use, see Arthanita.

CYCLE, *Cyclus,* from κυκλος, 'a circle.' A period or revolution of a certain number of years or days. The Methodists gave this name to an aggregate of curative means, continued during a certain number of days. Nine was the usual number.

CYCLE, HEBDOM'ADAL or HEPTAL. A period of seven days or years, which, according to some, either in its multiple or submultiple, governs an immense number of phenomena of animal life.

CYCLISCUS, Cyclismus.
CYCLIS'MUS. A *Troch, Trochis'cus.* The name, as well as *Cyclis'cus,* was also given to a circular kind of rasp. They have the same etymon as cycle.

CYCLOCEPH'ALUS, from κυκλος, 'a circle,' and κεφαλη, 'head.' A monster whose eyes are in contact, or united in one.

CYCLOPHOR'IA, from κυκλος, 'a circle,' and φερω, 'I bear.' The circulation of the blood or other fluids.

CYCLO'PIA. Same etymon as *Cyclops.* State of a monster that has both eyes united into one. Called, also, *Monops'ia* and *Rhinencephal'ia.*

CYCLOPIA GENISTOI'DES; *Nat. Ord.* Leguminosæ. A South African plant, the decoction and infusion of which are used as expectorants in chronic bronchitis and in phthisis.

CYCLOPS, κυκλωψ, from κυκλος, 'an orb or circle,' and ωψ, 'an eye.' *Monoc'ulus, Monops, Monophthal'mus, Monom'matus, Unioc'ulus, Unoc'ulus.* A monster having but one eye, and that placed in the middle of the forehead, like the fabulous Cyclops.

CYCLOTOME, Cyclot'omus, from κυκλος, 'a circle,' and τεμνειν, 'to cut.' An instrument, composed of a ring of gold and a cutting blade, by means of which the ball of the eye can be fixed, whilst the cornea is cut. It was invented by a surgeon of Bordeaux, named Guérin, for extracting the cataract. It is not used.

CYCLUS, Circulus.

CYDONIA, Pyrus cydonia — c. Maliformis, Pyrus cydonia—c. Vulgaris, Pyrus cydonia.
CYDONIA'TUM, *Cydona'tum, Dyacydonites.* A composition of the *Cydonia mala* or quinces, with the addition of spices.—Paulus of Ægina.
CYDONIUM MALUM, see Pyrus cydonia.
CYE'MA, κυημα, from κυω, 'I conceive.' *Conception.* Likewise the product of conception. See Embryo and Fœtus.
CYESIOGNO'MON, from κυησις, 'pregnancy,' and γνωμων, 'a sign, a token.' A sign of pregnancy.
CYESIOGNO'SIS, from κυησις, 'pregnancy,' and γνωσις, 'knowledge.' Diagnosis of pregnancy.
CYESIOL'OGY, *Cyesiolog''ia,* from κυησις, 'pregnancy,' and λογος, 'a description.' The doctrine of gestation.
CYESIS, Conception, Fecundation, Pregnancy.
CYESTEINE, Kiesteine.
CYLICH'NE, *Cylichnis.* A pill-box or earthenware pot, or small cup; from κυλιξ, 'a cup.' — Galen, Foësius.
CYLINDRI, see Villous membranes—c. Membranacei renum, see Calix.
CYL'INDROID, *Cylindroï'des,* from κυλινδρος, 'cylinder,' and ειδος, 'form.' Having the form of a cylinder. Chaussier calls the Cornu Ammonis, *Protubérance cylindroïde.*
CYLINDROIDES, Teres.
CYLLOEPUS, see Kyllosis.
CYLLOPODA, see Kyllosis.
CYLLOPODION, see Kyllosis.
CYLLO'SIS, κυλλωσις. Lameness, mutilation, or vicious conformation. — Hippocrates, Galen. See Kyllosis.
CYLLOSMUS; from κυλλος, 'crooked.' A malformation by defect, in which the fissure and eventration are lateral, chiefly in the lower part of the abdomen, the inferior extremity of the side affected with the fissure absent, or very little developed.—Vogel.
CYMATO'DES, *Undo'sus,* from κυμα, 'a wave,' and ειδος, 'resemblance.' The vacillating, undulatory character of the pulse in weak individuals.
CYMBA, Vulva.
CYMBALARIA ELATINE, Antirhinum elatine—c. Muralis, Antirhinum linaria.
CYMBALARIS, Cricoid.
CYMBIFORME OS, Scaphoid bone.
CYMBOPOGON SCHŒNANTHUS, Juncus odoratus.
CYMINUM, Cuminum cyminum.
CYNAN'CHĒ, *Angi'na,* from κυων, 'a dog,' and αγχω, 'I suffocate' (?), *Sore Throat, Paracynan'chē, Synan'chē, Prunel'la, Squinan'thia, Empres'ma Paristhmi'tis, Cauma Paristhmi'tis, Isthmi'tis, Paristhmi'tis, Inflammatio Fau'cium, 'Dog choak.'* Inflammation of the supradiaphragmatic portion of the alimentary canal, and of the lining membrane of the upper part of the air-passages:—(F.) *Angine, Esquinancie, Mal de Gorge, Synancie, Squinancie, Kinancie.* It comprises the following chief varieties.
CYNANCHE EPIDEMICA, Cynanche maligna—c. Externa, C. Parotidæa—c. Faucium, C. tonsillaris—c. Gangrænosa, Cynanche maligna—c. Laryngea, Laryngitis.
CYNANCHE MALIG'NA, *C. gangræno'sa, Angi'na ulcero'sa, Febris epidem'ica cum Angi'nâ, Empres'ma Paristhmi'tis Malig'na, Tonsilla'rum gangræ'na, Tonsil'læ pestilen'tes, Cynanchē epidem'ica, C. pur'puro-parotidæ'a, Cynanchē ulcero'sa, Epidem'ica gutturis lues, Pestilens fau'cium affec'tus, Pædan'chonē* (?)*, Gangræna Tonsilla'rum, Ulcus Syriacum, Garrotil'lo, Carbun'culus angino'sus, Angina ulcusculo'sa, A. epidem'ica, A. gangræno'sa, A. malig'na, A. fau'cium malig'na, Isthmoty'phus, Putrid, Ulcerous Sore Throat, Gangrenous Inflammation of the Pharynx,* (F.) *Angine gangréneuse, A. Maligne.* It is characterized by crimson redness of the mucous membrane of the fauces and tonsils; ulcerations, covered with mucus, and spreading sloughs, of an ash or whitish hue; the accompanying fever typhus. It is often epidemic, and generally contagious; and is frequently found accompanying scarlet fever,—giving rise to the variety, *Scarlatina maligna.* Cynanche maligna has been made to include both diphtheritic and gangrenous pharyngitis. See Pharyngitis, diphtheritic.
The general treatment is the same as in typhus; and stimulant antiseptic gargles must be used, consisting, for example, of the decoction of bark and muriatic acid.
CYNANCHE MAXILLARIS, c. Parotidæa—c. Œsophagea, Œsophagitis.
CYNANCHE PAROTIDÆ'A, *Empres'ma Paroti'tis, Parotitis, P. epidem'ica, P. erysipelato'sa, P. contagio'sa, P. spu'ria, P. sero'so-glu'tinē tu'mens, Parot'ia, Parotidi'tis, Cynan'chē Parotides, C. exter'na, Angina maxilla'ris, Gissa, Angina externa, Angi'na parotidæ'a exter'na, Erythrochœ'ras, Cynan'chē maxilla'ris, Genyocynan'chē, Gnathocynan'chē, Inflamma'tio paro'tidum, Infla'tio paro'tidum, Catar'rhus Bellinsula'nus, Branks* (Scotch), *Mumps,* (F.) *Inflammation de la Parotide, Oreillons, Ourles.* The characteristic symptoms are :—a painful tumour of the parotid gland, or of the cellular tissue surrounding it, or of both, not of the suppurative kind; frequently extending to the maxillary gland. It is very conspicuous externally, and is often accompanied with swelling of the testes in the male, and of the mammæ in the female; the testes being sometimes absorbed afterwards. It is generally epidemic, and apparently contagious. (?) The treatment is very simple; the adoption merely of the antiphlogistic plan, under which it usually soon disappears. When inflammation of the mammæ or testes supervenes, it must be treated as if idiopathic.
Epidem'ic Paroti'tis or *Mumps* is also termed *Paroti'tis polymor'pha, P. epidem'ica, P. specif'ica.*
CYNANCHE PHARYNGE'A, *Empres'ma Paristhmi'tis Pharyngea, Isthmi'tis, Pharyngi'tis, Inflamma'tio Pharyn'gis, Parasynan'chē, Angina inflammatoriæ, Sp. iv.*—(Boerhaave.) (F.) *Angine Pharyngée, Catarrhe pharyngien.* Inflammation of the pharynx.
This disease can hardly be said to differ, in pathology or treatment, from Cynanche tonsillaris. The same may be remarked of the *Cynanchē Œsophage'a, Œsophagi'tis.*
CYNANCHE PRUNELLA, C. Tonsillaris—c. Purpuro-parotidæa, Cynanche maligna—c. Simplex, Isthmitis—c. Stridula, C. trachealis.
CYNANCHE TONSILLA'RIS, *Empresma Paristhmi'tis Tonsilla'ris, Synan'chē, Cynan'chē faucium Amygdali'tis, Branci, Branchi, Hyan'chē, Tonsilli'tis, Cynanchē Prunel'la, Paristh'mia, Paristhmi'tis, Dyepha'gia inflammato'ria, Antiadi'tis, Angina inflammato'ria, A. cum tumo'rē, A. tonsilla'ris, A. Synocha'lis, A. Sanguin'ea, A. vera et legit'ima, Inflamma'tio Tonsilla'rum, Antiadon' cus inflammato'rius, Inflammatory Sore Throat, Common Squinancy, Squinsy or Quinsy,* (F.) *Amygdalite, Inflammation des Amygdales, Angine tonsillaire, Pharyngite tonsillaire, Esquinancie, Squinancie, Catarrhe guttural, Angine gutturale inflammatoire.* The characteristic symptoms of this affection are, swelling and florid redness of the mucous membrane of the fauces, and especially of the tonsils; painful and impeded deglutition, accompanied with inflammatory fever. It is generally ascribed to cold, and is one of the most common affections of cold and

temperate climates. It usually goes off by resolution, but frequently ends in suppuration.

Common sore throat is an affection of no consequence. It requires merely rest, and the observance of the antiphlogistic regimen. When more violent,—in addition to this,—bleeding, local or general, or both,—purgatives, inhalation of the steam of warm water; acid, or emollient gargles; rubefacients externally, or sinapisms or blisters. When suppuration must inevitably occur, the continued use of the inhaler must be advised, and an opening be made into the abscess as soon as pus shall have formed. If the patient be likely to be suffocated by the tumefaction, bronchotomy may be necessary.

CYNANCHE TRACHEA'LIS; the *Cynanche laryngea* of some, *Suffoca'tio strid'ula, Angi'na pernicio'sa, Asthma infan'tum, Cynanche strid'ula, Catar'rhus suffocati'vus Barbaden'sis, Angina polypo'sa sive membrana'cea sive pulpo'sa, Empresma Bronchi'tis, E. Bronchlemmi'tis, Angina inflammato'ria, A. suffocato'ria, A. strepito'sa, Angina canina, A. exsudato'ria, Laryngi'tis et Trachei'tis infan'tilis, Laryngos'tasis seu Laryngo-trachei'tis, Laryngo-tracheitis with diphtherit'ic exuda'tion, Laryngoc'acè, Orthopnœ'a cynan'chica, Cynanchorthopnœ'a, Pædanchonè (?), A. Trachea'lis, Morbus Strangulato'rius, Trachi'tis, Trachei'tis, Tracheli'tis, Diphtheri'tis trachea'lis, Expectora'tio Sol'ida, Cauma Bronchi'tis, Oroup, Roup, Hives, Choak, Stuffing, Rising of the lights*, (F.) *Angine laryngée et trachéale, Laryngite avec production de fausses membranes, Laryngite pseudo-membraneuse.* A disease characterized by sonorous and suffocative breathing; harsh voice; cough, ringing, or like the barking of a dog; fever, highly inflammatory. It is apt to be speedily attended with the formation of a false membrane, which lines the trachea beneath the glottis, and occasions violent dyspnœa and suffocation, but is sometimes expectorated. The dyspnœa, as in all other affections of the air-passages, has evident exacerbations. It differs in its character in different situations; being infinitely more inflammatory in some places than in others, and hence the success obtained by different modes of treatment. It chiefly affects children, and is apt to recur, but the subsequent attacks are usually less and less severe.

As a general rule, it requires the most active treatment; bleeding from the arm or neck, so as to induce paleness; leeches applied to the neck, &c., according to the age,—the warm bath, blisters to the neck or chest, and purgatives. Formidable as the disease may be, if this plan be followed *early*, it will generally be successful. Many specifics have been recommended, but the search has been idle and fruitless. The majority of cases of what are called croup are not of this inflammatory cast; but are more of a spasmodic character, and have been termed by the French *faux croups*, and with us are occasionally termed *spasmodic croup*. They generally yield to an emetic and the warm bath.

CYNANCHE TRACHEALIS SPASMODICA, Asthma acutum, A. Thymicum — c. Ulcerosa, Cynanche maligna.

CYNAN'CHICA. Medicines used in cases of quinsy were formerly so called.

CYANCHORTHOPNŒA, Cynanche trachealis.

CYNAN'CHUM. Same etymon. A genus of plants, *Nat. Ord.* Asclepiadaceæ, of which the following are used in medicine.

CYNANCHUM ARGEL, C. oleæfolium—c. Ipecacuanha, Asclepias asthmatica.

CYNANCHUM MONSPELIACUM, *Scam'mony of Montpellier.* The plant furnishes a blackish kind of gum-resin, which is purgative, and but little used.

CYNANCHUM OLEÆFO'LIUM, *C. argel, Solenostem'ma argel, Argel.* An Egyptian, Nubian and Arabian shrub, the leaves of which form a portion of most samples of Alexandrian senna. They resemble senna in their action.

CYNANCHUM VINCETOXICUM, Asclepias vincetoxicum.

CYNANCHUM VOMITO'RIUM, *Ipecacuan'ha of the Isle of France.* As its name imports, this plant resembles ipecacuanha in properties. It is emetic, in the dose of from 12 to 24 grains of the powder.

CYNANTHEMIS, Anthemis cotula.

CYNANTHRO'PIA, from κυων, 'dog,' and ανθρωπος, 'man.' A variety of melancholia, in which the patient believes himself changed into a dog; and imitates the voice and habits of that animal.

CYN'ARA, *C. Scol'ymus, Cin'ara scol'ymus.* The systematic name of the *Ar'tichoke, Alcoc'alum, Articoc'alus, Artiscoc'cus lævis, Costus nigra, Car'duus sati'vus non spino'sus, Cinara horten'sis, Scolymus sati'vus, Car'duus sativus, Carduus domest'icus cap'itĕ majo'rĕ, Carduus al'tilis,* (F.) *Artichaut.* Family, Carduaceæ. *Sex. Syst.* Syngenesia Polygamia æqualis. Indigenous in the southern parts of Europe. Much used as an agreeable article of diet. The juice of the leaves, mixed with white wine, has been given in dropsies.

CYN'ICUS, *Cyno'des,* from κυων, 'a dog.' *Cynic.* Relating to, or resembling a dog. *Cynic spasm* is a convulsive contraction of the muscles of one side of the face,—dragging the eye, cheek, mouth, nose, &c., to one side. See Canine.

CYNIPS QUERCÛS FOLII, see Quercus infectoria.

CYNOCOPRUS, Album græcum.
CYNOCRAMBE, Mercurialis perennis.
CYNOCTONON, Aconitum.
CYNOCYTISUS, Rosa canina.
CYNODEC'TOS, from κυων, 'a dog,' and δηκω, 'I bite.' One who has been bitten by a dog.—Dioscorides.
CYNODES, Cynicus.
CYNODESMION, Frænum penis.
CYNODESMUS, Frænum penis.
CYNODONTES, Canine teeth.
CYNOGLOS'SUM, from κυων, 'a dog,' and γλωσσα, 'a tongue.' *Cynoglos'sum officina'lĕ* seu *bi'color, Lingua Cani'na, Hound's tongue, Caballa'tion,* (F.) *Langue de Chien.* Family, Boragineæ. *Sex. Syst.* Pentandria Monogynia. It is aromatic and mucilaginous, and has been supposed to be possessed of narcotic properties.

CYNOLOPHOI, Spinous processes of the vertebræ.

CYNOLYSSA, Hydrophobia.
CYNOMETRA AGALLOCHUM, Agallochum.
CYNOMOIA, Plantago psyllium.
CYNOMO'RIUM COCCIN'EUM, from κυων, 'a dog,' and μοριον, 'the penis.' (F.) *Champignon de Malte.* Improperly called *Fungus Meliten'sis,* or *Fungus of Malta,* as it is not a fungus. The powder has been given as an astringent in hemorrhage, dysentery, &c.

CYNOREXIA, Boulimia.
CYNORRHODON, Rosa canina.
CYNOSBATOS, Rosa canina.
CYNOSORCHIS, Orchis mascula.
CYNOSPASTUM, Rosa canina.
CYON, κυων. The word sometimes signifies the frænum of the prepuce; at others, the penis.
CYOPHORIA, Pregnancy.
CYOT'ROPHY, *Cyotroph'ia, Embryot'rophy, Embryotroph'ia,* from κυος, 'embryo,' and τροφειν, 'to nourish.' Nutrition of the embryo. Fœtal nutrition.

CYPARISSUS, Cupressus sempervirens.
CYPERUS ANTIQUORUM, Lawsonia inermis—c. Indicus, Curcuma longa.
CYPE'RUS LONGUS, C. Roma'nus, from κυπαρος, 'a round vessel,' which its roots have been said to resemble. *Galangale*, (F.) *Souchet odorant.* It possesses aromatic and bitter properties, but is not used. See, also, Dorstenia contrayerva.
CYPERUS ODORUS, Dorstenia contrayerva — c. Peruanus, Dorstenia contrayerva — c. Romanus, C. longus.
CYPERUS ROTUN'DUS, *C. tetras'tachys*, the *Round Cype'rus*, (F.) *Souchet rond.* It is a more gratefully aromatic bitter than the *C. longus*.
CYPERUS TETRASTACHYS, C. rotundus.
CYPHO'MA, *Cyphos, Cypho'sis, Cyrto'ma, Cyrto'sis, Opisthocypho'sis*, from κυφος, 'gibbous.' Gibbosity of the spine. See Vertebral Column, &c. *Cyrtosis* forms a genus in the order *Dysthet'ica*, and class *Hæmat'ica* of Good, and is defined: 'head bulky, especially anteriorly; stature short and incurvated; flesh flabby, tabid, and wrinkled.' It includes *Cretinism*, and *Rickets*.
CYPHOSIS, Gibbositas, see Hump, and Kyphosis.
CYPRÈS, Cupressus sempervirens.
CYPRESS, Cupressus sempervirens—c. Tree, Liriodendron.
CYP'RINUM O'LEUM, *Oil of Cypress;* prepared of olive oil, cypress flowers, calamus, myrrh, cardamom, inula, bitumen of Judæa, &c. It was formerly employed in certain diseases of the uterus, pleurisies, &c., and was regarded to be both stimulant and emollient.
CYPRIPE'DIUM ACAU'LE, *Stemless Ladies' Slipper; Moccasin Flower;* indigenous; flowers in May and June. The roots are used by steamdoctors in nervous diseases, like valerian.
CYPRIPEDIUM CALCEOLUS, C. Luteum—c. Flavescens, C. Luteum.
CYPRIPE'DIUM LU'TEUM, *C. Calce'olus, C. Flaves'cens, C. Pubes'cens, C. Parviflo'rum, Yellow ladies' slipper, Moc'casin flower, Yellows, Bleeding heart, Amer'ican vale'rian, Yellow umbil, male Mervine, Noah's ark,* (F.) *Sabot de Vénus jaune.* An indigenous plant, *Nat. Order*, Orchidaceæ, which is found all over the United States; blossoming in May and June. The root is considered to be antispasmodic, and is used in the same cases as valerian.
CYPRIPEDIUM PARVIFLORUM, C. Luteum — c. Pubescens, C. Luteum.
CYPRIPEDIUM SPECTAB'ILE, *Showy ladies' slipper*, is the most beautiful of the genus.
CYPRIUM, Cuprum.
CYPSELE, Cerumen.
CYRCEON, Anus.
CYRTOIDES, Cuboid.
CYRTOMA, Curvature, Cyphoma.
CYRTONOSOS, Rachitis.
CYSSANTHEMON, Cyclamen.
CYSSARUS, Anus, Rectum.
CYSSOPHYLLON, Cyclamen.
CYS'SOTIS, from κυσος, 'the anus.' The lower part of the rectum : tenesmus.
CYST, Kyst.
CYSTAL'GIA, *Cystidal'gia*, from κυστις, 'the bladder,' and αλγος, 'pain.' Pain in the bladder.
CYSTANENCEPHA'LIA, from κυστις, 'a bladder,' and *anencepha'lia*, 'absence of brain.' A monstrosity, in which, in place of a brain, a bladder is found filled with fluid.—G. St. Hilaire.
CYSTAUCHENOTOM'IA, *Cystotrachelotom'ia, Cystidotrachelotom'ia*, from κυστις, 'a bladder,' αυχην, 'the neck,' and τομη, 'incision.' An incision into the neck of the bladder. See Lithotomy.
CYSTAUX'E, *Hypertroph'ia vesi'cæ urina'riæ, Callos'itas vesi'cæ;* from κυστις, 'bladder,' and αυξη, 'increase.' Hypertrophy of the coats of the urinary bladder.—Fuchs. See Cysthypersarcosis.

CYSTECTASY, Lithectasy.
CYSTENCEPH'ALUS, from κυστις, 'bladder,' and κεφαλη, 'head.' A monster having a head with a vesicular brain.—G. St. Hilaire.
CYSTEOL'ITHOS, from κυστις, 'the bladder,' and λιθος, 'a stone.' Stone in the bladder. Also, a medicine, employed to dissolve or break stone.
OYSTERETHIS'MUS, *Vesi'cæ Irritabil'itas;* from κυστις, 'the bladder,' and ερεθιζω, 'I irritate.' Irritability of the bladder.
CYSTHEPAT'ICUS, from κυστις, 'the bladder,' and 'ηπαρ, 'the liver.' Belonging to the gallbladder and liver. This name was given, formerly, to imaginary excretory ducts for the bile, which were supposed to pass directly from the liver to the gall-bladder.
CYSTHEPATOLITHI'ASIS, *Cystidepatolithi'asis, Cholelith'ia, Cholelithi'asis*, from κυστις, 'the bladder,' 'ηπαρ, 'the liver,' and λιθιασις, 'pain caused by a calculus.' The aggregate of phenomena caused by the presence of biliary calculi. See Calculi, biliary.
CYSTHITIS, Kysthitis.
CYSTHUS, Anus.
CYSTHYPERSARCO'SIS, from κυστις, 'bladder,' 'υπερ, 'over,' and σαρκωσις, 'a fleshy growth;' *Excrescen'tia Vesicæ urina'riæ*. A fleshy thickening of the coats of the bladder.
CYSTIC, *Cys'ticus*, from κυστις, 'a bladder.' Belonging to the gall-bladder.
CYSTIC ARTERY, *Arte'ria Cys'tica*, is given off from the right branch of the hepatic, and divides into two branches, which proceed to the gallbladder. It is accompanied by two *cystic veins*, which open into the vena porta abdominalis.
CYSTIO BILE. Bile contained in the gallbladder.
CYSTIC CALCULI. Calculi formed in the gallbladder.
CYSTIC DUCT, *Ductus cys'ticus, Mea'tus cys'ticus.* The duct proceeding from the gall-bladder, which, by its union with the hepatic, forms the *ductus communis choledochus*.
CYSTIC OXIDE CALCULI, see Calculi.
CYSTIC SARCO'MA, of AB'ERNETHY, *Emphy'ma Sarcoma cellulo'sum*. Tumour, cellulose or cystose; cells oval, currant-sized or grape-sized, containing serous fluid; sometimes caseous. Found in the thyroid gland (forming bronchocele,) testis, ovarium, &c.
CYS'TICA, *Cystic Remedies.* Such medicines as were formerly believed proper for combating diseases of the bladder.
CYSTICER'CUS, from κυστις, 'a bladder,' and κερκος, 'a tail.' A genus of entozoa of the family of the hydatids, distinguished by the caudal vesicle in which the cylindrical or slightly depressed body of the animal terminates. The *Cysticer'cus cellulo'sæ* seu *cellulo'sa, Hy'datis finna*, has been often found in the cellular membrane.
CYSTIDALGIA, Cystalgia.
CYSTIDELCO'SIS, from κυστις, 'bladder,' and 'ελκωσις, 'ulceration.' Suppuration or ulceration of the urinary bladder.
CYSTIDEPATICUS, Hepatocystic.
CYSTIDEPATOLITHIASIS, Cysthepatolithiasis.
CYSTIDOBLENNORRHŒA, Cystirrhœa.
CYSTIDOCATARRHUS, Cystirrhœa.
CYSTIDOCELE, Cystocele.
CYSTIDOPLEGIA, Cystoparalysis.
CYSTIDORRHAGIA, Cystorrhagia.
CYSTIDORRHEXIS, Cystorrhexis.

CYSTIDORRHŒA, Cystirrhœa.
CYSTIDOSOMATOTOMIA, Cystosomatotomia.
CYSTIDOSPASMUS, see Cystospastic.
CYSTIDOSTENOCHORIA, Stricture of the urinary bladder.
CYSTIDOTOMIA, Cystotomia.
CYSTIDOTRACHELOTOMIA, Cystauchenotomia.
CYSTINURIA, Urine, cystinic.
CYSTINX, Vesicula.
CYSTIPHLOGIA, Cystitis.
CYSTIRRHAG"IA, from κυστις, 'the bladder,' and ρηγνυω, 'I break forth.' *Hemorrhage from the bladder*, (F.) *Hémorrhagie de la Vessie.* By some used synonymously with cystirrhœa.
CYSTIRRHEUMA, Cystorrheuma.
CYSTIRRHŒ'A, from κυστις, 'the bladder,' and ρεω, 'I flow.' *Paru'ria Stillati"tia Muco'sa, Blennu'ria, Blennorrhœ'a urina'lis, B. vesi'cœ, Cysto-blennorrhœ'a, Cystorrhœ'a, Cystido-blennorrhœ'd, Ischu'ria, Cysto-phlegmat'ica, Tenes'mus Vesi'cœ Muco'sus, Uri'na muco'sa, Cystocatar'rhus, Cystido-catar'rhus, Cystidorrhœ'a, Urocystocatar'rhus, Dysu'ria Muco'sa, Pyu'ria Mucosa, P. vis'cida, P. sero'sa, Morbus cystophlegmat'icus, Catar'rhus vesi'cœ*, (F.) *Cystite muqueuse, Flux muqueux de la vessie, Catarrhe vésical*. A copious discharge of mucus from the bladder, passing out with the urine, and generally attended with dysuria. It is commonly dependent upon an inflammatory or subinflammatory condition of the lining membrane. The treatment must be regulated by the cause. If it be not produced by an extraneous body: the antiphlogistic plan,—the exhibition of warm diluents, and keeping the surface in a perspirable state, by wearing flannel, are indicated. Some of the turpentines may, at times, be given with advantage; and astringent or other appropriate injections be thrown into the bladder.
CYSTIS, Follicle, Urinary bladder—c. Choledochus, Gall-bladder—c. Fellea, Gall-bladder c. Serosa, Hygroma.
CYSTITE, Cystitis—c. *Muqueuse*, Cystitis.
CYSTI'TIS, from κυστις, 'the bladder.' *Inflamma'tio Vesi'cœ, Empres'ma Cysti'tis, Cysti'tis u'rica, Uro-cysti'tis, Cystiphlo'gia, Cystophlo'gia, Inflammmation of the bladder*, (F.) *Cystite, Inflammation de la vessie;* characterized by pain and swelling in the hypogastric region; discharge of urine painful or obstructed, and tenesmus. It may affect one or all of the membranes; but commonly it is confined to the mucous coat. In the chronic condition, it appears in the form of cystirrhœa. It must be treated upon the same energetic principles as are required in other cases of internal inflammation. Venesection, general and local, the warm bath, warm fomentations, warm, soothing enemata, diluents, &c. Cantharides must be avoided, even in the way of blisters, unless with precautions, as the disease is often occasioned by them.
CYSTITIS FELLEA, Cholecystitis—c. Urica, Cystitis.
CYSTITOME, Cystit'omus, Kibis'titome, from κυστις, 'the bladder,' and τεμνειν, 'to cut.' An instrument, invented by Lafaye, for dividing the anterior part of the capsule of the crystalline in the operation for extracting cataract. It was formed like the *Pharyngotome.*
CYSTOBLAST, Cytoblast.
CYSTO-BLENNORRHŒA, Cystirrhœa.
CYSTO-BUBONOCE'LE, from κυστις, 'the bladder,' βουβον, 'the groin,' and κηλη, 'a tumour.' Hernia of the bladder through the abdominal ring.
CYSTO-CATARRHUS, Cystirrhœa.
CYSTOCE'LE, *Cystoce'lia, Cistoce'lē, Cystido-*

ce'lē, from κυστις, 'the bladder,' and κηλη, 'a tumour,' *Her'nia vesi'cœ urina'ria, Hernia of the bladder*, (F.) *Hernie de la Vessie.* It is not common. It occurs, most frequently, at the abdominal ring; less so at the crural arch, perinæum, vagina, and foramen thyroideum. It may exist alone, or be accompanied by a sac, containing some abdominal viscus. The tumour is soft and fluctuating; disappears on pressure, and increases in size, when the urine is retained. It must be reduced and kept in position by a truss. *Vaginal cystocele* is kept in place by a pessary.
CYSTOCELE BILIOSA, Turgescentia vesiculæ felleæ.
CYSTODYN'IA, from κυστις, 'the bladder,' and οδυνη, 'pain.' Pain of the bladder; particularly rheumatic pain.
CYSTOID, *Cystoi'deus, Cyst-like*, from κυστις 'a bladder or cyst,' and ειδος, 'resemblance.' That which resembles a cyst, as 'cystoid tumour.
CYSTO-LITHIASIS, see Calculi, vesical.
CYSTO-LITH'IC, *Cystolith'icus*, from κυστις, 'the bladder,' and λιθος, 'a stone.' Relating to stone in the bladder.
CYSTOMA, see Kyst.
CYSTO-MEROCE'LE, from κυστις, 'the bladder,' μερος, 'the thigh,' and κηλη, 'hernia.' Femoral hernia, formed by the bladder protruding beneath the crural arch.
CYSTON'CUS, from κυστις, 'the bladder,' and ογκος, 'tumour.' Swelling of the bladder.
CYSTOPARAL'YSIS, *Cystidoparal'ysis, Cystidople'gia, Cystople'gia, Cystoplex'ia*, from κυστις, 'bladder,' and παραλυσις, 'palsy.' Paralysis of the urinary bladder. See Enuresis.
CYSTO-PHLEGMAT'IC, *Cystophlegmat'icus*, from κυστις, 'the bladder,' and φλεγμα, 'mucus, phlegm.' Belonging to the vesical mucus. *Morbus cystophlegmat'icus.* Cystirrhœa.
CYSTOPHLOGIA, Cystitis.
CYSTOPHTHI'SIS, *Phthisis vesica'lis*, from κυστις, 'the bladder,' and φθιω, 'I consume.' Consumption from ulceration of the bladder,— *Ul'cera seu Helco'sis vesi'cæ.*
CYSTOPLAS'TIC, *Cystoplas'ticus*: from κυστις, 'the bladder,' and πλασσω, 'I form.' An epithet for operations for the cure of fistulous openings into the bladder; sometimes restricted to the cure by translation of skin from a neighbouring part.
CYSTOPLEGIA, Cystoparalysis.
CYSTOPLEG"IC, *Cystopleg"icus.* Belonging to paralysis of the bladder; from κυστις, 'the bladder,' and πλησσω, 'I strike.'
CYSTOPLEX'IA, Cystoparalysis.
CYSTOPTO'SIS, from κυστις, 'the bladder,' and πιπτειν, 'to fall.' Relaxation of the inner membrane of the bladder, which projects into the canal of the urethra.
CYSTOPY'IC, *Cystopy'icus*, from κυστις, 'the bladder,' and πυον, 'pus.' Relating to suppuration of the bladder.
CYSTORRHAG"IA, *Hæmatu'ria cyst'ica, Hæmorrhag"ia vesi'cæ, Strangu'ria cruen'ta, San'guinis fluor vesi'cæ*, from κυστις, 'the bladder,' and ραγη, 'rupture.' A discharge of blood from the vessels of the urinary bladder.
CYSTORRHEU'MA, *Cystirrheu'ma, Rheumatis'mus vesi'cæ urina'riæ;* from κυστις, 'the bladder,' and ρευμα, 'defluxion,' rheumatism.' Rheumatism of the bladder.
CYSTORRHEX'IS, *Cystidorrhex'is;* from κυστις, 'bladder,' and 'ρηξις, 'rupture.' Rupture of the urinary bladder.
CYSTORRHŒA, Cystirrhœa.
CYSTOSARCO'MA, from κυστις, 'a bladder or cyst,' and *sarcoma*. A tumour consisting of a combination of cysts and cystoids, so called by J. Müller.

CYSTOSOMATOM'IA, *Cystosomatotom'ia, Cystidosomatotom'ia*, from κυστις, 'the bladder,' σωμα, 'body,' and τομη, 'incision.' An incision into the body of the bladder.

CYSTOSPASMUS, see Cystospastic.

CYSTOSPAS'TIC, *Cystospas'ticus*, from κυστις, 'the bladder,' and σπαω, 'I contract.' Relating to spasm of the bladder, and particularly of its sphincter;—*Cystidospas'mus, Spasmus Vesi'cæ, Ischu'ria spasmod'ica*, (F.) *Spasme de la Vessie*.

CYSTOSTENOCHO'RIA, *Cystidostenocho'ria, Strictu'ra vesi'cæ, Vesi'ca sacca'ta*. A stricture, narrowness, inequality or saccated condition of the urinary bladder.

CYSTOTHROM'BOID, *Cystothromboi'des*, from κυστις, 'the bladder,' and θρομβος, 'a clot.' Relating to the presence of clots in the bladder.

CYSTOTOME, *Cystot'omus*, from κυστις, 'the bladder,' and τεμνειν, 'to cut.' An instrument intended for cutting the bladder. Instruments of this kind have been more frequently, although very improperly, called *Lithotomes*.

CYSTOTOM'IA, *Cystidotom'ia*, same etymon. Incision of the bladder. *Sectio vesica'lis. Cystotomia* means cutting into the bladder for any purpose; (F.) *Incision de la vessie*. Commonly, it is applied to the puncturing of the bladder for the purpose of removing the urine; whilst *Lithotomy* has been employed for the incisions made with the view of extracting calculi from the bladder. See Lithotomy.

CYSTOTRACHELOTOMIA, Cystauchenotomia. See Lithotomy.

CYT'INUS, *Cytinus Hypocist'is, Hypocist'is, As'arum Hypocist'is*. A small parasitical plant, which grows in the south of France and in Greece, on the roots of the woody cistus. The juice of its fruit is acid, and very astringent. It is extracted by expression, and converted into an extract, which was called *Succus Hypocis'tidis*, and was formerly much used in hemorrhages, diarrhœa, &c.

CYTISI'NA, *Cytisine*. An immediate vegetable principle, discovered by Chevalier and Lassaigne, in the seeds of *Cytisus Labur'num* or *Bean-Trefoil tree. Family*, Leguminosæ. *Sex. Syst*. Diadelphia Decandria. Cytisine has analogous properties to emetine. In the dose of one or two grains, it produces vomiting and purging; and, in a stronger dose, acts as an acrid poison. The seeds of the *Cytisus Laburnum*, (F.) *Aubours*, have been long known to produce vomiting and purging.

CYTISMA ECZEMA, Eczema — c. Herpes, Herpes.

CYTISO-GENISTA, Spartium scoparium.

CYTISUS LABURNUM, see Cytisina — c. Scoparius, Spartium scoparium.

CYTITIS, *Scyti'tis, Dermati'tis, Dermi'tis, Cuti'tis, Corii'tis*, from κυτις, 'the skin,' and *itis*, 'denoting inflammation.' Inflammation of the skin.

CY'TOBLAST, *Cystoblast*, from κυτος, 'cell,' and βλαστος, 'germ.' *Cell-germ, Nu'cleus*, (F.) *Noyau*. A primary *granule*, from which all animal and vegetable bodies are presumed to be formed. When the nucleus or cytoblast forms a cell, and is attached to its walls, the *germinal cell*, thus formed, is called a *nucleated cell*. When the nucleus contains a simple granule, the latter is termed a *nucleolus*, (F.) *Nucléole, Nucléolule*.

CYTOBLASTE'MA; same etymon. *Intercel'lular substance, Hy'aline substance, Substan'tia vit'rea seu hyal'ina, Matrix*. The gum or mucus in the vegetable, and probably the liquor sanguinis after transudation from the vessels in the animal, in a state fully prepared for the formation of the tissues. — Schwann and Schleiden. By many, *Blastema* is preferred, inasmuch as it does not convey the idea of cellular development.

CYTTAROS, Glans.

D.

The figure of the Greek Δ, according to Galen, was the sign for quartan fever.

DABACH, Viscum album.

DACNE'RON, δακνηρον, from δακνειν, 'to bite.' An ancient name for a collyrium, composed of oxide of copper, pepper, cadmia, myrrh, saffron, gum Arabic, and opium.

DACRY, *Dac'ryma, Dac'ryon, δακρυ, δακρυμα, δακρυον*, 'a tear:' Hence:

DACRYADENAL'GIA, *Dacryoädenal'gia*, from δακρυω, 'I weep,' αδην, 'a gland,' and αλγος, 'pain.' Disease or pain in the lachrymal gland.

DACRYADENI'TIS, *Dacryoädeni'tis :* from δακρυω, 'I weep,' αδην, 'a gland,' and *itis*. Inflammation of the lachrymal gland.

DACRYALLŒO'SIS, from δακρυ, 'a tear,' and αλλοιωσις, 'change.' A morbid condition of the tears.

DACRYDION, Convolvulus scammonia.

DACRYGELO'SIS, from δακρυω, 'I weep,' and γελαω, 'I laugh.' A kind of insanity, in which the patient weeps and laughs at the same time.

DACRYHÆMOR'RHYSIS: from δακρυ, 'a tear,' and 'αιμορρυσις, 'hemorrhage.' A flow of bloody tears.

DACRYNOMA, Epiphora.

DACRYOÄDENALGIA, Dacryadenalgia.

DACRYOÄDENITIS, Dacryadenitis.

DACRYOBLENNORRHŒ'A, from δακρυω, 'I weep,' βλεννα, 'mucus,' and ρεω, 'I flow.' Discharge of tears mixed with mucus.

DACRYOCYSTAL'GIA, from δακρυω, 'I weep,' κυστις, 'a sac,' and αλγος, 'pain.' Disease or pain in the lachrymal sac.

DACRYOCYSTIS, Lachrymal sac.

DACRYOCYSTI'TIS, from δακρυον, 'a tear,' and κυστις, 'bladder.' Inflammation of the lachrymal sac.

DACRYOCYSTOSYRINGOKATAKLEI'SIS; from *dacryocystis*, the 'lachrymal sac,' συριγξ, 'a pipe, a fistula,' and κατακλεισις, 'a locking up.' A term, proposed by Dieffenbach for the healing of lachrymal fistulæ by transplantation. The operation consists in paring the edges of the fistula, loosening the borders, and assisting the requisite tegumental displacement by lateral incisions.

DACRYO'DES, *Lachrymo'sus*, from δακρυω, 'I weep.' Resembling tears:—hence, *Ulcus dac'ryo'des*. A sanious ulcer, a weeping sore.

DAC'RYOLITE, *Dacryol'ithus*, from δακρυω, 'I weep,' and λιθος, 'a stone.' A concretion found in the lachrymal passages.

DACRYOLITHI'ASIS; same etymon as the last. The formation of concretions in the tears.

DACRYO'MA. Same etymon. The effusion of tears, occasioned by an occlusion of the puncta lachrymalia.—Vogel.

DACRYON, Tear.

DACRYOPŒ'US, from δακρυω, 'I weep,' and ποιεω, 'I make.' A substance which excites the secretion of tears,—as the *onion, horse-radish, garlic,* &c.

DAC'RYOPS, from δακρυω, 'I weep,' and ωψ, 'the eye.' A weeping eye. A tumefaction of the lachrymal passages.

DACRYOPYORRHŒ'A, *Pyorrhœ'a via'rum lachryma'lium,* from δακρυ, 'a tear,' πυον, 'pus,' and ρεω, 'to flow.' A discharge of tears mixed with purulent matter.

DACRYORRHŒ'A, *Dacryrrhœ'a, Dacryor'rhysis, Dacryr'rhysis,* from δακρυ, 'a tear,' and ρεω, 'to flow.' A morbid flux of tears.

DACRYORRHYSIS, Dacryorrhœa.

DACRYOSOLENI'TIS, from δακρυ, 'a tear,' σωληυ, 'a canal,' and *itis,* denoting inflammation. Inflammation of the lachrymal ducts.

DACRYOSYRINX, Fistula lachrymalis.

DACRYRRHŒA, Dacryorrhœa.

DACRYRRHYSIS, Dacryorrhœa.

DACTYLE'THRA, *Dactyli'thra,* from δακτυλος, 'a finger.' A name given by the ancients to different topical applications, having the form of a finger, and proper for being introduced into the throat to excite vomiting.

DACTYLETUS, Hermodactylus.

DACTYL'ION, *Dactyl'ium,* from δακτυλος, 'a finger.' The union of the fingers with each other. This affection is generally congenital; but it may be owing to burns, ulcerations, inflammation of the fingers, &c.

DACTYL'IOS, from δακτυλος, 'a finger.' A troch or lozenge, when shaped like a finger. The anus.

DACTYLITIS, Paronychia.

DACTYLIUS, from δακτυλιος, *annulus,* 'a ring.'

DACTYL'IUS AGULEA'TUS. A worm of a light colour, annulated, cylindrical, but tapering slightly towards both extremities, from two-fifths to four-fifths of an inch long, which has been found in the urine.

DACTYLODOCHME, Dochme.

DACTYLOSYM'PHYSIS, from δακτυλος, 'a finger,' and συμφυσις, 'union.' Adhesion of the fingers to each other.

DACTYLOTHE'KE, from δακτυλος, 'a finger,' and θηκη, 'a case or sheath.' An instrument for keeping the fingers extended when wounded.—Ambrose Paré.

DAC'TYLUS, *Dig"itus,* 'a finger.' The smallest measure of the Greeks, the sixth part of a foot. Also, the Date.

DÆDA'LEA SUAVEOLENS, *Bole'tus* seu *Fungus Sal'icis, Boletus discoideus* seu *suaveolens, Fungus albus sali'geus,* (F.) *Agaric odorant, Bolet odorant.* A champignon, which grows on the trunks of old willows. It has a smell of anise, which is penetrating and agreeable; and has been recommended in phthisis pulmonalis in the dose of a scruple four times a day.

DÆDALUS, Hydrargyrum.

DÆDION, Bougie.

DÆMONOMANIA, Demonomania.

DÆS, Tædæ.

DAFFODIL, Narcissus pseudonarcissus.

DAFFY'S ELIXIR, Tinctura sennæ composita.

DAISY, Chrysanthemum leucanthemum, Erigeron Philadelphicum — d. Common, Bellis — d. Ox-eye, Chrysanthemum leucanthemum.

DALBY'S CARMIN'ATIVE. A celebrated empirical remedy, much used as a carminative for children. The following is a form for its preparation: (*Magnesiæ alb.* Ɖij; *ol. menthæ piper.* gtt. j; *ol. nuc. moschat,* gtt. iij; *ol. anisi,* gtt. iij; *tinct. castor.* gtt. xxx; *tinct. asafœtid.* gtt. xv; *tinct. opii,* gtt. v; *sp. pulegii,* gtt. xv; *tinct. cardam. c.* gtt. xxx; *aquæ menthæ pip.* ℥ij. M.)

A Committee of the Philadelphia College of Pharmacy recommend the following form:— (*Aquæ,* Ox; *Sacchar. alb.* ℥xxxij; *Carbon. Potass.* ℥ss; *Carb. Mag.* ℥xij; *Tinct. Opii.* f℥vj; *Ol. menth. pip., Ol. Anethi Fœnicul.* āā fƉij. M.)

DALTO'NIAN. An absurd name given to one who cannot distinguish colours; because the celebrated chemist Dalton had the defect. See Achromatopsia.

DALTONISM, Achromatopsia.

DAMSON, Prunum Damascenum — d. Mountain, Quassia simarouba — d. Tree, Prunus domestica.

DANCE, see Mania, dancing.

DANCING, *Salta'tio,* (F.) *Danse.* A kind of exercise and amusement, composed of a succession of motions, gestures, and attitudes, executed by measured steps to the sound of the voice or musical instrument. It is a healthy exercise.

DANCING MANIA, see Mania, dancing — d. Plague, see Mania, dancing.

DANDELION, Leontodon taraxacum.

DANDRIFF, Pityriasis.

DANDRUFF, Pityriasis.

DANDY, Dengue.

DANEVERT, MINERAL WATERS OF. A spring, a league and a half from Upsal, in Sweden. The waters contain carbonic acid, holding in solution carbonate of iron, sulphate of iron, sulphates of soda and lime, chloride of sodium, and silica. It is frequently employed in medicine.

DANEWORT, Sambucus ebulus.

DANICH; an Arabic word, signifying the weight of 8 grains.

DANSE, Dancing—*d. de St. Guy,* Chorea—*d. de St. Witt,* Chorea.

DAPHNE, Laurus.

DAPHNE ALPI'NA, *Chamæle'a, Chamælæ'a, Widow wail. Family,* Thymeleæ. *Sex. Syst.* Octandria Monogynia. A sort of dwarf-olive. An acrid, volatile, alkaline principle has been separated from the bark of this plant by M. Vauquelin, to which he has given the name *Daphnine.* The plants of the genus owe their vesicating property to this principle.

DAPHNÉ BOISGENTIL, Daphne mezereum — d. Flax-leaved, Daphne gnidium — *d. Garou,* Daphne gnidium.

DAPHNE GNID'IUM, *D. panicula'ta, Thymelæ'a, Th. Monspeliaca, Thymele'a, Cneo'ron, Spurge Flax, Flax-leaved Daphnè.* The plant which furnishes the *Garou Bark,* (F.) *Daphné Garou, Sain-bois.* It is chiefly used, when used at all, for exciting irritation of the skin. The *Granæ Gnid'ia,* (see *Cnid'ia grana,*) are acrid poisons, like all the plants of this genus, when taken in quantity. According to others, the garou bark and grana gnidia are obtained from the *daphne laureola.*

DAPHNE LAUREOLA, *D. major, Thymelæ'a lau're'ola.* The systematic name of the *Spurge Laurel, Laureola.* The bark of this plant has similar properties to the last.

DAPHNE LIOTTARDI, D. laureola—d. Major, D. laureola.

DAPHNE MEZE'REUM, *D. Liottar'di, Thymelæ'a meze'reum.* The systematic name of the *Meze'reon, Mezereum, Spurge olive,* (F.) *Daphné Boisgentil.* The bark of the mezereon, *Mezereum,* (Ph. U. S.) possesses analogous properties to the other varieties of Daphne. It is considered stimulant and diaphoretic; and, in large doses, is emetic. It has been employed in syphilitic cases, but its efficacy is doubtful. Soaked in vinegar,— like the other varieties of daphne, it has been employed to irritate the skin, especially to keep issues open.

DAPHNE PANICULATA, D. Gnidium.

DAPHNELÆ'ON, *O'leum Lauri'num*, from δαφνη, 'the laurel or bay tree,' and ελαιον, 'oil.' *Oil of Bay*.

DAPHNINE, see Daphne Alpina.

DARNEL, Lolium temulentum.

DARSENI, Laurus cinnamomum.

DARSINI, Laurus cinnamomum.

DARSIS, from δερω, 'I excoriate,' 'I skin.' The Greek physicians seemed to have used this word to designate the anatomical preparation, which consists in removing the skin for exposing the organs covered by it.

DARTA, Impetigo — d. Excoriativa, Herpes exedens—d. Maligna, Herpes exedens.

DARTOS. Same derivation; *Membra'na carno'sa, Tu'nica muscula'ris, T. rubicun'da scroti, Mares'pium musculo'sum;* from δαρτος, 'skinned.' A name, given to the second covering of the testicle, which the ancient anatomists conceived to be muscular, but which is merely areolar. Its external surface is towards the scrotum; the internal towards the tunica vaginalis. Frederick Lobstein and Breschet consider, that it proceeds from an expansion of the fibrous cord, known by the name *Gubernaculum Testis*.

DARTRE, Herpes, Impetigo, Pityriasis — d. *Crustacée,* Ecthyma impetigo — d. *Crustacée flavescente,* Porrigo lupinosa—d. *Croûteuse,* Impetigo —d. *Écailleuse,* Psoriasis—d. *Fongueuse,* Ecthyma—d. *Furfuracée arrondie,* Lepra, Lepra vulgaris—d. *Furfuracée volante,* Lichen, Pityriasis — d. *Phlycténoïde,* Herpes phlyctænoides — d. *Pustuleuse couperose,* Gutta rosea—d. *Pustuleuse disséminée,* Acne—d. *Pustuleuse mentagra,* Sycosis — d. *Rongeante,* Herpes exedens; see Esthiomenus — d. *Squammeuse humide,* Eczema — d. *Squammeuse lichénoïde,* Psoriasis — d. *Vive,* Eczema.

DARTREUX (F.), *Herpetic*. Participating in the characters of *Dartre* or *Herpes*. Also, one affected with dartre. Dartre has been used, at one time or other, for almost every disease of the skin. See Herpes.

DAS'YMA, from δασυς, 'rough,' 'hairy.' A disease of the eye — the same as trachoma, but less in degree.—Aëtius, Gorræus.

DAS'YTES. Same etymon. Roughness, particularly of the tongue and voice. Hairiness, *Hirsu'ties*.

DATE, *Pal'mula, Dac'tylus, Bal'anos, Phœ'nicos,* the fruit of the *Phœnix dactylif'era* seu *excel'sa, Palma dactylif'era,* (F.) *Datte*. The unripe date is astringent. When ripe, it resembles the fig. The juice of the tree is refrigerant.

DATE PLUM, INDIAN, Diospyrus lotus.

DATTE, Date.

DATURA, D. Stramonium.

DATU'RA SANGUIN'EA, *Red Thorn Apple;* called by the Indians of Peru *Huacacachu, Yerba de Huaca* (*huaca,* a grave) or *Grave-plant,* and *Bovachevo*. A plant from which the Peruvian Indians prepare a narcotic drink called *Tonga*.

DATU'RA STRAMO'NIUM, *Stramo'nium, Stramo'nia, Barycoc'calon, Sola'num fœ'tidum, Stramo'nium majus album,* seu *spino'sum* seu *vulga'tum* seu *fœ'tidum, Pomum* seu *Malum spino'sum, Nux methel, Datu'ra, Dutro'a, Daty'ra, Thorn Apple, Jamestown Weed, Jimston Weed, Stinkweed,* (F.) *Stramoine, Pomme épineuse*. The herbaceous part of the plant and the seeds are the parts used in medicine. They are narcotic and poisonous; — are given internally as narcotics and antispasmodics, and applied externally as sedatives, in the form of fomentation. The seeds are smoked like tobacco, in asthma. The dose of the powder is, gr. j to gr. viii.

DA'TURINE, *Daturi'na, Datu'ria, Datu'rium.* The active principle of the *Datura Stramonium,* separated by Brandes, a German chemist. It has not been rendered available in medicine.

DATURIUM, Daturine.

DATYRA, Datura stramonium.

DAUCI'TES VINUM. Wine, of which the *Daucus* or *Wild Carrot* was an ingredient. The seeds were steeped in must. It was formerly used in coughs, convulsions, hypochondriasis, diseases of the uterus, &c.

DAUCUS CANDIANUS, Athamanta cretensis.

DAUCUS CARO'TA. The systematic name of the *Carrot Plant; Daucus, Daucus sylves'tris* seu *vulga'ris* seu *sati'vus, Cauca'lis caro'ta, Pastina'ca sylvestris tenuifo'lia officina'rum, Ado'rion.* Order, Umbelliferæ. (F.) *Carotte*. The root, and seed, *Carota* — (Ph. U. S.) — have been used in medicine. The root is sweet and mucilaginous; and the seeds have an aromatic odour, and moderately warm, pungent taste. The *root* has been used as an emollient, to fetid and ill-conditioned sores. The *seeds* have been regarded as stomachic, carminative and diuretic; but they have little efficacy. The seeds of the *wild* plant are, by some, preferred to those of the *garden*.

DAUCUS CRETICUS, Athamanta cretensis — d. Cyanoides, Pimpinella magna — d. Sativus, D. carota — d. Seprinius, Scandix cerefolium — d. Sylvestris, D. carota—d. Vulgaris, D. carota.

DAUPHINELLE, Delphinium staphisagria.

DAVIDSON'S REMEDY FOR CANCER, see Conium maculatum.

DAVIER, Dentagra.

DAWLISH, CLIMATE OF. A town in Devonshire, frequented by phthisical invalids during the winter. It is well protected from northerly winds, and also from the violence of the south-westerly gales. It offers, however, but a confined space.

DAX, MINERAL WATERS OF. Dax is a city two leagues from Bordeaux, where there are four springs, that are almost purely thermal; containing only a very small quantity of chloride of magnesium, and sulphate of soda and lime. Temperature 76° to 133° Fahrenheit.

DAYMARE, Incubus vigilantium.

DAY-SIGHT, Hemeralopia—d. Vision, Hemeralopia.

DAZZLING, *Caliga'tio,* (F.) *Éblouissement*. A momentary disturbance of sight, occasioned either by the sudden impression of too powerful a light, or by some internal cause; as plethora.

DE VENTRE INSPICIENDO, 'of inspecting the belly.' Where there is reason to suppose, that a woman feigns herself pregnant, a writ *de ventre inspiciendo* may be issued to determine whether she be so or not. Until recently, in England, the decision was left to twelve matrons and twelve respectable men, according to the strict terms of the ancient writ.

DEAF-DUMBNESS, Mutitas surdorum.

DEAFNESS, from Anglo-Saxon ðeaf. *Sur'ditas, Copho'sis, Dysecoi'a, Dysecœ'a organ'ica, Baryecoi'a, Hardness of hearing, Hypocupho'sis, Subsur'ditas, Bradycoi'a, Bradyecoi'a,* (F.) *Surdité, Dureté de l'ouïe*. Considerable diminution or total loss of hearing. It may be the effect of acute or chronic inflammation of the internal ear, paralysis of the auditory nerve or its pulpy extremity, or of some mechanical obstruction to the sonorous rays. In most cases, however, the cause of the deafness is not appreciable, and the treatment has to be purely empirical. Syringing the ears, dropping in slightly stimulating oils, fumigations, &c., are the most likely means to afford relief.

DEAFNESS, TAYLOR'S REMEDY FOR, see Allium.

DEALBATIO, Paleness.

DEAMBULATIO, Walking.

DEARTICULATIO, Diarthrosis.

DEASCIATIO, Aposceparnismus.

DEATH, (Sax. ðɛaþ,) *Apobio'sis, Abio'sis, Extinc'tio, Ob'itus, Psychorag"ia, Psychorrhag"ia, Le'thum, Letum, Mors, Inter'itus, Than'atos, Death,* (F.) *Mort.* Definitive cessation of all the functions, the aggregate of which constitute life. *Real Death, Apothana'sia,* is distinguished from asphyxia or *apparent death:* — the latter being merely a suspension of those same functions. But it is often difficult to judge of such suspension, and the only certain sign of real death is the commencement of putrefaction. At times, therefore, great caution is requisite to avoid mistakes. Death is commonly preceded by some distressing symptoms, which depend on lesion of respiration, circulation, or of the cerebral function, and which constitute the *agony*. That which occurs suddenly, and without any, or with few, precursory signs, is called *sudden death*. It is ordinarily caused by disease of the heart; apoplexy; the rupture of an aneurism, or by some other organic affection. Death is *natural,* when it occurs as the result of disease: *violent,* when produced by some forcible agency. It may likewise affect the whole body, or a part only; hence the difference between *somatic* and *molecular* death.

The chief varieties of the modes of death may be thus given:—

Death beginning at the heart, { Suddenly—Syncope: Gradual—Asthenia.
" " in the lungs—Asphyxia.
" " in the brain—Apoplexy.
" " in the gray matter of the medulla, { Paralysis of pneumogastrics, &c.
" " in the blood—necræmia.

DEATH, APPARENT, Asphyxia.

DEATH, BLACK. The plague of the 14th century was so called, which is supposed to have proved fatal in Europe to 25,000,000 of people. — *Hecker.*

DEATH OF MAN, Cicuta maculata — d. Stiffening, Rigor mortis.

DEBILIS, Infirm.

DEBIL'ITANTS, *Debilitan'tia, Antidynam'ica, Philadynam'ica,* from *debilitare,* itself from *debilis,* quasi *dehabilis,* 'weak,' 'to weaken.' Remedies exhibited for the purpose of reducing excitement. Antiphlogistics are, hence, debilitants.

DEBILITAS, Debility—d. Erethisica, see Irritable—d. Nervosa, Neurasthenia, see Irritable—d. Visus, Asthenopia.

DEBIL'ITY, *Debil'itas, Astheni'a, Blaci'a, Anenerge'sia, Anenergi'a,* Weakness, (F.) *Faiblesse.* A condition, which may be induced by a number of causes. It must not be confounded with *fatigue,* which is temporary, whilst debility is generally more permanent.

Debility may be *real,* or it may be *apparent;* and, in the management of disease, it is important to attend to this. At the commencement of fever, for example, there is often a degree of apparent debility, which prevents the use of appropriate means, and is the cause of much evil. Excitement is more dangerous than debility.

DÉBOITEMENT, Luxation.

DÉBORDEMENT (F.), from *déborder,* (*de* and *border*) 'to overflow.' A popular term for one or more sudden and copious evacuations from the bowels. It is chiefly applied to bilious evacuations of this kind—*Débordement de Bile.*

DÉBRIDEMENT (F.). *Frœno'rum solu'tio,* from (F.) *débrider,* (*de* and *brider,*) 'to unbridle.' The removal of filaments, &c., in a wound or abscess, which prevent the discharge of pus. In a more general acceptation, it means the cutting of a soft, membranous or aponeurotic part, which interferes with the exercise of any organ whatever: thus, in paraphimosis, *débridement* of the prepuce is practised to put an end to the inflammation of the glans: in strangulated hernia, *débridement* of the abdominal ring is had recourse to, to remove the stricture of the intestine, &c.

DEC'AGRAMME, from δεκα, 'ten,' and γραμμα, 'a gramme.' The weight of ten grammes, 154.34 grains Troy.

DECAM'YRON, from δεκα, 'ten,' and μυρον, 'ointment.' An ancient cataplasm, composed of *malabathrum, mastich, euphorbium, spikenard, styrax calamita, carbonate of lime, common pepper, unguentum nardi, opobalsamum,* and *wax.*

DECANTA'TION, *Decanta'tio, Defu'sio, Metangism'os, Catach'ysis.* A pharmaceutical operation, which consists in pouring off, gently, by inclining the vessel, any fluid which has left a deposit.

DECAPITATIO ARTICULORUM, see Resection.

DECARBONIZATION, Hæmatosis.

DECESSIO, Ecpiesma.

DÉCHARNÉ, Demusculatus.

DÉCHAUSSEMENT (F.) (*de* and *chausser.*) The state, in which the gums have fallen away from the teeth, as in those affected by mercury, in old persons, &c. Also, the operation of lancing the gums. See Gum lancet.

DÉCHAUSSOIR, Gum lancet.

DÉCHIREMENT, Laceration.

DÉCHIRURE, Wound, lacerated.

DECIDENTIA, Cataptosis, Epilepsy.

DECIDUA, Decidua membrana.

DECID'UA MEMBRA'NA, *Decid'ua, Decid'uous Membrane,* from *decidere,* 'to fall off,' (*de,* and *cadere.*) So called on account of its being considered to be discharged from the uterus at parturition. A membrane, formerly defined to be the outermost membrane of the fœtus in utero; and still so defined by some—as by Dr. Lee. Chaussier calls it *Epicho'rion:* by others, it has been called *Membra'na cadu'ca Hunteri, M. flocculen'ta, M. cellulo'sa, M. sinuo'sa, M. commu'nis, M. præexis'tens,* Decidua externa, *Tu'nica exterior ovi, T. cadu'ca, T. crassa, Membra'na cribro'sa, Membra'na ovi mater'na, M. muco'sa,* Decidua *spongio'sa, Epio'nē, Placen'ta uteri succenturia'tus, Subplacen'ta, Membra'na u'teri inter'na evolu'ta, Indumen'tum, Anhis'tous membrane,* (F.) *Caduque, C. vraie, Membrane caduque, Épione, Périone.* Prior to the time of the Hunters, called *Cho'rion spongio'sum, C. tomento'sum, fungo'sum, reticula'tum,* &c., *Tu'nica filamento'sa, Shaggy Chorion, Spongy Chorion,* &c. Great diversity has prevailed, regarding this membrane and its reflected portion. It exists before the germ arrives in the uterus,—as it has been met with in tubal and ovarial pregnancies; and is occasioned by a new action, assumed by the uterine vessels at the moment of conception. Chaussier, Lobstein, Gardien, Velpeau and others consider it to be a sac, without apertures, completely lining the uterus, and that when the ovum descends through the tube, it pushes the decidua before it, and becomes enveloped in it, except at the part destined to form the placenta. That portion of the membrane, which covers the ovum, forms the *Membra'na decid'ua reflex'a,* (F.) *Caduque refléchie, Membrane caduque refléchie,* according to them;—the part lining the uterus being the *Decidua U'teri.* Towards the end of the fourth month, the decidua reflexa disappears. The very existence of a *Tunica decidua reflexa* has, however, been denied. This last membrane has received various names. Dr. Granville, regarding it as the external membrane of the ovum, has termed it *Cortex ovi*. It has also been termed *Involu'crum membrana'ceum, Membra'na retiform'is cho'rii, Membra'na filamento'sa, M. adventit'ia* and *M. crassa, Oculine* and *Decid'ua protru'sa*. To the membrane which, according to Bojanus and others, is situate between the placenta and the uterus, and which he considers to be produced at a later period than the decidua vera, he gave the name *membra'na decid'ua sero'tina*.

Histological researches seem to show, that the decidua is an altered condition of the lining membrane of the uterus, with a whitish secretion filling the uterine tubular glands. The decidua reflexa is probably formed by the agency of nucleated cells from the plastic materials thrown out from the decidua uteri; in the same manner as the chorion is formed in the Fallopian Tube from plastic materials thrown out from its lining membrane. That the decidua reflexa is not a mere inverted portion of the decidua uteri is shown by the fact, that the texture of the two is by no means identical.

DECIDUA PROTRUSA, Decidua reflexa.

DECIDUOUS MEMBRANE, Decidua (membrana).

DEC'IGRAMME, *Decigram'ma*, from *decimus*, 'the tenth part,' and γραμμα, 'gramme.' The tenth part of the gramme in weight; equal to a little less than two grains, French; 1.543 Troy.

DECIMA'NA FEBRIS, from *decem*, 'ten.' An intermittent, whose paroxysms return every 10th day or every 9 days. It is supposititious.

DECLAMA'TION, *Declama'tio*, from *de*, and *clamare*, 'to cry out.' The art of depicting the sentiments by inflections of the voice, accompanied with gestures, which render the meaning of the speaker more evident, and infuse into the minds of the auditors the emotions with which he is impressed. Declamation may become the cause of disease: the modification, produced in the pulmonary circulation,—accompanied by the great excitement, sometimes experienced,—is the cause of many morbid affections; particularly of pneumonia, hæmoptysis, and apoplexy. In moderation, it gives a healthy excitement to the frame.

DÉCLIN, Decline.

DECLINATIO, Decline.

DECLINE, *Declina'tio, Inclina'tio, Decremen'tum, Remis'sio, Parac'mē, Paracma'sis*, (F.) *Déclin*, from *de*, and *clinare*, 'to bend.' That period of a disorder or paroxysm, at which the symptoms begin to abate in violence. We speak, also, of the decline of life, or of the powers, (F.) *Déclin de l'age, L'age de déclin*, when the physical and moral faculties lose a little of their activity and energy. See Phthisis, and Tabes.

DÉCLIVE, (F.) *Decli'vis*, from *de*, 'from,' and *clivus*, 'acclivity.' Inclining downwards. This epithet is applied to the most depending part of a tumour or abscess.

DECOC'TION, *Decoc'tio*, from *decoquere*, 'to boil,' (*de* and *coquere*,) *Epse'sis, Apos'esis, Zesis, Hepse'sis, Aphepsis*, (F.) *Décoction*. The operation of boiling certain ingredients in a fluid, for the purpose of extracting the parts soluble at that temperature. Decoction, likewise, means the product of this operation, to which the terms *Decoctum, Zema, Aphepse'ma, Ap'osem, Apos'ema, Hepse'ma, Chylus* and *Epse'ma*, have been applied according to ancient custom, in order to avoid any confusion between the operation and its product;—as *præparatio* is used for the act of preparing; *præparatum*, for the thing prepared.

DECOCTION OF ALOES, COMPOUND, Decoctum aloes compositum — d. of Bark, Decoctum Cinchonæ — d. of Barley, Decoctum hordei — d. of Barley, compound, Decoctum hordei compositum — d. Bitter, Decoctum amarum — d. of Cabbage tree bark, Decoctum geoffrææ inermis — d. of Cassia, Decoctum cassiæ—d. of Chamomile, Decoctum anthemidis nobilis — d. of Cinchona, Decoctum Cinchonæ — d. of Cinchona, compound laxative, Decoctum kinæ kinæ compositum et laxans — d. of Colomba, compound, Decoctum Calumbæ compositum — d. of Dandelion, Decoctum Taraxaci—d. of Dogwood, Decoctum Cornûs Floridæ—d. of Elm bark, Decoctum ulmi—d. of Foxglove, Decoctum digitalis—*d. de Gayac composée*, &c., Decoctum de Guyaco compositum — d. of Guaiacum, compound, Decoctum Guaiaci compositum — d. of Guaiacum, compound purgative, Decoctum de Guayaco compositum — d. of Hartshorn, burnt, Mistura cornu usti—d. of Hellebore, white, Decoctum veratri — d. of Iceland moss, Decoctum cetrariæ — d. of Liverwort, Decoctum lichenis — d. of Logwood, Decoctum hæmatoxyli—d. of Marshmallows, Decoctum althææ — *d. de Mauve composée*, Decoctum malvæ compositum — d. of Oak bark, Decoctum quercûs — *d. d'Orge*, Decoctum hordei—*d. d'Orge composée*, Decoctum hordei compositum—d. of Pipsissewa, Decoctum chimaphilæ — d. of Poppy, Decoctum papaveris—d. of Quince seeds, Decoctum cydoniæ — *d. de Quinquina composée et laxative*, Decoctum kinæ kinæ compositum et laxans—*d. de Salsapareille composée*, Decoctum sarsaparillæ compositum — d. of Sarsaparilla, Decoctum sarsaparillæ—d. of Sarsaparilla, compound, Decoctum sarsaparillæ compositum—d. of Sarsaparilla, false, Decoctum araliæ nudicaulis—d. of Squill, Decoctum scillæ—d. of Uva ursi, Decoctum uvæ ursi — d. of the Woods, Decoctum Guaiaci compositum — d. of Woody nightshade, Decoctum dulcamaræ—d. of Zittmann, Decoctum Zittmanni.

DECOCTUM, Decoction — d. Album, Mistura cornu usti.

DECOCTUM AL'OES COMPOS'ITUM, *Balsam of Life, Compound Decoction of Aloes*. (*Ext. glyc.* ʒiv, *potass. subcarb.* Ðij, *aloes spicat. ext.*: *myrrhæ contrit.*: *croci stigmat.* āā ʒj, *aquæ* Oj. Boil to fʒxij : strain, and add *tinct. card. c.* fʒiv. *Pharm. L.*) The gum and extractive are dissolved in this preparation. The alkali is added to take up a little of the resin. The tincture prevents it from spoiling. It is gently cathartic. Dose, fʒss to ʒij.

DECOCTUM ALTHÆ'Æ, *D. altheæ officina'lis: Decoction of Marsh-mallows*, (F.) *Décoction de Guimauve*. (*Rad. altheæ* sicc. ʒiv. *uvar. passar.* ʒij, *aquæ*, Ovij. Boil to Ov. Pour off the clear liquor. *Pharm. E.*) It is used as a demulcent.

DECOCTUM AMA'RUM; *Bitter Decoction*. (*Rad. gent.* ʒj, *aquæ* Oijss. Boil for a quarter of an hour; add *species amaræ* ʒij. Infuse for two hours and filter, without expressing. *Pharm. P.*) It is tonic. Dose, fʒss to ʒij.

DECOCTUM ANTHEM'IDIS NOB'ILIS, *D. Chamæme'li; Decoction of Cham'omile*. (*Flor. anthemid. nobil.* ʒj, *sem. carui* ʒiv, *aquæ* Ov. Boil for fifteen minutes and strain. *Pharm. E.*) It contains bitter extractive and essential oil, dissolved in water. It is used, occasionally, as a vehicle for tonic powders, pills, &c., and in fomentations and glysters; but for the last purpose, warm water is equally efficacious. The Dublin college has a compound decoction.

DECOCTUM ARA'LIÆ NUDICAU'LIS; *Decoction of False Sarsaparilla*. (*Araliæ nudicaul.* ʒvj, *aquæ* Oviij. Digest for four hours, and then boil to four pints: press out and strain the decoction. Former Ph. U. S.) It is used as a stomachic, but it is an unnecessary and laborious preparation.

DECOCTUM CASSIÆ; *Decoction of Cassia.* (*Cassiæ pulp.* ℨij, *aquæ* Oij. Boil for a few minutes, filter without expression, and add *syrup. violar.* ℨj, or *mannæ pur.* ℨij. (*Pharm. P.*) It is laxative, in the dose of ℨvj.

DECOCTUM CETRA'RIÆ, *Decoction of Iceland Moss.* (*Cetrar.* ℨss, *aquæ* Oiss. Boil to a pint, and strain with compression. *Ph. U. S.*) Dose, fℨiv to Oss, and more.

DECOCTUM CHAMÆMELI, Decoctum anthemidis nobilis.

DECOCTUM CHIMAPH'ILÆ, *Decoction of Pipsissewa.* (*Chimaph. contus.* ℨj, *aquæ* Oiss. Boil to a pint, and strain. *Pharm. U. S.*) Dose, fℨiss.

DECOCTUM CINCHO'NÆ, Decoctum Cinchonæ, D. Cor'ticis Cinchonæ; Decoction of Cinchona, D. of Bark, Decoctum Kinæ Kinæ. (*Cinchon. cort. contus.* ℨj, *aquæ* Oj. Boil for ten minutes, in a slightly covered vessel, and strain while hot. *Pharm. U. S.*) It contains quinia and resinous extractive, dissolved in water. Long coction oxygenates and precipitates the extractive. It can be given, where the powder does not sit easy, &c. Dose, fℨj to ℨiv.

The Pharmacopœia of the United States has a *Decoctum Cinchonæ flavæ*, Decoction of yellow bark, and a *Decoctum Cinchonæ rubræ*, Decoction of red bark, both of which are prepared as above.

DECOCTUM COLOM'BÆ COMPOS'ITUM; *Compound Decoction of Colomba.* (*Colomb. contus., quassiæ,* āā ℨij, *cort. aurant.* ℨj, *rhej pulv.* ℈j, *potassæ carbonat.* ℨss, *aquæ* ℨxx. Boil to a pint, and add *tinct. lavand.* fℨss. Former *Ph. U. S.*) Given as a tonic, but not worthy an officinal station.

DECOCTUM COMMUNE PRO CLYSTERE, D. malvæ compositum—d. Cornu cervini, Mistura cornu usti.

DECOCTUM CORNÛS FLOR'IDÆ, *Decoction of Dogwood.* (*Cornûs Florid.* cont. ℨj, *aquæ* Oj. Boil for ten minutes in a covered vessel, and strain while hot. *Pharm. U. S.*) Dose, fℨiss.

DECOCTUM CYDO'NIÆ, *Mucila'go Sem'inis Cydo'nii Mali, M. Sem'inum Cydonio'rum; Decoction or Mu'cilage of Quince seeds.* (*Cydoniæ sem.* ℨij, *aquæ* Oj. Boil for ten minutes over a gentle fire, and strain. *Pharm. L.*) It is merely a solution of mucilage in water, and is used as a demulcent.

DECOCTUM DAPHNES MEZE'REI, *Decoction of Meze'rei, Decoction of Meze'reon.* (*Cort. rad. daphn. mezerei,* ℨij, *rad. glycyrrh.* cont. ℨss, *aquæ* Oiij. Boil over a gentle fire to Oij, and strain.) The acrimony of the mezereon and the saccharine mucilage of the liquorice root are imparted to the water. It is somewhat stimulant, and has been used in secondary syphilis; but is devoid of power. Dose fℨiij to ℨvj.

DECOCTUM DIAPHORETICUM, D. Guaiaci compositum—d. pro Enemate, D. malvæ compositum.

DECOCTUM DIGITA'LIS, *Decoction of Fox-glove.* (*Fol. digit. sicc.* ℨj, *aquæ* q. s. ut colentur fℨviij. Let the liquor begin to boil over a slow fire, and then remove it. Digest for fifteen minutes, and strain. *Pharm. D.*) It possesses the properties of the plant. Dose, fℨij to ℨiij.

DECOCTUM DULCAMA'RÆ, *Decoction of Woody Nightshade.* (*Dulcamaræ* cont. ℨj, *aquæ* Oiss. Boil to Oj, and strain. *Pharm. U. S.*) This decoction has been considered diuretic and diaphoretic, and has been administered extensively in skin diseases. It is probably devoid of efficacy.

DECOCTUM PRO FOMENTO, D. papaveris.

DECOCTUM GEOFFRÆ'Æ INERM'IS; *Decoction of Cabbage-Tree Bark.* (*Cort. geoffr. inermis* in pulv. ℨj, *Aquæ* Oij. Boil over a slow fire to a pint, and strain. *Pharm. E.*) It is possessed of anthelmintic, purgative, and narcotic properties, and has been chiefly used for the first of these purposes. Dose, to children, fℨij — to adults, fℨss to ℨij.

DECOCTUM GUAIACI COMPOS'ITUM, D. Guaiaci officina'lis compos'itum, Decoctum Ligno'rum, D. de Guyaco compos'itum, D. sudorif'icum, D. diaphoret'icum; *Compound decoction of Guaiacum, Decoction of the Woods.* (*Lign. guaiac. rasur.* ℨiij, *fruct. sicc. vitis vinifer.* ℨij, *rad. lauri. sassafr.* concis., *rad. glycyrrh.* āā ℨj, *aquæ* Ox. Boil the Guaiacum and raisins over a slow fire to Ov: adding the roots towards the end, then strain. *Pharm. E.*) It is possessed of stimulant properties, and has been given in syphilitic, cutaneous, and rheumatic affections. The resin of the guaiacum is, however, insoluble in water, so that the guaiac wood in it cannot be supposed to possess much, if any, effect. The Parisian Codex has a

DECOCTUM DE GUYACO COMPOS'ITUM ET PURGANS, (F.) *Décoction de Gayac Composée et Purgative; Compound purgative Decoction of Guaiacum.* (*Lign. guaiac. rasp., rad. sarsap.* āā ℨj, *potass. carbonat.* gr. xxv. Macerate for twelve hours, agitating occasionally, in *water* Oiv, until there remain Oiij. Then infuse in it *fol. sennæ* ℨij, *rhej* ℨj, *lign. sassafr., glycyrrh. rad.* āā ℨij, *sem. coriand.* ℨj. Strain gently, suffer it to settle, and pour off the clear supernatant liquor. The title sufficiently indicates the properties of the composition.

DECOCTUM HÆMATOX'YLI, *Decoction of Logwood.* (*Hæmatoxyl.* rasur. ℨj, *aquæ* Oij. Boil to a pint, and strain. *Pharm. U. S.*)

DECOCTUM HELLEBORI ALBI, D. veratri — d. Kinæ kinæ, D. Cinchonæ.

DECOCTUM HOR'DEI, *Decoctum Hordei Dis'tichi, Ptis'ana Hippocrat'ica, Tipsa'ria, Tapsa'ria, Aqua Hordea'ta, Hydrocri'thē, Barley Water, Decoc'tion of Barley,* (F.) *Décoction d'Orge, Tisane Commune.* (*Hord.* ℨij, *Aquæ* Oivss. Wash the barley well, boil for a few minutes in *water* Oss: strain this, and throw it away, and add the remainder, boiling. Boil to Oij, and strain. *Pharm. L.*) It is nutritive and demulcent, and is chiefly used as a common drink, and in glysters.

DECOC'TUM HORDEI COMPOS'ITUM, *Decoctum pectora'lē, Ptisana commu'nis;* Compound Decoction of Barley, (F.) *Décoction d'Orge composée.* (*Decoct. hord.* Oij, *caricæ fruct.* concis. ℨij, *glycyrrh. rad.* concis. et contus. ℨss, *uvarum pass.* demptis acinis. ℨij, *aquæ* Oj. Boil to Oij, and strain. *Pharm. L.*) It has similar properties to the last.

DECOCTUM KINÆ KINÆ COMPOS'ITUM ET LAXANS, *Décoction de quinquina composée et laxative; Compound lax'ative decoction of Cinchona.* (*Cort. cinchon.* ℨj, *aquæ* Oij. Boil for a quarter of an hour, remove it from the fire; then infuse in it for half an hour, *fol. sennæ, sodæ sulph.* āā ℨij: add *syrup de sennā* fℨj.) Its title indicates its properties.

DECOCTUM LICHE'NIS, *Decoctum Liche'nis Islan'dici; Decoction of Liv'erwort.* (*Lichen* ℨj, *aquæ* Oiss. Boil to a pint, and strain. *Pharm. L.*) It consists of bitter extractive and fecula, dissolved in water, and its operation is tonic and demulcent. Dose, fℨj to ℨiv. It is also nutrient, but hardly worthy of the rank of an officinal preparation.

DECOCTUM LIGNORUM, D. Guaiaci compositum.

DECOCTUM MALVÆ COMPOS'ITUM, *Decoctum pro enem'atē, Decoctum commu'nē pro clyste'rē; Compound Decoction of Mallow,* (F.) *Décoction de Mauve composée.* (*Malvæ exsicc.* ℨj, *anthe-*

mid. flor. exsicc. ℥ss, *aquæ* Oj. Boil for fifteen minutes and strain.) It consists of bitter extractive, and mucilage in water, and is chiefly used for clysters and fomentations. It is unworthy a place in the pharmacopœias.

DECOCTUM MEZEREI, D. daphnes mezerei—d. Pectorale, D. hordei compositum.

DECOCTUM PAPAV'ERIS, *Decoc'tum pro Fomen'to, Fotus commu'nis; Decoction of Poppy.* (*Papav. somnif. capsul.* concis. ℥iv, *aquæ* Oiv. Boil for fifteen minutes, and strain. *Pharm. L.*) It contains the narcotic principle of the poppy, and mucilage in water: is anodyne and emollient, and employed as such in fomentation, in painful swellings, ulcers, &c.

DECOCTUM POLYGALÆ SENEGÆ, D. Senegæ.

DECOCTUM QUERCÛS ALBÆ, *D. Quercûs Ro'boris; Decoction of White Oak Bark.* (*Quercûs cort.* ℥j, *aquæ* Oiss. Boil to a pint, and strain. *Pharm. U. S.*) It is astringent, and used as such, in injections, in leucorrhœa, uterine hemorrhage, &c., as well as in the form of fomentation to unhealthy ulcers.

DECOCTUM SARSAPARIL'LÆ, *D. Smi'lacis Sarsaparillæ; Decoction of Sarsaparilla.* (*Sarsaparill. rad.* concis. ℥iv, *aq. ferrent.* Oiv. Macerate for four hours, near the fire, in a lightly covered vessel; then bruise the root; macerate again for two hours; then boil to Oij, and strain. *Pharm. L.*) It contains bitter extractive, and mucilage in water; is demulcent, and has been used, although it is doubtful with what efficacy, in the sequelæ of syphilis. Dose, f℥iv to Oss.

DECOCTUM SARSAPARILLÆ COMPOS'ITUM; *Compound Decoction of Sarsaparil'la,* (F.) *Décoction de Salsapareille Composée.* (*Sarsaparill.* concis. et contus. ℥vj, *Sassafr. Cort.* concis., *Lign. Guaiac.* rasur., *Rad. Glycyrrhis.* contus. ää ℥j, *Mezerei,* concis. ʒiij, *Aquæ* Oiv. Boil fifteen minutes, and strain. *Pharm. U. S.*) This is considered to be possessed of analogous properties to the celebrated *Lisbon Diet-Drink, Decoc'tum Lusitan'icum,* which it resembles in composition.

DECOCTUM SCILLÆ; *Decoction of Squill.* (*Scillæ,* ʒiij, *juniper.* ℥iv, *Senegæ,* ℥iij, *Aquæ,* Oiv. Boil till one half the liquor is consumed; strain, and add *spirit of nitrous ether,* f℥iv. *Former Pharm. U. S.*) Dose, f℥ss.

DECOCTUM SEN'EGÆ, *D. Polyg'alæ Senegæ; Decoction of Senega.* (*Seneg.* cont. ℥j, *aquæ* Oiss. Boil to Oj, and strain. *Ph. U. S.*) It is reputed to be diuretic, purgative, and stimulant, and has been given in dropsy, rheumatism, &c.

DECOCTUM SMILACIS SARSAPARILLÆ, D. sarsaparillæ—d. Sudorificum, D. Guaiaci compositum.

DECOCTUM TARAX'ACI, *Decoction of Dandelion.* (*Taraxac.* contus. ℥ij, *aquæ* Oij. Boil to a pint, and strain. *Ph. U. S.*) Dose, f℥iss.

DECOCTUM ULMI, *D. Ulmi Campes'tris; Decoction of Elm Bark.* (*Ulmi cort. recent.* cont. ℥iv, *aquæ* Oiv. Boil to Oij, and strain. *Pharm. L.*) It is a reputed diuretic, and has been used in lepra and herpes; but, probably, has no efficacy. Dose, f℥iv to Oss.

DECOCTUM UVÆ URSI, *Decoction of uva ursi.* (*Uvæ ursi,* ℥j, *aquæ,* f℥xx. Boil to a pint and strain. *Ph. U. S.*) Dose, f℥iss.

DECOCTUM VERA'TRI, *Decoctum Helleb'ori albi; Decoction of White Hellebore.* (*Veratri rad.* cont. ℥j, *aquæ* Oij, *spir. rec.* f℥ij. Boil the watery decoction to Oj, and, when it is cold, add the spirit. *Pharm. L.*) It is stimulant, acrid, and cathartic; but is used only externally. It is a useful wash in *tinea capitis, psora,* &c. Should it excite intense pain on being applied, it must be diluted.

DECOC'TUM ZITTMAN'NI, *Zitt'mann's Decoction.* A most absurd farrago, extolled by Theden in venereal diseases, the formula for which, according to Jourdan, "some blockheads have lately reproduced among us as a novelty." It is composed of *sarsaparilla, pulvis stypticus, calomel* and *cinnabar,* boiled in *water* with *aniseed, fennel seed,* and *liquorice root.* A *stronger* and a *weaker* decoction were directed by Zittmann. Formulæ for its preparation are contained in Jourdan's Pharmacopœia Universalis; and in Lincke's Vollständiges Recept-Taschenbuch. Leipz., 1841.

DÉCOLLEMENT, (F.) *Deglutina'tio, Reglutina'tio,* (from *de* and *coller,* 'to glue.') The state of an organ that is separated from the surrounding parts, owing to destruction of the areolar membrane which united them. The skin is *décollée,* i. e. separated from the subjacent parts, by a burn, subcutaneous abscess, &c.

DÉCOLLEMENT DU PLACENTA is the separation or detachment of the whole or a part of the placenta from the inner surface of the uterus. *Décollement,* from *de,* 'from,' and *collum,* 'the neck,' *obtrunca'tio,* also means the separation of the head of the fœtus from the trunk, the latter remaining in the uterus.

DECOLORA'TION, *Decolora'tio, Discolora'tio,* from *de,* 'from,' and *colorare,* 'to colour.' Loss of the natural colour; *Parachro'sis.* Devoid of colour—*Achroma'sia.*

In Pharmacy, any process by which liquids, or solids in solution, are deprived wholly or in part of their colour,—as by bringing them in contact with animal charcoal.

DÉCOMPOSÉE, (F.) from *de,* 'from,' and *componere,* 'to compose.' *Decompo'sed, Dissolu'tus.* An epithet, applied to the face when extensively changed in its expression and colour; as in the choleric or moribund.

DECORTICA'TION, from *de,* 'from,' and *cortex,* 'bark.' An operation, which consists in separating the bark from roots, stalks, &c.

DECOS'TIS, *Apleu'ros,* from *de,* priv., and *costa,* 'a rib.' One who has no ribs.

DECREMENTUM, Decline.

DECREP'ITUDE, *Decrepitu'do, Ætas decrep'ita, Ul'tima senec'tus, Senec'ta decrep'ita seu extre'ma* seu *summa* seu *ul'tima,* from *decrepitus,* (*de,* and *crepare,* 'to creak,') 'very old.' The last period of old age, and of human life; which ordinarily occurs about the eightieth year. It may, however, be accelerated or protracted. Its character consists in the progressive series of phenomena which announce the approaching extinction of life.

DECRETORII DIES, Critical days.

DECU'BITUS, from *decumbere,* (*de,* and *cumbere,* 'to lie,') 'to lie down.' *Cuba'tio.* Lying down. Assuming the horizontal posture, *cu'bitus supi'nus;* (F.) *Coucher. Horâ decubitûs,* 'at bed time.' The French say — *Decubitus horizontal, sur le dos, sur le coté,* for, lying in the horizontal posture, on the back or side.

DECURTA'TUS, μειουρος, or μειουριζων, from *de,* and *curtus,* 'short,' 'shortened, curtailed,' 'running to a point.' When applied to the pulse, it signifies a progressive diminution in the strength of the arterial pulsations, which, at last, cease. If the pulsations return and gradually acquire all their strength, it is called *Pulsus decurta'tus recip'rocus.*—Galen.

DECUSSA'TION, *Decussa'tio, Chias'mos, Incrucia'tio, Intersec'tio, Intricatu'ra,* from *decussis,* that is, *decem asses;* also, the figure of the letter X. Union in the shape of an X or cross. Anatomists use this term chiefly in the case of the nerves — as the *decussation of the optic nerves,* which cross each other within the cranium.

18

DECUSSO'RIUM, from *decutio*, (*de*, and *quatio*,) 'I shake down.' An instrument used by the ancients, for depressing the dura mater, and facilitating the exit of substances effused on or under that membrane. It is described by Scultetus, Paré, &c. See Meningophylax.

DÉDAIGNEUR, Rectus superior oculi.

DEDENTITION, see Dentition.

DEDOLA'TION, *Dedola'tio*, from *dedolare*, (*de*, and *dolare*,) 'to cut and hew with an axe.' This word has been used by surgeons to express the action by which a cutting instrument divides obliquely any part of the body, and produces a wound with loss of substance. It is commonly on the head, that wounds by dedolation are observed. When there was a complete separation of a portion of the bone of the cranium, the ancients called it *Aposceparnis'mus*.

DEERBERRY, Gaultheria, Vaccinium stamineum.

DEERFOOD, Brasenia hydropeltis.

DEERS' TEARS, Bezoar of the Deer.

DÉFAILLANCE, Syncope.

DEFECA'TION, *Defœca'tio*, from *de*, and *fæces*, 'excrements.' The act by which the excrement is extruded from the body. *Caca'tio*, *Excre'tio alvi*, *E. alvi'na*, *E. fæcum alvina'rum*, *Dejec'tio alvi*, *Seces'sio*, *Expul'sio* vel *Ejec'tio fæcum*, *Apago'gē*, *Hypochore'sis*, *Ecchore'sis*, *Eccopro'sis*, *Eges'tio*. The fæces generally accumulate in the colon, being prevented by the annulus at the top of the rectum from descending freely into that intestine. In producing evacuations, therefore, in obstinate constipation, it is well, by means of a long tube, to throw the injection into the colon, as suggested by Dr. O'Beirne.

In *Pharmacy*, defecation means the separation of any substance from a liquid in which it may be suspended. See Clarification.

DEFECTIO ANIMI, Syncope.

DEFECTUS LOQUELÆ, Aphonia — d. Veneris, Anaphrodisia.

DÉFENSI'VUM, from *defendere*, (*de*, and *fendere*,) 'to defend.' A preservative or defence. The old surgeons gave this name to different local applications, made to diseased parts, for the purpose of guarding them from the impression of extraneous bodies, and particularly from the contact of air.

DEF'ERENS, from *defero*, (*de*, and *ferre*,) 'I bear away,' 'I transport.'

DEFERENS, VAS, *Ductus* seu *Cana'lis deferens*, *Vibra'tor*, (F.) *Conduit spermatique*, *Conduit déférent*, is the excretory canal of the sperm, which arises from the epididymis, describes numerous convolutions, and with the vessels and nerves of the testicle concurs in the formation of the spermatic chord, enters the abdominal ring, and terminates in the ejaculatory duct.

DEFIBRINATION, see Defibrinized.

DEFIB'RINIZED, (F.) *Défibriné*. Deprived of fibrin. A term applied to blood from which the fibrin has been removed, as by whipping. The act of removing fibrin from the blood has been termed *defibrination*.

DEFIGURATIO, Deformation.

DEFLAGRA'TION, *Deflagra'tio*, from *deflagrare*, (*de*, and *flagrare*, 'to burn,') 'to set on fire.' In pharmacy, the rapid combustion of a substance with flame; great elevation of temperature; violent motion, and more or less noise. Thus, we speak of the deflagration of nitrate, and of chlorate, of potassa, of gunpowder, &c.

DEFLECTENS, Derivative.

DEFLECTIO, Derivation.

DEFLORATION, Stuprum.

DEFLORA'TION, *Deflora'tio*, *Devirgina'tio*, *Virgin'itas deflora'ta*, from *deflorescere*, (*de*, and *florescere*,) 'to shed flowers.' The act of depriving a female of her virginity. Inspection of the parts is the chief criterion of defloration having been forcibly accomplished; yet inquiry must be made, whether the injury may not have been caused by another body than the male organ. Recent defloration is infinitely more easy of detection than where some time has elapsed.

DEFLUVIUM, Aporrhœa — d. Pilorum, Alopecia.

DEFLUXIO, Catarrh, Diarrhœa—d. Catarrhalis, Influenza.

DEFLUX'ION, *Deflux'io*, *Deflux'us*, *Catar'rhysis*, *Hypor'rhysis*, *Catar'rhus*. A falling down of humours from a superior to an inferior part. It is sometimes used synonymously with inflammation.

DEFLUXUS DYSENTERICUS, Dysentery.

DEFORMA'TION, *Deforma'tio*, *Cacomor'phia*, *Cacomorpho'sis*, *Dysmor'phē*, *Dysmor'phia*, *Dysmorpho'sis*, *Deform'itas*, *Defigura'tio*, *Disfigura'tion*, *Deform'ity*, *Inform'itas*, (F.) *Difformité*, from *de*, and *forma*. Morbid alteration in the form of some part of the body, as of the head, pelvis, spine, &c. A deformity may be natural or accidental.

DE'FRUTUM, (F.) *Vin cuit*, from *defrutare*, 'to boil new wine.' Grape must, boiled down to one-half and used as a sweetmeat. — Plin. Columell. Isidor. See Rob.

DEFUSIO, Decantation.

DEGENERATIO, Degeneration — d. Adiposa Cordis, Steatosis cordis.

DEGENERA'TION, *Degeneratio*, *Notheu'sis*, *Nothi'a*, from *degener*, 'unlike one's ancestors,' (*de*, and *genus*, 'family,') *Degen'eracy*, (F.) *Abatardissement*. A change for the worse in the intimate composition of the solids or fluids of the body. In pathological anatomy, *degeneration* means the change which occurs in the structure of an organ, when transformed into a matter essentially morbid; as a *cancerous*, or *tubercular*, degeneration.

Dégénérescence is, by the French pathologists, employed synonymously with Degeneration.

DÉGÉNÉRESCENCE, Degeneration — d. *Graisseuse du Foie*, Adiposis hepatica—d. *Granulée du Rein*, Kidney, Bright's disease of the— d. *Noire*, Melanosis.

DEGLUTINATIO, Décollement.

DEGLUTITIO, Deglutition—d. Difficilis, Dysphagia—d. Impedita, Dysphagia—d. Læsa, Dysphagia.

DEGLUTIT"ION, *Deglutit"io*, *Catap'osis*, from *de*, and *glutire*, 'to swallow.' The act by which substances are passed from the mouth into the stomach, through the pharynx and œsophagus. It is one of a complicated character, and requires the aid of a considerable number of muscles; the first steps being voluntary, the remainder executed under spinal and involuntary nervous influence.

DEGMUS, *Dexis*, *Morsus*, (F.) *Morsure*, — a bite in general, from δάκνω, 'I bite.' A gnawing sensation about the upper orifice of the stomach, which was once attributed to acrimony of the liquids contained in that viscus.

DÉGORGEMENT, Disgorgement.

DÉGOUT, Disgust.

DEGREE', from *degré*, originally from *gradus*, 'a step.' A title conferred by a college,—as the 'degree of Doctor of Medicine.' Galen used this expression to indicate the qualities of certain drugs. Both he and his school admitted *cold*, *warm*, *moist*, and *dry* medicines, and four different 'degrees' of each of those qualities. Thus, Apium was warm in the *first* degree, Agrimony in the *second*, Roche Alum in the *third*, and Garlic in the *fourth*. Bedegar was cold in the *first*, the flower of the Pomegranate in the *second*, the Sempervivum in the *third*, Opium in the *fourth*, &c. The French use the term *degré* to indicate, 1. The intensity of an affection: as a burn of the *first, second, third degree*, &c. 2. The particular stage of an incurable disease, as the *third degree* of phthisis, cancer of the stomach, &c.

DEGUSTA'TION, *Degusta'tio*, from *de*, and *gustare*, 'to taste.' *Gustation*. The appreciation of sapid qualities by the gustatory organs.

DEICTICOS, Index.

DEIRONCUS, Bronchocele.

DEJECTEDNESS, Depression.

DEJECTIO ALVI, Defecation — d. Alvina, Excrement.

DEJEC'TION, from *dejicere, dejectum, (de, and jacere,)* 'to cast down.' *Dejec'tio, Subduc'tio, Hypago'gè, Hypochore'sis, Hypecchore'sis, Apop'atus, Hypop'atus, Hypoph'ora*. The expulsion of the fæces;—*Ejec'tio, Eges'tio*. Also, a fæcal discharge or stool,—generally, however, with *alvine* prefixed,—as an *alvine Dejection, Alvus vir'idis, Dejectio alvi'na*. Also, depression of spirits.

DEJECTIONES NIGRÆ, Melæna.

DEJECTORIUM, Cathartic.

DELACHRYMATIO, Epiphora.

DELACHRYMATIVUS, Apodacryticus.

DELAPSIO, Prolapsus.

DELAPSUS, Prolapsus—d. Palpebræ, Blepharoptosis.

DELATIO, Indication.

DÉLAYANTS, Diluentia.

DELCROIX'S DEPILATORY, see Depilatory, Colley's.

DELETE'RIOUS, *Delete'rius, Pernicio'sus*, (F.) *Pernicieux*, from δηλεω, 'I injure.' That which produces destructive disorder in the exercise and harmony of the functions.

DELETERIUM, Poison.

DELIGATIO, Deligation, Ligature, see Bandage.

DELIGA'TION, *Deliga'tio, Epidei'sis, Deligatu'ra, Vul'nerum deliga'tio, Fascia'rum Applica'tio, Plaga'rum Vinctu'ra, Fascia'tio*, from *deligare, (de*, and *ligo*,) 'to bind.' The deligation of wounds formerly embraced the application of apparatus, dressings, &c., — the denomination *Beliga'tor Plaga'rum* being synonymous with *Medicus Vulnera'rius*, and in derivation, with the Wundarzt, 'wound physician' or surgeon, of the Germans. Deligation is hardly ever used now as an English word. In France, it is applied to the regular and methodical application of bandages, and to the ligature of arteries.

DELIGATURA, Deligation.

DELIQUES'CENT, *Deliques'cens*, from *deliquescere, (de*, and *liquescere*,) 'to melt,' 'to dissolve.' Any salt which becomes liquid by attracting moisture from the air. The deliquescent salts require to be kept in bottles, well stopped. Chloride of lime, acetate of potassa, and carbonate of potassa, are examples of such salts. The ancient chemists expressed the condition of a body, which had become liquid in this manner, by the word *Deliquium*.

DELIQUIUM ANIMI, Syncope.

DELIRANS, Delirious.

DÉLIRANT, Delirious.

DELIBATIO, Delirium—d. Senum, see Dementia.

DÉLIRE, Delirium—d. *Crapuleux*, Delirium tremens—d. *Tremblant*, Delirium tremens.

DELIRIA, Insanity.

DELIR'IOUS. Same etymon as DELIRIUM. *Deli'rans, Deli'rus, Excerebra'tus, Alloch'oüs,* *Alie'nus, Parale'rus, Raving*. (F.) *Délirant*. One who is in a state of delirium. That which is attended by delirium. The French use the term *Fièvre pernicieuse délirante* for a febrile intermittent, in which delirium is the predominant symptom.

DELIR'IUM, from *de*, 'from,' and *lira*, 'a ridge between two furrows:' *Parac'opè, Phreni'tis, Phledoni'a, Desipien'tia, Aphros'ynè, Paralere'ma, Paralere'sis, Paralog''ia, Phanta'sia, Paraphros'ynè, Emo'tio, Leros, Paranœ'a, Alloph'asis, Delira'tio*, (F.) *Délire, Égarement d'esprit*, &c., *Transport, Idéosynchysis*. Straying from the rules of reason; wandering of the mind. Hippocrates used the word μανια, *mania*, for *delirium sine febre*, and the Greek words given above for *delirium cum febre*. In different authors, also, we find the words, *Paraph'ora, Paraph'rotes, Paraphrene'sis, Paraphren'ia, Phrene'sis, Phreneti'asis*, &c., for different kinds of delirium. Delirium is usually symptomatic.

DELIRIUM EBRIOSITATIS, D. tremens — d. Epileptic, see Epilepsy — d. Furiosum, Mania — d. Maniacum, Mania—d. Potatorum, D. tremens— d. Tremifaciens, D. tremens.

DELIRIUM SENILE, see Dementia.

DELIRIUM TREMENS, *Ma'nia à Potû, Œnoma'nia, Ma'nia e temulen'tiâ, D. potato'rum, D. ebriosita'tis, D. tremifa'ciens, D. vig''ilans, Erethis'-mus ebrioso'rum, Dipsoma'nia, Meningi'tis seu Phreni'tis potato'rum, Tromoma'nia, Tromoparanœ'a, Potoparanœ'a, Pototromoparanœ'a*, (F.) *Encéphalopathie crapuleuse, Délire tremblant, D. crapuleux, Folie des Ivrognes*. A state of delirium and agitation, peculiar to those addicted to spirituous liquors, with great sleeplessness. It is preceded by indisposition, lassitude, watchfulness, headach, and anorexia; the delirium and tremors most commonly recurring in paroxysms. It is caused by the habitual and intemperate use of ardent spirits or of opium or tobacco; or rather by abandoning them after prolonged use. The treatment is various. Many have regarded stimulants, with large doses of opium to induce rest, to be indispensable. It is certain, however, that the expectant system will often, if not generally, be successful; and, it is probable, a cure effected in this manner will be more permanent than when produced by excitants.

DELIRUS, Delirious.

DÉLITESCENCE, see Repercussion.

DELITESCENTIA, see Repercussion.

DÉLIVRANCE, (F.) An expression, which, in common language, signifies the action of delivering, *libera'tio*, but in the practice of obstetrics, means the extrusion of the secundines, either spontaneously or by the efforts of art. This completion of delivery—*partus secunda'rius, secundina'rum expul'sio* vel *extrac'tio*, is produced by the same laws as the expulsion of the fœtus. Sometimes, the after-birth follows the child immediately; at others, it is retained; and requires manual interference to remove it. The following are the chief cases in which this becomes necessary. 1. Intimate adhesion between the placenta and paries of the uterus. 2. Spasmodic contraction of the orifice of the uterus. 3. Hour-glass contraction. 4. Torpor or hemorrhage after the expulsion of the child, and,—5. Insertion of the placenta at the orifice of the uterus.

DELIVERY, FALSE, False water.

DÉLIVRE, Secundines.

DELOCATIO, Luxatio.

DELPHIN'IUM, from δελφις, or δελφιν, 'a dolphin,' which the flowers resemble. *D. consol'ida* seu *Seg''etum* seu *Versic'olor, Calcitra'pa, Consol'ida Rega'lis, Branching Larkspur, Stag gerweed.* Family Ranunculaceæ. *Sex. Syst.* Polyandria Trigynia. (F.) *Pied d'alouette des champs.* It has been employed as a vermifuge. The flowers have been used in ophthalmia, and the seeds have the same property as those of *Stavesacre.*

DELPHINIUM CONSOLIDA, Delphinium — d. Segetum, Delphinium.

DELPHIN'IUM STAPHISA'GRIA. The systematic name of the *Staves'acre, Staphisagria, Phtheiroc'tonum, Phthei'rium, Staphis, Pedicula'ria,* (F.) *Staphisaigre, Herbe aux Poux, Dauphinelle.* The seeds have a disagreeable smell; a nauseous, bitterish, hot taste; and are cathartic, emetic, and vermifuge: owing, however, to the violence of their operation, they are seldom given internally, and are chiefly used in powder, mixed with hair powder, to destroy lice. The active principle of this plant has been separated, and received the name *Delphin'ia.* It is extremely acrid, and has been recently used, like veratria, in tic douloureux, paralysis and rheumatism. It is used in the form of ointment, or in solution in alcohol, (gr. x to xxx, or more, to ʒj,) applied externally.

DELPHINIUM VERSICOLOR, Delphinium.

DELPHYS, Uterus, Vulva.

DELTA, Vulva.

DELTIFORMIS, Deltoid.

DELTOID, *Deltoï'des, Delto'des, Deltoïdeus, Deltiform'is,* from the Greek capital letter Δ, δέλτα, and είδος, 'resemblance.' *Sous-acromio-clavi-huméral* of Dumas; *Sus-acromio-huméral* of Chaussier. A triangular muscle forming the fleshy part of the shoulder, and covering the shoulder-joint. It extends from the outer third of the clavicle, from the acromion and spine of the scapula, to near the middle and outer part of the os humeri, where it is inserted by means of a strong tendon. This muscle raises the arm directly upwards, when the shoulder is fixed, and carries it anteriorly or posteriorly, according to the direction of the fibres, which are thrown into action. If the arm be rendered immovable, the deltoid acts inversely and depresses the shoulder.

DELUSION, Hallucination.

DEM EL MUCA. A name given by Prosper Alpinus to a disease, which, he says, is proper to Egypt. He considers it to be inflammation of the brain; but others describe it as a pernicious intermittent.

DEMAGNETIZA'TION, *Demagnetisa'tio.* The act of removing the condition of magnetisation.

DÉMANGEAISON, Itching.

DEMANUS, Acheir.

DÉMENCE, Dementia—*d. Innée,* Idiotism.

DEMENTED, Insane.

DEMEN'TIA, *Amen'tia, Fatu'itas, Anœ'a, Anœ'sia, Deuteranœ'a, Eonœ'a, Paranœ'a, Mo'ria demens, Noësthenì'a, Incohe'rency, Imbecil'ity, Incohe'rent Insanity;* from *de,* 'from,' or 'out of,' and *mens,* 'mind,' or 'reason.' (F.) *Démence, Bêtise.* In common parlance, and even in legal language, this word is synonymous with insanity. Physicians, however, have applied it to those cases of unsound mind which are characterised by a total loss of the faculty of 'thought, or by such an imbecility of intellect that the ideas are extremely incoherent, there being at the same time a total loss of the power of reasoning. Mania and melancholy are apt to end in this, if possible, more deplorable state. *Dotage* is the *Dementia* of the aged—*Mo'ria demens lere'ma, Lere'ma, Lere'sis, Lerus, Delira'tio Senum, Amen'tia Seni'lis, Pueril'itas, Delir'ium Seni'lis, Anil'itas, Senile Insanity, Senile Dementia, Insanity of the aged,—*a form of moral insanity, in which the whole moral character of the individual is changed.

DEMI, Semi—*d. Bain,* Semicupium—*d. Épineux,* Semi-spinalis colli—*d. Épineux du dos,* Semi-spinalis dorsi—*d. Gantelet, Gantelet—d. Interosseux du pouce,* Flexor brevis pollicis manus—*d. Lunaire,* Semi-lunar—*d. Membraneux,* Semi-membranosus—*d. Orbiculaire,* Orbicularis oris—*d. Tendineux,* Semi-tendinosus.

DEMISSIO ANIMI, Depression.

DEMISSOR, Catheter.

DEMODEX FOLLICULORUM, (δημος, 'lard,' and δήξ, 'a boring worm,') Acarus folliculorum.

DEMONOMA'NIA, *Dæmonomania, Theoma'nia, Entheoma'nia,* from *δαιμων,* 'demon,' a spirit of good or evil, and *μανια,* 'madness.' Religious insanity. A variety of madness, in which the person conceives himself possessed of devils, and is in continual dread of malignant spirits, the pains of hell, &c.

DEM'ONSTRATOR, from *demonstrare,* (*de* and *monstrare,*) 'to show;' 'exhibit.' One who exhibits. The index finger.

DEM'ONSTRATOR OF ANAT'OMY. One who exhibits the parts of the human body. A teacher of practical anatomy.

DEMOTI'VUS LAPSUS, *Repenti'na mors,* from *demovere,* (*de* and *movere,*) 'to move off,' 'remove,' and *lapsus,* 'a fall.' Sudden death.

DEMUL'CENTS, *Demulcen'tia, Involven'tia, Obvolven'tia, Lubrican'tia,* from *demulcere,* (*de* and *mulcere,*) 'to soothe,' 'to assuage.' (F.) *Adoucissants.* Medicines supposed to be capable of correcting certain acrid conditions imagined to exist in the humours. Substances of a mucilaginous or saccharine nature belong to this class. Demulcents may act *directly* on the parts with which they come in contact; but in other cases, as in catarrh, their effect is produced by contiguous sympathy; the top of the larynx being soothed by them first, and *indirectly* the inflamed portion of the air-passages. In diseases of the urinary organs, they have no advantage over simple diluents.—See Diluents and Emollients. The following are the chief demulcents;—Acaciæ Gummi; Althææ Folia et Radix; Amygdalæ; Amylum; Avenæ Farina; Cera; Cetaceum; Cydoniæ Semina; Fucus Crispus; Glycyrrhiza; Hordeum; Lichen; Linum; Olivæ Oleum; Sassafras Medulla; Sesamum; Sevum; Tragacantha, and Ulmus.

DEMUSCULA'TUS, from *de,* and *musculus,* 'a muscle.' (F.) *Décharné.* Emaciated, devoid of flesh.

DENÆUS, Chronic.

DENA'RIUS; a Roman coin, equal in value to about 10 cents, or 8 pence English. It was marked with the letter X, to signify 10 asses.

Also, the 7th part of the Roman ounce.

DENDROLIBANUS, Rosmarinus.

DENERVATIO, Aponeurosis.

DEN'GUE, *Dingea, Dunga, Dandy, Bouquet* and *Bucket Fever, Rheumatis'mus febri'lis, Scarlati'na rheumat'ica, Exanthe'sis arthro'sia, Planta'ria, Febris exanthemat'ica articula'ris,* (F.) *Giraffe, Erup'tive artic'ular fever, E. rheumat'ic fever.* A disease, which first appeared in the years 1827 and 1828, in the West Indies, and in the southern states of North America. It was extremely violent in its symptoms, but not often fatal. It usually commenced with great languor, chilliness, and pain in the tendons about the smaller joints. To these symptoms succeeded burning heat and redness of the skin, pains in the muscles of the limbs or in the forehead, with vomiting or nausea. The fever continued for one, two or three days, and usually terminated by copious perspiration. In different places, it put on different appearances; but seems in all to have been a singular variety of rheumatic fever. The usual antiphlogistic treatment was adopted, and successfully.

DENIACH, MINERAL WATERS OF. Deniach is a village in Swabia, at the entrance of the Black Forest. The waters contain carbonic acid, carbonate of iron, carbonate of lime, sulphate of magnesia, and carbonate of soda.

DENIGRA'TIO, from *denigrare*, (*de*, and *niger*,) 'to become black.' The act of becoming black, as in cases of sphacelus, sugillation, &c.

DENS, Tooth — d. Leonis, Leontodon taraxacum.

DENS PRO'LIFER. A term used by Bartholin for a supernumerary tooth, which appears to grow upon a primitive or parent tooth.

DENT, Tooth — *d. de Sagesse*, see Dentition.

DENTAGOGUM, Dentagra.

DEN'TAGRA, *Den'ticeps, Dentar'paga, Dentidu'cum, Dentic'ulum, Dentago'gum, Denta'lis Jorfex, Forfex denta'ria, Odonthar'paga, Odon'tagra, Odontago'gon*, from *dens*, 'a tooth,' and *aypa*, 'a seizure.' (F.) *Davier*. A tooth-forceps.

DENTAL, *Denta'lis, Denta'rius, Denta'tus, Denticula'tus*, from *dens*, 'a tooth.' That which concerns the teeth. See Dentiformis.

DENTAL ARCHES, (F.) *Arcades dentaires*, are the arches formed by the range of alveoli in each jaw.

DENTAL AR'TERIES are those arteries which nourish the teeth. They proceed from several sources. The teeth of the upper jaw, e. g., receive their arteries from the *infraorbitar* and *superior alveolar*,—themselves branches of the *internal maxillary*. The teeth of the lower jaw receive their branches from the *inferior dental* or *inferior maxillary*, which is given off by the internal maxillary, and runs through the dental canal, issuing at the mental foramen, after having given numerous ramifications to the teeth and jaw.

DENTAL CANALS, (F.) *Conduits dentaires, Max'illary canals*. The bony canals, through which the vessels and nerves pass to the interior of the teeth.

DENTAL CAR'TILAGE, *Cartila'go denta'lis*. The cartilaginous elevation, divided by slight fissures, on the biting margins of the gums in infants, prior to dentition. It is a substitute for the teeth.

DENTAL CAV'ITY, (F.) *Cavité dentaire*. A cavity in the interior of the teeth in which is situate the *dental pulp*.

DENTAL FOL'LICLE, *Follic'ulus Dentis, Cap'sula dentis*, (F.) *Follicule dentaire*. A membranous follicle, formed of a double lamina, in which the teeth are contained before they issue from the alveoli, and which, consequently, aids in the formation of the alveolo-dental periosteum, and of the membrane that envelops the pulp of the teeth. The dental follicles are lodged in the substance of the jaws.

DENTAL GANGRENE, *Caries Den'tium, Odontalg''ia cario'sa, Odontonecro'sis, Odontosphacel'isis, Odontosphacelis'mus, Necro'sis Den'tium*, (F.) *Carie des Dents*. Gangrene or caries of the teeth. See Caries.

DENTAL NERVES, (F.) *Nerfs dentaires*. Nerves which pass to the teeth. Those of the upper incisors and canine are furnished by the infra-orbitar nerve, a branch of the superior maxillary; and those of the molares by the trunk of the same nerve. The teeth of the lower jaw receive the nerves from the inferior maxillary, which, as well as the superior maxillary, arises from the 5th pair.

DENTAL PULP, *Pulpa seu Nu'cleus seu Substan'tia pulpo'sa dentis, Germen denta'lè*, (F.) *Pulpe dentaire*. A pultaceous substance, of a reddish-gray colour, very soft and sensible, which fills the cavity of the teeth. It is well supplied with capillary vessels.

DENTAL SURGEON, Dentist.

DENTAL VEINS have a similar distribution with the arteries.

DENTALIS, Odontoid — d. Forfex, Dentagra.

DENTA'LIUM, from *dens*, 'a tooth,' the *dog-like tooth shell*. A genus of shells in the shape of a tooth. They formerly entered into several pharmaceutical preparations, but were useless ingredients; consisting — like shells in general — of carbonate of lime and gelatin.

DENTARIA, Anthemis Pyrethrum, Plumbago Europæa.

DENTARIUS, Dentist.

DENTARPAGA, Dentagra.

DENTATA VERTEBRA, Axis.

DENTATUS, Dental.

DENTELARIA, Plumbago Europæa.

DENTELÉ ANTÉRIEUR PETIT, Pectoralis minor — *d. Grand*, Serratus magnus — *d. Postérieur et inférieur, petit*, Serratus posticus inferior — *d. Supérieur, petit*, Serratus posticus superior.

DENTES, Teeth, see Tooth — d. Angulares, Canine teeth — d. Canini, Canine teeth — d. Clavales, Molar teeth — d. Columellares, Canine teeth — d. Ctenes, Incisive teeth — d. Cuspidati, Canine teeth — d. Dichasteres, Incisive teeth — d. Gelasini, Incisive teeth — d. Gomphii, Molar teeth — d. Incisores, Incisive teeth — d. Lactei, see Dentition — d. Laniarii, Canine teeth — d. Maxillares, Molar teeth — d. Molares, Molar teeth — d. Mordentes, Canine teeth — d. Oculares, Canine teeth — d. Primores, Incisive teeth — d. Rasorii, Incisive teeth — d. Sapientiæ, see Dentition — d. Serotini, see Dentition — d. Sophroretici, see Dentition — d. Sophronistæ, see Dentition — d. Sophronisteres, see Dentition — d. Tomici, Incisive teeth.

DENTICEPS, Dentagra.

DENTICULA'TUM, (*Ligamentum*,) diminutive of *dens*, 'a tooth.' *Ligamen'tum denta'tum, Membra'na denta'ta*. A slender cord, situate between the anterior and posterior fasciculi of the spinal nerves, and between the tunica arachnoidea and pia mater. It is attached to the dura mater, where that membrane issues from the cranium, and accompanies the spinal marrow to its inferior extremity. It sends off, from its outer edge, about twenty slender processes, in the form of *denticuli*, each of which passes outwards and connects itself with the dura mater in the intervals between the anterior and posterior roots of the nerves.

DENTICULATUS, Dental.

DENTICULUM, Dentagra.

DENTICULUS, Crena.

DENTIDUCUM, Dentagra.

DENTIER, (F.) from *dens*, 'a tooth.' *Denture*. A set or row of teeth, mounted on metal or ivory, to be adjusted to the alveolar margin. *Dentiers* are simple or double. To the latter, that is, to the full set, the name *Râteliers* is given.

DENTIFORM, *Dentiform'is*, from *dens*, 'a tooth,' and *forma*, 'form.' Resembling a tooth in shape.

DENTIFORMIS, Odontoid.

DEN'TIFRICE, *Dentifric''ium, Remed'ium dentifric''ium, Tooth powder, Tooth paste, Odontotrim'ma, Odontoemeg'ma*, from *dens*, 'a tooth.' and *fricare*, 'to rub;' a name given to different powders and pastes proper for cleansing the enamel of the teeth, and removing the tartar which covers them. Powdered bark and charcoal, united to any acidulous salt — as cream of tartar — form one of the most common *dentifrices*.

Electuaire ou *Opiate Dentifrice*, of the Codex, consists of *coral* ℨiv, *cuttlefish bones* and *cinnamon*, āā ℨij, *cochineal* ℨss, *honey* ℨx, *alum* gr. iv or v.

Poudre Dentifrice of the Parisian Codex is composed of *Bole Armeniac, red coral,* [prepared,] and *cuttlefish bones,* āā ℨvj, *dragon's blood* ℨiij, *cochineal* ℨj, *cream of tartar* ℨix, *cinnamon* Ɖij, *cloves,* gr. xij, well mixed.

Charcoal, finely powdered and mixed with chalk, forms as good a dentifrice as any.

DEN'TINAL, *Dentina'lis,* from *dens,* 'a tooth.' Relating to the dentine of the teeth.

DENTINE, see Tooth—d. Secondary, see Tooth.

DENTISCAL'PIUM, from *dens,* 'a tooth,' and *scalpere,* 'to scrape.' *Odonto'glyphum.* This word has been applied to the instrument used for scaling the teeth; to the *tooth-pick,* (F.) *Cure-dent;* and to the *gum lancet,*—the *déchaussoir* of the French.

DENT'IST, *Dentis'ta, Odontia'ter, Denta'rius, Dental Surgeon, Surgeon-Dentist.* One who devotes himself to the study of the diseases of the teeth, and their treatment.

DEN'TISTRY, *Odontotech'ny, Odontiatri'a, Odontotherapi'a, Dental Surgery.* The art of the dentist.

DENTITIO, Dentition—d. Difficilis, Dysodontiasis.

DENTIT"ION, *Dentit"io, Denti'tis, Odontophy'ia, Teething, Odonti'asis, Odonto'sis,* from *dentire,* 'to breed teeth.' The exit of the teeth from the alveoli and gums; or rather the phenomena which characterize the different periods of their existence. The germs of the first teeth, *dentes lac'tei* or *milk teeth,* (F.) *dens de lait,* are visible in the fœtus about the end of the second month; and they begin to be ossified from the end of the third to that of the sixth month. At birth, the corona of the incisors is formed, but that of the canine is not completed; and the tubercles of the molares are not yet all united. Gradually the fang becomes developed; and at about six or eight months begins what is commonly called, the *first dentit"ion, Odon'tia dentitio'nis lactan'tium.* The two middle incisors of the lower jaw commonly appear first; and, some time afterwards, those of the upper jaw; afterwards, the two lateral incisors of the lower jaw; and then those of the upper, followed by the four anterior molares: the *canine* or *eye-teeth,* at first, those of the lower, and, afterwards, those of the upper jaw, next appear; and, subsequently and successively, the first 4 molares—2 above and 2 below, 1 on each side. The whole number of the *primary, temporary, deciduous, shedding* or *milk-teeth,* (*dentes tempora'rii,*) (F.) *Dents de lait,* is now 20.

The eruption of the milk-teeth takes place, approximately, in the following order:

Central incisors........6th to 8th month.
Lateral incisors........7th to 10th month.
First molar............12th to 14th month.
Canines...............15th to 20th month.
Second molar..........20th to 30th month.

The *second dentition* or *shedding of the teeth, odon'tia dentitio'nis pueri'lis, Dedentit"ion,* begins about the age of 6 or 7. The germs or membranous follicles of these second teeth—to the number of 32—as well as the rudiments of the teeth themselves, are visible, even in the fœtus, with the exception of those of the small molares, which do not appear till after birth. They are contained in alveoli of the same shape as those of the first dentition. Their ossification commences at from 3 to 6 months after birth, in the incisors and first molares; at eight or nine months, in the canine; about three years, in the molares, 3¼ in the second great molares, and about 10 years in the last. As the alveolus of a new tooth becomes gradually augmented, the septum between it and that of the corresponding milk tooth is absorbed, and disappears. The root of the milk tooth is likewise absorbed; its corona becomes loose and falls out, and all the first teeth are gradually replaced by the *permanent teeth, Den'tes serot'ini.* This second dentition becomes necessary in consequence of the increased size of the jaws. The new teeth have neither the same direction nor the same shape as the old; and they are more numerous, amounting till the age of 25, (sooner or later,) to 28. About this period, a small molaris appears at the extremity of each jaw, which is called *Dens sapien'tiæ* or *wisdom tooth, Dens serot'inus, Dens sophroret'icus, D. sophronis'ta, D. sophronis'ter,* (F.) *Arrièredent, Dent de sagesse,* making the whole number of permanent teeth 32.

The eruption of the permanent teeth is remarkable for its general regularity; so that it constitutes an important means for ascertaining the age of the individual during the early period of life.

First molars................7th year.
Central incisors............8th year.
Lateral incisors............9th year.
First bicuspids............10th year.
Second bicuspids..........11th year.
Canines...................12th year.
Second molars............13th year.

The teeth of the lower jaw precede by a few weeks those of the upper.

During the period of dentition, that is, of the first dentition, the infant is especially liable to disease;—the irritation, produced by the pressure of the tooth on the superincumbent gum, sometimes occasioning pyrexia, convulsions, diarrhœa, &c., which symptoms are often strikingly relieved by a free division of the distended gum. This disordered condition is called *Teething, Odon'tia dentitio'nis, Odonti'asis, Odontal'gia dentitio'nis, Odaxis'mus.*

DENTITIS, Dentition.

DENTIUM CORTEX, Enamel of the teeth— d. Dolor, Odontalgia— d. Nitor, Enamel of the teeth— d. Scalptura, (Lancing the gums,) see Gum lancet—d. Vacillantia, Odontoseisis.

DENTO, from *Dens,* 'a tooth.' One whose teeth are prominent.

DENTOIDEUS, Odontoid.

DENTS BICUSPIDÉES, Bicuspid teeth—*d. Col des,* Collum dentium—*d. Conoïdes,* Canine teeth—*d. de Lait,* see Dentition—*d. Mâchelières,* Molar teeth—*d. Molaires,* Molar teeth—*d. Multicuspidées,* Molar teeth, great—*d. Œillières,* Canine teeth.

DENTURE, Dentier.

DENUDA'TION, *Denuda'tio, Gymno'sis,* from *denudare,* (*de,* and *nudare,*) 'to lay bare.' Condition of a part, deprived of its natural coverings, whether by wounds, gangrene, or abscess. It is particularly applied to the bones, when deprived of their periosteum, and to the teeth when they lose their enamel or dental substance.

DEOB'STRUENT, *Deob'struens, Dephrac'ticum, Deoppi'lans, Deoppilati'vum, Ecphrac'tic,* from *de,* and *obstruere,* (*ob,* and *struere,*) 'to obstruct.' (F.) *Désobstruant, Désobstructif, Désopilatif, Désopilant.* Medicines given with the view of removing any obstruction. The word corresponds to *aperient,* in its *general,* not in its par-

ticular sense. It is now almost abandoned, and, when used, conveys by no means definite ideas.

DEODORIZER, Antibromic.

DEONTOL'OGY, *Deontolog"ia;* from τα δέοντα, 'what is fitting or necessary,' and λόγος, 'a description.' A word introduced by Bentham to signify morals, or the science of duties.

MED'ICAL DEONTOL'OGY, *Deontolog"ia med'ica,* (F.) *Déontologie médicale, Medical ethics, Medical etiquette.* The duties and rights of medical practitioners.

DEOPPILATIVUM, Deobstruent.

DEPASCENS, Phagedenic.

DEPAUPERATUS, Impoverished.

DEPERDITIO, Abortion.

DEPHRACTICUM, Deobstruent.

DÉPILATIF, Depilatory.

DEPILATIO, Alopecia—d. Capitis, Calvities.

DEPILA'TION, *Depila'tio, Dropacis'mus, Made'sis, Mad'isis, Psilo'sis,* from *de,* and *pilus,* 'hair.' Loss of hair, either spontaneously or by art.

DEP'ILATORY, *Depilato'rium, Dropax, Psilo'thron, Ectillot'icus, Epilato'rium,* (F.) *Dépilatoire, Dépilatif.* Any thing which causes the loss of the hair. Depilatories are, usually caustic applications, in which quicklime or some other alkaline substance, sulphuret of iron, &c., enter.

DEPILATORY, COLLEY'S, seems to consist of *quicklime* and a portion of *sulphuret of potassa.*

A *pitch plaster, Pitch-cap,* is sometimes used as a *depilatory.* It of course pulls the hair out by the roots.

Delcroix's depilatory, and *Plenck's depilatory,* have a similar composition.

DEPI'LIS, same etymon. Devoid of hair. Hairless.

DEPLE'TION, *Deple'tio,* from *depleo,* 'I unload.' The act of unloading the vessels, by blood-letting and the different evacuants. Also, inordinate evacuation.

DEPLE'TORY, *Deple'ting.* Having relation to depletion:—as 'a *depletory* or *depleting* agent.'

DEPLUMA'TIO, *Ptilo'sis,* from *deplumis,* (de and *pluma,*) 'without feathers.' A disease of the eyelids, in which they are swollen, and the eyelashes fall out. See Madarosis.

DEPOS'IT, *Depos'itum,* from *depono,* (de and *pono,* 'to lay or put,') 'to lay or put down.' (F.) *Depôt.* Any thing laid or thrown down. In physiology and pathology, a structureless substance, separated from the blood or other fluid, as the typhous, tuberculous, purulent, melanic, and diphtheritic *deposits.*

DEPOS'IT, Feculence.

DEPOS'ITIVE, *Depositi'vus,* from *deponere,* (de and *ponere,*) to 'depose,' 'to put down.' An epithet used by Mr. Erasmus Wilson to express that condition of the membrane in which plastic lymph is exuded into the tissue of the derma, so as to give rise to the production of small hard elevations of the skin, or pimples. Under "*depositive inflammation of the derma,*" he comprises strophulus, lichen and prurigo.

DÉPÔT. Abscess, Sediment—*d. Laiteuse sur la Cuisse,* Phlegmatia dolens—*d. de l' Urine,* Sediment of the urine.

DEPRAVATION, *Deprava'tio,* from *de* and *pravus,* 'bad.' Perversion, corruption;—as depravation of the taste, &c.

DEPREHENSIO, Diagnosis, Epilepsy.

DEPRES'SION, *Depres'sio, Impres'sio,* from *deprimere, depressum (de,* and *premere,)* 'to depress;' *Esphla'sis.* In Anatomy, it means an excavation, hollow, or fossa. In Surgery, it is applied to a fracture of the cranium, in which the portions of fractured bone are forced inwards; (F.) *Subgrondation, Entablement;* called also, *Catapi'esis, Campsis Depres'sio, Thlasis Depres'sio. Depression,* (F.) *Abaissement,* means Couching.—See Cataract.

Depression also means *dejection* or *dejectedness* —*Ademon'ia, Ademo'synē, Demis'sio animi.*

DÉPRESSOIRE, Meningophylax.

DEPRESS'OR, (F.) *Abaisseur.* Same etymon. Several muscles have been so termed, because they depress the parts on which they act.

DEPRESSOR ALÆ NASI, *D. la'bii superio'ris alæque nasi, Incisi'vus me'dius, Myrtifor'mis, Depressor Labii superio'ris pro'prius, Constricto'res ala'rum nasi ac depresso'res la'bii superio'ris, Maxillo-alvéoli-nasal*—part of the *labialis,* (Ch.,) (F.) *Abaisseur de l'aile du nez.* It arises from the superior maxillary bone immediately above the junction of the gums with the two incisor and canine teeth; and passes upwards to be inserted into the upper lip and root of the ala nasi, which it pulls downwards.

DEPRESSOR AN'GULI ORIS, *Triangula'ris, Depressor labio'rum commu'nis, Depressor labiorum,* (F.) *Sousmaxillo-labial, Maxillo-labial* (Ch.), *Abaisseur de l'angle des lèvres* ou *Muscle Triangulaire.* A muscle, situate at the lower part of the face. Its form is triangular. It arises from the outer oblique line on the lower jawbone, and terminates in a point at the commissure of the lips, which it pulls downwards.

DEPRESSOR LA'BII INFERIO'RIS; *Quadra'tus, Quadra'tus menti, Depressor labii inferio'ris pro'prius,—Mentonnier-labial, Mento-labial* (Ch.), (F.) *Carré du Menton, Houppe du Menton, Abaisseur de la lèvre inférieure.* A small, thin, and quadrilateral muscle, which arises from the external oblique line of the lower jaw, and ascends to the lower lip, where it becomes confounded with the orbicularis oris. It pulls the lower lip downwards and outwards.

DEPRESSOR LABII SUPERIORIS PROPRIUS, D. Alæ nasi — d. Labiorum communis, D. Anguli oris—d. Oculi, Rectus inferior oculi.

DEPRESSOR PAL'PEBRÆ INFERIO'RIS. A fleshy bundle, which forms part of the palpebralis muscle. Heister describes it separately, but it is not admitted now.

DEPRESSORIUM, Meningophylax.

DEPRIMENS AURICULÆ, Retrahens auris — d. Maxillæ biventer, Digastricus—d. Oculi, Rectus inferior oculi.

DEPRIMENTIA, Sedatives.

DEPURAN'TIA, from *depurare, (de,* and *purus,)* 'to purify.' (F.) *Dépuratifs.* Medicines were formerly so called, which were supposed to possess the property of removing, from the mass of blood or humours, those principles which disturbed their purity; and of directing them towards some one of the natural emunctories. The juices of what were called anti-scorbutic herbs, sulphur, and many other medicines, were ranked under this class.

DÉPURATIFS, Depurantia.

DEPURA'TION, *Depura'tio.* Same etymon. *Catharis'mos, Munda'tio.* In *Pathology,* depuration has been used for the process by which nature purifies the animal economy, either by the agency of some eruptive disease, or some spontaneous evacuation, or by the assistance of medicine. See Clarification, and Depuratory.

DEPURATIVE, Depuratory.

DEP'URATORY. Same etymon. *Depurato'rius, Depurative.* That which causes depuration, as the *urinary* and *cutaneous depurations.* Applied, also, to diseases, which have been considered capable of modifying the constitution advantageously, by acting on the composition of the fluids — such as certain eruptions, intermittents, &c. The word is, also, appropriated to medicines and diet, by which the same effect is sought to be induced.

DER'ADEN, from δερη, 'the neck,' and αδην, 'a gland.' A gland in the neck.

DERADENI'TIS, from δερη, 'neck;' αδην, 'a gland;' and itis, denoting inflammation. Inflammation of the glands of the neck.

DERADENON'CUS, from δερη, 'the neck,' αδην, 'a gland,' and ογκος, 'a swelling.' Tumefaction of the glands of the neck.

DERANENCEPHA'LIA, from δερη, 'neck,' and anencephalia, 'absence of brain.' A monstrosity in which only a small portion of the brain exists, resting on the cervical vertebræ — more properly derencepha'lia.

DERANGED, Insane.
DERANGEMENT, Insanity.
DERBIA, Impetigo.
DERENCEPHALIA, Deranencephalia.

DERENCEPH'ALUS, from δερη, 'the neck,' and κεφαλη, 'head.' A monster whose brain is in the neck.—G. St. Hilaire.

DERIS, Cutis.
DERIVANS, Derivative.
DÉRIVATIF, Derivative.

DERIVA'TION, Deriva'tio, Deflec'tio, Parocheteu'sis, Antilep'sis, Antis'pasis, Revul'sion, Oura derivati'va seu revulso'ria, from de, and rivus, 'a river.' When a 'centre of fluxion' is established in a part, for the purpose of abstracting the excited vital manifestations from some other, a derivation is operated.

The term DERIVATION has likewise been applied to the suction power of the heart,—an agency in the circulation of the blood.

DERIV'ATIVE, Deflec'tens, Deri'vans, Derivato'rius, from derivare, 'to drain off.' Antispas'ticus, Revel'lent, Revul'sive, Revulsi'vus, Revulso'rius, (F.) Dérivatif, Révulsif. Same etymon. A remedy, which by producing a modified action in some organ or texture derives from the morbid condition of some other organ or texture. Revellents are amongst the most important remedies: they include, indeed, every physical and moral agent, which is capable of modifying the function of innervation, and therefore almost every article of the materia medica. The following is a list of the chief local Derivatives:

1. EPISPASTICS. — Acidum Aceticum, Acidum Nitricum, Acidum Sulphuricum, Allium, Ammonia, Ammoniacum, Asafœtida, Cantharis, Capsicum, Galbanum, Olea Essentialia, Pix Abietis, Sinapis, Caloric, Friction.

2. VESICANTS.—Ammonia, Argenti Nitras, Cantharis, Cantharis Vittata, Hydrargyri Iodidum rubrum, Ranunculus, Sinapis, Caloric.

3. SUPPURANTS. — Acida Mineralia, Antimonii et Potassæ Tartras, Cantharis, Mezereum, Pix Abietis, Sabina, Tiglii Oleum, Fonticulus, Setaceum.

4. — ESCHAROTICS. — A. Erodents. — Acidum Aceticum, Acida Mineralia, Alumen Exsiccatum, Argenti Nitras, Cupri Sub-Acetas, Cupri Sulphas, Sabina, Saccharum Purissimum.—

B. Actual Cauterants. — Caloric, White Hot Iron, Moxa.—

C. Potential Cauterants.—Acidum Arseniosum, Acidum Nitricum, Acidum Sulphuricum, Antimonii Murias, Argenti Nitras, Calx, Potassa, Potassa cum Calce, Zinci Chloridum.

DERIVATORIUS, Derivative.
DERMA, Cutis.
DERMAD, see Dermal Aspect.
DERMAL, Dermic, Derma'lis, Der'micus, from δερμα, 'the skin.' Relating or belonging to the skin.

DERMAL ASPECT. An aspect towards the skin or external surface.—Barclay. Dermad is used adverbially by the same writer to signify 'towards the dermal aspect.'

DERMAL'GIA, Dermatal'gia, Dermatodyn'ia, from δερμα, 'the skin,' and αλγος, 'pain.' Pain in the skin. Neuralgia of the skin. Rheumatic Dermalgia or Rheumatism of the skin is a form of neuralgia, which is referred, at times, to the nervous trunks, muscles, &c., but appears to be seated in the cutaneous nerves.

DERMATAGRA, Pellagra.
DERMATALGIA, Dermalgia.
DERMATAUXE, Dermatophyma.

DERMATIATRI'A, from δερμα, 'skin,' and ιατρεια, 'healing.' Healing of cutaneous diseases. The treatment of diseases of the skin. Diadermiatri'a, Dermatocrati'a.

DERMATITIS, Cytitis, Erysipelatous inflammation.
DERMATOCHOLOSIS, Icterus.
DERMATOCHYSIS, Anasarca.
DERMATOCRATIA, see Dermatiatria.
DERMATODES, Dermatoid.
DERMATODYNIA, Dermalgia.

DER'MATOID, Dermatoi'des, Dermato'des, Dermoi'des, Dermo'des, Dermoid, from δερμα, 'the skin,' and ειδος, 'form.' That which is similar to the skin. This name is given to different tissues, which resemble the skin. The dura mater has been so called by some.

Morbi dermato'des, chronic cutaneous diseases.

DERMATOL'OGY, Dermatolog''ia, Dermol'ogy, from δερμα, 'the skin,' and λογος, 'a discourse.' A discourse or treatise of the skin.

DERMATOPATHIA, Cutaneous disease.
DERMATOPERISCLERISMUS, Induration of the cellular tissue.
DERMATOPERISCLEROSIS, Induration of the cellular tissue.

DERMATOPHY'MA, Dermataux'ē, from δερμα, 'skin,' and φυμα, 'tumour.' A tumefaction of the skin.

DERMATOPHYMATA VENEREA, Condylomata.

DERMATORRHAG''IA, Dermatorrhœ'a, from δερμα, 'skin,' and ραγη, 'rupture.' A discharge of blood from the skin.

DERMATORRHŒA, Dermatorrhagia.
DERMATOSCLEROSIS, Callosity.
DERMATOSES, Cutaneous diseases.
DERMATOSIES VÉROLEUSES, Syphilides.
DERMATOSPASMUS, Horrida cutis.
DERMATOTYLOMA, Callosity.
DERMATOTYLOSIS, Callosity.
DERMATOTYLUS, Callosity.

DERMIC, Der'micus, Dermat'icus, Dermatinus, Dermatic, Dermal, Derma'lis; from δερμα, 'skin.' Relating to the skin.

DERMITIS, Cytitis.
DERMODES, Dermatoid.

DERMOG'RAPHY, Dermograph'ia, from δερμα, 'the skin,' and γραφω, 'I describe.' An anatomical description of the skin.

DERMOHÆ'MIA, from δερμα, 'skin,' and αιμα, 'blood.' Hyperæmia or congestion of the skin.

DERMOID, Dermatoid.
DERMOLOGY, Dermatology.
DERMO-SKELETON, see Skeleton.
DERMO-SYPHILIDES, Syphilides.

DERMOTOMY, Dermotom'ia, from δερμα, 'the skin,' and τεμνειν, 'to cut.' The part of anatomy which treats of the structure of the skin.

DERODYMUS, Dicephalus.
DERONCUS, Bronchocele.

DERTRON. This word, which is used by Hippocrates, signified, according to some, the omentum or peritoneum, but according to others, the small intestine. See Epiploon.

DÉSARTICULATION, (F.), from *de*, and *articulus*, 'a joint.' *Disjointing.* A word used to express the part of the operation, in amputation at an articulation, which consists in dividing the ligaments, and separating the articular surfaces. The word has, also, been used for that kind of anatomical preparation, the object of which is to separate the different bones of the skeleton, and especially those of the head.

DESCALORINÈSES, from *de*, 'from,' and *calor*, 'heat.' A name given by Baumes to diseases which are characterized by diminished heat.

DESCEMET, MEMBRANE OF, see Aqueous Humour, and Cornea.

DESCEMETI'TIS. A term improperly formed, and really signifying 'inflammation of Descemet.' Inflammation of the membrane of Descemet.

DESCENDENS NONI, see Hypoglossus.

DESCENSIO, Catabasis.

DESCENSUS, Catabasis—d. Testiculorum, Orchido-catabasis.

DESCENTE, Hernia—*d. de la Matrice*, Procidentia uteri.

DESECTUS, Castratus.

DÉSENFLURE, Détumescence.

DESICCANTIA, Desiccativa.

DESICCATIO, Draining.

DESICCATION, Drying.

DESICCATI'VA, *Desican'tia, Siccan'tia, Exsiccati'va*, from *desiccare*, (*de*, and *siccare*,) 'to dry up.' (F.) *Déssiccatifs.* Remedies, which, when applied externally, dry up the humours or moisture from a wound.

DESIPIENTIA, Delirium.

DESIRE, Libido — d. Venereal, Appetite, venereal, see Libido.

DES'MA, *Des'mē, Des'mus.* A bandage, a ligament. Hence:

DESMATUR'GIA, from δεσμα, 'bandage,' and εργον, 'work.' The doctrine of the application of bandages. Bandaging.

DESMEDION, Fasciculus.

DESMEUX, Ligamentous.

DESMI'TIS, *Desmophlogo'sis, Desmophlog''ia,* from δεσμη, 'a ligament,' and *itis*, denoting inflammation. Inflammation of ligaments.

DESMOCHAUNO'SIS, from δεσμος, 'ligament,' and χαυνωσις, 'relaxation.' Relaxation of an articular ligament.

DESMODYN'IA, from δεσμη, 'ligament,' and οδυνη, 'pain.' Pain in the ligaments.

DESMOG'RAPHY, *Desmograph'ia,* from δεσμος, 'a ligament,' and γραφη, 'a description.' An anatomical description of the ligaments.

DESMOID TISSUE, from δεσμος, 'a ligament,' and ειδος, 'shape.') *Ligamen'tous Tissue, Textus desmo'sus.* This tissue is very generally diffused over the human body; has a very close connexion with the areolar tissue, and is continuous with it in divers places. It constitutes the ligaments, aponeuroses, &c.

DESMOL'OGY, *Desmolog''ia,* from δεσμος, 'a ligament,' and λογος, 'a discourse,' 'a treatise.' That part of anatomy which describes the ligaments.

DESMOPHLOGIA, Desmitis.

DESMORRHEX'IS, from δεσμος, 'a ligament,' and ρηξις, 'rupture.' Rupture of an articular ligament.

DESMOS, Ligament.

DESMOSUS, Ligamentous.

DESMOT'OMY, *Desmotom'ia,* from δεσμος, 'a ligament,' and τεμνειν, 'to cut.' The part of anatomy which teaches the mode of dissecting the ligaments.

DÉSOBSTRUANT, Deobstruent.

DÉSOBSTRUCTIF, Deobstruent.

DÉSOPILATIF, Deobstruent.

DÉSORGANISATION, Disorganization.

DÉSOXYGENÈSES, from *de*, and *oxygen*. M. Baumes includes under this title an order of diseases, which he considers dependent upon a diminution in the quantity of the oxygen necessary for the animal economy.

DESPOTATS, (F.) Infirm soldiers, formerly charged with the office of removing the wounded from the field of battle: perhaps from *desporta'tor*, 'one who bears away.' The class of *Despotats* was introduced by Leo VI., at the commencement of the 9th century.

DESPUMA'TION, *Despuma'tio, Apaphris'mos, Epaphris'mos,* from *despumare*, (*de*, and *spuma*,) 'to skim' 'to remove the froth.' The separation of the froth and other impurities, which rise, by the action of the fire, to the surface of any fluid.

DESQUAMA'TION, *Desquama'tio Cutis, Eclep'isis, Aposyr'ma, Apolep'isis, Apolepis'mus, Moulting,* from *desquamare,* (*de*, and *squama*, 'a scale,') 'to scale off.' Exfoliation, or separation of the epidermis, in the form of scales, of a greater or less size. This affection is a common consequence of exanthematous diseases.

DESQUAMATORIUS, Exfoliative.

DESSÈCHEMENT, Atrophy, Draining.

DESSICATIFS, Desicativa.

DESTILLATIO, Coryza, Distillation—d. Pectoris, Catarrh.

DESTRUCTIO, Diaphthora.

DESUDA'TIO, *Ephidro'sis, Sudam'ina, Hidro'a,* from *desudare,* (*de*, and *sudare,* 'to sweat.') *Desudation* means a profuse and inordinate sweating, a mucksweat; but, most commonly, the term is applied to an eruption of small pimples, similar to millet seed, which appears chiefly on children, and is owing to want of cleanliness.

DÉSYMPHYSER, see Symphyseotomy.

DETENTIO, Catalepsy.

DETERGENS, Abstergent.

DETER'GENTS, from *detergere,* (*de*, and *tergere,* 'to clean,') 'to cleanse.' *Detergen'tia, Deterso'ria, Extergen'tia, Abstergen'tia, Absterri'va, Absterso'ria, Abluen'tia, Traumat'ica, Smec'tica, Emundan'tia, Mundificati'va, Mundifican'tia, Rhyp'tica, Abster'sives,* (F.) *Détersifs, Mundificatifs.* Medicines, which possess the power to deterge or cleanse parts, as wounds, ulcers, &c. They belong to the class of stimulants, or to that of emollients.

DETERMINA'TION, *Determina'tio,* from *de,* and *terminus,* 'a boundary.' Strong direction to a given point; — as 'a *determination* of blood to the head.'

DÉTERSIFS, Detergents.

DETERSORIA, Detergents.

DETERSO'RIUM, from *detergere,* 'to cleanse.' The place, in ancient bathing establishments, where the bather was cleansed and dried.

DETESTATIO, Castratio.

DÉTORSE, Sprain.

DETRACTIO SANGUINIS, Bloodletting.

DETRI'TUS, from *deterere,* (*de*, and *terere,*) 'to bruise or wear out.' The residuum, occupying the place of the organic texture of parts which have undergone disorganization.

DÉTROIT ABDOMINALE, Pelvis (brim)—*d. Inférieur,* Pelvis (outlet)—*d. Périnéal,* Pelvis (outlet)—*d. Supérieur,* Pelvis (brim.)

DÉTRONCATION, Detruncatio.

DETRUNCA'TION, *Detrunca'tio,* (F.) *Détroncation,* from *de,* and *truncus,* 'a trunk.' Separation of the trunk from the head of the fœtus, the latter remaining in the uterus.

DETRU'SION, *Detru'sio;* same etymon as the next. The act of thrusting or forcing down or away. Applied by Dr. Walshe to lateral displacement of the heart by extraneous pressure.

DETRU'SOR URI'NÆ, *Protru'sor,* from *detrudere, (de,* and *trudere,)* 'to thrust down or from.' The muscular coat of the urinary bladder was formerly so called. It was, also, named *Constrictor Vesi'cæ Urina'riæ.*

DÉTUMESCENCE (F.), *Detumescen'tia,* from *detumere, (de,* and *tumere,)* 'to cease to swell.' A diminution of swelling. This word has nearly the same signification as the French word *Désenflure.* The latter is, however, more particularly applied to the diminution of œdema or anasarca; the former, to the resolution of a tumour properly so called.

DEUNX. The ancient name of a weight of 11 ounces, supposing the pound to consist of 12.

DEURENS (FEBRIS,) Causus.

DEUS COPULATIONIS, Cupido.

DEUTERANŒA, Dementia.

DEUTERI'A, from δευτερος, 'the second.' Vogel has used this term for the symptoms produced by retention of the secundines. The word was also applied, by the Greeks, to a second or inferior wine.

DEUTERION, Secundines.

DEUTEROPATHI'A, *Hysteropathi'a, Morbus secunda'rius,* from δευτερος, 'the second,' and παθος, 'disease.' A secondary disease. One produced by another, and of which it is only, in some measure, symptomatic, or the sympathetic effect.

DEUTEROS'COPY, *Deuteroscop'ia,* from δευτερος, 'the second,' and σκοπεω, 'I view.' Second sight. A fancied power of seeing future things or events.

DEUTO, δευτερος, 'second.' A prefix denoting two, or double,—as *deutoxide,* having two degrees of oxidation.

DEVEL'OPMENT, *Evolu'tio,* from (F.) *développer,* 'to unfold.' In Physiology, it means growth or increase; and in Pathology, its signification is similar. By development of the pulse, e. g. is understood an increase in its strength and fulness. Diseases of development, *Morbi evolutio'nis,* are such as are peculiar to the period of growth.

'TAKING DEVELOPMENTS.' A term used by practical craniologists to signify the act of measuring prominences of the skull, which are regarded by them as indicating the size of corresponding cerebral organs.

DEVELOPMENT, VESICLE OF, see Vesicle of Development.

DEVERTICULUM, Diverticulum.

DEVIA'TION, *Devia'tio,* from *de,* 'from,' and *via,* 'the way.' Out of the way. By this word is meant—a vicious curvature of the spine or other bones;—faulty direction of the teeth or other part;—the passage of blood, bile, urine, milk, &c., into vessels not natural to them.

DÉVIATION DES RÉGLES, Menstruation (vicarious.)

DEVIL IN A BUSH, Nigella—d. Bit, Veratrum viride.

DEVIL'S BIT, Aletris farinosa, Scabiosa succisa. Chamælirium luteum—d. Bite, Liatris—d. Dung, Asafœtida—d. Shoestrings, Galega Virginiana.

DEVIRGINATIO, Defloration, Stuprum.

DÉVOIEMENT, Diarrhœa.

DEWBERRY, AMERICAN, see Rubus cæsius—d. Plant, Rubus cæsius.

DEWCLAWS, Crusta genu equinæ.

DEXIS, Degmus.

DEXOCAR'DIA, from δεξιος, 'right,' and καρδια, 'the heart.' A case in which the heart is found to beat on the right side. It is met with occasionally in pleurisy and pneumothorax.

DEX'TANS. A weight of 10 ounces, supposing the pound to consist of 12.

DEXTERINA, Dextrine.

DEXTRAD, from *dexter,* 'right-handed.' A term used adverbially by Dr. Barclay to signify 'towards the dextral aspect.' See Mesial.

DEXTRAL ASPECT, see Mesial.

DEXTRAL'ITY, from *dexter,* 'right.' The state of being on the right side. Right-handedness. The state of being right-handed.

DEXTRIN, *Dextrine, Dextri'num, Dexteri'na, British gum,* from *dexter,* 'right-handed.' So called, from its refracting the rays, in the polarization of light, more to the right hand than any substance known. A substance obtained by the continued action of diluted sulphuric acid upon starch at the boiling point. It is used in the treatment of fractures, by the 'immovable apparatus.' The bandages are soaked in a solution, in water, of the dextrine—previously moistened thoroughly with tincture of camphor, to prevent it from leaking when the water is added. The solution should be of the consistence of molasses.

DEXTRINUM, Dextrine.

DI, δι, δις, 'bis, twice, double.' Hence, *Dicrotus, Digastricus,* &c.

DIA, δια, in composition, 'through, asunder, out of, separated.' When prefixed to any therapeutical agent, it meant, in ancient pharmacy, a preparation into which that agent entered.

DIABEBOS, Astragalus, Malleolus.

DIABÈTE, Diabetes—*d. Chyleux,* Chyluria—*d. Faux,* see Diabetes—*d. Insipide,* see Diabetes—*d. Sucré,* Diabetes (mellitus.)

DIABE'TES, from δια, 'through,' and βαινω, 'I pass.' *Uri'næ proflu'vium, Hyperdiure'sis, Sipho uri'næ, Urorrhag''ia, Polyu'ria, Hydrops ad mat'ulam, H. Matel'læ, Polyure'sis, Uroze'mia, Ureorrhœ'a, Dip'sacos, Diarrhœ'a in Urind, D. urino'sa,* (F.) *Diabète, Flux d' Urine.* A disease, characterized by great augmentation and often manifest alteration in the secretion of urine; with excessive thirst, and progressive emaciation. Cullen has described two species: — *Diabetes insip'idus* and *D. Melli'tus;* the former, (F.) *Diabète faux* ou *insipide, Diabète,* being, simply, a superabundant discharge of limpid urine, of its usual, urinary taste: the latter, *D. Melli'tus,* called, also, *Paru'ria Melli'ta, Diabetes An'glicus, D. verus, Melitu'ria, Glucosu'ria, Glycyrrhœ'a urino'sa, Uroze'mia melli'ta, Saccharorrhœ'a urino'sa, Phthisu'ria, Uro-phthi'sis, Tabes diuret'ica* seu *diabe'tica, Dyspep'sia saccharig''ena, Apoceno'sis Diabetes Melli'tus, Sac'charine diabetes,* (F.) *Diabète sucré, Hyperurorrhée saccharine, Phthisurie sucrée,* — falls under the definition given above. The quantity of urine, discharged in the 24 hours, is sometimes excessive, amounting to 30 pints and upwards; each pint containing sometimes 2½ oz. saccharine matter. This replaces the urea, which is not found in quantity in the urine of those labouring under diabetes. Where the disease is situate is not clear. The whole system of nutrition, however, seems to be morbidly implicated. A part of the urine must be formed at the expense of the system, as the egesta frequently far exceed the solid and liquid ingesta. On dissection, no morbid appearance is met with, sufficient to enable us to fix on the seat of this distressing affection.

All the remedies that have been tried have usually been found insufficient in *D. Mellitus.*

D. insip'idus, Hyperure'sis aquo'sa, Hydru'ria, Hydrure'sis, Paru'ria incon'tinene aquo'sa, Diabe'tes spu'rius, Urorrhœ'a, U'real Diabetes, (F.) *Polyurie, Hyperurrorrhée, Diabète insipide, Faux diabète,* which occurs in hysterical habits, and has, hence, been called *D. hyster'icus,* is of comparatively trifling moment. Exclusive diet, and attention to the state of the cutaneous transpiration, which have sometimes produced good effects in D. Mellitus, have most commonly failed.

DIABETES ANGLICUS, see Diabetes — d. Chylosus, Chyluria — d. Insipidus, see Diabetes — d. Lactea, Chyluria — d. Mellitus, see Diabetes — d. Spurius, see Diabetes — d. Ureal, see Diabetes — d. Verus, Diabetes (mellitus.)

DIABET'IC, *Diabe'ticus.* Same etymon. Relating to diabetes.

DIABETIC SUGAR, Glucose.

DIABOT'ANUM, from δια, and βοτανη, 'an herb.' A medicine, prepared with herbs.—Galen.

DIABROSIS, Erosion, Corrosion.

DIABRO'TICUS, from δια, and βρωσκω, 'I eat or corrode.' A substance, capable of causing erosion of the part to which it is applied. It ordinarily means a medicine, whose activity places it between escharotics and caustics. See Corrosive.

DIACAR'YON, from δια, and καρυον, 'a nut.' *Rob nucum.* The rob of nuts or of walnuts.

DIACASSIA CUM MANNÂ, Confectio cassiæ.

DIACATHOL'ICON, *Diacathol'icum,* from δια, and καθολικος, 'universal.' The name of a purge, so called from its general usefulness. It was an electuary, and composed of the *pulp of cassia, tamarinds, leaves of senna, root of polypody, flowers of the violet, rhubarb root, aniseed, sugar, liquorice,* and *fennel.*

DIACAU'SIS, from διακαυω, 'I burn.' Excessive heat. Over-heating.

DIACAUST'IC, *Diacaust'icus.* Same etymon. That which is caustic by refraction; as a double convex lens, which has been sometimes used for cauterizing an ulcer by directing the sun's rays upon it.

DIACELTATESSON PARACELSI, Pulvis Cornachini.

DIACHALA'SIS, from διαχαλασιν, 'to be open or relaxed." Hippocrates uses this word for fracture of the bones of the skull; or for relaxation and separation of the sutures, in consequence of a wound of the head.—Hippocrates.

DIACHALCIT'EOS, from δια, and χαλκιτις, 'chalcitis or colcothar.' A plaster, whose composition is the same as that of the diapalma, except that, in place of the sulphate of zinc, a mixture of oil and colcothar is substituted.

DIACHEIRIS'MOS, *Diacheir'isis, Tracta'tio manua'ria,* from δια, and χειρ, 'the hand.' The preparation, administration, and dispensing of medicines.—Hippocrates.

DIACHORE'MA, *Diachore'sis,* from διαχωρεω, 'I separate from.' Every kind of excreted matter and excretion; but more particularly the fæces and alvine excretion. — Foësius, Gorræus. See Excrement.

DIACHOREMA XYSMATODES, see Ramenta intestinorum.

DIACHORESIS, Excretion.

DIACHRISIS, Inunction.

DIACHRIST'A, from δια, and χριω, 'I anoint.' Medicines, applied as abstergents to the velum palati, the palate itself, the tongue, &c. Probably gargles.—Paulus of Ægina.

DIACH'YLON, *Diach'ylum, Emplas'trum diach'ylon,* from δια, and χυλος, 'juice;' i. e. composed of juices. The plaster of this name was formerly made of certain juices. The term is now confined to the EMPLASTRUM PLUMBI or Lead Plaster.

DIACHYLON CUM GUMMI, Emplastrum gummosum—d. *Gommé,* Emplastrum cum gummi-resinis —d. Gum, Emplastrum gummosum—d. Magnum cum gummi, Emplastrum galbani comp.—d. Simplex, Emplastrum plumbi—d. White, Emplastrum plumbi—d. Yellow, Emplastrum gummosum.

DIACHYT'ICA, from δια, and χυω, 'I pour out.' Medicines which discuss tumours.

DIACINE'MA, from δια, and κινεω, 'I move.' A slight dislocation. — Celsus, Galen. A subluxation.

DIACLASIS, Refraction.

DIAC'LYSIS, *Diaclys'mus,* from δια, and κλυζειν, 'to wash out.' Rinsing or cleansing—especially of the mouth.

DIACLYSMA, Gargarism.

DIACOCCYMELON, Diaprunum.

DIACODION, Syrupus papaveris.

DIACO'DIUM, *Confec'tio ex Capit'ibus Papav'eris,* from δια, and κωδια, 'a poppyhead.' (F.) *Diacode.* The ancients had various forms for preparing it. The *Syrup of Poppies—Syr'upus Papav'eris seu Diaco'dion* — is now substituted for it.

DIACOPE, Abscission, Dissection, Intersection.

DIAC'OPE, *En'copē,* from δια, and κοπτειν, 'to cut.' A cut, incision, fissure, or longitudinal fracture. When used, since Galen, it generally signifies an oblique incision, made in the cranium by a sharp instrument, without the piece being removed. It is not now employed.

DIAC'OPE CRA'NII, *Præcis'io seu Dissec'tio Cra'nii.* Opening the head; and separation of the bones of the cranium.

DIACOPRÆ'GIA, from δια, κοπρος, 'excrement,' and αιξ, αιγος, 'a goat.' A name given, in Blancard's Lexicon, to a medicine, composed of goat's dung, which the ancients praised in diseases of the spleen, parotids, &c.

DIAC'RISES, from δια, and κρινω, 'I separate.' A class of diseases characterized by alterations of secretion.—Gendrin.

DIACRIT'ICA SIG'NA. Same etymon. Signs by which one disease can be accurately discriminated from another :—*differen'tial diagno'sis.*

DIACYDONITES, Cydoniatum.

DIADELPHIA DECANDRIA, Geoffræa vermifuga.

DIADE'MA, *Fascia cap'itis, Redimic'ulum,* from διαδεω, (δια, and δειν, 'to bind.') 'I surround.' A sort of bandage; advised in headach, in which relaxation of the sutures was apprehended.—Forestus.

DIADEX'IS, *Diad'ochē, Metatopto'sis,* from διαδεχομαι, (δια, and δεχομαι, 'to take or receive.') 'I transfer,' 'I succeed to.' A transformation of a disease into another, differing from the former both in its nature and seat.

DIADOCHE, Diadexis.

DIAD'OSIS, from διαδιδωμι, 'to distribute.' In some authors, it means the distribution of nutritive matter over the whole body,—in other words, *nutrition;* whilst, in others, it is synonymous with the remission or cessation of a disease.

DIÆDŒ'US, from δι, 'double,' and αιδοια, 'the parts of generation.' A monster whose organs of generation and urinary bladder are double. It has only been observed in animals.

DIÆ'RESIS, from διαιρεω, (δια, and αιρεω, 'I take away,') 'I divide,' 'I separate.' A division or solution of continuity. A surgical operation, which consists in dividing any part of the body. *Hæmorrhag"ia per diæ'resin* is hemorrhage owing to separation or division of vessels.

DIÆRESIS UNGULÆ, Onychoptosis.

DIÆRETICUS, Caustic.

DIÆTA, Diet—d. Lactea, Galactodiæta.

DIÆTE'MA has the same signification as diet, with most authors. Galen gives it a more extensive meaning, comprising, under it, what constitutes Hygiene.

DIÆTETICA, Dietetics.

DIAGNOSE, Diagnosticate.

DIAGNO'SIS, *Digno'tio, Diagnos'tica, Deprehen'sio*, from διά, and γινώσκω, 'I know.' *Discrimination*, (F.) *Diagnose, Diagnostique.* That part of medicine whose object is the discrimination of diseases, the knowledge of the pathognomonic signs of each. It is one of the most important branches of general pathology.

DIAGNOSIS, DIFFERENTIAL, see Diacritica signa.

DIAGNOS'TIC, *Discreti'vus, Diagnos'ticus;* same etymon. A symptom which is characteristic of a disease.

DIAGNOS'TICATE, — sometimes *diagnose*. To discriminate one disease or phenomenon from another.

DIAGRYDIUM, Convolvulus scammonia.

DIAGRYD'IUM CYDONIA'TUM, from *diagrydium*, 'scammony,' and *cydonium*, 'quince.' A pharmaceutical preparation, obtained by inspissating and drying, by means of heat, two parts of *scammony* and one of *quince juice*. It was formerly used as an energetic purgative.

DIAGRYD'IUM GLYCYRRHIZA'TUM. An analogous preparation, containing extract of liquorice in place of quince juice.

DIAGRYD'IUM SULPHURA'TUM. Scammony, which has been exposed to the vapour of burning sulphur. These *diagrydia* are not now used.

DIALEIPSIS, Apyrexia, Intermission.

DIALEIPYRA, Intermittent fever.

DIALEMMA, Apyrexia.

DIALEP'SIS, *Intercep'tio*, from διαλαμβάνω, 'I intercept.'—Hippocrates employs this word for the interstices, or intervals, left between the turns of a bandage.

DIALIPSIS, Apyrexia, Intermissio.

DIAL'YSIS, *Dissolu'tio*, from διά, and λύσις, 'solution.' A dissolution or loss of strength. *Resolu'tio vir'ium.* Weakness of the limbs. Also, a solution of continuity.

DIAMANT, Diamond.

DIAMASTEMA, Masticatory.

DIAM'BRÆ SPE'CIES. A name given by the ancients to powders, one of which bore the name—*Spe'cies diam'bræ sine odora'tis*,—the other, that of *Spe'cies diam'bræ cum odora'tis.* The *former* was composed of *cinnamon, angelica root, cloves, mace, nutmeg, galanga, cardamom,* and numerous other substances; the *latter*, besides, had *ambergris* and *musk*. These powders were used as tonics, in cases of debility of the stomach, and in certain nervous affections.

DIAMNES, Enuresis.

DI'AMOND, *Ad'amas*, from α, privative, and δαμάω, 'I conquer.' 'Invincible;' (F.) *Diamant.* So called from its hardness. It is the most precious of all stones, and was formerly conceived to possess extraordinary cordial virtues.

DIAMO'RUM, *Rob ex moris*, from διά, and μῶρον, 'a mulberry.' An ancient syrup prepared with honey and mulberry juice. It was employed as a gargle in sore throat.—Galen.

DIAMOTO'SIS, from μοτός, 'charpie,' 'lint.' The introduction of lint into an ulcer or wound.

DIANA, Argentum.

DIANANCAS'MUS, from διά, and ἀναγκάζω,

'I force.' Coaptation, reduction of a fractured or luxated limb.

DIANOEMA, Imagination.

DIAN'THUS CARYOPHYL'LUS, from Διός, 'Jove.' (?) ανθος, 'flower,' and *caryophyllum*, 'the clove.' *Clove Pink.* Also called *Caryophyl'lum rubrum, Tu'nica, Tu'nica horten'sis, T. rubra, Caryophyl'lus horten'sis, Clove July flower, Gil'liflower, Carna'tion.* Order, Caryophylleæ. (F.) *Œillet giroflée.* The flowers were once much used; but are now only employed in syrup, as a useful and pleasant vehicle for other medicines.

DIAPAL'MA, *Phœnic"ium Emplas'trum.* A plaster composed of equal parts of *litharge, olive oil, axunge, water*, a certain quantity of *sulphate of zinc* dissolved in water, and *white wax*. It is classed amongst the topical, desiccative, emollient, resolvent, detersive, and cicatrizing medicines. Mixed with a quarter of its weight of olive oil, it acquires the consistence of an ointment, and forms the *Cerate of Diapal'ma.*

DIAPASMA, Catapasma.

DIAPEDE'SIS, *Transuda'tio, Persuda'tio, Persulta'tio*, from διαπηδάω, 'I leap through.' Exhalation, as of blood, in the form of dew, at the surface of the skin, or of any membrane; *Sweating of blood*, (F.) *Sueur de Sang, Hæmorrhag"ia per diapede'sin, Hæmatopede'sis, Hæmidro'sis.*

DIAPENSIA CORTUSA, Sanicula.

DIAPEN'TES or DIAPENTE, from διά, and πέντε, 'five.' A medicine composed of five ingredients. See Diatessaron.

DIAPHŒ'NICON, *Diaphœ'nix, Medicamen'tum ex Pal'mulis*, from διά, and φοινιξ, 'a date.' A drastic electuary, of which the date was the chief excipient.

DIAPHORE'SIS, from διαφορέω, (διά, and φορέω, 'I convey,') 'I dissipate.' A greater degree of perspiration than natural, but less than in sweating. Every kind of cutaneous evacuation.

DIAPHORET'IC. Same etymon; *Diaphor'icus, Diaphoret'icus.* A medicine which excites diaphoresis. Diaphoretics are very uncertain as a class. The following is a list of the most reputed:—Ammoniæ Acetatis Liquor; Ammoniæ Carbonas; Antimonialis pulvis; Antimonii et Potassæ Tartras; Antimonii Sulphuretum præcipitatum; Asclepias tuberosa; Camphora; Contrayerva; Dulcamara; Eupatorium perfoliatum; Guaiaci Lignum; Guaiacum; Ipecacuanha; Mezereum; Opium, and its active principle Morphia; Sarsaparilla; Sassafras; Serpentaria; Spiritus Ætheris Nitrici; Sulphur; Xanthoxylum; Caloric; Exercise, (active;) and Friction.

The epithet *Diaphoretic* has also been given, by some, to continued fever, accompanied with constant perspiration.

DIAPHORETIC, MINERAL, Antimonium diaphoreticum.

DIAPHORETICUM JOVIALE, see Antihectic.

DI'APHRAGM, *Diaphrag'ma, Diaphrax'is, Respirato'rium Ventris, Discreto'rium, Phrenes, Septum transver'sum, Discri'men Thora'cis et Ventris, Disceptum, Cinc'tus, Diazo'ma, Præcinc'tus, Diazos'ma, Diazos'tra, Hypezo'cus, Hypozo'ma, Perizo'ma, Dissep'tum, Dissip'ium, Præcor'dia, Succin'gens membra'na vel mus'culus, Succinc'tus, Succinctu'ra,* the *Midriff,* from διά, 'between,' and φράσσω, 'I close;' A large, azygous muscle; stretched transversely between the thoracic and abdominal cavities, which it separates from each other; tendinous in the centre; thin, almost circular, and unequally convex, upwards. It is fleshy at its circumference, which is attached to the cartilago ensiformis, to the last six ribs, to the aponeurosis stretched from the last rib to the transverse process of the first lumbar vertebra; and, lastly, to the bodies of the first three or four lumbar vertebræ. When it contracts, its fibres become straight, the chest is enlarged, and the abdomen diminished. It is then an inspiratory muscle. It may, also, diminish the capacity of the chest, and be an expiratory muscle. This muscle plays an important part in sighing, yawning, coughing, sneezing, laughing, sobbing, crying, hiccoughing, singing, vomiting, the excretion of the fæces and urine, the expulsion of the fœtus, &c.

DIAPHRAGMA AURIS, see Tympanum—d. Cerebri, Tentorium—d. Narium, Septum narium d. Ventriculorum lateralium cerebri, Septum lucidum.

DIAPHRAGMAL'GIA, *Diaphragmatal'gia*, from διαφραγμα, 'the diaphragm,' and αλγος, 'pain.' Pain in the diaphragm.

DIAPHRAGMATALGIA, Diaphragmalgia.

DIAPHRAGMAT'IC, *Diaphragmat'icus*. Belonging to the diaphragm. A name given to several vessels and nerves.

DIAPHRAGMAT'IC or PHRENIC AR'TERIES. These are distinguished into *superior* and *inferior*. The *former*, called, also, *supradiaphragmat'ic*, are two in number, one on each side. They arise from the internal mammary, and descend along the phrenic nerve, to be distributed on the upper surface of the diaphragm. The latter, or *infradiaphragmat'ic*, are also two in number. They arise from the upper part of the abdominal aorta, or from the cœliac artery, and divide into two principal branches, which are distributed on the lower surface of the diaphragm and in its substance.

The *superior diaphragmat'ic veins* follow the same course as the arteries, and empty themselves—the *right*, into the vena cava superior; the *left*, into the corresponding subclavian vein. The two *inferior diaphragmatic veins* open into the vena cava inferior.

DIAPHRAGMAT'IC HER'NIA, *Phrenic Hernia, Diaphragmatoce'lè*. The abdominal viscera are occasionally protruded through the diaphragm, either through some of the natural apertures in the muscle, or through deficiencies, or wounds, or lacerations in it.

DIAPHRAGMAT'IC or PHRENIC NERVES, *Internal respiratory* of Sir Charles Bell, are two in number; one on the left side, the other on the right. They arise from the second and third nerves of the cervical plexus, about the middle of the neck, and receive two or three filaments from the brachial plexus, after which they descend into the chest at the sides of the pericardium, and are distributed on the diaphragm.

DIAPHRAGMAT'IC PLEX'USES are two in number; one right, and the other left. They arise from the upper part of the solar plexus, by a small number of branches, which are distributed to the diaphragm, following the branches of the inferior diaphragmatic arteries.

DIAPHRAGMAT'IC RING, (F.) *Anneau diaphragmatique* of Chaussier, is a name given to the irregularly quadrilateral aperture by which the vena cava inferior passes through the diaphragm.

DIAPHRAGMATITIS, Diaphragmitis.

DIAPHRAGMATOCELE, see Hernia.

DIAPHRAGMI'TIS, from διαφραγμα, 'the diaphragm,' and *itis*, a suffix denoting inflammation. *Diaphragmati'tis, Inflamma'tio septi transver'si, Paraphreni'tis, Empresma Pleuri'tis Diaphragmat'ica, Paraphrene'sis Diaphragmat'ica, Inflammation of the Di'aphragm*. The terms, *Paraphreni'tis* and *Paraphrene'sis* have been obtained from the Peripatetic philosophy, which supposed the seat of the φρην, or soul, to be the præcordia. The essential symptoms of diaphragmitis are:—painful constriction around the præcordia, with small, quick, laborious breathing. It is a rare disease.

DIAPHRATTON HYMEN, Mediastinum—d. Membrana, Mediastinum.

DIAPHRAXIS, Diaphragm.

DIAPH'THORA, *Destruc'tio*, from δια, and φθειρειν, 'to corrupt.' Corruption in general; more especially corruption of the fœtus in utero. Hippocrates. Also, corruption of the blood in the stomach.—Galen. See Abortion.

DIAPHYLACTIC, Prophylactic.

DIAPH'YSIS, from διαφυω, 'I rise between.' *Interstit"ium, Discrimina'tio:* 'an interstice, interval, division.' Any thing that separates two bodies. Also, the middle part or body of a long bone, *Corpus Ossis*. One of the ligaments of the knee.—Hippocrates, Paré.

DIA'PIA. Some lexicographers use this word synonymously with DIAPYESIS or SUPPURATION, others have employed it in opposition to MYOPIA.

DIAPLASIS, Conformation, Reduction.

DIAPLASMUS, Conformation, Reduction.

DIAPNEUSIS, Perspiration.

DIAPNOE, Perspiration.

DIAPNŒA, Perspiration.

DIAPNOGENOUS APPARATUS, see Perspiration.

DIAPNOICUS, Diaphoretic.

DIAPOPHYSES, Transverse processes of the vertebræ.

DIAPORE'MA. Anxiety, jactitation; from διαπορεω, 'I doubt.'

DIAPRU'NUM, *Diacoccyme'lon*. A purgative electuary, of which the *pulps of prunes* and *rhubarb* formed the basis. By adding to the *diaprunum simplex* a 24th part of powdered scammony, the *Diapru'num resoluti'vum seu composi'tum* was formed. It was more active than the former.

DIAPYEMA, Empyema, Suppuration.

DIAPYESIS, Suppuration—d. Oculi, Hypopyon.

DIAPYET'ICA, *Dyapye'mata*, from διαπυεω, διαπυησις, (δια, and πυον, 'pus,') 'suppuration.' Medicines which promote suppuration.

DIAPYETICUS, Suppurative.

DIARÆ'MIA, (F.) *Diarémie*, from δια, 'through,' ρεω, 'I flow,' and 'αιμα, 'blood.' A pathological condition, said to be common in sheep, in which the globules of the blood are diminished in quantity; the blood itself thinner, and transuding through the coats of the vessels into the cavities.—Delafore.

DIARÉMIE, Diaræmia.

DIARIA, Ephemera.

DIARRHAGE, Fracture.

DIARRHŒ'A, from δια, 'through,' and ρεω, 'I flow.' *Enterorrhœ'a, Incontinen'tia alvi, Alvi proflu'vium, A. fluxus aquo'sus, Ventris proflu'vium, Cœliorrhœ'a, Cœliol'ysis, Alvus cita, Cacato'ria, Coprorrhœ'a, Catar'rhus intestina'lis, Alvi fluxus, Rheuma, Epiph'ora Alvi, Fluxus alvi'nus, Lax'itas alvi, Deflux'io, Lax, Looseness, Purging,* (F.) *Diarrhée, Dévoiement, Catarrhe intestinal, Flux de Ventre, Cours de Ventre, Courante*. A disease characterised by frequent liquid alvine evacuations, and generally owing to inflammation or irritation of the mucous membrane of the intestines. It is commonly caused by errors in regimen, the use of food noxious by its quality or quantity, &c., constituting the *Diarrhœ'a stercora'ria, D. Crapulo'sa* of writers. It may be acute or chronic. Many varieties have been made by some nosologists—e. g. mucous,—*Diarrhœ'a muco'sa, Blennoche'sia, Blennoche'sia;* bañous,—*Ileo-cholo'sis, Diarrhœ'a bilio'sa;* serous, —*Hydroche'zia, Hydrodiarrhœ'a, Orrhoche'sia;* dependent upon the matters evacuated. Diarrhœa requires different treatment, according to its nature. If caused, as it often is, by improper matters in the intestinal canal, these must be evacuated; and the astringent plan of treatment must not be adopted, unless the discharges seem kept up by irritability of the intestines, or unless they are colliquative. The indiscriminate use of astringents is to be deprecated.

A very fatal diarrhœa prevails amongst the native inhabitants of India, to which Mr. Tytler has given the name *Diarrhœ'a hec'tica*, because, like hectic fever, it seems to obtain habitual possession of the constitution, to operate upon it with scarcely any perceptible intermission, and, in general, to defy the most powerful remedies.

DIARRHŒA ADIPOSA, *Gras-fondure*—d. cum Apepsiâ, Lientery—d. Arthritica, Cœliagra—d. Biliosa, see Diarrhœa—d. Carnosa, Dysentery—d. Chylosa, Cœliac flux—d. Chymosa, Cœliac flux—d. Crapulosa, see Diarrhœa—d. Cruenta, Hæmatochezia—d. Dyspeptica, Lientery—d. Hepatica, Hepatirrhœa—d. Ingestorum, Lientery—d. Lienteria, Lientery—d. Mucosa, see Diarrhœa—d. Purulenta, Pyochezia—d. Sanguinolenta, Hæmatochezia—d. Stercoraria, see Diarrhœa—d. in Urinâ, Diabetes—d. Urinosa, Diabetes.

DIARRHOÏS'CHESIS, from *Diarrhœa*, and σχεσις, 'arrest.' Arrest of a diarrhœa.

DIARTHRO'DIAL, *Diarthrodia'lis*. Relating to diarthroses or movable articulations; as *diarthro'dial articulation. Diarthro'dial cartilages* or *incrusting cartilages* are the cartilages which invest the articular extremities of bones.

DIARTHRO'SIS, from διαρθροω, (δια, and αρθροω,) 'I separate the limbs,' 'I articulate.' *Dearticula'tio, Prosarthro'sis, Aparthro'sis, Abarticula'tio, Coarticula'tio, Perarticula'tio, Rota'tio,* (F.) *Emboîture.* A movable articulation. One which permits the bones to move freely on each other in every direction, as in the case of the shoulder joint.

DIASATYR'ION, from δια, and σατυριον, 'the *orchis mas'cula.*' An electuary, of which this plant formed the basis. (?)—Myrepsus. The ancients attributed to it the faculty of exciting the organs of generation.

DIASCINCI ANTIDOTUS, Mithridate.

DIASCOR'DIUM, from δια, and σκορδιον, 'the water germander.' An electuary, so called because this plant entered into its composition. The Parisian codex has a formula for its preparation, under the title, *Electua'rium opia'tum astrin'gens* vel *diascor'dium.* (R. fol. scord. ℥iss, rosar. rubr., bistort. rad., gentianæ, tormentillæ, sem. berber. āā ℥ss, singib., piper. long. āā ʒij, cassiæ ligneæ, cinnamom., dictam. Cretens., styrac. calamit., galban., gum. acaciæ āā ℥ss, bol. oriental. præpar. ʒij, extract vinos opii. ʒij, mel. rosat. præp. ℔ij, vin. hispan. ℔ss: fiat electuarium.) In place of the *styrax calamita*, the balsam of tolu or benjamin may be used. The opium is, in this preparation, in the proportion of 1 to 184. The diascordium is employed in diarrhœa and dysentery, as a tonic, stomachic, and astringent. The common dose is from a scruple to a drachm and a half. See Pulvis cretæ compositus.

DIASOSTIC, Prophylactic.

DIASPASIS, Divulsio.

DIASPER'MATON. The ancient name of two cataplasms, composed of seeds.—Galen, Paulus.

DIASPHYXIS, Pulse. Also, a violent beat of the pulse.

DIASTAL'TIC, *Diastal'ticus*; from δια,

'through,' and στελλω, 'I contract.' An epithet applied by Dr. Marshall Hall to the reflex or excito-motory system of nerves; because the actions they induce are performed 'through' the spinal marrow as their essential centre.

DIASTALTICUS, Diastolic.

DIASTASÆ'MIA, (F.) *Diastasémie*, from διαστασις, 'separation,' and 'αιμα, 'blood.' A pathological condition, characterised by a separation of the elements of the blood globules;—the fibrin and albumen separating also from the colouring matter, whilst the fibrin attaches itself to the valves of the heart.—Delafore.

DIASTASE. Same etymon as the next but one. A vegetable principle, allied in its general properties to gluten, which appears in the germination of barley and other seeds and, by its presence, converts the starch into sugar and gum.

DIASTASÉMIE, Diastasæmia.

DIAS'TASIS, from δια, and ιστημι, 'to place,' 'separation,' 'distance.' *Diaste'ma, Dissiden'tia.* A separation of bones, and particularly of the bones of the cranium, from each other; of the radius from the ulna, and the fibula from the tibia. The ancients used this word to designate the three dimensions of the body,—length, breadth, and thickness; for the interval separating the patient from the physician; the swelling of varicose veins; the time at which some change occurred in disease, &c.

DIASTEMA, Diastasis, Interstice.

DIASTEMATELYT'RIA, from διαστημα, 'interstice,' and ελυτρον, 'vagina.' An organic deviation, characterized by a longitudinal division or fissure of the vagina.—Breschet.

DIASTEMATENCEPHA'LIA, from διαστημα, and εγκεφαλος, 'the brain.' An organic deviation, consisting in a longitudinal division of the brain. —Breschet.

DIASTEMA'TIA, from διαστημα. A term employed by Breschet for an organic deviation, characterized by the presence of a fissure in the mesial line of the body.

DIASTEMATOCAU'LIA, from διαστημα, and καυλος, 'trunk.' An organic deviation, characterized by a longitudinal division of the trunk.

DIASTEMATOCHEI'LIA, from διαστημα, and χειλος, 'the lip.' An organic deviation, consisting in a longitudinal division or fissure of the lip.

DIASTEMATOCRA'NIA, from διαστημα, and κρανιον, 'the cranium.' An organic deviation, consisting in a longitudinal deviation of the cranium.

DIASTEMATOCYS'TIA, from διαστημα, and κυστις, 'bladder.' An organic deviation, characterized by a longitudinal division of the urinary bladder.

DIASTEMATOGAS'TRIA, from διαστημα, and γαστηρ, 'the stomach.' An organic deviation, characterized by a longitudinal division of the stomach.

DIASTEMATOGLOS'SIA, from διαστημα, and γλωσσα, 'tongue.' An organic deviation, characterized by a longitudinal division or fissure of the tongue.

DIASTEMATOGNA'THIA, from διαστημα, and γναθος, 'jaw.' An organic deviation, characterized by a longitudinal division of the jaw.

DIASTEMATOME'TRIA, from διαστημα, and μητρα, 'womb.' An organic deviation, characterized by a longitudinal division or fissure of the womb.

DIASTEMATOPYEL'IA, from διαστημα, and πυελος, 'pelvis.' An organic deviation, characterized by a longitudinal division or fissure of the pelvis.

DIASTEMATORA'CHIA, from διαστημα, and ραχις, 'spine.' An organic deviation, characterized by a longitudinal division or fissure of the spine.

DIASTEMATORHI'NIA, from διαστημα, and ριν, 'the nose.' An organic deviation, characterized by a longitudinal division of the nose.

DIASTEMATOSTAPHYL'IA, from διαστημα, and σταφυλη, 'uvula.' An organic deviation, characterized by a longitudinal division of the uvula.

DIASTEMATOSTER'NIA, from διαστημα, and στερνον, 'the sternum.' An organic deviation, characterized by a longitudinal division of the sternum.

DIASTEMENTER'IA, from διαστημα, and εντερον, 'intestine.' An organic deviation, characterized by a longitudinal division of the intestine.

DIAS'TOLE, from διαστελλω, (δια and στελλω, 'I send,') 'I dilate,' 'I open.' *Relaxa'tio* seu *Remis'sio cordis et arteria'rum.* Dilatation of the heart and arteries, when the blood enters their cavities. It is the opposite movement to *systole*, in which the heart and arteries contract to send forth the blood. *Diastole* and *systole* are, consequently, successive movements. *Diastole, Motus cordis diastal'ticus*, occurs simultaneously in the two ventricles. The almost inappreciable time, which elapses between the diastole and systole has been called *perisys'tolē*, and that which succeeds to the diastole, *peridiastole*. When we speak of the *contraction* or *systole* of the heart, as well as of its *diastole* or *dilatation*, we mean that of the ventricles. This dilatation is active.

DIASTOLEUS, Dilator.

DIAS'TOLIC, *Diastol'icus, Diastal'ticus*; same etymon. Belonging to the diastole of the heart—as 'diastolic impulse of the heart.'

DIASTOLIC IMPULSE OF THE HEART, see Impulse, diastolic.

DIASTOMO'TRIS, from διαστομοω, (δια, and στομα, 'mouth.') 'I dilate an aperture.' Dilating instruments, such as the different kinds of specula for the mouth, anus, vagina, &c.

DIASTREMMA, Distortion, Perversion, Sprain.

DIASTROPHE, Distortion, Perversion, Sprain.

DIAT'ASIS, *Disten'sio*, from διατεινω, (δια, and τεινω, 'I stretch,') 'I distend.' *Tension.* The reduction of a fracture by extension and counter-extension.

DIATES'SARON, from δια, and τεσσαρες, 'four.' An electuary, into the composition of which entered four medicines; viz. the roots of *gentian, aristolochia rotunda,* and *bay-berries*, each ℥ij, *honey* ℔ij. The whole was incorporated with *extract of juniper.* The *diapentes* is nothing more than this electuary, mixed with two ounces of *ivory shavings.* The *diatessaron* is tonic, and it was formerly employed in cases of stings and bites of venomous animals. It was regarded as emmenagogue, alexiterial, and alexipharmic.

DIATH'ESIS, from διατιθημι, (δια, and τιθημι, 'to place,') 'I dispose.' Disposition, constitution, affection of the body: predisposition to certain diseases rather than to others;—(F.) *Imminence morbide.* The principal diatheses, mentioned by authors, are the *cancerous, scrofulous, scorbutic, rheumatic, gouty* and *calculous.*

DIATHESIS HÆMORRHOIDALIS, see Hæmorrhoids—d. Hemorrhagic, Hematophilia—d. Nervosa, Nervous diathesis—d. Rheumatic, see Rheumatic—d. Sthenica, Sthenia.

DIATRAGACAN'THUS. A powder composed of *gum tragacanth*, ℥ij, *gum Arabic*, ℥j and ℥ij, *starch*, ℥ss, *liquorice*, ℥iij, as much of the *seeds of the melon*, and *white poppy ; seeds of the water-melon, cucumber, and gourd,* and *sugar candy* ℥iij. It was used as a demulcent.

DIATRESIS, Perforation.

DIATRIMMA, Chafing.

DIATRINSANTALON, see Diatrion.

DIATRI'ON, *Diatri'um*, from δια, and τρεις, 'three.' A medicine composed of three ingredients. There were formerly two kinds. The first was called *Diatri'um Pipe'reon spe'cies,* and was formed of *black and long pepper, aniseed, thyme,* and *ginger.* It was highly stimulating. The second species was known under the name, *Diatrinsan'talon, Diatri'um Santalo'rum pulvis,* or *Powder of the three Sanders.* They were considered diaphoretic.

DIATRITA'RII. The Methodists were so called, who pretended to cure all diseases by subjecting the patients to treatment every third day.

DIAT'RITOS. Relating to every third day. A means used by the Methodists to cure disease.

DIAZOMA, Diaphragm.

DIAZOSMA, Diaphragm.

DIAZOS'TER, from διαζωννυμι, (δια, and ζωννυμι, 'to gird,') 'I surround.' The twelfth vertebra of the back, because it corresponds to the girdle, ζωστηρ.

DIAZOSTRA, Diaphragm.

DICEN'TRA CANADEN'SIS, *Squirrel corn, Colic weed. Family,* Fumariaceæ. An indigenous plant, growing from Maine to Wisconsin, which flowers in May, the flowers having the odour of hyacinths. It has been given internally in syphilis, and applied externally in syphilis and gonorrhœa.

DICEPHALIUM, Bicephalium.

DICEPH'ALUS, *Biceph'alus, Derod'ymus et Iod'ymus, Janus,* from δι, 'double,' and κεφαλη, 'head.' A monster with two heads.

DICERAS RUDE, Ditrachyceras rudis, see Worms.

DICHALCON. A weight, equal to a third part of the obolus.

DICHOPHY'IA, from διχα, 'double,' and φυω, 'I grow.' A disease of the hairs, in which they split and grow forked.

DICHROMOS, Verbena officinalis.

DICIATRIA, Medicine, legal.

DICLIDOSTO'SIS, from δικλις, 'a double door,' and οστωσις, 'ossification.' Ossification of valves—as of the heart.

DICLIS, Valve.

DICOR'YPHUS, *Dicra'nus,* from δι, 'double,' κορυφη, 'the crown of the head.' A monster with a double vertex or cranium.

DICORYPHUS DIHYPOGASTRIUS, Hemipages.

DICRANUS, Dicoryphus.

DI'CROTUS, *Bisfer'iens,* from δις, 'twice,' and κρυω, 'I strike.' An epithet given to the pulse, when it seems to beat twice as fast as usual. It is synonymous with the term *rebounding,* the artery rebounding after striking, so as to convey the sensation of a double pulsation. It has been considered, and with truth, to frequently foretell hemorrhage. In bad cases of typhus, it certainly announces such a tendency.

DICTAMNE, Dictamnus albus — *d. de Crète,* Origanum dictamnus.

DICTAM'NUS ALBUS, from Dictamnus, a town in Crete; *D. Fraxinel'la, Fraxinella Dictamnus, White Fraxinel'la, Bastard Dittany, Fraxinel'la,* (F.) *Dictamne, Fraxinelle.* The fresh root has been considered nervine, anthelmintic, emmenagogue. It is not used.

DICTAMNUS CRETICUS, Origanum dictamnus—d. Fraxinella, Dictamnus albus.

DICTYITIS, Retinitis.

DICTYON, Rete.

DIDELPHYS, Dihysteria.

DIDYMAL'GIA, from διδυμοι, 'the testicles,' and αλγος, 'pain.' Pain in the testicles.

DIDYMIS, Epididymis.

DIDYMITIS, Hernia humoralis.

DIDYMOS, Gemellus.

DIDYMUS, Testicle — d. Symphyogastrius, Gastrodidymus—d. Symphyohypogastricus, Hypogastrodidymus — d. Symphyoperinæus, Pygodidymus — d. Symphyothoracogastrius, Thoracogastrodidymus.

DIECBOL'ION, from δια, and εκβαλλω, 'I cast out.' A name given, by the ancients, to a remedy which they believed capable of producing abortion.

DIERENBACH, MINERAL WATERS OF. Dierenbach is a city in Bavaria, two leagues from which is a sulphurous spring.

DIERVIL'LA TRIF'IDA, *Bush honeysuckle.* An indigenous plant of the Honeysuckle tribe—Lonicereæ—whose flowers appear from June to August. It has been used as a diuretic; and in gonorrhœa and syphilis.

DIES, *He'mera, A day,* (F.) *Jour.* The day is, properly, the period during which the solar light illumines our horizon: but commonly, also, we designate by the word *day* the period of 24 hours or *Nycthe'meron*, which is frequently divided into four parts—morning, midday, evening, and midnight. In antiquity, great importance was attached to the observation of days in disease. The medical day is usually reckoned at 24 hours,—universally in estimating the duration of a disease. In parts of the United States, it comprises only the time when the sun is above the horizon, as regards the administration of medicine, so that if a medicine be ordered to be taken four times a day, it is understood to mean during the 12 hours of day.

DIES CANICULARES, see Canicula—d. Contemplabiles, Critical days—d. Contemplantes, Indicating days—d. Critici, Critical days—d. Decretorii, Critical days—d. Indicantes, Indicating days—d. Indicatorii, Indicating days—d. Indices, Indicating days—d. Internuntii, Critical days—d. Judicatorii, Critical days—d. Radicales, Critical days.

DIET, *Diæ'ta, Diæte'ma, Ra'tio victûs.* Originally, this word signified nearly the same thing as *Hygiene* and *Regimen*, that is, Diet was the employment of every thing necessary for the preservation of health and life. At the present day, it signifies a particular kind of food, and, at times, a privation of food and drink;—abstinence. To put any one upon diet, (F.) *mettre quelqu'un à la diète,* means to deprive him of his usual nourishment:—*milk diet* means a diet of milk, &c. See Aliment, Dietetics, Hygiene, and Regimen.

DIET SCALE. Every well regulated hospital has certain dietetic regulations. The following *Table of Dietary* shows the particular regimen selected for the sick, in certain hospitals.

DIET-TABLE OF DIFFERENT HOSPITALS OF GREAT BRITAIN, IRELAND, AND THE UNITED STATES.

I. ENGLAND.

LONDON HOSPITALS.

1. *London Hospital.*

	COMMON DIET.	MIDDLE DIET.	LOW DIET.	MILK DIET.
Per Day	12 oz. Bread. 1 pint Porter, *Men.* ½ pint do., *Women.*		8 oz. Bread.	12 oz. Bread.
Breakfast	Gruel.		Gruel.	Gruel.
Dinner	8 oz. Beef, with Potatoes, thrice a week. 8 oz. Mutton, with Potatoes, twice a week. 8 oz. Potatoes and Soup, with vegetables, twice a week.	The same, except that 4 oz. of Meat shall be given instead of 8 oz.	Broth.	1 pint Milk.
Supper	1 pint of Broth.		Gruel or Broth.	1 pint Milk.

2. *St. Bartholomew's Hospital.*

	COMMON DIET.	BROTH DIET.	THIN OR FEVER DIET.	MILK DIET.
Daily	Milk Porridge. 12 oz. Bread. 6 oz. Mutton or Beef. 1 pint Broth [with Peas or Potatoes, 4 times a week.] 2 pints Beer, *Men.* 1 pint, *Women.* 1 oz. Butter, twice a week.	Milk Porridge. 12 oz. Bread. 2 pints Broth. 1 pint Beer. 1 oz. Butter.	Milk Porridge. 12 oz. Bread. 1 pint of Milk, with Tapioca, Arrowroot, Sago, or Rice, as may be prescribed. Barley water.	Milk Porridge. 12 oz. Bread. 2 pts. Milk, with Tapioca, Arrow-root, Sago, or Rice, as may be prescribed. Barley water. 1 oz. Butter. Bread Pudding, three times a week, when ordered.

3. St. Thomas's Hospital.

	FULL DIET.	MILK DIET.	DRY DIET.	FEVER DIET.
Daily	2 pints Beer; 14 oz. Bread.	12 oz. Bread.	14 oz. Bread, 2 pints Beer.	12 oz. Bread; two pints Beer.
Breakfast	Water Gruel.	1 pint Milk.	Water Gruel.	Water Gruel.
Dinner	½ lb. of Beef when dressed, twice a week; 4 oz. Butter, or 6 oz. of Cheese, thrice a week; ½ lb. Mutton when boiled, thrice a week.	1 pint Milk, 4 times a week; Rice Pudding, thrice a week.	4 oz. Butter, 4 times a week; Rice Pudding and 4 oz. of Butter, three times a week.	½ lb. Beef, for tea.
Supper	1 pt. Broth, 4 times a week.	1 pint Milk.		

4. St. George's Hospital.

	EXTRA DIET.	ORDINARY DIET.	FISH DIET.	FEVER DIET.	BROTH DIET.	MILK DIET.
Daily	12 oz. Bread. *Men.* 2 pints Beer. *Women.* 1½ pint Beer.	12 oz. Bread. 1 pint Beer.	12 oz. Bread.	12 oz. Bread. Barley Water *ad libitum*.	12 oz. Bread.	12 oz. Bread.
Breakfast	1 pint Tea. ½ pint Milk.	1 pint Tea. ½ pint Milk.	1 pint Tea. ½ pint Milk.	1 pint Tea. ½ pint Milk.	1 pint Tea. ½ pint Milk.	1 pint Tea. ½ pint Milk.
Dinner	12 oz. Meat, roasted (weighed with the bone before it is dressed) four days,—boiled three days. ½ lb. Potatoes.	One-half of the meat allowed for extra diet. ½ lb. Potatoes.	4 oz. of plain boiled white fish (as Whiting, Plaice, Flounders, or Haddock.)	Arrow-root &c., must be specially directed.	1 pint Broth 6 oz. light Pudding.	1½ pint Rice. Milk four days. ½ lb. Bread or Rice Pudding three days.
Supper	1 pint Gruel. ½ pint Milk.	1 pint Gruel. ½ pint Milk.	1 pint Gruel. ½ pint Milk.	1 pint Tea. ½ pint Milk.	1 pint Gruel. ½ pint Milk.	½ pint Milk.

5. Guy's Hospital.

	FULL DIET.	MIDDLE DIET.	LOW DIET.	MILK DIET.	FEVER DIET.
Daily	14 oz. Bread. 1½ oz. Butter. 1 qt. Table Beer. 8 oz. Meat, when dressed.	12 oz. Bread. 1½ oz. Butter. 1 pt. Table Beer. 4 oz. Meat, when dressed, and ½ pint Broth.	12 oz. Bread. 1 oz. Butter. Tea and Sugar.	12 oz. Bread. 1 oz. Butter. 2 pints Milk.	6 oz. Bread. 1 oz. Butter. Tea and Sugar.

Half a pound of Beef, (for Beef-tea,) or Arrow-root or Sago, when ordered.
For each Diet, Gruel or Barley-water, as required.

6. Westminster Hospital.

	FULL DIET.	MIDDLE DIET.	LOW DIET.		SPOON, OR FEVER DIET.	INCURABLES' DIET.
			Fixed.	*Casual.*		
Daily	14 oz. Bread.	10 oz. Bread.	½ lb. Bread.	—	¾ lb. Bread.	¾ lb. Bread. ¼ lb. Meat. ½ lb. Potatoes. ½ pint Milk. 1 pint Porter.
Breakfast	1 pint Milk Porridge, or Rice Gruel.	1 pint Milk Porridge, or thin Gruel.	1 pint Tea, with Sugar and Milk.	—	1 pint Tea, with Sugar and Milk.	
Dinner	½ lb. Meat, roasted, boiled, or chops. ¾ lb. of Potatoes.	¼ lb. Meat, roasted, boiled, or chops. ½ lb. of Potatoes.	No fixed Diet for Dinner.	1 pint Broth, or ½ lb. of Bread, or Rice Pudding, or 1 pt. Beef Tea, or a Chop, or Fish.	Barley Water.	
Supper	1 pint Milk Porridge, or Rice Gruel.	1 pint Milk Porridge, or thin Gruel.	1 pint Tea, with Sugar and Milk.	—	1 pint Tea, with Sugar and Milk.	

7. *Middlesex Hospital.*

	DIÆTA CARNIS, OR MEAT DIET.	DIÆTA JUSCULI, OR SOUP DIET.	DIÆTA LACTIS, OR MILK DIET.	DIÆTA SIMPLEX, OR SIMPLE DIET.	CANCER DIET.
Daily	12 oz. Bread.	12 oz. Bread.	12 oz. Bread.	6 oz. Bread.	12 oz. Bread. ½ lb Meat. ½ lb. Potatoes. 1 pint Milk.
Breakfast	1 pint Milk.	1 pint Milk.	1 pint Milk.	1 pint Barley-water.	
Dinner	*Physician's Patients.* ½ lb. of Potatoes, 4 oz. dressed meat, (beef or mutton,) roast and boiled alternately, 4 days. 4 oz. Meat in Soup, 3 days. *Surgeon's Patients.* ¾ lb. of Potatoes, 4 oz. dressed meat, (beef or mutton,) roast and boiled alternately.	1 pint Soup, made with 4 oz. Beef, alternately with 1 pint of Broth with Barley.	½ pint of Milk with Rice-pudding, 4 days, and with Batter-pudding, 3 days.	1 pint Gruel.	
Supper	1 pint Gruel alternately with 1 pint of Barley-water.	1 pint Gruel.	½ pint Milk or 1 pint Gruel.	1 pint Gruel or Barley-water.	

8. *North London Hospital.*

	FULL DIET.	MIDDLE DIET.	LOW DIET.	MILK DIET.
Daily	16 oz. Bread. ¼ pint Milk. ½ lb. Meat and ½ lb. Potatoes 4 days. 1 pt. Soup or Rice 3 days.	16 oz. Bread. ¼ pint Milk. 1 pint Soup or Rice.	8 oz. Bread. ¼ pint Milk. Oatmeal for Gruel.	17 oz. Bread. 2 pints Milk.

9. *King's College Hospital.*

	FULL DIET.	MIDDLE DIET.	MILK DIET.	LOW DIET.	FEVER DIET.
Daily	1 pint Beer, or ½ pint Porter. 14 oz. Bread.	14 oz. Bread.	1 lb. Bread.	8 oz. Bread.	—
Breakfast	1 pt. Milk Porridge.	1 pt. Milk Porridge.	1 pint Milk.	1 pint Gruel.	1 pint Gruel.
Dinner	½ lb. Meat. ½ lb. Potatoes.	¼ lb. Meat. ½ lb. Potatoes.	1 pint Milk.	1 pint Broth.	2 pints Barley-water.
Supper	1 pt. Milk Porridge.	1 pt. Milk Porridge.	1 pint Gruel.	1 pt. Milk Porridge.	1 pt. Milk Porridge.

10. *Dreadnought Hospital Ship.*

	FULL DIET.	ORDINARY DIET.	LOW DIET.	MILK DIET.	FEVER DIET.
Breakfast	1 pint Tea. 1 lb. Bread.	Ditto. Ditto.	Ditto. ½ lb. Bread.	Ditto. 1 lb. Bread.	Ditto.
Dinner	¾ lb. Meat. ¾ lb. Potatoes. 2 pints Beer, (if ordered.)	½ lb. Meat. ½ lb. Potatoes. 1 pint Beer, (if ordered.)	1 pint of Beef Tea.	1 pint Milk.	Gruel.
Supper	1 pint Broth.	1 pint Broth or Gruel.	1 pint Gruel or Milk, (if ordered.)	1 pint Milk.	Gruel or Barley-water.

HOSPITALS.	ORDINARY DIET.	LOW DIET.
LIVERPOOL.	*Breakfast.*—A pint milk porridge, breaded every morn'g. *Dinner.*—(1, 5, 7*)—Boiled beef and vegetables.—(2)—Rice, milk, and bread.—(3)—Stewed beef and potatoes.—(4)—Pea soup and bread.—(6)—Ale, gruel, and bread. *Supper.*—A pint of broth and bread on Sunday and Thursday. A pint of milk and bread on the other days. FULL DIET.—The same as the ordinary diet.	Consists throughout the day of milk porridge, common batter, or rice, pudding. The ale and beer are bought.
BRISTOL.	*Breakfast.*—On Sunday, Tuesday, Thursday, and Saturday, milk porridge; Monday, Wednesday, and Friday, meat broth; 12 oz. of bread on meat days; 14 oz. on the other days. *Dinner.*—(1, 3, 5)—Three-fourths of a pound of meat, with vegetables; two pints of beer daily.—(2, 4, 6, 7)—A pint of gruel or pap. *Supper.*—A wine pint of gruel of meal broth on Sunday; 2 oz. of cheese for the men, one-fourth of an oz. of butter for the women, on Monday, Wednesday, Friday, and Saturday. FULL DIET.—The patients have meat every day.	*Breakfast.*--A wine quart of milk porridge or milk. *Dinner.*—A wine quart of weak broth. *Supper.*—The same as breakfast, 14 oz. of bread, and barley-water for common drink. 20 bushels of malt, 15 lbs. of hops to 14 gals. of strong ale; 21 bush. of malt, and 12 pounds of hops, to 360 gals. of ale; 11 bush. of malt, 7 pounds of hops, to 360 gals. of small beer.
BIRMINGHAM. Revised 1819.	*Breakfast.*—To each man a pint and a half of milk porridge, with 4 oz. of bread added to it. To each woman or child, one pint of milk porridge without bread. To each patient 2 oz. of bread daily. *Dinner.*—(1, 3, 5)—To each man 8 oz. of baked or boiled meat; to each woman or child, 6 oz. To each patient, 6 oz. of vegetables, and one pint of beer daily.—(2)—To each man, a quart of rice or barley broth, made with a variety of vegetables; to each woman or child, one pint and a half.—(4)—Twelve ounces of boiled rice or bread pudding.—(6)—Four oz. of boiled or baked meat, a pint of rice or barley broth, made with a variety of vegetables.—(7)—Six oz. of baked rice or bread pudding, or a pint of rice or barley broth, made with a variety of vegetables. *Supper.*—A pint of broth, milk porridge, or gruel. FULL DIET.—Breakfast the same as in ordinary diet. Dinner, 6 oz. of boiled or baked meat, 6 oz. of vegetables, 6 oz. of baked rice or bread pudding. Supper, the same as ordinary diet.	*Breakfast.*—The same as ordinary diet. *Dinner.*—A pint of broth or rice milk, 6 oz. of baked rice or bread pudding to each patient every day. *Supper.*—The same as ordinary diet.

II. SCOTLAND.

EDINBURGH.	*Breakfast.*—One mutchkin of porridge, three gills of milk or beer; or five and one-fourth ounces of fine bread, milk or beer. *Dinner.*—(1, 4)—One chopin of broth, 8 ounces of butcher's meat boiled in the broth, or beef-steak; five and one-fourth ounces of bread.—(2, 5, 7)—A chopin of broth made of beef and bones, barley, groats, potatoes, and vegetables; five and a-half ounces of bread.—(3, 6)—Potato soup, with beef and veal, or bones; bread as above. *Supper.*—As the breakfast each day. FULL DIET.—At discretion.	At discretion.
GLASGOW.	*Breakfast.*—Milk porridge, quantity not limited, with half a mutchkin of sweet milk, or one mutchkin of buttermilk or beer. *Dinner.*—(1)—Broth made of barley, vegetables, and the dripping of the meat roasted during the week, with a quartern loaf to a man, and half to a woman.—(2, 4)—Beef boiled: 8 oz. to the men, and 6 oz. to the women; a quartern loaf to a man, and half to a woman,—or vegetables.—(3, 6)—Broth, made with beef, barley, and vegetables; a quartern loaf to men, and half to women.—(5)—Potato soup, with cow heels, bones, &c.—(7)—Six oz. of cheese to men, 4 oz. to women; bread as above. *Supper.*—As the breakfast each day. FULL DIET.—At discretion.	At discretion.

* The figures in parentheses denote the days of the week.

III. IRELAND.

5. Hospitals of House of Industry.	*Per diem.*—Sixteen oz. of white bread, one quart of new milk, and one quart of buttermilk for whey. Full Diet.—Two ounces of bread *per diem*, one quart of broth, one quart of new milk.	One pint of flummery *per diem*, one quart of new milk, and one quart of buttermilk for whey.
Stephen's Hospital.	*Breakfast.*—Half a pound of bread, one pint of milk. *Dinner.*—(1, 2, 3, 5, 7)—One quart of soup, half a pound of bread, or two pounds of potatoes; one pint of milk or beer.—(4, 6) Twelve oz. of bread, one quart of sweetened gruel.	Daily, half a pound of bread, two quarts of new milk, and one quart of buttermilk.
Royal Hospital, Phœnix Park.	*Breakfast.*—One pint of oatmeal or rice gruel. *Dinner.*—Half a pound of meat, three-fourths of a pound of bread; one pound of potatoes. *Supper.*—One pint of oatmeal or rice gruel. Full Diet.—Three-fourths of a pound of meat, one pound of bread, half a pound of potatoes, one quart of beer.	*Breakfast.*—Tea. *Dinner.*—Half a pound of bread made into panada or pudding.
Richmond Hospital.	*Breakfast.*—One quart of stirabout, one pint of new milk. *Dinner.*—Bread, 8 oz.; soup, 1 quart. *Supper.*—Bread, 4 oz.; new milk, one pint. Full Diet.—Breakfast, bread, 8 oz.; new milk, one pint.—Dinner, bread, 8 oz.; mutton or beef, 8 oz.—Supper, bread, 4 oz.; new milk, one pint.	*Breakfast.*—Flummery, one pint; new milk, one pint. *Supper.*—Half a pound of bread, one pint of milk.
Belfast Hospital.	*Breakfast.*—One pint of stirabout, one pint of new milk. *Dinner.*—Half a pound of bread, one pint of new milk. *Supper.*—One pint of flummery, one pint of new milk. Full Diet.—Breakfast, one quart of stirabout, one pint of new milk.—Dinner, 2 lbs. of potatoes, one pint of milk.—Supper, one pint of flummery, one pint of new milk.	*Per diem.*—Quarter of a pound of bread, one quart of gruel, three pints of new milk, half a pint of flummery. Barley water at occasions.
Cork Fever Hospital.	*Breakfast.*—One half quartern loaf for every four, and one pint of new milk each. Under 12 years, half a quartern loaf for every eight. *Dinner.*—(1, 3, 5)—One pound of beef, and two pounds of potatoes. Under 12 years, half a pound of beef, and one pound of potatoes.—(2, 4, 6, 7)—Potatoes and milk. *Supper.*—One pint of milk and one of stirabout, for adults; half do. for children.	*Breakfast.*—One-fourth of a lb. of bread, with milk and water sweetened. *Dinner.*—Gruel, broth, wine, and porter, as ordered by the physician.

IV. UNITED STATES.

Pennsylvania Hospital, Philada.	*Breakfast.*—Tea, coffee, or chocolate, with sugar or molasses and milk, and common baker's bread at discretion. *Dinner.*—Soup always; meat of two kinds—mutton and beef, generally—pork frequently; vegetables, according to the season; potatoes and rice, always. *Supper.*—Tea and bread: no butter allowed either to breakfast or supper, unless prescribed.	Gruel, gum water, barley water, and other articles prescribed by the physician.
Philadelphia Hospital, (Blockley.)	House Diet.—Arrow-root, gruel, sago, tapioca, rice, beef tea, beef essence, chicken water, rice water, barley water, gum water, flaxseed tea, lemonade. (The diet on which the sick are placed on entering the house until otherwise directed.) Moderate Diet.—Tea, crackers, broth, rice, mush, milk, potatoes, &c. Full Diet.—Bread, coffee, tea, white meat, mutton, beef, ham, eggs, butter, soup, potatoes, &c.	The kind and quantity left to the physician. The House Diet may be regarded as low diet.
New York Hospital, N. York City.	*Breakfast.*—Bread and black tea, one ounce of tea to every six, and a pint of milk to every eight patients. *Dinner.*—Tuesdays, Wednesdays, Thursdays, and Saturdays, beef soup, with beef and potatoes, and bread. On Mondays, boiled rice, with one gill of molasses. *Supper.*—The same as breakfast.	Special diet is directed by the attending physician, and adapted to each case.

The *Diet Scale of the British Navy* allows from 31 to 35¼ ounces of dry nutritious matter daily; of which 26 ounces are vegetable, and the rest animal—9 ounces of salt meat, or 4½ ounces of fresh.

That of the Navy of the United States is as follows:—*Three days in the week*—Pork, 16 oz.; beans or peas, 7 oz.; biscuit, 14 oz.; pickles or cranberries, 1 oz.; sugar, 2 oz.; tea, ¼ oz.;—40¼ oz. *Two days in the week*—Beef, 16 oz.; flour, 8 oz.; fruit, dried, 4 oz.; biscuit, 14 oz.; tea and sugar, 2¼ oz.; pickles or cranberries, 1 oz.;— 45¼ oz. *Two days in the week*—Beef, 16 oz.; rice, 8 oz.; butter, 2 oz.; cheese, 2 oz.; biscuit, 14 oz.; tea and sugar, 2¼ oz.; pickles or cranberries, 1 oz.;—45¼ oz.

In the Edinburgh workhouse the total allowance of dry food is about 17 ounces—13 ounces vegetable, and 4 ounces animal. In the Edinburgh children's poor-house, the diet consists of milk and porridge, barley broth and bread, amounting to 13 ounces of vegetable food to 4 ounces of animal. These allowances have been found ample for the maintenance of health. Perhaps the case of the smallest quantity of food on which life was vigorously supported was that of Cornaro,—not more than 12 ounces a day, chiefly of vegetable matter, for a period of 58 years.

DIET DRINK. A decoction or potion, variously composed, and used in considerable quantity, for the purpose of purifying the blood. The *Decoc'tum Lusitan'icum* or *Lisbon Diet-drink*, is one of the most celebrated. See Decoctum Sarsaparillæ Compositum.

DIETARY, TABLE OF, see Diet Scale.

DIETET'ICS, *Diætet'icè*, *Diætet'ica*, *Medicina Diætet'ica*; same etymon. (F.) *Diététique*. A branch of medicine, comprising the rules to be followed for preventing, relieving, or curing diseases by diet. Dietetics is diet administered according to principle. It is an important part of Hygiene. A well regulated system of diet has great power in checking disease, and likewise in preventing it. A proper knowledge of dietetics is, indeed, as important as that of the Materia Medica, strictly so called.

Dietetics has been used, also, synonymously with *Hygiene*.

DIÉTÉTIQUE, Dietetics.

DIETET'ISTS, *Diætetis'tæ*. Physicians who apply only the rules of dietetics to the treatment of disease.

DIEU-LE-FILT, MINERAL WATERS OF. The waters of Dieu-le-filt, in France, are chalybeate, and much sought after.

DIEURYSMUS, Dilatation.

DIEX'ODOS, from διά, and εξοδος, 'an exit or way out.' *Di'odos*. Any opening by which an excretion takes place.

DIFFERENTIAL DIAGNOSIS, see Diacritica signa.

DIFFICULTAS INTESTINORUM, Dysentery.

DIFFLATIO, Perspiration.

DIFFORMITÉ, Deformation.

DIFFUSED BLOWING SOUND, see Murmur, respiratory.

DIFFU'SIBLE, (stimulants) from *diffundere*, (*dis*, and *fundere*, *fusum*, 'to pour,') 'to pour apart or abroad.' Those stimulating medicines are so called, which augment the action of the vascular and nervous systems in an acute but transitory manner.

DIGAS'TRICUS, from δις, 'twice,' and γαστηρ, 'a belly:' *Biven'ter*, B. *Maxill'æ*, *Dep'rimens Maxil'læ Biven'ter*, *Bigas'ter*, (F.) *Mastoïdohyogénien*, *Mastoïdo-génien*—(Ch.,) *Digastrique*, *Abaisseur de la machoire inférieure*. The name *Digastricus* was formerly given to several muscles. It is now restricted to one of the muscles of the superior hyoid region. The digastricus is thick and fleshy at its extremities, thin and tendinous at its middle. It is attached to the mastoid groove of the temporal bone, and to a fossette at the side of the symphysis menti. Its tendon passes through an aponeurotic ring, which is attached to the os hyoides.

The use of the digastricus is to depress the lower jaw, or to raise the os hyoides, and to carry it forwards or backwards, as in deglutition.

The strong double-bellied muscle, which forms the gizzard of birds, is also called *Digastricus*.

DIGASTRICUS CRANII, Occipito-frontalis.

DIGASTRIQUE, Digastricus.

DIGERENTIA, Digestives.

DIGES'TIBLE, *Concoc'tûs hab'ilis*. Capable of being digested. All food is not equally digestible, and some of the most nourishing is the least so:—the fat of meat, for example. Certain substances, again, are entirely rebellious. The following table exhibits the time required for the stomachal digestion of different alimentary substances, in a well-known case, which fell under the care of Dr. Beaumont. The table is extracted from the Author's Human Health, Philadelphia, 1844. The most digestible substances are taken as the standard, which has been arbitrarily fixed at 1,000; and accordingly, *aponeurosis*, the first article in the table, requiring 3 hours, whilst *pigs' feet soused*, rice, &c., require but one, its digestibility, compared with that of these aliments, is placed as 333 to 1000; and so of the others. It need scarcely be said, that all these tabular results apply, in strictness, to the individual concerned only; yet they afford useful comparative views, which with exceptions depending upon individual peculiarities, may be regarded as approximations applicable to mankind in general.

Aliments.	Form of preparation.	Time required for stomachal digestion.	Ratio of digestibility compared with the most digestible articles in the table.*	Aliments.	Form of preparation.	Time required for stomachal digestion.	Ratio of digestibility compared with the most digestible articles in the table.
		h.m.				h.m.	
Aponeurosis	boiled	3	333	Marrow, animal, spinal	boiled	2 40	375
Apples, mellow	raw	2	500	Meat and vegetables	hashed	2 30	400
Do. sour, hard	do.	2 50	352	Milk	boiled	2	500
Do. sweet, mellow	do.	1 50	545	Do.	raw	2 15	444
Barley	boiled	2	500	Mutton, fresh	roasted	3 15	307
Bass, striped, fresh	broiled	3	333	Do. do.	broiled	3	333
Beans, pod	boiled	2 30	400	Do. do.	boiled	3	333
Do. and green corn	do.	3 45	266	Oysters, fresh	raw	2 55	342
Beef, fresh, lean, rare	roasted	3	333	Do. do.	roasted	3 15	307
Do. do. do. dry	do.	3 30	285	Do. do.	stewed	3 30	285
Do. do. steak	broiled	3	333	Parsnips	boiled	2 30	400
Do. with salt only	boiled	2 45	363	Pig, sucking	roasted	2 30	400
Do. with mustard, &c.	do.	3 30	285	Pigs' feet, soused	boiled	1	1000
Do.	fried	4	250	Pork, fat and lean	roasted	5 15	190
Do. old, hard salted	boiled	4 15	235	Do. recently salted	boiled	4 30	222
Beets	boiled	3 45	266	Do. do.	fried	4 15	235
Brains, animal	boiled	1 45	571	Do. do.	broiled	3 15	302
Bread, corn	baked	3 15	302	Do. do.	raw	3	333
Do, wheat, fresh	baked	3 30	285	Do. do.	stewed	3	333
Butter†	melted	3 30	285	Potatoes, Irish	boiled	3 30	285
Cabbage, head	raw	2 30	400	Do. do.	roasted	2 30	400
Do. with vinegar	do.	2	500	Do. do.	baked	3 20	400
Do.	boiled	4 30	222	Rice	boiled	1	1000
Cake, corn	baked	3	333	Sago	do.	1 45	571
Do. sponge	do.	2 30	400	Salmon, salted	do.	4	250
Carrot, orange	boiled	3 15	302	Sausage, fresh	broiled	3 20	300
Cartilage	do.	4 15	235	Soup, barley	boiled	1 30	666
Catfish, fresh	fried	3 30	285	Do. bean	do.	3	333
Cheese, old, strong	raw	3 30	285	Do. beef, vegetables, and bread	do.	4	250
Chicken, full grown	fricasseed	2 45	363	Do. chicken	do.	3	333
Codfish, cured dry	boiled	2	500	Soup marrow bones	do.	4 15	235
Corn (green) and beans	boiled	3 45	266	Do. mutton	do.	3 30	285
Custard	baked	2 45	363	Do. oyster	do.	3 30	285
Duck, domesticated	roasted	4	250	Suet, beef, fresh	do.	5 30	181
Do. wild	do.	4 30	222	Do. mutton	do.	4 30	222
Dumpling, apple	boiled	3	333	Tapioca	do.	2	500
Eggs, fresh	hard boiled	3 30	285	Tendon, boiled	do.	5 30	181
Do. do.	soft boiled	3	333	Tripe, soused	do.	1	1000
Do. do.	fried	3 30	285	Trout, salmon, fresh	do.	1 30	666
Do, do.	roasted	2 15	444	Do. do.	fried	1 30	666
Do. do.	raw	2	500	Turkey, domestic	roasted	2 30	400
Do. do.	whipped	1 30	666	Do. do.	boiled	2 25	511
Flounder, fresh	fried	3 30	285	Do. wild	roasted	2 18	435
Fowls, domestic	boiled	4	250	Turnips, flat	boiled	3 30	285
Do. do.	roasted	4	250	Veal, fresh	broiled	4	250
Gelatin	boiled	2 30	400	Do. do.	fried	4 30	222
Goose, wild	roasted	2 30	400	Vegetables and meat hashed	warmed	2 30	400
Heart, animal	fried	4	250	Venison, steak	broiled	1 35	631
Lamb, fresh	boiled	2 30	400				
Liver, beef's, fresh	do.	2	500				

* Pigs' feet soused, rice, and tripe soused, being the most digestible articles in the table, are estimated at 1000.
† In the case of oils, and other substances of similar nature, which undergo little digestion in the stomach, the time merely indicates the period that elapses before they are sent into the duodenum.

DIGESTIO DEPRAVATA, Dyspepsia — d. Difficilis, Dyspepsia — d. Læsa, Dyspepsia.

DIGES'TION, *Digest'io*, from *digere*, 'to dissolve'; *Coctio, C. Cibo'rum, Pep'sis, Diges'tive Proc"ess.* Digestion is a function, by means of which alimentary substances, when introduced into the digestive canal, undergo different alterations. The object of this is to convert them into two parts; the one, a reparatory juice, destined to renew the perpetual waste occurring in the economy: the other, deprived of its nutritious properties, to be rejected from the body. This function is composed of a series of organic actions, differing according to the particular organization of the animal. In man they are eight in number, viz. 1. Prehension of food. 2. Mastication. 3. Insalivation. 4. Deglutition. 5. Action of the stomach. 6. Action of the small intestine. 7. Action of the large intestine. 8. Expulsion of the fæces.

DIGESTION is also a *pharmaceutical* operation, which consists in treating certain solid substances with water, alcohol, or other menstruum, at a slightly elevated temperature,—in a sand-bath, for example, or by leaving them exposed for some time to the sun.

DIGESTIVE. See Digestives — d. Principle, Pepsin—d. Process, Digestion.

DIGESTIVE TEXTURE. The particular organic condition of substances which affects their digestibility.

DIGESTIVE TUBE, Canal, alimentary.

DIGES'TIVES, *Digesti'va, Digeren'tia;* same etymon as Digestion. (F.) *Digestifs.* A term given, by surgeons, to substances, which, when applied to a wound or ulcer, promote suppuration; such as the *ceratum resinæ, warm cataplasms, fomentations,* &c.

DIG"ITAL, *Digita'lis;* from *digitus,* 'a finger;' having the shape of a finger; *digitated.* Belonging to the fingers.

The *Appen'dix vermifor'mis cæci* is sometimes called DIG"ITAL APPEN'DIX.

DIGITAL ARTERIES, VEINS, and NERVES are those distributed to the fingers.

DIGITAL BLANC, Clavaria.

DIGITAL CAVITY, An'cyroid cavity, Cornu descen'dens ventric'uli latera'lis. The occipital portion of the lateral ventricle of the brain.

DIGITAL HUMAIN, Clavaria.

DIGITAL IMPRESSIONS are the slight depressions observable on the inner surface of the bones of the cranium, which correspond to the cerebral convolutions.

DIGITA'LE. Same etymon. (F.) Doigtier. A finger stall. The term Doigtier d'Asdrubali has been given to a small iron instrument used for measuring the dimensions of the pelvis. Placed at the end of the index finger, it adds to its length and enables it to reach the promontory of the sacrum.

DIGITALINE, see Digitalis.

DIGITA'LIS, from digitus, 'a finger,' because its flower represents a finger; Digita'lis purpu'rea, Fox-glove, Bac'charis, Baccar (?); Family, Scrophularineæ. Sex. Syst. Didynamia Angiospermia. (F.) Digitale, Gants de notre dame, Doigtier. The leaves of this plant, which are indigenous in Great Britain, are powerfully sedative, diminishing the velocity of the pulse, diuretic, and sorbefacient. In over-doses, Digitalis causes vomiting, purging, dimness of sight, vertigo, delirium, hiccough, convulsions, and death: —all the symptoms, in short, which characterise the acro-narcotic class of poisons. Its active principle has been called Dig''italine. It is a hundred-fold stronger than the most active preparation of digitalis.

Digitalis has been administered in inflammatory diseases, phthisis, active hemorrhage, dropsy, &c.; but although it is a powerful remedy, it has not been as much employed as it probably would have been in particular cases, owing to the over-strained eulogiums, which many have passed upon it in almost all diseases. The average dose is one grain, in the form of pill, which may be repeated every six or eight hours.

DIGITALIS MINIMA, Gratiola officinalis.

DIGITA'TION, Digita'tio, Produc'tio denta'ta, Inser'tio denticula'ta, I. digita'ta. A division into processes having the form of fingers. Several muscles, as the serrati, exhibit digitations, similar to those which the fingers form, when held separate.

DIGITATIONES TUBARUM FALLOPII, see Tube, Fallopian.

DIGIT''IUM. Desiccation or atrophy of the fingers.—Linnæus. Sauvages calls the same affection Paronych'ia Digit''ium, see Paronychia.

DIGITORUM TENSOR, Extensor brevis digitorum pedis.

DIG''ITUS, Dac'tylos, Finger, (F.) Doigt. A name given to the prolongations which form the extremity of the hand. There are five on each hand: the first, the thumb, Anticheir, Pollex, Manus parva majo'ri adju'trix, Dig''itus primus, D. magnus, Pro'manus, (F.) Pouce; the second, the index; the third, D. médius, Impudi'cus, (F.) Doigt du milieu, middle finger or long finger; the fourth, the ring finger, Annula'ris, Param'esos, (F.) Annulaire; and the little finger, Oti'tes, Dig''itus auricula'ris, (F.) Auriculaire, Petit doigt. All of these have three phalanges, except the first, which has only two.

DIGITUS ANNULARIS, Annular finger—d. Auricularis, see Digitus—d. Index, Index—d. Indicatorius, Index—d. Magnus, Pollex, see Digitus —d. Medius, see Digitus.

DIG''ITUS PEDIS, Toe. (F.) Orteil. The toes are five in number, and distinguished numerically, reckoning from within to without. The first is, also, called great toe, (F.) gros orteil; the fifth, the little toe, petit orteil. They have nearly the same organisation as the fingers.

DIGITUS PRIMUS, Pollex, see Digitus—d. Salutatorius, Index—d. Secundus, Index.

DIG'NATHUS; from δι, 'double,' and γναθος, 'lower jaw.' A monster having two lower jaws. —Gurlt.

DIGNOTIO, Diagnosis.

DIHYPOGAS'TRIUS, from δι, 'double,' and 'υπογαστριον, 'the hypogastrium.' A monster whose pelvis, together with the lower portion of the abdomen, is double.

DIHYSTE'RIA, Dime'tra, Didel'phys, U'terus duplex, from δι, 'double,' and 'υστερη, 'uterus.' The state in which there is a double uterus.

DIJUDICATIO, Crisis.

DILACERATIO, Laceration.

DILATANTS, Dilating agents.

DILATATEUR, Dilator — d. Antérieur du larynx, Crico-thyroid muscle — d. Postérieur du larynx, Crico-arytenoid, posterior.

DILATATIO BRONCHIORUM, Bronchiectasis — d. Ventriculi, Gastrectasis — d. Intestinorum, Enterectasis.

DILATA'TION, Dilata'tio, from dilatare, (latum facere,) 'to enlarge;' Eurys'mus, Aneurys'mus, Dieurys'mus. Augmentation of the bulk of a body, occasioned by a separation of some of its molecules. Caloric has the property of dilating all bodies. In Surgery, it means the accidental or preternatural augmentation of a canal or opening; as in aneurisms, varices, &c., or the process of enlarging any aperture or canal. When used so as to obtain a view of parts, as by the speculum, it is termed Dioptris'mus.

DILATATOIRE, Dilator.

DILATATORIUM, Dilator.

DILATATORIUS, Dilator.

DILA'TING AGENTS, Dilatan'tia, (F.) Dilatants. Certain substances used in surgery, either to keep parts separate which have a tendency to unite — as after opening an abscess, to prevent the edges of the incision from uniting; or to increase and dilate openings of canals, either when natural, or formed accidentally or artificially. These agents differ from each other: the chief are — prepared sponge tents, gentian root, bougies, sounds, dried peas for issues, &c.

DILA'TOR, Dilatato'rius, Diastoleus, (F.) Dilatateur ou Dilatatoire. A muscle, whose office it is to dilate certain parts; such as the inspiratory muscles, which dilate the chest.

DILATOR, Dilatato'rium, (F.) Dilatateur. An instrument, used for dilating a wound, excretory canal, or other natural or artificial opening. When employed to obtain an inspection of internal parts, it is termed Spec'ulum, Diop'tra or Diop'tron. There are several instruments of this kind, each taking its name from the part to which it is applied; as Speculum Oris, S. Nasi, S. Uteri, &c.

DILATOR, ARNOTT'S. A modification of the old dilators for strictures of the urethra. It consists of a tube of oiled silk, lined with the thin gut of some small animal to make it air-tight, and fixed on the extremity of a small canula, by which it is distended with air or water, from a bag or syringe at the outer end, whilst a stop-cock or valve serves to keep the air or water in, when received. As soon as the bag is passed within the stricture or strictures, as much air is to be injected into it as the patient can easily bear. The instrument is not much used.

DILATORES ALARUM NASI, Compressor naris.

DILL, Anethum graveolens.

DILLY, Anthemis cotula.

DILUEN'TIA, from diluo, (dis, and luere,) 'I wash away.' (F.) Délayants. Medicines which have been conceived proper for augmenting the fluidity of the blood and other animal liquids. All aqueous drinks are diluents. They are administered, with great advantage, in various diseases. In fever, water, which is the most familiar diluent, may be freely allowed; the only precaution being to give it *hot* in the cold stage, *cold* in the hot, and *tepid* in the sweating. In diseases, where it is considered necessary to abstract blood largely, diluents should not be given too freely. The abstraction of blood occasions activity of absorption, and the mass is speedily restored. It is also obvious, that in cases of inflammation of the mammæ, in nurses, diluents should not be freely allowed, as they increase the secretion of milk, and add to the irritation. When *demulcents* are exhibited in cases of urinary disease, they act simply as diluents: their mucilaginous portion is digested in the stomach and small intestine,—the watery portion alone being separated by the kidney.

DILWEED, Anthemis cotula.
DIMETRA, Dihysteria.
DINANT, MINERAL WATERS OF. Dinant is a small town, six leagues from St. Malo, in France, where are mineral waters, containing carbonate of iron, chloride of sodium, &c. They are much esteemed.
DINGEE, Dengue.
DINICUS, Antidinic.
DINKHOLD, MINERAL WATERS OF. A rich carbonated water, situate near the junction of the Lahn with the Rhine, in the duchy of Nassau. It contains sulphate of soda, chloride of sodium, carbonate of soda, sulphate of lime, carbonate of lime, and sulphate of magnesia.
DINOMANIA, Tarantismus.
DINUS, Vertigo—d. Scotoma, Scotodynia—d. Vertigo, Vertigo.
DIOBOLON, Scruple.
DIOCRES, Pastil.
DIODOS, Diexodos.
DIŒCESIS, Dispensation.
DIONCO'SIS, from δια, and ογκος, 'a tumour.' The Methodists applied this name to a sort of tumefaction or plethora, occurring either directly from too great a quantity of fluid circulating in the system, or owing to the retention of substances which ought to be excreted. It is the antithesis to *symptosis*. See Intumescence.
DIONYSIA'NUS, from Διονυσος, 'Bacchus,' who is represented by the poets as wearing horns. One who has long or horn-like excrescences.
DIONYSIS'CUS, same etymon. One who has a long horn-like excrescence on the frontal region.—Vogel.
DIOPHTHALMUS, Binoculus.
DIOPTRA, Speculum, see Dilator.
DIOPTRISMUS, Dilatation.
DIOPTRON, Speculum, see Dilator.
DIORTHO'SIS, from διορθεω, 'I make straight.' The reduction of a fractured or luxated limb.
DIOSCOREA, see Yam.
Diosco'rea Villo'sa, *Wild Yamroot;* indigenous: *Order*, Dioscoriaceæ; flowering in July. A decoction of the root has been prescribed in bilious colic. It is said to be expectorant, diaphoretic, and, in large doses, emetic.
DIOSCURI, Parotis.
DIOSMA, D. crenata.
Dios'ma Crena'ta, from διος, 'divine,' and οσμη, 'odour.' *Barosma crena'ta, Agathos'ma crena'tum, Buchu Leaves, Diosma* (Ph. U. S., 1842, *Buchu*, 1851) *Buckho,* (F.) *Diosmée crénelée. Nat. Ord.* Diosmeæ. A South African plant, the powder of whose leaves is used by the Hottentots to perfume their bodies. It has been employed in chronic affections of the bladder and urinary organs in general. It has also been given in cholera. It is often adulterated in commerce, by the substitution of less potent plants of the same family, as *Diosma serratifo'lia,* and *Euplex'rum serrula'tum.*

DIOSMA SERRATIFOLIA, D. crenata.
DIOSMÉE CRÉNELÉE, Diosma crenata.
DIOS'PYROS LOTUS, apparently from διος, 'divine,' and πυρος, 'wheat,' but why is not clear; *Faba Græca, Indian Date Plum,* (F.) *Plaqueminier d'Europe.* This tree grows in some of the southern parts of Europe. Its fruit is very astringent, and has been recommended in dysentery and hemorrhages.
Dios'pyros Virginia'na, *Lotus Virginia'na, Persim'mon.* A common tree in the middle parts of the United States. The fruit, *Persim'mons, Yellow Plums, Winter Plums, Seeded Plums,* which is only eatable after frost, (when it is tolerable,) is sometimes made into cakes with bran. These, being dried in an oven, are kept to make beer. When bruised in water, fermentation takes place, The unripe fruit is distressingly acerb and astringent. The bark of the tree, *Diospyros,* (Ph. U. S.,) is extremely bitter, and may be used where bitters are indicated.
DIOTA, *Dyota,* from δις, and ους, genitive ωτος, 'ear.' Two-eared, two-handled. Applied to a wooden cup, lined with a composition of *resin, cinnamon, cloves,* and *ginger,* to give more flavour to beer. It was formerly much used in the north of Europe.
DIPHORUS, Diphrus.
DIPHRUS, *Di'phorus,* from δις, 'two,' and φερω, 'I carry.' Properly a seat for two. A close stool.
Diphrus Maieu'ticus, *Sella obstetric"ia.* An obstetric chair.
DIPH'RYGES; from δις, and φρυγω, 'I torrefy.' The oxide of copper, more or less pure. The ancients reckoned three kinds of diphryges, which they used as astringents.
DIPHTHERIA, Diphtheritis.
DIPHTHÉRITE BUCCALE, Stomatitis, pseudomembranous.
DIPHTHERI'TIS, *Diphther'ia, Diphtherit'ic Inflammation, Pellic'ular Inflammation,* from διφθερα, 'a membrane.' A name given by M. Bretonneau to a class of diseases, which are characterised by a tendency to the formation of false membranes, and affect the dermoid tissue,—as the mucous membranes, and even the skin.
Diphtheritis of the Throat, Angina pellicularis—d. Trachealis, Cynanche trachealis.
DIPLASIASMUS, Duplication.
DIPLECOIA, Double hearing.
DIP'LOË, from διπλοω, 'I double.' *Diplo'sis, Meditul'lium, Medium Calva'riæ Discri'men.* The cellular structure, which separates the two tables of the skull from each other. The ancients applied the term, also, to the proper coat of the uterus (?)—Rolfink, in Castelli.
The Diploë has the same use as the cellular structure of bones in general. See Cancelli.
DIPLOGEN'ESIS, διπλοος, 'double,' and γενεσις, 'generation.' An organic deviation, which is owing to the union of two germs.
DIPLOLEPIS GALLÆ TINCTORIÆ, see Quercus infectoria.
DIPLO'MA. Same etymon as Diploë. A letter or writing conferring some privilege; usually applied to the document, certifying that a person has obtained the title of Doctor. It was so called because formerly written on waxed tables, folded together. Diploma is also used in pharmacy for a vessel with double walls,—as a water-bath.
DIPLO'PIA, from διπλοος, 'double,' and ορραμαι, 'I see.' *Visus Duplica'tus, Ditto'pia, Distop'sia, Amphamphoterodiop'sia, Amphodiplo'pia, Double Vision,* (F.) *Bévue.* An affection of the

sight, in which two distinct sensations are produced by the same object, which consequently seems double. Sometimes more than two are seen; but still the disease is termed *Diplo'pia* and *Suffu'sio Mult'iplicans*. This affection arises from some derangement in the visual axes, in consequence of which, the images are not impressed on corresponding parts of the retina of each eye. The diplopia of both eyes has been termed *Amphodiplo'pia* and *Amphoterodiplo'pia*.

DIPLOSIS, Diploë, Duplication.

DIPLOSO'MA, from διπλοος, 'double,' and σωμα, 'body.' The *Diplosoma crena'ta* is an imperfectly described entozoon, which has been passed from the urinary bladder. It varies in length from four to six or eight inches, and is thinnest in the middle, where it is bent at an acute angle upon itself, so that the two halves hang nearly parallel, and give to it an appearance as if two worms had been tied together by their heads. It has been confounded with the *Spiroptera hominis*.

DIPNOOS, from δις, and πνεη, 'breath.' Having two vent holes; *Bispi'rus*. An epithet applied to wounds which pass through a part, and admit the air at both ends.—Galen.

DIPROSO'PUS, *Iriod'ymus* et *Opod'ymus*, from δι, 'double,' and προσωπον, 'countenance.' A monster having a double face.

DIPROSO'PUS DLÆDŒ'US, from δι, 'double,' and προσωπον, 'countenance;' and δι, 'double,' and αιδοια, 'parts of generation.' A double monster, in whom the duplication affects superiorly the face, and inferiorly the anterior pelvic region.— Barkow.

DIPROSO'PUS DIHYPOGAS'TRIUS, from δι, 'double,' and προσωπον, 'countenance,' and from δι, 'double,' and υπογαστριον, 'the hypogastrium.' A double monster in whom the duplication affects superiorly the face, and inferiorly the lower part of the body—four lower extremities being always present;—*Tetras'celus*.

DIPSA, Thirst.

DIPSACOS, Diabetes.

DIP'SACUS FULLO'NUM, *Herba Car'dui Ven'eris, Car'duus Ven'eris*, (F.) *Cardère cultivé, Chardon à foulon, Chardon à bonnetier*, has had similar properties ascribed to it. Both have been also regarded as stomachic.

DIP'SACUS SYLVES'TRIS, from διψα, 'thirst,' said to be so called owing to the leaves being so placed as to hold water. *Cultivated Teasel*, (F.) *Cardère*. The roots of this European plant are diuretic and sudorific. The water, which collects at the base of the leaves, has been recommended as an eye-water.

DIPSET'ICOS, from διψα, 'thirst.' A remedy believed to be capable of exciting thirst. See Alternative.

DIPSO'DES, *Sit"iens, Siticulo'sus*, from διψα, 'thirst,' and ειδος, 'resemblance.' Thirsty. Causing thirst.

DIPSOMANIA, from διψα, 'thirst,' and *mania*. Really, thirst-mania. Often, however, applied to habitual drunkenness and to delirium tremens. An insatiable desire for intoxicating liquors.

DIPSOP'ATHY, *Dipsopathi'a*, from διψα, 'thirst,' and παθος, 'disease.' A mode of treatment, which consists in abstaining from drinks.

DIPSO'SIS. Same etymon. *Morbid thirst*. The desire for drinking, excessive or impaired. A genus in the class *Cœliaca*, order *Enterica*, of Good.

DIPSO'SIS AVENS, Polydypsia — d. Expers, Adipsia.

DI'PYGUS, from δι, 'double,' and πυγη, 'the nates.' A double monster, the duplication being confined to the posterior portion of the lower end of the trunk—the coocygeal region.

DIPYRE'NON, from δις, 'twice,' and πυρην, 'a kernel.' A *specil'lum* or probe with two buttons or kernels—one at each end.

DIPYRITES, Biscuit.

DIPYROS, Biscuit.

DIRCA PALUS'TRIS, *Leatherwood, Swamp Leatherwood, Moosewood, Swampwood, Ropebark, Bois de plomb*, (Canada.) An indigenous shrub, which grows in boggy woods and low wet places throughout the United States. It is analogous to mezereon, in its action, — six or eight grains of the fresh bark producing violent vomiting, preceded by a sense of heat in the stomach, often followed by purging. Applied to the skin, the bark vesicates.

DIREC'TOR, *Itinera'rium*, from *dirigere, directum*, (dis, and *regere*, 'to rule,') 'to direct.' A *Conductor*. A grooved sound for guiding a knife, in dividing any part; (F.) *Sonde cannelée*.

DIRECTOR PENIS, Ischio-cavernosus.

DIRIBITORIUM, Mediastinum.

DIRT-EATING, Chthonophagia.

DIRUPTIO, Rhexis.

DIS, Di.

DISC, see Disk.

DISCEPTUM, Diaphragm.

DISCHARGE', (*dis*, and *charge*,) *Ec'roä, Fluxus, Proflu'vium*, (F.) *Écoulement*. In pathology, an increased discharge from any part, that naturally secretes a fluid.

DISCHROA, Dyschrœa.

DISCREET', from *discernere, discretum*, 'to separate.' *Discre'tus, Intertine'tus, Separated*, (F.) *Discret*. This epithet is given to certain exanthemata, in which the spots or pustules are separated from each other. It is opposed to confluent.

DISCRET, Discreet.

DISCRE'TA PURGA'TIO. The purgation or expulsion of some particular matter.

DISCRETIVUS, Diagnostic.

DISCRETORIUM, Diaphragm.

DISCRI'MEN, *Separation, Division*. A bandage, used in bleeding from the frontal vein; so called, because, in passing along the sagittal suture, it divides the head into two equal parts.

DISCRIMEN CALVARIÆ MEDIUM, Diploë — d. Narium, Septum N.

DISCRIMEN NASI; a bandage, in the form of the letter X, intended to support the nose, in transverse wounds of the organ.

DISCRIMEN THORACIS ET VENTRIS, Diaphragm.

DISCUS PROLIGERUS, Proligerous disc — d. Vitellinus, Proligerous disc.

DISCUSSIFS, Discutients.

DISCUSSIO, Resolution.

DISCUSSIVA, Discutients.

DISCUSSORIA, Discutients.

DISCU'TIENTS, *Discutien'tia, Resolven'tia, Discussi'va, Discusso'ria*, from *discutere*, 'to shake apart,' (*dis*, and *quatere*, 'to shake.') (F.) *Discussifs*. Substances which possess the power of repelling or resolving tumours.

DISEASE', old French *désaise*;—from *dis*, and *ease: Morbus, Nosos, Nose'ma, Noseu'ma, Nusus, Pathos, Pathe'ma, Lues, Malum, Passio, Ægritu'do, Ægrota'tio, Vit"ium, Arrhos'tia, Arrhoste'ma, Arrhosten'ia, Valetu'do adver'sa, Mal'ady, Complaint, Sickness, Distem'per*. (F.) *Maladie*. An opposite state to that of health, consisting in a change either in the position and structure of parts, or in the exercise of one or more of their functions, or in both.

By some, *Disease* is applied to structural change, whilst *Disorder* is restricted to functional derangement.

The following table, essentially that of Dr. C. J. B. Williams, comprises the chief elements of structural disease.

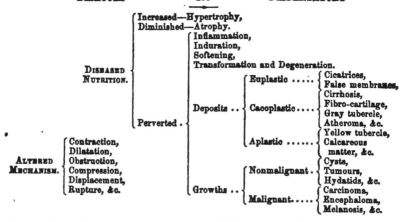

DISEASE, BLUE, Cyanopathy — d. of Bright, Kidney, Bright's Disease of the — d. English, Rachitis — d. Extrinsic, External disease — d. Family, see Hereditary — d. Fungoid, Encephaloid — d. Gastro-enteric, Gastro-enteritis — d. Hæmato-cerebriform, Encephaloid — d. Hereditary, see Hereditary — d. Pretended, Feigned disease — d. Simulated, Feigned disease — d. Surgical, External disease.

DISECOIA, Baryecoia.

DISFIGURATION, Deformation.

DISGORGE'MENT, (F.) *Dégorgement*, from *de*, and *gorge*, 'the throat.' An opposite condition to that of *Engorgement*. The discharge or abstraction of a certain quantity of fluid, which had previously collected in a part; as *Disgorgement of bile*. It also means particularly, a vomit.

DISGUST', from *de*, and *gustare*, 'to taste.' *Cibi fastid'ium*, *Aposit'ia*, *Asit'ia*, *Apoclei'sis*, *Abomina'tio*, *Siccha'sia*, *Horror Cibo'rum*, *Loathing*. An aversion for food. (F.) *Dégout*. Disgust is not the same as *Anorexia*. The latter is only a want of appetite; the former consists in real repugnance for food.

DISINFEC'TANT, *Disinfec'tans*, from *dis*, and *infect*. This term has been restricted by some to agents that are capable of neutralizing morbific effluvia; but the author includes under it, also, antiseptics or agents that are capable of removing any incipient or fully formed septic condition of the living body, or of any part of it.

DISINFECTING LIQUID, SIR WILLIAM BURNETT'S, see Burnett's Disinfecting Liquid — d. Liquid, Labarraque's, Liquor sodæ chlorinatæ — d. Liquid of Ledoyen, see Ledoyen's disinfecting liquid.

DISINFEC'TION, *Disinfec'tio*. The act of destroying miasmata, with which the air, clothing, &c., may be infected. Various means have been proposed for this purpose. Those most commonly employed are: — *chlorine*, *sulphurous* and *chlorohydric acid gases*, *vapours of vinegar*, *nitrous acid*; and, what is, perhaps, the most manageable of any, and equally efficacious, — *chlorinated lime*, or any of the chlorides of the alkalies. It is questionable if any chemical action occur between these agents and the miasmata, whence results a compound which is harmless. Disinfection also includes the action of antiseptics.

Chlorine or *Oxymuriat'ic Fumiga'tion*, *Solu'tio alexite'ria Gaubia'na*, *Fumiga'tio antiloim'ica Gau'bii*, *Alexite'rium chlo'ricum*, *Fumiga'tio Guytonien'sis*, is made by adding *common salt* ℥iij, to *black oxide of manganese* ℥j, *sulphuric acid* ℥j, and *water* f℥ij. This may be carried through an apartment, or be shut up in it.

Nitrous Fumiga'tion, *Alexite'rium Ni'tricum*, *Fumiga'tio Smythia'na*, may be formed by placing *nitrate of potass* ℥iv, and *sulphuric acid* ℥ij, in a saucer on hot sand.

DISJUNC'TI MORBI. (From *dis*, and *jungere*, *junctum*, 'to join.') *Disjoined diseases*. Fernelius has thus denominated diseases which occupy different organs, and are not produced by each other.

DISK, BLOOD, Globules of the blood — d. Intervertebral, Intervertebral Cartilage — d. Proligerous, see Proligerous Disk.

DISLOCATIO LIENIS SEU SPLENIS, Splenectopia.

DISLOCATION, Luxation.

DISOD'ICUS, from δις, 'twice,' and οδος, 'threshold.' Having a double opening.

DISORDER, see Disease.

DISORGANIZA'TION, *Organo'rum destructio*, (F.) *Désorganisation.* A complete morbid change in the structure of an organ, or even total destruction of its texture. In sphacelus, and sloughy ulcers, we have examples of this change.

DISPENSAIRE, Dispensary, Dispensatory.

DISPEN'SARY, *Dispensa'rium*, from *dispendere*, (*dis* and *pendere*, 'to weigh,') 'to take from a weight or mass,' 'to distribute.' The shop or place in which medicines are prepared. Also, an institution in which the poor are furnished with advice and necessary medicines. (F.) *Dispensaire*. This word is also used by the French synonymously with Dispensatory.

DISPENSA'TION, *Dispensa'tio*, *Diœce'sis*, *Epineme'sis*. The composition and distribution of medicines according to prescription. In France, it is more commonly applied to the weighing, measuring, and arranging of the articles, which have to enter into a formula, prior to combining them.

DISPENSATOR, Apothecary.

DISPEN'SATORY, *Dispensato'rium*; same etymon. *Antidota'rium*, *Liber Pharmaceut'icus*, (F.) *Dispensaire*. A book which treats of the composition of medicines. A Dispensatory differs from a Pharmacopœia, in containing the physical and medical history of the various substances; whilst the Pharmacopœia is mainly restricted to the mode of preparing them. The Pharmacopœia too, is published under the authority of, and by, the members of a college or association; whilst a dispensatory contains the whole of the Pharmacopœia or Pharmacopœias, with additions by the author, under whose authority, alone, it usually appears. The Pharmacopœia, in other words, is *officinal*; the Dispensatory, generally, *private*. Formerly, the words were used indiscriminately. See Formulary, and Pharmacopœia.

DISPLACED, see Percolation.

DISPLACEMENT, Percolation.

DISPOSIT"ION, *Disposit"io*, from *dis*, and *ponere*, 'to put or set.' A particular condition of the body, which renders it susceptible of altering, suddenly, to a state of health or disease; — of improving, or becoming changed for the worse. The *disposition* to phthisis pulmonalis is sometimes so strong, owing to original conformation, that the disease will make its appearance, notwithstanding every care. See Diathesis.

DISPUTATIO, Thesis.

DISQUE PROLIGÈRE, Proligerous Disk.

DISRUP'TIO, from *disrumpere*, 'to break off.' A puncture, which interests deep-seated parts.

DISSECTING ANEURISM, see Aneurism.

DISSECTIO, Dissection — d. Tendinum, Tenotomy.

DISSEC'TION, *Dissec'tio*, from *dissecare*, (*dis*, and *secare*, 'to cut,') 'to cut open;' *Diac'opē*, *Sec'tio Anatom'ica*, Practical Anatomy, *Necrot'-omy*. An operation, by which the different parts of the dead body are exposed, for the purpose of studying their arrangement and structure. Dissection has received various names, according to the organ concerned;—as *Osteotomy*, *Syndesmotomy*, *Myotomy*, *Angiotomy*, *Neurotomy*, *Desmotomy*, &c.

DISSEC'TOR, *Prosec'tor*, *Pro'tomus*, same etymon. (F.) *Prosecteur*. A practical anatomist. One who prepares the parts for the anatomical lecture.

DISSEPIMENTUM NARIUM, Septum narium—d. Thoracis, Mediastinum.

DISSEPTUM, Diaphragm.

DISSERTATION, INAUGURAL, Thesis.

DISSIDENTIA, Diastasis.

DISSIPIUM, Diaphragm.

DISSOLUTIO SANGUINIS, Hæmateclysis —d. Ventriculi, Gastromalacia.

DISSOLU'TION, *Dissolu'tio*, *Dial'ysis*, from *dissolvere*, (*dis*, and *solvere*,) 'to loosen,' 'to melt.' This word is in frequent use, in the writings of the humourists. It is employed, particularly, in speaking of the blood;—to designate, not its entire decomposition or putrefaction, but a diminution in its consistence.

DISSOLUTION, Solution.

DISSOLVANTS, Dissolventia.

DISSOLVEN'TIA, *Solvents*, (F.) *Dissolvants*. Medicines believed to be capable of dissolving swellings, concretions, &c. Discutients, Resolvents.

DISTAD; from *disto*, (*dis*, and *sto*,) 'to stand apart.' Away from a centre. Towards the far extremity. In anatomy, used by Dr. Barclay adverbially, to signify 'towards the distal aspect.'

DISTAL ASPECT. An aspect of a bone from the trunk, or towards the extremity.—Barclay.

DISTEMPER, Disease.

DISTEMPERANTIA, Dyscrasia.

DISTENSIO, Diatasis, Tension, Tetanus — d. Nervorum, Convulsion.

DISTENSION DE LA VÉSICULE DU FIEL, Turgescentia vesicæ felleæ.

DISTICHI'ASIS, *Distich'ia*, *Districh'ia*, *Districhi'asis*, *Distœ'chia*, *Distœchi'asis*, from δις, 'double,' and στιχος, 'a row.' An increased number of eyelashes; some tending towards the eye, and irritating the organ; whilst others preserve their natural direction.—Galen, Paulus of Ægina. See Entropion.

DISTILLATIO UTERI, Leucorrhœa.

DISTILLA'TION, *Destilla'tio*, *Stalag'mos*, from *destillare*, (*de*, and *stillare*,) 'to drop, little by little.' *Catastalag'mos*. An operation, by which—by the aid of heat and in close vessels—the volatile are separated from the fixed parts of bodies, with the view of collecting the former, when condensed in appropriate receivers. The ancients distinguished distillation *per latus*, *per ascen'sum*, and *per descen'sum*, according to the direction which the volatilized matters were made to take. In *distillation per latus*, the apparatus is so arranged, that the vapour passes horizontally through a succession of spaces before reaching the receiver. *Distillation per ascensum* is the ordinary method by the still. In *distillation per descensum*, the fire is applied above and around the top of the apparatus; and it is so arranged that the vapour must pass downwards. When dry organic matter is placed in an apparatus for distillation, and heat is applied until all volatile matter is driven out, the process is called *dry* or *destructive distillation*.

DISTILLATION, DESTRUCTIVE, see Distillation—d. Dry, see Distillation—d. Per Ascensum, see Distillation—d. Per Descensum, see Distillation—d. Per Latus, see Distillation.

DISTOC'IA, *Ditoc'ia*, from δις, 'twice,' and τοκος, 'birth.' Delivery of twins.

DISTŒCHIA, Distichiasis.

DISTŒCHIASIS, Distichiasis.

DIS'TOMA HEPAT'ICUM, from δις, and στομα, 'mouth.' *Fasci'ola hepat'ica*, *Plana'ria latius'cula*, *Fasciola huma'na*, *F. lanceola'ta*, *Gourd-worm*, *Fluke*, *Liver Fluke*, (F.) *Douve*, *D. du Foie*. An obovate, flat worm, an inch in length, and nearly an inch broad; sometimes found in the gall-bladder of man, whence it occasionally passes into the intestinal canal. It is one of the most common varieties of worms, infesting the livers of the sheep, goat, ox, stag, fallow-deer, horse, ass, hog, hare, &c. The treatment is like that required for other worms.

DISTOMA OC'ULI HUMA'NI. A parasite once observed in the eye of a child who had suffered from lenticular cataract.—Gescheidt.

DISTORSIO, Distortion, Sprain, Strabismus —d. Oris, Canine laugh.

DISTOR'TION, *Distor'sio*, *Intor'sio*, from *distorquere*, (*dis*, and *torquere*,) 'to wrest aside.' *Diastrem'ma*, *Dias'trophē*, *Ligys'ma*, (F.) *Distorsion*. Usually applied to the preternatural curvature of a bone; as *distortion of the spine, limbs*, &c. It signifies, also, a morbid state of the muscles of the eye, constituting squinting or strabismus.

DISTORTOR ORIS, Zygomaticus major.

DISTRIBUTORIA LACTEA THORACICA, Thoracic duct.

DISTRICHIA, Distichiasis.

DISTRICHIASIS, Distichiasis.

DISTRIX, from δις, 'double,' and θριξ, 'the hair.' *Trichio'sis distrix*, *Fissu'ra capillo'rum*. Hairs of the scalp, weak, slender, and splitting at their extremities.

DITOCIA, Distocia.

DITRACHYC'ERAS, from δις, 'two,' τραχυς, 'rough,' and κερας, 'horn.' A genus of intestinal worms. The *Ditrachyc'eras rudis*, *Dic'eras rudē*, (F.) *Bicorne rude*. This entozoon was first observed in the evacuations of a female, by M. Sulser of Strasburg. It is of a fawn colour, from 3 to 5 lines in length, with an oval head, flattened and terminating in a point posteriorly; contained in a membranous sac, and furnished, anteriorly, with a bifurcated, rugous horn. Laënnec considers it a vesicular worm or hydatid. See Worms.

DITTANDER, Lepidium sativum.

DITTANY, Cunila Mariana — d. American, Cunila Mariana—d. Bastard, Dictamnus albus

d. of Crete, Origanum dictamnus—d. Mountain, Cunila Mariana.

DITTECOIA, Double hearing.
DITTOPIA, Diplopia.
DITTOPSIA, Diplopia.
DIURESIÆSTHE'SIS, *Diureticoæsthe'sis, Uresiæsthe'sis;* from διουρειν, 'to pass the urine,' and αισθησις, 'feeling.' The desire or want to pass the urine.

DIURE'SIS, from διa, 'through or by,' and ουριω, 'I pass the urine.' An abundant excretion of urine.

DIURET'IC, *Diuret'icus, Ischuret'ic,* same etymon; *Uret'icus, Urina'lis.* A medicine which has the property of increasing the secretion of urine. Diuretics act by producing a discharge of the watery and other parts of the blood; and, by such discharge, indirectly promote absorption over the whole system. Hence, they are employed in dropsy. The following are the chief Diuretics:—Cantharis; Cantharis Vittata; Potassæ Acetas; Potassæ Liquor; Cahinca; Colchici Radix; Colchici Semen; Digitalis; Diosma Crenata; Juniperus; Oleum Terebinthinæ; Potassæ Nitras; Potassæ Bitartras; Scilla; Sodæ Sales, and Spiritus Ætheris Nitrici.

DIURETICA, Arnica Montana.
DIURETICO-ÆSTHESIS, Diuresiæsthesis.
DIVARICATIO, Ectropion.
DIVERSORIUM CHYLI, Receptaculum chyli.
DIVERTICULA SPIRITUUM ANIMALIUM, Ganglions, nervous.

DIVERTIC'ULUM, *Devertic'ulum.* 'A turning;' from *divertere, (di,* and *vertere,)* 'to turn aside.' A blind tube branching out from the course of a longer one. An organ which is capable of receiving an unusual quantity of blood, when the circulation is obstructed or modified elsewhere, is said to act as a diverticulum. Also, a malformation or diseased appearance of a part, in which it passes out of its regular course. It is sometimes applied to such a condition of the alimentary canal. Also, a hole to get out at. A by-passage. See Ectrope.

DIVERTIC'ULUM NUC'KII. The opening through which the round ligaments of the uterus pass.—Parr.

DIVERTICULUM PHARYNGIS, Pharyngocele.

DIVI'DING, *Div'idens,* from *di* or *dis,* and the Hetruscan verb *iduo,* 'to part or portion.' That which divides or separates.

DIVIDING BANDAGE, *Fas'cia div'idens,* (F.) *Bandage divisif,* is a bandage employed for the purpose of keeping parts separated from each other. It is used particularly to prevent improper union; as in cases of burns of the neck or other parts.

DIVINATIO, Mantia.

DIVISION, *Divis'io, Diæ'resis.* The accidental separation of parts naturally united; in other words, a wound or solution of continuity. Most frequently, however, it means an operation, which consists in cutting certain parts, with the view of fulfilling some therapeutical indication.

DIVUL'SIO, *Dias'pasis,* from *divellere, (dis,* and *vellere,)* 'to pull asunder.' A term used in Surgery, to express the rupture or laceration of organs by external violence.

DIVULSIO URINÆ, Cloudiness of urine.—See Enæorema.

DIXON'S ANTIBILIOUS PILLS, Pilulæ antibiliosæ.
DIYLISIS, Colatio.
DIYLISMUS, Colatio.
DIZZINESS, Vertigo.
DOCCIONE, MINERAL WATERS OF. This spring is at Lucca, in Italy. It is a thermal saline.

DOCH'MĒ, δοχμη. A measure of the Greeks, equal to about four fingers' breadth: *Dactylodoch'mē.*

DOCIMA'SIA, *Docimas'ticē, Docimasiolog"ia,* from δοκιμαζω, 'I try or prove the quality of any thing.' The act of assaying.

DOCIMA'SIA MEDICAMENTO'RUM ET VENENO'RUM. The testing of medicines and poisons.

DOCIMA'SIA PULMO'NUM, *D. Pulmona'lis, Pneobiomanti'a, Pneuobiomanti'a, Pneobioman'tica. Lung proof, Respiration proof.* Different proofs to which the organs of respiration of a new-born child are subjected, for the purpose of detecting whether it has or has not respired after birth; in other words, whether it was born alive or dead; —*Pneuobiogno'sis, Pneusiobios'copē.* These consist, chiefly, 1. In testing them with water, for the purpose of seeing whether the lungs are specifically heavier or lighter than that fluid. This is called *Docimasia Pulmonum hydrostat'ica* or the *Hydrostatic Test.* If lighter, it would be some evidence that the fœtus had respired: 2. In comparing the weight of the lungs with that of the whole body; the weight of lungs in which respiration has taken place being nearly twice as great. This is *Docima'sia Pulmo'num Stat'ica,* or Ploucquet's *Test;* and, 3. By measuring the circumference of the thorax and lungs; and comparing their dimensions with those of an infant which has not respired. This is *Daniel's Test.* These tests, singly, afford only probable evidence; but when united, the deductions may be more conclusive.

DOCIMASIOLOGIA, Docimasia.

DOCK, BLOODY, Rumex sanguineus—d. Blunt-leaved, Rumex obtusifolius—d. Cresses, Lapsana—d. Sour, Rumex acetosa—d. Sour, boreal, Oxyria reniformis—d. Water, Rumex hydrolapathum—d. Wild, sharp-pointed, Rumex acutus.

DOCNA SURA, MINERAL WATERS OF. This spring is in the Krapach mountains. The water contains sulphate of soda, carbonate of soda, chloride of sodium, carbonate of lime, silica, and iron.

DOCTOR, *Med'icus,* from *doctus,* 'learned;' '*un homme qui devrait être docte.*' A *Physician.* Frequently applied to any one who practises medicine; although properly confined to him who has received his degree of Doctor of Medicine.

DOCTRINA GALLIANA, Craniology—d. Soteria, Medicina.

DOCTRINE, MED'ICAL, *Doctri'na Med'ica.* The principles or positions of any medical sect or master. Medicine has been too full of doctrines. One of the first was that of Herodicus of Selivræa, who recommended gymnastic exercises in disease. The chief founders of doctrines have been Hippocrates, Serapion of Alexandria, Philinus of Cos, Herophilus, Asclepiades, Themison of Laodicea, Thessalus of Tralles, Soranus of Ephesus, Leonides of Alexandria, Athenæus of Attalia, Archigenes of Apamæa, Agathinus of Sparta, Galenus, Paracelsus, John Baptist van Helmont, Sylvius de le Boe, Keill, Hamberger, Pitcairne, H. Boerhaave, J. E. Stahl, Frederick Hoffmann, George Baglivi, Cullen, Darwin, John Brown, Beddoes, Girtanner, Reil, Rush, Raseri, and Broussais.

DOCTRINE, PHYSIOLOGICAL, Broussaism.

DODDER, Cuscuta glomerata—d. American, Cuscuta glomerata—d. of Thyme, Cuscuta epithymum.

DODECADACTYLITIS, Duodenitis.
DODECADACTYLON, Duodenum.
DODECAPHAR'MACUM, from δωδεκα, 'twelve,' and φαρμακον, 'a medicine.' An ancient name given to all medicines which con-

sisted of twelve ingredients. See Apostolorum Unguentum.

DODECATH'EON, from δώδεκα, 'twelve,' and τίθημι, 'I put.' An antidote, consisting of twelve simple substances.—Paulus of Ægina.

DODECATHEON, Sanicula—d. Plinii, Pinguicola vulgaris.

DODONÆA, Myrica gale.

DODONÆ'A THUNBERGIA'NA. A shrub of the Nat. Ord. Sapindaceæ, which grows at the Cape of Good Hope. A decoction of the root is used as a gentle cathartic in fever.

DODRANS, Spithama.

DOGCHOAK, Cynanche.

DOGDAYS, (F.) *Jours Caniculaires.* During these days, comprised between the 24th of July and the 23d of August, the temperature of the air in Europe is generally high and oppressive. They have received this name from the dogstar, *Canic'ula*, Σειριος, *Si'rius*—a very brilliant star in the constellation of the *great dog*, which rises and sets, at this time, with the sun. It was formerly believed to be a period particularly unpropitious to health; that it was dangerous to purge during it; and other phantasies were indulged in regard to it.

DOGGRASS, Triticum repens.

DOGMAT'IC, from the Greek δογμα, from δοκεω, 'I think.' *Dogmat'icus.* The name of an ancient medical sect; so called, because its members endeavoured, by reasoning, to discover the essence of diseases and their occult causes; whilst the *Empirics*, their rivals, confined themselves strictly to experience; i. e., to the observation of facts. The union of the two modes of investigation makes the rational physician. These sectarians are likewise called *Dog'matists*, and their doctrine *Dog'matism.* The founders of the sect were Hippocrates, Thessalus, Draco, and Polybius; and the most celebrated of its supporters were Diocles of Carysta, Praxagoras of Cos, Chrysippus of Soli, Herophilus, Erasistratus, &c.

DOGS' BANE, Apocynum androsæmifolium—d. Bane, bitter, Apocynum androsæmifolium.

DOGS' GRASS, Triticum repens.

DOGS' STONES, Orchis mascula.

DOGSTAR, Canicula.

DOGTREE, Cornus Florida.

DOGWOOD, Cornus Florida—d. Blueberried, Cornus sericea—d. Female, Cornus sericea—d. Florid, Cornus Florida—d. Great flowered, Cornus Florida—d. Jamaica, Piscidia erythrina—d. New England, Cornus sericea—d. Pond, Cephalanthus occidentalis—d. Silky-leaved, Cornus sericea—d. Virginian, male, Cornus Florida—d. Round-leaved, Cornus circinata—d. Swamp, Cornus sericea, Ptelea trifoliata.

DOIGT, Digitus—*d. Auriculaire*, Auricular finger—*d. Milieu*, see Digitus—*d. Petit*, see Digitus.

DOIGTIER, Digitale, Digitalis—*d. d'Asdrubali*, see Digitale.

DOLABRA, Ascia, Doloire.

DOLICHOCEPH'ALÆ (GENTES); from δολιχος, 'long,' and κεφαλη, 'head.' Longheads. Nations of men whose cerebral lobes completely cover the cerebellum—as the Kelts, Germans, negroes, &c.—Retzius.

DOL'ICHOS, from δολιχος, 'long.' A genus of plants of the leguminous family. It includes a number of species, generally indigenous in India or America. The *Dol'ichos Lablab*, or *Lablab*, is found in Egypt. (Prospero Alpini.) Its fruit is eaten there, like the haricot with us. The *Dol'ichos Sinen'sis*, is eaten in China, and is stored up as a provision for long voyages. The *Dol'ichos Tubero'sus*, (F.) *Pois Patate* of Martinique, has tuberous roots of the size of both fists, and has the consistence and taste of the turnip. The *Dol'ichos Bulbo'sus* of the West Indies resembles the turnip;—and from the *Dol'ichos Soja*, the Japanese prepare the well-known sauce *Soy*, which they term *Sooja.* The most important in medicine, is the

DOL'ICHOS PRU'RIENS, *Dol'ichos, Stizolo'bium, Mucu'na pru'riens, Negre'tia pru'riens, Cowhage, Cowitch, Adsaria Pala.* Order, Leguminosæ. (F.) *Pois à gratter.* The stiff hairs of the *Dolichos Pods*, called *Dolichos Pubes, D. Prurien'tis pubes, Dolichi Setæ Legu'minum, Lanu'go Sil'iquæ hirsu'tæ, Mucu'na,* (Ph. U. S.,) are the parts used in medicine. They excite an intolerable, prurient sensation when applied to the skin; but do not irritate the mucous membrane over which they pass, when administered internally. The Dolichos is a mechanical anthelmintic, and is useful in cases of ascarides lumbricoides, and oxyures vermiculares. Dose, gr. v to x, of the pubes, in molasses.

Mucu'na pruri'ta, a distinct species, but possessing similar properties, grows in the East Indies.

DOLOIRE (F.), *As'cia, Dol'abra,* 'a carpenter's axe.' *A Bandage en doloire* is one in which the turns are so placed, that each one covers two-thirds of that which is immediately beneath it. It has received the name *Doloire* from its representing the obliquity of the edge of the instrument whose name it bears. See Bandage.

DOLOR, Pain—d. Ani, Proctalgia—d. Capitis, Cephalalgia—d. Cephalicus, Cephalalgia—d. Colicus, Colic—d. Crucians faciei, Neuralgia, facial—d. Dentium, Odontalgia—d. Dentium à stridore, Hæmodia—d. Faciei, Neuralgia, facial—d. Ischiadicus nervosus, Neuralgia femoro-poplitæa—d. Lenis, Hypodynia—d. Mitis, Hypodynia—d. Nephreticus, Nephralgia—d. Pectoris externus, Pleurodynia—d. Pudendorum, Pudendagra—d. Rheumaticus et arthriticus, Rheumatism.

DOLORES AD PARTUM, Pains, labour—d. Intestinorum, Colic—d. Parturientis, Pains, labour—d. Post partum, Pains, after—d. Puerperarum, Pains, after—d. Rodentes, Pains, gnawing.

DOMBEY'A EXCEL'SA, *Arauca'ria Dombey'i.* A tree, which inhabits Chili, and furnishes *Dombeya turpentine*; a glutinous, milky-looking fluid of a strong odour and taste.

DOMES'TIC, *Domes'ticus*, from *domus*, 'a house.' The term *Domestic* or *Pop'ular Med'icine*, has been given to treatises written for the purpose of enabling those who are not of the profession to treat diseases, which may occur in their families, without the necessity of calling in a physician. The term, likewise, signifies—Medicine, when thus practised. It is probable, that such works have been attended with mischievous as well as advantageous results.

DOMINA'RUM AQUA. A medicine described by Myrepsus, which he considered emmenagogue.

DOMPTE-VENIN, Asclepias vincetoxicum.

DOMUS LEPROSARIA, Ladrerie.

DONDO, Albino.

DONESIS, Agitation.

DORADILLA, Asplenium ceterach.

DORCADIZON, Caprizans.

DOREA, Hemeralops.

DOREMA AMMONIACUM, see Ammoniac, Gum.

DORMITATIO, Somnolency.

DORMITIO, Sleep—d. Lucumoriana, see Lucumorianus.

DORONIC, Doronicum pardalianches—*d. d'Allemagne*, Arnica montana.

DORONICUM ARNICA, Arnica montana—d.

Cordatum, D. Pardalianches—d. Germanicum, Arnica montana—d. Officinale, D. Pardalianches—d. Oppositifolium, Arnica montana.

DORON'ICUM PARDALIAN'CHES, *D. Roma'num seu Corda'tum seu Officinale, Roman Leop'ard's Bane,* (F.) *Doronic, Mort aux Panthères.* The root of this plant resembles *Arnica Montana* in its properties.

DORONICUM ROMANUM, D. Pardalianches.

DORSAD, see Dorsal Aspect.

DORSAL, *Dorsa'lis,* from *dorsum,* 'the back.' *Notiæ'us, Notal, Tergal.* Relating to the back of the body, or of one of its parts; as the *Dorsal vertebræ, nerves,* &c.; *Dorsal artery of the tongue, penis,* &c.; *Dorsal region of the foot, hand,* &c.; *Dorsal Consumption,* &c.

DORSAL ASPECT. An aspect towards the *dorsum* or backbone.—Barclay. *Dorsad* is used by the same writer adverbially, to signify 'towards the dorsal aspect.'

DORSAL, LONG, Longissimus dorsi.

DORSALIS, Dorsal.

DORSA'LIS PENIS, (Nervus.) The branch of the internal pudic nerve, which is distributed to the upper part of the male organ; and to the clitoris of the female.

DORSO-COSTAL, Serratus posticus superior—d. *Lombo-costal,* Serratus posticus inferior—*d. Lombo-sacro-huméral,* Latissimus dorsi—*d. Sus-acromien,* Trapezius — *d. Trachélon - occipital,* Complexus.

DORSTENIA BRASILIENSIS, Caa-apla.

DORSTENIA CONTRAYER'VA, called after Dr. Dorsten; *Contrayer'va, Drake'na, Cype'rus longus, o'dorus seu Perua'nus, Bezoar'dica Radix, Dorste'nia Housto'nii, Lisbon Contrayer'va,* (F.) *Racine de Charcis, R. de Dracke, Racine des Philippines.* Family, Urticeæ. Sex. Syst. Tetrandria Monogynia. A plant of South America, whose root, *Contrayer'va* (Ph. U. S.), is aromatic, bitter, and astringent. It has been given as a tonic, stimulant and sudorific. Dose, gr. xij to ʒss.

DORSTENIA CORDIFOLIA, D. Brasiliensis — d. Placentoides, D. Brasiliensis—d. Vitella, D. Brasiliensis.

DORSUM, *Notos, Noton.* The back. *Metaph'renon, Tergum,* (F.) *Dos.* The posterior part of the trunk, extending from the inferior and posterior region of the neck as far as the loins. The *back of the foot, Dorsum pedis,* is the upper part of that organ, opposite the sole: the *back of the hand, Dorsum manûs,* the part opposed to the palm. In the same sense, we say *Dorsum penis, Dorsum nasi,* for the upper part of those organs.

DORSUM, Vertebral column — d. Manûs, Opisthenar.

DORYCIMUM, Costus creticus.

DOS, Dorsum.

DOSE, *Dosis, Præ'bium.* The quantity of any substance, which ought to form part of a compound medicine, or ought to be exhibited singly, to produce a desired effect. Many circumstances influence the doses of medicine. *Women* require smaller doses, as a general principle, than *men.* Habit has a great effect, as well as *climate, age,* and *idiosyncrasy:* all these, and other circumstances, must be taken into account; and every general rule on the subject will be found to have numerous exceptions. Some of the mechanical physicians laid it down as a rule, that the doses of medicines must always be as the *square of the constitution!*—A matter not easy of calculation.

The following Tables will exhibit an approximation to the proper doses (according to age) of most substances

TABLE OF DOSES ACCORDING TO AGE.

Age						
24	Let the full dose be			1		1 drachm.
18	will require				2-3ds.	2 scruples.
14	.	.	.	.	half.	⅓ drachm.
7	.	.	.	.	1-3d.	1 scruple.
4	.	.	.	.	1-4th.	15 grains.
3	.	.	.	.	1-6th.	10 grains.
2	.	.	.	.	1-8th.	8 grains.
1	.	.	.	.	1-12th.	5 grains.

The table of doses, according to age, recommended by Dr. Thomas Young, differs in some respects from the above. Either affords a sufficient general approximation. His rule is, that

For children, under twelve years of age, the doses of most medicines must be diminished in the proportion of the age to the age increased by twelve:

Thus, at two years, to 1-7th; i. e., $1\text{-}7\text{th} = \frac{2}{2+12}$.

At twenty-one the full dose is given.

DOSES, BROKEN. When an agent is given in small portions it is said to be in *broken doses,—refractis dosibus.*

DOSIOLOGIA, Posology.

DOSIS, Dose.

DOSSIL, *Bourdonnet.*

DOTAGE, Dementia.

DOTHIEN, Furunculus.

DOTHIENENTERIA, Dothinenteritis.

DOTHIENENTÉRIE, Dothinenteritis.

DOTHINENTERIA, Dothinenteritis.

DOTHIENTERI'TIS, properly *Dothienenteri'tis, Dothienenter'ia, Dothinenter'ia, Enteri'tis pustulo'sa, Enterodothie'nia, Helcenteri'tis, Follic'-ular Gastroënteri'tis,* from δοϑιην, 'a pustule,' and εντερον, 'intestine.' (F.) *Dothinentérite, Dothinentérie, Dothiénentérie, Dothiénentérite.* An inflammation and ulceration of the glands or follicles of Peyer and Brunner, which Bretonneau considers to be the essence of a large class of fevers, particularly of those of the typhoid character. See Typhus.

DOTHION, Furunculus.

DOTTRINA MEDICA ITALIANA, Controstimulus, (doctrine of.)

DOUBLE-CONSCIOUSNESS, see Consciousness, double.

DOUBLE-HEARING, *Dipleco'ia, Ditteco'ia, Paracu'sis duplica'ta, P. Imperfec'ta.* The action of the one ear unaccordant with that of the other: sounds heard doubly, and in different tones or keys.

DOUBLE-MONSTERS, see Duplication.

DOUCE AMÈRE, Solanum dulcamara.

DOUCHE, (F.) In Italian, *doccia;* modern Latin, *ducia; Cataclys'mus, Douse.* This term is applied to a column of fluid, of a determinate nature and temperature, let fall upon the body. *Pumping* is a variety of the *Douche.* In using this kind of bath, the fluid is directed upon the part on which we are desirous of acting. The *douches descendantes* are those in which the fluid falls from a height, — the *douches ascendantes,* those administered in diseases of the uterus, —the *douches horizontales,* where the fluid is impelled horizontally, &c. They may be *cold* or *warm,* according to circumstances. The apparatus consists of a reservoir of water having a pipe or plug, by means of which the water can be directed as the practitioner may desire. The *Douche* communicates a considerable and peculiar shock to the nervous system; and is one of the most successful means for taming the furious maniac. It is, also, useful in chronic rheumatism, stiff joints, &c.

Douch*es* of air are, also, occasionally used, as in cases of obstruction of the Eustachian tube by mucus. They are sent from an air-press—of which Deleau and Kramer have invented one each—through a catheter introduced through the nose into the tube.

DOULEUR, Pain—*d. de Côté,* Pleurodynia—*d. des Dents,* Odontalgia—*d. de l'Estomac,* Cardialgia—*d. Névralgique de l'Estomac,* Cardialgia—*d. Pulsative,* see Throbbing.

DOULEURS, Pains, labour—*d. Conquassantes,* see Conquassant.

DOUSE, *Douche.*

DOUVE, Distoma hepaticum — *d. du Foie,* Distoma hepaticum—*d. Petite,* Ranunculus flammula.

DRACHION, Pugillus.

DRACHM, *Drachma, Dram,* (F.) *Gros.* The ancient name of a piece of money, weighing the eighth part of an ounce. At the present day it is used for this weight.

DRACO MITIGATUS, Hydrargyri submurias —d. Sylvestris, Achillea ptarmica.

DRACOCEPH'ALUM CANARIEN'SE, *D. Moldav'icum, Melis'sa Tur'cica, Cedronel'la triphyl'la, Melis'sa Canariensis, Alpi'ni Bal'samum, Turkey Balsam, Cana'ry Balsam, Balm of Gil'ead Tree,* (F.) *Mélisse de Moldavie.* A Turkish and Siberian plant, which has an aromatic taste, joined with an agreeable flavour. It has been used as a tonic.

DRACONTHÆMA, see Calamus rotang.

DRACONTIUM, Dracunculus. See, also, Dracontium foetidum.

DRACON'TIUM FŒ'TIDUM, *Dracon'tium, Icto'des fœ'tidus, Symplocar'pus fœ'tida, Pothos fœ'tida, Arum America'num beta fo'lio, Pothos Puto'rii, Spathye'ma fœ'tida, Skunk-cabbage, Skunk-weed, Polecat-collard, Cow-collard, Collard, Itch-weed, Stink-poke, Swamp-cabbage, Pole'cat-weed, Hel'lebore, El'lebore, Irish cabbage. Nat. Ord.* Aroideæ. *Sex. Syst.* Tetrandria Monogynia. This indigenous plant, as some of its names import, is extremely fetid. The property on which its medical virtues are dependent, resides in a volatile principle, which is impaired by long keeping, especially in powder. Dose, of the dried root, *Dracontium,* (Ph. U. S.,) ten to twenty grains. It resembles asafoetida and other fetid gums in its properties; in other words, belongs to the class of reputed antispasmodics.

DRACONTIUM ANGUSTIS'PATHA, *Symplocar'pus Angustis'patha, Narrow-spathed Skunk-cabbage,* is possessed of similar properties.

DRACUN'CULUS, *Dracon'tium, Vena Medi'na Ar'abum, Vena seu Gor'dius Medinen'sis, Vermic'ulus Capilla'ris, Dracun'culus Gordius, Fila'ria Medinen'sis seu Guineen'sis, Malis Dracun'culus, Malis Gor'dii, Helminthon'cus Medinensis, Muscular Hairworm, Bichios, Bicho, Guinea Worm or Threadworm,* (F.) *Dragonneau, Ver de Guinée, Ver Filaire, V. de Médine, V. cutané, Veine de Médine.* A genus of worms, frequently met with in Indian and African climes. They are characterized by a filiform body, and are smooth and nearly of equal thickness throughout. The Guinea worm, when small, insinuates itself through the cutaneous pores, and penetrates into the areolar membrane and between the muscles; especially between those of the lower limbs, where it occasions a tumour like a boil, which subsequently suppurates, and the head of the worm appears and emerges gradually. The head must then be seized, and the worm be cautiously rolled round a small cylinder of linen or other substance. Care must be taken not to break it, as great pain and obstinate suppuration might be the consequence.

Considerable obscurity rests on this subject. Some even deny that the cases of Dracunculus, on record, are really those of worms.

DRACUNCULUS POLYPHYLLUS, Arum dracunculus—d. Pratensis, Achillea ptarmica.

DRAGÉES, (F.) Almonds or dried preserves, covered with white sugar; *Sugar-plums.*

DRAGÉES DE KEYSER. A pharmaceutical preparation, formerly much celebrated in syphilis. It was composed of *acetate of mercury, manna, starch, mucilage* and *gum tragacanth.*

DRAGMA, Pugillus.

DRAGMIS, Pugillus.

DRAGON (F.), *Dragon.* Some authors have given this name to opake spots on the cornea, and to cataract.

DRAGON CLAW, SCALY, Pterospora andromedea —d. Root, Arum triphyllum, Pterospora andromedea—d. Turnip, Arum triphyllum.

DRAGON'S BLOOD, see Calamus rotang.

DRAGONNEAU, Dracunculus.

DRAINING, *Desicca'tio,* (F.) *Dessèchement.* The act of drawing off the water from marshes, for the purpose of destroying the unhealthy emanations which proceed from them. It is a well known fact, that from marshes arise certain emanations or miasmata, with the nature of which we are, however, totally unacquainted, but which are the fertile source of intermittents and other diseases. Draining the soil and converting it into arable land changes its character, and the malaria ceases to be given off. It has happened, however, that although in some such situations intermittents have been got rid of, consumptions have taken their place.

DRAITSCH WATER, Godesberg, mineral waters of.

DRAKENA, Dorstenia contrayerva.

DRAPEAU, (F.) *Vexil'lum,* from *drap,* 'cloth.' A bandage, used in wounds, &c., of the nose, to keep the dressings *in situ.* It is composed of a small triangular compress, having two openings at its inferior part, corresponding to those of the nostrils. It is fixed by means of a bandage, passing from its superior angle over the head, and another passing round the head, under the orbits, so as to join the first at the nape of the neck. Also, Pterygion.

DRAP FANON, see Fanon.

DRASTIC, *Dras'ticus, Cenot'ic,* from δραω, 'I operate strongly.' Active. An epithet given to purgatives, which operate powerfully; as *elaterium, oil of croton,* &c.

DRAUGHT, *Haustus.* A term also applied by nurses to the sudden rush of blood to the mammæ, occasioned in the mother by the sight, or even thought, of her infant, and which occasions a greatly increased secretion of milk.

DRAUGHT, BLACK, see Infusum sennæ compositum.

DRAX, Pugillus.

DREAM, Somnium—d. Waking, Hallucination.

DRÈCHE, Malt.

DREGS, Feculence.

DREPANOIDES, Falciform.

DRESS, Vestitus.

DRESSER, from (F.) *dresser,* 'to put right.' An hospital assistant, whose office it is to dress wounds, ulcers, &c. He corresponds in function to the *Élève externe* of the French hospitals.

DRESSING, *Cura, Cura'tio,* (F.) *Pansement.* The methodical application of any remedy or apparatus to a diseased part. Also, the remedy or apparatus itself.

DRIBURG, MINERAL WATERS OF. At

the small town of Driburg, near Pyrmont, in Germany, there are nine springs, which are rich in saline ingredients, iron, and carbonic acid gas. Their action on the economy is like that of Pyrmont water. They contain chloride of sodium, sulphate of magnesia, sulphate of lime, carbonate of lime, carbonate of magnesia, carbonate of iron, chloride of calcium, and chloride of magnesium.

DRIMYPHA'GIA, from δριμυς, 'acrid,' 'aromatic,' and φαγω, 'I eat.' An aromatic and exciting diet.

DRIMYS WINTERI, Wintera aromatica.

DRINK, from Sax. drencan, *Poma, Po'tio, Potus, Bev'erage*, (F.) *Boisson*. Every liquid introduced into the alimentary canal for the purpose of repairing the loss of the fluid parts of the body. The necessity for its use is indicated by the sensation of thirst. Fluid, taken during a meal, aids in the digestion of the food. Some drinks are exciting and tonic, as the different varieties of beer, wine, and spirits, which we use at table. In a therapeutical point of view, drinks are used to appease the thirst which prevails in febrile affections, or to act as diluents in those and other cases.

The ordinary drinks, according to their chemical composition, are—1. *Water*, spring water, river water, well water, &c.—2. *Juices and infusions of Animal and Vegetable substances*, lemon juice, currant juice, whey, tea, coffee, mattee, &c.—3. *Fermented Liquors*, wines, ale, beer, cider, perry.—4. *Spirituous Liquors*, brandy, alcohol, ether, kirschwasser, rum, arack, gin, whiskey, ratafias, cordials, &c.

DRIVELLING, Slavering.

DROGUE, Drug.

DROGUIER, (F.) Same etymon as drug. A collection of different simple medicinal substances.

DROGUISTE, Druggist.

DROIT DE L'ABDOMEN, Rectus abdominis—d. *Antérieur de la cuisse*, Rectus femoris—d. *Antérieur de la tête*, Rectus capitis internus minor —d. *Antérieur de la tête, grand*, Rectus capitis internus major—d. *Externe de l'œil*, Rectus externus oculi—d. *Inférieur de l'œil*, Rectus inferior oculi—d. *Interne de la cuisse*, Gracilis—d. *Interne de l'œil*, Rectus internus oculi—d. *Latéral de la tête*, Rectus capitis lateralis—d. *Postérieur de la tête, grand*, Rectus capitis posticus major—d. *Postérieur de la tête, petit*, Rectus capitis posticus minor—d. *Supérieur*, Rectus superior oculi.

DROP, Gutta.

DROP, AGUE, TASTELESS, Liquor arsenicalis—d. Black, Guttæ nigræ—d. Red, Ward's, see Vinum antimonii tartarizati—d. Serene, Amaurosis.

DROPACISMUS, Depilation.

DROPAX, Depilatory.

DROPPED HANDS, see Hands, dropped.

DROPS, ABBÉ ROUSSEAU'S, Laudanum Abbatis Rousseau—d. Anodyne, Liquor morphinæ acetatis—d. Antiscorbutic, Marsden's, see Infusum gentianæ compositum—d. Anti-venereal, see Tinctura ferri muriatis—d. Chamomile, see Anthemis nobilis—d. Dutch, Balsam of sulphur, Balsam of Turpentine—d. Fit, Spiritus ammoniæ fœtidus, see Fuligo—d. Golden, de la Motte's, Tinctura seu alcohol sulfurico-æthereus ferri—d. Green's, see Liquor Hydrargyri oxymuriatis—d. Jesuit's, Tinctura benzoini composita—d. Lavender, Spiritus Lavandulæ compositus—d. Nitre, Spiritus ætheris nitrici—d. Norris's, see Antimonium tartarizatum—d. Norton's, Liquor Hydrargyri Oxymuriatis—d. Pectoral, Pectoral drops, Bateman's—d. Peppermint, Pastilli de menthâ piperitâ—d. Soot, see Fuligo—d. Wade's, Tinctura benzoini composita—d. White, Ward's, see Hydrargyri nitras.

DROPS, WARBURG'S. A secret preparation used in Demarara under the name of *Warburg's Fever Drops*. See Bebeeru.

DROPSICAL, Hydropicus.

DROPSY, Hydrops—d. of the Belly, Ascites—d. of the Brain, Hydrocephalus—d. of the Cellular Membrane, Anasarca—d. of the Chest, Hydrothorax—d. of the Eye, Hydrophthalmia.

DROPSY, FIBRINOUS. Dropsy in which the effused fluid contains fibrin.

DROPSY, GENERAL, Anasarca—d. of the Head, Hydrocephalus—d. of the Lachrymal Sac, Fistula lachrymalis, Lachrymal hernia—d. of the Pericardium, Hydropericardium—d. of the Peritoneum, Ascites—d. of the Pleuræ, Hydrothorax—d. Water of, Serum of Serous membranes—d. Wind, Emphysema—d. of the Womb, Hydrometra.

DROPWORT, Spiræa filipendula—d. Hemlock, Œnanthe—d. Water, Hemlock, Œnanthe—d. Western, Gillenia trifoliata.

DROS'ERA ROTUNDIFO'LIA. The systematic name of the *Sundew, Ros solis, Drosiobot'anon, Dro'sium, Rorel'la*, (F.) *Rossolis*. This plant has a bitter, acrid, and caustic taste. It has been used as a rubefacient, and to destroy warts and corns. It has, also, been regarded as a pectoral.

DROSIOBOTANON, Drosera rotundifolia.

DROSIUM, Drosera rotundifolia.

DROSOMELI, Fraxinus ornus.

DRUG, *Medicamen'tum*, (F.) *Drogue*. A name ordinarily applied to simple medicines, but, by extension, to every substance employed in the cure of disease. Ménage derives it from *droga*, and this from the Persian *droa*, 'odour;' because many drugs have a strong odour. It is, doubtless, from the Teutonic *trocken*, Sax. brigan, 'to dry.'

DRUG. To prescribe or administer drugs. Most commonly, perhaps, to dose to excess with drugs.

DRUG DISEASE. A morbid condition, which is—or is presumed to be—caused or kept up by the administration of drugs.

DRUG-GRINDER, see Pulverization—d. Mill, see Pulverization.

DRUGGIST, *Drugger, Drugster*. Same etymon. *Pharmacopo'la, Materialis'ta, Seplasia'rius, Pharmacopæ'us*, (F.) *Droguiste*. One who sells drugs.

DRUM OF THE EAR, Tympanum.

DRUM-SIEVE, see Cribration.

DRUNKENNESS, Temulentia.

DRYING, *Desicca'tion, Sicca'tio, Xeran'sis, Auan'sis, Desicca'tio, Exsicca'tio;* same etymon as Drug. Evaporation or removal of the superfluous humidity in a body.

DRYING OF PLANTS, *Desicca'tion of Plants*. Those which are very succulent should be dried quickly. They must be spread upon lattice work, covered from the light, and exposed to the heat of the sun or to that of a stove, not exceeding 110° Fahrenheit. The drying of less succulent plants can be effected at a lower temperature. *Flowers* must be dried very carefully, excluding light. *Seeds* are dried in a place where there is a free current of air. *Pulpy fruits* may be exposed to a gentle heat in a stove, which may be gradually elevated. *Roots* may also be dried in the stove: the tuberous require to be cut in slices.

DTHOKE, Framboesia.

DUAL'ITY, *Dual'itas*, from *duo*, 'two.' The state or quality of being two.

DUALITY OF THE MIND, OR BRAIN. As the organ consists of two hemispheres, they have been regarded by some as separately and distinctly concerned in the mental and moral manifestations.

DUCKFOOT, see Kyllosis.

DUCKSFOOT, Podophyllum montanum.

DUCT, ALIMENTARY, Canal, alimentary, Thoracic duct—d. of Bellini, Uriniferous tube—d. Nasal, Lachrymal duct — d. of Pecquet, Thoracic duct — d. Vitelline, see Vesicula umbilicalis —d. of Wirsung, see Pancreas.

DUCTIO PRÆPUTII, Masturbation.

DUCTOR CANALICULATUS, Gorget—d. Urinæ, Ureter.

DUCTUS, Canal, Meatus—d. Arteriosus, Arterial duct—d. Auris palatinus, Eustachian tube.

DUCTUS BARTHOLINIA'NUS, BARTHOLIN'S *Duct,* (F.) *Canal de* BARTHOLIN. The excretory duct of the sublingual gland.

DUCTUS BELLINIANI, Uriniferous tubes — d. Biliarii, Pori biliarii — d. Botalli, Arterial duct — d. Choledochus, Choledoch duct — d. Chyliferus, Thoracic duct — d. Cibarius, Canal, alimentary — d. Ferreini, Ferrein, canal of — d. Hepaticus, Hepatic duct — d. Incisivus, Palatine duct (anterior) — d. Intestinalis, Canal, alimentary — d. Lacteus, Thoracic duct—d. Lachrymalis, Lachrymal duct — d. Lacrumalis, Lachrymal duct—d. Nasalis orbitæ, Lachrymal or nasal duct —d. Nasalo-palatinus, Palatine duct (anterior)— d. ad Nasum, Lachrymal or nasal duct—d. Nutritii, Canals, nutritive—d. Omphalo mesentericus, see Vesicula umbilicalis—d. Pancreaticus, see Pancreas — d. Pecqueti, Thoracic duct — d. Punctorum lachrymalium, Lachrymal ducts—d. Riviniani, see Sublingual gland—d. Rorifer, Thoracic duct.

DUCTUS SALIVA'LIS INFE'RIOR, *Ductus Whartonia'nus,* (F.) *Canal de* WARTHON. The excretory duct of the submaxillary gland.

DUCTUS SALIVA'LIS SUPE'RIOR, *Ductus Stenonia'nus,* STENO'S *Duct,* (F.) *Canal de* STENON. The excretory duct of the parotid gland which opens into the mouth opposite the second upper molar tooth.

DUCTUS SEMI-CIRCULARES LABYRINTHI, Semicircular canals—d. Serosi, Lymphatic vessels—d. Spirales cochleæ, Scalæ of the cochlea—d. Stenonianus, Ductus salivalis superior — d. Thoracicus, Thoracic duct—d. Urinæ, Ureter—d. Urinarius, Urethra—d. Uriniferi Bellini, Uriniferous tubes — d. Varicosi uteri, Tubæ Fallopianæ — d. Venosus, Canal, venous — d. Vitellarius, see Vesicula umbilicalis—d. Vitello-intestinalis, see Vesicula umbilicalis — d. Waltheriani, see Sublingual gland — d. Whartonianus, Ductus salivalis inferior.

DUELECH, Dulech.

DUEL'LA. The ancient name of a weight, which was equivalent to eight scruples.

DUELLUM VENEREUM, Coition.

DUG, Nipple.

DULCAMARA, Solanum dulcamara—d. Flexuosa, Solanum dulcamara.

DULCEDO AMORIS, Clitoris.

DULECH, *Due'lech.* A term employed by Paracelsus and Van Helmont to designate a pretended tartarized substance, which forms in the human body, and produces acute pain, accompanied with great danger.

DULSE, Rhodomela palmata—d. Pepper, Laurentia pinnatifida.

DUMBNESS, Mutitas.

DUNBLANE, MINERAL WATERS OF. The springs of Dunblane, in Scotland, contain sulphate of soda, chlorides of sodium and calcium, and carbonate of iron.

DUNG, Fimus—d. Cow's, Fimus Vaccæ—d. Goose, Fimus anseris—d. Stone-horse, Fimus equinus.

DUNGA, Dengue.

DUODENI'TIS, *Dodecadactyli'tis.* A hybrid term, from *duodenum,* and *itis,* denoting inflammation. Inflammation of the duodenum, characterized by white tongue, bitter taste, anorexia, fulness and tenderness in the region of the duodenum, and often yellowness of skin, along with the ordinary signs of febrile irritation.

DUODE'NUM, *Ventric'ulus Succenturia'tus, Ec'physis seu Appen'dix seu Proces'sus Ventric'uli, Portona'rium, Dodecadac'tylon,* (from δωδεκα, 'twelve,' and δακτυλος, 'a finger.') The duodenum is the first part of the intestinal canal, commencing at the pyloric orifice of the stomach, and terminating in the jejunum. Its length is about twelve fingers' breadth, and as it is only partially covered by the peritoneum, it is susceptible of considerable dilatation; hence its name *Ventriculus succenturiatus.* In the duodenum, *chylification* takes place after the admixture of the biliary and pancreatic fluids with the chyme.

DUO-STERNAL. Béclard thus names the second osseous portion of the sternum, which corresponds to the second intercostal space.

DUPLICA'TION, (*duo,* 'two,' and *plicare,* 'to fold.') *Duplica'tio, Duplic''itas, Diplasias'mus, Diplo'sis.* A species of malformation or monstrosity, characterized by the parts concerned being doubled. *Double monsters.*—Meckel.

DUPLICATION OF THE FŒTUS, Evolution, spontaneous.

DU'PLICATURE, *Duplicatu'ra, Reflec'tum,* from *duplex,* 'double,' 'twofold.' The folding or reflection of a membrane upon itself; as *Duplicature* or *reflection of the pleura, peritoneum,* &c.

DUPON'DIUM. A weight of four drachms. —Galen.

DUR, Hard.

DURA MATER, *Crassa meninx, Dura meninx, Scleromc'ninx, Meninx exte'rior, Meninx sclera, M. pachei'a of* Galen, *Dura membra'na cer'ebrum am'biens, Cuticula'ris membra'na, M. dermato'des, Méninge,* (Ch.) It has been called *dura,* because of its great resistance; and *mater,* because it was believed to give rise to every membrane of the body. (F.) *Dure mère, Dure-taye* (Paré.) It is a fibrous semitransparent membrane, of a pearly-white colour, thick, and very resisting; lines the cavity of the cranium, and contains the spinal marrow; protects the brain and marrow; and, by its various expansions—the *falx cerebri, tentorium,* &c.,—supports the different parts of the cerebral mass. The largest artery of the dura mater is the *A. meningœ'a me'dia.*

DURA MATER, LATERAL PROCESSES OF THE, Tentorium — d. m. Testis, Albuginea.

DURATION OF LIFE, see Life—d. of Pregnancy, see Pregnancy.

DURE MÈRE, Dura mater.

DURE TAYE, Dura mater.

DURÉE DE LA VIE, see Longevity.

DURETÉ D'OREILLE, Baryecoia— *d. de l'Ouie,* Deafness.

DURILLON, Callosity.

DURUS, Hard.

DUSTING BAG. In pharmacy, a kind of sieve, which consists of a bag made of lawn or other like material, hung inside of a wide-mouthed bottle or tin canister, to the mouth of which it is secured. The powdered substance is put into the bag, and the mouth being closed with a cover, the apparatus is shaken, and the finer particles pass into the bottle or canister.

DUTROA, Datura stramonium.

DWARF, Nanus — d. Flag, Iris lacustris.

DWARFISH, see Nanus.

DWARFISHNESS, Nanosomus.

DYCTOIDES, Reticular.
DYERS' BROOM, Genista tinctoria—d. Weed, Genista tinctoria, Reseda luteola.
DYNAMETER, Dynamometer.
DYNAM'IC, *Dynam'icus,* (F.) *Dynamique,* same etymon. In Mechanics, *Dynam'ics* investigates the powers whereby bodies are put in motion, and the laws connected therewith. In Biology, that which relates to the vital forces, *Vital Dynamics.* The influences of agents on the organism, which are ascribable to neither mechanical nor chemical causes, are sometimes termed *dynamic.*
DYNAMIC DISEASES, see Organic.
DYNAMICS, VITAL, see Dynamic.
DYNAMICUS, Dynamic.
DYNAMIS, Faculty, Force.
DYNAMOM'ETER, *Myodynamiom'eter, Myodynamom'eter,* from δυναμις, 'force,' 'vital power,' and μετρον, 'measure.' An instrument, contrived by M. Regnier, for measuring the comparative muscular strength of man and animals. It consists of a spring, which, when pressed upon, causes a needle to move upon a portion of a circle, furnished with a scale of kilogrammes and one of myriagrammes. To measure the strength of the hands, the two branches of the spring are firmly grasped, and brought as near together as the force can carry them. This effort makes the needle traverse, and indicates, on the scale of kilogrammes, the strength of the experimenter's hands. A man, 25 or 30 years of age, exerts a force commonly equal to 50 kilogrammes or 100 pounds.
The strength of the loins of a man, about 30 years of age, as indicated by this instrument, is usually about 30 myriagrammes, or 265 pounds, which shows the weight he is capable of raising.
From experiments made by Peron, in his voyage, on 12 individuals of Van Diemen's Land, 17 of New Holland, 56 of the Island of Timor, 17 Frenchmen belonging to the expedition, and 14 Englishmen in the colony of New South Wales, he found their comparative strength, indicated by the dynamometer, to be as follows:

NATIVES OF	STRENGTH			
	of the arm.		of the loins.	
	Kilog.	lbs.	Myri.	lbs.
1. Van Diemen's Land.	50.6	101.2		
2. New Holland.	50.8	101.6	10.2	208.08
3. Timor.	58.7	117.4	11.6	238.64
4. France.	69.2	138.4	15.2	310.08
5. England.	71.4	142.4	15.2	332.52

DYNAMOMETER or DYNAMETER, MEDIC"INAL. An instrument, invented by Dr. Paris, for the purpose of showing the quantity of active matter contained in a given weight or measure of any officinal compound, with the dose of any preparation, which will be equivalent in strength to a given quantity of any other of the same class. The instrument is more ingenious than useful.
DYOTA, Diota.
DYS, δυς, in composition, 'difficult, faulty :' sometimes privative; mostly answering to the particles *dis, in, mis,* or *un,* in English. Hence :
DYSÆ'MIA, from δυς, 'with difficulty,' and αιμα, 'blood.' A morbid condition of the blood.
DYSÆSTHE'SIA, *Dysæsthe'sis,* from δυς, 'with difficulty,' and αισθανομαι, 'I feel.' Obscure, diminished, or even abolished sensation.
DYSÆSTHESIA AUDITORIA, Cophosis—d. Gustatoria, Ageustia—d. Interna, Amnesia—d. Olfactoria, Anosmia.
DYSÆSTHE'SIA VISUA'LIS, *Parov'sis.* Sense of sight vitiated or lost.
DYSÆSTHESIS, Dysæsthesia.
DYSANAGO'GOS, from δυς, 'with difficulty,' and αναγω, 'I bring up.' That which is expectorated with difficulty. An epithet given, by the Greek writers, to the sputa, when expectorated with difficulty, on account of their viscidity.
DYSANARRHOPHE'SIS,*Dysanarrhoph'ia;* from δυς, 'with difficulty,' and αναρροφησις, 'absorption.' Diminished absorption from morbid causes.
DYS'APHE, *Dysaph'ia,* from δυς, and αφη, 'feeling.' Morbid feeling.
DYSAPULO'TUS, *Dysapu'lus, Dysepulo'ticus, Dysulo'tus,* from δυς, and απουλουν, 'to heal.' Healing with difficulty.
DYSARTHRITIS, Gout, irregular.
DYSCATABROSIS, Dysphagia.
DYSCATAPOSIS, Dysphagia.
DYSCATAPO'TIA, from δυς, and καταπινω, 'I drink.' Difficulty of swallowing liquids. This term is recommended by Dr. Mead as a substitute for hydrophobia, which means dread of liquids. The dread seems to be partly caused by the difficulty of deglutition.
DYSCHE'ZIA; from δυς, and χεζειν, 'to go to stool.' Difficult and painful defecation.
DYSCHRŒ'A, from δυς, 'with difficulty,' and χροα or χροια, 'colour.' *Dischro'a.* Sickly and unhealthy colour of the skin. Used synonymously with the *maculæ* of Willan.
DYSCHROMATOPSIA, Achromatopsia.
DYSCHYMOSEN, Chymoplania.
DYSCINE'SIA, from δυς, 'with difficulty,' and κινεω, 'I move.' Difficulty or utter incapability of moving.—Galen.
DYSCOILIA, Constipation.
DYSCOPHO'SIS, from δυς, 'with difficulty,' and κοφοω, 'I am deaf.' A defect in the sense of hearing.—Hippocrates.
DYSCO'RIA, *Corometamorpho'sis,* from δυς, and κορη, 'the pupil.' Irregularity of shape of the pupil.
DYSCRA'SIA, from δυς, and κρασις, 'temperament.' *Intempe'ries, Distemperan'tia, Dys'crasy.* A bad habit of body.
DYSCRASIA SCROFULOSA, Scrofula—d. Tuberculosa, see Tubercle.
DYSCRASIACUM, Spanæmic.
DYSCRASIÆ, Dysthetica.
DYSCRASY, Dyscrasia—d. Biliosa, Cholosis, Icterus.
DYS'CRITOS, from δυς, 'with difficulty,' and κρισις, 'judgment.' That which it is difficult to judge of.—Hippocrates.
DYSDA'CRIA, *Dysdacryo'sis,* from δυς, and δακρυον, 'a tear.' A morbid condition of the tears.
DYSDACRYOSIS, Dysdacria.
DYSECCRIS'IA, from δυς, and εκκρισις, 'excretion.' Difficult or defective excretion.
DYSECŒA, Barycoia, Deafness.
DYSEL'CIA, *Dysepulo'tus,* from δυς, 'with difficulty,' and 'ελκος, 'an ulcer.' An ulcer difficult to heal.—Hippocrates, Foësius.
DYSEMESIA, Vomiturition.
DYSENTERIA, Dysentery—d. Biliosa, Colocholosis—d. Hæmatera, Dysentery—d. Hepatica, Hepatirrhœa—d. Maligna, Enterocace—d. Putrida, Enterocace—d. Scorbutica, Enterocace—d. Splenica, Melæna—d. Typhodes, Enterocace.
DYSENTER'IC, *Dysenter'icus, Dysen'terus,*

same etymon as Dysentery. Relating to dysentery.

DYSENTERIUM, Dysentery.

DYSENTERONERVIA, Colic—d. Saturnina, Colica metallica.

DYS'ENTERY, *Dysenter'ia, Dysenter'ium, Dysenter'ia hæmate'ra, Difficul'tas intestino'rum,* from δυς, and εντερον, 'an intestine;' *Dissolu'tus morbus, Diarrhœ'a carnosa, Coli'tis, Coloni'tis, Colo-recti'tis, Endocoli'tis, Esocoli'tis, Deflux'us Dysenter'icus, Febris Dysenter'ica, Flumen dysenter'icum, Fluxus dysenter'icus, F. cruen'tus cum Tenes'mo, Rheumatis'mus intestino'rum cum ul'cerè, Tor'mina Celsi, Tor'mina, Blennenter'ia, Morbus dissolu'tus, Sedes cruen'tæ, Lues dysenter'ica, Bloody Flux; Flux,* (F.) *Flux dysentérique, Flux de Sang.* Inflammation of the mucous membrane of the large intestine; the chief symptoms of which are:—fever, more or less inflammatory, with frequent mucous or bloody evacuations; violent tormina and tenesmus. When the evacuations do not contain blood, it has been called *Dysenter'ia alba* or *simple Dysentery.* The seat of the disease is, generally, in the colon and rectum. It occurs, particularly, during the summer and autumnal months, and in hot climates more than in cold: frequently, also, in camps and prisons, in consequence of impure air, and imperfect nourishment: and is often epidemic. Sporadic cases of dysentery are, generally, easily managed; but when the disease occurs epidemically, it often exhibits great malignancy. Generally, it yields to mild laxatives, as castor oil, combined with diaphoretic narcotics, such as the *pulvis ipecacuanhæ compositus,* and counter-irritants to the abdomen; but, at times, the inflammation runs on so speedily to ulceration, that, unless a new action be rapidly excited, death will be the consequence. In such cases, mercury must be rapidly introduced into the system, and narcotics may be combined with it. The whole management in acute dysentery must, of course, be strictly antiphlogistic.

DYSENTERY, BILIOUS, Colocholosis.

DYSEPULOTICUS, Dysapulotus.

DYSEPULOTOS, Dyselcia.

DYSGALACTIA, Dysgalia.

DYSGA'LIA, *Dysgalac'tia,* from δυς, and γαλα, 'milk.' An unhealthy condition or depravation of the milk.

DYSGENNE'SIA, from δυς, and γεννησις, 'generation.' Lesion of the generative organs or functions.

DYSGEU'SIA, *Disgeus'tia,* from δυς, and γευσις, 'taste.' A morbid condition of the sense of taste.

DYSHÆMORRHŒ'A, from δυς, 'αιμα, 'blood,' and ρεω, 'to flow.' Difficulty in the flow of blood, —according to some, of the hemorrhoidal flux. Also, symptoms occasioned by its diminution or suppression.—Sagar.

DYSHÆ'MIA, from δυς, and 'αιμα, 'blood.' A morbid condition of the blood.

DYSHAPH'IA, *Dysaph'ia,* from δυς, and 'αφη, 'touch.' A morbid condition of the sense of touch.

DYSHI'DRIA, *Dysi'dria,* from δυς, and 'ιδρως, 'sweat.' A morbid state of the perspiration.

DYSIA'TOS, δυσιατος, from δυς, 'with difficulty,' and ιαομαι, 'to heal;' *Cura'tu diffic"ilis.* Difficult of cure.—Hippocrates.

DYSLALIA, Balbuties, Bradylogia.

DYSLOCHI'A, *Col'ica lochia'lis, Hysteral'gia lochia'lis,* from δυς, and λοχιος; 'relating to parturition.' Diminution or suppression of the lochial discharge.

DYSMASE'SIS, *Dysmasec'sis, Bradymasec'sis,* from δυς, 'with difficulty,' and μασησις, 'mastication.' Difficult or impeded mastication.

DYSMENIA, Dysmenorrhœa.

DYSMENORRHÉE, Dysmenorrhœa.

DYSMENORRHŒ'A, *Dysme'nia, Parame'nia diffic"ilis, Menorrha'gia stillati"tia, Men'strua difficil'ia, M. Doloro'sa, Amenorrhœ'a diffic"ilis seu partia'lis, Menses dolorif"icæ, Menorrha'gia diffic"ilis, Menstrua'tio diffic"ilis, M. dolorif'ica, Labo'rious or Difficult Menstrua'tion,* (F.) *Dysmenorrhée, Menstruation difficile, Règles difficiles, Strangurie menstruelle.* Catamenia passed with great local pain, especially in the loins:— with sometimes a membranous discharge. Dysmenorrhœa is very difficult of removal, and prevents conception. In the married female, if she should be able to pass one period without pain, and subsequently become pregnant, the morbid action may be broken in upon by gestation, and a perfect cure be obtained. Change of air, soon after marriage, will sometimes give occasion to this desirable result. The affection generally depends upon erethism of the interior of the uterus, called into action at each catamenial period. The violence of the pain requires the liberal use of narcotics.

DYSMNE'SIA; from δυς, 'badly,' and μνησις, 'memory.' Defective memory.

DYSMORPHE, Deformation.

DYSMORPHIA, Deformation.

DYSMORPHOSIS, Deformation.

DYSNÉPHRONERVIE, Nephralgia.

DYSODES, Fetid.

DYSO'DIA, *Dysod'mia, Dysos'mia, Fœtor,* 'fœtor,' from δυς, 'badly,' and οζω, 'I smell.' (F.) *Puanteur.* Sauvages has given this generic name to all diseases, characterized by fetid emanations, from whatever part proceeding;—from the mouth, nasal fossæ, bronchia, stomach, axillæ, groins, &c. Also, a stench or stink, *Psoa.*

DYSODMIA, Dysodia.

DYSODONTI'ASIS, *Dentit"io diffic"ilis,* from δυς, 'with difficulty,' and οδοντιασις, 'dentition.' Difficult dentition.

DYSONEI'ROS, from δυς, 'with difficulty,' and ονειρος, 'a dream.' Insomnia, with restlessness.

DYSO'PIA, properly *Dysop'sia, Dysora'sis,* signifying 'shame,' from δυς, 'with difficulty,' and οπτομαι, 'I see.' Difficulty of seeing: obscurity of vision.

DYSOPIA DISSITORUM, Myopia.

DYSOPIA LATERA'LIS, *Parop'sis latera'lis, Skue-sight, Sight askew.* Vision only accurate when the object is placed obliquely. This state is generally caused by some opacity of the cornea.

DYSOPIA LUMINIS, Nyctalopia—d. Proximorum, Presbytia—d. Tenebrarum, Hemeralopia.

DYSOPSIA, Dysopia.

DYSORASIS, Dysopia.

DYSOREX'IA, *Inappeten'tia, Appeti'tus deflc"iens,* from δυς, 'with difficulty,' and ορεξις, 'appetite.' Diminution of appetite.

DYSOS'MIA, from δυς, 'with difficulty,' and οσμη, 'smell.' Diminution of smell.

DYSOSPHRE'SIA, *Dysosphre'sis, Dysosphra'sia, Dysphre'sis,* from δυς, and οσφρησις, 'the sense of smell.' A morbid state of the sense of smell.

DYSOSTO'SIS; from δυς, and οστεον, 'a bone.' A faulty conformation or morbid condition of bone.

DYSPATHIA, see Serious.

DYSPEPSIA, from δυς, 'with difficulty,' and πεπτω, 'I concoct.' *Limo'sis Dyspep'sia, Anorex'ia, Apep'sia, Bradypep'sia, Gastroatax'ia, Diges'tio deprava'ta, D. diffic"ilis, D. læsa, Gastro-ato'nia, Concoc'tio tarda, Stom'achi resolu'tio, Cru'ditas, Passio stomach'ica, Indigestion, Difficulty of Digestion.* A state of the stomach, in which its functions are disturbed, without the presence of other diseases, or when, if other diseases be present, they are of but minor importance. The symptoms of dyspepsia are very various. Those affecting the stomach itself are:— loss of appetite; nausea; pain in the epigastrium or hypochondrium; heart-burn; sense of fulness, or weight in the stomach; acrid or fetid eructations; pyrosis, and sense of fluttering or sinking at the pit of the stomach. The sympathetic affections are of the most diversified character. Dyspepsia, being generally of a functional nature, is devoid of danger. When arising from disease of the stomach itself, it is, of course, more serious.

It is usually dependent on irregularity of living; either in the quantity or quality of the food taken: and the most successful treatment is, to put the patient on a diet easy of digestion; to combat the causes, where such are apparent; and, by proper remedies and regimen, to strengthen the system in every practicable manner. A great error exists in regarding it as always a disease of debility. It is often connected with an inflammatory or subinflammatory condition of the mucous lining of the stomach, and of course a very different plan of treatment is required in the two cases. Dyspepsia is often attended with too great a secretion of the gastric acids; but, on other occasions, they would appear to be too small in quantity, so as to constitute *alkaline indigestion* or *neutral indigestion*.

DYSPEPSIA CHLOROSIS, Chlorosis — d. Hypochondriasis, Hypochondriasis — d. Pyrosis, Pyrosis.

DYSPEPSIODYNIA, Cardialgia.
DYSPEPSODYNIA, Cardialgia.
DYSPEP'TIC, *Dyspep'ticus, Dyspep'tus, Apep'tic, Apep'ticus;* same etymon. Having relation to dyspepsia, as '*dyspeptic* bread.' One who suffers from dyspepsia.
DYSPEPTICUS, Dyspeptic.
DYSPEPTODYNIA, Cardialgia.
DYSPEPTUS, Dyspeptic.
DYSPERMA'SIA, *Dyspermatis'mus*, from δυς, 'with difficulty,' and σπερμα, 'sperm.' Difficulty —sometimes incapacity—of voiding the sperm.
DYSPERMATISMUS, Bradyspermatismus.
DYSPHA'GIA, *Dyscatabro'sis, Dyscatap'osis, Deglutit"io diffic"ilis, D. læ'sa, D. impedi'ta,* from δυς, 'with difficulty,' and φαγω, 'I eat.' Difficulty of deglutition. Dysphagia is almost always symptomatic, either of inflammation or of other disease of the organs of deglutition, or of incomplete obstruction of the œsophagus, by some obstacle within it, or by a neighbouring tumour. At times, it is produced by spasm or paralysis of the œsophagus. The prognosis and treatment vary according to the cause.
DYSPHAGIA ATONICA, Pharyngoplegia.
DYSPHA'GIA CONSTRIC'TA, *D. Pharyngea, D. Œsophagea, D. Callo'sa, Strictu'ra Pharyn'gis seu Œsoph'agi vera, S. Œ. Callo'sa, Stenocho'ria Œsoph'agi, Œsophagiarc'tia, Læmosteno'sis.* Stricture of the pharynx and œsophagus is an affection which may be the result of pharyngitis or œsophagitis; but more frequently of malignant disease in the parietes of the tube. The only remedy is the bougie.
DYSPHA'GIA INFLAMMATORIA, Œsophagitis — d. Pharyngea, D. Constricta — d. Œsophagea, D. Constricta — d. Spasmodica, Œsophagismus — d. Callosa, D. Constricta — d. Paralytica, Œsophagoplegia, Pharyngoplegia — d. Nervosa, Œsophagismus — d. Torpida, Pharyngoplegia — d. Globosa, Angone — d. Hysterica, Angone — d. Inflammatoria, Cynanche tonsillaris — d. Linguosa, Paraglossa — d. Ranula, Ranula — d. Uvulosa, Staphylœdema — d. Scirrhosa, Læmoscirrhus — d. Spastica, Œsophagismus.

DYSPHO'NIA, from δυς, and φωνη, 'the voice.' Difficulty of producing and articulating sounds: voice imperfect or depraved. *Apho'nia*, (of some.)

DYSPHONIA IMMODULATA NASALIS, Rhinophonia — d. Immodulata palatina, Asaphia.

DYSPHOR'IA, *Inquietu'do, Ansta'sia*. Dissatisfaction; restlessness; suffering; indisposition; from δυς, and φερω, 'I bear.'

DYSPHORIA ANXIETAS, Anxiety — d. Nervosa, Fidgets — d. Simplex, Fidgets.

DYSPHOTIA, Myopia.
DYSPHRESIS, Dysosphresia.
DYSPIO'NIA, from δυς, and πιων, 'fat.' A morbid condition of the adipous substance.
DYSPLASMATIC, Cacoplastic.
DYSPLASTICUM, Spanæmic.
DYSPNŒ'A, from δυς, and πνεω, 'I breathe.' *Pseudo-asthma, Amphipneu'ma, Respira'tio diffic"ilis seu brevis et rara, Brachypnœ'a, Retentio ad'rea, Anhela'tion, Short breath, Difficulty of breathing,* (F.) *Courte Haleine.* Dyspnœa may be idiopathic or symptomatic. The latter accompanies almost all thoracic diseases. Urgent dyspnœa has been called *amphipneu'ma, αμφιπνευμα.* —Hippocrates.

DYSPNŒA CONVULSIVA, Asthma — d. Hydrothoracica, Hydrothorax — d. Physothoracica, Pneumothorax — d. Pinguedinosa, Pursiness — d. Pneumatica, Pneumothorax — d. Pyothoracica, Empyema.

DYSSIA'LIA, from δυς, and σιαλος, 'saliva.' A morbid condition of the saliva.

DYSSYN'ODUS, *Dyssynu'sia*, from δυς, and συνοδος, 'coition.' *Co'itus diffic"ilis.* Difficulty in coition.

DYSSYNUSIA, Dyssynodus.
DYSTHAN'ATOS, from δυς, and θανατος, 'death.' That which causes a slow and painful death. One who experiences this kind of death. —Hippocrates, Galen.

DYSTHELA'SIA, from δυς, and θηλαζω, 'I give suck.' Inaptitude for suckling.

DYSTHERAPEU'TOS, *Difficiliter cura'bilis;* from δυς, and θεραπεια, 'medical treatment.' That which is difficult of cure.

DYSTHE'SIA, from δυς, 'badly,' and τιθημι, 'I am situate.' *Dys'thesis, Cachex'ia.* Morbid habit. Bad humour. Impatience in disease. — Erotian.

DYSTHET'ICA, *Cachex'iæ, Cachexies;* same etymon. A morbid condition of the blood or blood-vessels; alone or connected with a morbid state of other fluids, producing a diseased habit. The fourth order in the class *Hæmatica* of Good, including *Plethora, Hæmorrhagia,* &c.

DYSTHYM'IA, from δυς, and θυμος, 'mind.' *Depression, Despondency.* A bad sign in acute diseases. Also, Melancholy.

DYSTOC'IA, *Mogostoc'ia, Bradytoc'ia, Reten'tio fœtûs,* from δυς, and τοκος, 'accouchement.' *A laborious accouchement, Labo'rious labour, Parodyn'ia, morbid labour, difficult labour, Partus diffic"ilis.* See Laborious.

DYSTOCIA ABORTIVA, Abortion—d. Dyscyesis, Pregnancy, morbid—d. Dyscyesis extra-uterina, see Pregnancy, preternatural.

DYSTŒCHI'ASIS, *Hispid'itas*, from δυς, 'bad,' and στοιχος, 'order.' Irregular position of the eye-lashes.—Forestus.

DYSTON'IA, from δυς, and τονος, 'tone.' Morbid condition of the tone of a tissue or organ.

DYSTROPH'IA, from δυς, 'with difficulty,' and τροφη, 'nourishment.' Imperfect or defective nutrition.

DYSULOTUS, Dysapulotus.

DYSURE'SIA, *Dysure'sis;* from δυς, and ουρησις, 'passing the urine.' Defective secretion and evacuation of the urine.

DYSU'RIA, *Uri'na diffic''ilis excre'tio*, from δυς, 'with difficulty,' and ουρον, 'urine.' *Stran'gury, (of some.)* Difficulty of passing the urine. In this affection the urine is voided with pain, and a sensation of heat in some part of the urethra. Dysuria is the first degree of retention of urine. It differs from strangury, in which the urine can only be passed in drops and with great straining.

DYSURIA CALCULOSA, Calculi, vesical — d. Irritata, Calculi, vesical — d. Mucosa, Cystirrhœa.

E.

EAGLE-STONE, Ætites.

EAR, *Auris, Ous, ους, Ac'oë*, Saxon, eaɲe, (F.) *Oreille.* The organ of audition. It is composed of a series of more or less irregular cavities, in which the sonorous rays are successively received and reflected, until they agitate the nerves which are destined to convey the impression to the brain. The ear is contained partly in the substance of the temporal bones; and a part projects externally, behind the joint of the lower jaw. It may be divided into three portions;—the *outer* or *external ear*, formed by the auricle and meatus auditorius; the *middle ear*, comprising the cavity of the tympanum and its dependencies; and the *internal ear*, comprehending the three semicircular canals, the cochlea and the vestibule; which, together, constitute the *osseous* labyrinth. Within the cavity of this labyrinth are contained membranes having nearly the shape of the vestibule and semicircular canals, but not extending into the cochlea. These membranes form the *membranous labyrinth*. Between the osseous and the membranous labyrinth is situate the liquor of Cotunnius, and within the membranous labyrinth is a fluid, termed, by De Blainville, *vitrine auditive*, from its supposed analogy to the vitreous humour of the eye. The form of the membranous vestibule is not an exact imitation of the osseous cavity, being composed of two distinct sacs, which open into each other,—the one termed the *Sac'culus vestib'uli;* the other *Sac'culus.* Each sac contains in its interior a small mass of white calcareous matter resembling powdered chalk, which seems to be suspended in the fluid of the sacs by means of a number of nervous filaments proceeding from the auditory nerve. These are the *otoconies* and *otolithes* of Breschet.

The auditory nerve is distributed to the cavities of the internal ear.

EAR-DOCTOR, Aurist — e. Flap, Proptoma auricularum.

EAR-PICK, *Otog'lyphis, Otog'lyphum, Coch'lear auricula'rē, Auriscal'pium*, (F.) *Cure-oreille.* A species of small scoop, used for extracting hardened cerumen from the meatus auditorius externus; or to remove foreign bodies from the ear. If carelessly used, it is apt to excite inflammation of the tube.

EAR-SURGEON, Aurist—e. Surgery, Otiatria.

EAR-TRUMPET, *Tubus acus'ticus, Acus'ticum Cornu*, (F.) *Cornet acoustique.* An instrument for collecting sound and increasing its intensity, used by those who are hard of hearing. It is, commonly, a kind of cone, formed of silver, tin, or elastic gum, the base of which is turned towards the person who is speaking, and the apex placed in the entrance of the meatus auditorius externus.

EARWAX, Cerumen.

EARWIG, Forficula auricularia.

EARTH CLUB, Orobanche Americana — e. Fuller's, Cimolia purpurescens — e. Gall, Veratrum viride—e. Heavy, Baryta—e. Japan, Catechu—e. Lemnian, Terra Lemnia—e. Nut, Pignut, Bunium balbocastanum—e. Ponderous, Baryta—e. Samian, Sami terra—e. Sealed, Terra sigillata —e Talc, Magnesia.

EATABLE, Esculent.

EAU, Water — *e. d'Aix-la-Chapelle*, see Aix-la-Chapelle.

EAU D'ALIBOUR. This compound is made of *sulphate of zinc*, and *sulphate of copper*, each ʒj; *camphor*, ten grains; *saffron*, four grains; *water*, four fluidounces. Employed in chronic inflammation of the eyelids, and as a vulnerary.

EAU DE L'AMNIOS, Liquor amnii — *e. d'Amandes amères*, Aqua amygdalarum concentrata.

EAU ANTIPUTRIDE DE BEAUFORT. Mineral lemonade prepared with sulphuric acid.

EAU D'ARMAGNAC, Tinctura cinnamomi composita—*e. de Balaruc*, Balaruc waters—*e. de Baréges*, Baréges water — *e. de Binelli*, Aqua Binellii — *e. Blanche*, Liquor plumbi subacetatis dilutus — *e. de Bonferme*, Tinctura cinnamomi composita—*e. de Bonnes*, Bonnes, mineral waters of—*e. de Boule*, see Ferrum tartarizatum—*e. de Bourbonne-les-Bains*, Bourbonne-les-Bains, mineral waters of—*e. de Brocchieri*, Aqua Brocchierii — *e. des Carmes*, see Melissa — *e. de Chaux*, Liquor calcis—*e. de Chaux composée*, Liquor calcis compositus.

EAU DE COLOGNE, Cologne water. A celebrated perfume, so called from the place where it is made. The following is one formula: *Oil of bergamot*, ʒiij; *Oil of lemon*, ʒij; *Oil of Lavender*, ʒiiss; *Oil of neroli*, ʒiiss; *Oil of origanum*, ʒij; *Oil of rosemary*, ʒj; *Essence of vanilla*, ʒij; *Musk*, ten grains; *Rectified spirit*, Oxiij; *Rosewater*, Oij; *Orange-flower water*, Oj. Macerate for fourteen days, and filter.

EAU DE CUIVRE AMMONIACALE, Liquor cupri ammoniati — *e. Distillée*, Water, distilled — *e. de Fontaine*, Water, spring — *e. des Fontaines de la Marégueric*, Rouen, mineral waters of—*e. contre la Gangrène*, Liquor hydrargyri nitrici—*e. de Goudron*, see Pinus sylvestris—*e. de Goulard*, Liquor plumbi subacetatis dilutus.

EAU HÉMASTATIQUE DE TISSERAND. A hemastatic water reputed to possess the same properties as the Aqua Brocchierii. It may be prepared by digesting *dragon's blood*, and *turpentine of the Vosges* in *water*.

EAU D'HUSSON, Vinum colchici — *e. des*

Hydropiques, Serum of serous membranes — *e. Hydrosulfurée simple*, Hydrosulphuretted water.
EAU DE JAVELLE, Bleaching liquid, Aqua alkali'na oxymuriat'ica, Labarraque's Solution, (Common salt, ℔ij; black oxide of manganese, ℔j; water, ℔ij. Put into a retort, and add, gradually, oil of vitriol, ℔ij. Pass the vapour through a solution of subcarbonate of potassa ℥iij in water ℥xxix, applying heat towards the last. S. g. 1.087.) It is stimulant, detergent, and antiseptic, —applied externally.
EAU DE LAC, Water, lake—*e. de Luce*, Spiritus ammoniæ succinatus—*e. Magnésienne*, Magnesia, fluid—*e. de Marais*, Water, marsh—*e. Médicinale d'Husson*, see Colchicum autumnale—*e. de Mer*, Water, sea — *e. Mercurielle*, Liquor hydrargyri nitrici—*e. Minérale*, Water, mineral—*e. de Monterossi*, Aqua Binellii—*e. de Naples*, Naples water, factitious — *e. de Neige*, Water, snow —*e. de Pluie*, Water, rain—*e. de Potasse*, Liquor potassæ—*e. de Puit*, Water, well—*e. de Rabel*, Elixir acidum Halleri—*e. Régale*, Nitro-muriatic acid—*e. de Source*, Water, well—*e. Styptique de Brocchieri*, Aqua Brocchierii—*e. Sucrée*, Hydrosaccharum—*e. Vegéto-minérale*, Liquor Plumbi subacetatis dilutus—*e. de Vichy*, Vichy water— *e. de Vie*, Brandy—*e. de Vie Allemande*, Tinctura jalapii composita — *e. de Vie camphrée*, Spiritus camphoræ.
EAUX, LES, Liquor amnii — *e. Hépatiques*, Waters, mineral, sulfureous—*e. Minérales artificielles*, Waters, mineral, artificial — *e. Minérales factices*, Waters, mineral, artificial—*e. Minérales ferrugineuses*, Waters, mineral, gaseous, &c.—*e. Minérales gaseuses ou acidules*, Waters, mineral, gaseous, &c.—*e. Minérales salines*, Waters, mineral, saline — *e. Minerales sulfureuses*, Waters, mineral, sulfureous—*e. Sulfurées*, Waters, mineral, sulfureous.
EBEAUPIN, MINERAL WATERS OF. An acidulous chalybeate, in the department of *Loire Inférieure*, near Nantes.
ÉBLOUISSEMENT, Dazzling.
EBRIECA'SUM. A term employed by Paracelsus to denote a disturbance of the reason, similar to what occurs in drunkenness.
EBRIETAS, Temulentia.
EBRIOSITAS, Temulentia.
EBULLITIO, Ebullition, Strophulus—*e. Stomachi*, Ardor ventriculi, Pyrosis.
EBULLIT"ION, *Ebullit"io, Æstuat"io, Anas'esis, Causis*, from *ebullire*, 'to bubble up.' *Boiling;* (F.) *Bouillonnement*. The motion of a liquid, by which it gives off bubbles of vapour, by heat or fermentation. The boiling point of liquids varies according to the pressure to which they are subjected. For the point of ebullition of different substances, see Heat.
Ebullition is used in France, in a vague manner, for every kind of transient eruption of the skin, occurring without fever or with a slight febrile attack.
EBULUS, Sambucus ebulus.
EBUR, Ivory.
EBURNIFICA'TION, *Eburnifica'tio*, from *ebur*, 'ivory,' and *fio*, 'to be made.' An incrustation of the articular surfaces of bones with phosphate of lime, which gives them the whiteness and hardness of ivory.
EC, (before a vowel, Ex,) εκ, εξ, 'out of, from, of.' Hence, Ecchymoma, Eclectic, &c.
ÉCAILLE, Scale.
ÉCAILLES D'HUITRES, Ostreæ testes.
ÉCAILLEUX, Squamous.
ECBALIA ELATERIUM, Momordica elaterium.
ECBESOMENON, Eventus.

ECBLOMA, see Abortion.
ECBOLE, Abortion.
ECBOLIC, Abortive.
ECBOLICUS, Abortive.
ECBOLIUM ELATERIUM, Momordica elaterium.
ECBOLIUS, Abortive.
ECBRAS'MATA, from εκβραζω, 'I boil up.' *Ecchym'ata*. Hippocrates uses the word for certain burning eruptions.
ECCATHARTICUS, Cathartic.
ECCEPHALO'SIS, *Excerebra'tio, Cephalotom'ia*, from εκ, 'out,' and κεφαλη, 'head.' The removal of the brain of the child to facilitate delivery.
ECCHELYSIS, Expectoration.
ECCHORESIS, Defecation.
ECCHYLOMA, Succus expressus.
ECCHYMATA, Ecbrasmata.
ECCHYMO'MA, *Ecchymo'sis, Pelidno'ma, Pelio'ma, Hyphæ'ma, Hypoæ'ma, Hypoæ'mia*, from εκ, 'out of,' and χυμος, 'juice,' 'humour;' *Effu'sio, Exsucca'tio, Suffu'sio san'guinis*. A livid, black, or yellow spot, *Livor sanguin'eus*, produced by blood effused into the areolar tissue from a contusion. Spontaneous effusions, occurring as the result of disease or after death, are called *suggillationes*.
ECCHYMOMA ARTERIOSUM, see Aneurism — *e.* Capitis recens natorum, Cephalæmatoma — *e.* Hyponychon, Hyponychon — *e.* Lymphaticum, Phlegmatia dolens—*e.* Melasma, Melasma.
ECCHYMOSIS, Ecchymoma.
ECCHYSIS, Effusion.
ECCLISIS, Luxation.
EC'COPE, *Ec'tomē, Ectom'ia*, from εκ, and κοπτειν, 'to cut.' The act of cutting out: also, a perpendicular division of the cranium by a cutting instrument. See *Entaille*.
ECCOP'EUS. Same etymon. A knife or instrument for cutting. An ancient instrument— the *raspatory*—used in trepanning.
ECCOPROSLÆSTHE'SIS, from εκ, κοπρος, 'excrement,' and αισθησις, 'sensation.' The sensation or desire to evacuate the bowels.
ECCOPROSIS, Defecation.
ECCOPROT'IC, *Eccoprot'icus, Ectoprot'ic*, from εξ, 'out of,' and κοπρος, 'excrement.' Mild purgatives or laxatives, whose operation is confined to simply clearing out the intestinal canal.
ECCORTHAT'ICUS, from εκ, 'out of,' and κορθαω, 'I collect.' An ancient epithet for remedies to which was attributed the property of evacuating collections of humours.
ECCRINOL'OGY, *Eccrinolog"ia, Eccrisiolog"ia*, from εκκρινω, (εκ, and κρινω,) 'I separate,' and λογος, 'a discourse.' A treatise on the secretions.
ECCRISIOLOGIA, Eccrinology.
ECCRISION'OSI, *Eccresionu'si*, from εκκρισις, 'excretion,' and νοσος, 'disease.' Diseases of excretion.
ECCRISIOS'CHESIS, from εκκρισις, 'excretion,' and σχεσις, 'retention.' Arrest or retention of excretions; or of a critical evacuation.
EC'CRISIS, Excretion.
ECCRIT'ICA. Diseases of the excernent function. The 6th class in Good's Nosology. Also, medicines that act on the excernent system.
ECCYESIS, Pregnancy, extra-uterine—*e.* Abdominalis, Pregnancy, abdominal — *e.* Ovaria, Pregnancy, ovarial—*e.* Tubalis, Pregnancy, tubal.
ECCYLIO'SIS, from εκ, 'out of,' and κυλιειν, 'to turn round.' *Morbus evolutio'nis*. A disease of evolution or development.
ECDEMIOMA'NIA, *Ecdemion'osus*, from εκδη-

sus, 'I travel about,' and μανια, 'mania.' A morbid desire to be travelling about.

ECDEMIONOSUS, Ecdemiomania.

EC'DORA, from εκ, and δερω, 'I flay.' *Anad'ora, Excoria'tio.* Excoriation in general, but more especially of the urethra.

EC'DYSIS, from εκδυω, (εκ, and δυω,) 'I put off.' Moulting of the skin of animals. Desquamation.

ÉCHALOTTE, *Eschalotte, Al'lium Ascalon'icum. Cepa Ascalon'ica. The shallot'.* A species of allium, employed in culinary preparations.

ÉCHANCRURE, (F.), *Emargina'tio, Emarginatu'ra, Incisu'ra.* A French word, employed by anatomists to designate depressions and notches of various shapes, observed on the surface or edges of bones.

ÉCHANCRURE ETHMOÏDALE is on the nasal bone, which unites with the ethmoid. See Ethmoid.

ÉCHANCRURE NASALE, *Nasal Notch*, belongs to the os frontis, and is articulated with the bones of the nose.

ÉCHANCRURE PAROTIDIENNE is a triangular space, comprised between the parotidean edge of the inferior maxillary bone and the mastoid process, so called because it lodges the parotid gland.

ÉCHANCRURE SCAPULAIRE, Notch, scapular—*é. Sciatique grande,* see Sciatic Notch—*é. Sciatique petite,* see Sciatic Notch.

ÉCHARDE, Splinter.

ÉCHARPE GRANDE, *et É. MOYEN,* see Sling—*é. de J. L. Petit,* see Sling—*é. Petite,* see Sling.

ÉCHAUBOULURES (F.), *Sudam'ina, Hidro'a.* A word whose meaning is not fixed. It is applied to any eruption on the surface of the body, accompanied with pricking and other uneasy sensations.

ÉCHAUFFANTS, Calefacients.

ÉCHAUFFEMENS, Chafing.

ÉCHAUFFEMENT (F.) *Calefac'tio, Excalefac'tio,* from (F.) *échauffer, (calefacere,)* 'to make warm.' Augmentation of heat in the animal economy; the symptoms of which are a more than ordinary sensation of heat, disposition to perspiration, great thirst, general indisposition, flushed countenance, &c. It goes off by the use of antiphlogistics and abstinence. In the vulgar language it is often used synonymously with *constipation,* and sometimes for simple gonorrhœa, and for chafing.

ECHECOL'LON, from εχω, 'I have,' and κολλα, 'glue.' *Echecollum.* Any topical glutinous remedy.—Gorræus, Galen.

ÉCHELLES DU LIMAÇON, Scalæ of the cochlea.

ECHENEIS, Remora Hildani.

ECHETROSIS, Bryonia alba.

ECHID'NA OCELLA'TA, *Brown ten-inch-long viper.* A most formidable viper in the forests of Peru, the bite of which is so rapidly fatal, that it kills a strong man in two or three minutes. Tschudi.

ECHINA'CEA PURPU'REA, *Purple Coneflower, Black Sampson,* of the *Composite* Family; indigenous in Ohio and westward; its dull purple flowers appearing in July. The root is aromatic, and used popularly as a carminative.

ÉCHINE, Vertebral column.

ECHINOCOCCUS HOMINIS, see Worms—*e. Humanus,* Hydatid.

ECHINODERMI, Porcupine men.

ECHINOGLOSSUM, Ophioglossum vulgatum.

ECHINOPHTHAL'MIA, from εχινος, 'a hedgehog,' and οφθαλμια, 'inflammation of the eye.' Ophthalmia of the eyelids, in which the cilia project like the quills of the hedgehog.

ECHI'NOPS, from εχινος, 'hedgehog,' and ωψ, 'appearance.' *Crocodil'ium, Acanthal'zuca, Scabio'sa carduifo'lia, Sphæroceph'ala ela'tior, Echi'nopus, Echinops Sphæroceph'alus. The globe thistle.* The root and seeds are reputed to be moderately diuretic.

ECHINOPUS, Echinops.

ECHINUS SCANDENS, Allamanda.

ECHOS, Sound, Tinnitus aurium.

ECHOSCOPE, Auscultation.

ECHOSCOPIUM, Stethoscope.

ECHTHYSTEROCYESIS, Pregnancy, extra-uterine.

ECLACTIS'MA, *Eclamp'sis, Eclamp'sia, Epilamp'sis, Effulgescen'tia,* from εκλακτιζω, 'I kick.' Epilepsy is often accompanied with flashings of light; and hence Hippocrates has used the last two words for epilepsy. They have all been applied to the convulsions of children.

ÉCLAIRE, Chelidonium majus—*é. Petite,* Ranunculus ficaria.

ECLAMP'SIA, Convulsion: also, the convulsions of children, *Eclamp'sia infan'tum, Epilep'sia acu'ta infan'tum, E. febri'lis infan'tum, E. pueri'lis,* (F.) *Convulsions des Enfans, Eclampsie.*

ECLAMP'SIA GRAVIDA'RUM ET PARTURIEN'TIUM; *Puerperal Convulsions,* (F.) *Convulsions des femmes enceintes et en couche.* Convulsions of pregnant and parturient women.

ECLAMPSIA INFANTUM, see Eclampsia—*e. Nutans,* Convulsion, Salaam—*e. Typhodes,* Raphania.

ECLAMPSIE DES ENFANS, Eclampsia infantum.

ECLEC'TIC, (PHYSICIANS,) *Eclec'tici Med'ici,* from εκλεγω, 'I choose.' A sect of physicians, who professed to choose, from other sects, all the opinions which appeared to them best founded. Agathinus of Sparta, master of Archigenes of Apamæa, in Syria, was its reputed founder; and Archigenes and Aretæus were its greatest ornaments. The doctrine was called *Eclec'tism, Eclectis'mus, Medici'na eclec'tica, Eclectic med'icine.* Every judicious physician must be an eclectic.

ECLECTISM, see Eclectic.

ECLEC'TOS, *Eclig'ma, Eligma, Eliz'is, Lombiti'cum, Linctus, Linctua'rium,* from εκλιχω, 'I lick.' (F.) *Looch.* A medicine, of a thick, syrupy consistence, chiefly used to allay cough, and consisting of pectoral remedies. It was formerly sucked from the end of a liquorice stick, made into a kind of pencil; hence its name *Linctus,* from *lingere,* 'to lick.' Although the linctus is usually exhibited in thoracic affections, it may have tonic virtues combined with it.

ECLEGMA ALBUM, Looch album—*e. Gummoso-oleosum,* Looch album.

ECLEIPISIS, Exfoliation.

ECLEPISIS, Desquamation.

ECLEPISITREPANON, Exfoliative trepan.

ECLIGMA, Eclectos.

ECLIMIA, Boulimia.

ECLIPSIS, Syncope.

ÉCLISSE, Splint.

ECLYSES, Adynamiæ.

EC'LYSIS, *Exsolu'tio;* from εκλυω, 'I loosen.' Resolution, prostration of strength; faintness.

ECLYSIS PNEUMO-CARDIACA, Asphyxia.

ECMYZESIS, Exsuctio.

ECNŒA, Dementia.

ÉCOLE, School.

ECON'OMY, *Œcono'mia,* from οικια, 'a house, a family,' and νεμω, 'I rule.' By the term ani-

mal œconomy is understood,—the aggregate of the laws which govern the organism. The word *œconomy* is, also, used for the aggregate of parts which constitute man or animals.

ÉCORCE, Cortex—*e. Cariocostine*, Canella alba—*é. de Saint Lucie*, Cinchonæ Caribææ cortex—*é. de Winter*, see Wintera aromatica—*é. Fausse de Winter*, Canella alba.

ÉCORCHURES, Chafing, Excoriation.

ÉCOULEMENT, Discharge, Gonorrhœa—*é. Blanc*, Leucorrhœa—*é. de Sang par l'Intestin*, Hæmatochezia.

ÉCOUVILLON, see *Écouvillonnement*.

ÉCOUVILLONNEMENT (F.), from *écouvillon*, 'a kind of mop, the sponge of a gun.' A term used by the French therapeutists for the act of cleansing or applying remedies to a part by means of a mop or brush fixed to the end of a piece of whalebone. Such mop or brush is termed *Ecouvillon*.

ECPHLOGOSIS, Inflammation.

ECPHLYSIS, Vesicula—*e. Herpes*, Herpes—*e. Herpes circinatus*, Herpes circinatus—*e. Herpes exedens*, Herpes exedens—*e. Herpes miliaris*, Herpes phlyctænodes—*e. Herpes zoster*, Herpes zoster—*e. Pompholyx*, Pompholyx—*e. Rhypia*, Rupia.

ECPHRACTIC, Deobstruent.

ECPHRAX'IS, from εκφρασσω, 'I remove obstruction.' The action of ecphractic or deobstruent remedies.

ECPHRONIA, Insanity—*e. Melancholia*, Melancholy.

ECPHYAS, Appendix vermiformis cæci.

ECPHYMA, Excrescence, Tumour—*e. Callus*, Callosity—*e. Caruncula*, Caruncle—*e. Clavus*, Corn—*e. Œdematicum*, Œdema, Phlegmatia dolens—*e. Physconia*, Physconia—*e. Trichoma*, Plica—*e. Verruca*, Verruca.

ECPHYMATA, Rubeola.

ECPHYSE'SIS, *Effla'tio*, *Effla'tus*, from εκφυσαω, 'I breathe through.' *Exsuffla'tio*. A quick and forced expulsion of air from the lungs.

ECPHYSIS, Apophysis—*e. Ventriculi*, Duodenum.

ECPIES'MA, from εκπιζω, 'I compress.' *Effractu'ra*, *Impac'tion*, *Deces'sio*. A fracture of the cranium, with depression of the fragments and compression of the brain.

ECPIES'MOS, *Expres'sio*, *Ex'itus*, *Ecpies'mon*, same etymon. Celsus uses these words to signify the forcing of the eye from the orbitar cavity, with apparent but not real augmentation of the organ. See Exophthalmia.

ECPLERO'MA, from εκ, and πλερωω, 'I fill.' *A cushion, a pad*. Hippocrates means, by this term, a small pad or ball of leather, or other substance intended to fill the hollow of the armpit; used probably in reducing luxations of the shoulder.

ECPLEXIA, Stupor.

ECPLEXIS, Stupor.

ECPNEUMATOSIS, Expiration.

ECPNEUSIS, Expiration.

ECPNOE, Expiration.

ECPTO'MA, *Ecpto'sis*, *Exciden'tia*; from εκπιπτω, 'I fall out.' This word has been used in various senses. 1. Synonymously with luxation. 2. For the separation of gangrenous parts. 3. For the expulsion of the secundines. 4. For the prolapsus of the womb: and 5. For intestinal or omental hernia, &c.

ECPTOSIS, Luxation.

ECPYCTICA, Incrassantia.

ECPYEMA, Abscess, Suppuration, Empyema.

ECPYESIS, Abscess, Empyema, Pustule—e.

Impetigo, Impetigo—*e. Porrigo*, Porrigo—*e. Porrigo crustacea*, Porrigo larvalis—*e. Porrigo favosa*, Porrigo favosa—*e. Porrigo furfuracea*, Porrigo furfurans—*e. Porrigo galeata*, Porrigo scutalata—*e. Porrigo lupinosa*, Porrigo lupinosa—*e. Scabies*, Psora.

ECPYETICUS, Suppurative.

ECPYISCONTUS, Suppurative.

ÉCREVISSE, Crab.

ECREX'IS, *Ruptu'ra*, from εκρηγνυμι, 'to break.' Rupture, laceration.

ECRHYTH'MUS, εκ, and ρυθμος, 'rhythm.' A term applied to the pulse, particularly when irregular.—Galen.

ECROE, Discharge.

ÉCROUELLES, Scrofula—*é. Mésentériques*, Tabes mesenterica.

EC'RYSIS, from εκρεω, 'I run from.' A discharge.

ECSARCO'MA, from εκ, and σαρξ, 'flesh.' A fleshy excrescence of various kinds. See Fungosity and Sarcoma.

ECSESMA, Eczema.

EC'STASIS, from εξισταμαι, 'I am beside myself.' An *ec'stasy* or trance, *Carus ec'stasis*, *Cat'ochus*, *Ex'stasis*, *Catalep'sia spu'ria*, *Hyperplexie*, (F.) *Extase*. A state in which certain ideas so completely absorb the mind, that the external sensations are suspended, the voluntary movements arrested, and even the vital action retarded. In catalepsy, there is, in addition, complete suspension of the intellectual faculties. This last condition is in general described as *trance*. See, also, luxation.

ECSTROPHE, Exstrophia.

ECTASIA, Aneurism—*e. Venarum*, Varix.

EC'TASIS, Extension, Expansion.

EC'TASIS I'RIDIS, is the extension or expansion of the iris, which occasions diminution of the pupil.

ECTEXIS, Colliquation.

ECTHÆTOBREPHOTROPHEUM, Brephotropheum.

ECTHLIM'MA, *Exulcera'tio*, from εκθλιβω, 'I express,' 'I bruise.' Attrition. Chafings, or excoriations, produced by external violence.—Hippocrates.

ECTHLIPSIS, Expression.

EC'THYMA or ECTHY'MA, from εκθυω, 'I break out.' *Ecpye'sis*, *Phlysis ecthyma*, *Phlyzacia a'gria*, *Sca'bies Vera*, *Furun'culi aton'ici*, (F.) *Dartre crustacée*, *D. fongueuse*. A cutaneous eruption, characterized by large round pustules, always distinct and seated upon an indurated and highly inflamed base. In the course of a day or two the pustules generally break, and olive-brown incrustations are formed which adhere firmly to the skin. These separate in about a fortnight. The disease requires the antiphlogistic treatment. Under the *Ecthymata*, Vogel has designated certain hard, unequal tumours, which appear transitorily on the skin. See Efflorescence, Exanthem, and Pustule.

ECTHYSTEROCYESIS, Pregnancy, extrauterine.

ECTILLOTICUS, Depilatory.

ECTILMOS, Evulsion.

ECTOME, Castration, Ecoope, *Entaille*, Excision.

ECTOMIA, Castration, Ecoope.

ECTOMIUS, Castratus.

ECTONION, Helleborus niger.

ECTOPARASITES, Epizoa.

ECTOP'IA, *Ectop'isis*, *Ectopismus*, *Entocœ'lē*, from εκτοπος, 'out of place.' Morbid displacement of parts. See Luxation.

ECTOPIA ANI, Proctocele.

ECTOPIA CORDIS, *Cardianas'trophē*. Displacement, dislocation, or unnatural position of the heart.

ECTOPIA HERNIOSA, Hernia.

ECTOPOCYS'TICUS, from εκτοπος, 'out of place,' and κυστις, 'bladder.' A disease dependent upon displacement of the bladder.

ECTOPROTIC, Eccoprotic.

ECTOZO'A, *Extozo'a*, *Extozoa'ria*, (F.) *Extozoaires*. Parasitic animals that infest the exterior of the body,—as lice. A term which, like *Helmin'thia errat'ica* and *Pseudohelmin'thes*, is applied to worms or larvae of insects that have been introduced into the intestinal canal by accident. Animalcules, most frequently swallowed, are the hairworm, leech, grub of the fly, caddy insect—*Phalæ'na penguina'lis*; the larve of the bee, the spider, the *triton palus'tris*, *lacer'ta aquat'ica*, &c. In animals, bots are produced by swallowing the ova of the *œstrus* or gadfly. See Helminthia erratica.

ECTRIM'MA, from εκτριβω, 'I rub off.' Ulceration of the skin; and particularly that which arises from the pressure of the bed on different parts of the body, after a protracted confinement.—Hippocrates.

ECTRODACTYL'IA; from εκτρωσις, 'abortion,' and δακτυλος, 'a finger.' A malformation, in which one or more fingers or toes are wanting.

ECTROMA, Abortion.

ECTRO'MELES; from εκτρωσις, 'abortion,' and μελος, 'a limb.' A genus of monsters, in which the limbs are nearly or altogether deficient, as in the ordinary cetacea.—J. G. St. Hilaire.

EC'TROPE, *Diverticu'ulum*, from εκτρεπω, 'I turn off,' 'divert.' Any duct by which peccant or morbific matter was supposed to be drawn off.—Hippocrates.

ECTROP'ION, same etymon. *Ectrop'ium*, *Ever'sio pal'pebræ*, *Blepharopto'sis Ectro'pium*, *Blepharoto'sis*, *Pal'pebra infe'rior extror'sum flexa*, *Divarica'tio seu Reflex'io seu Reclina'tio palpebra'rum*, (F.) *Éraillement des Paupières*, *Renversement des Paupières*. Eversion of the eyelids, so that they do not completely cover the globe of the eye. It happens more commonly to the lower than to the upper eyelid. It may be owing to the retraction of the skin, after the cure of an ulcer, wound, or burn of the eyelid; or it may depend on tumefaction or relaxation of the conjunctiva. In the majority of cases, removal of a portion of the conjunctiva will effect a cure; but there are many which defy the efforts of art. The ancients called Ectropion of the upper eyelid *lagophthalmia*.

ECTROSIS, Abortion.

ECTROSMOS, Abortion.

ECTROT'IC, from εκτρωμα, (εκ, and τιτρωσκω, 'I wound,') 'abortion.' *Ectrot'icus*, *Abortive*. An epithet applied to methods for preventing the development or causing the abortion of any disease — as of chancres by the use of caustic; small-pox pustules by the use of mercurial ointment, &c.

ECTYLOTICUS, Catheretic.

ECTYMPANOSIS, Tympanites.

ÉCUMEUX, Frothy.

ÉCUSSONS. 'Escutcheons or shields.' Plasters spread upon the skin; or small bags—*sachets*—of the shape of escutcheons, filled with odorous powders, which are applied on the skin. See Sachet.

EC'ZEMA, from εκζεω, 'I boil out,' 'I effervesce.' *Ecses'ma*, *Ecses'ma*, *Pus'tula ardens*, *Cytis'ma Eczema*, *Humid Tetter*, *Running Scall*, (F.) *Dartre squammeuse humide*, *D. vive*, *Gale épidémique*. Heat eruption. An eruption of small vesicles on various parts of the skin, usually set close or crowded together; with little or no inflammation around their bases, and unattended by fever.

EC'ZEMA MERCURIA'LE, *Ec'zema rubrum*, *Erythe'ma mercuria'le*, *E. ichoro'sum*, *Hydrargyr'ia*, *Hydrargyro'sis*, *Hydrargyri'asis*, *Morbus mercuria'lis*, *Mercu'rial lepra*. A variety of eczema, arising from the irritation of mercury. The treatment is chiefly palliative, consisting in ablution with mucilaginous infusions or decoctions; mild dressings, where the cuticle has exfoliated; avoiding all irritation; keeping the bowels open; with the use of sulphuric acid and cinchona. The *Ec'zema Impetigino'des*, *Gall*, or *Grocer's Itch*, is produced by the irritation of sugar.

ECZEMA OF THE FACE, at an advanced stage, and occurring in young children, has been described under the names *Crusta lactea* and *Porrigo larvalis*.

ECZEMA OF THE HAIRY SCALP is often confounded with other affections, under the names Porrigo and Tinea, which are pustular, not vesicular, in their form. It occurs during dentition, and even afterwards, and the discharge is so profuse, that the head appears as if dipped in some glutinous liquid. By and by, the secretion dries into crusts and mats the hair into little separate tufts. The scalp gives evidence of inflammatory excitement, and the lymphatic ganglions of the neck are apt to become inflamed and suppurate.

A variety of humid scalled head, in which the humour from the excoriated surface runs down upon the hairs, and encloses them in little silvery pellicles or sheaths, has received the name *Asbestos Scall*.

ECZEMA RUBRUM, Eczema mercuriale.

ECZEMATO'SES, (G.) Eczematosen, same etymon. A family of diseases, in the classification of Fuchs, including morbid conditions of the cutaneous secretions—as of the perspiration, sebaceous and colouring matters, &c., and hence many chronic cutaneous affections. His subdivisions are, *ephidroses*, *smegmorrhœa*, *acarpæ*, *polycarpæ* and *monocarpæ*.

ECZESIS, Effervescens.

ECZESMA, Eczema, Lichen tropicus.

EDEMATOUS, Œdematous.

EDENTATUS, Edentulus.

EDENTULI, Nefrendes.

EDEN'TULOUS, *Eden'tulus*, *Edenta'tus*, from *e*, and *dens*, *dentis*, 'a tooth.' *Ano'dus*, *Carens den'tibus*, *Nodes*, *Nodus*, (F.) *Édenté*. One without teeth. This defect can only be remedied by artificial means. See Nefrendes.

EDERA, Hedera helix.

EDIBLE, Esculent.

EDUCATIO INFANTUM, Pædia.

EDULCORA'TION, *Glycan'sis*, *Edulcora'tio*, from *edulcorare*, (*dulcis*, 'sweet,') 'to sweeten,' 'to render mild.' An operation, the object of which is to deprive a substance of its acrid and disagreeable taste, or at least to disguise it. Also, the addition of a saccharine substance to a medicine, whose taste it is desirable to modify agreeably.

ÉDULE, *Comestible*.

EDULIS, *Comestible*.

EF'FERENT, *Ef'ferens*, *Centrif'ugal*, *Exod'ic*, from *effero*, (*e*, and *ferro*,) 'I carry,' 'transport.' Conveying outwards, as from the centre to the periphery.

Vasa efferen'tia are those lymphatics, which issue from the lymphatic glands to convey their lymph to the thoracic duct; so called to distinguish them from those which pass to those glands, and which have been termed *vasa afferen'tia.* Also, nerves are so called that convey the nervous influence from the nervous centres to the circumference. See Afferent.

At the upper extremity of the mediastinum testis, the ducts of the rete testis terminate in from 9 to 30 small ducts, called *vasa efferentia,* which form the *Coni vasculo'si.*

EFFERVES'CENCE, *Effervescen'tia, Zesis, Ec'zesis,* from *effervescere,* (e, and *ferrescere,*) 'to grow hot.' That agitation, which is produced by the escape of gas through a liquid, independently of the heat of the mixture; such, for instance, as results from the mixture of acetic acid and carbonate of potassa.

In *Pathology* it has a similar signification. It expresses, in the language of the humourists, a sort of ebullition in the fluids of the living body, produced either by elevation of temperature or by the reaction on each other of the principles contained in the fluids in circulation.

EFFETUS, Impoverished.

EFFICA'CIOUS, *Ef'ficax,* from *efficere,* (e, and *facere,*) 'to accomplish.' That which produces a great effect,—as 'an *efficacious remedy.*'

Medici'na efficax, La Médecine efficace, is a term sometimes applied to surgery.

EFFILA, Ephelides.

EFFLATIO, Ecphysesis.

EFFLATUS, Ecphysesis.

EFFLORATIO, Exanthem.

EFFLORES'CENCE, *Efflora'tio, Efflorescen'tia,* from *efflorescere,* (e, and *florescere,*) 'to blow as a flower.' *Stribili'go, Ecthy'ma.* The conversion of a solid substance into a pulverulent state by exposure to the air. In salts this is generally owing to the loss of a part of their water of crystallization.

In *Pathology,* efflorescence has the same meaning as exanthema; and, in the nosology of Sauvages, the name is given to that order of diseases. Sometimes, it is confined to the *cutaneous blush,* the *exanthe'sis* of Good.

EFFLORESCENCE ÉRYSIPÉLATEUSE, Roseolæ.

EFFLORESCENTIA, Exanthem.

EFFLORESCENTIÆ, *Élévures.*

EFFLUVIUM, Emanation — e. Latrinarium, *Mitte*—e. Palustre, Miasm, Marsh.

EFFLUXION, Abortion.

EFFORT, (e, and *fortis,* 'strong.') *Nisus, Cona'tus,* Peira. A muscular contraction of greater or less strength, the object of which is, either to resist an external force, or to accomplish a function, which has become naturally laborious:— such are, the act of pushing away, or of drawing a body toward us, and the more or less painful efforts used by the mother to cause the expulsion of the fœtus. In France, the word *effort* is often used synonymously with hernia; and signifies, likewise, the painful twitches of muscles, occasioned by over-exertion, or by the rupture of some of their fleshy fibres. Sauvages calls *Efforts aux reins, Lumba'go à nisu,* the pain in the loins occasioned by bearing too heavy a burden.

EFFORT, Hernia—*e. des Reins,* see Effort.

EFFOSSIO, Exhumation.

EFFRACTURA, Ecpiesma.

EFFRACTU'RA CRANII, *Enthla'sis Cra'nii,* Fracture of the Cranium, with depression.—Paré.

EFFRENITATIO, Hypercatharsis.

EFFUSIO, Effusion—e. Seminis Ejaculation.

EFFU'SION, *Effu'sio, Ec'chysis,* from *effundere,* (e, and *fundere,*) 'to pour out.' (F.) *Épanchement,* (*Infiltration* is the term generally employed for effusion into the areolar membrane.) The pouring out of blood or of any other fluid into the areolar membrane, or into the cavities of the body. The *effusion of serum* or of *coagulable lymph,* for instance, is a common result of inflammation of serous membranes.

ÉGARÉ, Wild.

ÉGAREMENT D'ESPRIT, Delirium, Insanity.

EGER, MINERAL WATERS OF THE. In the valley of the Eger, at the western extremity of Bohemia, there are several acidulous springs. One of the most frequented of these is Franzensbad.

EGE'RIA. In ancient mythology, a nymph to whom pregnant females offered sacrifices *ut conceptus alvus facilius egeretur.* By some, supposed to have been identical with Lucina.

EGESTA, see Excretion.

EGESTAS, Want.

EGESTIO, Defecation, Dejection, Excretion.

EGG-BRANDY, see Ovum.

EGG PLANT, Solanum melongena—e. White of, Albumen ovi.

EGLANTIER DE CHIEN, Rosa canina—*e. Sauvage,* Rosa canina.

EGOBRONCHOPHONY, see Egophony.

ÉGOPHONE, Egophony.

EGOPH'ONIC, *Ægopho'nicus,* (F.) *Égophonique.* Same etymon as the next. Having the character of, or relating to, egophony.

ÉGOPHONIQUE, Egophonic.

EGOPH'ONY, *Ægopho'nia,* from αιξ, 'a goat,' and φωνη, 'voice.' *Caprilo'quium, Tragopho'nia, Goat's Voice, Bleating Voice,* (F.) *Voix chévrotante, V. égophonique, V. de Polichinelle, V. sénile, Pectoriloquie chévrotante.* Laënnec has designated by this name, the kind of resonance of the voice heard through the stethoscope, when we examine the chest of one labouring under moderate effusion into one of the pleuræ. The voice, which strikes the ear through the cylinder, is more sharp and harsh than usual, and tremulous and broken, like that of the goat. The patient himself is called *Égophone.* Bouillaud affirms that the 'bronchial and bleating voice,' (*égobronchophonie*) is the principal symptom of pleuropneumonia. Egophony exists, however, in cases of hepatization where there is no pleural disease.

EGREGOR'SIS, *Vigil'ia, Vigtli'æ, Vigilan'tia, Vigila'tio, Vigil'ium,* from εγρεγορω, 'I watch.' Watchfulness. A morbid want of sleep.—Galen.

EGRESSUS VENTRICULI, Pylorus.

EIDOS, ειδος, 'form, resemblance.' The ει is often changed into ω, at the termination of a word. Thus, *Hæmatoï'des* or *Hæmato'des.*

EILAMIDES, Meninges.

EILE'MA, from ειλεος, *Ileus,* (ειλεω, 'I roll,') 'a convolution.' Vogel has given this name to a fixed pain, occupying some portion of the intestinal canal, which the patient compares to the sensation that would be produced by a nail driven into the part.

EILEON, Ileon.

EILEUS, Ileus.

EILOID, (*Tumour,*) *Eiloi'des,* from ειλεω, 'I roll,' and ειδος, 'resemblance.' A morbid growth of the cutis, coiled or folded.

EILSEN, MINERAL WATERS OF. Eilsen is about six German miles from Hanover, at the foot of the Harrelberg. It has eleven springs, of which seven are sulphureous and four chalybeate.

EISANTHE'MA, *Exanthe'ma inter'num, Entanthe'ma,* from εις, 'within,' and ανθημα, 'efflorescence.' An eruption on a mucous membrane; —aphthæ, for example.

EISBOLE, Attack, Injection.
EISPNOE, Inspiration.
EJACULATIO, Ejaculation — e. Seminis Impedita, Bradyspermatismus.
EJACULA'TION, *Ejacula'tio*, from *e*, and *jaculare*,—itself from *jacere*, 'to throw.' *Gonobol'ia*, *Gonobolis'mus*, *Ejaculatio* seu *Profu'sio* seu *Effu'sio Sem'inis*, *Expatra'tio*, *Patra'tio*, *Spermob'olè*. The emission of sperm. The act, by which that fluid is darted out through the urethra.
EJAC'ULATOR. Same etymon. That which effects the emission of sperm. See Transversus perinæi.
EJACULATOR SEMINIS, Accelerator urinæ.
EJAC'ULATORY, *Ejacula'torius*, *Ejac'ulans*: same etymon. Concerned in the ejaculation of sperm.
EJACULATORY DUCTS or CANALS, (F.) *Conduits ou Canaux éjaculateurs*, are formed by the union of the vasa deferentia with the ducts of the vesiculæ seminales. They open at the lateral and anterior parts of the verumontanum, and convey into the urethra the sperm which is discharged from the vesiculæ, as well as that which comes directly from the testicle by the vas deferens. Between them there is often a depression, sometimes of a large size, which is termed *Utric'ulus*, *Vesi'ca* seu *vesic'ula prostat'ica* seu *Sinus pocula'ris*, which has been regarded as the analogue to the uterus in the female, and thence called *U'terus masculi'nus*.
EJECTIO, Excretion—e. Fæcum, Defecation.
EJEC'TION, *Ejec'tio*, from *ejicere*, (e, and *jacere*,) 'to throw out or eject.' The excretion of the fæces, urine, sputa, &c.
EL NISPERO, Sapota.
ELABORA'TION, *Elabora'tio*, from *e*, and *laborare*, 'to work.' This word is used, by physiologists, to signify the various changes which substances susceptible of assimilation undergo, through the action of living organs, before they are capable of serving for nutrition. The food is said to be *elaborated* in the stomach during the formation of chyme; the chyme is *elaborated* in the small intestine before it is chyle, &c.
ELÆA, Olea Europæa.
ELÆAGNUS, Myrica gale—e. Cordo, Myrica gale.
ELÆOCARPUS COPALIFERA, Copal.
ELÆOM'ELI, from ελαιον, 'oil,' and μελι, 'honey.' Dioscorides means, by this, an oil thicker than honey, and of a sweet taste, which flows from the trunk of a tree in Syria. It is acrid and purgative; and sometimes occasions serious symptoms, according to that author.— Gorræus.
ELÆOM'ETER, from ελαιον, 'oil,' and μετρον, 'measure.' A very delicate glass hydrometer, for testing the purity of olive or almond oil, by determining their densities. The 0 or zero of the scale is the point at which the instrument floats in the oil of poppy seeds. In pure olive oil, it floats at 50°, and the space between these points is divided into 50 equal parts, and numbered accordingly. It floats at 38° or 38½° in pure oil of almonds.
ELÆON, Oil.
ELÆOPH'ANES, from ελαιον, 'oil,' and φαινομαι, 'I appear.' That which has the appearance of oil; as *Uri'na elæoph'anes*.
ELÆO-SAC'CHARUM, from ελαιον, 'oil,' and σακχαρ, 'sugar.' *O'leo-Sac'charum, Bal'samo-Sac'charum.* A medicine, composed of essential oil and sugar. It was made by pouring upon an ounce of sugar, reduced to an impalpable powder, ʒss or ʒj of an essential oil; the mixture being triturated until the two substances were perfectly united.—Rolfink.
ELAIN, see Pinguedo.
ELAIS GUINEENSIS, see Cocos butyracea— e. Occidentalis, see Cocos butyracea.
ÉLAN, Cervus alces.
ÉLANCEMENT, see Lancinating.
ELAPHOBOSCUM, Pastinaca sativa.
ELAPHRIUM ELEMIFERUM, see Amyris elemifera—e. Tomentosum, Fagara octandra.
ELAPSUS, Luxation.
ELAS'MA, from ελαυνω, 'I drive up.' A clyster pipe.—Linden.
ELASTES, Elasticity.
ELASTIC"ITY, *Elastic"itas*, *El'ater*, *Elas'tes*, *El'ates*, *Vis elas'tica*, *Tone*, *Tonic"ity*, (F.) *Contractilité de Tissu*, *Contractilité par défaut d'extension*, from ελαυνω, 'I impel.' The property by which certain bodies return to their proper size and shape, where these have been modified by pressure or otherwise. It is possessed by the dead as well as by the living solid.
ELATE, Pinus picea—e. Theleia, Pinus rubra.
ELATER, Elasticity.
ELATERINE, see Momordica elaterium.
ELATERIUM, Extractum elaterii, Momordica elaterium—e. Cordifolium, Momordica elaterium.
ELATES, Elasticity.
ELATIN, see Momordica elaterium.
ELATINE, Antirhinum elatine—e. Cymbalaria, Antirhinum linaria—e. Hastata, Antirhinum elatine.
ELBOW, Sax, elboga, from *ell*, and *bow*; the bend of the ulna. *Cu'bitus, Ancon, Pechys, Ulna, Umbo*, (F.) *Coude*. This word, abstractedly, means the angle formed by the union of two straight bodies. It is particularly applied to the articulation of the arm with the forearm, and especially to the projection formed by the olecranon process at the posterior part of the joint.
ELBOW, MINERS', see Miners' Elbow.
ELCOMA, Ulcer.
ELCO'SIS, *Helco'sis, Elco'ma, Helco'ma*, from 'ελκος, 'an ulcer.' Ulceration in general. An ulcer. A deep ulceration of the cornea, in consequence of a blow or of violent inflammation.— Galen, Paré.
Sauvages applies the term to a state of the body, in which there are numerous ulcerations of an obstinate character, complicated with caries, putrescency, low fever, &c.
ELCUSTER, Embryulcus.
ELDER, Sambucus — e. Common, Sambucus Canadensis—e. Dwarf, Aralia hispida, Sambucus ebulus—e. Prickly, Aralia spinosa.
ELECAMPANE, Inula helenium.
ELECTRICITAS, Electricity — e. Animalis, Galvanism—e. Galvanica, Galvanism—e. Metallica, Galvanism.
ELECTRIC"ITY, *Electric"itas*, from ηλεκτρον, 'amber,'—the substance in which it was first noticed. Electricity is used medicinally as an excitant. It has been occasionally employed with success in paralysis, rheumatism, accidental deafness, amaurosis, amenorrhœa, &c., but it is uncertain, and not much used; and the cases are not always clear in which it could be of service. It may be communicated by means of the *electric bath — Bain électrique*, as it has been called; which consists in placing the patient upon an isolated stool, and connecting him with the prime conductor, of which he thus becomes a part. The fluid may be communicated by points, sparks, or by shocks, according to the required intensity.
ELECTRICITY, CHEMICAL, Galvanism — e. Contact, Galvanism — e. Magnetic, Electro-Magnetism—e. Voltaic, Galvanism.

ELEC'TRIFY, from *electric*, and *flo*, 'I make.' (F.) *Électriser*. To produce the electrical condition in a body, or to render it susceptible of producing electrical phenomena. It is often used to signify the act of communicating the electric fluid to man.

ÉLECTRISER, to electrify.

ELECTRO'DES, from ηλεκτρον, 'amber,' and ειδος, 'resemblance.' An epithet for evacuations, which shine like amber.—Hippocrates.—Foësius.

ELEC'TRO-MAG'NETISM, *Magnet'ic electric'ity*. An electro-magnetic apparatus is occasionally used in cases of paralysis. A convenient form consists of a battery of six curved permanent magnets, and an intensity armature, around whose cylinders 1500 yards of fine insulated copper wire are coiled. The ends of the wire communicate respectively, with a pair of directors, each of which holds a piece of sponge, dipped in vinegar or a solution of common salt. When the armature is rotated, and a portion of the body is interposed between the directors, a succession of shocks is received.

ELECTROPUNC'TURE, *Electropunctura'tion, Electrostix'is, Gal'vanopuncture*. The operation of inserting two or more wires, and then connecting them to the poles of the galvanic apparatus.

ELECTROSTIXIS, Electropuncture.

ELECTRUM, Succinum.

ELECTUAIRE DENTIFRICE, Dentifrice.

ELECTUA'RIUM, *Electa'rium;* an *Electuary*, from *eligere*, 'to make choice.' (F.) *Électuaire*. A pharmaceutical composition of a soft consistence, somewhat thicker than honey, and formed of powders, pulps, extracts, syrup, honey, &c. In the London and American Pharmacopœias, electuaries are called Confections.

ELECTUARIUM DE ALOE, Opiatum mesentericum—e. Aperiens, Confectio sennæ—e. Aromaticum, Confectio aromatica—e. Cassiæ, Confectio cassiæ—e. Cassiæ fistulæ, Confectio cassiæ — e. Cassiæ sennæ, Confectio sennæ—e. Cassiæ tamarindatum seu lenitivum, Confectio cassiæ — e. Catholicum communæ, Confectio sennæ—e. Cinchonæ, Opiatum febrifugum—e. de Croco emendatum, Confectio hyacinthi—e. Diaprunum, Confectio sennæ—e. Eccoproticum, Confectio sennæ — e. de Kinâ kinâ, Opiatum febrifugum — e. Laxativum, Confectio cassiæ — e. Lenitivum, Confectio sennæ — e. Opiatum, Confectio opii — e. Scammonii, Confectio Scammoniæ — e. è Scammonio, Confectio scammoniæ — e. Sennæ, Confectio sennæ — e. Sennæ compositum, Confectio sennæ—e. Sennæ cum pulpis, Confectio sennæ—e. Thebaicum, Confectio opii.

ELÉENCÉPHALE, from ελαιον, 'oil,' and εγκεφαλον, 'encephalon.' A fatty matter found by Couerbe in the encephalic neurine.

ELELISPHACOS, Salvia.

EL'EMENT, *Elemen'tum*, from ancient *eleo* for *oleo*, 'to grow,' (?) *Princip'ium, P. Primiti'vum, Stochei'on*. A simple, ultimate constituent or principle in the human body, which forms the basis of a fibre or tissue. Also, a constituent of a compound organ. The *inorganic elements* are simple principles. An *organic element, proximate principle or compound of organization*, results from the union of certain inorganic elements. Oxygen, hydrogen, carbon, and azote, are inorganic elements; fibrin, albumen, osmasome, &c., organic elements.

ELEMENTS, ORGANIC, Principles, immediate—e. Sarcous, see Sarcous.

ELEMENTARY CELL, see Cell.

ELEMENTUM ACIDIFICUM, Oxygen.

ELEMI, Amyris elemifera.

ELENIUM, Inula helenium.

ELEOSELINUM, Apium petroselinum.

ELEPHANTI'ASIS, *Elephanti'a, Elephantias'mus, El'ephas, Las'ari morbus* vel *malum, Phœnic'eus morbus, Phymato'sis Elephanti'asis*, from ελεφας, 'an elephant.' Various affections have been described under this name, by adding an epithet. It is ordinarily and generically applied to a condition, in which the skin is thick, livid, rugous, tuberculate, and insensible to feeling.

ELEPHANTIASIS OF THE ANTILLES, *Barba'does Leg, Glandular disease of Barbadoes,* (F.) *Jambes de Barbade*, is the Elephantiasis of many writers, *Bucne'mia*. It is characterized by the leg being enormously tumid and misshapen; skin thickened, livid, and rugose, often scaly; scrotum, arms, or other parts sometimes participates in the affection. The *Bucne'mia Trop'ica, Cochin leg*, is an affection of this kind.

ELEPHANTI'ASIS ARAB'ICA, *Maladie glandulaire, Ladrerie, Tyri'asis, El'ephas, Elephanti'asis, E. In'dica, Elephanti'a Ar'abum, Lepra Arabum*, (of some.) In this the tubercles are chiefly on the face and joints. There is loss of hair, except on the scalp; voice, hoarse and nasal; and the disease is said to be contagious and hereditary. It most frequently attacks the feet; and gives the lower extremity a fancied resemblance to the leg of an elephant, whence its name. The seat of the disease seems to be in the lymphatic vessels and glands, and in the subcutaneous areolar tissue: the inflammatory condition of which is accompanied with general morbid symptoms. Medicine has little or no effect on this loathsome complaint. See Lepra.

ELEPHANTIASIS OF CAYENNE, *Mal rouge de Cayenne*, seems to be a variety of Lepra, characterized by red and yellow spots, occupying the forehead, ears, hands, loins, &c., afterwards extending and becoming scaly, with deformity of the parts where they are seated, particularly of the face; and ultimately producing cracks, ulcers, caries, and sometimes death.

ELEPHANTIASIS OF THE GREEKS, *E. Grœco'rum*, is probably the same disease as Lepra.

ELEPHANTIASIS OF INDIA is characterized by red, livid, or yellowish spots, slightly prominent, to which succeed indolent tumours, formed in the areolar texture. At a more advanced period the phalanges swell, and become ulcerated; the bones of the nose carious, the lips thickened, and emaciation gradually carries off the patient. It likewise belongs to lepra.

ELEPHANTIASIS ITALICA, Pellagra.

ELEPHANTIASIS OF JAVA is likewise a variety of lepra, characterized by large white tumours on the toes and fingers, resembling scrofulous tumefactions. These tumours ulcerate, and the ulcerations spread from the extremities towards the trunk, destroying even the bones. Amputation can alone arrest its progress. The disease is often accompanied by alopecia, and by an eruption of red spots.

ELEPHANTI'NUM EMPLAS'TRUM, Ελεφαντινον. An ancient plaster, composed of 30 parts of *cerussa*, 45 of wax, *oil* ℔ss, *water* ℔j.— Castelli. Oribasius and Celsus both mention a plaster of this name, but they are by no means similar in composition.

ELEPHANTOMMA, Buphthalmia.

ELEPHAN'TOPUS, (F.) *Éléphantope;* from ελεφας, 'elephant,' and πους, 'foot.' One affected with elephantiasis.

ELEPHAS, Elephantiasis, Ivory.

ELETTARIA CARDAMOMUM, Amomum cardamomum.

ELEUTERIA, Croton cascarilla.

ÉLÉVATEUR, Elevator—*é. Commun de l'aile*

du nez et de la lèvre supérieure, Levator labii superioris alæque nasi—t. de l'Œil, Rectus superior oculi—t. de la Paupière supérieure, Levator palpebræ superioris.

ELEVA'TOR, from *elevare*, (*e*, and *levare*,) 'to lift up.' (F.) *Élévateur*. A muscle, whose function it is to raise the part into which it is inserted. See Levator.

ELEVATOR, *Elevato'rium, Vectis elevato'rius.* A name given to different surgical instruments employed for raising portions of bone which have been depressed, for raising and detaching the portion of bone separated by the crown of the trepan, and for removing stumps of teeth.

ELEVATOR ANI, Levator ani—e. Labii inferioris, Levator labii inferioris—e. Labii superioris proprius, Levator labii superioris proprius—e. Labiorum communis, Levator anguli oris—e. Oculi, Rectus superior oculi—e. Patientiæ, Levator scapulæ—e. Scapulæ, Levator scapulæ—e. Testiculi, Cremaster—e. Urethræ, see Transversus perinæi.

ELEVATOR, COMMON. This is a mere lever, the end of which is somewhat bent and made rough, in order that it may less readily slip away from the portion of bone which is to be raised. The instrument is used, by forming a fulcrum for it, either on the hand which holds it, or upon the fingers of the other hand; or by making a fixed point for it on the edge of the opening made with the trephine.

ELEVATOR OF LOUIS differed from the last only in the circumstance of the screw-peg being united to the bridge by a kind of pivot instead of hinge, so that greater extent of motion was permitted.

ELEVATOR OF PETIT consists of a lever mounted on a handle, and straight throughout its whole length, except at its very end, which is slightly curved, in order that it may be more conveniently put under the portion of bone intended to be elevated. The lever is pierced at various distances from its but-end with several holes, intended for the reception of a movable screw-peg, fixed on the top of a kind of bridge. This part of the instrument consists of an arch, the ends of which are long, and covered with small pads, and on its centre is the screw-peg already mentioned. By means of these holes the arm of the lever can be lengthened at pleasure.

ELEVATOR, TRIP'LOID, *Vectis triploi'des*. This was so called from its consisting of three branches, uniting above in one common trunk. The latter part was traversed by a long screw, having below a kind of hook, and above a handle for turning it. By turning the screw, the hook was drawn up, and the bone thus elevated.

The simple lever is the only one now used, owing to the want of facility and advantages in the use of the others.

ÉLÈVE EXTERNE, see House-surgeon—*t. Interne*, House-surgeon.

ÉLEVURES (F.), *Efflorescentiæ*. A generic name, including all the exanthemata, in which there is tumefaction of the tissue of the skin. See Exanthem.

ELIASTER, Ileeh.
ELICHRYSUM, Solidago virgaurea—e. Montanum, Antennaria dioica.
ELICOIDES, Capreolaris.
ELIGMA, Eclectos.
ELIQUATIO, Colliquation.

ELIXA'TIO, *Epse'sis*, from *elixus*, 'boiled,' 'sodden.' This word has been used synonymously with Decoction. The act of boiling.

ELIX'IR, *Isir, Ixir, Quelles, Alex'ir*. The etymology of this word is not clear. Lemery derives it from ἐλκω, 'I extract;' and also from ἀλείφω, 'I aid.' Others believe it to be from Arabic, *al-ecsir*, or *al-eksir*, 'chymistry.' An elixir is a medicine composed of various substances held in solution in alcohol. The name has been used, however, for preparations, which contain no spirit of wine.

ELIXIR AC"IDUM HALLERI seu DIPPEL'II, *Elixir Antipodag'ricum, E. Antinephret'icum, E. Sulphu'rico-ac"idum, Guttæ ac"idæ ton'icæ, Aqua Rabe'lii, Liquor ac"idus Halleri, Mistu'ra sulphu'rico-ac"ida, Æther sulphu'ricus ac"idus, Ac"idum sulphu'ricum alcoolisa'tum, A. vitriol'icum vino'sum, Al'cohol Sulphurica'tum, A. Sulphu'ricum*, is a mixture of concentrated sulphuric acid and alcohol;—in the *Eau de Rabel*, of one part of the former to three of the latter. It is employed as an astringent in hemorrhages, &c.

ELIXIR ALOES, Tinctura aloes composita—e. Anthelminticum Succorum, Tinctura jalapii composita.

ELIXIR, ANTI-ASTHMAT'IC, OF BOERHAAVE. This elixir is composed of *alcohol, aniseed, camphor, orris, asarabacca root, calamus aromaticus, liquorice,* and *elecampane*. It is given in asthma, in the dose of 20 or 30 drops.

ELIXIR ANTIHYPOCHONDRIACUM, Tinctura cinchonæ amara—e. Antinephreticum, E. acidum Halleri—e. Aperitivum, Tinctura aloes composita.

ELIXIR, ANTISCROF'ULOUS OF PEYRILHE; composed of weak *alcohol, subcarbonate of potassa,* and *gentian root*. It is administered in scrofula.

ELIXIR, BOERHAAVE'S, see Tinctura Aloes composita.

ELIXIR, CARMINATIVE, of Sylvius, Tinctura carminativa Sylvii—e. Daffy's, Tinctura sennæ comp.—e. Danorum, E. pectorale regis Daniæ—e. Fœtidum, Tinctura castorei composita—e. of Garus, Tinctura de croco composita—e. Guaiaci volatilis, Tinctura Guaiaci ammoniata—e. Jalapæ compositum, Tinctura jalapii composita—e. of Long Life, Tinctura aloes composita—*e. de Longue vie,* Tinctura aloes composita—*e. d'Or de M. le Général de la Motte,* Tinctura seu Alcohol sulfurico-æthereus—e. Paregoric, Edinburgh, Tinctura opii ammoniata—e. Paregoricum, Tinctura camphoræ composita—e. Pectorale dulce, E. pectorale regis Daniæ.

ELIXIR PECTORA'LE REGIS DA'NIÆ, *Elix'ir Dano'rum, E. Ringelman'ni, E. ex succo Glycyrrhi'zæ, E. pectora'lè dul'cè, E. è succo liquirit"ia*: (*Succ. glycyrrhiz.* p. 1; *Aq. Fœnicul.* p. 2. Alcohol ammoniat. p. 6. A formula in many of the Pharmacopœias of continental Europe.) With the addition of opium it constitutes the *Elixir ammoniato-opia'tum, Extractum theba'icum ammoniaca'le* of some Pharmacopœias.

ELIXIR PROPRIETATIS, Tinctura aloes composita—e. Purgans, Tinctura jalapii composita—e. Radcliffe's, see Tinctura aloes composita—e. Rhej dulce, Vinum rhej palmati—e. Ringelmanni, E. pectorale regis Daniæ—e. Roborans Whyttii, Tinctura cinchonæ amara—e. Sacrum, Tinctura rhej et aloes—e. Salutis, Tinctura sennæ comp.—e. Squire's, see Tinctura camphoræ composita—e. Stomachicum, Tinctura gentianæ composita—e. Stomachicus spirituosus, Tinctura cinchonæ amara—e. Stoughton's, see Tinctura gentianæ composita—e. ex Succo glycyrrhizæ, E. pectorale regis Daniæ—e. ex Succo liquiritiæ, E. pectorale regis Danorum—e. Sulphurico-acidum, E. acidum Halleri—e. Traumaticum, Tinctura Benzoini composita.

ELIXIR VITÆ OF MATHI'OLUS; composed of *alcohol* and 22 aromatic and stimulating substances. It was formerly employed in epilepsy.

ELIXIR OF VITRIOL, Sulphuric acid, dilute—e. Vitrioli, Sulphuricum acidum aromaticum—e. Vitrioli acido-aromaticum, Sulphuricum acidum aromaticum—e. Vitrioli dulce, Spiritus ætheris aromaticus, Sulphuricum acidum aromaticum—e. Vitrioli Edinburgensium, Sulphuricum acidum aromaticum—e. Vitrioli Mynsichti, Sulphuricum acidum aromaticum—e. of Vitriol, sweet, Spiritus ætheris aromaticus—e. Vitrioli cum tincturâ aromaticâ, Sulphuricum acidum aromaticum—e. of Vitriol, Vigani's, Spiritus ætheris aromaticus—e. Whyttii, Tinctura cinchonæ amara.

ELIXIRIUM ANTISEPTICUM DOCTORIS CHAUSSIER, Tinctura cinchonæ ætherea composita.

ELIXIS, Eclectos.

ELIXIVIATION, Lixiviation.

ELK, Cervus alces—e. Bark, Magnolia macrophylla—e. Tree, Andromeda arborea—e. Wood, Andromeda arborea, Magnolia macrophylla.

ELLEBORASTER, Helleborus fœtidus.

ELLEBORE, Dracontium fœtidum.

ELLEBORISMUS, Helleborismus.

ELLEBORUM ALBUM, Veratrum album.

ELLEBORUS ALBUS, Veratrum—e. Niger, Helleborus niger.

ELLIPTIC, Oval.

ELLYCHNIO'TOS, from ελλυχνιον, 'the wick of a lamp.' A sort of tent, used by the ancient surgeons, so called because it was shaped like a wick, or because it was made of a similar material.

ELM, COMMON, Ulmus—e. Red, Ulmus Americana—e. Rough-leaved, Ulmus Americana—e. Slippery, Ulmus Americana.

ELMINTHOCORTON, Corallina Corsicana.

ELO'DES, Helo'des, Paludal, Marshy, (F.) Marécageux. Febris elo'des seu helo'des seu paludo'sa, Helop'yra, Helopyr'etos, from 'ελος, 'a marsh,' and ειδος, 'resemblance.' Marsh fever. (F.) Fièvre intermittente paludéenne, Fièvre paludéenne. Also, a kind of fever, characterized by great moisture or sweating.

ELOME, Orpiment.

ELONGA'TION, Parathro'ma, Elonga'tio, from elongare, (e, and longus,) 'to lengthen,' 'extend.' An incomplete luxation, in which the ligaments of an articulation are stretched and the limb lengthened, without total luxation. The word has also been used for the extension required in the reduction of fractures and luxations, and for the increased length of limb, (F.) Allongement, in diseases and dislocations of the hip-joint.

ELUTRIATIO, Decantation, Elutriation.

ELUTRIA'TION, Elutria'tio; originally from eluo, (e, and luo, 'I wash,') 'I wash away, I rinse.' In pharmacy a process by which the finer particles of a powder are separated from the coarser. It consists in diffusing the powder in water, allowing the larger and heavier particles to subside, and decanting the liquor, that the finer particles may subside.

ELU'VIES, same etymon. An inordinate discharge of any fluid, and also the fluid itself. In the works of some authors it is particularly applied to the mucus which flows from the vagina in cases of leucorrhœa.

ELUXATION, Luxation.

ELYTRATRESIA, Colpatresia.

ELYTREURYNTER, Speculum vaginæ.

ELYTRITIS, Colposis, Leucorrhœa.

ELYTROBLENNORRHŒA, Leucorrhœa (vaginal).

EL'YTROCE'LE, from ελυτρον, 'a vagina or sheath,' and κηλη, 'a tumour.' Vogel has given this name to vaginal hernia, Colpoce'lè.

ELYTRODES (tunica), Vaginal coat of the testicle.

ELYTRŒDE'MA, Coleœde'ma, Colpœde'ma, from ελυτρον, 'a vagina or sheath,' and οιδημα, 'œdema.' Œdema of the vagina.

ELYTROITIS, Colposis.

EL'YTRON, from ελυω, 'I involve.' A sheath. The vagina. The membranes which envelope the spinal marrow are called elytra.

ELYTRON'CUS, Elytrophy'ma, from ελυτρον, 'a vagina or sheath,' and ογκος, 'a tumour.' A swelling of the vagina.

ELYTROPAP'PUS RHINOCERO'TIS. A South African bush, Nat. Ord. Compositæ, the whole of which is bitter and resinous. The tops of the branches, infused in wine or brandy, make excellent bitters. The tops are also given in powder to children affected with diarrhœa.

ELYTROPHYMA, Elytroncus.

ELYTROPTOSIS, Prolapsus vaginæ.

ELYTRORRHAGIA, Colporrhagia.

ELYTROR'RHAPHY, Elytrorrhaph'ia; Colpor'rhaphy, Kolpor'rhaphy; from ελυτρον, 'the vagina,' and ραφη, 'a suture.' The operation of closing the vagina by suture in cases of procidentia uteri.

EM and EN, εν, 'in, into, within.' Also 'excess;'—frequently used in this last sense by Dr. Good. A common prefix, generally answering to the prefixes im and in, in English. In composition, before β, π, φ, ψ, and μ, the ν is changed into μ; before γ, κ, ξ, and χ, into γ; before λ, into λ, and before ρ generally into ρ.

EMAC"IATE, Maces'cere, Tabes'cere, (F.) Amaigrir. To lose flesh, to become lean, to waste away.

EMACIA'TION, Emacia'tio, from emaciare, (e, and macies, 'to be lean,') 'to grow lean.' Extenua'tio, Ma'cies, Macritu'do, Macror, Marco'res, Skeleti'a, Leptysm'us, Leptyn'sis, Pingued'inis diminu'tio, (F.) Amaigrissement, Maigreur. That condition of the body, or of a part of the body, in which it grows lean. The state of one who is lean;—Leanness; Isch'notes.

ÉMAIL DES DENTS, Enamel of the teeth.

ÉMAILLOTAGE (F.), from maillot, 'swathing or swaddling clothes.' The 'wrapping up,' or 'packing up' in dry or wet sheets, which is practised in hydropathic establishments to induce sweating.

EMANA'TION, Emana'tio, Efflu'vium, from emanare, (e, and manare,) 'to issue or flow from.' The term is applied to a body which proceeds or draws its origin from other bodies; such as the light which emanates from the sun; the miasma which arise from the putrid decomposition of animal or vegetable substances, &c. See Miasm.

EMAN'SIO MEN'SIUM, from e, and manere, 'to stay.' This term has been applied to amenorrhœa or obstruction of the menses before they have been established. Some have used it for the retention which occurs even after they have been established. The former is the general acceptation.

EMARGINATIO, Échancrure, Notch.

EMARGINATURA, Échancrure, Notch.

EMASCULA'TION, Emascula'tio, from emasculare, (e, and masculus, 'a male,') 'to render impotent.' The act of removing or destroying the generative organs of a male animal.

EMASCULATUS, Castratus, Eunuch.

EMBALM'ING, from em, en, 'in,' and balsamum, 'balsam.' Balsama'tio, Smyrnis'mos, Cedeia, Pollinctu'ra, Necrocedi'a, Conditu'ra Cadav'erum, (F.) Embaument, Imbalsamation. An operation which consists in impregnating the dead body with substances capable of preventing it from becoming putrid, and thus putting it in a condition to be preserved.

EMBAM'MA, Apobam'ma, Bamma, from εμβαπτω, 'I immerse.' A medicated pickle or sauce. —Gorræus.

EMBARRAS, Emphraxis.

EMBARRAS GASTRIQUE (F.), *Gastric disorder* or *impediment*, *Collu'vies gas'trica, Sordes prima'rum via'rum, Status gas'tricus.* Disorder of the stomach, in which there is loss of appetite, with bitterness and clamminess of mouth, white and yellow tongue, feeling of oppression in the epigastrium, and sometimes pain in that region, nausea and bilious or bitter vomiting; this state being accompanied with headach, lassitude, and pain in the back and limbs.

EMBARRAS GASTRO-INTESTINAL, *Gastro-intesti'nal disorder.* Slight gastro-enteritis, according to the Broussaists, in which the symptoms of the *Embarras gastrique* and *E. intestinal* are united.

EMBARRAS INTESTINAL, *Intes'tinal disorder.* The principal characters assigned to this are: — tension of the abdomen, colic, borborygmi, discharge of flatus *per anum*, constipation or diarrhœa, &c.

EMBARRURE, Engisoma.

EMBAUMENT, Embalming.

EMBOÎTEMENT (F.). 'Encasing,' from *em*, 'in,' and *boîte*, 'a box.' *Enadelph'ia.* This term has been applied to the theory of generation which considers that the germs are encased in each other in the ovary of the female, in such sort that they are developed in succession after impregnation. It is the theory of *encasing of germs*, or of *monstrosity by inclusion*.

EMBOÎTURE, Diarthrosis.

EM'BOLE, from εμβαλλω, 'I put in place.' Reduction of a luxated bone. *Reposit"io*.

EMBOLIMOS, Intercalary.

EMBOLUM CEREBRI, Infundibulum of the brain.

EMBONPOINT, (F.) 'In good point or plight.' *Bona cor'poris habitu'do.* The state of the animal body when in full health. Excessive *embonpoint* constitutes corpulence and obesity, and may become a morbid condition.

EMBONPOINT EXCESSIF, Polysarcia adiposa.

EMBORISMA, Aneurism.

EMBROCATIO, Embrocation, Irrigation.

EMBROCA'TION, *Embroca'tio, Embreg'ma, Em'broché, Implu'vium*, from εμβρεχω, 'I sprinkle.' A fluid application to be rubbed on any part of the body. It is often used synonymously with liniment. Originally it was employed in the sense of *Fomentation*.

EMBROCATION, GUESTONIAN, see Oleum Terebinthinæ rectificatum.

EMBROCHE, Embrocation.

EMBRYEMA, Embrocation.

EM'BRYO, *Em'bryon*, from *εν*, 'in,' and *βρυω*, 'I grow.' *Oye'ma.* The fecundated germ, in the early stages of its development in utero. At a certain period of its increase, the name *fœtus* is given to it, but at what period is not determined. Generally, the *embryo state* is considered to extend to the period of quickening.

EMBRYOC'TONY, *Fœtûs trucida'tio*, from εμβρυον, 'the embryo,' and κτονος, 'destruction.' The act of destroying a fœtus in utero, when insurmountable obstacles — as certain deformities of the pelvis — oppose delivery.

EMBRYOG'RAPHY, *Embryogra'phia*, from εμβρυον, 'the embryo,' and γραφη, 'a description.' The part of anatomy which describes the embryo.

EMBRYOL'OGY, *Embryolog"ia*, from εμβρυον, 'the embryo,' and λογος, 'a description.' The doctrine of embryonic development.

EMBRYON'IC, *Embryon'icus*, (F.) *Embryonique, Embryonnaire*; same etymon as embryo. Relating or appertaining to an embryo: -- as 'embryonic life.'

EMBRYONIQUE, Embryonic.

EMBRYONNAIRE, Embryonic.

EMBRYOTHLAS'TA, *Embryothlas'tes, Embryothlas'tum*, (F.) *Embryotome*, from εμβρυον, 'the embryo,' and θλαω, 'I break.' An instrument for dividing the fœtus piecemeal, in order to effect delivery. A crotchet or other instrument, used, in certain cases of laborious parturition, to break the bones of the fœtus, for the purpose of extracting them with greater facility. — Hippocrates, Galen.

EMBRYOTOCIA, Abortion.

EMBRYOTOME, Embryothlasta.

EMBRYOT'OMY, *Embryotom'ia*, from εμβρυον, 'an embryo,' and τεμνειν, 'to cut.' A division of the fœtus into fragments, to extract it by piecemeal, when the narrowness of the pelvis or other faulty conformation opposes delivery.

EMBRYOT'ROPHY, *Embryotroph'ia*, from εμβρυον, 'the embryo,' and τροφη, 'nourishment.' Fœtal nutrition; *Cyot'rophy*.

EMBRYUL'CIA, *Embryusterul'cia*, from εμβρυον, 'embryo, fœtus,' and ελκω, 'I extract,' 'I draw.' A surgical operation, by which the fœtus is extracted by means of appropriate instruments, when faulty conformation or other circumstances prevent delivery by the natural efforts.

EMBRYUL'CUS, *Elcus'ter*, same etymon. An iron hook or crotchet, described by Fabricius ab Aquapendente, which was used to extract the fœtus in some cases of laborious labour.

EMBRYUSTERULCIA, Embryulcia.

EMENDANS, Corrigent.

ÉMERAUDE, Smaragdus.

EMESIA, Vomiturition.

EMESIS, Vomiting.

EMETATROPH'IA, from εμεω, 'I vomit,' and ατροφια, 'want of nourishment.' Atrophy induced by vomiting.

EMETIA, Emetine.

EMET'IC, *Emet'icum, Vomito'rium, Vom'itory, Vomit, Puke*, from εμεω, 'I vomit.' A substance capable of producing vomiting. (F.) *Émétique.* [This term is also restricted by the French to *tartarised antimony* — *the emetic*, as it were, par excellence.] *Vomitif.*

Tartarised antimony, emetine, ipecacuanha, and *sulphate of zinc*, are the chief emetics. They are valuable agents in disease, and may either act *primarily* on the stomach, or *secondarily* on other parts of the system, — the sympathy between the stomach and other parts of the body being very extensive, and an important object of study.

The following are the usual emetics: — Antimonii et Potassæ Tartras; Cupri Acetas; Cupri Sulphas; Emetina; Gillenia; Hydrargyri Sulphas Flavus; Ipecacuanha; Lobelia; Sanguinaria; Scilla; Sinapis, and Zinci Sulphas.

EMETIC ROOT, Euphorbia corollata — e. Tartar, Antimonium tartarizatum — e. Weed, Lobelia inflata.

EMETICOLOGIA, Emetology.

EM'ETINE, *Emeti'na, Emet'ia, Vom'itine.* A vegetable alkali, discovered by M. Pelletier in ipecacuanha, and to which it owes its emetic power. It is obtained from different ipecacuanhas, but chiefly from *psychot'ria emet'ica, callicoc'ca ipecacuan'ha*, and *vi'ola emet'ica.* It is in transparent scales, of a reddish-brown colour, almost inodorous, of a bitter, slightly acrid taste; is unchangeable in the air, soluble in water and alcohol, and insoluble in ether. Three grains of impure emetia or one grain of pure are equal to 18 of ipecacuanha. See Ipecacuanha.

ÉMÉTIQUE, Antimonium tartarizatum, Emetic.

EMETO-CATHARSIS, see Emeto-cathartic.

EM'ETO-CATHAR'TIC, *Em'eto-cathar'ticus*, from εμετος, 'vomiting,' and καθαρτικος, 'a purgative.' A remedy, which at the same time excites vomiting and purging—*Em'eto-cathar'sis*.

EMETOL'OGY, *Emetolog"ia, Emeticolog"ia*, from εμετος, 'vomiting,' and λογος, 'a discourse.' A treatise on vomiting, and on emetics.

EM'INENCE, *Eminen'tia, Protuberan'tia, Ex'oché, Exanthe'ma*. A projection at the surface of a healthy or diseased organ.

ÉMINENCE PORTE ANTÉRIEURE, Lobulus anonymus — *é. Porte postérieure*, Lobulus Spigelii—*é. Sus-pubienne*, Mons veneris.

ÉMINENCES BIGÉMINÉES, Quadrigemina corpora — *e. Latérales*, Corpora olivaria — *e. Pyramidales*, Corpora pyramidalia — *e. Vermiformes du cervelet*, Vermiformes processus.

EMINENTIA, Protuberantia — e. Annularis, Pons varolii—e. Pyramidalis, Crista vestibuli—e. Tympani, Pyramid.

EMINENTIÆ BIGEMINÆ, Quadrigemina tubercula—e. Candicantes, Mammillary Tubercles — e. Lenticulares, Corpora striata — e. Magnæ cerebri, Thalami nervorum opticorum — e. Medianæ Internæ, Corpora pyramidalia—e. Olivares, Corpora olivaria—e. Ovales Laterales, Corpora olivaria—e. Pyramidales, Corpora pyramidalia—e. Quadrigeminæ, Quadrigemina tubercula — e. Teretes, Processus teretes.

ÉMISSAIRE, Emunctory.

EMISSA'RIA SANTORI'NI. A name given to some small veins, which communicate with the sinuses of the dura mater, by apertures in the cranium. Such are the parietal, posterior condyloid, mastoid veins, &c.

EMISSIO, Emission — e. Seminis, Spermatismus.

EMIS'SION, *Emis'sio*, from *emittere*, (e, and *mittere*,) 'to send out,' 'drive out.' The act by which any matter whatever is thrown from the body. Thus, we say *Emission of urine, Emission of semen*, &c.

ÉMISSION SANGUINE, Bloodletting.

EMMEN'AGOGUES, *Emmenago'ga, Emmeniago'ga, Ame'nia*, from εμμηνα, 'the menses,' and αγω, 'I drive,' or 'expel.' *Men'agogues*. A name given to medicines believed to have the power of favouring the discharge of the menses. There is probably no substance which possesses this power directly. According to different conditions of the system, the most opposite remedies may act as emmenagogues. *Black hellebore, savin, madder, polygala senega*, and *ergot*, are reputed to be specific emmenagogues. The following list comprises the chief of them:—Cunila Pulegioïdes; Helleborus Niger; Mentha Pulegium; Rosmarinus; Rubia; Sabina; Secale Cornutum; Senega, and Tanacetum.

EMMENAGOLOG"IA, from εμμηναγωγα, and λογος, 'discourse.' A treatise of emmenagogues.

EMMENIA, Menses.

EMMENIAGOGA, Emmenagogues.

EMMENOLOG"IA. from εμμηνα, 'menses,' and λογος, 'a discourse.' A treatise on menstruation.

EMMENOLOG"ICAL, *Emmenolog"icus*: same etymon as the last. Relating or appertaining to menstruation.

EMMYXIUM ARTICULARE, Hydrarthrus.

EMOLLIENTIA, Emollients.

EMOL'LIENTS, *Emollien'tia, Malthac'tica, Relaxan'tia, Epiceras'tica, Malac'tica, Lubrican'tia, Malacopœ'a, Mollien'tia*, from *emollire*, (e, and *mollire*, 'to soften.') Substances which relax and soften parts that are inflamed, or too tense. They are used both internally and externally: as the former, however, consist of mucilaginous substances, they are generally reckoned as demulcents: the latter, or proper emollients, consist of oils, cataplasms, fomentations, &c. Oleaginous bodies, rubbed on a part, act by diminishing its cohesion. Fomentations, in cases of internal inflammation, act probably through contiguous sympathy. The following are the chief emollients:— Adeps; Amygdalæ Oleum; Avenæ Farina; Cera; Cetaceum; Linum; Olivæ Oleum; Sesamum; Tritici Farina, and Ulmus.

EMOLLITIES, Mollities—e. Morbosa, Mollities—e. Ossium, Mollities ossium—e. Uteri Morbosa, Hysteromalacia.

EMOLLITIO, Mollities—e. Ventriculi, Gastromalacia.

ÉMONCTOIRE, Emunctory.

EMOPTOE, Hæmoptysis.

EMOTIO, Delirium, Luxation, Passion.

EMO'TIONAL, from *emotio*, (e, 'from,' and *moveo, motus*, 'to move.') Relating to emotion or passion independently of the will: — hence an '*emotional* or *instinctive impulse*.'

EMPASMA, Cataplasma.

EMPÂTEMENT, from *empâter*, 'to render pasty or doughy.' A non-inflammatory engorgement, which retains, more or less, the impression of the finger.

EMPATHE'MA, *Ma'nia a pathe'maté*, (F.) *Manie sans délire;* ungovernable passion; from εμ, or εν, 'in,' and παθος, 'suffering.' Fixed delusion.

EMPEIRIA, Experience.

EMPETRUM, Herniaria glabra.

EM'PHLYSIS, from εμ, or εν, 'in,' and φλυσις, 'a vesicular tumour or eruption;' *Ich'orous Exan'them*. An eruption of vesicular pimples, filled progressively with an acrid and colourless, or nearly colourless, fluid; terminating in scurf or laminated scabs. A genus in the order *Exanthematica*, class *Hæmatica* of Good.

EMPHLYSIS APHTHA, Aphthæ, Stomatitis, aphthous — e. Erysipelas, Erysipelas — e. Miliaria, Miliary fever — e. Pemphigus, Pemphigus — e. Vaccina inserta, Vaccina—e. Varicella, Varicella.

EMPHRACTIC, Emphracticus.

EMPHRACTICA, Physconia.

EMPHRAC'TICUS, *Emphrac'tic*, from εμφρασσω, 'I close,' 'I obstruct.' *Emplas'ticus, Emplattom'enos*. Any substance which, when applied to the skin, was presumed to close the pores.

EMPHRAG'MA, same etymon. *Obturamen'tum, Impedimen'tum*. Anything that obstructs. Hippocrates uses this term to designate the obstacle to delivery on the part of the fœtus, when the presentation is preternatural.

EMPHRAGMA LACHRYMALE, Fistula lachrymalis—e. Salivare, Ranula.

EMPHRAX'IS, *Obstruc'tio, Obtura'tio, Oppila'tio, Infarc'tus, Farctus, Fartus*. Same etymon. 'Obstruction.' An *Embarras* or repletion of canals or cavities by any substance, which is either morbid from quantity or quality.

EMPHRAXIS HEPATIS, Hepatemphraxis.

EMPHYMA, Tumour — e. Encystis, Encystis — e. Encystis atheroma, Atheroma — e. Encystis ganglion, Ganglion, Testudo — e. Encystis meliceris, Meliceris — e. Encystis steatoma, Steatoma — e. Exostosis ossea, Exostosis—e. Exostosis periostea, Node—e. Sarcoma, Sarcoma—e. Sarcoma adiposum, Adipose sarcoma—e. Sarcoma cellulosum, Cystic sarcoma — e. Sarcoma mammarum, Mammary sarcoma — e. Sarcoma pancreaticum, Pancreatic sarcoma — e. Sarcoma scirrhosum, Scirrhous sarcoma — e. Sarcoma tuberculosum,

Tuberculate sarcoma — e. Sarcoma vasculosum, Sarcoma, vascular.

EMPHYSE′MA, from εμφυσαω, (εν, and φυσαω, 'I blow,') 'I inflate.' *Infla′tio, Empneumato′sis, Sarci′tes flatuo′sus, Emphyse′ma cellula′rē, Emphyse′ma pneumato′sis, Physon′cus, Tumor flatulen′tus, Pneumato′sis, Infla′tion, Wind-dropsy,* (F.) *Emphysème.* This term is commonly applied to any white, crepitant, shining, elastic, indolent tumour, caused by the introduction of air into the areolar texture. Injuries of the larynx, trachea, or lungs; fractures of the ribs, or wounds penetrating the chest, are the most frequent causes of this affection, which is owing to the air escaping from the air-passages and insinuating itself into the areolar texture surrounding the wound. There are some cases of emphysema, which are owing to internal causes; and hence a division has been made into the *accidental* and *symptomatic,* and the *spontaneous* and *idiopathic.*

EMPHYSEMA ABDOMINIS, Tympanites.

EMPHYSE′MA OF THE LUNGS, *E. Pulmo′num, Asthma aëreum ab Emphyse′matē Pulmo′num, Pneumato′sis Pulmo′num, Pneumonec′tasis, Pneumec′tasis,* (F.) *Pneumoëctasie, Emphysème du Poumon.* A considerable pressure or contusion of the chest, or any violent concussion of the lung, may produce a laceration in that viscus, without injury being done to the parietes of the thorax, and may give place to the infiltration of air into the areolar texture, *interlobular emphysema.* Laënnec has described another species of emphysema of the lungs, *Vesicular emphysema,* consisting in excessive dilatation of the air-cells, some of which become as large as hemp-seed, ultimately break, and give rise to irregular vesicles at the surface of the lung, some of which are as large as a hazel-nut. *Physical signs.* The thorax externally, generally or locally, appears unnaturally convex and prominent. The intercostal spaces are widened, but depressed. The inspiratory efforts are increased. The sound on percussion is morbidly clear, but not tympanitic. On auscultation, the inspiratory murmur is feeble or suppressed. The expiration, which is more frequently audible is prolonged, laborious and wheezing. There are no certain physical signs which can distinguish *interlobular emphysema* from the *vesicular.*

EMPHYSEMA PECTORIS, Pneumothorax — e. Scroti, Physocele — e. Tympanites, Tympanites — e. Uteri, Hysterophysis, Physometra.

EMPHYSEM′ATOUS, *Emphysemato′sus;* same etymon. Relating or appertaining to emphysema.

EMPHYSÈME, Emphysema — *e. du Poumon,* Emphysema of the lungs.

EMPHYTUM THERMUM, Biolychnium.

EMP′IRIC, *Empi′ricus,* from εμπειρια, (εν, and πειρα, 'a trial,') 'experience.' One who follows only experience. A sect of physicians, who rejected all theory, and took for their guide experience alone. It was opposed to the dogmatic sect. The Empiric sect prevailed till near the time of Galen. Among its most eminent members, after Philinus and Serapion, were Apollonius, Glaucias, Bacchius of Tanagra, and Zeuxis, both disciples of Herophilus, — Heraclides of Tarentum, Cleophantus, master of Asclepiades, Menodotus of Nicomedia, and Theudas of Laodicea. They occupied themselves, chiefly, with discovering the properties of drugs, and did important service, in this manner, to medicine.

At the present day, the word *Empiric* is only taken in a bad sense, being employed in nearly the same signification as *charlatan* or *quack.*

EMPIRICE, Empiricism.

EMPIR′ICISM; same etymon. *Empi′rica Ars, Empi′ricē,* (F.) *Empirisme.* Medicine founded on experience. It generally, at the present day, signifies *quackery.*

EMPIRISME, Empiricism.

EMPLAS′TICUS. Same etymon as the next. Also, a remedy which adheres, as a plaster, to the surface, and in this manner may obstruct the pores: an emphractic.

EMPLASTRO-ENDERMIC, Endermic.

EMPLAS′TRUM, from the Greek εμπλαττω, (εν, and πλασσειν, 'to form,') 'I spread upon,' (F.) *Emplâtre.* A solid and tenacious compound, adhesive at the ordinary heat of the human body. Some of the plasters owe their consistence to wax and resin; and others to the chemical union which takes place between the semivitreous oxide of lead and oil. Most of them become too consistent by age. When such is the case, they may be remelted by a gentle heat, and oil be added to them.

EMPLASTRUM ADHÆSIVUM, Emplastrum resinæ — e. Adhæsivum Woodstockii, see Sparadrapum Adhæsivum — e. Alexandri, Alexandrine — e. de Althææ, Unguentum de Althææ.

EMPLASTRUM AMMONI′ACI, *Ammoni′acum Plaster,* (Ammoniac. pur. ℥v, acidi acetici dil. Oss. Dissolve the ammoniac in the vinegar, and strain: then evaporate the solution by means of a water bath, stirring constantly until it acquires a proper consistence. — Ph. U. S.) It is used as a discutient plaster.

EMPLASTRUM AMMONI′ACI CUM HYDRAR′GYRO, *Ammoniacum plaster with mercury (Ammoniaci* ℔j, *hydrarg.* ℥iij, *olei oliv.* ℨj, *sulphur,* gr. viij. Rub the mercury with the oil until the globules disappear, then add the ammoniac, previously melted, and mix. *Ph. U. S.*

EMPLASTRUM ANDREÆ DE CRUCE, E. de pice et resinis glutinans — e. Anglicum, see Sparadrapum adhæsivum.

EMPLASTRUM AROMAT′ICUM, *Aromat′ic Plaster.* (*Thuris* ℥iij, *ceræ flavæ* ℥ss, *pulv. cort. cinnam.* ℨvj, *ol. ess. Piment., ol. ess. Limon.* ãã ℨij. Melt the frankincense and wax together, and strain; then add, as it cools, the cinnamon, previously rubbed with the oils, and form a plaster. *Ph. Dubl.*) Used as a stimulating plaster.

A spice plaster, made by incorporating powdered *cinnamon* and any other spices with melted *suet,* has been used in cholera infantum. It is spread on leather or linen, and is renewed twice in the twenty-four hours.

EMPLASTRUM ASAFŒ′TIDÆ, *Asafœtida plaster, E. antihyster′icum,* (*Emp. plumb., Asafœt.,* sing. ℔j, *Galban., Ceræ flavæ,* ãã ℔ss, *Alcohol. dilut.* Oiij. Dissolve the asafœtida and galbanum in the alcohol, in a water bath, strain while hot, and evaporate to the consistence of honey; add the lead plaster and wax previously melted together, stir the mixture well, and evaporate to the proper consistence. — *Ph. U. S.*) Used as an antispasmodic and anodyne plaster.

EMPLASTRUM ATTRAHENS, E. ceræ — e. Auriculare, Hypotium.

EMPLASTRUM BELLADON′NÆ, *Plaster of Belladon′na.* (*Empl. resin.* ℥iij, *Ext. Belladon.* ℥iss. Add the extract to the plaster, previously melted in a water bath, and mix. — *Ph. U. S.*)

EMPLASTRUM CALEFA′CIENS, *E. Picis cum canthar′idē,* (Ph. U. S.) *Calefa′cient plaster, Warm plaster,* (F.) *Emplâtre échauffant.* (*Cerat. can tharid.* (Ph. U. S.) ℔ss, *Picis abiet.* ℔ijss. Melt together, and form into a plaster. *Ph. U. S.*) It is rubefacient and stimulant.

EMPLASTRUM CANTHARIDIS, E. lyttæ — e. Cantharidis vesicatorii compositum, E. lyttæ comp. — e. Cephalicum, E. picis comp.

EMPLASTRUM CERÆ, *E. simplex, Wax plaster, E. At′trahens.* (*Ceræ flavæ, Sevi Præp.* ãã ℔ij, *resinæ flavæ* ℔j. Melt them together and strain.

Ph. L.) It has been considered drawing. It is stimulating.

EMPLASTRUM CICU'TÆ, *E. de Cicu'tâ, E. coni'i macula'ti, Unguen'tum sol'idum de cicu'tâ, Hemlock plaster*, (*F.*) *Emplâtre de Ciguë*. (*Resinæ abiet.* 960 p. *Ceræ flav.* 640 p. *Picis albæ,* 448 p. *Ol. cicutæ per decoct. præparat.* 128 p. *Fol cicut. recent.* 2000 p. Melt the resins, wax and oil; add the cicuta leaves, and boil; strain and add, after having dissolved it in vinegar of squills and cicuta juice, *gum ammoniac*. 500 p. *Ph. Par.*) It is used as a discutient, especially to scirrhous tumours.

EMPLASTRUM CITRINUM, Unguentum de althæâ e. Commune, E. Plumbi—e. Commune cum resinâ, E. resinæ—e. Conii, E. cicutæ.

EMPLASTRUM CUMI'NI, *Cummin plaster*. (*Cumin. semin., carui sem., lauri bacc.* sing. ℨiij, *picis aridæ* ℔iij, *ceræ flavæ* ℨiij. Melt the pitch and wax together, then add the other ingredients. *Ph. L.*) It is used as a warm, discutient plaster.

EMPLASTRUM DIACHYLON, Diachylon, E. plumbi —e. Divinum Nicolai, see Magnet—e. Emolliens, Unguentum de althæâ—e. Epispasticum, E. lyttæ.

EMPLASTRUM FERRI, *E. rob'orans, Iron Plaster, Strength'ening Plaster.* (*Ferri subcarb.* ℨiij, *Emp. plumbi,* ℔ij, *Picis abietis,* ℔ss. Add the subcarbonate of iron to the lead plaster and Burgundy pitch previously melted together, and stir constantly until they thicken upon cooling.—Ph. U. S.)

EMPLASTRUM FERRI RUBRI, E. oxidi ferri rubri—e. Flavum, Unguentum de althæâ—e. ad Fonticulos, Ceratum Galeni.

EMPLASTRUM GAL'BANI, *Galb'anum plaster*, (*Empl. litharg.* ℔ij, *gum. galban.* ℔ss, *ceræ flavæ* ℨiv. Melt the galbanum before adding the plaster and wax, then melt all together. *Ph. D.*) A stimulant and discutient.

EMPLASTRUM GAL'BANI COMPOS'ITUM. *E. li.har'gyri compos'itum, Diach'ylon magnum cum gummi, Compound galbanum plaster*. (*Galb. pur.* ℨviij, *Emp. plumbi,* ℔iij, *tereb. vulg.* ℨx, *abietis resin.* contus. ℨiij. Melt the galbanum and turpentine together, then mix in the resin, and afterwards the plaster, previously melted. It is a stimulant and discutient.

EMPLASTRUM GLUTINOSUM, see Sparadrapum udhæsivum—e. cum Gummatibus, E. gummosum.

EMPLASTRUM GUMMO'SUM, *Gum plaster, Emplastrum lithar'gyri cum gummi, E. cum gummat'ibus, E. e gummat'ibus resino'sis, E. Ox'ydi Plumbi semirit'rei gummo'sum, Yellow diach'ylon, Gum diachylon, Diachylon cum gummi.* (*Emp. oxid. plumbi semicitr.* p. viij, *g. resin. ammoniac., g. resin. bubon. galbani, ceræ flavæ,* āā, p. i. *Ph. E.*) Properties and uses like the last.

EMPLASTRUM E GUMMATIBUS RESINOSIS, E. gummosum.

EMPLASTRUM CUM GUMMI-RESI'NIS, (F.) *Emplâtre de gomme résine, Diachylon gommé, Plaster of gum resins.* (*Emplastr. simpl.* p. 1600, *ceræ flavæ,* p. 96, *picis albæ,* p. 96, *terebinth.* p. 96. Melt by a gentle heat, and add *gum ammoniac,* p. 32, *bdellium* 32, *galban.* 32, and *sagapenum*, p. 32. Dissolve in a sufficient quantity of *alcohol*, evaporate to the consistence of honey, and mix carefully all together. *Ph. P.*) A discutient.

EMPLASTRUM HYDRAR'GYRI, *Mercu'rial plaster, Emplastr. lithar'gyri cum hydrar'gyro.* (*Hydrarg.* ℨvj, *ol. oliv., resin.* āā ℨij, *emplast. plumbi,* ℔j. Melt the oil and resin together, and when cool rub the mercury with them till the globules disappear; then gradually add the lead plaster, previously melted, and mix all. *Ph. U. S.*) It is stimulant, resolvent, and discutient. Applied as a discutient to venereal and other tumours.

EMPLASTRUM HYDRAR'GYRI COMPOS'ITUM, *E. de hydrar'gyro compos'itum, E. de Vigo cum mercu'rio emenda'tum, Compound plaster of mer'cury.* (*Empl. simpl.* p. 1250, *ceræ flavæ,* p. 64, *resinæ,* p. 64. Melt, and before it congeals add *pulv. g. ammoniac,* p. 20, *bdellium,* p. 20, *oliban.* p. 20, *myrrh,* p. 20, *saffron,* p. 12. Mix carefully. Take of *mercury,* p. 380, *pure turpentine,* p. 64, *liquid* and *pure storax,* p. 192. Triturate in an iron mortar till the globules disappear: melt all together, and before congealing add *essential oil of Lavender,* p. 8. *Pharm. P.*) The same properties as the last.

EMPLASTRUM ICHTHYOCOLLÆ TELÆ INDUCTUM, see Sparadrapum adhæsivum—e. Irritans, E. lyttæ—e. Lithargyri, E. Plumbi—e. Lithargyri compositum, E. galbani compositum—e. Lithargyri cum gummi, E. gummosum—e. Lithargyri cum hydrargyro, E. hydrargyri—e. Lithargyri cum resinâ, E. resinæ—e. Lithargyricum cum resinâ pini, E. resinæ.

EMPLASTRUM LYTTÆ, *E. canthar'idis, E. cantharidis vesicato'rii, Plaster of the Spanish or blistering fly, Blistering Plaster, Fly Plaster, E. mel'oës vesicato'rii, E. vesicato'rium, E. epispas'ticum, E. e cantharid'ibus epispas'ticum solid'ius et tena'cius hærens, E. irri'tans, E. rubefi'ans.* (*Cantharides*, in powder, ℔j, *Emp. ceræ* ℔iss, *adipis. præp.* ℔j. Melt the plaster and lard together, and as the mixture becomes thick, on cooling, sprinkle in the flies, and mix. *Pharm. L.*) This is the common blistering plaster. Too much heat must not be used in its preparation. It requires to remain on six or eight hours before its full effect is induced, and it acts sufficiently well, provided even a piece of thin gauze or tissue paper be placed between it and the skin, whilst absorption of the flies is thus prevented. See Blister. The Blistering Plaster of the Pharmacopoeia of the United States, *Cera'tum Canthar'idis*, is made as follows:— *Cantharid.* in pulv. subtiliss., ℔j, *ceræ flavæ, resinæ*, āā ℨvij, *adipis*, ℨx. To the wax, resin, and lard, previously melted, add the Spanish flies, and stir the mixture constantly until cool.

EMPLASTRUM LYTTÆ COMPOS'ITUM, *E. canthar'idis vesicato'rii compos'itum, E. mel'oës vesicato'rii compos'itum, Compound plaster of canthar'ides* or *Spanish flies.* (*Resin. liq. pini laricis.* p. 18, *resinæ concret. pini abietis, meloës vesicat.* āā, p. 12, *ceræ flavæ,* p. 4, *subacet. cupri,* p. ij, *semin. sinapis alb., fruct. pip. nigr.* āā p. j. Melt the pitch and wax, then add the turpentine, and as these cool sprinkle in the other substances, in the form of powder, so as to make a plaster. *Ph. E.*) The same properties as the last, but more energetic and speedy in its action.

EMPLASTRUM MELOES VESICATORII, E. lyttæ— e. Meloes vesicatorii comp., E. lyttæ comp.—e. Mucilaginosum, Unguentum de althæâ—e. Nigrum of Augsburg, see Magnet.

EMPLASTRUM NORIMBERGEN'SE, *E. ex ox'ido plumbi rubro camphora'tum, Emplâtre de Nuremberg, Nuremberg plaster.* (*Oxid. plumb. rubr.* p. 300, *ol. oliv.* p. 600, *aquæ*, q. s. Boil until the oxide is dissolved, and almost to dryness. Remove the vessel from the fire and add *yellow wax*, p. 500. Put the vessel again on the fire, and after the wax is melted, add, before it congeals, *camphor,* p. 24: mix. *Ph. P.*) It is considered a desiccative, and has been employed in gangrene.

EMPLASTRUM NYGMATICUM, E. resinæ.

EMPLASTRUM OPII, *O'pium Plaster.* (*Opii* in pulv. ℨij, *Picis abiet.* ℨiij ; *emplastr. plumbi* ℔j, *aq. bullient.* f ℨiv. Melt together the lead plaster and Burgundy pitch; then add the opium previously mixed with the water, and boil over a gentle fire to the proper consistence.—*Ph. U. S.*) It is employed as an anodyne, and to give support.

EMPLASTRUM OX'IDI FERRI RUBRI, *E. Ferri rubri*, *E. Rob'orans*, *Plaster of red oxide of iron*, *Strength'ening plaster*. (*Empl. oxid. plumb. semivitr.* p. xxiv, *resinæ pin.* p. vi, *ceræ flavæ*, *olei oleæ Europ.* sing. p. iij, *oxidi ferri rubr.* p. viij. Rub the red oxide of iron with the oil, and add the other ingredients melted. *Ph. E.*) It is employed as a strengthening plaster.

EMPLASTRUM EX OXIDO PLUMBI SEMIVITREO, E. plumbi—e. Oxidi plumbi semivitrei, E. plumbi—e. Oxidi plumbi semivitrei gummosum, E. gummosum.

EMPLASTRUM PHŒNICEUM, Diapalma — e. ex Oxido plumbi rubro compositum, E. Norimbergense.

EMPLASTRUM PICIS BURGUN'DICÆ, *Emplastrum Picis*, *Burgundy Pitch Plaster*, *Pitch Plaster*, (*Picis Burgund.* ℔vj; *ceræ flavæ*, ℔ss.--Ph. U. S.)

EMPLASTRUM PICIS COMPOS'ITUM, *E. cephal'icum*, *Cephal'ic plaster*, *Compound pitch plaster*. (*Picis arid.* ℔ij, *abietis resinæ* ℔j, *resinæ flavæ*, *ceræ flavæ*, ā ā ʒiv, *myrist. ol.* ʒj, *ol. oliv., aquæ*, ā ā f ʒij. To the pitch, resin, and wax, melted together, add the other matters and mix. *Ph. L.*) It is stimulant and rubefacient. Sometimes used in headach,—applied to the temples. See Depilatory.

EMPLASTRUM PICIS CUM CANTHARIDE, E. Calefaciens.

EMPLASTRUM DE PICE ET RESI'NIS GLU'TINANS, *E. Andreæ de Cruce*, *Emplâtre d'André de la Croix*, *E. collant de poix et de résines*, *Adhesive plaster of pitch and resins*. (*Picis albæ*, p. 128, *resin elemi*, p. 32, *terebinth. pur.* p. 16, *ol. laur.* p. 16. Melt with a gentle heat, and pass through linen. *Ph. P.*) Used in contusions and fractures as a support.

EMPLASTRUM PLUMBI, *E. lythar'gyri*, *E. commu'ne*, *E. diach'ylum*, *E. ox'idi plumbi semivitrei*, *E. ex oxido plumbi semivitreo*, *Diach'ylon simplex*, *White Diach'ylon*, *Lead plaster*, *Diach'ylon plaster*. (*Plumbi oxid. semivitr.* in pulv. ℔v, *olei oliv.*, cong., *aquæ* Oij. Boil together over a slow fire, stirring constantly until the oil and oxide of lead cohere. *Ph. U. S.*)

EMPLASTRUM POLYCHRESTUM, E. resinæ.

EMPLASTRUM RESI'NÆ, *E. adhæsi'vum*, *E. lithar'gyri cum resi'nâ*, *E. resino'sum*, *E. nygmat'icum*, *Resin plaster*, *Adhe'sive* or *Sticking plaster*, *Emplastrum commu'ne cum resi'nâ*, *E. Polychrestum*, *E. lithargyr'icum cum resi'nâ pini*. (*Resin.* ℔ss. *emp. plumb.* ℔iij. Melt the plaster, with a gentle heat, add the resin, and mix. *Ph. U. S.*) Employed in wounds and ulcers.

Baynton's adhesive plaster is made by melting one pound of *lead plaster* and six drachms of *resin* together.

EMPLASTRUM RESINOSUM, E. Resinæ — e. Roborans, E. Ferri (Ph. U. S.), E. oxidi ferri rubri —e. Rubefians, E. lyttæ.

EMPLASTRUM SAPO'NIS, *E. sapona'ceum*, *Soap plaster*. (*Saponis concis.* ʒiv, *emplast. plumb.* ℔iij. Mix the soap with the melted plaster, and boil to a proper consistence. *Ph. U. S.*) It is a mild discutient. Applied to tumours, corns, &c.

EMPLASTRUM SIMPLEX, E. ceræ—e. Spermatis ceti, Ceratum cetacei.

EMPLASTRUM THURIS, *Frank'incense plaster*. (*Emp. lithargyri*, ℔ij, *thuris*, ℔ss, *oxid. ferri. rubr.* ʒiij. *Ph. D.*,) *Use:*—the same as the plaster of red oxide of iron.

EMPLASTRUM VESICATORIUM, Blister, E. lyttæ — e. de Vigo cum mercurio emendatum, E. hydrargyri compositum.

EMPLÂTRE, Emplastrum—e. *d'André de la Croix*, Emplastrum de pice et resinis glutinans—e. *de Ciguë*, Emplastrum cicutæ — e. *Collant de poix et de résines*, Emplastrum de pice et resinis glutinans—e. *de Gomme résine*, Emplastrum cum gummi-resinis — e. *de Nuremberg*, Emplastrum Norimbergense.

EMPLATTOMENOS, Emphracticus.

EMPNEUMATOSIS, Emphysema, Inspiration.

EMPOISONNEMENT, Poisoning.

EMPO'RIUM, *εμπoριον*, (*εμ* or *εν*, and *πορος*, 'a way,') 'a market or depôt.' The brain was so called, of old, because there all the mental affairs are transacted.

EMPORIUM SPIRITUUM, Sensorium.

EMPOSIS, Imbibition.

EMPREINTE, Impression.

EMPRESIS, Empresma.

EMPRES'MA, *Empres'mus*, *Empre'sis*, from *εμπρηθω*, 'I burn internally.' Inflammation. *Phlegma'tia membrano'sæ et parynchymato'sæ*, *Phlogis'tici*, *Febres continuæ inflammato'riæ*, *Inflamma'tio inter'na*, *Cau'ma*, *Inter'nal inflammation*. A genus in the class *hæmatica*, order *phlogotica*, of Good.

EMPRESMA BRONCHITIS, Cynanche trachealis—e. Bronchlemmitis, Cynanche trachealis—e. Carditis, Carditis—e. Cephalitis, Phrenitis—e. Cystitis, Cystitis—e. Enteritis, Enteritis—e. Gastritis, Gastritis—e. Hepatitis, Hepatitis—e. Hysteritis, Metritis—e. Nephritis, Nephritis—e. Orchitis, Hernia humoralis — e. Otitis, Otitis — e. Paristhmitis, Cynanche — e. Paristhmitis tonsillaris maligna, Cynanche maligna — e. Paristhmitis pharyngea, Cynanche pharyngea — e. Paristhmitis tonsillaris, Cynanche tonsillaris—e. Parotitis, Cynanche parotidæa—e. Peritonitis, Peritonitis—e. Peritonitis mesenterica, Mesenteritis—e. Peritonitis omentalis, Epiploitis—e. Picis cum Cantharide, E. calefaciens—e. Pleuritis, Pleuritis—e. Pleuritis diaphragmatica, Diaphragmitis—e. Pneumonitis, Pneumonia—e. Splenitis, Splenitis.

EMPRESMUS, Empresma.

EM'PRION, from *εν*, and *πριων*, 'a saw.' Serrated. Galen has given this name to the pulse, when the sensation produced by the artery under the fingers is analogous to that which would be caused by the unequal teeth of a saw.

EMPROSTHOCYRTOMA, Lordosis.

EMPROSTHOT'ONOS, *Emprosthoton'ia*, *Enta'sia tet'anus anti'cus*, *Tetanus anticus*, from *εμπροσθεν*, 'forwards,' and *τεινω*, 'I stretch,' 'I extend.' A variety of tetanus, in which the body is drawn forwards by the permanent contraction of the muscles.

EMPSYCHO'SIS, from *εμψυχοω*, (*εν*, and *ψυχη*, 'life,') 'I animate,' 'I vivify.' A word formerly used for the act of animating. The union of the soul with the body.

EMPTOE, Hæmoptysis.

EMPTOICA PASSIO, Hæmoptysis.

EMPTYSIS, Hæmoptysis.

EMPTYSMA, Sputum.

EMPYE, Empyema.

EMPYE'MA, *Empye'sis*, *Em'pyē*, from *εν*, 'in, and *πυον*, 'pus.' *Aposte'ma empye'ma*. A collection of blood or pus, and, conventionally, of other fluid, in some cavity of the body, and particularly in that of the pleura. Empyema is one of the terminations of inflammation of the pleura, and is called, also, *Pyotho'rax verus*, *Pleurorrhœ'a purulen'ta*, *Diapye'ma*, *Ecpye'ma*, *Ecpye'sis*, *Empye'sis pec'toris*, *Pyo'sis pec'toris*, *Hydrotho'rax purulen'tus*, *Dyspnœ'a pyothorac''ica*, *Pneumo'nia suppurato'ria*, *Absces'sus pec'toris*, *A. Thorac'is*, *Pleuraposte'ma*, *Pleuropye'sis*, (F.) *Pyopleurite.*

The operation for empyema properly means the making of an opening into the thorax for the purpose of giving issue to the matter collected in the cavity of the pleura, although it has been used for the operation required for the evacuation of any fluid from the chest, or synonymously with *Paracentesis thoracis.*

EMPYE'SIS; same etymon. Suppuration. An eruption of phlegmonous pimples, gradually filling with a purulent fluid, and terminating in thick scabs, frequently leaving pits or scabs. *Pus'tulous Exan'them.* A genus in the order *Exanthematica,* class *Hæmatica* of Good. See Empyema.

EMPYESIS OCULI, Hypopyon—e. Pectoris, Empyema—e. Variola, Variola.

EMPYMELIUM POLYSARCIA, Polysarcia adiposa.

EMPYOCE'LE, from εν, 'in,' πυον, 'pus,' and κηλη, 'tumour,' 'hernia.' A tumour, formed by an accumulation of pus in the scrotum. Different diseases have been described under this name, such as suppuration of the testicle, empyema of the tunica vaginalis, accumulation of pus in the cavity of a hernial sac, abscesses of different kinds formed in the cellular texture of the scrotum, &c.

EMPYOM'PHALUS, from εν, 'in,' πυον, 'pus,' and ομφαλος, 'the navel.' This word has been used to designate a suppurating tumour at the umbilicus; or, at times, umbilical hernia, the sac of which is filled with blood.

EMPYOS, Purulent.

EMPYREU'MA, from εμπυρευω, (εν, and πυρ, 'fire,') 'I kindle.' The burnt smell and acrid taste, which volatile products—gaseous and liquid —contract, when animal or vegetable substances are decomposed by a strong heat. The cause of this smell is seated in an oil, called *empyreumat'ic,* which does not exist in the substance subjected to the operation, but is the result of its decomposition. If the empyreuma occurs when the organic substance is placed in a still with a liquid, it is owing to the solid matter touching the bottom of the vessel to which the fire is applied.

EMPYREUMAT'IC, *Empyreumat'icus:* same etymon. Belonging to empyreuma, — as an *empyreumatic* odour.

EM'PYROS, *Febric"itans,* from πυρ, 'fire or fever.' One who has fever.—Hippocrates.

EMS, MINERAL WATERS OF. Celebrated springs on the river Lahn, duchy of Nassau. They are thermal (from 83 to 115° Fahrenheit,) and carbonated salines, containing carbonic acid, bicarbonate of soda, and chloride of sodium; and are much used in gastric and intestinal affections, &c.

EMUL'GENT, *Emul'gens,* from *emulgere,* (e, and *mulgere,*) 'to milk out,' 'to draw out.' A name given to the renal artery and vein, because the ancients imagined they milked, as it were, the urine through the kidneys. See Renal.

EMULSIN, see Amygdalin.

EMUL'SIO, *Emul'sion;* same etymon. A pharmaceutical preparation, of a milky-white opaque appearance, which is composed of oil, divided and held in suspension in water by means of mucilage. Emulsions have been divided into the *true* and *oily,* and into the *false* or *not oily;* the latter being composed of resinous substances, balsams, or camphor, rubbed up with dilute alcohol, mucilage, or yolk of egg.

EMULSIO ACA'CIÆ ARAB'ICÆ, *Emul'sio Arab'ica; Gum Ar'abic Emul'sion.* (*Nucleor. amygd. comm.* ℥j, *aquæ* ℔jss, *mucilay. acac.* ℥ij, *sacch.* ℥iv. While beating the decorticated almonds with the sugar and water, add the mucilage. — *Ph. E.*) Used in the same cases as the last.

EMULSIO AMYG'DALÆ, *Lac amyg'dalæ, Emul'sio simplex, Amygdala'tum, Mistu'ra amygdalæ, Emulsio* sive *Lac Amygdala'rum, Almond Emulsion, Almond Milk,* (F.) *Lait d'amandes.* (*Amygdal. dulc.* ℥ss; *Acaciæ,* in pulv. ℥ss; *Sacchar.* ℥ij; *Aquæ destillat.* f℥viij. Macerate the almonds in water, and having removed their external coat, beat them with the gum Arabic and sugar, in a marble mortar, till they are thoroughly mixed; then rub the mixture with the distilled water gradually added, and strain.— Ph. U. S.) It is used as a diluent and demulcent.

EMULSIO ANTIHYSTERICA, Mistura asafœtidæ —e. Arabica, Emulsio acaciæ Arabicæ.

EMULSIO CAM'PHORÆ, *E. Camphora'ta, Mistu'ra Camphoræ; Camphor Emulsion.* (*Camphoræ* ℈j, *amygd, com.* decortic., *sacch. dur.,* āā ℥iv, *aquæ* ℥vj.— *Ph. E.*) A convenient form for giving camphor.

EMULSIO GUAIACINA, Mistura guaiaci—e. Leniens, Looch ex ovo.

EMULSIO O'LEI AMYGDALA'RUM; *Emulsion of Oil of Almonds,* (*Ol. amygd.* ℥j, *gum acac. pulv.* ℥ij, *syrup.* ℥j, *aquæ destill.* ℥iv. Mix. A good pectoral or cough mixture.

EMULSIO O'LEI RIC'INI; *Castor Oil Emulsion* (*Ol. ricini* ℥ss, *vitelli ovi* q. s., *aquæ destillat.* ℥j.) An aperient draught.

EMULSIO O'LEI TEREBIN'THINÆ; *Emulsion of Oil of Tur'pentine,* (*Ol. tereb. rect.* ℈ij. *sacch. alb.* ℥ss. *vitell. ovi* j, *emuls. amygd.* vel *aquæ destillat.* ℥vj. Mix. In rheumatic and nephritic affections. Dose f℥iss.

EMULSIO OLEOSA, Looch ex ovo.

EMULSIO PURGANS CUM JALA'PÆ RESI'NA, *Purging Emulsion with Resin of Jalap.* (*Jalapæ resin.* gr. xij. *sacch. alb.* ℥ij. Triturate for some time, and add gradually half the yolk of an egg; continue to triturate, adding by degrees *emuls. simpl.* ℥v, *aq. flor, aurant.* ℥ij.—*Ph. P.*)

EMULSIO PURGANS CUM SCAMMO'NIO; *Purging Emulsion with Scammony.* It is prepared like the preceding, substituting only Scammony for the jalap.

EMULSIO SIMPLEX, E. Amygdalæ.

EMULSION, Emulsio—e. Almond, Emulsio amygdalæ—e. Camphor, Emulsio Camphoræ—e. Castor oil, Emulsio olei ricini—e. Gum Arabic, Emulsio acaciæ Arabicæ—e. *Huileuse,* Looch ex ovo—e. of Oil of Almonds, Emulsio olei amygdalarum—e. of Oil of Turpentine, Emulsio olei terebinthinæ—e. Purging with resin of jalap, Emulsio purgans cum jalapæ resinâ—e. Purging. with scammony. Emulsio purgans cum scammonio.

EMUL'SIVE, *Emulsi'vus;* same etymon. An epithet given to seeds whence oil may be extracted by expression; such as almonds, apricots, peaches, hemp, rape, melons, gourds; those of the nut kind, and cucurbitaceous and cruciferous plants in general.

EMUNCTORIUM, Emunctory — e. Cerebri, Nasus.

EMUNC'TORY, *Emuncto'rium,* from *emungere,* (e, and *mungere,*) 'to drain off,' 'to cleanse.' *Emissa'rium,* (F.) *Émonctoire, Émissaire.* Any organ whose office it is to give issue to matters which ought to be excreted. The ancients believed that some organs were more particularly destined to serve as emunctories of others: the nasal fossæ, for example, they believed to be the emunctories of the brain.

EMUNDANTIA, Detergents.

EMYS PALUS'TRIS, *Salt Water Ter'rapin.* This species of turtle is found exclusively in salt or brackish waters, near the sea shore, along the whole Atlantic coast. It is much prized by the epicure, and is nutritious and tolerably easy of digestion when dressed plain.

EN, see Em.

ENADELPHIA, *Emboîtement*.

ENÆMA, Hæmostatica.

ENÆMON, Styptic.

ENÆORE'MA, from εν, 'in,' and αιωρεω, 'I lift up,' 'that which hangs or floats in.' The *Neph'elē, Nubes, Sublimamen'tum, Sublima'tio, Subli'mē, Suspen'sum, S. Uri'næ, Suspen'sa, Nubec'ula* or cloud, which is suspended in the urine as it cools.

ENAM'EL OF THE TEETH, *Den'tium Nitor, Cortex, Cortex stria'ta, Substan'tia filamento'sa* of Malpighi, *S. Adaman'tina den'tium, Crusta Den'tium adaman'tina, Adamantine substance*. The substance which covers the coronæ of the teeth, and which has, also, been called the *vitreous substance, Substan'tia vit'rea*, (F.) *Substance vitrée* ou *émaillée, Émail des Dents*. The enamel is of a milky-white colour, and sufficiently hard to strike fire with steel. Its surface is very smooth and polished, and it forms a thicker layer towards the part where the teeth come in contact, and becomes thinner towards the cervix. The fibres of the enamel are perpendicular to the surface of the teeth, on the ivory of which they seem, as it were, planted. This gives them a velvety appearance, when examined by the microscope. The enamel has no blood vessels, and is not renewed when removed. It is formed of phosphate of lime, and a very small portion of animal matter.

ENANTHE'MA, same etymon as the next. A name recently given to certain eruptions of the mucous membrane, as exanthema is to certain eruptions of the skin.

ENANTHE'SIS, from εν, 'in,' and ανθεω, 'I flourish.' *Rash exan'them*. Eruption of red, level or nearly level patches, variously figured, irregularly diffused, often confluent, and terminating in cuticular exfoliations. A genus in the order *Exanthematica*, class *Hæmatica* of Cullen, including scarlet fever, measles, &c.

ENANTHESIS ROSALIA, Scarlatina — e. Urticaria, Urticaria.

ENANTIOPATHIC, Palliative.

ENARTHRO'SIS, *Inarticula'tio, Ball and Socket-joint*, from εν, 'in,' and αρθρωσις, 'an articulation.' A kind of diarthrodial articulation, in which the head of a bone is received into the cavity of another, and can be moved in all directions. The joint of the os femoris with the os innominatum is one of this character.

ENAR'THRUM, from εν, 'in,' and αρθρον, 'a joint.' A foreign body in a joint.

ENAUSMA, Fomites.

ENCAN'THIS, from εν, 'in,' and κανθος, 'the angle of the eye.' A tumour, formed by an increase in size, or a degeneration, of the caruncula lachrymalis. Any morbid growth in the inner angle of the eye.

ENCANTHIS BENIG'NA. Simple excrescence of the caruncula. It commonly yields to astringent collyria.

ENCANTHIS FUNGO'SA. A condition of the semilunar fold and lachrymal caruncle, in which they are the seat of morbid growths.

ENCANTHIS INFLAMMATO'RIA. Inflammation with enlargement — swelling — of the semilunar fold and lachrymal caruncle.

ENCANTHIS MALIG'NA has often a cancerous character, and requires extirpation before it has attained any considerable size.

ENCARPOS, Pregnant.

ENCASING, *Emboîtement*.

ENCATALEPSIS, Catalepsy.

ENCATHIS'MA, *Semicu'pium*. With the ancients *Encathis'ma*, εγκαθισμα, meant a vapour-bath taken sitting.

ENCAU'MA, from εν, 'in,' and καυω, 'I burn.' *Epicau'mis, Epicau'sis, Encau'sis*. A tumour produced by a burn. A burn. Also, an ulcer of the transparent cornea, occasioning loss of the humours.—Aëtius, Gorræus.

ENCAUSIS, Burn, Encauma, Moxibustion.

ENCAUSSE, MINERAL WATERS OF. Encausse is a village in the department of the Haute-Garonne, which possesses several saline, acidulous springs.

ENCA'VURE, Argema.

ENCEINTE, Pregnant.

ENCENS, Juniperus lycia.

ENCEPHALALGIA, Cephalalgia—e. Hydropica, Hydrocephalus internus.

ENCEPHAL'IC, *Encephal'icus*, from εν, 'in,' and κεφαλη, 'the head.' That which is situate in the head. A name given to several parts which relate to the encephalon, as, the *encephalic membranes, muscles*, &c.

ENCEPHALI'TIS: same etymon. This term has been used, by some nosologists, synonymously with *Cephali'tis* and *Phreni'tis*. By others, it has been appropriated to inflammation of the brain, in contradistinction to that of the membranes.

ENCEPHALITIS EXSUDATORIA, Hydrocephalus internus — e. Infantum, Hydrocephalus internus —e. Insolationis, *Coup-de-soleil*—e. Membranosa, Meningitis—e. Peripherica, Meningitis—e. Potatorum, Delirium tremens.

ENCEPHALIUM, Cerebellum.

ENCEPHALOCE'LE, from εγκεφαλον, 'the brain,' and κηλη, 'a tumour.' *Hernia Cer'ebri, Fungus Cerebri, Cranioce'lē, Hernia of the Brain*. This may be a *congenital* or *accidental* affection. In the former case, it is dependent upon tardy ossification of the fontanelles or some faulty conformation. In the latter, it is owing to some considerable loss of substance in the parietes of the cranium, produced by fractures, wounds with a cutting instrument, caries, the application of the trephine, &c. In slight congenital encephalocele, gentle pressure may be exerted upon the protruded portion. When the disease is of considerable extent, it is fatal. In accidental encephalocele, similar means must be used for confining the tumour, and preserving it from the action of external bodies.

ENCEPHALOCHYSIS, Hydrocephalus internus—e. Senilis, Apoplexy, serous.

ENCEPHALODYNIA, Cephalalgia.

ENCEPHALOHÆMIA, Cephalæmia.

ENCÉPHALOHÉMIE, Cephalæmia.

ENCEPH'ALOID, *Encephaloïdes, Ceph'aloid, Cephaloïdes, Cephalo'ma*, from εγκεφαλον, 'the brain,' and ειδος, 'resemblance.' Laënnec has given the term *Enceph'aloid* or *Cer'ebriform* matter to one of the morbid substances commonly formed by scirrhous or cancerous tumours. It is either encysted, in irregular masses without cysts, or infiltrated into the texture of the diseased organ. This name was given to it in consequence of its resemblance, when fully developed, to the medullary substance of the brain. It is also called *Fungus medulla'ris, F. Cancro'sus medulla'ris, Sarco'ma medulla'rē, Spongoid inflammation, Fungus cerebra'lis, Cancer cerebrifor'mē, Cancer mollis, C. Medulla'ris, Carcino'ma medulla'rē, C. Spongio'sum, Carci'nus spongio'sus, Myelo'ma, Myelomy'ces, Myelospon'gus, Tela accidenta'lis medulla'ris*, (F.) *Matière cérébriforme, Carcinome mou et spongeux, Tumeur encéphaloïde, Fongus médullaire, Carcinôme sanglant, Cancer mou; Milk-like tumour, Med'ullary sarcoma, Cel*-

lular cancer, Fungoid disease, Hæmatocer'ebriform disease. See Cancer.

ENCEPHALOID TUMOUR OF THE LUNG, Phthisis, cancerous.

ENCEPHALOLOG"IA, from εγκεφαλος, 'the encephalon,' and λογος, 'a description.' A description of the encephalon.

ENCEPHALOMALACIA, Mollities cerebri.
ENCEPHALOMALAXIS, Mollities cerebri.

ENCEPH'ALON, Enceph'alum, Enceph'alus, from εν, 'in,' and κεφαλη, the head.' That which is situate in the head. This name has generally been given to the brain, cerebellum, and mesocephalon. At times, it includes likewise the medulla spinalis, when it is also called the Cer'ebrospinal axis and Neural axis.

ENCEPHALOPATHI'A, from εγκεφαλος, 'the encephalon,' and παθος, 'disease.' A disease of the encephalon.

ENCEPHALOPATHIA PUERPERALIS, Mania, puerperal — e. Saturnina, see Encéphalopathie saturnine.

ENCÉPHALOPATHIE CRAPULEUSE, Delirium tremens.

ENCÉPHALOPATHIE SATURNINE, Encephalopathi'a Saturni'na, from εγκεφαλος, 'the encephalon,' παθος, 'disease,' and saturnus, 'lead.' Encephalic disorder occasioned by the poison of lead.

ENCEPHALOPHY'MATA, Phymato'ses seu Strumo'ses seu Tuber'cula cer'ebri. Tubercles of the brain.

ENCEPHALOPHTHISIS, see Encephalopyosis.

ENCEPHALOPYO'SIS, from εγκεφαλος, 'the brain,' and πυον, 'pus.' Aposte'ma seu Absces'sus seu Helco'sis cer'ebri. Suppuration of the brain. When accompanied with emaciation and hectic, it is called Encephalopthi'sis.

ENCEPHALORRHAGIA, see Apoplexy.
ENCEPHALOSCOPIA, Craniology.
ENCEPHALOSEPSIS, Mollities cerebri.
ENCEPHALOSIS OF THE LIVER, Hepatoscirrhus.

ENCEPHALOSISMUS, Concussion of the brain.

ENCEPHALOSTRUMOSIS, see Hydrocephalus internus.

ENCEPHALUM, Encephalon.
ENCEPHALUS OPISTHIUS, Cerebellum.
ENCEROSIS, Inceration.
ENCHARAXIS, Scarification.

ENCHEIRE'SIS, Enchire'sis, Enchei'ria, from εν, and χειρ, 'the hand.' Galen uses this term as a part of the title to one of his works, which treats of dissection. It means the manual treatment of any subject.

ENCHEIRIA, Encheiresis.
ENCHIFRÈNEMENT, Coryza.
ENCHIRESIS, Encheiresis.
ENCHONDROMA, Chondroma.
ENCHORIONOSUS, Endemic.
ENCHORIOS, Endemic.
ENCHRISTON, Liniment.
ENCHYLOSIS, Extraction.
ENCHYMA, Infusum, Plethora.

ENCHYMO'MA, Enchymo'sis, from εν, and χυω, 'I pour.' By the ancients, this word was used to designate the sudden effusion of blood into the cutaneous vessels which arises from joy, anger, or shame; in the last instance constituting blushing. It differs from enchymosis in there being, in the latter, extravasation of blood into the areolar texture, and its being produced by an external cause; a contusion, for example. — Hippocrates.

ENCHYSIS, Infusion.

ENCLAVÉE, Wedged.
ENCLAVEMENT, see Wedged.
ENCLUME, Incus.

ENCLYDAS'TICOS, intus fluc'tuans, from εγκλυδαζομαι, 'to float in.' Applied to liquids, e. g. to serum, pus, &c., contained in any cavity.

ENCLYSMA, Clyster, Enema.

ENCŒ'LIA, from εν, 'in,' and κοιλια, 'the belly.' The abdominal viscera. The entrails.

ENCŒLIALGIA, Tormina—e. Inflammatoria, Enceelitis.

ENCŒLI'TIS, Encœlii'tis, Encælialg"ia inflammato'ria, Inflamma'tio abdomina'lis, from εγκοιλια, 'the abdominal contents,' and itis, inflammation. Inflammation of any of the abdominal viscera.

ENCOLPIS'MUS, from εν, 'in,' and κολπος, 'the vagina.' Injection or introduction of any thing into the vagina.

ENCOPE, Diacope, Incision.
ENCRANION, Cerebellum.
ENCRANIS, Cerebellum.
ENCRE, Atramentum.
ENCYESIS, Fecundation, Pregnancy.
ENCYMON, Pregnancy.
ENCYMOSIA, Fecundation, Pregnancy.
ENCYSIS, Pregnancy.

ENCYST'ED, Cystidē obduc'tus, Sacca'tus, Saccula'tus, Sac'cated, Sac'culated, Pouched. Enclosed in a kyst or cyst, or pouch; from εν, 'in,' and κυστις, 'bladder.' (F.) Enkysté. An epithet given to certain tumours, or solid or fluid collections enclosed in a particular envelope or cyst. They are movable and often elastic to the touch.

ENCYS'TIS, Tumor tunica'tus, T. cys'ticus, Emphy'ma encys'tis. Same etymon. Lu'pia, Glan'dula Avicen'næ, Nodus. An encysted tumour.

ENDAN'GIUM; properly Endangi'on, from ενδον, 'within,' and αγγειον, 'a vessel.' The serous or lining membrane of vessels.

ENDEICTICOS, Indicant.

ENDEIXIOL"OGY, Endeixiolog"ia from ενδειξις, 'indication,' and λογος, 'a discourse.' The doctrine of indications.

ENDEIXIS, Indication.
ENDEMIA, Endemic.

ENDEM'IC, Endem'ical, Ende'mia, Regiona'lis morbus, Endem'icus, from εν, 'in,' and δημος, 'the people;' Encho'rios, Enchorion'osus, Vernac'ulus seu Endemius mor'bus, Endemy. A disease is said to be endemic, or to arise from endemic"ity, (F.) endémicité, when it is owing to some peculiarity in a situation or locality. Thus, ague is endemic in marshy countries; goître at the base of lofty mountains, &c. Some authors use the term in the same sense as epidemic. We have no accurate knowledge of the emanations or other circumstances which give occasion to endemic affections. We seem to know that some emanation from marshy lands does produce intermittents; but we are ignorant of the nature of such emanation.

ENDÉMICITÉ, see Endemic.
ENDEMICITY, see Endemic.

ENDEMIOL'OGY, Endemiolog"ia, from ενδημια, 'an endemic,' and λογος, 'a discourse.' The doctrine of endemic diseases.

ENDEMY, Endemic.
ENDEPIDERMIS, Epithelium.

ENDER'MIC, Ender'micus, Endermat'icus, Emplas'tro-endermic, from εν, 'in,' and δερμα, 'the skin.' An epithet given to the method of treating diseases by placing the therapeutical agent in contact with the skin, especially after the cuticle has been removed; Endermism, Endermis'mus, Endermo'sis, Meth'odus ender'mica seu en-

dermat'ica. Morphia, strychnia, &c., are often administered in this way.

ENDERMIS, see Endermic.

ENDERMISMUS, see Endermic.

ENDERMOSIS, see Endermic.

EN'DESIS, from *εν*, 'in,' and *δεω*, 'I bind.' A ligature, bandage, connexion. Hippocrates has so termed the ankle-joint.

ENDIVE, Cichorium endivia—e. Wild, Cichorium intybus.

ENDIVIA, Cichorium endivia.

ENDIXIS, Indication.

ENDO, from *ενδον*, 'within.' A common prefix, as in the following terms:

ENDO-AORTI'TIS, from *ενδον*, 'within,' and *aortitis*, 'inflammation of the aorta.' Inflammation of the lining membrane of the aorta.

ENDO-ARTERITIS, see Arteritis.

ENDOCAR'DIAC, *Endocar'dial, Endocardi'acus*: same etymon as the next. Relating to the endocardium, or to the interior of the heart; as '*endocardiac* sound or murmur,'—a sound produced within the cavities of the heart, in contradistinction to *exocardiac* or *exocardial* sounds or murmurs, which are induced by conditions of the external surface of the organ.

ENDOCARDI'TIS, *Cardi'tis inter'na, Inflamma'tio superfic"iei inter'næ cordis, Inter'nal Carditis, Inflamma'tion of the internal membrane of the heart*, from *Endocard'ium*, the lining membrane of the heart, and *itis*, inflammation. In this disease, the heart's action is visibly increased, and very manifest to the touch; the hand is strongly repelled, and, at moments, is sensible of a trembling vibratory motion. Percussion gives a dull sound over a surface of several inches, owing, according to Bouillaud, to the inflammatory turgescence of the heart, and the engorged state of its cavities. On auscultation a *bruit de soufflet* is generally heard, masking one or both sounds of the heart; and the ear is sensible of a metallic ringing with each systole of the ventricle. The pulsations are rapid as well as strong, and, with few exceptions, irregular, unequal and intermittent. The pulse, by the way, does not always indicate the force or number of the heart's contractions.

ENDOCAR'DIUM, from *ενδον*, 'within,' and *καρδια*, 'the heart.' The membrane that lines the interior of the heart.

ENDOCHORION, see Chorion.

ENDOCOLITIS, Dysentery.

ENDODONTI'TIS, (F.) *Inflammation de la Pulpe dentaire, Inflammation of the Dental membrane*, from *ενδον*, 'within,' *οδους*, 'a tooth,' and *itis*, denoting inflammation. Inflammation of the lining membrane of a tooth.

ENDO-ENTERITIS, see Enteritis.

ENDOGASTRI'TIS, *Esogastri'tis;* from *ενδον*, 'within,' and *gastritis*, 'inflammation of the stomach.' Inflammation of the lining membrane of the stomach.

ENDOGEN, see Endogenous.

ENDOG"ENOUS; from *ενδον*, 'within,' and *γενναω*, 'I engender.' A term first applied to plants—hence called *End'ogens*—in which the new woody matter is deposited within the old and towards the centre. In the animal, cells are often formed *endogenously*, or within the cells, as in the case of the sperm vesicles.

ENDOLYMPH, *Vitrine auditive.*

ENDOMETRI'TIS, from *ενδον*, 'within,' and *metritis*, 'inflammation of the uterus.' Inflammation of the lining membrane of the uterus.

ENDONARTERITIS, see Arteritis.

ENDOSIS, Remission.

ENDO-SKELETON, see Skeleton.

ENDOSMOSE, *Endosmo'sis, Imbibit"io, Imbibit"ion*, from *ενδον*, 'within,' and *ωσις*, 'impulse.' A term used by Dutrochet, to express the action by which fluids pass from without to within organic membranes. The action of two fluids on each other, when separated by a membrane. The general conditions of the phenomena are:—*first*, that they should have an affinity for the interposed membrane; and *secondly*, that they should have an affinity for each other, and be miscible.

At the present day, *endosmose* is generally used to signify the passage of the more transmissible fluid, whilst *exosmose* signifies that of the least transmissible. The rapidity with which endosmose is accomplished varies according to the nature of the septum or tissue and of the penetrating body, and to the penetrability of the tissue.

ENDOSMOT'IC, *Endosmot'icus;* same etymon. Belonging to endosmose:—as an '*endosmotic* current.'

ENDOSTEI'TIS, from *ενδον*, 'within,' *οστεον*, 'a bone,' and *itis*, denoting inflammation. Inflammation of the internal periosteum.

ENDOSTEUM, Medullary membrane.

ENDOÜTERITIS, see Metritis.

ENDUIT (F.), from *induere*, 'to put upon,' 'to put on.' A *coat;* a *fur*. This term is often applied to a layer of greater or less thickness which covers the surface of certain organs, and particularly of the tongue and the interior of the mouth. The *enduit* is designated variously, according to its appearance,—*enduit bilieux, jaune, blanc*, &c.—a *bilious, yellow, white coat* or *fur*, &c. It is at times owing to the evaporation of the watery portions of the secretions; at others, to a morbid condition of the secretions:—generally, to both causes combined.

ENDUIT CHOROIDIEN, see Choroid.

ENDURCISSEMENT, Induration—*e. du Cerveau*, Sclerencephalia—*e. Rouge*, see Hepatization—*e. du Cœur, Cardiosclérosie*—*e. du Tissu cellulaire*, Induration of the cellular tissue.

ENDYMA VENTRICULORUM, Ependyma ventriculorum.

ENECHEMA, Tinnitus aurium.

ENECIA, Synocha—e. Cauma, Synocha—e. Synochus Puerperarum, see Peritonitis—e. Synochus, Synochus.

EN'EMA, from *ενιημι*, (*εν*, and *ιημι*,) 'to inject.' *Clyema, Clyesmus, Enclys'ma, Lavamen'tum, Lo'tio*. An *Injection, Clyster*, (F.) *Clystère, Lavement*. A well-known form of conveying medicine into the intestinal canal. See Clyster.

ENEMA ANOD'YNUM, *Enema O'pii; An'odyne Clyster, Starch and Opium Clyster*. (*Gelat. amyli* Oss, *tinct. opii* gtt. 40 vel 60.) Exhibited in cases of severe diarrhœa or dysentery.

ENEMA CATHAR'TICUM; *Purging Clyster*. (*Mannæ* ℥j, *decoct. chamæm. comp.* ℥x, *olei oliv.* ℥j, *sulph. magnes.* ℥ss. Ph. D.)

ENEMA COMMU'NE; *Common Clyster, Domestic Clyster*. (*Water gruel, or molasses and water* Oss or Oj; *add a little oil or lard, and a spoonful of common salt*.) Given as a cathartic enema; and, without the common salt, as an emollient.

ENEMA FŒT'IDUM, *Fetid Clyster; Mis'tura asafœt'ida pro clys'mate, Clysma ton'icum et antispasmod'icum seu in'citans et sedans*, (F.) *Lavement antispasmodique*. (*The last, with the addition of* ℥j *of the tincture of asafœtida*. Ph. D.) Given as an antispasmodic and anodyne.

ENEMA NICOTIA'NÆ; *Tobac'co Clyster*. This generally consists of from half a pint to a pint of the *Infusum Tabaci*. It is employed in cases of strangulated hernia; but occasionally acts as a fatal poison when given in this way. The smoke *of tobacco* is sometimes thrown up the rectum to produce the same medicinal effects as the infusion.

ENEMA OPII, E. anodynum.

ENEMA TEREBIN'THINÆ; *Tur'pentine Clyster.* (*Ol. tereb.* f℥iij, *gruel* Oss, *one yolk of egg.*) Incorporate the turpentine with the yolk, then add the gruel.) To be administered in cases of ascarides, (*oxyures.*)

ENEPIDERM'IC, *Enepider'micus*, from εν, 'in,' επι, 'upon,' and δερμα, 'the skin.' An epithet given to the method of treating diseases, which consists in the application of medicines; as plasters, blisters, &c., to the skin.

ENEREISIS, Compression.

ENERGIA, Action, Force.

EN'ERGY, *Energi'a,* from ενεργεω, (εν, and εργον, 'action,') 'I act.' Action. Acting power. Also, vigour; as the '*muscular energy;*' the '*brain acts with energy.*'

ENERVATIO, Aponeurosis, Enervation.

ENERVA'TION, *Enerva'tio*, from *e*, 'out of,' and *nervus*, 'strength.' The act of weakening—the state of being weakened. See Debility.

ENERVATIONES TENDINEÆ, Inscriptiones tendineæ musculorum.

ENERVITAS, Inertia.

ENFANCE, Infancy.

ENFANT, Infans—*e. à Terme*, see Fœtus—*e. Légitime*, see Legitimate.

ENFLURE, Swelling, Œdema—*e. des Jambes et des cuisses de la femme accouchée*, Phlegmatia dolens.

ENFONCEMENT SCAPHOÏDE, Scaphoides fossa.

ENGASTERION, Laboratory.

ENGASTRIMISME, see Engastrimyth.

ENGASTRIMYSME, see Engastrimyth.

ENGAS'TRIMYTH; *Engastrimy'thus*, Englottogas'tor, Gastril'oquus, Ventril'oquus, Gastril'oquist, Eu'rycles, Eurycli'tus, Enteroman'tis, Gastroman'tis, from εν, 'in,' γαστηρ, 'the belly,' and μυθεομαι, 'I discourse.' A *Ventril'oquist.* (F.) *Ventriloque, Gastriloque.* One who possesses the art of modifying his natural voice, so that it seems to come from a greater- or less distance, and from different directions. It was formerly believed that such persons spoke from the belly; hence their name. It is an imitative art, and is called VENTRILOQUISM. (F.) *Engastrimisme, Engastrimysme.*

ENGEISOMA, Engisoma.

ENGELURE, Chilblain.

ENGHIEN MONTMORENCY, MINERAL WATERS OF. A hydrosulphurous water, four leagues from Paris, near Montmorency, which is possessed of some celebrity. It contains chloride of sodium, chloride of magnesium, sulphate of magnesia, sulphate of lime, carbonate of magnesia, carbonate of lime, silica, sulphohydrate of lime and magnesia, sulphohydric acid, carbonic acid and azote.

ENGISO'MA, *Engeiso'ma*, *Engizo'ma*, from εγγιζω, 'I approximate.' (F.) *Embarrure.* A species of fracture of the skull, in which a splinter passes beneath the sound portion of the bone, and compresses the brain.—Galen. Also, a kind of instrument used in fractures of the clavicle.

ENGLISH DISEASE, Rachitis.

ENGLOTTOGASTOR, Engastrimyth.

ENGOMPHOSIS, Gomphosis.

ENGORGEMENT, from *en*, 'in,' and *gorge*, 'the throat.' An obstruction occurring in the vessels of a part, giving rise to augmentation of volume. Congestion.

ENGORGEMENT DES MEMBRES ABDOMINAUX À LA SUITE DES COUCHES, Phlegmasia dolens—*e.* Hepatic, Hepatohæmia—*e. Laiteux des membres abdominaux*, Phlegmatia dolens.

ENGOUEMENT (F.), *Obstruc'tio, Iner'tia*, from *angere*, 'to choke.' Accumulation in a hollow organ, of the matters secreted by it or carried into it. There is said to be *Engouement des bronches*, when the mucus accumulates in the bronchia; and *Engouement des intestins*, when the matters which ought to pass through the intestines are detained; as in a case of strangulated hernia.

ENGOUEMENT DES POUMONS, *E. of the lungs*, in Pathological Anatomy, signifies that state of the lungs, in which a mixture of air and thin fluid escapes from them when cut into.

ENGOURDISSEMENT, Torpor.

ENGRENURE, Suture.

ENHÆMATOSIS, Hæmatosis.

ENIXA, Puerpera.

ENIXIO FŒTUS, Parturition.

ENIXUS FŒTUS, Parturition.

ENKYSTÉ, Encysted.

ENKYSTEMENT, Chatonnement.

ENNEAPHAR'MACOS, from εννεα, 'nine,' and φαρμακον, 'a medicine.' A medicine, composed of nine simple ingredients. A pessary, so formed.—Galen, Paulus. The *Antid'otus Heracli'dis*, described by Galen, and some plasters by Aëtius and Celsus, are, likewise, termed *Enneapharmaca.*—Gorræus.

ENOR'MON, ενορμων, *Hormon, Im'petum fa'ciens*, from εν, 'in,' and ορμαω, 'I rouse, excite.' A word used by Hippocrates in the same sense as *vital principle* is by modern physiologists.

ENOSIS, Insertion.

ENOSTOSIS, *Entosto'sis*, from εν, 'in,' and οστεον, 'a bone.' A morbid growth of bone inwards—the opposite to exostosis.

ENRYTH'MOS, from εν, and ρυθμος, 'number.' Having rhythm. An epithet applied to the pulse when its pulsations occur with some degree of order. It is opposed to *Aryth'mos*, and differs from *Eurythmos*, which signifies 'regular.'

ENROUEMENT, Raucedo.

ENS. A being. Paracelsus meant, by this term, the power exerted by certain beings on our body. He speaks of the *Ens Dei*, the *Ens Astro'rum*, the *Ens natura'lë*, the *Ens virtu'tis*, *Ens morbo'rum*, *Ens de poten'tibus spirit'ibus*, &c. These absurd denominations suggested to some of the ancient chymists a name for certain chemical preparations. The muriate of ammonia and iron was called *Ens martis;* the muriate of ammonia and copper, *Ens veneris;* and *Ens primum* was, with the alchymists, the name of a tincture which they considered possessed of the power of transmuting metals.

ENS MARTIS, Ferrum ammoniatum—*e.* Veneris Boylei, Ferrum ammoniatum.

EN'SIFORM, *Ensifor'mis*, from *ensis*, 'a sword,' and *forma*, 'form.' Sword-like.

ENSIFORM APOPH'YSES or PROC'ESSES are the lesser alæ of the sphenoid bone.

ENSIFORM APPEN'DIX or CAR'TILAGE is the xiphoid appendix of the sternum, &c. See Xiphoid.

ENSIFORMIS, Xiphoid.

ENSI-STERNAL. Relating to the ensiform process of the sternum. Béclard gave this name to the last osseous portion of the sternum. He also called it *l'os ultimi-sternal.* See Ultimosternal.

ENSOMATOSIS, Incorporation.

ENSTALAX'IS, Instillation.

EN'STROPHE, from εν, 'in,' and στροφη, 'I turn.' Inversion of a part, as of the eyelids.

ENTABLEMENT, Depression.

ENTAILLE (F.), from *en*, 'in,' and *tailler*, 'to cut.' *Excis'io, Ec'copē, Ec'tomē*. A deep wound made by a sharp instrument obliquely. *Entailles* and *Taillades* are, also, used to designate deep scarifications, made for the purpose of producing a speedy *dégorgement* of any tumefied part; such, for example, as are made in the tongue in certain cases of glossitis.

ENTANTHEMA, Eisanthema.

ENTASIA, Tonic spasm—e. Articularis, Contractura — e. Loxia, Torticollis — e. Priapismus, Priapismus—e. Systremma, Cramp—e. Tetanus, Tetanus—e. Tetanus anticus, Emprosthotonos—e. Trismus, Trismus.

ENTASIS, Tonic spasm.

ENTAT'ICUS, *Intensi'vus*, from εντεινω, 'I make tense.' A medicine which excites the venereal appetite.

ENTELIPATHIA, Nymphomania.

ENTELMINTHA, Worms.

ENTENDEMENT, Intellect.

ENTERAD'ENES, from εντερον, 'an intestine,' and αδην, 'a gland.' The mucous glands of the intestines. See Peyeri glandulæ.

ENTERADENOG'RAPHY, *Enteradenogra'phia*, from εντερον, 'intestine,' αδην, 'gland,' and γραφη, 'a description.' A description of the intestinal glands.

ENTERADENOL'OGY, *Enteradenolog"ia*, from εντερον, 'intestine,' αδην, 'gland,' and λογος, 'a treatise.' That part of anatomy which treats of the intestinal glands.

ENTERAL'GIA, *Enterodyn'ia*, from εντερον, 'intestine,' and αλγος, 'pain.' Pain in the intestines. Colic.

ENTERALGIA ACUTA, Enteritis — e. Inflammatoria, Enteritis—e. Saturnina, Colica metallica.

ENTERANGEMPHRAXIS, Enterangiemphraxis.

ENTERANGIEMPHRAX'IS, *Enterangemphrax'is*, from εντερον, 'intestine,' αγχω, 'I strangle,' and εμφρασσω, 'I obstruct.' Obstruction of the vessels of the intestines.

ENTERATROPH'IA, *Atroph'ia Intestino'rum*, from εντερον, 'intestine,' and *atrophia*, 'want of nutrition.' Atrophy of the coats of the intestines.

ENTERAUXE, from εντερον, 'intestine,' and αυξη, 'increase.' Hypertrophy of the muscular coat of the intestines.—Fuchs.

ENTERECHE'MA, *Son'itus intestina'lis*. The sound of the movement of the intestines, heard by the stethoscope.

ENTEREC'TASIS, *Dilata'tio Intestino'rum*, from εντερον, 'intestine,' and εκτασις, 'dilatation.' Dilatation of the intestines, as in tympanites.

ENTERELCO'SIS, *Enterhelco'sis, Enterohelco'sis*, from εντερον, 'intestine,' and 'ελκωσις, 'ulceration.' Ulceration of intestines — *Ulcera'tio intestina'lis, Ul'cera intestina'lia*.

ENTERELESIA, Ileus.

ENTERELOSIS, Ileus.

ENTEREMPHRAX'IS, *Infarc'tus Intestino'rum, Incarcera'tio intestino'rum inter'na*, (F.) *Étranglement des Intestins, É. Intestinale*, from εντερον, 'intestine,' and εμφραξις, 'obstruction.' Obstruction of the Intestines from accumulation of fæces or otherwise. Also, Enterangiemphraxis.

ENTEREN'CHYTA, *Enteren'chytes*, from εντερον, 'an intestine,' εν, 'in,' and χεω, 'I pour.' Any surgical instrument for administering injections.—Scultetus.

ENTEREPIPLOCELE, Enteroëpiplocele.

ENTEREPIPLOMPHALOCE'LE, from εντερον, 'intestine,' επιπλοον, 'omentum,' εμφαλος, 'navel,' and κηλη, 'rupture.' Hernia of the umbilicus with protrusion of the omentum and intestine.

ENTERHELCOSIS, Enterelcosis—e. Nervosa, Typhus (abdominal.)

ENTERHYPERTROPH'IA, *Hypertroph'ia intestino'rum*, from εντερον, 'intestine,' and *hypertrophia*, 'excessive nutrition.' Hypertrophy of the coats of the intestines.

ENTER'ICA, from εντερον, 'an intestine.' Diseases affecting the alimentary canal. Order I., Class I. (*Cœliaca*,) of Good. Also, medicines affecting the alimentary canal.

ENTÉRITE FOLLICULEUSE, see Typhus —e. *Typhohémique*, Typhoid fever.

ENTERI'TIS, from εντερον, 'an intestine,' and *itis*, denoting inflammation. Inflammation of the intestines. *Empres'ma Enteritis, Intestino'rum inflamma'tio, Ileo-coli'tis, Chordap'sus, Cauma Enteritis, Enterophlog"ia, Enterophlogo'sis, Co'lica acuta, C. inflammato'ria, Il'eus inflammato'rius, Enteral'gia acu'ta, E. Inflammato'ria, Febris intestino'rum, F. ili'aca inflammato'ria, Enterop'yra*, (F.) *Entérite, Inflammation des Intestins*. The essential symptoms of this disease are:— violent abdominal pain, increased on pressure; with vomiting and inflammatory fever. Enteritis may affect both the peritoneal and the mucous coat of the intestines; and, in violent cases, all the coats may be implicated. The structure of the mucous and peritoneal coats is different; so are their functions in health and disease. The inflammation of the serous coat, *Sero-enteritis*, resembles that of the cellular membrane; the inflammation of the mucous coat that of the skin. The former is usually, therefore, of a more active character. Inflammation of the mucous coat, *Eso-enteri'tis, Endo-enteri'tis, Muco-enteri'tis, Mucous Enteritis, Phlegmymeni'tis enter'ica*, is generally attended with diarrhœa, and its pathology is identical with that of dysentery. Inflammation of the peritoneal coat is, on the other hand, generally attended with constipation.

Enteritis of the peritoneal coat, for such usually is the meaning of the word in the abstract, requires the most active treatment. Copious bleeding, followed up by a large dose of opium — and, if the symptoms be not decidedly ameliorated, repeating the bleeding and opium—warm fomentations, and blisters, are the chief agents to be relied upon. Purgatives ought not to be exhibited until the inflammation and spasm are abated by the use of the bleeding and opium. When the physician is called early, this plan will usually succeed. Sometimes, Enteritis passes into a chronic state, requiring much careful management. Broussais considered inflammation of the mucous coat of the stomach and intestines as the proximate cause of the phenomena of fever.

ENTERITIS ARTHRITICA, Cœliagra — e. Colica, Colitis — e. Epiploitis, Epiploitis — e. Follicular, Typhoid fever — e. Folliculosa, see Typhoid — e. Mesenterica, Mesenteritis—e. Mucous, see Enteritis—e. Pustulosa, Dothinenteritis.

ENTERO, from εντερον, 'an intestine,' in compound words signifies intestine, as in the following:—

ENTEROBRO'SIS, *Enterorrhex'is, Perfora'tio Intestino'rum*, (F.) *Perforation des Intestins*, from εντερον, 'an intestine,' and βρωσις, 'the act of gnawing.' Perforation of the intestines.

ENTEROC'ACE, *Dysente'ria pu'trida* seu *typho'des* seu *scorbu'tica* seu *malig'na*, from εντερον, 'an intestine,' and κακος, 'evil.' Adynamic dysentery, accompanied by phenomena indicating a pseudo-membranous and gangrenous state of the lining membrane of the large intestine.

ENTEROCE'LE, *Hernia intestina'lis*, from εντερον, 'an intestine,' and κηλη, 'a hernia,' 'tumour.' Abdominal hernia, which contains only a portion of intestine, is so called.

ENTERO - CEPHALOPYRA INFANTUM, Hydrocephalus Internus.

ENTEROCŒ'LICUS, from εντερον, 'intestine,' and κοιλια, 'the cavity of the abdomen.' Relating to the cavity of the abdomen.

ENTEROCYSTOCE'LE, from εντερον, 'an intestine,' κυστις, 'a bladder,' and κηλη, 'a tumour.' Hernia formed by the bladder and a portion of intestine.

ENTERODAR'SIS, from εντερον, 'intestine,' and δαρσις, 'skinning.' Excoriation of the mucous membrane of the intestines.

ENTERODOTHIENIA, Dothinenteritis.

ENTERODYNIA, Enteralgia.

ENTERO-EPIPLOCE'LE, *Enterepiploce'lē, Her'nia intestina'lis omenta'lis*, from εντερον, 'intestine,' επιπλοον, 'the omentum,' and κηλη, 'tumour.' Hernia, formed by intestine and omentum.

ENTERO-EPIPLOM'PHALUS, from εντερον, 'intestine,' επιπλοον, 'the omentum,' and ομφαλος, 'the umbilicus.' Umbilical hernia, containing intestine and omentum. Almost all umbilical herniæ are of this kind.

ENTEROG'RAPHY, *Enterogra'phia*, from εντερον, 'intestine,' and γραφη, 'description.' The part of anatomy which describes the intestines.

ENTERO-HÆMORRHAGIA, Hæmatochezia.

ENTEROHELCOSIS, Enterelcosis.

ENTERO-HYDROCE'LE, from εντερον, 'intestine,' υδωρ, 'water,' and κηλη, 'tumour.' Intestinal hernia complicated with hydrocele.

ENTERO-HYDROM'PHALUS, from εντερον, 'intestine,' υδωρ, 'water,' and ομφαλος, 'the navel.' Umbilical hernia, in which the sac contains, along with a portion of intestine, a quantity of serum.

ENTERO-ISCHIOCE'LE, from εντερον, 'intestine,' ισχιον, 'ischium,' and κηλη, 'tumour.' *Ischiat'ic hernia*, formed of intestine.

ENTEROLITHI'ASIS, from εντερον, 'intestine,' and λιθιασις, 'the formation of stone.' The formation of concretions in the intestines.

ENTEROLITHUS, Calculi of the stomach and intestines — e. Bezoardus, Bezoar — e. Scybalum, Scybala.

ENTEROL'OGY, *Enterolog''ia*, from εντερον, 'intestine,' and λογος, 'a discourse.' The part of anatomy which treats of the intestines.

ENTEROMALA'CIA, *Enteromalax'is*, (F.) *Ramollissement de l'Intestin*, from εντερον, 'an intestine,' and μαλασσω, 'I soften.' Softening of the mucous or other coats of the intestine.

ENTEROMALAXIS, Enteromalacia.

ENTEROMANTIS, Engastrimyth.

ENTERO-MEROCE'LE, from εντερον, 'intestine,' μηρος, 'the thigh,' and κηλη, 'tumour.' Crural hernia, formed of intestine.

ENTERO-MESENTER'IC, *Entero-mesenter'icus*. Relating to the intestine and mesentery.

ENTERO-MESENTER'ICA FEBRIS. MM. Petit and Serres have given this name to the typhoid form of adynamic fever, in which the intestines are ulcerated, with enlargement of the corresponding mesenteric glands. See Typhus.

ENTÉRO-MÉSENTÉRITE, *Tabes mesenterica*—e. *Mésentérite typhoïde*, see Typhus.

ENTEROMOR'PHIA COMPRES'SA. One of the algæ, used by the Sandwich Islanders as an esculent.

ENTEROMPHALOCELE, Enteromphalus.

ENTEROM'PHALUS, *Enterompl.aloce'lē*, from εντερον, 'intestine,' and ομφαλος, 'umbilicus.' Umbilical hernia, formed of intestine.

ENTEROMYCODORI'TIS, from εντερον, 'intestine,' μυκος, 'slime,' δορα, 'skin,' and *itis*, denoting inflammation. Inflammation of the mucous membrane of the intestines.

ENTERON, Intestine.

ENTEROPARAL'YSIS, *Enterople'gia, Paral'ysis intestino'rum*, from εντερον, 'intestine,' παραλυσις, 'paralysis.' Paralysis of the Intestines.

ENTEROPARISAGOGE, Intussusceptio.

ENTEROPATHI'A, *Enterop'athy*, from εντερον, 'intestine,' and παθος, 'disease.' Disease of the intestines in general.

ENTEROPATHI'A CANCERO'SA, *Enteroscir'rhus, Enterosteno'sis scirrho'sa* seu *organ'ica, Enterosarco'mia, Indura'tio* seu *Scirrhus* seu *Cancer* seu *Carcino'ma Intestino'rum*, (F.) *Cancer des Intestins*. Cancer of the Intestines.

ENTEROPERIS'TOLE, *Enterosphig'ma, Hernia incarcera'ta, Incarcera'tio intestino'rum*, from εντερον, 'intestine,' and περιστιλλω, 'I contract.' Constriction or obstruction of the intestines, from a cause which acts either within the abdomen, or without it, as in strangulated hernia.

ENTEROPHLOGIA, Enteritis.

ENTEROPHLOGOSIS, Enteritis.

ENTEROPHTHI'SIS, from εντερον, 'intestine,' and φθισις, 'consumption.' Consumption of the bowels. Consumption owing to suppuration in the intestines.

ENTEROPHYMATA, Tubercula intestinorum.

ENTEROPLEGIA, Enteroparalysis.

ENTEROPYRA, Enteritis. Also, entero mesenteric fever.—Alibert.

ENTEROPYRA ASIATICA, Cholera — e. Biliosa, Fever, Bilious.

ENTERORRHAG"IA, from εντερον, 'intestine,' and ραγη. 'violent rupture.' Hemorrhage from the bowels.

ENTERORRHAGIA SIMPLEX, Hæmatochezia.

ENTERORRHA'PHIA, *Enteror'rhaphē*, from εντερον, 'intestine,' and ραφη, 'a suture.' Suture of the intestines, for the relief of injuries done to them.

ENTERORRHEU'MA, *Rheumatis'mus Intestino'rum*, from εντερον, 'intestine,' and ρευμα, 'defluxion, rheumatism.' Rheumatism of the intestines.

ENTERORRHEXIS, Enterobrosis.

ENTERORRHŒA, Diarrhœa, Melæna.

ENTEROSARCOCE'LE, from εντερον, 'intestine,' σαρξ, 'flesh,' and κηλη, 'a tumour.' Intestinal hernia, complicated with fleshy excrescence, or rather sarcocele.

ENTEROSARCOMIA, Enteropathia cancerosa.

ENTEROSCHEOCE'LE, *Enteroschoce'lē*, from εντερον, 'an intestine,' οσχεον, 'the scrotum,' and κηλη, 'tumour.' Scrotal hernia consisting of intestine.

ENTEROSCIRRHUS, Enteropathia cancerosa.

ENTERO'SES, from εντερον, 'an intestine.' A class of diseases, comprehending all those that are seated in the intestines.—Alibert.

ENTEROSPHIGMA, Enteroperistole.

ENTEROSTENO'SIS, from εντερον, 'intestine,' and στενωσις, 'stricture.' Stricture or constriction of the intestines. See Ileus.

ENTEROSTENOSIS VOLVULUS, Ileus — e. Organica, Enteropathia cancerosa — e. Scirrhosa, Enteropathia cancerosa.

ENTÉROTOME, Enterot'omus, from *εντερον*, 'intestine,' and *τεμνω*, 'I cut.' A name given by J. Cloquet to an instrument for promptly opening the intestinal canal through its whole extent. It consists of a pair of scissors, one blade of which is much longer than the other, and rounded at its extremity. This is passed into the intestine.

ENTEROTOM'IA, *Enterot'omy*, same etymon. In *anatomy*, it signifies dissection of the intestines. In *surgery*, it means an operation, little used, which consists in opening the intestines, in order to evacuate the fæcal matters accumulated in it; for example, in certain cases of hernia, accompanied with contraction of the intestinal canal; in operations for an artificial anus, performed on the new-born, where the rectum is imperforate or not existing, &c.

ENTEROTOMY, Enterotomia.
ENTEROTYPHUS, see Typhus.
ENTEROZOA, Worms.
ENTERYDROCE'LE, *Enterohydroce'lē*, from *εντερον*, 'intestine,' *ύδωρ*, 'water,' and *κηλη*, 'rupture.' Intestinal hernia with hydrocele.
ENTHELMINTHES, Worms.
ENTHEOMANIA, Demonomania.
ENTHLA'SIS, *Esphla'sis*, from *εν*, 'in,' and *θλαω*, 'I break.' A fracture of the cranium, with comminution, in which the bone is depressed, or has lost its level.

ENTHLASIS CRANII, Effractura Cranii.
ENTITÉ, Entity.
EN'TITY, *En'titas*, (F.) *Entité*, from *ens, entis*, 'a being.' The being or essence of anything. It has been used somewhat vaguely, in modern French medicine more especially, to signify apparently a general or essential disease, the nature and seat of which cannot be determined. — Nysten.

ENTOCELE, Ectopia.
ENTOCE'LE LENTIS. Dislocation of the crystalline into the anterior chamber of the eye.
ENTOGONYAN'CON, from *εντος*, 'within,' *γονυ*, 'the knee,' and *αγκων*, 'a bend.' Bending of the knees inwards. The state of being knock-kneed, or in-kneed.
ENTOHYALOID MUSCÆ, see Metamorphopsia.
ENTONIA, Tension, Tonic spasm.
ENTONIC, *Enton'icus*, from *εν*, denoting excess, and *τονος*, 'tone.' Having great tension or exaggerated action.
ENTONNOIR, Calix, Infundibulum — *e. du Ventricule Moyen du Cerveau*, Infundibulum of the brain.
ENTOPARASITES, Worms.
• ENTOPHTHAL'MIA, from *εντος*, 'within,' and *οφθαλμια*, 'inflammation of the eye.' Ophthalmia affecting the interior of the eye.
EN'TOPHYTE, *Entoph'yton*, from *εντος*, 'within,' and *φυτον*, 'a vegetable.' A vegetable parasite.
ENTOPHYT'IC, *Entophyt'icus*, same etymon. Of or belonging to an entophyte, — as 'an entophytic growth.'
ENTORSE, Sprain.
ENTOSTHETHIDIA, Entrails.
ENTOSTHIA, Entrails.
ENTOSTOSIS, Enostosis.
ENTOTORRHŒA, Otirrhœa.
ENTOTOZÆNA, Ozena.
ENTOXICISMUS, Poisoning.
ENTOXISMUS, Poisoning.
ENTOZOA, Worms.
ENTOZOAIRES, Worms.

ENTOZOARIA, Worms.
ENTOZOOGENESIS, Helminthiasis.
ENTOZOON FOLLICULORUM, Acarus Folliculorum.
ENTRAILLES, Entrails.
EN'TRAILS, *Splanchna, Encœ'lia, Viscera, Entosthid'ia, Entos'thia, Entosthethid'ia, Intera'nea*, from *enteralia*, a word of bad Latin, coming from *εντερον*, 'intestine.' It is used for the viscera enclosed in the splanchnic cavities, and especially for those in the abdomen; *Bowels, Guts*, (F.) *Entrailles, Viscères.*
ENTRE-FESSON, Chafing.
ENTRICHO'MA, from *εν*, 'in,' and *τριχωμα*, 'hair.' The tarsal cartilage, and the edge of the eyelids, in which the cilia are implanted.
ENTROP'ION, *Entrop'ium*, from *εν*, 'in,' and *τρεπω*, 'I turn.' *Inver'sio palpebra'rum, Capillit''ium, Trichi'asis, Introsuscep'tio entropium, Blepharelo'sis, Blepharopto'sis entropium, Tri'chia, Tricho'sis.* A name given to the inversion or turning inwards of the eyelids, so that the eyelashes are directed towards the globe of the eye; irritate and inflame it, and give rise to the affection called *Trichi'asis.*

The contact of the hair with the surface of the eye occasions considerable irritation of the conjunctiva, which is soon followed by chemosis, ulceration of the eye, and other symptoms, such as fever, watchfulness, &c.

If the disease be *entropion*, as above defined, that is, dependent upon the inversion of the eyelids, it must be remedied, — either by dispersing the œdema or swelling of the eyelids, or by cutting out a portion of the skin. When the disease is dependent on a vicious direction of the cilia, they must be plucked out and the bulbs be cauterized.

ENTROPIUM, Entropion.
ENTYPOSIS, see Glene.
ENUCLEA'TION, *Enuclea'tio*, from *enuclcare*, (*e*, and *nucleus*,) 'to take out a kernel.' This term has been proposed for the operation of removing tumours, &c., without cutting into them. — Percy.

The word is used in *Pharmacy*, for the operation of shelling or removing the kernels of any nut.

ENULA CAMPANA, Inula Helenium.
ENU'LON, from *εν*, 'in,' and *ουλον*, 'the gum.' The inner part of the gums. The external part was called *ουλον*, and that between the teeth *αρμος.* — Pollux.

ENURE'SIS, from *ενουρεω*, (*εν*, and *ουρεω*,) 'I void the urine in bed.' *Paru'ria iucon'tinens, Incontinen'tia uri'næ, Excre'tio Urinæ involunta'ria, Mic'tio involunta'ria, E. inopportu'sa, Uracra'tia, Urorrhœ'a, Perirrhœ'a, Strangu'ria,* (Galen,) *Aniachu'ria, Hyperure'sis, Diam'nes, Involuntary discharge of urine, Incontinence of urine.* This affection is most common in advanced life. It may depend on too great irritability of the bladder, or on distension, or injury of the fibres about its neck, paralysis of the organ, *Cysto-paral'ysis, Cysto-ple'gia*, the presence of an irregularly shaped calculus impacted in the urethra near its commencement; rupture of the bladder and urethra; renal disease; or on pressure exerted on the bladder by the distended womb or by a tumour. It often occurs after difficult labour, but generally yields, in the course of a week or ten days; the catheter being introduced twice a day in the mean time.

The treatment must of course vary according to the cause; and when the affection, on which it is dependent, cannot be removed, the discharge of urine may be prevented by exerting a degree of compression on the urethra, by means of appropriate instruments; or a urinal may be employed to receive the urine as it passes off.

ENVIE, Hangnail, Malacia, Nævus — e. de Vomir, Nausea.

ENYPNION, Somnium.

ENYSTRON, Abomasus.

ENZOÖTIA, Enzooty.

ENZOÖTY, *Enzoöt'ia*, (F.) *Enzoötie*, from εν, 'in,' and ζωον, 'animal.' An endemic disease attacking animals.

EP, EPH, EPI, επ, εφ, επι, 'upon, above;' in composition, generally means, 'augmentation, addition, increase, reciprocal action, repetition.' Hence:

EPACMAS'TICOS, from επι, and ακμαζω, 'I increase.' An epithet applied to fevers, *Febres epacmas'ticæ*, whose symptoms go on augmenting in violence, from the commencement to the termination. Such fevers are, also, called *Epanadidon'tes*.

EPAGOGIUM, Phimosis, Prepuce.

EPANADIPLOSIS, Anadiplosis.

EPANALEPSIS, Anadiplosis.

EPANASTASIS, Pustule. The formation of a tumour. The breaking out of an eruption — *Erup'tio exanthe'matis*.

EPANASTEMA, Exanthem, Swelling.

ÉPANCHEMENT, Effusion.

EPANESIS, Remission.

EPANETUS, Remittent — e. Hectica, Hectic fever — e. Malignus flavus, Fever, yellow — e. Mitis, Remittent fever.

EPANORTHOSIS, Restauratio.

EPANTHEMA, Exanthem.

EPANTHISMA, Exanthem.

EPAPHÆ'RESIS, from επαφαιρεω, 'I take away.' *Repeti'ta subla'tio* vel *evacua'tio*. A repeated abstraction or evacuation. It was formerly used synonymously with *repeated bloodletting; Phlebotom'ia itera'ta*.—Galen.

EPAPHRISMOS, Despumation.

EPARMA, Tumour.

EPARSIS, Tumour.

ÉPAULE, Humerus.

EPENCRANIS, Cerebellum.

EPENDYMA, Membrane.

EPEN'DYMA VENTRICULO'RUM, *En'dyma* seu *Indumen'tum ventriculo'rum*, from επι, 'upon,' and ενδυω, 'I enter;' hence, ενενδυμα, 'an upper garment or cloak.' The lining membrane of the ventricles of the brain, formed by a prolongation of the pia mater, and probably also of the arachnoid.

ÉPERON, Hippocampus minor — *é. des A téres*, Spur.

ÉPERVIER, Accipiter.

ÉPERVIÈRE DES MURAILLES, Hieracium murorum.

EPHEBÆ'ON, from επι, 'upon,' and 'ηβη, 'pubes.' The parts of generation: also, the region of the pubes, as well as the hair upon the pubes. It meant likewise a part of the ancient gymnasium in which the rhetoricians, philosophers, &c., disputed.

EPHEBEUM, Mons veneris.

EPHE'BIA, *Ephebi'a, Pubertas*. Same etymon. The age of puberty.

EPHEBOSYNE, Puberty.

EPHEBOTES, Puberty.

ÉPHE'BUS, *Pubens, Puber*, (F.) *Pubère, Éphèbe*. One who has attained the age of puberty.

EPHEDRANA, Nates.

EPHEL'CIS, from επι, 'upon,' and 'ελκος, 'an ulcer.' The crust or scab of an ulcer.

ÉPHÉLIDE SCORBUTIQUE, Chloasma.

EPHE'LIDES, from επι, 'upon,' and 'ηλιος, 'the sun.' *Epichro'sis, Mac'ula sola'ris, Mac'ulæ fuscæ, M. lenticula'res, Ephe'lis lentic'ula, Vitilig''ines, Phaci, Pannus lenticula'ris, Lentic'ula, Lenti'go, Ephelis Lenti'go, Ephelis à solè, Nigre'do à solè, Spilo'sis ephelis, Æsta'tes, Effila, Freckles, Sunburn*, (F.) *Taches de rousseure, Hale*. This term includes not only the yellow *lentigines*, which appear on persons of a fair skin, and the larger brown patches, which also arise from exposure to the direct rays of the sun, but also those large dusky patches which are very similar in appearance, but occur on other parts of the surface, that are constantly covered. See Chloasma. They do not extend farther than the skin. Many cosmetics have been recommended for their removal. Simple spirituous lotions or weak mineral acids, applied a few times in the day, are as effectual as any other means.

EPHELIS, see Ephelides — e. Lentigo, Ephelides — e. à Sole, Ephelides.

EPHELOTES, Leucoma.

EPHEM'ERA, *Dia'ria*, from επι, 'during,' and 'ημερα, 'a day.' That which continues a day. This epithet is given to diseases, and particularly to fevers, which last only a day.—*Febris dia'ria, Ephemerop'yra, Febris simplex, F. Ephe'mera, Febric'ula, Ephem'eral Fever, Di'ary Fever, Simple Fever*. The term *prolonged ephem'era* is sometimes used for fevers, which cease after two or three days' duration.

EPHEMERA ANGLICA PESTILENS, Sudor anglicus — e. Britannica, Sudor Anglicus — e. Maligna, Sudor Anglicus — e. Mortifera, Plague — e. Pestilentialis, Plague — e. Sudatoria, Sudor Anglicus.

EPHEMEROPYRA, Ephemera.

EPHEMERUS, Quotidian.

EPHIALTES HYPOCHONDRIACA, Incubus vigilantium — e. Nocturnus, Incubus — e. Vigilantium, Incubus vigilantium.

EPHIDRO'SES, (G.) *Ephidrosen*. A division of the family Ekzematosen of Fuchs, comprising morbid varieties of sweating.

EPHIDRO'SIS, from επι, 'upon,' and 'ιδρως, 'I sweat.' *Hidro'sis, Idro'sis*. A copious sweat.

EPHIDROSIS PROFU'SA, *E. sponta'nea, E. idiopath'ica, Hydropede'sis, Exsuda'tio, Exsuda'tio, Hyperephidro'sis, Hyperhydro'sis, Hydrorrhœ'a, Hidropede'sis*, (F.) *Flux de Sueur*. An excessive sweating, including debility and emaciation. A colliquative sweat. Such copious perspirations are generally owing to debility of the exhalants, and require the use of tonics, especially of the mineral acids, opium, &c.

EPHIDROSIS, Desudatio — e. Cruenta, Sudor cruentus — e. Saccharata, Sudor dulcis.

EPHIPPIUM, Pituitaria fossa, Sella Turcica.

EPH'ODOS, from επι, 'upon,' and 'οδος, 'a way,' 'a road or avenue to a place.' Hippocrates uses this word in three senses: 1. For the vessels or canals, which give passage to the excrements of the body. 2. For a periodical attack or accession of fever; and 3. For the approach of similar or dissimilar things which may be useful or hurtful to the body.—Castelli.

ÉPI, Spica.

EPI'ALOS, *Hepialos*. A name given by the ancients to fever, when the hot stage was mingled with irregular chills. Also, the cold stage of fever.

EPIALTES, Incubus.

EPIAMA, Lenitive.

EPIAN, Framboesia.

EPIBLEMA, Cataplema.

EPIBOLE, Incubus.

EPICANTHIS, Canthus.

EPICAN'THIS, from επι, 'upon,' and κανθος, 'the angle of the eye.' A defective formation, in which a fold of skin passes from the root of the nose over the inner canthus of the eye.

EPICAR'PIUM, *Pericar'pium,* from επι, 'upon,' and καρπος, 'the wrist.' An application made to the wrists or to the region of the pulse was so called.

EPICAUMA, Encauma.
EPICAUSIS, Encauma.
EPICERASTICA, Emollients.
EPICHOLOS, Bilious.
EPICHORDIS, Mesentery.
EPICHORION, Decidua.
EPICHORIUM, Epidermis.
EPICHRISIS, Inunctio.
EPICHRO'SIS, *Spilo'sis,* from επι, and χρωμα, 'colour.' Simple discoloration of the surface.— Good. Ephelides.

EPICHROSIS SPILI, see Nævus.
EPICHYSIS, Affusion.
EPICŒ'MASIS, from επικοιμαομαι, (επι, and κοιμαομαι,) 'to lie down to rest,' 'to sleep.' *Decu'bitus ad dormien'dum et Dormit"io.* The position of sleeping, as well as sleeping itself.

EPICOL'IC, from επι, 'upon,' and κωλον, 'the colon.' The *epicolic regions, regio'nes epicol'icæ,* are those parts of the abdomen which correspond to the colon.

EPICOLLESIS, Agglutination.
EPICON'DYLE, *Epicon'dylus,* from επι, 'upon,' and κονδυλος, 'a condyle.' A name given, by Chaussier, to an eminence at the outer part of the inferior extremity of the os humeri ; so called, because it is seated above the condyle. The epicondyle gives attachment to the outer lateral ligament of the elbow joint, and to a very strong tendon to which several of the muscles of the posterior part of the forearm are attached.

EPICONDYLO-CUBITALIS, see Anconeus— e. *Radial,* Supinator radii brevis — e. *Sus-métacarpien,* see Radialis — e. *Sus-phalangettien commun,* Extensor digitorum communis—e. *Sus-phalangettien du petit doigt,* Extensor proprius minimi digiti.

EPICOPHO'SIS, from επι, 'upon,' and κωφωσις, 'deafness.' Deafness supervening on another disease.

EPICRA'NIUM, from επι, 'upon,' and κρανιον, 'the cranium.' A name given to different parts seated on the cranium. The skin, aponeurosis between the occipital and frontal muscles, and the whole of the scalp, have been so called. Portal includes under this name the occipito-frontalis muscle, pyramidalis nasi, and superior and anterior auricular muscles. The pericranium.

EPICRANIUS, Occipito-frontalis.
EPICRA'SIS, *Contempera'tio,* from επικεραννυμι, (επι, and κεραννυμι, 'I mix,') 'I temper.' A term used by the humourists for *an amelioration of the humours.* They called *Cure by Epicrasis, —per epicrasin,* a mode of treatment by imagined alteratives, which they supposed to be possessed of the power of gradually correcting the vitiated humours.

EPICROUSIS, Percussion.
EPICTENIUM, Pubes.
EPICTETI MORBI, Acquired diseases.
EPICYEMA, see Superfœtation.
EPICYESIS, Superfœtation.
EPICYLIUM, see Palpebra.
EPICYSTOTOMIA, see Lithotomy.
EPIDEISIS, Deligation.
EPIDEM'IC, *Epide'mius, Epidem'icus,* (F.) *Epidémique.* Same etymon as Epidemy. Appertaining to an epidemy. An epidemy.

EPIDEMIC CONSTITUTION, Epidemy—e. *Disease,* Epidemy—e. *Influence,* see Epidemy.

EPIDEMICITÉ, see Epidemy.
EPIDEMICUS, Epidemy.
EPIDEMIOLOG"IA, from επι, 'upon,' δημος, 'the people,' and λογος, 'a description.' The doctrine of epidemics.

EPIDÉMIQUE, Epidemy.
EPIDEMIUS, Epidemy.
EP'IDEMY, *Epidem'ic, Epide'mia, Morbus pub'licus, M. popula'ris, E. epidem'icus seu epide'mius,* (F.) *Epidémie; Epidem'ic disease, Epidem'ic influence, Epidem'ic constitution;* from επι, 'upon,' and δημος, 'the people.' A disease which attacks at the same time a number of individuals, and which is depending upon some particular *constitutio aeris,* or condition of the atmosphere, with which we are utterly ignorant. It differs from *endemic,* the latter being owing to locality ; but it is obvious, that should a particular epidemic constitution of the air—*epidemic"ity,* (F.) *épidémicité*—exist along with a favouring endemic condition, these combined influences may act in the causation of several of those serious and fatal complaints, which at times visit a district, and are never afterwards met with, or at least not until after the lapse of a considerable period.

EPIDENDRUM VANILLA, see Vanilla.
EPID'ERIS, *Epider'rhis, Hypod'eris, Hypoder'mis, Hypoder'rhis,* from επι, 'upon,' and δερας, 'the skin.' This word, with some, means the nymphæ ; with others, the clitoris ; with others, again, the prepuce of the clitoris.

EPIDERMA, Epidermis.
EPIDERMATIS, Epidermis.
EPIDER'MIC, *Epiderm'icus, Epiderm'al, Epiderma'lis;* same etymon as epidermis. Belonging to the epidermis,—as

EPIDERMIC CELLS, see Cell, epidermic.
EPIDERMIDON'OSI, *Epidermidonu'si,* from επιδερμις, 'epidermis,' and νοσος, 'disease.' Diseases of the epidermis.

EPIDERMION, Epidermis.
EPIDER'MIS, *Epider'mion, Epider'matis, Epider'ma, Epicho'rium, Sum'mitas cutis, Cutic'ula, C. ex'tima, C. extre'ma, Cutis extima, C. summa, C. ul'tima, Pellis summa, Pellic'ula summa, P. supe'rior, Lam'ina prima cutis, Oper'culum cutis,* from επι, 'upon,' and δερμα, 'the true skin.' Scarf-skin, cuticle. (F.) *Surpeau, Cuticule.* A transparent, dry, thin membrane, devoid of nerves and vessels, which covers all the surface of the body, except the parts that correspond to the nails. It appears to consist of minute scales, placed one above the other. Chaussier considers it to be formed and reproduced by an excretory action of the true skin ; to act like a dry varnish, which prevents the immediate contact of bodies with the nervous papillæ, and consequently to deaden tactile impressions, which, without its intervention, might be painful. The *Epider'mic, Epider'meous,* or *Epider'moid* (as Bichat called it) *System,* in general anatomy, comprises three parts. 1. External Epidermis. 2. Epidermis spread over the mucous membranes. 3. The Nails and Hair.

EPIDERMIS LINGUÆ, see Tongue.
EPIDERRHIS, Epideris.
EPIDERRHITIS, Nymphitis.
EPIDESIS, see Bandage—e. *Hæmostasia,* Ligature.

EPIDESMIS, Epidesmus.
EPIDESMUM, Epidesmus.
EPIDES'MUS, *Epides'mis, Epides'mum, Superliga'men,* from επι, 'upon,' and δεω, 'I bind.' A Fascia, bandage or ligature, by which dressings are secured.—Hippocrates.

EPIDID'YMIS, from επι, 'upon,' and διδυμος, 'a testicle.' *Epidid'ymus, Did'ymis, Paras'tata,*

Testic'ulus acceso'rius, Caput testis, Corpus varico'sum seu *varicifor'mě testis, Supergemina'lis,* (F.) *Corpus variqueux* ou *variciforme.* That which is placed upon the testicle. A small, oblong, vermiform, grayish body, lying along the superior margin of the testicle. The Epididymis is a canal, formed by the union of all the seminiferous vessels folded several times upon themselves, after having traversed the *Corpus Highmoria'num.* Its lower portion or tail, *Cauda* vel *globus minor,* is curved upwards, and is continuous with the vas deferens; the opposite extremity is called the head, *globus major.* The length of this canal, folded as it is upon itself and describing numerous curvatures, is, according to Munro, 32 feet.

EPIDIDYMITIS, Parastatitis — e. Blennorrhagic, Hernia humoralis.

EPID'OSIS, from επι, 'upon,' and διδωμι, 'to give.' Augmentation, increase. A word applied to the natural increase of the body, or to the increase of a disease.

EPID'ROME, *Epidrom'ia, Epiph'ora,* from επιδρεμω, (επι, and ὀρεμω,) 'I run upon.' An afflux or congestion of humours.—Galen.

EPIDROMIA, Epidrome.

EPIFAGUS AMERICANUS, Orobanche Virginiana—e. Virginianus, Orobanche Virginiana.

EPIGÆ'A REPENS, *Trailing Ar'butus, Ground Laurel, Mayflower.* A small, trailing plant, of the *Family* Ericaceæ, which grows in sandy woods, or in rocky soil, especially in the shade of pines. Its flowers appear early in spring, and exhale a rich, spicy fragrance. The leaves and stems are prepared and used like uva ursi.

EPIGASTRAL'GIA, from επιγαστριον, 'the epigastrium,' and αλγος, 'pain.' Pain at the epigastrium.

EPIGAS'TRIC, *Epigas'tricus, Epigas'trius,* from επι, 'upon,' and γαστηρ, 'the stomach.' This name has been given to several parts.

EPIGASTRIC AR'TERY, *Arte'ria epigas'trica, A. sus-pubienne,* (Ch.) It arises from the *external iliac,* on a level with the crural arch; sometimes by a trunk proper to it, at others by one common to it and the *Obturator artery.* It ascends upwards and inwards, behind the spermatic cord, follows the outer edge of the rectus abdominis muscle, and anastomoses, towards the umbilicus, with the internal mammary. The epigastric artery anastomoses, also, with the obturator, spermatic, lumbar, and intercostal vessels.

EPIGASTRIC REGION, *Regio epigas'trica, R. cardi'aca, R. stomach'ica, R. stomacha'lis,* is the superior region of the abdomen, comprised between the false ribs on each side, and extending from the lower surface of the diaphragm to two fingers' breadth above the umbilicus. It is divided into three parts, one *middle,* the *epigas'trium,* — and two *lateral,* the *hypochon'dria.*

EPIGASTRIC VEIN follows nearly the same course as the artery.

EPIGASTRICUS, Epigastric.

EPIGAS'TRIUM. Same etymon. The belly; the epigastric region.

EPIGASTRIUS, Epigastric.

EPIGASTROCE'LE, from επι, 'upon,' γαστηρ, 'the stomach,' and κηλη, 'a tumour.' Hernia, formed by the stomach; *Gas'troce'lě.* This name has been given more especially to hernia, which occurs towards the upper part of the linea alba or in the epigastric region, whether formed or not by the stomach.

EPIGENEMA, Epigenesis.

EPIGEN'ESIS, from επι, 'upon,' and γενεσις, 'generation.' A theory of conception, according to which the new being is created entirely anew; and receives at once from each parent the materials necessary for its formation. Also, a new formation.

EPIGENESIS, as well as *Epigene'ma,* or *Epigene'ma,* is, also, applied to any symptom occurring during a disease, without changing its nature. An accessory symptom. *Epiginom'enos, Superve'niens,* has a similar acceptation.

EPIGINOMENOS, see Epigenesis.

EPIGLOT'TIC, *Epiglot'ticus:* same etymon. Relating to the epiglottis.

EPIGLOTTIC GLAND, *Periglot'tis, Caro glandulo'sa.* A collection of small, glandular granula, situate in the adipose, areolar texture at the base of the anterior surface of the epiglottis, in a triangular space, bounded anteriorly by the thyro-hyoid membrane and thyroid cartilage. It pours out an unctuous and mucous fluid, which lubricates the epiglottis, keeps it supple and movable, and prevents the larynx from being irritated by the constant passage of the air, in the act of respiration.

EPIGLOT'TIS, from επι, 'upon,' and γλωττις, 'the glottis.' *Epiglot'tic cartilage, Lig'ula, Oper'culum laryn'gis, Lingua Ex'igua, Lin'gula fis'tulæ, Sublin'guum, Superlig'ula.* A fibro-cartilage, situate at the upper part of the larynx, behind the base of the tongue. Its form is oval; texture elastic; thickness greater below than above, and greater in the middle than at the sides. By its smaller extremity, which is the lower, it is attached to the thyroid cartilage; its two surfaces are covered by the mucous membrane of the pharynx and larynx. The special use of the epiglottis would seem to be to cover the glottis accurately at the moment of deglutition, and, thus, to assist in opposing the passage of alimentary substances into the air tubes.

EPIGLOTTI'TIS, *Inflamma'tio Epiglot'tidis,* (F.) *Inflammation de l'Epiglotte, Angi'na epiglottide'a.* Inflammation of the epiglottis.

EPIGLOT'TUM. An instrument, mentioned by Paracelsus, for raising the eyelids. It resembled the epiglottis in shape.

EPIGLOU'TIS, from επι, 'upon,' and γλουτος, 'the buttocks.' The superior region of the nates.—Gorræus.

EPIGONATIS, Patella.

EPIG'ONĚ, *Gonē, Hypoph'ysis, Progen'ies, Proles, Sob'oles, Sub'oles,* from επι, 'upon,' and γονη, 'sperm.' Offspring. Progeny. Also, Superfœtation.

EPIGONION, Fœtus.

EPIGONIS, Patella.

EPIGONON, Superfœtation.

EPIGOUNIS, Patella.

EPIGUNIS, Patella.

EPILATORIUM, Depilatory.

EPILEMPSIS, Epilepsy.

EPILENTIA, Epilepsy.

EPILEPSIA, Epilepsy — e. Acuta Infantum, Eclampsia — e. Algetica, seo Algos — e. Febrilis infantum, Eclampsia—e. Nocturna, Incubus—e. Puerilis, Eclampsia infantum—e. Saltatoria, Chorea— e. Uterina, Lorind matricis.

ÉPILEPSIE, Epilepsy —e. *Utérine,* Hysteria —e. *Vertige,* see Epilepsia.

EP'ILEPSY, 'ιερη νουσος, σεληναια νουσος, *Epilep'sia, Epilep'sis, Epilemp'sis, Epilen'tia, Syspa'sia Epilepeia, Catalen'tia, Deciden'tia, Pas'sio cadi'va, Morbus comit"ialis, M. cadu'cus, M. Hercu'leus, Heracle'us morbus, M. sacer, M. astra'lis, M. sidera'tus, M. dæmoni'acus, M. Sancti Johan'nis, M. fœdus, Hieran'osus, M. pueri'lis, Deprehen'sio, Clonos epilep'sia, Hieran'osos, Prehen'sio, Perdit"io, Epilep'tica pas'sio, Morbus magnus, M. Major, M. Interlu"nius, M. divi'nus, M. dæmo'nius, M. son'ticus, M. seleni'acus, M.*

lunat'icus, M. mensa'lis, M. deif'icus, M. sceles'-tus, M. vitriola'tus, M. viridel'lus, M. Sancti Valenti'ni, Malum cadu'cum, Analep'sia, Catapto'sis, Insa'nia cadi'va, Apoplex'ia parva, Cadu'ca pas'sio, Lues divi'na, Vit''ium cadu'cum seu divi'num seu *Hercu'leum, Falling sickness,* (F.) *Mal caduc, Mal divin, Mal Saint-Jean, Mal de Terre, Haut-mal.* The word is derived from ετιλαμβανω, 'I seize upon.' It is a disease of the brain, which may either be idiopathic or symptomatic, spontaneous or accidental, and which occurs in paroxysms, with uncertain intervals between. These paroxysms are characterized by loss of sensation and convulsive motions of the muscles. Frequently, the fit attacks suddenly; at other times, it is preceded by indisposition, vertigo, and stupor. At times, before the loss of consciousness occurs, a sensation of a cold vapour is felt, hence called *aura epilep'tica.* This appears to rise in some part of the body, proceeds towards the head; and as soon as it has reached the brain the patient falls down. The ordinary duration of a fit is from 5 to 20 minutes. Sometimes it goes off in a few seconds; at others, it is protracted for hours. In all cases, there is a loss of sensation, sudden falling down, distortion of the eyes and face; countenance of a red, purple or violet colour; grinding of the teeth; foaming at the mouth; convulsions of the limbs; difficult respiration, generally stertorous; with, sometimes, involuntary discharge of fæces and urine. After the fit, the patient retains not the least recollection of what has passed, but remains, for some time, affected with head-ach, stupor, and lassitude.

The disease is in the brain, and is generally organic; but it may be functional and symptomatic of irritation in other parts, as in the stomach, bowels, &c. The prognosis, as to ultimate recovery, is unfavourable. It does not, however, frequently destroy life, but is apt to lead to mental imbecility. Dissection has not thrown light on its pathology.

To the attacks of epilepsy which are unaccompanied by convulsions, as is sometimes the case, the French give the name *Petit-mal,* and *Épilepsie Vertige.* When furious mania succeeds to a paroxysm, it is termed *Mania epileptica* and *Epileptic Delirium.*

In the *treatment,* the cause must be sought after, and if possible removed. In the paroxysm, but little can be done; but as the tongue is liable to be injured by the teeth, the jaws may be kept open by putting a cork or piece of wood between them. If the fit has been brought on by indigestible food, the stomach must be cleared. It is between the paroxysms that the great effort must be made. Generally, there is considerable irritability and debility of the nervous system, and hence tonics have been found the best remedies. Of these, perhaps the most powerful, in epilepsy, is the *argenti nitras,* given regularly and continued for months, if necessary. Preparations of iron, copper, and zinc, have also been used, and vegetable tonics and antispasmodics in general. Counter irritants, as blisters, moxa, &c., may be employed, if necessary, along with this course.

Unfortunately, in many cases, these means are found insufficient, and all that can be done is to palliate, removing carefully the exciting causes; such as the use of spirituous liquors, strong emotions, violent exercise, &c.; and regulating the diet.

EPILEP'TIC, *Epilep'ticus, Epilep'tus, Lunat'icus, Cadu'cans;* same etymon. One attacked with epilepsy. Any thing relating to epilepsy; as an *epilep'tic individual;* an *epilep'tic symptom.* Some authors also speak of *epileptic remedies.*

EPILEP'TOID, *Epileptoi'des;* same etymon. Resembling epilepsy—as '*epileptoid* symptoms.'

EPILO'BIUM AUGUSTIFO'LIUM, *Great Willow herb.* An indigenous plant, Order, Onagraceæ, which flowers in July. The root is emollient and slightly astringent.

EPILOBIUM COLORA'TUM, *Purple-veined Willow herb,* has similar properties.

EPILOBIUM VILLO'SUM, a South African plant, is used at the Cape of Good Hope as a domestic remedy for cleansing foul ulcers.

EPIM'ANES. A name given to a maniac when in a paroxysm.

EPIMELE'TAI, from επιμελεομαι, (επι, and μελω,) 'I take care of.' A name by which the ancient Persians called the *curers of wounds,* who followed their armies.

EPIMOR'IOS, 'unequal;' from επι, and μειρω, 'I divide.' An epithet applied to the pulse when unequal.—Galen.

ÉPINARD, Spinacia.—*t. Sauvage,* Chenopodium bonus Henricus.

ÉPINE, Spine—*é. du Dos,* Vertebral column—*é. Gutturale,* Nasal spine, inferior and posterior—*é. Sphénoïdale,* Sphenoidal spine—*é. Vinette,* Oxycantha Galeni.

EPINEMESIS, Dispensation.

EPINEPH'ELOS, *Nubilo'sus.* Presenting a cloud. Applied to the urine.—Hippocrates.

ÉPINEUX, Spinous—*é. du Dos, grand,* Spinalis dorsi major: see Interspinales dorsi et lumborum—*é. du Dos, petit,* see Interspinales dorsi et lumborum.

ÉPINGLE, Pin.

ÉPINIÈRE, Spinal.

EPINOTION, Scapula.

EPINYC'TIDES, from επι, 'upon,' and νυξ, 'the night.' Eruptions which appear on the skin in the night, and disappear in the day. *Pus'tula lirens et noc'tibus inquie'tans.*—Pliny.

EPINYCTIS PRURIGINOSA, Urticaria.

ÉPIONE, Decidua.

EPIPAROXYS'MUS. A paroxysm superadded to an ordinary paroxysm.

EPIPASTUM, Catapasmum.

EPIPE'CHU, επιπηχυ, from επι, 'upon,' and πηχυς, 'the elbow.' The upper part of the elbow.—Gorræus.

EPIPEPHYCOS, Conjunctiva.

EPIPHÆNOM'ENON, *Post appa'rens;* same etymon. Any kind of adventitious symptom which occurs during the progress of an affection: and which is not as intimately connected with the existence of the disease as the symptoms properly so called.

EPIPHA'NIA, from επι, 'upon,' and φαινω, 'I exhibit.' The external appearance of the body.—Castelli.

EPIPH'LEBUS, from επι, 'upon,' and φλεψ, 'a vein.' An epithet given to those whose veins are very apparent,—Hippoc., Aretæus.

EPIPHLEGIA, Inflammation.

EPIPHLOGISMA, Erysipelatous inflammation.

EPIPHLOGOSIS, Hyperphlogosis.

EPIPH'ORA, *Dacryno'ma, Lachryma'tio, Delachryma'tio, Illachryma'tio, Stillicid'ium lachryma'rum, Oc'ulus lach'rymans;* from επιφερω, (επι, and φερω,) 'I carry to.' Weeping. (F.) *Larmoiement.* The *watery eye;*—an involuntary and constant flow of tears upon the cheek. It is almost always symptomatic of some disease of the lachrymal passages, and occurs when the tears cannot pass into the *ductus ad nasum.* Occasionally, it is owing to the tears being secreted in too great quantity; as in certain cases of ophthalmia. The treatment must of course be directed to the removal of the cause.

EPIPHORA, Epidrome, Ophthalmia — e. Alvi, Diarrhœa — e. Ptyalismus, Salivation.

EPIPHYMATA, Cutaneous diseases.

EPIPH'YSIS, *Additamen'tum*, from επι, 'upon,' and φυω, 'I arise.' Any portion of a bone, separated from the body of the bone by a cartilage, which becomes converted into bone by age. The *epiphysis* of the fœtus becomes the *apophysis* of the adult.

EPIPHYSIS CRURIS LONGIORIS INCUDIS, Os orbiculare.

EP'IPHYTE, *Epiph'yton*, from επι, 'upon,' and φυτον, 'a plant.' A parasite derived from the vegetable kingdom. Epiphytes are divided by Vogel into 1. Vegetations in the human fluids, as the *tor'ula cerevis'iæ* in vomited fluids and fæcal evacuations, and the *sar'cina ventric'uli*, 2. Vegetations on the external skin and its appendages, as in tinea favosa, mentagra, herpes tonsurans and plica polonica, and, 3. Vegetations on the mucous membrane,—for example, in the aphthæ of children; in the cicatrices of the mucous membrane after typhus, &c.

EPIPLASMA, Cataplasm. Galen uses it especially for an application of wheaten flour, boiled in *hydrelæum*, and applied to wounds.

EPIPLE'GIA, from επι, 'above,' and πληγη, 'a stroke.' Paralysis of the upper extremities.

EPIPLERO'SIS, from επι, 'augmentative,' and πληρωσις, 'repletion.' Excessive repletion; distention.

EPIP'LOCE, from επι, 'upon,' and πλεκω, 'I twine.' Coition. Entanglement.

EPIP'LOCE INTESTINA'LIS, *Conglomera'tio intestino'rum*. Conglomeration of the intestines.

EPIPLOCE'LE, from επιπλοον, 'omentum,' and κηλη, 'tumour.' *Epip'loic her'nia, Zirba'lis hernia, Hernia omenta'lis, Omental hernia*, (F.) *Hernie de l'épiploon*. Omental hernia is recognised —but at times with difficulty—by a soft, unequal, pasty tumour, in which no gurgling sound is heard on pressing or reducing it. It is less dangerous than hernia of the intestines.

EPIPLO-ENTEROCE'LE, from επιπλοον, 'the omentum,' εντερον, 'intestine,' and κηλη, 'tumour.' Hernia, formed by the epiploon and a portion of intestine. It is more commonly called *En'tero-epiploce'lē*.

EPIPLOENTEROOSCHEOCE'LE, *Epiplo-enteroschoce'lē*, from επιπλοον, 'omentum,' εντερον, 'intestine,' οσχεον, 'scrotum,' and κηλη, 'rupture.' Hernia with omentum and intestine in the scrotum.

EPIP'LOIC, *Epiplo'icus*. Relating to the epiploon.

EPIPLOIC APPEN'DAGES; *Appendic'ulæ epi-plo'icæ, A. pinguedino'sæ, Fim'briæ carno'sæ coli, Supplemen'ta epiplo'ica*. Prolongations of the peritoneum beyond the surface of the large intestine, which are analogous in texture and arrangement to the epiploon.

EPIPLOIC AR'TERIES; *Arte'riæ Epiplo'icæ*. The arterial branches, which are distributed to the epiploon, and which are given off by the gastro-epiploicæ.

EPIPLO-ISCHIOCE'LE, from επιπλοον, 'the epiploon,' ισχιον, 'the ischium,' and κηλη, 'a tumour.' Hernia formed by the epiploon through the ischiatic notch.

EPIPLOÏ'TIS, from επιπλοον, 'the omentum,' and *itis*, denoting inflammation. Inflammation of the omentum; *Omenti'tis, Empresma perito-nitis omenta'lis, Omenti inflamma'tio, Enteri'tis epiploï'tis, Omente'sis*. A form of partial peritonitis.

EPIPLOMEROCE'LE, from επιπλοον, 'the omentum,' μηρος, 'the thigh,' and κηλη, 'a tumour.' Femoral hernia, formed by the epiploon.

EPIPLOMPHALOCELE, Epiplomphalon.

EPIPLOM'PHALON, *Epiploöm'phalon, Epiplomphaloce'lē, Hernia umbilica'lis*, from επιπλοον, 'the omentum,' and ομφαλος, 'the navel.' Umbilical hernia, formed by the epiploon.

EPIPLOM'PHRASIS, from επιπλοον, 'the epiploon,' and εμφρασσω, 'I obstruct.' Induration of the epiploon.

EPIPLOOCOMIS'TES, from επιπλοον, 'the epiploon,' and κομιζω, 'I carry.' One who has the omentum morbidly large. Also, one labouring under epiplocele.

EPIP'LOON, *Epiploum*, from επι, 'above,' and πλεω, 'I swim or float.' *Omen'tum, Retē, Retic'-ulum; Dertron; Zirbus, Gan'gamē, Gangamum, Operimen'tum intestino'rum, Saccus epiploïcus, Sage'na*. The *Caul*. A prolongation of the peritoneum, which floats above a portion of the intestines, and is formed of two membranous layers, with vessels and fatty bands distributed through it. Anatomists have described several epiploons. The uses of the omentum are but little known. The chief one seems to be, to retain the viscera *in situ*, and to give passage to vessels.

EPIPLOON, COLIC, *Colic Omentum, O. co'licum, Third Epiploon* or *Omentum*, is a duplicature of the peritoneum, situate along the ascending portion of the colon, as far as its junction with the transverse portion. It is behind the great epiploon, and fills up the angle formed by the junction of the ascending with the transverse colon. Its two laminæ are separated by colic arteries and veins.

EPIPLOON, GASTRO-COLIC, *Great Omentum, Omentum gastro-co'licum, Omentum majus, Peritonæ'um duplica'tum, Retē majus, Zirbus adipi'-nus*, consists of an extensive duplicature, which is free and floating on the folds of the intestines. It is quadrilateral, and longer on the left side than on the right:—its base being fixed, anteriorly, to the great curvature of the stomach; and, posteriorly, to the arch of the colon. It is formed of two laminæ, each consisting of two others. In this epiploon a number of vessels is distributed, and there is much fat.

EPIPLOON, GASTRO-HEPATIC, *Lesser Omentum, Omentum hep'ato-gas'tricum, Omentum minus, Membra'na macilen'tior*, is a duplicature of the peritoneum, which extends transversely from the right side of the cardia to the corresponding extremity of the fissure of the liver, and downwards from this fissure to the lesser curvature of the stomach, the pylorus and duodenum. Below it is the *foramen* or *hiatus* of WINSLOW; and between its laminæ are lodged the biliary and hepatic vessels. It contains but little fat. If air be blown in at the foramen of Winslow, the cavity of the omentum will be rendered perceptible.

EPIPLOON, GASTRO-SPLENIC, *Gastro-Splenic Omentum, O. Gastro-sple'nicum*. A reflection of the peritoneum, which passes between the concave surface of the spleen and the stomach, from the cardiac orifice to near its great curvature, and which lodges the vasa brevia and splenic vessels between its laminæ.

EPIPLOSARCOM'PHALUS, from επιπλοον, 'the epiploon,' σαρξ, 'flesh,' and ομφαλος, 'the navel.' Umbilical hernia, formed of indurated omentum.

EPIPLOSCHEOCE'LE, *Epiploschoce'lē*, from

επιπλοον, 'the epiploon,' οσχεον, 'the scrotum,' and κηλη, 'tumour.' Scrotal hernia, formed by a displacement of the epiploon.

EPIPLOUM, Epiploon.

EPIPNOIA, Afflatus.

EPIPORO'MA, from επιπωροω, (επι, and πωρος,) 'I harden.' A tophaceous concretion which forms in the joints. The callus of fracture.

EPIR'RHOE, *Epirrhæ'a*, from επι, 'upon,' and ρεω, 'I flow.' Afflux or congestion of humours.—Hippocrates.

EPIRRHŒA, Epirrhoe.

EPISARCIDIUM, Anasarca.

EPIS'CHESIS, Retention; from επισχνω, 'I restrain.' A suppression of excretions.

EPISCHET'ICUS; same etymon. *Sistens, Rep'rimens, Co'hibens*. 'Restraining.' An agent that diminishes—secretion, for example.

EPISCHION. Abdomen, Pubes, Pubis os.

EPISCOPALES VALVULÆ, Mitral valves.

EPISEION, Pubis (os), Vulva, Labium Pudendi, Tressoria.

EPISEMA'SIA, from επισημαινω, (επι, and σημα, 'a sign,') 'I afford some sign.' *Sema'sia*. It has been used synonymously with *sign*, and also with the invasion of an attack of fever. See Annotatio.

EPISIOCELE, see Hernia, vulvar.

EPISIŒDE'MA, from επισειον, 'the labia pudendi,' and οιδημα, 'œdema.' Œdema of the labia pudendi.

EPISION, Episeion.

EPISION'CUS, *Episiophy'ma*, from επισειον, (modern,) 'the labium pudendi,' and ογκος, 'a tumour.' *Tumor labio'rum*. A swelling or tumour of the labia pudendi.

EPISIOPHYMA, Episioncus.

EPISIORRHAG"IA, from επισειον, 'the labia pudendi,' and ραγη, 'rupture.' Hemorrhage from the labia pudendi.

EPISIOR'RHAPHY, *Episiorrhaph'ia*, from επισειον, (modern,) 'the labium pudendi,' and 'the vulva,' and ραφη, 'suture.' An operation practised in cases of prolapsus uteri, which consists in paring the opposing surfaces of the labia pudendi, bringing them together and uniting them by suture, so as to diminish the outlet of the vulva.

EPISOI'TIS, from επισειον, 'the labia pudendi,' and *itis*, denoting 'inflammation.' Inflammation of the labia pudendi.

EPISPA'DIA; *Hyperspa'dia*; same etymon as the next. The condition of an Epispadias.

EPISPA'DIAS, *Epispadiæ'us, Anaspa'dius, Anaspadiæ'us, Hyperspa'dias, Hyperspadiæ'us*, from επι, 'above,' and σπαω, 'I draw.' The opposite to Hypospadias. One who has a preternatural opening of the urethra at the upper part of the penis.

EPISPAS'TICS, *Epispas'tica, Ves'icants, Helc'tica*, (F.) *Épispastiques;* same etymon. An epithet for every medicinal substance which, when applied to the skin, excites pain, heat, and more or less redness, followed by separation of the epidermis, which is raised up by effused serum. Cantharides and mustard are epispastics. See Blister and Derivative.

EPISPASTICUM, Blister.

ÉPISPASTIQUES, Epispastics.

EPISPASTUM, Catapasma.

EPISPHÆ'RIA, from επι, 'upon,' and σφαιρα, 'a sphere.' Some physiologists have applied this term to the different convolutions and sinuosities presented by the external surface of the brain.

EPISPHAGISMOS, Signature.

EPISTACTIS'CHESIS, from επισταξις, 'epistaxis,' and ισχειν, 'to restrain.' Arrest of bleeding from the nose.

EPISTAPHYLINI, see Azygos Muscle.

EPIS'TASIS, *Insiden'tia*, from επι, 'upon,' and σταω, 'I rest.' A substance which swims at the surface of urine. It is opposed to the *hypostasis* or sediment. Epistasis has also been employed synonymously with suppression.

EPISTAX'IS, from επι, 'upon,' and σταζω, 'I flow drop by drop.' *Hæmorrhag"ia activa na'rium, H. narin'ea, H. na'rium, Epistax'is junio'rum, Epistax'is arterio'sa, Hæmorrhin'ia, Hæmorhinorrhag"ia, Hæmatis'mus, Choanorrhag"ia, Rhinorrhag"ia, Stillicid'ium seu Stilla'tio Sang'uinis e nar'ibus, Hemorrhage from the pituitary membrane, Bleeding at the nose, Noseblee*rd, (F.) *Hémorrhagie nasale, Saignement du nez, Hémorrhinie*. This is one of the most common varieties of hemorrhage; the organization of the Schneiderian membrane being favourable to it, as the blood-vessels are but slightly supported. It does not generally flow from both nostrils, and is very apt to recur. Puberty is the period at which it is most common. Its *exciting causes* are:—any thing that will induce local congestions, as running, coughing, blowing the nose, &c., provided there be a predisposition to it. A common case of epistaxis requires but little treatment, especially if in a young person. Light diet and a dose or two of the sulphate of magnesia will be sufficient. In more severe attacks, cold and astringent washes of alum, sulphate of zinc, weak sulphuric acid, or creosote, may be used, and the nostrils be plugged anteriorly; but if the bleeding goes on posteriorly, the posterior nares must be plugged likewise,—the patient being kept with the head raised. The flow of blood has been arrested by directing the patient to stand up with his head elevated, compressing the nostril whence the blood flows with the finger, raising the corresponding arm perpendicularly, and holding it in this position for about two minutes. A less vigorous circulation through the carotids appears to result from the increased force required to carry on the circulation through the upper extremities when raised.—Négrier. To prevent the recurrence, strict diet must be inculcated.

EPISTER'NAL, *Episterna'lis*, from επι, 'upon,' and στερνον, 'the sternum.' An epithet applied to two bones which form part of the sternum, and are situate upon its superior and lateral part. In the young subject, they are attached to the sternum by a synovial membrane, and a fibrous capsule. They have somewhat the appearance of the pisiform bones, but are of a greater size. According to Professor Owen, the piece of a segment of an articulate animal, which is immediately above the middle inferior piece or sternum.

EPISTHOT'ONOS, from εμπροσθεν, 'forwards,' and τεινω, 'I extend.' A spasm of the muscles, drawing the body forwards. The word *emprosthotonos* is more commonly employed.

EPISTROPHE, Relapse.

EPISTROPHEUS, Axis.

EPISTROPHUS, Axis.

EPISYNAN'CHE, (επι, and *synanche* or *cynanche*,) *Episynangi'na*. A Greek word, used by a modern writer for spasm of the pharynx, by which deglutition is prevented, and the solid and liquid food driven back towards the mouth or nasal fossæ.

EPISYNTHET'IC, *Episynthet'icus*, from επι, συντιθημι, (επι, συν, and τιθημι,) 'to collect, accumulate.' The name of a medical sect, whose object it was to reconcile the principles of the Methodists with those of the Empirics and Dogmatists. Leonides of Alexandria seems to have been one of the first partisans of this sect; of which we know little.

EPIT'ASIS, from επι, and τεινειν, 'to extend.' The period of violence of a fever, (*Febris inten'sio*,) attack or paroxysm; sometimes it is used in the same sense as epistasis, for '*suppression*.'

EPITELIUM, Epithelium.

EPITHE'LIAL, *Epithelia'lis*; same etymon as *epithelium*. Appertaining or relating to the epithelium,—as 'epithelial cells, or scales.'

EPITHE'LIUM, *Epite'lium*, *Epithe'lis*, *Endepiderm'is*, from επι, 'upon,' and θηλη, 'a nipple.' The thin layer of epidermis, which covers parts deprived of *derma*, properly so called,—as the nipple, mucous membranes, lips, &c. Modern histological researches have shown that it exists, in different forms, *pavement, cylinder* and *vibratile* or *ciliated epithelium*. *Tesselated epithelium* covers the serous and synovial membranes, the lining of blood-vessels, and the mucous membranes, except where cylinder epithelium exists. It is spread over the mouth, pharynx and œsophagus, conjunctiva, vagina, and entrance of the female urethra. *Cylinder epithelium* is found in the intestinal canal, beyond the cardiac orifice of the stomach; in the larger ducts of the salivary glands; in the ductus communis choledochus, prostate, Cowper's glands, vesiculæ seminales, vas deferens, tubuli uriniferi, and urethra of the male; and lines the urinary passages of the female, from the orifice of the urethra to the beginning of the tubuli uriniferi of the kidneys. In all these situations, it is continuous with tesselated epithelium, which lines the more delicate ducts of the various glands. For the uses of the *ciliated epithelium*, see Cilia.

EP'ITHEM, *Epith'ema* or *Epithe'ma*, from επι, 'upon,' and τιθημι, 'I put.' This term is applied to every topical application which cannot be classed either under ointments or plasters. Three sorts of epithems have been usually distinguished,—the *liquid, dry*, and *soft*, which comprise *fomentations, bags filled with dry substances*, and *cataplasms*.

EPITH'ESIS. Same etymon. The rectification of crooked limbs by means of instruments.

EPITHYM'IÆ, from επι, 'upon,' and θυμος, 'desire.' Morbid desires or longings.

EPITHYMIAMA, Fumigation.

EPITHYMUM, Cuscuta epithymum — e. Officinarum, Cuscuta Europæa.

EPITROCHI'LEA, from επι, 'upon,' and τροχαλια, 'a pulley.' That which is situate above a pulley. Chaussier gives this name to the unequal, round protuberance situate on the inside of the inferior extremity of the humerus above its articular trochlea. It is the part usually called the *inner* or *lesser condyle* of the humerus. From it originate several muscles of the forearm, to which it has given part of their names, according to the system of Chaussier.

ÉPITROCHLO-CARPI-PALMAIRE, Palmaris longus—*é. Cubito-carpien*, see Cubital muscles—*é. Métacarpien*. Palmaris magnus—*é. Phalanginien commun*, Flexor sublimis perforatus—*é. Radial*, Pronator radii teres.

EPIZO'A, (F.) *Epizoüires, Ectoparasites*, from επι, 'upon,' and ζωον, 'an animal.' Parasitic animals, which infest the surface of the body, or the common integument.

EPIZOÖTIA, *Epizoöty*. Same etymon. A disease which reigns amongst animals. It corresponds, in the veterinary art, to epidemy in medicine.

EPIZOÖT'IC, *Epizoöt'icus*, same etymon. Relating or appertaining to an epizoöty,—as an '*episoötic* aphtha.'

EP'OCHE, from επι, and εχω, 'to have or to hold.' Doubt, suspension of judgment—*Suspen'sa senten'tia*. Sometimes employed in the same sense as *epischesis* or suppression.

EPOCHETEUSIS, Derivation.

EPODE, Incantation.

EPO'MIS, *Superhumera'lī*, from επι, 'upon,' and ωμος, 'the shoulder.' The acromion. The upper part of the shoulder.—Hippocrates, Galen.

EPOMPHALICUM, Epomphalium.

EPOMPHALION, Uterus.

EPOMPHA'LIUM, *Epomphal'icum*, from επι, 'upon,' and ομφαλος, 'the navel.' A medicine, which, when placed upon the umbilicus, moves the belly.—Paulus of Ægina.

ÉPONGE, Spongia—*é. d'Eglantier*, Bedegar.

ÉPOQUES, Menses.

EPOSTOMA, Exostosis.

EPOSTOSIS, Exostosis.

ÉPREINTES, Tenesmus.

EPSEMA, Decoction.

EPSESIS, Decoction, Elixatio.

EPSOM, MINERAL WATERS OF. Epsom is a town in Surrey, about 15 miles from London. The water is a simple saline;—consisting chiefly of sulphate of magnesia, which has consequently received the name of *Epsom Salts*, though no longer prepared from the Epsom water.

ÉPUISEMENT, Exhaustion.

EPU'LIS, from επι, 'upon,' and ουλον, 'the gum.' *Odon'tia excres'cens, Sarco'ma epu'lis, Ulon'cus, Excrescen'tia gingi'væ*. An excrescence on the gum, sometimes ending in cancer.

EPULOSIS, Cicatrization.

EPULOTICA, Cicatrisantia.

EQUAL, *Æqua'lis*. An epithet applied particularly to the pulse and to respiration. The pulse and respiration are equal, when the pulsations and inspirations which succeed each other are alike in every respect.

EQUILIB'RIUM, from *æquus*, 'equal,' and *librare*, 'to weigh.' In medicine, this word is sometimes used to designate that state of organs, fluids, and forces, which constitutes health.

EQUINA CAUDA, see Cauda Equina.

EQUI'NIA, from *equinus*, 'belonging to a horse.' *Glanders*, (F.) *Morve*. A dangerous contagious disorder, accompanied by a pustular eruption, which arises from inoculation with certain diseased fluids generated in the horse, the ass and the mule. Two forms are met with,—*E. mitis*, contracted from horses affected with grease, and *E. glandulo'sa*, a dangerous and commonly fatal disease communicated to man, either in the acute or chronic form, from the glandered horse. The veterinary surgeons make two varieties of the disease in the horse—*Glanders, Ma'lia, Malias'mus, Ma'liī, Malis, Malleus; and Farcy glanders, Farcino'ma, Mal'leus farcimino'sus, Morbus farcimino'sus, Cachex'ia lymphat'ica farcimino'sa*, (F.) *Morve farcineuse*:—the *former* affecting the pituitary membrane and occasioning a profuse discharge from the nostrils, with pustular eruptions or small tumours, which soon suppurate and ulcerate, being attended by symptoms of malignant fever and by gangrene of various parts:— the *latter* being the same disease, but appearing in the shape of small tumours about the legs, lips, face, neck, &c. of the horse; sometimes very painful, suppurating and degenerating into foul ulcers. They are often seen together.

The mild cases require little treatment but rest; the more severe generally resist all remedies.

EQUISETUM ARVENSE, &c., see Hippuris vulgaris—e. Minus, Hippuris vulgaris.

EQUITATION, *Equita'tio, Hippei'a, Hippa'sia, Hippeu'sis*, from *equus*, 'a horse.' *Horseback exercise*. A kind of exercise, advisable in many diseases, although improper in others—in uterine affections, for instance. It has been much recommended in phthisis pulmonalis. It is less fatiguing than walking, and consequently more available in disease. But to prevent disease, where much exercise is required, the latter is preferable.

EQUIV'OROUS, *Equiv'orus, Hippoph'agous,* from *equus,* 'a horse,' and *voro,* 'I devour.' Feeding or subsisting on horseflesh.

EQUIV'OCAL, *Equiv'ocus,* from *æquus,* 'equal,' and *vox,* 'voice.' Those symptoms are occasionally so denominated which belong to several diseases. Generation is said to be 'equivocal,' when it is, or seems to be, spontaneous. See Generation.

EQUUS, Hippus.

ÉRABLE, Acer saccharinum.

ERADICA'TION, *Eradica'tio,* from *e,* 'from,' and *radix,* 'a root.' The act of rooting out, or completely removing a disease.

ERAD'ICATIVE, *Eradi'cans:* same etymon. Any thing possessed of the power of completely rooting out a disease.

ÉRAILLEMENT DES PAUPIÈRES, Ectropion.

EREBINTHUS, Acer arietinum.

ERECHTHI'TES HIERACIFO'LIA, *Sene'cio hieracifo'lius, Fireweed.* An indigenous plant, Order, Compositæ, which flowers from July to September. It is said to be an acrid tonic, and astringent, and in large doses emetic.

EREC'TILE TISSUE, *Tela erec'tilis,* from *erigere,* (*e,* and *rigere,*) 'to erect,' 'to become erect.' A tissue, whose principal character is:— to be susceptible of dilatation, i. e. of turgescence and increase of size. It is formed of a collection of arteries and veins, intermixed with nervous filaments; which form, by their numerous anastomoses, a spongy substance, whose areolæ communicate with each other. Smooth muscular fibres have been detected in it. This tissue exists in the corpora cavernosa of the penis and clitoris, at the lower and inner surface of the vagina, in the spongy part of the urethra, the lips, nipples, iris, &c. Sometimes it is developed accidentally, and constitutes a kind of organic transformation.

EREC'TION, *Erec'tio, Arrec'tio;* same etymon. The state of a part, in which, from having been stiff, it becomes stiff, hard, and swollen by the accumulation of blood in the areolæ of its tissue, as in the case of the penis;—*Styma, Stysis.*

ERECTOR CLITORIDIS, Ischio-cavernosus —e. Penis, Ischio-cavernosus.

EREMACAU'SIS, from *ερηρος,* 'waste,' and *καυσις,* 'combustion.' A term applied by Liebig to the slow combustion, oxidation, or decay of organic matters in the air.

EREMIA, Acinesia.

ERETHILYTICUM HÆMATOLYTICUM, Spanæmic.

ER'ETHISM, *Erethis'mus, Erethis'ia, Irritamen'tum, Irrita'tio,* from *ερεθιζω,* 'I irritate.' Irritation. Augmentation of the vital phenomena in any organ or tissue. *Orgasm.* Under this name, Mr. Pearson has described a state of the constitution produced by mercury acting on it as a poison. He calls it *Mercu'rial Erethis'mus.* It is characterized by great depression of strength; anxiety about the præcordia; irregular action of the heart; frequent sighing; tremors; small, quick, sometimes intermitting, pulse; occasional vomiting; pale, contracted countenance, and sense of coldness; but the tongue is seldom furred, nor are the vital and natural functions much disturbed. In this state any sudden exertion may prove fatal.

ERETHISMA, Rubefacient.

ERETHISMUS, Erethism, Irritation—e. Ebriosorum, Delirium tremens—e. Hydrophobia, Hydrophobia—e. Oneirodynia, Incubus, Paroniria— e. Simplex, Fidgets.

ERETHISTICUS. Erethiticus, Rubefacient.

ERETHIT'IC, *Erethit'icus, Erethis'ticus.* Belonging or relating to erethism,—as "erethitic phenomena," or phenomena of irritation.

EREUGMOS, Eructation.

EREUXIS, Eructation, Flatulence.

ERGASMA, Myrrha.

ERGASTERION SPIRITUS, Pulmo.

ERGASTERIUM, Laboratory.

ERGOT, (F.) *Ergot,* 'a spur.' *Er'gota, Seca'lē cornu'tum, Clavus secali'nus, Clavus seca'lis, Spermoë'dia clavus, Mater seca'lis, Calcar, Seca'lis mater, Seca'lē luxu'rians, Ustila'go, Clavus silig"inis, Frumen'tum cornu'tum, F. cornicula'tum, F. luxu'rians, F. tur'gidum, F. temulen'tum, Brisoderas, (?) Melanophy'ma, Spurred or Horned Rye, the Spur, Horneed,* (F.) *Seigle ergoté, Blé cornu.* Ergot is generally considered to be the result of a disease in rye, occurring most frequently when a hot summer succeeds a rainy spring. Decandolle, however, regards it as a parasitic fungus, and calls it, *Sclero'tium clavus;* whilst Leveillé esteems it to be a fungus giving a coating to the diseased grain; the medical virtues residing in the coating. This parasitic fungus he calls *Sphace'lia seg"etum.* More recently, it has been maintained, that it is a diseased state of the grain occasioned by the growth of a fungus not previously detected, to which the names *Ergota'tia abortans* seu *abortifa'ciens, Oidium abortifa'ciens, Ergot-mould,* have been given. It is found projecting from among the leaves of the spike or ear; and is a long, crooked excrescence, resembling the spur of a cock; pointed at its extremities; of a dark brown colour externally, and white within.

This substance has been long used in Germany to act on the uterus, as its names Mutterkorn and Gebärpulver (womb-grain, pulvis parturiens) testify. Upwards of forty years ago, it was recommended in this country, by Dr. John Stearns, of Saratoga County, New York, for accelerating parturition; and since that period, numerous testimonials have been offered in its favour. Half a drachm of the powder is gently boiled in half a pint of water, and one-third part given every 20 minutes, until proper pains begin. Some recommend the clear watery infusion; others advise the powder; others the oil, and others the wine. It is obvious, that in many cases the uterine efforts would return in the period which would necessarily elapse in the administration of ergot, so that several of the cases, at least, of reputed efficacy, may not have been dependent upon the assigned agent. Ergot also possesses—it is affirmed—narcotic virtues, which have rendered it useful in hemorrhagic and other affections of excitement.

Bread, made of spurred rye, has been attended with the effects described under ERGOTISM.

ERGOT, Hippocampus minor.

ERGOT-MOULD, see Ergot.

ERGOTA, Ergot.

ERGOTÆTIA ABORTANS, see Ergot—e. Abortifaciens, see Ergot.

ER'GOTIN, *Extrac'tum Er'gotæ, Extract of Ergot,* (F.) *Ergotine, Extrait hémostatique de Bonjean.* The extract of ergot has been found an excellent hemastatic in the dose of two grains several times a day. It has also been used externally.

ERGOTINE, Ergotin.

ER'GOTISM, *Ergoti'mus,* from *ergota,* 'ergot. *Morbus cerea'lis.* Poisoning by ergot. An affection produced by the use of spurred rye. At times, the symptoms are limited to vertigo, spasms, and convulsions. See Convulsio cerealis. Most commonly, there is torpor with numbness of the hands and feet, which waste away, lose sensation and the power of motion, and separate from the body by dry gangrene; *Ergotis'mus Sphacelo'sus, Sphac"elus cerea'lis, Necro'sis cerea'lis, Gangræ'na ustilagin'ea, Necrosis ustilagin'ea, Ergot or Mildew mortification,* (F.) *Ergotisme gangréneux, Gangrène des Solonois, Mal de Sologne.*

ERGOTISME CONVULSIVE, Convulsio cerealis.

ERGOTISMUS, Ergotism — e. Spasmodicus, Convulsio cerealis—e. Sphacelosus, Ergotism.

ERI'CA VULGA'RIS, *Callu'na vulga'ris* seu *Eri'ca, Common Heath,* (F.) *Bruyère vulgaire.* This has been regarded as diuretic and diaphoretic.

ERIG"ERON BELLIDIFO'LIUM, *Robin's plantain.* An indigenous plant of the Compositæ *family;* flowering in May. It is said to possess properties like the next.

ERIG"ERON PHILADEL'PHICUM, *Scabious, Skevisch, Philadelphia Flea-Bane, Skevisch Flea-Bane, Daisy, Cocash, Frostweed, Fieldweed, Squaw-weed,* (F.) *Vergerette de Philadelphie.* The plant has been used in decoction or infusion for gouty and gravelly complaints, and is said to operate powerfully as a diuretic and sudorific.

ERIGERON CANADEN'SE, *Can'ada Fleabane,* is considered to be allied in properties to the above, and the same may be said of *Erigeron Heterophyl"lum, Sweet Sca'bious* or *various-leaved Fleabane;* all of which are in the secondary list of the Pharmacopœia of the United States.

ERIGERUM, Senecio.

ÉRIGNE, Hook.

ÉRINE, Hook.

ERIOCEPH'ALUS UMBELLULA'TUS, *Wild Rose'mary.* A South African shrub, *Nat. Ord.* Compositæ, which is diuretic, and used by the farmers and Hottentots, in various forms of dropsy.

ERIOSPERM'UM LATIFO'LIUM. A South African plant, the tuber of which is musculent, and used externally in abrasions of the skin, and in superficial ulcers. It is also employed by the Mohammedans, in decoction, in amenorrhœa.

ERIX, ερίξ. This word signifies, in Galen, the upper part of the liver.

ERODENS, Caustic.

ERODIUM MOSCHATUM, Geranium moschatum.

EROMANIA, Erotomania.

ERON'OSUS, *Eronu'sos,* from ηρ, 'spring,' and *νοσος* or *νουσος,* 'disease.' A disease which appears chiefly in spring.

EROS, Love.

EROSIO, Corrosion — e. et Perforatio spontanea Ventriculi, Gastromalacia.

ERO'SION, *Ero'sio, Diabro'sis, Anabro'sis, Corro'sion,* from *erodere,* (e, and *rodere,*) 'to eat away.' The action of a corrosive substance, or the gradual destruction of a part by a substance of that kind. It is often employed in the same sense as ulceration, *spontaneous erosion.*

EROT'IC, *Ero'ticus,* from ερως, 'love.' That which is produced by love; — as *Erotic melancholy, E. delirium,* &c.

EROTICOMANIA, Erotomania.

EROTION, Melissa.

EROTOMA'NIA, *Eroma'nia, Ma'nia erot'ica,* from ερως, 'love,' and μανια, 'mania.' A species of mental alienation caused by love. *Erotic melancholy* is *Love melancholy.* Some authors write it *Erot'ico-mania.* Also, Nymphomania.

ERPES, Herpes.

ERRABUNDUS, Planetes.

ERRAT'IC, *Errat'icus, Atac'tos, At'ypos;* from *errare,* 'to err.' *Wandering, irregular.* That which disappears and recurs at irregular intervals. This name is given to intermittents, *Febres errat'icæ,* which observe no type. Most commonly, it is applied to pains or to any diseased manifestations which are not fixed, but move from one part to another, as in gout, rheumatism, erysipelas, &c.

ERREUR DE LIEU, Error loci.

ER'RHINE, *Errhi'num* or *Er'rhinum, Sternutato'rium, Ster'nutatory, Ptar'micum, Apophlegmat'isans per nares, Nasa'lē,* from εν, 'in,' and ριν, 'the nose.' A remedy whose action is exerted on the Schneiderian membrane, exciting sneezing and increased discharge. Errhines have been mainly used as local stimulants in head affections. The chief are: Asari Folia, Euphorbiæ gummi-resina, Hydrargyri sulphas flavus, Tabacum, and Veratrum album.

ERRHINUM, Sternutatory.

ER'RHYSIS, from εν, 'in,' and ρεω, 'I flow.' With some, a draining of blood. A trifling hemorrhage.

ERROR LOCI, *Apoplane'sis,* (F.) *Erreur de Lieu.* A term, frequently used by Boerhaave to express deviation of fluids, when they enter vessels not destined for them. Boerhaave admitted several orders of capillary vessels, the diameters of which went on decreasing. The largest received red blood: those which came next received only white: others only lymph; whilst the last of all were destined for yet more subtle fluids —for a kind of vapour. When the red globules entered vessels destined for the white, or the white those intended for the thinner fluids, there was, according to the theory of Boerhaave, an *error loci,* the proximate cause of inflammation and other mischiefs. See Aberration.

ERUCA, Brassica eruca, Sinapis—e. Barbarea, Erysimum barbarea—e. Fœtida, Brassica eruca— e. Sativa, Brassica eruca.

ERUCTA'TION, *Ructa'tio, Ereug'mus, Er'ygē, Eructa'tio, Ructus, Ructa'men, Ructua'tio, Ereux'is, Restagna'tio, Ruft,* (N. *of England,*) from *eructare,* (e, and *ructare,* 'to belch.') *Belching,* (F.) *Rot, Rapport.* A sonorous emission, by the mouth, of flatus proceeding from the stomach. When so frequent as to occasion a diseased condition, this is termed *Ructuo'sitas, Morbus ructuo'sus.*

ERUGATORIA, Tetanothra.

ÉRUGINEUX, Æruginous.

ERUPTIO, Eruption — e. Exanthematis, Epanastasis—e. Sanguinis, Hæmorrhagia.

ERUP'TION, *Erup'tio,* from *erumpere,* (e, and *rumpere,*) 'to issue with violence,' 'to break out.' This word has several meanings. 1. The sudden and copious evacuation of any fluid from a canal or cavity;—of serum, blood, pus, &c., for example. 2. The breaking out of an exanthem; and, 3, the exanthem itself, whether simply in the form of a rash, or of pustules, vesicles, &c.

ÉRUPTION ANOMALE, Roseolæ — e. Rosace, Roseolæ—e. Violet, Ionthus.

ERUP'TIVE, *Eruptivus.* That which is accompanied by an eruption. Thus small-pox, measles, scarlet fever, miliaria, &c., are *eruptive fevers.* The term *eruptive disease* is nearly synonymous with cutaneous disease.

ERVA DE SANCTA MARIA, Arum Dracunculus.

ERVALENTA, see Ervum.

ERVUM, E. *Ervil'ia, E. plica'tum, Vic"ia ervil'ia, Or'obus,* (F.) *Lentille Ers* ou *Orobe.* In times of scarcity, the seeds have been made into bread, but it is said not to be wholesome. The meal was one much used in poultices: it was formerly called *Orob'ion*, οροβιον. Under the name *Ervalent'a*, a secret preparation has been introduced into Paris. It is a vegetable powder, which, when mixed with milk and soup and taken night and morning, is said to have succeeded in removing old and obstinate obstructions! Buchner thinks it is bean-meal, Ditterich, the meal of the seed of Ervum Ervilia.—Aschenbrenner.

ERVUM ERVILIA, Ervum.

ERVUM LENS, *Cicer Lens, Lens esculen'ta, Phacos*, the *Lentil*, (F.) *Lentille*. The seed, *Phacê, Pha'cea, Phacus*, is eaten in many places like peas: they are flatulent and difficult of digestion.

ERVUM PLICATUM, Ervum.

ERYGE, Eructation.

ERYNGIUM, see E. Aquaticum.

ERYN'GIUM AQUAT'ICUM, *Water Eryn'go, Button Snake Root*. Nat. Order, Umbelliferæ. This root, *Eryn'gium*, (Ph. U. S.,) is nearly allied to the contrayerva of the shops, and acts more especially as a sudorific. It is a secondary article in the Pharm. U. S.

ERYNGIUM CAMPES'TRE, *E. vulga'rē, Centum Cap ita, Lyrin'gium, Aster inquina'lis, Capit'ulum Martis, Acus Ven'eris*, (F.) *Panicaut, Chardon-Roland*, is sometimes used for *E. maritimum*.

ERYNGIUM MARIT'IMUM seu MARI'NUM. The *Sea Holly* or *Eryngo, Æthe'rea Herba*, (F.) *Panicaut Maritime*. Eryngo root has a slightly aromatic odour, and sweetish and warm taste. It is considered to be diuretic and expectorant, but its powers are so weak, that it is scarcely ever used.

ERYNGIUM VULGARE, E. Campestre.

ERYNGO, SEA, Eryngium maritimum—e. Water, Eryngium aquaticum.

ERYS'IMUM, *Erys'imum officina'lē, Sisym'brium officina'lē, Chamæ'plion. Hedge-mustard*, (F.) *Vélar, Tortelle, Herbe aux Chantres*. This was, formerly, much used for its expectorant and diuretic qualities. The seeds greatly resemble mustard.

ERYSIMUM ALLIARIA, Alliaria.

ERYSIMUM BARBA'REA, *E. lyra'tum, Ar'abis barba'rea, Sisymbrium barba'rea, Eru'ca barba'rea, Barba'rea, B. stric'ta*, (F.) *Herbe de Sainte Barbe*, has been ranked amongst the antiscorbutic plants. See Alliaria.

ERYSIMUM CORDIFOLIUM, Alliaria—e. Lyratum, E. barbarea.

ERYSIPELA'CEA. Same etymon as the next. A family of eruptive diseases, comprising erysipelas, variola, rubeola, and scarlatina.

ERYSIP'ELAS, from ερυω, 'I draw in,' and πελας, 'near.' *Febris erysipelato'sa, Febris erysipela'cea, Erythrop'yra, Emphlysis Erysip'elas, St. Anthony's fire, Ignis Sancti Anto'nii, I. Columel'læ, Hieropyr, Icterit"ia rubra, Ignis sacer, Rose, Rubea icterit"ia, Vicinitra'ha, Vicinitrac'tus, Brunus, Lugdus*, (F.) *Érysipèle, Feu St. Antoine, Feu sacré, Mal Saint Antoine*. A disease, so called because it generally extends gradually to the neighbouring parts. Superficial inflammation of the skin, with general fever, tension and swelling of the part; pain and heat more or less acrid; redness diffused, but more or less circumscribed, and disappearing when pressed upon by the finger, but returning as soon as the pressure is removed. Frequently, small vesicles appear upon the inflamed part, which dry up and fall off, under the form of branny scales. Erysipelas is, generally, an acute affection: its medium duration being from 10 to 14 days. It yields, commonly, to *general* refrigerant remedies. Topical applications are rarely serviceable. At times, when the disease approaches the phlegmonous character, copious bleeding and other evacuants may be required, as in many cases of erysipelas of the face; but this is not commonly necessary.

In most cases, indeed, the general action seems deficient, and it becomes necessary to give tonics.

When erysipelas is of a highly inflammatory character, and invades the parts beneath, it is termed *Erysip'elas phlegmono'des*, (F.) *Érysipèle phlegmoneux*: when accompanied with phlyctenæ, and the inflammation terminates in gangrene, *Erysip'elas gangræno'sum*, (F.) *Érysipèle gangréneux*; and when associated with infiltration of serum *Erysip'elas œdemato'sum*, (F.) *Érysipèle œdemateux*.

ERYSIPELAS GANGRÆNOSUM, see Erysipelas — e. Œdematosum, see Erysipelas — e. Phlegmonodes, see Erysipelas — e. Periodica nervosa chronica, Pellagra — e. Phlyctenoides, Herpes zoster — e. Pustulosa, Herpes zoster — e. Zoster, Herpes zoster.

ERYSIPELATODES, Erysipelatous.

ERYSIPEL'ATOUS, *Erysipelato'des, Erysipelato'sus*. Belonging to erysipelas; as an *erysipel'atous affection*.

ERYSIPEL'ATOUS INFLAMMATION, *Inflamma'tio erysipelato'sa, Epiphlogis'ma, Cuti'tis, Dermati'tis*, is the character of inflammation which distinguishes erysipelas, *Erythe'ma erysipelato'sum*.

ÉRYSIPÈLE, Erysipelas — é. Ambulant, see Ambulant — é. *Gangréneux*, see Erysipelas — é. Œdemateux, see Erysipelas — é. *Phlegmoneux*, see Erysipelas — é. *Serpigineux*, see Serpiginous — é. *Pustuleux*, Herpes zoster.

ERYSOS, Erythema.

ERYTHE'MA, from ερυθαινω, ερυθρος, 'red, rose-coloured.' *Erythre'ma*, (F.) *Érythème*. This name is, sometimes, given to erysipelas, especially when of a local character. It is, also, applied to the morbid redness on the cheeks of the hectic, and on the skin covering bubo, phlegmon, &c. It forms the 6th genus of the 3d order, *Exanthemata*, of Bateman's classification of cutaneous diseases; and is defined, "a nearly continuous redness of some portion of the skin, attended with disorder of the constitution, but not contagious." Many varieties are described by dermatologists, — for example, *E. intertri'go, E. fugax, E. papula'tum, E. tubercula'tum, E. nodo'sum, E. læve, E. centrif'ugum, E. margina'tum*, and *E. acrodyn'ia*.

ERYTHEMA ACRODYNIA, Acrodynum — e. Ambustio, Burn — e. Anthrax, Anthrax.

ERYTHE'MA CENTRIF'UGUM. A variety of erythema affecting the face, commencing with a small red spot, and spreading around, so as, at times, to affect the whole face.

ERYTHEMA ENDEMICUM, Pellagra — e. à Frigore, Chilblain.

ERYTHE'MA FUGAX. Patches of erythema, that sometimes appear on the body in febrile diseases, teething children, &c., and which are of brief duration.

ERYTHEMA GANGRÆNOSUM, Anthrax — e. Ichorosum, Eczema mercuriale — e. Intertrigo, Chafing.

ERYTHE'MA LÆVE, (F.) *Érythème léger*. Slight erythema affecting the skin, as in œdema.

ERYTHE'MA MARGINA'TUM, (F.) *Érythème marginal*. A form in which the prominent patches of erythema are distinctly separated from the skin at their margins.

ERYTHEMA MERCURIALE, Eczema mercuriale.

ERYTHE'MA NODO'SUM, (F.) *Érythème noueux*. A more severe form of Erythema tuberculatum.

ERYTHE'MA PAPULA'TUM, (F.) *Érythème papuleux*. Patches of erythema, which are at first papulated, appearing on the face, neck, breast, &c., of females, and young persons more especially.

ERYTHEMA PELLAGRUM, Pellagra — e. Pernio, Chilblain.

ERYTHE'MA SOLA'RE. A name given by the Italians to Pellagra, owing to its being attended with an eruption of small red spots or patches on the parts that are exposed to the sun.

ERYTHE'MA TUBERCULA'TUM, *E. tuberculo'sum*, (F.) *Érythème tuberculeux*. A form of erythema in which the patches are in small lumps.

ERYTHEM'ATOUS, *Erythenat'ic, Erythemato'sus, Erythemat'icus*, (F.) *Erythémateux*. Appertaining or relating to Erythema.

ÉRYTHÈME, Erythema — *t. Léger*, Erythema læve — *t. Marginal*, Erythema marginatum — *t. Noueux*, Erythema nodosum — *t. Papuleux*, Erythema papulatum — *t. Tuberculeux*, Erythema tuberculatum.

ERYTHRÆA CENTAURIUM, Chironia centaurium — e. Chilensis, Canchalagua, Chironia Chilensis.

ERYTHRÆMIA, Plethora.

ERYTHRAN'CHE, *Angi'na erysipelato'sa*, from *ερυθρος*, 'red,' and *αγχω*, 'I suffocate.' Erysipelatous or erythematous sore throat.

ERYTHREMA, Erythema.

ERYTHRINA MONOSPERMA, Butea frondosa.

ERYTHROCHŒRAS, Cynanche parotidæa.

ERYTHRODANUM, Rubia.

ER'YTHROID, *Erythro'des, Erythroï'des*. Reddish.

ERYTHROID COAT. *Tu'nica erythro'des*. Vaginal coat of the testis.

ER'YTHROID VES'ICLE, *Vesic'ula Erythroïdea*. A vesicle of the fœtus described by Pockels and others. It is pyriform, and much longer than, although of the same breadth as, the umbilical vesicle. Velpeau, Weber, and others, doubt its being a physiological condition.

ERYTHRONIUM, E. Americanum.

ERYTHRO'NIUM AMERICA'NUM, *E. flavum, E. dens canis, E. lanceola'tum, E. longifo'lium, Common Erythro'nium, Yellow Snake-leaf, Yellow Adder's tongue, Adder-leaf, Dog vi'olet, Rattlesnake vi'olet, Lamb's tongue, Scrof'ula root, Yellow Snowdrop*. This plant is possessed of emetic properties, but is rarely, if ever, used. The root and herb, *Erythro'nium*, (Ph. U. S.,) are in the secondary list of the Pharmacopœia of the United States.

ERYTHRONIUM DENS CANIS, E. Americanum — e. Flavum, E. Americanum — e. Lanceolatum, E. Americanum — e. Longifolium, E. Americanum.

ERYTHROPYRA, Erysipelas.

ERYTHROSIS, Plethora.

ES'APHE, from *εσαφαω*, 'I touch with the fingers.' (F.) *Le Toucher*. The introduction of a finger or fingers into the vagina, for the purpose of examining the condition of the uterus. It is employed to verify the existence or non-existence of pregnancy and its different stages; to detect certain affections or faults of conformation in the genital organs and pelvis; and, during the process of accouchement, to examine into the progress of labour, &c.

ESCA, Aliment.

ESCARA, Eschar.

ESCARGOT, Limax.

ESCHALOTTE, *Échalotte*.

ESCHAR, *Es'chara, Es'char, a slough, a crust or scab*. The crust or disorganized portion, arising from the mortification of a part, and which is distinguishable from the living parts by its colour, consistence, and other physical properties. The inflammation which it excites in the contiguous parts, gives occasion to a secretion of pus between the living and dead parts, which ultimately completely separates the latter.

ESCHARA, Vulva.

ESCHAROT'IC, *Escharot'icum*, from *εσχαρα*, 'eschar.' Any substance, which, when applied upon a living part, gives rise to an eschar, such as *caustic potassa*: the concentrated mineral *acids*, &c.

ESCHAROTIC POISON, see Poison.

ESCHELLOHE, MINERAL WATERS OF. This water rises at the foot of a mountain near the convent of Etal in Bavaria. It is a sulpharosaline.

ESCHID'NA OCELLA'TA. A very poisonous viper, which inhabits the sugar-cane fields of Peru. Its bite is almost instantaneously fatal.

ESCORZONERA; Scorzonera.

ESCREVISSE, Crab.

ESCULAPIAN, Medical.

ES'CULENT, *Esculen'tus, Ed'ible, Eat'able*, from *esca*, 'food.' (F.) *Comestible*. Such plants or such parts of plants or animals as may be eaten for food.

ESO, *εσω*, 'within.' A prefix which signifies an affection of an internal part; as *Esoënteritis*, inflammation of the inner membrane of the intestines: — *Esogastri'tis*, inflammation of the inner membrane of the stomach, &c.

ESOCHAS, Esoche.

ES'OCHE, *Es'ochas*. A tumour—as a hemorrhoid—within the anus.

ESOCOLITIS, Desentery.

ESODIC, Afferent.

ESOËNTERITIS, see Enteritis.

ESOGASTRITIS, Endogastritis.

ESOTER'IC, *εσωτερος*, 'interior,' from *εσω*, 'within.' Private; interior; in contradistinction to *Exoter'ic*, public, exterior. Hence, we speak of '*esoteric* and *exoteric* causes of disease.'

ESOT'ERISM, MED'ICAL. Same etymon as Esoteric. A term used by M. Simon, in his *Déontologie médicale*, for that esotery, or mystery and secresy, with which the practitioner performs his daily duties, and which, he conceives, he is compelled to adopt by the prejudices and ignorance of his patients.

ESPACES INTERCOSTAUX, see Costa.

ESPÈCE, Powder, compound.

ESPÈCES VULNÉRAIRES, Falltranck.

ESPHLA'SIS, from *εις*, 'inwards,' and *φλαω*, 'I break, bruise,' &c. A fracture of the skull by comminution, the fragments being depressed. See Depression, and Enthlasis.

ESPRIT, Spirit — *e. d'Ammoniaque*, Spiritus ammoniæ — *e. d'Anis*, Spiritus anisi — *e. de Camphre*, Spiritus camphoræ — *e. de Cannelle*, Spiritus cinnamomi — *e. de Carvi*, Spiritus carui — *e. de Genièvre composé*, Spiritus juniperi compositus — *e. de Lavande*, Spiritus lavandulæ — *e. de Lavande composé*, Spiritus lavandulæ compositus — *e. de Menthe poivrée*, Spiritus menthæ piperitæ — *e. de Muscade*, Spiritus myristicæ — *e. de Pouliot*, Spiritus pulegii — *e. de Raifort composé*, Spiritus armoraciæ compositus — *e. de Romarin*, Spiritus rosmarini — *e. de Vin délayé*, Spiritus tenuior — *e. de Vin rectifié*, Spiritus rectificatus.

ESPRITS ANIMAUX, Nervous fluid.

ESQUILLE, Splinter.

ESQUINANCIE, Cynanche, Cynanche tonsillaris.

ESQUINE, Smilax China.

ES'SENCE, *Essen'tia*, corrupted from *existentia*, 'standing out.'(?) By some, used synonymously with *volatile oil*; by others, with *simple tincture*. The *oil of peppermint* is the oil obtained by distillation; the *essence*, the oil diluted with spirit. See Tinct. olei menthæ.

ESSENCE OF BARDANA, HILL'S, Tincturi guaiaci ammoniata — e. of Coltsfoot, see Tinctura bensoïni composita — e. of Musk, Tinctura moschi — e. of

Mustard Pills, Whitehead's, see Sinapis — e. of Mustard, Whitehead's, see Sinapis — e. of Peppermint, Tinctura olei menthæ piperitæ — e. of Spearmint, Tinctura olei menthæ viridis — e. of Spruce, see Pinus Abies.

ESSENCES, Olea volatilia.

ESSENTIA, Essence, Tincture — e. Abietis, see Pinus abies — e. Aloes, Tinctura aloes — e. Absinthii amara, Tinctura A. composita — e. Absinthii composita, Tinctura A. composita — e. Antimonii seu stibii, Vinum antimonii tartarizati — e. Antiseptica Huxhami, Tinctura cinchonæ composita — e. Aromatica, Tinctura cinnamomi composita — e. Castorei, Tinctura castorei — e. Catholica purgans Rothii, Tinctura jalapii composita — e. de Cedro, Oleum cedrinum — e. Chinæ, Tinctura cinchonæ composita — e. Cinnamomi, Tinctura cinnamomi — e. Neroli, see Citrus aurantium — e. Corticis Peruviani antiseptica Huxhami, Tinctura cinchonæ composita — e. Corticis Peruviana composita, Tinctura cinchonæ amara.

ESSEN'TIAL, *Essentia'lis*. The word *essential* has been applied to the immediate or active principles of vegetables, which were believed to be endowed with the properties of the plants from which they were extracted. *Essential oil* was so called because it was regarded as the only immediate principle which was *essential*. This expression is retained. *Essential salts* are true salts or extracts which exist, ready formed, in vegetables; and which are obtained by distillation, incineration, or some other process.

An *essential disease* is synonymous with a general disease; that is, one not depending on any local affection;—not symptomatic. See Entity.

ES'SERA, *Es'serā, Sora, Saire, Sare, Morbus porci'nus, Rosa saltans, Urtica'ria porcella'na*, (F.) *Ampoules, Porcelaine*. A species of cutaneous eruption, consisting of small, reddish tubercles over the whole body, accompanied by a troublesome itching. It seems to be a variety of lichen or urticaria. See Lichen tropicus.

ESSIEU, Axis.

ESSOUFFLEMENT, Anhelatio.

ESTHEMA, Vestitus.

ESTHESIS, Vestitus.

ESTHIOMÈNE, Esthiomenus.

ESTHIOM'ENUS, *Estiom'enus*, from εσθιω, 'I eat.' *Ex'edens*. (F.) *Esthiomène*. That which devours or eats away. Certain ulcers and eruptions—*Dartres rongeantes*—are so called.

ES'TIVAL, *Æsti'vus*; happening in summer, belonging to summer. This epithet is given to *summer diseases*, so called because they reign at that season, and appear to depend on the influence exerted by it on the animal economy. In the United States, the term *summer disease* or *complaint* means disorder of the bowels, as *diarrhœa, cholera morbus*, &c.

ESTOMAC, Stomach.

ESULA CYPARISSIAS, Euphorbia cyparissias — e. Major, Euphorbia palustris — e. Minor, Euphorbia cyparissias.

ESURIES, Hunger.

ESURIGO, Hunger.

ESURITIO, Hunger.

ESYCHIA, Acinesia.

ÉTAGE, Stage.

ÉTAIN, Tin — *é. de Glace*, Bismuth—*é. Gris*, Bismuth.

ÉTAT GRANULEUX DU REIN, Kidney, Bright's Disease of the.

ÉTERNUEMENT, Sneezing.

ETESTICULATIO, Castration.

ETHER, Æther, Æther sulphuricus—e. Acetic, see Æther.

ETHER, CHLORIC, Chloroform. Under the names *concentrated chloric ether* and *strong chloric ether*, a compound of pure *chloroform* and nearly absolute *alcohol*—in the proportion of one-third of the former to two-thirds of the latter—has been used as an anæsthetic by inhalation, in the same cases as sulphuric ether and chloroform. It is properly an *alcoholic solution* or *tincture of chloroform*.

ETHER, CHLOROHYDRIC, CHLORINATED, see Æther muriaticus—e. *Chlorohydrique chloré*, see Æther muriaticus.

ETHER, COMPOUND. A preparation consisting of a solution of *chloroform* in *sulphuric ether*, which has been used as an anæsthetic by inhalation, in the same cases as chloroform.

ETHER, HYDROCHLORIC, see Æther—e. Hydrocyanic, Æther hydrocyanicus—e. Muriatic, Æther muriaticus—e. Nitric, see Æther—e. Nitrous, see Æther—e. Phosphoric, see Æther—e. Rectified, Æther sulphuricus — e. Sulphuric, Æther sulphuricus — e. Terebinthinated, Æther terebinthinatus.

ETHEREAL, Æthereal.

ÉTHÉRÉE, Æthereal.

ETHEREOUS, Æthereal.

ETHERINE, HYDROCYANATE OF, Æther hydrocyanicus—e. Muriate of, Æther muriaticus.

ETHERIZA'TION, *Ætherisa'tio*. The aggregate of phenomena induced by the inhalation of ether.

E'THERIZED, *Ætherisa'tus*. Presenting the phenomena induced by the inhalation of ether.

ETHICS, MEDICAL, Deontology, medical.

ETHIOPIAN, see Homo.

ETHIOPS, see Æthiops.

ETHISIS, Filtration.

ETHISMUS, Filtration.

ETH'MOID, *Ethmo'des, Ethmoï'des, Ethmoï'deus*, from ηθμος, 'a sieve,' and ειδος, 'form.' Shaped like a sieve.

ETHMOID BONE, *Os ethmoïdeum, Os multifor'mē, Os spongio'sum, Os spongoï'des, Os cribro'sum, Os cribrifor'mē, Os cu'bicum, Os crista'tum, Os foraminulen'tum, Os colifor'mē, Os colato'rium*, (F.) *Os cribleux*. One of the eight bones which compose the cranium; so called, because its upper plate is pierced by a considerable number of holes. The ethmoid bone is situate at the anterior, inferior, and middle part of the base of the cranium. It seems to be composed of a multitude of thin, fragile, semi-transparent laminæ, which form more or less spacious cells, called the *Ethmoïdal labyrinth* or *cells*, distinguished into *anterior* and *posterior*. These communicate with the nose, and are lined by a prolongation of the pituitary membrane. The ethmoid bone is constituted of compact tissue, and is surrounded by the *Ethmoid suture*. It is articulated with the *frontal* and *sphenoidal bones*, the *cornua sphenoidalia*, the *superior maxillary bones*, the *palate bones*, the *ossa turbinata inferiora*, the *vomer*, the *proper bones of the nose*, and the *lachrymal bones*.

ETHMOID'AL, *Ethmoïda'lis*. Belonging to the ethmoid bone; as, *Ethmoïdal cells, E. suture*, &c. The *Ethmoï'dal apoph'ysis* or *process* is the advanced part of the sphenoid bone, which articulates with the ethmoid. The *ethmoidal arteries* are two in number, the anterior of which arises from the ophthalmic artery. The origin of the other varies. The *Échancrure ethmoïdale* of the os frontis receives the ethmoid bones. The *Ethmoïdal veins* correspond to the arteries.

ETHMOSYNE, Habit.

ETHMYPHE, Cellular tissue.

ETHMYPHI'TIS, *Inflamma'tio telæ cellulo'sæ*, from ηθμος, 'a sieve,' 'υφη, 'texture,' and *itis*, denoting inflammation. Inflammation of the cellular membrane.

ETHMYPHOTYLOSIS, Induration of the cellular tissue.

ETHOS, Habit.

ETHULE, CYANURET OF, Æther.

ÉTHUSE, Æthusa cynapium—é. Meum, Æthusa meum.

ETHYLE, CHLORIDE OF, Æther muriaticus.

ETIOLA'TION, Blanching, (F.) Étiolement. That state of plants which occurs in consequence of privation of light, when they become pale and watery. In pathology, it is sometimes used to denote the paleness produced in those persons who have been kept long without light; or a similar paleness, the result of chronic disease.

ÉTIOLEMENT, Etiolation.

ETIOLOGY, Ætiologia.

ETIQUETTE, MEDICAL, Deontology, medical.

ÉTISE, Hectisis—é. Mésentérique, Tabes mesenterica.

ÉTOILE, Stella.

ÉTONNÉE, Stunned.

ÉTOUFFEMENT, Suffocation.

ÉTOURDISSEMENT, Vertigo.

ÉTRANGLEMENT, Strangulation, Hysteria—é. des Intestins, Enteremphraxis.

ÉTRIER, Stapes.

ETRON, Abdomen, Hypogastrium.

ETRON'CUS, from ητρον, 'the lower belly,' and ογκος, 'a tumour.' A tumour of the lower belly.

ÉTUVE, Stove—é. Humide, Bath, vapour.

ÉTUVER, to Foment.

EU, ευ, 'good, proper,' when prefixed to words. Hence:

EUÆ'MIA, from ευ, 'well,' and 'αιμα, 'blood.' A good condition of the blood.

EUÆSTHE'SIA, from ευ, 'well,' and αισθησις, 'perception.' Vigorous perception. A good condition of the perceptive faculties.

EUÆSTHE'TOS. Same etymon. One whose senses are in full vigour.

EUANALEP'SIS, from ευ, 'good,' and αναληψις, 'recovery.' Rapid restoration to strength.

EUANTHEMON, Anthemis nobilis.

EUCALYPTUS RESINIFERA, see Kino.

EUCHRŒ'A, from ευ, 'good,' and χροια, 'colour.' A good or healthy colour of the skin. A good appearance of the surface.

EUCHYM'IA, from ευ, 'well,' and χυμος, 'juice.' A good state of the humours.

EUCRA'SIA, from ευ, 'well,' and κρασις, 'temperament.' A good temperament.

EUDIAPNEUS'TIA, from ευδιαπνευστος, 'one who breathes well.' Easy transpiration.

EUECTICA (medicina) Gymnastics.

EUEL'CES, from ευ, 'well,' and 'ελκος, 'an ulcer.' One in whom wounds and ulcers are readily healed.

EU'EMES, Euěm'etos, from ευ, 'well,' and εμεω, 'I vomit.' That which readily excites vomiting. One who vomits with facility.

EUETHES, Benign.

EUEX'IA, from ευ, 'well,' and 'εξις, 'constitution.' A good constitution.

EUFRAISE, Euphrasia officinalis.

EUGE'NIA CARYOPHYLLA'TA, called after Prince Eugene. Garrophyl'lus, Caryophyl'lus aromat'icus, Myrtus caryophyl'lus. The Indian tree which affords the clove. Order, Myrtaceæ. The Clove, Caryophyl'lus, C. aromat'icus, is the unexpanded bud, (F.) Girofle, Gérofle, Girophle. Its odour is strong, aromatic, and peculiar; taste, pungent and acrid. Like all substances, whose virtue depends upon essential oil, it is stimulant and carminative. It is generally used as a corrigent to other remedies, and in cases where substances containing the essential oils are demanded. The oil, (F.) Huile de Gérofle—Oleum caryophyl'li, Oil of Cloves—has the properties of the cloves.

EUGION, Hymen.

EULOPHIA, see Salep.

EUNUCH, Eunu'chus, from ευνη, 'the bed,' and εχω, 'I keep.' Hemian'drus, Hemianor, Hemianthro'pus, Semimas, Semimas'culus, Semivir, Thla'dias, Thla'sias, Thlib'ias, Castra'tus, Gallus, Excastra'tus, Evira'tus, Emascula'tus, Spado, Exsec'tus, Extesticula'tus, Extom'ius, Sem'ivir, Semimascula'tus. One whose organs of generation have been removed, or so altered, that he is rendered incapable of reproducing his species, or of exercising the act of venery. Eunuchs were common with the ancient Romans. In Italy, this horrible mutilation still takes place to improve the voice; and in the East, eunuchs have the surveillance of the seraglio.

EUNUCHISMUS, Castration.

EUNUCHIUM MECONIS, Lettuce.

EUNUCHUS, Castratus, Eunuch.

EUODES, Beneolentia.

EUONYMUS, Quassia simarouba.

EUON'YMUS AMERICA'NUS, Strawberry bush, Strawberry tree, Burning bush, Indian arrowwood. A shrub of the Nat. Ord. Celastraceæ, Sex. Syst. Pentandria monogynia, which, like the next, is found throughout the United States and Canada; flowering from May to June.

EUON'YMUS ATROPURPU'REUS, Burning bush, Spindle tree, Indian Arrow wood, flowers from June to July.

From these varieties of Euonymus the Wahoo or Whahoo bark is said to be obtained. It is diuretic, antiperiodic, tonic, and a hydragogue cathartic, and has been used in dropsy in infusion, in the proportion of an ounce to a pint of water.

EUPATHI'A, Euphor'ia, from ευ, 'well,' and παθος, 'suffering.' A disposition for being affected by pain easily. Also, a good state of health.

EUPATOIRE D'AVICENNE, Eupatorium cannabinum—e. Percefeuille, Eupatorium perfoliatum.

EUPATORIUM, Eupatorium perfoliatum.

EUPATO'RIUM AGERATOÏ'DES, White Snakeroot; indigenous; flowering in August and September; has the same properties as Eupatorium perfoliatum.

EUPATO'RIUM CANNAB'INUM, called after Mithridates Eupator, Eupato'rium, E. Arab'icum seu Japon'icum seu trifolia'tum, Cannab'ina aquat'ica, Hemp agrimony, Eupatorium of Avicenna, Herb of Saint Cunegonde, Trifo'lium cervi'num, Orig'anum aquat'icum, (F.) Eupatoire d'Avicenne. Family, Synantheræ; Sex. Syst. Syngenesia æqualis. The juice of this plant proves violently emetic and purgative, if taken in sufficient quantity. It has been considered diuretic, cathartic and emetic.

EUPATORIUM CONNATUM, E. perfoliatum — e. Guaco, Guaco—e. Japonicum, E. Cannabinum—e. Mesues, Achillea ageratum.

EUPATORIUM PERFOLIA'TUM, E. Conna'tum, Eupatorium—(Ph. U. S.) (F.) Eupatoire percefeuille; Boneset, Thor'oughwort, Thor'oughstem, Thor'ougwax, Vegetable antimony, Crosswort, Agueweed, Feverwort, Indian sage, Joe-pye, Teasel, Sweating plant, is a plant which grows in low, wet meadows throughout the United States. It is considered to be stimulating, tonic, emetic, purgative, diuretic, and sudorific. Dose, gr. xv. of the powder, as a gentle purgative.

EUPATORIUM, PURPLE-STALKED, E. purpureum.

EUPATORIUM PURPU'REUM, *Mohawk tassel, Purple-stalked Eupato'rium, Trumpet weed,* is used in similar cases, as well as

EUPATORIUM SESSILIFO'LIUM, Upland Boneset, and

EUPATORIUM TEUCRIFO'LIUM, *Wild horehound, Germander-leaved horehound.*

EUPATORIUM TRIFOLIATUM, E. Cannabinum.

EUPEP'SIA, from ευ, 'well,' and πεπτω, 'I digest.' A good digestion. The antithesis to *dyspepsia*.

EUPEP'TIC, *Eupep'tus, Eupep'ticus.* Same etymon. Relating to a good digestion. One endowed with a good digestion.

EUPHLO'GIA, from ευ, 'well,' and φλεγω, 'I burn.' Mild inflammation. Variola.

EU'PHONY, *Eupho'nia,* from ευ, 'well,' and φωνη, 'voice.' An agreeable or regular voice.

EUPHORBE CYPRÈS, E. cyparissias — *e. des Marais,* E. palustris — *e. Vomitive,* E. ipecacuanha.

EUPHOR'BIA CAPITA'TA, *Caa cica.* Ord. Euphorbiaceæ. A Brazilian plant, which is strongly astringent and not poisonous. It is considered to be one of the best remedies for the bites of serpents. It is, also, called *Colubri'na Lusitan'ica.*

EUPHORBIA COROLLA'TA, *Large flowering spurge, Milkweed, Snakes' milk, Ipecacuan'ha, Hippo, Picac, Ip'ecac, Milk purslain, Purge root, Emet'ic root, Bowman's root, Apple root, Indian Physic,* has similar properties to the last. The dose of the root is the same.

EUPHORBIA CYPARIS'SIAS, *Es'ula minor* seu *Cyparissias, Euphor'bia Cypressi'na, Tithym'alus Cyparis'sia.* The *Cypress spurge,* (F.) *Euphorbe cyprès.* This, like most of the spurges, is very acrimonious. Amongst the rustics, it was formerly called *poor man's rhubarb,* and was, consequently, a laxative. It is not used.

EUPHORBIA CYPRESSINA, E. Cyparissais.

EUPHORBIA HYPERICIFO'LIA. A native of the United States. It is astringent and tonic. Used in infusion—f℥ss to Oj of boiling water. Dose, a tablespoonful.

EUPHORBIA IPECACUAN'HA, *Anisophyllum Ipecacuanha, Ipecacuanha spurge,* (F.) *Euphorbe vomitive.* This species of spurge is common in the southern and middle parts of the United States. The root is a powerful emetic, in the dose of from five to fifteen grains: twenty grains act as a cathartic likewise. In large doses, it acts as a narcotico-acrid.

EUPHORBIA LATH'YRIS. The systematic name of the plant which affords the *lesser catapu'tia seeds, Catapu'tia minor, Caper spurge, Lath'yris, Gar'den spurge, Caper plant, Mole-plant, Tithym'alus latifo'lius* seu *la'thyris, Galarhœ'us Lath'yris.* The seeds possess cathartic properties, and an expressed oil of the seeds — *O'leum Euphor'biæ Lathyr'idis —* has been given as a cathartic in the dose of six to twelve drops.

EUPHORBIA OFFICINA'RUM. The systematic name of the plant which affords the *Euphorbium, Euphorbiæ gummi-resi'na, Gummi euphorbiæ,* in greatest abundance. The euphorbium is an inodorous gum-resin, in yellow tears, which have the appearance of being worm-eaten. It enters into the composition of some plasters, and has been used as an errhine.

EUPHORBIA PALUS'TRIS, *E. panicula'ta, Greater spurge, Es'ula major, Tithym'alus palus'tris, Galarha'us palus'tris, Marsh spurge,* (F.) *Euphorbe des marais.* The juice is given, in Russia, as a common purge. It is used, too, as an irritant in tinea, warts, &c.

EUPHORBIA PALUSTRIS and E. VILLOSA, or E. PILO'SA have been brought forward as preventives of hydrophobia — the bitten part being washed with a decoction, and, at the same time, the decoction being taken internally.

EUPHORBIA PANICULATA, E. palustris.

EUPHORBIA PARAL'IAS, *Tithym'alus paralias, Sea spurge.* This is violently cathartic and irritating, and is seldom used.

EUPHORBIA PILOSA, see Euphorbia palustris— e. Villosa, see Euphorbia palustris.

☞ All the spurges are vesicant and rubefacient, when applied externally.

EUPHORBIUM, Euphorbia officinarum.

EUPHORIA, Eupathia.

EUPHRAGIA, Euphrasia officinalis.

EUPHRA'SIA, *E. Officina'lis* seu *Min'ima* seu *Imbrica'ta, Ocula'ria, Euphra'gia, Ophthal'mica, Eyebright,* (F.) *Eufraise, Cassе-Lunette.* It has been recommended in diseases of the eye, but is unworthy of notice.

EUPLAS'TIC, *Euplas'ticus:* from ευ, 'well,' and πλασσω, 'I form.' Having the capacity of becoming organizable in a high degree,— as in false membranes resulting from acute inflammation in a healthy person.

EUPLEURUM SERRULATUM, Diosma crenata.

EUPNŒ'A, from ευ, 'well,' and πνεω, 'I respire.' Freedom or facility of respiration.

EURHYTH'MIA, from ευ, 'well,' and ρυθμος, 'rhythm.' Regularity of the pulse.

EURIBALI, Juribali.

EURODES, Carious.

EURODON'TICUS, from ευρος, 'caries,' and οδους, 'a tooth.' Suffering from carious teeth.

EURUS, ευρυς, 'mould, putrefaction,' *Mucor, Caries.* Corruption of the humours.

EURYCHORIA, Sinus.

EURYCLES, Engastrimyth.

EURYCLITUS, Engastrimyth.

EURYSMUS, Dilatation.

EURYTH'MIA, *Euryth'mus,* from ευ, 'well,' and ρυθμος, 'rhythm.' Regularity of pulse, both as regards quantity and quality.

EUSAR'CUS, from ευ, well,' and σαρξ, 'flesh.' One who is fleshy, robust, muscular.

EUSEMI'A, from ευ, 'well,' and σημειον, 'a sign.' A collection of good signs.

EUSPLANCH'NIA, from ευ, 'well,' and σπλαγχνον, 'a viscus.' A healthy state of the viscera.

EUSTA'CHIAN TUBE, *Tuba Eustachia'na, Syrin'ga, Syrinx, Mea'tus cæcus, Tuba Aristotel'ica, Ductus auris palati'nus, Iter a Pala'to ad Aurem,* (F.) *Trompe* ou *Conduit d'Eustache, Conduit guttural de l'oreille—*Ch. This tube was so called from its discoverer, Eustachius. It is partly bony and partly cartilaginous: extending from the cavity of the tympanum to the upper part of the pharynx. Its length is about two inches; the bony portion which belongs to the temporal bone, is about three-fourths of an inch long. It is lined, internally, by a prolongation of the lining membrane of the pharynx. Its nerves are furnished by the palatin branches of the ganglion of Meckel, and its vessels proceed from those of the pharynx and velum pendulum. The use of the tube seems to be, to permit the renewal of air in the cavity of the tympanum.

EUSTA'CHIAN VALVE, *Valve of Eusta'chius, Valvule d'Eustachi* ou *d'Eustache.* A membranous, semilunar fold, which corresponds to the opening of the vena cava inferior into the right auricle of the heart.

EUSTHENI'A, *Vigor, Exuberan'tia*, from ευ, 'well,' and σθενος, 'strength.' Flourishing, exuberant health.—Hippocrates.

EUSTOM'ACHUS, from ευ, 'well,' and στομαχος, 'stomach.' Digesting rapidly. Having a good stomach.

EUTAX'IA, from ευ, 'well,' and τασσω, 'I arrange.' *Euthe'sia.* A well-ordered constitution, in which every part has its proper relation. The ready return of a rupture, or of a luxated bone.

EUTHANA'SIA, from ευ, 'well,' and θανατος, 'death.' An easy death.

EUTHESIA, Eutaxia.

EUTHYENTERON, Rectum.

EUTHYENTEROSTENOMA, Stricture of the Rectum.

EUTHYM'IA, *An'imi tranquil'litas*, from ευ, 'well,' and θυμος, 'mind.' Tranquillity of mind. A good state of the mental faculties.

EUTHYPNOE, Orthopnœa.

EUTHYPNŒA, Orthopnœa.

EUTOC'IA, from ευ, 'well,' and τοκος, 'delivery.' An easy labour. Fecundity.

EUTROPH'IA, from ευ, 'well,' and τροφη, 'nourishment.' A good state of nutrition.

EUTROPH'IC, *Eutroph'icus*, same etymon. A term introduced into medical terminology, by the author, for an agent whose action is exerted on the system of nutrition, without necessarily occasioning manifest increase of any of the secretions.

The chief eutrophics are,—*mercurials*, the *preparations of iodine, bromine, cod liver oil, the preparations of gold and silver, sulphur, sugar,* and *sarsaparilla.*

EUZOODYNAMIA, Sanitas.

EVAC'UANTS, *Evacuan'tia*, from *e*, and *vacuare*, 'to empty.' (F.) *Évacuatifs.* Medicines are so called which occasion a discharge by some emunctory; such as purgatives, emetics, &c.

ÉVACUATIFS, Evacuants.

EVACUATIO, Evacuation, Excretion.

EVACUA'TION. Same etymon. The discharge of any matter whatever by the natural passages or by an artificial opening.

ÉVANOUISSEMENT, Syncope.

EVAN ROOT, Geum Virginianum.

EVAPORA'TION, *Evapora'tio, Vapora'tio, Exhala'tio*, from *e*, and *vaporare*, 'to emit a vapour.' Transformation of a liquid into vapour, in order to obtain the fixed matters contained in it dry and separate from the liquid. When the vapour is received in a proper vessel and condensed, the process is called distillation. Evaporation produces cold, and this is one of the processes by which the body is cooled, through the evaporation of the perspiratory fluid.

EVAUX, MINERAL WATERS OF. Evaux is situate in Auvergne, in France. The waters are hydrosulphurous and thermal.

EVENTRA'TION, *Eventra'tio, Hypogastrocœ'le*, from *e*, 'out of,' and *venter*, 'the belly.' A tumour, formed by a general relaxation of the parietes of the abdomen, and containing a great part of the abdominal viscera. Also, *ventral hernia*, or that which occurs in any other way than through the natural openings of the abdominal parietes. Lastly, any very extensive wound of the abdominal parietes, with issue of the greater part of the intestines.

EVEN'TUS, from *e*, 'out of,' and *venire*, 'to come.' *Apobai'non, Apobesom'enon, Ecbesom'enon, Termina'tio morbi.* The event or issue of a disease, either favourable or unfavourable.

EVERLASTING, DIŒCIOUS, Antennaria dioica.

EVERRIC'ULUM, *Specil'lum.* A sort of sound or scoop, used for extracting sand or fragments of stone or clots of blood from the bladder, after or during the operation of lithotomy.

EVERSIO PALPEBRÆ, Ectropion.

ÉVIGILATION, see Sleep.

EVIL, THE, Scrofula—e. King's, Scrofula.

EVIRATIO, Castration.

EVIRATUS, Castratus, Eunuch.

EVISCERATION, Exenterismus.

EVOLUTIO, Development—e. Spontanea, Evolution, spontaneous.

EVOLU'TION, SPONTA'NEOUS, *Ver'sio seu Evolu'tio sponta'nea*, from *e*, and *volvere*, 'to roll.' *Sponta'neous ver'sion, Sponta'neous expul'sion, Duplication of the fœtus.* A term, applied, by Dr. Denman, to what he considered to be a spontaneous turning of the fœtus in utero, in an arm presentation, in consequence of powerful uterine contractions forcing out the breech and feet, whilst the arm recedes. It is now usually considered to be a doubling of the fœtus, so that the arm changes its position but little, whilst the breech is forcibly expelled before the upper extremity; —the case becoming similar to a breech presentation.

EVOLUTION, VESICLE OF, Vesicle of development.

EVOMITIO, Vomiting.

EVONYMUS, Euonymus.

EVUL'SION, *Avulsion, Evul'sio*, from *evellere*, (*e.* and *vellere*,) 'to pluck out.' *Apotil'mos, Ectil'mos, Tilmos.* The action of plucking out; forcible extraction. (F.) *Arrachement.* This word is oftener used by the French than by the English surgeons, for the act of extracting certain parts, the presence of which is injurious,—as the teeth, &c.

EX MARIBUS, Castratus.

EXACERBATIO, Exacerbation, Paroxysm.

EXACERBA'TION, *Exacerba'tio, Exaspera'tio, Excrescen'tia*, from *exacerbare,* (*ex,* and *acerbus*,) 'to provoke.' (F.) *Rédoublement.* An increase in the symptoms of a disorder. Often used synonymously with paroxysm.

EXACUM SPICATUM, Coutoubea alba.

EXÆMATOSIS, Hæmatosis.

EXÆMIA, Anæmia.

EXÆMOS, Exanguious.

EXÆ'RESIS, from εξ, 'out of,' and αιρεω, 'I take away.' A surgical operation, which consists in drawing, extracting, or removing, from the human body, every thing that is useless, noxious, or extraneous. It is a generic term, which includes extraction, evulsion, evacuation, excision, ablation, amputation, &c.

EXÆRESIS, Extraction.

EXAGION. The sixth part of an ounce:— four scruples.—Actuarius.

EXAG'GERATED, *Exaggera'tus*,(F.)*Exagéré.* Heightened. Increased by expression. An epithet for sounds heard on auscultation and percussion; when much increased — *Hypereche'sis, Hypereche'ma.*

EXAL'MA, from εξ, out of,' and αλλομαι, 'I leap.' *Exalsis.* Hippocrates calls thus the displacement of the vertebræ.

EXALSIS, Exalma, Leap.

EXALTA'TION OF THE VITAL FORCES, *Exalta'tio vi'rium.* This expression has been used, by modern pathologists, to designate a morbid increase in the action of organs, and partly that which occurs in an inflamed organ. Some use *exaltation of the vital forces*, and *inflammation*, synonymously.

EXAMBLOMA, Abortion.

EXAMBLOSIS, Abortion.

EX'AMEN RIGORO'SUM. 'Rigorous examination.' An examination of a Candidate for the degree of Doctor of Medicine in the Prussian Universities, which, like the *Tentamen medicum*, is conducted in Latin, and takes place before the medical faculty on all branches of medicine.

EXANASTOMOSIS, Anastomosis.

EXANASTROPHE, Convalescence.

EXANGI'A, from εξαγγιζω, (εξ, and αγγος, 'a vessel,') 'I evacuate from a vessel.' *Exangei'a*. An enlargement or rupture of a blood-vessel, without external opening. A genus in the order *Dyæthetica*, class *Hæmatica* of Good. It comprises *aneurism* and *varix*.

EXANGIA ANEURISMA, Aneurism.

EXAN'GUIOUS, *Exæ'mos, Exsan'guis*, from *ex*, out of,' and *sanguis*, 'blood.' One who seems bloodless; as a female, who has suffered largely from uterine hemorrhage.

EXANIA, Proctocele.

EXANIMA'TION, *Exanima'tio*, from *ex*, 'out of,' and *anima*, 'the spirit.' This word has two acceptations. Sometimes, it means real death, corresponding with the Greek θανατος, *mors*. At others, it signifies apparent death, corresponding with the Greek αψυχια, εκψυχια, εκλυσις, *Ani'mi deli'quium*.

EXAN'THEM, *Exanthe'ma, Anthe'ma erup'tio, Epanthe'ma, Efflorescen'tia, Exanthis'ma, Ecthy'ma, Epanaste'ma, Epanthe'ma, Epanthis'ma, Efflora'tio*, from εξανθεω, (εξ, and ανθεω,) 'I flourish.' A rash. (F.) *Élevure*. Under this term, is comprehended, by some, every kind of eruption, of which the skin is the seat. Others comprehend by it those eruptions that are accompanied by fever, *Febres exanthemat'icæ*: including, under the head of the *major exanthemata*, those which attack a person but once in his life, and which are communicated by specific contagion; and, under the *minor exanthemata*, those which are not marked by these characteristics. Small-pox, measles, cow-pox, &c., belong to the major:— chicken-pox, herpes, lichen, &c., to the minor. The general acceptation of Exanthem is, however, a more or less vivid, circumscribed, or diffuse redness of the skin, which diminishes or disappears transiently under the pressure of the finger.

EXANTHEM, CARBUNCULAR, Anthracia—e. Ichorous, Emphlysis — e. Pustulous, Empyesis — e. Rash, Enanthesis.

EXANTHEMA, Eminence—e. Internum, Eisanthema.

EXANTHE'MA IŎD'ICUM. An eruption of darkred definite spots, of various sizes, spreading over the whole body, without the formation of scales, and disappearing only after a long time, which seems to be produced occasionally by the use of iodine.

EXANTHEMA MILIARIA, Miliary fever—e. Pestis, Plague,—e. Antivariolosum, Vaccina—e. Serosum, Pemphigus—e. Strophulus, Strophulus—e. Urticatum, Urticaria—e. Vaccina, Vaccina—e. Varicella, Varicella.

EXANTHEMAT'ICA. Same etymon. *Erup'tive fevers*. Cutaneous eruptions, essentially accompanied with fever; — the third order in the class *Hæmatica* of Good.

EXANTHEMATIS'CHESIS, *Exanthematos'chesis*, from εξανθημα, 'exanthem,' and ισχειν, 'to withhold.' Suppression of a cutaneous eruption.

EXANTHEMATOL'OGY, *Exanthematolog"ia*, from εξανθημα, 'exanthem,' and λογος, 'a discourse.' The doctrine of cutaneous eruptions.

EXANTHEMATOPHTHAL'MIA, *Ophthalm'ia exanthemat'ica*, from εξανθημα, 'exanthem,' and οφθαλμια, 'inflammation of the eye.' Ophthalmia in the course of, or succeeding to, a cutaneous eruption.

EXANTHÈME INTESTINALE, see Typhus.

EXANTHESIS, see Efflorescence—e. Arthrosia, Dengue, — e. Roseola, Roseola—e. Rubeola, Rubeola.

EXANTHISMA, Exanthem.

EXANTHROPIA, Misanthropia.

EXAPSIS, Inflammation.

EXARAG'MA, from εξαρασσω, 'I tear away,' 'I break.' Collision, violent fracture or friction.

EXARCHIA'TER. Chief of the archiatri or chief of physicians, a title, like that of *Comes Archiatro'rum*, given to the chief physician of an emperor or king. Archiater appears to have meant, at times, the same thing.

EXARMA, Swelling.

EXAR'SIO. A burning heat.

EXARTEMA, Amuletum.

EXARTERI'TIS, *Exarterii'tis*, from εξ, 'out of,' and *arteria*, 'an artery.' Inflammation of the outer coat of an artery.

EXARTHREMA, Luxation, Sprain.

EXARTHROMA, Luxation.

EXARTHROSIS, Luxatio, Sprain—e. Pareticus, see Pareticus.

EXARTICULATIO, Amputation, joint, Luxatio.

EXARYSIS, Exhaustion.

EXASPIRATIO, Exacerbation.

EXCÆCARIA AGALLOCHA, Agallochum.

EXCALEFACTIO, *Échauffement*.

EXCARNA'TION, *Excarna'tio*, from *ex*, and *caro*, 'flesh.' A mode of making anatomical preparations, which consists in separating injected vessels from the parts in which they are situate. This is done by means of corrosion by an acid or by putrefaction.

EXCASTRATIO, Castration, Eunuch.

EXCATHISMA, Bath, half, Semicupium.

EXCEREBRATIO, Eccephalosis.

EXCEREBRATUS, Delirious.

EXCERNENT, Secreting.

EXCIDENTIA, Ecptoma.

EXCIP'IENT, *Excip'iens*, from *excipere*, (*ex*, and *capere*,) 'to receive.' (F.) *Intermède*. A substance, which, in a medicinal prescription, gives form and consistence to it, and serves as a *vehicle* or *medium* for the exhibition of the other ingredients.

EXCIPULA, Cup.

EXCISIO, *Entaille*.

EXCIS'ION, *Excis'io*, from *excidere*, (*ex*, and *cædere*,) 'to cut off.' *Ec'tomē*. A surgical operation, by which parts of a small size are removed with a cutting instrument.

EXCITABIL'ITY, *Excitabil'itas*. Irritability. The faculty, possessed by living beings, of being sensible to the action of excitants. The doctrine of excitability forms an important part of the Brunonian system.

EXCITANT, Stimulant.

EXCITA'TION, *Excita'tio, Excite'ment;* same etymon; from *excitare*, (*ex*, and *citare*,) 'to excite.' The act of exciting; the state of an organ or organs excited. Excitement is, sometimes, used synonymously with augmented arterial action. The effect of the exciting powers acting on the excitability, according to Brown, constitutes *excitement*. Cullen used the term to express the restoration of the energy and action of the brain, which has been interrupted by sleep or some debilitating cause,—a state opposite to that of *collapse*. Not unfrequently it is employed in the sense of excessive action, — *Super-excita'tio* (F.) *Sur-excitation*.

EXCITED DISEASES, Feigned diseases.
EXCITO-MOTION, see Excito-motory.
EXCITO-MO'TORY. An epithet applied by Dr. Marshall Hall to a division of the nervous system—comprising the gray matter of the spinal marrow, with the afferent and efferent nerves connected with it;—all of which are concerned in *reflex* actions; or those by which impressions are transmitted to a centre, and reflected so as to produce muscular contraction without sensation or volition. See Nerves.

The term *excito-motion* has also been employed to signify motion no matter how excited, by the reflex nerves or by volition—C. J. B. Williams.

EXCORIATIO, Ecdora.
EXCORIA'TION, *Excoria'tio, Excoriatu'ra, Am'ychē,* from *ex,* and *corium,* 'skin.' (F.) *Écorchure.* A slight wound, which removes only the skin.
EXCORIATURA, Excoriation.
EXCREA'TION, *Excrea'tio, Exscrea'tio, Screa'tus, Rasca'tio,* from *ex,* and *screare,* 'to spit.' Act of spitting. (F.) *Orachement.* See Exspuitio.
EX'CREMENT, *Excremen'tum, Retrimen'tum, Excre'tum, Excre'tio, Perito'ma, Diachore'ma, Aph'odos, Aphodeu'ma, Apocho'reon, Apoc'risis, Ardas, Ar'daloe,* from *excernere, (ex,* and *cernere,)* 'to separate,' 'cleanse.' Every thing, which is evacuated from the body of an animal by the natural emunctories, as superfluous; such as the fæcal matters, the urine, perspiration, nasal mucus, &c. Generally, however, the term is restricted to the fæcal evacuations;—*Purgamenta, Hedra, Sedes, Fæces, Stercus, Caccē, Spat'ilē,* (especially when liquid,) *Dejec'tio alvi'na, O'nera alvi, Sordes ventris, Hypochore'ma, Cœ'lia, Hypochore'sis, Merda, Merdus, Catarrhex'is, Copros, Scor.*
EXCREMENT, HUMAN, Stercus humanum.
EXCREMENTIT"IAL, *Excrementit"ious, Excrementit"ius,* (F.) *Excrémenteux, Excrémentitiel.* That which is similar to excrement, and forms part of it. *Excrementitial humours* or *parts* are those destined to be evacuated as incapable of administering to the nutrition of the body.
EXCREMEN'TO-RECREMENTIT"IAL, *Excremento - recrementit"ious.* Animal fluids, intended to be partly absorbed and partly rejected.
EXCRES'CENCE, *Excrescen'tia, Ecphy'ma, Phymato'sis, Hypersarco'sis, Sarcophy'ia, Caro excres'cens,* from *excrescere, (ex,* and *crescere,)* 'to grow outwards.' (F.) *Excroissance.* A tumour, which forms at the surface of organs, and especially on the skin, mucous membranes, or ulcerated surfaces. Excrescences differ in size, shape, cause, &c., and each requires its own treatment. Warts, *condylomata, polypi, hemorrhoids,* belong to this head.
EXCRESCENTIA, Exacerbation, Protuberance, Tumour — e. Carnosa, Sarcoma — e. Fungosa, Fungosity—e. Gingivæ, Epulis—e. Vesicæ urinariæ carnosa, Cysthypersarcosis.
EXCRETA, see Excretion.
EXCRETIO, Excretion, Excrement—e. Alvina, Defecation—e. Fæcum alvinarum, Defecation—e. Urinæ involuntaria, Enuresis.
EXCRE'TION, *Excre'tio, Ec'crisis, Evacua'tio, Ejec'tio, Expul'sio, Eges'tio, Diachore'sis,* from *excernere, (ex,* and *cernere,)* 'to separate.' The separation or throwing off of those matters, *Excre'ta, Eges'ta, Ion'ta, Apion'ta,* from the body of an animal, which are supposed to be useless, as the urine, perspiration, and fæces.
EX'CRETORY, *Excreto'rius;* same etymon. An *Excretory vessel* or *duct* is one which transmits the fluid secreted by a gland, either externally or into the reservoirs into which it has to be deposited. The existence of an excretory duct was regarded as a distinctive character of the glands properly so called.

EXCRETORY ORGAN means any one charged with the office of excreting: thus, the skin is said to be an excretory organ, because through it the perspiration takes place.
EXCRETUM, Excrement.
EXCROISSANCE, Excrescence.
EXCU'TIA VENTRIC'ULI, *Stomach Brush.* An instrument, composed of iron or brass wire, at one of the extremities of which is a pencil of bristles. Some ancient authors proposed this to extract foreign bodies from the œsophagus, as well as to cleanse the stomach of viscid and tenacious matters adhering to it.
EXECHEBRONCHUS, Bronchocele.
EXECHEGLUTI, Exischioi.
EXEDENS, see Herpes exedens.
EXELCOSIS, see Ulceration.
EXELCYS'MOS, from *εξ,* 'from,' and *ελκοω,* 'I draw.' Extraction. Also the act of breaking out into ulcers.
EXELCYSMUS, Extraction.
EXENTERATION, Exenterismus.
EXENTERIS'MUS, *Exenter'isis, Exentera'tio, Exentera'tion, Eviscera'tion, Unbow'elling, Viscera'tion,* from *εξ,* 'out of,' and *εντερον,* 'an intestine.' The operation of disembowelling or eviscerating.
EXERA'MA, from *εξεραω,* 'I throw out.' Any thing cast out. Vomiting; or the matter vomited. —Hippocrates.
EX'ERCISE, *Exercita'tio, Exercit"ium, Asce'sis, Gymna'sion,* from *exercere,* 'to work.' Every motion of the body arising from the contraction of muscles subjected to the will. Also, the action of any organ whatever. Exercise may be *active* or *passive.* The passive are referred to, under the head of Gestation. The chief active exercises are:—walking, running, dancing, hunting, fencing, playing at ball, cricket, racket, quoits, swimming, declamation, singing, &c. Exercise is an important prophylactic, particularly for those disposed to be plethoric. It improves the digestion; augments the secretions; and, when used in moderation, gives strength to the body; but when carried to excess, produces debility and disease.
EXERRHO'SIS, from *εξ,* 'out of,' and *ρεω,* 'I flow.' The discharge which takes place by insensible perspiration.
EXFŒTATION, see Pregnancy.
EXFOLIA'TION, *Exfolia'tio, Desquama'tio, Eclep'isis,* from *ex,* and *folium,* 'a leaf.' By this is meant the separation of the dead portions of a bone, tendon, aponeurosis, or cartilage, under the form of lamellæ or small scales. Exfoliation is accomplished by the instinctive action of the parts, and its object is to detach the dead portions from those subjacent, which are still alive. For this purpose the latter throw out fleshy granulations, and a more or less abundant suppuration occurs, which tends to separate the exfoliated part,—now become an extraneous body. The ancients distinguished exfoliation into *sensible* and *insensible,* according as the dead portions of bone were detached in fragments of greater or less size, or in very thin pieces, and in an almost insensible manner. When the dead part embraces all or almost all the substance of a bone, it takes the name Sequestrum.
EXFO'LIATIVE, *Exfoliati'vus, Desquamato'rius.* That which takes away by leaves or scales. The term has been applied to certain medicines, which were regarded as proper to hasten exfoliation, such as alcohol, oil of turpentine, tincture of myrrh, &c.
EXFO'LIATIVE TREPAN, *Eclepisitrep'anum.* An

ancient raspatory, or instrument for scraping exfoliating portions of bone.
EXHALAISON, Exhalation.
EXHA'LANT, *Exha'lent, Exha'lans*, from *exhalare*, (*ex*, and *halare*, 'to breathe,') 'to exhale,' 'throw out.'
EXHALANT VESSELS, *Vasa exhalan'tia*, are very minute, and rise from the arterial capillary system. They are situate in every tissue of the body, and on the surface of the mucous and serous membranes and skin; on which each pours its particular fluid. Bichat distinguished three sets. 1. The *external*, terminating on the mucous and external dermoid system, where they pour the matter of perspiration. 2. The *internal*, comprising those of the areolar and medullary tissues, and of synovial surfaces; and, 3. The *nutritive exhalants*, which vary in each organ where they are found, and preside over the phenomena of composition and increase of every part of the body. The exhalants are the antagonists of the absorbents. They are imaginary vessels, inasmuch as they cannot be detected.
EXHALATIO, Evaporation.
EXHALA'TION, *Exhala'tio;* same etymon. *Anathymi'asis, Apopneu'sis*, (F.) *Exhalaison*. A function, by virtue of which certain fluids, obtained from the blood, are spread, in the form of dew, in the areolæ of the different textures, or at the surface of membranes; either for the sake of being thrown out of the body, or to serve certain purposes. The sweat is a *liquid, excrementitious exhalation;* the serous fluid of the pleura, a *liquid, recrementitious exhalation*.
Exhalation is, also, applied to that which exhales from any body whatever, organic or inorganic, dead or living.
EXHALATION, PULMONARY, see Perspiration.
EXHAUS'TION, *Exar'ysis, Vires exhaust'æ*, from *exhaurire*, (*ex*, and *haurire*,) 'to draw out.' (F.) *Épuisement*. Loss of strength, occasioned by excessive evacuations, great fatigue or privation of food, or by disease.
EXHIL'ARANT, *Exhil'arans*, from *ex*, and *hilaro*, 'I make merry.' An agent that exhilarates or enlivens.
EXHUMA'TION, *Exhuma'tio, Effos'sio*, from *ex*, and *humus*, 'the ground.' The disinterment of a corpse. The circumstances which render this necessary are:—1. Judicial investigations relative to the body of the person inhumed. 2. The removal of a body from one cemetery to another; and, 3. The evacuation of cemeteries or sepulchral vaults. The operation is attended with much unpleasant smell and annoyance, and requires the use of disinfecting agents, of which the most powerful is chlorinated lime. See Disinfection. The putrid effluvia from animal substances are not, however, found to excite endemic disease.
EXIDIA AURICULA JUDÆ, Peziza auricula.
EXISCHIUM. Same etymon as the next. Prominence of the hips.
EXIS'CHIUS, *Exis'chus*, from *εξ*, 'out of,' and *ισχιον*, 'the ischium.' A luxation of the os femoris. Those with large nates, and prominent hips, were formerly called *Exis'chioi* and *Exescheglu'ti*.
EXITU'RA. According to some, any abscess which discharges. Paracelsus calls thus every kind of putrid excrement.
EX'ITUS, from *exire*, 'to go out.' The outer termination or *exit* of a canal. The termination of a disease.

EXOARTERITIS, see Arteritis.
EXOCARDIAC, see Endocardiac.
EXOCARDIAL, see Endocardiac.
EXOCARDITIS, Pericarditis.

EX'OCHAS, *Ex'ochā*, from *εξω*, 'without,' and *εχω*, 'I have.' A soft tumour—as a hemorrhoid—without the anus. An outward pile.
EXOCHE, Eminence, Exochas.
EXOCHORION, see Chorion.
EXOCOLITIS, see Colitis.
EXOCULA'TIO, from *ex*, 'out of,' and *oculus*, 'an eye.' Want of eyes. Want of vision. Blindness.
EXOCYS'TE, *Exocys'tis*, from *εξ*, 'out of,' and *κυστις*, 'the bladder.' A prolapsus of the bladder into the urethra. Also called *Prolap'sus vesi'cæ*, *Ædopto'sis vesi'cæ*, (F.) *Renversement de la vessie*.
EXOCYS'TE NOELIA'NA. Protrusion of the inner membrane of the bladder. So called from M. Noel, who first accurately described it.
EXOCYS'TE SOLINGENIA'NA. Protrusion of the neck of the bladder. Called after M. Solingen, who first accurately described it.
EXŒDESIS, Swelling.
EXODIC, Efferent.
EXOG"ENOUS, from *εξ*, 'out of,' and *γενναω*, 'I engender.' A term first applied to plants—hence called *Ex'ogens*—in which the wood increases by annual additions to the outside.
In animal anatomy, processes which shoot out from every part are termed *exogenous*.
EXOGENS, see Exogenous.
EXOGOGE, Extraction.
EXOGONYAN'CON, from *εξω*, 'outwards,' *γονυ*, 'the knee,' and *αγκων*, 'an elbow.' Bowing of the knees outwards.
EXOINE, Exoène, from *ex*, 'out of,' and *idoneus*, 'fit,' or rather from *exonerare*, 'to exonerate.' In France, a certificate of excuse, exemption, or dispensation, given to those summoned to appear before a court of justice, and who are unable to do so.
EXOLCE, Extraction.
EXOLUTION, Syncope.
EXOMETRA, Prolapsus uteri.
EXOMOIOSIS, Assimilation.
EXOMPHALOCELE, Exomphalus.
EXOM'PHALUS, *Exumbilica'tio, Exom'phaloce'lē, Om'phaloce'lē, Hernia umbilica'lis, Omphalex'ochē, Omphalopropto'sis, Prolap'sus umbili'ci*, (F.) *Hernie ombilicale, H. du nombril, Umbilical hernia*, from *εξ*, 'out of,' and *ομφαλος*, 'the navel.' Hernia occurring at the navel. This affection happens more frequently in infants, and takes place by the umbilical ring. In adults, it occurs more commonly in females than in males; and, when it does so, the sac passes in the vicinity of the umbilicus. The organs, found in this kind of hernia, are particularly,— the epiploon, the jejunum, the arch of the colon, and sometimes the stomach. The tumour is, in general, round, and presents all the characters of hernia. It is, commonly, readily reducible, and not subject to strangulation. It must be reduced, and retained by an elastic bandage, made in the form of a girdle, and furnished with a pad at its middle part. When strangulated, the stricture may be divided upwards and towards the left side.
EXONCO'MA, *Exonco'sis*, from *εξ*, and *ογκος*, 'a tumour.' A large, prominent tumour. Used by Galen, for protuberance of the vertebræ after luxation.
EXONCOSIS, Exoncoma—e. Linguæ, Glossoncus.
EXONEIROGMUS, Pollution, nocturnal.
EXONEIROSIS, Pollution, nocturnal.
EXONEURISM, Magnetism, animal.
EXOPHTHAL'MIA, *Ptosis seu Prolap'sus seu Providen'tia Oc'uli seu Bulbi Oculi, Exorbitis'mus, Ophthalmoce'lē, Ophthalmopto'sis, Oculi totius prominen'tia*, from *εξ*, 'out of,' and *οφθαλμος*, 'eye.' (F.) *Procidence de l'œil*. A protru-

sion of the eye from its orbit, occasioned by an abscess or tumour in the areolar texture of the orbit; by exostosis of the parietes of the orbit, &c. In exophthalmia, the eye is pressed forwards; the eyelids are raised and separated, so that they can no longer cover the eye and defend it from the action of extraneous bodies: it becomes inflamed, and the sight is disturbed or destroyed. The treatment of course depends upon the cause.

EXOPHTHAL'MIA FUNGO'SA, Sarcosis bulbi—e. Sarcomatica, Sarcosis bulbi.

EXOPHTHALMUS, same etymon. One whose eyes are very prominent. The opposite to Cœlophthalmus.

EXORBITISMUS, Exophthalmia.

EXORMIA, Papula—e. Lichen, Lichen—e. Prurigo, Prurigo—e. Strophulus, Strophulus.

EXORTUS UNGUIUM, see Nail.

EXOSIS, Luxation.

EXO-SKELETON, see Skeleton.

EXOSMA, from ἐξ, 'out of,' and ωθεω, 'to move.' A luxated or dislocated limb or organ.

EXOSMOSE, *Exosmo'sis, Transuda'tion*, from ἐξ, 'out of,' and ωσμος, 'impulse.' The opposite to Endosmose. The act by which substances transude from within to without an animal or other membrane.

EXOSMOT'IC, *Exosmot'icus*: same etymon. Belonging to Exosmose:—as an *exosmotic* current.

EXOSSATIO, Exostosis.

EXOSTEMMA CARIBÆA, Cinchonæ caribææ cortex.

EXOSTOMA, Exostosis.

EXOSTOSE, Exostosis—*e. des Dents*, Exostosis dentium—*e. Sous-ungéale*, see Subungual.

EXOSTO'SIS, *Hyperosto'sis, Emphy'ma, Exosto'sis os'sea, Exosto'ma, Eposto'ma, Eposto'sis, Osteo'ma, Osto'ma, Osteoph'yta, Exossa'tio, Ossis Eminen'tia*, (F.) *Exostose, Osteophyte*; from ἐξ, 'out of,' and οστεον, 'a bone.' An osseous tumour, which forms at the surface of bones, or in their cavities. Various kinds have been enumerated. *I'vory Exosto'sis; E. eburnée*;—that which has the appearance and consistence of ivory. *Lam'inar Exosto'sis; E. Laminée*;—that which is formed of laminæ in superposition or of distinct filaments. The *Spongy Exosto'sis* is that whose structure is analogous to the spongy tissue of bones. Exostoses are sometimes distinguished into the *true*, which seem to be a projection of the osseous substance, and which have the same organization and hardness as that substance; and the *false* or osteo-sarcoma. Exostosis may depend on syphilis, scrofula, rickets, gout, &c. In such cases, it is important to get rid of the primary disease.

Those *exostoses*, which occur within the bones, have, by some, been called *Enostoses*.

EXOSTOSIS, Spina ventosa.

EXOSTOSIS DENTIUM, (F.) *Exostose des Dents*. Exostosis of the teeth.

EXOSTOSIS STEATOMATODES, Osteosteatoma—e. Subunguial, see Subungual.

EXOTERIC, see Esoteric.

EXOT'IC, *Exo'ticus*, from εξω, 'without.' That which comes from abroad. Plants or drugs which are procured from abroad are so called. It is opposed to indigenous.

EXOTICADE'NIA, from *Exotic*, and αδεω, 'I dislike.' Aversion for exotic drugs.

EXOTICHÆMATOSIS, Transfusion.

EXOTICOMA'NIA. The opposite to exoticadenia. Fondness for exotic remedies.

EXOTICOSYM'PHYSIS, from εξωτικος, 'foreign,' and συμφυσις, 'a growing together.' A union or growing together of foreign bodies, as of a foreign body with the human.

EXPANSIO, Expansion—e. Musculosa, Platysma myoides.

EXPAN'SION, *Expan'sio*, from *expandere*, (*ex* and *pandere*, 'to open,') 'to spread out.' A prolongation or spreading out, presented by certain organs. Thus, we say an *aponeurotic expansion*, &c.

EXPATRATIO, Ejaculation (of Sperm.)

EXPEC'TANT, *Expec'tans*, from *expectare*, (*ex* and *spectare*, 'to look,') 'to wait.' That which waits:—as *Expectant Medicine*,—*La Médecine expectante*. See Expectation.

EXPECTA'TION, *Expecta'tio*; same etymon. The word *expectation* has been applied, in medicine, to that method, which consists in observing the progress of diseases, and removing deranging influences, without prescribing active medicines, unless such shall be imperiously required. It consists, in fact, in leaving the disease almost wholly to the efforts of nature, and has been termed the *art of curing diseases by expectation* or *waiting*—*Ars sanan'di cum expectatio'ne*.

EXPEC'TORANT, *Expec'torative, Expec'torans, Anacathar'ticus, Ptys'magogue*, from *ex*, 'out of,' and *pectus*, 'the breast.' A medicine capable of facilitating or provoking expectoration. There is probably no such thing as a *direct* expectorant. They all act through the system, or by impressions made on parts at a distance, which, through the medium of general, continuous, or contiguous sympathy, excite the secretory vessels of the air-passages into action. The following are the chief reputed expectorants:—Ammoniacum; Asafœtida; Galbanum; Ipecacuanha; Myroxylon; Myrrha; Inhalations of Iodine, Stramonium, Tar, Burning Wool, Tobacco, &c.; Scilla; Senega, and Tolutanum.

EXPECTORATIO, Expectoration—e. Sanguinis, Hæmoptysis—e. Solida, Cynanche trachealis.

EXPECTORA'TION, *Expectora'tio, Ecchel'ysis, Bex hu'mida, Anap'tysis, Prop'tysis, Stethocathar'sis, Anacathar'sis, Anabex'is*, same etymon. The act of expelling from the chest matters or secretions there collected or existing. It is, likewise, used for the expectorated matter.

EXPECTORATION DE SANG, Hæmoptysis.

EXPECTORATION, PRUNE-JUICE, see Prune-juice.

EXPECTORATIVE, Expectorant.

EXPELLENS, Expulsive.

EXPE'RIENCE, *Experien'tia, Peira, Empei'ra*, from εξ, and πειρα, 'a trial.' A knowledge of things acquired by observation. In medicine, this knowledge can be obtained both by the practitioner's own experience, and by that obtained from tradition and from books. To profit by experience requires a mind capable of appreciating the proper relations between cause and effect; and hence it happens, that *false experience, Experien'tia fallax*, is extremely common; and that a man had better, in many instances, trust to that which he has learned from others, than to his own fallacious observation.

The union of accurate observation by the physician with that handed down by medical writers constitutes perfect experience, so far as it is attainable in any individual case.

EXPÉRIENCE, Experiment.

EXPERIMENT, *Experimen'tum*; same etymon. (F.) *Expérience*. A trial, made on the bodies of men or animals, for the purpose of detecting the effect of a remedy, or of becoming better acquainted with their structure, functions, or peculiarities. In a more general sense, it means any trial instituted with the intent of becoming better acquainted with any thing. By experiments on living animals, we have obtained much valuable information in the various departments of medicine; but particularly in physiology and toxicology.

EXPERIMENT OF MARIOTTE, see Mariotte.

EXPERS NUPTIARUM, Virgin.

EXPERT, (F.) *Exper'tus*, from *ex*, and *peritus*, 'skilled.' Skilful or of good experience. A physician, charged with the duty of making a report upon any case of legal medicine.

EXPIRA'TION, *Expira'tio*, *Exspira'tio*, *Ec'-pnoē*, *Ecpneumato'sis*, *Ecpneu'sis*, *Apopneu'sis*, *Apop'noē*, *Apopnœ'a*, from *exspirare*, (*ex*, and *spirare*,) 'to breathe out.' The act of expelling from the chest, the air received in during respiration.

EX'PIRATORY, *Expiratio'ni inser'viens*. Relating or appertaining to expiration. The expiratory muscles are all those which contribute to diminish the cavity of the chest, for the purpose of expelling the air contained in the lungs, or of producing expiration. These muscles are, chiefly, the intercostals, triangularis sterni, quadratus lumborum, serratus posticus inferior, the oblique and recti muscles of the abdomen, the sacro-lumbalis, &c.

EXPLORATIO, Exploration — e. Abdominis, Abdominoscopia.

EXPLORA'TION, *Explora'tio*, *Recognit"io*, from *explorare*, 'to search into.' The act of observing and attentively examining or investigating every thing connected with a case of disease. The word is chiefly used in this sense by the French practitioners.

EXPLORA'TOR, CHEST. An instrument, proposed by Dr. B. Babington for exploring the chest in cases of empyema. It consists of a needle, contained in the smallest sized canula. This is passed between the ribs into the chest. The needle is then withdrawn, and the escape of fluid indicates the nature of the case.

EXPLORATORIUM, Sound, Specillum.

EXPRES'SION, *Expres'sio*, *Ecpies'mos*, *Ecthlip'sis*, from *ex*, 'out of,' and *premere*, 'to press.' The act of compressing a substance, for the purpose of separating from it the fluids which it contains. Also, the manner in which impressions made upon us are depicted; especially in the traits of the countenance.

EXPRESSION OF SWEAT, (F.) *Sueur d'expression*, is a term given to the passive perspiration observable in very debilitated individuals.

EXPULSIO, Excretion—e. Fæcum, Defecation —e. Fœtûs, Parturition.

EXPULSION, SPONTANEOUS, Evolution, spontaneous.

EXPUL'SIVE, *Expel'lens*, *Expulso'rius*, from *expellere*, (*ex*, and *pellere*,) 'to drive away.' An *expulsive bandage*, (F.) *Bandage expulsif*, is one constructed with the view of compressing a part, from which we are desirous of expelling pus, serum, &c. Certain medicines were formerly called *expulsives*, which were believed to have the power of driving the humours towards the skin;—as diaphoretics, and sudorifics.

EXPULTRIX, see Vis Expultrix.

EXSANGUINITY, Anæmia.

EXSANGUIS, Exanguious. *Exsanguis* is used by Ausonius for one exhausted by venery;—as *sanguis* meant sperm as well as blood. See Sperm.

EXSARCOMA, Sarcoma.

EXSCREATIO, Excreation.

EXSECTIO VIRILIUM, Castration.

EXSECTUS, Castratus, Eunuch.

EXSICCATIO, Drying.

EXSICCATIVA, Desiccativa.

EXSOLUTIO, Eclysis.

EXSPIRATIO, Expiration.

EXSPUIT"ION, *Exspuit"io*, *Spuit"io*, *Sputa'tio*, *Anachremp'sis*, *Apochremp'sis*, *Chremp'sis*, *Ptysis*, *Anacine'ma*, *Anacine'sis*, (F.) *Sputation*, from *ex*, 'out of,' and *spuo*, 'I spit.' Rejection of the matters accumulated in the pharynx and larynx; spitting.

EXSTASIS, Ecstasis.

EXSTIRPATIO, Extirpation.

EXSTROPH'IA, *Ex'strophy*, *Ec'strophē*, from *ἐξ*, 'out of,' and *στροφή*, 'turning.' *Extrover'sio*, *Extrover'sion*. Eversion or turning out of a part —as of the eyelids. A term used by M. Chaussier for certain displacements of organs, and especially of the urinary bladder.

EXSTROPH'IA or EX'STROPHY OF THE BLADDER, (F.) *Renversement de la Vessie*, is a faulty conformation, in which the organ opens above the pubes; so that in the hypogastric region there is a red, mucous surface, formed by the inner coat of the bladder; on which two prominences are distinguishable, corresponding to the openings of the ureters.

EXSUCCATIO, Ecchymoma.

EXSUC'TIO, *Suc'tio*, *Ecmyze'sis*, from *ex*, 'out of,' and *succus*, 'a juice.' The action of sucking.

EXSUDATIO, Ephidrosis.

EXSUFFLATIO, Ecphysesis.

EXTEMPORA'NEOUS, *Extempora'neus*, *Extempora'lis*, from *ex*, and *tempore*, 'out of time.' Those prescriptions are called 'extemporaneous,' or 'magistral,' which are made on the spot, and composed according to the prescription of the physician.

EXTENSEUR COMMUN DES DOIGTS, Extensor digitorum communis — *e. Commun des orteils*, Extensor communis digitorum pedis — *e. Court du Pouce*, Extensor pollicis brevis—*e. Long du pouce*, Extensor longus pollicis — *e. Petit des orteils*, Extensor brevis digitorum pedis — *e. Propre du petit doigt*, Extensor proprius minimi digiti — *e. Propre de l'Index*, Extensor preprius indicis.

EXTENSIBIL'ITY, *Extensibil'itas*. A property, possessed by certain bodies, of being capable of extension or elongation.

EXTENSIO, Extension, Tetanus.

EXTEN'SION, *Exten'sio*, *Tasis*, *Ec'tasis*, *Catat'asis*, *Anat'asis*, from *extendere*, (*ex*, and *tendere*,) 'to stretch out.' An operation in surgery, in which either with the hands alone, or by straps, a fractured or luxated limb is pulled strongly, to restore it to its natural position. It is the opposite of *Counter-extension*.

EXTENSOR. Same etymon. (F.) *Extenseur*. A muscle, whose office is to extend certain parts.

EXTENSOR BREVIS DIGITO'RUM PEDIS, *Ped'icus*, *Calcanéo-phalanginien commun*, of DUMAS; (F.) *Muscle pédieux*, *Muscle petit extenseur des orteils*, *Calcanéo-sus-phalangettien commun*—(Ch.) *Carré du pied; Short Extensor of the Toes*. A muscle, situate on the dorsal region of the foot. It arises from the external surface of the calcaneum, and at the anterior edge of a ligament, which unites that bone to the astragalus. Anteriorly, each of its divisions terminates by a small tendon, which is fixed successively, at the superior part of the posterior extremity of the first phalanx of the great toe, and to the second and last phalanges of the next three toes. Its use is to extend the first four toes, and to direct them a little outwards.

EXTENSOR CARPI RADIALIS BREVIS, see Radialis — e. Carpi radialis longus, see Radialis — e. Carpi ulnaris, see Cubital muscles.

EXTENSOR COMMU'NIS DIGITO'RUM PEDIS, *E. Longus Digitorum Pedis*, *E. Digitorum longus*, *Péronéo-tibi-sus-phalangettien commun*, *Cnemodactyla'us*, *Péronéo-sus-phalangettien commun*, (F.)

Extenseur commun des Orteils. This muscle, also, is situate at the anterior part of the leg. It is long, thin, flattened, simple, and fleshy above, and divided into four tendons below. It arises from the outer tuberosity of the tibia and the anterior surface of the fibula, and is inserted into the superior part of the posterior extremity of the second and third phalanges of the last four toes. It extends the three phalanges of these toes.

EXTENSOR DIGITO'RUM COMMU'NIS, *Extensor digitorum communis manûs cum extenso'rē pro'prio auricula'ris, Digito'rum Tensor;* (F.) *Épicondylo-sus-phalangettien commun*—(Ch.,)—*Common Extensor of the Fingers, Extenseur commun des Doigts.* A long, flattened muscle; simple above, and divided into four portions inferiorly. It is situate at the posterior part of the forearm; arises from the external tuberosity of the humerus; from the aponeurosis of the forearm, and from the aponeurotic septa situate between it and the neighbouring muscles, and is inserted at the posterior surface of the second and third phalanges of the last four fingers. This muscle extends the phalanges of the last four fingers upon each other, and upon the metacarpal bone. It can, also, extend the hand on the forearm.

EXTENSOR DIGITORUM LONGUS, E. communis digitorum pedis — e. Longus digitorum pedis, E. communis digitorum pedis—e. Proprius hallucis, E. proprius pollicis pedis—e. Indicis, E. proprius indicis—e. Internodii ossis pollicis, E. longus pollicis — e. Primi internodii, Abductor longus pollicis.

EXTENSOR POL'LICIS BREVIS, *Exten'sor minor pol'licis manûs, E. primi interno'dii, E. pol'licis primus, E. Secun'di interno'dii,* (DOUGLAS,) *E. secun'di interno'dii ossis pol'licis;* (F.) *Cubito-sus-phalangien du pouce,*—(Ch.,) *Court extenseur du pouce.* Seated at the posterior and inferior part of the forearm. It is thin, long, and broader at its middle than at the extremities. It arises from the posterior surface of the ulna and the interosseous ligament, and is inserted behind the superior extremity of the first phalanx of the thumb. It extends the thumb, and aids in supination.

EXTENSOR POL'LICIS LONGUS; *Extensor major pol'licis manûs, Extensor secun'di interno'dii, Extensor pollicis secun'dus, Extensor ter'tii interno'dii* (DOUGLAS,) *Extensor interno'dii ossis pol'licis,* (F.) *Cubito-sus-phalangettein du pouce,*—(Ch.,) *Muscle long extenseur du pouce.* This muscle is long, flat, and fusiform; and is seated at the posterior part of the forearm. It arises from the posterior surface of the ulna and the interosseous ligament, and is inserted at the posterior part of the superior extremity of the first phalanx of the thumb. It extends the last phalanx of the thumb upon the first.

EXTENSOR PRO'PRIUS IN'DICIS, *E. proprius primi dig"iti manûs, E. In'dicis, Indica'tor, Extensor secun'di interno'dii in'dicis pro'prius,* (F.) *Cubito-sus-phalangettien de l'Index,*—(Ch.,) *Extenseur propre de l'Index.* This muscle is long and thin; broader in the middle than at the extremities; and is situate at the posterior part of the forearm. It arises from the posterior surface of the ulna, and is inserted at the posterior part of the upper extremity of the second and third phalanges of the index-finger. It extends the three phalanges of the index-finger; and has, besides, the same uses as the other extremities of the fingers.

EXTENSOR PRO'PRIUS MIN'IMI DIG"ITI, (F.) *Épicondylo-sus-phalangettien du petit doigt,*— (Ch.,) *Extenseur propre du petit doigt.* Situate on the inside of the *Extensor communis digito'rum.* It arises from the external condyle of the os humeri and the aponeurotic septa seated between it, the extensor communis digitorum, and the extensor carpi ulnaris; and is inserted into the last two phalanges of the little finger. Its use is to extend the little finger, and even the hand upon the forearm.

EXTENSOR PRO'PRIUS POL'LICIS PEDIS, *E. proprius Hal'lucis, E. Longus* (DOUGLAS), *E. pollicis longus, Péronéo-sus-phalangien du pouce, Péronéo-sus-phalangettien du pouce,*—(Ch.) This muscle is situate at the anterior part of the leg. It is fleshy, broad, flat above; small and tendinous below. It arises from the anterior part of the middle third of the fibula, and is inserted into the posterior part of the superior extremity of the last phalanx of the great toe. It extends the last phalanx of the great toe upon the first, and the first upon the first metacarpal bone.

EXTENSOR PRIMI INTERNODII, E. pollicis brevis — e. Secundi internodii, E. pollicis brevis, Extensor longus pollicis — e. Secundi internodii indicis proprius, E. proprius indicis—e. Tertii internodii, E. longus pollicis — e. Tertii internodii indicis, Prior annularis — e. Tertii internodii minimi digiti, Abductor minimi digiti — e. Ossis metacarpi pollicis manûs, Abductor longus pollicis—e. Pollicis longus, E. proprius pollicis pedis —e. Pollicis secundus, E. longus pollicis—e. Minor pollicis manûs, E. pollicis brevis—e. Primus pollicis, Abductor longus pollicis.

EXTENSOR TARSI MAGNUS, *E. Tarsi sura'lis.* A name given, by some anatomists, to the gastrocnemius and soleus combined.

EXTENSOR TARSI MINOR, Plantar muscle.

EXTENUATIO, Emaciation.

EXTERGENTIA, Detergents.

EXTER'NAL DISEASES, *Extrin'sic Diseases, Morbi extrin'seci, Surgical diseases,* (F.) *Maladies externes.* Those diseases which occupy the surface of the body, and form the object of surgical pathology, requiring, generally, external means, or surgical operations.

EXTERNAT. The post or office of an *externe.*

EXTERNE, see House-surgeon.

EXTERNUS AURIS, Laxator tympani — e. Mallei, Laxator tympani.

EXTESTICULATUS, Castratus, Eunuch.

EXTINCTIO, Death — e. Hydrargyri, Extinction of Mercury — e. Mercurii, Extinction of Mercury.

EXTINCTIO VOCIS, (F.) *Extinction de voix.* The French use this term for cases in which the voice is not wholly suppressed, but produces only feeble sounds:—*Incomplete aphonia.*

EXTINC'TION OF MER'CURY, *Extinc'tio Merou'rii vel Hydrar'gyri.* Trituration of mercury with lard or other substance, until the metallic globules disappear. The mercury is then so divided, that it forms a black powder, generally considered to be a protoxide of mercury, but, perhaps, erroneously.

EXTIRPATIO, Extirpation—e. Linguæ, Glossosteresis—e. Testiculorum, Castratio.

EXTIRPA'TION, *Extirpa'tio, Exstirpa'tio, Abla'tio, Aphæ'resis,* from *extirpare,* (*ex,* and *stirps,*) 'to root out.' The complete removal or destruction of any part, either by cutting instruments or the action of caustics. Thus, we speak of the extirpation of cancer, polypus, encysted tumour, &c.

EXTOMIUS, Eunuch.

EXTOZOA, Ectozoa.

EXTOZOAIRES. Ectozoa.

EXTOZOARIA, Ectozoa.

EXTRA-PELVIO-PUBI-TROCHANTÉ-RIEN, Obturator externus.

EXTRACT, Extractum — e. of Aconite, Extractum aconiti—e. of Aconite, alcoholic, Extractum aconiti alcoholicum — e. Alcoholic, see Extractum — e. of Aloes, purified, Extractum aloes purificatum—e. of Bark, Extractum cinchonæ—e. of Bark, resinous, Extractum cinchonæ resinosum—e. of Belladonna, Extractum belladonnæ—e. of Belladonna, alcoholic, Extractum belladonnæ alcoholicum — e. of Bittersweet, Extractum dulcamaræ — e. of Broom-tops, Extractum cacuminum genistæ — e. of Butternut, Extractum juglandis — e. of Cascarilla, resinous, Extractum cascarillæ resinosum — e. of Chamomile, E. anthemidis—e. of Cinchona, Extractum cinchonæ——e. of Colchicum, acetic, Extractum colchici aceticum — e. of Colocynth, Extractum colocynthidis e. of Colocynth, compound, Extractum colocynthidis compositum — e. of Cubebs, fluid, Extractum cubebæ fluidum—e. of Dandelion, Extractum taraxaci—e. of Elaterium, Extractum elaterii—e. of Ergot, Ergotin—e. Ethereal, see Extractum—e. of Gentian, Extractum gentianæ — e. of Hemlock, Extractum cicutæ — e. of Hellebore, black, Extractum hellebori — e. of Hemlock, alcoholic, Extractum conii alcoholicum — e. of Henbane, Extractum hyoscyami—e. of Henbane, alcoholic, Extractum hyoscyami alcoholicum — e. of Hops, Extractum humuli—e. of Jalap, Extractum jalapæ — e. of Lettuce, Extractum lactucæ — e. of Liquorice, Extractum glycyrrhizæ — e. of Logwood, Extractum hæmatoxyli — e. of Mayapple, Extractum podophylli—e. of Meat, saponaceous, Osmazome — e. of Oak-bark, Extractum corticis quercûs—e. of white Poppy, Extractum papaveris — e. of Quassia, Extractum quassiæ — e. of Quinia, Extractum quiniæ — e. of Rhatany, Extractum krameriæ — e. of Rhubarb, Extractum rhei — e. of Rhubarb, fluid, Extractum rhei fluidum — e. of Rue, Extractum rutæ — e. of Sarsaparilla, Extractum sarsaparillæ—e. of Sarsaparilla, fluid, Extractum sarsaparillæ fluidum — e. of Savine, Extractum foliorum sabinæ—e. of Senna, fluid, Extractum sennæ fluidum — e. of Spigelia and Senna, Extractum spigeliæ et sennæ—e. of Stramonium, Extractum stramonii — e. of Valerian, Extractum valerianæ — e. of Wormwood, Extractum cacuminum absinthii.

EXTRACTIF, Extractive.

EXTRAC'TION, *Extrac'tio, Exæ'resis, Exogo'gē, Exolcē, Exelcys'mus, Enchylo'sis*, from *extrahere*, (*ex*, and *trahere*,) 'to draw out.' The act of removing an extraneous substance from any part of the body. Thus, a splinter is said to be extracted. It is, also, applied to the removal of certain parts. The cataract is said to be *extracted*: a tooth is *extracted*, when carious, &c.

EXTRAC'TIVE, (F.) *Extractif*. Same etymon. A peculiar, immediate principle, which has been admitted in extracts. Thus, *bitter extractive* is the immediate principle of bitter vegetables, &c.

EXTRAC'TUM, *Extract, Ecchylo'ma*, (F.) *Extrait*. An extract is prepared by evaporating vegetable solutions, till a tenacious mass is obtained. When prepared from an infusion or decoction, it is called a *watery*, — from ether, an *ethereal*,—and from alcohol, an *alcohol'ic* or a *spirituous extract*. Both kinds contain all the principles of the vegetable, that are soluble in the menstrua with which they are prepared; but the volatile parts are dissipated, and some of the fixed parts are decomposed; the proper extractive is oxygenized, and the virtues of the vegetable substance consequently altered or destroyed. Extracts are *hard, soft*, or *fluid*: the consistence of the soft being such as to retain the pilular form without the addition of a powder. A patent was taken out many years ago, by a Mr. Barry, of London, for preparing them in vacuo; and, as the temperature is much lower than in the ordinary method, the virtues of the plant are less altered, and the extracts are generally green. Extracts are also prepared by displacement or percolation. They have, likewise, received different names, according to their predominant principle. The *gummy* or *mucous*, or *mucilaginous*, are those which are mainly composed of gum or mucilage. Gum tragacanth may be considered a pure gummy extract. *Gelatinous extracts* are those composed especially of gelatin; *resinous extracts*, those of a resinous character; *extractoresinous*, those composed of extractive or colouring matter and resin; *gum-resinous*, those containing gum and resin; and *sapona'ceous* or *sapona'ceous saline*, those containing a notable quantity of saline substances and a resinous matter, so combined with mucus and other soluble substances, that they cannot be separated.

EXTRACTUM ABSIN'THII CACU'MINUM, *Extract of Wormwood*. (A decoction defecated and evaporated.) The flavour is dissipated along with the essential oil. It is a bitter tonic. Dose, gr. x to ℈j, in pill.

EXTRACTUM ACONI'TI, *Extract of Aconite, Succus spissa'tus aconiti napelli*, (from the inspissated juice without defecation.) It is esteemed to be narcotic and diuretic; and has been given in the cases referred to under Aconitum. Dose, gr. j, gradually increasing it.

EXTRACTUM ACONI'TI ALCOHOL'ICUM, *Alcoholic Extract of Aconite*. (Aconit. in pulv. crass. ℔j; Alcohol. dilut. Oiv. Moisten the aconite with half a pint of diluted alcohol: let it stand for 24 hours: transfer it to a displacement apparatus, and gradually add the remainder of the diluted alcohol. When the last portion of this has penetrated the aconite, pour in from time to time water sufficient to keep the powder covered. Stop the filtration when the liquid which passes begins to produce a precipitate, as it falls, in that which has already passed. Distil off the alcohol, and evaporate to a proper consistence.— Ph. U. S.)

EXTRACTUM AL'OËS PURIFICA'TUM, *Pu'rified extract of aloes*. (The gummy part extracted by boiling water, defecated and inspissated.) Dose, gr. v to gr. xv.

EXTRACTUM ANTHEM'IDIS, *E. anthemidis no'bilis, E. chamæme'li, E. florum chamæme'li, Extract of Cham'omile*. The volatile oil is dissipated in this preparation. It is a pure, grateful bitter, and is tonic and stomachic. Dose, gr. x to gr. xx, in pills.

EXTRACTUM ASPARAGI, see Asparagus.

EXTRACTUM BELLADON'NÆ, *Succus spissa'tus at'ropæ belladon'næ, Extract of Belladon'na*, (an expressed juice inspissated.) Properties same as those of the plant. Dose, gr. ¼, gradually increased. It dilates the pupil when applied to the eye.

EXTRACTUM BELLADONNÆ ALCOHOL'ICUM, *Alcohol'ic extract of Belladonna*. (Prepared like the extractum aconiti alcoholicum.—Ph. U. S.)

EXTRACTUM CANNABIS, see Bangue.

EXTRACTUM CASCARIL'LÆ RESINO'SUM, *Res'inous extract of cascaril'la*. (*Cort. cascarillæ*, in pulv. crass. ℔j; *Sp. vini rect*. ℔iv. Digest for four days; then decant and strain; boil the residuum in ten pints of water to two; filter and evaporate the decoction, and distil the tincture in a retort, till both are thickened; then mix and evaporate to a pilular consistence.) Dose, gr. x to gr. xx, in pills.

EXTRACTUM CATHARTICUM, E. Colocynthidis compositum — e. Catechu, Catechu — e. Chamæmeli, E. Anthemidis—e. Cicutæ, E. Conii.

EXTRACTUM CATHOL'ICUM, (F.) *Extrait Catholique.* This epithet is given to pills composed of aloes, black hellebore, and colocynth, resin of jalap, and scammony. See, also, Extractum colocynthidis compositum.

EXTRACTUM CINCHO'NÆ, *Extract of Cincho'na, E. Cor'ticis Peruvia'ni, E. Cincho'næ Mollë, E. of Bark.* (*A decoction evaporated.*) The active principles are similar to those of the bark in substance; but it is not so effectual — owing to the chymical change induced in the drug during the boiling. When reduced, by drying, to a state fit for being powdered, it is called the *Hard Extract of Bark, Extrac'tum Cor'ticis Peruvia'ni durum, E. Cincho'næ durum.* Dose, gr. x to ʒss.

EXTRACTUM CINCHONÆ RESINO'SUM, *E. Cinchonæ lancifo'liæ, E. Cinchonæ Rubræ resino'sum, Res'inous Extract of Bark, E. Cincho'næ Resi'næ.* The aqueo-spirituous extract contains both the extractive and resin of the bark. Dose, gr. x to xxx.

Extractum Cinchonæ of the Pharmacopœia of the United States, (1842,) is directed to be prepared as follows: — *Peruvian Bark*, in coarse powder, ℔j; *Alcohol*, Oiv; *Water*, a sufficient quantity. Macerate the Peruvian bark with the alcohol for four days; then filter by a displacement apparatus, and when the liquid ceases to pass, pour gradually on the bark water sufficient to keep its surface covered. When the filtered tincture measures four pints, set it aside, and proceed with the filtration until six pints of infusion are obtained. Distil off the alcohol from the tincture and evaporate the infusion till the liquids are respectively brought to the consistence of thin honey; then mix and evaporate to form an extract.—Ph. U. S.

EXTRAC'TUM COL'CHICI ACE'TICUM, *Ace'tous* or *Ace'tic Extract of Colchicum.* (*Colchic. rad.* in pulv. crass. ℔j, *Acid. acet.* f℥iv, *Aquæ* q. s. To the acid add a pint of water, and mix this with the root. Put the mixture in a percolator, and pour on water until the liquid that passes has little or no taste. Evaporate to a proper consistence. Ph. U. S.) Dose, gr. j to gr. iij.

EXTRACTUM COLOCYN'THIDIS, *Extract of Col'ocynth.* A cathartic, in the dose of from gr. v to ʒss.

EXTRACTUM COLOCYN'THIDIS COMPOS'ITUM, *Ext, actum Cathar'ticum, E. Cathol'icum, E. Querceta'ni, Compound Extract of Colocynth.* (*Colocynth. pulp.* concis. ℥vj, *Aloes* pulv. ℥xij, *Scammon.* pulv. ℥iv, *Cardamom.* pulv. ʒj, *Saponis* ʒiij, *Alcohol.* dilut. cong. Macerate the pulp in the spirit at a gentle heat for four days; strain: add the aloes and scammony; then distil off the spirit and mix in the cardamom seeds. Ph. U. S.) It is a powerful cathartic, and is used in obstinate visceral obstructions, &c. Dose, gr. vj to ʒss.

EXTRACTUM CONI'I, *E. Cicu'tæ, Succus cicutæ spissa'tus, Extract of Hemlock, Succus spissatus conii macula'ti.* (*Expressed juice inspissated without defecation.*) Employed in the same cases as the conium. Dose, gr. iij to ƺj.

EXTRACTUM CONII ALCOHOL'ICUM, *Alcoholic Extract of Hemlock.* (Prepared like the Extractum aconiti alcoholicum.—Ph. U. S.)

EXTRACTUM CONVOLVULI JALAPÆ, E. jalapæ e. Corticis Peruviani, E. Cinchonæ.

EXTRACT'UM CUBEB'Æ FLU'IDUM, *Fluid Extract of Cubebs.* (*Cubebs exhausted by ether through percolation, and the solution evaporated.* Ph. U. S.)

EXTRACTUM DULCAMA'RÆ, *Extract of Bittersweet.* (Prepared by displacement from bittersweet in coarse powder.—Ph. U. S.)

EXTRACTUM ELATE'RII, *Elate'rium, Extract of Elaterium.* (*The fecula of the expressed juice.*) It is violently cathartic, hydragogue, and sometimes emetic. Dose, gr. ss. every hour till it operates.

EXTRACTUM ERGOTÆ, Ergotin.

EXTRACTUM GENIS'TÆ CACU'MINUM, *Extract of Broom Tops.* Diuretic and stomachic. Dose, ʒss to ʒj.

EXTRACTUM GENTIA'NÆ, *Ext. Gentia'næ lu'teæ, Ext. Radi'cis Gentia'næ, Extract of Gen'tian.* (*The evaporated decoction.*) Prepared also by displacement.—Ph. U. S.) Properties like those of Gentian. Dose, gr. x to ʒss.

EXTRACTUM GLYCYRRHI'ZÆ; *Extract of Liquorice, Succus Glycyrrhi'zæ inspissa'tus, Succus Liquirit''iæ.* (*The evaporated decoction.*) It is demulcent, taken *ad libitum.*

Refined Liquorice, which is sold in the form of cylinders, is made by gently evaporating a solution of the pure extract of liquorice with half its weight of gum Arabic, rolling the mass and cutting it into lengths, and then polishing, by rolling them together in a box.

EXTRAC'TUM GRAM'INIS, 'Extract of Grass.' An extract prepared from *Triticum repens.* It is considered by the Germans to be a mild tonic; and is greatly used, especially in convalescence from fever. It is probably devoid of all injurious properties, and as probably totally inefficacious.

EXTRACTUM HÆMATOX'YLI, *E. Hæmatox'yli Campechia'ni, E. Scobis Hæmatox'yli, Extract of Logwood.* (*The evaporated decoction.*) It is astringent. Dose, gr. x to ʒj.

EXTRACTUM RADI'CIS HELLEB'ORI NIGRI, *Ext. of Black Hell'ebore root, E. Hellebori nigri.* (*The evaporated decoction.*) In large doses, this is cathartic; in smaller, diuretic, resolvent (?) and emmenagogue (?). Dose, as a cathartic, gr. x to ƺj; as an emmenagogue, gr. iij to gr. x.

EXTRACTUM HELLEBORI, of the Pharmacopœia of the United States (1842), is prepared from Black Hellebore, in coarse powder, like the Extractum aconiti alcoholicum.

EXTRACTUM HU'MULI, *Extract of hops,* (*the evaporated decoction.*) It is tonic, anodyne (?), diuretic (?). Dose, gr. v to ʒj.

EXTRACTUM HYOSCY'AMI, *Extract of Henbane, Succus spissa'tus Hyoscyami nigri, Succ. Spiss. Hyoscyami.* (*The expressed juice, inspissated without defecation.*) Its virtues are narcotic. Dose, gr. v to ƺss.

EXTRACTUM HYOSCYAMI ALCOHOL'ICUM, *Alcoholic Extract of Henbane.* (Prepared from leaves of Hyoscyamus, in coarse powder, like the Extractum aconiti alcoholicum.—Ph. U. S.)

EXTRACTUM JALA'PÆ, *E. Convol'vuli Jalapæ, E. Jala'pii, Extract of Jalap, E. Jala'pi.* (*A spirituous tincture distilled; and an aqueous decoction evaporated; the residua being mixed together:* kept both soft and hard.) It is cathartic and hydragogue. Dose, gr. x to ƺj.

EXTRACTUM JALAPÆ of the Ph. U. S. is prepared like the Extractum cinchonæ, Ph. U. S.

EXTRACTUM JALAPÆ RESINO'SUM, *Res'inous Extract of Jalap.* This is cathartic.

EXTRACTUM JUGLAN'DIS, *Extract of Butternut.* (Prepared by displacement from butternut, in coarse powder.—Ph. U. S.)

EXTRACTUM KRAME'RIÆ, *Extract of Rhatany.* (Prepared by displacement from rhatany, in coarse powder.—Ph. U. S.)

EXTRACTUM LACTU'CÆ, *Extract of Lettuce, Succus spissa'tus Lactucæ sativæ.* (*Leaves of fresh lettuce* ℔j; beat them in a stone mortar, sprinkling them with water; then express the juice and evaporate, without allowing it to subside until it acquires a proper degree of consistence.) It is said to be narcotic and diaphoretic. Dose, gr. iij to gr. x.

An extract is, sometimes, made from the juice of the *wild lettuce*, *Lactuca viro'sa*, which is regarded as diuretic.

EXTRACTUM MARTIS ACETICUM, Ferri Acetas—e. Nucis Vomicæ, see Strychnos nux vomica.

EXTRACTUM O'PII, E. Opii aquo'sum, E. Theba'icum, Extract of Opium, E. Opii gummo'sum, Lau'danum opia'tum seu simplex, Opium cola'tum seu depura'tum. (*A watery solution defecated and evaporated.*) Dose, gr. ss to gr. v.

EXTRACTUM PANCHYMAGO'GUM. A drastic medicine, composed of *colocynth*, bruised with its *seeds*; *senna* bruised; *black hellebore root*, *Agaric*, *Scammony*, in powder, Extract of Aloes, and Powder of Diarrhodon.

EXTRACTUM PAPAV'ERIS, E. Papav'eris somnif'eri, E. Papaveris albi, Extract of white poppy. (*The decoction evaporated.*) It possesses nearly the same virtues as opium, but is weaker. Dose, gr. ij to ƷJ.

EXTRACTUM PIP'ERIS FLU'IDUM, Fluid Extract of Black Pepper. (*Black pepper* exhausted by *ether* through percolation, the solution evaporated, and the piperin in crystals separated by expression. Ph. U. S.)

EXTRACTUM PODOPHYL'LI, Extract of Mayapple. (Prepared from podophyllum, in coarse powder, in the same manner as the Extract of cinchona.—Ph. U. S.)

EXTRACTUM PURGANS, see Hedera helix—e. Quercetani, E. Colocynthidis compositum.

EXTRACTUM QUAS'SIÆ, Extract of Quassia. (Prepared by displacement from Quassia rasped. —Ph. U. S.)

EXTRACTUM COR'TICIS QUERCÛS, Extract of oak bark. (*The decoction evaporated.*) It is astringent and tonic.

EXTRACTUM QUI'NÆ, Quiniæ sulphas impu'rus. This is made by evaporating the liquor poured off the crystals of sulphate of quinia to the consistence of a pilular mass. Twenty-four grains will generally arrest an intermittent.

EXTRACTUM RHEI, Extract of Rhubarb. (*A solution in diluted alcohol evaporated.*) Uses like those of the powdered root. Dose, gr. x to ℨss.

EXTRACTUM RHEI FLU'IDUM, Fluid Extract of Rhubarb. (*Rhej* in pulv. crass. ℥viij, Sacchar. ℥v, Tinct. Zingib. f℥ss, Ol. fœnicul., Ol. anis. ȧȧ ♏iv; Alcohol. dilut. q. s. Digest the rhubarb, mixed with an equal bulk of coarse sand, with ℥xij of the diluted alcohol for 24 hours. Put the mass into the percolator, and pour on diluted alcohol until the liquid that passes has little odour or taste of rhubarb; evaporate to f℥v; dissolve it in the sugar, and mix the tincture of ginger and oils. Ph. U. S.)

EXTRACTUM RU'DII, Extract of Rudius, (F.) Extrait de Rudius. Pills made of *colocynth*, *agaric*, *scammony*, *roots of black hellebore and jalap*, *socotrine aloes*, *cinnamon*, *mace*, *cloves*, *and alcohol*.

EXTRACTUM RUTÆ GRAVEOLEN'TIS, E. folio'rum Rutæ, Extract of Rue, Extractum Rutæ. (*A decoction evaporated.*) Tonic, stomachic. The volatile oil being dissipated in the boiling, this is not a good preparation. Dose, gr. x to ƷJ.

EXTRACTUM FOLIO'RUM SABI'NÆ, Extract of Savine. (*A decoction evaporated.*) Tonic. The same remarks may be made on this preparation as on the last. Dose, gr. x to ℨss.

EXTRACTUM SARSAPARIL'LÆ, Extract of Sarsaparil'la. (*A strained decoction evaporated.*) Virtues the same as those of the powdered root. Dose, gr. x to ƷJ. *Extractum Sarsaparillæ* of the United States Pharmacopœia is prepared from Sarsaparilla, in coarse powder, like the Extractum aconiti alcoholicum.

EXTRACTUM SARSAPARILLÆ FLU'IDUM, Fluid Extract of Sarsaparilla. (*Sarsaparill.* concis. et contus. ℥xvj, *Glycyrrhis.* contus., *Sassafr. rad.* contus., ȧȧ ℥ij, *Mezerei* concis. ℨvj, *Sacchar.* ℥xij, *Alcohol. dilut.* Oviij. Macerate, with the exception of the sugar, for 14 days; express and filter; evaporate to f℥xij; and add the sugar. Ph. U. S.)

EXTRACTUM SATURNI, GOULARD'S, Liquor plumbi subacetatis—e. Scobis hæmatoxyli, E. hæmatoxyli.

EXTRACTUM SENNÆ FLU'IDUM, Fluid Extract of Senna. (*Sennæ* in pulv. crass. ℔ijss; *Sacchar.* ℥xx; *Ol. Fœnicul.* f℥j; *Sp. Æther. compos.* f℥ij; *Alcohol. dilut.* Oiv. Mix the senna and diluted alcohol; let the mixture stand for 21 hours; put it into a percolator, and gradually pour on water mixed with one third its bulk of alcohol, until a gallon and a half of liquid shall have passed; evaporate to f℥xx; add the sugar, and, when it is dissolved, the compound spirit of ether, holding the oil in solution.

EXTRACTUM SPIGE'LIÆ ET SENNÆ FLU'IDUM, Fluid Extract of Spigelia and Senna. (*Spigel.* in pulv. crass. ℔j; *Sennæ* in pulv. crass. ℥vj; *Sacchar.* ℔iss; *Potass. carbon.* ℨvj; *Ol. Carui, Ol. Anisi,* ȧȧ f℥ss; *Alcohol. dilut.* q. s. Pour on the spigelia and senna Oij of diluted alcohol; let it stand for 48 hours; place it in a percolator, and pour on gradually diluted alcohol until half a gallon has passed: evaporate to a pint; add the carbonate of potassa; and afterwards the sugar, previously triturated with the oils, and dissolve. Ph. U. S.)

EXTRACTUM STRAMO'NII, E. Stramo'nii foliorum, Extract of Stramo'nium, Extract of Stramonium leaves. (The expressed juice inspissated.) The *Extractum Stramonii Sem'inis*, Extract of Stramonium Seed, is made from the powdered seed by means of diluted alcohol, and with the aid of the percolator;—the solution being evaporated. Ph. U. S. Used as a narcotic in asthma and other spasmodic affections. Dose, gr. ij to gr. x.

EXTRACTUM TARAX'ACI, Ext. Herbæ et Radi'cis Tarax'aci, Extract of Dandeli'on. (*The strained juice evaporated.*) It has been considered deobstruent, laxative, and diuretic. Dose, gr. x to ƷJ.

EXTRACTUM THEBAICUM, E. Opii.

EXTRACTUM VALERIA'NÆ, Extract of Vale'rian. (*An expressed decoction evaporated.*) The virtues of the valerian being dependent upon its essential oil, this is an objectionable preparation. Dose, gr. x to ƷJ.

A *fluid extract of Valerian, Extractum Valeria'næ flu'idum,* has been introduced into the last edition of the Pharmacopœia U. S. (1851). It is prepared by exhausting the *valerian* by *ether* and *alcohol,* through the percolator, and evaporating.

There are some other extracts in the American and other Pharmacopœias, but they are prepared in the ordinary mode, and possess merely the virtues of the plants. They are besides, generally, of an unimportant character.

EXTRAIT, Extract—e. *Alcoholique de noix vomique,* see Strychnos nux vomica—e. *des Fruits,* Rob—e. *Hémostatique de Bonjean,* Ergotin.

EXTRA'NEOUS BODY, from *extra,* 'without.' Corpus extra'neum, C. exter'num, C. alie'num, (F.) Corps étranger. Any solid, liquid, or gaseous substance, inanimate or animate, proceeding from without, or formed in the body; and which constitutes no part of the body, but occupies, in the substance of the textures, or some of the cavities, a place foreign to it.

EXTRAVASA'TION, *Extravasa'tio*, from *extra*, 'out of,' and *vasa*, 'vessels.' Escape of a fluid—*extravasa'tum*—from the vessel containing it, and infiltration or effusion of the fluid into the surrounding textures.

EXTRAVASATUM, see Extravasatio.

EXTREM'ITY, *Extrem'itas*; from *extremus*, 'the outermost;' the end or termination of a thing. The limbs, *acrote'ria*, have been so called,—as the *upper and lower extremities*. It has been, also, used to express the last moments of life; as when we say, a patient is in 'extremity,' (F.) *le malade est à l'extrémité, à toute extrémité*. See Membrum.

EXTRIN'SIC, *Extrin'secus*. That which comes from without. This term has been used for muscles, which surround certain organs and attach them to the neighbouring parts; in order to distinguish them from other muscles, which enter into the intimate composition of these organs, and which have been named *intrinsic*. Thus, there are extrinsic and intrinsic muscles of the tongue, ear, &c.

EXTROVERSIO, Exstrophia.
EXTUBERANTIA, Protuberance.
EXTUBERATIO, Protuberance.
EXTUMEFACTIO, Swelling.
EXTUS'SIO, from *ex*, and *tussis*, 'a cough.' 'I cough with expectoration.'

EXU'BER, from *ex*, 'out of,' 'devoid of,' and *ubera*, 'breasts;' *Apogalac'tos*. 'A child which has been weaned.'

EXUDATION CORPUSCLES, see Corpuscles, exudation.

EXULCERATIO, Ecthlimma, Ulceration—e. Uteri, Hysterelcosis—e. Ventriculi, Gastrelcosis.
EXUMBILICATIO, Exomphalos.
EXUSTIO, Cauterization.
EXUTORIUM, Fonticulus.
EXUTORY, Fonticulus.

EYE, Sax. ea$_3$, Teuton. A u g e, *O'culus*, *Ops*, *Omma*, *Ophthal'mos*, *Illos*, *Op'tilos* (Doric,) *Viso'rium Org'anum*, (F.) Œil. The eye is the immediate organ of vision. It is seated in the orbit, while its dependencies, called by Haller *Tutam'ina Oc'uli*, occupy the circumference of the cavity, and are composed of the eyebrows, the eyelids, cilia, glands of Meibomius, &c. The *Ball*, *Globe*, or *Bulb* of the *Eye*, *Bulbus Oc'uli*, is covered anteriorly by the tunica conjunctiva; is moved by six muscles, four *straight*, two *oblique*, and is constituted of membranes, as the *sclerotic*, *cornea*, *choroid*, *tunica Jacobi*, *retina*, *iris*, *hyaloid*, and, in the fœtus, the *membrana pupillaris;* and of fluids, called *Humours*, or *Media*,—the *aqueous*, *crystalline*, and *vitreous*. The eyeball is invested with a membranous tunic, which separates it from the other structures of the orbit, and forms a smooth, hollow surface, by which its motions are facilitated. This investment has been called *cell'ular capsule of the eye*, *oc'ular capsule*, *tu'nica vagina'lis oc'uli*, *vag''inal coat*, and *submus'cular fascia of the eye*. The vessels of the eye proceed from the ophthalmic artery. The nerves, except the optic, are chiefly furnished from the ophthalmic ganglion. The following are the dimensions, &c., of the organ, on the authority of Petit, Young, Gordon, and Brewster:

Length of the antero-posterior diameter of the eye,	0.91
Vertical chord of the cornea,	0.45
Versed sine of the cornea,	0.11
Horizontal chord of the cornea,	0.47
Size of pupil seen through the cornea,	0.27 to 0.13
Size of pupil diminished by magnifying power of cornea to, from	0.25 to 0.12
Radius of the anterior surface of the crystalline,	0.30
Radius of posterior surface,	0.22
Principal focal distance of lens,	1.73
Distance of the centre of the optic nerve from the *foramen centrale* of Sömmering,	0.11
Distance of the iris from the cornea,	0.10
Distance of the iris from the anterior surface of the crystalline,	0.02
Field of vision above a horizontal line, 50° }	120°
Field of vision below a horizontal line, 70° }	
Field of vision in a horizontal plane,	150°
Diameter of the crystalline in a woman above fifty years of age,	0.378
Diameter of the cornea,	0.400
Thickness of the crystalline,	0.172
Thickness of the cornea,	0.042

EYE, APPLE, see Melum—e. Balm, Hydrastis Canadensis—e. Bright, Euphrasia officinalis, Lobelia—e. Cat's, amaurotic, see Amaurotic—e. Cellular capsule of the, see Eye—e. Drop, Tear.

EYE GLASS, *Scaphium oculare*, see Spectacles. Also, a glass adapted for the application of collyria to the eye.

EYE, GUM OF THE, *Chassie*—e. Lashes, Cilia—e. Lid, Palpebra—e. Lid, Granular, Trachoma—e. Melon, see Melum—e. Purulent, Ophthalmia, purulent, of infants—e. Salve, Singleton's, Unguentum Hydrargyri nitrico-oxydi; Eye-salve, Smellome's, see Cupri subacetas—e. Sight of the, Pupil.

EYE STONE. The shelly operculum of small turbinideæ. Used at Guernsey to get things out of the eyes. Being put into the inner corner of the eye, under the eyelid, it works its way out at the outer corner, and brings out any foreign substance with it.—*Gray*.

EYE TEETH, Canine teeth—e. of Typhon, Scilla—e. Water, Collyrium—e. Water, common, Liquor zinci sulphatis cum camphorâ—e. Water, blue, Liquor cupri ammoniati—e. Watery, Epiphora—e. White of the, see Sclerotic.

F.

FABA, Phaseolus, Vicia faba—f. Ægyptiaca, Nymphæa nelumbo—f. Cathartica, Jatropha curcas—f. Crassa, Sedum telephium—f. Febrifuga, Ignatia amara—f. Græca, Diospyros lotus—f. Indica, Ignatia amara—f. Major, Vicia faba—f. Pechurei, Tetranthera Pechurim—f. Pechurim, Tetranthera pechurim—f. Purgatrix, Ricinus communis—f. Sancti Ignatii, Ignatia amara—f. Suilla, Hyoscyamus—f. Vulgaris, Vicia faba.

FABÆ, Onisci aselli.
FABAGELLE, Zygophyllum fagabo.
FABARIA CRASSULA, Sedum telephium.
FABRICA ANDROGYNA, Hermaphrodeity.
FACE, *Facies*, *Vultus*, *Voltus*, *Proso'pon*, (F.) *Face*. The face is the anterior part of the head. It is formed of 13 bones, viz. the *two superior maxillary*, the *two malar*, the *two ossa nasi*, the *two ossa unguis*, the *vomer*, the *two ossa spongiosa inferiora*, the *two palate bones*, and the *inferior*

maxillary, without including the frontal portion of the os frontis, and the 32 teeth, which may be considered to form part of it. Its numerous muscles are chiefly destined for the organs of sight, hearing, taste, and smell. Its arteries proceed from the external carotid: its veins end in the jugular, and its nerves draw their origin immediately from the brain.

The face experiences alterations in disease, which it is important to attend to. It is yellow in jaundice, pale and puffy in dropsy; and its expression is very different, according to the seat of irritation, so that, in infants, by an attention to *medical physiognomy*, we can often detect the seat of disease.

Hippocrates has well depicted the change which it experiences in one exhausted by long sickness, by great evacuations, excessive hunger, watchfulness, &c., threatening dissolution. Hence this state has been called *Facies Hippocrat'ica, Facies Cadaver'ica, F. Tortua'lis.* In this, the nose is pinched; the eyes are sunk; the temples hollow; the ears cold, and retracted; the skin of the forehead tense, and dry; the complexion livid; the lips pendent, relaxed, and cold, &c.

The term *Face* (F.) is likewise given to one of the aspects of an organ; thus, we say, the *superior face of the stomach*.

FACE, INJECTÉE, see *Vultueux — f. Vultueuse*, see *Vultueux*.

FACET', (F.) *Facette*. Diminutive of *Face*. A small face. A small, circumscribed portion of the surface of a bone, as the *articular facette of a bone*.

FACHINGEN, MINERAL WATERS OF. These springs are at no great distance from those of Geilenau, and two miles north of Wisbaden. They contain free carbonic acid; carbonate, sulphate, and phosphate of soda; chloride of sodium, carbonate of lime, magnesia, and iron.

FA'CIAL, *Facia'lis*. Belonging to, or connected with, the face.

FACIAL ANGLE, see Angle, facial.

FACIAL ARTERY, *La'bial artery, An'gular or external max'illary artery, A. palato-labial* — (Ch.) is a branch of the external carotid, which rises beneath the digastricus, and is distributed to almost every part of the face. It furnishes the *inferior palatal, submental, superior labial, inferior labial*, and *dorsalis nasi*.

FACIAL LINE, see Angle, facial.

FACIAL NERVE, *Portio dura of the 7th pair, Ramus du'rior sep'timæ conjugatio'nis, Sympathet'icus minor, Res'piratory nerve of the face, Par sep'timum sive facia'lē, Commu'nicans faciei nervus.* This nerve arises from the inferior and lateral part of the tuber annulare, in the groove which separates it from the medulla oblongata, external to the corpora olivaria, and by the side of the auditory nerve. It issues from the cranium by the *meatus auditorius internus;* enters the aqueduct of Fallopius; receives a branch of the Vidian nerve; forms a gangliform swelling— *Intumescen'tia gangliform'is;* — sends off filaments to the internal muscles of the malleus and stapes; furnishes, according to many anatomists, that called *Chorda Tympani;* makes its exit at the foramen stylo-mastoideum, and divides into two branches—the *temporo-facial*, and *cervico-facial*. On the face it is termed, *Pes anseri'nus, Plexus nervo'rum anseri'nus*. See Portio Wrisbergii.

FACIAL VEIN, *Pal'ato-labial* — (Ch.,) arises between the skin and frontalis muscle, and bears the name *V. Fronta'lis*, (F.) *Veine frontale ou V. Préparate*. It then descends, vertically, towards the greater angle of the eye, where it is called *Angula'ris;* and afterwards descends, obliquely, on the face, to open into the internal jugular, after having received branches, which correspond with those of the facial artery. It is only in the latter part of its course that it is called *Facial Vein*. Chaussier calls the external carotid artery, *Facial Artery*.

FA'CIENT, *faciens*, 'making,' from *facio*, 'I make.' A suffix, as in *Calefacient, Rubefacient*, &c., 'warm making,' 'red making.'

FACIES, Face — f. Cadaverica, see Face — f. Concava pedis, Sole—f. Hippocratica, see Face—f. Inferior pedis, Sole—f. Tortualis, see Face.

FACTICE, Factitious.

FACTIT''IOUS, *Factit''ius*, (F.) *Factice*, from *facere*, 'to make.' Artificial. That which is made by art, in opposition to what is natural or found already existing in nature. Thus, we say, *factitious mineral waters*, for artificial mineral waters.

FACULTAS, Faculty—f. Auctrix, Plastic force—f. Formatrix, Plastic force—f. Nutrix, Plastic force—f. Vegetativa, Plastic force—f. Zotica, Vis vitalis.

FACULTATES NATURALES, see Function.

FAC'ULTY, *Facultas, Dy'namis, Power, Virtue*. The power of executing any function or act. The collection of the *intellectual faculties* constitutes the *understanding*. We say, also, *vital faculties* for *vital properties*, &c.

FÆCAL, Stercoraceous—f. Retention, Constipation.

FÆCES, Plural of *Fæx; Feces, Chersæ,* 'the dregs of any thing.' *Fec'ulence*, (F.) *Fèces*. The alvine evacuations are so called; (F.) *Garderobes;* the excrements, *Impurita'tes alvinæ, Fæcal matter*. See Excrement.

FÆCES INDURATÆ, Scybala.

FÆCOSITAS, Feculence.

FÆCULA, Fecula.

FÆCULENTIA, Feculence.

FÆCUNDATIO, Fecundatio.

FÆCUNDITAS, Fecundity.

FÆX, Feculence.

FAGA'RA OCTAN'DRA, *Elaph'rium tomento'sum, Am'yris tomento'sum*, from *fagus*, 'the beech,' which it resembles. The systematic name of the plant, which affords *Tacamaha'ca*, a resinous substance, that exudes from the tree *Tacamahaca*, which has a fragrant, delightful smell, was formerly in high estimation, as an ingredient in warm, stimulating plasters, and was given internally, like the balsams generally. The *East India Tacamahac, Bal'samum Vir'idē, O'leum Mar'iæ, Bal'samum Cal'aba, Balsamum mariæ, Baume vert*, is yielded by *Calophyl'lum inophyl'lum seu Balsama'ria Inophyl'lum*.

The name *Tacamahac* is also given to a resin furnished by *Pop'ulus balsamif'era seu tacamaha'ca*, which grows in the northern parts of America and Siberia.

FAGARA PIPERI'TA, (F.) *Fagarier poivré;* a native of Japan, possesses the qualities of pepper, and is used as such by the Japanese. It is, also, employed as a rubefacient cataplasm.

FAGARAS'TRUM CAPEN'SE. *Nat. Ord.* Xanthoxyleæ. A South African plant, the fruit of which is known to the Colonists as *wild Cardamom;* and, on account of its aromatic qualities, is prescribed in flatulency and paralysis.

FAGARIER POIVRÉ, Fagara octandria.

FAGOPYRUM, Polygonum fagopyrum.

FAGUS, F. sylvatica.

FAGUS CASTA'NEA. The systematic name of the *Chestnut Tree; Casta'nea, C. vulga'ris, Cas ta'nea vesca, Lo'pima, Mōta, Glans Jovis* THEOPHRASTI, *Ju'piter's Acorn, Sardin'ian Acorn;* the Common Chestnut, (F.) *Chataignier commun. Family*, Amentaceæ. *Sex. Syst.* Monœcia Polyandria. The Chestnut, *Casta'nea nux*, (F.) *Châtaigne*, is farinaceous and nutritious, but not easy of digestion.

FAGUS CASTANEA PU'MILA. The *Chin'capin* or *Chinquapin*, *Castanea Pumila*, (F.) *Chataignier nain*. The nut of this American tree is eaten like the chestnut. The bark, *Castanea*, (Ph. U. S.) has been used in intermittents.

FAGUS PURPUREA, F. sylvatica.

FAGUS SYLVAT'ICA. The systematic name of the Beech, *Fagus*, *F. sylves'tris seu purpu'rea*, *Orya*, *Balan'da*, *Valan'ida*; the *Beech Tree*, (F.) *Hêtre*. The *Beech-nut* or *Beech-mast*, (F.) *Faine*, affords an oil, by expression, which is of a palatable character, and is eaten in some places instead of butter. It has been supposed to be a good vermifuge, but it is no better than any mild oil.

FAGUS SYLVESTRIS, F. Sylvatica.

FAIBLESSE, Debility.

FAIM, Hunger — *f. Canine*, Boulimia — *f. de Loup*, Fames lupina.

FAINE, see Fagus sylvatica.

FAINTING, Syncope.

FAINTING-FIT, Syncope.

FAINTISHNESS, see Syncope.

FAINTNESS, Languor, Syncope.

FAIRBURN, MINERAL WATERS OF. The mineral waters at this place, which is in the county of Ross, in Scotland, are sulphureous, and frequented.

FAISCEAU, Fasciculus — *f. Intermédiaire de Wrisberg*, Portio Wrisbergii — *f. Petit*, Fasciculus.

FALCADINA, Scherlievo.

FAL'CIFORM, *Falcifor'mis*, *Drepanoï'des*, from *falx*, 'a scythe,' and *forma*, 'shape.' Having the shape of a scythe. This term has been applied to different parts. See Falx, and Sinus.

FALCIFORM EXPANSION OF THE FASCIA LATA is the scythe-shaped reflection of the fascia lata, which forms, outwards and upwards, the opening for the vena saphæna, and is attached to the crural arch by its superior extremity, forming the anterior paries of the canal of the same name.

FALLACIA, Hallucination.

FALLACIA OPTICA. An optic illusion.

FALLOPIAN TUBE, see Tube, Fallopian.

FALLTRANCK, Faltranck (G.), literally, *a drink against falls*. A vulnerary. It is a mixture of several aromatic and slightly astringent plants, which grow chiefly in the Swiss Alps, and hence the name — *Vulnéraire Suisse* — given to such dried plants cut into fragments. They are called, also, *Espèces Vulnéraires*, and *Thé Suisse*. Within the present century, in England, a kind of vulnerary beer was often prescribed, in country practice, in all cases of inward bruises. It bore the name *Cerevis'ia nigra*, or *black beer*, and was formed by infusing certain reputed vulnerary herbs in beer or ale.

The infusion of the *Falltranck* is aromatic, and slightly agreeable, but of no use in the cases for which it has been particularly recommended.

FALMOUTH, CLIMATE OF. The climate of Falmouth in Cornwall, England, resembles that of Penzance: and, like it, is in many respects, a favourable retreat for the phthisical during the winter months.

FALSA VIA, False passage.

FALSE, *Falsus*, *Nothus*, *Pseudo*, *Spu'rious*, *Bastard*, (F.) *Faux*, *Fausse*. This epithet has been frequently added to peripneumony, pleurisy, &c., to designate a disease similar to these, but less severe. Most commonly, a severe catarrh or pleurodynia has received the name. See Peripneumonia notha.

FALSE PASSAGE, *Falsa Via*, (F.) *Fausse Route*. An accidental passage, made in surgical operations, and particularly in introducing the catheter. The catheter is sometimes passed through into the rectum.

FALSE WATERS, *Hydrallan'tis*, *False Delivery*. Water, which sometimes collects between the amnion and chorion, and is commonly discharged before the birth of the child.

We say, also, *False Ribs*, *False Rhubarb*, &c.

FALSETTO VOICE, see Voice.

FALSIFICA'TION, *Adultera'tio*, from *falsus*, 'false,' and *facere*, 'to make.' A fraudulent imitation or alteration of. an aliment or medicine by different admixtures. *Manga'nium*, *Manganisa'tio*. It is synonymous with *adulteration* and *sophistication*.

TABLE OF COMMON FALSIFICATIONS OF SOME OF THE MOST USEFUL DRUGS, &c.

MEDICINES.	ADULTERATIONS.	MODE OF DETECTION.
ACACIÆ GUMMI.	*Gum Senegal*............	G. S. is clammy and tenacious. The A. G. is perfectly soluble in water, and its solution limpid.
ACETUM DESTILLATUM.	*Sulphuric Acid*........	Acetate of barytes causes a white precipitate.
	Nitric Acid.............	By evaporating it, the residuum deflagrates, when thrown on burning charcoal.
	Copper................	Supersaturate with ammonia — a blue colour is produced.
	Lead.................	Sulphuretted hydrogen causes a dark precipitate.
ACIDUM MURIATICUM.	*Sulphuric Acid*........	Deposites by evaporation the salts it may contain; precipitates with solution of hydrochlorate of baryta if it contains sulphuric acid.
——— NITRICUM.	*Muriatic and Sulphuric Acids.*	The presence of chlorine is indicated by a precipitate with nitrate of silver: that of sulphuric acid by the same result with hydrochlorate of baryta.
——— SULPHURICUM.	*Muriatic and Nitric Acids.*	The presence of muriatic and nitric acid is indicated by the smell, when the acid tested is strongly heated.
——— CITRICUM.	*Tartaric and Oxalic Acids.*	Their presence is indicated by forming a granular sediment in a concentrated solution of a neutral salt of potassa.

Medicines.	Adulterations.	Mode of Detection.
Æther Rectificatus.	Too dilute.	The S. G. detects this.
	Sulphuric Acid	By acetate of baryta. Precipitate white.
	Alcohol	With phosphorus a milky instead of limpid solution is formed.
Aqua Ammoniæ. Ammoniæ Carbonas.	Carbonic Acid	A precipitation occurs on adding a solution of muriate of lime. It should be capable of complete volatilization by heat.
Ammoniacum		The *Guttæ Ammoniaci* are white, clear, and dry. The *lump Ammoniacum, lapis Ammoniaci*, is often adulterated with common resin. It ought to be entirely volatilized by a red heat.
Ammonii Sulphuretum.	Lead.	Imparts a foliated texture, and is not vaporizable.
	Arsenic	A smell of garlic is emitted when thrown on live coals, &c.
	Manganese and Iron.	Are not vaporizable.
Argenti Nitras.	Copper	The solution assumes a blue colour, when supersaturated with ammonia. It may be suspected when the salt deliquesces.
	Nitrate of Potassa.	The adulteration with nitrate of potassa is easily recognised by the fracture of a stick of it, which is radiated when pure, and granular if adulterated; or by precipitating a solution of the salts with a sufficient quantity of muriatic acid, and evaporating the clear liquor: the nitrate of potassa or other salts will remain.
Arsenicum Album.	Chalk, Sulphate of Lime, Sulphate of Baryta.	Not volatizable by heat.
Balsamum Peruvianum.	A mixture of Resin and some Volatile Oil, with Benzoin.	Not easily detected.
Capsicum. Cayenne Pepper.	Chloride of Sodium	This disposes it to deliquesce.
	Red Lead	Digest in acetic acid, and add a solution of sulphuret of ammonia — a dark-coloured precipitate will be produced.
Castoreum. Castor.	A mixture of dried blood, gum ammoniac, and a little real castor, stuffed into the scrotum of a goat.	Smell and taste will generally detect the fraud.
	Earth or Peasmeal	May be suspected when the cake is brittle and colour grayish.
Cera Flava. Yellow Wax.	Resin	Put it in cold alcohol, which will dissolve the resin, without acting on the wax.
	Tallow	Is known by the greater softness and unctuosity, and its smell when melted. Turmeric is generally added in this case to obviate the paleness.
Cera Alba. White Wax.	White Lead	Melt the wax, the oxide will subside.
	Tallow	The cake has not its ordinary translucency.
Cinchona. Bark.	This is variously adulterated, but generally with the Carthagena and other inferior barks.	Can only be detected by practice, and examining into the quantity of quinia or cinchonia it contains.
Coccus. Cochineal.	Pieces of dough formed in moulds, and coloured with cochineal.	Throw it into water, the adulteration will appear.
Colomba.		The true is distinguishable from the false Colomba by adding to an infusion of the root, a few drops of solution of sulph. iron, which gives to the infusion of the false Colomba a greenish black colour; but produces no change in the other.
Copaiba. Balsam of Copaiva.	Oil	If it does not retain its spherical form when dropped into water, its adulteration may be inferred. Mix one part of strong liquid ammonia of 22°, with three parts of copaiba. If pure, the mixture will, in a few minutes, become transparent; if not, it will remain opake.
Crocus. Saffron.	Fibres of smoked Beef.	Affords an unpleasant odour when thrown on live coals.
	Petals of the Calendula officinalis, and Carthamus Tinctorius.	Infuse the specimen in hot water, and the difference will be perceptible.

Medicines.	Adulterations.	Mode of Detection.
Cubeba. *Cubebs.*	Turkey Yellow Berries, or the dried fruit of the Rhamnus Catharticus.	Detected by attentive examination.
Cusparlæ Cortex. *Angustura Bark.*	False Angustura sometimes sold for it.	The epidermis of the true Cusparia is characterized by being covered with a matter resembling the rust of iron.
Guaiaci Resina. *Resin of Guaiacum.*	Common Resin	Detected by the turpentine smell emitted when thrown upon hot coals.
	Manchineel Gum	Add to the tincture a few drops of spirit of nitre, and dilute with water; the guaiacum is precipitated—the adulteration floats in the white striæ.
Hydrargyri Chloridum Mite. *Calomel.*	Corrosive Sublimate, and Subnitrate of Bismuth.	A precipitation will be produced by the carbonate of potass, from a solution made by boiling the suspected sample with a small portion of muriate of ammonia in distilled water; or, the presence of deuto-chloride of mercury is indicated, by warming gently a small quantity of calomel in alcohol, filtering and adding to the clear liquor some lime-water, by which a reddish yellow precipitate is afforded. When calomel is rubbed with a fixed alkali, it ought to become intensely black, and not exhibit any orange hue.
Hydrargyri Oxidum Rubrum. *Red Precipitate.*	Red Lead	Digest in acetic acid: add sulphuret of ammonia, which will produce a dark coloured precipitate. It should be totally volatilized by heat.
Hydrargyri Sulphuretum Rubrum	Red Lead	Digest in acetic acid, and add sulphuret of ammonia—a black precipitate will be produced.
Hydrargyri Sulphuretum Nigrum.	Ivory Black	Throw a suspected portion on hot coals—the residuum will detect the fraud.
Iodine.	Plumbago, Charcoal, and Oxide of Manganese.	The tests of its purity are — that it is perfectly soluble in ether. Heated on a piece of glass or porcelain, it sublimes without residuum.
Jalapæ Radix. *Jalap Root.*	Bryony Root, spurious or false Jalap Root, and Liquorice Root.	Bryony root is of a paler colour, and less compact texture, and does not easily burn at the flame of a candle. Liquorice is detected by the taste.
Magnesia.	Lime	Detected by the solution in dilute sulphuric acid affording a precipitate with oxalate of ammonia.
	Sulphuret of Lime	Gives off when moistened, the smell of sulphuretted hydrogen.
Magnesiæ Subcarbonas. *Carbonate of Magnesia.*	Chalk	Detected by adding dilute sulphuric acid to the suspected substance, when, if chalk be present, there will be a white insoluble precipitate.
	Gypsum	Boil in distilled water, and test the solution by a barytic and oxalic reagent.
Manna.	A factitious article, consisting of honey or sugar, mixed with scammony, is sometimes sold for it.	The colour, weight, transparency and taste detect it.
Morphia et ejus Sales. *Morphia and its Salts.*	....	Morphia and its salts, when placed in contact with nitric acid, are coloured red; with persalts of iron, blue. They are perfectly soluble in warm alcohol, and acidulated warm water. When morphia is mixed with narcotina, the adulteration is ascertained by mixing them with sulphuric ether, which dissolves the narcotina, without sensibly affecting the morphia.
Moschus. *Musk.*	Dried Blood..........	The bag must not appear to have been opened. This may be suspected, if it emits a fetid smoke when inflamed.
	Asphaltum	Discovered by its melting and running, before it inflames.
	Fine particles of Lead ..	Rub with water. The metallic particles will subside.
Olea Destillata. *Essential Oils.*	Fixed Oils	Touch writing paper with it, and hold it before the fire: fixed oil leaves a stain of grease.
	Alcohol	Add water. A milkiness and increase of temperature occurs.
Oleum Ricini. *Castor Oil.*	Olive or Almond or Poppy Oil.	Alcohol S. G. ·820 will mix with any proportion of castor oil, whilst it dissolves very little of the others.

Medicines.	Adulterations.	Mode of Detection.
Opium.	Extract of Liquorice, Bullets and Stones sometimes in it; Extract of Poppy, of Chelidonium majus; G. Arabic, G. Tragacanth, Linseed Oil, Cow's Dung.	The best opium is covered with leaves and the reddish capsules of a species of *Rumex*. The inferior kinds have capsules adherent. It is bad when soft and friable, when intensely black or mixed with many impurities, and when sweet. The quantity of morphia affords the best test.
Potassii Iodidum. Iodide of Potassium.	Chlorides of Potassium and Sodium, Nitrate of Potassa.	The adulteration is ascertained by precipitating a solution of the salt with nitrate of silver, and treating the precipitate with ammonia, which dissolves the chloride of silver, without acting upon the iodide of this metal.
Quiniæ Sulphas. Sulphate of Quinia.	Mannite...............	Leaves no residue when submitted to calcination: is perfectly soluble in warm alcohol, and in water slightly acidulated with sulphuric acid.
Strychnlæ et ejus Sales. Strychnia and its Salts.	Brucia................	They are free from brucia when no colour is produced by contact with nitric acid.
Zinci Oxydum. Flowers of Zinc.	Chalk................. White Lead...........	Sulphuric acid excites an effervescence. Sulphuric acid forms an insoluble sulphate of lead.

FALTRANCK, Falltranck.

FALX. Anatomists have given this name to several membranous reflections having the shape of a falx or scythe.

FALX CEREBEL′LI, (F.) *Faux du cervelet, Falx minor, Septum médian du cervelet* (Ch.,) *Septum Cerebel′li, Proces′sus falcifor′mis Cerebel′li, Septum Parvum occipita′lē*, is a triangular process of the dura mater opposite the internal occipital protuberance. Its base is attached to the middle of the tentorium, and its top or apex bifurcates, to proceed to the sides of the foramen magnum. Its convex surface is towards the cranium, and its concave in the fissure or groove, which separates the two lobes of the cerebellum.

FALX CER′EBRI, *Septum Cerebri, Falx major, Ver′tical supe′rior longitu′dinal proc″ess, Mediasti′num cerebri*, (F.) *Faux du cerveau, Repli longitudinal de la méninge,* (Ch.,) *Proces′sus falciformis duræ matris*. The greatest process of the dura mater. It extends from the fore to the hind part of the skull, on the median line; is broad behind, and narrow before, and is lodged in the groove which separates the hemispheres from each other—the *interlobular fissure*. At its superior part is situated the longitudinal sinus (*superior,*) and at its lower, corresponding to the edge of the scythe, the inferior longitudinal sinus. Its anterior extremity is attached to the crista galli; its posterior is continuous with the tentorium cerebelli, and contains the straight sinus.

FALX MAJOR, Falx cerebri — f. Minor, Falx cerebelli.

FALX OF THE PERITONEUM, GREAT, *Falx peritone′i max′ima*, (F.) *Grande faux du péritoine, Faux de la Veine Ombilicale*, Falx of the umbilical vein, is a reflection of the peritoneum, which ascends from the umbilicus to the anterior and inferior surface of the liver.

FALCES OF THE PERITONE′UM, LESSER, *Falces Peritone′i min′imæ*, (F.) *Petites faux du péritoine*, are the lateral ligaments of the liver and the reflections which the peritoneum forms, raised up by the umbilical arteries.

FALX OF THE UMBILICAL VEIN, Falx, great, of the Peritoneum.

FAMEL′ICA FEBRIS, from *fames*, 'hunger.' Fever accompanied with insatiable hunger. — Sylvius.

FAMELICUS, Hungry.

FAMES, Hunger — f. Bovina, Boulimia — f. Canina, Boulimia.

FAMES LUPI′NA, *Lycorex′is*, (F.) *Faim de Loup*. Authors have described, under this name, a kind of boulimia, or depravation of the digestive function, in which the patient eats voraciously, and passes his food, almost immediately afterwards, *per anum*.

FAMEX, Contusio.

FAMIGERATIS′SIMUM EMPLAS′TRUM, from *fama*, 'fame,' and *gero*, 'I wear.' A plaster, extolled in ague, and made of aromatic, irritating substances. It was applied to the wrist.

FAMILIARICA SELLA, Close stool.

FAMILY DISEASES, see Hereditary.

FAMIS, Contusio.

FAMIX, Contusio.

FANCULUM, Anethum.

FANCY MARK, Nævus.

FANG, Radix.

FANON (F.) from (G.) *Fahne*, 'a banner,' 'ensign,' 'standard.' *Fer′ula, Lec′tulus stramin′eus, Thor′ulus stramin′eus*. A splint of a particular shape, employed in fractures of the thigh and leg to keep the bones in contact.

The *Fanons* were divided into *true* and *false*. The *true* consists of a cylinder of straw, strongly surrounded with a cord or riband, in the centre of which a stick is usually placed to ensure its solidity. The *false* consists of a thick piece of linen, made flat like a compress, and folded at the extremities. It was placed between the fractured limb and the true *fanon*. The *Drap-fanon* is a large piece of common cloth placed between the fractured limb, in which the fanons or lateral splints are rolled.

FANTOM, *Phantom*, from φάντασμα, 'a spectre.' (F.) *Phantôme, Fantôme, Mannequin, Man′nekin*. This word has two acceptations. It means the spectres and images which the imagination presents to the sick, when asleep or awake; and, also, the figure on which surgeons practise the application of bandages, or the accoucheur the manual part of midwifery, — *Phanto′ma obstet′ic″ium*.

FARCIMINALIS MEMBRANA seu TUNICA, Allantois.

FARCINOMA, Equinia.

FARCTU′RA, *Fartu′ra;* from *farcire*, 'to stuff.' The operation of introducing medicinal substances into the cavities of animals or of fruits, which have been previously emptied.

FARCTUS, Emphraxis.

FARCY GLANDERS, see Equinia.

FARD, Paint.

FARDEAU, Mole.

FARFARA, Tussilago—f. Bechium, Tussilago.

FARI'NA, *Al'phiton, Crimnon, Al'eton, Aleu'ron, Ale'ma,* from *far,* 'corn,' of which it is made. *Meal* or *flour.* The powder, obtained by grinding the seeds of the gramineous, leguminous, and cucurbitaceous plants in particular. It is highly nutritious, and is much used, dietetically as well as medicinally.

Leath's Alimen'tary Fari'na, or *Homœpath'ic Farina'ceous Food,* is said to consist principally of wheat flour, slightly baked, and sweetened with sugar, together with potato flour and a very small quantity of Indian corn meal and tapioca.

FARINA AMYGDALARUM, see Amygdala.

FARINA, COMPOUNDED, BASTER'S, is said to consist of wheat flour, sweetened with sugar.

FARINA, NUTRITIOUS, MAIDMAN'S, is said to consist of potato flour, artificially coloured of a pink or rosy hue, the colouring matter being probably rose pink.

FARINA TRIT'ICI, wheaten flour; *F. Seca'lis,* Rye flour or meal; *F. Hordei,* Barley meal; *F. Avena'cea,* Oat meal, &c. See Amylum.

FARINÆ RESOLVENT'ES, (F.) *Farines Résolutives.* This name was formerly given to a mixture of the farina of four different plants; the lupine, *Lupinus albus,* the *Ervum Ervilia,* the *Vicia faba,* and the Barley, *Hordeum distichum.* They were recommended to form cataplasms.

FARINA'CEOUS, *Farina'ceus, Farino'sus,* (F.) *Farineux, Mealy.* Having the appearance or nature of farina. A term given to all articles of food which contain farina. The term *Farinacea* includes all those substances, called *cerealia, legumina,* &c., which contain farina, and are employed as nutriment.

Hard's farinaceous food is fine wheat flour, which has been subjected to some heating process. *Braden's farinaceous food* is said to be wheat flour, baked.

In *Pathology,* the epithet *farinaceous,* (F.) *farineux,* is applied to certain eruptions, in which the epidermis exfoliates in small particles similar to farina.

FARINACEOUS FOOD, BRADEN'S, see Farinaceous—f. Food, Hard's, see Farinaceous—f. Food, Homœopathic, see Farinaceous.

FARINACEOUS FOOD, PLUMBE'S, is said to consist principally of bean or pea flour, most probably the former, with a little Tacca arrowroot, some potato flour, and a very little Maranta arrowroot.

FARINACEOUS FOOD, PRINCE ALBERT'S, "for infants and invalids of all ages," is said to consist entirely of wheat flour, slightly baked.

FARINARIUM, Alica.

FARINES RÉSOLUTIVES, Farinæ resolventes.

FARINEUX, Farinaceous.

FARINOSUS, Farinaceous.

FARRIER, Hippiater.

FART, Sax. ꝼꝥꞇ, from Teut. fahren, 'to go:'—fart, 'a voyage.' (G.) Furᴢ. *Bdellus, Bdolus, Bdelyg'mia, Bdelyg'mus, Porda, Physa, Physé, Flatus, Crep'itus,* (F.) *Pet.* A sonorous or other discharge of wind from behind. A low word, but of respectable parentage.

FARTURA, Farctura.

FARTUS, Emphraxis.

FAS'CIA, from *fascis,* 'a bundle.' *Liga'tio, Ligatu'ra, Alligatu'ra, Anades'mus, Vin'cula, Sparganon, Epides'mos, Vinctu'ra. A bandage,* *fillet, roller, ligature.* The aponeurotic expansions of muscles, which bind parts together, are, likewise, termed Fasciæ: — *Aponeuroses, Perimys'ia.* See, also, Tænia.

FASCIA APONEUROTICA FEMORIS, Fascia lata aponeurosis — f. Capitalis, Bonnet d'Hippocrate, Capelina—f. Capitis, Diadema—f. Cooperi, F. Transversalis.

FASCIA, CRIB'RIFORM, *Fascia Cribrifor'mis.* The sieve-like portion of the fascia lata; so called from its being pierced by numerous openings for the passage of lymphatic vessels.

FASCIA DENTA'TA, *Corps godronné* of Vicq d'Azyr. A band of gray matter seen beneath the tænia hippocampi on raising it up, which runs along the inner border of the cornu ammonis. It is, as it were, crenated by transverse furrows.

FASCIA DIGITALIS, *Gantelet*—f. Diophthalmica, Binoculus—f. Dividens, Dividing bandage—f. Heliodori, T bandage.

FASCIA ILI'ACA, *Il'iac aponeuro'sis.* An aponeurosis which proceeds from the tendon of the psoas minor, or which arises from the anterior surface of the psoas magnus, when the former muscle does not exist. It is attached, externally, to the inner edge of the crest of the ilium, below, and anteriorly — on one side, to the crural arch, sending an expansion to the fascia transversalis; and on the other, continuous with the deep-seated lamina of the fascia lata, which forms the posterior paries of the crural canal. Within and behind, the fascia iliaca is attached to the brim of the pelvis, and is continuens with the aponeurosis, which M. Jules Cloquet has called *Pelvian.* The iliac aponeurosis covers the iliac and psoas muscles, which it separates from the peritoneum.

FASCIA INGUINALIS, Spica.

FASCIA LATA. A name given by anatomists to an aponeurosis, and to a muscle.

FASCIA LATA APONEUROSIS, *Fascia aponeurot'ica fem'oris, Vagi'na fem'oris, Crural* or *Fem'oral Aponeurosis,* is the most extensive in the body, and envelopes all the muscles of the thigh. *Above,* it is attached to the outer edge of the ilia; *before,* it arises from the crural arch by two distinct laminæ, separated by the femoral vessels, and becoming confounded a little below the part where the great vena saphæna opens into the crural vein. Of these two laminæ, the one is more anterior and thicker than the other, and may be considered as a prolongation of the aponeurosis of the external oblique. It is intimately united to Poupart's ligament. The other, which is thinner, is behind, and deeper seated, and, after its union with the former, proceeds to be inserted into the pubis. *Inferiorly,* the fascia lata becomes confounded with the tendon of the triceps, and is attached to the external tuberosity of the tibia. The use of the fascia lata, like that of other aponeuroses, is to strengthen the action of the muscles, &c.

FASCIA LATA MUSCLE, *Tensor vagi'næ fem'oris, Fascia'lis, Membrano'sus, Mus'culus aponeuro'sis* vel *fasciæ latæ, Mus'culus fem'oris membrano'sus,* (F.) *Ilio-aponévrosi-fémoral, Ilio-aponévroti-fémoral*—(Ch.), *Tenseur de l'aponévrose fémorale.* A muscle, situate at the upper and outer part of the thigh. It arises, *above,* from the outer part of the anterior and superior spine of the ilium; and is inserted, *below,* between the two laminæ of the fascia lata, which it stretches and raises when it contracts.

FASCIA, OBTURATOR, see Pelvic aponeuroses— f. Pelvic, Internal, see Pelvic aponeuroses — f. Pelvic, Lateral, see Pelvic aponeuroses—f. Pelvic, Superior, see Pelvic aponeuroses.

FASCIA PRO'PRIA. A layer of areolar tissue derived from the sheath of the femoral vessels,—

er according to some from the cribriform fascia. It is one of the coverings of femoral hernia, and is generally pretty dense about the neck of the hernia; but thin or even wanting on its fundus.

FASCIA RSPENS, Spica—f. Scapularis, Scapulary—f. Sculteti, Bandage of separate strips—f. Semicircularis, Tænia semicircularis—f. Spiralis, Ascia—f. Stellata, Stella—f. Submuscular, see Vaginal, (of the eye.)

FASCIA, SUBPERITONE'AL, *Subperitone'al aponeuro'sis*. A thin tendinous layer on the outer surface of the peritoneum.

FASCIA SUPERFICIA'LIS, *Superficial aponeurosis of the abdomen and thigh*, (F.) *Aponévrose superficielle de l'abdomen et de la cuisse*. A very thin aponeurosis, which covers the muscles and aponeuroses of the abdomen; passes before the crural arch, to which it adheres with some degree of force; sends a membranous sheath, which surrounds the spermatic cord; and is continuous with the dartos, which it assists in forming. The fascia superficialis presents, beneath the crural arch, very distinct fibres, whose direction is parallel to the fold of the thigh. It is applied over the fascia lata aponeurosis, and is attached, internally, to the ascending ramus of the ischium, near the root of the corpus cavernosum. Before the descent of the testicle from the abdomen, the fascia superficialis is very manifestly continuous with the *Gubernaculum testis*.

FASCIA TFORMIS, T bandage—f. Tortilis, Tourniquet.

FASCIA TRANSVERSA'LIS, *F. Cooperi*. An aponeurosis, which separates the transversalis muscle from the peritoneum in the inguinal region. It arises above the posterior edge of the crural arch, where it seems to be continuous with the aponeurosis of the greater oblique muscle. Above, it is lost in the areolar tissue at the internal surface of the transversalis abdominis. Within, it is continuous with the outer edge of the tendon of the rectus muscle and Gimbernat's ligament; below, it is continuous with the aponeurosis of the greater oblique, and receives an expansion from the *Fascia Iliaca*. Towards its middle and a little above the crural arch, the fascia transversalis has the wide orifice of a canal, which is occupied, in the female, by the round ligament of the uterus; and, in man, furnishes an expansion, that serves as a sheath to the spermatic vessels.

FASCIÆ, Swathing clothes—f. Ligamentosæ Coli, see Colon.

FASCIALIS, Fascia lata muscle, Sartorius—f. Longus, Sartorius—f. Sutorius, Sartorius.

FASCIARUM APPLICATIO, Deligation.

FASCIATIO, Deligation, see Bandage—f. Cucullata, *Couvrechef*.

FASCIC'ULI INNOMINA'TI. Two large bundles of fibres in the interior of the medulla oblongata, behind the corpora olivaria, and more or less apparent between those bodies and the corpora restiformia. They ascend, and become apparent in the fourth ventricle, under the name *Fascic'uli seu Proces'sus ter'etes*.

FASCICULI, MEDIAN POSTERIOR, OF THE MEDULLA OBLONGATA, Funiculi graciles—f. Musculorum, see Muscular fibre—f. Pyramidales, Ferrein, pyramids of—f. Teretes, Processus teretes, see Fasciculi innominati—f. Teretes Cordis, Columnæ carneæ.

FASCIC'ULUS, *Phacel'lus, Pha'celus, Fas'cicle*, from *fascis*, 'a bundle;' *Desme'dion*, 'a small bundle.' In Anatomy, it is employed in this sense; as "a fasciculus of fibres." (F.) *Faisceau* ou *Petit Faisceau, Trousseau*. In Pharmacy, it means *manip'ulus, Cheirople'thes*, χειροπληθής, 'a handful:'—Musa Brassavolus says,—as much as can be held in two fingers.

FASCICULUS CUNEATUS, Reinforcement, fasciculus of—f. of Reinforcement, Reinforcement, F. of.

FASCINOSUS, Membrosus.

FASCINUM, Penis.

FASCIOLA, *Bandelette*—f. Cinerea, Tuberculum cinereum—f. Hepatica, Distoma hepaticum—f. Humana, Distoma hepaticum—f. Lanceolata, Distoma hepaticum.

FASELUS, Phaseolus vulgaris.

FASTID'IUM, abridged from *satis tædium*. *Fastidiousness, Squeamishness*, or the condition of a stomach that is readily affected with nausea.

FASTIDIUM CIBI, Asitia, Disgust.

FASTIGIUM, Acme.

FASTING, from Sax. fæstan, *Limo'sis expers protrac'ta, Anorex'ia mirab'ilis, Ine'dia, Jeju'nium*. Loss or want of appetite, without any other apparent affection of the stomach; so that the system can sustain almost total abstinence for a long time without faintness. Some wonderful cases of this kind are on record. See Abstinence.

FAT, *Pingue'do, Pim'elè, Piar, Piei'ron, Lipos, Stear, Adeps, Sevum, Sebum, Corpus adipo'sum, Axun'gia, Fat*, (F.) *Graisse*: from G. and A. S. Fett. A soft, white, animal substance; inodorous; insipid; oily; inflammable, easy to melt; spoiling in the air, and becoming rancid by union with oxygen: almost insoluble in alcohol; insoluble in water; soluble in fixed oils. Fat is formed of the immediate principles, *stearin, margarin* and *olein*, all of which are regarded as salts composed of stearic, margaric and oleic acids, and a common base, to which, from its sweetish taste, the name *Glyc"erin* has been given. To these are, almost always, joined an odorous and a colouring principle. Glycerin, *Glyceri'na*, has been introduced into the last edition of the Pharmacopœia of the U. S. (1851), in which it is directed to be prepared as follows:—*Lead plaster*, recently prepared and yet fluid; *boiling water*, of each a gallon; mix: stir briskly for 15 minutes; allow it to cool and pour off the liquid. Evaporate until it has the s. g. 1.15, and pass slowly through it a current of sulpho-hydric acid until a black precipitate is no longer thrown down. Filter and boil until the sulpho-hydric acid is driven off, and evaporate the liquid until it ceases to lose weight. Glycerin is a colourless or straw-coloured syrupy fluid; s. g. 1.25. It is soluble in water and in alcohol, but not in ether. It is used in the form of lotion, composed of half an ounce to ten fluidounces of water, in cutaneous diseases, as psoriasis, pityriasis, lepra and ichthyosis. It forms a kind of varnish, and might be useful in cases of burns.

Fat is found in a number of animal tissues, and is very abundant in the neighbourhood of the kidneys and in the epiploon. It is generally fluid in the cetacea; soft, and of a strong smell in the carnivora; solid, and inodorous in the ruminating animal; white, and abundant in young animals; and yellowish in old. It generally forms about a twentieth part of the weight of the human body. The fat, considered physiologically, has, for its function, to protect the organs; maintain their temperature; and to serve for nutrition in case of need; as is observed in torpid animals.

FAT, Corpulent—f. Cells, Fatty vesicles—f. Mackaw, see Cocos butyracea.

FATIGATIO, Copos.

FATIGUE, Copos.

FATTY, *Adipo'sus, Adipa'tus, Pimel'icus, Pimelo'des*, Sax. fæt; past participle of febán, to feed, *Ad'ipous, Pinguid, Pinguid'inous*. Relating to fat. Resembling or containing fat. The cellular membrane has been called *fatty* or *adipous*; from an opinion that, in its areolæ, the fat is deposited. The areolar membrane, however, merely lodges, between its lamellæ and filaments, the vesicles in which the fat is contained.

FATTY LIG'AMENT, *Ad'ipous ligament*. This name has been given to a reflection of the synovial membrane of the knee joint, which passes from the ligamentum patellæ towards the cavity that separates the condyles of the femur.

FATTY MEMBRANE, *Adipous membrane, Adipous tissue*. The subcutaneous areolar tissue, or that containing the fatty or adipous vesicles.

FATTY VES'ICLES, *Adipous vesicles, Sac'culi adipo'si, Fat cells*. This name is given to small bursæ or membranous vesicles which enclose the fat, and are found situate in the areolæ of the areolar tissue. These vesicles vary much in size. Generally, they are round and globular; and, in certain subjects, receive vessels which are very apparent. They form so many small sacs without apertures, in the interior of which are filaments arranged like septa. In fatty subjects, the adipous vesicles are very perceptible, being attached to the areolar tissue and neighbouring parts by a vascular pedicle. Raspail affirms that there is the most striking analogy between the nature of the adipose granules and that of the amylaceous grains.

FATTY VESSELS, *Adipous vessels*. The vessels connected with the fat. Some anatomists have called *Adipous canals*, (F.) *Conduits adipeux*, the vessels to which they attribute the secretion of fat.

FATTY DEGENERATION OF THE LIVER, Adiposis hepatica—f. Liver, Adiposis hepatica.

FATU'ITAS, *Moro'sis, Stultit''ia, Stupor mentis, Amen'tia;* from *fatuus*, 'foolish.' Mental imbecility. Idiotism. Dementia. One affected with fatuity is said to be *fat'uous*.

FATUOUS, see Fatuity.

FAUCES, Isthmus, Pharynx, Throat.

FAUCETTE VOICE, see Voice.

FAUNO'RUM LUDIB'RIA. *The sports of the Fauni*. Some authors have called thus the incubus; others, epilepsy.

FAUSSE, False.

FAUSSE COUCHE (F.), *Vanum partu'rium*. Some authors have used this term for the expulsion of different bodies constituting false conceptions; such as moles, hydatids, clots of blood, &c. Most accoucheurs use the term synonymously with abortion.

FAUSSE POSITION (F.), *False position*. The French use this term, in vulgar language, to indicate any attitude in which torpor, tingling, and loss of power over the motion of a part, are produced by too strong contraction or painful compression.

FAUSSE ROUTE, False passage.

FAUSTI'NI PASTIL'LI, *Faustinus's Lozenges*. These were once celebrated. They were composed of *burnt paper, quicklime, oxide of arsenic, sandarach, lentil, &c*.

FAUX, False —*f. du Cerveau*, Falx cerebri —*f. du Cervelet*, Falx cerebelli —*f. Grande du péritoine*, Falx, great, of the peritoneum —*f. Petite du péritoine*, Falx, lesser, of the peritoneum —*f de la Veine ombilicale*, Falx, great, of the peritoneum.

FAVEUX, Favosus.

FAVIFO'RMIS, Favosus.

FAVO'SUS. Similar to a honeycomb. *Favi form'is, Favous*, from *favus, cerion*, 'a honeycomb.' (F.) *Faveux*. An epithet given to a species of porrigo. *Cerion, Favus;* means also a state of ulceration, resembling a honeycomb.

FA'VULUS; diminutive of *favus*, 'a honeycomb.' *Favuli* is used by Dr. Morton, of Philadelphia, for the honeycomb-like depressions in the lining membrane of the stomach — the *stomach-cells* of Messrs. Todd and Bowman.

FAVUS, Porrigo, Porrigo favosa, see Favosus.

FEATHERFEW, Matricaria.

FEBRIC''ITANS, *Feb'riens, Enip'yros*. One attacked with fever; from *febricitare*, 'to have a fever.'

FEBRICITATIO, Feverishness.

FEBRICOSUS, Feverish.

FEBRIC'ULA, *Fe'veret*. Diminutive of *febris*, 'fever.' A term employed to express a slight degree of fever. Ephemera.

FEBRICULOSITY, Feverishness.

FEBRIENS, Febricitans, Feverish.

FEBRIFACIENT, see Feverish.

FEBRIF'EROUS, *Feb'rifer*, from *febris*, 'fever,' and *fero*, 'I carry.' Fever-bearing, as a *febriferous locality*.

FEBRIFIC, see Feverish.

FEB'RIFUGE, *Lexipyret'icus, Lexipyr'etus, Pyret'icus, Alexipyret'icus, Antifebri'lis, Antipyret'ic, Febrif'ugus*, from *febris*, 'a fever,' and *fugare*, 'to drive away.' A medicine which possesses the property of abating or driving away fever.

FEBRIFUGUM LIGNUM, Quassia.

FE'BRILE, *febri'lis*. Relating to fever, as *febrile movement, febrile pulse*, &c.

FEBRIS, Fever — f. Acmastica, Synocha — f. Acuta, Synocha—f. Acuta continua, Synocha—f. Adeno-meningea, Fever, adeno-meningeal — f. Adeno-nervosa, Plague—f. Africana, Fever, African—f. Agrypnodes, see Agrypnodes and Agrypnos—f. Alba, Chlorosis—f. Algida, see Algidus— f. Amatoria, Chlorosis, Hectic fever — f. Americana, Fever, yellow—f. Amphemera, Quotidian —f. Amphimerina hectica, Hectic fever—f. Amphimerina latica, Latica (febris)—f. Ampullosa, Pemphigus—f. Anabatica, Continued fever —f. Angiotenica, Synocha — f. Anginosa, Angina —f. Annua, see Annual diseases—f. Anomala, Fever, anomalous—f. Aphonica, Fever, aphonic —f. Aphthosa, Aphtha — f. Apoplectica, Fever, apoplectic—f. Ardens, Synocha—f. Arte promota, Fever, artificial—f. Arthritica, Gout—f. Asodes, Fever, bilious, see Asodes—f. Assidua, Continued fever—f. Asthenica, Fever, asthenic, Typhus— f. Asthmatica, Fever, asthmatic—f. Ataxo-adynamica, Fever, ataxo-adynamic—f. Azodes, see Asodes—f. Biliosa, Fever, bilious—f. Bullosa, Pemphigus — f. Cardialgia, Fever, cardialgic— f. Catarrhalis, Catarrh — f. Catarrhalis epidemica, Influenza — f. Caumatodes, Synocha — f. Causodes, Synocha—f. Cephalalgica, Fever, cephalalgic—f. Cephalica, Fever, cephalic—f. Cholepyretica, Fever, bilious — f. Cholerica, Fever, bilious, Fever, choleric — f. Chronica, Fever, chronic — f. Coalterna, see Coalternæ febres—f. Colliquativa, Fever, colliquative— f. Comatodes, Fever, apoplectic — f. Communicans, see Subintrantes F. — f. Confusa, see Confussæ febres—f. Continens, Typhus— f. Continens non putrida, Synocha — f. Continens putrida, Typhus—f. Continua inflammatoria, Empresma—f. Continua putrida, Synochus—f. Continua putrida icterodes Caroliniensis, Fever, yellow—f. Continua non putris, Synocha —f. Continua sanguinea, Synocha—f. Convulsiva, Fever, convulsive — f. Crymodes, see Crymodes, and Algid fever—f. Culicularis, Miliary fever—f. cum Delirio, Fever, delirious — f. Depuratoria, Fever, depuratory—f. Deurens, Synocha—f. Diaphoretica, Fever, diaphoretic— f. Diaria, Ephemera—f. Duodecimana, Fever, duodecimane—f. Dysenterica, Dysentery—f. Elodes, see Elodes— f. Elodes icterodes, Fever, yellow — f. Enterica, see Typhus — f. Enteromesenterica, Entero-mesenteric — f. Epacmastica, see Epacmasticos — f. Ephemera, Ephemera—f. Epidemica cum angina, Cynanche maligna—f. Epileptica, Fever, epileptic —f. Erotica, fever, erotic—f. Erratica, Fever, anomalous, Fever, erratic, see Erratic and Planetes—f. Erronea, see Planetes—f. Erysipelacea, Erysipelas—f. Erysipelatosa, Erysipelas—f. Esserosa, Miliary fever—f. Exquisita, Fever, regular—f. Exanthematica articularis, Dengue—f. Famelica, see Famelica Febris—f. Flava, Fever, yellow—f. Flava Americanorum, Fever, yellow—f. Gangrænodes, Fever, gangrenous—f. Gastrica, Fever, bilious, Fever, gastric—f. Gastrico-biliosa, Fever, gastric—f. Gastro-adynamica, Fever, gastro-adynamic—f. Hæmoptoica, Fever, hæmoptoic—f. Hebdomadana, Octana—f. Hectica, Hectic fever—f. Hectica infantum, Tabes mesenterica—f. Hectica maligna nervosa, Typhus mitior—f. Hemeresia, Quotidian—f. Hemitritæa, Hemitritæa—f. Hepatica, Fever, bilious—f. Hepatica inflammatoria, Hepatitis—f. Horrifica, see Algidus—f. Horrida, see Algidus—f. Humoralis, Fever, humoral—f. Hungarica, Fever, Hungarico—f. Hydrocephalica, Hydrocephalus internus—f. Hydrophobica, Fever, hydrophobic—f. Hysteretica, see Postpositio—f. Hysterica, Fever, hysteric—f. Icterica, Fever, icterico—f. Iliaca inflammatoria, Enteritis—f. Infantum remittens, Fever, infantile remittent—f. Inflammatoria, Synocha—f. Intensio, Epitasis—f. Intermittens, Intermittent fever—f. Intermittens cephalica larvata, Cephalalgia periodica—f. Intestinalis ulcerosa, see Typhus—f. Intestinorum, Enteritis—f. Irregularis, Fever, anomalous—f. Lactea, Fever, milk—f. Larvata, Fever, masked—f. Lenta, Fever, infantile remittent, Hectic fever, Synochus—f. Lenta nervosa, Typhus mitior, Fever, nervous—f. Lenticularis, Miliary fever—f. Lethargica, Fever, apoplectic—f. Lochialis, Fever, lochial—f. Lymodes, fever, singultous—f. Lyngodes, Fever, singultous—f. Maligna, Fever, malignant—f. Maligna biliosa Americæ, Fever, yellow—f. Maligna cum Sopore, Typhus—f. Maligna flava Indiæ occidentalis, Fever, yellow—f. Marasmodes, Hectic fever, Marasmopyra—f. Meningo-gastricus, Fever, gastric—f. Mesenterica, Fever, adeno-meningeal, Fever, mesenteric—f. Methemerina, Quotidian—f. Miliaris, Miliary fever—f. Minuta, Fever, syncopal—f. Morbillosa, Rubeola—f. Mucosa, Fever, adenomeningeal—f. Mucosa Verminosa, Fever, infantile remittent—f. Nautica pestilentialis, Typhus gravior—f. Nephritica, Fever, nephritic—f. Nervosa, Fever, nervous—f. Nervosa epidemica, Typhus—f. Nervosa enterica, see Typhus—f. Nervosa exanthematica, Typhus—f. Nervosa gastrica, see Typhus—f. Nervosa mesenterica, see Typhus—f. Nervosa petechialis, Typhus—f. Neurodes, Fever, nervous—f. Nocturnus, see Nocturnal—f. Nonana, Fever, nonane—f. Nosocomiorum, Typhus gravior—f. Nycterinus, see Nocturnal—f. Octana, Fever octane—f. Oscitans, Oscitant fever—f. Paludosa, see Elodes—f. Pannonica, Fever, Hungary—f. Pemphingodes, Pemphigus—f. Pemphygodes, Pemphigus—f. Pempts, Quintan—f. Periodica, Fever, periodic—f. Perniciosa, Fever, pernicious—f. Pestilens, Plague—f. Pestilens maligna, Typhus gravior—f. Pestilentialis, Fever, pestilential—f. Pestilentialis Europæ, Typhus gravior—f. Petechialis, Typhus gravior—f. Phthisica, Hectic fever—f. Planetes, see Planetes—f. Pleuritica, Pleuritis—f. Podagrica, Gout—f. Polycholica, Fever, bilious—f. Pneumonica, Fever, pneumonic, Pneumonia—f. Puerperalis biliosa, Metrocholosis—f. Puerperarum, Puerperal fever—f. Puncticularis, Miliary fever, Typhus gravior—f. Puerperalis, Fever, puerperal—f. Purpurate rubra et alba miliaris, Miliary fever—f. Purulenta, Fever, purulent—f. Putrida, Typhus gravior—f. Putrida nervosa, Typhus mitior—f. Quartana, Quartan—f. Querquera, see Algidus—f. Quinta, Quintan—f. Quintana, Fever, quintan, Quintan—f. Quotidiana, Fever, quotidian, Quotidian—f. Regularis, Fever, regular—f. Remittens, Remittent fever—f. Remittens infantum, Fever, infantile remittent—f. Rheumatica inflammatoria, Rheumatism, acute—f. Rubra, Scarlatina—f. Rubra pruriginosa, Urticaria—f. Sanguinea, Synocha—f. Sapropyra, Typhus gravior—f. Scarlatinosa, Scarlatina—f. Scorbutica, Fever, scorbutic—f. Semitertiana, Hemitritæa—f. Septana, Fever, septan—f. Sesquialtera, Hemitritæa—f. Sextana, Fever, sextan—f. Simplex, Ephemera, Fever, simple—f. Singultosa, Fever, singultous—f. Soporosa, Fever, apoplectic—f. Stercoralis, Fever, stercoral—f. Sthenica, Synocha—f. Stomachica inflammatoria, Gastritis—f. Subintrans, Fever, subintrant—f. Sudatoria, Fever, diaphoretic, Hydropyretus, Sudor anglicus—f. Syncopalis, Fever, syncopal—f. Syphilitica, Fever, syphilitic—f. Tabida, Fever, colliquative, Hectic fever—f. Tertiana, Fever, tertian, Tertian fever—f. Tonica, Synocha—f. Topica, Neuralgia, facial—f. Toxica, Fever, yellow—f. Tragica, Fever, tragic—f. Traumatica, Fever, traumatic—f. Tropica, Fever, yellow—f. Typhodes, Typhus—f. Urticata, Urticaria—f. Uterina, Metritis—f. Vaga, Fever, anomalous, see Planetes—f. Variolosa, Variola—f. Verminosa, Fever, infantile remittent, F. verminous, Helminthopyra—f. Vernalis, Fever, vernal—f. Vesicularis, Miliary Fever, Pemphigus—f. Virginum, Chlorosis.

FEB'RUA; from *februo*, 'I purge.' In ancient mythology, a goddess who presided over menstruation.

FECAL, Stercoraceous.

FÉCES, Fæces.

FÉCONDATION, Fecundation.

FÉCONDITÉ, Fecundity.

FEC'ULA, *Fæ'cula*, diminutive of *fæx*, 'lee.' An immediate principle of vegetables, composed of hydrogen, oxygen, and carbon. It exists in several plants, and has different names, according to that which furnishes it. When extracted from wheat or barley, it is called starch, *Am'ylum*. When from *Cycas circina'lis*, Sago;—from *Orchis mo'rio*, Salep. We say, also, Fecula of the Potato, Bryony, Arum, Manioc, &c.

FECULA, GREEN. This name is given to a green, solid matter, of variable character, which is believed to be resinous, and which renders turbid several kinds of juices, extracted from vegetables. It is, also, called *Chlorophyll*.

FECULA AMYLACEA, Amylum—f. Marantæ, Arrow-root—f. Tapioka, see Jatropha manihot.

FEC'ULENCE, *Fæculen'tia, Fæcos'itas, Fæx, Lemma, Fæ'ces, Lee, Deposit, Dregs*. In Pharmacy, feculent, albuminous, or other substances, which are deposited from turbid fluids.

FEC'ULENT, *Fæculen'tus, Hypot'rygus, Trygo'des*. 'Foul, dreggy, excrementitious;' as a *feculent fluid, feculent evacuations*, &c.

FEC'UND, *Fecun'dus, Fæcun'dus*, (F.) *Fécond*. Same etymon as the next. Fruitful, Prolific.

FECUNDA'TION, *Fæcunda'tio, Impregna'tio, Imprægna'tio, Ingravida'tio, Prægna'tio, Gravida'tio, Prægna'tus, Fructifica'tio, Cye'sis, Encye'sis, Encymo'sia, Procrea'tion*, (F.) *Fécondation*. The act by which, in organized beings, the material furnished by the generative organs of the female, unites with that prepared by those of the male, so that a new being results.

FECUN'DITY, *Eutoc'ia, Fæcun'ditas, Productiv'itas*, (F.) *Fécondité*. The faculty of reproduction, possessed by organized bodies.

It has been estimated that throughout a country, taking one marriage with another, not more than 4 children are the result; and in towns only 35 children to 10 marriages.

FEE, Sostrum.

FEET, BURNING OF THE. A singular cachectic disease, described by Mr. Malcolmson as occurring in India, the prominent symptom of which was a sense of burning in the feet.

FÉGARITE, Cancer aquaticus, Stomatitis, pseudo-membranous.

FEIGNED DISEASES, *Morbi dissimula'ti seu simula'ti seu cela'ti seu initia'ti seu pseuda'lei*, Sim'ulated diseases, Pretend'ed diseases, (F.) *Maladies dissimulées, M. simulées, M. feintes, M. supposées*. The tricks employed, by impostors, to induce a belief that they are attacked with diseases when they are not. These are generally assumed by beggars to obtain alms; by criminals to escape punishment; and by soldiers to be exempt from duty.

The following table exhibits the chief feigned diseases, with the means of detection.

A TABLE OF FEIGNED, PRETENDED, SIMULATED, OR EXCITED DISEASES OR DISQUALIFICATIONS.

Diseases, &c.	How Feigned.	How Detected.
1. Abortion.	By staining the clothes and body with borrowed blood.	
2. Abstinence.	....	By constant and minute attention.
3. Amaurotic Blindness.	By applying the extract of belladonna or datura stramonium to the eye.	Amaurosis is characterized by dilated pupil. Where these substances have been applied, the effects will go off in ten days or a fortnight.
4. Apoplexy.	By falling down as if deprived of sensation and consciousness.	By powerful stimulants; an electric shock; application of hot water, sternutatories, actual cautery, &c.
5. Cachexia, Anæmia, and Debility.	Using substances to make the face appear pale and livid. Indulging freely in wine, and privation of sleep prior to examination.	By examining if the pulse be strong, and the skin hot, and whether there be loss of appetite or of strength, or swelling of the limbs.
6. Excretion of Calculi.	Putting sand, pebbles, &c., into the urine.	By the aid of chymistry. We are acquainted with the chymical composition of urinary calculi.
7. Cancerous Ulcer.	By gluing on a portion of a spleen with the smooth side to the skin, leaving on the outside the appearance of an ulcerated surface.	By noticing whether there be signs of cachexia, and by attentive examination of the part.
8. Catalepsy.	By seeming to be suddenly motionless, the joints remaining flexible, and external objects making no impression.	By powerful stimulants, as recommended under apoplexy. Letting fall a drop of boiling water on the back. Proposing to use the actual cautery, and seeing whether the pulse rises.
9. Chorea.	By assuming the convulsive motions of a part which characterize chorea.	By examining the patient whilst he may imagine himself unobserved, and seeing whether the convulsive motions go on. By anæsthetics. (?)
10. Contraction of Joints in General.	....	Mode of discrimination sometimes so obscure as to deceive the most practised and attentive.
11. Contraction of the Fingers.	....	Introduce a cord between the fingers and the palm of the hand, and gradually apply weights so as to expand the fingers. Confine him so that he cannot obtain his food without using his clenched hand.
12. Convulsions.	....	When feigned, they do not present the rigidity of muscles or the rapidity of action which characterize the real. The mode of detection must be the same as in epilepsy.
13. Opake Cornea.	Produced by the application of a strong acid, by acrid powders, as quicklime, &c.	The existence of the opacity can be detected by attentive observation.
14. Cutaneous Diseases	Some articles of diet will bring on *urticaria* or *nettle-rash*, in particular individuals, as shell-fish, bitter almonds, &c. By acrids, acids, or any irritants applied to the surface. An ointment of tartarized antimony causes a painful pustular eruption. See Porrigo, in this list.	By careful examination on the part of practitioner and nurse.

Diseases, &c.	How Feigned.	How Detected.
15. Deaf-Dumbness.	....	The really deaf and dumb acquire an expression of countenance and gestures which it is difficult to assume.
16. Deafness.	It may be assumed or excited by putting a pea in the ear, or by inserting irritants, so as to induce inflammation and temporary loss of function.	Make a noise when not expected, and see if the countenance varies or pulse rises. Put to sleep by opium, and then fire a pistol close to the ear, when he may be thrown off his guard. Examine the ear to see if any trick has been played there.
17. Death.	Some persons possess the power of suspending or moderating the action of the heart.	If suspected, the plan recommended under apoplexy will be found most efficacious.
18. Debility, see Cachexia.		
19. Deformity.	....	Examine the part and its articulation, naked, and compare it with the opposite.
20. Delivery.	After enlargement produced artificially, a subsidence of the tumefaction; the parts being moistened by borrowed blood, and the child of another substituted as the female's own.	Can only be positively detected by examination *par vaginam*. Soon after delivery, the vagina will be relaxed and the lochial discharge be flowing in greater abundance, the shorter the time that may have elapsed since delivery.
21. Diarrhœa.	Said to have been caused by a mixture of vinegar and burnt cork. (?) May be occasioned by the use of any of the purgative roots, &c.	When diarrhœa is feigned by the lower classes, inspect the linen; if clean, the bowels are probably not much out of order. Let every individual have a close stool of his own; and inspect the evacuations, taking care that one suffering under the disease does not lend his evacuations to another.
22. Dropsy.	May be feigned, like pregnancy, by wearing pads. The anasarcous condition of the lower limbs has been caused by applying a ligature round them. By inflating the cellular membrane of the abdomen.	Can be detected by attentive examination. There will be a want of that leucophlegmatic habit which accompanies and characterizes dropsy.
23. Dysentery.	May be feigned, like diarrhœa, by adding a little blood to the evacuations, or by introducing a soap or some more irritating suppository.	Same rules as under diarrhœa.
24. Epilepsy.	The foaming of the mouth has been produced by keeping a piece of soap in it.	Sensation in epilepsy is totally abolished. If any remain, disease probably feigned. Incontractility of pupil, which occurs in epilepsy, cannot be feigned. Same means to be used as in feigned apoplexy.
25. Fever.	By various stimulants, as wine, brandy, pepper; swallowing a small quantity of tobacco, or introducing it into the anus. Flour or chalk used to whiten the tongue. Redness of skin, caused by friction with a hard brush.	This deceit is generally developed by a day or two's examination. Where flour or chalk has been used to whiten the tongue, the line of demarcation between the whitened part and the clean, healthy margin of the tongue, is too well marked to escape observation.
26. Fistula in Ano.	By making an incision near the verge of the anus, and introducing into it an acrid tent, such as the *root of white hellebore*, &c.	By careful examination.
27. Fractures.	There is generally nothing but the man's own testimony. He complains of pain in the part; if fracture of the skull be feigned, he states, perhaps, that he becomes deranged on tasting liquor.	By attentive examination.

Diseases, &c.	How Feigned.	How Detected.
28. Hæmatemesis.	By drinking the blood of some animal, or using some coloured liquid, and then throwing it up.	By cutting off the supply of the fluid and careful examination.
29. Hæmoptysis.	By secreting bullock's blood for the purpose of colouring the saliva; making small incisions in the mouth; using bole armeniac or paint of vermilion.	Blood from the lungs is frothy and light-coloured. Mouth and fauces must be carefully inspected, and the individual be observed.
30. Hæmorrhoids.	By introducing bladders of rats or of small fish partly into the rectum. The linen has also been stained with borrowed blood.	The means are obvious.
31. Heart, Diseases of, see Palpitation.		
32. Hepatitis.	....	Unless the person be a well-educated impostor, acute inflammation of the liver will be detected by the absence of marks of strong inflammatory action. *Chronic liver disease* is, frequently, not characterised by well-marked symptoms, and hence, when assumed, is difficult of detection.
33. Hernia.	In the same manner as hydrocele; — by inflation.	The detection is easy.
34. Hydrocele.	By puncturing the skin of the scrotum, and inflating the cellular membrane.	Do.
35. Hydrocephalus.	By opening the integuments of the head, near the vertex, e. g. and blowing in air.	Do.
36. Hysteria.	....	Does not easily resist the application of strong sternutatories to the nostrils. Attentive examination necessary.
37. Insanity.	....	The expression of countenance cannot easily be feigned. Nor can the affection be kept up so long as in real mental alienation. The individual cannot do so long without food, sleep, &c.
38. Jaundice.	By colouring the skin with an infusion of turmeric or tincture of rhubarb. *Clay-coloured stools* produced by taking daily a small quantity of muriatic acid. *High-coloured urine* by rhubarb taken internally.	The eyes cannot be coloured, although smoke has been used for this purpose. The skin must be washed to remove the colouring matter if any exist, and the supply of acid and rhubarb be prevented.
39. Lameness.	By keeping the limb in a contracted state, and resisting any efforts to move it.	By two persons taking hold of the individual and moving rapidly along with him; and when they are tired, having relays. The impostor will generally give in.
40. Menstruation.	By staining the clothes and body with borrowed blood.	By cutting off the supply.
41. Myopia. *Short-Sightedness.*	....	Present an open book, and apply the leaves close to the nose. If it cannot be read distinctly, when thus placed, or when glasses proper for short-sightedness are used, the disease is feigned.
42. Ophthalmia.	Excited by a variety of acrid and corrosive substances applied to the eye; as lime, &c. A portion of black muslin, spread over the cornea. The eyelashes are sometimes extracted, and caustic applied to excite disease in the palpebræ.	When ophthalmia is thus excited, its progress is ordinarily very rapid, arriving at its height within a few hours.
43. Ozæna.	By impregnating a piece of sponge with some offensive juices or oils, mixed with decayed cheese, and putting the imbued sponge into the nostrils.	

Diseases, &c.	How Feigned.	How Detected.
44. Palpitation.	White hellebore, given in the dose of 10 or 12 grains, and repeated, will occasion general indisposition, and undue action of the heart.	Cut off the supply.
45. Pains.	....	The detection is here often difficult. The non-existence of pain cannot be proved, and great pain may be present without any appearance externally. The imposition is more frequently detected by inconsistencies and contradictions in the patient's history of the case, than in any other manner.
46. Shaking Palsy.	....	May be suspected, if the person be in an ordinary state of vigour. Try violent remedies and means, recommended under Chorea.
47. Paralysis.	....	Violent remedies are here required. Cold affusion, actual cautery, electric shocks, &c.
48. Phthisis Pulmonalis.	Individuals with long necks and contracted shoulders have simulated phthisis, by covering the chest with blisters, cicatrices of issues, &c., and by taking drugs which cause paleness.	By attentive examination of the symptoms.
49. Polypus Nasi.	By introducing the testicle of a young cock, or the kidney of a rabbit, into the nostril, and retaining it there by means of a sponge fastened to it.	
50. Porrigo. Scalled Head.	By applying nitric acid to the head, after protecting the face with fatty substances; but the chronic state is imitated by the use of depilatories of different kinds applied sometimes in patches, so as to resemble the *Porrigo decalvans*.	
51. Pregnancy.	By wearing pads, and assuming the longing after particular articles of diet, &c.	By the absence of the areola; the presence of a pad; and, if necessary, by examination *per vaginam*.
52. Prolapsus Ani.	By a portion of the intestine of the ox, in which a sponge filled with a mixture of blood and milk is placed.	
53. Prolapsus Uteri.	By a similar fraud.	
54. Pulse, Weakness or Defect of.	By ligatures applied to the corresponding arm.	By examining whether the arteries of the two arms beat alike; and if a ligature be placed on the arm.
55. Chronic Rheumatism. See Pain.		
56. Scrofula.	By exciting ulcers below the angles of the jaw.	By examining the general habit, and observing whether the ulcerations be glandular, and the discharge of a scrofulous character.
57. Scurvy.	By covering the teeth with wax, and then applying acid, corrosive substances to the gums.	By examining the general habit; whether debilitated, cachectic, and possessing the usual general signs of scorbutus.
58. Stammering.	....	Simulators of this defect generally state, that it is connate, or ascribe it to a fit of apoplexy or severe fever. Where the organs of speech were perfect, and the moral evidence of the previous existence of the infirmity was not satisfactory, the French authorities used to confine the soldiers, and not supply them with food, until they called for it without stammering.

Diseases, &c.	How Feigned.	How Detected.
59. Stricture of the Urethra.	....	By passing a bougie.
60. Swelling of the Legs.	By ligatures round the thighs.	Examine the limbs uncovered.
61. Syncope.	Ligatures are sometimes used to prevent the pulse being felt. By applying lotions to the face to make it pale.	By using sternutatories. By the absence of some of the symptoms of syncope. Examine the naked arms. Wash the face.
62. Tympany.	Persons have possessed the power of swallowing air, so as to distend the stomach, and simulate tympany.	
63. Ulcer of the Ear.	By introducing a tent, imbued with blistering plaster into the ear, and repeating the application, until the tube becomes ulcerated, and a discharge of puriform matter is established. The fetid smell is imitated, by dropping into the ear a mixture of empyreumatic oil, asafœtida, and old cheese. Also, by introducing a little honey into the meatus.	By careful examination.
64. Ulcers of the Legs, &c.	By corrosives, or irritants. Sometimes by abrasion, by rubbing sand on the shin-bone. At others, they are pretended, by gluing on a piece of spleen or the skin of a frog.	Artificial ulcers have, usually, a more distinct margin, and are more readily healed than others; the latter being generally indicative of an impaired constitution.
65. Bloody Urine.	The fruit of the Indian Fig (*Cactus opuntia*) colours the urine as red as blood. Cantharides will cause it. Blood may also be procured and mixed with the urine.	By making the patient pass his urine in the presence of the physician, and examining the vessel before and after. By cutting off the supply of any substance, which could cause the appearance.
66. Incontinence of Urine.	....	Difficult, at times, of detection. Give the person a full dose of opium, and introduce the catheter when he is asleep. If there be urine, the incontinence is feigned.
67. Varicose Veins.	By a ligature, placed tightly round the limb. They may be excited in this manner, or aggravated if already existing.	By examining the limb.

FEL, Bile—f. Anguillæ, see Bile—f. Bovinum, Bile of the Ox — f. Bovis, see Bile — f. Naturæ, Aloes—f. Tauri, see Bile — f. Terræ, Ludus Helmontii—f. Ursi, see Bile—f. Vitri, see Vitrum.
FELDSCHEEREN, Bathers.
FELINEUS, Bilious.
FELLEUS, Biliary, Bilious.
FELLIDUCUS, Cholagogue.
FELLIS OBSTRUCTIO, Icterus — f. Superfusio, Icterus—f. Suffusio, Icterus.
FELON, Paronychia.
FELTING, from Anglo-Saxon ꝼelt, cloth or stuff made without *weaving*. Tangling. A term applied to the hair when inextricably interlaced, as occurs occasionally in women from inattention.
FÉLURE DE GLASER, Fissure, glenoid.
FELWORT, Gentiana lutea.
FEMALE, *Fœm'ina, Gynē*, (F.) *Femelle*, from φυω, 'I generate.' (?) In animals, the one that engenders and bears the young. It is, also, used adjectively;—as, the *Female Sex*, &c.
Female Parts, Vulva.
FEMELLE, Female.
FEMEN, Thigh, Vulva.
FEMINES'CENCE, *Fœminescen'tia*, from *fœmina*, 'a female.' The possession or assumption of certain male characteristics by the female. — Mehliss.
FEMME EN COUCHE, Puerpera.

FEM'ORAL, *Femora'lis*, from *femur*, 'the thighbone.' Belonging or relating to the thigh; as *Femoral artery, Femoral hernia*, &c. See Crural.
FEMORALIS, Triceps cruris.
FÉMORO-CALCANIEN PETIT, Plantar muscle—f. Popliteal, great, Sciatic nerve, great— *f. Popliti-tibial*, Popliteus muscle.
FEM'ORO-TIB'IAL, *Femoro-tibia'lis*. Belonging to the femur and tibia. The *Femorotibial articulation* is the knee-joint.
FEMUR, *Merus, Me'rium, Os fem'oris*. The *thigh bone*. (F.) *L'os de la Cuisse*. The strongest and longest of all the bones of the body, extending from the pelvis to the tibia, and forming the solid part of the thigh. The femur is cylindrical, slightly curved anteriorly, unsymmetrical and oblique downwards and inwards. The body of the bone is prismatic, and has, behind, a prominent ridge, the *linea aspera*.

Processes.	Upper or Pelvic Extremity.	Head supported on a column or neck. Great trochanter. Lesser trochanter.
	Inferior or Tibial Extremity.	External condyle. Internal condyle. External tuberosity. Internal tuberosity.

The femur ossifies from five points:—one on each process of the pelvis extremity; one in the body of the bone; and two on the condyles. It is articulated with the pelvis, tibia, and patella. See Thigh.

FÉMUR COL DU, Collum femoris—f. Moventium septimus, Iliacus internus—f. Moventium sextus, Psoas magnus—f. Summum, Vulva.

FENES'TRA. A *window.* (F.) *Fenêtre.* Anatomists have given this name to two apertures, situate in the inner paries of the cavity of the tympanum. The one of these is the *Fenest'ra ova'lis, F. vestibula'ris, Fora'men ova'lē.* It is oval-shaped; situate at the base of the stapes, and corresponds with the cavity of the vestibule. The other is the *Fenest'ra rotun'da, F. Cochlea'ris, Fora'men rotun'dum.* It is closed by a fine, transparent membrane, called *Membra'na Tympani secun'daria, Tympanum minus* seu *secunda'rium, Membra'na fenestræ rotun'dæ,* and corresponds to the inner scala of the cochlea.

FENESTRA OCULI, Pupil.

FENES'TRAL, *Fenestra'tus,* from *fenestra,* 'a window.' (F.) *Fenêtré* et *Fenestré.* Bandages, compresses, or plasters with small perforations or openings, are so called. The openings prevent the detention of the discharge.

FENESTRATUS, Fenestral.

FENESTRÉ, Fenestral.

FENÊTRE, Fenestra.

FENÊTRÉ, Fenestral.

FENNEL, Anethum—f. Dogs', Anthemis cotula—f. Flower, Nigella—f. Hog's, Peucedanum—f. Sweet, Anethum—f. Water, Phellandrium aquaticum.

FENOUIL, Anethum—*f. d'Eau,* Phellandrium aquaticum—*f. Marin,* Crithmum maritimum—*f. de Porc,* Peucedanum—*f. Puant,* Anethum graveolens.

FENTE, Fissure—*f. Capillaire,* see Pilatio—*f. Glénoidale,* Fissure, glenoid—*f. Orbitaire.* Orbitar fissure—*f. Orbitaire inférieure,* Sphenomaxillary fissure—*f. Sphéno-maxillaire,* Sphenomaxillary fissure—*f. Sphénoidale,* Sphenoidal fissure.

FÉNUGREC, Trigonella fœnum.

FENUGREEK, Trigonella fœnum.

FER, Ferrum—*f. Acétate de,* Ferri acetas—*f. Carbonate de,* Ferri protocarbonas—*f. Chaud,* Pyrosis—*f. Hydrate de, tritoxide de, Ætites*—*f. Iodure de,* Ferri iodidum, see Iodine—*f. Lactate de,* Ferri Lactas—*f. Limaille de,* Ferri limatura—*f. Peroxide de,* Ferri subcarbonas—*f. et de Potasse, tartrate de,* Ferrum tartarisatum—*f. et de Potassium, cyanure de,* Potassii Ferrocyanuretum—*f. et de Potassium, protocyanure de,* Potassii Ferrocyanuretum—*f. Réduit par l'hydrogène,* Ferri pulvis—*f. Sulphate de,* Ferri Sulphas—*f. Sulphure de,* Ferri Sulphuretum—*f. Tannate de,* Ferri tannas—*f. Valérianate de,* Ferri Valerianas.

FERALIS PEDICULUS, see Pediculus.

PERINE, *Feri'nus;* 'savage, brutal;' *The·rio'des.* A term, applied to any malignant or noxious disease. In France it is used only when joined to *Toux; Toux férine,* a dry, obstinate, and painful cough.

FERMENT, *Fermen'tum,* (quasi *fervimentum,*) *Zyma, Zymo'ma, Leven,* (F.) *Lévain.* The Iatrochymists applied this name to imaginary substances, *Fermen'ta mor'bi,* to which they attributed the power of producing disease, by exciting a fermentation in the humours.

FERMENTA'TION, *Fermenta'tio, Zymo'sis, Æstua'tio, Causis, Brasmos.* An intestinal movement, occurring spontaneously in a liquid; whence result certain substances, that did not previously exist in it.

The chemical physicians attributed all diseases to an imaginary fermentation of the humours.

FERMENTATION, PUTREFACTIVE, Putrefaction.

FERMENTUM CEREVISIÆ, Yest—f. Morbi, Ferment—f. Ventriculi, Gastric juice.

FERN, BUSH, Comptonia asplenifolia — f. Cinnamon, Osmunda cinnamomea — f. Eagle, Pteris aquilina — f. Female, Asplenium filix fœmina, Pteris aquilina—f. Gale, Comptonia asplenifolia—f. Male, Polypodium filix mas—f. Meadow, Comptonia asplenifolia—f. Rock, Adiantum pedatum—f. Root, Polypodium vulgare—f. Sweet, Adiantum pedatum, Comptonia asplenifolia—f. Sweet, shrubby, Comptonia asplenifolia.

FERNAMBUCO WOOD, Cæsalpinia echinata.

FERRAMEN'TUM, *Side'rion, Instrumen'tum fer'reum.* Any surgical instrument made of iron. By the vulgar, in France, the word *ferrements* means the *instruments* used in difficult labours.

FERRARIA, Scrophularia aquatica.

FERRATUS, Chalybeate.

FERREIN, CANAL OF, *Ductus Ferrei'ni.* A triangular channel, which Ferrein supposed to result from the approximation of the free edges of the eyelids applied to the globe of the eye; and which he considered adapted for directing the tears towards the puncta lachrymalia, during sleep. The canal is, probably, imaginary.

The same name is likewise given to the *cortical canals,*—the first portions of the uriniferous ducts, whilst still in the cortical substance of the kidney.

FERREIN, PYR'AMID OF, *Pyr'amis Ferrei'ni.* Each of the papillæ of the kidney, according to Ferrein, consists of, at least, 700 subordinate cones or pyramids. To these last the names '*pyramids of Ferrein,' Pyram'ides rena'les Ferrei'ni, Fascic'uli pyramida'les,* have been given.

FERRI ACE'TAS, *Extrac'tum martis ace'ticum, Ace'ticum martia'lē, Ac"etate of Iron, Iron Liquor,* (F.) *Acétate de fer.* A preparation of the Dublin Pharmacopœia, made by digesting 1 part of *carbonate of iron* in 6 parts of *acetic acid* for three days, and filtering. Dose, as a tonic and astringent, ♏v to ♏xx, in water.

FERRI ÆRUGO, F. Subcarbonas—f. et Ammoniæ murias, Ferrum ammoniatum—f. Ammoniochloridum, Ferrum ammoniatum.

FERRI ET ALU'MINÆ SULPHAS, *Sulphate of Iron and Alumina,* is made by treating *bicarbonated solution of soft iron* and *carbonated solution of pure washed alumina,* with *sulphuric acid.* It has been recommended as a valuable astringent. Dose, from five to ten grains.

FERRI AMMO'NIO-CITRAS, *Ammoniæ ferro-citras, Ferrum ammoni'aco-cit'ricum, Ammonio-citrate of iron, Citrate of ammonia and iron.* Prepared by adding *ammonia* to *citrate of iron,* so as to neutralize the excess of acid. Dose, gr. v. to gr. viij. A POTASSIO-CITRATE and a SODIO-CITRATE OF IRON have also been introduced; and a CITRATE of the MAGNETIC OXIDE OF IRON prepared by combining the *magnetic oxide* with *citric acid.*

FERRI AMMONIO-TARTRAS, *Ammonio-tartrate of Iron.* This salt is best made by dissolving to saturation freshly precipitated hydrated oxide of iron in a solution of bitartrate of ammonia, and evaporating to dryness. It is very soluble. The dose is five grains or more in pill or solution.

FERRI ARSENIAS, Arseniate of Iron—f. Borussias, Prussian blue—f. Bromidum, see Bromine—f. Carbonas, F. subcarbonas—f. Carbonas Saccharatum, see F. Protocarbonas—f. Carbonatum, Graphites—f. Carburetum, Graphites.

FERRI CITRAS, *Citrate of Iron.* Two citrates of iron are prepared—the *Sesquicitrate* or *Citrate of the Sesquioxide;* and the *Citrate of the Prot-*

oxide. The former is officinal in the Ph. U. S. They resemble, in their medical properties, the tartrate and the lactate of the metal.

FERRI CYANURETUM, Prussian blue—f. Deutocarbonas fúscus, F. subcarbonas—f. Deutoxydum nigrum, Æthiops martial—f. Ferrocyanas, Prussian blue—f. Ferrocyanuretum, Prussian blue—f. Hydriodas, F. Iodidum—f. Hydrocyanas, Prussian blue—f. Hypercarburetum, Graphites.

FERRI IO'DIDUM, *F. Iodure'tum, F. Hydri'odas, Iodide, Ioduret* or *Hydri'odate of Iron*, (F.) *Iodure de fer*, (*Iodin.* ℥ij, *Ferri rament.* ℥j, *Aq. destillat.* Oiss.) Mix the iodine with a pint of the distilled water, in a porcelain or glass vessel, and gradually add the iron filings, stirring constantly. Heat the mixture gently until the liquid acquires a light greenish colour; then filter, and, after the liquid has passed, pour upon the filter half a pint of the distilled water, boiling hot. When this has passed, evaporate the filtered liquor, at a temperature not exceeding 212°, in an iron vessel, to dryness; keep the dry iodide in a closely stopped bottle. (Ph. U. S.)

FERRI IODURETUM, F. Iodidum.

FERRI LACTAS, *Lactate of Iron, Lactate of Protox'ide of Iron*, (F.) *Lactate de Fer*. Prepared by digesting in a sand-bath, at a low temperature, diluted lactic acid with iron filings. It is employed in the same cases as the precipitated subcarbonate of iron, and especially in chlorosis. Twelve grains of the lactate may be given in the 24 hours, in the form of lozenges.

FERRI LIMATU'RA PURIFICA'TA, *Pu'rified Iron Filings:*—purified by means of the magnet, for internal use. The filings are, also, called *Ferri Scobs, F. Ramen'ta et Fila, Martis Limatu'ra, Spec'ulum In'dicum, Ferri in pul'verem resolu'tio*, (F.) *Limaille de Fer.* They are considered to possess the general properties of iron:—the iron becoming oxidized.

FERRI ET MAGNE'SIÆ CITRAS, *Citrate of iron and magne'sia*, is prepared by dissolving hydrated oxide of iron in a solution of citric acid, saturated with carbonate of magnesia, and evaporating to dryness. It is soluble in water, and does not constipate. Dose from four grains to fifteen, in solution.

FERRI NITRAS, see Liquor Ferri nitratis—f. Nitratis Liquor, see Liquor Ferri nitratis—f. Oxidum Fuscum, F. subcarbonas — f. Oxidum Nigrum, Oxydum ferri nigrum—f. Oxidum hydratum, Ferrum oxydatum hydratum—f. Oxidum rubrum, Colcothar, Ferri subcarbonas—f. Oxidum hydratum, Ferrum et Oxydum hydratum—f. Percyanidum, Prussian blue.

FERRI PHOSPHAS, *Phosphate of Iron*, (*Ferri Sulphat.* ℥v, *Sodæ Phosphat.* ℥vi, *Aquæ*, cong. Dissolve the sulphate of iron and phosphate of soda, severally, in four pints of the water; then mix the solutions, and set the mixture by, that the powder may subside; lastly, having poured off the supernatant liquor, wash the phosphate of iron with water, and dry it with a gentle heat.—Ph. U. S.) Dose, 5 to 10 grains as a chalybeate. Rarely used.

FERRI PILA, F. limatura—f. et Potassæ tartras, Ferrum tartarizatum—f. Potassio-citras, see Ferri ammonio-citras—f. Potassio-tartras, Ferrum tartarizatum.

FERRI PROTOCARBO'NAS, *Protocarbonate of Iron*, (F.) *Carbonate de Fer.* The protocarbonate of iron, thrown down from a solution of the sulphate of iron by the carbonate of soda, readily attracts oxygen and becomes converted into the sesquioxide. To prevent this, it may be associated with honey and sugar, and the mixture be reduced by evaporation to a pilular consistence. The mass constitutes the *Ferruginous Pills, Pi-* *lules ferrugineuses*, of Vallet, *Vallet's Pills*. See Pilulæ Ferri Carbonatis. The Edinburgh Pharmacopœia contains the *Ferri Car'bonas Saccha-ra'tum, Sac'charine Carbonate of Iron*, prepared in this manner. It is the *Ferrum Carbon'icum Saccharatum* of Klauer.

The protocarbonate is given in the same diseases as the lactate of iron; ten or fifteen grains in the course of the twenty-four hours.

FERRI PROTOSULPHAS VIRIDIS, F. Sulphas—f. Prussias, Prussian blue.

FERRI PULVIS, *Fer réduit, F. réduit par l'hydrogène, Ferrum metal'licum, Powdered iron;* prepared by passing a stream of *hydrogen gas* over the *sesquioxide of iron*, contained in an iron or porcelain tube heated to low redness. It is very liable to become oxidated, and must be kept in a dry, well-stopped bottle. It has been prescribed in anæmic, and especially in chlorotic cases. The ordinary dose is two grains three times a day, in pill made with sugar and gum. A formula for its preparation is given in the last edition of the Pharmacopœia of the United States (1851).

FERRI et QUI'NLÆ CITRAS, *Citrate of Iron and Qui'nia*, formed by the union of four parts of *citrate of iron* and one part of *citrate of quinia*, has been prescribed in cases where a combination of these tonics is indicated.

FERRI RAMENTA, F. limatura — f. Rubigo, F. Subcarbonas—f. Scobs, F. limatura—f. Sesquioxidum, F. subcarbonas præcipitatus.

FERRI SESQUINITRATIS, LIQUOR, see Tinctura Ferri muriatis—f. Sodio-tartras, see Ferri et ammonio-citras.

FERRI SUBCAR'BONAS, *F. Car'bonas, Ferrum præcipita'tum, Chal'ybis Rubi'go præpara'ta, Ferri Rubigo.* (The last two terms, as well as *Ferru'go*, are applied to the subcarbonate or rust, *Æru'go Ferri, Cacaferri*, formed by the action of moist air on metallic iron.) A protoxide of iron, oxidized by the decomposition of water; the carbonic acid being attracted from the air. Dose, gr. v to ʒss and more.

Ferri Subcarbonas may be precipitated from sulphate of iron by carbonate of soda. The following is the formula of the Pharmacopœia of the United States:—*Ferri sulph.* ℥viij; *sodæ carb.* ℥ix; *aquæ bullient.* cong. Dissolve the sulphate of iron and carbonate of soda severally in four pints of the water, then mix the solutions, and, having stirred the mixture, set it by that the powder may subside: having poured off the liquor, wash the subcarbonate with hot water, wrap it in bibulous paper, and dry with a gentle heat. It is, also, called *Ferri sesquiox'idum, Ox'idum ferri fuscum, Ox'idum ferri rubrum, Deuto-car'bonas Ferri fuscus, Crocus martis ape'riens, Sesquioxide* or *peroxide of iron*, (F.) *Peroxide de fer, Safran de Mars apéritif.*

FERRI SULPHAS, *Sal Martis, Vitriolum Martis, Vitriolum Ferri, Ferrum Vitriola'tum, Sulphas* vel *Protosulphas Ferri vir'idis, Caleadinum, Cal'cator, Cal'cotar, Chalcan'thum, Calcite'a, Atramen'tum auto'rium, Vit'riol, Vitriolum viride, An'ima Hep'atis, Sulphate of Iron, Green Vitriol, Copperas,* (F.) *Sulfate de fer.* The Pharmacopœia of the United States directs it to be made by the action of *sulphuric acid* ℥xviij, on *iron wire*, cut in pieces, ℥xij—*water*, a gallon—evaporating, crystallizing, and drying the crystals on bibulous paper. This salt is inodorous, and of a strong styptic taste. The crystals are light green, transparent, rhomboidal; and soluble in two parts of water. It is tonic and anthelmintic. Dose, gr. j. to vj and more.

FERRI SULPHAS CALCINATUM, Colcothar.

FERRI SULPHURE'TUM, *Sul'phuret of Iron, Iron pyri'tes*, (F.) *Sulfure de fer;* may be made by heating one part of *sublimed sulphur*, over three parts of *iron filings* in a crucible until the mass begins to glow. It is employed as a ready means for obtaining hydrosulphuric acid gas by the addition of sulphuric or chlorohydric acid.

FERRI TANNAS, *Ferrum tan'nicum, Tannate of Iron*, (F.) *Tannate de fer*. This salt is usually obtained by adding a solution of a *salt of sesquioxide of iron*, as the persulphate, to a *decoction of nut-galls*. It is possessed of tonic and astringent properties, and has been extolled especially in chlorosis.

FERRI TARTARUM, Ferrum tartarizatum — f. Tritoxydum, Colcothar.

FERRI VALERIA'NAS, *Ferrum Valeria'nicum, Vale'rianate of Iron*, (Fr.) *Valérianate de fer*. Formed by the action of *valerianic acid* on *oxide of iron*. It is a dark brick-red powder, insoluble in water, and has been given in hysteria complicating chlorosis. Dose, from two to four grains.

FERRICUS HYDRAS, Ferrum oxydum hydratum.

FERRUGINEUS, Chalybeate.

FERRUGINOUS, Chalybeate.

FERRUGO, Ferri subcarbonas, Ferrum oxydatum hydratum.

FERRUM, *Mars, Side'ros, Metal'lum hæmatopoiët'icum, Iron,* (F.) *Fer*. A metal of a bluish-gray colour; fibrous texture; brilliant and fine-grained fracture. Specific gravity 7.600 to 7.800; hard, ductile, malleable, and magnetic. The medicinal virtues of iron are tonic; producing fetid eructations, when it takes effect, owing to its meeting with acid in the stomach, which oxidizes it, and causes the evolution of hydrogen gas. When given in the metallic state, the filings are chiefly used; but the oxides and salts are most commonly employed.

FERRUM AMMONIACALE, F. ammoniatum — f. Ammoniaco-citricum, Ferri ammonio-citras.

FERRUM AMMONIA'TUM, *Mu'rias Ammo'niæ et Ferri, Ferri ammo'nio-chlo'ridum, Flores martia'les, Flores salis ammoni'aci martia'les, Ens martis, Ens Ven'eris Boy'lei, Sal martis muriat'icum sublima'tum, Sal ammoni'acum martia'lĕ, Ammo'nium muriat'icum martia'tum seu martia'lĕ, Aroph Paracel'si, Calen'dulæ minera'les, Ferrum ammoniaca'lĕ, Ammo'niated Iron, Ammo'nio-chloride of Iron,* (F.) *Muriate d'ammoniaque et de fer.* A mixture of the hydro-chlorates of ammonia and iron. (?) (*Ferri Subcarb.* ℥iij; *acid muriat.* f ℥x; *ammon. muriat.* ℔ijss; *aq. destillat.* Oiv. Mix the subcarbonate with the acid in a glass vessel and digest for two hours; then add the muriate, previously dissolved in distilled water, and having filtered the liquor, evaporate to dryness. Rub to powder.—Ph. U. S.) Dose, gr. iij. to gr. xv.

FERRUM BORUSSICUM, Prussian blue — f. Carbonicum Saccharatum, Ferri protocarbonas — f. Cyanogenatum, Prussian blue — f. Hæmatites, Hæmatites — f. Magnes attractorium, Magnet — f. Metallicum, Ferri pulvis.

FERRUM OXYDA'TUM HYDRA'TUM, *Ferri Oxidum Hydra'tum* (Ph. U. S.), *Ferru'go, Hydras Fer'ricus, Hydro-oxide of Iron, Hydrated Oxide of Iron, Hydrated peroxide of Iron, Hydrated Tritoxide of Iron*. It may be prepared by taking a solution of sulphate of iron, increasing its dose of oxygen by heating it with nitric acid, and precipitating the oxide by adding pure ammonia in excess, washing the precipitate, and keeping it moist.

The following is the formula adopted by the Pharmacopœia of the United States: *Ferri Sulph.* ℥iv; *acid. sulphuric.* f ℨiiiss; *acid. nitric.* f ℨvi, vel q. s., *Liq. ammoniæ* q. s., *aquæ* Oij. Dissolve the sulphate of iron in the water, and having added the sulphuric acid, boil the solution: then add the nitric acid in small portions, boiling the liquid for a minute or two after each addition, until the acid ceases to produce a dark colour. Filter the liquid, allow it to cool, and add the liquor ammoniæ in excess, stirring the mixture briskly; wash the precipitate with water, until the washings cease to yield a precipitate with chloride of barium, and keep it close in bottles with water sufficient to cover it.

It has been brought forward, of late, as an antidote to arsenic; and many cases of its efficacy have been published.

From 10 to 20 parts of the hydrated oxide would seem to be more than sufficient to convert 1 part of arsenious acid into the basic salt of iron.

FERRUM OXYDULATUM HYDROCYANICUM, Prussian blue—f. Potabile, F. tartarizatum—f. Præcipitatum, Ferri subcarbonas.

FERRUM TANNICUM, Ferri tannas.

FERRUM TARTARIZA'TUM, *Tartras Potas'sæ et Ferri, Tar'tarum Ferri, Ferri et Potassæ Tartras,* (Ph. U. S.) *Tar'tarus chalybea'tus, Mars solu'bilis, Tartras kal'ico-fer'ricus, Chalybs tartarisa'tus, Tartarus martia'lis, Ferri potassio-tartras, Tartras Potas'sæ ferrugino'sus, Ferrum potab'ilĕ, Globus martia'lis, Glob'uli Tar'tari martia'les seu martia'les solu'ti seu martia'ti seu tartra'tis ferri et lixiv'iæ, Boli Martis, Pyri martia'les, Tartarized Iron, Tartrate of Potassa and Iron,* (F.) *Tartrate de potasse et de fer, Boule de Mars, Boule de Nancy, B. de Molsheim, B. d'Acier.* (*Ferri subcarb.* ℥iij, *Acid. muriat.* f ℨx; *Liquor Potassæ,* Ovss; *Potass. Bitart.* ℥vijss, *Aquæ destillat.* cong. iss. Mix the subcarbonate of iron and the muriatic acid, and digest for two hours; pour the solution into a gallon of the distilled water; set aside for an hour, and pour off the supernatant liquor. To this add the liquor potassæ; wash the precipitate formed frequently with water, and, while yet moist, mix it with the bitartrate of potassa and half a gallon of the distilled water. Keep the mixture at the temperature of 140° for 30 hours, frequently stirring; filter the solution, and evaporate by means of a water bath, at the same temperature, to dryness.—(Ph. U. S.) It is one of the mildest of the salts of iron, and not unpalatable. Dose, gr. x. to ℨss.

The *Tinctu'ra Martis Aperiti'va, Tincture of Ludwig; Al'cohol cum Sulpha'tĕ Ferri tartarisa'tus; Tinctura Martis Glauberi* is, essentially, a solution of this salt. It is also called *Eau de Boule,* and is used in contusions.

Helvetius's Styptic was composed of the *filings of iron and tartar,* mixed to a proper consistence with French brandy. It was called in England *Eaton's Styptic;* but this is now formed of *Sulphate of Iron.*

FERRUM VALERIANICUM, Ferri valerianas — f. Vitriolatum, Ferri sulphas—f. Vitriolatum ustum, Colcothar — f. Zooticum, Prussian blue.

FERTILITY, Fecundity.

FER'ULA, *Fanon, Palette, Splint*—f. Africana, Bubon galbanum—f. Asafœtida, see Asafœtida—f. Graveolens, Anethum graveolens — f. Opoponax, Pastinaca opoponax — f. Persica, see Sagapenum.

FERUS, Homicidal.

FESSES, Nates.

FESSIER, Gluteal—*f. Grand,* Glutæus maximus—*f. Moyen,* Glutæus medius—*f. Petit,* Glutæus minimus.

FETID, *Fœ'tidus, Dyso'des, Caco'des, Bromo'sus, Graveolens*. Having a bad smell.

FETUS, Fœtus.

FEU ACTUEL, Canterium—*f. Persique,* Herpes zoster, see Anthrax—*f. Potential,* see Cauterium—*f. Sacré*, Erysipelas—*f. St. Antoine*, Erysipelas—*f. Sauvage*, Ignis sylvaticus—*f. Volage*, Ignis sylvaticus.

FEUX DE DENTS, Strophulus—*f. Volages*, Porrigo larvalis.

FÈVE, Vicia faba—*f. de Carthagène*, Habilla de Carthagena—*f. à Cochon*, Hyoscyamus—*f. Épaisse*, Sedum telephium—*f. des Marais*, Vicia faba—*f. de Sainte Ignace*, Ignatia amara—*f. Purgatif*, Ricinus communis.

FEVER, *Febris*, from *feritas*, 'wildness,' or from *fervor*, 'heat,' or from *februo*, 'I purify:' *Pyr, Pyr'etos*, πυρετος, (F.) *Fièvre*. One of the most frequent and dangerous affections to which the body is liable. A person has an attack of fever, when he is affected with rigors, followed by increased heat of skin, quick pulse, languor, and lassitude. Rigors, increased heat, and frequency of pulse have each been assumed as the essential character of fever. It is not characterized, however, by any *one*, but depends upon the coexistence of *many* symptoms. Fevers have been usually divided into *idiopathic* or *essential*, and into *symptomatic*. The idiopathic arise without any obvious local cause. The symptomatic are dependent upon local irritation. Idiopathic fevers may be divided into three classes: 1. Those attended with distinct paroxysms:—intermittents. 2. Remittent and continued fevers: and, 3. Fevers complicated with eruptions or the exanthematous. These divisions admit of great variety, owing to climate, season, soil, age, &c. All ages and climates are liable to fever; and its exciting causes are very numerous. These causes may be *common;* as irritations in the intestines; external injuries, stimulants, &c.; or they may be *specific;* as miasmata, contagion, &c. The greatest diversity has prevailed regarding the theory of fever. Its primary seat has been placed in the brain, mucous membrane of the stomach and intestines, skin, nerves, blood-vessels, liver, vena cava, pancreas, &c. It would seem, however, that although, in fever, the whole of the functions are morbidly impressed, the arguments in favour of the impression being first made on the nervous system and the system of nutrition are the strongest. The exciting cause of fever, whatever it may be, produces an irregular action in the system of nutrition, which is soon conveyed to the rest of the system, owing to the extensive sympathy which exists between every part of the body; and it is probable, that all those local inflammations and congestions are the consequence, rather than the cause, of this disordered condition of the system. The general character of fever is clearly shown by examination of the blood. When fever is devoid of inflammatory complication, the quantity of fibrin is in no case augmented. It frequently remains in the healthy proportion, and at times diminishes to an extent not met with in any other acute disease. The alteration of the blood in fevers, which consists generally in a diminution of the fibrinous element, is the reverse of what occurs in inflammation.

Many phenomena of fever are influenced by that *periodicity*, which we notice in the execution of several of the functions of the body. The types of intermittents are strong evidences of such an influence.

In the *treatment* of fever, it is important, 1. To bear in mind its tendency, particularly in the case of the exanthemata, to run a definite course, and terminate in restoration to health. 2. The disposition to local determination or hyperæmia:— the most frequent cause of the fatal termination of fever: a circumstance requiring the vigilant attention of the physician. 3. That the symptoms must be attentively studied, in order to deduce, as far as possible from them, the indications of cure. Lastly, attention must be paid to the prevalent epidemic. There are particular seasons in which fevers are very malignant; and others in which they are as mild; circumstances which necessarily have an effect upon the treatment.

FEVER AND AGUE, Intermittent Fever—f. Acclimating, F. strangers'.

FEVER, ADE'NO-MENINGE'AL, *Febris ade'nomeningea, Febris mesenter'ica* (BAGLIVI,) *Morbus muco'sus, Febris muco'sa; Mucous fever, Gastroduodenop'yra, Pitu'itous Fever, Catar'rhal Fever, Phlegmap'yra, Phlegmop'yra, Phlegmatop'yra, Gastro-Bronchi'tis*. Fever, accompanied with considerable mucous secretion; especially from the digestive tube.

FEVER, ADYNAM'IC, *Febris adynam'ica, Asthenicop'yra, Asthenicopy'retus, Asthenop'yra, Asthenopyr'etus*. Fever attended with great prostration of the vital powers—as Typhoid and Typhus fever.

FEVER, AFRICAN, *Febris Africa'na*. The malignant bilious remittent fever, which prevails on the Western Coast of Africa.

FEVER, ALGID, see Algidus.

FEVER, ANOM'ALOUS, *Febris anom'ala, F. errat'ica, F. irregula'ris, F. vaga*. A fever, whose progress and type are irregular.

FEVER, APHON'IC, *Febris apho'nica*. A variety of intermittent, in which the voice is lost during the paroxysm.

FEVER, APOPLEC'TIC, *Febris apoplec'tica, Com'atose Fever, Febris comato'des, F. Lethar'gica, F. soporo'sa*. An intermittent or continued fever, attended with apoplectic symptoms.

FEVER, ARTICULAR ERUPTIVE, Dengue—f. Articular rheumatic, Dengue.

FEVER, ARTIFIC''IAL, *Febris artificia'lis, Febris artē promo'ta*. Fever produced designedly by the internal or external use of stimulants.

FEVER, ASTHEN'IC, *Febris asthen'ica*. Fever accompanied with debility. It may include every variety of fever under certain circumstances, but is generally appropriated to typhus.

FEVER, ASTHMAT'IC, *Febris asthmat'ica*. A pernicious intermittent, accompanied with symptoms of asthma.

FEVER, ATAXO-ADYNAM'IC; *Febris atax'o-adynam'ica*. Fever characterized by symptoms of ataxia and adynamia.

FEVER, BARCELONA, FEVER, yellow — f. Bastard, Illegitimate fever.

FEVER, BIL'IOUS, *Febris bilio'sa, F. polychol'ica, Syn'ochus bilio'sa, F. aso'des, F. choler'ica, F. gas'trica, F. hepat'ica, Cholep'yra, Cholepyr'etus, Hepatogastrocholo'sis, Febris cholepyret'ica, Enterop'yra bilio'sa, Choloze'mia febri'lis*. The common remittent fever of summer and autumn; generally supposed to be owing to, or connected with, derangement of the biliary system.

FEVER, BILIOUS REMITTING, YELLOW, Fever, yellow — f. Bladdery, Pemphigus.

FEVER, BOA VISTA. A malignant bilious remittent fever, greatly resembling yellow fever, which was very fatal at Fernando Po, and in ships in its waters, in the year 1845.

FEVER, BONA. A malignant paludal fever, which prevailed amongst the troops of the garrison at Bona in Algeria, from 1832 to 1835.

FEVER, BONE, see Inflammation — f. Bouquet, Dengue — f. Brain, F. cerebral, Phrenitis — f. Brain, water, Hydrocephalus internus—f. Bucket, Dengue—f. Bulam, Fever, yellow—f. Camp, Typhus gravior.

FEVER, CARDIAL'GIC, *Febris cardial'gica*. A variety of pernicious intermittent, accompanied with violent cardialgia during the paroxysm.

FEVER, CARDIT'IC. Intermittent fever, accompanied with pain at the heart.

FEVER, CATARRHAL, F. adeno-meningeal.

FEVER, CEPHALAL'GIC, *Febris cephalal'gica.* A pernicious intermittent, accompanied with intense pain of the head. Also, intermittent cephalalgia.

FEVER, CEPHAL'IC, *Febris cephal'ica.* A febrile affection of children—intermediate between the acute form of active cerebral congestion and the chronic form — which is attended by fever, pain in the head, disorder, or more generally constipation of the bowels, and a train of phenomena often supposed to be premonitory of an attack of hydrocephalus.—Mauthner.

FEVER, CER'EBRAL, *Brain fever.* Fever, generally of an ataxic character, in which the brain is considerably affected.

FEVER, CHILDBED, Fever, puerperal, Puerperal Fever — f. Childbed, Low, see Peritonitis.

FEVER, CHOL'ERIC, *Febris choler'ica.* A variety of pernicious intermittent, accompanied with symptoms of cholera morbus.

FEVER, CHOLERIC, OF INFANTS, Cholera infantum.

FEVER, CHRONIC, *Febris chron'ica.* Some authors apply this name to protracted fevers; others to hectic fever.

FEVER, COLLIQ'UATIVE, *Febris tab'ida, Febris colliquati'va.* Fever, characterized by rapid emaciation, copious evacuations, and rapid prostration of strength.

FEVER, COMATOSE, F. apoplectic.

FEVER, CONGES'TIVE, *Febris congesti'va.* Fever accompanied by obscure symptoms; or by great oppression and depression; in which it is difficult — and often impossible — to induce reaction. Congestive fevers occur in various parts of this country, especially in the fall; and they are very common in India. The term congestive fever is often used in some parts of the south of the United States very indefinitely — to include winter typhus, and typhoid fevers, typhoid pneumonia, as well as intermittents and autumnal remittents.—Dickson.

FEVER, CONTINENT, see Continent and Continued fever — f. Continual, see Continued fever — f. Continued, common, Synochus.

FEVER, CONVUL'SIVE, *Febris convulsi'va.* A pernicious intermittent or remittent, accompanied by convulsions.

FEVER, DELIR'IOUS, *Febris cum delir'io,* (F.) *Fièvre délirante.* A pernicious intermittent, characterized by delirium in the paroxysms.

FEVER, DEP'URATORY, *Febris depurato'ria.* A fever, to which was attributed the property of purifying the blood; or which indicated, that such a supposed depuration had occurred.

FEVER, DIAPHORET'IC, *Febris diaphoret'ica, Febris sudato'ria.* A pernicious intermittent, with excessive sweating during the fit.

FEVER, DIARY, Ephemera.

FEVER, DIGES'TIVE. The chilliness, followed by increased heat and quickness of pulse, which frequently accompanies digestion.

FEVER, DOUBLE, (F.) *Fièvre double* ou *doublée.* An intermittent, which has two paroxysms in a given time, instead of one.

FEVER, DOUBLE-QUARTAN. A fever, whose paroxysms occur two days in succession, and fail the third day; the first paroxysm resembling the 4th; and the second the 5th.

FEVER, DOUBLE-QUOTIDIAN. An intermittent, whose paroxysms return twice every day at corresponding hours.

FEVER, DOUBLE-TERTIAN. An intermittent, whose paroxysms return every day; the first corresponding with the 3d, the second with the 4th, and so on.

FEVER, DUODEC''IMANE, *Febris duodecim'ana.* A supposititious intermittent, whose paroxysms recur on the 12th day, or every 11 days.

FEVER, DYNAMIC, Synocha — f. Endemial, Remittent F. — f. Endemic, Remittent F. — f. Endemical, Remittent F.—f. Enteric, see Typhus— f. Ephemeral, Ephemera.

FEVER, EPILEP'TIC, *Febris epilep'tica.* A variety of pernicious intermittent, accompanied with attacks of epilepsy.

FEVER, EROT'IC, *Febris erot'ica,* (F.) *Fièvre d'amour.* A chronic fever, occasioned by unpropitious love.

FEVER, ERRAT'IC, see Erratic — f. Eruptive, Exanthematica — f. Eruptive, articular, Dengue —f. Exacerbating, Remittent Fever.

FEVER, FAINTING, OF PERSIA. A singular and fatal epidemic, presenting some points of analogy with cholera, which prevailed at Teheran in the autumn of 1842.

FEVER, GAN'GRENOUS, *Febris gangræno'des.* Fever, accompanied by gangrene of various parts, and especially of the limbs and genitals. Sénac describes an intermittent of this kind.

FEVER, GASTRAL'GIC. An intermittent accompanied with acute burning lacerating pain at the stomach.

FEVER, GASTRIC, *Febris gas'trica, F. gas'trica bilio'sa, Gastrocholo'sis, Hepatogastrocholo'sis, Stomach'ic fever, Syn'ochus Bilio'sa.* A name, given by some to *bilious fever,* which has appeared to them to be dependent on an affection of the stomach. Also, called *Menin'go-gastric fever, Febris meningo-gas'trica, Meningo-gastri'tis, Harvest fever,* (F.) *Fièvre de la Moisson, F. Méningogastrique.*

FEVER, GASTRO-ADYNAM'IC, *Febris gastroadynam'ica.* A fever, in which the symptoms of bilious fever are joined with those of adynamic fever.

FEVER, GASTRO-ANGIOTEN'IC. A fever, in which the symptoms of bilious are united with those of inflammatory fever.

FEVER, GASTRO-ATAX'IC. A fever, in which the symptoms of bilious fever are united with those of ataxic fever.

FEVER, GIBRALTAR, Fever, yellow—f. Harvest, F. Gastric—f. Hæmagastric, F. yellow.

FEVER, HÆMOP'TOIC, *Febris Hæmopto'ica.* A variety of masked intermittent, in which periodical hæmoptysis is the chief symptom.

FEVER, HAY, *Catarr'hus æsti'vus, Summer Catarrh, Hay Asthma, Rose Catarrh, Summer Bronchi'tis.* A catarrh to which certain persons are subject in summer, and which has been ascribed in England to the effluvium of hay, but this is not the probable cause. It is a catarrh with sneezing, headach, weeping, snuffling and cough, with, at times, fever and general discomfort. It is not uncommon in this country. It disappears spontaneously, — to recur on subsequent years about the same period.

FEVER, HEBDOM'ADAL. A supposititious fever, whose paroxysms return weekly, and on the same day.

FEVER, HECTIC, see Consumption, and Hectic Fever.

FEVER, HEPAT'IC or HEPATAL'GIC. A pernicious intermittent, with violent pain in the right hypochondrium.

FEVER, HILL. A modification of remittent, occurring in the hilly districts of India.

FEVER, HOSPITAL, Typhus gravior.

FEVER, HU'MORAL, *Febris humora'lis.* Fever, in which an alteration or deterioration of the humours is suspected.

FEVER, HUN'GARY, *Febris Hungar'ica* seu *Pannon'ica* seu *Morbus Ungar'icus, Cephalon'osus, Vermis cer'ebri*, (F.) *Fièvre Hongroise ou de Hongrie*. An epidemic typhus, common amongst the soldiers in barracks, in Hungary.

FEVER, HYDROPHOB'IC, *Febris hydrophob'ica*. Pernicious intermittent with dread of liquids.

FEVER, HYSTER'IC, *Febris hyster'ica*. Hysteria, accompanied by fever. Hysteria, occurring with each paroxysm of intermittent.

FEVER, ICTER'IC, *Febris icter'ica*. Fever, accompanied by jaundice. Some intermittents exhibit this complication at each paroxysm.

FEVER, IN'FANTILE REMIT'TENT, *Febris infan'tum remit'tens, F. vermino'sa*, (of many), *Spurious worm fever, Remittent fever of children, F. muco'sa vermino'sa, Hec'tica infan'tilis, Febris lenta*. A fever occurring in childhood, which often assumes many of the characters of hydrocephalus. It appears generally to be dependent upon a morbid condition of the stomach and bowels.

FEVER, INFLAMMATORY, Synocha.

FEVER, INSID'IOUS. Fever, which, at first, seems devoid of danger, but subsequently becomes of a more or less malignant character.

FEVER, INTERMITTENT, see Intermittent fever — f. Jail, Typhus gravior — f. Jungle, see Jungle fever — f. Lenticular, Miliary fever — f. Irritative, Irritation, morbid.

FEVER, LO'CHIAL, *Febris lochia'lis*. That acceleration of the circulation which sometimes occurs during the discharge of the lochia.

FEVER, LUNG, Catarrh, Pneumonia.

FEVER, MALIG'NANT, *Febris malig'na*. Fever which makes its approaches insidiously, and subsequently becomes formidable. Any fever which exhibits a very dangerous aspect. *Typhus gravior*.

FEVER, MALIG'NANT PESTILENTIAL, Fever, yellow — f. Marsh, Elodes (febris.)

FEVER, MASKED, *Febris larva'ta*, (F.) *Fièvre larvée, Dead Ague, Dumb Ague*. Anomalous intermittent, the paroxysms of which have not the regular stages.

FEVER, MENINGO-GASTRIC, Fever gastric.

FEVER, MESENTER'IC, *Febris mesenter'ica*. A name given, by Baglivi, to a species of fever which appears to have belonged either to the *mucous* or *bilious*.

FEVER, MILK, *Febris lac'tea*, (F.) *Fièvre de lait* ou *laiteuse, F. lactée; Galactop'yra, Galactopyr'etus*. The fever, which precedes or accompanies the secretion of milk in women recently delivered. It comes on generally about the third day after delivery, and is characterized by quick pulse; increased heat; redness of face; diminution or temporary suspension of the lochial discharge; tumefaction and tension of the breasts. It commonly terminates in twenty-four hours, and often with profuse perspiration. It requires the use of antiphlogistics, with dry diet.

FEVER, MIXED, Synochus — f. Mucous, F. adeno-meningeal.

FEVER NEPHRIT'IC, *Febris nephrit'ica*. Intermittent fever, accompanied with nephritic pain during the paroxysm.

FEVER, NERVOUS, *Febris nervo'sa* seu *neuro'des, Febris lenta nervo'sa, Neurop'yra, Neuropyr'etus*. A variety of Typhus; the *Typhus mitior* of Cullen. By many, however, it is esteemed a distinct disease. See Typhoid fever.

FEVER, NERVOUS, WITH EXANTHEMATOUS ERUPTION, Typhus.

FEVER, NIGER. A malignant fever, of the bilious remittent kind, which proved fatal to many in the expeditions sent out by the British government to explore the Niger, in the years 1841-2, and previously.

FEVER, NON'ANE, *Febris nona'na*. A supposititious fever, whose paroxysms recur every ninth day, or every eight days.

FEVER, OC'TANE, *Febris octa'na*. An intermittent, whose paroxysms recur every eighth day.

FEVER, PALUDAL, Intermittent — f. Paroxysmal, Remittent fever — f. Periodic, Intermittent.

FEVER, PERIOD'ICAL, *Febris period'ica*. An intermittent or remittent fever.

FEVER PERNIC"IOUS, *Febris pernicio'sa*. Intermittent fever, when attended with great danger, and which destroys the majority of those affected by it in the first four or five paroxysms; sometimes in the very first.

FEVER, PESTILEN'TIAL, *Febris pestilentia'lis*. The *Plague*. Also a severe case of typhus. The yellow fever and sweating sickness have, likewise, been thus designated.

FEVER, PESTILENTIAL, OF CATTLE, Murr — f. Pituitous, F. adeno-meningeal.

FEVER, PLEURIT'IC. An intermittent or remittent, accompanied with inflammation of the pleura.

FEVER, PNEUMON'IC, *Febris pneumon'ica*. An intermittent, accompanied with inflammation of the lungs. Also, pneumonia.

FEVER POISON, see Poison.

FEVER, PSEUDO. Irritation, morbid.

FEVER, PUER'PERAL, *Febris puerpera'lis, Childbed fever*, (F.) *Fièvre puerpérale*. This name has been given to several acute diseases, supervening on delivery. It means, generally, a malignant variety of peritonitis, which runs its course very rapidly, and passes into a typhoid condition, unless met, at the very onset, by the most active depleting measures. By the generality of practitioners, it is esteemed to be eminently contagious; some, however, deny that it is so. See Peritonitis, and Puerperal fever.

FEVER, PUERPERAL ADYNAMIC or MALIGNANT, see Peritonitis.

FEVER, PUKING, Milk sickness.

FEVER, PU'RULENT, *Febris purulen'ta*. Fever, which accompanies suppuration.

FEVER, PUTRID, Typhus gravior.

FEVER, QUINTAN, *Febris quinta'na*. A fever, whose paroxysms return every fifth day. It is seen rarely, or never.

FEVER, QUOTIDIAN, see Quotidian — f. Red Tongue, see Typhus.

FEVER, REG'ULAR, *Febris regula'ris* seu *exquisi'ta*. An intermittent whose paroxysms follow a determinate type. It is opposed to *atypic*. Sometimes opposed to *anomalous*.

FEVER, REMITTENT, see Remittent Fever — f. Remittent, infantile, see Fever, infantile remittent — f. Remittent of children, F. infantile remittent — f. Rheumatic, Rheumatism, acute — f. Root, Triosteum perfoliatum.

FEVER, SCORBU'TIC, *Febris scorbu'tica*. The febrile movement, which sometimes accompanies scorbutus or scurvy.

FEVER, SEASONING, F., strangers'.

FEVER, SEC'ONDARY. A febrile condition, which recurs in certain affections after having ceased; such as the secondary fever, which comes on at the time of the maturation of the variolous pustules, or as the eruption of scarlatina, &c., disappears.

FEVER, SEPTAN, *Febris septa'na*. An intermittent, whose paroxysms recur every six days, and consequently on the seventh.

FEVER, SEXTAN, *Febris sexta'na*. A fever, which recurs every five days, and consequently on the sixth.

FEVER, SHIP, see Typhus.

FEVER, SIMPLE, *Febris Simplex*. Simple fever is that which has no predominant character—

bilious, inflammatory, or nervous; and which is unaccompanied by any local determination, hyperæmia, or complication. It may be continued, remittent, or intermittent.

FEVER, SIMPLE CONTINUED. This is the most favourable form of continued fever, and has a tendency to wear itself out, provided only the *lædentia* be avoided. The prognosis is consequently favourable, and the treatment simple; consisting in perfect repose of body and mind, abstinence, and relieving the thirst by cold drinks.

FEVER, SINGUL'TOUS, *Febris singulto'sa* seu *lygmo'des* seu *lyngo'des*. Fever, accompanied with singultus or hiccough.

FEVER, SPOTTED, Typhus gravior.

FEVER, STER'CORAL, *Febris stercora'lis*. Fever, produced by an accumulation of fæces in the intestines.

FEVER, STOMACHIC, Gastric Fever.

FEVER, STRANGERS', *Accli'mating* or *Seasoning fever*. Yellow, or remittent fever, which is endemic in certain places, and to which strangers are especially liable.

FEVER, SUBCONTINUAL, Remittent Fever.

FEVER, SUBINTRANT, *Febris subin'trans*. An intermittent, in which one paroxysm is scarcely finished before the other begins.

FEVER, SWEATING, Sudor Anglicus.

FEVER, SYN'COPAL, *Febris syncopa'lis, F. minu'ta*, (F.) *Fièvre syncopale*. A variety of pernicious intermittent, in which there is, in every paroxysm, one or more faintings.

FEVER, SYNOCHOID, Synochus.

FEVER, SYPHILIT'IC, *Febris syphilit'ica*. Fever, accompanying syphilis, or supposed to be owing to a syphilitic taint.

FEVER, TER'TIAN, *Febris tertia'na*. A fever, whose paroxysm returns on the third day, and consequently every two days.

FEVER, TRAG"IC, *Febris Trag"ica*. A low fever, in which the patient declaims like an actor during the delirium.

FEVER, TRAUMAT'IC, *Febris traumat'ica*. The fever, which supervenes on wounds or great surgical operations.

FEVER, TYPHOID, see Typhus — f. Typhoid, of India, Cholera—f. Typhous, Typhus.

FEVER, VER'MINOUS, *Febris vermino'sa, Helminthop'yra, Worm fever*. Fever, produced by the presence of worms in the digestive tube, or accompanied by their expulsion.

FEVER, VERNAL, *Febris verna'lis*. An intermittent or other fever occurring in the spring. Vernal intermittents were formerly considered salubrious.

"An ague in the spring
Is physic for a king."

FEVER, VESICULAR, Pemphigus.

FEVER, WAL'CHEREN, *Gall-sickness*. The remittents and intermittents to which the British troops were exposed, who were attached to the expedition to Walcheren, in 1809.

FEVER, WATER BRAIN, Hydrocephalus internus — f. Winter, see Tongue, black — f. Worm, Verminous F.—f. Worm, spurious, Fever, infantile remittent.

FEVER, YELLOW, *Febris flava, F. seu Pestis America'na, Cholo'sis America'na, Ochrotyphus, Loimocholo'sis, F. flava Americano'rum, Pestilen'tia hæmagas'trica, Pestis occidenta'lis seu intertrop'ica, Vom'itus niger, Epan'etus malignus flavus, Remitt'ens ictero'des, Tritæoph'ya America'na, Typhus ictero'des, F.trop'icus, F.contin'ua pu'trida ictero'des Caroliniensis, F. Elo'des ictero'des, Febris malig'na bilio'sa Amer'icæ, Ochrop'yra, Syn'ochus ictero'des, Fièvre matelote, Febris malig'na flava In'diæ Occidenta'lis, Ende'mial Causus of the West Indies, Causus trop'icus endem'icus, Bilious remitting yellow fever, Malignant pestilential fever, Fièvre jaune d'Amérique, Fièvre gastro-adynamique, Typhus miasmatique ataxique putride jaune, T. jaune, Vomito prieto, Vomito negro, Mal de Siam, Fièvre de la Barbade, F. de Siam, F. Ictérique, F. Gastro-hépatique, Hæmagas'tric Fever or Pes'tilence, Black vomit, Febris tox'ica, Febris trop'ica, Typhus d'Amérique, Bulam Fever, Gibraltar Fever, Barcelona Fever*. A very acute and dangerous febrile affection; so called, because complicated, in its second stage, with jaundice, and accompanied by vomiting of black matter. Sauvages, Cullen, and others regard it as a variety of typhus; and Pinel, as a species of gastro-adynamic, or bilious putrid fever. It occurs, endemically, only within the tropics; but it has been met with epidemically in the temperate regions. Broussais regards the disease as gastro-enteritis, exasperated by atmospheric heat; so that it runs through its stages with much greater rapidity than the gastro-enteritis of our climates. The yellow colour of the skin, according to him, is owing to the inflammation of the small intestine,—and especially of the duodenum, — augmenting the secretion of the liver, and at the same time preventing its discharge into the duodenum. The pathology of this affection, as well as its origin, is still unsettled. The treatment must generally be of the most active nature at the onset; consisting in bleeding largely, and exhibiting mercury, so as to excite a new action, if possible; — the other symptoms being combated according to general principles. It must vary, however, according to the epidemic.

FEVERBUSH, Laurus benzoin, Prinos.

FEVER DROPS, Warburg's, see Bebeeru.

FEVERET, Febricula.

FEVERFEW, Matricaria.

FE'VERISH, *Fe'verous, Feb'riens, Febrico'sus*, (F.) *Fièvreux*, from *febris*, 'fever.' That which causes fever or is *febrifa'cient* or *febrif'ic;* as *feverish food, feverish diathesis*, &c. Also, the state of one labouring under fever, *Feversick*.

FE'VERISHNESS, *Febricita'tio, Febriculos'ity*. The state of having fever. A slight febrile disorder.

FEVEROUS, Feverish.

FEVERROOT, Pterospora andromedea.

FEVERSICK, see Feverish.

FEVERTREE, Pinckneya pubens.

FEVERWOOD, Laurus benzoin.

FEVERWORT, Eupatorium perfoliatum, Triosteum.

FIBER, Castor fiber.

FIBRA, Fibre — f. Aurea, Coptis — f. Nervea, Nerve-fibre—f. Sanguinis, Fibrin.

FIBRÆ ARCIFORMES, see Arciform.

FIBRE, *Fibra, Is, Ctedon, Filum*. An organic filament, of a solid consistence, and more or less extensible, which enters into the composition of every animal and vegetable texture. The *simple* or *elementary fibre* of the ancients, from a particular assemblage and arrangement of which every texture of the body was conceived to be constituted, seems entirely ideal. The moderns usually admit, with Haller and Blumenbach, *three elementary fibres* or *tissues*. 1. The *cellular* or *laminated*, formed chiefly of thin plates, of a whitish colour and extensible, which seems to consist of concrete gelatin. 2. The *nervous, pulpy*, or *med'ullary*, formed of a soft substance, contained in a cellular sheath, and consisting of albumen united to a fatty matter. 3. The *muscular*, composed of round filaments, of a grayish or reddish colour, and formed of fibrin. Chaussier has added to these the *albugineous fibre*, but it seems to differ from the cellular fibre only in greater condensation of the molecules. See Fibrous.

A very small or ultimate fibre is called a *Fibril, Fibril'la.*

FIBRE, ALBUGINEOUS, see Albuginea.

FIBRES, CONVERG''ING. Nervous fibres, whose office it is to associate different portions of the nervous centres with each other. They form the *Commissures.*

FIBRES, DIVERG''ING. The fibres composing the columns of the medulla oblongata, which separate in their progress to the periphery of the cerebrum and cerebellum.—Gall and Spurzheim.

FIBRES, REMAK. Fibres described by Remak as peculiar to the sympathetic nerve, but which Valentin considers to be neurilemma, and to consist of fibro-cellular bundles.

FIBRIL, see Fibre.

FIBRILLA, Fibril — f. Muscularis, Muscular fibre.

FI'BRIN or *Fib'rin, Fibrine, Fibri'na, Fibri'nē, Fibra san'guinis, Mate'ria fibro'sa, Lympha plas'tica.* An immediate animal principle—solid, white, and inodorous; insipid; heavier than water; without action on the vegetable blues: elastic, when moist; hard and brittle when dry. It enters into the composition of the chyle and the blood, and forms the chief part of the muscles of red-blooded animals. In certain diseased actions, *Fibrin* or *Coagulable lymph, gluten,* is separated from the blood, and is found in considerable quantity on the surfaces of membranes, and in the cavities of the body. See Liquor Sanguinis.

Fibrin is likewise a proximate principle of vegetables, and differs but little in chemical composition from animal fibrin; nor does it differ much from albumen and casein. It is, however, more organizable than either. Albumen appears to be converted into fibrin, when it becomes eminently adapted for the formation of living tissue.

Fibrin is very nutritious.

FIBRINA'TION, *Fibrina'tio.* The act of adding fibrin to the blood. The opposite to *defibrination.*

FIB'RINOUS, *Fibrino'sus.* That which is composed of fibrin, or has the appearance of fibrin.

FIBRO-CAR'TILAGE, *Fibro-cartila'go.* An organic tissue, partaking of the nature of the fibrous tissue, and of that of cartilage. It is dense, resisting, elastic, firm, supple, and flexible. Fibro-cartilages are distinguished into,—1. *Membraniform,* or those which serve as moulds to certain parts, as the alæ nasi and eyelids. 2. *Vaginiform,* or those which form sheaths for the sliding of tendons. 3. *Interarticular,* those which are met with in the moveable articulations. 4. *Uniting,* (F.) *Fibro-cartilages d'union,* which form a junction between two bones, as the symphysis pubis. Fibro-cartilages are sometimes formed adventitiously, as the result of a morbid process in different organs.

FIBRO-CARTILAGES, TARSAL, see Tarsus.

FIBROMA, Tumour, fibrous.

FIBRO-MUCOUS, *Fibro-muco'sus.* Possessing the nature of fibrous and of mucous membranes. A term applied to fibrous membranes, which are intimately united with other membranes of a mucous nature, as the *pituitary membrane,* the *membrane of the urethra,* &c.

FIBRO-SEROUS, *Fibro-sero'sus.* Possessing the nature of fibrous and serous membranes. Membranes, composed of a fibrous, and a serous sheet, intimately united :— as the *Dura Mater, Pericardium, Tunica albuginea testis,* &c.

FI'BROUS, *Fibro'sus.* Composed of fibres. Certain membranes, as the dura mater, periosteum, ligamentous capsules of the joints, &c., are *fibrous.* The *fibrous system* of Bichat includes the system of organs formed by the *albugineous fibre* of Chaussier. It comprises, particularly, the periosteum and perichondrium; the articular capsules and ligaments; the tendons; the dura mater, pericardium, tunica sclerotica, tunica albuginea testis, outer membrane of the spleen, &c. Under *simple fibrous tissues,* certain writers have classed the *white* and *yellow fibrous tissues,* and areolar tissue. Both the yellow and the white may be detected in the areolar tissue. The *white* is said to exist alone in ligaments, tendons, fibrous membranes, aponeuroses, &c. The *yellow* exists separately in the middle coat of the arteries, the chordæ vocales, ligamentum nuchæ of quadrupeds, &c. It differs from the white in possessing a high degree of elasticity.

FIBROUS GROWTH, Tumour, fibrous — f. Matter of the Brain, see Cerebrum — f. Membranes, see Membranes, fibrous.

FIB'ULA, *Cruris ra'dius, Canna minor, Os per'onē, Perone'um, Fac''ilē minus, Sura, Arun'do minor, Fist'ula Cruris, Tib'ia min'ima, Os tib'iæ minus,* 'a clasp.' The *splinter bone* of the leg. (F.) *Péroné.* The long, small bone, situate at the outer part of the leg. The superior or tibial extremity of the fibula is rounded and forms the *caput* or *head.* It is articulated with the tibia. Its inferior or tarsal extremity is broader than the superior. It is articulated with the tibia and astragalus, and forms the *malleolus externus* or *uter ankle* by means of its *coronoid process.* The body of the bone has three faces, having more or less prominent edges. It is separated from the tibia by the interosseous space, and is developed by three points of ossification; one at the body, and one at each extremity. It prevents the foot from turning outwards.

FIBULAD, see Fibular Aspect.

FIBULAR, Peroneal.

FIBULAR ASPECT. An aspect towards the side on which the fibula is situated.—Barclay. *Fib'-ulad* is used by the same writer adverbially, to signify 'towards the fibular aspect.'

FIBULATIO, Infibulatio.

FIC, Ficus.

FICAIRE, Ranunculus ficaria.

FICARIA, Scrophularia aquatica—f. Communis, Ranunculus ficaria—f. Ranunculoides, Ranunculus ficaria—f. Verna, Ranunculus ficaria.

FICATIO, Ficus.

FICOSA EMINENTIA, Ficus.

FICUS, *Sycē, Sy'cea, Sycum, Syco'sis, Syco'-ma, Fica'tio, Fico'sus Tumor, Fico'sa eminen'tia, Marie'ca,* (F.) *Fic.* A fleshy excrescence, often soft and reddish, sometimes hard and scirrhous, hanging by a peduncle, or formed like a fig; occurring on the eyelids, chin, tongue, anus, or organs of generation. The fici seated on the last-mentioned parts are generally of a syphilitic character.

FICUS, F. Carica.

FICUS CAR'ICA, *F. commu'nis.* The systematic name of the fig tree; (F.) *Figuier. Carica, Ficus, Ficus vulga'ris, Ficus commu'nis, Sycē, surn,* (F.) *Figue:* the fig— *Ficus,* (Ph. U. S.)—is a pleasant fruit when ripe; as well as when dried in the state in which it is found in the shops. It is used, at times, in place of a cataplasm; especially in gum-boils.

FICUS COMMUNIS, F. Carica — f. Indiæ grana, Coccus cacti — f. Indica, Musa paradisiaca, see Caoutchouc and Lacca—f. Religiosa, see Lacca.

FIDERIS, MINERAL WATERS OF. These waters, in the Canton of the Grisons, are strong, acidulous, and alkaline and possess all the virtues of the class.

FIDGETS. Of doubtful etymology. *Dysphor'ia simplex, D. nervo'sa, Erethis'mus simplex, Tituba'tio*, (F.) *Frétillement*. General restlessness and troublesome uneasiness of the nerves and muscles; with increased sensibility, and inability of fixing the attention, accompanied with a perpetual desire of changing the position. See *Agacement des Nerfs*.

FIDICINALES, Lumbricales manus.

FIEL, Bile.

FIELDWEED, Anthemis cotula, Erigeron Philadelphicum.

FIÈVRE, Fever — *f. d'Accès*, Intermittent fever — *f. Adynamique*, Typhus — *f. Algide*, see Algidus — *f. d'Amour*, Fever, erotic — *f. Angeiotènique*, Synocha — *f. Annuelle*, see Annual Diseases — *f. Ardent*, Ardent fever, Synocha — *f. Ataxique*, Typhus — *f. de la Barbade*, Fever, yellow — *f. Bulleuse*, Pemphigus — *f. des Camps*, Typhus gravior — *f. Catarrhale*, Catarrh — *f. Catarrhale épidémique*, Influenza — *f. Cérébrale*, Cerebral fever — *f. Cérébrale des Enfans*, Hydrocephalus internus — *f. Cholérique*, Choleric fever — *f. de Consomption*, see Consumption — *f. Continente inflammatoire*, Synocha — *f. Délirante*, Fever, delirious — *f. Double*, Fever, double — *f. Doublée*, Fever, double — *f. Entéro-mesentérique*, Typhoid fever — *f. Étique*, Hectic fever — *f. Gastroadynamique*, Fever, yellow — *f. Gastro-hépatique*, Fever, yellow — *f. Hectique*, Hectic fever — *f. de Hongrie*, Fever, Hungario — *f. d'Hôpital*, Typhus gravior — *f. Ictérique*, Fever, yellow — *f. Inflammatoire*, Synocha — *f. Intermittente*, Intermittent fever — *f. Intermittente paludéenne*, see Elodes — *f. Irritative*, Synocha — *f. Jaune d'Amérique*, Fever, yellow — *f. Lactée*, Fever, milk — *f. de Lait*, Fever, milk — *f. Laiteuse*, Fever, milk — *f. Larvée*, Fever, masked — *f. Lenticulaire*, Typhus gravior — *f. du Levant*, Plague — *f. des Marais* — Intermittent Fever — *f. Matelote*, Fever, yellow — *f. Méningo-gastrique*, Fever, gastric — *f. Mésentérique*, see Typhus — *f. de la Moisson*, Fever, gastric — *f. Morbilleuse*, Rubeola — *f. Nerveuse*, Typhus mitior — *f. Nosocomiale*, Typhus gravior — *f. Ortiée*, Urticaria — *f. Oscitante*, Oscitant fever — *f. Paludéenne*, see Elodes — *f. Périodique*, Intermittent fever — *f. Péripneumonique*, Pneumonia — *f. Pernicieuse délirante*, see Delirious — *f. Pleurétique*, Pleurisy — *f. des Prisons*, Typhus gravior — *f. Pneumonique*, Pneumonia — *f. Pourprée*, Scarlatina — *f. Puerpérale*, Fever, puerperal, see Peritonitis — *f. Quarte*, Quartan — *f. Quotidienne*, Quotidian — *f. Rémittente*, Remittent fever — *f. Rhumatismale*, Rheumatism, acute — *f. Rouge*, Roseolæ, Scarlatina — *f. Sanguine*, Synocha — *f. Semitierce*, Hemitritæa — *f. de Siam*, Fever, yellow — *f. Suante*, Sudor Picardicus — *f. Syncopale*, see Fever syncopal, and Syncopal — *f. Tierce*, Tertian fever, *f. Typhoïde*, see Typhus — *f. Vésiculaire*, Pemphigus.

FIÉVREUX, Feverish.

FIG, INDIAN, Cactus opuntia.

FIGUE. see Ficus carica.

FIGUIER, Ficus carica — *f. d'Inde*, Cactus opuntia.

FIGURA VENOSA, Circulus venosus.

FIGURATIO, Imagination.

FIGURE, Countenance.

FIGURÉ, (F.) An epithet for a compressive bandage, applied over the head after bleeding from the frontal vein. It has also been called *bandage royal*.

FIGWORT, Scrophularia nodosa — f. Water, greater, Scrophularia aquatica.

FILACEOUS, Filamentous.

FILA NERVEA, Nerve-fibres.

FIL'AMENT, *Filum, Filamen'tum*, from *filum*, 'a thread.' This word is used synonymously with *fibril*; thus, we say, a *nervous* or *cellular filament* or *fibril*. Also, the glairy, thread-like substance, which forms in the urine in some diseases, and which depends on a particular secretion from the mucous membrane of the urinary passages.

FILAMEN'TOUS, *Filamento'sus*. Filaceous; threadlike; filiform. Containing threadlike substances, as the *tunica filamentosa* or decidua: — *Filamentous urine*; urine containing threadlike substances.

FILAMENTUM, Frænum.

FILARIA GUINEENSIS, Dracunculus — f. Hominis bronchialis, see Worms — f. Medinensis, Dracunculus — f. Oculi, see Worms.

FILBERT, Corylus avellana.

FILELLUM, Frænum.

FILET (DE LA LANGUE,) Frænum — *f. de la Verge*, Frænum penis — *f. Opération du*, see Frænum.

FILETUM, Frænum linguæ.

FILICULA, Polypodium filix mas — f. Dulcis, Polypodium vulgare.

FIL'IFORM, *Filiform'is*, from *filum*, 'a thread,' and *forma*, 'form;' having the shape of a thread; as the *filiform papillæ* of the tongue. See Papillæ.

FILING, Limatio.

FILIPENDULA, Spiræa filipendula.

FILIUS ANTE PATREM, Tussilago.

FILIX FŒMINEA, Pteris aquilina — f. Florida, Osmunda regalis — f. Mas, Polypodium filix mas — f. Non ramosa dentata, Polypodium filix mas — Nymphæa, Pteris aquilina — f. Pinnata, Polypodium filix mas — f. Veneris, Adiantum pedatum.

FILLE, Girl.

FILLET, Fascia, Laqueus.

FILTRA'TION, *Filtra'tio, Percola'tio, E'thisis, Ethis'mus*. A pharmaceutical operation, which consists in passing a fluid through a filter or strainer, for the purpose of clarifying it. In ancient physiology, it meant the action by which the different humours of the body are separated from the mass of the blood.

FILTRUM. A *filter*. Any porous material; such as *sand*, some kinds of *freestone*, powdered *charcoal*, pounded *glass, flannel*, unsized *paper*, &c., through which a fluid is passed for the purpose of separating it from the matters suspended in it.

FILUM, Filament — f. Musculare, Muscular fibre — f. Tæniaforme, Tæniola.

FILUM TERMINA'LE. A slender ligament, prolonged from the nervous sheath, formed by the spinal pia mater, which descends through the centre of the cauda equina, and is attached to the dura mater, lining the canal of the coccyx.

FIM'BRIA, *Parar'ma*. A band; a fringe; as the fimbria or fimbriated extremity of the Fallopian tube.

FIMBRIÆ CARNOSÆ COLI, Epiploic appendages — f. Tubarum Fallopii, see Tube, Fallopian.

FIMUS, *Bor'borus, Onthus, Stercus*. Dung: excrement.

FIMUS seu STERCUS AN'SERIS, *Goose-dung*, was applied as a poultice to the feet in malignant fever. See Chenocoprus.

FIMUS EQUI'NUS, *Stercus equi non castra'ti. Stone horse-dung*, was once thought anti-pleuritic.

FIMUS VACCÆ, *Cow-dung*, was employed as a cataplasm, especially in gout.

FINCKLE, Anethum.

FINGER, Digitus — f. Ring, Annular finger — f. Stall, Digitale.

FINIS ASPERÆ ARTERIÆ, Larynx.

FIOLE, Phiala.

FIR, MOSS, UPRIGHT, Lycopodium selago—f. Scotch, Pinus sylvestris—f. Spruce, Norway, Pinus abies—f. Tree, silver, European, Pinus picea—f. Yew-leaved, Pinus abies.

FIREDAMP, Hydrogen, carburetted—f. Persian, Anthracion—f. St. Anthony's, Erysipelas—f. Weed, Erechthites hieracifolia, Senecio.

FIRING, Cauterization.

FISHSKIN, Ichthyosis.

FISH-TONGUE. An instrument — so called from its shape—used by some dentists for the removal of the dentes sapientiæ.

FISSICULA'TIO, from *fissiculare*, 'to cut off,' 'open,' 'make incisions.' An old word for an opening made with a scalpel.

FISSIPARITÉ, see Generation.

FISSIPAROUS, see Generation.

FISSURA, Fissure—f. Capillorum, Distrix—f. Contrajacens, Contra-fissura—f. Cerebri longitudinalis, Fissure, longitudinal, of the Brain—f. Magna vulvæ, see Rima—f. Pilaris, Trichismus.

FISSU'RA LONGITUDINA'LIS, ANTE'RIOR ET POSTE'RIOR. Two vertical fissures in the median line, in front of, and behind, the medulla oblongata, which divide it superficially into two symmetrical lateral columns.

FISSURA TRANSVERSA MAGNA CEREBRI, Fissure, transverse, of the Brain.

FISSURE, *Fissu'ra, Schisma, Scissu'ra, Rhegē, Rhegma, Rhegmus*, from *findere*, 'to cleave;' a long and narrow cleft or opening in a bone—*Rhagē, payn, Ceasma, κεασμα*. (F.) *Fissure, Fente*.

FISSURE has various acceptations. 1. A fracture, *Catag'ma fissu'ra*, in which the bone is cracked, not separated, as in fracture. 2. A narrow, long, and superficial solution of continuity, around the external openings of the mucous membranes. A sort of chap, observed on the hands, particularly on the callous hands, of workmen, in certain mechanical employments. 3. Small, chapped ulcerations, sometimes noticed in young children, owing to the contact of the fæces and urine with the fine delicate skin of the thighs, nates, and genital organs. 4. Clefts of a more or less deep nature, occurring on the genital organs in the vicinity of the anus, in those labouring under syphilis. These are usually called *rhagades*. See Monster.

FISSURE OF BICHAT, Fissure, transverse, of the Brain—f. Capillary, see Pilatio.

FISSURE, CENTRAL. The aggregate of the cavities or ventricles of the brain. Meckel considers this but one cavity in the form of a cross.

FISSURE OF GLASER, Fissure, glenoid — f. of Glaserius, F. Glenoid.

FISSURE, GLENOID, *Fissure of Glaser* or *Glase'rius*, (F.) *Fissure ou Scissure de Glaser, Fente glenoïdale* ou *Félure de Glaser*, divides the glenoid cavity of the temporal bone into two parts, and gives passage to the chorda tympani, &c.

FISSURE OF THE HELIX. A small vertical fissure of the helix of the ear, a little above the tubercle for the attachment of the attrahens aurem muscle.

FISSURE, INFRAORBITAR, Suborbitar fissure.

FISSURE, LONGITUDINAL, OF THE BRAIN, *Fissu'ra cer'ebri longitudina'lis*. The space which separates the two hemispheres of the brain.

FISSURE, ORBITAR, see Orbitar fissure—f. Orbitar, inferior, Spheno-maxillary fissure — f. Orbitar, superior, Sphenoidal Fissure.

FISSURE OF ROLAN'DO. A transverse fissure placed between two superior cerebral convolutions, which are met with above the fissure of Sylvius.

FISSURE, SEMILU'NAR. A notch at the anterior edge of the cerebellum, where it receives fibres which connect it to the cerebellum and mesocephalon.

FISSURE OF SYL'VIUS, *Fissu'ra* vel *Fossa Magna Syl'vii*. A deep, narrow sulcus, which ascends obliquely backwards from the temporal ala of the sphenoid bone, near to the middle of the parietal bone, and which parts the anterior and middle lobes of the cerebrum on each side.

FISSURE OF SYLVIUS, Ventricle, fifth.

FISSURE OF THE TRAGUS. A fissure on the anterior surface of the tragus of the ear.

FISSURE, TRANSVERSE OF THE BRAIN, *Great transverse fissure, Fissure of Bichat, Fissu'ra seu Rima transver'sa magna cer'ebri*. A fissure, which passes beneath and behind the edge of the middle lobe of the brain, and extends beneath the hemisphere of one side to the same point of the opposite side.

FIST, A. S. ϝᵹᴛ, πυγμη, *Pygmē, Pugnus*, (F.) *Poing*. The clenched hand.

FIS'TULA, *Syrinx, Syrin'ga, Aulos*—when of a small size, *Aulis'cos*. A solution of continuity, of greater or less depth and sinuosity; the opening of which is narrow, and the disease kept up by an altered texture of parts, so that it is not disposed to heal. A fistula is *incomplete* or *blind*, when it has but one opening; and *complete* when there are two, the one communicating with an internal cavity, the other externally. It is lined, in its whole course, by a membrane, which seems analogous to mucous membranes. *Incomplete fistulæ* may be *internal* or *external*. The former are those which open *internally*; the latter those which open *externally*. *External incomplete fistulæ* are kept up by caries or necrosis of bones, by extraneous bodies in any of the living textures, or by purulent cavities, the walls of which have not become united. *Internal incomplete fistulæ* generally soon become complete, since the discharge that escapes from them into the cavities into which they open, has a constant tendency to make its way outwardly, and soon occasions ulceration of the integuments. Fistulæ have received different names, according to the discharge which they afford, and the organs in which they are seated, — as *lachrymal, biliary, salivary, synovial, urinary — Fis'tula uri'næ, U'rias*. The great object of treatment, in fistulous sores, is to bring on an altered condition of the parietes of the canal, by astringent or stimulating injections, caustics, the knife, pressure, &c. Those which are dependent on diseased bone, cartilage, tendon, &c., do not heal until after the exfoliation of the diseased part. Fistulæ of excretory ducts are produced either by an injury of the duct itself or by the retention and accumulation of the fluids to which they have to give passage. Thus, *Fis'tulu lachryma'lis, Dacryosyr'inx, Emphrag'ma lachryma'lē, Hydrops sacci lachryma'lis, Dropsy of the lachrymal sac*, commonly proceeds from the obliteration of the nasal ducts, or from atony of the lachrymal sac; which circumstances prevent the tears from passing into the nostrils.

FISTULA IN ANO, *Archosyr'inx*, generally occurs from some mechanical pressure or impediment. The principal indication in the treatment of these fistulæ of the excretory canals being to put a stop to the constant discharge of the secretions, &c., through the preternatural channel, the fistulous passage is at times laid open, and a communication established with the natural excretory canal; at others, strong pressure is employed to procure its obliteration.

FISTULA BELLINIANA, Uriniferous tube—f. Cibalis, Œsophagus—f. Cruris, Fibula—f. Duræ matris, Sinus of the dura mater—f. Lachrymalis, see Fistula—f. Nervorum, Neurilemma—f. Sacra,

Medulla spinalis, Vertebral column—f. Spiritalis, Trachea—f. Urinaria, Urethra—f. Ureterum renum, see Calix—f. Urinæ, see Fistula—f. Ventriculi, Œsophagus.

FISTULES STERCORAIRES,, see Stercoraceous.

FIS'TULOUS, *Fistulo'sus, Syring"icus, Syringo'des.* Relating to, or resembling, a fistula; as 'a *fistulous* opening.'

FIT-ROOT, Monotropa uniflora.

FITS, NINE DAY, Trismus nascentium.

FIVE FINGERS, Panax quinquefolium.

FIXATIO MONONŒA, Melancholy.

FIXED, *Fixus*, from *figere*, 'to fasten.' A body not capable of being volatilized by fire is said to be fixed. Thus, we say *fixed oils*, in contradistinction to *volatile oils*.

FIXEN, MINERAL WATERS OF. This spring is four leagues from Waldsassen, in Bavaria. It contains carbonic acid, holding in solution carbonates of lime and magnesia, chlorides of lime and magnesia, carbonate of soda and silica. In Bavaria, it replaces the Seltzer water.

FIXI DENTES. The teeth of the second dentition.

FLABELLA'TION, *Flabella'tio*, from *flabellare*, to agitate the air. An operation recommended by Ambrose Paré, which consists in keeping fractured limbs cool, as well as the dressings surrounding them, by the renewal of the air around them, either by the use of a fan, or the repeated change of position of the parts affected.

FLABELLUM ET VENTILABRUM CORDIS, Pulmo.

FLACCID'ITY, *Flaccid'itas*, from *flaccidus*, 'flabby,' 'soft.' Softness of a part, so as to offer little resistance on pressure.

FLAG, BLUE, Iris versicolor—f. Dwarf, Iris lacustris—f. Myrtle, Acorus calamus—f. Root, Acorus calamus.

FLAGELLATIO, Mastigosis.

FLAMBE, Iris Germanica—*f. Bâtard*, Iris pseudacorus.

FLAMBOISE, Ignis sylvaticus.

FLAME, VITAL, Vital principle.

FLAMMA, Fleam—f. Cordis, Biolychnium—f. Vitalis, Biolychnium.

FLAMME, Fleam—*f. Vitale*, Vital principle.

FLAMMETTE, Fleam.

FLAMMON, Lachesis rhombeata.

FLAMMULA, Fleam, *Ranunculus ficaria*—f. Cordis, Biolychnium—f. Jovis, Clematis recta—f. Vitalis, Animal heat, Biolychnium, Vital principle.

FLANCKS, Flanks.

FLANKS, *Il'ia, Il'ea, La'gones, Lap'ara, Ceneo'nes*, (F.) *Flancs, Les Îles*. The regions of the body which extend, on the sides, from the inferior margin of the chest to the *crista ilii*.

FLAP, (F.) *Lambeau*. A portion of the soft parts of the body separated from those beneath, but still attached by the base. Hence there may be '*flap wounds*,' (F.) *Plaies à lambeaux*, and '*flap* operations,' (F.) *Opérations à lambeaux*.

FLAP OPERATION OF AMPUTATION, Amputation à *lambeaux*.

FLAT TOP, Vernonia Neveboracensis.

FLATUARIUS, Alchymist.

FLAT'ULENCE, *Flatulen'tia, Flatus, Flatuos'itas, Aëriflux'us, Pneumato'sis ventric'uli et Pn. enter'ica, Pneumatosis, Bdes'ma, Hyperpneus'tia, Clydon, Physa, Polyphy'sia, Limo'sis Fla'tus, Ereux'is, Bombus, Flatuos'ity*, Wind, *Wind'iness, Ventos'ity, Vapour*, (F.) *Ventosité, Flatuosité*. Emission of wind by the mouth or anus, or accumulation of wind in the digestive tube.

FLATULENT, Windy.

FLATULENTIA, Flatulence.

FLATUOSITÉ, Flatulence.

FLATUOSITY, Flatulence.

FLATUS, Crepitation, Flatulence—f. Furiosus, Ambulo-flatulentus—f. Spinæ, Spina ventosa.

FLAVEDO CORTICUM CITRI, see Citrus medica.

FLAVOUR, from (F.) *flairer*, 'to smell.' The quality of a sapid body, which is appreciated by the taste and smell combined, and more especially by the latter. Some physiologists consider that flavour is effected through the smell alone.

FLAVUS, Yellow.

FLAX, COMMON, Linum usitatissimum—f. Purging, Linum catharticum—f. Seed, see Linum usitatissimum—f. Seed tea, Infusum lini compositum—f. Toad, Antirhinum linaria.

FLEA, COMMON, Pulex irritans.

FLEABANE, GREAT, Conyza squarrosa—f. Various-leaved, Erigeron heterophyllum—f. Bane, Canada, Erigeron Canadense—f. Philadelphia, Erigeron Philadelphicum—f. Skevish, Erigeron Philadelphicum.

FLEAM, *Flamma, Flam'mula, Schaste'rion, Fosso'rium, Phlebot'omum*. A surgical instrument used for the operation of phlebotomy. (F.) *Flamme, Flammette*. It consists of a small metallic box, containing a spear-pointed cutting instrument, which, by means of a spring, can be forced into the vein. It is much used in Germany and some other European countries, and is not unfrequently employed in America; but is scarcely ever seen in France or Great Britain.

FLEAWORT, Plantago psyllium.

FLÉCHISSEUR, Flexor—*f. Court commun des orteils*, Flexor brevis digitorum pedis—*f. Court du petit doigt*, Flexor parvus minimi digiti—*f. Court du petit orteil*, Flexor brevis minimi digiti pedis—*f. Profond des doigts*, Flexor profundus perforans—*f. Sublime des doigts*, Flexor sublimis perforatus—*f. Superficiel des doigts*, Flexor sublimis perforatus—*f. Court du gros orteil*, Flexor brevis pollicis pedis—*f. Grand commun des orteils*, Flexor longus digitorum pedis profundus perforans—*f. Long commun des orteils*, Flexor longus digitorum pedis profundus perforans—*f. Long du gros orteil*, Flexor longus pollicis pedis—*f. Court du Pouce*, Flexor brevis pollicis manûs.

FLECTENS PAR LUMBORUM, Quadratus lumborum.

FLEGMEN, Flemen.

FLEMEN, *Flegmen*. A tumour about the ankles. Also, a chap on the feet and hands.

FLERECIN, Gout.

FLESH, *Caro, Sarx*, (F.) *Chair*. Every soft part of an animal is so named; but more particularly the muscles, which are called *muscular flesh*.

FLESH, PROUD, Fungosity.

FLETUS, Lachrymatio.

FLEURS, Flowers, Menses—*f. Blanches*, Leucorrhœa—*f. de Muscade*, Mace—*f. de Soufre*, Sulphur sublimatum.

FLEXIBIL'ITY, *Flexibil'itas*, from *flectere*, 'to bend.' Capability of being bent. A physical property of the tissues, which varies greatly according to the structure. The tendons exhibit this property in a marked manner.

FLEXIO, Campsis, Flexion.

FLEX'ION, *Flex'io, Campe*, from *flectere*, 'to bend.' The state of being bent. The action of a flexor muscle.

FLEXOR. Same etymon. (F.) *Fléchisseur*. A muscle, whose office it is to bend certain parts.

FLEXOR BREVIS DIGITO'RUM PEDIS PERFORA'-TUS, *F. Subli'mis, Flexor brevis, Flexor digito'rum brevis sive perforatus pedis, Perfora'tus flexor secun'di interno'dii digito'rum pedis, Calcanéo-sous-phalangettien commun,—Calcanéo-sous-phalanginien commun,*—(Ch.) (F.) *Muscle court fléchisseur commun des orteils.* A muscle, placed at the middle of the sole of the foot. It is narrower and thicker behind than before, where it is divided into four portions. It arises from the posterior part of the inferior surface of the os calcis, and is inserted at the inferior surface of the second phalanx of the last four toes. It bends the second phalanges of the toes on the first, and the first on the metatarsal bones; in this manner augmenting the concavity of the vault of the foot.

FLEXOR BREVIS MINIMI DIGITI, F. parvus minimi digiti.

FLEXOR BREVIS MIN'IMI DIG"ITI PEDIS, *Parathenar minor*, (F.) *Court fléchisseur du petit orteil, Tarso-sous-phalangien du petit orteil*—(Ch.) A muscle, situate at the anterior and outer part of the sole of the foot. It arises from the posterior extremity of the fifth metatarsal bone, and is inserted into the posterior part of the first phalanx of the little toe, which it bends.

FLEXOR BREVIS POL'LICIS MANUS, *Flexor secun'di interno'dii, Thenar, Flexor primi et secun'di ossis pol'licis*, (F.) *Court fléchisseur du pouce, Carpophalangien du pouce*—(Ch.) *Demi-interosseux du pouce.* A muscle, situate at the outer part of the palm of the hand. It is divided into two portions by the tendon of the *Flexor longus pollicis.* It arises from the os magnum, the anterior annular ligament of the carpus and the third metacarpal bone; and is inserted into the superior part of the first phalanx of the thumb, and into the two ossa sesamoidea at the articulation of the first phalanx with the first metacarpal bone. Its use is to bend the first phalanx of the thumb on the first metacarpal bone, and the latter upon the trapezium.

FLEXOR BREVIS POL'LICIS PEDIS, *Flexor brevis, Flexor hal'lucis* vel *brevis pol'licis*, (F.) *Tarsophalangien du pouce, Court fléchisseur du gros orteil, Tarso-sous-phalangettien du premier orteil* —(Ch.) It is situate at the anterior and inner part of the sole of the foot; is thin and narrow behind, thick and divided into two portions before. It arises from the inferior part of the os calcis and the last two cuneiform bones, and is inserted at the inferior part of the base of the first phalanx of the great toe, and into the two sesamoid bones of the corresponding metatarso-phalangian articulation. It bends the first phalanx of the great toe on the first metacarpal bone.

FLEXOR CARPI RADIALIS, Palmaris magnus—f. Carpi ulnaris, see Cubital (muscles)—f. Hallucis, F. brevis pollicis pedis—f. Hallucis longus, F. longus pollicis pedis.

FLEXOR LONGUS DIGITO'RUM PEDIS PROFUN'DUS PER'FORANS; *Per'forane* seu *Flexor profun'dus, Perodactyle'us, Peronodactyl'ius, Peronodactyliæ'us, Peronedactyl'ius, Flexor digito'rum longus* sive *Perforans pedis, Perforans* seu *Flexor tertii internodii digito'rum pedis;* (F.) *Tibio-phalangettien*—(Ch.), *Grand* ou *long fléchisseur commun des orteils.* A muscle, situate at the posterior and deep-seated part of the leg. It is broader at its middle than at its extremities, the inferior of which is divided into four portions. It arises from the posterior surface of the tibia, and its tendons are attached to the posterior part of the lower surface of the three phalanges of the last four toes. It bends the three phalanges on each other, and the toes on the metatarsus, and extends the foot on the leg.

The *Accesso'rius Flexo'ris Longi Digito'rum Pedis, Caro quadra'ta Syl'vii, C. accesso'ria, Massa car'nea Jaco'bi Syl'vii, Planta'ris verus,*

(F.) *Accessoire du long fléchisseur commun des orteils, Carrée,* is a small muscle of the sole of the foot, which passes obliquely from the os calcis to the outer edge of the flexor longus, whose force it augments, and corrects its obliquity.

FLEXOR LONGUS POL'LICIS MANUS, *Flexor longus pollicis, Flexor tertii interno'dii, Flexor tertii internodii* sive *longis'simus pollicis;* (F.) *Radio-phalangettien du pouce,*—(Ch.) Situate at the anterior and profound part of the forearm. It arises from the upper three quarters of the anterior surface of the radius and interosseous ligament, and is inserted, by a tendon, into the anterior surface of the last phalanx of the thumb. It bends the second phalanx of the thumb on the first; the first on the corresponding metacarpal bone, and this upon the radius. It can, also, bend the hand on the forearm.

FLEXOR LONGUS POLLICIS PEDIS, *Flexor Hal'lucis* vel *Pollicis longus,* (F.) *Péronéo-phalangien du gros orteil, Long fléchisseur du gros orteil, Péronéo-sous-Phalangettien du pouce,*—(Ch.) It is situate at the posterior and profound part of the leg. It arises from the posterior surface of the fibula and the interosseous ligament, and is inserted, by means of a long tendon, into the inferior part of the first phalanx of the great toe. It bends the third phalanx on the first, and this upon the corresponding metatarsal bone. It augments the concavity of the sole of the foot, and extends the foot on the leg.

FLEXOR PARVUS MIN'IMI DIG"ITI, *Abduc'tor minimi digiti, Hypoth'enar Riola'ni, Flexor brevis minimi digiti manûs, Hypoth'enar minimi digiti,* (F.) *Carpo-phalangien du petit doigt*—(Ch.), *Court fléchisseur du petit doigt.* It arises from the anterior annular ligament of the carpus and the process of the os unciforme, and is inserted at the inner side of the superior extremity of the first phalanx of the little finger. It bends the first phalanx of the little finger.

FLEXOR PERFORANS, F. profundus perforans—f. Perforatus, F. sublimis perforatus—f. Primi internodii, Opponens pollicis—f. Primi internodii digitorum manus, Lumbricalis manus—f. Primi et secundi ossis pollicis, F. brevis pollicis manus.

FLEXOR PROFUN'DUS PER'FORANS, *F. Profundus, F. Per'forans, F. Per'forane* vulgo *profundus, Flexor ter'tii interno'dii digito'rum manûs* vel *Per'forans manûs;* (F.) *Cubito-phalangettien commun*—(Ch.,) *Fléchisseur profond des doigts.* A thick, flat, long muscle, seated beneath the *Flexor sublimis perforatus.* Its upper extremity is simple, and arises from the anterior surface of the ulna and from the interosseus ligament. Its inferior extremity terminates by four tendons, which, after having passed through the slits in the *sublimis,* are inserted into the anterior surface of the last phalanges of the four fingers. It bends the third phalanges on the second, and, in other respects, has the same use as the flexor sublimis perforatus.

FLEXOR SECUNDI INTERNODII DIGITORUM PEDIS, F. brevis digitorum pedis—f. Tertii internodii, F. longus pollicis manûs—f. Tertii internodii digitorum manûs, F. profundus perfori ns—f. Tertii internodii digitorum pedis, F. longus digitorum pedis profundus perforans—f. Ossis metacarpi pollicis, Opponens pollicis—f. Perforatus pedis, F. brevis digitorum pedis—f. Sublimis, F. brevis digitorum pedis.

FLEXOR SUBLI'MIS PERFORA'TUS, *F. Perfora'tus,* (F.) *Fléchisseur sublime* ou *superficiel des doigts, Epitroklo-phalanginien commun,*—(Ch.) It is a thick, flat, muscle, seated at the anterior part of the forearm. Its upper extremity, which is simple, arises from the internal condyle of the os humeri;— from the coronoid process of the ulna, and from the anterior edge of the radius. Its lower extremity divides into four tendons, which slide under the anterior annular ligament of the carpus, and are inserted into the second phalanges of the last four fingers, after having been slit to allow the tendons of the flexor profundus to pass through them., This muscle bends the second phalanges on the first; these on the carpal bones, and the hand on the forearm.

FLEXURA, Curvature—f. Sigmoides, Sigmoid flexure.

FLIXWEED, Sisymbrium sophia.

FLOCCI, see Villous membranes.

FLOCCILATION, Carphologia.

FLOCCILEGIUM, Carphologia.

FLOCCITATION, Carphologia.

FLOCCORUM VENATIO, Carphologia.

FLOCCULI, see Villous membranes.

FLOC'CULUS; diminutive of *floccus*, 'a lock of wool'—*Pneumogas'tric lob'ule, Lob'ulus pneumogas'tricus*. A long and slender prominence, extending from the side of the vallecula around the corpus restiforme to the crus cerebelli, lying behind the filaments of the pneumogastric nerves.

FLOR DE MISTELA, see Mistura.

FLORENCE, CLIMATE OF. This agreeable Italian city is by no means a favourable residence for the phthisical invalid. Sir James Clark affirms, indeed, that he does not know any class of invalids for whom Florence offers a favourable residence. It is subject to sudden vicissitudes of temperature, and to cold, piercing winds during the winter and spring.

FLORES BENZOES, Benjamin, flowers of— f. Boracis, Boracic acid—f. Macidos, see Myristica moschata—f. Macis, Mace—f. Martiales, Ferrum ammoniatum—f. Salis ammoniaci martiales, Ferrum ammoniatum.

FLORIDA, CLIMATE OF, see Saint Augustine.

FLORIDA, WATERS OF. Near Long Lake, in Florida, United States, which communicates with St. John's River by a small creek, there is a vast fountain of hot mineral water, issuing from a bank of the river. From its odour it would seem to be sulphureous.

FLORION, Influenza.

FLOS, *Anthos*. A flower. Also, the finest and noblest part of a body, and virginity.

FLOS, JOVIS, Crocus—f. Salis, Soda, subcarbonate of — f. Sanguineus monardi, Tropæolum majus — f. Trinitatis, Viola tricolor — f. Virginitatis, Hymen.

FLOUR, COLD, Pinoli.

FLOUR, PATENT, JONES'S. A farinaceous preparation, which is said to consist of wheat-flour, with tartaric acid and carbonate of soda.

FLOUR, POTATO, see Solanum tuberosum.

FLOWER DE LUCE, Iris Germanica.

FLOWERS, *Flores*, (F.) *Fleurs*. The ancient chymists gave this name to different solid and volatile substances obtained by sublimation. The term is not yet entirely banished from chymical and medical language, as *Flowers of Benjamin, Flowers of Sulphur*, &c.

FLOWERS, Menses.

FLOWERS, FOUR CARMIN'ATIVE, *Quat'uor flores carminati'vi*, were chamomile, dill, fever-few, and melilot.

FLOWERS, FOUR CORDIAL, *Quat'uor flores cordia'les*, were formerly, borage, bugloss, roses, and violets.

FLUCTUATIO, Fluctuation—f. Aurium, Tinnitus aurium.

FLUCTUA'TION, *Fluctua'tio*, from *fluctus*, 'a wave;' *Undula'tio*, (F.) *Ondulation*. The undulation of a fluid collected in any natural or artificial cavity, which is felt by pressure or by percussion, properly practised—*peripheric fluctuation*. In ascites, the fluctuation is felt by one of the hands being applied to one side of the abdomen, whilst the other side is struck with the other hand. In abscesses, fluctuation is perceived by pressing on the tumour, with one or two fingers alternately, on opposite points.

FLUCTUATION PERIPHERIC, see Fluctuation—f. Rhonchal, see Rhonchal — f. by Succussion, see Succussion.

FLUELLEN, Antirhinum elatine.

FLUELLIN, Veronica.

FLUEURS, Menses — *f. Blanches*, Leucorrhœa.

FLUID, *Flu'idus*, from *fluere*, 'to flow.' The human body is chiefly composed of fluids. If one, weighing 120 pounds, be thoroughly dried in an oven, the remains will be found not to weigh more than 12 or 13 pounds; so that the proportion of fluids to liquids in the body is about 9 or 10 to 1.

TABLE OF FLUIDS OF THE HUMAN BODY.

1. *Blood.*
2. *Lymph.*
3. *Exhaled or Perspiratory.* { Transpiration of the mucous, serous, and synovial membranes; of the areolar membrane; of the adipous cells; of the medullary membrane; of the interior of the thyroid gland; of the thymus; suprarenal capsules; eye; ear; vertebral canal, &c.
4. *Follicular.* { Sebaceous humour of the skin; cerumen; gum of the eye; mucus of the mucous glands and follicles; that of the tonsils, of the glands of the cardia, the environs of the anus, the prostate, &c.
5. *Glandular.* { Tears; saliva; pancreatic fluid; bile; cutaneous transpiration; urine; fluid of the glands of Cowper; sperm; milk; of the testes and mammæ of the new-born child.

FLUID, CEPHALO-RACHIDIAN, Cephalo-spinal fluid—f. Cephalo-spinal, Cephalo-spinal fluid—f. Cerebro-spinal, Cephalo-spinal fluid—f. of Scarpa, *Vitrine auditive*—f. Subarachnoidean, Cephalo-spinal fluid.

FLUIDE SÉMINAL, Sperm.

FLUIDUM NERVEUM, Nervous fluid — f. Cerebro-spinale, Cephalo-spinal fluid.

FLUKE, Distoma hepaticum—f. Liver, Distoma hepaticum.

FLUMEN DYSENTERICUM, Dysentery.

FLUMMERY, (Scotch) *Sowens*. A preparation of oatmeal, which forms a light article of food during convalescence. It may be made as follows:—Take of *oatmeal* or *groats*, a quart. Rub with two quarts of *hot water*, and let the mixture stand until it becomes sour; then add another quart of *hot water*, and strain through a hair sieve. Let it stand till a white sediment is deposited; decant, and wash the sediment with cold water. Boil this with fresh water till it forms a mucilage, stirring the whole time.

FLUOR, Flux—f. Albus Intestinorum, Cœliac flux—f. Albus malignus, Gonorrhœa impura—f. Muliebris, Leucorrhœa — f. Muliebris non Gallicus, Leucorrhœa — f. Sanguinis pulmonum, Hæmoptysis—f. Sanguinis vesicæ, Cystorrhagia.

FLUSH, *Flushing*, (F.) *Rougeurs*; from (G.) Fliessen, 'to flow. The redness produced by accumulation of blood in the capillaries of the face; as the sudden '*flush*' or '*blush* of emotion :' the '*flush* of hectic.'

FLUX, *Fluxus, Proflu'vium, Fluor,* from *fluere,* 'to flow.' A discharge. *Rhysis.* In nosology, it comprises a series of affections, the principal symptom of which is the discharge of a fluid. Generally it is employed for dysentery.

FLUX, BILIOUS, *Fluxus bilio'sus.* A discharge of bile, either by vomiting or by stool, or by both, as in cholera.

FLUX, BLOODY, Dysentery—*f. de Bouche,* Salivation—*f. Bronchique,* Bronchorrhœa—*f. Dysentérique,* Dysentery—*f.* Hemorrhoidal, see Hæmorrhois—*f. Hépatique,* Hepatirrhœa—*f.* Menstrual, Menses—*f. Muqueux,* Catarrh—*f. Muqueux de l'estomac,* Gastrorrhœa—*f. Muqueux de la vessie,* Cystirrhœa—f. Root, Asclepias tuberosa—*f. Salivaire,* Salivation—*f. de Sang,* Hæmorrhagia, Dysentery—*f.* Sebaceous, Stearrhœa—*f. de Sperme,* Spermatorrhœa—*f. de Sueur,* Ephidrosis—f. Weed, Sysimbrium sophia—*f. d'Urine,* Diabetes—*f. de Ventre,* Diarrhœa.

FLUXIO, Fluxion—f. Alba, Leucorrhœa—f. Arthritica, Gout—f. Vulvæ, Leuvorrhœa.

FLUX'ION, *Flux'io, Affiux'us* A flow of blood or other humour towards any organ with greater force than natural. A *determination.* Thus we say, in those disposed to apoplexy, there is a *fluxion* or *determination* of blood to the head.

FLUXION CATARRHALE, Catarrh—*f. sur les Dents,* Odontalgia.

FLUXION DE POITRINE, (F.) By this name, the French often understand *acute pulmonary catarrh,* or *pleurisy,* but most commonly peripneumony.

FLUXUS, Discharge—f. Alvinus, Diarrhœa—f. Chylosus, Cœliac flux—f. Cœliacus, Cœliac flux—f. Cœliacus per Renes, Chyluria—f. Cruentus cum tenesmo, Dysentery—f. Dysentericus, Dysentery—f. Hepaticus, Hepatirrhœa, see Hepateros—f. Lientericus, Lientery—f. Lunaris, Menses—f. Matricis, Leucorrhœa—f. Menstrualis, Menstruation—f. Menstruus, Menses—f. Muliebris, Leucorrhœa—f. Salivæ, Salivation—f. Splenicus, Melæna—f. Venereus, Gonorrhœa impura—f. Ventriculi, Gastrorrhœa.

FLYTRAP, Apocynum androsæmifolium.

FOC"ILE. This name was formerly given to the bones of the leg, as well as to those of the forearm.

FOCILE MAJUS, Tibia—f. Inferius seu majus, Ulna—f. Minus, Fibula—*f.* Minus seu superius, Radius.

FŒCUNDATIO, Fecundation.
FŒCUNDITAS, Fecundity.
FŒCUNDUS, Fecund.
FŒDI COLORES, Chlorosis.
FŒMEN, Perinæum.
FŒMINA, Female.
FŒMINESCENTIA, Feminescence.

FŒNICULUM, Anethum—f. Aquaticum, Phellandrium aquaticum—f. Erraticum, Peucedanum silaus—f. Marinum, Crithmum maritimum—f. Officinale, Anethum—f. Porcinum, Peucedanum—f. Vulgare, Anethum.

FŒNUGREEK, Trigonella fœnum.

FŒNUM CAMELORUM, Juncus odoratus—f. Græcum, Trigonella fœnum.

FŒTAB'ULUM. An encysted abscess.—Marcus Aurelius Severinus.

FŒTAL, *Fœta'lis.* Relating to the fœtus. A name, given to the parts connected with the fœtus. Thus we say—the *fœtal surface of the placenta,* in contradistinction to the *uterine* or *maternal* surface.

FŒTAL CIRCULATION differs from that of the adult in several respects. Commencing with the placenta, where it probably undergoes some change analogous to what occurs in the lungs in extra-uterine existence, the blood proceeds by the umbilical vein as far as the liver, where a part of it is poured into the vena porta; the other proceeds into the vena cava inferior; the latter, having received the suprahepatic veins, pours its blood into the right auricle. From the right auricle, a part of the blood is sent into the right ventricle; the rest passes directly through into the left auricle, by the foramen ovale. When the right ventricle contracts, the blood is sent into the pulmonary artery; but as the function of respiration is not going on, no more blood passes to the lungs than is necessary for their nutrition; the remainder goes directly through the ductus arteriosus into the aorta. The blood, received by the left auricle from the lungs, as well as that which passed through the foramen ovale, is transmitted into the left ventricle; by the contraction of which it is sent into the aorta, and by means of the umbilical arteries, which arise from the hypogastric, it is returned to the placenta.

FŒTAL HEAD. The diameters of this at the full period are as follows:—1. The *Biparietal* or *transverse,* extending from one parietal protuberance to the other, and measuring 3½ inches. 2. The *Temporal,* from one temple to another, 3 inches. 3. The *Occipito-mental,* from the occiput to the chin; the greatest of all, 5 inches. 4. The *Occipito-frontal* or *antero-posterior,* 4¼ or 4½ inches. 5. The *Cervico-bregmatic,* from the nape of the neck to the centre of the anterior fontanelle. 6. The *Fronto-mental,* from the forehead to the chin, about 3½ inches. 7. The *Trachelo-bregmatic,* from the front of the neck to the anterior fontanelle, 3½ inches. 8. The *Vertical diameter,* from the vertex to the base of the cranium.

FŒTAL NUTRITION, Cyotrophy.

FŒTATION, Pregnancy.

FŒ'TICIDE, *Fœticid'ium,* from *fœtus,* and *cædere,* 'to kill;' *Aborticid'ium.* Criminal abortion.

FŒTIDUS, Fetid.

FŒTOR, Dysodia—f. Oris, Breath, offensive.

FŒTUS, *Fetus, Cye'ma, Onus ventris, Sar'cina,* from *feo,* 'I bring forth.' The unborn child. By κυημα, *Cye'ma,* Hippocrates meant the fecundated, but still imperfect, germ. It corresponded with the term *embryo,* as now used; whilst *εηβρυον,* 'embryo,' signified the fœtus at a more advanced stage of utero-gestation. The majority of anatomists apply to the germ the name *embryo,* which it retains until the third month of gestation, and with some until the period of quickening; whilst *fœtus* is applied to it in its latter stages. The terms are, however, often used indiscriminately. When the ovule has been fecundated in the ovarium, it proceeds slowly towards, and enters the uterus, with which it becomes ultimately connected by means of the placenta. When first seen, the fœtus has the form of a gelatinous flake, which some have compared to an ant, a grain of barley, a worm curved upon itself, &c. The fœtal increment is very rapid in the first, third, fourth, and sixth months of its formation, and at the end of nine months it has attained its full dimensions—*Enfant à terme.* Generally, there is but one fœtus in utero; sometimes, there are two; rarely three. The fœtus presents considerable difference in its shape, weight, length, situation in the womb, proportion of its various parts to each other, arrangement and texture of its organs, state of its functions at different periods of gestation, &c. All these differences are important in an obstetrical and medico-legal point of view. The following table exhibits the length and weight of the fœtus at different periods of gestation, on the authority of different observers. Their discordance is striking. It is proper to remark, that the Paris pound — *Poid de Marc* — of 16 ounces, contains 9216 Paris grains, whilst the avoirdupois contains only 8532.5 Paris grains, and that the Paris inch is 1.065977 English inch.

	BECK.	MAYGRIER.	GRANVILLE.	BECK.	MAYGRIER.	GRANVILLE.
	Length.			Weight.		
At 30 days,	3 to 5 lines	10 to 12 lines		9 or 10 grains		
2 months,	2 inches	4 inches	1 inch	2 ounces	5 drachms	20 grains
3 "	3½ "	6 "	3 inches	2 to 3 "	2½ ounces	1½ ounces
4 "	5 to 6 "	8 "		4 to 5 "	7 or 8 "	
5 "	7 to 9 "	10 "		9 or 10 "	16 "	
6 "	9 to 12 "	12 "	9 inches	1 to 2 lbs.	2 pounds	1 pound
7 "	12 to 14 "	14 "	12 "	2 to 3 "	3 "	2 to 4 "
8 "	16 "	16 "	17 "	3 to 4 "	4 "	4 to 5 "

FŒTUS IN FŒTU, Cryptodidymus.
FŒTUS SEPTIMES'TRIS. A seven months' fœtus.
FŒTUS ZEPHYRIUS, Mole.
FOIE, Liver — *f. d'Antimoine*, Oxidum stibii sulphuretum — *f. de Soufre*, Potassæ sulphuretum.
FOLIA APALACHINES, see Ilex Paraguensis — f. Peraguæ, Ilex Paraguensis.
FOLIACEUM ORNAMENTUM, see Tuba Fallopiana.
FOLIE, Insanity — *f. des Ivrognes*, Delirium tremens.
FOLLETTE, Influenza.
FOL'LICLE, *Follic'ulus, Cystis*, diminutive of *Follis*, a bag. See Crypta.
FOLLICLES, CILIARY, Meibomius, glands of — f. of De Graaf, Folliculi Graafiani — f. of Liebermühn, see Intestine — f. Palpebral, Meibomius, glands of — f. Solitary, Brunner's glands — f. Synovial, Bursæ mucosæ.
FOLLIC'ULAR, *Follic'ulous, Follic'ulose, Folliculo'sus*, from 'follicle.' Relating or appertaining to a follicle, — as '*follicular* inflammation,' inflammation affecting crypts or follicles.
FOLLICULE, Crypta — *f. Ciliaire*, Meibomius, gland of — *f. Dentaire*, Dental follicle — *f. Palpébral*, Meibomius, gland of.
FOLLICULES DE GRAAF, Folliculi Graafiani.
FOLLIC'ULI GRAAFIA'NI, *Ova seu O'vula Graafia'na, Follicles* or *Vesicles of De Graaf, Ova'rian ves'icles*, (F.) *Follicules* ou *Vésicules de Graaf*. Small spherical vesicles in the stroma of the ovary, which have two coats; the outer termed *ovicapsule* and *tunic of the ovisac*; the latter *ovisac* and *membra'na propria; vésicule ovulifère* of M. Pouchet. They exist in the fœtus. The ovum — *ovule* of some — is contained in, and formed by, them.
FOLLICULI ROTUNDI ET OBLONGI CERVICIS UTERI, Nabothi glandulæ — f. Sanguinis, Globules of the blood — f. Sebacei, Sebaceous glands.
FOLLICULOSE GLAND, Crypta.
FOLLICULUS, Vulva.
FOLLIC'ULUS A'ERIS, *Air-chamber*. A space at the larger end of the bird's egg, formed by a separation of the two layers of the shell membrane, which is inservient to the respiration of the young being.
FOLLICULUS DENTIS, Dental Follicle — f. Fellis, Gall-bladder — f. Genitalis, Scrotum.
FOMENT, *Fove're*, (F.) *Étuver, Bassiner*. To apply a fomentation to a part.
FOMENTA'TION, *Fomenta'tio, Fotus, Py'ria, Thermas'ma, Chliss'ma, Æone'sis, Perfu'sio, Asper'sio, Fomen'tum*, (quasi *fovimentum*,) from *fovere* 'to bathe.' A sort of partial bathing, by the application of cloths which have been previously dipped in hot water, or in some medicated decoction. They act, chiefly, by virtue of their warmth and moisture, except in the case of narcotic fomentations, where some additional effect is obtained.

A *dry fomentation* is a warm, dry application to a part; — as a hot brick, wrapped in flannel; — a bag, half filled with chamomile flowers made hot, &c.

FOMENTATION HERBS, *Herbæ pro fotu*. The herbs, ordinarily sold under this title by the English apothecary, are — *southernwood, tops of sea wormwood, chamomile flowers*, each two parts; *bay leaves*, one part. ℥iijss of these to Ovj of water.
FOMENTUM, Fomentation.
FOMES MORBI, *Fomes mali*. The *focus* or seat of any disease. (F.) *Foyer*.
FOMES VENTRICULI, Hypochondriasis.
FOM'ITES, from *fomes*, 'fuel, any thing which retains heat.' *Enau'ma, Zop'yron*. A term applied to substances which are supposed to retain contagious effluvia; as woollen goods, feathers, cotton, &c.
FONCTION, Function.
FOND, Fundus.
FONDANT, Solvent.
FONGIFORME, Fungoid.
FONGOÏDE, Fungoid.
FONGOSITÉ, Fungosity.
FONGUS, Fungus — *f. Médullaire*, Encephaloid.
FONS, Fontanella — f. Lachrymarum, see Canthus — f. Medicatus, Water, mineral — f. Pulsans, Fontanella — f. Pulsatilis, Fontanella — f. Salutarius, Water, mineral — f. Soterius, Water, mineral — f. Vitalis, Centrum vitale.
FONSANGE, MINERAL WATERS OF. Fonsange is situated near Nismes in France. The water is sulphuretted.
FONTA'NA, CANAL OF. A canal of a triangular shape, at the inner side of the ciliary circle; partly formed by the groove at the inner edges of the cornea and sclerotica.
FONTANEL'LA. A *fontanel;* — diminutive of *fons*, 'a fountain.' *Fons pulsat'ilis, Fons pulsans, Vertex pal'pitans, Fons, Bregma, Fontic'ulus, Lacu'na*, Mould. The *opening of the head*. A name, given to a space occupied by a cartilaginous membrane, in the fœtus and new-born child, and situate at the union of the angles of the bones of the cranium. There are six fontanels. 1. The *great* or *sincip'ital* or *anterior*, situate at the junction of the sagittal and coronal sutures. 2. The *small* or *bregmat'ic* or *posterior*, situate at the part where the posterior and superior angles of the parietal bones unite with the upper part of the os occipitis. 3. The *two sphenoidal*, in the

25

temporal fossæ; and, 4. The *two mastoid*, or of Casserius, at the union of the parietal, occipital, and temporal bones.

FONTES, see Fons—f. Medicati Plumbarii, Plombières, mineral waters of—f. Sulphurei calidi, Waters, mineral, sulphureous.

FONTICULE À POIS, see Fonticulus.

FONTIC'ULUS, *Fontanel'la, Exuto'rium, Ex'utory, Issue,* (F.) *Fonticule, Cautère.* A small ulcer produced by art, either by the aid of caustics or of cutting instruments; the discharge from which is kept up with a view to fulfil certain therapeutical indications. The *Pea issue,* (F.) *Fonticule à pois,* is kept up by means of a pea placed in it. This *pea,* (F.) *Pois à cautère,* is sometimes formed of wax; at others, the young, blasted fruit of the orange is employed. The common dried garden pea answers the purpose. The seton is also an issue.

FOOD, Aliment—f. Farinaceous, see Farinaceous—f. of the Gods, Asafœtida.

FOOD, PRINCE OF WALES'S. A farinaceous preparation, which is used in the same cases as arrow-root, is said to consist entirely of potato-flour.

FOOL'S STONES, MALE, Orchis mascula.

FOOT, Pes—f. Flat, see Kyllosis—f. Griffon's, Gryphius pes.

FOOTLING CASE. A presentation of the foot or feet in parturition.

FORA'MEN, *Trema,* from *foro,* 'I pierce.' *Aulos,* (F.) *Trou.* Any cavity, pierced through and through. Also, the orifice of a canal.

FORAMEN ALVEOLARE ANTERIUS, see Palatine canals—f. Alveolare posterius, see Palatine canals—f. Amplum pelvis, Obturatorium foramen—f. Aquæductus Fallopii, F. stylomastoideum—f. Auditorium externum, see Auditory canal, external—f. Auditorium internum, see Auditory canal, internal—f. of Bichat, see Canal, arachnoid—f. of Botal, see Botal foramen—f. Cæcum ossis maxillaris superioris, see Palatine canals.

FORAMEN CÆCUM OF THE MEDUL'LA OBLONGATA or of VICQ. D'AZYR; (Fr.) *Trou borgne.* A tolerably deep fossa at the point where the medium furrow at the anterior surface of the medulla oblongata meets the pons.

FORAMEN CÆCUM OF THE TONGUE, see Cæcum foramen, and Tongue—f. Carotid, see Carotica foramina.

FORA'MEN CENTRA'LE ET LIMBUS LU'TEUS RET'INÆ. The *central foramen and yellow spot of the retina;* discovered by Sömmering. *Mac'ula lu'tea,* (F.) *Tache jaune.* It is situate about two lines to the outside of the optic nerve, and in the direction of the axis of the eye.

FORAMEN COMMUNE ANTERIUS, Vulva—f. Commune posterius, see Anus—f. Condyloid, see Condyloid—f. Conjugationis, see Conjugation—f. Ethmoideum, Orbitar foramen, internal—f. Incisivum, see Palatine canal—f. Infraorbitarium, see Suborbitar canal—f. Infrapubianum, Obturatorium foramen—f. Jugulare, Lacerum posterius foramen - -f. Lacerum in basi cranii, Lacerum posterius foramen—f. Lacerum inferius, Sphenomaxillary fissure—f. Lacerum superius, Sphenoidal fissure—f. Magnum, see Occipital bone—f. Mastoid, see Mastoid foramen—f. Mental, see Mental foramen.

FORAMEN OF MONRO. An opening behind the anterior pillar of the fornix, somewhat above the anterior commissure, by which the third ventricle communicates with the lateral ventricle.

FORAMEN OF MORGAGNI, see Cæcum foramen and Tongue—f. Obturatorium, Obturator foramen—f. Oculi, Pupil—f. Oodes, Ovale foramen—f. Orbitarium internum, Orbitar foramen, internal—f. Orbitarium superius, Orbitar foramen, superior, F. supraorbitarium—f. Ovale, Botal foramen, Fenestra ovalis, Obturatorium foramen, Ovale foramen—f. Palatinum anterius, see Palatine canals—f. Palatinum posterius, see Palatine canals—f. Palato-maxillare, see Palatine canals—f. Rotundum, Fenestra rotunda—f. Spheno-spinosum, Spinale foramen—f. Thyroideum, Obturatorium foramen—f. of Winslow, Hiatus of Winslow.

FORAM'INA THEBE'SII. Openings resembling vascular orifices, found below the orifice of the vena cava superior in the right auricle, which are supposed to be the openings of veins.

FORATIO, Trepanning.

FORCE, from *fortis,* 'strong.' *Vis, Poten'tia, Energi'a, Dy'namis, Cratos.* Any power which produces an action. Those powers which are inherent in organization are called *vital forces.* We say, also, *organic force,* and *muscular force,* to designate that of the organs in general, or of the muscles in particular. To the latter the word *Dynamis,* δυναμις, corresponds; and the absence of this force is termed *adyna'mia.* The *vital forces* have to be carefully studied by the pathologist. The doctrine of diseases is greatly dependent on their augmentation or diminution; freedom or oppression, &c.

FORCE OF ASSIMILATION, Plastic force—f. Catalytic, see Catalysis—f. of Formation, Plastic force—f. Germ, Plastic force—f. Metabolic, see Metabolic force—f. of Nutrition, Plastic force—f. of Vegetation, Plastic force—f. Vital, Vis vitalis—f. *Vitale,* Vis vitalis.

FORCE-REAL, MINERAL WATERS OF. The name of a mountain, situate four leagues from Perpignan in France. The water is chalybeate.

FORCEPS, quasi,*ferriceps,* from *ferrum,* 'iron,' and *capio,* 'I take.' *Pincers, Labis, Volsel'læ.* An instrument for removing bodies, which it would be inconvenient or impracticable to seize with the fingers. (F.) *Pinces, Pincettes.* There are various kinds of forceps, 1. The ordinary kind, contained in every dressing-case, for removing lint, &c. from wounds or ulcers. (F.) *Pinces à anneaux.* 2. *Dissecting* or *Lig'ature* or *Arte'rial Forceps,* (F.) *Pinces à dissection, P. à ligature,* to lay hold of delicate parts. 3. *Pol'ypus Forceps, Tooth Forceps, Forceps of Museux* for laying hold of the tonsils or other parts to be removed. 4. *The Bullet Forceps, Strombul'cus,* (Fr.) *Tireballe.* 5. The *Lithot'omy Forceps, Lithol'abon, Lithogo'gum, Tenac'ula, Volsel'la,* which resembles the *Craniotomy Forceps,* (F.) *Tenettes.*

Forceps is also an instrument used by obstetrical practitioners to embrace the head, and bring it through the pelvis. It consists of two branches, blades or levers; one of which, in the case of the *short forceps,* is passed over the ear of the child, and the other opposite to the former, so that the blades may lock. When the head is securely included between the blades, the operation of extraction can be commenced. See Parturition.

FORCEPS, see Corpus callosum—f. Anterior, see Corpus callosum—f. Arterial, see Forceps—f. Bullet, see Forceps—f. Craniotomy, see Forceps—f. Deceptoria, see Forceps—f. Lithotomy, see Forceps—f. of Museux, see Forceps—f. Polypus, see Forceps—f. Tooth, see Forceps.

FORD'S BALSAM OF HOREHOUND, see Balsam of horehound.

FOREARM, *Antibra'chium, Pygmè, Pars infe'rior bra'chii, Cu'bitus,* (F.) *Avant-bras.* The part of the upper extremity, comprised between the arm and the hand. It is composed of two bones—*radius* and *ulna*—and 20 muscles.

FOREHEAD, Front.

FORENSIC ANATOMY, see Anatomy—f. Medicine, Medicine, legal.

PORES, Genital organs.
FORESKIN, Prepuce.
FORFEX, Scissors—f. Dentaria, Dentagra.
FORFIC'ULA AURICULA'RIA, Earwig. An insect of the Order Orthoptera, which occasionally enters the meatus auditorius externus, and excites intense pain. It may be destroyed by tobacco-smoke, or by oil poured into the meatus.
FORGES, MINERAL WATERS OF. Forges is situate four leagues from Gournay, in the department of Seine Inférieure, France. There are three springs, which are acidulous chalybeates. These are called *Royal, Reinette*, and *Cardinal*, in honor of Louis XIII., Queen Anne of Austria, and Cardinal Richelieu, who used them.
FORMATIVE, Plastic.
FORMI'CA, *Myrmex*. The ant or pismire. (F.) *Fourmi*. It contains an acid juice and gross oil, which were formerly extolled as aphrodisiacs. The chrysalides of the animal are said to be diuretic and carminative; and have been used in dropsy. 2. Also the name of a black wart, *verru'ca formica'ria*, with a broad base and cleft surface; so called because the pain attending it resembles the biting of an ant, μυρμηκια, *myrme'cia*. — Forestus. 3. A varicose tumour on the anus and glans penis. 4. Also, miliary herpes.
FORMICA AMBULATORIA, Herpes circinatus — f. Corrosive, Herpes exedens.
FORM'ICANT, *Myrme'cizon, Formi'cans*, from *formica*, 'an ant.' (F.) *Fourmillant*. An epithet given to the pulse, *Pulsus formi'cans*, when extremely small, scarcely perceptible, unequal, and communicating a sensation like that of the motion of an ant through a thin texture.
FORMICA'TION, *Formica'tio, Myrmecias'mus, Myrmeci'asis, Myrmecis'mus, Myrmeco'sis, Stupor formi'cans*. Same etymon. (F.) *Fourmillement*. A pain, compared with that which would be caused by a number of ants creeping on a part.
FORMIX, Herpes esthiomenus.
FOR'MULA, from *forma*, 'a form.' (F.) *Formule, Ordonnance*. The receipt for the formation of a compound medicine; a prescription.
FORM'ULARY, *Formula'rium, Codex medicamenta'rius, Narthe'cia, Narthe'cium, Narthex*. A collection of medical formulæ or receipts.
FORMULE, Prescription.
FORMYL, PERCHLORIDE OF. Chloroform.
FORNIX, 'an arch or vault.' *For'nix cer'ebri, Cam'era, Fornix trilat'erus, Psalis, Psalid'ium, Testu'do cer'ebri, Arcus medulla'ris*, (F.) *Trigone cérébral* — (Ch.,) *Voûte à trois piliers, Triangle Médullaire*. A medullary body in the brain, below the corpus callosum and above the middle ventricle, on the median line. This body, which is curved upon itself, terminates anteriorly by a prolongation, which constitutes its *anterior pillar* or *crus*, (F.) *Pilier antérieur*, and posteriorly by two similar prolongations, called *posterior pillars* or *crura*. See Achicolum, and Vault.
FORNIX CEREBRI, Fornix.
FORPEX, Scissors.
FORTIFIANT, Corroborant, Tonic.
FORTRAITURE, Hysteralgia.
FOSSA, *Fo'vea*, from *fodio*, 'I dig.' *Scamma*. A cavity of greater or less depth, the entrance to which is always larger than the base. The fossæ of bones have been called *simple*, when they belong to one bone only, as the *parietal fossa*; and *compound*, (F.) *Fosses composées*, when several concur in their formation, as the *orbitar fossæ, temporal fossæ*, &c.
FOSSA AMYG'DALOID, *Amyg'daloid excava'tion*. The space between the anterior and posterior pillars of the fauces, which is occupied by the tonsils.

FOSSA AMYN'TÆ. A kind of bandage, used in fractures of the nose; so called, by Galen, from Amyntas of Rhodes, its inventor. It consisted of a long band, applied round the head, the turns of which crossed at the root of the nose.

FOSSA CANINA, Canine fossa.

FOSSA CEREBEL'LI, (F.) *Fosse cérébelleuse*. The inferior occipital fossa, which lodges the corresponding portion of the cerebellum.

FOSSA CORONA'LIS, *Coro'nal* or *frontal fossa*. A depression on the orbitar plate of the frontal or coronal bone, which supports the anterior lobe of the brain.

FOSSA CORONOI'DEA, *Cor'onoid fossa*. A cavity before the inferior extremity of the humerus, in which the coronoid process of the ulna is engaged during the flexion of the forearm.

FOSSA COTYLOIDEA, see Cotyloid.

FOSSA, DIGAS'TRIC, *Fossa digas'trica*. A deep groove on the mastoid portion of the temporal bone, which gives origin to the digastric muscle.

FOSSA ETHMOIDA'LIS, *Ethmoid fossa*. A shallow gutter on the upper surface of the cribriform plate of the ethmoid bone, on which is lodged the expanded portion of the olfactory nerve.

FOSSA GENU, Poples.

FOSSA GUTTURA'LIS, *Gut'tural fossa*. The depression which forms the guttural region of the base of the cranium, between the foramen magnum and posterior nares.

FOSSA HYALOIDEA, see Hyaloid (Fossa) — f. Iliac, see Iliac fossæ — f. Infra-orbitar, Canine fossa—f. Infra-spinous, see Infra-spinata fossa.

FOSSA INNOMINATA. The space between the helix and antihelix of the ear.

FOSSA, ISCHIO-RECTAL, Perineal fossa — f. Jugularis, Jugular fossa- f. Lachrymalis, Lachrymal fossa — f. Magna Muliebris, Vulva — f. Magna Sylvii, Fissura Sylvii.

FOSSA, MENTAL, *Fossa menta'lis*. A small depression on each side of the symphysis on the anterior surface of the body of the maxilla inferior, for the attachment of muscles.

FOSSA NAVICULARIS, Navicular fossa.

FOSSA OCCIPITA'LIS, *Occip'ital fossa*. The occipital fossæ are four in number; the *superior* or *cerebral*, and the *inferior* or *cerebellous*. They are separated by a groove, which lodges the lateral sinus.

FOSSA OVALIS, see Ovalis fossa — f. Palatina, Palate—f. Perinæi, Perineal fossa — f. Pituitaria, Sella Turcica.

FOSSA POPLITE'A, *Poplite'al fossa*. The hollow of the ham;—the popliteal region.

FOSSA SCAPHOIDES, Navicularis fossa—f. Suborbitar, Canine fossa.

FOSSA, SUBPYRAM'IDAL, *F. subpyramida'lis*. A deep fossa under the pyramid and behind the fenestra rotunda in the middle ear, remarkable for its constancy, and pierced by several foramina at the bottom.

FOSSA SUPRA-SPHENOIDALIS, Pituitaria fossa— f. of Sylvius, Ventricle, fifth—f. Umbilicalis, see Liver.

FOSSÆ CEREBRA'LES, *Cer'ebral fossæ*. Fossæ or excavations at the base of the cranium. They are nine in number; three occupy the median line, and three are placed at each side. They are distinguished into *anterior, middle*, and *posterior*.

FOSSÆ DIGITALES, see Impression.

FOSSE BASILAIRE, Basilary fossa — *f. Sous-épineuse*, Infra-spinata fossa — *f. Sus-épineuse*, Fossa supra-spinata.

FOSSES CONDYLOÏDIENNES, Condyloidea foramina—*f. Nasales, Ouvertures postérieures des*, Nares, posterior.

FOSSETTE, (F.) Diminutive of *fossa. Scrobic'ulus, Both'rion.* Several depressions are so called. A dimpled chin, *Fossette du menton,* consists in a slight depression, which certain persons have on the chin. 2. *A dimple of the cheek,* (F.) *Fossette des joues,* a depression which occurs on the cheeks of certain persons when they laugh. *Scrobic'ulus cordis, Anticar'dion, Præcor'dium,* (F.) *Fossette du cœur.* The depression observed on a level with the xiphoid cartilage at the anterior and inferior part of the chest. It is, also, called *pit of the stomach,* (F.) *Creux de l'estomac.*

FOSSETTE, *Fos'sula, A'nulus, Bothrium,* is also a small ulcer of the transparent cornea, the centre of which is deep.

FOSSETTE ANGULAIRE DU QUATRIÈME VENTRICULE, Calamus scriptorius—*f. du Cœur,* Scrobiculus cordis.

FOSSORIUM, Fleam.

FOSSULA, Argema, Fossa, *Fossette,* Fovea.

FOTHERGILL'S PILLS, see Pilulæ aloes et colocynthidis.

FOTUS, Fomentation—f. Communis, Decoctum papaveris.

FOU, Insane.

FOUGÈRE FEMELLE, Asplenium filix fœmina, Pteris aquilina—*f. Grande,* Pteris aquilina —*f. Mâle,* Polypodium filix mas.

FOULURE, Sprain.

FOUNDLING HOSPITAL, Brephotropheum.

FOURCHE, (F.), *fourché,* 'cleft;' from *furca,* 'a fork.' *Aposte'ma Phalan'gum.* A French provincial term for small abscesses which form on the fingers and hands of working-people. Also, an instrument, invented by M. J. L. Petit, for compressing the ranine artery in cases of hemorrhage from that vessel.

FOURCHETTE, *Furcil'la,* a little fork. *Fur'cula.* A surgical instrument used for raising and supporting the tongue, during the operation of dividing the frænum.

Fourchette, in anatomy, is, 1. The posterior commissure of the labia majora, called also, *Frænum* and *Fur'cula Labio'rum.* 2. The cartilago ensiformis: so called from its being sometimes cleft like a fork. Also, the semilunar notch at the superior or clavicular extremity of the sternum.

FOURMI, Formica.

FOURMILLANT, Formicant.

FOURMILLEMENT, Formication.

FOUSEL OIL, see Oil, fusel.

FO'VEA, diminutive, *Fove'ola,* from *fodio,* 'I dig.' *Bothros.* A slight depression. *Fos'sula.* The *pudendum muliebre;* see Vulva. Also, the *fossa navicularis.* A vapour-bath for the lower extremities.

FOVEA AXILLARIS, Axilla—f. Elliptica, see Crista Vestibuli — f. Hemisphærica, see Crista Vestibuli — f. Lacrymalis, Lachrymal fossa — f. Oculi, Orbit — f. Semi-elliptica, see Crista Vestibuli — f. Sulciformis, see Crista Vestibuli.

FOVEOLA, Fovea.

FOXBERRY, Arbutus uva ursi.

FOXGLOVE, Digitalis.

FOYER, Fomes morbi.

FRACTURA, Fracture — f. Dentis, Odontoclasis.

FRACTURE, *Fractu'ra,* from *frangere, fractum,* 'to break,' 'bruise.' *Catag'ma, Catag'ma Fractu'ra, Cataœ'is, Clasis, Clasma, Agmē, Agma, Diar'rhagē.* A solution of continuity in a bone, *Osteoc'lasis.* A *simple fracture* is when the bone only is divided. A *compound fracture* is a division of the bone with a wound of the integuments communicating with the bone,—the bone, indeed, generally protruding. In a *com'minuted fracture, Alphite'don,* αλφιτηδον, *Carye'don Catag'ma,* καρυηδον καταγμα, the bone is broken into several pieces; and in a *complicated fracture* there is, in addition to the injury done to the bone, a lesion of some considerable vessel, nervous trunk, &c. Fractures are also termed *transverse, oblique,* &c., according to their direction. The treatment of fractures consists, in general, in reducing the fragments when displaced; maintaining them when reduced; preventing the symptoms, which may be likely to arise; and combating them when they occur. The reduction of fractures must be effected by extension, counter-extension, and coaptation. The parts are kept in apposition by position, rest, and an appropriate apparatus. The position must vary according to the kind of fracture. Commonly, the fractured limb is placed on a horizontal or slightly inclined plane, in a state of extension; or rather in a middle state between extension and flexion, according to the case.

FRACTURE EN RAVE, Raphanedon.

FRACTURE OF THE RADIUS, BARTON'S, *Barton's Fracture.* A term applied to a fracture of the lower extremity of the radius, which commences at the articular surface, and extends upwards for an inch or more, to terminate on the dorsal aspect. Owing to the extensor muscles drawing up the separated portion of the bone, and with it the carpus, a deformity results, which has been confounded with simple dislocation. In consequence of the fracture having been well described by Dr. John Rhea Barton, of Philadelphia, it is often called after him.

FRACTURES PAR RÉSONNANCE, see Contrafissura.

FRÆNA EPIGLOT'TIDIS, Glosso-epiglottic ligaments — f. Morgagnii, F. of the Valve of Bauhin.

FRÆNA OF THE VALVE OF BAUHIN, (F.) *Freins de la valvule de Bauhin.* A name given by Morgagni to the projecting lines formed by the junction of the extremities of the two lips of the ileocœcal valve. They are also called *Fræna* and *Retinac'ula Morgagn'ii.*

FRÆNULUM, see Frænum, Bride — f. Clitoridis, Frænum clitoridis—f. Labiorum, *Fourchette* —f. Novum, Tænia semicircularis.

FRÆ'NULUM VELI MEDULLA'RIS ANTERIO'RIS. A narrow slip, given off by the commissure of the encephalic testes, which strengthens the junction of the testes with the valve of Vieussens.

FRÆNUM, *Fræ'num;* (F.) *Frein,* 'a bridle.' *Fræ'nulum, Filel'lum, Filamen'tum.* 'A small bridle.' A bridle. Names given to several membranous folds, which bridle and retain certain organs.

FRÆNUM CLITOR'IDIS, *Fræ'nulum Clitor'idis,* (F.) *Frein du Clitoris.* A slight duplicature formed by the union of the internal portions of the upper extremity of the nymphæ.

FRÆNUM GLANDIS, F. Penis.

FRÆNUM LABIO'RUM, (F.) *Frein des lèvres.* There are two of these; one for the upper, the other for the lower lip. They unite these parts to the maxillary bone, and are formed by the mucous membrane of the mouth. Also, the *Fourchette.*

FRÆNUM LINGUÆ, *Fræ'nulum* seu *Vin'culum Linguæ, Glossodes'mus, File'tum,* (F.) *Filet* ou *Frein de la langue,* is a triangular reflection, formed by the mucous membrane of the mouth, and situate between the inferior paries of that cavity and the inferior surface of the tongue. When the frænum extends as far as the extremity of the tongue, it cramps its movements, interferes with sucking, &c. This inconvenience is remedied by carefully snipping it with a pair of scissors. The French call this *l'opération du filet.*

FRÆNUM PENIS, *F.* seu *Fræ'nulum* seu *Vin'culum Præpu'tii, F. Glandis, Cynodes'mion, Cynodes'mus, Vin'culum Cani'num,* (F.) *Filet* ou *Frein de la verge,* is a membranous reflection which fixes the prepuce to the lower part of the glans. When too short, it prevents the prepuce from sliding over the glans.

FRÆNUM PRÆPUTII, F. Penis.

FRAGA'RIA, from *fragro,* 'I smell sweetly.' The *Strawberry, Fraga'ria vesca* seu *vulga'ris* seu *semper-florens, Chamæ'batos,* (F.) *Fraisier.* The fruit is agreeable and wholesome, and the roots have been used as tonic and slightly diuretic. The fruit is the *Fragrum, κομαρον* of the ancients; (F.) *Fraise.*

FRAGARIA ANSERINA, Potentilla anserina—f. Pentaphyllum, Potentilla reptans—f. Tormentilla officinalis, Potentilla tormentilla.

FRAGA'RIA VIRGINIA'NA, *Wild Strawberry.* An indigenous plant, which has astringent leaves.

FRAGILE VITREUM, Fragilitas ossium.

FRAGIL'ITAS, *Ruptibil'itas,* from *frango,* 'I break.' Fragility, Brittleness. The state of being easily broken or torn.

FRAGIL'ITAS OS'SIUM, *Osteopsathyro'sis, Brit'tleness of the bones, Friabil'ity of the bones, Paros'tia frag''ilis, Frag''ilis vit'reum.* Pathologists have given this name to the extreme facility with which bones break in certain diseases of the osseous texture. It is owing to a deficiency of the animal matter.

FRAGMENT, *Fragmen'tum, Fragmen, Ramen'tum,* from *frangere,* 'to break.' The French use this term for the two portions of a fractured bone; thus, they speak of the *superior* and the *inferior fragment.*

FRAGMENTS, PREC''IOUS. A name formerly given, in *Pharmacy,* to the garnet, hyacinth, emerald, sapphire and topaz. The Arabs falsely attributed to them cordial and alixiterial properties.

FRAGON, Ruscus.
FRAGUM, see Fragaria.
FRAISE, see Fragaria.
FRAISIER, Fragaria.

FRAMBŒ'SIA, *Frambœ'sia, Lepra fungif''era,* from *Framboise,* (F.) 'A raspberry.' *Syphilis In'dica, Anthra'cia ru'bula, Thymio'sis, Thymio'sis* seu *Lues In'dica, Vari'ola Amboinen'sis, Lepra fungif'era, Scroph'ula Molucca'na. The Yaws, Epian, Pian.* A disease of the Antilles and of Africa, characterised by tumours, of a contagious character, which resemble strawberries, raspberries, or champignons; ulcerate, and are accompanied by emaciation. The *Pian,* for so the Indians call it, differs somewhat in America and Africa.

Pian of *Amer'ica, Frambœ'sia America'na, Anthra'cia Bu'bula Americana,* occurs under similar circumstances with the next, and seems to be transmitted by copulation. The tumours have a similar form, and are greater in proportion to their paucity. In some cases they are mixed with ulcers.

Pian of *Guin'ea, Frambœ'sia Guineen'sis, Anthra'cia Ru'bula Guineen'sis,* is common amongst the negroes, especially in childhood and youth. It begins by small spots, which appear on different parts, and especially on the organs of generation and around the anus; these spots disappear, and are transformed into an eschar, to which an excrescence succeeds, that grows slowly, and has the shape above described.

The treatment is nearly the same in the two varieties. The tumours will yield to mercurial friction, when small. When large, they must be destroyed by caustic. In both cases, mercury must be given to prevent a recurrence.

An endemic disease resembling yaws was observed in the Feejee Islands by the medical officers of the United States' Exploring Expedition. It is called by the natives *Dthoke.*

FRAMBŒSIA ILLYRICA, Scherlievo—f. Scotica, Sibbens.

FRAMBOISE, Rubus idæus.
FRANCOLIN, Attagen.
FRANGES SYNOVIALES, Synovial glands.
FRANGULA ALNUS, Rhamnus frangula.
FRANKINCENSE, COMMON, see Pinus abies—f. True, Juniperus lycia.

FRANZENSBAD, FRANZBAD, or FRANZENSBRUNN, MINERAL WATERS OF. A celebrated water at Eger, in Bohemia, which contains sulphate of soda, carbonate of iron, and carbonic acid gas. The springs are also called Franzensbrunnen.

FRAPPER, Percuss.
FRASERA CAROLINIENSIS, see Calumba —f. Officinalis, see Calumba—f. Walteri, see Calumba.

FRATER UTERINUS, see Uterinus frater.
FRATERNITAS, Adelphixia.
FRATRATIO, Adelphixia.
FRAXINELLA DICTAMNUS, Dictamnus albus—f. White, Dictamnus albus.

FRAXINUS AMERICA'NA, *White Ash;* and FRAXINUS QUADRANGULA'TA, *Blue Ash,* indigenous; have bitter and astringent barks, and have been used as antiperiodics.

FRAXINUS APETALA, F. excelsior—f. Aurea, F. excelsior—f. Crispa, F. excelsior—f. Excelsa, F. excelsior.

FRAX'INUS EXCEL'SIOR. The systematic name of the *Ash tree, Frax'inus, Ornus* seu *Fraxinus sylves'tris, Fr. apet'ala* seu *au'rea* seu *crispa* seu *excel'sa* seu *pen'dula* seu *verruco'sa, Bume'lia* seu *Macedon'ica Fraxinus, Bumelia.* Ord. Oleaceæ. (F.) *Frêne.* The fresh bark has a moderately strong, bitterish taste. It has been said to possess resolvent and diuretic qualities, and has been given in intermittents. The seeds, called *Birds' tongues, Lingua avis, Ornithogloss'æ,* have been exhibited as diuretics, in the dose of a drachm. Its sap has been extolled against deafness.

FRAXINUS FLORIFERA, F. ornus—f. Macedonica, F. excelsior.

FRAXINUS ORNUS, *Fraxinus me'lia* seu *panicula'ta* seu *florif'era, Ornus mannif'era* seu *rotundifo'lia.* The systematic name of the tree whence manna flows. This substance is also called *Manna Calabri'na, Ros Calabri'nus, Aëromel'eli, Drosom'eli, Dryeom'eli, Mel aë'rium, Succus orni concre'tus.* In Sicily, not only the *Fraxinus Ornus,* but also the *F. rotundifolia* and *F. excelsior* are regularly cultivated for the purpose of procuring manna, which is their condensed juice. In the Ph. U. S. it is assigned to *Ornus Europæa.* Manna is inodorous, sweetish, with a very slight degree of bitterness; in friable flakes, of a whitish or pale yellow colour; opake, and soluble in water and alcohol. It is laxative, and is used as a purgative for children, who take it readily on account of its sweetness. More generally it is employed as an adjunct to other purgatives. Dose, ℥ss to ℥ij. Its immediate principle is called *Mannite* or *Mannin.* This has been recommended by Magendie as a substitute for manna. Dose, ℥ij, for children.

FRAXINUS PANICULATA, F. ornus—f. Quadrangulata, see F. Americana—f. Rotundifolia, F. ornus.

FRAYEUR NOCTURNE, Panophobia.
FRECKLES, Ephelides.
FREEMAN'S BATHING SPIRITS, see Linimentum saponis compositum.
FREIN, Frænum—*f. du Clitoris*, Frænum clitoridis—*f. de la Langue*, Frænum linguæ—*f. des Lèvres*, Frænum laborium—*f. de la Verge*, Frænum penis.
FREINS DE LA VALVULE DE BAUHIN, Frœna of the valve of Bauhin.
FREINWALDE, MINERAL WATERS OF. These springs are in Brandenburg, twelve leagues from Berlin. They contain chloride of sodium, sulphate of magnesia, chloride of magnesium, sulphate of lime, carbonates of lime and magnesia, iron, &c., and are used in asthenic diseases.
FRÉMISSEMENT, Shuddering.
FRÉMISSEMENT CATAIRE (F.), 'Cat's purr.' *Purring Tremor*. Laënnec has given this name to the agitation which is sensible to the hand, when applied on the præcordial region, and which he considers a sign of ossification or other contraction of the auriculo-ventricular openings. The name was chosen by him from the analogy of the sound to the purring of a cat.
FREMITUS, *Bruissement, Frémissement*, Shuddering.
The *Pec'toral* or *Vocal Frem'itus, Pectoral Vibra'tion, Tactile vibration*, is an obscure diffused resonance of the voice, which is felt when the hand is applied to the chest.
FRENA, Alveolus.
FRÊNE, Fraxinus excelsior—*f. Épineux*, Xanthoxylum clava Herculis.
FRENULUM, see Frænum.
FRENUM, Frænum.
FRET, Chafing, Herpes.
FRÉTILLEMENT, Fidgets.
FRICATIO, Friction.
FRICATORIUM, Liniment.
FRICĒ, *Fricum, Frico'sium*. A medicine which the ancients employed under the form of friction. They distinguish the *Fricē siccum* and *F. mollē*.—Gaubius.
FRICONIUM, Frice.
FRICTA, Colophonia.
FRICTIO, Friction—f. Humida, see Friction—f. Sicca, see Friction.
FRIC'TION, *Fric'tio, Frica'tio, Anat'ribē, Anatrip'sis, Trypsis, Chirap'sia*, from *fricare*, 'to rub.' The action of rubbing a part of the surface of the body more or less forcibly, with the hands, a brush, flannel, &c., constituting *Xerotrib'ia, Xerotrip'sis, Fric'tio sicca* or *dry friction;* or with ointments, liniments, tinctures, &c., constituting *moist friction, Fric'tio hu'mida*. It is a useful means for exciting the action of the skin.

FRICTION SOUND, *Bruit de frottement*.
FRICTRIX, *Tribade*.
FRICTUM, Liniment.
FRICUM, Frice.
FRIGEFACIENTIA, Refrigerants.
FRIGID, *Frig'idus*, (F.) *Froid:* same etymon as Frigidity. Cold. Not easily moved to sexual desire; *Imbel'lis ad ven'erem*. Impotent.
FRIGIDARIUM, Bath, cold.
FRIGID'ITY, *Frigid'itas*, from *frigidum*, 'cold.' A sensation of cold. Also, impotence, and sterility. *Frigidity of the stomach* is a state of debility of that organ, imputed to excessive venery,—the *Anorex'ia exhausto'rum* of Sauvages.
FRIGIDUS, Frigid.
FRIGORIF'IC, from *frigus*, 'cold,' and *fio*, 'I make.' That which has the power of producing cold. The best FRIGORIFIC MIXTURES are the following. Their effects are owing to the rapid absorption of heat when solids pass into the liquid state.

FRIGORIFIC MIXTURES WITH SNOW.

Mixtures.	Therm. falls.
Snow, or pounded ice, two parts by weight;	to—5°
Chloride of Sodium...... 1.	
Snow or pounded ice..... 5.	to—12°
Chloride of Sodium...... 2.	
Mur. of Ammonia......... 1.	
Snow or pounded ice.....24.	to—18°
Chloride of Sodium......10.	
Muriate of Ammonia...... 5.	
Nitrate of Potash........ 5.	
Snow or pounded ice.....12.	
Chloride of Sodium...... 5.	
Nitrate of Ammonia...... 5.	to—25°
Dilut. Sulph. Acid....... 2.	from +32°
Snow .... 3.	to—23°
Concentr. Mur. Acid..... 5.	from +32°
Snow .... 8.	to—27°
Concentr. Nitrous Acid.. 4.	from +32°
Snow .... 7.	to—30°
Chloride of Calcium..... 5.	from +32°
Snow .... 4.	to—40°
Crystall. Chloride of Calcium 3.	from +32°
Snow .... 2.	to—50°
Fused Potash............ 4.	from +32°
Snow .... 3.	to—51°

Frigorific Mixtures may also be made by the rapid solution of salts, without the use of snow or ice. The salts must be finely powdered and dry.

FRIGORIFIC MIXTURES WITHOUT SNOW.

Mixtures.	Therm. falls.
Mur. of Ammonia.......... 5.	from +50°
Nitrate of Potash.......... 5.	to—10°
Water.....................16.	
Mur. of Ammonia.......... 5.	
Nitrate of Potash.......... 5.	from +50°
Sulphate of Soda.......... 8.	to +10°
Water.....................16.	
Nitrate of Ammonia....... 1.	from +50°
Water..................... 1.	to + 4°
Nitrate of Ammonia....... 1.	
Carbonate of Soda........ 1.	from +50°
Water..................... 1.	to— 7°
Sulphate of Soda.......... 3.	from +50°
Dilut. Nitrous Acid....... 2.	to— 3°
Sulphate of Soda.......... 6.	
Mur. of Ammonia.......... 4.	from +50°
Nitrate of Potash.......... 2.	to—10°
Dilut. Nitrous Acid....... 4.	
Sulphate of Soda.......... 6.	
Nitrate of Ammonia....... 5.	from +50°
Dilut. Nitrous Acid....... 4.	to—14°
Phosphate of Soda......... 9.	from +50°
Dilut. Nitrous Acid....... 4.	to—12°
Phosphate of Soda......... 9.	
Nitrate of Ammonia....... 6.	from +50°
Dilut. Nitrous Acid....... 4.	to—21°
Sulphate of Soda.......... 8.	from +50°
Muriatic Acid............. 5.	to— 0°
Sulphate of Soda.......... 5.	from +50°
Dilut. Sulphuric Acid..... 4.	to— 3°

FRIGUS, Cold—f. Tenue, see Rigor.
FRISSON, Rigor.
FRISSONNEMENT, Horripilation.
FROGLEAF, Brasenia Hydropeltis.
FROG TONGUE, Ranula.
FROGS' SPAWN, Sperma ranarum.
FROID, Cold, Frigid—*f. Glacial*, Ice-cold.
FROISSEMENT, (F.) 'Rubbing, bruising.'
FROISSEMENT PULMONAIRE, Bruit de froissement pulmonaire, Pulmonary crumpling

sound. A name given by M. Fournet to a respiratory sound, which communicates to the ear the sensation of the rubbing (*froissement*) of a texture compressed against a hard body. It is by no means well defined.

FRÔLEMENT, (F.) 'Grazing or touching lightly.'

FRÔLEMENT PÉRICARDIQUE, *Bruit de frôlement péricardique*. Rustling noise of the pericardium. A sound resembling that produced by the crumpling of a piece of parchment or of thick silken stuff, accompanying the systole and diastole of the heart. It indicates roughness of the pericardium induced by disease.

FROMAGE, Cheese.

FROMENT, Triticum.

FRONCEMENT, Corrugation.

FRONCLE, Furunculus.

FRONDE, Funda.

FRONT, *Frons, Meto'pon*, Forehead, Brow. That part of the visage, which extends from one temple to the other, and is comprised in a vertical direction, between the roots of the hair and the superciliary ridges.

FRONTAL, *Fronta'lis*. Relating or belonging to the front. This name has been given to several parts. Winslow, Sömmering, and others, call the anterior part of the occipito-frontalis— the *frontal muscle* or *fronta'lis, Musculo'sa Frontis Cutem movens substan'tia Par* (Vesalius).

FRONTAL ARTERY, *A. supra-orbita'lis*, is given off by the ophthalmic, which is itself a branch of the internal carotid. It makes its exit from the skull at the upper part of the base of the orbit, and ascends the forehead between the bone and the orbicularis palpebrarum; dividing into three or four branches, which are distributed to the neighbouring muscles.

FRONTAL BONE, *Os frontis, Os corona'lè, Os inverecun'dum, Meto'pon, Os puppis, Os Ratio'nis.* A double bone in the fœtus, single in the adult, situate at the base of the cranium, and at the superior part of the face. It forms the vault of the orbit; lodges the ethmoid bone in a notch at its middle part; and is articulated, besides, with the sphenoid, parietal, and nasal bones, the ossa unguis, superior maxillary, and malar bones.

FRONTAL FURROW extends upwards from the frontal spine, and becomes gradually larger in its course, to lodge the upper part of the superior longitudinal sinus, and to give attachment to the falx cerebri.

FRONTAL NERVE, *Palpébro-frontal*— (Ch.,) is the greatest of the three branches of the ophthalmic nerve,— the first division of the 5th pair. It proceeds along the superior paries of the orbit, and divides into two branches:— the one, *internal*, which makes its exit from the orbitar fossa, passing beneath the pulley of the oblique muscle: —the other, *external*, issuing from the same cavity, by the foramen orbitarium superius.

FRONTAL PROTU'BERANCE, *Frontal tuberos'ity, Tuber fronta'lè, Suggrun'dium supercilio'rum*. The protuberance of the frontal bone above the superciliary arch.

FRONTAL SI'NUSES, *Fronta'les Sinus, Metopan'tra, Prosopan'tra, Sinus Supercilia'res, S. pituita'rii frontis, Cavern'æ frontis*, are two deep cavities in the substance of the frontal bone, separated from each other by a medium septum, and opening, below, into the anterior cells of the ethmoid bone.

FRONTAL SPINE, *Crista inter'na*, is situate in the middle of the under part of the bone, and is formed by the coalescence of the inner tables for the attachment of the falx cerebri.

Surgeons have given the name FRONTA'LIS to a bandage or topical application to the forehead. Such have, also, been called τρομετωπιδια and ανακολλημα.

FRONTAL TUBEROSITY, Frontal protuberance.

FRONTA'LÈ, from *frons*, 'the forehead.' A medicine applied to the forehead.

FRONTALIS ET OCCIPITALIS, Occipito-frontalis.

FRONTALIS VERUS, Corrugator supercilii.

FRONTODYMIA, see Cephalodymia.

FRONTO-ETHMOID FORAMEN, Cæcum foramen—*f. Nasal*, Pyramidalis nasi—*f. Sourcilier*, Corrugator supercilii.

FROSTBITE, Congelation.

FROSTWEED, Erigeron Philadelphicum, Helianthemum Canadense.

FROSTWORT, Helianthemum Canadense.

FROTH'Y, from Gr. αφρος, 'froth.' (?) *Spumo'sus*, (F.) *Spumeux, Écumeux, Mousseux*. An epithet given to the fæces or sputa, when mixed with air.

FROTTEMENT, see Bruit de frottement.

FROTTEMENT GLOBULAIRE. A name given by M. Simonnet, to the pulse in aortic regurgitation, when it is jerking, and, in well marked cases, appears as if the blood consisted of several little masses, which passed in succession under the finger applied to the artery.

FRUCTIFICATIO, Fecundation.

FRUCTUS HORÆI, Fruit, (summer)—f. Immaturus, Abortion.

FRUGIV'OROUS, *Frugiv'orus*, from *fruges*, 'fruits,' and *voro*, 'I eat.' One that eats fruits.

FRUIT, *Fructus*, from *frui*, 'to enjoy.' *Carpos*. In botany, the seed with its enclosing pericarp. In a medical sense it may be defined to be:— that part of a plant which is taken as food. The effects of fruits on the body, in a medical as well as a dietetical point of view, are various. They may be distinguished into classes: for, whilst the *Cerealia*, for example, afford fruits, which are highly nutritious, the *Summer Fruits* (*Fructus Horæ'i*,) which include strawberries, cherries, currants, mulberries, raspberries, figs, grapes, &c., are refrigerant and grateful, but afford little nourishment.

FRUIT-SUGAR, Glucose.

FRUMENT, *Fru'menty, Fur'menty*, from *frumentum*, 'wheat' or 'grain,' quasi *frugimentum;* from *fruges*, 'fruit.' Pottage made of wheat. Food made of wheat boiled in milk.

FRUMEN'TUM. Same etymon. *Sitos*. Any kind of grain from which bread was made;— especially wheat.

FRUMENTUM, Triticum—f. Corniculatum, Ergot —f. Cornutum, Ergot— f. Luxurians, Ergot— f. Temulentum, Ergot—f. Turgidum, Ergot.

FRUSTRATOIRE, (F.) Any liquor, taken a short time after eating, for the purpose of assisting digestion when difficult. Sugared water, *eau sucrée*, or water with the addition of a little brandy, or some aromatic substance, is commonly used for this purpose.

FRUTEX BACCIFER BRAZILIENSIS, Caaghivuyo—f. Indicus spinosus, Cara schulli.

FUCUS, F. vesiculosus, Paint.

FUCUS AMYLA'CEUS, *Jaffna Moss, Ed'ible Moss, Ceylon Moss, Ploca'ria can'dida, Gracila'ria lichenoï'des, Sphærococ'cus lichenoï'des, Gigarti'na lichenoï'des, Fucus lichenoï'des, Marine Moss*. This moss belongs to the natural order Algæ. It was introduced some years ago into England, from India. It is white, filiform and fibrous, and has the usual odour of sea-weeds. Its medical properties are similar to those of Irish moss.

FUCUS, BLADDER, F. vesiculosus.

FUCUS CRISPUS, *Lichen Carrageen, Chondrus,*

Ch. crispus, Sphærococ'cus crispus, Ulva crispa, Chondrus polymor'phus, Irish moss, Carrageen or Corrigeen moss, (F.) *Mousse d'Irlande, M. perlée.* This Fucus, of the Natural Family *Algæ,* is found on the coasts of England, Ireland, Western France, Spain, and Portugal, and as far as the tropics. It is also a native of the United States. In Ireland, it is used by the poor as an article of diet. As met with in America, it is of a light yellow colour, and resembles plates of horn, crisped and translucent. An agreeable jelly is obtained from it by boiling it in water or milk, which forms a good article of diet in consumptive cases. Its properties are indeed exactly like those of the *Iceland Moss.*

FUCUS HELMINTHOCORTON, Corallina Corsicana — f. Inflatus, F. vesiculosus — f. Lichenoides, F. amylaceus — f. Saccharine, Rhodomela palmata.

FUCUS VESICULO'SUS, *F. 'inflatus, Hal'idrys vesiculo'sa, Quercus Mari'na, Fucus, Bladder Fucus, Sea Oak, Sea Wrack, Yellow Bladder Wrack,* (F.) *Varec vésiculeux, Chêne marin.* It has been said to be a useful assistant to sea-water, in the cure of disorders of the glands. When the wrack, in fruit, is dried, cleaned, exposed to a red-heat in a crucible with a perforated lid, and is reduced to powder, it forms the *Æ'thiops vegetab'ilis*—the *Pulvis Quercûs Mari'næ* of the Dublin Pharmacopœia—which is used, like the burnt sponge, in bronchocele and other scrofulous swellings. Its efficacy depends on the iodine it contains. Dose, gr. x to ℈ij, mixed in molasses or honey. See Soda.

FUGA DÆMONUM, Hypericum perforatum.

FUGA'CIOUS, *Fugax,* from *fugere,* 'to fly.' An epithet given to certain symptoms, which appear and disappear almost immediately afterwards; as a *fugacious redness,*—a *fugacious swelling, Tumor fugax,* &c.

FUGAX, Fugacious.

FUGE, from *fugo,* 'I expel,' 'an expeller.' A common suffix. Hence, *Febrifuge, Vermifuge,* &c.

FU'GILE, *Fugil'la.* This term has several acceptations. It means, 1. The cerumen of the ear. 2. The nebulous suspension in, or deposition from, the urine. 3. An abscess near the ear.—Ruland and Johnson. 4. Abscess in general.

FUGILLA, Fugile.

FULGUR, Astrape.

FULIG"INOUS, *Fuligino'sus, Lignyo'des,* (F.) *Fuligineux,* from *fuligo,* 'soot.' Having the colour of soot. An epithet given to certain parts, as the lips, teeth, or tongue, when they assume a brownish colour, or rather, are covered with a coat of that colour.

FULI'GO, *Lignys, Soot,* (F.) *Suie,* &c. Woodsoot, *Fuligo Ligni,* consists of volatile alkaline salt, empyreumatic oil, fixed alkali, &c. A tincture, *Tinctu'ra Fulig"inis,* prepared from it, has been recommended as a powerful antispasmodic in hysterical cases. (*Fulig. lign.* ℥ij; *potass. subcarb.* ℔ss; *ammon. muriat.* ℨj; *aquæ fluviat.* Olij. Digest for three days.) This tincture bears the name *Soot drops* and *Fit drops.* An ointment of soot has been used in various cutaneous diseases.

FULIGO ALBA PHILOSOPHORUM, Ammoniæ murias.

FULIGO'KALI, from *fuligo,* 'soot,' and *kali,* 'potassa.' This is an analogous preparation to anthrakokali; soot being used in the place of coal. It is employed in the same diseases. What might be regarded as a weak solution of fuligokali has been used for many years in Philadelphia, under the names *medical lye, soot tea, alkaline solution,* and *dyspeptic lye.*

FULLERS' EARTH, Cimolia purpurescens.

FULMEN, Astrape.

FULMICOTON, see Collodion.

FULNESS, *Reple'tio, Plen'itude, Pletho'ra, Reple'tion.* The state of being filled. Also, a feeling of weight or distention in the stomach or other part of the system.

FUMA'RIA, *Fuma'ria officina'lis seu media, Fumus terræ, Capnos, Herba melancholif'uga, Fu'mitory, Common Fu'mitory, Fumiter'ra, Sola'men Scabioso'rum,* (F.) *Fumeterre.* The leaves are extremely succulent, and have a bitter, somewhat saline, taste. The infusion of the dried leaves and the expressed juice of the fresh plant have been extolled for their property of clearing the skin of many disorders of the leprous kind.

FUMA'RIA BULBO'SA, *F. cava seu major, Borckhausen'ia cava, Capnoi'des cava, Aristolochi'a faba'cea seu cava seu vulga'ris rotun'da, Coryd'alis bulbo'sa seu cava seu tubero'sa, Capnor'chis.* The root of this plant was formerly given as an emmenagogue and anthelmintic. (F.) *Fumeterre bulbeuse.*

FUMARIA CAVA, F. bulbosa — f. Major, F. bulbosa—f. Media, Fumaria—f. Officinalis, Fumaria.

FUMETERRE, Fumaria.

FUMIGATIO, Fumigation — f. Antiloimica Gaubii, see Disinfection — f. Guytoniensis, see Disinfection—f. Smythiana, see Disinfection.

FUMIGA'TION, *Fumiga'tio,* from *fumus,* 'smoke.' *Suffi'tus, Suffit"io, Suffumina'tio, Suffumig"ium, Suffimen'tum, Apocapnis'mus, Thymia'ma, Epithymia'ma, Hypothymia'ma, Hypothymia'sis, Thymia'sis, Capnis'mos, Hypocapnis'mos, Hypat'mus, Hypatmis'mus, Anathymia'sis.* An operation, the object of which is to fill a circumscribed space with gas or vapour; with the intention either of purifying the air, of perfuming it, or of charging it with a substance proper for acting upon a part of the surface of the human body. Hence, *fumigations* have been distinguished into *aqueous, aromatic, sulphureous, mercurial, disinfecting, Guytonian,* &c. Benzoin generally constitutes the chief ingredient in the *Fumigating Pastilles,* to which any variety of odoriferous substances may be added. The following is one formula:

℞. *Benzoin.* ℨj; *cascarillæ,* ℨss; *myrrh.* ℨj; *ol. myrist., ol. caryoph.* āā gtt. x; *potassæ nitrat.* ℨss; *carbon. lign.* ℨvj; *mucil. trag.* q. s.

FUMIGATION, CHLORINE, see Disinfection — f. Nitrous, see Disinfection — f. Oxymuriatic, see Disinfection.

FUMITERRA, Fumaria.

FUMITORY, Fumaria.

FUMUS ALBUS, Hydrargyrum—f. Citrinus, Sulphur—f. Terræ, Fumaria.

FUNAMBULA'TIO, from *funis,* 'a cord,' and *ambulare,* 'to walk.' An exercise with the ancients, which consisted in scaling ropes.

FUNC'TION, *Func'tio, Ac'tio,* (F.) *Fonction;* from *fungor,* 'I act,' 'perform.' The action of an organ or system of organs. Any act, necessary for accomplishing a vital phenomenon. A *function* is a special office in the animal economy, which has as its instrument, an organ or apparatus of organs. Thus, *respiration* is a function. Its object is the conversion of venous into arterial blood, and its instrument is the lungs. The ancient physiologists divided the functions into *vital, animal,* and *natural.* They called *vital functions* those which are essential to life, as innervation, circulation, respiration; *animal functions,* those which belong to the encephalon; viz.: the functions of the intellect, the affections of the mind, and the voluntary motions; and *natural functions, Faculta'tes* seu *Actio'nes natura'les,* those relating to assimilation, such as the actions of the abdominal viscera, of the absorbent and exhalant vessels, &c. Bichat divided the functions into those which relate to the preservation of the individual, and those that relate to the preservation of the species. The former he subdivided into *animal* and *organic*. The *animal functions* or *functions of relation* are those of the intellect, sensation, locomotion, and voice. The *organic functions* include digestion, absorption, respiration, circulation, secretion, nutrition, and calorification. The *functions*, whose object is the preservation of the species—the *organic, nutritive*, or *vegetative functions*—are all those that relate to generation;—such as conception, gestation, accouchement, &c. Each of these admits of numerous subdivisions in a complete course of *Physiology;*—for so the doctrine of the functions is called.

FUNCTIONAL DISEASES, see Organic Diseases.

FUNDA, *Sphen'donè*, (F.) *Fronde*. A bandage, composed of a fillet or long compress, cleft at its extremities to within about two inches of its middle. It is used in diseases of the nose and chin, and especially in cases of fracture of the lower jaw. In such case it has, also, been called *Mentonnière*, because placed beneath the chin; from (F.) *Menton*, 'the chin.'

FUNDAMENT, Anus—f. Falling down of the, Proctocele.

FUNDAMEN'TAL, from *fundare*, 'to lie deeply.' Some anatomists have called the sacrum *Os Fundamenta'lè*, because it seems to serve as a base to the vertebral column. The *sphenoid bone* has likewise been so denominated, from its being situate at the base of the cranium.

FUNDUS, (F.) *Fond*. The base of any organ which ends in a neck, or has an external aperture; as the Fundus vesicæ, F. uteri, &c. Also, the Vulva.

FUNDUS VAGINÆ, Laquear vaginæ.

FUNES CORDIS, Columnæ carneæ—f. Semicirculares, Semicircular canals.

FUNGIFORM PAPILLÆ, see Papillæ of the Tongue.

FUN'GOID, *Fungoï'des*, *Myco'des*, *Fungifor'mis*, *Fun'giform*, (F.) *Fongoïde, Fongiforme*, from *fungus*, 'a mushroom,' and ειδος, 'resemblance.' That which has the shape of, or grows in some measure like a mushroom, as the *fungoid* or *fungiform* papillæ of the tongue.

FUNGOID DISEASE, Encephaloid.

FUNGOS'ITY, *Fungos'itas, Caro luxu'rians, C. fungo'sa, Ecsarco'ma, Proud Flesh, Hypsersarco'ma, Hypsersarco'sis*, (F.) *Fongosité*. The quality of that which is fungous:—fungous excrescence, *Excrescen'tia fungo'sa*. The fungosities which arise in wounds or ulcers are easily repressed by gentle compression, dry lint, the sulphas cupri, or other gentle caustics. At times, the more powerful are necessary, and sometimes excision is required.

FUNGUS, *Myces*, (F.) *Fongus, Champignon*. The *mushroom* order of plants; *class* Cryptogamia, in the Linnæan system. In *Pathology*, the word is commonly used synonymously with fungosity, *myco'sis*. M. Breschet has proposed to restrict the term *fungosity* to vegetations which arise on denuded surfaces, and to apply the term *fungus* to the tumours which form in the substance of the textures, without any external ulceration. Fici and warts, for example, would be fungi of the skin.

FUNGUS ALBUS SALIGNEUS, Dædalea suaveolens—f. Articuli, Spina ventosa—f. Bleeding, Hæmatodes fungus—f. Cancrosus hæmatodes, Hæmatodes F.—f. Cancrosus medullaris, see Encephaloid—f. Cerebralis, see Encephaloid—f. Cerebri, Encephalocele—f. Chirurgorum, Lycoperdon —f. Cynosbati, Bedeguar—f. Hæmatodes, Hæma-todes fungus—f. Igniarius, Boletus igniarius—f. Laricis, Boletus laricis—f. of Malta, Cynomorion coccineum—f. Medullaris, see Encephaloid—f. Melanodes, Melanosis—f. Melitensis, Cynomorion coccineum—f. Petræus marinus, Umbilicus marinus—f. Quercinus, Boletus igniarius—f. Rosarum, Bedeguar—f. Salicis, Dædalea suaveolens—f. Sambucinus, Peziza auricula.

FUNIC BELLOWS' SOUND, see Bellows' Sound, funic.

FUNIC'ULI GRAC''ILES, *Poste'rior Me'dian Columns* or *Fascic'uli of the medul'la oblonga'ta*. Along the posterior border of each corpus restiforme, and separated from it by a groove, is a narrow white cord, separated from its fellow by the fissura longitudinalis posterior. The pair of cords are the *funiculi graciles*. Each funiculus forms an enlargement—*processus clavatus*—at its upper end, and is then lost in the corpus restiforme.

FUNIC'ULI SIL'IQUÆ. Longitudinal fibres seen in the groove which separates the corpus olivare from the corpus pyramidale and corpus restiforme. They enclose the base of the corpus olivare,—those which lie on its inner side forming the *funic'ulus inter'nus;* and those on its outer side the *funiculus externus*.

FUNICULUS, Cord—f. Externus, see Funiculi siliquæ—f. Internus, see Funiculi siliquæ—f. Spermaticus, Spermatic cord—f. Tympani, Chorda tympani.

FUNIC'ULUS UMBILICALIS, *Funis umbilica'lis, Intestin'ulum, Vin'culum umbilica'lè, Umbilical cord, Navel string*, diminutive of *Funis*, 'a cord.' (F.) *Cordon ombilicale*. A cord-like substance, which extends from the placenta to the umbilicus of the fœtus. It is composed of the chorion, amnion, an albuminous secretion called the *Jelly of the Cord*, cellular substance, an umbilical vein, and two umbilical arteries. The former conveys the blood from the placenta to the fœtus—the latter return it. All these parts are surrounded by a sheath—*Investitu'ra seu Vagi'na funic'uli umbilica'lis*. Its usual length is from 16 to 22 inches.

FUNICULUS VARICOSUS, Cirsocele.

FUNIS, Cord, Laqueus—f. Argenteus, Medulla spinalis—f. Hippocratis, Achillis tendo—f. Umbilicalis, Funiculus umbilicalis.

FUNNEL, see Infundibulum.

FUR, *Enduit*.

FURCELLA, *Fur'cula;* diminutive of *furca*, 'a fork.' The upper part of the sternum, the clavicle. The *Fourchette*.

FURCELLA INFERIOR, Xiphoid cartilage.

FURCHMUHL, MINERAL WATERS OF. These Bavarian springs contain carbonic acid, sulphuretted hydrogen, carbonates of lime and soda; chlorides of lime and magnesium, oxides of iron and magnesium, &c.

FURCILLA, *Fourchette*.

FURCULA, Furcella, Clavicle, *Fourchette*.

FUREUR UTÉRINE, Nymphomania.

FURFUR, *Bran, Pit'yron, Ach'yron, Apobras'ma, Lemma, Cantabru'no*, (F.) *Son*. The decoction is sometimes employed as an emollient.

FURFURA, Scarf.

FURFURA'CEOUS, from *furfur*, 'bran.' *Scurfy, Canica'ceous, Pithyri'nus, Pityroïdes, Pityro'des*. Resembling bran. A name given to eruptions, in which the epidermis is detached in small scales resembling bran. Also, a bran-like sediment observed at times in the urine;—*Urina furfura'cea, Sedimen'tum Uri'næ pityroïdes*.

FURFURATIO, Porrigo, Pityriasis.

FURFURISCA, Pityriasis.

FU'RIA INFERNA'LIS. A kind of vermiform insect, scarcely two lines long, common in

Sweden, which flies about and stings both man and animals, exciting the most excruciating torture.

FURIBUNDUS, Maniodes.
FURIOSUS, Maniodes.
FURIOUS, Maniodes.
FURMENTY, Frument.
FURNAS, MINERAL WATERS OF. A thermal chalybeate water in St. Michael's, Azores, which contains carbonic acid, and carbonate of iron.

FURONCLE, Furunculus.
FURONCLE GUÉPIER. A malignant boil, *Wasp's nest boil,* which generally attacks the nape and region of the neck, and rarely others than old people. Hence it has been called *Old People's boil.*

FUROR, Mania—f. Brevis, Rage—f. Mania, Mania—f. Uterinus, Nymphomania.
FURROW, MENTO-LABIAL, see Mento-labial furrow.
FURUNCULI ATONICI, Ecthyma—f. Ventriculus, see Furunculus.
FURUN'CULUS, from *furiare,* 'to make mad.' *Chi'adus, Chi'oli, Doth'ien, Dothion, Furun'culus suppurato'rius, F. Verus, F. benig'nus, Phyma furun'culus, Absces'sus nuclea'tus, a furuncle, a boil, a bile.* (F.) *Furoncle, Froncle, Clou.* A small phlegmon, which appears under the form of a conical, hard, circumscribed tumour, having its seat in the dermoid texture. At the end of an uncertain period, it becomes pointed, white or yellow, and gives exit to pus mixed with blood. When it breaks, a small, grayish, fibrous mass sometimes appears, which consists of dead areolar tissue. This is called the *Core, Setfast, Ventric'ulus* seu *Nucleus Furun'culi,* (F.) *Bourbillon.* The abscess does not heal until after its separation. The indications of treatment are,—to discuss by the application of leeches and warm fomentations;—or, if this cannot be done, to encourage suppuration by warm, emollient cataplasms. When suppuration is entirely established, the part may be opened or suffered to break, according to circumstances.

FURUNCULUS GANGRÆNOSUS, Anthrax—f. Malignus, Anthrax.

FUSÉE PURULENTE, (F.) The long and sinuous route which pus takes, in certain cases, in making its way to the surface. These *Fusées* almost always form beneath the skin between the muscles; or along aponeuroses, bones, tendons, &c.

FUSEL OIL, see Oil, fusel.
FUSIBLE, see Fusion.
FUSIBILITY, see Fusion.
FUSION, *Fu'sio, Melting, Liquefaction;* from *fundere, fusum,* 'to melt.' In chymistry, the transition of a solid body into a liquid by the aid of heat. Substances capable of such transition are said to be *fusible;* or to be possessed of *fusibility.*

FUSTIC TREE, Cladastris tinctoria.
FUTUTOR, Tribade.

G.

THE Greek G, Γ, with the ancient Greek physicians, signified an ounce.—Rhod. ad Scribonium.

GABALLA, Cabal.
GABELLA, Mesophryon.
GABIR'EA, γαβιρεα. A fatty kind of myrrh, mentioned by Dioscorides.
GÆOPHAGIA, Geophagism.
GÆOPH'AGUS, from γαια, 'earth,' and φαγω, 'I eat.' One who eats earth.
GAGEL, Myrica gale.
GAGUE SANG, Caque-sang.
GAHET, *Cagot.*
GAÏAC, Guaiacum.
GAILLET ACCROCHANT, Galium aparine —*g. Crochant,* Galium aparine—*g. Jaune,* Galium verum—*g. Vrai,* Galium verum.
GAÎNE, Vagina or sheath—*g. de l'Apophyse styloïde,* Vaginal process of the temporal bone—*g. de la veine porte,* Vagina or sheath of the vena porta.
GALA, γαλα, genitive γαλακτος, milk; hence:
GALACTACRA'SIA, from γαλα, 'milk,' and ακρασια, 'imperfect mixture.' A morbid mixture or constitution of the milk.
GALACTACRATIA, Galactia.
GALACTÆ'MIA, from γαλα, γαλακτος, 'milk,' and 'αιμα, 'blood.' A condition of the blood in which it contains milk.
GALACTAGOGA, Galactopoietica.
GALACTAPOSTEMA, Mastodynia apostematosa.
GALAC'TIA, *Galactirrhœ'a, Galactorrhœ'a,* from γαλα, 'milk.' *Lactis redundan'tia, Polygalac'tia, Galactoze'mia.* A redundant flow of milk, either in a female who is suckling, or in one who is not. It may occur without being provoked by suckling. When to a great extent, it sometimes causes wasting; *Tabes lac'tea, T. nutri'cum.* Dr. Good uses *Galac'tia,* in his Nosology, for 'morbid flow or deficiency of milk,' *Galactacrati'a.*

GALACTICUS, Lactic.
GALACTIFER, Galactophorous.
GALACTINE, Casein.
GALACTINUS, Lactic.
GALACTIRRHŒA, Galactia.
GALACTIS, Galaxias.
GALACTIS'CHESIS, *Galactos'chesis, Lactis reten'tio,* from γαλα, 'milk,' and ισχειν, 'to restrain.' Retention or suppression of milk.
GALACTITES, Galaxias.
GALACTOCATARACTA, Cataract, milky.
GALACTO'DES, from γαλα, 'milk,' and ειδος, 'resemblance.' In Hippocrates, the term signifies milkwarm, and likewise a milky colour, as of the urine—*uri'na galacto'des.*
GALACTODIÆ'TA, *Diæ'ta lac'tea,* from γαλα, 'milk,' and διαιτα, 'diet.' A milk diet.
GALACTODIARRHŒA, Cœliac Flux.
GALACTOGANGLION, Milk knot.
GALACTOHÆ'MIA, *Galacthæ'mia,* from γαλα, 'milk,' and 'αιμα, 'blood:' *Lactis sanguinolen'ti Excre'tio.* The secretion of bloody or bloodlike milk.
GALACTOMASTOPARECTOMA, Mastodynia apostematosa.
GALACTOM'ETER, *Lactom'eter,* from γαλα, 'milk,' and μετρον, 'measure.' An instrument for appreciating the quantity of cream in milk. It is a kind of graduated separatory or *éprouvette*—the degrees on the scale indicating the thickness of the layer of cream that forms on the surface of the milk.
GALACTON'CUS, *Tumor lac'teus,* from γαλα, 'milk,' and ογκος, 'a swelling.' A milk tumour.
GALACTOPH'AGOUS, *Galactoph'agus, Lactiv'orus,* sometimes used substantively; from

γαλα, 'milk,' and φαγω, 'I eat.' That which feeds on milk. A name given to certain people, with whom milk appears to constitute the chief nourishment.

GALACTOPHORA, Galactopoietica.

GALACTOPH'OROUS, *Galac'tifer, Lac'tifer, Lactif'erous*, from γαλα, 'milk,' and φιρω, 'I carry.' That which carries milk.

GALACTOPH'OROUS or LACTIF'EROUS DUCTS, are those which convey the milk, secreted by the mammary gland, towards the nipple, where their external orifices are situate. The *Lacteals* have also been so called.

GALACTOPH'ORUS. Some accoucheurs have given this name to an instrument intended to facilitate sucking, when the faulty conformation of the nipple prevents the child from laying hold of it.

GALACTOPH'YGUS, from γαλα, 'milk,' and φευγειν, 'to shun.' That which arrests or disperses the secretion of milk. Hence *Galactoph'yga Medicamen'ta*.

GALACTOPLA'NIA, *Metas'tasis seu Aberra'tio seu Viæ extraördina'riæ lactis, Galactorrhœa erro'nea*, from γαλα, 'milk,' and πλανη, 'wandering.' Extravasation of milk into the areolar membrane. Secretion of milk elsewhere than from the breasts.

GALACTOPLERO'SIS, from γαλα, 'milk,' and πληρωσις, 'repletion.' Redundance of milk.

GALACTOPOEA, Galactopoietica.

GALACTOPOESIS, Galactosis.

GALACTOPOIESIS, Galactosis.

GALACTOPOIET'ICA, *Galactoph'ora, Galactago'ga, Galactopœ'a*, from γαλα, 'milk,' and ποιεω, 'I make.' Substances, to which has been attributed the property of favouring the secretion of milk and augmenting its quantity.

GALACTOPO'SIA, from γαλα, 'milk,' and ποσις, 'drink.' The drinking of milk. Treatment of a disease by means of milk.

GALACTOP'OTES, *Galactop'otus, Lacti'potor*. Same etymon. A drinker of milk. One subjected to a milk diet.

GALACTOPYRA, Fever, milk.

GALACTOPYRETUS, Fever, milk.

GALACTORRHŒA, Galactia—g. Erronea, Galactoplania—g. Saccharata, Saccharorrhœa lactea.

GALACTOSACCHARUM, Saccharum lactis.

GALACTOSCHESIS, Galactischesis.

GALACTO'SIS, *Galactopoie'sis, Galactopoë'sis, Secre'tio lactis*, from γαλακτομαι, 'I am changed into milk.' The secretion or formation of milk.

GALACTOT'ROPHĒ, *Galactotroph'ia*, from γαλα, 'milk,' and τροφη, 'nourishment.' Nourishment by means of milk.

GALACTOZE'MIA, from γαλα, 'milk,' and ζημια, 'loss.' Loss of milk. Also, Galactia.

GALACTU'CHOS, from γαλα, 'milk,' and εχων, 'to have.' Suckling. Giving milk.

GALACTURIA, Chyluria.

GALANGA, Maranta galanga.

GALANGAL, Maranta galanga.

GALANGALE, Cyperus longus.

GALARHŒUS LATHYRIS, Euphorbia lathyris—g. Palustris, Euphorbia palustris.

GALARIPS, Allamanda.

GALAXIA, Thoracic duct.

GALAX'IAS, *Galacti'tes, Galac'tis*. A milk stone. A stone supposed to be capable of promoting the secretion of milk.

GALBANUM, see Bubon galbanum—g. Long-leaved, Bubon galbanum.

GAL'BULUS, from *galbus*, 'yellow.' A kind of congenital jaundice, in which the yellow colour continues through life. It is rather a defect in colour than a disease.—Vogel.

GALE, Myrica gale—*g. Odorant*, Myrica gale —g. Sweet, Myrica gale.

GALE, Psora—g. Canine, Psoriasis—*g. Épidémique*, Eczema—*g. Miliaire*, Psoriasis—*g. Sèche*, Lichen, Psoriasis.

GA'LEA. A helmet, from γαλη, 'a cat;' of the skin of which it was formerly made. A name given to the *amnios*, and, also, to the *bandage of Galen*. In *Pathology*, it indicates a headach affecting the whole head. See, also, Caul.

GALEA APONEUROT'ICA CAP'ITIS, *Ga'lea tendin'ea Santori'ni, Ga'lea cap'itis, Membra'na epicra'nia*. The tendinous expansion which unites the frontal and occipital portions of the occipito-frontalis muscle.

GALEAMAUROSIS, Amaurotic cat's eye.

GALEAN'CON, *Galian'con*, from γαλεα, 'a cat,' 'a weasel,' and αγκων, 'an elbow.' *Mustela'neus*. One who has two short arms.

GALEAN'THROPY, *Galeanthro'pia*, from γαλη, 'a cat,' and ανθρωπος, 'a man.' A variety of melancholy in which the patient believes himself changed into a cat. An affection similar to lycanthropy and cynanthropy.

GALE'GA, *G. officina'lis seu vulga'ris seu Per'sica, Ruta capra'ria*, Goat's Rue, (F.) *Rue de chèvre, Faux Indigo*. It is slightly aromatic, and was once used as a sudorific and alexiterial in malignant fevers, &c.

GALEGA PERSICA, Galega.

GALEGA VIRGINIA'NA, *Tephro'sia Virginia'na*, Turkey Pea, Hoary Pea, Devil's shoestrings, Virginia Goat's rue or cat-gut, is used in some parts of the United States as an anthelmintic. The decoction of the root is given.

GALEGA VULGARIS, Galega.

GALENE, Graphites.

GALENEA, Graphites.

GALEN'IC, *Galen'ical, Galen'icus, Gale'nius*, from *Galenus*. That which relates to the doctrine of Galen or to Galenism. Used, substantively, for drugs that are not chymical.

GALENIC MEDICINE, Galenism.

GA'LENISM, *Galen'ic med'icine*. The doctrine of Galen.

GA'LENIST, *Galenis'ta, Galenis'tes*. A follower of the doctrine of Galen.

GALENIUS, Galenic.

GALEOBDOLON, Galeopsis.

GALEOPDOLON, Galeopsis.

GALEOPSIS, Lamium album.

GALEOP'SIS, *Galiop'sis, Galeob'dolon, Galeop'dolon, La'mium rubrum, Urti'ca iners magna fœtidis'sima, Stachys fœ'tida*, Hedge nettle, (F.) *Ortie morte des bois*. This plant was formerly reckoned a vulnerary and anodyne.

GALEOPSIS ANGUSTIFOLIA, G. grandiflora—g. Dubia, G. grandiflora.

GALEOP'SIS GRANDIFLO'RA, *G. Ochroleu'ca seu la'danum seu angustifo'lia seu du'bia seu prostra'ta seu villo'sa, Tetrahit longiflo'rum, G. Seg'etum, Herba Sideri'tidis*. This plant is regarded in Germany as a bitter resolvent. It is the basis, also, of a celebrated nostrum, the *Blankenheimer Tea*, called, likewise, *Lieber's pectoral and phthisical herbs* (Liebersche Brust oder Auszehrungs-Krauter,) which has enjoyed great repute in pectoral complaints. The tops of the plant are given in decoction, (℥j, boiled in a pint of water for a quarter of an hour.) This quantity to be taken in a day.

GALEOPSIS LADANUM, G. grandiflora—g. Ochroleuca, G. grandiflora—g. Prostrata, G. grandiflora —g. Segetum, G. grandiflora.

GALEOP'SIS VERSIC'OLOR, is possessed of the same virtues.

GALEOPSIS VILLOSA, G. grandiflora.

GALEROPIA, Oxyopia.

GA'LIA. An ancient composition, in which galls were an ingredient; the *Galia pura.* There was, also, a *Galia aromat'ica, moscha'ta* vel *musca'ta*, which consisted of a mixture of several perfumes, such as musk.

GALIANCON, Galeancon.

GALIOPSIS, Galeopsis.

GALIPÆA FEBRIFUGA, Cusparia febrifuga —g. Officinalis, see Cusparia febrifuga.

GALIPOT, see Pinus sylvestris.

GA'LIUM, *Gal'lium,* (from γαλα, 'milk,' because some species curdle milk.) G. verum.

GALIUM ALBUM, G. Mollugo.

GA'LIUM APARI'NE, *G. infest'um* seu *aparinoï'des* seu *brachycarp'on* seu *scaber'rimum, Valan'tia apari'nē, Apari'nē his'pida, Aparinē, Lappa, Philanthro'pus, Ampelocar'pus, Omphalocar'pus, Ixus, Asphari'nē, Asper'ula,* Goose-grass, Cleaver's bees, Cleavers, Goose-share, Hayriff. Family, Rubiaceæ. *Sex. Syst.* Tetrandria Monogynia. (F.) *Gaillet accrochant, G. crochant, Gratteron.* The expressed juice has been given as an aperient diuretic in incipient dropsies; also, in cancer.

GALIUM APARANOIDES, G. aparine.

GA'LIUM ASPRELLUM, *Rough bed-straw, Rough ladies' bed-straw*: indigenous; has the diuretic properties of most of its genus.

GALIUM BRACHYCARPON, G. aparine—g. Caucasicum, G. verum.

GALIUM CIRCÆ'ZANS, *Wild Liquorice, Master of the Woods.* An indigenous plant, which flowers from June to August. It is demulcent and diuretic, and is a popular domestic remedy.

GALIUM INFESTE, G. aparine — g. Luteum, G. verum.

GALIUM MOLLU'GO, *Galium album* seu *Tyrolen'sē, Greater ladies' bed-straw, Alys'sum Plin'ii,* (F.) *Caillelait blanc.* The herb and flowers have been used, medicinally, in epilepsy.

GALIUM ODORATUM, Asperula odorata—g. Scaberrimum, G. aparine.

GA'LIUM TINCTO'RUM, an American species, closely allied in properties to G. verum.

GALIUM TYROLENSE, G. mollugo—g. Tuberculatum, g. Verum.

GA'LIUM VERUM, *Ga'lium, G. lu'teum* seu *Cauca'sicum* seu *tubercula'tum, Ladies' bed-straw, Cheese-rennet, Bed-straw, Cleavewort, Goose-grass, Savoyan, Clabber-grass, Milkweet, Poor Robin, Gravel-grass,* (F.) *Gaillet jaune, G. vrai, Vrai Caillelait.* The tops were used in the cure of epilepsy. The leaves and flowers possess the property of curdling milk.

GALL, Bile, see Eczema impetiginodes, Quercus infectoria, and Vitrum—g. of the earth, Prenanthes—g. Nut, see Quercus infectoria — g. of the Ox, see Bile—g. Sickness, Fever, Walcheren—g. Turkey, see Quercus infectoria.

GALL-BLADDER, *Vesic'ula fellis, Chol'ecyst, Cholecys'tis, Follic'ulus fellis, Cystis fel'lea, Vesi'ca fellea, Vesic'ula bilis. Vesi'ca bilia'ria, Follic'ulus fel'leus, Cystis choled'ochus,* (F.) *Vésicule du fiel* ou *Vésicule biliaire, Réservoir de la bile.* A membranous, pyriform reservoir, lodged in a superficial depression at the inferior surface of the right lobe of the liver. It receives, by the hepatic and cystic ducts, a portion of the bile secreted by the liver, when the stomach is empty, which becomes in it more acrid, bitter, and thick. It receives an artery, called the *cystic.* Its veins empty into the vena porta. Its nerves come from the hepatic plexus, and its lymphatic vessels join those of the liver.

GALLA, see Quercus infectoria—g. Maxima Orbiculata, see Quercus infectoria.

GALLÆ QUERCÛS, see Quercus infectoria— g. Tinctoriæ, see Quercus infectoria—g. Turcicæ, see Quercus infectoria.

GALLATURA, Molecule.

GALLI GALLINACEI CAPUT, Gallinaginis caput.

GALLINAG"INIS CAPUT, *Galli gallina'cei Caput, Caput gallina'ceum, Verumonta'num, Crista urethra'lis, Crête uréthrale,*—(Ch.,) from *Gallinago,* 'a woodcock.' An oblong, rounded projection, formed by the mucous membrane in the spongy portion of the urethra, at the sides of which the ejaculatory ducts open.

GAL'LIPOT. Perhaps from *gala,* 'finery.' (?) A pot painted and glazed or merely glazed, and commonly used to hold medicines.

GALLITRICHUM, Salvia sclarea.

GALLIUM, Galium.

GALLSTONES, Calculi, biliary.

GALLUS, Eunuch.

GALREDA, Gelatin.

GALVANISATION, Galvanization.

GAL'VANISM, *Galvanis'mus, Electric"itas anima'lis, E. Galvan'ica* vel *metal'lica, Irritamen'tum metallo'rum* vel *metal'licum, Vol'taism, Volta'ic* or *Chemical* or *Contact Electricity.* A series of phenomena, consisting in sensible movements, executed by animal parts, which are endowed with irritability, when placed in connexion with two metallic plates of different nature, between which a communication is established by direct contact or by means of a metallic wire. Galvanism has been employed medicinally in the same cases as electricity, and especially in neuralgic affections. It is often applied in the form of plates,—"*Mansford's plates.*" In asthma, for example, a small blister, the size of a dollar, may be placed on the neck over the course of the phrenic and pneumogastric nerves, and another on the side, in the region of the diaphragm. One metal is placed mediately or immediately over the vesicated surface on the neck, and another over that in the side. They are then connected by means of a wire. The new nervous impression, in this way induced, is often signally beneficial.

GALVANIZATION, *Galvanisa'tio,* (F.) *Galvanisation.* The act of affecting with galvanism.

GALVANOPUNCTURE, Electropuncture.

GAMBA, Patella.

GAMBARUS, Crab.

GAMBIER, see Nauclea gambir.

GAMBOGIA, Cambogia.

GAMMARUS, Crab.

GAM'MATA FERRAMEN'TA. Cauteries, having the shape of the Greek letter Γ; which were used for cauterizing herniæ.

GAMMAUT. The Italians, according to Scultetus, gave this name to a kind of crooked bistouri, used for opening abscesses.

GAMMISMUS, Psammismus.

GAMPHE, Gena.

GAMPHELE, Gena, Maxillary Bone.

GANGAME, Epiploon.

GANGAMUM, Epiploon.

GANGLIA CEREBRI POSTICA, Thalami nervorum opticorum—g. Formative, see Ganglion — g. Hemispherical, Hemispheres of the brain — g. of Increase, see Ganglion — g. Nervorum, Ganglions, nervous, see Ganglion—g. Sensory, see Sensory ganglia.

GANGLIAR, Ganglionic.

GANG'LIFORM, *Gang'lioform, Ganglifor'mis.* Having the shape of a ganglion. A name generally given to a knot-like enlargement, in the course of a nerve.

GANGLIOLUM, Diminutive of ganglion. A small ganglion.

GANG'LION, *Gang'lium*, 'a knot.' A name given to organs differing considerably from each other in size, colour, texture, functions, &c. They are divided into *glandiform, lymphatic*, and *nervous*. 1. *Glandiform ganglions*, called also *adenoid, vascular*, and *sanguineous ganglions, blind, aporic*, and *vascular glands, glandulæ spuriæ*, &c., are organs of whose functions we are, in general, ignorant; and which have the appearance of glands. They are formed of agglomerated globules, pervaded by blood-vessels, surrounded by areolar membrane, and contain a milky or yellowish fluid. To this class belong the spleen, thymus, thyroid, and supra-renal glands. 2. *Lymphatic ganglions*. See Conglobate. 3. *Nervous ganglions, Ganglia* seu *Nodi* seu *Nod'uli Nervo'rum, Ganglio'nes, Tumo'res* seu *Plexus gangliqform'es, Plexus glandiform'es, Tuber'cula nodo'sa Nervo'rum, Divertic'ula spirituum anima'lium, Ganglia of increase, Form'ative gang'lia*. Enlargements or knots in the course of a nerve. They belong, in general, to the system of the great sympathetic. One exists on the posterior root of every spinal nerve, and on one cerebral,— the 5th. Bichat regarded them as so many small brains, or centres of nervous action, independent of the encephalon, and intended exclusively for organic life. Being formed by the union of the cerebral and spinal nerves, they may send out the influence of both these nervous centres to the parts to which the nerves proceeding from them are distributed. Ganglia are chiefly composed of vesicular neurine; and appear to be concerned in the formation and dispensation of nerve power.

GANGLION. Same etymon. *Emphy'ma encys'tis ganglion*. A globular, hard, indolent tumour, without change in the colour of the skin; of a size varying from that of a pea, to that of an egg, and always situate in the course of a tendon. The tumour is formed of a viscid, albuminous fluid, contained in a cyst of greater or less thickness. The cyst is sometimes loose; but in the majority of cases it communicates, by a narrow footstalk, with the sheath of a tendon, or even with the synovial capsule of a neighbouring articulation. The *causes* are generally unknown. The *treatment* consists in compression, percussion, the use of discutients, extirpation, or incision.

GANGLION ABDOMINALE, G. semilunar—g. Adenoid, G. glandiform—g. of Andersch, Petrous ganglion—g. Annular, see Ciliary ligament—g. of Arnold, Oticum ganglion—g. Auricular, Oticum G.—g. Azygous, see Trisplanchnic nerve—g. Cardiac, Cardiac ganglion—g. Carotic or Carotid, see Carotid or Carotic nerve—g. Cavernous, see Carotid or Carotic nerve—g. Cerebelli, Corpus dentatum—g. Cerebral, anterior, Corpora striata—g. Cerebri Anterius, Corpora striata—g. *Cérébral inférieur, grand*, Thalami nervorum opticorum—g. Cerebral, posterior, Thalami nervorum opticorum—*g. du Cervelet*, Corpus dentatum—g. Ciliare, Corpus dentatum—g. Ciliary, Ophthalmic ganglion—g. Corpuscles, see Neurine.

GANGLION OF EHRENRITTER, *Ganglion nervi glosso-pharynge'i supe'rius, G. jugula'rs supe'rius, G. Ehrenritteri* seu *Mulleri*. A reddish-gray mass on the glosso-pharyngeal nerve in the foramen lacerum, above the ganglion of Andersch.

GANGLION OF GASSER, *Gan'glium* seu *Gan'glion Gasseri, Moles gangliform'is, Intumescen'tia gangliform'is* seu *semiluna'ris, Tæ'nia nervo'sa Halleri*. A semicircular knot on the 5th pair of nerves, before its division into three branches.

GANGLION, GLANDIFORM, see Ganglion—g. Globules, see Neurine—Impar, see Trisplanchnic nerve—g. Jugulare superius, G. of Ehrenritter—*g. Laiteux*, Milk-knot—g. of Laumonier, see Carotid or Carotic nerve—g. Lenticular, G. ophthalmic—g. Lymphatic, Conglobate gland—*g. Maxillotympanique*, Oticum G.—g. of Meckel, Sphenopalatine G.—g. Mulleri, G. of Ehrenritter—g. Nasopalatine, see Nasopalatine ganglion—g. Nervi glosso-pharyngei superius, G. of Ehrenritter—g. Ophthalmic, see Ophthalmic ganglion—g. Optic, Quadrigemina tubercula—g. Orbitar, G. ophthalmic—g. Oticum, Oticum G.—g. Petrosal, see Petrous ganglion.

GANGLION OF THE PNEUMOGAS'TRIC. A ganglionic structure in the pneumogastric as it passes through the foramen lacerum posterius.

GANGLION OF RIBES. A nervous ganglion upon the anterior communicating artery of the brain, and to be found at the point of junction of the right and left trunks of the sympathetic.

GANGLION, SANGUINEOUS, G. glandiform—g. Sensory, see Sensory ganglia—g. Solare, G. semilunare—g. Sphenoidal, Sphenopalatine ganglion—g. Splanchnicum, G. semilunare—*g. Supérieur du cerveau (grand,)* Corpora striata—g. of the Superior Laryngeal Branch, see Pneumogastric nerves—*g. Surrénal*, G. semilunare—g. Thyroid, see Trisplanchnic nerve—g. Transversum, G. semilunare—g. Vascular, G. glandiform—g. Vertebral, see Trisplanchnic nerve—*g. de Vieussens*, Cœliac plexus.

GANGLIONARY, Ganglionic.

GANGLIONES GANGLIOFORMES, Ganglions, nervous.

GANGLION'IC, *Ganglion'icus, Gan'glionary, Gan'gliar*. Relating to ganglia. Nerves are so called in the course of which ganglions are met with; as the greater part of the branches of the great sympathetic or trisplanchnic, the posterior roots of the spinal nerves, &c. *Ganglionics*, according to Dr. Pereira, are agents, which affect the ganglionic or great sympathetic system of nerves,(?)—as stimulants and sedatives.

GANGLIONIC NERVE, Trisplanchnic nerve—g. Nervous System, see Trisplanchnic nerve.

GANGLIONI'TIS, *Gangliï'tis*, from γαγγλιον, 'a ganglion,' and *itis*, denoting inflammation. Inflammation of a nervous ganglion. Sometimes used for inflammation of a lymphatic ganglion.

GANGLIONITIS PERIPHERICA et MEDULLARIS, Cholera.

GANGLIUM, Ganglion—g. Gasseri, Ganglion of Gasser.

GANGRÆ'NA ALOPECIA, Alopecia—g. Caries, Caries—g. Nosocomiorum, Hospital gangrene—g. Oris, Cancer aquaticus—g. Ossis, Spina ventosa—g. Ossium, Caries—g. Pottii, see Gangrene, and Gangrene of old people—g. Pulmonum, Necropneumonia—g. Senilis, Gangrene of old people—g. Sphacelus, Sphacelus—g. Tonsillarum, Cynanche maligna—g. Ustilaginea, Ergotism—g. Vaginæ, Colpocace.

GANGRÆNESCENTIA, Gangrænosis.

GANGRÆNICUS, Gangrenous.

GANGRÆNODES, Gangrenous.

GANGRÆNOPS'IS, Cancer aquaticus; also, gangrenous inflammation of the eyelids, *Blephari'tis gangræno'sa*.—Siebenhaar.

GANGRÆNO'SIS, *Gangrænescen'tia*, from γαγγραινα, 'gangrene.' The state of being gangrenous or of becoming gangrenous.

GANGRÆNOSUS, Gangrenous.

GANGRENE, *Gangræ'na, Cancre'na, Hot mortification*, (F.) *Gangrène, G. Chaude, Asphyxie des parties*. Privation of life or partial death of an organ. Authors have generally distinguished mortification into two stages; naming the first *incipient* or *gangrene*. It is attended with a sudden diminution of feeling in the part affected;

livid discoloration; detachment of the cuticle, under which a turbid fluid is effused; with crepitation, owing to the disengagement of air into the areolar texture. When the part has become quite black, and incapable of all feeling, circulation, and life, it constitutes the *second stage*, or *mortification*, and is called *sphac"elus*. Gangrene, however, is frequently used synonymously with mortification, — *local asphyxia* being the term employed for that condition, in which the parts are in a state of suspended animation, and, consequently, susceptible of resuscitation. When the part is filled with fluid entering into putrefaction, the affection is called *humid gangrene*, (F.) *Gangrène humide:* on the other hand, when it is dry and shrivelled, it constitutes *dry gangrene;* (F.) *Gangrène sèche*. To this class belongs the *gangræ'na seni'lis*, *G. Pot'tii*, *Presbyosphac"elus*, or *spontaneous gangrene* of old people, which rarely admits of cure. Whatever may be the kind of gangrene, it may be caused by violent inflammation, contusion, a burn, congelation, the ligature of a large arterial trunk, or by some internal cause inappreciable to us.

The treatment, both of external and internal gangrene, varies according to the causes which produce it. Gangrene from excessive inflammation is obviated by antiphlogistics; and that from intense cold by cautiously restoring the circulation by cold frictions, &c. When the gangrene has become developed, the separation of the eschars must be encouraged by emollient applications, if there be considerable reaction; or by tonics and stimulants, if the reaction be insufficient.

GANGRENE, HOSPITAL, see Hospital, Gangrene —g. of the Lungs, Necropneumonia.

GANGRÈNE DE LA BOUCHE, Cancer aquaticus — *g. Chaude*, Gangrene — *g. Froide* Sphacelus — *g. Humide*, see Gangrene — *g. Sèche*, see Gangrene — *g. Hôpital*, Hospital gangrene — *g. du Poumon*, Necropneumonia — *g. des Solonois*, Ergotism.

GAN'GRENOUS, *Gangræ'nicus, Gangræno'sus, Gangræno'des*. Affected with or relating to gangrene.

GANJAH, Gunjah.

GANTELET (F.), *Chirothe'ca, Fas'cia digita'lis, Gauntlet;* from (F.) *gant*, 'a glove.' A sort of bandage which envelops the hand and fingers, like a glove. It is made with a long roller, about an inch broad; and is applied so that the fingers are covered to their tips, when it is called *Gantelet entier* ou *complet*. The *Demigantelet* includes only the hand and base of the fingers. Both bandages are used in fractures and luxations of the fingers, burns of the hand, &c. See Chirotheca.

GANTS DES DAMES, Condom—*g. de Notre Dame*, Digitalis.

GAPING, Yawning.

GARANCE, Rubia.

GARCIN'IA CAMBO'GIA, *G. gutta, Cambogia gutta, Mangosta'na Cambogia*. A tree of Ceylon, *Family* Guttiferæ, which affords a concrete juice similar to Gamboge.

GARCINIA GUTTA, G. Cambogia.

GARCIN'IA MANGOSTA'NA, *Mangosta'na Garcin'ia*. The systematic name of the *Mangos'tan* or *Mangous'tan tree, Mangosta'na*. It grows in great abundance in Java and the Molucca islands. The fruit, which is about the size of an orange, is delicious, and is eaten in almost every disorder. The dried bark is used medicinally in dysentery and tenesmus; and a strong decoction has been much esteemed in ulcerated sore throat.

GARDE-MALADE, Nurse.

GARDEROBE, Artemisia abrotanum.

GARDEROBES, Fæces.

GARDINER'S ALIMENTARY PREPARATION, see Oryza.

GARDOUCHES, Vesiculæ seminales.

GARETUM, Poples.

GARGALISMUS, Gargalus.

GAR'GALUS, *Gar'galē, Gargalis'mus, Titilla'tio, Irrita'tio, Pruri'tus*. Titillation, irritation, itching. Also, masturbation; and, rarely, animal magnetism.

GARGAREON, Uvula.

GARGARISATIO, Gargarism.

GAR'GARISM, *Gargaris'mus, Gargaris'ma, Anagargalic'ton, Gargaris'mum, Collu'tio, Diaclys'ma, Anagargaris'ton, Anagargariem'us, Anaconchylis'mus, Anaconchylias'mus, Titillamen'tum,* from γαργαρίζω, 'I wash the mouth.' A gargle. Any liquid medicine, intended to be retained in the mouth, for a certain time, and to be thrown in contact with the uvula, velum pendulum, tonsils, &c. For this purpose, the liquid is agitated by the air issuing from the larynx, the head being thrown back. Gargles are employed in cynanche tonsillaris and other diseases of the fauces, and are made of stimulants, sedatives, astringents, refrigerants, &c., according to circumstances.

The process is termed *gargling, gargarisa'tio*. The term *colluto'rium* or *collutorium oris* is generally restricted to a wash for the mouth.

GARGET, Phytolacca decandra.

GARGLE, Gargarism.

GARGLING, see Gargarism.

GARGOUILLEMENT, Borborygmus, Gurgling. See *Râle muqueux*.

GARLIC, Allium—g. Hedge, Alliaria.

GAROSMUM, Chenopodium vulvaria.

GAROU BARK, Daphne gnidium.

GARRETUM, Poples.

GARROPHYLLUS, Eugenia caryophyllata.

GARROT (F.), from *garotter*, 'to tie fast.' A small cylinder of wood, used for tightening the circular band, by which the arteries of a limb are compressed, for the purpose of suspending the flow of blood in cases of hemorrhage, aneurism, amputation, &c.

GARROTILLO, Cynanche maligna.

GARRULITAS, Loquacity.

GARU'LEUM BIPINNA'TUM. A South African plant, *Nat. Ord.* Compositæ; known under the name *Snakeroot*, from its reputed effects as an antidote to the bites of venomous serpents. The root is a great favourite with the Boers in chest diseases—as asthma—and in affections in which a free secretion from the mucous membrane of the bronchia is indicated. It has diaphoretic properties, and acts as a diuretic in gout and dropsy. It is given in decoction or tincture. Dr. Pappe thinks the root ought to have a place in the Materia Medica.

GARUM, γαρον. The ancient Romans gave this name to a kind of pickle made by collecting the liquor which flowed from salted and half-putrefied fish. It was used as a condiment.—The *Geoponice*, Humelberg on Apicius, Martial, &c.

GAS, see Gaz — g. Ammoniacale, Ammonia— g. Animale sanguinis, G. sanguinis—g. Azoticum, Azote — g. Azoticum oxygenatum, Nitrogen, gaseous oxide of—g. Hepaticum, Hydrogen, sulphuretted — g. Hydrogenium sulphuretum, Hydrogen, sulphuretted—g. Intoxicating, Nitrogen, gaseous oxide of—g. Laughing, Nitrogen, gaseous oxide of — g. of the Lungs. Gas, pulmonary—g. Nitrous, dephlogisticated, Nitrogen, gaseous oxide of — g. Oxygenated muriatic acid, Chlorine — g. Oxymuriatic acid, Chlorine—g. Palustre, Miasm, marsh — g. Paradise, Nitrogen, gaseous oxide of —g. Sulphuris, Sulphurous acid.

GASCARILLA, Croton cascarilla.

GASTEIN, MINERAL WATERS OF. Gastein or Gasteiner Wildbad is in the Noric Alps, Austria. The waters are thermal. Temp. 106° to 118° Fah. They contain sulphate of soda, chloride of sodium, chloride of potassium, carbonate of soda, carbonate of lime, magnesia, manganese, iron, &c.

GASTER, γαστηρ. The abdomen. At times, but rarely, the uterus. Also, the stomach, in particular; Hence:

GASTERALGIA, Gastralgia.

GASTERANAX. A name given by Dolæus to a hypothetical vital principle, corresponding to the Archæus of Van Helmont, the seat of which he placed in the lower belly. See Bithnimalos.

GASTERANGEMPHRAXIS, Gasterangiemphraxis.

GASTERANGIEMPHRAX'IS, Gasterangemphrax'is, Gasteremphrax'is. Obstruction of the pylorus, from γαστηρ, 'stomach,' αγχω, 'I strangle,' and εμφρασσω, 'I obstruct.'—Vogel. Also, and properly, obstruction or congestion of the vessels of the stomach.

GASTERASE, Pepsin.

GASTERASTHENI'A, Imbecil'itas seu Aton'ia seu Lax'itas ventric'uli; from γαστηρ, 'stomach,' and ασθενεια, 'debility.' Debility of the stomach.

GASTERECHE'MA, Son'itus stomach'icus; from γαστηρ, 'the stomach,' and ηχημα, 'sound.' Sound presumed to be heard on auscultating the region of the stomach.

GASTEREMPHRAXIS, Gasterangiemphraxis.

GASTERHYSTEROTOMY, Cæsarean Section.

GASTRÆ'MIA; from γαστηρ, 'the stomach,' and 'αιμα, 'blood.' Determination of blood to the stomach.

GASTRALGIA, Cardialgia.

GASTRANEURYSMA, Gastrectasis.

GASTRATROPH'IA, from γαστηρ, 'the stomach,' and ατροφια, 'wasting.' Atrophy of the stomach.

GASTREC'TASIS, Gastrecta'sia, Gastraneurys'ma, Dilata'tio ventric'uli: from γαστηρ, 'the stomach,' and εκτασις, 'dilatation.' Dilatation of the stomach.

GASTRELCOBROSIS, Gastrobrosis ulcerosa.

GASTRELCO'SIS, Ulcera'tio seu Exulcera'tio seu Ul'cera ventric'uli, from γαστηρ, 'the stomach,' and 'ελκωσις, 'ulceration.' Ulceration of the stomach. When accompanied with hectic, it constitutes Gastrophthi'sis, Gastroph'thoë.

GASTRELYTROTOMIA, see Cæsarean Section.

GASTRENCEPHALO'MA, Gastromyelo'ma, Gastromyelo'sis, Gastroëncephalo'sis; from γαστηρ, 'the stomach,' and εγκεφαλος, 'the brain.' Encephaloid of the stomach.

GASTRENCHYTA, Stomach pump.

GASTRENTERIC, Gastroentericus.

GASTRENTERITIC, Gastroenteritic.

GASTRENTEROMALA'CIA, Gastrenteromalax'ia, from γαστηρ, 'stomach,' εντερον, 'intestine,' and μαλακια, 'softening.' Softening of the stomach and intestines.

GASTREPATICUS, Gastrohepatic.

GASTREPATI'TIS, Inflamma'tio ventric'uli et hep'atis; from γαστηρ, 'stomach,' and 'ηπαρ, 'liver.' Inflammation of the stomach and liver.

GASTREPIPLOICUS, Gastroëpiploic.

GASTRERETHIS'IA; from γαστηρ, 'stomach,' and ερεθιζω, 'I irritate.' Irritation of the stomach.

GASTRIC, Gas'tricus; from γαστηρ, 'the stomach.' Belonging or relating to the stomach.

GASTRIC AR'TERIES are three in number, Arte'ria gastro-epiplo'ica dextra, A. gastro-epiploi'ca sinis'tra, and A. corona'ria ventric'uli.

GASTRIC JUICE, Succus gas'tricus, Men'struum seu Fermentum Ventric'uli, (F.) Suc Gastrique, Gastric Acid. A fluid, secreted from the mucous membrane of the stomach. As met with, it is a mixture of the fluids secreted by that organ with those of the supra-diaphragmatic portion of the alimentary canal. Owing to such admixture, the most contrary properties have been assigned to it. That such a fluid is secreted, which concurs powerfully in digestion, is evident from many considerations, and has been positively proved by the author and numerous others. It was found by him to contain, in man, chlorohydric and acetic acids. The gastric fluid in cases of sudden death sometimes corrodes and perforates the stomach; giving rise to interesting questions in medical jurisprudence.

GASTRIC NERVES. The two cords by which the pneumogastric nerves terminate, and which descend on the two surfaces of the stomach; as well as the filaments of the great sympathetic, which accompany the gastric vessels.

GASTRIC PLEXUS, Plexus corona'rius ventric'uli. A nervous net-work, formed by the solar plexus. It accompanies the Arteria coronaria ventriculi, and passes along the lesser curvature of the stomach, to which it gives branches.

GASTRIC VEINS follow the same distribution as the arteries, and open into the Vena porta abdominis.

GAS'TRICISM, Gastricis'mus, from γαστηρ, 'the stomach.' A name by which is designated the medical theory, that refers all, or almost all, diseases to an accumulation of saburræ in the digestive passages.

GASTRILOQUE, Engastrimyth.

GASTRILOQUIST, Engastrimyth.

GASTRILOQUUS, Engastrimyth.

GASTRIMARGUS, Glutton.

GASTRINUM, Potash.

CASTRISMUS, Gluttony, see Saburra.

GASTRIT'IC, Gastrit'icus; same etymon as the rest. Relating to gastritis.

GASTRI'TIS, from γαστηρ, 'the stomach,' and itis, denoting inflammation. Ventric'uli inflamma'tio, Causma gastritis, Empres'ma gastritis, Inflamma'tio gastritis, Cardial'gia inflammato'ria, Febris stomach'ica inflammato'ria, Inflamma'tio ventric'uli, I. stom'achi, Phleg'monè ventric'uli, Inflammation of the stomach, (F.) Inflammation de l'Estomac, Gastrite, Catarrhe gastrique. A disease, characterized by pyrexia; great anxiety; heat and pain in the epigastrium, increased by taking any thing into the stomach; vomiting and hiccup. Gastritis may either be seated in the peritoneal or mucous coat. It is most frequently in the latter—Esogastri'tis, Endogastri'tis, Gastromycoderi'tis,—being excited directly by acrid ingesta. It requires the most active treatment; — bleeding, blistering, fomentations, diluents, &c. Some degree of inflammation of the mucous coat of the stomach was considered by the followers of Broussais to be present in almost all fevers; and the various forms of dyspepsia have been supposed by some to be nothing more than chronic endogastri'tis.

GASTRITIS ARTHRITICA, Cœliagra.

GASTRO-ARTHRITIS, Gout—g. Ataxia, Dyspepsia—g. Atonia, Dyspepsia—g. Bronchitis, Fever, adenomeningeal—g. Entérite intense Synocha—*g. Entérite*, with nervous affection of the brain, see Typhus—g. Enteritis, follicular, Dothinenteritis; see Typhus.

GASTROBRO'SIS, *Perfora'tio ventric'uli, Gastrorrhex'is,* (F.) *Perforation de l'Estomac;* from γαστηρ, 'the stomach,' and βρωσις, 'the act of gnawing.' Corrosion and perforation of the stomach.

GASTROBRO'SIS ULCERO'SA, *Gastrelcobro'sis.* Destruction and perforation of the coats of the stomach by ulceration.

GASTROCE'LE, from γαστηρ, 'the belly,' and κηλη, 'a tumour.' *Hernia of the stomach, Hernia ventric'uli,* (F.) *Hernie de l'Estomac.* Hernia, formed by the stomach through the upper part of the linea alba: a disease, the existence of which has been doubted by many. See Epigastrocele.

GASTRO-CEPHALI'TIS; from γαστηρ, 'the stomach,' κεφαλη, 'head,' and *itis,* denoting inflammation. Inflammation of the stomach and head,—a not uncommon concomitant of certain malignant fevers.

GASTROCHOLOSIS, Fever, gastric.
GASTROCNEME, Sura.
GASTROCNEMIA, Sura.
GASTROCNE'MII, from γαστηρ, 'the belly,' and κνημη, 'the leg.' The name of the two fleshy masses which occupy the posterior and superficial part of the leg, *Gemelli;* (F.) *Gastrocnémiens, Jumeaux de la jambe, Bifémoro-calcaniens*—(Ch.:) the two constituting the *Gastrocne'mius exter'nus,* of English anatomists. These muscles are distinguished into *internal* and *external,* which are distinct above, but united at their inferior extremity. They are long, flat, and thick; and arise—the *former* from the posterior part of the outer condyle of the femur; the *latter,* from the posterior part of the inner condyle of the same bone. The aponeurosis, which unites these muscles below, joins with that of the solaris, and forms with it, a large tendon, which, under the name *Tendo-Achillis,* is inserted at the posterior part of the calcaneum. These muscles extend the foot on the leg, and the leg on the foot. They can, also, bend the leg and the thigh reciprocally on each other. For the *Gastrocnemius internus,* see Soleus.

GASTROCNEMIUM, Sura.
GASTROCŒLIACUS, Cœliac.
GASTROCŒLICUS, Cœliac.
GASTROCOLIC, see Epiploon, gastrocolic.
GASTROCOLICA, Cardialgia.
GASTROCOLI'TIS, from γαστηρ, 'stomach,' and κωλον, 'colon.' Inflammation of the stomach and colon.

GASTROCOLPOTOMIA, see Cæsarean section.

GASTRODID'YMUS, *Did'ymus, Symphyogas'trius, Peod'ymus;* from γαστηρ, 'the belly,' and διδυμος, 'a twin.' A monstrosity in which twins are united by the abdomen.

GASTRODUODE'NAL, *Gastroduodena'lis;* from γαστηρ, 'stomach,' and *duodenum.* Relating to the stomach and duodenum.

GASTRODUODENOPYRA, Fever, adenomeningeal.
GASTRODYNE, Cardialgia.
GASTRODYNIA, Cardialgia—g. Flatulenta, Colica flatulenta.

GASTROËNTER'IC, *Gastroënter'icus, Gastrenter'ic, Gastrenter'icus,* from γαστηρ, 'the stomach,' and εντερον, 'intestine.' Relating to the stomach and intestine.

GASTROËNTÉRITE, Gastroenteritis.

GASTROËNTERIT'IC, *Gastroënterit'icus,* *Gastrenterit'ic, Gastrenterit'icus;* same etymon as the next. Relating to gastroenteritis.

GASTROËNTERI'TIS, *Inflamma'tio ventric'uli et Intestino'rum,* (F.) *Gastro-entérite, Gastroenter'ic disease,* from γαστηρ, 'the stomach,' εντερον, 'an intestine,' and *itis,* a suffix denoting inflammation. Inflammation of the stomach and small intestine. According to Broussais, the essential fevers of authors are gastro-enteritis, simple, or complicated.

GASTROËPIP'LOIC, *Gastro-epiplo'icus, Gastrepiplo'icus,* from γαστηρ, 'the stomach,' and επιπλοον, 'the epiploon.' That which relates to the stomach and epiploon.

GASTROËPIPLOIC ARTERIES, or *Gastric inferior,* are two in number, and distinguished into *right* and *left.* The *right,* also called *Gastro-hepatic, Gas'trica inferior dextra, Gastro-epiplo'ica dextra,* is furnished by the hepatic artery. It descends behind the pylorus, and passes from right to left, along the great curvature of the stomach. It gives branches to the pancreas, duodenum, stomach, omentum majus, and terminates by anastomosing with the *Gastro-epiplo'ica sinis'tra, Gas'trica sinis'tra, Gas'trica infe'rior sinis'tra.* This—the *left*—arises from the splenic artery. It is of considerable magnitude, and passes from left to right, along the great curvature of the stomach, distributing its branches more particularly to the stomach and omentum majus. It terminates by joining the right gastro-epiploic.

GASTROEPIPLOIC GANGLIONS are the lymphatic ganglions or glands, situate towards the great curvature of the stomach, between the two anterior laminæ of the omentum majus.

GASTROEPIPLOIC VEINS are distinguished, like the arteries, into *right* and *left.* They empty themselves;—the former, into the superior mesenteric: the latter, into the splenic vein.

GASTROHÆMORRHAGIA, Hæmatemesis.
GASTROHEPAT'IC, *Gastro-hepat'icus, Hep'ato-gas'tricus, Gastrepat'icus;* from γαστηρ, 'the stomach,' and 'ηπαρ, 'the liver.' Relating to the stomach and liver. This name has been given to several organs. See Epiploon, gastrohepatic, &c.

GASTROHYSTEROTOMY, Cæsarean section.
GASTROLIENALIS, Gastrosplenicus.
GASTROLITHI'ASIS, from γαστηρ, 'the stomach,' and λιθιασις, 'formation of stone.' The formation of concretions, *gastrol'ithi,* in the stomach.

GASTROMALACIA, Gastromalaxia.
GASTROMALAX'IA, *Gastro-mala'cia, Gastromalaco'sis, Malacogas'ter, Malax'is ventric'uli, Dissolu'tio ventric'uli, Emollit''io ventric'uli, Pseudophlogo'sis ventric'uli resoluti'va et colliquati'va, Metamorpho'sis ventric'uli gelatinifor'mis, Ero'sio et perfora'tio sponta'nea ventric'uli, Resolu'tio et diabro'sis ventric'uli,* (F.) *Ramollissement de l'Estomac,* from γαστηρ, 'the stomach,' and μαλαξις, 'softening.' Softening of the stomach, induced at times by the gastric secretions after death,—*Resolu'tio ventric'uli autopeptica.*

GASTROMANTIS, Engastrimyth.
GASTROMETROTOMIA, Cæsarean section.
GASTROMYCODERIS, see Stomach.
GASTROMYCODERITIS, see Gastritis.
GASTROMYELOMA, Gastroencephaloma.
GASTRONOSUS, Gastropathia.
GASTROPARAL'YSIS, *Gastrople'gia, Paral'ysis ventric'uli;* from γαστηρ, 'the stomach,' and παραλυσις, 'paralysis.' Paralysis of the stomach.

GASTROP'ATHY, *Gastropathi'a, Gastron'osus, Gastronu'sus,* from γαστηρ, 'the stomach,' and παθος, 'disease.' Disease of the stomach.

GASTROPERIODYN'IA; *Sool* (India.) A

violent periodical neuralgic pain at the pit of the stomach, not uncommon in Hindoostan.

GASTROPHREN'IC, *Gastro-phren'icus*, from γαστηρ, 'the stomach,' and φρενες, 'the diaphragm.' Belonging to the stomach and diaphragm.

GASTROPHRENIC LIGAMENT is a reflection of the peritoneum, which descends from the inferior surface of the diaphragm to the cardia.

GASTROPHTHISIS, Gastrelcosis.
GASTROPHTHOE, Gastrelcosis.
GASTROPLEGIA, Gastroparalysis.

GASTROR'APHY, *Gastrorrha'phia*, *Gastror'-rhaphê*, *Sutu'ra abdomina'lis*, from γαστηρ, 'the belly,' and ραφη, 'a suture.' The suture used for uniting wounds penetrating the abdomen, when they are too extensive or too unequal to be kept in contact by position, adhesive plaster, or appropriate bandages. The *interrupted* and *quilled* sutures are those chiefly employed.

GASTRORRHAGIA, Hæmatemesis.
GASTRORRHEXIS, Gastrobrosis.

GASTRORRHŒ'A, from γαστηρ, 'the stomach,' and ρεω, 'I flow.' *Blennorrhœ'a* seu *Fluxus ventric'uli*, (F.) *Flux muqueux de l'estomac, Catarrhe stomacal*. A morbid condition of the stomach, which consists in the secretion of an excessive quantity of mucus from the lining membrane of the stomach. Also, Cœliac flux.

GASTROSCIR'RHUS, *Indura'tio ventric'uli scirrho'sa*, *Scirrhus* seu *carcino'ma ventric'uli*. Scirrhous induration or cancer of the stomach.

GASTROSCOPIA, Abdominoscopia.

GASTRO'SIS. A generic name for diseases which are seated in the stomach.—Alibert.

GASTROSPLE'NIC, *Gastrosple'nicus*, *Gastroliena'lis*, from γαστηρ, 'stomach,' and σπλην, 'the spleen.' Relating to stomach and spleen.

GASTROSTENOSIS, Stricture of the stomach.

GASTROSTENOSIS CARDI'ACA et PYLOR'ICA; from γαστηρ, 'the stomach,' and στενος, 'narrow.' Narrowness of the cardiac and pyloric orifices of the stomach from cancer of that organ.

GASTROT'OMY, from γαστηρ, 'the belly,' and τομη, 'incision.' Several different operations have been so called. 1. The Cæsarean Section. 2. An incision made into the abdomen for the purpose of removing some internal strangulation or volvulus; or to reduce hernia, *Laparot'omy*: and, 3. The opening made in the stomach, to remove a foreign body which has passed into it through the œsophagus.

GASTRYPERNEU'RIA, from γαστηρ, 'stomach,' 'υπερ, 'above,' and νευρον, 'a nerve.' Morbidly increased activity of the nerves of the stomach.

GÂTEAU FÉBRILE, Ague cake.
GATTILIER, Vitex.
GAUDIA FŒDA, Masturbation.

GAULTHE'RIA, *G.* seu *Gualthe'ria procum'bens*, *Gaultie'ra repens*, Mountain Tea, Partridge Berry, Berried Tea, Grouseberry, Deerberry, Spies berry, Tea berry, Red berry, Wintergreen, Red berry Tea, Ground berry, Ground ivy, Ground holly, Hill berry, Box berry, Chequer berry. An American plant, which is one of the principle articles of the materia medica of some Indian tribes. The infusion of the leaves is stimulant and anodyne, and is said to have been used, with advantage, in asthma. The oil — *Oleum Gaultheriæ*, Ph. U. S.,—is used, chiefly on account of its pleasant flavour, to cover the taste of other medicines.

GAUNTLET, *Gantelet*.
GAUQUAVA, Smilax China.
GAUTIERA REPENS, Gaultheria.

GAY FEATHER, Liatris spicata.
GAYAC, Guaiacum.

GAYLUSSAC'IA RESINO'SA, *Vaccin'ium resino'sum*, Black Huckleberry. An indigenous plant, whose fruit is sweet and agreeable.

GAZ, *Gas, Air*. Van Helmont first designated by this name, — the etymology of which is unknown, — the carbonic acid developed in the vinous fermentation. Afterwards, the term was appropriated to every permanently elastic fluid; that is, which preserves its aëriform state at all temperatures: and ultimately it was extended to all aëriform bodies; — which were divided into *permanent* and *non-permaent gases*. The latter are generally termed vapours: — they return to the liquid state, when a portion of their caloric is abstracted. The permanent gases, or *gases* properly so called, are numerous, and may be divided into four sections with regard to their effects on the animal economy.

1. *Irrespirable gases.*	Carbonic acid, ammoniacal gas, muriatic acid gas, deutoxide of azote, nitrous acid gas, and chlorine.
2. *Negatively deleterious gases.*	Hydrogen, azote.
3. *Positively deleterious gases.*	Oxygen, protoxide of azote, carburetted hydrogen, carbonic oxide, sulphuretted hydrogen, and arseniuretted hydrogen.

It is proper to remark that the term *respirable* has been very differently employed by different writers. Sometimes it has meant the power of supporting life when applied to the blood in the lungs. At others, all gases have been deemed irrespirable, which are incapable of being introduced into the lungs by voluntary efforts,—without any relation to their power of maintaining vitality; and this is perhaps the best sense. The gases were, at one time, employed in medicine, under great expectations,—especially by the enthusiastic Beddoes; but they are now scarcely ever had recourse to. They differ, considerably, in their effects on the animal economy. Some, as oxygen, are exciting; others, as azote, depressing; whilst others, again, as the *Protoxide of azote or laughing gas*, produce the most singular effects.

GAZ, PUL'MONARY, *Gas of the lungs*. A name given to the expired air; which contains—besides common air, an increase of carbonic acid, water, and some animal matter.

GAZ SANG'UINIS, *Gas anima'li san'guinis, Hal'itus san'guinis, Aura san'guinis, Hæmat'mus*. The halitus, or vapour, given off by freshly drawn blood.

GAZELLE, Antilopus.
GÉANT, Giant.
GEBÄRPULVER, Ergot.

GEDE'OLA. The convex part of the liver.— Du Cange.

GEILNAU, MINERAL WATERS OF. Geilnau is a village in the grand duchy of Nassau, at no great distance from Frankfort. The waters contain carbonic acid, carbonate, sulphate, and phosphate of soda, chloride of sodium, carbonate of lime, magnesia, and iron.

GEISMAR, MINERAL WATERS OF. The mineral waters of Geismar, in Bavaria, are acidulous chalybeates.

GEISUM, *Geison*. The part of the frontal bone over the eyes.

GELAPPIUM, Convolvulus jalapa.
GELASINI DENTES, Incisive teeth.

GELASMUS, Canine laugh.

GEL'ATIN, *Gel'atine, Gelatina, Galreda*, from (F.) *Gelée*, 'gelly or jelly.' An immediate animal principle. It is semitransparent, insipid, inodorous, insoluble in cold water, very soluble in hot, which it thickens, and transforms into gelly on cooling. Gelatin is a very nutritious substance; and, when dissolved in a considerable quantity of water, forms an emollient fluid, much used in therapeutics, but not the most easy of digestion.

GELATIN OF WHARTON, *Gelatina Whartonia'na, Jelly of tee Cord*. A soft, dense, fluid, gelatinous substance, which envelops the umbilical cord, and is conceived, by some, to be inservient to the nutrition of the fœtus.

GELATINA AQUATICA, Brasenia hydropeltis.

GELATIO, Congelation.

GELÉE, Gelly.

GELLY. *Jelly, Jus gela'tum, Gelu, Jus coagula'tum*, (F.) *Gelée*. A substance of a soft consistence, tremulous, and transparent, which is obtained by an appropriate treatment, from animal and vegetable matters: hence the distinction into *animal* and *vegetable jelly*. The former is merely a concentrated solution of gelatin, left to cool.

Vegetable Jelly is found in the juice of the currant, mulberry, and of almost all acid fruits, when ripe. It is of itself colourless, but almost always retains a little colouring matter of the fruit which has furnished it. It has an agreeable taste; is scarcely soluble in cold water, but boiling water dissolves it readily: the jelly is, however, almost all deposited on cooling. If this aqueous solution be boiled for a long time, it becomes analogous to mucilage, and loses the property of being jellied on cooling.

GELSEMI'NUM NIT'IDUM, *Yellow Jes'samine*. The flowers, root, &c., of this shrub, are narcotic, and the effluvia from the former are said sometimes to induce stupor.

GELU, Gelly.

GELUS, Risus.

GEMELLI, Gastrocnemii, Ischio-trochanterianus, Testicles.

GEMEL'LUS, *Gem'inus, Did'ymus*, 'a twin.' (F.) *Jumeau, Jumelle, Besson, Bessonne*. One of two children, twins, born at the same accouchement, or gestation. Also, relating to twins, as "a twin conception."

GEMELLUS MUS'CULUS. Cowper applies this name to the long portion of the triceps brachialis united to the inner portion.

GEMINI, Ischio-trochanterianus, Testicles.

GEMINUM CENTRUM SEMICIRCULARE, Tænia semicircularis.

GEMINUS, Gemellus.

GEMIPOMA, Mamma.

GÉMISSEMENT, see Moaning.

GEMMA, Granulation—g. Oculi, Crystalline.

GEMMATION, GENERATION BY, see Generation.

GEMMIPARITÉ, see Generation.

GEMMIPAROUS, see Generation.

GEMUR'SA, a corn; also a name given by the ancients to a disease seated between the toes;—the nature of which is unknown to us.

GEN, *Gen'esis*, 'generation,' from γενναω, 'I make.' Hence Hydrogen, Osteogeny, &c.

GENA. The *Cheek, Genys, Parei'a, Gamphē, Gamphe'la, Gnathos, Gnathmus, Mala*, (F.) *Joue*. The cheeks form the lateral parts of the mouth. *Externally*, they have no precise limits: they are continuous, above with the lower eyelid; below, they descend as far as the base of the jaw; *before*, they terminate at the alæ nasi, and at the commissures of the lips; and *behind*, at the ear. Their thickness varies, according to the degree of fatness of the individual. They are formed of three layers;—one dermoid, another muscular, and the third mucous.

GENCIVES, Gingivæ.

GENEI'AS, *Lanu'go prima, Probar'bium*. The downy hairs, which first cover the cheek. Also, a bandage which passes under the chin.

GENEION, Beard, Mentum.

GENERAL ANATOMY, see Anatomy.

GÉNÉRALE, Influenza.

GENERATIO, Generation—g. Æquivoca, see Generation—g. Calculi, Lithia—g. Homogenea, see Generation—g. Primigena, see Generation—g. Primitiva, see Generation—g. Originaria, see Generation—g. Spontanea, see Generation.

GENERATION, *Genera'tio, Gen'esis, Genne'sis, Gonē, Gonus, Procrea'tio, Procreation, Breeding*, from γενω, or γενναω, 'I engender.' Under this name physiologists comprehend the aggregate of functions, which concur, in organized beings, towards the production of their kind. The *act of generation* means the union of the sexes. See Coition. The writers of antiquity believed, that all organized bodies are produced either by what is termed *univ'ocal* or *regular generation, Homogen'esis, genera'tio homogen'ea, propaga'tio*, which applies to the upper classes of animals and vegetables, or by *spontaneous generation, Autogon'ia, heterogen'esis, generatio heterogen'ea, æquiv'oca, primiti'va, primig''ena, origina'ria, sponta'nea, spontéparité* (Dugès), which they considered applicable to the very lowest classes only, as the mushroom, the worm, the frog, &c. There are still many distinguished naturalists who consider that beings low in the scale of animality, are produced in the latter way. Spontaneous generation and *equivocal generation* have been regarded by many to be synonymous. Others, however, mean by spontaneous generation, the production of a new being from the mere combination of inorganic elements: whilst by equivocal generation they understand the evolution of a new being from organized beings dissimilar to themselves, through some irregularity in their functions, or through the incipient decay or degeneration of their tissues. As to the mode in which regular generation is accomplished, there have been many views. According to the doctrine of Hippocrates, and of the ancient philosophers, the ovaries of the female furnish a prolific fluid, similar to that of the male; and the fœtus results from the mixture of the two seeds in copulation. Steno and others conceived, that the ovaries contain ova, which are not developed until vivified by the male sperm. Bonnet and Spallanzani believed in the pre-existence of germs, created since the origin of the world, but encased in each other, and becoming developed in succession; whence it would follow that the ovary of the first female must have contained the germs of all subsequent generations: and that the number of these germs must go on always diminishing, until ultimately extinct. This was the system of the *evolution of germs*. According to Leeuenhoek, the ovaries do not contain eggs, but vesicles destined to receive animalcules: which, in his view, live in the sperm. Thousands of these animalcules are thrown into the uterus during copulation, and the most expeditious and vigorous reaches the ovary, after having scattered and destroyed its competitors. Buffon — admitting the hypothesis of the two seeds — supposed that they were formed of molecules proceeding from every part of the body of each parent; and that, by a kind of elective affinity, those which were furnished by the head, the trunk, or the extremities of the male parent, could only unite with those proceeding from the same parts of the female. Before him, Maupertuis, admitting, with many of the ancient philosophers, the system of *Epigenesis*, and adopting, as regarded the composition of the sperm, a theory analogous to that of Buffon, had supposed that the molecules, capable of being organized, were attracted towards a centre; that the nose attracts the two eyes; the body, the arms; the arms, the hands, &c., nearly as the particles of a salt, dissolved in a liquid, arrange themselves in regular crystals around the same nucleus. These and various other systems have been successively proposed and abandoned, and the mystery of generation remains impenetrable.

The simplest kind of reproduction does not require sexual organs. The animal separates into several fragments, which form so many new individuals. This is *Fissip'arous generation*, *Fissiparism*, *G. from fission*, (F.) *Fissiparité*, *Scissiparité*. *Gemmip'arous generation*, (F.) *Gemmiparité*, consists in the formation of buds, sporules or germs on some part of the body, which at a particular period drop off and form as many new individuals. In *Ovip'arous generation*, (F.) *Oviparité*, the egg is hatched out of the body. In *ovovivip'arous generation*, the new being is hatched in the excretory passages. In *vivip'arous generation*, the new individual is born under its appropriate form; and in *marsu'pial* or *marsupiate generation*, the young being, born at a very early stage of development, is received and nourished in a *marsupium* or pouch. In *alternate generation*, the young not only do not resemble the parent at birth, but remain dissimilar during their whole life, so that their relationship is not apparent until a succeeding generation. Thus, the cercaria undergoes a change into the distoma.

All the acts comprising the function of generation in man may be referred to five great heads. 1. *Copulation*. 2. *Conception* or *fecundation*. 3. *Gestation* or *Pregnancy*. 4. *Delivery* or *Accouchement*: and, 5. *Lactation*.

GENERATION, ACT OF, see Generation—g. Equivocal, see Generation—g. by Fission, see Generation—g. Fissiparous, see Generation—g. by Gemmation, see Generation—g. Gemmiparous, see Generation—g. Marsupial, see Generation—g. Organs of, female, see Vulva—g. Oviparous, see Generation—g. Regular, see Generation—g. Spontaneous, see Generation—g. Univocal, see Generation—g. Viviparous, see Generation.

GEN'EROUS, *Genero'sus*. A name given to wines which contain a great quantity of alcohol.

GENESIOL'OGY, *Genesiolog"ia*, from γενεσις, 'generation,' and λογος, 'a discourse.' The doctrine of generation.

GÉNÉSIQUE, LE, Appetite, venereal.

GENESIS, Generation.

GENÊT, Spartium scoparium—*g. à Balai*, Spartium scoparium—*g. des Teinturiers*, Genista tinctoria.

GENETHLIACUS, from γενεθλιος, 'natal,' 'pertaining to nativity.' A name given by the ancients to certain astrologers, who, from the state of the heavens at the time of the birth of an individual, predicted his future character and the events of his life.

GENET'ICA, from γενεσις, 'origin,' 'rise.' Diseases of the sexual functions: the 5th class in Good's Nosology. Also, agents that act on the sexual organs.—Pereira.

GENETICOS, Genital.

GENEVA, Gin—g. Hollands, see Spirit.

GENÉVRIER, Juniperus communis.

GENGIVITE, Ulitis.

GÉNI, Genian.

GE'NIAN, *Genia'nus*, *Ge'nial*, from γενειον, 'the chin.' The *Genian apoph'ysis* or *Process*, (F.) *Apophyse génienne* ou *géni*, is situate at the posterior part of the symphysis menti, and is formed of four small tubercles.

GENICULATUM, see Corpora geniculata.

GÉNIE, *Ge'nius*. The French sometimes apply this term to diseases nearly synonymously with *nature*; as *Génie inflammatoire*, *G. bilieux*, *G. adynamique*. Some use it in the same sense as type; *Génie intermittent*. The unwonted predominance of any mental faculty is also so called.

GÉNIEN, Genian.

GENIÈVRE, Gin, Juniperis communis (the berry.)

GENI'OGLOSSUS, *Genio-hyoglos'sus*, from γενειον, 'the chin,' and λωσσα, 'the tongue.' *Mesoglossus*, *Mesoglot'tus*, Nonus lingua mus'culus. The name of a flat, triangular muscle, which extends from the genian apophysis to the inferior surface of the os hyoides and tongue, which it carries forward.

GENIOHYODES, Geniohyoideus.

GENIOHYOGLOSSUS, Genioglossus.

GENIOHYOIDES, Geniohyoideus.

GENI'OHYOIDEUS, *Geniohyo'des*, *Geniohyoï'des*, *Mento-bicorn'eus*, from γενειον, 'the chin,' and 'υοειδης, 'the hyoides.' A muscle which arises from the genian apophysis, and is inserted at the anterior part of the body of the os hyoides. Its use is to raise the os hyoides, and carry it forwards. It may, also, contribute to depress the lower jaw in contracting towards the os hyoides.

GENI'O-PHARYNGE'US, from γενειον, 'the chin,' and φαρυγξ, 'the pharynx.' A name given, by some anatomists, to a bundle of fibres which passes from the lower jaw to the sides of the pharynx, and forms part of the *constrictor pharyngis superior*.

GEN'IPA OBLONGIFO'LIA, *Huito*. A plant of Peru, with the juice of which the Indians paint their legs, to protect them against the stings of insects.

GENIPI ALBUM, Artemisia rupestris—*g. Blanc*, Artemisia rupestris—*g. Verum*, Achillea atrata.

GENISTA, Spartium scoparium—g. Canariensis, see Rhodium lignum—g. Hirsuta, Spartium scoparium—g. Scoparia, Spartium scoparium.

GENIS'TA SPINO'SA IN'DICA, *Bahel Schulli*. An oriental tree, a decoction of the roots of which is diuretic. The leaves boiled in vinegar have the same effect.—Ray.

GENIS'TA TINCTO'RIA, *Genistoï'des tincto'ria*, *Spar'tium tincto'rium*, *Dyers' broom*, *Dyers' weed*, *Green weed*, *Wood waxen*, (F.) *Genêt des Teinturiers*. A shrub cultivated in this country and in Europe. The flowering tops and seed have been used in medicine. It has the same properties as Spartium scoparium.

GENISTOIDES TINCTORIA, Genista tinctoria.

GEN'ITAL, *Genita'lis*, *Genet'icos*. Same etymon as Generation. That which belongs to generation.

GEN'ITAL ORGANS, *Sex'ual Organs*, *Puden'da*, *Natura'lia*, *Natu'ra*, *Ædœ'a*, *Me'zea*, *Me'sa*, *Mo'rion*, *Genital parts*, *Noble parts*, *Nat'ural parts*, *Private parts*, *Priv'ities*, *Privy parts*, *Privy Members*, *the Parts*, *Pars*, *Pars corporis seu obscæ'na*, *Fores*, *Partes genita'les seu genera'tio'ni inservien'tes*, *P. obscænæ*, *Me'dea*, *Verenda*, *Pedes*, *Inguen*, *Genita'lia*, *Gennet'ica*, *Gymna*,

Membra puden'da, Or'gana generatio'ni inservientia, (F.) *Organes génitaux, Parties génitales,* P. *honteuses,* P. *génitoires,* P. *nobles,* P. *sexuelles,* P. *naturelles, Les Parties.* The parts that are inservient to the reproduction of the species. These are very different in the male and female. In man, they are numerous; some *secreting the sperm,* as the testicles and their appendages; others *retaining it,* as the vesiculæ seminales; and another for *carrying it* into the organs of the female,—the penis. In the female, the parts of generation form an apparatus, perhaps more complicated than that of the male. Some are incervient to copulation, as the vulva, vagina, &c.; others to conception and the preservation of the product for a determinate time, as the uterus and its appendages; whilst others concur in the alimentation of the infant after birth, as the mammæ.

GENITALE, Sperm—g. Caput, Glans.

GENITALIA, Genital organs — g. Viri, Pudibilia.

GEN'ITO-CRURAL NERVE, *Nervus gen'ito-crura'lis, Subpu'bial nerve, Inter'nal in'guinal nerve.* A branch of the second lumbar nerve, which passes through the psoas muscle, and, approaching the femoral arch, divides into two branches,—an *internal, scrotal,* or *gen'ital, nervus spermaticus seu puden'dus exter'nus,* and an *external* or *femoral cutaneous branch, lumbo-inguinalis.*

GENITU'RA. That which is fecundated or engendered in the maternal womb. This word has been used synonymously with *embryo, fœtus,* and *infant.* Also, the sperm; and the penis. See GONE.

GENIUM, Mentum.

GENNESIS, Generation.

GENNETICA, Genital Organs.

GENNETICOCNES'MUS, from γεννητικος, 'genital,' and κνησμος, 'itching.' Itching of the genital organs.

GENNETICON'OSI, *Genneticonu'si,* from γεννητικος, 'genital,' and νοσος, 'disease.' Diseases of the genitals.

GENOA, CLIMATE OF. The climate of this Italian city and its vicinity has been often selected as favourable for the phthisical valetudinarian during the winter; but it is now admitted to be decidedly improper for pulmonary affections, being subject to frequent and rapid changes of temperature, and to dry cold winds from the north, alternately with warm moist winds from the south-east.—Sir James Clark.

GENONU'SI, *Morbi sexûs,* from γενος, 'sex,' and νουσος, 'disease.' Sexual diseases.

GENOS, Sex.

GENOU, Genu.

GÉNOUILLÉS, (Corps,) Corpora geniculata.

GENRE, Genus.

GENSANG, Panax quinquefolium.

GENTIA, Gentianina.

GENTIAN, Gentiana lutea, Triosteum — g. Blue, Gentiana catesbæi—g. Catesbian, Gentiana catesbæi — g. White, Laserpitium latifolium — g. Southern, Gentiana catesbæi — g. White, Triosteum—g. Yellow, Gentiana lutea, see Calumba.

GENTIANA, G. lutea—g. Alba, Laserpitium latifolium — g. Cachenlaguen, Chironia Chilensis —g. Centaurium, Chironia centaurium.

GENTIANA CATESBÆ'I; *G. Catesbia'na, Blue Gentian,* U. S., *Catesbian Gen'tian, Southern Gentian, Bluebells, Bitterroot.* It is a pure and simple bitter, and the root may be used wherever that of the *Gentiana lutea* is proper.

GENTIA'NA CHIRAYTA, *G. Chirayi'ta, Henrice'a Pharmacear'cha, Swer'tia, Chirayi'ta, Agatho'tes chirayi'ta, Ophe'lia chira'ta, Chiret'ta, Chirayi'ta, Chirae'ta.* A native of India, which has been much employed in that country, in dyspepsia, and as an antiperiodic in intermittents. It is preferred by some to sarsaparilla, where the latter is considered to be indicated,—as after large quantities of mercury have been taken, or where profuse salivation has been induced. It has also been advised in atonic leucorrhœa. It yields its virtues to alcohol and water.

GENTIANA CRINITA, see G. quinqueflora—g. Gerardi, Chironia centaurium.

GENTIA'NA LU'TEA. The systematic name of the officinal gentian; *Gentia'na, Gentia'na major, G. vet'erum, Gentia'na rubra, Swer'tia lu'tea, Aste'rias lu'tea, Yellow Gentian, Felwort.* Ord. Gentianeæ. (F.) *Gentiane jaune.* This is a plant common in the mountains of Europe. The root is almost inodorous, extremely bitter, and yields its virtues to ether, alcohol, and water. It is tonic and stomachic; and in large doses, aperient. Dose, gr. x. to ℈ij. It is most frequently, however, used in infusion or tincture.

GENTIANA MAJOR, G. lutea—g. Peruviana, Chironia Chilensis.

GENTIA'NA QUINQUEFLO'RA, *Five-flowered Gentian;* and GENTIA'NA CRINI'TA, *Fringed Gentian,* indigenous, are possessed of like virtues.

GENTIANA RUBRA, G. lutea — g. Veterum, G. lutea.

GENTIANE JAUNE, Gentiana lutea.

GENTIANI'NA, *Gentianine, Gentianin, Gentia'nia, Gentia.* A supposed neutral substance, obtained from gentian, and, by some, presumed to be its active principle. It is not so.

GENTILITIUS, Hereditary.

GENU, *Gony,* γονυ, (F.) *Genou.* The articulation of the leg with the thigh;—the *Femoro-tibial* or *knee-joint,* the *knee.* It is the most complicated in the body, and is formed by the inferior extremity of the femur, the superior extremity of the tibia, and the rotula. The articular surfaces of the bones are covered by layers of cartilage—more or less thick—and by the synovial membrane of the articulation. The soft parts of this joint are,—the *ligamentum patellæ,* two lateral ligaments, distinguished by the names *internal* and *external;* a posterior ligament, *Ligamen'tum posti'cum Winslow'ii;* two crucial ligaments, —the one anterior, and the other posterior; two interarticular fibro-cartilages; some albugineous fibres, which form an imperfect capsule, &c. The knee receives its arteries from the femoral and popliteal. They bear the name *articular.* Its veins have the same distribution as the arteries, and discharge their blood into the saphena and crural. Its nerves are furnished by the sciatic, popliteal, and crural. The joint is protected by the tendons and muscles which surround it.

The French use the term *Articulation en genou* for a joint, in which the head of a bone is received into a bony cavity of another, where it rolls and moves in all directions.

GENU CORPORIS CALLOSI, see Corpus callosum.

GENUGRA, Gonagra.

GENUINUS, Legitimate.

GENUS, (F.) *Genre.* A collection or group of species, analogous to each other, and which can be united by common characters. When a species cannot be referred to a known genus, it constitutes a distinct one.

GENUS CURATIONIS, Ratio medendi.

GENYANTRAL'GIA, from γενυσω, 'the maxilla,' αντρον, 'the antrum, and αλγος, 'pain.' Pain in the antrum of Highmore.

GENYANTRI'TIS, from γενυων, 'the maxilla,' αντρον, 'the antrum,' and *itis,* denoting inflammation. Inflammation of the antrum of Highmore.

GENYANTRUM, Antrum of Highmore.

GENYOCYNANCHE, Cynanche parotidæa.

GENYS, γενυς, 'the jaw;' also the chin. See Gena.

GEOFFRÆ'A INER'MIS, *G. racemo'sa seu Piso'nis seu Jamaicen'sis, Vouacap'oua America'na, Geoffræ'a, Geoffroy'a, Cabbag'ium, Cabbage Tree, Cabbage Bark Tree, Worm-Bark Tree, Andi'ra inerm'is seu racemo'sa. Nat. Ord.* Leguminosæ. *Sex. Syst.* Diadelphia Decandria. The odour of the bark is very unpleasant. It is anthelmintic and cathartic. Dose of the powder, ℈j to ℈ij.

GEOFFRÆA JAMAICENSIS, G. inermis—g. Pisonis, G. inermis—g. Racemosa, G. inermis.

GEOFFRÆ'A SURINAMEN'SIS, *Andi'ra Surinamen'sis*, has similar properties.

Huttenschmidt has separated their active principles, to which he has given the names *Jamaicine* and *Surinamine*. They are all alkaline.

GEOFFRÆA VERMIF'UGA, *Andira ibai, Arriba, Skolemo'ra Fernambucensis;* a South American plant has a fruit, the almond of which, called *angéline*, has a reputation at Rio Janeiro as a vermifuge. Dose, a grain to fifteen; or it may be given in infusion.

GEOFFROYA, Geoffræa inermis—g. Jamaicensis, G. inermis.

GEOG'RAPHY, MED'ICAL, *Geogra'phia Med'ica*. The description of the surface of the globe as regards the influence of situation on the health, vital functions, and diseases of its inhabitants—vegetable and animal; but principally on those of man.

GEOPH'AGISM, *Geophag"ia, Gæophag"ia*, from γη, 'earth,' and φαγω, 'I eat.' The act or practice of eating earth. See Chthonophagia.

GERÆOLOG"IA, *Geratolog"ia*, from γηρας, 'old age,' and λογος, 'a discourse.' The doctrine, or a description, of old age.

GER'ANIS, from γερανος, 'a crane,' which it resembled. A bandage, used by the ancients in cases of fractured clavicle. Some authors attribute it to Hippocrates; others, to Perigenes.

GERA'NIUM, same etymon, because its pistil is long, like the bill of the crane. The *Crane's Bill*.

GERANIUM FŒTIDUM, G. Robertianum—g. Maculatum, see Geranium, and G. Moschatum.

GERANIUM MOSCHA'TUM; *Erod'ium Moschatum*, (F.) *Bec de grue musqué*. A European plant, esteemed to be excitant and diaphoretic.

GERANIUM NOVEBORACENSE, G. Maculatum—g. Purpureum, G. Robertianum.

GERANIUM ROBERTIA'NUM; *G. fœ'tidum seu purpu'reum, Stinking Crane's Bill, Herb Robert*, (F.) *Herbe à Robert, Bec de Grue Robertin*. This plant was, at one time, used as an antispasmodic and slight stimulant, as well as for an external application in various painful sores and inflammations.

Most of the species of geranium have been used as astringents. In some of the northwestern parts of the United States, the root of the *Geranium macula'tum—Gera'nium*, (Ph. U. S.)—*G. Noveboracen'sě, Spotted Crane's Bill, Crowfoot, Alum root, Tormentil, Stork bill*—is called *Racine à Becquet*, after a person of that name. It is highly extolled by the Western Indians as an antisyphilitic.

GERAS, Senectus.

GERM, *Germen, Blastě, Blaste'ma*. The rudiment of a new being, not yet developed, or which is still adherent to the mother.

GERM FORCE, Plastic force.

GERMANDER, COMMON, Teucrium chamædrys—g. Creeping, Teucrium chamædrys—g. Marum, Teucrium marum—g. Small, Teucrium chamædrys—g. Water, Teucrium scordium.

GERMANDRÉE AQUATIQUE, Teucrium scordium—*g. Maritime*, Teucrium marum—*g. Officinale*, Teucrium chamædrys—*g. Scorodone*, Teucrium scordium.

GERME FAUX, Conception, false.

GERMEN, Germ, Sperm—g. Dentale, Dental Pulp—g. Falsum, Mole—g. Spurium, Conception, false.

GERMINAL CELL, see Cytoblast—g. Membrane and Vesicle; see Molecule—g. Nucleus, see Molecule—g. Spot, see Molecule—g. Vesicle, see Molecule.

GERMS, DISSEMINATION OF, Panspermia.

GEROBOS'CIA, *Gerontobos'cia*, from γηρας, 'old age,' and βοσκη, 'food.' Nourishment or maintenance proper for the aged.

GEROCOMEUM, Gerocomium.

GEROCO'MIA, *Gerocom'icē, Gerontocom'icē*, from γερων, 'an aged person,' and κομειν, 'to take care of.' The part of medicine whose object is the preservation of the health of the aged:—the hygiene of old people.

GEROCOMICE, Gerocomia.

GEROCOMI'UM, *Gerocome'um, Presbyodochi'um, Gerontocomi'um, Gerotrophe'um*, same etymon. An hospital for the aged.

GÉROFLE, see Eugenia caryophyllata.

GÉROFLÉE JAUNE, Cheiranthus cheiri.

GERONTATROPHIA, Marasmus senilis.

GERONTOBOSCIA, Geroboscia.

GERONTOCOMICE, Gerocomia.

GERONTOCOMIUM, Gerocomium.

GERONTO'PIA, from γηρας, 'old age,' and ωψ, 'the eye.' Weakness of sight of the aged.

GERONTOTOXON, Gerotoxon.

GERONTOXON, Gerotoxon.

GEROTOX'ON, *Gerontox'on, Gerontotox'on, Mac'ula cor'neæ arcua'ta, Arcus seni'lis;* from γερων, 'an old person,' and τοξον, 'a bow.' A bow-shaped obscurity at the under margin of the cornea, common to old people.

GEROTROPHEUM, Gerocomium.

GEROTROPHIA, Geroboscia.

GERSA, Plumbi suboarbonas—g. Serpentariæ, see Arum maculatum.

GESTA, 'things done,' from *gerere, gestum*, 'to do,' 'carry.' A Latin term, introduced by Halló into medical language, to designate, among the objects which belong to hygiene, the functions which consist in the voluntary movements of muscles and organs. In the class *Gesta* are found *sleep, the waking state, movements* or *locomotion*, and *rest*.

GESTA'TION, *Gesta'tio, Phora*, from *gestare*, 'to carry.' The time during which a female who has conceived carries the embryo in her uterus. See Pregnancy. Gestation, likewise, signifies the bearing or carrying of an individual; a kind of exercise easier than that in which he moves by virtue of his own powers. Thus, we speak of *gestation on horseback, in a carriage*, &c.

GESTATION, PROTRACTED. Pregnancy protracted beyond the usual period. See Pregnancy.

GESTICULA'TION, *Gesticula'tio*, same etymon. The act of making many gestures; a symptom in disease, which indicates great encephalic erethism. It is met with in numerous affections.

GETHYL'LIS SPIRA'LIS. A South African plant, *Nat. Ord.* Amaryllideæ, the orange-coloured fruit of which has a peculiar fragrance. An infusion in spirit or tincture is used in flatulence and colic.

GEUM, G. rivale—g. Caryophyllatum, G. ur

banum — g. Nutans, G. rivale — g. Palustre, G. rivale.

GEUM RIVALE, *G. palus'trē seu nutans, Caryophylla'ta aquat'ica seu nutans, Benedic'ta sylves'tris, Water avens,* (F.) *Benoîte aquatique, B. des Ruisseaux. Family,* Rosaceæ. *Sex. Syst.* Icosandria Polygynia. The root of this plant, *Geum* (Ph. U. S.), is astringent. It has been much extolled in the cure of intermittents, diarrhœa, hemorrhage, &c.

GEUM URBANUM, *G. caryophylla'tum, Caryophylla'ta, C. vulga'ris seu urba'na, Caryophyl'lus vulga'ris, Sanamun'da, Lagophthal'mus, Caryophyl'la, Janamun'da, Common avens, Herb Bennet, Herba benedic'ta,* (F.) *Benoîte.* The root of this plant has a smell not unlike that of cloves. Taste bitterish, austere; virtues yielded to water and alcohol. It has been used in intermittents, dysentery, chronic diarrhœa, debility, &c. Dose, ℨss to ℨj of the powder.

GEUM VERNUM, *Western early avens,* has the same properties as

GEUM VIRGINIA'NUM, *White avens, Avens, Evan root, Choc'olate root, Bennet, Throat root, Cureall,* (F.) *Benoîte de Virginie,* is common from Maine to Carolina and Kentucky, flowering in June and July. It has the same medical properties as Geum rivale.

GEUMA, Taste.

GEUSION'OSI, from γευσις, 'taste,' and νοσος, 'disease.' *Geusionu'si.* Diseases of the organ or sense of taste.

GEUSIS, Taste. Rarely, the root of the tongue—*Radix linguæ.*

GEUTHMOS, Taste.

GEZIR, see Pastinaca opoponax.

GÉZIT, Cagot.

GÉZITAIN, Cagot.

GHERKIN, see Cucumis sativus.

GHITTA JEMOCO, Cambogia.

GIALAPPA, Convolvulus Jalapa.

GIANT, *Gigas,* (F.) *Géant.* One much above the ordinary stature.

GIBBA, Hump.

GIBBER, Hump.

GIBBEROSITAS, Gibbositas.

GIBBOS'ITAS, *Gibberos'itas, Cypho'sis, Rhachio-cypho'sis,* from (F.) *Gibbeux,* (L.) *Gibbus,* 'something arched or vaulted; prominent.' *Gibbos'ity, Gib'bousness, Curvature of the spine, Hybo'ma.* A symptom which occurs in different diseases; particularly in rickets and caries of the vertebræ. See Hump.

GIBBOSITAS CARIOSA, Vertebral disease.

GIBBOUSNESS, Gibbositas.

GIBBUS, Hump—g. Pottii, Vertebral disease.

GIBLETS. According to Minsheu, from *Gobbet, Goblet;* but, according to Junius, from (F.) *Gibier,* 'game.' The word seems to be the old (F.) *Gibelez, Gibelet,* &c., i. e. *Gibier,* (L.) *Cibarium,* food, (F.) *Abattis.* It means, generally, the parts which are cut off from a goose before it is roasted. Also, the extremities of fowls, such as the head, wings, feet; to which are sometimes added, the liver, gizzard, &c. Soup, made from these, is moderately nutritious.

GIDDINESS, Vertigo.

GIDDY, Vertiginous.

GIGANTEUS, Gigantic.

GIGANTESQUE, Gigantic.

GIGAN'TIC, *Gigante'us, Giganto'des,* (F.) *Gigantesque.* Relating to one much above the ordinary stature.

GIGANTODES, Gigantic.

GIGARTINA HELMINTHOCHORTON, Corallina Corsicana—g. Lichenoides, Fucus amylaceus.

GIGARUS SERPENTARIA, Arum dracunculus.

GIGAS, Giant.

GILARUM, Thymus serpyllum.

GILEAD, BALM OF, see Amyris opobalsamum.

GILET DE FORCE, Waistcoat, strait.

GILL, Glechoma hederacea.

GILL-GO-BY-GROUND, Glechoma hederacea.

GILLA THEOPHRASTI, Zinci sulphas — g. Vitrioli, Zinci sulphas.

GILLE'NIA STIPULA'CEA, *Small-flowered In'dian Physic* has the same properties as

GILLE'NIA TRIFOLIA'TA, *Spiræ'a trifolia'ta, Common Gille'nia, Indian Physic, Western Dropwort, Indian Hippo, Ip'ecac, Bowman's root, Meadow sweet, Beaumont root. Nat. Ord.* Rosaceæ. *Sex. Syst.* Icosandria Pentagynia. The root of this shrub,—*Gille'nia,* (Ph. U. S.)—which grows plentifully in the United States, is a safe and efficacious emetic, in the dose of about 30 grains. It resembles ipecacuanha in its properties.

GILLIFLOWER, Dianthus caryophyllus.

GIM'BERNAT'S LIGAMENT. A fibrous, triangular expansion, which is detached from the posterior and inner part of the crural arch, and is inserted into the crest of the pubis. This ligament forms the inner part of the superior aperture of the crural canal. It is one of the most frequent causes of strangulation in crural hernia.

GIN, *Hollands, Gene'va,* (F.) *Genièvre.* This spirit, which is distilled from corn and juniper berries, or from some substitute for them, is largely used in Great Britain; and is extremely detrimental, to the lower classes particularly. It possesses the properties of other spirituous liquors, but is, in popular medicine, more used than other varieties, in cases of colic or intestinal pain of any kind. See Spirit.

GIN DRINKER'S LIVER, Liver, nutmeg — g. Liver, Liver, nutmeg.

GINGEMBRE, Amomum zingiber.

GINGER, Amomum zingiber—g. Beer powder, see Amomum zingiber—g. Indian, Asarum canadense — g. Jamaica, concentrated essence of, see Amomum zingiber — g. Preserved, see Amomum zingiber—g. Wild, Asarum Canadense.

GINGIBRA'CHIUM, from *gingivæ,* 'the gums,' and *brachium,* 'the arm.' A name given to the scurvy, because the gums and arms are chiefly affected by it. It has, also, been called *Gingipe'dium,* because the lower limbs are in many cases the seat of scorbutic spots. See Porphyra nautica.

GINGIPEDIUM, see Gingibrachium, Porphyra nautica.

GINGI'VÆ, from *gignere,* 'to beget,' because the teeth are, as it were, begotten in them. (?) The gums, ουλα, *U'la, Carnic'ula,* (F.) *Gencives.* The portion of the mucous membrane of the mouth which covers the maxillary bones to the level of the alveolar arches. The gums are formed of a red tissue, more or less solid, and of a fibro-mucous nature, which adheres strongly to the necks of the teeth, and transmits, between the roots and their alveoli, a very thin expansion,—the *alveolo-dental periosteum.* The gums fix the teeth and contribute greatly to their solidity. In the aged, after the loss of the teeth, they become fibrous and very solid, and are inservient to mastication.

GINGIVA'LIS, *Ulet'icus, U'licus;* from *gingivæ,* 'the gums.' Relating to the gums.

GING'LYMOID, *Ginglymoïdeus, Ginglymo'des,* from γιγγλυμος, 'a ginglymus,' and ειδος, 'resemblance.' Resembling a ginglymus or hinge. An epithet applied to joints which resemble a hinge, as a *ginglymoid joint.*

GIN'GLYMUS, *Cardinamen'tum, Cardo,* 'a

hinge.' (F.) *Charnière, Articulation en charnière.* A species of diarthrodial articulation, which only admits of motion in two directions, like a hinge, — as the knee-joint or elbow-joint.

GINSENG, Panax quinquefolium — g. Blue, Caulophyllum thalictroïdes — g. Yellow, Caulophyllum thalictroïdes — g. Horse, Triosteum — g. White, Triosteum.

GIRAFFE, Dengue.

GIRARD ROUSSIN, Asarum.

GIRDLE, Cingulum.

GIRL. This seems, formerly, to have been an appellation common to both sexes. Many etymologists deduce the word from the Su. Goth. Karl, 'a man.' It means a young female, (L.) *Filia*, from φιλεῖν, 'to love.' (F.) *Fille*.

GIROFLE, see Eugenia caryophyllata.

GIROFLÉE JAUNE, Cheiranthus cheiri.

GISSA, Cynanche parotidæa.

GIZZARD, Ventriculus callosus.

GLABELLA, Mesophryon.

GLABELLAD, see Glabellar.

GLABEL'LAR, from *glabella*, 'the space between the eyebrows.' An epithet for an aspect towards the glabella.—Barclay. *Glabellad* is used adverbially by the same writer to signify 'towards the glabellar aspect.'

GLABRITIES, Calvities.

GLACE, Ice.

GLACIALE, Mesembryanthemum crystallinum.

GLACIALIS HUMOR, Crystalline.

GLACIES, Ice.

GLADIOLUS, Machærion—g. Cæruleus, Iris Germanica.

GLADI'OLUS COMMU'NIS, *G. vulga'ris, Victoria'lis rotun'da, Cornflag, Victoria'lis feminea*, (F.) *Glayeul*. The root of this plant has been considered aphrodisiac. Applied in cataplasm, it has been extolled against scrofulous tumours.

GLADIOLUS LUTEUS, Iris pseudacorus—g. Vulgaris, G. communis.

GLADIUS, Penis.

GLAMA, Lippitudo, *Chassie*.

GLAND, *Glan'dula, Gran'dula*, from *glans*, 'an acorn, a kernel.' *Aden*. The ancient anatomists gave this name to a number of organs of a texture generally soft, and a shape more or less globular, but differing greatly in their nature and functions. They applied it, for instance, 1. To those organs which separate from the blood, any fluid whatever. When such organs were composed of several lobules, united by common vessels, they received the name *conglomerate glands*, as the parotid, pancreas, &c. 2. To the reddish and spongy, knot-like bodies, which are met with in the course of the lymphatics. These they called *conglobate glands;* — see Ganglion (*lymphatic;*) and 3dly and lastly, to various other organs, whose intimate texture and functions are still unknown, as the *Pineal gland, Pituitary gland, Glands of Pacchioni, Thyroid gland, Thymus gland. Supra-renal glands*, &c. Chaussier restricts the word *gland* to those softish, granular, lobated organs, composed of vessels, and a particular texture, of which there are in the human body, the *lachrymal, salivary*, and *mammary*, the *testicles*, the *liver, pancreas*, and *kidneys*. These *permanent glands*, or *glands with permanent ducts*, are all destined to draw from the blood the molecules necessary for the formation of new fluids; and to convey these fluids externally, by means of one or more excretory ducts. Several glands besides their excretory ducts, have especial reservoirs, in which the fluids, secreted by them, collect, remain for a greater or less space of time, and undergo slight modifications before being evacuated ; — such are, the gall-bladder for the liver, the urinary bladder for the kidneys, &c.

Each gland has an organization peculiar to it, but we know not the intimate nature of the glandular texture. — Malpighi believed that the vessels terminate in small, solid masses, to which he gave the name — *glandular grains* or *acini*. In these, he considered, the excretory ducts originate. Ruysch thought that the glands are entirely vascular, and that the excretory ducts are immediately continuous with the *vasa afferentia*, &c. The best view, perhaps, is, that the exhaling or secreting vessel is distributed on the animal membrane, which forms the blind extremity of the excretory duct, and that the secretion is effected through it by means of cells.

The term *glande* (F.) is sometimes appropriated to the tumour formed by inflammation or engorgement of a lymphatic ganglion.

GLAND, Glans—g. Accessory, of the Parotid, see Parotid—g. Globate, Conglobate gland—g. Prostate, Prostate—g. Salivary, abdominal, Pancreas.

GLANDAGE, Adenophyma.

GLANDE, Gland — *g. Thyroïde*, see Thyroid gland.

GLANDERS, Equinia—g. Farcy, see Equinia.

GLANDES BRONCHIQUES, Bronchial glands—*g. Conglobées*, Conglobate glands—*g. de Croissance*, Waxing kernels — *g. de Meibomius*, Meibomius, glands of.

GLANDIFORM CORPUSCLE, Acinus — g. Ganglion, see Ganglion.

GLANDIUM, Thymus.

GLANDS, see Quercus Alba — g. Accessory, Cowper's glands—g. Aggregate, Peyeri glandulæ —g. Agminated, Peyer's glands—g. Aporic, Ganglions, glandiform—g. Blind, Ganglions, glandiform — g. Diapnogenous, see Perspiration — g. Havers's, Synovial glands — g. of Bartholinus, Cowper's glands of the female—g. Cowper's, see Cowper's glands—g. of Duverney, Cowper's glands of the female — g. Lenticular, Lenticulares glandulæ—g. Lieberkühn's, Lieberkühn's glands, see Intestine—g. Miliary, Sebaceous glands—g. Oil, Sebaceous glands—g. Permanent, see Gland—g. Peyer's, Peyeri glandulæ — g. Renal, Capsules, renal — g. Sebaceous, see Sebaceous glands — g. Solitary, Brunner's glands—g. Sudoriparous, see Perspiration—g. Sweat, see Perspiration.

GLANDS, TEMPORARY, *Glands without permanent orifices*. Glands, that consist of a single primary vesicle or sacculus, which, having elaborated a secretion in its interior, bursts, discharges it, and disappears. Peyer's glands, and the Graafian vesicles afford examples of these.

GLANDS OF TYSON, Sebaceous glands of Tyson — g. Vascular, see Ganglion — g. of Vesalius, Bronchial glands—g. of Willis, Albicantia corpora, Mamillary tubercles.

GLANDULA, Gland—g. ad Aures, Parotid—g. Avicennæ, Encystis — g. Bartholiniana, Sublingual gland — g. Basilaris, Pituitary gland—g. Colli, Tonsil—g. Innominata Galeni, Lachrymal gland — g. Lachrymalis, Lachrymal gland — g. Mucosa, Conglobate gland — g. Pinealis, Pineal gland—g. Pituitosa, Pituitary gland—g. Riviniana, Sublingual gland — g. Salivalis abdominis, Pancreas — g. Socia Parotidis, see Parotid — g. Thymus, Thymus—g. Thyreoidea, Thyroid gland.

GLANDULÆ AGMINATÆ, Peyeri glandulæ — g. Articulares, Synovial glands — g. Assistentes, Prostate — g. Brunneri, Brunner's glands — g. Cervicis uteri, Nabothi glandulæ — g. Duræ matris, G. Pacchioni — g. Duræ meningis, G. Pacchioni — g. in Agmen congregatæ intestinorum, Peyeri glandulæ — g. Intestinales, Peyeri glandulæ — g. Meibomianæ, Meibomius, glands of—g. Mucosæ coagminatæ intestinorum, Peyeri glandulæ—g. Muciparæ racemtim congestæ intestinorum, Peyeri glandulæ — g. Myrtiformes, Carunculæ myrtiformes — g. Odoriferæ Tysoni, see Sebaceous glands — g. Peyerianæ, Peyeri glandulæ — g. Plexiformes, Peyeri G. — g. Prostatæ mulierum, see Corpus glandulosum mulierum — g. Sebaceæ ciliares, Meibomius, glands of — g. Solitariæ, Brunner's glands — g. Spuriæ, Peyeri glandulæ, Ganglions, glandiform—g. Sudoriferæ, see Perspiration—g. Suprarenales, Capsules, renal — g. Tysoni, Sebaceous glands of Tyson — g. Utriculares, Utricular Glands — g. Vasculosæ, Conglomerate glands — g. Vesalianæ, Bronchial glands.

GLANDULAIRE, Glandular.

GLAND'ULAR, *Glandula'ris, Glandulo'sus,* (F.) *Glandulaire, Glanduleux.* Having the appearance, form, or texture of *Glands;* as a *glandular* body, a *glandular* texture, &c.

GLANDULAR SUBSTANCE OF THE KIDNEY, see Kidney.

GLANDULE OF MALPIGHI, see Corpora Malpighiana.

GRANDULEUX, Glandular.

GLANDULO'SO-CARNEUS. Ruysch gives this epithet to fleshy excrescences which he found in the bladder.

GLANDULOSUS, Glandular.

GLANS, ('an acorn.') *Bal'anus, Cyt'taros, Cuspis, Caput, C. Penis, Genita'lē caput,* (F.) *Gland.* The extremity of the penis and of the clitoris. The *glans penis* is of a conical, slightly flattened shape. It is continuous with the urethra, which opens at its apex; and is circumscribed by a projecting edge, called the *Coro'na glandis.* It is covered by a thin mucous membrane; is furnished, at its base, with sebaceous follicles, called *glan'dulæ odorif'eræ Tyso'ni,* the secretion from which is termed *Smegma prepu'tii;* and can, almost always, be covered by the reflection of the skin, called the *prepuce.* Lastly, it is formed of a spongy texture, susceptible of being thrown into erection.

GLANS, Bronchocele, Pessary, Suppository.

GLANS CLITOR'IDIS is smaller. It is imperforate, and likewise covered with a sort of prepuce formed by the mucous membrane of the vulva.

GLANS JOVIS THEOPHRASTI, Fagus castanea—g. Ulnæ, Olecranon—g. Unguentaria, Guilandina moringa, Myrobalanus.

GLAREA, Gravel.

GLASS, Vitrum.

GLAUBER'S SALTS, Soda, Sulphate of.

GLAUCEDO, Glaucoma.

GLAUCO'MA, from γλαυκος, 'sea-green.' *Glauco'sis, Glauce'do, Cataract'a glauca, Oc'ulus cæ'sius, Cæ'sius, Phtharma glauco'ma, Parop'sis glauco'sis, Apoglauco'sis.* Amongst the older pathologists, this word was used synonymously with cataract. It is now ordinarily applied to opacity of the vitreous humour or of the tunica hyaloidea, which manifests itself by a grayish, or greenish spot, apparent through the pupil. The diagnosis is generally difficult; and the disease is almost always incurable.

GLAUCOMA WOULHOUSI, Cataract.

GLAUCOSIS, Glaucoma.

GLAYEUL, Gladiolus vulgaris — g. *Puant,* Iris fœtidissima.

GLECHO'MA HEDERA'CEA, *G. hirsu'tum, Heder'ula, Chamæcle'ma, O. hedera'cea, Calamin'tha hedera'cea, Calamin'ta humil'ior, Chamæcis'sus, Hed'era terres'tris, Nep'eta glecho'ma, Panace'a pec'toris, Ground-ivy, Gill, Gill-go-byground, Alehoof, Robin runaway,* (F.) *Lierre terrestre, Terrette.* This plant has a strong smell, and a bitterish, somewhat aromatic, taste. It has been considered expectorant and tonic.

GLECHON, Mentha pulegium.

GLECHONI'TIS. Wine, impregnated with the Glechon, γληχων, *mantha pulegium,* or pennyroyal.

GLECOMA HIRSUTUM, G. hederaceum.

GLEET, see Gonorrhœa.

GLEME, *Chassie,* Lippitudo.

GLENĒ, γληνη. The pupil. The anterior part of the eye. The eyeball. The eye. According to some, the crystalline lens. Also, a glenoid cavity.

GLENITIS, Phacitis.

GLENOID, Glene.

GLE'NOID, *Glenoid'al, Glenoïda'lis, Glenoï'des, Gleno'des, Glenoï'deus,* from γληνη, 'the pupil,' and ειδος, 'resemblance.' (F.) *Glénoïde, Glenoïdale.* Any shallow, articular cavity, Glenē, which receives the head of a bone; such as, 1. The *glenoid cavity* or *fossa* of the scapula, *Fossa glenoïdea, Omocot'ylē, Acetab'ulum hu'meri, Cav'itas hu'meri glenoïdes, Entypo'sis,* is situate at the anterior angle of the scapula; and is articulated with the head of the humerus. 2. The glenoid cavity or fossa of the temporal bone. It is seated between the two roots of the zygomatic process, and receives the condyle of the lower jaw.

GLENOID LIG'AMENT, (F.) *Ligament Glénoïdien,* is a fibro-cartilaginous ring or *bourrelet,* which seems formed by the expansion of the tendon of the long head of the biceps brachialis, and surrounds the glenoid cavity of the scapula, the depth of which it increases.

GLÉNOÏDALE, Glenoid.

GLISCHRAS'MA, *Glis'chrotes,* from γλισχραινω, (γλια, 'glue,') 'I become glutinous.' Lentor, viscidity.—Hippocrates.

GLISCHROCH'OLUS, from γλισχρος, 'viscid,' and χολη, 'bile.' An epithet for excrement which is glutinous and bilious.

GLISCHROTES, Glischrasma.

GLISOMARGO, Creta.

GLOBE, Bandage (head)—g. of the Eye, see Eye—g. Flower, Cephalanthus occidentalis.

GLOBULAIRE PURGATIVE, Globularia alypum.

GLOBULA'RIA AL'YPUM, *Globula'ria, Montpel'lier Turbith,* (F.) *Globulaire purgative, Turbith blanc.* The leaves of this plant are bitter, and have been used in intermittents and in constipation. See Alypon.

GLOB'ULE, *Glob'ulus, Sphæ'rion, Sphæ'rula.* A small globe.

GLOBULES OF THE BLOOD, *Blood globules, Blood-corpuscles, Blood-disks, Blood-vesicles, Glob'uli, Vesic'ulæ, Sphæ'rulæ seu Follie'uli san'guinis,* (F.) *Globules du sang,* are small, circular bodies, which are particularly observable when the transparent parts of cold-blooded animals are examined by the aid of the microscope; and are met with in the blood of all animals. They are circular in the mammalia, and elliptical in birds and cold-blooded animals; are flat in all animals, and generally composed of a central nucleus enclosed in a membranous sac. Chemically, they consist of hæmatin and globulin—*hæmato-globulin.*

SIZE OF THE GLOBULES.

Sir E. Home and Bauer, with colouring matter,	1.1700th part of an inch.
Eller,	1.1930
Sir E. Home and Bauer, without colouring matter,	1.2000
Müller,	1.2300 to 1.3500
Mandl,	1.2625 to 1.3150

Hodgkin, Lister, and Rudolphi,	1.3000
Sprengel,	1.3000 to 1.3500
Cavallo,	1.3000 to 1.4000
Donné,	1.3150 to 1.3280
Jurin and Gulliver,	1.3240
Blumenbach and Bénsé,	1.3330
Tabor,	1.3600
Milne Edwards,	1.3900
Wagner,	1.4000
Kater,	1.4000 to 1.5000
Prévost and Dumas,	1.4056
Haller, Wollaston, and Weber,	1.5000
Young,	1.6060

GLOBULE D'ARANTIUS, see Sigmoid valves—g. du Sang, Globule of the blood.

GLOBULES, GANGLION, see Neurine—g. Chyle, see Chyle—g. Lymph, see Lymph—g. Milk, see Milk—g. Mucous, see Mucus—g. Pus, see Pus—g. Pyoid, see Pus.

GLOBULI ARTERIARUM TERMINI, see Acinus—g. Sanguinis, Globules of the blood—g. Tartari martiales, Ferrum tartarizatum—g. Tartratis ferri et lixiviæ, Ferrum tartarizatum.

GLOB'ULIN, Glob'uline, Blood ca'sein. The colourless substance that remains after the abstraction of the colouring matter of the blood-corpuscle. It is a peculiar albuminous principle. The globulin of Berzelius consists of the envelopes of the blood globules, and of the part of their contents that remains after the extraction of the hæmatin. Lecanu regards it as identical with albumen; and, according to Mulder, it belongs to the combinations of protein.

The term globulin is likewise given by M. Donné to small granulations appertaining to the chyle, which are observable in the blood with the microscope. They are small white roundish, isolated or irregularly agglomerated grains; of about the 1-300 of a millimètre in diameter, and are regarded by M. Donné as the first elements of the blood globules. They are the white granulated corpuscles of Mandl.

GLOBULUS ARANTII, see Sigmoid valves—g. Nasi, see Nasus—g. Sanguineus, Punctum saliens—g. Stapedis Ossis, Os orbiculare.

GLOBUS HYSTER'ICUS, Nodus Hyster'icus, An'goné, Anad'romé. A sensation, experienced by hysterical persons, as if a round body were rising from the abdomen towards the larynx, and producing a sense of suffocation.

GLOBUS MAJOR, see Epididymis — g. Minor, see Epididymis — g. Martialis, Ferrum tartarisatum.

GLOBUS UTERI'NUS. A term applied by accoucheurs to the round tumour, formed by the uterus in the lower part of the abdomen, immediately after delivery.

GLOMERATE, Conglomerate.

GLOM'ERULE, Glomer'ulus; from glomus, 'a clew of thread.' A ball or clew, formed by an agglomeration of vessels; as Glomerule of Malpighi; see Corpora Malpighiana.

GLOSSA, Glotta, 'the tongue.' The power of speech. Speech. Hence:

GLOSSAGRA, Glossalgia.

GLOSSAL'GIA, Glos'sagra, from γλωσσα, 'the tongue,' and αλγος, 'pain.' Pain in the tongue.

GLOSSANIS'CHUM, Glossanoch'eus, Glossan'-ochum, from γλωσσα, 'tongue,' and ανιχειν, 'to hold up.' An instrument for holding up the tongue.

GLOSSANOCHEUS, Glossanischum.

GLOSSANOCHUM, Glossanischum.

GLOSSAN'THRAX, Pestis glossan'thrax, from γλωσσα, 'the tongue,' and ανθραξ, 'a carbuncle.' Carbuncle of the tongue. A disease more common in cattle than in man.

GLOSSEPIGLOT'TIC, Glossepiglot'ticus. Relating to the tongue and epiglottis, as Ligamen'tum glossepiglott'icum.

GLOSSIANUS, Lingual muscle.

GLOSSI'TIS, from γλωσσα, 'the tongue,' and itis, a suffix denoting inflammation. Glosson'cus inflammato'rius, Angi'na lingua'ria seu lingua'lis, Inflamma'tio Linguæ, Inflammation of the tongue, (F.) Inflammation de la Langue. When confined to the mucous membrane, it is of slight importance. That which affects the whole of the tongue is a serious disease, and requires the vigorous use of antiphlogistics. It is rare.

GLOSSOC'ACE, from γλωσσα, 'the tongue,' and κακος, 'evil.' Ulceration of the tongue, with symptoms of adynamic fever.

GLOSSOCARCINO'MA, Glossoscir'rhus, Carcino'ma Linguæ, from γλωσσα, 'the tongue,' and καρκινωμα, 'cancer.' Cancer of the tongue.

GLOSSOCAT'OCHUS, Glossocat'ochè, from γλωσσα, 'the tongue,' and κατιχω, 'I arrest.' Linguæ Deten'tor, Spec'ulum Oris, (F.) Abaisseur de la langue. An instrument, the invention of which is attributed to Paulus of Ægina, and which was employed to depress the tongue, in order to examine diseases of the fauces. It was composed of two branches; one of which had, at its extremity, a plate for depressing the tongue; whilst the other, shaped like a horse-shoe, was applied under the chin. The finger, or the handle of a spoon, or a spatula, is now alone used in similar cases. See Catagoglossum.

GLOSSOCE'LE, from γλωσσα, 'the tongue,' and κηλη, 'hernia,' 'tumour.' Hernia of the Tongue, Paraglos'sè, Prolap'sus linguæ, Glossomegis'tus, Glossopto'sis. Projection of the tongue from the mouth. It depends, generally, on an inflammatory swelling of the organ. At times, however, a chronic glossocele, or sort of œdematous engorgement, is met with; which proceeds to a great length, and deforms the dental arches, the lips, &c. Inflammatory glossocele must be combated by antiphlogistics. In the œdematous kind, such as is sometimes caused by excessive salivation, the infiltrated fluid may be pressed back by the hand of the practitioner, to get the tongue behind the teeth; and it may be kept there by a piece of gauze tied over the mouth. The chronic, elongated kind sometimes requires amputation of a portion of the organ.

GLOSSOCOMA, Glossospasmus.

GLOSSOC'OMON, Glossoc'omum, Glossocomi'-on, from γλωσσα, 'the tongue,' and κμεινο, 'to guard.' The ancients gave this name to a small case for holding the tongues of their wind-instruments. By extension, it was applied to the box or cradle in which fractured limbs were kept. We find, in the ancient writers, a Glossocomon of Hippocrates, of Nymphodorus, Galen, &c.

GLOSSODESMUS, Frænum linguæ.

GLOSSO-EPIGLOT'TICUS. That which belongs to the tongue and epiglottis. Some anatomists have so denominated certain fleshy fibres, which pass from the base of the tongue towards the epiglottis. These muscles are more evident in some of the mammalia than in man; and their use seems to be,—to raise the epiglottis, and to remove it farther from the glottis. Santorini, who described them after Eustachius, calls them Retracto'res Epiglot'tidis.

GLOSSO-EPIGLOT'TIC LIG'AMENTS, Fræna epiglot'tidis. Three folds of mucous membrane, which connect the anterior surface of the epiglottis with the root of the tongue.

GLOSSOG'RAPHY, Glossogra'phia, from γλωσσα, 'the tongue,' and γραφη, 'a description.' An anatomical description of the tongue.

GLOSSO-HYAL. A name given, by Geoffroy Saint-Hilaire, to the posterior cornua of the os hyoides.

GLOSSOL'OGY, *Glossolog''ia*, from γλωσσα, 'the tongue,' and λογος, 'a treatise,' 'a discourse.' A treatise on the tongue.

GLOSSOL'YSIS, *Glossople'gia, Paral'ysis linguæ*, P. *Nervi hypoglossi*, from γλωσσα, 'the tongue,' and λυσις, 'solution.' Paralysis of the tongue.

GLOSSOMANTI'A, *Progno'sis ex linguâ*, from γλωσσα, 'the tongue,' and μαντεια, 'divination.' Prognosis from the state of the tongue.

GLOSSOMEGISTUS, Glossocele, Paraglosse.

GLOSSON'CUS, from γωλσσα, 'the tongue,' and ογκος, 'tumour.' *Exonco'sis linguæ*. Swelling of the tongue.

GLOSSONCUS INFLAMMATORIUS, Glossitis.

GLOSSO-PALATINUS, Glosso-staphylinus—g. Pharyngeal, Pharyngo-glossal.

GLOSSO-PHARYNGEAL, Glosso-pharyngeus—g. p. Nerve, Pharyngo-glossal nerve.

GLOSSO-PHARYNGEUS, *Glosso-pharyngeal*, from γλωσσα, 'the tongue,' and φαρυγξ, 'the pharynx.' Belonging to the tongue and pharynx. Some anatomists thus designate certain fleshy bundles, which arise from the lateral parts of the base of the tongue, and are inserted into the parietes of the pharynx. They form part of the constrictor pharyngis superior.

GLOSSOPLEGIA, Glossolysis.

GLOSSOPTOSIS, Glossocele.

GLOSSOSCIRRHUS, Glossocarcinoma.

GLOSSOSCOP'IA, from γλωσσα, 'the tongue,' and σκοπεω, 'I view.' Inspection of the tongue as an index of disease.

GLOSSOSPAS'MUS, *Glossoco'ma, Spasmus lin'guæ*, from γλωσσα, 'the tongue,' and σπασμος, 'spasm.' Cramp or spasm of the tongue.

GLOSSOSPA'THA, *Spat'ula pro ore*, from γλωσσα, 'the tongue,' and σπαθη, 'spatula.' A spatula for pressing down the tongue to enable the fauces to be examined.

GLOSSO-STAPHYLI'NUS, from γλωσσα, 'the tongue,' and σταφυλη, 'the uvula.' *Glossopalati'nus, Pala'to-glossus, Constric'tor Isthmi Fau'cium*. A small, thin, narrow, and long muscle, which arises from the base of the tongue, and is inserted at the inferior and lateral part of the velum palati, in the anterior pillar of which it is situate. Its use is to contract the isthmus faucium, by depressing the venum palati, and raising the base of the tongue.

GLOSSOSTERE'SIS, *Linguæ extirpa'tio*, from γλωσσα, 'the tongue,' and στερησις, 'privation.' Extirpation of the tongue.

GLOSSOSTROPH'IA, from γλωσσα, 'tongue,' and στρεφω, 'I turn.' Doubling of the point of the tongue upwards and backwards,—said to have been a mode of suicide. (?)

GLOSSOT'OMY, *Glossotom'ia*, from γλωσσα, 'the tongue,' and τεμνειν, 'to cut.' Dissection of the tongue. Amputation of the tongue.

GLOSSYPERTROPH'IA, from γλωσσα, 'the tongue,' 'υπερ, 'over,' and τρεφειν, 'to nourish.' Hypertrophy or supernutrition of the tongue.

GLOTTA, Glossa, Tongue.

GLOTTIS, γλωττις, (also, the mouth-piece of a flute,') *Lig'ula*. A small oblong aperture, in the larynx, comprised between the *chordæ vocales*. It is narrow, anteriorly; wider, posteriorly; and is capable of being modified by muscular contraction, as may be required by the voice. It is by the chordæ vocales, that voice is produced. The glottis is nearly an inch long in the adult male: less in the female and child.

Glottis is, by some, used synonymously with ventricle of the larynx: with others, it includes the whole of the larynx.

GLOTTIS, LIPS OF THE, Thyreo-arytenoid ligaments.

GLOUGLOU D'UNE BOUTEILLE, Gurgling.

GLOUTERON, Arctium Lappa—*g. Petit*, Xanthium.

GLOUTIUS, Gluteal—g. Maximus et extimus, Glutæus maximus—g. Secundus et medius, Glutæus medius—g. Tertius et intimus, Glutæus minimus.

GLOUTON, Glutton.

GLOW WORM, Cicindela.

GLUANT, Glutinous.

GLUCOSE, from γλυκυς, 'sweet.' *Grape sugar, Fruit sugar, Starch sugar, Diabetic sugar, Honey sugar*. A variety of sugar, that occurs naturally in many vegetable juices, and in honey. Compared with cane sugar, it is much less soluble in water, and less disposed to crystallise; and, when injected into the blood-vessels, does not pass off to the like extent by the kidneys.

GLUCOSURIA, Diabetes mellitus.

GLUE BONE, Osteocolla.

GLUE FISH, Ichthyocolla.

GLUTÆUS MAGNUS, G. major—g. Major, G. Maximus.

GLUTÆ'US MAX'IMUS, *Glutæ'us major, Maximus et ex'timus glou'tius, G. magnus, Ilio-sacro-fémoral; Sacro-fémoral*, (Ch.,) (F.) *Muscle grand fessier*. This muscle is situate at the posterior part of the pelvis, and at the upper and posterior part of the thigh. It is large, thick, and quadrilateral; and is attached, *above*, to the posterior part of the crista ilii, to the part of the ilium comprised between the crista and the upper curved line, to the posterior surface of the sacrum, coccyx, and great sacro-sciatic ligament; and *below*, it terminates by a broad aponeurosis, which is inserted into the rugged surface that descends from the trochanter major to the linea aspera of the femur. This muscle extends the thigh on the pelvis, and rotates the thigh outwards. It is greatly concerned in station and progression.

GLUTÆ'US ME'DIUS, *Glou'tius Secun'dus et Mé'dius*, (F.) *Ilio-trochantérien: Grand Ilio-trochantérien*, (Ch.,) *Moyen Fessier*. This muscle is situate in part beneath the preceding; it is broad, very thick, radiated, and triangular; attached, *above*, to the crista ilii, and to the part of the outer surface of that bone comprised between the three anterior fourths of its crista, its upper curved line, and its lower; and *below*, it ends by a tendon, inserted at the upper edge of the great trochanter. It is an abductor of the thigh; but can turn the thigh outwards or inwards, according as its posterior or inferior fibres are thrown separately into contraction.

GLUTÆ'US MIN'IMUS, *Glutæ'us minor, Ilio-ischii-trochantérien, Ter'tius et In'timus Glou'tius* (F.) *Petit Fessier; — Petit Ilio-trochantérien* (Ch.) This muscle, which is situate beneath the preceding, is flat, triangular, and with radiated fibres. It is attached, *above*, to the external surface of the os ilii, from the inferior curved line to the acetabulum; and, *below*, is inserted into the anterior part of the great trochanter. It has the same uses as the preceding.

GLUTÆUS MINOR, G. minimus.

GLU'TEAL, *Glou'tius, Glutæ'us*, from γλουτος, 'the nates,' or 'buttocks.' (F.) *Fessier*. That which belongs or relates to the nates. This name has been given to many parts which compose the nates.

GLUTEAL APONEUROSIS. The upper and back part of the femoral fascia. In it is a remarkable opening, called the *gluteal arch*, for the passage of the gluteal vessels and nerves.

GLUTEAL ARCH, see Gluteal aponeurosis.

GLUTEAL ARTERY, *Posté'rior Il'iac Artery*, (F.) *Artère fessière*, is one of the largest branches of the hypogastric. It makes its exit from the pelvis at the upper part of the superior sciatic foramen; gains the posterior part of the pelvis, and divides into two branches;—the one *superficial*, the other *deep-seated*. The last subdivides into three secondary branches, whose ramifications are distributed particularly to the *Glutæi, Longissimus Dorsi, Sacro-lumbalis*, &c., and anastomose with the sciatic and internal circumflex arteries.

GLUTEAL NERVE, (F.) *Nerf Fessier*, is a large branch, furnished by the 5th pair of lumbar nerves. It is chiefly distributed to the glutæi muscles.

GLUTEAL VEIN, (F.) *Veine fessière*, follows the same march as the artery of the same name.

GLUTEN, *Glu'tinum, Lentor*, 'glue, paste.' *Veg''etable Gluten, Veg''etable Ca'sein*. An immediate principle of vegetables. It is soft, of a grayish white, viscid consistence, and very elastic. Exposed to the air, it becomes hard, brown, and fragile; and, in moist air, putrefies. Water and alcohol do not dissolve it. It is soluble in vegetable, and in weak mineral acids, at a high temperature. The farinæ, in which it is found, are those preferred for the preparation of bread; on account of the property it has of making the paste rise. It is a compound of protein, and hence has been ranged amongst the "*proteinaceous alimentary principles*" by Dr. Pereira. By washing wheaten dough with a stream of water, the gum, sugar, starch and vegetable albumens are removed: the ductile, tenacious, elastic, gray mass left is the gluten, *common gluten, Beccaria's gluten*. Pure gluten is the soluble portion on boiling common gluten in alcohol.

GLUTEN ARTICULORUM, Synovia—g. Beccaria's, see Gluten — g. Bread, see Bread, gluten — g. Common, see Gluten—g. Pure, see Gluten.

GLUTI, Nates.

GLUTIA, Nates, Quadrigemina corpora

GLUTINANS, Agglutinant.

GLUTINATIF, Agglutinant.

GLUTINATIO, Agglutination.

GLUTINEUX, Glutinous.

GLU'TINOUS, *Glutino'sus, Collo'des*, from *gluten*, 'paste, glue.' (F.) *Glutineux, Gluant*. An epithet given to substances taken from the animal or vegetable kingdom, and endowed with unusual viscidity. The decoctions of marshmallows, and figs, and the jelly of hartshorn, are said to be glutinous.

GLUTINUM, Gluten.

GLUTOI, Nates.

GLUTTON, same etymon as the next. *Gastrimar'gus, Hel'luo, Mando, Gulo'sus, Lurco*, (F.) *Glouton, Gourmand, Goulu*. An excessive eater.

GLUT'TONY, from *glutio*, 'I swallow,' *gluttus*, 'the gullet.' *Limo'sis Helluo'num, Gastris'mus*, (F.) *Gourmandise*. Excessive appetite, owing often to habitual indulgence.

GLUTTUS, Œsophagus.

GLUTUS, Trochanter major.

GLYCANSIS, Edulcoration.

GLYCAS'MA, from γλυκυς, 'sweet.' A sweet wine, prepared from must.—Linden.

GLYCERATON, Glycyrrhiza.

GLYCERIN, see Fat.

GLYCIPICROS, Solanum dulcamara.

GLYCISIDE, Pæonia.

GLYCYPHYTON, Glycyrrhiza.

GLYCYRRHI'ZA, from γλυκυς, 'sweet,' and ριζα, 'a root.' *Glycyrrhi'za Glabra* seu *Lævis, Liquorit''ia Scyth'ica, Glycera'tou, Glycyph'yton, Liq'uorice, Lic'orice, Adip'sos. Alcacas, Al'imos*, (F.) *Réglisse*. Ord. Leguminosæ. Sex. Syst. Diadelphia Decandria. The root of this southern European plant is inodorous; has a sweet taste; is mucilaginous; and leaves, when unpeeled, a degree of bitterness in the mouth. It is used as a demulcent, and chiefly in catarrh. The extract, made from it and sold in the shops, is known under the name *Spanish Liquorice or Liquorice Juice*, (F.) *Jus de Réglisse*.

Pectoral Balsam of Liquorice—a quack preparation—is said by Dr. Paris to consist chiefly of *Paregoric Elixir*, strongly impregnated with *Oil of Aniseed*.

GLYCYRRHŒ'A, from γλυκυς, 'sweet,' and ρεω, 'I flow.' A discharge of saccharine fluid from the system.

GLYCYRRHŒA URINOSA. Diabetes mellitus.

GLYSTER HERBS, *Herbæ pro Enem'ată*. The herbs ordinarily sold by the English apothecary under this title, are:—*mallow leaves*, one part; *chamomile flowers*, one part. (℥iss to Oj of water.)

GNAMPSIS, Curvature.

GNAPHALIUM DIOICUM, Antennaria dioica.

GNAPHALIUM MARGARITA'CEUM; *Cudweed, Life everlasting*. An indigenous plant, growing in woods and fields, and flowering in August. Its virtues are not defined, and the same may be said of

GNAPHALIUM POLYCEPH'ALUM; *Sweet-scented Life everlasting*.

GNATHALGIA, Neuralgia maxillaris.

GNATHANCYLO'SIS, from γναθος, 'the jaw,' and αγκυλωσις, 'stiffness of joint.' Ancylosis of the lower jaw.

GNATHI'TIS, *Inflamma'tio genæ*, from γναθος, 'the cheek, the jaw.' Inflammation of the cheek or upper jaw.

GNATHMUS, Gnathus.

GNATHOCEPH'ALUS, from γναθος, 'the jaw,' and κεφαλη, 'head.' A monster who has no head visible externally, but exhibits voluminous jaws. —G. St. Hilairo.

GNATHOCYNANCHE, Cynanche parotidæa.

GNATHONEURALGIA, Neuralgia maxillaris.

GNATHOPLAS'TICE, from γναθος, 'cheek,' and πλαστικος, 'formative.' The formation of an artificial cheek.

GNATHOPLE'GIA, *Gnathoparal'ysis*, from γναθος, and πληγη, 'a stroke.' Paralysis of the cheek. *Gnathoparalysis* is employed by Fuchs to signify paralysis of the lesser portion of the trifacial nerve, which supplies the muscles of mastication.

GNATHORRHAG''IA, from γναθος, and 'ρηγνυμι, 'to burst forth.' Hemorrhage from the internal surface of the cheeks.

GNATHOSPASMUS, Trismus.

GNATHUS, *Gnathmus*, from κναω, 'I scrape, rub.' The *cheek*, the *jaw*. Also, the part of the jaws in which the teeth are fixed.—Hippocrates, Foësius. See Bucca, Gena, and Maxillary Bone.

GNESIOS, Legitimate.

GNOME, Intellect.

GNOSIS, γνωσις, 'knowledge.' A common suffix, as in *Diagno'sis, Progno'sis*, &c.

GOACONAX, see Toluifera balsamum.

GOATS' BEARD, COMMON, Tragopogon.

GOATS' MILK, see Milk, goats'—g. Milk, artificial, see Milk, goats'—g. Thorn, Astragalus verus.

GOBELET ÉMÉTIQUE, Goblet, emetic.

GOBLET, EMETIC, *Poc'ulum emet'icum, Calix vomito'ria,* (F.) *Gobelet émétique.* A vessel, made by pouring melted antimony into a mould. By putting wine into this and allowing it to stand some time, it acquires the property of producing vomiting. This kind of emetic has been long rejected, as the practitioner could never be certain of the dose he exhibited.

GODESBERG, MINERAL WATERS OF. These waters at Godesberg, a German mile from Bonn, are an efficacious, acidulous chalybeate, formerly known by the name, *Draitsch Water.* They contain chloride of sodium, carbonate of soda, carbonate of lime, carbonate of magnesia, and carbonate of iron.

GODFREY'S COR'DIAL. A celebrated nostrum, for which Dr. Paris has given the following formula. Infuse ʒix of *sassafras* and of the seeds of *carraway, coriander,* and *anise,* each ʒj, in six pints of *water.* Simmer the mixture until reduced to ℔iv: then add ℔vj of *treacle,* and boil the whole for a few minutes. When cold, add ʒiij of *tincture of opium.* The following form is recommended by a committee of the Philadelphia college of Pharmacy. *Tinct. Opii,* Oiss; *Syrupi Nigri,* Oxvj; *Alcoholis,* Oij; *Aquæ,* Oxxvj; *Carbonatis Potassæ,* ʒijss; *Olei Sassafras,* fʒiv, M. It is anodyne.

GODRONNÉ, (CANAL,) *Cana'lis Petitia'nus, Couronne ciliaire, Canal de* PETIT, *Canal goudronné, Canal* or *Bul'lular Canal of Petit.* Petit gave this name (from (F.) *godron,* 'a plait or fold,') to the semicircular canal, formed by the tunica hyaloidea around the edge of the crystalline; because it appears, as it were, plaited or festooned.

GOGGLE-EYE, Strabismus.

GOITRE, Bronchocele — g. Leaf, see Laminaria.

GOITRE STICKS. In South America the stems of a seaweed are so called, because they are chewed by the inhabitants where goitre prevails.—Royle.

GOIT'ROUS, (F.) *Goîtreux.* Relating or appertaining to goitre. One affected by Goitre or Bronchocele,—*Goitred.*

GOLD, *Aurum, Chrysos, Sol, Rex metallo'rum,* (F.) *Or.* A solid, yellow, very brilliant, hard, very ductile, malleable, tenacious, and heavy metal; found in nature, either in its native state, or combined with a little silver, copper, or iron. S. g. 19·25.

Muriate of Gold, Chloride of Gold, Auri Chlo'ridum, A. Terchlo'ridum, A. Mu'rias, A. Chlorure'tum, Aurum Muriat'icum, A. Chlora'tum, A. Oxydula'tum muriat'icum, A. Sali'tum, (F.) *Chlorure d'or, Muriate d'or, Hydro-chlorate d'or* has been admitted into the Pharmacopœias of the United States, and into that of Paris, &c. The formulæ, however, differ. That of the United States is a muriate with two bases; and is prepared, according to the form of Dr. Chrestien, by dissolving the gold in a mixture of nitric and muriatic acids, and adding chloride of sodium to the residuum after evaporation; then redissolving and evaporating slowly to dryness. The Parisian formula for the *Muriate d'or, Murias seu Chlorure'tum Auri,* consists in simply dissolving the gold in the acids, and evaporating to dryness. It has been recommended as an antisyphilitic in old, rebellious, venereal affections, exostoses, and in venereal, scrofulous or cancerous glandular enlargements. Dose, gr. 1-8th to gr. ss, rubbed on the tongue or gums. Internally, one-sixteenth of a grain, in pill.

Various other preparations, as the *Cy'anide* or *Tercy'anide,* (Auri *Cyan'idum, A. Cyanure'tum, A. Tercyan'idum,* (F.) *Cyanure d'or;*) the metallic gold in a state of division (*Aurum metal'licum, Pulvis Auri,* (F.) *Or divisé,*) obtained by amalgamating gold with mercury and driving the latter off by heat; and in the form of filings (*Aurum lima'tum;* the *Chloride of Gold and Sodium,* (*Aurum muriat'icum natrona'tum, A. muriat'icum, A. chlora'tum natro'natum, Chlore'tum Au'ricum, Chlore'to na'trii, Mu'rias Au'rico-na'tricum, Chlorure'tum auri et natrii, So'dii auro-terchlo'ridum, Hydrochlorate* or *muriate of Gold and Soda,* (F.) *Chlorure d'or et de Sodium, Hydrochlorate* ou *muriate d'or et de Soude;* the *Nitromuriate of Gold,* (*Aurum Nitrico-muriat'icum, Auri nitromu'rias,* (F.) *Nitromuriate d'or;*) the *Oxide of Gold,* (*Auri Ox'idum, Aurum Oxida'tum, Auri terox'idum, Perox'ide of gold, Auric acid,* (F.) *Oxide d'or);* and the *Iodide of Gold,* (*Auri Io'didum, A. Iodure'tum,* (F.) *Iodure d'or,*) have been employed in the like affections, and with similar results.

GOLD-BEATER'S SKIN. The intestina recta of the ox, which have been beaten quite smooth, for the manufacture of gold leaf. Used as a defensive dressing for slight cuts, &c.

GOLD, CHLORIDE OF, see Gold—g. Cyanide of, see Gold—g. Hydrochlorate of, see Gold—g. Iodide of, see Gold—g. Muriate of, see Gold—g. Nitro-muriate of, see Gold—g. Oxide of, see Gold—g. Peroxide of, see Gold—g. Tercyanide of, see Gold—g. and Sodium, Chloride of oxide of, see Gold—g. and Soda, hydrochlorate of, see Gold—g. and Soda, muriate of, see Gold.

GOLD LEAF, *Aurum folia'tum, Aurum in libel'lis.* Used to gild pills and to plug carious teeth.

GOLD THREAD, Coptis.

GOLDEN ROD, Solidago virgaurea — g. r. Rigid, Solidago rigida — g. Seal, see Calumba, Hydrastis Canadensis.

GOLDENS, Chrysanthemum leucanthemum.

GOLDWASSER, see Spirit.

GOLFE, Sinus — g. *de la Veine jugulaire,* see Jugular veins.

GOLUNCHA, Menispermum cordifolium.

GOMME, Gumma, Gummi—*g. Adragant,* Tragacanth — g. *Ammoniaque,* Ammoniac gum—*g. Arabique,* Acaciæ gummi—*g. Astringente de Gambie,* see Butea frondosa—*g. Caragne,* Caranna—*g. Carane,* Caranna—*g. de Gaïac,* Guaiacum—*g. Gutte,* Cambogia—*g. de Lierre,* see Hedera helix—*g. du Pays,* Gummi nostras—*g. Séraphique,* Sagapenum.

GOMPHI'ASIS, *Gomphias'mus,* from γομφος, 'a nail.' A disease of the teeth, and particularly of the molares; looseness of the teeth in their sockets. *Agomphia'sis.* Pain in the teeth. Odontalgia.

GOMPHIASMUS, Gomphiasis.

GOMPHIOI, Molar teeth.

GOMPHOCAR'PUS CRISPUS. A South African plant, the root of which, formerly known to the Dutch apothecaries as *Radix Asclepiadis crispæ,* is extremely bitter and acrid; and, on account of its diuretic virtues, a decoction or infusion of it has been advised in various kinds of dropsy. A tincture of it is said to be valuable in colic.

GOMPHOMA, Gomphosis.

GOMPHO'SIS, *Cardinamen'tum, Clava'tio, Gompho'ma, Coagmenta'tio, Inclava'tio,* from γομφος, 'a nail.' *Engompho'sis.* An immovable articulation, in which one bone is received into another, like a nail or peg into its hole. Gomphosis is only met with in the articulations of the

teeth with the alveoli. It is, also, called *Articulation par implantation.*
GOMPHUS, Clavus.
GONACRASIA, Spermatorrhœa.
GONACRATIA, Spermatorrhœa.
GON'AGRA, *Gon'yagra,* from γονυ, 'the knee,' and αγρα, 'a prey.' "That which attacks the knees." Gout in the knees. Paracelsus calls it *Gen'ugra.*
GONAL'GIA, from γονυ, 'the knee,' and αλγος, 'pain.' *Pain in the knee. Gonyal'gia.* This is almost always produced by gout. It may, however, depend on some other disease, either of the knee or of another part—particularly of the hip-joint.
GONARTHRI'TIS, from γονυ, 'the knee,' αρθρον, 'joint,' and *itis,* denoting inflammation. Inflammation of the knee-joint.
GONARTHROCACE, Gonocace.
GONAURA, see Sperm.
GONDOLE OCULAIRE, Scaphium oculare.
GONDRET'S AMMONIACAL CAUSTIC, *Pommade de Gondret*—g. Counter-irritant, *Pommade de Gondret.*
GONĒ, *Gonos, Genitu'ra.* The semen; (hence, gonorrhœa)—the uterus, offspring. Hippocrates. See Epigone and Generation.
GONECYSTIDES, Vesiculæ seminales.
GONECYSTI'TIS, *Inflamma'tio vesicula'rum semina'lium,* from γονυ, 'sperm,' κυστις, 'bladder,' and *itis,* 'denoting inflammation.' Inflammation of the vesiculæ seminales.
GONEPŒUS, Spermatopœus.
GONEPOIETICUS, Spermatopœus.
GONFLEMENT, Swelling.
GONGRONA, Bronchocele.
GONGROPHTHISIS, Pthisis pulmonalis.
GONGYLIDIUM, Pilula.
GONGYLION, Pilula.
GONGYLIS, Pilula.
GONIOM'ETER, *Goniom'etrum;* from γωνια, 'an angle,' and μετρον, 'a measure.' An instrument for measuring angles.
A 'FACIAL GONIOMETER' has been invented by Mr. Turnpenny, of Philadelphia, which is well adapted for measuring the facial angle.
GONOBOLIA, Ejaculation, spermatic.
GONOC'ACĒ, *Gonarthroc'acē,* from γονυ, 'the knee,' and κακος, 'evil.' *Tumor genu albus.* White swelling of the knee. Hydrarthus.
GONOCELE, Spermatocele.
GONOĪ'DES, from γονυ, 'seed,' and ειδος, 'appearance.' *Genitu'ræ sim'ilis.* Similar to sperm. *Sperm'atoid, Spermatoi'des, Spermato'des.* A term appropriated to any substance which resembles sperm.
GONOPOIETICUS, Spermatopœus.
GONORRHÉE BÂTARDE, Gonorrhœa spuria.
GONORRHŒ'A. Erroneously called from γονυ, 'sperm,' and ρεω, 'I flow,' because the older writers believed it to be a flux of semen. *Blennorrhag"ia, Blennorrhœ'a, Blennure'thria, Phallorrhœ'a, Medorrhœ'a, M. viri'lis, Catar'rhus Gonorrhœ'a, C. ure'thra, Urethri'tis, Inflamma'tio ure'thra, Urethral'gia, Proflu'vium muco'sum ure'thræ, Blennorrhœ'a urethra'lis, Catarrhus urethra'lis,* (F.) *Écoulement, Uréthrite, Urétrite.* An inflammatory discharge of mucus from the membrane of the urethra in both sexes; and from that of the prepuce in man, and the vagina in woman. It may be excited spontaneously, or by irritants applied directly to the membrane; but is, usually, produced by impure connexion. Two great varieties have been generally reckoned.—1. GONORRHŒA PURA VEL BENIG'NA. That which does not follow an impure connexion; (F.) *Échauffement, Blennorrhag"ia benigna, Caulorrhœ'a benig'na, Catar'rhus Ure'thræ, Gonorrhœ'a catarrha'lis, G. non contagio'sa:*—and 2. GONORRHŒA IMPU'RA, *malig'na, contagio'sa, syphilit'ica, et virulen'ta; Fluor albus malig'nus, Fluxus vene'reus, Blennorrhœ'a luo'des, Myxio'sis, Lues gonorrho'ica, Scroph'ulæ gonorrho'icæ, Tuber'cula gonorrho'icа, Clap,* (F.) *Chaudepisse;* that which is the result of impure commerce. The French, also, distinguish the *Chaudepisse sèche,* or that unaccompanied with discharge; and the *Chaudepisse chordée, Gonnorrhœa corda'ta,* or that accompanied with chordee, and which, of course, occurs only in the male. It is the kind that most frequently engages the attention of the practitioner, and is characterized by mucous discharge from the urethra or vagina, intermixed with specific matter, and accompanied by burning pain on micturition. It is decidedly infectious. It is, however, a distinct disease from syphilis, and never produces it. Its duration is various, but the inflammatory symptoms usually subside in four or five weeks; leaving generally behind more or less of the gonorrhœa mucosa or gleet. Gonorrhœa of every kind, attended with any inflammatory symptoms, is best treated by the antiphlogistic regimen; avoiding every kind of irritation, and keeping the body cool by small doses of salts, and the urine diluted by the mildest fluids. After the inflammatory symptoms have subsided, cubebs, or the balsam of copaiba, exhibited in the dose of a teaspoonful, three times a day, will be found effectual: indeed, during the existence of the inflammatory symptoms, it often affords decided relief. Injections are rarely required.

Sometimes, gonorrhœa affects the glans; when it is called *Gonorrhœa Spu'ria, G. Bal'ani, Balanoblennorrhœ'a, Balannorrhœ'a, Balani'tis, Blennorrhag"ia spu'ria* vel *notha,* (F.) *Blennorrhagie du gland, Gonorrhée bâtarde, Fausse Blennorrhagie.* It requires only cleanliness and cooling lotions.

Some other varieties of gonorrhœa have been enumerated, but they are of little moment.

In consequence of repeated attacks of gonorrhœa, or of the debility induced by a single attack, it not unfrequently happens, as already remarked, that a constant, small discharge occurs, or remains behind, after all danger of infection is removed. The great difference between it and gonorrhœa is, that it is uninfectious. The discharge consists of globular particles, contained in a slimy mucus, and is generally devoid of that yellow colour which characterizes the discharge of gonorrhœa virulenta. It is unattended with pain, scalding, &c. To this state the names *Gleet, Gonorrhœ'a muco'sa, Blennorrhœ'a chron'- ica, Blennorrhœ'a,* &c., have been given. It is commonly a disease of some duration, and demands the use of the copaiba, astringent injections; and, if obstinate, the introduction of the bougie.

GONORRHŒA BALANI, G. spuria — g. Benigna, Leucorrhœa — g. Catarrhalis, G. pura — g. Chordata, Chordee.

GONORRHŒA DORMIEN'TIUM, *G. Oneirog'onos.* The seminal discharge which occurs during sleep, and is occasioned by libidinous dreams. See Pollution.

GONORRHŒA LAXO'RUM, *G. libidino'sa, Spermorrhœ'a aton'ica,* consists of a pellucid discharge from the urethra, whilst awake, without erection of the penis, but with venereal thoughts.

GONORRHŒA LAXORUM, Pollution, G. libidinosa — g. Mucosa, (gleet,) see Gonorrhœa — g. Noncontagiosa, G. pura — g. Notha inveterata, Leucor-

rhœa—g. Oneirogonos, G. dormientium, Pollution—g. Vera, Pollution, Spermatorrhœa.
GONOS, Gone.
GONOSTROMA, Proligerous disc.
GONY, *γονυ*, *Genu*, 'the knee;' hence:
GONYAGRA, Gonagra.
GONYALGIA, Gonalgia.
GONYC'ROTUS, from *γονυ*, 'the knee,' and *κροτω*, 'I strike.' One who is knock-kneed, or in-kneed. See Entogonyancon.
GONYON'CUS, from *γονυ*, 'the knee,' and *ογκος*, 'a tumour.' A swelling of the knee.
GOODYE'RA PUBES'CENS, *Tussa'ea reticula'ta*, *Satyr'ium*, *Neott'ia*, *Rattlesnake leaf*, *Rattlesnake Plantain*, *Networt*, *Netleaf*, *Scrofula weed*. An indigenous plant, used empirically in scrofula — the fresh leaves being applied to the sores. It is employed by the Indians.
GOOSEFOOT, Chenopodium anthelminticum—g. Angular-leaved, Chenopodium bonus Henricus—g. Stinking, Chenopodium vulvaria.
GOOSEGRASS, Galium aparine, G. verum.
GOOSESHARE, Galium aparine.
GOOSESKIN, Horrida cutis.
GORDIUS MEDINENSIS, Dracunculus.
GORGE, Throat—*g. Grosse*, Bronchocele—*g. Mal de*, Cynanche.
GORGERET, Gorget—*g. Lithotome*, Gorget, lithotomy—*g. à Repoussoir*, see Gorget.
GORGET, from (F.) *gorge*, 'the throat.' *Cana'lis canalicula'tus*, *Ductor canalicula'tus*, (F.) *Gorgeret*. An instrument representing a long gutter, in the shape of a throat, which is especially employed in the operations of lithotomy and fistula in ano.
GORGET, CUTTING, see Gorget, and Lithotomy.
GORGET, LITHOT'OMY, (F.) *Gorgeret Lithotome, Cutting Gorget*, is the one used in the operation for the stone, for the purpose of dividing the prostate and the neck of the bladder, so as to enable the surgeon to introduce the forceps and extract the stone. At the end of this gorget is a crest or beak, which fits the groove of the staff, and admits of the gorget being passed along it into the bladder. Besides *cutting*, there are also *blunt* gorgets, intended to be introduced into the wound — their concavity serving as a guide for the forceps into the bladder.
The chief modifications in the gorget have been made by Andouillet, Bell, Blicke, Bromfield, Cline, Desault, Foubert, Hawkins, Larrey, Lefèvre, Michaelis, Thomas, &c.
GORGET FOR FISTULA IN ANO consists of a semi-cylindrical wooden staff, four inches long, without including the handle, and furnished with a wide groove. This is introduced into the rectum, to prevent the point of the bistoury from injuring the intestine, when the internal orifice of the fistula is deeply situate, and it is desirable to perform the operation by incision. This instrument, invented by Marchettis, has been modified by Percy, Runge, &c.
Desault invented an instrument for conducting the wire by the anus, in the operation for fistula by ligature. He called it *Gorgeret à repoussoir*.
GORGO'NEI FONTES. Fountains described by Libavius as containing water which possessed a petrifying property; probably, water holding in solution supercarbonate of lime.
GORGOSSET, Pyrosis.
GOSIER, Pharynx, Throat.
GOSSUM, Bronchocele.
GOSSYP'IUM, *Gossyp'ium Herba'ceum; Gossyp'ion Xylon, Xylum, Bombax, Cotton*, (F.) *Coton*. Family, Malvaceæ. Sex. Syst. Monadelphia Polyandria. The seeds of the Cotton Tree, *Gossip'ium arbor'eum*, have been administered in coughs, on account of the mucilage they contain. The cotton wool is used in medicine for making moxas, &c.
GOTIUM, Bronchocele.
GOUDRON, see Pinus sylvestris.
GOUET, Arum maculatum.
GOUÊTRE, Bronchocele.
GOULARD'S LOTION, see Lotion, Goulard's.
GOULARD WATER, Liquor plumbi subacetatis dilutus.
GOULU, Glutton.
GOURD, Cucurbita — g. Bitter, Cucumis colocynthis—g. Bottle, Cucurbita pepo.
GOURD WORM, Distoma hepaticum.
GOURMANDISE, Gluttony.
GOURME, Porrigo larvalis. Vulgarly, in France, any cutaneous eruption.
GOUSSE, Legumen.
GOUT, *Arthri'tis, Arth'ragra, Arthral'gia, Morbus domino'rum, Malum articulo'rum, Morbus articula'ris, Gutta, Arthro'sia Pod'agra, Podal'gia, Pod'agra, Arthrit'icus verus, Arthri'tis Podagra, Podagra Arthri'tis, Flux'io arthrit'ica, Febris arthrit'ica, F. Podag'rica, Arthrodyn'ia podag'rica, Cauma podag'ricum, Flerecin, Gastro-arthri'tis, Misopto'chos*, (F.) *Goutte*. The gout was formerly regarded as a catarrh, and received its name from (F.) *goutte*, (L.) *gutta*, 'a drop;' because it was believed to be produced by a liquid, which distilled, *goutte à goutte*, 'drop by drop, on the diseased part.' This name, which seems to have been first used about the year 1270, has been admitted into the different languages of Europe. Gout is an inflammation of the fibrous and ligamentous parts of the joints. It almost always attacks, first, the great toe; whence it passes to the other smaller joints, after having produced, or been attended with, various sympathetic effects, particularly in the digestive organs: after this, it may attack the greater articulations. It is an affection which is extremely fugitive, and variable in its recurrence. It may be acquired or hereditary. In the former case, it rarely appears before the age of thirty-five; in the latter, it is frequently observed earlier. It is often difficult to distinguish it from rheumatism. A combination is, indeed, supposed to exist sometimes; hence called *Rheumatic gout*. During the paroxysm or fit, a burning, lancinating pain is experienced in the affected joint, attended with tumefaction, tension, and redness. One or more joints may be attacked, either at the same time or in succession; and, in either case, the attack terminates by resolution in a few days. This is the *Arthri'tis acu'ta, inflammato'ria* vel *regula'ris, Regular gout, Arthro'sia pod'agra regula'ris, Arth'ragra legit'ima* seu *vera* seu *genui'na* seu *norma'lis*, (F.) *Goutte régulière chaude*. At other times, pains in the joints exist, of more or less acute character; the swelling being without redness. These pains persist, augment, and diminish irregularly, without exhibiting intermission, and, consequently, without having distinct paroxysms. The disease is then called *aton'ic, asthen'ic, imperfect* or *irregular gout*, Chronic G., *Arthri'tis aton'ica* vel *asthen'ica, Arthro'sia Podagra larva'ta, Dysarthri'tis*. It is, also, commonly called in France *Goutte froide, Goutte blanche*. It may appear primarily, or succeed attacks of regular gout.
Gout does not always confine itself to the joints. It may attack the internal organs: when it is called *Arthritis aber'rans* seu *errat'ica* seu *planet'ica, Arth'ragra anom'ala, Pod'agra aber'rans, Vare'ni, Wandering, misplaced*, or *anomalous gout*, (F.) *Goutte vague*.
Ret'rograde gout, Arthritis retrog'rada, Podagra retrog'rada, Arthro'sia Podagra complica'ta,

Rece'dent, mispla'ced gout, (F.) *Goutte remontée, G. malplacée, G. rentrée*, is when it leaves the joints suddenly and attacks some internal organ, as the stomach, intestines, lungs, brain, &c.

Gout is also called, according to the part it may affect, *Podagra, Gonagra, Chiragra*, &c. It may be acute or chronic, and may give rise to concretions, which are chiefly composed of urate of soda. See Calculus, (arthritic.) It may, also, give occasion to nodosities, when it is called *Arthritis nodo'sa*, (F.) *Goutte nouée*.

The treatment is of the antiphlogistic kind, and the local disorder should be but little interfered with. Colchicum seems to have great power over the disease. It forms the basis of the *Eau médicinale d'Husson*, a celebrated French gout-remedy. The bowels must be kept regular by rhubarb and magnesia; and a recurrence of the disease be prevented by abstemious habits.

GOUT, DIAPHRAGMATIC, Angina pectoris.

GOUT, PAPER, so called, *Charta antiarthrit'ica, Charta antirheumat'ica*, is made by spreading a very thin layer of a mixture of an ethereal or spirituous extract of the bark of mezereon root, with wax, spermaceti, and oil, over the surface of paper.

GOUT, RHEUMATIC, see Rheumatism, acute—g. Weed, Ligusticum podagraria.

GOUT, Taste.

GOUTTE, Gout, Gutta — *g. Blanche*, Gout (atonic)—*g. Froide*, Gout (atonic)—*g. Malplacée*, Gout (retrograde)—*g. Nouée*, Gout (with nodosities) — *g. Régulière, chaude*, Gout (regular) — *g. Remontée*, Gout (retrograde)—*g. Rentrée*, Gout (retrograde)—*g. Rose*, Gutta rosea—*g. Sciatique*, Neuralgia femoro-poplitæa—*g. Sereine*, Amaurosis—*g. Vague*, Gout (wandering.)

GOUTTEUX, Arthritic, Podagric.

GOUTTIÈRE (F.), *Collic"iæ*. A gutter in a bone, like that used for carrying off rain. Some of these cavities are intended to facilitate the sliding of tendons, such as the *Gouttière Bicipitale* or *Bicip'ital groove*. Others, as the *Gouttière sagittale* or *Sagittal groove*, lodge bloodvessels and especially veins. Others, again, are merely intended for the support of certain organs; as the *Gouttière basilaire* or *Bas'ilary fossa*, which supports the medulla oblongata.

GOUTTIÈRE BASILAIRE, see *Gouttière—g. Bicipitale*, Bicipital groove — *g. Lacrymale*, Lachrymal groove — *g. Sacré*, Sacral groove — *g. Sagittale*, see *Gouttière*.

GOUTY RHEUMATISM, see Rheumatism, acute.

GOUVERNAIL DU TESTICULE, Gubernaculum testis.

GOWLAND'S LOTION, see Lotion, Gowland's.

GOWN, RED, Strophulus—g. Yellow, Icterus infantum.

GRACILARIA LICHENOÏDES, Fucus amylaceus.

GRAC''ILIS, Macer, Macilen'tus. Slender, lean. Also, the slender *Rectus inte'rior fem'oris sive Grac''ilis interior, Sous-pubio-créti-tibial, Sous-pubio-prétibial* (Ch.), *Droit ou grêle interne de la cuisse*. This muscle is situate at the inside of the thigh. It is thin and very long; and arises from the descending ramus of the pubis, to be inserted at the inner and inferior part of the tuberosity of the tibia. It bends the leg and causes abduction of the thigh. See *Grêle*.

GRACILIS, ANTERIOR, Rectus femoris.

GRAD'UATE, *Gradua'tus*, from *gradus*, 'a step,' 'a degree.' In medicine, one who has attained a degree, evidenced by a diploma—usually, the *degree* of doctor.

GRÆA, γραια. The pellicle, which forms on milk. The folds of skin round the umbilicus. An old woman.

GRAIN, *Granum*; the 60th part of a Troy, and the 72d part of a *Poids de marc* drachm.

GRAIN, OILY, Sesamum orientale.

GRAINE D'ÉCARLATE, Coccus cacti — *g. Musc*, Hibiscus abelmoschus—*g. de Turquie*, Zea mays — *g. d'Aspic*, see Phalaris Canariensis — *g. de Paradis*, Amomum granum paradisi — *g. de Perroquet*, Carthamus tinctorius (seed) — *g. de Santé*, see Pilulæ aloes et kinæ kinæ.

GRAISSE, Pinguede — *g. de Mouton*, Sevum — *g. d'Oie*, Adeps anserina—*g. Oxygénée*, Unguentum acidi nitrosi — *g. de Porc*, Adeps præparata.

GRAMEN ÆGYPTIACUM, G. Crucis cyperioidis—g. Caninum, Triticum repens.

GRAMEN CRUCIS CYPERIOÏ'DIS, *Gramen Ægyptiacum, Ægyp''tian Cock's foot grass*. The roots and plants possess the virtues of the *Triticum repens*, and have been recommended in the earlier stages of dropsy. They were, formerly, considered to possess many other properties.

GRAMEN DIOSCORIDIS, Triticum repens—g. Major, Sarsaparilla Germanica—g. Orientale, Juncus odoratus — g. Repens, Triticum repens — g. Rubrum, Sarsaparilla Germanica.

GRAMIA, *CHASSIE*, Lippitudo.

GRAMINIV'OROUS, *Graminiv'orus*, from *gramen*, 'grass,' and *voro*, 'I eat.' Feeding or subsisting on grass.

GRAMMARIUM, Scruple.

GRAMME, γραμμη. An ancient weight, equivalent to the 24th part of an ounce, or to 24 grains, or a scruple, avoirdupois. At the present day, the gramme is equal in weight to a cubed centimètre of water; or to 18 grains, poids de marc—15.434 grains, Troy.

GRAMME, Iris, Line.

GRANA, Hemicrania — g. Molucca, Croton tiglium—g. Moschi, Hibiscus abelmoschus—g. Orientis, see M...ispermum cocculus — g. Tiglii seu Tiglia, see Croton tiglium — g. Tilli, Croton tiglium.

GRANADILLA, APPLE-SHAPED, Passiflora maliformis.

GRANATI RADICIS CORTEX, see Punica granatum.

GRAND DORSAL, Latissimus dorsi.

GRANDEB'ALÆ. The hair which grows in the arm-pits.

GRANDINOSUM OS, Cuboid.

GRANDO, Chalaza.

GRANDULA, Gland.

GRANIV'OROUS, *Graniv'orus*, from *granum*, 'a grain,' and *voro*, 'I eat.' Feeding or subsisting on grain or seeds.

GRANTRISTUM, Anthrax.

GRANULA SEMINIS, see Sperm.

GRANULAR DEGENERATION or DISORGANIZATION OF THE KIDNEY, Kidney, Bright's disease of the—g. Conjunctiva, Trachoma —g. Eyelid, Trachoma—g. Liver, Cirrhosis— g. Tin, see Tin.

GRANULATED LIVER, Cirrhosis.

GRANULA'TION, *Granula'tio*, from *granum*, 'a grain.' *Gemma*, (F.) *Bourgeon, B. charnu*. Granulations are the reddish, conical, flesh-like shoots, which form at the surface of suppurating wounds and ulcers. They are the product of inflammatory excitement, and may be produced in indolent ulcers, by exciting the parts by proper stimulants. They form the basis of the cicatrix.

GRANULATION is, likewise, a name given by the modern French physicians to an organic lesion, consisting in the formation of small, round, firm, shining, semi-transparent tumours, of the size and shape of millet-seed, or of a pea; which are met with in the lungs particularly, and in considerable quantity; often without materially interfering with their functions.

In pharmacy, *granulation* is a process by which a metal is reduced to fine grains, by melting it, and causing it, whilst liquid, to pass through a kind of sieve into a vessel of water, — as in the making of shot : — or by shaking or rubbing the melted metal in an appropriate box or vessel,— as in the formation of granular tin or granulated zinc.

GRANULATIONS CÉRÉBRALES, Glandulæ Pacchioni.

GRANULA'TIONS MIL'IARY, or *Miliary tu'bercles*, are the small, transparent grains, of variable size, from that of a millet-seed to that of a grain of hemp, which are presumed to be the primitive state of tubercles.

GRAN'ULE, *Gran'ulum;* diminutive of *granum*, 'a grain.' A small grain; a small compact particle; a cytoblast.

GRAN'ULES SEM'INAL, *Gran'ula sem'inis.* Minute, rounded, granulated bodies, observable in the semen, which are, in all cases, much less numerous than the spermatozoids. See Sperm.

GRANVILLE'S LOTION, see Lotion, Granville's counter-irritant.

GRAPE, see Vitis vinifera — g. Sea-side, see Kino.

GRAPE-CURE, (F.) *Cure du raisin,* (G.) Traubencur. A mode of medication in Germany, which consists in the use of the grape for both meat and drink; nothing more at the farthest being allowed than a piece of dry bread. This diet is continued for weeks. Its effects are altogether revellent, and resemble in many respects those of hydropathy.

GRAPES, DRIED, Uvæ passæ.
GRAPHIDOIDES, Styloid.
GRAPHIODES, Styloid.
GRAPHIOIDES, Styloid.
GRAPHIS'CUS, *Graphis'cus Di'oclis.* An instrument invented by Diocles for extracting darts. It is described by Celsus.

GRAPHI'TES, *Plumba'go, Supercarbure'tum Ferri, Carbure'tum Ferri, Ferri Carbona'tum, F. Supercarbure'tum, Carbo minera'lis, Galena'a, Gale'né, Carburet of iron, Black lead, Wad,* (F.) *Crayon noir, Plombagine.* This substance has been esteemed slightly astringent and desiccative. It has been advised by Weinhold in the cure of herpes.

GRAPHOIDES, Styloid.
GRAPHOSPASMUS, Cramp, writers'.

GRAS DES CADAVRES, Adipocire — g. de Jambe, Sura — g. des Cimetières, Adipocire — g. de Jambe, Sura.

GRAS FONDURE (F.), *Diarrhœa adipo'sa,* literally, *molten grease.* A species of diarrhœa, referred to by old writers; accompanied with great emaciation, and in which the evacuations contain fat-like matter. According to Sauvages, the *Grasfondure* differs from colliquative diarrhœa in not being attended with hectic fever.

GRASS, Asparagus — g. Bitter, Aletris farinosa — g. Blue-eyed, Sisyrinchium Bermudianum — g. Brome, Bromus ciliatus — g. Brome, soft, Bromus ciliatus — g. Canary, cultivated, Phalaris Canariensis — g. Couch, Triticum repens — g. Dog, Triticum repens — g. Egyptian cock's foot, Gramen crucis cyperioides — g. Goat's, Scorzonera — g. Knot, Polygonum aviculare — g. Lily, Sisyrinchium Bermudianum — g. Physic, Sisyrinchium Bermudianum — g. Scurvy, Sisyrinchium Bermudianum — g. Sweet, Acorus Calamus — g. Vipers', Scorzonera — g. Yellow-eyed, Xyris bulbosa.

GRASSET, (F.) The anterior region of the thigh, bounded below by the patella.

GRASSEYEMENT (F.), *Sonus blæsus, Rotacis'mus,* from (F.) *gras,* 'thick.' 'Speaking thick.' According to Sauvages, a vicious pronunciation of the letter *r*. They who speak thick, like the inhabitants of Newcastle, in England, or of Havre, in France, have difficulty in pronouncing the *r*, and they frequently substitute for it the letter *l;* but this does not properly constitute *Grasseyement.* It consists in this: that, in words in which the letter.*r* is joined to another consonant, a sort of *burring* or guttural rolling is heard, nearly like that produced by gargling. See Rotacism.

GRASUS, Cinabra.
GRATELLE, Psoriasis.
GRATIA DEI, Gratiola officinalis.
GRATIOLA CENTAURIODES, G. officinalis.
GRATIO'LA OFFICINA'LIS, *Digita'lis min'ima, Gra'tia Dei, Gratiola Centaurioides, Hedge hyssop, Herb of Grace.* It is a native of the South of Europe. (F.) *Herbe au pauvre homme.* The plant is inodorous; taste strong, bitter, nauseous. It is possessed of anthelmintic, purgative, emetic, and diuretic properties. Dose, ten grains.

GRATTERON, Galium aparine.
GRATTOIR, Raspatorium.
GRAVATIF, Heavy.
GRAVE, Serious — g. Plant, Datura sanguinea.
GRAVEDO, Catarrh, Coryza — g. Neonatorum, Snuffles.

GRAVEL, *Lith'ia rena'lis areno'sa, Lithi'asis nephrit'ica, L. rena'lis,* (F.) *Gravelle.* A disease occasioned by small concretions, similar to sand or gravel, *Gla'rea,* (F.) *Gravier,* which form in the kidneys, pass along the ureters to the bladder, and are expelled with the urine. These concretions, which are commonly composed of uric acid and an animal matter, are deposited at the bottom of the vessel, immediately after the excretion of the urine; and, by their hardness and resistance under the finger, differ considerably from the ordinary sediment of that liquid. A vegetable diet and alkaline drinks are the best prophylactics. See Calculi, Urinary. *A fit of the Gravel, Nephral'gia calculo'sa seu areno'sa, Co'lica nephrit'ica,* is the excruciating suffering induced by the passage of gravel from the kidney to the bladder. It can only be relieved by anæsthetics, opiates, the warm bath, &c.

When the deposit is in fine particles, it is termed *Sand, Are'na, Are'nula, Psam'ma, Psammus.*

GRAVEL GRASS, Galium verum.
GRAVEL, PILEOUS or HAIRY, (F.) *Gravelle pileuse.* A species of gravel containing hairs, phosphate of lime, ammoniaco-magnesian phosphate, and a little uric acid. — Magendie.

GRAVELEUX, Calculous.
GRAVELLE, Chalaza, Gravel — g. Pileuse, Gravel, pileous.
GRAVEOLENS, Fetid.
GRAVID, Pregnant.

GRAV'IDINE; from *gravidus,* 'pregnant,' *gravis,* 'heavy.' A sediment in the urine of pregnant women, which by its decomposition gives rise to the pellicle kyestein. It differs from albumen, casein and gelatin. — Stark.

GRAVIDITAS, Fecundation, Pregnancy — g. Abdominalis, Pregnancy, abdominal — g. Extrauterina, see Pregnancy — g. Extra-uterina in Ovario, Pregnancy, ovarian — g. Extra-uterina Secundaria, Metacyesis — g. Interstitialis, Pregnancy, interstitial — g. Molaris, Mole — g. Spuria,

Pregnancy, false—g. Tubaria, Salpingo-cyesis—g. Uteri substantiâ, Pregnancy, interstitial—g. Uterina, Pregnancy.

GRAVIER, Gravel.

GRAVIMETER, Areometer.

GRAVIS, Heavy.

GRAV'ITY, SPECIF'IC, *Gravitas specif'ica*, (F.) *Pesanteur spécifique*. The relation between the weight of a body and its bulk; thus, supposing four bodies to be of the same size, but to weigh, one four, another three, another two, and the fourth one; the specific gravity of the first will be four times greater than that of the last. The specific gravities of different bodies are, therefore, as the weights, bulk for bulk. For solids, and liquids, water is taken as the unit; atmospheric air for the gases. Thus, water is 1.000; mercury at the common temperature, 13.58. Whence, we conclude mercury is between thirteen and fourteen times heavier than water.

GRAY MATTER OF THE BRAIN, Cortex cerebri, see Neurine.

GREASE, from (F.) *Graisse*, 'fat.' A specific inflammation, affecting the skin of the heels of the horse, which is especially interesting from the circumstance, that the matter, if inserted under the cuticle of an unprotected individual, may give rise to an affection — *grease-pox, variolæ equinæ*—which preserves the person from small-pox. (?)

GREASE, BARROW'S, Adeps suilla—g. Goose, Adeps anserina—g. Molten, *Gras-fondure*—g. Pox, see Grease.

GREENHEART, see Bebeeru.

GREENHOW'S TINCTURE FOR THE TEETH, Spiritus armoraciæ compositus.

GREEN SICKNESS, Chlorosis.

GREENWEED, Genista tinctoria.

GRÊLE (F.), *Grac"ilis*, 'long and thin.' This epithet is given by the French to various parts, as the

Apophyse Grêle du Marteau, the *slender apoph'ysis or process of the mal'leus*, a long process situate at the anterior part of the neck of the malleus, which passes out by the fissure of Glaserius. It is also called the *Apoph'ysis of Rau*, although it was already known to Fabricius ab Aquapendente and to Cæcilius Follius.

GRÊLE, *Chalaza—g. Interne de la Cuisse*, Gracilis.

GRÉMIL OFFICINALE, Lithospermum officinale.

GREMIUM, Vulva.

GRENADE, Influenza.

GRENADIER, Punica granatum.

GRENADIN, see Punica granatum.

GRENIERS, Vesiculæ seminales.

GRENOUILLE, Rana esculenta.

GRENOUILLETTE, Ranula.

GRÉOULX, MINERAL WATERS OF. Sulphuretted springs in the department of Basses-Alpes, France.

GRESSURA, Perinæum.

GRESSUS, Walking.

GREVEURE, Hernia.

GRIELUM, Apium petroselinum, Smyrnium olusatrum.

GRIFF, see Mulatto.

GRIFFO, see Mulatto.

GRINCEMENT DES DENTS, Brygmus.

GRINDERS, Molar teeth — g. Asthma, see Asthma, grinders'—g. Rot, Asthma, grinders'.

GRINDING MILL, see Pulverization.

GRIPES, Tormina, Colic.

GRIPES, WATERY. A popular name for a dangerous disease of infancy, common in England, which does not differ essentially from the cholera infantum of this country.

GRIPHOSIS, Onychogryphosis.

GRIPPE (F.), from *gripper*, 'to gripe,' 'catch hold of.' A vulgar name for several catarrhal diseases, which have reigned epidemically; as the influenza.

GRIPPÉ, Pinched.

GRITS, Groats, (Sax.) Sɲɪꞇꞇa; (G.) Gries, 'gravel, grits.'

GRIT GRUEL, *Water gruel*. This is made as follows:—Take three ounces of *grits*; wash them well in *cold water*, and, having poured off the fluid, put them into four pints of fresh water, and boil slowly until the water is reduced one-half; then strain through a sieve. It is a good demulcent, and is employed also as a vehicle for clysters.

GROAN, see Suspirium.

GROATS, German Grutze; *Grutum, Ave'na exsortica'ta*; (F.) *Gruau*, Oatmeal, (*Yorkshire.*) Oats, hulled, but unground, (*Lancashire.*) Hulled oats, half ground. Oats that have the hulls taken off; *Grits*. When crushed, they are termed *Embden groats*. In America, fine hominy is called *Grits*, and wheat prepared in the same way is likewise so designated. It is also called *wheaten hominy*.

GROATS, CRACOW, Semolina.

GROG-BLOSSOMS, Gutta rosea.

GROG-ROSES, Gutta rosea.

GROMWELL, Lithospermum officinale.

GROOVE, *Furrow, Sulcus*, (F.) *Rainure*. Icelandic, *grafa*, Sax. gɲaꝼan, 'to dig.' A channel or gutter, in a bone or surgical instrument. See *Coulisse*.

GROOVE, PRIMITIVE, *Primitive streak or trace, Nota primiti'va*. A bright streak in the long axis of the pellucid part of the area germinativa, after it presents a central pellucid and a peripheral opake part, and passes from the round to the pear shape.

GROOVED. Same etymon. *Sulca'tus, Stria'tus, Canalicula'tus*, (F.) *Cannelé* ou *Canelé* ou *Caniculé*; Canaliculated. Having a small channel or gutter.

GROS, Drachm—*g. Cou*, Bronchocele.

GROSEILLIER NOIR, Ribes nigrum—*g. Rouge*, Ribes rubrum.

GROSSE GORGE, Bronchocele.

GROSSESSE, Pregnancy—*g. Abdominale*, Pregnancy, abdominal—*g. Afœtale*, Pregnancy, afœtal—*g. Bigéminale*, Pregnancy, bigeminal—*g. Complexe*, Pregnancy, complex—*g. Composée*, Pregnancy, compound—*g. Contre-nature*, Pregnancy, extra-uterine—*g. Fausse* ou *apparente*, Pregnancy, false—*g. Fœtale*, Pregnancy, fœtal—*g. Gazo-hystérique*, Pregnancy, gazo-hysteric—*g. Hémato-hystérique*, Pregnancy, hemato-hysteric—*g. Hydro-hystérique*, Pregnancy, hydro-hysterio — *g. Inter-extra-utérine*, Pregnancy, complex—*g. Ovarienne*, Pregnancy, ovarial—*g. Sarco-hystérique*, Pregnancy, sarco-hysterio—*g. Sarcofœtale*, Pregnancy, sarcofœtal—*g. Simple*, Pregnancy, solitary—*g. Solitaire*, Pregnancy, solitary—*g. Trigéminale*, Pregnancy, trigeminal—*g. Triple*, Pregnancy, trigeminal—*g. Tubaire*, Pregnancy, tubal—*g. Utéro-abdominale*, Pregnancy, utero-abdominal—*g. Utéro-ovarienne*, Pregnancy, utero-ovarian—*g. Utéro-tubaire*, Pregnancy, utero-tubal.

GROSSULARIA NIGRA, Ribes nigrum—g. Non spinosa, Ribes nigrum—g. Rubra, Ribes rubrum.

GROUILLEMENT D'ENTRAILLES, Borborygmus.

GROUND BERRY, Gaultheria—g. Holly,

Gaultheria—g. Ivy, Gaultheria—g. Nut, Arachis hypogea, Pignut—g. Pine, Teucrium chamæpitys—g. p. French, Teucrium iva.

GROUNDSEL, Senecio.

GROUSEBERRY, Gaultheria.

GROWTH, from Dutch groeyen, *Crescentia, Anaplo'sis, Anaptyx'is*, (F.) *Croissance*. The development of the body; particularly in the direction of its height. Also, any adventitious tissue; thus, we speak of a *morbid growth* or *formation*.

GRUAU, Groats.

GRUB, Larve, see Ectozoa.

GRUEL, GRIT, see Grits—g. Water, see Avena, and Grits.

GRUFF, from Teutonic g e, and r u h, 'rough.' In pharmacy, the coarse residue, which will not pass through the sieve in pulverization.

GRUMEAU, Coagulum.

GRUMOUS, *Grumo'sus*, from *grumus*, 'a clot.' Clotted.

GRUMUS, Coagulum.

GRUTUM. 'Groats.' *Grutum Mil'ium, Mil'ium*. A hard white tubercle of the skin, resembling, in size and appearance, a millet-seed. It is confined to the face. See, also, Groats.

GRYPH'IUS PES. The *Griffon's foot*, (F.) *Pied de Griffon*. An instrument of which Ambrose Paré speaks, which was used for extracting moles from the uterus.

GRYPHOSIS, Onychogryphosis.

GRYPO'SIS, from γρυπόω, 'I incurvate.' *Incurva'tio*. Curvature or crookedness in general. Crookedness or incurvation of the nails. See *Onychogryposis*.

GRYPOTES, see Grypus.

GRYPUS. One who has a crooked or aquiline nose. The condition is termed *Gry'potes*.

GUA'CO, *Hua'co*. The name of a plant, *Eupato'rium Guaco*, described by Humboldt and Bonpland under the name *Mika'nia Guaco*, which grows in the valleys of Madalena, Rio-Cauca, &c., in South America. The negroes use the juice against the bites of poisonous reptiles;—both in the way of prevention and cure. It has been, of late, brought forward as a remedy in cholera.

GUAIAC, see Guaiacum.

GUAIACI LIGNUM, see Guaiacum — g. Resina, see Guaiacum.

GUAIACINE, see Guaiacum.

GUAI'ACUM, *G. Officina'lē*; *G. America'num, Lignum vitæ, L. sanctum, L. benedic'tum, Palus sanctus, Lignum In'dicum, Hagiox'ylum,* (F.) *Gayac, Gaïac*. The resin — *Guai'aci Resi'na, Guai'ac,* (F.) *Résine* ou *Gomme de Gaïac*—and the wood—*Guaiaci lignum*—are both used in medicine. Their odour is slightly fragrant; taste warm and bitter, of the resin more so than of the wood. The resin is concrete, brittle; colour, externally, greenish; internally grayish. Water dissolves about one-tenth; alcohol 95 parts. It is soluble, also, in *liquor potassæ* 15 parts, *liquor ammoniæ* 38 parts. The powder is whitish, but changes to green in the air. The base of the guaiacum is a peculiar resin, called *Guaiacine*.

Guaiacum is stimulant and diaphoretic; and in large doses, purgative. It is administered in chronic rheumatism, gout, cutaneous diseases, and the sequelæ of syphilis. Dose of resin, gr. v to xx.—to purge, gr. xx to xl.

GUALTHERIA, Gaultheria.

GUANO, — according to Tschudi, properly *Huanu*,—is formed of the excrements of different kinds of marine birds—mews, divers, sheerbreaks, & ., but especially of the *Sula variega'ta*. It is found in enormous layers in the South American islands of the Pacific, and is used as manure.

GUARANA, Paullinia.

GUARAPO. A fermented liquor made, in Peru, of sugar-cane pulp and water. It is a very favourite beverage of the negroes.—Tschudi.

GUARD (for a bed,) *Alèse*.

GUARERBA ORBA, Momordica elaterium.

GUAVA APPLE, Psidium pomiferum.

GUAYAVA, Psidium pomiferum.

GUBERNAC'ULUM DENTIS, (*Gubernaculum*, 'a rudder.') A cord, which passes from the follicle of the permanent tooth along a small long canal behind the alveolus of the milk tooth, and becomes continuous with the gum. The gubernaculum has been supposed to direct the permanent tooth outwards. The canal has been termed *Iter dentis*.

GUBERNACULUM TESTIS, *G. t. Hunteri, Ligamen'tum suspenso'rium Testis*, (F.) *Gouvernail du testicule*. A triangular, fibro-cellular cord; which, in the fœtus, arises from the ramus of the ischium and the skin of the scrotum, and proceeds to the posterior part of the testicle, before this organ issues from the abdomen. It has been supposed to be a continuation of the fascia superficialis with muscular fibres from the internal oblique muscle, which pass upwards to the testis when in the abdomen; and by their contraction draw the testis down and ultimately form the crevaster muscle.

GUÊPE, Wasp.

GUÉRISON, Cure.

GUÉRISSABLE, Curable.

GUI, Viscum album.

GUILANDI'NA MORIN'GA, *Hyperanthe'ra moringa*. A plant, which affords the *Ben nut*, and the *lignum nephriticum*. It is also called *Morin'ga Oleif'era* seu *Zeylan'ica* seu *Nux ben* seu *Pterygosper'ma*. The nut *Ben, Glans unguenta'ria, Ben Nux, Bal'anus Myrep'sica, San'dalum cæru'leum, Oily Acorn* or *Ben nut*, is a West India nut which furnishes an oil, *O'leum Balani'num*, that does not become rancid by age, and is hence used by perfumers. It is purgative. The wood of the Guilandina is called *Lignum Nephrit'icum*, and has been used in decoction, in affections of the urinary organs.

GUIMAUVE, Althæa—g. *Veloutée*, Hibiscus abelmoschus.

GULA, Œsophagus, Pharynx.

GULÆ IMBECILLITAS, Pharyngoplegia — g. Principium, Pharynx.

GULLET, Œsophagus.

GULOSUS, Glutton.

GUM ANIME, Anime—g. Arabic, Acaciæ gummi — g. Bassora, Bassora gum — g. British, Dextrin — g. Butea, see Butea frondosa — g. Caranna, Caranna — g. Dragon, Tragacantha — g. Elastic, Caoutchouc — g. Falling away of the, Ulatrophia — g. Hemlock, see Pinus Canadensis — g. Indigenous, Gummi nostras — g. Juniper, Sandarac—g. Orenburg, see Pinus larix—g. Red, Strophulus—g. Resin, Gummi resina—g. Sandarach, Sandarac— g. Seneca, Acaciæ gummi — g. Senega, Acaciæ gummi — g. Shrinking of the, Ulatrophia—g. Sweet, Liquidambar styraciflua— g. Tragacanth, Tragacanth—g. Tree, brown, see Kino—g. White, Strophulus—g. Yellow, Icterus infantum.

GUM-LANCET, *Dentiscal'pium, Odontog'lyphon*, (F.) *Déchaussoir*. An instrument for separating the gum from the cervix of the tooth, prior to extraction. It is formed much like a fleam. The operation itself is called *Lancing the gums, Den'tium scalptu'ra*, (F.) *Déchaussement*.

GUMBOIL, Parulis.

GUMMA, (F.) *Gomme*. An elastic tumour, formed in the periosteum, occupying particularly the cranium and sternum, and produced by the syphilitic virus, when it has been long in the constitution. It is so called, because, when opened, it contains a matter like gum.

GUMMI, *Commi*, κομμι, (F.) *Gomme*. An immediate principle of vegetables. It is a solid, uncrystallizable, inodorous substance, of a mawkish taste, unchangeable in the air, insoluble in alcohol, but soluble in water, with which it forms a mucilage. It is obtained from various species of *mimosa* and *prunus;* and consequently there are many varieties of gum. They are used in medicine as demulcents, emollients, and relaxants, particularly in catarrh, intestinal irritations, &c.; and in *Pharmacy*, they are employed in the formation of emulsions, pills, &c.

GUMMI ACACIÆ ARABICÆ, Acaciæ gummi — g. Acanthinum, Acaciæ gummi — g. Adstringens Fothergilli, Kino — g. Ammoniacum, Ammoniac — g. Anime, Anime — g. Arabicum, Acaciæ gummi — g. Astragali Tragacanthæ, Tragacantha — g. Bogia, Cambogia — g. Brelisis, Caranna — g. Copallinum, Copal — g. Elasticum, Caoutchouc — g. Euphorbiæ, see Euphorbia officinarum — g. Gamandræ, Cambogia — g. Gambiense, Kino — g. de Goa, Cambogia — g. Gutta, Cambogia — g. Hederæ, see Hedera helix — g. de Jemu, Cambogia — g. Juniperi, Sandarac — g. Laccæ, Lacca — g. Ladanum, see Cistus creticus — g. Lamac, Acaciæ gummi — g. Laricis, see Pinus larix — g. Leucum, Acaciæ gummi.

GUMMI NOSTRAS, (F.) *Gomme du Pays; Indig".-enous Gum.* These generic names are given to several species of gum, which flow spontaneously from certain indigenous fruit trees, — such as the almond, cherry, peach, apricot, &c. The indigenous gums have nearly the same properties as gum Arabic; but they are inferior to it.

GUMMI ORENBURGENSE, see Pinus larix — g. Panacis, see Pastinaca opoponax — g. ad Podagram, Cambogia.

GUMMI-RESINA, *Gum-Resin.* A milky juice, obtained by making incisions into the branches, stalks and roots of certain vegetables. Gum-resins are compounds of resins, gum, essential oil, and different other vegetable matters. They are solid, opake, brittle, of a strong odour, acrid taste, variable colour, and are heavier than water. Water dissolves a part of them, and alcohol another; hence proof spirit is the proper menstruum. The generality of the gum-resins are powerful stimulants to the whole or to parts of the economy. The chief are *asafœtida, gum ammoniac, euphorbium, galbanum, camboge, myrrh, olibanum, opoponax, scammony, aloes,* &c.

GUMMI RUBRUM ADSTRINGENS GAMBIENSE, Kino, see Butea Frondosa — g. Seneca, Senegal gum — g. Senega, Senegal, gum — g. Senegalense, Senegal, gum — g. Senica, Senegal, gum — g. Serapionis, Acaciæ gummi — g. Thebaicum, Acaciæ gummi — g. Tragacantha, Tragacantha — g. Uralense, see Pinus larix.

GUMMIODES, Mucilaginous.
GUMMIODES, Mucilaginous.
GUMMOSUS, Mucilaginous.
GUMS, Gingivæ.
GUN-COTTON, see Collodion — g. c. Ethereal solution of, Collodion.
GUNJAH, see Bangue.
GUNNERA PERPEN'SA. A South African plant, *Nat. Ord.* Urticaceæ; the decoction of which is taken as a domestic remedy by the farmers, as a tonic in dyspepsia. A tincture has been used in gravel. An infusion of the leaves is demulcent, and is employed in pulmonary affections. The leaves are applied fresh, to cure wounds and ulcers.

GURGITELLO, MINERAL WATERS OF. A thermal spring in the isle of Ischia. Temp. at its source, 176° Fah. It contains carbonic acid, carbonates of lime, magnesia, iron and soda, sulphates of lime and soda, chloride of sodium and silica.

GURGLING. 'Gushing with noise,' as water from a bottle. (F.) *Gargouillement*, same etymon as gargle. The rhonchus or *râle* heard on auscultation when there is a cavity in the lungs containing pus. It is the 'cavernous rattle or *rhonchus,' Râle caverneux.* The size of the bubbles heard varies, and hence the rhonchus has been called *cavernous* and *cavern'ulous*, (F.) *Râle cavernuleux.* If the cavern be large, this *râle* will nearly resemble the gurgling of a bottle (*glouglou d'une bouteille;*) if, on the contrary, the cavern be small, it will not differ from the *râle muqueux.*

GURGULIO, Penis, Uvula.
GUSTATIF, (*Nerf,*) see Lingual nerve.
GUSTATION, Degustation, Taste.
GUSTATORY NERVE, see Lingual Nerve.
GUSTUS, Taste — g. Depravatus, Parageustia.
GUT, Intestine — g. Blind, Cæcum.
GUTS, SLIPPERINESS OF THE, Lientery.
GUTTA, Apoplexy, Cambogia, Gout — g. Gamandræ, Cambogia — g. Gamba, Cambogia — g. Opaca, Cataract.

GUTTA. A *Drop, Stalag'ma, Alun'sel, Stilla,* (F.) *Goutte.* A quantity of liquid, generally valued, in pharmacy, at the weight of a grain. The weight, however, varies according to different circumstances, as the degree of tenacity of the fluid, and the extent of moist surface to which the suspended drop is attached before it falls; and it was found by Mr. Alsop to be influenced by the size of the bottle, and the angle of inclination at which it was held during the operation of dropping. The following are some of his results as to the number of drops required to measure a fluidrachm, when dropped from a large and a small bottle.

	From a large bottle.	From a small bottle.
(f℥j) Diluted sulphuric acid	24 drops	84 drops
Scheele's hydrocyanic acid	35	70
Distilled water	31	54
Solution of ammonia	40	48
Tincture of opium	84	135
Rectified spirits	100	130
Tincture of chloride of iron	100	150

GUTTA PERCHA. The concrete juice of a tree — *Isonan'dra gutta* — which is indigenous in Singapore and its vicinity, and belongs to the Natural order Sapotaceæ. Plunged in boiling water it softens, when it may be moulded like caoutchouc to any form, which it retains on cooling. Splints and other instruments have been made of it.

GUTTA ROSACEA SYPHILITICA, Crown of Venus.
GUTTA ROSEA, *Gutta Rosa'cea, Ion'thus corymb'ifer, Crusta serpigino'sa, C. prurigino'sa, Acnē rosa'cea, Rose'ola acno'sa, Thylacii'tis, Bacchia, Butiga, Carbuncled Face, Rosy Drop or Whelk, Copper-nose, Bottle-nose, Grog-blossoms, Grog-roses*, (F.) *Couperose, Goutte Rose, Bourgeons, Dartre pustuleuse couperose.* An eruption of small, suppurating tubercles, with shining redness, and an irregular granular appearance of the skin of the part of the face which is affected. The redness commonly appears first at the end of the nose, and then spreads on both sides. It is often produced by hard drinking. Its cure must be attempted by regular regimen, and cool

ing means internally: weak spirituous or saturnine lotions externally. The affection is usually very obstinate.

GUTTA SERENA, Amaurosis.

GUTTÆ ABBATIS ROUSSEAU, Laudanum abbatis Rousseau—g. Ammoniaci, see Ammoniac gum—g. Acidæ tonicæ, Elixir Acidum Halleri—g. Nervinæ, Alcohol sulfurico-æthereus ferri.

GUTTÆ NIGRÆ, *Ace'tum o'pii, Common Black Drop.* (*Opii* ℥viij, *aceti destillat.* ℔ij, Infuse.)

The celebrated *Black Drop, Lan'caster* or *Quaker's Black Drop*, may be made as follows. Take half a pound of *opium sliced;* three pints of *good verjuice*, (juice of the wild crab,) one and a half ounce of nutmegs, and half an ounce of saffron. Boil to a proper thickness, and add a quarter of a pound of sugar, and two spoonfuls of yeast. Set the whole in a warm place, near the fire, for six or eight weeks; then place it,in the open air until it becomes a syrup. Lastly, decant, filter, and bottle it up, adding a little sugar to each bottle. One drop is equal to three of laudanum; and it is nearly devoid of all the unpleasant exciting effects of the latter. An analogous formula is contained in the Pharmacopœia of the United States under the name *Ace'tum opii, Vinegar of Opium.*

GUTTALIS CARTILAGO, Arytenoid Cartilage.

GUTTERIA, Bronchocele.

GUTTUR. The throat; the larynx; the trachea.

GUTTUR GLOBOSUM, Bronchocele—g. Tumidum, Bronchocele.

GUT'TURAL, *Guttura'lis,* from *guttur,* 'the throat.' Relating or belonging to the throat.

The *Superior Thyroideal Artery* is sometimes called *Guttural Artery.*

A *Guttural Cough* is one occasioned by irritation of the larynx or trachea.

A *Guttural Sound* is one produced, as it were, in the throat.

GUTTURIS OS, Hyoïdes os.

GUTTURNIA, Arytenoid cartilages.

GYMNA, Genital Organs.

GYMNASION, Exercise.

GYMNA'SIUM, from γυμνος, 'naked.' *Palæs'tra.* An establishment amongst the ancients, intended for bodily exercises, as wrestling, running, &c.; a term now used in Germany, more especially for an academy or higher school.

GYMNAST, *Gymnas'tes, Gymnas'ta;* same etymon. The manager of a gymnasium. One, whose profession it is to prevent or cure diseases by gymnastics.

GYMNAS'TICS, *Gymnas'tica, Medici'na gymnas'tica* seu *euect'ica, Somacet'ice.* Same etymon. That part of hygienic medicine which treats of bodily exercises. It is called *Med'ical Gymnastics.* The ancients had also *Athlet'ic Gymnastics,* and *Mil'itary Gymnastics.* Herodicus, of Selivræa, first proposed gymnastics for the cure of disease.

GYMNOC'LADUS CANADEN'SIS, *Coffee Tree, Mahogany, Nicker Tree, Bondue.* An indigenous tree, which grows from Ohio to Louisiana. The leaves are cathartic, and said to contain cytisin. The seeds are a good substitute for coffee.

GYMNOGRAMME CETERACH, Asplenium ceterach.

GYMNOSIS, Denudation.

GYNÆ'CANER, from γυνη, 'a woman,' and ανηρ, 'a man.' *Vir effœmina'tus.* An effeminate man.

GYNÆCEA, Gynæceia.

GYNÆCEI'A, *Gynæci'a, Gynæce'a*, from γυνη, 'a woman.' The catamenia;—the lochia. The diseases of women in general.—Hippocrates, Galen, Foësius.

GYNÆCEUM, Antimonium, Vulva.

GYNÆCE'US, from γυνη, 'a woman.' Belonging to women. Female. Feminine.

GYNÆCIA, Gynæceia, Menses.

GYNÆCOLOG''IA, *Gynecol'ogy,* from γυνη, 'a woman,' and λογος, 'a description.' The doctrine of the nature, diseases, &c. of women.

GYNÆCOMA'NIA, from γυνη, 'woman,' and μανια, 'mania,' 'rage.' That species of insanity, which arises from love for women. Some have used the word synonymously with nymphomania.

GYNÆCOMAS'TUS, *Gynæcomas'thus*, from γυνη, 'woman,' and μαστος, 'a breast.' A man whose breasts are as large as those of a woman.—Galen, Ingrassias.

A considerable enlargement of the breasts of a female was formerly called *Gynæcomas'ton.*

GYNÆCOMYS'TAX, from γυνη, 'woman,' and μυσταξ, 'the beard.' The hair on the pubes of women.—Rolfink.

GYNÆCOPHO'NUS, from γυνη, 'a woman,' and φωνη, 'voice.' A man who has an effeminate voice.

GYNANDRIA, Hermaphrodeity.

GYNANDRUS, Gynanthropus.

GYNANTHRO'PUS, *Gynan'drus.* An hermaphrodite who belongs more to the male than to the female sex.

GYNATRE'SIA, from γυνη, 'a woman,' and ατρητος, 'imperforate.' Closure or imperforation of the external parts of generation of the female.

GYNE, Female.

GYNECOLOGY, Gynæcologia.

GYNIDA, Hermaphrodite.

GYNOARIUM, Ovarium.

GYNOPLAS'TIC, *Gynoplas'ticus,* from γυνη, 'a woman,' and πλασσω, 'I form.' The gynoplastic operation is employed for opening or dilating the closed or contracted genital openings of the female.

GYPSY-WEED, Lycopus sinuatus, and L. Virginicus.

GYRI CEREBRI, Anfractuosities (cerebral,) Convolutions (cerebral,)—g. Cochleæ, Scalæ of the Cochlea.

GYROMIA VIRGINICA, Medeola Virginica.

GYROPHLE, see Eugenia caryophyllata.

GYROPHORA, see *Tripe de Roche.*

GYRUS, Anfractuosity, Convolution.

GYRUS FORNICA'TUS, 'Arched convolution.' A large convolution of the brain, which lies horizontally on the corpus callosum, and may be traced forwards and backwards to the base of the brain, terminating by each extremity at the fissure of Sylvius. The surface of the hemisphere, where it comes in contact with the corpus callosum, is bounded by it.

H.

HAB-EL-KALIMBAT, Pistacia terebinthus.
HABBI, Hugenia Abyssinica.
HABE'NA. *A Bridle, Tel'amon*. A bandage for uniting the lips of wounds; which, in many instances, replaced the suture.—Galen.
HABENÆ OF THE PINEAL GLAND, see Pineal gland.
HABIL'LA DE CARTHAGE'NA, *Bejwio, Carthage'na Bean*, (F.) *Fève de Carthagène*. A kind of bean of South America, famed as an effectual antidote for the poison of all serpents, if a small quantity be eaten immediately.
HABIT, *Habitu'do*, from *habere*, 'to have or to hold;' *Assuetu'do, Mos, Usus, Consuetu'do, Ethos*, 'εξις, *Hexis, Ethmos'ynē*, (F.) *Habitude, Accoutumance*. Habit is the aptitude for repeating certain acts:— or, a facility, which results from the frequent repetition of the same act. It is, according to vulgar expression, 'a second nature.' Habit may predispose to certain diseases, or it may protect us against them. It ought not to be lost sight of, in attending to the progress of disease, or of its treatment.
HABIT OF BODY, *Constitu'tio, Hab'itus, Hab'itus Cor'poris, Catas'tasis, Hexis, Epiphani'a*, (F.) *Habitude extérieure, Habitude du corps*. The aggregate of the physical qualities of the human body.
HABITUDE, Habit—*h. du Corps*, Habit of body—*h. Extérieure*, Habit of body.
HABITUDO, Habit.
HABITUS, Habit of body — *h. Apoplecticus*, Apoplectic habit—*h. Corporis*, Habit of body.
HACHICH, see Bangue.
HACHISCH, Bangue.
HACKBERRY, Celtis occidentalis.
HÆMA, 'αιμα, 'αιματος, 'blood.'
HÆMACHROINE, Hæmatine.
HÆMACHRO'SES, ((G.) Hämachrosen,) from 'αιμα, 'blood,' and χρωσις, 'coloration.' A family of diseases in which the blood has its colour different from usual, as in purpura and cyanosis.—Fuchs.
HÆMACY'ANIN, from 'αιμα, 'blood,' and κυανος, 'blue.' A blue colouring matter, detected by Sanson in healthy blood, and in bile by some chemists, but not by others.
HÆMADON'OSUS, from 'αιμα, 'blood,' and νοσος, 'a disease.' *Hæmatangion'osus, Hæmatangionu'sus, Hæmatangio'sis*. Disease of the blood-vessels.
HÆMADOSTO'SIS, from 'αιμα, 'blood,' and οστωσις, 'a bony tumour.' Ossification of the blood-vessels.
HÆMADYNAMETER, Hæmadynamometer.
HÆMADYNAMOM'ETER, *Hæmatodynamom'eter, Hæmadynam'eter, Hæmom'eter, Hæmatom'eter*, (F.) *Hémadynamètre, Hémomètre*; from 'αιμα, 'blood,' δυναμις, 'power,' and μετρον, 'a measure.' An instrument for measuring the force of the blood in the vessels. It consists of a bent glass tube, the lower bent part of which is filled with mercury. A brass head is fitted into the artery, and a solution of carbonate of soda is interposed between the mercury and the blood, which is allowed to enter the tube for the purpose of preventing its coagulation. The pressure of the blood on the mercury in the descending portion of the bent tube causes the metal to rise in the ascending portion; and the degree to which it rises indicates the pressure under which the blood moves.
HÆMAGASTRIC PESTILENCE, Fever, yellow.
HÆMAGOGUM, Pæonia.
HÆMAGO'GUS, from 'αιμα, 'blood,' and αγω, 'I drive off.' A medicine which promotes the menstrual and hæmorrhoidal discharges.
HÆMAL, from 'αιμα, 'blood.' Relating to the blood or blood-vessels.
HÆMAL ARCH. The arch formed by the projections anteriorly from the body of the vertebræ of the ribs and sternum. It encloses the great blood-vessels.—Owen.
HÆMAL AXIS, Aorta—h. Spine, Sternum.
HÆMALO'PIA, Hæmophthalmia, Hæmalopis.
HÆMALOPIS, Hæmophthalmia.
HÆMALOPS, Hæmophthalmia.
HÆMAN'THUS COCCIN'EUS. A beautiful South African plant, *Nat. Ord*. Amaryllideæ, the bulb of which is employed as a diuretic. It is given as an exymel in asthma and dropsy. The fresh leaves are antiseptic, and applied to foul, flabby ulcers, and in anthrax.
HÆMAPERITONIRRHAG"IA, (F.) *Hémapéritonirrhagie*; from 'αιμα, 'blood,' περιτοναιον, 'peritoneum,' and ρηγη, 'a violent rupture.' An exhalation of blood into the peritoneum.
HÆMAPHÆ'IN, *Hæmatophæ'um, Hæmophæ'um*, from 'αιμα, 'blood,' and φαιος, 'of a dusky colour.' A term applied by Simon to the brown colouring matter of the blood, supposed by some to be nothing more than hæmatin modified by an alkali.
HÆMAPH'OBUS, *Hæmoph'obus*, from 'αιμα, 'blood,' and φοβος, 'dread.' One who has a dread of blood :—who cannot look at it without fainting.
HÆMAPOPHYSES, Costal cartilages,• see Costa.
HÆMAPOR'IA, *Hæmatapor'ia, Hæmatopo-'ia, Oligohæ'mia, Oligæ'mia*, from 'αιμα, 'blood,' and απορος, 'poor.' Paucity of blood. See Anæmia.
HÆMAPTYSIS, Hæmoptysis.
HÆMAS, 'αιμας, gen. 'αιμαδος. A blood-vessel.
HÆMASTATICA, Hæmatostatica.
HÆMASTAT'ICE, from 'αιμα, 'blood,' and ιστημι, 'I remain,' 'reside.' A science, which treats of the strength of the blood-vessels; *Hymastat'ics*.
HÆMATANGIONOSUS, Hæmadonosus.
HÆMATANGIOSIS, Hæmadonosus.
HÆMATAPORIA, Hæmaporia.
HÆMATAPORRHOSIS, Cholera.
HÆMATEC'LYSIS, *Hæmotex'ia, Hæmotex'is, Hæmatosep'sis, San'guinis dissolu'tio*; from 'αιμα, 'blood,' and εκλυσις, 'loosening.' Dissolution of the blood.
HÆMATELÆUM, see Blood.
HÆMATEM'ESIS, from 'αιμα, 'blood,' and εμεω, 'I vomit.' *Vom'itus cruen'tus, Hæmorrha'gia Hæmatem'esis, Vom'itus seu Vomit"io San'guinis, Gastrorrhag"ia, Gastro - hæmorrhag"ia, Hæmorrhag"ia ventric'uli, Hæmorrhœ'a ventric'uli, Vomiting of Blood*, (F.) *Hématémèse, Vomissement de sang*. Hæmatemesis is generally preceded by a feeling of oppression, weight, and dull or pungent pain in the epigastric and in the hypochondriac regions; by anxiety, and, occasionally, by syncope. Blood is then passed by vomiting, and sometimes, also, by stool,—the

blood being generally of a grumous aspect. Hæmatemesis may be active or passive, acute or chronic. The blood effused proceeds, almost always, from a sanguineous exhalation at the surface of the mucous mambrane of the stomach. It is often observed in females whose menstrual secretion is irregularly performed. It is not of much danger, except when connected with disease of some of the solid viscera of the abdomen. On dissection of those who have died from protracted hæmatemesis,—for the acute kind is comparatively devoid of danger,—the mucous membrane of the stomach is found red and inflamed, or black, and the vessels considerably dilated. Complete abstinence from food; rest; the horizontal posture; bleeding, if the hemorrhage be active; cold, acidulous drinks, &c., constitute the usual treatment.

HÆMATENCEPHALUM, Apoplexy.
HÆMATEPAGOGE, Congestion.
HÆMATERA, Hepatirrhœa.
HÆMATERUS, Sanguine.
HÆMATERYTHRUM, Hæmatin.
HÆMATEXOSTOSIS, Osteosarcoma.
HÆMATHIDROSIS, Sudor cruentus.
HÆMATHORAX, Hæmatothorax.
HÆMATIASIS, Hæmatonosus.
HÆMAT'ICA, from '*αιμα*, 'blood.' Diseases of the sanguineous function:—the third class in the nosology of Good. Also, medicines that act on the blood.—Pereira.
HÆMATICA DOCTRINA, Hæmatology.
HÆMATICUS, Sanguine.
HÆMATIDROSIS, Sudor cruentus.
HÆ'MATIN, *Hæmati'na, Hem'atine, Hæmatosin, Hem'atosine, Hæmater'ythrum, Hæmer'ythrum, Zoöhem'atin, Hemachro'in, Cru'orin, Rubrin, Glob'ulin* of some; from *αιμα*, 'blood.' The red colouring matter of the blood. It resides in distinct particles or globules, and, in the opinion of some observers, in the envelope of the globules. It appears to be of a peculiar character, and one that has not yet been determined by the chemist. That the colour of the blood is not owing to the peroxide of iron which it contains, is shown by the fact mentioned by Scherer, that he removed the iron by acids, and yet a deep red tincture was formed when alcohol was added to the residuum.
HÆMATIN'IC, *Hæmatin'icus*: from *hæmatin,* 'the red colouring matter of the blood.' An agent that augments the number of red corpuscles of the blood.—Pereira.
HÆMATINUS, Sanguine.
HÆMATIS'CHESIS, *Hæmis'chesis, Hæmocryph'ia,* from '*αιμα*, 'blood,' and *ισχειν,* 'to suppress.' The retention or suppression of a natural or artificial flow of blood.
HÆMATISMUS, Epistaxis, Hæmorrhagia.
HÆMATISTH'MUS, from '*αιμα*, 'blood,' and *ισθμος,* 'pharynx.' Hemorrhage into the pharynx.
HÆMATI'TES, *Hæmati'tis,* from '*αιμα,* 'blood.' Resembling blood. *Lapis Hæmati'tes.* A beautiful ore of iron, called also, *Bloodstone, O'chrea rubra, Ox'ydum fer'ricum crystalliza'tum nati'vum, Ferrum Hæmatites.* When finely levigated, and freed from the grosser parts, by frequent washings with water, it has been long recommended in hemorrhage, fluxes, uterine obstructions, &c., in doses of from one scruple to three or four. Also, a vessel that contains blood, '*αιματιτις φλεψ.*
HÆMATMUS, Gas sanguinis.
HÆMATOCATHAR'TICA, from '*αιμα,* 'blood,' and *καθαρσις,* 'purification or purgation.' Remedies for purifying the blood.
HÆMATOCE'LE, from '*αιμα,* 'blood,' and *κηλη,* 'tumour.' A tumour formed by blood. By some, this term has been applied to a tumour formed by blood, effused into the areolar texture of the scrotum. Others have used it for tumours arising from effusion of blood into the tunica vaginalis:—hæmatocele, according to them, differing from hydrocele, only in the character of the effusion.—Heister. Others, again, have applied it to effusions of blood into the interior of the tunica albuginea itself.—Richter. The first is the usual acceptation. It is most commonly caused by wounds or contusions; and requires the use of antiphlogistics, discutients, &c. Sometimes it is necessary to evacuate the effused blood.

HÆMATOCELE ARTERIOSA, Aneurism.
HÆMATO-CEREBRIFORM DISEASE, Encephaloid.
HÆMATOCHE'ZIA, from '*αιμα,* 'blood,' and *χιζω,* 'I go to stool.' *Sedes cruen'tæ, Catarrhœ'a vera, Enterorrhag"ia simplex, Diarrhœ'a cruenta seu sanguinolen'ta, Hæ'mato-diarrhœ'a, Hæmorrhag"ia intestino'rum, En'tero-hæmorrhag"ia,* (F.) *Hémorrhagie des intestins, Écoulement de sang par l'Intestin.* Discharge of blood by stool. See Melæna.
HÆMATOCHYSIS, Hæmorrhagia.
HÆMATOCŒ'LIA, from '*αιμα,* 'blood,' and *κοιλια,* 'the cavity of the abdomen.' Effusion of blood into the abdomen.
HÆMATOCOL'PUS, from '*αιμα,* 'blood,' and *κολπος,* 'vagina.' Effusion of blood into the vagina. Accumulation of blood owing to occlusion of the vagina.
HÆMATOCYANOSIS, Cyanopathy.
HÆMATOCYSTE, Hæmatoma saccatum.
HÆMATOCYST'IS, from '*αιμα,* 'blood,' and *κυστις,* 'bladder.' Hemorrhage into the bladder.
HÆMATO'DES, *Hæmatoï'des, Sanguin'eus, Hæ'matoid, He'matoid,* from '*αιμα,* 'blood,' and *ειδος.* 'appearance.' That which contains blood, or has the character of blood.
HÆMATODES FUNGUS, *Hæmatomy'ces, Fungus cancro'sus hæmato'des, Melæ'na fungo'sa carcino'des, Angidiospon'gus, Angiomy'ces, Hæmatospon'gus, Tumor fungo'sus sanguin'eus seu anom'alus, Spon'goïd inflammation, Pulpy* or *Med'ullary Sarco'ma, Carcino'ma Hæmato'des, Carcino'ma Spongio'sum, Bleeding Fungus, Soft Cancer,* (F.) *Carcinôme sanglant, Hématoncie fongoïde.* An extremely alarming carcinomatous affection, which was first described, with accuracy, by Mr. John Burns, of Glasgow. It consists in the development of cancerous tumours, in which the inflammation is accompanied with violent heat and pain, and with fungus and bleeding excrescences. Even when the diseased part is extirpated, at a very early period, recovery rarely follows; other organs being generally implicated at the same time. Fungus hæmatodes was the term first applied to the disease by Mr. Hey of Leeds. Mr. J. Burns called it *Spongoïd inflammation,* from the spongy, elastic feel, which peculiarly characterizes it, and continues even after ulceration has taken place. The disease has, most frequently, been met with in the eyeball, the upper and lower extremities, testicle and mamma; but it occurs in the uterus, ovary, liver, spleen, brain, lungs, thyroid gland, and in the hip and shoulder-joint.

Some French surgeons designate, by this name, those tumours which were formerly termed *anormales, caverneuses, variqueuses,* called *Erectiles* by Dupuytren, *Hématoncies,* by Alibert, and *Telangiectasiæ* by Gräfe.
HÆMATODIARRHŒA, Hæmatochezia.
HÆMATODYNAMOMETER, Hæmadynamometer.

HÆMATOGASTER, from *αιμα*, 'blood,' and γαστηρ, 'stomach.' Effusion of blood into the stomach.

HÆMATOGENETICA, Hæmatopoietica.

HÆMATOGLOBULIN, see Globules of the blood.

HÆMATOGRA'PHIA, *Hæmatog'raphy*, from *αιμα*, 'blood,' and γραφη, 'a description.' A description of the blood.

HÆMATOID, Hæmatodes.

HÆMATOL'OGY, *Hematol'ogy, Hæmatolog"ia, Hæmat'ica doctri'na*, (F.) *Hématologie*, from *αιμα*, 'blood,' and λογος, 'a discourse.' That part of medicine which treats of the blood.

HÆMATOLOGY, PATHOLOG"ICAL, (F.) *Hématologie pathologique*. Observation of the blood to detect its varying characters in disease.

HÆMATOL'YSES, (G.) Hämatolysen, from *αιμα*, 'blood,' and λυσις, 'solution.' An order of diseases in which there is diminished coagulability of the blood.—Fuchs.

HÆMATOLYTICUM, Spanæmic.

HÆMATO'MA, *Thrombus, Tumor sanguin'eus*. A bloody tumour, especially of the scalp of the new-born.

HÆMATO'MA SACCA'TUM. An encysted tumour containing blood—*Hæmatocys'tē*.

HÆMATOMANTI'A, from *αιμα*, 'blood,' and μαντεια, 'divination.' Judgment of disease from the appearance of the blood.

HÆMATOMATRA, Metrorrhagia.

HÆMATOMETACHYSIS, Transfusio sanguinis.

HÆMATOMETRA, Metrorrhagia.

HÆMATOMMA, Hæmophthalmia.

HÆMATOMPHALOCE'LE, *Hæmatom'phalum, Hæmatompha'lus*, from *αιμα*, 'blood,' ομφαλος, 'the navel,' and κηλη, 'a tumour.' Umbilical hernia, the sac of which encloses a bloody serum; or which has, at its surface, a number of varicose veins; constituting *Varicom'phalus*.

HÆMATOMPHALUM, Hæmatomphalocele.

HÆMATOMYCES, Hæmatodes fungus.

HÆMATON'CUS, (F.) *Hématoncie*, from *αιμα*, 'blood,' and ογκος, 'a tumour.' Alibert has given this name to the *Nævi mater'ni, Varicose tumours*. He admits three varieties:—the *H. fongoïde, H. framboisée,* and *H. tubéreuse*.

HÆMATON'OSUS, *Hæmati'asis, Hæmatopathi'a, Hæmopathi'a*, from *αιμα*, 'blood,' and νοσος, 'disease.' A disease of the blood. Blood-disease.

HÆMATOPATHIA, Hæmatonosus.

HÆMATOPEDESIS, see Diapedesis.

HÆMATOPERICAR'DIUM, from *αιμα*, 'blood,' and περικαρδιον, 'pericardium.' Effusion of blood into the pericardium.

HÆMATOPHÆUM, Hæmaphæin.

HÆMATOPHIL'IA, *Hæmophil'ia, Hæmorrhophil'ia, Idiosyncra'sia hæmorrhag"ica*, from *αιμα*, 'blood,' and φιλεω, 'I love.' A hemorrhagic diathesis.

HÆMATOPHLEBES'TASIS. Sudden suppression of a hemorrhage;—from στασις 'αιματος φλεβων,' 'suppression of the blood of the veins.'—Galen.

HÆMATOPHOB'IA, *Hæmophob'ia*, from *αιμα*, 'blood,' and φοβος, 'dread.' Dread or horror at the sight of blood, producing syncope, &c.

HÆMATOPHTHALMIA, Hæmopthalmia.

HÆMATOPH'THORES, (G.) Hämatophthoren; from *αιμα*, 'blood,' and φθορα, 'corruption.' An order of diseases in the classification of Fuchs, in which the blood is materially altered in its composition, as in typhus.

HÆMATOP'ISIS, (F.) *Hématopisie*. M. Capuron, of Paris, has applied the term *Hématopisie utérine*, from analogy with *Hydropisie utérine*, to a collection of blood which sometimes takes place in the uterus, when, owing to faulty conformation, the exit of the menstrual flux is prevented.

HÆMATOPLA'NIA, *Hæmatoplane'sis*, from *αιμα*, 'blood,' and πλανη, 'wandering.' A vicarious hemorrhage.

HÆMATOPLA'NIA MENSTRUA'LIS, Menstruation, vicarious.

HÆMATOPLETHORA, Plethora.

HÆMATOPŒA, Hæmatopoetica.

HÆMATOPOESIS, Hæmatosis.

HÆMATOPOËT'ICA, *Hæmatopœ'a, Hæmatogenet'ica*, 'bloodmakers,' from *αιμα*, 'blood,' and ποιεω, 'I make.' Agents that favour hæmatosis. Iron was called by the ancients *metal'lum hæmatopoet'icum*.

HÆMATOPOIESIS, Hæmatosis.

HÆMATOPORIA, Hœmaporia.

HÆMATOPS, Hæmophthalmia.

HÆMATOPSIA, Hæmophthalmia.

HÆMATOPTYSIA, Hæmoptysis.

HÆMATOPTYSIS, Hæmoptysis.

HÆMATORRHACHIS, Apoplexia myelitica.

HÆMATORRHAGIA, Hæmorrhagia.

HÆMATORRHŒA, Hæmorrhagia.

HÆMATORRHOSIS, Cholera.

HÆMATORRHYSIS, Hæmorrhagia.

HÆMATOSCHEOCE'LE, *Hæmoscheoce'lē, Hæmatos'cheum*, from *αιμα*, 'blood,' οσχεον, 'scrotum,' and κηλη, 'rupture.' Effusion of blood into the scrotum.

HÆMATOSCHEUM, Hæmatoscheocele.

HÆMATOSCOP'IA, *Hæmoscop'ia*, (F.) *Hémorhoscopie*, from *αιμα*, 'blood,' and σκοπεω, 'I view.' An examination of blood drawn.

HÆMATOSEPSIS, Hæmateclysis.

HÆMATOSIN, Hæmatin.

HÆMATO'SIS, *Exæmato'sis, Enhæmato'sis, Hæmatopoie'sis, Hæmatopoe'sis, Procrea'tio sanguinis; Decarboniza'tion, Atmospheriza'tion of the blood; Sanguifica'tion;* from *αιμα*, 'blood.' The transformation of the venous blood and chyle into arterial blood by respiration. Called, also, *Aëra'tion, Arterializa'tion of the blood*. Formation of blood in general.

HÆMATOSPILIA, Purpura hæmorrhagica.

HÆMATOSPONGUS, Hæmatodes fungus.

HÆMATOSTAT'ICA, from *αιμα*, 'blood,' and στατικη, 'statics.' *Ischæ'mia, Hæmastat'ica, Hæmatostat'ica, Hæmostat'ica, Enæ'ma*, (F.) *Hématostatiques, Hémastatiques, Hémostatiques*. The doctrine of the motion of the blood in living bodies. Also, remedies for stopping blood.—*Catastaltica*.

HÆMATOS'TEON, from *αιμα*, 'blood,' and οστεον, 'a bone.' Effusion of blood into the bones or joints.

HÆMATOSYMPHORESIS, Congestion.

HÆMATOSYNAGOGE, Congestion.

HÆMATOTELANGIOSIS, Telangiectasia.

HÆMATO'TIS, *Hæma'tus*, from *αιμα*, 'blood,' and ους, gen. ωτος, 'the ear.' Effusion of blood into the inner ear.

HÆMATOTHO'RAX, *Hæmatho'rax, Hæmotho'rax, Hæmop'tysis inter'na, Pleurorrhœ'a sanguin'ea, Pneumorrhag"ia inter'na, Hemorrhag"ie Pleu'risy, Pleural hem'orrhage*, from *αιμα*, 'blood,' and θωραξ, 'the chest.' Extravasation of blood into the chest.

HÆMATOX'YLON CAMPECHIA'NUM, *Aca'cia Zeylon'ica, Logwood*. The part of the tree, used in medicine, is the wood, *Hæmatox'yli Lignum, Lignum Campechen'sē, L. Campechia'-*

num, L. Campesca'num, L. In'dicum, L. Sappan, L. Brasilia'num rubrum, L. cœru'leum, (F.) Bois de Campêche. Family, Leguminosæ. Sex. Syst. Decandria Monogynia. Logwood is almost inodorous; of a sweetish, subastringent taste; and deep red colour. Its virtues are extracted both by water and alcohol. It is astringent and tonic, and is used in the protracted stage of diarrhœa and dysentery.

HÆMATURESIS, Hæmaturia.

HÆMATU'RIA, Hœmature'sis, from 'αιμα, 'blood,' and ουρεω, 'I make urine.' Voiding of blood by urine. Hœmorrhag''ia hœmatu'ria, H. ex viris urina'riis, Hœmure'sis, Hœmu'ria, Mictio cruen'ta, M. Sanguin'ea, Mictus Cruen'tus seu Sanguineus, Hœmorrha'a via'rum urinaria'rum, Sanguis in Uri'na, Bloody urine, (F.) Pissement de Sang, Hématurie. Hemorrhage from the mucous membrane of the urinary passages. Like other hemorrhages, it may be active or passive. It may proceed from the kidneys, bladder, or urethra. The essential symptoms are: — blood, evacuated by the urethra; preceded by pain in the region of the bladder or kidneys, and accompanied by faintness. Whencesoever it proceeds, hæmaturia usually takes place by exhalation. Rupture of vessels is by no means common in the mucous membranes. Active hœmaturia requires general or local blood-letting; diluent and cooling drinks; absolute rest, and the horizontal posture. The chronic kind is more troublesome. It requires acidulated or aluminous drinks; chalybeates and tonics in general. When hæmaturia is excessive, cold injections may be thrown into the rectum or into the vagina of women, and topical applications be made to the perinæum.

HÆMATURIA CYSTICA, Cystorrhagia—h. Ejaculatoria, Spermatocystidorrhagia — h. Seminalis, Spermatocystidorrhagia—h. Stillatitia, Urethrorrhagia.

HÆMATUS, Hæmatotis.
HÆMAXIS, Blood-letting.
HÆMENCEPHALUS, Apoplexy.
HÆMERYTHRUM, Hæmatin.
HÆMIDROSIS, see Diapedesis.
HÆMISCHESIS, Hæmatischesis.
HÆMI'TIS, from 'αιμα, 'blood,' and itis, a suffix denoting inflammation. Inflammation of the blood. (F.) Hémite. The alteration of the blood that occurs in inflammatory diseases.—Piorry.

HÆMO-ARTHRITIS, Rheumatism, (acute.)
HÆMOCARDIORRHAG''IA, Apoplex'ia cordis, Apoplexy of the heart, from 'αιμα, 'blood.' καρδια, 'the heart,' and 'ρηγνυμι, 'I break forth.' Effusion of blood into the substance of the heart.

HÆMOCERCH'NOS. This term has received two acceptations, owing to the different senses in which κερχνος is employed; signifying, sometimes, hissing; at others, dry. Consequently, the Hellenists have translated the compound word, at times, by spitting of blood, with hissing in the throat; at others, by evacuation of dry matters.

HÆMOCRYPHIA, Hæmatischesis.
HÆMODES, Sanguine.
HÆMO'DIA, Hœmodias'mus, Hemo'dia, Hebetu'do seu Stupor Den'tium, from 'αιμωδεω, ('αιμα, 'blood,' and οδους, 'a tooth,') 'I have pain in the teeth.' Pain in the teeth,—and more especially Agacement, or the setting on edge of those bodies by acid or acerb substances. It is also called Odon'tia Stupo'ris, Odontal''gia hœmo'dia, Dolor den'tium à strido'rē, Cataplex'is, Odontamblyog'mus, Odonthyperœsthe'sis, Tooth-edge.

HÆMODIASMUS, Hæmodia.
HÆMOIDES, Sanguine.
HÆMOPATHIA, Hæmatonosus.

HÆMOPERICAR'DIUM, Pericardi'tis exsudato'ria, from 'αιμα, 'blood,' and pericardium. Effusion of blood into the pericardium.

HÆMOPERITONÆ'UM, from 'αιμα, 'blood,' and περιτοναιον, 'peritoneum.' Effusion of blood into the peritoneum.

HÆMOPEX'IA, (G.) Hämopexien, from 'αιμα, 'blood,' and πηξις, 'coagulation.' An order of diseases in which there is increased coagulability of the blood.—Hyperino'sis san'guinis.—Fuchs.

HÆMOPHEUM, Hæmaphein.
HÆMOPHILIA, Hæmatophilia.
HÆMOPHOBIA, Hæmatophobia.
HÆMOPHTHAL'MIA, Hœmatophthal'mia, Hœmatop'sia, from 'αιμα, 'blood,' and οφθαλμος, 'eye.' Hœmalo'pia, Hœmalo'pis, Hœ'malops. Effusion of blood into the eye. When the extravasation is external, it is called H. exter'na, Hypospha'gma and Hœmalope exter'nus; when internal, Hœmophthal'mia inter'na, Hydrophthal'mus cruen'tus, Hypoch'ysis hœmato'des, Hœmatom'ma, and Hœ'malops inter'nus. A blood-shot eye.

HÆMOPLANIA MENSTRUALIS, Menstruation, vicarious.

HÆMOPLETHORA, Plethora.
HÆMOPROCTIA, Hæmorrhois.
HÆMOPTOE, Hæmoptysis—h. Laryngea et Trachealis, Tracheorrhagia.

HÆMOPTOSIS, Hæmoptysis.
HÆMOP'TYSIS, from 'αιμα, 'blood,' and πτυω, 'I spit.' Spitting of blood, Hœmorrhag''ia Hœmop'tysis, Hœmap'tysis, Hœmatoptys'ia, Hœmatop'tysis, Emp'toē, Emop'toē, Empto'ica pas'sio, Hœmoptys'mus, Hœmopto'sis, Sputum sang'uinis, San'guinis fluor pulmo'num, Emopto'ica pas'sio, Hœmotis'mus, Hœmorrhœ'a pulmona'lis, Cruen'ta exspui'tio, Hœmorrhag''ia pulmo'nis, Pas'sio hœmopto'ica, Rejec'tio sang'uinis è pulmo'nibus, Expectora'tio sang'uinis, Hœmorrhag''ia Bron'chica, Pneumorrhag''ia, Pneumonorrhag''ia, Pneumonorrhœ'a, Bronchorrhag''ia, Emp'tysis, Hœmop'toē, Sputum cruen'tum, (F.) Hémoptysie, Crachement de sang, Expectoration de sang. Hemorrhage from the mucous membrane of the lungs; characterised by the expectoration of more or less florid and frothy blood. It is generally preceded by cough; dyspnœa; sense of heat in the chest, &c. It is important to discriminate between hæmoptysis, produced by some accidental cause acting irregularly or periodically on the lungs; and that which is, as it were, constitutional, and dependent on some organic affection of the lungs, or some faulty conformation of the chest. These two varieties differ as much in their prognosis and method of treatment, as in their causes. Constitutional hæmoptysis is a serious disease, almost always announcing phthisis pulmonalis. The accidental variety is chiefly dangerous by frequent recurrence, or too great loss of blood.

The general causes of hæmoptysis are the same as those of other kinds of hemorrhage. It has, besides, particular causes; such as too great exercise of the lungs;—loud speaking, playing on wind instruments, breathing acrid vapours, &c. It usually occurs between puberty and the age of 35. A sudden and terrific kind of hæmoptysis is sometimes met with; consisting in a great afflux of blood to the lungs. This has been called Pul'monary Ap'oplexy, Apoplex'ia pulmona'lis, A. pulmo'num, Pneumorrhag''ia, Infarc'tus hœmorrhag''icus pulmo'num, (F.) Apoplexie pulmonaire, Hémoptysie foudroyante, Hémorrhagie interstitielle du Poumon. Infiltration of blood into the air-cells may occur without any hæmoptysis.

Physical signs. Percussion may not always aid us in hæmoptysis, but generally a circumscribed dulness will be perceived. The inspiratory murmur, on auscultation, is feeble or absent, locally; and is replaced by bronchial respiration and *bronchophony*. A fine liquid crepitus is detected around the affected part; and in the larger tubes, near the spine, a liquid bubbling rhonchus is usually heard. The value of these signs is determined by the nature of the expectoration. The treatment of hæmoptysis must be like that of internal hemorrhage in general.

HÆMOPTYSIS INTERNA, Hæmatothorax—h. Laryngea et Trachealis, Tracheorrhagia—h. Phthisis, Phthisis pulmonalis.

HÆMOPTYSMUS, Hæmoptysis.
HÆMORMESIS, Hyperæmia.
HÆMORRHACHIS, Apoplexia myelitica.
HÆMORRHAGE, Hæmorrhagia.
HÆMORRHAG″IA, from '*αιμα*,' 'blood,' and *ῥηγνυμι*, 'I break forth.' *San'guinis proflu'vium copio'sum, Sanguiflux'us, Hæmatoch'ysis, Aimorrhœ'a, Hæmorrhœ'a, Hæmatorrhag″ia, Hæmatis'mus, Hæmatorrhœ'a, Hæmator'rhysis, Hæmor'hysis, Proflu'vium* seu *Prorup'tio* seu *Eruptio sanguinis, Proflu'sio Sang'uinis, Hem'orrhage, Hæmorrhage, Bleeding, Loss of blood, Rupturing, bursting,* or *breaking* of a *blood-vessel,* (F.) *Hémorrhagie* ou *Hémorhagie, Perte de sang, Flux de sang.* Any discharge of blood from vessels destined to contain it; with or without rupture of their coats. Hemorrhages may be *spontaneous* or *traumatic*: the first belong to the domain of medicine, the latter to that of surgery. They may, also, be *internal* or *external; general*—as in scurvy—or *local*. The *hemorrhages by exhalation* —those which chiefly interest the physician— have been classed, by Pinel, as follows:—1. *Hemorrhage of the Mucous Membranes;* Epistaxis, Hæmoptysis, Hæmatemesis, Hæmorrhoids, Hæmaturia, Uterine Hemorrhage. 2. *Hemorrhage of the Tissues;* Cutaneous, Cellular, Serous, Synovial.

Hemorrhages have generally been distinguished into *active* and *passive*: in other words, into those dependent upon augmentation of the organic actions, and those dependent upon debility. According to Broussais, no spontaneous hemorrhage is passive; all are active,—that is, produced by increased action and excess of irritation of the blood-vessels: they may occur *with* debility, but not *from* debility. He calls those only *passive hemorrhages*, which are owing to an external lesion of the vessels. Hemorrhages have been, by some, divided into *constitutional*, or those depending on original conformation:—*accidental*, or those produced by some adventitious cause; *supplementary*, or those which succeed others; *symptomatic, critical, &c.*

When hemorrhage takes place into any tissue, or is *interstitial*, it receives the name, with many, of apoplexy.

Active Hemorrhage, Hemorrhag″ia acti'va, H. arterio'sa, Cauma hæmorrhag″icum, Angeiorrhag″ia, occurs chiefly in the young and plethoric. Good living; the use of fermented liquor— excessive exercise, or too sedentary a life, may perhaps be ranked as predisponent causes. It is commonly preceded by heaviness and pulsation in the part,—owing to the afflux of blood and consequent hyperæmia,—and by coldness of the extremities. The blood, evacuated, is generally of a florid red. In such active hemorrhages, the great indications of treatment will be, to diminish plethora where it exists, and to lessen the heart's action. Bleeding, purgatives, and cold, will be the chief agents.

Passive Hemorrhage, Hæmorrhag″ia passi'va, H. Veno'sa, Proflu'sio, P. hæmorrhag″ica, occurs in those of weak constitution; or who have been debilitated by protracted disease, poor diet, long watching, excessive evacuations, &c.

The direct *causes* may be:—previous active hemorrhage; scorbutus, or any thing capable of inducing atony or asthenic hyperæmia of the small vessels. These hemorrhages are not preceded by excitement or by any signs of local determination. They are usually accompanied by paleness of the countenance; feeble pulse; fainting, &c. The indications of treatment will be:— to restore the action of the small vessels and the general tone of the system: hence the utility of styptics and cold externally; and of tonics and astringents, creosote, mineral acids, &c., internally. Hemorrhage also occurs from mechanical hyperæmia, as when hæmoptysis is produced by tubercles in the lungs; hæmatemesis by disease of some of the solid viscera of the abdomen, &c.

In *Traumatic Hemorrhages*, or those which are the consequences of wounds of arterial or venous trunks, the blood is of a florid red colour, and issues by jets and pulses, if it proceed from an artery; whilst it is of a deeper red, issues slowly and by a continuous flow, if from a vein. If the capillary vessels be alone divided, the blood is merely effused at the surface of the wound. Of the means used for arresting these traumatic hemorrhages, some act mechanically as *absorbents, ligature,* and *compression;* others chymically, as *fire, caustics, creasote, astringents,* &c.

HÆMORRHAGIA ACTIVA NARIUM, Epistaxis — h. Bronchica, Hæmoptysis—h. Cerebri, Apoplexy —h. per Cutem, Sudor cruentus—h. per Diæresin, see Diæresis—h. per Diapedesin, Diapedesis— h. Faucium, Stomatorrhagia—h. Gingivarum, Ulorrhagia—h. Hæmatemesis, Hæmatemesis—h. Hæmaturia, Hæmaturia — h. Hæmoptysis, Hæmoptysis—h. Hepatica, Hepathæmorrhagia — h. Hepatis, Hepatorrhagia—h. Intestinorum, Hæmatochezia—h. Mucosa, see Hæmorrhois—h. Nabothi, see Parturition—h. Narinea, Epistaxis—h. Narium, Epistaxis—h. Oris, Stomatorrhagia—h. Penis, Stimatosis—h. Pulmonis, Hæmoptysis—h. Renum, Nephrorrhagia—h. Universalis, Purpura hæmorrhagica — h. Uterina, Metrorrhagia — h. Ventriculi, Hæmatemesis — h. Vesicæ, Cystorrhagia.

HÆMORRHINIA, Epistaxis.
HÆMORRHINORRHAGIA, Epistaxis.
HÆMORRHŒ'A, from '*αιμα*,' 'blood,' and *ῥεω*, 'I flow.' *Hæmorrhag″ia, Loss of blood.* Some writers have proposed to restrict this name to passive hemorrhages.

HÆMORRHŒA PETECHIALIS, Purpura hæmorrhagica—h. Pulmonalis, Hæmoptysis—h. Uterina, Metrorrhagia — h. Vasorum hæmorrhoidalium, Hæmorrhois — h. Ventriculi, Hæmatemesis — h. Viarum urinarium, Hæmaturia.

HÆMORRHOI'DAL, *Hemorrhoï'dal, Hæmorrhoïda'lis, Hæmorrhoïdeus.* Relating to hemorrhoids; as *hemorrhoidal flux, hemorrhoidal tumours,* &c.

HEMORRHOIDAL ARTERIES have been distinguished into *superior, middle,* and *inferior*. 1. The first is the termination of the inferior mesenteric artery, which assumes the name *superior hemorrhoidal,* when it reaches the upper and posterior part of the rectum. 2. The *middle hemorrhoidal* is furnished by the hypogastric or internal pudic. It ramifies on the inferior and anterior part of the rectum. 3. The *inferior hemorrhoidal* arteries are branches of the internal pudic, furnished to the inferior part of the rectum and to the muscles of the anus.

HEMORRHOIDAL NERVES. These emanate from the sciatic and hypogastric plexuses; and cover the rectum with their numerous filaments.

HEMORRHOIDAL VEINS follow the same distribution, and generally empty themselves into the lesser mesenteric. Some of them assist in the formation of the hypogastric vein.

HEMORRHOIDAL VESSELS, *Vasa seda'lia*, are those vessels which are distributed to the rectum —the seat of hemorrhoids.

HÆMORRHOIDALES NODI, Hæmorrhois.

HÆMORRHOIDES, see Hæmorrhois — h. Cæcæ, see Hæmorrhois — h. Fluentes, Hæmorrhois — h. Furentes, see Hæmorrhois — h. Mariscosæ, Hæmorrhois — h. non Fluentes, Hæmorrhois — h. Oris, Stomatorrhagia.

HÆMOR'RHOIS, *Aimor'rhois, Asclepias'mus*, from '*αιμα*, 'blood,' and *ρεω*, 'I flow.' *Aimor'rois, Proc'tica Maris'ca, Maris'ca, Proctal'gia Hæmorrhoïda'lis, Morbus Hæmorrhoidalis, Piles*, (F.) *Hémorrhoïdes*. The essential symptoms of this affection are: — Livid and painful tubercles or excrescences, (*Hemorrhoid'al Tumours*,) usually attended with a discharge of mucus or blood, (*Hæmorrhoid'al flux, Proctorrhœ'a, Hæmoproc'tia, Hæmorrhœ'a vasorum hæmorrhoïda'lium*, (F.) *Hémaproctie*.) The most common causes of piles are a sedentary life; accumulation of fæces in the rectum; violent efforts at stool; pregnancy, &c. The precursory symptoms are: — pains in the loins; stupor of the lower limbs; and uneasiness in the abdomen and rectum, with more or less gastric, cerebral, and indeed general disorder; — constituting the *Diath'esis Hæmorrhoida'lis, Motus* seu *Turba Hæmorrhoida'lis*, and *Moli'men Hæmorrhoida'lē*, of most of the writers of Continental Europe. To these symptoms follow one or more round, smooth, renitent, painful, pulsating, and erectile tumours, around the margin of the anus, or within the anus; some pouring out blood occasionally. After having remained, for a time, tense and painful, they gradually shrink and disappear. The chief symptoms, occasioned by hemorrhoidal tumours, when much inflamed, are; — constant pain, liable, however, to exacerbations, and obliging the patient to preserve the horizontal posture, and to become augmented by the least pressure, or by the passage of the fæces.

Hæmorrhoids have generally been distinguished into — *Hæmorrhoïdes Fluen'tes* seu *Marisco'sæ, Proc'tica Maris'ca cruen'ta, Bleeding* or *Open Piles;* and into *H. non fluen'tes, Proc'tica Maris'ca cæca, Hæmorrhoï'des cæcæ* seu *furen'tes, Hæmorrhoïda'les nodi, Shut* or *blind piles*. They have, also, been divided into *internal* or *occult*, and *external*, according to their situation; and into *accidental* or *constitutional*.

Hemorrhoidal Tumours are extremely troublesome, by their disposition to frequent recurrence; and they are apt to induce fistula; otherwise, they are devoid of danger. When anatomically examined, they are found not to consist in a varicose dilatation of the veins of the rectum; but to be formed of a very close, spongy, texture; similar to that which surrounds the orifice of the vagina; and to be erectile, like it. They are surrounded by a delicate membrane, and have no internal cavity. The treatment, in mild cases of hemorrhoidal tumours, is simple. Rest; the horizontal posture; the use of mild laxatives, as sulphur, castor oil, and emollient glysters, will be sufficient. If they be much inflamed, leeches may be applied; and warm cataplasms or cold lotions, according to circumstances, be prescribed, with abstinence, and cooling drinks. Afterwards, an ointment, composed of powdered galls and opium, may afford relief. It is in the relaxed kind, that such ointment, and the internal use of *Ward's Paste*, can alone be expected to afford much benefit. If, after repeated attacks, the tumours remain hard and painful, and threaten fistula, they may be removed.

By *Hemorrhoidal Flux, Fluxus hæmorrhoïdalis, Proctorrhag''ia*, is meant the hemorrhage which takes place from the rectum, owing to hemorrhoids. It is a common affection. The quantity of blood discharged is various: at times, it is very trifling; at others, sufficient to induce great debility, and even death. It is announced and accompanied by the same symptoms, as precede and attend hemorrhoidal tumours. Like other hemorrhages it may be *active* or *passive; accidental* or *constitutional*. The prognosis is rarely unfavourable. The affection may, almost always, be relieved by properly adapted means. These resemble such as are necessary in hemorrhages in general. Perfect quietude, — mental and corporeal, light diet, cooling drinks; bleeding if the symptoms indicate it; astringents, (if the disease be protracted and passive,) such as the *Tinctura Ferri Chloridi;* aspersions of cold water on the anus: astringent injections; plugging and compression. Such will be the principal remedial agents. When the hemorrhage has become habitual or is vicarious, some caution may be required in checking it; and, if inconvenience arise from a sudden suppression, its return may be solicited by the semicupium, sitting over warm water; aloetic purgatives, glysters, irritating suppositories, &c.; or leeches may be applied to the anus.

To the internal bleeding pile, a soft, red, strawberry-like elevation of the mucous membrane, Dr. Houston, of Dublin, gives the name *vascular tumour*. For its removal he recommends the application of nitric acid, so as to produce sloughing of its surface.

Some authors have described a species of *Leucorrhœ'a Ana'lis* or whitish discharge from the anus, which often attends ordinary hæmorrhoids. This they have called *Proctica maris'ca muco'sa, Hæmor'rhoïs alba, Hæmorrhag''ia muco'sa, Leucor'rhoïs*, &c. It requires no special mention.

HÆMORRHOIS AB EXANIA, Proctocele — h. Procedens, Proctocele.

HÆMORRHOÏS'CHESIS, from '*αιμορροις*, '*hæmorrhois*,' *ρεω*, 'I flow,' and *ισχω*, 'I restrain.' *Reten'tio fluxus hæmorrhoïda'lis*. Suppression or retention of the hemorrhoidal flux.

HÆMORRHOPHE'SIS, *Absorp'tio sang'uinis*, from '*αιμα*, 'blood,' and *ροφαω*, 'I sip up.' Absorption of blood.

HÆMORRHOPHILIA, Hæmatophilia.

HÆMORRHOSCOPIA, Hæmatoscopia.

HÆMORRHYSIS, Hæmorrhagia.

HÆMOSCHEOCELE, Hæmatoscheocele.

HÆMOSCOPIA, Hæmatoscopia.

HÆMOSPASIA, see Hæmospastic.

HÆMOSPAS'TIC, (F.) *Hémospasique*, from '*αιμα*, 'blood,' and *σπαω*, 'I draw.' An agent which draws or attracts blood to a part; as a cupping-glass. The operation is termed *Hæmospa'sia*, (F.) *Hémospasie*. It is generally applied to a process by which the air is exhausted over a considerable surface, as over one or more of the extremities, by an appropriate pneumatic apparatus.

HÆMOSTA'SIA, *Hæmos'tasis, Epid'esis, San'guinis stagna'tio*, (F.) *Hémostasie*, from '*αιμα*, 'blood,' and *στασις*, 'stagnation.' Stagnation of blood. This name has, also, been given to any operation, the object of which is to arrest the flow of blood.

HÆMOSTATICS, Hæmatostatica.

HÆMOTELANGIOSIS, Telangiectasia.

HÆMOTEXIA, Hæmateclysis.
HÆMOTEXIS, Hæmateclysis.
HÆMOTHORAX, Hæmathorax.
HÆMOTISMUS, Hæmoptysis.
HÆMOT'ROPHY, *Hæmotroph'ia;* from *'αιμα,* 'blood,' and *τροφη,* 'nourishment.' Excess of sanguineous nourishment.—Prout.

HÆMURIA, Hæmaturia.
HÆMURESIS, Hæmaturia.
HÆMYDOR, Serum of the blood.
HÆREDITARIUS, Hereditary.
HÆSITATIO, Balbuties.
HÆVEA GUIANENSIS, see Caoutchouc.
HAGARD, Haggard.

HAGE'NIA ABYSSIN'ICA, *Brayera anthelmin'tica, Bank'sia Abyssin'ica.* An Abyssinian tree of the *family* Rosaceæ; *Sexual system,* Icosandria Digynia, which the natives plant round their habitations, as an ornament. The infusion or decoction of its flowers is employed by them as an anthelmintic, especially in cases of tapeworm. It is called, there, *Cusso* or *Kosso,* and *Habbi.*

HAGGARD, (F.) *Hagard.* The French use the term *Air hagard, Œil hagard,* '*Haggard air,*' '*Haggard eye,*' for a physiognomy, in which there is at once an expression of madness and terror.

HAGIOSPERMUM, Artemisia santonica.
HAGIOXYLUM, Guaiacum.
HAIL, Chalaza.

HAIR, Sax. hær, *Crines, Pilus, Thrix, Pile,* (F.) *Poil.* A conical, corneous substance, the free portion or *shaft, scapus,* of which issues to a greater or less distance from the skin, to the tissue of which it adheres by a bulb, *Bulbus pili,* seated in the areolar membrane,—where alone it is sensible. The hair receives various names in different parts—as *Beard, Cilia, Eyebrows, Hair of the head* (*Capilli,*) &c.

HAIR, FALLING OFF OF THE, Alopecia—h. Matted, Plica—h. Muscular, Dracunculus—h. Plaited, Plica—h. Trichomatose, Plica—h. Worm, Seta equina, see Ectozoa.

HAIRY, Pileous.
HAL, Salt.
HALA'TION, *Hala'tium;* diminutive of *'αλς,* 'salt.' A pungent remedy, with the ancients, which contained salts.

HALCHEMI'A. The alchymists so called the art of fusing salts: from *'αλς,* 'salt,' and *χεω,* 'I pour out.'—Libavius.

HALCYON, Alcyon.
HALCYONIUM ROTUNDUM, Pila marina.
HALE, Ephelides.
HALEINE, Breath—*h. Courte,* Dyspnœa.

HALELÆ'ON, *Halelæ'um,* from *'αλς,* 'salt,' and *ελαιον,* 'oil.' *Oleum Sali mixtum.* A mixture of oil and salt, for removing swellings of the joints.—Galen.

HALÉTÉRATION, Alteration.

HALF-CASTE, *Half-Cast,* see Caste. A term applied, in India, to the offspring of a Hindoo and a European. Since, extended to the offspring of mixed races. The subjoined list from Tschudi's Travels in Peru, 1838—1842, shows the parentage of the different varieties of half-casts, and also the proper designations of the latter, as observed in South America.

PARENTS.	CHILDREN.
White Father and Negro Mother,	Mulatto.
White Father and Indian Mother,	Meztizo.
Indian Father and Negro Mother,	Chino.
White Father and Mulatta Mother,	Cuarteron.
White Father and Meztiza Mother,	Creole (only distinguished from the white by a pale brownish complexion.)
White Father and China Mother,	Chino-blanco.
White Father and Cuarterona Mother,	Quintero.
White Father and Quintera Mother,	White.
Negro Father and Mulatta Mother,	Zambo-negro.
Negro Father and Meztiza Mother,	Mulatto oscuro.
Negro Father and China Mother,	Zambo chino.
Negro Father and Zamba Mother,	Zambo-negro (perfectly black.)
Negro Father and Cuarterona or Quintera Mother,	Mulatto (rather dark.)
Indian Father and Mulatta Mother,	China-oscuro.
Indian Father and Meztiza Mother,	Mestizo-claro (frequently very beautiful.)
Indian Father and China Mother,	Chino-cholo.
Indian Father and Zamba Mother,	Zambo-claro.
Indian Father with China-chola Mother,	Indian (with rather short frizzy hair.)
Indian Father and Cuarterona or Quintera Mother,	Meztizo (rather brown.)
Mulatto Father and Zamba Mother,	Zambo (a miserable race.)
Mulatto Father and Meztiza Mother,	Chino (of rather clear complexion.)
Mulatto Father and China Mother,	Chino(rather dark.)

See Mulatto.

HALICA, Alica.
HALICACALUM, Physalis.
HALICES, Pandiculation.
HALIDRYS VESICULOSA, Fucus vesiculosus.

HALINA'TRUM, *Halini'trum, Haloni'trum;* from *'αλς,* 'salt,' and *natrum* or *natron.* A name given by the ancients to subcarbonate of soda, containing a little subcarbonate of ammonia, which is found, ready-formed, on the plaster of damp walls, in places inhabited by man or animals. Also, Potassæ nitras.

HALINITRUM, Halinatrum.
HALINUS, Saline.

HAL'ITUOUS, *Halituo'sus,* from *halitus,* 'vapour.' (F.) *Halitueux.* The skin is said to be *halitueuse,* when covered with a gentle moisture. The vapour, exhaled in all the cavities of the body, so long as the blood is warm, is called *Hal'itus.* The odorous vapour, exhaled by the blood itself whilst warm, is called *Hal'itus San'guinis.*

HALITUS, Breath—h. Oris Fœtidus, Breath, offensive—h. Sanguinis, Gas sanguinis. See Halituous.

HALL, MINERAL WATERS OF. The springs of Hall, in Upper Austria, contain iodine.

HALLUCINATIO HYPOCHONDRIASIS, Hypochondriasis—h. Vertigo, Vertigo.

HALLUCINA'TION, *Hallucina'tio, Halucina'tio, Falla'cia, Illu'sio sensûs, Socor'dia, Alu'sia, Illu'sio, Allucina'tio, Parora'sis, Somnia'tio in statu vig''ili, Ido'lum, Waking dream, Phan'tasm,* from *allucinari,* 'to err;' 'to be deceived.' A morbid error in one or more of the senses. Perception of objects, which do not in fact exert any impression on the external senses. Hallucination or *delusion* almost always, if not always, depends on disorder of the brain, but is not an index of insanity, unless the patient believes in the existence of the subject of the hallucination.

HALLUS, Pollex pedis.
HALLUX, Pollex pedis.
HALME, Muria.

HALMYRO'DES, *Salsugino'sus, Salsusig''inous,* from *'αλμυρις,* (*'αλμη,* 'sea-water,' *'αλς,* salt,') ' a salt liquor,' saltish. An epithet given to any affection, in which the heat feels pungent under the finger of the physician.—Hippocrates.

HALMYRUS, Saline.

HALO, Areola.

HALO SIGNA'TUS. The impression made by the ciliary processes on the anterior surface of the vitreous humour. So called from its consisting of a circle of indentations.—Sir C. Bell. Called by Haller, *Striæ ret'inæ subject'æ ligamen'to ciliɑ'ri.*

HALODERÆ'UM, from 'αλς, 'salt,' and δεραιον, 'a collar,' (δερη, 'neck.') *Colla'rium sali'num.* A collar of salt applied to the neck, as in cases of croup.

HALOGENE, Chlorine.

HALOIDUM OXYGENATUM, Potassæ murias hyperoxygenatus.

HALONIITIS, Induration of the cellular tissue.

HALONITRUM, Halinatrum.

HALOPE'GÆ, from 'αλς, 'αλος, 'salt,' and πηγη, 'a spring.' Mineral waters whose chief ingredient is common salt—chloride of sodium.

HALOS, Areola.

HALOT'YLE, *Cul'cita sali'na,* from 'αλς, 'salt,' and τυλη, 'a bolster.' A bolster or pillow of salt recommended in croup.

HALS, 'αλς,' 'salt;' hence *Halogene, Haloid,* &c.

HALTE'RES. Pieces of lead held in the hands by the ancients to assist them in leaping.

HALUCINATIO, Hallucination.

HALYCODES, Saline.

HALYCIS MEMBRANACEA, Bothriocephalus latus—h. Solium, Tænia solium.

· HAM, Poples.

HAMAME'LIS VIRGINIA'NA, *H. Virgin'ica, Witch hazel, Winter witch hazel, Snapping Haselnut, Winter bloom.* The bark of this tree, which is a native of the United States, is somewhat bitter and sensibly astringent; but it has not been much used. A cataplasm of the inner rind of the bark is said to have been found efficacious in painful inflammation of the eyes.

HAMARTHRI'TIS, *Holarthri'tis, Catholarthri'tis, Arthri'tis universa'lis,* from 'αμα, 'at once,' and αρθριτις, 'gout.' Gout in all the joints. Universal gout.

HAM'MA, *Nodus,* 'a tie.' A knot, used for retaining bandages on any part. — Hippocrates. A truss.

HAMPSTEAD, MINERAL WATERS OF. These waters, situate in the neighbourhood of London, are a good chalybeate.

HAMSTRING, To, see Hamstrings.

HAMSTRINGS, (F.) *Jarretiers.* The strings or tendons of the ham.

The HAMSTRING MUSCLES are the biceps femoris, whose tendon forms the *outer hamstring;* and the semimembranosus, semitendinosus, gracilis and sartorius, whose tendons form the *inner hamstring.*

'To hamstring' means to cut the strings or tendons of the ham.

HAMULAR PROCESS, see Hamulus.

HAM'ULUS. Diminutive of *hamus,* 'a hook.' A hook or crook: *Ancis'tron.* Also, any hook-like process; as the *hamulus* or *hamular process* of the pterygoid process.

HAMULUS LAMINÆ SPIRALIS, see Lamina spiralis.

HAMUS, see Hamulus.

HANCHE, Haunch.

HAND, Manus.

HANDS, DROPPED, *Hand-drop, Wrist-drop.* A popular term for the paralysis of the hand, induced by the action of lead.

HANGERS, Crusta genu equinæ.

HANGNAIL, (F.) *Envie.* A portion of epidermis, detached so as to tear the integument in the vicinity of the finger nails.

HANNEBANE, Hyoscyamus.

HAPANTIS'MUS, Badly formed from πας, or 'απας, 'all.' *Oblitera'tio comple'ta.* The matting or growing together of organic parts.

HAPHE, 'αφη, 'feeling, touch.' Hence:

HAPHON'OSI, *Haphonu'si,* from 'αφη, 'the touch.' *Morbi tactûs.* Diseases of the sense of touch.

HAPLOACNE, Acne simplex.

HAPLOPATHI'A, from 'απλος, 'simple,' and παθος, 'disease.' *Morbus simplex.* A simple or uncomplicated affection.

HAPLOTOM'IA, *Simplex sec'tio, Incis'io simplex, Opera'tio simplex,* from 'απλος, 'simple,' and τομη, 'incision.' A simple incision.

HAPSIS, Touch.

HAPTODYSPHOR'IA, *Tactus dolorif'icus;* from 'αφη, 'touch,' and δυσφορος, 'difficult to be borne.' Painful to the touch.

HAPTOT'ICA, *Haptot'icē,* from 'αφη, 'touch.' The doctrine of the phenomena of touch.

HARD, (G.) h a r t, *Durus, Scleros,* (F.) *Dur.* That which offers much resistance. In anatomy, the *hard parts* are those which compose the osseous basis of the body; in other words, the skeleton. See Pulse, hard.

HARD'S FARINACEOUS FOOD, see Farinaceous.

HARDESIA, Hibernicus lapis.

HARDHACK, Spiræa tomentosa.

HARE-LIP, *Lagochi'lus, Lagos'toma, Lagon'tomum, Lagen'tomum, La'bium Lepori'num, Olopho'nia Labii Loba'ta, Lepori'num rostrum,* (F.) *Bec de Lièvre.* A fissure or perpendicular division of one or both lips. It has been so called, in consequence of the upper lip of the hare being thus divided. Hare-lip is generally congenital; at other times it is *accidental,* or produced by a wound, the edges of which have not been brought into contact, and have healed separately. It is *simple,* when there is but one division; *double,* when there are two; and *complicated,* when there is, at the same time, a division or cleft of the superior maxillary bone and of the palate—*Cleft* or *fis'sured palate, Wolf's jaw, Rictus lupi'nus;* or a projection of the teeth into the separation of the lip.

In the *Hare-lip operation,* there are two indications to be fulfilled. First, to pare, with the knife or scissors, the edges of the cleft, and, afterwards, to preserve them in contact; in order to cause adhesion. This last object is accomplished by means of pins, passed through the edges of the division; in other words, by the twisted suture. The projecting teeth must, of course, be previously removed. If there be separation of the palate, it will become less and less after the union of the lip, or the operation of staphyloraphy may be performed upon it.

HARE'S EAR, Bupleurum rotundifolium—h. Eye, Lagophthalmia.

HARGNE, Hernia—h. *Anévrysmale,* Circocephalus.

HARICOT, Phaseolus vulgaris—h. *Grand de Perou,* Jatropha curcas.

HARMALIA, Aliment.

HARMONY, *Harmo'nia, Harmos,* primarily from αρω, 'I adjust.' Anatomists have called *Suture by Harmony* or simply *Harmony, Palæœ* or *superficial suture, Sutu'ra os'sium spu'ria, Compa'ges os'sium per lin'eam sim'plicem,* an immovable articulation, in which the depressions and eminences, presented by the bony surfaces, are but slightly marked; so that it might be presumed that the junction of the bones took place by simple apposition of their surfaces. An instance of harmony occurs in the union of the superior maxillary bones with each other.

HARMUS, Articulation, Harmony.

HAR'ROWGATE, MINERAL WATERS OF. The villages of High and Low Harrowgate are situate in the centre of the county of York, near Knaresborough, twenty miles from York, and fifteen from Leeds. Here are several valuable sulphurous and chalybeate springs. The *sulphureous springs* contain chloride of sodium, chloride of calcium, chloride of magnesium, bicarbonate of soda, sulphohydric acid, carbonic acid, carburetted hydrogen, and azote. The *chalybeate springs* contain protoxide of iron, chloride of sodium, sulphate of soda, chloride of calcium, chloride of magnesium, carbonic acid, azote, and oxygen. For the former, Harrowgate is celebrated and frequented.

HARROWGATE SALTS, ARTIFICIAL, are much employed, and not unfrequently by those who drink the genuine water, for the purpose of increasing its aperient power. They may be made as follows:—*Sulph. Potass. cum Sulph.* ʒvj ; *Potass. bitart.* ʒj ; *Magnes. Sulph.* in pulv. ʒvj. M. The usual dose is a teaspoonful, in a small tumblerful of tepid water, early in the morning.

HARROWGATE WATER, ARTIFICIAL, may be formed of *common salt*, ʒv ; *water*, Oiij ; impregnated with the gas from *sulphuret of potass*, and *sulphuric acid*, āā ʒiv. The following form has also been recommended. ℞. *Sulphat. Potass. cum sulph.* (Ph. Ed.) ʒj ; *Potass. bitart.* ʒss ; *Magnes. sulphat.* ʒvj ; *Aquæ destillat.* Oij. One-half to be taken for a dose.

HARTFELL, MINERAL WATERS OF. Hartfell Spa is about five miles from Moffat, in Scotland. The water is a chalybeate, and is much used.

HARTSHORN, Cervus, Cornu cervi, Liquor cornu cervi — h. Red, Spiritus lavandulæ compositus — h. and Oil, Linimentum ammoniæ carbonatis.

HARTS' TONGUE, Asplenium scolopendrium.

HARTWORT OF MARSEILLES, Seseli tortuosum.

HASCHICH, see Bangue.

HASTA, Penis — h. Nuptialis, Penis — h. Virilis, Penis.

HASTELLA, Splint.

HASTINGS, CLIMATE OF. This place has the reputation of being one of the mildest and most sheltered winter residences on the south coast of England. Owing to its low situation, and the height of the neighbouring cliffs, it is protected in a great degree from all northerly winds; and hence is found a favourable residence generally for invalids labouring under diseases of the chest.

HASTULA REGIS, Asphodelus ramosus.

HATFIELD'S TINCTURE, see Tinctura Guaiaci ammoniata.

HAUNCH, *Coxa, Coxen'dix*, of the Latins; εγχυ, or ισχιον, of the Greeks; *Ancha, Ischion, Osphys, Hip, Cossa*, (F.) *Hanche*. The region of the trunk which is formed by the lateral parts of the pelvis and the hip-joint, including the soft parts. In women, on account of the greater width of the pelvis, the haunches are more marked and prominent than in men.

HAUSTEL'LATE, *Haustella'tus*, from *haurio, haustus*, 'I drink up.' An epithet for the structure of mouth, which is adapted for drinking or pumping up liquids. Insects, which possess that kind of mouth, are so named. Ehrenberg refers the fancied spermatozoon to the haustellate entozoa.

HAUSTUS, *Po'tio, Potiun'cula*. A *Draught*. A liquid medicine, which can be taken at a draught.

HAUSTUS NIGER, see Infusum sennæ compositum.

HAUT MAL, Epilepsy.

HAVAN'A or HAVAN'NAH, CLIMATE OF. The climate of Cuba is often selected for the phthisical invalid during the winter months, and so far as regards elevation and comparative equability of temperature, it is more favourable for those of weak lungs than that of the United States. The mean annual temperature is high (78°), but the difference between the mean temperature of the warmest and coldest months is twice as great as at Madeira.

HAW, BLACK, Viburnum prunifolium.

HAWKNUT, Bunium bulbocastanum.

HAWKWEED, VEINY, Hieracium venosum.

HAWTHORN, WHITE, Mespilus oxyacantha.

HAY, CAMEL'S, Juncus odoratus—h. Asthma, Fever, Hay.

HAYRIFF, Galium aparine.

HAZEL, BEAKED, Corylus rostrata—h. Crotiles, Lichen pulmonarius—h. Nut, snapping, Hamamelis Virginiana—h. Nut tree, Corylus avellana—h. Witch, Hamamelis Virginiana.

HEAD, Sax. heapoð, heapð, *heaved;* the past participle of hea*p*an, 'to heave up.' *Caput, Cephalè, Cy'bē*, (F.) *Tête*. The head forms the upper extremity of the body, and tops the skeleton. It consists of the cranium and face. The first, which comprises all the superior and posterior part, has the encephalon in its cavity: the latter forms only the anterior part, and serves as the receptacle for the greater part of the organs of the senses.

HEAD, WATER IN THE, Hydrocephalus.

HEAD ACH, Cephalæa, Cephalalgia — h. Ach, intermittent, Cephalalgia periodica—h. Ach, sick, Cephalæa spasmodica.

HEADY, same etymon as Head. (F.) *Capiteux*. That which inebriates readily. An epithet, applied to wines, which possess this quality.

HEAL-ALL, Collinsonia Canadensis, Prunella vulgaris, Scrophularia nodosa.

HEALING, Curative—h. Art, Medicine.

HEALTH, Sanitas.

HEALTHY, Salutary.

HEARING, HARDNESS OF, Deafness—h. Perverse, Paracusis perversa.

HEART, Sax. heopτ, Germ. Herz, *Cor, Cear, Cer, Car'dia,* καρ, κηρ, καρδια, (F.) *Cœur*. An asygous muscle, of an irregularly pyramidal shape; situate obliquely and a little to the left side, in the chest;—resting on the diaphragm by one of its surfaces:—suspended by its base from the great vessels; free and movable in the rest of its extent, and surrounded by the pericardium. The right side of the body of the heart is thin and sharp, and is called *Margo acu'tus:* the left is thick and round, and termed *Margo obtu'sus*. It is hollow within, and contains four cavities; two of which, with thinner and less fleshy walls, receive the blood from the lungs and the rest of the body, and pour it into two others, with thick and very fleshy parietes, which send it to the lungs and to every part of the body. Of these cavities, the former are called *auricles*, the latter *ventricles*. The right auricle and right ventricle form the *Pulmonic* or *right* or *anterior heart*, (F.) *Cœur du poumon, C. du sang noir, C. droit, C. antérieur:* and the left-auricle and ventricle, the *systemic, corporeal, left,* or *aortic heart*, (F.) *Cœur du corps, C. gauche, C. aortique* ou *C. rouge*. In the adult, these are totally distinct from each other, being separated by a partition; — the *sep-*

tum cordis. Into the right auricle, the venæ cavæ,—superior and inferior,—and the coronary vein, open. The pulmonary artery arises from the right ventricle; the four pulmonary veins open into the left auricle, and the aorta arises from the left ventricle.

The mean weight of the heart, in the adult, from the twenty-fifth to the sixtieth year, is, according to Bouillaud, from eight to nine ounces. The dimensions, according to Lobstein and Bouilland, are as follows:— Length, from base to apex, five inches six lines; breadth, at the base, three inches; thickness of the walls of the left ventricle, seven lines; at a finger's breadth above the apex, four lines; thickness of the walls of the right ventricle, two and a quarter lines; at the apex, half a line; thickness of right auricle, one line; of the left auricle, half a line. The heart is covered, externally, by a very thin, membranous reflection from the pericardium. The muscular structure of which it is constituted is much thicker in the parietes of the ventricle than in those of the auricles. Its cavities are lined by a very delicate membrane, the *endocardium*, which is continuous with the inner membrane of the arteries, as regards the left cavities, and with that of the veins, as regards the right. Its arteries— the *coronary*—arise from the commencement of the aorta. Its nerves proceed, chiefly, from the pneumogastric and the cervical ganglions of the great sympathetic. The heart is the great agent in the circulation. By its contraction, the blood is sent over every part of the body. Its action does not seem to be *directly* owing to nervous influence received from the brain or spinal marrow, or from both. The circulation may, indeed, be kept up, for some time, if both brain and spinal marrow be destroyed.

When the ear is applied to the chest, a dull, lengthened sound is heard, which is synchronous with the arterial pulse. This is instantly succeeded by a sharp, quick sound, like that of the valve of a bellows or the lapping of a dog, and this is followed by a period of repose. The first sound appears to be mainly produced by the contraction of the ventricles; the second, by the reflux of the blood against the semilunar valves. These are what are called the *Sounds of the Heart.* Dr. C. J. B. Williams thinks that the word *lubb-dup* conveys a notion of the two sounds. The *Beating* or *Impulse of the heart, Heart-stroke*, against the parietes of the chest is mainly caused, perhaps, by the systole of the heart, which tends to project it forwards. It is doubted, however, by some, whether the impulsion be produced by the dilatation or the contraction of the ventricles.

The following table exhibits the different actions of the heart, and their coincidence with its sounds and impulse. It presumes, that the period from the commencement of one pulsation to that of another is divided into eight parts; and if the case of a person, whose pulse beats sixty times in a minute, be taken, each of these parts will represent the eighth of a second.

EIGHTHS OF A SECOND.

Last part of the pause,...1..Auricles contracting; ventricles distended.
First sound and impulse,.4..Ventricles contracting; auricles dilating.
Second sound,.........2..Ventricles dilating; auricles dilating.
Pause,................1..Ventricles dilating; auricles distended.

The heart is subject to different organic diseases; the chief of which are *aneurism, contraction of the apertures*, and *rupture of its parietes.*

HEART, ATROPHY OF THE, *Atroph'ia seu Aridu'ra Cordis, Phthisis Cordis, Cardiatroph'ia, Acardiotroph'ia.* A condition of the organ in which there is diminution in the thickness of the parietes of the whole organ.

HEART, BEATING OF THE, see Heart — h. Dilatation of the, see Aneurism—h. Displacement of the, Ectopia Cordis — h. Fatty, Steatosis cordis.

HEART, HY'PERTROPHY OF THE, *Hypertroph'ia Cordis, Hypercor'dia, Hypersarco'sis Cordis, Hypercardiotroph'ia, Cardiaux'ē, Aneurys'ma cordis acti'vum* (Corvisart), *Cor bori'num,* (F.) *Hypertrophie du Cœur.* Supernutrition of the muscular parietes of the heart, which are thicker than usual; the cavities being generally diminished. The *physical signs* which indicate it are the following. In cases of long standing, the præcordial region is generally prominent; the pulsations of the heart are visible over a greater extent than natural; and a marked vibration is communicated to the hand when placed on the cardiac region. The dull sound on percussion is more extensive than natural; and on auscultation there is a permanent increase of the force and extent of the heart's action; there is no increase, however, of frequency, and the rhythm is regular. The pulse is generally strong, full, and hard.

HEART, HYPERTROPHY WITH DILATATION OF THE, *Active an'eurism, Eccen'tric hy'pertrophy.* In this affection, the pulsations can be seen and felt over a larger space, and the apex is more to the left and lower down than natural. The impulse is less steady, but at times more violent than that which accompanies simple hypertrophy. Percussion gives more distinct evidence of the enlargement, the sound being more extensively dull. On auscultation, the impulse is often violent, but irregular: in extreme cases, it produces the sensation of a large mass of flesh rolling or revolving beneath the ear. The pulse is strong, full, and vibratory. The shock of the heart's action is often transmitted to the whole person, and to the bed on which the patient is lying.

HEART, CONCENTRIC HYPERTROPHY OF THE, *Cardiarctie,* is when the parietes augment at the expense of the cavities.

HEART, IMPULSE OF THE, see Heart—h. Neuralgia of the, Angina Pectoris—h. Rupture of the, Cardiorrhexis — h. Sounds of the, see Heart — h. Stroke, see Heart.

HEART'S EASE, Viola tricolor.

HEARTS, LYMPH, Lymphatic hearts — h. Lymphatic, Lymphatic hearts.

HEARTBURN, Ardor ventriculi, Cardialgia.

HEARTWORT, Laserpitium album.

HEAT, past participle of Sax. hætan, 'to make warm.' *Calor, Therma, Seψn.* (F.) *Chaleur.* The material cause, which produces the sensation—or the particular sensation itself—produced by a body of an elevated temperature, on our organs, especially on the organs of touch. Modern chymists have given the name *Calo'ric* to the principle, whatever may be its nature, which is the cause of heat. When we touch a body of a temperature superior to our own, a portion of caloric passes from the body to the hand, and produces the sensation of *heat.* If, on the contrary, we touch a body of a temperature inferior to our own, we communicate a portion of our caloric to it, and experience the sensation of *cold.* Our own sensations are but imperfect indexes of temperature. Two men meeting at the middle of a mountain,—the one ascending, the other descending,—will experience different sensations. The one ascending, passes from a warmer to a

HEAT 431 HEAT

colder atmosphere;—the one descending from a colder to a warmer. The chief instrument for measuring heat, used in medicine, is the thermometer. Of this there are three kinds:—that of Fahrenheit, that of Réaumur, and that of Celsius or the *Centigrade*. The following Table exhibits the correspondence of these different thermometric scales.

Fah.	Réau.	Centig.	Fah.	Réau.	Centig.	Fah.	Réau.	Centig.	Fah.	Réau.	Centig.
°	°	°	°	°	°	°	°	°	°	°	°
212a	80.00	100.00	148	51.55	64.44	85	23.55	29.44	22	− 4.44	− 5.55
211	79.55	99.44	147	51.11	63.88	84	23.11	28.88	21	− 4.88	− 6.11
210b	79.11	98.88	146	50.66	63.33	83	22.66	28.33	20u	− 5.33	− 6.66
209	78.66	98.33	145	50.22	62.77	82	22.22	27.77	19	− 5.77	− 7.22
208	78.22	97.77	144	49.77	62.22	81o	21.77	27.22	18	− 6.22	− 7.77
207	77.77	97.22	143	49.33	61.66	80	21.33	26.66	17	− 6.66	− 8.33
206	77.33	96.66	142g	48.88	61.11	79	20.88	26.11	16	− 7.11	− 8.88
205	76.88	96.11	141	48.44	60.55	78	20.44	25.55	15	− 7.55	− 9.44
204	76.44	95.55	140	48.00	60.00	77	20.00	25.00	14	− 8.00	−10.00
203	76.00	95.00	139	47.55	59.44	76p	19.55	24.44	13	− 8.44	−10.55
202	75.55	94.44	138	47.11	58.88	75	19.11	23.88	12	− 8.88	−11.11
201	75.11	93.88	137	46.66	58.33	74	18.66	23.33	11	− 9.33	−11.66
200	74.66	93.33	136	46.22	57.77	73	18.22	22.77	10	− 9.77	−12.22
199	74.22	92.77	135	45.77	57.22	72	17.77	22.22	9	−10.22	−12.77
198	73.77	92.22	134	45.33	56.66	71	17.33	21.66	8	−10.66	−13.33
197	73.33	91.66	133h	44.84	56.11	70	16.88	21.11	7v	−11.11	−13.88
196c	72.88	91.11	132	44.45	55.55	69	16.44	20.55	6	−11.55	−14.44
195	72.44	90.55	131	44.00	55.00	68	16.00	20.00	5	−12.00	−15.00
194	72.00	90.00	130	43.55	54.44	67	15.55	19.44	4	−12.44	−15.55
193	71.55	89.44	129	43.11	53.88	66	15.11	18.88	3	−12.88	−16.11
192	71.11	88.88	128	42.66	53.33	65	14.66	18.33	2	−13.33	−16.66
191	70.66	88.33	127	42.22	52.77	64	14.22	17.77	1	−13.77	−17.22
190	70.22	87.77	126	41.77	52.22	63	13.77	17.22	0	−14.22	−17.77
189	69.77	87.22	125	41.33	51.66	62	13.33	16.66	− 1	−14.66	−18.33
188	69.33	86.66	124	40.88	51.11	61	12.88	16.11	− 2w	−15.11	−18.88
187	68.88	86.11	123	40.44	50.55	60	12.44	15.55	− 3	−15.55	−19.44
186	68.44	85.55	122	40.00	50.00	59	12.00	15.00	− 4	−16.00	−20.00
185	68.00	85.00	121	39.55	49.44	58	11.55	14.44	− 5	−16.44	−20.55
184	67.55	84.44	120	39.11	48.88	57	11.11	13.88	− 6	−16.88	−21.11
183	67.11	83.88	119	38.66	48.33	56	10.66	13.33	− 7x	−17.33	−21.66
182	66.66	83.33	118	38.22	47.77	55	10.22	12.77	− 8	−17.77	−22.22
181	66.22	82.77	117	37.77	47.22	54	9.77	12.22	− 9	−18.22	−22.77
180	65.77	82.22	116	37.33	46.66	53	9.33	11.66	−10	−18.66	−23.33
179	65.33	81.66	115	36.88	46.11	52	8.88	11.11	−11y	−19.11	−23.88
178d	64.88	81.11	114	36.44	45.55	51	8.44	10.55	−12	−19.55	−24.44
177	64.44	80.55	113	36.00	45.00	50q	8.00	10.00	−13	−20.00	−25.00
176	64.00	80.00	112	35.55	44.44	49	7.55	9.44	−14	−20.44	−25.55
175	63.55	79.44	111	35.11	43.88	48	7.11	8.88	−15	−20.88	−26.11
174e	63.11	78.88	110i	34.66	43.33	47	6.66	8.33	−16	−21.33	−26.66
173	62.66	78.33	109	34.22	42.77	46	6.22	7.77	−17	−21.77	−27.22
172	62.22	77.77	108	33.77	42.22	45	5.77	7.22	−18	−22.22	−27.77
171	61.77	77.22	107	33.33	41.60	44	5.33	6.66	−19	−22.66	−28.33
170	61.33	76.66	106j	32.88	41.11	43	4.88	6.11	−20	−23.11	−28.88
169	60.88	76.11	105	32.44	40.55	42	4.44	5.55	−21	−23.55	−29.44
168	60.44	75.55	104k	32.00	40.00	41	4.00	5.00	−22	−24.00	−30.00
167f	60.00	75.00	103	31.55	39.44	40	3.55	4.44	−23	−24.44	−30.55
166	59.55	74.44	102l	31.11	38.88	39	3.11	3.88	−24	−24.88	−31.11
165	59.11	73.88	101	30.66	38.33	38	2.66	3.33	−25	−25.33	−31.66
164	58.66	73.33	100m	30.22	37.77	37	2.22	2.77	−26	−25.77	−32.22
163	58.22	72.77	99	29.77	37.22	36	1.77	2.22	−27	−26.22	−32.77
162	57.77	72.22	98n	29.33	36.66	35	1.33	1.66	−28	−26.66	−33.33
161	57.33	71.66	97	28.88	36.11	34	0.88	1.11	−29	−27.11	−33.88
160	56.88	71.11	96	28.44	35.55	33	0.44	0.55	−30	−27.55	−34.44
159	56.44	70.55	95	28.00	35.00	32r	0.00	0.00	−31	−28.44	−35.00
158	56.00	70.00	94	27.55	34.44	31	−0.44	−0.55	−32	−28.00	−35.55
157	55.55	69.44	93	27.11	33.88	30s	−0.88	−1.61	−33	−28.88	−36.18
156	55.11	68.88	92	26.66	33.33	29	−1.33	−1.66	−34	−29.33	−36.66
155	54.66	68.33	91	26.22	32.77	28t	−1.77	−2.22	−35	−29.77	−37.22
154	54.22	67.77	90	25.77	32.22	27	−2.22	−2.77	−36	−30.22	−37.77
153	53.77	67.22	89	25.33	31.66	26	−2.66	−3.33	−37	−30.66	−38.28
152	53.33	66.66	88	24.88	31.11	25	−3.11	−3.88	−38	−31.11	−38.88
151	52.88	66.11	87	24.44	30.55	24	−3.55	−4.44	−39s	−31.55	−39.44
150	52.44	65.55	86	24.00	30.00	23	−4.00	−5.00	−40	−32.00	−40.00
149	52.00	65.00									

a Water boils (*Barom.* 30 *inches.*)
b Heat of a stove, borne by Dr. Solander.
c Heat of a stove, borne for 10 minutes by Sir Joseph Banks and Dr. Solander.
d Water simmers.
e Alcohol boils.
f Very pure ether distils.
g Bees' wax melts.
h Spermaceti melts.

i Temperature at which liquids are often drunk.
j Heat observed in Scarlatina.
k Temperature of the common hen.
l Temperature of arterial blood. [?]
m Temperature of venous blood. Phosphorus melts.
n Ether boils. *o* Nitric ether boils.
p Muriatic ether boils.
q Medium temperature of the globe. *r* Ice melts.

s Milk freezes.
t Vinegar freezes.
u Strong wine freezes.
v A mixture of one part of alcohol and three of water freezes.
w Cold at the battle of Eylau, 1807
x A mixture of equal parts of alcohol and water freezes.
y A mixture of two parts of alcohol and one of water freezes.
z Melting point of quicksilver.

To reduce Centigrade degrees to those of Fahrenheit, multiply by 9, divide by 5, and add 32: thus, 40° Cent. × 9 ÷ 5 + 32 = 104° Fahr. To reduce Fahrenheit's degrees to those of Centigrade, subtract 32, multiply by 5, and divide by 9: thus, 104° Fahr. − 32 × 5 ÷ 9 = 40° Cent. To reduce Réaumur's degrees to those of Fahrenheit, multiply by 9, divide by 4, and add 32: thus, 32° Réaum. × 9 ÷ 4 + 32 = 104° Fahr. To reduce Fahrenheit's degrees to those of Réaumur subtract

32, multiply by 4, and divide by 9: thus, 104° Fahr. — 32 × 4 ÷ 9 = 32 Réaum. *To reduce Réaumur's degrees to those of Centigrade*, multiply by 5, and divide by 4: thus 32° Réaum. × 5 ÷ 4 = 40° Cent.; and, lastly, *to reduce Centigrade degrees to those of Réaumur*, multiply by 4, and divide by 5: thus, 40° Cent. × 4 ÷ 5 = 32° Réaum.

The human body can bear a high degree of heat diffused in the atmosphere. There are cases on record, where air of 400° and upwards, of Fahrenheit's scale, has been breathed with impunity for a short time. It can likewise withstand very severe cold. In the expedition of Capt. Back to the Arctic regions, the thermometer was as low as —70° of Fahr. Excessive heat disposes the body to gastric and intestinal diseases, and particularly to inflammation and enlargement of the liver; hence, the frequency of such affections within the torrid zone. Heat is often used therapeutically: the actual cautery, at a white heat, disorganizes the parts to which it is applied: a lesser degree occasions violent inflammation. Heat higher than that of the human body is excitant; of a lower degree, sedative. Excessive cold acts as a powerful sedative — inducing sleep, the tendency to which, after long exposure, becomes irresistible. See Cold. Many of the topical applications — as cataplasms — act wholly by virtue of their warmth and moisture.

HEAT, *Ardor vene'reus*, *Pruri'tus*, (F.) *Chaleur des Animaux*, *Rut*, is the periodical sexual desire experienced by animals, — *Œstrua'tion.* It is supposed by some to be owing to the periodical maturation and discharge of ova, — *Ovula'tion.*

HEAT, ACRID, see Acrid — h. Animal, see Animal Heat.

HEAT, INTER'NAL, (F.) *Chaleur interne*, is a sensation of heat felt by the patient, but not sensible to the touch. *External heat*, (F.) *Chaleur extérieure*, that which can be felt by others. Heat, *Ardor*, is called *moist*, (F.) *haliteuse*, when accompanied with moisture, like that felt after bathing; *dry*, (F.) *sèche*, when the skin has not its ordinary softness. It is called *acrid* and *pungent*, (F.) *âcre et mordicante*, when it conveys a disagreeable tingling to the fingers. The French employ the terms *nervous heat* and *errat'ic heat*, *Chaleur nerveuse* and *Chaleur erratique*, for that which comes by flushes, alternating with chills, and which moves rapidly from one part to another. M. Double has used the term *septic heat*, (F.) *Chaleur septique*, for that which produces a pungent sensation on the hand, similar to that of the acrid heat, but milder and more uniform, and which is accompanied with feebleness and frequency of pulse, &c.

HEAT, PRICKLY, Lichen tropicus.
HEATH, COMMON, Erica vulgaris.
HEAUTOPHONICS, see Autophonia.
HEAVINESS, Somnolency.
HEAVING, Vomiturition.
HEAVY, *Gravis*, (F.) *Gravatif*, from Sax. *heafan*, 'to heave.' An epithet given to any pain which consists in a sensation of weight or heaviness, or is accompanied by such sensation.
HEBDOMADAL CYCLE, see Cycle.
HEBDOMADARIA. Octana.
HEBE, 'ηβη, *Juven'ta*, *Juven'tas*, *Juben'tus*, *Hora.* In antiquity, the goddess of puberty. The word has been employed to designate, 1. The first hair that grows on the pubes, 2. The pubic region, and 3. Puberty.
HEBETES, Adolescens.
HEBETOR, Adolescens.
HEBETUDO ANIMI, Imbecility — h. Dentium, Hæmodia — h. Visus, Amblyopia, Caligo.

HEBRADENDRON CAMBOGIOIDES, see Cambogia.

HEBREWS, MED'ICINE OF THE. Medicine seems to have been at a very low ebb with the ancient Hebrews. Of anatomy they knew nothing. Their *physiology* was imperfect and filled with superstitions; and their *therapeutics* unsatisfactory. *Hygiene* appears to have been most attended to. Of the other departments of medicine we cannot judge of their knowledge.

HECATOMA PALUSTRIS, Ranunculus sceleratus.

HECATOMPHYLLUM, Rosa centifolia.

HEC'TEUS, 'εκτευς. A Greek measure, containing about 72 chopines or pints.

HECTIC FEVER, *Febris hec'tica*, *Hecticop'yra*, *Hecticopyr'etos*, *Hec'tica*, *Amphimer'ina hec'tica*, *Febris phthis'ica*, *Syntecop'yra*, *Syntecticop'yra*, *Febris marasmo'des*, *Marasmop'yra*, *Febris tab'ida*, *Leucopyr'ia*, *Epan'etus hec'tica*, *Febris lenta*, *F. amphimer'ina hec'tica*, *Febris amato'ria*, *Chloro'sis amato'ria*, (F.) *Fièvre Hectique*, *F. Étique*, from 'εξις, 'habit of body;' because in this disease every part of the body is emaciated; or, perhaps, from εκτηκω, 'I consume,' 'I am exhausted.' The name of a slow, continued, or remittent fever, which generally accompanies the end of organic affections, and has been esteemed idiopathic, although it is probably always symptomatic. It is the fever of irritation and debility; and is characterised by progressive emaciation, frequent pulse, hot skin, — especially of the palms of the hands and soles of the feet, — and, towards the end, colliquative sweats and diarrhœa. Being symptomatic, it can only be removed by getting rid of the original affection. This is generally difficult and almost hopeless in the disease, which it most commonly accompanies,—consumption.

HECTICA, Hectic Fever—h. Infantilis, Fever, infantile remittent.

HECTICOPYRA, Hectic fever.
HECTICOPYRETOS, Hectic fever.
HEC'TISIS, (F.) *Étisie*. Same etymon. The state of those who have hectic fever.

HEC'TOGRAMME, *Hectogram'ma*, from 'εκατον, 'a hundred,' and γραμμα. A measure of 100 grammes, i. e. 3 ounces, 1 drachm, and 44 grains, Troy.

HECTOLITRE. A measure containing 100 litres or 26.42 wine pints.

HECUSIUS, Voluntary.

HEDEO'MA, *Hedeo'ma pulegioi'des*, *Cuni'la pulegioi'des*, *Melis'sa pulegioides*, *Pennyroyal*, *Tickweed*, *Stinking Balm*, *Squawmint.* *Sex. Syst.* Diandria Monogynia; *Nat. Ord.* Labiatæ. An indigenous plant, common in all parts of the United States, and which, where it is abundant, perfumes the air for a considerable distance. It is employed in the same cases as the mints and the English pennyroyal. In popular practice it is used as an emmenagogue.

The *O'leum Hedeo'mæ* (Ph. U. S.) or *Oil of Pennyroyal* is used as a stimulating carminative, dropped on sugar. Dose, 2 to 6 drops.

HEDERA ARBOREA, H. Helix.

HED'ERA HELIX, *Hed'era arbo'rea*, *Bac'chica*, *Cissos*, κισσος, *Cittos*, κιττος, *Ed'era*, *Corymbe'tra*, *Corym'bos*, *Ivy*, (F.) *Lierre.* The taste of ivy *leaves* is bitter, styptic, and nauseous. They are not used in medicine. According to Haller, they were recommended in Germany against the atrophy of children; and the common people of England sometimes apply them to running sores and to keep issues open. The *berries* were supposed, by the ancients, to have an emetic and purgative quality; and a watery extract was made from them, called by Quercetanus *Extractum purgans*. From the stalk of the tree a resinous juice exudes, in warm climates, called *Gummi Hed'eræ*, (F.) *Gomme de lierre, Resine de lierre*. It is possessed of tonic and astringent properties, but is not used.

HEDERA TERRESTRIS, Glechoma hederacea.
HEDERULA, Glechoma hederacea.
HEDISARUM ALHAGI, Agul.
HEDRA, 'ἑδρα, 'ἑδρη, 'a vestige,' 'a seat.' A seat. A fracture of the bones of the cranium, in which the trace of the fracturing instrument is still perceptible. It was, also, used by the ancients, for the anus, the breech, excrement, a privy, a night-chair, and for the bottom of an abscess.

HEDROCELE, Proctocele.
HEDYCH'ROUM, from 'ηδυς, 'sweet,' and χροα, 'colour.' A remedy of a pleasant colour. Applied to certain trochs, the chief constituent of which was Theriac.

HEDYPHO'NIA, from 'ηδυς, 'sweet,' and φωνη, 'voice.' Sweetness of voice.
HEDYPNEUS'TUS, *Hedyp'nous*, from 'ηδυς, 'sweet,' and πνεω, 'I breathe.' Breathing sweetly or softly. Smelling sweetly.
HEDYPNOIS TARAXACUM, Leontodon taraxacum.
HEDYSARUM ALHAGI, Agul.
HEDYSMA, Condiment.
HEEL, see Calcaneum.
HELCENTERITIS, Dothinenteritis.
HELCO'DES, Ulcerated, Ulcerous.
HELCOL'OGY, *Helcolog"ia*; from 'ἑλκος, 'ulcer,' and λογος, 'discourse.' The doctrine of, or a treatise on, ulcers.

HELCOMA, Ulcer.
HELCOPHTHAL'MIA, *Ophthal'mia ulcero'sa*. Ophthalmia with ulceration.
HEL'COS, from 'ἑλκος, 'an ulcer.' Hence:
HELCOSIS, Elcosis, Ulceration — h. Cerebri, Encephalopyosis — h. Laryngis, Phthisis laryngea — h. Pulmonalis, Phthisis pulmonalis — h. Renalis, Nephrelcosis — h. Uteri, see Metrophthisis — h. Vesicæ, Cystophthisis.

HELCOSTAPHYLO'MA; from 'ἑλκος, 'ulcer,' and σταφυλωμα, 'staphyloma.' Staphyloma ending in ulceration.

HELCOXERO'SIS, from 'ἑλκος, 'ulcer,' and ξηρωσις, 'dryness.' The drying of an ulcer.
HELCTICA, Epispastics.
HELCUS, Ulcer.
HELCYD'RION, *Helcyd'rium*, 'ἑλκυδριον, *Ulcus'culum*, a small ulcer, a superficial ulceration of the cornea.—Galen, Paulus, Foësius.

HELCYS'TER, from 'ἑλκω, 'I draw.' An iron hook or crotchet for extracting the foetus. See Crotchet.

HELENIUM, Inula helenium.
HELEN'IUM AUTUMNA'LE, *False Sunflower, Sneezewort, Sneezeweed, Swamp Sunflower, Yellow star, Ox-eye*. An indigenous herb, with large golden-yellow compound flowers, which appear in August. All its parts are bitter and somewhat acrid, and when snuffed up the nostrils in powder are powerful sternutatories.

HELIAN'THEMUM CANADEN'SE, *Cistus Canaden'sis, Frostwort, Frostweed, Rock-rose*. An herbaceous plant, having large yellow flowers, which grows in all parts of the United States, and flowers, in the Middle States, in June. It has an astringent, slightly aromatic, and bitterish taste. It has been prescribed in scrofula, but probably is nothing more than an aromatic tonic.

HELIAN'THEMUM CORYMBO'SUM, *Rock rose*, an indigenous plant, is used in the same cases.

HELIASIS, Astrabolismus, Insolation.
HELICH'RYSUM NUDIFO'LIUM, *Caffer tea*. A South African plant, *Nat. Ord*. Compositæ, which is demulcent, and, in the form of infusion, is recommended in catarrh, phthisis, and other pulmonary affections.

HELICHRYSUM SERPYLLIFO'LIUM, *Hottentot's tea*, and HELICHRYSUM AURICULA'TUM have similar virtues.

HELICIA, Age.
HEL'ICINE, *Helic"inus, Helicoi'des, Helico'des*, from *helix*, 'the tendril of the vine.' Resembling the tendril of the vine.

HELICINE ARTERIES of the penis, as described by J. Müller, are short vessels given off from the larger branches, as well as from the finest twigs of the artery of the organ: most of those come off at a right angle, and project into the cavity of the spongy substance, either terminating abruptly or swelling out into a club-like process without again subdividing. Almost all these vessels are bent like a horn, so that the end describes half a circle or somewhat more. They have a great resemblance to the tendrils of the vine, whence their name. A minute examination of them, either with the lens or the microscope, shows that, although they at all times project into the venous cavities of the corpora cavernosa, they are not entirely naked, but are covered with a delicate membrane, which, under the microscope, appears granular.

HEL'ICIS MAJOR. A muscle of the ear, which originates from the anterior, acute part of the helix, upon which it ascends and is inserted into the helix. It pulls the part into which it is inserted a little downwards and forwards.

HELICIS MINOR. This muscle originates from the under and fore part of the helix, and is inserted into the helix, near the fissure in the cartilage, opposite the concha. Its use is to contract the fissure.

HELICOIDES, Helicine.
HELICOTRE'MA, from 'ἑλιξ, 'helix, cochlea,' and τρημα, 'a foramen.' The hole by which the two scalæ of the cochlea communicate at the apex.

HELIGMUS, Convolution.
HELIKIA, Age.
HELIONOSIS, Insolation.
HELIOSIS, Astrabolismus, Insolation.
HELIOTROPE, Heliotropium Europæum.
HELIOTROPION, Cichorium intybus.
HELIOTRO'PIUM EUROPÆ'UM, *H. erectum seu canes'cens seu supi'num, Verruca'ria*, The *He'liotrope*, (F.) *Tournesol, Herbe aux verrues*. This plant is considered to possess aperient properties; and to be capable of destroying cutaneous excrescences; hence one of its names.

HELIX, *Capre'olus*, from ειλειν, 'to envelop,' 'surround.' The fold is thus called, which forms the outer circumference or ring of the external ear.

HELIX, Limax.
HELIX POMA'TIA. A large kind of snail, transported from the south of Europe to England by Sir Kenelm Digby, for his lady when in a decline. It was considered highly restorative.
HELLEBORASTER, Helleborus fœtidus — h. fœtidus, Helleborus fœtidus.
HELLEBORE, Dracontium fœtidum—h. American, Veratrum viride—h. Black, Helleborus niger—h. *Blanc*, Veratrum album—h. *Noir*, Helleborus niger—h. Stinking, Helleborus fœtidus—h. Swamp, Veratrum viride—h. White, Veratrum album.
HELLEBORIS'MUS, *Elleboris'mus*. The method of treating disease, amongst the ancients, by hellebore. This comprised not only the choice, preparation, and administration of the medicine, but, likewise, the knowledge and employment of

preliminary precautions and remedies proper for aiding its action, and preventing the pernicious effects which it might occasion.

HELLEBORUS, H. niger—h. Albus, Veratrum album—h. Grandiflorus, H. niger—h. Trifolius, Coptis.

HELLEB'ORUS FŒ'TIDUS, *Helleboras'ter, H. fœ'tidus, Elleboraster, Stinking Hel'lebore* or *Bear's foot, Setterwort,* (F.) *Hellébore* ou *Ellébore fétide, Pied de Griffon.* The leaves of this plant are said to be anthelmintic. The smell of the fresh plant is extremely fetid, and the taste bitter and acrid. It usually acts as a cathartic.

HELLEBORUS NIGER, *H. grandiflo'rus, Elleb'orus niger, Melampo'dium, Melanorrhi'zum, Ectomon, Black Hel'lebore, Melampode, Christmas Rose,* (F.) *Hellébore noir.* The root of this European plant—*Helleborus,* (Ph. U. S.)—has a disagreeable odour, and bitter, acrid taste. It is possessed of cathartic properties, and has been recommended as an emmenagogue. It has been given in mania, melancholia, dropsy, suppressed menses, &c. Dose, gr. x to ℈j, as a cathartic.

HELLECEBRA, Sedum.
HELLENIA GRANDIFLORA, Costus.
HELMET-FLOWER, YELLOW, Aconitum Anthora.
HELMET POD, Jeffersonia Bartoni.
HELMINS, Plur. *Helmin'thes* seu *Elmin'thes,* from 'ελμινς, 'a worm.' A worm; an entozoon: —hence:
HELMINTHAGOGUE, Anthelmintic.
HELMINTHI, Worms.
HELMINTHIA, Helminthiasis—h. Alvi, Worms.

HELMIN'THIA ERRAT'ICA. Worms, introduced by accident and without finding a proper habitation in the stomach or intestines; producing spasmodic colic, with severe tormina, and occasionally vomiting or dejections of blood; the 12th genus of the order *Enterica,* class *Cœliaca,* of Good.

HELMINTHIA PODICIS, Worms.
HELMINTHI'ASIS, from 'ελμινς, 'a worm.' A generic name for the condition which gives occasion to the presence of intestinal worms. It is, also, called *Helmin'thia, Vermina'tio, Morbus vermino'sus, Status vermino'sus, Sabur'ra vermino'sa, Scoleci'asis, Scolece'sis, Entozöogen'esis, Parasitis'mus intestina'lis, Worm disease, Invermina'tion.* See Worms.

HELMINTHIC, Anthelmintic.
HELMINTHOCHORTUM, Corallina Corsicana.
HELMINTHOCOLICA, Colica verminosa.
HELMINTHOCORTON, Corallina Corsicana.
HELMINTHOL'OGY, *Helmintholog''ia,* from 'ελμινς, 'a worm,' and λογος, 'a description.' A treatise on worms.
HELMINTHONCUS, Malis—h. Medinensis, Dracunculus.
HELMINTHOP'YRA, *Helminthopyr'etos, Febris vermino'sa,* from 'ελμινς, 'a worm,' and πυρ, 'a fever.' Fever occasioned by worms. See Fever, verminous.
HELMINTHOPYRETOS, Helminthopyra.
HELMINTHUS GORDII, Seta equina.
HELODES, Elodes.
HELONIAS DIOICA, Chamælerium luteum—h. Lutea, Chamælerium luteum—h. Officinalis, see Veratrina.
HELOPYRA, Elodes (febris.)
HELOPYRETUS, Elodes (febris.)
HELOS, Clavus, Marsh.
HELO'SIS, *Helo'tis:* from 'ελω, 'I turn.' Eversion of the eyelids, and convulsions of the muscles of the eyes. Plica Polonica. Strabismus.
HELOTIS, Helosis, Plica.

HELUS, Clavus, Helos.
HELXINE, Parietaria.
HEMACHROIN, Hæmatin.
HÉMADYNAMÈTRE, Hæmadynamometer.
HÉMAPÉRITONIRRHAGIE, Hæmaperitonirrhag''ia; from 'αιμα, 'blood,' *peritonæum,* and ρηγνυμι, 'I break forth.' Hemorrhage into the peritoneum.
HÉMAPROCTIE, Hæmorrhois.
HÉMASTATIQUES, Hæmatostatica.
HÉMATIDROSE, Sudor cruentus.
HEMATIN, Hæmatin.
HÉMATO-ENCÉPHALIE, Apoplexy.
HEMATOID, Hæmatodes.
HÉMATOLOGIE, Hæmatology.
HEMATOLOGY, Hæmatology.
HÉMATOMYÉLIE, Hémorrhagie de la Moëlle Épinière.
HÉMATONCIE, Hæmatoncus, see Hæmatodes fungus—*h. Fongoïde,* Hæmatodes fungus.
HÉMATOPISIE, Hæmatops.
HEMATORRHACHIS, Apoplexia myelitica.
HEMATOSIN, Hæmatin.
HEMERA, 'ημερα, 'a day.' *Dies.* Hence:
HEMERALOPIA, see Nyctalopia.

HEMERALO'PIA, from 'ημηρα, 'the day,' and οπτομαι, 'I see.' *Hæmeralops, Dyso'pia tenebra'rum, Cali'go tenebra'rum, Parop'sis Noctif'uga, Visus diur'nus, Nyctalo'pia, (of some,) Nyctotyphlo'sis, Amblyo'pia crepuscula'ris, Cæcitas crepuscula'ris* seu *noctur'na, A'cies diur'na, Daysight, Day-vision, Hen blindness, Night blindness,* (F.) *Vue diurne, Aveuglement de Nuit.* A disease, in which the eyes enjoy the faculty of seeing, whilst the sun is above the horizon, but are incapable of seeing by the aid of artificial light. Its causes are not evident. The eye, when carefully examined, presents no alteration, either in its membranes or humours.

HEM'ERALOPS, *Dorea.* One labouring under hemeralopia. Also, Hemeralopia.
HEMERATYPHLOSIS, Nyctalopia.
HEMERODROMA, (febris) Ephemera.
HEMEROPATHI'A; from 'ημερα, 'a day,' and παθος, 'an affection.' A disease, which continues only a day; or, which is only observed during the day.
HEMI, 'ημι, 'ημισυς, 'half,' 'semi.' Hence:
HEMIAMAUROSIS, Hemiopia.
HEMIANDRUS, Eunuch.
HEMIANOR, Eunuch.
HEMIANTHROPIA, Mania.
HEMIANTHROPUS, Eunuch, Maniac.
HEMIAZYGA, (Vena) see Azygos vein.
HEMICEPHALÆA, Hemicrania.
HEMICEPHALÆUM, Sinciput.
HEMICEPHALIUM, Sinciput.
HEMICEPHALUM, Sinciput.

HEMICEPH'ALUS, *Semiceph'alus,* from 'ημι, 'half,' and κεφαλη, 'head.' One who has half a head.

HEMICRA'NIA, *Hemicephala'a, Migra'na, Grana, Hemipa'gia, Hemipe'gia, Heterocra'nia, Monopa'gia, Monope'gia, Cephala'a Hemicra'nia, Hemipathi'a, Megrim,* from 'ημισυς, 'half,' and κρανιον, 'cranium.' (F.) *Migraine.* Pain, confined to one half the head. It is almost always of an intermittent character;—at times, continuing only as long as the sun is above the horizon; and hence sometimes called *Sun-pain,*—and is cured by cinchona, arsenic, and the remedies adapted for intermittents.

HEMICRANIA IDIOPATHICA, Neuralgia, facial.
HEMIDES'MUS IN'DICUS, *Periplo'ca In'-*

dica, Ascle'pias Pseudosar'sa, Sarsaparil'la In'-dica, Nannari, Indian Sarsaparilla. A Hindoostanee plant, the root of which has a peculiar aromatic odour, and a bitterish taste. It is used in India as a substitute for sarsaparilla.

HEMIDIAPHORE'SIS, *Transpira'tio Unilat'era;* from *'ημι,* 'half,' and *διαφορησις,* 'perspiration.' Perspiration of one half the body.

HEMIEC'TON, *Hemiec'teon, Semisex'tum.* A vessel capable of containing 36 chopines or pints, and in which fumigations were made in diseases of the uterus and vagina.—Hippocrates.

HEMIM'ELES, from *'ημισυς,* 'one half,' and *μελος,* 'a limb.' A genus of monsters, in which the upper or lower extremities are very defective — mere stumps,—and the fingers and toes are entirely wanting or very imperfect.—G. St. Hilaire.

HEMIMŒ'RION, from *'ημισυς,* and *μοιρα,* 'a part.' 'One half.'—Foësius. Also, half a drachm. —Erotian.

HEM'INA. A Greek measure, answering to the *Cotyle, κοτυλη,* i. e. one half the sextarius, or about half a pint, English.

HEMIOBOL'ION, *Hemiob'olon.* Half the obolus. A weight of about five grains.—Gorræus.

HEMIO'LION. A weight of 12 drachms, or oz. 1½.—Galen. See Sescuncia.

HEMIO'PIA, *Hemiop'sis, Hemiopi'asis, Suffu'sio dimid'iana, Visus dimidia'tus, Marmor'ygē Hippoc'ratis, Hemiamauro'sis, Amauro'sis dimidia'ta,* from *'ημισυς,* 'one half,' and *οπτομαι,* 'I see.' Depraved vision, in which the person sees only one half of an object.

HEMIOPIASIS, Hemiopia.

HEMIOPSIS, Hemiopia.

HEMIPA'GES, *Dicor'yphus dihypogas'trius, Oc'topus synapheoceph'alus,* from *'ημι,* 'half,' and *πηγνυμι,* 'I fasten.' A monstrosity, in which twins are united from the navel to the vertex.— I. G. Saint Hilaire.

HEMIPAGIA, Hemicrania.

HEMIPATHIA, Hemicrania.

HEMIPEGIA, Hemicrania.

HEMIPHO'NIA, from *'ημι,* 'half,' and *φωνη,* 'voice.' Great weakness of voice.

HEMIPLE'GIA, *Hemiplex'ia, Paral'ysis Hemiplegia, Semiple'gia, Semi-sidera'tio,* from *'ημισυς,* 'one half,' and *πλησσω,* or *πληττω,* 'I strike.' Paralysis of one side of the body. See Paralysis. One so palsied is said to be *hemipleg"ic, semisidera'tus.*

HEMIPLEGIA FACIALIS, Paralysis, Bell's.

HEMIPLEXIA, Hemiplegia.

HEMIPROSOPLEGIA, Paralysis, Bell's.

HEMISPHÆRÆ CEREBRI, Hemispheres of the brain.

HEM'ISPHERE, *Hemisphæ'ra, Hemisphæ'rium,* from *'ημισυς,* 'one half,' and *σφαιρα,* 'a sphere.' One half of a sphere or of a body having a spheroidal shape.

HEMISPHERES OF THE BRAIN, *Hemisphæ'ræ cer'ebri, Hemispher'ical gan'glia,* are the upper spheroidal portions of the brain, separated from each other by the falx cerebri.

HEMISPHERICAL GANGLIA, Hemispheres of the brain.

HÉMITE, Hæmitis.

HEMITRITÆ'A, (FEBRIS,) *F. Semi-tertia'na, Febris sesquial'tera,* (F.) *Semi-tierce, Fièvre demitierce.* A semi-tertian fever, so called because it seems to possess both the characters of the tertian and quotidian intermittent. — Galen, Spigelius.

HEMIUNCIA, Hemiuncion.

HEMIUN'CION, *Hemiun'cia, Semun'cia, Sesun'cia.* Half an ounce.

HEMLOCK, Conium maculatum — h. American, Cicuta maculata—h. Bastard, Chærophyllum sylvestre — h. Common, Conium maculatum—h. Dropwort, Œnanthe — h. Gum, see Pinus Canadensis — h. Pitch, see Pinus Canadensis — h. Spruce, Pinus Canadensis—h. Water, American Cicuta maculata—h. Water, fine-leaved, Phellandrium aquaticum—h. Water, Cicuta aquatica—h. Wild, Cicuta maculata.

HÉMOCARDIOPLASTIES, see Polypus.

HEMODIA, Hæmodia.

*HÉMO-ENCÉPHALORRHAGIE,*Apoplexy.

HÉMOHÉPATORRHAGIE, Hepatorrhagia.

HÉMOMÈTRE, Hæmadynamometer.

HÉMOMYÉLORRHAGIE, Apoplexy, spinal.

HÉMOPTYSIE, Hæmoptysis — *h. Foudroyante,* see Hæmoptysis.

HEMORRHAGE, Hæmorrhagia—h. Accidental, see Hæmorrhagia—h. Active, see Hæmorrhagia—h. from the Bladder, Cystirrhagia—h. Constitutional, see Hæmorrhagia — h. Critical, see Hæmorrhagia—h. by Exhalation, see Hæmorrhagia—h. External, see Hæmorrhagia—h. General, see Hæmorrhagia — h. from the Intestines, Melæna—h. Internal, see Hæmorrhagia—h. Interstitial, Apoplexy—h. Local, see Hæmorrhagia—h. of the Mucous Membranes, see Hæmorrhagia —h. Passive, see Hæmorrhagia—h. from the Pituitary Membrane, Epistaxis—h. Pleural, Hæmatothorax—h. from the Skin, Sudor cruentus—h. Spinal, Apoplexy, spinal — h. Spontaneous, see Hæmorrhagia — h. Supplementary, see Hæmorrhagia—h. Symptomatic, see Hæmorrhagia—h. of the Tissues, see Hæmorrhagia—h. Traumatic, see Hæmorrhagia—h. Uterine, Metrorrhagia.

HEMORRHAGIC PLEURISY, Hæmatothorax.

HÉMORRHAGIE BUCCALE, Stomatorrhagia—*h. Cérébrale,* Apoplexy—*h. du Foie,* Hepatorrhagia — *h. Interstitielle,* Apoplexy—*h. Interstitielle du Poumon,* Hæmoptysis — *h. des Intestins,* Hæmatochezia — *h. de la Matrice,* Metrorrhagia — *h. Méningée,* Apoplexy, meningeal— *h, de la Moëlle épinière,* Apoplexia myelitica — *h. Nasale,* Epistaxis—*h. de la Vessie,* Cystirrhagia.

HEMORRHAGIP'AROUS, (F.) *Hémorrhagipare,* from *hæmorrhagia,* 'hemorrhage,' and *parire,* 'to bring forth.' That which gives occasion to hemorrhage: thus, softening of the neurine may be *hemorrhagiparous.*

HÉMORRHINIE, Epistaxis.

HÉMORRHOÏDAIRE, (F.) One who is subject to hemorrhoids.

HÉMORRHOÏDES, Hæmorrhois — *h. Aveugles,* Cæcæ hæmorrhoides. See Hæmorrhois.

HÉMORRHOSCOPIE, Hæmatoscopia.

HÉMOSPASIE, Hæmospasia.

HÉMOSPASIQUE, Hæmospastic.

HÉMOSTASIE, Hæmostasia.

HÉMOSTATIQUES, Hæmatostatica.

HEMP, INDIAN, Apocynum cannabinum, Bangue—h. Wild, Ambrosia trifida.

HEMPSEED, see Cannabis sativa.

HENBANE, Hyoscyamus.

HENBIT, Lamium amplexicaule.

HEN-BLINDNESS, Hemeralopia.

HENNÉ, Lawsonia inermis.

HENRICEA PHARMACEARCHA, Gentiana chirayita.

HENRICUS RUBENS, Colcothar.

HEPAR, *'ηπαρ,* 'genitive,' *'ηπατος,* 'liver.' A name for substances resembling liver in appearance. The ancient name for the *liver of sulphur, Hepar sul'phuris;* which is sometimes a compound of sulphur and potassium; at others, of sulphur and potassa. See Potassæ sulphuretum.

HEPAR ADULTERINUM, Spleen.

HEPAR ANTIMONIA'TUM is a compound of a sulphuret of antimony and an alkali. See Oxydum stibii sulphuretum.

HEPAR MARTIA'LE. A compound of sulphuret of potass and an oxide of iron.

HEPAR SANGUINIS, see Blood — h. Sinistrum, Spleen — h. Sulphuris salinum, Potassæ sulphuretum—h. Sulphuris volatile, Ammoniæ sulphuretum—h. Uterinum, Placenta.

HEPATAL'GIA, *Hepatodyn'ia, Neural'gia he'patis, Col'ica hepat'ica,* from 'ηπαρ, 'liver,' and αλγος, 'pain.' Pain in the liver. Neuralgia of the liver, (F.) *Névralgie du Foie.*

HEPATALGIA CALCULOSA, Colica hepatica—h. Petitiana, Turgescentia vesiculæ felleæ — h. Phlegmonoides, Hepatitis.

HEPATAPOSTE'MA, from 'ηπαρ, 'the liver,' and αποστημα, 'an abscess.' Abscess of the liver.

HEPATARIUS, Hepaticus.

HEPATATROPH'IA, *Atroph'ia* seu *Aridu'ra he'patis,* from 'ηπαρ, 'the liver,' and *atrophia,* 'atrophy.' Atrophy of the liver:—a general concomitant of *Cirrho'sis he'patis.*

HEPATAUXĒ, *Hypertroph'ia he'patis,* (F.) *Hyperhe'patotrophie, Hypertrophie du foie.* Hypertrophy of the liver.

HEPATECHE'MA, *Son'itus hepat'icus,* from 'ηπαρ, 'liver,' and 'ηχημα, 'sound.' Sound rendered by the liver on percussion.

HEPATEMPHRAX'IS, from 'ηπαρ, 'liver,' and εμφρασσω, 'I obstruct.' *Emphrax'is hepatis,* Hepatic obstruction.—Ploucquet.

HEPATENCEPHALO'MA, *Hepatomyelo'ma, Fungus he'patis medulla'ris,* from 'ηπαρ, 'liver,' and εγκεφαλος, 'encephalon.' Encephaloid of the liver.

HEPATE'RUS, *Hepat'icus, Jecora'rius.* A variety of diarrhœa, *Fluxus hepaticus.*—Gorræus.

HEPATHÆMORRHAG''IA, *Hæmorrhag''ia hepat'ica, Hepatorrhag''ia, Apoplex'ia hepat'ica,* (F.) *Hémorrhagie du foie, Hémohépatorrhagie,* from 'ηπαρ, 'liver,' and 'αιμορραγια, 'hemorrhage.' Hemorrhage from the liver.

HEPAT'IC, *Hepat'icus, Hepata'rius, Hepate'rus, Hepatoïdes, Hepato'des, Jecora'rius,* from 'ηπαρ, 'the liver.' Belonging or relating to or resembling liver.

HEPATIC AR'TERY, *Arte'ria Hepat'ica.* One of the three branches given off by the cœliac. It passes towards the inferior surface of the liver; where it divides into two branches, a *right* and a *left,* which proceed towards the corresponding parts of that organ. The right branch gives off the cystic artery. Before dividing, the hepatic artery sends off two considerable branches, the *A. pylorica* and *Gastro-epiploica dextra.*

HEPATIC DUCT, *Ductus hepat'icus,* (F.) *Canal hépatique,* is about three fingers' breadth in length, and of the size of a quill. It is formed by the union of the biliary ducts, and joins the cystic duct at a very acute angle, to form the ductus choledochus. Its function is to convey the bile from the liver towards the duodenum.

HEPATIC PLEXUS, *Plexus hepat'icus,* consists of nervous filaments, sent by the cœliac plexus to the liver, which accompany the hepatic artery.

HEPATIC VEINS, *Supra-hepatic Veins, Venæ cavæ hepat'icæ,* (F.) *Veines sus-hépatiques, Intralob'ular veins,* do not follow the course of the arteries of the same name. They arise in the substance of the liver; converge towards the posterior margin of that viscus, and open into the vena cava inferior. They convey away the blood carried to the liver by the hepatic artery and vena porta.

HEPAT'ICA. Medicines believed to be capable of affecting the liver.

HEPATICA, H. triloba—h. Americana, H. triloba—h. Fontana, Marchantia polymorpha—h. Nobilis, H. triloba—h. Stellata, Asperula odorata.

HEPATICA TRIL'OBA, *H. America'na, Anemo'ne hepat'ica* seu *nob'ilis, Herba trinita'tis, Hepat'ica, Hepat'icus flos, Trifo'lium hepat'icum, Trifo'lium au'reum, Liverwort, Liverweed, Trefoil, Noble Liverwort, Herb Trin'ity,* (F.) *Hépatique des jardins.* This plant—*Hepat'ica* (Ph. U. S.)—is a gentle astringent, but not possessed of much virtue.

HEPATICULA, Hepatitis, chronic.

HEPATICUS, Hepateros — h. Flos, Hepatica triloba.

HEPATIFICATIO, Hepatization.

HÉPATIQUE ÉTOILÉE, Asperula odorata—*h. des Fontaines,* Marchantia polymorpha—*h. des Jardins,* Hepatica triloba.

HEPATIRRHŒ'A, *Fluxus hepat'icus, Dysenter'ia hepat'ica, Diarrhœ'a hepat'ica, Hepatorrhœ'a, Hepatocholorrhœ'a, Hepatodysenter'ia, Hepatorrhag''ia, Hæmate'ra, Aimate'ra,* (F.) *Flux hépatique,* from 'ηπαρ, 'the liver,' and ρεω, 'I flow.' A species of diarrhœa in which the excreted matters seem to come from the liver, or are much mixed with bile.

HEPATIS EMUNCTORIA, Inguen—h. Suspensorium, Ligament, suspensory, of the liver.

HEPATISATIO, Hepatization — h. Pulmonum, Hepatization of the Lungs.

HÉPATISATION, Hepatization — *h. Grise,* see Hepatization—*h. Rouge,* see Hepatization.

HEPATITES VENA, Cava vena.

HEPATI'TIS, *Empres'ma hepati'tis, Cauma hepati'tis, Inflamma'tio he'patis, I. Jecino'ris, Febris hepat'ica inflammato'ria, Hepatal'gia phlegmonoi'des, Morbus jecino'ris, Hepatophlegmonē, Inflammation of the liver,* (F.) *Hépatite, Inflammation du foie, Pièce* (Provincial). It may be seated either in the peritoneal covering, *Sero-hepati'tis,* or in the substance of the liver, or in both, *Puro-hepati'tis,* and may be acute or chronic. The peculiar symptoms are:—pain in the right hypochondrium, shooting to the back and right shoulder, and increased on pressure; difficulty of lying on the left side; sometimes jaundice with cough, and synocha. Its termination is generally by resolution:—in tropical climates it often runs on to suppuration, *Jec'oris vom'ica, Hepati'tis apostemato'sa,* the abscess breaking either externally, or forming a communication with the intestines or chest, or breaking into the cavity of the abdomen. The *causes* are those of inflammation in general. Heat predisposes to it; hence its greater frequency in hot climates. On dissection of those who have died of it, the liver has been found hard and enlarged; colour of a deep purple; or the membranes have been more or less vascular; or adhesions, or tubercles, or hydatids, or abscesses, or biliary calculi may be met with. The treatment must be bold. Bleeding, general and local, fomentations, blisters, purgatives, and the antiphlogistic regimen. In hot climates especially, a new action must be excited by mercury as early as possible.

HEPATITIS APOSTEMATOSA, see Hepatitis.

HEPATITIS, CHRONIC, *Hepati'tis chron'ica, Inflamma'tio he'patis lenta, Hepatitis occul'ta, Hepatic'ula, Subinflamma'tio he'patis,* (F.) *Chronohépatite, Chronic liver disease,* is not as common as is believed. It may be suspected from the existence of the symptoms above mentioned, when in a minor degree; enlargement, constant dull pain in the region of the liver; sallow countenance; high-coloured urine; clay-coloured fæces, &c. The great object of treatment is to excite a new action by mercury and counter-irritants, and to keep the liver free by cathartics.

HEPATITIS CYSTICA, Cholecystitis—h. Occulta, H. chronic.

HEPATIZA'TION, *Hepatisa'tio, Hepatifica'tio,* from '*ηπαρ,* 'the liver.' Conversion into a liver-like substance. Applied to the lungs when gorged with effused matters, so that they are no longer pervious to the air;—*Hepatisa'tio pulmo'num, Carnifica'tio pulmo'num.* In such state, they are said to be *hepatised.*

HEPATIZATION, RED, (F.) *Hépatisation rouge, Endurcissement rouge, Ramollissement rouge,* characterises the first stage of consolidation of the lungs in pneumonia.

HEPATIZATION, GRAY, (F.) *Hépatisation grise, Induration grise, Ramollissement gris, Infiltration purulente,* characterises the third stage, or stage of purulent infiltration.

HEPATIZON, Chloasma.

HEPATOC'ACE, from '*ηπαρ,* 'liver,' and *κακος,* 'evil.' Gangrene of the liver.

HEPATOCE'LE, from '*ηπαρ,* 'the liver,' and *κηλη,* 'a tumour;' *Her'nia hepat'ica ; Hernia of the liver.* The liver has never been found entirely out of the abdominal cavity. Increase of its bulk, or injuries of the parietes of the abdomen, have been the sole cause of the protrusions which have been occasionally met with, especially in infants, in whom the upper part of the linea alba is very weak, and indeed scarcely seems to exist. Sauvages has distinguished two species of hepatocele :—the *ventral* (in the linea alba), and the *umbilical* or *hepatomphalum.*

HEPATOCHOLORRHŒA, Hepatirrhœa.

HEPATOCO'LICUM. A ligament of the liver, described by Haller, as passing from the gall-bladder and contiguous sinus portarum, across the duodenum to the colon. Another, termed *Hepato-renal,* descends from the root of the liver to the kidney. They are both peritoneal.

HEPATOCYS'TIC, *Hepatocys'ticus, Cystidepat'icus,* from '*ηπαρ,* 'the liver,' and *κυστις,* 'bladder.' Relating to the liver and gall-bladder.

HEPATOCYSTIC DUCT, *Ductus hepatocyst'icus.* The choledoch duct.

HEPATODYNIA, Hepatalgia.

HEPATODYSENTERIA, Hepatirrhœa.

HEPATOGASTRIC, Gastrohepatic.

HEPATOGASTROCHOLOSIS, Fever, bilious, Fever, gastric.

HEPATOG'RAPHY, *Hepatogra'phia ;* from '*ηπαρ,* 'the liver,' and *γραφη,* 'a description.' The part of anatomy which describes the liver.

HEPATOHÆ'MIA, *Hyperæ'mia he'patis, Hepatic Engorgement,* (F.) *Hyperémie du Foie,* from '*ηπαρ,* 'the liver,' and '*αιμα,* 'blood.' Sanguineous congestion of the liver.

HEPATODES, Hepatic.

HEPATOIDES, Hepatic.

HEPATOLITHI'ASIS, from '*ηπαρ,* 'the liver,' and *λιθιασις,* 'formation of stone.' The formation of concretions, *Hepatol'ithi,* in the liver.

HEPATOL'OGY, *Hepatolog''ia,* from '*ηπαρ,* 'the liver,' and *λογος,* 'a discourse,' 'treatise.' A treatise on the liver.

HEPATOMALA'CIA, *Malaco'sis he'patis,* (F.) *Ramollissement du Foie.* Softening of the liver.

HEPATOMYELOMA, Hepatencephaloma.

HEPATON'CUS, from '*ηπαρ,* ' the liver,' and *ογκος,* 'a tumour.' Tumefaction of the liver.

HEPATOPAREC'TAMA, from '*ηπαρ,* 'the liver,' and *παρεκταμα,* 'considerable extension.' Excessive enlargement of the liver.

HEPATOPATHI'A, from '*ηπαρ,* 'liver,' and *παθος,* 'suffering.' *Liver-Disease.* Disease of the liver.

HÉPATOPATHIE CANCÉREUSE, Hepatoscirrhus—*h. Tuberculeuse, Hépatostrumosie.*

HEPATOPHLEGMONE, Hepatitis.

HEPATOPHTHI'SIS, *Phthisis hepat'ica,* from '*ηπαρ,* 'the liver,' and *φθιω,* 'I consume.' Consumption from suppuration of the liver.

HEPATORRHAGIA, Hepatirrhœa, Hepathæmorrhagia.

HEPATORRHEX'IS, from '*ηπαρ,* 'liver,' and *ρηξις,* 'rupture.' Rupture of the liver.

HEPATORRHŒA, Hepatirrhœa.

HÉPATOSARCOMIE, Hepatoscirrhus.

HEPATOSCIR'RHUS, from '*ηπαρ,* 'liver,' and *σκιρρος,* 'cancerous induration.' *Scirrhus he'patis, Encephalo'sis of the liver, Carcinoma of the liver,* (F.) *Hépatosarcomie, Hépatopathie cancéreuse, Cancer du Foie.* Scirrhus or Cancer of the liver.

HÉPATOSTRUMOSIE, *Tuber'cula he'patis,* (F.) *Tubercules du Foie, Hépatopathie tuberculeuse ;* from '*ηπαρ,* 'the liver,' and *struma,* 'a tumour,' 'a scrophulous tumour.' Tubercle of the liver.

HEPATOT'OMY, from '*ηπαρ,* 'the liver,' and *τεμνω,* 'I cut.' Dissection of the liver.

HEPIALOS, Epialos.

HEPS, see Rosa canina.

HEPSEMA, Decoction.

HEPSESIS, Decoction.

HEPTAL CYCLE, see Cycle.

HEPTAL'LON GRAVEOLENS, *Hogwort, Bear's fright.* An indigenous plant, which has a fetid porcine smell ; and is said to be used by the Indians as a diaphoretic, cathartic, &c.

HEPTAPHAR'MACUM, from '*ἑπτα,* 'seven,' and *φαρμακον,* 'a remedy.' A medicine composed of seven substances ; cerusse, litharge, pitch, wax, colophony, frankincense, and bullock's fat. It was regarded as laxative, suppurating and healing.

HEPTAPHYLLUM, Tormentilla.

HEPTAPLEURON, Plantago major.

HERACLEUM, see H. lanatum — h. Branca, H. spondylium.

HERACLE'UM SPONDYL'IUM, *H. Bran'ca, Branca ursi'na, B. German'ica, Spondyl'ium, Sphondyl'ium, Cow Parsnep, All-heal,* (F.) *Berce, Brancursine bâtarde, Fausse Acanthe.* Family, Umbelliferæ. *Sex. Syst.* Pentandria Digynia. The root of this plant has a strong, rank smell ; and a pungent, almost caustic taste. It has been given as a tonic, stomachic and carminative ; both in powder and in decoction. The Russians, Lithuanians, and Poles obtain from its seeds and leaves, by fermentation, a very intoxicating spirituous liquor, which they call *Parst.*

The root of *Heracle'um Lana'tum, Masterwort, Cow parsnep,—Heracle'um* (Ph. U. S.)—is in the secondary list of the Pharmacopœia of the United States.

HERACLEUS MORBUS, Epilepsy.

HERB, *Herba, Bot'anē.* Any ligneous plant which loses its stalk during the winter.

HERB CHRISTOPHER, Actæa spicata.

HERB-DOCTOR, *Botan'ical Doctor, Botan'ical physic''ian.* One who treats diseases altogether by herbs ; as the—so called—"Thompsonians."

HERB OF GRACE, Gratiola officinalis—h. Mastich, common, Thymus mastichina— h. Mastich, Syrian, Teucrium marum—h. Robert, Geranium Robertianum — h. of Saint Cunegonde, Eupatorium cannabinum—h. Sophia, Sisymbrium sophia —h. Trinity, Hepatica triloba.

HERBA, Herb — h. Alexandrina, Smyrnium olusatrum—h. Althææ, Pelargonium cucullatum — h. Anthos, Rosmarinus — h. Benedicta, Geum urbanum—h. Britannica, Rumex hydrolapathum — h. Canni, Artemisia santonica — h. Cardiaca, Leonurus cardiaca—h. Cardui veneris, Dipsacus fullonum—h. Dorea, Solidago virgaurea—h. Felis, Nepeta—h. Genipi, Achillea atrata—h. Ignis, Lichen pyxidatus—h. Melancholifuga, Fumaria—h. Militaris, Achillea millefolium—h. Papillaris, Lapsana—h. Paralyseos, Primula veris—h. Paralytica, Primula veris—h. Patæ lapinæ, Leonurus cardiaca—h. Pulicaris, Plantago psyllium—h. Quercini, Lichen plicatus—h. Sacra, Verbena officinalis—h. Salivaris, Anthemis pyrethrum—h. Sideritidis, Galeopsis grandiflora—h. Tabaci, Nicotiana tabacum—h. Trinitatis, Anemone hepatica, Viola tricolor—h. Veneris, Adiantum pedatum—h. Ventis, Anemone pulsatilla—h. Vitri, see Salsola kali—h. Zazarhendi, Origanum.

HERBÆ PRO ENEMATE, Glyster herbs—h. pro fotu, Fomentation herbs.

HERBALIST, Herborist.

HERBA'RIUM, from *herba*, a plant. A collection of plants. Generally applied to a collection of dried plants—*Hortus siccus*. In Pharmacy, a plant that is used entire.

HERBARIUS, Herborist.

HERBE, Herb—*h. au Cancer*, Plumbago Europæa—*h. aux Chantres*, Erysimum—*h. aux Charpentiers*, Justitia pectoralis—*h. aux Chats*, Nepeta, Teucrium marum—*h. au Coq*, Tanacetum balsamita—*h. au Cuillers*, Cochlearia officinalis—*h. aux Écrouelles*, Scrophularia nodosa—*h. aux Écus*, Lysimachia nummularia—*h. à Éternuer*, Achillea ptarmica—*h. aux Gueux*, Clematis vitalba—*h. à la Houette*, Asclepias Syriaca—*h. d'Ivrogne*, Lolium temulentum—*h. aux Mamelles*, Lapsana—*h. aux Mouches*, Conyza squarrosa—*h. au Pauvre homme*, Gratiola officinalis—*h. aux Perles*, Lithospermum officinale—*h. à Pisser*, Pyrola umbellata—*h. à la Poudre de Chypre*, Hibiscus abelmoschus—*h. aux Poux*, Delphinium staphisagria—*h. aux Puces commune*, Plantago psyllium—*h. à Robert*, Geranium Robertianum.—*h. de Sainte Barbe*, Erysimum barbarea—*h. Sainte Christophe*, Actæa spicata—*h. de Saint Étienne*, Circæa lutetiana—*h. de Saint Jean*, Artemisia vulgaris—*h. de Saint Roch*, Inula dysenterica—*h. aux Sorciers*, Circæa lutetiana—*h. aux Verrues*, Heliotropium Europæum.

HERBIV'OROUS, *Herbiv'orus*, from *herba*, 'grass,' and *voro*, 'I eat.' An epithet applied to animals which feed on herbs.

HER'BORIST, *Herba'rius*. One who deals in useful plants. An *Herb'alist* or *Herb'arist*.

HERBORIZA'TION, *Herba'rum inquisit"io*. An excursion, made with the view of collecting plants. Such excursions are directed by the Apothecaries' Company of London, for the use of their apprentices, &c.

HERBS, FIVE CAP'ILLARY, *Quinque herbæ capilla'res*, were, anciently, hart's tongue; black, white, and golden maiden-hair, and spleenwort.

HERBS, FIVE EMOL'LIENT, *Quinque herbæ emollien'tes*, were, anciently, beet, mallow, marshmallow, French mercury, and violet.

HERCULES ALLHEAL, Pastinaca opoponax.

HERCULEUS MORBUS, Epilepsy.

HÉRÉDITAIRE, Hereditary.

HERED'ITARY, *Hæredita'rius, Heredita'rius, Gentilit"ius, Sym'phytos, Syn'genes*, (F.) *Héréditaire*, from *hæres*, 'an heir.' An epithet given to diseases, communicated from progenitors. Such diseases may exist at birth; or they may supervene at a more or less advanced period of existence. Hereditary diseases, *Morbi heredita'rii*, (F.) *Maladies héréditaires*, often prevail amongst several members of a family, or are *family diseases* or *complaints*.

HERMAPHRODE'ITY, *Hermaphrodis'ia, Hermaphroditis'mus, Hermaphrodis'mus, Fab'rica androg"yna, Androgyn'ia, Gynan'dria, Hermaph'rodism*; from Έρμης, 'Mercury,' and Ἀφροδιτη, 'Venus.' Appertaining to Mercury and Venus. Union of the two sexes in the same individual.

HERMAPHRODISIA, Hermaphrodeity.

HERMAPH'RODITE. Same etymon. *Hermaphrodi'tus, Gynida, Androg"ynus*. One who possesses the attributes of male and female: who unites in himself the two sexes. A term, applied to an animal or plant which is, at the same time, both male and female. True hermaphrodites are only met with in the lower degrees of the animal scale, amongst the zoophytes, mollusca, or gasteropoda. The individuals of the human species, regarded as hermaphrodites, owe this appearance to a vicious conformation of the genital organs; a kind of monstrosity, which renders them unfit for generation, although an attentive examination may exhibit the true sex. Hermaphrodites have, likewise, been described, which, instead of uniting the attributes of both sexes, cannot be considered male or female. These have been called *neutral hermaphrodites*.

HERMAPHRODITISMUS, Hermaphrodeity.

HERMAPHRODITUS, Hermaphrodite.

HERMET'ICA DOCTRI'NA, *Hermetica ars*, (F.) *Hermétique*. The doctrine of Hermes, a celebrated Egyptian philosopher, who is considered the father of alchemy. That part of chymistry, whose object was the pretended transmutation of the metals.

HERMODAC'TYLUS, *Dactyle'tus, An'ima articulo'rum*, from Έρμης, 'Mercury,' and δακτυλος, 'a finger;' or rather from *Hermus*, a river in Asia, upon whose banks it grows, and δακτυλος, 'a date;' or from Έρμης, 'Mercury,' and δακτυλος, 'a date;' (F.) *Hermodactyle, Hermoducte* ou *Hermodate*. The root of the Hermodactyl was formerly used as a cathartic. By some, it is supposed to be identical with the *Iris tubero'sa*. The best testimony seems to be in favour of its being a variety of the colchicum,—*Col'chicum Illyr'icum*.

HERMODATE, Hermodactylus.

HERMOPH'ILUS, from Έρμης, 'Mercury,' and φιλος, 'a lover.' One who is fond of mercury as a medicine.

HER'NIA, *Ramex, Ruptu'ra, R. hernio'sa, Crepatu'ra, Ectop'ia hernio'sa, Celē, Rupture, Burst*, (F.) *Hargne, Descente, Effort, Grecure, Rompeure*. Any tumour, formed by the displacement of a viscus or a portion of a viscus, which has escaped from its natural cavity by some aperture and projects externally. Herniæ have been divided into,—1. Hernia of the Brain; Encephalocele; 2. Hernia of the Thorax; Pneumocele; 3. Hernia of the Abdomen.

Abdom'inal Herniæ are remarkable for their frequency, variety, and the danger attending them. They are produced by the protrusion of the viscera, contained in the abdomen, through the natural or accidental apertures in the parietes of that cavity. The organs, which form them most frequently, are the intestines and the epiploon. These herniæ have been divided, according to the apertures by which they escape, into:

1. *Inguinal* or *Supra-Pu'bian Herniæ*. These issue by the inguinal canal: they are called *Bubonoce'lē*, when small; and *Scrotal Hernia* or *Oscheoce'lē*, in man, when they descend into the scrotum;—*Vulvar Hernia* or *Puden'dal* or *La'bial Hernia, Episioce'lē*, in women, when they extend to the labia majora. 2. *Crural* or *Fem'oral Hernia, Me'roce'lē*, when they issue by the crural canal. 3. *Infra-Pu'bian Hernia*, (F.) *Hernie sous-pubienne, Oădcoce'lē, Her'nia foram'inis ova'lis*, when the viscera escape through the opening, which gives passage to the infra-pubian

vessels. 4. *Ischiat'ic Hernia;* when it takes place through the sacro-sciatic notch. 5. *Umbil'ical Hernia, Exom'phalos, Omphaloce'lē;* when it occurs at the umbilicus or near it. 6. *Epigas'tric Hernia;*—occurring through the linea alba, above the umbilicus. 7. *Hypogas'tric* or *Infra-umbil'ical Hernia, Cœlioce'lē, Hypognstroce'lē,*—when it occurs through the linea alba below the umbilicus. 8. *Perinæ'al Hernia, Mesoscelocelē, Her'nia perinæ'i, Perinæoce'lē, Perineoce'lē*—when it takes place through the levator ani, and appears at the perineum. 9. *Vag"inal Hernia, Coleoce'lē* seu *Elytrocelē* — through the parietes of the vagina. 10. *Diaphragmat'ic Hernia, Diaphragmatoce'lē;* when it passes through the diaphragm. Herniæ are likewise distinguished,—according to the viscera forming them, — into *Enteroce'lē, Epiploce'lē, En'tero-epiploce'lē, Gastroce'lē, Cystoce'lē, Hepatoce'lē, Splenoce'lē,* &c.

When a hernia can be restored to its natural cavity, by the aid of pressure, &c., properly applied, it is said to be *reducible.* It is, on the contrary, *irreducible,* when adhesion, bulk, &c., oppose its return. When the aperture, which has given passage to the hernia, occasions more or less constriction on the protruded portion, the hernia is said to be *incarcerated* or *strangulated:* and, if the constriction be not removed, constipation, hiccough, vomiting, and all the signs of violent inflammation, followed by gangrene, supervene, with alteration of the features, small pulse, cold extremities, and death.

The therapeutical indications are, — 1. *As regards reducible hernia:* — to replace the viscera in the abdomen by the taxis; and to retain them there by the use of a *truss,* which, if properly adapted, may effect a radical cure. 2. *As regards irreducible hernia:* — to support the tumour by an appropriate suspensory bandage. 3. *As regards strangulated hernia:* — to have recourse to the taxis; blood-letting; warm bath; tobacco glysters; ice to the tumour; and, if these should not succeed, to perform an operation, which consists in dividing the covering of the hernia, and cutting the aponeurotic ring, which causes the strangulation; — reducing the displaced viscera, unless their diseased condition should require them to be retained without;—dressing the wound appropriately;—restoring the course of the fæces by means of gentle glysters:—preventing or combating inflammation of the abdominal viscera;— conducting the wound to cicatrization, by appropriate means; and afterwards supporting the cicatrix by a bandage.

The word *hernia* was also used, of old, for the scrotum, and, not unfrequently, for the testicle.

HERNIA, ANEURISMAL, Cirsomphalus — h. Arteriarum, see Aneurism—h. of the Bladder, Cystocele—h. Bronchialis, Bronchocele—h. Carnosa, Sarcocele — h. of the Cerebellum, Parencephalocele—h. Cerebri, Encephalocele.

HERNIA, CONGEN'ITAL, *Hernia congen'ita,* is a protrusion of some of the contents of the abdomen into the *Tunica vaginalis testis,* owing to a want of adhesion between its sides, after the descent of the testicle.

HERNIA CORNEÆ, Ceratocele — h. Crural, Merocele — h. Epiploic, Epiplocele — h. Femoral, Merocele — h. Foraminis Ovalis, see Hernia — h. Gutturis, Bronchocele — h. Hepatica, Hepatocele.

HERNIA HUMORA'LIS, *Empres'ma Orchi'tis, Didymi'tis, Orchi'tis, Orchidi'tis, Inflamma'tio tes'tium, Inflamma'tion of the Testicle, Swelled Testicle, Hernia Ven'eris, Orchioce'lē, Orchidoce'lē, Orchidon'cus,* (F.) *Inflammation du testicule, Orchite.* Swelling and inflammation of the testicle is a common symptom of gonorrhœa—*Chaudepisse*

tombée dans les Bourses; but it may arise from external injuries, or from other causes. It is a disease, which cannot be mistaken, and the treatment must obviously be strongly antiphlogistic, supporting the testicle during the treatment, and for some time afterwards: methodical compression has also been found useful. The disease is not generally of a serious character, going off as suddenly as it comes on. As it affects the epididymis more especially, when supervening on gonorrhœa or blennorrhœa, it is sometimes termed *blenorrhag"ic epididymi'tis.*

HERNIA INCARCERATA, Entero-peristole — h. Inguinalis, Bubonocele—h. Intestinalis, Enterocele—h. Intestinalis omentalis, Entero-epiplocele — h. Iridis, Ptosis Iridis — h. Ischiatica, Ischiocele—h. Lienalis, Splenocele.

HER'NIA LITT'RICA, *H. e Divertic'ulo Intesti'ni.* Hernia first described by Littre, in which the intestinal canal proper is not included in the hernial sac, the protruded portion of intestine consisting of a digital prolongation of the ileum, which Littre concluded was formed by the gradual extension of a knuckle of the bowel, that had been engaged in the inguinal canal.

HERNIA OF THE LIVER, Hepatocele—h. Omental, Epiplocele — h. Parorchido-enterica, Parorchido-enterocele — h. Perinæi, see Hernia — h. Pharyngis, Pharyngocele—h. Phrenic, Diaphragmatic hernia—h. Pinguedinosa Scroti, Liparocele — h. of the Pleura, Pleurocele — h. Pleurica et pulmonalis, Pleurocele — h. Pudendal, Pudendal hernia—h. Sacci lachrymalis, Lachrymal hernia, Mucocele—h. Scrotalis, Scrotocele—h. Seminalis scroti, Spermatocele — h. of the Stomach, Gastrocele—h. Suprapubian, II. inguinal—h. of the Tongue, Glossocele — h. Umbilicalis, Epiplomphalon, Exomphalos — h. Umbilici Aquosa, Hydromphalum—h. Urachi, Uromphalus—h. Uteri, Hysterocele — h. Varicose, Cirsocele — h. Varicosa, Varicocele — h. Venarum, Varix — h. Veneris, Hernia humoralis—h. Ventosa, Physocele — h. Ventral, see Ventral — h. Ventriculi, Gastrocele—h. Vesicœ Urinariæ, Cystocele—h. Zirbalis, Epiplocele.

HERNIAIRE, Hernial, Herniaria glabra.

HER'NIAL, *Hernia'rius,* (F.) *Herniaire.* Belonging to, or concerning hernia : — as *Hernial Bandage, Hernial Sac,* &c.

The (F.) *Hernié,* is applied to a part enveloped in a hernial sac. (F.) *Hernieux, Cele'ta, Celo'tes, Rup'tured, Burst, Bursten,* means one affected with hernia; and *Chirurgien herniaire,* one who devotes himself to the treatment of hernia.

HERNIA'RIA GLABRA, *H. vulga'ris* seu *hirsu'ta* seu *alpes'tris* seu *an'nua* seu *cine'rea* seu *frutico'sa, Milligra'na, Em'petrum, Rupture-wort,* from *hernia,* 'rupture.' (F.) *Herniaire, Tarquette, Herniole.* This plant, which, as its name imports, was formerly considered efficacious in the cure of hernia, seems destitute of all virtues.

HERNIARIUS, Hernial.

HERNIE CHARNUE, Sarcocele—*h. de l'Épiploon,* Epiplocele—*h. de l'Estomac,* Gastrocele—*h. Inguinale,* Bubonocele — *h. du Nombril,* Exomphalos—*h. Ombilicale,* Exomphalos—*h. de la Vessie,* Cystocele.

HERNIÉ, Hernial.

HERNIEMPHRAG'MUS, *Herniemphrax'is,* from *hernia,* and *εμφραγμος,* 'obstruction.' The mechanical obstruction of a hernial canal for the radical cure of the hernia.

HERNIEUX, Hernial.

HERNIOLE, Herniaria glabra.

HERNIOTOMY, Celotomia.

HERO'IC, *Hero'icus, Hero'ius, Hero'us,* from *ήρως,* 'a hero.' An epithet applied to remedies or practice of a violent character.

HERPEDON, Herpes.
HERPEN, Herpes.

HERPES, *Erpes*, *Herpe'don*, *Herpen*, *Serpens*, from ἕρπω, 'I creep;' because it creeps and spreads about the skin; *Eephly'sis Herpes*, *Cytisma Herpes*, *Tetter*, *Fret*, (F.) *Dartre*, *Olophlyctide*. A vesicular disease, which, in most of its forms, passes through a regular course of increase, maturation, decline, and termination in from 10 to 14 days. The vesicles arise in distinct, but irregular clusters, which commonly appear in quick succession, and near together, on an inflamed base; generally attended with heat, pain, and considerable constitutional disorder. The term, like all others which refer to cutaneous diseases, has not been accurately defined. The ancients had three varieties: the *miliary*, κεγχρίας; *vesicular*, φλυκταινώδης, and *ero'ding*, ἐσθιόμενος. Bateman has the following varieties: 1. HERPES PHLYCTÆNO'DES, *Herpes milia'ris*, *Eephly'sis Herpes Milia'ris*, (F.) *Dartre phlyctenoïde*, in which the vesicles are millet-sized; pellucid; clusters commencing on an uncertain part of the body, and being progressively strewed over the rest of the surface; succeeded by fresh crops. 2. HERPES ZOSTER, *Zoster*, *Zona ig'nea*, *Z. serpigino'sa*, *Ignis Per'sicus*, *Cinzilla*, *Sacer ignis*, *Eephly'sis Herpes zoster*, *Herpes peris'celis*, *Erysip'elas zoster*, *Erysip'elas phlyctænoi'des*, *E. pustulo'sa*, *Zona*, *Cir'cinus*, *Perizo'ma*, (F.) *Ceinture*, *C. dartreuse*, *Feu Persique*, *Érysipèle pustuleux*, *Shingles*, in which the vesicles are pearl-sized; the clusters spreading round the body like a girdle; at times confluent, and occasionally preceded by constitutional irritation. 3. HERPES CIRCINA'TUS, *Formi'ca ambulato'ria*, *An'nulus repens*, *Herpes Serpi'go*, *Serpi'go*, *Eephly'sis Herpes Circina'tus*, *Ringworm*, *Vesic'ular Ringworm*, consisting of vesicles with a reddish base, uniting in rings; the area of the rings slightly discoloured, often followed by fresh crops. 4. HERPES LABIA'LIS, and 5. HERPES PRÆPUTIA'LIS, *Aphthæ præpu'tii*, *Ulcus'cula præpu'tii*, appearing, respectively, on the lips and prepuce. 6. HERPES IRIS, *Iris*, *Rainbow-worm*, occurring in small circular patches, each of which is composed of concentric rings of different colours. To these may added, HERPES EX'EDENS, *Eephly'sis Herpes ex'edens*, *Herpes esthiom'enus*, *H. depas'cens*, *H. ferus*, *H. estiom'enus*, *H. ferox*, *Darta excoriati'va seu malig'na*, *Lupus vorax*, *Formi'ca corrosi'va*, *Formix*, *Pap'ula fera*, *Ul'cerative Ringworm*, *Nir'les*, *A'gria*, (F.) *Dartre rongéante*, in which the vesicles are hard; clusters thronged; fluid dense, yellow or reddish, hot, acrid, corroding the subjacent skin, and spreading in serpentine trails.

All the varieties demand simply an antiphlogistic treatment, when attended with febrile irritation. The *herpes circinatus*, alone, requires the use of astringent applications which have the power of repressing the eruption.

HERPES DEPASCENS, H. exedens — h. Esthiomenus, H. exedens—h. Estiomenus, H. exedens—h. Farinosus, Pityriasis—h. Ferox, H. exedens—h. Ferus, H. exedens—h. Furfuraceus, Pityriasis—h. Furfuraceus circinatus, Lepra, H. exedens — h. Miliaris, H. phlyctænoides — h. Periscelis, H. zoster — h. Serpigo, H. circinatus — h. Tonsurans, Porrigo decalvans.

HERPET'IC, *Herpet'icus*, (F.) *Dartreux*. Possessing the nature of herpes.

HERPETOG'RAPHY, *Herpetograph'ia*, from ἕρπης, 'herpes,' and γραφή, 'a description.' A description of the different forms of herpes.

HERPE'TON, *Herpet'icon*, from ἕρπειν, 'to creep.' A creeping eruption or ulcer.—Hippocrates.

HERPYLOS, Thymus serpyllum.
HERRENSCHWAND'S SPECIFIC, see Specific of Herrenschwand.
HESPERIS ALLIARIA, Alliaria.

HETERADELPH'IA, from ἕτερος, 'other,' and ἀδελφός, 'a brother.' A double monstrosity, in which the components of the double bodies are very unequal, and of which one portion may be regarded as the stem or trunk, to which another organized part, or even a whole body, less developed than itself, is affixed like a parasite.

HETEROCHRON'ICUS, *Heterochronus*, from ἕτερος, 'other,' and χρόνος, 'time.' Relating to difference of time.

Pulsus heterochron'icus. A pulse of varying rhythm. An irregular or intermittent pulse.

HETEROCHYMEU'SIS, from ἕτερος, 'other,' and χύμευσις, 'mixture.' A state of the blood in which it contains other matters than in health, as urea, bile, &c.

HETEROCLITE, see Homology, and Tissues.
HETEROCRANIA, Hemicrania.
HETEROCRIS'IA, from ἕτερος, 'other,' and κρίνω, 'I separate.' Modification in the situation of secretions.—Andral.

HETEROGENESIS, see Generation.
HETEROLALIA, Heterophonia.
HETEROLOGOUS TISSUES, see Tissues.
HETEROMORPH'ISM, *Heteromorphis'mus*, from ἕτερος, 'other,' and μορφή, 'shape.' A deviation from the natural shape of parts.

HETEROMORPHOUS, see Homology.
HETEROPATHIC, Allopathic.
HETEROPHO'NIA, from ἕτερος, 'other,' and φωνή, 'voice.' A cracked or broken voice. A change of the voice or speech—*Heterola'lia*.

HETEROPHTHAL'MIA, from ἕτερος, 'other,' and ὀφθαλμος, 'eye.' A difference in the two eyes, — as when one squints, or is of a different colour.

HETEROPLAS'TY, *Heteroplas'ticè*, *Heteropla'sia*, from ἕτερος, 'other,' and πλάσσω, 'I form.' Irregular plastic or formative operations, that do not admit of exact classification.

HETEROPROSO'PUS, from ἕτερος, 'different,' and πρόσωπον, 'countenance.' A monster having two faces.—Gurlt.

HET'EROPUS, from ἕτερος, 'other,' and πους, 'foot.' One who has one foot different from the other.

HETEROREXIA, Malacia.
HETERORRHYTH'MUS, from ἕτερος, 'other,' and ῥυθμος, 'rhythm.' Having another rhythm. An epithet given to the pulse, when it is such, in any individual, as is usually felt at a different age.

HETEROS, from ἕτερος, 'the one of two,' 'the other.' Hence:

HETEROSARCO'SES, from ἕτερος, 'other,' and σαρξ, 'flesh.' A class of diseases which consist in the formation of accidental tissues.—Gendrin.

HETEROTAX'IA, (F.) *Hétérotaxie*, from ἕτερος, and τάξις, 'order.' A malformation, which consists in the general transposition of organs. A change in the relation of organs.

HETEROTOP'IA, from ἕτερος, 'other,' and τόπος, 'place.' A deviation from the natural position of parts.

HÊTRE, Fagus sylvatica.

HEUCHERA, see H. cortusa — h. Acerifolia, H. cortusa.

HEUCHE'RA CORTU'SA, *H. America'na*, *H. Acerifo'lia*, *H. Vis'cida*, *Cortu'sa America'na*, *Alum*

Root, Amer'ican San'icle, Ground-maple, Cliff-weed, Split-rock. The root — *Heuchera* (Ph. U. S.) — is a powerful astringent, and is the basis of a *cancer powder*. The American Indians apply the powdered root to wounds, ulcers, and cancers. It is said to have been sold for colchicum.

HEUCHERA VISCIDA, H. cortusa.
HEUDELOTIA AFRICANA, see Bdellium.
HEVEA GUIANENSIS, see Caoutchouc.
HEXAGIUM, Sextula.
HEXATHYRIDIUM VENARUM, see Worms.
HEXIS, 'ἑξις. Habit, habit of body, constitution. Hence, *hectic, cachectic,* &c.
HIA'TUS, from χίαρε, 'to gape,' 'to open.' A foramen or aperture. Mouth. The vulva. Also, yawning.

HIATUS DIAPHRAG'MATIS AÖR'TICUS, *Semicir'culus exsculp'tus.* The opening in the diaphragm for the passage of the abdominal aorta.

HIATUS FALLOPII, see Aquæductus Fallopii — *h. Occipito-pétreux,* Lacerum posterius foramen — *h. Sphéno-pétreux,* Lacerum anterius foramen.

HIATUS OF WINSLOW, *Fora'men of Winslow.* An opening — situate behind the lesser omentum, and behind the vessels and nerves of the liver — which forms a communication between the peritoneal cavity and that of the omenta.

HIBER'NICUS LAPIS, *Teg'ula Hiber'nica, Arde'sia Hiber'nica, Harde'sia, Irish Slate.* A kind of slate or very hard stone, found in different parts of Ireland, in masses of a bluish-black colour, which stains the hands. It has been taken, powdered, in spruce-beer, against inward contusions.

HIBISCUS, Althæa.
HIBIS'CUS ABELMOS'CHUS, *Abelmos'chus mosha'tus.* The name of the plant, whose seeds are called *Grana Moschi* or *Muskseed.* It is the *Bel-mus'chus, Abelmos'chus, Granum Moschi, Ket'mia Ægyptiaca, Moschus Ar'abum, Ægyp'tia moscha'-ta, Bamix moscha'ta, Alce'a, Alcea Ind'ica, Alcea Ægyptiaca Villo'sa, Abelmosch, Abelmusk, Muskmallow,* (F.) *Graine de Musc, Herbe à la poudre de Chypre, Ambrette, Guimauve veloutée.* It is indigenous in Egypt and the Indies. The seeds are chiefly used as perfumes; and especially in the formation of *Cyprus Powder.*

HIBIS'CUS POPULE'US, - *Balimba'go.* A small Molucca tree. The fruit is full of a juice similar to camboge. The root is emetic. It is used in chronic diarrhœa, colic, dyspepsia, &c.

HICCOUGH, Singultus.
HICCUP, Singultus.
HICK'ORY. The name of several American trees of the genus *Carya;* Order, Juglandaceæ. The leaves are usually aromatic; and are reputed to be antispasmodic (?). The bark of those species that have bitter nuts, as *Carya ama'ra* and *C. porci'na,* is somewhat astringent. Some of them bear fruit that is much esteemed, as *Carya olivæ-formis, Pecan'* or *Pecean' nut,* and *C. sulca'ta, Shellbark.*

HIDDEN SEIZURES. An expression employed by Dr. Marshall Hall for obscure encephalic and spinal attacks, of an epileptoid character for example, which may be immediately owing to trachelismus.

HIDRISCHESIS, Hidroschesis.
HIDROA, Desudatio, *Echauboulures,* Hydroa, Sudamina.
HIDRON'OSUS, *Hidronu'sus,* from 'ίδρως, 'sweat,' and νοσος, 'a disease.' A disease accompanied by violent sweats. Sudor Anglicus.
HIDRONUSUS, Hidronosus.
HIDROPEDESIS, Ephidrosis.
HIDROPHOROS, Sudoriferous.
HIDROPOETICUM, Sudorific.

HIDROPYRA, Sudor Anglicus.
HIDROPYRETOS, Sudor Anglicus.
HIDRORRHŒA, Ephidrosis.
HIDROS, 'ἱδρως, *Sudor,* 'sweat.' Hence — *Hidropyra, Hidrosis,* &c.
HIDROS'CHESIS, *Hidris'chesis, Reten'tio sudo'ris,* from 'ίδρως, 'sweat,' and σχεσις, 'retention.' Suppression of perspiration.
HIDRO'SIS, *Hidro'sis, Suda'tio,* from 'ίδρως, 'sweat.' Sudation, Sweating, Ephidrosis.
HIDROTERION, Achicolum.
HIDROTERIUM, Sudorific.
HIDROTICUM, Sudorific.
HIDRO'TIUM, Diminutive of 'ίδρως, 'sweat.' A gentle sweat or perspiration.
HIDROTOPŒUM, Sudorific.
HIEBLE, Sambucus ebulus.
HI'ERA DIACOLOCYN'THIDOS, from 'ιερος, 'holy.' *Hiera of Colocynth.* An electuary, composed of 10 parts of *colocynth,* as much *agaric, germander, white horehound, stœchas:* — 5 parts of *opoponax,* as much *sagapenum, parsley, round birthwort root,* and *white pepper:* — 4 parts of *spikenard, cinnamon, myrrh,* and *saffron;* and 3 pounds, 3 ounces, and 5 drachms of *honey.*
HIERA OF COLOCYNTH, H. Diacolocynthidos — h. Logadii, Hiera picra.
HIERA PICRA, from 'ιερος, 'holy,' and πικρος, 'bitter.' *Holy bitter, Pulvis aloët'icus,* formerly called *Hiera loga'dii,* when made into an electuary with honey. It is now kept in the form of dry powder; — prepared by mixing *socotrine aloes* one pound, with 3 ounces of *canella alba.* See Pulvis aloes cum canellâ.
HIERA SYRINX, Vertebral column, Epilepsy.
HIERACI'TES, 'ιερακιτης, from 'ιεραξ, 'a hawk,' *Lapis Accip'itrum.* The ancient name of a precious stone, believed to be capable of arresting the hemorrhoidal flux. — Pliny, Galen, Paulus.
HIERACIUM LACHENALII, H. murorum.
HIERA'CIUM MURO'RUM, *H. Lachenalii, Pulmona'ria Gall'ica, Auric'ula mu'ris major,* (F.) *Épervière des murailles, Pulmonaire des Français.* A European plant, which is a slight tonic.
HIERACIUM OLERACEUM, Sonchus oleraceus.
HIERACIUM PILOSEL'LA. The systematic name of the *Auric'ula Muris, Pilosel'la, P. Alpi'na, Myoso'tis, Mouse-ear,* (F.) *Piloselle, Oreille de Souris.* This plant contains a bitter, lactescent juice, which has a slight degree of astringency. The roots are more powerful than the leaves.
HIERA'CIUM VENO'SUM, *Rattlesnakeweed, Veiny Hawkweed,* indigenous, has similar properties.
HIERANOSUS, Chorea, Epilepsy.
HIERAX, Accipiter.
HIEROBOTANE, Verbena officinalis.
HIEROGLYPH'ICA, from 'ιερος, 'holy,' and γλυφω, 'I carve.' A name given to the signs employed in medicine; and, also, to the folds in the hands, feet, and forehead, which afford chiromancy its pretended oracles.
HIEROPYR, Erysipelas.
HILL'S BALSAM OF HONEY, see Balsam of Honey, Hill's — h. Essence of Bardana, Tinctura guaiaci ammoniata.
HILLBERRY, Gaultheria.
HILL FEVER, see Fever, hill.
HILON, (F.) *Hilum,* improperly *Hilus.* A name given by some writers to a small blackish tumour, formed by the protrusion of the iris through an opening in the transparent cornea, so called from its comparison with the *hile* or black mark presented by the vicia faba at one of its extremities. In Botany, the *Hile* or *Hilum* is the cicatricula of a seed, which indicates the place by which it was attached in the cavity of the pericarp. It is the umbilicus of the seed. The fissure of the

spleen, kidney, &c., is, also, sometimes called *Hilus*.

HILUS, Hilon.
HILUS LIENA'LIS, *Incisu'ra liena'lis*. The concave part of the spleen.
HILUS RENA'LIS, *Incisu'ra rena'lis*. The concave part of the kidney.
HIMANTOMA, see Himas.
HIMANTOSIS, Himas.
HIMAS, 'ιμας, 'a thong of leather.' The uvula; likewise, elongation, and extenuation of the uvula. It is also called *Himanto'sis, Himanto'ma*. See Staphyloedema.
HIMEROS, Libido.
HIP, Haunch—h. Bone, Ischium—h. Disease, Coxarum morbus—h. Joint, Coxofemoral articulation—h. Tree, Rosa canina.
HIP'PACE, 'ιππακη, from 'ιππος, 'a horse.' *Ca'seus Equi'nus*. A cheese prepared from mare's milk.
HIPPANTHRO'PIA, from 'ιππος, 'a horse,' and ανθρωπος, 'a man.' A variety of melancholy, in which the patient believes himself changed to a horse. The Greek word 'ιππανθρωπος, means the fabulous Centaur.
HIPPASIA, Equitation.
HIPPEIA, Equitation.
HIPPEUSIS, Equitation.
HIPPIÄTER, *Hippiätros, Med'icus equa'rius*. A farrier. A horse doctor. Used also for one who treats the diseases of other domestic animals; *Veterina'rius, Mulomed'icus, Med'icus Veterina'rius, Zoiätrus*.
HIPPIATRI'A, *Hippiat'rica, Hippiat'ricē, Medici'na equa'ria*, from 'ιππος, 'a horse,' and ιατρικη, 'medicine,' (F.) *Hippiatrique*. A science, whose object is the knowledge of the diseases of the horse. It is sometimes made to include other domestic animals. See Veterinary art.
HIPPIATRIQUE, Hippiatria.
HIPPIATRUS, Hippiäter.
HIPPO, Euphorbia corollata—h. Indian, Gillenia trifoliata.
HIPPOCAMPE GRANDE, Cornu ammonis.
HIPPOCAMPUS MAJOR, Cornu ammonis.
HIPPOCAM'PUS MINOR, *Pes hippocam'pi minor, Pes hippopot'ami minor, Unguis, U. Avis, U. Halleri, O'crea, Collic'ulus ca'veæ posterio'ris ventriculo'rum latera'lium, Calcar a'vis, Un'ciform Em'inence*, (F.) *Ergot, Éperon*. A medullary tubercle or projection, observed in the posterior cornu of the lateral ventricle of the brain.
HIPPOCENTAUREA CENTAURIUM, Chironia centaurium.
HIPPOCRAS, Claret.
HIPPOCRATES, CAP OF, *Bonnet d'Hippocrate*—h. Sleeve, *Chausse*.
HIPPOCRAT'IC, *Hippocrat'icus*. Relating to Hippocrates, or concerning his doctrine,—as *Hippocratic doctrine, Hippocratic face*, &c.
HIPPOC'RATIST. A partisan of the Hippocratic doctrine.
HIPPOGONYOLEPUS, Crusta genu equinæ.
HIPPOLAPATHUM, Rumex patientia.
HIPPOLITHUS, Bezoard of the horse.
HIPPOMARATHRUM, Peucedanum silaus.
HIPPOPATHOL'OGY, *Hippopatholog"ia*, from 'ιππος, 'a horse,' παθος, 'a disease,' and λογος, 'a discourse.' The science of the diseases of the horse. Pathology of the horse.
HIPPOPHAGOUS, Equivorous.
HIPPOPUS, see Kyllosis.
HIPPOS, Equus.
HIPPOSELINUM, Smyrnium olusatrum.
HIPPOSTEOL'OGY, *Hipposteolog"ia*, from 'ιππος, 'a horse,' οστεον, 'a bone,' and λογος, 'a discourse.' Osteology of the horse.

HIPPOT'OMY, *Hippotom'ia*, from 'ιππος, 'a horse,' and τεμνειν, 'to cut.' Anatomy of the horse.
HIPPU'RIA, from 'ιππος, 'a horse,' and ουρον, 'urine,' because the urine contains hippuric acid, which is found in the urine of the horse. A pathological condition, in which there is an excess of hippuric acid in the urine.
HIPPURIC ACID, see Acid, hippuric.
HIPPU'RIS VULGA'RIS, from 'ιππος, 'a horse,' and ουρα, 'a tail.' The systematic name of the *Horse's Tail, Mare's Tail, Equise'tum minus, Equise'tum*, (F.) *Prêle, Presle, Asprêle*. It is an astringent, and frequently used, as tea, by the vulgar, in diarrhœa and hemorrhage. The same virtues are attributed to the *Equise'tum arven'sē, fluviat'ilē, limo'sum*, &c.
HIPPUS, *Equus, Nicta'tio*, from 'ιππος, 'a horse.' A disease of the eyes, in which, from birth, they perpetually twinkle, like those of a man on horseback. (?) Also, a tremulous condition of the iris, which occasions repeated alternations of contraction and dilatation of the pupil; *Iridot'romus, Tremor I'ridis*.
HIPS, Sax. heopa. The fruit of the dog-rose, *Rosa Cani'na:* chiefly used as a confection. See Confectio Rosæ Caninæ.
HIRCIS'MUS, *Hircus, Hirquus*, from *hircus*, 'a goat.' Stinking like a goat:—applied especially to the odour of the secretions of the axilla.
HIRCUS, Canthus (greater), Hircismus, Tragus—h. Alarum, Cinabra.
HIRQUITALITAS, from *hircus*, 'a goat,' *Parapho'nia pu'berum*. Goat's voice. See Egophony.
HIRQUUS, *Hircus*, Canthus (greater), Hircismus, Tragus.
HIRSU'TIES, *Das'yma, Das'ytes, Tricho'sis, Hirsu'ties, Hair'iness*. Growth of hairs on extraneous parts, or, superfluous growth on parts; as in cases of bearded women.—Good.
HIRU'DO, *The Leech, Sanguisu'ga, Bdella*. In medicine, the *Hiru'do Medicina'lis, Bdella Medicina'lis*, or *Medicinal Leech*, (F.) *Sangsue*, is employed. In the United States, *H. dec'ora* is used. The leech lives in fresh water, and feeds on the blood of animals, which it sucks, after having pierced the skin with its three sharp teeth. This habit has been taken advantage of, to produce local blood-letting. In applying the leech, the part must be wiped dry; and if there be difficulty in making it suck, a little milk or cream may be applied. When satiated, it will drop off, and by applying a little salt or vinegar to its head it will disgorge the blood. A good English leech will take about half an ounce of blood, including that which flows by fomenting the part subsequently. The American takes less.
HIRUDO ARTIFICIALIS, Antlia sanguisuga—h. Decora, see Hirudo—h. Medicinalis, Hirudo.
HIRUNDINARIA, Asclepias vincetoxicum, Lysimachia nummularia.
HIRUN'DO, *Chel'idon*, from *hærendo*, 'sticking;' because it sticks its nests against the houses. (?) *The Swallow*. The nests of the swallow were once employed as rubefacients, boiled in vinegar.
HISPANICUM VIRIDE, Cupri subacetas.
HISPIDITAS, Dystœchiasis, Phalangosis.
HISPIDULA, Antennaria dioicum.
HISSING RESPIRATION, see *Râle sibilant*.
HISTIOLOGY, Histology.
HISTODYAL'YSIS, from 'ιστος, 'organic texture,' and διαλυσις, 'dissolution.' A morbid dissolution of the tissues.
HISTOGEN'IA, *Histog"eny*, from 'ιστος, 'the organic texture,' and γενεσις, 'generation.' The formation and development of the organic textures.

HISTOLOGIA, Histology.
HISTOLOG"ICAL, *Histolog"icus*. Same etymon as the next. Relating to histology. Applied, also, at times, to the natural transformations that occur in the tissues in the embryo, in contradistinction to *morphological*, which applies to the alterations in the *form* of the several parts of the embryo.

HISTOL'OGY, *Histolog"ia, Histiol'ogy, Histiolog"ia*, from 'ιστος, 'the organic texture,' and λογος, 'a description.' Anatomy (general). The term is, also, more particularly appropriated to the minute anatomy of the tissues. See Anatomy.

HISTON'OMY, *Histonom'ia*, from 'ιστος' 'the organic texture,' and νομος, 'law.' The aggregate of laws, which preside over the formation and arrangement of the organic tissues.

HIS'TORY, MED'ICAL, *Histo'ria Medici'na*. A narration of the chief circumstances, and the persons connected with them, in the progress of medicine.

HIST'OS, 'ιστος, 'the organic texture.' *Tex-ta'ra seu Tela organ'ica*.

HISTOT'OMY, *Histotom'ia* from 'ιστος, 'organic texture,' and τομη, 'incision.' Dissection of the tissues.

HIVE SYRUP, Syrupus scillæ compositus.

HIVES, Cynanche trachealis, Urticaria, Varicella. In Scotland, according to Dr. Jameson, *Hives* or *Hyves* means any eruption of the skin, proceeding from an internal cause; and, in Lothian, it is used to denote both the red and the yellow gum. In the United States, it is vaguely employed: most frequently, perhaps, for Urticaria.

HIVES, BOLD, Urticaria.
HOARSENESS, Raucedo.
HOB-NAIL LIVER, Cirrhosis of the liver. Liver, nutmeg.
HOCK, Poples.
HOG-LICE, Onisci aselli.
HOGWORT, Heptallon graveolens.
HOLANENCEPHA'LIA, from 'ολος, 'entire,' and *anencephalia*, 'absence of brain.' Entire absence of brain,—the same as Anencephalia.—G. St. Hilaire.
HOLARTHRITIS, Hamarthritis.
HOLCÉ, 'ολκη, 'a dram.'—Galen.
HOL'CIMOS, 'ολκιμος, from 'ολκη, 'a weight,' A tumour of the liver.
HOLCUS SORGHUM, Panicum Italicum.
HOLERA, Cholera.
HOLLANDS, Gin.
HOLLY, AMERICAN, Ilex opaca—h. Common, Ilex aquifolium—h. Dahoon, Ilex vomitoria—h. Ground, Pyrola maculata—h. Ground, Pyrola umbellata—h. Sea, Eryngium maritimum.
HOLLYHOCK, COMMON, Alcea rosea.
HOLMES WEED, Scrophularia nodosa.
HOLMICOS, Alveolus.
HOLMOS, Mortar.
HOLOCYRON, Teucrium chamæpitys.
HOLONARCO'SIS, from 'ολος, 'whole,' and ναρκωσις' 'stupor.' Narcosis of the whole body. *Torpefactio universa'lis*.
HOLOPHLYCTIDES, Phlyctæna.
HOLOSTEUM ALSINE, Alsine media.
HOLOSTEUS, Osteocolla.
HOLOTETANUS, see Tetanus.
HOLOTONIA, Holotonicus, Tetanus.
HOLOTON'ICUS, 'ολος, 'the whole,' and τεινω, 'I stretch.' *Holoton'ia*. A spasm of the whole body. A variety of tetanus.—Sauvages.
HOL'YWELL, MINERAL WATERS OF. Holywell is a town in Wales, and takes its name from the famous well of St. Winifred. It is a simple cold water, remarkable for its purity.
HOMAGRA, Omagra.

HOMEOPATHY, Homœopathy.
HOMERDA, Stercus humanum.
HOME'RIA COLLI'NA. A poisonous South African plant, *Nat. Ord.* Irideæ, the bulb of which acts as a violent acro-narcotic, producing fatal results very speedily.
HOMESICKNESS, Nostalgia.
HOMICI'DAL, *Truculen'tus, Ferus*, from *homo*, 'man,' and *cædo*, 'I kill.' Pertaining or relating to homicide or the killing of man.
HOMICIDAL INSANITY, *Homici'dal Monoma'nia*, (F.) *Monomanie homicide*. Insanity, with an irresistible impulse to destroy life.
HOMILIA, Coition.
HOM'INY. A word of Indian derivation. Maize or Indian corn hulled and coarsely broken. It is prepared for food by being mixed with water and boiled.
HOMINY, WHEATEN, see Groats.
HOMIOSIS, Homoiosis.
HOMME, Homo.
HOMO, (F.) *Homme*, Man,—the chief and most perfect of the mammalia; in Greek, ανθρωπος, *Anthro'pos*, from ανα, 'upwards, and τρεπω, 'I turn;' because man, alone, of all animals, possesses the natural power of standing erect. He is, also, the only animal whose incisor teeth, wedged in a projecting jaw, are absolutely vertical. Man is especially distinguished from other mammalia by the faculty, which he possesses, of classing his ideas; comparing them with each other; and connecting, representing, and transmitting them by signs and articulate sounds. He possesses, in the highest degree, all the attributes of intelligence,—memory, judgment, and imagination. He inhabits all countries,—the burning regions of the torrid zone, and the chilling atmosphere of the polar climes. In different situations, he presents, in his figure, colour, and stature, differences which have caused mankind to be divided by naturalists into races or varieties. The number of such races can only be approximated. Blumenbach admits five, the *Caucasian, Ethiopian, Mongolian, Malay*, and *American*. Every division must necessarily be arbitrary, and the individuals composing each variety are far from being alike.
HOMO ALATUS, see Alatus.
HOMO CAUDA'TUS, 'Tailed man.' A fabulous, tailed variety of the human species, 'incola orbis antarctici,' admitted by Linnæus, although he is uncertain whether to rank them with men or apes!
HOMO FATUUS, Idiot.
HOMOËD'RUS, from ομου, 'together,' and εδρα, 'seat.' Having the same seat. *Morbi homoëdri*:—diseases that have the same seat.
HOMŒOMORPHOUS, see Homology.
HOMŒOPATH, Homœopathist.
HOMŒOPATH'IC, *Homœopath'icus, Homœop'athes*. Relating to homœopathy.
HOMŒOP'ATHIST, *Ho'mœopath, Homœopath'icus, Homœopathis'ta, Homœopathis'tes*. One who believes in homœopathy.
HOMŒOP'ATHY, *Homœopathi'a, Ars homœopath'ica, Homeop'athy*, from 'ομοιος, 'like,' and παθος, 'affection.' A fanciful doctrine, which maintains, that disordered actions in the human body are to be cured by inducing other disordered actions of the same kind, and this to be accomplished by infinitesimally small doses. often of apparently inert agents; the decilionth part of a grain of charcoal, for example, is an authorized dose.
HOMŒOZ'YGY, from 'ομοιος, 'like,' and ζυγος, 'I join together.' (F.) *Soi-pour-soi*. The law

-t association of organs, by which like parts adhere to like parts.—Serres.

HOMOETHNIA, Sympathy.

HOMOGENESIS, see Generation.

HOMOIOPATHIA, Sympathy.

HOMOIO'SIS, *Homio'sis*, from *ομοιοω*, 'I resemble,' 'I assimilate.' An elaboration of the nutritious juice, by which it becomes proper for assimilation.

HOMOLINON, see Apolinosis.

HOM'OLOGUE, *Homol'ogus*, same etymon as homology. A term applied to the same organ in different animals under every variety of form and function.

HOMOL'OGY, from *ομοιος*, 'like,' and *λογος*, 'a description.' The doctrine of similar parts. Thus, the two sides of the body are said to be 'homologous.' *Homol'ogous*, *homomorph'ous*, or *homœomorph'ous* tissues, are those that resemble others; in opposition to *heterol'ogous*, *het'eroclite*, or *heteromorph'ous*, which are new formations. Homology seems now to be accepted as the designation of the doctrine or study, the subject of which is the relations of the parts of animal bodies.—Owen.

HOMOMORPHOUS, see Homology.

HOMONOPAGIA, Cephalalgia.

HOMOPH'AGUS, from *ωμος*, 'raw,' and *φαγω*, 'I eat.' One who eats raw flesh.

HOMOPLAS'TY, *Homoöpla'sia*, from *ομοιος*, 'like,' and *πλασσω*, 'I form.' The formation of homologous tissues.

HOMOPLATA, Scapula.

HOMOT'ONOS, *Æqua'lis*, from *ομος*, 'equal,' and *τονος*, 'tone.' That which has the same tone. A continued fever, whose symptoms have an equal intensity during the whole course of the disease, has been so called. See Acmasticos, and Synocha.

HONESTY, Lunaria rediviva.

HONEWORT, FIELD, Sison amomum.

HONEY, Mel—h. Balsam of, Hill's, see Mel—h. Bloom, Apocynum androsæmifolium — h. of Borax, Mel boracis—h. Clarified, Mel despumatum — h. Prepared, Mel præparatum — h. of Roses, Mel rosæ—h. of Squill, compound, Syrupus scillæ compositus.

HONEYCOMB BAG, Reticulum.

HONEYSUCKLE, BUSH, Diervilla trifida.

HONEY SUGAR, Glucose.

HONGLANE, Coptis teeta.

HONOR CAPITIS, see Capillus.

HONORARIUM, Sostrum.

HONTEUX, Pudic.

HOODWORT, Scutellaria lateriflora.

HOOK, Sax. hoce, hooc, Dutch, hoeck, *Uncus*, *Unc"inus*, *Anc'yra*, (F.) *Érigne*, *Airigne* ou *Érine*. An instrument, consisting of a steel wire, flattened at the middle, and pointed. Some hooks are furnished with a handle at one extremity—the other having one or two hooks;—constituting the *single* or *double hook*. The hook is used by anatomists and surgeons to lay hold of, and raise up, certain parts, the dissection of which is delicate, or which would slip from the fingers.

The *Tenaculum* is a variety of the hook.

HOOK, BLUNT, *Ich'thya*, *Ich'thyē*, *Onyx*, *Unguis ferr'eus*. An instrument which is passed over the flexures of the joints to assist in bringing down the fœtus in parturition.

HOOP TREE, Melia azedarach.

HOOPER'S PILLS, Pilulæ Aloes et Myrrhæ.

HOOPING-COUGH, Pertussis — h. Roche's Embrocation for, see Roche.

HÔPITAL, Hospital.

HOPLOCHRIS'MA, from *οπλον*, 'a weapon,' and *χρισμα*, 'salve.' *Unguen'tum arma'rium*, *Arm'atory Unguent*. A salve which was supposed to cure wounds by sympathy,—the instrument with which the wound was inflicted being anointed with it.

HOPLOMOCH'LION, *οπλομοχλιον*, from *οπλον*, 'a weapon,' and *μοχλος*, 'a lever.' The name of an iron machine or apparatus, which embraced the whole body like armour. A figure of it is given by Fabricius ab Aquapendente.

HOP PILLOW, see Humulus lupulus — h. Plant, Humulus lupulus.

HOQUET, Singultus.

HORA, Hebe.

HORÆA, Menses.

HORÆOTES, Maturity.

HORDEI MALTUM, Malt.

HORDE'OLUM, diminutive of *Hordeum*, 'barley.' *Orde'olum*, *Pos'thia*, *Sclerophthal'mia*, *Crithē*, *Crithid'ion*, *Crythē*, *Stye*, *Styan*, (F.) *Orgelet*, *Orgeolet*. A small, inflammatory tumour, of the nature of a boil, which exhibits itself near the free edge of the eyelids, particularly near the inner angle of the eye.

HOR'DEUM, *Or'deum*, *Crithē*. The seeds of *Hordeum vulga'rē*, or *Scotch Barley*, are ranked amongst the *Cerealia*. (F.) *Orge*. They afford a mucilaginous decoction, which is employed as a diluent and antiphlogistic. The seeds of the *Hordeum dis'tichon*, *H. œsti'vum*, *Zeoc'riton dis'tichum*, and *H. hexas'tichon* possess similar properties. Barley is freed from its shells in mills, forming the *Hor'deum munda'tum* seu *decortica'tum* seu *excortica'tum*; and, at times, is rubbed into small, round grains, somewhat like pearls, when it is called *Hordeum perla'tum*, *Pearl Barley*, (F.) *Orge perlé*, and forms the *Hordeum denutatum* seu *perlatum*, the *Hordei sem'ina tu'nicis nuda'ta*, of the pharmacopœias, — *Hordeum* (Ph. U. S.)

HORDEUM CAUSTICUM, Veratrum sabadilla—h. Decorticatum, see Hordeum—h. Denudatum, see Hordeum — h. Excorticatum, see Hordeum — h. Galacticum, Oryza—h. Mundatum, see Hordeum — h. Perlatum, see Hordeum.

HOREHOUND, Marrubium — h. Black, Ballota fœtida — h. Germander-leaved, Eupatorium teucrifolium — h. Stinking, Ballota fœtida — h. Water, Lycopus sinuatus, Lycopus Virginicus—h. Wild, Eupatorium teucrifolium.

HORME, Instinct.

HORMINUM, Salvia horminum — h. Coloratum, Salvia horminum — h. Sativum, Salvia horminum.

HORMON, Enormon.

HORN, Cornu.

HORNSEED, Ergot.

HORNY EXCRES'CENCES, *Lepido'sis*, *Ichthyi'asis cornig"era*, *Cor'nua cuta'nea*, (F.) *Cornes de la Peau*. Certain excrescences, which occasionally form on some part of the skin, and resemble, in shape, the horns of an animal.

HORNY SUBSTANCE, see Tooth.

HORRENTIA, Horripilation.

HOR'RIDA CUTIS, *Goose-skin*, *Cutis anseri'na*, *Dermatospasmus*. A state of the skin accompanying the rigor of an intermittent.

HORRIPILA'TION, *Horripila'tio*, *Horror*, *Horren'tia*, *Phricē*, *Phricas'mus*, *Phrici'asis*, *Phri'cia*, from *horrere*, 'to bristle up,' and *pilus*, 'hair.' (F.) *Horripilation*, *Frissonnement*. General chilliness, preceding fever, and accompanied with bristling of the hairs over the body.

HORROR, Horripilation — h. Ciborum, Disgust for food.

HORSE BALM, Collinsonia Canadensis.

HORSE CANE, Ambrosia trifida.

HORSE CHESTNUT, Æsculus hippocastanum.
HORSE CRUST, Crusta genu equinæ.
HORSEFLY WEED, Sophora tinctoria.
HORSEMINT, Ambrosia trifida, Monarda coccinea and M. punctata — h. Sweet, Cunila mariana.
HORSE RADISH, Cochlearia armoracia.
HORSE'S TAIL, Hippuris vulgaris.
HORSEWEED, Ambrosia trifida, Collinsonia Canadensis.
HORTULUS CUPIDINIS, Vulva.
HORTUS, Vulva — h. Siccus, Herbarium.
HOS'PITAL, primarily from *hospes*, 'a guest.' *Nosocomi'um, Adynatocomi'um, Adynatodochi'um, Xenodoce'um, Xenodoche'um, Infirm'ary, Infirma'rium, Infirmato'rium, Nosodochi'um, Valetudina'rium*, (F.) *Hôpital*. An establishment for the reception of the sick, in which they are maintained and treated medically. Hospitals were first instituted about the end of the 4th century; a period at which the word νοσοκομειον was employed, for the first time, by St. Jerome. They may be *general*, receiving all cases; or *special*, admitting only the subjects of certain diseases.
HOS'PITAL GANGRENE, *Phageda'na gangræ- no'sa, Putrid* or *Malignant Ulcer, Gangræ'na Nosocomio'rum seu Nosocomia'lis, Sphac''elus nosocomia'lis, Hos'pital Sore, Gangræ'na contagio'sa, Putre'do*, (F.) *Pourriture* ou *Gangrène d'hôpital*. Gangrene, occurring in wounds or ulcers, in hospitals the air of which has been vitiated by the accumulation of patients, or some other circumstance. Hospital gangrene—many different varieties of which are met with, and always accompanied or preceded by fever — commonly commences with suppression of the suppuration of the wound, which becomes covered with a grayish and tenacious sanies. The gangrene then manifests itself. It extends from the centre of the ulcerated surface towards the edges; these become swollen, painful, and everted; and the patient dies with all the signs of typhus. The treatment must be varied according to circumstances. Sometimes, it requires the use of stimulating, acid, caustic, and antiseptic applications; with, occasionally, the actual cautery, aided by the exhibition of tonics, internally: — at others, the antiphlogistic regimen and emollient applications may be necessary.
HOSPITAL, LEPER, *Ladrerie.*
HOSTIARIUS, Pylorus.
HOT SPRINGS, see Virginia, mineral waters of.
HOUBLON, Humulus lupulus.
HOUGH, Poples.
HOUNDS' TONGUE, Cynoglossum.
HOUPPE NERVEUSE, see Papilla — h. *du Menton*, Depressor labii inferioris, Levator labii inferioris.
HOURGLASS CONTRACTION OF THE UTERUS, see *Chaton*.
HOUSELEEK, Sempervivum tectorum — h. Small, Sedum.
HOUSEMAID'S KNEE, see Knee, housemaid's.
HOUSE-PUPIL, see House-Surgeon.
HOUSE-SURGEON, *Resident Surgeon*. Usually a senior house-pupil or graduate, who attends in an hospital, to every accident and disease, in the absence of the attending physician or surgeon. It answers, in the British hospitals, to the *Élève interne* or *Interne* of the French. The *Élève externe* or *Externe* is a less advanced pupil; from whom *Internes* are chosen. In ordinary schools, *Élève externe* means a day-scholar: whilst *Élève interne* means a boarder.

HOUX, Ilex aquifolium — h. *Petit*, Ruscus — h. *Apalachine*, Ilex vomitoria.
HUACACACHU, Datura sanguinea.
HUACO, Guaco.
HUANU, Guano.
HUCKLEBERRIES, see Gaylussacia, and Vaccinium.
HUCKLEBONE, Ischion.
HUDSON'S PRESERVATIVE FOR THE TEETH AND GUMS, see Tinctura Myrrhæ.
HUILE, Oil — h. *d'Absinthe*, Artemisia absinthium (oil of) — h. *d'Acajou*, see Anacardium occidentale.
HUILE ACOUSTIQUE (F.), *Oleum acus'ticum*, Acoustic oil. An oil for deafness, prepared of *olive oil*, ℥ij; *garlic, ox-gall*, and *bay-leaves*, each ʒj; boiled for a quarter of an hour, and strained.
HUILE D'AMANDES, Oleum amygdalarum — h. *d'Aneth*, see Anethum graveolens — h. *Animale*, Oleum animale — h. *Animale de Dippel*, Oleum animale Dippelii — h. *Animalisée par infusion*, Oleum animalisatum per infusionem — h. *d'Anis*, see Pimpinella anisum — h. *Aromatique*, Oleum animalizatum per infusionem — h. *d'Aurone*, Artemisia abrotanum (oil of) — h. *de Cacao*, Butter of cacao — h. *de Cade*, see Juniperus oxycedrus — h. *de Carvi*, Carum (oil) — h. *de Cédrat*, Oleum cedrinum — h. *de petits Chiens*, Oleum animalisatum per infusionem — h. *de Corne de Cerf*, Oleum animale Dippelii — h. *de Foie de Morue*, Oleum Jecoris aselli — h. *de Gabian*, Petrolæum — h. *de Gérofle*, see Eugenia caryophyllata — h. *de Laurier*, Unguentum laurinum — h. *de Lin*, see Linum usitatissimum — h. *de Lis*, see Lilium candidum — h. *de Morelle*, see Solanum — h. *de Morue*, Oleum jecinoris aselli — h. *de Noix*, see Juglans cinerea — h. *d'Œillette*, Papaver (oil) — h. *de Ricin*, see Ricinus communis — h. *de Succin*, see Succinum — h. *Verte*, Balsam, green, of Metz — h. *de Vin douce*, Oleum æthereum.
HUILES ANIMALES, Olea animalia — h. *Empyreumatiques*, Olea empyreumatica — h. *Essentielles*, Olea volatilia — h. *Fixes* ou *Grasses*. Olea fixa — h. *Fugaces*, Olea fugacia — h. *Médicinales*, Olea medicinalia — h. *Volatiles*, Olea volatilia.
HUIT DE CHIFFRE. Figure of 8. A bandage in which the turns are crossed in the form of the figure 8. Such is the bandage used after bleeding from the arm.
HUITO, Genipa oblongifolia.
HUÎTRE, Ostrea.
HUM, VENOUS, *Bruit de diable.*
HUMBLE, Rectus inferior oculi.
HUMECTAN'TIA. A name formerly given to drinks, which appeared to possess the property of augmenting the fluidity of the blood.
HU'MERAL, *Humera'lis*. That which belongs to, or is connected with, the arm or humerus.
HU'MERAL AR'TERY, *Arte'ria humera'lis*, see Brachial artery.
HUMÉRO-CUBITAL, Brachialis anterior — h. *Sus-métacarpien*, see Radialis — h. *Sus-radial*, Supinator radii longus.
HU'MERUS, *Sca'pula, Omos, Armus*, (F.) *Épaule*. The most elevated part of the arm. The bones, which concur in forming it, are: — the scapula, head of the humerus, and the clavicle, united together by strong ligaments, and covered by numerous muscles.
HU'MERUS, *Os hu'meri, Os bra'chii, Os adjuto'rium, Os brachia'le, Bra'chium, Lacer'tus*, is the cylindrical, irregular bone of the arm; the upper extremity of which has a hemispherical head connected with the scapula; and two *tuberosities* or *tubercles*, a *greater* and *lesser*, for the attach-

ment of muscles, between which is the *Bicip'ital groove* or *Fossa*. At the inferior extremity may be remarked — the *inner condyle*, the *outer condyle;* the *small head*, which is articulated with the radius; the trochlea articulated with the ulna, &c. The humerus is developed by seven points of ossification: — one for the body; one for the head; one for the greater tuberosity; one for the trochlea; one for the epitrochlea; one for the epicondyle; and another for the lesser head.

HUMERUS SUMMUS, Acromion.

HUMEUR AQUEUSE, Aqueous humour — h. *Crystalline,* Crystalline — *h. Hyaloïde,* Corpus vitreum.

HUMEURS FROIDES, Scrofula.

HUMIDE RADICALE, Humidum radicale.

HUMIDUM NATIVUM, H. radicale—h. Nativum Articulorum, Synovia — h. Primigenium, H. radicale.

Hu'MIDUM RADICA'LE, *Hu'midum primige'nium seu Nati'vum seu Semina'le, Radical Moisture*, (F.) *Humide radicale.* Names formerly given to the liquid which was conceived to give flexibility and proper consistence to the different organic textures.

HUMIDUM SEMINALE, H. radicale.

HUMILIS, Rectus inferior oculi.

HUMILUS, Humulus lupulus.

HUMOR, Humour—h. Albugineous, Aqueous humour—h. Articularis, Synovia—h. Ceruminous, Cerumen — h. Doridis, Water, sea—h. Genitalis, Sperm—h. Glacialis, Crystalline, Corpus vitreum — h. Hyalinus seu Hyaloides, Corpus vitreum — h. Lacteus, Milk—h. Lachrymalis, Tear—h. Melancholicus, see Mercurialis— h. Mercurialis, see Mercurialis—h. Morgagnianus, Morgagni, humor of—h. Ovatus, Aqueous humour—h. Oviformis, Aqueous humour—h. Pericardii, see Pericardium —h. Purulentus, Pus—h. Seminalis, Sperm—h. Venereus, Sperm — h. Vitreus, Corpus vitreum.

HU'MORAL, *Humora'lis*, from *humere,* 'to moisten.' Proceeding from, or connected with, the humours.

HU'MORISM, *Hu'moral Pathol'ogy, Patholog"ia humera'lis.* A medical theory, founded exclusively on the parts which the humours were considered to play in the production of disease. Although traces of this system may be found in the most remote antiquity, the creation, or, at all events, the arrangement of it may be attributed to Galen, who enveloped it in metaphysical subtleties relating to the union between the elements and the four cardinal humours.

HU'MORISTS. The Galenical physicians, who attributed all diseases to the depraved state of the humours, or to vicious juices collected in the body.

HUMOUR, *Humor, Hygra'sia, Hygre'don, Hygrum.* Every fluid substance of an organized body; — as the blood, chyle, lymph, &c. The *Humours*, χυμοι, *Chymi, Humo'res*, differ considerably as to number and quality in the different species of organized beings; and even in the same species, according to the state of health or disease. The ancients reduced them to *four*; which they called *car'dinal humours:*—the blood, phlegm, yellow bile, and atrabilis or black bile. A modern classification of the humours is given under Fluid.

HUMP. Perhaps from *umbo,* 'the boss of a buckler.' *Hunch, Gibber, Gibbus, Gibba, Tuber*, (F.) *Bosse.* A prominence, formed by a deviation of the bones of the trunk. Commonly, it is formed by the spine or sternum, and is seated at the posterior or anterior part of the trunk. It may, also, be produced by deviation of the ribs or pelvis. The spine may be curved in three principal directions. 1. *Backwards*, the most common case; this the ancients called κυφωσις,

Cypho'sis, Gibbos'itas. 2. *Forwards,* λορδωσις, *Lordo'sis, Recurva'tio;* and, 3. *Laterally*, σκολιωσις, *Scolio'sis, Obstipa'tio.* Most curvatures occur at a very early age, and are caused by scrofula, rickets, &c.; and, not unfrequently, they are accompanied by caries of the vertebræ. See Vertebral disease.

HU'MULUS LU'PULUS, *Lu'pulus, L. scandens seu commu'nis seu salicta'rius, Humulus, Convol'vulus peren'nis,* the *Hop-plant. Nat. Ord.* Urticeæ. (F.) *Houblon, Vigne du nord.* Its cones or strobiles, *Hu'muli strob'ili* (Ph. L.), *Humulus* (Ph. U. S.), have a fragrant odour; and a bitter, aromatic taste, depending on a peculiar principle, named *Lu'pulin*, extractive and essential oil, which may be extracted, equally, by water and spirit, from the dried strobiles. The hop is employed as a tonic and hypnotic, and enters into the composition of ale and beer.

The *Hop pillow, Pulvi'nar Hu'muli,* has long been used for producing sleep.

HUNCH, Hump.

HUNGARICA FEBRIS, Fever, Hungary.

HUNGER, Anglo-Saxon, hunᵹer, *Fames, Limos, Peinâ, Peina, Esu'ries, Jeju'nium, Jeju'nitas, Esurit'io, Esuri'go,* (F.) *Faim.* The necessity for taking food. Hunger is an internal sensation, which some authors have attributed to the friction between the sides of the stomach in its empty state; others, to the compression of the nerves, when the organ is contracted; others, to the action of the gastric juice, &c. It is dictated by the wants of the system: — farther we know not. See Appetite.

HUNGER-CURE, Limotherapeia.

HUNGRY, *Famel'icus, Li'micus, Limo'des;* same etymon. Affected with hunger.

HURA BRASILIEN'SIS, *Assacou, Asencû, Ussacù.* A Brazilian tree, of the *Family* Euphorbiaceæ, which, in the form of the extract of the bark, is esteemed a specific in leprosy. It is, also, given in elephantiasis, and as an anthelmintic.

HYACINTH, WILD, Scilla esculenta.

HYACINTHUS MUSCARI, Bulbus vomitorius.

HYÆNAN'CHÊ GLOBO'SA. An arborescent shrub of South Africa, *Nat. Ord.* Euphorbiaceæ, the fruit of which, pounded, is used to destroy hyænas and other beasts of prey, and seems to contain strychnia.

HYALEUS, Hyaline.

HY'ALINE, *Hyali'nus, Hyale'us, Vit'reus, Vit'reous.* Glassy. Resembling glass.

HYALINE SUBSTANCE, Cytoblastema.

HYALI'TIS, *Inflamma'tio tu'nicæ hyaloïdeæ*, from *hyaloid,* and *itis,* denoting inflammation. Inflammation of the hyaloid membrane of the eye.

HY'ALOID, *Hyalo'des, Hyaloï'des,* from ὑαλος, 'glass,' and ειδος, 'resemblance.' Vitriform; resembling glass.

HYALOID CANAL, see Hyaloid membrane.

HYALOID FOSSA, *Fossa Hyaloidea*, is a cuplike excavation in the vitreous humour, in which the crystalline is imbedded.

HY'ALOID MEMBRANE, *Tu'nica Hyaloidea, Membra'na Arachnoï'dea, T. vit'rea,* is the extremely delicate membrane, which forms the exterior covering of the vitreous humour, and transmits within it prolongations, which divide it into cells. Fallopius discovered this membrane, and gave it the name *Hyaloid.* On a level with the entrance of the optic nerve into the eye, the hyaloid membrane has been described as forming, by reflection, a cylindrical canal, which pierces the vitreous humour from behind to before, as far as the posterior part of the crystalline. See Canal, hyaloid

HYALONIXIS, see Cataract.
HYALONYXIS, see Cataract.
HYALOS, Vitrum.
HYANCHE, Cynanche tonsillaris.
HYBOMA, Gibbositas.
HYBRID, (F.) *Hybride*, from the Greek, 'υβρις, 'υβριδος, 'mongrel.' A being born of two different species,—as the mule. The term is applied to plants as well as to animals. The result is termed *Hybridity*. Hybrid is often, also, used to designate words which are formed from two different languages,—as uter-*itis*, for inflammation of the uterus, in place of *metritis*.
HYBRIDITY, see Hybrid.
HYDARTHROSIS, Hydrarthrus.
HYDARTHRUS, Hydrarthrus.
HY'DATID, *Hy'datis, Bulla, Aqu'ula, Hydro'a, Hydrocys'tis, Hygrocys'tis, Tænia hydatig''ena, Echinococ'cus huma'nus*, from 'υδωρ, 'water.' This name was long given to every encysted tumour which contained an aqueous and transparent fluid. Many pathologists, subsequently, applied it to vesicles, softer than the tissue of membranes, more or less transparent, which are developed within organs, but without adhering to their tissue. It is by no means clear that these formations are really entozoa. They have been found in various parts of the body; sometimes in the uterus, occasioning signs nearly similar to those of pregnancy, but being sooner or later expelled. The expulsion is generally attended with more or less hemorrhage. See Acephalocystis.
Hydatis, Aqu'ula, Phlyctæ'nula, Verru'ca Palpebra'rum, Milium, also, meant a small, transparent tumour of the eyelids.—Galen, C. Hoffmann.
HYDATIDES CERVICIS UTERI, Nabothi glandulæ.
HYDATIDOCE'LE, *Hydatoce'lē*, from 'υδατις, 'hydatid,' and κηλη, 'a tumour.' Oscheocele containing hydatids; the *Oscheoce'lē hydatido'sa, Hydatidoscheoce'lē* of Sauvages.
HYDATIDOÏDES, Hydatoid.
HYDATIDO'MA, from 'υδατις, 'hydatid.' A tumour caused by hydatids.
HYDATIDOSCHEOCELE, Hydatidocele.
HYDATINUS, Hydatoid.
HYDATIS FINNA, Cysticercus cellulosæ.
HYDATIS'MUS, from 'υδωρ, 'water.' The noise caused by the fluctuation of pus contained in an abscess.—Aurelian, Foësius.
HYDATOCELE Hydatidocele, Hydrocele.
HYDATOCH'OLOS, from 'υδωρ, 'water,' and χολη, 'bile.' *Aquoso-bilious*. An epithet given to evacuated matters when mixed with water and bile.—Hippocrates, Foësius.
HYDATODES, Aqueous.
HY'DATOID, *Hydatoï'des, A'queous, Aquo'sus, Hydato'des, Hydat'inus, Hydatido'des, Hydatidoï'des*, from 'υδωρ, 'water,' and ειδος, 'resemblance.' Watery. Resembling water. This name has been given to the membrane of the aqueous humour; and, also, to the aqueous humour itself. *Vinum hydato'des*; wine and water.
HYDATONCUS, Anasarca, Œdema.
HYDATOPO'SIA, from 'υδωρ, 'water,' and ποσις, 'drinking. Water-drinking;—hence
HYDATOP'OTES. A water-drinker.
HYDERICUS, Hydropic.
HYDERODES, Hydropic.
HYDERONCUS, Anasarca, Œdema.
HYDEROS, Anasarca, Hydrops.
HYDOR, 'υδωρ, and *Hydas*, 'υδας, 'genitive,' 'υδατος, 'water.' Hence:
HYDRACHNIS, see Varicella.
HYDRADEN, Conglobate gland.

HYDRADENI'TIS, *Inflamma'tio glandula'rum lymphatica'rum*, from *Hydraden*, 'a lymphatic gland,' and *itis*, denoting inflammation. Inflammation of a lymphatic gland.
HYDRÆ'DUS, from 'υδωρ, 'water,' and αιδοια, 'genital organs.' Œdema of the female organs.
HYDRÆMIA, Hydroæmia.
HYDRAGOGA, Hydragogues.
HYDRAGOGIA, Hydragogues.
HYDRAGOGICA, Hydragogues.
HY'DRAGOGUES, *Hydrago'ga, Hydrago'gia, Hydrago'gica, Hydrop'ica, Hydrot'ica, Aquidu'ca*, from 'υδωρ, 'water,' and αγω, 'I expel.' Medicines believed to be capable of expelling serum effused into any part of the body. These are generally cathartics or diuretics.
HYDRAGOGUM BOYLEI, Argenti nitras.
HYDRALLANTE, False Waters.
HYDRALMÆ, Waters, mineral (saline).
HYDRAM'NIOS, from 'υδωρ, 'water,' and 'amnios.' An excessive quantity of the liquor amnii.
HYDRAN'GEA ARBORES'CENS, *Wild Hydran'gea, Bissum*. An indigenous plant, which flowers in July. The leaves are said to be tonic, sialagogue, cathartic, and diuretic.
HYDRANGEITIS, Angeioleucitis.
HYDRANGIA, Lymphatic vessels.
HYDRANGIOGRAPHIA, Angeiohydrography.
HYDRANGIOTOMIA, Angeiohydrotomy.
HYDRARGYRANATRIP'SIS, *Hydrargyrentrip'sis*, from 'υδραργυρος, 'quicksilver,' and ανατριψις, 'rubbing in.' The rubbing in of a preparation of quicksilver:—*Hydrargyrotrip'sis*.
HYDRARGYRENTRIPSIS, Hydrargyranatripsis.
HYDRARGYRI ACETAS, Hydrargyrus acetatus—h. Bichloridum, H. oxymurias—h. Bicyanidum, H. cyanuretum—h. Biniodidum, H. iodidum rubrum—h. Binoxydum, H. oxydum rubrum—h. Bisulphuretum, H. sulphuretum rubrum—h. Borussias, H. cyanuretum—h. Bromidum, see Bromine—h. Calx alba, Hydrargyrum præcipitatum—h. Chloridum, H. submurias—h. Chloridum corrosivum, H. Oxymurias—h. Chloridum mite, H. submurias.
HYDRAR'GYRI CYANURE'TUM, *H. Borus'sias, H. Bicyan'idum, Hydrar'gyrum Cyanogena'tum, H. Hydrocyan'icum, Prussias Hydrar'gyri, Cyan'uret* or *Prussiate of Mercury*, (F.) *Cyanure de Mercure*. (*Ferri Ferro-cyanuret*. ℨiv; *Hydrarg. oxid. rubr*. ℨiij, vel q. s.; *Aquæ destillat*. Oiij. Put the ferro-cyanuret and three ounces of the oxide of mercury, previously powdered and thoroughly mixed together, into a glass vessel, and pour on two pints of the distilled water. Boil the mixture, stirring constantly; and if, at the end of half an hour, the blue color remains, add small portions of the oxide of mercury, continuing the ebullition until the mixture becomes of a yellowish colour; then filter through paper. Wash the residue in a pint of the distilled water, and filter. Mix the solution and evaporate till a pellicle appears, and set the liquor aside, that crystals may form. To purify the crystals, subject it to resolution, evaporation, and crystallisation.—Ph. U. S.) This preparation has been strongly recommended as a powerful antisyphilitic, and is admitted into the Parisian codex. Twelve to twenty-four grains may be dissolved in a quart of distilled water, and three or four spoonfuls of the solution be taken daily, in a glass of any appropriate liquid.
HYDRARGYRI DEUTO-IODIDUM, H. Iodidum rubrum.

HYDRARGYRI DEUTO-IODURETUM, see Iodine—h. Hyperoxodes, Hydrargyri nitrico-oxydum.

HYDRARGYRI IOD'IDUM, *H. Protoiod'idum seu Proto-iodure'tum seu Subiod'idum, Hydrar'gyrum Ioda'tum flavum, Iod'idum seu Iodure'tum hydrargyro'sum, Hydrar'gyrum iodidula'tum, Protoïodure'tum mercu'rii, I'odide* or *Proti'odide of Mercury,* (F.) *Protiödure de Mercure,* (Hydrarg. ℨj, Iodin. ℨv, Alcohol q. s. Rub the mercury and iodine together, adding sufficient alcohol to form a soft paste, and continue the trituration till the globules disappear. Dry the iodide in the dark, with a gentle heat, and keep it in a well-stopped bottle, the light excluded.—Ph. U. S.) For properties and doses, see Iodine.

HYDRARGYRI, IODIDUM CHLORIDI, Mercury, iodide of chloride of.

HYDRARGYRI IODIDUM RUBRUM, *H. Biniod'idum seu Deuto-iod'idum seu Deuto-iodure'tum seu Period'idum, Hydrarg'yrum ioda'tum rubrum seu Biioda'tum seu Perioda'tum, Iode'tum seu Iod'idum Hydrargyr'icum, Deuto-iodure'tum mercu'rii, Red I'odide, Bini'odide, Deuti'odide* and *Peri'odide of Mercury,* (F.) *Deutiödure ou Periodure de Mercure.* (Hydrarg. corros. chlorid. ℨj, Potassii Iodid. ℨx, Aquæ destillat. Oij. Dissolve the chloride in a pint and a half, and the iodide of potassium in half a pint of distilled water, and mix the solutions. Collect the precipitate on a filter, and, having washed it with distilled water, dry it with a moderate heat, and keep it in a well-stopped bottle.—Ph. U. S.) For properties and doses, see Iodine.

HYDRARGYRI MURIAS BASI OXYDI IMPERFECTI, H. oxymurias—h. Murias corrosivum, H. oxymurias—h. Murias dulcis sublimatus, H. submurias—h. Oxygenatus, H. Oxymurias—h. Murias spirituosus liquidus, Liquor hydrargyri oxymuriatis—h. Murias suboxygenatus præcipitatione paratus, Hydrargyrum precipitatum.

HYDRARGYRI NITRAS, *Nitras Hydrar'gyri in crystallos concre'tus, Nitrate of Mercury.* It is employed in syphilis; and, externally, in fungous, obstinate ulcers.

It is used in the formation of the *Soluble Mercury* of Hahnemann.

An acid *nitrate of mercury, Liquor Hydrar'gyri supernitra'tis, Solution of supernitrate of mercury, Solution of supernitrate of deutoxide of mercury,* made by dissolving four parts of mercury in eight of *nitric acid,* and evaporating the solution to nine parts, has been used as a caustic in malignant ulcerations and cancerous affections.

Ward's White Drops,—a once celebrated antiscorbutic nostrum,—were prepared by dissolving *mercury* in *nitric acid,* and adding a solution of *carbonate of ammonia;* or, frequently, they consisted of a solution of *sublimate* with *carbonate of ammonia.*

HYDRARGYRI NI'TRICO-OXYDUM, *Hydrargyrus nitra'tus ruber, Mercu'rius corrosi'vus ruber, Mercurius præcipita'tus corrosi'vus, M. præcipita'tus ruber, Arca'num coralli'num, Mercurius coralli'nus, Pul'vis prin'cipis, Præcipita'tus ruber, Ox'ydum hydrar'gyri comple'tum, O. hydrargyr'icum, Panaoe'a mercu'rii rubra, Pulvis Joan'nis de Vigo, Oxo'des hydrargyri rubrum, Hyperoxo'des hydrargyri, Ox'ydum hydrar'gyri nit'ricum, Oxydum hydrargyri rubrum per ac'idum nit'ricum, Hydrar'gyri oxydum rubrum,* (Ph. U. S.) *Nitric oxide of mercury, Red precip'itate,* (F.) *Oxide nitrique de mercure.* (Hydrarg. ℨxxxv; Acid. nitric. f℥xviij; Aquæ Oij. Dissolve the mercury with a gentle heat, in the acid and water previously mixed, and evaporate to dryness. Rub into powder, and heat in a very shallow vessel till red vapours cease to rise.—Ph. U. S.) It is a stimulant and escharotic, and used as such in foul ulcers, being sprinkled on the part in fine powder, or united with lard into an ointment.

HYDRARGYRI OXODES RUBRUM, Hydrargyri nitrico-oxydum—h. Oxydi murias ammoniacalis, Hydrargyrum præcipitatum—h. Oxydulum nigrum, H. Oxydum cinereum.

HYDRARGYRI OXYDUM CINE'REUM, *Oxydum hydrargyri nigrum, Æthiops per se, Mercu'rius niger Mosca'ti, Oxydum hydrargyro'sum, Oxydum hydrargyr'icum præcipita'tum, Oxyd'ulum hydrar'gyri nigrum, Pulvis mercuria'lis cine'reus, Mercurius cine'reus, Turpe'thum nigrum, Mercurius præcipita'tus niger, Gray* or *Black oxide of Mercury,* (F.) *Oxide de mercure cendré, Oxide gris ou noir de mercure, Protoxide de mercure.* This oxide is made in various ways. It may be formed by boiling submuriate of mercury in lime water. The dose of this *Pulvis Hydrargyri cinereus* is from two to ten grains. There are four other preparations of it in estimation, viz:—*Plenck's solution,* made by rubbing mercury with mucilage. 2. By rubbing equal parts of sugar and mercury together. 3. A compound of honey or liquorice and purified mercury. 4. The blue pill and ointment. All these possess the usual properties of mercury.

The *Hydrargyri Oxidum Nigrum* of the Ph. U. S. is made as follows: — *Hydrarg. Chlorid. mit., Potassæ,* ℔ ℥iv, *Aquæ* Oj. Dissolve the potassa in the water, allow the dregs to subside, and pour off the clear solution. To this add the chloride, and stir constantly till the black oxide is formed. Pour off the supernatant liquor, wash the black oxide with distilled water, and dry with a gentle heat.

The *Mercurius solu'bilis* of Hahnemann is formed from a black oxide of mercury. It is the *Mercurius solu'bilis Hahneman'ni seu oxydum hydrargyri nigri median'te ammo'niâ ex protonitra'tâ hydrar'gyri præcipita'tum.* It is used in the same cases as the Hydrargyri oxydum cinereum.

HYDRARGYRI OXYDUM NIGRUM, H. oxydum cinereum—h. Oxydum nigrum mediante ammoniâ et protonitrate hydrargyri præcipitatum, see H. oxydum cinereum—h. Oxydum nitricum, Hydrargyri nitrico-oxydum.

HYDRARGYRI OXYDUM RUBRUM, *H. Binox'ydum, Mercurius calcina'tus, Hydrar'gyrus calcinatus,* (F.) *Oxide de Mercure rouge, Red oxide of mer'cury.* (Made by precipitation from a solution of bichloride of mercury by solution of potassa.) See Hydrargyri nitrico-oxydum.

It is stimulant and escharotic; and, in large doses, emetic. Owing to the violence of its operation, it is seldom given internally.

HYDRARGYRI OXYDUM RUBRUM PER ACIDUM NITRICUM, Hydrargyri nitrico-oxydum—h. Oxydum saccharatum, Hydrargyrum saccharatum—h. Oxydum sulphuricum, Hydrargyrus vitriolatus.

HYDRARGYRI OXYMU'RIAS, *H. Chlo'ridum Corrosi'vum,* (Ph. U. S.) *H. Bichlo'ridum, Hydrar'gyrus muria'tus, Mu'rias hydrargyri corrosi'vus, Murias hydrargyri oxygena'tus, Sublima'tus corrosivus, Mercurius corrosivus, Mercurius corrosivus sublima'tus, Hydrargyri permu'rias, Supermu'rias hydrargyri, Murias hydrargyri basi oxydi imperfec'ti, Murias hydrargyri corrosivum,* (F.) *Deutochlorure de mercure, Bichloride de mercure, Muriate oxygéné de mercure, Sublimé corrosif; Bichlo'ride of mercury, Oxymuriate of mercury, Corrosive sublimate, Corrosive muriate of mercury.* (Hydrarg. ℔ij, Acid. Sulphur. ℔iij, Sodii Chlorid. ℔iss. Boil the mercury with the sulphuric acid until the sulphate of mercury is left dry. Rub this, when cold, with the chloride of sodium, in an earthenware mortar; then sublime with a gradually increasing heat.—Ph. U. S.)

It is used as an antisyphilitic stimulant in venereal complaints, old cutaneous affections, &c. Gr. iij to Oj of water is a good gargle in venereal sore-throats, or an injection in gonorrhœa. Externally, it is applied in cases of tetter, and to destroy fungus, or stimulate old ulcers. Dose, gr. 1-16 to gr. 1-8, in pill, once in twenty-four hours. White of egg is the best antidote to it, when taken in an overdose.

HYDRARGYRI PERIODIDUM, H. Iodidum rubrum—h. Permurias, Hydrargyri oxymurias—h. Proto-iodidum, H. Iodidum—h. Proto-ioduretum, H. Iodidum—h. Proto-tartras, H. tartras—h. Prussias, H. cyanuretum—h. Saccharum vermifugum, Hydrargyrum saccharatum — h. Subchloridum, H. Submurias—h. Subiodidum, H. Iodidum.

HYDRARGYRI SUBMU'RIAS, *H. Chlor'idum, H. Subchlor'idum, H. Chlor'idum mitē* (Ph. U. S.), *Calom'elas, Calom'eli, Hydrar'gyrum muriat'icum mitē, C. Torqueti, Draco mitiga'tus, Submu'rias hydrargyri mitis, Submu'rias Hydrargyri sublima'tum, Mercu'rius dulcis, M. dulcis sublima'tus;*—when precipitated, *M. dulcis precipita'tus,—Panace'a Mercuria'lis* (when nine times sublimed), *Murias hydrargyri dulcis sublima'tus, Mercurius sublimatus dulcis, Mercu'rius Zo'ticus Hartmanni, Aq'uila, Manna Metallo'rum, Panchymago'gum minera'lē, P. Querceta'nus, mild Chloride, protochloride, submuriate, subchloride,* or *mild Muriate of Mercury, Cal'omel,* (F.) *Mercure doux, Protochlorure de mercure.* Mild chloride of mercury is thus directed to be prepared in the Pharmacopœia of the United States:—*Mercury,* ℔iv; *Sulphuric Acid,* ℔iij; *Chloride of Sodium,* ℔iiss; *Distilled water,* a sufficient quantity. Boil two pounds of the mercury with the sulphuric acid, until the sulphate of mercury is left dry. Rub this, when cold, with the remainder of the mercury, in an earthenware mortar, until they are thoroughly mixed. Then add the chloride of sodium, and rub it with the other ingredients till all the globules disappear: afterwards sublime. Reduce the sublimed matter to a very fine powder, and wash it frequently with boiling distilled water, till the washings afford no precipitate upon the addition of liquid ammonia; then dry it. *Properties.* Antisyphilitic and sialagogue: in large doses, purgative. *Dose:*—one or two grains given at night gradually excite ptyalism. Gr. v to xx, purge. Children bear larger doses than adults.

The BLACK WASH, *Lo'tio Hydrar'gyri nigra,* is formed of *calomel,* ℨij; *Lime-water,* Oj. Used for syphilitic sores.

HYDRARGYRI SUBMURIAS AMMONIATUM, Hydrargyrum præcipitatum—h. Subsulphas flavus, Hydrargyrus vitriolatus — h. Subsulphas peroxidati, Hydrargyrus vitriolatus — h. Sulphas, Hydrargyrus vitriolatus, H. S. flavus, Hydrargyrus vitriolatus.

HYDRARGYRI SULPHURE'TUM NIGRUM, *H. sulphure'tum cum sul'phurē, Hydrargyrus vel mercurius cum sul'phurē, Æthiops minera'lis, Hydrargyrus e sul'phurē, Pulvis hypnot'icus, Æthiops narcot'icus,* (F.) *Sulfure de mercure noir, Black sulphuret of mercury, Sulphuret of mercury with sulphur, Ethiops mineral.* (*Hydrarg., Sulphur,* āā ℔j. Rub together till the globules disappear.) Used chiefly in scrofulous and cutaneous affections. Dose, gr. x to ℨss.

HYDRARGYRI SULPHURE'TUM RUBRUM, *H. Bisulphuretum, Hydrargyrus sulphura'tus ruber, Min'ium purum, Minium Graco'rum, Magnes Epilep'siæ, Ammion, Purpuris'sum, Cinnab'aris, Mercurius Cinnabari'nus, Cinab'aris, Cinaba'rium, Bisulphuret or Red Sulphuret of Mercury, Cin'nabar, Vermil'ion,* (F.) *Sulphure de Mercure rouge, Cinabre.* (*Hydrarg.* ℨxl; *Sulphur.* ℨviij. Mix

the mercury with the sulphur melted over the fire; and as soon as the mass begins to swell remove the vessel from the fire, and cover it with considerable force to prevent combustion. Rub the mass into powder and sublime. (Ph. U. S.) It is an antisyphilitic, but is chiefly used in fumigation against venereal ulcers of the nose, mouth, and throat;—ℨss being thrown on a red-hot iron. This preparation is the basis of a nostrum, called *Boerhaave's Red Pill.*

HYDRARGYRI SUPERMURIAS, H. oxymurias.

HYDRARGYRI TARTRAS, *H. Proto-tartras, Tartrate of mercury.* Antisyphilitic. Dose, one or two grains twice a day.

HYDRARGYRI ET ARSENICI IODIDUM, Arsenic and Mercury, iodide of.

HYDRAR'GYRI ET QUI'NIÆ PROTO-CHLO'RIDUM, *Protochloride of Mercury and Quinia.* A combination of mild chloride of mercury and quinia, administered in obstinate cutaneous diseases.

HYDRARGYRIA, Eczema mercuriale.

HYDRARGYRI'ASIS, *Hydrargyro'sis, Mercurialis'mus,* from 'ὑδραργυρος, 'mercury.' A disease induced by the use of mercury; *Morbus Mercuria'lis.* Poisoning by mercury. Eczema mercuriale.

HYDRARGYRICUM, Mercurial.

HYDRARGYRIUM, Mercurial.

HYDRARGYROSIS, Eczema mercuriale, Hydrargyriasis.

HYDRARGYRO-STOMATITIS, see Salivation, mercurial, and Stomatitis, mercurial.

HYDRARGYROTRIPSIS, Hydrargyranatripsis.

HYDRAR'GYRUM, *Hydrar'gyrus,* from 'ὑδωρ, 'water,' and ἀργυρος, 'silver;' *Mercu'rius, Argentum vivum, A. mo'bilē, A. fusum, A. fugiti'vum, A. liq'uidum, Missadan, Fumus albus, Arca arcano'rum, Dæ'dalus, Mater metallo'rum, Mercury, Quicksilver,* (F.) *Mercure, M. cru, Vif Argent.* A fluid, brilliant metal; of a slightly bluish white colour; fluid above—39° of Fahr. and under 656°. S. g., when liquid, 13.568 (Cavendish); easily oxydized. Metallic quicksilver does not act on the body, even when taken into the stomach. When oxydized and combined with acids, it acts powerfully. It has been exhibited in cases of constriction of the bowels and in intussusception, from a notion that it must certainly pass through the bowels by its gravity. The water, in which mercury has been boiled, has been recommended as a vermifuge; but it probably enjoys no such property, as chemical tests do not exhibit the presence of the metal. When the crude metal is distilled in an iron retort, it forms the *Hydrar'gyrum purifica'tum.*

HYDRARGYRUM AMMONIATO-MURIATICUM, H. præcipitatum—h. Biiodatum, Hydrargyri iodidum rubrum—h. Biiodatum cum kalio iodato, Potassii hydrargyro-iodidum—h. Cyanogenatum, Hydrargyri cyanuretum.

HYDRARGYRI CUM CRETĀ (Ph. U. S.), *Hydrargyrus cum cretā, Mercurius alkalisa'tus, Mercury with chalk,* (F.) *Mercure avec la craie, Æ'thiops alcalisa'tus.* (*Hydrarg.* ℨiij; *Cretæ præparat.* ℨv. Rub them together till the globules disappear. Ph. U. S.) A protoxide of mercury, formed by trituration with carbonate of lime. It is somewhat uncertain: and consequently not much employed as a mercurial. It possesses the properties of the black oxide of mercury, and may be advantageously exhibited in cases of diarrhœa in children, dependent upon acidity and vitiated secretions. Dose, gr. v to ℨss, twice a day, in any viscid substance.

HYDRARGYRUM CUM MAGNE'SIĀ of the Dublin Pharmacopœia resembles it in properties.

HYDRARGYRUM HYDROCYANICUM, Hydrargyri cyanuretum—h. Iodatum, Hydrargyri iodidum—h. Iodatum cum chlorido Mercurii, Mercury, iodide of chloride of—h. Iodatum flavum, Hydrargyri iodidum—h. Iodatum rubrum, Hydrargyri iodidum rubrum—h. Iodidulatum, Hydrargyri iodidum—h. Muriaticum Mite, Hydrargyri submurias—h. Periodatum, Hydrargyri iodidum rubrum.

HYDRARGYRUM PRÆCIPITA'TUM, *H. ammonia'tum* (Ph. U. S.), *Hydrargyrum ammonia'to-muriat'icum, Hydrar'gyri ammo'nio-chlo'ridum, Mercurius cosmet'icus, Mu'rias oxidi hydrargyri ammoniaca'lis, Submu'rias ammoni'aco-hydrargyr'icus, Calx Hydrargyri alba, Submu'rias Hydrargyri ammoniatum, S. H. Præcipita'tum, Murias hydrargyri sub-oxygena'tus præcipitatio'ne para'tus, Præcipita'tum album, Ammo'nio-chloride of Mercury, White precip'itate of Mercury, White precipitate, Calcina'tum majus Pote'rii,* (F.) *Sous-muriate de mercure précipité ou Précipité blanc.* (Hydrarg. chlorid. corros. ℨvj; aquæ destillat. cong., Liquor ammoniæ, f℥viij. Dissolve the chloride in the water, with the aid of heat, and to the solution, when cold, add the solution of ammonia, frequently stirring. Wash the precipitate till it is tasteless, and dry it.—Ph. U. S.) A peroxide, combined with muriatic acid and ammonia, forming a triple salt. It is used in powder, to destroy vermin; and, united with lard, for the same purpose, as well as in scabies and some other cutaneous affections.

HYDRARGYRUM SACCHARA'TUM, *Æ'thiops sacchara'tus, Mercu'rius sacchara'tus, Ox'idum hydrargyri sacchara'tum, Sac'charum hydrargyri vermif'ugum.* A mild mercurial formula in several of the Pharmacopœias of continental Europe; formed by triturating one part of mercury with two of *white sugar.* It is used in the venereal affections of children.

HYDRARGYRUS, Hydrargyrum.

HYDRARGYRUS ACETA'TUS, *Sperma mercu'rii, Terra folia'ta mercurii, Mercurius aceta'tus, Hydrargyri Ace'tas, Acetas* vel *Proto-ace'tas Hydrargyri, Ac"etate of mercury.* This was the basis of *Keyser's pills,* and was once much celebrated in the cure of the venereal disease. The dose is from three to five grains, but it is not much used.

The formula for *Keyser's anti-venereal pills* was as follows:— Hydrarg. Acet. ℨiv; Mannæ, ℥xxx; Amyl. ℨij; Muc. G. Trag. q. s. into pills of gr. vj each. Dose, two pills.

HYDRARGYRUS CALCINATUS, Hydrargyri oxydum rubrum—h. cum Cretâ, Hydrargyrum cum cretâ—h. Muriatis, Hydrargyri oxymurias—h. Nitratus ruber, Hydrargyri nitrico-oxydum.

HYDRARGYRUS PHOSPHORA'TUS, *Phosphuret'ted mercury.* This preparation has been recommended in cases of inveterate venereal ulcers, but is now scarcely used.

HYDRARGYRUS SULPHURATUS RUBER, Hydrargyri sulphuretum rubrum — h. cum Sulphure, Hydrargyri sulphuretum nigrum — h. e Sulphure, Hydrargyri sulphuretum nigrum.

HYDRARGYRUS VITRIOLA'TUS, *Turpe'thum minera'lē, Mercurius emet'icus flavus, Calx mercurii vitriola'ta, Mercurius caus'ticus flavus, M. lu'teus, Hydrargyri sulphas, H. S. flavus* (Ph. U. S.), *Subsulphas Hydrargyri flavus, Oxydum hydrargyri sulphu'ricum, Subsul'phas hydrargyri peroxida'ti, Turbith min'eral,* (F.) *Sous-sulfate de mercure ou turbith minéral.* (Hydrarg. ℨiv; Acid. Sulph. ℥vj. Mix in a glass vessel, and boil in a sand-bath till a dry, white mass remains. Rub this into powder, and throw it into boiling water. Pour off the liquor, and wash the yellow, precipitated powder repeatedly with hot water; then dry it—Ph. U. S.) Two grains of this mercurial act on the stomach violently. It is sometimes recommended as an errhine in amaurosis.

HYDRARTHRON, Hydrarthrus.
HYDRARTHROS, Hydrarthrus.
HYDRARTHROSIS, Hydrarthrus.
HYDRAR'THRUS, *Hydarthrus, Hydrar'thrus synovia'lis, Hydrops articulo'rum, Hydrarthron, Hydrar'thros, Melice'ria, Spina vento'sa* of Rhases and Avicenna, *Arthri'tis Hydrar'thros, Hydarthrosis, Hydrarthro'sis, Emmyx'ium articula'rē, Tumor albus, White swelling;* from 'ὑδωρ, 'water,' and ἀρθρον, 'a joint.' (F.) *Tumeur blanche, T. lymphatique des articulations.* The French surgeons apply the term *Hydrarthrus* to dropsy of the articulations. White swelling is an extremely formidable disease. It may attack any one of the joints; but is most commonly met with in the knee, the haunch, the foot, the elbow, and generally occurs in scrofulous children. It consists, at times, in tumefaction, and softening of the soft parts and ligaments, which surround the joints; at others, in swelling and caries of the articular extremities of bones; or both these states may exist at the same time. The treatment consists in the employment of counter-irritants; the use of iodine internally and externally, &c. Also, Synovia.

HYDRAS'PIS EXPAN'SA, *Great freshwater Tortoise.* On the sandy banks of rivers in Peru this animal buries its eggs, from which the Indians extract oil. Its flesh supplies well-flavoured food. — Tschudi.

HYDRASTIS, H. Canadensis.
HYDRAS'TIS CANADEN'SIS, *Hydrastis, Warnera Canaden'sis, Hydrophyll'um verum, Yellow Root, Orange Root, Yellow Puccoon, Ground Rasp'berry, Yellow Paint, Golden Seal, In'dian Paint, Eyebalm.* It is used in Kentucky as a 'mouth water,' and as an outward application in wounds and local inflammations.

HYDRELÆ'ON, *Hydrolæ'um,* from 'ὑδωρ, 'water,' and ἐλαιον, 'oil.' A mixture of water and oil.

HYDRELYTRON, see Hydrocele.
HYDREMA, Œdema.
HYDRENCEPHALITIS, Hydrocephalus internus.
HYDRENCEPHALIUM, Hydrocephalus internus.
HYDRENCEPHALOCE'LĒ, *Hydrocephaloce'lē,* from 'ὑδωρ, 'water,' εγκεφαλος, 'the encephalon,' and κηλη, 'rupture, protrusion.' A monstrosity in which there is a fissure of the cranium, the integument of the head being present, and forming a hernial sac in which the brain lies outside the skull—the sac containing a large quantity of serous fluid. Also, Hydrocephalus chronicus.

HYDRENCEPHALON, see Hydrocephalus chronicus.
HYDRENCEPH'ALOID, from 'ὑδωρ, 'water,' εγκεφαλος, 'the brain,' and ειδος, 'resemblance.' Resembling hydrencephalus. *Hydrenceph'aloid disease, Spu'rious hydroceph'alus, Pseudo-encephali'tis.* Disorders of the bowels, and exhaustion in children, are at times attended with hydrencephaloid symptoms.

HYDRENCEPHALUS, Hydrocephalus internus.

HYDRENTEROCE'LE, from 'ὑδωρ, 'water,' εντερον, 'intestine,' and κηλη, 'a tumour.' Intestinal hernia, the sac of which encloses fluid.

HYDRENTEROMPHALOCE'LĒ, *Hydrenterom'phalus,* from 'ὑδωρ, 'water,' εντερον, 'intestine,' ομφαλος, 'umbilicus,' and κηλη, 'rupture.' Umbilical hernia with intestine and water in the sac.

HYDRENTEROMPHALUS, Hydrenteromphalocele.
HYDREPIGASTRIUM, see Ascites.
HYDREPIPLOCE'LE, from 'ὕδωρ,' 'water,' επιπλοον, 'omentum,' and κηλη, 'rupture.' Omental hernia, with water in the sac.
· HYDREPIPLOM'PHALUS, *Hydrepiplomphaloce'lē,* from 'ὕδωρ,' 'water,' επιπλοον, 'omentum,' and ομφαλος, 'umbilicus.' Umbilical hernia, with omentum and water in the sac.
HYDRETRUM, Ascites.
HYDRIASIS, Hydrosudotherapeia.
HYDRIATER, see Hydropathic.
HYDRIATRIA, Hydrosudotherapeia.
HYDRIATRICA ARS, Hydrosudotherapeia.
HYDRIATRICUS, see Hydropathic.
HYDRIATRUS, see Hydropathic.
HYDRIODAS KALICUS, see Potassæ hydriodas.
HYDRIODIC ACID, see Acid, hydriodic.
HYDRO'A, *Hidro'a, Aqu'ula, Boa, Planta noctis,* from 'ὕδωρ,' 'water.' An affection, which consists in an accumulation of water or serous fluid under the epidermis. Some have used *hydro'a* synonymously with *sudamina;* others with *pemphigus.* In the first case, it has generally, however, been written *hidro'a,* from 'ἱδρως,' 'sweat,' and in the latter *hydro'a.* See Hydatid.
HYDROÆ'MIA, *Hydræ'mia;* from 'ὕδωρ,' 'water,' and 'αιμα,' 'blood.' Anæmia. The state of the blood in which the watery constituents are in excess.
HYDROAËROPLEURIE, Hydropneumothorax.
HYDROÄ'RION, *Hydroöph'oron, Hydroü'rium, Hydroöva'rium, Hy'drops ova'rii, Asci'tes ovariis, A. sacca'tus,* (F.) *Hydropisie de l'ovaire,* from 'ὕδωρ,' 'water,' and ωαριον, 'ovarium.' Dropsy of the ovarium.
HYDROATA, Sudamina.
HYDROBLEPH'ARON, *Hy'drops Pal'pebræ, Blepharæde'ma aquo'sum, Œde'ma palpebra'rum.* An œdema or watery swelling of the eyelids; from 'ὕδωρ,' 'water,' and βλεφαρον, 'eyelid.'
HYDROCARDIA, Hydropericardium, see Pericardium.
HYDROCATARRHOPHE'SIS, *Hydrocatarrhoph'ia,* from 'ὕδωρ,' 'water,' and καταρροφειν, 'to sip up.' Absorption of water from without.
HYDROCE'LE, *Hydrops Scroti, H. testiculo'rum, Hydroscheoce'lē, Hydatoce'le, Hydros'cheum, Hydror'chis, Hydroschéonie,* (Alibert,) from 'ὕδωρ,' 'water,' and κηλη, 'a tumour.' A term generally applied to a collection of serous fluid in the areolar texture of the scrotum or in some of the coverings, either of the testicle or spermatic cord. To the first of these varieties the names — *External Hydrocele, H. œdemato'des,* (F.) *H. par infiltration* have been given; and to the second, those of *Hydroce'lē inter'na, H. tu'nicæ vaginа'lis tes'tis, Hydrel'ytron,* (F.) *H. par épanchement.* When the collection occurs in the envelope of the testicle, it is called *H. of the tunica vaginalis;* and the epithet *congenital* is added, when the interior of the membrane, in which it is situate, still communicates freely with the cavity of the abdomen. When it exists in the spermatic cord, it is called *encysted,* or *diffused Hydrocele of the spermatic cord,* as the case may be. The tumour of the distended scrotum is oblong: greater below than above; indolent and semi-transparent. When it becomes inconveniently large, the fluid may be evacuated by puncturing with a trocar, but, as it collects again, this operation can only be considered palliative. The radical cure consists, usually, in injecting, through the canula of the trocar, which has been left in, after puncturing, some irritating liquid, as wine. This is kept in the tunica vaginalis for a few minutes, and then withdrawn. The coat inflames; adhesion takes place, and the cavity is obliterated.

HYDROCELE OF THE NECK. A tumour, filled with a watery fluid, occupying some portion of the neck.
HYDROCELE PERITONÆI, Ascites — h. Spinalis, Hydrorachis.
HYDROCENO'SIS, from 'ὕδωρ,' 'water,' and κενωσις, 'evacuation.' The evacuation of water morbidly accumulated in the body.
HYDROCEPHALE, Hydrocephalus.
HYDROCÉPHALE AIGUË, Hydrocephalus internus.
HYDROCEPHALITIS, Hydrocephalus internus.
HYDROCEPHALIUM, Hydrocephalus.
HYDROCEPHALOCELE, Hydrencephalocele.
HYDROCÉPHALOËCTASIE, Hydrocephalus chronicus.
HYDROCEPH'ALUS, *Hydroceph'alum, Hydrocra'nia, Hydrocra'nium, Hydrocephal'ium, Hydroceph'alē, Hydrops Cap'itis, H. Cer'ebri,* from 'ὕδωρ,' 'water,' and κεφαλη, 'the head.' *Water in the head, Dropsy of the head, Dropsy of the brain.* A collection of water within the head. It may be *internal* or *external.*
HYDROCEPHALUS ACUTUS, H. internus — h. Acutus senum, Apoplexy, serous — h. Adnatus, see H. chronicus — h. Congenitus, see H. chronicus — h. Externus, H. chronicus — h. Meningeus, H. internus.
HYDROCEPHALUS CHRON'ICUS, *Hydrencephaloce'lē, Hydrops Cap'itis, Hydrocephalus externus,* (F.) *Hydrocéphale, Hydrocéphaloëctasie,* of some, may exist at birth. *Hydrenceph'alon, Hydrocephalus congen'itus* seu *adna'tus* commonly commences at an early period of existence, and the accumulation of fluid gradually produces distension of the brain, and of the skull, with separation of the sutures. It commonly proves fatal before puberty.
HYDROCEPHALUS EXTERNUS, *Œde'ma cap'itis, Cephalœde'ma* of some, is a mere infiltration into the subcutaneous cellular tissue of the cranium.
HYDROCEPHALUS INTER'NUS, *Hydroceph'alus acu'tus, H. meninge'us, Hydrops cer'ebri, Encephalal'gia hydrop'ica, Encephali'tis exsudato'ria, Encephali'tis* seu *Meningi'tis Infan'tum, Morbus cerebra'lis Whyt'tii, En'tero-cephalop'yra Infan'tum, Hydrophlogo'sis Ventriculo'rum cer'ebri, Encephaloch'ysis, Phrenic'ula hydrocephal'ica, Hydrenceph'alus, Hydrencephali'tis, Hydrencephal'ium, Hydrocephali'tis, Hydromeningi'tis, Febris Hydrocephal'ica, Apoplex'ia hydrocephal'ica, Carus hydroceph'alus, Water Brain Fever,* (F.) *Hydrocéphale aiguë, Fièvre cérébrale des Enfans,* is generally seated, according to modern observers, in the meninges and surface of the encephalon, and is a *tuber'cular meningi'tis, Meningi'tis tuberculo'sa, Encephalostrumo'sis,* (F.) *Méningite tuberculeuse* ou *granuleuse.* It is observed particularly in childhood. Its march is extremely acute and often very rapid; admitting, generally, however, of division into three stages. The symptoms of the *first stage* are those of general febrile irritation, with head-ach, intolerance of light and sound, delirium, &c. Those of the *second,* which generally denote that the inflammation has ended in effusion, are, great slowness of pulse, crying out as if in distress, moaning, dilated pupil, squinting, &c.; and lastly, in the *third* stage — profound stupor, paralysis, convulsions, involuntary evacuations, quick pulse, and frequently death. The disease is of uncertain duration; sometimes,

destroying in two or three days; at others, extending to two or three weeks. The prognosis is unfavourable. The treatment must be active during the stage of excitement, — precisely that which is necessary in phrenitis. In the second stage, the indication is;—to promote the absorption of the effused fluid. This must be done by counter-irritants, and mercury, chiefly. On dissection, water is generally found in the ventricles, or at the base of the brain; or there are evidences of previous vascular excitement, as effusions of coagulable lymph, &c.

HYDROCEPHALUS SPURIUS, Hydrencephaloid, (disease.)

HYDROCHAMAIMELUM, Infusum anthemidis.

HYDROCHEZIA, Diarrhœa serosa.

HYDROCHLORATE D'OR, see Gold.

HYDRO CHLORINAS NATRICUS, Soda, muriate of.

HYDROCHOLECYSTIS, Turgescentia vesiculæ felleæ.

HYDROCH'YSES, (G.) Hydrochysen, from '*ὑδωρ*,' 'water,' and *χυσις*, 'effusion.' A family of diseases, according to the classification of Fuchs, in which there is a sudden effusion of serous fluid, as in serous apoplexy; hydrocephalus, &c.

HYDROCIRSOCE'LÊ, *Hygrocirsoce'lê*, *Hygroce'lê*, from '*ὑδωρ*,' 'water,' *κιρσος*, 'varix,' and *κηλη*, 'tumour.' A tumour, formed by the varicose distention of the veins of the spermatic cord, and by the accumulation of serous fluid in the areolar texture of the scrotum.

HYDROCŒLIA, Ascites.

HYDROCOT'YLE CENTEL'LA. A South African plant, the roots and stalks of which are astringent; and used in diarrhœa and dysentery.

HYDROCOTYLE UMBELLATUM, Acaricoba.

HYDROCRANIA, Hydrocephalus.

HYDROCRANIUM, Hydrocephalus.

HYDROCRITHE, Decoctum Hordei.

HYDROCYAN'IC ACID, *Ac''idum Hydrocyan'icum*; from '*ὑδωρ*,' 'water,' and *κυανος*, 'blue.' *Prussic Acid, Ac''idum Prus'sicum, A. Borus'sicum, A. Zoöt'icum, A. Zoötin'icum, Cyanohy'dric Acid, Cyanhy'dric Acid,* (F.) *Acide Hydrocyanique* ou *Prussique*. This acid exists in a great variety of native combinations in the vegetable kingdom, and imparts to them certain properties, which have been long known and esteemed; as in the *bitter almond, Cherry laurel, leaves of the Peach tree, kernels of fruit, pips of apples,* &c. When *concentrated*, it is liquid, colourless, of a strong smell and taste, at first cool, afterwards burning. Its s. g. at 7° centigrade, is 0.7058. It is very volatile, and enters into ebullition at 80° Fahr. It speedily undergoes decomposition, sometimes in less than an hour, and consists of a peculiar gazeous and highly inflammable compound of carbon and azote, to which the name *Cyan'ogen* has been assigned; and of hydrogen, which acts as the acidifying principle: hence its name *Hydrocyanic acid*. In the Pharmacopœia of the United States, (1851,) two formulæ for the preparation of the *Ac''idum hydrocyan'icum dilu'tum — Ac''idum hydrocyan'icum*, Ph. U. S. of 1842 — are given; the one from the *Ferro-cyanuret of Potassium*; the other from the *Cyanuret of Silver*. According to Magendie, the acid, prepared after Scheele's method — the one in common use — is of irregular medicinal power: he, therefore, recommends Gay Lussac's acid, diluted with 6 times its volume, or 8.5 times its weight of distilled water, for medicinal purposes, and this he calls *Medic''inal Prussic Acid*. Dr. Ure has proposed, that the specific gravity should indicate that which is proper for medicinal exhibition; and, after comparative experiments of the gravity of the acids, obtained by different processes, he states, that the acid, usually prescribed, is of s. g. 0.996 or 0.997. Great caution is, however, necessary. One drop of pure prussic acid may instantly destroy, and the animal show hardly any traces of irritability, a few moments after death. It has been advised in laryngeal phthisis, in pulmonary phthisis, pulmonary inflammation and irritation, dyspepsia, uterine affections, hectic cough, cancer, chronic rheumatism, and mania, and as a local remedy in impetiginous affections; but, although possessed of powerful sedative properties, it is so unmanageable and the preparation so uncertain, that it is not much used. The *Dose* of Scheele's *Acid*, or of the *Medicinal Prussic Acid*, is from a quarter of a drop to two drops.

HYDROCYS'TIS, from '*ὑδωρ*,' 'water,' and *κυστις*, 'a bladder.' A cyst containing a watery or serous fluid. An hydatid. Also, saccated ascites.

HYDRODERMA, Anasarca.

HYDRODES, Aqueous.

HYDRODIARRHŒA, Diarrhœa, serous.

HYDRŒDEMA, Œdema.

HYDRO-ENCÉPHALORRHÉE, Apoplexy, serous.

HYDRO-ENTERO-EPIPLOCE'LE, *Hydroepiplo-enteroce'lê*; from '*ὑδωρ*,' 'water,' *εντερον*, 'intestine,' and *επιπλοον*, 'omentum.' Enteroepiplocele, the sac of which contains a serous fluid.

HYDRO-ENTERO-EPIPLOM'PHALUM, from '*ὑδωρ*,' 'water,' *εντερον*, 'an intestine,' *επιπλοον*, 'the caul,' and *ομφαλος*, 'the navel.' Umbilical hernia, the sac of which contains intestine, epiploon, and serum.

HYDRO-ENTEROM'PHALUM, *Hydrenterom'phalum*; from '*ὑδωρ*,' 'water,' *εντερον*, 'an intestine,' and *ομφαλος*, 'the umbilicus.' Hernia umbilicalis, the sac of which contains intestine and serum.

HYDRO-EPIPLOCE'LE, from '*ὑδωρ*,' 'water,' *επιπλοον*, 'omentum,' and *κηλη*, 'a tumour.' Hernia, formed by omentum, the sac of which contains serum.

HYDRO-EPIPLO-ENTEROCELE, Hydroentero-epiplocele.

HYDRO-EPIPLOMPH'ALUM, from '*ὑδωρ*,' 'water,' *επιπλοον*, 'the omentum,' and *ομφαλος*, 'the umbilicus.' Umbilical hernia, the sac of which contains epiploon and serum.

HYDROG'ALA, from '*ὑδωρ*,' 'water,' and *γαλα*, 'milk.' A mixture of water and milk.

HYDROGASTER, Ascites.

HY'DROGEN, *Hydrogen'ium, Inflam'mable air, Phlogis'ton, Princip'ium hydrogenet'icum, P. hydrot'icum, Mephi'tis inflammab'ilis,* (F.) *Hydrogène*, from '*ὑδωρ*,' 'water,' and *γενναω*, 'I produce.' This gas, when breathed, proves fatal from containing no oxygen. When diluted with two-thirds of atmospheric air, it occasions some diminution of muscular power and sensibility, and a reduction of the force of the circulation. It has been respired in catarrh, hæmoptysis, and phthisis.

HYDROGEN, CARBURETTED, *Inflammable air, Fire damp*, of miners — obtained by passing the vapour of water over charcoal, at the temperature of ignition, in an iron tube—has been found possessed of similar properties, when diluted, and has been used in like cases.

HYDROGEN, PROTOXIDE OF, Water.

HYDROGEN, SULPHURETTED, *Hydrosulph'uric acid, Hydrothion'ic acid, Hydrothi'on, Gas hepat'icum, Gas hydrogen'ium sulphura'tum, Mephi'tis hepat'ica,* (F.) *Acide hydrosulfurique*, may be disengaged from any of the sulphurets by the addition of a strong acid. It is a violent poison, but has been recommended to be inhaled, diluted, to allay the increased irritability which occasionally exists after diseases of the lungs. See Hydro-sulphuretted Water.

HYDROGENATION, see *Hydrogénèses.*

HYDROGÈNE, Hydrogen.

HYDROGÉNÈSES. Baumes gives this name to diseases which he fancifully considers to depend upon disturbed *hydrogenation.* In it he includes intermittent and remittent fevers.

HYDROGENO - SULPHURETUM AMMONIACÆ LIQUIDUM, Ammoniæ sulphuretum.

HYDROGLOSSA, Ranula.

HYDROGRAPHY, see Hydrology.

HYDROHÉMIE, Anæmia.

HYDROHYMENI'TIS, *Orrhohymeni'tis,* from 'υδωρ, 'water,' 'υμην, 'a membrane,' and *itis,* denoting inflammation. Inflammation of a serous membrane.

HYDROLÆUM, Hydrelæon.

HYDROLAPATHUM,Rumex hydrolapathum.

HYDROLATA, Aquæ destillatæ.

HYDROLATS, Aquæ destillatæ.

HYDROLÉS, see Hydrolica.

HYDROL'ICA, (F.) *Hydroliques,* from 'υδωρ, 'water.' Watery solutions of the active principles of medicinal agents. Those prepared by solution or admixture are termed, by the French, *Hydrolés;* those by distillation, *Hydrolats.*

HYDROLIQUES, Hydrolica.

HYDROL'OGY, *Hydrolog"ia,* from 'υδωρ, 'water,' and λογος, 'a discourse.' A treatise on water. By the term *Medical Hydrol'ogy* is meant that part of physics, whose object is the study of water, considered as it respects medicine ; and, consequently, embracing that of mineral waters. *Medical Hydrog'raphy* comprises the study of the influence exerted by the sea or by navigation on the health of man.

HYDROLOTIF, Lotion.

HYDROMA'NIA, from 'υδωρ, 'water,' and μανια, 'mania.' A name given by Strambi to pellagra, in which the patient has a strong propensity to drown himself.

HYDRO-MEDIASTI'NUM, *Hydrops mediasti'ni.* Effusion of serous fluid into the mediastinum.

HY'DROMEL, *Hydrom'eli,* from 'υδωρ, 'water,' and μελι, 'honey.' *Aqua mulsa, Meliti'tis, Mulsum, Melic'ratum, Mellic'ratum, Braggart, Medo.* A liquid medicine, prepared with an ounce and a half of *honey* and a pint of *tepid water.* It is used as a demulcent and laxative, and is generally known under the names *Simple hy'dromel, Vinous hy'dromel, Mead, Hydrom'eli vino'sum.* It is a drink made by fermenting honey and water, and is much used in some countries.

HYDROMENINGITIS, Hydrocephalus internus.

HYDROMETER, Areometer.

HYDROME'TRA, *Hydrome'tria, Hyster'ites, Hysteræde'ma, Hydrops u'teri,* from 'υδωρ, 'water,' and μητρα, 'the womb.' *Dropsy of the womb.* A disease characterized by circumscribed protuberance in the hypogastrium, — with obscure fluctuation, progressively enlarging, without ischury or pregnancy. If it ever occur, it must be a rare disease.

HYDROM'PHALUM, *Hydrops umbilica'lis, Exom'phalus aquo'sus, Her'nia umbili'ci aquo'sa,* from 'υδωρ, 'water,' and ομφαλος, 'the navel.' A tumour, formed by the accumulation of serum in the sac of umbilical hernia; or simply by distension of the navel in cases of ascites.

HYDROMYRIN'GA, *Hydromyrinx, Hydrops tym'pani,* from 'υδωρ, 'water,' and *myringa* or *myrinx,* 'the membrana tympani.' Dropsy of the drum of the ear; giving rise to difficulty of hearing, — *Dysecœ'a hydrop'ica.*

HYDROMYRINX, Hydromyringa.

HYDRONCUS, Anasarca, Œdema.

HYDRONEPHRO'SIS, (F.) *Hydronéphrose, Hydrorénale distension,* from 'υδωρ, 'water,' and νεφρος, 'kidney.' An accumulation in the kidney, owing to the obstruction of the tubes of the papillæ. — Rayer.

HYDRONOSUS, Hydrops.

HYDRONUSUS, Hydrops.

HYDROOPHORON, Hydroarion.

HYDROOVARIUM, Hydroarion.

HYDROPATH'IC, *Hydropath'icus, Hydriat'ricus,* from 'υδωρ, 'water,' and παθος, 'disease.' Relating to hydropathy or the water-cure, — as a hydropathic physician, *Hydriäter, Hydriätrus.*

HYDROPATHY, Hydrosudotherapeia.

HYDROPEDE'SIS, from 'υδωρ, 'water,' and πηδαω, 'I break out.' *Ephidro'sis.* Excessive sweating.

HYDROPEGE, Water, spring.

HYDROPELTIS PURPUREA, Brasenia hydropeltis.

HYDROPERICARDIA, Hydropericardium.

HYDROPERICARDITIS, Hydropericardium.

HYDROPERICAR'DIUM, *Hydropericar'dia, Hydropericardi'tis,* from 'υδωρ, 'water,' and *pericardium; Hydrops Pericar'dii, Hydrocar'dia, Dropsy of the pericar'dium,* (F.) *Hydropisie du Péricarde.* This is not a common disease. Palpitations; irregular or intermitting pulse; excessive dyspnœa, amounting often to orthopnœa, and dulness over a large space on percussion, will cause the pericardium to be suspected. The treatment is that of dropsies in general. It is, usually, however, of the active kind.

HYDROPÉRIONE, from 'υδωρ, 'water,' περι, 'around,' and ωον, 'an egg, or ovum.' The seroalbuminous substance, secreted by the lining of the uterus prior to the arrival of the impregnated ovum in that cavity. — Breschet.

HYDROPERITONEUM, Ascites.

HYDROPÉRITONIE, Ascites.

HYDROPHAL'LUS, from 'υδωρ, 'water,' and φαλλος, 'the male organ.' Œdema of the male organ.

HYDROPHIMOSIS, Phimosis œdematodes.

HYDROPHLEGMASIA TEXTÛS CELLULARIS, Phlegmasia alba.

HYDROPHLOGOSIS VENTRICULORUM CEREBRI, Hydrocephalus internus.

HYDROPHOB'IA, *Paraphob'ia, Parophob'ia, Phobodip'son, Pheu'gydron, Pheugophob'ia, Cynolys'sa, Cynolys'sum, Morbus hydrophob'icus* seu *hydroph'obus, Lycan'che, Lycan'chis, Aërophobia, Phreni'tis latrans, Lytta, Lyssa, Lyssa cani'na, Pantophob'ia, Rabies cani'na, Erethis'mus hydrophobia, Clonos hydrophobia, Hygrophobia, Aquæ metus, Canine madness,* (F.) *Rage;* from 'υδωρ, 'water,' and φοβος, 'dread.'

The term *Rabies* is more appropriate for the aggregate of symptoms resulting from the bite of rabid animals. Hydrophobia literally signifies a 'dread of water;' and, consequently, ought to be applied to one of the symptoms of rabies, rather than to the disease itself. It is a symptom which appears occasionally in other nervous affections. Rabies is susceptible of spontaneous development in the dog, wolf, cat, and fox, which can thence transmit it to other quadrupeds or to man; but it has not been proved that it can supervene, — without their having been previously bitten, — in animals of other species; or that the latter can, when bitten, communicate it to others. Many facts induce the belief, that the saliva and bronchial mucus are the sole vehicles of the rabid virus: the effects of which upon the economy sometimes appear almost immediately after the bite, and are, at others, apparently dormant for a considerable period. The chief symptoms are — a sense of dryness and constriction of the throat; excessive thirst; difficult deglutition; aversion for, and horror at, the sight of liquids as well as of brilliant objects; red, animated countenance; great nervous irritability; frothy saliva; grinding of the teeth, &c. Death most commonly happens before the fifth day. Hydrophobia has hitherto resisted all therapeutical means. Those which allay irritation are obviously most called for. In the way of prevention, the bitten part should always be excised, where practicable; and cauterized.

In some cases, symptoms like those which follow the bite of a rabid animal are said to have come on spontaneously. This affection has been termed *nervous* or *spontaneous hydrophobia.*

HYDROPHOBUS, Lyssodectus.

HYDROPHTHAL'MIA, from 'ὑδωρ, 'water,' and οφθαλμος, 'the eye.' *Hydrophthal'mus, Dropsy of the eye, Hydrops Oc'uli, Buphthal'mus, Zoöphthal'mus, Oc'ulus Bovi'nus, Oculus Bu'bulus, Oculus Elephan'tinus, Ophthalmopto'sis, Parop'sis Staphylo'ma simplex,* (F.) *Hydrophthalmie, Hydropisie de l'œil.* This affection is caused, at times, by an increase in the quantity of the aqueous, at others, of the vitreous, humour. In the former case, the iris is concave anteriorly, and pushed backwards: — in the latter, it is convex, and pushed forwards. Most commonly, the disease seems to depend on both humours at the same time. Hydrophthalmia sometimes affects both eyes; at others, only one. Children are more exposed to it than adults or old persons. The *treatment* must vary according to the cause; its longer or shorter duration; greater or less extent, &c. Hence, according to circumstances, hydragogue medicines, purgatives, general and local blood-letting, blisters, setons, moxa, cupping-glasses, fomentations, collyria, and fumigations of different kinds, have been employed. When all means fail, and the disease continues to make progress, the fluid may be evacuated, by a puncture made with a cataract needle at the lower part of the transparent cornea.

HYDROPHTHALMIA, CONICAL, Staphyloma of the cornea.

HYDROPHTHAL'MION. Same etymon. An œdematous swelling of the conjunctiva in hydropic persons.

HYDROPHTHALMUS, Hydrophthalmia — h. Cruentus, Hæmophthalmia.

HYDROPHYLLUM VERUM, Hydrastis Canadensis.

HYDROPHYSOCE'LE, *Hydropneumatoce'le,* from 'ὑδωρ, 'water,' φυσα, 'wind,' and κηλη, 'a tumour.' Hernia, which contains a serous fluid and gas.

HYDROPHYSOME'TRA, from 'ὑδωρ, 'water,' φυσαω, 'I inflate,' and μητρα, 'the womb.' A morbid condition of the womb, in which both fluid and air are contained in it.

HYDROP'IC, *Hydrop'icus, Hy'phydros, Hyder'icus, Hydero'des, Drop'sical,* (F.) *Hydropique.* One labouring under dropsy. Relating to dropsy. Also, an antihydropic, and a hydragogue.

HYDROPIPER, Polygonum hydropiper.

HYDROPISIA, Hydrops.

HYDROPISIE, Hydrops — *h. du Bas-ventre,* Ascites — *h. Cérébrale euraiguë,* Apoplexy, serous — *h. de l'Œil,* Hydrophthalmia — *h. de l'Ovaire,* Hydroarion — *h. du Péricarde,* Hydropericardium — *h. des Plèvres,* Hydrothorax — *h. de Poitrine,* Hydrothorax — *h. de la Vésicule du Fiel,* Turgescentia vesicæ felleæ.

HYDROPISIS, Hydrops — h. Vera, Anasarca.
HYDROPISMUS, Hydrops.
HYDROPLEURIE, Hydrothorax.
HYDROPNEUMATOCELE, Hydrophysocele.
HYDROPNEUMON, Hydropneumonia.

HYDROPNEUMO'NIA, *Hydropneu'mon, Œde'ma pulmo'num chron'icum, Hydrops pulmonum cellulo'sus, Anasar'ca pulmo'num, Hydrops pulmonum,* from 'ὑδωρ, 'water,' and πνευμων, 'the lung.' Dropsical infiltration of the lungs. See Œdema of the lungs.

HYDROPNEUMOSAR'CA, from 'ὑδωρ, 'water,' πνευμα, 'wind, air,' and σαρξ, 'flesh.' An abscess, containing water, air, and matters similar to flesh. — M. A. Severinus.

HYDROPNEUMOTHO'RAX, *Hydroaëropleurie,* from 'ὑδωρ, 'water,' πνευμων, 'the lung,' and θωραξ, 'the chest.' Pneumothorax with effusion of blood into the chest. See Pneumothorax.

HYDROPOÏ'DES, from 'ὑδωρ, 'water,' and ποιεω, 'I make.' An epithet for watery excretions, such as sometimes take place in hydropics.

HYDROP'OTA, *Hydrop'otes, Pota'tor Aquæ,* from 'ὑδωρ, 'water,' and ποτης, 'a drinker.' A *water drinker.* One who drinks only water, or drinks it in an extraordinary quantity.

HYDROPS, from 'ὑδωρ, 'water,' *Plegma'tia, Hy'deros, Affec'tus hydero'des, Hydrop'isis, Hydropis'ia, Hydropis'mus, Hydrop'sia, Hydrorrhœ'a, Hydrorrhoë, Hydrorrhoüs, Polyhy'dria, Hydron'osus, Hydronu'sus, Dropsy,* (F.) *Hydropisie.* A preternatural collection of a serous fluid in any cavity of the body, or in the areolar texture. When the cellular texture of the whole body is more or less filled with fluid, the disease is called *Anasar'ca* or *Leucoplegma'tia;* — and when this variety is local or partial, it is called *Œde'ma.* The chief dropsies, designated from their seat, are: — *Anasarca, Hydrocephalus, Hydrorachitis, Hydrothorax, Hydropericardium, Ascites, Hydrometra, Hydrocele,* &c.

Encyst'ed Dropsy, Hydrops sacca'tus, incarcera'tus vel cys'ticus, is that variety in which the fluid is enclosed in a sac or cyst; so that it has no communication with the surrounding parts. *Dropsy of the Ovarium, Hydrops Ova'rii, Asci'tes Ova'rii, Asci'tes sacca'tus,* is an instance of this variety.

Dropsy may be active or passive. The *former* consists in an increased action of the exhalants, so that those vessels pour out much more fluid than is absorbed: the *latter* arises from a state of atony of the absorbent vessels, which allows of an accumulation of fluid. It may also be *mechanical,* or produced by obstructions to the circulation, as in cases of diseased liver. Active dropsy, occurring accidentally in a sound individual, generally ends favourably. That which supervenes on other diseases, or is symptomatic of some internal affection, is rarely curable.

The treatment consists in the use of all those remedies which act on the various secretions: so that, the demand being increased, the supply will have to be increased accordingly; and in this manner some of the collected fluid may be taken up by the absorbents. To this end bleeding, if the dropsy be very active; purgatives, diuretics, sudorifics, sialogogues, &c., are the remedies chiefly depended upon.

HYDROPS ABDOMINIS, Ascites — h. Abdominis aereus, Tympanites — h. Abdominis saccatus, see Ascites — h. Anasarca, Anasarca — h. Anasarca acutus, see Anasarca — h. Articulorum, Hydrarthrus — h. Ascites, Ascites — h. Capitis, Hydrocephalus — h. Capitis, Hydrocephalus chronicus — h. Cavitatis columnæ vertebralis, Hydrorachis — h. Cellularis artuum, Œdema — h. Cellularis totius corporis, Anasarca—h. Cellulosus, Anasarca—h. Cerebri, Hydrocephalus, Hydrocephalus internus—h. Cutaneus, Anasarca—h. Cysticus, see Ascites, and Hydrops—h. Glottidis, Œdema of the Glottis—h. Incarceratus, see Hydrops—h. Intercus, Anasarca—h. Leucophlegmatias, Leucophlegmatia—h. ad Matulam, Diabetes—h. Mediastini, Hydromediastinum—h. Medullæ spinalis, Hydrorachis—h. Matellæ, Diabetes—h. Oculi, Hydrophthalmia—h. Ovarii, Hydroarion, see Hydrops—h. Palpebræ, Hydroblepharon—h. Pectoris, Hydrothorax—h. Pericardii, Hydropericardium—h. Pleuræ, Hydrothorax—h. Pulmonis, Hydrothorax—h. Pulmonum, Hydropneumonia, Œdema of the Lungs—h. Pulmonum cellulosus, Hydropneumonia—h. Saccatus, see Hydrops—h. Sacci lachrymalis, Fistula lachrymalis—h. Scroti, Hydrocele—h. Siccus et flatulentus, Tympanites—h. Spinæ, Hydrorachis—h. Spinæ vertebralis, Hydrorachis—h. Subcutaneus, Anasarca—h. Telæ cellulosæ, Anasarca—h. Testiculorum, Hydrocele—h. Thoracis, Hydrothorax—h. Tubarum Fallopii, Hydrosalpinx—h. Tympani, Hydromyringa—h. Tympanites, Tympanites—h. Umbilicalis, Hydromphalum—h. Uteri, Hydrometra—h. Vesicæ felleæ, Turgescentia vesiculæ felleæ.

HYDROPSIA, Hydrops.

HYDROPYR'ETOS, from *'ὕδωρ,* 'water,' and *πυρετος,* 'fever;' *Febris sudato'ria.* Fever with sweating. *Hidropyretos* would be more proper; from *'ἱδρως,* 'sweat.' See Sudor Anglicus.

HYDRORA'CHIS, from *'ὕδωρ,* 'water,' and *ῥαχις,* 'the spine.' *Hydrorrha'chis, Hydrorachi'tis, Hydrorrha'chia, Myeloch'ysis, Hydrops Cavita'tis Columnæ Vertebra'lis, H. Spinæ vertebra'lis, Hydrops medul'læ spina'lis, Hydroce'lē spina'lis, Hydrorachi'tis spino'sa, Hydrops spinæ.* An effusion of serum, often owing to inflammation of the spinal membranes — *myeli'tis exsudati'va*—and forming a soft, frequently transparent, tumour, constituted of the membranes of the spinal marrow, which are distended and projecting backwards from the vertebral canal, the posterior paries of which, when the affection is congenital, is wanting to a certain extent — *Spina bif'ida, Atelorachid'ia, Hydrora'chis dehis'cens seu congen'ita, Schistorrha'chis, Spi'nola.* The disease is often accompanied with paralysis of the lower extremities. It is congenital, and situate in the lumbar or sacral regions. It is almost always fatal:—the tumour rupturing, and death occurring instantaneously. On dissection, a simple separation or complete absence of the spinous processes of the vertebræ is perceived, with, at times, destruction or absence of spinal marrow. The treatment is the same as in *hydrocephalus chronicus;* and, as in it, advantage seems occasionally to have been derived by puncturing with a fine needle.

HYDRORACHIS DEHISCENS, see Hydrorachis.
HYDRORACHITIS, Hydrorachis.
HYDRORCHIS, Hydrocele.

HYDRORÉNALE DISTENSION, Hydronephrosis.

HYDRORRHACHIA, Hydrorachis.
HYDRORRHACHIS, Hydrorachis — h. Congenita, see Hydrorachis — h. Dehiscens, see Hydrorachis.

HYDRORRHAGIE, Apoplexy, serous.
HYDRORRHOE, Hydrops.
HYDRORRHŒA, Hydrops.
HYDRORRHOUS, Hydrops.

HYDROTHOPNŒ'A, from *'ὕδωρ,* 'water,' and *ορθοπνοια,* 'difficulty of breathing, except in the erect posture.' Orthopnœa, owing to a collection of water in the chest.

HYDROSAC'CHARUM, *Aqua sacchara'ta,* (F.) *Eau sucrée.* Sugared water.

HYDROSAL'PINX, *Hydrops tuba'rum Fallo'pii;* from *'ὕδωρ,* 'water,' and *σαλπιγξ,* 'a tube.' Dropsy of the Fallopian tube.

HYDROSAR'CA, from *'ὕδωρ,* 'water,' and *σαρξ,* 'flesh.' A tumour containing a fluid, as well as portions of flesh. Also, Anasarca.

HYDROSARCOCE'LE, from *'ὕδωρ,* 'water,' *σαρξ,* 'flesh,' and *κηλη,* 'a tumour.' *Sarcohydroce'lē.* A tumour, formed by a sarcocele, complicated with dropsy of the tunica vaginalis.

HYDROSCHEOCE'LE, *Oscheoce'lē aquo'sa,* from *'ὕδωρ,* 'water,' *οσχεον,* 'the scrotum,' and *κηλη,* 'rupture.' A collection of water in the scrotum. Hydrocele.

HYDROSCHÉONIE, Hydrocele.
HYDROSCHEUM, Hydrocele.
HYDROSIS, Hidrosis.

HYDROSTATIC TEST OF INFANTICIDE, see Docimasia.

HYDROSUDOPATHY, Hydrosudotherapeia.

HYDROSUDOTHERAPEI'A, *Hydrop'athy, Hydropathi'a, Hydrosudop'athy, Hydri'asis, Ars hydriat'rica, Hydriatri'a, Water cure,* (G.) *Wasserour,* from *'ὕδωρ,* 'water,' *sudo,* 'I sweat,' and *θεραπευω,* 'I remedy.' A badly compounded word, formed to express the mode of treating diseases systematically by cold water, sweating, &c.

HYDROSULPHURET'TED WATER, *Aqua hydrosulphura'ta simplex, Aqua hepat'ica,* (F.) *Eau hydrosulphurée simple.* (*Sulphuret of iron* 1000 parts, *sulphuric acid* 2000 parts, *distilled water* 4000 parts; add the water to the acid, and put the sulphuret of iron into a retort, to which a Wolff's apparatus of five or six vessels is adapted; the last containing about an ounce of potassa, dissolved in a quart of water. Pour the diluted acid gradually on the sulphuret, and, ultimately, throw away the water in the last vessel. *Ph. P.*) It is stimulant, diaphoretic, and deobstruent, (?) and is used in rheumatism, diseases of the skin, &c.

It has been, also, called *Ac"idum Hydrothion'icum liq'uidum.*

HYDROSULPHURETUM AMMONIACUM AQUOSUM, Ammoniæ sulphuretum—h. Ammoniacum, Ammoniæ sulphuretum.

HYDROTHION, Hydrogen, sulphuretted.

HYDROTHO'RAX, from *'ὕδωρ,* 'water,' and *θωραξ,* 'the chest.' *Hydrops Thora'cis, Hydrops pec'toris, Hydrops pulmo'nis, H. pleuræ, Stethoch'ysis, Pleurorrhœ'a lymphat'ica, Pl. sero'sa, Dyspnœ'a et Orthopnœ'a hydrothorac"ica.* (F.) *Hydropisie de Poitrine, H. des Plèvres, Dropsy of the Chest.* Idiopathic hydrothorax, termed by Laënnec *Hydropisie des plèvres, Dropsy of the Pleuræ,* — by Piorry, *Hydropleurie,*—is a rare disease, and difficult of diagnosis. It generally exists only on one side, which, if the fluid effused be considerable, projects more than the other. Dyspnœa, and fluctuation perceptible to the ear, are characteristic symptoms. When the chest is examined with the stethoscope, respiration is found to be wanting every where, except at the root of the lung. The sound is also dull on percussion.

Effusion into the chest, as a result of inflammation of some thoracic viscus, is as common as the other is rare. It is usually a fatal symptom. It has been called *symptomatic hydrothorax.*

In hydrothorax, the course of treatment proper in dropsies in general, must be adopted. Diuretics seem, here, to be especially useful; probably on account of the great activity of pulmonary absorption. Paracentesis can rarely be serviceable.

HYDROTHORAX CHYLOSUS, Chylothorax — h. Purulentus, Empyema.

HYDROTICA, Hydragogues.

HYDRO'TIS, from *'ὕδωρ,* 'water,' and *ους,* gen.

ωτος, 'the ear.' Dropsy of the ear. Properly, an accumulation of mucous or muco-purulent matter in the middle ear.

HYDRURESIS, Diabetes.

HYDRURIA, Diabetes, see Urine.

HYÈRES. This small town, agreeably situate on the declivity of a hill, about two miles from the Mediterranean, and twelve from Toulon, is the least exceptionable residence in Provence for the pulmonary invalid. It is in some measure protected from the northerly winds; but not sufficiently so from the *mistral* to render it a very desirable residence for the phthisical.—Sir James Clark.

HYGEA, *Hygiène*, Sanitas.
HYGEIA, Sanitas.
HYGEISMUS, Hygiene.
HYGEOLOGY, Hygiene.
HYGIANSIS, Sanitas.
HYGIASIS, Sanitas.
HYGIASMA, Medicament.
HYGIAS'TICA DOCTRI'NA. The doctrine of health. The doctrine of the restoration of health.
HYGIASTICUS, Salutary.
HYGIEA, Sanitas.
HYGIEIA, Hygiene, Sanitas.
HYGIEINUS, Salutary.
HYGIEIOLOGIA, Hygiene.

HYGIÈNE (F.), (generally Anglicised, and pronounced *hygeëne*) from 'υγιεια, 'health.' *Hygiene, Hygeis'mus, Hygiei'nē, Hygie'sis, Hygiei'a; Hygie'a, Hygei'a, Hygiene, Hygien'ice, Conservati'va medicina, Hygeolog''ia, Hygieiolog''ia, Hygeology, Hygiol'ogy*; from 'υγιης, 'healthy.' The part of medicine whose object is the preservation of health. It embraces a knowledge of healthy man, both in society and individually, as well as of the objects used and employed by him, with their influence on his constitution and organs. See Regimen.

HYGIEN'IC, (F.) *Hygiénique*. Same etymon. Relating to Hygiene — as '*hygienic* precautions, *hygienic* rules,' &c. &c.

HYGIENICS, Hygiene.

HYGIÉNIQUE, Hygienic.

HYGIÉ'NIST. One who understands the principles of hygiene.

HYGIERUS, Salutary.
HYGIESIS, Hygiene.
HYGIOLOGY, Hygiene.

HYGRA, from 'υδωρ, 'water,' or 'υγρος, 'humid.' Liquid plasters;—*Hygremplas'tra.*

HYGRASIA, Humour.

HYGRECHE'MA, from 'υγρος, 'humid,' and ηχημα, 'sound;' *Son'itus flu'idi*. The sound of fluid, heard by auscultation, or otherwise.

HYGREDON, Humour.

HYGREMPLASTRA, Hygra.

HYGROBLEPHAR'ICI, from 'υγρος, 'humid,' and βλεφαρον, 'eyelid;' *Hygrophthal'mici*. The excretory ducts of the lachrymal gland have been so called.

HYGROCATARAC'TA; from 'υγρος, 'humid,' and καταρακτης, 'cataract;' *Catarac'ta liq'uida*. Liquid or fluid cataract.

HYGROCELE, Hydrocirsocele.
HYGROCOLLYRIA, see Collyrium.
HYGROCYSTIS, Hydatid.

HYGROL'OGY, *Hygrolog''ia*, from 'υγρος, 'humid,' and λογος, 'a discourse.' The anatomy of the fluids of the body.

HYGRO'MA, from 'υγρος, 'humid.' *Tumor cys'ticus sero'sus, Cys'tis sero'sa*. Dropsy of the bursæ mucosæ.

HYGROM'ETRY, *Hygromet'ria, Hygrosco'-*

pia; from 'υγρος, 'humid,' and μητρον, 'measure.' The part of physics which concerns the measurement of the dryness or humidity of the atmosphere. It is probable, that diseases are as frequently caused by the varying moisture of the atmosphere as by changes in its weight or temperature. The *hygrometer* ought, consequently, to form part of every apparatus for medical meteorological observations.

HYGRON, Liquor.
HYGROPHOBIA, Hydrophobia.

HYGROPHTHAL'MIA, from 'υγρος, 'humid,' and οφθαλμια, 'inflammation of the eye.' Ophthalmia with much lachrymation.

HYGROPHTHALMICI, Hygroblepharici.
HYGROPISSOS, see Pinus sylvestris.
HYGROSCOPIA, Hygrometry.
HYGROTES, Humour, Liquor.
HYGRUM, Humour.

HY'LE, 'υλη, *Mate'ria*, 'Matter.' Wood. Materia Medica; also, the Philosopher's stone.

HYLE IATRICE, Materia Medica.
HYLISIS, Colatio.
HYLISMUS, Colatio.
HYLISTER, Colatorium.

HYLOPH'AGOUS, from 'υλη, 'wood,' and φαγω, 'I eat.' One that feeds upon the young shoots of trees, roots, &c. Hylophagous tribes yet exist in some parts of Africa.

HYMASTATICS, Hæmastatice.

HYMEN, 'υμην, which signifies 'marriage,' 'nuptial song,' 'membrane or pellicle.' *Claustrum seu Flos seu Sigil'lum seu Custo'dia seu Colum'na seu Zona virgina'tis, Flos virgina'lis, Virgin'ia, Cir'culus membrano'sus, Bucton, Intersep'tum virgina'lē, Cento virgina'lis, Argumen'tum Integrita'tis, Munimen'tum seu Zona Castita'tis, Pannic'ulus hgmenæ'us seu virgina'lis, Eugion, Val'vula ragi'næ, Membran'ula luna'ta vaginæ, Virginal membrane.* The semilunar, parabolic, or circular fold, situate at the outer orifice of the vagina in virgins, especially during youth, and prior to menstruation. This membrane is ordinarily ruptured by the first venereal act, and is effaced by accouchement; some irregular flaps remaining, to which the name *Carun'culæ Myrtifor'mes* has been given by reason of their resemblance to the leaves of the myrtle. Many circumstances of an innocent character may occasion a rupture or destruction of this membrane. It is often, indeed, found absent in children soon after birth; whilst it *may* remain entire after copulation. Hence the presence of the hymen does not absolutely prove virginity; nor does its absence prove incontinence; although its presence would be *primâ facie* evidence of continence.

HYMEN, Membrane — h. Diaphatton, Mediastinum.

HYMENÆA, see Copal — h. Courbaril, see Anime.

HYMEN'ICA AMENORRHŒ'A. Amenorrhœa occasioned by closure of the hymen.

HYMEN'ICUS, *Hymeno'des*, from 'υμην, 'hymen,' &c. Relating to the hymen. Also, membranous.

HYMENI'TIS, from 'υμην, 'a membrane,' and *itis*, denoting inflammation. Membranous inflammation. Inflammation of an internal membrane.

HYME'NIUM, *Membran'ula*, diminutive of 'υμην, 'a membrane.' A fine, delicate membrane.

HYMENODES, Hymenicus.
HYMENOGANGLIITIS, Cholera.

HYMENOG'RAPHY, *Hymenogra'phia*, from 'υμην, 'a membrane,' and γραφω, 'I describe.' That part of anatomy whose object is the description of the different membranes.

HYMENOL'OGY, *Hymenolog"ia*, from '*υμην*, 'a membrane,' and *λογος*, 'a description.' A treatise on the membranes.

HYMENOR'RHAPHY, *Hymenorrha'phia*; from '*υμην*, 'the hymen,' and *ραφη*, 'a suture.' A form of elytrorrhaphy, in which the operation is performed in the natural situation of the hymen.

HYMENOT'OMY, *Hymenotom'ia*, from '*υμην*, 'a membrane,' and *τεμνω*, 'I cut,' 'I dissect.' The part of anatomy which treats of the dissection of the membranes. The term has also been applied to the incision of the hymen, practised in certain cases of imperforation of the vagina, in order to give exit to the blood retained and accumulated in the cavity of the uterus.

HYMNIUM, Amnios.

HYO: in composition, an abridgment of Hyoides, os.

HYOBASIOGLOSSUS, Basioglossus.
HYOCHONDROGLOSSUS, Hyoglossus.
HYODEOGLOSSUS, Hyoglossus.
HYODEOTHYREODES, Thyreohyoideus.
HYODES, Hyoides.

HYO-EPIGLOT'TICUS, *Hyodepiglot'ticus*. Belonging to the os hyoides and epiglottis. Some anatomists have given the name *Hyo-epiglottic ligament* to a bundle of condensed areolar tissue, which passes from the posterior part of the body of the hyoid bone to the base of the epiglottic fibro-cartilage.

HYO-GLOSSO-BASI-PHARYNGIEN, Constrictor pharyngis.

HYOGLOS'SUS, *Hyodeo-glossus, Hyo-chondroglossus, Hypsiloglossus, Cer'ato-glossus* of Douglass and Cowper: *Basio-Cerato-Chondro-glossus*. A large, thin, quadrilateral muscle, situate at the anterior and superior part of the neck. Its insertions at three different points of the os hyoides permit it to be divided into three portions:—the *first*, (*Cerato-glossus* of Albinus) is attached to the great cornu of the os hyoides: the *second*, (*Basio-glossus* of Albinus,) arises from the superior part of the body of the same bone; and the *third*, (*Chondro-glossus* of Albinus,) arises from the lesser cornu and the cartilage, situate between the body and the greater cornu. The fibres of these three bundles are inserted into the lateral and inferior parts of the tongue. This muscle depresses the base of the tongue, or raises the os hyoides, when the tongue is fixed.

HYO-THYREOIDEUS, Thyreo-hyoideus.
HYO-THYROID, Thyreo-hyoid.
HYOID BONE, Hyoides, os.

HYOI'DES, OS, *Os Bicor'ne, Os hypsiloi'des, Os Lambdoi'des, Os Gut'turis, Os Linguæ, Os Lingua'lē, Upsiloi'des, Ypsiloïdes.* The *Hyoid Bone*; from the Greek *υ*, and *ειδος*, 'shape.' *Hyoi'deus, Hyo'des.* The hyoid bone is a very movable, osseous arch; of a parabolic shape; convex before, and suspended horizontally in the substance of the soft parts of the neck, between the base of the tongue and the larynx. This bone, separated entirely from the rest of the skeleton, is composed of five distinct portions, susceptible of motion on each other. The first, and most central, is the *body of the hyoid, Ossic'ulum me'dium Hyoi'dis*, which affords attachment to several muscles; the two others are lateral, and bear the name of *branches* or *greater cornua*. The last two are smaller, situate above the other, and are known under the name *lesser cornua* and *styloid cornua*, the *Ossa pisifor'mia lingua'lia* of Sömmering. The os hyoides is ossified from five points.

HYOIDES PRIMUS, Sterneo-hyoideus.
HYOIDEUS, Hyoides.

HYOIDIS QUARTUS MUSCULUS, Omohyoideus.

HYOSCY'AMUS, from '*υς*, 'a swine,' and *κυαμος*, 'a bean.' *Faba suil'la, Bengi, Jusquiamus, Hyoscyamus niger seu agres'tis, Apollina'ris, Alter'cum, Ag'onē, Altercan'genon, Henbane, Poison Tobac'co, Stinking nightshade*, (F.) *Jusquiaume, Fève a Cochon, Hannebane, Potêlée.* The leaves and seeds are the parts used in medicine. Their odour is narcotic and peculiar; taste insipid and mucilaginous. The virtues are yielded to proof spirit. Hyoscyamus is narcotic, anodyne, antispasmodic, and slightly stimulant. It is used as a substitute for opium, where the latter disagrees; and is applied, externally, as a cataplasm in cancer and glandular swellings. Dose, gr. iij to x of the powder.

HYOSCYAMUS AGRESTIS, Hyoscyamus.
HYOSCYAMUS ALBUS, *White Henbane*, possesses similar virtues.
HYOSCYAMUS LUTEUS, *Nicotiana rustica* — h. Niger, Hyoscyamus — h. Peruvianus, Nicotiana tabacum.

HYOSCYAMUS SCOPOLIA, *Scopoli'na atropoï'des.* The herb and root of this plant, which grows in Illyria, Hungary, Croatia, Gallizia, and Bavaria, are used in the same cases as belladonna. Dose of the powder, half a grain.

HYPACTICUS, Cathartic.

HYPÆ'MIA, from '*υπο*, 'beneath,' and '*αιμα*, 'blood;' *Oligæ'mia, Oligohæ'mia, Anæ'mia.* Deficiency of blood.—Andral. Also, extravasation of blood.

HYPAGOGE, Dejection.
HYPAGOGUS, Laxative.

HYPALEIM'MA, *Hypalim'ma, Hypaleïp'tum, Hypalip'tum*, from '*υπαλειφω*, 'I anoint.' An ointment or liniment to be rubbed or spread on a part.

HYPALEIPTRIS, Hypaleiptrum.

HYPALEIP'TRON, *Hypaleip'trum, Hypaleïptris, Hypaliptrum, Specil'lum, Spatha.* A sort of spatula for spreading ointments.—Hipp.

HYPALEIPTRUM, Hypaleiptron.
HYPALEIPTUM, Hypaleimma.
HYPALIMMA, Hypaleimma.
HYPALIPTRUM, Hypaleiptron.

HYPAMAURO'SIS, from '*υπο*, 'under,' and *amaurosis; Amauro'sis imperfec'ta.* Imperfect amaurosis; *Meramauro'sis*.

HYPAPOPLEX'IA, from '*υπο*, 'under,' and *apoplexia.* An incomplete attack of apoplexy.

HYPATMISMUS, Fumigation.
HYPATMUS, Fumigation.

HYPAUCHE'NIUM, from '*υπο*, 'under,' and *αυχην*, 'the neck.' A pillow or cushion for the neck.

HYPECCHORESIS, Dejection.
HYPECCHORETICUS, Laxative.
HYPELATUS, Cathartic, Laxative.
HYPENANTIOMA, Allopathy.
HYPENANTIOSIS, Allopathy.

HYPE'NĒ, '*υπηνη*. The beard which grows under the chin, according to some. Also, the upper lip.—Vesalius. See Mystax.

HYPER, '*υπερ*, 'above,' 'in excess.' Hence:

HYPERACU'SIS, *Oxyecoïa, Hyperac'oē, Phthongodyspho'ria*, from '*υπερ*, 'above,' and *ακοη*, 'audition.' Excessive sensibility of the organ of hearing.

HYPERADENO'SIS, *Hyperadeno'mia, Hypertroph'ia glandula'rum*, from '*υπερ*, 'in excess,' and *αδην*, 'a gland.' Hypertrophy of a gland.

HYPERÆ'MIA, *Hyperhæ'mia, Hæmorme'sis*, (F.) *Hyperémie, Angiohémie*, from '*υπερ*, 'above,' and 'αιηα, 'blood.' Preternatural accumulation of blood in the capillary vessels, more especially local plethora; congestion.—Andral. Various forms of hyperæmia are admitted by pathologists,—for example, the *active* or *sthenic;* as in the phlegmasiæ,—the *asthenic* or *passive*, from weakness of vessels; the *cadaveric*, or that which forms immediately before or after death; and the *hypostatic*, which occurs in depending parts.

HYPERÆMIA ABDOMINIS, Cœliæmia—h. Activa, Inflammation—h. Capitis, Cephalæmia—h. of the Brain, Stethæmia—h. Cerebri, Cephalæmia—h. Pectoris, Stethæmia—h. Pulmonum, Stethæmia—h. of the Lungs, Stethæmia—h. Hepatic, Hepatohæmia.

HYPERÆ'MIC, *Hyperæ'micus, Conges'ted, Bloodshot.* Affected with hyperæmia.

HYPERÆSTHESIA, Hyperæsthesis—h. Linguæ, Hypergeustia—h. Olfactoria, Hyperosphresia—h. Plexus cardiaci, Angina pectoris.

HYPERÆSTHE'SIS, *Hyperæsthæ'sia*, Oxyæsthe'sia, (F.) *Hyperesthésie,* from 'υπερ, 'above,' and αισθησις, 'the faculty of feeling.' Excessive sensibility, impressibility, or passibility.

HYPERÆSTHET'ICA, same etymon. Agents that are conceived to augment general sensibility—as strychnia, brucia, &c. Pereira.

HYPERANTHERA MORINGA, Guilandina moringa.

HYPERANTHRAXIS, see Cholera.

HYPERAPH'IA, *Oxyaphē, Oxyaph'ia,* from 'υπερ, 'in excess,' and 'αφη, 'touch.' Excessive acuteness of touch.

HYPERAPHRODIS'IA, from 'υπερ, 'in excess, and Αφροδιτη, 'Venus.' Excessive venereal desire.

HYPERASTHENI'A, from 'υπερ, 'in excess,' and ασθενεια, 'weakness.' Excessive debility.

HYPERAUXE'SIS, from 'υπερ, 'over,' 'above,' and αυξησις, 'augmentation.' *Hyperepid'osis.* Excessive increase or enlargement of a part;—as *Hyperauxe'sis Ir'idis*, an excessive enlargement of the iris, so as to stop up the pupil.

HYPERBOL'IC (*attitude*), from 'υπερ, 'above, over,' and βαλλω, 'I throw.' 'Excessive.' Galen, by this term, designates certain extraordinary attitudes, in which the limbs and vertebral column are in a state of complete extension or flexion.

HYPERBO'REAN, from 'υπερ, 'beyond,' and βορεας, 'the north wind.' A race of men found at the extreme north of the two continents, in the vicinity of the polar circle. It includes the Thibetans, Ostiaks, Kamtschadales, Laplanders, Samoiedes, Esquimaux, &c.

HYPERBU'LIA, from 'υπερ, 'in excess,' and βουλη, 'will.' Ungovernable will or volition.

HYPERCARDIA, Heart, hypertrophy of the.

HYPERCARDIOTROPHIA, Heart, hypertrophy of the.

HYPERCATAPINO'SIS, from 'υπερ, 'in excess,' and καταπινειν, 'to sip up.' Excessive activity of absorption.

HYPERCATHAR'SIS, *Hyperine'sis, Hyperinos, Superpurga'tio, Effrenita'tio,* from 'υπερ, 'in excess,' and καθαρσις, 'purgation.' Superpurgation.

HYPERCENO'SIS, from 'υπερ, 'in excess,' and κενωσις, 'evacuation.' Excessive evacuation, as of blood, bile, &c.

HYPERCERASIS, Staphyloma of the cornea.

HYPERCERATOSIS, Staphyloma of the cornea.

HYPERCHOLIA, Polycholia.

HYPERCINE'SIA, *Hypercine'sis,* from 'υπερ, 'above, over,' and κινησις (κινεω, 'I move,') 'motion.' Excessive motion. Under the term *hypercinesis*, Romberg includes the spasmodic neuroses.

HYPERCINESIA NERVOSA, see Irritable—h. Uterina, Hysteria.

HYPERCINESIS GASTRICA, Hypochondriasis.

HYPERCONJONCTIVITE, see Ophthalmia.

HYPERCORYPHO'SIS, from 'υπερ, 'above,' and κορυφη, 'the vertex;' the extreme point of anything. The lobes of the liver and lungs.—Hippocrates.

HYPERCRIN'IA, *Hyperdiac'risis, Chymose'mia,* from 'υπερ, 'above,' and κρινω, 'I separate.' A morbid increase in the quantity of the secretions.

HYPER'CRISIS, same etymon. *Superexere'tio, Superevacua'tio.* An excessive crisis, or evacuation; a flux.—A very violent, critical effort, or too copious critical evacuations.—Galen.

HYPERCYESIS, Superfœtation.

HYPERDERMATO'SIS, *Hyperdermato'ma, Hyperdermo'sis, Hyperdermo'ma,* from 'υπερ, 'in excess,' and δερμα, 'skin.' Hypertrophy of the skin.

HYPERDIACRISIS, Hypercrinia.

HYPERDIURESIS, Diabetes.

HYPERDYNAMIA, Hypersthenia.

HYPERDYNAM'IC, *Hyperdynam'icus,* from 'υπερ, 'in excess,' and δυναμις, 'strength.' Appertaining to or having the characters of hyperdynamia, or excessive strength—of the vital powers more especially.

HYPERECHEMA, see Exaggerated.

HYPERECHESIS, see Exaggerated.

HYPEREM'ESIS, *Hyperemes'ia; Vom'itus profu'sus,* from 'υπερ, 'in excess,' and εμεω, 'I vomit.' Excessive vomiting after an emetic.

HYPERÉMIE, Hyperæmia—*h. du Cerveau*, Cephalohæmia—*h. Cérébrale*, Cephalohæmia—*h. du Foie*, Hepatohæmia—*h. de la Moëlle épinière*, Hypermyelohæmia—*h. des Poumons*, Stethæmia.

HYPERENCÉPHALOTROPHIE; from 'υπερ, 'in excess,' εγκεφαλον, 'the encephalon,' and τροφη, 'nourishment.' Hypertrophy of the encephalon.—Piorry.

HYPERENCEPH'ALUS, from 'υπερ, 'above,' and κεφαλη, 'the head.' A monster whose excessive brain is situate in the skull.

HYPERENDOSMOSE, Inflammation.

HYPERENERGI'A, from 'υπερ, 'in excess,' and ενεργεια, 'activity.' Excessive activity, as of the nervous system.

HYPEREPHIDROSIS, Ephidrosis.

HYPEREPIDOSIS, Hyperauxesis.

HYPERERETHIS'IA, from 'υπερ, 'in excess,' and ερεθιζω, 'I excite.' Excessive irritability.

HYPERES'IA, 'υπερεσια, 'a ministry.' This word is sometimes applied to the organs;—when it means function.

HYPERESTHÉSIE, Hyperæsthesia.

HYPERETRIA, Midwife.

HYPERGEN'ESIS, from 'υπερ, 'in excess,' and γενεσις, 'generation.' The excess of formative power, which gives occasion to monstrosities by excess of parts.

HYPERGEUS'TIA, *Hypergeu'sis, Hyperæsthe'sia linguæ, Oxygeu'sia,* from 'υπερ, 'above,' and γευσις, 'taste.' Excessive sensibility of the organ of taste.

HYPERHÆMATOSIS, Inflammation.

HYPERHÆMIA, Hyperæmia.

HYPERHÉPATOTROPHIE, Hepatauxe.

HYPERHIDROSIS, Ephidrosis.

HYPERHO'RA, from 'υπερ, 'in excess,' and

'ωρα, 'time.' Premature development of the body, or of some part.

HYPERI'CUM BACCIF'ERUM, *Arbus'cula gummif'era, Brazilien'sis, Caa-opia.* A Brazilian tree, whose bark admits a juice, when wounded, which resembles gamboge.

HYPERICUM OFFICINALE, H. perforatum — h. Officinarum, H. perforatum.

HYPERICUM PERFORA'TUM, *Hypericum, H. officina'lë* seu *officina'rum* seu *vulga'rē* seu *Virgin'icum, Fuga Dæ'monum, Androsæ'mum, Co'rion, Perforated* or *Common St. John's Wort,* (F.) *Millepertuis ordinaire.* It is aromatic and astringent, and enters into a number of aromatic preparations; and, amongst others, into the *Falltrancks.* The *Oil of St. John's Wort, O'leum hyperici, Bal'samum hyperici sim'plex,* is made by infusing ʒiv. of the flowers in a quart of *olive oil.* It is vulnerary.

HYPERICUM VIRGINICUM, H. perforatum — h. Vulgare, H. perforatum.

HYPERIDROSIS, Ephidrosis.
HYPERINESIS, Hypercatharsis.
HYPERINOSIS, Hypercatharsis.
HYPERINO'SIS, *Hyperplus'ma,* from 'υπερ, 'above,' and ις, ινος, 'flesh.' The condition of the blood in which it contains an increase in the proportion of fibrin, a decrease of the corpuscles in proportion to the excess of fibrin, and an increase of the fat, — as in inflammation. In proportion to the increase of the fibrin and fat, and the decrease of the corpuscles, the whole solid residue will be diminished. Also, morbidly increased muscular activity.—Siebenhaar.

HYPERLYMPH'IA, (F.) *Hyperlymphie;* from 'υπερ, 'in excess,' and *lympha.* Excessive formation or accumulation of lymph.

HYPERMÉTROHÉMIE, Metrohæmia.
HYPERMNE'SIA, from 'υπερ, 'in excess,' and μναομαι, 'I recollect.' Excessive memory.

HYPERMYEOLOHÆ'MIA, (F.) *Hyperémie de la Moëlle Épinière, Congestion sanguine rachidienne,* from 'υπερ, 'in excess,' μυελος, 'marrow,' and 'αιμα, 'blood.' Hyperæmia of the spinal marrow.

HYPERNÉPHROTROPHIE, from 'υπερ, 'in excess,' νεφρος, 'kidney,' and τροφη, 'nourishment.' Hypertrophy of the kidney.

HYPERNEU'RIA, from 'υπερ, 'in excess,' and νευρον, 'a nerve.' Excessive nervous activity.

HYPERNEURO'MA, same etymon. Morbid development of the neurine or nervous masses.

HYPERO-PHARYNGEUS, Palato-pharyngeus.

HYPERO'A, from 'υπερ, 'upon,' and ωον, 'a high place.' The palatine arch,—the base of the cranium.

HYPEROA, Palate.
HYPEROI'TIS, *Inflamma'tio pala'ti, Angi'na Palati'na,* (F.) *Inflammation du Palais;* from *hyperoa,* 'the palate,' and *itis,* a suffix denoting inflammation. Inflammation of the velum palati.

HYPEROÖCHAS'MA, from 'υπερωα, 'the palate, and χασμα, 'an opening;' *Lycos'toma, Pala'tum fissum.* Fissure of the palate.

HYPEROPSIA, Oxyopia.
HYPEROS, Pilum.
HYPEROSMIA, Hyperosphresia.
HYPEROSPHRE'SIA, *Hyperos'mia, Hyperæsthe'sia olfacto'ria, Olfac'tus acu'tus,* from 'υπερ, and οσφρησις, 'smell.' Excessive acuteness of smell.

HYPEROSTOSIS, Exostosis.
HYPERPATHI'A, from 'υπερ, 'in excess,' and παθος, 'suffering.' Excessive sensibility in disease.

HYPERPHLEBO'SIS, from 'υπερ, 'in excess,' and φλεψ, 'a vein.' Too great development of the venous system; predominant venosity.

HYPERPHLEGMASIA, Hyperphlogosis.
HYPERPHLOGO'SIS, *Epiphlogo'sis, Hyperphlegma'sia, Inflamma'tio peracu'ta,* from 'υπερ, 'above,' and φλογωσις, 'inflammation.' A high degree of inflammation.

HYPERPHRÉNIE, Mania.
HYPERPIMELE, see Polysarcia.
HYPERPLASMA, Hyperinosis.
HYPERPLEXIE, Ecstasis.
HYPERPNEUSTIA, Flatulence.
HYPERPRESBYTIA, Presbytia.
HYPERSARCHIDIOS, Physconia.
HYPERSARCO'MA, *Hypersarco'sis, Hypersarx'is,* from 'υπερ, 'above,' and σαρξ, 'flesh.' A soft fungous excrescence, especially such as appears upon ulcerated parts. — A fungosity.

HYPERSARCOSIS, Excrescence, Fungosity, —h. Cordis, Heart, hypertrophy of the.

HYPERSARXIS, Hypersarcoma.
HYPERSPADIAS, Epispadias.
HYPERSPASMIA, Convulsion.
HYPERSPLÉNOTROPHIE, Splenoncus.
HYPERSPONGIA, Spina ventosa.
HYPERSTHENI'A, *Hyperdyna'mia, Hyperzoödyna'mia, Status inflammato'rius verus;* from 'υπερ, 'beyond,' and σθενος, 'strength.' Superexcitement. A morbid condition, characterized by over-excitement of all the vital phenomena.

HYPERSTHENIC, Stimulant.
HYPERSTHENICUS, Active, Stimulant.
HYPERTON'IA, 'υπερ, 'beyond,' and τονος, 'tone.' Excess of tone in parts. It is opposed to atony.

HYPERTROPHÆ'MIA, from 'υπερ, 'above,' τροφη, 'nourishment,' and 'αιμα, 'blood.' A state in which the plastic powers of the blood are increased.

HYPERTROPHIA CEREBRI, Phrenauxe — h. Cordis, Heart, hypertrophy of the — h. Glandularum, Hyperadenosis—h. Hepatis, Hepatauxe —h. Intestinorum, Enterhypertrophia—h. Lienis, Splenoncus — h. Splenis, Splenoncus — h. Uteri, Metrauxe — h. Vesicæ urinariæ, Cystauxe.

HYPERTROPHIE DU CŒUR, Heart, hypertrophy of the—*h. du Foie,* Hepatauxe—*h. de la Rate,* Splenoncus — *h. du Corps Thyroïde,* Bronchocele.

HYPERTROPHIED, see Hypertrophy.
HYPERTROPHOUS, see Hypertrophy.
HY'PERTROPHY, *Hypertroph'ia,* from 'υπερ, 'beyond,' and τροφη, 'nourishment.' The state of a part in which the nutrition is performed with greater activity; and which, on that account, at length acquires unusual bulk. The part thus affected is said to be *hypertrophied* or *hypertrophous.*

HYPERURESIS, Enuresis — h. Aquosa, Diabetes.

HYPERURORRHEE, Diabetes—*h. Saccharine,* Diabetes (Mellitus.)

HYPERZOODYNAMIA, Hypersthenia.
HYPEX'ODOS, 'υπεξοδος, from 'υπο, 'beneath,' and εξοδος, 'passing out.' An alvine discharge or flux. — Hippocrates.

HYPEZOCUS, Diaphragm, Pleura.
HYPHA, Texture.
HYPHÆMA, Ecchymoma.
HYPHÆMATO'SIS, from 'υπο, 'under,' and 'αιματωσις, 'sanguification.' Morbidly diminished hæmatosis. — *Sanguifica'tio debil'ior.*

HYPHÆMOS, Subcruentus.
HYPHE, Texture.

HYPHYDROS, Hydropic.

HYPINO'SIS, *Hypoplas'ma*, from 'υπο,' 'under,' and ις, ινος, 'flesh.' The condition of the blood in which the quantity of fibrin is frequently less than in health, or if it amounts to the usual quantity, its proportion to the blood corpuscles is less than in health: the quantity of corpuscles is either absolutely increased or their proportion to the fibrin is larger than in healthy blood; the quantity of solid constituents is also frequently larger than in health. Such is the condition of the blood in fevers, hemorrhages, and polyæmia. — Simon.

HYPNÆSTHESIS, Somnolency.

HYPNIA'TER, (F.) *Hypniatre*, from 'υπνος, 'sleep,' and ιατρος, 'a physician.' A name given to deluded or designing persons who have affirmed that they were able, during their 'magnetic sleep,' to diagnosticate disease and its appropriate treatment.

HYPNIC, *Hyp'nicus*, from 'υπνος, 'sleep.' An agent that affects sleep. — Pereira.

HYPNOBATASIS, Somnambulism.
HYPNOBATES, Somnambulist.
HYPNOBATESIS, Somnambulism.
HYPNOBATIA, Somnambulism.

HYPNO'DES, 'υπνωδης, from 'υπνο,' 'under,' and 'υπνος, 'sleep.' One in a state of slumber or somnolency.

HYPNODIA, Somnolency.

HYPNOLOG"ICA, *Hypnolog"icē*. The part of hygiene which treats of sleep.

HYPNOL'OGY, *Hypnolog"ia*, from 'υπνος, and λογος, 'a discourse.' Same etymon. A treatise on sleep. The doctrine of sleep.

HYPNONERGIA, Somnambulism.
HYPNOPOEUS, Somniferous.
HYPNOS, Sleep.
HYPNOSIS BIOMAGNETICA, Sleep, magnetic.
HYPNOTIC, Somniferous.
HYPNOTISM, Somnambulism, magnetic; see Magnetism, animal.
HYPNOTIZED, see Mesmerized.

HYPO, 'υπο, 'under,' 'sub.' In composition.
HYPO, Hypochondriasis.

HYPOÆMA, Ecchymoma.
HYPOÆMIA, Ecchymoma.

HYPOBLEPH'ARUM, from 'υπο, 'under,' and βλεφαρον, 'eyelid.' Tumefaction under one or both eyelids. Also, an artificial eye, placed under the eyelids.

HYPOCAPNISMA, Suffimentum.
HYPOCAPNISMUS, Fumigation.

HYPOCARO'DES, *Subsopora'tus*, from 'υπο, 'under,' and καρος, 'a heavy sleep.' One who is in a state approaching carus. — Hippocrates.

HYPOCATHAR'SIS, from 'υπο, 'beneath,' and καθαρσις, 'purgation.' Too feeble purgation. A word opposed to hypercatharsis.

HYPOCATHARTICUS, Laxative.

HYPOCAUS'TUM, from 'υπο, 'beneath,' and καιω, 'I burn.' A name given to a stove, or any such contrivance, to sweat in. Also, a furnace in any subterraneous place, used for heating baths: — 'υποκαυστον, *Balnea'rium, Vapora'rium*.

HYPOCEPHALÆ'UM, from 'υπο, 'under,' and κεφαλη, 'head.' A pillow for the head.

HYPOCERCHA'LEON, from 'υπο, and κερχαλεος, 'hoarse.' Roughness of the fauces affecting the voice. — Hippocrates.

HYPOCHLORETUM SULPHUROSUM, Sulphur, chloride of.

HYPOCHLOROM'ELAS, *sub-pal'lidē ni'gricans*, from 'υπο, χλωρος, 'green,' and μελας, 'black.' A term applied to one whose skin is pale, with a blackish hue. — Hippocr., Galen.

HYPOCHOILION, Abdomen.

HY'POCHONDRE, *Hypochon'drium, Subcartilagin'eum, Re'gio Hypochondri'aca, Hypochon'driac Region*, from 'υπο, 'under,' and χονδρος, 'a cartilage.' Each lateral and superior region of the abdomen is so called, because it is bounded by the cartilaginous margin of the false ribs, which forms the base of the chest. There is a *right* and a *left* hypochondrium.

HYPOCHON'DRIAC, *Hypochondri'acus, Hypochondri'acal, Va'poury, Va'pourish*, (F.) *Hypochondriaque*. Same etymon. Belonging to hypochondriasis. One labouring under hypochondriasis.

HYPOCHONDRIACISMUS, Hypochondriasis.
HYPOCHONDRIALGIA, Hypochondriasis.
HYPOCHONDRIAQUE, Hypochondriac.

HYPOCHONDRI'ASIS. Same etymon. *Alu'sia hypochondriasis, Morbus hypochondri'acus, M. Resiccato'rius, M. Ructuo'sus, Malum hypochondri'acum, Hallucina'tio hypochondriasis, Hypochondriacis'mus, Hypochondricis'mus, Dyspep'sia hypochondriasis, Pas'sio hypochondriaca, Affec'tio hypochondriaca, Anathymi'asis, Hypercine'sis gastrica, Splenes, Melancholia nervea, M. flatuo'sa, M. hypochondri'aca, Suffoca'tio hypochondri'aca, Morbus flatuo'sus, M. erudito'rum, Fomes ventric'uli, Hypochondrism, Hypo, Spleen, Vapours, English Malady, Low Spirits*, (F.) *Hypochondrie, Maladie imaginaire, Maladie Anglaise, Affection vaporeuse, Vapeurs*. This disease is probably so called, from the circumstance of some hypochondriacs having felt an uneasy sensation in the hypochondriac regions. The disease seems really to be, as Pinel has classed it, a species of neurosis, and of mental alienation, which is observed in persons who in other respects are of sound judgment, but who reason erroneously on whatever concerns their own health. Hypochondriasis is characterized by disordered digestion, without fever or local lesion; flatulence; borborygmi; extreme increase of sensibility; palpitations; illusions of the senses; a succession of morbid feelings, which appear to simulate the greater part of diseases; panics; exaggerated uneasiness of various kinds; chiefly in what regards the health, &c. Indigestion has usually been considered the cause of hypochondriasis. They are, unquestionably, much connected with each other: but there is every reason to believe, that the seat of the affection is really, though functionally, in the brain. The disease almost always appears at the adult age, most commonly in irritable individuals; and, in those exhausted, or rather in the habit of being exhausted, by mental labour, overwhelmed with domestic or public affairs, &c.

The treatment is almost entirely moral. The condition of the digestive function must, however, be accurately attended to.

HYPOCHONDRICISMUS, Hypochondriasis.
HYPOCHONDRISM, Hypochondriasis.
HYPOCHOREMA, Excrement.
HYPOCHORESIS, Dejection, Defecation, Excrement.
HYPOCHORETICUS, Cathartic.
HYPOCHYMA, Cataract.
HYPOCHYROSIS, Barycoia.
HYPOCHYSIS HÆMATODES, Hæmophthalmia.
HYPOCISTIS, Cytinus.

HYPOCLEP'TICUM, from 'υπο, 'beneath,' and κλεπτω, 'I steal.' A chymical vessel, formerly used for separating oil from water.

HYPOCŒLIS, Palpebra inferior.
HYPOCŒLIUM, Abdomen.

HYPOCŒLUM, Hypocoilon, Palpebra inferior.

HYPOCOI'LON, *Hypocœ'lon, Hypocœ'lum, Hypoœ'ylum*, from 'υπο, 'under,' and κοιλον, 'a cavity.' A cavity situate under the lower eyelid. The lower eyelid itself.

HYPOCOPHOSIS, Baryecoia, Deafness.

HYPOCRA'NIUM (APOSTEMA), from 'υπο, 'under,' and κρανιον, 'the cranium.' A collection of pus between the cranium and dura mater.

HYPOCYLUM, Hypocoilon, Palpebra inferior.

HYPOCYSTEOTOMIA, see Lithotomy.

HYPODERIS, Epideris.

HYPODERMAT'OMY, *Hypodermatom'ia,* from 'υπο, 'under,' δερμα, 'the skin,' and τομη, 'incision.' The section of subcutaneous parts, as of tendons and muscles.

HYPODERMIS, Clitoris, Epideris.

HYPODERRHIS, Epideris.

HYPODESMA, Bandage.

HYPODYNAMIC, Adynamic.

HYPODYN'IA, from 'υπο, 'under,' and οδυνη, 'pain.' *Dolor mitis* seu *lenis.* A slight pain.

HYPOGALA, Hypopyon.

HYPOGASTRAL'GIA, from 'υπογαστριον, 'the hypogastrium,' and αλγος, 'pain.' Pain in the hypogastrium.

HYPOGAS'TRIC, *Hypogas'tricus.* Relating or belonging to the hypogastrium.

HYPOGASTRIC ARTERY, *A. Ili'aca inter'na, A. Ili'aca poste'rior, A. pelvienne*—(Ch.), is the more internal of the two branches into which the primary iliac divides. It descends into the cavity of the pelvis, and gives off a considerable number of branches, which arise, at times, separately; at others, by common trunks. These branches are, 1. The *posterior*, i. e. the ilio-lumbar arteries, lateral, sacral, and gluteal. 2. The *anterior*, i. e. the umbilical, vesical, and obturator. 3. The *internal*, the middle hemorrhoidal arteries, uterine, and vaginal in women. 4. The *inferior*, i. e. the *ischiatic arteries*, and internal pudic.

HYPOGAS'TRIC GAN'GLION. A large nervous ganglion, described by Dr. Robt. Lee as seated on each side of the cervix uteri, immediately behind the ureter; which receives the greater number of the nerves of the hypogastric and sacral plexuses, and distributes branches to the uterus, vagina, bladder, and rectum.

HYPOGASTRIC OPERATION OF LITHOTOMY, (F.) *Taille hypogastrique.* The high operation, or that practised above the pubes.

HYPOGASTRIC PLEXUS, *Plexus sous-mésentérique* of Winslow, is situate at the lateral and posterior parts of the rectum and the *bas fond* of the bladder. It is formed by the sacral nerves and the inferior mesenteric plexus, and gives off numerous filaments, which accompany the arteries that pass to the rectum and genital organs.

HYPOGASTRIC VEIN furnishes nearly the same branches.

HYPOGASTRION, Abdomen, Hypogastrium.

HYPOGAS'TRIUM, *Hypogas'trion*, from 'υπο, 'under,' and γαστηρ, 'the stomach or belly;' *Etron, ητρον, Venter imus, V. parvus, Aqualic'ulus, Sumen, Rumen.* The lower part of the abdomen. The *Hypogastric region, Re'gio hypogas'trica* seu *hypogas'tria*, which extends as high as three fingers' breadth beneath the umbilicus, is divided into three secondary regions — one *middle* or *pubic*, and two *lateral* or *inguinal*.

HYPOGASTROCE'LE, from 'υπο, 'under,' γαστηρ, 'the stomach or belly,' and κηλη, 'a tumour.' Hernia in the hypogastric region, occurring through the separated fibres of the lower part of the linea alba. See Hernia, hypogastric.

HYPOGASTRODID'YMUS, *Did'ymus Symphyohypogas'tricus, Ischiopa'ges*, from 'υπο, 'under,' γαστηρ, 'the belly,' and διδυμος, 'a twin.' A monstrosity in which twins are united by the hypogastrium.—Gurlt.

HYPOGASTRORIXIS, Eventration.

HYPOGLOSSA, Hypoglottides.

HYPOGLOSSIA, Hypoglottides.

HYPOGLOSSIADENI'TIS, from 'υπο, 'under,' γλωσσα, 'tongue,' αδην, 'a gland,' and *itis*, denoting inflammation. *Inflamma'tio glandula'rum sublingua'lium.* Inflammation of the sublingual gland.

HYPOGLOSSIDIA, Hypoglottides.

HYPOGLOSSIS, Ranula.

HYPOGLOSSIUM, Ranula.

HYPOGLOSSUM, Ruscus hypoglossum, Ranula.

HYPOGLOS'SUS, from 'υπο, 'under,' and γλωσσα, 'the tongue.' That which is under the tongue.

HYPOGLOSSUS, *Hypoglossal Nerve, Nerf Hypoglosse* ou *Grand Hypoglosse, Hypoglossien* (Ch.), *Lingual N., Gustatory N., Lingua'lis Me'dius*, is the *ninth pair of nerves* of many anatomists. It arises by ten or twelve very fine filaments from the grooves, which separate the corpora pyramidalia from the C. olivaria; issues from the cranium by the foramen condyloideum anterius; and divides, near the angle of the jaw, into two branches; the one, the *cervica'lis descendens* or *descen'dens noni.* It forms, with the cervical plexus, a large anastomotic arch, and furnishes branches to several of the muscles of the neck. The other, the *lingual branch*, is the continuation of the principal trunk, and gives its numerous filaments to the muscles of the tongue and pharynx. The ninth pair communicates motion to the muscles to which it is distributed.

HYPOGLOTTIA, Hypoglottides.

HYPOGLOTT'IDES, (PILULÆ,) *Hypoglos'sia, Hypoglot'tia, Hypoglos'sa, Hypoglot'ta, Hypoglossid'ia, Pil'ulæ sublingua'les.* Pills placed under the tongue to dissolve there.

HYPOGLOTTIS, Ranula.

HYPOGLU'TIS, from 'υπο, 'under,' and γλουτος, 'the nates.' The lower and projecting part of the nates.— Gorræus.

HYPOGNATHADEN, Submaxillary gland.

HYPOGNATHADENI'TIS, *Hyposialadeni'tis*, from *hypognathaden*, the submaxillary gland, and *itis*, denoting inflammation. Inflammation of the submaxillary gland.

HYPOLEPSIOMANIA, Melancholy.

HYPO'MIA, from 'υπο, 'under, and ωμος, 'the shoulder.' The projecting part of the shoulder.—Castelli, Galen.

HYPOMIA, Axilla.

HYPOMNESIS, Memory.

HYPONARTHÉCIE, Hyponarthe'cia, from 'υπο, 'under,' and ναρθηξ, 'a splint.' A term used by M. Mayor for his mode of treating fractures by position only, — the limb resting upon a properly cushioned board or splint.

HYPONEU'RIA, from 'υπο, 'under,' and νευρον, 'a nerve.' Morbidly diminished nervous energy.

HYPON'OMOS, *Ulcus subtus depas'cens*, from 'υπο, 'under,' and νεμω, 'I feed.' A deep fistula or ulcer.

HYPON'YCHON, from 'υπο, 'under,' and ονυξ, 'the nail.' *Ecchymo'ma Hyponychon.* Effusion of blood under a nail.

HYPOPATHI'A, *Subaffec'tio*, from 'υπο, 'under,' and παθος, 'disease.' A disease of a slight character.

HYPOPATUS, Dejectio.

HYPOPE'DIUM, from 'υπο, 'under,' and πους, 'the foot,' A cataplasm for the sole of the foot.

HYPOPH'ASIS, from 'υπο, 'under,' and φαινω, 'I appear.' The state of the eyes in which the white only is seen through the opening of the eyelids. — Hippocrates.

HYPOPHLEGMASIA, Subinflammatio.

HYPOPH'ORA, from 'υπο, 'under,' and φερω, 'I carry;' *Ulcus sinuo'sum seu fistulo'sum.* A fistulous ulcer. — Galen. A dejection.

HYPOPHTHALMIA, Hypopyon.

HYPOPHTHAL'MION, from 'υπο, 'under,' and οφθαλμος, 'the eye.' That part under the eye where œdema generally commences in chronic diseases and in cachexia. — Hippocrates.

HYPOPHYSIS, Cataract, Epigone — h. Cerebri, Pituitary gland.

HYPOP'ITYS LANUGINO'SA, *American Pine-sap, False Beech-drops, Birds' Nest.* Indigenous; flowering from June to August. Order, Ericaceæ. Used as a nervine in the form of the powdered root.

HYPO'PIUM, from 'υπο, 'under,' and ωψ, 'eye.' The part of the face under the eye: — a black eye.

HYPOPIUM Os, Malæ os.

HYPOPLASMA, Hypinosis.

HYPOPLASTÆ'MA, from 'υπο, 'under,' πλαστικος, 'formative,' and 'αιμα, 'blood.' Diminished plasticity of the blood.

HYPOPLEURIUS, Pleura.

HYPOPO'DIA, *Supplanta'lia, Suppeda'nea,* from 'υπο, 'under,' and πους, 'the foot.' Remedies, as sinapisms, which are applied under the foot.

HYPOP'YON, *Hypop'yum, Hypophthal'mia, Pyophthal'mia, Empye'sis seu Diapye'sis Oc'uli, Oc'ulus purulen'tus, Lunella, Hypog'ala, Hypopyum lac'teum, Pyo'sis, Abscessus Oc'uli, Parop'sis Staphylo'ma purulentum;* from 'υπο, 'under,' and πυον, 'pus;' because the pus is under the cornea. This name has been given to small abscesses between the laminæ of the cornea, as well as to different purulent collections in the chambers of the eye; hence, some pathologists have distinguished *Hypop'yon of the chambers* from *Hypop'yon of the Cor'nea.* In abscesses of the chambers, the purulent matter is mixed with the aqueous humour, which it renders turbid; and is deposited particularly at the lower part of the eye; forming behind the cornea a kind of whitish crescent, that rises more or less before the pupil, and closes it entirely or in part. It requires the use of local and general antiphlogistics, and sorbefacients. At times, it is necessary to puncture the cornea and evacuate the pus.

HYPOPYUM LACTEUM, Hypopyon.

HYPORIN'ION, *Hyporrhin'ium,* from 'υπο, 'under,' and ριν, 'the nose.' That part of the beard which grows beneath the nose. The mustaches. Also, the upper lip.

HYPORRHYSIS, Defluxion, Prolapsus.

HYPOSA'PRUS, *Subputris, Putres'cens.* Growing putrid. Slightly putrid.

HYPOSAR'CA, from 'υπο, 'under,' and σαρξ, 'flesh.' *Hyposarcid'ius,* Anasarca. In Linné's and in Cullen's Nosology, it is synonymous with *Physconia.*

HYPOSARCIDIUS, Anasarca, Hyposarca.

HYPOSARCO'SIS, from 'υπο, 'under,' and σαρκωσις, 'a fleshy growth.' A small, fleshy growth: — a wart.

HYPOSIAGONARTHRI'TIS, from 'υπο, 'under,' σιαγων, 'the jawbone,' αρθρον, 'a joint,' and *itis,* denoting inflammation; *Inflamma'tio artic'uli maxill'æ inferio'ris.* Inflammation of the joint of the lower jaw.

HYPOSIALADENITIS, Hypognathadenitis.

HYPOSPA'DIA, from 'υπο, 'under,' and σπαω, 'I draw.' A malformation, in which the canal of the urethra, instead of opening at the apex of the glans, terminates at its base, or beneath the penis, at a greater or less distance from the symphysis pubis. When the orifice of the urethra is very near the root of the penis, the scrotum is divided, as it were, into two great labia; and this malformation has often been taken for a case of hermaphrodism. Hypospadias is ordinarily incurable; and an idea has been entertained that it is the cause of impotence. It is not exactly so; but it renders impregnation less probable.

HYPOSPA'DIAS, *Hypospadiæ'us, Hypospad'icus.* One affected with hypospadia.

HYPOSPHAG'MA, from 'υπο, 'under,' and σφαζω, 'I kill.' The coagulated blood, which is collected when an animal is killed and used for food. Also, an effusion of blood, especially under the conjunctiva.

HYPOSPHAGMA, Hæmophthalmia.

HYPOSTAPHYLE, Staphylœdema.

HYPOSTAPHYLITIS, Staphylœdema.

HYPOS'TASES, from 'υπο, 'under,' and στασις, 'the act of placing.' Morbid depositions in the body.

HYPOSTASIS, Sediment.

HYPOSTAT'IC, *Hypostat'icus,* from 'υπο, 'under,' and στασις, 'stagnation.' Relating to hypostases, sediments or depositions.

HYPOSTATIC HYPERÆ'MIA. A congestion of blood in the vessels of a part caused by its depending position.

HYPOSTEMA, Sediment.

HYPOSTHENIC, Contrastimulant.

HYPOS'TROPHE, 'υποστροφη, 'change of position,' from 'υπο, and στρεφω, 'I turn.' Act of a patient turning himself. Also, a relapse or return of a disease. — Hippoc., Foësius.

HYPOSYPH'ILIS, from 'υπο, 'under,' and *Syphilis.* A mild form of syphilis.

HYPOTH'ENAR, *Sub'vola,* from 'υπο, 'under,' and θεναρ, 'the palm of the hand or sole of the foot.' *Hypothenar Eminence.* The fleshy projection of the palmar surface of the hand, which corresponds with the little finger, and is supported by the fifth metacarpal bone. This eminence is formed of four muscles: the *Palmaris brevis, Adductor minimi digiti, Flexor brevis minimi digiti,* and *Opponens minimi digiti.* The name *Hypothenar* has also been given to different muscles of the hand. The *Hypothenar min'imi digiti* of Riolan comprehended the *Abductor, Flexor brevis* and *Opponens minimi digiti;* and his muscle, *Hypothenar pol'licis,* corresponded to the *Abductor,* and a portion of the *Flexor brevis pollicis.* Winslow called *muscle petit hypothénar* ou *hypothénar du petit doigt,* the *Adductor minimi digiti.*

HYPOTHENAR MINIMI DIGITI, Flexor parvus minimi digiti — h. Minor metacarpeus, Abductor minimi digiti — h. Riolani, Flexor parvus minimi digiti.

HYPOTHETON, Suppository.

HYPOTHYMIAMA, Fumigation.

HYPOTHYMIASIS, Fumigation.

HYPO'TIUM, (*Emplastrum ;*) from 'υπο, 'under,' and ους, 'the ear.' *Emplastrum auricula'rē ;* a plaster applied behind or under the ear.

HYPOTROPE, Relapse.

HYPOTROPH'IA, from 'υπο, 'under,' and τροφη, 'nourishment.' Scanty nourishment, or nutrition.

HYPOTROPIASMUS, Relapse.

HYPOTRYGUS, Feculent.

HYPOUTRION, Abdomen.

HYPOX'YS EREC'TA, *Stargrass;* indigenous; *Order*, Amaryllidaceæ. The root is eaten, and has been used as a vulnerary; and in chronic ulcers and agues.

HYPOZO'MA, from 'υπο, 'under,' and ζωννυμι, 'I bind round;' *Membrana succin'gens.* A membrane or septum, as the mediastinum, diaphragm, &c.

HYPPOCRAS, Claret.
HYPSELOGLOSSUS, Basioglossus.
HYPSILODES, OS, Hyoides, os.
HYPSILOGLOSSUS, Hyoglossus.
HYPSOPHO'NUS, from 'υψος, 'high,' and φωνη, 'voice.' One who has a clear loud voice.
HYPSOSIS, Sublimation.
HYPTIASMA, Supination.
HYPTIAS'MOS, from 'υπτιαζω, 'I lie with the face upwards.' Lying in a supine posture. Also, inversion of the stomach, as in nausea, regurgitation, or vomiting.—Hippocr., Galen.

HYPU'LUS, from 'υπο, and ουλη, 'cicatrix.' Imperfectly cicatrized.

Ulcera Hypu'la. Ulcers healed at the top, but not at the bottom.

HYRA'CEUM. A substance found in the Cape Colony, which Thunberg and other travellers mistook for a kind of bitumen; but, according to Dr. Pappe, it is obtained from the urine of the *Klipdas* or *Hyrax Capensis*, which, when passed, is thick and of a glutinous nature. The animal is in the habit of evacuating the urine at one spot, where its aqueous parts evaporate in the sun—the more tenacious adhering to the rock and hardening.

In smell, and medical properties, it most resembles castor, which, according to Dr. Pappe, it may replace. It is used by the Cape farmers in nervous and spasmodic affections.

HYRAX CAPENSIS, see Hyraceum.
HYRTOCHEILIDES, Labia pudendi.
HYSSOP, Hyssopus—h. Hedge, Gratiola officinalis.

HYSSOPI'TES. Ancient name of a wine, of which hyssop was the chief ingredient, and which Dioscorides extolled in chronic inflammation of the chest. It was regarded as diuretic and emmenagogue.

HYSSO'PUS, from the Hebr. *Azob, Cassi'la, Hyssopus officina'lis, Common hyssop.* It has been chiefly used as an aromatic, stimulant, and pectoral, in the form of infusion.

HYSTERA, 'υστερα, 'υστερη, 'the uterus.' Hence: HYSTERA, Secundines.

HYSTERAL'GIA, *Hysterodyn'ia*, (F.) *Fortraiture*, from 'υστερα, 'the uterus,' and αλγος, 'pain.' Pain in the uterus. *Irritable uterus*, (F.) *Névralgie de l'uterus.* Hippocrates uses the epithet *Hysteral'ges*, υστεραλγης, for any thing that excites uterine pain; and, especially, for vinegar.

HYSTERALGIA CATARRHALIS, Metrorrheuma—h. Galactica, Phlegmatia alba dolens—h. Lochialis, Dyslochia—h. Rheumatica, Metrorrheuma.

HYSTERATRE'SIA, from 'υστερα, 'the uterus,' and ατρητος, 'imperforate.' Imperforation of the os uteri.

HYSTERELCO'SIS, from 'υστερα, 'uterus,' and 'ελκος, 'an ulcer.' *U'teri exulcera'tio, U'teri ulcus.* Ulceration of the uterus.

HYSTERELOSIS, Hysteroloxia.
HYSTEREMPHYSEMA, Physometra.
HYSTE'RIA, *H. vaga, Hystericis'mus, Hysterismus, Hysterias, Hysteri'asis, Hysteropathi'a, Hyperoinesia uteri'na, H. hyste'ria, Uteri adscensus, Suffoca'tio hyster'ica, S. uteri'na, S. Mulie'rum, Asthma u'teri, Prafoca'tio matri'cis seu uteri'na, Syspa'sia hysteria, Malum hyster'icum, M. hystericohypochondri'acum, Vapo'res uteri'ni,*

Affec'tio hyster'ica, Passio hysterica, Morbus hyster'icus, Strangula'tio uteri'na, S. Vulvæ, Vapours, Hyster'ics, Hysteric fit, (F.) *Hystérie, Mal de Mère, Maladie imaginaire, Passion hystérique, Suffocation utérine, Etranglement, Épilepsie utérine, Vapeurs, Maux de Nerfs,* from 'υστερα, 'the uterus.' A species of neurosis, classed amongst the spasmi by Sauvages and Cullen, and in the *Névroses de la génération,* by Pinel. It received the name of *hysteria*, because it was reputed to have its seat in the uterus. It generally occurs in paroxysms; the principal characters of which consist in alternate fits of laughing and crying, with a sensation as if a ball set out from the uterus and ascended towards the stomach, chest, and neck, producing a sense of strangulation. If the attack be violent, there is, sometimes, loss of consciousness (although the presence of consciousness generally distinguishes it from epilepsy) and convulsions. The duration of the attacks is very variable. It appears to be dependent upon irregularity of nervous distribution in very impressible persons, and is not confined to the female; for well marked cases of hysteria are occasionally met with in men. During the fit,—dashing cold water on the face; stimulants applied to the nose or exhibited internally, and antispasmodics form the therapeutical agents. Exercise, tranquillity of mind, amusing and agreeable occupations constitute the prophylactics. See Mania, dancing.

HYSTERIA CATALEPTICA, Catalepsy—h. Vaga, Hysteria.
HYSTERIAS, Hysteria.
HYSTERIASIS, Hysteria.
HYSTERICA, see Hysterical.
HYSTERICAL, *Hyster'icus, Va'pourish, Va'pouring*, (F.) *Hyste'rique.* Same etymon as hysterical. Relating to, or affected with hysteria.

The word *hysterica* was used by Martial for a female affected with nymphomania or with strong sexual desires.

HYSTERICISMUS, Hysteria.
HYSTERICS, Hysteria.
HYSTÉRIE, Hysteria.
HYSTERISMUS, Hysteria.
HYSTERITES, Hydrometra.
HYSTERITIS, Metritis, Hydrometra.
HYSTEROCARCINOMA, Metrocarcinoma.
HYSTEROCE'LE, from 'υστερα, 'the womb,' and κηλη, 'hernia.' *Hernia uteri, Hernia of the womb.* This is a rare disease. The womb may protrude through the inguinal or the crural canal, or through the lower part of the linea alba.

HYSTEROCELE NUDA, Prolapsus uteri.
HYSTEROCOLICA, Colica uterina.
HYSTEROCNES'MUS; from 'υστερα, 'uterus,' and κνησμος, 'itching.' Pruritus of the uterus or genitals.

HYSTEROCYESIS, Pregnancy.
HYSTERO-CYSTIC, *Hys'terocys'ticus,* from 'υστερα, 'the uterus,' and κυστις, 'the bladder.' Relating to the uterus and bladder. Some authors have called *Hystero-cystic Retention of urine,* that which is caused by the compression of the bladder by the uterus, during pregnancy.

HYSTERO-CYSTOCE'LE, from 'υστερα, 'the womb,' κυστις, 'the bladder,' and κηλη, 'a tumour.' Hernia of the uterus complicated with displacement of the bladder.

HYSTERODYNIA, Hysteralgia.
HYSTERŒDEMA, Hydrometra.
HYS'TEROID, *Hystero'des, Hysteroi'des,* from 'hysteria,' and ειδος, 'resemblance.' Resembling hysteria;—as a hysteroid disease, symptom, &c.

HYSTEROL'OGY, *Hysterolog''ia,* from 'υστερα, 'the uterus,' and λογος, 'a description.' A treatise on the sound and morbid uterus.

HYSTEROLOX'IA, *Hysterelo'sis, Oliq'uitas u'teri, Situs obli'quus uteri, Flexio seu Versio incomple'ta uteri, Inclina'tio uteri, Metrolox'ia, Metrocampe'is, Uterus obli'quus, U. Inclina'tus;* from '*υστερα*,' 'the uterus,' and '*λοξος*,' 'oblique.' An oblique position of the uterus, occurring during pregnancy. *Anteversion of the uterus, Hysterolox'ia anterior, Anteversio uteri, Prona'tio uteri, Venter propendens;* and *Retroversion of the uterus, Hysterolox'ia posterior, Retrover'sio uteri, Reflex'io uteri completa,* are varieties.

HYSTEROMALA'CIA, *Hysteromalaco'sis, Hysteromalaco'ma, Metromalaco'sis, Metromalaco'ma, Malaco'sis uteri, Emollit"ies uteri morbosa, Putrescen'tia u'teri grav'idi,* from '*υστερα*,' 'the uterus,' and *μαλακια*, 'softness.' Softness of the uterus during pregnancy, which renders it liable to rupture in labour.

HYSTEROMALACOMA, Hysteromalacia.

HYSTEROMANIA, Nymphomania.

HYSTEROMOCHLIUM, Lever.

HYSTERON'CUS, from '*υστερα*,' 'the uterus,' and *ογκος*, 'tumour.' *Tumor uteri.* A tumour of the uterus.

HYSTERO-PARAL'YSIS, from '*υστερα*,' 'the uterus,' and *παραλυσις*, 'paralysis.' Paralysis of the uterus.

HYSTEROPATHI'A, from '*υστερα*,' 'the uterus,' and *παθος*, 'suffering.' Disease or suffering in the uterus. Also, hysteria, and deuteropathia.

HYSTEROPHYSE, Physometra.

HYSTEROPH'YSIS, from '*υστερα*,' 'the uterus,' and *φυση*, 'wind.' Distention of the uterus with air; *Emphysema uteri.*

HYSTEROPLEGIA, Hysteroparalysis.

HYSTEROPOLYPUS, Metropolypus.

HYSTEROPSOPHIA, Physometra.

HYSTEROPTO'SIS, from '*υστερα*,' 'the womb,' and *πτωσις*, 'fall;' *Prolapsus uteri.* Also *Inversio uteri, Anas'trophê uteri.* In a general sense, a protrusion of any of the genital organs or of excrescences from them into the genital passages; *Ædoptosis.*

HYSTEROPTOSIS, Prolapsus uteri—h. Vaginæ prolapsus, Prolapsus vaginæ.

HYSTERORRHAGIA SANGUINEA, Metorrhagia.

HYSTERORRHEXIS, Uterus, rupture of the.

HYSTERORRHŒA, Metrorrhagia—h. Mucosa, Leucorrhœa.

HYSTEROSALPINX, Tube, Fallopian.

HYSTEROSCIRRHUS, Metroscirrhus.

HYS'TEROSCOPE, from '*υστερα*,' 'the uterus,' and *σκοπεω*, 'I view.' A metallic mirror, used in inspecting the state of the os uteri for throwing the rays of a taper to the bottom of the speculum uteri.—Colombat de l'Isère.

HYSTEROSTOMA, Os uteri.

HYSTEROSTOMAT'OMUS, from '*υστερα*,' 'the womb,' *στομα*, 'orifice,' and *τεμνειν*, 'to cut.' An instrument invented by Coutouly for dividing the os uteri, when it is important to deliver immediately, as in cases of convulsions.

HYSTEROSTOMIUM, Os uteri.

HYSTEROTOM'IA, *Hysterot'omy.* Same etymon as Hysterotomus. Cæsarean section. Also, dissection of the uterus.

HYSTEROTOMOTOCIA, Cæsarean section.

HYSTEROT'OMUS, from '*υστερα*,' 'the womb,' and *τεμνειν*, 'to cut.' An instrument for dividing the womb through the vagina. It is a kind of *Bistouri caché,* and is intended to divide the cervix uteri.

HYSTREMPHYSEMA, Physometra.

HYSTRIASIS, Hystriciasis.

HYSTRICI'ASIS, *Hystri'asis, Hys'trix, Hystricis'mus, Osrostro'sis, Tricho'sis seto'sa,* from '*υστριξ*, 'a hedgehog or porcupine.' A disease of the hairs, in which they stand erect like the quills of the porcupine.

HYSTRICISMUS, Hystriciasis.

HYSTRIX, Hystriciasis.

HYVES, Hives.

I.

IAMA, Medicament.

IAMATOLOGY, Materia medica.

IAMATOSYNTAXIOLOGIA, see Prescription.

IAMATOSYNTAXIS, see Composition.

IAMATOTAXIOLOGIA, see Prescription.

IASIMOS, Curable.

IASIS, Curation.

IATERIA, Medicina.

IATERIUS, Medicinal.

IATRALEIP'TICÊ, *Iatralipticê (Ars), Iatraleiptic method;* same etymon. The method of treating diseases adopted by the Iatraleiptes,— that is, by friction chiefly.

IATRALEP'TES, *Iatraleip'tes, Iatralip'ta, Iatroleip'tes, Med'icus Unguenta'rius;* from *ιατρος*, 'a physician,' and *αλειφω*, 'I anoint.' One who treats diseases by unguents, frictions, and by external means generally. Prodicus, a disciple of Æsculapius, was the chief of the Iatraleptes.

IATRALIPTES, Iatraleiptes.

IATRALIPTICE, Iatraleiptice.

IATREUSIOLOG"IA, from *ιατρευσις*, 'the exercise of the art of healing,' and *λογος*, 'a description.' The doctrine of the exercise of the healing art.—Reil.

IATREUSIS. The exercise of the healing art.

IATRIA, Medicine.

IATRICE, Medicina.

IATRI'NÊ, Medicina. Also, a female practitioner of medicine; a midwife.

IATRI'ON, *Iatre'on, Iätron.* The house or office of a physician or surgeon. Also, the physician's fee or *honorarium.*

IATROCHEMIA, Chymiatria.

IATROCHYMIA, Chymiatria.

IATROGNOM'ICA, *Iatrognom'icê;* from *ιατρος*, 'a physician,' and *γινοσκω*, 'I know.' A knowledge of medical objects.—Hufeland.

IATROLEIPTES, Iatraleiptes.

IATROLOG"IA, *Iatrol'ogy,* from *ιατρος*, 'a physician,' and *λογος*, 'a description.' A treatise on physic and physicians.

IATRO-MATHEMATICAL PHYSICIANS, *Iatromathemat'ici.* Mechanical physicians.

IATROMECHANICI, Mechanical physicians.

IATRON, Iatrion.

IATROPHYSICS, Physics, medical.

IATROSOPHIS'TA, from *ιατρος*, 'a physician,' and *σοφιστης*, 'one skilled in an art or science.' A learned, or theoretically educated physician.

IATROTECH'NA, *Iatrotech'nes;* from *ιατρος*,

'a physician,' and τεχνη, 'art.' A practical physician or surgeon.

IATROTECHNICE, Medicina, Therapeutics.

IATRUS, Physician; also, a surgeon.

IBERIS, Lepidium iberis.

IBE'RIS AMA'RA, *Bitter candytuft*, (F.) *Passerage*. A small herbaceous plant, *Ord.* Cruciferæ, indigenous in Europe, which was employed, of old, in gout, rheumatism, &c. The seeds have been used, in the dose of one to three grains, in asthma, bronchitis, dropsy, and hypertrophy of the heart. It is said to possess acro-narcotic properties; but it is not much used.

IBERIS BURSA PASTORIS, Thlaspi bursa — i. Campestris, Thlaspi campestre — i. Sophia, Cardamine pratensis.

IBICUIBA, *Becuiba, Becuiba nux*. A species of nut from Brazil, the emulsive kernel of which is ranked amongst balsamic remedies.

IBIS, ιβις. A bird held sacred by the Egyptians. When sick, it is asserted that it was wont to inject the water of the Nile into its fundament: whence, according to Langius, was learned the use of glysters.

IBISCHA MISMALVA, Althæa.

IBISCUS, Althæa.

IBIXUMA, Saponaria.

ICE, Sax. iſ, *Gla'cies, Frozen water*, (F.) *Glace*. Iced water is much used internally, as the best refrigerant in fever. It is, also, applied externally, in cases of external inflammation, as well as in phrenitic and hernial affections, &c.

ICE-COLD, *Icy cold*, (F.) *Froid glacial*. A very strong morbid sensation of cold, compared by the patient to that which would be produced by the application of pieces of ice.

ICELAND, MINERAL WATERS OF. Hot springs are found in every part of Iceland. The most noted of these is one called Geyser, two days' journey from Hecla, and near Skalholt. The diameter of the basin is 59 feet; and the height to which the water is thrown is often more than 100. The heat of the water is 212°.

ICE-PLANT, Mesembryanthemum crystallinum, Monotropa uniflora.

ICHNUS, ιχνος. The foot. The sole of the foot. The heel.

ICHOR, ιχωρ, *Ichos*. The serum of the blood, *Sanies, Sordes, Virus, Pus malig'num, Tabum*. A thin, aqueous, and acrid discharge.

ICHOROIDES, Ichorous.

ICH'OROUS, *Ichoro'sus, Ichoroi'des, Sanio'sus, Sa'nious*. Belonging to or resembling ichor.

ICHTHYA, Hook, blunt.

ICHTHYOCOL'LA, from ιχθυς, 'a fish,' and κολλα, 'glue.' *Colla Pis'cium, l'singlass, Fishglue*, (F.) *Ichthyocolle, Colle de Poisson*. A name given to the dried fish-bladder of the *Acipenser huso*, and other species of acipenser, which is almost wholly composed of gelatin, and is employed in medicine in the formation of nutritive jellies. It is, also, occasionally used in anatomical injections. The *English Court Plaster* is made with it.

ICHTHYOPH'AGISTS, *Ichthyoph'agi*, from ιχθυς, 'a fish,' and φαγω, 'I eat.' People who feed habitually on fish;—generally the most uncivilised of mankind.

ICHTHYOPHAGOUS, Piscivorous.

ICHTHYOSE, Ichthyosis.

ICHTHYO'SIS, from ιχθυς, 'a fish,' from the resemblance of the scales to those of a fish. *Lepido'sis Ichthyi'asis, Lepra Ichthyo'sis, Lepido'sis Ichthyo'sis, Alvaras nigra* (Arab.), *Impeti'go excorticati'va*, (F.) *Ichthyose ; Fishskin, Porcupine Disease*. A permanently harsh, dry, scaly, and, in some cases, almost horny texture of the integuments of the body, unconnected with internal disorder. Willan and Bateman have two varieties, *I. simplex* and *I. cornea*. Alibert has three, the *I. nacrée* or *pearly*, the *I. cornée*, and the *I. pellagre* or *Pellagra*.

ICHTHYOSIS PELLAGRA, Pellagra.

ICHTHYOSIS SEBA'CEA, *Seba'ceous Ichthyo'sis*. A morbid incrustation of a concrete sebaceous substance upon the surface of the epidermis, confounded, according to Mr. E. Wilson, with ichthyosis, to which it bears a close resemblance. In many cases there is neither redness nor heat, nor is the affection often accompanied by constitutional symptoms.

ICHTHYOTOX'ICUM, from ιχθυς, 'a fish,' and τοξικον, 'a poison.' Fish poison.

I'CICA ARACOUCHI'NI. *Aracouchini* is a balsam, extracted by incision, from this tree in Guyana. The Galibis use it for healing wounds.

ICICA ICICARIBA, see Amyris elemifera.

IOTÈRE, Icterus — *i. Bleu*, Cyanopathy — *i. des Nouveau-nés*, Icterus infantum — *i. Noire*, Melæna.

ICTERIC FEVER, REMITTING, see Relapse.

ICTERICUS, Antiicteric. Also, relating to, or resembling Icterus,—*Ictero'des*.

ICTERITIA ALBA, Chlorosis—i. Flava, Icterus—i. Rubea, Erysipelas—i. Rubra, Erysipelas.

ICTERODES, Icterious.

IC'TERUS, *Ic'terus flavus, I. verus*, from ικτις, a species of weasel, whose eyes are yellow (?) *Morbus arcua'tus* vel *arqua'tus, Auru'go, Auri'go, Morbus regius, Morbus lute'olus, Cholelith'ia icterus, Cholihæ'mia, Cholæ'mia, Cholopla'nia, Cholo'sis, Dermatocholo'sis, Suffu'sio aurigino'sa* seu *fellis* seu *bilis, Icteritia flava, Il'eus flavus, I. Icteroïdes, Cachex'ia icter'ica, Fellis suffu'sio, Fellis obstruc'tio, F. Superfu'sio, Bil'ious Dyscrasy, Jaundice, Yellows*, (F.) *Ictère, Jaunisse, Bile répandue*. A disease, the principal symptom of which is yellowness of the skin and eyes, with white fæces and high-coloured urine. It admits of various causes; in fact, any thing which can directly or indirectly obstruct the course of the bile, so that it is taken into the mass of blood and produces the yellowness of surface; — the bile being separated by the kidneys, causes yellowness of urine, and its being prevented from reaching the intestine occasions the pale-coloured fæces. The prognosis, in ordinary cases, is favourable;—when complicated with hepatic disease, unfavourable. The treatment is simple: — an emetic or purgative, given occasionally so as to elicit the return of the bile to its ordinary channels; light tonics; unirritating diet; cheerful company, &c.

ICTERUS ALBUS, Chlorosis.

ICTERUS INFAN'TUM, *I. Neonato'rum, Pædict'erus, Auri'go neophyto'rum, Yellow gum, Yellow gown*, (F.) *Ictère des nouveau-nés*, is a common affection and frequently dependent upon obstruction of the choledoch duct by the meconium. It requires time; and castor oil, occasionally.

ICTERUS MELAS, Melæna — i. Neonatorum, I. infantum—i. Niger, Melæna.

ICTERUS SATURNI'NUS, *Lead jaundice*. The earthy-yellow hue in saturnine cachexy.

ICTODES FŒTIDUS, Dracontium fœtidum.

ICTUS. 'A stroke or blow;' *Plegê, Plaga, Ictus solis*, a stroke of the sun. See *Coup de soleil. Ictus*, also, means the pulsation of an artery, and the sting of a bee or other insect.

ICTUS, Blow—i. Cordis et arteriarum, Pulse — i. Sanguinis, Apoplexy—i. Solis, *Coup de soleil*.

IDE'A, *I'dea, Ido'lum, Ideach* (? Paracelsus) (F.) *Idée*. The image or representation of an object in the mind; from ειδω, 'I see.'

IDE'A, FIXED or PREDOM'INANT, *I'dea fixa, Ideopeg'ma*. Tension of the mind on one notion; often observed in insanity.

I'DEA MORBI. Knowledge or idea of a disease.
IDEACH, Idea.
IDEAGENOUS, Sentient.
IDE'AL, *Idea'lis.* Mental, notional, fancied. *Morbi ideales.* Ideal diseases. Diseases of the imagination.
IDÉE, Idea.
IDEN'TITY (PERSONAL), *Iden'titas*, from *idem*, 'the same.' *Sameness.* It is sometimes a question in legal medicine to decide upon personal identity: that is, whether an individual be the same he represents himself to be. Physical marks form the great criteria.
IDEOL'OGY, *Ideolog"ia*, from ειδω, 'I see,' and λογος, 'a discourse.' The science of ideas. Intellectual philosophy.
IDEOPEGMA, Idea, fixed.
IDÉOSYNCHYSIE, Delirium.
IDIANŒA, Idiotism.
IDIOCRASIS, Idiosyncrasy.
IDIOCTONIA, Suicide.
IDIO-MIASMATA, see Miasm.
IDIOPATHI'A, *Idiopathei'a, Protopathi'a, Pro'prius affectus, Morbus idiopath'icus* seu *proprius* seu *prima'rius* seu *protopath'icus* seu *origina'lis, Malum prima'rium*, from ιδιος, 'peculiar, proper,' and παθος, 'an affection.' A primary disease; one not depending on any other.
IDIOPATH'IC, *Pro'prio hab'itu* seu *Constitutio'ne pro'priâ pendens, Idiopath'icus, Idiop'athes.* Primary affections and their symptoms are so denominated.
IDIOPTCY, Achromatopsia.
IDIOPTS, see Achromatopsia.
IDIOSYNCRASIA, Idiosyncrasy—i. Hæmorrhagica, Hæmatophilia— i. Olfactoria, Parosmia.
IDIOSYN'CRASY, *Idioc'rasy, Idiosyn'crasis, Idiosyncra'sia, Idiotroph'ia, Idioc'rasis, Idiosyncris'ia*, from ιδιος, 'peculiar,' συν, 'with,' and κρασις, 'temperament.' A peculiarity of constitution, in which one person is affected by an agent which, in numerous others, would produce no effect. Thus shell-fish, bitter almonds, produce urticaria in some, by virtue of their idiosyncrasies. Others faint at the sight of blood, &c.
ID'IOT, *Idio'ta*, 'foolish, stupid, ignorant.' Now used for one who is fatuous, or who does not possess sufficient intellectual faculties for the social condition, and for preserving himself from danger,— *Homo fat'uus*. In law, one who has been without understanding from his birth, and whom the law presumes to be never likely to attain any.
IDIOTIA, Idiotism.
IDIOTIE, Idiotism.
ID'IOTISM, *Idiotis'mus, Idioti'a, Idianœ'a, Imbecil'litas mentis; Mo'ria demens, Anœ'a, Mo'ria, Moro'sis, Meio'sis, Fatu'itas, Amen'tia, Stupid'itas, Vecor'dia, Imbecill'itas Inge'nii, Id'iocy, Id'iotcy, Fatu'ity.* (F.) *Démence innée, Idiotisme, Idiotie.* Same etymon. A species of unsound mind, characterized by more or less complete obliteration of the intellectual and moral faculties. It may supervene on mania and melancholia, when it is termed *Demen'tia*, but more commonly it depends upon original conformation. It may also, be symptomatic of organic disease of the brain, which has come on after birth. Idiotism exists in various degrees. Some idiots are mere automata, exhibiting scarcely any sensibility to external impressions; others are capable of articulating a few words, and possess certain mental emotions to a limited extent. The physiognomy is usually vacant, step unsteady, and articulation imperfect or broken. The affection is almost always incurable; but it may often be palliated.
IDIOTISME, Idiotism.
IDIOTROPHIA, Idiosyncrasy.

IDOLUM, Hallucination, Idea.
IDROSIS, Ephidrosis.
IF, Taxus baccata.
IFFIDES, Plumbi subcarbonas.
IGDE, Mortar.
IGDIS, Mortar.
IGNA'TIA AMA'RA, *Strychnos Igna'tii, Ignatia'na Philippin'ica.* The systematic name of the plant which affords *St. Ignatius's Bean. Faba In'dica, Faba Sancti Igna'tii, Faba febrif'uga*, (F.) *Ignatie, Fève de Saint Ignace.* The seeds are bitter and poisonous, containing Strychnia; which see.
IGNATIE, Ignatia amara.
IGNAVIA, Inertia—i. seu Ignavitas partium genitalium, Impotence.
IGNIS, 'fire.' Hence:
IGNIS ACTUALIS, Cauterium—i. Animalis, Animal heat.
IGNIS CAL'IDUS. 'A hot fire.' A violent inflammation, about to degenerate into gangrene.
IGNIS COLUMELLÆ, Erysipelas.
IGNIS FRIG"IDUS. 'A cold fire.' Sphacelus.
IGNIS NATURALIS, Animal heat.
IGNIS PERSICUS, Anthrax, Herpes zoster—i. Philosophicus, Phosphorus—i. Potentialis, see Cauterium—i. Sacer, Erysipelas, Herpes zoster—i. Sancti Antonii, Erysipelas.
IGNIS SAPIEN'TIUM. The ancient name for the heat of horses' dung.
IGNIS SYLVAT'ICUS, *I. sylves'tris, I. volat'icus, I. vola'grius, Stroph'ulus sylves'tris, S. volat'icus,* (F.) *Feu sauvage, F. volage, Flamboiss.* Probably, the *Porri"go larva'lis* or *Crusta lactea* of infants. Also, a transient redness of the face and neck, sometimes observed in hysterical and chlorotic females.
IGNIS SYLVESTRIS, I. sylvaticus— i. Vitalis, Animal heat— i. Volagrius, I. sylvaticus— i. Volaticus, I. sylvaticus.
IGNIVOROUS, Pyrophagus.
IGNYE, Poples.
IGNYS, Poples.
ILAPHIS, Arctium lappa.
ILEA, Flanks.
ILECH, *Y'lech, Ilei'as, Ilias'ter, Ylia'ter, Elias'ter, Ilias'trum, Ilei'ados, Ilei'dos, Ilei'adum, Ili'adus.* Terms used by Paracelsus to designate the first matter:— the beginning of every thing.
ILEIADOS, Ilech.
ILEIADUM, Ilech.
ILEIAS, Ilech.
ILEIDOS, Ilech.
ILEI'TIS; from *ileum*, 'the intestine ileum,' and *itis*, a suffix denoting inflammation. Inflammation of the ileum.
ILEO-CHOLOSIS, Diarrhœa, bilious.
IL'EO-COLIC, *Ileo-col'icus.* Relating to the fleum and colon :— as the ileo-colic valve or valve of Bauhin.
ILEO-COLITIS, Enteritis.
ILEO-DICLIDITE, see Typhus.
ILEO-LUMBAR, *Ileo-lumba'lis, Ilio-lumba'ris.* Belonging to the ilium and lumbar region.
ILEO-LUMBAR ARTERY, *Ilio-lumbar artery, Iliaco-mus'cular*, (Ch.) is given off by the hypogastric, opposite the base of the sacrum. It ascends behind the psoas muscle, and divides into two branches;—an *ascending* and a *transverse*, which give off numerous ramifications to the neighbouring parts.
ILEO-LUMBAR LIGAMENT, *Ilio-lumbar Lig'ament, Ilio-lumbo-ver'tebral ligament, Vertebro-iliac ligament*, is a broad, membraniform, triangular ligament, extending horisontally from the transverse process of the 5th lumbar vertebræ to

the upper and posterior part of the iliac crest. It unites the vertebral column with the pelvis.

IL'EON, *Il'eum, Eil'eon, Il'ium, Intesti'num circumvolu'tum,* from ειλειν, 'to turn,' 'to twist.' Anatomists have given this name to the longest portion of the small intestine, which extends from the jejunum to the cæcum. It was so called, from its forming a considerable number of convolutions.

ILEOPYRA, see Typhus.
ILEOSIS, Ileus.
ILEO-TYPHUS, see Typhus.
ILES, Flanks.

IL'EUS, *Eil'eos,* from ειλεω, 'I twist or contract.' *Co'lica Ileus, Enterele'sia, Enterelo'sis, Colica spasmod'ica, Ileus spasmod'icus, Chordap'sus, Passio Ili'aca, Iliac Passion, Vol'vulus, Ileo'sis, Misere'rē mei, Convol'vulus, Tormen'tum, Intercep'tio Intestino'rum, Enterosteno'sis volvulus,* (F.) *Colique de Miséricorde, C. de Miserere.* A disease, characterized by deep-seated pain of the abdomen, stercoraceous vomiting, and obstinate constipation. It is occasioned by hernia or other obstruction to the passage of the fæces through a part of the intestinal canal, *Enterosto'sis.* The term Ileus has been applied to various affections —to simple nervous colic, intussusception, and to strangulation of the small intestine, &c. Various remedies have been employed;—the majority for the purpose of procuring alvine evacuations,—as purgatives, in draught, pill, or glyster; suppositories, tobacco glysters; pure mercury; leaden bullets; antispasmodics and narcotics; blisters to the epigastrium; ice by the mouth, or injected into the rectum. Some of these have, occasionally, succeeded, — especially the tobacco glyster, and ice to the tumour, where the disease has been occasioned by strangulated hernia. It is very dangerous.

ILEUS FLAVUS, Icterus—i. Icteroides, Icterus—i. Inflammatorius, Enteritis.

ILEX AQUIFO'LIUM. The systematic name of the *Common Holly, Aquifo'lium, Agrifo'lium,* (F.) *Houx, H. commun* ou *Chêne vert.* The leaves of this plant have been recommended as tonic, astringent, and antiseptic, and have been prescribed in atonic gout; intermittents; dyspepsia, &c. *Il'icine,* the active principle, has also been advised. It is obtained by dissolving the alcoholic extract of the leaves of the holly in water, and successively treating it with the subacetate of lead, sulphuric acid, and carbonate of lime. The filtered and evaporated product is then dissolved in alcohol; and the mixture filtered and evaporated in shallow vessels.

ILEX CASSINE, Ilex vomitoria.
ILEX MAJOR. From the berries of this tree, called by the Spaniards *Bellotas,* a juice may be expressed, which forms a slightly astringent emulsion with water, and has been recommended by some Spanish physicians in humid cough, hæmoptysis, &c.

ILEX MATE, Ilex paraguensis.
ILEX OPA'CA, *American Holly,* grows throughout the Atlantic portion of the United States. It is said to possess the same properties as the European variety.

ILEX PARAGUEN'SIS, *Vibur'num læviga'tum* seu *Cassinoï'des, Cassi'nē Perag'ua* seu *Carolinia'na, I. Matē;* a native of Paraguay, which affords the celebrated *Mattee,* or *Matē, Folia Apalachines* seu *Per'aguæ,* is drunk in place of the Chinese tea by the people of Paraguay.

ILEX VOMITO'RIA, *Ilex Casi'ne, Cassi'na, Dahoon holly, Apalach'inē Gallis, South-Sea Tea, Ev'ergreen Cassi'nē, Cassee'na, Yaupon, Yopon,* (F.) *Thé des Apalaches, Houx Apalachine, Apalachine, Thé de la Mer du Sud.* A tree, indigenous in the southern parts of the United States. The leaves, when dried, are aromatic, stimulant, stomachic, and expectorant, and are used as a tea. When fresh, they are emetic and cathartic.

ILIA, Flanks.

ILIAC, *Ili'acus,* from *Ilia,* 'the flanks.' Relating to, or connected with, the flanks.

ILIAC ARTERIES, *Arte'riæ Iliacæ.* This term has been given to several arteries. The *Primary Iliacs,* (F.) *A. Iliaques primitives,—Pelvicrurales,* (Ch.) arise from the bifurcation of the aorta, opposite the body of the 4th lumbar vertebra, and descend, in a divergent manner; until, opposite the sacro-iliac symphysis, they divide into two considerable trunks,—the *internal Iliac* or hypogastric (which see) and the *external Iliac—Portion Iliaque de la crurale,* (Ch.) This proceeds from the sacro-iliac juncture as far as the crural arch, when it assumes the name *Femoral Artery.* Before passing under the arch it gives off two pretty considerable branches, — the *Epigastric,* and the *Circumflexa Ilii.* This last, which is called, also, *anterior Iliac* by some anatomists,—*Circonflexe de l'Ilium;* (Ch.) leaves the external iliac at the crural arch. It ascends along the outer edge of the iliacus muscle, and divides into two branches—an *internal* and an *external.*

The *Iliaca Inter'na Minor* vel *Ilio-lumbal'is* is a small artery, which sometimes arises from the hypogastric; at others, from the beginning of the gluteal. It is sent, chiefly, to the psoas and iliacus internus muscles.

ILIAC CREST, *Crista Il'ii,* is the upper margin of the ilium. (F.) *Crête Iliaque.* It is very thick, and curved like the Italic *S.* It affords attachment to the broad muscles of the abdomen.

ILIAC FOSSÆ are two in number; the *internal,* the depression presented by the ilium on its interior, and at the upper part in which the *Iliacus internus* is lodged:—and the *external,* an excavation on the outer surface of the same bone, occupied by the *Glutæi muscles.*

ILIAC MUSCLE, INTERNAL, *Ili'acus internus Muscle, Iliacus, Iliaco-trochantérien* (Ch.); *Femur moven'tium sep'timus, Iliac muscle,* is situate in the fossa iliaca, and at the anterior and superior part of the thigh. It is broad, radiated, triangular; and is attached, *above,* to the two upper thirds of the fossa iliaca, and to the internal part of the iliac crest:—*below,* it terminates by a tendon, which is common to it and the psoas magnus, and is fixed into the lesser trochanter. When this muscle contracts, it bends the pelvis on the thigh, and conversely. It is also a rotator of the thigh outwards, and prevents the trunk from falling backwards.

ILIAC PASSION, Ileus.
ILIAC REGIONS, *Regio'nes ili'acæ, Inan'ia,* are the sides of the abdomen between the ribs and the hips.

ILIAC SPINES, *Spinous Proc''esses of the Ilium,* are four in number. They are distinguished into *anterior* and *posterior.* Of the *anterior,* one is *superior.* It bounds the crista ilii anteriorly, and affords origin to the sartorius muscle. The other is *inferior,* and receives the tendinous origin of the rectus femoris.

The two *Posterior Iliac Spines* are divided, like the anterior, into *superior* and *inferior.* They afford insertion to strong ligaments, which unite the ilium with the sacrum.

ILIACO-TROCHANTÉRIEN, Iliacus internus.

ILIACUS, I. internus—i. Externus, Pyramidalis.

ILIADUS, Ilech.
ILIASTER, Ilech.
ILIASTRUM, Ilech.

ILINGOS, Vertigo.

ILIO-ABDOMINAL, Obliquus internus abdominis—*i. Aponévrosi-fémoral*, Fascia lata muscle—*i. Costal*, Quadratus lumborum—*i. Cresti-tibial*, Sartorius—i. Femoral, Coxo-femoral—i. Hypogastricus (nervus), Musculo-cutaneous nerve, superior—i. Inguinal, Musculo-cutaneous nerve, inferior—*i. Ischii-trochantérien*, Glutæus minimus—*i. Lombo-costo-abdominal*, Obliquus internus abdominis—i. Lumbalis, Ileo-lumbar, see Iliac arteries—*i. Lumbi-costal*, Quadratus lumborum—i. Lumbo-vertebral ligament, Ileo-lumbar ligament.

IL'IO-PECTINEA, belonging to the ilium and to the pecten or pubis.

ILIO-PECTINEAL EMINENCE is so called from being formed by the junction of the ramus of the ilium with that of the pubis. It affords attachment to the psoas minor.

ILIO-PECTINEA LINEA, *Linea innomina'ta*, is the projecting line or ridge of the ilium and pubis, which forms part of the brim of the pelvis.

ILIO-PRÉTIBIAL, Sartorius.

ILIO-PSOI'TIS, from *Ilium*, 'the ilion,' ψοας, 'the loins,' and *itis*, denoting inflammation. Inflammation of the ilium and psoas muscle.

ILIO-PUBO-COSTO-ABDOMINAL, Obliquus externus abdominis—*i. Rotulien*, Rectus femoris—i. Sacral, Sacro-iliac—i. Sacral articulation, Sacro-iliac articulation—*i. Sacro-femoral*, Glutæus major—i. Scrotal nerve, Musculo-cutaneous, superior—*i. Trochantérien*, Glutæus medius—*i. Trochantérien petit*, Glutæus minimus.

IL'ION, *Il'ium, Il'eum, Haunch bone.* The largest of the three bones which constitute the os innominatum in the fœtus and child. It was probably so called from its seeming to support the intestine ilion; or, perhaps, because its crest is curved upon itself, from ιλεω, 'I twist,' 'I roll.' This portion of the os innominatum is usually so called in the adult. The posterior surface is called *Dorsum*, the internal *Venter*. The upper semicircular edge is the *Crista* or *Spine*, at the anterior part of which is the *anterior and superior spinous process*; and, below, the anterior and inferior spinous process. At the back part of the spine are two *spinous processes*, the *posterior and superior*, and *posterior and inferior.* See Iliac.

ILITHYI'A, Ειλειθυια, *Luci'na, Juno Lucina.* The goddess who presided over parturient females, with the Greeks and Romans.

ILIUM, Ileum, Ilion.

ILKESTON, MINERAL WATERS OF. Ilkeston is in Derbyshire, England, about eight miles from Nottingham. The water contains carbonates of lime and soda, chloride of calcium, sulphate of magnesia, sulphate of soda, carbonic acid, sulphohydric acid, and a little iron.

ILLACHRYMATIO, Epiphora.

ILLECEBRA, Sedum—i. Major, Sedum telephium.

ILLECEBRUM VERMICULARE, Sedum.

ILLEGIT'IMATE, *Illegit'imus*, from *il, in*, 'negation or opposition,' and *legitimus*, 'legitimate;' from *lex, legis*, 'law.' That which is contrary to law: which has not the conditions required by law,—as an illegitimate birth—one out of wedlock.

ILLEGITIMATE OR BASTARD FEVERS are those whose progress is anomalous.

ILLIC"IUM ANISA'TUM, *Yellow-flowered Anise, An'iseed Tree, Star Anise, Ani'sum stella'tum, Anisum Sinen'sé, Semen Badian*, (F.) *Anis de la Chine, A. étoilé, Badiane.* Fam. Magnoliaceæ. *Sex. Syst.* Polyandria Polygynia. The seeds are used like the aniseed. The same tree is supposed to furnish the aromatic bark, called *Cortex Ani'si Stella'ti, Cortex Lavola.*

Illicium Anisatum is said to furnish much of the so called *Oil of Anise*, used in the United States.

ILLICIUM FLORIDA'NUM, *Florida Anise Tree, Star Anise, Sweet Laurel.* An evergreen shrub, the bark, leaves, &c., of which have a spicy odour like anise, and might be used for it.

ILLICIUM PARVIFLO'RUM, a shrub of the hilly regions of Georgia and Carolina, has a flavour closely resembling that of sassafras root.

ILLINITIO, Inunction.

ILLITIO, Inunction.

ILLITUS, Inunction.

ILLOS, Eye, see Strabismus.

ILLO'SIS, *Ilo'sis*, from ιλλος, 'the eye.' Distortion of the eyes. Strabismus.

ILLUSIO SENSUS, Hallucination.

ILLUSION, Hallucination.

ILLUTAMENTUM, see Illutatio.

ILLUTA'TIO, from *il, in*, 'upon,' and *lutum*, 'mud.' A word used, by the ancients, for the act of covering any part of the body with mud,—*illutamen'tum*—with therapeutical views.

ILOSIS, Illosis.

IMAGINA'TION, *Imagina'tio, Figura'tio, Phanta'sia, Dianoë'ma*, from *imago*, 'image.' The faculty of forming in the mind an assemblage of images and combinations of ideas which are not always in connexion with external objects.

IMBALSAMATION, Embalming.

IMBECIL'ITY, *Imbecil'litas, Stupid'itas, Hebetu'do an'imi.* Weakness, especially of the intellect; incoherency; *Imbecil'litas mentis*.

IMBECILLIS, Infirm.

IMBECILLITAS INGENII, Idiotism, Imbecility—i. Mentis, Idiotism, Imbecility—i. Ventriculi, Gasterasthenia.

IMBELLIS AD VENEREM, Frigid.

IMBER'BIS, *Imber'bus, Agenei'os, Apo'gon*, from *im, in*, 'negation,' and *barba*, 'beard.' One devoid of beard.

IMBIBITIO, Absorption, Imbibition.

IMBIBIT"ION, *Imbibit"io, Emp'osis, Endosmose, Aspiration*, from *imbibere* (*in*, and *bibere*), 'to drink, to imbibe.' The action, by which a body becomes penetrated by a liquid. See Endosmose. Many of the phenomena of absorption are owing to imbibition.

IMBREX NARIUM, Septum narium.

IMBRICARIA SAXATILIS, Lichen saxatilis.

IMMERSUS, Subscapularis muscle.

IM'MINENCE, *Imminen'tia*, from *im*, and *manere*, 'to stay.' Staying over, or upon; impending. Some authors have designated, by this term, the period which precedes the invasion of a disease; when certain indications foretell its approach.

IMMINENCE MORBIDE, Diathesis, Predisposition.

IMMISSIO CATHETERIS, Catheterismus.

IMMISSOR, Catheter.

IMMOBILITAS, Acinesia—i. Pupillæ, Amaurosis.

IMMODERANTIA, Intemperance.

IMMODERATIO, Intemperance.

IMMOVABLE APPARATUS, see Apparatus, immovable.

IMMUTANS, Alterative.

IMPAC'TION, *Impac'tio*, from *impingere* (*in*, and *pangere*), 'to strike against.' A fracture of the cranium, ribs, or sternum, with depression of some of the fragments and projection of others externally. See Eopiesma.

IMPA'TIENS BALSAMI'NA, *Balsam weed, Touch-me-not.* This probably resembles the other species in its properties.

IMPA'TIENS FULVA and I. PAL'LIDA, *Touch-me-not, Jewel weed, Balsam weed, Slippers, Cel'-andine, Quick-in-the-hand, Weath'ercocks.* Indigenous plants, having tender, juicy, almost transparent stems, and yellow flowers, which appear in July and August. It is found in low, moist ground, in every part of the Union. The properties are probably the same as those of

IMPA'TIENS NOLI-ME-TAN'GERE of Europe, which has an acrid taste, and acts as an emetic, cathartic, and diuretic.

IMPEDIMENTUM, Emphragma.

IMPERATO'RIA, *I. Ostru'thium, Seli'num ostru'thium, S. Imperato'ria, Angel'ica officina'lis, Astruthium, Ostruthium, Astran'tia, Magistran'tia, Masterwort*, (old F.) *Austruche.* The roots of this plant were formerly considered *divinum remedium*. They are merely aromatic and bitter, and are not used.

IMPERATORIA SYLVESTRIS, Angelica sylvestris.

IMPERFORATE, Atretus.

IMPERFORATIO, Imperforation — i. Ani, Atresia ani adnata, Proctatresia — i. Pupillæ, Synezixis — i. Uteri, Metratresia.

IMPERFORA'TION, from *im*, 'in,' *per*, 'through', and *forare*, 'to bore.' *Imperfora'tio, Atre'sia, Atretis'mus, Cap'etus.* Absence of a natural aperture; as, of the mouth, anus, vulva, nostrils, &c. It is congenital, being dependent upon faulty conformation.

IMPERFORATION DE L'ANUS, Atresia ani adnata.

IMPE'RIAL. A pleasant, cooling drink, formed of *bitartrate of potassa*, ℥ss; one *lemon*, cut into slices; *white sugar*, ℔ss; and *water*, Oiij. Let the mixture stand for half an hour, and strain.

IMPETIGINOSITAS, Impetigo.

IMPETI'GO, from *impeto*, 'I infest.' *Impetiginos'itas, Darta, Der'bia, Im'petus, Peti'go, Ec-pye'sis impeti'go, Phlysis impeti'go, Lepra squam-mo'sa, Running Scall* or *Tetter, Crusted Tetter, Pustular* or *Humid Tetter, Scall, Couvrap,* (F.) *Dartre, D. crustacée, D. croûteuse, Lèpre humide, Mélitagre.* A word used in various acceptations. With some writers it is synonymous with itch. In others, it means a variety of herpes. Sauvages employs it as a generic term, under which he comprises syphilis, scorbutus, rachitis, elephantiasis, the itch, tinea, scrofula, &c. It forms, also, a genus in the class *Cachexiæ* of Cullen. In Bateman, it is the first genus of the 5th order, *Pustulæ*, and is defined — *the humid* or *running tetter;* consisting of small pustules, denominated *Psydracia.* It is unaccompanied by fever; not contagious, or communicable by inoculation. He has five species: — the *I. figura'ta, I. sparsa, I. erysipelato'des, I. scab'ida,* and *I. rodens.* See Psoriasis.

IMPETIGO EXCORTICATIVA, Ichthyosis — i. Figurata, Porrigo lupinosa — i. Pellagra, Pellagra — i. Ulcerata, Zerna.

IMPETUM FACIENS, Enormon.

IMPETUS, Impetigo, Paroxysm.

IMPLICATIONES RETICULARES NERVORUM, Plexus nervorum.

IMPLIC"ITI MORBI, *Implica'ti seu compli-ca'ti Morbi.* Diseases, which exist in an organ; and produce, concurrently, disorders in other organs.

IMPLUVIUM, Embrocation, Bath, shower.

IMPOSTHUME, Abscess.

IM'POTENCE, *Acrati'a, Impoten'tia, I. gene-ran'di, Agenne'sia, Agen'nesis, Igna'via* seu *Ig-nav'itas partium genita'lium,* (F.) *Impuissance;* from *im*, 'priv.,' and *potens*, 'able.' Loss of power over one or more of the members. Commonly, it means want of sexual vigour; incapacity for copulation; and chiefly on the part of the male. *Asty'sia, Astyph'ia, Asyno'dia, Adynamia viri'lis.* It has, also, been used synonymously with *sterility*. Impotence may be *absolute* or *relative*, *constitutional* or *local*, *direct* or *indirect*, *permanent* or *temporary*.

IMPOTENTIA, Adynamia, Impotence — i. Generandi, Impotence.

IMPOV'ERISHED, *Effe'tus, Depaupera'tus,* (F.) *Appauvri.* 'Having become poor;' originally from (L.) *pauper*, 'poor.' The Humorists applied this epithet to a humour, deprived of a part of its constituents, and particularly to the blood. This fluid was considered to be impoverished when it was pale, without the proper consistence, and abounding in serum. It was, on the contrary, rich, in their opinion, when of a scarlet colour; possessing consistence; when it coagulated promptly, and the quantity of serum, compared with that of the clot, was by no means considerable.

IMPRÆGNATIO, Fecundation, Pregnancy.

IMPREGNATION, Fecundation, Pregnancy.

IMPRESSIBILITY, GREAT, Hyperæsthesis.

IMPRES'SION, *Impres'sio* (*in*, and *premere*, *pressum*, 'to press'), *Pros'bolê,* (F.) *Empreinte.* A more or less deep indentation which certain organs seem to make on others. Inequalities observable on the bones, which appear to be made by the subjacent organs.

IMPRES'SIONS DIG"ITAL, *Impressio'nes digita'tæ cra'nii, Fossæ digita'les,* are the depressions of various forms, observable at the inner surface of the cranium, which look, at first view, as if they were made with the fingers.

IMPU'BER, *Impu'bes, Impu'bis, Ane'bus, Capilla'tus*, from *in*, 'negation,' and *pubertas*, 'puberty.' (F.) *Impubère.* One who has not attained the age of puberty.

IMPUBES, Impuber.

IMPUDICUS, see Digitus.

IMPUISSANCE, Impotence.

IMPULSE, DIAS'TOLIC, *Back stroke of the heart.* A jog or stroke which has been termed the 'back stroke,' felt at the end of each pulsation, and which would seem to be owing to the refilling of the ventricles.

IMPULSE OF THE HEART, see Heart.

IMPURITATES ALVINÆ, Fæces.

INANIA, Iliac regions.

INANITIATED, see Inanitiation.

INANITIA'TION, *Inanitia'tio*, same etymon. The act of being exhausted for want of nourishment. One so exhausted is said to be *inanitiated*.

INANIT"ION, *Inanit"io, Inan'itas*, from *inanire*, 'to empty.' *Ceno'sis.* Exhaustion for want of nourishment. To die from inanition is to die from exhaustion.

INAPPETENTIA, Anorexia, Dysorexia.

INARTICULATIO, Enarthrosis.

INAURA'TION, *Inaura'tio*, from *in*, and *aurum*, 'gold.' The gilding of pills or boluses.

INCANTAMENTUM, Charm.

INCANTA'TION, *Incanta'tio, Incantamen'tum, Ep'odē*, from *in*, and *cantare*, 'to sing,' — for example, a magical song. A mode of curing diseases by charms, &c., defended by Paracelsus, Van Helmont, and others.

INCARCERA'TIO, *Chatonnement*, Incarceration — i. Intestinorum interna, Enteremphraxis — i. Intestinorum, Enteroperistole.

INCARCERA'TION, *Incarcera'tio*, from *in*, 'in,' and *carcer*, 'prison.' Hernia is said to be *incarcerated, Hernia incarcera'ta*, when, owing to constriction about the neck of the hernial sac or elsewhere, it cannot be reduced with facility

Incarceration is sometimes used in the same sense as strangulation.

INCAR'NANS, *Incarnati'vus, Sarco'ticus, Stal'ticus, Plero'ticus, Anaplero'ticus, Sarcot'ic,* from *in,* and *caro, carnis,* 'flesh.' Medicines, which were fancied to promote the regeneration of the flesh. Certain bandages and sutures have, also, been so called.

INCARNATIO, Incarnation — i. Unguium, Onychogryphosis.

INCARNA'TION, *Incarna'tio,* same etymon. Growth of flesh or granulations.

INCARNATUS, Carneous.

INCEN'DIUM, from *incendere (in,* and *candere),* 'to burn.' *Pyrcæ'a, πυρκαια, Causis, Phlogo'sis.* A burning fever or any burning heat. — *Incen'dium febri'lē, Incen'sio.* — Willis. Inflammation, Phlegmon.

INCENDIUM SPONTANEUM, Combustion, human.

INCENSIO, Incendium.

INCENTIVUM, Stimulant.

INCERA'TION, *Incera'tio, Encero'sis,* from *cera,* 'wax.' The act of incorporating wax with some other body; or, rather, the operation whose object is to communicate to a dry substance the consistence of wax.

INCERNIC'ULUM, from *incernere (in,* and *cernere),* 'to sift.' A strainer or sieve.

INCESSIO, Bath, half, Semicupium.

INCESSUS, Walking.

INCIDEN'TIA, from *incidere (in,* and *cædere),* 'to cut.' (F.) *Incisifs.* This name was formerly given to medicines to which was attributed the property of cutting thick or coagulated humours. The fixed alkalies, hydrosulphurets of alkalies, sulphurous water, &c., were considered to belong to this class.

INCINERA'TION, *Incinera'tio, Cinefac'tio,* from *cinis, cineris,* 'ashes.' In pharmacy, a process by which animal or vegetable substances are reduced to ashes.

INCINCTA, Pregnant.

INCISIFS, Incidentia.

INCISIO, Cut, Incision—i. Simplex, Haplotomia.

INCIS'ION, *Incis'io, En'copē, Incisu'ra, Inci'sus, Tomē,* (F.) *Taillade.* A methodical division of soft parts with a cutting instrument.

INCI'SIVE, *Incisi'vus, Inciso'rius, Fossa incisi'va, F. myrtifor'mis,* is a depression in the superior maxillary bone, above the incisor teeth.

INCISIVE BONE, Intermaxillary bone—i. Canal, see Palatine canals.

INCISIVE NERVE, *Nervus incisi'vus.* A branch of the inferior dental nerve, which supplies the incisor teeth.

INCISIVE TEETH, *Inci'sor Teeth, Den'tes inciso'res, tom'ici, ctenes, dichasteres, gelasi'ni, primo'res, raso'rii.* The teeth which occupy the anterior part of the upper and lower jaws are so called, because they are used for *cutting* the food in the manner of cutting instruments.

INCISIVUS, MUSCULUS, Levator labii superioris proprius—i. Inferior, Levator labii inferioris — i. Lateralis et pyramidalis, Levator labii superioris alæque nasi—i. Medius, Depressor alæ nasi.

INCISOR TEETH, Incisive teeth.

INCISO'RIUM, *Tomi'on.* An operating table. A scalpel.

INCISORIUS, Incisive.

INCISURA, *Echancrure,* Incision—i. Crucialis, Crucial Incision—i. Ischiadica Major, Sciatic notch, greater—i. Ischiadica Minor, Sciatic notch, lesser — i. Lienalis, Hilus lienalis — i. Renalis, Hilus renalis—i. Scapularis, Notch, scapular — i. Septi, see Ventricles of the brain.

INCISU'RA TRAG'ICA, *Notch of the Concha.* A wide, deep and rounded notch, which separates the tragus from the antitragus.

INCISURES DE SANTORINI, Santorini, fissures of.

INCISUS, Incision.

INCITABILITY, Irritability.

INCITAMENTUM, Stimulus.

INCITANS, Stimulant.

INCITATIO, Stimulation.

INCLAVATIO, Gomphosis, see Wedged.

INCLINATIO, Decline — i. Cœli, Climate.

INCLUSION, MONSTROSITY BY, *Emboîtement.*

INCLUSUS, Wedged.

INCOCTUS, see Crudity.

INCOHE'RENCE, *Incohe'rency,* (F.) *Anacoluthie, Rêvasserie;* from *in,* negative, *co, con, cum,* 'with,' and *hærere,* 'to stick.' Want of dependence of one part on another. The condition of the mental manifestations in dementia, &c.

INCOMPAT'IBLE, from *in,* 'negation,' and *competere,* 'to agree.' A substance, which cannot be prescribed with another, without interfering with its chemical composition or medicinal activity.

INCONTINEN'TIA, from *in,* 'negation,' and *contineo,* 'I contain;' *Anepis'chesis.* 'Incontinence.' 'Inability to retain the natural evacuation.' Abuse of the pleasures of love.

INCONTINENTIA ALVI, Diarrhœa — i. Urinæ, Enuresis, Scoracrasia.

INCORPORA'TION, *Incorpora'tio, Corpora'tio, Ensomato'sis, Metensomato'sis,* from *in,* and *corpus,* 'a body.' An operation, by which medicines are mixed with soft or liquid bodies, in order to give them a certain consistence. Also, the thorough admixture of various substances.

INCRASSAN'TIA, *Incrassati'va, Inviscan'tia, Spissan'tia, Ecpyo'tica, Condensan'tia, Pachyn'tica, Pycnot'ica, Pycnicmas'tica,* from *in,* and *crassus,* 'thick.' Medicines which were formerly believed to possess the power of thickening the humours, when too thin. All mucilaginous substances were so regarded.

INCRASSATIVA, Incrassantia.

IN'CREASE, *Incremen'tum, Auxis, Auxe'sis,* from *in,* and *crescere,* 'to grow.' (F.) *Accroissement.* Augmentation of the size or weight of a body, by the application of new molecules around those which already exist.

INCREMENTUM, Augmentation, Increase.

INCRUCIATIO, Decussation.

INCRUSTA'TION, *Incrusta'tio,* from *in,* and *crusta,* 'a crust;' *Coni'asis.* The act of forming a crust on the surface of a body, as well as the crust itself. Also, the calcareous deposites or cartilaginous plates, which sometimes form in organs.

INCUBA'TION, *Incuba'tio, Incubit"io, Incu'bitus,* from *incubare, (in,* and *cubare,)* 'to lie upon.' This word, which is used in natural history for the sitting of birds upon their eggs, is employed, figuratively, in medicine, for the period that elapses between the introduction of a morbific principle into the animal economy and the invasion of the disease.

INCUBITIO, Incubation.

INCUBITUS, Incubation.

INCUBO, Incubus.

IN'CUBUS. Same etymon. *In'cubo, Epial'tes, Ephial'tes noctur'nus, Ephial'tes, Epilep'sia nocturna, Asthma noctur'num, Pnigal'ion, Suc'cubus, Oneirodyn'ia gravans, Erethis'mus oneirodyn'ia, Noctur'na oppres'sio, Epib'olē, Babusica'rius, Nightmare,* (F.) *Cauchemar, Cauchevicille, Cochemar, Oneirodynia gravatives.* Same etymon. A sensation of a distressing weight at the epigastrium during sleep, and of impossibility of motion, speech or respiration; the patient at length awaking in terror, after extreme anxiety. Nightmare is often the effect of difficult digestion or of an uneasy position of the body. At other times, it occurs in consequence of severe emotions. The sensation of suffocation was formerly ascribed to the person's being *possessed*, and the male spirits were called *incubes*—the female *succubes*. The disease requires no particular treatment. The causes must be avoided.

INCUBUS VIGILAN'TIUM, *Ephial'tes vigilan'tium, E. hypochondri'aca, Daymare.* This is produced during wakefulness; the sense of pressure being severe and extending over the abdomen; respiration frequent, laborious, and constricted; eyes fixed; sighing, deep and violent; intellect, undisturbed.

INCUNABULA, Swathing clothes.

INCUNEATIO, see Wedged.

INCU'RABLE, *Incurab'ilis, Rem'ediless, Irresme'diable, Insanab'ilis, Anal'thes, Anaces'tos, Atherapeu'tus,* from *in*, negative, and *cura*, cure. Not susceptible of cure;—applied to both patients and diseases.

INCURIA, Acedia.

INCURSUS ARTERIARUM, Pulse.

INCURVATIO, Gryposis.

INCUS, (*in*, and *cudo*, 'I hammer,') 'an anvil.' *Acmon, Os incu'di sim'ilē, Ossic'ulum Incudi seu mola'ri denti compara'tum,* (F.) *Enclume.* One of the small bones of the ear, so called from its fancied resemblance to a smith's anvil. It is situate in the cavity of the tympanum, between the malleus and orbiculare. Its body is articulated with the malleus; its *horizontal ramus*, which is the shortest, corresponds with the entrance of the mastoid cells; and its *vertical ramus* is articulated with the os orbiculare. The incus is composed of a compact tissue, and is developed from a single point of ossification.

INDEX, *Dig"itus index seu secun'dus seu salutator'ius, Demonstra'tor, Indica'tor, Indicato'rius, Lich'anos, Deic'ticos,* from *indicare*, 'to point out.' The forefinger, index finger. See Digitus.

INDIAN ARROW WOOD, see Euonymus—i. Paint, Hydrastis Canadensis—i. Physic, Gillenia trifoliata—i. Physio, small-flowered, Gillenia stipulacea.

INDIA'NA, MINERAL WATERS OF. A medicinal spring, near Jeffersonville, is much frequented. Its waters are strongly impregnated with sulphur and iron.

IN'DICANT, *In'dicans, Endeic'ticos,* (F.) *Indicatif.* Same etymon as *index*. Any thing which, in the course of a disease or in what precedes or accompanies it, concurs in pointing out the means to be used for its cure.

INDICATIF, Indicant.

IN'DICATING DAYS, *Dies In'dices, D. Indicato'rii seu Indican'tes, D. contemplan'tes,* (F.) *Jours indicateurs.* Hippocrates and others have thus called the middle day of the septenary; because they imagined, that indications were sometimes given then of the crisis which would occur in the last day of the septenary.

INDICA'TION, *Indica'tio, Accusa'tio, Dela'tio, Endeix'is, Endex'is, Boëthemat'icum Semei'on.* The object proposed in the employment of any means which are had recourse to for the cure of disease. It may also be defined—the manifestation afforded by the disease itself of what is proper to be done for its removal.

INDICATOR, Extensor proprius indicis, see Digitus, and Index.

INDICUM, Indigo.

INDICUS COLOR, Indigo.

INDIGENCE, Want.

INDIG"ENOUS, *Indig"ena.* Whatever is native in a country, in opposition to *exotic*; as an *indigenous remedy, indigenous disease,* &c.

INDIGESTION, Dyspepsia—i. Alkaline, see Dyspopsia—i. Neutral, see Dyspepsia.

INDIGITATIO, Intussusceptio.

INDIGNABUNDUS, Rectus externus oculi.

INDIGNATORIUS, Rectus externus oculi.

IN'DIGO, *Indigum, In'dicum, Indicus color, Pigmen'tum In'dicum.* A dye-stuff, in small solid masses, of a deep azure blue colour, and devoid of smell and taste. It is obtained, by a fermentative process, from *Indigof'era anil,* (*I. suffruticо'sa,*) *I. argen'tea,* (*I. articula'ta seu tincto'ria seu glau'ca seu colora'ta,*) and *I. tincto'ria seu In'dica,* and is sometimes used by the apothecary for colouring certain preparations. It has likewise been administered internally, of late, in spasmodic diseases, especially in epilepsy. The dose may be at first grains, but it may be elevated to drachms.

INDIGO, FALSE, (TALL WHITE,) see Sophora tinctoria.

INDIGO, FAUX, Galega officinalis—i. Weed, Sophora tinctoria—i. Wild, Sophora tinctoria—i. Yellow, Sophora tinctoria.

INDIGOFERA, see Indigo, Sophora tinctoria.

INDIGUM, Indigo.

INDISPOSIT"ION, *Mala disposit"io, Dysphor'ia,* (F.) *Malaise.* A slight functional disturbance, which may scarcely bear the name of disease. A feeling of sickness—*sensus ægritu'dinis.*

IN'DOLENT, *In'dolens,* from *in*, privative, and *dolere*, 'to be in pain.' Exhibiting little or no pain. An epithet particularly applied to certain tumours.

INDOLENTIA, Anodynia.

IN'DOLES. A natural disposition or character.

INDOLES AN'IMI. The natural disposition or character of mind.

INDOLES MORBI. The nature or character of a disease.

INDOSYNCLONUS, Beriberi.

INDUC'TIO, *Apago'gē,* from *inducere,* (*in,* and *ducere,* 'to lead.') A word used especially for the action of extending a plaster upon linen.

INDUCULA, Waistcoat, strait.

INDUMENTUM CORDIS, Pericardium—i. Nervorum, Neurilema—i. Ventriculorum, Ependyma ventriculorum.

IN'DURANS, (*in* and *durus,*) *Sclerot'icus, Sclerun'ticus, Scleryn'ticus.* A medicine which hardens the parts to which it is applied.

INDURATIO, Induration—i. Intestinorum, Enteropathia cancerosa—i. Maligna, Scirrhus—i. Renum, Nephroscleria—i. Telæ cellulosæ neonatorum, see Induration—i. Ventriculi scirrhosa, Gastroscirrhus.

INDURA'TION, *Indura'tio, Sclerys'ma, Sclerys'mus, Callos'itas, Indurescen'tia, Poro'ma, Poro'sis,* (F.) *Endurcissement.* The hardness which supervenes, occasionally, in an inflamed part. It is one of the terminations of inflammation, and is owing to a change in the nutrition of the part.

INDURATION OF THE CELLULAR TISSUE, *Indura'tio seu Oppila'tio telæ cellulo'sæ neonato'rum, Ethmyphotylo'sis, Œde'ma neonato'rum, Compact Œde'ma of Infants, Cat'ochus Infan'tum, Induratio cellulo'sa, Sclere'mia, Sclere'ma, Sclero'ma, Scleroder'ma, Cutis tensa chron'ica, Dermatoperisclero'sis, Dermatoperiscleryemus, Ethmyphotylosis, Halonii'tis, Phlegmasia cellula'ris, Scirrhosar'ca neonato'rum, Scleri'asis neonato'rum, Scleroʼsis, Stipa'tio telæ cellulo'sæ Infan'tum, Skinbound Disease,* (F.) *Endurcissement du tissu cellulaire; Œdème du tissu cellulaire des nouveau-nés, Asphyxie lente des nouveau-nés,* is a disease which attacks infants a few days after birth, and which Chaussier proposed to call *Sclérème,* from σκληρος, 'hard.'

The Induration of the cellular tissue of the adult, *Sclerosteno'sis cuta'nea,* has been regarded as the result of inflammation of the corium, *Chorioni'tis.*

INDURATION OF THE BRAIN, Sclerencephalia—*i. Grise,* see Hepatization.

INDURESCENTIA, Induration.

INDU'SIUM, *Chitonis'cos.* Strictly, 'a shirt,' 'a small tunic;' but some have so called the amnion.

INE'BRIANT, *Ine'brians, Phantas'ticus;* from *in* and *ebrio,* 'I intoxicate.' Intoxicating. An agent that intoxicates.

INEBRIATION, Temulentia.

INEDIA, Fasting.

INER'TIA, from *in,* 'privative,' and *ars, artis,* 'art,' (?) *Igna'via, Ener'vitas.* Sluggishness, inactivity.

INER'TIA OF THE WOMB, (F.) *Inertie de la matrice.* The diminution and even total cessation of the contractions of the uterus during labour; as well as the species of languor into which it sometimes falls after the expulsion of the fœtus.

INERTIE PAR EPUISEMENT, see Parturition—*i. de la Matrice,* Inertia of the womb.

INESIS, Cenosis.

INETHMOS, Cenosis.

IN'FANCY, *Infun'tia,* from *in,* 'negation,' and *fans,* from *fari,* 'to speak.' Early childhood. Childhood; *Nepiot'es, Paidi'a,* (F.) *Enfance.* It generally includes the age from birth till the seventh year. See Age.

INFANS, *Pai'dion, Ne'pios,* (F.) *Enfant.* An infant; a child; one in infancy. In law, one who has not attained the age of legal capacity; which is, in general, fixed at twenty-one years.

INFANS RECENS NATUS, *Nouveau-né.*

INFANTIA, Infancy.

INFAN'TICIDE, *Infantici'dium, Tecnocton'ia, Child-murder,* from *infans,* 'a child,' and *cædere,* 'to kill.' The murder of a child newly born, or on the point of being born. It may be perpetrated by the mother, or by some other person, either by *commission,* that is, in consequence of a direct, voluntary act; — or by *omission* of those cares which are necessary for the preservation of the new-born.

INFARCTUS, Emphraxis — i. Intestinorum, Enteremphraxis—i. Lactei extremitatum, Phlegmatia dolens—i. Lienis, Splenoncus.

INFARC'TUS MAMMÆ LAC'TEUS, *Laetis concretio'nes, Nodi* seu *Thrombi lactei, Trichi'asis lactea.* Knotty tumours of the female mammæ, owing to the accumulation and arrest of milk in the galactophorous ducts.

INFARCTUS UTERI, Metremphraxis.

INFECTION, see Contagion.

INFECUNDITY, Sterility.

INFECUNDUS, Sterile.

INFER'NAL, *Infer'nus;* 'relating to hell.' A name applied to caustic—*Lapis Inferna'lis*—on account of its strong burning properties.

INFIBULA'TIO, *Fibula'tio, Infibula'tion, Ancterias'mus;* from *fibula,* 'a clasp.' (F.) *Bouclement.* An operation, formerly practised, which consisted in passing a ring through the prepuce, after having drawn it over the glans; — in order to prevent coition. The ancients employed infibulation with their gladiators, to preserve all their strength by depriving them of venery. In the women, to preserve their chastity, the ring was passed through the labia majora.

INFILTRA'TION, *Infiltra'tio,* from *filtrare,* 'to filter.' Effusion. The accumulation of a fluid in the areolæ of any texture, and particularly of the areolar membrane. The fluid effused is ordinarily the *Liquor sanguinis,* sound or altered, — sometimes blood or pus, fæces, or urine. When infiltration of a serous fluid is general, it constitutes *anasarca;* when local, *œdema.*

INFILTRATION PURULENTE, see Hepatization.

INFIRM, *Infirm'us, Imbecillis, Deb'ilis, As'thenes,* from *in,* negative, and *firmus,* 'firm.' Not firm or sound; weak; feeble.

INFIRMARIUM, Hospital.

INFIRMARY, Hospital.

INFIRMATORIUM, Hospital.

INFIRMIER (F.), from *infirmus,* (*in,* negative, and *firmus.*) *Infirma'rius, Nosoc'omus, Cura'tor infirmo'rum.* One employed in an hospital or infirmary to take care of the sick.

INFIRM'ITY, *Infirm'itas, Astheni'a, Arrhos'tia, Invaletu'do.* Any disease which has become habitual, either owing to its chronic character, or its numerous relapses.

INFLA'MED, *Inflamma'tus,* (F.) *Enflammé,— Phlogo'sed,* according to some. Same etymon as inflammation. Affected with inflammation.

INFLAMMABLE AIR, Hydrogen, carburetted.

INFLAMMATIO, Inflammation, Phlegmon—i. Abdominalis, Encœlitis — i. Articuli Maxillæ Inferioris, Hyposiagonarthritis—i. Auris, Otitis—i. Bronchiorum, Bronchitis—i. Cæci, Typhlo-enteritis—i. Capsulæ lentis, Phacohymenitis—i. Cerebelli, Cerebellitis — i. Clitoridis, Nymphitis—i. Conjunctivæ, see Ophthalmia — i. Corneæ, Ceratitis—i. Coxæ, Osphyitis—i. Cystidis felleæ, Cholecystitis—i. Epiglottidis, Epiglottitis — i. Erysipelatosa, Erysipelatous inflammation — i. Faucium, Cynanche, Isthmitis — i. Gastritis, Gastritis —i. Genæ, Gnathitis — i. Genarum, Melitis — i. Gingivæ, Ulitis—i. Glandularum lymphaticarum, Hydradenitis — i. Glandularum lymphaticarum, Lymphadenitis — i. Glandularum sublingualium, Hypoglossiadenitis — i. Gulæ, Œsophagitis — i. Hepatis, Hepatitis — i. Hepatis lenta, Hepatitis (chronic) — i. Interna, Empresma — i. Intestinorum, Enteritis — i. Iridis, Iritis—i. Jecoris, Hepatitis—i. Laryngis, Laryngitis—i. Lienis, Splenitis —i. Ligamentorum, Syndesmitis — i. Linguæ, Glossitis—i. Mediastini, Mesodmitis—i. Medullæ Spinalis, Myelitis—i. Musculi pecas, Psoitis — i. Musculorum, Myositis — i. Musculorum abdominalium, Myocœliitis — i. Nervorum, Neuritis—i. Oculorum, Ophthalmia—i. Œsophagi, Œsophagitis—i. Omenti, Epiploitis—i. Ossis, Ostalgitis—i. Ovarii, Oaritis—i. Palati, Hyperoitis—i. Pancreatis, Pancreatitis—i. Parenchymatica, Parenchymatitis—i. Parotidum, Parotitis, Cynanche parotidæa — i. Pectoris acuta, Pneumonia — i. Peracuta, Hyperphlogosis, Hyperphlegmasia—i. Pericardii, Pericarditis — i. Periostei, Periostitis — i. Periostei orbitæ, Periorbitis—i. Peritonæi, Peritonitis — i. Pharyngis, Cynanche pharyngea — i. Phrenitis, Phrenitis — i. Pleuræ, Pleuritis — i. Pneumonica, Pneumonia — i. Pulmonum, Pneumonia — i. Renum, Nephritis — i. Renum succenturiatorum, Paranephritis—i. Retinæ, Dictyitis, Retinitis—i. Scleroticæ, Sclerotitis—i. Scroti, Oschitis — i. Septi transversi, Diaphragmitis — i. Sinuum frontalium, Metopantritis — i. Stomachi, Gastritis—i. Superficiei internæ cordis, Endocarditis — i. Telæ cellulosæ, Ethmyphytis — i. Telæ fibrosæ, Inohymenitis — i. Testium, Hernia humoralis—i. Tonsillarum, Cynanche tonsillaris—i. Tunicæ hyaloideæ, Hyalitis — i. Tympani, Tympanitis — i. Urethræ, Gonorrhœa — i. Uteri, Metritis—i. Uteri catarrhalis, see Metritis—i. Uteri et Peritonæi, Metroperitonitis—i. Uvulæ, Uvulitis—i. Vasorum, Angoitis—i. Vasorum lymphaticorum, Angeioleucitis—i. Ventriculi, Gastritis—i. Ventriculi et intestinorum, Gastro-enteritis—i. Vesicæ, Cystitis—i. Vesicæ felleæ, Cholecystitis.

INFLAMMATION, *Inflamma'tio*, from *in*, 'within,' and *flamma*, 'flame,' 'fire;' *Phleg'monè*, *Phlogo'sis*, *Ecphlogo'sis*, *Epiphleg''ia*, *Exap'sis*, *Phlegma'sia*, *Causo'ma*, *Empres'ma*, *Phlo'gia*, *Hyperendosmose* (Dutrochet), *Incen'dium*, *Hyperhæmato'sis*, *Hyperæ'mia acti'va*, *Phleboplero'sis ecphrac'tica*, (F.) *Angii'te*, is so called in consequence of the acute or burning pain, felt in a part affected with it. An irritation in a part of the body is occasioned by some stimulus;—owing to which the blood flows into the capillary vessels in greater abundance than natural, and those vessels become over-dilated and enfeebled; whence result pain, redness, heat, tension, and swelling; symptoms which appear in greater or less severity, according to the structure, vital properties, and functions of the part affected, and its connexion with other parts, as well as according to the constitution of the individual. The inflammations of the areolar and serous membranes greatly agree;— and those of the mucus and skin; the former being more active, and constituting the *phlegmonous* variety;—the latter, the *erythematic* or *erysipelatous*. Of this variety is the *diffusive inflammation* produced by morbid poisons; as during dissection, where solutions of continuity exist on the fingers of the operator. It is seen, too, in workers in bone, and hence has been called *bone fever*. Preparatory to the turning of bones, it is customary to macerate them in water. The fluid soon becomes putrid, and if the hands be kept in it diffusive inflammation results. Inflammation may end by resolution, suppuration, gangrene, adhesion, effusion, or induration. Each of the inflammations of internal organs has received a name according to the organ affected;— as, *gastritis*, *cephalitis*, *enteritis*, *hepatitis*, &c. Besides the above inflammations, there is considered to be an instinctive kind established for the union of parts which have been divided, whether the union takes place *immediately*, or by the aid of an intermediate body. This is the *adhesive inflammation*. See Adhesion, Callus, Cicatrix. Broussais considered that the term *inflammation* should include every local exaltation of the organic movements which is sufficiently great to disturb the harmony of the functions, and disorganize the texture in which it is situate. He farther extended the name *inflammation* to irritations which do not induce disorganization of the textures, and which had been previously, and are still, called *fevers*.

Examination of the blood drawn always exhibits an increase of the fibrinous element — the average proportion of which, in healthy blood, is about three in the thousand. In inflammation, it at times rises as high as ten. In fevers unaccompanied with inflammation, the proportion is natural, or below the average; but whenever inflammation supervenes, it immediately rises.

External inflammation is easily detected by the characters already mentioned:—*internal*, by disturbance of function and pain upon pressure; but the last sign is often not available. Both forms require the removal of all irritation, and the reduction of vascular excitement and nervous irritability; hence, blood-letting—local and general — sedatives, refrigerants, and counter-irritants become valuable remedies in almost all cases of inflammation.

INFLAMMATION DES AMYGDALES, Cynanche tonsillaris — *i. des Artères*, Arteritis— i. of the Bladder, Cystitis — *i. de la Bouche*, Stomatitis — *i. des Bronches*, Bronchitis — *i. du Cæcum*, Typhlo-enteritis—i. of the Cæcum, Typhlo-enteritis—*i. du Cerveau et du Cervelet*, Phrenitis *i. du Cœur*, Carditis — *i. du Colon*, Colitis—*i. de la Conjonctive*, see Ophthalmia — i. of the Diaphragm, Diaphragmitis—i. Diffusive, see Inflammation—i. Diphtheritic, Diphtheritis — i. of the Ear, Otitis—*i. de l'Épiglotte*, Epiglottitis—*i. de l'Estomac*, Gastritis—i. of the Eye, Ophthalmia— *i. du Foie*, Hepatitis — *i. des Gencives*, Ulitis—i. General, Synocha—i. of the Internal Membrane of the Heart, Endocarditis—i. Internal, Empresma—*i. des Intestins*, Enteritis—i. of the Iris, Iritis—i. of the Kidney, Nephritis—*i. de la Langue*, Glossitis—i. of the Larynx, Laryngitis—i. of the Liver, Hepatitis—*i. de la Luette*, Uvulitis—i. of the Lungs, Pneumonia—i. of the Malpighian Bodies, Kidney, Bright's disease of the—*i. des Mamelles*, Mastitis—*i. de la Matrice*, Metritis—*i. de la Membrane alvéolo-dentaire*, Periodontitis — *i. de la Membrane séreuse céphalo-rachidienne*, Meningitis—i. of the Mesentery, Mesenteritis—*i. de la Moëlle épinière ou rachidienne*, Myelitis— i. of the Mouth, pseudo-membranous, Stomatitis, pseudo-membranous—i. of the Mouth, pultaceous, Aphthæ — *i. des Muscles*, Myositis — *i. des Nerfs*, Neuritis—*i. de l'Œil*, Ophthalmia—*i. de l'Oreille*, Otitis—*i. de l'Ovaire*, Oaritis—*i. du Palais*, Hyperoitis—*i. du Parenchyme pulmonaire*, Pneumonia — *i. de la Parotide*, Cynanche parotidæa—i. Pellicular, Diphtheritis — *i. du Péricarde*, Pericarditis — i. of the Pericardium, Pericarditis — *i. du Péritoine*, Peritonitis — i. of the Peritonæum, Peritonitis — i. of the Pleura, Pleuritis — *i. de la Plèvre*, Pleuritis — *i. des Poumons*, Pneumonia—*i. du Muscle psoas*, Psoitis—*i. de la Rate*, Splenitis—*i. des Reins*, Nephritis—i. Spongoid, Hæmatodes Fungus, see also Encephaloid— i. of the Stomach, Gastritis — *i. de la Testicule*, Hernia humoralis—i. of the Testicle, Hernia humoralis — *i. des Tissus blancs*, Angeioleucitis—i. of the Tongue, Glossitis — *i. des Vaisseaux Lymphatiques*, Angeioleucitis—*i. des Veines*, Phlebitis—*i. de la Vésicule du Fiel*, Cholecystitis—*i. de la Vessie*, Cystitis—i. of the Womb, Metritis.

INFLAMMATIUN'CULA, *Subinflamma'tio*. A superficial and often insignificant inflammation of the skin, as in many cutaneous affections.

INFLAM'MATORY, *Inflammato'rius; Phlog''icus, Phlogo'des, Phlogis'ticus, Phlogis'tic*, belonging to inflammation;—as, *inflammatory* tumour, *inflammatory* fever, &c. The blood is said to be *inflammatory* when cupped or buffy.

INFLATIO, Emphysema, Puffiness, Colica flatulenta—i. Parotidum, Cynanche parotidæa— i. Uteri, Physometra.

INFLEXIO, Campsis.

INFLUENCE, Influenza.

INFLUENTIA, Influenza.

INFLUENZA. The Italian for 'Influence.' *Influenza Europæ'a, Influen'tia, Catar'rhus epidem'icus, Febris catarrha'lis epidem'ica, Catar'rhus à conta'gio, Rheuma epidem'icum, Morbus Verveci'nus, M. Catarrha'lis, Syn'ochus catarrha'lis, Deflux'io catarrha'lis, M. Arie'tis, Cephalal'gia contagio'sa* (epidemics of the 16th and 17th centuries): (F.) *Tac, Ladendo, Quinte, Florion, Coqueluche, Baraquette, Générale, Grippe, Follette, Grenade, Coquette, Cocote, Petite Poste, Petit Courier, Allure, Fièvre catarrhale épidémique; Influence, Epidemic catarrh*. A severe form of catarrh occurring epidemically, and generally affecting a number of persons in a community. See Catarrh, epidemic. Gluge, from his investigations, considers that the following is the chronological order of the return of the influenza:—14th century, 1323, 1326—15th century, 1410, 1411, 1414—16th century, 1510, 1557, 1562, 1574, 1580, and 1593—17th century, 1658, 1649, 1675, 1693—18th century, 1708, 1712, 1729, 1732,

1733, 1742, 1743, 1761, 1762, and 1775—19th century, 1800, 1803, 1831, and 1833. To these may be added 1837, and 1843.

INFLUENZA EUROPÆA, Influenza.

INFLUEN'ZOÏD, *Influenzoï'des.* An expressive but hybridous compound: from *influensa,* and *eidos,* 'resemblance.' Resembling influenza.—Dr. T. Thompson.

INFORMITAS, Deformation.
INFORTUNIUM, Contrafissura.
INFRA-ATLOIDÆUS, Sub-atloidæus.
INFRA-AXOIDÆUS, Sub-axoidæus.
INFRA-COSTALES, see Intercostal muscles.
INFRA-MAXILLARIS, Sub-maxillary.
INFRAMAXILLOSTERNODYMIA, Cephalosomatodymia.
INFRA-ORBITAR, Sub-orbitar.
INFRAPUBIAN LIGAMENT, Triangular ligament.
INFRA-SCAPULARIS, Subscapularis.
INFRA-SPINALIS, Infra-spinatus.
INFRA-SPINA'TUS, *Infraspina'lis,* from *infra,* 'beneath,' and *spina,* 'a spine.' Situate beneath the spine of the scapula;—*Infra Spina'lis.*

INFRA-SPINA'TA FOSSA, (F.) *Fosse sous-épineuse.* A large excavation on the posterior surface of the scapula, beneath its spine. It is filled by the

INFRA-SPINATUS *Muscle, Grand Scapulo-trochitérien, Superscapula'ris inferior* (Ch.), (F.) *Sous-épineux,* which is broad, flat, and triangular. It is attached, by its base, to the three inner quarters of the fossa; and is inserted, by a long tendon, into the middle part of the great tuberosity of the os humeri (*Trochiter*). It turns the arm outwards, and, when the arm is elevated, carries it backwards.

INFRINGENS, Corrigent.

INFUNDIB'ULUM, (*in,* and *fundere,* 'to pour out.') A Latin word signifying a *Funnel,*— *Choa'nè, Chonos,* (F.) *Entonnoir,*— of which various kinds are employed in pharmaceutical operations. A name, given to many parts which, more or less, resemble a funnel. It is particularly appropriated to the following organs:—

INFUNDIB'ULUM OF THE BRAIN, *Infundib'ulum seu Pelvis seu Choa'na seu Choa'na seu Cy'athus seu Scyphus seu Concha seu Lacu'na seu Em'bolum seu Aquæduc'tus seu Labrum seu Concav'itas conchula'ris seu Processus orbicula'ris Cer'ebri,* (F.) *Entonnoir du ventricule moyen du cerveau, Tige Pituitaire, Tige sus-sphénoïdale.* A depression in the inferior paries of the middle ventricle, above the pituitary gland. It was, anciently, regarded as a canal by which the fluid collected in the ventricles of the brain was evacuated, and poured into the nasal fossæ.

INFUNDIB'ULUM CEREBRI, I. of the Brain.

INFUNDIBULUM OF THE COCHLEA, *I. Coch'lea, Scyphus Vieussen'ii, S. audito'rius, Cucul'lus, Ca-no'lis Scala'rum commu'nis.* This, with the modiolus, forms the nucleus around which the gyri of the cochlea pass. It is an imperfect funnel, the apex of which is common with that of the modiolus; and the base is covered with the apex of the cochlea, termed *Cu'pola.*

In *Surgery,* infundibula are used to direct steam or vapours; to conduct the actual cautery to certain morbid parts, &c.

INFUNDIBULUM OF THE ETHMOID BONE, or OF THE NASAL FOSSÆ. One of the anterior cells of that bone, which is broad and expanded above, and narrow below; opening, above, into the frontal sinus; below, into the anterior part of the middle meatus of the nasal fossæ.

INFUNDIBULUM OF THE HEART, Conus arteriosus—i. of the Kidney, see Calix—i. Lachrymale, Lachrymal Sac—i. Tubarum Fallopii, see Tube, Fallopian—i. Ventriculi, Œsophagus.

INFU'SION, *Infu'sio, En'chysis,* from *infundere* (*in,* and *fundere*), 'to pour in,' 'to introduce.' A pharmaceutical operation, which consists in pouring a hot or cold fluid upon a substance whose medical virtues it is desired to extract. *Infusion* is, also, used for the product of this operation. In *Surgery,* infusion — *Chirur'gia infuso'ria, Ars clysma'tica nova* — is the act of introducing into the veins medicinal substances, by aid of an instrument called *Infusor.* This mode of introducing medicines was called *Ars infuso'ria.*

INFUSION OF ANGUSTURA, Infusum Cuspariæ —i. of Bark, Infusum cinchonæ—i. of Buchu, Infusum Diosmæ — i. of Calumba, Infusum calumbæ — i. of Cascarilla, Infusum cascarillæ — i. of Catechu, Infusum catechu compositum — i. of Cayenne pepper, Infusum capsici — i. of Chamomile, Infusum anthemidis — i. of Cinchona, Infusum cinchonæ—i. of Cloves, Infusum caryophyllorum — i. of Cusparia, Infusum cuspariæ — i. of Dandelion, Infusum Taraxaci — i. of Foxglove, Infusum digitalis—i. of Gentian, compound, Infusum gentianæ compositum—i. of Ginger, Infusum Zingiberis — i. of Hops, Infusum humuli —i. of Horseradish, compound, Infusum armoraciæ compositum — i. of Binseed, Infusum lini compositum — i. of Mint, compound, Infusum menthæ compositum — i. of Orange-peel, compound, Infusum aurantii compositum—i. of Pinkroot, Infusum spigeliæ — i. of Quassia, Infusum quassiæ—i. of Rhatany, Infusum Krameriæ—i. of Rhubarb, Infusum rhei — i. of the Rose, Infusum rosæ compositum — i. of Sarsaparilla, Infusum sarsaparillæ — i. of Sassafras pith, Infusum sassafras medullæ — i. of Senna, Infusum sennæ compositum — i. of Simarouba, Infusum simaroubæ — i. of Slippery elm, Infusum ulmi — i. of Thoroughwort, Infusum eupatorii—i. of Tobacco, Infusum tabaci—i. of Valerian, Infusum valerianæ—i. of Virginia snakeroot, Infusum serpentariæ — i. of Wild cherry, Infusum pruni Virginianæ.

INFUSOIR (F.), same etymon. An instrument for injecting medicinal substances into the veins. It was a kind of funnel, the elongated apex of which was stopped by a metallic rod, which could be withdrawn when the apex was introduced into a vein.

INFU'SUM, *En'chyma.* The product of an infusion.

INFUSUM ACACIÆ CATECHU, I. catechu compositum—i. Amarum vinosum, Vinum gentianæ compositum — i. of Angustura, I. cuspariæ.

INFUSUM ANTHEM'IDIS, *Hydrochamaime'lum, Infusion of Cham'omile.* (*Anthemid. flor.* ℥ss; *aq. bullient.* Oj. Macerate for ten minutes in a covered vessel, and strain.—*Ph. L.*) Dose, f℥j to f℥iss.

INFUSUM ARMORA'CIÆ COMPOS'ITUM, *Infusum Armoraciæ* (Ph. U. S.), *Compound infusion of Horseradish.* (*Armorac. rad. concis., sinapis* cont. sing. ℥j; *aquæ bullient.* Oj. Macerate for two hours, and strain.) Dose, f℥j to f℥iij.

INFUSUM AURAN'TII COMPOS'ITUM, *Compound Infusion of Orange Peel.* (*Aurant. cort. sicc.* ℥ij; *limon. cort. recent.* ℥j; *caryoph.* cont. ℥ss; *aq. fervent.* Oss. Macerate for fifteen minutes, and strain.—*Ph. L.*) Dose, f℥iss to f℥ij.

INFUSUM BRASIL, Wort—i. Buchu, Infusum Diosmæ—i. Bynes, Wort.

INFUSUM CALUM'BÆ, *I. Calom'bæ, I. Colombæ, Infusion of Columba.* (*Calumb. rad. concis.* ℥ss; *aq. fervent.* Oj. Macerate for two hours, and strain.—Ph. U. S.) Dose, f℥iss to f℥iij.

INFUSUM CAP'SICI, *Infusion of Cayenne Pepper.* (*Capsic.* in pulv. crass. ℥ss; *aq. bullient.* Oj.

INFUSUM 475 INFUSUM

Macerate for two hours, and strain.—Ph. U. S.) Dose, f℥iss.

INFUSUM CARYOPHYL'LI, *Infusion of Cloves.* (*Caryoph.* contus. ℨij; *aq. bullient.* Oj. Macerate for two hours, and strain.) Dose, f℥iss to f℥ij.

INFUSUM CASCARIL'LÆ, *Infusion of Cascarilla.* (*Cascarill.* contus. ℨj; *aq. bullient.* Oj. Macerate for two hours, and strain.) Dose, f℥iss to f℥ij.

INFUSUM CASSIÆ SENNÆ, I. sennæ compositum.

INFUSUM CAT'ECHU COMPOS'ITUM, *Infusum Catechu, I. Aca'ciæ Catechu, Infusion of Catechu.* (*Catechu*, in pulv. ℨss; *cinnam.* cont. ℨj; *aq. bullient.* Oj. Macerate for an hour, and strain.) Dose, f℥iss to f℥ij.

INFUSUM CINCHO'NÆ, *I. Cinchonæ lancifo'liæ, Infusion of Cinchona.* (*Cinch.* contus. ℨj; *aq. fervent.* Oj. Macerate for two hours, and strain.) This infusion may also be made from the same quantity of bark in coarse powder by the process of displacement with hot or cold water. Dose, f℥j to f℥iij. The Pharmacopœia of the United States has an *Infu'sum Cincho'næ flavæ, Infusion of yellow bark*, and an *Infusum Cinchonæ rubræ, Infusion of red bark*, which are prepared in the same manner. It has also an *Infu'sum Cincho'næ Compositum*, which is made as follows: (*Cinchon. rubr.* in pulv. ℨj; *Acid. Sulph. aromat.* fℨj; *aquæ*, Oj. Macerate for twelve hours, occasionally shaking, and strain.) Dose, same as the last.

INFUSUM CINCHONÆ COMPOSITUM, see Infusum Cinchonæ.

INFUSUM CINCHONÆ FLAVÆ, see Infusum Cinchonæ.

INFUSUM COLOMBÆ, I. calumbæ.

INFUSUM CUSPA'RIÆ, *I. Angustu'ræ, Infusion of Cuspa'ria.* (*Cuspar. cort.* contus. ℨss; *aq. bullient.* Oj. Macerate for two hours, and strain.) Dose, f℥j to f℥iij.

INFUSUM DIGITA'LIS, *I. Digitalis purpu'reæ, Infusion of Foxglove.* (*Digital.* ℨj; *aq. bullient.* Oss : *tinct. cinnamomi*, f℥j. Macerate, and add *sp. cinnam.* f℥j.) Dose, f℥j.

INFUSUM DIOS'MÆ, Ph. U. S., 1842, *Infusum Buchu*, Ph. U. S., 1851, *Infusion of Buchu.* (*Diosm.* ℨj; *aq. bullient.* Oj. Macerate for four hours in a covered vessel, and strain.—Ph. U.S.) Dose, f℥iss.

INFUSUM EUPATO'RII, *Infusion of Thoroughwort.* (*Eupator.* ℨj; *aq. bullient*, Oj. Macerate for two hours, and strain.—Ph. U. S.) Dose, f℥ij.

INFUSUM GENTIA'NÆ COMPOS'ITUM, *Compound Infusion of Gentian.* (*Gentian.* cont. ℨss; *Aurant. cort., Coriandr.* contus. āā ℨj; *alcohol. dilut.* f℥iv; *aquæ*, f℥xij. First pour on the acohol, and three hours afterwards, the water; then macerate for twelve hours, and strain.—Ph. U. S.) Dose, f℥j to f℥ij.

Marsden's Antiscorbu'tic Drops, an empirical preparation, consist of a solution of *corrosive sublimate* in an *infusion of gentian*.

INFU'SUM HU'MULI, *Infusion of Hops.* (*Humul.* ℨss; *aq. bullient.* Oj. Macerate for two hours, and strain.—Ph. U. S.) Dose, f℥iss to f℥iij.

INFU'SUM KRAME'RIÆ, *Infusion of Rhat'any.* (*Kramer.* contus. ℨj; *aq. bullient*, Oj. Macerate for four hours, and strain.—Ph. U. S.) Dose, f℥iss.

INFUSUM LINI, I. L. compositum.

INFUSUM LINI COMPOS'ITUM (Ph. U. S., 1851), *I. Lini* (Ph. U. S., 1842), *I. Lini usitatis'simi, Infusion of Linseed, Flaxseed Tea.* (*Lini sem.* cont. ℨss; *glycyrrh. rad.* cont. ℨij; *aquæ bullient.* Oj. Macerate for four hours, and strain.) Dose, a teacupful. *ad libitum.*

INFUSUM MALTI, Wort.

INFUSUM MENTHÆ COMPOS'ITUM, *Compound Infusion of Mint.* (*Fol. menth. sat.* sicc. ℨij; *aq. fervent.* q. s. ut. colentur. f℥vj. Macerate for half an hour; and, when cold, strain : then add — *sacch. alb.* ℨij; *ol. menth. sat.* gtt. iij, dissolved in *tinct. card. c.* f℥ss.—*Ph. D.*) Dose, f℥j to f℥iij.

INFUSUM PICIS EMPYREUMATICÆ LIQUIDÆ, see Pinus sylvestris — i. Picis liquidum, see Pinus sylvestris.

INFUSUM PRUNI VIRGINIA'NÆ, *Infusion of Wild Cherry Bark.* (*Prun. Virginian.* cont. ℨss; *aquæ*, Oj. Macerate for two hours, and strain.— Ph. U. S.)

INFUSUM QUASSIÆ, *I. Quassiæ excel'sæ, Infusion of Quassia.* (*Quassiæ lign.* conc. ℨij; *aq.* Oj. Macerate for two hours, and strain.) Dose, f℥j to f℥iv.

INFUSUM RHEI, *An'ima Rhei, Infusion of Rhubarb.* (*Rhei*, cont. ℨj; *aq. ferv.* Oss. Macerate for two hours, and strain.) Dose, f℥j to f℥iv.

INFUSUM ROSÆ COMPOS'ITUM, *I. Rosæ Gal'licæ, Infusion of the Rose.* (*Ros. Gallic.* ℨiv; *aq. bullient.* Oiiss; *acid. sulph. d.* f℥iij; *sacch. purif.* ℨiss. Add the water, and afterwards the acid;— macerate for half an hour; strain, and add the sugar.) Dose, f℥iss to Oss.

INFUSUM SARSAPARIL'LÆ, *Infusion of Sarsaparilla.* (*Sarsaparill.* contus. ℨj; *aquæ bullient.* Oj. Digest for two hours in a covered vessel, and strain.—Ph. U. S.) It may also be prepared by displacement. Dose, f℥ij to f℥iv.

INFUSUM SASSAFRAS, *Infusion of Sassafras Pith, Mu'cilage of Sassafras Pith.* (*Sassafras medull.* ℨj; *aquæ*, Oj. Macerate for three hours, and strain.) An emollient collyrium; and demulcent drink.

INFUSUM SENNÆ, *I. S. Compos'itum, I. Cassiæ Sennæ, I. Sennæ simplex, Infusion of Senna.* (*Sennæ*, ℨj; *coriandr.* cont. ℨj; *aq. bullient.* Oj. Macerate for an hour, and strain.) Dose, f℥j to f℥iv.

The *Black Draught, Black Dose, Haustus niger*, is usually formed of this infusion. It may be made of *infus. sennæ*, f℥v; *aq. cinnam.* f℥j; *mannæ*, ℨiv; *magnes. sulph.* ℨvj. Dose, a wineglassful.

Selway's Prepared Essence of Senna is a concentrated infusion of the leaves in combination with an alkali.

INFUSUM SENNÆ COMPOSITUM, I. sennæ.

INFUSUM SERPENTA'RIÆ, *Infusion of Virginia Snakeroot.* (*Serpentar.* ℨss; *aq. bullient.* Oj. Macerate for two hours, and strain.—Ph. U. S.) Dose, f℥iss.

INFUSUM SIMAROU'BÆ, *Infusion of Simarouba.* (*Simaroub. cort.* cont. ℨss; *aq. fervent.* Oss. Macerate for two hours, and strain.—*Ph. L.*) Dose, f℥ij.

INFU'SUM SPIGE'LIÆ, *Infusion of Pinkroot.* (*Spigel.* ℨss; *aq. bullient.* Oj. Macerate for two hours, and strain.—Ph. U. S.) Dose, f℥iv to Oss.

INFUSUM TAB'ACI, *Infusion of Tobacco.* (*Tabaci fol.* ℨj; *aq. ferv.* Oj. Macerate for an hour, and strain.—Ph. U. S.)

INFUSUM TARAX'ACI, *Infusion of Dandelion.* (*Taraxac.* contus. ℨij; *aq. bullient.* Oj. Macerate for two hours, and strain.— Ph. U. S.) Dose, f℥iss, as a diuretic, &c.

INFUSUM ULMI, *Infusion of Slip'pery Elm, Slippery Elm Tea.* This preparation, in the Pharmacopœia of the United States, is made by infusing one ounce of *slippery elm bark* in a pint of *boiling water*.

INFUSUM VALERIA'NÆ, *Infusion of Vale'rian.* (*Rad. valerian.* in crass. pulv. ℨss; *aq. bullient.* Oj.

Macerate for an hour, and strain.—*Ph. D.* and *U. S.*) Dose, ℨiss to ℨij.

INFUSUM ZINGIB'ERIS, *Infusion of Ginger, Ginger Tea.* (*Zingib.* contus. ℨss; *aq. bullient.* Oj. Macerate for two hours, and strain.— Ph. U. S.) Dose, f ℨiss, as a carminative.

INGE'NIUM (*Morbi*). The genius of a disease. This word is employed, especially by the French, synonymously with *nature.* They speak, for instance, of *Génie inflammatoire, bilieux,* &c. Some, also, use *génie* in the place of *type* of an intermittent.

INGES'TA, from *in,* and *gerere, gestum,* 'to bear or carry into.' Substances, introduced into the body by the digestive passages; as food, condiments, drinks, &c.

INGLU'VIES, *Aples'tia, Victûs intemperan'tia:* — Gluttony, Insatiableness; also, the *Crop* or *Craw* of Birds, (F.) *Jabot;* and the *first stomach* or *paunch* of ruminant animals—*Pen'ula, Rumen, Venter magnus.* Also, the Pharynx.

INGRAS'SIAS, APOPH'YSES OF. The lesser alæ of the sphenoid bone.

INGRAVIDATIO, Fecundation, Pregnancy.

INGRAVIDATION, Fecundation, Pregnancy.

INGRESSUS SUPERIOR, Cardia.

INGUEN, *Bubon, Bubo,* 'the groin.' *Ædœ'on,* αιδοιον, *He'patis emuncto'ria,* (F.) *Aine.* The oblique fold or depression which separates the abdomen from the thigh. It is only, properly speaking, a line that extends from the anterior and superior spinous process of the ilium to the middle part of the horizontal ramus of the pubis. Also, the genital organs.

IN'GUINAL, *Inguina'lis,* from *inguen,* 'the groin.' Belonging or relating to the groin. This epithet has been given to various parts met with in the region of the groin or inguinal region.

INGUINAL ARTERY is that portion of the femoral artery situate immediately beneath the crural arch in the inguinal region.

INGUINAL CANAL is a canal, about two inches in length, proceeding obliquely downwards, inwards and forwards at the lower part of the abdomen; through which passes the spermatic cord, in men, and the round ligament of the uterus in women. This canal is formed, inferiorly and anteriorly, by the aponeurosis of the greater oblique muscle; posteriorly by the *fascia transversalis,* which is joined to the preceding aponeurosis, and forms with it a deep channel, into which are received the lesser oblique and transversalis muscles. The inguinal canal has two apertures; the one, the *lower* and *inner,* is called the *inguinal* or *abdominal ring.* It is bounded by two strong tendinous pillars, which fix it — the innermost to the symphysis, the outermost to the spine of the pubis. The *upper and outer aperture* is formed by the fascia transversalis. From the edge of this aperture arises a membranous funnel, — a prolongation of the fascia transversalis, — which receives the spermatic vessels; forms their proper sheath, and accompanies them as far as the testicle. On its inside lies the epigastric artery. Above it, is the lower edge of the transversalis muscle: and, below, it is bounded by the channel of the greater oblique. By following the oblique direction of this canal, and passing, consequently, on the outside of the epigastric artery, the viscera are displaced, so as to constitute internal inguinal hernia.

IN'GUINAL RE'GION, *Re'gio inguina'lis, Bubo, Inguen.* The region of the groin.

INGUINAL RING, *Abdom'inal Ring, An'nulus abdom'inis,* (F.) *Anneau Inguinal,* is the inferior aperture of the inguinal canal.

IN'GUINO-CUTA'NEUS. A name given by Professor Chaussier to the middle ramus of the anterior branch of the first lumbar nerve; because it sends its numerous filaments to the groin, scrotum, and to the skin of the superior part of the thigh.

INHÆRENS, Inherent.

INHALATIO, Absorption, Inhalation — i. Cutis, see Absorption.

INHALA'TION, *Inhala'tio;* from *in* and *halare,* 'to breathe.' The act of drawing air or vapour into the lungs — *Inhala'tio pulmona'lis.* Also, absorption.

INHA'LER. Same etymon. An apparatus for inhalation. *Mudge's Inhaler* is an apparatus for inhaling the steam of hot water, in affections of the air-passages. It consists of a pewter tankard provided with a lid, into which a flexible tube is inserted. Through this, the vapour is inhaled.

INHE'RENT, *Inhærens,* (*in,* and *hærens.*) That which adheres, or which is joined or united to any thing.

INHERENT CAUTERY, (F.) *Cautère inhérent,* is the actual cautery, left in contact with a part until it is reduced to the state of a deep eschar.

INHUMA'TION, *Inhuma'tio,* from *inhumo,* (*in,* and *humus,*) 'I put into the ground.' *Inhuma'tio.* The *sepulture of the dead.* This belongs to the subject of medical police.

INIAD, see Inial.

IN'IAL, from ινιον, the ridge of the occiput. An epithet, proposed by Dr. Barclay, for an aspect towards the plane of the ridge of the occiput. *Iniad* is employed by him adverbially to signify 'towards the inial aspect.'

INIODYMUS, Diprosopus.

INION, ινιον. Some of the Greek physicians give this name to the occiput, or the ridge of the occiput; others to the back part of the neck, and the muscles of the occiput. Blanchard says it is the commencement of the spinal marrow.

INI'TIS, *Inohymeni'tis,* from ις, gen. ινος, 'a fibre,' and *itis,* a suffix denoting inflammation. Fibrous inflammation.

INITIUM, Arche — i. Asperæ arteriæ, Larynx — i. Extuberans Coli, Cæcum.

INIUM, ινιον. The nucha. Also, the muscles at the back of the neck. See Inion.

INJACULA'TIO. A term employed by Van Helmont to designate an acute pain of the stomach, with rigidity and immobility of the body.

INJECT'ED, *Injec'tus,* from *injicere,* (*in,* and *jacere,* 'to throw into.' The face and other parts are said to be *injected,* when the accumulation of blood in the capillary vessels gives them an evident red colour. A subject or part of a subject, is also said to be *injected,* when its vessels have been filled, by the anatomist, with an appropriate composition.

INJEC'TION, *Injec'tio, Eis'bolē:* same etymon. The act of introducing, by means of a syringe or other instrument, a liquid into a cavity of the body. The liquid injected is also called an *injection.* Anatomists use injections — *Injectio'nes anatom'icæ* — for filling the cavities of vessels, in order that they may be rendered more apparent, and their dissection be facilitated. For this purpose, they employ syringes of different dimensions, and various materials. The most common injections are made of soot, wax, and turpentine, coloured with lamp-black, vermilion, &c. There are three kinds chiefly used by anatomists, — the *coarse,* the *fine,* and the *minute.* The following are formulæ for each.

COARSE INJECTION.

No. 1.

Pure yellow wax, oz. xvj.
Bleached rosin, oz. viij.
Turpentine varnish, by measure, oz. vj.

No. 2.
Yellow rosin, lb. ij.
Yellow wax, lb. j.
Turpentine varnish, a sufficient quantity to make the mixture flexible when cold.

No. 3.
Tallow, lb. ij.
White wax, oz. x.
Common oil, oz. vj.
Venice turpentine, oz. iv.
Mix and liquefy over a slow fire or over boiling water.

To make any of these mixtures.
Red — add *vermilion*, oz. iij.
Yellow — *King's yellow*, oz. iiss.
White — *best flake white*, oz. vss.
Pale-blue { *best flake white*, oz. iiiss.
           { *fine blue smalt*, oz. iiiss.
Dark-blue — *blue verditer*, oz. xss.
Black — *lamp-black*, oz. j.
Green { *powdered verdigris*, oz. ivss.
      { *best flake white*, oz. iss.
      { *powdered gamboge*, oz. j.

Fine Injection.

Brown spirit varnish, oz. iv.
White spirit varnish, oz. iv.
Turpentine varnish, oz. j.

To make this mixture,
Red — add *vermilion*, oz. j.
Yellow — *King's yellow*, oz. j¾.
White — *best flake white*, oz. ij.
Light-blue { *fine blue smalt*, oz. iss.
           { *best flake white*, oz. j¾
Dark-blue — *blue verditer*, oz. iv.
Black — *lamp-black*, oz. ss.

Minute Injection.

Take of *transparent size*, broken to pieces, or *Isinglass*, oz. viij.
Water, lb. iss. Dissolve.

To make this mixture,
Red — add *vermilion*, oz. v.
Yellow — *King's yellow*, oz. iv.
White — *best flake white*, oz. v.
Blue — *fine blue smalt*, oz. viij.
Green { *powdered verdigris*, oz. iij.
      { *best flake white*, dr. ij.
      { *powdered gamboge*, dr. j.
Black — *lamp-black*, oz. j.

Beautiful injections are made with ether as the menstruum.

Cold Injection.

White lead and *red lead*, each, oz. iv; *linseed oil*, enough to form a thick paste when they are rubbed well together. Liquefy this paste with *turpentine varnish*, oz. viij.

The advantage of this mixture is, that the subject need not be heated.

In order to inject the arteries, the injection must be forced from the great trunks towards their ultimate ramifications. To inject the veins, on the contrary, it is indispensable, on account of their valves, to send the injection from the smaller divisions towards the greater. The lymphatics are usually injected with mercury. The practitioner injects, by forcing with a syringe, liquids, such as emollient, narcotic, stimulant, and other decoctions or infusions, into different hollow organs, as the rectum, vagina, nasal fossæ, urethra, tunica vaginalis, auditory canal, &c., to fulfil various therapeutical indications.

The following injection has been strongly recommended by Dr. Horner to preserve the dead body.

Take of *Liverpool St. Ubes*,
or *Turk's Island Salt*,   oz. 36 avoird.
Nitrate of potassa,   " 19
Carbonate of soda,   " 8
Molasses (Sugar-house,)   " 4 by meas.
Water,   six pints.

The saline constituents to be dissolved first of all in boiling hot water; the molasses to be afterwards stirred in: the starch to be mixed well with half a pint of cold water, and then to be stirred in with the other articles. As soon as it begins to boil, the whole mass swells up, when it must be removed from the fire. On the proper reduction of temperature it is fit for use.

INJECTION, MATTHEWS'S, see Tinctura cantharidis.

INJECTIONES ANATOMICÆ, see Injection.

INK, Atramentum.

IN-KNEED, Entogonyankon.

IN'NATE, from *in*, and *natus*, 'born.' Inborn.

INNATE DISEASES, *Morbi conna'ti, M. congen'iti*, (F.) *Maladies innées*. Diseases with which the infant is born. They are not always hereditary, as hereditary diseases are not always innate.

INNERLEITHEN, MINERAL WATERS OF. These springs, situate near the Tweed, and supposed to be the scene of "St. Ronan's Well," contain chlorides of sodium and calcium, and carbonate of magnesia.

INNERVA'TION, *Innerva'tio*, from *in*, 'in,' and *nervus*, 'a nerve.' By this term is meant — the nervous influence, necessary for the maintenance of life and the functions of the various organs; — an influence of whose character and source we are ignorant. It seems to resemble the galvanic or electric agencies. See Nerves.

INNOMINA'TUM, *Anon'ymum*, from *in*, priv. and *nomen*, 'a name.' (F.) *Anonyme*. Having no name.

INNOMINA'TA ARTE'RIA, *Brachio-cephal'ic artery, A. brachio-céphalique* (Ch.),—*Arte'ria anon'yma, Right Subclavian*, (F.) *Artère innominée*, is the trunk common to the right primitive carotid and to the subclavian. It arises from the anterior part of the arch of the aorta, ascends obliquely to the right, along the trachea; and, after a course of about an inch in length, divides into two trunks, which go off at right angles. The one is *external* — the *right subclavian proper;* the other *superior* — the *primitive carotid*, of the same side.

INNOMINATA CARTILAGO, Cricoid.

INNOMINATA CAV'ITAS. A cavity of the outer ear, between the *helix* and *anthelix*.

INNOMINATUM FORA'MEN. A foramen, near the middle of the anterior surface of the pars petrosa of the temporal bone, leading backwards for the passage of the Vidian nerve, reflected from the 2d branch of the 5th to the portio dura of the 7th pair.

INNOMINATA FOSSA, see Fossa.

INNOMINATA LINEA, see Ilio-pectinea Linea.

INNOMINATI vel ANONYMI NERVI. Some anatomists have thus called the nerves of the fifth pair.

INNOMINATUM OS, *Os Coxen'dicis, Os Coxæ, Os anon'ymum, Os pelvis latera'lè*, (F.) *Os innominé, Os Coxal, Os anonyme*, &c. A very large, flat bone, which forms the anterior and lateral paries of the pelvis. It is curved upon itself in two opposite directions. In the first periods of life, it is composed of three portions; — the *ilium, ischium*, and *pubis*, which join each other in the acetabulum. It is articulated *before* with its fellow, — *behind*, with the sacrum; and *laterally* with the femur.

INNOMINATA MINO'RA OSSA, — *Lesser Ossa innominata, Ossic'ula innomina'ta*. Some anatomists have given this name to the three cuneiform bones of the tarsus.

INNOMINATA OSSICULA, Innominata minora ossa—i. Tunica Oculi, Sclerotic.

INNOMINATÆ VENÆ OF VIEUSSENS. Vieussens has given this name to two or three veins, which arise on the anterior surface and right margin of the heart, and open into the auricle towards its right margin. The term VENÆ INNOMINATÆ OF MECKEL is given to the *brachiocephalic* veins, which are generally included in the description of the subclavian vein, and correspond to the arteriæ innominatæ, being formed by the union of the internal jugular vein and the subclavian properly so called, which correspond to the common carotid and subclavian arteries.

INNOMINATUS, Anonymous.

INNUTRITIO OSSIUM, Rachitis.

INOCULA'TION, *Inocula'tio, Insit"io, Insit"io variola'rum,* from *inoculare,* (in, and *oculus,* 'an eye,') 'to ingraft.' Any operation by which small-pox, for example, may be artificially communicated, by introducing the virus of the particular disease into the economy, by means of a puncture or scratch made in the skin. When the word inoculation is used alone, it usually means that for the small-pox,— *Variola'tion.*

INOCULATION, COWPOX, Vaccination—i. Jennerian, Vaccination.

INOC'ULATOR, Same etymon. *In'sitor.* One who practises inoculation.

INODULAR TISSUE, see Tissue, inodular.

INODULE, Tissue, inodular.

INOHYLOMA, Tumor, fibrous.

INOHYMENI'TIS: from ις, gen. ινος, 'a fibre;' ὑμην, 'a membrane,' and *itis,* denoting inflammation. *Inflamma'tio telæ fibro'sæ.* Inflammation of the fibrous tissue.

INOPOLYPUS, see Polypus.

INORGAN'IC, *Inorgan'icus, Unor'ganized,* (Fr.) *Inorganique;* from *in,* priv. and *organum,* 'an organ.' A term applied to bodies which have no organs;—such as minerals. At the present day, naturalists admit of but two classes of bodies,—the *organized* and *inorganic.* Parts of the body which, like the epidermis, are devoid of blood-vessels and nerves, have been called *anorganic.*

INOSCLERO'MA, from ις, gen. ινος, 'a fibre,' and σκληρωμα, 'induration.' Induration of the fibrous tissue.

INOSCULATIO, Anastomosis.

INQUIES, Inquietude.

INQUIETATIO, Inquietude.

INQUI'ETUDE, *Inquietu'do, In'quies, Inquieta'tio, Jactita'tio,* from *in,* priv. and *quies,* 'rest.' Agitation or trouble, caused by indisposition. Restlessness.

INQUINAMENTUM, Miasm.

INQUISITIO MEDICO-LEGALIS, see Medico-legal.

INSALIVA'TION, *Insaliva'tio,* from *in,* and *saliva.* The mixture of the food with the saliva, and other secretions of the mouth.

INSALU'BRIOUS, *Insalu'bris, Nose'ros, Noso'des.* That which is unhealthy,—which injures the health.

INSANABILIS, Incurable.

INSANE, *Insa'nus;* from *in,* 'un,' and *sanus,* 'sound;' *Aliena'tus, Crazy, Mad, Non-sane, Demented, Deranged,* (F.) *Aliéné, Fou, Insensé.* One affected with mental aberration, or of unsound mind.

INSANIA, Mania—i. Cadiva, Epilepsy—i. Lupina, Lycanthropia—i. Puerperarum, Mania, puerperal.

INSAN'ITY, *Insa'nia;* from *in,* privative, and *sanus,* 'sound;' *Mental aliena'tion, Abaliena'tio seu Alienatio Mentis, Arrep'tio, Unsound Mind,* *Derange'ment, Deranged intellect, Cra'siness, Aphros'ynē, Ecphro'nia, Ecphros'ynē, Paral'lagē, Parallax'is, Delir'ia, Vesa'niæ, Delir'ium,* (Crichton,) *Insipien'tia,* (F.) *Folie, Égarement d'Esprit, Paraphrénie.* This term includes all the varieties of unsound mind, — Mania, Melancholia, Moral Insanity, Dementia, and Idiocy. A slight degree of insanity is sometimes popularly called "*a kink in the head;*" in Scotland, "*a bee in the bonnet.*"

INSANITY, HOMICIDAL, see Homicidal—i. Incoherent, Dementia — i. Moral, Pathomania — i. Puerperal, Mania, puerperal—i. Senile, Delirium senile—i. Suicidal, see Suicide.

INSANUS, Insane.

INSCRIPTION, see Matriculate.

INSCRIPTIO'NES TENDIN'EÆ MUSCULO'RUM, *Intersectio'nes seu Enervatio'nes tendin'eæ musculo'rum, Interme'dia ligamenta'lia seu ner'vea.* The tendinous portions which cross several muscles, and especially the straight muscles of the abdomen.

INSENESCENTIA, Agerasia.

INSENSÉ, Insane.

INSENSIBIL'ITY, *Anæsthe'sia, Insensibil'itas.* Loss or absence of sensibility. It is very common in cerebral affections, and may extend to every part, or be limited to one or more. Some organs are much more sensible than others. The bones, cartilages, ligaments, &c., are insensible in health, but acutely sensible in disease.

INSEN'SIBLE, *Sensibilita'tē carens.* That which is devoid of sensibility. This word is applied, also, to phenomena which cease to be appreciable to the senses. Thus, we say, the pulse becomes *insensible.*

INSER'TION, *Inser'tio, Symph'ysis, Enc'sis,* from *inserere,* (in, and *serere,* 'to join or knit,') 'to ingraft.' (F.) *Attache.* The attachment of one part to another. Insertions occur chiefly on bones, cartilages, and fibrous organs; thus, we speak of the insertion of muscular fibres into a tendon or aponeurosis; the insertion of a tendon, aponeurosis, or ligament, into a cartilage or bone. The word *insertion* has likewise been used by pathologists, for the act of inoculating or introducing a virus into the body.

INSES'SIO, from *insidere,* (in, and *sedere,*) 'to sit in.' This term is, sometimes, applied to a vapour bath, the person being seated in a perforated chair, beneath which a vessel, filled with hot water, or the hot decoction of some plant, is placed. See Semicupium.

INSESSUS, Bath, half.

INSIDEN'TIA, *Epis'tasis.* Any thing which swims on or in the urine. It is opposed to the *Hypos'tasis* or *subsiden'tia.*

INSIPIENTIA, Insanity.

INSISIO CILIORUM, Blepharoplastice.

INSITIO, Inoculation—i. Dentis, Transplantatio Dentis—i. Variolarum, Inoculation.

INSOLA'TION, *Insola'tio,* from *in,* and *sol,* 'the sun;' *Aprica'tio, Helio'sis, Heli'asis, Helieno'sis, Siri'asis.* Exposure to the sun. Exposure of a patient to the rays of the sun is, sometimes, had recourse to, with the view of rousing the vital forces when languishing, or of producing irritation of the skin. Insolation is occasionally used in the same sense as *coup de soleil.*

In *Pharmacy, insolation* means the drying of chemical and pharmaceutical substances.

INSOLAZIONE DE PRIMIVERA, Pellagra.

INSOM'NIA, *Insom'nitas, Sahara, Zaara, Pervigil'ium, Pernocta'tio, Aǵp'nia, Agryp'nia, Ahyp'nia, Anyp'nia, Typhoma'nia, Sleeplessness, Vig"ilance,* from *in,* privative, and *somnus,* 'sleep,' 'absence of sleep.' ' This may exist alone, and constitute a true disease; or it may be connected with another affection. It is an unequivocal sign of suffering in some organ; even when the patient experiences no pain.

INSOMNIUM, Somnium.

INSPECTIO MEDICO-LEGALIS, see Medico-legal.

INSPIRATEUR, Inspiratory.

INSPIRA'TION, *Inspira'tio, Empneumato'sis, Eisp'noē, Adspira'tio, Aspira'tio*, from *in*, 'in,' and *spiro*, 'I breathe.' The action by which the air penetrates into the interior of the lungs. A movement opposed to that of expiration. As regards the average quantity of air received into the lungs at each inspiration, there is much discrepancy amongst observers. The following table sufficiently exhibits this:—

	Cubic inches at each inspiration.
Rell	42 to 100
Menzies, Sauvages, Hales, Haller, Ellis, Sprengel, Sömmering, Thomson, Bostock,	40
Jurin	35 to 38
Fontana	35
Richerand	30 to 40
Dalton	30
Jeffreys	26
Herbst	24 to 30
Herholdt	20 to 29
Jurine and Coathupe	20
Allen and Pepys	16½
J. Borelli	15 to 40
Goodwyn	14
Sir H. Davy	13 to 17
Abernethy and Mojon	12
Kentsch	6 to 12

INSPIRATION OF VENOUS BLOOD. By this is meant the aspiration of blood towards the heart, occasioned by the approach to a vacuum produced by the dilatation of the thorax during inspiration.

IN'SPIRATORY. Same etymon. *Inspiratio'ni inser'viens*, (F.) *Inspirateur*. A name given to muscles, which, by their contraction, augment the size of the chest, and thus produce inspiration. The diaphragm and intercostal muscles are the chief agents of inspiration. In cases where deep inspirations are necessary, the action of these muscles is aided by the contraction of the pectoralis major and pectoralis minor, subclavius, serratus major anticus, scaleni, serratus posticus superior, &c. Most of these muscles become inspiratory, by taking their fixed point at the part which they ordinarily move, and elevating the ribs.

INSPISSA'TIO, *Pycno'sis*, from *in*, and *spissare*, 'to thicken.' The act of rendering thick; as in the formation of an extract—*Succus Inspissa'tus*.

INSTEP, *Collum pedis*, (F.) *Coude-pied, Cou du pied*. The projection at the upper part of the foot, near its articulation with the leg—the *tarsus*.

INSTILLATIO, Instillation.

INSTILLA'TION, *Enstalax'is, Instilla'tio*, from *in*, 'into,' and *stilla*, 'a drop.' The act of pouring a liquid drop by drop.

INSTINCT, (L.) *Instinc'tus*, (in, and *stinguo*, 'I sting,') 'inwardly moved.' *Bru'tia, Hormē*. The action of the living principle, whenever manifestly directing its operations to the health, preservation, or reproduction of a living frame or any part of such frame — *Moli'men natu'ræ saluta'rium*. The law of instinct is, consequently, the law of the living principle, and instinctive actions are the actions of the living principle. Instinct is natural. Reason is acquired.

INSTINC'TIVE, *Instinc'tus*. Same etymon. Relating to or caused by instinct; as *instinctive actions*. See Emotional. Those instinctive actions of animals which are owing to impressions made on the sensory ganglia, exciting respondent motor influences that are propagated to the various muscles of the body, are termed *consensual*.

INSTITUTES OF MEDICINE, see Theory of medicine.

INSTITUTUM ORTHOPÆDICUM, Orthopedic institution.

IN'STRUMENT, *Instrumen'tum, Or'ganum*. A tool, an agent.

INSTRUMENTA, Pudibilia.

INSTRUMEN'TUM CHIRUR'GICUM. A surgical tool or instrument.

INSTRUMENTUM DIGESTIONIS. The digestive apparatus.

INSTRUMENTUM INSTRUMENTORUM, Manus.

INSUFFIC''IENCY, from *in*, and *sufficient*. Inadequateness to any end or purpose,— as *Insufficiency of the valves of the heart*; (F.) *Insuffisance des valvules du Cœur*;—a condition in which they are not adapted, as in health, to properly close the apertures.

INSUFFISANCE DES VALVULES DU CŒUR, Insufficiency of the valves of the heart.

INSUFFLA'TION, *Insuffla'tio*, from *in*, *sub*, and *flare*, 'to blow.' The act of blowing a gas or vapour into some cavity of the body; as when tobacco smoke is injected into the rectum; or when air is blown into the mouths of new-born children to excite the respiratory functions.

INSULA, Insula cerebri.

IN'SULA CER'EBRI, *Island* or *In'sula of Reil*. The intermediate lobe of the brain, *Lobus intermedius cer'ebri*. A remarkable group of convolutions within the fissure of Sylvius. It is called, by Cruveilhier, *Lobule of the Fissure of Sylvius, Lobule of the corpus striatum*. The 'island' of Reil, with the substantia perforata, forms the base of the corpus striatum.

INSULA SANGUINIS, see Blood.

INSULTUS, Attack, Paroxysm.

INSURANCE OF LIFE, see Life Insurance.

INTEGRITAS, Sanitas, Virginity.

INTEG'UMENT, *Integumen'tum, Tegumen'tum, Teg'umen, Teg'imen, Tegmen, Involu'crum seu Velamen'tum corp'oris commu'nē; Vela'men seu Velamentum nati'vum*, from *in* and *tegere*, 'to cover.' (F.) *Tégument*. Any thing which serves to cover, to envelop. The *skin*, including the cuticle, rete mucosum, and cutis vera is the *common integument* or *tegument* of the body.

INTEGUMEN'TA FŒTŪS. The membranes surrounding the fœtus in utero.

IN'TELLECT, *Intellec'tus, Nous, Mens, Gnomē, Noos, Nūs, Noe'sis, Syn'esis*, from *intelligere*, (*inter*, 'between,' and *legere*, 'to choose;') 'to understand,' 'conceive,' 'know.' (F.) *Entendement, Intelligence*. The aggregate of the intellectual faculties — perception, formation of ideas, memory, and judgment.

INTELLECT, DERANGED, Insanity.

INTELLIGENCE, Intellect.

INTEM'PERANCE, *Intemperan'tia; Immoderan'tia, Immodera'tio, Acra'sia, Acola'sia, Plesmonē, Amet'ria, Aples'tia*, from *in*, 'negation,' and *temperare*, 'to temper.' Immoderate use of food and drink, especially the latter; — a fruitful source of disease.

INTEMPER'IES. Same etymon. *Dyscra'sia.* Derangement in the constitution of the atmosphere and of the seasons; bad constitution; derangement or disorder in the humours of the body.

INTENSIVUS, Entaticos.

INTEN'TION, *Inten'tio,* from *in,* and *tendere,* 'to stretch.' *Propos'itum.* The object which one proposes. In *surgery,* a wound is said to heal *by the first intention, Reu'nio per primam intentio'nem,* when cicatrization occurs without suppuration; union by *the second intention, Reu'nio per secun'dam intentio'nem,* being that, which does not occur until the surfaces have suppurated. To obtain union by the first intention, the edges of a recent wound must be brought in apposition and kept together by means of adhesive plasters and a proper bandage. Delpech has substituted for those expressions, *Réunion primitive,* and *Réunion secondaire.*

INTERANEA, Entrails.

INTERARTIC'ULAR, *Interarticula'ris.* Parts situate between the articulations are so called; as *interarticular* cartilages, *interarticular* ligaments, &c.

INTERCA'DENCE, *Intercaden'tia, Interciden'tia,* from *inter,* 'between,' and *cadere,* 'to fall.' Disorder of the arterial pulsations, so that, every now and then, a supernumerary pulsation occurs. The pulse, in such case, is said to be *intercurrent.*

INTER'CALARY, *Intercala'ris, Inter'cidens,* from *intercalare,* 'to insert.' *Embol'imos, Interpola'tus, Provocato'rius.* The days which occur between those that are critical. The term has, also, been applied to the days of apyrexia in intermittent fevers.

INTERCEL'LULAR PAS'SAGES. A term given by Mr. Rainey to irregular passages through the substance of the lung, which form the terminations of the bronchial tubes, are clustered with air-cells, and not lined by mucous membrane.

INTERCELLULAR SUBSTANCE, see Cytoblastema.

INTERCEP'TIO, from *inter,* 'between,' and *capere,* 'to take.' A bandage, by the aid of which the ancients proposed to arrest the progress of the material cause of gout and rheumatism; and which consisted in covering the affected limbs with carded wool; surrounding them, afterwards, with broad bandages, applied from the fingers to the axilla, or from the toes to the groin.

INTERCEPTIO INTESTINORUM, Ileus.

INTERCERVICAUX, Interspinales colli.

INTERCIDENS, Intercalary.

INTERCIDENTIA, Intercadence.

INTERCILIUM, Mesophryon.

INTERCLAVIC'ULAR, *Interclavicula'ris,* from *inter,* 'between,' and *clavicula,* 'a clavicle.' That which is placed between the clavicles.

INTERCLAVICULAR LIG'AMENT is a fibrous bundle, placed transversely above the extremity of the sternum, between the heads of the two clavicles. This ligament is flat. Its fibres, which are always longer above than below, are separated by small apertures, which are traversed by vessels. It prevents the separation of the two clavicles in the forced depression of the shoulder.

INTERCOS'TAL, *Intercosta'lis,* from *inter,* 'between,' and *costa,* 'a rib.' *Mesopleu'rus, Mesopleu'rius.* That which is situate between the ribs. (F.) *Sous-costal.*

INTERCOSTAL AR'TERIES vary in number. There is constantly, however, a *supe'rior, Arte'ria Intercosta'lis supe'rior* vel *Intercosta'lis subcla'via,* which is given off from the posterior part of the subclavian, and which sends branches into the first two or three intercostal spaces; and, generally, eight or nine *inferior* or *aortic intercostals.* These arise from the lateral and posterior parts of the pectoral aorta, and ascend obliquely in front of the vertebral column, to gain the intercostal spaces, where they divide into a *dorsal* branch and an *intercostal,* properly so called.

INTERCOSTAL MUSCLES are distinguished into *internal,* — *inter-plévrocostaux* of Dumas, — and *external.* The *former* are inserted into the inner lip, the *latter* into the outer lip of the edge of the ribs. The fibres of the *external intercostals* are directed obliquely downwards and forwards; and those of the *internal* downwards and backwards. Both are inspiratory or expiratory muscles, according as they take their origin on the upper or lower rib. Some small, fleshy fibres, seen occasionally at the inner surface of the thorax, descending obliquely from one rib to another, have been called *Infracostales.*

INTERCOSTAL NERVE, Trisplanchnic nerve.

INTERCOSTAL NERVES, *Branches souscostales* (Ch.), *Costal* or *Dorsal nerves,* proceed from the anterior branches of the dorsal nerves. They are twelve in number, and are distributed especially to the muscles of the parietes of the chest and abdomen.

INTERCOSTAL SPACE, *Interval'lum* seu *Interstit''ium intercosta'lè, Mesopleu'rum, Mesopleu'rium,* is the interval which separates one rib from that immediately above or below it.

INTERCOSTAL VEINS are distinguished like the arteries. The *right superior intercostal vein* is often wanting. When it exists, it opens into the back part of the subclavian. The same vein of the left side is very large. It communicates with the demi-azygos, receives the left bronchial vein, and opens into the corresponding subclavian. The *right inferior intercostal veins* open into the vena azygos; and those of the left into the demi-azygos.

INTERCOS'TO-HU'MERAL NERVES. So called from their origin and distribution. They are the cutaneous branches of the second and third intercostal nerves.

INTERCUR'RENT, *Intercur'rens,* from *inter,* 'between,' and *currere,* 'to run.' Diseases are so called which supervene at different seasons of the year, or which cannot be considered as belonging to any particular season. — Sydenham. A disease is likewise so termed which occurs in the course of another disease, as *Intercurrent Pneumonia.*

INTERCUTANEUS, Subcutaneous.

INTERDEN'TIUM, from *inter,* 'between,' and *dens,* 'a tooth.' The interval between teeth of the same order. — Linden.

INTERDIGITAIRE, Interdigital.

INTERDIG''ITAL, *Interdigita'lis,* (F.) *Interdigitaire,* same etymon as the next. That which relates to the spaces between the fingers. *Interdigital space,* (F.) *Espace interdigitaire,* is used, also, for the commissure between the fingers.

INTERDIGIT''IUM, from *inter,* 'between,' and *digitus,* 'a finger.' A corn or wart, which grows between the fingers and toes, especially between the latter. — Pliny.

INTERÉPINEUX CERVICAUX, Interspinales colli.

INTERFINIUM NARIUM, Septum narium.

ENTERFŒMINEUM, Perinæum, Vulva.

INTERFORAMINEUM, Perinæum.

INTERGANGLION'IC, *Interganglionicus,* from *inter,* 'between,' and *ganglion,* 'a knot.' An epithet for nervous cords, placed between ganglia, which they connect together.

INTERITUS, Death.

INTERLOB'ULAR, *Interlobula'ris,* from *inter,*

'between,' and *lobulus*, 'a small lobe.' That which is between lobes, — as of the lungs.

INTERLOBULAR FISSURE. The interval between the lobules of the liver. See Liver.

INTERLOBULAR PLEXUS OF THE BILIARY DUCTS. See Liver.

INTERLOBULAR SPACES. The angular interstices formed in the liver by the apposition of several lobules.

INTERLOB'ULAR TISSUE, *Textum interlobula're, Ligamen'ta interlobula'ria pulmo'num.* The cellular tissue between the pulmonary lobules.

INTERLOBULAR VEINS, see Liver.

INTERMAX'ILLARY, *Intermaxilla'ris*, from *inter*, 'between,' and *maxilla*, 'a jaw.' That which is situate between the maxillary bones.

INTERMAXILLARY BONE, *Inci'sive, Pal'atine,* or *Labial bone*, is a bony portion, wedged in between the two superior maxillary bones, which supports the upper incisors. This bone is found in the mammalia; and, also, in the human fœtus.

INTERMÈDE, Excipient.

INTERMEDIA LIGAMENTALIA seu NERVEA, Inscriptiones tendineæ musculorum.

INTERMÉDIAIRE DE WRISBERG, Portio Wrisbergii.

INTERMEDIATE VASCULAR SYSTEM, Capillary system.

INTERMENT, PREMATURE, Zoothapsis.

INTERMIS'SION, *Intermis'sio, Dialeip'sis, Dialip'sis, Tempus intercala'rē, Interval'lum,* from *inter*, 'between,' and *mittere*, 'to put or send.' (F.) *Intermittence*. The interval which occurs between two paroxysms of an intermittent or other disease — during which the patient is almost in his natural state. There is said to be *intermission* of the pulse, when, in a given number of pulsations, one or more may be wanting.

INTERMITTENCE, Intermission.

INTERMIT'TENT, *Intermit'tens*. Same etymon. That which has intermissions.

INTERMITTENT FEVER, *Febris intermit'tens, Dialeip'yra, Intermittens, An'etus, Pyretolypo'sis, Ague, Ague and Fever, Fever and Ague, Palu'dal Fever, Period'ic Fever*, (F.) *Fièvre intermittente, F. d'Accès, F. des marais, F. Périodique,* is a fever consisting of paroxysms, with a complete state of apyrexia in the intervals. The chief types are the *Quotidian, Tertian,* and *Quartan*. The symptoms of intermittents are those of a decided and completely marked *cold stage:* (F.) *Stade de froid*, attended with paleness; collapse; impaired sensibility; and coldness, more or less diffused, followed by general rigors. After this occurs the *hot stage; Stade de la Chaleur*, the heat returning partially and irregularly, and at length becoming universal, and much above the standard of health. The pulse is now hard and strong; tongue white; urine high-coloured; thirst considerable. At length, the *sweating stage*, (F.) *Stade de Sueur*, makes its appearance; the moisture usually beginning on the forehead, face, and neck, and soon extending universally; the heat abating; thirst ceasing; the urine throwing down a sediment, and the functions being gradually restored to their wonted state. The tertian type is the most common, and the quartan the most severe. The quotidian more readily changes into a remittent and continued fever. The quartan has, generally, the longest cold stage, the tertian the longest hot. The chief *exciting cause* is marsh miasmata. Ague, also, occurs in districts where there are no marshy emanations. Such districts are, generally, of a volcanic nature; farther we know not. When the disease has once attacked an individual, it is apt to recur. The *prognosis* is, in general, favourable, as far as regards life; but long protracted intermittents are apt to induce visceral obstructions and engorgements, which may end in dropsy. In some countries, the disease is of a very pernicious character. The indications of treatment are, 1. To abate the violence of the paroxysm; and, 2. To prevent its return. The first indication requires the adoption of the general principles and remedies required in ordinary fever. The *second* is the most important. The period of apyrexia is that for action. The means for fulfilling this indication are: — the use of emetics, purgatives, cinchona, quinia, &c., arsenic, and forcible impressions made on the mind of the patient.

INTERMUS'CULAR, *Intermuscula'ris*, from *inter*, 'between,' and *musculus*, 'a muscle.' That which is placed between muscles.

INTERMUS'CULAR APONEURO'SES are aponeurotic laminæ or septa, situate between muscles, to which they often give attachment.

INTER'NAL, *Inner, Inter'nus*. That which is placed on the inside. This epithet is given to parts that look towards an imaginary central plane, which divides the body into two equal and symmetrical portions, as well as to those which correspond with a cavity. Thus, we say—the *inner surface of the arm* or *thigh*—the *inner surface of the skull,* &c.

INTERNAL DISEASES, *Morbi inter'ni*, are those which occupy the inner parts of the body. Their investigation belongs to the physician; *external* diseases falling under the management of the surgeon.

INTERNAT. The post or office of an *interne*.

INTERNE, see House-Surgeon.

INTERNODIA DIGITORUM MANUS, Phalanges of the fingers — i. Digitorum pedis, Phalanges of the toes.

INTERNO'DIUM, *Mesagon'ium*, from *inter*, 'between,' and *nodus*, 'a knot.' The part of the fingers between the joints. A phalanx.

INTERNUN'CIAL, *Internuncia'lis*, from *inter*, 'between,' and *nuncius*, 'a messenger.' Relating or belonging to a messenger between parties. A term applied by Mr. Hunter to the function of the nervous system.

INTERNUNTII DIES, Critical days.

INTERNUS AURIS, Tensor tympani—i. Mallei, Tensor tympani.

INTEROS'SEI PEDIS,*Métatarso-phalangien-latéral*, (Ch.) The number, arrangement, shape, and uses of these are the same as in the case of the preceding muscles. Four are *dorsal*, and three *plantar:* six belong to the three middle toes and one to the little toe. The great toe is devoid of them. As in the hand, they are distinguished, in each toe, into abductor and adductor.

INTERROS'SEOUS, *Interos'seus*. That which is situate between the bones; from *inter*, 'between,' and *os*, 'a bone.'

INTEROSSEOUS AR'TERIES OF THE FOREARM AND HAND. Of these there are several. 1. The *common interosseous artery* arises from the posterior part of the ulnar, a little below the bicipital tuberosity of the radius; passes backwards and divides into two branches: the one called *anterior interosseous* descends vertically, anterior to the interosseous ligament; the other, called *posterior interosseous*, passes above that ligament, appears at its posterior part and divides into two great branches, — the *posterior recurrent radial* and the *posterior interosseous*, properly so called. In the hand, — 1. The *dorsal metacarpal interosseous arteries* are given off by the *dorsalis carpi*, a division of the radial artery. 2. The *Palmar interosseous arteries*, which arise from the convexity of the deep palmar arch, and give off the

middle interosseous arteries. 3. The *dorsal interosseous of the index*, proceeding directly from the radial artery. In the foot, are distinguished:—
1. The *dorsal interosseous arteries*, three in number, which arise from the artery of the metatarsus, a branch of the dorsalis tarsi. 2. The *plantar interosseous arteries*, which are, also, three in number, and arise from the plantar arch.

INTEROSSEOUS LIG'AMENTS. Ligaments seated between certain bones, which they unite; such are the ligaments between the radius and ulna, and between the tibia and fibula.

INTEROSSEOUS MUSCLES. These occupy the spaces between the bones of the metacarpus and metatarsus; and, consequently, belong,—some to the hand, others to the foot.

INTEROSSEOUS NERVE is a branch, given off by the median nerve, which descends before the interosseous ligament, accompanying the artery of the same name.

INTEROSSEOUS VEINS have the same arrangement as the arteries.

INTEROSSEUS MANÛS, (F.) *Muscle interosseux de la main.—Métacarpo-phalangien-latéral suspalmaire et métacarpo-phalangien latéral*, (Ch.) These muscles are seven in number; two for each of the three middle fingers, and one for the little finger. Four are situate on the back of the hand, and three only in the palm. They are inserted into the metacarpal bones, and send a tendon to the tendon of the extensor communis. According to their office, they are, to each finger, an *adductor* and an *abductor*. The *index* has a dorsal abductor and a palmar one. The *middle finger* has two dorsal muscles for adductor and abductor; the *ring finger* has a dorsal adductor and a palmar abductor; and the *little finger* has only one interosseous abductor, which is palmar. These muscles produce abduction and adduction of the fingers, which they can also extend, owing to their connexion with the extensor tendons.

INTEROSSEUS SECUNDUS, Prior medii digiti—i. Quartus, Prior annularis.

INTEROSSEUX DE LA MAIN, Interosseus manûs.

INTERPARIE'TAL BONE, *Os Interparieta'lē.* A bone found in the skulls of the children of the Peruvian races. It lies in the situation of the upper angle of the occipital bone, where the parietal bones separate from each other; and is the analogue of the interparietal bone of ruminants and carnivora.—Tschudi.

INTERPELLA'TUS, (*Morbus*,) from *interpello*, 'I interrupt.' A term, by which Paracelsus designated those diseases whose progress is unequal, and paroxysms irregular.

INTERPLÉVRO-COSTAUX, Intercostal muscles.

INTERPOLATUS, Intercalary.

INTERRUPTIO MENSTRUATIONIS, Amenorrhœa.

INTERSCAP'ULAR, *Interscapula'ris*, (*inter*, and *scapula*.) That which is between the shoulders; as the *interscapular region*. The *interscapular cavities*, *Cavita'tes interscapula'res*, are the depressions between the scapulæ and the spinous processes of the vertebræ.

INTERSCAPU'LIUM. The spine of the scapula.

INTERSECTIO, Decussation, Intersection.

INTERSEC'TION, *Intersec'tio*, *Diac'opē*, from *inter*, 'between,' and *seco*, 'I cut.' The point where two lines meet and cut each other. The name *aponeurot'ic intersection* is given to fibrous bands, which certain muscles present in their length, and by which they seem interrupted. Aponeurotic intersections are found in the recti muscles of the abdomen; in the semi-membranosus, complexus, sterno-thyroideus, &c.

INTERSECTIONES TENDINEÆ MUSCULORUM, Inscriptiones tendineæ musculorum.

INTERSEPIMENTUM THORACIS, Mediastinum.

INTERSEPTA HORIZONTALIA PACCHIONI, Tentorium.

INTERSEP'TUM, from *inter*, 'between,' and *septum*, 'a partition.' *Cion, κιων*. The uvula; also, the septum narium. The diaphragm.

INTERSEPTUM NARIUM, Septum narium—i. Virginale, Hymen.

INTERSPI'NAL, *Interspina'lis*, from *inter*, 'between,' and *spina*, 'the spine.' That which is seated between the spinous processes.

INTERSPI'NAL LIG'AMENT, *Membra'na interspina'lis*, (F.) *Ligament interépineux*. These occupy the intervals between the spinous processes in the back and loins. In the neck, they are replaced by the muscles of the same name. They prevent the too great flexion of the spine, and keep the spinous processes *in situ*.

INTERSPINA'LES COLLI, *Spina'les Colli mino'res*, *Spina'ti*, (F.) *Interépineux-cervicaux, Intercervicaux*, (Ch.) These are twelve in number, and occupy, in two parallel rows, the intervals between the spinous processes of the cervical vertebræ, from that of the atlas and vertebra dentata, to that between the last cervical and first dorsal vertebræ. They are flat, thin, and quadrilateral. These muscles contribute to the extension of the neck and to throwing the head backwards.

INTERSPINALES DORSI ET LUMBO'RUM; portions of the *Transversaire-épineux* of Boyer, and the *sacro-spinal* of Chaussier. These muscles are of two kinds. The one (*Muscle grand épineux du dos*, of Winslow) representing fleshy bundles of different lengths, applied upon the lateral surfaces of the spinous processes, from the third dorsal vertebra to the second lumbar. The other (*Muscle petit épineux du dos*, Winslow) covered by the preceding. They are situate on each side of the interspinal ligament, in the form of small, short flat bundles, which pass from one spinous process to the second, third or fourth above it. These muscles aid in extending the vertebral column; and incline it a little to one side, when they act on one side only.

IN'TERSTICE, *Interstit''ium, Areo'ma*, from *inter*, 'between,' and *sto*, 'I stand.' *Diaste'ma, Interval'lum*. Anatomists have given this name to the intervals between organs. The *iliac crest, crista ilii*, for example, has two *lips* and an interstice between them, which affords attachment to the lesser oblique muscle of the abdomen.

INTERSTICE, Pore.

INTERSTIT''IAL, *Interstitia'lis*, same etymon. Applied to that which occurs in the interstices of an organ, — as '*interstitial* absorption,' '*interstitial* pregnancy,' &c.

INTERSTITIUM, Interstice—i. Ciliare, Ciliary ligament—i. Intercostale, Intercostal space—i. Jugulare, Throat.

INTERTINCTUS, Discreet.

INTERTRACHÉLIENS, Intertransversales colli.

INTERTRANSVERSAIRES DES LOMBES, Intertransversales lumborum.

INTERTRANSVERSA'LIS, *Intertransversa'rius*. That which is placed between the transverse processes of the vertebræ.

INTERTRANSVERSALES COLLI, (F.) *Intertransversaires cervicaux, Intertrachéliens*, (Ch.) These are small, muscular bundles; quadrilateral; thin and flat; situate, in pairs, in the intervals between the transverse processes of the neck, except between the first and second, where there is only one. They are distinguished into *anterior* and *posterior*. The former are six in number; the latter five. These muscles bring the transverse processes of the neck nearer each other, and contribute to the lateral flexion of the neck.

INTERTRANSVERSALES LUMBO'RUM, *Musculi intertransversi lumbo'rum*, (F.) *Intertransversaires des lombes*. These are almost entirely fleshy, and ten in number; five on each side. They are similar to the preceding in general arrangement; except that they are more marked, and not placed in two rows. Each intertransverse space contains only one. They are quadrilateral, and flat. The first occupies the space between the transverse processes of the first lumbar and the last dorsal vertebra; and the last is between that of the fourth and fifth lumbar vertebræ. These muscles incline the lumbar regions laterally; and straighten it when inclined to one side.

INTERTRIGO, Chafing—i. Podicis, Chafing.

INTERVAL, LUCID, see Lucid.

INTERVALLUM, Intermission, Interstice—i. Intercostale, Intercostal space.

INTERVENIUM, Mesophlebium.

INTERVER'TEBRAL, *Intervertebra'lis*, (*inter*, and *vertebra*.) That which is situate between the vertebræ.

INTERVERTEBRAL CAR'TILAGES, *Intervertebral fibro-cartilages, Intervertebral discs, Ligamen'ta intervertebra'lia*. These organs are of a fibro-cartilaginous nature; sections of a cylinder; flexible; whitish; resisting; and situate between the bodies of the vertebræ,—from the space between the second and third as far as that between the last vertebra and sacrum. Their form is accommodated to that of the vertebra with which they are in connexion; so that, in the neck and loins, they are oval, whilst in the dorsal region they are nearly circular.

INTERVERTEBRAL DISCS, Intervertebral cartilages — I. fibro-cartilages, Intervertebral cartilages.

INTESTABILIS, Castratus.

INTESTATUS, Castratus.

INTESTIN, Intestine.

INTES'TINAL, *Intestina'lis*, from *intus*, 'within.' That which belongs to the intestines, — as *intestinal* canal, &c. Bordeu uses the term *Pouls intestinal* for a pulse, which he conceived to announce an approaching crisis by the intestines.

INTESTINAL JUICE, Succus entericus.

INTESTINAL TUBE or TRACT, *Cana'lis* seu *Tractus intestino'rum*. The canal formed by the intestines from the pyloric orifice of the stomach to the anus.

INTES'TINE, *Intesti'num, En'teron, Chorda, Gut, Nedy*ia (pl.), *Pan'tices* (pl.), *Boel'li* (pl.), *Bowel*, (F.) *Intestin, Boyau*. A musculo-membranous canal, variously convoluted, which extends from the stomach to the anus, and is situate in the abdominal cavity; the greater part of which it fills. In man, its length is six or eight times that of the body. It is divided into two principal portions, called *small intestine* and *large intestine*. The former, *Intesti'num ten'uĕ, I. grac'ilĕ*, (F.) *Intestin grêle*, constituting nearly four-fifths of the whole length, begins at the stomach and terminates in the right iliac region. It is divided into *duodenum, jejunum* and *ileum*. Some anatomists give the name *small intestine* to the last two only; which are kept in place by the mesentery, and form a large *paquet*, occupying the umbilical and hypogastric regions, a part of the flanks, of the iliac regions, and of the cavity of the pelvis. It is composed of, 1. A serous membrane, which is peritoneal. 2. Of a muscular coat, whose fibres are very pale, and are placed, in part, longitudinally; but the greater part transversely. 3. Of a whitish, mucous membrane; villous, and forming folds or valves — *valvulæ conniventes* — at its inner surface, and furnished with a considerable number of mucous follicles, called *glands* of Lieberkühn, (*Crypts* or *Follicles of Lieberkühn*,) and Brunner, and, with those of Peyer. The arteries of the small intestine proceed from the superior mesenteric; its veins open into the vena porta. Its nerves proceed from the superior mesenteric plexus. The large intestine, *Intesti'num crassum, Megaloca'lia*, (F.) *Gros intestin*, forms a sequence to the small. It is much shorter, and is solidly attached in the regions of the abdomen which it occupies. It begins in the right iliac region; ascends along the right flank, till beneath the liver, when it crosses the upper part of the abdomen, descends into the left iliac fossa, and plunges into the pelvic cavity, to gain the anus. The great intestine is usually divided into three portions,—the *cæcum, colon* and *rectum*. It receives its arteries from the superior and inferior mesenterics. Its veins open into the vena porta. Its nerves are furnished by the mesenteric plexuses. Its lymphatic vessels, which are much less numerous than those of the small intestine, pass into the ganglions or glands seated between the different reflections of the peritoneum, which fix it to the abdominal parietes. The use of the intestines is,—in the *upper* part, to effect the chylification of the food and the absorption of the chyle;—in the *lower*, to serve as a reservoir, where the excrementitious portion of the food collects; and, also, as an excretory duct, which effects its expulsion.

INTESTINORUM LÆVITAS, Lientery.

INTESTINULA CEREBRI, Anfractuosities (cerebral)—i. Meibomii, Meibomius, glands of.

INTESTINULUM, Funiculus umbilicalis.

INTESTINUM CELLULATUM, Colon—i. Circumvolutum, Ileon — i. Crassum, Colon, see Intestine — i. Gracile, see Intestine — i. Grande, Colon — i. Laxum, Colon — i. Majus, Colon — i. Medium, Mesentery—i. Plenum, Colon—i. Rectum, Rectum—i. Tenue, see Intestine.

INTIMUM UNGUIS, Nail, root of the.

INTONATIO INTESTINALIS, Borborygmus.

INTORSIO, Distorsion.

INTOXICATIO, Poisoning—i. Arsenicalis, Arsenicismus—i. Opiaca, Meconismus—i. Saturnina, Saturnismus.

INTOXICATION, Poisoning, Temulentia—*i. des Marais*, see Miasm.

INTOXICATION SATURNINE. Lead poisoning; saturnine cachexy. The aggregate of symptoms which present themselves prior to an attack of lead colic. — Tanquerel des Planches.

INTRALINGUAL SALIVARY GLANDS, see Salivary glands.

INTRALOB'ULAR, *Intralobula'ris*; from *intra*, 'within,' and *lobulus*, 'a lobule.' Relating to the space within a lobule:—as the "*intralobular veins*," *venæ* seu *ven'ulæ intralobula'res* seu *centra'les*, of the liver: — veins which communicate with the interlobular veins, and are the radicles of the hepatic veins.

INTRA-PELVIO TROCHANTÉRIEN, Obturator internus.

INTRA-U'TERINE, *Intraüteri'nus*; from *intra*, 'within,' and *uterus*, 'the womb.' That which takes place within the womb — as '*intra-uterine* life.'

INTRICATURA, Decussation.

INTRIN'SIC, *Intrin'secus*; from *intra*, 'within,' and *secus*, 'towards.' Applied to the internal muscles of certain organs; as those of the ear, tongue, and larynx. Linnæus gave the name *Intrin'seci* to internal diseases.

INTROITUS PELVIS, see Pelvis—i. Vaginæ, Rima vulvæ.

INTROMIS'SION, *Intromis'sio;* from *intro*, 'within,' and *mitto*, 'I send.' The act of introducing one body into another, as *Intromissio Penis*, (F.) *Intromission de la Verge*.

INTROSUSCEPTIO, Intussusceptio — i. Entropium, Entropion.

INTUBUM, Cichorium endivia—i. Erraticum, Cichorium intybus.

INTUMES'CENCE, *Intumescen'tia, Onco'sis, Dionco'sis*, from *intumescere*, (*in*, and *tumescere*,) 'to swell.' Augmentation of size in a part or in the whole of the body. Sauvages uses the word *Intumescen'tia* for an order of diseases, in which he comprehends polysarcia, pneumatosis, anasarca, œdema, physconia, and pregnancy.

INTUMESCENTIA GANGLIFORMIS, Ganglion of Gasser, see Facial nerve—i. Lactea Mammarum, Sparganosis — i. Lienis, Splenoncus — i. Semilunaris, Ganglion of Gasser.

INTUS INVERSUS, Transposition of the viscera.

INTUSSUSCEP'TIO, from *intus*, 'within,' and *suscipio*, 'I receive.' *Introsuscep'tio.* In *physiology*;—the mode of increase peculiar to organized bodies. In *pathology*, like *Convol'vulus, Vol'vulus intestino'rum, Suscep'tio intestino'rum, Chordap'sus, Enteroparisago'gē, Parisago'gē intestino'rum, Indigita'tio, Tormen'tum*, and *Invagina'tio*, it means the introduction of one part of the intestinal canal into another, which serves it as a sort of *vagina* or sheath. Generally, it is the upper part of the small intestine, which is received into the lower, when the intussusception is said to be *progres'sive*. At times, however, it is *ret'rograde*. As the disease cannot be positively detected by the symptoms, it must be treated upon general principles. At times, the invaginated portion has separated and been voided per anum,—the patient recovering. The disease is, however, of a very dangerous character.

INTYBUM, Cichorium endivia.

INTYBUS HORTENSIS, Cichorium endivia.

INULA, see Inula helenium — i. Britannica, I. dysenterica — i. Common, I. helenium — i. Conyzæa, I. dysenterica.

IN'ULA DYSENTER'ICA. The systematic name of the *Lesser Inula, I. Britan'nica seu Conyzæ'a, Aster dysenter'icus seu undula'tus, Pulica'ria dysenter'ica, Cony'sa, C. media, Ar'nica Sueden'sis, Ar'nica spu'ria, Cuni'la mas'cula seu me'dia, Cunila'go,* (F.) *Aunée antidysentérique, Herbe de Saint Roch. Nat. Ord.* Compositæ. This plant was once considered to possess great antidysenteric virtues. The whole plant is acrid and somewhat aromatic.

INULA HELEN'IUM. The systematic name of the *El'ecampane, En'ula, E. campa'na, Elen'ium, Necta'rium, Helinium, Aster helen'ium* seu *officina'lis, Corvisar'tia helen'ium, Ommum Inula,* (F.) *Aunée.* The root *In'ula* (Ph. U. S.) was formerly in high esteem in dyspepsia, cachexia, pulmonary affections, &c. It is now scarcely used.

INULA LESSER, Inula dysenterica — i. Squarrosa, Conyza squarrosa.

INUNCTIO, Inunction, Liniment.

INUNC'TION, *Inunc'tio, Perunc'tio, Illit''io, Illi'tus, Illinit''io, Oblinit''io, Chrisis, Catach'risis, Diach'risis, Epich'risis, Unctio.* An ointment or a liniment. Also, the act of rubbing in; unction, (F.) *Onction*.

INUNDATIO, Depuration.

INUSTIO, Cauterization, Cauterium.

INUSTORIUM, Cauterium.

INVAG''INATED, *Invagina'tus*, from *in*, and *vaginæ*, 'a sheath.' Applied to a part which is received into another, as into a sheath.

The *invaginated* or *slit and tail bandage* is one in which strips or tails pass through appropriate slits or button-holes.

INVAGINATIO, Intussusceptio.
INVALETUDO, Infirmity.
INVALID, Valetudinary.
INVALIDUS, Valetudinary.
INVASIO, Arche, Attack, Paroxysm.
INVERMINATION, Helminthiasis.
INVERSIO PALPEBRARUM, Entropion—i. Uteri, Hysteroptosis, Uterus, inversion of the.

INVERSION DE LA MATRICE, Uterus, inversion of the.

INVERTENTIA, Absorbents, Antacids.
INVESTITURA FUNICULI UMBILICALIS, see Funiculis umbilicalis.
INVETERATUS, Chronic.
INVISCANTIA, Incrassantia.

INVISCA'TIO OC'ULI. A morbid adhesion of the eyelids to each other, or to the globe of the eye. Also, gluing together of the eyelids by a viscid secretion.

INVOLU'CRUM, *Involumen'tum*, from *involvere*, 'to fold in.' A covering; hence *Involu'cra cer'ebri*, the membranes of the brain. *Involu'cra nervo'rum*, the sheaths of the nerves.

INVOLUCRUM CORDIS, Pericardium—i. Corporis commune, Integument—i. Linguæ, see Tongue— i. Membranaceum, Decidua reflexa—i. Nervorum, Neurilema—i. Reti comparatum, Retina.

INVOLUMENTUM, Involucrum.
INVOLVENTIA, Demulcents.
IODE, Iodine.
IODES, Æruginous.
IODETUM HYDRARGYRICUM, Hydrargyri iodidum rubrum.

IODHYDRARGYRITE DE CHLORURE MERCUREUX, Mercury, iodide of chloride of.

IODIC, *Iod'icus*, (F.) *Iodique*. Same etymon as Iodine. Containing iodine.

IODIDUM HYDRARGYRI CHLORIDI, Mercury, iodide of chloride of — i. Hydrargyricum, Hydrargyri iodidum rubrum — i. Hydrargyrosum, Hydrargyri iodidum.

I'ODINE, *Io'dina; Io'dinum, Iodin'ium, Io'dum, Io'dium, Io'nium, Io'num,* (F.) *Iode;* from ιώδης, *viola'ceus*, 'of a violet colour,' so called from the violet flavour it exhales when volatilized. It is contained in the mother waters of certain fuci, and is obtained by pouring an excess of concentrated sulphuric acid on the water obtained by burning different fuci, lixiviating the ashes and concentrating the liquor. The mixture is placed in a retort to which a receiver is attached, and is boiled. The iodine passes over and is condensed. It is solid, in the form of plates; of a bluish gray colour, of a metallic brightness, and smell similar to that of the chloride of sulphur. Its s. g. is 4.946. When heated, it becomes volatilized, and affords the vapour which characterizes it. With oxygen it forms *Iodic* acid, and with hydrogen *Hydriodic* acid. The tincture of iodine and the iodides have been employed with great success in the treatment of goître and of some scrofulous affections. It must be administered in a very small dose and for a long period. It is said to be apt, however, to induce cholera morbus, signs of great nervous irritability, and emaciation of the mammæ. When these symptoms, collectively termed *I'odism, Iodo'sis,* and *Iodin'ia*, are urgent, the dose may be diminished, or it may be wholly discontinued, and afterwards resumed.

Various preparations of iron are employed in medicine.

IODOGNO'SIS, (F.) *Iodognosie;* from *iodine,* and γνωσις, 'knowledge.' A knowledge of iodine in its various relations.—Dorvault.

IODINIA, see Iodine.
IODINIUM, Iodine.
IODINUM, Iodine.
IODIQUE, Iodic.
IODISM, see Iodine.
IODIUM, Iodine.

I'ODOFORM, *Iodofor'mum,* (F.) *Iodoforme,* so called from its analogy to chloroform. It is obtained by the reaction on each other of iodine, bicarbonate of potassa, water, and alcohol. It is in crystalline plates, of a beautiful citrine colour; and may be given in the same cases as the other preparations of iodine. Dose, one grain three times a day. It is the sesqui-oxide of carbon. See Carbonis sesqui-iodidum.

IODOHYDRARGYRATE OF POTASSIUM, see Iodine.
IODOSIS, see Iodine.
IODUM, Iodine.
IODURE PLOMBIQUE, Plumbi iodidum.
IODURETUM AMMONIÆ, see Iodine — i. Amyli, see Iodine — i. Hydrargyrosum, Hydrargyri iodidum — i. Sulphuris, see Iodine.
IODYMUS, Dicephalus.
ION, Viola.
IONIA, Teucrium chamæpitys.
IONID'IUM MARCUCCI, *Cinchunchulli* — a South American plant. *Sex. Syst.* Pentandria Monogynia; *Nat. Ord.* Violariæ; said to be extremely efficacious in the Mal de San Lazaro of Colombia.
IONIUM, Iodine.
IONTA, see Excretion.
ION'THUS, *Varus, Violet Eruption,* from ιον, 'the violet,' and ανθος, 'a flower,' or ονθος, 'foulness.' An unsuppurative, tubercular tumour; stationary; chiefly on the face. A genus in the class *Hæmatica,* order *Phlogotica* of Good.
IONTHUS CORYMBIFER, Gutta rosea — i. Varus, Acne.
IONUM, Iodine.
IOTACIS'MUS, from the Greek letter *Iota.* Defective articulation, — the patient not being able to pronounce the palatals *j* and *g* soft.
IPECAC, Apocynum androsæmifolium, Euphorbia corollata, Gillenia trifoliata, Ipecacuanha, Triosteum.
IPECACUAN'HA. In common parlance, often abridged to *Ipecac.* The pharmacopœial name of the *Cephaë'lis ipecacuan'ha, Callicoc'ca Ipecacuan'ha, Cagosanga. Nat. Ord.* Cinchonaceæ. It is also obtained from the *Psycho'tria emet'ica* of Peru. The odour of the root, *Ipecacuan'ha root, Ipecacacuan'hæ radix, Radix Brazilien'sis,* — *Ipecacuanha,* (Ph. U. S.) — is faint and peculiar; taste bitter, subacrid, and mucilaginous; both water and alcohol extract its virtues, which depend on a peculiar principle, called *Emet'ia.* It is emetic in large doses; sudorific in smaller. *Dose,* as an emetic, gr. xx to xxx, — alone, or united with gr. i to ij. of tartarized antimony.
IPECACUANHA, Euphorbia corollata.— i. Bastard, Asclepias curassavica, Triosteum perfoliatum—*i. Blanc de l'Ile de France,* Asclepias asthmatica —*i. Blanc de St. Domingue,* Asclepias curassavica — i. of the Isle of France, Cynanchum vomitorium.
IPECACUAN'HA, WHITE, is obtained from different species of *Richardsonia* and *Ionidium. Vi'ola ipecacuan'ha* seu *Solea ipecacuan'ha* seu *Pomba'lea ipecacuan'ha,* also affords it. It is weaker than the gray.
IPO, Upas.

IPOMŒA JALAPA, Convolvulus jalapa — i. Macrorrhiza, Convolvulus Jalapa.
IRA, Rage.
IRACUNDUS, Rectus externus oculi.
IRAL'GIA; *Ireal'gia, Iridal'gia,* from ιρις, 'the iris,' and αλγος, 'pain.' Pain in the iris.
IRASCIBLE, Rectus externus oculi.
IREALGIA, Iralgia.
IREONCION, Iriancistron.
IRIANCIS'TRON, *Iridancist'ron, Ireon'cion,* from ιρις, and αγκιστρον, 'a hook.' A hooked instrument, used by Schlagintweit in the formation of an artificial pupil.
IRIDÆ'A EDU'LIS. One of the Algæ, eaten in Scotland and the southwest of England.
IRIDALGIA, Iralgia.
IRIDANCISTRON, Iriancistron.
IRIDAUXE'SIS, from *Iris, I'ridis,* and αυξησις, 'augmentation;' *Staphylo'ma I'ridis, Staphylo'ma U'veæ, Iridonco'sis, Lymphon'cus I'ridis.* Exudation of fibrin into the tissue of the iris.
IRIDECTOMEDIALYSIS, see Coretomia.
IRIDECTOMIA, Coretomia.
IRIDENCLEISIS, see Coretomia.
IRIDENCLEISMUS, see Coretomia.
IRIDERE'MIA, from ιρις, and ερημος, 'deprived of;' *Iridostere'sis.* Absence of iris, either apparent or real.
IRIDOCELE, Ptosis iridis.
IRIDOCOLOBOMA, Coloboma iridis.
IRIDODIALYSIS, Coretomia.
IRIDOMALA'CIA, from ιρις, 'the iris,' and μαλακια, 'softness.' Mollescence or softening of the iris.
IRIDOMELANO'MA, *Iridomelano'sis,* from ιρις, 'the iris,' and μελανειν, 'to colour black.' The deposition of black matter on the tissue of the iris.
IRIDONCO'SIS, *Iridon'cus, Hyperonco'sis Iridis,* from ιρις, 'the iris,' and ογκος, 'a swelling.' Tumefaction or thickening of the iris. Also, Iridauxesis.
IRIDONCUS, Iridoncosis.
IRIDOPERIPHAKI'TIS; from ιρις, 'the iris,' περι, 'around,' and *phacitis,* inflammation of the lens. Inflammation of the anterior hemisphere of the capsule of the lens.
IRIDOPTOSIS, Ptosis iridis.
IRIDOR'RHAGAS, *Iridorrho'gē, Iridor'rhox, Iridoschis'ma, Fissu'ra I'ridis,* from ιρις, 'iris,' and ραγας, 'a fissure.' Fissure of the iris.
IRIDORRHOGE, Iridorrhagas.
IRIDORRHOX, Iridorrhagas.
IRIDOSCHISMA, Iridorrhagas.
IRIDOSTERESIS, Irideremia.
IRIDOTENCLEISIS, Coretomia.
IRIDOTOMIA, Coretomia.
IRIDOTROMUS, Hippus.
IRIS, (gen. I'ridis) *Grammē.* So called from its resembling the rainbow in a variety of colours. A membrane, stretched vertically at the anterior part of the eye, in the midst of the aqueous humour, in which it forms a kind of circular, flat partition, separating the anterior from the posterior chamber. It is perforated by a circular opening called the *pupil,* which is constantly varying its dimensions, owing to the varying contractions of the fibres of the iris. Its posterior surface has been called *uvea,* from the thick, black varnish which covers it. The greater circumference of the iris is adherent to the ciliary processes and circle. It has an external plane of radiated fibres and an internal one of circular fibres, which serve — the one to dilate, the other to contract the aperture of the pupil. The iris receives the irian nerves. Its arteries are furnished by the long ciliary arteries which form two

circles by their anastomoses; the one very broad, near the great circumference; the other, smaller, and seated around the circumference of the pupil. The veins of the iris empty themselves into the *Vasa vorticosa*, and into the long ciliary veins. The use of the iris seems to be, — to regulate by its dilatation or contraction, the quantity of luminous rays necessary for distinct vision. The different colours of the iris occasion the variety in the colours of the human eye.

IRIS, see Herpes Iris — i. Common, I. Germanica — *i. Commun*, I. Germanica — *i. de Florence*, I. Florentina.

IRIS FLORENTI'NA, *Florentine iris* or *orris*, (F.) *Iris de Florence*. The rhizoma of this plant is extremely acrid in its recent state; and, when chewed, excites a pungent heat in the mouth, that continues for several hours. When dried, the acrimony is lost, or nearly so, and the smell is very agreeable. It is indebted to its agreeable flavour for its retention in the pharmacopœias, although it is ranked as an expectorant.

IRIS FŒTIDIS'SIMA, *I. fœ'tida, Spath'ula fœ'tida, Xyris, Stinking iris*, (F.) *Iris puant, Glayeul puant*. The root has been esteemed antispasmodic and narcotic.

IRIS GERMAN'ICA. The systematic name of the *Flower-de-Luce, Iris nostras, Aier'sa, Iris vulga'ris, Common iris* or *orris, Gladi'olus cœru'leus*, (F.) *Iris commun, Flambe*. The fresh roots have a disagreeable smell and an acrid, nauseous taste. They are powerfully cathartic, and are given in dropsies, where such remedies are indicated.

IRIS LACUS'TRIS, *Dwarf-flag, Dwarf lake-iris;* has the properties of I. versicolor.

IRIS, LAKE, DWARF, I. lacustris — i. Lutea, I. pseudacorus.

IRIS DES MARAIS, I. pseudacorus — i. Nostras, I. Germanica — i. Palustris, I. pseudacorus.

IRIS PSEUDAC'ORUS. The systematic name of the *Yellow water-flag, Iris palus'tris* seu *lu'tea, Gladi'olus lu'teus, Ac'orus vulga'ris* seu *adulteri'nus* seu *palus'tris, Pseudac'orus, Bu'tomon*, (F.) *Iris des marais, Faux acore, Flambe bâtard, Acore bâtard*. The root has an acrid, styptic taste. It is an errhine, sialogogue, and acrid astringent. The expressed juice is diuretic, and said to be a useful application to serpiginous and other cutaneous affections. Rubbed on the gums, or chewed, it is said to cure toothache.

IRIS PUANT, I. fœtidissima — i. Stinking, I. fœtidissima.

IRIS VERSIC'OLOR, *Blue flag*. The rhizoma of this is an active cathartic, and has been much used, as such, by the American Indians. It is reputed to be diuretic.

IRIS VULGARIS, I. Germanica.

IRISITIS, Iritis.

IRI'TIS, *Inflammation of the iris, Inflamma'tio I'ridis, Irisi'tis*. The chief symptoms are; — change in the colour of the iris; fibres less movable; tooth-like processes shooting into the pupil; pupil irregularly contracted, with the ordinary signs of inflammation of the eye. If the inflammation do not yield, suppuration takes place; and, although the matter may be absorbed, the iris remains immovable. It is often caused by syphilis. The general principles of treatment are, to deplete largely and exhibit mercury freely; along with attention to other means advisable in ophthalmia. The free use of quinia is sometimes serviceable. When the inflammation is seated in the serous covering of the iris, it is termed *Iritis sero'sa*.

IRON, Ferrum — i. Acetate of, Ferri acetas — i. and Alumina, sulphate of, Ferri et aluminis sulphas — i. Ammoniated, Ferrum ammoniatum — i. Ammonio-citrate of, Ferri ammonio-citras — i. Ammonio-chloride of, Ferrum ammoniatum — i. Ammonio-tartrate of, Ferri ammonio-tartras — i. and Ammonia, citrate of, Ferri ammonio-citras — i. and Quinia Hydriodate of, see Iodine — i. Bromide of, see Bromine — i. Carbonate of, saccharine, Ferri proto-carbonas — i. Carburet of, Graphites — i. Black oxide of, Oxydum ferri nigrum — i. Citrate of, Ferri citras — i. Citrate of the magnetic oxide of, see Ferri ammonio-citras — i. Ferrocyanuret of, Prussian blue — i. Ferroprussiate of, Prussian blue — i. Filings, purified, Ferri limatura purificata — i. Hydrated oxide of, Ferrum oxydatum hydratum — i. Hydrated peroxide of, Ferrum oxydatum hydratum — i. Hydrated tritoxide of, Ferrum oxydatum hydratum — i. Hydriodate of, Ferri iodidum — i. Hydro-oxide of, Ferrum oxydatum hydratum — i. Iodide of, see Iodine — i. Iodide of, Ferri iodidum — i. Ioduret of, Ferri iodidum — i. Lactate of, Ferri lactas — i. Liquor, Ferri acetas — i. and Magnesia, citrate of, Ferri et Magnesiæ citras — i. Nitrate of, solution of, see Tinctura Ferri muriatis — i. Peroxide of, Ferri subcarbonas — i. Phosphate of, Ferri phosphas — i. Pills of, compound, Pilulæ ferri compositæ — i. Potassio-citrate of, see Ferri ammonio-citras — i. Protocarbonate of, Ferri protocarbonas — i. Protoxide of, lactate of, Ferri lactas — i. Pyrites, Ferri sulphuretum — i. and Quinia, citrate of, Ferri et Quiniæ citras — i. and Quinia, hydriodate of, see Quinia, iodide of, iodhydrate of — i. Sesquinitrate of, Solution of, see Tinctura ferri muriatis — i. Sesquioxide of, Ferri subcarbonas — i. Sodio-citrate of, see Ferri ammonio-citras — i. Sulphate of, Ferri sulphas — i. Sulphuret of, Ferri sulphuretum — i. Tannate of, Ferri tannas — i. Tartarised, Ferrum tartarizatum — i. Ternitrate of, solution of, see Tinctura ferri muriatis — i. Trito-hydro-ferrocyanate of, Prussian blue — i. and Potass, tartrate of, Ferrum tartarizatum — i. Valerianate of, Ferri valerianas — i. Weed, Vernonia Noveboracensis.

IRREDU'CIBLE, (F.) *Irréducible*. An epithet given to fractures, luxations, herniæ, &c., when they cannot be reduced.

IRRÉDUCIBLE, Irreducible.

IRREG'ULAR, *Irregula'ris, Anom'alous;* from *im*, 'privative,' and *regula*, 'a rule.' A term chiefly applied to the types of a disease; and, also, to the pulse, when its beats are separated by unequal intervals.

IRREG'ULAR PRACTIT''IONER. One who does not practise his profession according to rules sanctioned by law or custom.

IRREMEDIABLE, Incurable.

IRREPTIO, Attack.

IRRIGA'TION, *Irriga'tio, Embroca'tio, Irrora'tio:* 'the act of watering or moistening.' The methodical application of water to an affected part, to keep it constantly wet.

IRRITABILITAS, Irritability — i. Morbosa, see Subsultus tendinum — i. Vesicæ, Cysterethismus.

IRRITABIL'ITY, *Irritabil'itas*, from *irrito*, (*in*, 'privative,' and *ritus*, 'the usual manner,') 'I provoke.' *Vis irritabilita'tis, Vis Vitæ, Vis in'sita* of Haller, *Vis vita'lis* of Gorter, *Oscilla'tio* of Boerhaave, *Tonic power* of Stahl, *Vita pro'pria, Inherent power, Contractil'ity, Excitabil'ity*, &c. A power, possessed by all living, organised bodies, of being acted upon by certain stimuli, and of moving responsive to stimulation. It is the ultimate vital property.

IR'RITABLE, *Irritab'ilis*. That which is endowed with irritability. Every living organised tissue is irritable; that is, capable of feeling an appropriate stimulus, and of moving responsive to such stimulus. Irritable is often used in the same sense as *impressible*, as when we speak of an irritable person, or habit, or temper. This last condition has been variously termed — *Debilitas nervo'sa*, D. *Erethis'ica*, *Hypercine'sia nervo'sa*, *Neurastheni'a*, *Neurostheni'a*, *Sensibil'itas anom'ala*, S. *Morbo'sa*, S. *aucta*.

IRRITAMEN, Irritant, Stimulus.

IRRITAMENTUM, Erethism, Irritant, Stimulus — i. Metallicum, Galvanism.

IR'RITANT, *Irri'tans, Irrita'men, Irritamentum*. That which causes irritation or pain, heat and tension; either *mechanically*, as punctures, acupuncture, or scarification; *chemically*, as the alkalies and acids; or in a *specific manner*, as cantharides.

Irritants are of great use in the treatment of disease.

IRRITATING POISON, see Poison.

IRRITATIO, Erethism, Gargale, Irritation.

IRRITA'TION, *Irrita'tio, Erethis'mus*. The state of a tissue or organ, in which there is excess of vital movement; commonly manifested by increase of the circulation and sensibility. Broussais defines irritation to be; — the condition of an organ, the excitation of which is carried to so high a degree, that the equilibrium resulting from the balance of all the functions is broken. In this signification, he also uses the word *sur-irritation*, which he considered as a higher degree, and as the essential cause of fever. Irritation is the precursor of inflammation.

IRRITA'TION, MORBID, *Constitu'tional irritation, Ir'ritative fever, Pseudo-fever*, is that excitement which occurs after injuries done to the body, or to any part thereof; — constituting cases of *diseased sympathy*.

IRRITATIVE FEVER, Irritation, morbid.

IRRORATIO, Irrigation.

IS, Fibre.

ISA'TIS TINCTO'RIA, *Woad, Pastel*. A European plant, whose leaves have a fugitive pungent smell, and an acrid durable taste. They are not used, however, in medicine at the present day; but are the source of the dye-stuff, *woad*.

ISCA, Boletus igniarius.

ISCHÆ'MIA, from ισχω, 'I retain,' and 'αιμα, 'blood.' Morbid retention or suppression of an habitual flux of blood, as of the hemorrhoidal or menstrual flux or of epistaxis. See Hæmatostatica.

ISCHÆ'MON, *Ischæ'mum*. Same etymon. A medicine which restrains or stops bleeding.

IS'CHESIS, from ισχειν, 'to retain.' Suppression or retention of a discharge or secretion.

IS'CHIA, MINERAL WATERS OF. In this volcanic isle, five miles from Naples, there are several thermal waters, one of which — that of Gurgitello — raises the thermometer of Fahr. to 167°.

ISCHIACUS, Ischiatic.

ISCHIADICUS MORBUS, Neuralgia femoropoplitæa — i. Nervus, Sciatic nerve.

ISCHIADOCELE, Ischiocele.

ISCHIAGRA, *Is'chias, Ischial'gia*, from ισχιον, 'the haunch,' and αγρα, 'a seizure.' A name given to ischiatic gout. *Femoro-popliteal neuralgia* has, also, been so called.

ISCHIALGIA, Ischiagra, Neuralgia femoropoplitæa.

ISCHIAS, Ischiagra — i. Nervosa Antica, Neuralgia femoro-prætibialis — i. Nervosa Cotunnii, Neuralgia femoro-poplitæa — i. Nervosa digitalis, Neuralgia cubito-digitalis — i. Nervosa postica, Neuralgia femoro-poplitæa — i. à Sparganosi, Phlegmatia dolens.

ISCHIAT'IC, *Ischiad'ic, Ischiat'icus, Ischiad'icus, Ischiacus, Sciat'ic*, from ισχιον, 'the haunch;' whence the word *Sciatic*. An epithet given to parts connected with the ischium. The SCIATIC NOTCHES, (F.) *Échancrures Ischiatiques*, are formed by this bone; the ISCHIATIC SPINE belongs to it, and gives attachment to the small sacrosciatic ligament. The TUBEROS'ITY OF THE ISCHIUM, *Os sedenta'rium, Tuber Is'chii*, (F.) *Tuberosité sciatique*, is formed by it. It receives the insertions of different muscles of the thigh, and forms the projection on which the body rests when seated.

ISCHIATIC ARTERY, *Sciat'ic Ar'tery*, (F.) *Artère Fémoro-Poplitée* (Ch.) arises singly from the hypogastric, or with the gluteal; and seems to be really a continuation of the trunk of the hypogastric. It issues from the pelvis, at the lower part of the great sciatic notch; and, afterwards, divides into a considerable number of branches, which are distributed particularly to the posterior and superior region of the thigh.

ISCHIATIC REGION, *Sciat'ic region; Regio ischiad'ica*. The region of the hip.

ISCHIATIC VEIN presents the same arrangement as the artery.

ISCHIATICUS, Sciatic.

ISCHIATOCELE, Ischiocele.

ISCHIDRO'SIS, *Sudo'ris suppres'sio, Oligid'ria*, from ισχω, 'I restrain,' and 'ιδρως, 'sweat.' Suppression of perspiration.

ISCHIOBLEN'NIA, *Ischoblen'nia*, from ισχω, 'I restrain,' and βλεννα, 'mucus.' The suppression of a morbid but habitual discharge of mucus.

ISCHIO-CAVERNO'SUS. Belonging to the ischium and corpus cavernosum.

ISCHIO-CAVERNOSUS muscle, *Collatera'lis, Direc'tor penis, Erec'tor penis, Sustenta'tor Penis, Ischio-uréthral* (Ch.) is a small, long, flat muscle, which surrounds the origin of the corpus cavernosum. It is fixed *below* to the inner side of the tuberosity of the ischium, and *above* to the root of the penis, where it is confounded with the fibrous membrane of the corpus cavernosum. It draws the root of the penis downwards and backwards.

ISCHIO-CAVERNOSUS of the female, *Erectorclitor'idis, Sustenta'tor clitor'idis, Superior rotun'dus clitor'idis*, (F.) *Ischio-clitoridien, Ischio sous-clitorien*, (Ch.), is arranged nearly as in the male, but is less bulky. It arises, by aponeurosis, from the tuberosity of the ischium, and terminates by embracing the corpus cavernosum of the clitoris, to the erection of which it appears to contribute.

ISCHIOCE'LĒ, *Ischiatoce'lē, Ischiadoce'lē, Hernia ischia'tica;* from ισχιον, 'the ischium,' and κηλη, 'tumour.' *Ischiatic hernia*. One in which the viscera issue by the great sciatic notch. It is a rare disease. The protruded parts must be reduced—the patient being placed in a favourable position, and they must be retained by a bandage.

ISCHIO-CLITORIA'NUS. That which is connected with the ischium and clitoris.

ISCHIO-CLITO'RIAN ARTERY of Chaussier is a division of the internal pudic, which furnishes the two arteries of the clitoris — the *superficial* and *deep-seated*.

ISCHIO-CLITORIAN NERVE, of the same professor, is the superior branch of the pudic nerve, which is distributed to the clitoris.

ISCHIO-CLITORIDIEN, Ischio-cavernous — i. Coccygeus, Coccygeus — *i. Crêti-tibial*, Semi-tendinosus, — i. Femoralis, Adductor magnus — *i. Fémoro-péronier*, Biceps flexor cruris — *i. Périneal*, Transversus perinæi — *i. Popliti-fémoral*, Semi-membranosus — *i. Popliti-tibial*, Semi-membranosus — *i. Prétibial*, Semi-tendinosus — *i. Sous-clitorien*, Ischio-cavernosus — *i. Sous-trochantérien*, Quadratus femoris — *i. Spino-trochan-*

rien, Ischio-trochanterianus — *i. Uréthral*, Ischio-cavernosus.

ISCHIODYMIA, see Somatodymia.

IS'CHION, *Ischium, Os ischii, Os coxen'dicis, Hip-bone, Huckle-bone, Seat-bone*, (F.) *Os de l'assiette*. The lowermost of the three portions which compose the os innominatum in the fœtus and young individual. The inferior region of the same bone has, also, been called *ischium*, in the adult. According to Hesychius, the ancients designated by the word *ischion*, the capsular ligament of the coxo-femoral articulation, as well as the articulation itself. Some derive the word from ιοχις, the lumbar region; others from the verb ιοχω, 'I arrest,' 'I retain ;'—because that bone serves as a base or support for the trunk, when we are seated.

ISCHION, Haunch,

ISCHIOPA'GES, from *Ischion*, and παγω, 'I fasten.' A monstrous union of two fœtuses, in which they are attached to each other by the ischia. — Geoffroy St. Hilaire. See Hypogastrodidymus.

ISCHIOPHTHI'SIS, *Tabes coxa'ria seu ischiad'ica, Phthisis ischiad'ica*, from ιοχιον, 'ischium,' and *phthisis*. Phthisis in consequence of suppuration of the hip joint.

ISCHIO-PROSTAT'ICUS. Winslow, Sanctorini, Albinus, and Sömmering, have given this name to the fibres of the transversus perinæi muscle, which go towards the prostate.

ISCHIO-RECTAL FOSSA, Perineal fossa.

ISCHIOSIS, Neuralgia femoro poplitæa.

ISCHIO-TROCHANTERIA'NUS, *Gem'ini, Gemel'li*. Part of the *Marsupia'lis* of Cowper; *Car'neum Marsu'pium, Ischio-spini-trochantérien, Secun'dus et ter'tius quadrigem'inus*, (F.) *Muscle cannelé, Accessoire à l'obturateur interne*. Two small, fleshy bundles, long and flat, which arise, — the *superior* on the outside of the sciatic spine; the *inferior* behind the tuberosity of the ischium. Both pass horizontally outwards, and are attached to the tendon of the obturator internus, which they accompany into the fossa of the trochanter. These muscles are rotators of the lower limb outwards. They can, also, turn the pelvis on the femur, in standing on one foot.

ISCHIUM, Ischion.

ISCHL, MINERAL WATERS OF. These springs, which are in Upper Austria, contain iodine and bromine.

ISCHNOPHO'NIA, from ιοχνος, 'slender,' and φωνη, 'voice.' Slenderness of voice. — Hippocrates, Galen.

ISCHNOTES, Emaciation.

ISCHO, ιοχω, 'I keep back,' 'I restrain,' 'I hold firm.' Hence:

ISCHOBLENNIA, Ischioblennia.

ISCHOCENO'SIS, from ιοχω, 'I arrest,' and κενωσις, 'evacuation.' Retention or suppression of a natural evacuation — as of the menses.

ISCHOCHOL'IA, from ιοχω, 'I arrest,' and χολη, 'bile.' *Reten'tio bilis*. Retention or suppression of the biliary secretion.

ISCHOCOILIA, Constipation.

ISCHOCOPRIA, Constipation.

ISCHOGALAC'TIA, *Reten'tio lactis*, from ιοχω, and γαλα, 'milk.' Want of milk in the mammæ.

ISCHOLO'CHIA or *Ischolochi'a, Lochios'chesis, Suppres'sio lochio'rum*, from ιοχω, 'I restrain,' and λοχια, 'the lochial discharge.' *Reten'tio lochio'rum*. Suppression of the lochial discharge.

ISCHOMENIA, Amenorrhœa.

ISCHONEURALGIA, Neuralgia femoro-poplitæa.

ISCHOPHONIA, Balbuties.

ISCHOSPER'MIA, from ιοχω, 'I retain,' and σπερμα, 'sperm ;' *Sem'inis reten'tio*. Retention or suppression of the spermatic secretion.

ISCHURET'IC, *Ischuret'icum*. Same etymon as the next. A medicine for relieving suppression of urine. A diuretic.

ISCHU'RIA, *Uri'næ suppres'sio, Stoppage of urine, Suppres'sio lo'tii, Paru'ria retentio'nis*; from ιοχω, 'I arrest,' 'I retain,' and ουρον, 'urine.' Impossibility of discharging the urine. Generally restricted to suppression of the secretion, or to renal Ischuria or *Anu'ria, Anure'sis*.

Ischuria Vera is that in which the urine having accumulated in the bladder, the patient is unable to pass it, notwithstanding the inclination which constantly distresses him. In *false ischuria, Paru'ria inops, Paru'ria retentio'nis rena'lis, Ischuria notha* seu *spu'ria*, of some, (F.) *Suppression d'Urine*, owing to some disease of the kidney or uterus, the urine cannot reach the bladder.

Ischuria has likewise received various other names, according to the seat and character of the obstacle which opposes the exit of the urine: hence the expressions — *Renal, Ureteric, Vesical, Urethral*, and *Calculous Ischuria*. *Vesical Ischuria* is synonymous with Retention of urine, which see.

ISCHURIA CYSTO-PHLEGMATICA, Cystirrhœa — i. Phimosica, see Phimosicus — i. Spasmodica, Cystospasmus — i. Spuria, see Ischuria — i. Urethralis à phimosi, see Phimosicus — i. Vera, see Ischuria — i. Vesicalis, Retention of urine.

ISINGLASS, Ichthyocolla.

ISIR, Elixir.

ISIS NOBILIS, see Coral.

ISLAND OF REIL, Insula cerebri.

ISLE OF WIGHT, CLIMATE OF. This beautiful island is a favourable summer retreat for invalids. Undercliff is the situation chosen as a winter residence for phthisical valetudinarians. Cowes, Niton, Sandown, Shanklin, and Ryde, are delightful summer residences.

ISOCH'RONOUS, *Isoch'ronus, Isochron'ius, Isod'romus*, from ισος, 'equal,' and χρονος, 'time.' That which takes place in the same time, or in equal times. The pulsations of the arteries, in various parts of the body, are nearly isochronous.

ISOCH'RYSON, *Auro compar;* from ισος, 'equal,' and χρυσος, 'gold.' A collyrium, described by Galen as worth its weight in gold. Libavius has also given this name to an amalgam, made with equal parts of antimony and mercury.

ISOC'RATES, from ισος, 'equal,' and κεραννυμι, 'I mix.' A mixture of equal parts of wine and water. — Hippocrates.

ISODROMUS, Isochronous.

ISOLUSINE, see Polygala senega.

ISOM'ERIC, *Isomer'icus, Isom'erus, Isomœ'rus, Isom'orus*, from ισος, 'equal,' and μερος, 'part.' An epithet applied to different bodies which agree in composition, but differ in properties. The condition is termed *Isom'erism*.

ISOMERISM, see Isomeric.

ISOMORPHISM, see Isomorphous.

ISOMOR'PHOUS, *Isomor'phus, Isomor'phicus*, from ισος, 'equal,' and μορφη, 'form.' An epithet applied to different bodies which have the same crystalline form. The condition is called *Isomorphism*.

ISONANDRA GUTTA, see Gutta percha.

ISOPATHI'A, *Isop'athy*, from ισος, 'equal,' and παθος, 'disease.' This term has been used by some of the German writers to signify the cure of diseases by the disease itself, or its products ; — under the hypothesis, that every contagious disease contains in its contagious matter the means for its cure;—thus, that variola may be cured by homœopathic doses of variolous matter; syphilis, with venereal matter, &c., &c. Others have given to isopathy another form;—maintaining, that every diseased organ has its remedy in the same organ,—that eating liver, for example, will remove disease of the liver!

Isopathia has been used by an American writer—Dr. J. M. B. Harden, of Georgia—to mean "*Parallelism of Diseases;*" "the disposition of diseases to 'anastomose with each other,' or to wear each other's livery."

ISSUE, Fonticulus—i. Peas, Aurantia curassaventia, see Fonticulus.

ISTHME DU GOSIER, Isthmus of the fauces.

ISTHMION, Isthmus, Pharynx.

ISTHMI'TIS, *Inflamma'tio Fau'cium, I. pala'ti, Angi'na simplex, Cynan'chê simplex, Angi'na mitis, A. faucium, Angor fau'cium*, (F.) *Angine simple*. Inflammation of the fauces. See Cynanche pharyngea, and Angina.

ISTHMOCATAR'RHUS; from ισθμος, 'the fauces,' and καταρροος, 'catarrh.' Catarrh of the fauces.

ISTHMODYN'IA, from ισθμος, 'the fauces,' and οδυνη, 'pain.' Pain in the fauces.

ISTHMOPLE'GIA; from ισθμος, 'the fauces,' and πληγη, 'a stroke.' Paralysis of the fauces.

ISTHMOS, Pharynx.

ISTHMOTYPHUS, Cynanche maligna.

ISTHMUS, *Isth'mion*. A tongue of land joining a peninsula to a continent, or which separates two seas. Anatomists have given the name *Fauces, Isthmus of the Fauces, Isthmus Fau'cium, Claustrum Gut'turis*, (F.) *Isthme du gosier*, to the strait which separates the mouth from the pharynx. It is formed above by the velum palati and uvula; at the sides, by the pillars of the fauces and the tonsils; and below, by the base of the tongue.

ISTHMUS OF THE FOSSA OVA'LIS; *Isthmus Vieussen'ii, Striga cartilagino'sa cordis*, is the prominent arch formed above the fossa ovalis by the union of the two pillars which bound the cavity.

ISTHMUS OF THE THYROID GLAND is a narrow band that unites the two chief lobules composing the thyroid gland.

ISTHMUS HEPATIS, see Lobulus anonymus—i. Urethræ, see Urethra—i. Vieussenii, Isthmus of the fossa ovalis, see Ovalis fossa.

ITALICUS MORBUS, Syphilis.

ITCH, Psora—i. of Animals, Scabies ferina—i. Bakers', see Psoriasis—i. Barbers', Sycosis.

ITCH, COWPOX. A cutaneous eruption, observed and described by Gölis, which appeared after the fourteenth day from vaccination, and consisted of isolated vesicles, often filled with a puriform fluid.

ITCH, GROCERS,' see Psoriasis—i. Insect, see Psora—i. Weed, Veratrum viride.

ITCHING, *Parap'sis pruri'tus, Autal'gia prurigino'sa, Pruri'tus, Pruri'go, Cnesmos, Cnesma*, (F.) *Prurit, Demangeaison*. A sensation, more inconvenient than painful, seated especially at the surface of the body, which provokes the patient to scratch the part. It may be either an external or an internal sensation: that is, produced by an external body, or by some modification in the organic actions of the part to which it is referred.

ITEA, Salix.

ITER DENTIS, see Gubernaculum dentis—i. Femineum, Perinæum—i. ad Infundibulum, Vulva—i. a Palato ad Aurem, Eustachian tube—i. ad Quartum ventriculum, Aquæductus Sylvii—i. ad Tertium ventriculum, Vulva—i. Urinæ, Urethra—i. Urinarium, Urethra.

ITHYPHAL'LUS, from ιθυς, 'straight,' and φαλλος, 'penis.' An amulet, in the form of a penis, anciently worn round the neck, to which were attributed alexiterial properties.

ITINERARIUM, Conductor, Director.

ITIS, from ιτης, 'bold,' 'rash.' A suffix denoting inflammation;—as encephal*itis*, inflammation of the encephalon;—Pleur*itis*, inflammation of the pleura.

IVA, Teucrium iva—i. Arthritica, Teucrium chamæpitys—i. Moschata Monspeliensium, Teucrium iva—i. Pecanga, Smilax sarsaparilla.

IVETTE MUSQUÉE, Teucrium iva—*i. Petite*, Teucrium chamæpitys.

IVOIRE, Ivory.

IVORY, *Ebur, El'ephas*, (F.) *Ivoire*. The tusk of the elephant. It is chiefly composed of phosphate of lime, and is used for the fabrication of pessaries, artificial teeth, handles of instruments, &c. Formerly, when calcined to whiteness, it entered into some pharmaceutical preparations. It was regarded as astringent and anthelmintic, and was called *Spodium*.

The *dentine* is the ivory of the human tooth. See Tooth.

IVRAIE, Lolium temulentum.

IVRESSE, Temulentia.

IVY, Hedera helix, Kalmia angustifolia—i. American, Ampelopsis quinquefolia—i. Big, Kalmia latifolia—i. Fine-leaved, Ampelopsis quinquefolia—i. Ground, Glecoma hederaceum.

IXIA, Varix, Viscum album.

IXINE, Atractylus gummifera.

IXIR, Elixir.

IXOS, Viscum album.

IXUS, Galium aparine.

IXYOMYELI'TIS, from ιξυς, 'the lumbar region,' μυελος, 'marrow,' and *itis*, denoting inflammation. Inflammation of the spinal marrow in the lumbar region.

IXYS, *Ix'ya, Ix'yê*. Used by different authors for the ilia, flanks, and loins; most frequently for the last.—Hippocrates.

J.

JABOT, Ingluvies.

JACA INDICA, Thymus mastichina.

JACEA, Tricolor, Viola Tricolor—j. Ramosissima, Centaurea calcitrapa.

JACENS, Sick.

JACK IN THE HEDGE, Alliaria.

JACKSON'S BATHING SPIRITS, Linimentum saponis compositum.

JACOBÆA, Senecio Jacobæa.

JACOBÉE, Senecio Jacobæa.

JACOB'S LADDER, FALSE, Polemonium reptans.

JACOBSON'S ANASTOMOSIS, see Petrosal ganglion.

JACTA'TION, *Jactita'tion, Jacta'tio, Jacta'tus, Rhiptas'mos, Jactita'tio*, from *jactare*, 'to toss about.' Extreme anxiety; excessive restlessness;—a symptom observed in serious diseases.

JACTITATIO, Inquietude.
JADE NÉPHRITE ou *ORIENTALE*, Nephreticus lapis.
JAGRE, see Tari.
JALAP, Convolvulus jalapa, Phytolacca decandra — j. Cancer root, Phytolacca decandra — j. Wild, Convolvulus panduratus.
JALAPA, Convolvulus jalapa.
JALAPINE, see Convolvulus jalapa.
JALAPIUM, see Convolvulus jalapa.
JALAPPA, Convolvulus jalapa — j. Alba, Convolvulus mechoacan.
JALEYRAC, MINERAL WATERS OF. These waters are situate two leagues from Mauriac in France, on the road from Clermont in Auvergne. The waters contain lime and carbonate of soda, and are esteemed to be tonic, aperient, &c.
JALOPA, Convolvulus jalapa.
JAMAICA, see West Indies — j. Bark tree, Bursora gummifera.
JAMAICINE, see Geoffræa inermis.
JAMBES DE BARBADE, see Elephantiasis — *j. du Cervelet*, Corpora restiformia.
JAMBIER, Tibial — *j. Antérieur*, Tibialis anticus — *j. Grèle*, Plantar muscle — *j. Postérieur*, Tibialis posticus.
JAMES'S ANALEPTIC PILLS, see Analeptica.
JAMESTOWN WEED, Datura stramonium.
JANAMUNDA, Geum urbanum.
JANIPHA MANIHOT, Jatropha manihot.
JANITOR, Pylorus.
JANITRIX, Porta vena.
JANON-TARENTISME, Tarantismus.
JANUS, Dicephalus.
JACQUIER, Artocarpus.
JARRET, Poples.
JARRETIER, Popliteus muscle, Hamstring.
JARRETIÈRE (F.), *Peris'celis*, a garter, from *garetum* or *garretum*, in low Latin, the *ham*. A kind of furfuraceous herpes, which occupies the part of the leg where the garter is worn.
JASMIN, Jasminum officinale.
JASMINUM ARABICUM, Coffea Arabum.
JASMI'NUM OFFICINA'LE, *Jasminum, Jesemi'num*, the *Jes'eamine*, (F.) *Jasmin*. The flowers of this beautiful plant have a very fragrant smell, and a bitter taste. They afford, by distillation, an essential oil; which is much esteemed in Italy, for rubbing paralytic limbs, and in the cure of rheumatic pains.
JASPER, Jaspis.
JASPIS, *Jasper*. A precious stone, supposed by the ancients to be capable of arresting hemorrhage when worn as an amulet.
JATAMANSI, Sumbul.
JAT'ROPHA CURCAS, *Rici''inus major, Ricinoï'des, Pi'neus purgans, Pinho'nes In'dici, Faba cathar'tica, Avella'na cathar'tica, Nux cathar'tica America'na, Nux Barbaden'sis, Physic Nut*, (F.) *Pignon d'Inde, Médicinier cathartique, Grand haricot de Pérou, Pignon de Barbarie, Noix cathartique, N. Américaine* ou *des Barbades*. *Nat. Order*, Euphorbiaceæ. The seeds of this plant afford a quantity of oil, given, in many places, like the castor oil; to which, indeed, it is nearly allied. They contain a peculiar acid, the *Jatrophic* or *Igasuric*.
The seeds of JATROPHA MULTIF'IDA are called *Purging Nuts*, and give out a similar oil.
JATROPHA ELASTICA, see Caoutchouc.
JATROPHA MAN'IHOT, *Jan'ipha Man'ihot*. The plant affording the *Cassa'da* or *Cassa'va Root, Caca'vi, Cassa'vè, Casabi, Pain de Madagascar, Ric''inus Minor, Man'ioc, Magnoc, Maniot, Yucca,*

Maniibar, Aipi, Aipima coxera, Aipipoca, Janipha. The juice of the root is extremely acrid and poisonous. What remains, after expressing it, is made into cakes or meal; of which the cassada or cassava bread is formed. This bread constitutes a principal food of the inhabitants of those parts where it grows.
The fecula of the root forms Tapioca, *Cipipa, Fec'ula Tapio'ka, Am'ylum manihot'icum*, which is very nutritious. It may be prepared in the same manner as sago.
A factitious Tapioca is met with in the shops, which is in very small, smooth, spherical grains, and is supposed to be prepared from potato starch. It is sold under the name *pearl tapioca*.
JAUNDICE, Icterus — j. Black, Melæna — j. Lead, Icterus saturninus — j. Red, Phenigmus.
JAUNE, Yellow — *j. d'Œuf*, see Ovum.
JAUNISSE, Icterus.
JAW BONE, Maxillary Bone.
JAW-DISEASE, PHOSPHORUS, see Phosphorus.
JEAN-DE-GLAINES, ST., MINERAL WATERS OF. These waters are situate two leagues from Billom in Auvergne. They contain chloride of calcium, and carbonate of magnesia; dissolved in an excess of carbonic acid.
JECINUS, Liver.
JECORARIA, Marchantia polymorpha.
JECORARIUS, Hepateros, Hepatic.
JECORIS VOMICA, see Hepatitis.
JECTIGA'TIO. A word used by Van Helmont for a species of epilepsy or convulsion.
JECUR, Liver — j. Uterinum, Placenta.
JEFFERSO'NIA BARTONI, *J. Diphyl'la, Common Twinleaf, Yellow Root, Helmet Pod, Ground Squirrel Pea*. An indigenous plant, belonging to *Nat. Ord*. Berberideæ, *Sex. Syst*. Octandria Monogynia; which possesses medical properties analogous to those of hydrastis.
JEJUNITAS, Hunger.
JEJUNI'TIS; a term of hybrid formation, — from *Jejunum*, 'the intestine jejunum,' and *itis*, a suffix denoting inflammation. Inflammation of the jejunum.
JEJUNIUM, Hunger, Fasting.
JEJU'NUM, from *jejunus*, empty;' *Nestis, νηστις, Nesti'a*. The part of the small intestine comprised between the duodenum and ileum. It has been so called, because it is almost always found empty in the dead body.
JELLY, Gelly — j. of the Cord, Gelatin of Wharton — j. Rice, see Oryza — j. Water, Brasenia hydropeltis.
JENKINSONIA ANTIDYSENTERICA, Pelargonium antidysentericum.
JERGON, see Arrow-poison.
JERKING RESPIRATION, Respiration, jerking.
JERKS, see Mania, dancing.
JERSEY, CLIMATE OF. Jersey is the largest of the islands of the British Channel, and is most frequented by invalids. Its climate closely resembles that of the south-west coast of England, and especially of Penzance, and it is adapted to the same class of invalids.
JERUSALEM OAK OF AMERICA, Chenopodium anthelminticum.
JESEMINUM, Jasminum officinale.
JESSAMINE, Jasminum officinale — j. Yellow, Gelseminum nitidum.
JEUNESSE, Adolescence.
JEWEL WEED, Impatiens balsamina.
JEW'S EAR, Peziza auricula — j. Harp, Trillium latifolium.
JIGGER, Chique.
JIMSTON WEED, Datura stramonium.
JOANNESIA PRINCEPS, Anda.

JOANNETTE, MINERAL WATERS OF. Several springs are found at Joannette, about five leagues from Angers, in France. The waters are both cold and warm, and contain sulphate of lime; subcarbonate of soda; chloride of sodium; some iron; chloride of calcium, and, sometimes, a kind of saponaceous matter. They are chiefly used as a tonic in chlorosis, leucorrhœa, &c.

JOE PYE, Eupatorium perfoliatum.

JOHNE, MINERAL WATERS OF. Johne is a village near Dol in Franche-Comté, France, where is a mineral spring, which contains subcarbonate of soda, and subcarbonates of magnesia and iron. It is used chiefly as a bath in certain diseases of the skin, and in atonic affections.

JOINT, Articulation—j. Ball and Socket, Enarthrosis—j. Dove-tail, Suture—j. Stiff, Ankylosis.

JONAS, MINERAL WATERS OF. This spring is situate to the south-west of Bourbon-l'Archambault, in France. The waters contain chloride of calcium and sulphate of lime; chloride of sodium, and sulphate of soda; carbonate of iron, and carbonic acid gas. They are tonic and aperient.

JOUAN, ST., MINERAL WATERS OF. St. Jouan is a village, near Saint-Malo, in France. The water is a cold chalybeate.

JOUBARBE ÂCRE, Sedum—*j. des Toits*, Sempervivum tectorum—*j. des Vignes*, Sedum telephium.

JOUE, Gena.

JOULOS, Julus.

JOUR, Dies.

JOURS CANICULAIRES, Dog days—*j. Critiques*, Critical days—*j. Indicateurs*, Indicating days.

JOVIS FLOS, Crocus—j. Glans, Juglans.

JUCATO CALLELOE, Phytolacca decandra.

JUDÆ'US, *Juda'icus (Lapis,) Phœnici'tes Lapis, Tecol'ithos*, (F.) *Pierre Judaique*. A stone, found in Judæa, Palestine, &c. Called, also, *Lapis Syriacus*. It was formerly esteemed to be diuretic and lithontriptic.

JUDGMENT, *Judic"ium*, (F.) *Jugement*. The faculty of the intellect, by which ideas are compared with each other, and their relative worth appreciated.

JUDICATORII DIES, Critical days.

JUDICIUM, Judgment.

JUGAL, Zygomatic—j. Process, Zygomatic process.

JUGAL REGION, *Re'gio juga'lis*. The region of the cheek-bone.

JUGALE OS, Malæ os.

JUGALIS, Zygomatic.

JUGALIS SUTU'RA, from ζυγον, 'a yoke.' The suture which unites the *Os Malæ* or *Os Juga'lé* with the superior maxillary bone. Also, the sagittal suture.

JUGEMENT, Judgment.

JUGLANS CINER'EA (*Jovis glans*), *Butter Nut, Oil Nut, White Walnut*. The inner bark of the root of this tree, *Juglans* (Ph. U. S.), which is abundant in the United States, is used in medicine, in the form of extract, as an efficacious and mild laxative, in doses of from 10 to 20 grains. It is in the secondary list of the Pharmacopœia of the United States.

JUGLANS RE'GIA, *Juglans, Nux Juglans, Carya basil'ica*, καρυα, *Carya*. The *Walnut*, (F.) *Noyer*, the tree; *Noix*, the nut, καρυον, *Car'yon*. The unripe fruit, in the state in which it is pickled, was formerly esteemed to be anthelmintic. The *putamen* or green rind of the walnut has been celebrated as a powerful antisyphilitic, and used as a sort of diet drink. The *kernel* is an agreeable article of dessert; but, like all nuts, is difficult of digestion. The expressed oil, *Huile de Noix*, is used in France as an aliment, and, like other fixed oils, is laxative.

Various preparations of the leaves have been recommended in scrofulous affections.

JUG'ULAR, *Jugula'ris*, from *jugulum*, 'the throat.' Relating to the throat.

JUGULAR FOSSA, *Fossa Jugula'ris*, is a cavity in the *petro-occipital* suture. It is formed by the petrous portion of the temporal bone, and by the occipital bone, and lodges the origin of the internal jugular vein. It is, sometimes, called *thimble-like cavity*.

JUGULAR VEINS, *Venæ Jugula'res, V. sphagit'-ides, V. apoplec'ticæ, V. sopora'les*. These are situate at the lateral and anterior parts of the neck. They are two on each side; one *external*, the other *internal*. 1. The *External Jugular Vein, Trachélo-sous-cutanée*, (Ch.) is of less size than the internal. It descends, almost vertically, along the anterior and lateral part of the neck, from the cervix of the lower jaw to the subclavian vein, into which it opens, a little above the internal jugular. It is formed by the *internal maxillary, superficial temporal*, and *posterior auricular veins*. It is this vein which is commonly opened in bleeding in the neck. 2. The *Internal Jugular Vein, V. Céphalique* (Ch.), *Vena apoplec'tica*, is much larger, and more deeply seated than the preceding. It descends, vertically, along the anterior and lateral part of the neck, from the posterior part of the foramen lacerum posterius as far as the subclavian vein. It commences at the *sinus* of the *jugular vein*, (F.) *Golfe de la veine jugulaire*, and receives the blood, which returns by the *sinus of the dura mater*, and that of the *facial, lingual, pharyngeal, superior thyroid, occipital*, and *diploic veins*.

JUGULUM, Clavicle, Throat—j. Uteri, Collum uteri.

JUGUM PENIS, *Presse-urèthre*.

JUICE, EXPRESSED, see Succus.

JUJUBE, *Jujuba, Ziz'yphum, Baccæ jujubæ, B. Ziz'yphi*. The fruit of *Rhamnus Ziz'yphus, Ziz'yphus vulga'ris* seu *jujuba* seu *sati'va*, a native of the south of Europe. It was formerly ranked amongst the pectoral fruits. It has an agreeable sweet taste. The fruits of two other species of Zizyphus—*Z. jujuba, Rhamnus jujuba, Mansana arbo'rea*, a native of the East Indies, and *Z. lotus, Rhamnus lotus, Zizyphus nit'ida* seu *sati'va* seu *sylves'tris*, growing in North Africa, possess similar properties to Zizyphus vulgaris.

JUJUBE PASTE, Paste of jujubes.

JULAPIUM, Julep—j. Camphoræ, Mistura Camphoræ.

JULEB, Julep.

JULEP, *Jula'pium, Jule'pus, Zula'pium, Juleb* of the Persians. A sweet drink. A demulcent, acidulous or mucilaginous mixture.

JULEP, CAMPHOR, Mistura camphoræ—*j. Camphré*, Mistura camphoræ—j. Mint, see Mint julep.

JULUS, *Julos, Ioulos*, ιουλος. The first down that appears upon the chin.—Rufus of Ephesus.

JUMEAU, Gemellus.

JUMEAUX DE LA JAMBE, Gastrocnemii.

JUMELLE, Gemellus.

JUMENTOUS URINE, *Urine jumenteuse*.

JUNCTURA, Articulation.

JUNCUS ODORA'TUS, *Andropo'gon schœnan'thus* seu *bicor'nis* seu *citra'tus* seu *citriodo'-rus, Cymbopo'gon schœnan'thus, Fœnum camelo'rum, Juncus aromat'icus, Camel's hay, Sweet rush, Schœnan'thus, Schœnan'thum, Scœnan'thum, Cal'amus odora'tus, Squinan'thus, Gramen orienta'li, (F.) *Jonc odorant.* The dried plant, which is generally procured from Turkey and Arabia, has an agreeable smell, and a warm, bitterish taste. It was formerly used as a stomachic and deobstruent.

JUNGLE FEVER. A variety of remittent occurring in the jungle districts of India.

JUNIPER TREE, Juniperus communis.

JUNIP'ERUM VINUM. Wine impregnated with juniper berries.

JUNIP'ERUS COMMU'NIS, *J. Suecica, Arceu'thos, Ju'niper tree; Akat'alis, Akat'era. Family,* Coniferæ. *Sex. Syst.* Diœcia Monadelphia. The tops and berries, *Junip'erus* (Ph. U. S.), are ordered in the pharmacopœias. Their odour is strong, but not unpleasant. Taste warm, pungent. Properties dependent upon essential oil, which they yield to both water and alcohol. Dose, ℈j to ℨss, rubbed with sugar. In Holland, juniper berries are used for flavouring gin. The oil, *O'leum junip'eri,* possesses the virtues of the plant. It is called, by Ruland, *Targar.* (F.) *Genévrier* (the plant), *Genièvre* (the berry).

JUNIPERUS LYCIA. This plant—*T'hu'rea, T'h. virga, Arbor thurif'era*—has been supposed to afford the *true frankincense, Cedros Olib'anum, Thus Libano'tos, Libano'tum, Lib'anos, Thus mas'culum, Thus verum,* (F.) *Encens.* By some, however, it is supposed to be the produce of an *Am'yris,* and by others of *Boswel'lia serra'ta.* The odour of olibanum is peculiar and aromatic; taste bitterish and slightly pungent; partly soluble in alcohol, and forming a milky emulsion, when triturated with water. It was formerly used in dysentery and hæmoptysis, but is now never employed except as a perfume in a sick room.

JUNIPERUS OXYCE'DRUS, (F.) *Cade, Oxicèdre, Oxycèdre,* grows in the south of Europe, Siberia, &c. By combustion of the wood, a liquid tar, *O'leum ca'dinum, Junip'eri o'leum empyreumat'icum, Huile de Cade* ou *de Genévrier,* is obtained, which is employed externally in various chronic cutaneous and other diseases.

JUNIPERUS SABI'NA, *Sabi'na, Savi'na, Sabi'na ster'ilis, Bruta, Cedrus baccif'era, Common or barren savin; Brathu, Brathys, Ba'rathron, Bo'rathron,* (F.) *Sabine, Savinier.* The odour of savin leaves is strong and disagreeable. Taste hot, acrid, and bitter, depending on an essential oil. Their operation is stimulant, emmenagogue, anthelmintic, and abortive; externally, escharotic. Dose, internally, gr. v to x of the powder. As an escharotic, they are applied in powder or formed into a cerate. The essential oil, *O'leum Sabi'næ* (Ph. U. S.), has the virtues of the savine. Dose, two to five drops.

JUNIPERUS SUECICA, J. communis.

JUNIPERUS VIRGINIA'NA, *Red cedar.* This tree is known throughout the United States by the name of *savine,* and is often used for the same purposes.

JUNK, Pad.

JUNO LUCINA, Ilithyia.

JUPITER, Tin.

JURIBALI, *Euribali.* A tree in the forests of Pomeroon. *Fam.* Meliaceæ. *Class,* Octandria. *Nat. Order,* Monogynia. The bark is febrifuge, and may be given in powder or infusion, (ℨj ad aq. bullient. Oij.)

JURISPRU'DENCE, MED'ICAL, from *jus, juris,* 'law,' and *prudentia,* 'knowledge.' *Jurispruden'tia Med'ica.* This word is often used synonymously with *Legal Medicine.* It is now, as frequently, perhaps, employed for the embodied laws and regulations that relate to the teaching and practice of medicine.

JURY OF MATRONS. A jury formed of women empanelled under a writ *de ventre inspiciendo,* to try the question, whether a woman be with child or not.

JUS, *Zomos, Zomid'ium, Sorbit"io, Sor'bitum.* Soup, broth, *Jus'culum* or *bouillon.*

JUS BOVINUM, Beef-tea—j. Coagulatum, Gelly.

JUS D'HERBES, (F.) The juice of certain vegetables administered as depuratives; as that of fumitory, burdock, water trefoil, &c.

JUS JELATUM, Gelly—*j. de Réglisse,* see Glycyrrhiza—*j. de Viande,* see Bouillon.

JUSCULUM, see Jus.

JUSQUIAMUS, Hyoscyamus.

JUSQUIAUME, Hyoscyamus.

JUSTICIA BIVALVIS, Adulasso—j. Adhatoda, Adhatoda.

JUSTIC"IA ECBOL'IUM, *Carim curini.* A Malabar plant, the root of which, and the leaves, in decoction, are considered in the country to be lithontriptic.

JUSTICIA PECTORA'LIS. A West India plant, which is slightly astringent. (F.) *Carmantine, C. Pectorale, Herbe aux Charpentiers.*

JUVANS, *Auxil'ium, Remed'ium.* A medicine or substance of any kind, which relieves a disorder. An adjuvant.

JUVENIS, Adolescens.

JUVENTA, Adolescence, Hebe.

JUVENTAS, Adolescence, Hebe.

JUVENTUS, Adolescence, Hebe.

JUXTAPOSIT"ION, *Jaxtaposit"io,* from *juxta,* 'near to,' and *ponere, positum,* 'to place.' The mode of increase proper to minerals; which consists in the successive application of new molecules upon those that form the primitive nucleus. It is opposed to *intussusception.*

K.

N. B.—Most of the terms under K, derived from the Greek, are found under the letter C.

K. This letter was formerly used to designate a compound of gold.

KAATH, Catechu.

KAAWY. Ancient name of an Indian drink, prepared from maize.

KABALA, Cabal.

KÆMPFERIA GALANGA, see Maranta galanga.

KÆMPFE'RIA ROTUN'DA. Called after Kæmpfer, the naturalist; *Zedoa'ria, Z. rotun'da, Amo'mum zedoa'ria, Col'chicum Zeylan'icum, Cur'cuma aromat'ica, Zed'oary,* (F.) *Zédoaire rond.* The roots of this Ceylonese plant have a fragrant smell, and warm, bitterish, aromatic taste. They are in wrinkled, gray, ash-coloured, heavy, firm, short pieces; of a brownish-red colour within; and are stimulant and carminative. Dose, ℈j to ℨj of the powder.

According to some, the *round zedoary* is furnished by *Curcuma zerumbet;* the *long, Zedoa'ria longa,* by *Cur'ouma zedoa'ria.*

KAHINCÆ RADIX, Cainces radix.

KAIB, *Kayl.* A word employed by the alchemists for sour and coagulated milk.
KAJEPUT, Cajeput.
KAKOCHYMIA, Cacochymia.
KALI, Potash, Potassa— k. Acetas, Potassæ acetas — k. Aeratum, Potassæ carbonas — k. Bichromicum, Potassæ bichromas — k. Causticum, Potassa fusa — k. Causticum cum calce, Potassa cum calce—k. Chloricum, Potassæ murias hyperoxygenatus—k. Chromicum acidum, Potassæ bichromas—k. Chromicum flavum, Potassæ bichromas—k. Chromicum rubrum, Potassæ bichromas — k. Chromicum neutrale, Potassæ chromas— k. Hydriodinicum, see Potassæ hydriodas — k. Inermis, see Salsola kali — k. Nitricum, Potassæ nitras—k. Oxalicum acidulum, Potassa, oxalate of — k. Præparatum, Potassæ subcarbonas k. Præparatum e tartaro, see Potash—k. Purum, Potassa fusa — k. Soda, see Salsola kali — k. Spinosum cochleatum, Salsola kali—k. Subcarbonas, Potassæ subcarbonas — k. Sulphas, Potassæ sulphas—k. Sulphuricum, Potassæ sulphas—k. Sulphuretum, Potassæ sulphuretum — k. Tartarizatum, Potassæ tartras—k. e Tartaro, see Potash— k. Vitriolatum, Potassæ sulphas.
KALICUM HYDRAS, Potassa fusa.
KALIUM IODATUM, see Potassæ hydriodas —k. Iodatum Hydrargyratum, Potassii hydrargyro-iodidum.
KALMIA ANGUSTIFO'LIA. Called after Kalm, the botanist. *Ivy, Narrow-leaved Kalmia* or *Laurel, Dwarf Laurel, Sheep Laurel.* This plant has the same virtues as K. latifolia. So also has
KALMIA GLAUCA, *Swamp Laurel.*
KALMIA, BROAD-LEAVED, K. latifolia.
KALMIA LATIFO'LIA, *Broad-leaved Kalmia, Cal'ico bush, Laurel, Mountain Laurel, Rose Laurel, Big Ivy, Spoonwood, Lambkill, Sheep-poison, Broad-leaved Laurel.* This plant kills sheep and other animals. The Indians use it as a poison. The powdered leaves have been applied successfully in tinea capitis; and a decoction of it has been used for the itch. The powder, mixed with lard, has been applied in herpes.
KALMIA, NARROW-LEAVED, K. angustifolia.
KALO, Arum esculentum.
KAMPHUR, Camphor.
KAPHUR, Camphor.
KARABE, Asphaltum.
KARABITUS, Phrenitis.
KARCINOSEN, Carcinoses.
KARENA, Carena.
KASSADER, Convolvulus panduratus.
KASSAUDER, Convolvulus Panduratus.
KATASARCA, Anasarca.
KATASTALTICA, Astringents.
KAVA, Ava.
KAVIAC, Caviare.
KAYL, Kaib.
KEITA, Monsonia ovata.
KELOID, Cancroid.
KELOTOMIA, Celotomia.
KELP, *Varec.* The impure mineral alkali obtained by burning certain marine plants. See Soda.
KENNELWORT, Scrophularia nodosa.
KENTUCKY, MINERAL WATERS OF. The Olympian Springs in this state are near the sources of Licking River. There are three different kinds, in the space of half a mile. One of them is saline, impregnated with sulphur;—another is chalybeate, and a third a sulphureous spring. In various parts of Kentucky, there are saline waters, which are frequented by invalids. The *Salines* at Bigbone, formerly employed in the manufacture of salt, are now resorted to. A spring, near Harrodsburg, in Mercer County, is strongly impregnated with sulphate of magnesia.
KERATITIS, Ceratitis.
KERATO-GLOSSUS, Cerato-glossus.
KERATO-IRITIS, Aquo-membranitis.
KERATONYXIS, Ceratonyxis.
KERATO-PHARYNGEUS, Cerato-pharyngeus.
KERATO-STAPHYLINUS, Cerato-staphylinus.
KERATOTOMUS, Ceratotomus, Knife, cataract.
KERMES, *Chermes, Alkermes.* One of the species of the genus kermes lives on a green oak, and is called *Coccus il'icis, Kermes animal, Coccum, Cocci granum, Coccum baph'icum seu infecto'rium, tincto'rum, scarlati'num,* &c. The oak, to which allusion has been made, is known by botanists under the name *Quercus coccif'era,* and grows abundantly in the uncultivated lands of southern France, Spain, and in the islands of the Grecian Archipelago. The kermes inhabiting it has the appearance of a small, spherical, inanimate shell. Its colour is reddish-brown, and it is covered with a slightly ash-coloured dust. This is the kermes of the shops. It is now only used in dyeing; but was formerly reputed to possess aphrodisiac, analeptic, anti-abortive, and other virtues.
KERMES MINERAL, see Antimonii sulphuretum præcipitatum.
KERNEL, Tubercle.
KERNELS, WAXING, see Waxing kernels.
KERUA, Ricinus communis.
KETCHUP, *Catchup.* A pickle prepared from the liquor of the mushroom, walnut, tomato, &c.
KETMIA ÆGYPTIACA, Hibiscus abelmoschus.
KEY, Sax. cæg, *Clavis, Cleis, Clavis An'glica,* (F.) *Clef de Garangeot.* An instrument, used for extracting teeth. It consists of a firm handle, with a claw at right angles to it, and moving upon a pivot. This claw embraces the tooth. It has undergone several modifications, and hence various instruments are used under this denomination. The French have the *Clef à pompe, Clef à pivot,* and *Clef à noix.*
KEYRI CHEIRI, Cheiranthus cheiri.
KHALA MIMUC, Bit noben.
KIAS'TER, *Chiaster,* from χιαζειν, 'to cross.' A species of bandage, having the form of the Greek letter χ, which the ancients used for approximating, and maintaining in contact, the fragments of the patella, in cases of fracture of that bone. It was applied in the form of the figure 8.
KIBISTITOME, Cystitome.
KIDNEY. Its etymology is uncertain. Serenius derives it fancifully from Su. Goth. *qued,* the belly; and *nigh,* (quasi, *quidney.*) *Ren, Nephros, Protme'sis,* (F.) *Rein.* The kidneys or *reins* are the secretory organs of the urine. They are two glands, situate deeply,—the one on the right, and the other on the left side,—in the hypochondres: at the sides of the lumbar vertebræ; behind the peritoneum; and in the midst of an abundant, fatty areolar tissue, *Tu'nica adipo'sa.* The kidney is of a reddish-brown colour; oval form; and flattened on two surfaces. It has, at its internal margin, a deep fissure, by which the renal vessels and nerves enter or quit the organ, and the ureter issues. It resembles, pretty accurately, the haricot or kidney-bean. Two *substances* are readily distinguishable in it;—the outer, *secerning, cortical, glandular* or *vascular, Substan'tia cortica'lis, S. glandulo'sa,* which secretes the urine; and the inner, *tubular, medullary, uriniferous, conoidal* or *radiated, Substan'tia medul*

la'ris, S. Tubulo'sa, S. Fibro'sa, which appears under the form of small cones or unequal *papillæ*, each resulting from the union of small capillary tubes, adherent by one of their extremities to the cortical substance; and opening, by the other, at the summit of the cone, into *calices*, a species of membranous tubes, more or less numerous, which transmit the urine of the papillæ to the *pelvis*. By the *pelvis* is meant a small, membranous sac, of an irregularly oval shape, at the base of which are the orifices of the calices, and the other extremity of which is continuous with the ureter. The kidney is surrounded by a fibrous membrane proper to it, *Perineph'rus*. It has been shown by Mr. Bowman and others that the renal artery is distributed to the corpora Malpighiana, where the watery portion of the urine is separated. The blood then becomes venous, and is distributed by different veins—*portal veins* of the kidney—to the convoluted tubes through which the proper urine is secreted. Hence the blood passes into the renal vein. The intermediate vessels between the Malpighian bodies and the convoluted tubes, have been termed the *Portal System of the Kidney*.

KIDNEY, BRIGHT'S DISEASE OF THE, *Morbus Bright'ii, M. albuminen'sis, Nephri'tis albumino'sa, Neph'ria, Uroso'mia albumino'sa, Cachec'tic nephri'tis, Nephri'tis socia'ta, Asso'ciated nephritis, Inflammation of the Malpig'hian cor'puscles, Disease of Bright, Gran'ular Degenera'tion or Disorganiza'tion of the Kidney, Granular Kidney* of Bright, (F.) *Maladie de Bright, Néphrite albumineuse, État Granuleux* ou *Dégénérescence granulée du Rein, Albuminurrhée*. A granular disease of the cortical part of the kidney, which gives occasion to the secretion of urine that contains albumen, and is of less specific gravity than natural, and which destroys by inducing other diseases. It was first described by Dr. Bright of London.

KIDNEY, GRANULAR, OF BRIGHT, Kidney, Bright's disease of the.

KI'ESTEINE, *Ki'estein*, properly *Ky'esteine, Ky'estein, Kystein, Cy'esteine* or *Cy'estein*, from κυειν, 'to be pregnant,' and εσθης, 'a garment or pellicle.' A peculiar pellicle, which forms on the urine of a pregnant female when allowed to stand for a few days. It is whitish, opalescent, slightly granular, and may be compared to the fatty substance that swims on the surface of soups, after they have been allowed to cool. When taken in conjunction with other phenomena, it is a valuable aid in the diagnosis of early pregnancy.

KIESTIN'IC, *Kiestin'icus ;* same etymon. Relating or appertaining to kiesteine; as '*kiestinic urine*.'

KILBURN, MINERAL WATERS OF. These springs contain carbonic acid, sulphohydric acid; carbonates of lime, magnesia, and iron; sulphates of soda, lime, and magnesia, and chloride of sodium.

KILOGRAMME, *Chiliogram'ma*, from χιλιοι, 'a thousand,' and γραμμα, 'a gramme.' The weight of a thousand grammes; — two pounds eight ounces, one drachm, and twenty-four grains, Troy.

KILOLITRE, from χιλιοι, 'a thousand,' and λιτρα, 'a litre.' A measure containing a thousand litres.

KINA KINA, Cinchona.
KINANCIE, Cynanche.
KINCOUGH, Pertussis.
KINDCOUGH, Pertussis.
KINESIP'ATHY, *Kinesitherapi'a*, from κινησις, 'motion,' and παθος, 'disease.' A mode of treating disease by gymnastics or appropriate movements.

KINETIC, Motory.
KINGCURE, Pyrola maculata.
KING'S EVIL, Scrofula.
KINICI ACETAS, Quinia, acetate of.
KININUM, Quinina.
KINK IN THE HEAD, see Insanity.
KINKINA, Cinchona.
KINO, *Gummi Gambien'sē, Gummi rubrum adstrin'gens Gambien'sē, Af'rican kino, East India kino, Amboy'na kino, Gummi adstrin'gens Fothergil'li*. The trees, whence one variety of this resin is obtained, are not botanically ascertained. The London college ascribe it to *Pterocar'pus erina'cea ;* the Edinburgh to *Eucalyp'tus resinif'era, Metroside'ros gummif'era ;* and the Dublin to *Butea frondo'sa*. The Pharmacopœia of the United States, (1842,) defines it to be "an extract obtained from an uncertain plant;" that of 1851 states it to be the inspissated juice of *Pterocarp'us marsu'pium* (De Candolle) and of other plants. On wounding the bark, the kino flows drop by drop. A West India variety is said to be derived from *Coccoloba uvif'era* or *Sea-side Grape ;* and a Botany Bay kino is said to be the concrete juice of *Eucalyp'tus resinif'era* or *brown gum-tree* of New Holland. *Sex. Syst.* Icosandria Monogynia. *Nat. Ord.* Myrtaceæ. Kino consists chiefly of tannic and gallic acids, oxide of iron, and colouring matter. It is inodorous; the taste a sweetish bitter; and it is sometimes gritty between the teeth. It comes to us in fragments of a dark ruby red colour, and is easily pulverized. Its properties are powerfully astringent. Dose, gr. x to gr. xx in powder.

KIONORRHAPHIA, Staphyloraphy.
KI'OTOME, *Kiot'omus*, from κιων, 'a pillar,' 'support,' and τεμνειν, 'to cut.' (F.) *Coupebride*. An instrument invented by Desault, to cut any accidental *brides* or filaments in the rectum and bladder; and which he afterwards used for the removal of the tonsils. It is composed of a flat, silver sheath, open at one edge. This sheath is provided with a cutting blade, which can be forced through the opening, and thus all the parts can be divided with which it comes in contact.

KIPPERNUT, Bunium bulbocastanum.
KIRATE. A weight of four grains, according to Blancard.
KIRKLAND'S NEUTRAL CERATE, see Cerate, Kirkland's Neutral.
KIRRHONOSIS, Cirrhosis.
KIRRHOSIS, Cirrhosis.
KIRSCHWASSER, (G.) '*Cherry water.*' An alcoholic liquor, obtained from cherries bruised with their stones, by subjecting them to distillation, after having caused them to ferment. See Spirit.
KISSINGEN, MINERAL WATERS OF. These Bavarian springs have been long frequented. There are three, — two chalybeate, and one alkaline and acidulous.
KIST. A weight of 14 grains.—Paracelsus.
KLAPROTHII SULPHAS, Cadmii sulphas.
KLAPROTHIUM SULPHURICUM, see Cadmii sulphas.
KLEPTOMA'NIA, *Cleptoma'nia, Klopema'nia, Clopemania ;* from κλεπτω, 'I steal,' and *mania*. Insanity, with an irresistible propensity to steal.
KLIPDAS, see Hyrax Capensis.
KLOPEMANIA, Kleptomania.
KNARESBOROUGH, MINERAL WATERS OF, see Harrogate, mineral waters of.
KNEADING, Shampooing.
KNEE, Genu.
KNEE, HOUSEMAID'S. An inflammation of the bursa, which in most individuals is in front of the patella, and is apt to inflame and enlarge from

effusion in those in whom it is subjected to much pressure. Hence its name. It is a form of capsular rheumatism.

KNEE-JOINT, Genu.

KNEE-SCAB, Crusta genu equinæ—k. Encircled hoof, Crusta genu equinæ.

KNIFE. Sax. cnif. Swed. Knif. Dan. Kniv. (F.) *Canif. Culter, Smilé, Cultell'us, Tomei'on, Tome'us, Machæ'ra, Machæ'rion, Machæ'ris*, (F.) *Couteau*. A cutting instrument, used in surgery to divide the soft parts, and which only differs from the bistouri or scalpel in being usually larger.

The most common knives are the following:

KNIFE, AMPUTA'TION, (F.) *Couteau à amputation, C. droit, Culter rectus*. This is the largest of the knives used in surgery. Formerly, they were curved; now they are straight, and provided with one or two edges.

KNIFE, CAT'ARACT, *Ceratot'omus, Keratot'omus*, (F.) *Couteau à cataracte*. The cataract knives of Richter, Wenzel, Ward, and others, being intended to perform the section of the transparent cornea, are so shaped as to exactly fill the small wound made by them; and thus to prevent the discharge of the aqueous humour, until the section is completed. The blade of the knives of Wenzel and Ward resembles a very narrow lancet, blunt in the posterior five-sixths of one of its edges. The blade of that of Richter is pyramidal, cutting through the whole length of its inferior edge, and also blunt in the five-sixths of the upper.

KNIFE, CHES'ELDEN'S. A knife with a fixed handle; very convex on its edge, concave on the back, which was used by Cheselden in *lithotomy*.

KNIFE, CROOKED, *Culter falca'tus, Culter curvus*, (F.) *Couteau courbe*. A knife, which is crooked and concave on its cutting edge. It was formerly employed in amputation of the limbs.

KNIFE, CROTCHET, *Cultel'lus uncus*, (F.) *Couteau à crochet*. A steel instrument, composed of a round staff, furnished with a handle at one extremity, and at the other with a curved knife. It was formerly used to cut to pieces monstrous fœtuses in utero, and to open the head when necessary.

KNIFE, DOUBLE-EDGED, *Anceps cultel'lus, Amphis'mela, Amphis'milé, Catling*, (F.) *Couteau à deux tranchans, Couteau désarticulateur, C. interosseux*. A knife, the blade of which is straight and sharp on both sides. It is used for disarticulating bones; and for cutting the soft parts situate between the bones, in amputation of the leg and forearm.

KNIFE *EN SERPETTE*, (F.) *Couteau en serpette*. A sort of knife, of the shape of a *serpette* or pruning-knife, invented by Desault for dividing the bony paries of the maxillary sinus, for the purpose of extracting fungi from it.

KNIFE, LENTIC'ULAR, *Culter lenticula'ris*, (F.) *Couteau lenticulaire*. An instrument, used in the operation of trepanning, for removing inequalities in the inner table of the skull, which may have been left by the crown of the trephine around the opening made by it. It is formed of a lenticular button, fixed at the extremity of an iron staff, which is convex on one side, flat on the other; sharp at both edges, and mounted on an ebony handle.

KNIFE, LITHOT'OMY, (F.) *Couteau lithotome*. A name, given by Foubert to a large knife, the narrow blade of which, four and a half inches in length, was sharp in its whole extent, and made an obtuse angle with the handle. He used it in the lateral operation.

KNIFE, ROOT-CUTTING. In Pharmacy, a knife moving on a joint at its pointed extremity, by which roots and other ligneous matters are divided in pharmaceutical processes.

KNOCK-KNEED, Entogonyancon.

KNOT, Tubercle.

KNOT, PACKER'S, (F.) *Nœud d'emballeur*. A compressive bandage, used for arresting hemorrhage from the temporal artery or its branches. The *nœud d'emballeur* is made with a double-headed roller, five ells long. A graduated compress is placed over the opening in the artery, and the bandage is applied over it; the balls of the roller being carried horisontally round to the opposite temple, where they are crossed obliquely and carried back to the part where the compress is situate. The hands are then changed with the rollers, crossing them so as to form a knot, and taking one above the head; the other beneath the chin. They are then crossed again, so as to form several knots, one above the other. This bandage is called, by some surgeons, *Solar* or *oblique chevestre* or *capistrum*.

KNOT, SURGEON'S, *Nodus chirur'gicus*, (F.) *Nœud du chirurgien*. A double knot made by passing the thread twice through the same noose. This knot is used frequently in the ligature of arteries, the umbilical cord, &c.

KNOTBERRIES, Rubus chamæmorus.

KNOTGRASS, Polygonum aviculare.

KNOTROOT, Collinsonia Canadensis.

KNOTWEED, Collinsonia Canadensis, Polygonum aviculare.

KNOWLTON'IA VESICATO'RIA. *Nat. Order, Ranunculaceœ*. An acrid plant of South Africa, used by the Cape colonists as a blister in rheumatism.

KOINO-MIASMATA, see Miasm.

KOLERUS, a name given by Paracelsus to a dry ulcer.

KOLPORRHAPHY, Elytrorrhaphy.

KOLTO, Plica.

KOOCHLA TREE, Strychnos nux vomica.

KOPYOPIA, see Copyopia.

KORIS, Cimex.

KOSSO, Hagenia Abyssinica.

KOUMIS, Kumyss.

KRAME'RIA, *Ratan'hia, Rhatan'ia, Rat'anhy*, (F.) *Ratanhie*. Krameria, *Krameria triandra*,— *Sex. Syst.* Tetrandria Monogynia, *Nat. Ord.* Polygaleæ,—is a native of Java. The root has a bitter taste; and is astringent, diuretic, and detergent. Dose, ℨj to ℨj.

KRAME'RIA IXI'NA or *Ratanhy of the Antilles* has similar virtues.

KREASOTON, Creasote.

KREATIC NAUSEA, see Nausea.

KREATINE, Creatine.

KREATININE, see Creatine.

KREOSOTON, Creasote.

KRETINISMUS, Cretinism.

KRIEBELKRANKHEIT, Convulsio cerealis.

KUA KAHA, Curcuma longa.

KUMYSS, *Koumyss, Koumis*. A beverage used in families by the people of Yakutz. It resembles sour buttermilk, without being greasy. According to Sir George Simpson, it is prepared in a very simple way from mare's milk, which is merely allowed to stand for some days in a leathern churn till it becomes sour. It is then bottled for use. This drink is rather nutritious than exhilarating; but from the same material the Burats and the Kirghes prepare an intoxicating spirit in which they indulge to excess.

KUSSAUDER, Convolvulus panduratus.

KUTKULEJA, Cæsalpinia bonducella.

KUTOOKURUNJA, Cæsalpinia bonducella.

KUTUBUTH. An Arabic name for a species of melancholy in which the patient is never quiet at any one place, but wanders about here and there. Also, the name of an insect, which lives at the surface of stagnant waters, and is in a constant state of agitation. Some lexicographers imagine that it is on account of this last circumstance, that the name of the insect has been given to the disease.

KYANOSIS, Cyanopathy.
KYAPUTTY, Caieput.
KYESTEINE, Kiesteine.
KYESTINIC, Kiestinic.
KYLLO'SIS, from κυλλος, 'crooked,' 'lame.' *Cyllo'sis.* Professor Chaussier so calls congenital distortion of the feet, *Clubfoot, Tal'ipes,* (F.) *Pied bot.* Of this there are many varieties. In one, the foot, instead of resting on the soil, by the whole plantar surface, touches it only with the metatarso-phalangian articulations. It seems as if turned backwards and broken upon the leg, (*Pes seu Tal'ipes Equi'nus, Hip'popus, Oxypo'dia.*) In other cases the foot is twisted inwards, (*Varus, Tal'ipes varus, Blæsop'odes, Blæ'sopus, Cylloepus, Cyllop'oda, Cyllopod'ion, Lo'ripes,* (F.) *Cagneux,*) so that it rests only on the ground on its outer edge; or it may be twisted outwards, (*Valgus, Tal'ipes Valgus,*) or rest only on its inner edge. In the *flatfoot* or *splayfoot, Duck-foot, Sar'apus, Plat'ypus, Platypod'ia,* (F.) *Pied plat,* the plantar surface of the foot is flattened instead of being concave.

These deformities are rarely accidental. They are almost always congenital, and may be rectified, at an early period, by proper mechanical means to strengthen the foot gradually and restore it to its proper shape and direction; and if these means fail, the tendons and muscles concerned in the deformity may be divided.

KYMOGRAPH'ION; from κυμα, 'wave,' and γραφω, 'I describe.' 'A wave describer or measurer.' An instrument invented by Ludwig, which is self-registering, and exhibits the relation between the waves of the pulse and the undulations produced by respiration. (Müller's Archiv., 1847, s. 242.)

KYNA, Pastinaca opoponax.
KYPHOSIS, see Cyphosis—k. Inflammatoria, Vertebral disease — k. Paralytica, Vertebral disease.

KYST, *Cyst, Kystis, Cystis,* from κυστις, 'a bladder,' 'pouch.' (F.) *Kyste.* This term is generally applied to a pouch or sac,—*Cysto'ma,*—without opening, and commonly of a membranous nature, which is accidentally developed in one of the natural cavities, or in the substance of organs. Many theories have been successively emitted to explain the formation of cysts, but none are entirely satisfactory. Some are formed by a thin, translucent membrane, having scarcely the thickness of the arachnoid; others of a whitish, fibrocellular membrane, more or less thick. Some contain cartilaginous or bony flakes. The greater part have but one cavity; others, on the contrary, have several, separated by complete or imperfect septa, as is frequently seen in those developed in the ovaries. The matter contained in cysts is sometimes limpid, serous, yellowish white, reddish, and, at others, more or less thick, albuminous, adipous, or caseous. The tumour, formed by them, is called Encysted.

KYSTE, Kyst—k. *Anévrysmal,* Aneurismal sac.
KYSTEIN, Kiesteine.
KYSTHI'TIS, *Cysthi'tis,* from κυσθος, 'the vagina.' Inflammation of the vulva and of the mucous membrane of the vagina.
KYSTHOPTO'SIS, from κυσθος, the 'vagina,' and πιπτω, 'I fall.' Prolapsus or inversion of the vagina.
KYTTARRHAG"IA, from κυτταριον, 'an alveolus,' and ρηγνυμι, 'I break forth.' Discharge of blood from an alveolus.

L.

LABARIUM, from *labi,* 'to fall.' Looseness of the teeth.
LABDACISMUS, Lallation.
LABDAMEN, Cistus creticus.
LABDANUM, see Cistus creticus.
LABE, λαμβανω, 'I seize,' 'I take,' 'the act of grasping.' Invasion. Also, employed to denote the first paroxysm of fevers.—Galen, Hippocrates.
LABEO, Chilon.
LABES, Chilon, Macula.
LABIA CUNNI, Lips of the vulva—l. Interna seu Minora, Nymphæ—l. Majora, Lips of the vulva—l. Pudendi, Lips of the vulva—l. Pudendi minora, Nymphæ.
LABIAL, *Labia'lis,* from *labium,* 'a lip.'
LABIAL, Orbicularis oris.
LABIAL ARTERY. Haller and Sabatier call thus the *facial artery* of the majority of anatomists. The *labial arteries,* properly so called, *coronary arteries of the lips,* (F.) *Coronaires des lèvres,* are two in number. The *superior* arises from the facial, above, and very close to, the commissure of the lips. It is large and tortuous, and is distributed to the upper lip. The *lower* arises from the facial, at a considerable distance from the commissure, and proceeds, in a serpentine course, into the substance of the lower lip, to which it is distributed.

LABIAL GLANDS. This name is given to a multitude of muciparous follicles, of some size, round, prominent, and separate from each other, which are found on the inner surface of the lips, below the mucous membrane.

LABIAL VEINS are distinguished, like the arteries, into *superior* and *inferior.* They open into the facial vein;—a division of the internal jugular.
LABIALIS, Orbicularis oris.
LABIDOMETER, Labimeter.
LABIM'ETER, (F.) *Labimètre* ou *Labidomètre,* from λαβις, λαβιδος, 'forceps,' and μετρον, 'measure.' A scale adapted to the handles of the forceps, which indicates the distance of the blades from each other, when applied to the head of the child *in utero.*
LABIS, Forceps.
LABIUM, Lip—l. Leporinum, Harelip—l. Uteri, Amphideum.
LABLAB, Dolichos lablab.
LABORANS, Sick.
LABORATOIRE, Laboratory.
LABORATORIUM, Laboratory—l. Chymicum seu pharmaceuticum, Pharmacopœia.
LAB'ORATORY, *Laborato'rium, Ergaste'rion,* (F.) *Laboratoire,* from *laborare,* 'to work.' A work-shop. A place for preparing chemical or pharmaceutical products, &c.
LABORIOSUS, Sick.
LABO'RIOUS. Delivery is said to be labo-

rious, *Partus laborio'sus, Mogostoc'ia*, (F.) *Accouchement laborieux*, when attended with more difficulty and suffering than usual. With some, *laborious labour* means one that requires the use of instruments. See Dystocia.

LABOUR, Parturition.

LABOUR CHAIR, *Obstet"ric chair*. A chair, in which a parturient woman is placed during delivery.

LABOUR, DIFFICULT, Dystocia—l. Dry, *Partus siccus*—l. Morbid, Dystocia—l. Pains, see Pains—l. Powerless, see Parturition—l. Premature, Parturition, (premature)—l. Preternatural, Metatocia, see Parturition—l. Show, see Parturition.

LABRISULCIUM, Cheilocace, Stomacace.

LABRUM, Lip—l. Cerebri, Infundibulum of the brain.

LABRUSCA, Bryonia alba.

LAB'YRINTH, *Labyrinth'us, Antrum buccino'sum*. A place, full of turnings, the exit of which is not easily discoverable. Anatomists have given this name to the aggregate of parts, constituting the internal ear, *Labyrinth'us auris in'timæ, In'tima pars or'gani audi'tûs, Labyrinth'ic cavity of the ear*. The Labyrinth is situate between the tympanum and meatus auditorius internus. It is composed of several cavities, which communicate with each other in the dried bone; as the *vestibule, cochlea, semicircular canals*, &c. It is lined by periosteum, and also by a *pulpy membrane*, constituting the *membranous labyrinth*, on which the auditory nerve is regularly dispersed. This membrane forms two sacs in the vestibule, called *sac'culus vestib'uli* and *sac'culus*, respectively, which resemble in shape that of the bony cavities containing them. Each sac contains calcareous matter, constituting the *Otolithes* and *Otoconies*. When the sac is laid open, upon the upper and outer part, a partition appears, partaking of the nature of the sac, and called by Meckel, *Septum vestib'uli nervo'somembrana'ceum*.

LABYRINTH, MEMBRANOUS, see Labyrinth.

LABYRINTHIC CAVITY OF THE EAR, Labyrinth.

LABYRINTHUS, Labyrinth—l. Auris Intimæ, see Labyrinth.

LAC, Milk, *Lacca*—l. Ammoniaci, Mistura ammoniaci—l. Amygdalæ, Emulsio amygdalæ—l. Asafœtidæ, Mistura asafœtidæ—l. Avis, Albumen ovi—l. Guaiaci, Mistura Guaiaci—l. Gum, Lacca—l. Lunæ, Marga candida—l. Maris, Sperm—l. Primum Puerperæ, Colostrum—l. Seed, Lacca—l. Shell, Lacca—l. Stick, Lacca—l. Sulphuris, Sulphur præcipitatum—l. Terræ, Magnesiæ carbonas—l. Virginis, Virgin's milk.

LACCA, from *lakah*, Arab. *Gummi laccæ, Stick-lac, Gum-lac, Seed-lac, Shell-lac*, (F.) *Laque*. Lac is a substance formed by an insect, and deposited on different species of trees, chiefly in the East Indies,—for example, on *Croton laccif'erum*, and two species of Ficus, — *Ficus religio'sa*, and *F. In'dica*. The various kinds, distinguished in commerce, are *stick-lac*, which is the substance in its natural state, investing the small twigs of the tree; and *seed-lac*, which is the same broken off. When melted, it is called *shell-lac*.

Lac was, at one time, used in the form of tincture, as a tonic and astringent; and it still forms part of particular dentifrices.

LACERA'TION, *Lacera'tio, Rhegē, Rheg'mus, Rhegma, Ruptu'ra, Rupture*, from *lacerare*, 'to tear:'—*Dilacera'tio, Sparag'ma*, (F.) *Arrachement, Déchirement, Dilaceration, Broiement*. The act of tearing or rending. The breach made by tearing or rending; as a *lacerated wound, Treesis vulnus lacera'tum, Laceratu'ra, Vulnus laceratum*.

LACERATURA, see Laceration.

LACERTA, Lizard — l. Aquatica, see Ectozoa.

LACERTI CORDIS, Columnæ carneæ—l. Musculorum, see Muscular fibre.

LACERTULI CORDIS, Columnæ carneæ.

LACERTUS, Brachium, see Muscular fibre.

LAC"ERUM. Same etymon as Laceration. Any thing torn, or appearing as if torn.

LAC"ERUM FORA'MEN ANTE'RIUS, (F.) *Trou déchiré antérieur, Hiatus spheno-pétreux*, (Ch.) is an irregular opening, formed by the sphenoid and petrous portion of the temporal bone. This foramen transmits the third, fourth, and sixth pairs of nerves and the first branch of the fifth pair to the eye and its appendages.

LACERUM FORAMEN POSTE'RIUS, *Foramen jugula'rē, F. lacerum in Basi Cra'nii*, (F.) *Trou déchiré postérieur, Hiatus occipito-pétreux*, (Ch.) is formed by the occipital bone, and the inferior edge of the petrous portion of the temporal bone. Through it, the internal jugular vein, the eighth pair of nerves, and accessory nerve pass out of the cranium.

LACHESIS PICTA, see Arrow-poison.

LACHESIS RHOMBEA'TA, *Flammon*. A poisonous serpent common in the lower forests of Peru.

LACHRYMA, Tear; see, also, Vitis vinifera.

LACH'RYMAL, *Lacryma'lis*, from *lacryma*, 'a tear.' Belonging to the tears. This epithet is given to various parts.

LACHRYMAL ARTERY proceeds from the ophthalmic; and distributes its principal branches to the lachrymal gland.

LACHRYMAL CANAL or DUCT, *Nasal Canal or duct, Cana'lis lacryma'lis, Canalis or'bitæ nasa'lis, Ductus nasa'lis orbitæ, Cana'lis sacci lacryma'lis, Ductus ad Nasum*, is formed by the superior maxillary bone, os unguis, and os turbinatum inferius; and is seated in the outer paries of the nasal fossæ. It is lined by a prolongation of the mucous membrane of the lachrymal sac; and its inferior orifice is furnished with a valvular duplicature. This duct transmits the tears, which have been absorbed at the great angle of the eye by the puncta lacrymalia, into the nasal fossæ.

LACH'RYMAL CARUNCLE, see Caruncula lacrymalis.

LACHRYMAL FOSSA, *Fossa seu Fo'vea lacryma'lis*, is a slight depression at the upper part of the orbit, which lodges the lachrymal gland.

LACHRYMAL GLAND, *Glan'dula lacryma'lis* seu *innomina'ta Gale'ni*, is seated in a depression of the frontal bone at the upper, anterior, and outer part of that orbit. It is of about the size of an almond; and of an oval shape, flattened above and below:—its great diameter being the anteroposterior. It is composed of several small lobules, united by areolar tissue, and separated by it as well as by vessels and nerves which creep in the intervals. This gland has seven or eight excretory ducts, which open behind the upper eyelid. Its *use* is to secrete the tears, and pour them on the globe of the eye by the excretory ducts.

LACHRYMAL GROOVE, (F.) *Gouttière lacrymale*, is the bony channel, which lodges the lachrymal sac. It is seated at the anterior and inner part of the orbit, and is formed by the os unguis and the ascending process of the upper jaw bone.

LACHRYMAL HERNIA, *Lach·ymal Tumour, Her'nia Sacci Lacryma'lis*, is when the tears enter the puncta, but cannot pass to the nose, and accumulate. By Anel, this was called *Dropsy of the Lachrymal Sac*.

LACHRYMAL NERVE is the smallest of the three branches formed by the ophthalmic nerve. It is distributed, particularly, to the lachrymal gland and to the upper eyelid. In its course it gives off a *spheno-maxillary* and a *malar* filament.

LACHRYMAL PAPILLA, see Lachrymal Puncta.

LACHRYMAL PASSAGES, *Viæ lacryma'les*, (F.) *Voies lacrymales*. The organs concerned in the secretion of tears, in spreading them over the eye, and taking them up again to transmit them into the nasal fossæ. The lachrymal passages are composed of the *lachrymal gland*, *caruncle*, *puncta*, *ducts*, *lachrymal sac*, and *nasal duct*.

LACHRYMAL PUNCTA, *Puncta Lacryma'lia*, *Spiram'ina Palpebra'rum*, (F.) *Points lacrymaux*, are two small, round, and contractile openings, situate in the centre of a tubercle or papilla, *Papilla lacryma'lis*, *Tuber'culum lacryma'lē*, about a line and a half distant from the inner commissure of the eyelids, and continuous with the lachrymal ducts. These ducts, *Lacryma'les Canalic'uli*, *Cana'les* seu *Ductus lacryma'les*, *Ductus lacrymales latera'les*, *D. puncto'rum lacryma'lium*, *Cor''nua lacryma'lia* seu *lima'cum*, *Collic''iæ puncto'rum lacryma'lium*, *Canalic'uli lima'cum*, *Cornua Lima'cum*, (F.) *Conduits lacrymaux*, are two in number — a *superior* and an *inferior* — which extend from the puncta to the lachrymal sac. They seem formed by a very delicate prolongation of the conjunctiva, which is continuous with the mucous membrane of the *lachrymal sac*, (F.) *Reservoir des larmes* : — the *Saccus* seu *Sinus* seu *Lacus lacryma'lis*, *Dacryocys'tis*, *Infundib'ulum lacryma'lē*, *Saccus lacryma'lis*.

LACHRYMAL TUBERCLE, see Lachrymal puncta.

LACHRYMAL VEINS accompany the artery of the same name, and open into the ophthalmic and palpebral veins.

LACHRYMA'TIO, Epiphora. Also, a profuse secretion of tears from any cause : — weeping, *Fletus*, *Plora'tio*, *Plora'tus*.

LACINIÆ TUBARUM FALLOPII, see Tube, Fallopian.

LACIS, Plexus.

LACMUS TINCTORIUS, Lichen roccella.

LACONICUM, Vaporarium, see Stove.

LACQ, Laqueus.

LACRIMA, Tear.

LACRUMA, Tear.

LACRYMA, Tear.

LACTANS, Nurse.

LACTA'TION, *Lacta'tio*, *Thela'sis*, *Thelas'mus*, from *lacteo*, (*lac*, ' milk,) ' I suckle,' ' I give milk.' *Suckling:* — the *giving of suck*, (F.) *Allaitement*. The French make four varieties of lactation. 1. *Allaitement maternel* — Maternal Lactation, when the mother suckles the child. 2. *A. étranger mercenaire*, — when another suckles it. 3. *A. artificiel*, when the child is brought up by hand. 4. *A. animal*, when the child is suckled by an animal.

LACTEALS, Chyliferous vessels.

LACTENS, Sucking child.

LACTES, Mesentery, Pancreas.

LACTEUS, Lactic.

LACTIC, *Lac'teus*, *Galac'ticus*, *Galac'tinus*, *milky*, from *lac*, ' milk.' Appertaining to milk.

LACTIC ACID, *Ac''idum Lac'teum*, *Acid of milk*, *Acidum Lactis*, (F.) *Acide Lactique*. This has been recommended as a therapeutical agent in atonic dyspepsia, owing to its being presumed to be one of the gastric acids secreted in health. It is given either in the form of lemonade or of lozenges. The acid is obtained either from milk or from the juice of the red beet.

LACTICA, Typhoid.

LACTICANS, Nurse.

LACTICINIA, Parotid.

LACTIFÈRE, Lactiferous.

LACTIF'EROUS, *Galactoph'orous*, *Lac'tifer*, (F.) *Lactifère*, from *lac*, ' milk,' and *fero*, ' I carry.' Milk-conveying.

LACTIFEROUS VESSELS, *Lactiferous Ducts*, *Tub'uli lactiferi* vel *Ductus lactiferi* seu *lac'tea*, (F.) *Vaisseaux* ou *conduits lactifères*, are the excretory ducts of the mammary gland.

LACTIFEROUS or LACTEAL SWELLING. A tumefaction of the breast, supposed by Sir Astley Cooper to arise from a large collection of milk in one of the lactiferous tubes, the result of chronic inflammation of the tube near the nipple, with closure of its aperture, and obliteration of the canal for an inch or more. The tube requires to be punctured.

LACTIF'UGA, *Lac'tifuge*, from *lac*, ' milk,' and *fugo*, ' I drive away.' Medicines which dispel milk.

LACTIGO, Porrigo larvalis.

LACTINE, Sugar of milk.

LACTIN'IA, from *lac*, ' milk.' Food prepared with milk.

LACTIPOTOR, Galactopotes.

LACTIS CONCRETIONES, Infarctus Mammæ lacteus.

LACTIS REDUNDANTIA, Galactia — l. Retentio, Galactischesis — l. Sanguinolenti Excretio, Galactohæmia.

LACTISUGIUM, Antlia lactea.

LACTIVORUS, Galactophagous.

LACTOMETER, Galactometer.

LACTU'CA, from *lac*, ' milk;' so called, from its milky juice. *Lactuca Sati'va*, Lettuce, *Garden Lettuce*, *Euns'chium Meco'nis*, *Thridax*, *Cherbas*, (F.) *Laitue ordinaire*, is used as a wholesome salad. The seeds possess a quantity of oil, which, when formed into an emulsion, has been advised in ardor urinæ, &c.

The inspissated juice, *Lactuca'rium*, *Thrid'acē*, resembles, in odour and appearance, that of opium, and is, like it, narcotic, but uncertain. Dose, gr. j to x and more.

LACTUCA ELONGATA, see L. virosa — l. Graveolens, L. virosa — l. Floridana, Mulgedium Floridanum.

LACTUCA SCARI'OLA, *L. Sylves'tris*, *Scariola*, (F.) *Laitue Scariole*, *L. Sauvage*, possesses a stronger degree of bitterness than L. sativa. It has similar virtues with *Z. virosa*.

LACTUCA SYLVESTRIS, L. scariola — l. Villosa, Mulgedium acuminatum.

LACTUCA VIRO'SA, *L. graveolens*, *Strong-scented Lettuce*, (F.) *Laitue vireuse*. The odour of this plant, the leaves of which are used in medicine, is strongly narcotic, and the taste bitter. They are narcotic, diuretic, and aperient; and have been used in dropsies. *Lactu'ca elonga'ta*, *Wild Lettuce* of the United States, has been employed for L. virosa.

LACTUCIMEN, Aphthæ.

LACTUCIMINA, Aphthæ.

LACTUMEN, Porrigo larvalis.

LACTUMINA, Aphthæ.

LACU'NA, *Canalic'ulus*, from *lacus*, ' a lake or deep ditch. A *Fossa* or *Ditch*. A small cavity in a mucous membrane, the parietes of which secrete a viscid humour. It is used synonymously with *crypt*.

LACUNA, Crypta, Fontanella — l. Cerebri, Infundibulum of the brain, Pituitary gland.

LACUNA seu SULCUS seu SUL'CULUS LABII SUPERIORIS, *Amab'ilē*, *Amato'rium*, *Philtrum*, *Phile'trum*. The hollow of the upper lip under the nose.

LACUNA MAGNA, see Urethra.

LACUNÆ, see Urethra.

LACUNÆ OF BONE. Certain dark stellate spots with thread-like lines radiating from them, seen under a high magnifying power. These were at first believed to be solid *osseous* or *bone corpuscles*, *Corpus'cula os'sium* — *Corpuscles of Purkinje;* but are now regarded as excavations in the bone — *Sac'culi chalicoph'ori* — with minute tubes or *canaliculi* proceeding from them, and communicating with the Haversian canals. The lacunæ and canaliculi are fibres concerned in the transit of nutrient fluid through the osseous tissue.

LACUNÆ GRAAFIA'NÆ, L. *muco'sæ vulvæ.* The mucous follicles of the vagina.

LACUNÆ MUCOSÆ VULVÆ, L. Graafianæ—L Palpebrarum, Meibomian, glands of.

LACU'NAR, *La'quear,* 'an arched roof.' The roof of a chamber. Hence,

LACU'NAR OR'BITÆ. The roof of the orbit.

LACUNAR VENTRICULI QUARTI SUPERIOR, Valvula Vieussenii.

LACUNE DE LA LANGUE, Cæcum foramen.

LACUS LACRYMALIS, Lachrymal sac.

LACUS LACRYMA'RUM. A small space in the inner angle of the eye between the lids, towards which the tears flow, and at which the triangular canal formed between the closed lids terminates.

LADA, Piper nigrum.

LADANUM, see Cistus creticus.

LADENDO, Influenza.

LADIES MANTLE, Alchemilla.

LADIES' SLIPPER, SHOWY, Cypripedium spectabile—l. Slipper, stemless, Cypripedium acaule—l. Slipper, yellow, Cypripedium luteum.

LADIES' SMOCK, Cardamine pratensis.

LADRERIE (F.) from *ladre,* 'a leper.' (F.) *Léproserie, Maladrerie.* A vulgar name for elephantiasis, or lepra. Also, an hospital for the reception of the leprous, *Leprosa'rium, Domus leprosa'ria, Leper hospital.*

LADYBIRD, Coccinella septempunctata.

LADYBUG, Coccinella septempunctata.

LADYCOW, Coccinella septempunctata.

LADY CRESPIGNY'S PILLS, see Pilulæ Aloes et Kinæ Kinæ.

LADY HESKETH'S PILLS, see Pilulæ Aloes et Kinæ Kinæ.

LADY WEBSTER'S PILLS, see Pilulæ Aloes et Kinæ Kinæ.

LÆMOPARALYSIS, Œsophagoplegia.

LÆMOS, Pharynx.

LÆMOSCIR'RHUS, *Cancer pharyn'gis et œsoph'agi, Læmosteno'sis* seu *Dyspha'gia scirrho'sa;* from λαιμος, 'the pharynx or œsophagus.' Cancer of the pharynx or œsophagus.

LÆMOSTENOSIS, Dysphagia constricta — l. Scirrhosa, Læmoscirrhus.

LÆSIO, Lesion.

LÆTIFICAN'TIA, from *lætifico (lætus,* and *facio),* 'I make glad.' Medicines formerly used as cordials, in depression of spirits, &c.

LÆVIGATIO, Levigation.

LÆVITAS INTESTINORUM, Lientery.

LAGENTOMUM, Harelip.

LAGNEA, Coition, Satyriasis, Sperm.

LAGNEIA, Coition, Satyriasis, Sperm.

LAGNESIS, Furor Femininus, Nymphomania — l. Furor masculinus, Satyriasis — L. Salacitas, Satyriasis.

LAGNEUMA, Coition, Sperm.

LAGNIA, Satyriasis.

LAGNOSIS, Satyriasis.

LAGOCHEILUS, Harelip.

LAGONES, Flanks.

LAGONOPONOS, Pleurodynia.

LAGONTOMUM, Harelip.

LAGOPHTHAL'MIA, from λαγος, 'a hare,' and οφθαλμος, 'an eye.' *Lagophthal'mus, Hare's Eye; Lepori'nus Oc'ulus,* (F.) *Œil de Lièvre.* A vicious arrangement of the upper eyelid, which is so retracted that it cannot cover the globe of the eye during sleep. It has been asserted that this condition of the eye is natural in the hare when asleep.

LAGOPHTHALMUS, Lagophthalmia, Geum urbanum.

LAGOSTOMA, Harelip.

LAICHE, Sarsaparilla Germanica—*l. des Sables,* Sarsaparilla Germanica.

LAIT, Milk—*l. Adoucissant:,* Looch ex ovo—*l. d'Anesse,* Milk, asses'—*l. d'Amandes,* Emulsio amygdalæ — *l. d'Asafœtida,* Mistura asafœtidæ—*l. de Beurre,* Buttermilk—*l. de Brebis,* Milk, ewes'—*l. Caillé,* Curds—*l. de Chèvre,* Milk, goats'—*l. Épanché, L. répandu*—*l. de Femme,* Milk, human—*l. de Jument,* Milk, mares'—*l. de Poule,* see Ovum.

LAIT RÉPANDU, (F.) *Lait épanché.* A popular expression in France, under which is comprehended every kind of disease (and particularly vague pains) occurring after delivery; all being ascribed to diffusion or deposition of milk.

LAIT DE VACHE, Milk of the cow—*l. Virginal,* Virgin's milk.

LAITERON DOUX, Sonchus oleraceus.

LAITIAT, (F.) Sour whey, in which different wild fruits have been macerated. Said to be much used in the Jura as a refreshing drink.

LAITUE ORDINAIRE, Lettuce—*l. Sauvage,* Lactuca scariola—*l. Scariole,* Lactuca scariola—*l. Vireuse,* Lactuca virosa.

LAKEWEED, Polygonum hydropiper.

LALIA, Voice, articulated.

LALLA'TION, *Lalla'tio, Lambdacis'mus, Labdacis'mus, Lul'laby speech.* Sauvages uses this term for a vicious pronunciation, in which the letter L is improperly doubled, or softened, or substituted for R.

LAMAC, Acaciæ gummi.

LAMBDACISMUS, Lallation.

LAMBDOID, *Lambdoïd'al, Lambo'ïdes, Lambdo'des, Lambdoïdeus,* from the Greek letter Λ, λαμβδα, and ειδος, 'shape,' 'resemblance.' Anatomists have given the name LAMBDOIDAL SUTURE, *Sutu'ra Lambdoïda'lis* seu *lambdoïdes* seu *lambdoïdea, S. Proræ,* to the suture, formed by the parietal bones and the occipital, because it resembles the letter Λ, lambda, of the Greeks. It is the *Occipito-parietal suture*—*Suture occipitale,* (Ch.) In this suture, the ossa Wormiana are most frequently met with; and the denticulations are most distinctly marked.

LAMBEAU, Flap.

LAMBITIVUM, Eclectos.

LAMBKILL, Kalmia latifolia.

LAME, Lamina—*l. Cornée,* Tænia semicircularis—*l. Ruyschienne,* Ruyschiana tunica.

LAMELLA, Lamina.

LAMEL'LAR, *Lamello'sus, Lam'inated,* (F.) *Lamelleux, Lamineux,* composed of thin laminæ or leaves—as the *Lamellar* or *laminated tissue;* i. e. the areolar tissue.

LAMELLEUX, Lamellar.

LAMENESS, Claudication.

LAM'INA, *Lamel'la,* (F.) *Lame.* A thin, flat part of a bone; a plate or table, as the cribriform lamina or plate of the ethmoid bone. *Lamina* and *Lamella* are generally used synonymously; although the latter is properly a diminutive of the former.

LAM'INA CINER'EA. A thin layer of gray substance, which forms the anterior part of the inferior boundary of the third ventricle of the brain.

LAM'INA COR'NEA, *Tæ'nia Tari'ni.* A yellowish band or a thickening of the lining membrane of the ventricle, by which the vena corporis striati is overlaid in the lateral ventricle of the brain.

LAMINA CRIBROSA, Cribriform lamella.

LAMINA CRIBROSA OSSIS ETHMOÏDEI, see *Criblé*—l. Medullaris triangularis cerebri, Lyra.

LAMINA PERITONÆI EXTERNA. The outer lamina or fold of the peritonæum.

LAMINA PRIMA CUTIS, Epidermis.

LAMINA SPIRA'LIS, *Septum scala, Septum cock'leæ auditoria.* A partition between the scalæ of the cochlea. The largest part of this next the modiolus is formed of bone. The remainder, or that part next the opposite side of the scalæ, is composed of a cartilaginous membrane, called, by Valsalva, *Zona* seu *Zo'nula Coch'leæ.* By some anatomists, the lamina is divided into a *Zona os'sea* and *Z. mollis.* By others, it is considered to consist of four laminæ, when examined with a strong glass: a *Zona os'sea,* next to the modiolus — a *Zona coria'cea,* on the outer side of this: a *Zona vesicula'ris* — and a *Zona membrana'cea,* which is, perhaps, the lining membrane of the cochlea. At the apex of the cochlea, the lamina spiralis terminates by a pointed hook-shaped process, *ham'ulus lam'inæ spira'lis.*

LAM'INÆ DORSA'LES, *Dorsal laminæ.* Two oval masses on each side of the primitive groove of the embryo, which approach so as to form a groove, in which are lodged the future brain and spinal marrow.

LAMINÆ SPONGIOSÆ NASI, Turbinated bones.

LAM'INÆ VENTRA'LES, *L. viscera'les.* Thickened prolongations of the serous layer of the germinal membrane, which, by their union, form the anterior wall of the trunk of the new being.

LAMINA'RIA DIGITA'TA, *Tangle.* One of the Algæ eaten in Scotland, and hawked about the streets with the Pepper-dulse.

The leaf of a sea-weed — a species of Laminaria — is employed in the Himalayas under the name of *goître leaf,* so called because chewed by the inhabitants, where goître prevails.

LAMINATED, Lamellar.

LAMINEUX, Lamellar.

LA'MIUM ALBUM, *L. folio'sum, Urti'ca mor'- tua, Galeop'sis* Archangel'ica, *Dead Nettle, White Arch'angel Nettle,* (F.) *Ortie blanche, Ortie morte.* Infusions of this plant have been recommended in uterine hemorrhage, and leucorrhœa. It is not used.

LA'MIUM AMPLEXICAU'LE, *Dead Nettle, Henbit;* naturalized; flowering from May to October; is regarded as tonic, diaphoretic, and laxative.

LAMIUM FOLIOSUM, L. album — l. Montanum, Melittis melissophyllum—l. Plinii, Melittis melissophyllum — l. Rubrum, Galeopsis.

LAMOTTE, MINERAL WATERS OF. These thermal springs are in the department of Isère, France. Temperature, 184°.

LAMPOURDE, Xanthium.

LAMPROPHO'NUS, from λαμπρος, 'clear,' and φωνη, 'voice.' One who has a clear voice.

LAMPSANA, Lapsana.

LAMPYRIS, Cicindela.

LANA PHILOSOPHORUM, Zinci oxydum.

LANARIA, Saponaria, Verbascum nigrum.

LANCE DE MAURICEAU, (F.) An instrument invented by Mauriceau for perforating the head of the fœtus. A perforator.

LANCEOLA, Lancet.

LANCET, *Lance'ola, Lancet'ta, Schaste'rion, Scalpum chirur'gicum,* (F.) *Lancette,* — diminutive of *lancea,* 'a lance.' A surgical instrument, used in the operation of phlebotomy. It is composed of two parts, the handle, (F.) *Chasse,* and the blade, (F.) *Lame.* The former is made of two small plates of ivory, bone, or shell, moveable on the blade for whose preservation they are intended. The blade is formed of well-polished steel. Lancets are made of different shapes; some being *broad-shouldered* — others, *spear-pointed.* The French distinguished three kinds: 1. *Lancette à grain d'orge,* which, on account of the almost oval shape of its point, makes a large opening. 2. The *L. à langue de serpent,* which is very narrow towards the point; and, 3. The *L. à grain d'avoine,* which holds a medium station between the two former, and is generally preferred.

The *Abscess Lancet* is merely a large lancet for the purpose of opening abscesses.

LANCETTA, Lancet.

LANCETTE, Lancet.

LANCETTIER, (F.) A lancet-case.

LANCINANT, Lancinating.

LAN'CINATING, *Lan'cinans,* from *lancinare* (*lancea,* 'a lance'), 'to strike or thrust through.' (F.) *Lancinant,* (substantive *Élancement.*) A species of pain, which consists in lancinations or shootings, similar to those that would be produced by the introduction of a sharp instrument into the suffering part. It is especially in cancer that this kind of pain is felt.

LAND'S END, CLIMATE OF. The climate of the Land's End, in England, resembles that of the south of Devonshire, but is more relaxing. It is considered to be most likely to prove beneficial in consumptive cases, in which the disease is accompanied by an irritated state of the pulmonary mucous membrane, producing a dry cough. Where the system is relaxed, and the secretion from the lungs considerable, the climate, it is conceived, will generally prove injurious. As a brumal retreat, the southern coast of Devonshire would seem to be preferable to it.

LANGEAC, MINERAL WATERS OF. Acidulous, mineral waters at Langeac, in the department of Haute-Loire, France. They are employed as refrigerant, aperient, and diuretic. They contain carbonic acid, carbonates of soda and magnesia, and a little iron.

LAN'GII AQUA EPILEP'TICA, *Epilep'tic Water of Langius,* formerly employed against epilepsy. It was composed of the flowers of *convallaria* and *lavender, Spanish wine, cinnamon, nutmeg, mistletoe, peony* and *dittany roots, long pepper, cubebs,* and *rosemary flowers.*

LANGUE, Tongue — *l. Abaisseur de la,* Glossocatochus — *l. de Carpe,* see Lever — *l. de Cerf,* Asplenium scolopendrium — *l. de Chien,* Cynoglossum— *l. de Serpent,* Ophioglossum vulgatum.

LANGUEUR, Languor.

LANGUOR, *Aph'esis, Faintness,* (F.) *Langueur.* A species of atony, depression, or debility, which generally comes on slowly.

LANTA'NA, *Sage Tree, Blueberry,* (F.) *Cailleau.* The leaves of this indigenous plant form a fine-scented tea, like *L. Camara* or *Bahama Tea,* and *L. Pseudothe'a* or *Brazil Tea.* The tea is used as a diaphoretic.

LANU'GO, *Pili cutis, Pluma,* from *lana,* 'wool.' The soft, fine hair on different parts of the body, especially of the young.

LANUGO PRIMA, Geneias — l. Pudendorum, Pubes—l. Siliquæ hirsutæ, see Dolichos pruriens.

LANUVIUM, Vulva.

LAONI'CA CURA'TIO seu CURA. A mode of treating the gout, which consisted in the employment of local applications, proper for evacuating the morbific matter.(?)

LAOS, Tin.

LAPACTICUS, Cathartic, Laxative.

LAPARA, Abdomen, Flanks, Lumbi.

LAPAROCE'LE, from λαπαρα, 'the lumbar region,' and κηλη, 'rupture.' *Lumbar Hernia,* through a separation of the fibres of the quadratus lumborum, and a protrusion of the aponeurosis of the transverse muscle on the outside of the mass common to the sacro-lumbalis and longissimus dorsi. — Cloquet.

LAPAROCYSTOTOMIA, see Lithotomy.

LAPARO-ELYTROTOMIA, Cæsarean Section.

LAPARO-ENTEROT'OMY, *Lap'aro-entero-*

tom'ia, from λαπαρα, 'the lumbar region,' the 'abdomen,' εντερον, 'intestine,' and τομη, 'incision.' The operation of opening the abdomen and intestinal canal, for the removal of disease.

LAPAROSCOPIA, Abdominoscopia.

LAPAROTOMY, see Gastrotomy.

LAPATHOS, Rumex acutus — l. Aquaticum, Rumex hydrolapathum — l. Chinense, Rheum — l. Orientale, Rheum — l. Sanguineum, Rumex sanguineus — l. Unctuosum, Chenopodium bonus Henricus.

LAPATHUM, Rumex acutus—l. Acutum, Rumex acutus — l. Hortense, Rumex patientia — l. Pratense, Rumex acetosa — l. Scutatum, Rumex scutatus — l. Sylvestre, Rumex acutus, R. obtusifolius.

LAPE, Mucus.

LAPIDIL'LUM, from *lapis*, 'a stone.' Blasius has given this name to a kind of scoop, used for extracting stone from the bladder.

LAPILLATIO, Lithia.

LAPILLI GLANDULÆ PINEALIS, see Pineal gland.

LAPIL'LUS, diminutive of *lapis*, 'a stone.' A small stone; gravel; a grain of sand.

LAPIS, Calculus — l. Accipitrum, Hieracites — l. Aerosus, Calamina — l. Ammoniaci, see Ammoniac gum — l. Animalis, Blood — l. Armenius, Melochites — l. Aureus, Urine — l. Bezoardicus, Bezoar — l. Cæruleus, Cupri sulphas — l. Calaminaris, Calamina — l. Carneolus, Cornelian — l. Causticus, Potassa cum calce, Potassa fusa — l. Collymus, Ætites — l. Contrayervæ, Pulvis contrayervæ compositus — l. Cyanus, L. lazuli.

LAPIS DIVI'NUS, *L. Ophthal'micus* seu *Ophthal'micus Sti. Ivesii*. (*Cupri sulphat., Alumin., Potass. nitrat.* āā ℥j. Melt together, adding at the end *Camphor*, ℨjs.) Employed to make an eyewater, ℨij ad *aquæ* ℨiv.

LAPIS FULMINEUS, Ceraunion — l. Hematites, Hæmatites—l. Heracleus, Magnet—l. Infernalis, Argenti nitras — l. Infernalis alkalinus, Potassa fusa — l. Infernalis sive septicus, Potassa cum calce—l. Judaicus, Judæus (lapis).

LAPIS LAZU'LI, *Lapis Cy'anus, Asulci, Las'ulite*, (F.) *Pierre d'azur, Outremer*. A stone, of a beautiful blue colour; opake; and close-grained; fracture, dull. It is composed of silex; alumine; carbonate and sulphate of lime; oxide of iron, and water. It was formerly looked upon as a purgative and emetic, and given in epilepsy.

LAPIS MALUCENSIS, Bezoard of the Indian porcupine — l. Nauticus, Magnet — l. Ophthalmicus, L. Divinus — l. Ophthalmicus St. Ivesii, L. Divinus — l. Phœnicites, Judæus (lapis) — l. Porcinus, Bezoard of the Indian porcupine — l. Prunellæ, Potassæ nitras fusus sulphatis paucillo mixtus — l. Sardius, Cornelian — l. Septicus, Causticum commune, Potassa fusa — l. Specularis, S. lucidum — l. Syderitis, Magnet — l. Syriacus, Judæus (lapis) — l. Vini, Potassæ supertartras impurus.

LAPPA, Arctium lappa, Galium aparine, Lippitudo — l. Minor, Xanthium.

LAPPULA HEPATICA, Agrimony.

LAP'SANA, *Lampsa'na, Na'pium, Papilla'ris herba, Dock-cresses, Nipple-Wort*, (F.) *Lampsane, Herbe aux Mamelles*. This plant is a lactescent bitter. It has been chiefly employed, however, as an external application to sore nipples, &c.

LAPSUS PILORUM, Alopecia.

LAQ, Laqueus.

LAQUE, Lacca.

LAQUEAR, Lacunar.

LA'QUEAR VAGI'NÆ, *Fundus Vaginæ*. The part of the vagina in which the cervix uteri terminates.

LA'QUEUS, *Funis*. A cord, ligature or bandage, with running knots;—a *Noose*, a *loop*. A *fillet, Brochos, Pach'etos*, (F.) *Lag* ou `*Lacq*. The term is applied to a bandage or fillet of any kind, attached by means of a loop upon any part, with the view of fixing it; as in certain cases of labour, where a hand or foot presents; or to facilitate extension in luxations and fractures.

Also:—A prominent band in the brain, behind the brachium posterius of the corpora quadrigemina, which marks the course of the superior division of the fasciculus olivaris.

LAQUEUS GUT'TURIS, 'Noose of the throat.' Violent inflammation of the tonsils, in which the patient appears as if suffocated by a noose. According to some, gangrenous cynanche.

LARCH, Pinus larix.

LARD, Adeps.

LARDACÉ, Lardaceous.

LARDA'CEOUS, *Larda'ceus, Lar'deus, Lard'iform, Lardifor'mis*, (F.) *Lardacé;* from *lardum*, 'lard,' the fat of bacon. An epithet given to certain organic alterations in the textures, whose aspect and consistence resemble lard. (F.) *Tissu lardacée*.

LARDEUS, Lardaceous.

LARDIFORM, Lardaceous.

LARGE, Broad.

LARIX, Pinus larix — l. Communis, Pinus larix—l. Decidua, Pinus larix — l. Europæa, Pinus larix—l. Pyramidalis, Pinus larix.

LARKSPUR, BRANCHING, Delphinium consolida.

LARME, Tear.

LARMOIEMENT, Epiphora.

LA-ROCHE POSAY, MINERAL WATERS OF. Simple sulphurous waters in the department of Vienne, France.

LARVA, Mask. Also the *larve, grub*, or vermiform condition of an insect: the first change it experiences after leaving the ovum. Larves of insects are occasionally developed in the intestinal canal from ova swallowed. See Ectozoa.

LARYNGÉ, Laryngeal.

LARYNGE'AL, *Larynge'us*, (F.) *Laryngé, Laryngien*. Same etymon as LARYNX. That which belongs to the larynx.

LARYNGEAL ARTERIES are given off from the thyroid arteries.

LARYNGEAL NERVES, (F.) *Nerfs Laryngés*, are two in number;—a *superior* and an *inferior*. The *superior laryngeal nerve* is given off from the trunk of the pneumogastric, at the upper and deep part of the neck. It passes downwards and inwards, behind the internal carotid artery, and divides into two secondary branches; the one, *external*, which distributes its filaments, on the outside of the larynx, to the sterno-thyroid, hyo-thyroid, constrictor inferior, crico-thyroid muscles, &c. The other, the *internal*, which crosses the thyro-hyoid membrane, and gives filaments to the epiglottis, the mucous membranes of the pharynx and larynx, to the arytenoid gland, the arytenoid and crico-thyroid muscles, and ultimately anastomoses with the inferior laryngeal nerve. The *inferior laryngeal nerves* or *recur'rents, Nervi reversi'vi, Rameaux Trachéaux* (Chaus.,) arise from the trunk of the pneumogastric within the thorax. They ascend in the furrow, which separates the trachea from the œsophagus, to be distributed on the neck, after having been reflected;—the left around the arch of the aorta; the right, around the corresponding subclavian. They send off filaments to the cardiac plexuses; to the parietes of the œsophagus, and trachea; to the thyroid gland: to the inferior constrictor of the pharynx; the posterior and lateral crico-arytenoid and thyro-arytenoid muscles; and to the mucous membrane of the pharynx and larynx.

LARYNGEAL PHTHISIS, Phthisis, laryngeal — l. Sound, Laryngeche.

LARYNGEAL VEINS open into the internal jugular. Winslow gives the name *laryngeal* to the *superior thyroid artery*.

LARYNGEAL VOICE, see Voice.

LARYNGE'CHE, from λαρυγξ, 'the larynx,' and ηχη or ηχος, 'sound.' The *laryngeal sound* heard by the stethoscope during breathing and speaking.

LARYNGIEN, Laryngeal.

LARYNGISMUS STRIDULUS, Asthma thymicum.

LARYNGITE, Laryngitis—*l. Muqueuse*, Laryngitis (simple)—*l. Œdémateuse*, Œdema of the glottis—*l. Œdémateuse et séro-purulente*, Œdema of the glottis—*l. avec Production de Fausses membranes*, Cynanche trachealis—*l. Pseudo-membraneuse*, Cynanche trachealis—*l. avec Sécrétion de Pus*, Phthisis laryngea—*l. Sus-glottique*, Œdema of the glottis—*l. Striduleuse*, Asthma thymicum—*l. Sous-muqueuse*, Œdema of the glottis.

LARYNGI'TIS, from *Larynx*, and *itis*, a suffix denoting inflammation; *Inflamma'tio Laryn'gis, Cynanchè laryngë'a, Angi'na laryngea*, (F.) *Laryngite, Catarrhe laryngien, Angine laryngé, Inflammation of the Larynx*. This disease, in some measure, resembles croup; but is usually devoid of that peculiar sonorous inspiration, which attends the latter. There is, also, pain upon pressing the larynx; and, whilst laryngitis is a disease of more advanced life, croup attacks children. The membraniform exudation is, also, absent; probably, because the inflammation, being seated above the glottis, the coagulable lymph is readily expectorated. It requires the most active treatment.

Simple Laryngitis is called by some *mucous Laryngitis, Laryngitis acu'ta, L. muco'sa acuta*, (F.) *Laryngite muqueuse*, to distinguish it from *submucous Laryngitis* or Œdema of the glottis.

Chronic Laryngitis is generally regarded as synonymous with laryngeal phthisis; but it may exist independently.

LARYNGITIS ACUTA, Laryngitis — l. Chronic, see Phthisis Laryngea—l. Mucosa acuta, Laryngitis — l. Mucous, Laryngitis (simple) — l. Œdematous, Œdema of the glottis—l. Seropurulenta, Œdema of the glottis — l. Submucous, Œdema of the glottis—l. et Tracheitis chronica, see Phthisis laryngea — l. et Tracheitis infantilis, Cynanche trachealis.

LARYNGOCACE, Cynanche trachealis.

LARYNGO-CATAR'RHUS, *Catarrhus Laryngeus et trachea'lis*. Catarrh affecting the larynx and trachea more especially, as indicated by alteration of the voice — hoarseness — itching and sensation of burning in those parts; short cough and expectoration, &c.

LARYNGO-ET-TRACHEO-PHTHISIS, Phthisis laryngea.

LARYNGOG'RAPHY, *Laryngogra'phia*; from λαρυγξ, 'the larynx,' and γραφη, 'a description.' An anatomical description of the larynx.

LARYNGOL'OGY, from λαρυγξ, 'the larynx,' and λογος, 'treatise.' A treatise on the larynx.

LARYNGOPARALYSIS, see Aphonia.

LARYNGOPH'ONY, *Tracheoph'ony, Laryngë'al voice, Tracheal voice;* from *Larynx*, and φωνη, 'voice.' The sound heard in health, when the stethoscope is placed over the larynx or trachea, at the time a person speaks. The voice appears to pass immediately up to the ear of the auscultator. A similar physical sign exists when there is a cavity in the lungs, and the instrument is placed over it whilst the patient speaks. See Pectoriloquy.

LARYNGOPHTHISIS, Phthisis laryngea.
LARYNGOSPASMUS, Asthma thymicum.
LARYNGOSTASIS, Cynanche trachealis.
LARYNGOSTENO'SIS; from λαρυγξ, 'the larynx,' and στενωσις, 'contraction.' Contraction or narrowness of the larynx.

LARYNGOT'OMY, *Laryngotom'ia*, from λαρυγξ, 'the larynx,' and τεμνειν, 'to cut.' A surgical operation, which consists in opening the larynx, either to extract a foreign body, or to remedy an obstruction of the glottis. The operation is, sometimes, erroneously called *Bronchotomy*, and *Tracheotomy*.

LARYNGO-TRACHEITIS, Cynanche trachealis — l. Tracheitis with Diphtheritic exudation, Cynanche trachealis.

LAR'YNX, λαρυγξ, ('a whistle.') *Caput seu Oper'culum seu Init"ium seu Finis supe'rior seu Ter'minus superior seu Pars prima as'peræ arte'riæ*. The apparatus of voice is situate at the superior and anterior part of the neck; and at the top of the trachea, with which it communicates. It is composed of four cartilages, — the thyroid, cricoid, and two arytenoid; is moved by a number of muscles, and lined by a mucous membrane, having certain membranous reflections, constituting the *superior ligaments of the glottis*, &c.

PARTS COMPOSING THE LARYNX.

1. *Cartilages*		Thyroid.
		Cricoid.
		Two arytenoid.
		Epiglottis.
2. *Muscles*.	Extrinsic,	Sterno-thyroid.
		Constrictors of the pharynx.
		All the muscles of the hyoid region.
	Intrinsic,	Crico-thyroid.
		Crico-arytenoid, posterior.
		Cryco-arytenoid, lateral.
		Thyro-arytenoid.
		Arytenoid.
3. *Mucous Membrane*.		
4. *Glands*		Epiglottic.
		Arytenoid.
		Thyroid.
5. *Membranes*		Thyro-hyoid.
		Crico-thyroid.
6. *Ligaments*		Crico-arytenoid.
		Thyro-arytenoid.

The vessels and nerves of the larynx are called *Laryngeal*.

The larynx is destined to give passage to the air, in the act of respiration, and to impress upon it certain modifications, which constitute voice. Its dimensions vary in different individuals. In men, it is always larger, and situate lower, than in women.

LARYNX, PELLICULAR or PLASTIC INFLAMMATION OF THE, Cynanche trachealis.

LAS'ANUM, *Sella familiar'ica*, (F.) *Chaise percée*. A close stool.

LASCIVIA, Satyriasis.
LASCIVITAS, Satyriasis.
LASCIVUS, Libidinous.

LASER, Laserpitium — *l. à Larges feuilles*, Laserpitium latifolium.

LASERPIT″IUM, *Laser, Sil′phium, σπες σιλ-φιον.* A term applied, anciently, both to a plant and its juice, regarding the nature of neither of which we possess any precise information. Bentley, Laurence, Geoffroi, &c., regard it to have been the same as asafœtida:—Theophrastus, Dioscorides, and the ancient scholiast of Aristophanes, however, by assigning a sweet and agreeable flavour to the laserpitium, discountenance the idea. From whatever plant obtained, it was so rare, and consequently so costly, that the Romans deposited it in the public treasury. It was obtained from Cyrene—*Succus Cyrena′icus*—and likewise from Persia—the latter being the most valuable. The Laserpitium is called by Avicenna, *Altihit.*

LASERPITIUM ASPERUM, L. latifolium.

LASERPITIUM LATIFO′LIUM, *L. as′perum, Gentia′na alba, White Gentian, Cerva′ria alba;* (F.) *Laser à larges feuilles.* The root of this plant is bitter and tonic.

LASERPITIUM MONTANUM, L. siler.

LASERPITIUM SILER, *L. trifolia′tum* seu *monta′num, Ses′eli, Siler monta′num* seu *lancifo′lium, Heart-wort, Sermountain.* The seeds and roots are possessed of aromatic properties.

LASERPITIUM TRIFOLIATUM, L. siler.

LASSITUDE OCULAIRE, Copyopia.

LASSITUDO, Copos.

LATENS IN ORE, Pterygoideus internus.

LATENT, *Latens,* from *latere,* 'to lie hid.' 'Lying hid,' 'concealed.' An epithet applied to certain diseases or states of disease, in which the symptoms are so concealed and obscure, *morbi occul′ti,* as to escape the observation of the physician. Thus, we say *latent inflammation, latent period of small-pox.*

LAT′ERAD, from *latus, lateris,* 'the side.' A term used adverbially by Dr. Barclay to signify 'towards the lateral aspect.'

LATERAL ASPECT, see Mesial.

LATERIT″IOUS, *Laterit″ius, Lateric″ius,* from *later,* 'a brick.' An epithet applied to the brick-like sediment, occasionally deposited in the urine of people afflicted with fever; *Sedimen′tum uri′næ lateric″ium.*

LATESCENTIS CHORDÆ (Musculus), Palmaris longus.

LATEX NIVEUS, Milk.

LATHYRIS, Euphorbia lathyris.

LATIB′ULUM, from *lateo,* 'I lie hid.' The *foyer* of a febrile poison; whence it spreads to every part to induce a paroxysm. See *Clapier.*

LAT′ICA. Same etymon. *Amphimer′ina lat′ica* of Sauvages. A species of quotidian remittent, whose paroxysms are very long, and which is accompanied with *latent* heat (?), whence its name.

LATICES LACTEI, Receptaculum chyli.

LATIS′SIMUS COLLI, Platysma myoides.

LATIS′SIMUS DORSI, *Aniscalp′tor, Brachium movens quartus,* (F.) *Lombo-huméral* (Ch.), *Dorsi-lombo-sacro-huméral, Muscle grand dorsal, M. très large du dos.* A flat muscle; broad, especially below; thin; quadrilateral; and situate at the posterior, lateral, and inferior region of the trunk. It is attached to the posterior half of the outer lip of the crest of the ilium; to the posterior surface of the sacrum; to the spinous processes of the six or seven last dorsal vertebræ, to all those of the loins, and to the last four false ribs, and is inserted by a strong tendon at the posterior edge of the bicipital groove of the humerus. Its upper fibres are almost horizontal; the middle very long and oblique upwards and outwards; and the anterior almost vertical. This muscle carries the arm backwards, depressing it, and making it turn on its axis. It also draws backwards and downwards the prominence of the shoulder. When, suspended by an arm, we make an effort to raise ourselves, it draws the trunk towards the arm. It can, also, raise the ribs by assuming its fixed point on the humerus, and become an inspiratory muscle.

LATITUDO HUMERI, Scapula.

LATTICE WORK, Cancelli.

LATUS, Broad—l. Ani, Levator ani.

LAU, see Spirit.

LAUCA′NIA, *Leuca′nia, Lau′chanĕ,* from λαυω, 'I enjoy,' 'I take.' The fauces and œsophagus. Also, the chin.—Gorræus.

LAUCHANE, Laucania.

LAUD′ANUM or LAUDA′NUM. Perhaps, from *laus,* 'praise;' *lauda′tum,* 'praised.' Every preparation of opium, solid or liquid, but more particularly the extract and tincture, and especially the latter.

LAUDANUM ABBA′TIS ROUSSEAU, *Guttæ Abbatis Rousseau, Vinum opia′tum fermentatio′nĕ para′tum, Abbé Rousseau′s Drops.* (*Mel. Narbonnens.,* ℥xij; *aquæ calidæ,* Oiij. Set in a warm place, and, as soon as the mixture ferments, add *opium,* ℥iv, dissolved in *water,* f℥xij. Let it ferment for a month, and evaporate to f℥x: strain, and add *rectified spirit of wine,* ℥ivss.

LAUDANUM, FORD's, Vinum opii — l. Liquid, Tinctura opii — l. Liquidum Hoffmanni, Vinum opii — l. Liquidum Sydenhami, Vinum opii — l. Opiatum, Extractum opii — l. Simplex, Extractum opii.

LAUGH, Risus — l. Sardonic, Canine laugh.

LAUGHING, Risus.

LAUGHTER, Risus.

LAUREL, Kalmia latifolia, Magnolia macrophylla — l. Broad-leaved, Kalmia latifolia — l. Cherry, Prunus lauro-cerasus — l. Common, Prunus lauro-cerasus — l. Dwarf, Kalmia angustifolia — l. Great, Rhododendron maximum — l. Ground, Epigæa repens — l. Mountain, Kalmia latifolia, Rhododendron — l. Narrow-leaved, Kalmia angustifolia — l. Poison, Prunus lauro-cerasus — l. Rose, Kalmia latifolia — l. Sheep, Kalmia angustifolia — l. Swamp, Kalmia glauca — l. Sweet, Illicium Floridanum — l. Water, see Prunus lauro-cerasus — l. White, Magnolia glauca.

LAURENT, SAINT, MINERAL WATERS OF. A thermal spring, five leagues from Joyeuse in France. Temp. 127° Fahr.

LAUREN′TIA PINNATIF′IDA, *Pepper-dulse.* One of the Algæ, eaten in Scotland, and hawked about the streets of Edinburgh along with *Lamina′ria digita′ta* or Tangle.

LAUREOLA, Daphne laureola.

LAURIER, Laurus — *l. Alexandrin,* Ruscus hypoglossum — *l. Amandier,* Prunus lauro-cerasus — *l. Cérise,* Prunus lauro-cerasus — *l. Rose,* Nerium oleander.

LAURO-CERASUS, Prunus lauro-cerasus.

LAURUS, *Laurus nob′ilis, Daph′nĕ, Sweet Bay. Nat. Ord.* Laurineæ. (F.) *Laurier.* The leaves and berries have a sweet, fragrant smell, and an aromatic, astringent taste. Sweet bay has been advised as a stomachic and carminative, but is now rarely used. It is, sometimes, employed as a fomentation and in glysters; and the berries are an ingredient in the *Emplastrum Cumini.*

LAURUS ÆSTIVALIS, L. benzoin — l. Alexandrina angustifolia, Ruscus hypoglossum — l. Camphora, see Camphor.

LAURUS BEN′ZOIN, *Benzoin odorif′erum, Laurus Pseudo-benzoin* seu *æstiva′lis, Spice wood, Spice bush, Allspice bush, Wild allspice, Spice berry, Fever wood, Fever bush.* An indigenous shrub, growing in moist, shady places in all parts of the United States; flowering early in spring. All parts of the shrub have a spicy, agreeable flavour, which is strongest in the bark and berries. An infusion or decoction of the small branches is used in popular practice as a vermifuge, and agreeable drink in low fevers. The bark has been used in intermittents; the berries, dried and powdered, for allspice. The oil of the berries is used as an excitant.

LAURUS CANELLA, L. Cassia.

LAURUS CAS'SIA, *L. canel'la, Per'sea cassia*. The species of laurus which yields the *Cassia lig'nea, Cassia, Cassia cinnamo'mea, Cortex Canel'læ Malabar'icæ, Cassia lignea Malabar'ica, Xylo-cassia, Canel'la Malabarica et Javen'sis, Canella Cuba'na, Arbor Juda'ica, Cassia Canel'la, Canellif'era Malabar'ica, Cortex cras'sior, Cinnamo'mum Malabar'icum seu In'dicum seu Sinen'se, Calihac'ha canel'la,* Wild Cinnamon, *Malabar Cinnamon, Cassia,* (F.) *Cannelle de Malabar ou de Java ou de la Chine ou des Indes ou de Coromandel, C. fausse, C. matte, Casse en bois, Casse aromatique*. The bark and leaves abound with the flavour of cinnamon, for which they may be substituted; but they are much weaker. The unopened flower-buds are used in the same manner.

LAURUS CINNAMO'MUM, *Per'sea cinnamo'mum, Cinnamo'mum, C. Zeylan'icum, Darse'ni, Darsi'ni, Cinnamon, Xylo-cinnamomum, Cuurdo Canel'la,* (F.) *Cannelle, Baume de Cannelle, Cannelle officinale.* Cinnamon bark, which is obtained, also, from the *Cinnamo'mum aromat'icum,* is stimulant and carminative, and is employed, chiefly, as a grateful aromatic, to cover the taste of nauseous remedies. Dose, gr. x to ℨj. The *Flowers,* called *Cassiæ Flores* in the shops, possess aromatic and astringent virtues, and may be used wherever cinnamon is required. The volatile oil of the bark — *O'leum Cinnamo'mi* — *Oil of Cinnamon,* is officinal in the Pharm. U. S.

LAURUS CUBEBA, Piper cubeba — l. Cullaban, L. Culilawan.

LAURUS CULIL'AWAN, *L. Culil'aban seu Caryophyl'lus, Cinnamo'mum Culilawan.* The tree that affords the *Cortex Culilawan seu Culilaban, Culilawan, Culitlawan, Cortex caryophylloïdes, C. Caryophylloïdes Amboinen'sis.* This bark resembles the sassafras in appearance and properties, and is used in Java as a condiment.

LAURUS MALABATHRUM, see Malabathrum — l. Nobilis, Laurus — l. Pseudobenzoin, L. Benzoin.

LAURUS SAS'SAFRAS, *Per'sea sas'safras, Sassafras, Cornus mas odora'ta, Anhuiba, Ague-free.* Indigenous in the United States. Sassafras wood and root, and especially the bark of the root, *Sassafras Radi'cis Cortex* (Ph. U. S.), have been considered stimulant, sudorific, and diuretic. The virtues depend upon essential oil, *Oleum Sassafras,* the odour of which is not unlike that of fennel. It has been used in cutaneous diseases, chronic rheumatism, &c.

The pith of the stems, *Sassafras medul'la,* abounds in gummy matter, which it readily imparts to water, forming a limpid mucilage, which is much employed as a collyrium in ophthalmia, and as a drink in dysentery, catarrh, &c. (one dram of the pith to a pint of boiling water).

LAUTIS'SIMA VINA. (*Lautus,* 'elegant.') Wines were formerly so called, which were strongly impregnated with myrrh.

LAVAMENTUM, Clyster, Enema.

LAVANDE, Lavendula.

LAVANDULA, Lavendula.

LAVEMENT, Clyster, Enema — *l. Antispasmodique,* Enema fœtidum.

LAVENDER, COMMON, Lavendula — l. Sea, Statice limonium, Statice Caroliniana.

LAVEN'DULA, from *lavo,* 'I wash;' so called from being used in baths. *Laven'dula spica seu latifo'lia,* Spica, *L. vera, Lavan'dula* (Ph. U. S.), Common Lavender, (F.) *Lavande, Aspic, Spic.* The odour of lavender flowers is fragrant and agreeable; taste warm and bitterish — depending upon an essential oil. It has been used as a stimulant; particularly in the form of the oil, — *O'leum laven'dulæ.* The dried leaves have been employed as an errhine.

The French use the LAVENDULA STŒCHAS, *Stœchas et Stichas Arab'ica, French Lavender,* of which they have a compound syrup, *Syru'pus de stœ'chadē compos'itus:* given as a pectoral.

LAVENDULA LATIFOLIA, Lavendula.

LAVER GERMANICUM, Veronica beccabunga — l. Odoratum, Sisymbrium nasturtium.

LAVIPEDIUM, Pediluvium.

LAW MEDICINE, Medicine, legal.

LAWSONIA ALBA, L. Inermis.

LAWSO'NIA INER'MIS, *L. alba, Alcan'a vera, A. Orienta'lis, Cyperus antiquo'rum, Ligus'trum Ægyptiacum,* Smooth *Lawso'nia,* (F.) *Henné.* An East Indian and African plant, the root of which is slightly astringent.

In India, the root of the *Lawso'nia spinosa* is employed in lepra and other cutaneous affections.

LAX, Diarrhœa.

LAXANS, Laxative, Relaxant.

LAX'ATIVE, *Laxati'vus, Laxans, Le'niens,* from *laxare,* 'to loosen;' *Minorati'vus, Soluti'vus, Alvid'ucus, Hypecchoret'icus, Hypago'gus, Hypel'atus, Hypocathar'ticus, Lapac'ticus.* A medicine which gently opens the bowels; such as tamarinds, manna, &c.

LAXATIVUS INDICUS, Cambogia.

LAXATOR AURIS INTERNUS, L. tympani.

LAXATOR TYMPANI, *L. major tym'pani, Exter'nus mallei, Ante'rior mallei, Obli'quus auris, Externus auris* vel *Laxator inter'nus, Eusta'chii mus'culus,* (F.) *Antérieur du marteau, Sphéni-salpingo-mallien.* A muscle which arises from the spine of the sphenoid bone and from the cartilage of the Eustachian tube, and is inserted, by a tendon, into the apophysis of Rau. It relaxes the membrana tympani.

LAXA'TOR TYM'PANI MINOR. A very small muscle which extends from the upper part of the external auditory canal, and is inserted at the inferior part of the process of the handle of the malleus. Its existence is denied by most anatomists.

LAXITAS, Atony — l. Alvi, Diarrhœa — l. Ingestorum, Lientery — l. Intestinorum, Lientery — l. Scroti, Rhacosis — l. Ventriculi, Gasterasthenia.

LAX'ITY, *Lax'itas, Laxness.* Condition of a tissue, when loose or relaxed; or of one which wants tone. We say *laxity of fibre, laxity of skin,* to express, that those parts have lost some of the tenseness proper to them.

LAYER, ANIMAL, see *Tache embryonnaire* — l. Mucous, see *Tache embryonnaire* — l. Serous, see *Tache embryonnaire* — l. Vascular, see *Tache embryonnaire* — l. Vegetative, see *Tache embryonnaire.*

LAYERS OF THE BLASTODERMA, see *Tache embryonnaire.*

LAZARET'TO, *Lazaret, Lazar-house,* from (I.) *lazzero,* 'a leper.' A solitary edifice in most seaports of magnitude, intended for the disinfection of men and goods proceeding from places where contagious diseases are prevailing.

LAZULITE, Lapis lazuli.

LEAD, Plumbum — l. Black, Graphites — l. Chloride of, Plumbi chloridum — l. Colic, see Colica metallica — l. Iodide of, Plumbi iodidum — l. Nitrate of, Plumbi nitras — l. Oxyd of, semi-vitrified, Plumbi oxydum semivitreum — l. Paralysis, see Palsy, lead — L. Red, Plumbi oxidum rubrum.

LEAD RHEU'MATISM, *Lead Neural'gia, Arthral'gia* of M. Tanquerel. The neuralgic and spasmodic pains caused by the poison of lead.

LEAD, SUBCARBONATE OF, Plumbi superacetas — l. Tannate of, see Tannin — l. White, Plumbi subcarbonas.

LEAD-POISONING, *Molybdo'sis, Morbus plumbeus, Cacochym'ia plumbea,* (F.) *Intoxication saturnine.* Morbid phenomena induced by lead received into the system.

LEADWORT, Plumbago Europæa.

LEAF, SOUR, Andromeda arborea.

LEAMINGTON, MINERAL WATERS OF. Saline waters at Leamington, about two miles east of Warwick, England, which contain chloride of sodium, sulphate of soda, and chlorides of calcium and magnesium.

LEANNESS, Emaciation.

LEAP, Sax. hlæpan, *Sultus, Salit"io, Exalsis,* (F.) *Saut;* Bound, Jump, — the act of leaping. Muscular movement or movements, by which the body is detached from the soil by the forcible and sudden extension of the lower limbs, previously flexed upon the pelvis.

LEAPING AGUE. This disease is said by the Scotch writers to be characterized by increased efficiency, but depraved direction, of the will, producing an irresistible propensity to dance, tumble, and move about in a fantastic manner, and often with far more than the natural vigour, activity, and precision! See Mania, dancing.

LEATHER FLOWER, Clematis viorna — l. Wood, Dirca palustris.

LEB'ANON, MINERAL WATERS OF. The spring at Lebanon, 26 miles east of Albany, New York, is an almost pure thermal. Temp. 72° Fahr.

LECHENEION, Torcular Herophili.

LECHO, Puerpera.

LECHOPYRA, Puerperal fever.

LE CRAN, Cochlearia armoracia.

LECONTIA, Peltandra Virginica.

LECTISTER'NIUM, from *lectus,* 'a bed,' and *sternere,* 'to spread.' The arrangement of a bed so as to adapt it to a particular disease. Also, a supplication, with the Romans, in times of public danger, when beds or couches were spread for the gods, as if they were about to feast, and their images were taken down from their pedestals and placed upon these couches around the altars. The lectisternium was first introduced in the time of a pestilence. — Livy.

LECTUA'LIS, from *lectus,* 'a bed.' An epithet applied to a protracted disease.

LÈDE SAUVAGE, Ledum sylvestre.

LECTULUS STRAMINEUS, *Fanon.*

LEDOYEN'S DISINFECTING LIQUID. A solution of nitrate of lead, (*Plumb. nitrat.* ℥j ad *aquæ* f ℥j,) used as an antiseptic and antibromic.

LE DUM LATIFO'LIUM, *Labrador' Tea,* grows in damp places, in Canada and the United States. The leaves have a pleasant odour and taste, and have been used as tea. They have also been esteemed pectoral and tonic.

LEDUM PALUS'TRE, *Rosmari'nus sylves'tris, Anthos sylves'tris, Marsh Tea,* (F.) *Lède* ou *Romarin sauvage. Nat. Ord.* Ericineæ. *Sex. Syst.* Decandria Monogynia. This plant has a bitter, subastringent taste, and was formerly used in Switzerland in place of hops: the virtues are equivocal.

LEE, Feculence, Lixivium, Ley, Lye.

LEECH, Hirudo, see Ectozoa.

LEEK, Allium porrum.

LEES, SOAP, Liquor potassæ.

LEG, (Danish,) *Orus, Scelos, Cnemâ.* The portion of the lower extremity, which extends from the knee to the foot. It consists of three bones; *Tibia, Fibula,* and *Patella,* and also of a great number of muscles, vessels, and nerves. The projection, formed by the muscles at the back part of the leg, has received the name of *Calf of the leg.* It is the special attribute of man, and proves that he is destined to be biped.

LEG, SWELLED, Phlegmatia dolens — l. Cochin, see Elephantiasis.

LEGIT'IMATE, *Legit'imus,* from *lex, legis,* 'law;' *Genui'nus, Gne'sios.* An epithet applied to things which are according to rule. A *legitimate child,* (F.) *Enfant légitime,* is one conceived or born during marriage. *Legitimate diseases,* (F.) *Maladies légitimes,* are those which follow a regular march.

LEGNA, from λεγνον, 'a fringed edge.' The orifice of the pudendum muliebre, or of the uterus.

LÉGUME, Legumen.

LEGU'MEN, from *lego,* 'I gather:' (F.) *Légume, Gousse.* So called because it is usually gathered by the hand, instead of being reaped. All kinds of *pulse,* as peas, beans, &c., are thus termed.

LEGUMIN, Casein.

LEICHEN, Lichen.

LEI'OPUS, *Li'opus, Planeus, Plautus, Plotus,* from λειος, 'smooth,' and πους, 'a foot.' One who is affected with *flat-footedness, splay-footedness, Leiopod'ia, Liopod'ia.* One, the soles of whose feet are flat, instead of having the concavity which they commonly present.

LEIOSIS, Comminution.

LEIPHÆ'MIA, *Liphæ'mia:* same etymon as Leiphæmos. Poverty or paucity of blood.

LEIPHÆMOI, Achroi.

LEIPHÆ'MOS, *Liphæ'mos,* (F.) *Leiphème,* from λειπω, 'I want,' and 'αιμα, 'blood.' A word sometimes used adjectively; at others, substantively, either for a vicious state of the blood — or rather for a sort of anæmia — or for the patient who labours under this condition.

LEIPHÈME, Leiphæmos.

LEIPO, Lipo.

LEIPODERMIA, Aposthia.

LEIPODER'MOS, *Lipoder'mos,* from λειπω, 'I want,' and δερμα, 'skin.' One who wants a part of his skin. It is especially applied to one who wants the prepuce. See Apella and Aposthia.

LEIPOMERIA, Lipomeria.

LEIPOPSYCHIA, Syncope.

LEIPOTHYMIA, Syncope.

LEIPYR'IAS, from λειπω, 'I want,' and πυρ, 'fire,' or 'heat.' A species of continued fever, referred to by the Greek physicians, in which there is burning heat of the internal parts and coldness of the extremities. Avicenna described, under this name, a kind of hemitritæa.

LEMA, *Chassie.*

LEME, Lippitudo.

LEMITHOCORTON, Corallina Corsicana.

LEMMA, Cortex, Feculence, Furfur, Sedimentum.

LEMNISCUS, Pessary, Tent.

LEMON GROUND, Podophyllum montanum — l. Juice, see Citrus medica — l. Juice, artificial, see Citrus medica — l. Peel, see Citrus medica — l. Tree, Citrus medica — l. Wild, Podophyllum montanum.

LEMONADE', *Limona'da,* (F.) *Limonade.* Lemon juice diluted with water and sweetened. See Citrus medica.

LEMONADE, DRY, (F.) *Limonade sèche.* Citric or tartaric acid reduced to powder and mixed with sugar. *Lemonade Powders* may be made as follows: — Pound ℥jß *of citric acid* with a few drops of essence of lemon-peel and ℥j or more of lump sugar. Divide into six papers, each of which will make a glass of lemonade. See Citric acid.

Limonade Gazeuse, (F.) is an agreeable drink prepared by adding syrup of lemons, raspberry, &c., to water saturated with carbonic acid.

LEMONADE, MAGNESIAN, Magnesiæ citras.

LEMONADE, NITRIC. Nitric acid considerably diluted with water, and sweetened.

LEMONADE, SULPHURIC, and LEMONADE, TARTARIC, are made with the sulphuric and tartaric acids.

LEMOSITAS, *Chassie*, Lippitudo.
LENIENS, Laxative, Lenitive.
LENIS, Lenitive.
LEN'ITIVE, *Leniti'vus, Lenis, Len'iens, Epia'ma, Mit'igans*, from *lenio*, 'I assuage.' A medicine, which allays irritation or palliates disease; also, a laxative medicine. A *lenitive electuary* is one that purges gently.

LENOS, Torcular Herophili.
LENS, Ervum lens—l. Crystalline, Crystalline—l. Esculenta, Ervum lens.
LENTIC'ULA. Dim. of *lens*, 'a lentil.' A freckle. Also, the eruption of lenticular fever. See Ephelides.
LENTICULAR GANGLION, Ophthalmio G.
LENTICULA'RES GLAN'DULÆ, *Lentic'ular glands*. Mucous follicles, having the shape of a lentil, which are observed especially towards the base of the tongue.
LENTIGO, Ephelides.
LENTIL, Ervum lens.
LENTILLE, Ervum lens—l. *Crystalline*, Crystalline—l. Ers, Ervum ervilia.
LENTIS'CINUM VINUM. Wine impregnated with mastich; from *Lentiscus*, 'the mastich tree.'
LENTISCUS VULGARIS, Pistacia lentiscus.
LENTITIA, Lentor.
LENTITIS, Phacitis.
LENTITUDO, Lentor.
LENTOR, *Lentit"ia, Lentitu'do*, from *lentus*, 'clammy.' A viscidity or siziness of any fluid. See Gluten.
LENUM, Torcular Herophili.
LEONO'TIS LEONU'RUS. A South African plant, which has a peculiar smell and nauseous taste, and is said to produce narcotic effects if incautiously used. It is employed in decoction in chronic cutaneous diseases. The Hottentots smoke it like tobacco, and take a decoction of its leaves as a strong cathartic. It is also given as an emmenagogue. In the eastern districts of the Cape Colony, *Leonotis ova'ta* is used for the same purpose.

LEONTI'ASIS, *Leon'tion*, from λέων, 'a lion.' A name given to lepra of the face, from some fancied resemblance between the countenance of those labouring under it and that of the lion. To this kind of lepra the epithets *le'onine* and *le'ontine* have been given.

LEON'TICE THALICTROIDES, Caulophyllum thalictroïdes.
LEONTION, Leontiasis.
LEON'TODON TARAX'ACUM, *L. officina'lē, seu vulga'rē, Tarax'acum officina'lē, Dens Leo'nis, Hedyp'nois tarax'acum, Urina'ria, Caput Mon'achi, Dandeli'on, Piss-a-bed, Puffball*, (F.) *Pissenlit, Liondent*. Order, Compositæ. The young leaves are sometimes eaten as salad. The roots are, also, roasted and used as a substitute for coffee. The root, *Tarax'acum*, (Ph. U. S.,) is, moreover, reputed to be aperient and diuretic; hence its vulgar name. Its efficacy is doubtful.

LEONOTIS OVATA, see Leonotis leonurus.
LEONTOPODIUM, Alchemilla.
LEONU'RUS, from λέων, 'a lion,' and ουρα, 'a tail.' *Lion's Tail*.

LEONURUS CARDI'ACA, *Agripal'ma Gallis, Marru'bium, Cardi'aca crispa seu triloba'ta seu vulga'ris, Herba cardiaca, H. Patæ lapi'næ, Motherwort, Throatwort*, (F.) *Agripaume*. Its properties are those of a nauseous bitter; and hence it has been used in hysteria and other nervous affections.

LEONURUS LANATUS, Ballota lanata.
LEOPARD'S BANE, ROMAN, Arnica montana, Doronicum pardalianches.
LEPAS, *Lepis*, λεπας, gen. λεπαδος; λεπις, gen. λεπιδος, 'a scale.'
LEPER, see Leprous.
LEPER HOSPITAL, *Ladrerie*.
LEPIA CAMPESTRIS, Thlaspi campestre—l. Sativa, Lepidium Iberis.
LEPID'IUM, from λεπις, 'a scale;' so called from its supposed usefulness in cleansing the skin from scales and impurities. *Pepper-wort*.
LEPIDIUM CAMPESTRE, Thlaspi campestre.
LEPID'IUM IBE'RIS, *Ibe'ris, Cardaman'tica, Sciat'ica cresses*. This plant possesses a warm, penetrating, pungent taste, like other cresses, and is recommended as an antiscorbutic, antiseptic, and stomachic.
LEPIDIUM SATI'VUM, *Lep'ia sati'va, Thlaspi nastur'tium seu sati'vum, Nastur'tium horten'sē seu sati'vum, Garden cress, Dittander*, (F.) *Cresson alénois, Cresson des Jardins*. This plant possesses warm, stimulating properties, and is used like the last.
LEPIDIUM SQUAMATUM, Cochlearia coronopus.
LEPIDODES, Squamous.
LEPIDOIDES, Squamous.
LEPIDOSARCO'MA, *Tumor squamifor'mis carno'sus*. A fleshy tumour, covered with scales; from λεπις, 'a scale,' and σαρκωμα, 'a fleshy tumour.' Marcus Aurelius Severinus describes tumours of this kind in the interior of the mouth.
LEPIDOSIS, Scaly diseases.
LEPIDOSIS ICHTHYIASIS, Ichthyosis—l. Ichthyiasis cornigera, Horny excrescences—l. Lepriasis, Lepra—l. Pityriasis, Pityriasis—l. Psoriasis, Psoriasis.
LIPIDOTIS CLAVATA, Lycopodium clavatum
LEPIRA, Lepra.
LEPIS, Scale.
LEPORINUM LABIUM, Harelip—l. Rostrum, Harelip.
LEPORINUS OCULUS, Lagophthalmia.
LEPRA, *Lep'ira*, from λεπις, 'a scale.' *Lepido'sis Lepri'asis, Lepro'sis, Lepro'sitas, Vitili'go, Lepra Græco'rum, Herpes furfura'ceus circina'tus, Leprosy*, (F.) *Lèpre, Mal Saint-Main, Dartre furfuracée arrondie*. This term has been applied to various affections, very different in character. 1. To the *Leprosy of the Jews, Leuce, Lepido'sis, Lepriasis canes'cens, Lepra Mosa'ica seu Hebræo'rum*,—a variety of the *Alphos* or *Lepra alphoï'des*. The leuce was, generally, not scaly, but consisted of smooth, shining patches, on which the hair turned white and silky, and the skin, with the muscular flesh, lost its sensibility. It was incurable. To the *Elephantiasis* or *Lepra of the Arabs*, see Elephantiasis; and 3. To the *Lepra of the Greeks*, which includes all the varieties met with at the present day. It is characterised by scaly patches of different sizes, but having always nearly a circular form. Bateman and Willan describe three chief varieties of this lepra.

1. *Lepra alphoï'des, Lepido'sis Lepri'asis al'bida, Alphos, Morphæ'a alba, Vitili'go alphus, Al'barus alba, Albarēs, Albaros, Lèpre écailleuse* of Alibert, *White leprosy*. An affection, characterized by white patches, surrounded by a rose-coloured areola, which appears here and there on the surface; depressed in the middle.

2. *Lepra ni'gricans, Lepra melas, Vitili'go melas, V. Nigra, Morphæ'a nigra, Lepra maculo'sa nigra, Al'baras nigra, Melas, Lepido'sis lepri'asis ni'gricans, Black leprosy;* in which the scales are livid; the size of half a dollar; and diffused over the body, but less widely than in the *Alphoides.* The French pathologists usually admit three species of lepra, to which they give the epithets *scaly, (squameuse,) crustaceous, (crustacée,)* and *tubercular, (tuberculeuse,)* according as the skin may be covered with scales, crusts, or tubercles.

3. *Lepra vulga'ris, Lepido'sis lepri'asis vulga'ris, Dartre furfuracée arrondie,* of Alibert, characterized as follows: scales glabrous, whitish, size of a crown piece; preceded by smaller reddish and glossy elevations of the skin, encircled by a dry, red, and slightly elevated border; often confluent; sometimes covering the whole of the body except the face.

Lepra appears to be endemic in Egypt, in Java, and certain parts of Norway and Sweden. Imperfect and faulty nutriment appears to contribute to its development. The means, best adapted for its removal, are:—a mild, unirritating diet, emollient fomentations—sulphureous baths, fumigations, &c.; but, often, all remedial agents will be found ineffectual.

LEPRA ARABUM, Elephantiasis Arabica—l. Borealis, Radzyge—l. Fungifera, Frambœsia—l. Græcorum, Lepra—l. Hebræorum, see Lepra—l. Ichthyosis, Ichthyosis—l. Lombardica, Pellagra—l. Maculosa nigra, L. Nigricans—l. Mediolanensis, Pellagra—l. Mercurial, Eczema mercuriale—l. Mosaica, see Lepra—L. Norvegica, Radzyge—l. Squamosa, Impetigo—l. Taurica, *Mal de Crimée.*

LÈPRE, Lepra—*l. des Cosaques, Mal de Crimée—l. Écailleuse,* Lepra alphoides—*l. Humide,* Impetigo.

LEPRICUS, Leprous.
LEPROSARIUM, Ladrerie.
LÉPROSERIE, Ladrerie.
LEPROSIS, Lepra.
LEPROSITAS, Lepra.
LEPROSY, Lepra—l. Black, Lepra nigricans—l. Norwegian, see Radzyge—l. White, Lepra alphoides.
LEP'ROUS, *Lepro'sus, Leprot'icus, Lep'ricus, Lepro'des.* Relating to or resembling or affected with leprosy; a *leper.*
LEPSIS, Attack.
LEPTAN'DRA VIRGIN'ICA, *Veroni'ca Virgin'ica, Culver's physic.* An indigenous plant, which grows throughout the United States, and flowers in August. The flowers are white, and terminate the stem in a long spike. A variety with purple flowers has been described, as

LEPTANDRA PURPU'REA, *Physic root, Black root, Whorlywort, Culvert root, Brinton root, Bowman root.* The root is bitter and nauseous, and when fresh is emetic and cathartic. In the dried state it is more uncertain. Dose of the powder, gr. xx to ʒj.

LEPTO, LEPTOS, λεπτος, 'thin,' 'light.' Hence:

LEPTOCHRO'A, *Lep'tochros,* from λεπτος, 'thin, fine,' and χροα, χροια, 'the colour of the skin: the skin.' Fineness, thinness of skin.

LEPTOCHYM'IA, from λεπτος, 'thin,' and χυμος, 'a juice.' Morbid thinness of the juices.

LEPTOHYME'NIA, from λεπτος, 'thin,' and 'υμην, 'a membrane.' Thinness, delicacy of membrane.

LEPTOMER'IA, from λεπτος, 'thin, fine,' and μερος, 'a part.' Fineness, delicacy of bodily formation.

LEPTONTIQUES, Attenuants.

LEPTOPHONIA, Oxyphonia.
LEPTOSPERMUM LEUCADENDRUM, Melaleuca cajaputi.
LEPTOTHRIX, Leptotrichus.
LEPTOT'RICHUS, *Leptothrix,* from λεπτος, 'fine,' and θριξ, 'hair.' One who has fine hair.
LEPTOTROPH'IA, *Microtroph'ia, Microtrapex'ia,* from λεπτος, 'light,' and τροφη, 'nourishment.' Light nutrition.
LEPTYNSIS, Emaciation.
LEPTYNTICA, Attenuants.
LEPTYSMOS, Emaciation.
LEREMA, seo Dementia.
LERESIS, see Dementia.
LERUS, Delirium, see Dementia.
LE'SION, *Læ'sio,* from *læsus,* 'hurt,' 'injured.' Derangement, disorder; any morbid change, either in the exercise of functions or in the texture of organs. *Organic lesion* is synonymous with *organic disease.*
LESSIVE, Lixivium.
LESSIVE DES SAVONNIERS, Liquor potassæ. Also, a solution of caustic soda in water, containing about 3 parts of soda to 8 of water.
LESSIVE DE TARTRE, Liquor potassæ subcarbonatis.
LETALITAS, Mortality.
LETHALIS, Lethiferous, Mortal.
LETHALITAS, Mortality.
LETHAR'GIC, *Lethar'gicus, Veterno'sus,* (F.) *Léthargique.* Relating to lethargy; affected with lethargy.
LÉTHARGIQUE, Lethargic.
LETH'ARGY, *Lethar'gia, Lethar'gus, Carus lethargus, Veter'nus, Obliv'io iners,* from ληθη, 'oblivion,' and αργια, 'idleness.' A constant state of stupor from which it is almost impossible to arouse the individual; and, if aroused, he speedily relapses into his former condition.
LE'THEON, from ληθη, 'oblivion.' A name given by some to sulphuric ether, when inhaled as an anæsthetic agent.
LETHIF'EROUS, *Le'thifer, Letha'lis, Lethif'icus, Mor'tifer, Mortif'erous,* from ληθη, 'death,' and φερω, 'I bear.' Death-bearing; deadly.
LETHUM, Death.
LETTUCE, Lactuca—l. Blue, Mulgedium acuminatum—l. False, Mulgedium Floridanum—l. Indian, see Calumba—l. Strong-scented, Lactuca virosa—l. White, Nabalus albus—l. Wild, Lactuca elongata.
LETUM, Death.
LEUCADES, see Sclerotic.
LEUCÆ'MIA, *Leukæ'mia,* from λευκος, 'white, and 'αιμα, 'blood.' A condition of the blood in which it is deficient in colouring matter.
LEUCÆTHIOPIA, see Albino.
LEUCÆTHIOPS, Albino.
LEUCANIA, Laucania.
LEUCANTHEMUM, Anthemis nobilis, Matricaria chamomilla—l. Vulgare, Chrysanthemum leucanthemum.
LEUCE, Lepra (of the Jews.)
LEUCELECTRUM, Succinum (album.)
LEUCITIS, Sclerotitis.
LEUCOCYTHÆ'MIA, from λευκος, 'white,' κυτος, 'cell,' and 'αιμα, 'blood.' A condition of the blood, which consists in a superabundant development of the white corpuscles, a disease which has been observed at times to be accompanied by enlargement of the spleen and liver, and at others by increased size of the lymphatic glands.
LEUCODENDRON, Melaleuca cajaputi.
LEUCŒNUS, see Wine.
LEUCOIUM, Lunaria rediviva—l. Luteum, Cheiranthus cheiri.

LEUCOLEIN, Leukoleinum.

LEUCO'MA, from λευκος, 'white.' *Oculo'rum albu'go, Leucom'ma, Leuco'sis, Albu'go, Al'bula, Ceratoleuco'ma, Ephel'otes.* Leucoma and Albugo are often used synonymously to denote a white opacity of the cornea. Both are essentially different from nebula of the cornea; nebula being usually the result of chronic ophthalmy and an effusion of a milky serum into the texture of the delicate continuation of the conjunctiva over the cornea;—the others are the result of violent, acute ophthalmia. In this state, a thick, coagulable lymph is extravasated from the arteries, sometimes superficially, at other times deeply into the substance of the cornea. On other occasions, the disease consists of a firm, callous cicatrix on this membrane,—the effect of a wound or ulcer with loss of substance. The affection is more difficult of cure in proportion to its duration and to the age of the individual; the activity of the absorbents being greater in youth. If inflammation still exist, antiphlogistics must be persevered in, and, afterwards, gentle stimulants be used to excite absorption; along with the internal use of mercury or iodine.

LEUCOMA, Albumen—l. Margaritaceum, see Margaritaceus.

LEUCOMMA, Leucoma.

LEUCOMORIA, Cuttubuth.

LEUCONECRO'SIS, from λευκος,, 'white,' and νεκρωσις, 'death.' A form of dry gangrene,—the opposite in appearance to anthraconecrosis.

LEUCONYMPHÆA, Nymphæa alba.

LEUCOPATHIA, see Albino, Chlorosis.

LEUCOPHAGIUM, *Blanc-manger*.

LEUCOPHLEGMASIA, Leucophlegmatia—l. Dolens puerperarum, Phlegmatia dolens.

LEUCOPHLEGMA'TIA, *Leucophlegmasia, Hydrops leucophlegma'tias, Tumescen'tia pituito'sa,* from λευκος, 'white,' and φλεγμα, 'phlegm.' A dropsical habit. Some writers use the word synonymously with *anasarca* and *œdema*; others with *emphysema*.

LEUCOPHLEGMATIA ÆTHIOPUM, Chthonophagia.

LEUCOPIPER, Piper album.

LEUCOPYRIA, Hectic fever.

LEUCORRHÉE, Leucorrhœa.

LEUCORRHŒ'A, *Fluxus* vel *Fluor mulie'bris, Proflu'vium mulie'bre, Cursus matri'cis, Fluxus matri'cis, Elytri'tis, Coleosi'tis, Colpi'tis, Destilla'tio u'teri, Fluxio alba, F. Vul'væ, Ulcus u'teri, Catar'rhus genita'lium, Hysterorrhœ'a muco'sa, Catame'nia alba, Menses albi, Men'strua alba, Menorrhag''ia alba, Fluor mulie'bris non Gal'licus, Blennelyt'ria, Gonorrhœ'a benig'na notha invetera'ta, Purga'tio mulie'bris alba, Alba purgamen'ta, Cachex'ia uteri'na, Rheuma u'teri, U'teri Cory'sa, Medorrhœ'a femina'rum insons, Blennorrhœ'a* seu *Blennorrhag''ia genita'lium, Ædœoblennorrhœ'a* seu *Medoblennorrhœ'a femina'rum; The whites;* (F.) *Fleurs* ou *Flueurs blanches, Pertes blanches, Écoulement blanc, Catarrhe utérin, Perte utérine blanche,* from λευκος, 'white,' and ρεω, 'I flow.' A more or less abundant discharge of a white, yellowish, or greenish mucus; resulting from acute or chronic inflammation or from irritation of the membrane lining the genital organs of the female. *Vag''inal Leucorrhœa* has been termed *Blennorrhœa* seu *Fluor albus vagi'næ, Leucorrhœ'a, Medorrhœ'a vaginæ, Vagini'tis, Elytroblennorrhœ'a, Colporrhœ'a*. *Uterine Leucorrhœa* has received the names *Fluor albus uteri, Leucorrhœ'a* seu *Medorrhœ'a uteri, Metroblennorrhœ'a*, (F.) *Leucorrhée utérine, Catarrhe utérin*. It is often attended with pain and a sense of heaviness in the loins, abdomen and thighs; disordered digestive functions, &c., so that, at times, the health suffers largely, although there are few females who are not occasionally subject to moderate leucorrhœa. Attention to the general health, change of air, keeping up a perspirable state of the surface by flannel worn next the skin, the horizontal posture, &c., do more than pharmaceutical agents; which are almost entirely confined to astringent injections. These may be employed, when the discharge is so great as to require them.

LEUCORRHŒA ANALIS, see Hæmorrhois—l. Nabothi, see Parturition.

LEUCORRHOIS, see Hæmorrhois.

LEUCO'SES; from λευκος, 'white.' In the nosology of M. Alibert, all the diseases of the lymphatic apparatus. The 7th family in his *Nosologie*. In that of Fuchs, it is a family of diseases, (G.) Leukosen, which includes the various forms of anæmia.

LEUCOSIS, Leucoma, Paleness.

LEUK or LOCCHE, MINERAL WATERS OF. Saline, chalybeate waters, about six leagues distant from Sion. They contain chloride of sodium, with a little sulphate of magnesia; sulphate of lime, carbonate of magnesia, carbonic acid, and protoxide of iron.

LEUKÆMIA, Leucæmia.

LEUKOLEIN'UM, *Chinolein'um, Leukol, Leu'coleine, Leu'colein, Chi'nolein, Chi'nolin*. This substance is the product of the dry distillation of coal; mixed with picolin, anilin and other substances, in mineral tar. It is procured, also, by heating *quinia, cinchonia* and *strychnia*, with as concentrated a ley of *potassa* as can be made. Its specific gravity is 1.081; and it is slightly soluble in water, and miscible in all proportions with alcohol, ether and essential oils.

LEVAIN, Ferment.

LEVA'TOR AN'GULI ORIS, *Abdu'cens labio'rum, Eleva'tor labiorum commu'nis, Cani'nus,* (F.) *Sus maxillo-labial, Petit sus-maxillo-labial* (Ch.), *Muscle canin.* A small, flat, long, quadrilateral muscle, which arises from the fossa canina, and is inserted at the commissure of the lips, where it is confounded with the triangularis. It raises the corner of the mouth, and draws it towards the ear.

LEVATOR ANI, *Levator magnus* seu *internus, Latus ani, Eleva'tor ani, Sedem attol'lens,* (F.) *Pubio-coccygien annulaire, Sous pubio-coccygien* (Ch.), *Releveur de l'anus*. A muscle, situate at the lower part of the pelvis. It is broad, flat, quadrilateral, and broader above than below. It represents a kind of membranous partition, which closes the outlet of the pelvis, and the upper concavity of which is opposed to that of the diaphragm. It is attached, above, to the posterior surface of the body of the pubis, to the upper part of the obdurator foramen, and to the spine of the ischium; and is inserted into the coccyx, into an aponeurotic line common to it and its fellow, and into the lateral parts of the rectum. This muscle supports the rectum; raises it, and carries it upwards during the evacuation of the excrement. It can, also, compress the bladder and vesiculæ seminales, and thus favors the expulsion of the urine and sperm.

LEVATOR ANI PARVUS, Transversus perinæi—l. Auris, Attollens aurem—l. Coccygis, Coccygeus.

LEVATOR GLAN'DULÆ TYROI'DEÆ. A muscle occasionally found connected with the upper border or isthmus of the thyroid gland; and attached superiorly to the body of the os hyoides, or to the thyroid cartilage.

LEVATOR MENTI, Levator labii inferioris—l.

Oculi, Rectus superior oculi—l. Proprius scapulæ, L. scapulæ.

LEVATOR LABII INFERIO'RIS, *Levator menti, Elevator labii inferio'ris, Incisi'vus infe'rior, Elevator labii inferioris pro'prius, Mus'culus penicilla'tus,* (F.) *Houppe du menton, Releveur de la lèvre inférieur, Releveur du menton.* A portion of the *mento-labial* of Chaussier. A small muscle situate before the symphysis menti. It is thick, conical; and attached by its apex to a fossette at the side of the symphysis in the inferior maxillary bone. Its fibres proceed diverging and vanishing in the manner of a *tuft,* (F.) *Houppe,* on the skin of the chin. This muscle raises the chin, and pushes upwards the lower lip.

LEVATOR LABII SUPERIO'RIS ALÆQUE NASI, *Incisi'vus latera'lis et pyramida'lis,* (F.) *Grand sus-maxillo-labial* (Ch.,) *Elévateur commun de l'aile du nez et de la lèvre supérieure.* This muscle is a fleshy, thin, triangular bundle, situate at the sides of the nose. It arises from the ascending process of the superior maxillary bone: thence its fibres descend in a diverging manner, a part being inserted into the ala of the nose, and a part losing themselves in the upper lip. This muscle raises the upper lip and ala nasi, which it draws a little outwards.

LEVATOR LABII SUPERIORIS PROPRIUS, *Musculus incisi'vus, Elevator labii superioris proprius,* (F.) *Moyen sus-maxillo-labial,* (Ch.,) *Orbito-maxillo-labial.* This thin, flat, quadrilateral muscle is situate at the middle and inner part of the face. It arises from the os malæ and the os maxillare superius, and is inserted into the upper lip, which it raises, at the same time carrying it a little outwards.

LEVATOR PALA'TI, *Levator Palati Mollis, Petrosalpin'go-staphyli'nus, Salpin'go-staphyli'nus inter'nus, Salpingo-staphylinus, Pter'ygo-staphylinus externus, Spheno-staphylinus, Spheno-palati'nus, Peristaphylinus internus superior, Pétro-staphylin,* (Ch.) This muscle is long, narrow, and almost round above; broader and flatter inferiorly. It arises from the lower surface of the *pars petrosa;* from the cartilage of the Eustachian tube; and is inserted into the substance of the velum palati. Its use is to raise the velum palati.

LEVATOR PAL'PEBRÆ SUPERIO'RIS, *Palpebræ superioris primus, Apertor Oc'uli, Ape'riens Palpebra'rum rectus, Reclu'sor palpebra'rum,* (F.) *Orbito-palpébral* (Ch.), *Orbito-sus-palpébral, Élévateur de la paupière supérieure.* A long, small, thin muscle, situate at the upper part of the orbitar cavity. By its posterior extremity it is inserted into the little ala of the sphenoid bone, immediately in front of the foramen opticum, and, by its anterior extremity, which is expanded, it terminates at the upper margin of the tarsal cartilage of the eyelid. This muscle raises the upper eyelid, draws it backwards, and sinks it into the orbit.

LEVATOR PROS'TATÆ, (F.) *Releveur de la prostate.* Santorini has given this name to the anterior fibres of the levator ani, which embrace the prostate.

LEVATOR SCAP'ULÆ, *Eleva'tor scapulæ, Elevator sou Mus'culus Patien'tiæ, Angula'ris vulgo Levator pro'prius,*—(F.) *Trachélo-scapulaire* (Ch.), *Angulaire de l'omoplate, Releveur de l'omoplate.* This muscle is so called, because it is attached to the upper and internal angle of the scapula. It is situate at the posterior and lateral part of the neck, and at the upper part of the back. It is long, flat, and broader above than below. In this *latter* direction, it is inserted into the superior internal angle of the scapula; and, in the *former,* into the tops of the transverse processes of the first four cervical vertebræ. It depresses the prominence of the shoulder, by raising the posterior angle of the scapula, on which it impresses a kind of rotary motion. It can, also, draw the head to one side.

LEVATOR URE'THRÆ, (F.) *Releveur de l'Urèthre.* Santorini describes under this name a portion of the transversus perinæi muscle.

LEVATORES COSTARUM, Supracostales.

LEVEN, Ferment.

LEVER, from *levare,* 'to lift up.' *Vectis, Mochlus, Porrec'tum.* An inflexible rod, turning round a fixed point, and used for moving bodies, bearing burdens, or raising them. The point on which the lever moves is called the *Fulcrum, Hypomoch'lion.* The force which moves the lever is called the *power;* and the weight to be moved, the *resistance.* There are three kinds of levers. A *lever of the first kind* has the *fulcrum* between the power and resistance. A *lever of the second kind* has the *resistance* between the fulcrum and power; whilst a *lever of the third kind* has the *power* between the fulcrum and resistance. In the locomotive system of the human body, we have examples of all the three kinds. The bones represent *levers:* the muscles of locomotion are *powers;* the weight of parts to be moved constitutes the *resistance.* The *fulcra* are, at times, the joints; at others, the ground, &c. The head moves on the neck, as a lever of the first kind; the first cervical vertebra forming the fulcrum. We rise on tiptoe by a lever of the second kind, the fulcrum being the ground under the toes; and we have examples of a lever of the third kind in the flexion of the fore-arm on the arm, in the elevation of the arm, &c.

LEVER, *Hystero-moch'lium, Mochlis'cus, Vectis obstetric''ius, Vectis,* (F.) *Levier,* is an instrument curved at the extremity, and having a fenestra. It is used to assist the extraction of the child's head, when instrumental aid is necessary. Levers are, also, used by the dentist for extracting stumps, &c. The *Levier de l'Écluse, Langue de Carpe, Trivelin* or *Punch,* is employed for extracting the molar teeth.

LEVI'ATHAN PENIS, *Pria'pus Ceti, Bale'nas.* The penis of the whale. This singular medicine was, at one time, given, in powder, in cases of dysentery and leucorrhœa.

LEVIER, Lever—*l. de l'Écluse,* see Lever.

LEVIGA'TION, *Læviga'tio,* from *lævigare,* (*lævis,* 'smooth,') 'to polish.' *Porphyrisa'tion.* An operation, by which bodies are reduced to very fine powder. It is performed by putting substances, already pulverised, into water; the coarser parts are not long in being deposited, whilst the finer molecules remain suspended in the water. The liquor is decanted into another vessel, and suffered to remain at rest, until the fine particles are collected at the bottom. The fluid part is then separated by decantation.

LEVISTICUM, Ligusticum levisticum.

LÈVRE, Lip.

LÈVRES GRANDES, Labia pudendi—*l. Petites,* Nymphæ—*l. de la Vulve,* Labia pudendi.

LEVURE, Yest—*l. de la Bière,* Yest.

LEXIPHARMACUS, Alexipharmic.

LEXIPYRETICUS, Febrifuge.

LEY, Lixivium, Lye—l. Soap, Liquor potassæ.

LEYS'SERA GNAPHALOI'DES. A South African plant, *Nat. Ord.* Compositæ, which is emollient, and highly recommended at the Cape, in catarrh, cough, and even in phthisis.

LÉZARD, Lizard.

LIA'TRIS SPICA'TA, *Gayfeather, Button snakeroot.* An indigenous plant, growing in meadows and moist grounds in the middle and southern states. Its beautiful purple compound flowers are in a spike. They appear in August. The root has been considered diuretic.

LIA'TRIS SCARIO'SA and L. SQUARRO'SA, *Throatwort, Sow-wort, Backache root, Devilsbite, Blasing star, Prairie pines, Rough root,* are called, from their reputed powers in bites from the rattlesnake, *Rattlesnake's master.* The roots, bruised, are applied to the wound, and the decoction, in milk, is given internally.

LIBANOTIS ANNUA, Athamanta cretensis —l. Coronaria, Rosmarinus—l. Cretensis, Athamanta cretensis—l. Hirsuta, Athamanta cretensis.

LIBANOTUS, see Juniperus lycia.

LIBANUS, Juniperus lycia.

LIBER PHARMACEUTICUS, Dispensatorium.

LIBIDINIS SEDES, Clitoris.

LIBIDINOSUS, Libidinous.

LIBID'INOUS, *Libidino'sus; Lasci'vus, Veneriv'agus;* from *libido,* 'lust.' Lewd; lustful.

LIBI'DO. Desire, necessity. Authors speak of *Libido uri'næ, Libido intesti'ni.* Some employ it synonymously with *Prurigo;* others, with *Salac"itas, Lubi'do, Hi'meros.*

LIBOS, from λειβω, 'I distil.' A defluxion from the eyes.—Galen.

LIBRA, Pound.

LICHANOS, Index, see Digitus.

LICHEN, λειχην or λιχην, (pronounced *li'ken,*) *Exor'mia Lichen, Leichen, Serpi'go, Volat'ica, Pap'ulæ, P. siccæ, Peti'go, Pustulæ siccæ, Sca'bies sicca, S. a'gria, Licheni'asis adulto'rum, Li'chenous rash,* (F.) *Gale sèche, Dartrs furfuracée volante, Poussée.* The cutaneous affection described under this name by the Greek writers, is not clearly defined. Some have believed it to be *Impetigo,* but this is doubtful. The name is, now, generally applied to a diffuse eruption of red pimples, accompanied by a troublesome sense of tingling or pricking. Drs. Willan and Bateman define it,—"an extensive eruption of papulæ affecting adults, connected with internal disorder, usually terminating in scurf; recurrent, not contagious." One of their varieties, however, the *Lichen Tropicus,* does not accord well with this definition; for it affects children as well as adults, and is unconnected with internal disorder.

LICHEN A'GRIUS, *Exor'mia Lichen ferus, Pap'ula a'gria,* is distinguished by pimples in clusters or patches, surrounded by a red halo; the cuticle growing gradually harsh, thickened, and chappy, often preceded by general irritation. In addition to antiphlogistics, a cooling ointment may be used, to allay itching.

LICHEN BARBATUS PLICATUS, L. plicatus.

LICHEN CIRCUMSCRIP'TUS is characterized by clusters or patches of papulæ, having a well defined margin, and an irregularly circular form: continuing for six or eight weeks. These varieties require but little medical treatment. The antiphlogistic plan is all that is necessary.

LICHEN LIV'IDUS. The papulæ have a dark red or livid hue, without any fever. They are more permanent in this variety. It requires the mineral acids and bark.

LICHEN PILA'RIS, *Exor'mia Lichen pilaris,* is merely a modification of the preceding; the papulæ appearing at the roots of the hair.

LICHEN SIMPLEX, *Exor'mia Lichen simplex,* consists of an eruption of red papulæ, appearing first on the face or arms, and afterwards extending over the body; preceded for a few days by slight febrile irritation, which usually ceases when the eruption appears,—with an unpleasant sense of tingling during the night. It generally dies away in ten days or a fortnight.

LICHEN TROP'ICUS, *Exormia Lichen tropicus,*

Ecses'ma, Es'sera (?), *Sudam'ina* (?), *Prickly Heat, Summer Rash.* The pimples are bright red, and of the size of a small pin's head; with heat, itching, and pricking, as if by needles. It is local; produced by excessive heat; and disappears when the weather becomes cooler, or the individual is inured to the climate.

LICHEN URTICA'TUS, *Exor'mia Lichen urtico'sus,* is another variety. The *Nettle Lichen* consists of papulæ, accompanied by wheals like those of nettle rash.

LICHEN ARBORUM, Lichen pulmonarius—*l. Blanc de Néige,* L. caninus—*l. Bottier,* L. pyxidatus.

LICHEN CANINUS, seu *spu'rius* seu *terres'tris* seu *veno'sus* seu *ciner'eus terres'tris, Muscus cani'nus, Phys'cia niva'lis, Peltig"era cani'na, Peltid'ea cani'na* seu *leucorrhi'za* seu *mala'ces* seu *amplis'sima* seu *spu'ria, Ash-coloured Ground Liverwort,* (F.) *Lichen contre-rage, Lichen blanc de néige.* This cryptogamous plant was, for a long time, considered capable of preventing and curing *Rabies canina.* It has, also, been used in mania and in spasmodic asthma.

LICHEN CINEREUS TERRESTRIS, L. caninus—l. Carrageen, Fucus crispus—l. Cocciferus. L. pyxidatus—*l. contre Rage,* L. caninus—*l. Entonnoir,* L. pyxidatus—l. Eryngifolius, L. islandicus—l. Floridus hirtus, L. plicatus—l. Hirtus, L. plicatus.

LICHEN ISLAN'DICUS, *L. eryngifo'lius, Lichenoï'des Island'icum, Loba'ria Islan'dica, Muscus Islandicus, M. cathar'ticus, Clado'nia Islan'dica, Phys'cia Islandica, Cetra'ria Islandica; Parme'lia Islan'dica, Iceland Lichen* or *Liverwort* or *Moss,* (F.) *Lichen d'Islande.* This plant is inodorous, with a bitter and mucilaginous taste. It is esteemed to be tonic, demulcent, and nutrient. Dose, ʒj to ivʒ, being first steeped in water holding in solution some carbonate of potassa to extract the bitter, and then boiled in milk. A bitter principle has been extracted from it, termed *Cetrarin, Cetrari'num, Cetra'rium,* which has been given in intermittents.

LICHEN LACINIATUS, L. saxatilis.

LICHEN PLICA'TUS seu *hirtus* seu *barba'tus plica'tus* seu *Floridus hirtus, Parme'lia plica'ta, Li'uea plica'ta* seu *Flor'ida hirta* seu *hirta, Muscus arbo'reus* seu *albus* seu *quernus, Querci'ni Herba.* This plant is applied, by the Laplanders, as an astringent, to bleeding vessels; and to parts which are excoriated after long journeys.

LICHEN PULMONA'RIUS, *Lichen ar'borum* seu *reticula'tus, Parme'lia pulmona'cea, Reticula'ria officina'lis, Muscus pulmonarius querci'nus, Pulmona'ria arbo're, Loba'ria pulmonaria, Sticta pulmona'cea, Oak Lungs, Tree Lungwort, Hazel Crottles,* (F.) *Lichen pulmonaire.* This plant is sub-astringent, and rather acid. It was once in high repute for curing diseases of the lungs.

LICHEN PYXIDA'TUS, *Muscus Pyxida'tus, Scyphoph'orus pyxida'tus, Mus'culus pyxoï'des terres'tris, Lichen pyxida'tus major, Lichen coccif'erus, Herba Ignis, Cup Moss,* (F.) *Lichen entonnoir, Lichen Bottier, L. Pyxide.* This plant is sub-astringent, and has been used in decoction in hooping-cough.

LICHEN RETICULATUS, L. pulmonarius.

LICHEN ROCCEL'LA, *Parme'lia roccel'la, Roccella, R. tincto'ria, Seta'ria roccella, Litmus, Lacmus tincto'rius, Orchill, Casa'ry Archell, Chinney Weed, Herb Archell,* (F.) *Orseille.* The chief use of this plant is as a blue dye. It has been employed to allay cough in phthisis, &c.

LICHEN SAXAT'ILIS, *L. tincto'rius* seu *lacinia'tus, Parme'lia saxat'ilis, Inbrica'ria saxat'ilis, Loba'ria saxat'ilis, Muscus Cra'nii huma'ni, Li'nea.* This moss, when found growing on a human skull, was formerly in high estimation against head affections, &c.

LICHEN SPURIUS, L. caninus—l. Stellatus, Marchantia polymorpha—l. Tinctorius, L. Saxatilis.

LICHENIASIS ADULTORUM, Lichen—l. Strophulus, Strophulus.

LICHENOIDES ISLANDICUM, Lichen Islandicus.

LICORICE, Glycyrrhiza.

LIEBENSTEIN, MINERAL WATERS OF. These waters, situated in the duchy of Saxe-Meiningen, are amongst the strongest acidulous chalybeates in Germany. They contain sulphate of soda, chloride of sodium, sulphate of lime, chloride of calcium, carbonate of lime, chloride of magnesium, and carbonate of iron.

LIEBERKÜHN'S GLANDS or FOLLICLES, so called from their first describer, are fine, capillary, blind sacs, the openings of which are from 1-20th to 1-30th of a line in diameter, so closely placed over the whole of the small intestine as to give the mucous membrane a general sieve-like or perforated appearance. They secrete the *succus entericus*.

LIEBERSCHE AUSZEHRUNG'S KRAUTER, see Galeopsis grandiflora—l. Brustkrauter, see Galeopsis grandiflora.

LIEBWERDA, MINERAL WATERS OF. Liebwerda is a Bohemian village, near the Silesian frontier. The springs are much frequented. There are four, all of which are rich in carbonic acid and contain but little saline matter.

LIÈGE, Suber.

LIEN (F.), *Vin'culum*. A band, strap or garter, used in certain operations; as to tie patients during the operation of lithotomy; to fix the apparatus in fracture, &c. Also, the spleen.

LIEN ACCESSORIUS, Lienculus—l. Ingens, Splenoncus—l. Succenturiatus, Lienculus.

LIEN'CULUS, diminutive of *lien*, 'spleen.' *Lien succenturia'tus seu accesso'rius*. A supernumerary spleen.

LIENOSUS, Splenic.

LI'ENTERY, *Lienter'ia*, from λειος, 'smooth,' and εντερον, 'intestine.' *Læ'vitas seu Lax'itas intestino'rum, Diarrhœ'a lienter'ia, Fluxus Lienter'icus, Chymorrhœ'a seu Lax'itas ingesto'rum, Bromatoëc'crisis, Diarrhœ'a Dyspep'tica, D. cum apepsiâ, D. Ingesto'rum, Slip'periness of the Guts*. Frequent liquid evacuations, the food only half digested. This condition is always symptomatic of great irritation in the intestinal canal, the sensibility of which is so much augmented that it cannot bear the sojourn of the food in it.

LIERRE, Hedera helix—l. *Terrestre*, Glechoma hederacea.

LIFE, Sax. liḟ, lyḟ, *Vita, Bios, Bi'otē, Zoē, Pneuma, Spir'itus*, (F.) *Vie*. The state of organized beings, during which, owing to the union of an unknown principle with matter, they are capable of performing functions different from those that regulate other natural bodies; all of which functions, however numerous and diversified, work to one end. Life has only a limited duration; beyond which,—the organic functions ceasing to be executed,—the body is given up to the agency of chemical affinity. Hence Bichat has defined life to be—*the aggregate of the functions which resist death*. On account of the difference that exists among the vital functions, he has applied the term *Organic Life* to the functions subservient to composition and decomposition;—as digestion, respiration, circulation, calorification, absorption, secretion, and nutrition; and *Animal Life*, to the functions which connect man and animals with external bodies; as the understanding, sensations, locomotion and voice.

LIFE, DURATION OF, see Longevity—l. Everlasting, Gnaphalium margaritaceum — l. Everlasting, sweet-scented, Gnaphalium polycephalum—l. Expectation of, see Longevity.

LIFE-INSU'RANCE. A contract entered into, usually by an *insurance company*, to pay a certain sum of money on a person's death, on the condition of his paying an annual premium during his life. The medical practitioner may be applied to to certify that the life of the insurer is one that is insurable according to the rules of the company.

LIFE, VALUE OF, see Longevity, and Mortality.

LIFE'S BLOOD, Cillo.

LIG'AMENT, *Ligamen'tum;* from *ligare*, 'to bind;' *Desmos, Syndes'mos, Colliga'men, Cop'ula*. A name given to fibrous structures, which serve to unite bones, and to form articulations; hence the division into *interosseous* and *articular* ligaments. They are of a white, close texture; are but little extensible, and difficult to break. The name *ligament* has, also, been given to any membranous fold, which retains an organ in its situation.

TABLE OF THE PRINCIPAL LIGAMENTS.

1. *Of the Lower Jaw.*	Capsular ligament. Suspensory ligament of the stylo-glossus. Lateral ligament.
2. *Connecting the Head with the first and second Vertebræ, and these with each other.*	Two capsular ligaments between atlas and head. Circular ligament. Two capsular between atlas and axis. Perpendicular ligament. Two lateral or moderator ligaments. Transverse ligament and its appendices.
3. *Of the other Vertebræ.*	Anterior common. Crucial intervertebal. Ligaments running from the edge of the bony arch and spinous process of one vertebra to that of the next. Interspinous ligament. Ligamentum nuchæ. Intertransverse. Capsular. Posterior or internal common.
4. *Of the Ribs, Sternum, &c.*	Capsular of the heads of ribs. Capsular of the tubercles. Ligamenta transversaria interna. Ligamenta transversaria externa. Ligamenta cervicis costarum externa. Ligamentous fibres running from the margins of the extremities of the ribs to the corresponding cartilages. Radiated ligaments from cartilage of ribs to the sternum. Capsular ligaments of the cartilages of the ribs. Proper membrane of sternum. L. of cartilago-ensiformis. Tendinous expansions over the intercostales, &c.
5. *Of the Pelvis.*	Two transverse,—one superior, one inferior. Ilio-sacral. Capsular of the sacro-iliac synchondrosis. Two sacro ischiatic,—posterior and anterior, with the superior and inferior appendices. Longitudinal of os coccygis Inguinal ligament Capsular of symphysis pubis. Ligament of foramen thyroideum.

6. *Of the Clavicle.*	Radiated ligament Capsular. Interclavicular. Ligamentum rhomboideum. Claviculo-acromial. Conoid. Trapezoid.	
7. *Of the Scapula.*	Anterior triangular. Proper posterior.	
8. *Of the Shoulder-Joint.*	Capsular.	
9. *Of the Elbow-Joint.*	Capsular. Brachio-ulnar. Brachio-radial. Coronary of the radius. Anterior and posterior accessory. Intermuscular of the os humeri.	
10. *Carpal Extremity of Radius and Ulna, and between those bones.*	Interosseous ligament. Oblique or chorda transversalis cubiti. Capsular.	
11. *Between Fore-arm and Wrist.*	Capsular. Two lateral. Mucous.	
12. *Of the Carpus.*	Annular. Capsular. Short ligaments, — oblique, transverse, capsular, and proper.	
13. *Between Carpal and Metacarpal bones.*	Articular lateral. Straight, perpendicular, &c.	
14. *Between the extremities of the Metacarpal bones.*	Interosseous, at the bases and heads, — dorsal, lateral, palmar.	
15. *At the base of the Metacarpal bone of the Thumb, and at the first joint of the Fingers.*	Capsular. Lateral.	
16. *Of the first and second joints of the Thumb, and second and third joints of the Fingers.*	Capsular. Lateral.	
17. *Retaining the Tendons of the Muscles of the Hand and Fingers in situ.*	Annular. Vaginal or flexor tendons. Vaginal or crucial of the phalanges. Accessory of the flexor tendons. Posterior annular. Vaginal of extensors. Transverse of extensors.	
18. *Connecting the Os Femoris with the Os innominatum.*	Capsular and accessory slips. Round or teres ligament. Cartilaginous ligament. Double cartilaginous ligament. Ligamenta mucosa.	
19. *Of the Knee-Joint.*	Lateral, — internal and external. External short lateral ligament. Posterior ligament. Ligament of the patella. Capsular. Ligamentum alare, — majus et minus. Ligamentum mucosum. Two crucial, — anterior and posterior. Transverse.	
20. *Connecting Fibula and Tibia.*	Capsular. Interosseous. Anterior superior. Posterior superior.	
21. *Connecting the Tarsal with the Leg Bones.*	Anterior ligament of the fibula. Posterior of fibula. Deltoides of tibia. Capsular.	
22. *Of the Tarsus.*	Capsular. Short ligaments. Capsular, broad superior, and lateral ligaments, connecting astragalus and naviculare. Superior, lateral, and inferior, fixing os calcis to os cuboides. Long, oblique, and rhomboid forming the inferior ligaments. Superior superficial, interosseous and inferior transverse ligaments, fixing the os naviculare and os cuboides. Superior lateral, and plantar, which fix the os naviculare and cuneiform. Superior superficial and plantar, connecting the os cuboides, and os cuneiforme externum. Dorsal and plantar, uniting the ossa cuneiformia. The proper capsular of each bone.	
23. *Between Tarsus and Metatarsus.*	Capsular. Dorsal, plantar, lateral, straight, oblique, and transverse.	
24. *Connecting the Metatarsal Bones.*	Dorsal, plantar, and lateral, connecting the metatarsal bones. Transverse ligaments	
25. *Of the Phalanges of the Toes.*	Capsular. Lateral.	
26. *Retaining the Tendons of the Muscles of the Foot and Toes in situ.*	Annular. Vaginal of the tendons of the peronei. Laciniated. Vaginal of the tendon of the flexor longus pollicis. Vaginal and crucial of the tendons of the flexors of the toes. Accessory of the flexor tendons of the toes. Transverse of the extensor tendons.	

LIGAMENT, ANTERIOR, OF THE BLADDER. A name given by the older anatomists to a portion of the superior pelvic aponeurosis, which becomes attached to the front of the neck of the bladder.

LIGAMENT ARTÉRIEL, Arterial ligament —l. Camper's, Perineal fascia—l. Cervical supraspinal, see Supraspinosa ligamenta—*l. Ciliaire,* Ciliary ligament.

LIGAMENT, COR'ONARY, OF THE LIVER, is a reflection formed by the peritoneum, between the posterior margin of the liver, and the lower surface of the diaphragm. See Falx.

LIGAMENT, COSTO-XIPHOID, Xiphoid ligament —l. Dorso-lumbo-supraspinal, see Supra-spinosa ligamenta—l. of Fallopius, Crural arch—l. Gimbernat's, see Gimbernat's ligament—l. Glosso-epiglottic, see Glossoepiglottic—l. Infra-pubian, Triangular ligament—*l. Interépineux,* Interspinal ligament—l. of the Ovary, see Ovarium—l. Palmar inferior, Metacarpal ligament—l. Poupart's, Crural arch—*l. Rond,* Ligamentum teres—*l. Sur-épineux cervical,* see Supra-spinosa ligamenta—*l. Sur-épineux-dorso-lombaire,* see Supraspinosa ligamenta.

LIGAMENT, SUSPEN'SORY, OF THE LIVER, *Ligamen'tum latum, Suspenso'rium He'patis,* is a large triangular reflection, formed by the peritoneum between the superior surface of the liver and the diaphragm. It is constituted of two layers, and is continuous, below, with another reflection, called the *Falx of the Umbilical Vein.* See Falx.

LIGAMENT, TRIANGULAR, Perineal fascia.

LIGAMENTA INTERLOBULARIA PULMONUM, Interlobular tissue—l. Intervertebralia, Intervertebral cartilages—l. Lata uteri, see Uterus—l. Rotunda uteri, Round ligaments of the uterus—l. Tarsea lata, see Tarsea lata (ligamenta).

LIGAMENTEUX, Ligamentous.

LIGAMENTOSUS, Ligamentous.

LIGAMEN'TOUS, *Ligamento'sus, Desmous, Desmo'sus,* (F.) *Ligamenteux, Desmeux.* Having the character, or relating to, a ligament.

LIGAMENTS, BROAD, OF THE UTERUS, see Uterus—*l. Croisés*, Crucial ligaments, *l. Cruciformes*, Crucial ligaments—*l. Jaunes*, Yellow ligaments—*l. Larges de l'utérus*, see Uterus—l. of the Larynx, inferior, Thyreo-arytenoid ligaments—*l. Ronds de l'utérus*, Round ligaments of the uterus.

LIGAMENTUM DENTATUM, Denticulatum ligamentum—l. Iridis, Ciliary ligament—l. Nuchæ, Cervical ligament—l. Posticum Winslowii, see Genu—l. Suspensorium hepatis, Suspensory ligament of the liver—l. Suspensorium testis, Gubernaculum testis.

LIGATIO, Fascia, Ligature—l. Linguæ, Aphonia.

LIGATION, see Ligature.

LIGATURA, Ligature, Fascia—l. Glandis, Phimosis.

LIG'ATURE, *Ligatu'ra, Liga'tio, Alligatu'ra, Deliga'tio, Vinctu'ra, Fascia, Epid'esis*, from *ligo*, 'I bind.' This word has various acceptations. It means, 1. The thread with which an artery or vein is tied, to prevent or arrest hemorrhage. 2. The cord, or thread, or wire, used for removing tumours, &c. 3. The bandage used for phlebotomy. *Ligature* is, also, sometimes applied to the act of tying an artery or considerable vessel —*Liga'tion*. When the artery alone is tied, the ligature is said to be *immediate;* when any of the surrounding parts are included, it is said to be *mediate*. The ligature occasions obliteration or adhesion of the arterial parietes, by cutting through the middle and internal coats; the adhesion being favoured by the formation of a coagulum, which acts, in some degree, as a barrier against the impulse of the blood, and subsequently disappears by absorption.

LIGHT, Sax. leohč, lihč, (G.) L i c h t — *Lux, Lumen, Phos*, (F.) *Lumière*. An extremely rare fluid; diffused over the universe; emanating from the sun and fixed stars; traversing more than four millions of leagues in a minute; passing through transparent bodies, which refract it according to their density and combustibility; and arrested by opake bodies, by which it is reflected at an angle equal to the angle of incidence. It is the cause of colour in all bodies, being entirely reflected by white surfaces and absorbed by black. It is decomposed in passing through a transparent prism into seven rays—red, orange, yellow, green, blue, purple, and violet.

Light acts upon the body as a gentle and salutary stimulus. It urges to exercise, whilst privation of it induces sleep and inactivity, and disposes to obesity. Hence it is, that, in rural economy, animals which are undergoing the process of fattening are kept in obscurity. When vegetables are deprived of light, their nutrition is interfered with, and they become *etiolated*. To a certain extent this applies to animals, and there is every reason to believe, that want of light prevents the due development of organized bodies. It has been found that, when tadpoles were deprived of light, they did not undergo the perfect metamorphosis into the frog, but that monstrosities from arrest of development were induced.

LIGHTNING, Astrape.

LIGHTS, RISING OF THE, Cynanche trachealis.

LIGNE, Line—*l. Âpre*, Linea aspera—*l. Blanche*, Linea alba—*l. Courbe*, Curved line—*l. Médiane de l'abdomen*, Linea alba—*l. Sous-trochantérienne*, Linea aspera.

LIGNIN, from *Lignum*, 'wood.' Ligneous or woody fibre; the fibrous structure of vegetable substances.

LIGNUM ALOES, Agallochum—l. Aspalathi, Agallochum—l. Benedictum, Guaiacum—l. Brasilianum rubrum, Hæmatoxylon campechianum—l. Cæruleum, Hæmatoxylon campechianum—l. Campechense, Hæmatoxylon campechianum—l. Campechianum, Hæmatoxylon campechianum—l. Campescanum, Hæmatoxylon campechianum—l. Colubrinum, see Strychnos — l. Febrifugum, Quassia — l. Hæmatoxyli, Hæmatoxylon campechianum—l. Indicum, Guaiacum, Hæmatoxylon campechianum—l. Infelix, Sambucus—l. Nephriticum, Guilandina Moringa (the wood)—l. Pavanæ, Croton tiglium—l. Quassiæ, see Quassia—l. Sanctum, Guaiacum — l. Sandalinum, see Pterocarpus santalinus—l. Sappan, Hæmatoxylon campechianum—l. Serpentum, Ophioxylum serpentinum—l. Vitæ, Guaiacum.

LIGNYODES, Fuliginous.

LIGNYS, Fuligo.

LIG'ULA, *Lin'gula*. The clavicle; also, the glottis and epiglottis. A measure containing 3 drachms and a scruple, or about half an ounce. Also, a species of bandage or ligature.—Scribonius.

LIGUSTICUM CAPILLACEUM, Æthusa meum — l. Carvi, Carum — l. Fœniculum, Anethum.

LIGUS'TICUM LEVIS'TICUM, from Λιγυστικος, appertaining to Liguria. *Levis'ticum, Laserpitium German'icum, Ligusticum, Angel'ica levis'ticum seu paludapifo'lia*, Lovage, (F.) *Livêche, Ache des montagnes*. The properties of this plant are said to be stimulant, carminative, emmenagogue, &c.

LIGUSTICUM MEUM, Æthusa meum—l. Phellandrium, Phellandrium aquaticum.

LIGUSTICUM PODAGRA'RIA, *Podagra'ria ægopo'dium, Ægopo'dium podagraria, Sison podagra'ria, Pimpinel'la angelicafo'lia, Sium vulga'rě, Tragoseli'num angel'ica, Ses'eli ægopo'dium, Angel'ica sylvestris, Gout-weed*. A British plant, once considered useful in cases of gout.

LIGUSTICUM SILAUS, Peucedanum silaus.

LIGUSTRUM ÆGYPTIACUM, Lawsonia inermis.

LIGUS'TRUM VULGA'RE, *Privet, Privy,* (F.) *Troëne*. A shrub, which grows wild both in Europe and the United States, usually in hedges. The leaves are astringent and bitter; and the flowers, which are snow-white, and of an agreeable odour, have been employed in decoction in sore throat, and ulcerous stomatitis. The berries are said to be cathartic.

LIGYSMA, Distortion.

LILAC, COMMON, Syringa vulgaris—l. Vulgaris, Syringa vulgaris.

LILI, Lilium Paracelsi.

LILIA'GO. Dim. of *Lil'ium*, the *lily; Spiderwort; Liliae'trum*. This plant was formerly said to be alexipharmic and carminative.

LILIASTRUM, Liliago.

LIL'IUM CAN'DIDUM, *L. album*, Orinon. The *white lily*. (F.) *Lis blanc*. The infusion of the flowers of the lily in olive oil is emollient, and often applied externally, under the name of *Lily oil*, (F.) *Huile de lis*. The scales of the bulb, roasted, are sometimes employed as maturatives.

LILIUM CONVALLIUM, Convallaria maialis.

LILIUM PARACEL'SI, *Tinctu'ra Metallo'rum, Lili*. A medicine employed by Paracelsus. It was prepared by melting in a crucible four ounces of each of the following alloys: *Antimony and iron, antimony and tin, antimony and copper*, previously mixed with eighteen ounces of nitrate of potassa and as much salt of tartar. The melted mass, when pulverized, was treated with rectified alcohol, which really dissolved only the potassa set at liberty by the decomposition experienced by the nitre and salt of tartar. The *Lilium Paracelsi* was used as a cordial. It entered into the composition of the theriacal elixir, &c.

LILY, GROUND, Trillium latifolium—l. May, Convallaria maialis—l. Pond, Nelumbium luteum—l. Pond, White, Nymphæa odorata—l. Toad, Nymphæa odorata—l. of the Valley, Convallaria maialis—l. Water, little, Brasenia hydropeltis—l. Water, sweet, Nymphæa odorata—l. Water, sweet-scented, Nymphæa odorata—l. Water, white, Nymphæa alba—l. Water, yellow, Nymphæa lutea—l. White, Lilium candidum, Nelumbium luteum.

LIMA, CLIMATE OF. The climate of Peru does not appear to be favourable to the generation of consumption; and Lima would seem to be a good residence for the phthisical valetudinarian. Many have been benefited by a residence there; but when they have gone farther south, as to Chili, the effect, according to Dr. M. Burrough, has generally been fatal.

LIMA DENTARIA, Scalprum dentarium.

LIMAÇIEN (F.), from limaçon, the cochlea of the ear. A branch of the acoustic or labyrinthic nerve sent to the cochlea.

LIMAÇON, Cochlea, Limax—l. Rampes du, see Cochlea.

LIMACUM CORNUA, see Lachrymal puncta.

LIMANCHIA, Abstinence.

LIMA'TIO, from lima, 'a file.' Filing: an operation employed by the dentist more especially to prevent immediate contact of the teeth with each other.

LIMATURA FERRI, Ferri Limatura.

LIMAX, Helix, Slug or Snail, (F.) Limaçon, Colimaçon, Escargot. A syrup has been prepared from these animals, which has been given in phthisis, &c. The raw snails have also been taken in consumption. They have been used as food.

LIMB, Membrum.

LIMBUS ALVEOLARIS, Alveolar border—l. Luteus retinæ, see Foramen centrale—l. Posterior corporis striati, Tænia semicircularis.

LIME. A fruit like a small lemon, the juice of which is strongly acid, and much used for making punch. It is, also, used in long voyages as an antiscorbutic, &c. It is a species of lemon, the fruit of Citrus acida.

LIME, Calx—l. Carbonate of, Creta—l. Chloride of, Calcis chloridum—l. Chlorite of, Calcis chloridum—l. Chloruret of, Calcis chloridum—l. Hydrate of, see Calx—l. Hypochlorite of, Calcis chloridum—l. Muriate of, solution of, see Calcis marias—l. Oxymuriate of, Calcis chloridum—l. Slaked, see Calx—l. Sulphuret of, Calcis sulphuretum—l. Tree, Tilia—l. Water, Liquor calcis—l. Water, compound, Liquor calcis compositus.

LIMICUS, Hungry.

LIMITROPHES, see Trisplanchnic nerve.

LIMNE, Marsh.

LIMNE'MIC, Limnæ'mic, Limnhe'mic, Limnæ'micus, Limnhæ'micus, from λιμνη, 'a marsh,' and 'αιμα, 'blood.' An epithet given to affections induced by paludal emanations; (F.) Affections limnhémiques.

LIMOCTON'IA, Abstinence. Abstinence to death. Death from hunger; from λιμος, 'hunger,' and κτονος, 'death.' Suicide by hunger.

LIMODES, Hungry.

LIMON, see Citrus medica.

LIMONADA, Lemonade.

LIMONADE, Lemonade—l. Gazeuse, see Lemonade—l. Sèche, Lemonade, dry; see Citric acid.

LIMONIUM, Statice limonium—l. Malum, see Citrus medica.

LIMONUM BACCA, see Citrus medica.

LIMOS, λιμος, 'hunger.' Hence:

LIMO'SIS, Stomach disease, Morbid appetite. A genus in the class Cœliaca, order Enterica, of Good.

LIMOSIS CARDIALGIA MORDENS, Cardialgia—l. Cardialgia sputatoria, Pyrosis—l. Dyspepsia, Dyspepsia—l. Expers, Anorexia—l. Expers protracta, Fasting—l. Flatus, Flatulence—l. Helluonum, Gluttony—l. Pica, Malacia.

LIMOTHERAPEI'A, Nestitherapei'a, Nestotherapei'a, Nestiatri'a, Peinotherapi'a, Curatio morbi per ine'diam, from λιμος, 'hunger,' and θεραπεια, 'treatment.' Hunger-cure. Cure by fasting.

LIMUS, Limos.

LIN, Linum usitatissimum—l. Graines de, see Linum usitatissimum—l. Purgatif, Linum catharticum.

LINAIRE, Antirhinum linaria.

LINAMENTUM, Linteum.

LINARIA, Antirhinum linaria—l. Cymbalaria, Antirhinum linaria—l. Elatine, Antirhinum elatine—l. Vulgaris, Antirhinum linaria.

LINCTUARIUM, Eclectos.

LINCTUS, Eclectos—l. Albus, Looch album—l. Amygdalinus, Looch album—l. ad Aphthas, Mel boracis—l. de Borace, Mel boracis—l. Communis, Looch album.

LINDEN TREE, Tilia.

LINE, Lin'ea, Grammē, (F.) Ligne. Extent in length, considered without regard to breadth or thickness. As a measure, it means the 12th part of an inch.

MEDIAN LINE OF THE BODY is an imaginary line supposed to set out from the top of the head and to fall between the feet, so as to divide the body vertically into two equal and symmetrical parts.

LINEA, Line.

LINEA ALBA, L. A. Abdom'inis, (F.) Ligne blanche, Ligne médiane de l'abdomen (Ch.), Candid'ula abdom'inis lin'ea, Lin'ea centra'lis. A tendinous, strong, and highly resisting cord; extending from the ensiform cartilage of the sternum to the symphysis pubis, with the umbilicus near its middle. The linea alba is formed by the decussation of the aponeurosis of the abdominal muscles; and its use is to limit the movement of the chest backwards; to prevent it from separating too far from the pelvis, and to furnish a fixed point for the muscles of the abdomen in their contraction.

LINEA AS'PERA, (F.) Ligne âpre, Ragged ridge, Ligne sous-trochantérienne, (Ch.) A rough projection at the posterior surface of the femur, which gives attachment to muscles.

LINEA CANDIDULA ABDOMINIS, L. alba—l. Centralis, L. alba—l. Innominata, Ilio-pectinea Linea.

LINEÆ SEMILUNA'RES are the lines, which bound the outer margin of the recti muscles of the abdomen. They are formed by the union of the abdominal tendons. The lines which cross these muscles are called Lineæ transver'sæ.

LINEÆ TIB'IÆ, An'guli tib'iæ. Sharp lines on the tibia.

LINEÆ TRANSVERSÆ, see L. semilunares, and Processus teretes.

LINÉAIRE, Linear.

LIN'EAMENT, Lineamen'tum, from linea, 'a line.' A delicate trait observed on the countenance, which constitutes its special character, enables us to preserve its image, and is the cause of resemblance to others. A feature.

Bonnet gave the name Linéament to the first traces of organization in the embryo of man and animals.

LIN'EAR, *Linea'ris, Linea'rius.* Same etymon. (F.) *Linéaire.* Pathologists apply the epithet *linear* to fractures which are very narrow, and in which the fragments are scarcely separated.

LINE'OLA; a diminutive of *linea,* 'a line.' A small line.

LINE'OLÆ MAMMA'RUM. The white lines on the breasts.

LINGUA, Tongue — l. Bovis, Anchusa officinalis — l. Canina, Cynoglossum — l. Cervina, Asplenium scolopendrium — l. Exigua, Epiglottis — l. Prognosis ex, Glossomantia — l. Serpentaria, Ophioglossum vulgatum.

LINGUÆ AVIS, see Fraxinus excelsior — l. Detentor, Glossocatochus — l. Exoncosis, Glossoncus — l. Scalpium, *Cure-langue.*

LIN'GUAL, *Lingua'lis,* from *lingua,* 'the tongue.' Relating or belonging to the tongue.

LINGUAL AR'TERY, *Arte'ria lingua'lis,* arises from the external carotid; and, after several tortuosities, reaches the base of the tongue, becomes horizontal, and, under the name *Ranine,* advances to the tip, where it anastomoses with its fellow. In its course, it gives off the *Dorsalis linguæ* and *sublingual.*

LINGUAL MUSCLE, *Lingua'lis, Basio-glossus* (Cowper), *Glossia'nus,* is a small, long, fasciculus of fibres, hidden beneath the sides of the tongue, between the hyoglossus and styloglossus muscles, which are on the outside, and the genioglossus, within. This muscle passes from the base to the tip of the tongue; and, at its sides, is confounded with the muscles just referred to. It shortens the tongue, depresses its point, and can carry it to the right or left side.

LINGUAL NERVE is a name which has been given to the ninth pair or hypoglossus. It is, also, a term applied to a branch given off from the *Inferior maxillary,* or third branch of the fifth pair. Near its origin it anastomoses with, or simply runs close to, the chorda tympani. It afterwards gives off a considerable number of filaments, which are distributed to the tongue, and some of which are said to have been even traced as far as the papillæ; — a distribution which has occasioned it to be regarded as the *Gustatory nerve,* (F.) *Nerf gustatif.*

LINGUAL SALIVARY GLANDS, see Salivary glands.

LINGUAL VEIN follows nearly the same distribution as the artery. It opens into the internal jugular.

LINGUALIS, Lingual muscle.

LINGUETTA LAMINOSA, Lingula.

LINGULA, Ligula.

LIN'GULA, *Linguet'ta lamino'sa.* A thin, transversely grooved lobule of gray substance, derived from the anterior border of the cerebellum, which, for a short distance, lies over the velum medullare anterius.

LINGULA FISTULÆ, Epiglottis.

LINI USITATISSIMI SEMINA, see Linum usitatissimum.

LIN'IMENT, *Linimen'tum, Litus, Enchris'ton, Catachris'ton, Perich'risis, Perichris'ton, Aleiph'a, Aleim'ma, Enchris'ta, Frictum, Fricato'rium, Inunc'tio,* from *linire,* 'to anoint gently,' 'to anoint.' An unctuous medicine, containing usually oil or lard, which is used externally in the form of friction.

LINIMENT AMMONIACAL, Linimentum ammoniæ — *l. de Carbonate d'Ammoniaque,* Linimentum ammoniæ carbonatis.

LINIMENT ANTIHÉMORRHOÏDALE DE SIEUR ANDRY, (F.) This is formed of *Narbonne honey, Olive oil,* and *Turpentine.*

LINIMENT ANTIPARALYTIQUE, (F.) Composed of *subcarbonate of ammonia, alcoholized oil, black soap,* and *oil of rosemary.*

LINIMENT, ANTISCROF'ULOUS, OF HUFELAND. It is composed of *fresh ox-gall, White Soap, Unguentum althæ'æ, Volatile oil of petroleum, Carbonate of ammonia,* and *Camphor.*

LINIMENT CALCAIRE, Linimentum aquæ calcis — l. Camphor, Linimentum camphoræ — *l. Camphré,* Linimentum camphoræ — l. of Cantharides, camphorated, Linimentum e cantharidibus camphoratum — *l. Cantharide camphré,* Linimentum e cantharidibus camphoratum — *l. d'Eau de chaux,* Linimentum aquæ calcis — l. of Limewater, Linimentum aquæ calcis — *l. de Mercure,* Linimentum hydrargyri — l. Mercurial, Linimentum hydrargyri — *l. Oléo-calcaire,* Linimentum aquæ calcis.

LINIMENT RÉSOLUTIF DE POTT, composed of *oil of turpentine* and *muriatic acid.* Used in rheumatism, swellings, &c.

LINIMENT, SAINT JOHN LONG'S. A liniment used by a celebrated empiric at the commencement of the second quarter of the 19th century. It is said to have consisted of *oil of turpentine* and *acetic acid,* held in suspension by yolk of egg. It was a powerful counter-irritant.

LINIMENT DE SAVON, Linimentum saponis compositum — *l. de Savon opiacé,* Linimentum saponis et opii.

LINIMENT SAVONNEUX HYDROSULFURE DE JADELOT. Composed of *sulphuret of potass,* ʒvj; *white soap,* ℔ij; *oil of poppy,* ℔iv; *oil of thyme,* ʒij. Used in itch.

LINIMENT, SIMPLE, Linimentum simplex — l. Soap, Linimentum saponis — l. Soap and opium, Linimentum saponis et opii — l. Soap, compound, Linimentum saponis compos. — l. Turpentine, Linimentum terebinthinæ — l. of Verdigris, Linimentum æruginis — *l. de Vert-de-gris,* Linimentum æruginis — *l. Volatil,* Linimentum ammoniæ fortius.

LINIMENTUM, Liniment.

LINIMEN'TUM ÆRU'GINIS, *Ox'ymel Æru'ginis, Unguen'tum Ægyptiacum, Melli'tum de aceta'tā cupri, Linimentum of verdigris,* (F.) *Liniment de Vert-de-gris, Miel d'acétate de cuivre.* (*Ærugin.* cont. ʒj; *acet.* ʒvij; *mellis despum.* pond. ʒxiv. Liquefied, strained, and inspissated by boiling. — *Ph. L.*) It is used as an escharotic and detergent; — diluted, as a gargle in venereal ulcerations and in foul ulcers.

LINIMENTUM ALBUM, Ceratum cetacei, Unguentum cetacei — l. ad Ambustiones, L. aquæ calcis.

LINIMENTUM AMMO'NIÆ, *Sapo ammoniaca'lis, Linimen'tum ammonia'tum* seu *ammo'nicum* seu *Anglica'num, Sapo ammo'niæ olea'ceus, Unguen'tum album resol'vens, Oleum ammonia'tum, Linimentum ammo'niæ, Strong liniment of ammonia,* (F.) *Liniment volatil* ou *ammoniacal, Savon ammoniacal.* (*Liq. ammon.* f ʒj; *olei olivæ,* f ʒij. Mix. — *Ph. U. S.*) A stimulating and rubefacient soap.

LINIMENTUM AMMO'NIÆ CARBONA'TIS, *Liniment of subcarb'onate of ammo'nia, Linimentum ammo'niæ, Linimentum volat'ilē, Hartshorn and oil,* (F.) *Liniment de carbonate d'ammoniaque.* (*Solut. subcarb. ammon.* f ʒj; *olei oliv.* f ʒiij. Shake till they unite.) A stimulating liniment, mostly used to relieve rheumatic pains, bruises, &c.

LINIMENTUM AMMONIATUM seu AMMONICUM, L. ammoniæ fortis — l. Anglicanum, L. Ammoniæ fortis — l. ad Aphthas, Mel boracis.

LINIMENTUM AQUÆ CALCIS, *Linimentum Calcis* (Ph. U. S.), *Oleum lini cum calce, Sapo calca'rius, Linimentum ad ambustio'nes, Liniment of limewater,* (F.) *Liniment d'eau de chaux, Savon calcaire, Liniment calcaire, Liniment oléo-calcaire.*

(*Olei lini, aquæ calcis*, āā f℥ij. Misce.) A cooling and emollient application to burns and scalds.

LINIMENTUM ARCÆI, Unguentum elemi compositum — l. de Borate, Mel boracis — l. Calcis, L. aquæ calcis.

LINIMENTUM CAM'PHORÆ, *Oleum Camphora'tum, Solu'tio camphoræ oleo'sa, Camphor liniment*, (F.) *Liniment Camphré*, (*Camphoræ*, ℥iv; *olei olivæ*, f℥ij. Dissolve.) It is used as a stimulant and discutient.

LINIMENTUM CAM'PHORÆ COMPOS'ITUM, *Ward's essence for the headach, Compound camphor liniment.* (*Camphor*, ℥ij; *liq. ammoniæ*, f℥ii; *spirit. lavand.* Oj.—*Ph. L.*) It is stimulant and anodyne.

LINIMENTUM CANTHAR'IDIS, *Liniment of Spanish Flies.* (*Cantharid.* in pulv. ℥j; *Ol. Terebinth.* Oss. Digest for three hours by means of a water bath, and strain.—Ph. U. S.) Used as an excitant liniment in typhus, &c.

LINIMENTUM E CANTHARID'IBUS CAMPHORA'TUM, *Camph'orated liniment of canthar'ides*, (F.) *L. cantharide camphré.* (*Tinct. cantharid.* ℥ss; *ol. amygd. dulc.* ℥iv; *sapon. amygd.* ℥j; *camphor.* ℥ss. Dissolve the camphor in the oil, and add this mixture to the tincture and soap. — *Ph. P.*) Rubefacient, and discutient.

LINIMENTUM HYDRAR'GYRI, *Mercu'rial liniment*, (F.) *L. de Mercure.* (*Ung. Hyd. fort., adip. præp.* āā ℥iv; *camphoræ*, ℥j; *sp. rect.* gtt. xv; *liquor ammon.* f℥iv. Rub the camphor with the spirit; add the ointment and lard; and, lastly, gradually add the solution.—*Ph. L.*) It is used as a stimulant and discutient to venereal swellings, &c.

LINIMENTUM PLUMBATUM, Unguentum plumbi superacetatis — l. Saponaceum opiatum, L. saponis et opii.

LINIMENTUM SAPONA'CEUM HYDROSULPHURA'TUM. (*Common Soap*, 500 p. Liquefy in a water bath in an earthen vessel; and add *white poppy oil*, 250 p. Mix intimately, and add dry *sulphuret of potass*, 100 p. Beat together, and add *oil of poppy-seed*, 750 p.—*Ph. P.*) In cutaneous affections, as psora, herpes, &c.

LINIMENTUM SAPONATO-CAMPHORATUM, L. Saponis camphoratum.

LINIMENTUM SAPO'NIS, *Tinctu'ra saponis camphora'ta* (Ph. U.S.), *Camphorated Tincture of Soap, Soap Liniment.* (*Saponis* concis. ℥iv; *camphor.* ℥ij; *Ol. Rosmarin.* f℥ss; *alcohol*, Oij. Digest the soap and alcohol in a water bath, until the former is dissolved; filter, and add the camphor and oil.—Ph. U. S.) Used in sprains, bruises, and as an embrocation.

LINIMENTUM SAPO'NIS CAMPHORA'TUM, *L. S. compos'itum, L. Sapona'to-camphora'tum, Bal'samum opodel'doc, Tinctura saponis camphora'ta* (Ph. U. S.), *Opodel'doch, Steer's opodeldoch*, (F.) *L. de Savon. Compound Soap Liniment.* (*Sapon.* rasur. ℥iv; *Camphor.* ℥ij; *Ol. Rosmarini*, f℥ss; *Aquæ*, f℥iv; *Alcohol.* Oij. Mix the alcohol and water; digest the soap in the mixture by means of a water bath, until it is dissolved; filter, and add the camphor and oil.—(Ph. U. S.) Stimulant and anodyne; in bruises, local pains, &c.

Freeman's Bathing Spirits consist of *lin. sapon comp.* coloured with *Daffy's elixir*.

Jackson's Bathing Spirits differ from Freeman's in the addition of some essential oils.

LINIMENTUM SAPO'NIS ET OPII, *L. sapona'ceum opia'tum, Soap and opium liniment, Bates's anodyne balsam, Balsamum anod'ynum, Tinctura saponis et opii,* (F.) *L. de Savon opiacé.* (*Saponis* duri. ℥iv; *opii*, ℥j; *camphoræ*, ℥ij; *olei rorismarin.* f℥ss; *alcohol*, Oij.—*Ph. E.*) Anodyne; in chronic rheumatism and local pains in general.

LINIMENTUM SIMPLEX, *Simple Liniment.* (*Ol. oliv.* 4 p.; *ceræ albæ*, 1 p. fiat linimentum.—*Ph. E.*) Emollient; used in chaps, &c.

LINIMENTUM SIMPLEX, Unguentum ceræ.

LINIMENTUM TEREBIN'THINÆ, *Turpen'tine liniment.* (*Cerat. resinæ*, ℔j; *ol. terebinth.* Oss. Melt the cerate and stir in the oil.) A stimulant; applied to burns, &c.

LINIMENTUM VOLATILE, L. ammoniæ carbonatis.

LINNÆ'A, *L. Borea'lis.* This plant, called after Linnæus, has a bitter, sub-astringent taste; and is used, in some places, in the form of fomentation, in rheumatic pains. An infusion in milk is used in Switzerland for the cure of sciatica.

LINOSPERMUM, see Linum usitatissimum.

LINSEED, see Linum usitatissimum.

LINT, Carbasus, Linteum.

LINTEAMEN, Linteum, Pledget.

LIN'TEUM, *L. carptum* seu *rasum, Lintea'men, Oth'oně, Othon'ion, Car'basus, Car'basa, Car'pia, Motos, Motě, Motum, Linamen'tum, Tilma, Xystos, Xysma, Achně, Lint*, (F.) *Charpie.* A soft, flocculent substance, made by scraping old linen cloth, (F.) *Charpie râpée*, or by unravelling old linen cut into small pieces—(F.) *Charpie brute;* and employed in surgery as a dressing to wounds, ulcers, &c., either simply or covered with ointment.

LINTEUM CARPTUM, see Linteum — l. Rasum, see Linteum.

LINUM, see Linum usitatissimum—l. Arvense, L. usitatissimum.

LINUM CATHAR'TICUM, *L. min'imum, Chamæli'num, Purging flax* or *Mill mountain*, (F.) *Lin purgatif.* This plant is possessed of cathartic properties, and has a bitterish, disagreeable taste. Dose, ℥j, in substance.

LINUM CRUDUM, see Apolinosis — l. Minimum, L. Catharticum.

LINUM USITATIS'SIMUM, *L. arven'se, Common flax*, (F.) *Lin.* The seed, *Linum* (Ph. U. S.), *Sem'ina lini usitatis'simi, Linosper'mum, Linseed, Flaxseed*, (F.) *Grains de lin*, are inodorous, and almost tasteless; yielding mucilage to warm water, and oil by expression. They are demulcent and emollient. Linseed, when ground into powder, forms a good emollient poultice. It is only necessary to stir the powder into boiling water. The oil, *Oleum lini, Flaxseed oil*, (F.) *Huile de Lin*, is emollient and demulcent.

LIONDENT, Leontodon taraxacum.

LION'S FOOT, Nabalus albus, Prenanthes—l. Tail, Leonurus.

LIOPODIA, Leiopodes.

LIOPUS, Leiopus.

LIP, Sax. and Germ. Lippe, *Cheilos, La'bium, Labrum*, (F.) *Lèvre.* [In Entomology, *labium* means the lower lip,—*labrum*, the upper.] The lips are composed of different muscular fasciculi, nerves, and vessels, covered by the skin and mucous membrane of the mouth. They circumscribe the anterior aperture of that cavity; and are inservient to mastication, pronunciation, &c. They are distinguished into *upper* and *lower* — *Anochei'lon*, and *Catochei'lon* — and are placed in front of each jaw, forming between them the anterior aperture of the mouth. They unite at each side, and form what are called the *angles* or *commissures* of the mouth—*Chal'ini.* Their free edge is covered with a mucous membrane, of a more or less livid red, according to the individual. They receive their arteries from the external carotid. Their veins open into the two jugulars. Their lymphatic vessels descend into the ganglions situate beneath the chin. Their nerves are derived from the infra-orbitar, mental, and facial.

LIPS, *La'bia*, (F.) *Lèvres de la vulve*, are folds belonging to the genital organs of the female, and distinguished into—1. *Labia puden'di* seu *Cunni* seu *majo'ra*, *Episi'a*, *Alæ puden'di mulie'bris*, *Hytrochei'lides*, *Rupes*, *Alæ majo'res*, *Crem'noi*, (F.) *Grandes Lèvres*. These are two membranous folds, thicker above than below, which limit the vulva laterally, and extend from the inferior part of the mons veneris to the perinæum. They unite anteriorly and posteriorly, forming commissures; the posterior of which is called *Fourchette*. Their outer surface is convex; formed of skin and covered with hair. The inner surface is white, and covered by a mucous membrane, continuous with that lining the other parts of the vulva. The space between the skin and mucous membrane is filled with a fatty tissue and fibrous bands, some fibres of the constrictor vaginæ muscle, vessels, and nerves.

We speak, also, of the *lips of a wound, ulcer,* &c., when alluding to the edges of these solutions of continuity.

LIPA, λιπα, fat; also, Lippitudo.

LI'PARA, from λιπαρος, 'fatty,' and λιπα, 'fat.' Plasters, containing much oil or fat.

LIPARIA, see Polysarca.

LIPAROCE'LE, *Lipoce'lē*, from λιπαρος, 'fatty,' and κηλη, 'tumour.' *Lipo'ma*, or fatty tumour of the scrotum, *Her'nia pinguedino'sa scroti*.

LIPAROLÉ, Pomatum, *Pommade*.

LIPAROTES, see Polysarcia.

LIPAROTRICH'IA, from λιπαρος, 'fat,' and θριξ, 'hair.' Too great oiliness of the hair.

LIPASMA, see Polysarcia.

LIPEMANIA, Melancholy, see Lypemania.

LIPHÆMIA, Leiphæmia.

LIPHÆMOS, Leiphæmos.

LIPO or LEIPO, λειπω, 'I leave,' 'I forsake.' Hence, *Leipopsychia*, *Leipothymia*.

LIPOCELE, Liparocele.

LIPODERMIA, Aposthia.

LIPODERMOS, Leipodermos.

LIPO'MA, *Lypo'ma*, from λιπος, 'fat,' 'fatty tumour.' A fatty tumour of an encysted or other character.

LIPOME'RIA, *Leipome'ria*, from λειπω, 'I leave,' and μερος, a 'part.' Monstrosity from arrest of development, or from defect. Deficiency of one or more of the parts of the body; for example, where a person has only four fingers.

LIPOPSYCHIA, Syncope.

LIPOS, Pinguedo.

LIPOSIS, see Polysarcia.

LIPOTHYMIA, Syncope.

LIPPA, *Chassie*.

LIPPIA, Adali.

LIPPITU'DO, *Ophthal'mia chron'ica* of some, *Lippitude, Blear-eye, Lappa, Lipa, Xerophthal'mia, Lema, Lemē, Lemos'itas, Glemē, Glama, Gra'mia*. A copious secretion of the sebaceous humour of the eyelids, which renders them gummy. It is owing to a state of chronic inflammation of the tarsal margins; the eyelids being generally red, tumefied, and painful.

LIPPITUDO NEONATORUM, see Ophthalmia.

LIPPUS, *Chassieux*.

LIPSIS ANIMI, Syncope.

LIPSOTRICHIA, Alopecia, Calvities.

LIQUAMU'MIA, *Adeps huma'nus*. Human fat — Ruland and Johnson.

LIQUARIUM, Syrupus simplex.

LIQUATIO, Liquefaction.

LIQUEFA'CIENT, *Liquefa'ciens*, from *liquidus*, 'liquid,' and *facere*, 'to make.' A medicinal agent, which seems to have the power of liquefying solid depositions. To this class mercury, iodine, &c., have been referred by some.

LIQUEFAC'TION, *Liqua'tio*, *Liquefac'tio*; (same etymon.) Transformation of a solid substance into a liquid. It is used particularly in speaking of metals and fatty bodies, see Fusion.

LIQUEUR D'ALUMINE COMPOSÉE, Liquor aluminis compos. — *l. Arsénicale*, Liquor arsenicalis — *l. Fumante de Boyle*, Ammoniæ sulphuretum, Liquor fumans Boylii — *l. Volatile de corne de cerf*, Liquor volatilis cornu cervi — *l. de Cuivre ammoniacal*, Liquor cupri ammoniati — *l. de Fer alcaline*, Liquor ferri alkalini — *l. de Sous-acétate de plomb*, Liquor plumbi subacetatis — *l. de Potasse*, Liquor potassæ — *l. de Sous-carbonate de potasse*, Liquor potassæ subcarbonatis.

LIQUID, ADHESIVE, MAYNARD'S, Collodion—l. Disinfecting, Burnett's, see Burnett's disinfecting liquid — l. Disinfecting, Labarraque's, Liquor sodæ chlorinatæ — l. Disinfecting, Ledoyen's, see Ledoyen's disinfecting liquid.

LIQUIDAMBAR ASPLENIFOLIA, Comptonia asplenifolia—l. Officinalis, see Styrax—l. Peregrina, Comptonia asplenifolia.

LIQUIDAM'BAR STYRACIF'LUA, *Liquidam'bra, Sweet gum*. The name of the tree which affords the *Liquid amber* and *Storax liquida*, *Styrax liquida* or *Liquid storax*. Liquid amber is a resinous juice of a yellow colour, inclining to red; at first of about the consistence of turpentine; by age, hardening into a solid, brittle mass. It is not used medicinally.

Styrax Liquida is obtained from this plant by boiling. There are two sorts, — one more pure than the other. It is used, occasionally, as a stomachic, in the form of plaster.

LIQUIDUM NERVEUM, Nervous fluid.

LIQUIRITIA, Glycyrrhiza.

LIQUOR, *Liqua'men, Hygron', Hy'grotes*, (F.) *Liqueur*. A name given to many compound liquids, and especially to those the bases of which are water and alcohol.

LIQUOR ACIDUS HALLERI, Elixir acidum Halleri — l. Æthereus, Ether — l. Æthereus sulphuricus, Spiritus ætheris sulphurici.

LIQUOR ALU'MINIS COMPOS'ITUS, *Aqua alu'minis compos'ita, Aqua alumino'sa Batea'na, Compound solu'tion of Alum*, (F.) *Liqueur d'alumine composée*. (*Aluminis, zinci sulphat.* sing. ℥ss, *aquæ fervent.* Oij. Dissolve and filter through paper.) Detergent and stimulant. Used as a collyrium, when properly diluted, in ophthalmia; as an injection in gleet, leucorrhœa, &c.

LIQUOR AMMO'NIÆ, *Liq. ammoniæ puræ, Al'cali ammoni'acum flu'idum, Ammo'nia liq'uida, A. caus'tica liquida, A. pura liquida, Lixiv'ium ammoniaca'lē, Spiritus salis ammoniaci aquo'sus, Aqua ammoniæ, Aqua ammoniæ caus'ticæ, Liquid ammonia, Solution of ammonia*, (F.) *Ammoniaque liquide*. (Directed to be made in the Pharm. U. S. from *muriate of Ammonia*, in fine powder; and *Lime*, each a pound; *distilled water* a pint; *water*, nine fluidounces. The water is employed to slake the lime; this is mixed with the muriate of ammonia and put into a glass retort in a sand-bath. Heat is applied so as to drive off the ammonia, which is made to pass into a quart bottle containing the distilled water. To every ounce of the product three and a half fluidrachms of distilled water are added, or as much as may be necessary to raise its s. g. to 0.96. This Liquor Ammoniæ may also be made by mixing one part of liquor ammoniæ fortior with two parts of distilled water. (Ph. U. S. 1842.) Its s. g. is 0.960. LIQUOR AMMONIÆ FORTIOR, *Stronger solution of ammonia* (Ph. U. S.) is an aqueous solution of ammonia of the s. g. 0.882. Liquor ammoniæ is stimulant, antacid, and rubefacient. Dose gtt. to xx, in water or milk.

LIQUOR AMMONIÆ ACETA'TIS, *Al'cali ammoni'-acum aceta'tum, Alcali volat'ilĕ aceta'tum, Aqua aceta'tis ammo'niæ, Solution of acetate of ammonia, Aqua ammo'niæ aceta'ta, Ace'tas ammoniæ, Spirit of Mindere'rus, Sal ammoni'acum vegetab'ilĕ, Spir'itus ophthal'micus Mindere'ri, Sal aceto'sus ammoniaca'lis.* (*Acid. acetic. dilut.* Oij, *Ammon. carbonat.* in pulv. add the salt to the acid until it is saturated. Ph. U. S. 1851.) A sudorific; *externally,* cooling. Dose, f℥ij to f℥iss.

LIQUOR AMMONIÆ SUBCARBONA'TIS, *Solu'tio subcarbonatis ammoniæ, Aqaa carbonatis ammoniæ, Solution of subcarbonate of ammonia.* (*Ammoniæ carbon.* ℥iv, *aquæ destillat.* Oj. Dissolve and filter through paper.) *Use;* — the same as that of the carbonate of ammonia.

LIQUOR AMMONII HYDROTHIODIS, Ammoniæ sulphuretum — l. ex Ammoniâ et oleo succini, Spiritus ammoniæ succinatus — l. Ammonii vinosus, Spiritus ammoniæ.

LIQUOR AM'NII, *Aqua amnii.* The liquor of the amnios. (F.) *Eaux de l'amnios.* The fluid exhaled by the amnios, and which envelops the fœtus during the whole period of utero-gestation. It is often simply called the *waters,* (F.) *Les Eaux.* Its relative quantity diminishes as pregnancy advances, although its absolute quantity continues to increase till the period of delivery. In some women only five or six ounces are met with : in others, it amounts to pints. It is limpid, yellowish, or whitish; exhales a faint smell, and has a slightly saline taste. It contains water in considerable quantity; albumen; chloride of sodium; phosphate of lime; an alkaline substance; and a particular acid. It facilitates the dilatation of the uterus, and aids delivery by acting as a soft wedge enclosed in its membranes, *Poche dex Eaux,* &c. It is probably inservient to useful purposes in the nutrition of the fœtus.

LIQUOR AMNII, FALSE. The fluid contained between the amnion and chorion in the early periods of fœtal existence.

LIQUOR, ANODYNE, HOFFMANN's, Spiritus ætheris sulphurici compositus — l. Anodynus martialis, Alcohol sulphurico-æthereus ferri.

LIQUOR ANOD'YNUS TEREBINTHINA'TUS. A formula prescribed by Rademacher in cases of gallstone, and of obstructions and indurations of the liver and spleen. It was composed of *Hoffmann's anodyne liquor* ℥j; *rectified oil of turpentine* ∂ij. Dose 5 to 10 drops. It resembles the *Remède de Durand.*

LIQUOR ARSENICA'LIS, *L. potas'sæ arseni'tis* (Ph. U. S.), *Solu'tio arsenicalis, S. arsenica'ta, S. arseni'tis kal'icæ, Arsen'ical solution, Min'eral solvent, Ar'senis potas'sæ liq'uidus, Ar'senis potassæ aquo'sus, Fowler's solution of arsenic, Solvens minera'lĕ, Ital'ian poison, Aqua Tofa'na, Aqua Toffa'nia, Acqua della Toffana, Acqua di Napoli, Acquet'ta* (?), *Tasteless ague drop,* (F.) *Liqueur arsénicale.* (*Acid. Arsenios.* in frustulis, *potassæ carbonatis pur.,* sing. gr. lxiv., *aquæ destillat.* q. s. Boil together the arsenious acid and carbonate of potassa with twelve fluidounces of distilled water, in a glass vessel, until the arsenic is dissolved. When the solution is cold, add *Spirit. lavand. c.* f℥iv, and as much *distilled water* as will make the whole one pint. *Ph. U. S.*) f℥j contains gr. ss of the arsenious acid. Dose, gtt. xx.

LIQUOR ARSENICI ET HYDRARGYRI IODIDI, see Arsenic and Mercury, Iodide of — l. Barlii chloridi, Baryta, muriate, solution of — l. Bellosti, L. Hydrargyri nitrici — l Calcii chloridi, see Calcis murias.

LIQUOR CALCIS, *Solu'tio calcis, Aqua calcis, Aqua benedic'ta, Calca'ria pura liq'uida, Aqua calca'riæ ustæ, Solution of Lime, Lime Water,* (F.) *Eau de chaux.* (*Calcis* ℥iv. *aq. destill.* cong. Pour the water on the lime, and stir. Let it stand in a covered vessel three hours; bottle the lime and water in stopped bottles, and use the clear solution.) It is astringent, tonic, and antacid; and is used in diarrhœa, diabetes, heartburn, &c., and as a lotion to foul and cancerous ulcers, &c. Dose, ℥ij to Oss, in milk.

LIQUOR CALCIS COMPOS'ITUS, *Aqua calcis composita, Compound lime water, Aqua benedic'ta composita,* (F.) *Eau de chaux composé.* (*Lign. guaiac. ras.* ℔ss, *rad. glycyrrh.* ℥ j, *cort. sassafras,* ℥ss; *semin. coriand.* ℥ij, *liquor calcis,* Ovj. Macerate for two days, and filter.) It is stimulant, diaphoretic, and astringent, and is used in cutaneous affections.

LIQUOR CALCIS MURIATIS, see Calcis murias — l. Cereris, Cerevisia — l. Chloreti natri, L. sodæ chlorinatæ — l. Chlorini, see Chlorine — l. Chlorureti natri, L. Sodæ chlorinatæ — l. Chlorureti sodæ, L. sodæ chlorinatæ.

LIQUOR CUPRI AMMONIA'TI, *Aqua cupri ammonia'ti, Aqua sapphari'na, Blue eyewater, Solution of ammoniated copper;* (F.) *Liqueur ou Eau de cuivre ammoniacal.* (*Cupri ammoniat.* ℥j. *aquæ destill.* Oj. Dissolve and filter the solution through paper. *Ph. L.*) Corrosive and detergent. Used externally to foul ulcers; and diluted with an equal part of distilled water, it is applied by means of a hair pencil to specks and films, on the eye.

LIQUOR CUPRI SULPHA'TIS COMPOS'ITUS, *Aqua cupri vitriola'ti composita.* (*Cupri sulphat., alumin. sulphat.* āā ℥iij, *aquæ puræ* Oij, *acid sulph.* ℥ij. Boil the salts in the water until they are dissolved; then filter the liquor, and add the acid.) Used as an astringent in epistaxis, &c. It was also called *Aqua Styp'tica.*

LIQUOR CYRENIACUS, Benjamin — l. Excitans, Spiritus ammoniæ succinatus.

LIQUOR FERRI ALKALI'NI, *Solution of Alkaline Iron,* (F.) *Liqueur de fer alcaline.* (*Ferri* ℥iss, *acid. nitric.* ℥ij, *aquæ destillat.* f℥vj. *liq. potass. subcarb.* f℥vj. To the acid and water mixed, add the iron; and, after the effervescence, add the clear solution, gradually, to the *liq. potassæ subcarb.;* shaking it occasionally till it assumes a deep brown-red colour, and the effervescence stops. After six hours' settling, pour off the clear solution. *Ph. L.*) It is tonic, like other preparations of iron. Dose, f℥ss to f℥iss.

LIQUOR FERRI IO'DIDI, *Solution of Iodide of Iron, Syru'pus Ferri io'didi, Syrup of Iodide of Iron.* (*Iodin.* ℥ij, *Ferri ramant.* ℥j, *Sacchar. pulv.* ℥xij, *Aquæ destillat.* q. s. Mix the iodine with f℥x of the distilled water, in a porcelain or glass vessel, and gradually add the iron filings, constantly stirring. Heat the mixture gently until the liquor acquires a light greenish colour; then, having added the sugar, continue the heat a short time, and filter. Lastly, pour distilled water upon the filter, and allow it to pass until the whole of the filtered liquor measures twenty fluidounces. Keep the solution in closely stopped bottles. — Ph. U. S.) Dose, 10 to 30 drops.

LIQUOR FERRI MURIATIS, Tinctura ferri muriatis.

LIQUOR FERRI NITRA'TIS, *L. F. Sesquinitra'tis seu ternitra'tis, Solu'tio Ferri nitra'tis. Solution of nitrate, ternitrate of sesquioxide, or sesquinitrate of iron,* has been recommended in chronic diarrhœa and dysentery. Its virtues exactly resemble those of chloride of iron. It is prepared as follows: — *Ferri fili,* incis. ℥j, *Acid. nitric.* f℥iij, *Aq. destillat.* q. s. Mix the acid and a pint of distilled water, until gas ceases to be given off; filter, and add distilled water to make f℥xxx. — Ph. U. S.) Dose, 10 to 20 drops.

LIQUOR FUMANS BOY'LII, *Sulphure'tum Ammo'-niæ Hydrogena'tum, Hydrosulphure'tum Ammoniæ, Tinctu'ra Sul'phuris Volat'ilis, Aqua Sulphure'ti Ammoniæ, Boyle's Fuming liquor*, (F.) *Liqueur fumante de Boyle*. It is possessed of nauseating and emetic properties, and has been given in diabetes and diseases of excitement as a *deoxygenizer!*

LIQUOR FUMING, BOYLE'S, Liquor fumans Boylii—l. Fuming, of Libavius, Tin, muriate of—l. Genital, Sperm—l. of Hartshorn, volatile, Liquor volatilis cornu cervi—l. Hydrargyri Bichloridi, Liquor hydrargyri oxymuriatis—l. Hydrargyri chloridi corrosivi, L. hydrargyri oxymuriatis—l. Hydrargyri et arsenici iodidi, see Arsenic and Mercury, iodide of.

LIQUOR HYDRAR'GYRI NITRICI, *L. Bellosti*, (F.) *Eau mercurielle, Eau contre la gangrène, Remède du Duc d'Antin, R. du Capucin*, (*Hydrarg.* 120 p., *acid nitr.* (33°,) 150 p. Dissolve, and add to the solution, *distilled water*, 900 p. *Ph. P.*) Dose, two or three drops in a glass of water. Not much used.

LIQUOR HYDRAR'GYRI OXYMURIA'TIS, *Liquor Hydrar'gyri Chlo'ridi corrosi'vi, L. Hydrar'gyri bichloridi, Solu'tion of Oxymuriate of Mercury, Liquor Swietenii, L. Syphilit'icus Turneri, Mu'rias hydrargyri spirituo'sus liq'uidus, Solutio Muria'tis hydrar'gyri oxygenati, Liquor or Solution of Corro'sive Sub'limate or of Van Swieten.* (*Hyd. oxym.* ℈j, *aquæ destill.* f℥xv, *sp. rect.* f℥j. Dissolve in the water and add the spirit. *Ph. P.*) Dose, f℥ss, or f℥j.

Norton's Drops, Green's Drops, and *Solomon's Anti-Impetig''ines*—all nostrums—seem to be disguised solutions of *Corrosive Sublimate*.

LIQUOR HYDRARGYRI SUPERNITRATIS, see Hydrargyri nitras—l. Hydriodatis Arsenici et Hydrargyri, Arsenic and mercury, iodide of.

LIQUOR IO'DINI COMPOS'ITUS, (Ph. U. S. 1842,) *Liquor Iodin'ii compos'itus*, (Ph. U. S. 1851,) *Solu'tio Potas'sii Io'didi Iodure'ta, Compound Solution of Iodine, Lugol's Solution.* (*Iodin.* ℈j, *Potass. iodid.* ℈iss, *Aquæ destillat.* Oj. Dissolve the iodine and iodide of potassium in the water. — Ph. U. S.) Dose, gtt. vj. ad xij, in sugared water.

LIQUOR LITHARGYRI SUBACETATIS, L. plumbi subacetatis—l. Lithargyri subacetatis compositus, Liquor plumbi subacetatis dilutus.

LIQUOR OF MONRO, *Solution of Monro*. A solution, used by Monro for the preservation of anatomical preparations. It was composed of alcohol at 22° or 24°, with a drachm of nitric acid to each pint.

LIQUOR MORGAG'NII. The small quantity of fluid contained within the capsule of the crystalline lens.

LIQUOR MORPHI'NÆ seu MORPHIÆ ACETA'TIS, *Solution of Acetate of Morphia, An'odyne Drops.* (*Acetate of morphia*, gr. xvj, *distilled water*, f℥vj, *dilute acetic acid*, f℥ij.) Dose, from six to twenty-four drops.

LIQUOR MORPHI'NÆ seu MOR'PHIÆ SULPHA'TIS, *Solution of Sulphate of Morphia*. (*Morphiæ sulphat.* gr. viij, *aquæ destillat.* Oss. Dissolve the sulphate of morphia in the water.—Ph. U. S.) Dose, f℥j to f℥ij—containing from an eighth to a quarter of a grain.

LIQUOR NATRI OXYMURIATICI, L. Sodæ chlorinatæ—l. Nervinus Bangii, Tinctura ætherea camphorata—l. Oleosus Sylvii, Spiritus ammoniæ aromaticus—l. Opii sedativus, (Haden's,) see Tinctura opii.

LIQUOR OPII SEDATI'VUS. An empirical preparation by a London druggist of the name of Battley. It is said to be an aqueous solution of opium, evaporated to dryness to get rid of the acid resin, re-dissolved in water, and a small portion of alcohol added to give it permanence.—Redwood. It is devoid of many of the narcotic effects of opium.

LIQUOR OVI ALBUS, Albumen ovi—l. Pancreaticus, see Pancreas—l. Pericardii, see Pericardium—l. Plumbi acetatis, L. P. subacetatis—l. Plumbi diacetatis, Liquor Plumbi subacetatis.

LIQUOR PLUMBI SUBACETA'TIS, *Liquor Subaceta'tis Lithar'gyri, Solution of Subacetate of Lead, Liquor Plumbi Aceta'tis, L. P. Diaceta'tis*, Goulard's *Extrac'tum Satur'ni, Lithar'gyri Acc'tum*, (F.) *Liqueur de sous-acétate de Plomb*. (*Plumb. acet.* ℥xvj, *Plumb. oxid. semivitr.* in pulv. subtil. ℥ixss, *aq. destillat.* Oiv. Boil together in a glass or porcelain vessel, for half an hour, occasionally adding distilled water, so as to preserve the measure. Filter through paper, and keep the solution in closely stopped bottles.—Ph. U. S.) It is used externally as a cooling astringent, and discutient, when diluted with distilled water.

LIQUOR PLUMBI SUBACETA'TIS DILU'TUS, *Liquor Subaceta'tis Lithar'gyri Compos'itus, Aqua Satur'ni, Ace'tas Plumbi dilu'tum alcohol'icum, Diluted Solu'tion of Subac''etate of Lead, Aqua veg''eto-minera'lis, Tinctu'ra plumbo'sa, Aqua Lithar'gyri Aceta'ti compos'ita, Liquor Plumbi Aceta'tis dilu'tus, Goulard water*, (F.) *Eau, blanche, Eau de Goulard, Eau végéto-minérale, White Wash, Royal Preventive.* (*Liq. plumbi subacet.* f℥ij, *aquæ destillat.* Oj. Ph. U. S.) Properties the same as the last, but feebler.

LIQUOR POTAS'SÆ, *Aqua Potas'sæ, Aqua Kali Caust'ici, Solution of Potash or of Potassa, Lixiv'ium magistra'lè, L. Sapona'rium, Soap Lees, Aqua Kali puri, Soap Ley, Lixiv'ium cau'sticum, Potas'sa liq'uida*, (F.) *Eau, solution ou liqueur de Potasse, Potasse liquide, Lessive des Savonniers.* (*Potassæ carb.* ℔j, *calcis* ℔ss, *aquæ destill. fervent.* congium. Dissolve the alkali in Oij of the water, and add the remainder of the lime. Mix the whole: set aside in a close vessel, and, when cold, filter through calico. Ph. L.) It is antilithic in cases of uric acid calculi, and antacid. Externally, stimulant and escharotic. Dose, gtt. x to xx.

LIQUOR POTASSÆ ARSENITIS, L. arsenicalis—l. Potassæ Carbonatis, L. P. Subcarbonatis.

LIQUOR POTASSÆ CITRA'TIS, *Solution of Citrate of Potassa, Neutral Mixture, Saline Mixture.* (*Succ. Limon.* Oss, *Potass. Bicarbonat.* q. s.) saturate by the carbonate of potassa, and filter; or, *Acid. Citric* ℥ss; *Ol. Limon.* ♏. ij; *Aquæ* Oss, *Potass. Bicarbonat.* q. s.; dissolve, saturate by the carbonate of potassa, and filter. Ph. U. S.) Used in fever, but probably of little or no efficacy.

LIQUOR POTASSÆ SUBCARBONA'TIS, *L. P. Carbonatis* (Ph. U. S.), *Aqua Subcarbonatis Kali, O'leum Tar'tari per deliq'uium, Aqua Kali, Lixiv'ium Tartari, Aqua Kali præpara'ti, Oil of Tartar, Saline oil of Tartar, Solu'tion of Subcar'bonate of Potass*, (F.) *Liqueur de sous-carbonate de Potasse, Lessive de Tartre*, (*Potass. subcarb.* ℔j, *aquæ destillat.* f℥xij. Dissolve and filter.) Dose, gtt. x to xxx.

LIQUOR POTASSII IODIDI seu POTASSÆ HYDRIODA'TIS, *Solution of Iodide of Potassium or of Hydriodate of Potass.* (*Potassii iodid.* gr. 36, *aquæ destillat.* f℥j.) Dose, gtt. xx, three times a day.

LIQUOR, PROPAGATORY, Sperm—l. Prostaticus, Prostatic liquor—l. Puris, see Pus.

LIQUOR SANG'UINIS. A term given by Dr. Babington to one of the constituents of the blood, the other being the red particles. He considers, from his experiments that fibrin and serum do not exist as such in circulating blood, but that the *Liquor Sanguinis — Plasma*, of Schultz, *Coagulable* or *plastic Lymph*, the *Mucago* or *Mucilage* of Harvey, Hewson and others— when removed from the circulation and no longer subjected to the laws of life, has then, and not before, the property of separating into fibrin and serum. It is the oxyprotein of the liquor sanguinis, after the red particles have subsided, and, according to Mulder, forms the buffy coat of inflammatory blood.

LIQUOR OF SCARPA, *Vitrine auditive.*

LIQUOR SEM'INIS. The homogeneous, transparent fluid, in which the spermatozoa and seminal granules are suspended.—Wagner. See Sperm.

LIQUOR SODÆ CHLORIDI, L. sodæ chlorinatæ.

LIQUOR SODÆ CHLORINA'TÆ, *L. sodæ chlo'ridi, L. sodæ oxymuriat'icæ, L. chlore'ti natri, L. chlorureti natri, L. chloreti sodæ, L. chlorure'ti sodæ, Natrum chlora'tum liq'uidum, L. natri oxymuriat'ici, Aqua natri oxymuriat'ici, Labarraque's Disinfecting Liquid, Solution of Chlorinated Soda.* (*Culcis Chlorinat.* ℔j; *Sodæ Carbonat.* ℔ij; *Aquæ* cong. iss. Dissolve the carbonate of soda in three pints of the water, with the aid of heat. To the remainder of the water add, by small portions at a time, the chlorinated lime, previously well triturated, stirring the mixture after each addition. Set the mixture by for several hours, that the dregs may subside; decant the clear liquid, and mix it with the solution of carbonate of soda. Lastly, decant the clear liquor from the precipitated carbonate of lime, pass it through a linen cloth, and keep it in bottles secluded from the light; Ph. U. S.) Used in the same cases as the chloride of lime. Internally, 10 drops to a fluidrachm, for a dose. Diluted with water, it is an excitant and disinfectant in various *morbi externi.*

LIQUOR SODÆ EFFERVESCENS, Acidulous water, simple — l. Sodæ Oxymuriaticæ, L. sodæ chlorinatæ—l. Stypticus Ruspini, Styptic, Ruspini's—l. Sulphuricus Alcoolisatus, Spiritus ætheris sulphurici — l. Swietenis, L. hydrargyri oxymuriatis — l. Syphiliticus Turneri, L. hydrargyri oxymuriatis—l. Tartari emetici, Vinum antimonii tartarizati — l. of Van Swieten, L. hydrargyri oxymuriatis.

LIQUOR VOLAT'ILIS CORNU CERVI, *L. volat'ilis Cornu Cervi'ni, Vol'atile Liquor of Hartshorn, Spir'itus Lumbrico'rum, Spir'itus Millepeda'rum, Spir'itus Cornu Cervi, Liquor volat'ilis os'eium; Hartshorn, Spirit of Hartshorn, Bone Spirit,* (F.) *Liqueur volatile de Corne de cerf.* This is a solution of subcarbonate of ammonia, impregnated with empyreumatic oil. It possesses the same virtues as the subcarbonate of ammonia. It is in common use to smell at, in faintings, &c.

LIQUOR VOLATILIS OSSIUM, L. volatilis cornu cervi.

LIQUOR ZINCI SULPHA'TIS CUM CAMPH'ORÂ, *Aqua Zinci vitriola'ti cum Camphorâ, Aqua vitriol'ica camphora'ta, Aqua ophthal'mica, Common Eye Water.* (*Zinci sulph.* ʒss, *camphor,* ʒij, *aq. bullient.* Oij; dissolve and filter.) Used as a lotion for ulcers; or, diluted with water, as a collyrium.

LIQUORICE, Glycyrrhiza — l. Bush, Abrus precatorius — l. Juice, see Glycyrrhiza — l. Refined, Extractum glycyrrhizæ — l. Spanish, see Glycyrrhiza—l. Wild, Aralia nudicaulis, Galium circæzans.

LIQUORITIA, Glycyrrhiza.

LIRIODEN'DRON, *Liriodendron tulipif'era, Tulipif'era Lirioden'dron, Old wife's shirt, Tulip Tree, Poplar Tree, Tulip-bearing Poplar, American Poplar, White Wood, Cypress Tree,* (New England,) (F.) *Tulipier.* The bark — Lirioden*dron* (Ph. U. S.)—especially of the root, of this noble forest tree, which is indigenous in the United States, is a strong aromatic bitter, and has been employed advantageously as a tonic. An active principle was separated from it by Professor J. P. Emmet of the University of Virginia, and has been called *Lirioden'drin.* It is not used in medicine.

LIS BLANC, Lilium candidum—*l. Asphodèle,* Asphodelus ramosus.

LISERON, GRAND, Convolvulus sepium — *l. des Haies,* Convolvulus sepium—*l. Mechameck,* Convolvulus panduratus.

LISTON'S ISINGLASS PLASTER, see Sparadrapum adhæsivum.

LITE, λιτη. A plaster, formerly made of verdigris, wax, and resin.— Galen.

LITHAGO'GUM, from λιθος, 'a stone,' and αγω, 'I expel.' A remedy which was supposed to possess the power of expelling calculi. Also, a lithotomy forceps.

LITHANTHRAX, Carbo fossilis.

LITHANTHROKOKALI, Anthrakokali.

LITHARGE, Plumbi oxydum semivitreum—l. of Gold, see Plumbi oxydum semivitreum—l. of Silver, see Plumbi oxydum semivitreum.

LITHARGYRI ACETUM, Liquor plumbi subacetatis.

LITHARGYRUM, Plumbi oxydum semivitreum.

LITHARGYRUS, Plumbi oxydum semivitreum.

LITHAS, Urate.

LITHATE, Urate—l. of Soda, Urate of soda.

LITHEC'TASY, from λιθος, 'a stone,' and εκτασις, 'dilatation;' *Cystec'tasy.* An operation which consists in extracting stone from the bladder by dilating the neck of the organ, after making an incision in the perineum, and opening the membranous portion of the urethra.

LITH'IA, *Lithi'asis, Lithogen'ia, Uri'asis, Urolithi'asis, Cachex'ia calculo'sa, Cal'culi Morbus, Lapilla'tio, Genera'tio cal'culi,* from λιθος, 'a stone.' The formation of stone, gravel, or concretions in the human body. Also, an affection in which the eyelids are edged with small, hard, and stone-like concretions.

LITH'IA, CAR'BONATE OF, *Lith'iæ Car'bonas,* (F.) *Carbonate de Lithine.* A salt found in certain mineral waters, which have been serviceable in lithuria. Hence, it has been suggested in that morbid condition.

LITHIA RENALIS ARENOSA, Gravel—l. Renalis, Nephrolithiasis — l. Vesicalis, Calculi, vesical.

LITHIÆ CARBONAS, Lithia, carbonate of.

LITHIASIS, Lithia—l. Cystica, Calculi, vesical — l. Nephretica, Gravel, Nephrolithiasis.

LITHI'ASIS PULMO'NUM, *Pulmo'nes tartariza'ti.* The formation of concretions in the lungs, occasioning at times *Phthisis calculo'sa, Phthisis calculeuse,* of Bayle.

LITHIASIS RENALIS ARENOSA, Gravel — l. Renalis, Nephrolithiasis — l. Vesicalis, Calculi, vesical.

LITHIC, *Lith'icus.* Same etymon. Belonging to lithio or uric acid, or to stone: hence *Lithic Diath'esis.* Also, an antilithic.

LITHIC ACID, Uric acid—l. Acid diathesis, Lithuria—l. Diathesis, Lithuria—l. Sediments, see Lithuria.

LITHINE, CARBONATE DE, Lithia, carbonate of.

LITHIURIA, Lithuria.

LITHOCENOSIS, Lithotrity.

LITHOCYSTOTOMY, Lithotomy.

LITHODIALYSIS, Lithotrity.

LITHODRAS'SIC, *Lithodras'sicus,* (F.) *Litho-*

drassique, from λιθος, 'a stone,' and δρασσειν, 'to seize hold of.' An epithet given to a form of stone forceps—*Pince lithodrassique*—used in the operation of lithotrity, by MM. Meirieu and Tanchou.

LITHOGENIA, Lithia.

LITHOID, *Litho'des, Lithoï'des;* from λιθος, 'stone,' and ειδος, 'resemblance.' Of the nature of stone, or resembling stone: as

LITHOIDES OS, see Temporal bone.

LITHOLABE, (F.) *Lithol'abum*. An instrument, employed for laying hold of a stone in the bladder, and keeping it fixed, so that lithotritic instruments can act upon it.

LITHOLABON, Forceps, (Lithotomy.)

LITHOL'ABUM, from λιθος, 'a stone,' and λαμβανω, 'I seize.' An instrument concerned in extracting stone from the bladder. It had various shapes.— Fabricius ab Aquapendente, Hildanus. See Litholabe.

LITHOME'TRA, from λιθος, 'a stone,' and μητρα, 'the uterus.' Osseous, or other concretions of the uterus.

LITHONLYTIC, Lithontriptic.

LITHONTHRYPTIC, Lithontriptic.

LITHONTRIP'TIC, *Lithontrip'ticus, Lithonthryp'tic, Lithonlyt'ic, Calculif'ragus, Saxif'ragus*, from λιθος, 'a stone,' and θρυττω, 'I break in pieces.' A remedy believed to be capable of dissolving calculi in the urinary passages. There is not much reliance to be placed upon such remedies. By *antilithics*, exhibited according to the chemical character of the calculus (see Calculi, urinary,) the disease may be prevented from increasing; but most of the vaunted lithontriptics for dissolving the calculus already formed have been found unworthy of the high encomiums which have accompanied their introduction.

LITHOPÆ'DION, *Infans lapide'us, Osteopæ'dion*, from λιθος, 'a stone,' and παις, 'a child.' A fœtus, petrified in the body of the mother.

LITHOPRINIE, Lithotrity.

LITHOPRIONE, from λιθος, 'a stone,' and πριων, 'a saw.' An instrument proposed by M. Leroy for preventing the fragments of a calculus, when subjected to lithotrity, from falling into the bladder. It is a variety of *litholabe*.

LITHORINEUR, from λιθος, 'a stone,' and ρινειν, 'to file.' An instrument, proposed by MM. Meirieu and Tanchou for filing down calculi in the bladder.

LITHOS, Calculus.

LITHOSPER'MUM OFFICINA'LE, *Mil'ium Solis, Ægon'ychon, Gromwell, Bastard Al'kanet,* (F.) *Grémil officinal, Herbe aux Perles*. The seeds of this plant were formerly supposed, from their stony hardness, (λιθος, 'a stone,' and σπερμα, 'seed,') to be efficacious in calculous affections. They have, also, been considered diuretic.

LITHOSPERMUM VILLOSUM, Anchusa tinctoria.

LITHOTERE'THRUM, from λιθος, 'stone,' and τερειν, 'to rub.' A lithotritor.

LITHOTHRYPSIS, Lithotrity.

LITHOTHRYPTORS, see Lithotrity.

LITHOTOME, Lithot'omus, from λιθος, 'a stone,' and τεμνω, 'I cut.' This name has been given to a number of instruments of different shapes and sizes, which are used in the operation for the stone, to cut the neck or body of the bladder. They ought, with more propriety, to be called *Cystotomes*.

The *Lithotome Caché* of Frère Côme is the most known, and is still occasionally used. It is composed of a handle, and a flattened sheath, slightly curved: in this there is a cutting blade, which can be forced out, by pressing upon a *bas-cule* or lever, to any extent that may be wished by the operator.

A *Double Lithotome* was used by Dupuytren in his bilateral operation. See Lithotomy.

LITHOT'OMIST. Same etymon. *Lithot'omus*. One who devotes himself entirely to operating for the stone. One who practises lithotomy.

LITHOT'OMY, *Lithotom'ia, Cystotom'ia, Urolithotom'ia, Sectio vesica'lis, Lithocystot'omy*, same etymon. (F.) *Taille*. The operation by which a stone is extracted from the bladder. The different methods, according to which this operation may be practised, are reducible to five principal; each of which has experienced numerous modifications.

1. The *Method of Celsus, Meth'odus Celsia'na, Cystotom'ia cum appara'tu parvo, Appara'tus Minor, Cutting on the Gripe*. This consisted in cutting upon the stone, after having made it project at the perinæum by means of the fingers introduced into the rectum. This method was attended with several inconveniences; such as the difficulty of dividing the parts neatly, injury done to the bladder, as well as the impossibility of drawing down the stone in many persons. It is sometimes, also, called *Meth'odus Guytonia'na;* from Guy de Chauliac having endeavoured to remove from it the discredit into which it had fallen in his time. It was termed *Apparatus Minor,* (F.) *Le petit appareil,* from the small number of instruments required in it.

2. *Apparatus Major*. This method was invented, in 1520, by John de Romani, a surgeon of Cremona, and communicated by him to Mariano-Santo-di-Barletta, whence it was long called *Mariano's Method, Sec'tio Maria'na*. It was called, also, *Apparatus Major,* and *Cystotom'ia* vel *Meth'odus cum appara'tu magno,* (F.) *Le grand appareil,* from the number of instruments required in it. An incision was made on the median line; but the neck of the bladder was not comprehended in it. It was merely dilated. The greater apparatus was liable to many inconveniences, such as ecchymoses; contusion; inflammation of the neck of the bladder; abscesses; urinary fistulæ; incontinence of urine; impotence, &c.

3. The *High Operation, Apparatus altus, Cystotom'ia cum apparatu alto, C. Hypogas'trica, Epicystotom'ia, Laparocystotom'ia, Sectio seu Meth'odus Franconia'na, S. Hypogas'trica, S. alta,* (F.) *Haut appareil, Taille Hypogastrique, Taille sus-pubienne,* was first practised by Peter Franco, about the middle of the 16th century. It consisted in pushing the stone above the pubis by the fingers introduced into the rectum. Rousset afterwards proposed to make the bladder rise above the pubis by injecting it. The method had fallen into discredit, when Frère Côme revived it. It is used when the calculus is very large. It was practised by opening first the membranous part of the urethra upon the catheter passed into the canal. Through this incision, the *Sonde à dard* — a species of catheter, having a spearpointed stilet — was introduced into the bladder. An incision was then made into the linea alba, above the symphysis pubis, of about four or five fingers' breadth, and the peritoneum detached to avoid wounding it. The stilet was pushed through the bladder, and used as a director for the knife, with which the bladder was divided anteriorly, as far as the neck; and the stone extracted. It was performed in England by Douglass, in 1719, and since by others, with various modifications.

4. The *Lateral Operation, Hypocystotom'ia, Cystotom'ia latera'lis, Cystauchenotom'ia, Cysto-

trachelotom'ia, Urethrocystauchenotom'ia, Ure-throcysteotrachelotom'ia, Sec'tio latera'lis, Appa-ra'tus latera'lis, (F.) *Appareil lateralisé,* so named from the prostate gland and neck of the bladder being cut laterally, was probably invented by Peter Franco. It was introduced into France by Frère Jacques de Beaulieu. He performed it with rude instruments, invented by himself, and improved by the suggestions of some of the Parisian surgeons. In England, it received its earliest and most important improvements from the celebrated Cheselden. It is the method practised at the present day, according to different modes of procedure. In this method, the patient is placed upon a table; his legs and thighs are bent and separated; the hands being tied to the feet. The perinæum is then shaved, and a staff is introduced into the bladder; the handle being turned towards the right groin of the patient. An oblique incision is now made from the raphe to the middle of a line drawn from the anus to the tuberosity of the ischium of the left side; and taking the staff for a guide, the integuments, areolar tissue of the perinæum, membranous portion of the urethra, transversus perinæi muscle, bulbo-cavernosus, some fibres of the levator ani, the prostate and neck of the bladder, are successively divided. For this latter part of the operation, the knife, the beaked bistoury, *Bistouri* ou *Lithotome Caché,* cutting gorget, &c., is used, according to the particular preference. The forceps are now introduced into the bladder, and the stone extracted. In the operation, care must be taken not to injure the rectum, or the great arterial vessels, distributed to the perinæum.

A variety of the *Lateral Apparatus,* called by the French *Appareil latéral,* consisted in cutting into the *bas-fond* of the bladder, without touching the neck of that organ: but it was soon abandoned, on account of its inconveniences.

The method of Le Cat and of Pajola—*Urethrocysteo-aneurysmatotom'ia*—consists in dividing the prostate in part only,—the enlargement of the wound being effected by a peculiar dilator.

The *Bilateral Operation* is founded on that of Celsus. It consists in making an incision posterior to the bulb of the urethra, and anterior to the anus, involving both sides of the perinæum by crossing the raphe at right angles: an incision is then made through the membranous part of the urethra, and the prostate may be cut bilaterally, either with the double lithotome of Dupuytren, or the prostatic bisector of Dr. Stevens, of New York.

5. *Lithotomy by the Rectum, Proctocystotom'ia, Sec'tio recto-vesica'lis,* (F.) *Taille par le Rectum, Taille postérieure, T. Recto-vésicale.* This was proposed by Vegetius in the 16th century; but it was never noticed until M. Sanson, in the year 1817, attracted attention to it; since which time it has been successfully performed in many instances. It consists in penetrating the bladder through the paries corresponding with the rectum, by first cutting the sphincter ani and rectum about the root of the penis, and penetrating the bladder by the neck of that organ, dividing the prostate,—or by its *bas-fond.*

Lithotomy in women, from the shortness of the urethra, is a comparatively insignificant operation.

LITHOTOMY BY THE RECTUM, see Lithotomy—L. by the Vagina, see Lithotomy.

LITHOTRESIS, Lithotrity.
LITHOTRIPSIS, Lithotrity.
LITHOTRIPSY, Lithotrity.
LITHOTRIPTORS, see Lithotrity.
LITHOTRITES, see Lithotrity.
LITHOTRITEURS, see Lithotrity.

LITHOTRITOR, see Lithotrity.
LITHOT'RITY, *Lithotri'tia, Lithotrypsy, Lithotripsy. Lithothrip'sy, Lithothryp_is, Lithotre'sis, Lithotripsis, Lithoceno'sis, Lithodial'ysis, Lithoprinie,* from λιθος, 'a stone,' and τρηβω, 'I break.' The operation of breaking or bruising the stone in the bladder. It has been performed, of late years, with success, by French, and, after them, by English and American surgeons. The instruments employed for this purpose are called, in the abstract, *Lithotrites, Lithotriteurs. Lithotritors, Lithotriptors,* and *Lithothryptors.* The most celebrated are those of Civiale, Jacobson, Heurteloup and Weiss. See *Brise-Pierre articulé,* and *Percuteur à Marteau.*

LITHOXIDU'RIA, from λιθος, 'a stone,' *oxide,* and ουρον, 'urine.' The discharge of urine containing lithic or xanthic oxide.

LITHU'RIA, *Lithiu'ria, Lithourorrhée* (Piorry;) from λιθος, 'a stone,' and ουρον, 'urine.' *Lithic Diath'esis, Lithic Acid Diathesis.* The condition of the system and of the urine in which deposits of lithic acid and the lithates—*Lithic sediments*—take place from the urine. See Urine.

LITHUS, Calculus.
LITMUS, Lichen roccella.
LITRA, Pound.
LITRE, *Litra.* A measure containing a cubed decimètre, which is equal nearly to 2.1135 pints. The ancients gave the name *litra,* λιτρα, to a measure capable of containing 16 ounces of liquid.

LITSÆA CUBEBA, Piper cubeba—L. Piperita, Piper cubeba.

LITUS, Liniment.
LIVÈCHE, Ligusticum levisticum.

LIVER, Sax. lipep, *Hepar, Jecur, Jec"inus,* (F.) *Foie.* The liver is the largest gland in the body. It is an azygous organ; unsymmetrical; very heavy; and of a brownish-red colour; occupying the whole of the right hypochondrium, and a part of the epigastrium. *Above,* it corresponds to the diaphragm; *below,* to the stomach, transverse colon, and right kidney; *behind,* to the vertebral column, aorta, and vena cava; and *before,* to the base of the chest. Its upper surface is convex; the lower, irregularly convex and concave, so that anatomists have divided the organ into three lobes,—a *large* or *right* or *colic lobe;*—a *lesser lobe, lobule,* or *inferior lobe,* the *Lobulus Spigelii,*—and a *middle* or *left lobe.* At its inferior surface, are observed:—1. A *Sulcus* or *Furrow* or *Fissure,* called *horizontal* or *longitudinal, Great fissure, Fossa Umbilica'lis,* (F.) *Sillon horizontal, longitudinal, S. de la veine ombilicale, Sulcus antero-posterior Jec'oris, S. horisonta'lis Jec'oris, S. longitudina'lis Jecoris, S. sinis'ter Jecoris, S. Umbilica'lis,* which lodges, in the fœtus, the umbilical vein and ductus venosus. 2. The *Principal Fissure,* termed *Sulcus Transversus* vel *Sinus Porta'rum, Fissure of the Vena porta, Portal Fissure,* (F.) *Sillon transversal ou de la veine porte,* which receives the sinus of the vena porta. 3. The *Fissure of the Vena Cava infe'rior, Sillon de la veine cave inférieure,* situate at the posterior margin of the organ, and lodging the vena cava inferior. 4. The *Lobulus Spige'lii,* or *posterior portal eminence.* 5. The *anterior portal eminence, Auri'ga* vel *Lobulus anon'ymus.* 6. Depressions corresponding to the upper surface of the stomach, gall-bladder, arch of the colon, right kidney, &c. Continued from the fossa umbilicalis is a small fossa, called *Fossa Ductûs Veno'si,* between the left lobe and Lobulus Spigelii. The posterior margin of the liver is very thick; much more so than the anterior. The liver is surrounded by a serous or peritoneal covering, which forms for it a *suspensory* or *broad ligament* and two *lateral* and *triangular* ligaments. See Falx. The blood-vessels of the liver are very numerous. The hepatic artery and vena porta furnish it with the blood necessary for its nutrition and the secretion of bile. The hepatic veins convey away the blood, which has served those purposes. The lymphatic vessels are very numerous; some being superficial; others deep-seated. The nerves are, also, numerous, and proceed from the pneumogastric, diaphragmatic, and from the hepatic plexuses.

The intimate structure of the parenchyma of the liver has been well studied. When cut, it presents a porous appearance, owing to the division of a multitude of small vessels. When torn, it seems formed of granulations;—the intimate structure of which has given rise to many hypotheses. In these granulations are contained the radicles of the excretory ducts of the bile; the union of which constitutes the hepatic duct. According to M. Kiernan, the intimate structure consists of a number of lobules composed of *intralobular* or hepatic veins, which convey the blood back that has been inservient to the secretion of bile. The *interlobular* plexus of veins is formed by branches of the vena porta, which contain both the blood of the vena porta and of the hepatic artery; both of which, according to Mr. Kiernan, furnish the pabulum of the biliary secretion. The biliary ducts form likewise an *interlobular plexus*, having an arrangement similar to that of the interlobular veins. Mr. Kiernan's views are embraced by many anatomists; but are denied by some.

The liver is the only organ, which, independently of the red blood carried to it by the hepatic artery, receives black blood by the vena porta. The general opinion is, that the vena porta is the fluid which furnishes bile, whilst that of the artery affords blood for the nutrition of the liver. It is probable, however, that bile is secreted by the latter vessel.

The liver is liable to a number of diseases. The principal are — *Hepati'tis* or *inflammation*, cancer, *biliary calculi*, *encysted* and other *tumours* or *tubercles, hydatids*, &c.; and it has, at times, been the *fashion* to refer to it as the cause of symptoms with which it is in no wise connected.

LIVER, *Hepar*. Under this name the ancients designated several substances, having a brownish colour, analogous to that of the liver; and composed of sulphur and some other body. See Potassæ Sulphuretum, *Liver of Sulphur*.

LIVER *of Antimony* is the semi-vitreous sulphuret, &c.

LIVER DISEASE, Hepatopathia—l. Fatty, Adiposis hepatica—l. Gin, L. nutmeg—l. Gin-drinkers', L. nutmeg—l. Granulated, Cirrhosis of the liver.

LIVER-GROWN, *Tu'mido jec'oră præ'ditus*. Having a large liver.

LIVER, HOBNAIL, Cirrhosis of the liver — l. Mammillated, Cirrhosis of the liver.

LIVER, NUTMEG, *Tu'beriform liver*. An appearance of the liver when cut across, resembling that of the section of a nutmeg; supposed by some to be the result of intemperance in the use of alcoholic drinks; but occurring under other causes. The terms *whisky liver, gin-drinkers' liver*, and *gin liver*, occasionally applied to it, are, consequently, not distinctive.

LIVER SPOT, Chloasma — l. Tuberculated, Cirrhosis of the liver — l. Tuberiform, L. nutmeg — l. Weed, Hepatica triloba—l. Whisky, L. nutmeg—l. Wort, Hepatica triloba, Marchantia polymorpha—l. Wort, ground, ash-coloured, Lichen caninus — l. Wort, Iceland, Lichen Islandicus — l. Wort, noble, Hepatica triloba.

LIVIDUS MUSCULUS, Pectinalis.
LIVOR, Suggillation — l. Sanguineus, see Ecchymoma.
LIVRE, Pound.
LIXIVIA TARTARIZATA, Potassæ tartras — l. Vitriolata, Potassæ sulphas — l. Vitriolata sulphurea, Potassæ sulphas cum sulphure.
LIXIVIÆ seu KALICUM ACETAS, Potassæ acetas.
LIXIV'IAL, *Lixivio'sus*, from *lixivium*, 'lee.' (F.) *Lixivial, Lixivieux*. An ancient term for salts obtained by washing vegetable ashes,—such as the fixed alkalies.
LIXIVIA'TION, *Elixivia'tion, Lixivia'tio*. Same etymon. An operation which consists in washing wood-ashes with water, so as to dissolve the soluble parts. The filtered liquor is the *lee*.
LIXIV'IUM, *Lixiv'ia, Con'ia, Lee, Ley, Lye*, (F.) *Lessive*. Any solution containing potass or soda — *Sal lixivio'sum* — in excess; from *lix*, 'potash.'
LIXIVIUM AMMONIACALE, Liquor ammoniæ — l. Ammoniacale aromaticum, Spiritus ammoniæ aromaticus — l. Causticum, Liquor potassæ — l. Magistrale, Liquor potassæ — l. Saponarium, Liquor potassæ — l. Tartari, Liquor potassæ subcarbonatis.
LIZARD, *Lacer'ta, Lacer'tus*, said to be so called in consequence of its limbs resembling the arms (*lacerti*) of man (?). *Saura, Sauros*, (F.) *Lésard*. Lizards were formerly employed in medicine as sudorifics; and were, at one time, extolled in syphilis, cutaneous affections, and in cancer.
LIZARD'S TAIL, Saururus cernuus.
LOADSTONE, Magnet.
LOATHING, Disgust.
LOBARIA ISLANDICA, Lichen Islandicus — l. Pulmonaria, Lichen pulmonarius — l. Saxatilis, Lichen saxatilis.
LOBE, *Lobus*. A round, projecting part of an organ. The liver, lungs, and brain, for example, have lobes.
LOBE OF THE EAR, *Lob'ule of the Ear*, is a soft, rounded prominence, which terminates the circumference of the pavilion inferiorly, and which is pierced in those who wear rings.
The under surface of the brain is divided into *two anterior, two lateral, two posterior*, and *two intermediate lobes* or *processes*. These Chaussier calls *lobules* of the brain: the cerebral hemispheres he terms *lobes*.
LOBE, BIVEN'TRAL. A wedge-shaped lobe of the cerebellum, situate behind the amygdala.
LOBE DOUDÉNAL, Lobulus Spigelii — *l. Pancréatique*, Lobulus Spigelii — *l. Petit du foie*, Lobulus Spigelii — *l. de Spigel*, Lobulus Spigelii.
LOBELIA, BLUE, L. syphilitica.
LOBE'LIA CARDINA'LIS, *Lobelia coccin'ea, Trache'lium Ameri'canum, Car'dinal Plant, Car'dinal Flower, Scarlet Lobelia*. This species is also indigenous in the United States. It blooms in autumn, having beautiful carmine flowers. The root is a reputed anthelmintic with the Indians.
LOBELIA COCCINEA, L. Cardinalis.
LOBE'LIA INFLA'TA, *Indian Tobac'co, Wild Tobac'co, Puke Weed, Asthma Weed, Eyebright, Emet'ic Weed, Lobe'lia* (Ph. U. S.) The prominent virtues of this American plant are those of an emetic. In smaller doses it is sedative, and has been given as a pectoral in croup, asthma, &c. It is, also, sudorific and cathartic, and is an acronarcotic poison. Twenty grains act as an emetic.
LOBELIA PINIFO'LIA. A South African plant, *Nat. Ord.* Campanulaceæ, the root of which is excitant and diaphoretic. A decoction of it is

sometimes used in the Cape Colony as a domestic remedy in cutaneous affections, chronic rheumatism, and gout.

LOBELIA, SCARLET, L. Cardinalis.

LOBELIA SYPHILIT'ICA, *Lobelia reflex'a, Ranun'culus Virginia'nus, Rapun'tium Syphilit'icum, Blue Lobelia, Blue Car'dinal Flower*. The root of this plant, which is indigenous in the United States, is an emetic and drastic cathartic. It has been used in syphilis; hence its name. The mode of preparing it is to boil ℥ss of the dried root in Oxij of water, until the fluid is reduced to Oviij. Dose, Oss.

LOBES, CEREBRAL, see *Lobe*.

LOBES OF THE LIVER, *Pinnæ* seu *Lobi* seu *Pin'nulæ He'patis*. See Lobule.

LOBES, OPTIC, Quadrigemina tubercula.

LOBI HEPATIS, Lobes of the liver — l. Pulmonum, see Pulmo.

LOB'ULAR, *Lobula'ris*. Same etymon as Lobule. Relating to or belonging to a lobule: — as *lobular pneumonia*, (F.) *Pneumonie lobulaire, P. mamelonnée, P. disséminée*. Pneumonia anatomically characterized by nuclei of red or gray hepatization disseminated in variable numbers in one or both lungs.

LOBULAR BILIARY PLEXUS. The plexus formed of lobular hepatic ducts, which are derived chiefly from the interlobular. This plexus forms the principal part of the substance of the lobule.

LOBULAR VENOUS PLEXUS. The plexus interposed between the interlobular portal veins, and the intralobular hepatic vein.

LOB'ULE, *Lob'ulus*, diminutive of *Lobus*. A little lobe. Mr. Kiernan uses the term *lobule* for an *acinus* of the liver of many anatomists.

LOBULE OF THE CORPUS STRIATUM, Insula cerebri — l. of the Ear, Lobe of the Ear — l. of the Fissure of Sylvius, Insula cerebri — l. Pneumogastric, Flocculus.

LOBULE DU FOIE, Lobulus Spigelii.

LOBULUS ACCESSORIUS ANTERIOR QUADRATUS, L. anonymus.

LOB'ULUS seu LOBUS ANON'YMUS, *L. accesso'rius ante'rior quadra'tus, L. quadra'tus*, (F.) *Éminence porte antérieure*. This is situate in the liver between the passage for the round ligament and the gall-bladder, and is less prominent, but broader, than the *Lobulus caudatus*. From the lobulus anonymus a bridge runs across the passage for the round ligament. It is called *Pons vel Isthmus he'patis*.

LOBULUS seu LOBUS CAUDA'TUS, *Proces'sus caudatus*. This is merely the root or one of the angles of the lobulus Spigelii, advancing towards the middle of the lower side of the great lobe, and representing a kind of tail. Also, the termination of the helix and anthelix of the ear, which is separated from the concha by an extensive fissure.

LOB'ULUS CENTRA'LIS. A small lobule or prominence of the superior vermiform process of the cerebellum, situate in the incisura anterior.

LOBULUS NASI, see Nasus — l. Pneumogastricus, Flocculus—l. Posterior, L. Spigelii—l. Posticus papillatus, L. Spigelii — l. Quadratus, L. anonymus.

LOBULUS seu LOBUS SPIGE'LII, *L. poste'rior, L. posti'cus papilla'tus*, (F.) *Éminence porte postérieure, Lobule* ou *Petit lobe du foie, Lobe de Spigel, Lobe duodénal, L. pancréatique*, is situate near the spine, upon the left side of the great lobe of the liver, and is of a pyramidal shape, projecting, like a nipple, between the cardia and vena cava, at the small curvature of the stomach.

LOBUS, Lobe, see Lobulus.

LOCAL, *Loca'lis, Top'icus, Mer'icus, Partia'lis, Top'ical*, (F.) *Locale, Topique*. An affection is called *local — Morbus Loca'lis*, — when confined to a part, without implicating the general system; or, at all events, only secondarily. *Local* is thus opposed to *general*. A *local* or *topical application* is one used externally. See Topical.

LOCH, Looch.

LOCHADES, see Sclerotic.

LOCHI'A or LO'CHIA, *Purgamen'ta Puerpe'rii* seu *U'teri, Purga'tio puerpe'rii, Lyma*, from λοχος, 'a woman in childbed;' (F.) *Suites de couches, Vidanges*. The *cleansings*. A serous and sanguineous discharge following delivery. During the first two or three days, it is bloody; but afterwards becomes green-coloured, and exhales a disagreeable and peculiar odour. The duration, quantity, and character of the discharge vary according to numerous circumstances. It flows from the part of the uterus which formed a medium of communication between the mother and fœtus, and continues, usually, from 14 to 21 days. See Parturition.

LOCHIOCŒLIITIS, Puerperal fever.

LOCHIODOCHIUM, Lochodochium.

LOCHIOPYRA, Puerperal fever.

LOCHIORRHAG"IA, from λοχεια, and ῥηγνυμι, 'I make an irruption.' An immoderate flow of the lochia. Hemorrhage from the uterus in the child-bed state.

LOCHIORRHŒ'A, from λοχεια, 'the lochia,' and ῥεω, 'I flow.' Discharge of the lochia.

LOCHIORUM RETENTIO, Ischolochia.

LOCHIOSCHESIS, Ischolochia.

LOCHOCH, Looch,

LOCHODOCHI'UM, *Lochiodochium*, from λοχος, 'a female in childbed,' and δεχομαι, 'I receive.' An institution for the reception of pregnant and childbed females. A *Lying-in-hospital*.

LOCHOS, Puerpera.

LOCI, Uterus — l. Muliebres, Uterus, Vulva.

LOCKED JAW, Trismus.

LOCOMOTILITY, see Locomotion.

LOCOMO'TION, *Locomo'tio*, from *locus*, 'a place, and *movere*, 'to move.' An action peculiar to animal bodies, by which they transport themselves from place to place. It, as well as *muscula'tion*, has also been used for the function of animal movements. The faculty is sometimes called *Locomotiv'ity* and *Locomotil'ity*.

LOCOMOTION OF AN ARTERY, is the movement produced in a vessel with a curvature, by the impulse of the blood sent from the heart, which tends to straighten the artery, and causes the movement in question.

LOCOMOTIVITY, see Locomotion.

LOCUS NIGER, see Peduncles of the Brain.

LOCUS PERFORA'TUS ANTI'CUS. A triangular flat surface of the brain, which corresponds to the posterior extremity of each olfactory process.

LOCUS PERFORATUS POSTICUS, Tarini pons.

LOCUST, BLACK, Robinia Pseudo-acacia — l. Eaters, Acridophagi—l. Plant, Cassia Marilandica—l. Tree, Robinia Pseudo-acacia—l. Yellow, Cladrastis tinctoria.

LODOICEA, see Coco of the Maldives.

LOECHE, MINERAL WATERS OF, Leuk, mineral waters of.

LŒME, Plague.

LŒMIA, Plague.

LŒMICUM, see Lœmology.

LŒMOCHOLOSIS, Fever, yellow.

LŒMOGRAPHY, Loimography.

LŒMOLOGIUM, see Lœmology.

LŒMOL'OGY, *Lœmolog"ia*, from λοιμος, 'plague,' and λογος, 'a description.' The doctrine of plague and pestilential diseases. A treatise on the same, — *Lœ'micum, Lœmolog"ium*.

LŒMOPHTHALMIA, see Ophthalmia.
LÆMOPYRA, Plague.
LŒMOS, Plague.
LOGADES, Sclerotic.
LOGADITIS, Sclerotitis.
LOGIATROS, *Logiater;* from λογος, 'a word,' and ιατρος, 'a physician.' In the bad sense, a physician without experience; a mere theorist. In the good sense, a rational physician; one who treats disease according to theoretical or scientific principles.
LOGOS, Reason.
LOGWOOD, Hæmatoxylon Campechianum.
LOG"Y, λογος, 'a description.' A suffix denoting 'a treatise or description.' Hence, Angio*logy* and Neuro*logy*, &c.
LOHOCH, Looch.
LOIMOCHOLOSIS, Fever, yellow.
LOIMOG'RAPHY, *Loimograph'ia, Lœmog'raphy*, from λοιμος, 'plague,' and γραφω, 'I describe.' A description of the plague and pestilential diseases.
LOIMOLOGY, Lœmology.
LOIMOS, Plague.
LOINS, Lumbi.
LOLIACEUM RADICE REPENTE, Triticum repens.
LOLIUM ANNUUM, L. temulentum.
Lo'lium Temulent'um, *L. an'nuum, Crepa'lia temulen'ta, Bromus temulen'tus,* Darnel (F.) *Herbe d'Ivrogne.* A species of the genus *Lolium,* (F.) *Ivraie; Fam.* Gramineæ; *Sex. Syst.* Triandria digynia, which has decidedly poisonous properties; occasioning, when mixed in bread or beer, intoxication, vertigo, nausea, and vomiting.
LOMBAIRE, Lumbar.
LOMBO-ABDOMINAL, Transversalis abdominis — *l. Costal,* Serratus posticus inferior — *l. Costo-trachélien,* Sacro-lumbalis—*l. Dorso-spinal,* Transversalis dorsi—*l. Dorso-trachélien,* Longissimus dorsi — *l. Huméral,* Latissimus dorsi — *l. Sacré,* Lumbo-sacral.
LOMBRIC, Ascaris lumbricoides.
LOMBRICOÏDE, Ascaris lumbricoides.
LONCHADES, see Sclerotic.
LONCHADITIS, Sclerotitis.
LONCHITIS, Polypodium filix mas.
LONG, *Longus, Macros.* That which is much greater in length than in breadth; as the *long bones.* The epithet is, also, applied to several muscles, to distinguish them from others of similar function, when the latter are shorter. We say, for instance, *long* flexors, and *long* extensors, in opposition to *short* flexors, and *short* extensors.
LONG DU COU, Longus colli — *l. du Dos,* Longissimus dorsi.
LONGÆVUS, Macrobiotic.
LONGANON, Rectum.
LONGAON, Rectum.
LONGAS, Rectum.
LONGEV'ITY, *Longæ'vitas, Macrobio'sis, Macrobi'otes.* The prolongation of existence to an advanced age. Haller collected examples of more than one thousand centenarians. He had knowledge of sixty-two persons aged from 110 to 120 years; of twenty-nine, from 120 to 130 years; and of fifteen, who had attained from 130 to 140 years. Beyond this advanced age, examples of longevity are much more rare and less sufficiently attested.

The following list of instances of very advanced ages has been given:

	Lived. Age.
Apollonius of Tyana, A. D.	99..130
St. Patrick	491..122
Attila	500..124
Llywarch Hên	500..150
St. Coemgene	618..120
Piastus, King of Poland	861..120
Thomas Parr	1635..152
Henry Jenkins	1670..169
Countess of Desmond	1612..145
Thomas Damme	1648..154
Peter Torten	1724..185
Margaret Patten	1739..137
John Rovin and wife	1741..172 and 164
St. Monagh or Kentigen	1781..185

Longevity also means *length* or *duration of life* (F.) *Durée de la vie.* The mean age at death (F.) *Vie moyenne,* of different classes and professions enables an estimate to be formed of the expectation or *value of life* in each.
LONGIS'SIMUS DORSI, *Semi-spina'tus,* (F.) *Lombo-dorso-trachélien, Portion costo-trachélienne du sacro-spinal,* (Ch.,) *Long dorsal, Long du dos,* is situate vertically at the posterior part of the trunk, and fills, in a great measure, the vertebral furrows. It is thick and almost square below; thin and pointed above. It is attached to the posterior surface of the sacrum, to the transverse processes of all the lumbar and dorsal vertebræ, and to the inferior margin of the last 7 or 8 ribs. It maintains the vertebral column in a straight position; straightens it when bent forwards, and can even carry it back. It also assists in the rotatory motion of the trunk.
Longissimus Femoris, Sartorius — 1. Oculi, Obliquus superior oculi.
LONG-SIGHTEDNESS, Presbytia.
LONGUS COLLI, (F.) *Pré-dorso-cervical, Pré-dorso-atloïdien,* (Ch.,) *Long du cou.* This muscle is situate at the anterior and superior part of the vertebral column. It is long, flat, and broader at its middle than at its extremities, which are pointed. It is attached to the anterior surface of the bodies of the first three dorsal and last six cervical vertebræ; to the intervertebral ligaments; to the anterior edge of the transverse processes of the last five cervical vertebræ; and to the tubercle on the anterior arch of the first. This muscle bends the cervical vertebræ upon each other and upon the dorsal vertebræ. If the upper portion acts on one side only, it occasions the rotation of the atlas on the vertebra dentata; and, consequently, of the head on the neck.
LONICERA GERMANICA, L. Periclymenum — l. Marilandica, Spigelia Marilandica.
Lonice'ra Periclym'enum, *L. German'ica, Periclym'enum, P. vulga'ré, Caprifo'lium, C. Periclym'enum seu sylvat'icum seu distinct'um, Common Woodbine,* (F.) *Chèvre-feuille.* This common plant is slightly astringent and tonic, and was formerly much used in gargles.
LOOCH, *Lohoch, Loch, Lochoch, Look.* A linctus. See Eclegma and Eclectos.
Looch absque Emulsio'ne Para'tum, *Looch préparé sans émulsion; Looch prepared without emulsion.* (Pulv. g. trag. gr. xvj — gr. xxx, ol. amygd. dulc. ℨss., sacchar. ℨj, aquæ ℨiij, aquæ flor. aurant. ℨij. Mix by rubbing in a marble mortar.) Demulcent.
Looch Album, *Looch amygdali'num, Linctus albus, L. amygdalinus, L. commu'nis, Eclegma album, Eclegma gummo'so-oleo'sum,* (F.) *Looch blanc, L. b. amygdalin, L. b. pectoral.* (Amygd. dulc. ℨss, amygd. amar. No. ij, sacchar. alb. ℨiv. Make an emulsion by gradually adding ℨiv of water. Then take *pulv. tragacanth.* gr. xvj, ol. amygd. dulc. recent. ℨss, sacch. ℨij. Add the almond milk gradually to this, and afterwards aq. flor. aurant. ℨij, Ph. P.) It is demulcent and pectoral.
Looch Amygdalinum, L. album — *l. Blanc,* L.

album—l. cum Croco et pistaciis, L. viride—l. of Egg, L. ex Ovo.

LOOCH EX OVO, *Potio seu emul'sio seu mistu'ra len'iens* seu *oleo'sa, Looch pectora'lē len'iens, Looch of Egg,* (F.) *Look d'œuf, Looch rouge, Emulsion huileuse, Mixture calmante, Potion pectorale, Lait adoucissant.* (*Vitell. ovi. recent.* ℨss, *ol. amygd. dulc.* ℨiss, *syrup. althæa,* ℨj. Rub in a mortar, and add by degrees, *aq. flor. aurant.* ℨj, *aq. papav. rhœad.* ℨij. *Ph. P.*) Virtues the same as the preceding.

LOOCH ROUGE, L. ex Ovo—l. Vert, L. viride.

LOOCH VIR'IDE, *Look cum croce et pista'ciis,* (F.) *Looch vert.* (*Syrup. Violar.* ℨj, *tinct. croci* gtt. xx. *aquæ* ℨiv. Mix, and add *pistacia semin. sicc.* ℨvj. *Ph. P.*) Virtues like the last.

LOOK, Looch — *l. d'Œuf,* Looch ex ovo — *l. Préparé sans émulsion,* Looch absque emulsione paratum.

LOOSE STRIFE, CREEPING, Lysimachia nummularia—l. s. Four-leaved, Lysimachia quadrifolia.

LOOSENESS, Diarrhœa — l. of the Teeth, Odontoseisis.

LOPEZ RADIX, *Radix lopezia'na, Radix In'dica lopezia'na.* The root of an unknown Indian tree, not possessed of any remarkable smell or taste, or of any appearance of resinous matter. It has been extolled, notwithstanding, in cases of colliquative diarrhœa. Gaubius compares its action to that of simarouba, but thinks it more efficacious.

LOPHADIA, Lophia.

LOPHIA, *Lopha'dia.* The first vertebra of the back — *Ver'tebra dorsi prima.* — Gorræus.

LOPIMA, Fagus castanea.

LOQUAC"ITY, *Garru'litas;* from *loquor,* 'I speak.' (F.) *Babillement.* The act of speaking with volubility. It is sometimes a symptom of disease, and is observable in hysteria, &c.

LOQUELA, Voice, articulated — l. Abolita, Aphonia — l. Blæsa, Balbuties—l. Impedita, Baryphonia.

LORDO'SIS, *Lordo'ma,* from λορδός, 'curved,' 'bent;' *Repanda'tio, Repan'ditas.* A name given to curvatures of the bones in general; and particularly to that of the vertebral column forwards; *Spina dorsi intror'sum flexa, Emprosthocyrto'ma.* This gives rise to the projection of the sternum called *chicken-breasted* or *pigeon-breasted.*

LORIND MATRI'CIS, *Epilep'sia uteri'na, Convulsi'ous u'teri morbus.* A barbarous name given to a pretended epilepsy of the womb.

LORIPES, see Kyllosis.

LOT, Urine.

LOTIO, Enema, Lotion — l. Saponacea, see Sapo.

LO'TION, *Lo'tio, Lotu'ra,* from *lavare, lotum,* 'to wash.' (F.) *Hydrolotif.* A fluid external application. Lotions are ordinarily applied by wetting linen in them and keeping it on the part affected.

LOTION, BARLOW'S, *Lotion of Sulph'uret of potassium.* (℞. *Potassii sulphur.* ℨiij. *Sapon.* ℨiss, *Aq. Calcis,* f℥viss, *alcohol. dilut.* f℥ij. M.) Used in various chronic cutaneous diseases.

LOTION, GOWLAND'S. An empirical preparation. (*Bitter almonds,* ℨj, *sugar,* ℨij, *distilled water,* ℔ij. Grind together, strain, and add *corrosive sublimate,* ∋ij, previously ground with *sp. vini rect.* ℨij.) Used in obstinate eruptions.

LOTION, GRANVILLE'S COUNTER-IRRITANT, *Granville's Lotion, Granville's antid'ynous lotion.* Of this lotion, Dr. Granville gives two forms — a milder, and a stronger. The *milder* is made as follows: *Liq. ammon. fort.* f℥j, *Sp. Rosmarin.* f℥vj, *Tinct. camphor,* f℥ij, M.

The *stronger* is made as follows: *Liq. ammon.*

fort. f℥x, *Spir. Rosmar.* f℥ss, *Tinct. camphor,* f℥ij, M.

The stronger lotion vesicates rapidly. A piece of cotton or linen folded six or seven times, or a piece of thick flannel may be imbued with them, and laid for a few minutes on the part to be irritated.

LOTION, HANNAY'S, *Preven'tive wash.* This famous nostrum, for the prevention of venereal infection, was nothing more than a solution of caustic potass.

LOTION, HYDROCYAN'IC, *Lotio Ac"idi Hydrocyan'ici.* (*Hydrocyanic acid,* f℥iv, *rectified spirit of wine,* f℥j, *distilled water,* f℥xss.) Used with much success in impetigo, &c.

LOTION, STRUVE'S, FOR HOOPING-COUGH. (*Antim. et Potass. tart.* ℨj, *Aquæ,* ℨij. Add *tinct. cantharid,* ℨj.)

LOTIUM, Urine.

LOTURA, Lotion.

LOTUS SYLVESTRIS, Trifolium melilotus — l. Virginiana, Diospyros Virginiana.

LOUCHEMENT, Strabismus.

LOUCHES, see Strabismus.

LOUPE, Wen.

LOUSE, Pediculus.

LOUSINESS, Phtheiriasis.

LOUSY DISEASE, Phtheiriasis.

LOUTRON, Bath.

LOVAGE, Ligusticum levisticum.

LOVE, *Eros, Amor,* from Sax. lufian, (G.) lieben, 'to love.' (F.) *Amour.* A tender and elevated feeling, which attracts one sex to the other. Love is occasionally a cause of disease, especially of insanity.

LOVE APPLE PLANT, Solanum lycopersicum — l. Pea, Abrus precatorius.

LOW SPIRITS, Hypochondriasis.

LOWER, TUBERCLE OF, *Tuber'culum Loweri.* Anatomists have given this name to a small projection, the existence of which is by no means constant, and which is found in the sinus venosus, between the superior and inferior cava.

LOXAR'THRUS, *Loxar'thrum,* from λοξός, 'oblique,' and αρθρον, 'articulation.' (F.) *Perversion de la tête des os et des muscles.* A vicious deviation or direction of the joints, without spasm or luxation, — as in *clubfoot.*

LOXIAS, Torticollis.

LOXOPHTHALMUS, Strabismus.

LOZANGIA, Lozenge.

LOZENGE, Tabella.

LOZENGES, BARK, Tabellæ cinchonæ — l. of Catechu and magnesia, Tabellæ antimoniales Kunckelii — l. Faustinus's, Faustini pastilli — l. for the Heart-burn, Trochisci carbonatis calcis — l. Magnesiæ, Tabellæ de magnesiâ — l. of Marshmallows, Tabellæ de altheâ — l. of Oxalic acid, Tabellæ acidi oxalici — l. Pectoral, black, Trochisci glycyrrhizæ glabræ — l. Pectoral, of emetine, Trochisci emetinæ pectorales — l. Rhubarb, Tabellæ de rheo — l. of Scammony and senna, compound, Tabellæ de scammonio et sennâ — l. Spitta's, see Trochisci glycyrrhizæ cum opio — l. Steel, Tabellæ de ferro — l. of Steel, aromatic, see Tabellæ de ferro — l. Sulphur, simple, Tabellæ de sulphure simplices — l. Sulphur, compound, Tabellæ de sulphure compositæ — l. of Sulphuret of antimony, Tabellæ antimoniales Kunckelii — l. Wistar's, Trochisci glycyrrhizæ cum opio — l. Worm, Ching's, see Worm losenges, (Ching's.)

LUBIDO, Libido — l. Intestini, Voluntas descendendi.

LUBRICANTIA, Demulcents, Emollients.

LUBRICUM CAPUT, Penis.

LUCCA, MINERAL WATERS AND CLIMATE OF. The baths and waters, near this ancient Italian city, have been long celebrated.

They are thermal, and resemble, in properties, those of Plombières in France, and of Bath in England. They contain carbonic acid, sulphates of alumina, soda, magnesia, and iron. There are ten different sources, the temperature of which varies from 94° to 130° Fahr.

Lucca is much frequented in summer; partly on account of its mineral waters, but more on account of the coolness of the situation.

LUCID, *Lu'cidus*. In medicine, the word *lucid* is particularly applied to the *intervals, Interval'la lu'cida*, of apparent reason, which occur in mental alienation.

LUCIF'UGUS, from *lux, lucis*, 'light' and *fugere*, 'to shun.' *Photoph'obus, Photophob'icus*. Dreading or avoiding the light.

LUCINA, Ilithyia.

LUCOMANIA, Lycanthropia.

LUCUMA, (S.) A fruit which grows in the southern provinces of the coast of Peru, and the north of Chili. It is round; and the gray-brown husk encloses a fibrous, dry, yellow-coloured fruit with its kernel. — Tschudi.

LUCUMORIA'NUS, probably from *lux*, 'light,' and *morari*, 'to tarry.' Continuing for several days: hence, *Dormit"io lucumoria'na*. A morbid sleep persisting for several days.

LUDUS HELMON'TII, *L. Paracel'si, Fel terræ*. A calcareous stone, the precise nature not known, which was used by the ancients in calculous affections. The term was also applied to every species of calculous concretion occurring in the animal body.

LUDUS PARACELSI, L. Helmontii.

LUES, Disease, Plague, Syphilis — l. Divina, Epilepsy — l. Dysenterica, Dysentery — l. Gonorrhoica, Gonorrhœa impura — l. Gutturis epidemica, Cynanche maligna — l. Indica, Frambœsia — l. Inguinaria, Plague — l. Polonica, Plica — l. Sarmatica, Plica — l. Syphilis, Syphilis — l. Syphilodes, Syphilis pseudo-syphilis — l. Trichomatica, Plica — l. Venerea, Syphilis — l. Scorbutica, see Purpura.

LUETTE, Uvula — *l. Vésicale*, see Urinary bladder.

LUGDUS, Erysipelas.

LUJULA, Oxalis acetosella.

LULLABY SPEECH, Lallation.

LUMBA'GO, from *lumbi*, 'the loins.' *Arthro'sia lumbo'rum, Lumbago rheumat'ica, Nephral'gia rheumat'ica, Rachirrheu'ma, Rachiorrheu'ma, Rheumatis'mus dorsa'lis, Osphyrrheu'ma*. Rheumatism affecting the lumbar region.

Lumba'go psoad'ica, L. apostemato'sa, L. ab arthroc'acê. Pain in the loins from abscess. See Psoitis.

LUMBAGO A NISU, see Effort.

LUMBAR, *Lumba'ris* vel *Lumba'lis*, (F.) *Lombaire*. Belonging or having reference to the loins.

LUMBAR ABSCESS, *Psoas abscess, Aposte'ma psoat'icum, Absces'sus lumbo'rum, Morbus psoad'icus*. This abscess is so called from the matter being found on the side of the psoas muscle, or betwixt that and the iliacus internus. Between these muscles is a quantity of loose, areolar substance; and, when an abscess takes place there, it can find no outlet except by a distant course. Generally, it descends along the psoas muscle, forming a swelling immediately beneath Poupart's ligament; at times, however, it extends down the thigh under the fascia. Severe hectic follows the bursting of the abscess, and often death. Its causes are, — scrofula, injury to the loins, &c.

When, from the pain of the back continuing for some time, with other symptoms, the disease is suspected, caustics, or the moxa, applied opposite the transverse processes of the lumbar vertebræ, may be recommended; and, when the abscess is ready for opening, it may be emptied by repeated discharges of the matter, through a small opening, made with a lancet, or small, lancet-pointed trocar. The medical treatment consists in supporting the system, under the great restorative efforts required of it.

LUMBAR ARTERIES are four or five in number on each side. They arise from the sides of the abdominal aorta, and pass behind the muscles situate in front of the lumbar portion of the spine, to gain the broad muscles of the abdomen. They give off, 1. Spinal branches. 2. Anterior, posterior, and external muscular branches.

LUMBAR NERVES are five in number, and issue from the vertebral column by the spinal foramina of the loins. The first lumbar nerve gives off three branches:—the *external* or *ilio-scrotal;* the *middle* or *inguino-cutaneous*, and the *internal* or *infra-pubian*. Along with the three pairs below it, it forms the lumbar plexus.

LUMBAR PLEXUS, *Portion lombaire du plexus crural* (Ch.), *Plexus Lombo-abdominal*. This plexus is formed by the union of the *Rami communican'tes* of the anterior branches of the first four lumbar nerves. It is situate behind the psoas muscle, and before the transverse processes of the lumbar vertebræ. It furnishes, besides the branches which proceed from the first pair, several filaments, that are distributed to the psoas muscle, to the iliacus, the integuments, and glands of the groin; and three great branches—the *crural, obdurator*, and *lumbo-sacral*.

LUMBAR REGION, Lumbi.

LUMBAR VEINS have an arrangement analogous to that of the arteries of the same name. They communicate with the vertebral sinuses, azygous veins, &c., and pass into the vena cava inferior.

LUMBARIS EXTERNUS, Quadratus lumborum — l. Internus, Psoas magnus.

LUMBI, *The loins*, the *Lumbar region, Re'gio lumba'lis, Lap'ara, Psoæ, Osphys, Reins*. The posterior regions of the abdomen, comprised between the base of the chest and the pelvis. The parts which enter into the formation of the lumbar region are, — the skin; a considerable quantity of areolar texture; broad and strong aponeuroses;—the *Latissimus Dorsi, Obliquus externus*, and *Obliquus internus abdominis, Transversalis abdominis, Quadratus lumborum*, and the mass common to the *Sacro-lumbalis, Longissimus dorsi*, and *Multifidus spinæ*. These muscles surround the lumbar region of the vertebral column. The vessels, nerves, &c., of the loins, are called *lumbar*.

LUMBO-SACRAL. Belonging to the lumbar and sacral regions. (F.) *Lombo-sacré*. Bichat calls thus a very large nerve, given off from the anterior branch of the fifth lumbar pair, which descends into the pelvis before the sacrum to join the sciatic plexus.

LUMBRICA'LIS, *Vermicula'ris*. Resembling a *lumbricus*, or 'earthworm.' A name given to small muscles, met with in the palm of the hand and sole of the foot.

LUMBRICALES MANÛS, *Fidicina'les, Flexor primi interno'dii digito'rum manûs* vel *perfora'tus lumbrica'lis*, (F.) *Annuli-tendino-phalangiens, Palmi-phalangiens*. Four small, fleshy, thin, round, long, fusiform fasciculi, situate in the palm of the hand, and distinguished into first, second, third, and fourth, counting from without to within. They arise from the tendons of the flexor communis digitorum, and are inserted at the outer and posterior side of the superior extremity of the first phalanges of the last four fingers. These muscles bend the fingers on the metacarpus, and fix the tendons of the flexor digitorum communis.

LUMBRICALES PEDIS, (F.) *Planti-tendino-phalangiens, Planti-sous-phalangiens,* (Ch.) They are analogous to those of the hand in form, number, and arrangement. They increase the flexion of the toes, and draw them inwards.

LUMBRICUS, Ascaris lumbricoides — l. Latus, Bothriocephalus latus, Tænia solium — l. Teres hominis, Ascaris lumbricoides.

LUMBUS VENERIS, Achillea millefolium.

LUMEN, Light, Pupil — l. Constans, Phosphorus.

LUMIÈRE, Light.

LUNA, Argentum, Moon — l. Albini, Sciatic notch, lesser — l. Imperfecta, Bismuth — l. Potabilis, Argenti nitras.

LUNAR, Lunatic.

LUNA'RE OS, *Os semiluna'ri.* The second bone in the upper row of the carpus.

LUNARIA, Menses.

LUNA'RIA REDIVI'VA, *Leucoïum, Bulbonach, Satin, Honesty.* Said, by Ray, to be a warm diuretic.

LUNARIS, Lunatic.

LU'NATIC, *Lunat'icus, Luna'ris, Luna'rius, Lunar,* from *luna,* 'the moon.' Relating to the moon. An epithet given to diseases which are supposed to appear at certain phases of the moon, or to those who are affected by them. The term *lunatic* is restricted to one labouring under lunacy, or mental alienation; — *Moonstruck, Selenoble'tus.* In law, a lunatic is one who has had an understanding, but by disease, grief, or other accident, has lost the use of his reason.

LUNATICUS, Epileptic, Lunatic, Somnambulist.

LUNATISMUS, Somnambulism.

LUNE, Moon.

LUNELLA, Hypopyon.

LUNES, Menses.

LUNETTES ORDINAIRES, Spectacles.

LUNG, Pulmo — l. Black, of coal miners, Anthracosis — l. Cancer of the, Phthisis, cancerous — l. Fever, Catarrh, Pneumonia.

LUNG, PERFORATING ABSCESS OF THE. A purulent collection, which forms exterior to the lung, and afterwards perforates its tissue, so that it is evacuated through the bronchial tubes.

LUNG PROOF, Docimasia pulmonum — l. Wort, Pulmonaria — l. Wort, cow's, Verbascum nigrum — l. Wort, tree, Lichen pulmonarius.

LUNULA UNGUIUM, see Nail — l. Scapulæ, Notch, scapular.

LUPIA, Encystis, Wen — l. Junctura, Spina ventosa.

LUPI'NUS. Under this term the *white lupin, Lupi'nus al'bus seu sati'vus,* is meant, in some pharmacopœias. The seeds, which were much eaten in the days of Pliny and of Galen, are now neglected. The meal is, however, occasionally used as an anthelmintic, and as a cataplasm.

LUPULI'NA, *Lu'pulin, Lupulin'ic glands.* A substance which exists in the *humulus lupulus* or hop. It is in the form of small, shining, yellowish grains, which cover the base of the scales of the hop; is pulverulent, and of an aromatic odour. When analyzed, it is found to contain resin, volatile oil in small quantity, and a bitter principle. It is aromatic and tonic, and — according to some — narcotic.

LUPULINIC GLANDS, Lupulina.

LUPULUS, l. humulus — l. Communis, L. humulus — l. Salictarius, L. humulus — l. Scandens, L. humulus.

LUPUS, 'the wolf.' So named from its rapacity. *Ulcus Tuberculo'sum, Cancer lupus, Noli me tangere, Phymato'sis lupus.* Tubercular excrescences, with ragged, spreading ulcerations, chiefly about the alæ nasi, where they destroy the skin, &c., for some depth. Sometimes they appear in the cheek, circularly, or in the shape of a sort of ringworm, destroying the substance, and leaving a deep and deformed cicatrix. The knife or caustic should be used to separate the sound from the morbid parts. Arsenic has been given internally with advantage. See, also, Herpes exedens, and Lycoides.

LUPUS CANCROSUS, Cancer — l. Varicosus, Nævi — l. Vorax, Herpes exedens.

LURCO, Glutton.

LURID, *Lu'ridus.* Pale, yellow, sallow; — applied to the complexion.

LUROR, Paleness.

LUSCIOSITAS, Luscitas, Myopia.

LUSCIOSUS, *Borgne,* Myops.

LUS'CITAS, *Luscios'itas, Luscit"ies.* Strabismus. The term has also been given to all those cases of obliquity in which the eye is fixed in an unnatural position. — Beer.

LUSCITIES, Luscitas.

LUSTRAMENTUM, Cathartic.

LUSCUS, *Borgne.*

LUT, Lute.

LUTE, *Lutum,* ('mud,') *Cæmen'tum.* (F.) *Lut.* A composition employed either for closing apertures in a pharmaceutical instrument, or for covering the surface of retorts, tubes, &c., which have to support a great degree of heat. Lutes are composed differently, according to the object to be accomplished. Commonly they are made of linseed meal and starch. The *fat lute* is formed of clay and drying oil. Sometimes, the white of egg and lime are used; and that which is employed for covering vessels, intended to be strongly heated, is made of clay, sifted sand, and water.

LUTEOLA, Reseda luteola.

LUTEUS, Yellow.

LUTRON, λουτρον. A bath. Also, an ophthalmic medicine. — Galen.

LUX, Light.

LUXATIO, Luxation — l. Imperfecta, Sprain.

LUXA'TION, *Eluxa'tion,* from *luxare,* 'to put out of place.' *Disloca'tion, Olisthe'ma, Apoped'asis, Luxa'tio, Disloca'tio, Ec'clisis, Strem'ma, Luxatu'ra, Ectop'ia, Ecpto'sis, Elap'sus, Lygis'mus, Emo'tio, Ec'stasis, Exarthre'ma, Exarthro'ma, Exarthre'ma luxa'tio, Exarthro'sis, Exo'sis, Exothe'sis, Paratop'ia, Streblo'sis, Deloca'tio, Exarticula'tio,* (F.) *Luxation, Dislocation, Déboîtement.* A displacement of a part from its proper situation. A putting out of joint. A displacement of two or more bones, whose articular surfaces have lost, wholly, or in part, their natural connexion; either owing to external violence, (*accidental luxation,*) or to disease of some of the parts about the joint (*spontaneous luxation.*) Luxation is *complete* when the bones have entirely lost their natural connexion; *incomplete,* when they partly preserve it; and *compound,* when a wound communicates with the luxated joint. The general indications of treatment, are; — 1 To reduce the protruded bone to its original place. 2. To retain it *in situ.* 3. To obviate any attendant or consequent symptoms.

To reduce requires extension, counter-extension, and coaptation.

LUXEUIL, MINERAL WATERS OF. Saline waters, at the town of Luxeuil, at the foot of the Vosges, in the department of Haute Saône. Five springs are thermal, and two cold. They seem to contain carbonic acid, carbonates of iron and lime, and chloride of sodium; and are employed as aperient, tonic, and stimulant.

LYCAN'CHE, Lycan'chis, from λυκος, 'a wolf,' and αγχω, 'I strangle.' *Wolf quinsy, Wolf choak;* — as *Cynanche* means *Dog choak.* Also, hydrophobia. See Lycoïdes.

LYCANCHIS, Lycanche.

LYCANTHROPE, see Lycanthropia.

LYCANTHRO'PIA, from λυκος, 'a wolf,' and ανθρωπος, 'a man:' *Lyca'on, Insa'nia lupi'na, Lycoma'nia.* A variety of melancholy, in which the person believes himself to be changed into a wolf, and imitates the voice and habits of that animal. One so circumstanced is called a *Ly'canthrope, Lycanthro'pus.*

LYCANTHROPUS, see Lycanthropia.

LYCAON, Lycanthropia.

LYCHNIDIUM, Biolychnium.

LYCHNIS OFFICINALIS, Saponaria—l. Sylvestris, Saponaria.

LYCHNIUM, Biolychnium.

LYCOÏ'DES, *Lyco'des,* from λυκος, 'a wolf,' and ειδος, 'form.' *Lupo sim'ilis.* An epithet for a species of cynanche, called, also, *Lupus,* and *Strangula'tor,* and absurdly attributed to excessive retention of sperm in its reservoirs and its passage into the blood (?).—Galen.

LYCOPE DE VIRGINIE, Lycopus Virginicus.

LYCOPER'DON, from λυκος, 'a wolf,' and περδω, 'I break wind;' *L. Bovis'ta* seu *Arrhi'zon* seu *Globo'sum, Crep'itus Lupi, Fungus Chirurgo'rum, Puff-ball, Bull Fists, Mol'lipuffs, Bovis'ta,* (F.) *Vesseloup.* The puff-ball dries into a very fine, light brownish dust, which is sometimes used as a mechanical styptic to arrest hemorrhage.

LYCOPERDON ARRHIZON, Lycoperdon—l. Globosum, Lycoperdon—l. Gulosorum, L. Tuber.

LYCOPER'DON TUBER, *L. Guloso'rum, Tuber Agriocas'tanum, Trubs, Tuber ciba'rium* seu *Guloso'rum* seu *Nigrum, Tu'bera Terræ, Truffle,* (pronounced *troofle,) Tuckaho,* (F.) *Truffe.* A fleshy, firm body, unknown in its mode of reproduction, which is found under ground, especially in different parts of France, Italy, &c., and is much esteemed as an aliment. It seems to belong to the champignons, and has a particular perfume. Aphrodisiac virtues have been ascribed to it.

LYCOPERSICUM ESCULENTUM, Solanum lycopersicum—l. Pomum amoris, Solanum lycopersicum—l. Tuberosum, Solanum tuberosum.

LYCOPO'DIUM, from λυκος, 'a wolf,' and πους, 'a foot.' *L. Clava'tum* seu *Officina'lě, Lepido'tis clava'ta, Cingula'ria, Muscus clava'tus, Club-moss, Wolf's-claw.* This is the largest of the European mosses. The dust, which fills the capsules of its spikes, is very inflammable, and hence has been called *Vegetable Sulphur;* — and, also, *Fari'na* seu *Pulvis* seu *Semen* seu *Sulphur Lycopo'dii.* It is used in France to roll pills and boluses in; and in medicine is a desiccative, in the excoriations to which infants are liable. It is collected chiefly in Switzerland and Germany for commerce.

LYCOPO'DIUM COMPLANA'TUM, *Common Club-moss, Ground Pine;* indigenous; has the same properties as Lycopodium selago.

LYCOPO'DIUM OFFICINALE, L. clavatum—l. Recurvum, L. Selago.

LYCOPODIUM SELA'GO, *L. Recur'vum, Planan'thus fastiga'tus* seu *sela'go, Muscus erec'tus* seu *Cathar'ticus, Sela'go, Upright Club-moss, Fir Club-moss, Upright Fir-moss.* A decoction of this plant acts violently as an emetic and purgative; and was formerly, on this account, used as an abortive. It is also employed to kill vermin.

LY'COPUS, *L. Virgin'icus, Bugleweed, Water Bugle, Water Horehound, Gypsy Weed, Paul's Bet'ony,* (F.) *Lycope de Virginie.* This indigenous herb, *Sex. Syst.* Diandria Monogynia, *Nat. Ord.* Labiatæ, grows throughout the greater part of the United States. The whole herb is said to be slightly narcotic. It is given in infusion, (*Lycop.* ʒj; *aq. fervent.* Oj.)

LYCOPUS SINUA'TUS, *Water Horehound, Gypsy Weed, Paul's Bet'ony,* indigenous, has similar properties.

LYCOPUS VIRGINICUS, Lycopus.

LYCOREXIS, Fames lupina.

LYCOSA TARENTULA, see Tarantula.

LYCOSTOMA, Hyperoöchasma.

LYE, Lixivium, Ley—l. Dyspeptic, see Fuligokali—l. Medical, see Fuligokali.

LYGISMUS, Luxation.

LYGMODES, Singultous.

LYGMUS, Singultus.

LYGODES, Singultous.

LYING-IN STATE, Parturient state.

LYMA, Lochia.

LYMPH, *Lympha,* from νυμφη, 'water,' by changing ν into λ. *White blood, Lympha Nutrit"ia.* A name given to the fluid contained in the lymphatic vessels and thoracic duct of animals, which have been made to fast for 24 hours. According to Chevreul, the lymph of the dog contains water, fibrin, albumen, common salt, subcarbonate of soda, phosphates of lime and magnesia, and carbonate of lime. The properties and composition of lymph vary somewhat according to the part whence the lymphatic vessels obtain it. Generally, it is under the form of a transparent, slightly alkaline fluid, sometimes of a madder-red or yellowish colour,—of a spermatic odour, and saline taste; soluble in water,—the solution becoming turbid, when mixed with alcohol. When left to itself, it coagulates. The clot or solid portion becomes of a scarlet red, if put in contact with oxygen; and of a purple red, if placed in carbonic acid.

Like the blood, the lymph consists of a fluid in which *lymph corpuscles* or *globules* are suspended. The lymph is probably the product of internal absorption in different parts of the body: it then flows along the lymphatic vessels, uniting with the chyle, and is poured with it into the veins; thus becoming one of the materials of the blood. According to others, the blood, when it reaches the arterial radicles, is divided into two portions, —the one red, which is carried to the heart,— the other serous or white, which is absorbed by the lymphatic vessels, and constitutes the lymph. By others, again, the lymphatics are considered to be the vessels of return for the white blood sent to certain tissues. White blood, however, has probably no existence.

The word lymph is sometimes used erroneously by the surgeon to signify liquor sanguinis.

LYMPH, COAGULABLE, Fibrin, Liquor sanguinis—l. Corpuscles, see Lymph—l. Globules, see Lymph—l. Hearts, Lymphatic hearts—l. Plastic, Liquor sanguinis.

LYMPHA, Lymph—l. Arborum, see Sap—l. Muculenta narium, Nasal mucus—l. Nutritia, Lymph—l. Pancreatis, see Pancreas—l. Pericardii, see Pericardium—l. Plastica, Fibrin.

LYMPHADENI'TIS: from *lympha,* 'lymph, and *adeni'tis,* 'inflammation of a gland.' *Inflamma'tio glandula'rum lymphatica'rum, Adeni'tis lymphat'ica,* (F.) *Adénite lymphatique.* Inflammation of a lymphatic gland or ganglion.

LYMPHÆDUCTUS, Lymphatic vessels.

LYMPHANGEITIS, Angeioleucitis.

LYMPHANGIA, Lymphatic vessels.

LYMPHANGIEC'TASIS, *Lympheurys'ma;*

from *lymph*, αγγειον, 'a vessel,' and εκτασις, 'dilatation.' Dilatation of lymphatic vessels.

LYMPHANGITIS, Angeioleucitis.

LYMPHANGIOG'RAPHY, *Lymphangiograph'ia;* from *lymph*, αγγειον, 'a vessel,' and γραφη, 'a description.' A description of the lymphatic vessels.

LYMPHANGIOITIS, Angeioleucitis.

LYMPHANGIOL'OGY, from *Lymphangion*, 'a lymphatic,' and λογος, 'a description.' A treatise on the lymphatics.

LYMPHANGIOT'OMY, *Lymphangiotom'ia;* from *lymph*, αγγειον, 'a vessel,' and τομη, 'incision.' The anatomy or dissection of the lymphatic vessels.

LYMPHANGON'CUS, *Lymphon'cus;* from *lymph*, αγγειον, 'a vessel,' and ογκος, 'a tumour.' Tumefaction of the lymphatics.

LYMPHAT'IC, *Lymphat'icus.* That which relates to lymph.

LYMPHATIC HEARTS. *Lymph Hearts.* The frog and several other animals are provided with large receptacles for the lymph immediately underneath the skin, which exhibit distinct and regular pulsations like the sanguiferous heart. Their use appears to be—to propel the lymph.

LYMPHATIC SYSTEM is that particular system of organs which is inservient to the formation and circulation of lymph. These organs are:

1. LYMPHATIC GANGLIONS or GLANDS, see 'Conglobate.

2. LYMPHATIC VESSELS, *Lymphæduc'tus, Lymphangi'a, Lymphange'a, Venæ lymphat'icæ, Ductus sero'si, Vasa lymphatica, V. resorben'tia, Vasa hydrago'ga, Hydrangi'a.* These are very numerous. Arising at the surface of membranes and in the tissue of the organs, they carry into the veins the lymph from those parts. Lymphatic vessels are found in every part of the body. Wherever they are met with, however, they form two orders,— one *superficial,* the other *deep-seated;*—the two orders frequently communicating with each other. Lymphatic vessels are generally smaller than arteries and veins. They are very thin, diaphanous, and cylindrical; but present, here and there, more or less considerable dilatations, caused by valves in their interior. They are slightly tortuous in their course; their anastomoses are very numerous, and they often cross each other, forming successive plexuses. Of the arrangement of the extreme radicles we are ignorant. All the branches, before joining the principal trunks, pass through lymphatic ganglions, in which they are convoluted, or subdivide almost *ad infinitum.* They are formed of an outer cellular membrane and an internal coat, similar to that of the veins; of the latter, the valves are formed. All the lymphatics of the body ultimately discharge themselves into the subclavian and internal jugular veins. Two of these trunks are considerably larger than the others, — the *thoracic duct,* and the great trunk of the right side, (F.) *La grande veine lymphatique droite.* The *former* receives the lymphatics of the abdomen, of the lower extremities, the left side of the thorax, the left upper extremity, and the corresponding side of the head and neck; the *latter* receives those of the right upper extremity, and of the right side of the head, neck and thorax.

LYMPHATITIS, Angeioleucitis.

LYMPHE DE COTUGNO, Cotunnius, liquor of.

LYMPHEURYSMA, Lymphangiectasis.

LYMPHITIS, Angeioleucitis.

LYMPHIZA'TION. A term used by Professor Gross to signify effusion of coagulable lymph. It is not a happy word, inasmuch as lymph has another meaning, whilst the term 'coagulable lymph' is now almost abandoned.

LYMPHOCHE'ZIA, from *lympha*, 'lymph,' and χεζω, 'I go to stool.' Serous diarrhœa.

LYMPHONCUS, Lymphangoncus — l. Iridis, Iridauxesis.

LYMPHOPYRA, Fever, adeno-meningeal.

LYMPHO'SIS. The preparation or elaboration of lymph.

LYMPHOT'OMY, from *lympha*, 'lymph,' and τεμνω, 'I cut.' Dissection of the lymphatics.

LYNCH'S EMBROCA'TION. An emollient nostrum, formed of *olive oil* impregnated with *bergamot* and other essences, and coloured with *alkanet root.*

LYNGODES, Singultous — l. Febris, Fever, singultous.

LYNGYODES, Singultous.

LYNN WAHOO, Ulmus alata.

LYNX, Singultus.

LYPE, Athymia.

LYPEMANIA, Melancholy.

LYPE'RIA CRO'CEA. A South African plant, *Nat. Ord.* Scrophulariaceæ, the flowers of which closely resemble saffron in smell and taste, and possess similar medical virtues.

LYPEROPHRÉNIE, Melancholy.

LYPOMA, Lipoma.

LYPOTHYM'IA, from λυπη, 'sadness,' and θυμος, 'heart, courage.' Very great sadness or despondency.

LYRA, λυρα, 'the lyre.' *Psalter, Psalte'rium, Corpus Psalloi'des, Lyra Da'vidis, Lam'ina medulla'ris triangula'ris cer'ebri, Spa'tium tri'gonum.* The under surface of the posterior part of the body of the fornix is impressed with numerous transverse and oblique lines, which have been so called from some resemblance they bear to the ancient lyre.

LYRINGIUM, Eryngium campestre.

LYSIA, Lysis.

LYSIMA'CHIA NUMMULA'RIA, *L. nemorum, Nummula'ria, Hirundina'ria, Centimor'bia, Creeping Loose Strife, Money Wort,* (F.) *Herbe aux écus.* This plant was formerly accounted vulnerary. It has been considered to possess antiscorbutic and astringent qualities, and has been used in leucorrhœa.

LYSIMACHIA PURPUREA, Lythrum salicaria.

LYSIMA'CHIA QUADRIFO'LIA, *Four-Leaved Loose Strife, Crosswort,* an indigenous plant, is astringent; and has been used as a stomachic and antiperiodic.

LYSIS, *Lysia,* from λυω, 'I dissolve.' Solution. A common suffix; also, a name given to solutions or terminations of disease, which are operated insensibly; that is, gradually and without *critical* symptoms.

LYSSA, Hydrophobia — l. Canina, Hydrophobia.

LYSSAS, Maniodes.

LYSSETER, Maniodes.

LYSSODEC'TUS, from λυσσα, 'canine madness,' and δακνω, 'I bite.' *Hydroph'obus; Canis rab'ido morsus.* One who has been bitten by a mad dog, or is actually labouring under hydrophobia.

LYSSODEG'MA, *Lyssodeg'mus, Lyssodexis,* same etymon. The bite of a mad dog.

LYSSODEXIS, Lyssodegma.

LYTE'RIOS, λυτηριος, (from λυω, 'I dissolve,') 'solving.' An epithet given to those signs which announce the solution of a very violent disease.

LYTHRUM SALICA'RIA, *Lysima'chia purpu'rea, Salica'ria vulga'ris seu spica'ta;* — the *Common* or *Purple Willow Herb.* The herb, root, and flowers possess a considerable degree of astringency, and are used, occasionally, in the cure of diarrhœa and dysentery, leucorrhœa, hæmoptysis, &c.

LYTTA VESICATORIA, Cantharis.

LYTTA RU'FIPES. A variety of Lytta, peculiar to Chili, which is more active as a vesicant than the cantharis, or the lytta next described.

LYTTA VITTA'TA, Can'tharis vittata, Pota'to Fly, (F.) Cantharide tachetée. Four species of meloe that blister are found in the United States. The lytta vittata feeds principally upon the potato plant, and, at the proper season of the year, may be collected in immense numbers. The potato fly resembles the cantharides in every property, and is fully equal to them.

M.

M. This letter signifies, in prescriptions, *manipulus*, 'a handful.' Also, *misce*, 'mix.' See Abbreviation.

MACAPATLI, Smilax sarsaparilla.

MACARO'NI. An alimentary paste, moulded of a cylindrical shape, and formed of rice or wheaten flour. It is eaten — when boiled — in soup — prepared with cheese, &c.

Also, a name formerly given to a pulverulent compound of sugar and glass of antimony, carried into France by the Italian monks, and employed at the hospital *La Charité* in the treatment of painters' colic.

MACE, see Myristica moschata — m. Reed, Typha latifolia.

MACEDONISIUM, Smyrnium olusatrum.

MACER, Gracilis.

MACERA'TION, *Macera'tio*, from *macero*, 'I soften by water.' An operation which consists in infusing, usually without heat, a solid substance in a liquid, so as to extract its virtues.

MACERONA, Smyrnium olusatrum.

MACES, see Myristica moschata.

MACESCERE, Emaciate.

MACHÆRA, Culter, Knife, Penis.

MACHÆRIDION, Machærion.

MACHÆ'RION, *Machæ'ris*, *Machærid'ion*, *Glad'iolus*. A knife. An amputating knife. Rufus of Ephesus asserts, that the Aruspices gave this name to a part of the liver of animals.

MACHÆRIS, Knife, Novacula.

MACHA'ON, from $\mu\alpha\chi\alpha\omega$, 'I desire to fight.' The son of Æsculapius, and a celebrated physician.

MACHAÖ'NIA seu MACHAÖN'ICA ARS. Medicine. The *Healing Art:* — so called after Machaon, the son of Æsculapius.

MACHI'NAL, *Mechan'icus*. This epithet is added especially by French writers to the word *movement*, to express that the will takes no part in it.

MACHINE', *Mach'ina*, *Machinamen'tum*, *Me'chané*, *Mechane'ma*. A more or less compound instrument, used in physics and chymistry to put a body in motion, or to produce any action whatever. Physiologists sometimes use it for the *animal body;* — as the *machine* or *animal machine*.

MACHLOSYNE, Nymphomania.

MACHOIRE, Maxillary bone — m. *Diacranienne*, Maxillary bone, lower — m. *Syncranienne*, Maxillary bone, superior.

MACIES, Atrophy, Emaciation — m. Infantum, Tabes mesenterica.

MACILENTUS, Gracilis.

MACIS, see Myristica moschata.

MACRAU'CHEN, from $\mu\alpha\kappa\rho\sigma\varsigma$, 'long,' and $\alpha\nu\chi\eta\nu$, 'the neck.' *Longo collo præ'ditus.* One who has a long neck. — Galen.

MACRE FLOTTANTE, Trapa natans.

MACRITUDO, Emaciation.

MACROBIOSIS, Longevity.

MACROBIOTES, Longevity.

MACROBIOT'IC, *Macrobiot'icus*, *Macrobi'otus*, *Macro'bius*, *Longæ'vus*, from $\mu\alpha\kappa\rho\sigma\varsigma$, 'great,' 'long,' and $\beta\iota\sigma\varsigma$, 'life.' That which lives a long time. The *macrobiotic art* is the art of living a long time.

MACROBIOTUS, Macriobiotic.

MACROBIUS, Macrobiotic.

MACROCEPH'ALUS, from $\mu\alpha\kappa\rho\sigma\varsigma$, 'great,' 'long,' and $\kappa\epsilon\phi\alpha\lambda\eta$, 'head.' *Qui magnum habet caput.* 'One who has a large head.' This epithet is given to children born with heads so large that they seem to be hydrocephalic; but in which the unusual development is owing to a large size of the brain. Such are supposed to be more than ordinarily liable to convulsions.(?) The term has also been applied by Hippocrates to certain Asiatics who had long heads. See Capitones.

MACROCO'LIA, from $\mu\alpha\kappa\rho\sigma\varsigma$, 'great,' and $\kappa\omega\lambda\sigma\nu$, 'a limb.' Great length of limbs in general, and of the lower limbs in particular.

MACRODAC'TYLUS, from $\mu\alpha\kappa\rho\sigma\varsigma$, 'great,' and $\delta\alpha\kappa\tau\upsilon\lambda\sigma\varsigma$, 'a finger.' Having long fingers.

MACROGASTER PLATYPUS, Acarus folliculorum.

MACROGLOSSA, see Macroglossus.

MACROGLOS'SUS, from $\mu\alpha\kappa\rho\sigma\varsigma$, 'large,' and $\gamma\lambda\omega\sigma\sigma\alpha$, 'tongue.' One who has a very large or prolapsed tongue. See Paraglossa.

MACRONOSIÆ, Chronic diseases.

MACROPHAL'LUS, from $\mu\alpha\kappa\rho\sigma\varsigma$, 'large,' and $\phi\alpha\lambda\lambda\sigma\varsigma$, 'the male organ.' A large size of the male organ.

MACROPHO'NUS, from $\mu\alpha\kappa\rho\sigma\varsigma$, 'great,' and $\phi\omega\nu\eta$, 'voice.' One who has a strong voice.

MACROPHYSOCEPH'ALUS, from $\mu\alpha\kappa\rho\sigma\varsigma$, 'long,' $\phi\upsilon\sigma\alpha$, 'air,' and $\kappa\epsilon\phi\alpha\lambda\eta$, 'head.' A word used by Ambrose Paré to designate an augmentation of the head of the fœtus, produced by a sort of emphysema [?], which retards delivery.

MACROPIPER, Piper longum.

MACROPNŒ'A, from $\mu\alpha\kappa\rho\sigma\varsigma$, 'long,' and $\pi\nu\epsilon\omega$, 'I breathe.' A long and deep respiration.

MACROP'NUS, *Macrop'noos.* One who breathes slowly: — a word met with in some authors. — Hippocrates.

MACROP'ODUS, *Mac'ropus*, from $\mu\alpha\kappa\rho\sigma\varsigma$, 'great,' and $\pi\sigma\upsilon\varsigma$, 'foot.' One who has a large foot.

MACROR, Emaciation.

MACROR'RHIS, from $\mu\alpha\kappa\rho\sigma\varsigma$, 'great,' and $\rho\iota\varsigma$ or $\rho\iota\nu$, 'nose.' One who has a long nose.

MACROS, Long.

MACROS'CELES, *Crura longa habens;* from $\mu\alpha\kappa\rho\sigma\varsigma$, 'long,' and $\sigma\kappa\epsilon\lambda\sigma\varsigma$, 'the leg.' One who has long legs.

MACROSIÆ, Chronic diseases.

MACRO'TES, from $\mu\alpha\kappa\rho\sigma\varsigma$, 'great,' and $\sigma\upsilon\varsigma$, 'an ear.' One who has long ears.

MACROTRYS RACEMOSA, see Actæa racemosa.

MAC'ULA. A spot. *Dyschro'a, Celis, Labes,* (F.) *Tache.* A permanent discoloration of some portion of the skin, often with a change of its texture. *Ephelis, Nævus, Spilus, &c.,* belong to Maculæ.

MACULA, Molecule — m. Corneæ, Caligo — m. Corneæ arcuata, Gerotoxon — m. Corneæ margaritacea, Paralampsis — m. Cribrosa, see Auditory canal, internal — m. Fusca, Ephelides — m. Germinativa, see Molecule — m. Hepatica, Chloasma materna, Nœvus — m. Lenticularis, Ephelides — m. Lutea retinæ, see Foramen centrale — m. Matricalis, Nævus—m. Matricis, Nævus—m. Solaris, Ephelides.

MACULÆ ANTE OCULOS VOLITANTES, Metamorphopsia.

MACULOSUS, *Sablé.*

MAD, Insane.

MADAR, Mudar.

MADARO'SIS, from μαδος, 'bald.' *Madaro'ma, Made'sis, Madar'otes, Made'ma, Mad'isis, Depluma'tio, Milphæ, Milpho'sis, Ptilo'sis, Calvi'ties.* Loss of the hair, particularly of the eyelashes.

MADAROTES, Madarosis.

MADDER, DYERS', Rubia.

MADEIRA, CLIMATE OF. This island is much frequented by pulmonary invalids, on account of the mildness and equability of its climate. Owing, indeed, to the mildness of the winter, and the coolness of the summer, together with the remarkable equality of the temperature during day and night, as well as throughout the year, it has been considered that the climate of Madeira is the finest in the northern hemisphere. Sir James Clark is of opinion that there is no place on the continent of Europe, with which he is acquainted, where the pulmonary invalid could reside with so much advantage, during the whole year, as in Madeira.

MADELEON, Bdellium.

MADEMA, Madarosis.

MADESIS, Depilation, Madarosis.

MADISIS, Depilation, Madarosis.

MADISTE'RIUM, *Madiste'rion, Trichola'lium, Trichol'abis, Volsel'la.* Tweezers. An instrument for extracting hairs.

MADNESS, CANINE, Hydrophobia — m. Raving or furious, Mania.

MADOR, Moisture. A cold sweat.

MADREPORA OCULATA, see Coral.

MADWEED, Scutellaria lateriflora.

MAEA, Midwife.

MAEEIA, Obstetrics.

MAEIA, Obstetrics.

MAEUTRIA, Midwife.

MAGDA'LIA, *Magda'leon, Magdalis.* Crumb of bread. Any medicine, as a pill, formed of crumb of bread. A roll of plaster.

MAGEIRICE, Culinary art.

MAGGOT PIMPLE, see Acne.

MAGIS, μαγις, 'a cake.' A sort of cake, composed of cloves, garlic and cheese, beaten together. — Hippocrates.

MAGISTERIUM, Magistery — m. Bismuthi, Bismuth, subnitrate of — m. Jalapæ, Resin of Jalap — m. Marcasitæ, Bismuth, subnitrate of — m. Plumbi, Plumbi subcarbonas — m. Sulphuris, Sulphur lotum — m. Tartari purgans, Potassæ acetas.

MAG"ISTERY, *Mayiste'rium,* from *magister,* 'a master.' Certain precipitates from saline solutions were formerly so called; as well as other medicines, the preparation of which was kept secret.

MAGISTERY OF BISMUTH, Bismuth, subnitrate of.

MAG"ISTRAL, *Magistra'lis.* Same etymon. *Extempora'neous.* Medicines are so called which are prepared extemporaneously; *officinal* medicines being such as have been prepared for some time before they are prescribed.

MAGISTRANTIA, Imperatoria.

MAGMA, μαγμα, (F.) *Marc.* The thick residuum, obtained after expressing certain substances to extract the fluid parts from them. The grounds which remain after treating a substance with water, alcohol, or any other menstruum. Also, a salve of a certain consistence.

MAGMA or MARC OF OLIVES is the residuum after the greatest possible quantity of oil has been extracted from olives by making them ferment. It was formerly employed as a stimulant, under the form of a *bath* — to which the name *Bain de Marc* was given by the French.

MAGMA or MARC OF GRAPES, *Bry'tia,* was once employed for the same purposes.

MAGMA RÉTICULÉ, 'reticulated magma.' The gelatiniform substance found between the chorion and amnion in the early period of embryonic existence.

MAGNES, Magnet.

MAGNES ARSENICA'LIS. (*Sulphur, white arsenic,* and *common antimony,* of each equal parts. Mix by fusion.) It is corrosive. See Magnetic plaster.

MAGNES EPILEPSIÆ, Hydrargyri sulphuretum rubrum.

MAGNE'SIA, *Abarnahas, Chambar, Terra ama'ra, Magnesia terra, Talc earth;* from *magnes,* 'the magnet;' because it was supposed to have the power of attracting substances from the air. Its metallic base is *magne'sium.*

MAGNESIA, *M. usta, M. calcina'ta, Cal'cined Magnesia, Oxide of magne'sium,* (F.) *Magnésie brulée, Magnésie, M. Caustique.* This is obtained by exposing carbonate of magnesia to a strong heat. It is inodorous; taste very slightly bitter; in the form of a white, light, spongy, soft powder. S. g. 2.3; requiring 2000 times its weight of water for its solution. It is antacid, and laxative when it meets with acid in the stomach. Dose, gr. x to ʒj in water or milk.

MAGNESIA AERATA, Magnesiæ carbonas — m. Alba, M. carbonas — m. Calcinata, M. usta — m. Citrate of, Magnesiæ citras — m. Edinburgensis, M. carbonas.

MAGNESIA, EFFERVESCING, MOXON'S. (*Magnes. carb.; M. sulphat.; Sodæ bicarbon., Acid tartaric.* āā partes æquales; to be pulverized, well dried, mixed, and enclosed in bottles hermetically sealed.) Dose, a teaspoonful in half a tumbler of water, drunk in a state of effervescence.

MAGNESIA, FLUID. Under this name a preparation is designated, which consists of a solution of carbonate of magnesia in carbonated water. It is also termed *carbonated magnesia water, aërated magnesia water,* and *condensed solution of magnesia,* (F.) *Eau magnésienne.*

MAGNESIA, HENRY'S, Magnesiæ carbonas — m. Mitis, Magnesiæ carbonas — m. Muriate of, Magnesii chloridum — m. Nigra, Manganese, black oxide of.

MAGNESIA OPALI'NA. A name given by Lémery to a mixture of equal parts of *antimony, nitrate of potass,* and *chloride of sodium,* (decrepitated.) It has emetic properties, but is not used.

MAGNESIA SALIS AMARI, Magnesiæ carbonas — m. Salis Ebsdamensis, Magnesiæ carbonas — m. Saturni, Antimonium — m. Solution of, condensed, M. fluid — m. Subcarbonate of, Magnesiæ carbonas — m. Subcarbonate of, Hydrated, Magnesiæ carbonas — m. Terra, Magnesia — m. Vitriolata, Magnesiæ sulphas — m. and Soda, sulphate of, see Soda, sulphate of — m. Usta, Magnesia.

MAGNESIÆ CAR'BONAS, *M. Subcar'bonas, Magnesia,* (Dublin,) *M. aëra'ta, M. carbon'ica, M. alba, Subcar'bonate of Magnesia, Hy'drated Subcar'bonate of Magnesia, Henry's Magnesia, M. Subcarbon'ica, M. Mitis, M. Edinburgen'sis, M. Salis Ebsdamen'sis, M. Salis ama'ri, Car'bonas magne'sicum, Lac terræ, Hypocar'bonas magne'siæ, T. amara aëra'ta, T. absor'bens minera'lis, T. Talco'sa oxyanthraco'des,* (F.) *Sous-carbonate ou carbonate de Magnésie, Magnésie aérée, M. blanche, M. crayeuse, M. douce, M. effervescente, M. moyenne, Poudre de Sentinelli, P. de Valentini, P. du Comte de Palme.* Prepared from sulphate of magnesia by subcarbonate of potass. It is inodorous; insipid; light; white; spongy; opake; effervescing with acids; insoluble in water. Properties the same as the last; but the carbonic acid, when set free, sometimes causes unpleasant distension.

MAGNESIÆ CITRAS, *Citrate of Magnesia,* (F.) *Citrate de Magnésie.* A saline preparation, formed by saturating a solution of *citric acid* with either *magnesia* or its *carbonate.* Dose, an ounce. It is devoid of the bitter taste of the magnesian salts.

A solution in water, or in mineral water, sweetened with syrup, and acidulated with citric acid, makes an agreeable purgative. A simple solution in water has been called *magnesian lemonade.* In the effervescing state, it is the *effervescing magnesian lemonade.* The Pharmacopœia of the United States (1851) has a form for the LIQUOR MAGNESIÆ CITRA'TIS, *Solution of Citrate of Magnesia.* Take of Carbonate of magnesia, ʒv; citric acid, ʒviiss; Syrup of citric acid, fʒij; Water, a sufficient quantity. Dissolve the citric acid in fʒiv of water, and add ʒiv of the carbonate of magnesia, previously rubbed with fʒiij of water. When the reaction has ceased, filter into a strong fʒxij glass bottle, into which the syrup of citric acid has been previously introduced. Rub the remaining carbonate of magnesia with fʒij of water, and pour the mixture into the bottle, which must be well corked, and secured with twine; and shake the mixture occasionally until it becomes transparent.

MAGNESIÆ HYPOCARBONAS, M. carbonas — m. Subcarbonas, M. carbonas — m. Vitriolicum, Magnesiæ sulphas.

MAGNESIÆ SULPHAS, *Sulphas Magnesiæ purifica'ta, Magnesia vitriola'ta, Sal cathar'ticus ama'rus, Sal catharticum amarum, Sal ama'rum, S. Anglica'num, Sulphate of Magnesia, Sal Epsomen'sis, Sal catharticus Anglica'nus, Sal Sedlicen'sis, Sal Ebsdamen'sě, S. Seydschutzen'sě, Terra ama'ra sulphu'rica, Vitriol'icum Magne'siæ, Epsom Salt, Bitter purging Salt,* (F.) *Sulfate de magnésie, Sel admirable de Lémèry, Sel d'égra.* Generally obtained from sea-water. Its taste is bitter and disagreeable. It is soluble in an equal quantity of water at 60°. It is purgative and diuretic. Dose, as a cathartic, ʒss to ʒij.

MAGNESIAN LEMONADE, Magnesiæ citras.

MAGNÉSIE AÉRÉE, Magnesiæ carbonas — *m. Blanche,* Magnesiæ carbonas — *m. Brulée,* Magnesia usta — *m. Carbonate de,* Magnesiæ carbonas — *m. Caustique,* Magnesia usta — *m. Citrate de,* Magnesiæ citras — *m. Crayeuse,* Magnesiæ carbonas — *m. Douce,* Magnesiæ carbonas — *m. Effervescente,* Magnesiæ carbonas — *m. Moyenne,* Magnesiæ carbonas — *m. Souscarbonate de,* Magnesiæ carbonas — *m. Sulfate de,* Magnesiæ sulphas.

MAGNE'SII CHLO'RIDUM, *Chloride of Magne'sium, Muriate of Magnesia.* This bitter deliquescent salt has been given as a mild and effective cholagogue cathartic, in the dose of half an ounce to the adult. Being deliquescent, it may be kept dissolved in its weight of water.

MAGNESIUM, see Magnesia — m. Chloride of, Magnesii chloridum — m. Oxide of, Magnesia usta.

MAGNET, *Magnes, Magne'tes, Ferrum magnes attracto'rium, Sideri'tes, Sideri'tis, Lapis heracle'us, L. Syderi'tis, L. nau'ticus, Magni'tis,* so called from Magnes, its discoverer, or from *Magnesia,* whence it was obtained; (F.) *Aimant;* The *magnet* or *loadstone.* An amorphous, oxydulated ore of iron, which exerts an attraction on unmagnetized iron, and has the property of exhibiting poles; that is, of pointing by one of its extremities to the north. This ore, by constant or long rubbing, communicates its properties to iron; and thus artificial magnets are formed. Magnetic ore is found in many countries, and particularly in the island of Elba. The magnet is sometimes used to extract spicula of iron from the eye or from wounds. It has been employed as an antispasmodic; but acts only through the imagination. The powder has been given as a tonic. In *Pharmacy,* it is used to purify iron filings. It attracts the iron, and the impurities remain behind. It formerly entered, as an ingredient, into several plasters, to draw bullets and heads of arrows from the body — as the *Emplastrum divinum Nicolai,* the *Emplastrum nigrum* of Augsburg, the *Opodeldoch,* and *Attractivum* of Paracelsus, &c.

MAGNETES, Magnet.

MAGNET'IC, *Magnet'icus.* Same etymon. That which belongs or relates to magnetism; — mineral or animal.

MAGNETIC FLUID. A name given to the imponderable fluid to which the magnet owes its virtues. By analogy it is applied to a particular principle, supposed to be the source of organic actions, which affects, it is conceived, the nervous system principally, and is susceptible of being transmitted from one living body to another, by contact or simple approximation, and especially under the influence of fixed volition. See Magnetism, Animal.

MAGNETIC PLASTER. A plaster, at present, not used. It had for its base a mixture, called *Magnes arsenica'lis;* formed of equal parts of antimony, sulphur and arsenic melted together in a glass cucurbit. The name *Magnetic plaster* was, likewise, given to such as contained powdered magnet.

MAGNETINUS, Potassæ supertartras impurus.

MAG'NETISM, AN'IMAL, *Mes'merism, Path'etism, Neuroga'mia, Bioga'mia, Biomagnetis'mus, Zoömagnetis'mus, Exon'eurism* (proposed by Mr. H. Mayo,) *Telluris'mus, Anthropomagnetis'mus, Gar'galê, Gargalis'mus, Gar'galus.* Properties attributed to the influence of a particular principle, which has been compared to that which characterizes the magnet. It is supposed to be transmitted from one person to another, and to impress peculiar modifications on organic action, especially on that of the nerves. The discussions, to which this strange belief has given rise, are by no means terminated. There is no evidence whatever of the existence of such a fluid. Highly impressible persons can be thrown into a kind of hysterio or 'magnetic' sleep and somnambulism, (designated by Mr. Braid, *hyp'notism, neuro-hyp'notism,* and *nervous sleep*); but farther than this, the efforts of the magnetizer cannot reach. It is a mode of action upon the nerves through the medium of the senses.

MAGNETIZATION, Mesmerisation.
MAGNETIZED, Mesmerized.
MAGNETIZER, Mesmerizer.
MAGNITIS, Magnet.
MAGNITUDO CORPORIS, Stature.
MAGNOC, Jatropha manihot.
MAGNOLIA FRAGRANS, M. glauca.

MAGNO'LIA GLAUCA, *M. fragrans*, Small Magnolia, Magnolia, Swamp *Sas'safras*, Elk Bark, Indian Bark, White Laurel, Sweet Bay, Beaver Wood, White Bay, Cinchona of Virginia, Castor Bay, Sweet maynolia. The bark is possessed of tonic properties, resembling those of cascarilla, canella, &c. The same may be said of the *Magnolia tripet'ala* or *Umbrel'la tree;* the *M. acumina'ta* or *Cu'cumber tree*, the *M. grandiflo'ra* and *M. macrophyl'la*, Laurel, Elk wood, Silverleaf, Big leaf, White Bay, Beaver Tree, Elk bark, Big bloom.

MAGNUM DEI DONUM, Cinchona.
MAGNUM Os. The third bone of the lower row of the carpus, reckoning from the thumb. It is the largest bone of the carpus; and is, also, called *Os capita'tum;* (F.) *Grand Os.*

MAGRUMS. A popular name in the State of New York for a singular convulsive affection, which resembles chorea. It rarely, however, occurs before the adult age; never ceases spontaneously, and, when fully developed, is devoid of any paroxysmal character.

MAGUEY, Agave Americana.
MAHMOUDY, Convolvulus scammonia.
MAHOGAN FÉBRIFUGE, Swietenia febrifuga.
MAHOGANY, Gynocladus Canadensis — m. Mountain, Betula lenta — m. Tree, Swietenia mahogani.
MAIANTHEUM, Convallaria maialis.
MAIDENHAIR, Adiantum capillus veneris — m. American, Adiantum pedatum — m. Canada, Adiantum pedatum — m. Common, Asplenium trichomanoides — m. Golden, Polytrichum—m. White, Asplenium ruta muraria.
MAIDENHEAD, Virginity.
MAIDENHOOD, Virginity.
MAIEIA, Obstetrics.
MAIEUSIS, Parturition.
MAIEUTA, see Parturition.
MAIEUTER, *Accoucheur.*
MAIEUTES, *Accoucheur.*
MAIEUTICA ARS, Obstetrics.
MAIGREUR, Emaciation.
MAILLET, Mallet.
MAILLOT, Swathing clothes.
MAIN, Manus.
MAIRANIA UVA URSI, Arbutus urva ursi.
MAÏS, Zea mays.
MAJOR HEL'ICIS. A narrow band of muscular fibres situate upon the anterior border of the helix of the ear, just above the tragus.
MAJORANA, Origanum majorana — m. Hortensis, Origanum majorana — m. Syriaca, Teucrium marum.
MAL D'AMOUR, Odontalgia.
MAL DES ARDENS. A name given to a species of pestilential erysipelas or *Saint Anthony's fire*, which reigned epidemically in France, in 1130.
MAL D'AVENTURE, Paronychia — *m. di Breno, Scherlievo*—*m. Caduc*, Epilepsy.
MAL DE CRIMÉE (F.), *Lèpre des Cossaques, Lepra Tau'rica.* A variety of lepra in the Crimea.
MAL DE DENT, Odontalgia—*m. d'Estomac*, Chthonophagia — *m. Divin*, Epilepsy — *m. d'Enfant*, Pains (Labour)—*m. di Fiume*, Scherlievo—*m. Français*, Syphilis—*m. de Gorge*, Cynanche—

m. Haut, Epilepsy—*m. de Machoire*, Trismus—*m. de Mer*, Nausea marina—*m. de Mère*, Hysteria—*m. de Misère*, Pellagra—*m. de Naples*, Syphilis—*m. Petit*, Epilepsy—*m. du Roi*, Scrofula—*m. Rouge de Cayenne*, Elephantiasis of Cayenne—*m. Saint Antoine*, Erysipelas—*m. Saint Jean*, Epilepsy—*m. Saint Main*, Lepra, Psora—*m. di Scherlievo, Scherlievo*—*m. de Siam*, Fever, yellow.

MAL DE SAN LAZARO, Cocobay. A leprous disease, common in Colombia, S. America.

MAL DEL SOLE, Pellagra—*m. de Sologne*, Ergotism — *m. de Terre*, Epilepsy — *m. à Tête*, Cephalalgia—*m. del Valle*, Proctocace—*m. Vat*, see Anthrax.

MALA, Gena—m. Aurea, see Citrus aurantium.
MALABATH'RINUM. Ancient name of an ointment and a wine, into which the *malabathrum* entered.

MALABA'THRUM, *Cadeji-Indi.* The leaves of a tree of the East Indies. These leaves entered into the theriac, mithridate, and other ancient electuaries. They are believed to be from a species of laurel—*Laurus Cassia;* but, according to others, from *Laurus Malabathrum.* The *O'leum Malabathri* is obtained from it.

MALACCÆ RADIX, Sagittarium alexipharmacum.
MALACHE, Malva rotundifolia.
MALA'CIA, from μαλακια, 'softness.' A depravation of taste, in which an almost universal loathing is combined with an exclusive longing for some particular article of food. If the patient desires substances that are not eatable or noxious, it constitutes *Pica, Pisso'sis, Pitto'sis, Heterorex'ia, Heterorrhex'ia, Cissa, Citto'sis, Citta, Limo'sis Pica, Allotriopha'gia, Picacis'mus, Pica'tio, Deprav'ed ap'petite,* (F.) *Envie.* These symptoms accompany several nervous affections,—those of females in particular. In pregnancy it is common, and is termed *Longing.*

MALACIA AFRICANORUM, Chthonophagia — m. Cordis, Cardiomalacia.
MALACISMUS, Mollities.
MALACOGASTER, Gastromalaxia.
MALACOPHO'NUS, from μαλακια, 'softness,' and φωνη, 'voice.' One who has a soft voice.
MALACOPŒA, Emollients.
MALACORIUM, see Punica granatum.
MALACOSAR'COS, from μαλακος, 'soft,' and σαρξ, 'flesh.' One of a soft constitution: *hab'itê cor'poris mollio'ri præ'ditus.*—Galen.
MALACOSIS, Mollities—m. Cerebri, Mollities cerebri—m. Cordis, Cardiomalacia— m. Hepatis, Hepatomalacia—m. Uteri, Hysteromalacia.
MALACOSTEON, Mollities ossium.
MALACTICA, Emollients.
MALACTICUM, Relaxant.
MALADE, Sick.
MALADIE, Disease—*m. Anglaise*, Hypochondriasis — *m. Bleue*, Cyanopathy — *m. de Bright*, Kidney, Bright's disease of the—*m. de Ourveilheir*, see Brash, weaning— *m. Cuculaire*, Pertussis—*m. Glandulaire*, Elephantiasis Arabica—*m. Imaginaire*, Hypochondriasis, Hysteria.

MALADIE DES MINEURS. Anæmia occurring in the workers in mines.

MALADIE NOIRE, Melæna— *m. du Pays*, Nostalgia— *m. Pédiculaire*, Phtheiriasis — *m. de Pott*, Vertebral disease—*m. Typhoïde*, see Typhus—*m. Vénérienne*, Syphilis—*m. de Vénus*, Syphilis *m. de Werlhof*, Purpura hæmorrhagica.

MALADIES ACQUISES, Acquired diseases—*m. Annulles*, Annual diseases—*m. Chroniques*, Chronic diseases—*m. Connées*, Connate diseases—*m. Dissimulées*, Feigned diseases—*m. Externes*, External diseases—*m. Feintes*, Feigned diseases—*m. Héréditaires*, Hereditary diseases—*m. Innées*, Innate

diseases—m. *Légitimes*, see Legitimate—m. *Nerveuses*, Nervous diseases — m. *Simulées*, Feigned diseases — m. *Supposées*, Feigned diseases — m. *Venteuses*, Pneumatosis.
MALADIF, Sickly.
MALADRERIE, Ladrerie.
MALADY, ENGLISH, Hypochondriasis.
MALÆ, OS, from *malum*, 'an apple;' so called from its roundness. *Os mala'rē, Os Juga'lē, Os Jugamen'tum, Os Genæ, Zygo'ma, Os Zygomat'icum, Os Hypo'pium, Os Subocula'rē, Os Pud'icum*, (F.) *Os Malaire, Os Zygomatique, Os de la Pommette*. The *cheek* or *malar bone*. This bone is situate at the lateral and superior part of the face; and constitutes the zygomatic region of the cheek. It is irregularly quadrilateral. Its *outer* surface is convex, covered by muscles and skin, and pierced with canals, called *malar*, through which vessels and nerves pass. Its *upper* surface is concave, and forms part of the orbit. Its *posterior* surface is concave, and enters into the composition of the temporal fossa. This bone is thick and cellular. It is articulated with the frontal, temporal, sphenoid, and superior maxillary bones, and is developed by a single point of ossification.
The part of the face rendered prominent by it, the French call *Pommette*.
MALAG'MA, from μαλασσω, 'I soften.' An emollient cataplasm, and, in general, every local application which enjoys the property of softening organic tissues.
MALAISE, Indisposition
MALAKIEN, Mollities.
MALAMBO BARK, Matias.
MALANDRIA. A species of lepra or elephantiasis.— Marcellus Empiricus.
MALANDRIO'SUS, *Leprous*. Affected with a species of lepra.
MALAR, *Mala'ris*, from *mala*, 'the cheek.' Belonging to the cheek,—as the *malar* bone.
MALAR PROCESS, Zygomatic process.
MALARE OS, Malæ os.
MALARIA, Miasm.
MALA'RIOUS, *Mala'rial*. Owing to, or connected with Malaria,— as a *malarious soil, malarious disease,* &c.
MALASSIMILA'TION, *Malassimila'tio;* from *mala*, 'bad,' and *assimilatio*, 'assimilation.' Imperfect or morbid assimilation or nutrition.
MAL'AXATE, *Molli'rē, Subig''erē, Malacissa'rē*, (F.) *Malaxer*, from μαλασσω, 'I soften.' To produce softening of drugs, by kneading them. The process is called *Malaxa'tion, Malaxa'tio.*
MALAXATION, see Malaxate.
MALAXIA VENTRICULI, Gastromalaxia.
MALAXIS, Mollities — m. Cordis, Cardiomalacia.
MALAY, see Homo.
MALAZISSA'TUS, *Malacissa'tus*, from *malacisso*, 'I soften.' One in whom the testicles have not descended. It has, also, been used synonymously with *emascula'tus* and *muliera'tus*.—Castelli.
MALCE, Chilblain.
MALE, *Mas, Mas'culus*. Of the sex that begets young. Not female. What belongs to the male sex; as the *male organs of generation.*
MALE, Axilla — m. Organ, Penis.
MALEFICIUM, Poisoning.
MALFORMA'TION, *malforma'tio, malconforma'tio;* from *mala*, 'bad,' and *forma*, 'form.' A wrong formation; or irregularity in the structure of parts. See Monster.
MALIA, see Equinia.
MALIASMUS, Malis, see Equinia.
MALICHORIUM, see Punica granatum.
MALICORIUM, see Punica granatum.
MALIE, Equinia.

MALIG'NANT, *Malig'nus*, (F.) *Malin*. A term applied to any disease whose symptoms are so aggravated as to threaten the destruction of the patient. A disease of a very serious character, although it may be mild in appearance;—*Morbus malignus.*
MALIN, Malignant.
MALING'ERER; from (F.) *malingre*, 'sickly.' A simulator of disease, so termed in the British military service.
MALIS, *Malias'mos, Cuta'neous vermina'tion, Helminthon'cus*. The cuticle or skin infested with animalcules, — *Phthiri'asis, Parasitis'mus superfic''iei*. In Persia, this affection is produced by the Guinea worm; in South America, by the Chigre; and in Europe, occasionally by the Louse. See Equinia, and Phtheiriasis.
MALIS DRACUNCULUS, Dracunculus—m. Gordii, Dracunculus—m. Pediculi, Phtheiriasis.
MALLE'OLAR, *Malleola'ris*, from *malleolus*, 'the ankle.' Belonging or relating to the ankles.
MALLEOLAR ARTERIES are two branches furnished by the *anterior tibial* about the instep; the one—the *internal*—passes transversely behind the tendon of the tibialis anticus, to be distributed in the vicinity of the malleolus internus; — the other — the *external* — glides behind the tendons of the *extensor communis digitorum pedis* and the *peroneus brevis*, and sends its branches to the parts which surround the outer ankle, as well as to the outer region of the tarsus.
MALLE'OLUS. Diminutive of *malleus*, 'a mallet, or hammer;' *Raece'ta, Raste'ta, Rascha, Rasetta, Rase'ta, Sphyra, Talus, Diab'ebos, Tale'olus, Peza*, the *Ankle*, (F.) *Malléole, Cheville du Pied*. The two projections formed by the bones of the leg at their inferior part. The *inner* belongs to the tibia; the *outer* to the fibula. The ankles afford attachment to ligaments; and each has a sort of gutter, in which certain tendons slide. See Malleus.
MALLET, *Malle'olus*, (F.) *Maillet*. A kind of hammer, used with a gouge for removing or cutting bones, in certain surgical and anatomical operations.
MAL'LEUS, *Malle'olus, Ossic'ulum Malleolo assimila'tum*, (F.) *Marteau*. The longest and outermost of the four small bones of the ear. It is situate at the outer part of the tympanum, and is united to the membrana tympani. It has, 1. An ovoid head, which is articulated behind with the incus, and is supported by a narrow part called the neck: this has, anteriorly, a *long apophysis*, which is engaged in the glenoid fissure, and is called the *Apophysis* or *Process, Proces'sus grac''ilis*, of Rau. It affords attachment to the *anterior mallei* muscle. 2. A *handle*, which forms an obtuse angle with the neck, and corresponds to the membrane of the tympanum, which it seems to draw inwards. It is furnished at its upper extremity with a process—the *processus brevis*, to which the *internus mallei* is attached. This bone is developed by a single point of ossification.
MALLEUS, Equinia—M. farciminosus, see Equinia — m. Slender Process of the, *Grêle apophyse du marteau.*
MALLOW, COMMON, Malva—m. Compound decoction of, Decoctum malvæ compositum — m. Yellow, Abutilon cordatum.
MALMEDY, MINERAL WATERS OF. Malmedy is a town in Rhenish Prussia, between Spa and Coblenz. In its immediate vicinity are several acidulous chalybeate springs.
MALO DI SCARLIEVO, *Scherlievo.*
MALOGRANATUM, Punica granatum.
MALPIGHI, ACINI OF, Corpora Malpighiana.
MALPIG'HIA MOUREL'LA, (F.) *Mourrilier, Simarouba faux.* The bark of this shrub

a native of Cayenne — is reputed to be febrifuge, and useful in diarrhœa.

MALPIGHIAN BODIES, Corpora Malpighiana—m. b. Inflammation of the, Kidney, Bright's disease of the—m. b. of the Spleen, see Spleen.

MALPRAX'IS, *Mala praxis*, *Malum reg''imen*. Bad management or treatment.

MALT, Sax. mealō, Dutch m o u t, Teut. m a l t; from μαλαττω, 'I soften;' [?] *Bynē*, *Maltum*, *Hor'dei maltum*, *Bra'sium*, (F.) *Drêche*. Barley made to germinate, for the purpose of forming beer. It has been recommended in medicine, as antiscorbutic, antiscrofulous, &c.

MALT SPIRIT. A spirit distilled from malt. It is the basis of most of the spirituous cordials.

MALTA, CLIMATE OF. The climate of Malta is pretty equable, the range of temperature in the twenty-four hours being rarely more than 6°. The air is almost always dry and clear. The most disagreeable wind is the sirocco, which is the source of more or less suffering to the pulmonary invalid. The winter climate is favourable. Dr. Liddell thinks that no place which he has seen in the south of Europe can compete with Malta, for a mild, dry, bracing air in November, December, and part of January; and during the other winter and spring months, he thinks it is equal to any of them.

MALTHA, *Malthē*, from μαλαττω, 'I soften.' Wax, particularly soft wax.

MALTHACTICA, Emollients.

MALTHAXIS, Mollities.

MALUM, Disease, Melum — m. Articulorum, Gout—m. Caducum, Epilepsy—m. Caducum pulmonum, Asthma—m. Canum, see Pyrus cydonia —m. Coense, Averrhoa carambola—m. Cotoneum, see Pyrus cydonia — m. Hypochondriacum, Hypochondriasis—m. Hystericum, Hysteria—m. Insanum, see Solanum Melongena—m. Ischiadicum, Neuralgia femoro-poplitæa—m. Lazari, Elephantiasis—m. Lycopersicum, Solanum lycopersicum.

MALUM MOR'TUUM. A species of lepra, in which the affected portions of skin seem to be struck with death.

MALUM PILARE, Trichosis—m. Pottii, Vertebral disease—m. Primarium, Idiopathia—m. Regimen, Malpraxis—m. Spinosum, Datura stramonium— m. Terrestre, Atropa Mandragora—m. Venereum, Syphilis.

MALUS, Pyrus malus — m. Aurantia major, Citrus aurantium—m. Communis, Pyrus malus— m. Dasyphylla, Pyrus malus.

MALUS IN'DICA, *Bilumbi biting-bing* of Bontius. The juice of this East India tree is cooling, and is drunk as a cure for fevers. The leaves, boiled and made into a cataplasm with rice, are famed in all sorts of tumours. The juice, mixed with arrack, is drunk for the cure of diarrhœa. The ripe fruit is eaten as a delicacy; and the unripe is made into a pickle for the use of the table.

MALUS LIMONIA ACIDA, see Citrus medica—m. Medica, see Citrus medica—m. Sylvestris, Pyrus malus.

MALVA, *Malva sylves'tris* seu *vulga'ris*, Common Mallow, (F.) *Mauve sauvage*. The leaves and flowers are chiefly used in fomentations, cataplasms, and emollient enemata. Its properties are demulcent.

Malva rotundifo'lia, *Mal'achē*, *Mal'ochē*, has like virtues; as well as the other varieties.

MALVAVISCUM, Althæa.

MALVERN, WATERS OF. The village of Great Malvern, (pronounced *Maw'vern*,) in Worcestershire, England, has for many years been celebrated for a spring of remarkable purity, which has acquired the name of the *Holy well*. It is a carbonated water; containing carbonates of soda and iron, sulphate of soda, and chloride of sodium; and is chiefly used externally, in cutaneous affections.

MAMA-PIAN. An ulcer of a bad aspect, which is the commencement of the pian; and which, after having destroyed the flesh, extends to the bones. It is also called the *Mother of Pians*;—*La mère des pians*.

MAMEI, *Mamoe*, *Momin* or *Toddy tree*. From incisions made in the branches of this West Indian tree, a copius discharge of pellucid liquor occurs, which is called *momin* or *Toddy wine*. It is very diuretic, and is esteemed to be a good antilithic and lithontriptic.

MAMELLE, Mamma.

MAMELON, Nipple.

MAMELONNÉ, Mammillated.

MAMELONS DU REIN, Papillæ of the kidney.

MAMILLA, see Mamma.

MAMMA, from *mamma*, one of the earliest cries of the infant, ascribed to a desire for food. *Masthos*, *Mastus*, *Mazos*, *Thelē*, *Titthos*, *Rusa*, *Uber*, *Nutrix*, *Gemip'oma*. The *female breast*, (*Mammil'la*, *Mamilla* being the male breast;) (F.) *Mamelle*. A glandular organ, proper to a class of animals — the *mammalia* — and intended for the secretion of milk. The mammæ exist in both sexes, but they acquire a much greater size in the female; especially during pregnancy and lactation. In women, before the age of puberty, the breasts are but little developed. At this period, however, towards the central part of each breast, the skin suddenly changes colour, and assumes a rosy tint. It is of a reddish brown in women who have suckled several children. This circle has a rugous appearance, owing to the presence of sebaceous glands, and is called *Are'ola* or *Aure'ola*. These glands—*Tubercles of the Areola*, of Sir Astley Cooper—furnish an unctuous fluid for defending the nipple from the action of the saliva of the sucking infant. In the midst of the aureola is the nipple, a conoidal eminence, of a rosy tint, susceptible of erection, and at the surface of which the galactophorous ducts open. Besides the skin covering them, the breasts are, also, composed of a layer of fatty areolar tissue, more or less thick; of a large gland; excretory ducts; vessels, nerves, &c. See Mammary.

The breasts are called the *bosom*, *sinus*, (F.) *Sein*. Mamma also means a nurse.

MAMMAL, plural *Mamma'lia*, *Mam'mifer*, *mammif'erous animal*; from *mamma*, 'a breast.' An animal that suckles its young.

MAM'MARY, *Mamma'rius*, from *mamma*, 'the breast.' Relating to the breasts.

MAMMARY ABSCESS, Mastodynia apostematosa.

MAMMARY ARTERIES are three in number. They are distinguished into — 1. The *Internal Mammary*, *Arte'ria sterna'lis*, *A. Sous-sternal* (Ch.), *Internal thorac''ic*. It arises from the subclavian, and descends obliquely inwards, from its origin to the cartilage of the third rib. Below the diaphragm it divides into two branches; the one *external*, the other *internal*. From its origin until its bifurcation, it gives branches to the muscles and glands of the neck, to the thymus, mediastinum, pericardium, and œsophagus. In each intercostal space, it gives off *internal* and *external musculo-cutaneous* branches, and also, on each side, the *superior diaphragmatic*. Its two ultimate branches are distributed on the parietes of the abdomen, and anastomose with the external mammary, intercostal, lumbar, circumflexa ilii, and epigastric arteries. 2. The *External Mammary Arteries* are two in number, and are distinguished into *superior* and *inferior*. The *superior external mammary*, *First of the thoracics*

(Ch.,) *Superior external thoracic, Superior thoracic*, is furnished by the axillary artery. It descends obliquely forwards between the pectoralis major and pectoralis minor, to which it is distributed by a considerable number of branches. The *inferior external mammary*, the *second of the thoracics* (Ch.,) *Long* or *inferior thoracic*, arises from the axillary artery, a little below the preceding. It descends vertically over the lateral part of the thorax; curves, afterwards, inwards; becomes subcutaneous and divides into a number of branches, which surround the breast. It gives branches to the pectoralis major, serratus major anticus, the intercostal muscles, the glands of the axilla, and the integuments of the breast.

MAMMARY GLAND is the secretory organ of the milk. It is situate in the substance of the breast, to which it gives shape and size. The tissue of this gland results from the assemblage of lobes of different size, united intimately by a dense areolar tissue. Each of these is composed of several lobules, formed of round granulations, of a rosy white colour, and of the size of a poppy seed. The glandular grains give rise to the radicles of the excretory canals of the mamma, which are called *galactophorous* or *lactiferous*. These excretory vessels unite in ramusculi, rami, and in trunks of greater or less size; collect towards the centre of the gland; are tortuous, very extensible and semi-transparent. All terminate in sinuses, situate near the base of the nipple, which are commonly from 15 to 18 in number. These sinuses are very short, conical, and united by areolar tissue. From their summits, a fasciculus of new ducts sets out, which occupy the centre of the nipple and open separately at its surface. The arteries of the mammary gland come from the thoracic, axillary, intercostal, and internal mammary. The veins accompany the arteries; the nerves are furnished by the intercostals, and brachial plexus; the lymphatic vessels are very numerous, and form two layers. They communicate with those of the thorax, and pass into the axillary ganglions.

MAM'MARY SARCO'MA, *Mastoid sarcoma* of Abernethy, *Emphy'ma sarcoma mamma'rum*. A tumour, of the colour and texture of the mammary gland; dense and whitish; sometimes softer and brownish; often producing, on extirpation, a malignant ulcer with indurated edges. Found in various parts of the body and limbs.

MAMMARY VEINS follow the same course as the arteries, and have received the same denominations. The *internal mammary vein*, of the right side, opens into the superior cava; that of the left, into the corresponding subclavian vein. The *external mammary veins* open into the axillary vein.

MAMME'A AMERICA'NA. The systematic name of the tree on which the *mammee* fruit grows. This fruit has a delightful flavour when ripe; and is much cultivated in Jamaica, where it is generally sold in the markets as one of the best fruits of the island.

MAMMEA'TA, *Mammo'sa*, from *mamma*, 'the breast.' One who has large breasts.

MAMMELLA, Nipple.
MAMMIFER, Mammal.
MAMMIFEROUS ANIMAL, Mammal.
MAMMIFORM, Mastoid.
MAMMILLA, Mamma (male,) Nipple.
MAMMILLÆ MEDULLARES, see Mammillary.
MAMMILLARIS, Mastoid.
MAM'MILLARY, *Mammilla'ris*, from *Mammilla*, 'a small breast, a nipple.' See Mastoid.
MAMMILLARY EM'INENCE is a name given, 1. To more or less marked prominences on the inner surface of the bones of the cranium, which correspond to the anfractuosities of the cranium. 2. To white, round, medullary tubercles, of the size of a pea, situate at the base of the brain, behind the gray substance from which the *Tige pituitaire*, of the French anatomists, arises. These *Mammillary Tubercles, Cor'pora albican'tia, C. Candican'tia, C. Mammilla'ria, C. Pisiforʼmia, Bulbi forʼnicis, Mammillæ medulla'res, Prominentiæ albican'tes, Proces'sus mammilla'res cer'ebri, Protensioʼnes glandula'res, Eminen'tiæ candican'tes, Prio'rum crurum for'nicis bulbi, Willis's Glands*, (F.) *Bulbes de la voûte à trois piliers, Tubercles pisiformes* (Ch.), are united to each other by a small grayish band, which corresponds with the third ventricle. They receive the anterior prolongations of the fornix. Some ancient anatomists, taking the nervous trunks, to which Willis first gave the name of *olfactory nerves*, for simple appendages of the brain, called them, on account of their shape, *Carun'culæ mammilla'res*. Vesalius, Fallopius, Columbus, and several others, termed them *Proces'sus mammilla'res cer'ebri ad nares*.

MAM'MILLATED, (F.) *Mamelonné*, from *mamma*, 'the female breast.' That which has mammiform projections on its surface.

MAMMILLATED LIVER, Cirrhosis.
MAMMOSA, Mammeata.
MAMOE, Mamei.
MAN, Aner, Anthropos, Homo.
MAN-IN-THE-GROUND, Convolvulus panduratus.
MANCHE D'HIPPOCRATE, Chausse.
MANCURANA, Origanum.
MANDIBULA, Maxillary bone.
MANDIBULARIS MUSCULUS, Masseter.
MANDO, Glutton.
MANDRAGORA, Atropa mandragora — m. Acaulis, Atropa mandragora — m. Officinalis, Atropa mandragora — m. Vernalis, Atropa mandragora.
MANDRAGORI'TES, from μανδραγόρα, the *At'ropa mandrag'ora* or mandrake. Wine in which the roots of mandrake have been infused.
MANDRAKE, Atropa mandragora, Podophyllum peltatum, P. montanum.
MANDUCATIO, Mastication — m. Difficilis, Bradymasesis.
MAN'DUCATORY, *Manducato'rius;* from *Manducatio*, 'mastication.' Appertaining or relating to mastication; — as,
MANDUCATORY NERVE, see Trigemini.
MANGANESE, BLACK OXIDE OF, *Mangane'sii ox'idum, M. Binox'idum, Tetrox'ide of manganese, Magne'sia nigra, Mangane'sium vitrario'rum, M. oxydu'tum nati'vum seu nigrum, Mangane'sium ochra'ceum nigrum, M. oxydu'tum nati'vum, Man'ganum oxyda'tum nativum, Molybdæ'num magne'sii, Oxo'des man'gani nati'va, Perox'ydum mangane'sii nigrum nativum, Superox'ydum mangan'icum*, (F.) *Oxyde noir de manganèse*. This oxide is not much used in medicine. It has been advised to dust the affected parts, in tinea capitis, with the powder.
MANGANESE, SALTS OF, see Manganese, sulphate of.
MANGANÈSE, OXYDE NOIR DE, Manganese, black oxide of.
MAN'GANESE, SULPHATE OF, *Mangane'sii Sulphas, M. Protox'idi Sulphas, Sulphate of Protox'ide of Man'ganese*. A rose-coloured and very soluble salt, isomorphous with sulphate of magnesia. It is prepared on a large scale for the use of the dyer, by heating, in a close vessel, peroxide of manganese and coal, and dissolving the im-

pure protoxide thus obtained in sulphuric acid, with the addition of a little chlorohydric acid towards the end of the process. The solution is evaporated to dryness, and again exposed to a red heat, by which the persulphate of iron is decomposed. Water then dissolves the pure sulphate of manganese, leaving the oxide of iron behind. This salt has been recommended as a cholagogue, in doses of a drachm or two.

The *salts of manganese* have been recommended in chlorosis and amenorrhœa, and as substitutes for chalybeates generally. The subcarbonate and the oxide have been chiefly employed.

MANGANESE, TETROXIDE OF, M. Black oxide of.
MANGANESII BINOXIDUM, Manganese, black oxide of—m. Oxidum, Manganese, black oxide of—m. Peroxydum nigrum nativum, Manganese, black oxide of—m. Protoxidi sulphas, Manganese, sulphate of—m. Sulphas, Manganese, sulphate of.

MANGANESIUM OCHRACEUM NIGRUM, Manganese, black oxide of—m. Oxydatum nativum seu nigrum, Manganese, black oxide of—m. Vitrariorum, Manganese, black oxide of.

MANGANI OXODES NATIVA, Manganese, black oxide of.

MANGANICUM SUPEROXIDUM, Manganese, black oxide of.

MANGANUM OXYDATUM NATIVUM, Manganese, black oxide of.

MANGE, Scabies ferina.

MANGIF'ERA IN'DICA, *M. domes'tica.* The *Mango tree*, (F.) *Manguier*. A tree cultivated over Asia, and in South America. Mangos, when ripe, are juicy, of a good flavour, and so fragrant as to perfume the air to a considerable distance. They are eaten, either raw or preserved with sugar. From the expressed juice a wine is prepared; and the remainder of the kernel can be reduced to an excellent flour for bread.

MANGO TREE, Mangifera Indica.
MANGONISATIO, Falsification.
MANGONIUM, Falsification.
MANGOSTAN, Garcinia mangostana.
MANGOSTANA, Garcinia mangostana — m. Cambogia, Garcinia cambogia—m. Garcinia, Garcinia mangostana.
MANGOUSTAN, Garcinia mangostana.
MANGUIER, Mangifera Indica.
MANHOOD, Adult age.
MANI, Arachis hypogæa.
MA'NIA, *Furor, Hemianthro'pia, Furor mania, Insa'nia, Delir'ium mani'acum, Ecphro'nia mania, Delir'ium mania, D. furio'sum, Mania universa'lis, Vesa'nia mania,* (F.) *Manie, Hyperphrénie, Raving or furious madness;* from μαίνομαι, 'I am furious.' With some, it means *insanity*. Disorder of the intellect, in which there is erroneous judgment or hallucination, which impels to acts of fury. If the raving be not directed to a single object, it is mania properly so called; if to one object, it constitutes *monomania*, which term is, however, usually given to melancholy. Mania attacks adults chiefly; and women more frequently than men. The prognosis is unfavourable. About one-third never recover; and they who do are apt to relapse. *Separation* is one of the most effective means of treatment, with attention to the corporeal condition and every thing that can add to the mental comfort of the patient, and turn his thoughts away from the subjects of his delusion. In the violence of the paroxysms, recourse must be had to the strait waistcoat, the shower bath, &c. Separation should be continued for some weeks during convalescence, with the view of preventing a relapse.

MANIA, DANCING. *Dancing plague*. A form of convulsion, which has appeared, at various times, epidemically under the form of St. Vitus's dance, St. John's dance, Tarantism, Hysteria, Tigretier (in Abyssinia), and diseased sympathy; and which has been fully described by Hecker in his 'Epidemics of the Middle Ages.' See *Convulsionnaire*.

A form of convulsion, induced by religious phrenzy, has been vulgarly called the *Jerks*.

MANIA EPILEPTICA, see Epilepsy—m. Erotica, Erotomania—m. Lactea, M. puerperal—m. Melancholica, Melancholy—m. a Pathemate, Empathema—m. a Potû, Delirium tremens.

MANIA, PUER'PERAL, *Ma'nia puerpera'rum acu'ta, M. puerpera'lis, M. lac'tea, Insa'nia puerpera'rum, Encephalopathi'a puerpera'lis, Puerperal Insanity.* Mania which supervenes in the childbed state.

MANIA PURPERARUM ACUTA, M. puerperal—m. *sine Delirio*, Pathomania—m. a Temulentiâ, Delirium tremens—m. Pellagria, Pellagra.

MANIACAL, Maniodes.
MANIACUS, Maniodes.
MANICA HIPPOCRATIS, *Chausse*.
MANIE, Mania—*m. sans Délire*, Empathema.
MANIGUETTA, Amomum grana paradisi.
MANIIBAR, Jatropha manihot.
MANILU'VIUM, *Manulu'vium*, from *manus*, 'the hand,' and '*lavo*, 'I wash.' A bath for the hands. It may be rendered stimulating, by means of muriatic acid, mustard, &c.

MANIOC, Jatropha manihot.
MANIO'DES, *Mani'acus, Mani'acal*. One labouring under mania; *Hemianthro'pus, Furio'sus, Furibun'dus, Lyssas, Lysse'ter*.

MANIPULA'TION, from *manus*, 'a hand.' Mode of working in the arts.

MANIP'ULUS, (F.) *Poignée*. The quantity of a substance capable of filling the hand. A handful. See Fasciculus.

MAN-MIDWIFE, Accoucheur.
MANNA, see Fraxinus ornus—m. Briançon, see Pinus larix—m. Brigantina, see Pinus larix—m. Calabrina, see Fraxinus ornus—m. Croup, Semolina—m. Laricea, see Pinus larix—m. Metallorum, Hydrargyri submurias.

MANNEQUIN, Fantom.
MANNEKIN, Fantom.
MANNIN, see Fraxinus ornus.
MANNITE, see Fraxinus ornus.
MANŒUVRE (F.), pronounced *manew'ver*; from *main*, 'the hand,' and *œuvre*, 'work.' A dexterous movement. Applied in France to the practice of surgical or obstetrical operations on the dead body or phantom; *Opera'tio chirur'gica vel obstet'rica*.

MANSANA ARBOREA, see Jujube.
MANSFORD'S PLATES, see Galvanism.
MANSORIUS, Buccinator.
MANSTUPRATIO, Masturbation.
MANTELE, Bandage (body).
MANTI'A, *Man'tica, Man'ticè*, in English. *mancy*; a common suffix, denoting 'divination;' *Divina'tio, Prædivinatio, Præsa'gium*.

MANTILE, Bandage (body).
MANTLE, Panniculus carnosus.
MANU'BRIUM, from *manus*, 'a hand.' The handle of any thing:—as *manu'brium mal'lei, petiolus mal'lei*, 'the handle of the malleus.'

MANUBRIUM, *Chasse*—m. Manûs, Radius.
MANUBRIUM STERNI. The uppermost broad part of the sternum.

MANULUVIUM, Bath, hand, Maniluvium.
MANUS, *Cheir, Chir, Instrumentum Instrumentorum, Hand, Paw*, (F.) *Main*. The part which terminates the upper extremity in man, and which is inservient to prehension and touch. It extends from the fold of the wrist to the extremity of the fingers. The hand is sustained by a

bony skeleton, composed of a number of pieces, movable on each other; of muscles, tendons, cartilages, ligaments, vessels, nerves, &c. It is divided into three parts—the *carpus* or wrist, the *metacarpus*, and *fingers*. Its concave surface is called the *palm;* the convex surface the *back of the hand*. The facility of being able to oppose the thumb to the fingers in order to seize objects forms one of the distinctive characters of the human hand.

MANUS CHRISTI PERLA'TA. A name anciently given to troches, prepared of pearls and sugar of roses. They were called *Manus Christi sim'plices*, when pearls were not employed.

MANUS DEI. An ancient plaster, prepared of *wax, myrrh, frankincense, mastich, gum ammoniac, galbanum, oil*, &c. See Opium.

MANUS HEPATIS, Porta vena—m. Jecoris, Porta vena—m. Parva majori adjutrix, see Digitus.

MANUSTUPRATIO, Masturbation.

MANUSTUPRATOR, Masturbator.

MANYPLIES, Omasum.

MAPLE, Acer saccharinum—m. Ground, Heuchera cortusa.

MARAIS, Marsh.

MARANTA ARUNDINACEA, Arrow-root.

MARAN'TA GALAN'GA, *Alpi'nia galan'ga, Amo'mum galanga, Galanga*. The *smaller galan'gal*. Two kinds of galangal are mentioned in the pharmacopœias ; the *greater*, obtained from *Kæmpferia galanga*, and the *smaller*, from the root of *Maranta galanga*. The dried root is brought from China, in pieces, from one to two inches in length, but scarcely half as thick; branched; full of knots and joints, with several circular rings, of a reddish brown colour, on the outside, and brownish within. It was formerly much used as a warm stomachic bitter, and generally ordered in bitter infusions.

MARASCHINO, see Spirit.

MARASMOP'YRA, *Febris marasmo'des*, from μαρασμος, 'marasmus,' and πυρ, 'fever.' Fever of emacination in general. Hectic fever.

MARASMUS, Atrophy — m. Lactantium, Pædatrophia—m. Phthisis, Phthisis pulmonalis.

MARASMUS SENI'LIS, *Tabes senum, Gerontatroph'ia*. Progressive atrophy of the aged.

MARASMUS TABES, Tabes — m. Tabes dorsalis, Tabes dorsalis.

MARATHRI'TES, from μαραθρον, 'fennel.' Wine impregnated with fennel.

MARATHROPHYLLUM, Peucedanum.

MARATHRUM, Anethum—m. Sylvestre, Peucedanum.

MARAUGIA, Metamorphopsia.

MARBLE, Marmor.

MARBRE, Marmor.

MARC, Magma.

MARCASITA, Bismuth — m. Alba, Bismuth, subnitrate of—m. Plumbea, Antimonium.

MARCASITÆ MAGISTERIUM, Bismuth, subnitrate of.

MARCHAN'TIA POLYMOR'PHA, *M. stella'ta seu umbella'ta, Hepat'ica fonta'na, Lichen stella'tus, Jecora'ria, Liv'erwort*, (F.) *Hépatique des fontaines*. This plant is mildly pungent and bitter. It is recommended as aperient, resolvent, and antiscorbutic; and is used in diseased liver, &c.

MARCHE LA, Walking.

MARCHIO'NIS PULVIS, *Powder of the Marquis*. A powder, formerly considered to be antiepileptic; and composed of *Male pæony root, Mistletoe, Ivory shavings, Horn of the hoof of the stag, Spodium, Tooth of the monodon, coral*, &c.

MARCORES, Atrophy, Emaciation.

MARCORY, Stillingia.

MARÉCAGEUX, Elodes.

MAREO, Puna.

MARE'S TAIL, Hippuris vulgaris.

MARGA CAN'DIDA, *Lac lunæ*. An ancient name for a variety of spongy, white, friable marl, which was employed as an astringent and refrigerant.

MARGARETIZZA, *Scherlievo*.

MARGARITA, Pearl.

MARGARITA'CEOUS, *Margarita'ceus, Na'creous*, (F.) *Nacré;* from *Margarita*, 'pearl, mother of pearl.' Resembling, or of the nature of, mother of pearl, — as *Leuco'ma Margarita'ceum;* Pearl-like leucoma.

MARGARON, Pearl.

MARGELIS, Pearl.

MARGELLIUM, Pearl.

MARGINI-SUS-SCAPULO-TROCHITERIEN, Teres minor.

MARGO, *Bord*—m. Dentatus, see Retina—m. Orbitalis, see Orbit.

MARGUERITE PETITE, Bellis — *m. des Prés, grande*, Chrysanthemum leucanthemum.

MARIENBAD, MINERAL WATERS OF. Celebrated springs in Bohemia. The Kreuzbrunn contains sulphate of soda, carbonate of iron, and carbonic acid.

MARIGOLD, DIAMOND FIG, Mesembryanthemum crystallinum — m. Garden, Calendula officinalis — m. Single, Calendula officinalis — m. Wild, Calendula arvensis.

MARIOTTE, EXPERIMENT OF. A celebrated experiment of the Abbé Mariotte, which consists in placing two small round spots on a wall at some distance from each other, standing opposite the left-hand object, and looking at it with the right eye, the left being closed. By walking backwards, until the distance from the object is about five times as great as the distance between the two objects, the latter will be found to disappear. Mariotte and, after him, many ophthalmologists, inferred that the optic nerve, on which the ray doubtless falls in this experiment, is insensible; and hence that the choroid may be the seat of vision,—not the retina. The inference is illogical; for it doubtless falls on the part of the optic nerve where the central artery enters, and the central vein leaves the eyeball, and where there is necessarily no neurine.

MARIS, μαρις. Ancient name of a measure, containing 83 pints and 4 ounces.

MARISCA, Ficus, Hæmorrhois.

MARJOLAINE, Origanum majorana.

MARJORAM, COMMON, Origanum—m.Wild, Origanum—m. Sweet, Origanum majorana.

MARJORANA, Origanum majorana—m. Mancurana, Origanum.

MARMALADE, Marmelade.

MARMARYGE, see Metamorphopsia.

MARMARYGO'DES, 'brilliant.' An epithet, joined particularly to the word οφθαλμος, to indicate a brilliant eye, a flashing eye. An eye which transmits the image of imaginary objects. See Metamorphopsia.

MAR'MELADE, *Marmela'da, Marmela'ta, Marmalade, Miva*. Parts of vegetables, confected with sugar, and reduced to a pultaceous consistence.

MARMELADE OF APRICOTS. A marmelade, prepared with two parts of ripe apricots deprived of their stones, and one part of white sugar.

MARMELADE OF FERNEL, M. of Tronchin.

MARMELADE OF TRONCHIN, or OF FERNEL. A kind of thick looch, of an agreeable taste, prepared with *two ounces of oil of sweet almonds*, as much *syrup of violets, manna* in tears, very fresh *pulp of cassia*, 16 grains of *gum tragacanth*, and two drachms of *orange flower water*. It is used as a laxative, demulcent, and pectoral.

MARMELATA, Marmelade.

MARMOR, *Marble, Calcis Car'bonas durus*, (F.) *Marbre*. White granular carbonate of lime. Used in pharmacy for the preparation of a pure lime, and the disengagement of carbonic acid.

MARMORATA AURIUM, Cerumen.

MARMORYGE, see Metamorphopsia—m. Hippocratis, Hemiopia.

MAROUTE, Anthemis cotula.

MAR'RIOTT, DRY VOMIT OF. This once celebrated emetic, called *dry*, from its being exhibited without drink, consisted of equal portions of *tartarized antimony* and *sulphate of copper*.

MARRONIER D'INDE, Æsculus Hippocastanum.

MARROW, *My'elos, Medul'la, M. ossium, Med'ullary Juice, Axun'gia de Mum'ia*, Sax. mepʒ, (F.) *Moëlle, Suc médullaire*. The oily, inflammable, whitish or yellowish juice, which fills the medullary canal of the long bones, the cancellated structure at the extremities of those bones, the diploë of flat bones, and the interior of short bones. The marrow is furnished by the exhalation of the medullary membrane. It is fluid during life, and appears under the form of small points or brilliant grains after death. It is enveloped in the medullary membrane.

MARROW, SPINAL, Medulla spinalis — m. Vertebral, Medulla spinalis.

MARRUBE BLANC, Marrubium — m. *Noir*, Ballota fœtida.

MARRU'BIUM, *Marrubium vulga'rĕ* seu *album* seu *German'icum* seu *apulum, Pra'sium, Phrasum, Horehound*, (F.) *Marrube blanc*. The leaves have a moderately strong, aromatic smell; and a very bitter, penetrating, diffusive, and durable taste. It has often been given in coughs and asthmas, united with sugar. Dose, ℥ss to ℥j, in infusion; dose of extract, gr. x to ℥ss.

FORD'S BALSAM OF HOREHOUND, is made as follows :—*horehound, liquorice root*, āā ℔iij and ℥viij; *water*, q. s. to strain ℔vj. Infuse. To the strained liquor add :—*proof spirit* or *brandy*, ℔12; *camphor*, ℥j and ℥ij; *opium* and *benjamin*, āā ℥j; *dried squills*, ℥ij; *oil of aniseed*, ℥j; *honey*, ℔iij and ℥viij.—Gray. It is pectoral.

MARRUBIUM, Leonurus cardiaca — m. Album, Marrubium—m. Apulum, Marrubium — m. Germanicum, Marrubium — m. Nigrum, Ballota fœtida—m. Vulgare, Marrubium.

MARS, Ferrum—m. Solubilis, Ferrum tartarisatum.

MARSEILLES, (CLIMATE OF.) The remarks made upon the climate of Montpelier apply even in greater force to that of Marseilles. It possesses all the objectionable qualities of the climate of southeastern France.

MARSH, *Limnē, Helos, Palus*, Sax. meɲɼc, (F.) *Marais*. Marshy districts give off emanations, which are the fruitful source of disease and the cause of great insalubrity in many countries. The chief disease, occasioned by the malaria or miasm, is intermittent fever. Hence it becomes important to drain such regions, if practicable. Some marshy countries are not so liable to phthisis pulmonalis, and it has been found, that where intermittents have been got rid of by draining, consumption has, at times, become frequent. The most unhealthy periods for residence in a marshy district are during the existence of the summer and autumnal heats; at which times the water becomes evaporated, and the marshy bottom is more or less exposed to the sun's rays. This postulatum seems necessary for the production of the miasmata: for whilst the marsh is well covered with water, no miasma is given off.

MARSH POISON, Miasm (marsh)—m. Mallow, Althæa—m. Root, Statice Caroliniana—m. Tea, Ledum palustre.

MARSHALL'S CERATE, see Cerate, Marshall's.

MARSHY, Elodes.

MARSIPIUM, Marsupion.

MARSUM, *Mar'sium, Mar'sicum*. An ancient wine of Marsia, in Italy, which was used as an astringent in certain diseases of the mouth.

MARSUPIAL, see Marsupion.

MARSUPIALIS, Ischio-trochanterianus, Obturator internus.

MARSUPIATE, see Marsupion.

MARSU'PION, *Marsyp'ion, Marsip'pon, Marsu'pium, Marsip'ium, Sac'culus*. A sac or bag, with which any part is fomented. Also, the abdominal pouch in the kangaroo, opossum, &c., into which the young, born at a very early stage of development, are received and nourished with milk secreted from glands which open into the pouches. Such animals are termed *Marsu'pial, Marsu'piate, Marsupia'lia*. See Generation.

MARSUPIUM, Scrotum — m. Musculosum, Dartos.

MARSYPION, Marsupion.

MARTEAU, Malleus.

MARTIAL, Chalybeate.

MARTIALIS, Chalybeate.

MARTIANA POMA, see Citrus aurantium.

MARTIA'TUM UNGUEN'TUM, (F.) *Onguent de Soldat, Soldier's ointment*. This was composed of *bay berries, rue, marjoram, mint, sage, wormwood, basil, olive oil, yellow wax*, and *Malaga wine*. It was invented by Martian; and was employed by soldiers as a preservative against cold.

MARTIS LIMATURA, Ferri limatura.

MARUM CORTUSI, Teucrium marum — m Creticum, Teucrium marum—m. Syriacum, Teucrium marum — m. Verum, Teucrium marum — m. Vulgare, Thymus mastichina.

MAS, Male, Modiolus.

MASCARPIO, Masturbator.

MASCHALE, Axilla.

MASCHALIÆUS, Axillary.

MASCHALIATRI'A, from μασχαλη, 'the axilla,' and ιατρεια, 'healing.' Treatment of disease by applications made to the axilla.

MASCHALIS, Axilla.

MASCHALISTER, Axis.

MASCHALON'CUS, *Maschalopa'nus*, from μασχαλη, 'the axilla,' and ογκος, 'a tumour.' A tumour or bubo or swelling in the axilla.

MASCHALOPANUS, Maschaloncus.

MASCULA, *Tribade*.

MASCULUS, Male.

MASESIS, Mastication.

MASHUA, (S.) A tuberous root, of a flat, pyramidal shape, which is cultivated and cooked like the potato by the Serranos of Peru. It is watery and insipid, but nevertheless is much eaten by them. The Indians use the mashua as a medicine in dropsy, dyspepsia, and dysentery. The plant is unknown to botanists. — Tschudi.

MASK, *Larva*, (F.) *Masque*. A bandage applied over the face, as a sort of mask, in cases of burns, scalds, or erysipelas. It serves to preserve the parts from the contact of air, and to retain topical applications *in situ*. It is made of a piece of linen, of the size of the face, in which apertures are made corresponding to the eyes, nose, and mouth, and which is fixed by means of strings stitched to the four angles.

MASLACH, *Moslich, Am'phion, An'fion*. A

medicine much used by the Turks, and into the composition of which opium enters. It is excitant.

MASQUE, Mask.

MASS, μαζα, *Massa, Massa,* from μασσω, 'I mix.' The compound, from which pills have to be formed.

MASSA, Mass — m. Carnea Jacobi Sylvii, see Flexor longus digitorum pedis profundus perforans — m. de Dactylis, Paste, date — m. de Extracto glycyrrhizæ, Pasta glycyrrhizæ, &c. — m. de Gummi Arabico, Paste, marshmallow — m. de Zizyphorum fructu, Paste of jujubes.

MASSAGE, Shampooing.

MASSE D'EAU, Typha latifolia.

MASSEMA, Mastication.

MASSEMENT, Shampooing.

MASSES APOPHYSAIRES, see Vertebræ.

MASSESIS, Mastication.

MASSE'TER, from μασαομαι, 'I eat,' 'I chew.' *Mus'culus mandibula'ris,* (F.) *Zygomato-maxillaire.* A muscle situate at the posterior part of the cheek, and lying upon the ramus of the lower jaw-bone. It is long, quadrilateral, and is attached, *above,* to the inferior edge and to the inner surface of the zygomatic arch; *below,* it terminates at the angle of the jaw, and at the outer surface and inferior margin of the ramus of that bone. It is composed of an intermixture of fleshy and aponeurotic fibres. Its office is to raise the lower jaw, and to act in mastication.

MASSETER INTERNUS, Pterygoideus internus.

MASSETER'IC, *Mas'seterine, Masseter'icus, Masseteri'nus.* Relating or belonging to the masseter muscle.

MASSETERINE ARTERY arises from the trunk of the internal maxillary or temporalis profunda posterior, and is distributed to the masseter muscle, after having passed, horizontally, through the sigmoid notch of the lower jaw-bone.

MASSETERINE NERVE is given off from the inferior maxillary branch of the fifth pair. It passes through the sigmoid notch, and is distributed on the inner surface of the masseter. In luxation of the lower jaw, this nerve is strongly stretched, and considerable pain, consequently, produced.

MASSETERINE VEIN has the same distribution as the artery. It opens into the internal maxillary vein.

MASSETERINUS, Masseteric.

MASSETTE, Typha latifolia.

MASSICOT, Plumbi oxydum semivitreum.

MASSING, Shampooing.

MASSULA, Molecule.

MASTADENITIS, Mastitis.

MASTALGIA, Mastodynia.

MASTAX, Mystax.

MASTEMA, Masticatory.

MASTER OF THE WOODS, Galium circæzans.

MASTERWORT, Angelica atropurpurea, Heracleum lanatum, Imperatoria.

MASTESIS, Mastication.

MASTHELCOSIS, Mastodynia apostematosa.

MASTHOS, Mamma.

MASTICA'TION, *Mastica'tio, Mass'sis, Masse'sis, Masse'ma, Maste'sis, Manduca'tio, Commanduca'tio, Manduca'tion,* from μαστιχαω, 'I chew.' The action of chewing or bruising food, to prepare it for the digestion it has to undergo in the stomach. This is executed by the joint action of the tongue, cheeks, and lips, which push the alimentary substance between the teeth; and by the motions of the lower jaw it is cut, torn, or bruised.

MAS'TICATORY, *Masticato'rium, Maste'ma, Diamaste'ma.* Same etymon. Chewing. Relating or appertaining to mastication or chewing. Also, a substance, chewed with the intention of exciting the secretion of saliva.

MASTICATORY NERVE, see Trigemini.

MASTICH, see Pistacia lentiscus — m. Herb, common, Thymus mastichina—m. Herb, Syrian, Teucrium marum — m. Tree, Pistacia lentiscus.

MASTICHINA GALLORUM, Thymus mastichina.

MASTIGODES HOMINIS, Trichocephalus.

MASTIGO'SIS, *Flagella'tio.* Flagellation, scourging; employed by the ancients as a remedy in many diseases.

MASTI'TIS, *Mastoi'tis, Masoi'tis, Inflamma'tio Mammæ, Mastadeni'tis,* (F.) *Inflammation des Mamelles,* from μαστος, 'the breast,' and *itis,* denoting inflammation. Inflammation of the breast. Inflammation of the mammary gland of the pregnant or parturient female is vulgarly called a *weed,* and a *weed in the breast.*

MASTITIS APOSTEMATOSA, Mastodynia apostematosa.

MASTITIS PUERPERA'LIS. Inflammation of the mamma in the childbed woman.

MASTIX, see Pistacia lentiscus.

MASTODES, Mastoid.

MASTODYN'IA, *Mastal'gia, Mazodyn'ia,* from μαστος, 'the breast,' and οδυνη, 'pain.' Pain in the breasts; a form of neuralgia. See Neuralgia mammæ.

MASTODYN'IA APOSTEMATO'SA, *Phleg'monē Mammæ, Masthelco'sis, Masti'tis apostemato'sa, Galactapostē'ma, Galactomastoparecto'ma, Absces'sus Mammæ,* A. lac'teus, *Phleg'monē Mastodyn'ia, Abscess of the Breast, Mam'mary Abscess, Milk-abscess.* Phlegmonous inflammation of the breasts, running on to suppuration, generally in the childbed female. It is one of the best examples of acute phlegmonous inflammation, and requires the active use of appropriate treatment.

MASTODYNIA POLYGALA, Sparganosis—m. Polygala, Mastospargosis.

MASTOID, *Mastoi'des, Masto'des, Mastoideus, Mammilla'ris, Papil'li-au-tmammilli-formis, Mammiform'is, Mam'miform,* from μαστος, 'a breast,' and ειδος, 'form, resemblance.' Having the form of a nipple. Also, that which relates to the mastoid process, *Mastoi'deus.*

MASTOID APERTURE:—the opening of communication between the cavity of the tympanum and the mastoid cells.

MASTOID CELLS, *Antrum mastoi'deum, Mastoid Sinuses.* These are situate in the mastoid process; communicate with each other, and open into the cavity of the tympanum. Their use seems to be to increase the intensity of sound.

MASTOID FORAMEN is situate behind the mastoid process, and gives passage to a small artery of the dura mater, as well as to a vein which opens into the lateral sinus.

MASTOID FOSSA, (F.) *Gouttière mastoïdienne,* is a depression at the inner surface of the mastoid portion of the temporal bone, which forms part of the lateral sinus.

MASTOID or DIGASTRIC GROOVE, (F.) *Rainure mastoïdienne ou digastrique,* is a groove, situate at the inner side of the mastoid process, which affords attachment to the posterior belly of the digastric muscle.

MASTOID MUSCLE, POSTERIOR, Splenius.

MASTOID or MAM'MIFORM or MAM'MILLARY PROCESS, *Pars mastoïdea,* is situate at the inferior and posterior part of the temporal bone, and gives attachment to the digastric and mastoid muscles.

MASTOIDEUS, Sterno-cleido-mastoideus—m. Lateralis, Complexus minor.

MASTOÏDO-CONCHINIEN, Retrahens auris.—m. *Génien*, Digastricus—m. *Hyogénien*, Digastricus—m. *Oriculaire*, Retrahens auris.

MASTON'CUS, *Thelon'cus*, from μαστος, 'the breast,' and ογκος, 'a tumour.' A tumefaction of the nipple, or of the breast itself.

MASTONCUS POLYGALACTICUS, Mastospargosis.

MASTOPATHI'A, from μαστος, 'the breast,' and παθος, 'disease.' An affection of the breast.

MASTORRHAG"IA, from μαστος, 'the breast,' and ρηγνυμι, 'to flow.' An unusual flow of milk.

MASTOS, Mamma.

MASTOSPARGO'SIS, *Mastodyn'ia polyg'ala, Maston'cus polygalac'ticus*, from μαστος, 'the breast,' and σπαργαω, 'I am full to bursting.' Fulness of the breasts with milk, so that they are ready to burst.

MASTRUPATIO, Masturbation.

MASTURBA'TION, *Cinæ'dia, Gar'galē, Gar'galus, Gargalis'mus, Mastupra'tio, Manustupra'tio, Manustupra'tio*, from *manus*, 'the hand,' and *stupro*, 'I ravish;' *Ona'nia, On'anism, Ædœogargaris'mus, Ædœogar'galus, Anaplas'mus, Gau'dia fœda, Duct'io præpu'tii, Vol'untary Pollution, Self Pollution, Self-abuse*, (F.) *Abus de soi-même, Attouchement*. Excitement of the genital organs by the hand.

MASTURBA'TOR, *Mastupra'tor, Manustupra'tor, Mascar'pio*: same etymon. One given to masturbation.

MASTUS, Mamma.

MAT, (F.) Dull.

MAT SON, (F.) A *dull sound*. The obscure noise, afforded in certain diseases when any part, as the chest, is percussed. It has been compared to that produced when the thigh is struck. It is opposed to the *Son clair*, or 'clear sound.'

MATE, see Ilex Paraguensis.

MATER. Uterus—m. Dura, Dura mater—m. Herbarum, Artemisia vulgaris—m. Metallorum, Hydrargyrum—m. Mollis, Pia mater—m. Perlarum, see Pearl—m. Pia, Pia mater—m. Secalis, Ergot—m. Tenuis, Pia mater.

MATERIA, Matter—m. Fibrosa, Fibrin.

MATE'RIA MED'ICA, *Pharmacolog"ia, Pharmacol'ogy, Acol'ogy or Akol'ogy or Aceolog"ia, Hylā Iatricē, Iamatolog"ia, Iamatol'ogy*, (F.) *Matière Médicale*. The division of medical science which treats of the knowledge of medicines; their action on the animal economy, and mode of administration. The study of the Materia Medica is one of great importance;—it is a study of the tools with which the practitioner has to work in the cure of disease. Much labour has been spent in contriving classifications of the Materia Medica. Some have arranged the articles according to their natural resemblances; others, according to their real or presumed virtues: others, according to their active constituent principles. The Pharmacopoeias place them alphabetically. Perhaps the best classification would be one founded on the agency exerted by the articles on the different tissues; but this arrangement, in the present state of science, is by no means easy; and, moreover, ideas in regard to the action of medicines are so associated with certain terms,—as narcotics, tonics, sedatives, &c., employed to denote certain operations, which they are esteemed capable of producing, that, to abandon them, would be to throw obstacles in the way of the student, without the ultimate advantage accruing to him of possessing a better knowledge of the *modus operandi* of medicines than when a classification, somewhat resembling those usually embraced, is adopted.

The following is the classification adopted by the Author, in his "General Therapeutics and Materia Medica," 4th edit., Philad., 1850:—

1. Agents that affect prominently the alimentary canal or its contents, { Emetics, Cathartics, Anthelmintics.

2. Agents that affect prominently the respiratory organs, { Expectorants.

3. Agents that affect prominently the follicular or glandular organs, { Errhines, Sialogogues, Diuretics, Antilithics, Diaphoretics.

4. Agents that affect prominently the nervous system, { Narcotics, Tetanics, Antispasmodics.

5. Agents that affect prominently the organs of reproduction, { Emmenagogues, Parturifacients.

6. Agents that affect various organs, { Excitants, Tonics, Astringents, Sedatives, Refrigerants, Revellents, Eutrophics.

7. Agents whose action is prominently chemical, { Antacids, Antalkalies, Disinfectants.

8. Agents whose action is prominently mechanical, { Demulcents, Diluents.

Of old, the Materia Medica consisted of more articles than at present. The tendency, indeed, is, and must be, to diminish it still further; to get rid of those articles which possess no advantages over others equally common, or whose properties are doubtful. In a dictionary, it becomes necessary to insert all that have been reputed to possess virtues; but the majority are unnecessary. The catalogue might be largely reduced, with impunity.

MATERIA MEDICA, DYNAMICAL, Pharmacodynamics.

MATERIA MORBO'SA, *M. Peccans, Mate'ries Morbi*. Morbid matter. The matter or material which is the cause of disease.

MATERIA OSSEA, Terra Ossea—m. Peccans, M. Morbosa—m. Salina, see Saliva—m. Testacea dentium, see Tooth—m. Urinosa, Urea.

MATERIALISTA, Druggist.

MATÉRIAUX IMMÉDIATS, Principles, immediate.

MATERIES, Matter—m. Morbi, Materia morbosa.

MATHEW'S PILLS, Pilulæ ex helleboro et myrrha.

MA'TIAS. The bark of a South American tree, not yet determined. It is used in its native country in intermittents, and as a tonic generally. Its principal characteristic constituent is a bitter resinous matter. It is probably the same as the *Malambo bark*.

MATI'CO, (pronounced *matee'co*,) *Yerba del Soldado*, or *Soldier's weed*. A South American herb—*Piper angustifolium, Artan'thē elonga'ta*—which is possessed of astringent virtues, and is used both internally and externally. It is given in *infusion* made of one ounce of the leaves to a pint of boiling water, of which the dose is f℥iss, or in *tincture*, made of ℥iiss of the leaves to a pint of dilute alcohol.

MATIÈRE, Matter—m. *Cérébriforme*, Encephaloid—m. *Extractive du Bouillon*, Osmazome—m. *Médicale*, Materia Medica—m. *Perlée de Kerkring*, Antimonium diaphoreticum—m. *Pulmonaire noire*, see Pulmo.

MATLOCK, MINERAL WATERS OF. Matlock is a village in Derbyshire, England, at which there is a mineral spring of the acidulous class. Temperature 66°. It differs but little, except in temperature, from good spring-water. It is generally used as a tepid bath.

MATONIA CARDAMOMUM, Amomum cardamomum.

MATORIUM, Ammoniac, gum.

MATRACIUM, Matrass, Urinal.

MATRASS, *Matra'cium*. A glass vessel with a long neck; and a round, and sometimes oval, body. It may be furnished with tubulures, or not. It is used in *Pharmacy* for distillation, digestion, &c.

MATRES CEREBRI, Meninges.

MATRICAIRE, Matricaria.

MATRICA'LIS, *Matrica'rius*, from *matrix*, 'the uterus.' Relating to the uterus.

Matricalia are remedies for diseases of the uterus.

MATRICA'RIA, from *matrix*, 'the womb;' so called from its reputed virtues in affections of that organ. *Matrica'ria Parthe'nium, Parthe'nium febrif'ugum, Py'rethrum parthe'nium, Chrysanth'emum parthe'nium, Argyroche'ta, Chrysoc'alis, Fever-few, Feather-few, Mother-wort*, (F.) *Matricaire. Nat. Ord.* Compositæ. It resembles, in its properties, chamomile and tansy; and, like them, has been esteemed tonic, stomachic, resolvent, emmenagogue, vermifuge, &c. It is not much used.

MATRICARIA, Anthemis nobilis.

MATRICA'RIA CHAMOMIL'LA, *M. Suav'eolens, An'themis vulga'ris, Chamæme'lum Vulga'rē, Chamomil'la nostras, Leucan'themum* of Dioscorides, *Wild Corn, Dog's Cham'omile, German Chamomile,* (F.) *Camomille vulgaire.* It resembles Matricaria in properties.

MATRICA'RIA GLABRA'TA. A South African plant, known at the Cape as *Wild Chamomile*, has the same properties as the other species of matricaria.

MATRICARIA LEUCANTHEMUM, Chrysanthemum Leucanthemum—m. Suaveolens, M. Chamomilla.

MATRICE, Uterus — m. *Col de la*, Collum uteri.

MATRIC'ULATE, from *matricula*, diminutive of *matrix*, 'a roll,' originally 'an army roll or register.' One who is admitted into a university or college, by enrolling or having his name enrolled on the register of the institution. In France, *prendre inscription* means 'to matriculate;' and, in the university regulations of that country, it is required, that the *inscription* shall be made every three months, until the termination of the prescribed period of study; the student having to take his inscription within the first fortnight of each *trimestre* or of every three months, and to present himself within the last fortnight of the *trimestre* to establish the fact of his attendance.

In this country, it is only necessary to matriculate at the commencement of each session.

One who has thus enrolled himself in an institution is called a *Matriculate*.

MATRISYLVA, Asperula odorata.

MATRIX, Cytoblastema, Uterus — m. Unguis, see Nail.

MATRONA, Midwife.

MATRONALIS, Viola.

MATTEE, see Ilex Paraguensis.

MATTER, *Mate'ria, Hylē, Mate'ries*, (F.) *Matière*. Any substance which enters into the composition of a body. In *Medicine*, it is sometimes applied to the substance of evacuations; and is also used synonymously with pus.

MATTING OF PARTS, Hapantismus.

MATULA, Urinal.

MATURA'TION, *Matura'tio*, from *maturare*, 'to ripen.' *Pepda'mos, Pepan'sis.* Progression of an abscess towards maturity. The state of maturity. Coction.

MATURATIF, Maturative.

MAT'URATIVE, *Matu'rans, Pepanticos*, (F.) *Maturatif.* A medicine which favours the maturation of an inflammatory tumour.

MATURATUS, Concocted.

MATU'RITY, *Matu'ritas, Horæ'otes.* The state of fruits and seeds, when comparatively developed. State of an abscess, in which the pus is completely formed.

MATURITY, PRECOCIOUS, Præotia.

MAUDLIN, Achillea ageratum — m. Tansey, Achillea ageratum — m. Wort, Chrysanthemum leucanthemum.

MAUVE SAUVAGE, Malva.

MAUX DE NERFS, Hysteria.

MAXILLA, Maxillary Bone.

MAX'ILLARY, *Maxilla'ris*, (F.) *Maxillaire*, from *maxilla*, 'a jaw.' Relating or belonging to the jaws; from μασσαω, 'I chew.'

MAXILLARY ARTERIES are three in number. 1. *External maxillary*. See Facial. 2. *Internal maxillary — A. Gutturo-maxillaire*, (Ch.) This arises from the external carotid with the temporal. It is remarkable for its complex course, and for the number of branches which it transmits to the deep-seated parts of the face. Immediately after its origin, it buries itself under the neck of the lower jaw, curving inwards and downwards. It then advances directly inwards; proceeding in the space between the two pterygoid muscles towards the *maxillary tuberosity*. It turns again, becomes vertical, and ascends into the bottom of the zygomatic fossa, until, having arrived at the floor of the orbit, it takes a horizontal and transverse direction; enters the spheno-maxillary fossa, and divides into several branches. See Artery, (table.)

MAXILLARY BONE, *Maxil'la, Mandib'ula, Gam'phelē, Gnathus, Mola, Siagon,* 'jaw.' (F.) *Machoire.* A name given to two bones, which support the teeth, and, by means of them, are inservient to the cutting, bruising, and tearing of alimentary substances.

The maxillary bones are two in number.

MAXILLARY BONE, INFERIOR, *Lower jaw-bone, Os Maxilla'rē inferius, Machoire diacranienne, Maxil'la inferior*, (F.) *Os maxillaire*, (Ch.,) is a symmetrical, nearly parabolic bone, the middle portion of which is horizontal, and called the *body;* and the posterior is vertical, the angular portions being termed *Rami* or *branches*. These have behind a *parotidean edge*, which forms — by uniting with the base — *the angle of the jaw*. The branches terminate above by two processes, separated by the *sigmoid notch* or *fossa;* the anterior of which is called the *coronoid;* the posterior, the *condyloid* process or *maxillary condyle*, supported by a *Cervix, Collum*, or *Neck*. The chief parts observed on the lower jaw are — 1. *Externally,* — the *Sym'physis menti, Apoph'ysis menti, Mental foramen*, and the *external oblique line.* 2. *Internally,* — the *Geniapoph'ysis*, the *internal* or *Myloid oblique lines*, and the *entrance of the dental canal.* The lower jaw has, also, an *alveolar edge*, which contains alveoli for the reception of the teeth. The lower jaw-bone is developed by two points of ossification, which unite at the symphysis of the chin. It is articulated with the temporal bone and with the teeth.

MAXILLARY BONE, SUPERIOR, *Upper jaw-bone, Maxil'la superior, Os maxilla'rē supe'rius, Maxil'la syncra'nia,* (F.) *Os sus-maxillaire*, (Ch.,) *Machoire syncranienne.* The upper jaw-bones are to the face what the sphenoid bone is to the cranium. They are articulated with all the portions composing it. They determine, almost alone, the shape of the face, and give it solidity. Their size is considerable; form unequal. They occupy the middle and anterior part of the face; and enter into the composition of the nasal fossæ, orbit, and mouth. The chief parts observable in the upper jaw are:— 1. *Externally,* — the *Nasal process,* (F.) *Apophyse montante,* the *Fora'men infra-orbita'rium, Zygomat'ic process, Canine fossa, Myr'tiform fossa.* 2. *Internally,* — the *Pal'atine process, Ante'rior pal'atine canal,* and the *Antrum of Highmore.* Its circumference is very unequal, and it has behind a round, unequal prominence, called the *Maxillary tuberosity,* which is pierced by the *posterior dental canal.* Anteriorly, there is a notch, which forms part of the anterior aperture of the nasal fossæ, and beneath, an eminence, called the *anterior nasal spine.* The lower part of this circumference forms the *alveolar margin.* Each superior maxillary bone is articulated with the ethmoid, frontal, nasal, lachrymal, palatine, inferior, spongy, vomer, its fellow, the teeth of the upper jaw, and sometimes the sphenoid bone. It is developed by four or five points of ossification.

MAXILLARY NERVES are two in number, and formed of the second and third branches of the fifth pair. The SUPERIOR MAXILLARY NERVE, *Nerf sus-maxillaire* (Ch.), arises from the middle of the gangliform enlargement of the fifth pair; passes forwards, and issues from the cranium through the foramen rotundum of the sphenoid bone; enters the spheno-maxillary fossa, which it crosses horizontally; passes into the infraorbitar canal, which it traverses; and makes its exit to vanish on the cheek. It gives off the following branches, — the *orbitar,* a branch which goes to the *spheno-palatine ganglion; posterior dental branches; the anterior dental,* — and terminates in the *infra-orbitar* nerves, which are divided into *superior, inferior,* and *internal.* The *inferior maxillary nerve, Nerf maxillaire* (Ch.), is the largest of the three branches furnished by the fifth pair. It issues from the cranium by the foramen ovale of the sphenoid. Having reached the zygomatic fossa, it divides into two trunks; the one *superior* and *external,* which gives off the *temporales profundi, masseterine, buccal,* and *pterygoids;* — the other — *inferior* and *internal* — the larger of the two, which furnishes the *inferior dental, lingual,* and *auricular.*

MAXILLARY VEINS present the same arrangement as the arteries they accompany.

MAXILLO-ALVÉOLI-NASAL, Depressor alæ nasi — m. *Labial,* Depressor anguli oris — m. *Narinal,* Compressor naris — m. *Palpébral,* Orbicularis palpebrarum — m. *Scléroticien,* Obliquus inferior oculi.

MAY APPLE, Podophyllum peltatum — m. a. Mountain, Podophyllum montanum — m. Flower, Anthemis cotula — m. Weed, Anthemis cotula.

MAYELLA, Curcuma longa.

MAYNARD'S ADHESIVE LIQUID, Collodion.

MAYS, Zea mays — m. Americana, Zea mays — m. Zea, Zea mays.

MAZA, Mass, Placenta.

MA'ZICUS, from *maza,* 'placenta.' Relating to the placenta.

MAZISCH'ESIS, from *maza,* 'the placenta,' and σχισις, 'holding,' 'retention.' Retention of the placenta.

MAZODYNIA, Mastodynia.

MAZOITIS, Mastitis.

MAZOL'YSIS, from *maza,* 'placenta,' and λυσις, 'solution.' Separation of the placenta.

MAZOPATHI'A, from *maza,* 'placenta,' and παθος, 'disease.' A disease of the placenta. One originating from the placenta.

MAZOS, Mamma.

MEAD, Hydromeli, Melizomum.

MEADOW BLOOM, Ranunculus acris — m. Fern, Comptonia asplenifolia — m. Pride, see Calumba — m. Rue, Thalictron — m. Saffron, Vinegar of, Acetum colchici — m. Sweet, Gillenia trifoliata, Spiræa ulmaria — m. Sweet, red, Spiræa tomentosa.

MEALY TREE, Viburnum dentatum.

MEASLES, Rubeola — m. Black, see Rubeola — m. False, Roseolæ — m. French, Roseolæ.

MEASLY, Morbillous.

MEASUREMENT, Mensuration.

MEASURING, MEDICAL, Mensuration.

MEAT BISCUIT, see Biscuit, meat.

MEAT, EXTRACTIVE OF, Osmazome.

MÉAT, Meatus.

MEA'TUS, *Ductus, Cana'lis, Porus,* (F.) *Méat.* A passage or canal.

MEATUS AUDITORIUS EXTERNUS, Auditory canal, external — m. Auditorius internus, Auditory canal, internal — m. Cæcus, Eustachian tube — m. Narium, see Nasal fossæ — m. Seminales uteri, Tubæ Fallopianæ — m. Seminarius, Corpus Highmori — m. Urinarius, Urethra.

MECHAMECK, Convolvulus panduratus — m. Bindweed, Convolvulus panduratus.

MECHANE, Machine.

MECHANEMA, Machine.

MECHAN'ICAL, *Mechan'icus,* from μηχανη 'a machine.' An epithet given to irritating bodies, which do not act chymically — as a *mechanical irritant.*

MECHANICAL or IATRO-MATHEMATICAL PHYSICIANS, *Iätro-mechan'ici seu Iätromathemat'ici,* are such as refer every function, healthy or morbid, to mechanical or mathematical principles; — *Medici'na mechan'ica.*

MECHAN'ICS, AN'IMAL. That part of physiology whose objects are to investigate the laws of equilibrium and motion of the animal body.

MECH'ANISM. The structure of a body; the collection or aggregate of the parts of a machine; the mode in which forces produce any effect, &c.

MÈCHE, Tent. This term is usually applied in French surgery to a collection of threads of charpie, cotton or raw silk united together, which are used for deterging sinuous or fistulous ulcers; or to keep open or enlarge natural or artificial apertures. They are generally applied by means of an instrument called *Porte-mèche.*

MECHOACANA NIGRA, Convolvulus jalapa — m. Nigricans, Convolvulus jalapa.

MECHOACANÆ RADIX, Convolvulus mechoacan.

MECHOACAN DU CANADA, Phytolacca decandra.

MECOM'ETER, (F.) *Mécomètre;* from μηκος, 'length,' and μετρον, 'measure.' A kind of graduated compass, — *compas de proportion,* — used at the Hospice de Maternité of Paris, to measure the length of new-born infants.

MECON, Meconium, Opium, Papaver.

MECONICUM, Opiate.

MECONIS'MUS, *Intoxica'tio opia'ca;* from μηκων, 'the poppy.' Poisoning by opium.

MECO'NIUM, same etymon. *Poppy juice, Papaver'culum, Purgamen'ta Infantis, Mecon.* The excrement passed by the infant a short time after birth, which had accumulated in the intestines during pregnancy. It is of a greenish or deep black colour, and very viscid. It seems formed of the mucous secretions of the intestines mixed with bile. See Opium.

MECONOLOG"IA, *Opiolog"ia;* from μηκων, 'a poppy,' and λογος, 'a description.' A treatise on opium.

MECONOPSIS DIPHYLLA, Stylophorum diphyllum.

MEDEA, Genital organs.

MÉDECIN, Physician — *m. Consultant,* Consulting physician.

MÉDECINE, Medicina — *m. Expectante,* Expectation — *m. Légale,* Medicine, legal — *m. Opératoire,* Surgery, operative — *m. Perturbatrice,* Perturbatrix (Medicina.)

MEDELA, Curation.

MEDEOLA VERTICILLIFOLIA, M. Virginica.

MEDE'OLA VIRGIN'ICA, *M. verticillifo'lia, Gyro'mia Virgin'ica, Indian cu'cumber.* An indigenous herb, growing in every part of the United States, the root of which resembles a small cucumber. It has been thought to be diuretic.

MEDIAN, *Media'nus;* from *medium,* 'the middle.' That which is situate in the middle.

MEDIAN LINE. A vertical line, supposed to divide a body longitudinally into two equal parts; the one right, the other left. Chaussier calls the *linea alba* the *ligne médiane* of the abdomen.

MEDIAN NERVE, *Médian digital,* (Ch.) This nerve arises chiefly from the anterior branches of the last two cervical nerves and first dorsal. The fifth and sixth cervical pairs also send it a branch, which separates from the musculo-cutaneous nerve. The median nerve descends the inner part of the arm along the biceps muscle. Opposite the elbow joint it buries itself behind the aponeurosis of that muscle, and engages itself between the two fasciculi of the pronator teres. Lower down, it is situate between the flexors — sublimis and profundus — and passes, with their tendons, under the anterior annular ligament; it then divides into five branches, which are distributed to the muscles of the thenar eminence, to the lumbricales, the integuments of the thumb, the index, middle finger, and outer part of the ring finger. This nerve gives no branches to the arm. In the forearm, it furnishes filaments to all the pronator and flexor muscles; and one of them accompanies the anterior interosseous artery. It also gives off a filament to the integuments of the palm of the hand.

MEDIAN VEINS. Three of the superficial veins of the forearm are so called. The *median basilic* — the *median cephalic* and *common median* or *funis brachii.* See Basilic and Cephalic.

MEDIANUM, Mediastinum, Mesentery.

MEDIAS'TINAL, *Mediastina'lis.* Relating to the Mediastinum.

MEDIASTINAL ARTERIES are very delicate arterial branches, distributed in the areolar texture of the mediastinum. They are distinguished, according to their situation, into anterior and posterior.

MEDIASTINITIS, Mesodmitis.

MEDIASTI'NUM, *Mediasti'nus,* quasi, in *medio stans,* as being in the middle; *Mesod'ma, Media'num, Mesotœ'chium, Mesotœ'chum, Septum thora'cis, Hymen Diaphrat'ton, Membra'na Diaphratton, Membra'na thora'cem intersep'iens, Intersepimen'tum thora'cis, Diribito'rium, Dissipimen'tum thora'cis.* A membranous septum formed by the approximation of the pleuræ, dividing the chest into two parts, the one right, the other left. The mediastinum, formed by a double reflection of the pleura, extends from the spine to the posterior surface of the sternum. Its anterior part, called *Anterior mediastinum, Mediastinum pecto-*

ra'lě, lodges, at its upper part, the thymus gland in the fœtus, and is filled below with fatty, areolar tissue. Its posterior part, parallel to the spine, is occupied by the œsophagus, vena azygos, thoracic duct, the lower part of the windpipe, the origin of the bronchia and a number of lymphatic glands. This part is called the *posterior mediastinum — Mediastinum dorsa'lě.*

MEDIASTINUM AURIS, see Tympanum — m. Cerebri, Falx cerebri, Septum lucidum — m. Testis, Corpus Highmori.

MEDIASTINUS, Mediastinum.

MEDICABILIS, Curable.

MEDICABLE, Curable.

MED'ICÆ. Sworn midwives, whose duty it was, of old, to inspect women in cases of suspected pregnancy.

MED'ICAL, *Medica'lis, Iät'ricus, Pæon'ius, Pæon'icus, Phys'ical, Escula'pian,* (F.) *Médical.* Same etymon as Medicament. Appertaining or relating to medicine or to medicines.

MEDICAL JURISPRUDENCE, Medicine, legal.

MEDICALIS, Medical.

MED'ICAMENT, *Medicamen'tum, Remed'ium, Ace'sis, Aces'ma, Aces'tium, Aces'tys, Althos, Hygias'ma, Ia'ma, Acos, Medica'men, Phar'macum, Pharmaceu'ma, Alkar, Auxil'ium, Boëthe'ma, Med'icine, Physic, Rem'edy,* (F.) *Remède;* from *medicare,* 'to cure or heal.' A medicine. Any substance exhibited with the view of curing or allaying morbid action. Medicines are obtained from the three kingdoms of nature, and are divided into *internal* and *external,* according as they are administered internally or applied externally.

MEDICAMENTAL, Medicinal.

MEDICAMENTO'SUS LAPIS, *Medic"inal stone,* (F.) *Pierre médicamenteuse.* A name formerly given to a mixture of *peroxyd of iron, litharge, alum, nitre, sal ammoniac,* and *vinegar;* evaporated and calcined at a red heat for an hour. The product was regarded as eminently astringent.

MEDICAMENTUM, Drug — m. ex Palmulis, Diaphœnicon.

MEDICAS'TER, *Medicastra.* An ignorant practitioner. A charlatan.

MEDICA'TION, *Medica'tio,* from *mederi,* 'to remedy.' The change in the animal economy produced by the operation of remedies. Treatment by medicine.

MEDICI'NA, *Ars med'ica, Res medica, Ars Machaö'nia, A. Machaön'ica, Iat'ricě, Iate'ria, Iätri'a, Iatri'ně, Pæos'yně, Pæon'icě, Iatrotech'nicě, Acesto'ria, Scien'tia med'ica seu medendi, Sote'ria doctri'na, Med'icine, The healing art, Physic,* (F.) *Médecine.* A science, the object of which is the cure of disease and the preservation of health. Occasionally, it is used to comprehend all the branches of the healing art; at others to comprise one great division, in contradistinction to *surgery* and *obstetrics.* Medicine, in this sense, includes many branches; — the chief of which are, Anatomy, Physiology, Pathology, Therapeutics, Hygiene, Materia Medica, and Pharmacy.

MEDICINA CONSERVATIVA, Hygiene — m. Diætetica, Dietetics — m. Eclectica, see Eclectic — m. Efficax, Surgery — m. Equaria, Hippiatria — m. Eueotica, Gymnastus — m. Forensis, Medicine, legal — m. Gymnastica, Gymnastics — m. Hermetica, see Spagyrists — m. Judiciaria, Medicine, legal — m. Mechanica, see Mechanical — m. Methodica, see Methodists — m. Operativa, Surgery — m. Paracelsistica, see Spagyrists — m. Perturbatrix, see Perturbatrix — m. Politica, Police, medical — m. Sinica, Chinese medicine — m. Spagyrica, Chymiatria; see Spagyrists — m. State, Police medi cal—m. Tristitiæ; Orocus—m. Veterinaria, Veterinary art.

MEDICINABLE, Medicinal.

MEDIC"INAL, *Medicina'lis, Medicament'al, Medic"inable, Med'ical, Iäter'ius, Reme'dial, Reme'diate.* Having a remedial power;—as medicinal plants, &c. Relating to medicine, as

MEDICINA'LES DIES, *Medic"inal days.* Days on which the ancients considered that remedies might be administered; and especially evacuants. Such days were not esteemed critical.

MEDICINE, Medicament, Medicina.

MEDICINE is, also, used in the same sense as Medicament, and for a purging potion.

To MEDICINE was formerly used for "to restore or cure by medicine."

MEDICINE, CLINICAL, see Clinical—m. Eclectic, see Eclectic—m. Empirical, Arcanum—m. Galenic, Galenism.

MEDICINE, LEGAL, *Medical jurispru'dence of some, Law med'icine, Foren'sic medicine, Medici'na foren'sis, M. judicia'ria, Diciatri'a,* (F.) *Médecine légale.* The application of medical knowledge to the solution of every question connected with the preservation of the species, and the administration of justice.

MEDICINE, PATENT, see Patent medicine—m. Political, Police, medical—m. Quack, Arcanum.

MÉDICINIER CATHARTIQUE, Jatropha curcas.

MEDICO-CHIRURG"ICAL, *Med'ico-Chirur'gicus.* Relating or appertaining to medicine and surgery;—as '*medico-chirurgical* society.'

MEDICO-CHIRURGICAL ANATOMY, see Anatomy.

MEDICO-LEGAL, *Med'ico-lega'lis.* Relating to legal medicine; as '*a medico-legal* inquiry, *Inquisit"io medico-lega'lis*—'a *medico-legal* inspection,' *Inspec'tio med'ico-lega'lis.*

MEDICO-STATISTICAL, see Statistics, medical.

MEDICUS, Doctor, Physician—m. Equarius, Hippiater—m. Ocularius, Oculist—m. Unguentarius, Iatraleptes—m. Vulnerarius, see Deligation—m. Veterinarius, Hippiater—m. Vulnerum, Surgeon.

MEDIM'NUS, *Medim'nos, μέδιμνος.* An ancient measure, capable of containing about 4 pecks and 6 pints.

MEDITULLIUM, Diploë.

MEDIUM MUSCULI, see Muscle.

ME'DIUS, Middle, Median.

MIDDLE FINGER, (F.) *Doigt du Milieu,* is between the index and ring finger.

MEDLAR, Mespilus.

MEDO, Hydromeli.

MEDOBLENNORRHŒA, Leucorrhœa.

MEDORRHŒA, Gonorrhœa—m. Feminarum Insons, Leucorrhœa—m. Virilis, Gonorrhœa.

MEDULLA, Marrow—m. Cerebri, see Cerebrum—m. Dorsalis, m. Spinalis—m. Dorsualis, M. Spinalis—m. Nervorum, Neurine.

MEDUL'LA OBLONGA'TA, *Cer'ebral protu'berance, Nervous system of the senses,* (Gall,) *Cer'ebrum elonga'tum,* (F.) *Mésocephale, Moëlle allongée, Mésencéphale,* (Ch.) The medullary substance that lies within the cranium upon the basilary process of the occipital bone. The anterior surface which rests in the basilary groove, is impressed by the basilary artery. At the upper extremity, and on its posterior surface are the *Tubercula quadrigemina.* At the same extremity, the medulla gives rise to two prolongations, the *peduncles of the brain,* separated from each other by the mammillary eminences, and becoming lost in the optic thalami. The lower extremity is called the *tail* or *Rachid'ian bulb, Bulbus rachid'icus,* and is continuous with the medulla spinalis. It is to this part only that some anatomists apply the name *Medulla oblongata.* From the posterior angles two other prolongations arise, called *Peduncles* of the cerebellum. The medulla oblongata has several eminences—the *Pons varolii, Corpora pyramidalia, C. olivaria,* &c.—and it has a longitudinal fissure before, and another behind, called the *anterior* and *posterior medium fissures.* The vesicular neurine in the centre of the medulla is the nervous centre of respiration and deglutition: hence it has been called *centrum vitale.*

MEDULLA OSSIUM, Marrow—m. Spinæ, M. spinalis.

MEDUL'LA SPINA'LIS seu *Spinæ* seu *dorsua'lis* seu *dorsa'lis, Corda spina'lis, Funis argenteus, Rhache'trum, My'elus, M. rhachi'tes* seu *notiæ'us* seu *diauche'nius* seu *paoi'tes, My'elon, Notomy'elus, Rhachi'tes, Æon, Medul'la vertebra'lis, Proces'sus rachidia'nus, Sacra fis'tula, Spinal prolonga'tion, Ver'tebral marrow, Spinal cord, Nervous system of voluntary motion and tactile impression* (Gall), *Spinal marrow,* (F.) *Moëlle épinière, Moëlle vertébrale,* called by Ch., *Prolongement rachidien* of the encephalon, is the continuation of the medulla oblongata. It commences at the foramen magnum of the occipital bone, and descends in the vertebral canal as low as the 2d lumbar vertebra, without filling it; presenting, in its course, several evident enlargements. It is grooved on both its anterior and posterior surfaces by a furrow, which divides it, in its whole length, into two great nervous cords, intimately united with each other. It terminates by an oval tubercle, whence a number of nerves set out called *Cauda equi'na,* (F.) *Queue de cheval,* from its resemblance to a horse's tail. The spinal marrow has no analogy, as regards its structure, with the marrow of long bones. It is formed of two substances; one white, the other gray, presenting an inverse arrangement to that which they have in the brain, the white being external, the cineritious at the centre. It is enveloped by a yellowish, fibrous membrane, very resisting, which seems to be continued insensibly from the pia mater, and by two other membranes, which are merely prolongations of the arachnoid and dura mater. See Nerve.

MEDULLA VERTEBRALIS, M. spinalis.

MEDULLÆ, Sperm.

MED'ULLARY, *Medulla'ris,* from *medulla,* 'marrow.' Relating to the marrow or analogous to marrow.

MEDULLARY AR'TERIES. The arteries, which enter bones and pass to the marrow.

MEDULLARY CANAL, see Canal, medullary—m. Cells, see Medullary Membrane—m. Juice, Marrow—m. Matter of the brain, see Cerebrum.

MEDULLARY MEMBRANE, *Periosteum Inter'num, Endos'teum.* A vascular, areolar web of extreme tenuity, which envelops the marrow and lines the inner surface of the medullary canal of the long bones. This membrane has been considered as a species of internal periosteum of those bones. It has numerous vessels, which bury themselves in the thickness of the marrow; and others which nourish the innermost plates of the bone. The cells formed by it are termed *Cel'lulæ* seu *Sac'culi medulla'res.*

MEDULLARY NEURINE, see Neurine—m. Sarcoma, Encephaloid, Hæmatodes fungus.

MEDULLARY SUBSTANCE OF THE KIDNEY, see Kidney—m. s. of Schwann, see Nerve-fibre.

MEDULLARY SYSTEM. Bichat gives this name to the marrow and its membranes. He distinguishes two species of medullary *systems;* the one occupies the cellular tissue at the extremities of the long bones and that of the flat and short bones; the other is found merely in the central canal of long bones.

MEDULLARY TUMOUR OF THE LUNGS, Phthisis, cancerous.

MEDULLITIS, Myelitis.

MEGALANTHROPOGEN'ESIS, from μεγας, 'great,' ανθρωπος, 'man,' and γενεσις, 'birth.' A term used by a French physician, named Robert, to designate the art of procreating great men; men of mind; men of genius. He considered that they may be perpetuated by always taking care to have talented men united to clever women!

MEGALOCAR'DIA, from μεγας, 'great,' and καρδια, 'heart.' The state of having a very large heart.

MEGALOCŒLIA, Intestine, great, Megalosplanchnia.

MEGALOPHO'NIA, from μεγας, μεγαλη, 'great,' and φωνη, 'voice.' The condition of having a full, strong voice.

MEGALOPHTHAL'MUS; from μεγας, μεγαλη, 'great,' and οφθαλμος, 'eye.' A congenital deformity, in which the eye is inordinately large.

MEGALOSPLANCH'NUS, from μεγαλος, 'great,' and σπλαγχνον, 'a viscus.' Megalocœ'lia. Hippocrates applies the epithet to those in whom a viscus, or the viscera, are tumid. Some have used the substantive Megalosplanch'nia for the tumour itself.

MEGALOSPLENIA, Splenoncus.

MEGETHOS, Stature.

MEGRIM, Hemicrania.

MEIBO'MIUS, GLANDS OF, Fol'licles of M., Pal'pebral Fol'licles, Cil'iary F., Glandulæ seba'ceæ cilia'res seu Meibomia'næ, Intestin'ula Meibo'mii, Lacu'næ palpebra'rum, (F.) Follicules palpébraux ou ciliaires, Glandes de Meibomius. Small, sebaceous follicles, called after Henry Meibomius, although known long before his description of them. They are situate in special grooves in the tarsal cartilages; and are ranged by the side of each other, in the form of yellowish, parallel, and vertical lines; sometimes straight, at others, tortuous. They may be seen at the inner surface of the eyelids, through the conjunctiva, and secrete a sebaceous humour, called Lippitu'do, Gum, (F.) Chassie.

MEIO'SIS, Meo'sis, Mio'sis, Imminu'tio, Minuthe'sis, Minitho'sis, from μειοω, 'I lessen.' The period of a disease, in which the symptoms begin to diminish; — the decline. Remission. Also, idiotism.

MEIUROS, Decurtatus, Myurus.

MEL, Meli, Nili'acum, Honey, (F.) Miel. A substance of a muco-saccharine nature, prepared by the Apis mellifi'ca, or common bee, which collects it from the nectaries of flowers. Honey is employed as aliment, condiment, and medicine. It is demulcent and aperient; and is prescribed as an adjunct to gargles in cynanche tonsillaris, &c. It is, at times, used as a detergent to foul ulcers. Virgin Honey, Mel vir'ginum seu virgin'eum, (F.) Miel vierge, is that which flows from the wax spontaneously.

HILL'S BALSAM OF HONEY is formed of balsam of tolu. ℔j, honey, ℔j, rectified spirit, one gallon. It was long a celebrated empirical pectoral.

HONEY WATER is a mixture of essences coloured with saffron. A little honey is added to communicate a clamminess; the effect of which is to make it retain the scent the longer. It is used as a scent.

MEL ACETATUM, Oxymel — m. Ægyptiacum, Ægyptiacum — m. Aërium, Fraxinus ornus — m. Arundinaceum, Saccharum.

MEL BORA'CIS, Mel subbora'cis, Colluto'rium adstrin'gens, Linimen'tum de Bora'te, L. ad aphthas, Mel Boraxa'tum, Linctus de Bora'ce, L. ad aphthas, Honey of Borax. (Boracis contrit. ʒj, mellis despumati ʒj, Ph. L.) Detergent. Applied to the mouth in aphthous affections.

MEL CANNÆ, Saccharum (non purificatum) — m. Coctum, Pelicide.

MEL DESPUMA'TUM, Clar'ified Honey, Anaphrom'eli, (F.) Miel Clarifié. Melt the honey in a water-bath, and remove the scum. Uses the same as honey.

MEL PRÆPARA'TUM, Prepared Honey. (Mel. despumat. Oss. Alcohol. dilut. Oj. Cretæ præparat. ʒss. To the honey and diluted alcohol, mixed, add the prepared chalk, and let the mixture stand for two hours, occasionally stirring. Then heat to ebullition, filter, and by means of a waterbath, evaporate the clear liquor to the specific gravity 1.32. Ph. U. S.)

MEL ROSÆ, Mel rosa'tum, Melli'tum de Rosis, Rhodom'eli, Rhodostac'ton, Honey of Roses, (F.) Miel rosat, Mellite de Roses. (Rosæ gallic. ʒij, aquæ bullient. fʒxij, mellis despum. fʒxx. Macerate the roses in fʒviij of boiling water for four hours; press out as much fluid as possible and set aside. Macerate the residue in fʒiv of boiling water for half an hour, and again express. Reserve fʒiv of the first infusion; mix the remainder with the infusion last obtained; add the honey, and evaporate to a pint. Lastly, add the reserved infusion, and strain. Ph. U. S.) Astringent and detergent. Used chiefly in gargles and washes for aphthæ, &c.

MEL SCILLÆ, Oxymel scillæ — m. Scillæ compositum, Syrupus scillæ compositus.

MEL VINOSUM, Œnomel — m. Virginum, see Mel.

MELÆ'NA, Melanorrhag"ia, Melænorrhag"ia, Ic'terus niger, Melanchlo'rus, Melanic'terus, Melas Ic'terus, Morbus niger Hippoc'ratis, Enterorrhœ'a, Black Jaundice, Morbus niger, (F.) Muladie noire, Méline, Ictère noire; from μελας, 'black.' A name given to vomiting of black matter, ordinarily succeeded by evacuations of the same character. It seems to be often a variety of hæmatemesis. The Black Vomit in yellow fever is owing to a morbid secretion from the lining membrane of the stomach and small intestine. Melæna also signifies hemorrhage from the intestines; Fluxus sple'nicus, Dysenter'ia sple'nica, Dejectio'nes nigræ, Seces'sus niger, Hem'orrhage from the Intes'tines.

MELÆNA FUNGOSA CARCINODES, Hæmatodes fungus.

MELÆNORRHAGIA, Melæna.

MELALEU'CA CAJAPUTI, M. Minor seu Leucoden'dron, Myrtus Leucaden'dron, Leptospermum Leucaden'drum. This plant affords the Cajeput Oil, (see Cajeput.) The leaves are esteemed diuretic, stomachic, and emmenagogue.

MELALEUCA LEUCODENDRON, M. Cajaputi — m. Minor, M. Cajaputi.

MELAMPHO'NUS; from μελας, 'obscure,' and φωνη, 'voice.' Having a hoarse or indistinct voice.

MELAMPHYLLUM, Acanthus mollis.

MELAMPODE, Helleborus niger.

MELAMPODIUM, Helleborus niger.

MELANÆMA, Suffocation.

MELANÆMIA, Venosity.

MEL'ANAGOGUE, Melanago'gus, from μελας, 'black,' and αγω, 'I expel.' A medicine which the ancients believed adapted for expelling black bile or melancholy.

MELANCHLO'RUS, from μελας, 'black,' and χλωρος, 'green.' The ancients gave this name to certain dark-coloured topical remedies. See Melæna.

MELANCHOLE, Atrabilis.

MELANCHOLIA, Melancholy — m. Autochirica, Suicide — m. Errabunda, Cuttubuth — m. Flatuosa, Hypochondriasis — m. Hypochondriaca, Hypochondriasis — m. Nervea, Hypochondriasis — m. Pleonectica, see Pleonectica — m. Saltans, Chorea — m. Suicidium, Suicide — m. Uterina, Nymphomania — m. Zoanthropia, Melancholy.

MEL'ANCHOLIC, *Melanchol'icus, Melan'cholus, Melancholo'des,* from μελας, 'black,' and χολη, 'bile.' One labouring under melancholy. That which belongs or relates to melancholy. In popular language, one of a gloomy disposition.

MELANCHOLINESS, Melancholy.

MELANCHOLODES, Melancholic.

MELANCHOLUS, Melancholy.

MEL'ANCHOLY, *Melancho'lia,* same etymon. *Lypema'nia, Ecphro'nia Melancho'lia, Mania Melanchol'ica, Mania Melancho'lia, Tristema'nia, Baryth'mia, Hypolepsioma'nia, Anœ'sia adstric'ta, Fixa'tio mononœ'a, Melancholiness;* (F.) *Mélancholie, Lyperophrénie.* A disease supposed, by the ancients, to be caused by black bile. A variety of mental alienation, characterized by excessive gloom, mistrust, and depression, generally, with insanity on one particular subject or train of ideas, *Monoma'nia, Monomo'ria. Panophobia, Demonomania, Erotomania, Nostalgia,* &c., may be referred to this head. *Melancholy* is also used for unusual gloominess of disposition.

MELANCHOLY, EROTIC, Erotomania — m. Love, Erotomania.

MELAN'CHRUS, *Melan'ochrus,* from μελας, 'black,' and χρως, 'a colour.' One attacked with black jaundice. It is probably an abbreviation of Melanchlorus.

MÉLANCOLIE, Melancholy.

MÉLANGE PECTORAL, Mistura acidi hydrocyanici.

MELAN'IC, *Melan'icus, Melanot'ic, Melanot'icus;* from μελας, 'black.' Of or belonging to Melanosis; — as *Melanic deposit,* a black colouring matter deposited from the blood under special circumstances; — see Melanosis.

MELANIC DEPOSIT, Melanosis.

MELANICTERUS, Melæna.

MELANOCHRUS, Melanchrus.

MELANOMA, Melanosis.

MELANOMA PULMONUM, see Melanosis.

MELANOMYCES, Melanospongus.

MELANOPATHI'A, from μελας, 'black,' and παθος, 'affection.' *Ni'gritism, Nigrit"ies.* A disease of the skin, which consists in augmentation of black pigment; generally in patches.

MELANOPHYMA, Ergot.

MELANOPIPER, Piper nigrum.

MELANOPNEUMON, see Melanosis.

MELANORRHAGIA, Melæna.

MELANORRHIZUM, Helleborus niger.

MÉLANOSE, Melanosis.

MELANO'SIS, *Melan'sis, Melano'ma, Nigritu'do, Carcino'ma melanot'icum, Cancer mela'neus, Fungus melano'des,* (F.) *Dégénérescence noire, Mélanose, Cancer mélane, Black cancer, Black tubercle,* from μελας, 'black.' An organic affection, in which the tissue of the parts is converted, owing to a *melan'ic depos'it,* into a black, hard, homogeneous substance, near which ulcers or cavities form; — owing to the softening, either of the substance itself, or of some other morbid tissue, — of tubercles especially. This morbific change affects the lungs particularly; when it is called *Melano'sis* seu *Melano'ma* seu *Anthraco'sis Pulmo'num, Melanopneu'mon, Nigritu'do* seu *Carcino'ma melanot'icum* seu *Melan'sis Pulmonum, Pneumonomelano'sis,* (F.) *Mélanose Pulmonaire.* It is, also, met with in the liver and areolar texture. Its causes are very obscure. Melanosis of the lungs constitutes one of the species of phthisis of Bayle; but it is impossible to distinguish it from the other species during life.

In the classification of Fuchs, **Melanosen** (G.) forms a family of diseases.

MELANOSIS PULMONUM, see Melanosis — m. Universalis, Venosity.

MELANOSMEGMA, see Sapo.

MELANOSPON'GUS, *Melanomyces;* from μελας, 'black,' and σπογγος, 'sponge.' The tuberiform variety of melanosis of the lungs.

MELANOTIC, Melanic — m. Cancer, Cancer, melanotic.

MEL'ANOTHRIX, *Atricapill'us,* from μελας, 'black,' and θριξ, 'hair.' Having black hair.

MELANSIS, Melanosis — m. Pulmonum, Melanosis pulmonum.

MELANTHIUM, Nigella, M. Virginicum.

MELAN'THIUM VIRGIN'ICUM, *Melanthium, Quofadil;* indigenous; *Order,* Melanthaceæ, flowering in July, is said to be a sure but severe remedy for itch.

MELAS, Lepra nigricans — m. Icterus, Melæna.

MELAS'MA, *Ecchymo'ma Melas'ma, Nigror,* from μελας, 'black.' A black spot or ecchymosis, occurring on the lower extremities of old people especially. Also a cutaneous affection analogous to chloasma, differing from it only in the dark colour of the morbid pigment. It is also called *Pityriasis nigra.*

MELAS'SES, *Molas'ses, Melus'tum, Theriaca commu'nis, Syru'pus empyreumat'icus* seu *niger, Treacle.* The syrup, which remains after the juice of the sugar-cane has been subjected to all the operations for extracting sugar from it. In the United States, the syrup, made in the process of forming common sugar, is called *molasses;* that remaining after the refinement of sugar being termed *sugar-house melasses* or *treacle.*

MELASSES SPIRIT, Rum.

MELATROPH'IA, from μελος, 'a limb,' and ατροφια, 'wasting.' Wasting of the limbs.

MELCA, μελκα. Food made of acidulated milk.

MELE, Specillum.

MELEA, Pyrus malus.

MELEGUETTA, Amomum grana paradisi.

MELEI'OS, μηλειος, *Meli'nus, Melias.* A species of alum found in the island of Melos.

MÉLÈZE, Pinus larix.

MELI, Mel.

MELIA, Fraxinus ornus.

ME'LIA AZED'ARACH, *Azedara'cha ama'ra, Poison Berry Tree, Azed'arach, Pride of India, Pride of China, Pride tree, Hop tree, Bead tree. Nat. Ord.* Meliaceæ; *Sex. Syst.* Decandria Monogynia. The bark of the root — called in India *Neem Bark, Azedarach,* (Ph. U. S.), is usually given in decoction, in the proportion of three or four ounces of the bark of the fresh root to a quart of water, boiled down to a pint. The dose is one or two table-spoonfuls, every two or three hours, till purging is induced. It is given in this manner as an anthelmintic. It is sometimes formed into an ointment, and used in tinea capitis. The tree is a native of Syria, Persia, and the north of India, and is abundant in the southern states of the Union.

MELIA TERRA, Creta.

MELIAN'THUS MAJOR, *Nat. Ord.* Zygophylleæ. A south African plant, a decoction of whose leaves is a good external remedy in tinea capitis, crusta serpiginosa, necrosis and foul ulcers. It is also useful as a gargle and lotion in sore throat and diseases of the gums. The bruised leaves applied to ulcers promote granulation.

MELICERA, Porrigo favosa.
MELICERIA, Hydrarthrus, Porrigo favosa.
MELICE'RIS, *Melifa'vium*, from μελι, 'honey,' and κηρος, 'wax.' *Emphy'ma encys'tis melice'ris*. An encysted tumour filled with a substance resembling honey. Also, Porrigo favosa.
MELIC"EROUS, *Melicer'itous*: same etymon. Having the characters of meliceris,—as a *melicerous* tumour.
MELICERUM, Porrigo favosa.
MELICHEIUM, from μελι, 'honey,' and χεω, 'I pour out.' A honey-like discharge from an ulcer.
MELICRATUM, Hydromeli.
MELIFAVIUM, Meliceris, Porrigo favosa.
MELIGEI'ON, from μελι, 'honey.' A fetid humour of the consistence of honey, discharged from ulcers, accompanied with caries of a bone.
MÉLILOT, Trifolium melilotus.
MELILOTUS, Trifolium melilotus.
MELIME'LUM, from μελι, 'honey,' and μηλον, 'an apple.' A name given to two compounds:—one of honey and quince, the other of honey and apples.
MÉLINE, Melæna.
MELINI SULPHAS, Cadmii sulphas.
MELI'NUM, μηλινον. The ancient name of an ointment, and of several plasters, described by Dioscorides and Galen: so called from their resembling the μηλον, or quince, in colour.
MELINUM SULPHURICUM, Cadmii sulphas.
MELINUS, Meleios.
MELIPHYLLUM, Melissa.
MELIS'SA, from μελισσα, 'a bee,' because bees gather honey from it. *Melissa officina'lis* seu *Roma'na* seu *hirsu'ta* seu *cit'rina* seu *citra'ta* seu *horten'sis*, *Citra'go*, *Citra'ria*, *Melitei'a*, *Melissob'otos*, *Melitæ'na*, *Melissobot'anum*, *Melissophyl'lum*, *Meliphyl'lum*, *Mentha citra'ta*, *Melit'tis*, *Cedronel'la*, *Apias'trum*, *Melissa cit'rina*, *Ero'tion*, *Balm*, (F.) *Mélisse*, *La Citronelle*; Nat. Ord. Labiatæ. The leaves of balm, *Melissa* (Ph. U. S.), have a pleasant odour; and an austere and aromatic taste. Balm was formerly much used in nervous diseases, but is now only employed when made into a tea, as a diluent, in febrile affections. It is the basis of a celebrated preparation,—the *Eau des Carmes*.
MELISSA CALAMIN'THA, *Calamin'tha*, *C. vulga'ris* seu *officina'rum* seu *grandiflo'ra*, *Thymus calamin'tha*, *Cal'amint*, (F.) *Calament*. This plant smells like wild mint, though more agreeably. It is used, popularly, as a tea in dyspepsia; flatulent colic; hysteria; uterine obstructions, &c.
MELISSA CANARIENSIS, Dracocephalum Canariense—m. Citrata, Melissa—m. Citrina, Melissa.
MELISSA GRANDIFLO'RA, *Thymus grandiflo'rus*, *Calamin'tha magno flore*, *C. monta'na*, *Mountain Cal'amint*. This plant resembles the last in virtues.
MELISSA HIRSUTA, Melissa—m. Hortensis, Melissa—m. Humilis, Melittis melissophyllum.
MELISSA NEP'ETA, *Thymus nep'eta* seu *multiflorus*, *Calamin'tha An'glica* seu *Pulb'gii odo'ræ* seu *nep'eta* seu *parviflo'ra* seu *trichot'oma*, *Nep'eta agres'tis*, *Field Cal'amint*, *Spotted Cal'amint*. Formerly used as an aromatic.
MELISSA PULEGIOIDES, Hedeoma—m. Romana, Melissa—m. Tragi, Melittis melissophyllum—m. Turcica, Dracocephalum Canariense.

MÉLISSE DES BOIS, Melittis melissophyllum—m. *de Moldavie*, Dracocephalum Canariense.
MELISSOBOTANUM, Melissa.
MELISSOBOTOS, Melissa.
MELISSOPHYLLUM, Melissa, Melittis melissophyllum.
MÉLISSOT, Melittis melissophyllum.
MELITÆ'MIA, from μελι, 'honey,' and 'αιμα, 'blood.' A condition of the circulating fluid, in which it contains an unusual quantity of saccharine matter.
MELITÆNA, Melissa.
MÉLITAGRE, Impetigo.
MELITEIA, Melissa.
MELITHOCORTON, Corallina Corsicana.
MELI'TIS, *Inflamma'tio gena'rum*; from μηλον, 'the cheek,' and *itis*, denoting inflammation. Inflammation of the cheek.
MELITITES, Hydromeli.
MELITTA, Bee.
MELITTIS, Melissa.
MELIT'TIS MELISSOPHYL'LUM, *La'mium monta'num*, *Melissa hu'milis* seu *sylves'tris*, *Melissa Tragi*, *La'mium Plin'ii*, *Melissophyl'lum*, *Bastard Balm*, (F.) *Mélisse des Bois*, *Mélissot*. This plant was formerly employed, like the balm, in uterine obstructions.
MELITTIS SYLVESTRIS, M. Melissophyllum.
MELITURIA, Urine, diabetic, see Diabetes.
MELI'TUS, *Melli'tus*, from *mel*, 'honey.' Appertaining to honey. Of the nature of honey.
MELIZO'MUM, from μελι, 'honey,' and ζωμος, 'broth;' *Mead*, *Melli'na*, *Metheg'lin*. A drink prepared with honey.
MELLA'GO, from *mel*, 'honey.' Any medicine having the consistence of honey. A fluid extract.
MELLICRATUM, Hydromeli.
MELLIFAVIUM, Porrigo favosa.
MELLINA, Melizomum.
MELLITE DE ROSES, Mel rosæ.
MELLI'TUM, from *mel*, 'honey.' A prepared honey:—a medicated honey.
MELLITUM DE ACETATE CUPRI, Linimentum Æruginis.
MELLITUM DE MERCURIA'LI COMPOS'ITUM, (F.) *Miel de mercuriale composé*, *Syrop de longue vie* (Succ. purif. mercurialis ℔ij, boraginis, anchusæ officinalis, ää ℔ss, iris pseudacori radicis recent. ʒij, rad. sicc. gentianæ ʒj, mellis ℔iij, vini albi ʒxiij. Macerate the bruised roots in the wine for 24 hours; strain; mix the juices and honey; boil slightly, and filter: then add the two liquors, and boil to the consistence of syrup. Ph. P.) Cathartic, stomachic, &c.
MELLITUM DE ROSIS, Mel rosæ.
MELLITUM SIMPLEX, *Syru'pus de Melle*, *Syrup of Honey*. (Mellis ℔vj, aquæ ℔iss, carbonat. calcis. præparat. ʒiij. Mix the honey, water, and carbonate of lime in a silver vessel: boil the mixture, stirring, at the same time, for 2 or 3 minutes: then add *prepared animal charcoal* ʒvj, *two whites of eggs*, mixed in a pint of water. Mix all, and boil to the consistence of syrup: remove from the fire; let the syrup rest for 15 minutes, and pass through a cloth. Ph. P.) Demulcent.
MELLITUS, Melitus.
MELOÆ'MIA, from μελας, 'black,' and 'αιμα, 'blood.' A state of blood, characterized by its incoagulability, black colour, and septic properties.
MELOCHI'TIS, *Lapis Arme'nius*, *Armeni'tes*, *Arme'nian Stone*. A variety of blue carbonate of copper. It is found in Germany, the Tyrol, and especially in Armenia. It was formerly em-

ployed as a cardiac, and as proper for purging away melancholy.

MEL'OE NIGER, *M. Pennsylvan'icus.* A blistering fly, native of the United States. It feeds upon *Prunel'la vulga'ris* or *Self-heal,* and *Ambro'sia trif'ida* or *Stick-weed.* These flies resemble the Spanish flies in properties.

MELOE PENNSYLVANICUS, M. niger.

MELOE PROSCARABÆ'US, *Cantarel'lus,* was anciently used as a diuretic and anti-hyhrophobic.

MELOE VESICATORIUS, Cantharis.

MELON, μηλον, 'an apple.' A disorder of the eye, in which it protrudes out of the socket. See Exophthalmia.—Castelli.

MELON, Cucumis melo—m. *d'Eau,* Cucurbita citrullus—m. Plant, Cucumis melo—m. Water, Cucurbita citrullus.

MELONGENA, Solanum melongena.

MELOPLACUNTIUM, Meloplacus.

MELOPLA'CUS, *Meloplacun'tium,* from μηλον, 'an apple,' 'a quince.' A compound obtained by boiling *wine, honey, quince, pepper,* &c., together. —Galen.

MELOPLAS'TIC, *Meloplas'ticus;* from μηλον, 'the cheek,' and πλασσω, 'I form.' The operation for forming a new cheek when any part of it has been lost.

MELOS, μελος, *Membrum.* A member. An organized part, composed of other parts.—Castelli.

MELO'SIS, *Catheteris'mus, Cenembate'sis,* from μηλη, 'a probe.' The act of probing a wound, ulcer, &c.—Hippocrates. Catheterism.

MELOTHRUM, Bryonia alba.

MELO'TIS, *Melo'tris, Specil'lum minus.* A small probe,—a probe for the ear. See Apyromele.

MELOTRIS, Melotis.

MELTING, Fusion.

MELUM, μηλον, *Malum.* An apple. Fruit in general. Also, a round, firm female breast. The cheek. The *apple-eye* or *melon-eye;* an apple-formed projection of the eye from the orbit.

MELUM ARMENIACUM, Prunus armeniaca—m. Cydonium, see Pyrus cydonia.

MELUSTUM, Melasses.

MEMBRA PUDENDA, Genital organs.

MEMBRANA, Membrane—m. Abdominis, Peritonæum—m. Adiposa, Cellular membrane—m. Adventitia, Decidua reflexa—m. Agnina, Amnios —m. Amphiblestrodes, Retina—m. Arachnoidea, Hyaloid membrane—m. Capsularis testis, Albuginea—m. Carnosa, Dartos—m. Cellulosa, Cellular membrane—m. Cellulosa, Decidua—m. Cerebri tenuis, Pia mater—m. Cerebri mollis, Pia mater—m. Cerebri propria, Pia mater—m. Circumossalis, Periosteum—m. Communis, Decidua —m. Circumplexa, Pericardium—m. Cordis, Pericardium—m. Costalis, Pleura—m. Costas succingens, Pleura—m. Crassa, Decidua reflexa— m. Cribrosa, Decidua—m. Cuticularis, Dura mater—m. Decidua serotina, see Decidua—m. Demuriana, see Aqueous humour, and Cornea—m. Dentata, Denticulatum ligamentum—m. Dermatodes, Dura mater—m. Descemetii, see Aqueous humour, and Cornea—m. Diaphratton, Mediastinum—m. Dura cerebrum ambiens, Dura mater— m. Epicrania, Galea aponeurotica capitis—m. Externa dentium, Tapetum alveoli—m. Farciminalis, Allantois—m. Fenestræ rotundæ, see Fenestra—m. Filamentosa, Decidua reflexa—m. Flocculenta, Decidua—m. Fœtum involvens, Amnios.

MEMBRA'NA GRANULO'SA, *Gran'ular membrane,* (F.) *Membrane granuleuse, Couche celluleuse* (Coste). A layer of yellow, granular matter, which lines the inner layer of the Graafian follicle.

MEMBRANA INTERSPINALIS, Interspinal ligament—m. Intestinalis, Allantois—m. Linguæ, see Tongue—m. Macilentior, Epiploon, gastrohepatic—m. Mucosa, Decidua, see Membrane— m. Nervorum, Neurilema—m. Nictitans, Valvula semilunaris—m. Olfactoria, Pituitary membrane —m. Ossis, Periosteum—m. Ovi materna, Decidua—m. Ovuli corticalis, Oiocalymma—m. Pellucida, Amnios—m. Pinguedinosa, see Cellular membrane—m. Pinguis intestinorum, Mesentery —m. Pituitaria, Pituitary membrane, see Membrane—m. Pituitosa, see Membrane—m. Pleuretica, Pleura—m. Præexistens, Decidua—m. Propria, Basement membrane, and Folliculi Graafiani, see Cortex ovi—m. Pupillaris, Pupillary membrane.

MEMBRA'NA PUTAM'INIS, (*putamen*, 'a shell or husk.') The membrane adherent to the inner surface of the eggshell.

MEMBRANA RETIFORMIS CHORII, Decidua reflexa—m. Ruyschiana, Choroid (inner layer.)

MEMBRANA SACCIFORM'IS. A separate synovial membrane for the inferior radio-cubital articulation, which covers the upper surface of the triangular ligament, and the sort of incomplete ring which circumscribes the head of the ulna.

MEMBRANA SEMIPELLUCIDA, Caligo—m. Sinuosa, Decidua—m. Subcostalis, Pleura—m. Succingens, Diaphragm, Pleura.

MEMBRANA TESTÆ, *Shell membrane.* The membrane that lines the shell of the bird's egg:— a simple membrane.

MEMBRANA THORACEM INTERSEPIENS, Mediastinum—m. Tympani, see Tympanum—m. Tympani secundaria, see Fenestra—m. Urinaria, Allantois—m. Uteri interna evoluta, Decidua—m. Uvea, Uvea—m. Vasculosa cerebri, Pia mater— m. Verricularis, Retina.

MEMBRA'NA VERSIC'OLOR. A peculiar membrane—according to Mr. Fielding, of Hull— situate immediately behind the retina, and in connexion with it. It is separable into distinct layers from the choroid, and is supplied with blood-vessels.

MEMBRANA WACHENDORFIANA, Pupillary membrane.

MEMBRANACEOUS, Membranous.

MEMBRANE, *Membra'na, Hymen, Meninx, Epen'dyma.* A name, given to different thin organs, representing a species of supple, more or less elastic, webs; varying in their structure and vital properties, and intended, in general, to absorb or secrete certain fluids; and to separate, envelop, and form other organs. Bichat has divided the membranes into simple and compound.

Simple membranes comprise three orders. 1. A *Mucous membrane, Membrana mucosa seu pituito'sa seu pituita'ria, Phleg'mymen, Phlegma'lymen, Membrane folliculeuse* (Ch.), is so called, on account of the mucous fluid by which they are constantly lubricated. They line the canals, cavities, and hollow organs, which communicate externally by different apertures on the skin. Bichat refers the mucous membranes to two great divisions—the *gastro-pulmonary,* and the *genitourinary.* The mucous membranes have a striking analogy with the cutaneous tissue, in organization, functions, and diseases. They are composed of chorion, papillæ, and epidermis; and are furnished with a multitude of follicles, which secrete a viscid humour—mucus. They receive a quantity of arterial vessels, veins, lymphatics, and nerves. 2. The *Serous membranes, M. villeuses simples* (Ch.), are transparent, thin, and composed of one lamina. One surface adheres to other textures; the other is smooth, polished, and moistened by a serous fluid. They are arranged—in the form of sacs without apertures—as great, intermediate reservoirs for the exhalant and absorbent systems, in which the serous fluid in passing from one system tarries some time before it enters the other. The serous membranes resemble the areolar membrane in structure and diseases. They facilitate the motion on each other of the organs which they envelop. They may be divided into (a) *Serous membranes*, properly so called; as the arachnoid, pleura, peritoneum, and tunica vaginalis. (b) *Synovial membranes* or *capsules;* which belong to joints, tendons, aponeuroses, &c. These membranes—mucous and serous—are constituted of similar layers — epithelium, basement membrane, condensed areolar tissue; and a looser form of areolar tissue, termed *submucous* in one case, — *subserous* in the other. 3. *Fibrous membranes*, Membranes albugineuses (Ch.) These are almost all continuous, and terminate at the periosteum — their common centre. They have been divided into two sections. 1. *Enveloping aponeuroses, Aponeuroses of insertion, Fibrous capsules of the joints*, and *Fibrous sheaths of tendons*. 2. The *Periosteum, Dura mater, Sclerotica, Tunica albuginea testis, Fibrous membrane of the spleen*, &c. The fibrous membranes are not free or moistened by any particular fluid. They adhere by both surfaces to the neighbouring parts; are firm, resisting, but slightly elastic, and of a white colour; sometimes pearly and glistening. Their vessels are numerous, in some, as in the dura mater and periosteum; in others, scarcely perceptible, as in the aponeuroses. The presence of nerves has never been proved, although several circumstances, regarding their sensibility, render their existence probable. The fibrous membranes serve, in general, to augment the solidity of the organs which they envelop; to retain the muscles in their respective positions; to favour the motion of the limbs, and that of the muscles and skin; to form canals and rings for the passage of different organs, &c.

Bichat admits three species of *Compound Membranes*. 1. The *Sero-fibrous*, formed of a serous and fibrous lamina, intimately adherent to each other;—as the pericardium, dura mater, and tunica albugineus. 2. The *Sero-mucous*, formed of a serous and mucous lamina;—as the *gall-bladder* at its lower part. 3. The *Fibro-mucous*, constituted of the union of a fibrous and mucous membrane; as *the mucous membrane of the nasal fossæ, gums*, &c. Chaussier admits six kinds of membranes. 1. The *laminated*. See Cellular Tissue. 2. The *serous* or *simple villous*. 3. The *follicular* or *complicated villous*. 4. The *muscular* or *fleshy*. 5. The *albugineous*. 6. The *albuminous*.

MEMBRANE, ACCIDENTAL, M. false — m. *Accidentelle*, M. false — m. *Adnée*, Conjunctiva — m. Adventitious, M. false — m. Anhistous, Decidua.

MEMBRANE, BASEMENT, *Pri'mary membrane, Membra'na pro'pria*. A delicate, structureless lamella of membrane found beneath the epidermis or epithelium, on all the free surfaces of the body.

MEMBRANE CADUQUE, Decidua — m. *Caduque réfléchie*, Decidua reflexa — m. *de Demours*, see Aqueous Humour, and Cornea — m. *de Descemet*, see Aqueous Humour, and Cornea.

MEMBRANE, FALSE, *Acciden'tal membrane, Adventi'tious membrane, Pseudo-membrane, Pseud'ymen, Pseudome'ninx*, (F.) *Fausse membrane, M. accidentelle*. Membranous productions, which form on all the free natural surfaces, and on every free accidental surface are so called. They are, in general, produced by the exudation of a fibrinous matter, susceptible of organization, which takes place in consequence of inflammation of the various tissues. These accidental membranes occur on the skin after the application of a blister; on mucous surfaces, as in croup; on the parietes of inflamed veins and arteries, &c. The cicatrices of wounds are formed of them.

MEMBRANE FAUSSE, Membrane false — m. Germinal, see Molecule — m. Granular, Membrana granulosa — m. *Granuleuse*, Membrana granulosa — m. Primary, Membrane, basement — m. Pseudo, M. false — m. Hyaloid, see Hyaloid membrane — m. *Ruyschienne*, Choroid (inner layer), Ruyschiana tunica — m. Shell, Membrana testæ — m. *du Tympan*, see Tympanum — m. Virginal, Hymen — m. Vitellary, Zona pellucida — m. *Vitelline*, Zona pellucida.

MEMBRANES ALBUGINEUSES, Membranes, fibrous, see Albuginea — m. *Folliculeuses*, Membranes, mucous — m. *Veloutées*, Villous membranes — m. *Villeuses simples*, Membranes, serous.

MEMBRANES OF THE FŒTUS, *Membra'næ fœtum involven'tes, Velamen'ta infan'tis*. The membranes which immediately envelop the fœtus in the cavity of the uterus, and the rupture of which gives rise to the discharge of the liquor amnii. These membranes are the *decidua, chorion*, and *amnion*.

MEMBRANEUX, Membranous.

MEMBRAN'IFORM, *Membraniform'is*, from *membrana*, and *forma;*—resembling a membrane. A name given to thin and flat parts, which resemble membranes.

MEMBRANIFORM MUSCLES. Very broad and thin muscles, as the platysma myoides, obliquus abdominis, &c.

MEMBRANOSUS, Fascia lata muscle.

MEM'BRANOUS, *Membrano'sus, Membrana'ceus, Hymeno'des*, (F.) *Membraneux*. Having the nature of membrane. Formed of membrane.

MEMBRANULA, Hymenium — m. Coronæ ciliaris, see Ciliary — m. Lunata vaginæ, Hymen — m. Nervorum, Neurilema — m. Semilunaris conjunctivæ, Valvula semilunaris.

MEM'BRANULE, *Membran'ula*, diminutive of *membrana*, 'a membrane.' A small membrane.

MEMBRE, Membrum — m. *Viril*, Penis.

MEMBRO'SUS, *Membro'sior, Mentula'tus, Mutonia'tus, Nasa'tus, valdè Mentula'tus, Fascino'sus, Psolon*, from *membrum*, 'the male organ.' One whose penis is very large.

MEMBRUM, *Artus, Melos, Colon*, a limb, a member, (F.) *Membre*. The *limbs* or *extremities* or *members* of animals are certain parts exterior to the body, which are more or less apparent, long, and moveable. It is by means of their limbs, that animals transport themselves from one place to another; and that they defend themselves, or attack others. The limbs are arranged on each side of the trunk, with which they are articulated. In man, they are four in number: —two *upper* or *thoracic*, and two *lower*, *pelvic* or *abdominal*. Also, the male organ.

MEMBRUM GENITALE VIRORUM, Penis — m. Muliebre, Clitoris — m. Seminale, Penis — m. Virile, Penis.

MÉMOIRE, Memory — m. *Perte de*, Amnesia.

MEMORIA DELETA, Amnesia.

MEM'ORY, *Memo'ria, Mnemè, Hypomne'sis, Recorda'tio, Recorda'tus*, (F.) *Mémoire*. The cerebral faculty, by virtue of which past impressions are recalled to the mind.

MEMPHI'TES LAPIS. A sort of stone, found in the environs of Memphis; which was formerly esteemed narcotic.

MENAGOGUES, Emmenagogues.

MENDESION, Ægyptiacum.

MENE, Moon.

MENECRATIS ACCIPITER, Accipiter.

MENES, Menses.
MÉNESPAUSIE, see Menses.
MENFRIGE, see Pistacia lentiscus.
MENINGARTHROC'ACE, *Inflamma'tio membrana'rum articulatio'nis, Arthromeningi'tis*, from μηνιγξ, 'membrane,' αρθρον, 'a joint,' and κακος, 'disease.' Inflammation of the membranes of a joint.
MÉNINGE, Dura mater.
MENINGÉ, Meningeal.
MENIN'GEAL, *Menin'geus*, from μηνιγξ, 'a membrane.' (F.) *Méningé*. Relating to the meninges, or merely to the dura mater.
MENINGEAL APOPLEXY, see Apoplexy.
MENINGEAL ARTERY, MIDDLE, *Arte'ria menin'gea me'dia, A. Sphæno-spino'sa, A. Duræ Matris me'dia max'ima, A. Sphæno-spina'lis, Spinal Artery,* (F.) *Artère méningée moyenne, A. Sphénoépineuse, A. Épineuse*, is the largest of the branches given off by the internal maxillary artery. It enters the cranium by the foramen spinale, and distributes its branches chiefly to the dura mater.
MENINGEAL VESSELS, *Vasa menin'gea*. The vessels of the membranes of the brain.
MENIN'GES, *Eilam'ides, Matres* seu *Involu'cra Cer'ebri, Omen'ta* seu *Velamen'ta cerebra'lia*, from μηνιγξ, 'a membrane.' The three membranes which envelop the brain—*Dura mater, Arachnoid*, and *Pia mater*.
MÉNINGETTE, Pia mater.
MENINGI'NA, (F.) *Méningine*. Same etymon. A name given by Chaussier to the pia mater, united to the cerebral layer of the arachnoid.
MENINGINA, INNER LAMINA OF THE, Pia mater.
MÉNINGINE, Meningina.
MENINGINI'TIS, from *meningina*, and *itis*, denoting inflammation. Inflammation of the meningina.
MENINGION, Arachnoid membrane.
MENINGIS CUSTOS, Meningophylax.
MÉNINGITE, Meningitis—m. *Granuleuse*, Hydrocephalus internus—m. *Rachidienne*, Meningitis, spinal—m. *Tuberculeuse*, Hydrocephalus internus.
MENINGI'TIS, *Encephali'tis peripher'ica, E. membrano'sa*, (F.) *Inflammation de la membrane séreuse céphalo-rachidienne, Méningite*. Inflammation of the meninges or membranes of the brain. See Phrenitis.
MENINGITIS ARTHRITICA, Cephalagra—m. Infantum, Hydrocephalus internus—m. Membranosa, M. spinal.
MENINGI'TIS MESENCEPHAL'ICA. Inflammation of the meninges of the medulla oblongata and pons varolii more especially.
MENINGITIS PERIPHERICA, M. spinal—m. Potatorum, Delirium tremens—m. Rachidian, M. spinal.
MENINGITIS, SPINAL, *M. Rachid'ian, M. Spina'lis* seu *peripher'ica* seu *membrano'sa, Perimyeli'tis*, (F.) *Méningite rachidienne*. Inflammation of the meninges of the spinal marrow.
MENINGITIS, TUBERCULAR, see Hydrocephalus internus—m. Tuberculosa, Hydrocephalus internus.
MENIN'GIUM. Diminutive of μηνιγξ, 'a membrane.' A fine, delicate membrane. The tunica arachnoidea of the brain.
MENINGO-CEPHALI'TIS, *Meningo-encephali'tis, Ceph'alo-meningi'tis*, from μηνιγξ, 'a membrane,' κεφαλη, 'head,' and *itis*, a suffix denoting inflammation. Inflammation of the membranes and brain.
MENINGOGASTRITIS, Fever, gastric.
MENINGOMALA'CIA, from μηνιγξ, 'membrane,' and μαλακια, 'softening.' Softening of membranes in general.
MENINGOPH'YLAX, *Custos menin'gis, Depresso'rium*, (F.) *Dépressoire*, from μηνιγξ, 'a membrane,' the dura mater; and φυλαξ, 'a preserver.' An instrument for depressing the dura mater, and guarding it from injury, whilst the bone is cut or rasped.
MENINGORRHŒ'A, from μηνιγξ, 'membrane,' and ρεω, 'I flow.' Effusion of blood upon or between the membranes of the brain.
MENINGO'SIS. Same etymon. The union of bones by means of membrane; e. g. the articulation of the bones of the cranium in the fœtus. Meningosis is a variety of Syndesmosis.
MENINGOSYM'PHYSIS; from μηνιγξ, 'membrane,' and συμφυσις, 'growing together.' Adhesion of or by membrane. Adhesion of the membranes of the brain to each other, or to the brain.
MENINX, Membrane—m. Choroides, Pia mater—m. Crassa, Dura mater—m. Dura, Dura mater—m. Exterior, Dura mater—m. Interior, Pia mater—m. Media, Arachnoid membrane—m. Pacheia, Dura mater—m. Sclera, Dura mater.
MENISCHESIS, see Amenorrhœa.
MENISPERMUM ANGULATUM, M. Canadense.
MENISPERM'UM CANADEN'SE, *M. angula'tum*, from μηνη, 'the moon,' and σπερμα, 'seed.' A climbing plant, growing in various parts of the United States. Said to be used in Virginia as a substitute for sarsaparilla in scrofula. It is an excitant tonic.
MENISPERM'UM COC'CULUS, *M. glaucum, Anamir'ta Coc'culus, A. panicula'ta, Coc'culus subero'sus*, so called from the shape of its seed. Family Menispermeæ. *Sex. Syst.* Diœcia Dodecandria. The systematic name of the plant, the berries of which are well known by the name of *Coc'culus In'dicus, Indian Berries, Baccæ Piscato'riæ, Coc'culus subero'sus, Indian Cockles, Coccus In'dicus, Cocculæ officina'rum, Cocci orienta'les, Grana Orien'tis*, (F.) *Coque du Levant, Coque levant*. These berries are remarkable for their inebriating and destructive quality to fish. The deleterious principle appears to reside in the kernel, and in the active principle called *Picrotox'ine*. Cocculus Indicus has been used in decoction to kill vermin. It has, at times, been added to beer, by fraudulent tradesmen, to render it more inebriating.
MENISPERMUM GLAUCUM, M. cocculus—m. Palmatum, Calumba.
MENISPERM'UM TUBERCULA'TUM, *M. Verruco'sum, Coc'culus crispus*. A Chinese plant, an extract from the root of which is tonic to the stomach and bowels, and possesses some astringency. Dose, 5 to 10 grains.
The same may be said of *Menisper'mum cordifo'lium*—the *Goluncha*, of Bengal.
MENISPERMUM VERRUCOSUM, M. tuberculatum.
MENOCRYPHIA, Amenorrhœa.
MENOLIPSIS, see Menses.
MENOPAUSIS, see Menses.
MENOPHANIA, see Menses.
MENOPLANIA, Menstruation, vicarious.
MENORRHAG''IA, from μην, 'a month,' and ρηγνυμι, 'I flow fiercely.' Flow of the menses. Frequently, the word is used synonymously with uterine hemorrhage or *metrorrhagia*, or for immoderate flow of the menses—*profuse menstruation, Parame'nia super'flua, P. profu'sa, Menorrhag''ia rubra, Catamenio'rum fluxus immod'icus, Menstrua immod'ica, M. super'flua, Menorrha'a*.
MENORRHAGIA, Menstruation, Metrorrhagia—m. Alba, Leucorrhœa—m. Difficilis, Dysmenorrhœa—m. Erronea, Menstruation, erroneous—m. Stillatitia, Dysmenorrhœa.

MENORRHŒ'A, from μην, 'month,' and ρεω, 'I flow.' Too long continuing, or too often returning, menstruation. Also, menorrhagia.

MENOSCHESIS, see Amenorrhœa.

MENOSTASIA, Amenorrhœa.

MENOS'TASIS, from μην, 'month,' and στασις, 'stasis,' 'stagnation.' This word, according to some, signifies the retention of the menses and their accumulation in the uterus. According to others, it means the acute pain which, in some females, precedes each appearance of the menses: a pain which has been presumed to proceed from the stasis of blood in the capillary vessels of the uterus.

MENOXEN'IA, *Menoxeno'sis,* from μην, 'a month,' and ξενος, 'foreign.' Irregular menstruation.

MENOXENOSIS, Menoxenia.

MENS, Anima, Intellect.

MENSA, 'a table.' The upper superficial part of the jaw teeth.

MENSES, (*Mensis,* 'a month;') *M. Mulie'bres, Mulie'bria, Menes, Fluxus men'struus, F. luna'ris, Pro'fluvium mulie'bră, P. genita'lă muliebre, Consuetu'do menstrua, Catame'nia, Men'strua, Emme'nia, Tribu'tum luna'ră seu men'struum, Purgatio'nes, P. menstruæ, Gynæcci'a, Aphedri'a, Oursus men'struus, Horæ'a, Luna'ria, Courses, Menstrual flux, Monthly courses, M. periods, Flowers, Turns, Terms, the Reds, Troubles,* (F.) *Mois, Règles, Lunes, Flueurs, Affaires, Époques, Ordinaires, Purgations, Fleurs, Menstrues.* The sanguineous evacuation from the uterus, *Sanguis menstruus,* the monthly occurrence of which constitutes *menstruation.* The first appearance of the menses — *menopha'nia* — is usually preceded by the discharge of a fluid whitish matter from the vagina; by nervous excitement, and by vague pains and heaviness in the loins and thighs; numbness of the limbs, tumefaction and hardness of the breasts, &c. More or less indisposition and irritability also precede each successive recurrence of the *menstrual flux.* In temperate climates, each period ordinarily continues from three to six days; and the quantity lost varies from four to eight ounces. The menses continue to flow from the period of puberty till the age of 45 or 50. At the term of its natural cessation, *Menolip'sis, Ménespausie* (Gardanne,) *Menopau'sis,* the flux becomes irregular; and this irregularity is occasionally accompanied with symptoms of dropsy, glandular tumours, &c, constituting the *Parame'nia cessatio'nis* of Good, and what is called the *critical time* or *turn of life;* yet it does not appear that the mortality is increased by it. With the immediate causes of menstruation we are unacquainted. We express only our ignorance, when we assert it to depend upon periodicity; the discharge comes from the vessels of the uterus and vagina, and differs from ordinary blood by its peculiar odour, and by its not coagulating. It is evidently connected with the condition of the ovaries, and appears to be connected with the periodical discharge of ova from them. It is arrested, as a general principle, during pregnancy and lactation. In warm climates, women usually begin to menstruate early, and cease sooner than in the temperate regions. The quantity lost is also greater. In the colder regions, the reverse of this holds as a general rule.

MENSES ALBI, Leucorrhœa — m. Anomalæ, Paramenia — m. Devii, Menstruation, vicarious — m. Dolorifici, Dysmenorrhœa — m. Retention of the, see Amenorrhœa — m. Suppression of the, Amenorrhœa.

MENSIUM RETENTIO, see Amenorrhœa.

MENSTRUA, Menses — m. Alba, Leucorrhœa — m. Difficilia, Dysmenorrhœa — m. Dolorosa, Dysmenorrhœa — m. Immodica, Menorrhagia — m. Superflua, Menorrhagia.

MENSTRUAL, Catamenial — m. Flux, Menses.

MENSTRUANT, *Men'struans,* from *menstrua,* 'the catamenia.' One subject to the catamenia.

MENSTRUATIO ANOMALA, Paramenia — m. Difficilis, Dysmenorrhœa — m. Dolorifica, Dysmenorrhœa — m. Impedita, see Amenorrhœa — m. Per insolitas Vias, Menstruation, vicarious.

MENSTRUA'TIO RECIDI'VA. Menstruation, when protracted beyond the usual age.

MENSTRUATIO RETENTA, Amenorrhœa, Paramenia — m. Suppressa, Amenorrhœa, Paramenia.

MENSTRUA'TION, *Menstrua'tio, Chronogu'nea, Menorrhag''ia, Fluxus menstrua'lis.* The flow of the menses.

MENSTRUATION DIFFICILE, Dysmenorrhœa — m. Difficult, Dysmenorrhœa — m. Laborious, Dysmenorrhœa — m. Profuse, Menorrhagia.

MENSTRUATION, VICA'RIOUS, is that which occurs from other parts than the uterus. It is called *Parame'nia erro'ris, Menorrhag''ia erro'nea, Mensium per alie'na loca excre'tio, Menses de'vii, Aberra'tio men'sium* seu *menstruo'rum, Menstrua'tio per insol'itas vias, Hæmatopla'nia* seu *Hæmopla'nia menstrua'lis, Menopla'nia,* (F.) *Deviation des Règles, Règles déviées.* At times, the secreted fluid has all the characters of the menstrual secretion; at others, it appears to be mere blood.

MENSTRUEL, Catamenial.

MENSTRUES, Menses.

MENSTRUOUS, Catamenial. Also, one affected with the menses or catamenia.

MEN'STRUUM, (F.) *Menstrue.* Same etymon; — the menstruum being, of old, usually continued in action for a *month.* This name was formerly given to every substance which possesses the property of dissolving others slowly and with the aid of heat. At present, it is used synonymously with *solvent.* Thus — water, alcohol, ether, acids, oils, &c., are menstrua.

MENSTRUUM AURI, Nitro-muriatic acid — m. Ventriculi, Gastric juice.

MENSU'RA MED'ICA. A measure of 48 ounces.

MENSURA'TION, *Meta'tio,* from *mensura,* 'measure.' *Measurement, Medical meas'uring.* One of the means used for exploring the state of the thoracic and other cavities. It consists in a comparative measurement of each side of the chest, by means of a riband extended from the median line of the sternum to the spine. When effusion exists on one side, the measurement is usually greater than on the other. When, on the other hand, a portion of a lung has ceased, for some time, to exert its respiratory functions, the corresponding side of the chest becomes smaller, in consequence of the contraction of the pleura, retraction of the pulmonary tissue, and greater approximation of the ribs.

MENTA, Mentha, Penis.

MENTAGRA, Mentulagra, Sycosis — m. Infantum, Porrigo lupinosa.

MEN'TAGRAPHYTE, *Men'tagrophyte,* from *mentagra,* and φυτον, 'a plant.' A name proposed by M. Gruby, of Vienna, for a cryptogamic plant, which he found in the eruption of mentagra.

MENTAL, *Menta'lis,* from *mens,* 'mind;' belonging or relating to the mind, as *mental phenom'ena, mental diseases* (*Morbi menta'les,*) &c.

In Anatomy, Mental, *Menta'lis,* (F.) *Mentonnier,* signifies that which relates to the chin; from *mentum,* 'the chin.'

MENTAL AR'TERY, (F.) *Artère mentonnière,*

This is given off by the inferior dental, and issues at the mental foramen to be distributed on the lower lip.

MENTAL FORA'MEN, (F.) *Trou mentonnier, Anté'rior maxillary F.*, is the outer orifice of the inferior dental canal. It is situate on the outer surface of the lower jaw-bone, opposite the second incisor, or the canine tooth, and gives passage to the vessels and nerves.

MENTAL FOSSA, see Fossa, mental.

MENTAL NERVE, (F.) *Nerf mentonnier*, is furnished by the inferior dental nerve. It issues by the mental foramen, and is distributed, in numerous filaments, to the muscles of the lower lip.

MENTAL REGION, *Re'gio menta'lis*. The region of the chin.

MENTHA seu MENTA AQUAT'ICA, *Menthas'trum, Sisym'brium menthastrum, Mentha palus'tris seu hirsu'ta seu rotundifo'lia palus'tris, Bal'samus palus'tris, Watermint*, (F.) *Menthe aquatique, M. rouge. Nat. Ord.* Labiatæ. This is less agreeable than the *Mentha viridis*, and more bitter and pungent. It is used like *spearmint*.

MENTHA BALSAMEA, M. piperita.

MENTHA CAPEN'SIS, which grows at the Cape of Good Hope, possesses the medical properties of the *mints*.

MENTHA CERVI'NA, *Hart's pennyroyal, Hyssop-leaved mint, Pule'gium cervi'num*, (F.) *Menthe cervine*. Possesses the properties of pennyroyal, but is very unpleasant.

MENTHA CITRATA, Melissa.

MENTHA CRISPA, *M. hercyn'ica, Colymbif'era minor, Curled Mint*, (F.) *Menthe frisée, Menthe crêpue, Baume d'eau à feuilles ridées*. Possesses the properties of peppermint.

MENTHA GENTILIS, M. viridis — m. Hercynica, M. crispa — m. Hirsuta, M. Aquatica — m. Lævigata, M. viridis — m. Officinalis, M. piperita — m. Palustris, M. Aquatica.

MENTHA PIPERI'TA, *Mentha Piperi'tis seu offi-cina'lis seu balsame'a, Peppermint*, (F.) *Menthe poivrée*. The odour of this variety is strong and agreeable. Taste, pungent, aromatic, and producing a sensation of coldness in the mouth. Virtues depend upon essential oil and camphor. It is stomachic and carminative. It is chiefly used in the form of essential oil—the *oleum menthæ piperitæ*.

Essence of Peppermint consists of *ol. menthæ pip.* ʒij, *sp. vin. rectif.*, coloured with *spinach leaves*, Oij. See Tinctura olei menthæ piperitæ.

MENTHA PULE'GIUM, *Pulegium, Pulegium rega'lê, Pulegium latifo'lium, Glechon, Pennyroyal, Pudding grass*, (F.) *Pouliot*. The oil — *O'leum pule'gii* — possesses the virtues of the plant. It resembles the mints in general in properties. Amongst the vulgar, it is esteemed an emmenagogue.

MENTHA ROMANA, Balsamita suaveolens, Tanacetum balsamita — m. Rotundifolia palustris, M. aquatica — m. Saracenica, Balsamita suaveolens, Tanacetum balsamita — m. Sativa, M. viridis — m. Spicata, M. viridis.

MENTHA VIR'IDIS, *M. Sati'va seu vulga'ris seu gentilis seu spica'ta seu læviga'ta, Spearmint*, (F.) *Menthe sauvage, Baume des jardins, Menthe verte, Menthe des jardins*. Odour strong, aromatic; taste, warm, austere, bitterish. Virtues the same as those of the peppermint. The *Oleum menthæ viridis* is obtained from it.

MENTHA VULGARIS, M. viridis.

MENTHASTRUM, Mentha aquatica.

MENTHE AQUATIQUE, Mentha aquatica — *m. Cervine*, Mentha cervina — *m. Coq*, Tanacetum balsamita — *m. Crêpue*, Mentha crispa — *m. Frisée*, Mentha crispa — *m. des Jardins* — Mentha viridis — *m. Poivrée*, Mentha piperita — *m. Rouge*, Mentha aquatica — *m. Sauvage*, Mentha viridis — *m. Verte*, Mentha viridis.

MENTIGO, Porrigo larvalis, Sycosis.

MENTISME, from *mens, mentis*, 'mind.' Any irregular movement of the mind, whether from emotion or a vivid imagination. — Baumes.

MENTOBICORNEUS, Geniohyoideus.

MENTO-LABIAL, *Mento-labia'lis*. Under this name Chaussier has united the Levator labii inferioris, and Quadratus muscles. See Depressor labii inferioris.

MENTO-LABIAL FURROW: a transverse depression situate between the lower lip and the chin, which is remarkable for the perpendicular direction of the hairs growing upon it.

MENTON, Mentum.

MENTONNIER, Mental — *m. Labial*, Depressor labii inferioris.

MENTONNIÈRE, see Funda.

MENTULA, Penis — m. Muliebris, Cercosis, Clitoris — m. Parva, Pipinna.

MEN'TULAGRA, *Men'tagra*. A hybrid word, from *mentula*, 'the penis,' and *αγρα*, 'a seizure.' A convulsive erection of the mentula or penis; such as is said to be sometimes observed in eunuchs. See Pudendagra.

MENTU'LATUS, Membrosus.

MENTUM, *Genei'on, Geni'um, Anthe'reon*, 'the chin.' (F.) *Menton*. The inferior and middle part of the face, situate below the lower lip. The chin is formed of skin, areolar tissue, muscles, vessels, nerves, and the os maxillare inferius.

MENYAN'THES TRIFOLIA'TA, *Minyan'thes, Trifo'lium paludo'sum seu aquat'icum seu palus'trê seu fibri'num, Menyan'thes, Water trefoil, Buckbean, Bogbean. Nat. Ord.* Gentianeæ. (F.) *Trèfle d'eau*. The taste is intensely bitter, and is extracted by water. It is tonic, anthelmintic, diuretic, cathartic, and, in large doses, emetic. In some countries, it is used as a substitute for hops in making beer.

MENYAN'THES VERNA, *American buck bean, Marsh trefoil, Water shamrock, Bitter root*, has similar properties.

MEOSIS, Meiosis.

MEPHIT'IC, *Mephit'icus;* from a Syriac word, signifying 'to blow, to breathe.' Any thing possessed of an unwholesome property; chiefly applied to exhalations.

MEPHITIS, see Mephitism — m. Hepatica, Hydrogen, sulphuretted — m. Inflammabilis, Hydrogen — m. Urinosa, Ammonia.

MEPH'ITISM. Same etymon. Any pernicious exhalation. *Mephi'tis* and *Mophe'ta*, (F.) *Mofette* ou *Moufette*, are old names for azote; and, in general, for all exhalations and gases that are unfit for respiration.

MERACUS, Merus.

MERAMAUROSIS, Hypamaurosis.

MERANÆSTHE'SIS, *Meranæsthe'sia*, from μέρος, 'a part,' αν, 'privative,' and αισθησις, 'sensation.' Insensibility of a part of the body.

MERATROPH'IA, from μέρος, 'a part,' and ατροφια, 'want of nourishment.' Atrophy of some part of the body.

MERCURE, Hydrargyrum — *m. Bichlorure de*, Hydrargyri oxymurias — *m. avec la Craie*, Hydrargyrum cum cretâ — *m. Cru*, Hydrargyrum — *m. Cyanure de*, Hydrargyri cyanuretum — *m. Deutiodure de*, Hydrargyri iodidum rubrum — *m. Deuto-chlorure de*, Hydrargyri oxymurias — *m. Doux*, Hydrargyri submurias — *m. Gommeux de Plenck*, Syrupus de mercurio mediante gummi — *m. Muriate oxygéné de*, Hydrargyri oxymurias — *m. Oxide de, cendré*, Hydrargyri oxydum cinereum — *m. Oxide gris de*, Hydrargyri oxydum cinereum — *m. Oxide nitrique de*, Hydrargyri nitrico-oxydum — m. *Oxide noir de*, Hydrargyri oxydum cinereum — m. *Oxide rouge de*, Hydrargyri oxydum rubrum — m. *Periodure de*, Hydrargyri Iodidum rubrum — m. *Protiodure de*, Hydrargyri iodidum — m. *Protochlorure de*, Hydrargyri submurias — m. *Protoxide de*, Hydrargyri oxydum cinereum—m. *Sous-muriate de, précipité,* Hydrargyrum præcipitatum — m. *Sous-sulfate de*, Hydrargyrus vitriolatus—m. *Sulphure de, noir*, Hydrargyri sulphuretum nigrum — m. *Sulphure de, rouge*, Hydrargyri sulphuretum rubrum.

MERCU'RIAL, *Mercuria'lis, Hydrargyr'icum, Hydrargyr'ium.* That which contains mercury. A preparation of mercury.

MERCURIA'LIS, *Mercuria'lis an'nua, French mercury.* It has been esteemed cathartic, hypnotic and cosmetic, and has been chiefly used by way of *lavement.* See Chenopodium Bonus Henricus.

MERCURIALIS HUMOR, *Humor melanchol'icus.* A supposititious humour with the older physicians, out of which they presumed that *morbi melanchol'ici* seu *mercuria'les* arose.

MERCURIALIS PEREN'NIS, *Cynocram'bē, Cani'na bras'sica, M. monta'na, M. Sylves'tris, Dog's mercury.* This plant is possessed of acro-narcotic properties.

MERCURIALISMUS, Hydrargyriasis.

MERCU'RIALIST, *Mercurialis'ta;* from *mercurius,* 'mercury.' One inordinately addicted to prescribing mercury.

MERCURIALIZA'TION. Same etymon. The state of being affected by mercury. One under the influence of mercury is said to be *mercurialized.*

MERCURII CALX VITRIOLATA, Hydrargyrus vitriolatus — m. Deuto-ioduretum, Hydrargyri iodidum rubrum — m. Proto-ioduretum, Hydrargyri iodidum—m. Sperma, Hydrargyrus acetatus—m. Terra foliata, Hydrargyrus acetatus.

MERCURIUS, Hydrargyrum — m. Acetatus, Hydrargyrus acetatus — m. Alkalisatus, Hydrargyrum cum cretâ — m. Calcinatus, Hydrargyri oxydum rubrum—Causticus flavus, Hydrargyrus vitriolatus — m. Cinereus, Hydrargyri oxydum cinereum—m. Cinnabarinus, Hydrargyri sulphuretum rubrum — m. Corallinus, Hydrargyri nitrico-oxydum — m. Corrosivus, Hydrargyri oxymurias — m. Corrosivus ruber, Hydrargyri nitrico-oxydum — m. Corrosivus sublimatus, Hydrargyri oxymurias — m. Cosmeticus, Hydrargyrum præcipitatum — m. Dulcis, Hydrargyri submurias — m. Emeticus flavus, Hydrargyrus vitriolatus — m. Gummosus Plenckii, Syrupus de mercurio mediante gummi—m. Luteus, Hydrargyrus vitriolatus—m. Mortis, Algaroth — m. Niger Moscati, Hydrargyri oxydum cinereum — m. Præcipitatus corrosivus, Hydrargyri nitrico-oxydum—m. Præcipitatus niger, Hydrargyri oxydum cinereum — m. Saccharatus, Hydrargyrum saccharatum — m. Solubilis of Hahnemann, see Hydrargyri oxydum cinereum — m. Sublimatus dulcis, Hydrargyri submurias — m. cum Sulphure, Hydrargyri sulphuretum nigrum — m. Terrestris, Polygonum hydropiper — m. Vitæ, Algaroth — m. Zoticus Hartmanni, Hydrargyri submurias.

MERCURY, Hydrargyrum — m. Acetate of, Hydrargyrus acetatus — m. Acid, nitrate of, see Hydrargyri nitras — m. Ammoniated, Hydrargyrum præcipitatum — m. Ammonio-chloride of, Hadrargyrum præcipitatum — m. Bichloride of, Hydrargyri oxymurias — m. Biniodide of, Hydrargyri iodidum rubrum, see Iodine — m. Bisulphuret of, Hydrargyri sulphuretum rubrum — m. Bromide of, see Bromine — m. with Chalk, Hydrargyrum cum cretâ— m. Chloride of, mild, Hydrargyri submurias—m. Cyanuret of, Hydrargyri cyanuretum — m. Deuto-iodide of, see Iodine —

m. Dog's, Mercurialis perennis—m. English, Chenopodium bonus Henricus — m. French, Mercurial—m. Iodide of, Hydrargyri Iodidum—m. Iodide of, red, Hydrargyri Iodidum rubrum.

MERCURY, IODIDE OF CHLORIDE OF, *Iod'idum Hydrar'gyri chlo'ridi, Hydrar'gyrum ioda'tum cum chlorido mercurii,* (F.) *Iodhydrargyrite de chlorure mercureux.* Made by the reaction of *iodine* on *mild chloride of mercury.* Two iodides may be prepared — the *iodide* and the *biniodide.* Both are violent irritants: the biniodide, especially, is a powerful caustic. Both have been given in scrofula. The biniodide is only used externally like nitrate of silver in scrofulous and certain syphilitic ulcerations. An ointment of the iodide (gr. xv ad adipis ℥ij) is rubbed on scrofulous tumefactions.

MERCURY, IODO-ARSENITE OF, Arsenic and Mercury, iodide of—m. Muriate of, corrosive, Hydrargyri oxymurias — m. Muriate of, mild, Hydrargyri submurias — m. Nitrate of, Hydrargyri nitras — m. Nitric oxyd of, Hydrargyri nitrico-oxydum — m. Oxide of, black or gray, Hydrargyri oxydum cinereum — m. Oxide of, red, Hydrargyri oxydum rubrum — m. Oxymuriate of, Hydrargyri oxymurias — m. Periodide of, Hydrargyri iodidum rubrum — m. Phosphuretted, Hydrargyrus phosphoratus — m. Precipitate of, white, Hydrargyrum præcipitatum — m. Protochloride of, Hydrargyri submurias — m. Protoiodide of, see Hydrargyri iodidum, and Iodine—m. Prussiate of, Hydrargyri cyanuretum — m. Soluble, Hydrargyri nitras — m. Subchloride of, Hydrargyri submurias—m. Submuriate of, Hydrargyri submurias—m. Sulphuret of, black, Hydrargyri sulphuretum nigrum — m. Sulphuret of, red, Hydrargyri sulphuretum rubrum, Realgar — m. Sulphuret of, with Sulphur, Hydrargyri Sulphuretum nigrum — m. Supernitrate of, Solution of, see Hydrargyri nitras—m. Tartrate of, Hydrargyri tartras—m. Three-seeded, Acalypha Virginica.

MERCURY AND ARSENIC, IODIDE OF, Arsenic and Mercury, Iodide of — m. and Quinia, Protochloride of, Hydrargyri et Quiniæ Protochloridum.

MERDA, Excrement.
MERDIVOMUS, Copremetus.
MERDUS, Excrement.
MÈRE DES PIANS, Pian.
MEREMPHRAX'IS, from μερος, 'a part,' and εμφραξις, 'obstruction.' Obstruction or infarction of an organ.
MERICUS, Local.
MERIDRO'SIS, *Sudor partia'lis* seu *loca'lis;* from μερος, 'a part,' and 'ιδρωσις, 'sweating.' A partial perspiration.
MERIMNA, Cura.
MERIMNE, Cura.
MERISIER, Prunus avium.
MEROBALÁNEUM, Bath, partial.
MEROBALNEUM, Bath, partial.
MEROCE'LĒ, *Miroce'lē, Merorix'is, Merorrhex'is,* from μερος, 'the thigh,' and κηλη, 'tumour;' *Hernia cruralis* seu *femora'lis, Femoral* or *crural hernia,* (F.) *Hernie crurale* ou *fémorale.* In this hernia, the viscera issue from the abdomen through the crural canal; or through an opening immediately on the outer side of Gimbernat's ligament, which gives passage to lymphatic vessels. This affection is more frequent in the female than in the male, and especially in those who have had children. The tumour, formed by merocele, is generally small, round, and more or less difficult of reduction. In other respects, it possesses all the characters of hernia. The neck of the sac has, close on the outside, the epigastric artery; above, the spermatic cord and spermatic

artery in the male — the round ligament in the female; on the inside, Gimbernat's ligament; and, below the pubes. When the obturator artery arises from the epigastric, it generally passes on the outside of and below the orifice of the sac; sometimes, however, it takes a turn above, and then to the inside of the opening. J. Cloquet asserts, that of 134 cases, in one only did he find the epigastric artery on the inside of the orifice of the sac.

The operation, required in strangulation of this variety, may be practised on the aponeurotic opening, by cutting downwards and inwards, on the side of Gimbernat's ligament.

MEROCOXALGIA, Coxalgia.

MERO'PIA, from μερος, 'a part,' and ωψ, 'the eye.' A partial obscurity of vision.

MERORIXIS, Merocele.

MERORRHEU'MA, *Rheumatis'mus partia'lis, Rh. loca'lis, Rh. Membro'rum singulo'rum;* from μερος, 'a part,' and ρευμα, 'defluxion, rheumatism.' Rheumatism affecting a part. Topical or local rheumatism.

MERORRHEXIS, Merocele.

MEROS, Femur, Thigh.

MERRY-ANDREW. An itinerant quack, who exposes his nostrums for sale at fairs and markets. See CHARLATAN.—So called from Dr. Andrew Boorde, who lived in the reigns of Henry VIII., Edward VI., and Queen Mary, and who was in the habit of frequenting fairs and markets at which he harangued the populace.

MERULIUS AURICULA, Peziza auricula.

MERUS, *Mera'cus, A'cratos,* 'pure, genuine;' as *Vinum merum,* unmixed wine.

MERUS, Femur, Thigh.

MERVINE MALE, Cypripedium luteum.

MERYCISMUS, Rumination.

MERYCOLOG"IA, from μερυκω, 'I ruminate,' and λογος, 'a description.' Any work on rumination may be so termed.

MESA, Genital organs.

MESARÆUM, Mesentery.

MESARAIC, Mesenteric.

MESEMAR, Mismar.

MESEMBRYANTHEMUM COPTICUM, see Soda.

MESEMBRYAN'THEMUM CRYSTAL'LINUM, *M. ficoi'des, Di'amond fig-maryyold, Ice-plant,* (F.) *Glaciale, Crystalline. Nat. Ord.* Ficoideæ: a plant common in the neighbourhood of Cape Town. It has been recommended in dysuria, ischuria, and some other affections of the urinary organs.

MESEMBRYANTHEMUM EDU'LE; and *M. acinaciforme,* South African plants, are much used as domestic remedies at the Cape. The expressed juice of the leaves acts as an astringent in dysentery, and as a mild diuretic. It is also used as an antiseptic gargle in malignant sore throat, violent salivation and aphthæ, and as a lotion to burns and scalds.

MESEMBRYAN'THEMUM TORTUO'SUM, also a South African plant, is said to possess narcotic properties.

MÉSENCÉPHALE, Medulla oblongata, Pons Varolii.

MES'ENTERIC, *Mesara'ic, Mesenter'icus, Mesara'icus, Mesaræ'icus;* from μεσεντεριον, or μεσαραιον, 'the mesentery.' That which relates or belongs to the mesentery.

MESENTERIC ARTERIES are two in number, and distinguished into, 1. The *Superior mesenteric,* which arises from the anterior part of the abdominal aorta, below the cœliac. It immediately descends to the left, forwards, behind the pancreas, and in front of the third portion of the duodenum,—to gain the superior extremity of the mesentery, where it makes a long curvature, the convexity of which is turned forwards and to the left. Towards the termination of the ileum, it ends by anastomosing with a branch of the *A. colica dextra inferior.* At its concavity, it gives off the three *Arteriæ colicæ dextræ,* which belong to the great intestine; and, at its convexity, it sends off fifteen or twenty branches, which are distributed to the small intestine, after having formed numerous arches by their anastomoses.

2. The *Inferior Mesenteric Artery* arises from the anterior part of the abdominal aorta, an inch and a half before its termination. It descends, on the left side, behind the peritoneum; engages itself in the substance of the iliac mesocolon, forming a considerable curvature, whose convexity faces the left side. When it reaches the brim of the pelvis, it passes along the posterior separation of the mesorectum, and attains the neighbourhood of the anus, under the name *Superior hemorrhoidal artery.* It gives off no branch at its concave part; but, from the convex, the three *Arteriæ colicæ sinistræ* arise.

MESENTERIC DISEASE, Tabes mesenterica.

MESENTERIC GLANDS are the lymphatic ganglions of the mesentery. Through them, the chyliferous vessels pass to the thoracic duct. Their uses are unknown. When diseased, nutrition is interfered with, and atrophy produced.

MESENTERIC HERNIA. If one of the layers of the mesentery be torn by a blow, whilst the other remains in its natural state, the intestines may insinuate themselves into the aperture, and form a kind of hernia. It is not known during life.

MESENTERIC PLEXUSES are furnished by the solar plexus, and have been distinguished into *superior* and *inferior;* like the mesenteric arteries which they accompany.

MESENTERIC or MESARAIC VEINS are two in number, and belong to the vena porta. They are distinguished into, 1. The *Superior mesenteric* or *mesaraic* or *great mesaraic.* This trunk receives, from above to below and on the right side, the three *venæ colicæ dextræ* and the *Gastro-epiploica dextra.* Into its left side, the veins of the small intestine open. It passes in front of the transverse portion of the duodenum; and, behind the pancreas, unites with the splenic vein to concur in the formation of the vena porta.

The *inferior* or *lesser mesenteric vein* corresponds to the artery of the same name, and opens into the splenic, near the union of that vein with the superior mesenteric, and behind the pancreas.

MESENTERIITIS, Mesenteritis.

MESENTERI'TIS, *Mesenterii'tis, Empres'ma peritoni'tis mesenter'ica, Enteri'tis mesenter'ica, Inflamma'tion of the mesentery.* The pain is here deeper seated and more immediately in the mesenteric region. The external tenderness is less than in some of the other varieties of peritonitis. See Tabes Mesenterica.

MESENTERIUM, Mesentery—m. Crassum, Mesocolon.

MESENTERON, Mesentery.

MES'ENTERY, *Mesenter'ium, Mesarai'cα, Mesaræ'um, Media'num, Membra'na pinguis intestino'rum, Lactes, Mesen'teron, Mesera'um, Mesoræ'um, Medium intesti'num, Epichor'dis,* from μεσος, 'in the middle,' and εντερον, 'intestine.' (F.) *Mésentère.* A term in anatomy, applied to several duplicatures of the peritoneum, which maintain the different portions of the intestinal canal in their respective situations; allowing, however, more or less motion. They are formed of two laminæ, between which are contained the corresponding portion of intestine and the vessels that pass to it. One only of these duplicatures has received the name *mesentery*, properly so called. This belongs to the small intestine, which it suspends and retains *in situ*. Its posterior margin, which is the smallest, is straight, and descends obliquely from the left side of the body of the second lumbar vertebra to the right iliac fossa. Its anterior margin is curved, undulating, plaited, and corresponds to the whole length of the small intestine. The mesentery contains, between the two laminæ which form it, a number of lymphatic ganglions; the trunks and branches of the mesenteric vessels; the nervous plexuses accompanying them, and many lacteals and lymphatics.

MESERA, Tutia.
MESERÆUM, Mesentery.
MESERAION, Mesentery.
ME'SIAL, from μεσος, 'in the middle.' Relating or appertaining to the middle.

MESIAL PLANE, an imaginary *plane*, dividing the head, neck, and trunk into similar halves, towards right and left. Every aspect towards this plane is *mesial;* and every aspect towards right or left is *lateral;* every lateral aspect being *dextral* or *sinistral*.

MESIAMUM, Aniceton.
MESMER'IC, *Mesmer'icus*. Relating to mesmerism or animal magnetism:—as the 'mesmeric state,' 'mesmeric sleep,' &c. &c.
MESMERISM, Magnetism, animal.
MES'MERIST. A practiser of, or believer in, mesmerism.
MESMERIZA'TION, *Magnetiza'tion*. The act of mesmerizing. The state of being mesmerized.
MES'MERIZED, *Mesmeriza'tus, Mag'netized*. Affected with mesmerism or animal magnetism. When the person is in a state of 'magnetic sleep,' he is said to be *hyp'notized*.
MES'MERIZER, *An'imal Magneti'zer, Magneti'zer*. One who practises mesmerism.
MESO, μεσος, 'in the middle.' A prefix to certain words.
MESOBREGMATE, see Cranium.
MESOCÆ'CUM. A name given to a duplicature of the peritoneum, (in some persons only,) at the posterior part of the cæcum.
MÉSOCÉPHALE, Medulla oblongata, Pons Varolii.
MESOCHON'DRIAC, *Mesochondri'acus;* from μεσος, and χονδρος, 'cartilage.' A name given by Boerhaave to fleshy fibres situate between the cartilaginous rings of the trachea.
MESOCOL'IC HERNIA. Hernia is so named by Sir Astley Cooper, when the bowels glide between the layers of the mesocolon.
MESOCO'LON, *Mesoco'lum, Mesenter'ium crassum*, from μεσος, and κωλον, 'the colon.' A name given to the duplicatures of the peritoneum, which fix the different parts of the colon to the abdominal parietes. It has received different names, according to its situation. The *right lumbar mesocolon* fixes the ascending colon to the corresponding lumbar region. The *transverse mesocolon* arises from the concave arch of the colon, and forms a septum between the epigastric and umbilical regions. Its inferior portion is continuous with the mesentery. The *left lumbar mesocolon*, which contains the ascending colon, is continuous below with the *Iliac mesocolon*. The last includes between its layers the sigmoid flexure of the colon, and ends in the mesorectum. Under the right kidney, it is narrow and firm, and forms the *right lig'ament of the colon:* at the under end of the left kidney, it forms the *left lig'ament of the colon*.
MESOCRANIUM, Sinciput.

MESOCRANUM, Sinciput.
MESODERMUM, Corpus mucosum.
MESODME, Mediastinum.
MESODMI'TIS, from μεσοδμη, 'the mediastinum,' and *itis*, 'inflammation.' *Mesotœchi'tis, Mediastini'tis, Inflamma'tio mediasti'ni*. Inflammation of the mediastinum.
MESOGASTRIUM, Umbilical region.
MESOGLOSSUS, Genioglossus.
MESOGLOTTUS, Genioglossus.
MESOGONIUM, Internodium.
MESOLO'BAR. Belonging to the *Mésolobe* or *Corpus callo'sum*.
MESOLOBAR ARTERIES, *Arte'riæ mesolob'icæ, A. cor'poris callo'si cer'ebri*, are the arteries of the corpus callosum.
MÉSOLOBE, Corpus callosum.
MESOMER'IA, from μεσος, and μηρος, 'the thigh.' The parts of the body situate between the thighs or hips.
MESOMERION, Perinæum.
MESOMPHALUM, Umbilicus.
MESOPHLEB'IUM, from μεσος, 'in the middle,' and φλεψ, 'a vein;' *Interve'nium*. The space between two veins.
MESOPH'RYON, *Glabell'a, Gabel'la, Intercil'ium, Meto'pium, Nasal eminence*. The part between the eyebrows; from μεσος, 'the middle,' and οφρυα, 'the eyebrows.'
MESOPLEURIUM, Intercostal space.
MESOPLEURIUS, Intercostal.
MESORÆUM, Mesentery.
MESOR'CHIUM, from μεσος, 'the middle,' and ορχις, 'a testicle.' A duplicature of the peritoneum, which supports the testicle in its passage from the abdomen into the scrotum. — Seiler.
MESOREC'TUM. A hybrid word; from μεσος, and *rectum*, 'the intestine rectum.' A triangular reflection, formed by the peritoneum, between the posterior surface of the rectum and the anterior surface of the sacrum. Between the two layers of which the mesorectum is composed are found much areolar tissue, and the termination of the inferior mesenteric vessels.
MESOS, Meso.
MESOSCELOCELE, Hernia, perineal.
MESOSCELON, Perinæum.
MESOSCELOPHY'MA, from *Mesoscelon*, 'perinæum,' and φυμα, 'swelling.' A tumour of the perinæum.
MESOTH'ENAR, from μεσος, and θεναρ, 'the thenar,' 'the palm of the hand.' A muscle, which carries the thumb towards the palm. Winslow applied the term to the adductor pollicis, united to the deep-seated portion of the flexor brevis pollicis.
MESOT'ICA, from μεσος, 'middle.' Diseases affecting the parenchyma. Pravity in the quantity or quality of the intermediate or connecting substance of organs; without inflammation, fever, or other derangement of the general health. The first Order, class *Eccritica* of Good.
MESOTŒCHITIS, Mesodmitis.
MESOTŒCHIUM, Mediastinum.
MESOTŒCHUM, Mediastinum.
MES'PILUS, *Mespilus German'ica seu domes'tica*. The *medlar*, (F.) *Néflier*. The fruit, (F.) *Nèfle*, and seeds of the medlar have both been used medicinally:—the immature fruit as an astringent, and the seeds in nephritic diseases. See Cratægus Aria and Sorbus acuparia.
MESPILUS ARIA, Cratægus aria—m. Domestica, Mespilus, Sorbus domestica—m. Germanica, Mespilus — m. Intermedia, Mespilus oxyacantha — m. Lævigata, Mespilus oxyacantha.
MESPILUS OXYACAN'THA, *M. Oxyacanthoi'des*

seu *interme'dia* seu *læviga'ta*, *Oxyacantha, Spina alba, White Hawthorn,* (F.) *Aubepine.* The flowers of this uncommon European plant are sometimes used in infusion as a pectoral.

MESPILUS OXYACANTHOIDES, Mespilus oxyacantha.

META, μετα, *Meth', μεθ',* 'with,' 'together with,' 'after,' 'change of form and place.' A common prefix to words. Hence:

METAB'ASIS, *Tran'situs, Metab'olē, Metabol'ia, Metal'lagē, Metallax'is,* from μεταβαινω, 'I digress.' A change of remedy, practice, &c.—Hippocrates.

METABOLE, Metabasis, Transformation.

METABOLEL'OGY, *Metabolelog"ia;* from μεταβολη, 'change,' and λογος, 'a description.' A description of the changes which supervene in the course of a disease.

METABOLIA, Metabasis.

METABOL'IC, *Metabol'icus,* from μεταβολη, 'change.' Appertaining to change or transformation.

METABOL'IC FORCE. A term employed by Schwann for the power possessed by living cells of changing the character of the substances brought in contact with them.

METACAR'PAL, *Metacarpia'nus,* (F.) *Métacarpien.* Relating or belonging to the metacarpus.

METACARPAL ARTERY, *Arte'ria dorsa'lis metacar'pi,* arises from the radial, at the moment it engages itself in the upper extremity of the abductor indicis. It descends obliquely upon the back of the hand. Its branches are distributed to the abductor indicis, and the integuments: some communicate with the dorsalis carpi.

METACARPAL ARTICULA'TIONS are those by which the last four metacarpal bones are united together at their upper extremity.

METACARPAL BONES, or bones which compose the metacarpus, are five in number; and distinguished into *first, second, third,* &c., beginning from the outer or radial side. They are articulated by their superior extremity with the bones of the second range of the carpus; and by the lower with the first phalanges.

METACARPAL LIG'AMENT, *Infe'rior palmar Lig'ament,* is a fibrous band, stretched transversely before the inferior extremities of the last four metacarpal bones, which it keeps in their respective positions.

METACARPAL PHALANGES are the first phalanges of the fingers; so called, because they are articulated with the bones of the metacarpus.

METACARPAL RANGE or row of the carpal bones, (F.) *Rangée métacarpienne du carpe,* is the lower row of carpal bones; so called because they are articulated with the bones of the metacarpus. It is composed of the trapezium, trapezoides, magnum, and unciforme.

METACARPEUS, Abductor metacarpi minimi digiti.

MÉTACARPIEN, Metacarpal — *m. du Petit doigt,* Opponens minimi digiti—*m. du Pouce,* Opponens pollicis.

METACARPION, Metacarpus.

METACARPO-PHALANGÆUS POLLICIS, Adductor pollicis manus.

METACAR'PO-PHALAN'GIAN, *Metacarpophalangia'nus, Metacarpo-phal'angal,* (F.) *Métacarpo-phalangien.* That which belongs to the metacarpus and phalanges.

METACARPO-PHALANGIAN or METACARPO-PHALANGAL ARTICULATIONS are formed by the bones of the metacarpus and the corresponding phalanges. In these articulations, the bony surfaces are incrusted with cartilage, covered by a synovial membrane, and kept in connexion by means of an anterior and two lateral ligaments.

MÉTACARPO-PHALANGIEN LATÉRAL SUS-PALMAIRE, ET MÉTACARPO-PHALANGIEN LATÉRAL, Interosseus manus.

METACAR'PUS, from μετα, 'after,' and *carpus,* 'the wrist;' *Metacar'pion, Postbra'chia'lē, Postcar'pium, Torus manûs,* (F.) *Métacarpe.* The part of the hand comprised between the carpus and fingers. It is composed of five parallel bones, called *metacarpal;* forming the back of the hand, externally, and the palm internally.

METACERASMA, Cerasma.
METACHEIRIXIS, Surgery.
METACHIRISIS, Surgery.
METACHIRISMUS, Surgery.
METACHORESIS, Metastasis.
METACINEMA, Metastasis.
METACINESIS, Metastasis.
METACONDYLE, see Phalanx.

METACYE'SIS, from μετα, 'after,' and κυησις, 'pregnancy;' *Gravid'itas extra-uteri'na secunda'ria.* Extra-uterine pregnancy in which the fœtus is at first in the uterus, but subsequently in some other place.

METADERMATO'SIS, from μετα, 'after,' and δερμα, 'skin.' A morbid development of the epidermis or epithelium.

METAL, *Metal'lum.* A class of simple, combustible bodies; distinguished from others by considerable specific gravity; a particular splendour; almost total opacity; insolubility in water; and the property they have of ringing when struck. Metals have no effect, except of a mechanical nature, when taken into the stomach; unless they have already undergone, or undergo in the stomach, oxidation or union with an acid; when several most deleterious compounds may be formed. Copper cents; half-pence; quicksilver; lead, have frequently been swallowed in the metallic state with impunity. Tin and mercury are the only metals prescribed for a mechanical effect; the former as an anthelmintic, — the latter, idly enough, in cases of fancied intussusception.

MÉTAL DES CLOCHES, Bell-metal.
METALLAGE, Metabasis.
METALLAXIS, Metallage.
METALLIC VOICE, *Tintement métallique.*

METALLODYN'IA, from μεταλλον, 'a metal,' and οδυνη, 'pain.' Pain owing to the injurious influence of a metal—as lead, quicksilver, &c.

METALLUM, Metal — m. Hæmatopoieticum, Ferrum.

METAMORPHOP'SIA, *Phantasmascop'ia, Phantasmatoscop'ia,* from μεταμορφοω, (μετα, and μορφη, 'form,') 'I transform,' and ωψ, 'the eye.' *Suffu'sio, Suffu'sio Oculo'rum, Suffu'sio metamorpho'sis, S. Myo'des, Imagination* (Maître-Jean): *Crupsia, Marmar'ygē, Marmor'ygē, Mac'ulæ ante oc'ulos volitan'tes, Marau'gia, Oc'uli marmaryco'des, False sight,* (F.) *Berlue.* Aberration of the sense of sight, which transmits the image of imaginary objects. This affection sometimes depends on a slight opacity in the transparent parts of the eye; the cornea, crystalline, or vitreous humour, when it is symptomatic and of no consequence. At other times, it appears to be idiopathic; and occurs particularly in those who have been in the habit of constantly fixing their eyes on very brilliant or small bodies. The objects fancied to be seen are various. They are sometimes circular, perpetually moving, or shining or black spots, cobwebs, insects, or pieces of wood—when they are often termed *Muscæ volitan'tes,* (F.) *Mouches volantes,* and the condition

Visus musca'rum, Scotom'ata, Suffu'sio Myo'des, Myiodeop'sia, Myodeopsia, Visus musca' rum. These appearances sometimes continue for a few days; being dependent on the state of the nerves of the individual at the time; or they may exist for life, and ultimately impair the sight. Certain of them change their position, and appear to be seated in the humours of the eye, and — it has been supposed — in the vitreous humour more especially: hence the term *entohy'aloid musca* applied to them.

If the affection be symptomatic, it is of but little moment. If idiopathic, and connected with any excitement of the brain, which is not often the case, attention will have to be paid to that organ.

METAMORPHOSIS VENTRICULI GELATINIFORMIS, Gastromalacia.
METANGISMOS, Decantation.
METAPEDIUM, Metatarsus.
METAPHRENON, Dorsum.
METAPHYTEIA, Transplantatio.
METAPODIUM, Metatarsus.
METAPOROPŒ'IA, *Metaporopoie'sis,* from μετα, 'after,' πορος, 'a pore,' and ποιειν, 'to make.' The change produced in the minute pores, in the capillary extremities of vessels,—when they pass from the morbid to the healthy condition.—Galen.

METAPTO'SIS, *Metaschematis'mus, Metaschemat'isis.* Mutation, change; from μεταπιπτω, (μετα, and πιπτω, 'I fall,) 'I digress.' Any change in the form or seat of a disease. Transformation.

METARRHŒ'A, *Metar'rhysis,* from *meta,* 'change of form or place,' and ρεω, 'I flow.' Reflux. The transfer of a disease from without to within, or from one part to another.

METARRHYSIS, Metarrhœa.
METASCHEMATISIS, Metaptosis.
METASCHEMATISMUS, Metaptosis.
METAS'TASIS, *Metachore'sis, Metacine'ma, Metacine'sis,* from μεθιστημι, (μετα, and στασις, place,') 'I change place.' *Displace'ment, Transla'tion.* A change in the seat of a disease; attributed, by the Humorists, to the translation of the morbific matter to a part different from that which it had previously occupied: and by the Solidists, to the displacement of the irritation. It has also been used in the same extensive sense as Metaptosis. Disputes have often been indulged, whether a case of metastasis ought not rather to be esteemed one of extension of the disease. The phenomena of goût and acute rheumatism are in favour of metastasis occasionally supervening.

METASTASIS LACTIS, Galactoplania, Phlegmatia dolens.

METASTAT'IC, *Metastat'icus.* Belonging or relating to metastasis. A *metastatic crisis* is one produced by metastatis;—a *metastatic affection,* one caused by metastasis, &c. See Abscess, metastatic.

METASYN'CRISIS, from συγκρινω, 'I compose,' and μετα, which indicates a change. *Recomposi"tion.* A word employed by some disciples of Asclepiades. This physician supposed, that all animals are formed by the union or assemblage of atoms. He designated all bodies by the word συγκριματα, which signifies 'assemblage.' Συγκρινεσθαι, 'to be assembled,' was, with him, synonymous with '*to exist;*' and διακρινεσθαι, '*to separate,*' was, with him, synonymous with '*to dissolve,*' '*to cease to exist.*' The word *Metasyncrisis* was invented to express the recomposition of bodies after their momentary dissolution. Some have rendered the word by the Latin *Recorpora'tio.*

METASYNCRIT'IC, *Metasyncrit'icus, Recorporati'vus.* Belonging or relating to metasyncrisis. A name formerly given to medicines to which was attributed the virtue of producing the metasyncrisis or regeneration of the body, or some of its parts.

METASYNCRITIC CYCLE meant a determinate series of remedies employed for this purpose.

METATAR'SAL, *Metatar'seus,* (F.) *Métatarsien.* Relating or belonging to the metatarsus.

METATARSAL ARTERY, *Artère sus-métatarsienne* of Chaussier, arises from the *Arteria dorsa'lis Tarsi;* passes transversely over the back of the foot; and furnishes, at its convexity, which is anterior, three branches, called *A. interos'seæ dorsa'les Pedis.* These branches are distributed in the interosseous spaces.

METATARSAL ARTICULA'TIONS are those resulting from the junction of the metatarsal bones with each other. They are strengthened, *behind,* by *dorsal* and *plantar* ligaments; and *before,* by a *transverse metatarsal ligament,* which is plantar, and has the greatest analogy to the *inferior transverse metacarpal ligament.*

METATARSAL BONES, (F.) *Os métatarsiens,* are five in number, and distinguished by their number; *first, second, third,* &c., reckoning from the outer side.

METATARSAL PHALANGES are the first phalanges of the toes; so called because they are united to the metatarsus.

METATARSAL Row—(F.) *Rangée métatarsienne* — of the bones of the tarsus, is the second row, or that contiguous to the metatarsus; comprehending the cuboides and three cuneiform bones: some add the scaphoides.

METATARSEUS, see Abductor minimi digiti pedis.

MÉTATARSIEN, Metatarsal.
METATARSO-PHALAN'GIAN, *Metatarsophalangia'nus, Metatarso-phalangal.* Relating to the metatarsus and phalanges.

METATARSO-PHALANGIAN or METATARSO-PHALANGAL ARTICULATIONS are formed by the bones of the metatarsus and the corresponding phalanges. They bear the greatest analogy to the *metacarpo-phalangian articulations.*

MÉTATARSO-PHALANGIEN-LATÉRAL, see Interossei pedis — *m. Sous-phalangien transversal du premier orteil,* Transversus pedis.

METATAR'SUS, *Metatar'sium, Metape'dium, Metapo'dium, Præcor'dium seu So'lium pedis, Vestig"ium pedis,* from μετα, 'after,' and ταρσος, 'the tarsus.' That part of the foot which is situate between the tarsus and toes, corresponding with the metacarpus. It is composed of five parallel bones; one to each toe. Like the metacarpal bones, they are developed from two points of ossification.

METATH'ESIS, from μετατιθημι, (μετα, and τιθημι, 'to place,') 'I change place.' *Transposit"io.* An operation, by which a morbific agent is removed from one place to another, where it may produce less disturbance in the exercise of the functions:—as, for example, in the operation of depressing cataract, or when calculus in the urethra is pushed back into the bladder. Also, Derivation.

METATIO, Mensuration.
METATOC'IA, from μετα, 'change of form or place,' and τοκος, 'birth.' Parturition in a preternatural manner. Preternatural labour.
METATOPTOSIS, Diadexis.
METENSOMATOSUS, Incorporation.
METEORISMUS, Sublimation, Tympanites.
METEOROL'OGY, *Meteorolog"ia,* from μετεωρος, 'a meteor,' and λογος, 'a discourse.' The

science, whose object is a knowledge of the origin, formation, appearance, &c. of meteors. The state of the atmosphere has a most important bearing upon the health of animals. The whole range of epidemic affections have their causes seated there. Meteorological affections have, hence, ever been attended to by the physician for the purpose of detecting the precise character of any particular epidemic influence. The barometer, thermometer, and hygrometer are the instruments used with this intent — to detect, as well the varying weight or pressure, and the temperature, as the moisture. Perhaps, of the three conditions, the last exerts more influence in the production of disease than either of the others. Our knowledge, however, of this part of physics is extremely limited and unsatisfactory.

METER, μετρον, 'a measure,' a suffix to words denoting 'a measure,' as in *Barometer, Pleximeter,* &c.

METHÆMACHYMIA, Transfusion.

METHÆ'MATA; from μεθ', 'change of form,' and 'αιμα, 'blood.' The capillary or intermediate system of vessels in which the blood undergoes the change from venous to arterial, and conversely.—Marshall Hall. See Capillary vessels.

METHE, Temulentia.

METHEGLIN, Melizomum.

METHEMERINUS, Quotidian.

METHOD, *Meth'odus*, from με', 'with,' and 'οδος, 'way.' This word has different acceptations in the sciences. In medicine, *curative method, meth'odus meden'di*, is the methodical treatment of disease.

METHOD OF COUNTING, Method, numerical.

METHOD, MARIANO'S, see Lithotomy.

METHOD, NUMER'ICAL, *Method of Observation or of Counting*, of Louis, (F.) *Méthode numérique*, consists in observing every case and every symptom of a case numerically, so as to ensure, as far as practicable, accuracy of observation; and to enable us, by the analysis and collation of such facts, to deduce general laws and conclusions. Also, the application of numbers to the study of disease. See Statistics, Medical.

MÉTHODE NUMÉRIQUE, Method, numerical, Statistics, medical—*m. Perturbatrice,* Perturbatrix (Medicina.)

METHODICS, Methodists.

MÉTHODIQUES, Methodists.

METH'ODISTS, *Method'ical sect, Method'ics,* (F.) *Méthodistes, Méthodiques.* A sect of physicians whose doctrine was in vogue after that of the Empirics and Dogmatists, towards the end of the first century. According to the Methodists, of whom Themison was the chief, almost every disease is dependent on contraction or relaxation—*strictum* or *laxum.* To these two causes, they added a third—*mixed* or *compound*—to include those affections which partook of the two characters. The doctrine, *medici'na method'ica*, resembled, in some respects, that of Brown.

METHODOL'OGY (MEDICAL), *Methodolog''ia Med'ica,* from μεθοδος, 'method,' and λογος, 'a discourse.' A word used, by the French more especially, to signify *method* applied to the study of any science. *Medical Methodology*, consequently, means method applied to the study of medicine

METHODUS CATALEPTICA, see Cataleptic — m. Celsiana, see Lithotomy — m. Curatoria, Therapeutics.

METHODUS DERIVATO'RIA. The derivative or revellent system of treatment.

METHODUS ENDERMAT'ICA seu ENDERM'ICA, see Endermic — m. Franconiana, see Lithotomy —

m. Guytoniana, see Lithotomy — m. Medendi, Method of cure, Therapeutics.

METHOMA'NIA, from μεθη, 'drunkenness,' and μανια, 'mania.' An irresistible desire for intoxicating substances. Temulentia.

METHYSMUS, Temulentia.

METHYS'TICUS, from μεθη, 'drunkenness.' That which causes, or pertains to, drunkenness.

METHYSTOPHYL'LUM GLAUCUM. A South African plant, *Nat. Ord.* Amyridaceæ, an infusion of whose leaves is pleasant to the taste, and is used in bronchitis, asthma, and other thoracic diseases. With the Bushmen and others, it is a favourite beverage, and is called by them *Boschjeemansthee,* 'Bushman's tea.' It is, also, chewed.

METODONTI'ASIS, from μετα, 'in the sense of change,' and οδοντιασις, 'dentition.' Faulty development of the teeth.

METOPAGES, Symphyocephalus.

METOPANTRA, Frontal sinuses.

METOPANTRAL'GIA, from μετωπον (μετα, and ωψ, 'the eye') 'the forehead,' αντρον, 'a cavity,' and αλγος, 'pain.' Pain in the frontal sinuses.

METOPANTRI'TIS, *Inflamma'tio si'nuum fronta'lium,* from μετωπον, 'the forehead,' αντρον, 'a cavity,' and *itis*, denoting inflammation. Inflammation of the frontal sinuses.

METOPION, Bubon galbanum.

METOPIUM, Mesophryon.

METOPODYNIA, Neuralgia frontalis.

METOPON, Front, Frontal bone.

METOPOS'COPY, *Metoposcop''ia,* from μετωπον, 'the forehead,' and σκοπειν, 'to view.' The art of knowing the temperament and character of a person by inspecting the traits of his forehead or face. See Physiognomy.

METRA, Uterus.

METRÆMORRHAGIA, Metrorrhagia.

METRAL'GIA, *Metrodyn'ia,* from μητρα, 'the womb,' and αλγος, 'pain.' Pain in the uterus.

METRANASTROPHE, Uterus, inversion of the.

METRATRE'SIA, *Imperfora'tio u'teri,* from μητρα 'the womb,' and ατρησια, 'imperforation.' An unnatural closure of the uterus.

METRATROPH'IA, from μητρα, 'the uterus,' *a*, 'privative,' and τροφη, 'nourishment.' Atrophy or want of development of the uterus.

METRAUX'E, *Hypertroph'ia* seu *Sarco'sis u'teri*, from μητρα, 'the uterus,' and αυξη, 'increase.' Hypertrophy of the uterus.

METRELCO'SIS, *Metrhelco'sis,* from μητρα, 'the womb,' and 'ελκος, 'an ulcer.' Ulceration of the uterus.

METREMPHRAX'IS, from μητρα, 'the uterus,' and εμφρασσω, 'I obstruct.' Obstruction of the womb or of the vessels of the womb— *Infarc'tus u'teri.* A name under which some authors have confounded chronic inflammation of that viscus, and the different degenerations to which it is exposed.

METREMPHYSEMA, Physometra.

METREN'CHYTA, *Metren'chytes,* from μητρα, 'the uterus,' and εγχυω, 'I inject.' Injection of the uterus. Substances injected into the uterus are called *Metren'chyta.*

METREURYS'MA, from μητρα, and ευρυς, 'dilated.' A morbid dilatation of the womb.

METRHELCOSIS, Metrelcosis.

METRHYMENITIS, see Metritis.

METRIOPATHI'A, from μετριος, 'tempered,' and παθος, 'affection.' State of an individual whose passions are temperate.

METRI'TIS, from μητρα, 'the womb.' Febris uteri'na, Hysteri'tis, Empres'ma Hysteri'tis, Inflamma'tio U'teri, Metrophlogo'sis, Inflammation of the Uterus or Womb, (F.) Inflammation de la matrice. The characteristic symptoms of this affection are:—pain, swelling, and tenderness in the hypogastric region; with heat, pain, and tenderness of the os uteri; vomiting, smallness, and frequency of pulse. It occurs most frequently after delivery, when there is generally suppression of the lochial discharge. The treatment must be vigorous, — bleeding early, so as to make a decided impression; followed by a full dose of opium, fomentations, blisters, &c.

Acute inflammation of the womb, seated in its internal membrane, Endo-metri'tis, Metrhymen'itis, has been called Inflamma'tio catarrha'lis u'teri or Acute catarrh, (F.) Catarrhe aigu, of that viscus. It is known by the discharge of a clear, stringy fluid per vaginam; preceded by pains, which, from the hypogastric region, shoot to the thighs, groins, &c., with more or less fever. It requires the antiphlogistic treatment. Chronic metritis sometimes succeeds the acute. To it must be referred the indurations, observed in the uterus, and many of the leucorrheal discharges to which females are subject.

METRITIS RHEUMATICA, Metrorrheuma — m. Septica, Metrocace — m. Venosa, see Phlebitis.

METROBLENNORRHŒA, Leucorrhœa uteri.

METROC'ACE, Metri'tis sep'tica, from μητρα, 'the womb,' and κακος, 'evil.' Putrescency or gangrene of the uterus.

METROCAMPSIS, Hysteroloxia.

METROCARCINO'MA, Hysterocarcino'ma, U'teri carcino'ma, Cancer u'teri, from μητρα, 'the uterus,' and καρκινωμα, 'cancer.' Cancer of the uterus.

METROCELIDES, Nævus.

METROCHOLO'SIS, from μητρα, 'the uterus,' and χολος, 'bile.' Febris puerpera'lis bilio'sa.

METRODYNIA, Metralgia.

METROHÆ'MIA, Hypermetrohémie, from μητρα, 'the uterus,' and 'αιμα, 'blood.' Hyperæmia or congestion of blood in the uterus.

METROHEMORRHAGE, Metrorrhagia.
METROLOXIA, Hysteroloxia.
METROMALACOMA, Hysteromalacia.
METROMALACOSIS, Hysteromalacia.
METROMANIA, Nymphomania.

METROPARAL'YSIS, from μητρα, 'the uterus,' and παραλυσις, 'paralysis.' Paralysis of the uterus.

METROPATHI'A, from μητρα, 'the womb,' and παθος, 'affection.' An affection of the womb.

MÉTRO-PÉRITONITE PUERPÉRALE, see Peritonitis.

METROPERITONI'TIS, from μητρα, 'the uterus,' and 'peritonitis.' Inflamma'tio u'teri et peritonæi. Inflammation of the uterus and peritoneum. Puerperal Fever. See Peritonitis.

METROPHLEBI'TIS, from μητρα, 'the uterus,' φλεψ, 'a vein,' and itis, denoting inflammation. Inflammation of the veins of the uterus.

METROPHLEBITIS PUERPERALIS, see Phlebitis.

METROPHLOGOSIS, Metritis.

METROPHTHI'SIS, Phthi'sis uteri'na, from μητρα, 'the uterus,' and φθιω, 'I consume.' Consumption from ulceration of the uterus — Ul'cera seu Helco'sis u'teri.

METROPOL'YPUS, Hys'tero-pol'ypus, Polypus U'teri, from μητρα, 'the uterus,' and polypus. Polypus of the uterus.

METROPROPTOSIS, Prolapsus uteri.
METROPTOSIS, Prolapsus uteri.

METRORRHAG''IA, Metræmorrhag''ia, Hæmorrhagia uteri'na, H. u'teri, Sanguiflux'us uteri'nus, San'guinis stillicid'ium ab U'tero, Fluor. uteri'ni san'guinis, Proflu'vium San'guinis ex u'tero, Hysterorrhag''ia sanguin'ea, Hysterorrhœ'a, Hæmorrhœ'a uteri'na (of some), Menorrhag''ia (of some), Uterine Hemorrhage, Hemorrhage from the Womb, Metrohemorrhage, Hæmatome'tra, Hæmatoma'tra, (F.) Hémorrhagie de la Matrice, Pertes, Pertes utérines rouges, P. de sang; from μητρα, 'the womb,' and ρηγνυμι, 'I break forth.' An effusion of blood from the inner surface of the uterus, either at the menstrual or other periods; but in a greater quantity than proper. Uterine hemorrhage may be caused by those influences which produce hemorrhage in general. It happens, however, more frequently during pregnancy, and during or after delivery, when the vascular system of the uterus is so circumstanced as to favour its occurrence more than at other periods. The termination of metrorrhagia is usually favourable. Should it, however, be very copious, or frequently recur; or should it happen to a great extent after delivery, death may occur very speedily; and, in some cases, without the discharge being perceptible; constituting internal hemorrhage.

Uterine hemorrhage may be active or passive; requiring obviously a different treatment. The general management is similar to that of hemorrhage in general;—the horizontal posture; acid drinks; free admission of cool air; cold applications to the loins, thighs, and abdomen; injection of cold water, even of iced water, into the vagina; plugging the vagina, so as to prevent the discharge per vaginam, and thus induce a coagulum in the mouths of the bleeding vessel. Such will be the special plan adopted where the hemorrhage has occurred in one not recently delivered. In uterine hemorrhage after delivery, the same cooling plan must be followed; but, as the flow of blood is owing to the uterus not contracting so as to constringe its vessels, pressure must be made on the abdomen to aid this; and, if necessary, the hand must be introduced into the uterus to stimulate it to contraction. Should the female be excessively reduced, so as to render the accoucheur apprehensive that she may expire from loss of blood, brandy may be exhibited. The profuse exhibition of opium in such cases, is, at least, a doubtful plan.

Transfusion has, at times, been practised as a last resource.

METRORRHEU'MA, Rheumatis'mus U'teri, Hysteral'gia rheumat'ica seu catarrha'lis, Metri'tis rheumat'ica, (F.) Rheumatisme de l'utérus; from μητρα, 'the womb,' and ρευμα, 'defluxion,' rheumatism.' Rheumatism of the uterus.

METRORRHEXIS, Uterus, rupture of the.

METRORRHŒ'A, from μητρα, 'the uterus, and ρεω, 'I flow.' A protracted discharge of any fluid from the uterus.

METROSCIR'RHUS, Hysteroscir'rhus, Scirrhus seu Carcino'ma u'teri, from μητρα, 'the womb,' and σκιρρος, 'scirrhus.' Scirrhus of the uterus.

MET'ROSCOPE, Metroscop'ium, from μητρα, 'the uterus,' and σκοπεω, 'to view.' An instrument, invented by M. Nauche, for listening to the sounds of the heart of the fœtus in uterogestation, when the sounds and movements are imperceptible through the parietes of the abdomen. The extremity of the instrument — the first notion of which was given to M. Nauche by the stethoscope of Laënnec — is introduced into the vagina and applied against the neck of the uterus.

METROSIDEROS GUMMIFERA, see Kino.

METROSTERE'SIS, from μητρα, 'the uterus,' and στερησις, 'privation.' Extirpation of the uterus. Want of uterus.

METROTOMIA, Cæsarean section.

MEU, Æthusa meum.

MEULIÈRE, Molar.

MEUM, Æthusa meum — m. Anethifolium, Æthusa meum — m. Athamanticum, Æthusa meum.

MEURTRISSURE, Contusion.

MEVIUM, Syphilis.

MEZEA, Genital organs.

MEZEREON, Daphne mezereum.

MIAMMA, Miasma.

MIANSIS, Miasma.

MIARIA, Miasma.

MIAS'MA, *Miasm, μιασμα*, 'a stain,' from μιαινω, 'I contaminate.' *Miam'ma, Mian'sis, Mia'ria, Mias'mus, Inquinamen'tum, Molyn'sis, Conta'gium*. The word *miasm* has, by some, been employed synonymously with contagion. It is now used more definitely for any emanation, either from the bodies of the sick, or from animal and vegetable substances, or from the earth, especially in marshy districts, (*Marsh poison, Efflu'vium palus'tre, Gas palus'tre*, (F.) *Intoxication des Marais,*) which may exert a morbid influence on those who are exposed to its action. To these terrestrial emanations — the *Koino-mias'mata* of Dr. E. Miller, of New York — the Italians give the name *aria cattiva*, but, more commonly, *mala'ria;* a word which has been adopted into other languages. The deleterious effluvia, originating from the decomposition of matter derived from the human body, have been called by Dr. Miller, *Idiomias'mata;* the epithets *Koino* and *Idio* being derived respectively from κοινος, 'common,' and ιδιος, 'personal.' Of the miasms which arise either from the animal body or from the most unhealthy situations, we know, chemically, nothing. All that we do know is, that, under such circumstances, emanations take place, capable of causing disease in many of those who are exposed to their action.

MIASMAT'IC, *Miasmat'icus*. Belonging or relating to miasmata. Sauvages, in his classification of diseases according to their etiology, has a class under the name *Morbi miasmat'ici*. A fever that arises from marsy miasms, is styled *mala'rious, palu'dal, Helop'yra, Helopyr'etus*, &c.

MIASMUS, Miasma.

MICÆ PANIS, see Triticum.

MICATIO CORDIS, Systole.

MICHE'LIA CHAM'PACA, *Champaca, Michelia Tsjampaca*. An Oriental tree, much prized for the odour and beauty of its flowers. The oily infusion of the flowers is employed in the Moluccas in headach.

MICLE'TA: A medicine used by Mesue for arresting hemorrhage; perhaps, according to Siebenhaar, from the Arabic, *michnata*, "proved by experience."

MICOSIS, Frambœsia.

MICRENCEPHALIUM, Cerebellum.

MICRENCEPHALON, Cretinism.

MICRENCEPHALUM, Cerebellum.

MICROCEPH'ALUS, *Microcra'nius*, from μικρος, 'small,' and κεφαλη, 'head.' One who has a small head. A monster having a small imperfect head, or a small imperfect cranium.

MICROCORIA, Myosis.

MI'CROCOSM, *Microcos'mus*, from μικρος, 'little,' and κοσμος, 'world.' A little world. Some philosophers have given this appellation to man, whom they consider as the epitome of all that is admirable in the world. The world they call *Macrocosm*.

MICROCOSMETOR, Vital principle.

MICROCOSM'ICA MACHI'NA. The organism of man.

MICROCOSMICA SCIENTIA, Physiology.

MICROCOSMICUM SAL, with the ancients meant the salts of the urine, — *Sal uri'næ*.

MICROCOSMOGRAPHIA, Physiology.

MICROCOUST'IC, *Microcus'ticus*, from μικρος, 'small,' and ακουω, 'I hear.' This word, as well as *Microphonous*, from μικρος, 'small,' and φωνη, 'voice,' means any thing that contributes to increase the intensity of sound — as the speaking trumpet — by collecting the sonorous rays.

MICROCRANIUS, Microcephalus.

MICROGLOS'SIA, from μικρος, 'small,' and γλωσσα, 'tongue.' Original smallness of tongue.

MICROLEUCONYMPHÆA, Nymphæa alba.

MICROM'ELUS, *Hemim'eles*, from μικρος, 'small,' and μελος, 'a limb.' A monster having imperfectly developed extremities.

MICROMMATUS, Microphthalmus.

MICROPHONOUS, Microcoustic.

MICROPHTHAL'MUS, *Microm'matus*, from μικρος, 'little,' and οφθαλμος, 'eye.' One who has small eyes. A monster with too small, or imperfectly developed eyes. A small eye, — *Ophthalmid'ium, Ophthal'mium*.

MICROPODIA, Micropus.

MICROPROSO'PUS, *Aproso'pus*, from μικρος, 'small,' and προσωπον, 'face.' A monster in which a part of the face is absent.

MI'CROPUS, from μικρος, 'small,' and πους, 'foot.' One who has small feet. The condition is called *Micropo'dia*.

MICROR'CHIDES; from μικρος, 'small,' and ορχις, 'a testicle.' They who have very small testicles.

MI'CROSCOPY, *Microscop'ium;* from μικρος, 'small,' and σκοπη, 'a view.' Observation by the microscope; an important agency in the examination of the healthy and morbid tissues.

MICROSPHYC'TUS, same etymon as the next. One who has a small pulse.

MICROSPHYX'IA, from μικρος, and σφυγμος 'pulse.' Smallness or weakness of pulse.

MICROS'TOMUS; from μικρος, 'small,' and στομα, 'mouth.' One who has a small mouth.

MICROTE'SIA, *Par'tium organica'rum par'vitas morbo'sa;* from μικροτης, 'smallness.' Morbid smallness of organic parts.

MICROTRAPEZIA, Leptotrophia.

MICROTRICH'IA; from μικρος, 'small,' and θριξ, 'hair.' Fineness or shortness of hair.

MICROTROPHIA, Leptotrophia.

MICTIO, Micturition — m. Cruenta, Hæmaturia — m. Inopportuna, Enuresis — m. Involuntaria, Enuresis — m. Sanguinea, Hæmaturia.

MICTION, Micturition.

MICTURIT''ION, *Mic'tio, Mictus, Ure'sis, Uri'asis, Omiche'sis*, (F.) *Miction*, from *micturio*, 'I make water.' The act of making water. Also, morbid frequency of passing the water.

MICTUS, Micturition — m. Cruentus, Hæmaturia.

MIDRIFF, Diaphragm.

MIDWIFE, from mið, 'with,' and ƿif, 'wife,' or, from mið, 'meed,' 'recompense,' and ƿif, 'wife.' *Matro'na, Obstet'rix, Hypere'tria, Mæa, Mæas, Mæu'tria, Aces'toris, Aces'tria. Aces'tris,* (F.) *Sage femme, Accoucheuse*. A female who practises obstetrics.

MIDWIFERY, Obstetrics.

MIEL, Mel—*m. d'Acétate de Cuivre*, Linimentum æruginis — *m. Mercuriale composé*, Mellitum de mercuriali compositum.
MIEUTER, Accoucheur.
MIGMA, Mistura.
MIGRAINE, Hemicrania.
MIGRANA, Hemicrania.
MIKANIA GUACO, Guaco.
MILFOIL, Achillea millefolium.
MILIAIRE, Miliary fever.
MILIARIA, Miliary fever — m. Sudans, Miliary fever — m. Sudatoria, Miliary fever.
MILIARIS SUDATORIA, Sudor anglicus, S. picardicus.
MIL'IARY (FEVER,) *Emphly'sis milia'ria, Miliaria, M. sudans, Milia'ris, M. sudato'ria, Sudor, S. milia'ris, Pap'ula milia'ris, Febris miliaris, Exanthe'ma miliaria, Syn'ochus miliaria, Aspre'do milia'cea, Febris essero'sa, F. puncticula'ris, F. culicula'ris, F. vesicula'ris, F. lenticula'ris, Pur'pura puerpera'rum, P. milia'ris, Febris purpura'tē rubra et alba milia'ris, Pap'ula sudo'ris, Millet-seed rash*, (F.) *Miliaire, Millot, Pourpre blanc, Millet*. It is so called from the eruption resembling the seed of the *milium* or *millet*. Fever, accompanied by an eruption of small, red, isolated pimples, rarely confluent, but almost always very numerous, slightly raised above the skin, and presenting, at the end of 24 hours, a small vesicle filled with a white transparent fluid; which quickly dries up, and separates in the form of scales. Miliary fever is now rare, in consequence of the cooling practice in fevers and other states of the system. It is almost always brought on by external heat, and hence the prevention is obvious. The treatment is simple. It requires merely the antiphlogistic regimen, in ordinary cases.
MILIARY GRANULATIONS OR TUBERCLES, see Granulation.
MILII SEMINA, Panicum Italicum.
MILIOLUM. Diminutive of *milium*, 'millet.' *Cenchrid'ion*. A small tumour on the eyelids, resembling, in size, a millet-seed.
MILITARIS HERBA, Achillea millefolium.
MILIUM, Grutum, Panicum miliaceum, see Hydatid—m. Esculentum, Panicum miliaceum— m. Indicum, Panicum Italicum—m. Panicum, Panicum miliaceum — m. Solis, Lithospermum officinale.
MILK, Sax. melc, *Lac, Gala, Humor lac'teus, Latex ni'veus*, (F.) *Lait*. A fluid secreted by the mammary glands of the mammalia. The skimmed *milk of the cow*, (F.) *Lait de Vache*, contains water, caseous matter, traces of butter, sugar of milk, chloride of sodium, phosphate, and acetate of potass, lactic acid, lactate of iron, and earthy phosphate. The *cream* is formed of butter, casein, and whey, in which there is sugar of milk and salts. When examined by the microscope, milk is seen to contain a large number of particles, of irregular size and shape, varying from $\frac{1}{12500}$th to $\frac{1}{8045}$th of an inch in diameter. They consist of oily matter, surrounded by a delicate pellicle, and are the *milk globules*.
Cow's milk is employed for the preparation of cream, butter, cheese, whey, sugar of milk, and frangipane. It is useful in a number of cases of poisoning; either by acting as a demulcent, or by decomposing certain poisons, or by combining with others so as to neutralize them. It is constantly employed as aliment, and may be regarded as an emulsion in which butter and casein are found in suspension. When taken into the stomach, it is coagulated by the gastric fluids, and the coagulum is digested like any other solid. The watery parts are absorbed.

Between milk, flour, and blood, there is great similarity of composition. The following table is given by Dr. Robert Dundas Thomson:

Milk.	Flour.	Blood.
Curd or Casein, { Fibrin, Albumen, Casein, Gluten.	Fibrin, Albumen, Casein, Colouring matter.
Butter............	Oil.	Fat.
Sugar	{ Sugar, Starch,	} Sugar.
Chloride of potassium, ——— sodium, Phosphate of soda, ——— lime, ——— magnesia, ——— iron,	Do.	Do.

From a considerable number of experiments, Messrs. Deyeux and Parmentier class the six kinds of milk, which they examined, according to the following table, as regards the relative quantity of materials they contain.

Casein.	Butter.	Sugar of Milk.	Serum.
Goat Sheep Cow	Sheep Cow Goat	Woman Ass Mare	Ass Woman Mare
Ass Woman Mare	Woman Ass Mare	Cow Goat Sheep	Cow Goat Sheep

MILK ABSCESS, Mastodynia apostematosa— m. Almond, Emulsio amygdalæ.
MILK AND SODA WATER. An agreeable mode of taking milk in cases where it lies heavily on the stomach. Heat, nearly to boiling, a teacupful of *milk;* dissolve in it a teaspoonful of *sugar*, put it into a large tumbler, and pour over it two-thirds of a bottle of *soda water*.
MILK, ASSES', (F.) *Lait d'Anesse*, considerably resembles human milk, of which it has the consistence, smell, and taste: but it contains a little less cream, and more soft, caseous matter. It is often used by those labouring under pulmonary affections.
Artificial Asses' Milk may be made by taking *gelatin* ℨss; dissolving it, by the aid of heat, in *barley water* Oij; adding *refined sugar* ℨj; pouring into the mixture new *milk* Oj; and beating the whole with a whisk.
It may also be prepared by dissolving *sugar of milk* ℨij in tepid skimmed *cow's milk* Oj.
MILK, EWES', (F.) *Lait de Brebis*. It affords more cream than cows' milk; but the butter is softer. The caseum, on the contrary, is fatter, and more viscid. It contains less serum than cow's milk. The Roquefort cheeses are made from it.
MILK FEVER, see Fever, milk — m. Glass, Breast glass — m. Globules, see Milk.
MILK, GOATS', (F.) *Lait de Chèvre*, resembles cows' milk: the butyraceous matter, however, which enters into its composition, is more solid than that of the cow.
Artificial Goats' Milk may be made by taking fresh *suet* ℨj; cutting it into small pieces; tying it in a muslin bag, large enough to leave the morsels free from compression; and boiling in a quart of *cows' milk*, sweetened with a quarter of an ounce of *white sugar candy*.
Used as a diet in scrofulous cases, and also in phthisis.

MILK, HUMAN, (F.) *Lait de femme*,—contains more sugar, milk, and cream, and less caseum, than cows' milk. Its composition differs according to the distance of time from delivery.

MILK KNOT, *Galacto-gan'glion;* (F.) *Ganglion laiteux.* The knots often observed in the breast after inflammation of the organ, or for some time after the suppression of the secretion. They generally end by resolution.

MILK LEG, Phlegmatia dolens — m. Males', Sperm.

MILK, MARES', (F.) *Lait de Jument*,—contains only a small quantity of fluid butyraceous matter; a little caseum, softer than that of cows' milk, and more serum.

MILK SCALL, Porrigo larvalis.

MILK SICKNESS, *Sick stomach, Swamp sickness, Tires, Slows, Stiff joints, Puking fever, River sickness*. A disease occasionally observed in the states of Alabama, Indiana, and Kentucky, which affects both man and cattle, but chiefly the latter. It is attributed in cattle to something eaten or drunk by them; and in man to the eating of the flesh of animals labouring under the disease. Owing to the tremors that characterize it in animals, it is called the *Trembles*. It is endemic. The symptoms of the disease are such as are produced by the acro-narcotic class of poisons — vomiting, purging, extreme nervous agitation, &c.: and the approved indications of treatment appear to be—gentle emetics and laxatives, with quiet, and mucilaginous drinks.

MILK, SNAKES', Euphorbia corollata—m. Spots, Strophulus—m. Stone, Morochthus—m. Sugar of, Sugar of milk—m. of Sulphur, Sulphur præcipitatum—m. Sweet, Galium verum—m. Teeth, see Dentition—m. Thrush, Aphthæ—m. Vetch, Astragalus verus—m. Vetch, stemless, Astragalus exscapus—m. Weed, Apocynum androsæmifolium, Asclepias Syriaca, Euphorbia corollata—m. Weed, long-leaved, green, Acerates longifolia—m. Weed, smooth, Asclepias Sullivantii—m. Wort, bitter, Polygala amara—m. Wort, common, Polygala—m. Wort, dwarf, Polygala paucifolia—m. Wort, rattlesnake, Polygala.

MILKY, Lactic.

MILL MOUNTAIN, Linum catharticum.

MILLEFEUILLE, Achillea millefolium.

MILLEFOLIUM, Achillea millefolium.

MILLEMORBIA SCROPHULARIA, Scrophularia nodosa.

MILLEPEDES, Onisci aselli.

MILLEPERTUIS ORDINAIRE, Hypericum perforatum.

MILLET, Aphthæ, Miliary fever—m. Barbadoes, Panicum Italicum—m. Common, Panicum miliaceum—m. Indian, Panicum Italicum—m. *des Oiseaux*, Panicum Italicum—m. *Ordinaire*, Panicum miliaceum.

MILLET-SEED RASH, Miliary fever.

MILLIGRAMME, from *mille*, 'a thousand,' and γραμμα, 'a gramme.' The thousandth part of a gramme;—about 0.0154 Troy grain.

MILLIGRANA, Herniaria glabra.

MILLIMÈTRE, Millim'eter, from *mille*, 'a thousand,' and μετρον, 'measure.' The thousandth part of the metre;—equal to 0.03937 English inch, or about two-fifths of a line.

MILLOT, Miliary fever.

MILPHÆ, Madarosis.

MILPHOSIS, Madarosis.

MILT-LIKE TUMOUR, Encephaloid.

MILTUS, Plumbi oxydum rubrum.

MILTWASTE, Asplenium

MIMOSA CATECHU, Catechu—m. Cochliacarpa, see Cortex adstringens Brasiliensis—m. Leucophlea, see Spirit (Arrack)—m. Nilotica, see Acaciæ gummi—m. Scandens, Cashang-parang—m. Senegal, see Senegal, gum—m. Virginalis, see Cortex adstringens Brasiliensis.

MIND, ABSENCE OF, Aphelxia socors—m. Abstraction of, Aphelxia intenta—m. Unsound, Insanity.

MINERALIUM, Antimonium.

MINER'S ELBOW. An enlargement of a bursa over the olecranon, occurring in such as are in the habit of leaning much upon it; and, therefore, often seen in those who work on the side in low-roofed mines.

MINIM'ETER; badly compounded from *minimum* and μετρον, 'measure.' An instrument for measuring minims, invented by Mr. Alsop. It consists of a glass tube, graduated from the conical point into minims; and having a piston, by the elevation of which, fluid may be drawn into the tube, and by its depression be forced from it.

MIN'IMUM, a *minim*, 'the least part or portion.' The 60th part of a fluidrachm. This measure has been introduced by the London College of Physicians, in consequence of the uncertainty of the size of the drop, (see Gutta.) The subdivision of the wine pint has, accordingly, been extended to the 60th part of the fluidrachm: and glass measures, called "minim-measures," have been adopted by the London College. The proportion between the minims and the drops of various fluid preparations is exhibited in the following table. The results were obtained by Mr. Durand, a skilful *pharmacien* of Philadelphia, under circumstances, as regards the different articles, as nearly identical as possible.

TABLE OF THE NUMBER OF DROPS OF DIFFERENT LIQUIDS EQUIVALENT TO A FLUIDRACHM.

Acid Acetic, crystallizable	120
Acid Hydrocyanic (medicinal)	45
——— Muriatic	54
——— Nitric	84
——— ——— diluted (1 to 7)	51
——— Sulphuric	90
——— ——— aromatic	120
——— ——— diluted (1 to 7)	51
Alcohol (rectified Spirit)	135
Alcohol, diluted (proof Spirit)	120
Arsenite of Potassa, solution of	57
Ether, Sulphuric	150
Oils of Aniseed, Cinnamon, Cloves, Peppermint, Sweet Almonds, Olives	120
Tinctures of Asafœtida, Foxglove, Guaiac, Opium	120
Tincture of Chloride of Iron	132
Vinegar, distilled	78
——— of Colchicum	78
——— of Opium (black drop)	75
——— of Squill	75
Water, distilled	45
Water of Ammonia (strong)	54
Do do. (weak)	45
Wine (Teneriffe)	78
——— Antimonial	72
——— of Colchicum	75
——— of Opium	78

MINISTER GYMNASTÆ, Pædotribes.

MINITHOSIS, Meiosis.

MINIUM, Plumbi oxydum rubrum—m. Græcorum, Hydrargyri sulphuretum rubrum—m. Purum, Hydrargyri sulphuretum rubrum.

MINOR HEL'ICIS. A muscle situate on the posterior border of the helix of the ear, at its commencement in the fossa of the concha.

MINORATIVUS, Laxative.

MINT, COCK, Tanacetum balsamita—m. Curled, Mentha crispa—m. Cat, Nepeta—m. Horse, Monarda coccinea and M. punctata—m.

Horse, hairy, Blephilia hirsuta—m. Horse, Ohio, Blephilia hirsuta—m. Horse, sweet, Cunila Mariana—m. Hyssop-leaved, Mentha cervina.

MINT JULEP. A drink, consisting of brandy, sugar, and pounded ice, flavoured by sprigs of mint. It is an agreeable alcoholic excitant.

MINT, MOUNTAIN, Monarda coccinea—m. Mountain, common, Pyonanthemum incanum—m. Pepper, Mentha piperita — m. Spear, Mentha viridis —m. Squaw, Hedeoma — m. Stone, Cunila Mariana—m. Water, Mentha aquatica.

MINUTHESIS, Meiosis.
MINYANTHES, Menyanthes.
MIOSIS, Meiosis.
MIROCELE, Merocele.
MISADIR, Ammoniæ murias.
MISANTHRO'PIA, *Misan'thropy, Exanthro'-pia, Phyganthro'pia*, from μισος, 'hatred,' and ανθρωπος, 'man.' Aversion to man and society;— a symptom of melancholy, and hypochondriasis.
MISCARRIAGE, Abortion.
MISERERE MEI, Ileus.
MISHME TEETA, Coptis teeta.
MISMAR, *Mesemar.* A name given by Avicenna to a kind of nodus, which forms on the toes as the sequel of contusion or inflammation of those parts.
MISOPTO'CHUS, from μισος, 'hatred,' and πτωχος, 'poor.' That which has hatred for the poor. The gout has been so called by some, because it commonly affects the rich.
MISSADAN, Hydrargyrum.
MISSIO SANGUINIS, Bloodletting.
MISTIO, Mistura.
MISTLETOE, Viscum album—m. Yellowish, Viscum flavescens.
MISTU'RA, *Migma, Mis'tio, Mix'tio, Mixtu'ra,* a *mixture;* from *miscere, mixtum,* 'to mix.' A mingled compound, in which different ingredients are contained in the fluid state; suspended or not by means of mucilaginous or saccharine matter. In this sense, it is synonymous with the French *Potion.* In France, however, the word *mixture* is more frequently understood to mean a liquid medicine, which contains very active substances, and can only be administered by drops. A mixture, in other words, in the French sense, may be regarded as a *potion* deprived of watery vehicle.

MISTURA, (S.) A fragrant yellow-coloured water, used as a perfume by the ladies of Peru. It is prepared from gillyflower, jasmine, and *flor de mistela* (Talinum umbellatum). See Campomanesia lineatifolia.

MISTURA AC'IDI HYDROCYAN'ICI, *Mixture of Prussic acid, Mélange pectoral* (Magendie). (*Medicinal prussic acid*, ʒj, *distilled water,* ℥xiv, *pure sugar,* ℥iss.) A dessert-spoonful every morning and evening, as a pectoral, &c.

MISTURA AMMONI'ACI, *Lac ammoniaci, Mixture of ammoniac.* (*Ammoniac.* ʒij, *aquæ* Oss. Rub the ammoniacum: adding the water gradually until they are perfectly mixed.) Dose, fʒss to ℥j.

MISTURA AMYGDALÆ, Emulsio amygdalæ.

MISTURA ASAFŒ'TIDÆ, *Lac asafœtidæ, Emulsio antihyster'ica, Mixture of asafœtida,* (F.) *Lait d'asafœtida.* (*Asafœtidæ* ʒij, *aquæ* Oss. Rub together, adding the water by degrees.) Used where pills cannot be swallowed, and as a glyster in irritations during dentition, and in ascarides. Dose, fʒss to fʒiss.

MISTURA ASAFŒTIDÆ PRO CLYSMATE, Enema fœtidum.

MISTURA CAM'PHORÆ, *Aqua camphoræ* (Ph. U. S.), *Camphor mixture, Camphor julep, Mistura camphora'ta, Jula'pium e camphorâ seu camphoratum,* (F.) *Julep camphré.* (*Camphor,* ʒij, *alcohol,* ♏xl, *magnes. carb.* ℥iv, *aquæ* Oij. Rub the camphor with the alcohol, and afterwards with the magnesia, add the water, and filter.) Virtues like those of camphor. See Emulsio camphoræ.

MISTURA CORNU USTI, *Decoc'tum cornu cervi'ni, Decoc'tum album, Decoction of burnt hartshorn, Mixture of burnt hartshorn.* (*Cornuum ust.* ℥ij, *acaciæ gum. cont.* ʒj, *aquæ* Oiij. Boil to Oij, constantly stirring, and strain. Ph. L.)

MISTURA CRETÆ, *Potio carbona'tis calcis, Mistura creta'cea, Mucila'go cretica, Chalk mixture, Creta'ceous mixture,* (F.) *Mixture de Craie.* (*Oretæ* pp. ℥ss, *sacchar., acaciæ gum.* in pulv., āā ʒij, *aquæ cinnam., aquæ,* āā f℥iv. Mix. Ph. U. S.) Antacid and absorbent. Dose, fʒj to ℥ij.

MISTURA DIABOL'ICA. A mixture under this name is kept in military hospitals for malingerers. It is made of sundry nauseous ingredients, as aloes, asafœtida, castor, &c., and is given so as to keep up a disagreeable impression on the gustatory nerves.

MISTURA EMETI'NÆ VOMITO'RIA, *Emetic mixture of emetine.* (*Emetine* 4 gr., *orange flower water* ℥ij, *syrup* ℥ss; M.) A dessert-spoonful every half hour till it acts.

MISTURA FERRI COMPOS'ITA, *Compound mixture of iron,* (F.) *Mixture de fer composée, Griffith's mixture.* (*Myrrh* cont. ʒj, *potassæ* carb. gr. xxv, *aquæ rosæ* f℥viiss, *ferri sulph.* in pulv. ♅j, *sp. lavand.* ℥ss, *sacchar.* ʒj. Rub together the myrrh, subcarbonate of potassa, and sugar; then add, while triturating, the rose-water, spirit of nutmeg; and, lastly, the sulphate of iron. Pour the mixture directly into a glass bottle, and stop it close. Ph. U. S.) It is tonic and emmenagogue, and is useful wherever iron is indicated.

MISTURA GLYCYRRHI'ZÆ COMPOS'ITA, *Compound mixture of Liq'uorice, Brown Mixture.* (*Extract. Glycyrrhiz.* pulv., *Acaciæ* pulv., *Sacchar.,* āā ℥ss; *Tinct. opii camphorat.* f℥ij; *Vin. antimon.* f℥j; *Spirit. æther. nitric.* f℥ss; *Aquæ* f℥xij. Rub the liquorice, gum arabic, and sugar with the water, gradually poured upon them; add the other ingredients and mix. Ph. U. S.) A popular cough medicine, but not deserving of being made officinal. Dose, a tablespoonful or f℥ss.

MISTURA GUAI'ACI, *Mixture of guai'ac, Lac guaiaci, Emul'sio guaiaci'na, Mistura guaiaci gummo'sa, M. gummi gua'iaci Bergeri, Solu'tio guaiaci gummo'sa, S. resi'næ guaiaci aquo'sa,* (F.) *Mixture de Guyac.* (*Guaiac. g. resin.* ℥iss, *sacch. pur.* ʒij, *muc. acaciæ gum.* ʒij, *aq. cinnam.* f℥viij. Rub the guaiacum with the sugar; then with the mucilage. Add, gradually, the cinnamon water. Ph. L.) Dose, f℥ss to f℥ij.

MISTURA GUMMI GUAIACI BERGERI, Mistura Guaiaci—m. Leniens, Looch ex ovo.

MISTURA MOSCHI, *Musk mixture, Mistura moscha'ta.* (*Moschi, acaciæ gum.* contus., *sacch. purif.,* sing. ʒj, *aq. rosæ* f℥vj. Rub the musk with the sugar; add the gum, and, by degrees, the rose-water. Ph. L.) Dose, f℥ss to f℥ij.

MISTURA STRYCH'NIÆ, *Mixture of strych'nia.* (*Distilled water,* ℥ij, *very pure strychnia,* 1 gr., *white sugar,* ʒij; M.) Dose, a dessert-spoonful.

MISTURA SULPHURICO-ACIDA, Elixir acidum Halleri — m. Vulneraria acida — *Arquebusade, Eau d'.*

MITCHEL'LA REPENS, *Partridge berry.* A pretty little indigenous trailing evergreen, of the Cinchona *family*—Cinchoneæ,—which flowers from June to July. It has been considered an expectorant, emmenagogue, and diuretic; and has been prescribed in dropsy and gout.

MITELLA, Sling.

MITH'RIDATE, *Mithridati'um, Mithridat'icum medicamen'tum, Antid'otum Mithrida'tium, Diascin'ci antid'otus, Confec'tio Damoc'ratis.* A very compound electuary, into which entered — *Myrrh* of Arabia, *Saffron, Agaric, Ginger, Cinnamon, Frankincense, Garlic, Mustard, Birthwort, Galbanum, Castor, Long pepper, Opoponax, Bdellium, Gum Arabic, Opium, Gentian, Orris, Sagapenum, Valerian, Acacia, Hypericum, Canary wine, Honey,* &c. It was invented by Mithridates, king of Pontus and Bithynia, and was formerly regarded as alexipharmic. It is little used at the present day, and, from its heterogeneous nature, should be wholly abandoned.

MITHRIDATICUM MEDICAMENTUM, Mithridate.

MITIGANS, Lenitive.

MITRA HIPPOCRATICA, *Bonnet d'Hippocrate.*

MITRAL, *Mitra'lis.* Having the form of a mitre; resembling a bishop's mitre.

MITRAL VALVES, *Val'vulæ mitra'les, V. Cordis mitra'les, V. episcopa'les, V. bicuspida'les.* Two triangular valves at the opening of communication between the left auricle of the heart and the corresponding ventricle. These valves are formed by the inner membrane of the left cavities of the heart; and are retained on the side of the ventricle by tendinous cords, proceeding from the columnæ carneæ. They form a species of valve, which permit the blood to pass from the auricle into the ventricle and oppose its return.

MITRIUM, Sling.

MITTE (F.), *Efflu'vium Latrina'rium.* An emanation exhaled from privies, which strongly irritates the eyes. It consists of ammonia, united to the carbonic and hydro-sulphuric acids.

MIUAMARU, see Arrow poison.

MIXIS, Coition.

MIXTIO, Mistura.

MIXTURA, Mistura.

MIXTURE, Mistura — m. of Ammoniac, Mistura ammoniaci — m. of Asafœtida, Mistura asafœtidæ — m. Brown, Mistura glycyrrhizæ composita — m. *Calmante,* Looch ex ovo — m. Camphor, Mistura camphoræ — m. Chalk, Mistura cretæ — m. *de Craie,* Mistura cretæ — m. Cretaceous, Mistura cretæ — m. of Emetine, emetic, Mistura emetinæ vomitoria — m. *de Fer composée,* Mistura ferri composita — m. *de Goyac,* Mistura Guaiaci — m. Griffith's, Mistura ferri composita — m. of Guaiac, Mistura Guaiaci — m. of Hartshorn, burnt, Mistura cornu usti — m. of Iron, compound, Mistura ferri composita.

MIXTURE, HOPE'S. A mixture recommended by Mr. Hope, in diarrhœa and dysentery. It is essentially a nitrate of morphia. Although the proposer employed the acidum nitrosum of the Edinburgh Pharmacopœia, nitric acid is generally used. (*Acid. nitros.* f℥j; *Aquæ camphor.* f℥viij; *Tinct. opii* gtt. xl.; M.) Dose, a fourth part every three or four hours.

MIXTURE OF LIQUORICE, COMPOUND, Mistura glycyrrhizæ composita.

MIXTURE, MUSK, Mistura moschi — m. Neutral, Liquor potassæ citratis — m. of Prussic acid, Mistura acidi hydrocyanici.

MIXTURE, SCUDAMORE'S. A mixture recommended by Sir C. Scudamore in gouty and rheumatic affections, and much prescribed in the United States. *Magnes. sulph.* ℥j — ℥ij; *Aquæ menthæ* f℥x; *Aceti colchic.* f℥j — f℥iss; *Syrup croci* f℥j; *Magnes.* ℥viij. M. Dose, one, two, or three tablespoonfuls, repeated every two hours in a paroxysm of gout, until from four to six evacuations are produced in the twenty four hours.

MIXTURE OF STRYCHNIA, Mistura strychniæ.

MNEMÈ, Memory.

MNEME CEPHAL'ICUM BAL'SAMUM. A very compound medicine, into which entered *Balm,* *Lily, Rosemary, Lavender, Borage, Broom, Roses, Violet, Saffron, Thyme, Storax, Galbanum,* &c.

MNEMONEUTICE, Mnemonics.

MNEMON'ICS, *Mnemon'icē, Mnemoneu'ticē,* from μναομαι, 'I recollect.' The art of aiding the memory by signs; and of forming, in some sort, an artificial memory.

MOANING, from Sax. mænan, 'to grieve.' *Respira'tio luctuo'sa, Mychthis'mos.* A plaintive respiration, in which the patient utters audible groans — *moans,* (F.) *Gémissemens.*

MOBILE, see Saint Augustine.

MOBIL'ITY, *Mobil'itas,* from *mob'ilis,* contraction of *movibilis,* 'that can be moved.' The power of being moved. In *physiology,* great nervous susceptibility, often joined to a disposition to convulsion. Greatly developed excitability.

MOCCASIN FLOWER, Cypripedium acaule, C. luteum.

MOCH'LIA. Reduction of a luxated bone; from μοχλος, a lever.

MOCHLICUS, Purgative.

MOCHLISCUS, Lever.

MOCHLUS, Lever.

MOCHTHUS, Agony.

MOCK-KNEES, Crusta genu equinæ.

MODELLING PROCESS. A term proposed by Dr. Macartney, of Dublin, to signify the mode in which wounds are healed without inflammation or suppuration, by a deposite of plastic matter from the surface of the wound, by which the gap is more rapidly filled, — portion being laid upon portion, without waste, after the manner of clay in the hands of the sculptor: — hence the term.

MODI'OLUS, 'the nave of a wheel.' *Pyr'amis* seu *Axis coch'leæ.* A hollow cone in the cochlea of the ear, forming a nucleus, axis, or central pillar, round which the gyri of the cochlea pass. The modiolus forms the inner and larger portion of the central pillar, and is the cavity seen at the bottom of the meatus auditorius internus. It lodges a branch of the auditory nerve. The central portion of the modiolus contains a number of minute canals, and is called in consequence *Tractus spira'lis foraminulo'sus.* Into these the nerves of the cochlea enter, and pass out at right angles between the bony plates forming the zona ossea of the lamina spiralis, to be expanded on the membranous portion of the lamina.

MODIOLUS, *Mas,* also means the crown of the trepan.

MO'DIUS. A dry measure, the third of an amphora, equal to the bushel. — Varro.

MODUS OPERAN'DI, 'mode of operating.' This term is applied to the general principles upon which remedies act in morbid states of the body; — a subject of much interest, although involved in considerable obscurity.

The following classification will convey some idea of the ways in which different organs may be excited into action.

1. By actual or immediate contact of the remedy, and by absorption or mediate contact.
2. By an impulse conveyed by the nerves, through an impression made on the stomach or elsewhere.
3. By contiguous or continuous sympathy, or by mere proximity or continuity of parts.

MOËLLE, Marrow — m. *Allongée,* Medulla oblongata — m. *Épinière,* Medulla spinalis — m. *Vertébrale,* Medulla spinalis.

MŒNIA DENTIUM, Alveoli dentium.

MŒROR, Athymia.

MOFETTE, see Mephitism.

MOFFAT, MINERAL WATERS OF. Moffat

is a village situate about 56 miles S. W. of Edinburgh. The water is a cold sulphureous; containing, in a wine gallon, 36 grains of chloride of sodium, 5 cubic inches of carbonic gas, 4 of azote, and 10 of sulphohydric acid. It resembles Harrowgate water in its properties.

A strong chalybeate spring was discovered there about the year 1828, which contains sesquisulphate of peroxide of iron, sulphate of alumina, and uncombined sulphuric acid.

MOGIGRAPHIA, Cramp, writers'.

MOGILA'LIA, *Parala'lia*, from μογις, 'with difficulty,' and λαλειν, 'to speak.' This word is inaccurately written by Paul Zacchias,—*Mola'lia*, and *Molila'lia*. Difficult or defective articulation. Impediment of speech. See Balbuties.

MOGOSTOCIA, Dystocia, Laborious labour.

MOGUS, Agony.

MOHAWK TASSEL, Eupatorium purpureum.

MOHRIA THURIF'RAGA. A South African fern, *Nat. Ord.* Filices, the dry leaves of which, pulverized and made into an ointment with fat, are serviceable in burns and scalds.

MOIGNON, Stump.

MOIS, Menses.

MOISTURE, *Mador*, (F.) *Motteur*, anciently *moisteur*. Simple humidity of the skin. The skin is said to be *moist* or in a state of moisture, when there is slight perspiration.

MOÎTEUR, Moisture.

MOLA, Maxillary bone, Molar tooth, Mole, Patella.

MOLAGOCODI, Piper nigrum.

MOLAIRE, Molar.

MOLALIA, Mogilalia.

MOLAR, *Mola'ris, My'licus*, (F.) *Molaire, Meulière*. That which bruises or grinds; from *molaris*, 'a grindstone,' or *mola*, 'a millstone.'

MOLAR GLANDS. Two small bodies formed by a collection of mucous crypts; seated in the substance of the cheeks, between the masseter and buccinator muscles, and whose excretory ducts open into the mouth opposite the last molar tooth.

MOLAR TEETH, *Grinders, Jaw Teeth, Mola'res permanen'tes dentes, Dentes molares seu maxilla'res seu gom'phii seu clara'les, Molæ, Gomphioi, My'lacri, My'lodontes, My'lodi, Momis'ci*, (F.) *Dents molaires* ou *mâchelières*, occupy the farther part of each alveolar arch. Their coronæ are broader than they are high: unequal, tuberculated; and the roots are more or less subdivided. They are 20 in number, 10 in each jaw. The first two pairs of molar teeth in each jaw have been called *lesser molares* or *bicuspid, Dentes bicuspida'ti*. The coronæ have two tubercles; the outer being more prominent and larger than the inner. The root is commonly simple; sometimes bifurcated. The other three pairs have been termed, *Great molares—Dents multicuspidées* (Ch.) Their coronæ are cubical, rounded, and have, at the upper surface, four or five tubercles, separated by deep furrows. The root is divided into two, three, four, and five *fangs*, which are more or less curved. The third great molaris appears a long time after the others, and hence has been called *Dens sapien'tiæ* or *Wisdom tooth*.

MOLASSES, Melasses.

MOLE, *Mola*, from *moles*, 'mass.' *Mylē, Zephyr'ius fœtus, Germen falsum, Pseudocye'sis molaris, Gravid'itas molaris, Mooncalf*, old French, *Fardeau*. A fleshy, insensible, at times, soft—at others, hard—mass; of variable and determinate size, which forms in the uterus, and is slightly united by vessels to that organ; from which its feeble vitality is derived. It has been conceived by some to be always owing to imperfect conception; but moles may form in the undoubted virgin. They seem to be owing to a morbid process; and certainly are generally connected with conception. At times, they contain parts of the fœtus; but commonly do not. At very different periods, in different women, the diseased mass is expelled from the uterus, with ordinary symptoms of abortion; and the case requires similar management. See, also, Nævus and Conception, (false.)

MOLE PLANT, Euphorbia lathyris.

MOLEC'ULAR, *Molecula'ris*. Of or belonging to molecules or minute portions of any thing. Hence *molecular* death, in contradistinction to *somatic* death.

MOL'ECULE, *Molec'ula, Mass'ula;* diminutive of *moles*, 'a mass.' A minute portion of any body. Also, the *cicatric'ula, ma'cula, gallatu'ra, gelat'inous molecule, tread of the cock*, or embryo part of the impregnated ovum, observable by the microscope before the ovum has left the ovarium of the hen. It lies under the epidermic coats of the yelk, and upon its proper coat. If the ovum, according to Valentin, be lacerated and its contents minutely examined, the cicatricula is found like a grayish white disk, which in its whole periphery is dense, granulous, and opake; but in the centre presents a clear, nongranulous, and perfectly diaphanous point. Purkinje found, that when he removed the dark granulous mass by suction with a small tube, there remained a perfectly transparent vesicle filled with a pellucid lymph, which had a decidedly spherical form, but, being extremely delicate, was easily lacerated, and then its fluid escaped. As he found this, which later naturalists have named—after its discoverer—the *Purkin'jean ves'icle*, in the ova of the ovary, but could not see it in ova, which had already entered the oviduct, he gave it the name *germinal vesicle, vesic'ula prolif'era* seu *germinati'va*, (F.) *Vésicule germinative*. Besides a perfectly colourless fluid, this contains one or more dark corpuscles, which appear as a nucleus through the including membrane in the shape of opake spots—the *germinal spot, macu'la germaniti'va* seu *ger'minans, nu'cleus germaniti'vus*, (F.) *Tache germinative*. The granulous membrane—its thickened portion, the so called 'cicatricula,' —and the germinal vesicle, constitute those parts of the ovum which pass immediately into the original foundation of the embryo, the *blastoderma* or *germinal membrane, vesic'ula blastodermat'ica, blastoder'mic vesicle*.

MOLECULE, GELATINOUS, Molecule.

MOLÈNE, Verbascum nigrum.

MOLES GANGLIFORMIS, Ganglion of Gasser.

MOLIBDUS, Plumbum.

MOLILALIA, Mogilalia.

MOLI'MEN, pl. MOLIMINA, from *molior*, 'to move or stir.' An attempt, a struggle. Hence:

MOLIMEN CRIT'ICUM. An impulsion towards a sudden solution or crisis of a disease.

MOLIMEN HÆMORRHAG'ICUM. The hemorrhagic diathesis or impulsion.

MOLIMEN HÆMORRHOIDA'LE. The hemorrhoidal diathesis or impulsion. See Hæmorrhois.

MOLIMEN MENSTRUA'LE. The menstrual diathesis or impulsion.

MOLIMEN NATURÆ SALUTARIUM, Instinct.

MOLLESCENCE, Mollities.

MOLLET, Sura.

MOLLIPUFFS, Lycoperdon.

MOLLIS MATER, Pia mater.

MOLLIT'IES, *Molles'cence, Malacis'mus, Mollit''ia, Mollitu'do, Emollit''ies, Emollities morbo'sa, Mollitio, Malax'is, Malaco'sis, Malthax'ia*, (F.) *Ramollissement;* (G.) Malakien (Fuchs);

from *mollis*, 'soft.' Preternatural softness of an organ or part of an organ.

MOLLITIES CER'EBRI, *Malaco'sis Cer'ebri, Encephalomala'cia, Encephalomalax'is, Necrenceph'alus* (W. Farr,) *Cerebromala'cia, Encephalosep'sis, Molles'cence* or *softening* or a kind of liquefaction of the cerebral substance; the remainder preserving its ordinary consistency. (F.) *Ramollissement du cerveau*. The neurine often contains small clots of blood, giving rise to what has been termed *Apoplexie capillaire*, (Cruveilhier.) The symptoms denoting it are equivocal.

MOLLITIES CORDIS, Cardiomalacia.

MOLLITIES MEDUL'LÆ SPINA'LIS, *Myelomala'cia*, (F.) *Ramollissement de la Moëlle Épinière*. Softening of the spinal marrow.

MOLLITIES OS'SIUM, *Malacosteo'sis, Malacosteon, Emollit''ies os'sium, Paros'tia flex'ilis, Osteomalaco'sis, Rachi'tis* seu *Rachi'tis adulto'rum, Spina vento'sa* (of some), *Osteomala'cia, Softening of the bones*, (F.) *Ostéo-malacie, Ostéo-malaxie, Ostéo-malakie, Ramollissement des os*. A rare affection in which the bones are deprived of their salts, particularly of the phosphate of lime, and consist only, or mainly, of gelatin; hence they acquire a degree of suppleness which renders them unfit for the performance of their functions. The disease generally affects all the bones; but it is especially remarkable during life in the long bones, which assume any curvature that may be wished. Very violent pain is often experienced in them; and the urine frequently contains an enormous proportion of calcareous phosphate. The patient is compelled to remain in the horizontal posture; the bones no longer being fixed points for the muscles to act upon. The disease has, hitherto, always terminated fatally, and dissection has exhibited the gelatinous nature of the bones; which, by desiccation, have become transparent, as if they had been macerated in acid.

Experience has afforded no means of relief in this dreadful affliction. The alkaline salts, earthy phosphates, &c. are of little or no use.

MOLLITIO, Mollities.

MOLLITUDO, Mollities.

MOLLUS'CUM, *Athero'ma*. A cutaneous affection, so called in consequence of its resemblance to certain molluscous animals. It consists of numerous tumours, varying in size from that of a pea to that of a pigeon's egg, filled with an atheromatous matter, which are developed in the substance of the derma, and are of various shapes, some having a large base,—others adherent by means of a pedicle.

Molluscum contagio'sum, a singular variety, is characterized by the presence of hard, round, tubercles, which are smooth and transparent, and when pressed, pour out from an orifice in their summits a little opake or milky fluid.

The disease is probably seated in the sebaceous follicles.

If internal treatment be adopted at all, it must consist of eutrophics, as arsenic, iodine, &c. The external treatment consists in the employment of measures calculated to excite the tubercles to inflammation, as by touching them with potassa.

MOLOCHE, Malva rotundifolia.

MOLOPES, Vibices.

MOLYBDÆNUM MAGNESII, Manganese, black oxide of.

MOLYBDOS, Plumbum.

MOLYBDOSIS, Lead-poisoning.

MOLYNE, Anus.

MOLYNSIS, Miasma.

MOMIE, Mummy.

MOMIN, Mamei.

MOMISCI, Molar teeth.

MOMOR'DICA, *M. Balsami'na, Balsami'na, Nevrosper'ma cuspida'ta, Balm-apple, Balsam apple*, (F.) *Balsamine, Pomme de merveille*. The fruit of this oriental tree, *Pomum mirab'ile* seu *hierosolymita'num*, was formerly considered vulnerary.

MOMORDICA ASPERA, M. Elaterium.

MOMOR'DICA ELATE'RIUM: *M. as'pera, Elate'rium, Ecba'lia Elate'rium, Cu'cumis agres'tis* seu *asini'nus, C. sylvestris, Elate'rium officina'rum* seu *cordifo'lium, Charan'tia, Bouba'lios, Guarerba orba, Wild* or *Squirting cu'cumber, Ecbol'ium elate'rium*, (F.) *Concombre Sauvage, Momordique. Nat. Order*, Cucurbitaceæ. The dried sediment from the juice is the elaterium of the shops. (See Extractum Elaterii.) It is a most powerful cathartic, and, as such, has been used in dropsies. Its active principle is the *Elatin, Elaterin* or *Elaterium*. Dose, gr. ¼ to gr. j. until it operates.

MOMORDIQUE, Momordica elaterium.

MONAD, from *monas*, 'unity.' A simple particle, or atom, or unit.—Leibnitz. The smallest of all visible animalcules. A primary cell or germ.

MONÆ, Nates.

MONAR'DA COCCIN'EA, *Scarlet Rose balm, Mountain mint, Oswego Tea, Mountain Balm, Horsemint, Square stalk, Red Balm;* a beautiful indigenous plant, having the excitant properties of Monarda punctata.

MONAR'DA FISTULO'SA, *Purple monar'da*. The leaves have a fragrant smell; and an aromatic, somewhat bitter taste. They are reputed to be nervine, stomachic, and deobstruent.

MONAR'DA PUNCTA'TA, *Horsemint. Sex. Syst.* Diandria Monogynia. *Nat. Ord.* Labiatæ. Indigenous in the United States. Stimulant and carminative. The *Oleum monardæ* is officinal in the United States.

MONARDA, **PURPLE**, M. fistulosa.

MONDER (F.), from *mundus*, 'cleanly.' To render clean or pure. In *Pharmacy*, it means to separate any substance from its impure or useless portion. In surgery, *monder* ou *mondifier* une *plaie*, is to clean or deterge a wound.

MONDIFICATIFS, Detergents.

MONDIFIER UNE PLAIE, see *Monder*.

MONE'MERON, *Monoë'meron, Monohe'meron;* from μονος, 'one,' and 'ημερα, 'a day.' A name given to several collyria, which were supposed to be capable of curing diseases of the eyes in a day.

MONENTERUM, Colon.

MONE'SIA. A vegetable extract imported into Europe from South America, in hard, thick cakes. It is prepared from the bark of a tree, whose botanical name is uncertain—probably *Chrysophyl'lum glycyphlæ'um*. It is very friable, and its fracture very much resembles that of a well-torrefied cocoanut. It is wholly soluble in water; and its taste—which is at first sweet like liquorice—sometimes becomes astringent. It is on account of its astringent properties that it has been prescribed in chronic bronchitis, hæmoptysis, diarrhœa, leucorrhœa, uterine hemorrhage, &c. It has been applied locally, in the form of ointment, (*Moses.* p. 1, *Adipis*, p. vij.

The dose of Monesia is from 12 to 40 grains a day.

MONEYWORT, Lysimachia nummularia.

MONGO'LIAN. Anthropologists give the name *Mongolian* race to a variety of the human species, spread over a great part of the north of Asia, in China, India, Thibet, the Moluccas, &c. The individuals composing it have the skin of a brown red, forehead flat, nose broad, cheeks prominent, and lips large. See Homo.

MONISM; *Monis'mus;* from μονος, 'alone.' The doctrine, which declares matter and mind to be identical.

MONK PHYSICIANS AND SURGEONS. A class of practitioners of whom Frère Cosme and Jacques Beaulieu in France, and Pravetz in Germany, were the most distinguished.

MONKSHOOD, Aconitum—m. Common, Aconitum napellus—m. Salutary, Aconitum anthora.

MONNI'NA POLYSTA'CHIA. A beautiful South American plant. *Nat. Ord.* Polygaleæ. *Sex. Syst.* Diadelphia Octandria. The bark of the root is a powerful astringent, and much used in South America in diseases of the bowels.

MONOBLEP'SIS, from μονος, 'one,' and βλεψις, 'sight.' An affection in which vision is confused, imperfect, and indistinct, when both eyes are employed; but perfect or nearly so, when either eye is used singly.

MONOCAR'PÆ; from μονος, 'alone,' 'single,' and καρπος, 'fruit.' A division of cutaneous affections, of the family of Ecxematosen of Fuchs, which includes strophulus, psydracia, and ecthyma.

MONOCEPH'ALUS, from μονος, 'one,' and κεφαλη, 'head.' A compound monster having two bodies with a single head.

MONOCOLON, Cæcum, Rectum.

MONOCRA'NUS, from μονος, 'one,' 'single,' and κρανον, κρανιον, 'cranium.' A monster with one cranium, but with the face in part double — Gurlt.

MONOCULUM, Cæcum.

MONOC'ULUS, *Mon'ocle, Monophthal'mus, Unioc'ulus, Unoc'ulus,* from μονος, 'one,' and *oculus,* 'an eye.' A bandage employed to maintain topical applications over one of the eyes. This bandage, called by some surgeons *Simplex oc'ulus,* (F.) *Œil simple,* is made of a roller three or four ells long, rolled into a single ball. See Cyclops.

MONODIPLO'PIA; from μονος, 'alone,' διπλους, 'double,' and ωψ, 'eye.' Double vision with one eye.

MONOEMERON, Monemeron.

MONOGAS'TRIC, *Monogas'tricus*; from μονος, 'one,' and γαστηρ, 'stomach.' That which has but one stomach. Man is *monogastric*; ruminating animals, on the contrary, are *polygastric.*

MON'OGRAPH, MED'ICAL, *Monograph'ia med'ica*; from μονος, 'one,' and γραφη, 'description.' An *ex professo* treatise on a single class of diseases, or on a single disease.

MONOHEMERON, Monemeron.

MONOMACHON, Cæcum.

MONOMACUM, Cæcum.

MONOMANIA, see Melancholy — m. Homicidal, Homicidal insanity—m. Incendiary, Pyromania.

MONOMANIE, Melancholy — m. *Homicide,* Homicidal insanity.

MONOMMATOS, Cyclops.

MONOMORIA, see Melancholy.

MONOPAGIA, Clavus hystericus, Hemicrania.

MONOP'ATHY, *Monopathi'a,* from μονος, 'one,' and παθος, 'disorder.' A state in which one organ or function is disordered. Applied to melancholy or monomania; which is said to be a *monopathic* affection.

MONOPEGIA, Clavus hystericus, Hemicrania.

MONOPHTHALMUS, Cyclops, Monoculus.

MONOPLAS'TIC, *Monoplas'ticus*: from μονος, 'one,' and πλασσω, 'I form.' That which has one form. A *monoplastic element,* in histology, is one which retains its primary form. — Gerber.

MONOPODIA, Sympodia.

MONOPS, Cyclops.

MONOPSIA, Cyclopia.

MONOPUS, Symmeles.

MONOR'CHIS, from μονος, 'one,' and ορχις, 'testicle.' One who has only one testicle.

MONOSI'TIA, from μονος, 'one,' and σιτος, 'food,' 'repast.' The habit of taking only one meal in the day.

MONOT'ROPA UNIFLO'RA, *Indian pipe, Iceplant, Pipe-plant, Nest root, Fit root.* An indigenous plant, whose juice, mixed with water, has been extolled by the Indians in ophthalmia. The dried root in powder has been given in epilepsy and nervous diseases.

MONROIA'NUM FORA'MEN. A foramen at the anterior part of the lateral ventricles of the brain, by which they communicate with each other, is so called from the second Monro.

MONS VEN'ERIS, *Montic'ulus Ven'eris, Ephebe'um,* (F.) *Mont de Vénus, Pénil, Motte, Éminence sus-pubienne.* The more or less projecting eminence, situate at the base of the hypogastrium, above the vulva and in front of the os pubis. At the period of puberty it becomes covered with hair, formerly called *Tresso'ria.*

MONSO'NIA OVA'TA, *Keita,* of the Hottentots. A plant of the *Nat. Ord.* Geraniaceæ, which grows at the Cape of Good Hope. The root and herb are very astringent, and are used successfully in dysentery.

MONSTER, *Monstrum, Teras, Pelor, Pelo'ria, Pelo'rium, Pelo'rum.* Any organized being, having an extraordinary vice of conformation, or a preternatural perversion of every part, or of certain parts only.

The following classification embraces the main varieties of malformations — *Vitia primæ conformatio'nis.*—1. Those in which certain parts of the normal body are absent or defective—*monstra deficientia.* 2. These produced by fusion or coalition of organs — *coalitio partium, symphysis.* 3. Those, in which parts, united in the normal state are separated from each other — *clefts, fissures.* 4. Those in which normal openings are occluded — *atresia.* 5. Those by excess, or in which certain parts have a disproportionate size—*monstra abundantia.* 6. Those, in which one or many parts have an abnormal position—*situs mutatus.* 7. Those affecting the sexual organs — *hermaphroditism*; and to these " true malformations" Vogel adds 8. Diseases of the fœtus, and abnormal states of its envelopes.

Amongst the numerous hypotheses entertained on the origin or cause of monsters, or of monstrosity—*terato'sis, monstros'itas,* (F.) *monstruosité,* as the state has been called — three only are worth mentioning. They have been attributed, 1. To the influence of the maternal imagination on the fœtus in utero. 2. To accidental changes, experienced by the fœtus at some period of its uterine existence: and 3. To a primitive defect in the germs. The second seems to be the only one that is philosophical.

As a medico-legal question, monsters, if capable of action as individuals, have the same rights as other persons.

MONSTERS, DOUBLE, see Duplication — m. Triplet, see Triplet.

MONSTRA ABUNDANTIA, see Monster — m. Deficientia, see Monster — m. Trigemina, see Triplet—m. Triplica, see Triplet.

MONSTROSITAS, see Monster.

MONSTROSITY, see Monster.

MONSTRUM, Monster.

MONSTRUOSITÉ, see Monster.

MONT DE VÉNUS, Mons Veneris.

MONTBRISON, MINERAL WATERS OF. Montbrison is a town in France, in the department of the Loire, fifteen leagues from Lyons. There are three cold springs here, which are highly acidulous, and used as refrigerants and aperients.

MONT-DE-MARSAN, MINERAL WATERS OF. Mont-de-Marsan is a small French town, 10 leagues from Dax; where there is a chalybeate spring, somewhat frequented.

MONT-D'OR, MINERAL WATERS OF. Mont d'Or is a village seven leagues from Clermont, (Puy-de-Dôme,) at which are several mineral springs, cold and thermal. Those of the Fountain *La Madelaine*, and of the *Great Bath*, are thermal, temp. 112° Fahr., and contain carbonic acid, subcarbonate and sulphate of soda, chloride of sodium, subcarbonate of lime and magnesia, alumine and oxide of iron. Those of *St. Margaret* are cold, and contain much carbonic acid.

MONTECATI'NI, MINERAL WATERS OF. This town is situate near Borgo-Buggiano, in Tuscany. The springs are thermal; ranging from 78° to 118° Fahrenheit.

MONTHLY COURSES, Menses — m. Periods, Menses.

MONTICULUS CEREBELLI, see Vermiform processes of the Cerebellum — m. Veneris, Mons veneris.

MONTPELLIER, CLIMATE OF. This seat of a celebrated medical school in the S. E. of France was at one time renowned for its climate, and especially in regard to its adaptation to consumptive cases. This is now exploded, and it is at present esteemed an unfit residence for them. The climate possesses the general characters of that of south-eastern France—being dry, hot, and irritating; subject to frequent vicissitudes, and especially to blasts of keen, cold, northerly winds. It is, indeed, most injurious in pulmonary diseases.

MOON, *Luna*, *Sele'nē*, *Menē*, Sax. Mona, (G.) Mond, (F.) *Lune*. The moon has been supposed to exert considerable influence over the human body, in health and disease. Such influence has been grossly exaggerated. Not many years ago, it would have been heretical to doubt the exacerbation of mania at the full of the moon; yet it is now satisfactorily shown, that if the light be excluded at this period, the *lunatic* is not excited more than ordinarily.

MOONSTRUCK, Lunatic.
MOONCALF, Mole.
MOORBERRY, Vaccinium oxycoccos.
MOORSHEAD, Alembic.
MOORWORT, BROAD-LEAVED, Andromeda mariana.
MOOSEWOOD, Dirca palustris.
MOPHETA, see Mephitism.
MORBEUX, Morbid.

MORBI, see Morbus — m. Acquisiti, Acquired diseases — m. Acuti, see Acuto — m. Adventitii, Acquired diseases—m. Anniversarii, Annual diseases—m. Annui, Annual diseases—m. Asthenici, Adynamiæ — m. Celati, Feigned diseases — m. Chronici, Chronic diseases — m. Cognati, Innate diseases — m. Complicati, see Complication, Impliciti morbi—m. Congeniti, Innate diseases—m. Connati, Connate diseases — m. Connexi, Conjuncti morbi — m. Consequentes, Conjuncti morbi — m. Constrictorii, see Spasmoticus—m. Dermatodes, see Dermatoid—m. Dispersi, Sporadic diseases — m. Dissimulati, Feigned diseases — m. Epicteti, Acquired diseases—m. Evolutionis, see Development — m. Hereditarii, Hereditary diseases — m. Homoedri, see Homoëdrus — m. Infitiati, Feigned diseases—m. Interni, Internal diseases—m. Melancholici, see Mercurial—m. Mercuriales, see Mercurial — m. Nervosi, Nervous diseases — m. Occulti, see Latent — m. Olfactūs, Osmcnosi — m. Perplexi, see Complication — m. Pseudalei, Feigned diseases — m. Recidiva, Relapse—m. Recursus, Palindromia — m. Sexuales, see Sexual—m. Sexûs, Genonusi—m. Simulati, Feigned diseases — m. Sparsi, Sporadic diseases —m. Spasmotici, see Spasmoticus—m. Subacute, see Acute — m. Tactus, Haphonosi — m. Tropici, Troponusi.

MORBID, *Mor'bidus*, *Morbo'sus*, *Pathic*, *Path'ical*, *Path'icus*, (F.) *Morbeux*, *Morbide*; from *morbus*, 'a disease.' Diseased, or relating to disease.

MORBID ANATOMY, see Anatomy.

MORBIF'IC, *Morbif'icus*, (F.) *Morbifique*; from *morbus*, 'a disease,' and *facere*, 'to make.' Causing or producing disease — as *morbific* emanations.

MORBILITY, Disease.
MORBILLEUX, Morbillous.
MORBILLI, Rubeola — m. Confluentes, Scarlatina — m. Ignei, Scarlatina.
MORBILLOSUS, Morbillous.
MORBILLOUS, *Morbillo'sus*, *Measly*, (F.) *Morbilleux*. Affected or connected with measles.
MORBOSUS, Sickly.

MORBUS, Disease, see Morbi — m. Ampullaceus, Pemphigus — m. Anglicus, Rachitis — m. Aphrodisius, Syphilis — m. Arcuatus, Icterus — m. Arietis, Influenza — m. Arquatus, Icterus — m. Articularis, Gout — m. Astralis, Epilepsy — m. Attonitus, Apoplexy — m. a. Celsi, Catalepsy — m. Brightii, Kidney, Bright's disease of the — m. Bullosus, Pemphigus — m. Caducus, Epilepsy — m. Cœruleus, Cyanopathy — m. Calculi, Lithia — m. Cardiacus, Cardialgia — m. Catarrhalis, Influenza — m. Catoxys, see Catoxys — m. Cerealis, Ergotism — m. Cerebralis Whytii, Hydrocephalus Internus — m. Cirrhorum, Plica — m. Cœliacus, Cœliac flux — m. Comitialis, Epilepsy—m. Costalis, Pleuritis—m. Coxarius, Coxarum morbus — m. Croatus, Scherlievo — m. Cucullaris, Pertussis — m. Cucullis, Pertussis — m. Cystophlegmaticus, Cystirrhœa—m. Dæmoniacus, Epilepsy—m. Dæmonius, Epilepsy—m. Deificus, Epilepsy—m. Dissolutus, Dysentery—m. Divinus, Epilepsy—m. Dominorum, Gout—m. Endemius, Endemic—m. Epidemicus, Epidemy—m. Epidemicus gutturis Foresti, Scarlatina—m. Eruditorum, Hypochondriasis—m. Extrinsecus, External disease— m. Farciminosus, see Equinia — m. Febrilis, Pyreticosis — m. Fellifluus, Cholera — m. Flatuosus, Hypochondriasis — m. Fluminiensis, Scherlievo — m. Fœdus, Epilepsy — m. Frigidus, Atrophy — m. Gallicus, Syphilis — m. Gesticulatorius, Chorea—m. Gravis, see Serious — m. Hæmorrhoidalis, Hæmorrhois — m. Heracleus, Epilepsy — m. Herculeus, Epilepsy — m. Hispanicus, Syphilis — m. Hydrophobicus, Hydrophobia — m. Hypochondriacus, Hypochondriasis — m. Hystericus, Hysteria — m. Idiopathicus, Idiopathia — m. Indicus, Syphilis — m. Interlunius, Epilepsy —m. Ischiadicus, Neuralgia femoro-poplitæa—m. Italicus, Syphilis — m. Jecinoris, Hepatitis — m. Lateralis, Pleuritis — m. Lazari, Elephantiasis — m. Lunaticus, Epilepsy — m. Luteolus, Icterus—m. Maculosus hæmorrhagicus Werlhofii, Purpera hæmorrhagica—m. Magnus, Epilepsy—m. Major, Epilepsy — m. Mensalis, Epilepsy — m. Mercurialis, Eczema mercuriale, Hydrargyriasis — m. Metallicus, Colic, metallic — m. Mucosus, Fever, adeno-meningeal — m. Nauticus, Nausea marina — m. Neapolitanus, Syphilis—m. Niger, Melæna —m. Originalis, Idiopathia—m. Œsophagi, Œsophagopathia—m. Oryzeus, Cholera—m. Pallidus, Chlorosis—m. Pancœnus, Pandemic—m. Parthenius, Chlorosis — m. Pandemius, Pandemic — m. Pedicularis, Phtheiriasis — m. Peracutus, see Catoxys—m. Phœniceus, Elephantiasis—m. Pilaris, Trichiasis—m. Pleuriticus, Pleuritis — m. Plumbeus, Lead-poisoning — m. Porcinus, Essera — m.

Popularis, Epilepsy—m. Primarius, Idiopathia—m. Proprius, Idiopathia—m. Protopathicus, Idiopathia—m. Proteiformis, see Proteiformis—m. Psoadicus, Lumbar abscess—m. Publicus, Epidemy—m. Puerilis, Epilepsy—m. Pulicularis, Typhus gravior—m. Pustulosus Finnicus, see Anthrax—m. Recidivus, Relapse—m. Recidivus, Palindromia—m. Regionalis, Endemic—m. Regius, Icterus—m. Resiccatorius, Hypochondriasis—m. Ructuosus, Hypochondriasis—m. Ructuosus, see Eructation—m. Sacer, Epilepsy—m. Saltatorius, Chorea—m. Sancti Joannis, Epilepsy—m. Sancti Valentini, Epilepsy—m. Scarlatinosus, Scarlatina—m. Scelestus, Epilepsy—m. Scrophulosus, Scrofula—m. Secundarius, Deuteropathia—m. Seleniacus, Epilepsy—m. Sideratus, Epilepsy—m. Silesiacus, Raphania—m. Simplex, Haplopathia—m. Solstitialis, *Coup-de-Soleil*—m. Sonticus, Epilepsy—m. Spasmodicus malignus seu popularis, Raphania—m. Strangulatorius, Cynanche trachealis—m. Sudatorius, Sudor Anglicus—m. Truculentus infantum, Cynanche trachealis—m. Tuberculosus, see Tubercle and Tubercular cachexia—m. Ungaricus, Fever, Hungaric—m. Verminosus, Helminthiasis—m. Vernaculus, Endemic—m. Vervecinus, Influenza—m. Vesicularis, Pemphigus—m. Virgineus, Chlorosis—m. Viridellus, Epilepsy—m. Vitriolatus, Epilepsy—m. Vocis, Phononosus—m. Vulpis, Alopecia.

MORCEAU DU DIABLE, see Tuba Fallopiana—*m. Frangé*, see Tuba Fallopiana.

MOR'DICANT, *Mor'dicans, Calor mor'dicans.* A morbid heat, causing a disagreeable pungent sensation in the fingers of the physician.

MORDICES, Teeth : see Tooth.

MOREA, Morus nigra.

MORELLE, Boletus esculentus—*m. à Fruit noir*, Solanum—*m. Furieuse*, Atropa belladonna—*m. en Grappes*, Phytolacca decandra—*m. Grimpante*, Solanum dulcamara.

MORETARIUM, Mortar.

MORE'TUS, *More'tum*, from *morum*, 'the mulberry.' Ancient name of a cordial julep, into the composition of which the syrup of mulberries entered.—Schröder.

MORGAGN'I, HUMOUR OF, *Humor Morgagnia'nus.* A peculiar, transparent, slightly viscid fluid, found between the crystalline and its capsule.

MORGELINE, Alsine media.

MORGUE, (F). A dead-house, wherein persons, found dead, are exposed with the view of being recognized by their friends.

MORIA, Idiotism—m. Demens, Idiotism, Dementia—m. Demens Ierema, see Dementia—m. Imbecilis amnesia, Amnesia.

MORIBUND, Psychorages.

MORINGA NUX BEN, Guilandina moringa—m. Oleifera, Guilandina moringa—m. Pterygosperma, Guilandina moringa—m. Zeylanica, Guilandina moringa.

MORION, Genital organ, Penis.

MORIOPLAS'TICE, *Chirur'gia curto'rum, Ch. Anaplas'tica, Restitu'tio organ'ica seu par'tium deperdita'rum, Transplanta'tio, Autoplas'ticē, Anaplas'tic Surgery, Autoplas'ty or Autoplastic or Plastic Surgery, Chirur'gia plas'tica*, from μοριον, 'a part,' and πλαστικος, 'forming.' The restoration of lost parts. The operations for this purpose have various names, according to the part concerned, as *Cheiloplastice, Ceratoplastice, Rhinoplastice*, &c.

MORO, from *morum*, 'a mulberry :'—*Morum*, (F.) *Mure.* A small abscess resembling a mulberry. A small tumour, of a similar appearance, particularly on the genital organs after impure coition.

MOROCH'THUS, *Morock'tus, Morochi'tes, Morochi'tes, Meroc'tes, Galax'ia, Leucograph'ia*, (F.) *Pierre au lait, Milk stone.* An Egyptian stone, used by the ancients as an application to the intertrigo of children : probably a variety of fuller's earth, inasmuch as it appears to have been used by fullers.

MOROCHITES, Morochthus.
MOROCHTUS, Morochthus.
MOROCOMIUM, Morotrophium.
MORODOCHIUM, Morotrophium.
MOROSIS, Fatuitas, Idiotism.

MOROSITA'TES, from μωρια, 'folly.' A generic name given by Linnæus to an order of Vesaniæ, in which he included pica, bulimia, polydipsia, antipathia, nostalgia, panophobia, satyriasis, nymphomania, tarentismus, and hydrophobia.

MOROTROPH'IUM, *Morocomi'um, Morodochi'um*, from μωρος, 'fatuous,' and τροφη, 'support.' An *insane establishment ; a lunatic asylum ; a mad-house.* Under proper management, a valuable institution ; but liable to various abuses.

MORPHÆA, Morphew—m. Alba, Lepra alphoides—m. Nigra, Lepra nigricans.

MORPHÉE, Morphew.

MORPHEW, *Morphœ'a*, (F.) *Morphée.* A term vaguely applied to scurfy eruptions on the face. *Morphæa* was formerly applied to squamous diseases in general.

MORPHIA, Morphina—m. Acetate of, Morphinæ acetas—m. and Zinc, double iodide of, Zinc and Morphia, double iodide of—m. Citrate of, see Morphina—m. Muriate of, see Morphina—m. Sulphate of, Morphinæ sulphas.

MORPHIÆ ACETAS, Morphinæ acetas—m. Sulphas, Morphinæ sulphas.

MOR'PHICA, from μορφη, 'shape.' Monstrosities of birth. The 3d order, class *Typhica* of Good.

MORPHI'NA, *Mor'phia, Mor'phium, Morphi'nā, Morphine*, from *Morpheus*, the 'god of sleep.' A solid, colourless alkali ; crystallizable in beautiful pyramids, truncated and transparent ; soluble in alcohol, and slightly so in boiling water. It exists, combined with meconic acid, in opium. It may be obtained by decomposing, by means of ammonia or calcined magnesia, an aqueous solution of opium made in the cold.

The following is the process of the Pharm. U. S. *Opium*, sliced, ℔j ; *distilled water, alcohol, animal charcoal*, each a sufficient quantity ; *solution of ammonia*, f℥vj. Macerate the opium with four pints of distilled water for 24 hours, and having worked it with the hand, digest for 24 hours, and strain. Macerate the residue twice successively with distilled water, and strain. Mix the infusions ; evaporate to six pints, and filter ; then add first five pints of alcohol, and afterwards three fluidounces of the solution of ammonia, previously mixed with half-a-pint of alcohol. After 24 hours, pour in the remainder of the solution of ammonia, mixed as before with half-a-pint of alcohol ; and set the liquor aside for 24 hours, that crystals may form. To purify these, boil them with two pints of alcohol till they are dissolved ; filter the solution, while hot, through animal charcoal, and set it aside to crystallize.

Morphia dissolves perfectly in the acids, which it saturates ; and with which it forms very crystallizable salts, with the exception of the acetate. All these salts have a bitter taste, and act upon the animal economy in the same manner as opium, but more powerfully. The *acetate* is the salt commonly employed in medicine. It was, at one time, supposed that Morphia is the purely sedative part of opium, divested of its irritating properties; but experience has not confirmed this. On the contrary, it will generally disagree where opium does. Dose of morphia, ¼ to ½ of a grain.

MORPHI'NÆ ACE'TAS, *Mor'phiæ Acetas, Ac''etate of Morphine, Acetate of Morphia.* A salt formed by saturating morphia with acetic acid. (*Morphia*, in powder, freed from narcotina by boiling with sulphuric ether, ℥j; *distilled water*, Oss; *acetic acid*, a sufficient quantity. Mix the morphia with the water; then carefully drop in the acid, constantly stirring until the morphia is saturated and dissolved. Evaporate the solution in a water-bath to the consistence of syrup. Lastly, dry the acetate with a gentle heat and rub it into powder.—Ph. U. S.) Dose, from ¼ of a grain to a grain.

MORPHI'NÆ SULPHAS, MOR'PHIÆ SULPHAS, *Sulphate of Morphia.* A salt, formed by saturating morphia with sulphuric acid, evaporating, and crystallizing. Dose, the same as of the acetate.

Muriate and *Citrate of Morphia* have likewise been used; but they possess no advantages over the other salts. The sulphate and muriate are officinal in the Ph. U. S.

MORPHIUM, Morphina.

MORPHOLOG''ICAL, *Morpholog''icus,* from μορφη, 'shape,' and λογος, 'a description.' That which has relation to the anatomical conformation of parts. Applied, at times, to the alterations in the *form* of the several parts of the embryo, in contradistinction to *histological*, which is applied to the transformation by which the tissues are gradually generated. In comparative anatomy, it is applied to the history of the modifications of forms, which the same organ undergoes in different animals.

MORPHOLOGY, Anatomy.

MORPHOLY'SIS, from μορφη, 'shape,' and λυσις, 'solution.' Destruction of organization. An agent, that occasions such destruction, is called a *morpholyt'ic.*

MORPHOLYTIC, see Morpholysis.

MORPHON'OMY, *Morphonom'ia:* from μορφη, 'shape,' and νομος, 'a law.' The laws of organic formation. The department of anatomical science which teaches the laws of organic configuration.

MORPHOTOMY, see Anatomy.

MORPIO, see Pediculus.

MORPION, Crab-louse, see Pediculus.

MORS, Death — m. Apparens, Asphyxia — m. Putativa, Aphyxia — m. Repentina, Demotivus lapsus — *m. du Diable,* Scabiosa succisa.

MORSELLUS, Tabella.

MORSULI ANTIMONIALES, Tabellæ antimoniales Kunckelii — m. Stibii, Tabellæ antimoniales Kunckelii.

MORSULUS, Tabella.

MORSURE, Degmos.

MORSUS, Degmos—m. Diaboli, Scabiosa succisa, see Tuba Fallopiana — m. Gallinæ, Alsine media—m. Stomachi, Cardialgia—m. Ventriculi, Cardialgia.

MORT, Death—*m. Apparente,* Asphyxia — *m. du Chien,* Cholera — *m. aux Chiens,* Colchicum autumnale—*m. aux Panthères,* Doronicum pardalianches.

MORTA, Pemphigus.

MORTAL, *Morta'lis,* from *mors, mortis,* 'death.' *Letha'lis, Leta'lis, Thanato'des, Thanas'imus,* (F.) *Mortel.* That which is subject to death; — that which causes death : — as, *man is mortal; a disease is mortal.* Of old, it was the custom to have a division of *mortal* wounds, which gave rise to many errors in medico-legal investigations, as the mortality of wounds depends upon various circumstances; and it is often a matter of extreme difficulty to pronounce whether or not a wound is necessarily mortal.

MORTAL'ITY, *Mortal'itas, Lethal'itas, Letal'itas,* (F.) *Mortalité.* This word, taken in an extended sense, expresses the condition of all organized bodies,—of being subject to the cessation of life. In the sense in which it is most frequently employed, it signifies,—the proportional quantity of individuals who, in a certain population, die in a given time. If we assume the population of the earth to be one thousand millions, and a generation to last thirty-three years; in that space of time the one thousand millions must all die, and, consequently, the number of deaths will be, by approximation,

Each year 30,000,000
Each day 82,109
Each hour 3,421
Each minute 57
Each second .... 1 nearly.

If, on the other hand, as has been supposed, the number of deaths is to that of the births as TEN to TWELVE: there will be born,

Each year 36,000,000
Each day 98,356
Each hour 4,098
Each minute 68
Each second .... 1 & 2-15ths.

It has been estimated that the average mortality of the Pays du Vaud, is 1 in 49; of Sweden and Holland, 1 in 48; of Russia, 1 in 41; of France, 1 in 40; of Austria, 1 in 38; of Prussia and Naples, 1 in 33 to 35; of England, 1 in 45; and of South America, 1 in 30. The same rate of mortality has been given to the United States as to France; but the statistical details on all this matter have been inadequate, and—it is not improbable—inaccurate. The following has been given as the annual mortality of some of the chief cities of this country and Europe: (See the author's Human Health, p. 101: Philadelphia, 1844.) Philadelphia, 1 in 45.68; Glasgow, 1 in 44; Manchester, 1 in 44; Geneva, 1 in 43; Boston, 1 in 41.26; Baltimore, 1 in 41; London, 1 in 40; New York, 1 in 37.83; St. Petersburgh, 1 in 37; Charleston, 1 in 36.50; Leghorn, 1 in 35; Berlin, 1 in 34; Paris, Lyons, Strasburg, and Barcelona, 1 in 32; Nice and Palermo, 1 in 31; Madrid, 1 in 29; Naples, 1 in 28; Brussels, 1 in 26; Rome, 1 in 25; Amsterdam, 1 in 24; and Vienna, 1 in 22½.

In the cities, the mortality under two years of age bears a large ratio. This is exhibited by the following table:

Ages.	London.	Philad.	Baltimore.
Under 1 year,	28.52	22.7	24.11
From 1 to 2,		8.6	8.55
2 to 5,	9.97	7.3	11.18
5 to 10,	4.33	4.	5.
10 to 20,	4.03	5.	6.3
20 to 30,	6.64	12.	9.87
30 to 40,	8.08	12.	10.58
40 to 50,	8.89	10.	8.88
50 to 60,	8.89	7.2	5.78
60 to 70,	9.15	5.	4.5
70 to 80,	7.83	3.5	3.
80 to 90,	3.18	1.9	1.67
90 to 100,	0.40	0.5	0.36
100 to 110,	——	0.09	0.18
110 to 120,	——	0.013	

It would not be proper to regard the *value of life* in different countries, or in different periods in the same country, to be indicated by the average mortality; inasmuch as in one case a greater mortality may occur amongst children, and in another amongst adults.

MORTALITY, BILLS OF, *Bills of Necrol'ogy, Mor'tuary Reg'isters,* (F.) *Tables de Mortalité.* Tables, instituted for the purpose of exhibiting the number of deaths, &c. in a given time. Well-kept bills of mortality are of great use to the physician and political economist. Those of London were proverbial for their inaccuracy and insufficiency; especially as regards the complaints of which the persons have died. They were formerly made out by the parish clerks, and the information was conveyed to them by two old women, who were appointed in each parish, and were called *Searchers;* — their duty being to see that the deceased had died a natural death. This miserable system has, however, been abolished; and the Registrar-General's annual reports of births, deaths, and marriages, exhibit how admirably vital statistics are now conducted in Great Britain.

MORTAR, *Morta'rium, Moreta'rium, Morto'rium, Piso, Ac'onē, Pila, Holmos, Igdē, Igdus,* (F.) *Mortier.* A vessel for reducing to powder different solid substances, and for making certain mixtures. Various substances are employed in the construction of mortars;—iron, marble, glass, wedgewood ware, &c.

MORTARIOLUM, Alveolus.

MORTEL, Mortal.

MORTIER, Mortar.

MORTIFER, Lethiferous.

MORTIFICATIO, Mortification — m. Pulmonum, Necropneumonia.

MORTIFICA'TION, *Mortifica'tio, Necro'sis, Sphacela'tion,* from *mors,* 'death,' and *fio,* 'I become.' The loss of vitality in a part of the body. The incipient stage of mortification, when the case is still recoverable, is called Gangrene; when totally destroyed, Sphacelus. Mortification of a bone is called Necrosis.

MORTIFICATION, COLD, Sphacelus — m. Ergot, Ergotism — m. Hot, Gangrene — m. Mildew, Ergotism.

MORTOOTH, Cupri sulphas.

MORTUARY REGISTERS, Mortality, bills of.

MORUM, see Morus nigra — m. Palpebræ internæ, Trachoma carunculosum.

MORUS NIGRA, *M. lacinia'ta, Mul'berry Tree, More'a, Sycami'nos,* (F.) *Mûrier Noir.* The fruit of the mulberry tree, *Morum, Sycami'num,* (F.) *Mûre,* is pleasant, sweet, subacid, and abounds with a deep violet-coloured juice. A syrup is directed in the London Pharmacopœia. The bark of the root has been regarded as an anthelmintic.

MORUS RUBRA, *Red Mulberry, Wild Mulberry;* indigenous. The root has been used to destroy tænia.

MORVE, Mucus, Nasal mucus; see Equinia — m. *Farcineuse,* see Equinia.

MOS, Habit.

MOS MORBI BENIG'NUS, seu MALIG'NUS. The benign, or malignant character of a disease.

MOSCHARDI'NA, *Muscer'da,* from μοσχος, 'musk.' A lozenge for the mouth, composed of musk, ambergris, and other aromatics.

MOSCHELÆ'ON, *Moscolæ'a.* A compound aromatic oil, containing musk.

MOSCHUS, Musk—m. Arabum, Hibiscus abelmoschus—m. Factitious, Musk, artificial.

MOSCOLÆA, Moschelæon.

MOSLICH, Maslach.

MOSQUITA, see Mosquito.

MOSQUI'TO (S.) Diminutive of (S.) *mosca,* 'a fly.' *Musquito.* A very troublesome insect in warm, moist situations. Curtains, called *Mosquito curtains,* are used in India, by way of protection. The entrance of mosquitos into the bedchamber may also be prevented, to a certain extent, by keeping the doors and windows closed until the lights are extinguished. The pain and itching from the bites are alleviated by washing them with hartshorn.

MOSQUITA is a name given, by the Portuguese, to small, red pimples on the skin, resembling the bites of the musquito.

MOSS BERRY, Vaccinium oxycoccos — m. Ceylon, Fucus amylaceus—m. Club, Lycopodium —m. Cup, Lichen pyxidatus—m. Iceland, Lichen Islandicus—m. Irish, Fucus crispus—m. Marine, Fucus amylaceus.

MOTA, Fagus castanea.

MOTAMEN, Motion.

MOTATIO, Motion.

MOTE, Carbasus, Linteum.

MOTEUR, Motory.

MOTHER'S MARKS, Nævus — m. Spots, Nævus.

MOTHERWORT, Leonurus cardiaca, Matricaria.

MOTIL'ITY, *Motil'itas,* from *motus,* 'movement.' (F.) *Motilité, Motricité.* Faculty of moving; moving power; contractility.

MOTION, *Motus, Mo'tio, Mota'tio, Mota'men, Commo'tio, Permo'tio, Cine'sis, Movement,* (F.) *Mouvement.* The act of changing place. The various motions may be divided into,—*First,* the *voluntary* or those that are executed under the influence of the brain. *Secondly,* the *involuntary,* which may be subdivided into, 1, The *excited,* of the *reflex function* of Dr. Marshall Hall and others,—as the closure of the larynx on the contact of acrid vapours, of the pharynx on that of the food,—a function of the spinal marrow; and 2. Those that are executed under the organic and other nerves of involuntary function. It is probable, too, that every living tissue is capable of moving responsive to its appropriate irritant. See Irritability.

MOTION, CILIARY, see Cilia — m. Involuntary, see Automatic — m. Vibratory, see Ciliary — m. Voluntary, Autocinesis.

MOTIVE, Motory.

MOTOR, Motory.

MOTOR OCULI EXTER'NUS, *Nervus tim'idus,* (F.) *Nerf oculo-musculaire externe* (Ch.), *Nerf moteur oculaire externe, Sixth pair of nerves,* arises from the furrow which separates the pons Varolii from the medulla oblongata. It enters the cavernous sinus; anastomoses on the outside of the carotid artery with two filaments furnished by the superior cervical ganglion; enters the orbit by the sphenoidal fissure, and is lost on the rectus externus oculi. This pair is, also, called *Abducentes.*

MOTO'RES OCULO'RUM, *Moto'rii Oculorum, Ocula'res commu'nes, Ophthal'mici exter'ni, Common Oculo-muscular Nerves,* (F.) *Nerfs moteurs oculaires communs,* (Ch.,) The *third pair of nerves.* This nerve arises from a depression at the inner side of the peduncles of the brain, between the tuber annulare and corpora mammillaria. It enters the outer part of the cavernous sinus, and passes into the orbitar cavity. Behind the sphenoidal fissure, it divides into two branches; the one *superior,* and the other *inferior.* The *former* is lost on the rectus superior oculi and the levator palpebræ superioris; the *latter*—the larger of the two—divides into three branches, which pass to the rectus internus, rectus inferior, and lesser oblique. The last furnishes a filament, which passes to the ophthalmic.ganglion.

MOTORIAL, Motory.

MO'TORY, *Motive, Motor, Moto'rial, Motrix, Kinet'ic* or *Cinet'ic,* (F.) *Moteur.* That which moves or causes movement, as *motor nerves*, in contradistinction to *sensory*.

MOTOS, Linteum, Tent.

MOTO'SIS, μοτος, 'charpie.' The application of charpie to a wound.

MOTRICITÉ, Motility.

MOTRIX, Motory.

MOTTE, Mons veneris.

MOTUM, Carbasus, Linteum.

MOTUS, Motion — m. Assimilationis, Plastic force — m. Automaticus, see Automatic — m. Compressorius, Peristole — m. Cordis diastalticus, Diastole — m. Hæmorrhoidalis, Hæmorrhois — m. Intestinorum, Borborygmus — m. Involuntarius, see Autocinesis — m. Peristalticus, Peristole — m. Testudineus, Peristole — m. Vermicularis, Peristole — m. Voluntarius, Autocinesis.

MOUCHE, Cantharis — *m. d'Espagne*, Cantharis.

MOUCHER L'ACTION DE, Munctio.

MOUCHES, see Pains, labour — *m. Volantes*, see Metamorphopsia.

MOUCHETURE, see Scarification.

MOUCHOIR EN TRIANGLE, Couvrechef, see Bandeau.

MOUFETTE, see Mephitism.

MOULD, Fontanella.

MOULE, Mytilus edulis.

MOULEUR, Muller.

MOULTING, Desquamation.

MOUREILLER, Malpighia mourella.

MOURON DES OISEAUX, Alsine media — *m. Rouge*, Anagallis.

MOUSE-EAR, Alsine media, Hieracium pilosella.

MOUSE-SIGHT, Myopia.

MOUSSE DE CORSE, Corallina Corsicana — *m. d'Island*, Fucus crispus — *m. Perlée*, Fucus crispus.

MOUSSERON, see Agaric.

MOUSSEUX, Frothy.

MOUSTACHE, Mystax.

MOÛT DE LA BIÈRE, Wort.

MOUTARDE, Sinapis.

MOUTH, Sax. muð, *Os, Cavum Oris, Stoma*, (F.) *Bouche*. This word sometimes signifies the cavity situate between the jaws, and containing the tongue, &c.; — at others, the outer orifice of that cavity. The mouth, in the first acceptation, *Cav'itas* seu *Spa'tium Oris*, is the cavity ; bounded, *above*, by the palatine arch; *below*, by the tongue; *before*, by the lips; and *behind*, by the velum palati and pharynx. The sides of the mouth and the organs it contains are lined by a mucous membrane. The *anterior* aperture of the mouth is, sometimes, called *facial* — the posterior, *pharyngeal*. In the mouth are the teeth, gums, alveolar margins, tongue; the excretory ducts of the salivary glands, and those of a number of mucous follicles, &c. It is in this cavity that the food is cut, torn, or bruised by the teeth; is impregnated with saliva, and formed into a mass or *bolus*, which is then subjected to the act of deglutition. The mouth contains the organs of taste; and it serves in respiration, articulation, expectoration, suction, &c.

The condition of the mouth requires to be attended to in *Semeiology*. The state of the mucous membrane, like that of the tongue, indicates the condition of the membrane of the alimentary canal generally.

MOUTH, *Os, Apertura, Orific"ium, Hia'tus, Peristo'mium*, is, also, applied to the open extremities of vessels or other canals.

MOUTH ROOT, Coptis — m. Sore, Aphthæ — m. Watering, see Salivation.

MOUVEMENT, Motion.

MOVEMENT, Motion.

MOXA, *Moxibu'rium*. A word by which the Chinese and Japanese designate a cottony substance, which they prepared by beating the dried leaves of the *Artemisia moxa*, — a kind of mugwort. With this down they form a cone, which is placed upon the part intended to be cauterized, and is set fire to at the top. The heat and pain gradually increase, in proportion as the combustion proceeds downwards, until ultimately an eschar may be formed. In Europe and this country, the same operation is usually practised with a cylinder of cotton-wool, or with one formed from the pith of the greater sun-flower. This mode of cauterization is employed as a powerful counter-irritant; which it assuredly is. Sloughing may be in some measure prevented, according to Baron Larrey, by the application of liquid ammonia to the burnt part.

The term moxa has been extended to any substance, which by gradual combustion on or near the skin is employed as a counter-irritant.

MOXIBURIUM, Moxa.

MOXIBUS'TION, *Moxibus'tio, Encau'sis*. Mode of cauterization by means of moxa.

MOXON'S EFFERVESCING MAGNESIA, see Magnesia, effervescing, Moxon's.

MUCAGO, Liquor sanguinis, Mucilage.

MUCARUM, Mucharum.

MUCCINIUM, Mucilage.

MUCEDO, Mucilage.

MUCHA'RUM, *Muca'rum*. A barbarous term, formerly used for an aqueous infusion of roses, sweetened, and evaporated to the consistence of syrup.

MUCIFIC, Blennogenous.

MU'CIFORM, *Muciform'is, Myxo'des, Blenno'des, Blennoï'des, Blennoï'deus*, from *mucus*, and *forma*, 'form.' Resembling mucus in character or appearance.

MU'CILAGE, *Mucila'go, Muca'go, Muce'do, Muccin'ium*, from the Lat. *mucus*, — itself presumed to be from *mungere*, 'to wipe the nose.' A mixture of gum and a small quantity of matter analogous to mucus, which is found in abundance in linseed, quince-seed, &c. It is obtained by beating with water the parts, or products, of plants which contain it. It is much used in the preparation of emollient cataplasms and the greater part of the demulcent *tisanes*.

MUCILAGE, see Liquor sanguinis — m. Animal, Mucus — m. of Quince-seeds, Decoctum cydoniæ — m. of Rice, see Oryza — m. of Sassafras Pith. Infusum sassafras medullæ — m. Starch, Mucilago amyli.

MUCILAGINEUX, Mucilaginous.

MUCILAG"INOUS, *Mucilagino'sus, Gummo'sus, Gummio'des, Gummido'des*, (F.) *Mucilagineux*. Gummy. Resembling gum. That which possesses the character of mucilage.

MUCILAGO, Mucilage, Synovia.

MUCILAGO ACA'CIÆ, *M. Acaciæ Arab'icæ, M. Gummi Arab'icæ, Mucilage of aca'cia, M. of gum Arabic*. (*Acaciæ gum.* contus. ʒiv ; *aq. bullient.* Oss. Rub the gum with the water gradually added.) Demulcent. To allay cough ; but, chiefly, to suspend insoluble matters in water, &c.

MUCILAGO AM'YLI, *Starch mucilage*. (*Amyli*, ʒiij ; *aquæ*, Oj. Rub the starch with the water gradually added ; then boil till it forms a mucilage. — *Ph. L.*) Demulcent. Generally given per anum.

MUCILAGO ARTICULORUM seu JUNCTURARUM, Synovia.

MUCILAGO ASTRAG'ALI TRAGACAN'THÆ, *M. tragacanthæ* (Ph. U. S.), *M. gummi tragacanthæ, Mucilage of tragacanth*. (*Gummi tragacanth.* ʒj ; *aquæ bullient.* Oj. Macerate for 24 hours; triturate till the gum is dissolved, and press through linen.) For pharmaceutical purposes.

MUCILAGO CRETICA, Misturæ cretæ—m. Gummi Arabici, M. acaciæ—m. Seminis cydonii mali, Decoctum cydonii—m. Gummi tragacanthæ, M. astragali tragacanthæ—m. Tragacanthæ, M. astragali tragacanthæ.

MUCIN, Mucus.

MUCIP'AROUS, *Mucip'arus*, from *mucus*, and *pario*, 'I bring forth.' Mucous-producing; as *muciparous* glands or follicles.

MUCKSWEAT, Desudatio.

MUCOCE'LE, *Hernia sacci lacryma'lis*, from *mucus*, and *κηλη*, 'rupture.' An enlargement or protrusion of the mucous membrane of the lachrymal passages, giving occasion to fistula lacrymalis. Also, dropsy of the lachrymal sac.

MUCO-ENTERITIS, see Enteritis.

MUCO-PU'RULENT, *Muco-purulen'tus, Pyoblen'nicus*, from *mucus*, and *pus*. Having the character or appearance of mucus and pus.

MUCOR, Euros, Mucus—m. Narium, Nasal mucus.

MUCOSITAS, Mucus.

MUCOS'ITY, *Mucos'itas*. A fluid, which resembles mucus, or contains a certain quantity of it.

MUCOUS, *Muco'sus*. An epithet for all bodies containing mucilage or mucus. It is, also, sometimes used synonymously with gummy. In *pathology*, it is occasionally employed to express the seat of a disease, as *mucous disease, mucous phlegmasia;* that is, having its seat in a mucous membrane.

MUCOUS CORPUSCLES, see Mucus—m. Layer, see *Tache embryonnaire*—m. Membranes, see Membranes—m. Web, Corpus mucosum.

MUCRO, Apex.

MUCRO seu *Cor'yphé* seu *Fundus* seu *Vertex Cordis.* The apex or point of the heart.

MUCRO HUMERI, Acromion.

MUCRONATA CARTILAGO, Xiphoid cartilage.

MUCRONATUM OS, Xiphoid cartilage.

MU'CULENT, *Muculen'tus*, from *mucus*. Slimy, viscid.

MUCUNA, see Dolichos pruriens—m. Pruriens, Dolichos pruriens—m. Prurita, see Dolichos.

MUCUS, *Mucor, Muco'sus humor, Mucos'itas, Myxa, Mycus, Lapé, Pitui'ta, Zoömy'cus, Zoomyx'a, Pit'uite, Animal mucus, Blenna, Animal mucilage,* (F.) *Muqueux animal, Morve, Mucilage animal,* presumed to be from *mungere,* 'to wipe the nose.' A substance, analogous to vegetable mucilage; from which, however, it differs, by affording subcarbonate of ammonia on distillation. Mucus exudes through the skin, in a state of combination with a peculiar oily matter; and, drying, forms the epidermis. It constitutes, in part, the different epidermeous productions, as the hair, nails, wool, and horn of animals, feathers of birds, and scales of fish. It is found at the surface of the mucous membranes, and presents some difference in its composition and properties, according to the particular mucous membrane from which it is obtained. Its chief organic constituent is an albuminous compound, — *mucin*. Mucus preserves the membranes moist, and in a state best fitted for the performance of their functions. The French give the term *glaire* to the thick, stringy mucus, secreted by the mucous membranes when in a state of disease.

When mucus is examined with the microscope it is found to contain numerous epithelial scales or flattened cells; together with round, granular bodies, which are commonly termed *mucous corpuscles* or *mucous globules.*

MUCUS CARPHODES, see Carphodes—m. Catharticus, Lichen Islandicus—m. Malpighii, Corpus mucosum—m. Narium, Nasal mucus.

MUD-APPLE PLANT, Solanum melongena.

MUDAR, *Madar*. The *Calotropis mudarii seu madarii;* or, according to the generality of authorities, the *C. gigante'a* or *Ascle'pias gigante'a.* In the Hindoo practice of physic, the bark of the root, as well as the concrete juice of the plant, enters into various compound formulæ for the cure of elephantiasis and many other disorders. Experiments instituted by Dr. Duncan, jr., exhibit its properties to be like those of ipecacuanha.

MUDGE'S INHALER, see Inhaler.

MUGUET, Aphthæ, Convallaria maialis—*m. des Bois*, Asperula odorata—*m. de Mai*, Convallaria maialis.

MUGWORT, Artemisia vulgaris.

MULÂTRE, Mulatto.

MULATTO, (F.) *Mulâtre*, (S.) *Mulata*. An individual of the human species engendered of a white and black race; from *mulus,* 'a mule.' The following table exhibits the proportion of white blood in the various castes,—arising from the hybridous admixture of white and black,—according to the principles sanctioned by usage.

PARENTS.	OFFSPRING.	DEGREE OF MIXTURE.	
Negro and White,	Mulatto,	1-2 White,	1-2 black.
White and Mulatto,	Terceron,	3-4 ——	1-4 ——
Negro and Mulatto,	{ Griffo, Griff, or Zambo, òr Black Terceron, }	1-4 ——	3-4 ——
White and Terceron,	Quarteron or Quadroon,	7-8 ——	1-8 ——
Negro and Terceron,	Black Quarteron or Quadroon,	1-8 ——	7-8 ——
White and Quarteron,	Quinteron,	15-16 ——	1-16 ——
Negro and Black Quarteron,	Black Quinteron,	1-16 ——	15-16 ——

The last two were considered to be respectively white and black, in the British West India Islands; and the former, prior to modern changes, were white by law, and consequently free. See Half-caste.

MULBERRY CALCULUS, see Calculi, urinary—m. Rash, see Typhus—m. Red, Morus rubra—m. Tree, Morus nigra—m. Wild, Morus rubra.

MULES (F.), *Mulæ*. Chilblains on the heels.

MULGE'DIUM ACUMINA'TUM, *Lactu'ca villo'sa, Blue Lettuce;* and

MULGE'DIUM FLORIDA'NUM, *Lactu'ca Florida'na, Sonchus Florida'nus, False Lettuce;* indigenous plants; *Order,* Compositæ; have the reputation of curing the bites of rattlesnakes.

MULIEBRIA, Menses, Vulva.

MULIEBRITY, Mulieritas.

MULIEBROS'ITAS, *Philogyn'ia*, from *mulier,* 'a woman,' *muliebra,* 'appertaining to women.' Fondness for women. Hence, *Muliebro'sus, Muliera'rius,* and *Muliero'sus;* one who is fond of women.

MULIEBROSUS, see Muliebrositas

MULIERARIUS, see Muliebrositas.
MULIE'RITAS, *Mulieb'rity, Womanhood*, from *mulier*, 'a woman.' The state of puberty in the female.
MULIEROSUS, see Muliebrositas.
MULIER PLENA, Pregnant.
MULLED WINE, see Wine.
MULLEIN, BLACK, Verbascum nigrum—m. Broad-leaved, great, Verbascum nigrum — m. Yellow, Verbascum nigrum.
MULLER, (F.) *Mouleur*. A moulder. A stone held in the hand, with which any powder is ground upon a flat horizontal stone. It is sometimes called *mullet*, (F.) *Mollette*.
MULLIGRUBS, Tormina, Colic.
MULOMEDICINA, Veterinary art.
MULOMEDICUS, see Hippiater.
MULSA ACIDA, Oxyglycus.
MULSUM, Hydromeli—m. Vinosum, Œnomel.
MULTIFIDUS SPINÆ, Transversalis dorsi.
MULTIFŒTA'TION, *Multifœta'tio*, from *multus*, 'many,' and *fœtus*. Pregnancy with more than two fœtuses.
MULTILOC'ULAR, *Multilocula'ris*, from *multus*, 'many,' and *loculus*, 'a cell.' Having many cells or cavities.
MULTIMAM'MÆ, from *multus*, 'many,' and *mamma*, 'a breast.' A variety of hypergenesis, in which there are supernumerary mammæ.
MULTIP'AROUS, (F.) *Multipare*, from *multus*, 'many,' and *parire*, 'to bring forth.' One that brings forth several young at the same time. Such a birth is called *plural*.
MULTITUDO, Plethora.
MULTIVORANTIA, Polyphagia.
MUMIA, Mummy.
MUMMIFICA'TION, from *mummy*, and *fio*, 'to make.' *Sceleteu'sis*. The mode of preparing a mummy.
MUMMY, *Mumia*, Arab. *Moumya*, from *mum*, 'wax.' *Rebolea*, *Rebona*, (F.) *Momie*. A dead body simply dried, or dried after having been embalmed. The latter acceptation is the most common. Formerly, the Egyptian mummy was extolled as useful in contusions. It was presumed, also, to have healing, tonic, and resolvent properties. It is now only regarded as an archaical curiosity.
MUMPS, Cynanche parotidea.
MUNC'TIO, *Apomex'is*, (F.) *l'Action de moucher*. The act of blowing the nose.
MUNDIFICANTIA, Detergents.
MUNDIFICATIVA, Detergents.
MUND'TIA SPINO'SA. A plant of the *Nat. Ord.* Polygaleæ, which grows in Southern Africa, and a decoction of whose branches is used in atrophy, phthisis, &c.
MUNGOS RADIX, Ophiorrhiza mungos.
MUNIMENTUM CASTITATIS, Hymen.
MUQUEUX ANIMAL, Mucus.
MUR, Coryza.
MURAL, *Mura'lis*, from *murus*, 'a wall.' Vesical calculi are so called when rugous and covered with tubercles or asperities. They are composed of oxalate of lime.
MURE, Moro, see Morus nigra.
MU'RIA, *Halmē*, *Salsila'go*, *Brine*, (F.) *Saumure*. This was formerly used as a glyster in dysentery, in certain inveterate neuralgiæ, &c.
MURIA, Soda, muriate of.
MURIAS AURICO-NATRICUM, see Gold.
MURIATE D'AMMONIAQUE, Ammoniæ murias—m. *d'Ammoniaque et de fer*, Ferrum ammoniatum—m. *d'Or*, Gold, muriate of, see Gold.
MURIAT'IC AC''ID, from *muria; Ac''idum salis, Spir'itus salis mari'ni, Sp. salis Glaube'ri, Acidum mari'num concentra'tum, Acidum salis culina'ris, Acidum salis marini, Spir'itus salis ac''idus* seu *fumans, Acidum hydrochlor'icum* seu *muriaticum, Spirit of salt*, (F.) *Acide hydrochlorique* ou *muriatique*. An aqueous solution of chlorohydric acid gas of s. g. 1.16. The odour of muriatic acid is suffocating; taste very acid and caustic. It is nearly colourless when pure; but commonly of a pale yellow; volatile; the fumes visible. Muriatic acid is possessed of tonic and antiseptic properties. It is used in typhus; cutaneous eruptions; in gargles for inflammatory and putrid sore throats, (gtt. xxx to f℥vj of water,) &c. When added to a pediluvium, it renders it stimulating.
ACIDUM MURIAT'ICUM DILU'TUM of the *Ph. U. S.* contains four ounces, by measure, of muriatic acid to twelve ounces of distilled water.
MURIDE, Bromine.
MURIER NOIR, Morus nigra.
MURIGENE, Chlorine.
MURINA, Bromine.
MURMUR, (F.) *Murmure*. A word existing both in the Romanic and Teutonic languages, and probably a variety of onomatopœia;—*mur mur* expressing the kind of sound which the word indicates. A low continued or continuously repeated sound, as that of flame, or of a stream running over a stony bottom.
MURMUR AURIUM, Tinnitus Aurium—m. Intestinale seu intestinorum seu Ventris, Borborygmus.
MURMUR, RES'PIRATORY. The noise heard during inspiration and expiration, especially the former. It is produced by the passage of the air through the bronchial tubes and into the air-cells. It has been also called *murmur of the expansion of the lungs;* and, when distinctly vesicular, *Respiration of the cells* or *vesicular respiration*, (F.) *Respiration vésiculaire*. Vesicular respiration is of course absent when the cells of the lungs have been obliterated from any cause. We may then have the *Respiration nulle, Absence du bruit respiratoire, Silence*, and *Respiration silencieuse* of the French writers.
At times, it is rude during inspiration or expiration, or both — the *Respiration rude* or *R. râpeuse* of the French. At others, there is a *blowing* sound, (F.) *Souffle, Respiration soufflante*, as if some one were blowing into the auscultator's ear through a tube. This is heard in the healthy state over the larynx, trachea, and about the bifurcation of the bronchia; but when it proceeds from the lungs it denotes disease. It may be *tubular* or *diffused*. In the former, the *whiffing murmurs* appear to occur in a space limited to the immediate neighbourhood of the part examined. In the latter, they are produced with but moderate intensity, and sometimes at a distance from the ear, over a tolerably extended space.
The respiration, perceived over the trachea and bronchia in health, is called *tracheal* or *bronchial* or *tubal*, (F.) *Respiration bronchique, Souffle tubaire*, according to the situation in which it is heard.
MURMUR, UTERINE, *Bruit placentaire* — m. Utero-placental, *Bruit placentaire*.
MURMUR, WHIFFING, see Murmur, respiratory.
MURR, *Murrain*, from A. S. mȳrnhan, 'to destroy,' or from (L.) *mori*, 'to die.' (F.) *Clavean, Clavelée, Pestilential Fever*. An epizootic, perhaps contagious, disease, having some resemblance to small-pox, which affects cattle — especially sheep; and is said to have been transferred to man.
MURRAIN, Coryza, Murr.
MURREN, Coryza.
MUSA, M. Paradisiaca — m. Cliffortiana, M. Paradisiaca—m. Mensaria, M. Paradisiaca.
MUSA PARADISI'ACA, *Musa, M. Mensa'ria* seu

Cliffortia'na, Amusa, Palma hu'milis, Ficus In'dica, Bata, Plat'anus. The *Plantain tree.* Family, Musaceæ. *Sex. Syst.* Hexandria Monogynia. It grows in many parts of India and South America. The fruit, which is largely eaten for bread, consists of a mealy substance. It is clammy; has a sweetish taste, and will dissolve in the mouth without chewing. The whole spike of fruit often weighs forty or fifty pounds. The leaves of the tree serve the Indians for tablecloths and napkins. Being smooth and soft, they are also employed as dressings for blisters. The water from the soft trunk is astringent, and sometimes used in diarrhœa.

MUSA SAPIEN'TUM. The *Bana'na tree, Baco'ba*, (F.) *Bananier, Bacove.* This differs somewhat from the last. The fruit, *Bana'na*, (S.) *Platano*, is shorter, straighter, and rounder; the pulp softer and of a more luscious taste. When ripe, it is very agreeable; it is eaten like the plantain, and relished by all ranks of people in the West Indies. Both varieties are natives of Guinea.

MUSC, Musk.
MUSCA HISPANICA, Cantharis.
MUSCÆ ENTO-HYALOID, see Metamorphopsia—m. Volitantes, see Metamorphopsia.
MUSCADE, see Myristica moschata.
MUSCADIER, Myristica moschata.
MUSCERDA, Moschardina.
MUSCLE, *Mus'culus, Torus, Mys, Myon*, from μυς, 'a rat;' because, say some etymologists, the ancients compared the muscles to flayed rats. According to Diemerbroeck, Douglass, Chaussier, &c., μυων comes rather from μυειν, 'to close,' 'to move,' &c., a function proper to muscles. This etymon is the more probable. Muscles have been divided into those of *Animal life* or *of the life of relation — voluntary muscles —* which execute movements under the influence of the will; as the muscles of the limbs, head, trunk, &c., and into those of *organic life—involuntary muscles—* which contract under the influence of certain special stimuli; as the heart, fleshy fibres of the stomach, &c. *Mixed muscles* are those which belong partly to each of these divisions;—as the muscles of respiration; the sphincters, &c. Muscles that act in opposition to each other are called *antagonists;* thus, every extensor has a flexor for an antagonist, and conversely. Muscles that concur in the same action are termed *congenerous.* The muscles present numerous varieties in form, size, situation, use, &c., and have been divided, by some, into *long, broad,* and *short.* Each of these divisions comprises *simple* and *compound* muscles. *Simple* or *rectilinear muscles* have all their fibres in a similar direction, and only one body—as the *Sartorius, Pronator quadratus,* &c. *Compound muscles* are those which have only one belly and several tendons, as the flexors of the fingers and toes; or several bellies and several tendons,—as the biceps flexor cubiti, sacro-lumbalis, &c. To the compound muscles belong, also, the *radiated muscles.* Their fibres set out from a common centre, and are arranged like the radii of a circle;—such are the diaphragm, iliacus, temporal, &c. *Pennated* or *Penniform Muscles.* Their fibres are arranged in two rows, which are united at a median line, at greater or less angles; nearly as the feathers are inserted into a quill. The palmaris longus is one of these. *Semi-penniform muscles:* their fibres are oblique, as in the last case; but they are inserted only on one side of the tendon. *Hollow Muscles* are,— the heart, intestines, urinary bladder, &c.

Much difference has existed in the enumeration of muscles. Some authors reckon them at upwards of 400. Chaussier admits only 368. The greater part of them are in *pairs.* Very few are *asygous.*

TABLE OF THE MUSCLES, ARRANGED AFTER THE MANNER OF DR. BARCLAY, ACCORDING TO THEIR ACTIONS.

THE HEAD IS MOVED

Forwards by	*Backwards by*	*To either side by*
Platysma myoides, Sterno-mastoideus, Rectus anticus major, " " minor,	Part of trapezius, Splenius capitis, Complexus, Trachelo-mastoideus, Rectus posticus major, " " minor, Obliquus capitis superior.	Platysma myoides, Sterno-mastoideus, Part of trapezius, Splenius capitis, " colli, Trachelo-mastoideus, Complexus.
Assisted (when the lower jaw is fixed) by		
Mylo-hyoideus, Genio-hyoideus, Genio-hyo-glossus, Digastrici.		

THE NECK IS MOVED

Forwards by	*Backwards by*	*Laterally by*
Platysma myoides, Sterno-mastoideus, Digastricus, Mylo-hyoideus, Genio-hyoideus, Genio-hyo-glossus Omo-hyoidei, Sterno-hyoidei, Thyro-hyoidei, Rectus anticus minor, Longus colli.	Part of trapezius, Rhomboideus minor, Serratus posticus superior, Splenius capitis, " colli, Complexus, Trachelo-mastoideus, Transversalis colli, Inter-spinales colli, Semi-spinales colli, Rectus posticus major, " " minor, Obliquus capitis superior, " " inferior, Scaleni postici, Levator scapulæ.	Various combinations of those muscles which separately move it forwards and backwards, assisted by the scaleni, intertransversales, and recti laterales.

THE TRUNK IS MOVED

Forwards by
Rectus abdominis,
Pyramidalis,
Obliquus externus abdominis,
Obliquus internus,
Psoas magnus,
" parvus,

Assisted (when the arms are carried forwards) by
Pectoralis major,
" minor,
Serratus magnus.

Backwards by
Trapezius,
Rhomboideus major,
Latissimus dorsi,
Serratus posticus superior,
" " inferior,
Sacro-lumbalis,
Longissimus dorsi,
Spinales dorsi,
Semi-spinales dorsi,
Multifidus spinæ,
Inter-transversales dorsi et lumborum.

Laterally by
Obliquus externus,
" internus,
Quadratus lumborum,
Longissimus dorsi,
Sacro-lumbalis,
Serrati postici,
Latissimus dorsi

THE SCAPULA IS MOVED

Upwards by
Trapezius,
Levator scapulæ,
Rhomboidei.

Downwards by
Lower part of trapezius,
Latissimus dorsi,
Pectoralis minor.

Forwards by
Pectoralis minor,
Serratus magnus.

Backwards by
Part of trapezius,
Rhomboidei,
Latissimus dorsi.

THE HUMERUS IS MOVED

Forwards by
Part of deltoid,
Part of pectoralis major,

Assisted in some circumstances by
Biceps,
Coraco-brachialis.

Backwards by
Part of deltoid,
Teres major,
" minor,
Long head of triceps,
Latissimus dorsi.

Inwards by
Part of pectoralis major,
Latissimus dorsi.

Rotated inwards by
Subscapularis,

Assisted occasionally by
Pectoralis major,
Latissimus and teres major.

Outwards by
Supra-spinatus,
Infra-spinatus,
Teres minor.

THE FORE-ARM IS MOVED

Forwards by
Biceps,
Brachialis anticus,
Pronator teres,

Assisted by
Flexor carpi radialis,
" sublimis,
" ulnaris,
Supinator longus.

Backwards by
Triceps,
Anconeus.

Rotated inwards by
Pronator teres,
Flexor carpi radialis,
Palmaris longus,
Flexor sublimis,
Pronator quadratus,

Outwards by
Biceps,
Supinator brevis,
Extensor secundi internodii.

THE CARPUS IS MOVED

Forwards by
Flexor carpi radialis,
Palmaris longus,
Flexor sublimis,
" carpi ulnaris,
" profundus,
" longus pollicis.

Backwards by
Extensor carpi radialis longior,
Extensor carpi radialis brevior,
Extensor secundi internodii,
Indicator,
Extensor communis digitorum,
Extensor proprius pollicis.

Outwards by
Flexor carpi radialis,
Extensor carpi radialis longior,
Extensor carpi radialis brevior,
Extensor ossis metacarpi,
Extensor primi internodii.

Inwards by
Flexor sublimis,
" carpi ulnaris,
" profundus,
Extensor communis digitorum,
Extensor minimi digiti,
Extensor carpi ulnaris.

THE THUMB IS MOVED

Inwards and forwards, across the palm, by
Opponens pollicis,
Flexor brevis,
" longus

Outwards and backwards by
Extensor ossis metacarpi pollicis,
Extensor primi internodii,
Extensor secundi internodii.

Upwards and forwards, away from the other fingers, by
Abductor,

Assisted by part of the
Flexor brevis.

Backwards and inwards to the other fingers, by
Adductor,
Extensor primi internodii,
Extensor secundi internodii.

THE FINGERS ARE MOVED

Forwards, or flexed, by
Flexor sublimis,
" profundus,
Lumbricales,
Interossei,
Flexor brevis digiti minimi,
Abductor digiti minimi.

Backwards, or extended, by
Extensor communis,
" minimi digiti,
Indicator.

Outwards, to radial border, by
Abductor indicis,
" digiti minimi,
Interossei.

Inwards by
Abductor digiti minimi,
Interossei.

THE THIGH IS MOVED

Forwards by
Psoas magnus,
Iliacus,
Tensor vaginæ femoris,
Pectineus,
Adductor longus,
" brevis.

Backwards by
Gluteus maximus,
Part of gluteus medius,
Pyriformis,
Obturator internus,
Part of adductor magnus,
Long head of biceps,
Semi-tendinosus,
Semi-membranosus.

Inwards by
Psoas magnus,
Iliacus,
Pectineus,
Gracilis,
Adductor longus,
" brevis,
" magnus,
Obturator externus,
Quadratus femoris.

Outwards by
Tensor vaginæ femoris,
Gluteus maximus,
" medius,
" minimus,
Pyriformis.

THE THIGH IS ROTATED

Inwards by
Tensor vaginæ femoris,
Part of gluteus medius,

And, when the leg is extended, by
Sartorius,
Semi-tendinosus.

Outwards by
Gluteus maximus,
Part of gluteus medius,
Pyriformis,
Gemellus superior,
Obturator internus,
Gemellus inferior,
Quadratus femoris,
Obturator externus,
Psoas magnus,
Iliacus,
Adductor longus,
" brevis,
" magnus,
Biceps cruris, slightly.

THE LEG IS MOVED

Backwards, or flexed, by
Semi-tendinosus,
Biceps,
Semi-membranosus,
Gracilis,
Sartorius,
Popliteus.

Extended by
Rectus,
Crureus,
Vastus externus,
" internus.

THE FOOT IS MOVED

Forwards, or flexed, by
Tibialis anticus,
Extensor proprius pollicis,
Extensor longus digitorum,
Peroneus tertius.

Backwards, or extended by
Gastrocnemius,
Plantaris,
Soleus,
Flexor longus digitorum,
" longus pollicis,
Tibialis posticus,
Peroneus longus,
" brevis.

Inclined inwards by
Extensor proprius pollicis,
Flexor longus digitorum,
" longus pollicis,
Tibialis posticus.

Outwards by
Peroneus longus,
" brevis,
Extensor longus digitorum,
Peroneus tertius.

THE TOES ARE MOVED

Backwards, or flexed, by
Abductor pollicis,
Flexor brevis digitorum,
Abductor minimi digiti,
Flexor longus pollicis,
" digitorum,
" accessorius,
Lumbricales,
Flexor brevis pollicis,
Adductor pollicis,
Flexor brevis minimi digiti,
Interossei.

Forwards, or extended, by
Extensor longus digitorum,
Extensor proprius pollicis,
" brevis digitorum.

Inclined inwards by
Abductor pollicis,
Interossei.

Outwards by
Adductor pollicis,
" digiti minimi,
Interossei.

Muscles have been variously named. 1. *According to their uses*, as diaphragm, buccinator, extensors, flexors, adductors, abductors, levators, depressors, &c. 2. *According to their position*, as interspinales, interossei, subclavius, popliteus, anconeus, cubitalis, iliacus, temporalis, &c. 3. *According to their shape*, as trapezius, splenius, lumbricalis, serratus, digastric, deltoid, scalenus, rhomboides, &c. 4. *According to their dimensions*, as pectoralis major, rectus capitis anticus major, pectoralis minor, glutæus maximus, medius, and minimus. 5. *According to their direction*, as obliquus abdominis, transversalis abdominis, rectus femoris, rectus abdominis, &c. 6. *According to their composition*, as semi-membranosus, semi-tendinosus, complexus, &c. 7. *According to their attachments*, or the different points of the skeleton to which they are connected by means of tendons or aponeuroses; as sterno-cleido-mastoideus, sterno-hyoideus, &c. On this is grounded the nomenclature of M. Dumas, and that of Chaussier.

The end of the muscle, which adheres to the most fixed part, is usually called the *origin* or *head*, (F.) *Tête;* and that which adheres to the more moveable part, the *insertion* or *tail*, (F.) *Queue;* the intervening part or *body* of the muscle being called the *venter* or *belly, Venter mus'culi, Me'dium mus'culi:* hence the names gastrocnemii, digastricus, biceps, and triceps; according as they have two bellies, two or three heads, &c.

Muscles are formed,— 1. Essentially of the *muscular* or *fleshy fibre*, (see Muscular Fibre.) 2. Of *Areolar tissue*, which unites together the fibres. This areolar tissue is not very visible between the fine and loose fibres; but becomes more so, when they unite in more considerable fasciculi. It forms, moreover, to each muscle, an external envelope, which unites it to the neighbouring parts, and admits of its motion. This envelope was formerly called *Tu'nica propria musculo'rum.* 3. Of *Arteries.* These proceed from neighbouring trunks, and are, generally, very large. Their size and number are always in proportion to the bulk of the muscle. With the exception of some viscera, as the lungs and the kidneys, there are few organs that receive as much blood as the muscles. 4. Of *Veins.* They follow the same course in the muscles as the arteries. Bichat asserts that they are generally devoid of valves. 5. Of *Lymphatics.* Of these we know little, and cannot easily follow them between the fleshy fibres. 6. Of *Nerves.* These are numerous, and of different sizes. They, almost all, proceed from the encephalon; some, however, issue from ganglions, and accompany the arteries. In general, they penetrate the fleshy tissue along with the vessels, to which they are narrowly united. After they have entered the muscles, they divide and subdivide until they are lost sight of.

MUSCLE CANIN, Levator anguli oris — *m. Cannelé*, Ischio-trochanterianus.

MUSCLE OF GAVARD. The oblique muscular fibres of the stomach.

MUSCLE GRAND FESSIER, Glutæus major—m. of Guthrie, Compressor Urethræ—m. of Herner, Tensor Tarsi—m. of Houston, Compressor venæ dorsalis penis — *m. très Large du dos*, Latissimus dorsi—m. of Wilson, Compressor urethræ.

MUS'CULAR, *Muscula'ris, Musculo'sus, Toro'sus.* That which belongs or relates to the muscles. Well furnished with muscles.

MUSCULAR AR'TERIES. Arteries that are distributed to the muscles. The name, *Muscular Arteries of the eye*, has been especially given to two branches sent off by the ophthalmic artery: —the one, *inferior*, which furnishes branches to the rectus inferior oculi, lachrymal sac, &c., and some of the anterior ciliary arteries: the other —the *superior*, which is sometimes wanting; but, when it exists, gives branches to the rectus superior oculi and levator palpebræ superioris.

MUSCULAR CONTRAC'TION. The exertion of the power, possessed by muscles, of shortening themselves, or of contracting to produce motion:— *muscular motion* being the change in the situation and relation of organs, induced by muscular contraction. When a muscle contracts, its fibres assume more the zigzag direction, and the extremities approximate; but the bulk of the whole muscle is not augmented. This contraction takes place, at times, with extreme velocity: a single thrill, in the letter R, can be pronounced in the 1-30,000th part of a minute. The *force* of contraction, *Myody'namis*, depends upon the healthy physical condition of the muscle, combined with due energy of the brain. The *duration*, in voluntary motion, is for a certain time dependent upon the will:—contractions, excited involuntarily, cannot be so long maintained.

MUSCULAR FIBRE, *Fleshy fibre, Filum muscula'rē, Fibril'la muscula'ris.* A name given to the filaments, which, by their union, form the muscles. This fibre is flat, soft, downy, linear, little elastic, more or less red; and arranged in zigzag according to its length, which is variable. It is firmer in adults than in the young or the aged; of the same size in the great and small muscles; and runs its course without bifurcation or ramification. It is but slightly resisting in the dead body, tearing readily; but during life it supports very great efforts without laceration. It is, itself, composed of a considerable number of fibrils, similar to each other, and subdividing almost *ad infinitum.* The ultimate filaments into which the fibre can be decomposed by mechanical means seem to be hollow or tubular. The fibre exists under two forms, the *striated* or *striped*, and the *non-striated, smooth* or *unstriped;* the muscles composed of the former ministering, as a general rule, to the *animal functions,—* the latter always, perhaps, to the *organic.* The colour of the muscular fibres is red in man, and white in several animals. A greater or less number, — united in fasciculi, *Fascic'uli seu Lacer'ti musculo'rum*, approximated to each other, and forming a distinct mass, of very variable size and shape, the extremities being attached to bones by means of tendons,—constitutes a muscle. In this are included areolar membrane, vessels and nerves. See Muscle.

MUSCULAR NERVES. The nerves distributed to the muscles are so named. Winslow calls the 4th pair of nerves — *Nerf musculaire oblique supérieur.*

MUSCULAR SYSTEM. A term given to the aggregate of the muscles of the body.

MUSCULAR VEINS. These bring back the blood, which has been carried to the muscles by the muscular arteries.

MUSCULARIS, Corroborant.

MUSCULA'TION, see Locomotion.

MUSCULI ACCESSORII AD SACRO-LUMBALEM, see Sacro-lumbalis—m. Papillares, Columnæ carneæ—m. Pectinati, Pectinated muscles.

MUS'CULO-CUTA'NEOUS, *Mus'culo-cuta'neus*, from *musculus*, 'a muscle,' and *cutis*, 'skin.' That which appertains to muscles and skin.

MUSCULO-CUTANEOUS NERVE. This name is especially given to two nerves;— the one, the *External cutaneous nerve*, furnished by the brachial plexus (see Cutaneous:—) the other, given off from the popliteus externus, (F.) *Nerf Scia-*

teus, Poplité externe, Prétibio digital, (Ch.) It descends on the anterior and outer part of the leg,—at first, hid among the muscles; becomes superficial about the middle of the leg; and divides into two branches, which pass superficially on the back of the foot. Two musculo-cutaneous nerves—superior and inferior—proceed from the first lumbar. The *superior musculo-cutaneous — il'io-scrotal, il'io-hypogas'tricus* — which divides into two branches,—abdominal and scrotal. The *inferior musculo-cutaneous* is smaller than the superior, and is distributed as its name, *il'io-in'-guinal,* indicates.

MUSCULO-RACHIDÆ'US. Belonging or relating to muscles and to the spine. A name given to branches, furnished behind by the intercostal, lumbar, and sacral arteries, which are distributed to the spine and to the muscles of the neighbourhood.

MUSCULOSA EXPANSIO, Platysma myoides.

MUSCULO-SPIRAL NERVE, Radial nerve.

MUSCULOSUS, Muscular.

MUSCULUS ACCLIVIS, Obliquus internus abdominis—m. Auxiliarius, Pyramidalis abdominis—m. Constrictorius, Sphincter—m. Cutaneus, Platysma myoides—m. Eustachii, Laxator tympani—m. Fallopii, Pyramidalis abdominis—m. Femoris membranosus, Fascia lata—m. Patientiæ, Levator scapulæ—m. Penicillatus, Levator labii inferioris—m. Pyxoides terrestris, Lichen pyxidatus—m. Scandularius, Parathenar—m. Subcutaneus, Platysma myoides—m. Succenturiatus, Pyramidalis abdominis—m. Succingens, Diaphragm—m. Supercilii, Corrugator supercilii—m. Testicondus, Cremaster—m. Testis, Cremaster—m. Tubæ novæ, Circumflexus.

MUSCUS ARBOREUS, Lichen plicatus—m. Caninus, Lichen caninus—m. Cathartious, Lycopodium selago—m. Clavatus, Lycopodium—m. Corallinus, Corallina Corsicana—m. Cranii humani, Lichen saxatilis—m. Erectus, Lycopodium selago—m. Helminthocortos, Corallina Corsicana—m. Islandicus, Lichen islandicus—m. Marinus, Corallina Corsicana—m. Maritimus, Corallina—m. Pulmonarius quercinus, Lichen pulmonarius—m. Pyxidatus, Lichen pyxidatus—m. Villosus, Peristroma.

MUSEAU DE TANCHE, Os uteri.

MUSEUM ANATOM'ICUM, *Supel'lex anatom'ica.* An anatomical museum.

MUSHROOM, Fungus.

MUSIC, *Mu'sica,* (F.) *Musique,* from μουσα, *musa,* 'a song.' The art of producing harmonious and cadenced sounds; an art, which has, at times, been beneficially used in diseases, particularly in those of the mind; or on which the mind could act in a salutary manner.

MUSICOMA'NIA, *Musoma'nia,* from *music,* and *mania,* A variety of monomania in which the passion for music is carried to such an extent as to derange the intellectual faculties.

MUSING, LISTLESS, Aphelxia otiosa.

MUSIQUE, Music.

MUSK, *Moschus, Mosch* (Arab.), (F.) *Musc.* A peculiar concrete animal substance, of a very diffusible odour, bitter taste, and a deep brown colour: solid, and enclosed in a sac found near the anus of the *Moschus moschif'erus* or *Musk Deer.* It is possessed of stimulant and antispasmodic properties. Dose, gr. v to ʒj in bolus.

MUSK, ARTIFIC"IAL, *Moschus factit"ius, Resi'na Suc'cini.* (*Ol. succini rectif.* 1 part, *acid. nitric.* 4 parts. Digest;—a black matter will be deposited, which must be well washed with water.)

MUSKGRAPE FLOWER, Bulbus vomitorius.

MUSKMALLOW, Hibiscus abelmoschus.

MUSKROOT, Sumbul.

MUSKSEED, see Hibiscus abelmoschus.

MUSKWOOD, Thymiama.

MUSOMANIA, Musicomania.

MUSQUITO, Mosquito.

MUSSÆN'DA FRONDO'SA, *Belil'la, Bele'son.* A decoction of this plant has been esteemed refrigerant.

MUSSEL, Mytilus edulis.

MUSSITA'TIO, *Mussita'tion,* from *mussitare,* itself from *mussare,* 'to murmur.' A condition, in which the tongue and lips move, as in the act of speaking, but without sounds being produced. This sort of murmuring is an unfavourable sign in disease, as indicating great cerebral debility.

MUSTA'CEUM: from *Mustacea,* a kind of laurus used in making it. A kind of weddingcake used by the ancients, which consisted of meal, aniseed, cummin, and several other aromatics; its object—it has been conceived—being to prevent or remove the indigestion occasioned by too great indulgence at the marriage feast.

MUSTACHE, Mystax.

MUSTARD, BLACK, Sinapis—m. Clammy, Polanisia graveolens—m. Essence of, Whitehead's, see Sinapis—m. False, Polanisia graveolens—m. Hedge, Erysimum—m. Mithridate, Thlaspi campestre—m. Stinking hedge, Alliaria—m. Treacle, Thlaspi arvense—m. White, Sinapis alba—m. Wild, Sinapis arvensis.

MUSTELANEUS, Galeancon.

MUSTUM, Wort.

MUTACIS'MUS, *Mu'tacism,* from μυτακισμ, 'I use the letter m too frequently.' A vicious pronunciation; consisting, according to Sauvages, in the frequent repetition of the letters B, P, and M, which are substituted for others.

MUTA'TIO SEXÛS. A change or conversion of sex. A notion prevailed in antiquity that such a conversion was possible.

MUTEO'SIS. Under this name is comprehended every phenomenon of expression, voluntary and involuntary, which impresses the sight or touch.

MUTILA'TION, *Mutila'tio, Maiming,* from *mutilus,* 'broken.' The removal or privation of a limb, or of some other external part of the body. In all countries, this crime has been punished with severity.

MUTINUS, Penis.

MUTISME, Mutitas.

MU'TITAS, *mutus,* 'dumb.' *Obtumescen'tia, Ala'lia, Anau'dia, Dumbness, Speech'lessness,* (F.) *Mutisme, Mutité.* Impossibility of *articulating* sounds; although they can be elicited. Dumbness is often congenital, and united with deafness, of which it is an effect. In some cases it is accidental.

MUTITAS SURDO"RUM, *Apho'nia Surdorum, Surdomu'titas, Deaf-dumbness.* Speechlessness from deafness; congenital, or produced during infancy. The subjects of this affection are called *deaf-dumb,* (F.) *Sourds-muets.*

MUTITÉ, Mutitas.

MUTO, Penis.

MUTONIATUS, Membrosus.

MUTTERKORN, Ergot.

MUTTON TEA. Prepared from a pound of *mutton,* freed from the fat and cut into thin slices; and a pint and a half of boiling soft *water* poured over them, as in the case of beef tea; except that it requires to be boiled for half an hour after the maceration, before it is strained through a sieve.

MUTUNNUS, Priapus.

MYACANTHA; Ruscus.

MYALGIA, Cramp.

MYASTHENI'A, from μυς, 'a muscle,' and ασθενεια, 'debility.' Muscular debility.

MYCE, Occlusion.

MYCES, Fungus.
MYCHMUS, Suspirium.
MYCHTHISMUS, Moaning, Suspirium.
MYCODERM'A, *My'coderm;* from μυκης, 'a mushroom,' and δερμα, 'skin.' A cryptogamous growth, which constitutes the crusts of favus. See Porrigo favosa.
MYCODERMA CEREVISIÆ, Torula cerevisiæ.
MYCODES, Fungoid.
MYCORTHOPNŒ'A; from μυκος, 'mucus,' and ορθοπνοια, 'difficulty of breathing except when in the erect attitude.' Orthopnœa from excessive secretion of mucus in the air-passages —*Orthopnœa pituito'sa.*
MYCOSIS, Fungus.
MYCTERES, Myxæ, Nares.
MYCTEROPHONIA, Rhinophonia.
MYCTEROXE'ROTES; from μυκτηρες, 'the nares,' and ξηροτης, 'dryness.' *Na'rium sic'citas.* Dryness of the interior of the nose.
MYCUS, Mucus.
MYDE'SIS, from μυδαω, 'I abound with moisture.' In its most general sense, it means *corruption.* By some, it is used for a mucous discharge from inflamed eyelids.
MYDON, μυδων. Same etymon. Fungous or putrid flesh in certain fistulous ulcers. — Pollux. Also, flesh putrid from mouldiness.
MYDRI'ASIS, *Platycor'ia, Platycori'asis, Amydri'asis.* A name given by several writers to morbid dilatation of the pupil; and, by others, to weakness of sight, produced by hydrophthalmia; from μυδος, 'moisture.'
MYDRIAT'ICUS, *Mydriat'ic.* Relating to or causing dilatation of the pupil. Pereira.
MYELAL'GIA; from μυελος, 'the spinal marrow,' and αλγος, 'pain.' Pain in the spinal marrow.
MYELAPOPLEXIA, Apoplexia myelitica.
MYELATELI'A; from μυελος, 'the spinal marrow,' and ατελια, 'want of end or finish.' Incompleteness of the spinal marrow.
MYELATROPHIA, Tabes dorsalis.
MYÉLITE, Myelitis.
MYELI'TIS, *M. parenchymato'sa, M. spina'lis, Inflamma'tio medul'læ spina'lis, Spini'tis, Spinodorsi'tis, Notomyeli'tis, Rachiomyeli'tis, Rachialgi'tis,* (of some,) (F.) *Myélite, Inflammation de la moëlle épinière ou rachidienne,* from μυελος, 'the marrow,' and *itis,* denoting inflammation. Inflammation of the spinal marrow or its membranes;—indicated by deep-seated burning pain in the spine, with various nervous and vascular irregularities of function. It is not common. Dr. Marshall Hall proposes to call inflammation of the membranes of the brain *Meningitis;* that of the substance of the brain *Myelitis.*
MYELITIS SPINALIS, Myelitis — m. Exsudativa, Hydrorachis — m. Parenchymatosa, Myelitis.
MYELOCHYSIS, Hydrorachis.
MYELOGANGLIITIS, Cholera (sporadic.)
MYELOMA, see Encephaloid.
MYELOMALACIA, Mollities medullæ spinalis.
MYELOMYCES, see Encephaloid.
MYELON, Medulla spinalis.
MYELOPARALYSIS, Paraplegia.
MYELOPHTHISIS, Tabes dorsalis—m. Sicca, Tabes mesenterica.
MYELOPHY'MATA, *Tuber'cula medullæ spina'lis,* from μυελος, 'marrow,' and φυμα, 'a tubercle.' Tubercles of the spinal marrow.
MYELORRHAGIA, Apoplexia myelitica.
MYELOSPONGUS, see Encephaloid.
MYELUS, Marrow, Medulla spinalis — m. Dischenius, Medulla spinalis — m. Dorsites, Medulla spinalis — m. Notiæus, Medulla spinalis — m. Psoitæs, Medulla spinalis.

MYENERGI'A, from μυς, 'a muscle,' εν, and εργον, 'work.' Muscular strength.
MYGMUS, Suspirium.
MYIOCEPHALUM, Staphyloma.
MYIODEOPSIA, Metamorphopsia.
MYITIS, Myositis, Rheumatism, acute.
MYLACRI, Molar teeth.
MYLACRIS, Patella.
MYLE, Patella, Mole.
MYLICUS, Molar.
MYLODI, Molar teeth.
MYLODONTES, Molar teeth.
MYLO-GLOSSUS, from μυλη, 'the jaw,' and γλωσσα, 'the tongue.' Winslow has given this name to muscular fibres, which pass from the posterior part of the myloid line of the lower jaw, and from the sides of the base of the tongue to the parietes of the pharynx. These fibres belong to the constrictor superior pharyngis.
MYLO-HYOID LINE, see Mylo-hyoideus.
MYLO-HYOID FURROW OR GROOVE. A furrow which passes from the superior orifice of the inferior dental canal of the lower jaw, in the same direction as the canal, and lodges the *mylo-hyoid nerve,* a branch of the inferior-dental.
MYLO-HYOID NERVE, see Mylo-hyoid furrow.
MYLO-HYOIDEUS, from μυλη, 'the jaw,' and 'υοειδης, 'the os hyoides.' *Mylua'des,* (F.) *Mylohyoïdien.* The *Mylo-pharyngeus* of Morgagni and Santorini. This muscle is situate at the upper and anterior part of the neck, behind the lower jaw. It is broad, flat, and has the form of a truncated triangle. It arises from the *internal oblique. internal maxillary* or *mylo-hyoid line* of the lower jaw bone, and is inserted at the fore part of the body of the os hyoides. Its innermost fibres unite with those of the opposite side to form a raphe on the median line. The mylohyoideus raises the os hyoides and carries it forward, or it depresses the lower jaw.
MYLO-PHARYNGEUS, Constrictor pharyngis, Mylo-hyoideus.
MYLUODES, Mylo-hyoideus.
MYOCARDITIS, Carditis.
MYOCEPHALI'TIS, *Myi'tis cephal'ica;* from μυς, or μυων, 'a muscle,' κεφαλη, 'head,' and *itis,* denoting inflammation. Inflammation of the muscles of the head.
MYOCEPHALON, Staphyloma.
MYOCŒLIAL'GIA, from μυων, 'muscle,' κοιλια, 'abdomen,' and αλγεω, 'I suffer.' Pain in the muscles of the abdomen.
MYOCŒLI'TIS, *Myocœlii'tis, Inflamma'tio musculo'rum abdomina'lium,* from μυων, 'muscle,' κοιλια, 'lower belly,' and *itis,* denoting inflammation. Inflammation of the muscles of the abdomen.
MYODEOP'SIA, Metamorphopsia.
MYO'DES, from μυς, 'a muscle,' and ειδος, 'resemblance.' Like unto muscle. Muscular.
MYODESOPSIA, Metamorphopsia.
MYODYNA'MIA, *Vis muscula'ris;* from μυς, 'a muscle,' and δυναμις, 'power.' The force or power of a muscle.
MYODYNAMICS, see Muscular contraction.
MYODYNAMIOMETER, Dynamometer.
MYODYNAMOMETER, Dynamometer.
MYODYN'IA, from μυων, 'muscle,' and οδυνη, 'pain.' Pain in the muscles,—rheumatismal or other. Rheumatism.
MYODYNIA INFLAMMATORIA, Myositis.
MYOG'RAPHY, *Myogra'phia,* from μυων, 'muscle,' and γραφειν, 'to describe.' An anatomical description of the muscles.
MYOLEM'MA, *Myole'ma,* from μυων, 'a muscle,' and λεμμα, 'a coat.' The membranous tube

of each muscular fibre. It has also the same signification as Sarcolemma.

MY'OLINE, from μυων, 'a muscle.' A name given by Mr. Erasmus Wilson to a transparent substance that fills the cells, which, he conceives, by their juxtaposition form the ultimate muscular fibril.

MYOL'OGY, *Myolog"ia, Sarcolog'ia, Myosiolog"ia;* from μυων, 'a muscle,' and λογος, 'a discourse.' That part of anatomy which treats of the muscles.

MYON, Muscle.

MYONARCO'SIS, from μυων, 'a muscle,' and ναρκη, 'stupor.' Numbness of the muscles.

MYONITIS, Myositis.

MYON'OSUS, *Myonu'sos, Myopathi'a,* from μυων, 'a muscle,' and νοσος, 'disease.' A disease of the muscles.

MYOPALMUS, Subsultus tendinum.

MYOPATHIA, Myonosus.

MYOPE, Myops.

MYOPHO'NIA, from μυων, 'a muscle,' and φωνη, 'voice.' The sound of muscular contraction, — as that of the ventricles of the heart, during the systole of that organ.

MYO'PIA, *Myopi'asis, Luscios'itas, Myo'sis, Parop'sis propin'qua, Amblyo'pia dissito'rum, Dyso'pia dissito'rum, Dyspho'tia, Visus ju'venum,* from μυω, 'I close,' or from μυς, 'a mouse,' and ωψ, 'the eye;' *My'opy, Short-sightedness, Near-sightedness, Mouse-sight, Purblindness,* (F.) *Vue courte.* Persons who can only see objects very near. The defect is owing to the too great convexity of the eye, or too great density of the humours, and is palliated by wearing concave glasses.

MYOPI'C, *Myop'icus;* same etymon. *Short-sighted, Poreblind, Purblind.* Relating or appertaining to myopia.

MYOPODIORTHO'TICON, from μυωψ, 'one that is short-sighted,' and διορθωτικον, 'having power to correct.' An apparatus for the cure of short-sightedness. — A. A. Berthold.

MYOPS, *Luscio'sus, Myo'pus, My'ope.* Same etymon. One affected with myopia or short-sightedness.

MYOPY, Myopia.

MYORRHEX'IS, from μυς, 'a muscle,' and ρηξις, 'rupture.' Rupture of a muscle.

MYO'SIS, from μυω, 'I close.' *Microcor'ia.* Smallness of the pupil. *Phthi'sis pupilla'ris.* Permanent contraction of the pupil. It is usually caused by iritis, and is extremely difficult to cure. When it exists to such an extent as to obliterate the pupil, it is called *Synizesis.* Also, Myopia.

MYOSITÉ, Myositis.

MYOSIT'IC; *Myosit'icus,* from *Myosis.* Causing contraction of the pupil, — as opium. — Pereira.

MYOSI'TIS, *Myi'tis, Mysi'tis, Myoni'tis, Sarci'-tis, Rheumatis'mus phlegmono'des, Myodyn'ia inflammato'ria, Phlegma'sia myoïca, Inflammatio seu Phlegmonē Musculo'rum,* (F.) *Myosite, Inflammation des muscles,* from μυων, 'a muscle.' A name proposed by Sagar for inflammation of the muscles. Also, Rheumatism.

MYOSOTIS, Hieracium pilosella, Rheumatism, Rheumatism, acute.

MYOSPASMUS, Cramp.

MYOTIL'ITY, *Myotil'itas,* from μυων, 'a muscle.' Muscular contractility. — Chaussier.

MYOT'OMY, *Myotom'ia,* from μυων, 'a muscle,' and τεμνειν, 'to cut.' The part of practical anatomy which treats of the dissection of the muscles. Also, the surgical operation of the division of muscles to remove deformity.

MYOTYRBE, Chorea.

MYRAC'OPUM, from μυρον, 'an ointment,' and κοπος, 'fatigue.' An ointment used by the ancients in cases of fatigue.

MYREPSUS, Unguentarius.

MYR'IAGRAMME, from μυρια, '10,000,' and γραμμα, 'gramme.' A weight equal to 10,000 grammes, or to 26 pounds, 9 ounces, and 6 drachms Troy.

MYRIAMÈTRE. A measure of 10,000 mètres; equal to 16 miles, 1 furlong, 156 yards, and 14 inches.

MYRICA ASPLENIFOLIA, Comptonia asplenifolia — m. Cerifera, see Cera flava et alba, and Wax, myrtle.

MYRI'CA GALE, *Myrtus Braban'tica seu Ang'-lica, Myri'ca palus'tris, Myrtifo'lia Bel'gica, Gale, Gagel, Rhus sylves'tris, Ac'aron, Elæag'nus, E. Cordo, Chamælæog'nus, Dodonæ'a, Dutch myrtle, Sweet gale, Sweet willow, Candleberry myrtle,* (F.) *Piment Royal, Thé de Simon Pauli, Gale odorant.* Family, Amentaceæ. *Sex. Syst.* Diœcia Tetrandria. The leaves, flowers, and seeds have a strong, fragrant smell, and a bitter taste. They are used for destroying moths and cutaneous insects. The infusion is given internally as a stomachic and vermifuge.

MYRICA PALUSTRIS, M. Gale.

MYRINGA, see Tympanum.

MYRINGI'TIS, *Inflamma'tio tym'pani;* from *Myringa,* 'the membrana tympani;' and *itis,* denoting inflammation. Inflammation of the membrana tympani; and, also, of the tympanum.

MYRINX, see Tympanum.

MYRIS, *Myrothē'cē, Narthe'cia, Narthe'cium, Narthex,* from μυρον, 'a perfumed oil or ointment.' A perfumed oil or ointment box or jar.

MYRIS'TICA, *M. Moscha'ta, M. aromat'ica seu officina'lis seu fragrans, Comacon. Nat. Ord.* Myristiceæ. The tree which produces the nutmeg and mace. (F.) *Muscadier.* The *Nutmeg, Myristica,* (Ph. U. S.) *Myris'ticæ nu'cleus, Myris'ticæ moscha'tæ nu'cleus, Nux moscha'ta seu unguenta'ria, Nucis'ta, Nux myris'tica, Chrysobal'-anus Gale'ni, Unguenta'ria, As'sala, Nux aromat'ica,* (F.) *Muscade,* is the seed or kernel. It has a fragrant, aromatic odour; an agreeable pungent taste, and is much used for culinary purposes. Alcohol extracts its active matter. It has the properties of aromatics in general; being stimulant and stomachic. The oil—*O'leum myris'ticæ*—possesses the virtues of the nutmeg. Dose of the nutmeg, gr. v. to ℈j;—of the oil gtt. iij to gtt. vj.

Mace, Macis, Maces, Flores macis seu ma'cidos, (F.) *Fleurs de muscade,* is the involucrum of the fruit. It is membranous, with the odour and taste of the nutmeg, and is possessed of similar qualities. The *O'leum macis* is a fragrant, sebaceous substance, expressed in the East Indies. It is only used externally.

MYRISTICÆ NUCLEUS, see Myristica moschata.

MYRMECIA, Formica.

MYRMECIASIS, Convulsio cerealis, Formication.

MYRMECIASMUS, Convulsio cerealis, Formication.

MYRMECISMUS, Convulsio cerealis, Formication.

MYRMECIZON, Formicant.

MYRMECOSIS, Convulsio cerealis, Formication.

MYRMEX, Formica.

MYROBAL'ANUS, from μυρον, 'an ointment,' and βαλανος, 'a nut;' so called, because formerly used in ointment; *Angeloc'ucos, Myro'balan, Glans unguenta'ria, Palma unguentario'rum.* A dried

Indian fruit, of the plum kind, of different species of *Termina'lia.* Of this there are several varieties—the *M. Bellir'ica* or *Belliric myrobalan, Bellegu, Bellerigi, Belnileg:*—the *M. cheb'ula* or *Chebule myrob'alan;* the *M. cit'rina* or *Yellow myrobalan, Ara'ra;* the *M. Em'blica* or *emblic myrobalan,* and the *M. In'dica, As'uar, Indian* or *Black myrobalan.* All the myrobalans have an unpleasant, bitterish, very austere taste; and strike an inky blackness with a solution of steel. They are said to possess laxative as well as astringent properties.

MYRON, Myrum, Unguentum.

MYROPISSOCE'RON. A topical application in alopecia, referred to by Galen; from μυρον, 'ointment,' πισσα, 'pitch,' and κηρος, 'wax.'

MYROPŒUS, Unguentarius.

MYROPOLES, Apothecary, Unguentarius.

MYROSPERMUM FRUTESCENS, Myroxylum Peruiferum—m. Peruiferum, see Myroxylon Peruiferum.

MYROXYLON, see M. Peruiferum.

MYROX'YLON PERUIF'ERUM, *Myrosperm'um frutes'cens,* from μυρον, 'an ointment,' and ξυλον, 'wood;' *Caburei'ba. Nat. Ord.* Leguminosæ. The tree which affords the *Peru'vian balsam, Bal'samum Peruvia'num, Putzochill, Myrox'yli Peruiferi bal'samum, Myrox'ylon, Balsamum Perua'num, Cabureiciba, Indian, Mexican,* or *American balsam,* (F.) *Baume de Pérou.* This balsam consists of benzoic acid, resin, and essential oil. Its odour is fragrant and aromatic; taste hot and bitter: it is soluble in alcohol, and miscible in water by the aid of mucilage. It is stimulant and tonic, and considered to be expectorant: as such, it has been employed in paralysis, chronic asthma, chronic bronchitis and rheumatism, gleet, leucorrhœa, &c., and externally, for cleansing and stimulating foul indolent ulcers. Dose gtt. v to gtt. xxx.

White Balsam of Peru, Natural balsam, Bal'samum album, Styrax alba, Balsamelaon, is obtained by incision from *Myrosper'mum peruif'erum.*

MYROXYLON TOLUIFERUM, Toluifera Balsamum.

MYRRHA, Heb. מר; *Bola, Stactē, Ergas'ma, Myrrh, Calo'nia, Smyrna, Myrrha rubra,* (F.) *Myrrhe.* The exudation of an unknown plant of Abyssinia or Arabia Felix, said to be the *Balsamaden'dron myrrha.* This gum-resin has a fragrant, peculiar odour; and bitter aromatic taste. It is in reddish-yellow, light, brittle, irregular tears; partially soluble in distilled water when aided by friction. S. G. 1.360. It is stimulant; and has been used in cachectic affections, humoral asthma, chronic bronchitis, &c. Dose, gr. x to ℨj.

MYRRHA IMPERFECTA, Bdellium.

MYRRHINE, Myrtus.

MYRRHIS ANNUA, Athamanta Cretensis—m. Major, Chærophyllum odoratum—m. Odorata, Chærophyllum odoratum.

MYRSINE, Myrtus.

MYRSINELÆ'ON, from μυρσινη, 'the myrtle,' and ελαιον, 'oil.' Oil of myrtle.—Dioscorides.

MYRSINI'TES, μυρσινιτης. Wine in which branches of myrtle have been macerated.

MYRTACANTHA, Ruscus.

MYRTE COMMUN, Myrtus.

MYRTID'ANON, μυρτιδανον. An excrescence, growing on the trunk of the myrtle, and used as an astringent. Also, a wine — *Vinum Myrtid'anum* — made from wild myrtle berries.

MYRTIFOLIA BELGICA, Myrica gale.

MYR'TIFORM, *Myrtiform'is, Myrto'des,* from *myrtus,* 'a myrtle,' and *forma,* 'shape.' Having the shape of a leaf of myrtle. A name given to a muscle (depressor alæ nasi), to the fossa incisiva; and to certain caruncles, &c.

MYRTIFORMIS, Compressor naris, Depressor alæ nasi.

MYRTI'TES. A name given to a medicine prepared with honey and myrtle berries.

MYRTLE, Myrtus—m. Berry, Vaccinium myrtillus—m. Candleberry, Myrica gale—m. Dutch, Myrica gale—m. Wild, Ruscus.

MYRTOCHEILIDES, Nymphæ.

MYRTOCHILA, Nymphæ.

MYRTODES, Myrtiform.

MYRTON, Clitoris.

MYRTUS, *Myr'tus commu'nis, M. communis Ital'ica, Myrei'nē, Myrrhi'nē, The Myrtle,* (F.) *Myrte Commun.* The berries of this plant have been recommended in alvine and uterine fluxes and other disorders of relaxation and debility. They are moderately astringent and somewhat aromatic.

MYRTUS ANGLICA, Myrica gale—m. Brabantica, Myrica gale.

MYRTUS CARYOPHYLLA'TA, *Calyptran'thes caryophylla'ta, Cassia caryophylla'ta, Canel'la caryophyllata,* (F.) *Capelet, Cannelle girofée.* The tree which is considered to afford the *Clove bark; Cortex caryophylla'tus seu caryophyllata.* This bark is a warm aromatic; resembling clove with an admixture of cinnamon. It may be used with the same views as cloves or cinnamon.

MYRTUS CARYOPHYLLUS, Eugenia caryophyllata—m. Leucodendron, Melaleuca cajaputi.

MYRTUS PIMEN'TA. The tree which bears the *Jamaica pepper, Pimen'tæ baccæ, Pimento berries, Pimento, Piper caryophylla'tum, Coc'culi Indi aromat'ici, Piper chia'pæ, Amo'mum pimenta, Fructus pimenti, Carive, Caryophyl'lus America'nus seu Pimen'ta, Piper odora'tum Jamaicen'sē, Allspice, Piper Jamaicen'sē, Piper tabas'cum,* (F.) *Poivre de Jamaique, Toute épice, Assourou.* The unripe berries—*Pimenta* (Ph. U. S.)—have an aromatic odour; resembling a mixture of cinnamon, nutmeg, and cloves; the taste is pungent, but mixed, like the odour. Like other peppers, this is stimulant and carminative. The oil—*O'leum Pimen'tæ*—possesses the virtues of the berries. The powdered fruit has been called *Quatre épices* or *Four spices.* Dose gr. v to ℨij.

MYRUM, Myron, μυρον. A perfumed oil or ointment. A liquid perfume. The spontaneously exuding juice of many plants, especially of that from which myrrh is obtained.

MYS, Muscle.

MYSIOLOGIA, Myology.

MYSITIS, Myositis.

MYSTAX, *Mastax.* The hair growing on each side of the upper lip in men. The *mustache* or *mustachio,* (F.) *Moustache.* Also, the upper lip.

MYSTE'RION, μυστηριον, 'a mystery.' An arcanum, nostrum, or secret preparation in general. Also, an antidote referred to by Galen and others.

MYSTRON, μυστρον. A Greek measure, which held about three drachms.

MYT'ILUS EDU'LIS. The *common mussel,* (F.) *Moule.* A bivalve, the flesh of which, when at all in a state of decomposition, is highly poisonous. When fresh, it is an agreeable, but not very digestible article of diet.

MYU'RUS, *Meiu'ros.* A pulse is so called when it sinks progressively and becomes smaller and smaller like a rat's tail; from μυς, 'rat,' and ουρα, 'tail.' *Pulsus myurus recip'rocus,* a pulse, which, after having become gradually weaker, resumes, by degrees, its former character.

MYXA, Mucus, Sebestina.
MYXÆ, Mycteres.
MYXEOSIS, Gonorrhœa impara.
MYXODES, Muciform.
MYXOR'RHOOS, μυξορροος, from μυξα, 'mucus,' and ρεω, 'I flow.' One who is subject to mucous discharge. Applied to an infant, that discharges a considerable quantity of mucous and saliva.
MYXOSARCO'MA, from μυξα, 'mucus,' and σαρξ, 'flesh.' A tumour which is mucosarneous; partly mucous and partly fleshy.
MYXOTER, Nasus.
MYZESIS, Sucking.

N.

N. This letter, in prescriptions, is an abridgment of *Numero*, 'by number.'

NAB'ALUS ALBUS, *Prenan'thes serpenta'ria, White Lettuce, Lion's Foot, Rattlesnake's Master, Rattlesnake root.* An indigenous plant, of the *order* Compositæ, which, with several other species of the genus, is reputed to possess the power of curing the bites of serpents. The root has been used in dysentery.

NABOT, Saccharum candidum.

NABO'THI GLAN'DULÆ, *O'vula seu Ova Nabothi* seu *Nabothia'na, Ova'rium Nabothi, Fol- li'culi rotun'di et oblon'gi, Vesic'ulæ seu Bullæ rotun'dæ cervi'cis u'teri, Vesic'ulæ semina'les mu- lie'rum, Cor'pora globo'sa, Corpus'cula globo'sa, Glandulæ* seu *Hydat'ides cervi'cis uteri.* Small, mucous crypts or follicles situate in the interstices of the duplicatures of the lining membrane of the cervix uteri. Naboth, from noticing them in a morbid condition, mistook them for ova; and hence they received the name *Ovula Nabothi.*

NACRA, *Nakra, Nasa.* A kind of influenza common in the East Indies.

NACRÉ, Margaritaceous.

NACREOUS, Margaritaceous.

NÆVI, see Nævus.

NÆVUS, Plural *Nævi; Nævus mater'nus,* N. *Sigil'lum, Nota mater'na, Nevus, Mac'ulæ matri'- cis, M. Mater'næ* seu *matrica'les, Notæ infan'tum, Lupus varico'sus, Stig'mata, Metrocel'ides, Con- gen'itæ notæ, Mother's Marks, Fancy marks, Mo- ther's spots,* (F.) *Envie, Tache de Naissance.* Spots of various kinds on the skin of children when born, which have been attributed to the influence of the maternal imagination on the fœtus in utero. They are of various appearances, some much better supplied with blood than others. Some are merely superficial or stain-like spots: others are prominent; and often have long, irregular hairs growing from them. These have usually been called *Moles, Spili, Spilo'ma, Epichro'ses spili,* &c.

When nævi are superficial, without any disposition to enlarge or spread, they need not be meddled with: but all those that partake of the character of aneurism by anastomosis had better be removed, where practicable.

NÆVUS SIGILLUM, Nævus.

NAFDA, Naphtha.

NAIL, Sax. nægl, (G.) N a g e l, *Unguis, Onyx,* (F.) *Ongle.* A whitish transparent substance, similar to horn, which covers the dorsal extremity of the fingers. Three portions are distinguished in it; the *extremity,* which is free, at the end of the finger;—the *body* or middle portion adherent by its inner surface; and the *root, Radix* seu *Matrix unguis, In'timum unguis.* The last presents two distinct parts; the one, terminated by a thin, serrated edge, is buried in a duplicature of the skin; the other, called *Lu'nula* seu *Semi- lu'nula* seu *Sele'nē* seu *Arcus* seu *Exor'tus* seu *Anat'olā* seu *Albe'do un'guium,* is whitish and of a semilunar shape, and is situate above the part where the epidermis terminates. The nails are composed of a horny tissue, of the same nature as that which forms the hoofs, horns, and scales of different animals. When the nail has been torn off, the papillæ of the skin become covered by a soft, whitish lamina, whose consistence gradually augments. New laminæ are then formed underneath, and give the nail the thickness it ought to possess. The corneous substance, being thus constantly produced at the extremity of each of these laminæ, the whole of the nail is pushed forwards, and it would grow indefinitely, were it not cut or worn by friction.

The nails protect and support the extremities of the fingers against the impression of hard bodies. They are, also, useful in laying hold of small bodies; and dividing those that have but little consistence.

NAIN, Nanus.

NAKRA, Nacra.

NANNARI, Hemidesmus Indicus.

NANNYBERRY, Viburnum lentago.

NANOCEPH'ALUS, from νανος, 'a dwarf,' and κεφαλη, 'head.' A monstrous state in which the whole head or certain of its parts are too small, whilst the trunk and extremities are normal.

NANOCOR'MUS, from νανος, 'a dwarf,' and κορμος, 'a trunk.' A monstrous condition in which the trunk is too small, whilst the head possesses its normal size.

NANOM'ELUS, from νανος, 'a dwarf,' and μελος, 'a limb.' A monstrous condition in which some part of an extremity is too small, and tne whole limb too short.

NANOSO'MUS, from νανος, 'a dwarf,' and σωμα, 'body.' *Dwarf'ishness.* A state in whica the entire body with all its parts is smaller than common.

NANUS, *Pumil'io, Pu'milo, Pusil'lus,* 'a dwarf.' (*Pu'milus, Pumi'lius,* 'dwarfish.') (F.) *Nain.* One who is much below the usual stature. The term is applicable to all organized beings from man to the vegetable. Trees have their dwarfs, as the human species have theirs. Some curious authenticated instances of human dwarfs are on record. Bebe, the dwarf of Stanislaus, king of Poland, was 33 inches (French) long, and well proportioned. The Polish nobleman, Borwlaski, who was well made, clever, and a good linguist, measured 28 Paris inches. He had a brother, 34 inches high, and a sister 21. A Friesland peasant, at 26 years of age, had attained 29 Amsterdam inches. C. H. Stöberin, of Nürnberg, was under three feet high at 20, yet he was well proportioned and possessed of talents. General Tom Thumb, so called, was seen by the Author in 1847. He was said to be 15 years old; measured 28 inches in height, and when weighed at the mint was found to weigh 20 pounds and 2 ounces. See Pygmy.

NAPE OF THE NECK, Nucha.
NAPELLUS VERUS, Aconitum napellus.
NAPHÆ FLORES, see Citrus aurantium.
NAPHTHA, Acetone.
NAPHTHA, *Nafda, Napta, Napta'lius, O'leum petræ album;* from a Chaldaic and Syriac word signifying *bitumen.* A bituminous substance, found in Persia, Calabria, Sicily, &c. It is liquid, limpid, of a yellowish white colour, a smell slightly resembling that of oil of turpentine, and lighter than water. It resembles petroleum in its properties, and has been chiefly used as an external application; although, occasionally, as an anthelmintic, and in inhalation in phthisis pulmonalis.
NAPHTHA, COAL TAR, LIGHT, see Anæsthetic.
NAPHTHA VITRIOLI, Æther sulphuricus—n. Vitrioli camphorata, Tinctura ætherea camphorata—n. Vitrioli martialis, Tinctura seu Alcohol sulphurico-æthereus ferri—n. Wood, Acetone.
NAPH'THALINE, *Naphthali'na, Naph'thalin.* When coal-tar is subjected to distillation, naphthaline passes over after coal naphtha. It is a white, shining, concrete, crystalline substance, fusible at 176° and boiling at 423°. It is soluble in alcohol, ether, naphtha and the oils, but insoluble in water. It has been used as an excitant expectorant, in the dose of 8 to 30 grains, in emulsion or syrup, and repeated. It has also been used as an anthelmintic; and, when made into an ointment, in psoriasis, lepra vulgaris, &c.
NAPIFORM, Bunioid.
NAPIUM, Lapsana, Sinapis.
NAPLES, (CLIMATE OF.) The climate of Naples in its general characters resembles that of Nice, but it is more changeable: the sirocco too, which is little known in Nice, is severely felt at Naples. It is not a good residence for the phthisical invalid: Sir James Clark, indeed, considers it altogether unsuitable.
NAPLES, MINERAL WATERS OF. In the Quarter Santa Lucia, near the coast, is a cold spring, rich in sulphuretted hydrogen and carbonic acid. It is much used as an aperient tonic, and in cutaneous affections.
NAPLES WATER, FACTIT''IOUS, (F.) *Eau de Naples, Aqua Neapolita'na, Aqua acid'ula hydrosulphura'ta.* (Acidulous water, containing four times its bulk of carbonic acid, ℥xv, and ℨiij; hydrosulphuretted water, ℨix; carbonate of soda, gr. viij; carbonate of magnesia, gr. x. M. Ph. P.)
NAPTA, Nanus, Nata.
NAPTALIUS, Nanus.
NAPUS, Sinapis—n. Leucosinapis, Sinapis alba—n. Sylvestris, Brassica napus.
NAPY, Sinapis.
NARCAPHTE, Thymiama.
NARCAPH'THON, *Nascaph'thon.* The bark of an aromatic tree formerly brought from India. By some, supposed to be that of the tree which affords the olibanum. It was used in fumigation, in diseases of the lungs.
NARCE, Narcosis.
NARCEMA, Narcosis.
NARCESIS, Narcosis.
NARCISSE FAUX, Narcissus pseudo-narcissus—*n. des Prés,* Narcissus pseudo-narcissus—*n. Sauvage,* Narcissus pseudo-narcissus.
NARCIS'SUS PSEUDO-NARCIS'SUS, *N. festa'lis seu glaucus seu grandiflo'rus seu hispan'icus seu major seu serra'tus seu sylves'tris, Bulboco'dium, Pseudo-narcissus, Daf'fodil,* (F.) *Narcisse sauvage, Narcisse des prés, Faux narcisse.* The root is emetic and cathartic, in the dose of ℨij. The flowers are antispasmodic. Dose, 24 grains.
NARCODES, Narcotized.

NARCO'SIS, *Nar'cotism, Narcé, Narce, Narce'ma, Narce'sis,* from ναρκοω, 'I benumb.' *Torpe'do, Torpor, Stupor, Stupefac'tio.* The aggregate effects produced by narcotic substances. At times, narcotism is confined to a state of more or less profound stupor; and constitutes, in certain cases, a useful remedial condition; at others, it is a true poisoning, characterized by vertigo, nausea, a state of intoxication or apoplexy, constant delirium, convulsive motions, &c. Emetics in strong doses, and not much diluted with water; purgatives and glysters are the first means to be used in this condition. The stupor may afterwards be combated by the use of exciting and stimulating drinks.
NARCOSIS FOLLICULO'RUM. A state of the scalp, which Mr. Erasmus Wilson conceives to be dependent upon torpid action of the hair follicles, and in which the scalp and hair are found covered with a yellowish, dirty-looking powder, composed of an admixture of granular particles and furfuraceous scales.
NARCOSPAS'MUS, from ναρκη, 'stupor,' and σπασμος, 'spasm.' Stupor combined with spasm.
NARCOTIA, Narcotine.
NARCOTIC POISON, see Poison.
NARCOTICO-ACRID, see Poison.
NARCOT'ICS, *Narcot'ica, Carot'ica, Obstupefacien'tia, Stupefacien'tia, Stupefa'cients,* (F.) *Stupéfactifs, Stupéfiants.* Same etymon. Substances, which have the property of stupefying;—as opium, stramonium, hyoscyamus, belladonna, &c. They are used in medicine as soothing agents; exerting their special influence on the brain and tubular matter of the spinal marrow. In small doses, as a general rule, narcotics stimulate; in large, they act as sedatives. The following is a list of the chief narcotics:—Aconitum, Ætherea, Belladonna, Camphora, Cannabis, Conium, Digitalis, Humulus, Hyoscyamus, Lactucarium, Opium and Morphia, Stramonii Folia, Stramonii Semina, Mental Narcotics, (Appropriate Music, Monotonous sounds, or any succession of monotonous impressions.)
NAR'COTINE, *Narcoti'na, Narcot'ia, Narcotin, Anarcoti'na, Opia'num;* same etymon; (F.) *Sel de Déroene, Opiane, Sel d'opium, Principe crystallizable de Déroene.* A solid, white, inodorous, and insipid substance; by some considered to be alkaloid; by others neuter; crystallizable in straight prisms with a rhomboidal base; fusible like the fats; soluble in boiling alcohol and ether, and scarcely soluble in water. Narcotine produces all the unpleasant effects of opium; but, at the same time, throws the animal into a state of stupor. It is not used in medicine, on account of these objections. The salts, which are very bitter, have been used successfully in India for the cure of intermittents.
NARCOTISM, Narcosis.
NAR'COTIZED, *Tor'pidus, Narco'des.* Affected with stupor, as from the use of a narcotic.
NARD, CELTIC, Valeriana Celtica—n. Indica, Nardus Indica—*n. Indien,* Nardus Indica—*n. Indique,* Nardus Indica—*n. Petit,* Aralia nudicaulis—*n. Sauvage,* Asarum.
NARDUM GALLICUM, Valeriana Celtica.
NARDUS AMERICANUS, Aralia nudicaulis—n. Celtica, Valeriana Celtica—n. Montana, Asarum.
NARDUS IN'DICA, *Spica nardi, Spica In'dica, Andropo'gon nardus seu citriodo'rus, Indian nard, Spikenard.* The root of this plant is one of the ingredients in the mithridate and theriaca. It is moderately warm and pungent, and has a flavour by no means disagreeable. It is used by the Orientals as a spice:—(F.) *Nard Indien, N. Indique.* An ointment was formerly used, called

Unguen'tum nardi'num. It was prepared of Nard, Malabathrum leaves, Oil of worms, Costus, Amomum, Myrrh, &c., and was used as a detergent.

NARDUS RUSTICA, Asarum.

NARES, *Rhines, Cav'itas Na'rium, Cavum* seu *Ca'vea* seu *Caver'na na'rium, Nasus inter'nus, Mycte'res, Na'rium ad'itus, Ocheteu'mata. The nostrils,* (F.) *Narines.* Two elliptical apertures, situate beneath the nose, and separated from each other by the cartilaginous septum seu colum'na nasi. These apertures are continually open, and give passage to the air we breathe, and to the mucous fluids secreted in the nasal fossæ.

NARES INTERNÆ, Nasal fossæ.

NARES POSTERIOR, *Nares postre'mæ, Extre'mæ nares, Os'tia posterio'ra* seu *Choa'næ na'rium, Na'rium Ex'itus,* (F.) *Arrières narines, Ouvertures postérieures des fosses nasales,* are the posterior apertures of the nasal cavities, which establish a communication between those cavities and the pharynx. They are bounded, *above,* by the body of the sphenoid bone; *below,* by the palate bone, and the base of the velum pendulum; and, on the *outside,* by the internal ala of the pterygoid process. They are separated from each other by a septum, of which the vomer is the bony part.

NARIFUSO'RIA, from *nares,* 'the nostrils,' and *fundere, fusum,* 'to pour.' Medicine dropt into the nostrils.

NARINES, Nares.

NARIUM ADITUS, Nares—n. Siccitas, Mycteroxerotes.

NARTHECIA, Formulary, Myris.

NARTHECIUM, Formulary, Myris.

NARTHEX, Formulary, Myris, Splint—n. Asafœtida, see Asafœtida.

NASA, Nacra, Nata.

NASAL, *Nasa'lis,* from *nasus,* 'the nose.' That which relates to the nose.

NASAL ARTERY. This is the largest of the two branches in which the ophthalmic artery terminates. It issues from the orbit, above the tendon of the orbicularis palpebrarum, passes above the side of the root of the nose, and anastomoses with the last extremity of the facial. Haller gave the name *nasal* to the spheno-palatine. He also called the dorsales nasi, furnished by the external maxillary, *Nasa'les latera'les.*

NASAL BONES, *Ossa nasi, Ossa nasa'lia, Ossic'ula nasi, Ossa maxil'læ superio'ris quarta* seu *quinta* seu *secun'da,* (F.) *Os naseaux, Os propres du nez.* These bones are situate beneath the nasal notch of the os frontis, and occupy the space between the nasal or angular processes of the superior maxillary bone. Their shape is nearly quadrilateral. They have an *external* or *cutaneous* surface, an *internal* or *nasal,* and four margins. Each is articulated with its fellow, with the os frontis, ethmoid, and superior maxillary bones. They ossify from a single point.

NASAL CAR'TILAGE, *Cartila'go triangula'ris Nasi.* A cartilage formed of three portions, which unite at the dorsum nasi, and are distinguished into the *cartilage of the septum,* and the *lateral cartilages.* This cartilage is continuous, *above,* with the ossa nasi, and, *inferiorly,* with membranous fibro-cartilages, which form the supple and movable part of the nostrils. They are two in number—the one before, the other behind.

NASAL DUCT, Lachrymal duct—n. Eminence, Mesophryon.

NASAL FOSSÆ, *Cavi na'rium, Nares inter'næ.* Two large, anfractuous cavities, situate between the orbits below the cranium, and lined by the pituitary or Schneiderian membrane. These cavities have no communication with each other; but the various sinuses in the neighbouring bones —the ethmoidal, sphenoidal, superior maxillary, &c.—all communicate with them. The general cavity of each nostril is divided by the ossa spongiosa into three *meatus* or *passages,* which run from before backwards. 1. The *Meatus narium supe'rior,* placed at the upper, inner, and back part of the superior spongy bone. 2. The *Meatus me'dius,* situate between the superior and inferior spongy bones; and 3. The *Meatus infe'rior,* situate between the inferior spongy bone and the bottom of the nose. The Schneiderian membrane receives the first pair of nerves, and various branches from the fifth pair. The arteries are furnished by the branches of the *internal maxillary,* known under the names of spheno-palatine, infra-orbitar, superior alveolar, palatine, pterygo-palatine; by the supra-orbitar, and ethmoidal branches of the ophthalmic artery, by the internal carotid, superior labial, and dorsales nasi. Its veins are little known, and generally follow the course of the arteries. The lymphatics are almost unknown. The nasal fossæ are the seat of smell; they aid, also, in repiration and phonation.

NASAL MEATUS, see Nasal fossæ.

NASAL MUCUS, *Mucus na'rium, Phlegma na'rium crassum, Mucor* seu *Pitui'ta* seu *Blenna* seu *Lympha muculen'ta na'rium, Apomyx'ia,* vulgarly called *Snot,* (F.) *Morve,* is the mucus secreted by the Schneiderian membrane.

NASAL NERVE, *Naso-palpébral* (Ch.), *Nasoocula'ris* (Sömmering), *Naso-cilia'ris.* One of the three branches of the ophthalmic nerve of Willis. It enters the orbit by the sphenoidal fissure, passes along the inner paries of that cavity, and divides, opposite the internal and anterior orbitar foramen, into two branches. 1. The *internal* and *posterior,* which passes into the *Foramen orbitarium internum anterius,* enters the cranium beneath the dura mater, and passes into the nasal fossæ, through an aperture at the side of the *Crista galli.* It afterwards divides into several filaments: one of them—the *Naso-lobar,* of Chaussier—is very small, and descends on the posterior surface of the os nasi, and ramifies on the integuments of the ala nasi. A second terminates near the septum; others descend along the outer paries of the nasal fossæ. 2. The other is *external* and *anterior,* and is called the *external nasal nerve.* It is distributed to the outside of the orbit. Before dividing, the nasal nerve communicates with the ophthalmic ganglion, and gives off two or three ciliary nerves: the *Posterior Nasal Nerve.* Sömmering has given this name to the nerves, which arise from the internal part of the spheno-palatine ganglion.

NASAL NOTCH, (F,) *Échancrure nasale.* A semicircular notch, situate between the nasal prominence of the frontal bone, and articulated with the nasal bones and the nasal processes of the superior maxillary bones.

NASAL PROCESS, Maxillary bone, superior.

NASAL PROM'INENCE, (F.) *Bosse nasale.* A prominence, situate on the median line, at the anterior surface of the os frontis, between the two superciliary arches.

NASAL REGION, *Re'gio nasa'lis.* The region of the nose.

NASAL SPINES. These are three in number. 1. The *Supe'rior nasal spine* of the os frontis, occupying the middle of its nasal notch, and articulated before with the nasal bones, behind with the ethmoid. 2. The *infe'rior* and *ante'rior nasal spine,* situate at the inferior part of the anterior opening of the nasal fossæ. It is formed by the two superior maxillary bones; and 3. The *infe'rior* and *poste'rior nasal spine, Épine gutturale* (Ch.), a process, formed on the median line by the two palate bones at the posterior part of the palatine arch.

NASALE, Errhine.

NASALIS, Compressor naris.

NASA'LIS LA'BII SUPERIO'RIS. A small muscular slip, which runs up from the middle of the orbicularis and the lip to the tip of the nose. It lies exactly in the furrow, and is occasionally a levator of the upper lip, or a depressor of the tip of the nose.

NASAS, Nata.

NASATUS, Membrosus.

NAS'CALE. A kind of pessary, made of wool or cotton, which was formerly introduced into the vagina, after being impregnated with oil, ointment, or some other proper medicament.

NASCAPHTHON, Narcarphthon.

NASDA, Nata.

NASI, see Oryza.

NASITAS, Rhinophonia.

NASITIS, Rhinitis—n. Postica, Angina nasalis.

NASO, Nasu'tus, from nasus, 'the nose.' One who has a long nose.

NASOCILIARIS (Nervus), Nasal nerve.

NASO-LA'BIAL, Naso-labialis; from nasus, 'the nose,' and labium, 'a lip.' Relating to the nose and lip.

NASO-LABIAL LINE. A line or furrow, which separates the lip from the cheek, and commences at the ala nasi.

NASO-LABIA'LIS. A muscular fasciculus described by Albinus, which arises from the anterior extremity of the septum nasi, and terminates in the orbicularis oris.

NASO-PAL'ATINE, Naso-palati'nus. That which belongs to the nose and velum palati.

NASO-PALATINE GANGLION is situate in the foramen palatinum anterius. Its greater extremity receives the two naso-palatine branches; whilst the smaller gives off two or three filaments, which reach the palatine vault, where they ramify on the membrane of the same name, anastomosing with filaments of the great palatine nerve.

NASO-PALATINE NERVE is furnished by the spheno-palatine, which proceeds from the ganglion of Meckel. It traverses the vault of the nasal fossæ, and proceeds upon the septum between the two layers of the pituitary membrane. It enters the anterior palatine canal, and terminates at the superior angles of the naso-palatine ganglion, without attaining the mouth.

NASO-PALPÉBRAL, Orbicularis palpebrarum.

NASTA, Nata.

NASTURTIUM AMPHIBIUM, see Sisymbrium—n. Aquaticum, Cardamine pratensis, Sisymbrium nasturtium—n. Bursa pastoris, Thlaspi bursa—n. Hortense, Lepidium sativum—n. Indicum, Tropæolum majus—n. Officinale, Sisymbrium nasturtium—n. Palustre, see Sisymbrium—n. Peruvianum, Tropæolum majus—n. Pratense, Cardamine pratensis—n. Sativum, Lepidium sativum.

NASUM DILATANS, Pyramidalis nasi.

NASUS, The Nose, Rhin, Rhis, Or'ganon olfactûs seu odora'tûs seu olfacto'rium, Promonto'rium faciei, Myxo'ter, Emuncto'rium cer'ebri, Snout, (F.) Nez. The nose is a pyramidal eminence, situate above the anterior apertures of the nasal fossæ, which it covers; and, consequently, occupying the middle and upper part of the face, between the forehead and upper lip, the orbits and the cheeks. Its lateral surfaces form, by uniting angularly, a more or less prominent line, called Dorsum seu Rhachis seu Spina Nasi, (F.) Dos du nez. This line terminates, anteriorly, by the lobe,—Lob'ulus. The sides are called Alæ Nasi, Pinnæ Naris, (F.) Ailes du nez. The columna is the inferior part of the partition. Its apex or tip has been called Glob'ulus nasi.

The chief varieties of the nose are the aq'uiline, the flat nose, (F.) Nez camarret ou épaté, and the snub nose, (F.) Nez retroussé. The nose is formed, besides its bones, of fibro-cartilage, cartilage, muscles, vessels, and nerves; and its use seems to be to direct odours to the upper part of the nasal fossæ.

NASUS INTERNUS, Nares.

NASUTUS, Naso.

NATA, Natta, Nasa, Nasda, Nasta, Nenes, Napta. A fleshy, indolent excrescence, having the shape of the nates.

NATARON, Natron.

NATA'TION, Nata'tio, from natare, itself from nare, 'to swim.' Swimming. The action of swimming, or of supporting one's self, or moving upon the water. Swimming resembles the horizontal leap in its physiology—the medium being water instead of air. The difference between the specific gravity of the human body and that of water is not great; so that but little exertion is required to keep a part of the body above water. Swimming is a healthy gymnastic exercise, combining the advantages of bathing.

NATES, Ephed'rana, Nat'ulæ, Sca'phia, Clunes, Glutoi, Gluti, Glu'tia, Sedi'lia, Pygē, Monæ, the Bottom, Backside, Poste'riors, Buttocks, &c., (F.) Fesses. Two round projections, at the inferior and posterior part of the trunk, on which we sit. Amongst the mammalia, man alone has the nates prominent and round. They are formed chiefly by the skin, and a thick layer of areolar tissue, which covers the three glutæi muscles.

NATES CEREBRI, see Quadrigemina corpora—n. et Testes, Quadrigemina corpora.

NATRIUM, Sodium.

NATROCRENÆ, Natropegæ.

NATRON, Natrum, Nat'aron, Nitrum, Anatrum, Aphronitrum, from Natron, a lake in Judæa. A saline compound, very abundant in Egypt, which is almost wholly formed of subcarbonate of soda.

NATRONIUM, Sodium.

NATROPE'GÆ, Natrocre'næ, from Natron, and πηγη, 'a spring.' Soda springs.

NATRUM, Natron—n. Chloratum liquidum, Liquor sodæ chlorinatæ—n. Muriaticum, Soda, muriate of—n. Muriatum, Soda, muriate of—n. Præparatum, Soda, subcarbonate of—n. Tartarizatum, Soda, tartrate of—n. Vitriolatum, Soda, sulphate of—n. Nitricum, Soda, nitrate of—n. Oxymuriaticum, Soda, chloride of—n. Oxyphosphorodes, Soda, phosphate of—n. Sulphuricum, Soda, sulphate of.

NATTA, Nata.

NATULÆ, Nates.

NATU'RA, from nasci, 'to be born or arise.' Physis. Nature. Also, genital organs.

NATU'RA MORBI. The essence or condition of a disease.

NATURAL PARTS, Genital organs.

NATURALIA, Genital organs.

NA'TURISM, Nat'uralism. A view which attributes every thing to nature, as a sage, prescient, and sanative entity.—Nysten. See Expectation.

NA'TURIST. A physician who scrupulously investigates, interprets, and follows the indications presented by nature in the treatment of disease.

NAU'CLEA GAMBIR, Unca'ria gambir. A plant of the family and tribe Cinchonaceæ, a native of the Malayan Peninsula and Indian Archipelago, which yields large quantities of the kind of Catechu known by the names Terra Japon'ica and *Square Catechu*, and which, in Indian commerce, is called *Gambeer*. It is a powerful astringent, much used in tanning, and in medicine, as a substitute for the Catechu of the Acacia.

NAU'SEA, *Nau'sia, Nausi'asis, Nausio'sis, Nau'tia, Queasiness, Squeasiness*, (F.) *Nausée, Envie de vomir;* from ναῦς, *navis*, 'a ship;' because those unaccustomed to sailing are so affected. Sickness. Inclination to vomit.

NAUSEA, KREAT'IC, (κρεας, κρεατος, 'flesh.') The sickness and vomiting, excited, in some nervous patients, by the smallest portion of animal food.

NAUSEA MARI'NA, *Morbus nau'ticus, Vom'itus navigan'tium* seu *mari'nus, Sea-sickness*, (F.) *Mal de mer.* The sickness, vomiting, &c., experienced at sea by those unaccustomed to a sea-life; and from which those who are accustomed are not always exempt. It generally ceases when the person becomes habituated to the motion of the vessel, and not till then.

NAU'SEANT, *Nau'seans*. An agent that excites nausea, which is a state of diminished action. Nauseants are, hence, valuable remedies in diseases of excitement.

NAUSIA, Nausea.

NAUSIASIS, Nausea.

NAUSIO'SIS. This word, besides being synonymous with nausea, has been used to express the state of venous hemorrhage, when blood is discharged by jets.

NAUTIA, Nausea.

NAVEL, Umbilicus — n. String, Funiculus umbilicalis — n. Wort, Cotyledon umbilicus — n. Wort, Venus's, Cotyledon umbilicus.

NAVET, Brassica rapa.

NAVETTE, Brassica rapa.

NAVIC'ULAR, *Navicula'ris, Navifor'mis*, from *navicula*, 'a little ship.'

NAVIC'ULAR FOSSA, *Fossa Navicula'ris, F. Scaphoi'des, Navic'ula, Scaph'ula.* See Scaphoid. This name has been given, 1. To a small depression between the entrance of the vagina and the posterior commissure of the labia majora or fourchette. 2. To a perceptible dilatation, presented by the urethra in man, near the base of the glans. 3. To the superficial depression which separates the two roots of the helix. This is also called *Scapha*.

NAVICULARE OS, Scaphoides os.

NAVIFORMIS, Navicular.

NAVIS, Vulva.

NEAR-SIGHTEDNESS, Myopia.

NEB'ULA, *Nubes, Nubec'ula, Nephos, Neph'elē, Nephe'lion,* (F.) *Nuage, Ombrage.* A slight speck on the cornea. A mist or cloud suspended in the urine. See Caligo.

NEBULOUS, Nepheloid.

NEC"ESSARY, *Necessa'rius,* (*ne,* and *cessare.*) The *Necessaries of Life, Vitæ necessita'tes,* (F.) *Besoins de la vie,* include every thing requisite for the maintenance of life, and particularly food.

NECK, DERBYSHIRE, Bronchocele — n. Swelled, Bronchocele — n. Stiff, Torticollis — n. Wry, Torticollis.

NECKLACE, AN'ODYNE. These are formed of the roots of hyoscyamus, Job's tears, allspice steeped in brandy, or the seeds of the wild liquorice vine, to suit the fancy of the prescriber. They are employed to facilitate dentition in children, and to procure sleep in fever.(!)

NECKWEED, Veronica beccabunga, V. peregrina.

NECRÆ'MIA, from νεκρος, 'death,' and 'αιμα, 'blood.' Death of the blood. Death beginning with the blood.

NECRENCEPHALUS, Mollities cerebri.

NECROCEDIA, Embalming.

NECRODES, Cadaverous.

NECROLOGY, BILLS OF, Mortality, bills of.

NEC'ROMANCY, *Necromanti'a, Negromanti'a, Necyomanti'a, Nigromanti'a,* from νεκρος, 'death,' and μαντεια, 'divination.' Divination by the dead.

NECROMANTIA, Necromancy.

NECRON, Cadaver.

NECRONARCEMA, Rigor mortis.

NECROPHOB'IA, from νεκρος, 'death,' and φοβος, 'fear.' Exaggerated fear of death. This symptom occurs in patients where the disease is not mortal; as in hypochondriasis. In fevers, it is not a good symptom.

NECROPNEUMO'NIA, *Pneumo'nia gangræno'sa* seu *typho'sa, Gangræ'na* seu *Mortifica'tio* seu *Anthrax* seu *Carbun'culus Pulmo'num, Pneumosep'sis, Pneumoc'acē,* (F.) *Gangrène du Poumon;* from νεκρος, 'death,' and *pneumonia.* Gangrenous inflammation of the lungs. This may be *diffused* or *circumscribed.* The only pathognomonic symptom is the extraordinary and repulsive odour of the breath and expectoration. The treatment consists in the use of the chlorides internally, or of chlorine by inhalation; allaying irritation by opium, and supporting the patient by wine-whey, and nourishing diet.

NECROPSIA, Autopsia cadaverica.

NECROPSY, Autopsia cadaverica.

NECROSCOPIA, Autopsia cadaverica.

NECROSCOPY, Autopsia cadaverica.

NECRO'SIS, from νεκροω, 'I kill.' Mortification. State of a bone or of a portion of a bone deprived of life. *Osteoganyræ'na, Osteonecro'sis.* Necrosis may take place without the surrounding soft parts being struck with gangrene. It is to the bones what gangrene is to the soft parts. The part of the bone affected with necrosis becomes a foreign body, similar to the gangrenous eschar, and its separation must be accomplished by the efforts of nature, or by art. When necrosis occurs in the centre of long bones, it never extends to their articular extremities. The exterior layers of bone form a canal round the dead portion or *sequestrum;* between these swollen layers and the sequestrum, suppuration takes place; the matter presses against the bony canal; perforates it, and is discharged by apertures, which become fistulous.

In the treatment, the exit of the sequestrum must be facilitated by proper incisions, by the application of the trepan to the bone, &c.

NECROSIS CEREALIS, Ergotism — n. Dentium, Dental gangrene — n. Ustilaginea, Ergotism.

NECROTOMY, Dissection.

NECTANDRA RODIEI, see Bebeeru.

NECTAR, from νη, 'a particle of negation,' and κταω, 'to kill.' A pleasant liquor, feigned by the poets to have been the drink of the gods, and to have rendered immortal those who partook of it. A name given, by the ancients, to many drinks; and particularly to one made with wine, evaporated, and sweetened with honey.

NECTARIUM, Inula helenium.

NECUSIA, see Wound.

NECYOMANTIA, Necromancy.

NEDYIA, Intestines.

NEDYS, νηδυς. The belly, abdomen, stomach, uterus.

NEEDLE, Sax. neðl, næðl, from Teut. neten, 'to sew.' *Acus, Bel'onē, Raphis, Raph'ion, Aces'tra,* (F.) *Aiguille.* A steel instrument, used in many professions. In *Surgery,* a steel, gold, silver, or platina instrument, that may be round, flat, or triangular, straight, or curved, supported or not by a handle, but having *always* a point, by means of which it penetrates the textures; and *often* having, either near the point, or, more commonly, near the other extremity, an aperture or eye for the reception of a thread or tape, which

It introduces into the parts. The *Aiguille à appareil* of the French is the ordinary sewing needle used in the making of bandages, &c.

NEEDLE, ACUPUNCTURE, (F.) *Aiguille à Acupuncture*, An inflexible gold or silver needle; conical, very delicate, four inches long, furnished with a handle, and, at times, with a canula shorter than it by about half an inch. An ordinary needle, waxed at the head, will answer as a substitute for this. See Acupuncture.

NEEDLE, CATARACT, *Acus ophthal'mica*, (F.) *Aiguille à cataracte*. Needles of gold, silver, and steel have been used; the latter, alone, at the present day. The cataract needle is employed to depress or tear the crystalline when opake. This needle is usually made from 15 to 24 lines long; and is attached to a fine handle. The extremity may be, as in Scarpa's and Langenbeck's, pointed, prismatic, triangular, and curved; in Dupuytren's and Walther's, flat, curved, and sharp-edged; in Hey's, flat, with a semicircular and sharp end; or, as in Beer's, Siebold's, Schmidt's, Himly's, Von Gräfe's, &c., straight and spear-pointed. A mark is generally placed upon the handle to inform the operator, — when the instrument is engaged in the eye,—what side corresponds to the crystalline.

NEEDLE FOR A COUNTER-OPENING, *Acus invagina'ta*, (F.) *Aiguille à Contre-ouverture, Aiguille engainée, Aiguille à gaine*, — a long, narrow instrument of steel; the point of which is fine and sharp on both sides;—the heel (*talon*) having an aperture to receive a thread, tape, &c., provided with a flat, silver sheath, shorter than the blade, the point of which it covers when passing through parts that have to be respected.

NEEDLE, DESCHAMP'S, *Paupe's needle*, (F.) *Aiguille de Deschamps, Aiguille à manche*, &c., is the last described needle, fixed to a handle. The eye is placed near the point. It is employed in the ligature of deep-seated arteries.

NEEDLE, FIS'TULA, (F.) *Aiguille à Fistule*. A long, flat, flexible, silver instrument; having an aperture near one extremity; blunt at the other. This was formerly used for passing a seton into fistulous ulcers. On one of its sides was a groove for guiding a bistouri in case of necessity.

Also, a long, steel instrument, terminated by a point like that of a trocar, which Desault employed for penetrating the rectum, when operating for fistula that had no internal aperture.

NEEDLE, HARE-LIP, (F.) *Aiguille à Bec de Lièvre*. A small, silver canula, to which is attached a spear-point, that can be readily withdrawn. This needle, armed with the point, is introduced at one side of the fissure in the lip, and through the other. The twisted suture is then applied, and the pin withdrawn.

NEEDLE, LIG'ATURE, (F.) *Aiguille à ligature*. A long, steel instrument, sharp towards one extremity, with an eye near the other, which was formerly used for suspending the circulation of blood prior to amputation, by being passed through the limb, so as to include the principal artery and a part of the muscles and integuments.

Also, a steel instrument of various dimensions, round towards one of its extremities, which was straight, and furnished with an aperture; curved and flat towards the opposite, which was pointed, and had a slight ridge on its concave side. At the commencement of the last century, this instrument was used to pass ligatures around vessels.

Also, a steel instrument of various dimensions, flat, regularly curved in the form of a semicircle, with a sharp or lance point, and a long eye, used with advantage in place of the last.

NEEDLE, SETON, (F.) *Aiguille à Seton*. A long, narrow, steel blade; pointed and sharp at one extremity; pierced at the other by an aperture. The *Aiguille à contre-ouverture* may be used for the same purpose.

NEEDLE, SUTURE, (F.) *Aiguille à Suture*. For the twisted suture, the hare-lip needle is used; for the others, the straight or curved needle: the straight needle is preferable for stitching up the abdomen, &c., in dissection. In the suture of the tendons, a curved needle has been used; flat on both sides, and cutting only at the concave edge, in order that the instrument may pass between the tendinous fibres without dividing them.

NEEDLE-BEARER, *Porte-aiguille*.
NEEDLE-CARRIER, *Porte-aiguille*.
NÈFLE, Mespilus (the fruit.)
NÉFLIER, Mespilus.
NEFREN'DES, properly, 'sucking pigs.' — Varro. *Nodoi, Eden'tuli (vn, privative, and odovç, 'a tooth.')* Persons devoid of teeth. Young children, for instance, who have not cut them; or aged persons, who have lost them. This state is called *Nefrendie, Nodo'sia, Odon'tia eden'tula*.

NEGOTIUM PARTURITIONIS, Parturition.
NÈGRE BLANC, Albino.
NEGRETIA PRURIENS, Dolichos pruriens.
NEGRO, *Ni'grita*. One of the Æthiopian race. See Homo and Mulatto.
NEGROMANTIA, Necromancy.
NEIÆ'RA, *Nei'ra, Imus Venter*. The lower part of the belly. — Hippocrates.
NEIGE, Snow.
NEIRA, Neiæra.
NELUM'BIUM LU'TEUM, *Yellow ne'lumbo, Yellow water lily, Pond lily, Water shield, Water nuts, Water chin'capin, Rattle nut, Sacred bean*. A beautiful water plant, common in the United States, and belonging to *Nat. Ord.* Nymphaceæ; *Sex. Syst.* Polyandria Polygynia. The leaves are cooling and emollient when applied to the surface. The roots, leaves, and nuts are eaten. The last are called by the Indians and others *water chincapins*.

NELUMBO, YELLOW, Nelumbium luteum.
NENDO, Angelica lucida.
NENNDORF, MINERAL WATERS OF. Nenndorf is a village three and a half German miles from Hanover. Its cold sulphureous spring is much celebrated.
NENUPHAR, Nymphæa alba — *n. Blanc,* Nymphæa alba — *n. Jaune*, Nymphæa lutea — *n.* Lutea, Nymphæa lutea — *n. Odorant*, Nymphæa odorata.
NEOARTHRO'SIS, from *νεος*, 'new,' and *αρθρον*, 'a joint.' A new joint; an artificial joint.
NEOG'ALA, from *νεος*, 'new,' and *γαλα*, 'milk.' Milk secreted immediately after the colostrum. Also, the colostrum.
NEOGENES, *Nouveau-né*.
NEOGILUS, *Nouveau-né*.
NEOGNUS, *Nouveau-né*.
NEONATUS, *Nouveau-né*.
NE'OPLASTY, *Neoplas'tice*: from *νεος*, 'new,' and *πλασσω, πλαττω*, 'I form.' An operative process for the formation of new parts. It includes autoplasty, cicatrization of wounds, and the formation of adhesions. — Burdach.
NEOTTIA, Goodyera pubescens.
NEP, Nepeta.
NEPEN'THA DESTILLATO'RIA, *Bandu'ra*, A Ceylonese plant, the root of which is astringent.
NEPEN'THES, from *νη*, negative particle, and *πενθος*, 'grief.' A remedy much extolled by the ancients against sadness and melancholy.

The women of Thebes, according to Diodorus

Siceliotes, alone possessed the secret of its composition; and, according to Homer, Helen introduced it from Egypt. Some suppose it to have been opium.

NEPENTHES, Bangue—n. Opiatum, Pilulæ opiatæ.

NEP'ETA, *N. Cata'ria seu vulga'ris Cata'ria vulga'ris, Herba felis, Nep* or *Catmint,* (F.) *Herbe aux Chats*,—so called, because cats are fond of it. The leaves, *Cata'ria* (Ph. U. S.), have a smell and taste like those of an admixture of spearmint and pennyroyal. It has been recommended in uterine disorders, dyspepsia, flatulency, &c., like pennyroyal; and is much used in domestic medicine, on the American continent, in flatulencies, &c., of children.

NEPETA AGRESTIS, Melissa nepeta—n. Glechoma, Glechoma hederacea—n. Vulgaris, Nepeta.

NEPHALIOTES, Temperance.
NEPHELE, Enæorema, Nebula.
NEPHELION, Nebula.
NEPH'ELOID, *Nephelo'i'des, Nephelo'des, Neb'ulous, Nubilo'sus.* An epithet applied to urine when it is cloudy — *Uri'na nephelo'des.*
NEPHOS, Nebula.
NEPHRAL'GIA, *Dolor Nephret'icus, Neural'gia Renum,* (F.) *Névralgie des Reins, Dynéphronervie,* from νεφρος, 'a kidney,' and αλγος, 'pain.' Pain and neuralgia in the kidney.
NEPHRALGIA ARENOSA, see Gravel—n. Calculosa, see Gravel—n. Rheumatica, Lumbago.
NEPHRAPOS'TASIS, *Nephropyo'sis, Absces'sus rena'lis,* from νεφρος, 'kidney,' and αποστασις, 'abscess.' Renal abscess.
NEPHRATON'IA, from νεφρος, 'kidney,' and ατονια, 'want of tone.' *Renum aton'ia seu paral'ysis.* Atony of the kidney.
NEPHRELCO'SIS, *Nephropyo'sis, Helco'sis rena'lis,* from νεφρος, 'kidney,' and 'ελκωσις, 'ulceration.' Ulceration of the kidney.
NEPHRELMIN'TIC, *Nephrelmin'ticus,* from νεφρος, 'a kidney,' and 'ελμινς, 'a worm.' That which is owing to the presence of worms in the kidney.
NEPHREMPHRAX'IS, from νεφρος, 'a kidney,' and εμφρασσω, 'I obstruct.' A name given by Plouquet to obstruction of the kidneys.
NEPHRET'IC, *Nephrid'ius, Nephrit'ic, Nephrit'icus,* from νεφρος, 'a kidney.' That which relates to the kidney. Applied, especially, to pain, &c., seated in the kidney.
NEPHRET'ICUM, in *Materia Medica,* means a medicine employed for the cure of diseases of the kidney.
NEPHRETICUM LIGNUM, Guilandina moringa.
NEPHRET'ICUS LAPIS, *Talcum nephrit'icum,* (F.) *Pierre néphretique, Jade néphrite* ou *oriental.* A green, fatty kind of stone, — once used as an amulet against epilepsy; an absurd name, as there can be no such remedy.
NEPHRID'ION, *Pingue'do rena'lis.* The fat which surrounds the kidneys. — Hippocrates.
NEPHRIDIUM, Capsule, renal.
NEPHRIDIUS, Nephretic.
NÉPHRITE, Nephritis—n. Albumineuse, Kidney, Bright's disease of the.
NEPHRITES, Asphaltites.
NEPHRITIC, Nephretic.
NEPHRITICUM LIGNUM, Guilandina moringa.
NEPHRITIS, Asphaltites.
NEPHRITIS, *Empres'ma Nephritis,* from νεφρος, 'kidney,' and *itis,* 'denoting inflammation;' *Renum inflamma'tio, Nephro-phleg'monē,— Inflammation of the Kidney,* (F.) *Néphrite, Inflammation des Reins,* is characterized by acute pain; burning heat, and a sensation of weight in the region of one or both kidneys; suppression or diminution of urine; fever; dysuria; ischuria; constipation, more or less obstinate; retraction of the testicle, and numbness of the thigh of the same side. It may be distinguished into *simple* and *calculous nephritis.* In the latter, the urine often contains small particles of uric acid or of urate of ammonia. The most common causes of nephritis are,—excess in irritating and alcoholic drinks; abuse of diuretics; blows or falls on the region of the kidneys; the presence of renal calculi, &c. It may be distinguished from lumbago by the pain which attends the latter on the slightest motion, &c. It usually terminates by resolution in from one week to two or three. It may, however, end in suppuration—*pyonéphrite;* or may become chronic—*chrononéphrite,* (Piorry.) In the treatment, antiphlogistics, as bleeding, baths, &c., are required to the full extent; with the use of diluents, opiates, &c.

NEPHRITIS ALBUMINENSIS, Kidney, Bright's disease of the—n. Albuminosa, Kidney, Bright's disease of the—n. Associated, Kidney, Bright's disease of the—n. Cachectic, Kidney, Bright's disease of the—n. Sociata, Kidney, Bright's disease of the.

NEPHRODES, Nephroid.
NEPHRODIUM FILIX MAS, Polypodium filix mas.
NEPHROG'RAPHY, from νεφρος, 'a kidney,' and γραφη, 'a description.' An anatomical description of the kidney.
NEPHROHÆ'MIA, from νεφρος, 'kidney,' and 'αιμα, 'blood.' Hyperæmia or congestion of the kidney.
NEPH'ROID, *Nephroi'des, Nephro'des, Reniform'is,* from νεφρος, 'kidney,' and ειδος, 'form, resemblance.' Reniform. Having a resemblance to a kidney — as *'nephroid cancer,'* so called because the morbid growth resembles the kidney in structure.
NEPHROLITHI'ASIS, from νεφρος, 'a kidney,' and λιθος, 'a stone.' The disease of calculus in the kidney; *Lith'ia rena'lis, Lithi'asis nephrit'ica, L. Rena'lis.* See Gravel.
NEPHROLITH'IC, same etymon. Belonging to calculi in the kidneys. This epithet has been applied to ischuria, occasioned by calculi formed in the kidneys.
NEPHROL'OGY, *Nephrolog"ia,* from νεφρος, 'kidney,' and λογος, 'a treatise.' A treatise on the kidneys. Dissertation on the kidneys and their functions.
NEPHROMALA'CIA, from νεφρος, 'kidney,' and μαλακια, 'softness.' Softening of the kidney.
NEPHROMETRÆ, Psoæ.
NEPHRON'CUS, *Tumor rena'lis,* from νεφρος, 'kidney,' and ογκος, 'a tumour.' A tumefaction of the kidney.
NEPHROPHLEGMAT'IC, *Nephro-phlegmat'icus,* from νεφρος, 'kidney,' and φλεγμα, 'phlegm.' A name given, by some authors, to ischuria produced by mucus contained in the urine.
NEPHROPHLEGMONE, Nephritis.
NEPHROPHTHI'SIS, from νεφρος, 'kidney,' and φθισις, 'consumption.' Phthisis from suppuration of the kidney.
NEPHROPLETHOR'IC, *Nephro-plethor'icus,* from νεφρος, 'a kidney,' and πληθωρα, 'plethora.' Belonging to plethora of the kidneys. An epithet given to ischuria dependent upon this cause.
NEPHROPY'IC, *Nephro-py'icus,* from νεφρος, 'a kidney,' and πυον, 'pus.' Belonging to suppuration of the kidney.

NEPHROPYOSIS, Nephrapostasis, Nephrelcosis.

NEPHRORRHAG"IA, *Hæmatu'ria rena'lis, Hæmorrhag"ia renum*, from νεφρος, 'kidney,' and ῥαγη, 'rupture;' *Profu'vium san'guinis e re'nibus.* Hemorrhage from the kidney.

NEPHROS, Kidney.

NEPHROSCLE'RIA, from νεφρος, 'kidney,' and σκληρια, 'hardness;' *Indura'tio renum.* Induration of the kidneys.

NEPHROSPAS'TIC, *Nephrospas'ticus,* from νεφρος, 'a kidney,' and σπαω, 'I draw.' That which depends upon spasm of the kidney. An epithet given to a variety of ischuria.

NEPHROTHROM'BOID, *Nephro-thromboï'des,* from νεφρος, 'a kidney,' and θρομβος, 'a clot.' That which depends upon clots of blood, contained in the kidneys or their ducts. An epithet for a species of ischuria.

NEPHROT'OMY, *Nephro-lithot'omy, Nephrotom'ia, Nephro-lithotom'ia, Sectio rena'lis, S. re'nis,* from νεφρος, 'a kidney,' and τεμνειν, 'to cut.' Dissection of the kidney. Also, an operation proposed with the view of extracting calculi formed in the kidney, by means of an incision into the tissue of that organ.

NEPHRUS, Kidney.

NEPIOS, Infans.

NEPIOTES, Infancy.

NEPTA, Asphaltum.

NERANTIA, see Citrus aurantium.

NERF, Nerve—*n. Circonflexe,* Axillary nerve—*n. Dentaire,* Dental nerve—*n. Fessier,* Gluteal nerve—*n. Glosso-pharyngien,* Pharyngo-glossal nerve—*n. Gustatif,* see Lingual nerve—*n. Gustatif innominé,* Trigemini—*n. Guttural,* Palatine (middle) nerve—*n. Gutturo-palatin,* Palatine nerve—*n. Honteux,* Pudic nerve—*n. Irien,* Ciliary nerve—*n. Ischio-clitorien,* Pudic nerve—*n. Ischiopénien,* Pudic nerve—*n. Labyrinthique,* Auditory nerve—*n. Mentonnier,* Mental nerve—*n. Moteur oculaire externe,* Motor oculi externus—*n. Oculo-musculaire externe,* Motor oculi externus—*n. Oculo-musculaire interne,* Pathetious nervus—*n. Pathétique,* Pathetious nervus—*n. Péronière branche,* Popliteal nerve, external—*n. Pharyngoglossien,* Pharyngo-glossal nerve—*n. Première paire trachélienne,* Occipital nerve—*n. Vertébrodigital,* Musculo-cutaneous nerve—*n. Prétibiodigital,* Musculo-cutaneous nerve—*n. Prétibio susplantaire,* Tibial nerve, anterior—*n. Radiodigital,* Radial nerve—*n. Sciatique grand,* Sciatic nerve, great—*n. Sciatique petit,* Sciatic nerve, lesser—*n. Sciatique poplité externe,* Musculocutaneous nerve—*n. Sous-occipital,* Occipital nerve—*n. Sous-pubio-fémoral,* Obturator nerve—*n. Spino-cranio-trapézien,* Spinal nerve—*n. Sus-maxillaire,* Maxillary superior nerve—*n. Suspubien,* Supra-pubian nerve—*n. Tibiale branche,* Popliteal internal—*n. Trachéal,* Laryngeal inferior nerve—*n. Trachélo-dorsal,* Spinal nerve—*n. Trijumeau,* Trigemini—*n. à Trois cordes,* Trigemini—*n. Tympanique,* Chorda tympani.

NERFS BRONCHIQUES, Bronchial nerves—*n. Ciliaires,* Ciliary nerves—*n. Moteurs oculaires communs,* Motores oculorum—*n. Sacrés,* Sacral nerves—*n. Sous-costales,* Intercostal nerves.

NÉRIS, MINERAL WATERS OF. Néris is on the high road from Moulins to Limoges, eighty leagues from Paris. There are four springs, the water of which is clear, inodorous, tasteless, and has an unctuous feel. It contains carbonic acid gas, carbonate of soda, and sulphate of soda, chloride of sodium, silex and an animal matter to which its 'oleaginous' property is probably owing. The waters are generally used in the form of thermal baths.

NERIUM, N. oleander.

NE'RIUM ANTIDYSINTER'ICUM, *Wright'ia antidysenter'ica.* The tree which affords the *Codaga'pala Bark, Cones'si cortex, Tillicher'ry cortex, Cortex proflu'vii.* Family, Apocyneæ. *Sex. Syst.* Pentandria Monogynia. (F.)*Codagapale, Cropale.* The bark of this Malabar tree is of a black colour, externally, and is generally covered with a white moss or scurf. It has an austere, bitter taste, and has been recommended as an astringent in diarrhœa, dysentery, &c.

NE'RIUM OLEAN'DER, *Ne'rium, Rhododaph'nis Rosa'go,* (F.) *Laurier rose.* The leaves are reputed to be narcotic. The infusion is employed internally, in herpetic affections, and the powder, incorporated with lard, is used in the itch.

NERONIA'NA (PHLEBOTOM'IA.) An epithet given, for some cause, to phlebotomy, when more than one vein was opened on the same day.

NERPRUN PURGATIF, Rhamnus.

NERVE, *Nervus, Neuron,* νευρον, 'a string.' (F.) *Nerf.* Neuron and Nervus meant also, with the ancients, the tendons and ligaments, *Partes nervo'sæ;* and hence the different acceptations of 'nervous;'— a man of nerve — a strong, *nervous* man; and a weak, *nervous* woman. The nerves are tubular cords of the same substance as that which composes the encephalon and spinal marrow. They extend from one or other of the nervous centres to every part of the body, communicating, frequently, with each other; forming *plexuses,* and, occasionally, *ganglions;* and being, at length, lost in the parenchyma of organs. There are 42 pairs, and, according to their origin, they are termed *Cranial* or *Encephalic,* and *Spinal.* Each nerve is composed of several filaments or cords placed alongside each other, and is surrounded by a neurilemma. The encephalic nerves, in general, have only one root in the brain, whilst the spinal arise from the marrow by two roots: the one from an anterior fasciculus of filaments, the other from a posterior, separated from each other by the *Ligamentum denticulatum;* uniting outside this ligament, and presenting, near the intervertebral foramen, a ganglion formed only by the posterior root. The two roots make, afterwards, but one nerve; and, like the encephalic nerves, proceed to their destination, subdividing into rami and ramusculi, until they are finally lost in the texture of the organs. The trunks first formed are commonly round, and proceed alone, or accompany the great vessels, being placed in the areolar spaces which separate the organs, and are thus protected from injury. Their manner of termination we are not acquainted with; whether the nervous pulp, for instance, be distributed or lost in a membrane, as seems to be the case with the nerves of sight, hearing, and smell, — or are looped. Certain it is, that there is considerable difference in the organs, as respects the quantity of nerves that terminate in them; and the particular arrangement of the nervous extremities. Some organs have numerous nerves; others seem to have none: a circumstance which influences considerably the sensibility of parts.

The *Encephalic Nerves* arise from the encephalon, or are inserted into it; (according as we consider the brain the origin or termination of the nerves;) and make their exit by foramina at the base of the skull. They are 12 in number. The spinal nerves are 30 in number, 8 *cervical,* 12 *dorsal,* 5 *lumbar,* and 5 or 6 *sacral :* the four inferior cervical being much larger than the superior, because they furnish the nerves of the upper extremities.

SYNOPTICAL TABLE OF THE NERVES.

I. Cranial or Encephalic Nerves.

1. *Olfactory* (1st pair.)	Divided into internal, external, and middle branches, which are distributed on the Schneiderian membrane.
2. *Optic* (2d pair.)	Terminate in the retina.
3. *Motores Oculorum.* (3d pair.)	*Superior Branch.* To the rectus superior oculi and levator palpebræ superioris. *Inferior Branch.* To the rectus internus, rectus inferior and lesser oblique muscles; a filament which goes to the ophthalmic ganglion.
4. *Patheticl* (4th pair.)	To the greater oblique muscle of the eye.
5. *Par Trigeminum.* (5th pair.)	*Ophthalmic Branch.* Divided into three branches. 1. The *lachrymal branch,* to the lachrymal gland and upper eye-lid. 2. *Frontal branch,* to the forehead and upper eyelid. 3. *Nasal branch,* to the eyelids, nasal fossæ, and nose. *Superior Maxillary Branch.* 1. The *orbitar branch,* to the orbit. 2. The *posterior and superior dental,* to the last three molar teeth and gums. 3. The *anterior dental,* to the incisor, canine, and two lesser molares. 4. *Infra-orbitar,* to the upper lip, cheek, and nose. *Inferior Maxillary Branch.* 1. *Temporal* profound branches, to the temporal muscle. 2. *Masseterine* branch, to the masseter muscle. 3. *Buccal,* to the inner surface of the cheek. 4. *Pterygoid,* to the internal pterygoid muscle. 5. *Lingual,* to the mucous membrane of the tongue. 6. *Inferior dental,* to the teeth of the lower jaw, and to the lower lip. 7. *Auricular* branch, to the pavilion of the ear and forehead.
6. *Abducentes* (6th pair.)	To the rectus externus oculi.
7. *Facial* (Portio dura of the 7th pair.)	1. At its exit from the cranium, the *posterior auricular, stylohyoid,* and *inframastoid,* to the pavilion of the ear, the mastoid process, the digastricus, and the muscles attached to the styloid process. 2. Near the parotid gland, the *temporal, malar, buccal, supra-maxillary,* and *infra-maxillary* to the whole superficies of the face.
8. *Auditory* (Portio mollis of the 7th pair.)	To the vestibule, semi-circular canals, and cochlea.
9. *Glosso-pharyngeal.* (Portion of the 8th pair.)	To the base of the tongue and pharynx.
10. *Par Vagum* (8th pair.)	1. *IN THE NECK,*—a *pharyngeal* branch to the pharynx; *superior laryngeal* branch to the larynx, and to some muscles of the inferior hyoid region. *Cardiac* branches to the cardiac plexus. 2. *IN THE CHEST,*—the *inferior laryngeal* branch to the larynx: *pulmonary* branches, which form the plexus of the same name: *œsophageal* branches to the œsophagus. 3. *IN THE ABDOMEN.*—*gastric* branches to the parietes of the stomach: filaments which go to the neighbouring plexuses.
11. *Spinal* or *Accessory of* Willis.	At its exit from the cranium—the *accessory of the pneumogastric nerve* anastomosing with this nerve. In the neck—filaments to the trapezius muscles.
12. *Hypoglossal.* (9th pair.)	*Cervicalis descendens,* to the muscles of the inferior hyoid region, and to the cervical nerves. Filaments to the muscles of the tongue.

II. Spinal or Vertebral Nerves.

1. Cervical Nerves.

1st Cervical Pair	*Anterior Branch.* Anastomosing *par arcade* with the second pair.
2d Cervical Pair	*Anterior Branch.* A branch anastomosing with the first pair: a branch which goes to the cervical plexus.
3d and 4th Cervical Pairs.	*Anterior Branch.* Concurring in the cervical plexus.
	The *Posterior Branch* of these four pairs ramifies on the occiput and muscles of the superficial and deep-seated cervico-occipital regions.
Cervical Plexus	DESCENDING BRANCHES.—1. *Internal descending,* anastomosing with a branch of the hypoglossus. 2. *Phrenic branch,* to the diaphragm. 3. *External descending branches,* dividing into supra-clavicular, supra-acromial, infra-clavicular, and cervicales profundi, to the muscles and integuments of the upper part of the chest and shoulder, to the trapezius, levator scapulæ, rhomboideus, &c. ASCENDING BRANCHES.—1. *Mastoid,* to the posterior and lateral part of the head and the inner surface of the pavilion of the ear. 2. *Auricular,* to the parotid gland and pavilion of the ear. *Superficial Cervical Branches.* (2.) To the platysma myoides, diga tricus, the integuments of the neck, &c. *Anterior Branches.* Assisting in the formation of the brachial plexus.
5th, 6th, and 7th Cervical Pairs.	*Posterior Branches* To the muscles and integuments of the posterior part of the neck and upper part of the back.
Brachial Plexus	1. *Thoracic Branches,* (2.) to the anterior and lateral parts of the chest. 2. *Supra-scapulary* branch to the muscles of the posterior scapular region. 3. *Infra-scapulary* branches (3.) to the subacapularis, teres major, teres minor, and latissimus dorsi. 4. The *brachial interna cutaneous,* to the integuments of the palmar and dorsal surfaces of the forearm, near the ulnar margin. 5. The *brachial external cutaneous,* principally to the integuments of the palmar and dorsal surfaces of the forearm, near the radial margin. 6. The *median nerve,* to the forearm, hand, and palmar surface of all the fingers. 7. The *cubital nerve,* to the last two fingers. 8. The *radial,* to the first three. 9. The *axillary,* around the shoulder-joint, and to the neighbouring muscles.

II. Spinal or Vertebral Nerves.—Continued.

2. Dorsal Nerves, (Nervi dorsales.)

- **1st Dorsal Pair.** — *Anterior Branch.* To the brachial plexus.
- **2d and 3d Dorsal Pairs.** — *Anterior Branches.* An intercostal and brachial branch.
- **4th, 5th, 6th, and 7th Dorsal Pairs** — *Anterior Branches. Internal* branches, to the intercostals, triangularis sterni, pectoralis major, and to the skin. *External* branches to the integuments of the chest, the obliquus externus abdominis, and the skin of the abdomen.
- **8th, 9th, 10th, and 11th Dorsal Pairs.** — *Anterior Branches. Internal* branches, to the transversalis, obliquus internus, and rectus muscles, and to the skin of the abdomen. *External* branches, to the integuments of the chest, and to the muscles and skin of the abdomen.
- **12th Dorsal Pair** — *Anterior Branch.* To the first lumbar nerve, and to the muscles and skin of the abdomen as far as the iliac crest.

The *Posterior Branches* of the dorsal nerves are distributed to the muscles and integuments of the back and loins.

3. Lumbar Nerves.

- **1st, 2d, 3d, and 4th Lumbar Pairs** — *Anterior Branches.* Concurring to form the lumbar plexus.
- **5th Pair** — *Anterior Branch.* Aiding in forming the sciatic plexus.

The *Posterior Branches* of the lumbar nerves are distributed to the loins, sacrum, and nates.

- **Lumbar Plexus** — 1. *Musculo-cutaneous Branches,* to the number of three. One *superior,* to the muscles of the abdomen, to the fold of the groin, and the scrotum: a *middle,* to the integuments and muscles of the abdomen: and an *inferior,* to the skin of the thigh. 2. A *genito-crural* branch to the integuments of the scrotum, the groin, and the thigh. 3. The *crural* nerve, to the integuments and muscles of the thigh, skin of the leg, and foot. 4. The *obturator* nerve, to the muscles at the inner part of the thigh. 5. The *lumbo-sacral,* to the sciatic plexus. It gives off the *gluteal* nerve to the glutæi muscles.

Sacral Nerves.

- **1st, 2d, 3d, and 4th Sacral Pairs** — *Anterior Branches.* They form by their union the sciatic plexus.
- **5th and 6th Pairs** — *Anterior Branches.* To the parts in the vicinity of the coccyx.

The *Posterior Branches* ramify on the muscles and integuments of the nates.

- **Sciatic Plexus** — 1. *Hemorrhoidal nerves,* to the rectum. 2. *Vesical,* to the bladder. 3. *Uterine* and *vaginal,* to the vagina and uterus. 4. *Inferior gluteal,* to the gluteal muscles, perinæum, and integuments of the posterior part of the thigh. 5. *Pudic,* to the perinæum, penis, or vulva. 6. *Sciatic,* divided into the *external popliteal,* which ramifies on the integuments and muscles of the external side of the leg, on the dorsum of the foot, and the dorsal surface of the toes; and into the *internal popliteal,* distributed on the dorsal surface of the two last toes, to the muscles of the foot, and on the plantar surface of all the toes.

Classifications of the nerves have been recommended according to their uses, in preference to the ordinary anatomical arrangement. It has been remarked that the encephalic nerves have generally one root; the spinal two. Now, experiments and pathological facts have proved, that the anterior fasciculus of the narrow and the anterior roots of the spinal nerves are inservient to volition or voluntary motion: and that the posterior fasciculus and roots are destined for sensibility. Hence the spinal nerves, which have two roots, must be the conductors both of motion and feeling; whilst the encephalic, which, with but few exceptions, have but one, can possess but one of these properties:—they must be either *sensitive* or *motive,* according as they arise from the posterior or anterior fasciculus of the medulla: and, consequently, three classes of nerves may be distinguished.

1. **Sensory** — Arising, by a single root, from the posterior fasciculus of the medulla oblongata or spinal marrow.
2. **Motor** — Arising, by a single root, from the anterior fasciculus of the same parts.
3. **Sensory and Motor** — Which have two roots: one from the anterior, and one from the posterior fasciculus.

According to Sir Charles Bell, the medulla oblongata is composed of three fasciculi on each side; an *anterior,* a *middle,* and a *posterior.* Whilst the anterior and posterior fasciculi produce the nerves of motion and sensation respectively; the middle, according to Sir Charles, gives rise to a third set of nerves — the *respiratory.* To this order belong:—

1. The accessory nerve of Willis, or *superior respiratory.*
2. The par vagum.
3. The glosso-pharyngeal.
4. The facial or *respiratory of the face.*
5. The phrenic.
6. A nerve which has the same origin as the phrenic;—the *external respiratory.*

When a horse has been hard-ridden, every one of these nerves is in action.

This division is now, however, generally abandoned, and there does not seem to be a third column, especially destined for respiration.

Sir C. Bell, again, has reduced the system of nerves to two great classes. 1. Those that are *regular, primitive, symmetrical,* and common to all animals, from the worm to man; which have double roots, and preside over sensibility and motion: and, 2. The *irregular* or *superadded,* which are added to the preceding, in proportion as the organization of animals offers new or more complicated organs. To the first class belong all the spinal nerves and one encephalic—the 5th pair;—to the second, the rest of the nervous system.

Dr. Marshall Hall has proposed a division of the nervous system, which is calculated to explain many of the anomalous circumstances we so frequently witness. He proposes to divide all the nerves into, 1. The *cerebral* or the sentient and voluntary. 2. The *true spinal* or excito-motory. 3. The *ganglionic* or *cyclo-ganglionic*,—the nutrient and secretory. If the sentient and voluntary functions be destroyed by a blow upon the head, the sphincter muscles will still contract when irritated, because the irritation is conveyed to the spine, and the reflex action takes place to the muscle so as to throw it into contraction. But if the spinal marrow be now destroyed, the sphincters remain entirely motionless, because the centre of the system is destroyed. Dr. Hall thinks that a peculiar set of nerves constitutes, with the true spinal marrow as their axis, the second subdivision of the nervous system; and as those of the first subdivision are distinguished into sentient and voluntary, these may be distinguished into the *excitor* and *motory*. The *first*, or the excitor nerves, pursue their course principally from internal surfaces, characterized by peculiar excitabilities, to the true medulla oblongata and medulla spinalis; the *second*, or the motor nerves, pursue a reflex course from the medulla to the muscles, having peculiar actions concerned principally in ingestion and egestion. The motions connected with the first or cerebral subdivision are sometimes, indeed frequently, *spontaneous;* those connected with the true spinal are, he believes, *always excited*. Dr. Hall thinks, too, that there is good reason for viewing the fifth, and posterior spinal nerves as constituting an external ganglionic system for the nutrition of the external organs; and he proposes to divide the *ganglionic* subdivision of the nervous system into, 1. The *internal* ganglionic, which includes that usually denominated the sympathetic, and probably filaments of the pneumogastric; and, 2. The *external* ganglionic, embracing the fifth and posterior spinal nerves. To the *cerebral* system he assigns all diseases of sensation, perception, judgment, and volition—therefore all painful, mental, and comatose, and some paralytic diseases. To the true *spinal, excito-motory, reflex*, or *diastaltic nervous system*, belong all spasmodic and certain paralytic diseases. He properly adds, that these two parts of the nervous system influence each other both in health and disease, as they both influence the ganglionic system.

The main views of Dr. Hall on the excito-motory function have been generally embraced.

The following tabular view of the arrangement and connexions of the nerves and nervous centres is given by Dr. Carpenter.

TABULAR VIEW OF THE NERVOUS CENTRES.

Afferent fibres derived from Sensory Ganglia; efferent fibres transmitted to motor centres.	CEREBRAL GANGLIA, the seat of the formation of Ideas, and the instrument of the Reasoning processes and Will; participating also with the Sensory Ganglia in the formation of the Emotions; and thus the original source of *Voluntary* and *Emotional* movements.	Afferent fibres derived from Sensory Ganglia; efferent fibres transmitted to motor centres.
Afferent fibres derived from posterior column of spinal cord; efferent fibres transmitted into posterior column.	CEREBELLIC GANGLIA, for harmonisation of muscular actions; including also the ganglionic centre of the sexual sense (?).	Afferent fibres derived from posterior column of spinal cord; efferent fibres transmitted into motor column.
	CRANIO-SPINAL AXIS, or centre of *Automatic* actions; including—	
Radiating fibres to Cerebral Ganglia:—Nerves of Common and Special Sensation; — Motor nerves forming part of general motor system.	SENSORY GANGLIA, the seat of Sensation, and centre of *Consensual* (or Instinctive) movements, or of Automatic actions involving sensation.	Radiating fibres to Cerebral Ganglia:— Nerves of Common and Special Sensation; — Motor nerves forming part of general motor system.
Afferent and motor nerves of Respiration, Deglutition, &c.	Fibrous strands, connecting the Spinal Cord and Sensory Ganglia. / RESPIRATORY and STOMATO-GASTRIC GANGLIA, forming the true centres of the *Medulla Oblongata;* instruments of *Reflex* movements or automatic actions independent of sensation. / Fibrous strands, connecting the Spinal Cord and Sensory Ganglia.	Afferent and motor nerves of Respiration, Deglutition, &c.
Afferent and motor fibres, forming Trunks of Spinal Nerves.	Fibrous strands, connecting different segments with each other; and with Medulla Oblongata and Sensory Ganglia. / SPINAL GANGLION, or *True Spinal Cord,* consisting of a coalesced series of segmental ganglia, the instruments of *Reflex* operations, or Automatic actions independent of Sensation. / Fibrous strands, connecting different segments with each other; and with Medulla Oblongata and Sensory Ganglia.	Afferent and motor fibres, forming Trunks of Spinal Nerves.

The nerves are covered and united to the neighbouring parts by an abundant layer of fatty areolar texture, which sends, inwards, prolongations that separate the nervous cords and filaments from each other. The arterial trunks, which furnish them, transmit branches into their interior. The veins follow the same course as the arteries. Absorbents are not easily traced even on the greatest trunks.

NERVE, ACCESSORY, OF WILLIS, Spinal nerve — n. Articular, Axillary nerve— n. Buccinator, Buccal nerve—n. Cells, see Neurine—n. Femoral cutaneous, see Genito-crural nerve—n. Femoropopliteal, lesser, Sciatic nerve, lesser.

NERVE FIBRES, *Fila ner'vea, Tu'buli ner'vei, Fibræ ner'veæ.* The minute fibrils or tubules, full of nervous matter, that constitute the nerves. There is a difference between the central and peripheral portion:—the former has been called the *axis cylinder* and *primitive band;* the latter, the *medullary* or *white substance of Schwann,*—being that to which the peculiarly white aspect of cerebrospinal nerves is principally due.

NERVE, GENITAL, see Genito-crural nerve—n. Genito-crural, see Genito-crural nerve — n. Gluteal of the Sacral plexus, Sciatic nerve, lesser— n. Gustatory, Hypoglossal nerve—n. Inguinal, internal, Genito-crural nerve — n. of Jacobson, see Petrosal ganglion—n. Lateral nasal, Sphenopalatine nerve—n. Lingual, Hypoglossal nerve— n. Naso-ocularis, Nasal nerve — n. Naso-palpebral, Nasal nerve—n. Orbito-frontal, Ophthalmic nerve — n. Ocular, Optic nerve — n. of Organic life, Trisplanchnic nerve—n. Palpebro-frontal, Frontal nerve — n. Popliteal internal, Tibial nerve, posterior—n. Power, Nervous power—n. Respiratory, of the face, Facial nerve—n. Respiratory, superior, Spinal nerve—n. Scapulo-humeral, Axillary nerve — n. Scrotal, see Genito-crural nerve—n. Spiral, Radial nerve—n. Spiral, muscular, Radial nerve — n. Sub-occipital, Occipital nerve—n. Sub-pubian, Genito-crural nerve — n. Superficial temporal, Auricular nerve — n. Sympathetic, Trisplanchnic nerve — n. Temporal cutaneous, Auricular nerve — n. Ulnar, Cubital nerve—n. Vidian, Pterygoid nerve—n. of Wrisberg, see Cutaneous nerves—n. Zygomato-auricular, Auricular nerve.

NERVES, COSTAL, Intercostal nerves — n. Dorsal, Intercostal nerves — n. Eighth pair of, Pneumogastric—n. Encephalic, first pair, Olfactory nerves—n. Encephalic, eleventh pair, Spinal nerves—n. Ethmoidal, Olfactory nerves—n. Fifth pair, Trigemini — n. Fourth pair of, Patheticus nervus — n. Infra-orbitar, Sub-orbitar nerves—n. Ninth pair of, Hypoglossal nerve—n. Oculo-muscular, common, Motores oculorum — n. Phrenic, Diaphragmatic nerves—n. Recurrent, Laryngeal inferior nerves—n. Sixth pair of, Motor oculi externus—n. Spinal, Vertebral nerves — n. Tenth pair of, Pneumogastric — n. Third pair of, Motores oculorum.

NERVI ACROMIALES, Acromial nerves — n. Anonymi, Innominati nervi—n. Claviculares, Clavicular nerves—n. Outanei clunium inferiores, see Sciatic nerve, lesser—n. Divisi, Trigemini— n. Entobænontes, Afferent nerves—n. Gustatorii, Trigemini.

NERVI MOLLES. 'Soft nerves.' The anterior branches of the superior cervical ganglion of the great sympathetic, which accompany the carotid artery and its branches, around which they form intricate plexuses, and, here and there, small ganglia. They are called *molles* from their softness, and *subru'fi,* from their reddish hue.

NERVI ODURATORII, Olfactory nerves — n. Reversivi, Laryngeal inferior nerves — n. Subrufi, Nervi molles—n. Vulneratio, Neurotrosis.

NERVINE, *Nervi'nus, Neurot'ic, Neurit'ic, Antineurotic, Antineuropath' ic.* A medicine which acts on the nervous system.

NERVOUS, *Nervo'sus, Neuro'des, Ner'vens, Neu'ricus.* Relating or belonging to the nerves. Strong. Also, weak, irritable.

NERVOUS ATTACK, (F.) *Attaque des nerfs,* is an affection accompanied with spasm, pain, and different nervous symptoms, to which impressible individuals are liable.

NERVOUS CENTRES, see Centres, nervous.

NERVOUS DIATH'ESIS is termed *Atax'ia spirituum, Anoma'lia nervo'rum, Status nervo'sus, S. erethit'icus, Diath'esis nervo'sa, Constitu'tio nervo'sa, Nervousness.* Medically, *nervousness* means unusual impressibility of the nervous system. Formerly, it signified strength, force, and vigour. Recently, it has been applied to a hypochondriacal condition verging upon insanity, occasionally occurring in those in whom the brain has been unduly tasked;—a condition termed by some *cerebrop'athy;* by others, *brain-fag.*

NERVOUS DISEASES, *Morbi nervo'si,* (F.) *Maladies nerveuses.* Affections seated in the nervous system. To purely functional disease of the nerves, Dr. Laycock has given the name *neuræ'mia,* and to the class of diseases he applies the epithet *neuræ'mic.*

NERVOUS FLUID, *Nervous principle, Flu'idum ner'veum, Liq'uidum nerveum, Succus nerveus, Spir'itus vita'lis.* The fluid which is supposed to circulate through the nerves, and which has been regarded as the agent of sensation and motion. Of this fluid we know nothing, except that it resembles, in many respects, the electric or galvanic. It was formerly called *Animal spirits, Spir'itus anima'les,* (F.) *Esprits animaux.*

NERVOUS PAIN, Neuralgia.

NERVOUS POWER, *Nerve power, Vis nervo'sa seu nervo'rum, Neurodyna'mia, Neurody'namia.* The power of the nerves as exhibited in the living organism.

NERVOUS PRINCIPLE, N. fluid.

NERVOUS SYSTEM. The nerves of the human body considered collectively. See Nerves.

NERVOUS SYSTEM OF THE AUTOMATIC FUNCTIONS, Trisplanchnic nerve — n. System, ganglionic, see Trisplanchnic nerve — n. System, organic, see Trisplanchnic nerve—n. System of the senses, Medulla oblongata—n. System of voluntary motion, &c., Medulla spinalis.

NERVOUSNESS, Nervous diathesis.

NERVUS, see Nerve, Penis—n. Ambulatorius, Pneumogastric nerve — n. Anonymus, Trigemini n. Caroticus, Carotid nerve — n. Cervico-facialis, Cervico-facial nerve — n. Communicans faciei, Facial nerve — n. Cutaneus internus, see Saphenous nerves — n. Cutaneus internus longus, see Saphenous nerves—n. Decimus, Pneumogastric— n. Genito-cruralis, Genito-crural nerve.

NERVUS IMPAR. A prolongation of the neurilemma below the lower extremity of the spinal cord, as a fibrous filament, which is inserted into the base of the coccyx. It was formerly regarded as a nerve :—hence its name.

NERVUS INCISIVUS, Incisive nerve — n. Innominatus Trigemini—n. Ischiadicus, Sciatic nerve —n. Juvenilis, menis—n. Latus, Achillis tendo— n. Lingualis lateralis, Pharyngo-glossal nerve— n. Lingualis Pedius, Hypoglossal nerve—n. Lumbo-inguinalis, Genito-crural nerve — n. Mixtus, Trigemini — n. Musculi pterygoidei, Pterygoid nerve—n. Naso-ciliaris, Nasal nerve—n. Opticus, Optic nerve—n. Pneumogastricus, Pneumogastric — n. Pudendus externus, see Genito-crural nerve—n. Quintus, Trigemini—n. Spermaticus, see Genito-crural nerve—n. Subcutaneus malæ, Orbitar nerve—n. Sympatheticus medius, Trigemini, Pneumogastric—n. Sympatheticus minor, Facial nerve—n. Sympathicus medius, Trigemini—n. Temporo-facialis, Temporo-facial nerve—n. Timidus, Motor oculi externus—n. Tremellus, Trigemini—n. Trochlearis, Patheticus nervus—n. Vagus cum accessorio, Spinal nerve.

NESTIA, Jejunum.

NESTIATRIA, Limotherapeia.

NESTIS, Jejunum.

NESTITHERAPEIA, Limotherapeia.

NESTOTHERAPEIA, Limotherapeia.

NESTROOT, Monotropa uniflora.

NETLEAF, Goodyera pubescens.

NETTLE, ARCHANGEL, WHITE, Lamium album—n. Dead, Lamium album, L. amplexicaule—n. Dwarf, Urtica urens—n. Hedge, Galeopsis—n. Pill-bearing, Urticaria pilulifera—n. Rash, Urticaria—n. Stinging, common, Urtica.

NETWORT, Goodyera pubescens.

NEURADYNAMIA, Neurasthenia.

NEURÆMIA, see Nervous diseases.

NEURÆMIC, see Nervous diseases.

NEURAL; from νευρον, 'a nerve.' Relating to a nerve or to the nervous system.

NEURAL ARCH. The arch formed by the posterior projections connected with the body of the vertebra, which protect the medulla.

NEURAL AXIS. see Encephalon—n. Spines, Spinous processes.

NEURAL'GIA, from νευρον, 'a nerve,' and αλγος, 'pain.' *Rheumatis'mus spu'rius nervo'sus, Neurodyn'ia*, (F.) *Névralgie, Névrodynie, Nervous pain*. A generic name for a certain number of diseases, the chief symptom of which is a very acute pain, exacerbating or intermitting, which follows the course of a nervous branch, extends to its ramifications, and seems, therefore, to be seated in the nerve. The principal neuralgiæ have been distinguished by the names *facial* (of which the *infra-orbitar, maxillary*, and *frontal* are but divisions)—the *ilio-scrotal, femoro-popliteal, femoro-pretibial, plantar*, and *cubito-digital*. A division of *anomalous* neuralgiæ has likewise been admitted.

All varieties of neuralgia are obstinate, and the greatest diversity of means has been made use of:—bleeding, general and local,—emetics, purgatives, rubefacients, vesicants, actual cautery, narcotics, mercurial frictions, electricity; destruction of a portion of the nerve, &c. The most successful remedy, perhaps, is the carbonate of iron, given in doses of some magnitude; as, for instance, ʒss or ƷJij, twice or thrice a day, in molasses. This plan of treatment, continued for a month or two, will generally relieve, and ultimately remove this much dreaded affection. The mode in which it acts is by no means clear; but it is almost as certain as any other remedy used in disease in producing its salutary effects. The bowels must be kept free; and all inflammatory symptoms removed during its administration.

NEURAL'GIA, ANOM'ALOUS. Under this name Chaussier has included different neuroses, some of which are characterized by acute pains circumscribed within a short compass, or extending by irradiations, but not having their seat in the course of a nerve; and others which are occasioned by tumours in the course of a nerve, or which succeed contusions or incomplete divisions of nerves.

NEURALGIA BRACHIALIS, Brachialgia—n. Brachio-thoracica, Angina pectoris—n. Cruralis, N. femoro-tibialis.

NEURALGIA CU'BITO-DIGITALIS, *Is'chias nervo'sa digita'lis*. In this variety the pain extends from the part where the nerve passes under the inner condyle to the back of the hand and to its cubital edge.

NEURALGIA DENTALIS, Odontalgia nervosa.

NEURALGIA, FA'CIAL, *Neuralgia fa'ciei, Trismus maxilla'ris, T. Dolorif'icus, Opsial'gia, Dolor cru'cians faciei, Hemicra'nia idiopath'ica, Autal'gia doloro'sa, Tic douloureux, Dolor faciei, Dolor faciei typ'ico characte'rē, D. F. Fothergilli, Trismus clon'icus, T. dolorif'icus, Rheumatis'mus cancro'sus, Rhematis'mus larva'tus, Prosopal'gia, Prosopodyn'ia, Dolor faciei period'icus, Febris top'ica, Ophthalmodyn'ia period'ica, Tortu'ra Oris, Affectus spasmodico-convulsi'vus Labio'rum*, is characterized by acute lancinating pains, returning at intervals; and by twinges in certain parts of the face, producing convulsive twitches in the corresponding muscles. It may be seated in the frontal nerve, in the infra-orbitar, or in the maxillary branch of the fifth pair.

Metopodyn'ia, Brow-ague, Neural'gia fronta'lis, Ophthalmodyn'ia, Tic douloureux, Dolor period'icus, &c., commences at the superciliary foramen and extends along the ramifications of the frontal nerve that are distributed on the forehead, upper eyelid, caruncula lacrymalis, and nasal angle of the eyelids. Sometimes it is felt particularly in the orbit.

Neuralgia infra-orbita'ria, Dolor faciei atrox, Rheumatis'mus cancro'sus, Trismus clon'icus, Prosopal'gia, Febris top'ica, Odontal'gia remit'tens at intermit'tens, Hemicra'nia sæva, Infra-orbitar neuralgia, Tic douloureux, is chiefly felt in the infra-orbitar foramen, whence it passes to the cheek, upper lip, ala nasi, lower eyelid, &c.

In *Neuralgia maxilla'ris, Gnathal'gia, Gnathoneural'gia, Tic douloureux, Trismus catarrha'lis maxillaris*, the pain usually sets out from the mental foramen and passes to the chin, lips, temple, teeth, and tongue.

NEURALGIA, FALSE. A term assigned to pains along a nerve or its ramifications, produced by some body compressing it,—those pains terminating with the removal of the compressing cause.

NEURALGIA FEM'ORO-POPLITÆ'A, *Sciat'ica, Schias, Malum ischiad'icum, Morbus ischiad'icus, Passio ischiad'ica, Ischiagra, Ischial'gia, Ischio'sis, Coxal'gia, Neural'gia Ischiadica, Dolor Ischiad'icus nervo'sus, Is'chias nervo'sa Cotugnii vel Cotunnii, Neurisch'ias, Ischias nervo'sa posti'ca, Is'chias, Cox'agra, Ischias rheumat'icum, Ischiat'ica, Ischoneural'gia*, (F.) *Sciatique, Goutte sciatique*. This is characterized by pain following the great sciatic nerve from the ischiatic notch to the ham, and along the peroneal surface of the leg to the sole of the foot.

NEURALGIA FEM'ORO-PRÆTIBIA'LIS, *N. crural, Ischias nervo'sa anti'ca, Scelal'gia anti'ca*. In this, the pain, setting out from the groin, spreads along the fore part of the thigh, and passes down, chiefly, on the inner side of the leg, to the inner ankle and back of the foot.

NEURALGIA OF THE HEART, Angina pectoris—n. Hepatica, Hepatalgia.

NEURALGIA ILIO-SCROTAL has been rarely observed. It is characterized by a very acute pain, in the course of the branches of the first lumbar pair; this pain follows the crista ilii and accompanies the spermatic vessels to the testicle, which is often painfully retracted.

NEURALGIA, LEAD, see Lead rheumatism—n. Lienis, Splenalgia.

NEURAL'GIA MAMMÆ, *Ir'ritable breast*. An exceedingly painful affection of the female mamma, unaccompanied by inflammation.

NEURALGIA PLANTA'RIS. This is rare; and the pain is confined to the course of the plantar nerves.

NEURALGIA RENUM, Nephralgia— n. Spinalis, Spinal irritation— n. Testis, Orchidalgia.

NEURASTHENI'A, *Neuradyna'mia, Debilitas nervo'sa.* Debility or impaired activity of the nerves; from νευρον, 'a nerve,' and ασθενεια, 'debility.'—See Irritable.

NEURICUS, Nervous.

NEURILEMM'A, *Neurile'ma, Neurily'ma, Neu'rymen, Perineu'rion, Fis'tula* seu *Tu'bulus* seu *Cap'sula* seu *Involu'crum nervo'rum, Membra'na* seu *Membran'ula* seu *Tu'nica* seu *Indumen'tum nervo'rum, Vagi'na nervo'rum;* (F.) *Névrilemme;* from νευρον, 'a nerve,' and λεμμα, 'a coat.' The fine transparent, and apparently fibrous membrane that surrounds the nerves—to every filament of which it forms a true canal.

NEURILEMMATITIS, Neurilemmitis.

NEURILEMMI'TIS, *Neurilemmati'tis, Neurolemmati'tis, Neurili'tis,* (F.) *Névrilemmite.* Same etymon. Inflammation of the neurilemma.

NEURILITIS, Neurilemmitis.

NEURILYMA, Neurilemma.

NEURINE, *Medull'a nervo'rum,* (F.) *Névrine.* The substance of which the nervous system is composed. It consists chiefly of albumen and a peculiar fatty matter, associated with phosphorus. There are two kinds of neurine—the one *vesicular* or consisting essentially of *nerve vesicles* or *nerve cells* or *corpuscles,* or, as they are sometimes called, from their prevailing in the ganglia —*ganglion corpuscles* and *ganglion globules;* the other, the *tubular;* formed—as the word imports —of tubules. The former is the *cineritious* or *cortical* nervous matter of the older anatomists;— the latter, the *white* or *medullary.* The *vesicular* neurine appears to be concerned in the production and distribution of nerve-power; the *tubular,* in its conduction.

NEURISCHIAS, Neuralgia femoro-poplitæa.

NEURITIC, Nervine.

NEURI'TIS, *Inflamma'tio nervo'rum, Neurophlogo'sis, Neurophleg'monē,* (F.) *Inflammation des Nerfs, Névrite,* from νευρον, 'a nerve,' and *itis,* a suffix denoting inflammation. Inflammation of a nervo.

NEUROBLACI'A, from νευρον, 'a nerve,' and βλακεια, 'stupor.' Insensibility of the nerves.

NEUROCHONDRO'DES, from νευρον, 'a sinew,' χονδρος, 'a cartilage,' and ειδος, 'resemblance.' A hard substance between a sinew and a cartilage.

NEURODES, Nervous.

NEURODYNAMIA, Nervous power.

NEURODYNAMIS, Nervous power.

NEURODYNIA, Neuralgia.

NEUROGAMIA, Magnetism, animal.

NEUROG'RAPHY, *Neurograph'ia;* from νευρον, 'a nerve,' and γραφη, 'a description.' The part of anatomy which describes the nerves.

NEURO-HYPNOTISM, see Magnetism, animal.

NEUROLEMMATITIS, Neurilemmitis.

NEUROL'OGY, *Neurolog"ia,* (F.) *Névrologie,* from νευρον, 'a nerve,' and λογος, 'a discourse.' That part of anatomy which treats of the nerves.

NEURO'MA, (F.) *Névrôme,* from νευρον, 'a nerve.' A morbid enlargement of a nerve. Applied to subcutaneous, circumscribed, and highly painful tumours formed on the tissue of the nerves; and likewise to small, hard, grayish tumours of the size of a pea, which are observed in the course of nerves, and appear to be formed from the neurilemma.

NEUROMALA'CIA; from νευρον, 'a nerve,' and μαλακια, 'softening.' Softening of nerves.

NEUROMETRES, Psoæ.

NEUROMYELITIS, from νευρον, 'a nerve,' μυελος, 'marrow,' and *itis,* denoting inflammation. Inflammation of the medullary matter of the nerves.

NEURON, see Nerve.

NEURON'OSOS, *Neuroso'sos,* from νευρον, 'a nerve,' and νοσος, 'a disease.' A disease of the nerves.

NEURONYG'ME, *Neuronyg'mus, Neuronyx'is,* from νευρον, 'a nerve,' and νυγμα, 'puncture;' *Punc'tio nervi.* Puncture of a nerve.

NEUROPATH'IC, *Neuropath'icus,* from νευρον, 'a nerve,' and παθος, 'a disease.' Belonging to disease of the nerves, to *Neuropathia* or *Neuron'osos.*

NEUROPHLEGMONE, Neuritis.

NEUROPHLOGOSIS, Neuritis.

NEUROPLAS'TY, *Neuroplas'ticē,* (F.) *Néuroplastie,* from νευρον, 'a nerve,' and πλασσειν, 'forming.' M. Serres applies this term to a ganglionary alteration of the peripheral nerves.

NEUROPYRA, Fever, nervous, Typhus mitior.

NEUROPYRETUS, Fever, nervous, Typhus mitior.

NEURO'SES, (F.) *Névroses,* from νευρον, 'a nerve.' A generic name for diseases supposed to have their seat in the nervous system, and which are indicated by disordered sensation, volition, or mental manifestation; without any evident lesion in the structure of the parts, and without any material agent producing them. Such is the usual definition. Broussais attributes them to a state of irritation of the brain and spinal marrow.

NEURO-SKELETON, see Skeleton.

NEUROSPASMI, see Spasm.

NEUROSTHENI'A, (F.) *Névrosthénie,* from νευρον, 'a nerve,' and σθενεια, 'strength.' Excess of nervous irritation. Nervous irritation.

NEUROTHELIC APPARATUS, Corpus papillare.

NEUROTIC, Nervine.

NEUROT'ICA. Diseases of the nervous function. The 4th class of Good's Nosology.

NEUROTOME, *Neurot'omus;* from νευρον, 'a nerve,' and τεμνω, 'I cut,' 'I dissect.' An instrument used by anatomists to dissect the nerves. It is a long and very narrow scalpel, having two edges.

NEUROT'OMY, *Neurotom'ia,* (F.) *Névrotomie.* Same etymon. Dissection of the nerves. Also, an incised wound of a nerve.

NEUROTRO'SIS, *Neurotros'mus,* from νευρον, 'a nerve,' and τρωσις, 'wounding.' *Nervi vulnera'tio.* Wound or wounding of a nerve.

NEUROTROSMUS, Neurotrosis.

NEURYMEN, Neurilemma.

NEUTA, *Neutha.* A membrane, according to Paracelsus, which covers the eyes and ears of the fœtus in utero.

NEUTRAL, from *neuter,* 'neither.' Belonging to neither in particular.

NEUTRAL SALTS, *Sec'ondary salts,* (F.) *Sels neutres.* Salts, composed of two primitive saline substances, combined together, and not possessing the characters of acid or of base.

NEVIS, MINERAL WATERS OF. Thermal springs in the department of Allier, France. Temperature, 136° to 148° Fahrenheit.

NÉVRALGIE, Neuralgia—*n. du Foie,* Hepatalgia—*n. des Reins,* Nephralgia—*n. de l'Utérus,* Hysteralgia.

NÉVRILEMME, Neurilemma.

NÉVRILEMMITE, Neurilemmitis.

NÉVRINE, Neurine.

NÉVRITE, Neuritis.
NÉVRODYNIE, Neuralgia.
NÉVROLOGIE, Neurology.
NÉVROME, Neuroma.
NÉVROSE DU CŒUR, Angina pectoris.
NÉVROSES, Neuroses.
NÉVROSTHÉNIE, Neurosthenia.
NÉVROTOME, Neurotome.
NÉVROTOMIE, Neurotomy.
NEVUS, Nævus.
NEW JERSEY, MINERAL WATERS OF. In the upper part of Morris county and in the county of Hunterdon, near the top of Musconetcong mountain, there are chalybeate springs, which are resorted to. See Schooley's Mountain.
NEW YORK, MINERAL WATERS OF. The chief waters are those of Ballston, Saratoga, and Sharon.
NEXUS STAMINEUS OCULI, Ciliary body.
NEZ, Nasus.
NIANDRIA ANOMALA, Anisodus luridus.
NICARAGUA WOOD, see Cæsalpinia.
NICE, CLIMATE OF. The climate of Nice possesses some advantages over the neighbouring climates of Provence and Italy, being free from the sirocco of the latter, and protected from the mistral of the former. Spring is the most unfavourable season. The climate is very dry. It has been a great winter retreat for the consumptive; but does not deserve the encomiums that have been passed upon it.
NICKAR TREE, Gymnocladus Canadensis.
NICODE'MI O'LEUM, *Oil of Nicode'mus.* An oil made by digesting, for some time,—in a mixture of white wine and olive oil,—old turpentine, litharge, aloes, saffron, oxyd of zinc, &c.
NICOTIANA, N. tabacum—n. Minor, N. rustica.
NICOTIA'NA RUS'TICA, called after Nicot, who carried it to Europe; *N. minor, Priapei'a, Hyoscy'amus lu'teus, English Tobacco.* The leaves possess the properties of tobacco, but are milder.
NICOTIANA TAB'ACUM, *Nicotia'na, Herba tabaci, Tabacum, Petum, Petun, Hyoscy'amus Peruvia'nus, Tobacco, Virgin'ia tobacco,* (F.) *Tabac, Nicotiane.* Tobacco is a violent acro-narcotic; its properties seeming to depend upon a peculiar principle, *Nicotin* or *Nicotianin.* It is narcotic, sedative, diuretic, emetic, cathartic, and errhine. In incarcerated hernia, it is injected, in the form of smoke or infusion, but requires great caution. It is extensively and habitually used as an errhine and sialogogue. The infusion is used to kill vermin, and in some cutaneous eruptions.
NICOTIANE, Nicotiana tabacum.
NICOTIANIN, see Nicotiana tabacum.
NICOTIN, see Nicotiana tabacum.
NICTATIO, Hippus, Nictatio.
NICTA'TION, *Nicta'tio, Nictita'tio,* from *nictare,* 'to wink.' *Clonus nictita'tio, Blepharism'us, Palpebra'tio, Twinkling of the eye,* (F.) *Clignotement, Clignement, Cillement, Souris.* A rapid and repeated movement of the eyelids, which open and shut alternately. As occasionally performed, it is physiological; if repeatedly, a disease. It seems to be executed chiefly by the motor 7th pair of nerves; but it is necessary that the excitor 5th pair should likewise be in a state of integrity.
NIDAMENTUM, Decidua.
NIDOREUX, Nidorous.
NI'DOROUS, *Nidoro'sus,* (F.) *Nidoreux,* from *Nidor, Cnissa,* 'the smell of any thing burnt,' &c. Having the smell of burnt or corrupt animal matter.
NIDUS, Nidus hirundinis.

NIDUS HIRUN'DINIS, *Nidus, Swallows' Nest.* A deep fossa in the cerebellum — so called from its fancied resemblance — situate between the velum medullare posterius in front, and the nodulus and uvula behind.
NIEDERBRONN, MINERAL WATERS OF. Saline waters in the department of Bas-Rhin, France, which contain chloride of sodium, sulphate of magnesia, and carbonic acid.
NIELLE, Nigella.
NIGELLA, Coptis.
NIGEL'LA, *N. Sati'va, Melan'thium, Cumi'num Nigrum, Fennel flower, Nutmeg flower, Devil in a bush,* (F.) *Nigelle, Nielle.* This small southern European and Syrian plant was formerly used medicinally as an expectorant and deobstruent, errhine, sialogogue, &c.
NIGELLE, Nigella.
NIGHT-BLINDNESS, Hemeralopia.
NIGHT EYES, Crusta genu equinæ—n. Mare, Incubus.
NIGHTSHADE, AMERICAN, Phytolacca decandra—n. Bittersweet, Solanum dulcamara— n. Common, Solanum — n. Deadly, Atropa belladonna — n. Enchanter's, Circæa Lutetiana — n. Garden, Solanum — n. Palestine, Solanum sanctum — n. Stinking, Hyoscyamus niger — n. Vine, Solanum dulcamara — n. Woody, Solanum dulcamara.
NIGREDO À SOLE, Ephelides.
NIGRITA, Negro.
NIGRITIES, Melanopathia — n. Ossium, Caries.
NIGRITISM, Melanopathia.
NIGRITUDO, Melanosis—n. Pulmonum, Melanosis pulmonum.
NIGROMANTIA, Necromancy.
NIGROR, Melasma.
NIGRUM OCULI, Pupil.
NIHIL ALBUM, Zinci oxydum—n. Griseum, Zinci oxydum.
NILIACUM, Mel.
NINDSIN, Sium ninsi.
NINE-DAY FITS, Trismus nascentium.
NINSI, Sium ninsi.
NINSING, Panax quinquefolium.
NINZIN, Sium ninsi.
NIPPLE, Sax. nypele. The *Teat, Tit, Dug, Pap, Acromas'tium, Uber, Staph'ylis, Staphyl'ium, Bubona, Mammil'la, Mammel'la, Papil'la, Thelē, Tit'thē, Titthos, Tit'thion, Titthis,* (F.) *Mamelon.* The conical tubercle, situate at the centre of the breast. Towards the central part of each breast the skin changes colour, and assumes a rosy tint in young females, or a reddish brown in those who have suckled several children. The circle is called the *Areola* or *Aureola of the nipple.* The nipple is capable of erection on being excited.
NIPPLEWORT, Lapsana.
NIRLES, Herpes exedens.
NISUS, *Nixus, Peira, Straining,* from Lat. *nitor,* 'to endeavour.' A voluntary retention of the breath, so as to force down the diaphragm; the abdominal muscles being at the same time contracted forcibly. In this manner the contents of the abdomen are compressed; and the evacuation of the fœces, urine, &c., is effected.
NISUS, Effort — n. Formativus, Plastic force.
NISUS PARTURIENTIUM. The efforts or forcing during parturition.
NITEDULA, Cicindela.
NITON, MINERAL WATERS OF. These springs in the Isle of Wight contain iron, and sulphate of alumina and potassa.
NITRAS KALICUM, Potassæ nitras—n. Lixiviæ, Potassæ nitras—n. Natricum, Soda, nitrate of — n. Plumbicus, Plumbi nitras — n. Potassæ

cum sulphure fusus, Potassæ nitras fusus sulphatis paucillo mixtus — n. Sub-bismuthicum, Bismuth, sub-nitrate of.

NI'TRATE, *Nitras.* A salt, formed of a base and nitric acid. Several nitrates are employed in medicine.

NITRATE D'AMMONIAQUE, Ammoniæ nitras — *n. D'Argent,* Argenti nitras.

NITRE, Potassæ nitras — n. Cubic, Soda, nitrate of.

NITRIC ACID, *Acidum ni'tricum, A. azo'ticum, A. sep'ticum, A. nitri, Aqua fortis, Nitrous acid, Spir'itus nitri duplex, Sp. nitri fumans, Sp. nitri Glaube'ri, Azot'ic acid, Dephlogisticated nitrous acid, Oxysepton'ic acid, Spir'itus nitri ac"idus,* (F.) *Acide nitrique.* Nitric acid is obtained from nitre—*Nitrate of potassa.* Its odour is suffocating; taste very acid and caustic. It is corrosive, liquid, colourless, and transparent. S. g. 1.500.

Strong nitric acid is rarely used except as an application to foul, indolent ulcers, or to warts. When given internally, it is in the form of the *Acidum ni'tricum dilu'tum, Spir'itus nitri simplex, Sp. nitri vulga'ris*—the *Diluted nitric acid,* which, in the Pharmacopœia of the United States, consists of *nitric acid,* ʒj, *water,* ʒix, by measure. Diluted largely with water, it is used, as a drink, in fevers of the typhoid kind; in chronic affections of the liver, syphilis, &c.; but, in the latter affections, it is not to be depended upon.

NITROGEN, Azote.

NI'TROGEN, GASEOUS OXIDE OF, *Nitrous oxide, Protox'ide of nitrogen* or of *azote, Paradise gas, Intoxicating gas, Laughing gas, Dephlogisticated nitrous gas, Gas azot'icum oxygena'tum.* This gas, when respired, produces singular effects; great mental and corporeal excitement; and, generally, so much exhilaration as to render the appellation, "*laughing gas*" by no means inappropriate. It has not been much used in medicine, although recommended in paralysis. Its effects are too violent and too transient to render it a valuable remedial agent; and, in the delicate, it has been productive of unpleasant effects, inducing palpitation, fainting, and convulsions.

NITROGEN, PROTOXIDE OF, Nitrogen, gaseous oxide of.

NITROGÈNE, Azote.

NITROGENIUM, Azote.

NI'TROGENIZED, *A'zoted, A'zotised.* Containing nitrogen or azote:—as a *nitrogenised, azoted,* or *azotised* aliment.

NITRO-MURIAT'IC ACID, *Ac"idum nitromuriat'icum, Nitro-hydrochlor'ic acid, Hydrochloro-nitric acid, Aqua regia, Aqua styg"ia, Chrysulca, Aqua regis, Acidum muriaticum nitro'so-oxygena'tum, Mens'truum auri,* (F.) *Eau régale.* A mixture of the nitric and muriatic acids, has been used in diseases of the liver, in the form of a bath for the feet and legs made sharply acidulous. It has, also, been employed, and with more uniform results, in cutaneous affections. Whatever advantage it may possess in internal diseases — and these advantages are doubtful — they are probably dependent upon the chlorine formed by the mixture, or upon the properties possessed by the mineral acids in general. See Chlorine.

The *Acidum nitro-muriaticum* of the Pharmacopœia of the United States is formed by mixing four fluidounces of nitric acid with eight of muriatic acid.

NITROUS OXIDE, Nitrogen, gaseous oxide of.

NITRUM, Natron, Potassæ nitras — n. Antiquorum, Soda — n. Cubicum, Soda, nitrate of — n. Factitium, Borax — n. Flammans, Ammoniæ nitras — n. Lunare, Argenti nitras — n. Rhomboidale, Soda, nitrate of — n. Saturninum, Plumbi nitras — n. Vitriolatum Schroederi, Potassæ sulphas — n. Tabulatum, Potassæ nitras fusus sulphatis paucillo mixtus — n. Vitriolatum, Potassæ sulphas.

NIX, Snow — n. Fumans, Calx viva — n. Zinci Zinci oxydum.

NIXUS, Nisus — n. Parturientium, Nisus parturientium.

NOAH'S ARK, Cypripedium luteum.

NOBLE, *Nob'ilis, Prin'cipal, Essen'tial.*

NOBLE PARTS, *Partes essentia'les.* Some anatomists have given this name to parts, without which life cannot exist; such as the heart, liver, lungs, brain, &c. The organs of generation have, likewise, been so called.

NOCAR, *νωκαρ, Torpor Soporif'icus.* Lethargic torpor.

NOCTAMBULATIO, Somnambulism.

NOCTAMBULISMUS, Somnambulism.

NOCTAMBULUS, Somnambulist.

NOCTILUCA, Cincindela.

NOCTISURGIUM, Somnambulism.

NOCTUI'NI OC'ULI Gray or blue eyes.— Castelli.

NOCTURNA BELLA, Coitus.

NOCTUR'NAL, *Noctur'nus, Nycter'inus,* from *nox,* 'night.' Relating to night, as *Febris nocturn'na* seu *nycter'ina.* A fever occurring in the night.

NODDING, Annuitio.

NODDLEPOX, Syphilomania.

NODE, *Nodus, Emphy'ma exosto'sis perios'tea,* (F.) *Nodosité, Nœud;* from Hebr. בן, 'a heap.' A hard concretion or incrustation, which forms around joints attacked with rheumatism or gout. Some include, under this name, exostoses, articular calculi, ganglions, and even the chronic swellings of the joints, known under the name of white swellings.

NODES, Edentulus.

NODI DIGITORUM MANUS, Phalanges of the fingers — n. Lactea, Infarctus mammæ lacteus — n. Nervorum, Ganglions, nervous — n. Hæmorrhoidales, see Hæmorrhois.

NODOI, Nefrendes.

NODOSIA, see Nefrendes.

NODOSITÉ, Node.

NOD'ULI ARAN'TII, *Noduli Morgagn"ii, Cor'pora Aran'tii.* The small sesamoid bodies situate on the periphery of the semilunar valves of the aorta and pulmonary artery, for the better occlusion of the artery.

NODULI MORGAGNII, Noduli Arantii — n. Nervorum, Ganglions, nervous.

NOD'ULUS, diminutive of *nodus,* 'a knot.' A small knot. A small prominence or lobule in the portion of the cerebellum, which forms the posterior boundary of the fourth ventricle. The nodulus is on the median line, and before the uvula. See Vermiform process, inferior.

NODUS, Articulation, Edentulus, Encystis, Hamma — n. Cerebri, Pons Varolii — n. Chirurgicus, Knot, surgeon's — n. Encephali, *Nœud de l'Encéphale,* Pons Varolii — n. Hystericus, Globus hystericus — n. Vitæ, Centrum vitale.

NOESIS, Intellect.

NŒUD, Node — *n. du Chirurgien,* Knot, surgeon's — *n. Emballeur,* Knot, packer's.

NŒUD DE L'ENCÉPHALE (F.), *Nodus Enceph'ali.* M. Cruveilhier, under this name, includes the pons Varolii, peduncles of the cerebrum and cerebellum, and the tubercula quadrigemina.

NŒUD VITAL, Centrum vitale.

NŒUDS, Calculi, arthritic.

NOISETIER, Corylus avellana.

NOISETTE, Corylus avellana (nut.)

NOIX, Juglans regia (nux) — *n. Américaine*, Jatropha curcas — *n. des Barbades*, Jatropha curcas — *n. Cathartique*, Jatropha curcas — *n. d'Eau*, Trapa natans — *n. de Galle*, see Quercus infectoria — *n. de Serpent*, see Thevetia Ahouai — *n. Vomique*, see Strychnos nux vomica.

NOLA CULINARIA, Anemone pulsatilla.

NOLI ME TANGERE, Lupus, see *Chancreux (Bouton.)*

NOMA, Cancer aquaticus — n. Pudendorum, Colpocace infantilis.

NOM'AD, Nom'ade, Nomas, from νομη, 'pasturage.' An epithet given to people who have no fixed habitation, and who travel, with their flocks, from country to country, for pasturage. Such are the Tartars. By analogy, the word *Nomad'ic* has been applied to spreading ulcer.

NOMBRIL, Umbilicus — *n. de Vénus*, Cotyledon umbilicus.

NOME, Cancer aquaticus, Phagedenic ulcers.

NO'MENCLATURE, *Nomencla'tio, Nomenclatu'ra, Onomatolog"ia, Onomatocle'sis, Termon'ology, Terminol'ogy, Orismol'ogy*, from ονομα, 'name,' and καλεω, 'I call.' A collection of terms or words peculiar to a science or art. In all sciences, nomenclature is an object of importance; and each term should convey to the student a définite meaning. The Lavoisierian nomenclature was a valuable gift to chemistry; and anatomy has derived advantage from the labours of Barclay, Dumas, and Chaussier, who have given names to parts indicative of their situation. See Musclo. The nomenclature of pathology has required the greatest attention; and although repeated attempts have been made to improve it, the barbarous terms that disgrace it are still frequently adopted. It consists of Hebrew and Arabic terms; Greek and Latin, French, Italian, Spanish, German, English, and even Indian, African, and Mexican; often barbarously and illegitimately compounded. A want of principle in founding the technical terms of medicine is every where observable. They have been formed: —
1. From *colour*; as *Melæna, Melas, Atrabilis, Leuce, Alphos, Chlorosis, Rubeola, Scarlatina, Purpura*, &c. 2. From *duration*; as *ephemeral, quotidian, tertian*, and *quartan, continued*, and *intermittent*, &c. 3. From *Birds, Beasts, Fishes, Insects*, and *Plants*; as *Rabies canina, Cynanche, Boulimia, Pica, Hippopyon, Elephantiasis, Urticaria, Lichen, Ichthyosis*, &c. 4. From *Persons* or *Places*; as *Morbus Herculeus, Facies Hippocratica, Lepra Arabum, Plica Polonica, Sudor Anglicus, Morbus Gallicus, Ignis Sancti Antonii, Chorea Sancti Viti*, &c.

NOMUS, Cancer aquaticus.

NON-NAT'URALS, *Non natura'lia*. Under this term the ancient physicians comprehended air, meat, and drink, sleep and watching, motion and rest, the retentions and excretions, and the affections of the mind. They were so called, because they affect man without entering into his composition, or constituting his *nature*; but yet are so necessary that he cannot live without them.

NON-SANE, Insane.

NON-STRIATED MUSCULAR FIBRE, see Muscular fibre.

NONUS HUMERI PLACENTINI, Teres minor — n. Linguæ musculus, Genio-glossus — n. Vesalii, Peronæus tertius.

NOOS, Intellect.

NORMA VERTICALIS, see Normal.

NORMAL, *Norma'lis*, from *norma*, 'a perpendicular,' 'a rule.' According to rule; perpendicular.

The *normal line, norma vertica'lis*, of Blumenbach, is a vertical line let fall from the prominence of the frontal bone and shaving the superior maxillary, so as to mark the projection of the latter bone beyond the arch of the forehead.

NORRIS'S DROPS, see Antimonium tartarizatum.

NORTON'S DROPS, Liquor hydrargyri oxymuriatis.

NOSACERUS, Sickly.

NOSE, Nasus — n. Bleed, Epistaxis — n. Running at the, Coryza.

NOSELI'A, *Nosocome'sis, Nosocomia*, from νοσος, 'disease.' Care of the sick.

NOSEMA, Disease.

NOSENCEPH'ALUS, from νοσος, 'disease,' and εγκεφαλος, 'brain.' A monster whose skull is open only on the frontal and parietal regions, the posterior fontanelle being distinctly present.

NOSEROS, Insalubrious, Sick.

NOSEUMA, Disease.

NOSOCOMESIS, Noselia.

NOSOCOMIA, Noselia.

NOSOCO'MIAL, *Nosocomia'lis*, from *nosocomium*, 'an hospital.' Relating to an hospital, — as '*nosocomial* or hospital fever.'

NOSOCOMIUM, Hospital.

NOSOCOMUS, *Infirmier*.

NOSODES, Insalubrious, Sick, Sickly.

NOSODOCHIUM, Hospital.

NOSOGENESIS, Pathogeny.

NOSOGENIA, Pathogeny.

NOSOGENY, Pathogeny.

NOSOG'RAPHY, *Nosograph'ia*, from νοσος, 'a disease,' and γραφω, 'I describe.' A description of diseases.

NOSOL'OGY, *Nosolog"ia*, from νοσος, 'a disease, and λογος, 'a discourse. A name given to that part of medicine whose object is the classification of diseases. The most celebrated nosological systems have been those of Sauvages (1763), Linnæus (1763), Vogel (1764), Sagar (1776), Macbride (1772), Cullen (1772), Darwin (1796), Selle, Crichton (1804), Parr (1809), Swediaur (1812), Pinel (1813), Young (1813), Good (1817), Hosack (1818), &c. Besides these general nosographies, others have been published on *Surgery* exclusively, none of which are particularly worthy of enumeration amongst nosological systems. Nosological arrangements have, also, been formed of single families or groups of diseases. Plenck, of Baden, is the author of two different treatises of this kind: the one, a methodical arrangement of the diseases of the eyes, and the other, of cutaneous diseases. Dr. Willan published an arrangement of cutaneous diseases, which was completed by Dr. Bateman, and adopted into the Nosology of Dr. Hosack. Mr. Abernethy, also, published a methodical classification of tumours, and many other partial nosological classifications might be enumerated. Also, Pathology.

NOSON'OMY, *Nosonom'ia*, from νοσος, 'a disease,' and ονομα, 'name.' The nomenclature of diseases.

NOSOPH'YTA, from νοσος, 'disease,' and φυτον, 'a plant.' A disease supposed to be produced by, or to consist in the development of parasitic plants — as porrigo, mentagra, &c. — Gruby.

NOSOPŒ'US, *Nosopoët'icus*, from νοσος, 'disease,' and ποιεω, 'I make.' That which causes disease.

NOSOS, Disease.

NOSOTAX'Y, *Nosotax'ia*, from νοσος, 'a disease,' and ταξις, 'arrangement.' The distribution and classification of diseases.

NOSOTHEO'RIA, from νοσος, 'disease,' and θεωρια, 'doctrine.' The doctrine or theory of disease.

NOSTAL'GIA, from νοσος, 'return,' 'a journey home,' and αλγος, 'pain.' *Nostoma'nia, Nos-*

tras'ia, Apodemial'gia, Pathopatridal'gia, Patopatridal'gia, Philopatridal'gia, Philopatridoma'nia, Ademon'ia, Ademos'yne, Home-sickness, (F.) *Nostalgie, Maladie du pays*. An affection produced by the desire of returning to one's country. It is commonly attended by slow wasting, and sometimes by hectic, which may speedily induce death. M. Pinel properly regards it as a variety of melancholy.

NOSTOMANIA, Nostalgia.
NOSTRASSIA, Nostalgia.
NOSTRILS, Nares.
NOSTRUM, Arcanum.
NOSTRUM, CHITTICK'S. An empirical remedy for stone in the bladder, said to be a solution of alkali in veal-broth.
NOTA MATERNA, Nævus — n. Primitiva, Groove, primitive.
NOTÆ INFANTUM, Nævi.
NOTAL, Dorsal.
NOTAL'GIA, *Notial'gia*, (*Nostalgia*, improperly, of Köchlin and others,) from νωτος, 'the back,' and αλγος, 'pain.' Pain in the back. Spinal irritation.
NOTANENCEPHALIA, see Notencephalus.
NOTCH, Teut. Nocke, Ital. *Nocchia, Emargina'tio, Emarginatu'ra*, (F.) *Échancrure*. A depression or indentation of different shape and size, observed on the circumference or edges of certain bones.
NOTCH OF THE CONCHA, Incisura tragica.
NOTCH, ETHMOID'AL, (F.) *Échancrure ethmoïdale*, is situate on the frontal bone, and joins the ethmoid.
NOTCHES, ISCHIAT'IC, (F.) *Échancrures Ischiatiques*, are two in number:—the *greater* and the *less*. The *former* is large, situate at the inferior part of the pelvis, and formed by the sacrum and ilium. It gives passage to the sciatic nerve, pyramidalis muscle, and to the superior gluteal vessels and nerves. The *latter* is much smaller than the other, from which it is separated by the sciatic spine. It gives passage to the tendon of the obturator internus, and to the internal pudic vessels and nerves.
NOTCH, PAROT'ID, (F.) *Échancrure parotidienne*, is the triangular space comprised between the parotid edge of the inferior maxillary bone and the mastoid process; so called, because it lodges the parotid gland. The notches in soft parts are generally called Fissures.
NOTCH, SCAP'ULAR, *Incisu'ra scapula'ris, Lu'nula scap'ulæ*, (F.) *Échancrure scapulaire*. The notch on the superior edge or *costa* of the scapula, which is converted into a foramen by means of a ligament, and gives passage to the suprascapular nerve.
NOTCH, SEMILUNAR OF THE STERNUM, Fourchette.
NOTENCEPHALIA, see Notencephalus.
NOTENCEPH'ALUS, from νωτος, 'the back,' and εγκεφαλον, 'the head.' A monster whose head, with the brain, is on the back. The condition is termed *Notencepha'lia* and *Notanencepha'lia*.—G. St. Hilaire.
NOTHEUSIS, Degeneration.
NOTHIA, Degeneration.
NOTHROTES, Torpor.
NOTHUS, False.
NOTIÆUS, Dorsal — n. Myelus, Medulla spinalis.
NOTIALGIA, Notalgia.
NOTOMYELITIS, Myelitis.
NOTOMYELUS, Medulla spinalis.
NOTON, Dorsum.
NOTOS, Dorsum, Vertebral column.
NOUAGE DE LA CORNÉE, Caligo.

NOUÉ, (*Bandage*) (F.); 'knotted,' from *nodus*, 'a knot.' A bandage which has a considerable number of knots placed above each other. It is made with a roller, 6 or 7 ells long, rolled into two balls, and is used to compress the parotid region, after the extirpation of the parotid gland.
Also, an epithet applied to children in whom the disease of rickets has swollen the articulations.
It is, likewise, applied to the gout, when it has caused nodes on the joints.
NOUET (F.), *Nod'ulus*. A bag filled with medicinal substances, and infused in a liquid to communicate their properties to it.
NOUFFER'S, MADAME, REMEDY, Polypodium filix mas.
NOURRICE, Nurse.
NOURRICIER, Nutritious.
NOURRITURE, Aliment.
NOUS, Intellect.
NOUURE, Rachitis.
NOUVEAU-NÉ (F.), *Neona'tus, superrime Natus, Neog'enes, Neog'ilos, Neog'ilus, Neog'nus, Infans recens natus*. That which has been just born. A new-born infant.
NOVACULA, Razor.
NOYAU, see Cytoblast.
NOYAU CENTRAL DES PÉDONCULES DU CERVELET, Corpus dentatum.
NOYER, Juglans regia — n. *de Ceylon*, Adhatoda.
NUAGE, Nebula.
NUBECULA, Enæorema, Nebula.
NUBES, Enæorema, Nebula.
NU'BILE, *Nu'bilis*, 'marriageable,' 'fit to marry.' Generally, the period of puberty is considered to be the age at which both sexes are *nubile*. They are truly nubile, however, only when they are fitted to procreate healthy and vigorous children, and are competent to discharge their duties as parents.
NUBIL'ITY, *Nubil'itas*, (F.) *Nubilité;* same etymon. The state of being nubile or marriageable.
NUBILOSUS, Nepheloid.
NUCES AQUATICÆ, see Trapa natans — n. Quercūs, see Quercus alba.
NUCHA, *In'ium*, (F.) *Nuque*. The *nuke*, hinder part, or *nape* of the neck. The part where the spinal marrow begins.
Ligamen'tum Nuchæ. A strong ligament from the neck, proceeding from one spinous process to another, and inserted into the occipital bone. It is very strong in quadrupeds. It is called in them *Paxywaxy, Paxwax*, and *Packwax*.
NUCHAL RE'GION, *Re'gio nuchæ seu occipita'lis infe'rior*. The region of the nucha or nape of the neck.
NUCISTA, see Myristica moschata.
NUCK, CANAL OF. A small prolongation of the peritoneum often sent into the inguinal canal of the female fœtus. So called from Nuck, who first described it.
NU'CLEATED, *Nuclea'tus*, from *nucleus*, 'a kernel.' Having a nucleus or central particle. Applied to the elementary cells of organized tissues; the vital properties of which are seated in the nucleus. See Cytoblast.
NUCLEATED CELL, see Cytoblast.
NUCLEI CEMBRÆ, see Pinus Cembra — n. Ossei, Ossification, points of — n. Pineæ, see Pinus pinea.
NUCLEOLE, see Cytoblast.
NUCLEOLULE, see Cytoblast.
NUCLEOLUS, see Cytoblast.
NUCLEUS, see Cytoblast — n. Blastodermatis, *Tache embryonnaire* — n. Centralis, Corpus dentatum — n. Cicatriculæ, *Tache embryonnaire* — n.

Dentatus, Corpus dentatum — n. Dentis, Dental pulp — n. Encased, Cytoblast — n. Fimbriatus, Corpus dentatum — n. Furunculi, see Furunculus — n. Germinal, see Molecule — n. Germinativus, see Molecule — n. Olivæ, Corpus dentatum — n. Ossificationis, Ossification, point of — n. Rhomboidalis, see Corpus dentatum.

NUCULA TERRESTRIS, Bunium bulbocastanum.

NUKE, Nucha.

NUMERICAL METHOD, see Method, numerical.

NUM'MULAR, *Nummula'ris*. Relating to money, from *nummus*, 'money.' An epithet applied to the sputa in phthisis, when they flatten at the bottom of the vessel, like a piece of money.

NUMMULARIA, Lysimachia nummularia.

NUPHUR LUTEUM, Nymphæa lutea.

NUQUE, Nucha.

NURSE, Sax. nojuce, *Nutrix*, (from *nourish*, itself from *nutrire*,) *Tithe'nē*, *Trephou'sa*, *Lactans*, *Lac'ticans*, *Nu'triens*, *Thelas'tria*, *Mamma*, (I.) *Nutrice*, (F.) *Nourrice*. One who suckles her own child or another's. One that has the care of a sick person, (F.) *Garde-malade*.

NURSE, DRY. One who gives every care to a child, but does not suckle it.

NURSE, WET. A female, who suckles the child of another.

To '*nurse artificially*,' is to bring up a child by the hand.

NŪS, Intellect.

NUSUS, Disease.

NUT, BUTTER, Juglans cinerea—n. Cembros, see Pinus cembra—n. Physic, Jatropha curcas—n. Pine, see Pinus picea—n. Pistachio, see Pistacia vera—n. Poison, see Strychnos nux vomica—n. Purging, see Jatropha—n. Rattle, Nelumbium luteum—n. Soap, see Sapindus saponaria—n. Tree, Malabar, Adhatoda—n. Vomic, see Strychnos nux vomica—n. Zirbel, see Pinus picea.

NUTA'TION, *Nuta'tio*, from *nutare*, 'to nod.' Constant oscillation of the head, by which it moves involuntarily in one or more directions.

NUTATOR CAPITIS, Sterno-cleido-mastoideus.

NUTMEG, see Myristica moschata—n. Flower, Nigella—n. Liver, Liver, nutmeg.

NUTRICATIO, Nutrition.

NUTRICIER, Nutritious.

NUTRICIUS, Nutritious.

NUTRIENS, Aliment, Nurse.

NUTRIMEN, Aliment.

NUTRIMEN'TAL, *Nutrimenta'lis*, *Aliment'al*, *Alimenta'lis*, from *nutrimen*, 'aliment.' Having the qualities of food or nutriment.

NUTRIMENTUM, Aliment, Pabulum.

NUTRIT''ION, *Nutrit''io*, *Nutrica'tio*, *Nutri'tus*, *Alitu'ra*, *Threpsis*, from *nutrire*, 'to nourish.' Nutrition is that function by which the nutritive matter already elaborated by the various organic actions, loses its own nature, and assumes that of the different living tissues,—to repair their losses and maintain their strength. Sometimes the word is used in a more extended signification, to express the whole series of actions by which the two constant movements of composition and decomposition are accomplished, in organized bodies. Nutrition, then, would comprehend digestion, absorption, respiration, circulation, and assimilation; the latter being *nutrition*, properly so called, and being operated in the intermediate system over the whole of the body,— the cells of the tissues attracting from the blood the elements necessary for their reparation.

NUTRITION, FORCE OF, Plastic force.

NUTRIT''IOUS, *Nutric''ius*, *Nu'tritive*, *Alib'ilis*, *Trophi'mos*, *Tropho'des*, (F.) *Nourricier*,

Nutricier. Having the quality of nourishing: as nutritious food, nutritious lymph, &c.

NUTRITIOUS or NUTRITIVE ARTERIES, (F.) *Artères nutricières*. Arterial branches which enter the *foramina nutricia* of long bones, and penetrate to the medullary membrane.

NU'TRITIVE, Nutritious. Also, relating to nutrition: hence the '*nutritive* functions,' or those that are concerned in nutrition.

NUTRITUS, Aliment, Nutrition.

NUTRIX, Mamma, Nurse.

NUTS, WATER, Nelumbium luteum.

NUX AROMATICA, see Myristica moschata —n. Avellana, Corylus avellana (nut)—n. Barbadensis, Jatropha curcas—n. Becuiba, Ibicuiba— n. Cathartica Americana, Jatropha curcas — n. Gallæ, see Quercus cerris — n. Juglans, Juglans regia—n. Medica, Coco of the Maldives—n. Metella, Strychnos nux vomica—n. Methel, Datura stramonium — n. Moschata, see Myristica moschata—n. Myristica, see Myristica moschata—n. Pistacia, see Pistacia vera—n. Unguentaria, see Myristica moschata—n. Vomica, Strychnos nux vomica.

NYCTALOPE, see Nyctalopia.

NYCTALOPEX, see Nyctalopia.

NYCTALO'PIA, from νυξ, 'night,' and ωτομαι, 'I see;' *Parop'sis Lucif'uga*, *Nyctalopi'asis*, *Cœcitas diur'na*, *Visus noctur'nus*, *Oxyo'pia*, *Hemeralo'pia* (moderns,) *Amblyo'pia meridia'na*, *Hemeratyphlo'sis*, *Photophob'ia*, *Photophobophthal'mia*, *Dyso'pia lu'minis*, *Visus a'crior*, *Nyc'talopy*, (F.) *Vue nocturne*, *Aveuglement de Jour*. The faculty of seeing during the night, with privation of the faculty during the day. It affects both eyes at once when idiopathic. Its duration is uncertain, and treatment very obscure. It is, however, a disease of nervous irritability, and one of excitement of the visual nerve in particular. The indications of cure will consequently be — to allay direct irritation in every way; to excite counter-irritation by blisters; and to gradually accustom the eye to the impression of light.

One labouring under this affection is called a *Nyc'talope*, *Nyc'talope*, *Nyctalo'pex*.

NYCTALOPS, see Nyctalopia.

NYCTALOPY, Nyctalopia.

NYCTERINUS, Nocturnal.

NYCTHEMERON, see Dies.

NYCTHE'MERUM, from νυξ, 'night,' and 'ημερα, 'day.' The space of 24 hours, or of a day and night. Certain complaints continue only so long.

NYCTOBADIA, Somnambulism.

NYCTOBASIS, Somnambulism.

NYCTOBATESIS, Somnambulism.

NYCTOBATIA, Somnambulism.

NYCTOTYPHLOSIS, Hemeralopia.

NYGMA, Wound, punctured.

NYGMATICUM EMPLASTRUM, Emplastrum resinæ.

NYMPHA, Clitoris.

NYMPHÆ, from νυμφη, 'a water nymph.' *Alæ inter'næ mino'res clitor'idis*, *Carun'culæ cuticula'res*, *Alæ mino'res*, *A. mulie'bres mino'res*, *Cristæ clitor'idis*, *Collic'uli vagi'næ*, *Myrtochi'la*, *Myrtocheil'ides*, *Labia mino'ra seu inter'na*, *L. puden'di mino'ra*, (F.) *Nymphes*, *Petites lèvres*. Two membranous folds, which arise from the lateral parts of the prepuce of the clitoris, and descend on the inner surface of the labia majora: terminating, by becoming gradually thinner, about the middle of the circumference of the orifice of the vagina. They are formed each of two folds of the mucous membrane of the vulva; and contain, in their substance, a thin layer of spongy, erectile tissue. Their use seems to be,—not, as was once supposed, to direct the course of the urine, which notion gave rise to their name, but to favour the elongation and dilatation of the vagina in pregnancy and labour.

The word νυμφη, *Nymphè*, has also been used synonymously with clitoris by Oribasius, Aëtius, &c.

NYMPHÆ'A ALBA, *Leuconympha'a, Nenu'-phar, Microleuconympha'a, Casta'lia specio'sa, White Water Lily,* (F.) *Nénuphar blanc. Nat. Ord.* Ranunculaceæ. *Sex. Syst.* Polyandria Monogynia. Formerly employed as a demulcent, antaphrodisiac, emollient, and slightly anodyne remedy.

NYMPHÆA INDICA, N. nelumbo — n. Major lutea, N. lutea.

NYMPHÆA LU'TEA, *N. major lutea, N. umbilica'lis, Nuphar lu'teum, Nenu'phar lutea, Nyphozanthus vulga'ris, Yellow Water Lily,* (F.) *Nénuphar jaune.* Used for the same purposes.

NYMPHÆA NELUM'BO, *Faba Ægyptiaca, Cyamus Ægyptiacus, Nympha'a In'dica; Pontic* or *Ægyptian Bean.* The fruit of this is eaten raw in Egypt and some of the neighbouring countries; and is considered to be tonic and astringent.

NYMPHÆ'A ODORA'TA, *Sweet-scented Water Lily, Sweet water lily, White pond lily, Toad Lily, Cow Cabbage, Water Cabbage,* (F.) *Nénuphar odorant.* An indigenous plant, growing in most parts of the United States in fresh water ponds, and on the borders of streams, and having large white, beautiful, sweet-scented flowers. The root is very astringent and bitter. It is sometimes made into a poultice and used as a discutient.

NYMPHÆA UMBILICALIS, N. lutea.
NYMPHE, Clitoris.
NYMPHES, Nymphæ.
NYMPHI'TIS; from νυμφη, 'the clitoris,' and *itis,* denoting inflammation. *Epiderrhi'tis, Inflamma'tio Clitor'idis.* Inflammation of the clitoris.
NYMPHOCLUIA, Nymphomania.
NYMPHOMA'NIA, from νυμφη, 'a bride,' and *mania,* 'fury;' *Furor uteri'nus, Uteroma'nia, Lagne'sis furor femini'nus, Metroma'nia, Ædæogargalus, Ædæogaris'mus, Thelygon'ia, Erotoma'nia, Ædæoma'nia, Aidoioma'nia, Melancho'lia uteri'na, Nymphoclu'ia, Sympto'ma turpitu'dinis, Androma'nia, Gynæcoma'nia, Machlos'yne, Entelipathi'a, Tenti'go vene'rea, Hysteroma'nia, Salac"itas vulvæ, Uteri pruri'tus, Bracku'na, Aras'con, Arsa'tum, Œstroma'nia,* (F.) *Nymphomanie, Fureur utérine.* An irresistible and insatiable desire, in females, for the venereal act. It occurs in those particularly, who possess a nervous temperament, and vivid imagination, especially if excited by improper language, masturbation, &c. Its course, as described, is as follows. In the commencement, the sufferer is a prey to perpetual contests between feelings of modesty and impetuous desire. At an after period, she abandons herself to the latter, seeking no longer to restrain them. In the last stage the obscenity is disgusting; and the mental alienation, for such it is, becomes complete. The treatment consists in the use of the same means as are required in the satyriasis of man. When the mental alienation is complete, solitude is indispensable.

NYMPHON'CUS, from νυμφη, 'the nympha,' and ογκος, 'a tumour.' A morbid tumefaction of the nymphæ.

NYMPHOT'OMY, *Nymphotom'ia, Nympha'rum Sec'tio,* from νυμφη, 'nympha,' and τεμνειν, 'to cut.' An operation, known and practised for a long time, which consists in the excision of the nymphæ. The operation is had recourse to, when they are attacked with scirrhus, cancer, fungus, or gangrene; or when they are so large as to interfere with walking or coition. *Nymphotomy* is the circumcision of the female. It is practised in some countries.

Some authors have used the term *Nymphotomy* for amputation of the clitoris.

NYPHOZANTHUS VULGARIS, Nymphæa lutea.

NYSTAG'MUS. A partial rotatory movement of the eyeball from side to side. Also, Coma vigil.
NYXIS, Puncture.

O.

OAK, BLACK, Quercus tinctoria — o. Common, Quercus robur — o. Jerusalem, Chenopodium botrys — o. Lungs, Lichen pulmonarius — o. Poison, Rhus toxicodendron — o. Red, Quercus rubra montana — o. Sea, Fucus vesiculosus — o. Spanish, Quercus rubra montana — o. White, Quercus alba.

OARIOCYESIS, Pregnancy, ovarian.
OARION, Ovary.
OARION'CUS, *Oariophy'ma, Ova'rium tu'midum, Tumor Ova'rii,* from ωαριον, 'the ovarium,' and ογκος, 'swelling.' Ovarian tumour.

OARIOPAREC'TAMA, *Oophoraux'è,* from ωαριον, 'ovarium,' and παρεκτεινειν, 'to extend.' Enlargement of the ovary.

OARIORRHEX'IS, from ωαριον, 'ovarium,' and ρηξις, 'rupture.' *Ruptu'ra Ova'rii.* Rupture of the ovary.

OARIOT'OMY, *Oariotom'ia, Ovariotom'ia, Ovariot'omy,* from ωαριον, 'the ovarium,' and τομη, 'incision.' The operation for removing the ovary.

OARI'TIS, *Oöphori'tis, Oori'tis, Inflamma'tio Ova'rii, Ovari'tis,* (F.) *Inflammation de l' Ovaire,* from ωαριον, 'the ovarium, and *itis,* the termination denoting inflammation. Inflammation of the ovarium.

OARIUM, Ovary.
OARTHROC'ACE, formed by contraction from *omo-arthrocace.* Said to be used by. Rust to designate inflammation of the scapulo-humeral articular surfaces. — Nysten.
OATMEAL, see Avena.
OATS, Avena.
OBAUDITIO, Baryecoia.
OBAUDITUS, Baryecoia.
OBCÆCATIO, Cæcitas.
OBDORMIT"IO, from *ob,* and *dormio,* 'to sleep.' The state of the limbs being asleep. *Stupor ar'tuum.*
OBDUCTIO, Autopsia cadaverica legalis.
OBELÆA RAPHE, Sagittal suture.
OBESITAS, Polysarcia — o. Colli, Struma adiposa — o. Nimia, Pimelosis — o. Viscerum, Physconia adiposa.
OBÉSITÉ, Polysarcia.
OBESITY, Polysarcia.
OBESUS, Corpulent.
OBFUSCATIO, Amaurosis.

OBITUS, Death.

OBJECT'IVE CONE. The cone of light proceeding from an object, the apex of which is on the object, and the base on the cornea.

OBJECTIVE SENSATIONS, see Sensation.

OBLINITIO, Inunction.

OBLIQUE', *Obli'quus.* Any thing inclined, or which deviates from the vertical line. Anatomists have given this name to certain muscles, which have an oblique direction as regards the plane that divides the body into two equal and symmetrical halves. These are:—

OBLIQUE MUSCLES OF THE ABDOMEN. They are two in number, and distinguished into: 1 *Obliquus Exter'nus, Abdom'inis, O. descen'dens exter'nus, O. descendens, O. major,* (F.) *Ilio-pubo costo-abdom'inal, Costo-abdom'inal* (Ch.), *Grand oblique, Oblique externe.* One of the broadest muscles of the body. It is situate at the lateral and anterior part of the abdomen; and is flat and quadrilateral. It is attached, *above,* to the outer surface and lower edge of the 7 or 8 last ribs: *below,* to the anterior third of the external lip of the crista ilii: *before,* it terminates at the linea alba by means of a broad and strong aponeurosis, which covers the rectus, and presents towards its inferior part two very solid fibrous fasciculi, which are inserted, — the one at the symphysis, the other at the spine of the pubis, — under the name of *Pillars of the Abdominal Ring.* These pillars leave between them an opening, which forms the inferior orifice of the inguinal canal. The obliquus externus abdominis depresses the ribs, and carries them backwards during a strong expiration. It impresses on the chest a movement of rotation, and bends the thorax upon the pelvis, and conversely. It contracts, also, the abdominal cavity. 2. *Obliquus Inter'nus Abdominis, M. aocli'vis, O. ascendens, O. minor, O. internus, O. ascendens internus,* (F.) *Ilio-lombo-costo-abdominal, Ilio-abdominal* (Ch.), *Muscle petit oblique* ou *oblique interne,* is broad, especially before; thin, and irregularly quadrilateral, like the preceding, beneath which it is situate. It is attached, above, to the inferior edge of the cartilages of the 5th, 4th, 3d, and 2d false ribs; below, to the anterior two-thirds of the interstice of the crista ilii, to the posterior part of the crural arch, and to the pubis; behind, to the spinous processes of the last two lumbar vertebræ, and to those of the first two portions of the sacrum; before, to the linea alba. Its upper fibres run obliquely upwards and forwards; the middle are horizontal; and the lower pass obliquely downwards and forwards.

These last, in the male, are dragged down through the inguinal ring, when the testicle descends, and form the two fasciculi of the cremaster.

The obliquus internus resembles the O. externus in function.

OBLIQUE MUSCLES OF THE EYE, *Amato'rii, Circumagen'tes, Rotato'res Oc'uli,* are two in number. They are distinguished into: 1. *Obliquus Superior Oculi, Amato'rius mus'culus, Trochlea'ris, Trochlea'tor, Obliquus major, Circumductio'nis op'ifex, Longi'ssimus oc'uli,* (F.) *Optico-trochlei scléroticien, Grand trochléateur* (Ch.), *Grand oblique de l'œil, O. supérieur de l'œil, Amoureux (Muscle),* is situate at the inner and upper part of the orbit. It is small, round, fusiform, and reflected upon itself in the middle of its course. Behind, it is attached to the inside of the foramen opticum; and when it arrives opposite the internal orbitar process, it becomes a small, round tendon, which slides in a cartilaginous pulley fixed to the os frontis, and is reflected, at an acute angle, to proceed downwards and outwards, and to attach itself to the outer and back part of the globe of the eye. This muscle carries the globe of the eye forwards and inwards; making it experience a movement of rotation, which directs the pupil downwards and inwards. This is conceived to be an involuntary muscle as well as the next. In sleep, according to Sir C. Bell, when the power over the straight or voluntary muscles of the organ is nearly lost, the eye is given up to the oblique muscles, which lodge the transparent cornea under the upper eyelid. At the approach of death, the same thing is observable; hence, the turning up of the eye, at such a time, is not an evidence of agony or suffering, but of insensibility. 2. *Obli'quus Infe'rior Oc'uli, O. minor oculi,* (F.) *Maxillo-scléroticien, Petit Trochléateur* (Ch.), *Petit oblique* ou *oblique inférieur de l'œil,* is situate at the anterior and inferior part of the orbit. It is flat and attached to the inner and anterior part of the orbitar surface of the superior maxillary bone, on the outside of the lachrymal gutter; from thence it passes outwards and backwards, and terminates by an aponeurosis, at the posterior and inner part of the globe of the eye. It carries the globe of the eye inwards and forwards; and directs the pupil upwards and outwards.

OBLIQUE MUSCLES OF THE HEAD. These are two in number. 1. *Obliquus Superior Cap'itis, O. minor capitis,* (F.) *Trachélo-atloïdo-occipital, Atloïdo-sous-mastoïdien* (Ch.), *Muscle oblique superior* ou *petit oblique de la tête.* This muscle is situate at the sides of, and behind, the articulation of the head: it is flat and attached, on the one hand, to the top of the transverse process of the atlas; and, on the other, terminates at the occipital bone, beneath the inferior curved line, and sometimes, also, at the mastoid region of the temporal bone. It extends the head, — inclining it to one side. 2. *Obliquus Inferior Capitis, Obliquus major,* (F.) *Spini-axoïdo-trachéli-atloïdien, Axoïdo-atloïdien* (Ch.), *Oblique inférieur* ou *grand oblique de la tête,* is situate at the posterior part of the neck and head. It is round, fusiform; attached to the spinous process of the axis, and proceeds to terminate behind and below the summit of the transverse process of the atlas. It impresses, on the first vertebra and the head, a movement of rotation, which turns the face to one side.

OBLIQUE PROCESSES, see Vertebræ.

OBLIQUE EXTERNE, Obliquus externus abdominis — *o. Grand,* Obliquus externus abdominis — *o. Grand de l'œil,* Obliquus superior oculi — *o. Grand de la tête,* Obliquus inferior capitis — *o. Inférieur de l'œil,* Obliquus inferior oculi — *o. Inférieur de la tête,* Obliquus inferior capitis — *o. Interne,* Obliquus internus abdominis — *o. Petit,* Obliquus internus abdominis — *o. Petit de l'œil,* Obliquus inferior oculi — *o. Petit de la tête,* Obliquus superior oculi — *o. Supérieur de l'œil,* Obliquus superior oculi — *o. Supérieur de la tête,* Obliquus superior capitis.

OBLIQUITÉ DE LA MATRICE, Retroversio uteri.

OBLIQUUS ASCENDENS, O. internus abdominis — *o.* Auris, Laxator tympani — *o.* Descendens externus, O. externus abdominis — *o.* Major, O. externus abdominis, O. inferior capitis, O. superior oculi — *o.* Minor, O. internus abdominis — *o.* Minor capitis, O. superior capitis — *o.* Minor oculi, O. inferior oculi.

OBLIT'ERATED, *Oblitera'tus;* from *obliterare,* 'to efface,' *(literæ,* 'letters.'?) A vessel or duct is said to be obliterated, when its parietes have approximated and contracted such an adhesion to each other that the cavity has completely disappeared.

OBLITERATIO COMPLETA, Hapantismus.

OBLIVIO, Amnesia — o. Iners, Lethargy.
OBLOBIUM, Antilobium.
OB'OLUS, *Onoloeat.* A weight of 9 or 10 grains.
OBSCŒNÆ PARTES, Genital organs.
OBSCURCISSEMENT DE LA VUE, Caligo.
OBSERVA'TION, *Observa'tio,* (from *ob,* and *servare,* 'to keep,' e. g. in sight.) *Tere'sis, Symparatere'sis.* Act of examining a thing by means of the external senses. This word is employed in several acceptations. It expresses — 1. The action of observing — 2. The aggregate of knowledge, afforded by observation. In French — but not in English — it means the *case* or history of the phenomena presented by a patient in the course of a disease.
OBSERVATION, Case — o. Method of, Numerical method.
OBSTET'RIC, *Obstet'ricus;* same etymon as obstetrics. Relating or appertaining to obstetrics, — as '*obstetric* auscultation,' '*obstetric* exploration,' &c.
OBSTETRIC CHAIR, Labour-chair.
OBSTETRICANS, Accoucheur.
OBSTET'RICS, from *Obstetrix,* 'a midwife.' *Tokol'ogy, Tocol'ogy, Maieï'a, Maeei'a, Maei'a, Maeeu'tica ars, Ars obstetric''ia, Obstet'ricy,* (F.) *Obste'trique.* The art of midwifery. Midwifery in general.
OBSTETRICY, Obstetrics.
OBSTÉTRIQUE, Obstetrics.
OBSTETRIX, Midwife.
OBSTIPATIO, Constipation — o. Tenesmus, Tenesmus.
OBSTIPATIO, see Hump.
OBSTIPITAS, Torticollis — o. Capitis seu Colli, Torticollis.
OBSTRUCTIO, Emphraxis, Stegnosis — o. Alvi, Constipation — o. Ductûs Alimentarii, Constipation — o. Ductûs Stenoniani, Stenostenosis — o. Intestinalis, Constipation — o. Recti Spastica, Stricture of the Rectum, spasmodic — o. Pulmonum pituitosa febrilis, Peripneumonia notha.
OBSTRUCTION OF THE INTESTINES. Enteremphraxis.
OB'STRUENS, from *obstruo,* (*ob,* and *struere,* 'to build,') 'I stop up by building against.' *Oppilati'vus.* A medicine which closes the orifices of ducts or vessels.
OBSTUPEFACIENTIA, Narcotics.
OBTONDANT, Obtundens.
OBTUMESCENTIA, Mutitas.
OBTUN'DENS, (F.) *Obtondant,* from *obtundere* (*ob* and *tundere,* 'to beat,') 'to beat against,' and therefore to blunt the edge. An epithet applied to remedies that were supposed, according to an erroneous theory, to be possessed of the power of blunting the acrimony of the humours. A demulcent is one of these.
OBTURAMENTUM, Emphragma.
OBTURATEUR DU PALAIS, Palate, artificial.
OBTURATIO, Emphraxis.
OBTURA'TOR, *Obturato'rius,* (F.) *Obturateur,* from *obturare,* 'to close,' 'stop up the entrance.' A name given to several parts.
OBTURATOR ARTERY, *Arteria obturato'ria, A. obturatrix,* (F.) *Sous-pubio fémorale* (Ch.), *Artère obturatrice,* arises, most commonly, from the hypogastric. It is, however, frequently given off from the epigastric; a matter of importance to be determined in cases of femoral hernia. Of 500 obturator arteries examined by Mr. J. Cloquet, 348 were furnished by the hypogastric, and 152 by the epigastric or crural. When it arises from the hypogastric, it passes forwards and outwards, and then turns horizontally into the cavity of the pelvis, to issue from this cavity by the opening left at the upper part of the obturator membrane. When, on the contrary, the obturator artery arises from the epigastric or the crural, it descends obliquely inwards, behind the os pubis, to the obturator foramen. At its exit from the pelvis, the artery divides into two branches, a *posterior* and an *anterior,* which are distributed to the muscles of the anterior and superior part of the thigh.

OBTURA'TOR FORA'MEN, *Fora'men Obturato'rium, F. infra-pubia'num, Fora'men ovale, F. thyroïdeum, F. Thyroï'des, F. Amplum Pelvis,* (F.) *Trou sous-pubien.* A large opening, of an oval or triangular form, in the anterior part of the os innominatum, on the outside of the symphysis pubis and beneath the horizontal ramus of the os pubis. This foramen is closed by a membranous ligament.

OBTURATOR LIGAMENT OR MEMBRANE, *Subpubic membrane,* is a fibrous membrane, fixed to the whole circumference of the obturator foramen, except above, where an opening remains for the passage of the vessels and nerves of the same name.

OBTURATOR MUSCLES, *Obturato'res, Rotato'res fem'oris.* These are two in number. They are divided into
a. Obturator Exter'nus, Extra-pelvio-pubi-trochantérien, Sous-pubio-trochantérien externe (Ch.) A muscle, situate at the anterior and inner part of the thigh. It is broad, flat, and triangular; and is attached, on the one hand, to the anterior surface of the os pubis, to that of the ischium, and to the anterior surface of the obturator ligament. Its fleshy fibres converge to the tendon, which proceeds to be inserted at the inferior part of the cavity of the great trochanter. This muscle rotates the thigh outwards.
b. Obturator Inter'nus, Marsupia'lis, Bursa'lis, Intra-pelvio-trochantérien, Sous-pubio-trochantérien interne (Ch.) is seated, almost entirely, in the pelvis. It arises from the inner surface of the obturator ligament, and from the posterior part of the circumference of the obturator foramen, and is inserted, by means of a strong tendon, running between the two portions of the gemini, into the cavity at the root of the great trochanter; after having turned upon the ischium, which forms for it a kind of pulley. This muscle also rotates the thigh outwards.

OBTURATOR NERVE, *Sous-pubio-fémoral,* (Ch.), proceeds principally from the 2d and 3d lumbar nerves. It descends into the pelvis; gains the obturator foramen; gives branches to the obturator muscles, and divides, behind the adductor primus and pectinalis, into two branches; one *anterior,* whose branches are distributed to the first two adductors, gracilis, and integuments; the other, *posterior,* distributing its ramifications to the obturator externus and third adductor.

OBTURATOR VEIN has, ordinarily, the same arrangement as the artery. It is common, however, to find it arising from the epigastric; whilst the corresponding artery proceeds from the hypogastric, and conversely.

OBTURATORES, Obturator muscles.
OBVOLVENTIA, Demulcents.
OCA, Oxalis tuberosa.
OCCÆCATIO, Cæcitas.
OCCIP'ITAL, *Occipita'lis.* That which belongs to the occiput.
OCCIPITAL ARTERY. This arises from the posterior part of the external carotid, beneath the parotid. It proceeds backwards, passes between the mastoid process and the transverse process of the atlas; reaches the occipital bone and divides into two branches, which may be called ascending posterior and anterior, and are distributed to the neighbouring muscles and ligaments.

OCCIP'ITAL BONE, *Os occip'itis* seu *occipit'ii* seu *occipita'lē, Os sphæno basila'rē, Os memo'ria, Os nervo'sum, Os basila'rē, Os prora, Os pyx'idis* seu *sextum cra'nii* seu *lambdoi'des* seu *lambdæ* seu *laudæ* seu *puppis* seu *nervo'sum* seu *fibro'sum* seu *pelvicephal'icum*, (F.) *Os occipital*, is situate at the posterior and inferior part of the cranium, which it assists in forming. It is flat, symmetrical, and curved upon itself. It presents, 1. An *occipital* or *posterior surface*, which is convex, and has, upon the median line, the *basilary surface*, the *foramen magnum*, through which passes the spinal marrow with its membranes and vessels,—the *external occipital crest*, the *external occipital protuberance*; and, at the sides, the *upper curved line, large rough arched ridge* or *transverse arch* or *linea semicircularis*, the *lower curved line*, the *posterior condyloid fossæ*, the *condyles* for the articulation of this bone with the atlas; and the *anterior condyloid fossæ*, pierced by a foramen for the passage of the ninth pair of nerves. 2. A *cerebral* or *anterior surface*. On the median line are: the *basilary fossæ*, the *inner orifice* of the foramen magnum, the *internal occipital crest*, the *internal occipital protuberance*, the *cruciform spine*; a *channel*, which lodges the termination of the straight sinus, and on each side, the *occipital fossæ* distinguished into *superior* or *cerebral*, and *inferior* or *cerebellous*, and separated by a groove which lodges the lateral sinus. 3. The surfaces of the occipital bone are separated by four ridges and four angles. The two superior edges are articulated with the parietal bones; the two lower join the temporal; and the anterior angle, under the name *basilary process*, is united to the sphenoid.

The occipital bone is developed from four points of ossification; and sometimes from a greater number.

OCCIPITAL MUSCLE, *Occipita'lis.* Many anatomists have given this name to the posterior fasciculus of the occipito-frontalis.

OCCIPITAL NERVE, *Sub-occipital nerve*, (F.) *Première paire trachélienne* (Ch.), *Nerf occipital ou sous occipital.* It arises from the upper part of the spinal marrow by eight or ten filaments, united in two fasciculi. Thus formed, it passes between the foramen magnum and the posterior arch of the atlas; and, at this place, forms a long ganglion, afterwards dividing into two branches. Of these, the *anterior*, which is long and small, makes a turn above the transverse process of the atlas, and forms an anastomotic noose with a branch of the second cervical nerve. The *posterior* branch, larger and shorter, divides into seven or eight branches, which are distributed to the muscles of the upper and back part of the neck.

OCCIPITAL REGION, Occiput.

OCCIPITAL VEIN. Its roots follow exactly the course of the branches of the artery, and unite into a single trunk, which opens into the internal jugular vein, and sometimes into the external.

OCCIPITIUM, Occiput.

OCCIP'ITO-AT'LOID, *Occipito - atloīdeus*, (F.) *Occipito-atloīdien.* That which has reference to the occiput and atlas.

OCCIPITO-ATLOID ARTICULATION is the articulation of the condyles of the occipital bone with the superior articular cavities of the atlas. It is strengthened by two ligaments; the one *anterior*, the other *posterior*, called *occipito-atloid ligaments*: the one extends from the anterior, the other from the posterior, arch of the atlas, to the corresponding portion of the circumference of the foramen magnum.

OCCIP'ITO-AX'OID, *Occipito-axoīdeus*, (F.) *Occipito-axoīdien.* That which relates to the occipital bone and the axis or second vertebra.

OCCIPITO-AXOID ARTICULATION is the connexion of the occipital bone with the axis or second vertebra, although these bones are not really articulated, but are merely retained in apposition by three strong ligaments, the posterior of which is called the *occipito-axoid*, and the two others *odontoid*.

OCCIPITO-FRONTA'LIS, *Digas'tricus cra'nii, Epicra'nius, Fronta'lis et occipitalis.* The majority of anatomists call by this name the whole of the fleshy plane, with the epicranial or coronal aponeurosis, (see *Calotte*,) which covers the head from the occiput to the forehead. It is attached, by its posterior fasciculus, to the two outer thirds of the upper curved line of the occipital bone, and to the outer surface of the mastoid portion of the temporal; and, by its anterior fasciculus, it terminates at the eyebrow, where it becomes confounded with the superciliaris, pyramidalis nasi, and orbicularis palpebrarum.

The occipito-frontalis, by the contraction of its anterior fasciculus, draws forward a part of the integuments of the cranium. It wrinkles the skin of the forehead transversely, and may, also contribute to open the eye by its decussation with the orbicularis palpebrarum. The posterior fasciculus of the muscle draws backwards a part of the skin of the cranium, and assists in stretching the common aponeurosis.

OCCIP'ITO-MENINGE'AL. That which belongs to the occipital bone, and to the meninge or dura mater.

OCCIPITO-MENINGEAL ARTERY, in Chaussier's nomenclature, is a branch of the vertebral, given off to the dura mater at its entrance into the cranium.

OC'CIPUT, *Occipit'ium, Regio occipita'lis, In'ion*, from *ob*, and *caput, Opisthocra'nium, Opisthoceph'alon, Prora, Occipi'tium.* The back part of the head, formed by the occipital bone.

OCCIPUT, SOFT, Craniotabes.

OCCLU'SION, *Occlu'sio, Mycē*, from *occludere*, 'to shut up.' Sometimes this word signifies, simply, the transient approximation of the edges of a natural opening—the *occlusion of the eyelids*, for example; at others it is synonymous with imperforation, as *occlusion of the pupil, vagina, &c.*

OCCULT DISEASES, see Latent.

OCHEMA, Vehicle.

OCHETEUMATA, Nares.

OCHETOS, Canal.

OCHEUS, Scrotum.

OCHLE'SIS, from *οχλος*, 'a crowd.' A term, applied by Dr. George Gregory to a morbid condition induced by the crowding together of sick persons under one roof.

OCHREA RUBRA, Hæmatites.

OCHRIASIS, Paleness.

OCHROMA, Paleness.

OCHROPYRA, Fever, yellow.

OCHROTES, Paleness.

OCHROTYPHUS, Fever, yellow.

OCHTHODES, Callous.

OCIMUM ADSCENDENS, O. Basilicum.

OC'IMUM BASIL'ICUM, *O. adscen'dens* seu *pilosum* seu *racemo'sum, Basil'icum, Beren'daroa, Basil'icum majus, B. citra'tum, Oci'mum citra'tum, Common* or *Citron basil*, (F.) *Basilic commun. Nat. Ord.* Labiatæ. *Sex. Syst.* Didynamia Gymnospermia. This herb has a fragrant odour and aromatic taste. It is used as a condiment, and has been supposed to possess nervine properties.

OCIMUM CARYOPHYLLA'TUM, *O. min'imum, Small* or *Bush basil*. Possesses properties similar to the former. It is sometimes used as snuff.

OCIMUM CITRATUM, O. Basilicum—o. Pilosum, O. Basilicum—o. Racemosum, O. Basilicum.

OCOTEA PICHURIN, see Pichurim beans.
OCREA, Hippocampus minor, Shin.
OCTA'NA, *Hebdomada'ria, Febris hebdomada'ria*, from *octo*, 'eight.' A fever whose paroxysms recur every week. A supposititious case.
OCTA'RIUS. The eighth part of a wine-gallon. It contains sixteen fluidounces, (Ph. U. S.) to 20 fluidounces imperial measure.
OCTOPUS, Synapheocephalus, Hemipages.
OCTUNX. A weight of eight ounces.
OC'ULAR, *Ocula'ris;* from *oculus,* 'an eye.' Of or belonging to the eye.
OCULAR CONE. The cone formed within the eye by a pencil of rays proceeding from an object; the base of the cone being on the cornea, —the apex on the retina.
OCULARES COMMUNES, Motores oculorum —o. Dentes, Canine teeth.
OCULARIA, Euphrasia officinalis.
OCULI MARMARYGODES, Metamorphopsia — o. Palpebrarum scabies pruriginosa, Ophthalmia tarsi.
OC'ULIST, *Oculis'ta, Ophthalmia'ter, Med'icus ocula'rius.* One who occupies himself, chiefly, with the management of diseases of the eye.
OCULISTIQUE, Ophthalmology.
OCULO-MUSCULAR NERVES, COMMON, Motores oculorum.
OCULUM MOVENS PRIMUS, Rectus internus oculi — o. Movens quartus, Rectus inferior oculi—o. Movens secundus, Rectus externus oculi — o. Movens tertius, Rectus superior oculi.
OCULUS, Eye—o. Bovinus, Hydrophthalmia — o. Bovis, Chrysanthemum leucanthemum — o. Bubulus, Hydrophthalmia—o. Cæsius, Glaucoma — o. Duplex, Binoculus — o. Elephantinus, Hydrophthalmia—o. Genu, Patella—o. Lacrymans, Epiphora — o. Purulentus, Hypopyon — o. Simplex, see Monoculus—o. Typhonis, Scilla.
OCYMUM, see Ocimum — o. Sylvestre, Clinopodium vulgare.
OCYODYNIC, Ocytocic.
OCYPH'ONUS, from οκυς, 'quick,' and φονος, 'murder.' An agent that kills speedily.
OCYTOCEUS, Ocytocic.
OCYTOC'IC, *Oxytocic, Ocytoc'eus, Ocytoc'ius, Ocyt'ocus, Ocyody'nic, Odinago'gus,* from οξυς, 'quick,' and τοκος, 'labour.' Any thing that expedites parturition.
OCYTOCIUS, Ocytocic.
OCYTOCUS, Ocytocic.
ODAXIS'MUS, *Odazes'mus, Odontocne'sis, Odontocnesmus,* from οδους, 'a tooth.' The painful itching of the gums which precedes the appearance of the teeth. Dentition.
ODES. A suffix, see Eidos.
ODEUR, Odour.
ODIN, Pains, (labour.)
ODINAGOGUS, Ocytocic.
ODINOL'YSIS, from ωδιν, 'labour pains,' and λυσις, 'solution.' Mitigation of labour pains.
ODINOPŒ'A, from ωδιν, 'labour pains,' and ποιεω, 'I make.' Agents that encourage labour pains.
ODIS, Pains, labour.
ODME, Odour.
ODONTAGOGON, Dentagra.
ODON'TAGRA, from οδους, 'a tooth,' and αγρα, 'a seizure.' A rheumatic or gouty pain in the teeth. Dentagra.
ODONTAL'GIA, from οδους, 'a tooth,' and αλγος, 'pain.' *Odon'tia, Den'tium dolor, Toothach, Odon'tia doloro'sa, Gomphi'asis, Gomphias'mus, Odontodyn'ia,* (F.) *Douleur des dents, Fluxion sur les dents, Mal de dent, Mal d'amour.* A disease dependent upon a variety of causes affecting the cavity of the tooth; but generally owing to caries, which exposes the cavity to the action of the air, and to extraneous matters in general. Hence, the treatment consists in plugging the tooth, or destroying the sensibility of the nerve, by powerful stimulants; and, if these means fail, in extracting the tooth.
ODONTALGIA CARIOSA, Dental gangrene — o. Dentitionis, Dentition — o. Hæmodia, Hæmodia.
ODONTALGIA NERVOSA, *Neural'gia Denta'lis.* Neuralgia of the teeth. Characterized by periodical pain, shooting with the utmost violence along the branches of the fifth pair distributed to the affected jaw.
ODONTALGIA REMITTENS ET INTERMITTENS, Neuralgia infra-orbitaria.
ODONTALGIC, Anti-odontalgic.
ODONTAMBLYOGMUS, Hæmodia.
ODONTHÆMODIA, Hæmodia.
ODONTHARPAGA, Dentagra.
ODONTHYPERÆSTHESIS, Hæmodia.
ODONTIA, Odontalgia.
ODONTIA DEFOR'MIS. Deformity of the teeth from error of shape, position, or number.—Good.
ODONTIA DENTITIONIS LACTANTIUM, see Dentition (first)—o. Dentitionis puerilis, see Dentition (second) — o. Edentula, see Nefrendes — o. Excrescens, Epulis — o. Incrustans, Odontolithos — o. Stuporis, Hæmodia.
ODONTIASIS, Dentition.
ODONTIATER, Dentist.
ODONTIATRIA, Dentistry.
ODONTIC, Anti-odontalgic.
ODONTI'TIS, *Odontopthleg'monè,* from οδους, 'a tooth,' and *itis,* denoting inflammation. Inflammation of the teeth.
ODONTOBOTHRI'TIS, *Odontophatni'tis, Inflamma'tio alveolo'rum,* from *odontobothrium,* 'alveolus,' and *itis,* denoting inflammation. Inflammation of the alveoli.
ODONTOBOTHRIUM, Alveolus.
ODONTOCLA'SIS, from οδους, 'a tooth,' and κλασις, 'fracture;' *Fractu'ra den'tis.* Fracture of a tooth.
ODONTOCNESIS, Odaxismus.
ODONTOCNESMUS, Odaxismus.
ODONTODES, Odontoid.
ODONTODYNIA, Odontalgia.
ODONTOG"ENY, *Odontogen'ia;* from οδους, οδοντος, 'a tooth,' and γενεσις, 'generation.' Generation or mode of development of the teeth.
ODONTOGLYPHON, Dentiscalpium, Gum lancet.
ODONTOGLYPHUM, Dentiscalpium, Gum lancet.
ODONTOG'RAPHY, *Odontograph'ia,* from οδους, 'a tooth,' and γραφη, 'a description.' A description of the teeth.
ODON'TOID, *Odontoï'des, Odonto'des, Dentiform'is, Denta'lis, Dentoideus, Pyrenoï'des,* from οδους, 'a tooth,' and ειδος, 'shape,' 'resemblance.' This epithet is given to the *Processus dentatus* of the second vertebra or axis.
ODONTOID LIG'AMENTS, (F.) *Ligaments odontoïdiens,* are two strong and short conical fasciculi, whose truncated summits embrace the sides of the odontoid process, and whose bases are fixed in the fossæ at the inner side of the condyles of the occipital bone. Their direction is obliquely outwards and slightly upwards. They enter into the composition of the occipito-axoid articulation; strengthen the junction of the head with the vertebral column, and limit the movement of rotation of the atlas on the axis.
ODONTOL'ITHOS, from οδους, 'a tooth,' and λιθος, 'a stone.' A sort of incrustation, of a yellowish colour, which forms at the base of the teeth, and is called *Tartar, Tar'tarus Dentium,*

Odon'tia incrus'tans, Cal'culus denta'lis, (F.) *Tartre des Dents.* It consists of seventy-nine parts of phosphate of lime; twelve and a half of mucus; one of a particular salivary matter, and seven and a half of animal substance, soluble in chlorohydric acid. Infusoria have been found in it.

ODONTOL'OGY, *Odontolog''ia*, from ὀδούς, 'a tooth,' and λογος, 'a discourse.' An anatomical treatise of the teeth.

ODONTONECROSIS, Dental gangrene.

ODONTOPARALLAX'IS, from ὀδούς, 'a tooth,' and παραλλαξις, 'deviation.' Irregularity and obliquity of the teeth.

ODONTOPHATNĒ, Alveolus.

ODONTOPHATNITIS, Odontobothritis.

ODONTOPHYIA, Dentition.

ODONTOPRISIS, Brygmus, Stridor dentium.

ODONTOSEI'SIS, *Odontoseis'mus, Den'tium vacillan'tia.* Looseness of the teeth.

ODONTOSEISMUS, Odontoseisis.

ODONTOSMEGMA, Dentifrice.

ODONTOSPHACELISIS, Dental gangrene.

ODONTOSPHACELISMUS, Dental gangrene.

ODONTOSTERE'SIS, from ὀδούς, 'a tooth,' and στερησις, 'privation.' Loss of the teeth.

ODONTOSYNERISMUS, from ὀδούς, 'a tooth,' and συνεριζειν, 'to strike together.' (F.) *Claquement.* Chattering of the teeth.

ODONTOTECHNY, Dentistry.

ODONTOTHERAPIA, Dentistry.

ODONTOTRIMMA, Dentifrice.

ODORAMENTUM, Odoriferum.

ODORAT, Olfaction.

ODORATIO, Olfaction.

ODORATUS, Olfaction — o. Deperditus, Anosmia.

ODORIF'ERUM, from *odor*, 'odour,' and *fero*, 'I carry;' *Odoramen'tum.* A medicine that gives odour or flavour. A scent. A perfume.

ODOS, Way.

O'DOUR, *Odor, Odmē, Osmē*, (F.) *Odeur.* A smell. Odours are subtle particles, constantly escaping from the surface of certain bodies. They act, in some manner, by actual contact with the nerves of the Schneiderian membrane, and give occasion to the sense of smell or olfaction.

ODOUS, Teeth.

OD'YNE, ὀδυνη, 'pain,' *Dolor, Odyne'ma.* A very common suffix to words; as in Pleurodyne.

ODYNEMA, Odyne.

ŒCONOMIA, Economy — œ. Animalis, Physiology.

ŒDALICUS, Œdematous.

ŒDALIUS, Œdematous.

ŒDE'MA, from οἰδεω, 'I am swollen.' *Hydron'cus, Œdemat'ia, Hyderon'cus, Hydaton'cus, Hydrocæde'ma, Hydrede'ma, Hydrops cellula'ris ar'tuum, Phlegma'tia, Leucophlegma'tia, Ecphy'ma œdemat'icum*, (F.) *Œdème, Œdématie, Enflure.* Swelling produced by the accumulation of a serous fluid in the interstices of the areolar texture. This swelling is soft; yields under the finger; preserves the impression for some time, and is pale and without pain. It presents the same characters as anasarca, which is general œdema. Its etiology and treatment are also the same. See Anasarca.

ŒDEMA ACUTUM, see Anasarca.

ŒDEMA ARSENICA'LIS. The swelling of the eyelids and face, induced by continued use of the preparations of arsenic.

ŒDEMA CALIDUM, see Anasarca — œ. Capitis, Hydrocephalus externus.

ŒDE'MA CER'EBRI, (F.) *Œdème du cerveau.* Œdema of the brain. A condition of the cerebral pulp, in which there is an infiltration of serous fluid into it, so that it appears more moist or watery than common; and, when sliced or pressed, small drops of water are seen to ooze out.

ŒDEMA, COMPACT, Induration of the cellular tissue — œ. Cruentum, Suggillation — œ. Febrile, see Anasarca — œ. Fugax, Anathymiasis — œ. Hystericum, Anathymiasis.

ŒDEMA OF THE GLOTTIS, *Œdem'atous Laryngi'tis*, L. *submuco'sa* sou *œdemato'sa* seu *seropurulen'ta, Œde'ma glot'tidis, Hydrops glot'tidis, Angi'na aquo'sa*, A. *larynge'a œdemato'sa, Submu'cosa Laryngi'tis, Œdem'atous angi'na*, (F.) *Laryngite œdémateuse*, L. *œdémateuse et séro-purulente*, L. *susglottique*, L. *sous-muqueuse, Angine laryngée œdémateuse, Œdème de la glotte.* A disease consisting of serous or sero-purulent infiltration into the submucous tissue of the glottis. The symptoms resemble those of croup; but the disease attacks the adult rather than the child. The age is, indeed, a principal means of diagnosis between the two affections.

The disease is almost always fatal. The treatment has to vary according to the accompanying general symptoms.

ŒDEMA LACTEUM, Phlegmatia dolens.

ŒDEMA OF THE LUNGS, *Œde'ma pulmo'num, Pneumoch'ysis, Pneumonœde'ma, Hydrops Pulmo'num, Hydropneumo'nia, Anasar'ca Pulmo'num*, (F.) *Œdème du poumon.* Laënnec has so called the infiltration of serum into the tissue of the lung, carried to such an extent as to diminish its permeability to air. It is not an uncommon sequela of pneumonia, and the major exanthemata. The respiration is laborious; the respiratory murmur scarcely perceptible, although the thorax is largely expanded, and there is a slight *râle crepitant*, particularly at the base and inferior part of the lung. The sound on percussion is clear, and on both sides equally so. The cough is attended with aqueous expectoration. In some cases the respiration becomes puerile in a small portion of the summit of the lung.

ŒDEMA NEONATORUM, Induration of the cellular tissue — œ. Palpebrarum, Hydroblepharon — œ. Puerperarum, Phlegmatia dolens—œ. Pulmonum, Œdema of the lungs — œ. Pulmonum chronicum, Hydropneumonia — œ. Scroti aquosum, Oschydrœdema—œ. Scroti cruentum, Œschæmatœdema—œ. Scroti purulentum, Oscheopyœdema — œ. Scroti urinosum, Urecele — œ. Spasticum, Anathymiasis — œ. Uvulæ, Staphylœdema.

ŒDEMATIA, Œdema.

ŒDÉMATIÉ, Œdema.

ŒDEMATOSARCA, Œdemosarca.

ŒDEMATOSCHEOCE'LĒ, *Œdemoscheoce'lē, Oscheoce'lē œdemat'ica.* Oscheocele with œdema of the scrotum.

ŒDEM'ATOUS, *Œdemato'sus, Œdemat'icus, Œdemato'des, Œdal'ius, Œdal'icus, Edem'atous.* Affected with œdema.

ŒDÈME, Œdema — œ. *du Cerveau*, Œdema cerebri — œ. *Douloureux des femmes en couche*, Phlegmatia dolens—œ. *des Nouvelles accouchées*, Phlegmatia dolens — œ. *actif des Nouvelles accouchées*, Phlegmatia dolens — œ. *de la Glotte*, Œdema of the glottis — œ. *de la Glotte*, Angina œdematosa — œ. *du Tissu cellulaire des nouveaunés*, Induration of the cellular tissue.

ŒDEMOSAR'CA, *Œdematosar'ca.* A species of tumour mentioned by M. A. Severinus, which holds a middle place between œdema and sarcoma.

ŒDEMOSCHEOCELE, Œdematoscheocele.

ŒIL, Eye—œ. *de Bœuf*, Anthemis tinctoria— œ. *Double*, Binoculus—œ. *de Lièvre*, Lagophthalmus — œ. *Simple*, see Monoculus.

ŒILLET GIROFLÉE, Dianthus caryophyllus.

ŒILLIÈRE, Scaphium oculare.

ŒNAN'THE, Œ. croca'ta, Œ. chærophyl'li fo'liis, Hemlock dropwort, Hemlock water-dropwort. Nat. Ord. Umbelliferæ. Sex. Syst. Pentandria Digynia. A violent poison of the acro-narcotic class. Its juice has been recommended in certain cutaneous diseases; but it is scarcely ever used. It is employed in fomentations.

ŒNANTHE AQUATICA, Phellandrium aquaticum—œ. Phellandrium, Phellandrium aquaticum—œ. Striata rigida, Seseli tortuosum.

ŒNELÆ'ON, from οινος, 'wine,' and ελαιον, 'oil.' A mixture of oil and wine.—Galen. Also, rectified spirit or alcohol.

ŒNOG'ALA, οινογαλα, from οινος, 'wine,' and γαλα, 'milk,'—'a mixture of wine and milk.' According to some, wine as warm as new milk.

ŒNOG'ARON, Garum vino mistum. Wine mixed with garum.—Aëtius.

ŒNOIDES, Vinous.

ŒNOMA'NIA, Oinoma'nia, from οινος, 'wine,' and mania. Delirium tremens. Properly, wine-mania. An insatiable desire for intoxicating liquors.

ŒNOMEL, Œnom'eli, from οινος, 'wine,' and μελι, 'honey.' Mel vino'sum, Mulsum Vino'sum. Honey wine. Wine mead.

ŒNOPHLYGIA, Temulentia.

ŒNOPHLYXIS, Temulentia.

ŒNOS, Wine.

ŒNOSTAGMA, Spiritus vini rectificatus.

ŒNOTHE'RA BIEN'NIS, Œ. Mollis'sima seu murica'ta seu gauroï'des, On'agra, Evening Primrose, Tree Primrose, Primrose tree, Cure-all, Scabish. An indigenous plant, common on the borders of fields, and in natural hedges. Sex. Syst. Octandria Monogynia. Its properties are mucilaginous and slightly acrid. A decoction has been used in cases of infantile and other eruptions.

ŒNOTHERA GAUROIDES, O. biennis — œ. Muricata, O. biennis.

ŒSOPHAGE'AL, Œsophaga'us, (F.) Œsophagien. Relating or belonging to the œsophagus.

ŒSOPHAGEAL AP'ERTURE OF THE DI'APHRAGM, (F.) Ouverture œsophagienne du diaphragme. An opening in the diaphragm for the passage of the œsophagus.

ŒSOPHAGEAL APERTURE OF THE STOMACH. A name given to the superior or cardiac orifice of the stomach, to distinguish it from the inferior or pyloric.

ŒSOPHAGEAL MUSCLE, Œsophaga'us. Some anatomists have given this name to the transverse muscular fibres which surround the œsophagus at its upper extremity.

ŒSOPHAGEAL TUBE, see Tube, œsophageal.

ŒSOPHAGEURYS'MA, Œsoph'agus succenturia'tus, from οισοφαγος, 'the œsophagus,' and ευρυσμα, 'dilatation.' Dilatation of the œsophagus.

ŒSOPHAGIALGIA, Œsophagismus.

ŒSOPHAGIARCTIA, Dysphagia constricta.

ŒSOPHAGIEN, (muscle,) Constrictor œsophagi.

ŒSOPHAGIS'MUS, Œsophagis'mum. A name given by Vogel to spasm of the œsophagus, Dyspha'gia spasmod'ica, D. Spas'tica, Œsophago-spasm'us, D. Nervo'sa, Strictu'ra œsoph'agi spasmod'ica, Œsophagial'gia, Tenes'mus Gulæ, (F.) Ténesme de l'œsophage. By some used synonymously with œsophagitis, dysphagia, and contraction of the œsophagus.

ŒSOPHAGI'TIS, Angi'na œsophaga'a, Cynan'chê œsophaga'a, Dyspha'gia inflammato'ria, Inflamma'tio œsoph'agi, I. Gulæ, (F.) Angine œsophagienne. Inflammation of the œsophagus.

ŒSOPHAGODYN'IA, from οισοφαγος, 'the œsophagus,' and οδυνη, 'pain.' Pain in the œsophagus.

ŒSOPHAGOPATHI'A, Morbus Œsoph'agi, from οισοφαγος, 'the œsophagus,' and νοσος, 'disease.' A morbid condition of the œsophagus.

ŒSOPHAGOPLE'GIA, Dyspha'gia paralyt'ica, Læmoparaly'sis, from οισοφαγος, 'the œsophagus,' and πληγη, 'a stroke.' Paralysis of the œsophagus.

ŒSOPHAGORRHAG"IA, from οισοφαγος, 'the œsophagus,' and ραγη, 'a rupture.' Hemorrhage from the œsophagus.

ŒSOPHAGORRHŒ'A from οισοφαγος, 'the œsophagus,' and ρεω, 'I flow.' Discharge of blood or mucus from the œsophagus.

ŒSOPHAGOSPASM'US, from οισοφαγος, 'the œsophagus,' and σπασμος, 'spasm.' Spasm of the œsophagus.

ŒSOPHAGOT'OMY, Œsophagotom'ia, from οισοφαγος, 'the œsophagus,' and τεμνειν, 'to cut.' An incision made into the œsophagus for the purpose of extracting foreign bodies from it.

ŒSOPH'AGUS, from οιω, 'I carry,' and φαγω, 'I eat;' Gula, Fis'tula ciba'lis, Via stom'achi et ventris, Fis'tula vel Infundib'ulum Ventric'uli, Gluttus. The Gullet. A musculo-membranous canal, cylindrical, and depressed from before to behind, which extends from the inferior extremity of the pharynx to the upper orifice of the stomach. At its origin, it is situate in the median line; but, beneath the larynx, it deviates to the left, and in the chest experiences different inflections. In its cervical portion, it corresponds, behind, with the spine; before, with the larynx and trachea; and, at the sides, it is close to the primitive carotids, internal jugular veins, par vagum, recurrent nerves, &c. In its inferior or thoracic portion, the œsophagus is entirely contained in the posterior mediastinum; and enters the abdomen through the œsophageal aperture of the diaphragm. The œsophagus is composed of a very strong muscular layer, sometimes called Tunica vagina'lis gulæ; formed, itself, of two sets of fibres, the external being general longitudinal, the internal transverse or annular. 2. Of a mucous membrane which is soft, fine, thin, and white, especially at its lower part. It is continuous, above, with the mucous membrane of the pharynx. The mucous follicles, found beneath it, are not numerous, and have been called Œsophageal glands. The arteries of the œsophagus proceed, in the neck, from the thyroid; in the chest, from the bronchial arteries and directly from the aorta;—in the abdomen, from the inferior phrenic, and coronaria ventriculi. Its veins empty themselves into the inferior thyroid, the vena cava superior, the internal mammary, azygos, bronchial, phrenic, and coronaria ventriculi. Its lymphatics pass into the ganglia surrounding it. Its nerves are afforded by the pharyngeal and pulmonary plexuses; by the cardiac nerves; the thoracic ganglia, and, especially, by the pneumogastrics and their recurrent branches.

ŒSOPHAGUS SUCCENTURIATUS, Pharyngocele.

ŒSTROMANIA, Nymphomania.

ŒSTRUATION, Orgasm, see Heat.

ŒSTRUM, Clitoris.

ŒSTRUM VEN'ERIS, Œstrum vene'reum, Œstrus vene'reus; from οιστρος, œstrus, 'a violent impulse or desire.' A vehement desire for sexual intercourse. With some, œstrum signifies Clitoris.

ŒSTRUS, Clitoris — œ. Venereus, Œstrum venereum.

ŒSYPUS, from οἶς, 'a sheep,' and πῶρος, 'dirt' [?]. The greasy matter of unwashed wool; formerly employed in friction in diseased joints.

ŒUFS, Ova.

OFFICE, PHYSICIAN'S or SURGEON'S, Iatrion.

OFFICINA, Pharmacopolium.

OFFIC"INAL, *Officina'lis*, from *officina*, 'a shop.' An epithet for medicines found in the shop of the apothecary, ready prepared — *usua'lia;* in opposition to *magistral* or *extemporaneous*, — those prepared after the prescription of the physician.

OFFIUM, Affion, Opium.

OFFSPRING, Epigone.

OFFUSCATIO, Amaurosis.

OGLA, Oogala.

OGNON, a Corn — o. *Marin*, Scilla.

OHI'O, MINERAL WATERS OF. *Yellow Spring* is a chalybeate, situate in Greene county, 64 miles from Cincinnati. It is somewhat frequented.

OIDIUM ABORTIFACIENS, see Ergot.

OIE, Sorbus domestica.

OIGNON, Allium cepa.

OIL, *O'leum, Ela'on,* (F.) *Huile;* from ἐλαία, 'the olive.' A collective name, under which two classes of fluids are included, very different from each other: those belonging to the one class, are viscid, mawkish or almost insipid; those of the other are nearly devoid of viscidity, and are caustic and very volatile. The former are called *fat* or *fixed oils;* the latter *volatile* or *essential oils*, or *essences*.

Oil of Almonds, Oleum amygdalarum — o. of Amber, rectified, see Succinum — o. Animal, Oleum animale — o. Animal, of Dippel, Oleum animale Dippelii — o. of Bay, Daphnelæon — o. of Bays, Oleum laurinum — o. of Beeswax, Unguentum ceræ — o. of Benjamin or Benzoin, Oleum benzoini — o. Benne, see Sesamum orientale.

Oil, British. An empirical preparation often used in cases of sprains.

A committee of the Philadelphia College of Pharmacy recommend the following form for its preparation. — *Ol. Terebinth., Ol. Lini. usitatiss.* āā. f℥iij, *Ol. Succini., Ol. Juniper.* āā. f℥iv, *Petrol. Barbadens.* f℥iij, *Petrol. American.* (*Seneca Oil,*) f℥j. M.

Oil of Cacao, Butter of Cacao — o. of the Cashew nut, see Anacardium occidentale — o. Castor, see Ricinus communis — o. of Chabert, Oleum animale empyreumaticum Chaberti — o. of Cinnamon, see Laurus cinnamomum — o. of Cloves, Eugenia caryophyllata — o. Cod, O. Jecoris aselli o. Codliver, O. Jecoris aselli — o. of Copaiba, Oleum Copaibæ — o. of Cubebs, see Piper cubeba — o. of Cypress, Cyprinum oleum — o. of Dill, see Anethum graveolens — o. Dippel's, Oleum animale Dippelii — o. of Egg, see Ovum — o. Ethereal, Oleum Æthereum — o. Flaxseed, see Linum usitatissimum.

Oil, Fusel, *Al'cohol amyl'icum,* (Ph. D.) *Fousel oil, Pota'to oil.* An acrid volatile oil, formed in the manufacture of potato brandy, and which is not easily separable from it. Its chemical constitution is analogous to that of alcohol. It exhales a powerful and peculiarly suffocating odour. S. g. .818. In small doses it is highly stimulating, — acting like narcotics in general. In large doses it destroys the mucous membranes of the stomach.

Oil, Haerlem. An empirical preparation supposed to consist chiefly of petroleum, turpentine, and balsam of sulphur. Used internally in renal and rheumatic affections.

Oil, Krumholz, see Pinus mughos — o. of Lemons, see Citrus medica — o. Lily, see Lilium candidum — o. of Mucilages, Oleum e mucilaginibus — o. Neatsfoot, Oleum bubulum — o. of Nicodemus, Nicodemi oleum — o. Nut, Juglans cinerea — o. of Nutmegs, see Myristica moschata — o. Olive, Oleum olivæ — o. Palm, see Cocos butyracea — o. Paper, Pyrothonide — o. of Pennyroyal, see Hedeoma pulegioides — o. of Pike, Oleum lucii piscis — o. Rock, Petrolæum — o. Potato, Oil, Fusel — o. Rag, Pyrothonide — o. Rayliver, sce Oleum Jecoris aselli — o. of Roses, see Rosa centifolia — o. of Rue, Peganelæon, see Ruta — o. of Spike, Oleum terebinthinæ — o. of St. John's Wort, see Hypericum perforatum — o. Salad, Oleum olivæ — o. of Scorpion, see Scorpion — o. Sulphuretted, Balsamum sulphuris simplex — o. of Tartar, Liquor potassæ subcarbonatis — o. of Tobacco, Oleum tabaci — o. of Turpentine, Oleum terebinthinæ — o. of Turpentine, rectified, Oleum terebinthinæ rectificatum — o. of Valerian, Oleum valerianæ — o. of Vitriol, Sulphuric acid — o. of Wine, Oleum æthereum.

Oils, Animal, Olea animalia — o. Distilled, Olea volatilia — o. Empyreumatic, Olea empyreumatica — o. Essential, Olea volatilia — o. Ethereal, Olea volatilia — o. Expressed, Olea fixa — o. Fatty, Olea fixa — o. Fixed, Olea fixa — o. Fugacious, Olea fugacia — o. Medicinal, Olea medicinalia — o. Volatile, Olea volatilia.

OILY, Oleaginous — o. Grain, Sesamum orientale.

OINOMANIA, Œnomania.

OINTMENT, Unguentum — o. of Antimony, tartarized, Unguentum antimonii tartarizati.

Ointment, Arsen'ical, of *Sir Astley Cooper.* This is made of *arsenious acid* ℨj; *sulphur,* ℨj; *spermaceti cerate,* ℨj. It is spread on lint, and applied to cancerous sores.

Ointment, Basilicon, Unguentum resinæ — o. Bay, Unguentum laurinum — o. of Belladonna, Unguentum belladonnæ — o. Blister, Cerate of cantharides — o. Blistering, green, Unguentum lyttæ medicatum — o. Blistering, milder, Unguentum lyttæ — o. Blistering, yellow, Unguentum lyttæ medicatum aliud — o. Blue, Unguentum hydrargyri — o. Citrine, Unguentum hydrargyri nitratis — o. of Creasote, Unguentum creasoti — o. Cyrillo's, Unguentum muriatis hydrargyri oxygenati medicatum — o. Digestive, simple, Unguentum digestivum simplex — o. Edinburgh, see Unguentum veratri — o. Elder, Unguentum sambuci — o. of Elemi, Unguentum elemi compositum — o. for the Eyes, (Smellome's,) see Ceratum resinæ — o. Golden, Unguentum hydrargyri nitrico-oxidi — o. Golden, Singleton's, see Singleton's golden ointment — o. Goulard's, Ceratum plumbi compositum — o. Green, Unguentum sambuci — o. Hellebore white, Unguentum veratri — o. of Iodide of potassium, Unguentum potassæ hydriodatis — o. of Iodide of Sulphur, Unguentum sulphuris iodidi — o. of Iodine, Unguentum Iodini — o. of Iodine, compound, Unguentum iodini compositum — o. Itch, Unguentum sulphuris compositum — o. Itch, Bateman's, see Unguentum sulphuratum alcalinum ad scabiem — o. Itch, Bailey's, see Unguentum sulphuratum ad scabiem — o. Itch, Helmerick's, Unguentum sulphuratum alcalinum ad scabiem — o. Issue, Dr. Physick's, see Unguentum lyttæ medicatum aliud — o. of white oxide of Lead, Unguentum oxidi plumbi albi — o. of Lydia, Bacaris — o. Marshmallow, Unguentum de Althææ — o. Mercurial, Unguentum hydrargyri — o. of nitrate of Mercury, Unguentum hydrargyri nitratis — o. of gray oxide of Mercury, Unguentum oxidi hydrargyri cinerei — o. of nitric oxyd of Mercury, Unguentum hydrargyri nitrico-oxydi — o. of Nitrous acid, Unguentum acidi nitrosi —

o. Plunkett's, for cancer, Plunkett's ointment—o. red Precipitate, Unguentum hydrargyri nitrico-oxydi—o. of white Precipitate, Unguentum hydrargyri præcipitati albi—o. Resin, Ceratum resinæ flavæ—o. Resin, black, Unguentum resinæ nigræ—o. of Rosewater, Unguentum aquæ rosæ—o. Soldier's, Martiatum unguentum—o. of Spanish flies, Cerate of Cantharides, Unguentum lyttæ—o. Spermaceti, Unguentum cetacei—o. of Stramonium, Unguentum stramonii—o. of Subacetate of copper, Unguentum subacetatis cupri—o. of Sugar of lead, Unguentum plumbi superacetatis—o. Sulphur, Unguentum sulphuris—o. Sulphur, compound, Unguentum sulphuris compositum—o. Tar, Unguentum picis liquidæ—o. Tobacco, Unguentum Tabaci—o. Tutty, Unguentum oxidi zinci impuri—o. Verdigris, Unguentum subacetatis cupri—o. Wax, Unguentum ceræ—o. White, Unguentum oxidi plumbi albi—o. Zinc, Unguentum zinci—o. of impure oxide of Zinc, Unguentum oxidi zinci impuri.

OIOCALYM'MA, *Oiocalyp'trum;* from ωιον, 'egg,' and καλυπτειν, 'to cover;' *Membra'na O'vuli cortica'lis.* The membrane of the eggshell.

OLD AGE, Senectus.

OLD MAN, Artemisia abrotanum.

OLD WIFE'S SHIRT, Liriodendron.

OLEA ANIMA'LIA, *Animal oils,* (F.) *Huiles animales.* A name given to fixed oils holding in solution the mucilaginous and gelatinous principles of certain animals, as the *Oil of frogs, Oil of scorpions, Oil of spiders,* &c. Sometimes, also, the term *animal oils* is given to empyreumatic oils, produced during the decomposition of animal substances by heat.

OLEA DESTILLATA, O. volatilia.

OLEA EMPYREUMAT'ICA, *Empyreumat'ic oils,* (F.) *Huiles empyreumatiques.* Oils which have an empyreumatic or burnt smell. They are obtained by treating vegetable or animal matters by heat, in close vessels. They do not exist in organised bodies, but are formed during their decomposition by fire. The animal oil of Dippel is an empyreumatic oil.

OLEA EUROPÆ'A, *O. sati'va seu lancifo'lia* seu *polymor'pha* seu *Gall'ica, Oli'va, Olive tree,* ελαια, *Ela'a,* (F.) *Olivier,* (Fruit) *Olive. Nat. Ord.* Jasmineæ. *Sex. Syst.* Diandria Monogynia. The leaves of the olive are bitter, and an extract prepared from them, and a substance called *olivi'na,* the bitter principle of the leaves, have been given in Italy as antiperiodics. The fruit, when pickled, is extremely grateful to some stomachs. Olives, as met with in the shops, are prepared from the green, unripe fruit, repeatedly steeped in water. To this, some quicklime or alkaline salt is added, and, afterwards, they are washed and preserved in a pickle of common salt and water. From this fruit is prepared the *Olive oil* or *Salad oil* of the Pharmacopœias, which is obtained by grinding and pressing the olives, when thoroughly ripe. The finer and purer oil issues first by gentle pressure, and the inferior sort on heating what is left, and pressing it more strongly. See Oleum Olivæ. In Calabria, an odorous resin exudes from its trunk, which is employed as a perfume by the Neapolitans.

A gum flows from certain wild olives, in warm countries, which consists, according to Pelletier, of a resin, a little benzoic acid, and a peculiar substance, called *Olivile.* It is in yellow masses, of a slightly acrid taste, and of a vanilla smell. It is called *Olea gummi, O. resi'na,* and *O. bals'amum,* (F.) *Gomme olivier,* and is esteemed astringent and detersive.

OLEA FIXA VEL PIN'GUIA, *Expressed oils, Fixed oils, Fatty oils,* (F.) *Huiles fixes* ou *grasses.* All the oils obtained from the seeds or pericarps of vegetables, without distillation, and which are viscid, but slightly odorous and sapid; lighter than water, and insoluble in alcohol. The rancidity of oils depends on the absorption of oxygen, and therefore they should be kept in bulk as much as possible; and in narrow-necked bottles, so that a very small surface only can be exposed to the air. All the fixed oils are emollient, and, in a certain dose, they act as purgatives and emetics. They are prepared by expressing the fruit or seed containing them.

OLEA FUGA'CIA, *Fuga'cious oils,* (F.) *Huiles fugaces.* A name given to oils which are so volatile that, in order to obtain them, recourse must be had to a different process from that employed for other essential oils. Such are the oils of jessamine, lily, violet, &c.

OLEA GALLICA, O. Europæa—o. Lancifolia, O. Europæa.

OLEA MEDICINA'LIA, *Medic''inal oils,* (F.) *Huiles Medicinales.* A name given to oils prepared by macerating, infusing, or boiling medicinal substances in olive or any other fixed oils. These oils may then be regarded as oily solutions of certain medicinal substances; whence they can never be simple. They have, however, been divided into *simple* and *compound medicinal oils.* To the former belong the *Oils of St. John's wort,* of the *Solanum nigrum,&c.;* to the other—which have often been called *Oily balsams,* (F.) *Baumes huileux*—the *Balsams of Fioraventi, Metz,* &c. Medicinal oils are, almost always, employed externally.

OLEA POLYMORPHA, O. Europæa—o. Sativa, O. Europæa.

OLEA VOLATIL'IA, *Olea destilla'ta, Vol'atile oils, Æthero'lea, Ethe'real oils, Essential oils, Distil'led oils, Es'sences,* (F.) *Huiles volatiles, H. essentielles.* Oils found in aromatic vegetables, and in every part of them, except in the interior of the seeds. The majority are obtained by distillation; but some by expression. They possess unctuosity, inflammability, and viscidity, like the fixed oils; but they are generally odoriferous, pungent, and acrid. The greater part are lighter than water; but some are heavier, and congeal at a moderate temperature. They dissolve, in small quantity, in distilled water, by simple agitation. Almost all are soluble in alcohol. The odour and taste are the usual tests of their goodness. To preserve them, they should be kept in a cool place, in small bottles, quite full and well corked. Volatile oils are possessed of the aromatic properties of the plants whence they are obtained. They are all, when applied externally, stimulant and rubefacient.

OLEAG''INOUS, *Oleagino'sus, Oleo'sus.* Oily: containing oil,—as 'an *oleaginous* or *oily* mixture.'

OLEA'MEN, *Oleamen'tum.* Any soft ointment prepared of oil.—Scribonius.

OLEANDER, Rhododendron chrysanthemum.

OLECRANARTHRI'TIS, from ωλεκρανον, 'the olecranon,' αρθρον, 'joint,' and *itis,* denoting inflammation. Inflammation of the elbow joint.

OLECRANOID CAVITY, see Ulna.

OLEC'RANON, *Olecra'non, Olec'ranum, Olec'ranon mob'ile;* from ωλενη, 'the elbow,' and κρανον, 'the head.' *Acrole'nion, Additamen'tum seca'tum, Ancon, Proces'sus anconeus, Glans seu Coro'na* seu *Coro'na posterior* seu *Additamen'tum unca'tum Ulnæ, Vertex Cu'biti, Patel'la fixa, Rostrum exter'num* seu *poste'rius, Top of the cubit.* Head or projection of the elbow. A large process at the upper extremity of the ulna, on which we lean. When this process is fractured, it is apt to be drawn up by the triceps, and much care is required to keep the parts in apposition.

OLECRANARTHROC'ACE, from ὠλένη, 'the elbow,' κρανον, 'the head,' and *arthrocace*. A name given by Rust to inflammation of the articular surfaces of the elbow.

OLEFIANT GAS, CHLORIDE OF, see Anæsthetic.

OLENE, Ulna.

OLEO-CERATUM AQUÂ SUBACTUM, Ceratum Galeni.

OLEO-SACCHARUM, Elæo-saccharum.

OLEOSUS, Oleaginous.

OLETTE, MINERAL WATERS OF. At Olette, in the department Pyrénées Orientales, is a thermal spring, which raises the thermometer to 190° Fahr. It is the hottest in France.

OLEUM, Oil—o. Abietis, see Pinus picea—o. Absinthii, Artemisia absinthium, (oil of)—o. Acusticum, *Huile acoustique.*

OLEUM ÆTHE'REUM, *Æthe'real oil (formed in the distillation of ether), Oleum vini, Oil of wine,* (F.) *Huile douce de vin.* A peculiar oleaginous matter, obtained by continuing the distillation, after the whole of the sulphuric ether has passed over in the process for the preparation of the latter. It is used only as an ingredient in the compound spirit of ether. It is officinal in the Ph. U. S.

OLEUM AMMONIATUM, Linimentum ammoniæ fortius.

OLEUM AMYGDALA'RUM, *Oleum amyg'dalæ, Oil of Almonds,* (F.) *Huile d'amandes. (Expressed from both sweet and bitter almonds,—Amygdalus communis.* ℨxvj of almonds yield ℨv of oil.) It is inodorous, insipid, and of a pale straw colour, and is employed as a demulcent and emollient.

OLEUM ANACARDII, see Anacardium occidentale.

OLEUM ANIMA'LE, *An'imal oil,* (F.) *Huile animale.* An oil obtained by the decomposition of the immediate principles of animals, subjected to the action of heat. It is fetid, and always contains a certain quantity of subcarbonate of ammonia. See Olea Empyreumatica. The name *animal oil* is sometimes also given to the fat contained in the fatty vesicles. The composition of this fat does not, indeed, differ from that of the fixed oil.

OLEUM ANIMA'LE DIPPE'LII, *Animal oil of Dippel, Oleum cornu cervi, O. C. C. rectifica'tum, Animal oil, Dippel's oil, Oleum pyro-anima'lĕ depura'tum, O. anima'lĕ æthe'reum, Pyro'leum os'sium rectifica'tum,* (F.) *Huile animale de Dippel, Huile de corne de cerf,* is obtained by distilling animal matters, especially hartshorn, on the naked fire. The subcarbonate of ammonia, which it contains, renders it partly soluble in water, and communicates to it the stimulant properties for which it is used in medicine. It is employed as an antispasmodic.

OLEUM ANIMA'LE EMPYREUMAT'ICUM CHABER'-TI, *O. Empyreumat'icum seu anthelmin'ticum seu contra tæ'niam Chaber'ti, Empyreumat'ic oil of Chabert, Oil of Chabert,* is made by adding one part of *animal oil* to three parts of *oil of turpentine,* leaving them to combine for four days, and then distilling three parts. An effective anthelmintic. Dose, a tea-spoonful three times a day.

OLEUM ANIMALIZA'TUM PER INFUSIO'NEM, (F.) *Huile animalisée par infusion, Huile aromatique, H. de petits chiens.* A preparation, formerly esteemed tonic and cephalic. It was obtained by boiling new-born puppies in oil, first depriving them of their blood, skin, and intestines. When the decoction was cold, origanum, thyme, pennyroyal, St. John's-wort, and marjoram were added.

OLEUM ANISI, see Pimpinella anisum—o. An-thelminticum Chaberti, Oleum animale empyreumaticum Chaberti—o. Aurantii, see Citrus aurantium—o. Balaninum, Guilandina moringa (oleum) —o. Balsami, see Amyris opobalsamum.

OLEUM BENZO'INI, *Oil of Benzoin or Benjamin.* An oil obtained by heating, in a sand-bath, the matter which remains after benzoic acid has been separated from benzoin by the aid of heat. It has been regarded as balsamic and sudorific.

OLEUM BERGAMII, see Bergamote.

OLEUM BU'BULUM, *Neat's-foot oil.* The oil prepared from the bones of *Bos Domesticus.* It is obtained by boiling in water for a long time the feet of the ox, previously deprived of the hoof. It is introduced into the officinal list of the Ph. U. S. as an ingredient of the ointment of nitrate of mercury.

OLEUM CACAO SPISSATUM, Butter of Cacao — o. Cadinum, see Juniperus oxycedrus—o. Cajuputi, Caieput (oil)—o. Camphoratum, Linimentum camphoræ—o. Cari seu Carui, Carum (oleum) —o. Caryophylli, see Eugenia caryophyllata.

OLEUM CED'RINUM, *Essentia de cedro,* (F.) *Huile de cédrat.* The oil of the peel of citrons, obtained in Italy in a particular manner, without distillation.

OLEUM CHABERTI, O. animale empyreumaticum Chaberti—o. Chenopodii, see Chenopodium anthelminticum—o. Cicinum, see Ricinus communis—o. Cinnamomi, see Laurus cinnamomum— o. Contra Tæniam Chaberti, Oleum animale empyreumaticum Chaberti.

OLEUM COPA'IBÆ, *Oil of Copa'iba. (Copaib.* ḃij; *Aquæ,* cong. iv. Distil three gallons; separate the oil; return the water to the copaiba, and again distil three gallons. Separate the oil, and add it to the other. Ph. U. S.) Dose gtt. x to xxx.

OLEUM CORNU CERVI, O. animale Dippelii—o. Cubebæ, see Piper cubebæ—o. Euphorbiæ lathyridis, see Euphorbia lathyris—o. Fixum nucum cocos butyraceæ, see Cocos butyracea—o. Fœniculi, see Anethum—o. Gabianum, Petrolæum—o. Gallinæ, Alkale—o. Gaultheriæ, see Gaultheria —o. Hedeomæ, see Hedeoma pulegioides—o. Hyperici, see Hypericum perforatum—o. infernale, O. Ricini.

OLEUM JEC'ORIS ASELLI, *O. Mor'rhuæ, O. Jecino'ris Aselli, Azun'gia Ga'di, A. Pisci'na mari'na, Codliver oil, Cod oil.* (F.) *Huile de morue, Huile de Foie de morue.* The animal oil, which appears under this name in commerce, is obtained from several of the species belonging to the genus Gadus. The clearest sorts are generally used. It appears to have no sensible effect upon the economy; but has been given in strumous affections, rheumatism, chronic cutaneous diseases, and tumours of the mammæ. The dose for an adult is from fℨij to fℨiss.

Rayliver oil, O'leum raiæ, is used in the same cases and doses.

OLEUM JUNIPERI, see Juniperis communis—o. Juniperi empyreumaticum, see Juniperus oxycedrus—o. de Kervâ, see Ricinus communis—o. Kervinum, see Ricinus communis.

OLEUM LAURI'NUM, *Oleum lauri, Oil of bays.* An oil obtained from bayberries, and sometimes used in sprains and bruises, unattended with inflammation.

OLEUM LAURINUM, Daphnelæon, Unguentum L.—o. Lavendulæ, see Lavendula—o. Lentiscinum, Schinelæon—o. Limonis, see Citrus medica —o. Lini, see Linum usitatissimum—o. Lini cum calce, Linimentum aquæ calcis.

OLEUM LU'CII PISCIS, *Oil of Pike.* From the liver of the *Esox lucius* an oil is spontaneously separated, which is used in some countries to destroy specks on the cornea.

OLEUM MALABATHRI, see Malabathrum—o.

Mariæ, see Fagara octandra — o. Melaleucæ leucodendri, Caieput (oil) — o. Menthæ piperitæ, see Mentha piperita — o. Menthæ viridis, Mentha viridis — o. Monardæ, Monarda punctata — o. Morrhuæ, O. jecoris aselli.

OLEUM E MUCILAGIN'IBUS, *Oil of Mu'cilages.* (*Rad. althææ rec.* ℔ss; *sem. lini, sem. fænugræci,* āā ℨiij; *aquæ,* Oij. Boil for half an hour; add *ol. oliv.* Oiv; continue the boiling till the water is nearly consumed, and pour off the oil.) Emollient.

OLEUM MYRISTICÆ, see Myristica moschata — o. Neroli, see Citrus aurantium.

OLEUM OLI'VÆ, *O. oliva'rum, Olive oil, Salad oil.* An inodorous, insipid, and transparent oil; obtained by expression from the olive, when ripe. It is demulcent and emollient, — possessing the qualities of the fixed oils in general.

An inferior kind, obtained by boiling olives in water, and skimming the oil from the surface, is also used in Pharmacy. See Olea Europæa.

OLEUM OMPHACINUM, Omotribes — o. Origani, see Origanum — o. Oxydi cupri viride, Balsam, green, of Metz — o. de Palmâ Christi, see Ricinus communis — o. Palmæ, see Cocos butyracea — o. Palmæ liquidum, see Ricinus communis — o. Petræ, Petrolæum — o. Petræ album, Naphtha — o. Picinum, Brutia, Pisselæum — o. Pimentæ, see Myrtus pimenta — o. Pini purissimum, O. terebinthinæ rectificatum — o. Pulegii, see Mentha pulegium — o. Pyro-animale, O. animale Dippelii — o. Raiæ, see Oleum Jecoris Aselli — o. Ricini, see Ricinus communis — o. Rosæ, see Rosa centifolia — o. Rosarum, Rhodelæon — o. Rutaceum, Peganelæon — o. Rosmarini, see Rosmarinus — o. Rutæ, see Ruta — o. Sabinæ, see Juniperus Sabina — o. Sassafras, see Laurus Sassafras — o. Sesami, see Sesamum orientale — o. Sinapis, see Sinapis — o. Spicæ vulgaris, O. terebinthinæ — o. Succini, see Succinum — o. Succini rectificatum, see Succinum.

OLEUM SULPHURA'TUM, *Bal'samum sulph'uris simplex, Sulph'urated oil.* (Sulph.ur. lot. ℨij; *olivæ olei,* ℔j. Heat the oil in a large iron pot, and throw in the sulphur by degrees; stirring the mixture after each addition till they unite.) It is stimulating, and was formerly much used in coughs, asthma, &c., and, externally, to foul ulcers.

OLEUM TAB'ACI, *Oil of Tobacco.* An empyreumatic oil, obtained from coarsely powdered tobacco by heating the retort to dull redness. Ph. U. S.

OLEUM TARTARI PER DELIQUIUM, Liquor potassæ subcarbonatis — o. Templinum, see Pinus mughos.

OLEUM TEREBIN'THINÆ, *Oil of Turpentine.* The volatile oil of the juice of pinus palustris, and other species of pinus.

OLEUM TEREBIN'THINÆ RECTIFICA'TUM, *Oleum pini puris'simum, Rectified oil of turpentine, Oleum terebin'thinæ æthe'reum, Sp. of turpentine.* Common oil of turpentine is also called *Common oil of Spike, Oleum spicæ vulga'rĕ.* (*Olei terebinth.* Oj; *aquæ,* Oiv. Distil over the oil.) It is stimulant, diuretic, anthelmintic, and rubefacient. Dose, ℨss to ℨj.

Guestonian Embrocation for rheumatism consists of *ol. terebinth., ol. oliv.* āā ℨiss; *acid. sulph. dil.* ℨiij.

OLEUM THEOBROMÆ CACAO EXPRESSUM, Butter of cacao — o. Tiglii, Croton tiglium.

OLEUM VALERIA'NÆ, *Oil of Vale'rian.* The distilled oil of the root of *Valeriana officinalis.* — Ph. U. S.

OLEUM VINI, O. æthereum — o. Vitrioli, Sulphuric acid.

OLFAC'TION, *Olfac'tus,* from *olfacere* for *odefacere* (*odor,* and *facere*), *Osphre'sis, Osphra'sia, Osphre'sia, Osme'sis, Odora'tio, Odora'tus, Sensus osmomet'ricus, Sense of smell, Smelling,* (F.) *Odorat.* The sense by which we perceive the impressions made on the olfactory nerves by the odorous particles suspended in the atmosphere. The olfactory nerve or first pair has usually been considered the great nerve of smell; and it is probably the nerve of special sensibility, general sensibility being communicated by the branches of the fifth pair, distributed on the pituitary membrane of the nose and sinuses.

OLFAC'TORY, *Olfacti'vus, Olfacto'rius, Osphran'ticus, Osphrante'rius, Osphre'ticus,* from *olfactus,* 'the smell.' That which belongs or relates to the sense of smell.

OLFACTORY BULB, see Olfactory nerves.

OLFAC'TORY FORAM'INA, (F.) *Trous olfactifs,* are the holes in the cribriform plate of the ethmoid bone, through which the olfactory nerve passes.

OLFACTORY LOBE, see Olfactory nerves.

OLFAC'TORY NERVES, *Ethmoid'al nerves, Par primum Nervo'rum cer'ebri, Nervi odorato'rii, Proces'sus mamilla'res* seu *Papilla'rum, Processus mamillares cer'ebri ad nares, P. papilla'res, Carun'culæ mamilla'res,* — *the first pair of encephal'ic nerves.* This nerve, which probably arises from the medulla oblongata, is observed to leave the brain, opposite the inner part of the fissure of Sylvius, by three roots; which, by their union, form a triangular knot or expansion. When it reaches the ethmoid fossa it expands and forms a triangular ganglion, or grayish, soft bulb, — *Bulbus olfacto'rius* — *Olfactory bulb, tubercle,* or *lobe,* — which furnishes, from its inferior surface, the branches that have to be distributed to the nasal fossæ. These filaments are very numerous; they pass through the foramina in the cribriform plate and enter the nasal fossæ. They are distinguished into the *internal, external,* and *middle.* The former are distributed over the mucous membrane, covering the outer paries of the nasal fossæ; the second descend upon the septum, and the third are lost, almost immediately, on the portion of the pituitary membrane that lines the vault of the fossæ.

OLFACTORY TUBERCLE, see Olfactory nerves.

OLFACTUS, Olfaction — o. Acutus, Hyperosphresia — o. Amissio, Anosmia — o. Deficiens, Anosmia — o. Depravatus, Parosmia.

OLIBANUM, see Juniperus lycia — o. Sylvestre, see Pinus abies — o. Vulgare, see Pinus abies.

OLIGÆMIA, Anæmia, Hæmaporia, Hypæmia.

OLIGIDRIA, Ischidrosis.

OLIGOBLEN'NIA, from ὀλίγος, 'few,' and βλέννα, 'mucus.' A deficiency of mucus.

OLIGOCHOL'IA, from ὀλίγος, 'few,' and χολή, 'bile.' Paucity of bile.

OLIGOCH'YLUS, from ὀλίγος, 'little,' and χυλός, 'juice,' 'chyle.' An epithet for food which is but little nutritive; which furnishes little chyle.

OLIGOCOP'RIA, from ὀλίγος, 'few,' and κόπρος, 'excrement.' Scantiness of alvine evacuations.

OLIGODAC'RYA, from ὀλίγος, 'little,' and δάκρυ, 'a tear.' Paucity of lachrymal secretion.

OLIGOGALACTIA, Agalactia.

OLIGOGALIA, Agalaxis.

OLIGOHÆMIA, Anæmia, Hæmaporia, Hypæmia.

OLIGOPO'SIA, from ὀλίγος, 'little,' and πόσις, 'drink.' Diminution in the quantity of drinks.

OLIGOSIA'LIA, from ὀλίγος, 'little,' and σίαλον, 'saliva.' Paucity of saliva.

OLIGOSPER'MIA, from ολιγος, 'little,' and σπερμα, 'sperm.' Paucity of spermatic secretion.
OLIGOSPOND'YLUS, from ολιγος, 'few,' 'small,' and σπονδυλος, 'a vertebra.' A monster with defective vertebræ. — Gurlt.
OLIGOTRICH'IA, from ολιγος, 'little,' and θριξ, 'hair.' Want of hair. Paucity of hair.
OLIGOTROPH'IA, Par'cior nutrit"io, from ολιγος, 'little,' and τρεφω, 'I nourish.' Deficient nourishment.
OLIGURE'SIA, Oligure'sis, Oligoure'sis, Oligoure'sia, from ολιγος, 'little,' and ουρεω, 'I pass urine.' Morbidly diminished urinary secretion.
OLISTHEMA, Luxation.
OLIVA, Olea Europæa.
OLIVÆ, Corpora olivaria.
OLIVAIRE CAUTÈRE, of the French surgeons, is a cautery whose extremity is terminated by a button having the shape of an olive.
OLIVARIS, Olive-shaped.
OLIVARY, Olive-shaped — o. Bodies, Corpora olivaria.
OL'IVARY PROC"ESS, Proces'sus Oliva'ris, is a small ridge, running transversely between, and a little behind, the roots of the anterior clinoid processes of the sphenoid bone, and by some considered as the fourth clinoid process.
OLIVE, see Olea Europæa — o. Tree, Olea Europæa.
OLIVE-SHAPED, Oliva'ris, Olivifor'mis, Ol'ivary, from oliva, 'an olive.' Resembling an olive. See Corpora olivaria.
OLIVES, PICKLED, Colymbades.
OLIVIER, Olea Europæa.
OLIVIFORMIS, Olive-shaped.
OLIVINA, see Olea Europæa.
OLLA CAPITIS, Cranium.
OLMITELLO, MINERAL WATERS OF. A thermal spring in the isle of Ischia. Temperature, 100° Fahrenheit.
OLOPHLYCTIDE, Herpes.
OLOPHO'NIA, from ολλω, ολλυω, 'I lose,' and φωνη, 'voice.' Congenital misconstruction of the vocal organs. — Good.
OLOPHONIA LABII LOBATA, Harelip — o. Linguæ frænata, see Ankyloglossum.
OM'AGRA, Hom'agra, from ωμος, 'the shoulder,' and αγρα, 'a seizure.' Gout in the shoulder.
OMAL'GIA, from ωμος, 'the shoulder,' and αλγος, 'pain.' Pain in the shoulder.
OMARTHRI'TIS, from ωμος, 'the shoulder,' αρθρον, 'a joint,' and itis, denoting inflammation. Inflammation of the shoulder-joint.
OMARTHROC'ACE, from ωμος, 'shoulder,' αρθρον, 'a joint,' and κακος, 'bad.' Arthrocace of the shoulder-joint. Caries or suppuration of the shoulder-joint.
OMA'SUM, Omasus, Manyplies. The third stomach of ruminant animals.
OMBILIC, Umbilicus.
OMBILICALE, Umbilical.
OMBRAGE, Nebula.
OMENTA, Meninges.
OMENTESIS, Epiploitis.
OMENTITIS, Epiploitis.
OMENTULA, Appendiculæ pinguedinosæ.
OMENTUM, Epiploon — o. Colicum, Epiploon, colic — o. Gastro-colicum, Epiploon, gastro-colic — o. Gastro-splenic, Epiploon, gastro-splenic — o. Great, Epiploon, gastro-colic — o. Hepato-gastricum, Epiploon, gastro-hepatic — o. Lesser, Epiploon, gastro-hepatic — o. Majus, Epiploon, gastro-colic — o. Minus, Epiploon, gastro-hepatic — o. Ossium, Periosteum — o. Third, Epiploon, colic.
OMICHESIS, Micturition.

OMICHMA, Urine.
OMI'TIS, from ωμος, 'the shoulder,' and itis, denoting inflammation. Inflammation in or about the shoulder-joint.
OMMA, Eye, Vision.
OMNIPHAGUS, Omnivorous.
OMNIVORE, Omnivorous.
OMNIV'OROUS, Omnivorus, Omniph'agus, Pantoph'agus, (F.) Omnivore, from omnis, 'all,' and voro, 'I eat.' An epithet for animals — Pantophagists — which eat every kind of food, animal or vegetable.
OMO. In composition, an abridgment of omos or omus, the humerus.
OMO-CLAVICULAR, see Coraco-clavicular.
OMOCOTYLE, see Glene.
OMO-HYOÏDEUS, Cor'aco-hyoïdeus, Scapulo-hyoïdien, Omo-hyoïdien, Omoplat-hyoïdien, Hyoïdis Quartus Mus'culus. This muscle is situate obliquely at the sides and front of the neck. It is slender, long, and flat. It arises from the superior costa of the scapula, near the semi-lunar notch, and from the ligament that runs across it, and is inserted at the sides of the inferior margin of the body of the os hyoides. It consists of two fasciculi, united by a common tendon, and is a true digastric muscle. It depresses the os hyoides, carrying it a little backwards, and to one side, except when it acts with its fellow, when the bone is depressed, and drawn obliquely backwards.
OMOPHAG"IA, Omosit"ia, from ωμος, 'raw,' and φαγω, 'I eat.' Fondness for raw food. Eating of raw food.
OMOPLATE, Scapula — o. Col de l', Collum scapulæ.
OMOPLAT-HYOÏDIEN, Omo-hyoideus.
OMOS, Crude, Humerus.
OMOSITIA, Omophagia.
OMOTAR'ICHOS, from ωμος, 'the shoulder,' and ταριχος, 'pickled.' Salsamen'tum crudum; Salted Tunny Fish, in particular. Properly, the neck or shoulder-piece of a salted animal. Once much recommended against the bites of vipers, and in hydrophobia.
OMOTES, Crudity.
OMOTOCIA, Abortion.
OMOT'RIBES, Omphac"inum O'leum, from ωμος, 'crude,' and τριβω, 'I bruise.' Oil expressed from unripe olives.
OMPHA'CION, ομφακιον, from ομφακος, 'an unripe grape;— Succus uvæ acer'bæ, Ompha'cium. The juice of unripe grapes. Also, Verjuice.
OMPHACI'TES (VINUM). A name given to wine prepared from the unripe grape. Omphaci'tis is also the name of a small gall. — Dioscorides.
OMPHACIUM, Verjuice.
OMPHACOM'ELI, from ομφακος, 'an unripe grape, and μελι, 'honey.' A sort of oxymel, made of the juice of unripe grapes and honey.
OMPHALELCO'SIS, from ομφαλος, 'the navel,' and 'ελκος, 'an ulcer.' Ulceration of the navel.
OMPHALEX'OCHÉ, Exomphalus.
OMPHALOCARPUS, Galium aparine.
OMPHALOCELE, Exomphalos.
OMPHALOMANTI'A, from ομφαλος, 'the navel,' and μαντεια, 'prophecy.' A species of divination, practised by credulous matrons, who pretend to be able to know the number of children a female will have, by the number of knots in the navel-string of the child.
OM'PHALO-MESENTER'IC, Omphalo-mesenter'icus, Om'phalo-mesara'icus; from ομφαλος, 'the navel,' and mesenterium, 'the mesentery.'
OMPHALO-MESENTERIC VESSELS, Vitel'lo-me-

enter'ic, Vit'elline vessels. Haller gave this name to two very fine vessels, which spread their ramifications on the parietes of the umbilical vesicle. There is an *omphalo-mesenteric artery* and *vein.* The *omphalo-mesenteric artery* is a branch of the superior mesenteric;—the vein empties itself into the trunk, or into one of the branches of the superior mesenteric. Velpeau affirms, that they inosculate with a branch of the second or third order of those great vessels, with those in particular that are distributed to the cæcum, and he regards them to be the vessels of nutrition of the umbilical vesicle. They are occasionally met with in the fœtus, at the full period, under the form of whitish filaments, which extend from the mesenteric vessels to the umbilicus.

OMPHALO-MESERAIC, Omphalo-mesenteric.

OMPHALONCUS, Omphalophyma.

OMPHALONEURORRHEXIS, Omphalorrhexis.

OMPHALOPHY'MA, *Omphaloncus*, from ομφαλος, 'the navel,' and φυμα, 'tumour.' A tumefaction of the navel.

OMPHALOPROPTOSIS, Exomphalus.

OMPHALORRHAG"IA, *Omphalor'rhagĕ*, from ομφαλος, 'the umbilicus,' and ρηγνυμι, 'I break out.' Hemorrhage from the umbilicus, in the new-born in particular.

OMPHALORRHEX'IS; from ομφαλος, 'navel,' and ρηξις, 'rupture.' *Omphaloneurorrhexis.* Rupture of the navel string.

OMPHALOS, Umbilicus.

OMPH'ALOSITE, from ομφαλος, 'the navel,' and σιτος, 'nourishment.' A monster that possesses an imperfect kind of life, which ceases when the umbilical cord is divided.

OMPHALOT'OMY, *Omphalotom'ia*, from ομφαλος, 'the umbilicus,' and τεμνω, 'I cut.' The division of the navel string.

OMPHALUS, Umbilicus.

OMUS. Crude, Humerus.

ONAGRA, Œnothera biennis.

ONANIA, Masturbation.

ONANISM, Masturbation.

ONCOS, Tumour.

ONCO'SES, from ογκος, 'a tumour.' Tumours, as diseases.

ONCOSIS, Intumescence.

ONCOT'OMY, *Oncotom'ia, Onkotomy*, from ογκος, 'a tumour,' and τομη, 'incision.' The opening of an abscess with a cutting instrument, or the excision of a tumour.

ONCTION, Inunction.

ONCUS, Swelling, Tumour.

ONDULATION, Fluctuation.

ONEBERRY, Paris.

ONEIROCRIT'ICUS, *Oneiroc'rites*, from ονειρος, 'a dream,' and κρισις, 'judgment.' One who judges according to dreams.

ONEIRODYN'IA, from ονειρος, 'a dream,' and οδυνη, 'pain.' Painful dreams. *Incubus* and *Somnambulism* are oneirodyniæ.

ONEIRODYNIA ACTIVA, Paroniria, Somnambulism—o. Gravans, Incubus.

ONEIRODYNIE GRAVATIVE, Incubus.

ONEIROG'MUS, *Oneirog'ynĕ, Oneiropol'esis,* from ονειρος, 'a dream.' A lascivious dream; pollution; nocturnal pollution.

ONEIROGONORRHŒA, Pollution, nocturnal.

ONEIROGONOS, Pollution.

ONEIROL'OGY, *Oneirolog"ia*, from ονειρος, 'a dream,' and λογος, 'a description.' The doctrine of dreams.

ONEIROMANTI'A, from ονειρος, 'a dream,' and μαντεια, 'divination.' The art of divining by dreams; or of interpreting dreams.

ONEIRON'OSUS; from ονειρος, 'a dream,' and νοσος, 'a disease.' *Somnia'tio morbo'sa.* Morbid, uneasy dreaming.

ONEIROPOLESIS, Oneirogmus.

ONERA ALVI, Excrement.

ONGLADE, Paronychia.

ONGLE, Nail.

ONGLÉE, (F.) *Digito'rum stupor à gelu.* Painful numbness at the extremities of the fingers, caused by cold.

ONGLET, Pterygion.

ONGUENT, Unguentum — *o. d'Althéa,* Unguentum de Althæâ—*o. de Blanc de baleine,* Unguentum cetacei — *o. Blanc de Rhazes,* Unguentum plumbi subcarbonatis — *o. de Cerusse,* Unguentum plumbi subcarbonatis—*o. Citrin contre la gale,* Unguentum hydrargyri nitras—*o. Digestif simple,* Unguentum digestivum simplex — *o. Gris,* Unguentum oxidi hydrargyri cinereum—*o. de Guimauve,* Unguentum de althæâ—*o. de Laurier,* Unguentum laurinum — *o. Mercuriel,* Unguentum hydrargyri—*o. Napolitain,* Unguentum hydrargyri—*o. de Nitrate de mercure,* Unguentum hydrargyri nitratis — *o. de Poix et de cire,* Basilicon—*o. de Soldat,* Martiatum unguentum—*o. de Sureau,* Unguentum sambuci—*o. de Tornamira,* Unguentum plumbi subcarbonatis.

ONION, COMMON, Allium cepa — *o.* Sea, Scilla.

ONIS'CUS, *Asel'lus, Cu'tio, Porcel'lio, Porcel'lus, Por'culus,* Diminutive of *ονος,* 'a small ass.' A genus of insects very common in cellars and dark and moist places.

ONISCI ASELLI, *Millep'edes, Aselli, Millep'edes, Fabæ, Wood-lice, Slaters, Hog-lice,* (F.) *Cloportes ordinaires,* had, at one time, a place in the pharmacopœias. They were considered stimulant and diuretic, and useful in jaundice.

ONITIS, Origanum dictamnus.

ONKOTOMY, Oncotomy.

ONOLOSAT, Obolus.

ONOMATOCLESIS, Nomenclature.

ONOMATOLOGIA, Nomenclature.

ONONIS ANTIQUORUM, O. spinosa.

ONO'NIS ARVEN'SIS, (F.) *Bugrane des champs,* has properties like the next.

ONONIS SPINO'SA, *Ano'nis, Resta bovis, Arres'ta bovis, Rem'ora Ara'tri, Ononis antiquo'rum, Rest harrow,* (F.) *Arrête-bœuf, Bugrande épineuse, Bugrane.* *Nat. Ord.* Leguminosæ. *Sex. Syst.* Diadelphia Decandria. The root of this plant was once used as a diuretic.

ONOPORDON ACAN'THIUM, *Onopor'dum acan'thium, Car'duus tomento'sus, Acan'thium, Ac'anos, A. spina, Spina alba, Cotton Thistle,* (F.) *Chardon aux Ânes.* *Family,* Cinarocephalæ. *Sex. Syst.* Syngenesia Polygamia æqualis. The expressed juice has been recommended as a cure for cancer applied externally.

ONOPORDUM ACANTHIUM, Onopordon acanthium.

ONTHUS, Fimus.

ONYCHAUXÊ, from ονυξ, ονυχος, 'a nail,' and αυξη, 'increase.' Unusual increase of the size and thickness of the nails.

ONYCHEXALLAX'IS; from ονυξ, 'a nail,' and εξαλλαξις, 'change.' A morbid condition of the nails.

ONYCHIA, Paronychia.

ONYCHI'TIS; from ονυξ, 'nail,' and *itis*, denoting inflammation. Inflammation of a nail.

ONYCHOC'LASIS; from ονυξ, 'a nail,' and κλασις, 'fracture.' Fracture of a nail.'

ONYCHOCRYPTOSIS, Onychogryphosis.

ONYCHOGRYPHO'SIS, *Onychogrypu'sis,*

Onychogrypto'sis, Onychocrypto'sis, Gripho'sis, Grypho'sis, Onyx'is, from *ονυξ*, 'the nail,' and *gryposis,* 'crookedness.' Curvature of the nails; such as occurs in hectic individuals. Also, growing in of the nails; *Incarna'tio* seu *Adunca'tio* seu *Arctu'ra un'guium.*

ONYCHON'OSI, *Onychonu'si,* from *ονυξ,* 'a nail,' and *νοσος,* 'a disease.' Disease of the nails.

ONYCHOPH'THORA, *Onychophtho'ria, Onycoph'thora, Onycophtho'ria,* from *ονυξ,* 'the nail,' and *φθορα,* 'degeneration.' A degenerate condition or destruction of the nails.

ONYCHOPHY'MA, from *ονυξ,* 'the nail,' and *φυμα,* 'a tumour.' A painful degeneration of the nails, which become thick, rough, and crooked. It occurs as a symptom of syphilis and of lepra.

ONYCHOPTO'SIS, *Piptonyc'hia, Dia'resis Un'gulæ,* from *ονυξ,* 'a nail,' and *πτωσις,* 'falling.' The falling off of the nails.

ONYCOPHTHORA, Onychophthora.

ONYX, Hook, blunt, Nail, Pterygion. Also, a collection of purulent matter between the laminæ of the cornea, having the shape of a nail.

ONYXIS, Onychogryphosis.

ONYXITIS, see Paronychia.

OOCYESIS, Pregnancy, ovarian.

OODEOCELE, see Hernia (foraminis ovalis.)

OODES, Aqueous humour, Oval.

OÖG'ALA, *Oög'la, Ogla, Puls ex Ovis et Lacté.* Milk of eggs. A preparation of eggs and milk.

OOGLA, Oogala.

OOIDES, Aqueous humour, Oval.

OOLEMMA PELLUCIDUM, Zona pellucida.

OÖLOG"IA, *Ovolog''ia, Ovol'ogy,* from *ωον,* 'an ovum or egg,' and *λογος,* 'a discourse,' 'a description.' A description of the ovum.

OON, Ovum.

OONINE, Albumen.

OOPHORAUXE, Oarioparectama.

OOPHORITIS, Ooritis.

OOPHORON, Ovary.

OORITIS, Oaritis.

OPAC"ITY, *Opac''itas, Opa'couness;* from *opacare,* 'to obscure.' Quality of that which is opake. The property possessed by some bodies of not allowing the light to traverse them. It is opposed to transparency. *Opacity of the cornea* constitutes *albugo* or *leucoma;* — opacity of the crystalline causes cataract.

OPAKE', *Opa'cus, Opa'cous.* An epithet given to bodies, which do not permit the passage of rays of light. The *opake cornea* is the sclerotica, in contradistinction to the *transparent* cornea or true cornea.

OP'ALINE. That which resembles the opal. A fluid is said to be opaline, when milky, and when it presents an appearance more or less like that of the opal.

OPERATIO, Action, Operation — o. Chirurgica, see Operation—o. Chymica seu pharmaceutica, Operation, chymical, &c. — o. Simplex, Haplotomia.

OPERA'TION, *Opera'tio,* from *opus, operis,* 'work.' The application of instruments to the human body with the view of curing disease. The object of an operation, *opera'tio chirur'gica,* is generally to divide or reunite parts, to extract extraneous or noxious bodies, and to replace organs that are wanting, by different instruments or artificial means. The principal operatory methods have been called *Synthesis, Diæresis, Exæresis,* and *Prothesis.* Frequently, the most difficult subject connected with an operation is to decide when it is absolutely called for or advisable, and when improper.

OPÉRATION. A LAMBEAU, see Flap.

OPERATION, BILATERAL, see Lithotomy—o. Cæsarienne, Cæsarean section.

OPERATION, CHYM'ICAL or PHARMACEU'TICAL, *Opera'tio chym'ica* seu *pharmaceu'tica,* is any process whose object is the preparation of medicines; their combinations with each other, analysis, and decomposition; — such are, *solution, distillation, sublimation, evaporation, digestion, maceration, infusion, decoction, calcination, &c.* Some of these operations are mechanical; others, really chymical.

OPERATION, HIGH. see Lithotomy—o. Lateral, see Lithotomy—o. Sigaultian, Symphyseotomy.

OP'ERATOR. A surgeon who is in the habit of practising the greater operations. One who performs any operation. To be a good operator, the surgeon must be well acquainted with anatomy, and be possessed of strong nerve. See Surgeon.

OPER'CULUM, *Operto'rium, Operimen'tum,* from *operire,* 'to cover.' A cover or lid. In fishes, the gill cover.

OPERCULUM ASPERÆ ARTERIÆ, Larynx—o. Cutis, Epidermis—o. Ilei, Bauhin, valve of—o. Laryngis, Epiglottis—o. Oculi, Palpebra.

OPERCULUM PAPILLA'RUM. A shield for the nipple.

OPERIMENTUM, Operculum—o. Intestinorum, Epiploon—o. Prætensum abdominis, Peritonœum.

OPERTORIUM, Operculum.

OPHELIA CHIRATA, Gentiana chirayta.

OPHIASIS, Calvities, Porrigo decalvans.

OPHIOGLOS'SUM VULGA'TUM, *O. ora'tum* seu *echinoglos'sum, Lingua serpenta'ria, Adder's Tongue,* (F.) *Langue de Serpent. Family,* Filicoideæ. *Sex. Syst.* Cryptogamia. This plant was formerly considered to be vulnerary.

OPHIOPH'AGUS, from *οφις,* 'a serpent,' and *φαγω,* 'I eat.' An epithet for animals which feed on serpents. Pliny has called certain African tribes by this name.

OPHIORRHI'ZA, *O. mungos,* from *οφις,* 'a serpent.' and *ριζα,* 'root.' *Family,* Gentianeæ. *Sex. Syst.* Pentandria Digynia. The name of the plant whose root has been called *Radix Serpen'tum, Mungos Radix.* The bitter root is much esteemed in Java, Sumatra, &c., for preventing the effects that usually follow the bite of the *naja,* a venomous serpent; with which view it is eaten by the natives. It is, also, a reputed anthelmintic.

OPHIOXYLON, Ophioxylum.

OPHIOX'YLUM, from *οφις,* 'a serpent,' and *ξυλον,* 'wood.' *Ophioxylum* seu *Ophioxylon serpenti'num* seu *trifolia'tum, Acawe'ria, Lignum serpentum,* has been recommended in the bites of serpents, and in intermittents. It is said to be very bitter.

OPHIS, Serpent.

OPHI'TES, from *οφις,* 'a serpent.' *Serpenti'nus, Ser'pentine* or *Black Por'phyry.* This rock was formerly worn as an amulet, to cure diseases of the head.

OPHROSTAPHYLON, Bryonia alba.

OPHRYS, Supercilium.

OPHTHALMAL'GIA, from *οφθαλμος,* 'the eye,' and *αλγος,* 'pain.' Pain in the eye. Neuralgia of the eye.

OPHTHALMEMPASMA, Collyrium siccum.

OPHTHAL'MIA, *Ophthalmi'tis,* from *οφθαλμος,* 'the eye.' *Oculo'rum inflamma'tio, Cauma ophthalmi'tis, Ophthalmopo'nia, Inflamma'tion of the Eye, Ophthalmy,* (F.) *Ophthalmie, Ophthalmite, Inflammation de l'œil, Catarrhe oculaire.* Three great varieties of ophthalmia, independently of the *acute* and *chronic* (which conditions occur in all inflammations,) may be reckoned:—the *Ophthalmia membranarum, O. purulenta,* and *O. tarsi.* The first is characterized by the general symptoms of ophthalmia;—pain and redness of the eye or its appendages; with intolerance of light, and unusual flow of tears; the inflammation being seated chiefly in the coats of the eyeball. It is the *Hymeuophthal'mia, Ophthalmia tarax'is, Conjunctivi'tis, Inflamma'tio conjuncti'væ, Symphymeni'tis, Syndesmi'tis, Catarr'hal ophthalmia, Ophthalmo-conjunctivi'tis, O. hu'mida, O. vera, Epiph'ora* (Galen), *Conjunctival Ophthal'mia, Tarax'is* (Paulus of Ægina), *Chemo'sis* (Aëtius), *O. Chemosis, Lach'rymose Ophthalmia,* (F.) *Conjonctivite, Inflammation de la conjonctive.* In the second,—*Ophthalmia purulen'ta, O. puriform'is, Blennorrhœa, Bleph'aroblennorrhœ'a, Ophthalmoblennorrhœa, Blennorrhœa oc'uli*—the internal surface of the palpebræ associates in the inflammation of the eye-ball; and there is a copious secretion of a purulent fluid. An epidemic and contagious(?) variety of this is the *Ægyptian Ophthalmia, Ophthalmia epidem'ica, O. purulen'ta epidem'ica, O. contagio'sa, O. Catarrha'lis bel'lica, Lœmophthal'mia, O. bel'lica, O. Asiat'ica, Blennorrhœ'a Oculi Ægyptiaca, Conjunctivi'tis puro-muco'sa contagio'sa* vel *Ægyptiaca, Blepharo'tis glandula'ris contagio'sa, Adeni'tis pulpebra'rum contagiosa, O. purulenta contagio'sa, Conjunctivi'tis puro-muco'sa contagio'sa, Suppurative ophthalmia, Epidemic contagious ophthal'mia*—called *Egyptian,* from its prevalence in Egypt during the British Expedition under Sir Ralph Abercrombie. The inflammation is rapid and destructive; granulations shoot from the tunica conjunctiva, and occasionally there is intolerable pain, often succeeded by delirium. In newborn children, a species of purulent ophthalmia, *O. purulen'ta infan'tum, O. Neonato'rum, Blepharophthalmia neonato'rum, Lippitu'do neonato'rum, Blennorrhœ'a Oc'uli neonato'rum, Ophthal'moblennorrhœ'a neonato'rum, Blepharo-blennorrhœ'a neonato'rum, Blepharo-pyorrhœa neonato'rum, Pyophthalmia neonato'rum, Psorophthalmia neonato'rum,* (F.) *Ophthalmie puriforme des nouveaunés,* in which the palpebræ are florid and peculiarly tumid, is by no means uncommon. It seems to be caused by acrid discharges from the mother, applied to the eye of the infant during its exit; or to the stimulus of the light, when the child first opens its eyes. A severe form of purulent ophthalmia—*Hyperconjonctivite* (Piorry) —is produced by the application of gonorrhœal matter to the eye. It is the *Ophthalmia gonerrho'ica, Blennorrhœ'a oculi gonorrho'ica, Conjunctivi'tis blennorrhag''ica, C. gonorrho'ica, Gonorrhœ'al Ophthal'mia,* (F.) *Ophthalmie blennorrhagique, Conjonctivite blennorrhagique.*

Ophthalmia is likewise modified by the condition of the constitution, and hence we have *strumous, variolous,* and other inflammations of the conjunctiva.

The third variety—the *Ophthalmia Tarsi, O. glutino'sa, Blepharophthal'mia, Blepharotis, Blepharoti'tis, Blephari'tis, Blepharadeni'tis, Psorophthal'mia, Oc'uli palpebra'rum sca'bies prurigino'sa, Adenophthalmia*—is seated chiefly in the tarsus; the sebaceous crypts secreting a viscid and acrid fluid, that glues and ulcerates its edges, and irritates the eye.

The different forms of inflammation of the conjunctiva are thus classed by M. Desmarres:

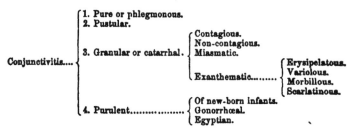

Conjunctivitis, when slight, requires little treatment: the antiphlogistic regimen—and, particularly, avoiding exposure to light,—being all that is necessary. When more severe, along with this, general and local blood-letting, especially by leeches to the side of the septum narium, must be employed so as to make a decided impression on the system; with nauseating doses of antimony, purgatives, blisters (at some distance from the organ), refrigerants; and astringents, cold or warm, according to circumstances, to the eye. In *Purulent Ophthalmy,* these measures must be still more actively employed, otherwise disorganization will speedily follow:—the granulations, which form on the adnata of the eyelids may be removed with the scissors, and the sore be touched with a solution of alum. *Ophthalmia Tarsi* must be treated on general principles, when severe. It usually, however, requires merely the antiphlogistic regimen, with the occasional use, especially at night, of a slightly stimulating ointment, such as the unguentum hydrargyri nitrico-oxydi, considerably reduced with lard. The ointment prevents the eyelids from being glued together during the night, and thus obviates the irritation caused by attempts at separating them.

OPHTHALMIA, ÆGYPTIAN, see Ophthalmia—o. Asiatica, see Ophthalmia—o. Bellica, see Ophthalmia—o. Biliosa, Ophthalmocholosis—o. Catarrhal, see Ophthalmia—o. Catarrhalis bellica, see Ophthalmia—o. Chronica, Lippitudo—o. Conjunctival, see Ophthalmia—o. Contagiosa, see Ophthalmia—o. Epidemica, see Ophthalmia—o. Glutinosa, see Ophthalmia—o. Gonorrhoica, see Ophthalmia—o. Gonorrhœal, see Ophthalmia—o. Humida, see Ophthalmia—o. Lachrymosa, see Ophthalmia—o. Membranarum, see Ophthalmia—o. Neonatorum, see Ophthalmia—o. Phlyctenular, see Ophthalmia—o. Puriformis, see Ophthalmia—o. Purulenta, see Ophthalmia—o. Purulenta contagiosa, see Ophthalmia—o. Purulenta epidemica, see Ophthalmia—o. Purulenta infantum, see Ophthalmia—o. Rheumatic, Sclerotitis —o. Sicca, Xerophthalmia—o. Suppurative, see Ophthalmia—o. Taraxis, see Ophthalmia—o. Tarsi, see Ophthalmia—o. Ulcerosa, Helcophthalmia—o. Varicose, Cirsophthalmia—o. Vera, see Ophthalmia.

OPHTHALMIATER, Oculist.

OPHTHALMIATRI'A, *Ophthalmiatrotech'nica, Ophthalmotherapi'a;* from ὀφθαλμός, 'the eye,' and ιατρος, 'a physician.' The art of the oculist. Treatment of diseases of the eye.

OPHTHALMIATROTECHNICA, Ophthalmiatria.

OPHTHAL'MIC, *Ophthal'micus*, from οφθαλ-μος, 'the eye.' That which relates or belongs to the eye.

OPHTHALMIC ARTERY, *A. orbitaire*, (Ch.) arises from the internal carotid, and issues from the cranium by the foramen opticum. At first, it is situate at the outer and lower side of the optic nerve, but ascends above this nerve, and passes towards the inner angle of the orbit. It furnishes, in its course, the *lachrymal, centralis retinæ, infra-orbitars, ciliaries, anterior ciliaries, inferior and superior musculars, anterior and posterior ethmoidals,* and *superior and inferior palpebrals.* After having given off these, it divides into two branches — the *frontal* and *nasal,* which furnish a number of ramifications, — some superficial, others deep-seated.

OPHTHAL'MIC GANG'LION, *Lentic'ular G., Cil'iary ganglion, G. orbitaire* (Ch.), is one of the smallest ganglions of the body, and formed by the 5th and 3d pairs of encephalic nerves. It is situate at the outer side of the optic nerve near the bottom of the orbit; is irregularly quadrilateral and flat: its colour of a reddish gray. Behind, it communicates by its posterior angles—by means of nervous filaments—with the nasal nerve of the ophthalmic and the motor oculi. Each of its anterior angles furnishes a fasciculus of small nerves. These are the ciliary nerves.

OPHTHALMIC NERVE, *Ophthalmic Nerve* of Willis, *Or'bito-frontal,* (Ch.) is the smallest and first of the three branches given off by the 5th pair. It proceeds along the external paries of the cavernous sinus, and enters the orbit by the sphenoidal fissure. It divides into three branches: one, *external*—the lachrymal nerve; another, *superior* — frontal nerve; and the last, *internal* — the nasal nerve. See Lachrymal, Frontal, Nasal.

OPHTHALMIC or OPTIC REMEDY, *Ophthal'micum seu Op'ticum,* (F.) *Topique ophthalmique,* is a medicine employed in ophthalmia.

OPHTHALMIC SINUS, see Cavernous Sinus.

OPHTHALMIC VEIN has the same arrangement as the artery, which it accompanies in all its divisions. It issues from the orbit at the inner part of the sphenoidal fissure, and discharges its blood into the cavernous sinus.

The name *Facial Ophthalmic* has been given to the branch by which the facial vein communicates with the ophthalmic.

OPHTHALMICA, Euphrasia officinalis.

OPHTHALMICI EXTERNI, Motores oculorum.

OPHTHALMICUM. Ophthalmic remedy.

OPHTHALMIDIUM. Microphthalmus.

OPHTHALMIE PURIFORME DES NOUVEAU-NÉS, see Ophthalmia — *o. Blennorrhagique,* see Ophthalmia.

OPHTHALMITE, Ophthalmia.

OPHTHALMI'TIS, Ophthalmia. This term is occasionally restricted to inflammation of the globe of the eye, in which, both the external and internal structures are involved.

OPHTHALMIUM, Microphthalmus.

OPHTHALMO-BLENNORRHŒA, Ophthalmia (purulent)—o. Neonatorum, see Ophthalmia (purulenta infantum.)

OPHTHALMO-CARCINO'MA, from οφθαλμος, 'the eye,' and καρκινωμα, 'cancer.' Cancer of the eye.

OPHTHALMOCELE, Exophthalmia.

OPHTHALMOCHOLO'SIS, from οφθαλμος, 'the eye,' and χολη, 'bile;' *Ophthal'mia bilio'sa.* Ophthalmia from biliary excitement.

OPHTHALMOCHROÏTES, see Choroidea tunica.

OPHTHALMO-CONJUNCTIVITIS, see Ophthalmia.

OPHTHALMODULI'A, from οφθαλμος, 'the eye,' and δουλεια, 'servitude.' Eye-service. The title of a book by Bartisch on diseases of the eye.

OPHTHALMODYN'IA, from οφθαλμος, 'the eye,' and οδυνη, 'pain,' especially rheumatic pain of the eye. Plenck has given this name to neuralgia of the frontal nerve, in which the pain radiates particularly towards the bottom of the orbit. See Neuralgia, Frontal.

OPHTHALMODYNIA PERIODICA, Neuralgia, facial.

OPHTHALMŒDE'MA; from οφθαλμος, 'the eye,' and οιδημα, 'œdema.' Œdema of the conjunctiva.

OPHTHALMOG'RAPHY, from οφθαλμος, 'the eye,' and γραφη, 'a description.' The part of anatomy which gives a description of the eye. An anatomical description of the eye.

OPHTHALMOL'OGY, *Ophthalmolog"ia, Ophthalmotol'ogy,* (F.) *Oculistique,* from οφθαλμος, 'the eye,' and λογος, 'a discourse.' The part of anatomy which treats of the eye. An anatomical treatise on the eye. A description of the eye in health and disease.

OPHTHALMOM'ETER, from οφθαλμος, 'the eye,' and μετρον, 'measure.' An instrument of the nature of compasses, invented by F. Petit, for measuring the capacity of the anterior and posterior chambers of the eye in anatomical experiments.

OPHTHALMOMYI'TIS, *Ophthalmomyosi'tis,* from οφθαλμος, 'the eye,' μυς, 'a muscle,' and *itis,* denoting inflammation. Inflammation of the muscles of the eye.

OPHTHALMOPARALYSIS, Ophthalmoplegia.

OPHTHALMOPHLEBOTOM'IA, from οφθαλμος, 'the eye,' φλεψ, 'a vein,' and τομη, 'incision.' Bleeding from the vessels of the conjunctiva.

OPHTHALMOPHTHAR'SIS, *Ophthalmophthi'sis,* from οφθαλμος, 'the eye,' and φθαρσις, 'corruption.' Destruction of the eyeball.

OPHTHALMOPHTHISIS, Ophthalmophtharsis.

OPHTHALMOPLE'GIA, *Ophthalmoparal'ysis,* from οφθαλμος, 'the eye,' and πλησσω, 'I strike.' Paralysis of one or more of the muscles of the eye.

OPHTHALMOPONIA, Ophthalmia.

OPHTHALMOPTO'SIS, from οφθαλμος, 'an eye,' and πτωσις, 'a prolapse.' A word employed by some authors in the sense of exophthalmia, by others, in that of hydrophthalmia.

OPHTHALMORRHAG"IA, from οφθαλμος, 'the eye,' and ρηγνυμι, 'I break forth.' Hemorrhage from the tunica conjunctiva. It is rare.

OPHTHALMOS, Eye.

OPHTHALMOSCOP'IA, *Ophthalmoscopy,* from οφθαλμος, 'the eye,' and σκοπεω, 'I regard attentively.' The art of judging of the temper, &c. of a person by examining his eyes. The art of judging of health or disease by inspection of the eyes. Exploration of the eyes in order to a diagnosis.

OPHTHALMOSTA'TUM, (F.)*Ophthal'mostat,* from οφθαλμος, 'the eye,' and στασις, 'station;' *Spec'ulum Oc'uli.* An instrument for fixing the eye.

OPHTHALMOTHERAPIA, Ophthalmiatria.

OPHTHALMOTOLOGY, Ophthalmology.

OPHTHALMOT'OMY, *Ophtholmotom'ia,* from οφθαλμος, 'the eye,' and τεμνω, 'I cut.' The part of anatomy which treats of the dissection of the eye. It has, also, been applied to extirpation of the eye.

OPTHALMOXEROSIS, Xerophthalmia.

OPHTHALMOX'YSIS, from οφθαλμος, 'the eye,' and ξυω, 'I scrape.' A name given to the scarification sometimes practised on the conjunctiva, in cases of ophthalmia.

OPHTHALMOXYS'TRUM, *Ophthalmoxys'ter, Ophthalmoxyste'rium, Xystrum ophthal'micum.* An instrument for scraping the eye. Name given to a small brush, with barbs like an ear of barley or rye, intended to scarify the eyelids in certain cases of ophthalmia.

OPHTHALMUS, Eye.

OPHTHALMYMENI'TIS, *Ophthalmohymeni'tis*, from οφθαλμος, 'eye,' ὑμην, 'membrane,' and *itis*, denoting inflammation. Inflammation of one or more of the membranes of the eye.

OPIACÉ, Opiate.

OPIACUM, Opiatum.

OPIANE, Narcotine.

OPIANUM, Narcotine.

OPIAT, Opiate — o. *Dentifrice*, Dentifrice.

O'PIATE, *Opia'tum, Opia'cum, Papavera'ceum, Meco'nicum*, (F.) *Opiat, Opiacée,* from οπιον, (οπος, 'juice,') 'opium.' A medicine containing opium. A medicine that procures sleep. An *electuary;* — formerly, an electuary, which contained opium.

O'PIATED, *Opia'tus.* Impregnated with opium. Affected by opium.

OPIATUM FEBRIF'UGUM, *Electua'rium de Kinâ Kinâ; Elec'tuary of Cincho'na.* (Pulv. cinch. ʒxviij, ammon. muriat. ʒj, mellis, syrup. absinth. āā ʒij. Make into an electuary. Ph. P.) Given, when cinchona is indicated.

OPIATUM MESENTER'ICUM, *Electua'rium de A'loë, Muria'tē Hydrar'gyri, et Ferro.* (Gum. ammon. ʒss, sennæ ʒvj, hydrargyri submuriat., rad. ari., aloës socotrin. āā ʒij, pulv. scammon. comp. (vulg. de tribus,) rhej. rad. āā ʒiij, ferri limatur. porphyrisat. ʒss. Bruise and mix together, add of *compound syrup of apples* double the weight of the other matters, and make into an electuary. Ph. P.) Dose, ʒss to ʒij, in obstructions of the liver, mesentery, &c.

OPIATUS, Opiated.

OPION, Opium.

OPISMA, Succus.

OPIS'THENAR, *Dorsum manûs*, from οπισθι, 'backwards,' and θεναρ, 'the flat of the hand.' The back of the hand.

OPISTHOCEPHALON, Occiput.

OPISTHOCRANIUM, Occiput.

OPISTHOCYPHOSIS, Cyphoma.

OPISTHOLOB'IUM, *Opisthot'ium*, from οπισθι, 'behind,' and λοβιον, 'the lobe of the ear.' Any agent applied behind the ear.

OPISTHOTIUM, Opistholobium.

OPISTHOT'ONOS, *Raptus posterga'nens, Tet'anus dorsa'lis, T. posti'cus, T. posterga'neus,* from οπισθι, 'backwards,' and τεινω, 'I stretch.' A species of tetanus, in which the body is bent backwards.

OPIUM, see Papaver — o. *Colatum*, Extractum opii — o. *Depuratum*, Extractum opii — o. *Eaters*, Theriaki.

OPOBALSAMUM, see Amyris opobalsamum.

OPOCARPASON, Carpasium (juice.)

OPODELDOC, Opodeldoch.

OPODEL'DOCH, *Opodel'toch, Opodeldoc.* An unmeaning term, frequently used by Paracelsus. Formerly, it signified a plaster for all external injuries; now, it is applied to the Linimentum Saponis Compositum.

OPODELDOCH, STEER'S. A liniment, called after the inventor. There are many formulæ for its preparation. The following is one. *Sap. alb.* ℔j, *camphor* ʒij, *ol. rorismarini* f ʒiv, *spiritus vini rectificati* Oij. See Linimentum Saponis Compositum.

OPODYMUS, Diprosopus.

OPOPIOS, Optic.

OPOPONACUM, Pastinaca opoponax.

OPOPONAX, see Pastinaca opoponax.

OPOPONAXWORT, Pastinaca opoponax.

OPO'RICE, from οπωρα, 'autumnal fruits.' A medicine, composed of several autumnal fruits, particularly of quinces, pomegranates, &c. and wine. It was formerly administered in dysentery, diseases of the stomach, &c.

OPOS, *Succus expressus* — o. Silphion, Laserpitium.

OPPIDULUM, Vulva.

OPPILATIO, *Emphraxis* — o. Telæ Cellulosæ, Induration of the cellular tissue.

OPPILATIVUS, Obstruens.

OPPO'NENS, (F.) *Opposant*, from *ob*, and *ponere*, 'to place.' That which faces or is put in opposition to something. The name has been given to two muscles of the hand.

OPPONENS MIN'IMI DIG"ITI, *Carpo-m/tacarpien du petit doigt* (Ch.), *Métacarpien du petit doigt,* (F.) *Opposant du petit doigt.* This muscle has the same shape and arrangement as the preceding, but is of less size. It is situate in the hypothenar eminence. Its fibres are inserted into the anterior annular ligament of the carpus, and terminate on the whole length of the inner edge of the 5th metacarpal bone. This muscle carries the 5th metacarpal bone forwards and outwards, and thus augments the concavity of the palm of the hand.

OPPONENS POL'LICIS, *Flexor ossis metacar'pi pollicis, Opponens pollicis manûs, Flexor primi interno'dii* (Douglass,) *Antith'enar sive semi-interosseus pollicis,* (F.) *Carpo-métacarpien du pouce* (Ch.) *Métacarpien du pouce, Opposant du Pouce.* A small, flat, triangular muscle, situate in the substance of the thenar eminence. It is attached, on the one hand, to the anterior annular ligament of the carpus and to the trapezium; and, on the other, to the whole of the outer margin of the first metacarpal bone. This muscle impresses on the first bone of the metacarpus a movement of rotation, which opposes the thumb to the other fingers.

OPPOSANT, Opponens — o. *du Petit doigt.* Opponens minimi digiti — o. *du Pouce,* Opponens pollicis.

OPPRESSIO, *Catalepsy, Oppression* — o. *Nocturna*, Incubus.

OPPRESSION, *Oppres'sio, Thlipsis, Catathlipsis,* from *opprimere* (*ob*, and *premere.* *pressum*,) 'to press against.' A state, in which the patient experiences a sensation of weight in the part affected. When employed abstractedly, it means, particularly, *Oppression of the chest — Oppressio Pec'toris,* (F.) *O. de Poitrine.*

OPPRESSION, *Oppres'sio vir'ium,* (F.) *Oppression des forces,* is, also, used for that condition, at the commencement of fevers, &c., in which the system is oppressed rather than debilitated, and where the vascular action rises, as the obstruction to free circulation is relieved by bleeding, purging, &c.

OPS, Eye.

OPSEONUSI, Opsionusi.

OPSIALGIA, Neuralgia, facial.

OPSIONU'SI, *Opseonu'si,* from ωψις, 'vision.' and νουσος, 'a disease;' *Morbi visûs.* Diseases of vision.

OPSIOTOC'IA, from οψε, 'too late,' and τοκος, 'birth;' *Partus sero'tinus.* Parturition after the usual period. See Pregnancy.

OPSIS, Pupil, Vision.

OPSOMA'NIAC, *Opsom'anes,* (F.) *Opsomane,* from ο ἰ ορ, 'aliment,' and μανια. One who loves some particular aliment to madness.

OPTESIS, Assatio.

OPTIC, *Op'ticus, Opo'pios,* from οπτομαι, 'I see.' That which relates to vision.

OPTIC CENTRE, *Centrum op'ticum.* The optic centre of the crystalline is the point at which the various rays proceeding from an object cross in their way to the retina.

OPTIC COMMISSURE, see Chiasmus.

OPTIC FORAMEN, *Fora'men op'ticum,* (F.) *Trou optique.* A round opening in the sphenoid bone, near the base of its lesser ala, through which the optic nerve passes.

OPTIC GANGLIA, Quadrigemina tubercula.

OPTIC GROOVE. A transverse groove on the superior surface of the sphenoid bone, on which the commissure of the optic nerve rests, and which is continuous on each side with the optic foramen.

OPTIC LOBES, Quadrigemina tubercula.

OPTIC NERVE, *Nervus op'ticus, Par secun'dum seu op'ticum seu viso'rium, Nerve of the 2d pair, Nervus visi'vus seu viso'rius, Ocular nerve* of Chaussier. The optic nerves are remarkable for their size; for their running a longer course within than without, the cranium; and for their furnishing no branch from their origin to their termination. They do not seem to arise, as was long supposed, from the optic thalami, but from the tubercula quadrigemina. Immediately after their origin the *optic tracts, Tractus op'ticus,* proceed forwards; are, at first, broad and flat; but afterwards become narrower and round. In front of the fossa pituitaria, they unite and decussate, each nerve proceeding through the optic foramen with the ophthalmic artery. The nerve passes to the back part of the globe of the eye, becomes narrower, and enters that organ to give rise to the nervous expansion called the retina. Besides its neurilemma, the optic nerve is surrounded by a sheath, furnished by the dura mater. This accompanies it as far as the eye.

The optic nerve is the nerve of special sensibility of the eye.

OPTIC REMEDY, see Ophthalmic remedy.

OPTIC THALAMI, Thalami nervorum opticorum —o. Tracts, see Optic nerve.

OPTICO-TROCHLÉI-SCLÉROTICIEN, Oblique, superior of the eye.

OPTICUM, Ophthalmic remedy.

OPTILOS, Eye.

OPTOM'ETER, from οπτομαι, 'I see,' and μετρον, 'a measure.' An instrument for measuring the distance of distinct vision.

OPUNTIA, Cactus opuntia.

OR, Gold—o. *Cyanure, d',* see Gold—o. *Divisé,* see Gold—o. *Hydrochlorate d',* see Gold—o. *Iodure d',* see Gold—o. *Nitromuriate d',* see Gold—o. *Oxide d',* see Gold—o *et de Sodium, chlorure d',* see Gold—o. *et de Soude, Hydrochlorate d',* see Gold—o. *et de Soude, Muriate d',* see Gold.

ORA SERRATA, see Ciliary (Body.)

ORACH, STINKING, Chenopodium vulvaria.

ORAL, (F.) *Oral, Vocal,* from *os, oris,* 'a mouth.' Relating to the mouth or to speech.

ORANGE, FLOWERS OF THE, see Citrus aurantium — o. Root, Hydrastis Canadensis — o. Tree, Citrus aurantium.

ORANGEADE. A drink, made with orange juice diluted with water. It is antiphlogistic, and often recommended in acute diseases.

ORANGES, see Citrus aurantium — o. Curassos, Aurantia curassaventia.

ORBES CARTILAGINOSI TRACHEÆ, see Trachea.

OBICULAIRE DES LÈVRES, Orbicularis oris — *o. des Paupières,* Orbicularis palpebrarum.

ORBIC'ULAR, *Orbicula'ris,* from *orbis,* 'a circle.' Spherical, circular.

ORBICULAR BONE, *Os orbicula'rē seu lenticula'rē seu Sylvii seu orbicula'rē Syl'vii, Glob'ulus stap'edis ossis, Epiph'ysis cruris longio'ris in'cudis, Ossic'ulum orbicula'rē seu squamo'sum seu cochleare seu quartum,* is the smallest of the four bones of the ear. It is scarcely perceptible, round, convex on two surfaces, and situate between the long ramus of the incus and the head of the stapes.

ORBICULAR MUSCLES are muscles with circular fibres surrounding some natural opening of the body. 1. *Orbicula'ris Oris, Sphincter Labio'rum, Semi* vel *Demi-orbicula'ris, Supra-semi-orbicula'ris, Constric'tor Oris, Labia'lis, Osculato'rius, Basia'tor,* (F.) *Labial, Orbiculaire des lèvres.* A muscle situate in the substance of the lips, and extending from one commissure to the other. It is formed of two very distinct portions, of a semi-oval shape; one belonging to the upper lip, the other to the lower. Their extremities cross at the commissures, and are confounded with the other muscles of the parts. The use of this fleshy muscle is to bring the lips together, and to close the aperture of the mouth, by making it represent a sort of *bourrelet* with radiated wrinkles. It is an antagonist to every other muscle of the lips. 2. *Orbicularis Palpebra'rum, Orbicularis oc'uli, Orbicularis palpebra'rum cilia'ris, Palpebra'rum duo mus'culi, Maxil'lo-palpébral, Palpebra'lis, Constrict'or palpebra'rum, Sphincter Palpebra'rum seu Oculi,* (F.) *Naso-palpébral* (Ch.), *Palpébral, Orbiculaire des paupières.* A muscle common to both the eyelids, and seated in their substance. It is broad, thin, transversely oval, and cleft in its great diameter. It is attached to the nasal process of the superior maxillary bone; to the internal angular process of the frontal bone, and to the orbitar process of the superior maxillary bone. From these origins the muscle passes outwards, under the skin of the eyelids, surrounding the orbit in a circular manner, extending somewhat beyond it, and covering the upper part of the cheek. It is inserted into the skin of the eyelids, its upper and inner edge being intimately connected with the frontal and corrugator muscles. Its use is to close the eye, by bringing the eyelids together. The part of the orbicularis which covers the cartilages of the eyelids, and which is remarkably thin, is the *Musculus Ciliaris* of some authors.

ORBICULARIS OCULI, Orbicularis palpebrarum, see Orbicular muscles — o. Oris, see Orbicular muscles — o. Palpebrarum, see Orbicular muscles — o. Palpebrarum ciliaris, see Orbicular muscles — o. Recti, Sphincter ani externus.

ORBICULUS CILIARIS, Ciliary ligament, Ciliary zone.

ORBIS GENU, Patella.

ORBIT, *Or'bita, O. oc'uli, Troch'ia, Conchus seu Cav'itas seu Fo'vea seu Pelvic'ula oc'uli,* from *orbis,* 'a circle.' The circular cavities are so called, which lodge the organs of sight. The *orbits* or *orbitar fossæ* or *cavities,* conchi, κογχοι, are situate at the upper part of the face, and are composed of seven bones, viz.: — the *frontal,* above: the *palate* and *superior maxillary,* below; the *sphenoid* and *malar,* externally; and the *ethmoid* and *lachrymal,* internally. The orbit is filled by the globe of the eye, with its different accessory parts — muscles, nerves, vessels, the lachrymal gland, &c. Its margin is termed *margo orbita'lis.*

ORBITA. Orbīt — o. Oculi. Orbit.
ORBITAL FISSURE, INFERIOR, Sphenoidal fissure — o. Fissure, superior, Maxillary fissure.
OR'BITAR, *Orbita'rius, Orbita'lis, Or'bital.* Same etymon. Relating or belonging to the orbit.

ORBITAR APOPH'YSES or PROC"ESSES terminate the two extremities of the orbitar arch. The *external* is much more prominent, and is articulated with the cheek-bone; the *internal* is thinner, and joins the os unguis.

ORBITAR ARCH, (F.) *Arcade orbitaire,* is the projecting, round margin, which separates the *frontal* and *orbitar* surfaces of the os frontis, and forms a part of the circumference of the orbit.

OR'BITAR FISSURES, (F.) *Fentes orbitaires.* These are situate in the orbit. They are two in number: one *superior,* the Sphenoidal; the other *inferior,* the Spheno-maxillary.

ORBITAR FORAM'INA. Of these there are several: — 1. The *Foramen orbitarium superius,* (F.) *Trou orbitaire supérieur,* which is situate at the junction of the inner third of the orbitar arch with its two outer thirds, and gives passage to the frontal nerve. 2. The *Foram'ina orbita'ria interio'ra* vel *inter'na, Foram'ina Ethmoidea.* These are situate at the upper part of the internal paries of the orbit, are formed by the union of two notches of the os frontis with two similar ones of the ethmoid; and are distinguished into *anterior* and *posterior*. The former gives passage to the ethmoidal filament of the nasal nerve and to a small artery.

ORBITAR NERVE, *Nervus orbita'lis* seu *orbita'rius* seu *subcuta'neus malæ,* is a branch given off from the superior maxillary. It enters the orbit by the spheno-maxillary fissure, and divides into two filaments; the one — *malar* — which passes over the cheek-bone, is distributed to the orbicularis palpebrarum, and anastomoses with the facial nerve; the other — *temporal* — which passes to the temporal fossa, and anastomoses with the inferior maxillary and facial, to become afterwards subcutaneous.

ORBITO-EXTUS-SCLÉROTICIEN, Rectus externus oculi — o. *Intus-Scléroticien,* Rectus internus oculi — o. *Maxillo-labial,* Levator labii superioris proprius — o. *Palpébral,* Levator palpebræ superioris — o. *Sus-palpébral,* Levator palpebræ superioris.

ORCANETTE, Anchusa officinalis.
ORCHALGIA, Orchidalgia.
ORCHAS, Scrotum.
ORCHEI'TIS, *Oschi'tis, Oschei'tis, Inflamma'tio scroti,* from οϱχας, 'the scrotum,' and *itis,* denoting inflammation. Inflammation of the scrotum.

ORCHEITIS, Hernia humoralis.
ORCHEOCATABASIS, Orchidocatabasis.
ORCHEOCELE, Orchiocele.
ORCHEOTOMY, Castration.
ORCHESTROMANIA, Chorea.

ORCHIDAL'GIA, *Orchal'gia, Orchidodyn'ia,* from οϱχις, 'a testicle,' and αλγος, 'pain.' Pain of the testicle. Neuralgia of the testicle. Irritable testicle. A form of neuralgia.

ORCHIDATROPH'IA, *Atroph'ia testic'uli,* from οϱχις, οϱχιδος, 'a testicle,' and *atrophia,* 'atrophy.' Atrophy or wasting of the testicles.

ORCHIDITIS, Hernia humoralis.

ORCHIDOCATAB'ASIS, *Orcheocatab'asis, Descen'sus testiculo'rum,* from οϱχις, 'the testicle,' and καταβασις, 'descent.' The descent of the testes into the scrotum.

ORCHIDOCELE, Hernia humoralis.
ORCHIDODYNIA, Orchidalgia.

ORCHIDONCUS, Hernia humoralis.
ORCHIDOTOMY, Castration.
ORCHILL, Lichen roccella.

ORCHIOCE'LE. *Orcheoce'lē,* from οϱχις, 'the testicle,' and κηλη, 'a rupture.' A tumour of the testicle. Scrotal hernia. Hernia humoralis. A name given to several diseases of the testicle and its envelopes, essentially differing from each other.

ORCHIOCE'LE SCIRRHO'SA, *Scirrhoce'lē.* A malignant tumour of the testis.

ORCHIS, Testicle — o. Butterfly. Orchis bifolia.

ORCHIS MAS'CULA, *Satyr'ion, Male Orchis, Testic'ulus cani'nus, Cynosor'chis, Dogs' stones, Male Fools' stones, Twinroot.* This root has had a place in some pharmacopœias, on account of the glutinous, slimy juice it contains. The root of the *Orchis bifolia* or *Butterfly orchis,* has likewise been collected. It has been used as a demulcent. Its fancied aphrodisiac virtues seem to be owing to its resemblance to οϱχις, 'a testicle,' whence its name.

Salep is obtained from this variety of the orchis; — and from the *Orchis morio,* &c. See Salep.

ORCHIS, ROUND-LEAVED, LARGE, Platanthera orbiculata.
ORCHITE, Hernia humoralis.
ORCHITIS, Hernia humoralis.
ORCHOI, see Tarsus.
ORCHOTOMIA, Castration. Also, removal of the tarsi.
ORDEOLUM, Hordeolum.
ORDEUM, Hordeum.
ORDINAIRES, Menses.
ORDONNANCE, Formula, Prescription.
OREILLE D'HOMME, Asarum — o. *de Souris,* Hieracium pilosella.
OREILLETTE, Asarum, Auricle of the heart.
OREILLONS, Parotis, Cynanche parotidæa.
ORELIA GRANDIFLORA, Allamanda.
ORELLANA, see Terra Orleana.
OREOSELINUM, Athamanta aureoselinum — o. Africanum, Bubon galbanum — o. Legitimum, Athamanta aureoselinum — o. Nigrum, Athamanta aureoselinum.
OREXIS, Appetite, Pyrosis — o. Cynodes, Boulimia.

ORGAN, *Or'ganum, Or'ganon.* 'An instrument.' Part of an organized being, destined to exercise some particular function. Thus — the eyes are organs of sight; the muscles are organs of motion, &c. The collection of organs, which concur in any function, is called *apparatus*.

ORGANA GENERATIONI INSERVIENTIA, Genital organs — o. Sudoripara, see Perspiration.

ORGANES GÉNITAUX, Genital organs.

ORGAN'IC, *Organ'icus.* Relating to an organ or organs, and to beings possessed of organs. Hence, ORGANIC FUNCTIONS are those possessed by both animals and vegetables. It is also used synonymously with *vital,* in contradistinction to *physical.*

ORGANIC CHEMISTRY, see Chymistry.

ORGANIC DISEASES or LESIONS are such as concern the organ itself, in contradistinction to *functional, rat"ional,* or *dynam'ic,* which merely concern the function. Of course, organic diseases of a part are always more serious than *functional.*

ORGANIC NERVOUS SYSTEM, see Trisplanchnic nerve.

ORGANICISM, *Organicism'us,* from οϱγανον, 'an organ.' The doctrine of the localization of disease. A modern term, but not much used.

ORGANISATIO, Organization.

ORGANISATUS, Organized.

OR'GANISM. Same etymon. The living economy. Many physiologists have used this word synonymously with organization; but more especially to designate the aggregate of vital actions in organized beings, animals as well as vegetables. The collection of parts composing an organized body, and the laws which govern it.

ORGANIZABIL'ITY, from *organisatio*, and *habilis*, 'suitable.' Capability of organization or of being formed into living tissue. Substances possessed of such capability—as fibrin—are said to be organizable.

ORGANIZABLE, see Organizability.

ORGANIZA'TION, *Organisa'tio*, from οργανον, 'an organ.' The manner of structure proper to different beings. It is also employed in the sense of the structure of a part; as, the *organization of the heart*, &c.

ORGANIZATION, COMPOUNDS OF, Principles, immediate.

OR'GANIZED, *Or'ganis instruc'tus, Organisa'tus*. That which is composed of organs.

ORGANIZED BODIES, (F.) *Corps organisés*, are those endowed with life; i. e. animals and vegetables: in contradistinction to *inorganic* bodies, which comprise the mineral kingdom. See Corpus.

ORGANOCHEMIA, Chymistry, organic.

ORGANOG"ENY, *Organogen'ia*, from οργανον, 'an organ,' and γενεσις, 'generation.' The doctrine of the formation of different organs.

ORGANOGNO'SIA, from οργανον, 'organ,' and γνωσις, 'knowledge.' The knowledge and discrimination of organized bodies.

ORGANOG'RAPHY, *Organograph'ia*, from οργανον, 'an organ,' and γραφη, 'a description.' A description of the organs of a living body.

ORGANOLOGY, Anatomy, Craniology.

ORGANON OLFACTÛS, Nasus.

ORGANONOM'IA, from οργανον, 'an organ,' and νομος, 'a law.' The doctrine of the laws of organic life.

ORGANOZOONOMIA, Zoonomia.

ORGANUM, Instrument.

ORGASM, *Orgas'mus, Orgo'sis*, from οργαω, 'I desire ardently,' 'I am excited.' *Œstrua'tion.* A strong impulse or desire for something. State of excitement and turgescence of any organ whatever. Erethism. Applied particularly to the height of venereal excitement in sexual intercourse.

ORGASMUS, Turgescence.

ORGAS'TICA. Same etymon. The second order of the class *Genetica* of Good. Defined: diseases affecting the orgasm; organic or constitutional infirmity disordering the power or the desire of procreating.

ORGE, Rage.

ORGE, Hordeum — *o. Perlé*, see Hordeum.

ORGEAT, Syrupus amygdalæ.

ORGELET, Hordeolum.

ORGEOLET, Hordeolum.

ORGOSIS, Orgasm.

ORICHALCUM, Brass.

ORICULAR, Auricular.

ORICULE, Auricle, Pavilion of the ear.

ORIFICIUM, Mouth—o. Dextrum Ventriculi, Pylorus—o. Uteri, Os uteri—o. Ventriculi Sinistrum, Cardia.

ORIG'ANUM, *Origanum vulga'rē, Cuni'la bu'bula, Marjora'na mancura'na, O. heracleot'icum, Zasarhen'di herba, Wild marjoram, Common marjoram, Mancura'na*, (F.) *Pied de lit. Family,* Labiatæ. *Sex. Syst.* Didynamia Gymnospermia. This plant resembles marjoram in smell; and has a pungent taste, much like thyme. It is aromatic and stimulant; and its oil possesses the properties of the essential oils in general. The oil, *oleum origani* (Ph. U. S.), is very pungent, and is rarely given internally. It is used in toothach.

ORIGANUM AQUATICUM, Eupatorium cannabinum—o. Creticum, O. dictamnus.

ORIGANUM DICTAM'NUS, *Dictamnus Cret'icus, O. Creticum, Amar'acus tomento'sus, Oni'tis, Dit'any of Crete*, (F.) *Dictamne de Crète*. The leaves of this plant were once recommended as emmenagogue and alexipharmic.

ORIGANUM HERACLEOTICUM, Origanum.

ORIGANUM MAJORA'NA, *Marjora'na, O. majoranoi'des, Majorana, M. horten'sis, Sweet marjoram, Samp'sucus, Agriorig'anum, Amar'acus*, (F.) *Marjolaine*. Its odour is strong and fragrant; taste aromatic and bitterish. Its properties are those of a stomachic and errhine. It is chiefly used, however, for culinary purposes, and as a snuff in headach.

ORIGANUM SYRIACUM, Teucrium marum.

ORIGINAIRE (F.), from *origo*, 'origin.' This term has been used, by French writers, in the same sense as *congenital*. It is particularly applied to affections depending upon faulty conformation, or to faulty conformation itself.

ORIGO, Arche.

ORISMOLOGY, Terminology.

ORLEANA, see Terra Orleana.

ORME, Appetite.

ORME, Ulmus.

ORMSKIRK MEDICINE. A celebrated antilyssic remedy, supposed to consist of *Pulv. Cretæ*, ℨss; *Bol. Armen.* ℨiij; *Alumin.* gr. x; *Pulv. Inulæ*, ℨj; *Ol. Anisi*, gtt. vj.

This is taken for a dose every morning for six times, in a glass of water, with a small proportion of fresh milk.

ORNAMENTUM FOLIACEUM, see Tube, Fallopian.

ORNITHOG'ALUM ALTIS'SIMUM. A South African plant, *Nat. Ord.* Asphodeleæ, the fleshy bulb of which is diuretic. An oxymel is prepared of it, which is given in catarrh, asthma, phthisis, and hydrothorax. It resembles squill in its medical properties.

ORNITHOGALUM MARITIMUM, Scilla—o. Squilla, Scilla.

ORNITHOGLOSSÆ, see Fraxinus excelsior.

ORNUS EUROPÆA, see Fraxinus ornus—o. Mannifera, Fraxinus ornus — o. Rotundifolia, Fraxinus ornus — o. Sylvestris, Fraxinus excelsior.

OROBAN'CHE VIRGINIA'NA, *Epifa'gus America'nus, E. Virginia'nus, Virgin'ia broomrape, Beech-drops, Cancer-root. Family,* Orobanchoideæ. This parasitic plant is astringent, and a peculiar and extremely nauseous bitter. It is most powerful when fresh. It has been used in dysentery; and, externally, to obstinate ulcers.

OROBAN'CHE AMERICA'NA, and *O.* UNIFLO'RA, have the same properties, and are, likewise, called *Cancer-root, Earth-club,* and *Clapwort*.

OROBE, Ervum ervilia.

OROBION, see Ervum ervilia.

OROBOÏ'DES, from οροβος, 'the orobus,' and ειδος, 'form.' *Orobo'des*. Having the shape of the orobus. A name given to urine, *Urina orobo'des seu oroboï'des*, when depositing a substance of a fawn colour, like the meal of the orobus.

OROBUS, Ervum ervilia—o. Faba, Vicia faba.

ORONGE, see Agaric.

OROPHALL'US, from ορος, or οῤῥος, 'the rump,' and φαλλος, 'the male organ.' A monster having a second male organ originating from the rump.—Gurlt.

OROS, *Oroupion*, Serum.

OR'PIMENT, *Auripigmen'tum, Orpin, Rini-gal'lum, Rissigallum, Cloanx, Elomē, Sira, Lempniae, Spec'ulum cit'rinum, Yrideø, Yride.* The native yellow sulphuret of arsenic. It is poisonous, but less so than the oxide. It is, also, called *Adarigo, Adarnech, Akusal, Althanacha, Azarnet.* The Turks prepare a depilatory with it, which they call *Rusma.*

ORPIN, Orpiment — *o. Brûlant*, Sedum — *o. Grand*, Sedum telephium — *o. Reprise*, Sedum telephium.

ORPINE, Sedum telephium.

ORRHOCHEZIA, Diarrhœa, serous.

ORRHOCYST'IS, from *oppos*, 'serum,' and *κυστις*, 'a bladder.' An encysted tumour containing a serous fluid.

ORRHOHYMENITIS, Hydrohymenitis.

ORRHOPYG'ION. The inferior extremity of the vertebral column; from *opos*, 'extremity,' and *πυγη*, 'the nates.' The os coccygis. Also, the raphe, extending from the penis to the anus, and separating the scrotum into two parts.

ORRHORRHŒ'A, from *oppos*, 'serum,' and *ῥεω*, 'I flow.' A morbidly increased secretion of a serous fluid.

ORRHOS, *Croupion*, Serum.

ORRIS, Iris Florentina — *o. Common*, Iris Germanica.

ORSEILLE, Lichen roccella.

ORTEIL, Digitus pedis.

ORTHOCO'LUM, from *opθos*, 'straight,' and *κωλον*, 'limb.' Stiffness of the limb, so that it is kept quite straight.

ORTHODO'RON. A measure with the Greeks, equal to eleven finger-breadths.

ORTHOG'NATHOUS, from *opθos*, 'right, straight,' and *γναθος*, 'jaw.' Having a vertical jaw. A term applied to the form of head in which the facial angle approaches the right angle.

ORTHOMORPHIA, Orthopædia.

ORTHOMORPHOSIS, Orthopædia.

ORTHONTROPIA, Orthopædia.

ORTHOPÆDI'A, *Orthopæ'dicē, Orthomor'phia, Orthomorpho'sis, Orthontrop'ia, Orthoped'ics*, from *opθos*, 'right,' and *παις*, 'a child.' The part of medicine whose object is to prevent and correct deformity in the bodies of children. Often used, however, with a more extensive signification, to embrace the correction or prevention of deformities at all ages. *Orthosomat'ice, Orthosomat'icē*, from *opθos*, 'right,' and *σωμα*, 'body,' has been proposed as a preferable term.

ORTHOPE'DIC, *Orthopæ'dicus*; same etymon. Relating to orthopædia, — as *Orthopedic Institution, Institu'tum orthopæ'dicum seu orthopæ'dium:* an institution for the correction or prevention of deformities in children.

ORTHOPEDICS, Orthopædia.

ORTHOPE'DIST, *Ortho'ter, Orthopæ'dicus*, same etymon. One who practises orthopædia.

ORTHOPHREN'IC, *Orthophren'icus*, from *opθos*, 'right,' and *φρην*, 'mind.' Relating to sound mind.

ORTHOPNŒ'A, *Suffoca'tio, Strangula'tio, Præfoca'tio, Pnix, Pnigmus, Euthyp'noē, Euthyp·æ'a, Angor, Apnœ'a*, from *opθos*, 'right,' 'straight,' and *πνεω*, 'I respire.' Impracticability of breathing in the horizontal posture. Necessity of being in the erect posture, in order to respire.

ORTHOPNŒA CARDIACA, Angina Pectoris — *o.* Convulsiva, Asthma — *o.* Cynanchica, Cynanche trachealis — *o.* Hydrothoracica, Hydrothorax — *o.* Hysterica, Angone — *o.* Pituitosa, Myoorthopnœa — *o.* Tussiculosa, Pertussis.

ORTHOSOMATICE, Orthopædia.

ORTHOSOMATIQUE, Orthopædia.

ORTHOTER, Orthopedist.

ORTHYSTEROPTOMA, Prolapsus uteri.

ORTHYSTEROPTOSIS, Prolapsus uteri.

ORTIE, Urtica — *o. Blancke*, Lamium album — *o. Brûlante*, Urtica urens — *o. Morte*, Lamium album — *o. Morte des Bois*, Galeopsis — *o. Romaine*, Urtica pilulifera.

ORTYX, Tetrao coturnix.

ORUS, *Croupion*, Serum.

ORVALE, Salvia sclarea.

ORVIETA'NUM. From the Italian *Orvietano.* An electuary regarded as an invaluable antidote, and composed of *Old theriac, Dried vipers, Scorzonera, Carlina, Imperatorium, Angelica, Bistort, Rosemary, Juniper, Cinnamon, Cloves, Mace, Honey*, and a crowd of other substances. Its medical properties resembled, in some respects, those of the theriac. It was so called, according to some, because invented by Orvietano, a celebrated charlatan; or, according to others, from Orvieto, a town in Italy.

ORY'ZA, from *Orez*, (Arab.,) *Ory'za sati·va, Rice*, (F.) *Riz. Family*, Gramineæ. *Sex. Syst.* Hexandria Monogynia. A plant, almost aquatic, and indigenous in China, one of the richest productions of Egypt, and which prospers in the warmer regions of the four quarters of the globe. The grain inclosed in the husk is called by the Malays *Paddy, Padi, or Paddie;* when deprived of the husk, *Bras*, and when boiled *Nasi.* Its amylaceous seeds, *Ory'za, Ory'zum, Hordeum galac'ticum*, nourish more men than those of wheat and rye together. Besides being alimentary, they are demulcent and emollient. *Gardiner's alimentary preparation* is very finely ground rice-meal.

Mucilage of Rice, Rice water, may be formed by taking one ounce of *rice*, and, having washed it, macerating it for three hours in a quart of tepid soft *water*, in a pan placed upon a stove; then boiling the whole slowly for another hour, and straining through a sieve.

It may be sweetened and acidulated, or be prepared with milk, like arrow-root, and be used as a demulcent.

Rice Jelly is made by macerating a sufficient quantity of clean *rice* in as much *water* as will cover it; boiling slowly, adding water as it evaporates, until the rice is reduced to a pap, sweetening and flavouring with *lemon-juice* or *vanilla*, and passing through a fine sieve into a form or mould. It may be eaten alone or with milk; and is a good diatetic preparation for those of weak digestive powers.

Ground rice. Take a tablespoonful of *ground rice*; a pint and a half of milk, and half an ounce of *candied lemon-peel*. Rub the rice smooth with the milk: then add the lemon-peel cut into small pieces; boil for half an hour, and strain whilst the milk is hot. It is used in the same cases as rice jelly.

OS, Bone, Mouth, see Ossiculum — *o.* Acromii. Acromion — *o.* ad Cubitale, Radius — *o.* Adjutorium, Humeri os — *o.* Alæforme. Sphenoid — *o.* Alagas, Coccyx, Sacrum — *o.* Amphideon, Os uteri — *o. Anonyme*, Innominatum os — *o. Anonymum*, Innominatum os — *o.* Anticum, *Avant bouche — o.* Arcuale, Temporal bone — *o.* Armale, Temporal bone — *o.* Asser, Sternum — *o. de l'Assiette*, Ischion — *o.* Azygos, Sphenoid — *o.* Ballistæ, Astragalus — *o.* Basilare, Occipital bone, Palate bone. Sacrum, Sphenoid — *o.* Baxillare, Sphenoid — *o.* Bicorne, Hyoides os — *o.* Brachiale, Humeri os — *o.* Brachii, Humeri os — *o.* Calcis, Calcaneum — *o.* Capitatum, Magnum os — *o.* Caudæ, Occipital bone — *o.* Clunium, Sacrum — *o.* Coccygis, Coccyx — *o.* Colatorium, Ethmoid bone — *o.* Coliforme, Ethmoid—o. Convolutum superius, Turbinated bone, middle— o. Coronale, Frontal bone — o. Coxæ, Innominatum os — o. Coxal, Innominatum os, Ischion — o. Cribleux, Ethmoid — o. Cribriforme, Ethmoid — o. Cribrosum, Ethmoid—o. Cristatum, Ethmoid—o. Crochu, Os uniciforme.

OS CROTOPHALE. A name given by M. Béclard to a bone sometimes met with at the anterior and inferior angle of the parietal bone; from κροταφος, 'the temple.'

Os CROTAPHITICUM, Temporal bone — o. Cubicum, Ethmoid bone—o. Cubiti Inferius, Ulna—o. de la Cuisse, Femur—o. Cuneiforme, Sphenoid — o. Cuneo comparatum, Sphenoid—o. Cymbiforme, Scaphoid bone — o. Disciforme, Patella — o. Durum, Temporal bone—o. Ensiforme, Sternum.

OS ÉPACTALE. A name given to one of the ossa Wormiana; particularly to one met with in the posterior fontanelle, and which has been described by G. Fischer, under the name Os Epactale seu Goëthian'um.

OS ÉPACTAUX, Wormiana ossa.

Os EXTERNUM. The entrance into the vagina, in contradistinction to the Os inter'num or Os u'teri.

Os EXTRA ORDINEM CARPI, Os pisiforme — o. Fibrosum, Occipital bone — o. Foraminulentum, Ethmoid — o. Frontis, Frontal bone — o. Genæ, Malæ os—o. Gladioli, Sternum—o. Grand, Magnum os—o. Grand, col du, Collum ossis magni— o. Grandinosum, Cuboid—o. Gutturis, Hyoides os —o. Hamatum, Os unciforme — o. Hors du rang, Os pisiforme—o. Hypopium, Malæ os—o. Hypseloides, Hyoides os — o. Inconjugatum, Sphenoid —o. Incudi similis, Incus—o. Inferius ventriculi, Pylorus—o. Innominé, Innominatum os—o. Intercalés, Wormiana ossa—o. Internum, Os uteri—o. Inverecundus, Frontal bone—o. Ischii, Ischion — o. Interparietale, Interparietal bone — o. Jugale, Malæ os — o. Jugamentum, Malæ os — o. Juguli, Clavicle — o. Lacrymale, Unguis os—o. Lambda, Occipital bone—o. Lambdoides, Hyoides os, Occipital bone—o. Lapideum, Temporal bone —o. Latum, Sacrum—o. Latum humeri, Scapula, — o. Lenticulare, Os orbiculare, Os pisiforme—o. Lepidoides, Temporal bone—o. Linguæ, Hyoides os—o. Linguale, Hyoides os—o. Lithoides, Temporal bone—o. Magnum, neck of the, Collum ossis magni — o. Malaire, Malæ os — o. Malare, Malæ os — o. Maxillæ superioris undecimum, Vomer—o. Maxillaire inférieure, Collum mandibulæ—o. Memento mori, Temporal bone — o. Memoriæ, Occipital bone — o. Mendosum, Temporal bone — o. Morsus Adami, Thyroid cartilage — o. Mucronatum, Xiphoid cartilage — o. Multangulum majus, Trapezium os — o. Multangulum minus, Trapezoides os — o. Multiforme, Ethmoid, Sphenoid — o. Nasauz, Nasal bones—o. Naviculare, Os scaphoides — o. Nervale, Temporal bone — o. Nervosum, Occipital bone — o. Occipiti, Occipital bone — o. Orbiculare, Os pisiforme — o. du Palais, Palate bone — o. Palati, Palate bone — o. Palatin, Palate bone — o. Papillare, Sphenoid — o. Parietale inferius, Temporal bone—o. Paxillare, Sphenoid — o. Pectinis, Pubis, os — o. Pectoris, Sternum — o. Pelvi-cephalicum, Occipital bone — o. Pelvis laterale, Innominatum os — o. Perone, Fibula—o. Petrosum, Temporal bone — o. Polymorphon, Sphenoid—o. de la Pommette, Malæ os—o. Posterum, Pharynx — o. Præruptæ rupi assimilatum, Temporal bone — o. Procubitale, Ulna — o. Propres du nez, Nasal bones—o Proræ, Occipital bone—o. Pudicum, Malæ os—o. Puppis, Frontal bone, Occipital bone—o. Pyramidale carpi, Trapezoides os—o. Pyxidis, Occipital bone—o. Rationis, Frontal bone — o. du Rayon, Radius — o. Sacrum, Sacrum — o. Saxeum, Temporal bone — o.

Scutiforme, Patella—o. Sedentarium, see Ischiatic —o. Semilunare, Lunare os—o. Sextum cranii, Occipital bone — o. du Sinciput, Parietal bones, see Sinciput—o. Sous-ethmoïdal, Turbinated bone, inferior—o. Sphœno-basilare, Occipital bone—o. Sphecoides, Sphenoid—o. Sphenoidale, Sphenoid —o. Sphenoides, Sphenoid—o. Spongiosum, Ethmoid—o. Spongiosum inferius, Turbinated bone, inferior — o. Spongiosum medium, Turbinated bone, middle—o. Spongiosum superius, Turbinated bone, middle, Turbinated bone, superior—o. Spongoides, Ethmoid—o. Squamosum, Temporal bone — o. Suboculare, Malæ os — o. Surnuméraires, Wormiana ossa — o. Susmaxillaire, Maxillary (superior) bone—o. Sylvii, Os orbiculare—o. Temporis, Temporal bone—o. Tessera, Cuboid— o. Thyreoides, Patella—o. Tibiæ minus, Fibula — o. Tincæ, Os uteri — o. Triangulaires, Wormiana ossa — o. Turbinatum, Turbinated bone, middle — o. Turbinatum inferius, Turbinated bone, inferior—o. Uncinatum, Os unciforme—o. Upsiloides, Hyoides os — o. Varium, Cuboid — o. Vespiforme, Sphenoid — o. Vomeris, Vomer — o. Wormiens, Wormiana ossa — o. Xiphoides, Sternum — o. Ypseloides, Hyoides os — o. Zygomaticum, Malæ os.

Os U'TERI, Os tincæ, Protos'porus, Os inter'num, Os amphid'eon seu amphid'eum, Os'cheon, Hysteros'toma, Os'culum u'teri, Hysterostom'ium, Orific''ium u'teri, (F.) Museau de Tanche. The mouth of the womb, see Uterus.

OSCEDO, Yawning.

OSCHÆMATŒDE'MA, Oschæmatœde'ma, Œde'ma scroti cruen'tum; from οσχεον, 'scrotum,' αιμα, 'blood,' and οιδημα, 'œdema.' Effusion of blood into the scrotum.

OSCHÆMŒDEMA, Oschæmatœdema.

OSCHE, Scrotum.

OSCHEITIS, Orcheitis, Oschitis.

OSCHEOCARCINOMA, Cancer, chimneysweepers'.

OSCHEOCE'LE, Oschoce'lè, from οσχεον, 'the scrotum,' and κηλη, 'tumour;' Scrotal hernia, see Bubonocele. Sauvages uses it in the sense of Dropsy of the scrotum, see Hydrocele.

OSCHEOCELE AQUOSA, Hydroscheocele—o. Flatulenta, Physocele—o. Hydatidosa, Hydatidocele —o. Œdematica, Œdematoscheocele—o. Seminalis, Spermatocele—o. Urinalis, Urocele—o. Varicosa, Varicocele.

OSCHEON, Scrotum, Os uteri.

OSCHEON'CUS, Oschon'cus, Oscheophy'ma, Oschophy'ma, from οσχεον, 'scrotum,' and ογκος, 'a tumour.' A preternatural swelling of the scrotum.

OSCHEOPHYMA, Oscheoncus.

OSCHEOPLAS'TIC, Oscheoplas'ticus, from οσχεον, 'the scrotum,' and πλασσω, 'I form.' An epithet given to the operation for restoring the scrotum when lost.

OSCHEOPYŒDE'MA, Oschopyœde'ma, Œde'ma scroti purulen'tum. Purulent tumefaction of the scrotum.

OSCHEUS, Scrotum.

OS'CHION. The raised margin of the os uteri. According to some, an excrescence from the os uteri.

OSCHI'TIS, Orchei'tis, Oschei'tis, Inflamma'tio scroti, from οσχεον, 'the scrotum,' and itis, 'inflammation.' Inflammation of the scrotum.

OSCHOCARCINOMA, Cancer, chimneysweepers'.

OSCHOCELE, Oscheocele.

OSCHONCUS, Oscheoncus.

OSCHOPHYMA, Oscheoncus.

OSCHOPYŒDEMA, Oscheopyœdema.

OSCHURŒDE'MA; from οσχιον, 'scrotum,' ουρον, 'urine,' and οιδημα, 'œdema.' Œdema from effusion of urine into the scrotum.

OSCHUS, Scrotum.

OSCHYDRŒDE'MA, from οσχιον, 'scrotum,' 'ὑδωρ, 'water,' and οιδημα, 'œdema.' Œdema scroti aquo'sum. Watery œdema of the scrotum.

OSCILLA'TIO, Irritability, Oscillation.

OSCILLA'TION, Oscilla'tio; from oscillum, 'an image perhaps of Bacchus, hung on ropes, and swung up and down in the air.' Vibration, Vibra'men, Vibra'tio, Vibra'tus. Also, a partial rotatory movement of the eyeball to and from its antero-posterior axis.

OS'CITANT (FEVER), Febris os'citans, (E.) Fièvre oscitante, from oscitare, 'to yawn.' A fever, in which the patient is continually yawning.

OSCITATIO, Yawning.

OSCULATORIUS, Orbicularis oris.

OSCULUM UTERI, Os uteri.

OSCUS, Scrotum.

OSEILLE, Rumex acetosa — o. Boucher, Rumex scutatus — o. Petite, Rumex scutatus — o. Ronde, Rumex scutatus — o. Rouge, Rumex sanguineus.

OS'MAZOME, Os'mozome, Osmazo'ma, Osmoso'ma, Zomod'mum, (F.) Matière extractive du Bouillon; Extrac'tive of meat, Saponaceous extract of meat; from οσμη, 'smell,' and ζωμος, 'soup.' M. Thénard gave this name to an extractive matter, contained in muscular flesh and in the blood of animals, which he considers of a peculiar nature. It has an agreeable smell and taste, and is found in Bouillons of meat, in the proportion of one part to seven of gelatin. Vauquelin discovered in it some fungi. It is the substance which gives the flavour of meat to soups, and hence its name. It has been prescribed in the dose of ʒss to ʒj, in broth or in powder, with aromatics, as a stimulant to the digestive actions and a restorer of appetite in convalescence. An Osmazome chocolate, Chocola'ta cum osmazo'ma, has been introduced as an analeptic article of diet. It consists of chocolate ℔j to osmazome ʒj.

OSME, Odour.

OSMESIS, Olfaction.

OSMIDRO'SIS, from οσμη, 'odour,' and 'ιδρως, 'sweat.' Perspiration of an unusual odour.

OSMITOPS'IS ASTERISCOÏ'DES, Bellis. A plant, of the Cape of Good Hope, which, from its smell and taste, seems to contain camphor; hence its antispasmodic virtues. In infusion, it is often beneficially employed in cough, hoarseness, and diseases of the chest generally, and is said to be serviceable in flatulent colic. Infused in spirit, spir'itus bellidis, it has been used successfully as an external remedy in paralysis.

OSMOMETRICUS SENSUS, Olfaction.

OSMON'OSI, Osmonu'si, Morbi olfac'tûs, from οσμη, 'odour,' and νοσος, 'a disease.' Diseases of olfaction.

OSMONOSOLOG'IA, from οσμη, 'odour,' νοσος, 'disease,' and λογος, 'description.' The doctrine of, or a treatise on, the diseases of the sense of smell.

OSMORRHI'ZA LONGIS'TYLIS, Sweet Cic"ely. An indigenous plant, Order Umbelliferæ, which flowers in May and June. It is an agreeable aromatic, having much of the flavour of anise.

OSMOZOME, Osmazome.

OSMUND, ROYAL, Osmunda regalis.

OSMUN'DA CINNAMO'MEA, Cinnamon Fern. Indigenous; Order, Filices; is regarded to be demulcent, subastringent, and tonic. Boiled in milk, it yields a fine mucilage, which is useful in d'arrhœa.

OSMUN'DA REGA'LIS, Filix Flor'ida, Osmundroyal. This plant was once thought to possess astringent and emmenagogue virtues.

OSORON, Opium.

OSPHRANTERICUS, Olfactory.

OSPHRANTICOS, Olfactory.

OSPHRASIA, Olfaction.

OSPHRESIOL'OGY, Osphresiolog"ia, from οσφρησις, 'odour,' and λογος, 'a discourse.' A treatise on olfaction and odours.

OSPHRESIS, Olfaction.

OSPHRETICUS, Olfactory.

OSPHRIS'TICE, from οσφρησις, 'olfaction.' The doctrine of the phenomena of odours.

OSPHYALGEMA, Coxalgia.

OSPHYALGIA, Coxalgia.

OSPHYARTHRITIS, Osphyitis.

OSPHYARTHROCACE, Coxarum morbus.

OSPHYI'TIS, Osphy'tis, Osphyarthri'tis, Inflamma'tio coxæ, from οσφυς, 'the hip,' and itis, denoting inflammation. Inflammation of the parts about the hip.

OSPHYRRHEUMA, Lumbago.

OSPHYS, Haunch, Lumbi.

OSPHYTIS, Osphyitis.

OSSA BREGMATIS, Parietal bones—o. Convoluta inferiora, Turbinated bones, inferior — o. Digitorum manûs, Phalanges of the fingers — o. Digitorum pedis, Phalanges of the toes—o. Epactalia, Wormiana ossa — o. Maxillæ superioris quarta seu quinta seu secunda, Nasal bones — o. Nasalia, Nasal bones—o. Nasi, Nasal bones — o. Nervalia, Parietal bones—o. Pisiformia lingualia, see Hyoides os—o. Raphogeminantia, Wormiana ossa — o. Sesamoidea, Sesamoid bones — o. Sincipitis, Parietal bones—o. Spongiosa, Turbinated bones—o. Suturarum, Wormiana ossa—o. Tertia maxillæ superioris, Turbinated bones — o. Tetragona, Parietal bones—o. Triangularia, Sphenoidal cornua — o. Triangularia Blasii, Wormiana ossa — o. Triquetra, Wormiana ossa — o. Turbinata, Turbinated bones—o. Verticalia, Parietal bones.

OSSELETS DE L'OREILLE, Ossicula auditûs.

OSSEOUS, Os'seus, Osto'des, Ostoï'des, (F.) Osseux; from os, 'a bone.' Bony. Resembling bone.

OSSICLE, Ossiculum.

OSSICULA, see Ossiculum.

OSSIC'ULA AUDI'TUS, Ossic'ula Auris, (F.) Osselets de l'oreille, O. de l'ouie. The small bones situate in the cavity of the tympanum, and forming an uninterrupted chain from the membrane of the tympanum to that of the fenestra ovalis. They are four in number; and their series, from without to within, is as follows: Malleus, Incus, Os orbiculare, Stapes.

OSSICULA BERTINI, Sphenoidalia cornua—o. Innominata, Innominata minora ossa — o. Nasi, Nasal bones — o. Sesamoidea, Sesamoid bones.

OSSIC'ULUM, (plural Ossic'ula,) Osta'rion, Os'sicle. Diminutive of os, 'a bone.' A small bone. See Os.

OSSICULUM COCHLEARE, Orbicular bone — o. Incudi Comparatum, Incus — o. Malleolo assimilatum, Malleus — o. Molari denti comparatum, Incus—o. Orbiculare, Orbicular bone — o. Quartum, Orbicular bone — o. Squamosum, Orbicular bone.

OSSIFICA'TION, Ossifica'tio, from os, 'a bone,' and facere, 'to make.' Osteogen'ia, Osteogen"sis, Osteo'sis, Osto'sis. Formation of bone. Development, or increase of the osseous system. Ossification takes place in the same manner as the nutrition of other organs. The bones are, at first, mucous, and afterwards cartilaginous; the cartilage, at length, receives the phosphate of lime, and is, at the same time, replaced by a gelatinous parenchyma, when the bone has acquired the whole of its development.

OSSIFICATION, POINTS OF, *Puncta* seu *Nu'clei ossificatio'nis*, *Nu'clei ossei*, are the points where the ossification of a bone commences, whence it extends to other parts. Almost all the bones present a greater or less number of points of ossification. Besides the natural ossification, which we observe in the fœtus and in the first periods of life, there are also *acciden'tal ossifications*, such as those frequently remarked after the inflammation of serous membranes, in the parietes of arteries, and to which the terms *Osthex'ia*, *Incrusta'tion* and *Petrifac'tion* have, sometimes, been applied.

OSSIFRAGA, Osteocolla.
OSSIS SACRI ACUMEN, Coccyx.
OSSISANA, Osteocolla.
OSSIV'OROUS, from *os*, 'a bone,' and *voro*, 'I devour.' A species of tumour, mentioned by Ruysch, which destroys bone.

OS'TAGRA, *Os'teagra*, from *osteon*, 'a bone,' and *agra*, 'seizure.' A forceps to cut or remove portions of bone.

OSTALGIA, Osteocopus.
OSTALGI'TIS, *Osti'tis*, *Ostei'tis*, from *osteon*, 'a bone,' and *itis*. *Inflamma'tio Ossis.* Inflammation of bone; characterized by violent shooting and lancinating pains in the bone.

OSTARIUM, Ossiculum.
OSTARTHRITIS, Arthrophlogosis.
OSTARTHROCACE, Spina ventosa.
OSTEAGRA, Ostagra.
OSTEALGIA, Osteocopus.
OSTEITES, Osteocolla.
OSTEITIS, Ostalgitis.

OSTEMPYE'SIS. *Osteëmpye'sis*, *Ostempyo'sis*, from *osteon*, 'a bone,' and *empyesis*, 'effusion of pus.' An abscess in the interior of a bone.

OSTEMPYOSIS, Ostempyesis.

OSTEOCE'LE, from *osteon*, 'a bone,' and *kele*, 'a tumour.' A hernia in which the sac is cartilaginous and bony:—a rare case. Also, osseous induration of one or both testicles.

OSTEOCLASIS, Fracture.

OSTEOCOL'LA, from *osteon*, 'a bone,' and *kolla*, 'glue.' *Glue-bone*, *Stone* or *Bone binder*, *Ossif'raga*, *Holos'teus*, *Ossisa'na*, *Ostri'tes*, *Ostei'tes*, *Amos'teus*, *Osteol'ithos*, *Stelochi'tes*. A name given to petrified carbonate of lime, found in some parts of Germany and other portions of the globe; so called, because it has been supposed to possess the power of favouring the formation of *callus* in fractures. It is the *Chaux carbonatée concretionnée incrustante* of Haüy. Not used.

OSTEOC'OPUS, *Osteal'gia*, *Ostal'gia*, *Osteodyn'ia*, from *osteon*, 'a bone,' and *kopos*, 'fatigue.' *Boneach.* Pain in the bones.

OSTEODENTINE, see Tooth.
OSTEODYNIA, Osteocopus.
OSTEOGANGRÆNA, Necrosis.
OSTEOGENIA, Ossification.
OSTEOG'RAPHY, *Osteogra'phia*, from *osteon*, 'a bone,' and *graphein*, 'to describe.' Description of the bones. The part of anatomy which describes the bones.

OSTEOLITHOS, Osteocolla.
OSTEOL'OGY, *Osteolog''ia*, from *osteon*, 'a bone,' and *logos*, 'a discourse.' The part of anatomy which treats of bones.

OSTEOMA, Exostosis.
OSTEOMALACIA, Mollities ossium — o. Infantum, Rachitis.
OSTEOMALACOSIS, Mollities ossium.
OSTEON, Bone—o. Hieron, Sacrum.
OSTEONABRO'SIS, from *osteon*, 'a bone,' *a*,

priv., and βρωσις, 'nutriment.' Atrophy of the osseous texture marked by diminution of volume.

OSTEON'CUS, from *osteon*, 'a bone,' and *onkos*, 'a tumour.' A bony tumour.

OSTEONECROSIS, Necrosis.

OSTEON'OSI, *Osteonu'si*, from *osteon*, 'a bone,' and *nosos*, 'a disease.' *Mor'bi os'sium.* Diseases of the bones.

OSTEOPÆDION, Lithopædion.

OSTEOPALIN'CLASIS, from *osteon*, 'a bone,' παλιν, 'again,' and κλασις, 'fracture.' The breaking again of a bone which has united unfavourably.

OSTEOPHYMA, Osteoncus.

OSTEOPH'YTA, *Os'teophyte*, *Exosto'sis*. Under this name, Rokitansky, of Vienna, describes a deposition of bony matter, found by him on the inner surface of the parietes of the skull of pregnant women.

OSTEOPLEU'RA, *Pleurosto'sis*, from *osteon*, 'a bone,' and πλευρον, 'a rib.' Ossification of the cartilages of the ribs.

OSTEOPORO'SIS, *Osteosclero'sis*, from *osteon*, 'a bone,' and πωρωσις, 'induration.' Induration of a bone, from the deposition of too much bony matter.

OSTEOPSATHYROSIS, Fragilitas ossium.

OSTEO-SARCO'MA, *Osteo-sarco'sis*, *Sarcosto'sis*, *Hæmatexosto'sis*, from *osteon*, 'bone,' and *sarx*, 'flesh.' Disease of the bony tissue, which consists in softening of its laminæ, and their transformation into a fleshy substance, analogous to that of cancer; accompanied with general symptoms of cancerous affection. The word has often, also, been used synonymously with spina ventosa.

OSTEOSARCOSIS, Osteosarcoma.
OSTEOSCLEROSIS, Osteoporosis.
OSTEOSIS, Ossification.

OSTEO-STEATO'MA, *Exosto'sis steatomato'des*, from *osteon* 'a bone,' and *stear*, 'suet or fat.' A name given to bony tumours or degenerations, which sometimes belong to osteo-sarcoma; at others, to spina ventosa, exostosis, &c.

OSTEOT'OMIST, *Osteotomis'ta*. Same etymon as the next. An instrument, invented by Dr. D. Davis, for cutting the bones of the fœtal cranium, where it becomes necessary to greatly reduce the size of the head in parturition.

OSTEOT'OMY, *Osteotom'ia*, from *osteon*, 'a bone,' and *temnein*, 'to cut.' The part of practical anatomy whose object is the dissection of bones.

OSTEOTOPHUS, Tophus.
OSTEOTYLUS, Callus.
OSTEULCUM, Bone-nippers.
OSTEUM, Bone.
OSTHEXIA, see Ossification.
OSTIA ATRIO-VENTRICULARIA, see Ostium.
OSTIARIUS, Pylorus.
OSTIOLUM, from *osteon*, 'a mouth or opening.' A small door or gate.
OSTIOLA CORDIS, *Val'vulæ cordis*, *Pellic'ulæ cordis*. The valves of the heart.
OSTITIS, Ostalgitis.

OS'TIUM, *Orific''ium*, a door or gate,—of the heart, for example. The opening—*Os'tia atrio-ventricula'ria*—between the auricle and ventricle of each side; *Os'tium veno'sum*, that of the right side; *Os'tium arterio'sum*, that of the left.

OSTIUM ABDOMINALE, see Tube, Fallopian—o. Internum, see Ostium uteri.

OSTIUM U'TERI. The vulva; the vagina. The term *Os'tium inter'num* has been applied to the inferior opening of the uterus, which establishes a free communication between the cavities of the body and neck, and which is often obliterated in old women.—Cruveilheir. The neck of the uterus; the mouth of the uterus.

OSTIUM UTERINUM, see Tube, Fallopian — o. Ventriculi Duodenale seu Pyloricum seu Dextrum seu Inferius, Pylorus.

OSTODES, Bony.

OSTOIDEA SUBSTANTIA, see Tooth.

OSTOIDES, Bony.

OSTOMA, Exostosis.

OSTOSIS, Ossification.

OS'TREA, Os'treum, (F.) Huître. The oyster. The oyster is a wholesome article of diet, often advised as analeptic and easy of digestion. The shells, Testæ Os'treæ, Testa (Ph. U. S.), (F.) Écailles d'huîtres, have been received into the Pharmacopœias, and used medicinally. Their virtues are similar to those of the carbonate of lime. See Creta.

OSTREUM, Ostrea.

OSTRITES, Osteocolla.

OSTRUTHIUM, Imperatoria.

OSYRIS, Antirhinum linaria.

OTACOUS'TIC, Otacous'ticus; from ους, ωτος, 'the ear,' and ακουω, 'I listen.' Any instrument is so called which improves the sense of hearing, —as the different species of trumpets.

OTAGRA, Otalgia.

OTAL'GIA, Ot'agra, Otod'ynē, Otal'gy, from ους, ωτος, 'the ear,' and αλγος, 'pain.' Pain in the ear; Dolor au'rium, Spas'mus au'rium, Ear-ache. See Otitis.

OTAL'GIC, Otal'gicus. An epithet for remedies used in otalgia.

OTECHUS, Tinnitus aurium.

OTEMPLAS'TRUM, Otoplas'ta, Otoplas'trum, from ους, 'the ear,' and εμπλαστρον, 'a plaster.' A plaster put behind the ears.

OTEN'CHYTES, Otenchyta, from ους, ωτος, 'the ear,' εν, 'into,' and χυω, 'I pour.' Sipho auricula'ris. A species of syringe, used for injecting the ear.

OTHELCO'SIS, from ους, ωτος, 'the ear,' and 'ελκωσις, 'ulceration.' Ulceration or suppuration of the ear.

OTHONE, Linteum.

OTHONION, Linteum.

OTHYGROTES, Otirrhœa.

OTIATER, Aurist.

OTIATRI'A, Otiat'rice, from ους, ωτος, 'the ear,' and ιατρεια, 'medicine.' The business of the aurist. The management of diseases of the ear. Aural Medicine and Surgery, Ear Surgery.

OTIATRICE, Otiatria.

OTIATRUS, Aurist.

O'TIC, O'ticus, from ους, ωτος, 'the ear.' Belonging or relating to the ear. A medicine employed in diseases of the ear.

OTIC GANGLION, Otogan'glium, Gang'lion auricula'rē, Ganglion o'ticum, Auric'ular ganglion, Ganglion of Arnold, (F.) Ganglion maxillo-tympanique. This is a small ganglion, although more than double the size of the ophthalmic, ash-coloured and pulpy like the ganglions of the sympathetic. It is situate in advance of the ganglion of Gasser, on the lower surface of the inferior maxillary nerve, at the inner margin of the foramen ovale of the sphenoid bone. See Petrous ganglion.

OTIRRHŒ'A, Otorrhœ'a, Othy'grotes, Blennotorrhœ'a, (F.) Ontarrhe de l'Oreille, from ους, 'the ear,' and ρεω, 'I flow.' Discharge of a purulent or puriform liquid, from the meatus auditorius externus, Pyorrhœ'a au'rium, Otopyorrhœ'a, Pya-otorrhœ'a, Otorrhœ'a purulen'ta. It is a symptom of chronic otitis. Some authors have, indeed, used the term synonymously with chronic otitis. When it extends to the brain, it is termed cer'ebral otorrhœ'a; and when from the middle or internal ear, it is termed internal otorrhœa, Otorrhœ'a inter'na, and Entotorrhœ'a.

OTIRRHŒA, CEREBRAL, see Otirrhœa.

OTITES, see Digitus.

OTI'TIS, Otophleg'monē, Empres'ma otitia, Inflamma'tio auris, Inflammation of the ear, (F.) Inflammation de l'oreille. Inflammation of the mucous membrane of the ear, characterized by excruciating pain; intolerable humming in the ear, with a discharge of mucus generally from the meatus externus or from the Eustachian tube. When the inflammation is restricted to the lining membrane of the meatus, it is termed otitis catarrha'lis. Otitis is divided into external and internal, according as it affects the meatus auditorius, or the cavity of the tympanum or internal ear. It may be acute or chronic. Acute otitis commonly terminates in a few days in a favourable manner, with the aid of antiphlogistics. Chronic otitis, otirrhœ'a, is almost always accompanied by a purulent discharge from the meatus auditorius. It is often incurable, and may ultimately give occasion to disease of the internal ear, and even of the brain.

OTITIS CATARRHALIS, see Otitis.

O'TIUM, Ota'rium, from ους, ωτος, 'the ear.' A small ear. The auricle or pavilion of the ear.

OTOCEPH'ALUS, Mono'tia, from ους, ωτος, 'the ear,' and κεφαλη, 'head.' A monster, whose ears are in contact, or united into one.

OTOCONIES, see Otolithi.

OTODYNE, Otalgia.

OTOGLYPHIS, Earpick.

OTOGLYPHUM, Earpick.

OTOG'RAPHY, Otogra'phia, from ους, ωτος, 'the ear,' and γραφη, 'a description.' The part of anatomy which describes the ear.

OT'OLITHS, Otol'ithi, (F.) Otolithea, from ους, ωτος, 'the ear, and λιθος, 'a stone.' White calcareous substances contained in the membranous vestibule, and seeming to be suspended in the fluid of the vestibule by means of a number of nervous filaments proceeding from the auditory nerve. Their universal presence in the ear of the mammalia would seem to show that they are inservient to audition. When of a looser consistence, they are called Otocon'ia, (F.) Otoconia, from ους, 'the ear,' and κονια, 'dust.'

OTOL'OGY, Otolog'ia, from ους, ωτος, 'the ear,' and λογος, 'a discourse.' The part of anatomy which treats of the ear. An anatomical treatise on the ear.

OTOPATHEMA, Otopathy.

OTOP'ATHY, Otopathi'a, Otopathe'ma, from ους, ωτος, 'the ear,' and παθος, 'a disease.' A diseased condition of the ear.

OTOPHLEGMONE, Otitis.

OTOPLASTA, Otemplastrum.

OTOPLAS'TICE, from ους, ωτος, 'the ear,' and πλαστικος, 'forming.' The operation for restoring a lost ear.

OTOPLASTRUM, Otemplastrum.

OTOPYORRHŒA, Otirrhœa.

OTORRHAG"IA; from ους, ωτος, 'the ear,' and ραγη, 'rupture.' Bleeding from the ear or ears.

OTORRHEUMATIS'MUS, from ους, ωτος, 'the ear, and ρευματισμος, 'rheumatism;' Otal'gia rheumat'ica. Rheumatic ear-ache.

OTORRHŒA, Otirrhœa—o. Cerebral, see Otirrhœa—o. Interna, see Otirrhœa—o. Purulenta, Otirrhœa.

OTOSCOP'IUM, from ους, ωτος, 'the ear,' and σκοπη, 'examination.' An instrument for examining the condition of the external ear.

OTOT'OMY, *Ototom'ia*, from ους, ωτος, 'the ear,' and τεμνειν, 'to cut.' The part of practical anatomy which teaches the mode of dissecting and preparing the ear.

OULA, Gingivæ.

OULE, Cicatrix.

OUNCE, *Un'cia*. A weight equal to the 16th part of a pound avoirdupois, the 12th of a pound troy. It is composed of 8 drachms. See Weights and Measures.

OURAQUE, Urachus.

OURARY, Curare.

OUREMA, Urine.

OURLES, Parotis, Cynanche parotidæa.

OURON, Urine.

OUS, Ear.

OUTRE MER, Lapis lazuli.

OUVERTURE CADAVÉRIQUE, Autopsia cadaverica.

OVA GRAAFIANA, Folliculi Graafiani — o. Nabothi, Nabothi glandulæ.

OVAL, *Ova'lis, Oö'des, Oöi'des, Ova'tus*, from *ovum*, 'an egg.' Egg-shaped; elliptic. That which is round and oblong like an egg.

OVALE FORA'MEN, Foramen oö'des, (F.) *Trou ovale*. The foramen obturatorium; also, the foramen in the inner paries of the middle ear, which opens into the vestibule; the foramen in the sphenoid bone, through which the third branch of the fifth pair issues from the cranium; and the aperture, in the fœtus, between the auricles of the heart. See Botal Foramen.

OVALIS FOSSA, *Val'vula* seu *Vestig"ium Foram'inis ovalis*, is a depression observed in the right auricle of the heart, on the septum, which separates it from the left auricle. It has thick and strong edges, at its upper and fore part, called *Colum'næ foram'inis ova'lis, Isthmus seu An'nulus Vieusse'nii* seu *An'nulus fossæ ovalis*: in the fœtus called *An'nulus foram'inis* vel *fossæ ova'lis*. The fossa ovalis, in the adult, replaces the inter-auricular aperture in the septum auricularum of the fœtus.

OVA'RIAN, *Ova'rial, Ovaria'nus*, from *ovarium*, ωαριον, 'the ovary.' Relating to the ovary —as Ovarian pregnancy.

OVARIAN ARTERY, Spermatic artery—o. Nerves, Spermatic plexus of nerves — o. Pregnancy, see Pregnancy, ovarian—o. Veins, Spermatic veins— o. Vesicles, Folliculi Graafiani.

OVARIOTOMY, Oariotomy.

O'VARISTS, *Ovists*. Same etymon as Ovarian. Those physiologists who think that the phenomena of generation, in the human species and in every species of animal, result from the development of the ova or ovula of the female, merely incited by the male. Not many of the physiologists of the present day can be classed among the ovarists.

OVARITIS, Oaritis.

OVA'RIUM. Same etymon. The *O'vary, Testis mulie'bris, T. femineus, Oa'rion, Ooph'o-ron, Gynoa'rium, Vesica'rium*, (F.) *Ovaire*. The ovaries are the organs in which the ova are formed in oviparous animals. By analogy, the name has been given to the organs which the ancients called the *testicles* of the female. They are two ovoid bodies, almost as large as the testicles in men, placed on each side of the uterus, between the Fallopian tube and round ligament, and in the substance of the broad ligament. Their outer extremity gives attachment to one of the projections of the fimbriated extremity of the Fallopian tube; and the internal is fixed to the uterus by a small ligamentous cord, called *Ligamen'tum rotun'dum ova'rii, Lig'ament of the O'vary*. The ovaries are composed of a very close,

spongy texture—*stroma*,—and of small vesicles— *Follic'uli Graafiani*,— filled with a clear fluid: these vesicles contain ovules, which detach themselves from the ovarium before and after fecundation, and are carried into the cavity of the uterus by the Fallopian tube.

OVARIUM TUMIDUM, Oarioncus — o. Nabothi, Nabothi glandulæ.

OVATUS, Oval.

OVER-EATING, COLIC FROM, Colica crapulosa.

OVERO BUTUA, Pareira brava.

OVICAPSULE, see Folliculi Graafiani.

OVIDUCTUS MULIEBRIS, Tuba Fallopiana.

OVIG"EROUS, *O'viger, Ovig"erus ;* from *ovum*, 'an egg,' and *gero*, 'I bear.' Containing or producing ova or eggs.

OVIPARITÉ, see Oviparous.

OVIP'AROUS, *Ovip'arus ;* from *ovum*, 'an egg,' and *pario*, 'I bring forth.' An epithet applied to animals which are hatched from eggs outside of the body. The condition may be termed *Ovip'arousness*, (F.) *Oviparité*. See Generation.

OVIPAROUSNESS, see Oviparous.

OVISAC, see Folliculi Graafiani—o. Tunic of the, see Folliculi Graafiani.

OVISTS, Ovarists.

OVOLOGY, Oologia.

OVO-VIVIP'AROUS, from *ovum*, 'an egg,' *vivus*, 'living,' and *pario*, 'I bring forth.' Oviparous animals, whose ova are hatched within the mother,—vipers, for example. See Generation.

OVULA GRAAFIANA, Folliculi Graafiani— o. Nabothi, Nabothi glandulæ.

OVULA'TION; from *ovulum*, diminutive of *ovum*, 'an egg.' The formation of ova in the ovary, and the discharge of the same.

SPONTANEOUS OVULATION, (F.) *Ovulation spontanée*, is the spontaneous formation and discharge of ova which takes place in the female of the mammalia. See Heat.

OVULINE, Decidua reflexa.

O'VULUM, *O'vule ;* diminutive of *ovum*, 'an egg.' A small egg. That which has the appearance of a small egg. See Ovum.

OVUM, ωον, *Oön*, an egg. The eggs of poultry are chiefly used as food. The different parts are, likewise, employed in medicine. The shell, *Auran'cum, Auran'tum*, (F.) *Coque d'œuf, Coquille d'œuf*, calcined, is esteemed an absorbent. The *Oil of the egg* is emollient, and is used, externally, to burns and chaps. The *Yolk* or *Yelk of the egg*— *Vitel'lum* seu *Vitel'lus ovi*—renders oils, &c., miscible with water. Eggs, when light boiled, are easy of digestion; but, when very hard-boiled or fried, they are more rebellious.

Egg brandy is made by taking of Brandy f℥iv; *Cinnamon water*, f℥iv ; the yolks of two *eggs ; Sugar*, ℥ss ; and *Oil of cinnamon*, gtt. ij. Mix the yolks of the eggs first with the water, the oil and the sugar, stirring constantly. Then add the brandy little and little, until a smooth fluid is formed. It is an agreeable mode of giving brandy in adynamic states.

In *Pharmacy, white of egg*, which consists chiefly of albumen, is used for clarifying syrups, &c. *Yolk of egg*, (F.) *Jaune d'œuf*, beaten up with warm water and sugar, and aromatized with orange-flower water, forms an emulsion, which is emollient, and known under the name *Lait de poule* or *chicken's milk*.

Anatomists give the name *Ova, O'vula, O'vules*, (F.) *Œufs*, to round vesicles, containing a humour similar to the yolk of egg, which are situate in the ovaries of the female, and, when fecundated, constitute the rudiments of the fœtus. During gestation, the embryo and its enveloping membranes retain the name *Ovum*, (F.) *Œuf*. The changes induced in the mammalia after impregnation greatly resemble those in the bird.

Ovum, Testiclo—o. Hystericum, see Clavus hystericus.

OXALAS SUBPOTASSICUS, Potass, oxalate of.

OXALAT'IC, *Oxalat'icus*. Relating to *oxalates*: hence *Oxalat'ic* or *Oxalic acid Diath'esis* is the habit of body which favours the formation and deposition of oxalates from the urine.

OXAL'IC ACID, *Acidum oxali'num, A. sac-chari'num, A. hydro-carbon'icum, A. acetosel'læ, A. oxal'icum, Acidum sac'chari, Acid of sugar, Acid of sorrel, Car'bonous acid*, from οξαλις, 'sorrel.' An acid found in sorrel. It crystallizes in long, colourless, quadrangular prisms, and is generally found, in nature, united with lime or potassa. It has been proposed, in a diluted state, as a refrigerant, but it is unnecessary; and, besides, in quantity, it is a virulently acrid poison. It is largely employed for cleaning boot-tops; and, as it strongly resembles the sulphate of magnesia, has often been taken for it. Several fatal cases are, indeed, on record. For its antidotes, &c., see Poison.

OXALIC ACID DIATHESIS, see Oxalatic.
OXALIDE, Oxalis acetosella.
OXALIS ACETOSA, Rumex acetosa.

Ox'ALIS ACETOSEL'LA. *O. America'na, Oxys alba*. The systematic name of the *Woodsorrel, Cuckowbread, Sour Tref'oil, White sorrel, Mountain Sorrel, Trifo'lium aceto'sum, Oxitriphyl'lum, Lujula, Allelu'ja, Acetosel'la, Oxyphyl'lon, Oxytriphyl'lon, Panis cu'culi*, (F.) *Surelle, Oxalide, Pain a Coucou, Alleluia*. Family, Geraniæ. Sex. Syst. Decandria Decagynia. This plant has a gratefully acid taste, and is used in salads. It has been esteemed refrigerant, antiscorbutic, and diuretic.

OXALIS AMERICANA, O. acetosella.

OXALIS TUBERO'SA, *Oca*. A tuberous plant, whose oval-shaped root is used as food by the Peruvians. It is watery, has a sweetish taste, and is much liked.

OXALIUM, Potass, oxalate of.

OXAL'MĒ, from οξυς, 'acid,' and 'αλς, 'salt.' A mixture of vinegar and salt.

OXALU'RIA, Urine, oxalic.

OXELÆ'ON, from οξυς, 'acid,' and ελαιον, 'oil.' A mixture of vinegar and oil, used as a condiment.

OX EYE, Helenium autumnale—o. Gall, Bile of the ox.

OXICÊDRE, Juniperus oxycedrus.
OXID, Oxyd.
OXIDATION, Oxydation.
OXIDE, Oxyd.
OXIDUM, Oxyd, see Oxydum.
OXI'NES, οξινης, (οινος,) from οξυς, 'acid.' Wine already sour, but not yet vinegar.
OXITRIPHYLLUM, Oxalis acetosella.
OXODES, Acidulous.
OXOIDES, Acidulous.
OXOS, Acetioum acidum.
OXYA, Fagus sylvatica.
OXYÆSTHESIA, Hyperæsthesis.
OXYAPHE, Hyperaphia.
OXYAPHIA, Hyperaphia.
OXYBAPHON, see Acetabulum.
OXYBOL'IA, from οξυς, 'quick,' and βολη, 'jection.' Too rapid emission of sperm.
OXYCANTHA, Mespilus oxyacantha.
OXYCAN'THA GALE'NI, *Ber'beris, Ber'beris vulga'ris, Spina so''ida, Crespi'nus*, (F.) *Épine vinette, Vinettier*. Family, Berberideæ. Sex. Syst. Hexandria Monogynia. The *Barberry*. The fruit of the berries, *Barberries, Pipperidges*, is gratefully acid, and moderately astringent. By preparing an alcoholic extract of the root and adding water to it, a pulverulent brown substance is thrown down, which, when dissolved in alcohol and evaporated, yields the bitter principle, *Berberin*, which is an excellent stomachic in the dose of 2, 5, or 10 grains.

The American Barberry, *Bar'beris Canaden'sis, Pipperidge Bush, Sowberry*, differs slightly from the European. It flourishes on mountains and hilly districts from Canada to Virginia.

OXYCÈDRE, Juniperus oxycedrus.

OXYCOCCOS, Vaccinium oxycoccos—o. Palustris, Vaccinium oxycoccos.

OX'YCRATE, *Oxycra'tum*, from οξυς, 'acid,' and κραω, 'I mix;' *Posca, Phusca*. A mixture of vinegar and water; frequently used in medicine as a refrigerant and antiseptic.

OXYCRO'CEUM EMPLASTRUM, from οξυς, 'acid,' and κροκος, 'saffron.' A plaster, composed of *saffron, pitch, colophony, yellow wax, turpentine, galbanum, gum ammoniac, myrrh, olibanum*, and *mastic*. It was employed as a strengthening plaster.

OXYCUM, Oxygen.

OXYD, *Oxid, Oxide, Oxyde, Ox'ydum, Ox'idum*, from οξυς, 'acid.' A combination, not acid, of a simple body with oxygen.

OXYDA'TION, *Oxyda'tio, Oxida'tion, Oxygena'tion*. The action of oxydizing a body; that is, of combining it with oxygen; a combination from which results an oxyd.

OXYDE, Oxyd.

OXYDE, CYSTIC. A species of urinary calculus, having the shape of confused, yellowish, semi-transparent, insipid, very hard crystals. When distilled, it furnishes subcarbonate of ammonia, like all nitrogenised matters. It dissolves in the nitric, sulphuric, phosphoric, and oxalic acids.

OXYDE D'ANTIMOINE SULFURÉ, Oxydum stibii sulphuratum.

OXYDER'CIA, *Oxydor'cia, Visus a'cies*, from οξυς, 'quick,' and δερκεσθαι, 'to see.' Sharpness of vision.

OXYDER'CICUS, *Oxyder'ces*, from οξυ, 'sharp,' and δερκω, 'I see.' A medicine which sharpens the sight.

OXYDORCIA, Oxydercia.

OXYDUM, Oxid—o. Antimonii cum phosphate calcis, Antimonial powder.

OXYDUM FERRI NIGRUM, *Ferri ox'idum nigrum, Black oxyd of iron*. The scales, which fall from iron, when heated, consist of iron, combined with oxygen. They have been used like the chalybeates in general.

OXYDUM FERRICUM CRYSTALLIZATUM NATIVUM, Hæmatites—o. Hydrargyri completum, Hydrargyri nitrico-oxydum—o. Hydrargyricum, Hydrargyri nitrico-oxydum—o. Hydrargyricum præparatum, Hydrargyri oxydum cinereum—o. Hydrargyrosum, Hydrargyri oxydum cinereum.

OXYDUM STIBII SULPHURA'TUM, *Hepar antimo'nii, Cro'cus metallo'rum, Crocus antimo'nii*, (F.) *Oxyde d'antimoine sulfuré, Foie d'Antimoine*. This was formerly exhibited in the cure of fevers, but it is now rarely employed.

OXYDUM URICUM, Uric oxide.

OXYECOIA, Hyperacusis.

OXYG'ALA, from οξυς, 'sour,' and γαλα, 'milk.' Sour milk. The *Oxygala equi'num, Caracos'mos*, is reckoned amongst the delicacies of the Tartars.

OXYG'ARON, from οξυς, 'acid,' and γαρον, 'garum.' A composition of garum and vinegar.

OX'YGEN, *Oxygen ium, Empy'real air, Pure*

air, Vital air, Dephlogis'ticated air, Oxyg"enes, Ox'ycum, Princip'ium oxyg"enans seu oxygenet'-icum seu acid'ificans seu ac"idum, Elemen'tum acidif'icum, (F.) Oxygène, Air du feu; from οξυς, 'acid,' and γεινομαι, 'I engender,' that is, generator of acids; and such it was believed to be, exclusively, at the period when the name was given to it. This is now known not to be the case. Oxygen is largely distributed in nature. It exists in the air, in water, in several acids, in all the oxyds, and in vegetable and animal substances, &c. It is obtained by decomposing the peroxyd of manganese or the chlorate of potassa by heat in close vessels. Although oxygen, in the state of admixture in which it is found in the atmosphere, is of vital importance, it cannot be respired in a pure state with impunity. Animals die in it long before the whole of the oxygen is consumed. The properties of oxygen seem to be stimulant. It increases the force and velocity of the pulse, and has, accordingly, been used in cases of chronic debility, chlorosis, asthma, scrofula, dropsy, paralysis, &c. It requires to be diluted with from 10 to 20 parts of atmospheric air; one to two quarts being given during the day.

OXYGENATION, Oxydation.

OXYGÈNE, Oxygen.

OXYGÉNÈSES. A name given by Baumes to diseases which he attributed to disordered oxygenation.

OXYGEUSIA, Hypergeustia.

OXYG'LICUS, Oxyg'lices, from οξυς, 'acid,' and γλυκυς, 'sweet;' Mulsa acida, Ace'tum mulsum dulce. Prepared by macerating and boiling honey-comb (from which the greater part of the honey has been taken) in water, and adding vinegar. An Oxymel.

OXYLAPATHUM, Rumex acutus.

OX'YMEL, Apom'eli, Mel aceta'tum, from οξυς, 'acid,' and μελι, 'honey.' Honey and vinegar boiled to a syrupy consistence.

OXYMEL ÆRUGINIS, Linimentum Æruginis.

OXYMEL COL'CHICI, Oxymel of meadow saffron, (F.) Oxymel colchiqué. (Rad. colch. recent. in laminas tenues sectæ ʒj, aceti destillati ℔j, mellis despumat. pond. ℔ij. Macerate in a gentle heat for 48 hours. Press and boil the liquor with the honey to the thickness of a syrup; stirring with a wooden spoon. Ph. D.) It is expectorant and diuretic. Dose, fʒj, in gruel.

OXYMEL COLCHIQUÉ, O. colchici — o. of Meadow saffron, O. colchici.

OXYMEL SCILLÆ, Oxymel of squills, Mel scillæ, Oxymel scillit'icum. (Mellis. despumat. Oiss, aceti scillæ Oij. Boil in a glass vessel over a gentle fire to a proper consistence.) It is reputed to be expectorant and diuretic. Dose, ʒj.

OXYMEL, SIMPLE, Oxymel simplex, is prepared as follows: (Mellis despumati ℔ij, acidi acetici ℔j. Boil in a glass vessel, over a slow fire, to a proper thickness. Ph. L.) It is cooling;— externally detergent.

OXYMEL OF SQUILL, O. scillæ.

OXYMYRRHINE, Ruscus.

OXYMYRSINE, Ruscus.

OXYNGIUM, Adeps suillus.

OXYNI'TRON, from οξυς, 'acid,' and νιτρον, 'nitre.' Name of a plaster, composed chiefly of vinegar and nitre, and recommended by Aëtius.

OXYNOSEMA, Acute disease.

OXYNOSOS, Acute disease.

OXYNUSOS, Acute disease.

OXYO'PIA, Galero'pia, Hyperop'sia, Suffu'sio excla'rans, Acies visûs, from οξυς, 'quick,' and ωψ, 'sight.' Excessive acuteness of the sense of sight. Instances have occurred where persons could see the stars in the day time. The cause is seated in great sensibility of the retina. The term has been used synonymously with nyctalopia.

OXYOSPHRE'SIA, Oxyosphra'sia, from οξυς, 'acute,' and οσφρησις, 'smell.' Excessive acuteness of the sense of smell.

OXYPHLEGMA'SIA, οξυφλεγμασια, Acu'ta et ve'hemens inflamma'tio. A violent inflammation.

OXYPHŒNICON, Tamarindus.

OXYPHO'NIA, Vox acu'ta; from οξυς, 'sharp,' and φωνη, 'voice;' Parapho'nia clangens, P. ulcero'sa, Clangor, Vox clango'sa, Leptopho'nia. A shrill and squalling voice;—frequently, a symptom of morbid affection of the larynx.

OXYPHYLLON, Oxalis acetosella.

OXYPODIA, see Kyllosis.

OXYPROTEIN, see Corium phlogisticum.

OXYREG'MIA, Ructus ac"idus, from οξυς, 'sour,' and ερευγω, 'I belch.' Acid eructation.

OXYR'IA RENIFORM'IS, Rumex dig"ynus, Boreal sourdock, Mountain Sorrel, Welsh sorrel. A plant, Sex. Syst. Diandria digynia, which grows in the northern parts of America and Europe; blossoming in the spring. It possesses the same properties as oxalis acetosella.

OXYRRHOD'INON, Ace'tum rosa'tum, from οξυς, 'acid,' and ῥοδον, 'a rose.' A composition of vinegar and roses. (Ol. rosat. ʒij, acet. rosat. ʒj.) Used as a liniment in herpes and erysipelas.

OXYS, Acetum, Acid, Acute — o. Alba, Oxalis acetosella.

OXYSAC'CHARUM, from οξυς, 'acid,' and σακχαρον, 'sugar.' A mixture of sugar and vinegar. It was called Oxysac'charum vomiti'vum, when it held in solution the glass of antimony; and Oxysac'charum scillit'icum, when it contained squills.

OXYSAL DIAPHORET'ICUM AN'GELI SALÆ. A preparation of Angelo Sala. Acetate of potass exposed to the atmosphere; and consequently fallen into a state of deliquium.— Orfila.

OXYTARTARUS, Potassæ acetas.

OXYTES, Acidities.

OXYTOC'IA. Same etymon as the next. Rapidity of parturition. Too great rapidity of birth.

OXYTOC'IC, Oxyt'ocus, from οξυς, 'quick,' and τικτω, 'I bring forth.' A medicine which promotes delivery.

OXYTRIPHYLLON, Oxalis acetosella.

OXYURE VERMICULAIRE, Ascaris vermicularis.

OYSTER ROOT, Tragopogon — o. Shells, Ostreæ testæ—o. Prepared, Testa præparata.

OZÆ'NA, Coryza enton'ica, C. purulen'ta, Pyorrhœa nasa'lis, Entozæ'na, C. ozæno'sa, C. ulcero'sa, Coryza virulen'ta, C. malig'na, Rhini'tis ulcero'sa, Ulcus na'rium fœtens, from οζω, 'I smell of something.' (F.) Ozène, Punaisie. An affection of the pituitary membrane, which gives occasion to a disagreeable odour, similar to that of a crushed bed-bug; hence the name Punais, by which the French designate one labouring under ozæna. It is, sometimes, owing to caries of the bones; but is, perhaps, most frequently dependent upon syphilitic ulceration of the pituitary membrane, with or without caries of the bones of the nose.

OZÆNA BENIGNA, Coryza, chronic.

OZE, Breath, offensive.

OZEMAN, Albumen.

OZÈNE, Ozæna.

OZONE: same etymon as Ozæna. The powerfully odorous matter produced when a current of ordinary electricity passes from pointed bodies into the air.—Schönbein.

P.

P. A contraction of *Pugillus.*
P. Æ. A contraction of *Partes æquales.* See Abbreviation.
P. P. A contraction of *Pulvis patrum.*

PAB'ULUM, *Trophē, Phorbē, Alimen'tum, Nutrimen'tum.* Food, aliment. The *animal heat* and *animal spirits*—unmeaning terms—were formerly considered the *Pabulum vitæ.*

PACAY, Prosopis dulcis.

PACCHIO'NI, GLANDS OF, *Glan'dulæ Duræ Matris, G. duræ Menin'gis, Tuber'cula parva duræ matris, Cor'pora glandifor'mia duræ matris,* (F.) *Granulations cérébrales.* Small, whitish, or yellowish bodies, sometimes separate, at others united like a bunch of grapes, which are observed in several parts of the dura and pia mater. They receive vessels, but apparently no nerves. Their texture and uses are unknown. A considerable number is observed in the longitudinal sinus, covered by the internal membrane.

PACHÆ'MIA, *Pachyæ'mia, Pachæ'ma, Pachyæ'ma,* from παχυς, 'thick,' and 'αιμα, 'blood.' Too great thickness of the blood.

PACHEABLEPHARO'SIS, *Pacheablepha'ara, Pachyblepha'aron, Pachyblepharo'sis, Pach'ytes,* from παχυς, 'thick,' and βλεφαρον, 'an eyelid.' A name given, by some authors, to a thickening of the eyelids, produced by tubercles or excrescences formed on their margins. It is the same affection as that which Sauvages designates *Cali'go à Pacheablepharo'si.*

PACHETOS, see Laqueus.

PACHULOSIS, Pachylosis.

PACHYÆMIA, Pachæmia.

PACHYBLEPHARON, Pacheablepharosis.

PACHYCHOL'IA, from παχυς, 'thick,' and χολη, 'bile.' Morbid thickness of the bile.

PACHYLO'SIS, *Pachulo'sis,* from παχυς, 'thick.' An inordinate production of the epidermis dependent upon hypertrophy of the papillæ of the skin.—E. Wilson.

PACHYNSIS, Polysarcia adiposa.

PACHYNTICA, Incrassantia.

PACHYSMUS, Polysarcia adiposa.

PACHYTES, Pacheablepharosis.

PACINIAN CORPUSCLES, see Corpuscles.

PACKING, OF THE HYDROPATHISTS; *Emaillotage.*

PACKWAX, see Micha.

PAD, (S.) *Pajado,* from *paja,* 'straw.' *Plumace'olus, Pulvil'lus, Pulvin'ulus, Parvum pulvi'nar ;*—a cushion, a *little cushion;* a *junk ;* (F.) *Coussinet.* A small bag, filled with feathers, wool, hair, bran, chaff, &c. It is used to compress or support parts. In the treatment of certain fractures, soft pads or cushions, called by the French *Remplissages,* are placed between the splints and the fractured limb, in order that the prominent parts may not be chafed by the splints.

PADDIE, see Oryza.

PADDY, see Oryza.

PADNOON, Bit noben.

PAD'UA, MINERAL WATERS OF. Near Padua, in Italy, there are several thermal, sulphureous springs; the hottest of which is 188° Fahr. The chief establishments are Abano, Battaglia, and Montegrotto.

PADUS, Prunus padus — p. Avium, Prunus padus — p. Lauro-cerasus, Prunus lauro-cerasus.

PÆDAN'CHONE, from παις, παιδος, 'a child,' and αγχω, 'I strangle ;' *Angi'na Sicca.* Name of a fatal species of cynanche, mentioned by M. A. Severinus; probably the *Cynanche Trachealis,* or *Cynanche Maligna.*

PÆDARTHROCACE, Spina ventosa.

PÆDATROPH'IA, *Atrophia infan'tilis, Maras'mus lactan'tium,* from παις, παιδος, 'a child,' a, privative, and τροφη, 'nourishment.' Atrophy of children. Tabes mesenterica.

PÆDATROPHIA GLANDULOSA, Scrofula.

PÆDERAS'TIA, *Pædogo'gium, Pædica'tio, Cinæ'dia,* from παις, 'a boy,' and ερως, 'love.' The love of boys. A disgraceful passion, common in ancient times, but now unknown. These terms are likewise applied to the crime of sodomy.

PÆDI'A, παιδια, 'learning.' *Educa'tio infan'tum.* The bringing up or education — physical as well as moral — of children.

PÆDIATRI'A, *Pædiat'rica,* from παις, 'a child,' and ιατρεια, 'medical management.' Treatment of the diseases of children.

PÆDICATIO, Pæderastia.

PÆDICTERUS, Icterus infantum.

PÆDOBAROMACROMETER, Baromacrometer.

PÆDOGOGIUM, Pæderastia.

PÆDOMETER, Baromacrometer.

PÆDON'OSUS, from παις, παιδος, 'a child,' and νοσος, 'disease.' A disease of childhood.

PÆDOPHLEBOTOM'IA, from παις, 'a child,' φλεψ, 'a vein,' and τομη, 'incision.' *Venæsec'tio puero'rum.* Bleeding performed on children.

PÆDOT'RIBES, *Min'ister Gymnas'tæ,* from παις, 'a child,' and τριβω, 'I train.' In ancient gymnastics, the officer acquainted with all the prescribed exercises, and who carried them into effect, according to the directions of the superior.

PÆO'NIA, *P. officina'lis* seu *mas'cula* seu *nemora'lis* seu *fem'ina* seu *loba'ta, Glyce'idā, Hemago'gum, Pe'ony,* or *Pi'ony, male and female.* (F.) *Pivoine, Pione.* The root, flowers, and seeds were long esteemed powerful medicines. They are feebly astringent, and have been considered to be narcotic and antispasmodic. They have been given, particularly, in intermittents and epilepsy, but are not now used. The flowers are called *Rosæ benedic'tæ, R. re'giæ.*

PÆONICE, Medicine.

PÆONICUS, Medical.

PÆONIUS, Medical.

PÆOSYNE, Medicine.

PAGAPOPLEX'IA, from παγειν, 'to nail fast,' and αποπληξια, 'apoplexy.' Apoplexy from cold.

PAIDIA, Infancy.

PAIDION, Infans.

PAIGIL, Primula veris.

PAIN, (old F.) *painer,* 'to torment ;' Sax. *pinan,* 'to torture.' *Dolor, Algos, Alge'ma, Alge'do, Alge'sis, Od'ynē,* (F.) *Douleur.* A disagreeable sensation, which scarcely admits of definition. It is generally symptomatic, and is called *acute,* (F.) *aiguē,* when very violent; *pungent,* (F.) *pongitive,* when it resembles that which would be produced by a sharp instrument run into the part: *heavy,* (F.) *gravative,* when attended with a sensation of weight; *tensive,* when the part seems distended: *lan'cinating,* when occurring in shoots: *lac'erating* or *tearing,* when the part seems to be tearing: *burning,* (F.) *brûlante,* when resembling that produced by a burn, &c.

PAIN, SUN, Hemicrania.
PAIN, see Triticum—p. à *Coucou*, Oxalis acetosella—p. *de Madagascar*, Jatropha manihot—p. *de Pourceau*, Cyclamen.
PAINS, AFTER, see P. labour.
PAINS, GNAWING, *Dolo'res roden'tes*. Pains resembling what might be produced by the gnawing of an animal.
PAINS, Labour pains, Throes, Throws, *Parturien'tis dolo'res, Odin, Odis, Dolo'res ad partum, Torm'ina parturientium*, (F.) *Mal d'Enfant, Douleurs*. The uneasy sensations that accompany labour, and are owing to uterine contraction. The pains that precede actual delivery, and are simply employed in dilating the os uteri, are called *grinding*; those which extrude the child, *forcing*. Those which take place in the first days after delivery, and are employed in forcing away coagula, &c., are termed *After pains, Dolo'res* seu *Tormina post partum, D. puerpera'rum*, (F.) *Tranchées utérines*.
"To take a pain,"—"To try a pain,"—is to make an examination *per vaginam*, during labour, to discover its progress, character, &c.
The French term the pains, which precede and announce labour, *mouches*; those which accompany it, *douleurs*; and those which occur immediately afterwards, *tranchées* ou *coliques*.
PAINT, from *pingere, pinctum*, 'to paint,' (I.) *pinto*, (F.) *peint*; *Pigmen'tum, Fucus*, (F.) *Fard*. A name given to different substances, employed for embellishing the complexion or rendering the skin softer. The substances most commonly used for this purpose are:—the *Subnitrate of Bismuth*, (F.) *Blanc de fard*. A spirituous solution of benzoin, precipitated by water, and forming *Virgin's milk*, (F.) *Lait virginal*; the red or *rouge* of the carthamus; *Spanish white*; the oxides of lead, tin, and mercury, vermilion, red saunders, &c. All paints may be said to be noxious. They injure the skin; obstruct perspiration; and, thus, frequently lay the foundation for cutaneous affections. See Cosmetic.
PAINT, INDIAN, Hydrastis Canadensis, Sanguinaria Canadensis—p. Yellow, Hydrastis Canadensis.
PALÆSTRA, Gymnasium.
PALAIS, Palate.
PALATAL, Palatine.
PALATE, *Pala'tum, Hypero'a, Hyperö'um, Urani'cos, Roof of the mouth, Fossa Palati'na, Palatum stab'ilä, Hard Palate*, (F.) *Palais*. The upper part of the cavity of the mouth; a kind of parabolic vault, formed by the two superior maxillary bones, and the two palate bones covered with a thick and dense mucous membrane: bounded, before and at the sides, by the superior dental arch; and, behind, by the velum palati. A whitish line runs along the middle, from before to behind; at the anterior extremity of which is a tubercle corresponding to the inferior orifice of the anterior palatine canal. The arteries of the palate and corresponding gums proceed from the palatine, alveolar, infra-orbitar, labial, and buccal branches. The veins follow a similar course. The nerves are given off from the palatine, facial, infra-orbitar, superior dental, and from the naso-palatine ganglion.
PALATE, ARTIFIC"IAL, (F.) *Obturateur du Palais*. A plate of tortoise-shell, silver, &c., used to close a deficiency of the palate.
PALATE BONE, *Os Pala'ti, Os basila'ré*, (F.) *Os Palatin, Os du Palais*, is a small bone, of an irregular shape, situate at the posterior part of the nasal fossæ and palate. It seems formed by the union of two bony plates joined at right angles to each other; so that one is *inferior* and *horizontal*;—the other, *superior* and *vertical*. The *horizontal* or *palatine portion, Arch of the palate*, is quadrilateral. Its upper surface forms part of the nasal fossæ; the lower forms part of the palatine arch, and contains the inferior orifice of the *posterior palatine canal*. Its *anterior* edge is articulated with the palatine process of the superior maxillary bone; the *posterior* is free and sharp. It gives attachment to the velum palati, and presents an eminence, which, when joined with one on the opposite side, forms the posterior nasal spine. Its inner edge is articulated with the corresponding bone; its outer is confounded with the vertical portion. The *vertical* or *ascending portion* has the form of a long square. The inner surface forms part of the outer paries of the nasal fossæ. Its outer surface is unequal, and is articulated with the superior maxillary bone; behind, it presents a vertical groove, which forms part of the posterior palatine canal; and, above, a small free surface, which looks into the zygomatic fossa. Its anterior edge is united with the superior maxillary bone; the posterior is unequal, and rests on the internal ala of the pterygoid process. The angle, which it forms by uniting with the posterior edge of the horizontal portion, presents a very prominent pyramidal eminence, called the *tuberosity of the palate bone*. Its upper margin is surmounted by two eminences;—the one, anterior, called the *orbitar process*;—the other posterior, the *sphenoid process*. These two processes are separated by an almost circular notch, which the sphenoid bone forms into a foramen, called the *spheno-palatine*.
This bone appears to be developed from a single point of ossification. It is articulated, with the sphenoid, ethmoid, the cornua sphenoidalia, superior maxillary bone, the inferior spongy bone, the vomer, and its fellow.
PALATE, CLEFT, see Harelip—p. Falling down of, the Uvulitis—p. Fissured, see Harelip—p. Hard, Palate—p. Soft, Velum pendulum palati.
PAL'ATINE, *Pal'atal, Palati'nus, Pal'atic*, from *palatum*, 'the palate.' Relating or belonging to the palate.
PALATINE or PALATAL ARTERIES are two in number. They are distinguished into, 1. The *superior palatal* or *palatine, Palati'na descen'dens* or *Pal'ato-max'illary*, which leaves the internal maxillary behind the top of the orbit; descends into the pterygo-maxillary fissure, and enters the posterior maxillary canal. Its branches are distributed to the velum palati and the nasal fossæ. 2. The *inferior* or *ascending palatine* or *palatal*, which is very small, and separates from the facial near its origin. It passes along the lateral and superior part of the pharynx, between the pillars of the velum palati, and divides into a number of ramusculi, which are distributed to the pharynx, the corresponding tonsil, the Eustachian tube, and the velum palati.
PALATINE CANALS or DUCTS. These are two in number. The *anterior, Ductus incisi'vus* vel *Nasa'lo-palati'nus, Inci'sive canal*, is situate at the anterior part of the palatine arch, and is formed by the two superior maxillary bones. It is single beneath, but opens above by two apertures, one into each nasal fossa. The foramen is called *Fora'men incisi'vum* vel *F. Palatinum ante'rius, F. Alveola'ré ante'rius*, and *F. cæcum ossis maxilla'ris superio'ris*. The *posterior palatine canal* is situate at the posterior part of the palate. It is formed by the palate and superior maxillary bones, ascends between these two bones; and, in its course, gives rise to two or three small accessary palatine canals, which open above the tuberosity of the palate bone. It transmits the nerves and vessels which bear its name. The foramen

is called, *F. Palati'num poste'rius, F. Palato-maxilla'rē, F. alveola'rē poste'rius.*

PALATINE MEMBRANE is the fibro-mucous membrane that lines the palate or roof of the mouth.

PALATINE or PALATAL NERVES, *Gutturo-palatins,* (Ch.) are three in number; and arise from the inferior part of the spheno-palatine ganglion. 1. The *great palatine, Palatin inférieur,* (Ch.) is situate anteriorly to the two others, and descends into the posterior palatine canal; gives a *nasal* filament and a *staphyline* filament, and is distributed on the palate. 2. The *middle palatine, Guttural,* (Ch.,) which arises behind the preceding; enters one of the accessory palatine canals, and is distributed to the tonsils and velum palati. 3. The *little palatine nerve,* situate still more backward than the last, which loses itself by several filaments in the uvula, tonsils, and follicles of the palatine membrane.

PALATITE, Isthmitis.

PALATITIS, Uranisconitis.

PALATO-GLOSSUS, Glossostaphylinus.

PALATO-PHARYNGEUS, *Pharyn'go-staphyli'nus, Staphyli'no-pharyngeus, Thyro-pharyn'-go-staphyli'nus,* part of the *Hypero-pharyngeus,* (F.) *Palato-pharyngien, Stylo-pharyngien* (Ch.) A membranous muscle, broader at its middle than at its extremities, and situate vertically in the lateral paries of the pharynx and velum palati. It includes the perystaphylo-pharyngeus, pharyngo-staphylinus, and thyro-staphylinus of Winslow. When the two palato-pharyngei contract together, they depress the velum. They elevate and shorten the pharynx, and act principally in deglutition.

PALATO-PHARYNGIEN, Palato-pharyngeus — p. Salpingeus, Circumflexus — *p. Salpingien,* Circumflexus.

PALATOSTAPHYLINI, see Azygos muscle.

PALATUM FISSUM, Hyperoochasma — p. Molle, Velum pendulum palati — p. Pendulum, Velum pendulum palati.

PALE, Pollen.

PALENESS, *Pallor, Och'rotes, Ochro'ma, Ochri'asis, Leuco'sis, Dealba'tio, Luror,* (F.) *Pâleur.* Whiteness of complexion. It appears to be owing to a diminution or alteration of the blood circulating in the capillary vessels, and is often a sign of disease.

PÂLES COULEURS, Chlorosis.

PALETTE, (F.) *Pal'mula, Fer'ula.* An instrument of percussion. It has the shape of a spatula with a long handle; is made of very light, white wood, and has been proposed, by Mr. Percy, for what is called the *Massage,* a kind of pressure or kneading, exerted by the hand on the body and limbs to excite the tone of the skin and subjacent tissues.

Palette also means a cup for bleeding, and the xiphoid cartilage (?).

PALETTE À PANSEMENT. A small splint of thin, scooped wood, having the shape of the hand, and used to support the hand in certain cases—when burnt, for example—in order to prevent the fingers from being deformed by the cicatrices.

PALETTE DE CABANIS. An instrument, invented by Cabanis of Geneva to draw out the extremity of the stylet when passed into the nose, in the operation for fistula lachrymalis. It is composed of two plates of silver, pierced with several holes, and movable on each other. To use it, the instrument must be carried into the nose, so that the holes of the two plates correspond. When the end of the stylet is received into one of these holes, it is pinched, by sliding one of the plates on the other, and is easily withdrawn.

PÂLEUR, Paleness.

PALI PLAGUE, see Plague.

PALILLO, Campomanesia lineatifolia.

PALIMPISSA, see Pinus sylvestris.

PALINCOTESIS, Recrudescentia.

PALINDROME, Palindromia.

PALINDROM'IA, *Palin'dromē,* from παλιν, 'again,' and δρομος, 'a course.' This word signifies, with some, a reflux of fluids from the exterior towards the interior; and, according to others, the relapse of an affection — the recurrence — *Recur'sio, Repetit''io* — of a paroxysm or disease, — *Morbus recidi'vus, Morbi recur'sus.*

PALINGENESIA, Regeneration.

PALLIA'TION, *Pallia'tio,* from *palliare,* 'to cover, mask;' from *pallium,* 'a mantle.' The act of palliating — that is, of causing the symptoms of a disease to mitigate, without curing it. The medical art can frequently only moderate the symptoms of a disease, prevent it from making progress, prolong the days of the patient, and diminish his sufferings. This is a *palliative treatment.*

PAL'LIATIVE, *Palliati'vus, Antipath'ic, Enantiopath'ic.* A remedy or mode of treatment, which only relieves a disease, without curing it. The *palliative* treatment — *Cura palliati'va,* is placed in antithesis to the radical, *Cara radica'lis;* see Radical.

PALLIDULUS, *Blafard.*

PALLIDUS MORBUS, Chlorosis.

PALLOR, Paleness — p. Virginum, Chlorosis.

PALM, *Palma, Vola, V. manūs, Plate'a, Thenar, Ages, Agos'tus, Poc'ulum, Pat'era, Supellex* seu *Supellec'tilē Diog''enis,* (F.) *Paume* ou *Creux de la main.* The hollow or inside of the hand. It is limited, *without,* by the thenar eminence, which answers to the thumb; *within,* by the hypothenar eminence, which answers to the little finger; *above,* by the wrist-joint; and, *below,* by the four fingers.

PALMA CHRISTI, Ricinus communis — p. Cocos, Cocos nucifera — p. Dactylifera, Date tree — p. Humilis, Musa paradisiaca — p. Unguentariorum, Myrobalanus.

PALMÆ U'TERI PLICA'TÆ, *Arbor vita uteri'nus, A. u'teri viv'ificans.* The arborescent striæ in the interior of the cervix uteri.

PALMAIRE CUTANÉ, Palmaris brevis — p. Grand, Palmaris magnus — *p. Grêle,* Palmaris longus — p. Long, Palmaris longus.

PALMAR, *Palma'ris,* from *palma,* 'the palm of the hand.' That which concerns the palm of the hand. The palm has, sometimes, been divided into three regions, called *palmar.* 1. The *external palmar region* corresponds to the thenar eminence. 2. The *internal palmar region* is formed by the hypothenar eminence: and, 3. The *middle palmar region* is the hollow of the hand, (F.) *Creux de la main.*

PALMAR APONEURO'SIS, *Palmar fas'cia.* A strong triangular aponeurosis, which arises from the inferior tendon of the palmaris brevis, and the anterior annular ligament of the carpus. It covers the whole palm of the hand, and adheres, somewhat strongly, to the skin of the part. The *palmar ligaments* are small, very numerous, fibrous fasciæ, which unite the different bones of the carpus and metacarpus.

PALMAR ARCHES, (F.) *Arcades* ou *Crosses palmaires.* The curved extremities of the radial and cubital arteries in the palm of the hand. There are two palmar arches: — the one *cubital* or *superficial,—grande Arcade palmaire* of Chaussier, furnishes, at its convexity towards the fingers, the collateral arteries of the fingers, and the internal collateral of the thumb; the other, the *radial, profound,* or *deep-seated,— petite Arcade palmaire* of Chaussier, is deep in the palm of the hand beneath the tendons of the flexor muscles of the fingers. It gives some small branches only to the surrounding parts. The palmar veins accompany the corresponding arteries.

PALMAR ARTERIES, see Palmar arches—p. Fascia, P. aponeurosis.

PALMAR MUSCLES. These are three in number. 1. *Palma'ris Magnus, Flexor carpi radia'lis, Radia'lis intern'us,* (F.) *Épitrochlo-métacarpien* (Ch.), *Palmaire grand, Radial antérieur.* A long fusiform muscle, which passes obliquely from the inner tuberosity of the humerus to the upper extremity of the second metacarpal bone. It bends the hand. 2. *Palmaris longus, Latescen'tis chorda, Ulna'ris grac''ilis,* (F.) *Épitrochlo-carpi-palmaire* (Ch.), *Palmaire long, P. grêle.* This muscle is situate on the inner side of the last. It is very slender, and passes from the inner tuberosity of the humerus to the anterior annular ligament of the carpus, and to the palmar aponeurosis, which it seems to form by the vanishing of its fibres. It stretches the palmar aponeurosis, and bends the hand. 3. *Palmaris Brevis, Caro quadra'ta, Carpiæ'us,* (F.) *Palmaire cutané.* A small, thin, quadrilateral muscle; situate before the thenar eminence. It passes from the annular ligament of the carpus to the integuments of the palm of the hand, which it wrinkles by its contractions.

PALMAR VEINS, see Palmar arches.

PALMARIS BREVIS, see Palmar muscles—p. Longus, see Palmar muscles—p. Magnus, see Palmar muscles.

PALMETTO, SAW, Chamærops serratula.

PALMI-PHALANGIENS, Lumbricales manus.

PALMISTRY, Chiromancy.

PALMOSCOP'IA, from παλμος, 'palpitation,' and σκοπεω, 'I view.' Investigation of the beating of the heart and pulse. Prognosis from the beating of the heart and pulse.

PALMULA, Date, *Palette.*

PALMUS, Palpitation—p. Cordis, Palpitation—p. Plumbarius, Colic, metallic—p. Vomitus, Vomiting.

PALO DE CALENTURAS, Calenturas.

PALOS DE CALENTURA, Cinchona.

PALPA'TION, from (F.) *palper,* to feel. The sense of touch. It is also used for the mode of exploring disease by feeling or pressing upon the diseased organ.

PAL'PEBRA, supposed to be from *palpitare,* 'to palpitate,' owing to its frequent motion (?) *Bleph'aron, Oper'culum* seu *Coöper'culum oc'uli, Eyelid,* (F.) *Paupière.* The eyelids are two movable vela, situate in front of the eye; which by their separation permit the organ to receive the impression of light, or by their greater or less occlusion protect it from the influence of too great light, or from the action of extraneous bodies. They are separated, above, from the forehead, by the eyebrows; and, below, are confounded with the cheeks. They are distinguished into *upper, Palpebra major* seu *superior, Epicyl'ium,*—and *lower, Palpebra minor* seu *inferior, Hypocæ'lis, Hypocæ'lum, Hypoc'ylum.* The former is much broader and more movable than the latter. They are separated by a transverse cleft; and their edges are thick, and furnished with the cilia or eyelashes. Supported by the tarsal cartilages, they unite at the extremities of the transverse diameter of the orbit, forming two angles, the innermost being called the *greater angle of the eye,* or *inner* or *greater canthus;* the other, the *lesser* or *external angle* or *canthus.* They are formed, 1. Of a thin dermoid texture: 2. Of a muscular membrane,—a portion of the orbicularis: 3. Of a particular fibrous membrane: 4. Of the tarsi: 5. Of a mucous membrane,—a part of the tunica conjunctiva.

Their vessels and nerves are called Palpebral.

PALPEBRA INFERIOR EXTRORSUM FLEXA, Ectropion—p. Tertia, Valvula semilunaris.

PALPEBRÆ SUPERIORIS PRIMUS, Levator palpebræ superioris.

PAL'PEBRAL, *Palpebra'lis,* from *palpebra,* 'the eyelid.' That which belongs or relates to the eyelid.

PALPEBRAL ARTERIES are those distributed to the eyelids. They are two in number; an *upper* and a *lower.* The *former* arises from the ophthalmic, a little beyond the cartilaginous pulley of the greater oblique muscle, and descends towards the upper eyelid, over which it is distributed. The *latter* arises at the side of, and a little behind, the preceding, and sends its ramifications to the lower eyelid and the neighbouring parts. The palpebral veins have a similar arrangement; except that some of them open into the temporal and labial veins.

PALPEBRAL FLUX, PURIFORM. A puriform discharge, furnished by the glands of Meibomius, when inflamed; and to which Scarpa attributes fistula lachrymalis, in many cases.

PALPEBRAL LIGAMENTS are distinguished into *superior* and *inferior.* Some anatomists, with Winslow, have described, under this name, the fibrous layer which is attached,—on the one hand, to the outer part of the circumference of the orbit; on the other, to the tarsal cartilages.

PALPEBRAL NERVES, *Nerves of the eyelids,* arise, particularly, from the frontal and lachrymal branches; from the ophthalmic nerve of Willis; and from the facial, nasal, and infraorbitar branch of the superior maxillary nerve.

PALPEBRALIS, Orbicularis palpebrarum.

PALPEBRARUM APERIENS RECTUS, Levator palpebræ superioris—p. Duo musculi, Orbiculares palpebrarum.

PALPEBRATIO, Nictation.

PALPITATIO, Palpitation—p. Arteriarum, see Palpitation—p. Cordis trepidans, Cardiotromus.

PALPITATIO MEMBRO'RUM. A term used by Gaubius for involuntary shaking of the legs.

PALPITA'TION, *Palpita'tio, Palmus, P. Cordis, Palpita'tio* seu *Pulsa'tio Cordis, Tremor Cordis, Vibra'tio Cardi'aca* seu *Cordis, Cardiog'mus, Cardiopal'mus, Subsul'tio, Clonus Palpita'tio,* (F.) *Palpitation, P. du Cœur.* A name given to the pulsations of the heart, when they become stronger, more extensive, or more sensible to the individual, than ordinarily. Palpitations occur in a number of affections. They are, sometimes, owing to organic diseases of the heart, hypertrophy, inflammation, &c.; at others, to a disease in some other viscus; whilst, frequently, they are merely nervous.

PALPITATION is sometimes felt in the arteries, constituting *Palpitatio Arterio'sa.*

PALPITATION DU CŒUR, Palpitation.

PALSIED, Paralytic.

PALSY, Paralysis—p. Bell's, Paralysis, Bell's.

PALSY, LEAD, *Paral'ysis saturni'na, P. metal'lica,* (F.) *Paralysie saturnine, Metal'lic Palsy, Painters' Palsy.* The paralysis of the upper extremities especially, induced by the poison of lead.

PALSY, METALLIC, see Palsy, lead—p. Painters', P. lead—p. Shaking, Paralysis agitans—p. Trembling, Paralysis agitans.

PALTA, Persea gatissima.

PALUDAL, Elodes.

PALUDAPIUM, Apium graveolens.

PALUDOSUS, Elodes.

PALUS, Marsh, Penis—p. Sanctus, Guaiacum.
PAMBIOMA, Panbioma.
PAMOISON, Syncope.
PAMPINIFORM PLEXUS, Corpus pampiniforme.
PAMPINIFORME CORPUS, see Corpus pampiniforme.
PAMPLE'GIA, *Panplegia*, from παν, 'all,' and πληγω, 'I strike.' General paralysis. Palsy of the whole body.
PANACE'A, *Cathol'icon*, *Cathol'icum*, from παν, 'all,' and ακεομαι, 'I cure.' *Universa'lě reme'dium*, *Panchres'tos*. A pretended universal remedy. There is no such thing in existence.
PANACEA DUCIS HOLSATIÆ, Potassæ sulphas—p. Duplicata, Potassæ sulphas—p. Lapsorum, Arnica montana—p. Mercurialis, Hydrargyri submurias—p. Mercurii rubri, Hydrargyri nitrico-oxidum—p. Pectoris, Glechoma hederacea—p. Vegetabilis, Crocus.
PANA'DA, diminutive of Ital. *pane*, 'bread,' (Lat. *panis*,) *Pana'ta*, *Panatel'la*. Bread, boiled in water to the consistence of pap. Sometimes administered to the sick.
SIMPLE BREAD PANADA may be made by putting any quantity of grated stale *bread* into enough *water* to form a moderately thick pulp; covering it up, and leaving it to soak for an hour; then beating it up with two tablespoonfuls of *milk*, and a small portion of *refined sugar*, and boiling the whole for ten minutes, stirring all the time.
PANARIS, Paronychia.
PANARITIUM, Paronychia.
PANARIUM, Paronychia.
PANATA, Panada.
PANATELLA, Panada.
PANAX COSTINUM, Pastinaca opoponax—p. Heracleum, Pastinaca opoponax—p. Pastinacea, Pastinaca opoponax.
PANAX QUINQUEFO'LIUM, *Aurelia'na Canaden'sis*, *Ara'lia Canaden'sis*, Ginseng, Ninsing, Genseng, Redberry, Five-fingers. Family, Araliaceæ. *Sex. Syst.* Polyandria Monœcia. This plant grows in Tartary and North America. The root is about the thickness of the little finger; an inch or two in length, often dividing into two branches; of a whitish-yellow colour; wrinkled on the surface, and of a compact, almost horny, texture. It has no smell, but a very sweet taste, combined with a slight degree of aromatic bitterness. It is much esteemed by the Chinese, who pay a high price for it. It is a gentle and agreeable stimulant.
PANBIO'MA, *Pambio'ma*, from παν, 'all,' and βιος, 'life.' The original animating principle. The general principle of life.
PANCHRESTOS, Panacea.
PANCHYMAGO'GUM, *Pantago'gon*, from παν, 'all,' χυμος, 'juice,' and αγω, 'I drive away.' A medicine which the ancients believed capable of purging away all sorts of humours.
PANCHYMAGOGUM MINERALE, Hydrargyri submurias.
PANCŒNOSUS, Pandemic.
PANCŒNUS (MORBUS), Pandemic.
PANCRATIUM, Pancreas.
PAN'CREAS, from παν, 'all,' and κρεας, 'flesh;' i. e. 'quite fleshy.' *Callic'reas*, *Panera'tium*, *Pan'creum*, *Lactes*, *Pulvi'nar ventri'culi*, *Totum carno'sum*, *Gland'ula saliva'lis abdom'inis*, *Pancré'ně*. A gland, deeply seated in the abdomen, and lying transversely on the vertebral column, between the three curvatures of the duodenum, behind the stomach, and to the right of the spleen. Its left extremity is called the *tail* of the pancreas; it is smaller than the right, which is called the *head*. At its right portion, it has, almost

always, a greater or less prolongation; called, by Winslow, and some others, the *lesser pancreas*, (F.) *Petit pancréas*, *Pancreas of Aselli*, *Pancreas minus*. The pancreas resembles the salivary glands in structure, and has been called the *Abdominal Salivary Gland*. It is composed of lobes and granulated lobules, distinct, and united by areolar tissue. From each of the granulations of these lobes arise the radicles of its excretory duct, which are very delicate, and united like veins. The duct itself, *Ductus Pancreat'icus*, *Canal* or *Duct of Wirsung* or *Wirsungs*, (F.) *Canal pancréatique*, proceeds in a serpentine course through the substance of the organ; and when it has reached behind the second portion of the duodenum, it becomes free, and is of the size of a crow's quill. It opens at an acute angle into the choledoch duct, or proceeds close to it, opening separately into the duodenum. The *Pancreatic arteries* are very numerous and small. They proceed from the cœliac, splenic, superior mesenteric, right gastro-epiploic, coronaria ventriculi, and left capsular. Its *veins* open into the radicles of the vena porta; and, particularly, into the splenic and lesser mesenteric. Its *nerves* emanate from the solar plexus, and its lymphatics pass into ganglions, to which it gives its name. The pancreas secretes the *Pancreatic juice*, *Succus* seu *Liquor Pancreat'icus*, *Lympha Pancrea'tis*, which resembles the saliva.
PANCREAS OF ASELLI, see Pancreas—p. Minus, see Pancreas—p. Petit, see Pancreas—p. Second, Brunner's glands.
PANCREATAL'GIA, from παγκρεας, 'the pancreas,' and αλγος, 'pain.' Pain or disease of the pancreas.
PANCREATEMPHRAX'IS, from παγκρεας, 'the pancreas,' and εμφρασσω, 'I obstruct.' Obstruction of the pancreas.
PANCREAT'IC, *Pancreat'icus*. Same etymon as *Pancreas*. Relating to or affecting the pancreas.
PANCREATIC ARTERIES, see Pancreas—p. Duct, see Pancreas—p. Juice, see Pancreas—p. Nerves, see Pancreas—p. Veins, see Pancreas.
PANCREAT'IC SARCO'MA OF AB'ERNETHY, *Emphy'ma sarco'ma pancreat'icum*. A tumour, in irregular masses, connected by loose fibrous substance, like the irregular masses of the pancreas. Found in the areolar substance; but, more usually, in lymphatic glands, chiefly in the female breast.
PANCREATI'TIS, *Inflamma'tio pancrea'tis*, (F.) *Inflammation du Pancréas*. Inflammation of the pancreas;—an affection, the phenomena of which are not well known.
PAN'CREATOID, from παγκρεας, 'the pancreas,' and ειδος, 'appearance.' *Pancreatoi'des*. A tumour resembling the pancreas in structure.
PANCREATON'CUS, from παγκρεας, 'the pancreas,' and ογκος, 'a swelling.' Tumour of the pancreas.
PANCRENE, Pancreas.
PANCREUM, Pancreas.
PANDA'LEA, *Panda'leum*. A kind of lozenge used by the Arabian physicians.
PANDALEUM, Pandalea.
PANDALITIUM, Paronychia.
PANDEMIA, Pandemic.
PANDEM'IC, *Pan'demy*, *Pande'mia*, *Morbus Pande'mius* seu *Pande'mus* seu *Pancœ'nus*, *Pancœno'sus*, (F.) *Pandémie;* from παν, 'all,' and δημος, 'people.' An epidemic which attacks the whole population.
PANDÉMIE, Pandemic.
PANDEMY, Pandemic.

PANDICULA'TION, *Pandicula'tio, Scordine'ma, Scordinis'mus, Clonus Pandicula'tio,* from *pandere,* 'to stretch out.' *Stretching, Hal'osis,* (pl.) An action, which consists in elevating the upper limbs, and throwing the head and trunk backwards, at the same time that the lower limbs are extended. This series of motions of the extensor muscles is in some measure independent of the will, and is accompanied with yawning, which is equally involuntary. In the state of health, stretching occurs before and after sleep; especially when we are fatigued. It is also observed at the onset of certain paroxysms of fever, hysteria, &c.

PANDOCE'UM, *Pandochi'um, Pandoci'um,* from παν, 'all,' and δεχεσθαι, 'to receive.' An inn that receives all classes. A general hospital, or one that admits all cases.

PANDOCHIUM, Pandoceum.
PANDOCIUM, Pandoceum.

PANHIDRO'SIS, from παν, 'all,' and 'ιδρωσις, 'sweating.' *Sudor universa'lis.* Sweating over the whole body.

PANHYPERÆMIA, Plethora.

PANICAUT, Eryngium campestre—p. *Maritime,* Eryngium maritimum.

PANIC GRASS, ITALIAN, Panicum Italicum.
PAN'ICUM ITAL'ICUM, *Ital'ian Panic Grass, Indian Millet, Guinea Corn, Barbadoes Millet, Mil'ium In'dicum, Sorghum, Holcus Sorghum,* (F.) *Millet des oiseaux. Nat. Ord.* Gramineæ. The seed—*Mil'ii Sem'ina*—are much esteemed in Italy, being a constant ingredient in soups, and made into a variety of forms for the table.

PANICUM MILIA'CEUM, *P. mil'ium, Common Millet, Milium, M. Pan'icum seu Esculentum, Cenchron, Cenchrus,* (F.) *Millet ordinaire.* Millet-seed are esteemed a nutritious article of diet, and are often made into puddings.

PANICUM MILIUM, P. miliaceum.

PANIS CANICACEUS, see Canicæ—p. *Cibarius seu secundarius,* Syncomistos — p. Cuculi, Oxalis acetosella — p. Porcinus, Cyclamen.

PANIV'OROUS, *Paniv'orus,* from *panis,* 'bread,' and *voro,* 'I devour.' Subsisting on bread.

PANNI, Swathing clothes.
PANNICULE CHARNU, Panniculus carnosus.

PANNIC'ULUS, diminutive of *pannus,* cloth. A piece of fine cloth. Pterygion.

PANNICULUS ADIPOSUS, Cellular membrane.

PANNICULUS CARNO'SUS, *Tu'nica carnosa, Muscular Web, Mantle,* (F.) *Panniculecharnue,* is a general covering found in the quadruped, and formed by a thin, subcutaneous muscle, which serves to move the skin. It exists only in certain parts of the human body, — as in the forehead, where it is formed by the occipito-frontalis; in the neck, by the platysma myoïdes; and, in the scrotum, by the cremaster muscle.

PANNICULUS CORDIS, Pericardium — p. Hymenæus, Hymen — p. Virginalis, Hymen.

PANNUS. A piece of cloth. This word has several other meanings, many of which are equivocal. It means a tent for a wound, and, also, an irregular nævus or mark on the skin. — Castelli. Modern ophthalmologists apply it to an opake and vascular condition of the anterior membrane of the cornea, almost invariably produced by the continuance of purulent or strumous ophthalmia, or by chronic inflammation of the cornea. This part becomes nebulous, covered with red vessels, and opake. At times, the sclerotic conjunctiva undergoes a similar change to that which occurs in the corneal portion.

PANNUS HEPATICUS, Chloasma—p. Lenticularis, Ephelides.

PANOCHIA, Bubo.
PANOPHO'BIA, *Pantopho'bia, Panpho'bia, Pavopho'bia, Athym'ia, Pavor,* (F.) *Frayeur nocturne, Souci,* from Παν, 'the god Pan,' and φοβος, 'fear.' A panic or fear inspired by the god Pan, according to the opinion of the ancients. Some derive it from παν, 'all,' and φοβος, 'fear.' This is sometimes morbid, and is a symptom of melancholy.

PANOPHTHALMI'TIS, from παν, 'all,' and *ophthalmitis,* 'inflammation of the eye.' Inflammation of the whole eye.

PANPHOBIA, Panophobia.
PANPLEGIA, Pamplegia.
PANSCLERO'SIS, from παν, 'all,' and σκληρωσις, 'hardness.' Complete induration of a part.
PANSEMENT, Dressing.
PANSIES, Viola tricolor.
PANSPER'MIA, from παν, 'all,' and σπερμα, 'sperm.' The theory of *Dissemination of Germs,* according to which, ova or germs are disseminated over all space, undergoing development under favourable circumstances.

PANTAGOGON, Panchymagogum.
PANTANENCEPHA'LIA, from παν, παντος, 'all,' and *anencepha'lia,* absence of brain. Entire absence of brain—the same as anencephalia. —G. St. Hilaire.

PANTATROPH'IA, from παν, 'all,' and ατροφια, 'atrophy.' Universal atrophy.

PANTHOD'IC, *Panthod'icus,* from πας, παντος, 'all,' and 'οδος, 'a way.' An epithet applied by Dr. Marshall Hall, to a course of nervous action proceeding from one point in all directions to every other.

PANTICES, Intestine.
PANTING, Anhelatio.
PANTOGANGLIITIS, Cholera.
PANTOPHAGISTS, see Omnivorous.
PANTOPHAGUS, Omnivorous.
PANTOPHOBIA, Hydrophobia, Panophobia.
PANTOZOOTIA, Panzootia.
PANUS, Phygethlon — p. Faucium, Stomatopanus — p. Inguinalis, Bubo.

PANZOÖT'IA, *Pantozoötia;* from παν, 'all,' and ζωον, 'animal.' An endemic or epidemic disease affecting animals generally.

PAP, Nipple. Also, a soft food made of bread boiled or softened with water.
PAP, OF THE THROAT, Uvula.
PAPAS AMERICANUS, Solanum tuberosum.
PAPA'VER, *P. somnif'erum, Mecon.* The *White Poppy, Papaver sati'vum,* (F.) *Pavot des Jardins. Family* Papaveraceæ. *Sex. Syst.* Polyandria Monogynia. The CAPSULE OF THE WHITE POPPY, *Co'dia,* κωδια or κωδεια, *Sca'phion, Papav'eris Caput* vel *Cap'sula, Mecon, Poppyhead,* is used in fomentation as an anodyne and relaxant, to inflamed or ulcerated parts. The expressed oil of the seeds is called by the French *Huile d' Œillette.* It is from the poppy that OPIUM — called, also, *Opium Theba'icum, Meco'nium, Opion, Manus Dei, Affion, Amphian, Aflum, Ocoron, Lau'danum, Mecon, Sopio*—is procured. It is the milky juice obtained after the flowering of the plant, by making longitudinal incisions in the capsules and stalks. It is commonly obtained from the Levant or India, where the poppy grows abundantly. Opium is a compound of morphia, narcotina, meconic acid, codeia, narcein, meconin, caoutchouc, fecula, resin, oil, and several other substances. *Turkey Opium* is of a heavy and slightly fetid odour. Its taste is nauseous, bitter, acrid, and warm: it is in flat pieces; solid and tenacious; of a dark brown colour, and yellowish when powdered; making a light brown, interrupted streak on paper. In *East India Opium,*

the odour is the same, and empyreumatic; the taste is less bitter, but more nauseous, and the colour darker. The varieties of opium known in commerce are the *Smyrna*, the *Constantinople*, the *Egyptian*, the *Persian*, and the *Indian*. Opium is stimulant in small doses; sedative, in large; narcotic and anodyne; operating through the nervous system. It is a most valuable remedy in all painful affections, and inflammations, when given so as to produce its full, sedative effects, especially in peritonitis. In diarrhœa and dysentery, it acts as an astringent; in intermittents, it will often prevent the paroxysm. In typhus, in small doses, it acts as a cordial; in larger, it allays irritation and produces sleep. When applied externally, its narcotic effects are developed: and, hence, it is a useful application to irritable sores, painful tumours, &c. Dose, gr. ¼ to ½ as a stimulant; gr. j to iv as a sedative.

PAPAVER CEREALE, P. rhœas — p. Corniculatum, Chelidonium majus—p. Erraticum, P. rhœas —p. Luteum, Chelidonium majus.

PAPAVER NIGRUM. This is merely a variety of the white poppy, producing black seeds.

PAPAVER RHŒAS. The systematic and pharmacopœial name of the *Red corn-poppy, Corn rose, Papaver errat'icum, P. cerea'lē, P. rubrum, Rhœas*, (F.) *Coquelicot*. The heads of this species, also, contain a milky juice of a narcotic quality. A syrup of its flowers has been directed, which has been esteemed diaphoretic and slightly soothing; but is more admired for its colour than for any other property.

PAPAVERACEUM, Opiate.
PAPAVERCULUM, Meconium.
PAPAVERINUM, Codeine.
PAPAW TREE, Carica papaya.
PAPAYER, Carica papaya.
PAPER, BLISTERING, see Sparadrapum vesicatorium.

PAPIER EPISPASTIQUE, see Sparadrapum vesicatorium.

PAPIL'LA, *P. Mammæ, Thelē, U'beris apex:* —diminutive, perhaps, from *papa*, one of the earliest cries of the infant, ascribed to a craving for food. The end of the breast, the nipple. An eminence similar to a nipple. A name given to small eminences more or less prominent, at the surface of several parts, particularly of the skin and mucous membranes, in which latter situation they are also called Villous. See Villous. They appear formed by the ultimate expansion of the vessels and nerves, and are susceptible, in some cases, of a kind of erection. They are also called *Papillæ nervo'sæ* seu *Ner'veæ, P. Pyramida'les, Nervous papillæ*, (F.) *Papilles* ou *Papilles nerveuses, Houppes nerveuses.*

PAPILLA LACHRYMALIS, see Lachrymal puncta —ƫ. Mammæ, Papilla.

PAPILLÆ CALYCIFORMES, see Papillæ of the tongue—p. Capitatæ, see Papillæ of the tongue - -p. Circumvallatæ. see Papillæ of the tongue— p. Conical, see Papillæ of the tongue—p. Conoidal, see Papillæ of the tongue—p., Corpuscles, Pacinian—p. Filiform, see Papillæ of the tongue — p. Fungiform, see Papillæ of the tongue—p. Fungoid, see Papillæ of the tongue.

PAPILLÆ OF THE KIDNEY, (F.) *Mamelons du rein*, are the projections into the pelvis of the kidney of the apices of the cones—*Pyramids of Malpighi, Pyram'ides Malpighia'næ* — of the tubular substance of the organ. They are also called *Proces'sus mamilla'res, Carun'culæ papilla'res*, and *Papill'æ renum*.

PAPILLÆ, LENTICULAR, see Papillæ of the tongue — p. Maximæ, see Papillæ of the tongue —p. Mediæ, see Papillæ of the tongue—p. Minimæ, see Papillæ of the tongue—p. Mucosæ, see Papillæ of the tongue—p. Nerveæ, Corpuscles, Pacinian, see Papillæ—p. Nervous, see Papilla— p. Pyramidal, see Papillæ of the tongue—p. Pyramidales, see Papillæ—p. Renum, see Papillæ of the kidney—p. Semilenticulares, see Papillæ of the tongue.

PAPILLÆ OF THE TONGUE are very numerous and marked. They are observed, particularly, at the upper surface of the organ, and are distinguished into—1. The *Lentic'ular papillæ, Papillæ muco'sæ, P. max'imæ, P. capita'tæ, P. valla'tæ, P. circumvalla'tæ, P. trunca'tæ, P. calyci'for'mes*. They are arranged at the base of the tongue in two oblique lines having the shape of the letter V; and united angularly at the foramen cæcum. They have, in general, an ovoid or spherical shape, and have seemed to be mucous follicles similar to those of the palate, lips, &c. 2. The *Fun'giform* or *Fungoid papillæ, Papillæ me'diæ, P. Semilenticula'res*, are of indeterminate number, but always more numerous than the preceding. They are irregularly disseminated near the edges and the point of the tongue; have a rounded and flattened head, supported by a short and narrow footstalk. Their tint is whitish. Of their real nature we are ignorant. 3. The *Con'ical, Conoid'al* or *Pyram'idal papillæ, P. min'imæ, P. villo'sæ*, are the most numerous of all. Their arrangement is more regular in the forepart of the tongue than behind. They resemble small cones; the base being towards the tongue and the apex free. The anterior are very small, and have been called *Fil'iform papil'læ*. They appear to be produced by the terminations of the filaments of the lingual nerve, and are surrounded by an evident vascular network.

PAPILLÆ TRUNCATÆ, see Papillæ of the tongue —p. Vallatæ, see Papillæ of the tongue—p. Villosæ, see Papillæ of the tongue.

PAP'ILLARY, *Papilla'ris, Pap'illous*, from *papilla*. Of or belonging to the nipple or to the papillæ.

PAPILLARY BODY, Corpus papillare.
PAPILLI-AUT-MAMMILLI-FORMIS, Mastoid.
PAPILLOUS, Papillary.
PAPOOSE ROOT, Caulophyllum thalictroides.
PAPPEA CAPEN'SIS. A small tree of the *Nat. Ord.* Sapindaceæ, common in Cafferland, the fruit of which is called *Wild Plums*. It furnishes a vinous beverage, and excellent vinegar. Its kernel contains an oil, which, although eatable, is somewhat cathartic, and is recommended as an external application in tinea capitis, alopecia, &c.

PAPPUS AMERICANUS, Solanum tuberosum.

PAP'ULA. A *pimple, Exor'mia*, (F.) *Bouton, Bourgeon*. A small, acuminated elevation of the cuticle, with an inflamed base; very seldom containing a fluid, or suppurating, and commonly terminating in scurf or desquamation.

Papulæ form the first order of Willan and Bateman's arrangement of cutaneous diseases.

PAPULA AGRIA, Lichen agrius—p. Fera, Herpes exedens—p. Miliaris, Miliary fever.

PAPULÆ, Lichen—p. Siccæ, Lichen—p. Sudoris, Miliary fever—p. Sudorales, Sudamina.

PAP'ULOSE, *Papulo'sus, Pap'ulous, Papula'tus, Pimpled*, from *papula*. Of or belonging to, resembling, or covered with, papulæ or pimples.

PAQUERETTE VIVACE, Bellis.

PAR NERVO'RUM, *Sys'ygi nervo'rum*. A pair of nerves.

PAR OPTICUM NERVORUM, Optic nerve—p. Primum nervorum cerebri. Olfactory nerves—p. Quintum nervorum cerebralium, Trigemini—p.

Secundum nervorum, Optic nerve—p. Septimum sive faciale, Facial nerve—p. Trigeminum, Trigemini—p. Trium funiculorum, Trigemini—p. Vagus, Pneumogastric—p. Visorius, Optic nerve.

PARA, παρα, a common prefix, 'by, near, contrary to, through,' (per;) 'above and beyond,' (ultra:) 'besides,' (præter.) In certain terms, as in Paracusis, Parapsis, Parabysma, &c., used by Dr. Good, para means a defective or morbid condition.

PARABAL'ANUS, from παραβαλλειν, (παρα, and βαλλειν, 'to cast,') 'to expose one-self.' A name given, by the ancients, to a person who devoted himself to the service of the sick in hospitals; and particularly during epidemics and the plague.

PARABYS'MA, from παρα, and βυειν, 'to stuff.' Infarction or engorgement of an organ—as *Parabysma Lie'nis*, Engorgement of the spleen.

PARABYSMA MESENTERICUM, Tabes mesenterica.
PARABYS'TIA, same etymon. Engorgement or infarction of an organ with blood.

PARACELSIS'TA, *Paracel'sist, Paracel'sian;* from Paracelsus. A follower of Paracelsus.

PARACELSISTICA MEDICINA, see Spagyrists.

PARACENTE'RIUM. Same etymon as the next. Woolhouse has given this appellation to a small trocar, employed by Nuck for puncturing the eye in cases of dropsy of that organ.

PARACENTE'SIS, *Perfora'tio, Punc'tio, Punctu'ra, Cenembate'sis, Cente'sis, Compunc'tio:* from παρακεντεω, (παρα, and κεντεω, 'I pierce,') 'I pierce through.' Puncture. The operation of *tapping* to evacuate the collected fluid in ascites, ovarial dropsy, &c.

PARACENTESIS, Puncturing—p. Thoracis, Thoracocentesis.

PARACENTETERION, Trocar.
PARACENTICION, Trocar.
PARACHRŒ'A, from παρα, and χροα, 'colour.' Morbid change of colour of the surface, especially of the face.

PARACHROMA, Achromatopsia.
PARACHROSIS, Decoloration.
PARACINE'SES, (G.) Parakinesien, from παρα, 'defective,' and κινησις, 'motion.' Diseases of the motor nerves; morbid movements of voluntary muscles.

PARACMASIS, Decline.
PARACMAS'TIC, *Paracmas'ticus*, from παρακμαζω, 'I decrease.' Decreasing. An epithet for a distemper, which gradually decreases. Also, according to Galen, the period of life when a person is said to grow old, which he places at from 35 to 49, after which he is said to be old — a definition that would not suit us at the present day.—Gorræus, and Castelli.

PARACMASTICOS, see Acmasticos.
PARACME, Decline.
PARACOE, see Cophosis, Paraeusis.
PARAC'OPE, *Paraph'ora, Paracru'sis*, from παρακοπτω, 'I strike falsely.' Delirium. In Hippocrates, it means the slight delirium which sometimes occurs in febrile diseases.

PARACOUSIA, see Cophosia.
PARAC'RISES, (G.) Parakrisien: from παρα, 'defective, morbid,' and κρισις, 'secretion.' Diseases of the secretory function.—Fuchs.

PARACRUSIS, Paracope.
PARACUSIS, Cophosis. Also, perverted audition.

PARACU'SIS ACRIS, *Audi'tus a'crior, Paracu'sis oxycoi'a*, from παρα, 'defective,' and ακουσις, 'the act of hearing.' The hearing painfully acute, and intolerant of the lowest sounds; a symptom in otalgia, epilepsy, cephalitis, and febrile affections.

PARACUSIS DUPLICATA, Double hearing—p. Imaginaria, Tinnitus aurium—p. Imperfecta, Double hearing, P. perversa—p. Obtusa, Baryecoia—p. Oxycoia, P. acris.

PARACUSIS PERVER'SA, *P. Willisia'na, P. imperfec'ta, Perverse hearing.* The ear only sensible to articulate sounds, when excited by other and louder sounds intermixed with them.— Good.

PARACUSIS SURDITAS, see Cophosis—p. Willisiana, Paracusis perversa.

PARACYCLE'SES, (G.) Parakyklesen, from παρα, 'defective, morbid,' and κυκλησις, 'circulation.' Diseases of the blood as regards its distribution and motion.— Fuchs.

PARACYESIS, Pregnancy, morbid, Pregnancy, preternatural—p. Abortus, Abortion—p. Tubaria, Salpingo-cyesis.

PARACYNAN'CHE, (para and cynanche.) Inflammation of the external muscles of the larynx. According to others, a slight cynanche.

PARÆSTHESIA, Paresthesis — p. Olfactoria, Parosmia.

PARÆSTHESIS, Paresthesis — p. Auditûs flacca, Proptoma auricularum.

PARÆTHENAR, Parathenar.
PARAGEUSIS, Ageustia. Also, perversion of taste, *Parageu'sia, Parageust'ia, Allotriogeus'tia, Gustus deprava'tus.*

PARAGEUSTIA, Parageusis.
PARAGLOSSA, *Paraglos'sis,* from παρα, and γλωσσα, 'the tongue;' Swelling of the tongue; *Dyspha'gia Linguo'sa, Glassomegis'tus, Macroglos'sa, Prolap'sus linguæ.* Sauvages, under the term *Paraglossa deglutito'ria,* means a pretended doubling of the tongue into the pharynx, (F.) *Renversement de la langue.* See Glossocele.

PARAGOGE, Abduction, Coaptation.
PARAGOMPHO'SIS, *Paragomphosis cap'itis,* from παρα, 'by,' 'near,' and γομφωσις, 'a nailing.' Incomplete wedging of the head of the child in the pelvis during labour.

PARAKINESIEN, Paracineses.
PARAKRISIEN, Paracrises.
PARAKYKLESEN, Paracycleses.
PARALALIA, Mogilalia — p. Nasalis, Rhinophonia.

PARALAMP'SIS, παραλαμψις, from παραλαμπω, (παρα and λαμπω, 'I shine,') 'I shine at the side of;' *Mac'ula corneæ margarita'cea, Perla.* A cicatrix on the transparent part of the eye.— Hippocrates.

PARARELEMA, Delirium.
PARALLAGE, Insanity.
PARALLAGMA, *Chevauchement.*
PARALLAXIS, *Chevauchement,* Insanity.
PARALLE'LA. A kind of scurfy, cutaneous eruption, affecting the palms of the hands, in parallel lines, and symptomatic of the venereal disease.— Forestus.

PARALLELISM OF DISEASES, Isopathia.
PARALOGIA, Delirium.
PARALOPH'IA, from παρα, 'near,' and λοφια, 'the first vertebra of the back.' The lower and lateral part of the neck, near the vertebræ.—Keil.

PARALYSÉ, Paralytic.
PARALYSIE, Paralysis—p. Saturnine, Palsy, lead.

PARAL'YSIS, *Par'esis, Resolu'tio membro'rum, R. nervo'rum, Carus paralysis, Catal'ysis,* (F.) *Paralysie, Résolution des membres; Palsy,* from παραλυω, (παρα and λυω, 'I loosen,') 'I relax.' Abolition or great diminution of the voluntary motions, and sometimes of sensation, in one or more parts of the body.

Palsy is said to be *local,* when it affects only a few muscles. When it extends to half the body, vertically or horizontally, it is called *Hemiplē-*

gia or *Paraple'gia*. It is commonly symptomatic of disease of the brain or of the nerves themselves, and is a frequent accompaniment, precursor, or successor of apoplexy,—*Phrenoparal'ysis*. The immediate cause is, generally, pressure, either by blood effused, or by serum, or by vascular turgescence. At its onset, therefore, bloodletting may be advisable; but, afterwards, the disease becomes one of nervous debility, and requires stimulants — to the paralyzed parts, or to the mucous membranes, — frictions, sinapisms, blisters, the moxa, baths, electricity, galvanism, purgatives, and the nux vomica, which last has the property of exciting movements where the will has no longer power. The disease generally admits only of palliation, and is extremely apt to recur.

PARALYSIS, Primula veris.

PARAL'YSIS AG"ITANS, *P. trem'ula, Syn'clonus ballis'mus, Scelotyr'bē festi'nans, Tremor, Tromos, Shaking Palsy, Trembling Palsy*. A variety of tremor, in which the muscles are in a perpetual alternation of contraction and relaxation.

PARALYSIS, BELL'S, *Bell's Palsy, Paral'ysis facia'lis, Prosoparal'ysis, Trismus dias'trophē Sauvage'sii, Dias'trophē Gale'ni, Hemiple'gia faoia'lis, Oris tortu'ra paralyt'ica Linnœ'i, Hemiprosople'gia*. The paralysis of the face induced by a lesion of the portio dura, has been called Bell's Palsy, owing to Sir Charles Bell having been one of the first to investigate it minutely.

PARALYSIS BERIBERIA, Beriberi — p. Extremitatum, Acro-paralysis — p. Facialis, Paralysis, Bell's — p. Hemiplegia, Hemiplegia — p. Intestini recti, Proctoparalysis — p. Intestinorum, Enteroparalysis — p. Linguæ, Glossolysis — p. Medullaris, Paraplegia — p. Metallica, Palsy, lead — p. Nervi hypoglossi, Glossoplegia — p. Nervi vagi in parte thoracicâ, Asthma — p. Nervorum thoracis, &c., Stethoparalysis — p. from Poisons, p. Venenata — p. Rachialgia, Colic, metallic — p. Saturnine, Palsy, lead — p. Scorbutica, Pellagra — p. Spinalis, Paraplegia — p. Tremula, Paralysis agitans,

PARAL'YSIS VENENA'TA, *Paralysis e vene'nis, Paralysis from poisons*. Paralysis, the result of poisonous substances—as of lead, mercury, arsenic, ergot, &c.

PARALYSIS E VENENIS, P. Venenata — p. Ventriculi, Gastroparalysis.

PARALYT'IC, *Paralyt'icus, Paraly'zed, Pal'sied*, (F.) *Paralysé*. Same etymon as Paralysis. Affected with or causing paralysis.

PARALYTIC STROKE, see Stroke, paralytic.

PARALYZED, Paralytic.

PAREME'NIA, from παρα, 'badly,' and μην, 'a month;' *Menstrua'tio anom'ala, Menses anom'ala, Mismenstruation*. Difficult menstruation. Disordered menstruation.

PARAMENIA DIFFICILIS, Dysmenorrhœa — p. Erroris, Menstruation, vicarious — p. Obstructionis, see Amenorrhœa — p. Profusa, Menorrhagia — p. Superflua, Menorrhagia.

PARAME'RIA, παραμηρια, from παρα, 'about,' and μηρος, 'the thigh.' The internal parts of the thigh.

PARAMESOS, Annular finger, see Digitus.

PARANEPHRI'TIS, from παρα, and νεφριτις, 'inflammation of the kidney.' Inflammation of the renal capsules, *Inflamma'tio renum succenturiato'rum*.

PARANŒA, Delirium, Dementia.

PARANYMPH'US, from παρα, 'near,' and νυμφη, 'a young spouse,' 'a bride.' A name given by the ancients to him who led the bride to the house of her husband. The term was adopted into the ancient schools of medicine, to designate the usual discourse pronounced at the end of the prescribed period of study for licentiate, in which the qualifications and merits of the candidate were described.

PARAPATHIA, Pathomania.

PARAPECHYON, Radius.

PARAPHIA, Parapsis.

PARAPHIMO'SIS, *Periphimo'sis, Circumligatu'ra, Phimo'sis circumliga'ta, Penis lipoderm'us*, from παρα, 'about,' and φιμοω, 'I bridle.' Strangulation of the glans penis, owing to the opening of the prepuce being too narrow. It frequently happens in persons affected with phimosis, when the prepuce has been pushed violently behind the base of the glans, during copulation, &c. In paraphimosis, the narrow and resisting aperture of the prepuce forms, behind the corona glandis, a kind of ligature, which strangulates the part, causes it to swell and inflame, and even to become gangrenous. Attempts must be made to bring back the prepuce. These excite considerable pain, yet they must be persevered in for some time; and should they not succeed, the rings, formed by the tumefied prepuce, must be cut transversely, and the antiphlogistic treatment be adopted.

PARAPHOBIA, Hydrophobia.

PARAPHO'NIA, from παρα, and φωνη, 'the voice.' Affection of the voice, when its character or *timbre* is less agreeable.

PARAPHONIA CLANGENS, Oxyphonia — p. Gutturalis, Asaphia — p. Nasalis, Rhinophonia — p. Puberum, Hirquitalitas — p. Rauca, Raucedo — p. Ulcerosa, Oxyphonia.

PARAPHORA, Delirium, Paracope.

PARAPHRENESIS, Paraphrenitis — p. Diaphragmatica, Diaphragmitis.

PARAPHRÉNIE, Insanity.

PARAPHRENI'TIS, from παρα, 'near,' and φρενες, 'the diaphragm;' *Paraphrene'sia*. A name given to inflammation of the diaphragm, (see Diaphragmitis,) which was supposed always to produce delirium:—as well as to the delirium itself accompanying that affection. See Phrenitis.

PARAPHROSYNE, Delirium.

PARAPHROTES, Delirium.

PARAPLAS'TIC: *Paraplast'icus*, from παρα, and πλαστικος, 'formative.' Possessed of depraved formative powers,—as Carcinoma, Encephaloma, Melanosis, &c.

PARAPLE'GIA, *Paraplex'ia, Rachioparal'ysis, Rhachiople'gia, Rhachioparal'ysis, Myeloparal'ysis, Paral'ysis spina'lis, P. Medulla'ris, Carus paralysis paraple'gia*, from παρα, dim. particle, and πλησσω, 'I strike.' Palsy of the lower half of the body, including the bladder and rectum. It is, generally, owing to disease of some part of the cerebro-spinal axis; especially of the spinal portion. The ancients sometimes used the term for incomplete apoplexy. Some authors have, also, made a distinction between *paraplegia* and *paraplexia*,—using the former for *partial apoplexy*—the latter for *general* or *complete apoplexy*.

PARAPLEURITIS, Pleurodynia.

PARAPLEXIA, Paraplegia.

PARAP'OPLEXY, *Parapoplex'ia*, from παρα, dim., and αποπληξια, 'apoplexy.' False apoplexy; a soporous state, resembling apoplexy; and especially that which occurs in the paroxysms of pernicious intermittents.

PARAP'SIS, *Paroph'ia*, from παρα, 'defectively,' and απτομαι, 'I touch.' Sense of touch or general feeling vitiated or lost.— Good.

PARAPSIS ACRIS TENERITUDO, Soreness — p. Expers, Torpor, Anæsthesia — p. Illusoria, Pseudæsthesia — p. Pruritus, Itching.

PARARMA, Fimbria.

PARARRHYTHMICUS, Pararrhythmus.

PARARRHYTH'MUS, *Pararrhyth'micus*, from παρα, 'dim.,' and ρυθμος, 'rhythm.' An epithet for the pulse, when it has not the rhythm proper to the age and constitution of the individual.

PARARTHRE'MA, *Pararthro'ma*, *Pararthre'sis*, *Pararthro'sis*, *Parec'tasis*, *Parastrep'sis*, from παρα, and αρθρον, 'a joint.' Incomplete luxation; subluxation.

PARACEPAS'TRA, from παρα, and σκεπζω, 'I cover.' A cap or bandage, which covers the whole head.—Galen.

PARASCEUE, Apparatus.

PARAS'CHIDES, from παρα, and σκιζω, 'I cleave.' Fragments or splinters of a broken bone.

PAR'ASITE, *Parasi'tus*, from παρα, 'near,' and σιτος, 'corn,' 'food.' Parasites are plants which attach themselves to other plants; and animals which live in or on the bodies of other animals,— so as to subsist at their expense. The mistletoe is a parasitic plant;—the louse a parasitic animal. The chief parasitic animals are the *Pedic'ulus huma'nus corp'oris*, *P. cap'itis*, *P. pubis*, *Pulex irri'tans*, *P. pen'etrans*, and the *Ac'arus Sca'biei*.

PARASIT'IC, *Parasit'icus*, *Par'asitoid*, *Parasitoï'des*. Same etymon. Having the nature of, or resembling a parasite, as 'parasitic growths,' tubercles, cancer, &c.

PARASITICIDE, Antiparasitic.

PARASITISMUS INTESTINALIS, Helminthiasis—p. Superficiei, Malis.

PARASITOID, Parasitic.

PARASPA'DIA, from παρα, and σπαω, 'I draw.' A preternatural opening of the urethra at the side of the penis. One whose urethra opens in this manner is called *Paraspadiæ'us* and *Paraspadias*.

PARASPADIÆUS, see Paraspadia.

PARAS'PHAGIS, from παρα, 'near,' and σφαγη, 'the throat.' The part of the neck contiguous to the clavicles.

PARAS'TATA, *Paras'tates*, from παριστημι, (παρα, and ιστημι,) 'I stand near.' The prostate. In Hippocrates, it means the epididymis. The epididymes were called by Herophilus and Galen *Varico'sæ parastatæ* to distinguish them from *glandulo'sæ parastatæ* or *prostate*. Rufus of Ephesus called the Tubæ Fallopianæ *Parastatæ varico'sæ*.

PARASTATA ADENOIDES, Prostate—p. Glandula, Prostate—p. Glandulosa, Prostate.

PARASTATES, Parastata.

PARASTATI'TIS, *Epididymi'tis*; from *parastata*, 'epididymis,' and *itis*, denoting inflammation. Inflammation of the epididymis.

PARASTREM'MA, *Paras'trophē*, from παραστρεφω, (παρα, and στρεφω, 'I turn,') 'I distort or pervert.' Convulsive distortion, especially of the face, the soft parts being drawn laterally.

PARASTREPSIS, Pararthrema.

PARASTROPHE, Parastremma.

PARASYNANCHE, Cynanche parotidæa.

PARASYSTOLE, Acinesia.

PARATH'ENAR, *Paræ'thenar*, from παρα, 'near,' and θεναρ, 'the sole of the foot.' Winslow called *grand parathénar*, *parathenar major*, a portion of the abductor of the little toe, *musculus scandula'rius*; and *petit parathénar*, *parathenar minor*, the short flexor of that toe.

PARATHENAR MAJOR, Abductor minimi digiti pedis—p. Minor, Flexor brevis minimi digiti pedis.

PARATHROMA, Elongatio.

PARATONIA, see Spasm.

PARATOPIA, Luxation.

PARATOP'IÆ; from παρα, in the sense of change, and τοπος, 'place.' Diseases in which organs are removed from their proper position. See Ectopia.

PARATRIMMA, Chafing.

PARATROPE, Apotrope.

PARAT'ROPHY, *Parat'rophē*, *Paratroph'ia*, from παρα, 'dim,' and τροφη, 'nourishment.' Misnutrition.

PARDALIANCHES, Aconitum.

PARDALIANCHUM, Aconitum.

PAREC'TAMA, *Parec'tasis*, from παρα, 'beyond,' εκ, 'out of,' and τεινω, 'I stretch.' Immoderate extension or dilatation of a part—as of the heart.

PARECTASIS, Pararthrema, Parectama.

PAREGOR'IC, *Paregor'icus*, *So'piens*, from παρηγορεω (παρα, and αγορευω), 'I soothe, I calm.' That which soothes or assuages—as paregoric elixir. An anodyne.

PAREIA, Gena.

PAREIRA, see P. brava.

PAREI'RA BRAVA, *Cissam'pelos Pareira*, *Pareyra*, *Butua*, *Pariera brava*, *Abu'ta*, *Albu'tua*, *Botou*, *Caa-peba*, *Overo butua*, *Wild vine*, *Velvet leaf*. Family, Menispermeæ. Sex. Syst. Diœcia Monadelphia. The root of this plant—*Pareira* (Ph. U. S.)—a native of South America and the West Indies, has a sweet taste with considerable bitterness and slight roughness. It has been recommended in nephritic and calculous affections; but it is not much used.

PARELLE, Rumex hydrolapathum.

PARENCEPHALIS, Cerebellum.

PARENCEPHALITIS, Cerebellitis.

PARENCEPHALOCE'LE, from παρεγκεφαλις, (παρα, and εγκεφαλος, 'the brain,') 'the cerebellum,' and κηλη, 'a rupture.' *Hernia of the cerebel'lum*; a very rare disease. It occurs under the form of a soft, indolent, or slightly painful tumour, without change in the colour of the skin, and is situate in the occipital region. It is constituted of the cerebellum, which escapes through an aperture in the occipital bone. Great attention must be paid not to mistake it for an ordinary tumour, as its extirpation would be attended with fatal consequences.

PARENCEPHALUS, Cerebellum.

PAREN'CHYMA, *Caro parenchymat'ica seu vis'cerum seu viscera'lis seu viscero'sa*, *Substan'tia parenchymato'sa*, *Procheu'ma*. The texture of glandular and other organs, composed of agglomerated globules united by areolar tissue, and tearing with more or less facility. Such is the texture of the liver, kidneys, &c. Παρεγχυμα signifies in Greek, effusion, (παρα, εν, and χυω, 'I pour,') and it was believed, that this tissue consisted of effused blood or other fluid.

PARENCHYMA TESTIS, Pulpa testis.

PAREN'CHYMAL, *Parenchym'atous*, *Paren'chymous*, *Parenchyma'lis*, *Parenchymat'icus*; same etymon. Belonging or relating to the parenchyma of an organ.

PARENCHYMATI'TIS; from παρεγχυμα, 'parenchyma,' and *itis*, denoting inflammation. *Inflamma'tio parenchymat'ica*. Inflammation of the substance of an organ.

PARENCHYMATOUS, Parenchymal.

PAR'ESIS, from παριημι, 'I relax.' Paralysis. According to some, a slight, incomplete paralysis, affecting motion, not sensation.

PARESTHE'SIS, *Paræsthe'sis*, or *Paresthe'sia*, *Sensus imperfec'tus*, from παρα, 'defective,' and αισθησις, 'sensation.' Congenital misconstruction of the external organs of sense. A genus in the nosology of Good. Also, perversion of sensibility.

PARET′ICA EXARTHRO′SIS. Luxation from relaxation of the ligaments of a joint.

PARETICUS, Relaxant.

PARFUM, Suffimentum.

PARIERA BRAVA, Pareira brava.

PARIES, Table.

PARI′ETAL, *Parieta′lis*, from *paries, parietis*, 'a wall.'

PARIETAL ARTERY, see P. Bones.

PARIETAL BONES, *Ossa parieta′lia, Ossa vertica′lia, Ossa ver′ticis, Ossa sincip′itis, Ossa breg′matis, Ossa nerva′lia, Ossa tetrag′ona*, are two fellow-bones, occupying the lateral and upper parts of the cranium, in the formation of which they assist. They have a quadrilateral shape: their external surface is convex, and presents, at its middle part, an eminence called the *Parietal protuberance*, (F.) *Bosse pariétale*. Their inner or cerebral surface, which is concave, has a depression that corresponds with the preceding eminence, and which is called the *Parietal fossa, Fossa parieta′lis*. Above and behind, near the superior edge of these bones, is a foramen, which does not always exist, called the *Parietal foramen, Fora′men parieta′lĕ*, through which passes a vein — *parietal vein* — that opens into the superior longitudinal sinus of the dura mater, and an artery — *parietal artery* — a branch of the occipital, which ramifies on the same sinus. Each parietal bone is articulated *above*, with its fellow; *below*, with the temporal bone; *before*, with the frontal; *behind*, with the occipital, and by the anterior and inferior angle with the great ala of the sphenoid. Each parietal bone is developed from a single point of ossification.

PARIETAL FORAMEN, see P. Bones — p. Fossa, see P. Bones — p. Protuberance, see P. Bones — p. Veins, see P. Bones.

PARIETA′RIA, *P. officina′lis, Helx′inĕ, Vitra′ria, Wall pel′litory*, (F.) *Pariétaire commune*. Family Urticeæ. *Sex. Syst.* Polygamia Monœcia. This plant grows on old walls, and contains much nitrate of potassa. It is diuretic, but is not much used.

PARIETA′RIA PENNSYLVAN′ICA, *Amer′ican Pel′litory*, a small weed, flowering from June to August, has been used in juice or decoction as a diuretic, deobstruent (?) and emmenagogue.

PARI′ETES, Plural of *Paries*, 'a wall,' (F.) *Parois*. A name given to parts which form the enclosures — the limits of different cavities of the body, as the *Parietes of the cranium, chest*, &c.

PARIS, *P. quadrifo′lia, Sola′num quadrifo′lium, Uva inver′sa seu lupi′na seu vulpi′na, Oneberry, Truelove*, (F.) *Parisette, Raisin de Renard*. It possesses narcotic properties, and was formerly considered a powerful love philter. It is emetic, and is sometimes used externally as a resolvent and anodyne.

PARISAGOGE INTESTINORUM, Intussusceptio.

PARISETTE, Paris.

PARISTH′MIA, παρα, and ισθμος, 'the throat.' A word employed to designate the tonsils, and, likewise, inflammation of the tonsils. *Cynanche tonsillaris*, and Cynanche in general.

PARISTHMIOT′OMUS, from παρισθμια, 'the tonsils,' and τεμνω, 'I cut.' An instrument with which the tonsils were formerly scarified.

PARISTHMITIS. Cynanche, C. tonsillaris.

PARISTHMIUM, Tonsil.

PARISWORT, Trillium latifolium.

PARMACITY, Cetaceum.

PARMELIA ISLANDICA, Lichen Islandicus — p. Plicata, Lichen plicatus — p. Pulmonacea,

Lichen pulmonarius — p. Roccella, Lichen roccella — p. Saxatilis, Lichen saxatilis.

PAROCHETRUSIS, Derivation.

PARODON′TIDES, from παρα, 'near,' and οδους, 'a tooth.' Tumours on the gums; parulis, &c.

PARODYNIA, Dystocia — p. Perversa, Presentation, preternatural.

PAROIS, Parietes.

PAROLE, Voice, articulated.

PAROMPHALOCE′LĔ, from παρα, 'near,' ομφαλος, 'the navel,' and κηλη, 'rupture.' Hernia near the navel.

PARONIR′IA, from παρα, and ονειρον, 'a dream.' Depraved, disturbed, or morbid dreaming; *Oneirodyn′ia acti′va, Erethis′mus oneirodyn′ia*. The voluntary organs connected with the passing train of ideas, overpowered by the force of the imagination during dreaming, are involuntarily excited to their natural or accustomed actions, while the other organs remain asleep. — Good.

PARONIRIA AMBULANS, Somnambulism — p. Salax, Pollution.

PARONY′CHIA, *Paron′ychis, Paronychi′tis, Pan′aris, Redu′via, Redio′ia, Relu′via, Vermis dig″iti, Panarit″ium, Pteryg′ium dig″iti, Digitium, Pandalit″ium, Passa, Dactyli′tis, Pana′rium, Onych′ia*, (F.) *Onglade*, from παρα, 'near,' and ονυξ, 'the nail.' The ancients gave this name to an inflammatory tumour, — *Onyxi′tis* (Gross), — seated near the nail, and involving the pulp or matrix. Some of the moderns have extended it to inflammation of the hand, and even of the forearm. It usually means every phlegmonous tumour of the fingers or toes, and especially of the first phalanx. Four kinds of paronychia are commonly pointed out: 1. That seated between the epidermis and skin, called in France *Tourniole*. 2. That seated in the subcutaneous areolar tissue. 3. That occupying the sheath of a tendon; and 4. That considered to be seated between the periosteum and bone. The last three are only different degrees of the same disease, constituting *Whitlow*, (F.) *Mal d'aventure*: — the worst kinds, in English, are called *Felon*. The inflammation generally commences in the subcutaneous areolar tissue, and spreads to other parts, occasioning excessive, lancinating pain, owing to the parts being put upon the stretch; hence, the necessity of dividing them freely, — even down to the bone, when there is reason to believe that the affection belongs to the fourth division, — making use of emollient applications, the antiphlogistic treatment, and opiates to relieve pain.

PARONYCHIA, Asplenium ruta muraria — p. Digitium, Digitium.

PARONYCHIS, Paronychia.

PARONYCHITIS, Paronychia.

PAROPHOBIA, Hydrophobia.

PAROPIA, Canthus (lesser.)

PAROPLEXIA, Paraplegia.

PAROPSIS, Dysæsthesia visualis — p. Amaurosis, Amaurosis — p. Cataracta, Cataract — p. Glaucosis, Glaucoma — p. Illusoria, Pseudoblepsia — p. Lateralis, Dysopia lateralis — p. Longinqua, Presbytia — p. Lucifuga, Nyctalopia — p. Noctifuga, Hemeralopia — p. Propinqua, Myopia — p. Staphyloma, Staphyloma — p. Staphyloma purulentum, Hypopyon — p. Staphyloma simplex, Hydrophthalmia — p. Strabismus, Strabismus — p. Synezisis, Synezisis.

PAROPTE′SIS, from παρα, dim., and οπτω, 'I roast.' Forcing a sweat by placing a patient before the fire or putting him in a dry bath.

PARORA′SIS, from παρα, dim., and οραω, 'I

see.' Perversion of sight, which prevents the person from judging accurately of the colour of objects. *Achromatop'sia.* Hallucination.—Galen.

PARORCHID'IUM, from *παρα,* dim., ' something wrong,' and *ορχις,* ' testicle.' Any position of one or both testicles, different from that which they ought to occupy in the scrotum ;— whether they may not have descended through the abdominal ring, or are drawn up to the groins by the cremaster muscle.

PAROR'CHIDO-ENTEROCE'LE, *Hernia paror'chido-enter'ica.* Intestinal hernia complicated with displacement of the testicle. — Sauvages.

PAROSMIA, Anosmia. Also, perversion of smell; *Parœsthe'sia olfacto'ria, Olfac'tus depravа'tus, Idiosyncra'sia olfacto'ria.*

PAROS'TIA, from *παρα,* 'defectively,' and *οστεον,* 'a bone.' Bones untempered in their substance, and incapable of affording proper support. — Good.

PAROSTIA FLEXILIS, Mollities ossium—p. Fragilis, Fragilitas ossium.

PAROTIA, Cynanche parotidæa.

PAROT'ID, *Gland'ula parotidea, G. ad Aures, Paro'tis, Animel'læ, Alimel'læ, Lacticin'ia;* from *παρα,* 'about,' and *ους,* 'the ear.' The largest of the salivary glands, seated under the ear, and near the angle of the lower jaw. It is composed of many separate lobes, giving rise to excretory ducts, which unite to form one canal, called the *Parotid duct, Steno's canal*—the *Ductus superior* or *Superior salivary canal* of some. This duct, after having advanced horizontally into the substance of the cheek, proceeds through an opening in the buccinator muscle, and terminates in the mouth opposite the second upper molaris. About the middle of its course, it sometimes receives the excretory duct of a glandular body, situate in its vicinity, and called the *Ac'cessory Gland of the Parotid, So'cia Parot'idis, Gland'ula so'cia parot'idis.* In the substance of the parotid are found—a number of branches of the facial nerve, of the transverse arteries of the face, and the posterior auricular. It receives, also, some filaments from the inferior maxillary nerve, and from the ascending branches of the superficial cervical plexus. Its lymphatic vessels are somewhat numerous, and pass into ganglions situate at its surface or behind the angle of the jaw. The parotid secretes saliva, and pours it copiously into the mouth.

PAROTID, ACCESSORY GLAND OF THE, see Parotid.

PAROTID APONEURO'SIS. A sheath of great thickness, continuous, below, with the cervical fascia. It forms a frame-work to the parotid by means of fibrous prolongations from its deep surface. Its density accounts for the pain of parotitis, and for the difficulty with which pus makes its way to the surface.

PAROTID ARTERIES, see Parotid — p. Duct, see Parotid — p. Veins, see Parotid.

PAROTIDE, Parotis.

PAROTIDON'CUS, *Tumor paro'tidis, T. glan'dulæ parotideæ,* from *παρωτις,* ' the parotid,' and *ογκος,* 'a tumour.' Swelling of the parotid.

PARO'TIS, *Phleg'monē parotidea, Inflamma'tio paro'tidum, Cynan'chē parotidæ'a, Paroti'tis, Dioscu'ri,* (F.) *Parotide,* is the name of a tumour seated under the ear; which is reddish, hard, and attended with obtuse pain; the progress to suppuration being slow and difficult. Sometimes it is of a malignant character, sloughing, and long protracted. Some French pathologists restrict the term *parotide* to symptomatic parotitis — as to that which occurs in plague; whilst they apply the terms *Oreillons* or *Ourles* to Cynanche parotidæa or Mumps.

PAROTIS CONTAGIOSA, Cynanche parotidæa — p. Epidemica, Cynanche parotidæa — p. Serosa glutine tumens, Cynanche parotidæa — p. Spuria, Cynanche parotidæa.

PAROTITIS, Cynanche parotidæa, Parotis — p. Epidemica, Cynanche parotidæa — p. Erysipelatosa, Cynanche parotidæa — p. Polymorpha, Cynanche parotidæa — p. Specifica, Cynanche parotidæa.

PAROVA'RIUM: from *παρα,* ' near;' and *ωαριον,* 'the ovary.' A body closely analogous in structure to the epididymis, which is seated between the Fallopian tube and the ovary in the broad ligament. The Corpus Wolffianum concurs in its formation. — Kobelt.

PAR'OXYSM, *Paroxys'mus,* from *παροξυνω, (παρα,* and *οξυνειν,* ' to render sharp.') 'I irritate ;' *Im'petus, Insul'tus, Inva'sio, Exacerba'tio, Acces'sio, Acces'sus,* (F.) *Exacerbation, Redoublement, Accès.* The augmentation which supervenes at equal or unequal intervals in the symptoms of acute diseases. Also, a periodical exacerbation or fit of a disease.

PAROXYS'MAL, *Paroxysma'lis;* same etymon. (F.) *Paroxystique.* Of or belonging to a paroxysm ; — as a *paroxysmal* day, (F.) *Jour paroxystique ;* a day on which a paroxysm of disease occurs.

PAROXYSMUS FEBRILIS, Pyrexia.

PAROXYSTIQUE, Paroxysmal.

PARS, Genital organs — p. Corporis, Genital organs — p. Inferior Pedis, Sole — p. Intermedia, see Corpus spongiosum urethræ — p. Mastoidea of Temporal Bone, Mastoid process — p. Naturalis medicinæ, Physiology—p. Obscœna, Genital organs—p. Petrosa, see Temporal Bone—p. Prima asperæ arteriæ, Larynx — p. Pyramidalis ossis temporis, see Temporal Bone — p. Squamosa, see Temporal Bone — p. Urethræ membranacea, see Urethra — p. Vaga, Pneumogastric — p. Virilis, Penis.

PARSLEY, COMMON, Apium petroselinum — p. Fool's, Æthusa cynapium — p. Macedonian, Bubon Macedonicum—p. Mountain, black, Athamanta aureoselinum — p. Poison, Conium maculatum — p. Spotted. Conium maculatum — p. Water, Cicuta maculata.

PARSNEP, COW, Heracleum spondylium, Heracleum lanatum — p. Garden, Pastinaca sativa — p. Meadow, Thaspium Barbinode — p. Water, common, Sium latifolium.

PART, see Parturition — *p. Légitime et illégitime,* see Parturition.

PARTES GENERATIONI INSERVIENTES, Genital organs — p. Genitales, Genital organs — p. Laterales nasi, Scapulæ nasi—p. Nervosæ, see Nerve — p. Obscœnæ, Genital organs.

PARTHENEIA, Virginity.

PARTHENIUM FEBRIFUGA, Matricaria — p. Mas, Tanacetum.

PARTHEN'IUS, *(Morbus ;)* from *παρθενος,* 'a virgin.' A disease in a young female. Also, chlorosis.

PARTHENOGEN'ESIS; from *παρθενος,* ' a virgin,' and *γενεσις,* ' generation.' The successive production of procreating individuals from a single ovum. — Owen.

PARTHENOL'OGY, *Parthenolog''ia,* from *παρθενεια,* ' virginity,' and *λογος,* 'a description.' A description or consideration of the state of virginity in health or disease.

PARTHENUS, Virgin.

PARTIALIS, Local.

PARTICLES, PRIMITIVE, OF MUSCLES, Sarcous Elements.

PARTIES, LES, Genital organs — p. *Génitales*, Genital organs — p. *Honteuses*, Genital organs — p. *Génitoires*, Genital organs — p. *Naturelles*, Genital organs — p. *Nobles*, Genital organs — p. *Sexuelles*, Genital organs.

PARTIO, Parturition.

PARTRIDGE-BERRY, Gaultheria, Mitchella repens.

PARTS, THE, Genital organs.

PARTURA, Parturition.

PARTU'RIENT, *Partu'riens*, from *parturire*, itself from *parere*, 'to bring forth.' Bringing forth, or about to bring forth, or having recently brought forth. — Young.

The *Parturient, Puer'perous, Childbed*, or *Lying-in-state, Puerpe'rium*, requires careful management, and is subject to various diseases.

A *Partu'rient* or *Parturifa'cient* is a medicine which induces or promotes labour; as ergot, and, perhaps, borate of soda, see Abortive.

PARTURIFACIENT, Parturient.

PARTURIGO, Parturition.

PARTURIT"ION, *Puerpe'rium, Partus, Partio, Parturit''io, Parturi'go, Partu'ra, Tocos, To'cetos, Texis, Lochi'a, Apocye'sis, Maeeu'sis, Maieu'sis, Nego'tium* seu *Actus parturitio'nis, Enix'us* seu *Enix'io fœtûs, Expul'sio fœtûs, Apol'ysis, Labour, Child-bearing, Child-birth, Trav'ail*, (F.) *Accouchement, Couche, Travail d'Enfant*. The delivery of the fœtus and its appendages. Labour is the necessary consequence of conception, pregnancy, and the completion of gestation. It does not take place, at the full time, until after nine months of utero-gestation,—the causes producing it being the contraction of the uterus and abdominal muscles. By different authors, the stages of labour have been variously divided. We may, perhaps, admit of four. The *first stage* comprises the precursory signs. One, two, or three days before labour, a mucous discharge, streaked with blood, takes place from the vagina, which is called the *Signum, Leucorrhœ'a Nabo'thi, Hæmorrhag''ia Nabothi, Labour-show*, or *Show*; and, along with this, trifling grinding pains, called by the French *Mouches*, are felt in the loins and abdomen. *Second stage*:—Peculiar pains, which extend from the lumbar region towards the uterus; tension and dilatation of the neck and orifice of that organ; protrusion into the vagina of the envelopes of the fœtus, forming the *bag of waters*, (F.) *Poche des eaux*; and rupture or breaking of the waters. *Third stage*:—Contractions of the uterus and abdominal muscles; forcing pains; the head of the fœtus becomes engaged in the pelvis; the occiput being commonly situate above the left acetabulum, passes beneath the arch of the pubis. *Fourth stage*:— the head now presents at the vulva, the perineum being considerably distended; at length it clears the external parts, and the rest of the body is easily disengaged. The child still continues attached to the mother by the umbilical cord, which has to be divided. In the course of fifteen or twenty minutes, trifling pains occur, and the secundines are expelled. This completes delivery. In by far the majority of cases, the head is the presenting part, the occiput directed anteriorly, and the face posteriorly. Of 12,633 children, born at the Hospital *La Maternité*, in Paris, from the 10th of December, 1797, to the 31st of July, 1806, the following were the presentations:

The head, with the face posteriorly... 12,120
The head anteriorly............................ 63
The breech....................................... 198
The feet... 147
The knees.. 3
Other positions.................................. 102

          12,633

The following table, drawn up from data furnished by Velpeau, gives an approximative view of the comparative number of presentations, according to the experience of the individuals mentioned:

TABLE, EXHIBITING THE RATIO OF PRESENTATIONS IN 1000 CASES.

	ACCORDING TO						
	Merriman.	Bland.	Madame Boivin.	Madame Lachapelle.	N'ægle.	Lovati.	Hospital of the Faculté.	Boër.
Regular, or of the vertex	924	944	969	933	933	911	980	
I. *Occipito-anterior*...............	908		944	910		895		
a. Occipito-cotyloid (left)........			760	717		537		
Do. (right)			179	209				
b. Occipito pubian			0.29					
II. *Occipito-posterior*			9.4	9				
a. Fronto-cotyloid (left).........			5.3	7.3				
b Do. (right)			4.4	2.9				
Face presentation	2.2	2.6	3.6	4.6				8.8
Mento-iliac (right)................				2.6				
Of the pelvis	36	28	29	36	47			29
Of the foot	12.7	9.4		14				10.3
Of the knees			0.19	0.40				
Of the breech....................	23	13	18	22				19
Of the trunk			4.6	5.3	4.8			
Requiring Forceps	6.6	4.7	4.6	3.4	36			5.7
" Turning	10	4.7		7.8	7.2			5.9
" Cephalotomy	3.3	5.2	4.77	0.53	2.4			1.5

Labour has received different names, according to the period of pregnancy at which it occurs, and the mode in which it takes place. It is called *miscarriage* or *abortion*, prior to the seventh month; *premature labour, Omotoc'ia, Partus præ'cox* seu *præmatu'rus*, between this and eight months and a half; and *labour at the full period*, (F.) *Accouchement à terme*, when it happens at the end of nine months. Labours have likewise been variously divided by different authors. Perhaps the one into *Natural, Preternatural*, and *Laborious*, is as common as any; — *natural Labour* meaning that which would occur without manual assistance; *preternatural*, requiring the assistance of art, but by the hand solely: and *laborious*, requiring instrumental assistance; which M. Capuron calls *Accouchement Méchanique, Powerless labour*, the *Inertia par épuisement* of Madame La Chapelle, is that in which the muscular powers from exhaustion are unable to accomplish delivery.

The French use the term *Part, Partus*, at

times, synonymously with *delivery;* at others, with *fœtus, Maieu'ma, Maeeu'ma. Suppression de part* means concealment of delivery; *Part légitime,* a fœtus which comes into the world with the condition necessary for its enjoying advantages granted by law; and *Part illégitime,* one that does not fall under those conditions.

TABLE OF THE COURSE AND MANAGEMENT OF DIFFERENT KINDS OF LABOURS.

I. NATURAL LABOURS,
Or those in which Delivery can be effected without Assistance.

HEAD PRESENTING. (Four Positions.)	1. *Occiput towards the Left Acetabulum.*	The head with the chin bent upon the breast clears the brim of the pelvis. Motion of rotation produced by the inclined planes of the pelvis; the occipital protuberance is carried behind the symphysis pubis, and the face towards the hollow of the sacrum.
	2. *Occiput towards the Right Acetabulum.*	The head attains the outlet: clears it; the occiput being first disengaged, and the face afterwards, which passes successively along the whole of the hollow of the sacrum. The shoulders enter the brim diagonally; and execute the movement of rotation. The one behind first clears the outlet. The same thing occurs with the nates.
	3. *Occiput towards the Right Sacro-iliac Symphysis.*	The same course is here followed: except that after the rotary movement, the face passes behind the symphysis pubis, and the occiput into the hollow of the sacrum. The occiput is first extruded; — the face next.
	4. *Occiput towards the Left Sacro-iliac Symphysis.*	When the chin presents and is turned forwards, the face is first expelled; the head is thrown backwards. This presentation is uncommon. If the chin present and be thrown backwards, natural delivery cannot be effected.
LOWER EXTREMITY PRESENTING. (Four Positions of the Feet, Knees, and Breech.)	1. *Heel, Tibia, or Sacrum towards the Left Acetabulum.*	The nates enter the brim diagonally; movement of rotation: the one passes behind the symphysis pubis; the other towards the hollow of the sacrum. The one behind is first extruded.
	2. *Heel, Tibia, or Sacrum towards the Right Acetabulum.*	The same thing happens to the shoulders. The chin is bent upon the chest to clear the brim: movement of rotation: the occiput passes behind the symphysis pubis, and the face towards the hollow of the sacrum. The face clears the outlet first; the occiput last.
	3. *Heel, Tibia, or Sacrum towards the Right Sacro-iliac Symphysis.*	The same progress, except that after the movement of rotation, the face is towards the pubis, and the occiput towards the sacrum. The face is here again delivered first.
	4. *Heel, Tibia, or Sacrum towards the Left Sacro-iliac Symphysis.*	

II. PRETERNATURAL LABOURS,
Or those which require Manual Assistance only.

I. PRESENTATION OF THE HEAD, UPPER EXTREMITIES, BACK, ABDOMEN, &c.	1. When the labour is without any serious complication, and the head is not in a good position at the brim of the pelvis, endeavours are to be made to place it in its natural position: the hand to be introduced with the fingers united, and the long diameter of the head to be placed diagonally in the brim, if possible. Or the lever may be fixed over the occiput, and, by drawing it down, a closer approximation of the chin and chest may be effected; the position of the head to the pelvis being at the same time attended to.
	2. If complicated with syncope, convulsions, hemorrhage, want of uterine action, &c., the feet must be laid hold of, and the child *turned*. For this purpose, empty the rectum and bladder; and turn, if possible, prior to the escape of the liquor amnii. The female may be placed on her back or left side, with the breech over the edge of the bed. Use the right or left hand, according as the feet of the child are to the right or left side of the pelvis; always so introducing the hand, that the child shall be in its palm, and the back of the hand opposed to the inner surface of the uterus. The hand and arm to be introduced during an interval of pain; and they must be flattened and tranquil whilst the uterus is contracting forcibly. If both feet cannot be readily brought down, seize one, and tie a fillet around it.
	3. If the toes point to the vertebral column, or to the abdomen of the mother, the head, in its descent, will not enter the pelvis: the chin and occiput will be hitched on the pubis and promontory of the sacrum. In such case, grasp the nates as soon as they have passed the os externum; and, during a pain, endeavour to direct the toes towards either sacro-iliac synchondrosis. When the fingers can be passed along the body of the child, and over the shoulders to the bend of the elbows, draw down the arms successively. When the body is expelled, and the head filling up the brim, the termination of labour must be accelerated by passing two fingers over the shoulder of the child; using moderate and steady extracting power, whilst one finger of the other hand, passed into the mouth, depresses the chin on the sternum. In this way, the head may be extracted.

III. INSTRUMENTAL LABOURS,
Or those requiring the Assistance of appropriate Instruments.

GENERAL OBSERVATIONS.	If the pains become feeble, or inadequate from any cause;—or if the presenting part be firmly wedged in the pelvis; or the woman be becoming exhausted, instrumental assistance may be required. In all such cases, place the female on the back or left side, empty the bladder and rectum; wait till the os uteri is in a fit state; afford assistance during the pains; introduce the instrument during the intervals between the pains; have the patient on her left side (generally); and extract according to the axes of brim and outlet, as the case may be.

1. Short Forceps.	Apply these to the sides of the head of the child, so that the ears and parietal protuberances may be within the fenestræ. Introduce the left-hand blade first; the index and middle fingers of the right hand guiding it to the ear. With the right hand pass the other in an opposite line, corresponding with the course of the first blade, guided by the fore and middle fingers of the left hand; the third and little fingers being employed to retain the left-hand blade in place; humour the instrument so as to allow the blades to lock. The handles may now be tied gently together. The force used must be from blade to blade, with a gentle, tractile effort.
2. Long Forceps.	Applicable where the head does not enter the brim. The long forceps must be applied, in most cases, over the occiput and face of the child, so that the convex edges of the blades may be towards the hollow of the sacrum. When used, the power may be exerted from side to side, with moderate traction.
3. Lever or Vectis.	The lever is applicable to the same cases as the forceps. It must not be used strictly as a lever, but as a hook with which to draw downwards. It may be applied to any part of the head, but is generally hitched on the occiput.
4. Fillet and Blunt Hook.	In certain cases of breech and knee presentation, where the hand is insufficient, it may be necessary to pass over the joint a fillet, or the blunt hook, with which to exert some force of traction. The operation is very simple.
Embryulcia.	Disproportionate size of head, or distorted or deformed pelvis, may require the child to be destroyed, and its bulk lessened; or the Cæsarean section or symphysotomy, or the induction of premature labour may be called for. The instruments required here, are the *Perforator, Crotchet*, and *Craniotomy Forceps*. Make a steady pressure on the abdomen; pass two fingers of the left hand up to the head: feel for a suture or fontanelle; introduce the perforator and bore through, until the progress of the instrument is arrested by its *shoulders*. Open the handles, and turn the instrument in different directions, so that the opening may be large enough to admit the perforator, with which the brain must be broken down. If, after this, delivery cannot be accomplished without further aid, pass up the craniotomy forceps; open the handles slightly, and introduce the blade without teeth within the cranium. On closing the forceps, a hold is obtained; and a tractile force can now be exerted during the pains, and the extrusion of the child be effected. Should great difficulty exist at the brim, the bones at the top of the head may have to be removed, until the base alone remains. The chin must then be brought through first. The crotchet is often used instead of the craniotomy forceps, being passed into the opening made by the perforator, and hooked upon some bony projection in the interior of the skull; but it is not a good instrument. In presentations of the face demanding perforation of the cranium, the perforator should be introduced just above the nose, in the sagittal suture. When it is necessary to open the head after the lower extremities have been expelled, the perforation must be made behind the ear.
Symphysotomy and Cæsarean Section.	In cases of great narrowness of the pelvis, the operation of *Symphysotomy* has been adopted by French practitioners,—rarely by British or American; and, in extreme cases, recourse has been had to the *Cæsarean Section*.
Separation of the Head of the Fœtus from the Body.	If the body of the fœtus has been forcibly separated, and the head left in the uterus, it must be laid hold of with one hand, and the forceps be applied: or the head be opened and delivered, as under embryulcia. Should the head have been brought away, and the body left behind, the feet must be brought down.
Induction of Premature Labour.	In cases of narrowness of the pelvis, where the fœtus, at the full term, cannot be born alive, delivery may be brought about at an earlier period, or as soon as the child is capable of carrying on its functions independently of the mother. The most advisable plan for accomplishing this object is merely to pass the finger round and round within the os and cervix uteri, so as to detach the decidua;—the membranes being thus left entire, and the life of the child not so much endangered, as where the membranes are punctured, and the waters evacuated. Parturition usually follows within forty-eight hours.

The laying of eggs by animals is termed in French *ponte*. The term has been applied to the periodical discharge—*ponte périodique*—of ova, (F.) *Chute des Œufs*, which is supposed to take place from the ovaries at each menstrual period.

PARTURITION, DRY, Partus Siccus.

PARTURIUM VANUM, *Fausse couche*.

PARTUS, Parturition — p. Abactio, Abortion — p. Abactus, Abortion — p. Cæsareus, Cesarean section — p. Difficilis, Dystocia — p. Laboriosus, Dystocia, Laborious labour — p. Præcox, Parturition (premature) — p. Præmaturus, Parturition (premature) — p. Serotinus, Opsiotocia.

PARTUS SICCUS, *Dry labour or parturition*. Labour, which is neither preceded nor attended by a discharge of the liquor amnii.

PARU'LIS, from παρα, 'near,' and ουλον, 'the gum.' *Aposte'ma parulis* vel *paroulis, Phleg'monē Parulis, Gum Boil*. Small abscesses are so called which form in the gums, sometimes without any known cause, but which often depend upon carious teeth.

PARU'RIA, from παρα, 'defectively,' and ουρεω, 'I pass urine.' Morbid secretion or discharge of urine.

PARURIA INCONTINENS, Enuresis — p. Incontinens aquosa, see Diabetes — p. Inops, Ischuria, false — p. Mellita, Diabetes — p. Retentionis, Ischuria — p. Retentionis renalis, Ischuria — p. Retentionis vesicalis, Retention of urine — p. Stillatitia, Strangury — p. Stillatitia mucosa, Cystirrhœa.

PARVITAS MORBOSA PARTIUM ORGANICARUM, Microtesia.

PAR'YGRON, from παρα, and 'υγρος, 'humid.' A liquid or moist preparation for allaying topical inflammation.

PAS D'ÂNE, Tussilago.

PASMA, Catapasma.

PASQUEFLOWER, Anemone pulsatilla.

PASSA, Paronychia.

PASSÆ CORINTHIACÆ, see Vitis Corinthiaca.

PASSAGES, DIGESTIVE, Ways, digestive — p. Second, Ways, second.

PASSE-PIERRE, Crithmum maritimum.

PASSERAGE, Iberis amara—*p. Sauvage*, Cardamine pratensis.

PASSIBILITY, GREAT, Hyperæsthesia.

PASSIFLO'RA LAURIFO'LIA, *Bay-leaved Passion Flower.* A native of Surinam. The fruit has a delicious smell and flavour, and quenches thirst, abates heat of the stomach, increases the appetite, &c.

PASSIFLORA MALIFOR'MIS, *Apple-shaped Granadil'la.* The fruit of this species is esteemed a delicacy in the West Indies, where it is served up at table in desserts.

Some of the genus are said to possess narcotic and emetic properties.

PASSIO, Disease, Passion — p. Æmoptoica, Hæmoptysis—p. Cadiva, Epilepsy—p. Cardiaca, Cardialgia— p. Cœliaca, Cœliac flux — p. Cholerica, Cholera—p. Felliflua, Cholera—p. Hæmoptoica, Hæmoptysis— p. Hypochondriaca, Hypochondriasis — p. Hysterica, Hysteria — p. Iliaca, Ileus — p. Ischiadica, Neuralgia femoro-poplitæa — p. Pleuritica, Pleuritis — p. Stomachica, Dyspepsia — p. Ventriculosa, Cœliac flux — p. Vomicoflua, Phthisis pulmonalis.

PASSION, *Pas'sio, An'imi Pathe'ma, Affec'tus, Emo'tio,* from *patior, passus,* 'to suffer.' An active affection or emotion of the mind; as rage, terror, love, hatred, &c.

PASSION FLOWER, BAY-LEAVED, Passiflora laurifolia—*p. Hystérique,* Hysteria—p. Iliac, Ileus.

PASSIONES ANIMI, Affections of the mind.

PASSIVE, *Passi'vus.* Same etymon as Passion. An epithet for diseases which seem owing to a greater or less diminution of the strength, or which are without apparent reaction. Thus, passive hemorrhages are such as supervene in debilitated individuals, or under conditions in which increased action of the arteries can scarcely be presumed. The term *passive* has, also, been given to aneurisms of the heart with extenuation of the parietes; in opposition to *active* aneurisms, with thickness of the parietes — hypertrophy.

PASSULÆ MAJORES, see Vitis vinifera — p. Minores, see Vitis Corinthiaca.

PASSULA'TUM, *Uvæ passæ,* 'raisins, dried grapes.' A medicine in which the pulp of raisins is a chief ingredient.

PASSY, MINERAL WATERS OF. This village is in the vicinity of Paris. There are several springs, containing sulphates of lime, iron, and magnesia, alum, common salt, carbonate of iron, carbonic acid, &c. They are employed as a tonic and astringent.

PASTA DE ALTHÆA, Paste, marshmallow — p. Amygdalina, Confection (almond) — p. de Dactylis, Paste, date — p. Emulsiva, Confection (almond) — p. de Jujubis, Paste of jujubes — p. Regia, Confection (almond).

PASTA GLYCYRRHI'LÆ GUMMA'TA ET ANISA'TA *seu Massa de extracto glycyrrhi'zæ.* A compound of *extract of liquorice, gum Senegal, sugar, Florence orris-root,* and *volatile oil of aniseed.* Demulcent.

PASTE, *Pasta,* (F.) *Pâte.* A compound medicine, like the pastil, but less consistent, flexible, less saccharine, and more mucilaginous.

PASTE, DATE, *Massa* seu *Pasta de dac'tylis.* Composed of *dates, sugar, gum Arabic, water,* and *orange-flower water.*— Ph. P. Demulcent.

PASTE OF JU'JUBES, *Pasta de ju'jubis, Massa de zizypho'rum fructû.* Composed of *jujubes, gum Senegal, sugar, water,* and *tincture of lemon-peel.* Demulcent.

PASTE, MARSHMAL'LOW, *Massa de gummi Arab'ico, Pasta de althæ'æ.* A compound of *gum Arabic, sugar, white of egg,* and *orange-flower water.*— Ph. P. It is demulcent.

PASTE, TOOTH, Dentifricium — p. Vienna, see Powder, Vienna — p. Ward's, Confectio piperis nigri.

PASTEL, *Pastil'lus, Diocres, Avic'ula Cip'ria, Cande'la fuma'lis, Phthois, Phthois'cus.* A compound of aromatic substances in various shapes; used as a fumigating material when set fire to. See Fumigation.

The French use the term *Pastille,* (L.) *Pastillus,* for a solid, dry, round, oblong, square, or triangular compound, whose base is essential oil, and sugar the excipient. These pastilles are in fact small lozenges, and only differ from the *tablette* in their smaller size.

PASTEL, Isatis tinctoria.

PASTÈQUE, Cucurbita citrullus.

PASTILLE, see Pastel.

PASTILLES DIGESTIVES D'HAUTE-RIVE-VICHY, see Trochisci Sodæ bicarbonatis — p. Fumigating, see Fumigation — *p. de Vichy,* see Trochisci Sodæ bicarbonatis.

PASTILLI DIGESTIVI DARCETII, see Trochisci Sodæ bicarbonatis — p. Emetinæ Pectorales, Trochisci emetinæ pectorales.

PASTIL'LI DE MENTHÂ PIPERI'TÂ, *Peppermint drops. (Sacch. alb., aquæ menthæ pip., aq. destillat.* āā ʒij. Boil to the consistence of an electuary. Take of fine *white sugar* in powder, ʒiv; *volatile oil of peppermint,* ʒss. Mix, and add the electuary whilst warm. Drop it then on marble, and dry the *drops.*— Ph. P.)

PASTILLUS, Pastel.

PASTINACA ALTISSIMA, P. opóponax—p. Anethum, Anethum graveolens — p. Graveolens, Anethum graveolens—p. Opaca, P. sativa.

PASTINA'CA OPOP'ANAX. The name of the plant which furnishes the *Opopanax.* The plant, whence the gum resin is obtained, has, also, been called *Fer'ula opop'onax, Pastina'ca altiss'ima, Laserpit'ium chiro'nium, Seli'num opop'onax, Opopana'cum, Panax heracle'um, Panax costi'num, Pastina'cea, Kyna, Hercules-all-heal, Opop'-anaxwort.*

Opopanax, Opopana'cis gummi-resi'na, Gesir, Pop'anax, Gummi Pana'cis, exudes from the roots when wounded. Its odour is strong and peculiar; taste, bitter and acrid. It is met with in the shops, in lumps of a reddish-yellow colour, without; white within. It has been recommended as an antispasmodic and emmenagogue; but is seldom used. Dose, gr. x. to ℈j in powder.

PASTINACA PRATENSIS, P. sativa.

PASTINA'CA SATI'VA, *Elaphobos'cum, Pastinaca sylves'tris* seu *opa'ca* seu *praten'sis, Ana'thum pastina'ca, Seli'num pastina'ca, Ban'ica, Garden parsnep.* The root is sweet and nutritious, and is in esteem as an article of food. It has been used as a diuretic and demulcent in calculous affections, &c.

PASTINACA SYLVESTRIS, P. sativa—p. Sylvestris tenuifolia officinarum, Daucus carota.

PÂTE, Paste—*p. Arsénicale,* Arsenical paste.

PATELLA, *Rot'ula, R. genu, Epigon'atis, Epigon'tis, Acromy'lē, Epigou'nis* seu *Epigou'nis* seu *Epig'onis, Mola* seu *Concha* seu *Oc'ulus* seu *Orbis* seu *Scutum genu, Os scutifor'mē* seu *disciformē* seu *thyreoi'des, Supergenua'lis, Caucaloi'des, My'lacris, Mylē, Gamba, Oleo'ranon mob'ilē,* (F.) *Rotule.* Diminutive of *patina,* 'a dish,' so called from its shape. A sort of sesamoid, flat, short, thick, rounded bone, situate in front of the knee, and enveloped in the substance of the tendon common to the extensor muscles of the leg. The posterior surface of the patella is divided into two *facettes,* united angularly, which are encrusted with cartilage, and each of which is articulated with one of the condyles of the femur. The patella is developed by a single point of ossification. When the patella is fractured, it is difficult to produce bony union. This can only be accomplished by keeping the fractured extremities closely in apposition.

PATELLA, Cup—p. Fixa, Olecranon.

PATENT MED'ICINE, *Médecine brevetée* ou *patentée, Remède breveté* ou *patenté*. A medicinal compound, for the sale of which the proposer obtains from government an exclusive privilege. A specification of his *invention* must be registered in the Patent Office, and, hence, it differs from a secret medicine.

PATER OMNIUM VIVENTIUM, Penis.
PATERA DIOGENIS, Palm.
PATHEMA, Affection, Disease.
PATHEMATOLOGY, Pathology.

PATHET'IC, *Pathet'icus*, from παθειν, 'to feel.' That which moves the passions. A name given to the *superior oblique muscle of the eye*, and, also, to a nerve.

PATHETIC MUSCLE, Oblique superior of the eye.

PATHETIC NERVE, *Nervus Pathet'icus*, *N. trochlea'ris* seu *trochleato'rius* seu *trochlea'tor*, the *4th pair of nerves*, (F.) *Oculo-musculaire interne* (Ch.), *Nerf pathétique*, is the smallest encephalic nerve. It arises behind the inferior part of the tubercula quadrigemina (*testes*) at the lateral parts of the valvula Vieussenii. Its roots unite into one thin round cord, which makes a turn upon the peduncles of the brain, and passes into a canal of the dura mater near the posterior clinoid process. It enters the orbit by the broadest part of the sphenoidal fissure, and terminates in the superior oblique muscle of the eye, by dividing into several filaments.

PATHETISM, Magnetism, animal.
PATHIC, Morbid.
PATHICAL, Morbid.
PATHICUS, Morbid.
PATHNE, Alveolus.

PATHOGENET'IC, *Pathogenet'icus*, *Pathogen'icus*. Same etymon as the next. Relating to pathogeny.

PATHOGENETIC PHYSIOLOGY, *Physiolog''ia pathogenet'ica*. That part of physiology which relates to the origin of disease.

PATHOGENICUS, Pathogenetic.

PATHOG''ENY, *Pathogen'ia*, *Nosogen'esis*, *Nosogen'ia*, from παθος, 'a disease,' and γενεσις, 'generation.' The branch of pathology which relates to the generation, production and development of disease.

PATHOGNOMON'IC, *Pathognomon'icus*, *Signum conjunc'tum* seu *characteris'ticum* seu *morbi essentia'lè;* from παθος, 'an affection,' and γινωσκω, 'I know.' A *characteristic symptom* of a disease.

PATHOG'RAPHY, *Pathograph'ia*, from παθος, 'disease,' and γραφω, 'I describe.' A description of disease.

PATHOLOGIA, Pathology — p. Humoralis, Humorism—p. Solidaris, Solidism.

PATHOLOG''ICAL, *Patholog''icus*, *Pathol'ogus;* same etymon as pathology. Relating to pathology. Often used in the sense of pathical.

PATHOLOGICAL ANATOMY, see Anatomy.

PATHOL'OGIST, *Pathol'ogus*. Same etymon. One versed in pathology.

PATHOL'OGY, *Pathematol'ogy*, *Patholog''ia*, *Pathematolog''ia*, *Patholog''icë*, from παθος, 'a disease,' and λογος, 'a discourse.' The branch of medicine whose object is the knowledge of disease. It has been defined *diseased physiology*, and *physiology of disease*. It is divided into *general* and *special*. The *first* considers diseases in common;—the *second*, the particular history of each. It is subdivided into *internal* and *external*, or *medical* and *surgical*.

PATHOLOGY, HUMORAL, Humorism.

PATHOMA'NIA, *Parapathi'a*, *Moral Insanity*, from παθος, 'a disease,' and *mania*. *Ma'nia sine Delir'io*. A morbid perversion of the natural feelings, affections, inclinations, temper, habits, moral disposition, and natural impulses, without any remarkable disorder or defect of the intellect or knowing and reasoning faculties, and particularly without any insanity or hallucination.

PATHOMYOTOM'IA; from παθος, 'affection,' μυς or μυων, 'muscle,' and τομη, 'incision.' The title of a work by Dr. John Bulwer (1649), being "a dissection of the significative muscles of the affections of the mind."

PATHOPATRIDALGIA, Nostalgia.

PATHOS, Affection, Disease.

PATIENCE, Rumex patientia — p. d'Eau, Rumex hydrolopathum—p. Garden, Rumex patientia—p. Rouge, Rumex sanguineus — p. Sauvage, Rumex acutus.

PATIENT, see Sick.

PATIENTIA, Rumex patientia.

PATIENTIÆ MUSCULUS, Levator scapulæ.

PATNE, Alveolus.

PATOPATRIDALGIA, Nostalgia.

PATOR NA'RIUM. The cavity or the opening of the nostrils.

PATRATIO, Ejaculation, (of sperm.)

PATTE D'OIE (F.), 'Goose's foot.' An aponeurotic expansion, which covers the internal surface of the tibia at its upper part, and consists of the expansion formed by the tendons of the sartorius, gracilis, and semi-tendinosus muscles.

PATURSA, Syphilis.

PAU, (CLIMATE OF.) Pau is the capital of the department of the Lower Pyrenees, and is about 150 miles from Bordeaux, and 50 from Bayonne. The climate corresponds with that of the south-west of France generally; its great quality is the comparative mildness of its spring, and exemption from cold winds. It is regarded as a favourable winter residence for invalids labouring under chronic affections of the mucous membranes. It is too changeable for the consumptive; and to be avoided by the rheumatic.

PAULLIN'IA. This is an extract from a plant of the same name in Brazil. It is prepared by the Indians, and appears to possess excitant powers. In Brazil, and the neighbouring countries, it is given in the form of tisane—the powder being mixed with cocoa — in diarrhœa and dysentery. It has been employed also as a tonic. An extract is prepared in Brazil from *Paullinia sor'bilis*, known there under the name of *Guarana*, which is administered in similar pathological cases.

PAUME DE LA MAIN, Palm.
PAUNCH, Ingluvies.
PAUONTA, Sedatives.
PAUPIÈRE. Palpebra.

PAUSIME'NIA, from παυσις, 'cessation,' and μηνες, 'menses.' Cessation of the menses.

PAVANA WOOD, Croton tiglium.

PAVIL'ION. The French give the name *pavillon*, to the expanded extremity of a canal or cavity,—for example, of a catheter, sound, &c.

PAVILION OF THE EAR, *Auric'ula*, *Pinna*, *O'tium*, *Ala*, (F.) *Auricule* ou *Oricule*, *Pavillon de l'oreille*, is seated behind the cheeks, beneath the temple, and anterior to the mastoid process. Its size varies in individuals. It is free above, behind, and below. Anteriorly and within, it is continuous with the neighbouring parts. Its outer surface has several prominences, the *Helix*,

Antaelix, Tragus, Antitragus, and *Lobe;* and several cavities—the *groove of the Helix,* the *fossa navicularis* seu *scaphoides,* and the *Concha.* The skin which covers the pavilion is very fine, and studded with a number of sebaceous follicles. The auricle is fixed to the head by three fibro-areolar ligaments;— a *superior, anterior,* and *posterior.*

PAVILLON DE L'OREILLE, Pavilion of the ear—*p. de la Trompe,* see Tuba Fallopiana.

PAVIMENTUM CEREBRI, Base of the brain.

PAVINA, Æsculus hippocastanum.

PAVITA'TIO, *Tremor;* from *pavor,* 'dread.' Trembling for fright.

PAVOPHOBIA, Panophobia.

PAVOR, (L.), Dread. Great fright. Panophobia.

PAVO'RES NOCTUR'NI SEU DORMIEN'TIUM. Fear during sleep.

PAVOT, Papaver.

PAW, Manus.

PAXWAX, see Nucha.

PAXYWAXY, see Nucha.

PAZAHAR, Bezoar.

PEA, Pisum — p. Garden, Pisum—p. Ground Squirrel, Jeffersoniana Bartoni—p. Hoary, Galega Virginiana—p. Love, Abrus precatorius—p. Nut, Arachis hypogea—p. Partridge, Cassia chamæcrista—p. Pisum—p. Turkey, Galega Virginiana.

PEACH BRANDY, Amygdalus Persica—p. Tree, Amygdalus Persica—p. Wood, see Cæsalpinia.

PEAGLE, Primula veris.

PEAR, see Pyrus malus.

PEARL, *Perla, Mar'garon, Margari'ta, Margel'lium, Marge'lis, U'nio,* (F.) *Perle.* A roundish concretion of a silvery white colour, and brilliant polish, found in several shells, and especially in the *Avic'ula margaritif'era,* which has, hence, been called *Mater perlarum, Margari'ta,* and *Mother of pearl,* and is much used in the fabrication of handles for surgical instruments, &c. Pearls were formerly given in powder as astringents and antacids. They consist of lime and an animal matter.

PEARL ASH, Potash of commerce—p. Mother of, see Pearl—p. White, Bismuth, subnitrate of.

PEAU, Cutis.

PEAUCIER, Platysma myoides.

PECAN or PECCAN NUT, see Hickory.

PECCANT, *Peccans,* from *peccare,* 'to sin.' Morbid, not healthy. An epithet given by the humourists to the humours when erring in quality or quantity. See Materia Morbosa.

PECHEDEON, Perinæum.

PECHER, Amygdalus Persica.

PECHIAGRA, Pechyagra.

PECHU'RIM seu PICHU'RIM CORTEX. A highly aromatic bark, the produce of a species of laurus. It is extremely fragrant, like that of cinnamon, which it greatly resembles in its properties. In Portugal it is used in the cure of dysentery, &c. See Pichurim beans.

PECH'YAGRA, *Pech'iagra, Ancon'agra, Pectihagra,* from πηχυς, 'the elbow,' and *sypa,* 'a seizure.' Gout affecting the elbow.

PECHYS, Elbow.

PECHYTYRBE, Porphyra nautica.

PECTE, Cheese.

PECTEN, Pubes. Also, a comb.

PECTEN DENTIUM, Sepes dentium—p. Veneris, Scandix cerefolium.

PECTIHAGRA, Pechyagra.

PECTIN, from πηκτις, 'a coagulum.' A name given by Braconnot to a principle which forms the basis of vegetable jelly. It is extensively diffused in the juices of pulpy fruits and roots, especially when they are mature; and occasions these juices to coagulate when they are mixed with alcohol or boiled with sugar.

It is the basis of one of the classes of elementary principles of Dr. Pereira—the *pectinaceous.*

PECTINACEOUS, Pectinous.

PECTINA'LIS, from *pecten,* 'the pubes;' *Pectina'us, Mus'culus liv'idus, Pectina'tus,* (F.) *Pubio-fémoral, Suspubio-fémoral* (Ch.), *Pectiné.* This muscle is situate at the inner and upper part of the thigh. It is long, flat, and triangular; is attached, above, to the space which separates the ileo-pectineal eminence from the spine of the os pubis; and, below, by a flat tendon, to the oblique line which descends from the lesser trochanter to the linea aspera. The pectinalis bends the thigh on the pelvis, and carries it outwards in adduction and rotation. It may also bend the pelvis on the thigh.

PEC'TINATED, *Pectina'tus, Pectin'iform, Pectinate,* (F.) *Pectiné,* from *pecten,* 'a comb.' Having the shape of the teeth of a comb.

PECTINATED MUSCLES, *Pectina'ti mus'culi.* The fascicular texture observed in the right auricle of the heart: — *Mus'culi Auric'ulæ Pectina'ti.* Their main use probably is—to prevent the over dilatation of the auricles.

PECTINATUS, Pectinalis.

PECTINÉ, Pectinalis, Pectinated.

PECTINEUS, Pectinalis.

PECTINIFORM, Pectinated.

PEC'TINOUS, *Pectina'ceus, Pectino'sus, Pectina'ceous,* from *pectin.* Of or belonging to pectin or vegetable jelly,—as a *pectinous* or *pectinaceous* vegetable principle.

PEC'TORAL, from *pectus,* 'the breast.' Relating to the breast. See Pectorals.

PECTORAL, GRAND, Pectoralis major.

PECTORALE, Corset.

PECTORALIS INTERNUS, Triangularis sterni.

PECTORA'LIS MAJOR, from *pectus,* 'the breast.' *Pectora'lis, Sterno-cleido-brachia'lis,* (F.) *Sterno-costo-clavio-huméral, Sterno-huméral* (Ch.), *Grand Pectoral.* A large, flat, triangular muscle, situate at the anterior part of the chest, before the axilla. It is attached, on the one hand, by means of aponeurotic fibres, to the inner half of the anterior edge of the clavicle; to the anterior surface of the sternum, and to the cartilages of the first six true ribs;— on the other, by a strong tendon, which is inserted at the anterior edge of the bicipital groove of the humerus. The use of this muscle is, to move the arm in various directions. If it be hanging by the side of the body, it carries it inwards and a little forwards. When the arm is raised, it depresses it and carries it inwards. It can, also, move it in rotation inwards. If the humerus be raised and fixed, the pectoralis major draws the trunk towards the upper extremity.

PECTORA'LIS MINOR, *Serra'tus anti'cus minor,* (F.) *Costo-coracoïdien* (Ch.), *Petit Pectoral, Petit dentlé antérieur.* This muscle is situate beneath the preceding, at the anterior and upper part of the chest. It is flat and triangular; is attached by its base, which appears digitated, to the upper edge and outer surface of the 3d, 4th, and 5th true ribs, and is inserted at the anterior part of the coracoid process. The pectoralis minor draws the scapula forwards and downwards, and makes it execute a rotatory motion, by virtue of which its inferior angle is carried backwards, and the anterior depressed. When the shoulder is fixed, it elevates the ribs to which it is attached, and aids in the dilatation of the chest.

PEC'TORALS, *Pectora'lia, Thorac''ica.* Medicines considered proper for relieving or removing affections of the chest.

PECTORAL DROPS, BATEMAN'S, consist chiefly of *tincture of castor*, with some *camphor* and *opium*, flavoured by *aniseed*. Gray gives the following formula: *Castor*, ℥j; *ol. anisi*, ℨj; *camph.* ʒv; *cocci*, ʒiss; *opii*, ʒvj; *proof spirit*, a gallon.

A form, advised by a committee of the Philadelphia College of Pharmacy, is the following:— *Alcohol. dil.* cong. iv; *Santal. rubr. ras.* ℥j; digere per horas xxiv; cola, et adde *Pulv. opii, Pulv. catechu, Camphoræ*, ā ā ℥ij; *Ol. anisi*, ʒiv. Digest for ten days.

PECTORILOQUE, from *pectus*, 'the chest,' and *loqui*, 'to speak.' Laënnec calls thus one who presents the phenomenon of *Pectoriloquism*. Also, a stethoscope.

PECTORILOQUIE, Pectoriloquy—p. *Chévrotante*, Egophony.

PEC'TORILOQUY, *Pectoril'oquism, Cav'ernous voice, Pectorilo'quia*, (F.) *Pectoriloquie, Voix caverneuse, V. articulée*. Same etymon. Speech or voice coming from the chest. Laënnec has designated, by this name, the phenomenon often presented by consumptive individuals, when their chests are examined with the stethoscope. The voice seems to issue *directly* from the chest, and to pass through the central canal of the cylinder, — a phenomenon owing to the voice resounding in the anfractuous cavities, produced in the lungs by the suppuration or breaking down of tubercles, which constitute *abscesses* or *ulcers of the lungs*.

PECTUS, Sternum, Thorax — p. Carinatum, see Carina.

PECULIUM, Penis.

PEDAGRA, Potassæ supertartras impurus.

PEDAL, *Peda'lis*, from *pes, pedis*, 'the foot.' Relating to the foot: — as

PEDAL APONEURO'SIS, (F.) *Aponévrose pédieuse*. A thin, aponeurotic layer, which invests the extensor brevis digitorum pedis, and separates the tendons of the foot from each other.

PEDES, Genital Organs.

PEDESIS, Pulsation.

PEDETHMOS, Pulsation.

PEDIAL'GIA, *Pedional'gia, Pedioneural'gia*, from πεδίον, 'the sole of the foot,' and αλγος, 'pain.' Pain in the sole of the foot. Neuralgia of the foot in general.

PEDICLE, VITELLINE, see Vesicula umbilicalis.

PEDICULARIA, Delphinium staphisagria.

PEDICULATIO, Phtheiriasis.

PEDIC'ULUS, *Phtheir*, the *Louse*, (F.) *Pou*. A genus of parasitic insects. The human body is infested with three kinds: the *Body-louse*, or *Clothes-louse*, *Pedic'ulus vestimen'ti*, (F.) *Pou de corps*; the *Head-louse*, *Pedic'ulus cap'itis*, (F.) *Pou de la tête*, which lives in the hair; the *Crab-louse, Mor'pio, Fera'lis pedic'ulus, Plat'ula, Phthi'rius inguina'lis, Pedic'ulus Pubis*, (F.) *Morpion*, which infests the hair of the pubes. Infusion of tobacco, or mercurial ointment, or ointment of white precipitate of mercury, or the white or red precipitate of mercury, readily destroys them. The louse occurring in phtheiriasis, *pedic'ulus tabescen'tium*, differs from the common louse. —Vogel.

PEDICULUS CAPITIS, see Pediculus — p. Pubis, Crab-louse — p. Tabescentium, see Pediculus — p. Vestimenti, see Pediculus.

PÉDICURE, Chiropodist.

PEDICUS, Extensor brevis digitorum pedis.

PÉDIEUX (muscle), Extensor brevis digitorum pedis.

PEDIGAMBRA, Ysambra.

PEDILU'VIUM, from *pedes*, 'the feet,' and *lavo*, 'I wash.' *Lavipe'dium*, (F.) *Bain de pied*. A bath for the feet. See Bath.

PEDION, Sole.

PEDIONALGIA, Pedialgia.

PEDIONEURALGIA, Pedialgia.

PEDIUM, Tarsus.

PÉDONCULES DU CERVELET, Corpora restiformia.

PEDORA. The sordes of the eyes, ears, and feet.

PED'UNCLE, *Pedun'culus*. This term has been applied to different prolongations or appendices of the encephalon, from *pes, pedis*, 'a foot.' Thus, the *Peduncles of the brain* are the *Crura cerebri*; the *Peduncles of the cerebel'lum*, the *Crura cerebelli*.

PEDUNCLES OF THE BRAIN, *Pedun'culi cer'ebri*, called, also, *Crura anterio'ra medul'læ oblonga'tæ*, are two white cords, about ⅔ths of an inch in diameter, on the outside of the corpora albicantia. They arise from the medullary substance of the brain, and gradually approach, till they join the tuber annulare. They are formed, internally, of a mixture of cineritious and medullary matter; the former of which, being of a darker colour at one part than in any other part of the brain, has been called *Locus niger crurum cerebri*.

PEDUNCLES OF THE CEREBELLUM, *Pedun'culi cerebel'li*, called, also, *Crura posterio'ra*, are six in number, three on each side — a *superior*, a *middle*, and an *inferior*. The superior peduncles are generally known as the *Processus cerebelli ad testes, Crura cerebel'li ad cor'pora quadrigem'ina, Bra'chia copulati'va*; the inferior are the *Processus cerebelli ad medullam oblongatam*; and the middle are called, also, *Cerebel'lar ped'uncles — Proces'sus* seu *Crura cerebel'li ad pontem, Bra'chia pontis*.

PEDUNCLES, INFERIOR OF THE CEREBELLUM, Corpora restiformia — p. of the Medulla Oblongata, Corpora restiformia.

PEDUNCLES OF THE PINEAL GLAND are two medullary bands or strips, which seem to issue from the pineal gland, and proceed on each side upon the upper and inner region of the optic thalami.

PEDUNCULI CEREBELLI, Peduncles of the Cerebellum — p. Cerebri, Peduncles of the Brain — p. Medullæ Oblongatæ, Corpora restiformia.

PEDUNCULUS, Peduncle.

PEGA, Canthus (lesser).

PEGANELÆON, *Oleum ruta'ceum, O'leum rutæ*, from πηγανον, 'rue.' Oil of Rue.

PEGANUM, Ruta.

PEINE, Hunger.

PEINOTHERAPIA, Limotherapeia.

PEIRA, Effort, Experience, Nisus.

PELADA. A word of uncertain origin, applied to alopecia, especially to that resulting from syphilis.

PELA'GIA. A kind of scaly erysipelas of the hands — sometimes of the legs, at others, of the face. Pellagra.(?)

PELAGRA, Pellagra.

PELARGO'NIUM ANCEPS, *Peris'tera anceps*. A South African plant, *Nat. Ord*. Geraniaceæ; the decoction of which is used by the Malays in amenorrhœa, and to promote parturition and abortion.

PELARGONIUM ANTIDYSENTER'ICUM, *Jenkinso'nia antidysenter'ica*. This South African plant is used by the natives in dysentery. It is boiled in milk.

PELARGO'NIUM CUCULLA'TUM. Common along the side of the Table Mountain. It has been recommended in decoction as an enema in colic, nephritis, and suppression of urine. It is an excellent emollient, and was formerly exported to Holland under the name *Herba Althææ.*

PELARGO'NIUM TRISTE, *Polyac'tium tristē.* The root of this plant, which grows at the Cape of Good Hope, is somewhat astringent, and is used there in diarrhœa and dysentery, and as an anthelmintic.

PEL'ICAN, *Pelica'nus, Peleca'nus, Pel'ecan, Pel'ecas.* An instrument, curved at the end like the beak of a pelican. Its use is to extract teeth.

PELICIDE, *Pelu'dē, Mel coctum.* Boiled honey. — Ruland and Johnson.

PELICOMETER, Pelvimeter.

PELIDNOMA, Ecchymoma, Pelioma.

PELIO'MA, *Pelidno'ma,* from πελος, 'black.' A livid ecchymosis. — Forestus. See Ecchymoma.

PÉLIOSE, Purpura.

PELIOSIS, Purpura hæmorrhagica — p. Rheumatica, see Purpura simplex.

PELLA, Cutis, Prepuce.

PEL'LAGRA, *Pel'agra, Ichthyo'sis Pellagra, Elephanti'asis Ital'ica, Tuber Pellagra, Lepra Mediolanen'sis,* L. *Lombard'ica, Scorbu'tus alpi'nus, Ma'nia pella'gria, Erythe'ma endem'icum* seu *pel'lagrum, Insolazione de Primavera, Mal del Sole, Dermat'agra, Erysip'elas period'ica nervo'sa chron'ica, Mal de misère, Paral'ysis scorbu'tica, Scurvy of the Alps, Impeti'go Pellagra,* (F.) *Scorbut des Alpes;* from πελλα,(?) 'skin,' and αγρα, 'seizure.' A disease, particularly noticed among the Milanese, which consists in the skin becoming covered with wrinkles, and assuming a scaly appearance, especially in the parts exposed to the air. The strength diminishes, the intellectual faculties and sensations become obscure, and cramps, convulsions, and other lesions of muscular contractility supervene. It is a singular endemic affection, and has been supposed to follow every where the introduction of Indian corn: hence the name *Rapha'nia mais'tica,* given to it by some of the Italian physicians.

PELLENS, from *pellere,* 'to drive.' Driving; impelling.

PELLEN'TIA MEDICAMEN'TA are medicines that promote the occurrence of the menstrual or hæmorrhoidal flux.

PELLICULA SUMMA, Epidermis — p. Superior, Epidermis.

PELLÍCULÆ CORDIS, Ostiola cordis.

PELLIS, Cutis — p. Summa, Epidermis.

PELLITORY, Xanthoxylum fraxineum — p. American, Parietaria Pennsylvanica — p. Bastard, Achillea ptarmica — p. of Spain, Anthemis pyrethrum — p. Wall, Parietaria.

PELMA, Sole.

PELOR, Monster.

PELORIA, Monster.

PELORIUM, Monster.

PELORUM, Monster.

PELOTE DE MER, Pila marina.

PELTALIS seu PELTATUS CARTILAGO, Thyroid cartilage, Xiphoid cartilage.

PELTAN'DRA VIRGIN'ICA, *Arum Virgin'icum, Lecon'tia, Rensselæ'ria, Arrow Arum, Taraho, Wampee;* indigenous; of the *Order* Araceæ. The fresh roots and seeds are acrid stimulants, like Arum.

PELTIDEA AMPLISSIMA, Lichen caninus — p. Canina, Lichen caninus — p. Leucorrhiza, Lichen caninus — p. Malacea, Lichen caninus — p. Spuria, Lichen caninus.

PELTIGERA CANINA, Lichen caninus.

PELUDE, Pelicide.

PELVIC, *Pel'vicus, Pelvi'nus.* Belonging or relating to the pelvis.

PELVIC APONEUROSIS, (F.) *Aponévrose pelvienne.* A tendinous lamina, given off from the sides of the pelvis, and from the entire circumference of the brim, which passes into and lines the pelvis, and is soon divided into two distinct layers; — one *external,* the *lateral pelvic* or *obturator fascia,* which continues to line the sides of the pelvis, and covers the obturator internus muscle; the other, *internal* or *superior,* which passes inwards upon the side of the prostate, bladder, and rectum in the male, and of the bladder, vagina, and rectum in the female, in order to form the floor of the pelvis.

PELVIC CAVITY, (F.) *Cavité pelvienne.* The cavity of the pelvis.

PELVIC MEMBERS. The lower extremities.

PELVIC SURFACE OF THE IL'IUM. That which faces the pelvic cavity.

PELVICULA OCULI, Orbit.

PELVI-TROCHANTE'RIAN, *Pelvi-trochanteria'nus.* That which relates to the pelvis and great trochanter. The *Pelvi-trochante'rian region* is formed by the muscles — *pyramidalis, two obturators, gemini,* and *quadratus femoris,* which pass from the pelvis to the digital cavity of the great trochanter.

PELVIM'ETER, *Pelycom'eter, Pelyom'eter, Pelicom'eter, Pyelom'eter,* from *pelvis,* and μετρον, 'a measure.' A barbarous hybrid. This name has been given to different instruments, invented for measuring the diameters of the pelvis, and particularly the antero-posterior or fore-and-aft diameter of the brim. Two have been chiefly employed, especially by French practitioners: — the *Compas d'épaisseur,* and the *Pelvimeter* of Coutouly. 1. The *Compas d'épaisseur* or *Cal'lipers* of Baudelocque, is formed like a pair of compasses — with blunt extremities — the branches of which can be moved at will. One of these is applied to the symphysis pubis, and the other on the sacrum. About three inches must be deducted from this measurement for the thickness of the mons veneris, pubis, and the base of the sacrum. 2. The *Pelvimeter* of *Coutouly* resembles the instruments used by shoemakers for measuring the length of the foot. The two branches are introduced, in a state of approximation, into the vagina; and then separated, so that one touches the promontory of the sacrum, the other comes behind the os pubis. It is a barbarous contrivance, and its introduction ought never to be attempted on the living subject. It does not, indeed, seem possible to introduce it without mischief.

The finger is, decidedly, the best pelvimeter, and by it we can judge whether the base of the sacrum be unusually prominent. Measurement of the pelvis by the hand has been called *Pelycochirometre'sis;* from πελυξ, 'the pelvis,' χειρ, 'the hand,' and μετρον, 'measure.'

PELVIS, *Cho'ana, Py'elos,* (F.) *Bassin;* so called, because fancied to be shaped like an ancient basin. The part of the trunk which bounds the abdomen below. It is a large, bony, irregular, canoidal cavity, — open above and below, — which supports and contains a part of the intestines, and the urinary and genital organs; and serves, at the same time, as a fixed point for the articulation of the lower limbs, the attachment of their muscles, and the execution of their movements. The pelvis supports, behind, the vertebral column, and is sustained, before, by the ossa femorum. It is situate, in the adult, near the middle part of the body, and is composed of four broad, flat, unequally thick bones, differing much in their shape, size, and arrangement, which touch, are articulated at some part of their surface, and intimately united by means of a number of ligamentous fasciæ. Of these bones, two are behind, on the median line, — the sacrum and the coccyx; the two others are before and at the sides,—the ilia. They are fellows, and unite, before, with each other. The most important parts of the pelvis, in an obstetrical point of view, are the *brim* and the *outlet*. The BRIM, *Angus'tia abdomina'lis, Intro'itus, Apertu'ra pelvis supe'rior, Upper Opening* or *strait of the Cavity of the Pelvis*, (F.) *Détroit supérieur, D. abdominal*, is the narrow part which separates the greater pelvis from the less—the *false* from the *true, Pelvis vera seu minor*. In the well-formed woman it is elliptical, and slightly inclined forwards. Its *antero-posterior* or *sacro-pubic diameter*, in a *standard pelvis*, measures 4½ inches, but with the soft parts, 3¾ inches; its *transverse* or *iliac* or *lateral*, 5¼ inches, but with the soft parts 4 inches; and its *oblique* with the soft parts, 4⅜ inches. The OUTLET, *Ex'itus, Inferior opening* or *strait, Angus'tia perinæa'lis*, (F.) *Détroit inférieur, D. périnéal*, forms the lower aperture of the pelvis. The antero-posterior diameter is here, on account of the mobility of the coccyx, 5 inches: the lateral, 4 inches. The AXIS OF THE PELVIS is important to be known in obstetrics. The *Axis of the Brim* is indicated by a straight line drawn from the umbilicus to the apex of the coccyx;—the *Axis of the Outlet* by a line drawn from the first bone of the sacrum to the entrance of the vagina. An imaginary curved line which indicates the direction of the canal of the pelvis, has occasionally been termed the *curve of Carus*, in consequence of its having been pointedly described by the German obstetrician.

PELVIS AURIUM, Cochlea—p. Cerebri, Infundibulum of the brain.

PELVIS OF THE KIDNEY, *Pelvis rena'lis* seu *renum, Sinus, Venter* seu *Alvus Renum*, (F.) *Bassinet*. This is a small, membranous pouch, occupying the posterior part of the fissure of the kidney. It is placed behind the renal artery and vein; is elongated from above to below; flattened from before to behind; irregularly oval in figure; and, below, contracts considerably, to be continuous with the ureter. It receives the orifices of the infundibula, which pour the urine secreted in the kidney into its cavity.

PELVIS MINOR, Pelvis—p. Ocularis, Scaphium oculare—p. Renalis, Pelvis of the kidney—p. Renum, Pelvis of the kidney—p. Vera, Pelvis.

PELYCOMETER, Pelvimeter.

PELYOMETER, Pelvimeter.

PEMMICAN. Meat cured, pounded, and mixed with fat. It has been much used as nutriment on long overland journeys.

PEM'PHIGUS, *Emphly'sis Pem'phigus, Pom'pholyx*, from πεμφιξ, 'a blister;' *Febris bullo'sa, vesicula'ris, ampullo'sa* seu *pemphigo'des* seu *pemphingo'des, Exanthe'ma serosum, Morta, Pem'phigus morta, Pemphigus Helveticus, Pemphigus major, Pemphigus minor, Morbus bullosus* seu *vesicula'ris* seu *ampulla'ceus, Pem'phinx, Pemphix, Pemphyx, Typhus vesicula'ris, Vesic'ular Fever, Bladdery Fever*, (F.) *Fièvre bulleuse, F. Vésiculaire*. A disease, defined to consist of vesicles, scattered over the body; transparent, filbert-sized, with a red, inflamed edge, but without surrounding blush or tumefaction; on breaking, disposed to ulcerate; fluid, pellucid or slightly coloured; fever, typhous. It is doubtful whether any such idiopathic fever have ever existed: the probability is, that the fever and vesications have been an accidental complication. Cullen thinks the *Pemphigus Helveticus* must have been malignant sore throat. If, however, such a distinct disease did exist, it was probably only as an endemico-epidemic.

PEMPHIG· & HUNGARICUS, see Anthrax—p. Major, Pemphigus—p. Minor, Pemphigus—p. Morta, Pemphigus—p. Variolodes, see Varicella.

PEMPHINX, Pemphigus.
PEMPHIX, Pemphigus.
PEMPHYX, Pemphigus.
PEMPTÆA FEBRIS, Quintan.
PENÆA MUCRONATA, see Sarcocolla—p. Sarcocolla, Sarcocolla.
PENCIL-LIKE PROCESSES, Styloid processes.
PENDULOUS ABDOMEN, Physconia.
PENDULUM PALATI, Velum pendulum palati.
PEN'ETRATING, *Pen'etrans*, from *penetrare*, (*penitus intrare*,) 'to go into.' A wound is so called which penetrates one of the great splanchnic cavities — *Vulnus penetrans*.
A medicine is, also, so called, which is supposed to pass through the pores, and stimulate.
PENICILLUM, Compress, Penicillus.
PENICIL'LUS, *Penicill'um*, 'a painter's brush;' diminutive of *penis*, 'a tail.' A tent or pledget. The secreting glandiform extremities of the venæ portæ, (*Ac''ini bilio'si*) have been so termed, as well as the villous textures.
PENICILLUS, Tent.
PENICULUM, Compress.
PENICULUS, Tent.
PENIDES, Saccharum hordeatum.
PENID'IUM, *Penidium sacchara'tum*. A kind of clarified sugar, made up into rolls. *Barley sugar*. It is demulcent; see Saccharum hordeatum.

PÉNIL, Mons veneris.

PENIS, 'a tail,' from *pendere*, 'to hang down:' *Caulis, Coles, Caules, Caulos, Men'tula, Menta, Phall'us, Posthè, Pros'thium, Crithè, Cor'ynè, Femer, Pater om'nium viven'tium, Pria'pus, Virga, V. viri'lis, V. genita'lis, Vere'trum, Sathè, Membrum viri'lè, Membrum, Verbus, Viri'lè, Pars Viri'lis, Membrum seminalè* seu *genitalè viro'rum, Morion, Cyon, Sic'ula, Tentum, Hasta, H. nuptia'lis, H. viri'lis, Vas, Vas'culum, Pecu'lium, Virgula, Vir, Thyrsus, Tensus, Clavus, Cauda salax, Cauda, Fas'cinum, F. viri'lè, Muto, Nervus, N. fistulo'sus* seu *fistula'ris* seu *juveni'lis, Per'tica per se, Scapus, Leco, Curcu'lio, Vena, Contus, Telum, Gurgu'lio, Sceptrum, Arma, Gla'dius, Lubricum Caput, Muti'nus, Palus, Pes'culus, Radix, Ramus, Rutab'ulum, Arma Ventris, Columna existans inguin'ibus, Columna, Pyr'amis, Trala, Spina, Catapulta viri'lis, Verpa, Macha'ra, Taurus*; the *Yard, Male organ*, &c. (F.) *Verge, Membre viril*. This organ, the use of which is to carry the seminal fluid into the female organs of generation, is cylindroid, long, and erectile, and situate before and beneath the symphysis pubis. In the ordinary state, it is soft and pendent in front of the scrotum. During erection, it becomes elongated, upright, and assumes a triangular shape. Its upper surface is called the *Dorsum penis*, (F.) *Dos de la verge*; and, at its anterior surface, there is a longitudinal projection formed by the canal of the urethra. The two sides of the penis are round, and its posterior extremity or root is attached to the pelvis. Its anterior extremity is free, and presents the glans, prepuce, and orifice of the urethra. The penis is formed of the corpora cavernosa, the principal seat of erection; the corpus spongiosum of the urethra for the conveyance of the urine and sperm, and of the glans, which terminates the canal. The *Arteries* of the penis are branches of the internal pudic. The *Veins* correspond with the arteries. The *Nerves* are from the internal pudic.

PENIS CEREBRI, Pineal gland—p. Femineus, Clitoris—p. Lipodermus, Paraphimosis—p. Muliebris, Clitoris.

PENNATUS, Penniform.

PEN'NIFORM, *Pennifor'mis, Penna'tus*, from *penna*, 'a pen,' and *forma*, 'form.' An epithet for muscles whose fleshy fibres are inserted on each side of a middle tendon, like the feathers of a pen on their common stalk.

PENNYCRESS, Thlaspi.

PENNYROYAL, Mentha pulegium, Hedeoma pulegioides—p. Hart's, Mentha cervina.

PENSACOLA, see Saint Augustine.

PENSÉE, Viola tricolor — *p. Sauvage*, Viola tricolor.

PENSILIA, Pudibilia.

PENTAMY'RON, *Pentamœ'ron*, from πεντε, 'five,' and μυρον, 'ointment.' An ancient ointment, consisting of five ingredients. These are said to have been — storax, mastich, wax, opobalsam, and unguentum nardinum.—Paulus, and Aëtius.

PENTAPHAR'MACON, from πεντε, 'five,' and φαρμακον, 'remedy.' Any medicine consisting of five ingredients.

PENTAPHYLLUM, Potentilla reptans.

PEN'TATEUCH, (SURGICAL,) *Pentateu'chus*, from πεντε, 'five,' and τευχος, 'a book,' which signifies the five books of Moses—Genesis, Exodus, Leviticus, Numbers, and Deuteronomy. By analogy, some surgeons have given the name *Surgical Pentateuch* to the division of external diseases into five classes: — wounds, ulcers, tumours, luxations, and fractures.

PENTATH'ETUM, from πεντε, 'five,' and τιθεναι, 'to place.' An ancient plaster consisting of five ingredients.

PENULA, Ingluvies.

PENZANCE, CLIMATE OF. This is the chief residence of invalids in Cornwall, England, during the winter. It is situated on Mount's Bay, about ten miles from the Land's End. It is 5½° warmer in winter than London; 2° colder in summer; scarcely 1° warmer in the spring, and only about 2½° warmer in the autumn. It is a very favourable winter residence for the phthisical invalid.

PEONY, Pæonia.

PEPANSIS, Coction, Maturation.

PEPANTICOS, Maturative.

PEPASMOS, Coction, Maturation.

PEPAS'TIC, *Pepas'ticus*, from πεπαινω, 'I concoct.' A medicine supposed to have the power of favouring the concoction of diseases. Maturative.

PEPEIRUS, Concocted.

PEPINO, (S.) A *cucurbitacea*, which is cultivated in great abundance in the fields of Peru. The pulp or edible part is solid, juicy, and well flavoured; but is apt to disagree.

PEPO, Cucurbita pepo—p. Lagenarius, Cucurbita lagenaria—p. Vulgaris, Cucurbita pepo.

PEPPER, BLACK, Piper nigrum—p. Cayenne, Capsicum annuum—p. Cubeb, Piper cubeba—p. Guinea, Capsicum annuum—p. Jamaica, Myrtus Pimento—p. Long, Piper longum—p. Poor-man's, Polygonum hydropiper—p. Tailed, Piper cubeba —p. Turnip, Arum triphyllum—p. Water, Polygonum hydropiper—p. Water, of America, Polygonum punctatum—p. Wall, Sedum — p. White, Piper album.

PEPPERWORT, Lepidium.

PEPSIN, *Peps'inum, Chy'mosin, Gas'terase, Diges'tive Prin'ciple*, from πεψις, 'coction.' A peculiar organic matter, which in combination with the gastric acids, is considered to form the proper digestive solvent. Its chemical constitution is unknown. It would appear that its presence is necessary to induce changes in the elements of the food, which may enable the gastric acids to act upon them so as to form chyme.

PEPSINUM, Pepsin.
PEPSIS, Coction, Digestion.
PEPTIC, *Pep'ticus*, from πεπτω, 'I ripen.' An agent that promotes digestion, or is digestive. Also, applied adjectively to an article of food that is easy of digestion.

PEPTIC PERSUADER, see Pilulæ aloes et Kinæ Kinæ.

PERACUTUS, Catoxys.
PERARTICULATIO, Diarthrosis.
PERATODYNIA, Cardialgia.
PERCE-CRANE, Perforator.
PERCE-FEUILLE, Bupleurum rotundifolium.
PERCE-MOUSSE, Polytrichum.
PERCE-PIERRE, Crithmum maritimum.
PERCEP'TA, from *percipere*, 'to perceive,' 'receive.' A word used by some writers on hygiene to indicate, in a general manner, the effects of the nervous action on the animal economy; in other words, the sensations, the functions of the mind, and their deterioration or privation.

PERCEP'TION, *Percep'tio*. The appreciation which the brain has of an impression made upon an organ of sense.

PERCEPTIV'ITY. Same etymon. The power of perception.

PERCOLATIO, Filtration, Percolation.

PERCOLA'TION, *Percola'tio*, from *percolare*, (*per* and *colare*,) 'to strain through.' The terms percolation and *displacement* are applied in pharmacy to an operation which consists in placing any substance, the virtues of which have to be extracted by a menstruum, in a funnel-shaped instrument, having a septum perforated with holes, or its tube stuffed with cotton or tow, and pouring fresh portions of the menstruum upon it until all its virtues have been extracted. The operation is used in the formation of certain infusions, extracts, tinctures, &c.

An instrument used for this purpose is called a *displacer* or *per'colator*.

PERCOLATOR, see Percolation.

PERCUSS. *Percu'terĕ*, (F.) *Percuter, Frapper*. Same etymon as the next. To strike upon with the view of appreciating the resulting sound. To practise percussion.

PERCUS'SION, *Epicrou'sis, Percus'sio*, from *percutere*, (*per*, and *quatere*,) 'to strike.' When *immediate* or direct percussion is made on the chest or abdomen, the more or less perfect resonance is an index of the state of the contained organs; and the physician is thus aided in his diagnosis. For this purpose the chest may be struck with the fingers, gathered into a bundle, and their tips placed upon a level. It is better, however, to employ *mediate percussion*, which consists in interposing, between the point of the fingers and the chest, the finger of the other hand, or a *Plexim'eter*, and striking this instead of the naked chest.

PERCUSSION, AUSCULTATORY, see Acouophonia.

PERCUTER, Percuss.

PERCUTEUR COURBE À MARTEAU, (F.) An instrument used by Baron Heurteloup in the operation of lithotomy, in which a hammer is employed instead of a screw, to force together the blades of the instrument on the foreign body.

PERDO'NIUM. A medicated wine of herbs. — Paracelsus.

PERETERIUM, Trepan.
PERETORIUM, Trepan.
PER'FORANS, from *perforare*, (*per*, and *forare*,) 'to bore through.' A name given to different muscles, whose tendons pass through intervals between the fibres or tendons of other muscles; thence called *perforated*. See Flexor

Longus Digitorum, &c. Under the name *Perforating Arteries*, are included, 1. *In the hand*—arterial branches, given off by the profound palmar arch, which traverse the muscles and interosseous spaces. 2. *In the thigh*—three or four arteries, furnished by the profunda, which pass through the openings of the abductor magnus. 3. *In the foot*—the anterior and superior branches of the plantar arch.

PERFORANS CASSERII, see Cutaneous — p. Manūs, Flexor profundus perforans — p. Profundus, Flexor longus digitorum pedis profundus perforans.

PERFORATED SPOT, Locus perforatus.

PERFORATING ARTERIES, see Perforans.

PERFORATIO, Perforation — p. Cranii, see Perforator — p. Intestinorum, Enterobrosis — p. Ventriculi, Gastrobrosis.

PERFORA'TION, *Perfora'tio, Anatre'sis, Diatre'sis*, from *perforare*, 'to pierce.' An accidental opening in the continuity of organs, either from an external or internal cause.

PERFORATION, Paracentesis — *p. de l'Estomac,* Gastrobrosis — *p. des Intestins*, Enterobrosis — p. Uteri, Uterus, rupture of the.

PER'FORATOR, *Perforato'rium*, (F.) *Percecrane*. An instrument for opening the head of the foetus in utero, when it is necessary to diminish its size. The operation is called *Cephalotom'ia, Perfora'tio cra'nii*.

PERFORATORIUM, Perforator.

PERFORA'TUS. That which is pierced. Anatomists have given this name to muscles whose fibres or tendons separate to suffer other parts to pass through them. Such are the *Flexor brevis digitorum pedis, F. sublimis perforatus*, and *Coraco-brachialis*. Also, to parts that are perforated for any purpose — as the *substan'tia perfora'ta* of the brain.

PERFORATUS CASSERII, Coraco-brachialis.

PERFRIC'TIO, *Perfrige'rium, Catapsyx'is, Peripsyx'is*, from *perfrigere*, (*per*, and *frigere*,) 'to shiver with cold.' Considerable refrigeration. Great sense of cold: — shivering.

PERFRIGERATIO, see Rigor.

PERFRIGERIUM, Perfrictio.

PERFUSIO, Fomentation — p. Frigida, see Affusion.

PERI, περι, 'about, on all sides, round about.' An augmentative prefix. Hence:

PERIÆRE'SIS, from περι, 'about,' and αιρεω, 'I take away.' A sort of circular incision, which the ancients made in the neighbourhood of large abscesses. The periæresis is now only practised in some cases of tumours.

PERIAL'GIA, from περι, 'on all sides,' and αλγος, 'pain.' A very violent pain.

PERIAMMA, Amuletum.

PERIAPTON, Amuletum.

PERIBLEMA, Catablema.

PERIBLEP'SIS, from περι, 'around,' and βλεπω, 'I look.' The wild look that accompanies delirium. — Foësius.

PERIB'OLE, from περιβαλλω, 'I surround.' The dress of a person. The pericardium. Also, 'the translation of morbific matters towards the surface of the body.

PERIBRO'SIS, *Pericro'sis*, from περιβρωσκω, (περι, and βρωσκω, 'I eat,') 'I eat around.' Ulceration or erosion at the corners of the eyelids.

PERICAR'DIAC, *Pericar'dial, Pericardi'acus;* same etymon as the next. Relating to the pericardium, — as '*pericardial* murmur,' '*pericardial* effusion,' '*pericardial* arteries, veins,' &c., &c.

PERICARDIAL, Pericardiac.

PERICARDI'TIS, from περικαρδιον, 'the pericardium,' and *itis*, denoting inflammation; *Inflamma'tio Pericar'dii, Pleuri'tis pericar'dii, Cardi'tis exter'na seu aero'sa seu membrano'sa, Exocardi'tis, Inflamma'tion of the pericardium*, (F.) *Péricardite, Inflammation du Péricarde*. This is, probably, the proper appellation for most of those cases which have received the names of *Carditis, Cardipericardi'tis*, and *Cardiopericardi'tis*. Along with signs of pyrexia, the local symptoms resemble those of pneumonia. Those which point out that the pericardium is the seat of disease, are the following: — pain, referred to the region of the heart, or scrobiculus cordis, — sometimes pungent, at others, dull and heavy: palpitation, accompanied with spasmodic twitchings in the neighbourhood of the heart, shooting up to the left shoulder; pulsation, and sometimes soreness of the carotids, with tinnitus aurium and vertigo; the breathing is by catches; dyspnœa considerable; pulse jarring, jerking, peculiar: the tongue white, covered with a mucous coat, and the skin often bathed in sweat, as in acute rheumatism. The *physical signs* during the first period are as follows. The action of the heart is generally evident to the eye, and may be felt by the hand. There is soreness to the touch over the intercostal spaces, and over a small surface in the epigastric region, when the pressure is directed upwards towards the pericardium. Percussion is usually natural, but at times there is dulness. On auscultation, the cardiac movements are found to be frequent, abrupt, jerking, and tumultuous; often irregular and intermittent. The pulse presents corresponding characters. When effusion of lymph has occurred, percussion may be negative, or be but slightly affected. On auscultation, in addition to the preceding signs, there may be one or more of the rubbing or friction *bruits* resembling the rustling of parchment, or of a sawing or rasping character. In some cases, the sound is like the creaking of new leather. This has been supposed to be pathognomonic of effused lymph. The most important point in the pathology of pericarditis is its connexion with acute rheumatism; and it forms one of the most dangerous occurrences in the latter disease. It may be *acute* or *chronic*: in either case, it is, of course, formidable. The most active depletion must be used; with large doses of opium, counter-irritants, and all the means required in the most violent internal inflammations.

PERICARDITIS EXSUDATORIA SANGUINOLENTA, Hæmopericardium.

PERICAR'DIUM, *Pericar'dion, Perib'olē. Membra'na Cor circumplex'a, Involu'crum seu Ar'cula seu Capsa seu Cap'sula seu Cam'era seu Indumen'tum seu Pannic'ulus seu Membra'na seu Theca seu Saccus seu Sac'culus seu Scrotum seu Vagi'na seu Vesi'ca seu Arca seu Thal'amus regal'is seu Amphico'ma seu Bursa Cordis. Sac* or *Capsule of the Heart,* (F.) *Péricarde;* from περι, 'around,' and καρδια, 'the heart.' The pericardium is a membranous sac, which envelopes the heart, and the arterial and venous trunks that pass from or into it. It is seated in the separation of the mediastinum, above the central aponeurosis of the diaphragm, to which it strongly adheres. Its shape is triangular, like that of the heart; to which it is fitted. The pericardium is composed of two membranes: — the one — *external* — fibrous; the other — *internal* — serous. The latter, having lined the inner surface of the external layer, is reflected over the heart, and covers it entirely; without, however, having the least within it; in which arrangement it resembles other serous membranes. The pericardium envelops the heart; retains it in position, and facilitates its movements by means of the serous fluid, *Liquor* seu *Aqua* seu *Humor* seu *Lympha* seu *Uri'na Pericar'dii, Hydrocar'dia*, which it contains in greater or less quantity.

The *arteries* of the pericardium are small, and derived from the superior phrenic, anterior mediastinal and bronchial. The *veins* accompany them, and open into the brachio-cephalic. No nerves have been traced to it. The *lymphatics* enter the lymphatic glands that surround the vena cava superior.

PERICARPIUM. Epicarpium.

PERICHOLIA, Polycholia.

PERICHONDRI'TIS, *Inflamma'tio perichon'drii*, from *perichondrium*, and *itis*, denoting inflammation. Inflammation of the perichondrium: hence *Perichondri'tis laryn'gea;* — Inflammation of the perichondrium covering the larynx.

PERICHON'DRIUM, from περι, 'around,' and χονδρος, 'a cartilage.' A membrane of a fibrous nature, which covers cartilages that are non-articular, and bears considerable analogy to the periosteum in organization and uses.

PERICHRISIS, Circumlitio, Liniment.

PERICHRISTON, Circumlitio, Liniment.

PERICLA'SIS, from περι, 'about,' and κλαω, 'I break.' A comminuted fracture, with denudation of the bone. — Galen, Foësius.

PERICLYMENUM, Lonicera periclymenum — p. Vulgare, Lonicera periclymenum.

PERICNE'MIA, from περι, 'about,' and κνημη, 'the leg.' The parts surrounding the tibia; — the tibia itself.

PERICRANICEDE'MA, from *pericranium*, and οιδημα, 'a swelling.' Œdema of the head, owing to fluid effused under the pericranium.

PERICRA'NIUM, *Pericra'nion, Pericra'nia*, from περι, 'around,' and κρανιον, 'the cranium.' The periosteum, which covers the cranium externally.

PERICRASIS, Peribrosis.

PERIDE'RIA, from περι, 'around,' and δερη, 'the neck.' Twisting of the cord round the neck of the child.

PERIDES'MIC, *Perides'micus;* from περι, 'around,' and δεσμος, 'a ligament.' Some nosologists have given this name to ischuria caused by a ligature round the penis or by stricture of the urethra.

PERIDES'MIUM; from περι, 'around,' and δεσμος, 'ligament.' The delicate areolar tissue covering a ligament.

PERIDIASTOLE, see Diastole.

PERID'ROMUS, from περι, 'about,' and δρομος, 'a course.' The extreme circumference of the hairs of the head. — Gorræus.

PERIESTICOS, Salutary.

PERIGLOTTIS, Epiglottic gland: see Tongue.

PERIG'RAPHE, from περιγραφω, (περι, and γραφω, 'I write,') 'I circumscribe.' The aponeurotic intersections of the rectus abdominis are so called. — Vesalius.

PERILYMPH, Cotunnius, liquor of.

PERIMYELITIS, Meningitis, spinal.

PERIMYS'IUM, *Fas'cia*, from περι, 'around,' and μυς, 'a muscle.' The areolar membrane or sheath — *vagi'na muscula'ris* — that surrounds a muscle, or its fasciculi. The sheath of the whole muscle is termed *Perimysium externum;* of the fasciculi, *Perimysium internum*.

PERIN, *Peris*, from περα, 'a sac or pouch.' With some, this means the scrotum; with others, the testicle; with others, the vagina; with others, the peritonæum; and with others, the anus.

PERINÆOCELE, Hernia, perineal.

PERINÆ'UM, *Interfemin'eum, Interfæmin'eum, Interfæmin'ium, Interfæ'mina, Iter femin'eum, Peris, Perin, Perinæum, Gressu'ra, Plochas, Am'phiplex, Peche'deon, Mesos'celon, Mesos'celus, Perine'on, Perinæ'os, Perine'os, Tramis, Tauros, Interforamine'um, Cocho'ne, Plichos, Mesome'rion, Fœmen, Re'gio Perinæ'i*, (F.) *Périnée*. The space at the inferior region of the trunk, between the ischiatic tuberosities, anus, and genital organs. It is smaller in the female than in the male; has a triangular shape, and is divided into two equal parts by a median line, called *Raphé*. It is occasionally ruptured in labour. At times, it has been made to extend posteriorly as far as the os coccygis. The part between the pudendum and anus is sometimes called *ante'rior perinæ'um*, to distinguish it from that which extends from the anus to the coccyx, called *poste'rior perinæ'um*.

PERINÆUS, Perineal.

PERINE'AL, *Perinæ'us, Perinæa'lis, Perinea'lis*. That which relates or belongs to the perinæum; as *Perineal artery, P. hernia*, &c.

PERINEAL APONEUROSIS, P. Fascia.

PERINEAL ARTERY, *Arte'ria perinæa'lis, Superficial artery of the Perinæ'um*. A branch of the internal pudic distributed to the perinæum.

PERINEAL CUTANEOUS NERVE, see Sciatic nerve, lesser.

PERINEAL FAS'CIA, *F. Perinæ'i, Perine'al aponeuro'sis*. The fasciæ, — *superficial* and *deepseated*—*Perine'al lig'ament* — *Camper's ligament, Trian'gular lig'ament,*—which belong to the perinæum.

PERINE'AL FOSSA, *Fossa perinæ'i, Ischio-rectal fossa*. A conical fossa, the base of which corresponds with the skin; is formed anteriorly by the transversus perinæi muscle; behind, by the inferior border of the glutæus maximus; internally, by the levator ani; and externally, by the tuber ischii. It is filled up with fat and fibrous striæ.

PERINEAL ISCHURIA, *Ischu'ria Perinea'lis*. A name given by Sauvages to retention of urine, caused by a tumour seated in the perinæum.

PERINEAL LIGAMENT, see P. fascia.

PERINEAL NERVE. A branch of the internal pudic; which is mainly distributed to the perinæum and scrotum of the male; and to the vulva and perinæum of the female.

PERINEAL REGION, Perinæum.

PÉRINÉE, Perinæum.

PERINEPHRI'TIS, (F.) *Phlegmon périnéphrétique*, from περι, 'around,' νεφρος, 'kidney,' and *itis*, denoting inflammation. Inflammation of the external areolar and fibrous membranes of the kidney, or of their investing adipose areolar tissue.

PERINEPHRUS, see Kidney.

PERINEURION, Neurilemma.

PERINYC'TIDES, περι, and νυξ, 'night.' An eruption appearing at night and disappearing by day. — Erotian.

PE'RIOD, *Periodus, Periodei'a, Periodeu'sis, Sta'dium, Circu'itus*, from περι, 'about,' and 'οδος, 'way;' *Circuit*. Periods are the different phases or revolutions of a disease,—the epochs which are distinguishable in the course of a disease. Three periods are commonly enumerated. 1. The *augmentation, increase,* or *progress*, (*Incremen'tum ;*) 2. The *acme* or *height*, (F.) *État (Status ;)* and, 3. The *decline* (*Decrementum*.) Some authors reckon only the *invasion* and *termination*.

Period is sometimes used in describing an intermittent, for the time between the commence ment of a paroxysm and that of the next, including the fit as well as interval.

PERIODS, MONTHLY, Menses.

PERIODEIA, Period.

PERIODEUSIS, Period.
PERIODEUTES, Charlatan.
PERIODIC"ITY, *Periodic"itas,Rhythm;* same etymon. The aptitude of certain physiological and pathological phenomena, in health or disease, to recur at particular periods, after longer or shorter intervals, during which they cease completely. Diseases, thus recurring, are called *Periodical* or *rhyth'mical — Typo'ses.*

PERIODOL'OGY, *Periodolog"ia;* from περιοδος, 'a course or circuit,' and λογος, 'a discourse.' The doctrine of periodicity in health and disease.

PERIODONTI'TIS, (F.) *Périodontite, Inflammation de la Membrane alvéolo-dentaire,* from περι, 'about,' and οδους, 'a tooth.' Inflammation of the membrane that lines the socket of a tooth.
PERIODONTITIS GINGIVARUM, Ulitis.

PERIOD'OSCOPE; from περιοδος, 'a period,' and σκοπεω, 'I view.' An instrument, proposed by Dr. Tyler Smith, for the ready calculation of the periodical functions of the sex. It consists of a movable circular dial, upon which the months and days are engraved, fixed on a pivot in the centre of a large plate on which are numbered the different conditions of the reproductive system, as conception, abortion, premature labour, hemorrhage, labour, &c. By a knowledge of the date of conception, say November 14th, and fixing the movable plate opposite the point on the fixed plate which indicates conception, the observer is enabled, at once, to see, that, allowing 280 days for gestation, labour may be expected about the 20th of August. The dial is made of card-board, and is affixed to a small volume, in which its uses and applications are explained.

PERIODUS MORBI, Type — p. Sanguinis, Circulation.

PERIODYN'IA, from περι, and οδυνη, 'pain.' A violent and extensive pain.

PÉRIONE, Decidua.

PERIOR'BITA, *Perios'teum or'bitæ,* from περι, 'around,' and *orbita,* 'the orbit.' An appellation used, by some, for the periosteum lining the orbit, which is a continuation of the dura mater. The inflammation of this periosteum is termed *Periorbi'tis* or *Periorbiti'tis,* and *Inflamma'tio perios'tei or'bitæ.*

PERIORBITIS, see Periorbita.
PERIORBITITIS, see Periorbita.
PERIOSTEITIS, see Periostitis.

PERIOS'TEUM, *Perios'teon, Periosteos, Perios'tium, Circumossea'lē, Membra'na ossis, Omen'tum os'sium, Circumossea'lis Membra'na,* from περι, 'around,' and οστεον, 'a bone.' The periosteum is a fibrous, white, resisting medium which surrounds the bones every where, except the teeth at their coronæ, and the parts of other bones that are covered with cartilage. The external surface is united, in a more or less intimate manner, to the neighbouring parts by areolar tissue. Its inner surface covers the bone, whose depressions it accurately follows. It is united to the bone by small, fibrous prolongations; and, especially, by a prodigious quantity of vessels, which penetrate their substance. The periosteum unites the bones to the neighbouring parts. It assists in their growth, either by furnishing, at its inner surface, as M. Béclard demonstrated, an albuminous exudation, which becomes cartilaginous, and at length ossifies; — or by supporting the vessels, which penetrate them to carry the materials of their nutrition. See Medullary membrane.
PERIOSTEUM INTERNUM, Medullary membrane — p. Orbitæ, Periorbita.

PERIOSTI'TIS, *Periostei'tis, Inflamma'tio perios'tei,* from *periosteum* and *itis,* denoting inflammation. Inflammation of the periosteum.

PERIOSTO'SIS. Tumour of the periosteum. Tumours are so called which are developed on bones, and formed by their outer membrane. These tumours are more rapidly developed, have a less degree of consistence, and sooner disperse than exostoses, which they resemble greatly.

PERIPHERAL, see Peripheral aspect.
PERIPH'ERAL, *Periph'eric, Peripher'ical;* from περι, 'around,' and φερω, 'I bear.' Relating or appertaining to the periphery or circumference.

PERIPHERAL ASPECT. An aspect towards the circumference of an organ.—Barclay. *Periph'erad* is used by the same writer adverbially to signify 'towards the peripheral aspect.'

PERIPHERAL VASCULAR SYSTEM, Capillary system.
PERIPHIMOSIS, Paraphimosis.
PERIPLEUMONIA, Peripneumonia.
PERIPLOCA INDICA, Hemidesmus Indicus.

PERIP'LYSIS, from περι, and πλυσις, 'the act of washing;' *Proflu'vium.* A copious discharge from any part, especially from the bowels.

PERIPNEUMO'NIA, *Peripleumo'nia, Peripneumoni'tis, True peripneu'mony,* from περι, 'around,' and πνευμων, 'the lung.' Inflammation of the substance of the lungs. — See Pneumonia.

PERIPNEUMONIA BILIO'SA. Inflammation of the lungs, accompanied with bilious fever.

PERIPNEUMO'NIA CATARRHA'LIS. Bronchitis or pulmonary catarrh, with pain in some part of the chest. Peripneumonia notha.

PERIPNEUMO'NIA NOTHA, *P. spu'ria, P. pituito'sa, P. catarrha'lis, Pneumo'nia notha, Pseudoperipneumonia, Pseudo-pneumoni'tis, Bronchoc'ace, Blennotho'rax, Obstruc'tio pulmo'num pituito'sa febri'lis, Bronchi'tis asthen'ica, False* or *Bastard Peripneu'mony.* (F.) *Péripneumonie bâtarde* ou *fausse.* An inexact name, under which some affections are comprised that resemble pneumonia; and, especially chronic bronchitis with pleurodynia. — See Bronchitis (chronic.)

PERIPNEUMONIA PITUITOSA, P. notha.
PERIPNEUMONITIS, Peripneumonia.
PERIPNEUMONY, Pneumonia — p. Bastard, Peripneumonia notha.

PERIPNEUMONY, LATENT. Peripneumony whose symptoms are so obscure as to be recognised with difficulty.

PERIPSYXIS, Catapsyxis, Perfrictio.
PERIPYE'MA, from περι, 'about,' and πυον, 'pus.' Suppuration around an organ; — a tooth, for example.

PERIRRHŒ'A, *Perir'rhoē,* from περι, 'about,' and ρεω, 'I flow.' Afflux of fluids from every point of the body towards an organ which has to remove them from the economy. Also, enuresis.

PERIS, Perin.
PERISCELIS, *Jarretière.*
PERISCYPHISMUS, Periscythismus.

PERISCYTHIS'MUS, *Periscy'thisis, Perys'cytis'mus, Periscy'tisis, Periscy'phisis, Periscyphismus, Scalping,* from περι, 'around,' and Σκυθης, 'a Scythian,' that is, 'scalping after the manner of the Scythians.' An operation described by Paulus of Ægina. It consisted of an incision made around the cranium, and was employed in habitual weakness of the eyes, pains of the head, &c.

PERISPHAL'SIS, *Circumduc'tio,* from περι, 'about,' and σφαλλω, 'I move.' A circular motion impressed on a luxated bone, for the purpose of reducing it.

PERISSODACTYLUS, Polydactylus.

PERISTALTIC, Systaltic — p. Action, Peristole.

PERISTAPHYLINUS EXTERNUS, Circumflexus musculus — p. Inferior, Circumflexus musculus — p. Internus, Levator palati.

PERISTERA ANCEPS, Pelargonium anceps.

PERISTERIUM, Verbena officinalis.

PERISTER'NA, from περι, 'about,' and στερνον, 'the sternum.' The lateral parts of the chest.

PERIS'TOLĒ, *Motus Perital'ticus, M. compresso'rius* seu *vermicula'ris* seu *testudin'eus*, from περι, 'around,' and στελλω, 'I contract,' 'I close.' The *peristaltic action* of the intestines, *Motus peristal'ticus*. It consists of a kind of undulation or vermicular movement, in appearance irregular, but in which the circular fibres of the muscular membrane of the intestine contract successively, from above downwards, in proportion as the chyme advances in the alimentary canal; so that, being compressed above, it is pushed into the next portion of the intestine, whose fibres are in a state of relaxation. When the fibres contract inversely, they occasion an *antiperistaltic action*. The peristaltic action is involuntary, and is not under the immediate influence of either brain or spinal marrow. It continues for some time after death.

PERISTOMA, Peristroma.

PERISTOMIUM, Mouth.

PERISTRO'MA, *Peris'toma, Mus'cus villo'sus, Crusta membrana'cea, Crusta vermicula'ris*, from περι, 'around,' and στρωννυμι, 'to spread.' The villous or mucous coat of the intestines.—Castelli.

PERISYS'TOLĒ, from περι, 'about,' and συστολη, 'contraction.' The interval that exists between the systole and diastole of the heart, which is only perceptible in the dying.—Bartholine.

PERITERION, *Trépan perforatif*.

PERITESTIS, Albuginea.

PÉRITOINE, Peritonæum.

PERITOME, Circumcision.

PERITONÆRIX'IS, *Peritonæorex'is*, from περιτοναιον, 'the peritonæum,' and ρηγνυω, 'I break.' Hernia formed by the rupture of the peritonæum.

PERITONÆ'UM, *Peritone'um, Peritonæ'on, Peritonei'on, Peritonæ'os, Peritoni'on, Peritoneos, Velamen'tum abdomina'lē, Tu'nica prætension'ea* seu *Operimen'tum prætensum* seu *Membra'na abdominis, Siphar, Syphar, Zepach, Ziphac*, (F.) *Péritoine*, from περι, 'around,' and τεινω, 'I stretch.' A serous membrane, which lines the abdominal cavity; extends over the greater part of the organs contained there; envelops them wholly or in part, and maintains their respective relations by means of different prolongations and ligamentous folds:—the *mesentery, epiploon, mesocolon*, &c. Like all the serous membranes, the peritonæum is a sort of sac without aperture, which covers the abdominal organs, without containing them within it, and the internal surface of which is smooth, and lubricated by a serous fluid. In the male fœtus, the peritonæum furnishes a prolongation, which accompanies the testicle at the time of its descent, and, in the female fœtus, forms the *Canal of Nuck*. Below the neck of the gall-bladder, the peritonæum has a triangular opening, called the *Foramen* or *Hiatus of Winslow*, through which it proceeds behind the stomach, to form a sort of secondary cavity, called the *posterior cavity of the peritonæum*, (F.) *Arrière cavité péritonéale* ou *Cavité des Epiploons*.

PERITONÆUM DUPLICATUM, Epiploon, gastrocolic.

PÉRITONITE, Peritonitis — *p. Puerpérale*, see Peritonitis.

PERITONI'TIS, *Empres'ma Peritonitis, Peritonæi'tis, Cauma Peritonitis, Inflamma'tio Peritonæ'i, Phleg'monē peritonæ'i, Phlegma'sia* or *Inflammation of the Peritonæ'um*, from *peritoneum*, and *itis*, denoting 'inflammation.' (F.) *Péritonite, Inflammation du Péritoine*. The characteristic signs of acute inflammation of the peritonæum are, — violent pain in the abdomen, increased by the slightest pressure, often by the simple weight of the bed-clothes. It generally occurs in the parturient state; and begins on the second or third day after delivery. At times, a malignant epidemic, and perhaps contagious, variety has made its appearance, and destroyed numbers of females. This has been described under the name *Puer'peral Fever, Metroperitoni'tis, Ene'cia Syn'ochus Puerpera'rum*, (F.) *Péritonite puerpérale, Métropéritonite puerpérale, Fièvre puerpérale, Typhus puerpéral, Erythemat'ic* or *Nonplas'tic Puerperal Peritonitis, Typhohæ'mic Peritoni'tis, Adynam'ic* or *Malig'nant Puer'peral Fever, Low Fever of Childbed*. It is, according to some, a malignant inflammation of the peritonæum and uterus; according to others, a *Uterine Phlebitis*. In any form it requires active treatment, early employed. The appearances on dissection are such as occur whenever a serous membrane has been inflamed, and such inflammation has produced death :— effusion of fluid with flakes of coagulable lymph in it; appearances of vascularity, &c., in the membrane. The treatment—in *active peritonitis*—must consist of the same course as recommended under Enteritis. In the *chronic* kind, symptoms must be combated as they arise, and it may be advisable to excite a new action in the system by means of mercury. In the epidemic and malignant variety, unless bleeding be freely employed at the very outset, it does harm. If used early, it is of decided advantage. Every thing depends upon arresting the morbid process at the outset.

PERITONITIS, ERYTHEMATIC, see Peritonitis — p. Nonplastic, see Peritonitis — p. Puerperal, see Peritonitis — p. Typhohæmic, see Peritonitis.

PERITTOMA, Excrement.

PERITYPHLI'TIS; from περι, 'around,' and *typhlitis*, inflammation of the cæcum. Inflammation of the areolar substance surrounding the cæcum. See Typhlo-enteritis.

PERIWINKLE, LESSER, Vinca minor.

PERIZO'MA, from περιζωννυμι, (περι, and ζωννυμι, 'to gird,') 'to gird around.' A bandage; a girdle. In Fabricius Hildanus, a truss. Herpes zoster. The diaphragm.

PER'KINISM. A therapeutical means, first employed by Dr. Elisha Perkins, of Norwich, Connecticut, towards the termination of the last century, and named after him. It consisted in drawing over affected or other parts the pointed extremities of two metallic rods, called *Metallic Tractors*, each made of a different metal. The success obtained, was through the influence of the imagination; and, consequently, as a remedial agent, it ranks as high as animal magnetism, but no higher. The operation was, also, called *Tractora'tion*.

PER'KINIST. A believer in and practiser of Perkinism.

PERKINIS'TIC. Relating or belonging to Perkinism.

PERLA, Pearl, Paralampsis.

PERLĒ, Pearl.

PERMISTIO, Coition.

PERMIXTIO, Coition.

PERMOTIO, Motion.
PERNICIEUX, Deleterious.
PERNICIOSUS, Deleterious.
PERNIO, Chilblain.
PERNOCTATIO, Insomnia.
PEROCEPH'ALUS, from πηρος, 'deficient,' and κεφαλη, 'head.' A monster with a defective head.
PEROCOR'MUS, *Oligospon'dylus*, from πηρος, 'defective,' and κορμος, 'trunk.' A malformation in which the trunk is defective, and too short, from the absence of one or more vertebræ, — the head and limbs being normal.
PERODACTYLEUS, Flexor longus digitorum pedis profundus perforans.
PERODYNIA, see Cardialgia.
PEROMEL'IA, from πηρος, 'wanting,' and μελος, 'a limb.' Congenital misconstruction, or mutilation of the limbs. A genus in the nosology of Good.
PEROM'ELUS. A monster possessed of the deformity mentioned above.
PÉRONÉ, Fibula— *p. Col du*, Collum fibulæ.
PERONE'AL, *Peronœ'us, Fibula'ris, Fib'ular*, from περονη, 'the fibula.' Belonging or relating to the fibula.
PERONEAL ARTERY, *Fib'ular A.*, arises from the popliteal, and is situate deeply in the posterior and outer part of the leg. It gives off branches of little importance. Near the outer ankle, it divides into two branches. 1. The *posterior peroneal*, which descends behind the lower joint of the fibula, on the outer surface of the calcaneum. 2. The *anterior peroneal*, which crosses the inferior extremity of the interosseous ligament, to be distributed on the dorsal surface of the foot.
PERONEAL MUSCLES are three in number. 1. *Peronæus Brevis, P. Secundus, P. anti'cus, P. Me'dius, Semi-fibulæ'us*, (F.) *Grand-péronéo-sus-métatarsien, Court péronéo-latéral, Moyen Péronier*. A muscle, situate beneath the peronæus longus. It is attached above, to the outer surface of the fibula, and terminates, below, at the posterior extremity of the 5th metatarsal bone, after having been reflected beneath the malleolus externus. It extends the foot upon the leg, at the same time raising a little the outer edge. It may, also, act upon the leg, and extend it upon the foot. 2. *Peronæus Longus, Peronæus primus seu posti'cus, P. max'imus seu poste'rior*, (F.) *Tibi-péronéo-tarsien, Long péronier latéral, Péronéo-sous-tarsien*, (Ch.,) *Muscle grand péronier*. This muscle is situate at the outer part of the leg. It is long, thick, and triangular above; thin, narrow, and flat below. It is attached above to the outer edge of the upper extremity of the fibula, and to the upper third of the outer surface of that bone. Below, it terminates at the outer part of the posterior extremity of the first metatarsal bone. This muscle extends the foot on the leg, turning its point outward, and raising its outer edge. It acts, also, upon the leg, which it extends on the foot. 3. *Peronæus Tertius, Nonus Vesa'lii*, (F.) *Péronier antérieur, Petit péronéo-sus-métatarsien* (Ch.,) *Petit Péronier*. A muscle, situate at the anterior, outer, and inferior part of the leg. It is long and flat, and is attached, above, to the inferior third of the anterior margin and inner surface of the fibula; terminating, below, at the posterior extremity of the 5th metatarsal bone. This muscle bends the foot on the leg, by raising its outer edge. It can, also, bend the leg on the foot.
PERONEAL NERVE, see Popliteal nerves.
PERONEAL VEIN follows the same course as the artery.

PERONE DACTYLIUS, Flexor longus digitorum pedis profundus perforans.
PÉRONÉO-LATÉRAL COURT, Peronæus brevis — *p. Phalanginien du gros orteil*, Flexor longus pollicis pedis — *p. Sous-phalangettien du pouce*, Flexor longus pollicis pedis — *p. Sous-tarsien*, Peronæus longus — *p. Sus-métatarsien*, Peronæus tertius — *p. Sus-métatarsien, grand*, Peronæus brevis — *p. Sus-phalangettien du pouce*, Extensor proprius pollicis pedis — *p. Tibi sus-phalangettien commun*, Extensor communis digitorum pedis — *p. Sus-phalangien du pouce*, Extensor proprius pollicis pedis.
PERONEUM, Fibula.
PÉRONIER, GRAND, Peronæus longus — *p. Latéral, long*, Peronæus longus — *p. Moyen*, Peronæus brevis — *p. Petit*, Peronæus tertius.
PERONODACTYLIÆUS, Flexor longus digitorum pedis profundus perforans.
PERONODACTYLIUS, Flexor longus digitorum pedis profundus perforans.
PEROSO'MUS, from πηρος, 'mutilated,' and σωμα, 'body.' A monster, whose whole body is imperfectly developed. — Gurlt.
PEROSPLANCH'NICA, from πηρος, 'wanting,' and σπλαγχνον, 'a viscus.' Congenital misconstruction of the viscera. A genus in the nosology of Good.
PERPENDICULUM HEPATIS, Suspensory ligament of the liver.
PERPERACU'TUS. 'Extremely acute.' An epithet applied to very violent and rapid diseases.
PERPLEXI MORBI, see Complication.
PERPLICA'TION, *Perplica'tio*; from *per*, 'through,' and *plico*, 'I fold.' A method of tying arteries, which consists in making a small incision in the side of the artery, near its bleeding orifice, introducing a small pair of forceps, seizing the open extremity, and drawing it backward, through the aperture made in the side of the vessel, so as to form a kind of knot.
PERROSIN, see Pinus abies.
PERSEA CAMFORA, See Camphor — p. Cassia, Laurus cassia — p. Cinnamomum, Laurus cinnamomum — p. Cubeba, Piper cubeba.
PER'SEA GATIS'SIMA, *Palta tree*. A slender, very high tree of Peru, with a small dome-like top, which grows on the eastern declivity of the Andes, and rises, at times, to the height of more than 60 feet. Its fruit, — (S.) *Palta* — which is pear-shaped, is generally much liked. It dissolves, like butter, on the tongue, and hence is called, in some of the French colonies, *beurre végétale*.
PERSEA PICHURIM, see Pichurim beans — p. Sassafras, Laurus sassafras.
PERSIAN FIRE, Anthracion.
PERSICA VULGARIS, Amygdalus Persica.
PERSICAIRE DOUCE, Persicaria.
PERSICARIA, Polygonum Persicaria — p. Minor, Polygonum Persicaria — p. Mitis, Polygonum Persicaria — p. Urens, Polygonum hydropiper — p. Wandspiked, Polygonum Virginianum.
PERSIL, Apium petroselinum — p. d'Ane. Chærophyllum sylvestre — p. Faux, Æthusa cynapium — p. de Macédoine, Bubon Macedonicum — p. de Montagne, Athamanta aureoselinum.
PERSIMMON, Diospyros Virginiana.
PERSOLATA, Arctium lappa.
PERSOLLATA, Arctium lappa.
PERSOLUTA, Arctium lappa.
PERSPICILLUM, see Spectacles.
PERSPIRABILE SANCTORIANUM, Perspiration.
PERSPIRA'TION, *Perspira'tio, Transpira'tio, Diffla'tio, Diap'noë, Diapnœ'a, Diapœu'sis. Perspirab'ile Sanctoria'num*, from *per*, 'through,'

and *spirare,* 'to breathe, exhale.' The *insensible transpiration* or exhalation continually going on at the surface of the skin and membranes. Sensible perspiration is called *sweat.* The perspiratory fluid is secreted by an appropriate glandular apparatus, termed by Breschet *diapnog"enous*, or *sudorip'arous glands, Gland'ulæ sudorip'aræ, Or'gana sudorip'ara, sweat glands,* consisting of a secreting parenchyma, situate beneath the true skin, and of spiral ducts, which open obliquely under the scales of the epidermis. A certain portion of the perspired fluid is thrown off by ordinary physical evaporation.

The *Pulmonary exhalation* or *transpiration* is that which takes place into the bronchia, and is sent out with the expired air.

PERSUDATIO, Diapedesis.
PERSULTATIO, Diapedesis.
PERTE, Metrorrhagia — *p. d'Appetit*, Anorexia— *p. de la Mémoire*, Amnesia—*p. de l'Odorat*, Anosmia—*p. de Sang*, Hæmorrhagia—*p. de la Voix*, Aphonia — *p. de la Vue*, Cæcitas.

PERTÉRÉBRANT, Perter'ebrans; from *per,* 'through,' and *terebrare,* 'to bore.' The French give this epithet to an acute pain — *Douleur pertérébrante*—which occasions a sensation like that which would be produced by an instrument penetrating and lacerating a part; — the pain from whitlow, for example.

PERTES BLANCHES, Leucorrhœa — *p. de Sang,* Metrorrhagia — *p. Séminales,* Spermatorrhœa — *p. Utérines,* Metrorrhagia — *p. Utérines rouges,* Metrorrhagia—*p. Utérines blanches,* Leucorrhœa.

PERTICA PER SE, Penis.
PERTURBATIONES ANIMI, Affections of the mind.
PERTURBA'TRIX, *(Medici'na)* .*Per'turbating Treatment,* (F.) *Méthode* ou *Médecine perturbatrice.* A mode of treatment in which very active means are employed, and such as impress upon diseases a different course from that natural to them. It is the antithesis to the *Medicina expectans.* Much evil has resulted from such treatment, especially in febrile diseases.

PERTUS'SIS, from *per,* a prefix denoting excess, and *tussis,* 'a cough.' *Tussis feri'na, T. convulsi'va, T. pu'eros strang'ulans, T. quinta, T. stomacha'lis, T. an'hela clamo'sa, T. stran'gulans, T. delas'sans, T. suf'focans, T. amphemer'ina, T. tussiculo'sa, T. spasmod'ica, T. asini'na, T. cani'na, Bronchi'tis convulsi'va, Bronchocephali'tis, Pneusis pertus'sis, Amphemer'ina, Orthopnœ'a tussiculo'sa, clango'sa, suffocati'va, clamo'sa, spasmod'ica, Ouculus, Bechorthopnœ'a, Bex convulsi'va, Bex therio'des, Hooping-cough, Whooping-cough, Chin-cough, Kin-cough, Kind-cough,* (Germ. Kind, 'a child,') (F.) *Coqueluche, Catarrhe* ou *Bronchite convulsive, Toux convulsive, T. quinteuse, T. bleue, Maladie cuculaire.* A violent convulsive cough, returning by fits, (F.) *Quintes,* at longer or shorter intervals; and consisting of several expirations, followed by a sonorous inspiration or *whoop.* The fits of coughing generally recur more frequently during the night, morning, and evening, than in the day. It is esteemed to be contagious, and attacks the young more particularly. It is rare for it to affect an individual for the second time. The duration is various,—six or eight weeks or more. Although the paroxysms are very violent, it is not a dangerous disease. It may, however, give rise to other affections, as convulsions, pneumonia, &c., when the complication is very dangerous, as the cause cannot be removed. Those children suffer the least, who evacuate the contents of the stomach during the fit. In the treatment, all that can be done is to palliate. It must be borne in mind, that the disease will, in time, wear itself out. If there be much tensive pain of the head, or fever, bleeding may be required, but it is seldom necessary. Narcotics occasionally afford relief, but it is temporary. Gentle emetics, given occasionally, when the paroxysms are long and dry, give decided relief, and aid in the expectoration of the morbid secretions. After the disease has continued for some weeks, and persists in part from habit, change of air is essential, and this, even should the change be to an atmosphere that is less pure.

PERU, see Lima.
PERUNCTIO, Inunction.
PERVENCHE, Vinca minor.
PERVER'SION, *Perver'sio,* from *per* and *vertere,* 'to turn.' *Dias'trophě, Diastrem'ma.* One of the four modifications of function in disease: the three others being augmentation, diminution, and abolition. The humourists used this term also to designate disorder or morbid change in the fluids.

PERVERSION DE LA TÊTE DES OS ET DES MUSCLES, Loxarthrus.
PERVIGILIUM, Insomnia, Coma vigil.
PES, πους, *Ichnus,* (F.) *Pied,* 'the foot.' The inferior extremity of the abdominal member, representing a bony arch, an elastic vault, which transmits the weight of the body to the ground. It is divided into three parts;—the *tarsus, metatarsus,* and *toes.*

PES ALEXANDRINUS, Anthemis pyrethrum—p. Anserinus, Chenopodium bonus Henricus, Facial nerve—p. Cati, Antennaria Dioica—p. Equinus, see Kyllosis — p. Hippocampi major, Cornu ammonis—p. Hippocampi minor, Hippocampus minor—p. Hippopotami major, Cornu ammonis—p. Hippopotami minor, Cornu ammonis—p. Leonis, Alchemilla.

PÉSANTEUR, Weight—*p. Spécifique,* Gravity, specific.
PÈSE-ACIDE, Acidometer—*p. Liqueur,* Areometer—*p. Sirop,* Saccharometer.
PES'SARY, *Pessa'rium,* from πεσσος, 'a small stone.' *Pessus, Pessum, Pes'sulus, Supposito'rium uteri'num, Glans, Lemnis'cus.* A solid instrument, composed of cork, ivory, or elastic gum, which is introduced into the vagina to support the uterus, in cases of prolapsus or relaxation of that organ; to keep vaginal hernia reduced, &c. The ancients made use of medicated pessaries, which they distinguished into emollient, astringent, aperient, &c. The form of pessaries is very variable;— round, oval, &c., according to circumstances.

PESSARY, EGYPTIAN, Ægyptius pessus.
PESSULUS, Pessary, Penis.
PESSUM, Pessary.
PESSUS, Pessary.
PEST, Plague.
PESTE, Plague.
PESTICHIÆ, Petechiæ.
PESTICIÆ, Petechiæ.
PES'TILENCE, *Pestilen'tia, Pestil'itas,* from *pestis,* 'a pest.' A malignant spreading disease; —applied especially to plague.

PESTILENCE, CHOLERIC, Cholera spasmodica— p. Glandular, Plague — p. Hæmagastric, Fever. yellow—p. Septic, Plague.
PESTILENT-WORT, Tussilago petasites.
PESTILENTIA, Plague — p. Hæmagastrica, Fever, yellow.
PESTILENT'IAL, *Pestilentia'lis, Pestilentia'rius, Pestilentio'sus, Pestilen'tus,* from *pestis,* 'a pest.' Relating to the plague. *Pestilential diseases* are those that bear some resemblance to the

plague, in respect to mode of propagation, symptoms, danger, &c.

PESTILITAS, Plague.

PESTIS, Plague—p. Acutissima, Plague — p. Adeno-septica, Plague — p. Americana, Fever, yellow—p. Bellica, Typhus—p. Britannica, Sudor Anglicus — p. Bubonaria orientalis, Plague — p. Contagiosa, Plague—p. Glandulosa, Plague — p. Glossanthrax, Glossanthrax — p. Inguinaria, Plague—p. Intertropica, Fever, yellow—p. Occidentalis, Fever, yellow — p. Orientalis, Plague—p. Septica, Plague—p. Variolosa, Variola.

PESTLE, Pilum—p. Spring, see Pilum.

PET, Fart.

PETALE, Phtheiriasis.

PETASITES, Tussilago petasites — p. Hybrida, Tussilago petasites—p. Officinalis, Tussilago petasites—p. Vulgaris, Tussilago petasites.

PETAURUM. A seat suspended by ropes, in which a person taking the exercise sat, and was tossed about by assistants.—Juvenal and Martial.

PETE'CHIÆ, *Petio'ulæ, Pestich'iæ, Pestic''iæ, Punctic'ulæ, Pur'pura malig'na, Por'phyra Græco'rum.* Small spots, similar in shape and colour to flea-bites, which occur spontaneously upon the skin, in the course of severe fevers, &c. They are, under such circumstances, signs of great prostration.

PETECHIÆ SINE FEBRE, Purpura simplex.

PETECHIAL SCURVY, Purpura simplex.

PETECHIANOSIS, Purpura hæmorrhagica.

PET'ELA TRIFOLIA'TA, *Shrubby Tre'foil, Swamp dogwood, Stinking Pra'irie Bush, Stinking ash, Wing-seed.* A tall indigenous shrub—family, Xanthoxylaceæ—which flowers in June. It has been used as a tonic and antiperiodic.

PETER'S PILLS, Pilulæ Aloes et Cambogiæ — p. Worm lozenges, see Worm lozenges, Sherman's.

PETICULÆ, Petechiæ.

PETIGO, Impetigo.

PETINA, Sole.

PETIOLUS, *Pediolus,* diminutive of *pes,* 'a foot. A footstalk or leafstalk of a plant. A petiole.

PETIOLUS EPIGLOTTIDIS. The root of the epiglottis.

PETIOLUS MALLEI, Manubrium mallei.

PETIT COURIER, Influenza—*p. Lait,* Serum lactis—*p. Lait d'Hoffmann,* Serum lactis Hoffmanni — *p. Mal,* see Epilepsy — *p. Sus-maxillolabial,* Levator anguli oris.

PETITE POSTE, Influenza.

PETRÆLEUM, Petroleum.

PETRÆUM, Solidago virgaurea.

PETRAPIUM, Bubon Macedonicum.

PÉTRÉOLE, Petroleum.

PÉTREUX, (OS,) see Temporal bone.

PETRO DEL PORCO, Bezoar of the Indian porcupine.

PÉTROLE, Petroleum.

PETRO'LEUM, *Petrolæ'um, Petrœleum, Petræoleum, Bitu'men Petroleum, Pissela'um In'dicum, Rock Oil, Petroleum Barbaden'sè, Barbadoes Tar,* (F.) *Pétrole* ou *Pétréole,* from πετρος, 'rock,' and ελαιον, 'oil.' A bituminous substance of a fetid odour, and bitter, acrid taste. It is semi-liquid, tenacious, semi-transparent; of a reddish-brown colour; insoluble in water and alcohol; combines with fixed and essential oils and sulphur; and is partially soluble in ether. The petroleum found at Gabian, near Béziers, in France, has been called *Oleum Gabia'num,* (F.) *Huile de Gabian, Petroleum ruorum.*

PETRO-OCCIP'ITAL, *Petro-occipitalis.* Belonging to the petrous portion of the temporal bone and to the occipital bone.

PETRO-OCCIPITAL SUTURE is formed by the junction of the petrous portion of the temporal to the occipital bone. It is a deep groove separating the bones, which have between them a thin layer of cartilage.

PETRO-SALPIN'GO-PHARYNGEUS. A fleshy fasciculus, which extends from the sphenoid bone, from the petrous portion of the temporal bone, and from the Eustachian tube to the upper part of the pharynx. See Constrictor.

PETRO-SALPINGO-STAPHYLINUS, Circumflexus—p. Salpingo-staphylinus, Levator palati—*p. Staphylin,* Levator palati.

PETRO-SPHENOID'AL, *Petro-sphenoida'lis.* Belonging to the petrous portion of the temporal bone and to the sphenoid bone.

PETRO-SPHENOIDAL SUTURE;— a name given to the small suture which is formed by the anterior edge of the petrous portion of the temporal bone and the posterior edge of the sphenoid.

PETROLEUM BARBADENSE, Petroleum.

PETROLEUM SULPHURA'TUM, *Bal'samum Sulphuris Barbaden'sè,*—(Composed of *petrol. Barbad.* ʒxvj, *flor. Sulph.* ʒiv) has been used as a pectoral; and as a detergent to ulcers. It has been accounted antispasmodic and sudorific. Dose, gtt. x to xxx. Externally, it is used as a stimulant and discutient.

PETROSAL, Petrous.

PETROSELINUM, Apium petroselinum — p. Macedonicum, Bubon Macedonicum.

PETROSUM, OS, see Temporal.

PETROUS, *Petro'sus, Petro'sal,* from πετρος, 'a stone.' Resembling stone; having the hardness of stone.

PETROUS GAN'GLION, *Petro'sal Ganglion, Ganglion of Anderech,* is formed by the glosso-pharyngeal nerve, shortly after it emerges from the jugular fossa. From this ganglion, M. Jacobson of Copenhagen traced an anastomosing loop through the cavity of the tympanum, which left branches there, and was thence reflected downwards to join the Vidian nerve.— See Otic Ganglion. This has been called the *Nerve of Jacobson, Tympan'ic branch of the glosso-pharyngeal,* and the inosculation, *Jacobson's Anastomo'sis.*

PETROUS PORTION OF TEMPORAL BONE, see Temporal Bone—p. Process, see Temporal Bone.

PETROUS SI'NUSES, *Petro'sal Sinuses,* are two venous sinuses of the dura mater, connected with the petrous portion of the temporal bone, and distinguished on each side, into: — 1. The *superior petrosal sinus.* It arises from the cavernous sinus; follows the upper edge of the petrous portion which affords it a gutter; passes into the great circumference of the tentorium cerebelli, and opens into the lateral sinus where the latter experiences a bend near the base of the pars petrosa. Its form is triangular. 2. The *inferior petrosal sinus* arises from the cavernous sinus at the same point as the last, with which it communicates at the moment of its origin. It descends between the inferior edge of the pars petrosa and the basilary process; and terminates in the lateral sinus, at the sinus or gulf of the internal jugular vein. It is triangular, and broader at its extremities than at the middle.

PETUM, Nicotiana tabacum.

PEUCE, Pinus sylvestris.

PEUCEA BALSAMEA, see Pinus abies.

PEUCEDANUM, *P.officina'lè,P.aloat'icum seu altis'simum seu panicula'tum seu terna'tum, Si'linum peuced'anum, Mar'athrum sylves'trè, Marathrophyl'lum, Pinastel'lum, Fænic'ulum porci'num, Bonus Ge'nius, Hog's Fennel, Sulphurwort,* (F.) *Queue de Pourceau, Fenouil de Porc, Family.* Umbelliferæ. *Sex. Syst.* Pentandria Digynia. The root has a strong, fetid smell—somewhat resembling that of sulphureous solutions—and an acrid, unctuous, bitterish taste. It has been recommended as antihysteric and nervine.

PEUCEDANUM ALSATICUM, Peucedanum—p. Altissimum, Peucedanum—p. Officinale, Peucedanum—p. Oreoselinum, Athamanta aureoselinum—p. Paniculatum, Peucedanum—p. Pratense, P. silaus.

PEUCEDANUM SILAUS, *P. praten'sĕ, Ses'eli praten'sĕ, Sium sil'aüs, Ligus'ticum sil'aüs, Cnid'ium sil'aüs, Saxif'raga vulga'ris, S. An'glica, Hippomar'athrum, Fœnic'ulum er'raticum, English* or *Meadow Sax'ifrage,* (F.) *Sĕsĕli des prés.* The roots, leaves, and seeds have been recommended as aperients, diuretics, and carminatives. Rarely used.

PEUCEDANUM TERNATUM, Peucedanum.
PEUPLIER NOIR, Populus.
PEXIS, Concretion.
PEY'ERI GLAN'DULÆ, *G. Peyeria'næ, Pey'eri Plexus glandulo'si, Gland'ulæ muco'sæ coagmina'tæ* seu *agmina'tæ* seu *mucip'aræ racema'tim conges'tæ intestino'rum, G. intestina'les* seu *plexifor'mes* seu *spu'riæ, Corpus'cula glandula'rum simil'ia* seu *Gland'ulæ in agmen congrega'tæ intestino'rum, Enterade'nes, Peyer's Glands, Ag'minated* or *aggregate glands.* Small glands or follicles, situate beneath the villous coat of the intestines. They are clustered together, having a honey-comb appearance—*Plaques gaufrées*—and are extremely numerous. They occur most numerously in the lower portion of the ileum. Their structure and functions are not well known.

PEZA, πέζα, Doric and Arcadian for πους, 'a foot.' The foot: according to some, the sole of the foot; and to others, the astragalus. The ankle.

PEZI'ZA seu PEZE'ZA AURIC'ULA, *Tremell'a auric'ula, Auricula Judæ, Auricula'ria sambu'ci* seu *sambu'cina, Exid'ia auric'ula Judæ, Meru'lius auric'ula, Fungus sambu'cinus, Agar'icus Auric'ulæ formâ, Jew's Ear.* This fungus is said to be astringent; but has chiefly been used as a gargle in relaxed sore throat.

PFEFFERS or PFÄFFERS, MINERAL WATERS OF, *Thermæ Piperi'næ, Th. faba'riæ.* These springs, which are in the Swiss Alps, are simply thermal: temperature 100° of Fahrenheit.

PHACE, *Pha'cea, Phacus,* φακη; a grain of the lentil, *Ervum lens.* Also, chloasma; the crystalline lens; and a flask for the application of heat, so called owing to its flattened lens-like shape.

PHACELLUS, Fasciculus.
PHACELUS, Fasciculus.
PHACHYMENITIS, Phacohymenitis.
PHACI, Ephelides.
PHA'CICUS, *Phaco'tus, Phaco'des;* from φακη, 'lens.' Lens-shaped, lenticular.

PHACI'TIS, *Phacoïdeï'tis, Lentī'tis, Crystalli'tis, Glenī'tis,* from φακος, 'a lens,' and *itis,* a termination denoting inflammation. Inflammation of the crystalline lens. Inflammation of the capsule of the lens is termed *Capsī'tis, Capsulī'tis,* and *Crystal'lino-capsulī'tis.*

PHACO'DES, Phacicus.
PHACOHYMENI'TIS, *Phakomeni'tis, Phachymeni'tis, Inflamma'tio cap'sulæ lentis;* from φακος, 'a lens,' 'υμην, 'a membrane,' and *itis,* denoting inflammation. Inflammation of the capsule of the crystalline.

PHACOIDEITIS, Phacitis.
PHACOMALACIA, Cataract, soft.
PHAC'OPIS, *Phaco'tus;* from φακη, 'lens,' and κοπις, 'a knife;' *Scalpel'lum lenticula'rĕ.* A lenticular-shaped knife.
PHACOPS'IS, from φακη, 'lens,' and οψις, 'vision.' The state of one who has chloasma or freckles on the face.

PHACOPTIS'ANA, *Pha'cium;* from φακη, 'lens,' and πτισανη, 'drink.' A drink of lentils. A poultice of lentils.

PHACOS, *Ervum lens.*
PHACOSCOTOMA, Cataract.
PHACOTUS, Phacicus, Phacopis.
PHACUS, Phace.
PHADARODES, Trachoma tuberculosum.
PHADAROSIS, Trachoma tuberculosum.
PHÆNIGMUS, Phenigmus.
PHÆNOMENOLOGIA, Semeiology.
PHÆNOMENON, Phenomenon.
PHAGÆNA, Boulimia.
PHAGEDÆNA, Boulimia, Phagedenic ulcer—p. Sloughing of the mouth, Cancer aquaticus—p. Gangrænosa, Hospital gangrene.

PHAGEDEN'IC, *Phagedæ'nicus, Depas'cens,* from φαγω, 'I eat.'
PHAGEDENIC ULCER, *Nomĕ, Phageda'na, Ulcus depas'cens* seu *obam'bulans* seu *feri'num,* is one which rapidly eats and corrodes the neighbouring parts.

Phageden'ic, in Materia Medica, is a substance used for destroying fungous granulations in ulcers, &c.

PHAKOHYMENITIS, Phacohymenitis.
PHALACRA, Calvities.
PHALACROMA, Calvities.
PHALACROSIS, Calvities.
PHALACROTIS, Alopecia.
PHALÆNA PINGUINALIS, see Ectozoa.
PHALAIA. A barbarous term, employed by Basil Valentine to designate a universal medicine or panacea.

PHALAN'GAL, *Phalan'gian, Phalangia'nus.* Having relation to a phalanx.
PHALANGARTHRI'TIS, from φαλαγξ, 'a phalanx,' αρθρον, 'a joint,' and *itis,* denoting inflammation. Gout in the fingers. Inflammation of the joints of the fingers.

PHALANGE, Phalanx.
PHALANGES DES DOIGTS, see Phalanx—p. of the Fingers, see Phalanx—*p. des Orteils,* see Phalanx—p. of the Toes, see Phalanx.
PHALANGETTES, see Phalanx.
PHALANGETTIEN. Professor Chaussier uses this term for any thing relating to the third phalanx of the fingers or toes,—*Phalangien,* for what relates to the first, — and *Phalanginien,* to the second.

PHALANGIAN, Phalangal.
PHALANGIEN, see *Phalangettien.*
PHALANGINES, see Phalanx.
PHALANGINIEN, see Phalangettien.
PHALANGIUM ESCULENTUM, Scilla esculenta.

PHALANGO'SIS, *Hispid'itas,* from φαλαγξ, 'a row of soldiers.' An affection of the eyelids in which the lashes are arranged in two or three rows. See *Trichiasis.* Also, dropping of the upper eyelid, from paralysis of the levator palpebræ superioris muscle.

PHALANX, *Phalan'gĕ, Phalango'ma.* Same etymon. A name given to the small bones which form the fingers and toes, because placed alongside each other like a phalanx. They are distinguished into the *Phalanges of the fingers, Ossa* seu *Ag'mina* seu *A'cies* seu *Artic'uli* seu *Scutic'ula* seu *Scu'tula* seu *Nodi* seu *Interno'dia* seu *Scytal'ides* seu *Con'dyli Digito'rum Manûs;* and the *Phalanges of the Toes, Ossa* seu *Artic'uli* seu *Interno'dia Digito'rum Pedis.* I. *Phalanges of the fingers,* (F.) *Phalanges des doigts.* They are, in each hand, fourteen,—three to each finger, and two to the thumb; and are situate one above the other. They are distinguished, numerically, reck-

owing from the base towards the tip of the finger.
1. The *first* or *metacarpal*, *Procon'dyli*, (F.) *Premières phalanges* ou *Phalanges métacarpiennes*.
2. The *second* or *middle phalanges*, (F.) *Secondes phalanges* ou *Phalanges moyennes, Phalangines*, (Ch.) 3. The *third phalanges, Metacon'dyli, Phalan'ges un'guium*, (F.) *Troisièmes phalanges* ou *Phalanges unguéales, unguifères, unguinales, Phalangettes* (Ch.), which terminate each finger, and support the nail. II. *Phalanges of the Toes*, (F.) *Phalanges des Orteils*. They are the same in number as those of the fingers, but much smaller, and of a very different shape.

The phalanges of a finger or toe are united with each other; and the first with the metacarpal or metatarsal bone. They are developed from two points of ossification; one for the superior extremity, and the other for the body and inferior extremity.

PHAL'ARIS CANARIEN'SIS, *P. ova'ta, Cul'tivated Canary Grass*, (F.) *Alpiste*. Family, Gramineæ. *Sex. Syst.* Triandria Digynia. The seed of this grass, *Canary seed*, (F.) *Graines d'aspic*, afford a nourishing meal. The ancients recommended them for allaying pains in the kidney and bladder.

PHALLAL'GIA, P*hallodyn'ia*, from φαλλος, 'the male organ,' and αλγος, 'pain.' Pain in the male organ.

PHALLANCYLOSIS, Chordee.

PHALLI'TIS, *Priapi'tis*, from φαλλος, 'the male organ,' and *itis*, a suffix denoting inflammation. Inflammation of the male organ.

PHALLOCAMPSIS, Chordee.

PHALLOCARCINO'MA, from φαλλος, 'the male organ,' and καρκινωμα, 'cancer.' Carcinoma or cancer of the penis.

PHALLODYNIA, Phallalgia.

PHALLON'CUS, from φαλλος, 'the male organ,' and ογκος, 'swelling.' Tumefaction of the male organ.

PHALLOPSOPH'IA, from φαλλος, 'the male organ,' and ψοφος, 'a noise.' Discharge of wind from the male urethra.

PHALLORRHAG"IA, from φαλλος, 'the male organ,' and ρηγνυμι, 'I break out.' Hemorrhage from the male urethra. Stimatosis.

PHALLORRHŒA, Gonorrhœa.

PHALLORRHOÏS'CHESIS, from φαλλος, 'the male organ,' ροη, 'discharge,' and ισχειν, 'to withhold.' Sudden arrest of a gonorrhœal discharge.

PHALLUS, Penis.

PHANEROG'AMOUS, *Phanerogam'ic*, *Phanerogam'icus*, from φανερος, 'evident,' and γαμος, 'marriage.' An epithet used by botanists for plants whose sexual organs are apparent. It is, consequently, the opposite to *cryptogamous*.

PHANTASIA, Delirium, Imagination.

PHANTASM, *Phantas'ma, Phanto'ma, Phasma*, from φανταζω, 'I make appear.' A phantom, false appearance, apparition. Hallucination. Derangement of the sense of sight or of the intellectual faculties, causing objects to be perceived, which are not before the eyes.

PHANTASMA, Pseudoblepsia.

PHANTASMATICUS, Phantasticus.

PHANTASMATOSCOPIA, Metamorphopsia.

PHANTASMOSCOPIA, Metamorphopsia.

PHANTAS'TICUS, Inebriant. Creating phantasms—*phantasmat'icus*.

PHANTOM, Fantom.

PHANTOMA, Phantasma—p. Obstetricium, Fantom.

PHARMACEIA, Poisoning.

PHARMACEUM, Apotheca.

PHARMACEUS, Apothecary.

PHARMACEUTA, Apothecary.

PHARMACEU'TIC, *Pharmaceu'ticus*, from φαρμακον, 'a medicine.' An epithet for every thing belonging to pharmacy. Thus, we say, *Pharmaceutical preparations*, &c.

PHARMACEUTICE, Pharmacy.

PHARMACEUTIST, Apothecary.

PHARMACIEN, Apothecary.

PHARMACOCATAGRAPHOLOG"IA. *Catagrapholog"ia, Ars for'mulas concinnan'di*, from φαρμακον, 'a medicine,' κατα, 'beneath,' γραφω, 'a writing,' and λογος, 'a description.' The art of writing prescriptions.—J. J. Plenck.

PHARMACOCHYMIA, Chymistry, pharmaceutical.

PHARMACODYNAM'ICS, from φαρμακον, 'a medicine,' and δυναμις, 'power.' *Pharmacodynam'icè, Dynam'ical Materia Medica, Pharmacodynam'ica doctri'na, Pharmacodynamiolog"ia*. A division of pharmacology, which considers the effects and uses of medicines.

PHARMACODYNAMIOLOGIA, Pharmacodynamics.

PHARMACOGNOS'IA, *Accognos'ia, Acognos'ia*, from φαρμακον, 'a medicine,' and γνωσις, 'knowledge.' A division of pharmacology, which treats of simples, or unprepared medicines.

PHARMACOLOGIA, Materia medica.

PHARMACOMA'NIA, from φαρμακον, 'a medicine,' and μανια, 'mania.' One who has a mania for prescribing or for taking medicine.

PHARMACON, Poison.

PHARMACOPŒ'IA, *Pharmacopœ'a*, (F.) *Pharmacopée*, from φαρμακον, 'a medicine,' and ποιεω, 'I make.' A work, containing a collection of formulæ for the preparation, &c., of medicines: generally published by authority. Formerly, a chemical laboratory, *Laborato'rium chym'icum* seu *pharmaceut'icum*.

PHARMACOPŒUS, Apothecary, Druggist.

PHARMACOPOLA, Apothecary, Druggist.

PHARMACOPOLE, Apothecary, Druggist.

PHARMACOPOLI'UM, *Apothe'ca, Offici'na, Taber'na Med'ica*. The shop of the druggist or apothecary, from φαρμακον, 'a medicine,' and πωλεω, 'I sell.'

PHARMACOPOS'IA, from φαρμακον, 'a medicine,' and ποσις, 'a potion.' A liquid medicine, especially one that is cathartic.

PHARMACO'SA MEDICAMEN'TA, from φαρμακον, 'a poison.' Medicines that contain poisonous substances.—Fallopius.

PHARMACOTHE'CA, φαρμακοθηκη, from φαρμακον, 'a medicine,' and τιθημι, 'I place.' A case for medicines.

PHARMACOTHERAPI'A, from φαρμακον, and θεραπεια, 'treatment.' Cure of diseases by remedies.

PHARMACTER, Apothecary.

PHARMACUM, Medicament, Poison—p. Ægyptiacum, Ægyptiacum—p. Amatorium, Philter.

PHAR'MACUM AD AURES, *Ægyp'tium Medicamen'tum ad Aures*. A name given to a medicine, composed of bitter almonds, white pepper, saffron, myrrh, opium, frankincense, castor, verjuice, sulphate of iron, vinegar, pomegranate-bark, unguentum nardinum, &c. It was believed to be useful for cleansing fetid ulcers in the ears.

PHARMACURGICUS, Apothecary.

PHARMACURGUS, Apothecary.

PHAR'MACY, *Pharmaci'a, Pharmaceu'ticè, Pharmax'is*, from φαρμακον, 'a medicine.' The art which teaches the knowledge, choice, preservation, preparation, and combination of medicines. It was formerly divided into *Galen'ical* and *Chym'ical*. The former, called after Galen, embraced the operations undertaken on medicines without chymistry; — the latter, *Chymical Pharmacy* or *Pharmaceu'tic Chymistry, Pharmacochym'ia*, comprised the preparation of medicines, founded on the chymical action of their principles.

PHARMAXIS, Pharmacy.

PHARNA'CEUM LINEA'RE. A South African plant, *Nat. Ord.* Paronychiaceæ, employed at the Cape in pulmonary affections. It is generally given in infusion.

PHARUS, Pharynx.

PHARYGATHRON, Pharynx.

PHARYGETHRUM, Pharynx.

PHARYNGÆ'UM (SAL.), from *pharynx*. A compound of cream of tartar, nitrate of potassa, burnt alum, and distilled vinegar. It was formerly employed, united with honey and plantain-water, to make gargles, which were advised in quinsy.

PHARYNGÉ, Pharyngeal.

PHARYNGE'AL, *Pharyngæ'us*, (F.) *Pharyngé, Pharyngien*. That which relates to the pharynx. A name given to the muscles, vessels, and nerves of the pharynx.

PHARYNGEAL ARTERIES. These are two in number. The one—*superior* or *pterygo-palatine, Ramus Pharyngæ'us supe'rior* of Haller — arises from the internal maxillary at the base of the zygomatic fossa, passes through the pterygo-palatine canal, and proceeds to be distributed to the pharynx and the corresponding part of the Eustachian tube. The other — the *inferior — Pharyngæ'a ascen'dens* of Haller — arises from the external carotid, on a level with the facial. It ascends along the lateral and posterior part of the pharynx, and divides into two branches: the one — the *pharyngeal*, properly so called — is distributed to the pharynx; the other — the *meningeal* — gives its branches particularly to the dura mater.

PHARYNGEAL NERVE. A branch sent by the pneumogastric to the pharynx. It descends behind the internal carotid; communicates with the glosso-pharyngeal; and divides, opposite the middle constrictor of the pharynx, into a great number of filaments, which anastomose, in a multitude of different directions, with filaments of the glosso-pharyngeal nerve, of the superior laryngeal branch, and of the first cervical ganglion. These different nervous filaments united constitute the *pharyngeal plexus*, the irregular meshes of which send numerous ramifications to the pharynx.

PHARYNGEAL VOICE, see Voice.

PHARYNGEMPHRAXIS, from φαρυγξ, 'the pharynx,' and εμφραξις, 'obstruction.' Obstruction of the pharynx.

PHARNGETHRON, Pharynx.

PHARYNGEURYSMA, Pharyngocele.

PHARYNGICUS, Pharyngeal.

PHARYNGIEN, Pharyngeal.

PHARYNGITE, Cynanche pharyngea — p. *Tonsillaire*, Cynanche tonsillaris.

PHARYNGITIS, Cynanche pharyngea.

PHARYNGITIS APOSTEMATO'SA. Abscess of the pharynx.

PHARYNGI'TIS, DIPHTHERIT'IC, *Angi'na pseudo-membrana'cea, A. membrana'cea, A. pellicula'ris, A. plas'tica, A. diphtherit'ica, A. malig'na, A. pseudo-membrano'sa, A. pestilentia'lis, Pharyngoc'ace, Pseudo-membranous Inflammation of the Throat,* (F.) *Angine couenneuse, A. gutturale couenneuse, A. pseudo-membraneuse, A. plastique, A. diphthéritique*. Diphtheritic inflammation of the pharynx. See Cynanche maligna.

PHARYNGI'TIS, FOLLIC'ULAR, *Follicular Inflammation of the Pharynx, Angi'na folliculo'sa of the Pharynx, Acne of the Throat*. Inflammation and enlargement of the follicles of the pharynx, occasionally extending to the larynx. Sometimes termed *Clergyman's Sorethroat, Tubercles of the Larynx* and *Fauces*, and *Tuber'cular Sorethroat*.

PHARYNGI'TIS, GANGRENOUS, Cynanche maligna.

PHARYNGOCACE, Pharyngitis, diphtheritic.

PHARYNGOCE'LE, *Pharyngeurys'ma, Divertic'ulum* seu *Hernia* seu *Prolap'sus Œsoph'agi* vel *pharyn'gis, Œsoph'agus succenturia'tus*, from φαρυγξ, 'the pharynx,' and κηλη, 'a tumour.' An enlargement at the upper part of the gullet, in which the food sometimes rests in considerable quantity.

PHARYNGODYN'IA, from φαρυγξ, 'the pharynx,' and οδυνη, 'pain.' Pain in the pharynx.

PHARYNGOGLOSSAL, *Glossopharyngeal, Pharyngoglossia'nus*. That which belongs to the pharynx and tongue.

PHARYNGOGLOSSAL NERVE, *Glossopharyngeal Nerve, Lingua'lis latera'lis*, (F.) *Nerf Glossopharyngien, Pharyngoglossien* — a portion of the eighth pair—arises from the superior and lateral parts of the spinal marrow, between the facial and pneumogastric nerves, by several filaments, which soon unite into a single cord, that passes out of the cranium by the foramen lacerum anterius; goes downwards and forwards, and gains the posterior and inferior part of the tongue. Immediately after its exit from the cranium, it gives a branch to the meatus auditorius externus, and receives a filament from the facial, and another from the pneumogastric nerve. It then furnishes two other filaments, which descend upon the carotid artery, and unite at the bottom of the neck with branches from the cervical ganglions and cardiac nerves, and give two filaments to the stylo-pharyngeus muscle. The glossopharyngeus, after sending a twig or two to the tonsil, to the upper part of the pharynx and membrane of the epiglottis, divides into many branches, which run partly to the margin, and partly to the middle of the root of the tongue; supplying, especially, the papillæ majores, and the parts in their neighbourhood.

By some, this nerve is regarded as the controller of the associated motions of the tongue and pharynx. By others, it is esteemed to be the special nerve of gustation.

PHARYNGOG'RAPHY, *Pharyngogra'phia*, from φαρυγξ, 'the pharynx,' and γραφη, 'a description.' An anatomical description of the pharynx.

PHARYNGOL'OGY, *Pharyngolog''ia*, from φαρυγξ, 'the pharynx,' and λογος, 'a discourse.' The part of anatomy which treats of the pharynx.

PHARYNGOLYSIS, Pharyngoplegia.

PHARYNGOPARALYSIS, Pharyngoplegia.

PHARYNGOPLE'GIA, from φαρυγξ, 'the pharynx,' and πλησσω, 'I strike.' *Dyspha'gia paralyt'ica, D. tor'pida, D. aton'ica, Angi'na paralyt'ica, Astheni'a Deglutitio'nis, Pharyngol'ysis, Pharyngoparal'ysis Paral'ysis Œsogph'agi, Gulæ Imbecil'litas*. Paralysis of the pharynx or œsophagus: commonly a symptom of general paralysis, or of approaching dissolution.

PHARYNGORRHAG''IA; from φαρυγξ, 'the pharynx,' and ραγη, 'rupture.' Hæmorrhage from the vessels of the pharynx.

PHARYNGOSPAS'MUS; from φαρυγξ, 'the pharynx,' and σπασμος, 'spasm.' Spasm or cramp of the pharynx.

PHARYNGOSTAPHYLINUS, Palato-pharyngeus.

PHARYNGOTOME, *Pharyngot'omus*, from φαρυγξ, 'the pharynx,' and τεμνω, 'I cut.' An instrument, invented by J. L. Petit, used to scarify inflamed tonsils, and to open abscesses, which form in the parietes of the pharynx. It is composed of a long, narrow blade with a lancet point, enclosed in a sheath or canula of silver slightly curved. This instrument is carried to the part to be cut, and the point of the blade is made to pass out of the sheath, by pressing on a button at the end of the pharyngotome. A spring causes the blade to re-enter as soon as the pressure is removed.

PHARYNGOT'OMY, *Pharyngotom'ia*; same etymon. Some authors have used this word synonymously with œsophagotomy. It means, also, scarification of the tonsils, or an incision, made for opening abscesses there, &c.

PHARYNX, *Pharyx*, *Pharus*, *Gula*, *Lœmos*, *Fauces*, *Pharyg'ethrum*, *Pharyn'gethron*, *Pharyn'gethros*, *Pharygathron*, *Isthmos*, *Isth'mion*, *Inglu'vies*, *Princip'ium Gulæ*, *Os pos'terum*, (F.) *Arrière-bouche*, *Gosier*. A species of musculo-membranous, symmetrical canal, on the median line, irregularly funnel-shaped, and situate between the base of the cranium and the œsophagus, in front of the vertebral column. It is very narrow above; but dilates in the middle, and again contracts below, at its junction with the œsophagus. Into the anterior paries of the pharynx open, successively, from above to below,—the posterior orifices of the nasal fossæ; the Eustachian tubes; the posterior aperture of the mouth, and the top of the larynx. The pharynx is formed, externally, of a muscular coat, and, internally, of a mucous membrane, which is continuous, above, with the Schneiderian membrane; and in the middle, with that of the mouth; below, with that of the œsophagus; and, at the sides, with that of the Eustachian tubes. This membrane has no villi, and presents only a few inequalities, which are owing to the presence of muciparous follicles. The muscular coat of the pharynx is composed of the constrictor muscles, stylopharyngei, and pharyngostaphylini. The vessels and nerves are called *pharyngeal*. The pharynx serves as a common origin for the digestive and respiratory passages. It gives passage to the air, during respiration; and to the food at the time of deglutition.

PHARYNX, FOLLICULAR INFLAMMATION OF THE, Pharyngitis, follicular.

PHARYX, Pharynx.

PHASELUS, Phaseolus.

PHASE'OLUS, *P. Vulga'ris*, *Phasi'olus*, *Phase'lus*, *Fase'lus*, *Fase'olus*, *Bona*, *Boona*, *Faba*; the *Kidney Bean*; the *French Bean*, (F.) *Haricot*. Family, Leguminosæ. *Sex. Syst.* Diadelphia Decandria. When young and well boiled, this is easy of digestion, and delicately flavoured. It is less flatulent than the pea.

PHASEOLUS CRETICUS, *Cajan*, *Cayan*. A decoction of the leaves, according to Ray, restrains the hemorrhoidal flux when excessive.

PHASEOLUS VULGARIS, Phaseolus.

PHASIA'NUS GALLUS, so called from the river Φασις, in Colchis, near the Black Sea: (F.) *Coq* The parts of generation of the cock, dried and pulverized, were formerly regarded as proper for increasing the quantity of semen. The fat was used as emollient and resolvent; the brain, in diarrhœa; the gall, in freckles and diseases of the eyes. These phantasies are now abandoned.

PHASIOLUS, Phaseolus.

PHASMA, Phantasm.

PHATNE, Alveolus.

PHATNION, Alveolus.

PHATNORRHAG"IA, *Stomatorrhag"ia* alveolo'rum, from φατνιον, 'an alveolus,' and ρηγνυμι, 'I break forth.' Hemorrhage from the alveoli.

PHAUSIN'GES, φαυσιγγες, plural of φαυσιγξ, from φαυζω, 'I roast.' Spots or blisters on the legs, produced by heat; and, in a more extensive signification, by any other cause. Also, a pustule.—Foësius.

PHELLANDRE, Phellandrium aquaticum.

PHELLAN'DRIUM AQUAT'ICUM, *Phellandrium*, *Œnan'thē phellan'drium seu aquat'ica*, *Ligus'ticum phellan'drium*, *Fœnic'ulum aquat'icum*, *Cicuta'ria aquatica*, *Water Fennel*, *Fine-leaved Water Hemlock*, (F.) *Phellandre*, *Fenouil d'eau*, *Ciguë d'eau*. Family, Umbelliferæ. *Sex. Syst.* Pentandria Digynia. This plant is stimulant and narcotic. It has been used in intermittents and dyspepsia. It has, also, been given in phthisis pulmonalis, and in cases of scrofulous atonic ulcers.

PHENIG'MUS, *Pharnig'mus*, *Pharnig'mus*, from φοινιξ, 'red.' *Red Jaundice*. A cutaneous affection, consisting of redness diffused over the skin, without fever. Sauvages makes it a genus of his order *Icteritiæ*. Also, the act of irritating a part by a stimulating application.

PHÉNOMÈNE, Phenomenon.

PHENOM'ENON, *Phænom'enon*, (P.) *Phénomène*, from φαινομαι, 'I appear. An extraordinary and unexpected event. In *Medicine*, it means any change, appreciable by our senses, which supervenes in an organ or function:—as the *phenomena* of the circulation, respiration, &c. It is used in pathology, synonymously with symptom.

PHEUGOPHOBIA, Hydrophobia.

PHEUGYDRON, Hydrophobia.

PHI'ALA, *A Phial* or *Vial*, (F.) *Fiole*. A small bottle, in which apothecaries are in the habit of sending out their mixtures, draughts, &c.: hence called *Med'icine Vials*, (F.) *Fioles à Médecine*. They are usually sold in grosses, and assorted into vials of oz. 8; oz. 4; oz. 3; oz. 2; oz. 1½; oz. 1; and oz. ½.

PHILADYNAMICA, Debilitants.

PHILANTHROPUS, Galium aparine.

PHILETRON, Philter.

PHILETRUM, Lacuna labii superioris.

PHILIATROS, φιλιατρος, from φιλεω, 'I love,' and ιατρικη, 'medicine.' An amateur of medicine. One who studies medicine; *Studio'sus medici'næ*.

PHILOBIO'SIS, (F.) *Philobiosis:* from φιλεω, 'I love,' and βιος, 'life.' The love of life.

PHILŒ'NIA, from φιλεω, 'I love,' and οινος, 'wine.' Love of wine. Addiction to wine.

PHILOGYNIA, Muliebrositas.

PHILONIUM LONDINENSE, Confectio opii.

PHILOPATRIDALGIA, Nostalgia.

PHILOPATRIDOMANIA, Nostalgia.

PHILOSOPHER'S STONE, see Alchymy.

PHILOSOPHIA CORPORIS VIVI, Physiology—p. Hermetica, Alchymy—p. per Ignes. Chymistry.

PHILTER, from φιλεω, 'I love.' *Philtrum*, *Phil'etron*, *Phar'macum* vel *Poc'ulum amato'rium*, *Amato'rium venefic"ium*, (F.) *Philtre*. A medicine or drink considered capable of causing love.

PHILTRUM, Lacuna labii superioris.

PHILYRA, Tilia.

PHIMA, Phyma.

PHIMOS, Capistrum.

PHIMO'SICUS. Relating to Phimosis. Sauvages calls *Ischu'ria phimo'sica*, *Ischu'ria urethra'lis à phimo'si*, the retention of urine which depends upon phimosis.

PHIMO'SIS, *Phymo'sis*, *Capistra'tio*, *Epspas'gium*, *Ligatu'ra glandis*, *Strictu'ra præpu'tii*,

Redúc'tio præpu'tii impedi'ta, from φιμοω, 'I bind up.' A disease which consists in a preternatural narrowness of the opening of the prepuce, so that it cannot be carried behind the corona glandis. This affection is most commonly congenital. Sometimes it is accidental, and dependent upon tumefaction of the glans, or of the prepuce, as occurs in syphilis. To remedy this state, the prepuce may be divided by means of a bistoury and director; or circumcision may be practised.

PHIMOSIS ADNATA seu CONGENITA seu PUERILIS, Congenital phimosis—p. Circumligata, Paraphimosis—p. Congenita, P. adnata.

PHIMO'SIS ŒDEMATO'DES, *Hydrophimo'sis*. Phimosis with œdematous swelling of the prepuce.

PHIMOSIS PUERILIS, Ph. adnata.

PHLASMA, Contusion.

PHLEBARTERIODIALYSIS, see Aneurism.

PHLEBECTA'SIA, *Phlebec'tasis*, from φλεψ, 'a vein,' and εκτασις, 'dilatation.' Dilatation of a vein, or of a portion of a vein.—Alibert.

PHLÉBECTIARCTIE. A mongrel term, from φλεψ, 'a vein,' and *arcto*, 'I contract.' Contraction of a vein.

PHLEBES, (Arteries.) See Artery.

PHLEBEURYSMA, Varix.

PHLEB'ION, diminutive of φλεψ, 'a vein.' A vein.—Hippocrates. A small vein,— *Ve'nula*.

PHLEBIS'MUS; from φλεψ, φλεβις, 'a vein.' A term employed by Dr. Marshall Hall for the turgescence of veins, produced by impeded return of the blood. See Trachelismus.

PHLEBI'TIS, *Inflamma'tio vena'rum*, (F.) *Inflammation des veines*, from φλεψ, 'a vein,' and *itis*, the termination for inflammation. Inflammation of the inner membrane of a vein, which sometimes follows blood-letting, and extends from the small wound made in that operation to the neighbouring parts of the venous system. The symptoms are, first, inflammation in the punctured part; and, afterwards, a knotty, tense, painful cord, following the direction of the vessel, and accompanied with more or less fever, according to the extent of the inflammation, the nervous symptoms, &c. Phlebitis, also, sometimes supervenes on the ligature or excision of varices; after amputation, gun-shot wounds, delivery (*Uterine Phlebitis, Metro-phlebi'tis puerpera'lis, Phlebi'tis uteri'na, Metri'tis veno'sa*), the ligature of the umbilical cord, &c. It may terminate by resolution, suppuration, ulceration, or gangrene.

PHLEBITIS, CRURAL, Phlegmatia dolens — p. Uterina, see Peritonitis, and Phlebitis.

PHLEBOG'RAPHY, *Phlebogra'phia*, from φλεψ, 'a vein,' and γραφη, 'a description.' A description of the veins.

PHLEB'OLITE, *Phlebol'ithus, Vein stone*, from φλεψ, 'a vein,' and λιθος, 'a stone.' A loose concretion, varying in size from that of a currant to that of a pea, occasionally found in the veins. It would seem to be formed in the blood.

PHLEBOLITHUS, Phlebolite.

PHLEBOL'OGY, *Phlebolog"ia*, from φλεψ, 'a vein,' and λογος, 'a discourse.' The part of anatomy which treats of the veins.

PHLEBOPA'LIA, from φλεψ, 'a vein,' and παλλω, 'I palpitate.' With the ancients, *pulsation*, which they conceived to be produced by the veins. See Pulsus venarum.

PHLEBOPHTHALMOTOM'IA, *Ophthalmophlebotom'ia*, from φλεψ, 'a vein,' οφθαλμος, 'the eye,' and τεμνω, 'I cut.' Blood-letting in the eye.

PHLEBOPLERO'SIS ECPHRACTICA, Inflammation.

PHLEBORRHAG"IA, from φλεψ, 'a vein,' and ρηγνυμι, 'I break out.' Rupture of the veins; and, in a more extensive sense, venous hemorrhage.

PHLEBORRHEX'IS, from φλεψ, 'a vein,' and ρηξις, 'rupture.' Rupture of a vein. Also, hemorrhage from a vein, *Phleborrhag"ia*.

PHLEBOSTENO'SIS; from φλεψ, 'a vein,' and στενωσις, 'contraction.' Constriction or contraction of a vein.

PHLEBOT'OMIST, from φλεψ, 'a vein,' and τεμνω, 'I cut.' A bleeder. One who practises particularly the art of phlebotomy. See Blood-letting.

PHLEBOTOMUM, Fleam.

PHLEBOTOMY, see Blood-letting.

PHLEBS, Vein.

PHLEDONIA, Delirium.

PHLEGM, *Phlegma, Pitui'ta, Pit'uite, Mucus*, (F.) *Pituite*. One of the four natural humours of the ancients, which, according to them, was cold and moist, as atrabilis was cold and dry. It predominated, especially, in winter.

Pituita was afterwards applied to every aqueous or excrementitious humour, such as the saliva, nasal and intestinal mucus, serum, &c. The terms *phlegm* and *pituita* are no longer used in physiology,—the different humours having received particular names; but the vulgar still use *phlegm* to designate a stringy mucus, expectorated, or rejected by vomiting. The ancient chymists gave the name 'phlegm' to aqueous, insipid, and inodorous products obtained by subjecting moist vegetable matters to the action of heat.

PHLEGMA NARIUM CRASSUM, Nasal mucus—p. Vitrioli, Sulphuric acid (very dilute.)

PHLEG'MAGOGUE, *Phlegmago'gus*; from φλεγμα, 'phlegm,' and αγω, 'I expel.' A medicine, formerly believed capable of "*cutting*" or removing phlegm.

PHLEGMAPYRA, Fever adeno-meningeal.

PHLEGMASIA, Inflammation, Phlegmon—p. Adenosa, Adenitis—p. Alba dolens puerperarum, Ph. dolens — p. Cellularis, Induration of the cellular tissue—p. Glandulosa, Adenitis—p. Myoica, Myositis—p. of the Peritoneum, Peritonitis.

PHLEGMA'TIA, from φλεγμα, 'phlegm.' Œdema, Anasarca, Hydrops.

PHLEGMA'TIA DOLENS, *P. lac'tea, P. dolens puerpera'rum, P. alba dolens puerpera'rum, Leucophlegmasia dolens puerperarum, Scelon'cus, Scelal'gia puerpera'rum, Anasar'ca sero'sa, Ecphy'ma œdemat'icum, Spargano'sis puerperarum, Ecchymo'ma lymphat'icum, Is'chias a spargano'si, Œde'ma puerperarum, Œd. lacteum, Infarc'tus lac'tei extremita'tum, Metas'tasis lactis, Hysteral'gia galac'tica, Hydrophlegma'sia textûs cellulo'si, Crural Phlebi'tis, White leg, Swelled leg, Milk leg, White swelling of lying in women*, (F.) *Œdème des nouvelles accouchées, Œdème douleureux des femmes en couche, Dépôt laiteux sur la cuisse, Œdème actif des nouvelles accouchées, Enflure ou Engorgement des jambes et des cuisses de la femme accouchée, E. laiteux des membres abdominaux*. It occurs, for the most part, in the second or third week after delivery:—is limited to the lower extremity, and chiefly to one side; exhibiting to the touch a feeling of numerous irregular prominences under the skin. It is hot, white, and unyielding; and is accompanied, sooner or later, with febrile excitement. After a few days, the heat, hardness, and sensibility diminish, and the limb remains œdematous for a longer or shorter period. The disease frequently, if not generally, consists in the obstruction of the iliac or other veins. Owing to the pressure of the gravid uterus — the flow of blood being obstructed—the serous part of it is thrown into the cellular membrane of the limb. Sometimes the vein is found completely obliterated.

The treatment consists in the use of antiphlogistics:— the application of leeches or cuppingglasses near the groin: fomentations to the limb, &c.; and, when the active state has subsided, the use of a roller, applied gently at first, but, afterwards, gradually tightened.

PHLEGMATIA LACTEA, P. dolens.

PHLEGMATIÆ, see Empresma—p. Membranosæ et parenchymatosæ, Empresma.

PHLEGMATOPYRA, Fever, adeno-meningeal.

PHLEGMATORRHAG"IA, *Phlegmatorrhœ'a, Catarrh*, from φλεγω, 'phlegm,' and ρεω, 'I flow.' Stahl and his partisans gave this name to a copious secretion, by the nostrils, of a limpid and thin mucus, without inflammation. It is the *Cory'za Phlegmatorrhag''ia* of Sauvages. See Coryza.

PHLEGMHYMENITIS, Phlegmymenitis.

PHLEGM'ON, from φλεγω, 'I burn.' *Phlogo'sis phleg'monē, Phleg'monē, Phlegma'sia, Incen'dium, Inflamma'tio.* Inflammation of the areolar texture accompanied with redness, circumscribed swelling, increased heat and pain; which is, at first, tensive and lancinating; afterwards, pulsatory and heavy. It is apt to terminate in suppuration. It requires the antiphlogistic treatment, until suppuration seems inevitable, when the suppuration must be encouraged as the next favourable termination to resolution.

PHLEGMON PÉRINÉPHRÉTIQUE, Periphrenitis.

PHLEGMONE, Inflammation—p. Mammæ, Mastodynia apostematosa—p. Mastodynia, Mastodynia apostematosa—p. Parotidæa, Parotis—p. Peritonæi, Peritonitis—p. Parulis, Parulis—p. Musculorum, Myositis—p. Ventriculi, Gastritis.

PHLEGMONODES, Phlegmonous.

PHLEGMONOID, Phlegmonous.

PHLEG'MONOUS, *Phlegmono'des, Phleg'monoid*, from φλεγμονη, 'a phlegmon,' and ειδος, 'resemblance.' That which relates or belongs to or resembles phlegmon.

PHLEGMONOUS INFLAMMATION is the active inflammation of the areolar membrane; in contradistinction to erysipelatous inflammation, or that of the skin.

PHLEGMOPYRA, Fever, adeno-meningeal.

PHLEGMORRHAGIA, Blennorrhœa.

PHLEGMORRHAGIE PULMONAIRE, Bronchorrhœa.

PHLEGMORRHŒA, Blennorrhœa.

PHLEGMYMENI'TIS, *Phlegmhymeni'tis*, from φλεγμα, 'phlegm,' 'υμην, 'a membrane,' and *itis*, the termination for inflammation. Inflammation of a mucous membrane.

PHLEGMYMENITIS ENTERICA, see Enteritis.

PHLEPS, Vein.

PHLOGIA, Inflammation.

PHLOGICUS, Inflammatory.

PHLOGISTIC, Inflammatory.

PHLOGISTICI, Empresma.

PHLOGISTON, Hydrogen.

PHLOGMUS, Verbascum thapsus.

PHLOGO'DES, from φλοξ, 'flame,' and ειδος, 'resemblance.' *Infla'med, Inflamma'tus, Inflammato'rius,* Inflammatory. An epithet employed particularly to express the red colour of the face.

PHLOGOPYRUS, Synocha.

PHLOGOSED, Inflamed.

PHLOGO'SIS, *Incen'dium, Inflamma'tion.* Some writers use this word exclusively for external inflammation — phlegmon; others, for that which is superficial or erysipelatous.

PHLOGOT'ICA, *Inflammations.* The second order in the class *Hæmatica* of Good.

PHLOIOS, Cortex.

PHLOMUS, Verbascum thapsus.

PHLOOS, Cortex.

PHLOR'IDZINE, *Phloridzi'na, Phloridzin,* from φλοος, 'inner bark,' and ριζα, 'root.' The bitter or active principle of the root and trunk of the apple, pear, cherry, and plum tree. It is deposited from the decoction on cooling; crystallizes in silky spicula of a dead white colour, when in masses, or in long slender prisms or tables, when crystallized with care. 1000 parts of water, at a temperature of from 32° to 71°, only dissolve about one part; but at from 70° to 212°, it is dissolved in all proportions. It is very soluble in pure alcohol, but only slightly so in ether; s. g. 1.429. It has been administered successfully in intermittents,—10 to 20 grains being generally required to arrest the paroxysm. It may be given either in the form of pill or powder.

PHLOUS, Cortex.

PHLOX, Verbascum thapsus.

PHLYCTÆ'NA, *Phlyctæ'nis, Phlyctis, Phlyza'cion, Ampullæ, Holophlyc'tides, Phlyc'tides, Phlysis,* from φλυζω, 'I boil.' Tumours formed by the accumulation of a serous fluid under the epidermis.

PHLYCTÆNULA, see Hydatid.

PHLYC'TENOID, *Phlyctenoi'des.* Resembling phlyctænæ. An epithet for a variety of herpes.

PHLYCTEN'ULAR, same etymon as Phlyctæna. Of or belonging to phlyctænula,—as *phlyctenular ophthalmia,* inflammation of the eye, accompanied with phlyctænulæ on the cornea.

PHLYCTIDES, Phlyctæna.

PHLYCTID'IUM, same etymon. A circular or annular spot of inflammation of the corium, encircled by a red ring or zone, within which suppuration takes place. The genuine small-pox pustule, and that produced by the application of tartar emetic ointment, are examples of it.

PHLYCTIS, Phlyctæna.

PHLYSIS, from φλυζω, 'I am hot,' 'I boil.' A cutaneous eruption. An ulcerative, subcutaneous tumour: flat, tensive, glabrous; diffused, hot, throbbing; at length fluctuating, with an acrid ichor. — Good.

PHLYSIS, Phlyctæna — p. Ecthyma, Ecthyma — p. Impetigo, Impetigo — p. Porrigo, Porrigo — p. Scabies, Psora.

PHLYZACIA, Ecthyma.

PHLYZACION, Phlyctæna.

PHOBODIPSON, Hydrophobia.

PHOCOM'ELES, from φωκη, 'a seal,' and μελος, 'a limb.' A genus of monsters, in which the limbs are shortened; the hands and feet appearing to exist alone, and to be inserted immediately on the trunk, as in the seals and the herbivorous cetacea. — J. G. St. Hilaire.

PHŒNICISMUS, Rubeola.

PHŒNIGMUS, Phenigmus — p. Petechiæ, Purpura simplex.

PHŒNIX DACTYLIFERA, Date tree — p. Excelsa, Date tree.

PHONA'TION, *Phona'tio,* from φωνη, 'voice.' The physiology of the voice.

PHONE, Voice.

PHO'NICA, φωνικα, from φωνη, 'voice.' The first order of the class *Pneumatica,* in Good's Nosology. Defined: diseases affecting the vocal avenues: — the passage of the voice impeded, or its power suppressed or depraved.

PHONON'OSI, *Phonono'si,* from φωνη, 'the voice,' and νοσος, 'a disease.' *Phonopathi'a, Morbi vocis.* Diseases of the voice.

PHONOPATHIA, Phononosi.
PHORA, Gestation.
PHORBE, Pabulum.
PHORONOM'IA, from φορεομαι, or φερομαι, 'I put myself in motion,' and νομος, 'law.' The doctrine of muscular motion.
PHOROUS, from φερω, 'I carry.' A suffix denoting conveyance. Hence, Galactophorous, &c.
PHOS, Light.
PHOSPHAS CALCICUM STIBIATUM, Antimonial powder—p. Calcis stibiatus, Antimonial powder—p. Natricum, Soda, phosphate of.
PHOSPHAT'IC, *Phosphat'icus*, from *Phosphorus*. Relating to the phosphates; hence the *Phosphat'ic Diath'esis* is the habit of body which favours the deposition of the phosphates from the urine.
PHOSPHÈNE, Photopsia.
PHOSPHORE, Phosphorus.
PHOSPHORÉNÈSES. M. Baumes unites, under this generic name, diseases which he attributes to disordered phosphorization; i. e. to excess or deficiency of calcareous phosphate or its decomposition. Amongst these affections he ranks rachitis, osteo-malacia, and gout.
PHOSPHORES'CENCE, *Phosphorescen'tia*. The properties possessed by certain bodies of being luminous in obscurity, or under particular circumstances.
PHOS'PHORIC ACID, *Ac''idum phosphor'icum*, (F.) *Acide phosphorique*. A solid, colourless compound; highly sapid; very soluble in water, and vitrifiable by fire. It exists in bones combined with lime. It has been employed in medicine in the form of lemonade, in passive hemorrhage, typhus, phthisis, marasmus, &c., and in injection in cases of cancer of the uterus. It does not seem preferable to other acids.
PHOSPHORURIA, Urine, phosphorescent.
PHOS'PHORUS, *Phos'phorum*, *Autophos'phorus*, *Ignis philosoph'icus*, *Lumen constans*, from φως, 'light,' and φερω, 'I carry.' (F.) *Phosphore*. 'A light carrier.' An elementary or undecomposed substance; not metallic; solid; transparent or semitransparent; colourless; brilliant; flexible; of a sensible garlic odour; very inflammable, and susceptible of combining with the oxygen of the atmosphere, at even the ordinary temperature. It does not exist pure in nature, but is found frequently united to other bodies. Its fumes in the manufacture of lucifer and congreve matches have caused, it is said, necrosis of the lower jaw—'*phosphorus jaw disease*.'
Phosphorus has been used in medicine, dissolved in ether or suspended in the yolk of egg, as a stimulant; but the greatest precautions are necessary in its administration: hence it is rarely employed.
PHOSPHORUS JAW DISEASE, see Phosphorus.
PHOSPHURIA, Urine, phosphorescent. See Urine.
PHOTODAMPSIS, Refraction.
PHOTOMA'NIA, from φως, 'light,' and *mania*. Insane delirium induced by light.
PHOTOPHO'BIA, from φως, φωτος, 'light,' and φοβος, 'fear.' Aversion to light:—intolerance of light. Nyctalopia.
PHOTOPHOBICUS, Lucifugus.
PHOTOPHOBOPHTHALMIA, Nyctalopia.
PHOTOPHOBUS, Lucifugus.
PHOTOP'SIA, *Visus lu'cidus*, from φως, 'light,' and ωψ, 'the eye.' (F.) *Phosphène*. A false perception of light, as of sparks, flashes of fire, &c., occasioned by certain conditions of the retina and brain, and by pressure on the eyeball. When pressure does not induce the luminous appearance, the existence of amaurosis may be inferred. See Metamorphopsia.

PHOTU'RIA, from φως, 'light,' and ουρον, urine.' A luminous condition of the urine.
PHRAGMOS, φραγμος, from φρασσω, 'I enclose.' A row of teeth.
PHRASIS, Voice, articulated.
PHRASUM, Marrubium.
PHREN, φρην, 'the mind.' Also, the diaphragm and scrobiculus cordis.
PHRENAUX'É, *Hypertroph'ia cer'ebri*; from φρην, 'the mind, the organ of mind,' and αυξη, 'increase.' Hypertrophy of the brain.
PHRENATROPH'IA, *Atroph'ia cer'ebri*; from φρην, 'the mind, the organ of mind,' α, priv., and τροφη, 'nourishment.' Wasting or atrophy of the brain.
PHRENES, Diaphragm.
PHRENESIA, Phrenitis.
PHRÉNÉSIE, Phrenitis.
PHRENESIS, Delirium, Phrenitis.
PHRENETIASIS, Delirium, Phrenitis.
PHRENETISMUS, Phrenitis.
PHRENIC, Diaphragmatic.
PHRE'NICA, from φρην, 'the mind.' Diseases affecting the intellect; characterized by error, perversion, or debility of one or more of the mental faculties, (*Phrenopathi'a*.) The first order of the class *Neurotica* of Good. Also, remedies that affect the mental faculties—*Phren'ics*. Pereira.
PHRENICS, see Phrenica.
PHRENICULA HYDROCEPHALICA, Hydrocephalus internus.
PHRENISMUS, Phrenitis.
PHRENI'TIS, *Phren'esis*, *Phrene'sia*, *Phreneti'asis*, *Phrenis'mus*, *Phrenetis'mus*, *Cephali'tis*, *Cephalal'gia inflammato'ria*, *Karabitus* (Arab.), *Sibare*, *Sphacelis'mus cer'ebri*, *Empres'ma cephali'tis*, *Siri'asis*, *Seiri'asis*, *Sidera'tio*, *Inflammatio phreni'tis*, *Encephali'tis*, *Cauma phreni'tis*, *Phrensy*, *Delirium*, *Brain Fever*, (F.) *Phrénésie*, *Inflammation du cerveau et du cervelet*, from φρην, 'the mind,' and *itis*, denoting inflammation. A disease characterized by violent pyrexia, pain in the head, redness of the face and eyes, intolerance of light and sound, watchfulness, and delirium, either furious or muttering. Its causes are the same as those of other inflammations: sometimes, however, it is induced by a *Coup de soleil*; by inebriation; violent mental emotions, &c. Some authors have given the name *Phrenitis* and *Meningitis* to inflammation of the membranes of the brain; and that of *Cephalitis, Encephalitis*, or *Cerebritis* to inflammation of the substance of the brain; but there are no pathognomic symptoms, which can lead us to refer the seat of the disease to either of those parts exclusively. Phrenitis is, of course, a very dangerous affection, from the importance of the organ concerned. The most active treatment must necessarily be pursued. Repeated bleeding; purging; the application of ice to the shaved head; a position in which the head is raised; and the avoiding of irritation of every kind;—form the remedial means during the violent stage. After this has yielded, counter-irritants to the nape of the neck or to other parts of the body will be useful adjuvants. When the brain and meninges were affected only symptomatically, as in inflammation of the diaphragm, the disease was formerly called *Paraphrenitis*.
Hydrocephalus acutus is a variety of phrenitis.
PHRENITIS CALENTURA, *Coup-de-soleil*—p. Latrans, Hydrophobia—p. Potatorum, Delirium tremens—p. Verminosa, Vercoquin.
PHRENOLOGY, Craniology.
PHRENO-MAG'NETISM, *Phreno-mesmer-*

ism. A term applied to the condition of a mesmerized person, in which, when any cerebral or phrenological organ—so called—is touched, the functions of the organ are manifested. It has been established, that no such phenomena can be elicited in children, or in those who have never seen a phrenological cast or picture.

PHRENOPARALYSIS, see Paralysis.
PHRENOPATHIA, see Phrenica.
PHRENOPATHI'A ÆTHE'REA. The aggregate of encephalic phenomena induced by the inhalation of ether.
PHRENSY, Phrenitis.
PHRICASMUS, Horripilation.
PHRICE, Horripilation.
PHRICIA, Horripilation.
PHRICIASIS, Horripilation.
PHRICO'DES (FEBRIS,) from φρικη, 'a shivering;' *Horrif'ica.* A fever in which the chill is very intense and prolonged.
PHRYAGMA, Shuddering.
PHRYCTE, Colophonia.
PHRYG"IUS (LAPIS.) An earthy matter, found in Phrygia and Cappadocia, and formerly employed as an astringent.— Gorræus.
PHTHARMA CALIGO, Caligo—p. Cataracta, Cataract—p. Glaucoma, Glaucoma.
PHTHEIR, Pediculus.
PHTHEIRE'MIA; from φθειρω, 'I corrupt,' and 'αιμα, 'blood.' A state in which the plastic powers of the blood are deteriorated.
PHTHEIRI'ASIS, *Phthiriasis,* from φθειρ, 'a louse;' *Morbus pediculo'sus, M. pedicula'ris, Pruri'go pedicula'ris, Pedicula'tio, Malis pedic'uli, Peta'lē, Lousiness, Lousy disease,* (F.) *Maladie pédiculaire, Phthiriase.* A disease which consists in the excessive multiplication of lice on the human body, under conditions in which it does not ordinarily take place, and in spite of cleanliness. It has been asserted that the affection has often caused death. Simple and medicated baths have been recommended for its removal; lotions of the decoction or infusion of tobacco and stavesacre, mercurial frictions, &c.
PHTHEIRIUM, Delphinium staphisagria.
PHTHEIROCTONUM, Delphinium staphisagria.
PHTHINAS, Phthisis.
PHTHINODES, Phthisicus.
PHTHIRIASE, Phtheiriasis.
PHTHIRIASIS, Malis, Phtheiriasis.
PHTHIRIUM SCABIEI, see Psora.
PHTHIRIUS, Antiparasitic — p. Inguinalis, see Pediculus.
PHTHIROCTONUS, Abortive.
PHTHIROPORON, Autumn.
PHTHISES: same etymon as Phthisis. In the classification of Fuchs, diseases attended with ulceration, hectic fever, and emaciation.
PHTHISIC, Phthisis.
PHTHISICAL, Phthisicus.
PHTHIS'ICUS, *Phthino'des, Phthis'ical, Tis'ical,* (F.) *Poitrinaire;* same etymon as phthisis. Belonging to phthisis. Also, one labouring under phthisis.
PHTHISIE, Phthisis pulmonalis—*p. Calouleuse,* Calculi, pulmonary, see Lithiasis pulmonum—*p. Carcinomateuse,* Phthisis, cancerous—*p. avec Mélanose,* Anthracosis pulmonum—*p. Mésentérique,* Tabes mesenterica.
PHTHISIOL'OGY, *Phthisiolog"ia,* from φθισις, and λογος. A treatise on phthisis.
PHTHISIOSIS, Tubercular consumption.
PHTHISI-PNEUMONIA, Phthisis pulmonalis.
PHTHISIS, *Phthoë, Phthinas, Tabes, Te'cedon, Consumption, Decline, Phthis'ic, Tis'ic;* from φθιω, 'I dry, I fade.' This word, taken in a general sense, means progressive emaciation of every part of the body. It is usually, however, restricted to phthisis pulmonalis.

PHTHISIS, BLACK, see Anthracosis.
PHTHISIS, BRON'CHIAL, *Phthisis bronchia'lis.* Phthisis occasioned by the pressure of enlarged tuberculous bronchial glands, which, not unfrequently, communicate with caverns in the lungs, or with the bronchia.
PHTHISIS CALCULOSA, Lithiasis pulmonum.
PHTHISIS, CAN'CEROUS, *Scirrhus, Carcinoma et Fungus Pulmo'num, Med'ullary or Enceph'aloid Tumour of the Lung,* (F.) *Cancer du Poumon.* Cancer of the lung, which gives rise to carcinomatous phthisis, (F.) *Phthisie carcinomateuse,* of Bayle.
PHTHISIS CONSUMMATA, see Ph. pulmonalis—p. Dorsalis, Tabes Dorsalis — p. Dyspeptic, see Phthisis — p. Exulcerata, Ph. pulmonalis — p. Hepatica, Hepato-phthisis—p. Ischiadica, Ischiophthisis.
PHTHISIS LARYNGE'A, *Chronic Laryngi'tis, Laryngi'tis et Trachei'tis chron'ica, Tuberculo'sis laryn'gis et trache'æ, Laryn'go et Tracheophthisis, Laryngophthisis, Ul'cera seu Helco'sis Laryngis,* (F.) *Phthisie laryngée, Ulcère du larynx, Laryngite avec sécrétion de Pus,* is a species of consumption analogous to phthisis pulmonalis, produced by inflammation and ulceration of the interior of the larynx, and sometimes by caries of the cartilages. *Phthisis trachea'lis, Tracheophthi'sis,* is a similar affection, seated in the trachea. Chronic inflammation of the larynx and trachea may exist, however, without tubercles or phthisis.
PHTHISIS MESERAICA, Tabes mesenterica—p. Nodosa, Ph. pulmonalis — p. Notias, Tabes dorsalis.
PHTHISIS PULMONA'LIS, *Ph. pulmo'num, Ph. pulmona'lis vera seu tuberculo'sa seu scrophulo'sa seu tuberculo-ulcera'ta seu purulen'ta exulcera'ta seu exulcera'ta, Maras'mus phthisis, Hec'tica phthisis, Hæmop'tysis phthisis, Ph. Pulmona'ris* seu *nodo'sa, Passio vomicof'lua, Phthisi-pneumo'nia, Tabes pulmona'lis* seu *pulmo'num, Ulcus pulmonum, Helco'sis pulmona'lis, Pneumonophthi'sis, Pneumonoph'thoë, Phthisis scrophulo'sa, Pneumop'thoë, Pulmo'nia, Phthisis tuberculo'sa, Tuberculo'sis Pulmo'num, Gongrophthi'sis, Tuberculous disease of the lungs, Pulmonary consumption, Consumption, Decline, Phthisic, Tisic,* (F.) *Phthisie, P. pulmonaire, Crachement de pus.* Occasionally, this formidable disease occurs accidentally: but, usually, it is caused by a conformation obtained from progenitors. This, at least, predisposes to it; and but a slight exciting cause may be required to rouse the predisposition into action. It is less a disease of the torrid zone; and, in the temperate regions of the globe, its pathology is often intimately allied with that of scrofula. It consists in the formation of tubercles in the lungs, which sooner or later inflame and break down. In such a constitution, ulcerations of the lungs do not readily heal; and hectic fever—the universal attendant upon irritability and debility—is established. This persists, and gradually wears down the patient, till he ultimately expires, exhausted by the irritative fever. The chief symptoms are the following. The patient feels a sense of uneasiness in the chest, with severe fits of coughing, or a short and dry cough with dyspnœa. This may be considered the incipient stage. The cough then becomes extremely troublesome, especially in the morning; and dyspnœa is increased on the slightest exertion. The expectoration is evidently purulent, with fever in the evening, and circumscribed redness of the cheeks; wasting and colliquative sweats early in the morning. This must

be considered the confirmed stage,—*Phthisis consumma'ta, Pneumophthi'sis.* In the third, or last stage, the hectic is constant, with small pulse, pungent heat, colliquative sweats, and diarrhœa. The weakness becomes extreme, and the patient exhausted. *Physical Signs.*— 1. In the first stage, whilst there are yet scattered miliary tubercles,—the only appreciable change at the exterior of the chest, and this is not constant, is a want of freedom in the movements under one or both clavicles. Percussion will generally discover a slight diminution of sound corresponding to the summit of one lung. In the same situation, auscultation shows that the inspiratory murmur is either weaker, rougher, or confused. The sound of expiration is more distinct. The voice and cough are rather more resonant, and wheezing or mucous *râles* are occasionally heard in the same region. 2. When the tubercular deposition has become more abundant, the motion of the chest is more markedly diminished under one or both clavicles. The loss of sound on percussion is more distinct, the inspiration, on auscultation, is bronchial, the expiration louder and more superficial, and the resonance of the voice and cough is increased. The rest of the lung is perhaps healthy, or the respiration may be puerile. 3. When the tubercles are undergoing softening, —in addition to the preceding signs, auscultation exhibits a subcrepitant *râle* around the apex of the lung, decreasing from above downwards. It is most distinct during or after the cough, and at the close of a deep inspiration. As the disease proceeds, the bubbling becomes successively larger, and ultimately *gargouillement* is heard. The inspiration and expiration are cavernous or tracheal. The voice and cough indicate unusual resonance and pectoriloquy. The intercostal spaces are often depressed locally, and percussion may become gradually clearer and even tympanitic as the cavern increases.

It is only in the incipient state of this formidable disease, that advantage can be expected from any plan of treatment; and of all means that can be devised, that of removing to a climate in which air and exercise can be daily enjoyed during the autumnal, winter, and spring months is the best. See Climate. If this be impracticable, the patient must be kept in a regulated temperature, taking care that the chamber be duly ventilated; and gestation in the open air be used, whenever the atmosphere, although cold, is dry. The other indications will be: 1. To moderate inflammatory action: 2. To support the strength; and, 3. To palliate urgent symptoms. The whole treatment indeed is palliative. Counter-irritants relieve pain: demulcents and mild opiates alleviate the cough: the mineral acids, united with opium, relieve the colliquative sweats; and chalk and opium the diarrhœa.

Dr. Wilson Philip has pointed out a particular species of phthisis, which is characterized, in the early stage, by a deranged state of the digestive organs; flatulent, irregular bowels; furred tongue; impaired appetite; unnatural fæces; and the epigastric region more or less full and tender on pressure. The affection of the lungs is here secondary. He calls it *Dyspeptic phthisis.*

Phthisis Pulmonalis Purulenta Exulcerata, Phthisis pulmonalis — p. Pulmonalis scrofulosa, Phthisis pulmonalis — p. Pulmonalis tuberculosa, Phthisis pulmonalis — p. Pulmonalis tuberculosa-ulcerata, Phthisis pulmonalis — p. Pulmonalis vera, Phthisis pulmonalis — p. Pupillæ, Synezisis — p. Pupillaris, Myosis — p. Scrophulosa, Phthisis pulmonalis — p. Sicca, Tabes dorsalis — p. Tuberculosa, Phthisis pulmonalis — p. Uterina, Metrophthisis — p. Vesicalis, Cystophthisis.

PHTHISURIA, Diabetes.
PHTHISURIE, Diabetes—*p. Sucrée,* Diabetes mellitus.
PHTHOË, Phthisis.
PHTHOIS, Pastil, Trochiscus.
PHTHOISCOS, Pastil, Trochiscus.
PHTHONGODYSPHORIA, Hyperacusis.
PHTHORA, Abortion, Corruption, Plague.
PHTHORIUS, Abortive.
PHTHOROCTONUS, Abortive.
PHUCAGROSTIS MINOR, Pila marina.
PHUSCA, Oxycrate.
PHYGANTHROPIA, Misanthropia.
PHYGETH'LON, *Panus, Phypella,* from φυω, 'I grow.' Inflammation of the superficial lymphatic glands, not ending in suppuration.
PHYLACTERION, Amuletum.
PHYLACTE'RIUM, from φυλασσω, 'I preserve.' A *Phylac'tery.* An amulet:—a prophylactic.
PHYLAXIS, Conservation.
PHYLLAN'THUS URINA'RIA, *Binkohumba.* A plant employed in Ceylon, in decoction, as a diuretic.
PHYLLITIS, Asplenium scolopendrium — p. Muraria, Asplenium ruta muraria — p. Rotundifolia, Asplenium trichomanoides.
PHYMA, *Phima,* from φυομαι, 'I spring up.' With the ancients, this word was used with great latitude: sometimes, in the sense of phlegmon, for tumours larger than a boil, and perfectly suppurative. In the nosology of Sauvages, *Phymata* is an order of diseases, to which he refers erysipelas, œdema, phlegmon, emphysema, scirrhus, &c. In that of Dr. Good it is a genus, including hordeolum, furunculus, sycosis, and anthrax.
Phyma Anthrax, Anthrax — p. Anthrax terminthus, Terminthus — p. Sycosis, Sycosis.
PHYMATO'SES, from φυμα, 'a hard tumour.' Tuberculous diseases. — Fuchs.
PHYMATOSIS, Excrescence—p. Cerebri, Encephalophymata — p. Elephantiasis, Elephantiasis — p. Lupus, Lupus — p. Verrucosa, Verruca.
PHYMOSIS, Phimosis.
PHYPELLA, Phygethlon.
PHYSA, Crepitation.
PHYSAGOGA, Carminatives.
PHY'SALIS, *P. Alkeken'gi seu halicac'abum, Sola'num vesica'rium, Alchachen'gi, Alkeken'gi, Halicac'abum, Winter Cherry,* (F.) *Alkekenge, Coqueret. Family,* Solaneæ. *Sex. Syst.* Pentandria Monogynia. The berries are recommended as a diuretic, from 6 to 12 for a dose, in dropsical and calculous cases.
Physalis Alkekengi, Physalis—p. Halicacabum, Physalis—p. Stramonium, Anisodus luridus.
PHYSCIA ISLANDICA, Lichen islandicus — p. Nivalis, Lichen caninus.
PHYSCO'NIA, from φυσκη, 'a bladder.' *Ventros'itas, Ecphy'ma physco'nia, Hyposar'ca, Emphrac'tica, Visco'nia, Hypersarchid'ios, Potbelly, Pendulous abdo'men, Swagbelly.* A generic term, under which Sauvages has comprised every large tumour developed in the abdomen, that is neither fluctuating nor sonorous. Linnæus calls it Hyposarca.
Physco'nia Adipo'sa, *Obes'itas seu Polysar'cia vis'cerum.* Accumulation of fat in the intestines.
Physconia Biliosa, Turgescentia vesiculæ felleæ.
Physconia Emphysemat'ica. Accumulation of air in the areolar tissue, or between the coats of particular viscera.
Physconia Lienis, Splenoncus — p. Mesenterica, Tabes mesenterica— p. Splenica, Ague cake.
Physconia Strumo'sa, *Scrofula abdomina'lis*

inter'na. Tumid abdomen from scrophulous enlargement of the glands.

PHYSCONIE MÉSENTÉRIQUE, Tabes mesenterica.

PHYSEMA, Tympanites, Physesis.

PHYSE'SIS, *Physe'ma,* from φυσαω, 'I inflate.' An emphysematous tumour. Tympanites.

PHYSETER MACROCEPHALUS, see Cetaceum.

PHYSIATRICE, Vis medicatrix naturæ.

PHYSIAUTOCRATIA, Vis medicatrix naturæ.

PHYSIC, Medicament, Medicina — p. Indian, Euphorbia corollata, Gillenia trifoliata—p. Root, Leptandria purpurea.

PHYSICAL, Medical.

PHYSIC"IAN, *Med'icus, Iatros, Aces'tor, Aces'ter, Althæus;* from φυσις, 'nature. (F.) *Médecin.* One who has received his degree from an incorporated Institution, as Doctor of Medicine. The French formerly used the word *physicien* in the same sense. It is now appropriated to the natural philosopher.

PHYSICIAN, FAMILY. One regarded as the regular attendant on a family.

PHYSICIAN, LEARNED, Iatrosophista—p. Practical, Iatrotechna — p. Priest, see Asclepiadæ.

PHYSICIEN, Physician.

PHYSICS, MED'ICAL, *Iatrophys'ics.* Physics directly applied to medicine, — either to the explanation of the vital phenomena, the preservation of individuals, or the treatment of disease.

PHYSIOAUTOCRATIA, Vis medicatrix naturæ.

PHYSIOG'NOMY, *Physiognom'ia, Physiognom'ica, Physiognom'icē, Physionom'ia, Physiognomon'ia, Physiognom'onē, Physiognomos'ynē, Physiognomosia, Anthroposcop'ia, Prosopomanti'a, Prosopolog"ia, Semiot'icē fa'ciei, Physiognomon'ica, Physiognom'ony, Metopos'copy, Prosopo'sis,* from φυσις, 'nature,' and γνωμη, 'knowledge.' The art of knowing the dispositions of men from their external appearance; especially from the features. Every inference of this kind must necessarily be extremely fallacious, and cannot be reduced to rule, as was attempted by Lavater and others. In infantile diseases, numerous shades of expression are evident, which experience teaches how to appreciate; and which afford useful guides in understanding the pathology of that period of existence.

PHYSIOLOGIA PATHOGENETICA, see Pathogenetic.

PHYSIOLOGICAL ANATOMY, see Anatomy — p. Doctrine, Broussaism.

PHYSIOLOGICE, Physiology.

PHYSIOL'OGY, *Physiolog"ia, Biol'ogy, Bion'omy, Biot'ice, Biophænomenolog"ia, Physiolog"icē, Œconom'ia anima'lis, Anatom'ia viva, Anat'omē anima'ta, Anthropolog"ia, Microcosmogra'phia, Microcos'mica scien'tia, Cognit"io physiolog"ica, Pars natura'lis medici'næ, Philosoph'ia cor'poris vivi;* from φυσις, 'nature,' and λογος, 'a description.' Formerly, Physiology meant the same as Physics, in its extensive signification, now does. At the present day, it includes the science which treats of the functions of ánimals or vegetables; an acquaintance with the phenomena the aggregate of which constitute life. It is *the science of life.* It is divided into *animal—Zoöphysiologia,* and *vegetable — Phytophysiolog"ia,* according as it considers the life of animals or of vegetables singly. *Comparative physiology* comprises both. Physiology is, also, *general* or *special,* according as it treats of life in the abstract or in some particular species. To the latter belongs the *Physiology of Man.* — called also, *Hygienic Physiology* to distinguish it from *Pathological Physiology* or *Pathology.*

PHYSIOLOGY, PATHOGENETIC, see Pathogenetic.

PHYSIONOMIA, Physiognomy.

PHYSIONOMIE ÉGARÉE, see Wild.

PHYSIS, Natura, Sex.

PHYSOCE'LE, *Pneumatoce'lē, Hernia vento'sa; Oscheoce'lē flatulen'ta, Emphyse'ma Scroti,* from φυσαω, 'I insufflate,' and κηλη, 'a tumour.' An emphysematous tumour of the scrotum; probably a case of intestinal hernia, containing much flatus.

PHYSOCEPH'ALUS, from φυσαω, 'I inflate,' and κεφαλη, 'the head.' *Physoceph'alus.* Emphysematous tumefaction of the head.

PHYSOCŒLIA, Tympanites.

PHYSO'DES; from φυσαω, 'I inflate,' and ειδος, 'resemblance.' Full of air; apparently full of air — applied to tumours, &c.

PHYSOME'TRA, *Emphyse'ma U'teri, Hysteroph'ysē, Hysteropsoph'ia, Hysteremphyse'ma, Hystremphyse'ma, Metremphyse'ma, Ædiopsoph'ia uteri'na, Emphyse'ma uteri'num, Infla'tio U'teri, Tym'pany of the Womb, U'terine tympanites,* from φυσαω, 'I inflate,' and μητρα, 'the womb.' A light, tense, circumscribed protuberance in the hypogastrium, obscurely sonorous, with wind occasionally discharged through the os uteri.

PHYSON, Flatulence.

PHYSONCUS, Emphysema.

PHYSOPSOPH'IA; from φυσαω, 'I inflate,' and ψοφος, 'a noise.' A discharge of air with noise.

PHYSOSPASMUS, Colica flatulenta.

PHYSOTHORAX, Pneumothorax.

PHYTIVOROUS, Phytophagous.

PHYTOALOPECIA, Porrigo decalvans.

PHYTO-CHYMISTRY, see Chymistry.

PHYTOLAC'CA DECAN'DRA, *P. vulgaris. Poke Weed, Amer'ican Night Shade, Cancer root. Poke, Skoke, Jucato Caleloe,* (?) *Jalap, Pigeon Berries, Jalap cancer root, Sola'num racemo'sum America'num, S. magnum Virginia'num rubrum, Blitum America'num, Garget,* (F.) *Raisin d'Amérique, Phytolaque à dix étamines, Morelle en grappes, Mechoacan du Canada. Family, Chenopodeæ. Sex. Syst.* Decandria Decagynia. The leaves, berries, and roots are employed. The young stems, when boiled, are sometimes eaten at table; but when old, they must be cautiously used, as the plant is emetic and cathartic. It is most celebrated as a remedy in chronic rheumatism; and is given in the form of tincture of the ripe berries. It is, also, used in cutaneous eruptions; tinea capitis, itch, cancerous ulcers, &c. The root is gathered and dried in the fall.

PHYTOLAQUE À DIX ÉTAMINES, Phytolacca decandra.

PHYTOLOGIA MEDICA, Botany, medical.

PHYTOPH'AGOUS, *Phytoph'agus; Phytivorous, Phytiv'orus;* from φυτον, 'a plant,' and φαγω, 'I eat.' Feeding or subsisting on vegetables.

PHYTOPHYSIOLOGIA, see Physiology.

PHYTOSPERM'A, (F.) *Phytosperme;* from φυτον, 'a vegetable,' and σπερμα, 'sperm.' Particles similar to the spermatozoids of animals, observed in vegetables, and presumed to possess a similar agency in reproduction.

PHYTOTOMY, see Anatomy, (vegetable.)

PHYTOZOON, Zoophyte.

PIA MATER, *Pia seu mollis seu ten'uis Mater, Pia meninx, Meninx inte'rior, Meninx cho'roï'des, Inner lam'ina of the Méningine,* (Ch.) *Membra'na vasculo'ea Cer'ebri, Membra'na Cer'ebri ten'uis seu mollis seu pro'pria,* (F.) *Pie mère, Méningette.* The pia mater is a very delicate membrane, which covers the brain immediately, penetrates into its anfractuosities, and envelops, also, the cerebellum and the spinal prolongation, &c. Bichat does not regard it as a membrane, properly so called, but as a net-work of blood-vessels, united by a lax areolar tissue. The *Pia Mater exterior* is the portion of membrane which covers the exterior of the encephalon, and faces the arachnoid externally. The *Pia Mater interior* is that which lines the cerebral fossæ, into which it penetrates by a cleft situate between the posterior part of the corpus callosum and the fornix; and by two other fissures, situate between the corpora fimbriata and thalami nervorum opticorum. The pia mater contains a great number of granulations similar to the *Glandulæ Pacchioni*.

PIA MATER TESTIS, Tunica vasculosa—p. Meninx, P. Mater.

PIAN, Framboesia.

PIANS, MOTHER OF, Mama-pian.

PIAR, Fat.

PIARHÆ'MIA; from πιαρ, 'fat,' and 'αιμα, 'blood.' Fat in the blood. — Simon.

PICA, Malacia—p. Africanorum, Chthonophagia.

PICAC, Euphorbia corollata.

PICACISM'US, *Pica'tio*, from *pix*, 'pitch.' Depilation by means of a pitch plaster. Also, Malacia.

PICATIO, Malacia, Picacismus.

PICEA, Pinus abies.

PICERION, Butter.

PICHU'RIM BEANS. The seed of a tree, supposed to be *Persea pichurim*, *Oco'tea pichu'-rim*, which grows in Brazil, Guiana, Venezuela, and other parts of South America. They are of an elliptical shape; flat on one side, convex on the other; of an aromatic odour between that of nutmegs and sassafras, and of a spicy, pungent taste. The medical properties are the same as those of other aromatics. For the bark, see Pechurim cortex.

PICKERELWEED, SHOVEL, Unisema deltifolia.

PICOTE, Variola.

PICOTEMENT, Pricking.

PICRÆNA EXCELSA, Quassia.

PICRIA, Bitterness.

PICRIUM SPICATUM, Coutoubea alba.

PICROCHOLOS, Bilious.

PI'CROMEL, *Bilin;* from πικρος, 'bitter,' and μιλι, 'honey.' A name given by Thénard to a colourless, soft substance, of an acrid, bitter, saccharine taste, nauseous smell, and very soluble in water.

It forms part of the bile, and is classed amongst the animal immediate principles.

PICROPE'GÆ, from πικρος, 'bitter,' and πηγη, 'a spring.' Mineral waters; bitter from the presence of chloride of magnesium.

PICROS, Amarus.

PICROTOX'INE, *Picrotox'ina*, *Picrotox'in*, from πικρος, 'bitter,' and τοξινον, 'poison.' A vegetable alkali, discovered by M. Boullay in the *Menispermum Cocculus*. It crystallizes in quadrangular, white, brilliant, semitransparent prisms; which are excessively bitter, soluble in three parts of alcohol, and in fifteen of boiling water.

The Cocculus Indicus owes its poisonous properties to this principle.

PIE MÈRE, Pia mater.

PIE-MÉPITE, *Inflamma'tio piæ matris*. A miserably compounded term, employed by M. Grisolle, to express inflammation of the pia mater:— from (F.) *pie mère*, 'the pia mater,' and *ite*, *itis;* a termination denoting inflammation.

PIÈCE, Hepatitis.

PIÈCES D'ANATOMIE ARTIFICIELLES, see Artificial.

PIED, Pes — p. *d'Alexandre*, Anthemis pyrethrum — p. *d'Alouette des champs*, Delphinium consolida—p. *Bot*, see Kyllosis—p. *de Chat*, Antennaria dioica— p. *de Cheval marin*, Cornu ammonis — p. *de Griffon*, Gryphius pes, Helleborus foetidus— p. *de Lion*, Alchemilla—p. *de Lit*, Origanum—p. *d'Ours*, Acanthus mollis—p. *Plat*, see Kyllosis — p. *de Veau*, Arum maculatum — p. *de Veau Triphylle*, Arum triphyllum.

PIEIRON, Fat.

PIERRE, Calculus — p. *d'Aigle*, Ætites — p. *d'Azur*, Lapis lazuli — p. *Calaminaire*, Calamine — p. *à Cautère*, Potassa cum calce—p. *Infernale*, Argenti nitras — p. *Judaique*, Judæus (lapis) — p. *au Lait*, Morochthus — p. *Médicamenteuse*, Medicamentosus lapis — p. *Néphrétique*, Nephreticus lapis — p. *Ponce*, Pumex.

PIERRES CRAYEUSES, Calculi, arthritic — p. *au Fiel*, Calculi, biliary — p. *Stercorales*, Calculus of the Stomach and Intestines—p. *Urinaires*, Calculi, urinary.

PIESTER, Press.

PIESTERION, Press.

PIESTRON, from πιεζω, 'I press.' An instrument recommended by Hippocrates for breaking the bones of the foetal head when too large to be extracted otherwise.

PIGAMON JAUNÂTRE, Thalictron.

PIGEON BERRIES, Phytolacca decandra — p. Breasted, see Lordosis — p. Tree, Aralia spinosa.

PIGMENT CELLS, see Cell, pigment.

PIGMEN'TAL, from *pigmentum*, 'paint.' Having relation to pigment or colouring matter.

PIGMENTAL APPARA'TUS, (F.) *Appareil pigmental*. The apparatus concerned in the coloration of the skin of the coloured varieties of man. — Flourens.

PIGMENTARIUS, Apothecary, Unguentarius.

PIGMENTUM, Paint—p. Indicum, Indigo— p. Nigrum, see Choroid — p. Uracu, Terra Orleana.

PIGMY, Pygmy.

PIGNEROLE, Centaurea calcitrapa.

PIGNON DE BARBARIE, Jatropha curcas — p. *d'Inde*, Jatropha curcas.

PIGNUT, *Earthnut*, *Groundnut*. The bulbous root of *Bu'nium Bulbocas'tanum*. Called *pignuts*, from the fondness of the pig for them. They have been considered to possess a styptic quality; and are deemed serviceable in atonic affections of the kidney. — Hooper.

PIGNUT, Bunium bulbocastanum.

PIG'S FLARE, Adeps suillus.

PILA, *Sphæra*, *Ball*. A gymnastic exercise, much used by the ancients as well as moderns.— Galen. Also, a mortar and a pestle—*Ac'onē*.

PILA, Mortar, Pillar — p. Damarum, Ægagropila—p. Rupicaprarum, Ægagropila.

PILA MARI'NA, *Sphæra Marina*, *Sphæra Thalas'sia*, *Halcyo'nium rotun'dum*, (F.) *Pelote de Mer*. Certain light, round, depressed, or oblong masses—inodorous and insipid—in which rushes, hairs, and the *débris* of shells are met with. These are found on the sea-shores, and have been regarded by Spielmann as consisting chiefly of the roots of the *Zos'tera Mari'na seu Marit'ima*, *Alga Mari'na*, *Phucagros'tis minor*. Iodine is detected in the ashes, which accounts for their success in goître. They have, also, been given as a vermifuge.

PILARE MALUM, Trichosis.

PILA'TIO, from *pilus*, 'a hair.' Fracture of the cranium in which the fissure is narrow, and has the appearance of a hair—a *cap'illary fissure*, (F.) *Fente capillaire*.

PILE, Hair.
PILEA PUMI'LA, *Rickweed, Clearweed, Coolweed;* indigenous; *Order,* Urticaceæ; flowering from July to September; has been used as a wash in poisoning by Rhus. It has a strong, grateful smell.
PILEOLUM, *Calotte.*
PILEOLUS, Caul, Pileus.
PI'LEOUS, *Pilo'sus, Pilose, Pilous,* (F.) *Pileux.* That which relates to the hair. Hairy.
PILEOUS SYSTEM of Bichat is that formed by the hair. It comprises the different species of hair of the human body.
PILES, BLIND, Cæcæ hæmorrhoïdes, see Hæmorrhois.
PILEUS, 'a hat, cap, or bonnet for the head.' *Pile'olus.* A shield. A nipple-like instrument, formed of various materials, and used by females for protecting the nipple during the child's sucking, when the part is painful. Also, a caul.
PILEUS, Cucupha — p. Hippocraticus, *Bonnet d'Hippocrate.*
PILEUX, Pileous.
PILEWORT, Ranunculus acris, and R. ficaria.
PILI CAPITIS, see Capillus — p. Cutis, Lanugo — p. Palpebrarum, Cilia — p. Pudendorum, Pubes.
PILIER, Pillar.
PILIMICTIO, see Trichiasis.
PILL, Pilula — p. Abernethy's, see Pilulæ hydrargyri — p. of Aloes and Camboge, Pilulæ aloes et cambogiæ — p. of Aloes and cinchona, Pilulæ aloes et kinæ kinæ — p. of Aloes and colocynth, Pilulæ aloes et colocynthidis — p. of Aloes and fetid gums, Pilulæ de aloe et fœtidis—p. of Aloes and ginger, Pilulæ aloes et singiberis — p. Aloes and myrrh, Pilulæ aloes et myrrhæ — p. Aloetic, Pilulæ aloeticæ — p. Aloetic and assafœtida, Pilulæ aloes et assafœtidæ — p. Aloetic, compound, Pilulæ aloes compositæ — p. of Ammoniuret of copper, Pilulæ ammoniureti cupri—p. Analeptic, James's, see Analeptica — p. Anderson's, see Pilulæ aloes et jalapæ—p. Anodyne, Pilulæ opiatæ —p. Antibilious, Barclay's, Pilulæ antibiliosæ — p. Antibilious, Dixon's, Pilulæ antibiliosæ — p. Asiatic, Pilulæ Asiaticæ — p. Assafetida, Pilulæ Assafœtidæ—p. Bacher's, Pilulæ ex helleboro et myrrhâ—p. Barbarossa's, Barbarossæ pilulæ—p. Barthez, see Pilulæ aloes et myrrhæ.
PILL, BLAIR'S. An empirical preparation of colchicum, much used in England in cases of gout.
PILL, BLAUD'S. These pills, proposed by M. Blaud as antichlorotic, are formed as follows : — Take of *gum tragacanth,* in powder, six grains; *water,* one drachm. Macerate in a glass or porcelain mortar, until a thick mucilage is formed, and if it be desired to prevent the formation of peroxide of iron, and to make the pill similar to those of Vallet, substitute a drachm of powdered sugar for the mucilage. Add afterwards of *sulphate of iron,* in powder, half an ounce. Beat well until the mixture is homogeneous, and add *subcarbonate of potass,* half an ounce. Beat until the mass becomes of a deep-green colour, and of a soft consistence. Divide into 48 (?) pills. Dose, one a day; gradually increasing to two, and afterwards to three.
PILL, BLUE, Pilulæ hydrargyri—p. Brandreth's, Pilulæ aloes et cambogiæ —[p. Calomel, Pilulæ hydrargyri chloridi mitis — p. Camboge, Pilulæ cambogiæ compos.—p. Camboge, compound, Pilulæ cambogiæ compositæ — p. of Carbonate of iron, Pilulæ ferri carbonatis — p. Cathartic, compound, Pilulæ catharticæ compositæ — p. Common, Pilulæ aloes et myrrhæ — p. Dinner, see Pilulæ aloes et kinæ kinæ.
PILL, DINNER, OF MR. MAYO. This is composed of *P. Rhej,* gr. iv; *Sodæ Carb.* gr. j.

PILL, EVERLASTING. A pill once in vogue, and said to be composed of metallic antimony. It was believed to have the property of purging as often as it was swallowed. A lady having swallowed one of these pills, became seriously alarmed at its not passing. "Madam," said her physician, "fear not; it has already passed through a hundred patients without any difficulty."— Paris.
PILL, FEMALE, Pilulæ de aloe et fœtidis — p. Ferruginous, of Vallet, see Ferri protocarbonas —p. Fothergill's, see Pilulæ aloes et colocynthidis — p. Frank's see Pilulæ aloes et kinæ kinæ — p. Fuller's, see Pilulæ de aloe et fœtidis — p. Galbanum, compound, Pilulæ galbani compositæ — p. Griffitt's, see Pilulæ rhej compositæ—p. Gum, Pilulæ galbani compositæ — p. of Hellebore and myrrh, Pilulæ ex helleboro et myrrhâ—p. Hooper's, see Pilulæ aloes et myrrhæ—p. of Iodide of Iron, Pilulæ ferri iodidi—p. James's Aanaleptic, see Analeptica — p. Keyser's, see Hydrargyrus acetatus — p. Lady Crespigny's, Pilulæ aloes et kinæ kinæ—p. Lady Hesketh's, see Pilulæ aloes et kinæ kinæ — p. Lady Webster's, Pilulæ aloes et kinæ kinæ.
PILL, LARTIGUES', *Pil'ulæ Col'chici et Digita'lis.* (*Ext. Coloc. e.* ʒss; *Ext. Sem. Colchic. alcoholic., Extract. Digital. alcohol.* āā gr. iss; f. massa in pilul. x dividend.) Dose, two, three, or more, in the 24 hours, in gout.
PILL MACHINE, *Pilulier* — p. Matthews's, see Pilulæ ex helleboro et myrrhâ — p. Mercurial, Pilulæ hydrargyri — p. of mild chloride of Mercury, Pilulæ hydrargyri chloridi mitis — p. Moffat's, Pilulæ aloes et cambogiæ — p. Morrison's, Pilulæ aloes et cambogiæ, see Pilulæ cambogiæ compositæ—p. Moseley's, Pilulæ rhej compositæ —p. Night, common, Pilulæ opiatæ—p. Opiate, Pilulæ opiatæ—p. Peter's, see Pilulæ aloes et cambogiæ—p. Plummer's, Pilulæ hydrargyri submuriatis compositæ — p. of Sulphate of Quinia, Pilulæ quiniæ sulphatis—p. Red, Pilulæ hydrargyri submuriatis compositæ—p. Red, Boerhaave's, see Hydrargyri sulphuretum rubrum—p. of Rhabarb, Pilulæ rhej — p. of Rhubarb, compound, Pilulæ rhei compositæ—p. Rufus's, Pilulæ aloes et myrrhæ — p. Rush's, see Pilulæ aloes et cambogiæ — p. Scotch, Pilulæ de aloe et fœtidis —p. of Soap and opium, Pilulæ saponis cum opio—p. Speediman's, see Pilulæ aloes et myrrhæ — p. Squill, compound, Pilulæ scillæ compositæ — p. Starkey's, see Pilulæ ex helleboro et myrrhâ — p. Storax, Pilulæ e styrace—p. of Strychnia, Pilulæ strychniæ — p. of Submuriate of mercury, compound, Pilulæ hydrargyri submuriatis compositæ—p. Tanjore, Pilulæ Asiaticæ — p. Turpentine, Pilulæ de terebinthinâ—p. Vallet's, see Ferri protocarbonas, and Pilulæ ferri carbonatis — p. Webster's, Pilulæ aloes et kinæ kinæ—p. Whytt's, see Pilulæ de aloe et fœtidis.
PILLAR, *Pi'la, Colum'na, Columel'la,* (F.) *Pilier.* A name given to several parts; as the *pillars of the velum palati, diaphragm, &c.*
PILON, Pilum.
PILOSELLA, Hieracium pilosella— p. Alpina, Hieracium pilosella.
PILOSUS, Pileous.
PILOUS, Pileous.
PIL'ULA, plural *Pil'ulæ.* Diminutive of *pila,* 'a ball.' *Sphærid'ion, Catapo'tion, Catop'otum, Sphæ'rion, Gongyl'ion, Gon'gylis, Gongylid'ion.* A pill. (F.) *Pilule.* A simple or compound medicine, weighing from one to five grains, of a firm consistence and spherical form; intended to be swallowed at once, without chewing. The *Pill* differs from the *Bolus,* the latter being softer and larger.
Medicines are often given in the form of pill,

on account of their disagreeable taste and odour. *Pilula*, also, means a *Pilular mass*.

PILULÆ EX ALOE, P. aloes compositæ—p. de Aloe et cambogiâ, P. aloes et cambogiæ.

PILULÆ ALOËS, *P. Aloet'icæ, Pilulæ ex Aloë et Sapo'në, Aloet'ic Pill*, (F.) *Pilules d'aloes ou aloëtiques*. (*Aloes in pulv.; saponis*, sing. ℥j; *syr*. q. s. to form 240 pills.—Ph. U. S.) Dose, gr. x to xx, in habitual costiveness.

PILULÆ ALOES ET ASSAFŒ'TIDÆ, *Aloetic and Assafœtida Pills*. (*Aloes, assafœtidæ, saponis*, sing. ℥ss; *aquæ*, q. s. to form 180 pills.— Ph. U. S.) Purgative and stomachic. Dose, gr. x.

PILULÆ ALOES ET CAMBO'GIÆ, *P. de Aloë et Cambo'giâ, P. Hydrargo'gæ Bon'tii, Pill of Aloes and Camboge*. (*Aloes, cambog., gum. ammoniat.*, āā p. æ. Make into a powder. Dissolve in vinegar; pass through a cloth; express the residuum strongly; and afterwards evaporate, in a waterbath, to a pilular consistence. P. P.) Purgative; used in dropsy. Dose, gr. xij to xxx.

Peter's Pills—a nostrum—are formed of *aloes, jalap, scammony*, and *camboge*, of each equal parts.

The basis of *Morrison's Pills*, often called *Hygiène Pills*, of *Brandreth's Pills*, and *Moffat's Pills*, is said to be aloes, with camboge, scammony, &c.

Rush's Pills were formed of *calomel, aloes*, and *camboge*, with *oil of mint*.

PILULÆ ALOES ET COLOCYN'THIDIS, *P. ex Colocynth'idĕ cum aloĕ, P. Aloes cum Colocynthidĕ, P. coc'cinæ, P. cocchii, P. colocyn'thidis compos'itæ, P. cocciæ mino'res, Pill of Aloes and Colocynth*. (*Pulp. coloc.* ℥ss; *aloes hepat., scammon*, āā ℥j; *sapon.* ℥ij; *ol. caryoph.* ℥j; *syrup.* q. s.— Ph. D.) Cathartic. Dose, gr. v to x or more.

Foth'ergill's Pills consist of *aloes, scammony, colocynth*, and *oxide of antimony*.

PILULÆ ALOES COMPOS'ITÆ, *Pilulæ ex Aloē, Compound Aloetic Pills*. (*Aloes spic. extract. cont.* ℥j; *ext. gentianæ*, ℥ss; *olei carui*, gtt. xl; *syr*. q. s.— Ph. L.) These are sometimes, also, called *Family pills, Antibilious pills*, &c.

PILULÆ DE ALOE ET FŒ'TIDIS, *P. Benedic'tæ Fulleri, Pill of aloes and fetid gums, Pilulæ ecphrac'ticæ, Female pills, Pilula aloes martia'les,* (F.) *Pilules bénites de Fuller*. (*Aloes socotr., sennæ, assafœtidæ, galbani*, āā ℥ij; *myrrh*, ℥iv; *croci, macis*, āā ℥j; *ferri sulphat.* ℥iss. Reduce to powder separately, and add *ol. succin.* gtt. viij; *syr. artemisiæ*, q. s.— Ph. P.) Purgative, and given in hysteria. Dose, gr. xv to xx.

Whytt's Pills, given in similar cases, consisted of chloride of iron, aloes, extract of horehound, and assafœtida.

PILULÆ ALOES ET JALAP'Æ, commonly called *Anderson's pills, Anderson's Scots' pills, Scotch pills*. (*Aloes Barbad.* ℔j; *rad. helleb. nigr., rad. jalapæ, potassæ subcarb.* āā ℥j; *ol. anisi*, ℥iv; *syrup. simpl.* q. s.—Gray.) Dose, gr. x to xxx.

A committee of the Philadelphia College of Pharmacy recommend the following: *Aloes Barbadens.* ℥xxiv; *saponis*, ℥iv; *colocynthid.* ℥j; *cambogiæ*, ℥j; *ol. anis.* f℥ss.

PILULÆ ALOES ET KINÆ KINÆ, *P. stomach'icæ P. ante cibum, Pill of aloes and cinchona*, (F.) *Pilules gourmandes*. (*Aloes socotr.* ℥vj; *ext. cinchon.* ℥iij; *cinnam.* ℥j; *syrup. absinth.* q. s.— Ph. P.) Stomachic and laxative. Dose, gr. x to xx.

Lady Crespigny's pills, Lady Webster's pills, Lady Hesketh's pills, and the *Pilula stomach'icæ Mesuës* (Ph. L. 1635), resemble these.

Frank's pills, much employed, also, as '*dinner pills*,' or, — to use the language of the eccentric Kitchener — as '*peptic persuaders*,' are said to be much used, under the name *Graines de santé*, in various parts of Europe. They consist of *aloes, jalap*, and *rhubarb*, with *syrup of wormwood* as an excipient.

PILULÆ ALOES MARTIALES, P. de aloe et fœtidis.

PILULÆ ALOES ET MYRRHÆ, *P. aloes cum myrrhâ, P. de aloë et myrrhâ, Rufus's* or *Rufus's pills, Common pills, Pilulæ Rufi* seu *Ruffi, P. commu'nes, Pills of aloes and myrrh*. (*Aloes*, ℥ij; *croci*, in pulv. ℥ss; *myrrh*, ℥j; *syr*. q. s. to form 480 pills.— Ph. U. S.) Cathartic and emmenagogue. Dose, gr. x to xx.

Hooper's pills—possessed of similar properties —according to one of Gray's formulæ, are made as follows; *Ferri sulph., aquæ*, āā ℥viij. Dissolve. Add *aloes Barbad.* ℔ij and ℥viij; *canellæ albæ*, ℥vj; *gum myrrh*, ℥ij; *opopanacis*, ℥iv. The committee of the Philadelphia College of Pharmacy recommend the following form: *Aloes Barbadensis*, ℥viij; *ferri sulphatis exsiccat.* ℥ij, ℥iss, vel *ferri sulph. crystall.* ℥iv; *ext. helleb. nigr.* ℥ij; *myrrh*, ℥ij; *saponis*, ℥ij; *canellæ*, in pulv. tritæ, ℥j; *zingib.* in pulv. tritæ, ℥j.

Speediman's pills consist of *aloes, myrrh, rhubarb, extract of chamomile*, and *essential oil of chamomile;* and the *Pills of Barthes*, of *aloes, myrrh, musk, camphor*, and *balsam of Peru*.

PILULÆ DE ALOE ET SAPONE, P. aloeticæ.

PILULÆ ALOES CUM ZINGIB'ERÆ, *Pill of aloes and ginger*. (*Aloes hepat.* ℥j; *rad. zingib.* in pulv. ℥j; *sapon. Hispan.* ℥ss; *ol. ess. menthæ pip.* ℥ss.— Ph. D.) In habitual costiveness. Dose, gr. x to xx.

PILULÆ AMMONIURE'TI CUPRI, *Pills of Ammoniuret of copper, Pilulæ cupri*, (F.) *Pilules d'ammoniure de cuivre*. (*Ammoniur. cupri*, in pulv. ten. trit. gr. xvj; *micæ panis*, ℈iv; *aquæ carbonatis ammoniæ*, q. s. Beat into a mass, and divide into xxxij pills.— Ph. E.) Tonic and antispasmodic, in epilepsy, &c. Dose, one pill twice daily; gradually increasing the dose.

PILULÆ ANTE CIBUM, P. aloes et kinæ kinæ.

PILULÆ ANTIBILIO'SÆ, *Barclay's Antibil'ious pills*. (*Extract de colocynth*, ℥ij; *resin of jalap*, ℥j; *almond soap*, ℥iss; *guaiac*, ℥iij; *emetic tart.* gr. viij; *oils of juniper, carraway, and rosemary*, āā iv drops; *syrup of buckthorn*, q. s. to form 64 pills.) Dose, two or three.

Dixon's Antibilious pills are formed of *aloes, scammony, rhubarb*, and *tartarized antimony*.

PILULÆ ANTIHERPETICÆ, Pilulæ hydrargyri submuriatis comp.—p. Antihystericæ, P. galbani compositæ.

PILULÆ ANTISCROPHULO'SÆ, *P. ex ox'ido stib'ii et hydrar'gyri sulphure'to nigro compos'itæ*. (*P. scammon., hydrarg. sulphur. nigr.* āā ℥ij; *antimonii oxidi albi, milleped., sapon. amygdalin.* āā ℥iij; *extract. glycyrrh.* ℥v. Make into a mass.— Ph. P.) Dose gr. iv to xx.

PILULÆ ANTISPASTICÆ, P. galbani compositæ —p. Assafœtidæ compositæ, P. galbani compositæ.

PILULÆ ASIAT'ICÆ, *Asiat'ic pills, Tanjore pills*. (*Acid. arsenios.* gr. lv; *piper. nigr.* pulv. ℥ix; *acaciæ*, q. s. ut fiant pil. 800. Each pill contains about one-fifteenth of a grain of arsenious acid. These pills are employed in India for the cure of syphilis and elephantiasis.

PILULÆ ASSAFŒ'TIDÆ, *Assafet'ida pills*. (*Assafœtid.* ℥iss; *saponis*, ℥ss. Beat with *water* so as to form a mass to be divided into 240 pills.— Ph. U. S.)

PILULÆ BALSAM'ICÆ, *P. Docto'ris Morton*. (*Milleped*, pulverisat. ℥xviij; *gum. ammon.* ℥xj; *acid. benzoic.* ℥vj; *croci, balsam. Peruv.* āā ℥j; *balsam. sulph. anisat.* ℥vj. Mix.— Pb P.) Tonic, expectorant, and balsamic.

PILULÆ BENEDICTÆ FULLERI, P. de aloe et fœtidis.

PILULÆ CAMBO'GIÆ COMPOS'ITÆ, *P. de guttâ gamam'drâ, P. hydrago'gæ, Gamboge pills, Pilulæ gummi guttæ aloet'icæ, Compound camboge pills,* (F.) *Pilules de gomme gutte composées.* (*Cambogiæ contritæ, aloes spicat. extrat. contriti., pulv. cinnam. comp.* sing. ℈j; *saponis,* ℈ij.—Ph. L.) Cathartic. Dose, gr. x to xx.

Morrison's pills are said by Dr. Paris to be nothing more than the above, with the addition of a small portion of *cream of tartar.*

PIL'ULÆ CATHAR'TICÆ COMPOS'ITÆ, *Compound cathartic pills.* (*Ext. colocynth. comp.* in pulv. ℨss; *ext. jalapæ,* in pulv., *hydrarg. chlorid. mit.* āā ℈iij; *gambog.* in pulv. ℈ij. M. Form into a mass with *water,* and make into 180 pills.—Ph. U. S.) Three for a dose.

PILULÆ COCCHII, P. aloes et colocynthidis—p. Cocciæ minores, P. aloes et colocynthidis—p. Coccinæ, P. aloes et colocynthidis—p. Colchici et digitalis, P. Lartigues'—p. Colocynthidis compositæ, P. aloes et colocynthidis—p. ex Colocynthide cum aloe, P. aloes et colocynthidis—p. Communes, P. aloes et myrrhæ—p. Cupri, P. ammoniureti cupri.

PILULÆ COPA'IBÆ, *Pills of copaiba.* (*Copaib.* ℈ij; *magnesiæ,* recenté præpar. ℈j. Mix, and set aside till it concretes into a pilular mass, to be divided into 200 pills.—Ph. U. S.) Each pill contains nearly five grains of copaiba. Two to six for a dose.

PILULÆ DE CYNOGLOS'SO, *P. de extrac'to o'pii.* (*Pulv. rad. cynogloss., semin. hyoscyam. alb., extract. opii vinos.* āā ℨiv; *pulv. myrrh.* ℨvj; *oliban.* ℈v; *croci., castor.,* āā ℈iss; *syrup opii,* q. s.—Ph. P.) Anodyne. In cough, &c. Dose, gr. iv to gr. viij.

PILULÆ DEPURANTES, P. hydrargyri submuriatis compos.—p. Ecphracticæ, P. de aloe et fœtidis.

PILULÆ FERRI CARBONA'TIS, *Pills of carbonate of iron, Vallet's pills, Vallet's ferru'ginous pills.* (*Ferri sulph.* ℨviij; *sodæ carbonat.* ℨx; *Mel. despumat.* ℨiij; *sacchar.* ℨij; *aquæ bullientis,* Oij; *syrup.* q. s. Dissolve the sulphate of iron and carbonate of soda, each in a pint of the water, and to each solution add a fluidounce of syrup; then mix the two solutions in a bottle just large enough to contain them; close it accurately with a stopper, and set it by, that the carbonate of iron may subside. Pour off the liquid, and having washed the precipitate with warm water, sweetened with syrup in the proportion of f℈j of the latter to Oj of the former, until the washings no longer have a saline taste, place it upon a flannel cloth, and express as much water as possible; then mix it with the honey and sugar. Lastly, heat the mixture in a water-bath, until it attains a pilular consistence.— Ph. U. S.)

PILULÆ FERRI COMPOS'ITÆ, *Compound pills of iron, Pilulæ ferri cum myrrhâ,* (F.) *Pilules de fer composées.* (*Myrrh,* in pulv. ℈ij; *sodæ subcarb., ferri sulph.* āā ℈j; *syrup,* q. s. Mix, to form 80 pills.— Ph. U. S.) Tonic. Dose, gr. x to xx.

PILULÆ FERRI IOD'IDI, *Pills of iodide of iron.* (*Ferri sulphat.* ℈j; *Potass. iodid.* ℈iv; *traganth.* pulv. gr. x; *sacchar.* pulv. ℨss. Beat with syrup int. a mass, to form 40 pills.— Ph. U. S.) Dose, one to three, where a tonic and eutrophic is indicated.

PILULÆ FERRI CUM MYRRHÂ, P. Ferri compositæ—p. Fœtidæ, P. galbani compositæ.

PILULÆ GAL'BANI COMPOS'ITÆ, *P. assafœtidæ compos'itæ, P. fœ'tidæ, P. gummo'sæ, P. e gummi, Compound galbanum pill, Pilulæ antispas'ticæ, P. antihyster'icæ, P. myrrhæ compos'itæ, Gum pill.* (*Galban., myrrhæ,* āā ℈vj; *assafœtidæ,* ℈ij; *syrup.* q. s. to form 240 pills.— Ph. U. S.) Antispasmodic and emmenagogue. Dose, gr. x to xx.

PILULÆ GUMMI, P. galbani compositæ—p. Gummi guttæ aloeticæ, P. cambogiæ compositæ —p. Gummosæ, P. galbani compositæ—p. de Guttâ gamandrâ, P. cambogiæ compositæ.

PILULÆ EX HELLEB'ORO ET MYRRHÂ, *P. ton'icæ, Backer's pills, Tonic pills of Backer, Pills of hellebore and myrrh.* (*Ext. helleb. nig., myrrh.* āā ℈j; *fol. cardui benedict.* in pulv. ℈iij. M.— Ph. P.) Tonic and emmenagogue. In dropsical, cutaneous, and verminous affections. Dose, gr. iv to gr. viij.

Matthews's pills,— Starkey's pills, are formed of *rad. helleb. nigr., rad. glycyrrh., sapon. Castill., rad. curcumæ, opii purif., syrup. croci,* āā ℨiv; *ol. tereb.* q. s. ut fiat massa.— Gray.

PILULÆ HYDRAGOGÆ, P. cambogiæ compositæ—p. Hydragogæ Bontii, Pilulæ aloes et cambogiæ.

PILULÆ HYDRAR'GYRI, *P. mercuria'les, Mercurial pill, Blue pill,* (F.) *Pilules de Mercure.* (*Hydrarg. purif.* ℈j; *conf. rosæ,* ℨiss; *glycyrrh.* pulv. ℨss. Rub the quicksilver with the confection, until the globules disappear; then add the liquorice powder, and beat the whole into a uniform mass, to be divided into 480 pills.— Ph. U. S.) Antisyphilitic; mercurial;—in large doses, purgative.

A purgative pill, much prescribed by Mr. Abernethy, and called *Abernethy's pill,* consisted of *pil. hydrarg.* gr. x; *jalap,* pulv. gr. xx; *syrup rhamni,* q. s. ut fiant pil. vj. Two were given at night, and the next morning a wineglassful of *infusum sennæ.*

PILULÆ HYDRAR'GYRI CHLO'RIDI MITIS, *Pills of mild chloride of mercury, Calomel pills.* (*Hydrarg. chlorid. mit.* ℨss; *acaciæ,* in pulv. ℈j; *syrup.* q. s. ut fiant pil. 240.— Ph. U. S.) Each pill contains one grain.

PILULÆ DE HYDRARGYRO, SCAMMO'NIO ET ALOE, vulgo MERCURIA'LES, (F.) *Pilules Mercurielles ou de Mercure, Scammonée et Aloes.* (*Hydrarg. purif.* ℈j; *mellis,* ℨxj. Rub until the globules disappear; then add *aloes Socot., scammon.* āā ℈ij; *macis, cinnam.* āā ℈ij. Make into a mass.— Ph. P.) Uses, same as the last, but they are more purgative. Dose, gr. viij to xxx. These pills are nearly the same as the *Pastilles de Renaudot.*

PILULÆ EX HYDRARGYRO MURIATICO MITI CUM SULPHURE STIBIATO AURANTIACO, Pilulæ hydrargyri submuriatis compositæ.

PILULÆ HYDRARGYRI SUBMURIATIS COMPOSITÆ, *Pilulæ ex stib'io et hydrar'gyro,* (F.) *antihyper'icæ, P. ex hydrargyro muriat'ico cum sul'phure stibia'to auriantiaco, P. resolven'tes cum mercurio, P. depurantes, P. hydrargyri submuriatis, Compound pills of submuriate of mercury, Calomel pills, Plummer's pills, Red pill.* (*Hydrarg. submur., antimon. sulphur. precipitat.* sing. ℈ij; *guaiac. gum resin. contrit.* ℨiv; *spirit rect.* ℨss. Beat together.— Ph. L.) Mercurial, and reputed to be diaphoretic and alterative. Dose, gr. v to x.

Leake's pilula saluta'ria resembles these. It is used in syphilis.

PILULÆ MERCURIALES, P. hydrargyri, P. de hydrargyro, scammonio et aloe—p. Doctoris Morton, P. balsamicæ — p. Myrrhæ compositæ, P. Galbani compositæ.

PILULÆ OPIA'TÆ, *P. Theba'icæ, Opiate pill, Common night pills, Anodyne pills, Nepen'thes opia'tum,* (F.) *Pilules opiacées.* (*Opii,* p. 1; *ext. glycyrrh.* p. 7; *fruct. myrt. piment.* p. 2. Mix.— Ph. E.) Five grains contain gr. ss of opium.

PILULÆ OPII, P. saponis cum opio—p. de Extracto opii, P. de cynoglosso—p. ex Oxido stibii et hydrargyri sulphureto nigro compositæ, Pilulæ antiscrophulosæ — p. Resolventes cum mercurio, P. hydrargyri submuriatis compos. — p. de Rhabarbaro, Pilulæ rhei compositæ.

The stomachic nostrum, sold under the name of *Moseley's pills*, consists merely of *rhubarb* and *ginger*.

PILULÆ QUI'NLÆ SULPHA'TIS, *Pills of sulphate of quinia*. (*Quin. sulph.* ʒj; *acaciæ*, in pulv. ʒij; *mel.* q. s. ut fiant pilulæ 480.—Ph. U. S. Each pill contains a grain of the sulphate of quinia.

PILULÆ RHEJ, *Pills of rhubarb*. (*Rhej*, pulv. ʒvj; *saponis*, ʒij. M. et fiant pil. 120. — Ph. U. S.) Each pill contains three grains of rhubarb.

PILULÆ RHEI COMPOS'ITÆ, *P. de Rhabar'baro, Compound rhubarb pills*. (*Rhei*, pulv. ʒj; *aloes*, pulv. ʒvj; *myrrh.* pulv. ʒiv; *ol. menthæ* pip. fʒss. Beat into a mass, with *syrup of orange-peel*, to form 240 pills. — Ph. U. S.) Laxative and stomachic. Dose, gr. x to xx.

Griffitt's pills, so called after Dr. S. P. Griffitts, of Philadelphia, who prescribed them as a tonic aperient, were formed as follows: — *Rhej*, pulv. ʒiss; *ferri sulph.* ʒss; *saponis*, Đij; *aquæ*, q. s. ut fiat massa in pil. xl dividenda. Dose, three or four at bedtime.

PILULÆ RUFI, P. aloes et myrrhæ — p. Salutariæ, Leake's, see Pilulæ hydrargyri submuriatis compositæ— p. Saponaceæ, P. saponis cum opio — p. Saponis compositæ, P. saponis cum opio.

PILULÆ SAPO'NIS CUM O'PIO, *P. sapona'ceæ, Pills of soap and opium, P. sapo'nis compos'itæ*, (F.) *Pilules de savon et d'opium*. (*Opii*, ʒss; *sapon.* ʒij. M.—Ph. U. S.) Five grains contain one of opium.

The Pharmacopœia of the United States has a form for the *Pilulæ opii, Opium pills*, as well as for the *Pilulæ saponis compositæ*; the only difference between them being in the proportion of the ingredients. The following is the formula for the Pilulæ opii:—*Opii*, pulv. ʒj; *saponis*, gr. xij. Beat with water into a mass to form 60 pills.

PILULÆ E SCILLÂ, P. scillæ compositæ.

PILULÆ SCILLÆ COMPOS'ITÆ, *P. scillit'icæ, P. scillæ cum zinzib'ere, P. e scillâ, Compound squill pill.* (*Scillæ*, pulv. ʒj; *zingib.* pulv., *ammoniac.* pulv. ăă ʒij; *saponis*, ʒiij; *syrup.* q. s. ut fiant pil. 120. — Ph. U. S.) Dose, two pills. Expectorant and diuretic. Dose, gr. x to xx.

PILULÆ SCILLÆ CUM ZINGIBERE, P. scillæ compositæ—p. Scilliticæ, P. scillæ compositæ—p. ex Stibio et hydrargyro, P. hydrargyri submur. compos.—p. Stomachicæ, P. aloes et kinæ kinæ.

PILULÆ STRYCH'NLÆ, *Pills of Strychnia*. (Very pure *strychnine*, 2 gr.; *conserve of roses*, ʒss. Make into 24 pills.) One or two for a dose.

PILULÆ E STY'RACE, *Storax Pills*. (*Styracis* pur. ʒiij, *opii purif., mellis, croci*, sing. ʒj. Ph. D.) Six grains contain one of opium.

PILULÆ SUBLINGUALES, Hypoglottides.

PILULÆ DE TEREBIN'THINÂ, *Turpentine Pills*. Made of turpentine boiled in 3 times its weight of water, until, when thrown into cold water, it forms a soft paste, which has the properties of turpentine, and has been administered in gleet, &c.

PILULÆ THEBAICÆ, P. opiatæ—p. Tonicæ, P. ex Helleboro et myrrhâ.

PIL'ULAR, *Pilula'ris*; from *pilula*, 'a pill.' Relating to pills,—as 'a *pilular mass*,' '*pilular* form,' &c.

PILULES, Pilulæ—*p. Agrégatives*, see Aggregate—*p. d'Aloes ou aloétiques*, Pilulæ aloeticæ—*p. d'Ammoniure de cuivre*, Pilulæ ammoniureti cupri—*p. Bénites de Fuller*, Pilulæ de aloe et fœtidis—*p. de Fer composées*, Pilulæ ferri compositæ—*p. Ferrugineuses de Vallet*, see Ferri protocarbonas—*p. Gourmandes*, Pilulæ aloes et kinæ kinæ—*p. de Mercure*, Pilulæ hydrargyri—*p. de Mercure*, &c., Pilulæ de hydrargyro, et scammonio et aloe—*p. Mercurielles*, Pilulæ de hydrargyro, scammonio et aloe—*p. Opiacées*, Pilulæ opiatæ—*p. de Savon et d'Opium*, Pilulæ saponis cum opio.

PILULIER (F.) *Pill Machine*. An instrument invented by the Germans for rolling and dividing pills. Also, the earthen pot in which pills are preserved.

PILUM, *Pistil'lus, Pistillum, Hyp'eros, Cer'cis*, (F.) *Pilon*. A pestle. A wooden, iron, bellmetal, marble, agate, porcelain, or glass instrument for beating or dividing substances in a mortar.

A *spring pestle* is one attached above to a spring, so as to take off the weight, and thus lessen the labour of pounding.

PILUS, Capillus, Caul, Hair.

PIMELE, Fat.

PIMELECCHYSIS, Pimelorrhœa.

PIMELICUS, Fatty.

PIMELI'TIS, from πιμελη, 'fat,' and *itis*, denoting inflammation. Inflammation of the adipous tissue.

PIMELODES, Fatty.

PIMELO'MA, from πιμελη, 'fat.' A fatty swelling.

PIMELORRHŒ'A, *Pimelec'chysis*, from πιμελη, 'fat,' and ρεω, 'I flow.' A morbid discharge or disappearance of fat.

PIMELORTHOPNŒ'A, *Piorthopnœ'a*; from πιμελη, 'fat,' ορθος, 'upright,' and πνειν, 'to breathe.' Dyspnœa, practicable only in the erect attitude, owing to fat.

PIMELO'SIS, *Obes'itas nim'ia*, from πιμελη, 'fat.' Conversion into, or formation of, fat,—as *Pimelo'sis hepat'ica*, 'fatty degeneration of the liver.'

PIMELOSIS HEPATICA, Adiposis hepatica—p. Nimia, see Polysarcia.

PIMENT, Capsicum annuum—*p. Royal*, Myrica gale.

PIMENTA, see Myrtus pimenta.

PIMENTÆ BACCÆ, see Myrtus pimenta.

PIMENTO, see Myrtus pimenta.

PIMIACULA, Labia pudendi.

PIMPERNEL, BLUE, Scutellaria lateriflora —p. Red, Anagallis—p. Scarlet, Anagallis arvensis—p. Water, Veronica beccabunga.

PIMPILIM, Piper longum.

PIMPINEL, see Pimpinella—p. Italian, Sanguisorba officinalis.

PIMPINELLA ALBA, P. saxifraga—p. Angelicæfolia, Ligusticum podagraria.

PIMPINEL'LA ANI'SUM, *Anise plant, Anisum, A. officina'lě seu vulga'rě, Sison ani'sum, A'pium ani'sum, Sola'men intestino'rum, Ane'sum*, (F.) *Anis. Family*, Umbelliferæ. *Sex. Syst.* Pentandria Digynia. A native of Egypt. The seeds, *Ani'sum*, (Ph. U. S.) *Sem'ina Ani'si, An'iseed*, have an aromatic odour; and a sweetish, warm, grateful taste. They are carminative, and used in dyspepsia and in tormina of infants. Dose, gr. xv to ʒj, bruised. The oil,—OLEUM ANI'SI, (F.) *Huile d'anis*—is officinal. Dose, gtt. v tu xv. Most of the oil used in this country under the name of *Oil of Anise* is said to be obtained from *Illicium Anisatum*.

PIMPINELLA, GREATER, P. magna—p. Hircina, P. Saxifraga—p. Laterifolia, Sion ammi.

PIMPINEL'LA MAGNA seu *nigra* seu *major* seu *rubra; Greater Pimpinel'la; Tragoseli'num magnum* seu *majus, Daucus, Cyan'opus*, (F.) *Boucage majeur*. The root has been extolled as diuretic and resolvent, as well as in erysipelatous ulcerations, tinea capitis, rheumatism, &c.

PIMPINELLA MAJOR, P. magna—p. Nigra, P. magna—p. Nostras, P. saxifraga—p. Officinalis, Sanguisorba officinalis—p. Rubra, P. magna.

PIMPINELLA SAXIF'RAGA, *Sax'ifrage, Burnet sax'ifrage, Pote'rium sanguisor'ba, Sorbastrel'la, Tragoseli'num, T. saxif'raga, Pimpinel'la hirci'na seu umbellif'era seu alba seu nostras,* (F.) *Boucage mineur, Petit B., Pimprenelle.* The root has an unpleasant smell, and hot, pungent, bitterish taste. It has been recommended as a stomachic; and as a stimulating gargle in paralysis of the tongue.

PIMPINELLA UMBELLIFERA, P. saxifraga.
PIMPLE, Papula.
PIMPLED, Papulose.
PIMPRENELLE, Pimpinella saxifraga—*p. Noire,* Sanguisorba officinalis.

PIN. Perhaps from *pennum,* low Latin; or from *spina; Spina fer'rea, Acus capita'ta,* (F.) *Épingle.* An iron or brass instrument, generally of a small size, pointed at one extremity, and having a head at the other. It is used, in Surgery, to fix rollers and dressings; and occasionally in sutures.

PIN À PIGNON, see Pinus picea.
PINASTELLUM, Peucedanum.
PINASTER, Pinus sylvestris.
PINCÉ, Pinched.
PINCE LITHODRASSIQUE, see Lithodrassic.
PINCÉE, Pugillus.
PINCERS, Forceps.
PINCETTES, Forceps.
PINCHED, *Contrac'tus,* (F.) *Pincé, Grippé.* An epithet applied to the face, when the features are contracted or shrunken; as in violent abdominal affections, or during intense pain.

PINCKNE'YA PUBENS, *P. Pubes'cens, Georgia Bark, Bitter Bark, Florida Bark, Fever tree.* This bark has been used in Georgia in the cure of intermittents, and successfully. It is a powerful bitter. Dose of the powder, ʒj.

PINDARS, Arachis Hypogea.
PINE APPLE, Bromelia ananas—p. Aphernousli, Pinus cembra—p. Ground, Lycopodium complanatum—p. Ground, stinking, Camphorosma Monspeliaca—p. Mountain, see Pinos mughos —p. Mugho, see Pinus mughos—p. Sap, American, Hypopitys lanuginosa—p. Stone, Pinus pinea—p. Sugar, see Arrow Root.
PINEA, Pinus pinea.
PINE'AL, *Pinea'lis,* from *pinus,* 'a pine.' That which resembles a pine-apple.

PINEAL GLAND, *Glandula pinea'lis, Cerebral epiph'ysis, Cona'rium, Conoi'des corpus, Penis cer'ebri, Corpus turbina'tum, Virga seu Turbo cer'ebri,* is a small body, of a conical shape; pale red or grayish colour; and soft consistence; situate between the fornix and the tubercula quadrigemina. It almost always contains sabulous particles, *Sab'ulum cona'rii:* when these are grouped together over the base of the gland, they form the *Acer'vulus Cer'ebri* of Sömmering, A. seu *Lapil'li glan'dulæ pinea'lis.* From its anterior part arise two medullary striæ, which proceed over the posterior commissure; coast along the optic thalami, and unite at the anterior pillar of the fornix,—the *habe'næ* or *reins of the pineal gland.*

The uses of the pineal gland are unknown. Descartes supposed it to be the seat of the soul!
PINEI, see Pinus pinea.
PINEOLI, see Pinus pinea.
PINEUS PURGANS, Jatropha curcas.
PINGUEC'ULA, *Pteryg'ium pinguë seu lar-da'ceum,* from *pinguis,* 'fat,' 'fatty.' A small, whitish-yellow tumour in the sclerotic conjunctiva and subjacent areolar tissue, close to the margin of the cornea on its nasal or temporal side; so called from its being supposed, but erroneously, to be of a fatty nature.

PINGUE'DO, Fat—p. Renalis, Nephridion.
PINGUIC'ULA VULGA'RIS, *P. alpi'na, Sanic'ula monta'na, S. Eboracen'sis, Vi'ola palustris, Dodecath'eon Plin'ii, Butter-wort, Yorkshire San'icle.* Family, Personneæ. *Sex. Syst.* Diandria Monogynia. The unctuosity of this plant has caused it to be applied to chaps, and as a pomatum to the hair. Decoctions of the leaves, in broths, are used by the common people in Wales as a cathartic.

PINGUID, Fatty.
PINGUIDINOUS, Fatty.
PINGUIN, Bromelia pinguin.
PINGUITUDO, Polysarcia adiposa.
PINHOLE PUPIL, see Pupil, pinhole.
PINHONES INDICI, Jatropha curcas.
PINK, CAROLINA, Spigelia Marilandica.
PINK DYE. *Stripped safflower,* ʒj, *subcarb. of potass.* gr. xviij, *spirit of wine* ʒvij; digest for two hours; add *distilled water* ʒij: digest for two hours more, and add *distilled vinegar* or *lemon juice* q. s., to reduce it to a fine rose-colour. Used as a cosmetic.

PINK, GROUND, Silene Virginica—p. Indian, Spigelia Marilandica—p. Wild, Silene Virginica.
PINNA, Ala, Pavilion of the ear—p. Marina, see Bissus.
PINNACULUM FORNICIS GUTTURALIS, Uvula.
PINNÆ HEPATIS, Lobes of the liver—p. Naris, see Nasus.
PINNULA, *Aileron.*
PINNULÆ HEPATIS, Lobes of the liver.
PINO'LL. (S.) A preparation used for subsistence on long journeys in the West. It is parched corn, beaten or ground very fine, and sweetened with sugar, to be used with water, and drunk on the march. It is the *cold flour* of the Indians, and early Western pioneers.
PIÑONCILLO TREE, Castiliognia lobata.
PINUS A'BIES, *P. excel'sa* seu *picea, A'bies Abies rubra* seu *excelsa* seu *picea, El'atë thele'a, Pice'a, Norway Spruce Fir, Yew-leaved Fir. Nat. Ord.* Coniferæ. *Sex. Syst.* Monœcia Monadelphia. The tops are used in making *Spruce Beer.*

Essence of Spruce, Essen'tia Abie'tis, is a fluid extract, prepared by decoction from the twigs of this species of fir. From this is made *Spruce Beer.*

This fir affords the Burgundy pitch and common frankincense. 1. *Bur'gundy Pitch, White pitch, Pix Burgun'dica, Pix alba, Resi'na abie'tis hu'mida, Resi'na alba humida, Pinë abie'tis resina spontë concre'ta, Pix ar'ida, Pix abieti'na, P. abietis* (Ph. U. S.,) (F.) *Poix blanche, Poix grasse, P. jaune, P. de Bourgogne.* This prepared concrete juice is of a close consistence, rather soft, of a reddish-brown colour, and not unpleasant smell. It is very adhesive to the skin; and, consequently, forms excellent plasters for remaining upon the part for some time;—as in cases of affections of the chest. 2. *Abie'tis Resi'na,* (Ph. L. since 1809.) *Thus, Common Frankincense, Perrosin, Thus fœmin'eum, T. vulga'rë, Olib'anum vulgarë* seu *sylves'trë, Resina abietis sicca, Resin of the Spruce Fir.* It is solid, dry, brittle; externally, brownish-yellow: internally, whitish. Used in plasters like the last.

PINUS ABIES, see P. picea—p. Alba, P. picea.
PINUS BALSAME'A, *A'bies balsamea* seu *bal-*

ramif'era, Peu'cea balsame'a. The tree which affords the *Canada Balsam, Balsamum Canaden'sě seu de Can'ada, Resina strobili'na, Terebinth'ina Canaden'sis, Pini balsame'a, Canada Turpentine* or *Balsam, Balsam of Fir,* (F.) *Baume de Canada,* is one of the purest turpentines. It has the common properties of those substances.

PINUS CANADEN'SIS, *Abies Canaden'sis, Hemlock Spruce.* A tree, which is abundant in Canada, Nova Scotia, and the more northern parts of New England, and is found in the elevated and mountainous regions of the Middle States. The pitch—*Pix Canadensis, Canada Pitch, Hemlock Pitch*—obtained from it is commonly known under the name *Hemlock Gum.*

PINUS CANDICANS, P. Picea.

PINUS CEMBRA, *P. Monta'na, Aphernous'li Pine.* It yields an agreeably scented turpentine:—the *Carpa'thian Balsam, Bal'samum Carpath'icum, B. Lib'ani, Carpath'icum, Briançon Tur'pentine.* The nuts, *Cembro nuts, Nu'dei Cembræ,* have an eatable kernel, and yield oil. The shoots yield *Riga Balsam* by distillation.

PINUS DAMAR'RA, *Ag'athis Damarra,* grows in the East India Islands. The juice speedily concretes into a very hard resin,—the *Damarra turpentine.*

PINUS EXCELSA, P. abies—p. Gallica, P. picea.

PINUS LARIX *A'bies larix, Larix, L. commu'nis* seu *decid'ua* seu *Europæ'a* seu *pyramida'lis.* The *Larch,* (F.) *Mélèze.* From this tree exudes *Or'emberg gum, Bri'ançon manna, Gummi lar'icis* seu *Oremburgen'sě* seu *Uralen'sě, Manna Briganti'na* seu *larice'a.* It also yields, by boring, *Common Venice Turpentine, Resina Lar'icis, Terebinthina Ven'eta* seu *larici'na, Pini Lar'icis resi'na liq'uida,* (F.) *Térébenthine de Vénise, M. de Mélèze.* It is usually thinner than the other sorts of turpentine.

PINUS MUGHOS. The *Mountain* or *Mugho Pine, Pinus Pumil'io.* From the extremities of the branches exudes the *Resina Strobili'na,* of the Germans, or *Hungarian Balsam.* It is also obtained, by expression, from the cones. By distillation, the Hungarian balsam affords the *Krumhols oil, Oleum Templinum.*

PINUS PALUSTRIS, see Pinus sylvestris.

PINUS PICE'A, *P. Abies, A'bies, A. pice'a* seu *pectina'ta* seu *Gal'lica* seu *alba* seu *can'dicans* seu *vulga'ris* seu *taxifo'lia, European Silver Fir Tree, El'ate,* (F.) *Sapin commun.* By piercing the tubercles of the bark of this fir, the *Strasburg Turpentine* is obtained : — the *Resi'na Abie'tis,* (Ph. L. before 1809,) *Oleum Abietis, Terebinth'ina Argentoraten'sis.*

PINUS PINASTER, see P. sylvestris.

PINUS PI'NEA, *Stone Pine, Pinea, Pinus, P. uber'rima* seu *sati'va.* The nuts, *Zirbel nuts, Nu'clei Pi'neæ, Pinei, Pine'oli,* (F.) *Pin à pignons,* are eaten raw, or preserved like almonds. They are, also, used in emulsions.

PINUS PUMILIO, see Pinus Mughos—p. Sativa, P. pinea.

PINUS SYLVES'TRIS, *Pinas'ter, Peucě, Scotch Fir.* This pine, as well as *P. marit'ima,* (*P. Pinaster*) and other species of Pinus, affords common turpentine and its oil, resin, tar, and pitch. 1. *Common Turpentine of Europe, Terebinth'ina, T. vulga'ris, T. commu'nis, Resina pini, Bijon, Horse Turpentine, Bordeaux Turpentine,* (F.) *Térébinthine de Bordeaux, Térébinthine commune,* is obtained by wounding the tree in hot weather. It is used, chiefly, as a dressing for wounds, &c., in horses, and for the distillation of the oil, (see Oleum Terebinthinæ.) The *white Turpentine,* or *common Turpentine of America*—*Terebinth'ina,* Ph. U. S.—is produced chiefly from *Pinus palustris* and *P. tæda,* and perhaps from other species inhabiting the Southern States. When the oil is distilled with water, yellow resin, or *Rosin,* (*Resi'na,* Ph. U. S.)—*Resina flava*—is left, which is only used in the formation of ointments and plasters: if without the addition of water, the residuum is common resin or Colophony. 2. When the cold begins to check the exudation of the common turpentine, part of it concretes in the wounds. This is called, in France, *Gallipot, Barras;* and *White Rosin, Resina alba,* when hardened after long exposure to the air. 3. When the old trees are subjected to distillation, in a coarse manner, Tar is obtained — *Hygropissos, Pissa, Pix ce'dria, Resi'na pini empyreumat'ica liq'uida, Terebinth'ina empyreumat'ica, Alchitram, Alchitu'ra, Cedria, Pix liquida,* (F.) *Goudron, Brai liquide.* Tar water, *Aqua Picea, A. Picis, Infu'sum Picis liq'uidæ* seu *Picis empyreumaticæ liquidæ, Po'tio pice'a,* (F.) *Eau de Goudron,* was, at one time, a fashionable remedy in numerous complaints, and its use has been revived, since its virtues have been presumed to be owing to creasote. It is employed chiefly in pulmonary affections, and the vapour has been recommended in phthisis and other diseases of the lungs. It is used externally as a detergent. 4. *Common Pitch, Pix nigra, Black Pitch, Burnea, Burnia, Stone Pitch, Pix sicca, P. atra, P. nava'lis, Topissa, Palimpis'sa, P. ar'ida* (Ph. L. before 1809), (F.) *Poix navale, P. noire,* is obtained by inspissating tar. It is used only as a resolvent in plasters.

PINUS TÆDA, see P. sylvestris — p. Taxifolia, P. picea — p. Uberrima, Pinus pinea—p. Vulgaris, P. picea.

PIONE, Pæonia.

PIONY, Pæonia.

PIORTHOPNŒA, Pimelorthopnœa.

PIOULQUES. (F.) A kind of sucking-pump, invented by Louis, for extracting water that had entered internal cavities, in cases of drowning. A useless instrument.

PIPE-PLANT, Monotropa uniflora.

PIPER, see Piper nigrum.

PIPER ALBUM *Leucopiper, White Pepper,* is black pepper freed from its cuticle.

PIPER AUGUSTIFOLIUM, Matico—p. Aromaticum, P. nigrum—p. Betel, Betel—p. Brazilianum, Capsicum annuum—p. Calecuticum, Capsicum annuum.

PIPER CAPEN'SE, a South African species, has all the properties of the peppers, and, in appearance and taste, greatly resembles cubebs. It possesses, too, similar virtues.

PIPER CARYOPHYLLATUM, see Myrtus pimenta —p. Caudatum, P. cubeba—p. Chiapæ, see Myrtus pimenta.

PIPER CUBEB'A, *Per'sea cubeba, Laurus cubeba, Litsæa cubeba* seu *piperi'ta.* A native of Java and Guinea. The odour of these berries — *Cubeba, Com'peper, Compeba, Cubal sini, Piper cauda'tum, Baccæ Piperis glabri, Cubeb Pepper, Tailed Pepper, Cuma'mus,* (F.) *Poivre-à-queue, Quabebe* — is aromatic ; taste at first cooling, afterwards pungent. The active principle is an essential oil — *Oleum Cubebæ,* oil of cubebs — which is officinal in the Pharm. U. S. The properties of the cubeb are stimulant and purgative. It is used only in gonorrhœa, Dose, from ℈j to ʒj, in powder, three or four times a day; of the volatile oil, 10 or 12 drops.

'Turkey yellow berries,'—the dried fruit of the *Rhamnus Catharticus*—are often substituted for cubebs.

PIPER GUINEENSE, Capsicum annuum—p. Hispanicum, Capsicum —p. Indicum, Capsicum annuum—p. Jamaicense, see Myrtus pimenta.

PIPER LONGUM, *Macrop'iper, Acapat'li, Catutrip'ali, Pim'pilim, Long Pepper,* (F.) *Poivre long*. As we receive the berries, they consist of the unripe fruit dried in the sun; and are small, round grains, disposed spirally on a cylindrical receptacle. They are stimulant, carminative, and tonic, like the other peppers. Dose, gr. v to ℈j.

PIPER LUSITANICUM, Capsicum annuum — p. Murale, Sedum.

PIPER METHISTICUM, see Ava.

PIPER NIGRUM, *Melanop'iper*, *Molagoco'di*, *Lada*, *Piper aromat'icum*, Piper (Ph. U. S.), *Black Pepper*, (F.) *Poivre noir*. Black pepper is the unripe fruit dried in the sun. *Virtues*, same as those of the other peppers.

PIPER ODORATUM JAMAICENSE, see Myrtus pimenta — p. Tabascum, see Myrtus pimenta — p. Turcicum, Capsicum annuum.

PIPERI'NA, *Piperi'num*, *Pip'erine*, *Piperin*. A resinoid substance, obtained from the piper nigrum by M. Œrstadt, in which a part of the virtues of the pepper resides. It has been employed, like the quinia, in intermittents, and successfully.

PIP'EROID, *Piperoï'dum*, *Zingib'erin*. A yellow syrupy mass obtained by exhausting ginger root by ether. It is soluble in ether, alcohol, and oils, and may be given in tincture, sugar, lozenge, or syrup, in cases where ginger is indicated.

PIPEROPAS'TUS; from πέπερι, 'pepper,' and πάσσειν, 'to strew.' Strewed with pepper,—socks, for example, where it is desirable to excite the surface of the feet.

PIPETTE. 'A small pipe.' In Pharmacy, a small tube terminating in a perforated point, which is passed into a liquid to be removed, from the surface of a precipitate, for example. The liquid is drawn into the tube by applying the mouth to the free extremity.

PIPIN'NA, *Men'tula parva*. A small penis.

PIPPERIDGE BUSH, see Oxycantha Galeni.

PIPSISSEWA, Pyrola umbellata — p. Spotted, Pyrola maculata — p. White, Pyrola maculata.

PIPTONYCHIA, Onychoptosis.

PIQUETÉ, see *Sablé*.

PIQURE, Puncture, Wound, punctured.

PISA, (CLIMATE OF.) Pisa has long been celebrated as one of the most favourable climates in Italy for the consumptive. It is genial, but somewhat oppressive and damp. It is softer than that of Nice, but not so warm; less soft, but less oppressive than that of Rome.

PISCIARELLI, MINERAL WATERS OF. A spring at Monte Secco, in Italy, between Lake Agnano and Solfatara. It is thermal (100° Fahr.), sulphureous, and carbonated, and is chiefly used in old ulcers, leucorrhœa, chronic diarrhœa, and in cutaneous affections.

PISCID'IA ERYTHRI'NA, *Jamaica Dogwood*. A small branching tree, common in most of the West India Islands; — Diadelphia Decandria of Linnæus. It is used in the West Indies to poison fish. It appears to be an acro-narcotic, and has been used in the form of a tincture of the bark of the root in toothach.

PISCINA, *Baignoire*.

PISCIV'OROUS, *Pisciv'orus*, *Ichthyoph'agous*, *Ichthyoph'agus*, from *piscis*, 'a fish,' and *voro*, 'I eat.' Feeding or subsisting on fish.

PIS'IFORM, *Pisiform'is*, from *pisum*, 'a pea,' and *forma*, 'shape.'

PISIFORM'E, OS, *Os lenticula'rĕ*, *Os orbicula'rĕ*, *Os extra or'dinem carpi*, (F.) *Os hors du rang*, is the fourth bone of the first row of the carpus. It is round, and gives attachment to the tendon of the cubitalis anterior, and to the anterior transverse ligament of the carpus. It is articulated, behind, with the os cuneiforme.

PISO, Mortar.

PISSA, see Pinus sylvestris.

PISSASPHAL'TUS, *Pissasphal'tum*, *Mineral Pitch*, from πίσσα, 'pitch,' and ασφαλτος, 'bitumen.' (F.) *Poix minérale*. A thicker kind of Petroleum or Rock oil; formerly employed as a vulnerary. It is synonymous with *Glu'tinous bitu'men*, *Malta bitu'men*, and *Mineral tar*.

PISSELÆ'UM, *Oleum Pici'num*, from πίσσα, 'pitch,' and ελαιον, 'oil.' An oily matter obtained from boiling pitch, and used for the same purposes as tar.

PISSELÆUM INDICUM, Petroleum.

PISSEMENT DE SANG, Hæmaturia.

PISSENLIT, Leontodon taraxacum.

PISSE'ROS, from πίσσα, 'pitch.' Ancient name of a cerate, prepared of *olive oil*, *oil of roses*, and *dried pitch*. It was, also, called *Cera'tum pica'tum*, and *C. tetraphar'macum*. — Hippocrates.

PISSI'TES, *Vinum pica'tum*. Same etymon. A wine prepared from tar and the must of the grape. It was regarded to be stomachic.

PISSOSIS, Malacia.

PISSWEED, Anthemis cotula.

PISTACHIO NUTS, see Arachis hypogæa, Pistacia vera.

PISTACIA CHIA, P. lentiscus.

PISTA'CIA LENTIS'CUS, *P. Chia*, *Terebin'thus lentiscus*, *Lentiscus vulga'ris*; the *Mastich Tree*. Family, Terebinthaceæ. The wood of this tree abounds with the resinous principles of mastich; and a tincture made from it has been used in the cure of dyspeptic affections, gout, and dysentery. It yields, by incision, the resin *Mastich*, *Ren'na Lentisci'na*, *Men'frigĕ*, *Masti'chĕ*, *Mastix*, *Pistaciæ Lentis'ci Resi'na*. This resin has an agreeable smell when heated: is almost insipid; in globular, irregular, yellowish, semi-transparent masses; soluble in ether; partially so in alcohol. It is stimulant, and has been used in old coughs, and gleet, and is chewed to sweeten the breath. It is sometimes, also, employed, to stop holes in carious teeth.

PISTACIA NARBONENSIS, P. lentiscus — p. Reticulata, P. lentiscus.

PISTACIA TEREBIN'THUS, *P. Narbonen'sis seu reticula'ta seu vera*, *Turpentine Tree*, *Hab-el-Kelimbat*, *Terebinthus vulga'ris*, *Terminthos*. The tree which affords the *Cyprus Turpentine*, *Res'na Terebin'thi*, *Terebinth'ina vera*, *T. Chia*, *T. Cyp'ria*, (F.) *Térébinthine de Chio*. This substance is classed amongst the resins. It is procured by wounding the bark of the trunk. The best Chio turpentine is of about the consistence of honey; very tenacious, clear, and almost transparent; of a white colour inclining to yellow, and of a fragrant smell; moderately warm to the taste, but free from acrimony and bitterness. It resembles in virtues the other turpentines.

PISTACIA VERA. Name of the tree which affords the *Nux Pistacia*. *Pista'chio nuts* have a sweetish, unctuous taste, resembling that of sweet almonds. Like these, they afford an oil, and may be formed into an emulsion.

PISTILLUM, Pilum.

PISTOLOCHIA, Aristolochia pistolochia.

PISTORIENSIS GLADIUS, *Bistouri*.

PISUM, *Pisum sati'vum*, *Pea*, *Garden pea*, (F.) *Pois*, *P. cultivé*. The seeds of the pea, Fam. Leguminosæ, Sex. Syst. Diadelphia decandria, are much employed as an aliment, both in the fresh and dried state. They are farinaceous, and, when dried, not easy of digestion.

PIT, Pock mark — p. of the Stomach, *Fossette de cœur*.

PITAY'A BARK. This bark is preferred in Colombia to any other. It contains a new vegetable alkali, to which the name *Pitayine* has been given.

PITAYINE, see Pitaya bark.

PITCAITHLEY, MINERAL WATERS OF. These saline springs, at Pitcaithley, about four miles from Perth, Scotland, contain chlorides of sodium and calcium.

PITCH, Colophonia—p. Black, see Pinus sylvestris—p. Burgundy, see Pinus abies—p. Canada, see Pinus Canadensis.

PITCH CAP, see Depilatory.

PITCH, COMMON, Pinus sylvestris—p. Hemlock, see Pinus Canadensis—p. Jew's, Asphaltum—p. Mineral, Pissasphaltum.

PITCH PLASTER, see Depilatory, Emplastrum picis.

PITCH, STONE, see Pinus sylvestris — p. White, see Pinus abies.

PITHYRIASIS, Pityriasis.

PITHYRINUS, Acerosus, Furfuraceous.

PITTA'CIUM. A pitch plaster, from πίττα, 'pitch.'

PITTING, Pock mark.

PITTOSIS, Malacia.

PITTO'TA. Medicines in which pitch is the chief ingredient.

PITTSBURG, MINERAL WATERS OF. A chalybeate mineral spring, situate about four miles south-west of Pittsburg, in Pennsylvania. It contains chloride of sodium, chloride of magnesium, oxide of iron, sulphate of lime, and carbonic acid.

PITUITA, Mucus, Phlegm—p. Narium, Nasal mucus.

PITU'ITARY, *Pituita'rius*, from *pituita*, 'phlegm.' Concerned in the secretion of mucus or phlegm. A name given to several parts.

PITUITARY BODY, P. Gland.

PITUITARY FOSSA, *Fossa Pituita'ria*. A depression on the cerebral surface of the sphenoid bone, which lodges the pituitary gland. It is called, on account of its shape, *Sella Turc"ica*, *Ephip'pium*. Chaussier calls it *Fossa supra-sphenoida'lis*, from its situation.

PITU'ITARY GLAND, *Glan'dula Pituito'sa* vel *pituita'ria*, *Glandula basila'ris*, *Lacu'na* vel *Appendic'ula cer'ebri*, *Hypoph'ysis* seu *Appendix cer'ebri*, *Pituitary body*, *Corpus pituita'rē* ;— *Appendice sus-sphenoïdale du cerveau*, (Ch.) A small, round body; the anterior portion of which is of a cineritious yellow hue, and the posterior, which is smaller, is whitish and pulpy. Its functions are unknown.

PITUITARY MEMBRANE, *Schneide'rian Membrane*, *Membra'na pituita'ria*, *M. olfacto'ria*. The mucous membrane which lines the nasal fossæ, and extends to the different cavities communicating with the nose. In the nasal fossæ, the membrane appears formed of two layers, intimately united;—the one in contact with the bone is fibrous;—the other is free at one surface. The latter is a mucous membrane, on which papillæ are not easily distinguishable, but which contains them, as well as a number of very small mucous follicles, that open into the cavity of the nares. On penetrating the maxillary, frontal, sphenoidal, and ethmoidal sinuses, the membrane becomes very thin, transparent, less vascular, and seems reduced to its mucous layer. The pituitary membrane receives the impression of odours, by means of the expansion of the olfactory nerves upon it. It is the seat of smell.

PITU'ITOUS, *Pituito'sus;* from *pituita*, mucus or phlegm. Consisting of, or resembling, or full of mucus or phlegm.

PITYRI'ASIS, from πιτυρον, 'bran;' *Lepido'sis Pityriasis*, *Pityris'ma*, *Pithyri'asis*, *Herpes furfura'ceus*, *H. farino'sus*, *Porri'go* (of some,) *Tin'ea furfura'cea*, *T. porrigino'sa*, *Furfura'tio*, *Furfuris'ca*, *Dandriff*, *Dandruff*, (F.) *Teigne*, *Dartre*, *Dartre furfuracée volante ;* — a very superficial affection; characterized by irregular patches of thin scales, which repeatedly exfoliate and recur; but which never form crusts, or are accompanied with excoriations. It is not contagious. It occurs under three or four varieties of form.

PITYRIASIS, Porrigo — p. Nigra, Melasma — p. Versicolor, Chloasma.

PITYRISMA, Pityriasis.

PITYROIDES, Furfuraceous.

PITYRON, Furfur.

PIVOINE, Pæonia.

PIV'OTING. In dentistry, an operation, which consists in fastening in a new crown upon the root of a tooth by means of a piece of gold wire, called 'a *pivot*.'

PIX, Sperm — p. Abietina see Pinus abies — p. Abietis, see Pinus abies — p. Alba, see Pinus abies — p. Arida see Pinus abies, and Pinus sylvestris—p. Atra, see Pinus sylvestris—p. Brutia, Brutia—p. Burgundica, see Pinus abies—p. Canadensis, see Pinus Canadensis — p. Cedria, see Pinus sylvestris—p. Græca, Colophonia—p. Liquida, see Pinus sylvestris—p. Navalis, see Pinus sylvestris — p. Nigra, see Pinus sylvestris — p. Sicca, see Pinus sylvestris.

PLACE'BO, 'I will please.' A medicine, prescribed rather to satisfy the patient than with any expectation of its effecting a cure.

PLACEN'TA. A Latin word, signifying a *Cake*. P. *uteri* seu *uteri'na* seu *uteri car'nea*, *Hepar* seu *Jecur uteri'num*, *Caro* seu *Affu'sio orbicularis*, *Maza*. A soft, spongy, vascular body, adherent to the uterus, and connected with the fœtus by the umbilical cord. It is not in existence during the first period of the embryo state, but its formation commences perhaps with the arrival of the embryo in the uterus. It is generally considered to have two portions, one *fœtal*, and the other *maternal*. The fœtal consists of highly vascular villi and tufts, which contain the inosculating loops of the umbilical arteries and umbilical vein of the fœtus. The maternal portion is considered by Dr. Reid to consist, essentially, of a large sac formed by the inner coat of the vascular system of the mother, into which the maternal blood is poured by the curling arteries of the uterus, and from which it is returned by the utero-placental veins. The tufts and villi of the fœtal placenta are ensheathed by this inner coat of the maternal vascular system; and, according to Prof. Goodsir, two distinct sets of nucleated cells—one maternal and the other fœtal—separate the maternal and fœtal portions where they come in contact, one set of which are probably, he thinks, concerned in the separation of nutritive matter from the maternal blood, and the other destined to convey it into the vessels of the fœtus. The placenta is formed of several *lobes* or *cotyledons*, which can be readily distinguished from each other on the uterine surface; but towards the fœtal surface are confounded into one mass. It is composed of the umbilical vessels, areolar tissue, and whitish, resisting filaments, which are vascular ramifications obliterated. Lymphatic vessels have also been presumed to exist in it; and nerves have been traced, proceeding from the great sympathetic of the fœtus.

The main function of the placenta appears to be like that of the lungs in the adult. It admits of the blood of the fœtus being *shown* to that of the mother, and undergoing requisite changes. It may, also, be an organ for nutritive absorption, as observed above.

PLACEN'TA CRUORIS, see Blood — p. Febrilis.

Ague cake — p. Oblata, P. prævia — p. Obvia, P. prævia.

PLACEN'TA PRÆ'VIA, (from *præ*, 'before,' and *via*, 'way,') *P. ob'via, P. obla'ta.* Presentation of the placenta; a condition which gives rise to *unavoidable hemorrhage* from the uterus. The safety of the female depends upon speedy delivery.

PLACENTA SANGUINIS, see Blood — p. Uteri Succenturiata, Decidua.

PLACEN'TAL, *Placenta'lis.* Relating, or appertaining to, the placenta.

PLACENTI'TIS, *Placunti'tis, Placoï'tis, Inflamma'tio placen'tæ.* A hybrid word — from *placenta*, and *itis*, a suffix denoting inflammation. Inflammation of the placenta.

PLACEN'TULA, 'a little cake.' A rudimentary placenta. The placenta of an abortion.

PLACOITIS, Placentitis.

PLACUNTITIS, Placentitis.

PLADAROMA, Pladarosis.

PLADARO'SIS, *Pladaro'ma, Pladar'otes*, from πλαδαρος, 'soft.' A soft tumour on the eyelid, unaccompanied with redness or pain.

PLADAROTES, Pladarosis.

PLAFOND DES VENTRICULES DU CERVEAU, Corpus callosum.

PLAGA, Ictus, Wound.

PLAGIOBOL'IA, *Planobol'ia*, from πλαγιος, 'to one side,' and βαλλειν, 'to throw.' Imperfect emission of sperm into the vagina. Emission to one side; sometimes practised to render impregnation less probable.

PLAGUE, from πληγη, *plaga*, 'a stroke.' *Pestis, P. orienta'lis, P. bubona'ria orientalis seu inguina'ria, P. contagio'sa, P. acutiss'ima, P. sep'tica, P. Glandulo'sa, P. Ade'no-septica, P. inguinaria, Pestil'itas, Ephem'era pestilentia'lis, E. mortif'era, Lues inguina'ria, Clades glandula'ria, Phthora, Pestilen'tia, Lues, Loimos, Febris ade'no-nervo'sa, Læmos, Læmē, Læ'mia, Læmop'yra, Chaosda, Anthra'cia Pestis, Anthracotyphus, Febris pes'tilens, Syn'ochus pestilentia'lis, Typhus pestis, T. pestilentia'lis, T. gravis'simus, T. anthra'cicus, T. Bubon'icus, Exanthe'ma pestis*, the Pest, Levant plague, Septic or glan'dular pes'tilence, (F.) *Peste, Typhus d'Orient, Fièvre du Lévant.* An eminently malignant disease; endemic in the Levant; frequently epidemic, and destroying at least two-thirds of those it attacks. It is a fever of the most aggravated kind, with affection of the lymphatic glands of the groin or axillæ, and carbuncles. Its miasmata — it has been conceived — adhere to different organic textures, to woollen goods, clothing and furniture; and may thus be transported to a considerable distance; but this is not certain. The mean duration of the disease is six or seven days; some die in twenty-four hours, others not till ten or twelve days. Pathological anatomy has afforded little light with respect to it. Various means have been used for arresting it, but none have seemed to be pre-eminently distinguished. The great point is, to watch the indications as they develop themselves; and to treat the case, in general, like one of typhus gravior. It is universally agreed that the suppuration of the buboes should be aided as far as practicable. For preventing the importation and spread of the plague, the *Quar'antine Laws* have been instituted; and when the disease has actually appeared, a *cordon sanitaire* has been drawn round the infected district, so as to prevent all communication.

PLAGUE, COLD. A severe form of congestive fever, seen in the Southern States. Bilious pneumonia, in which there is no reaction, has been, also, so called.

PLAGUE MARK, Plague token.

PLAGUE, PALI. A malignant fever, greatly resembling Plague, which prevailed in Rajpootana after July, 1836.

PLAGUE SPOT, Plague token.

PLAGUE TOKEN, *Plague mark, Plague spot.* A mark by which one struck with the plague was known. Perhaps the early stage of carbuncle in unfavourable cases. It is described as a small tubercle — *Bossa* — somewhat resembling a wart, callous and more or less deficient in sensibility, varying in size from that of a millet-seed to that of a bean.

PLAGULA, Compress, Pledget, Splint.

PLAIE, Wound — *p. d'Arme à feu*, Wound, gunshot — *p. d'Arquebusade*, Wound, gunshot — *p. Contuse*, Wound, contused — *p. Envenimé*, Wound, poisoned — *p. par Arrachement*, Wound, lacerated — *p. à Lambeaux*, see Flap.

PLANANTHUS FASTIGATUS, Lycopodium selago — p. Selago, Lycopodium selago.

PLANARIA LATIUSCULA, Distoma hepaticum.

PLANCHER (F.), 'floor.' In anatomy, the inferior wall or boundary of a cavity.

PLANCHER DU CERVEAU, Tentorium.

PLANCUS, Leiopus.

PLANE, Plexus — p. Mesial, see Mesial.

PLANET-STRUCK, see Sideratio.

PLANE'TES, *Plane'ticus, Plan'icus, Errabun'dus, Errat'ic.* An epithet given to diseases, whose returns are irregular — especially to intermittent fever; *Planetes Febris, F. Errat'ica, F. Erro'nea, F. Vaga.*

PLANETICA ARTHRITIS, Gout, wandering.

PLANICUS, Planetes.

PLANIPEDES, Steganopodes.

PLANITIES PEDIS, Sole.

PLANOBOLIA, Plagiobolia.

PLANTA NOCTIS, Hydroa, Sudamina — p. Pedis, Sole — p. Prima pedis, Tarsus.

PLANTA'GO, *P. Major, Centiner'via, Arnoglos'sum, Septiner'via, Polyneu'ron, Heptapleu'ron, Planta'go latifo'lia* seu *major* seu *vulga'ris*, (F.) *Plantain commun*. Family, Plantagineæ. Sex. Syst. Tetrandria Monogynia. The leaves have been said to be refrigerant, attenuant, substyptic, and diuretic.

PLANTAGO AQUATICA, Alisma plantago.

PLANTAGO CORON'OPUS, *Coronopo'dium, Cornu cervi'num, Stella terræ, Plantago, Buckshorn Plantain.* Properties like the last.

PLANTAGO NITIDA, P. psyllium.

PLANTAGO PSYL'LIUM, *P. nit'ida, Psyl'lium, P. erec'tum, Pulica'ris herba, Crystal'lion, Cracmoi'a, Branching Plantain, Fleawort*, (F.) *Herbe aux puces commune.* The seeds have a nauseous, mucilaginous taste, and no remarkable smell. The decoction of the seeds is recommended in hoarseness and roughness of the fauces.

PLANTAGO VULGARIS, Plantago.

PLANTAIN, BRANCHING, Plantago psyllium — p. Buckshorn, Plantago coronopus — p. Commun, Plantago — p. d'Eau, Alisma plantago — p. Rattlesnake, Goodyera pubescens — p. Robin's, Erigeron bellidifolium — p. Tree, Musa paradisiaca — p. Water, Alisma plantago, Unisema deltifolia.

PLANTAIRE, Plantar muscle — p. Grêle, Plantar muscle.

PLANTAR, *Planta'ris*, from *planta*, 'the sole of the foot.' That which relates or belongs to the sole of the foot. This name has been given to several parts.

PLANTAR APONEURO'SIS, *P. fas'cia.* A thick, dense, resisting aponeurosis; of a triangular shape, and superficially situate, which occupies the middle and sides of the sole of the foot, and furnishes insertions to several of the muscles of the region, either directly or through the medium of septa, which it sends between them.

PLANTAR ARCH, see Plantar arteries.

PLANTAR ARTERIES. These are two in number, and arise from the extremity of the posterior tibial artery. They are distinguished into:—The *internal plantar artery*, situate above the abductor pollicis pedis. It extends from the termination of the posterior tibial to the trunk of one of the collaterals of that toe. The *external plantar artery* is larger than the preceding, and ought to be considered as the termination of the posterior or tibial. Situate above the flexor communis digitorum pedis, it extends from beneath the calcaneum to the posterior extremity of the last metatarsal space. When it has reached this part, it turns from without inwards; advances towards the posterior extremity of the first metatarsal bone, and anastomoses with the perforating branch of the *dorsalis tarsi*. In the first part of its course, it furnishes calcaneal, articular, muscular, and adipous branches. The second portion of the artery is called the *Plantar Arch* or *Cross*. It gives branches in all directions. The inferior and posterior have received no name. The superior—three in number—are the *posterior perforating arteries*. The anterior branches are larger, and there are commonly four. They furnish the *anterior perforating*, and the *collaterals* of the last four toes.

PLANTAR CROSS, see Plantar arteries—p. Fascia, P. aponeurosis.

PLANTAR LIGAMENTS. A name given to the inferior ligaments, which unite the bones of the tarsus and metatarsus, to distinguish them from the superior, called *dorsal*.

PLANTAR MUSCLE, *Planta'ris, P. grac"ilis, Tibia'lis grac"ilis, Exten'sor tarsi minor,* (F.) *Plantaire, P. Grêle, Jambier grêle, Petit fémorocalcanien,* (Ch.) A muscle, situate at the posterior part of the leg. It is long, thin, and narrow. Above, it is attached to the posterior part of the external condyle of the os femoris: below, it terminates by a long tendon, which is attached to the posterior and inner part of the calcaneum. This muscle extends the leg on the foot, and conversely. It can, also, assist in the flexion of the leg on the thigh.

PLANTAR NERVES. These are two in number, and are furnished by the termination of the posterior tibial nerve. They are distinguished into —1. The *internal plantar nerve*, which extends from the inferior part of the tibial nerve to both sides of the first three toes, and the inner side of the fourth. It furnishes, also, branches to the abductor of the great toe; to the short flexor of the toes; to the accessory; to the short flexor of the great toe, the lumbricales, &c. 2. The *external plantar nerve* proceeds from the termination of the posterior tibial to the posterior extremity of the 5th metatarsal bone, and gives branches to the flexor brevis digitorum pedis, the accessory and the abductor of the little toe. This trunk subsequently divides into two branches;—the one—*profunda*—is distributed to the short flexor of the great toe: the interosseous and abductor pollicis pedis: the other—*superficialis*—sends filaments to the short flexor of the little toe, the two sides of that toe, the outer side of the 4th, and the last lumbricalis.

PLANTAR REGIONS or SURFACES are different regions or surfaces of the sole of the foot. Three are generally reckoned, — the *internal, middle,* and *external.*

PLANTAR VEINS follow a similar arrangement.

PLANTARIA, Dengue.

PLANTARIS, Plantar, P. muscle—p. Superficies pedis, Sole—p. Verus, see Flexor longus digitorum pedis profundus perforans (accessorius.)

PLANTARIUM, Pubes.

PLANTE DU PIED, Sole.

PLANTI-SOUS-PHALANGIENS, Lumbricales pedis—*p. Tendino-phalangiens,* Lumbricales pedis.

PLANUM AFONEUROTICUM DIAPHRAGMATIS. The tendinous expansion of the diaphragm.

PLANUM OS, from *planus,* 'soft, smooth.' The papyraceous or orbitar plate of the ethmoid bone was formerly so called.

PLANUM PEDIS, Sole.

PLANUM SUPE'RIUS LINGUÆ. The upper surface of the tongue.

PLANU'RIA, from πλανος, 'wandering, false,' and ουρον, 'urine.' Discharge of urine through unwonted ways.

PLAQUEMINIER D'EUROPE, Diospyros lotus.

PLAQUES GAUFRÉES, Peyeri glandulæ— p. *Laiteuses,* see *Taches laiteuses.*

PLASMA, Liquor sanguinis.

PLASMEXHIDRO'SIS, from *plasma,* the *liquor sanguinis;* εξ, 'out of,' and 'ιδρωσις, 'perspiration.' Exudation of the plasma of the blood from the vessels.

PLASTER, Emplastrum — p. Adhesive, Emplastrum resinæ, Sparadrapum adhesivum — p. Adhesive, Baynton's, see Emplastrum resinæ—p. Adhesive, of pitch and resins, Emplastrum de pice et resinis glutinans — p. Ammoniacum, Emplastrum ammoniaci—p. Ammoniacum with mercury, Emplastrum ammoniaci cum hydrargyro—p. Aromatic, Emplastrum aromaticum — p. Asafœtida, Emplastrum asafœtidæ — p. of Belladonna, Emplastrum belladonnæ — p. Blister, Blister—p. Blistering, Emplastrum lyttæ—p. of Blistering fly, Emplastrum lyttæ — p. Calefacient, Emplastrum calefaciens — p. of Cantharides, compound, Emplastrum lyttæ compositum — p. Cephalic, Emplastrum picis comp.— p. Corn, Sparadrapum viride — p. Corn, Kennedy's, Sparadrapum viride — p. Court, English, see Ichthyocolla, Sparadrapum adhesivum — p. Cummin, Emplastrum cumini—p. Defensive, Sparadrapum Galteri—p. Diachylon, Emplastrum plumbi—p. Fly, Emplastrum lyttæ — p. Frankincense, Emplastrum thuris—p. Galbanum, Emplastrum galbani — p. Galbanum, compound, Emplastrum galbani compositum—p. Gum, Emplastrum gummosum — p. of Gum-resins, Emplastrum cum gummi-resinis—p. Hemlock, Emplastrum cicutæ — p. Iron, Emplastrum ferri — p. Isinglass, see Sparadrapum adhæsivum — p. Issue, Sparadrapum pro fonticulis—p. Lead, Emplastrum plumbi —p. Machine, *Sparadrapier*—p. Mercurial, Emplastrum hydrargyri—p. of Mercury, compound, Emplastrum hydrargyri compositum—p. Nuremberg, Emplastrum Norimbergense — p. Opium, Emplastrum opii — p. Pitch, see Depilatory — p. Pitch, comp., Emplastrum picis compositum—p. Resin, Emplastrum resinæ — p. of Red oxide of iron, Emplastrum oxidi ferri rubri — p. Soap, Emplastrum saponis — p. of Spanish flies, compound, Emplastrum lyttæ compositum— p. Sticking, Emplastrum resinæ—p. Strengthening, Emplastrum ferri, Emplastrum oxidi ferri rubri — p. Warm, Emplastrum calefaciens — p. Wax, Emplastrum ceræ.

PLASTIC, *Plas'ticus, Formati'vus, Form'ative,* from πλασσω, 'I form.' That which forms, or serves to form.

PLASTIC ELEMENT. One which bears within it the germs of a higher form. — Gerber.

PLASTIC FORCE. The generative or formative power in organized bodies. It is also called *Nisus formati'vus, Vis seu Virtus plas'tica seu formati'va, Vis essentia'lis seu reproductiva, Fac'ultas formatrix seu nutrix seu auctrix seu vegetati'va; Blas alterati'vum, Motus assimilationis, An'ima vegetati'va, Plasticism'us, Virtus formatrix, Plas"tic"itas, Plastic"ity, Force of Nutrition, F. of assimilation, Force of Form'ation, Force of vegeta'tion, Puissance du moule intérieur* (Buffon), Bildungstrieb, *Germ-force* of the Germans.

PLASTIC LYMPH, Liquor Sanguinis—p. Surgery, Morioplastice.

PLASTICIMUS, Plastic Force.
PLASTICITAS, Plastic Force.
PLASTICITY, Plastic Force.
PLASTILYTIC, Antiplastic.
PLASTILYTICUM (HÆMATOLYTICUM), Spanæmic.
PLATA, Scapula.
PLATANO, Musa Sapientum.
PLATANTHE'RA ORBICULA'TA, *Large round-leaved Orchis*; indigenous. Order Orchidaceæ; flowering in July. The leaves are large, soft and fleshy, and are used, in certain places, for dressing blisters.
PLATANUS, Musa paradisiaca.
PLATEA, Bothriocephalus latus.
PLATES, MANSFORD'S, see Galvanism.
PLATIAS'MUS, from πλατυς, 'broad.' Excessive development of the lips, causing the articulation to be imperfect.
PLATINA, Platinum.
PLAT'INUM, *Plat'ina*, from (S.) *plata*, 'silver.' The preparations of platinum resemble in their therapeutical properties those of gold. The BICHLO'RIDE, *Plat'ini Bichlo'ridum*, made by dissolving *platinum* in *aqua regia*, and the DOUBLE CHLORIDE of PLATINUM and SODIUM, *So'dii chloroplat'inas, Chloroplat'inate of So'dium*, prepared by dissolving *bichloride of platinum* and pure *chloride of sodium*, in proper proportions, in water, evaporating and crystallizing,—are the preparations used. They are not much prescribed.
PLATULA, see Pediculus.
PLATYBREGMATE, see Cranium.
PLATYCORIA, Mydriasis.
PLATYCORIASIS, Platycoria.
PLATYNO'SIS, from πλατυς, 'broad.' *Amplifica'tio.* Morbid extension of parts.
PLATYOPHTHALMON, Antimonium.
PLATYPOLIA, see Kyllosis.
PLATYPUS, see Kyllosis.
PLATYS'MA, from πλατυς, 'broad.' Any thing broadly extended. A spread plaster.
PLATYS'MA MYOÏDES, *P. Myo'des, Mus'culus cuta'neus, M. subcuta'neus* (Winslow), *Quadra'tus genæ* vel *latis'simus colli, Expan'sio musculo'sa, Tetrago'nus, Stomoman'icon*, (F.) *Thoraco-maxillo facial, Thoraco-facial* (Ch.), *Peaucier*. A muscle situate superficially on the lateral parts of the neck. It is flat, broad, and quadrilateral. Its fibres, which are all parallel to each other, pass obliquely downwards, and from without inwards. They arise from the areolar tissue, which covers the anterior and superior part of the chest; pass before the clavicle, and proceed to attach themselves at the interior part of the symphysis menti, at the external oblique line of the jaw, and at the commissure of the lips. The fibres of this last insertion form a distinct fasciculus, called by some anatomists *Mus'culus Riso'rius Santori'ni*. The platysma myoïdes depresses the commissure of the lips, and carries it outwards. It contributes, also, to the depression of the lower jaw. When it contracts, it wrinkles the skin of the neck transversely.

PLATYSTER'NOS, from πλατυς, 'broad,' and στερνον, 'the sternum.' One who has a broad well developed chest.—D. Peehlin.
PLATYS'TOMUS; from πλατυς, 'broad,' and στομα, 'mouth.' One who has a broad mouth.
PLAUTUS, Leiopus.
PLECHAS, Perinæum.
PLECTANÆ, Cornua uteri.
PLEC'TANE, *Plica, Plegma, Plexus.* A fold; a plexus. Also, a cornu of the uterus.
PLEC'TRUM. The styloid process of the temporal bone. Also, the uvula, and the tongue. —Castelli.
PLEDGET, (D.) Plagghe, *Plumace'olus, Lintea'men, Plag'ula*, (F.) *Plumaceau, Plumaseau.* A small compress or *gâteau* of lint—(the filaments arranged parallel to each other)—flattened between the hands after the extremities have been cut off or folded down. It is applied over wounds, ulcers, &c., to preserve them from the contact of the air, to retain dressings *in situ*, and to absorb the discharges.
PLEGE, Blow, Ictus.
PLEGMA, Plectane, Plexus.
PLEGOMETER, Pleximeter.
PLEIN, (F.) 'Full.' The middle part of a roller.
PLEIOMASTHUS, Polymasthus.
PLEIOMAZIA, see Polymasthus.
PLENA MULIER, Pregnant.
PLENITUDE, Fulness.
PLENITUDO, Plethora.
PLENCK'S DEPILATORY, see Depilatory, Colley's.
PLEONEC'TICA ATHYM'IA SEU MELAN-CHO'LIA. A form of insanity characterized by a desire for gain or by covetousness.
PLEONEC'TICUS, from πλεον, 'more,' and εχειν, 'to have.' Covetous. Desirous to acquire; hence *mania pleonectica*.
PLERO'SIS, from πληρης, 'full;' also *Reple'tio, Refec'tio, Reple'tion.* Restoration of flesh after sickness. Plethora.
PLEROTICUS, Incarnans.
PLES'MONE, *Plenitu'do, Sati'etas, Sati'ety.* Intemperance. A condition the opposite to that of hunger.
PLESSER, Plexor.
PLESSIMETER, Pleximeter.
PLETHOMER'IA, from πληθος, 'many,' and μερος, 'a part.' Superabundance of parts, as in the case of six fingers to one hand.
PLETHO'RA, from πληθω, 'I fill.' *Polyæ'mia, Polyhyperhæ'mia, Panhyperæ'mia, Polychyn'ia sanguin'ea, Angeioplero'sis, Angioplero'sis, Erythræ'mia, Erythro'sis, Hæmatopletho'ra, Hæmopletho'ra, Plenitu'do, Multitu'do, Redundan'tia, Reple'tio, En'chyma, Comple'tio, Pleth'ory, Reple'tion, San'guineness, Fulness*, (F.) *Abondance, Rédondance.* The word *plethora*, which means repletion, *Plero'sis*, expresses a superabundance of blood in the system, or in some part of it:—hence the division of plethora into *general* and *local*; the latter being called, according to its seat, *cerebral, pulmonary, uterine*, &c. The principal symptoms of plethora exist in the circulatory system; such as redness of the surface, swelling of the veins, increase in the fulness of the pulse, in the strength of the heart's pulsations, &c., with spontaneous hemorrhages occasionally. With these are usually united general heaviness, torpor, lassitude, vertigo, tinnitus aurium, flushes of heat, &c. The blood of plethoric persons differs from healthy blood in the smaller ratio of water which it contains, and especially in the augmentation of the red corpuscles.
The tendency to plethora, or its actual existence, must be obviated by purgatives, proper diet,

exercise, &c.; and, if the danger from it be pressing, by blood-letting. This is, however, a doubtful remedy for general plethora, as it increases hæmatosis.

PLETHORA, LOCAL, Hyperæmia.

PLETHOR'IC, *Pletho'ricus, Polyæ'mic, Polyæ'micus, Sanguine, Sanguineous,* (F.) *Pléthorique.* Same etymon. Full of blood. Relating to or affected with plethora.

PLETHORICUS, Plethoric.

PLETHORY, Plethora.

PLETHOS, Satiety.

PLEUMON, Pulmo.

PLEUMONIA, Pneumonia.

PLEURA, *Pleurum, Pleuro'ma,* 'the side, a rib.' *Membra'na pleurit'ica succin'gens* seu *costas succin'gens, Membra'na* seu *Tu'nica costalis* seu *subcosta'lis, Hypopleu'rios,* (F.) *Plèvre* ou *Pleure.* The pleuræ are two thin, diaphanous, perspirable membranes, which line each side of the chest, and are reflected thence upon each lung. Like all serous membranes — to which class they belong—each represents a sac without aperture. From the junction of the pleura of each side the mediastina are formed. That portion of the pleura which lines the parietes of the chest is called *Pleura Costa'lis;* the portion that covers the lungs, *Pleura Pulmona'lis.* The arteries of the pleuræ are from the intercostals, internal mammaries, phrenic, inferior thyroid, &c. The veins correspond with the arteries. They are, also, supplied with lymphatics, but nerves are not traceable in them.

Pleura is also used for *Cavity of the Pleura, Saccus Pleuræ.*

PLEURÆ. The sides of the chest.

PLEURAL, *Pleura'lis, Pleu'ricus, Pleu'rites.* That which concerns the pleura; — as a *pleural* fistula;—*pleural* cavity, *pleural* hemorrhage, &c.

PLEURALGIA, Pleurodyne.

PLEURAPOPHYSES, Costæ veræ, see Costa.

PLEURAPOSTEMA, Empyema.

PLEURARTHROC'ACÉ, from πλευρα, 'a rib,' αρθρον, 'a joint,' and κακος, 'bad.' Caries of the ribs.

PLEURE, Pleura.

PLEURESIA, Pleuritis.

PLEURÉSIE, Pleurisy.

PLEURESIS, Pleuritis.

PLEURÉTIQUE, Pleuritic.

PLEURICUS, Pleural.

PLEURIS, Pleuritis.

PLEURISY, Pleuritis.

PLEURISY, BILIOUS, *Pleuri'tis bilio'sa.* Pleurisy accompanied with bilious symptoms;—the effect of duodenitis or duodeno-hepatitis.

PLEURISY, FALSE, Pleurodynia.

PLEURISY, HEAD. A ridiculous term, occasionally used by the vulgar, in the Southern States especially, for bilious pneumonia before the pneumonitic phenomena are developed, and whilst the head is prominently affected.

PLEURISY, HEMORRHAGIC, Hæmatothorax — p. Rheumatic, Pleurodynia — p. Root, Asclepias tuberosa.

PLEURISY, TYPHOID, *Pleuri'tis typhoi'des* seu *typho'des* seu *typho'sa.* Pleurisy accompanied by adynamic symptoms.

PLEURITES, Pleural.

PLEURIT'IC, *Pleurit'icus, Pleurit'ical,* (F.) *Pleurétique;* same etymon as *pleuritis.* Relating or appertaining to pleuritis — as '*pleuritic* pain.'

PLEURI'TIS, from πλευρα, 'the pleura;' *Morbus latera'lis, M. pleurit'icus, M. Costa'lis, Empres'ma Pleuritis, Pleuris, Pleure'sis, Pleure'sia, Pleuritis costa'lis* seu *vera, Pleurit'ica Febris, Cauma Pleuri'tis, Passio pleurit'ica, Inflamma'tio Pleuræ, Pleurisy, Inflamma'tion of the Pleura,* (F.) *Pleurèse, Fièvre pleurétique, Inflammation de la Plèvre,* may be acute or chronic. Perhaps the most violent of all internal inflammations is the active form; known by acute, lancinating pain in one side of the chest, increased by inspiration, by coughing, and often by pressure; dyspnœa, the inspirations short and frequent; cough dry, or with little expectoration; and difficulty of lying on the affected side. Symptoms, attending the phlegmasiæ in general, strongly marked.

Physical Signs. There is seldom any perceptible alteration in the exterior of the chest. When effusion has taken place to a great extent, the signs will be similar to those of chronic pleurisy. The motion of the affected side is diminished, and the vibrations of the voice cannot be detected by the hand. There is more or less dulness of sound on percussion, the dulness diminishing or disappearing by change of position. On auscultation, the inspiration is feeble, distant, or inaudible; but change of position modifies it. Egophony is usually present, when the effusion is in moderate quantity, and is best heard over a portion of the thoracic parietes, represented by a band of three inches, running from below the inferior margins of the scapula in the direction of the ribs to the sternum. Simple pleurisy rarely attacks both sides at once: when such is the case, the presence of tubercles may be suspected.

Formerly, a *true pleurisy* meant one seated in the pleura: a *mediastinal pleurisy,* one situated in the anterior mediastinum; and *false pleurisy* or *rheumatismal pleurisy,* that which occupies the intercostal muscles. The last has received the name *Pleurodyn'ia;* that of *pleurisy* being exclusively appropriated to inflammation of the pleura. Pleurisy has also been distinguished into *dry* and *humid,* according as it is or is not accompanied by expectoration. *Humid* or *moist pleurisy* is now properly regarded as a complication of pleurisy with pulmonary catarrh. It is the *catar'rhal pleurisy* of some. The majority of the species of pleurisy, admitted by Sauvages, consist of complications.

The causes of pleurisy are like those of other internal inflammations. It may terminate by resolution, effusion, or suppuration.

CHRONIC PLEURISY, which has been particularly described by Bayle, Broussais, and Laënnec, most commonly terminates by a serous or purulent effusion, which sometimes simulates hydrothorax; at others, phthisis pulmonalis. It may form slowly, without evident symptoms; or it may succeed acute pleurisy. In the former case, vague pains are felt in the chest, with small, dry cough, oppression at intervals, shivering, irregular febrile symptoms, and hardness of pulse.

Physical Signs. The affected side is smoother, more rounded and motionless; the intercostal spaces are dilated and filled up, or may even protrude slightly. In very chronic cases, however, the affected side may be smaller. The triangular space above the clavicle and the depression immediately above the sternum are often drawn downwards on the diseased side. No vibration is experienced by the hand when the patient speaks. The parietes of the thorax are sometimes œdematous, and fluctuation may be occasionally felt between the ribs. On percussion the sound is dull, or if clear, only so in the upper portions of the chest. On auscultation, there is an absence of the usual sounds over the affected parts, excepting occasionally transmitted sounds. There are no physical signs that can enable us to know whether pus or serum is effused into the chest. The introduction of a grooved needle through the intercostal space, as recommended by Dr. Thomas Davies, would of course settle the question.

On *dissection* of those who have died of pleurisy, the pleura is found thickened, red, inflamed, and covered with membranous exudations or false membranes. Sometimes it seems cartilaginous and ossified. Its cavity frequently contains serous or sero-purulent effusions.

The acute form of the disease requires the most active treatment. General blood-letting, to such an extent as to make a very decided impression on the system, and repeated if necessary. This is the most important agent. After the violence of the disease has been got over, counter-irritants will be found highly beneficial; as well as when it has passed into the chronic state. The cough may be relieved by demulcents.

Sauvages has given the name PLEURI'TIS VENTO'SA, and Pringle that of PLEURODYN'IA VENTO'SA, to a pain behind the false ribs, attributed to the presence of air in the intestines.

PLEURITIS BRONCHIALIS, Bronchitis — p. Costalis, Pleuritis — p. Diaphragmatica, Diaphragmitis — p. Humida, Bronchitis — p. Muscularis, Pleurodynia — p. Notha, Pleurodynia — p. Pericardii, Pericarditis — p. Pulmonis, Pleuropneumonia — p. Rheumatica, Pleurodynia — p. Spuria, Pleurodynia — p. Spuria simulata, Pleurodynia — p. Typhoides, see Pleuritis, (biliosa) — p. Vera, Pleuritis.

PLEUROCE'LE, from πλευρα, 'the pleura,' and κηλη, 'a tumour.' *Hernia of the pleura, Hernia pleu'rica et pulmona'lis.* This name, employed by Sagar, is inaccurate, as the pleura never protrudes alone. It only forms a hernia, when it serves as an envelope to the lung, to tumours, or to purulent collections, which have protruded from the thoracic parietes.

PLEUROCOLLE'SIS, from πλευρα, 'the pleura,' and κολλαω, 'I glue.' An adhesion between the pleura costalis and pleura pulmonalis.

PLEURODYNE, Pleurodynia.

PLEURODYN'IA, *Pleural'gia, Pseudo-pleuri'tis, Pseudo-pleurisy, Pleurod'yně, Autal'gia doloro'sa, A stitch, Pain in the side, Stitch in the side, Parapleuri'tis; Stethorrheu'ma, Rheumatis'mus pec'toris, Pleuri'tis rheumat'ica, P. muscula'ris, P. spu'ria, False Pleurisy, Rheumat'ic or rheumatis'mal pleurisy, Pleuri'tis notha* seu *spu'ria* seu *spu'ria simula'ta, Pneumo'nia exter'na, Lagonop'onos, Thoracod'yně, Dolor Pec'toris exter'nus,* (F.) *Point de côté, Douleur de côté*; from πλευρα, 'the side or pleura,' and οδυνη, 'pain.' A spasmodic or rheumatic affection, generally seated in the muscles of the chest, and, ordinarily, in the intercostals. It is usually augmented by outward pressure, inspiration, coughing, exertion, moving the thorax, and sometimes even the corresponding arm. It is unaccompanied by fever, cough, or dyspnœa, excepting under the form of a *stitch*, when dyspnœa exists. It is, generally, by no means obstinate, and yields promptly to warm applications and to cupping or leeches. If it still resist, a blister will, almost always, remove it.

PLEURODYNIA VENTOSA, Pleuritis ventosa.
PLEUROMA, Costa, Pleura.

PLEUROPATHI'A, from πλευρα, 'the pleura,' and παθος, 'a disease.' A disease of the pleura.

PLEUROPERIPNEU'MONY, *Pleuroperipneumo'nia, Pleuropneumo'nia, Pneumonopleure'sis, Pneumonopleuri'tis, Pleuritis pulmo'nis, Pneumo'nia pleuritis.* Inflammation occupying the pleura and the lung at the same time. Pleurisy and peripneumony existing simultaneously. *Physical signs.* A dull sound is yielded by percussion for a variable extent over the more dependent portions of the affected side. The loss of sound is partially modified by change of position. The respiratory murmur on auscultation is very feeble or absent inferiorly; higher up, the crepitation or bronchial respiration of pneumonia may be detected; round the root of the lung, and near the inferior angle of the scapula, egophony is generally present. There is seldom much enlargement of the affected side, or displacement of the adjacent organs, as in the case of simple chronic pleurisy.

PLEUROPNEUMA, Pneumathorax.
PLEUROPNEUMONIA, Pleuroperipneumony.
PLEUROPNEUMONITIS, Pleuroperipneumony.
PLEUROPYESIS, Empyema.
PLEURORRHŒ'A, from πλευρα, 'the side,' and ρεω, 'I flow.' Accumulation of fluid in the pleura.

PLEURORRHŒA CHYLOSA, Chylothorax—p.Lymphatica, Hydrothorax — p. Purulenta, Empyema — p. Sanguinea, Hæmatothorax—p. Serosa, Hydrothorax.

PLEURORTHOPNŒ'A, from πλευρα, 'the side,' ορθος, 'erect,' and πνεω, 'I respire.' Pain of the side, which does not permit the patient to breathe, except when in the vertical position.

PLEUROSO'MUS, from πλευρα, 'side,' and σωμα, 'body.' A malformation in which the fissure is somewhat lateral, with eventration extending chiefly upon the upper part of the abdomen and upon the chest; the upper extremity of the fissured side being more or less atrophied. —Vogel.

PLEUROSTO'SIS, from πλευρα, 'the pleura,' and οστεον, 'a bone.' Ossification of the pleura, or in the cavity of the pleura. *Osteopleu'ria.*

PLEUROTETANUS, Pleurothotonos.
PLEUROTHOT'ONOS, *Pleurot'onos, Pleurotet'anus, Tetanus latera'lis,* from πλευροθεν, 'laterally,' and τονος, 'tension.' A variety of tetanus, in which the body is curved laterally by the stronger contraction of the muscles of one side of the body.

PLEUROTONOS, Pleurothotonos.
PLEURUM, Costa, Pleura.
PLÈVRE, Pleura.

PLEXIM'ETER, *Plexom'eter, Plegom'eter, Plessim'eter,* from πληοσω, 'I strike,' and μετρον, 'measure,' 'a measure of percussion.' An ivory plate of a circular or ovoid shape, from an inch and a half to two inches in diameter, and about one-sixth of an inch in thickness. It has either a raised rim or edge, or projecting handles on its upper side, to permit its being held between the finger and thumb of the left hand, whilst it is struck with the right. It is used in percussion of the chest. A piece of metal, a coin, or the finger of the left hand may be used with equal advantage.—See Percussion, mediate.

PLEXOMETER, Pleximeter.

PLEXOR, from πληοσω, 'I strike.' *Plessor.* Any instrument employed in percussion. The ends of the fingers of the right hand brought together are the best *plexor;* as the finger of the left is, perhaps, the best *pleximeter.*

PLEXUS, *Plegma, Plec'tană, Plană, Retě,* from *plecto,* 'I interlace,' 'I entwine.' (F.) *Lacis.* A network of blood vessels or of nerves. The nervous plexuses, *Implicatio'nes reticula'res* seu *Textus nervorum* belong — some to the system of encephalic nerves—*others* to that of the great sympathetic; whilst some, as the pharyngeal, seem to be formed of the two sets. The plexuses represent complex networks, with more or less loose meshes, formed by the numerous and diversified anastomoses of the nervous filaments; from which proceed other branches, that are distributed to organs, or to other plexuses.

PLEXUS, CARDIAC, Cardiac plexus—p. Carotid, see Carotid nerve — p. Choroides, see Choroid—p. Ciliaris, Ciliary ligament—*p. Cœliaque,* Cœliac plexus—p. Coronarius ventriculi, Gastric plexus —p. Coronary, see Cardiac plexus, and Coronary plexus — p. Gangliformis semilunaris, Cœliac plexus—p. Ganglioformes, Ganglions, nervous—p. Glandiformes, Ganglions, nervous—p. Glandulosi Peyeri, Peyeri glandulæ — p. Hederaceus, Corpus pampiniforme — p. Hepaticus, Hepatic plexus—p. Infra-thyroideal, see Thyroideal veins —*p. Lombo-abdominal,* Lumbar plexus — p. Median, Cœlic plexus — p. Mesenterii proprius et maximus, Cœliac plexus — p. Nervorum anserinus, Facial nerve — *p. Opistogastrique,* Cœliac plexus—p. Pampiniformis, Corpus pampiniforme —p. Pharyngeal, see Pharyngeal nerve—p. Pneumogastricus, see Pneumogastric nerves—p. Retiformis, Corpus cavernosum vaginæ—p. Reticularis, Bulbus vestibuli, Choroides plexus—p. Solar, Cœliac plexus — *p. Sous-mésentérique,* Hypogastric plexus—*p. Testiculaire,* Spermatic plexus—*p. Trachélo-sous-cutané,* Cervical plexus—p. Vasculosus funiculi spermatici pampiniformis, Corpus pampiniforme.

PLICA, from *plicari,* 'to be knit together.' *Tricho'sis plica, Tricho'ma, Tricæ, T. Incuborum, T. Scrofo'rum,* Plica *Polonica, P. Polon'ica Judæ'ica, P. Cacheo'tica, P. Saxon'ica, Affec'tio Sarmat'ica,* Matted hair, Plaited hair, *Trichom'atose* hair, *Lues Sarmat'ica, L. Polon'ica, L. Trichomat'ica, Helo'sis, Helo'tis, Cir'ragra, Cir'rhagra, C. Polono'rum,* Plica *caput Medu'sæ, Morbus Cirrho'rum,* Plica *caput Medu'sæ,* Plica *longicau'da latera'lis, Coma Cæsa'rea, Kolto, Rhopalo'sis, Plica'tio, Plicatu'ra,* (F.) *Plique, P. Polonaise.* A disease endemic in Poland, Lithuania, and other parts of Northern Europe; so called on account of its being characterized by interlacing, twisting, and agglutination or matting of the hair. By some it has been regarded as a disease; by others, as the want of attention to cleanliness. However this may be, it generally appears upon the hair of the head, but sometimes in that of other parts, as the beard, the hair on the axilla, pubes, &c. Alibert admits three species of plica. 1. *Plica multiform'is* or *Plica caput Medu'sæ,* in which the hairs are mixed and agglutinated in greater or less masses; and this has been again subdivided into two varieties, according as the meshes are almost straight (*P. C. M. lacinia'ta,* (F.) *Plique en lanières*) or much twisted (F.) *P. en vrilles.*) 2. *Plica longicau'da,* (F.) *Plique solitaire ou à queue;* when the hair is united into a single long mass, and 3. *Plica cæspito'sa,* (F.) *Plique en masse,* in which the hairs are matted into one large, shapeless mass. Pinel places this disease amongst the *Cutaneous phlegmasiæ;* but it is far from demonstrated, that it is the result of inflammation of the skin. Certain it is, however, that the tangling of the hair is symptomatic of an affection—*sui generis*—of the dermoid system. The idea that it is entirely owing to want of cleanliness, as has been conceived by some, is not tenable.

PLICA, Plectane — p. Cachectica, Plica — p. Caput Medusæ, Plica—p. Longicauda lateralis, Plica — p. Lunata, Valvula semilunaris — p. Polonica Judaica, Plica — p. Saxonica, Plica — p. Semilunaris, Valvula semilunaris.

PLICATIO, Plica.
PLICATURA, Plica.
PLICATURÆ CEREBRI, Gyri cerebri.
PLICHOS, Perinæum.

PLIN'THIUM, πλινθιον. A machine invented by one Nileus, which was formerly employed in the reduction of fractures and luxations. Soultetus describes it in his *Armamentarium Chirurgicum.*

PLIQUE, Plica—*p. Polonaise,* Plica.
PLOCARIA CANDIDA, Fucus amylaceus.
PLOMB, Plumbum.
PLOMB, (F.) The sulphuretted gas disengaged from privies, which proves fatal at times to the nightmen, (F.) *Vidangeurs,* engaged in emptying them.

PLOMB, ACÉTATE ACIDE DE, Plumbi superacetas—*p. Blanc,* Plumbi subcarbonas—*p. Blanc de,* Plumbi subcarbonas — *p. Carbonate de,* Plumbi subcarbonas — *p. Chlorure de,* Plumbi chloridum — *p. Iodure de,* Plumbi iodidum — *p. Nitrate de,* Plumbi nitras — *p. Oxide de, fondu,* Plumbi oxydum semivitreum—*p. Oxide rouge de,* Plumbi oxydum rubrum—*p. Oxide semi-vitreux de,* Plumbi oxydum semivitreum.

PLOMBAGINE, Graphites.
PLOMBIÈRES, MINERAL WATERS OF, *Fontes medica'ti Plumba'rii, Thermæ Plumbariæ.* Plombières is a town in the department of the Vosges, 17 leagues from Nancy, and two from Remiremont. Here are several sources of thermal water. That which is called *Saponaceous* (F.) *Savonneuse,* is formed of the subcarbonate and sulphate of soda, chloride of sodium, silica, carbonate of lime, and much vegeto-animal matter. This last component, when held in solution by means of the subcarbonate of soda, gives to the water an unctuous character. This is the origin of its name. The waters of Plombières are employed as solvents in engorgements of the abdominal viscera, and as alteratives in chronic diseases of the skin.

PLORATIO, Lachrymatio.
PLORATUS, Lachrymatio.
PLOTUS, Leiopus.
PLUGGING (Sw.) *Plugg,* (F.) *Tamponnement.* The act of stopping a hole. The introduction of a plug of lint or rag into a wound or natural cavity—as the uterus or vagina—to arrest hemorrhage; or of some substance into a carious tooth to prevent toothache.

PLUM, Prunum, Prunus domestica—p. Assyrian, Sebestina.
PLUMA, Lanugo.
PLUMACEAU, Pledget.
PLUMACEOLUS, Pad, Pledget.
PLUMASSEAU, Pledget.
PLUMBAGO, Graphites, Persicaria.
PLUMBA'GO EUROPÆ'A, *P. lapathifo'lia* seu *undula'ta, Denta'ria, Crepanel'la, Squama'ria, Dentela'ria, Leadwort,* (F.) *Dentelaire, Herbe au Cancer.* Family, Plumbagineæ. *Sex. Syst.* Pentandria Monogynia. The root was formerly much esteemed as a cure for the toothache, like the *Pel'litory of Spain,* which is also called *Dentaria.*

PLUMBI ACETAS, P. superacetas—p. Acetas dilutum alcoholicum, Liquor plumbi subacetatis dilutus — p. Acidulus siccus, Plumbi superacetas —p. Carbonas, P. Subcarbonas.

PLUMBI CHLO'RIDUM, *Chloride of Lead,* (F.) *Chlorure de Plomb.* This salt of lead has been used in the form of lotion and ointment in cancerous ulcerations.

PLUMBI DEUTOXYDUM RUBRUM, P. oxydum rubrum — p. Hydriodas, P. Iodidum — p. Iodhydras, P. Iodidum.

PLUMBI IOD'IDUM, *Plumbi Iodure'tum* seu *Hydri'odas* seu *Hydroi'odas* seu *Iodhydras, Plumbum ioda'tum* seu *Hydroiod'icum, I'odide* or *Iod'uret of Lead,* (F.) *Iodure de Plomb, Iodure plombique.* This salt is formed by the double decomposition of *iodide of potassium* and *nitrate*

and resolvent, as well as in erysipelatous ulcerations, tinea capitis, rheumatism, &c.

PIMPINELLA MAJOR, P. magna—p. Nigra, P. magna—p. Nostras, P. saxifraga—p. Officinalis, Sanguisorba officinalis—p. Rubra, P. magna.

PIMPINELLA SAXIF'RAGA, *Sax'ifrage, Burnet sax'ifrage, Pote'rium sanguisor'ba, Sorbastrel'la, Tragoseli'num, T. saxif'raga, Pimpinel'la hirci'na seu umbellif'era seu alba seu nostras*, (F.) *Boucage mineur, Petit B., Pimprenelle*. The root has an unpleasant smell, and hot, pungent, bitterish taste. It has been recommended as a stomachic; and as a stimulating gargle in paralysis of the tongue.

PIMPINELLA UMBELLIFERA, P. saxifraga.

PIMPLE, Papula.

PIMPLED, Papulose.

PIMPRENELLE, Pimpinella saxifraga—*p. Noire*, Sanguisorba officinalis.

PIN. Perhaps from *pennum*, low Latin; or from *spina; Spina fer'rea, Acus capita'ta*, (F.) *Épingle*. An iron or brass instrument, generally of a small size, pointed at one extremity, and having a head at the other. It is used, in Surgery, to fix rollers and dressings; and occasionally in sutures.

PIN À PIGNON, see Pinus picea.

PINASTELLUM, Peucedanum.

PINASTER, Pinus sylvestris.

PINCÉ, Pinched.

PINCE LITHODRASSIQUE, see Lithodrassic.

PINCÉE, Pugillus.

PINCERS, Forceps.

PINCETTES, Forceps.

PINCHED, *Contrac'tus*, (F.) *Pincé, Grippé*. An epithet applied to the face, when the features are contracted or shrunken; as in violent abdominal affections, or during intense pain.

PINCKNE'YA PUBENS, *P. Pubes'cens, Georgia Bark, Bitter Bark, Florida Bark, Fever tree*. This bark has been used in Georgia in the cure of intermittents, and successfully. It is a powerful bitter. Dose of the powder, ʒj.

PINDARS, Arachis Hypogea.

PINE APPLE, Bromelia ananas—p. Aphernousli, Pinus cembra—p. Ground, Lycopodium complanatum—p. Ground, stinking, Camphorosma Monspeliaca—p. Mountain, see Pinos mughos—p. Mugho, see Pinus mughos—p. Sap, American, Hypopitys lanuginosa—p. Stone, Pinus pinea—p. Sugar, see Arrow Root.

PINEA, Pinus pinea.

PINE'AL, *Pinea'lis*, from *pinus*, 'a pine.' That which resembles a pine-apple.

PINEAL GLAND, *Glandula pinea'lis, Cerebral epiph'ysis, Cona'rium, Conoi'des corpus, Penis cer'ebri, Corpus turbina'tum, Virga seu Turbo cer'ebri*, is a small body, of a conical shape; pale red or grayish colour; and soft consistence; situate between the fornix and the tubercula quadrigemina. It almost always contains sabulous particles, *Sab'ulum cona'rii*: when these are grouped together over the base of the gland, they form the *Acer'vulus Cer'ebri* of Sömmering, *A.* seu *Lapil'li glan'dulæ pinea'lis*. From its anterior part arise two medullary striæ, which proceed over the posterior commissure; coast along the optic thalami, and unite at the anterior pillar of the fornix,—the *habe'næ* or *reins of the pineal gland*.

The uses of the pineal gland are unknown. Descartes supposed it to be the seat of the soul!

PINEI, see Pinus pinea.

PINEOLI, see Pinus pinea.

PINEUS PURGANS, Jatropha curcas.

PINGUEC'ULA, *Pteryg'ium pingué seu lar-*

da'ceum, from *pinguis*, 'fat.' 'fatty.' A small, whitish-yellow tumour in the sclerotic conjunctiva and subjacent areolar tissue, close to the margin of the cornea on its nasal or temporal side; so called from its being supposed, but erroneously, to be of a fatty nature.

PINGUE'DO, Fat—p. Renalis, Nephridion.

PINGUIC'ULA VULGA'RIS, *P. alpi'na, Sanic'ula monta'na, S. Eboracen'sis, Vi'ola palus'tris, Dodecath'eon Plin'ii, Butter-wort, Yorkshire San'icle*. *Family*, Personneæ. *Sex. Syst*. Diandria Monogynia. The unctuosity of this plant has caused it to be applied to chaps, and as a pomatum to the hair. Decoctions of the leaves, in broths, are used by the common people in Wales as a cathartic.

PINGUID, Fatty.

PINGUIDINOUS, Fatty.

PINGUIN, Bromelia pinguin.

PINGUITUDO, Polysarcia adiposa.

PINHOLE PUPIL, see Pupil, pinhole.

PINHONES INDICI, Jatropha curcas.

PINK, CAROLINA, Spigelia Marilandica.

PINK DYE. Stripped *safflower*, ʒj, *subcarb. of potass*. gr. xviij, *spirit of wine* ʒvij; digest for two hours; add *distilled water* ʒij: digest for two hours more, and add *distilled vinegar* or *lemon juice* q. s., to reduce it to a fine rose-colour. Used as a cosmetic.

PINK, GROUND, Silene Virginica—p. Indian, Spigelia Marilandica—p. Wild, Silene Virginica.

PINNA, Ala, Pavilion of the ear—p. Marina, see Bissus.

PINNACULUM FORNICIS GUTTURALIS, Uvula.

PINNÆ HEPATIS, Lobes of the liver—p. Naris, see Nasus.

PINNULA, *Aileron*.

PINNULÆ HEPATIS, Lobes of the liver.

PINO'LI. (S.) A preparation used for subsistence on long journeys in the West. It is parched corn, beaten or ground very fine, and sweetened with sugar, to be used with water, and drunk on the march. It is the *cold flour* of the Indians, and early Western pioneers.

PIÑONCILLO TREE, Castiliognia lobata.

PINUS A'BIES, *P. excel'sa seu picea, A'bies, Abies rubra seu excelsa seu picea, El'atē thelei'a, Pice'a, Norway Spruce Fir, Yew-leaved Fir. Nat. Ord*. Coniferæ. *Sex. Syst*. Monœcia Monodelphia. The tops are used in making *Spruce Beer*.

Essence of Spruce, Essen'tia Abie'tis, is a fluid extract, prepared by decoction from the twigs of this species of fir. From this is made *Spruce Beer*.

This fir affords the Burgundy pitch and common frankincense. 1. *Bur'gundy Pitch, White pitch, Pix Burgun'dica, Pix alba, Resi'na abie'tis hu'mida, Resi'na alba humida, Pini abie'tis resina sponte concre'ta, Pix ar'ida, Pix abieti'na. P. abietis* (Ph. U. S.), (F.) *Poix blanche, Poix grasse, P. jaune, P. de Bourgogne*. This prepared concrete juice is of a close consistence, rather soft, of a reddish-brown colour, and not unpleasant smell. It is very adhesive to the skin; and, consequently, forms excellent plasters for remaining upon the part for some time;—as in cases of affections of the chest. 2. *Abie'tis Resi'na*, (Ph. L. since 1809.) *Thus, Common Frankincense, Perrosin, Thus fœmini'num, T. vulga'rē, Olib'anum vulgarē seu vulgar'trē, Resina abietis sicca, Resin of the Spruce Fir*. It is solid, dry, brittle; externally, brownish-yellow; internally, whitish. Used in plasters like the last.

PINUS ABIES, see P. picea—p. Alba, P. picea.

PINUS BALSAME'A, *A'bies balsame'a* seu *bal-*

amif'era, *Peu'cea balsame'a*. The tree which affords the *Canada Balsam*, *Balsamum Canaden'sě* seu de *Can'ada*, *Resina strobili'na*, *Terebinth'ina Canaden'sis*, *Pini balsame'a*, *Canada Turpentine* or *Balsam*, *Balsam of Fir*, (F.) *Baume de Canada*, is one of the purest turpentines. It has the common properties of those substances.

PINUS CANADEN'SIS, *Abies Canaden'sis*, *Hemlock Spruce*. A tree, which is abundant in Canada, Nova Scotia, and the more northern parts of New England, and is found in the elevated and mountainous regions of the Middle States. The pitch—*Pix Canadensis*, *Canada Pitch*, *Hemlock Pitch*—obtained from it is commonly known under the name *Hemlock Gum*.

PINUS CANDICANS, P. Picea.

PINUS CEMBRA, *P. Monta'na*, *Aphernous'li Pine*. It yields an agreeably scented turpentine:—the *Carpa'thian Balsam*, *Bal'samum Carpath'icum*, *B. Lib'ani*, *Carpath'icum*, *Briançon Tur'pentine*. The nuts, *Cembro nuts*, *Nu'dei Cembræ*, have an eatable kernel, and yield oil. The shoots yield *Riga Balsam* by distillation.

PINUS DAMAR'RA, *Ag'athis Damarra*, grows in the East India Islands. The juice speedily concretes into a very hard resin,—the *Damarra turpentine*.

PINUS EXCELSA, P. abies—p. Gallica, P. picea.

PINUS LARIX *A'bies larix*, *Larix*, *L. commu'nis* seu *decid'ua* seu *Europæ'a* seu *pyramida'lis*. The *Larch*, (F.) *Mélèze*. From this tree exudes *Or'emberg gum*, *Bri'ançon manna*, *Gummi lar'icis* seu *Oremburgen'sě* seu *Uralen'sě*, *Manna Briganti'na* seu *larice'a*. It also yields, by boring, *Common Venice Turpentine*, *Resina Lar'icis*, *Terebinthina Ven'eta* seu *larici'na*, *Pini Lar'icis resi'na liq'uida*, (F.) *Térébenthine de Vénise*, *M. de Mélèze*. It is usually thinner than the other sorts of turpentine.

PINUS MUGHOS. The *Mountain* or *Mugho Pine*, *Pinus Pumil'io*. From the extremities of the branches exudes the *Resina Strobili'na*, of the Germans, or *Hungarian Balsam*. It is also obtained, by expression, from the cones. By distillation, the Hungarian balsam affords the *Krumhols oil*, *Oleum Templinum*.

PINUS PALUSTRIS, see Pinus sylvestris.

PINUS PICE'A, *P. Abies*, *A'bies*, *A. pice'a* seu *pectina'ta* seu *Gal'lica* seu *alba* seu *can'dicans* seu *vulga'ris* seu *taxifo'lia*, *European Silver Fir Tree*, *El'ate*, (F.) *Sapin commun*. By piercing the tubercles of the bark of this fir, the *Strasburg Turpentine* is obtained:—the *Resi'na Abie'tis*, (Ph. L. before 1809,) *Oleum Abietis*, *Terebinth'ina Argentoraten'sis*.

PINUS PINASTER, see P. sylvestris.

PINUS PI'NEA, *Stone Pine*, *Pinea*, *Pinus*, *P. uber'rima* seu *sati'va*. The nuts, *Zirbel nuts*, *Pine nuts*, *Nu'clei Pi'neæ*, *Pinei*, *Pine'oli*, (F.) *Pin à pignons*, are eaten raw, or preserved like almonds. They are, also, used in emulsions.

PINUS PUMILIO, see Pinus Mughos—p. Sativa, P. pinea.

PINUS SYLVES'TRIS, *Pinas'ter*, *Peucē*, *Scotch Fir*. This pine, as well as *P. marit'ima*, (*P. Pinaster*) and other species of Pinus, affords common turpentine and its oil, resin, tar, and pitch. 1. *Common Turpentine of Europe*, *Terebinth'ina*, *T. vulga'ris*, *T. commu'nis*, *Resina pini*, *Bijon*, *Horse Turpentine*, *Bordeaux Turpentine*, (F.) *Térébinthine de Bordeaux*, *Térébinthine commune*, is obtained by wounding the tree in hot weather. It is used, chiefly, as a dressing for wounds, &c., in horses, and for the distillation of the oil, (see Oleum Terebinthinæ.) The *white Turpentine*, or *common Turpentine of America*—*Terebinth'ina*, Ph. U. S.—is produced chiefly from *Pinus palustris* and *P. tæda*, and perhaps from other species inhabiting the Southern States. When the oil is distilled with water, yellow resin, or *Rosin*, (*Resi'na*, Ph. U. S.)—*Resina flava*—is left, which is only used in the formation of ointments and plasters: if without the addition of water, the residuum is common resin or Colophony. 2. When the cold begins to check the exudation of the common turpentine, part of it concretes in the wounds. This is called, in France, *Gallipot*, *Barras*; and *White Rosin*, *Resina alba*, when hardened after long exposure to the air. 3. When the old trees are subjected to distillation, in a coarse manner, Tar is obtained—*Hygrupissos*, *Pissa*, *Pix ce'dria*, *Resi'na pini empyreumat'ica liq'uida*, *Terebinth'ina empyreumat'ica*, *Alchitram*, *Alchitu'ra*, *Cedria*, *Pix liquida*, (F.) *Goudron*, *Brai liquide*. Tar water, *Aqua Picis*, *A. Picis*, *Infu'sum Picis liq'uidæ* seu *Picis empyreumaticæ liquidæ*, *Po'tio pice'a*, (F.) *Eau de Goudron*, was, at one time, a fashionable remedy in numerous complaints, and its use has been revived, since its virtues have been presumed to be owing to creasote. It is employed chiefly in pulmonary affections, and the vapour has been recommended in phthisis and other diseases of the lungs. It is used externally as a detergent. 4. *Common Pitch*, *Pix nigra*, *Black Pitch*, *Burnea*, *Burnia*, *Stone Pitch*, *Pix sicca*, *P. atra*, *P. nava'lis*, *Topissa*, *Palimpis'sa*, *P. ar'ida* (Ph. L. before 1809), (F.) *Poix navale*, *P. noire*, is obtained by inspissating tar. It is used only as a resolvent in plasters.

PINUS TÆDA, see P. sylvestris — p. Taxifolia, P. picea — p. Uberrima, Pinus pinea—p. Vulgaris, P. picea.

PIONE, Pæonia.

PIONY, Pæonia.

PIORTHOPNŒA, Pimelorthopnœa.

PIOULQUES. (F.) A kind of sucking-pump, invented by Louis, for extracting water that had entered internal cavities, in cases of drowning. A useless instrument.

PIPE-PLANT, Monotropa uniflora.

PIPER, see Piper nigrum.

PIPER ALBUM *Leucopiper*, *White Pepper*, is black pepper freed from its cuticle.

PIPER AUGUSTIFOLIUM, Matico—p. Aromaticum, P. nigrum—p. Betel, Betel—p. Brazilianum, Capsicum annuum—p. Calecuticum, Capsicum annuum.

PIPER CAPEN'SE, a South African species, has all the properties of the peppers, and, in appearance and taste, greatly resembles cubebs. It possesses, too, similar virtues.

PIPER CARYOPHYLLATUM, see Myrtus pimenta—p. Caudatum, P. cubeba—p. Chiapæ, see Myrtus pimenta.

PIPER CUBEB'A, *Per'sea cubeba*, *Laurus cubeba*, *Litsæa cubeba* seu *piperi'ta*. A native of Java and Guinea. The odour of these berries — *Cubeba*, *Com'peper*, *Compeba*, *Cubal sini*, *Piper cauda'tum*, *Baccæ Piperis glabri*, *Cubeb Pepper*, *Tailed Pepper*, *Cuma'mus*, (F.) *Poivre-à-queue*, *Quabebe* — is aromatic; taste at first cooling, afterwards pungent. The active principle is an essential oil — *Oleum Cubebæ*, oil of cubebs — which is officinal in the Pharm. U. S. The properties of the cubeb are stimulant and purgative. It is used only in gonorrhœas, Dose, from ℈j to ʒj, in powder, three or four times a day; of the volatile oil, 10 or 12 drops.

'Turkey yellow berries,'—the dried fruit of the *Rhamnus Catharticus* — are often substituted for cubebs.

PIPER GUINEENSE, Capsicum annuum—p. Hispanicum, Capsicum—p. Indicum, Capsicum annuum—p. Jamaicense, see Myrtus pimenta.

PIPER LONGUM, *Macrop'iper*, *Acapat'li*, *Catutrip'ali*, *Pim'pilim*, *Long Pepper*, (F.) *Poivre*

disease which we can always subdue. Great extent of inflammation; very considerable oppression; orthopnœa, and difficult expectoration are unfavourable symptoms. The most active treatment is of course necessary. General bleeding forms the sheet-anchor,—employed so as to make a decided impression on the system, and repeated, if necessary; local blood-letting; nauseating doses of antimonials; purgatives; and when the violence of the inflammation has been got under, — counter-irritants, &c. Chronic pneumonia sometimes succeeds the acute, and, at others, occurs accidentally. It must be managed on general principles. Small bleedings, especially locally; and counter-irritants of all kinds are indicated.

PNEUMONIA BILIOSA, P. bilious.
PNEUMONIA, BILIOUS, *Pneumo'nia bilio'sa, Pneumocholo'sis*. Inflammation of the lungs, accompanied by gastric fever, and not uncommonly by typhoid symptoms;—*Pneumotyphus, Pneumo'nia typhoï'des* seu *typho'des* seu *typho'sa*, Putrid, typhoid, adynamic, or erysipel'atous *pneumo'nia*.

PNEUMONIA, ERYSIPELATOUS, P. bilious — p. Gangrænosa, Necropneumonia — p. Hypostatica, Pneumonypostasis — p. Intermittens, Pneumotyposis — p. Lobular, see Lobular — p. Notha, Peripneumonia notha — p. Pleuritis, Pleuropneumonia — p. Putrid, P. bilious — p. Typhodes, P. bilious — p. Typhoid, P. bilious — p. Typhosa, P. bilious, Necropneumonia — p. Vesicular, Bronchitis, vesicular.

PNEUMONIC, Pulmonic.
PNEUMON'ICA. Diseases affecting the lungs, their membranes or motive power; characterized by irregular, impeded, or painful respiration. The second order of the class Pneumatica of Good.

PNEUMONIC'ULA, diminutive of pneumonia. A slight inflammation of the lung.
PNEUMONICUS, Pulmonic.
PNEUMONIE, Pneumonia — *p. Disséminée*, see Lobular — *p. Lobulaire*, see Lobular — *p. Melonnée*, see Lobular.
PNEUMONIE DES AGONISANTS, Pneumonie hypostatique. The hyperæmic engorgement, which takes place in the lungs during the last moments of life, has been so termed. It would seem to be hyperæmia rather than inflammation.

PNEUMONIT'IC, *Pneumonit'icus*. Of, or belonging to pneumonitis, or inflammation of the lungs.
PNEUMONITIS, Pneumonia.
PNEUMONOCARCINO'MA, from πνευμων, 'the lung,' and καρκινωμα, 'cancer.' Cancer of the lungs.
PNEUMONOCE'LE, from πνευμων, 'the lung,' and κηλη, 'rupture.' Hernia of the lung.
PNEUMONOCE'LE DIAPHRAGMAT'ICA INTER'NA. Hernia of the lung through the diaphragm.
PNEUMONOCELE EXTER'NA seu THORAC''ICA, Hernia through the parietes of the chest.
PNEUMONOCELE THORACICA, Pn. externa.
PNEUMONŒDEMA, Œdema of the lungs.
PNEUMONOMELANOSIS, see Melanosis.
PNEUMONOPHTHISIS, Phthisis pulmonalis.
PNEUMONOPHTHOE, Phthisis pulmonalis.
PNEUMONOPLEURESIS, Pleuroperipneumony.
PNEUMONOPLEURITIS, Pleuroperipneumony.
PNEUMONORRHAGIA, Hæmoptysis.
PNEUMONORRHŒA, Hæmoptysis.
PNEUMONOSCIR'RHUS, from πνευμων, 'the lung,' and σκιρρος, 'induration.' Induration of the lungs.
PNEUMONOSES, Pneumoses.

PNEUMONY, Pneumonia.
PNEUMONYPOS'TASIS, *Pneumo'nia hypostat'ica*. Pneumonia in a depending portion of the lung, caused by lying on the back.
PNEUMOPÉRICARDE, Pneumo-pericardium.
PNEUMO-PERICARD'IUM, *Pneumo-pericardi'tis*, (F.) *Pneumo-péricarde*, from πνευμα, 'air,' and περικαρδιον, 'pericardium.' Laënnec designates, under this name, the effusion of air into the cavity of the pericardium.
PNEUMOPHTHISIS, Phthisis pulmonalis.
PNEUMOPHYMATA, Tubercles of the lungs.
PNEUMOPLEURESIS, Pleuroperipneumony.
PNEUMOPTHOE, Phthisis pulmonalis.
PNEUMORRHAGIA, Hæmoptysis — p. Interna, Hæmatothorax.
PNEUMOSEPSIS, Necropneumonia.
PNEUMOSES, from πνευμων, 'the lung.' A term under which Alibert comprises every morbid affection of the lungs.
PNEUMOTHO'RAX, *Pneumatho'rax, Pneumatotho'rax, Emphyse'ma pec'toris, Asthma aërium, A. emphysemat'icum, Dyspnœ'a pneumat'ica, D. physothorac''ica, Physothorax, Aërothorax, Aëropleurie* (Piorry), from πνευμα, 'air,' and θωραξ, 'the thorax.' An accumulation of air in the cavity of the pleura. A complaint generally sudden in its invasion and fatal in its character. In many instances, along with the air, a liquid is effused,—*Hydropneumothorax*. The disease may be spontaneous and simple, but in a large proportion of cases it is complicated with pleurisy and pulmonary tubercles. The signs vary according as there is, or is not, a communication between the pleura and the bronchia. The affected side gives a hollow, tympanitic sound, even where the thickness of the parietes of the thorax is great. When the effusion is considerable, the affected side is dilated, but there is no *râle* of any kind. When a gaseous and a liquid effusion are present at the same time, the sound on percussion is found to be clear at the superior part of the thorax, but dull inferiorly; hence, by varying the position of the patient, and by consequence that of the contained fluids, the seats of the clear and the dull sound will be varied. When the gaseous effusion is owing to a fistulous communication between the pleura and bronchia, the metallic respiration and resonance are heard; and if there be both gaseous and liquid effusion, with a fistulous communication, in addition to these signs there is the *tintement métallique*. The presence of liquid can always be ascertained by succussion. See Emphrysema of the lungs.
PNEUMOT'OMY, *Pneumotom'ia*, from πνευμων, 'the lung,' and τεμνω, 'I cut.' Dissection of the lungs.

PNEOMOTYPHUS, Pneumonia, typhoid.
PNEUMOTYPO'SIS, *Pneumo'nia intermittens*, from πνευμων, 'the lung,' and τυπος, 'a stamp, a type.' Pneumonia characterized by periodicity.
PNEUOBIOMANTIA, Docimasia pulmonum.
PNEUSIOBIOGNOSIS, Docimasia pulmonum.
PNEUSIOBIOSCOPE, Docimasia pulmonum.
PNEUSIS, Respiration — p. Pertussis, Pertussis — p. Singultus, Singultus — p. Tussis, Tussis.
PNEUSOMETER, Spirometer.
PNIGALION, Incubus.
PNIGMOS, Orthopnœa, Strangulation.
PNIGOPHOBIA, Angina pectoris, Suffocation.
PNIX, Orthopnœa, Strangulation.
PNOE, Aura.
PNŒUM. A nostrum of Dr. Samuel Hahnemann, the founder of the 'Homœopathic System,' which consisted — it is said — of borax only!

PNOOCOLYTICUS, Asthmatic.

POCHE DES EAUX, see Liquor Amnii, and Parturition.

POCK, from Teut. *pocca*, '*pock* or little pouch.' A pustule of smallpox.

POCK, KINE, Vaccina.

POCKFRETTEN, see Pockmark.

POCKHOLE, Pockmark.

POCKMARK, *Pockhole*, *Scrobic'ulus Vari'olæ*, *Cica'trix Variolæ*. The mark or *pit* or *pitting* left from a smallpox pustule. One pitted with smallpox is said to be *pockfretten*.

POCKY. Infected with, or appertaining to, or resembling, smallpox or syphilis.

POC'ULUM ABSINTHIA'TUM: This was regarded, in remote ages, as a wholesome beverage; the *absinthium*, or 'wormwood,' being supposed to act as an antidote to drunkenness.

POCULUM AMATORIUM, Philter — p. Diogenis, Palm — p. Emeticum, Goblet, emetic.

POD'AGRA, *Podarthri'tis*, *Podorrheu'ma*, *Podal'gia*, from πους, 'the foot,' and αγρα, 'seizure.' Pain which attacks the feet. Gout, situate in the articulations of the foot. It has, also, been used in a more extensive signification synonymously with *gout*.

PODAGRA ABERRANS, Gout, (wandering) — p. Arthritis, Gout — p. Retrograda, Gout, (retrograde.)

PODAGRARIA, Ligusticum podagraria — p. Ægopodium, Ligusticum podagraria.

PODAGRIC, *Podag'rical*, *Podag'ricus*, *Arthrit'icus*, *Arthrit'ic*, *Gouty*, (F.) *Goutteux*. Relating or belonging to gout. Affected with gout.

PODALGIA, Gout, Podagra.

PODALYRIA TINCTORIA, Sophora tinctoria.

PODANENCEPHALIA, see Podencephalus.

PODARTHRITIS, Podagra.

PODARTHROC'ACE, from πους, 'the foot,' αρθρον, 'an articulation,' and κακος, 'bad.' Caries of the articulation of the foot.

PODENCEPHALIA, see Podencephalus.

PODENCEPH'ALUS, *Podanenceph'alus*, from πους, 'the foot,' and κεφαλη, 'the head.' A monster whose brain is placed outside the skull, and seems to be supported on a pedicle, which traverses the summit of the skull. This state of monstrosity is termed *Podanencepha'lia*, or more properly, *Podencepha'lia*.— G. St. Hilaire.

PODEX, Anus.

PODŒ'MA; from πους, 'foot,' and οιδημα, 'a swelling.' Œdema of the foot.

PODOL'OGY, *Podolog"ia*, from πους, 'the foot,' and λογος, 'a discourse.' A description of the foot. A treatise on the foot.

PODOPHYL'LUM PELTA'TUM, *Podophyl'lum*, *Anapodophyll'um Canadensē*, *May-apple*, *Mandrake. Family*, Podophylleæ. *Sex. Syst.* Polyandria Monogynia. A common plant throughout North America. The fruit is eatable, and esteemed by many. The leaves are said to be poisonous. The root or rhizoma, *Podophyllum* (Ph. U. S.), is purgative in the dose of 20 grains. It has also been used as an anthelmintic.

PODOPHYLLUM MONTA'NUM, *Mountain May-apple*, *Mandrake*, *Wild Lemon*, *Duckfoot*, *Raccoon Berry*, *Yellow Berry*, *Ground Lemon*, has the same properties.

PODORRHEUMA, Podagra.

PODOTHE'CA, from πους, 'a foot,' and θηκη, 'a receptacle, a sheath.' The cuticle of the foot. An anatomical preparation. *Chirothe'ca*, has been used for the cuticle of the hand.

POËLETTE, Cup.

POË'PHAGUS; from ποη, or ποα, 'a plant, an herb,' and φαγω, 'I eat.' One who subsists on herbs or vegetables. The act of subsisting or feeding on herbs or vegetables is called *Poëphag"ia*. Hence Strabo calls the Irish ποηφαγοι.

POGON, Beard.

POGONI'ASIS, *Pogo'nia*, from πωγων, 'the beard.' A female beard. Also, great strength or quantity of beard. A female having a beard —*Vira'go*.

POGO'NIUM, diminutive of πωγων, 'beard.' A weak or small beard.

POHON ANTIAR, Upas.

POI. A favourite aliment in the Sandwich Islands. It is a sort of paste made from the root of the Kalo—*Arum esculen'tum*.

POIDS ET MÉSURES, Weights and measures.

POIGNÉE, Manipulus.

POIGNET, Carpus.

POIL, Hair.

POILETTE, Cup.

POILS, see Typha latifolia.

POING, Fist.

POINT, Stitch.

POINT, BLISTERING. A name given by Dr. Rush to an indeterminate period in the course of a continued fever, intermediate between the stages of high excitement and collapse, in which blisters will—he thought—usually produce unequivocally good effects.

POINT DE COTÉ, Pleurodynia.

POINTS LACRYMAUX, Lachrymalia puncta.

POIRE, see Pyrus communis.

POIREAU, Allium porrum.

POIRIER, Pyrus communis.

POIS, Pisum—*p. à Cautère*, see Fonticulus — *p. Chiche*, Cicer arietinum—*p. Cultivé*, Pisum— *p. à Gratter*, Dolichos pruriens—*p. Patate*, Dolichos tuberosus.

POISON, *Phar'macon*, *Phar'macum*, *Tox'icum*, *Vene'num*, *Virus*, *Delete'rium*, *Venena'tion*, (F.) *Poison*. A generic name for all substances which, when introduced into the animal economy, either by cutaneous absorption, respiration, or the digestive canal, act in a noxious manner on the vital properties or the texture of organs. Hence we speak of *fever poison*, *cholera poison*, &c. Poisons exist in the three kingdoms of nature; but those which proceed from animals are often called *venoms*, as the venom of the viper, scorpion, tarantula, &c.; whilst those that are the products of disease have the name *virus*. In common parlance, therefore, *poison* is restricted to deleterious articles, furnished by the mineral and vegetable kingdoms. Orfila has divided poisons into four classes. 1. ACRID, IRRITATING, CORRO'SIVE, or ESCHAROT'IC, such as the concentrated acids and alkalies; mercurial, arsenical, cupreous, and antimonial compounds, cantharides, &c. 2. NARCOT'IC; those that act particularly upon the brain; as hyoscyamus, opium, &c., but without inflaming the organ with which they come in contact. 3. NARCOT'ICO-ACRID or ACRO-NARCOT'IC;—those that act on the brain, but, at the same time, irritate the parts to which they are applied; as aconite, belladonna, &c. 4. SEPTIC or PUTRES'CENT;—those furnished by the animal kingdom. See Venom and Virus. Various classifications, of a similar character, have been recommended by different toxicologists; but they are liable to the objection, that they throw substances together whose physiological action on the system is very different. It is, indeed, difficult to avoid unnatural compression of matters into places not properly belonging to them, in all such arrangements.

The following table, which exhibits a *coup d'œil* of the chief poisons, with most of the circumstances of importance connected with them, is not free from these objections.

TABLE, EXHIBITING THE SYMPTOMS, TREATMENT, AND MODE OF DETECTING THE VARIOUS POISONS, MINERAL, VEGETABLE AND ANIMAL.

N. B. In all cases the Stomach-Pump should be used as soon as possible.

I. INORGANIC POISONS.

Poisons.	Symptoms.	Treatment.	Tests.
ACIDS. *Acetic Acid.* *Citric Acid.* *Muriatic Acid.* *Nitric Acid.* *Sulphuric Acid.* *Tartaric Acid.* *Oxalic Acid.*	The acids, generally, are strong corrosive poisons. Sour, acrid taste, burning in the throat, which is increased by pressure, swallowing, or coughing; eructation, and excruciating pain in the stomach; more or less corrugation of the lining membranes of the mouth and primæ viæ; excoriation about the mouth or such other parts of the skin as the acid may have touched. The matter vomited effervesces with carbonate of lime. The countenance becomes glazed, extremities cold and clammy; convulsions and death. Nitric acid occasions yellow stains, and sulphuric acid, black.	The carbonates of soda, potassa, lime and magnesia, are all antidotes to the acids; calcined magnesia also. They are to be used with the following restrictions: for the acetic, citric, muriatic, sulphuric, and tartaric acids, they may be used indiscriminately. For the nitric and oxalic, carbonates of magnesia and lime can alone be employed with safety. In the case of sulphuric acid, water should not be drunk, on account of the great heat which is produced by their mixture. Subsequent inflammation to be treated by ordinary means. The carbonates of the alkalies and of magnesia and lime have the inconvenience, that a large quantity of gas is extricated in the stomach.	*Sulphuric acid* is known by a white precipitate with any salt of baryta, insoluble in nitric acid. *Muriatic acid* is known by a white precipitate with nitrate of silver, insoluble in nitric acid, which turns black by the action of light. *Nitric acid* gives rise to orange-coloured fumes, when copper is placed in it, and an ability to dissolve gold when mixed with muriatic acid. *Acetic acid* exhales the odour of vinegar. *Citric acid* blackens when heated. *Tartaric acid* precipitates crystals, with a solution of potassa and a white precipitate is thrown down by lime-water. *Oxalic acid* gives a white precipitate with lime-water, which, when heated, is converted into carbonate of lime.
Prussic Acid. *Oil of Bitter Almonds.* *Laurel Water.*	Is a sedative poison; nausea, giddiness, debility, hurried pulse, weight and pain in the head; eructations having the flavour of the acid; spasms, tetanus, contractile pupil; convulsions, death.	Ammonia is an antidote; but it should not be employed in a very concentrated form. Liquid chlorine has also been found efficacious. The cold douche to the head has been recommended.	*Prussic acid* exhales the odour of peach-kernels; forms a white precipitate with nitrate of silver neutralized with an alkali, gives a blue precipitate with the per-salts of iron.
ALKALIES and their SALTS. Ammonia, Strong Liquor or Water of. Muriate of Ammonia or Sal Ammoniac. Potassa. Caustic Potassa, and Liquor Potassa.	Violent, caustic, acrid taste; great heat in the throat, with destruction of its lining membrane; difficult and painful deglutition; vomiting of bloody matter, which turns the yellow of turmeric brown; acute pain in the stomach; cold sweats, weakness, hiccough; violent colic pains, with purging of bloody stools and membranous flakes; death.	The vegetable acids, such as vinegar, lemon juice, citric and tartaric acid in solution are antidotes to the alkalies and their carbonates. The fixed oils, such as castor, linseed, almond and olive, form soaps with the free alkalies, and therefore destroy their caustic effects.	The alkalies are known by their action on turmeric paper: restoring the colour of litmus, which has been reddened by an acid. Carbonates are known by their effervescence with an acid; some of them affect the turmeric paper. Sal ammoniac gives out the pungent odour of ammonia, when mixed with quicklime.
Carbonate of Potassa, or Pearl Ash, and Salt of Tartar. Nitrate of Potassa or Saltpetre. Sulphuret of Potassium or Liver of Sulphur. Soda.	The nitrate of potassa will not manifest the effect with turmeric paper. The carbonates, when vomited, will effervesce with acids; and the liver of sulphur will give rise to eructations of sulphuretted hydrogen.	Poisoning by nitrate of potassa to be treated on general antiphlogistic principles; mucilaginous drinks. Liver of sulphur is said to be decomposed and neutralized by common salt. The liquid chloride of soda will also decompose it.	Nitrate of potassa decrepitates and deflagrates when thrown on hot coals. Liver of sulphur emits the odour of sulphuretted hydrogen when dissolved, or when treated with an acid.
EARTHS and COMPOUNDS. Baryta. Carbonate of Baryta. Chloride of Barium. Nitrate of Baryta. Lime.	Analogous to those of the corrosive metals. Violent burning in the stomach, vomiting, gripes, diarrhœa; excessive muscular debility, headache, convulsions, death. Lime differs from baryta in being a pure irritant.	The sulphates of soda and magnesia are prompt and effective antidotes to all the poisonous salts of baryta. Phosphate of soda will also counteract their effects. Lime may be neutralized by dilute acids. Carbonic acid, in soda-water, effervescing draught or yeast, it is supposed, would answer a good purpose. The fixed oils may be employed either for baryta or lime, when not in a compound state.	Baryta and its salts invariably give a white precipitate, insoluble in acid, with a soluble sulphate. Lime, when dissolved, gives a white precipitate with oxalic acid. Also with carbonic acid or a soluble carbonate. The same as baryta.

Poisons.	Symptoms.	Treatment.	Tests.
ALCOHOL. Brandy, Wines, and all Spirituous Liquors.	Intoxication, and when taken very freely, complete insensibility, with apoplexy or paralysis of one side; the countenance swollen and of a dark-red colour; the breathing difficult, and often stertorous, with a peculiar puffing out of the lips; the breath smells of liquor, which will distinguish the symptoms from those of spontaneous apoplexy.	A powerful emetic of white vitriol, or tartar emetic, should be got into the stomach as soon as possible; and if the person has lost the power of swallowing, a flexible catheter or tube should be the means of conveying it thither. The vomiting should be encouraged as much as possible with warm water; and large and active glysters of salt and water should be thrown up. The patient should be placed erect, and if the countenance and other appearances be not improved after these means have been used, the jugular vein may be opened, and cold wet cloths applied to the head, particularly if the body be hotter than natural. If the extremities become cold, warmth and friction should be perseveringly used.	
VOLATILE OILS. Creasote. Dippel's Animal Oil. Oil of Tar. Oil of Tobacco. Oil of Turpentine. Fusel Oil.	General action, that of irritant poisons. Burning pain, vomiting, pungent taste, purging, &c. The oils of turpentine and tobacco affect the nervous system; the peculiar odour of each oil will be manifested in the matter vomited.	Creasote is immediately coagulated by albumen. Dippel's animal oil may be counteracted with dilute acids and the fixed oils. The other oils have no particular antidotes, and their effects must, therefore, be counteracted upon general principles.	No better mode of recognising these substances exists, than that derived from their peculiar odour. Dippel's oil has the pungent odour of ammonia; creasote and oil of tar, a peculiar smell of smoke; the odour of tobacco and turpentine are well known; and fusel oil has a peculiar, offensive, suffocating odour.
GASES. Carbonic Acid, or Fixed Air. Carbonic Oxide. Fumes of Burning Charcoal. Chlorine. Sulphuretted Hydrogen.	Chlorine produces, when inhaled, violent irritation of the organs of respiration; cough, bloody expectoration, inflammation of the lungs, and permanent pulmonary disease. The other gases, although producing some effect on the respiratory organs, act as poisons, in consequence of their sedative agency. The symptoms, therefore, are those of apoplexy, or narcotic poisoning.	The antidotes to chlorine are the cautious inhalation of ammonia, or sulphuretted hydrogen. The inflammatory symptoms from chlorine to be treated on general principles. For the other gases, cold affusions to the head, blood-letting, artificial respiration.	Chlorine is recognised by its peculiar odour and bleaching properties. Sulphuretted hydrogen, by its fetid smell, and the rapid blackening of lead. Carbonic acid, by its occasioning turbidness in lime-water placed in its atmosphere. Carbonic oxide, by the blue colour of its flame.
IODINE. Iodide of Potassium.	Irritant symptoms; burning pain in the throat, lacerating pain in the stomach, and fruitless efforts to vomit; suffusion of the eyes; excessive pain and tenderness of the epigastrium.	Iodine combines with starch, and forms an insoluble compound. The prompt administration of starch, wheat flour, or other vegetable matter containing fecula, beat up in water, is recommended. Iodide of potassium has no antidote. Vomiting should be promoted by draughts of warm water, and inflammation be subdued by general treatment.	Iodine is known by its odour, and the formation of a blue precipitate, when brought in contact with a cold solution of starch. Iodide of potassium gives a crystalline precipitate, with tartaric acid in excess. The supernatant fluid will give the blue colour to starch.
METALS. Antimony. Tartar Emetic. Chloride, or Butter of Antimony. Oxide of Antimony.	Vomiting. If vomiting do not occur promptly, violent irritant effects are produced. Burning pain in the pit of the stomach; Purging; colicky pains, sense of tightness in the throat, violent cramps; repeated recurrence of vomiting.	If vomiting have not been produced, it should be brought about by tickling the fauces, and administering copious draughts of warm water. Astringent infusions, such as of galls, oak bark, Peruvian bark, act as antidotes, and should be given promptly; powdered yellow bark may be used, until the infusion is prepared.	Antimony in solution is best distinguished by the peculiar orange-red precipitate, which it forms with sulphuretted hydrogen or solutions of the hydrosulphates. Free alkalies produce white precipitates. The muriate is known by a white precipitate, when it is poured into water. In its solid form, it may be known by the formation of white fumes, when heated, which redden litmus. It may also be converted into chloride, and then precipitated by adding water.

Poisons.	Symptoms.	Treatment.	Tests.
Arsenic. *Arsenious Acid, or White Arsenic.* *Orpiment, or Yellow Sulphuret of Arsenic.* *King's Yellow.* *Realgar, or Red Sulphuret of Arsenic.* *Fly Powder.* *Fowler's Solution.* *Arsenical Paste.* *Arsenical Soap.* *Arsenite of Copper, Scheele's Green.*	Violent burning pain in the region of the stomach and bowels; tenderness on pressure; retching: vomiting; sense of dryness and tightness in the throat; thirst; hoarseness and difficulty of speech; the matter vomited, greenish or yellowish, sometimes streaked with blood; diarrhœa; tenesmus; sometimes excoriation of the anus; urinary organs occasionally affected with violent burning pains and suppression; convulsions and cramps; clammy sweats; lividity of the extremities; countenance collapsed; eyes red and sparkling; delirium; death.	The hydrated peroxide of iron diffused through water; or the precipitated carbonate; or the rubigo ferri, in very fine powder, to be administered every five or ten minutes, until relief is obtained. This is particularly efficacious when the *white arsenic* has been swallowed. If the arsenic have been taken in the form of Fowler's Solution, lime-water, in copious draughts, may be given. For either of the other forms, emetics of sulphate of zinc; diluents; demulcents, such as flaxseed tea, infusion of slippery elm, &c. Counter-irritants may be used to relieve the spasm, and violent pain in the stomach. Bleeding, as promoting absorption, should not be employed until the stomach is completely evacuated.	If the suspected substance can be obtained free from organic matter, the presence of arsenic may readily be shown by boiling it in distilled water, filtering, and testing with, 1st. Ammoniaco-sulphate of copper. 2d. Ammoniaco-nitrate of silver. (*Hume's Test*) 3d. Sulphuretted hydrogen gas. The first will produce a *green* precipitate; second, a *pale yellow* precipitate; third, a *bright yellow* precipitate, if arsenic be present. A portion of the powder, or one of these precipitates, carefully and thoroughly dried, is then to be mixed with charcoal and exsiccated carbonate of soda, to be placed in a small glass tube, closed at one end, and then to be heated to a red heat in the flame of a lamp. The arsenic will be reduced, and sublime in the upper part of the tube, forming a dark crust, having considerable lustre on its exterior surface, resembling polished steel. By gently heating this crust in a very small flame, crystals of white arsenic will be formed, having a high adamantine lustre. If organic matter be present, it must be entirely destroyed, by heating the substance with nitro-muriatic acid. After this has been done, and a clear, transparent solution in distilled water has been obtained, the subsequent process is as above indicated. If arsenious acid be submitted to the action of nascent hydrogen, it is deoxidized, and the metallic arsenic thereby obtained, combining with hydrogen, forms arseneuretted hydrogen gas. (*Marsh's Test.*) Add to a suspected solution a few drops of pure chlorohydric acid, and place in it a slip of bright copper; no change occurs until the liquid is brought to the boiling point, when, if arsenic be present, even in small quantity, the copper acquires an iron-gray coating from the deposit of that metal. Remove the slip of copper; wash it in water, dry it and gradually heat it in a reduction tube, when arsenious acid will be sublimed in minute octohedral crystals. The test succeeds with powdered arsenic, the arsenites, arsenic acid, the arseniates, and orpiment. It will even separate the arsenic from arsenite of copper, and from common lead-shot. *Reinsch's Test.*
Bismuth. *Nitrate of Bismuth.* *Pearl Powder.* *Oxide of Bismuth.*	Similar to those produced from other irritant poisons. General inflammation of the whole alimentary canal; suppression of urine; hiccough, disagreeable metallic taste; vomiting; cramps; delirium; death.	Milk, and sweet mucilaginous drinks are recommended. Leeches, general bleeding; glysters; fomentations to be employed on the general principles of treatment for inflammatory symptoms.	Bismuth is known by the formation of a white precipitate, when its solution in nitric acid is poured into water; and by the formation of a black precipitate with sulphuretted hydrogen gas and hydrosulphates in solution.
Copper. *Sulphate of Copper, Blue Vitriol.* *Acetate of Copper, Verdigris.* *Carbonate of Copper, Blue Verditer.* *Arsenite of Copper, Scheele's Green.* *Food cooked in dirty copper vessels, or pickles made green by copper.*	Very similar to those produced by arsenic. Coppery eructations and taste. Fatal cases are generally terminated by convulsions, palsy, insensibility.	Albumen to be administered in either of its forms which can be most readily obtained, as milk or whites of eggs. Vinegar should not be given. The inflammatory symptoms are to be treated on general principles, and so of the nervous.	The presence of copper is readily shown in solutions. By ammonia a beautiful bluish precipitate is thrown down, which dissolves in an excess of the precipitant, and the solution has a rich blue colour. A bright iron bar, introduced into solutions of copper, occasions the separation of the copper, in a metallic form, which deposits itself upon the iron.

Poisons.	Symptoms.	Treatment.	Tests.
GOLD. *Chloride of Gold.* *Fulminating Gold.*	Very analogous to those of other irritant poisons. This substance communicates a pink stain to the flesh, and patches of that colour may be found about the lips, and inside the mouth.	The salts of gold are decomposed by sulphate of iron; and this has, therefore, been recommended as an antidote. Inflammatory symptoms to be treated on general principles.	Chloride of gold is very readily decomposed, and the gold separated in a metallic state. Protosulphate of iron, nitrate of silver and protochloride of tin, all answer this purpose. The precipitated powder will be found insoluble, except in nitro-muriatic acid.
IRON. *Sulphate of Iron, Copperas, Green Vitriol.* *Chloride of Iron.*	Symptoms of irritant poisoning; colic pains, constant vomiting and purging. Violent pain in the throat, tension of the epigastrium, coldness of the skin, and feebleness of the pulse.	Carbonate of soda would be a most excellent antidote to either of these substances. Mucilaginous drinks might also be employed; and particular symptoms relieved by general treatment.	Iron is recognised by a bluish-black precipitate, with tincture of galls; rich blue, with prussiate of potassa; and a greenish or reddish precipitate, with the free alkalies or their carbonates.
LEAD. *Acetate of Lead, Sugar of Lead. Carbonate of Lead, White Lead. Red Oxide, or Red Lead. Litharge.* *Wines sweetened by Lead.* *Water which has been kept in Leaden vessels.* *Acid food, cooked, or left standing in vessels glazed with Lead.*	Irritation of the alimentary canal; spasm; nervous symptoms; paralysis, either partial or complete. When taken for some time, in small quantity, violent and obstinate colic; rigidity of abdominal muscles, cramps; remission of pain; obstinate constipation, urine diminished, saliva increased; countenance anxious and gloomy. If relief be not promptly obtained, giddiness, debility, torpor, coma, convulsions and death. The paralysis affects generally the upper extremities.	Sulphate of magnesia and phosphate of soda are both good antidotes for the soluble salts of lead. For the solid forms, dilute sulphuric acid may be drunk. These are applicable to the irritant forms of poisoning by lead. In the chronic form, or colica pictonum, purgatives and anodynes are resorted to; venesection; and external applications to relieve the cramps. The use of strychnia is recommended for the paralysis.	Soluble salts of lead yield a white precipitate with sulphates and carbonates in solution. Salts of chromic acid and iodide of potassium occasion a yellow precipitate. Sulphuretted hydrogen, a black precipitate. If solid, the lead may be converted into a state of solution by nitric acid, and the dilute solution be tested as above.
MERCURY. *Corrosive Sublimate.* *Cyanide of Mercury.* *Nitrate of Mercury.* *White Precipitate.* *Red Oxide,* or *Red Precipitate.* *Sulphate,* or *Turbith Mineral.* *Vermilion,* or *Red Sulphuret.*	Violent symptoms of irritant poisoning; harsh metallic astringent taste; burning pain in the stomach; vomiting and purging frequently of bloody matter; often irritation of the urinary organs, and sometimes suppression; tightness and burning in the throat, occasionally so great as to prevent speech; countenance not always pale, but sometimes flushed; tendency to doze; stupor, convulsions and death.	Albumen, in some form, must be promptly administered; either white of eggs beaten up with water, milk, or wheat flour beaten up. The inflammatory symptoms to be counteracted by the usual means. Gold, finely mixed in dust, with fine iron filings. (?)	The free alkalies differ in their precipitates from solutions of mercury. Potassa gives, with corrosive sublimate, a yellowish one; ammonia, a white; lime-water, an orange; and sulphuretted hydrogen, a black. If a drop of the solution be placed on a piece of gold, and touched with a knife or key, the mercury will be reduced, which amalgamates with the gold, producing a white spot. The nitrate of mercury gives a black precipitate with the free alkalies. All the solid forms of mercury are volatile, and may be reduced by heating them in a glass tube with charcoal and carbonate of soda, when the metallic mercury will sublime, and may be collected in a globule.
SILVER. *Nitrate of Silver,* or *Lunar Caustic.*	Those of other irritant poisons.	Chloride of sodium, or common salt, immediately decomposes this substance, and destroys its activity. Antiphlogistic treatment is to be employed for the inflammatory symptoms.	Nitrate of silver is distinguished by the formation of a white precipitate, insoluble in nitric acid, with chloride of sodium; a gray precipitate with ammonia, which is redissolved in an excess of ammonia; yellow precipitate with phosphate of soda. The precipitate of chloride of silver, obtained by adding muriate of soda to the nitrate of silver, is readily reduced, and the metallic silver obtained, by mixing it with dilute sulphuric acid and granulated zinc.
TIN. *Chloride of Tin. Solution of Tin, used by Dyers. Oxide of Tin,* or *Putty Powder.*	The same as those from other irritant poisons, and a peculiar tanned appearance of the villous coat of the stomach.	Milk to be given copiously, and the subsequent treatment to be regulated by the symptoms.	The chloride precipitates vegetable colouring matter; also albumen and gelatin. The white oxide is precipitated from its solution by free alkalies; with sulphuretted hydrogen gas, a brown precipitate.
ZINC. *Oxide of Zinc.* *Sulphate of Zinc, White Vitriol.* *Acetate of Zinc.*	Violent vomiting; astringent taste, burning pain in the stomach; pale countenance; cold extremities; dull eyes; fluttering pulse. Death seldom ensues, in consequence of the emetic effects.	The vomiting may be relieved by copious draughts of warm water. Carbonate of soda, administered in solution, will decompose the sulphate of zinc. Milk and albumen also act as antidotes. General principles to be observed in the subsequent treatment.	A white precipitate is thrown down by the free alkalies from the soluble salts of zinc, which becomes yellow when strongly heated—recovering its white colour on cooling. Sulphuretted hydrogen occasions a white precipitate.

Poisons.	Symptoms.	Treatment.	Tests.
PHOSPHORUS.	Symptoms of irritant poisoning; pain in the stomach and bowels; vomiting, diarrhœa, tenderness and tension of the abdomen.	An emetic to be promptly administered; copious draughts containing magnesia in suspension; mucilaginous drinks; general treatment for inflammatory symptoms.	Phosphorus is known by its ready inflammability, luminousness at ordinary temperatures, and alliaceous odour.
GLASS, or ENAMEL.	If taken in very coarse powder, it produces irritation and inflammation of the bowels.	Large quantities of crumb of bread should be eaten, to envelop the particles. (?) An emetic of sulphate of zinc should then be given, and vomiting be promoted by demulcent drinks.	

II. ORGANIC POISONS.
I. VEGETABLE POISONS.

Irritant Poisons.	Symptoms.	Treatment.
Anemone *pulsatilla*. Wind Flower. Arum *maculatum*. Wake Robin. Bryonia *dioica*. Bryony. Caladium *seguinium*. Dumbcane. Calla *palustris*. Water Arum. Caltha *palustris*. Marsh Marigold. Chelidonium *majus*. Celandine. Clematis *vitalba*. Virgin Bower. Convolvulus *jalapa*. Jalap. Convolvulus *scammonia*. Scammony. Croton *tiglium*. Purging Croton. Cucumis *colocynthis*. Colocynth. Cyclamen *Europæum*. Sow Bread. Daphne *gnidium*. Spurge Flax. Daphne *mezereum*. Mezereon. Delphinium *staphisagria*. Stavesacre. Dioica *palustris*. Swamp leather-wood. Equisetum *hyemale*. Scourgrass. Euphorbia *officinarum*. Euphorbium. Spurge. Gratiola *officinalis*. Hedge Hyssop. Hippomane *mancinella*. Manchineel. Hura *crepitans*. Sand Box. Hydrocotyle *vulgaris*. Marsh Pennywort. Jatropha *curcas*. Indian Nut. Jatropha *manihot*. Cassada. Juniperus *sabina*. Savin (oil of). Juniperus *Virginiana*. Red Cedar (oil of.) Momordica *elaterium*. Squirting Cucumber. Narcissus *pseudo-narcissus*. Daffodil. Pastinax *sativa*. Common Parsnep. Pedicularis *palustris*. Marsh Lousewort. Phytolacca *decandra*. Poke. Piper *cubeba*. Cubebs. Plumbago *Europæa*. Toothwort. Ranunculus *acris*, and other species. Crowfoot. Rhododendron *chrysanthemum*. Oleander. Ricinus *communis*. Castor Oil Plant. Sambucus *ebulus*. Elder. Sedum *acre*. Stone Crop. Stalagmitis *cambogioides*. Gamboge. Tanacetum *vulgare*. Tansy (oil of.) ACRO-NARCOTIC. Æthusa *cynapium*. Common Fool's Parsley. Aconitum *napellus*. Monkshood. Agaricus, five species. Mushrooms (poisonous). Amanita *muscaria*. Truffles (poisonous). Anagallis *arvensis*. Meadow Pimpernel. Anda *Gomesii*. Apocynum *androsæmifolium*. Dogsbane. Aristolochia *clematitis*. Birthwort. Arnica *montana*. Leopard's bane. Asclepias *Syriaca*. Swallowwort. Atropa *belladonna*. Deadly Night Shade. Æsculus *Ohioensis*. Buckeye. Brucea *antidysenterica*. False Angustura Bark. Cerbera, three species. Cerbera. Chærophyllum *sylvestre*. Bastard Hemlock.	The general effects of this class of vegetable poisons are; — an acrid pungent taste, with more or less of bitterness, excessive heat, great dryness of the mouth and throat, with sense of tightness there; violent vomiting, the efforts being continued even after the stomach is emptied; purging, with great pain in the stomach and bowels; pulse strong, frequent, and regular; breathing often quick and difficult; appearances of intoxication; the pupil of the eye frequently dilated, insensibility resembling death; the pulse becomes slow and loses its force, and death closes the scene. If applied externally, many of them produce violent inflammation of the skin, with vesications or eruptions of pustules.	If vomiting have been occasioned by the poison, and the efforts are still continued, they may be rendered easier by large draughts of warm water, or thin gruel; but if symptoms of insensibility have come on without vomiting, it ought to be immediately excited by the sulphate of zinc, or some other active emetic substance, and after its operation a sharp purgative should be given. After as much as possible of the poison is got rid of, a very strong infusion of coffee, or vinegar diluted with water, may be given with advantage. Camphor mixture with ether may be taken frequently, and if insensibility be considerable, warmth, frictions, and blisters, may be employed. If inflammation or other dangerous consequences have been induced, they are to be treated upon general principles. The fruit of Feuillea Cordifolia has been recommended as a powerful antidote against vegetable poisons; it is to be used in as recent a state as possible. (?) N. B. Bromine, chlorine, and iodine are said to be antidotes to the alkaloids generally.

IRRITANT POISONS.	SYMPTOMS.	TREATMENT.
Charlotia toxicana. Ratbane. Chenopodium murale. Wormseed. Cicuta maculata. American Hemlock. Cicuta virosa. Water Hemlock. Cissus. Cissus. Cocculus Indicus. Fish berries. Colchicum autumnale. Meadow saffron. Conium maculatum. Hemlock. Coriaria myrtifolia. Myrtle-leaved Sumach. Curare. Indian War Poison. Cynanchum erectum. Cynanchum. Cytisus laburnum. Laburnum. Datura stramonium. Thorn Apple. Digitalis purpurea. Foxglove. Ergot. See Secale. Ervum ervilia. Bitter Vetch. Gaultheria procumbens. Wintergreen (oil of). Hæmanthus toxicarius. Helleborus niger. Black Hellebore. Hypophyllum sanguinaria. Paddock Stool. Ipecacuanha. Ipecacuanha. Lathyrus cicera. Lathyrus. Laurus camphora. Camphor. Lobelia inflata. Indian Tobacco. Lolium temulentum. Darnel. Melia azedarach. Pride of China. Mercurialis perennis. Mountain Mercury. Nerium oleander. Common Oleander. Nicotiana tabacum. Tobacco. Œnanthe crocata. Hemlock Dropwort. Passiflora quadrangularis. Barbadine. Piscidia erythrina. Jamaica Dogwood. Polygala venenosa (of Java). Rhus radicans. Poison Vine. Rhus toxicodendron. Poison oak, or Sumach. Robinia pseudo-acacia. Locust Tree. Ruta graveolens. Rue. Sanguinaria Canadensis. Blood Root. Scilla maritima. Squill. Sea Onion. Secale cornutum. Ergot. Spurred Rye. Sium latifolium. Procumbent Water Parsnep. Spigelia Marilandica. Pink Root. Strychnos Ignatii. St. Ignatius's Bean. Strychnos nux vomica. Nux vomica. Symplocarpus fœtida. Skunk Cabbage. Ticunas. Extract of various plants — South America. Tieuté. Upas Tieuté. Tree of Java. Triticum Hybernum. Wheat (diseased.) Upas antiar. Tree in Java. Veratrum album. White Hellebore. Veratrum viride. American Hellebore. Woorara. War Poison of Guiana. Zea mays. Maize (diseased). NARCOTIC. Actæa spicata. Baneberry. Amygdalus communis. Bitter Almond. Amygdalus Persica. Peach. Gelseminum nitidum. Yellow Jessamine. Helonias erythrosperma. Fly Poison. Hyoscyamus albus. White Henbane. Hyoscyamus niger. Black Henbane. Kalmia latifolia. Mountain Ivy. Lactuca virosa. Strong scented Lettuce. Opium, and its proximate principles. Papaver somniferum. Poppy. Paris quadrifolia. Herb Paris. Prunus Caroliniana. Wild Orange. Prunus lauro-cerasus. Cherry Laurel. Prunus nigra. Black Cherry. Prunus padus. Cluster Cherry. Prunus Virginiana. Wild Cherry. Solanum dulcamara. Bitter-sweet. Sorbus acuparia. Mountain Ash. Taxus baccata. Yew.	The narcotic vegetable poisons, if taken into the stomach or applied to a wound, occasion the following effects:— stupor; numbness; heaviness in the head; desire to vomit, slight at first, but afterwards insupportable; a sort of intoxication, stupid air, pupil of the eye dilated; furious or lively delirium, sometimes pain; convulsions of different parts of the body, or palsy of the limbs. The pulse is variable, but at first generally strong and full; the breathing is quick, and there is great anxiety and dejection, which, if not speedily relieved, soon ends in death.	The stomach to be effectually evacuated, by giving four or five grains of tartar emetic, or from ten to twenty of the sulphate of zinc, repeated every quarter of an hour, till the full effect is produced. These means may be assisted by tickling the throat with a feather or the finger. Large and strong glysters of soap dissolved in water, or of salt and gruel, should be speedily administered, to clear the bowels, and assist in getting rid of the poison; and active purgatives may be given after the vomiting has ceased. When as much as possible of the poison has been expelled, the patient may drink, alternately, a tea-cupful of strong hot infusion of coffee, and vinegar diluted with water. If the drowsiness, which is sometimes extreme, and the insensibility bordering on apoplexy, be not remedied by these means, blood may be taken from the jugular vein, blisters may be applied to the neck and legs, and the attention be roused by every means possible. If the heat declines, warmth and frictions must be perseveringly used. Vegetable acids are on no account to be given *before* the poison is expelled, and it is desirable that but little fluid of any kind should be administered. N. B. Bromine, chlorine, and iodine are said to be antidotes to the alkaloids generally.
POISONOUS MUSHROOMS. Agaricus muscarius. Fly Agaric. Agaricus piperatus. Pepper Agaric. Agaricus necator. Deadly Agaric. Agaricus bulbosus. Bulbous Agaric. Agaricus chantarellus. Champignon.	Nausea, heat, and pain in the stomach and bowels, with vomiting and purging; thirst; convulsions, and faintings; pulse small and frequent; delirium; dilated	The stomach and bowels to be cleared by an emetic of tartarized antimony, followed by frequent doses of Glauber's or Epsom salt, and large, stimulating glysters. After the poison is evacuated, ether may be administered, with small

POISONS.	SYMPTOMS.	TREATMENT.
	pupil, and stupor; cold sweats, and death. Poisonous mushrooms may be distinguished from the edible by their botanical characters, and by the following criteria. The former grow in wet, shady places, have a nauseous odour; are softer, more open, and porous; have a dirty-looking surface, sometimes a gaudy colour, or many very distinct hues, particularly if they have been covered with an envelope; they have soft, bulbous stalks, grow rapidly, and corrupt very quickly.	quantities of brandy and water; but if inflammatory symptoms manifest themselves, such stimuli should be omitted, and other appropriate means be had recourse to.

2. ANIMAL POISONS.

	SYMPTOMS.	TREATMENT.
POISONOUS FISH. Balistes *monoceros*. Old wife. Cancer *astacus*. Crawfish. Cancer *ruricolus*. Land Crab. Clupea *thryssa*. Yellow-billed Sprat. Coracinus *fuscus major*. Gray Snapper. Coracinus *minor*. Hyne. Coryphæna *splendens*. Dolphin. Morinyra. Blue Parrot Fish. Muræna *major*. Conger Eel. Mytilus *edulis*. Mussel. Ostracion *globellum*. Smooth Bottle Fish. Perca *major*. Barracuda. Perca *venenosa*. Grooper. Perca *venenata*. Rock Fish. Physalia. Portuguese Man of War. Scomber *cæruleus*. Spanish Mackerel. Scomber *maximus*. King Fish. Scomber *thynnus*. Bonetta. Sparus *chrysops*. Porgee. Tetrodon *scelleratus*. Tunny. Tetrodon *ocellatus*. Blower.	In an hour or two, or often in a much shorter time, after the fish has been eaten, a weight at the stomach comes on, with slight vertigo and headache, sense of heat about the head and eyes, considerable thirst, and often an eruption of the skin (urticaria), and in many cases death.	An emetic should be speedily administered, or, in the absence of it, vomiting may be excited, by tickling the throat with the finger, and taking large draughts of warm water. After full vomiting, an active purgative should be given, to remove any of the noxious matter that may have found its way into the intestines. Vinegar and water may be drunk after the above remedies have operated, and the body may be sponged with the same. Water, made very sweet with sugar, to which ether may be added, may be drunk freely as a corrective, and a very weak solution of alkali has been recommended to obviate the effects of the poison. If spasm ensue; after evacuations, laudanum, in considerable doses, is necessary. If inflammation should occur, the usual means of removing it must be employed.
POISONOUS SERPENTS. Boa *crotaloides*. Copperhead. Cenchris *mockeson*. Mockeson. Cerastes *nasicornis*. Horned Viper of Western Africa. Coluber *berus*. Viper. Coluber *præster*. Black Viper. Crotalus, (5 species.) Rattle Snake Scytale *piscivorus*. Water Viper.	A sharp pain in the wounded part, which soon extends over the limb or body; great swelling, at first hard and pale, then reddish, livid, and gangrenous in appearance; faintings, vomitings, convulsions, and sometimes jaundice; pulse small, frequent, and irregular; breathing difficult, cold sweats, the sight fails, and the intellectual faculties are deranged. Inflammation, and often, extensive suppuration and gangrene, followed by death.	A cupping-glass to be applied over the wound, or a moderately tight ligature above the bites, and the wound left to bleed after being well washed with warm water; the actual cautery, lunar caustic, or butter of antimony, to be then applied freely to it, and afterwards covered with lint, dipped in equal parts of olive oil and spirit of hartshorn. The ligature to be removed if the inflammation be considerable. Warm, diluting drinks, and small doses of ammonia or hartshorn, to cause perspiration; the patient to be well covered in bed, and a little warm wine given occasionally. If gangrene be threatened, wine may be given more freely, and the bark should be had recourse to. Arsenic, the principal ingredient in the Tanjore Pill, has been strongly recommended.
CANTHARIS VESICATORIA. Spanish, or Blistering Fly. Lytta *vittata*. Potato Fly.	Nauseous odour of the breath; acrid taste; burning heat in the throat, stomach, and abdomen; frequent vomitings, often bloody, with copious bloody stools; excruciating pain in the stomach; painful and obstinate priapism, with heat in the bladder, and strangury or retention of urine; frightful convulsions, delirium and death.	Vomiting to be excited by drinking sweet oil, sugar and water, milk, or linseed tea, very freely. Emollient glysters should be administered, and if symptoms of inflammation of the stomach, kidney, or bladder supervene they must be subdued by appropriate treatment. Camphor dissolved in oil may be rubbed over the belly and the thighs.
VENOMOUS INSECTS. Tarantula. Scorpio. Scorpion. Vespa *crabro*. Hornet. Vespa *vulgaris*. Wasp Apis *mellifica*. Bee. Culex *pipiens*. Gnat. Œstrus *bovis*. Gad-fly	In general, the sting of these insects occasions only a slight degree of pain and swelling; but occasionally the symptoms are more violent, and sickness and fever are produced by the intensity of the pain.	Hartshorn and oil may be rubbed on the affected part, and a piece of rag, moistened in the same, or in salt and water, may be kept upon it till the pain is removed. A few drops of hartshorn may be given frequently in a little water, and a glass or two of wine may be taken. The sting may, in general, be removed by making strong pressure around it with the barrel of a small watch-key.

	SYMPTOMS.	TREATMENT.
SALIVA OF THE RABID DOG.	At an uncertain interval after the bite, generally, however, between the twentieth day and three or four months, pain or uneasiness occurs in the bitten part, though the wound may have been long healed. Anxiety, uneasiness, languor, spasms, horror, disturbed sleep, difficult respiration succeed, and are soon very much increased; violent convulsions affect the whole body, hideously distorting the muscles of the face; the eyes are red and protruded, the tongue swells and often hangs out, and viscid saliva flows from the mouth; there is pain in the stomach, with bilious vomitings, a horror of fluids, and impossibility of drinking them. All these symptoms are aggravated till the sufferer is relieved by death.	Hydrophobia is more easily prevented than cured; indeed, it is doubted whether it ever has been cured. Mercury, arsenic, opium, musk, camphor, acids, wine, vegetable and mineral alkali, oil, various herbs, and many other remedies whose effects are quite opposite, have been employed, but none can be relied on. Large blood-lettings, the warm and cold bath, and almost every other remedial agent, have been tried without success. The bitten part should be completely cut out, even after it has healed, if the symptoms have not yet come on; the part should then be immersed in warm water, or be washed with it as long as it will bleed, and, after the most persevering ablution, caustic should be applied to every part of the surface, and then the wound covered with a poultice, and suffered to heal by granulation. No milder discipline can ensure safety.

The most energetic poisons are used therapeutically, and often with considerable advantage. They have, of course, to be administered in extremely small doses; to avoid producing poisoning.

POISON, ARROW, see Arrow poison—p. Sausage, Allantotoxicum.

POISON-BERRY TREE, Melia azedarach—p. Italian, Liquor arsenicalis — p. Morbid, Virus—p. Oak, Rhus toxicodendron—p. Root, Cicuta maculata — p. Vegetable, Upas — p. Vine, Rhus radicans.

POISONING, *Venefic"ium, Toxica'tio, Intoxica'tio, Entoxis'mus, Entoxicis'mus, Pharmacei'a, Malefic"ium, Venena'tion,* (F.) *Empoisonnement, Intoxication.* The art of applying a poisonous substance to any of the textures in a dose capable of occasioning more or less serious symptoms. Rigorously speaking, therefore, if a physician, in treating any case, employs a deleterious medicine in a small dose, which, owing to particular circumstances, produces unpleasant symptoms, he may be said to have poisoned. The term is, however, generally restricted to poisoning by design.

Poisoning has also been used, by a few, to denote the series of symptoms resembling those produced by certain poisons, which occasionally follow the use of substances that are generally innoxious. Overloading the stomach with indigestible food, has, for example, given occasion to symptoms resembling those produced by a narcotic poison, and the effect has been termed *poisoning*.

Secret poisoning was, at one time, practised as an art. It consisted in administering medicines, which should act as *slow poisons*, and gradually undermine the strength and life. Its agency was far from being so extensive as was imagined.

POI'SONOUS, *Tox'ical, Nox'ius;* having the qualities of a poison.

POISONS, ACRO-NARCOTIC, P. narcotico-acrid—p. Corrosive, P. acrid—p. Escharotic, P. acrid — p. Irritating, P. acrid—p. Putrescent, P. septic.

POITRINAIRR, Phthisicus.

POITRINE, Thorax.

POIVRE D'EAU, Polygonum hydropiper—p. *de Guinée,* Capsicum annuum—p. *d'Inde,* Capsicum annuum—p. *de Jamaique,* see Myrtus pimenta—p. *Long,* Piper longum—p. *Noir,* Piper nigrum—p. *Petit,* Vitex — p. *à Queue,* Piper cubeba—p. *Sauvage,* Vitex.

POIX BLANCHE, see Pinus abies — p. *de Bourgogne,* see Pinus abies—p. *Grasse,* see Pinus abies — p. *Jaune,* see Pinus abies — p. *Minérale,* Pissasphaltum — p. *Navale,* see Pinus sylvestris —p. *Noire,* see Pinus sylvestris.

POKE, Phytolacca decandra — p. Indian, Veratrum viride—p. Stink, Dracontium foetidum—p. Weed, Phytolacca decandra, Veratrum viride.

POLANIS'IA GRA'VEOLENS, *Clammyweed, Stinkweed, Wormweed, Clammy Mustard, False mustard.* An indigenous plant, *Nat. Ord.* Capparideæ; *Sex. Syst.* Dodecandria Monogynia—which blossoms in summer, and is found in every part of North America. To the whole plant have been ascribed anthelmintic properties.

POLECAT WEED, Dracontium foetidum.

POLEMO'NIUM REPTANS, *False Jacob's Ladder, Greek Vale'rian, Sweat-root.* Order, Polemoniaceæ; indigenous, flowering in May; has been used as a diaphoretic and expectorant.

POLENTA, Alphiton.

POLES, Chalazæ.

POLEY MOUNTAIN, OF CANDY, Teucrium Creticum—p. Mountain of Montpelier, Teucrium capitatum.

POLIATER, from πολις, 'a town,' and ιατρος, 'a physician.' A physician exercising his profession in a town, by the appointment of the government. —Castelli.

POLICE', MED'ICAL, *Politi'a med'ica, Politobiotherapi'a, Medici'na polit'ica, State med'icine, Polit'ical med'icine.* Hygienic rules established, or to be established, for the prevention of disease, and to contribute to the progress of medicine. The salubrity of districts, especially during the existence of spreading disease, is greatly ensured by an efficient medical police.

POLICLIN'ICA, from πολις, 'a town,' and κλινη, 'a bed.' Treatment of diseases in a town.

POLIO'SIS, *Tricho'sis polio'sis, Spilo'sis polio'sis, Canit"ies.* Hair prematurely gray or hoary. The state of becoming gray.

POLITIA MEDICA, Police, medical.

POLITOBIOTHERAPIA, Police, medical.

POLIUM CAPITATUM, Teucrium capitatum.

POLIUM CRETICUM, Teucrium Creticum—p. Montanum, Teucrium capitatum.

POLLEN, (L.) *Pollen, Pollis*, παλη, 'dust.' The fecundating dust contained in the anthers of flowers, which is dispersed on the stigma.

POLLEX, *An'ticheir, Prom'anus, Dig''itus primus seu magnus*, from *pollere*, 'to have much strength.' (F.) *Pouce*. The first of the fingers in size and strength. It is asserted that the term *poltroon* is derived from *Pol'licē truncā'to*;—the Romans who were desirous of being exempted from military service being accustomed to cut off the thumb, and thus render themselves unfit to handle arms.

POLLEX, see Digitus.
POLLEX PEDIS, *Hallus, Hallux*. The great toe.
POLLINC'TOR, *Pollinc'ter*, (L.) In antiquity, an anointer, dresser, or embalmer of the dead.
POLLINCTURA, Embalming.
POLLIS, Pollen.
POLLOD'IC, *Pollod'icus*; from πολυς, 'many,' and 'οδος, 'a way.' An epithet proposed by Dr. Marshall Hall for a course of nervous action proceeding from one point in many directions to every other.
POLLOM, LITTLE, Polygala paucifolia.
POLLU'TION, *Pollu'tio*, from *polluo*, 'I profane.' The excretion of the seminal liquor or sperm at other times than during coition. When occasioned by a voluntary act, it is called simply *Pollution* or *Masturbation*; when excited during sleep, by lascivious dreams, it takes the name *Nocturnal pollution, Exoneiro'sis, Oneirog'mos, Oneirog'onos, Oneirogonorrhœ'a, Exoneirog'mus, Spermatoelem'ma, Spermatoclep'sis, Spermatolep'-sis, Spermatolip'sis, Gonorrhœa dormien'tium, G. oneirog'onos*, G. *vera, G. libidino'sa, Proflu'vium sem'inis, Spermatorrhœ'a, Paronir'ia salax, Night pollution*, (F.) *Pollution involontaire*.

POLLUTION INVOLONTAIRE, Pollution—p. Nocturnal, Pollution—p. Self, Masturbation—p. Voluntary, Masturbation.

POLY, *Polys*, πολυς, 'many, full.' Hence—
POLYACTIUM TRISTE, Pelargonium triste.
POLYÆMIA, Plethora.
POLYÆMIC, Plethoric.
POLYÆMICUS, Plethoric.
POLYANHÆMIA, Anæmia.
POLYANHÉMIE, Anæmia.
POLYANTH'ES TUBERO'SA, *Amarucachu*. The root is cut into slips and laid upon the bites of serpents by the Peruvian Indians.
POLYBLEN'NIA, from πολυς, 'much,' and βλεννα, 'mucus.' Excessive secretion of mucus.
POLYBREPHIA, Pregnancy, complex.
POLYCARP'Æ, from πολυς, 'many,' and καρπος, 'fruit.' A division of cutaneous diseases of the family Eczematosen, of Fuchs, including Psoriasis, Lichen, Herpes, and Impetigo.
POLY'CERAS, from πολυς, 'many,' and κερας, 'horn.' A monstrous animal having many horns.—Gurlt.
POLYCHO'LIA, *Pericho'lia, Hypercho'lia*, from πολυς, 'much,' and χολη, 'bile.' Superabundance of bile; such as is supposed to exist in bilious fevers.
POLYCHREST'US, from πολυς, 'much,' and χρηστος, 'useful.' Having many virtues. An ancient name for certain medicines considered to be useful in many diseases.
POLYCHRONIUS, Chronic.
POLYCHY'LIA, from πολυς, 'much,' and χυλος, 'juice.' *Polychy'mia*. Fulness of juices.
POLYCHYMIA, Polychylia— p. Sanguinea, Plethora.
POLYCLIN'ICA, from πολυς, 'much,' and κλινη, 'bed.' Provided with many beds;—as an hospital.

POLYCOR'IA, from πολυς, and κορη, 'the pupil.' The state in which there is more than one pupil.—Von Ammon.

POLYCYE'SIA, *Polycye'sis*, from πολυς, 'many,' and κυησις, 'pregnancy.' Frequent or quickly recurring pregnancies: also, compound pregnancy.

POLYDAC'TYLUS, *Perissodac'tylus*, from πολυς, 'many,' and δακτυλος, 'a finger.' One who has a supernumerary finger or fingers, or toes.

POLYDIP'SIA, from πολυς, 'much,' and διψα, 'thirst;' *Sitis morbo'sa seu inten'sa, Polypo'sia, Dipso'sis avens, Excessive thirst*, (F.) *Soif excessive*. A constant desire for drinking, with a sense of dryness in the mouth and throat. It is mostly symptomatic of fever, inflammation, dropsy, excessive discharges, &c., and is so much a part of diabetes, that it has been called Polydipsia.

POLYG'ALA, from πολυς, 'much,' and γαλα, 'milk;' *P. vulga'ris, Common Milkwort. Family*, Rhinanthoideæ. *Sex. Syst.* Diadelphia Octandria. The leaves are bitter, and are used in the same cases as the polygala amara.

POLYGALA AMA'RA, *P. amarel'la* seu *vulga'ris, Bitter Milkwort*. A powerful bitter; and, consequently, tonic. Its reputed virtues are balsamic, demulcent, and corroborant. The *Polygala rubel'la*, or *Bitter Polygala* of the United States, has the same virtues.

POLYGALA AMARELLA, P. amara — p. Bitter, see P. amara—p. Grandiflora, P. senega.

POLYG'ALA PAUCIFO'LIA, *Triclisper'ma grandiflo'ra, Dwarf Milkwort, Little Pollom, Evergreen Snakeroot*, (F.) *Polygale naine*, possesses the same properties as P. Senega.

POLYG'ALA SEN'EGA, *P. Virginia'na* seu *grandiflo'ra, Sen'eka, Rattlesnake Milkwort, Seneca* or *Rattlesnake root*, (F.) *Polygale de Virginie* ou *de Seneka*. The bark is the active part of the root. Its taste is at first acrid, and afterwards very hot and pungent. It was once esteemed to be specific against the poison of the rattlesnake and in pleurisy, pneumonia, &c., after the inflammatory action had been got under. It has been given also in humoral asthma, chronic rheumatism, dropsy, croup, amenorrhœa, &c. According to Peschier, it contains three particular principles, *Polyg'aline* or *Sen'egine, Isol'usine*, and *Polyg'alic Acid*. Dose, gr. 30 to 40 of the powder.

POLYGALA SERPENTA'RIA. A shrub of Caffraria, the root of which is considered by the natives as a sure antidote against the bites of venomous serpents.

POLYGALA VIRGINIANA, P. senega—p. Vulgaris, P. amara.

POLYGALAC'TIA, *Polyga'lia*, from πολυς, 'much,' and γαλα, 'milk.' Superabundant secretion of milk; galactia.

POLYGALE NAINE, Polygala paucifolia—*p. de Virginie*, Polygala Virginiana.

POLYGALIA, Polygalactia.
POLYGALINE, see Polygala senega.
POLYGONATUM, Convallaria polygonatum—p. Anceps, Convallaria polygonatum—p. Multiflorum, Convallaria multiflora — p. Uniflorum, Convallaria polygonatum—p. Vulgare, Convallaria polygonatum.

POLYG'ONUM, *P. avicula'rē*, from πολυς, 'much,' and γονυ, 'seed.' *P. centino'dium* seu *erec'tum, Centino'dia, Centumno'dia, Biadewed, Sanguina'lis Corrig'iola, Sanguina'ria, Knotgrass, Knotweed*, (F.) *Renouée, Trainasse, Centinode*. *Family*, Polygoneæ. *Sex. Syst.* Octandria Trigynia. This grass is said to be a feeble astringent.

POLYGONUM ACRE, P. hydropiper.

POLYGONUM BISTOR'TA, *P. bistortoï'des, Bistorta, Colubrina, Offic''inal Bistort, Great Bistort* or *Snakeweed.* The root is a powerful astringent and tonic; and, as such, has been used in internal hemorrhage, atonic diarrhœa, ague, &c. Dose, gr. xv to ʒj.

POLYGONUM BISTORTOIDES, P. bistorta—p. Centinodium, P. aviculare.

POLYGONUM DIVARICA'TUM; *Eastern Buckwheat plant.* The roots, reduced to a coarse meal, are said to be much used as an article of diet by the Siberians.

POLYGONUM ERECTUM, P. aviculare.

POLYGONUM FAGOP'YRUM, *Fagop'yrum, F. esculen'um, Trit'icum Fagi'num, Buckwheat,* (F.) *Sarrasin, Blé noir.* The grain of this plant constitutes a principal article of food with the inhabitants of Russia, Germany, and Switzerland. It is much used in the United States.

POLYGONUM HYDROP'IPER, *P. acrē, Hydropiper, Persica'ria urens, Mercu'rius terres'tris, Poor Man's Pepper, Biting Arse-smart, Lakeweed, Water-pepper,* (F.) *Poivre d'eau.* The leaves of this plant have an acrid, burning taste, and resemble those of the arum. They have been recommended as possessing antiseptic, aperient, and diuretic virtues. The fresh leaves have been applied externally as a stimulating cataplasm.

POLYGONUM HYDROPIPEROIDES, P. punctatum.

POLYGONUM PERSICA'RIA, *Persicaria, P. minor seu mitis, Plumba'go, Arse-smart,* (F.) *Persicaire douce.* This plant is said to possess vulnerary and antiseptic qualities. It has been given in wine to arrest gangrene.

POLYGONUM PUNCTA'TUM, *P. hydropiperoï'des, Water pepper* of America, *Smartweed,* possesses similar properties to Polygonum hydropiper, and is occasionally used internally in gravel, and externally in chronic ulcers. A fluidrachm of the saturated tincture has been extolled in amenorrhœa.

POLYG'ONUM VIRGINIA'NUM, *Wand-spiked Persica'ria Virgin'ia Bistort;* indigenous; is astringent, diuretic, and tonic.

POLYGROMA Staphyloma.

POLYHI'DRIA, *Polyï'dria, Polyīdro'sis,* from πολυς, 'much,' and 'ιδρως, 'sweat.' Excessive sweating.

POLYHYDRIA, Hydrops.

POLYHYPERHÆMIA, Plethora.

POLYIDRIA, Polyhidria.

POLYIDROSIS, Polyhidria.

POLYLYMPHIA, Anasarca.

POLYMASTH'US, *Pleiomas'thus,* from πολυς, 'many,' and μασθος, 'breast.' A monster having several breasts.—Gurlt. The condition has been called *Polyma'sia,* and *Pleioma'sia.*

POLYMAZIA, see Polymasthus.

POLYMERIA, Polymerismus—p. Promiscua translativa, Transposition of the viscera.

POLYMERIS'MUS, *Polymer'ia,* from πολυς, 'much,' and μερος, 'a part.' A monstrosity, which consists in the existence of supernumerary organs; as a sixth finger of the hand.

POLYNEURON, Plantago.

POLYOP'SIA, *Pol'yopy,* from πολυς, 'much,' and οψις, 'sight.' Vision is so called, when multiple.

POLYOPY, Polyopsia.

POLYOREX'IA, from πολυς, 'much,' and ορεξις, 'appetite.' Excessive appetite or hunger. A genus in the gastroses of M. Alibert.

POLYPE'RIA, from πολυς, 'much,' and πηρος, 'mutilated.' Congenital misconstruction of various parts or organs.—Good.

POLYPHA'GIA, *Multivoran'tia,* from πολυς, 'much,' and φαγω, 'I eat.' Voracity. Faculty of eating or subsisting on many kinds of food. See Boulimia.

POLYPH'AGOUS. Relating or appertaining to polyphagia.

POLYPHARMACI'A, *Polypharm'acy;* from πολυς, 'much,' and φαρμακον, 'a medicine.' The prescribing of too many medicines. A prescription, consisting of a number of medicines; hence the name *Polyphar'macus,* given to one who is in the habit of prescribing a number of medicines, and whose prescriptions are loaded with ingredients. The term is taken in bad part.

POLYPHYSIA, Flatulence.

POLYPIFORM CONCRETIONS, see Polypus.

POLYPIONIA, see Polysarcia — p. Infantum, see Polysarcia.

POLYPLAS'TIC, *Polyplas'ticus,* from πολυς, 'much,' and πλασσω, 'I form.' That which has many shapes.

POLYPLASTIC ELEMENT, in histology, is one which does not retain its primary shape; but undergoes transformation into others.—Gerber.

POLYPODITES. Wine impregnated with polypody.

POLYPO'DIUM, *P. Vulga'rē, P. Virginia'num seu pinnatif'idum, Filic'ula dulcis, Common Pol'ypody, Fern root, Rock Brake, Brake root.* This fern grows in the clefts of rocks, walls, &c., in both hemispheres. It was formerly regarded as a cholagogue, and was given in head diseases. It is not used now.

POLYPODIUM ADIANTIFORME, see Calaguala radix — p. Ammifolium, see Calagualæ radix — p. Argenteum, see Calagualæ radix — p. Calaguala, Calagualæ radix — p. Coriaceum, see Calagualæ radix — p. Dentatum, Asplenium filix fœmina—p. Filix fœmina, Asplenium filix fœmina.

POLYPO'DIUM FILIX MAS, *Aspid'ium Filix Mas, A. depas'tum seu ero'sum, Filix pinua'ta, Pteris, Athyr'ium Filix Mas, Blechnon, Pulyrrhï'zon, Blanenon Oriba'sii, Lonchi'tis, Filic'ula, Male Polypody* or *Fern, Filix mas, F. non ramo'sa denta'ta, Nephro'dium crena'tum, N. Filix mas, Polys'ticum callip'teris, P. filix mas,* (F.) *Fougère mâle. Nat. Ord.* Filices. *Sex. Syst.* Cryptogamia Filices. The rhisoma of this plant has been much extolled as an anthelmintic, and in cases of tænia. It was the basis of a once celebrated remedy—*Madame Nouffer's,* but, perhaps, more of the efficacy was to be attributed to the active purgatives by which it was followed than to the fern. Dose, ʒij to ʒiij of the powdered solid part of the root; followed in the morning by a strong cathartic of camboge or jalap. An ethereal extract has been proposed by Dr. Peschier, of Geneva.

POLYPO'DIUM INCA'NUM, *Pol'ypody, Rock Brake;* indigenous; has been considered demulcent, cathartic and anthelmintic.

POLYPO'DIUM INCISUM, Asplenium filix fœmina —p. Molle, Asplenium filix fœmina—p. Pennatifidum, P. vulgare — p. Politum, see Calagualæ radix — p. Trifidum, Asplenium filix fœmina—p. Virginianum, P. vulgare — p. Vulgare, Polypodium.

POLYPODY, Polypodium incanum—p. Common, Polypodium vulgare—p. Male, Polypodium filix mas.

POL'YPOID, *Polypoï'des;* from polypus, and ειδος, 'form.' Having the shape of, or resembling, a polypus.

POLYPORUS IGNIARIUS, Boletus igniarius —p. Officinalis, Boletus laricis.

POLYPOSIA, πολυποσια, from πολυς, 'much,' and ποσις, 'drink.' Great thirst—desire for drink. Polydipsia.

POLYPOUS, *Polypo'sus:* same etymon as the next. Relating, or belonging to, or resembling polypus.

POL'YPUS, *Pseudometamorpho'sis polypo'sa*, from πολυς, 'many,' and πους, 'a foot.' A name given to tumours, which occur in mucous membranes especially; and which have been compared to certain zoophytes. Polypi may form on every mucous membrane. They are most commonly observed in the nasal fossæ, pharynx, and uterus; more rarely in the stomach, intestines, bronchial tubes, bladder, and meatus auditorius externus. They vary much in size, number, mode of adhesion, and intimate nature. Accordingly, they have received various appellations; *mucous, soft, vesic'ular,* when their substance has been soft, spongy, vesicular, and, as it were, gorged with fluid. Others have been called *hard;* and these have been distinguished into *fibrous* or *fleshy,* and into *scirrhous* or *cancerous*. Fibrous polypi, *Pol'ypi fibro'si, Inopol'ypi,* are of a dense, compact texture, and whitish colour. They contain few vessels, and do not degenerate into cancer. The *scirrhous* or *carcinom'atous* are true cancerous tumours, painful and bleeding. They present all the pathological changes which belong to cancerous affections, and the prognosis is of course unfavourable.

The mode of treating polypi must differ according to their character. The means used to destroy them have been, 1. To subject them to the action of certain astringent powders or solutions, to obtain their resolution. 2. *Cauterisation* or the application of the actual cautery or caustics. 3. *Excision* or ablation with a cutting instrument. 4. *Extirpation* with the fingers or with the polypus forceps. 5. A *ligature,* put round them so as to prevent their nutrition. A seton has, also, been sometimes used to gradually destroy the pedicle.

The term POLYPI, *Pseudopol'ypi, Cardi'tis polypo'sa, Pol'ypiform Concre'tions,* (F.) *Concrétions polypeuses* ou *polypiformes* ou *sanguines du Cœur, Hémocardioplasties,* (Piorry,) has likewise been applied to collections of blood—fibrinous concretions—found in the heart or great vessels after dissolution. These were once, erroneously, regarded as morbid. The presence of these concretions may be suspected, when in the course of an acute or chronic affection of the heart, or at the close of chronic diseases in general—especially those of the lungs—the heart's action becomes suddenly tumultuous, obscure, and accompanied with a soft bellows' murmur, whilst the general symptoms indicate the effects of obstructed circulation. The right cavities are most frequently affected.

POL'YPUS BRONCHIA'LIS, *Bronchlemmi'tis, Bronchi'tis membrana'cea, B. plastic, Bronchial Croup, Chronic Croup* (?) *Pseudo-mem' branous Bronchitis.* A membraniform secretion in the bronchial tubes of a diphtheritic character, having the shape, when unexpectorated, of the bronchia. It is the result of inflammation of the lining membrane of those tubes.

POLYPUS CARNOSUS, Sarcoma—p. Fibrosus, see Polypus—p. Uteri, Metropolypus.

POLYRRHIZON, Polypodium filix mas.

POLYRRHŒA, Profluvium.

POLYSAR'CIA, *Polysarco'sis*, from πολυς, 'much,' and σαρξ, 'flesh.' *Carnos'itas, Polysoma'tia, Adelipa'ria, Corpulen'tia, Steati'tes.* Excessive corpulency. Authors have distinguished two varieties of this:— POLYSARCIA CARNO'SA, *Cor'pulency,* and P. ADIPO'SA, *Polypio'nia, Pimelo'sis nim'ia, Pachys'mus, Pachyn'sis, Obes'itas, Hyperpım'elē, Lipa'ria, Adipo'sis, Polysar'cia faginc'sa, Empyme'lium pinguar'cia, Baryso'mia, Barysomat'ica, Lıpo'sis, Lipar'otcs, Lipas'ma, Pinguitu'do, Pin'guitude, Obes'ity,* (F.) *Obésité, Embonpoint excessif.* A severe regimen and exercise are the best preventives. Children are occasionally met with of unusual fatness, in spite of every care. This morbid deposition has been termed *Polypio'nia infantum,* and *Chloro'sis gigante'a*.

POLYSARCIA VISCERUM, Physconia adiposa.
POLYSARCOSIS, Polysarcia.
POLYSIA'LIA; from πολυς, 'much,' and σιαλον, 'saliva.' Excessive discharge of saliva.
POLYSOMATIA, Polysarcia.
POLYSPAS'TON, from πολυς, 'much,' and σπαω, 'I draw.' A powerful instrument for reducing luxations.—Gorræus.
POLYSPER'MIA; from πολυς, 'much,' and σπερμα, 'sperm.' Richness or fulness of sperm.
POLYSTICUM CALLIPTERIS, Polypodium filix mas—p. Filix Mas, Polypodium filix mas.
POLYSTOMA PINGUICOLA, see Worms— —p. Venarum, see Worms.
POLYTRIC, Asplenium trichomanoides.
POLYT'RICHUM, from πολυς, 'much,' and θριξ, 'hair.' *Polyt'ricon, Polyt'richum vulga'ré, Adian'tum au'reum, Golden Maiden-hair,* (F.) *Perce-mousse.* It is possessed of astringent properties, and was formerly given in diseases of the lungs, and in calculous affections.
POLYTRICHUM COMMUNE, Asplenium trichomanoides.
POLYTROPH'IA, from πολυς, 'much,' and τρεφω, 'I nourish.' Abundant or excessive nutrition.
POLYURESIS, Diabetes.
POLYURIA, Diabetes.
POLYU'RICUS, from πολυς, 'much,' and ουρον, 'urine.' Sauvages calls—*Ischu'ria polyu'rica*—a kind of ischuria, caused by accumulation of urine in the bladder.
POMA, Drink—p. Chinensis, see Citrus aurantium.
POMACEUM, Cider.
POMA'TUM, *Pomma'tum,* (F.) *Pommade, Liparolé.* A pharmaceutical preparation, employed only externally; which differs but little from an ointment, except in having generally less consistence. It is usually made aromatic, and coloured to render it more agreeable.
Common Pomatum is made of *lard,* 12℔s; *suet,* 4℔s; *essence,* ℨviij.
POMATUM AD LABIA DEMULCENDA, Cerate for the lips—p. Epispasticum flavum, Unguentum lyttæ medicatum aliud—p. Epispasticum viride, &c., Unguentum lyttæ medicatum—p. for the Lips, Cerate for the lips—p. Nitricum vel oxygenatum, Unguentum acidi nitrosi—p. Satarai, Unguentum plumbi superacetatis.
POMBALEA IPECACUANHA, see Ipecacuanha.
POMEGRANATE, Punica granatum.
POMILIUS, see Nanus.
POMMADE, Pomatum—*p. d'Alyon,* Unguentum acidi nitrosi—*p, Antipsorique de Jasser,* Unguentum sulphuris compositum—*p. d'Autenrieth,* Unguentum antimonii tartarizati—*p. de Cyrille,* Unguentum muriatis hydrargyri oxygenato medicatus—*p. Épispastique jaune,* Unguentum lyttæ medicatum aliud—*p. Épispastique vert,* Unguentum lyttæ medicatum—*p. de Garou,* Unguentum epispasticum de daphne gnidio.
POMMADE DE GONDRET, P. ammoniacale de Gondret (F.), *Gondret's Counterirritant, Gondret's ammoniacal Caustic. Liq. ammon. p. ij; Sevi,* p. j; *Ol. amygdal.* p. j; M. Used to excite a speedy revulsion in cases of chronic affections of the brain, incipient cataract, amaurosis, &c., as well as to cauterise the integuments deeply.
The above formula, is that of the French Codex, but, according to M. Trousseau, it is much too hard for use, unless the weather is warm.

He proposes *two formulæ*, one for summer, the other for winter. In the *former* he directs three parts of *lard*, one of *suet*, and four of *liquor ammoniæ;* in the *latter*, equal parts of *lard* and *liquor ammoniæ*.

POMMADE POUR LES LÈVRES, Cerate for the lips—*p. Ophthalmique* (Regent's,) Unguentum ophthalmicum — *p. Oxygénée*, Unguentum acidi nitrosi — *p. Stibiée*, Unguentum antimonii tartarizati.

POMME, see Pyrus malus — *p. d'Adam*, Pomum *Adami*—*p. d'Amour*, Solanum lycopersicum — *p. Epineuse*, Datura stramonium — *p. de Merveille*, Momordica balsamica — *p. Mousseuse*, Bedegar—*p. de Terre*, Solanum tuberosum.

POMMES HÉMORRHOÏDALES, see Viscum album.

POMMETTE, see Malæ os.

POMMIER, Pyrus malus.

POMPH'OLYX, from πομφος, 'a bladder.' A small vesicle on the skin. An eruption of *bullæ* or *blebs*, appearing without any inflammation around them, and without fever. It is the *Ecphlysis Pompholyx* of Good. See Pemphigus.

POMPHOLYX, Tutia, Zinci oxydum.

POMPION, Cucurbita pepo.

POMUM ADA'MI, (F.) *Pomme d'Adam*, *Adam's Apple*. The projection formed by the thyroid cartilage in the neck—of males particularly. It is so called from a notion that it was caused by the apple sticking in the throat of our first parent.

POMUM AMORIS, Testicle—p. Hierosolymitanum, Momordica balsamina—p. Melongenæ, see Solanum melongena — p. Mirabile, Momordica Balsamina — p. Spinosum, Datura stramonium.

PONCTION, Puncturing.

POND SHOVEL, Unisema deltifolia.

PONDERA ET MENSURÆ, Weights and measures.

PONDUS, Pudibilia—p. Pharmaceuticum, see Weights and Measures.

PONGITIF, Pungent.

PONS CEREBELLI, Pons Varolii — p. Hepatis, see Lobulus anonymus — p. Sylvii, Quadrigemina Tubercula — p. Tarini, Tarini pons.

PONS VARO'LII, *Pons Cerebel'li*, *Corpus annula'rĕ*, *Proces'sus annularis*, *Prominen'tia annula'ris cer'ebri*, *Eminen'tia annularis*, *Varo'li's bridge*, *Nodus enceph'ali* vel *Cer'ebri*, *Cerebral protu'berance*, *Protuberan'tia annula'ris Willisii*, (F.) *Protubérance cérébrale*, *P. annulaire*, *Mésencéphale*, *Mésocéphale*, *Pont de Varole*, *Annular protuberance*. An eminence at the upper part of the medulla oblongata, first described by Varolius. It is formed by the union of the crura cerebri and crura cerebelli.

PONS ZYGOMATICUS, Zygomatic arch.

PONTE, see Parturition — *p. Périodique*, see Parturition.

PONTEDERIA CORDATA, Unisema deltifolia.

PONTICUM ABSINTHIUM, Artemisia Pontica.

POPLAR, AMERICAN, Liriodendron — p. Balm of Gilead, Populus Candicans — p. Black, Populus—p. Tree, Liriodendron — p. Tulip-bearing, Liriodendron.

POPLES, *Gare'tum*, *Garretum*, *Ignys*, *Ig'nyĕ*, *Suffra'go*, *Fossa genu*, *Fossa poplitæ'a*, the *Ham*, the *Hough*, *Hock*, (F.) *Jarret*, from *post*, and *plico*, 'I fold.' The posterior part of the knee joint. The ham forms what is called the *popliteal region* or *space*.

POPLITÆUS, Popliteal muscle.

POPLITÉ, Popliteus muscle.

POPLITEAD, see Popliteal aspect.

POPLITE'AL, *Poplitæ'us*, *Poplit'ic*, from *poples*, 'the ham.' That which relates to the ham. A name given to various parts.

POPLITEAL ARTERY — *Popliteal portion of the crural*, — (Ch.) is really a continuation of the femoral, which changes its name on passing through the adductor magnus muscle. It descends a little obliquely outwards into the hollow of the ham, and extends from the commencement of the lower third of the thigh to the end of the upper quarter of the leg, where it terminates by dividing into the *posterior tibial* and peroneal arteries. In the ham, it gives off the three *superior articular arteries;* and, at the top of the leg, the arteries of the gemini muscles or *gemini branches*, (F.) *branches jumelles*, the *two inferior articular arteries*, and the *tibialis antica*.

POPLITEAL ASPECT. An aspect towards the side on which the *poples* or ham is situated. Barclay. *Poplite'ad* is used by the same writer adverbially, and signifies 'towards the popliteal aspect.'

POPLITEAL FOSSA, Poples.

POPLITE'AL GLANDS, *Glan'dulæ poplitææ*. Lymphatic glands, four in number, seated in the popliteal region or space.

POPLITEAL MUSCLE, *Poplitæus Muscle*, *Muscle Jarretier*, *Fémoro-popliti-tibial*, (Ch.,) *Subpoplitæus*, (F.) *Muscle poplité*, is seated in the popliteal region. It is triangular, long, flat; and is inserted, on the one hand, by means of a strong tendon, into the tuberosity at the outer condyle of the femur, terminating below at the upper part of the posterior surface of the tibia. This muscle bends the leg on the thigh, and, reciprocally, the thigh on the leg. When the leg is bent, it causes it to turn, in rotation, inwards.

POPLITEAL NERVES. They result from the bifurcation of the sciatic, and are two in number, viz. 1. The *external popliteal*, Peroneal nerve, *Branche péronière*, (Ch.) It is smaller than the internal; turns to the outside of the fibula at the upper part of the leg, and divides into the *musculo-cutaneous branch*, *nerf prétibio-digital*, (Ch.) and the *anterior tibial*, *nerf prétibio-susphalangétaire*, (Ch.) 2. The *inter'nal poplite'al nerve*, *Branche tibiale*, (Ch.) which is larger than the other, and seems to be the real continuation of the sciatic nerve. It descends vertically into the hollow of the ham; and passes beneath the aponeurotic arch of the solaris muscle, beyond which it takes the name *tibial nerve*. It furnishes the *external saphena nerve*, and a number of branches, that are distributed to the posterior muscles of the leg. It then passes to the sole of the foot to be divided into two branches, called *Plantar nerves*.

POPLITEAL REGION, Poples—p. Space, Poples.

POPLITEAL VEIN has the same arrangement as the artery behind which it is situate.

POPLITIC, Popliteal.

POPONAX, see Pastinaca opoponax.

POPPY, CELANDINE, Stylophorum diphyllum — p. Corn, red, Papaver rhœas — p. Heads, see Papaver—p. Horn, Stylophorum diphyllum—p. Juice, Meconium—p. Prickly, Argemone Mexicana—p. Spotling, Cucurbalus Behen—p. Thorn, Argemone Mexicana — p. White, Papaver — p. White, capsule, see Papaver.

POP'ULUS, *Populus nigra*, *Ægei'ros*, *Achero'is*, *Black poplar*, (F.) *Peuplier noir*. The young *buds*, *oculi* or rudiments of the leaves, which appear in the beginning of spring, were formerly used in an officinal ointment — the *unguen'tum popule'um*. It was, also, recommended in chronic affections of the lungs.

The bark of *Pop'ulus Tremuloï'des*, *American aspen*, of P. TREM'ULA seu pen'dula, *European aspen*, and of POPULUS CAN'DICANS, *Balm of Gilead*

Poplar, is antiperiodic, and furnishes *salicin* and *populin*, in which the properties probably reside.

POPULUS BALSAMIFERA, see Fagara octandra—p. Candicans, see Populus—p. Pendula, P. tremula —p. Tacamahaca, see Fagara octandra— p. Tremula, see Populus—p. Tremuloides, see Populus.

PORCELAINE, Essera, Urticaria.

PORCELLIO, Oniscus.

PORCELLUS, Oniscus.

PORCULUS, Oniscus.

PORCUPINE DISEASE, Ichthyosis.

PORCUPINE MEN, *Echinoder'mi*. Persons have been so called in whom the cuticle is produced in the form of pointed prolongations, as if it had been moulded on the papillæ, like the shorter and blunter quills of the porcupine.

PORCUS, Vulva.

PORDE, Crepitation.

PORE, *Porus*, *In'terstice*, πορος, 'a passage.' Anatomists have given this name to the openings at the extremities of vessels at the surface of different membranes. EXHALANT PORES have been supposed to exist in the exhalants, to transmit the fluids exhaled. — ABSORBENT PORES are employed in taking up parts that have to enter the circulation. Pores exist in the cuticle; yet Humboldt, with a powerful magnifying-glass, was unable to observe them. The pores of the skin have also been called *spira'cula*.

POREBLIND, Myopie.

PORI BILIA'RII, *Ductus bilia'rii*, *Sur'culi fell'ei*. Ducts which receive the bile from the penicilli of the liver, and convey it to the hepatic duct.

PORI CUTA'NEI, P. *Exhalan'tes* seu *Sudorif'eri* seu *Resorben'tes*. The pores of the skin.

PORI EXHALANTES, P. cutanei—p. Pulmonum, Cellules, bronchic—p. Resorbentes, P. cutanei— p. Sudoriferi, P. cutanei.

POROCE'LE, from πυρος, callus,' and κηλη, 'a tumour.' A hard tumour of the testicle or its envelopes.

POROMA, Induration.

POROMPHALOCELE, Poromphalon.

POROM'PHALON, *Poromph'alus*, *Poromphaloce'lē*, from πυρος, 'hard,' and ομφαλος, 'the navel.' Umbilical hernia with hard and thickened parietes.

POROS, Canal.

POROSIS, Chalaza, Induration.

POROT'IC, *Porot'icus*, from πυρος, 'callus.' A remedy believed to be capable of assisting the formation of callus.

PORPHYRA, Purpura— p. Græcorum, Petechiæ— p. Hæmorrhagica, Purpura hæmorrhagica.

PORPHYRISMA, Scarlatina.

PORPHYRISMUS, Scarlatina.

PORPHYRIZATION, Levigation.

PORPHYRO-TYPHUS, see Typhus.

PORPHYRU'RIA, *Porphyu'ria*; from πορφυρα, 'purple,' and ουρον, 'urine.' A state of the urine — *pur'puric urine* — in which it deposits the remarkable colouring matter— *pur'purine*—in association with urate of ammonia.

POR'PHYRY, *Porphyri'tes*, from πορφυρα, 'purple.' A species of very hard, compound rock, susceptible of considerable polish, and used in the fabrication of mortars and slabs for the apothecary.

PORPHYRY, BLACK, Ophites.

PORPHYURIA, Porphyruria.

PORRACÉ, Porraceous.

PORRA'CEOUS, *Porra'ceus*, *Pra'sinus*, from *porrum*, 'a leek.' (F.) *Porracé*. Having the green colour of the leek. An epithet given to certain excreted matters,— the sputa, bile and fæces particularly.

PORREAU, Allium porrum.

PORRECTUM, Lever.

PORRET, Allium porrum.

PORRIGINE, Porrigo favosa.

PORRIGINEUX, Porriginous.

PORRIGINOSUS, Porriginous.

PORRIG"INOUS, *Porrigino'sus*, (F.) *Porrigineux*. Appertaining to porrigo.

PORRI'GO (L.), 'scurf or scall in the head.' *Tin'ea*, *Favus*, *Furfura'tio*, *Fur'fures*, *Ecpyē'sis porrigo*, *Phlysis porrigo*, from *porrigere*, 'to spread.' (F.) *Teigne*, *Rache*. Some of the varieties are contagious. It is principally characterised by an eruption of the pustules, called favi and achores, unaccompanied by fever.

PORRIGO DECAL'VANS, *Tricho'sis a'rea*, *Area*, *Alope'cia area'ta*, *A. partia'lis*, *A. circumscrip'ta*, *Phytoalope'cia*, *Tyr'ia*, *Tyro'ma*, *Ophi'asis*, *Tin'ea tondens*, *Herpens tonsu'rans*, *Limited or partial Baldness*, consists of patches of baldness without decay or change of colour in the surrounding hair, the exposed parts of the scalp being glabrous, white, and shining. The morbid condition sometimes spreads, so that the patches coalesce, rendering the baldness extensive. To a vegetable growth found at the roots of the hair in Tinea tondens, Malmstèn of Stockholm has given the name *Trichoph'yton tonsu'rans*. The treatment consists in keeping the scalp cleared by constant shaving, and in the steady application of some stimulating liniment or ointment.

PORRIGO FAVO'SA, *Ce'rion*, *Favus*, *Ecpyē'sis porrigo favosa*, *Tinea favosa*, *Sca'bies cap'itis favosa*, *Melice'ra*, *Melice'rum*, *Melice'ris*, *Mellifa'vium*, *Porrigophyte*, *Honey-comb Scall or Tetter*, (F.) *Teigne faveuse*, *Porrigine*. This consists in an eruption of pustules common to the head, trunk, and extremities, pea-sized, flattened at the top, in clusters, often uniting; discharge, fetid; scabs, honey-combed; the cells filled with fluid. It occurs both in early and adult life. Modern researches have satisfied some observers, that the crusts of favus are of vegetable nature, and formed of a parasitic plant, belonging to the genus *mycoderm'a*, for which Remak has proposed the name *Achorion Schönleini*. The point is not, however, settled. The treatment of this variety must consist in the exhibition of laxatives and the mildest stimulating ointments, such as the *Ung. zinci*, *Ung. hydrargyri præcipitat. alb.*, &c. Eczema of the hairy scalp is often confounded with Porrigo.

PORRIGO FUR'FURANS, *Ecpyē'sis porrigo furfura'cea*, *Tinea furfuracea*, *Tinea porrigino'sa*, *Pityri'asis Tricho'sis furfura'cea*, *Teigne furacée* (Alibert), commences with an eruption of small achores, the fluid of which soon concretes and separates in innumerable, thin, laminated scabs, or scale-like exfoliations. It is attended with a good deal of itching and some soreness of the scalp, to which the disease is confined. It occurs chiefly in adults. In the treatment the scalp must be kept shaved. The part must be washed repeatedly with soap and water, and an oiled silk cap worn. The nature of the ointments used must vary according to the period of disease and the irritability of the part affected. *Lead ointment;*— one made with the *Cocculus indicus*; — the *Sulphur ointment;* — *Citrine ointment* and *Ung. hydrargyri nitrico-oxydi; Tar ointment* and *Nitric acid ointment* have all been found useful. Should inflammation or discharge arise, these applications must of course be intermitted.

PORRIGO LARVALIS, P. lupinosa.

PORRIGO LARVA'LIS, *Crusta lac'tea*, *Ecpyē'sis*

Porrigo crusta'cea, Menti'go, Achor, Tin'ea lac'-tea, T. Fa'ciei, Milky scall or *Tetter, Lactu'men, Lacti'go,* (F.) *Croûte de lait, Croûte laiteuse, Feux volages, La Graine.* This is, almost exclusively, a disease of infancy. It commonly appears first on the forehead and cheeks, in an eruption of numerous, minute, whitish achores on a red surface. These break and discharge a viscid fluid, which becomes incrusted in thin, yellowish, or greenish scabs. The patches spread, until the whole face becomes, as it were, enveloped in a mask; hence the epithet *larvalis*. The disease is rather a variety of Eczema. Sometimes the eruption appears on the neck and breast; and, occasionally, on the extremities. In general, the health of the child does not suffer, but the eruption is always attended with much itching and irritation. The treatment consists in mild, tepid ablution, and the application of gently stimulating ointments, as of the oxydum zinci. The bowels must be kept in a soluble state by small doses of calomel, or by rhubarb and magnesia.

PORRIGO LUPINO'SA, *Tin'ea lupi'na, Scabies cap'itis, Ecpye'sis porrigo lupino'sa, Porri'go larva'lis, Impeti'go figura'ta, Tin'ea granula'ta, T. musco'sa, Crusta lactea* (of some), *Ment'agra infan'tum,* (F.) *Teigne, Dartre crustacée flavescente,* consists of minute pustules in small patches, mostly commencing on the scalp; the patches terminate in dry, delving scabs, resembling lupine seeds; the interstices often covered with a thin, whitish, and exfoliating incrustation. It occurs chiefly in early life, and requires the same treatment as the last.

PORRIGO SCUTULA'TA, *Tin'ea granula'ta, Ecpye'sis porrigo galea'ta, Tinea fico'sa, Acho'res seu Sca'bies cap'itis, Ringworm of the Scalp, Scalled head,* (F.) *Teigne annulaire, T. en anneau, T. nummulaire.* It commences with clusters of small, light, yellow pustules, which soon scab off; and, if neglected, become hard by accumulation. If the scabs be removed, the surface is left red and shining, but studded with slightly elevated points. If not attended to, it involves the whole head. It occurs in children three or four years of age, and is very unmanageable. The rules laid down under *Porrigo furfurans* must be here still more perseveringly enforced. The whole tribe of stimulating ointments may be used in succession. No one will always succeed, and hence the necessity of change, provided advantage should not seem to follow any particular application. The *Unguentum ad Scabiem,* of Banyer, sometimes cures, when others fail.

PORRIGOPHYTE, Porrigo favosa.

PORRUM, Allium porrum, Thymion.

PORRUS, Sarcoma, Thymion.

PORTA, πυλη, *Pylē,* 'a gate.' The part of the liver where its vessels enter as by a gate. Also, the Vulva.

PORTA JECORIS, Porta vena.

PORTA VENA, *Vena portæ, V. porta'rum seu porta'lis, Rama'lis vena, Jan'itrix, Vena magna seu quæ ad portas est seu stelechia'a seu lac'tea seu ostia'ria, Porta Jec'oris, Porta, Vena arterio'sa* seu *arteria'lis, Manus Jec'oris* seu *he'patis, Vena ad portas.* The *System of the vena porta* or the *Abdom'inal venous system,* (F.) *Veine porte, Porte veine,* is a vascular apparatus of black blood, situate in the abdomen, and resulting from two distinct orders of vessels, united into one common trunk. 1. One of these trunks, much more extensive than the other, has received the name *Vena porta abdomina'lis,* because it arises from all the organs enclosed in the cavity of the abdomen, except the kidneys and bladder; and in the female, the uterus. The *Abdominal vena porta* has two principal roots, the *splenic vein* and the *superior mesenteric,* which have their ramifications in all the digestive organs. 2. The other trunk, destined solely to the liver, has been called the *Hepat'ic vena porta*. It appears to be a continuation of the abdominal vena porta, and proceeds towards the inferior surface of the liver. Opposite to the transverse fissure of that organ, it divides, like an artery, into two branches, which, by their union, seem to form a canal or duct, called by some the *Sinus of the vena porta.* These branches are distributed in the substance of the liver, whither they are accompanied by a prolongation of the fibrous capsule of that organ, —the capsule of Glisson. The different branches of the vena porta are devoid of valves. See Liver.

PORTAL, from *porta,* 'a gate.' Relating to the porta of the liver, — as the *portal* system, or system of the vena porta. By extension, the term has been applied to an analogous system of vessels in the kidney. See Kidney.

PORTAL FISSURE, see Liver — p. System of the Kidney, see Kidney — p. Veins of the Kidney, see Kidney.

PORTE-AIGUILLE, *Acutenac'ulum, Needle-carrier, Needle-bearer,* from (F.) *porter,* 'to carry,' and *aiguille,* 'a needle.' An instrument for accurately laying hold of a needle, and giving it greater length, when it is so fine and small that it cannot be held by the fingers. It is of steel or silver, about two inches long, and throughout the whole, almost, of its length, divided into two branches, so as to form a kind of forceps, capable of being closed by means of a sliding ring. A modification of this instrument was devised by Dr. Physick for taking up deep-seated arteries beyond the reach of a tenaculum or common needle. It consists of a forceps so constructed as to hold in its extremity a needle armed with a ligature. The handles of the forceps are fastened together, temporarily, by a spring or catch; and, when the needle is fairly deposited beneath the vessel, it is disengaged from the forceps and drawn out, leaving the ligature behind, which can be tied without difficulty.

PORTE-BOUGIE, (F.) A silver canula similar to that of a trochar, except that it is longer. It is used for conducting bougies into the urethra.

PORTE-CAUSTIQUE, *Porte-pierre—p. Feuille,* Subscapularis.

PORTE-LIGATURE, from *porter,* 'to carry,' and *ligature.* An instrument for conveying a ligature to deep-seated parts.

PORTE-MÈCHE (F.), from *porter,* 'to carry,' and *mèche,* 'a tent.' An instrument for carrying tents or *mèches* deeply into fistulous openings, or sinuses, to the bottom of ulcers, &c. It is a wire of silver or steel, four or five inches long, having a notch at one extremity, and a button at the other.

PORTE-MOXA, (F.) A small instrument for keeping the moxa applied to a part to be canterized. It consists of a metallic ring—separated from the skin by three supports of ebony— to which a handle is adapted.

PORTE-NŒUD (F.), from *porter,* 'to carry,' and *nœud,* 'a knot.' An instrument for carrying a ligature round the base or pedicle of a tumour.

PORTE-PIERRE (F.), *Porte-caustique, Caustic bearer.* An instrument similar to a *porte-crayon* for carrying lunar caustic.

PORTE-SONDE, (F.) An instrument resembling a porte-crayon, employed for holding the style or *sonde,* and inserting it more readily into the nasal duct, during the operation for fistula lachrymalis.

PORTE-VEINE, Porta Vena.

PORTER, Cerevisia.

PORTIO DURA, Facial nerve — p. Inter duram et mollem, Portio Wrisbergii—p. Intermedia Wrisbergii, Portio Wrisbergii—p. Media inter portionem duram et portionem mollem, Portio Wrisbergii.

PORTIO MOLLIS, Auditory nerve.

POR'TIO WRISBER'GII, *Portio interme'dia Wrisber'gii, Portio media inter portionem duram et portionem mollem, Portio inter duram et mollem,* (F.) *Faisceau intermédiaire de Wrisberg, Intermédiaire de Wrisberg.* A small, white fasciculus, intermediate between the portio mollis and portio dura of the seventh pair of nerves, which was first described by Wrisberg. The Chorda Tympani is supposed by some to emanate from this nerve.

PORTION COSTO-TRACHÉLIENNE DU SACRO-SPINAL, Longissimus dorsi—p. *Écailleux ou squameux du temporal,* Squamous portion of the temporal — p. *Lombaire du plexus crural,* Lumbar plexus.

PORTION GODRONNÉE DE LA CORNE D'AMMON. A name given by Vicq d'Azyr to a small, denticulated cord, of a compact tissue and granular appearance, which unites the cornu ammonis to the paries of the lateral ventricle.

PORTONARIUM, Pylorus, Duodenum.

PORTULA'CA, *Andrach'nē, Al'lium Gal'licum, Portula'ca olera'cea, Purslane,* (F.) *Pourpier cultivé.* This plant abounds with a watery and somewhat acid juice; and is often put into soups or pickled with spices. It is regarded as antiseptic and aperient.

POROUS, Callus, Meatus — p. Acusticus, Auditory canal, internal.

PORUS OP'TICUS. An opening in the centre of the cribriform lamella of the sclerotic, through which the central artery of the retina enters the eyeball.

POSCA, Oxycrate.

POSE, Coryza.

POSIMOS, Potable.

POSITION, FALSE, False position.

POSOL'OGY, *Posolog"ia, Dosiolog"ia,* from ποσος, 'quantity,' and λογος, 'a discourse.' Indication of the doses in which the different articles of the materia medica ought to be exhibited.

POSSET, *Posse'tum,* from (L.) *posca,* 'sour wine and water.' Milk curdled with wine, or any acid, or treacle. A preparation of beer and milk; *Zythog'ala.*

POSSET, SACK, see Sack—p. Sago, see Sago.

POSSETING, Regurgitation (of Infants).

POSTBRACHIALE, Metacarpus.

POSTCARPIUM, Metacarpus.

POSTE'RIOR ANNULA'RIS. An external, interosseous muscle, which arises from the corresponding sides of the metacarpal bones of the ring-finger and little finger, and is inserted into the inside of the tendon on the back of the ring-finger. Its *use* is to draw the ring-finger inwards.

POSTERIOR AURIS, Retrahens auris.

POSTERIOR IN'DICIS MANŪS. An internal, interosseous muscle, which arises from the inner or ulnar side of the metacarpal bone of the forefinger, and is inserted into the inside of the tendon on the back of the fore-finger. Its *use* is to draw the fore-finger inwards.

POSTERIOR INDICIS PEDIS, *Abduc'tor Indicis Pedis* An external, interosseous muscle, which arises from the contiguous sides of the metatarsal bones of the fore-toe, and second of the small toes, and is inserted into the outside of the root of the first bone of the fore-toe. Its *use* is to pull the fore-toe outwards.

POSTERIOR ME'DII DIG"ITI MANŪS. An external, interosseous muscle, which arises from the corresponding sides of the metacarpal bones of the middle and ring-fingers; and is inserted into the inside of the tendon on the back of the middle finger. Its *use* is to draw the middle finger inwards.

POSTERIOR MEDII DIG"ITI PEDIS, *Abductor medii digiti pedis.* An external, interosseous muscle, which originates from the contiguous sides of the metatarsal bones of the second and third of the small toes, and is inserted into the outside of the root of the first bone of the second of the small toes. Its *use* is to pull the toe outwards.

POSTERIOR TER'TII DIG"ITI, *Adductor tertii digiti.* An external, interosseous muscle, which arises from the contiguous sides of the metatarsal bones of the third and fourth of the small toes, and is inserted into the outside of the root of the first bone of the third of the small toes. Its *use* is to pull the toe outwards.

POSTHE, Penis, Prepuce.

POSTHET'OMIST, *Posthet'omus,* from ποσθη, 'prepuce,' and τομη, 'incision.' One who performs the operation of circumcision.

POSTHETOMY, Circumcision.

POSTHIA, Hordeolum.

POSTHIOPLAS'TIC, *Posthioplas'ticus,* from ποσθη, 'the prepuce,' and πλασσω, 'I form.' An epithet applied to the operation for restoring the prepuce.

POSTHI'TIS, from ποσθη, 'the prepuce, the penis,' and *itis,* the termination for inflammation. Inflammation of the prepuce or penis.

POSTHIUM, Prepuce.

POSTHON'CUS, from ποσθη, 'the prepuce or penis,' and ογκος, 'a tumour.' Swelling of the prepuce or penis.

POSTHOPLAS'TICA, from ποσθη, 'prepuce,' and πλαστικος, 'formative.' The art of making a new prepuce.

POST'HUMOUS, from *post,* 'after,' and *humus,* 'the ground.' Occurring after death.

POSTHUMOUS CHILD. One born after the death of its father, or taken from the dead body of its mother, as by the Cæsarean section.

POST-MORTEM. 'After death;' as 'a *post mortem* or necroscopic examination.'

POST-NATUS. In the old law writers, the second son.

POST-PARTUM. 'After delivery.' As '*post partum* hemorrhage.'

POSTPOSIT"IO. Delay in the return of a paroxysm. It is opposed to *anticipatio,* which means the return of a paroxysm earlier than its accustomed hour.

In this sense, we speak of an *anticipating,* and a *postponing (Febris hysteret'ica)* intermittent.

POSTREMA, Uterus.

PO'TABLE, *Potab'ilis,* from *potare,* 'to drink.' *Pot'imos, Potos, Pos'imos,* 'drinkable.' Water is said to be potable, when it contains atmospheric air; is not brackish; and has no mineral impregnation of consequence.

POTASH. So called from the pots or vessels in which it was made;— *Vegetable alkali, Gastrinum.* Also, Potassa.

POTASH OF COMMERCE, *Potassa impu'ra, Impure potassa, Alu'men cati'num, Cin'eres Ru'ssi, Subcar'bonas potas'sæ impu'rus, Potas'sæ carbonas impurus,—*the Pearlash of commerce, is prepared from the ashes of land-plants by calcination, solution in water, filtration, and evaporation. It usually consists of subcarbonate of potass, sulphate of potassa, chloride of potassium, silex, oxide of iron, &c.

From the ashes of lees of wine, and from vine-twigs, a much purer alkali is obtained. It is called *Cinis infecto'rius, C. fæcum, Cin'eres clavella'ti, Alu'men fæcum, Cin'eres gravella'ti,* (F.) *Cendres gravélées, Cendres de sarment.*

Another variety of the alkali is afforded by burning argol in a crucible; afterwards powdering and calcining it, till it is nearly white; then dissolving in water, filtering, and evaporating. It is called *Salt of Tartar, Sal Tar'tari, Kali præpara'tum e tar'taro, Kali e tartaro, Subcar'bonas potassæ puris'simus, Potas'sæ subcar'bonas e tar'taro.* Lastly, when wormwood is burnt to ashes, dissolved in water, filtered, and evaporated to dryness, it affords another variety of vegetable alkali, the *Sal absin'thii* or *Salt of wormwood.*

Impure potash is used for preparing the subcarbonate for medical use.

POTASS, Potassa, Potassa fusa, Potash. The protoxide of potassium.

POTASSA, ACETATE OF, Potassæ acetas—p. Bichromate of, Potassæ bichromas—p. Bisulphate of, Potassæ supersulphas—p. Bitartrate of, Potassæ supertartras—p. Carbonate of, Potassæ carbonas—p. Carbonate of, pure, see Potassæ subcarbonas—p. Chlorate of, Potassæ murias hyperoxygenatus—p. Chromate of, Potassæ chromas—p. Chromate of, neutral, Potassæ chromas—p. Chromate of, yellow, Potassæ chromas.

POTAS'SA CUM CALCE, *Potass with lime, Calx cum cali puro, Caus'ticum commu'nē for'tius, Lapis inferna'lis* sive *sep'ticus, Kali caus'ticum cum calcē, Potas'sa opē calcis para'ta et ignē fusa, Lapis caus'ticus,* (F.) *Potasse préparée avec la chaux, P. à la Chaux, Pierre a cautère.* (*Potassæ, Calcis* āā ʒj. Rub together, and keep in a well-stopped bottle. Ph. U. S.) Used for the same purposes as the next, but more manageable; being less deliquescent.

POTASSA, EUCHLORATE OF, Potassæ murias hyperoxygenatus—p. Ferrocyanate of, Potassii ferrocyanuretum—p. Ferroprussiate of, Potassæ cyanuretum.

POTASSA FUSA, *Potassa, Kali caus'ticum, Fused potass, Caus'ticum commu'nē acer'rimum, Kali purum, Al'kali vegetab'ilē fixum caus'ticum, Causticum alkali'num, C. commu'nē, C. Potentia'lē, C. Sali'num, Hydras ka'licum, Hydras potas'sæ puræ fusæ, Potassæ hydras, Lapis caus'ticus, Lapis causticus chirurgo'rum, Lapis inferna'lis alcali'nus, L. sep'ticus, Rupto'rium commu'nē, Fixed veg''etable alkali, Hydrate of Potassa,* (F.) *Potasse caustique.* (Prepared by evaporating solution of potass to dryness in an iron vessel.) This preparation is generally run into cylindrical moulds, covered with paper, and kept in well-corked vessels. It is powerfully escharotic, and is used for forming issues, curing strictures, &c.

POTASSA, FUSED, Potassa fusa—p. Hydriodate of, Potassæ hydriodas—p. Hydrobromate of, see Bromine—p. Hydrocyanate of, Potassii cyanuretum—p. Hyperoxalas, Potass, oxalate of—p. Hypertartras, P. supertartras—p. Impura, Potash of commerce—p. and Iron, tartrate of, Ferrum tartarizatum—p. with Lime, Potassa cum calce—p. Liquida, Liquor potassæ—p. Mephite of, Potassæ subcarbonas—p. Monochromate of, Potassæ chromas—p. Muriate of, Potassæ murias—p. Nitrate of, Potassæ nitras—p. Ope calcis parata et igne fusa, Potassa cum calce—p. Oxymuriate of, Potassæ murias hyperoxygenatus—p. Prussiate of, Potassii ferrocyanuretum—p. and Soda, Tartrate of, Soda, tartrate of—p. Subcarbonate of, Potassæ subcarbonas—p. Sulphate of, Potassæ sulphas—p. Sulphate of, acid, Potassæ supersulphas—p. Sulphuret of, Potassæ sulphuretum—p.

Supercarbonate of, Potassæ carbonas—p. Supersulphate of, Potassæ supersulphas—p. Supertartrate of, Potassæ supertartras—p. Tartrate of, Potassæ tartras.

POTASSÆ ACE'TAS, *Acetas kali, Oxytar'tarus, Acetas liciv'iæ* seu *ka'licum, Al'kali tar'tari ace'to satura'tum, Alcali vegetab'ilē cum acetō, Magiste'rium tartari purgans, Terra folia'ta Tartari, Kali aceta'tum, Sal diuret'icus, Sal Senner'ti, Ac''etate of potass, Arca'num tartari,* (F.) *Acétate de potasse.* (*Acid. acetic.* Oj, *Potassæ carbon,* q. s. Mix and add, by degrees, enough acetic acid to saturate the alkali. Then filter and evaporate till a pellicle is formed, which is to be dried upon bibulous paper; evaporate again in a water-bath, and, removing the pellicles, dry. — Ph. U. S.)

It is cathartic and diuretic. Dose, ʒj to ʒij, or more.

POTASSÆ ET ALUMINÆ SULPHAS, Alumen — p. Biantimonias, Antimonium diaphoreticum — p. Bicarbonas, Potassæ carbonas.

POTAS'SÆ BICHRO'MAS, *Kali chro'micum rubrum* seu *ac''idum* seu *bichro'micum, Bichro'mate of potas'sa.* Procured by adding *sulphuric, nitric,* or *acetic* acid to a solution of the *neutral chromate,* and setting it aside to crystallize. It is a violent irritant poison; and has been used as a caustic in cases of morbid growths, in the proportion of from half a drachm to a drachm of the salt to from an ounce to an ounce and a half of water.

POTASSÆ BISULPHAS, P. supersulphas — p. Bitartras, P. supertartras.

POTASSÆ CAR'BONAS, *Kali aëra'tum, Bicar'bonas potassæ, Potas'sæ bicar'bonas* (Ph. U. S.) *Deutocarbonas potassii, Carbonate, bicar'bonate,* or *supercar'bonate of potassa.* This is not caustic, like the subcarbonate of potass, and hence, has been preferred to relieve acidity. (*Potass. carbon.* ℔iv, *Aquæ destillat.* Ox. Pass carbonic acid through the solution until it is saturated, and filter. Evaporate at a heat not exceeding 160°, and dry the crystals on bibulous paper. Carbonic acid is obtained from marble by the addition of dilute sulphuric acid. — Ph. U. S.) Dose, gr. x to ʒss. It is used in forming the soda powders, as well as for its antacid properties.

POTASSÆ CARBONAS, P. subcarbonas — p. Carbonas impurus, P. subcarbonas — p. Carbonas purus, see P. subcarbonas — p. Chloras, P. murias hyperoxygenatus — p. Chloruretum oxydatum, P. murias hyperoxygenatus.

POTAS'SÆ CHROMAS, *Kali chro'micum flavum* seu *neutra'lē, Neutral yellow Chromate,* or *Monochromate of potassa.* Prepared by igniting a mixture of four parts of native *chromite of iron* (chrome-iron ore) and one part of *nitre;* dissolving out the chromate of potassa by *water,* and crystallizing. It has been used as an emetic, expectorant and diaphoretic. Dose, as an emetic, from two to four grains; as an expectorant, from ¼th to ½ grain. In the proportion of one drachm to 32 ounces of water, it has been used as an antiseptic wash — called by Jacobson, *Liquor conserva'trix.*

POTASSÆ CITRAS, *Citrate of potassa.* (*Acid. citric.* ʒx, *Potass. bicarb.* ʒxiv, *Aq.* q. s. Dissolve the acid in the water; and after effervescence has ceased, strain and evaporate to dryness. The salt is deliquescent, and must be kept in well-stopped bottles. Ph. U. S.) It possesses the refrigerant properties of the neutral salts, and may be given in fever, when to do little or nothing is the most advisable course. Dose, gr. x to ʒss.

POTASSÆ ET FERRI TARTRAS, Ferri tartarizatum — p. Hydras, Potassa fusa.

POTASSÆ HYDRI'ODAS, *Potassæ Protohydri'o-*

das, *Potas'sii protoxi'di hydri'odas*, *Kali Hydriodin'icum*, *K. Hydriod'icum*, *Hydriodas Ka'licus*, *Hydri'odate of potass*, (F.) *Hydriodate de potasse*. If a solution of potass be poured on iodine, an iodate and hydriodate are formed. These may be separated by means of alcohol, which only dissolves the latter of these salts. The hydriodate, or rather the *Iodide of Potas'sium*, *Kalium Ioda'tum*, *Potassii Ioduretum* seu *Io'didum*, (F.) *Iodure de potassium*, may be obtained by evaporation. When the *Iodide of potassium* is dissolved in water, it becomes the *Hydriodate of Potassa*. The following is the formula in the Ph. U. S. *Potass.* ℥vj; *Iodin.* in pulv. ℥xvj; *Carbon. ligni* in pulv. subtiliss. ℥ij; *Aq. bullient.* Oiij. Dissolve the potassa in the water; add the iodine gradually, stirring until the solution becomes colourless, and continue the additions until the liquid remains slightly coloured from excess of iodine. Evaporate to dryness, stirring in the charcoal towards the close. Rub to powder, and heat to dull redness in an iron crucible, keeping up the temperature for 15 minutes. When cool, dissolve out the saline matter with pure water, filter the solution, evaporate and set aside to crystallize. By evaporating and crystallizing as before, an additional quantity of crystals may be obtained. Virtues, — those of iodine.

POTASSÆ MU'RIAS, *Sal Digesti'vus* vel *Sal febrif'ugus Syl'vii*, *Muriate of Potass*, *Spir'itus salis mari'ni coagula'tus*. Bitter and refrigerant.

POTASSÆ MU'RIAS HYPEROXYGENA'TUS, *Potassæ Chloras*, *P. oxymu'rias*, *Oxymu'riate* or *hyperoxymu'riate of potass*, *Chlorate of potas'sa*, *Euchlo'rate of potass*, *Alcali vegetab'ile sali'todephlogistica'tum*, *Chlorure'tum potas'sæ oxyda'tum*, *Haloi'dum oxygena'tum*, *Oxyge'no-Chlorure'tum potas'sii*, *Protochlo'rate of potas'sium*, *Kali chlo'ricum*, *Chloras Ka'licus depura'tus*, (F.) *Chlorate de potasse*. It has been regarded as antineuropathic, and as an alterative purifier of the blood and humours. It is of doubtful efficacy. Dose, 3 to 6 grains or more.

POTAS'SÆ NITRAS, *Nitrate of Potass*, *Nitrum*, *Sal nitrum*, *Nitre*, *Saltpetre*, *Sal petræ*, *Salse'do nucrum*, *Sanguin'ea*, *Berenic'ium*, *Halini'trum*, *Protoni'trate of Potas'sium*, *Nitrate of protox'ide of Potassium*, *Kali ni'tricum*, *Nitras ka'licum*, *Nitras lixiv'iæ*, (F.) *Nitrate de potasse*. Obtained from the putrefaction of animal matters, in contact with calcareous or alkaline earths, by elixiviation; adding, if necessary, wood-ashes to supply the alkaline basis. It is formed, in an impure state, by nature, in warm climates. It is diuretic and refrigerant, and, in large doses, purgative; externally, cooling and detergent. Dose, gr. x to ℨss. In large doses it is an acrid poison.

POTASSÆ NITRAS FUSUS SULPHA'TIS PAUCIL'LO MIXTUS, *Sal prunel'læ*, *Crystal'lus minera'lis*, *Nitras potas'sæ cum sul'phure fusus*, *Nitrum tabula'tum*, *Lapis Prunel'læ*, *Sore-throat salt*, *Min'eral crystal*, *Anod'ynum minera'lē*. Nitrate of potass, mixed with a little sulphate of potass and run into moulds. Its properties are those of nitre.

POTASSÆ OX'ALAS, *Superox'alate of Protox'ide of Potas'sium*, *Ox'alas Acid'ulum Potas'sæ* seu *Potas'sæ acid'ulus* seu *ba'sicus*, *Superox'alas ka'licum*, *S. Potassæ*, *Hyperoxalas Potassæ*, *Sal Acetosel'læ*, *Oxa'lium*, *Kali oxal'icum acid'ulum*, *Ox'alas subpotas'sicus*, *Oxalate of Potass*, *Salt of Sorrel*. Prepared from the juice of wood sorrel. It is refrigerant, and is used to make lemonade, &c.

POTASSÆ OXALAS ACIDULUM, Potass, oxalate of—p. Oxymurias, P. murias hyperoxygenatus—p. Protohydriodas, P. hydriodas—p. Puræ fusæ hydras, Potassa fusa—p. et Sodæ tartras, Soda, tartrate of.

POTASSÆ SUBCAR'BONAS, *P. Car'bonas* (Ph. U. S.), *Subcar'bonas Kali*, *Car'bonas Potassæ*, *Kali præpara'tum*, *Sal Herba'rum*, *Calca'reous Tartar*, *Sal Planta'rum*, *Subcarbonate of Potassa*, *Sal Tar'tari*, *Sal Absin'thii*, *Mephite of Potass*, &c. (See Potash.) A filtered solution of the impure subcarbonate, *Potas'sæ car'bonas impu'ra* (Ph. U. S.) *Pearl-ash* (see Potash,) evaporated to dryness. This deliquescent salt is given in the same cases as the potassæ carbonas, than which it is more caustic and disagreeable.

The Parisian codex has a *Subcar'bonas Potas'sæ ex tar'taro combus'to*, vulgo *Sal Tartari* or *Salt of Tartar*—it is the *Potassæ carbonas purus*, *Pure Carbonate of Potassa*, Ph. U. S.; a *Subcarbonas Potassæ ex deflagran'tibus simul tar'trate acid'ulo et Nitrate Potassæ paratus*, vulgo *Nitrum ex tartaro fixum*; and a *Subcarbonas potassæ ex deflagran'tē cum Carbo'nibus Nitra'tē Potassæ paratus*, vulgo *Nitrum fixum*. They are all used like the preceding.

POTASSÆ SUBCARBONAS IMPURUS, Potash of commerce.

POTASSÆ SULPHAS, *Kali vitriola'tum*, *Sulphas Kali*, *Kali sulphu'ricum*, *Lixiv'ia vitriola'ta*, *Nitrum vitriolatum Schroederi*, *Sal Sapien'tiæ*, *Sal Tar'tari Sulphura'tum*, *Specif'icum Paracel'si*, *Spi'ritus vitrioli coagula'tus Mynsichti*, *Protosulph'ate of Potas'sium*, *Al'kali vegeta'bilē vitriolatum*, *Sal de duobus*, *Arca'num duplica'tum*, *Nitrum vitriola'tum*, *Tar'tarum vitriolatum*, *Panace'a Ducis Holsa'tiæ*, *Panace'a duplica'ta*, *Sal Polychres'tus*, *Sulphate of Potass*, (F.) *Sulfate de potasse*. (The salt, that remains after the distillation of nitric acid, dissolved; the excess of acid saturated with subcarbonate of potass and crystallized.) Purgative and diuretic. Dose, ℨss to ℨj as a laxative. In a large dose it has proved an irritant poison.

POTASSÆ SULPHAS CUM SUL'PHURE: *Sal Polychres'tus Glase'ri*, *Lixiv'ia Vitriola'ta Sulphu'rea*. (Formed by deflagrating nitrate of potass with sublimed sulphur.) Same virtues as the last. Dose, gr. xv to xxx.

POTASSÆ SULPHURE'TUM, *Potas'sii Sulphure'tum*, *P. tersulphure'tum*, *Kali sulphuretum*, *Hepar Sulph'uris sali'num*, *H. sulphu'ris vulga'rē*, *Sulphure'tum lixiv'iæ*, *S. ka'licum*, *Hepar Sulphuris*, *Liver of Sulphur*, *Sulphuret of Potass*, (F.) *Sulfure de potasse*, *Sulfure de potassium sulfuré*, *Foie de Soufre*. (*Sulphur.* ℨj, *Potassæ carb.* ℨ). Rub them together, and place the mixture in a covered crucible upon the fire until they unite. It has been employed in affections of the chest, as an expectorant, in the dose of from ℨss to ℨj; largely diluted; but it is chiefly used as a bath or wash in cases of itch, tinea capitis, and other cutaneous affections.

POTASSÆ SUPEROXALAS, Potassæ oxalas.

POTASSÆ SUPERSUL'PHAS. *P. Bisulphas*, *Sienix'um*, *Supersulphate of Potass*, *Sal febrifugus of Lem'ery*, *Acid Sulphate of Potassa*, *Binphate of Potass*, *Super-protosulphate of Potassium*, (F.) *Bisulfate, de Potasse*. (The salt remaining after the distillation of nitric acid dissolved, strained, and crystallized.) It is refrigerant and purgative. Dose, ℨss to ℨij.

POTASSÆ SUPERTAR'TRAS IMPU'RUS, *Tartarus crudus*, *Tar'tarum*, *Lapis vini*, *Magnet'iam*, *Fædagra*, *Tartar*, (F.) *Tartre cru*, *T. brut*. It is called, also, *Tartarum rubrum* and *Red Argol*, when obtained from red wines; *Tartarum album* or *White Argol*, when from white wines. Tartar is the saline deposit from wines as they become aged; which attaches itself to the sides of the casks and bottles in which they are kept. It consists of a considerable quantity of acidulous tartrate of potass, tartrate of lime, silica, alumen, oxyd of iron, manganese, and a red colouring matter, if the wine be red. It is chiefly used for the preparation of cream of tartar.

POTASSÆ SUPERTAR'TRAS, *Crystal'li Tar'tari, Tartras Acid'ulus Potassæ purus, Supertar'trate of Protox'ide of Potas'sium, Potas'sæ Bitar'tras* (Ph. U. S.), *P. tartras ac"ida, Bitartrate* or *Supertartrate of Potass, Hypertartras Potassæ, Tartras superpotas'sicus, T. subpotas'sicus, Crystals of Tartar, Cremor Tar'tari, Cream of Tartar* (when in powder,) *Supertar'trate of Potass,* (F.) *Tartrate acide de potasse, Crème de Tartre.* (The tartar of wine purified.) It requires 120 parts of water at 60° to dissolve it. It is mildly purgative, refrigerant and diuretic. Dissolved in water, with a small quantity of white wine, some sugar and lemon-peel, it forms an agreeable beverage in febrile diseases, under the name of *imperial.* Dose, as a diuretic, ℨj to ℨij; as a purgative, ℨss to ℨj.

POTASSÆ TARTRAS, *Kali tartariza'tum, Al'cali fixum tartarisatum, Tar'tarum solu'bilĕ, Tartarus tartariza'tus, Lixiv'ia Tartariea'ta, Sal Panchres'tum, Tartras Kalinus, T. lixiv'iæ, Sal vegetab'ilis, Alkali vegetab'ilĕ tartarisatum, Tartrate of Potass, Soluble Tartar,* (F.) *Tartrate de Potasse.* (*Potassæ carbon.* ℨxvj; *Potassæ Bitartrat.* in pulv. subtiliss. ℔iij, vel q. s., *aquæ bullientis,* cong. Dissolve the carbonate of potassa in the water, add the bitartrate to saturation, and boil; filter, evaporate till a pellicle forms, and set aside to crystallize. Pour off the liquid; dry the crystals on bibulous paper, and keep in closely-stopped bottles. — Ph. U. S.) A saline cathartic in the dose of ℨij to ℨj.

POTASSÆ TARTRAS ACIDA, P. supertartras—p. Tartras acidulus purus, P. supertartras—p. Tartras stibialis seu stibiosus, Antimonium tartarizatum.

POTASSE, ACETATE DE, Potassæ acetas — p. Bisulphate de, Potassæ supersulphas — p. Caustique, Potassa fusa — p. à la Chaux, Potassa cum calce — p. Chlorate de, Potassæ murias hyperoxygenatus — p. Hydriodate de, Potassæ hydriodas—p. Liquide, Liquor potassæ—p. Nitrate de, Potassæ nitras — p. Préparée avec la chaux, Potassa cum calce — p. et de Soude, tartrate de, Soda, tartrate of—p. Sulfate de, Potassæ sulphas, p. Sulfure de, Potassæ sulphuretum—p. Tartrate de, Potassæ tartras—p. Tartrate, acide de, Potassæ supertartras.

POTAS'SII BRO'MIDUM, *Potas'sæ hydrobro'mas,* (F.) *Bromure de Potassium, Bromide of potassium.* (*Bromin,* ℨij; *Ferri fili,* ℨj; *Potass. carbon.* ℨij and ℨj, vel q. s.; *Aq. destillat.,* Oiv. Add the iron filings and bromine to a pint and a half of the water; stirring for half an hour. Apply a gentle heat, and when the liquor assumes a greenish colour, add gradually the carbonate of potassa, dissolved in Oiss of the water, until it ceases to cause a precipitate. Continue the heat for half an hour, and filter. Wash the precipitate with the remaining water, boiling hot, and filter. Mix the liquors and crystallize by evaporation. Ph. U. S.) Virtues: — those of iodide of iron.

POTASSII CYANIDUM, P. Cyanuretum.

POTAS'SII CYANURE'TUM, *P. Cyan'idum, Cyanuret of Potassium, Hydrocy'anate of Potassa,* (*Potassii Ferrocyanur.,* in pulv. ℨviij; *Potass. Carbonat.,* ex siccat., ℨiij. Mix intimately and throw into a deep iron crucible, heated to redness; keep up the heat till effervescence ceases, and the fused mass concretes, of a pure white colour, upon a warm glass rod dipped into it; then pour out the liquid carefully into a shallow dish, to solidify, stopping before the salt becomes contaminated with the precipitated iron. Break up the mass whilst warm, and preserve in well-stopped bottles. Ph. U. S.) Used in the same cases as the hydrocyanic acid. Dose, a quarter of a grain.

POTASSII DEUTO-CARBONAS, Potassæ carbonas.

POTASSII FERROCYANURE'TUM, *P. Ferrocyan'idum, Ferrocy'anide* or *Ferrocyan'uret of Potassium, Ferrocy'anate of Potassa, Ferroprussiate of Potassa, Prussiate of Potassa,* (F.) *Protocyanure jaune de fer et de potassium, Cyanure de fer et de potassium.* The yellow double cyanuret of potassium and iron, the salt from which the cyanuret of potassium is obtained by calcination. It is not much used in medicine. It has been advised as an astringent in the colliquative sweats of phthisis, in leucorrhœa, &c.; but it does not seem to be possessed of much activity. Dose, 10 or 15 grains every four or five hours.

POTASSII HYDRARGYRO-IODIDUM, *Potassæ Iodohydrar'gyras, Hydrargyrum biiodatum cum kalio iodato, Kalium iodatum hydrargyratum, Iodhydrar'gyrate of Potassium, Hydrargyro-iodide of Potassium.* This salt is made by the combination of *iodide of potassium* with *red iodide of mercury.* Its properties are similar to those of the iodides of mercury, but in a less degree.

POTASSII IODIDUM, Potassæ hydriodas—p. Ioduretum, Potassæ hydriodas — p. Oxygeno-chloruretum, Potassæ murias hyperoxygenatus — p. Protoxidi hydriodas, Potassæ hydriodas—p. Sulphuretum, Potassæ sulphuretum—p. Tersulphuretum, Potassæ sulphuretum.

POTASSIUM. Same etymon as potash. The metallic base of potassa.

POTASSIUM, BROMURE DE, see Bromine —p. Cyanuret of, Potassii cyanuretum—p. Ferrocyanide of, Potassii ferrocyanuretum — p. Ferrocyanuret of, Potassii Ferrocyanuretum—p. Iodide of, Potassæ hydriodas — p. Iodohydrargyrate of, Potassii hydrargyro-iodidum — *p. Iodure de,* Potassæ hydriodas — p. Oxide of, Potass — p. Protoarsenite of, Arsenite of protoxide of potassium—p. Protochlorate of, Potassæ murias hyperoxygenatus — p. Protonitrate of, Potassæ nitras — p. Protoxide of, Potass—p. Protoxide of, nitrate of, Potassæ nitras — p. Protoxide of, superoxalate of, Potass, oxalate of—p. Protoxide of, supertartrate of, Potassæ supertartras — p. Protosulphate of, Potassæ sulphas—*p. Sulfure de, sulfaté,* Potassæ sulphuretum — p. Sulphuret of, Potassæ sulphuretum—p. Superprotosulphate of, Potassæ supersulphas.

POTATO, Solanum tuberosum—p. Fly, Lytta vittata—p. Hog, Convolvulus panduratus — p. Spanish, Convolvulus batatas—p. Sweet, Convolvulus batatas — p. Vine, wild, Convolvulus panduratus—p. Wild, Convolvulus panduratus.

POTBELLY, Physconia.

POTELÉE, Hyoscyamus.

POTENTIA, Force.

POTEN'TIA seu POTES'TAS COËUN'DI, Capability of copulation.

POTENTIA GENERAN'DI. The power of procreation.

POTENTIA IRRITANS, Stimulus.

POTEN'TIAL, *Potentia'lis;* from *potens,* 'able.' An epithet for remedies which, although energetic, do not act till some time after their application. The caustic alkalies, for instance, are called Potential cauteries in contradistinction to the hot iron, which is termed *actual.*

POTENTILLA, P. reptans.

POTENTIL'LA ANSERI'NA, *P. argenti'na* seu *impo'lita* seu *neglec'ta, Argenti'na vulga'ris, Fraga'ria anseri'na, Ar'gentine, Chenobos'con, Argenta'ria, Anseri'na, Silver Weed, Wild Tansy,*

(F.) *Argentine, Potentille.* The leaves are mildly astringent and tonic.

POTENTILLA ARGENTINA, P. anserina — p. Impolita, P. anserina — p. Neglecta, P. anserina.

POTENTILLA NORVEG"ICA, *Norway Cinque-foil,* an indigenous plant, is possessed of similar properties.

POTENTILLA PALUSTRIS, Comarum palustre.

POTENTIL'LA REPTANS, *Pentaphyl'lum, Fraga'ria pentaphyl'lum, Potentil'la, Quinquefo'lium, Q. majus, Common cinquefoil,* (F.) *Quintefeuille.* The roots are possessed of astringent properties.

POTENTILLA TORMENTILLA, Tormentilla.

POTERIUM SANGUISORBA, Pimpinella saxifraga.

POTESTAS COEUNDI, Potentia coeundi — p. Generandi, Potentia generandi.

POTEX, Anus.

POTHOS FŒTIDA, Dracontium fœtidum — p. Putorii, Dracontium fœtidum.

POTIMOS, Potable.

POTIO, Drink, Haustus, Potion — p. Calcis carbonatis, Mistura cretæ — p. Effervescens antiemetica, Potion of Riverius — p. Leniens, Looch ex ovo — p. Oleosa, Looch ex ovo — p. Picea, see Pinus sylvestris.

POTION (F.), *Potio;* from *poto,* 'I drink.' A liquid medicine, from 4 to 8 ounces or more in quantity, the composition of which varies, and which is administered in divided doses. It corresponds to the English *mixture.*

POTION PECTORALE, Looch ex ovo.

POTION OF RIVE'RIUS. A mixture of *Lemon Juice* and *Subcarbonate of Potass,* — generally given in a state of effervescence. It is the *Potio efferves'cens anti-emet'ica dicta Rive'rii,* of the Parisian codex. The name in the codex indicates its use.

POTIONIS DESIDERIUM, Thirst.

POTIRON, Cucurbita pepo.

POTIUNCULA, Haustus.

POTOPARANŒA, Delirium tremens.

POTOS, Potable.

POTOTROMOPARANŒA, Delirium tremens.

POTT'S DISEASE, Vertebral disease.

POTUS, Drink — p. Hippocraticus, Claret.

POU, Pediculus.

POUCE, Pollex, see Digitus.

POUCHED, Encysted.

POUDRE, Powder, Pulvis — p. *Absorbante et anti-acide,* p. Pulvis de magnesiâ compositus — p. *d'Alun composée,* Pulvis sulphatis aluminæ compositus — p. *Antiarthritique amère,* Pulvis de amaris compositus — p. *Antiasthmatique,* Pulvis de sulphure et scillâ — p. *Antimoniale composée ou de James,* Antimonial powder — p. *Aromatique,* Pulvis cinnamomi compositus — p. *d'Asarum composée dite sternutatoire,* Pulvis asari compositus — p. *Balsamique,* Pulvis myrrhæ compositus — p. *de Birckmann,* Pulvis de aro compositus — p. *de Blanchement,* Calcis chloridum — p. *de Cannelle composée,* Pulvis cinnamomi compositus — p. *Cathartique,* Pulvis scammoneæ compositus — p. *de Chypre,* see Cladonia rangiferrina — p. *du Comte de Palme,* Magnesiæ carbonas — p. *Cornachine,* Pulvis cornachini — p. *de Corne brulée avec opium,* Pulvis cornu usti cum opio — p. *de Craie composée avec opium,* see Pulvis cretæ compositus cum opio — p. *de Dower,* Pulvis ipecacuanhæ compositus — p. *de Dupuytren,* Powder of Dupuytren — p. *Gasifère laxative,* Powders, Seidlitz — p. *Gasifère simple,* Powders, soda — p. *de Gomme adragant composée,* Pulvis tragacanthæ compositus — p. *de Gomme gutte,* Pulvis e gummi guttâ — p. *Hydragogue,* Pulvis e gummi guttâ — p. *Incisive,* Pulvis de sulphure et scillâ — p. *d'Ipecacuanha et opium,* Pulvis ipecacuanhæ compositus — p. *de Jalap composée,* Pulvis jalapæ compositus — p. *de Kino composée,* Pulvis kino compositus — p. *de Pérard,* Pulvis de sennâ, scammonio et lignis — p. *de Quercetanus,* Pulvis e gummi guttâ — p. *de Saint Ange,* Pulvis asari compositus — p. *de Savon végétale,* Pulvis gummosus alkalinus — p. *de Scammonée composée,* Pulvis scammoneæ compositus — p. *de Sedlitz,* Powders, Seidlitz — p. *de Séné composée,* Pulvis sennæ comp. — p. *de Satinelli,* Magnesiæ carbonas — p. *Styptique,* Pulvis sulphatis aluminæ compositus.

POUDRE SUBTIL DE DELCROIX. A fashionable depilatory "for removing superfluous hair in less than ten minutes." It is said to consist of *Quicklime* and *Sulphuret of Arsenic,* with some vegetable powder. — Paris.

POUDRE TEMPÉRANTE DE STAHL, Pulvis de Sulphate potassæ compositus — p. *de Tennant,* Calcis chloridum — p. *de Valentini,* Magnesiæ carbonas — p. *Vermifuge mercurielle,* Pulvis e sulphureto hydrargyro nigro et scammonio — p. *Vermifuge sans mercure,* Pulvis ex helminthocorro compositus.

POUGUES, MINERAL WATERS OF. These alkaline waters are in the department of Nièvre, France. They contain carbonic acid, carbonates of soda, lime, and magnesia; chloride of sodium, alumina, and silica, with protoxide of iron.

POULAIN, Bubo.

POULET, VIN DE (F.), *Pullet Wine.* A disgusting preparation, made by infusing the excrement of the pullet in white wine. According to Nysten, it is employed by the vulgar in France in a number of diseases, and especially in falls, contusions, &c.

POULIOT, Mentha pulegium.

POULS, Pulse — p. *Abdominal,* Pulsus inferior — p. *des Adultes,* Pulse, natural — p. *Agité,* Pulsus fortis — p. *Bas,* Pulse, low — p. *Capital,* Pulse, nasal — p. *Combiné,* Pulse, complex — p. *Compliqué,* Pulse, complex — p. *Composé,* Pulse, complex — p. *Concentré,* Pulse, contracted — p. *Défaillant,* Pulsus deficiens — p. *Deprimé,* Pulse, depressed — p. *de la Diarrhée,* Pulse, intestinal — p. *Dur,* Pulse, hard — p. *Élevé,* Pulse, ardent — p. *Embarrassé,* Pulsus intricatus — p. *de l'Estomac,* Pulse, stomachal — p. *Étroit,* Pulsus strictus — p. *de l'Expectoration,* Pulse, pectoral — p. *Faible,* Pulse, feeble — p. *du Foie,* Pulse, hepatic — p. *Grand,* Pulse, large — p. *Insensible,* Pulsus deficiens — p. *Intercadent,* Pulse, intermittent — p. *des Intestins,* Pulse, intestinal — p. *Languissant,* Pulse, languid — p. *Lent,* Pulse, slow — p. *de la Matrice,* Pulsus uterinus — p. *Modéré,* Pulse, natural — p. *Mou,* Pulse, soft — p. *de Nez,* Pulse, nasal — p. *Ondoyant,* Pulse, undulating — p. *Ondulant,* Pulse, undulating — p. *Palpitant,* Pulse, tremulous — p. *Parfait,* Pulse, natural — p. *Petit,* Pulse, small — p. *Plein,* Pulse, full — p. *Précipité,* Pulse, frequent — p. *Profond,* Pulse, deep — p. *Prompt,* Pulse, sharp — p. *Rare,* Pulse, slow — p. *Rebondissant,* Pulsus dicrotus — p. *Redoublé,* Pulsus dicrotus — p. *des Règles,* Pulsus uterinus — p. *Roide,* Pulse, tense — p. *Serratile,* Pulsus serrinus — p. *Serré,* Pulse, contracted — p. *de la Sueur,* Pulsus sudoralis — p. *Tardif,* Pulse, slow — p. *Tendu,* Pulse, tense — p. *Tremblant,* Pulse, tremulous — p. *de l'Urine,* Pulsus urinalis — p. *Véhément,* Pulsus fortis — p. *Ventral,* Pulsus inferior — p. *Vide,* Pulsus vacuus — p. *Vif,* Pulse, sharp — p. *Vite,* Pulse, sharp.

POULTICE, see Cataplasm.

POUNCE, Sandarac.

POUND, Libra, Litra, λιτρα, Lat. *Pondo, Bage'dia* (of twelve oz.), *Barda'dia,* (F.) *Livre,* from *pondere,* 'to weigh.' A weight, consisting of twelve ounces Troy, — sixteen ounces avoirdupoise. See Weights and Measures.

POURPIER CULTIVÉ, Portulaca.

POURPRE BLANC, Miliary fever.

POURRITURE, Putrefaction — p. *d'Hôpital*, Hospital gangrene.

POUS, Pes.

POUSSE, Pursiness.

POUSSÉE, Lichen.

POUSSIÈRE TUBERCULEUSE (F.), 'Tuberculous Dust.' A name given by MM. Rilliet and Barthez to fine white or yellow minute points of tuberculous matter occurring in myriads, so as to be likened to dust.

POWDER, Pulvis.

POWDER OF ÆTHIO'PIA, GUY'S. A once celebrated anthelmintic, which consisted of pure *rasped tin, mercury*, and *sulphur*, triturated together.

POWDER OF ALOES, COMPOUND, Pulvis aloes compositus, Pulvis sulphatis aluminæ compositus — p. of Aloes with canella, Pulvis aloes cum canellâ — p. Antimonial, Chenevix's, Antimonial powder — p. Aromatic, Pulvis aromaticus.

POWDER, ARSENICAL, OF CÔME, *Côme's powder* — a caustic — is formed of *arsenious acid*, gr. x; *red sulphuret of mercury*, gr. xl; powdered *animal charcoal*, gr. x. It is made into a paste with mucilage.

POWDER OF ARUM, compound, Pulvis de aro compositus — p. of Asarabacca, compound, Pulvis asari compositus — p. of Bladder-wrack, yellow, Pulvis quercûs marinæ — p. Bleaching, Calcis chloridum — p. Camboge, Pulvis e gummi guttâ — p. Cardinal del Lugo's, Cinchona — p. of Chalk, compound, Pulvis cretæ compositus — p. of Chalk with opium, compound, Pulvis cretæ compositus cum opio — p. of Cinnamon, compound, Pulvis cinnamomi compositus — p. Côme's, Powder arsenical of Côme — p. of Contrayerva, compound, Pulvis contrayervæ compositus — p. Countess's, Cinchona — p. Countess of Kent's, Cantianus pulvis — p. Cyprus, Hibiscus abelmoschus — p. Dover's, Pulvis ipecacuanhæ compositus.

POWDER OF DUPUYTREN (CAUSTIC;) (F.) *Poudre de Dupuytren*, formed of 1 part of arsenious acid and 200 parts of mild chloride of mercury. A mild and manageable caustic for causing an eschar on exposed surfaces, and in lupus, &c.

POWDER, EARL OF WARWICK'S, Pulvis cornachini — p. of Ethiopia, Powder of Æthiopia.

POWDER OF FAYNARD. A celebrated powder for arresting hemorrhage, said to be nothing more than the charcoal of beech wood finely pulverized.

POWDER, FEVER, SCHWANBERG'S, Antimonial powder.

POWDER-FOLDER. In Pharmacy, an apparatus by which papers containing powders are folded of the desired length.

POWDER, GINGER-BEER, see Amomum zingiber — p. Gout, Duke of Portland's, Pulvis Ducis Portlandiæ — p. of Burnt hartshorn with opium, Pulvis cornu cervi cum opio — p. Ipecacuanha compound, Pulvis ipecacuanhæ compositus — p. of Jalap, compound, Pulvis jalapæ compositus — p. James's, factitious, Antimonial powder — p. Jesuit's, Cinchona — p. of Kino, compound, Pulvis kino compositus — p. of Lemonade, see Lemonade — p. of Magnesia, compound, Pulvis de magnesiâ compositus — p. of the Marquis, Marchionis pulvis — p. Mead's, against the bite of a Mad dog, Pulvis antilyssus — p. Myrrh, compound, Pulvis myrrhæ compositus — p. Portland, Pulvis Ducis Portlandiæ — p. of the three Sanders, see Diatrium — p. Scammony and aloes, Pulvis scammonii cum aloe — p. Scammony compound, Pulvis scammoniæ compositus — p. of Senna, compound, Pulvis sennæ compositus — p. Sneezing, see Veratrum album — p. Spruce beer, see Spruce beer —

p. Tennant's, Calcis chloridum — p. Tooth, Dentifricium — p. Tragacanth, compound, Pulvis tragacanthæ compositus.

POWDER, VIEN'NA, is composed of equal parts of quicklime and potassa cum calce. In using it, it is made into a paste — *Vienna paste*, (F.) *Caustique de Vienne* — with spirits of wine, and is applied on the diseased part, previously circumscribed by a hole cut in a sticking plaster.

To be left on from 10 to 20 minutes, according to the depth of the eschar required. Used in cases of lupous ulceration.

By fusing the potass and lime, and raising the heat so as to cause ebullition, the caustic may be run into cylinders: — when it is called *Caustique-Filhos, Caus'ticum Viennen'sè fusum Filhos*, from the name of the author of the process.

POWDERS, CASTILLON, so called from the name of the physician who first proposed them. They are formed of *sago*, in powder; *salep*, in powder; *tragacanth*, in powder, each, four parts; *prepared oyster-shells*, one part, *cochineal*, half a part, divided into powders of one drachm each; one of which is given three or four times a day as a demulcent in diarrhœa and dysentery.

POWDERS, SODA, *Pul'veres effervescen'tes*, (F.) *Poudres gasifères simples. (Sodæ carb.* ʒss, in each *blue* paper; *tartaric acid*, gr. xxv in each *white* paper; for half a pint of water.) A pleasant, cooling drink; taken during the effervescence.

Seidlitz Powders, (F.) *Poudres gasifères laxatives* ou *Poudres de Seidlitz*, contain one or two drachms of tartrate of potassa and soda, added to the alkali in the blue paper.

POWER, Faculty — p. Inherent, Irritability — p. Tonic, Irritability.

POX, Syphilis, Variola — p. Chicken, Varicella — p. Doctor, Syphilidiater — p. French, Syphilis — p. Grease, see Grease — p. Noddle, Syphilomania — p. Small, Variola — p. Swine, see Varicella — p. Water, see Varicella.

POZZUOLI, MINERAL WATERS OF. Pozzuoli is in the neighbourhood of Naples. The springs are, 1. *Acqua della pietra*, Temp. 91° Fah. 2. *Acqua di Cavalcanti*, Temp. 100°. *A. di subveni homini*, Temp. 102°; *A. del cantarello*, Temp. 86 to 89°; and that of the Temple of Serapis in Pozzuoli, Temp. 102 to 107°. The last contains carbonic acid, carbonates of lime, magnesia, alumina, and iron, carbonate of soda, chloride of sodium, sulphate of lime, and silica.

PRACTICE OF PHYSIC, Therapeutics.

PRACTITIONER, GENERAL, Surgeon apothecary — p. Irregular, see Irregular — p. Regular, see Regular — p. Routine, Routinist.

PRÆBIUM, Dose.

PRÆCAUTIO, Prophylaxis.

PRÆCIPITANS MAGNUM, Sepia.

PRÆCIPITATUM ALBUM, Hydrargyrum præcipitatum.

PRÆCIPITATUS RUBER, Hydrargyri nitrico-oxydum.

PRÆCISIO PRÆPUTII, Circumcision.

PRÆCOCIA, Prunus Armeniaca.

PRÆCOCITY, Præotia.

PRÆCOGNITIO, Prognosis.

PRÆCORD'IA, from *præ*, 'before,' and *cor*, 'the heart.' The diaphragm; also, the thoracic viscera, and the epigastrium.

PRÆCOR'DIAL or PRECORDIAL REGION, *Re'gio præcordiaca* seu *præcordia'lis*, is the epigastric region. Also, and more properly, the region of the heart. A line drawn from the inferior margins of the third ribs across the sternum, passes over the valves of the pulmonary artery a little to the left of the mesial line, and those of the aorta are behind them, but about half an inch lower down. A vertical line, coinciding with the left margin of the sternum, has about one-third of the heart, comprising the upper portion of the right ventricle, on the right,—and two-thirds, comprising the lower portion of the right ventricle and the whole of the left, on the left. This is the præcordial region.

PRÆCORDIUM, *Fossette du cœur*—p. Pedis, Metatarsus.

PRÆCOX MATURITAS, Præotia.

PRÆCUSTODIA, Prophylaxis.

PRÆDICTIO, Prognosis.

PRÆDISPOSITIO, Predisposition.

PRÆDIVINATIO, Mantia.

PRÆDOMIN'IUM; from *præ*, 'before,' and *dominus*, 'a lord.' Predominance of one thing over another.

PRÆDOMIN'IUM AQUÆ. A predominance of watery fluid,—*Tenu'itas aquo'sa*.

PRÆDOMINIUM SAN'GUINIS ARTERIO'SI. A predominance of arterial blood, *Arterios'itas san'guinis*.

PRÆDOMIN'IUM SAN'GUINIS VENO'SI, *Venos'itas San'guinis*. Predominance of venous blood.

PRÆFOCATIO, Orthopnœa, Suffocation — p. Faucium, Angone—p. Matricis, Angone—p. Uterina, Angone.

PRÆFOCATION, Strangulatio uterina.

PRÆGNANS, Pregnant.

PRÆGNAS, Pregnant.

PRÆGNATIO, Fecundation, Pregnancy.

PRÆGNATUS, Fecundation, Pregnancy.

PRÆGNAX, Pregnant.

PRÆGUSTATIO, *Avant-gout*.

PRÆHENSIO, Prehensio.

PRÆLIN'GUA. The anterior part or tip of the tongue.

PRÆLIUM, Coition, Press, Tourniquet—p. Arteriale, Tourniquet.

PRÆLUMBARIS, Prelumbar.

PRÆNOTIO, Prognosis.

PRÆNUNTIATIO, Prognosis.

PRÆPARATIO, Preparation—p. Chyli, Chylification.

PRÆPARATUM, Preparation.

PRÆPOTEN'TIA, from *præ*, 'before,' and *potens*, 'powerful.' Great power or strength.

PRÆPOTEN'TIA VIRI'LIS. Great, or too great procreative power on the part of the male.

PRÆPOTIO, Propotismos.

PRÆPUTIALIS, Preputial.

PRÆPUTIUM, Prepuce.

PRÆSAGIUM, Mantia.

PRÆSCIENTIA, Prognosis.

PRÆSCITIO, Prognosis.

PRÆSCRIPTIO, Prescription.

PRÆSEPIOLUM, Alveolus.

PRÆSEPIUM, Alveolus.

PRÆSERVATIO, Prophylaxis.

PRÆSERVATIVUM, Amuletum.

PRÆSERVATO'RIA INDICA'TIO. A preservative indication; one proper for preventing the development of disease.

PRÆSERVATORIUS, Prophylactic.

PRÆSPINALIS, Prespinal.

PRÆTIBIALIS, Pretibial.

PRAIRIE BUSH, STINKING, Ptelea trifoliata—p. Pines, Liatris.

PRASINUM VIRIDE, Cupri subacetas.

PRASINUS, Porraceous.

PRASI'TES, from *prasium*, 'horehound.' Wine in which the leaves of horehound have been infused.

PRASIUM, Marrubium.

PRASUM, Allium Prasum.

PRAXIS, Action.

PRAXIS MED'ICA. The practical exercise of the healing art.

PRECIPITATE, RED, Hydrargyri nitrico-oxydum — p. White, Hydrargyrum præcipitatum.

PRECIPITA'TION, *Præcipita'tio*, (F.) *Précipité*, from *præcipitare*, (*præ*, 'before,' and *caput*, 'the head,') 'to throw *headlong*.' The action by which a body abandons a liquid in which it is dissolved, and becomes deposited at the bottom of the vessel. The matter, so thrown down or precipitated, is called a *precipitate*.

PRÉCIPITATION DE LA MATRICE, Procidentia uteri.

PRÉCIPITÉ BLANC, Hydrargyrum præcipitatum.

PRECORDIAL, Præcordial.

PRECUR'SORY, *Præcurso'rius*; from *præ*, 'before,' and *curro*, *cursum*, 'I run.' That which precedes.

PRECUR'SORY or PREMON'ITORY SIGNS or SYMPTOMS, (F.) *Signes précurseurs*, S. *avant coureurs*, are those which indicate an approaching disease.

PREDISPONENT CAUSES, see Causes, predisponent.

PREDISPOSIT''ION, *Prædisposit''io*, *Semin'ia morbo'rum* (Gaubius); from *præ*, 'before,' and *disponere*, 'to dispose.' (F.) *Imminence morbide*. That constitution or condition of the body, which disposes it to the action of disease under the application of an exciting cause. Thus, in hereditary diseases, the conformation is such, that but a slight exciting cause may be required to produce them. When the disease arises solely from the predisposition, or under the additional influence of an extremely slight exciting cause, it is, by some, termed a *disposition*.

PREDOR'SAL, *Prædorsa'lis*, from *præ*, 'before,' and *dorsum*, 'the back.'

PRÆDORSAL REGION of the vertebral column is the anterior surface of the dorsal region.

PRÉ-DORSO-ATLOÏDIEN, Longus colli.

PRÉ-DORSO-CERVICAL, Longus colli.

PREG'NANCY, *Prægna'tio*, *Pregna'tus*, *Impregna'tio*, *Ingravida'tio*, *Ingravida'tion*, from *præ*, 'before,' and *genere*, 'to beget.' *Hysterocye'sis*, *Gravid'itas*, *G. uteri'na*, *En'cymon*, *Cye'sis*, *Encye'sis*, *En'cyesis*, *Encymo'sia*, *Cyopho'ria*, *Gestation*, *Fœta'tion*, *Utero-gesta'tion*; (F.) *Grossesse*. The state of a female who has within her a fecundated germ, which gradually becomes developed in or out of the uterus. When placed in the cavity of the uterus,—by virtue of the vital principle which animates it, it becomes attached to the inner surface of that viscus, and obtains from it indirectly the nutriment necessary for its gradual development, during the space of ten lunar months or two hundred and eighty days — the ordinary term or *duration of gestation*, although the period may be protracted to 300 days or upwards,—at the expiration of which parturition occurs. Pregnancy is commonly limited to a single fœtus: at times, the uterus contains two or three.—See Reproduction. Occasionally, one or two moles—the degenerated products of conception—alone occupy the uterus :—at other times, a fœtus likewise exists. In certain cases, and owing to accidental circumstances, the fecundated ovum remains in the ovarium, or is arrested in the Fallopian tube. Pregnancy has, accordingly, been distinguished into, 1. *Natural* or *uterine*, when the fœtus is carried in the cavity of the womb: and, 2. *Præternatural* or *extra-uterine*, *Exfœta'tion*. *Conceptio vitio'sa*, *Paracye'sis* seu *Ecrye'sis*, *Ecthyaterocye'sis*, *Echthysterocye'sis*, *Dyato'cia*, *Dysoye sis* seu *Gravid'itas extra-uteri'na*, (F.) *Grossesse-contre-nature*,—when it occurs in the ovarium, tube, or cavity of the abdomen.

During pregnancy, the female experiences remarkable changes in the condition of her organs and functions. The genital apparatus is, of course, most affected. The uterus changes its shape, situation, size, and texture. The usual signs of pregnancy are,—suppression of the catamenia; the abdomen gradually enlarging and forming a hard tumour; the umbilicus prominent in the latter months; the breasts increasing in size; the areola round the nipple becoming darker and the follicles more developed; kyestein in the urine from an early period; a bluish tint of the vagina after the fourth week; about the fifth month, the evidence by *ballottement*, and the placental *souffle* and sound of the fœtal heart heard on auscultation; the motion of the fœtus perceptible, and the neck of the uterus diminishing in length at the advanced periods.

PREGNANCY, ABDOM'INAL, *Eccye'sis abdomina'lis, Cœliocye'sis, Gravid'itas abdomina'lis,* (F.) *Grossesse abdominale.* That in which the ovum has escaped into the cavity of the abdomen.

PREGNANCY, AFŒ'TAL, *Pregnancy without a fœtus,* (F.) *Grossesse afœtale, G. sans fœtus.* Pregnancy produced by a false or degenerate conception, or any other affection, which has given place to unusual development of the uterus. Madame Boivin includes in this class, *sarco-hysteric, hydro-hysteric, gazo-hysteric,* and *hemato-hysteric pregnancies.*

PREGNANCY, BIGEM'INAL, (F.) *Grossesse bigéminale, Double pregnancy.* Pregnancy in which there are twins in utero.—Madame Boivin.

PREGNANCY, COMPLEX, (F.) *Grossesse complexe, G. inter-extra utérine,* is when the womb, besides a fœtus, contains much water, hydatids, a mole, &c.

PREGNANCY, COMPOUND, *Polybreph'ia, Polycye'sia. Polycye'sis,* (F.) *Grossesse composée,* is when there are two or three fœtuses in the cavity of the uterus.

PREGNANCY, DOUBLE, Pregnancy, bigeminal—p. Duration of, see Pregnancy—p. Extra-uterine, see Pregnancy.

PREG'NANCY, FALSE, *Gravid'itas spuria,* (F.) *Grossesse fausse* ou *apparente, Pseudocye'sis.* Authors have called thus different affections of a more or less serious character, which resemble pregnancy; so as, at times, to impose upon the best-informed practitioners. These diseases may be seated in the uterus or its dependencies, in the intestines or some other part of the abdomen. They may be;—a mole, hydatids, water, blood, or polypus distending the parietes of the uterus; — chronic enlargement of the uterus; development of tumours, &c., in its substance;—scirrhus; dropsy of the ovaria; ascites; tympanites, &c.

PREGNANCY, FŒTAL, (F.) *Grossesse fœtale.* Pregnancy in which there is a fœtus, or more than one, in the uterus or out of it. Madame Boivin puts in this class—the *solitary, bigeminal, trigeminal,* and *sarco-fœtal* pregnancies, which form the first order; and the *tubal, ovarial,* and *abdominal,* which constitute the second.

PREGNANCY, GAZO-HYSTER'IC, (F.) *Grossesse Gazo-hystérique.* Afœtal pregnancy, caused by development of air or gas in the cavity of the womb.—Madame Boivin.

PREGNANCY, HÆMATO-HYSTERIC, (F.) *Grossesse hémato-hystérique.* Afœtal pregnancy, caused by accumulation of blood in the uterus.—Madame Boivin.

PREGNANCY, HYDRO-HYSTERIC, (F.) *Grossesse hydro-hystérique.* Afœtal pregnancy, occasioned by the secretion and accumulation of serous fluid in the uterus.

PREGNANCY, INTERSTIT"IAL, *Gravid'itas in uteri substan'tiâ, Gravid'itas interstitia'lis.* The development of the embryo in the proper substance of the uterus. The case generally terminates fatally at an early period of gestation; the thin external paries of the uterus being ruptured, and the ovum passing into the abdominal cavity.

PREGNANCY, MORBID, *Paracye'sis, Dysto'cia, Dyscye'sis.* The progress of pregnancy disturbed or endangered by the supervention of general or local disorder.— Good.

PREGNANCY, OVA'RIAN, (F.) *Grossesse ovarienne* ou *de l'ovaire, Eccye'sis ova'ria, Oäriocye'sis, Oöcye'sis, Gravid'itas extra-uteri'na in ova'rio.* Pregnancy in which the fœtus is developed in the interior of the ovary.

PREGNANCY, PLEA OF. A plea, which a woman, capitally convicted, may set up in arrest of execution until she is delivered. See Jury of Matrons, and De ventre inspiciendo.

PREGNANCY, PRETEND'ED. The criminal act of a female, who, not having been delivered, presents an infant as having been born of her. (F.) *Supposition de part.* (This term, in French, likewise includes the case of a female, who, having been delivered of a dead child, substitutes for it a living child which is not hers.)

PREGNANCY, SARCO-FŒTAL, (F.) *Grossesse sarco-fœtale.* Pregnancy in which there are one or more fœtuses, and one or more moles.—Madame Boivin.

PREGNANCY, SARCO-HYSTERIC, (F.) *Grossesse sarco-hystérique.* Afœtal pregnancy formed by moles, hydatids, or a false conception.—Madame Boivin.

PREGNANCY, SOL'ITARY, (F.) *Grossesse solitaire* ou *simple.* Pregnancy in which there is a single fœtus.—Madame Boivin.

PREGNANCY, TRIGEM'INAL, (F.) *Grossesse trigéminale* ou *triple.* Pregnancy in which there are three fœtuses in the cavity of the uterus.—Madame Boivin.

PREGNANCY, TUBAL, (F.) *Grossesse tubaire, Eccye'sis tuba'lis.* Pregnancy where the fœtus remains and is developed in the Fallopian tube.

PREGNANCY, UTERINE, see Pregnancy.

PREGNANCY, UTERO-ABDOM'INAL, (F.) *Grossesse utéro-abdominale.* Pregnancy consisting of two fœtuses; one in the uterus—the other in the abdominal cavity.—Madame Boivin.

PREGNANCY, UTERO-OVA'RIAL, (F.) *Grossesse utéro-ovarienne.* Pregnancy with two fœtuses, one in the womb, the other in the ovary.

PREGNANCY, UTERO-TUBAL, (F.) *Grossesse utéro-tubaire.* Pregnancy in which there is at the same time a fœtus in the womb and another in the Fallopian tube.

PREGNANT, *Prægnans, Prægnas, Prægnax, Encar'pos, Grav'ida, Plena mu'lier, Incinc'ta, Gravid, Breeding,* (F.) *Enceinte.* One in a state of pregnancy;—one with child.

PREHENSIO, Catalepsy, Epilepsy.

PREHEN'SION, *Prehen'sio,* from *prehendere,* 'to lay hold of.'

PREHENSION OF FOOD is the act of carrying it to the mouth, and introducing it into that cavity. It is, also, called *Assump'tio, Proslep'sis, Pros'phora.*

PRÊLE, Hippuris vulgaris.

PRÉLOMBAIRE, Prelumbar.

PRÉLOMBO-PUBIEN, Psoas parvus — p. Trochantin, Psoas magnus.

PRELUM, Press — p. Arteriale, Tourniquet.

PRELUM'BAR, *Prælumba'ris,* (F.) *Prélombaire,* from *præ,* 'before,' and *lumbi,* 'the loins.' That which is placed before the loins. The prelumbar surface of the spinal column is the anterior surface of the lumbar portion.

PREMONITORY, see Precursory.

PRENAN'THES, *Gall of the Earth, Dewis Snakeroot, Lion's Foot.* There are many species of this indigenous plant, whose root and milky juice are very bitter. They are used in popular practice in dysentery; and in the form of cataplasm to bites of serpents.

PRENANTHES SERPENTARIA, Nabalus albus.
PRENDRE INSCRIPTION, see Matriculate.
PREPARA'TION, *Præpara'tio*, from *præ*, 'before,' and *parare*, *paratum*, 'to get ready.' The act of making ready any substance whatever that has to be employed for any purpose.

Also, the product of any pharmaceutical operation;—*Præpara'tum*.

Any part of the human body, preserved for the uses of the anatomist, is so called.

PREP'UCE, *Præpu'tium*, perhaps from πρός, and ποσθή, 'the foreskin.' *Epago'gium*, *Posthē*, *Pella*, *Pos'thium*, *Pu'tium*, *Foreskin*. The prolongation of the integuments of the penis, which covers the glans. The prepuce is composed of two membranous layers: one external or cutaneous; the other internal or mucous, separated by areolar membrane. The mucous membrane lines the inner surface of the cutaneous layer till beyond the glans, when it is reflected over the latter; forming, behind the corona, a small cul-de-sac above the corpora cavernosa, which is interrupted by a triangular duplicature of the mucous membrane, called the *frænum*, fixed in the furrow at the inferior part of the glans, and terminating at a little distance from the orifice of the urethra. The clitoris is covered by a semilunar fold formed by a continuation of the skin of the labia. It is called *Præpu'tium clitor'idis*.

PREPU'TIAL, *Præputia'lis*; same etymon. Belonging or relating to the prepuce;—as the 'preputial secretion,'—or that which takes place from the lining of the prepuce covering the glans.

PRESBYODOCHIUM, Gerocomium.

PRESBYON'OSI; from πρεσβυς, 'old,' and νοσος, 'disease.' Diseases of old age.

PRESBYOPIA, Presbytia.

PRESBYSPHACELUS, Gangrene of old people.

PRESBYT'IA, *Presbyo'pia*, *Amblyo'pia proximo'rum*, *Visus seni'lis*, *Pres'byopy*, (F.) *Vue longue;* from πρεσβυς, 'an old person.' A very high degree is termed *Hyperpresbyt'ia*. A condition of vision, common in old persons, which consists in the circumstance of near objects being confusedly seen, whilst those at a greater distance are clearly distinguished. It is supposed to depend generally on diminution of the convexity of the cornea; whence results an alteration in the convergency of the rays, so that they form a focus behind the retina. This defect is remedied by the use of convex glasses, which augment the convergence of the luminous rays. It is, also, called *Long-sightedness*, *Parop'sis longin'qua*, *Dyso'pia proximo'rum*.

PRESCRIP'TION, *Præscrip'tio*, *Anag'raphē*, from *præ*, 'before,' and *scribere*, 'to write.' *For'mula med'ica*, *Præscrip'tio med'ica*, *Recep'tum*, (F.) *Formule*, *Ordonnance*. The formula which the physician writes for the composition of medicine adapted to any case of disease. A prescription should be as simple as possible, and should bear upon its face the evidence of the objects to be fulfilled by it. No article should form part of it, unless adapted for serving some useful purpose. A compound prescription has been divided into four parts:—the *basis* or principal ingredient of the prescription; the *ad'juvans*, or that which is designed to promote the action of the former; the *cor'rigens*, or that intended to correct its operation, or obviate any unpleasant symptom which it may be apt to produce; and the *constit'uens*, *excip'ient*, or substance which gives to the other ingredients consistence or form. All these are seen in the following formula for cathartic pills:

Aloes.....................ʒj.............Basis.
Hyd. Chlorid. mit. gr. x.............Adjuvans.
Olei Carui ....gtt. v ....Corrigens.
Syrupi...................q. s...........Constituens.
M. et fiant. Pilulæ xx. See Symbol.

It is obvious, however, that most prescriptions are more simple than this. The basis, for example, may require neither adjuvant, corrigent, nor constituent.

Dr. Paris has given the following synopsis of the principles of medicinal combination, *Iamatotaxiolog''ia*, *Iamatosyntaxiolog''ia*, which may serve as an instructive guide to the prescriber:—

OBJECT I.
TO PROMOTE THE ACTION OF THE BASIS.

A. By combining the several different forms or preparations of the *same substance*. B. By combining the basis with substances which are of the same nature; i. e., which are individually capable of producing the same effects, with less energy than when in combination with each other. C. By combining the basis with substances of a *different nature*, and which do not exert any chemical influence upon it, but are found by experience, or inferred by analogy, to be capable of rendering the stomach or system more susceptible of its action.

OBJECT II.
TO CORRECT THE OPERATION OF THE BASIS BY OBVIATING ANY UNPLEASANT EFFECTS IT MIGHT BE LIKELY TO OCCASION, AND WHICH WOULD PERVERT ITS INTENDED ACTION, AND DEFEAT THE OBJECT OF ITS EXHIBITION.

A. By *chymically* neutralizing or *mechanically* separating the offending ingredient. B. By adding some substance calculated to guard the stomach or system against its deleterious effects.

OBJECT III.
TO OBTAIN THE JOINT OPERATION OF TWO OR MORE MEDICINES.

A. By uniting those medicines which are calculated to produce the *same ultimate results*, but by modes of operation totally different. B. By combining medicines which have entirely different powers; and which are required to obviate different symptoms, or to answer different indications.

OBJECT IV.
TO OBTAIN A NEW AND ACTIVE REMEDY, NOT AFFORDED BY ANY SINGLE SUBSTANCE.

A. By combining medicines which excite different actions in the stomach and system, in consequence of which *new* or *modified* results are produced. B. By combining substances which have the property of acting *chymically* upon each other; the results of which are:—a. The formation of new compounds; b. The decomposition of the original ingredients, and the development of the more active elements. C. By combining substances, between which no other change is induced than a diminution or increase in the *solubility* of the principles in which their medicinal virtues reside. a. By the intervention of substances that act *chymically*. b. By the addition of ingredients whose operation is entirely mechanical.

OBJECT V.
TO AFFORD AN ELIGIBLE FORM.

a. By which the *efficacy* of the remedy is enhanced. b. By which its *aspect* or *flavour* is rendered more agreeable, or its mode of administration more convenient. c. By which it is *preserved* from the spontaneous decomposition to which it is liable.

[The vocabulary in the author's "Medical Student," Philad. 1844, will aid the student, not only in translating, but in writing his prescriptions *more solito*.]

PRESENTA'TION, from (Lat.) *præsens*, (*præ*, 'before,' and *ens*, 'being.') The part of a fœtus which is felt *presenting*, on examination *per vaginam*. When the head presents, and especially the vertex, or the feet, knees, or breech, the presentation is said to be *natural*: when any other part, *preternatural*, and the labour is styled *perverse* or *preternatural*, *Parodyn'ia perver'sa*, *Dysto'cia perver'sa*, *Cross-birth*, (F.) *Accouchement contre nature*. When any part besides the head, feet, knees, or breech presents, the operation of *turning* becomes necessary. See Parturition.

PRESIS, Swelling.

PRÈSLE, Hippuris vulgaris.

PRESMA, Swelling.

PRESPI'NAL, *Præspina'lis*, from *præ*, 'before,' and *spina*, 'the spine.' That which is situate before the spine. The prespinal surface of the vertebral column is the anterior surface.

PRESS, *Præ'lium*, *Præ'lium*, *Presso'rium*, *Piester*, *Pieste'rion*, (F.) *Pressoir*, *Presse*. An instrument for subjecting matters to considerable pressure, for the purpose of separating the liquid from the solid portion.

PRESS OF HEROPHILUS, Torcular Herophili.

PRESSE-ARTÈRE. An instrument invented by Deschamps for the immediate compression of arteries. It is composed of a plate six or seven lines long, and three broad, and of a rod or stem two inches long, placed perpendicularly above the plate and riveted. At each extremity of the plate is a hole, through which each of the ends of the ligature, to be placed upon the artery, is passed. The ligature is then to be tightened by drawing the ends, and fixing them to the perpendicular rod. This *presse-artère* or *serre-artère*, surrounded with charpie, remains in the wound, until there is no longer danger of hemorrhage. The ligature is then cut, and the instrument withdrawn. It is an unnecessary instrument.

PRESSE-URÈTHRE, *Jugum Penis*. A kind of forceps of elastic iron, the branches of which, padded, may be approximated or separated by means of a screw. The penis is introduced between the branches, one of them being applied to the urethra, and the screw is tightened so as to exercise a degree of pressure sufficient to bring the parietes of the canal in contact. This instrument is sometimes used in incontinence of urine, to prevent the constant discharge of that fluid.

PRESSIO, Pressure.

PRESSION ABDOMINALE, Pressure, abdominal.

PRESSOIR, Press—*p. d'Hérophile*, Torcular Herophili.

PRESSORIUM, Press.

PRESSURE, *Pres'sio*, from *premo*, *pressum*, 'I press.' The action of pressing.

PRESSURE, ABDOM'INAL, (F.) *Pression abdominale*. A mode of examination by means of which the sensibility, size, suppleness, or hardness of any morbid abdominal viscus may be compared, in these respects, with its healthy condition. Bichat proposed, with the view of exploring the state of the thoracic organs, to exert a pressure from below upwards on the abdominal organs, so as to crowd them upon the diaphragm, and thus to diminish the dimensions of the cavity of the chest, noticing to what extent respiration was affected by this action. No great information can of course be derived from it.

PRETENDED DISEASES, Feigned diseases.

PRETIB'IAL, *Prætibia'lis*, from *præ*, 'before,' and *tibia*, 'the tibia.' That which is situate before the tibia; as the *ilio-pretibial* and *ischiopretibial* muscles.

PREVEN'TIVE, ROYAL, from *prævenire*, (*præ*, and *venire*,) 'to come before.' An empirical preparation, used as a prophylactic against the venereal virus. It is a solution of *acetate of lead*,—the Liquor Plumbi Subacetatis dilutus.

PREVER'TEBRAL APONEURO'SIS. The aponeurosis which covers the muscles of the prevertebral region.

PREVERTEBRAL ARTERY. A ramus of the meningeal branch, and sometimes even of the trunk, of the pharyngeal artery, which is distributed to the prevertebral region.

PREVERTEBRAL MUSCLES, see Cervical region, anterior — p. Region, Cervical region, anterior.

PRIAPEIA, Nicotiana rustica.

PRIAPIS'COS. Same etymon as the next. Name of a piece of wood which forms part of the *scamnum Hippocraticum*. Paulus of Ægina calls thus a tent of linen shaped like a penis.

PRIAPIS'MUS, *Tenti'go*, *T. Penis*, *Pri'apism*, *Horn-colic* (vulg.), *Enta'sia Priapis'mus*, *Rhopalis'mus*, *Satyri'asis*, *Styma*, *Stysis*, from Πριαπος, Priapus, 'the male organ.' Constant and distressing erection, without any voluptuous idea or desire for venery. It is often symptomatic; and sometimes the immediate result of morbific causes,—of the action of cantharides, for example. The application of cold liquids to the penis, and the internal use of opium and camphor, are the means usually had recourse to for its removal.

PRIAPITIS, Phallitis.

PRIA'PUS, *Mutun'nus*. In ancient mythology the deity who presided over gardens and the parts of generation, so called *propter deformitatem et membri virilis magnitudinem*.

PRIAPUS, Penis—p. Cervi, see Cervus—p. Ceti, Leviathian penis.

PRICKING, Sax. ppiccian, (D.) pricken, (F.) *Picotement*. A variety of pain, compared to that which pointed bodies would occasion.

PRIDE OF CHINA, Melia azedarach—p. of India, Melia azedarach—p. Tree, Melia azedarach.

PRIEST-PHYSICIANS, see Asclepiadæ.

PRIEST'S PINTLE, Arum maculatum.

PRIMA CELLA COLI, Cæcum.

PRIMÆ VLÆ. The *first passages*. The stomach and intestinal canal:—the lacteals being the *secun'dæ vi'æ* or *second passages*. See Ways, digestive.

PRIMARY CELL, see Cell.

PRIMEVÈRE, Primula veris.

PRIMIP'ARA, *Primipartu'riens*, from *primus*, 'first,' and *parere*, 'to bring forth.' A name given to a female who brings forth for the first time.

PRIMIPARTURIENS, Primipara.

PRIMI-STERNAL, *Primi-sterna'lis*, from *primus*, 'the first,' and *sternum*, 'the sternum.' M. Béclard has called *os primi-sternal* or *clavi-sternal*, the bony portion of the sternum.

PRIMIT"IÆ. The *first waters*, or *the waters* discharged before the extrusion of the fœtus.

PRIMITIVE BAND, see Nerve fibres—p. Streak, Groove, primitive.

PRIMORDIAL CELL, see Cell.

PRIMORDIUM, Arche.

PRIMROSE, EVENING, Œnothera biennis—p. Tree, Œnothera biennis.

PRIMULA OFFICINALIS, P. veris—p. Variabilis, P. veris.

PRIM'ULA VERIS, *P. officina'lis seu variab'ilis*, from *prim'ulus*, 'the beginning.' So called, because it flowers in the beginning of the spring. *Verbas'culum, Paral'ysis, Herba paralys'eos seu paralyt'ica*, the *Cowslip, Paigil* or *Peagle*, (F.) *Primevère. Family*, Primulaceæ. *Sex. Syst.* Pentandria Monogynia. The flowers have been considered to be mildly tonic, antispasmodic, and anodyne.

PRIMULA VULGA'RIS. The leaves and roots of this plant have been used as sternutatories.

PRINCEPS, Rectum.

PRINCEPS CERVI'CIS (*Artery*), *Cervical Artery*. A branch of the occipital artery, which descends between the splenius and complexus muscles, and may be followed down to the lower part of the neck.

PRINCEPS POL'LICIS (*Arteria*), *Arte'ria magna pol'licis*. When the two collateral arteries of the thumb take origin from a common trunk—the trunk is the *Princeps pollicis*.

PRINCIPE CRYSTALLIZABLE DE DÉROSNE, Narcotine.

PRINCIPES IMMEDIATS, Principles, immediate.

PRINCIPIUM, Arche, Element — p. Acidificans, Oxygen—p. Adstringens, Tannin—p. Byrsodepsicum, Tannin — p. Coriaceum, Tannin—p. Hydrogeneticum, Hydrogen — p. Hydroticum, Hydrogen—p. Oxygenans, Oxygen—p. Salivale, see Saliva— p. Scytodepsicum, Tannin—p. Urinosum, Urea.

PRIN'CIPLE, COL'OURING, OF THE BLOOD. A name, given to the immediate principle in animals, to which the blood owes its red colour. It is solid, inodorous, and insipid. When recently separated from blood, it has a purplered colour. When distilled, it furnishes, amongst other products, a purple oil. It is insoluble in water; but, if diluted with that liquid, acquires a vinous-red hue. It communicates a red colour to the albumen of the blood, and affords, on analysis, iron, to which the colour has been ascribed. See Hæmaphæin, and Hæmatin.

PRINCIPLE, DIGESTIVE, Pepsin — p. Vital, see Vital principle.

PRINCIPLES, IMME'DIATE, (F.) *Principes immédiats, Matériaux immédiats*. A name given to a considerable number of substances, composed of at least three elements, and which are obtained from animals and vegetables without alteration, by simple processes, and, in some measure, *immediately*.

PRINCIPLES, IMMEDIATE, OF ANIMALS, *Proximate principles, Organic Elements, Compounds of Organization*. These are divided into acid principles, fatty principles, and principles which are neither fat nor acid. The first include the *uric, rosacic, purpuric, allantoic, caseic, butyric*, &c. The fatty principles are: — *stearin, elain, cholesterin*, &c.; and the last division includes the most important compounds of organization: —*fibrin, gelatin, albumen, casein, osmazome*, &c.

PRINCIPLES, PROXIMATE, P. immediate.

PRINOS, *P. verticilla'tus, Alcan'na major latifo'lia dentu'ta, Aquifo'lium fo'liis decid'uis, Prinos Grono'vii, Prinos padifolius, Black Alder, Virginia Winterberry, Whorled Winterberry, Feverbush*, (F.) *Apalachine à feuilles de Prunier*. *Ord.* Aquifollaceæ. *Sex. Syst.* Hexandria Monogynia. The bark of this common shrub of the United States is astringent, bitter, and pungent. The berries are, likewise, bitter. The bark has been used as a substitute for the cinchona, in intermittents, and as a tonic.

PRINOS GRONOVII, Prinos.

PRINOS LÆVIGA'TUS, Smooth Winterberry. Indigenous; has the same properties as PRINOS PADIFOLIUS, Prinos.

PRION, Saw.

PRIONO'DES, from πρίων, 'a saw,' and εἶδος, 'shape.' *Serra'ted*. Applied to the sutures of the head.

PRIOR ANNULA'RIS, *Interos'seus quartus* of Winslow. An internal interosseous muscle, which arises from the outside of the metacarpal bone of the ring-finger, and is inserted into the outside of the tendon on the back of the ring-finger. Its use is to draw the ring-finger outwards.

PRIOR IN'DICIS, *Exten'sor ter'tii interos'dii in'dicis*, (P.) *Sous-métacarpo-latéri-phalangien*. It arises from the outer or radial side of the metacarpal bone of the fore-finger, and is inserted into the outside of the tendon on the back of the fore-finger. *Action:* — to draw the finger outwards, towards the thumb.

PRIOR INDICIS PEDIS, *Adductor In'dicis pedis*. An external, interosseous muscle of the foot, which arises from the contiguous sides of the metatarsal bones of the great and fore toes, and is inserted into the inside of the root of the first bone of the fore-toe. *Action:* — to pull the fore-toe inwards.

PRIOR MEDII, Prior medii digiti.

PRIOR ME'DII DIG"ITI, *Prior Medii, Second interos'seous* of Douglas. An external, interosseous muscle of the hand, which arises from the corresponding sides of the metacarpal bones of the fore and middle fingers, and is inserted into the outside of the tendon on the back of the middle finger. *Action:* — to draw the middle finger outwards.

PRIOR MEDII DIGITI PEDIS, *Adductor medii digiti pedis*. An internal, interosseous muscle of the foot, which arises from the inside of the metatarsal bone of the middle toe, and is inserted into the inside of the root of the first bone of the middle toe. *Use:*—to pull the middle toe inwards, or towards the inner side of the foot.

PRIOR MIN'IMI DIGITI, *Adduc'tor min'imi dig'iti*. An internal, interosseous muscle of the foot, which originates from the inside of the metatarsal bone of the little toe, and is inserted into the inside of the root of the first bone of the little toe. *Action:* — to pull the little toe inwards.

PRIOR TERTII DIGITI PEDIS, *Adduc'tor tertii dig"iti pedis*. An internal, interosseous muscle of the foot, which arises from the inner and under part of the metatarsal bone of the third of the small toes, and is inserted into the inside of the root of the first bone of the third of the small toes. *Action:* — to pull the third of the small toes inwards.

PRISIS, Brygmus, Trepanning.

PRISMA, Scobs.

PRISMUS, Brygmus, Trepanning.

PRIVATE PARTS, Genital organs.

PRIVET, Ligustrum vulgare.

PRIVITIES, Genital organs.

PRIVY, Ligustrum vulgare—p. Members, Genital organs — p. Parts, Genital organs.

PRO, πρό, 'before.' A common prefix to words, as in *Procatarctic, Prostate*, &c.

PROAGOREUSIS, Prognosis.

PROBANG, *Detruso'rium ex bale'na*. A long slender rod of whalebone, with a piece of sponge at its extremity, intended to push down extraneous bodies, arrested in the œsophagus, into the stomach. A similar instrument is called by J. L. Petit, *Repoussoir d'arêtes*.

PROBARBIUM, Geneias.

PROBASCANIUM, Amuletum.

PROBASCANTIUM, Amuletum.

PROBE, Catheterize, Specillum — p. Eyed, see Specillum.
PROBING, see Melosis.
PROBOLE, Processus.
PROCARDIUM, Scrobiculus cordis.
PROCÉDÉ, Process.
PROCEDURE, *Procédé*.
PROCEPHALI, Capitones.
PROCERUS NASI, Pyramidalis nasi.
PROCÈS CILIAIRES, Ciliary processes.
PROCESS, Apophysis, Processus.
PROC"ESS, Ratio, (F.) *Procédé*, from *procedere*, to march forwards. Procedure,—method of performing any operation, chemical, pharmaceutical, or surgical.
PROCESS, CUNEIFORM, Basilary process — p. Modelling, see Modelling Process — p. of Rau, see Malleus — p. Vertical superior longitudinal, Falx cerebri.
PROCES'SUS. *A process;* same etymon; *Projectu'ra, Prob'olē*. An apophysis or eminence of a bone; see Apophysis. Also, any part which seems prolonged beyond others with which it is in connexion; as the *Ciliary processes*.
PROCESSUS ANCONEUS, Olecranon — p. Annularis, Pons Varolii — p. Belenoides, see Belenoid — p. Caudatus, Lobulus caudatus — p. à Cerebello ad medullam oblongatam, Corpora restiformia — p. Cerebelli ad pontem, Peduncles of the cerebellum — p. Cerebelli ad testes, Peduncles of the cerebellum — p. Cerebri lateralis, Cornu ammonis — p. Ciliares, Ciliary processes — p. Clavatus, see Funiculi graciles — p. Cochleariformis, see Tympanum — p. Cuneiformis ossis occipitis, Basilary process — p. Enteroidei cerebri, Convolutions (cerebral) — p. Falciformis cerebelli, Falx cerebelli — p. Falciformis duræ matris, Falx cerebri — p. Gracilis of Rau, see Malleus — p. Laterales uteri, Tubæ Fallopianæ — p. Mamillares, Papillæ of the kidney, Olfactory nerves — p. Mamillares cerebri, Mamillary tubercles — p. Olivaris, Olivary Process — p. Orbicularis cerebri, Infundibulum of the brain — p. Papillares, Olfactory nerves — p. Papillarum, Olfactory nerves — p. Rachidianus, Medulla spinalis — p. Sterni xiphoideus, Xiphoid.
PROCES'SUS TER'ETES, *Eminen'tiæ seu Fascic'uli ter'etes.* Two slightly convex bodies forming the anterior wall or floor of the fourth ventricle of the brain. They are separated by a longitudinal groove, which is continuous, inferiorly, with the sulcus longitudinalis posterior of the spinal cord. They are crossed transversely by several white and gray fasciculi—*lineæ transver'sæ, striæ medulla'res*—the origin of the auditory nerves.
PROCESSUS AD TESTES, see Valvula Vieussenii — p. Transversus duræ matris, Tentorium — p. Uvifer, Uvula — p. Ventriculi, Duodenum — p. Xiphoides, Xiphoid cartilage — p. Xipho-sternalis, Xiphoid cartilage — p. Zygomaticus, Zygomatic process.
PROCHEILA, Antelabia.
PROCHEILIDION, Procheilon.
PROCHEI'LON, *Procheilid'ion, Prola'bium, Antila'bium.* The extreme projecting part or margin of the lips.
PROCHEUMA, Parenchyma.
PROCIDENCE DE L'ŒIL, Exophthalmia.
PROCIDENTIA, Prolapsus — p. Ani, Proctocele — p. Intestini recti, Proctocele — p. Iridis, Staphyloma of the Iris — p. Oculi, Exophthalmia — p. Sedis, Proctocele — p. Uteri, Prolapsus uteri.
PROCNEME, Tibia.
PROCNEMIUM, Tibia.
PROCŒ'LIUS, *Procœ'lus*, from προ, 'before,' and κοιλια, 'belly.' One who has a large pendulous abdomen.
PROCŒLUS, Procœlius.

PROCON'DYLUS, προκονδυλος, from προ, 'before,' and κονδυλος, 'a knot.' The first joint of the fingers; the second being called κονδυλος; and the third μετακονδυλος.
PROCREATIO, Generation — p. Sanguinis, Hæmatosis.
PROCREATION, Fecundation, Generation.
PROC'TAGRA, from πρωκτος, 'anus,' and αγρα, 'seizure.' Gout in the rectum. Proctalgia.
PROCTAL'GIA, *Proc'tica simplex, Proc'tagra, Dolor ani, Proctodyn'ia*, from πρωκτος, 'the anus,' and αλγος, 'pain.' Pain in the anus: generally symptomatic of disease, as of hemorrhoids, scirrhus, &c.
PROCTALGIA, Clunesia — p. Hæmorrhoidalis, Hæmorrhois — p. Inflammatoria, Rectitis — p. Intertriginosa, Chafing — p. Rheumatica, Proctorrheuma.
PROCTATRE'SIA, *Imperfora'tio ani*, from πρωκτος, 'the anus,' and ατρησια, 'imperforation.' Imperforate state of the anus.
PROC'TICA. Pain or derangement about the anus, without primary inflammation. A genus in the class *Cœliaca*, order *Enterica*, of Good.
PROCTICA EXANIA, Proctocele — p. Marisca, Hæmorrhois — p. Simplex, Proctalgia — p. Tenesmus, Tenesmus.
PROCTISIS, Proctitis.
PROCTI'TIS, *Proc'titis, Archi'tis, Clune'sia, Cysso'tis*, from πρωκτος, 'the anus.' Inflammation of the anus and rectum. Rectitis.
PROCTITIS GANGRÆNOSA, Proctocace.
PROCTOC'ACE, *Procti'tis gangræno'sa*, from πρωκτος, 'the anus,' and κακος, 'evil.' A disease of the rectum, so called by Fuchs, which, according to him, is common in Peru, in the neighbourhood of Quito and Lima, on the Honduras and Mosquito coasts, in Brazil, and on the Gold coast, &c. It is called by the Portuguese, *Bicho*, and *Bicho di Culo;* by the people of Quito, *Mal del Valle*, from its prevalence in the valleys; and in Africa, *Bitios de Kis*. It is an adynamic, inflammatory condition, frequently ending in gangrene. It has been attributed to bad food, and the use of spices.
PROCTOCE'LE, from πρωκτος, 'the anus,' and κηλη, 'hernia.' *Prolap'sus Ani, Proctopto'ma, Proctopto'sis, Procto'sis, Hedroce'lē, Archecpto'ma, Archecpto'ma, Archopto'ma, Archeoce'lē, Archopto'sis, Exa'nia, Hæmor'rhois procc'dens, Hæmor'rhois ab exa'niā, Prociden'tia Ani, P. intesti'ni recti, P. sedis, Ecto'pia Ani, Sedes procid'ua, Falling down of the Fundament, Coming down of the Body*, (F.) *Chute du rectum, C. du Fondement, Renversement du rectum*. Inversion and prolapse of the mucous coat of the rectum, from relaxation of the sphincter with more or less swelling. In the treatment, the application of cold water and astringent lotions must be recommended: and if other means fail, one of the radii of skin, which converge at the anus, may be snipped off. On cicatrizing, the verge of the anus will be contracted, and the cure probably complete. In the way of palliation, the parts may be retained by an appropriate bandage.
PROCTOCYSTOTOMIA, see Lithotomy.
PROCTODYNIA, Proctalgia.
PROCTON'CUS, from πρωκτος, 'anus,' and ογκος, 'swelling.' Swelling of the anus.
PROCTOPARAL'YSIS, *Proctople'gia, Paral'ysis Intesti'ni Recti*. Paralysis of the muscles of the rectum.
PROCTOPLEGIA, Proctoparalysis.
PROCTOPTOMA, Proctocele.
PROCTOPTOSIS, Proctocele.
PROCTORRHAGIA, Hæmorrhoidal flux.

PROCTORRHEU'MA, from πρωκτος, 'anus,' and ρευμα, 'defluxion.' Rheumatism of the anus.

PROCTORRHŒ'A, from πρωκτος, 'the anus,' and ρεω, 'I flow.' A discharge of blood or slime from the anus. See Hæmorrhois.

PROCTOS, Anus.

PROCTOSIS, Proctocele.

PROCTOSPASMUS, Tenesmus.

PROCTOSTENOSIS ORGANICA, Stricture of the rectum.

PROCTOTOREU'SIS, from πρωκτος, 'anus,' and τορυειν, 'to perforate.' Perforation of a closed anus.

PROCTUS, Anus.

PROCURATIO ABORTÛS. The promotion of abortion.

PROD'ROMUS, from προ, 'before,' and δρομος, 'course.' *Sta'dium opportunita'tis* seu *prodromo'rum;* in contagious diseases, *Sta'dium laten'tis conta'gii.* The period immediately preceding an attack of disease; in which the *precursory signs* occur.

PROD'UCT, from *produco*, 'I produce.' (F.) *Produit.* The result sought to be attained by any pharmaceutical operation.

PRODUCTIO, Prolapsus—p. Uvulæ à pituitâ, Staphylœdema.

PRODUC'TION, *Produc'tio;* same etymon. This word is used, especially by the French, synonymously with *prolongation.* The mesentery is, in this sense, a production of the peritoneum.

PRODUCTION ACCIDENTELLE. An accidental or adventitious structure.

PRODUCTIVITAS, Fecundity.

PRODUIT, Product.

PROEGUMENÆ CAUSÆ, Causes, predisponent.

PRŒLIUM, Press, Tourniquet.

PROËM'INENT, *Proëm'inens,* from *pro,* 'forwards,' and *eminere,* 'to project.' Some anatomists call the 7th cervical vertebra the *proeminent vertebra,* on account of the length of its spinous process, which passes the level of that of the neighbouring vertebræ.

PRŒO'TIA, *Proï'otes,* πρωιοτης, or προιοτης, from πρωι, 'early.' 'Precocity.' *Præcox matu'ritas, Preco'cious matu'rity.* Premature development of sexual organization or power.—Good.

PROFLUVII CORTEX, Nerium antidysentericum.

PROFLU'VIUM, *Discharge, Fluxus, Polyrrhœ'a, Flux;* from *profluo,* 'I run down.' A term under which some nosologists have comprised all morbid discharges or fluxes:—others, increased excretions attended by fever.

PROFLUVIUM ALVI, Diarrhœa—p. Genitale muliebre, Menses—p. Mucosum urethræ, Gonorrhœa —p. Muliebre, Leucorrhœa, Menses—p. Sanguinis, Hæmorrhagia—p. Sanguinis è Renibus, Nephrorrhagia—p. Sanguinis ex Ore, Stomatorrhagia —p. Sanguinis ex Utero, Metrorrhagia—p. Seminis, Pollution—p. Ventris, Diarrhœa.

PROFUN'DUS, (*pro,* and *fundus,* 'base.') *Altus,* 'having a deep base.' A name given to different parts, which are seated profoundly as regards others.

PROFUNDA ARTE'RIA FEM'ORIS, *A. vasta poste'rior* seu *muscula'ris fem'oris, Artère-grande musculaire de la cuisse.* (Ch.) This large branch arises commonly from the posterior part of the crural, between the pubis and lesser trochanter. It descends deeply, situate before the adductors; passes through the third adductor above the opening in it for the trunk of the femoral; and terminates in the short portion of the biceps. The *muscularis profunda* gives off, 1. The *external circumflex:* 2. The *internal circumflex:* and, 3. The three *perforantes.*

PROFUNDA ARTE'RIA HU'MERI, *P. supe'rior, Arte'ria spira'lis,* (F.) *Artère humérale profonde, A. collatérale externe, Grand musculaire du bras,* (Ch.) Its origin is variable. When it arises from the brachial artery, it is given off opposite the groove of the humerus destined for the radial nerve, and descends backwards between the three portions of the triceps, accompanied by the nerve; giving branches to that muscle and to the humerus. When it reaches the posterior part of the bone, it divides into two branches, which are distributed to the triceps, supinator longus, &c.

PROFUNDA ARTERIA INFERIOR vel MINOR is often a branch of the last; but, commonly, is given off from the brachial, near the middle of the arm. It gives off branches to the muscles, &c., about the inner side of the os humeri. It is, also, called *large communicating ulnar* or *profundo-ulnar.*

PROFUNDA ARTERIA PENIS. Chaussier has given this name to the *cav'ernous ar'tery,* which arises from the artery of the penis, furnished by the internal pudic.

PROFUNDA ARTERIA SUPERIOR, Profunda humeri.

Certain muscles are distinguished by the names *profound* or *deep-seated,* and *superficial.* Thus, we speak of the *superficial* and *deep-seated* muscles of the neck, &c.; the *Flexor profundus perforans,* &c.

PROFUSIO, Hæmorrhagia.

PROFUSIO AQUÆ. The discharge or breaking of the waters at birth.

PROFUSIO SANGUINIS, Hæmorrhagia—p. Seminis, Ejaculation — p. Subcutanea,. Purpura simplex.

PROGAS'TOR, from προ, 'before,' and γαστηρ, 'belly.' One who has a pendulous belly.

PROGENIES, Epigone.

PROGENY, Epigone.

PROGLOS'SIS, from προ, 'before,' and γλωσσα, 'the tongue;' *Apex linguæ.* The extremity or tip of the tongue.

PROG'NATHOUS, from προ, 'before,' and γναθος, 'the jaw.' Having a projecting jaw. A term applied to the form of the head in which there is a prolongation or forward extension of the jaws, as in the negro.

PROGNO'SIS, *Proägoreu'sis, Prorrhe'sis, Præcognit"io, Prognos'ticè, Prænoʼtio, Præsentia'tio, Præscien'tia, Præscit"io, Prona'a, Progl'asis, Prædic'tio,* (F.) *Prognostic, Pronostic,* from προ, 'before,' and γνωσις, 'knowledge.' A judgment formed by the physician regarding the future progress and termination of any disease.

PROGNOSIS, GENERAL. The opinion formed of a disease in the abstract. Thus, we say, the *General prognosis* of *Cynanche tonsillaris* is favourable;—of *Phthisis pulmonalis,* unfavourable, &c.

PROGNOSIS, PARTICULAR. The opinion formed of any particular case of disease. The *particular prognosis* of one case of typhus, for example, may be favourable, whilst that of another may be unfavourable.

PROGNOSIS EX LINGUÂ, Glossomantia.

PROGNOSTIC, Prognosis.

PROGNOSTICE, Prognosis.

PROGRESSIO, Augmentation.

PROGRESSUS, Augmentation.

PROIOTES, Præotia.

PROJECTURA, Process.

PROLABIUM, Procheilon.

PROLAP'SUS, from *prolabor, prolapsus,* (*pro* and *labor, lapsus,* 'to slide,') 'I slip down.' *Proci'den'tia, Delap'sio, Delap'sus, Hyporrhysis, Propto'ma, Propto'sis, Produc'tio, Propendentia,*

Prominen'tia, Ptosis, Casus, (F.) *Chute; a protrusion; a falling down.* A genus of diseases in the class *Locales* and order *Ectopiæ* of Cullen, distinguished by the falling down of a part through the orifice with which it is naturally connected.

PROLAPSUS ANI, Proctocele — p. Bulbi oculi, Exophthalmia — p. Corneæ, Staphyloma of the cornea—p. Iridis, Ptosis iridis—p. Linguæ, Glossocele, Paraglossa — p. Œsophagi, Pharyngocele — p. Palpebræ, Blepharoptosis — p. Pharyngis, Pharyngocele—p. Umbilici, Exomphalus.

PROLAPSUS U'TERI, *Exome'tra, Metropto'sis, Metropropto'sis, Orthysteropto'sis, Orthysteropto'ma, Falling down of the womb, Ædopto'sis u'teri, Hysteropto'sis, Hysteroce'lē nuda, Prociden'tia u'teri,* (F.) *Abaissement de la matrice, Chute de la matrice, Descente de la matrice, Précipitation de la matrice.* Some use the term, 'Procidentia Uteri' for a minor degree of the affection than prolapsus;—*Relaxatio uteri* expressing the slightest state of all. A falling down of the uterus, owing to relaxation of the parts about the uterovaginal region. In the treatment, the horizontal posture must be insisted upon; the injection of astringent substances *per vaginam* be advised; and if the affection be not remedied by these means, a pessary may be employed as a palliative, or the operation of *Episioraphy* be performed.

PROLAPSUS UVULÆ, Staphylœdema.

PROLAPSUS VAGI'NÆ, *Hysteropto'sis Vagi'næ, Prolapsus Ædoptosis Vaginæ, Coleopto'sis, Colpopto'sis, Elytropto'sis* — Protrusion of the upper part of the vagina into the lower. This, like the descent of the uterus, may be *relaxation, procidentia, prolapsus,* or complete *inversion.*

PROLAPSUS VESICÆ, Exocyste.

'PROLECTA'TIO; from *pro,* and *legere, lectum,* 'to gather.' Action of separating the finer parts of a body from the grosser.

PROLEP'TICS, *Prolep'ticē,* from προ, 'before,' and λαμβανω, 'I seize hold of.' A term proposed by Dr. Laycock to signify the art and science of predicting in medicine.

PROLEPTICUS, Anticipating.

PROLES, Epigone.

PROL'ICIDE, *Prolicid'ium;* from *proles,* 'offspring,' and *cædere,* 'to kill.' Destruction of offspring: a term, which includes fœticide as well as infanticide.

PROLIF'IC, *Prolif'icus;* from *proles,* 'offspring,' and *facio,* 'I make.' That which has the faculty of engendering. Applied to man, and animals, and to their sperm or seed; as well as to remedies, which, by strengthening the genital organs, increase the secretion of sperm.

PROLIG"EROUS, *Pro'liger, Prolig"erus,* from *proles,* 'offspring,' and *gero,* 'I carry.' That which is connected with carrying the offspring.

PROLIGEROUS DISC or LAYER, *Discus prolig"erus, Discus vitellinus, Stratum prolig"erum, Gonostro'ma,* (F.) *Disque proligère.* A granular layer, situate generally towards the most prominent part of the ovarian vesicle, in the centre of which the true ovum or ovule exists.—Von Baer.

PROLONGEMENT RACHIDIEN, Medulla spinalis — p. *Sous-occipital,* Basilary process.

PROMALACTE'RIUM, from προ, 'before,' and μαλασσω, 'I soften.' The room, in the ancient gymnasium, in which the body was softened and anointed. One of the operations in bathing.

PROMANUS, see Digitus, Pollex.

PROMETOPIDIA, Frontal bandages.

PROMETO'PIS, *Prometopid'ion,* from προ, 'before,' and μετωπον, 'the forehead.' The skin of the forehead.

PROMINENTIA, Prolapsus, Protuberance — p. Annularis Cerebri, Pons Varolii — p. Corneæ, Ceratocele — p. Ossis Continua, Apophysis.

PROMINENTIÆ ALBICANTES, Mammillary tubercles—p. Semiövales Medullæ Oblongatæ, Corpora olivaria.

PROMONTORIUM, Promontory — p. Faciei, Nasus.— p. Ossis Sacri, see Sacrum.

PROM'ONTORY, *Promonto'rium,* (from *pro* and *mons, montis,* 'a mountain,') seu *Tuber* seu *Tubero'sitas Tym'pani.* A small projection at the inner paries of the cavity of the tympanum, which corresponds to the external scala of the cochlea, and especially to the outer side of the vestibule.

PROMONTORY OF THE SACRUM, see Sacrum.

PRONATEUR CARRÉ, Pronator radii quadratus—*p. Grand ou rond,* Pronator radii teres—*p. Petit,* Pronator radii quadratus.

PRONA'TION, *Prona'tio,* from *pronus,* 'inclined forwards.' Anatomists understand, by pronation, the motion by which the inferior extremity of the radius passes before the ulna, and thus causes the hand to execute a kind of rotation from without inwards.

PRONA'TOR. That which produces the motion of pronation. This name has been given to two of the muscles of the forearm.

PRONATOR OBLIQUUS, P. radii teres — p. Quadratus, P. radii quadratus.

PRONATOR RA'DII QUADRA'TUS, *P. quadratus, Quadratus ra'dii, P. quadratus* seu *transvers'us* (Winslow), *Pronator radii brevis* seu *quadratus* (Cowper,) (F.) *Cubito-radial* (Ch.), *Petit* ou *carré pronateur.* This muscle is situate at the anterior, inferior, and profound part of the forearm. It is flat and square, and is attached, within, to the inferior quarter of the anterior surface of the ulna; and, without, to the inferior quarter of the anterior surface of the radius. It produces the motion of pronation.

PRONATOR RADII TERES, *P. teres* sive *obli'quus* (Winslow), (F.) *Épitrochlo-radial* (Ch.), *Grand* ou *rond pronateur.* A muscle seated at the upper and anterior part of the forearm. It is long, flat, and larger above than below. It is attached, above, to the inner tuberosity of the humerus and to the coronoid process of the ulna. From thence it passes obliquely downwards and outwards, and terminates at the middle of the outer surface of the radius. It causes the radius to turn on the ulna, to produce the motion of pronation. It can, also, bend the forearm on the arm, and conversely.

PRONATOR TERES, P. radii teres.

PRONAUS, Vestibulum.

PRONERVATIO, Aponeurosis, Tendon.

PRONŒA, Prognosis.

PRONOSTIC, Prognosis.

PROPENDENTIA, Prolapsus.

PROP'ERTIES, PHYSICAL, OF THE TISSUES. These are *flexibility, extensibility* and *elasticity, racornissement* and *imbibition.*

PROPERTIES, VITAL. Those which depend upon organization, as *contractil'ity.*

PROPHASIS, Prognosis.

PROPHYLAC'TIC, *Prophylac'ticus, Diaphylac'tic, Diasos'tic, Synteret'icus, Præservato'rius,* from προ, and φυλασσω, 'I defend.' A preservative.

PROPHYLAX'IS, *Prophylacē, Prophylac'ticē, Syntere'sis.* Same etymon. *Præserva'tio, Præcau'tio, Præcusto'dia.* Preservative or preventive treatment.

PROP'OLIS, from προ, 'before,' and πολις, 'city;' literally, 'that which is before the city.' *Ceranthe'mus, Commo'sis, Bee-bread.* A red, resinous matter, with which the bees cover the bottom of the hive. Its fume has been esteemed antiasthmatic.

PROP'OMA, from προ, 'before,' and πομα, 'a drink.' Ancient name of a medicine, composed of seven parts of *honey* and four of *wine*. It was drunk before a meal.—Paulus of Ægina.

PROPORTIO, Symmetry.

PROPOSITUM, Intention.

PROPOTIS'MOS. Same etymon. *Præpo'tio.* An ancient name for medicines which were given to the patients before purging them, and, in some sort, to prepare them.

PROPRIUS AURIS EXTERNÆ, Retrahens auris.

PROPTOMA, Prolapsus.

PROPTO'MA AURICULA'RUM, *Paræsthe'sis audi'tûs flacca*, Flap Ear. Lobe of the ear broad, loose, and pendent from birth.—Good.

PROPTOMA SCROTI, Rachosis.

PROPTOSIS, Prolapsus—p. Palpebræ, Blepharoptosis—p. Uvulæ, Staphylœdema.

PROPTYSIS, Expectoration.

PRORA, Occiput.

PRORRHESIS, Prognosis.

PRORUPTIO SANGUINIS, Hæmorrhagia.

PROS, προς. In composition, this prefix generally signifies 'in addition to,' 'over and above,' 'besides.'

PROSARTHROSIS, Diarthrosis.

PROSBOLE, Impression.

PROSCHYSIS, Affusion.

PROSCOLLESIS, Adherence, Agglutination.

PROSECTEUR, Dissector.

PROSECTIO, Anatomy.

PROSECTOR, Dissector.

PROSLEPSIS, Prehension.

PROSODOS, Aditus.

PROSOPALGIA, Neuralgia, facial.

PROSOPANTRA, Frontal sinuses.

PROSOPANTRI'TIS, from *prosopantra*, the frontal sinuses, and *itis*, denoting inflammation. Inflammation of the frontal sinuses.

PROSOPARALYSIS, Palsy, Bell's.

PROSO'PIS DULCIS. A tree of rather large size, native of Peru. The fruit—*Pacay*—is a pod, from 20 to 24 inches long, containing black seeds imbedded in a white, soft, flaky substance; which last is eaten by the Limeños with pleasure.—Tschudi.

PROSOPODYNIA, Neuralgia, facial.

PROSOPODYSMOR'PHIA, from προσωπον, 'the face,' δυς, 'with difficulty,' and μορφη, 'shape.' Malformation or atrophy of the face,—as where the process of nutrition suffers from diminished nervous influence.

PROSOPOLOGIA, Physiognomy.

PROSOPOMANTIA, Physiognomy.

PROSOPON, Face.

PROSOPORRHEU'MA, *Rheumatis'mus faciei*, from προσωπον, 'face,' and ρευμα, 'defluxion,' 'rheumatism.' Rheumatism affecting the face.

PROSOPOSIS, Physiognomy.

PROSOPOSPASMUS, Canine Laugh.

PROSOPOSTERNODYMIA, see Cephalosomatodymia.

PROSPERITAS VALETUDINIS, Sanitas.

PROSPHORA, Prehension.

PROS'PHYSIS, *Adnascen'tia, Coalit"io*, 'adhesion, adherence, connexion,' from προς, and φυω, 'I grow.' In a more limited sense, this word means morbid adhesion of the eyelids, either between themselves, or with the globe of the eye; *Ankylobleph'aron.*

PROS'TASIS, προστασις, (προ, and στασις, 'station,') 'superiority, preponderance;' same etymon as *Prostata*. A predominance or abundance of *excrementitious* humour.—Hippocr.

PROSTATA, Prostate—p. Bartholini, Cowper's glands in the female—p. Muliebris, Cowper's glands in the female.

PROSTATÆ, Prostate.

PROSTATAL, Prostatic.

PROSTATAL'GIA, from προστατα, 'the prostate,' and αλγος, 'pain.' Pain in the prostate.

PROSTATAUXE, Prostatoparectasis.

PROSTATE, προστατα, from προ, 'before,' *ισταημι*, 'I stand.'—*Pros'tata, P. gland'ula, Pro[...] P. glandulo'sæ, Paras'tata adenoïdes seu g[...] lo'sa, Adstans, Paras'tatæ, P. gland'ula, P[...] tæ adenoi'des, Testis minor, Corpus glan[...] seu glando'sum, C. adeniform'è, C. gland[...] C. glandulo'sum, C. adenoi'des, Assisten[...] dulæ, Ads'tites glandulosi;* the *Prostate g[...]* A glandular, cordiform body, of the size of a chestnut, situate before the neck of the bladder, behind the symphysis pubis, and surround[...] first portion of the urethra. Its excretory [...] lets, to the number of 10 or 12, open into the [...] of the urethra that traverses it, and pour [...] a whitish viscid humour, intended to lubri[...] interior of the urethra, and to serve as a vehicle for the sperm in its ejaculation.

PROSTATELCO'SIS, from προστατα, 'prostate,' and 'ελκος, 'an ulcer.' Ulceration of the prostate.

PROSTATES INFÉRIEURES, Cowper's glands—p. *Petites*, Cowper's glands.

PROSTAT'IC, *Prostat'icus, Pros'ta'al*. That which relates to the prostate. Wins[...] named—*Superior Prostatic Muscles*—li[...] which pass from the pubis to the lateral part of the prostate. He, also, calls—*Inferior p[...] muscles*—the fleshy fibres, which, from the lower parts of the urethra, near its membranous portion, pass to be inserted into the pubis.

PROSTATIC BISEC'TOR. An instrument employed by Dr. Stevens, of New York, in the lateral operation of lithotomy. In form [...] bles a large olive, with a beak at the extremity, with cutting edges at the sides parallel [...] longest axis, and with a straight handle.

PROSTATIC LIQUOR, *Liquor prostat[...]* fluid secreted by the prostate, which mixes [...] sperm during emission.

PROSTATIC PORTION OF THE URETHRA. part of the canal of the urethra included by the prostate: it is about 15 lines long.

PROSTATIC SINUS, see Sinus, prostatic.

PROSTATICUS SUPERIOR, Compr[...] prostatæ.

PROSTATI'TIS, *Inflamma'tio Pros[...]* προστατα, 'the prostate,' and *itis*, denoting [...] mation. Inflammation of the prostate.

PROSTATOCELE, Prostatoncus.

PROSTATON'CUS, *Prostatoce'le*, [...] *tatæ*, from προστατα, 'the prostate,' and ο[...] tumour.' Swelling of the prostate.

PROSTATOPAREC'TASIS, from [...] 'prostate,' and παρεκτασις, 'to exten[...] largement of the prostate; also, indurati[...] same, *Prostatoscir'rhus, Prostataux'è.*

PROSTATOSCIRRHUS, see Prost[...] tasis.

PROSTERNID'IUM, from προ, 'be[...] στερνον, 'the sternum.' Any agent appl[...] anterior part of the chest; a plaster to th[...]

PROSTHESIS, Prothesis.

PROSTHETA, Subdita.

PROSTHIUM, Penis.

PROSTOM'IA, *Commissu'ra labio'r[...]* προ, 'before,' and στομα, 'mouth.' The c[...] sure of the lips.

PROSTRA'TION, *Prostra'tio vi'ri[...] Prostration des forces, Abattement.* Great pression of strength. Almost total loss of power over the muscles of locomotion.

PRO'TEA MELIFE'RA. A South African plant, *Nat. Ord.* Proteaceæ, whose involucra and flowers, at the time of inflorescence, are filled with a sweet watery liquid, which contains a great deal of honey. By inspissation it forms a delicious syrup—*Syru'pus Pro'teœ*, which is much used in pulmonary affections.

PROTEA LEPIDOCARPON, and some other Proteæ, supply the same kind of juice.

PRO'TEAN, *Pro'teiform, Proteiform'is*, from *Proteus*, who could assume various shapes. Assuming different shapes.

PROTEIFORMIS, Protean.

PROTEIFORM'IS MORBUS. A disease which assumes various characters.

PRO'TEIN, *Proteine, Protei'na*: from πρωτευω, 'I take first rank.' A product of the decomposition of albumen, &c., by potassa. When animal albumen, fibrin or casein is dissolved in a moderately strong solution of caustic potassa, and the solution is exposed for some time to a high temperature, these substances are decomposed. The addition of acetic acid causes, in all three, the separation of a gelatinous translucent precipitate which has exactly the same characters and composition. This is protein.— Mulder.

Protein is the basis of animal and vegetable fibrin, albumen, and casein, and of gluten, which have been, consequently, classed under the "proteinaceous alimentary principle," by Dr. Pereira.

PROTEINACEOUS, Proteinous.

PRO'TEINOUS, *Proteina'ceous, Proteino'sus*, (F.) *Protéique*. Of, or belonging to protein;— as "a proteinous alimentary principle."

PROTÉIQUE, Proteinous.

PROTENSIONES GLANDULARES, Mammillary eminences.

PROTH'ESIS, *Pros'thesis, Adjunc'tio, Adjec'tio, Apposi"tio*, 'addition, application;' from προς, 'in addition to,' and τιθημι, 'I put.' That part of surgery whose object is to add to the human body some artificial part, in place of one that may be wanting, as a wooden leg, an artificial eye, &c.

PROTMESIS, Umbilicus, Kidney.

PROTOGALA, Colostrum.

PROTOIATROS, Archiater.

PROTOMEDICUS, Archiater.

PROTOMUS, Dissector.

PROTOPATHIA, Idiopathia.

PRO'TOPHYTE, *Protoph'yton*, from πρωτος, 'first,' and φυτον, 'a plant.' A vegetable production at the foot of the scale; as a cryptogamous plant, — a fungus.

PROTOSPOROS, Os uteri.

PROTOZÖ'ON, from πρωτος, 'first,' and ζωον, 'an animal.' An animal low in the scale;— as a monad.

PROTRUSION, Prolapsus.

PROTU'BERANCE, *Protuberan'tia, Extubera'tio, Prominen'tia, Excrescen'tia, Extuberan'tia*, from *pro*, 'before,' and *tuber*, 'a projection.' (F.) *Bosse*. A name given to rough, unequal protuberances, seen at the surface of certain organs; the *parietal protuberances, occipital protuberances, annular protuberances*, &c.

PROTUBERANCE, ANNULAR, Pons Varolii — p. Cerebral, Medulla oblongata, Pons Varolii — p. *Cylindroïde*, Cornu ammonis.

PROTUBERANTIA, Eminence—p. Annularis Willisii, Pons Varolii — p. Cylindrica, Cornu ammonis.

PROTRUSOR, Detrusor urinæ.

PROULIMATE'SIS. A word employed by Forestus for hernia of the stomach.

PROUNE, Prunus domestica.

PROVENTRIC'ULUS, *Bulbus glandulo'sus, Infundibu'lum, Second stomach;* from *προ,* 'before,' and *ventriculus,* 'the stomach.' A bulbous expansion at the termination of the œsophagus, immediately above the gizzard of birds, the walls of which are thickly studded with a layer of glands or follicles which secrete a digestive fluid.

PROVERBS, MED'ICAL. A proverbial expression frequently contains sound sense in its directions. In medicine, the greatest collection is in the *Regimen of Health of the School of Salernum,* composed in the 11th century, by John of Milan. Yet, although good sense is often inculcated, we frequently meet with the reverse.

Most of the proverbs are hygienic. The following are a few.

1. *Qu' après la soupe un coupe d'excellent vin*
   Tire un écu de la poche du médecin.

2. *Surge quintâ, prande nonâ, cœna quintâ, dormi nonâ, nec est morti vita prona.*

3. *Nunquam rectè corpus exerceri sine animo, neque animum sine corpore posse.*

4. *Viande bien machée est à demi digérée.*

5. *Optimum condimentum fames.*
   Appetite is the best sauce.

6. *Plures occidit gula quam gladius.*

7. Early to bed and early to rise,
   Makes a man healthy, wealthy, and wise.

8. One man's meat's another man's poison.

9. An ounce of prevention is better than a pound of cure.

PROVERSIO, Anteversion.

PROVINS, MINERAL WATERS OF. Chalybeate springs in the department of Seine et Marne, France, which contain carbonic acid and iron.

PROVOCATORIUS, Intercalary.

PROX'IMAD, see Proximal aspect.

PROX'IMAL, from *proximus,* 'next.' Proximate; nearest; next.

PROXIMAL ASPECT. An aspect towards the trunk, in the course of an extremity. — Barclay. *Proximad* is used by the same writer adverbially to signify 'towards the trunk.'

PRUNA, Anthrax.

PRUNE, Prunum.

PRUNE JUICE EXPECTORA'TION or SPUTA. The sputa resembling prune juice, which occur in the third or purulent stage of pneumonia.

PRUNELLA, Angina pectoris, Aphthæ, Cynanche, Pupil.

PRUNEL'LA, *P. vulga'ris* seu *officina'lis, Brunel'la, Consol'ida minor, Sym'phytum minus, Self-heal, Heal-all, Bugle,* (F.) *Prunelle, Brunelle; Family,* Labiatæ. *Sex. Syst.* Didynamia Gymnospermia. This plant has been recommended as an astringent, in hemorrhages and fluxes; and, also, in gargles against aphthæ, and in inflammation of the fauces.

PRUNELLÆ SAL, Potassæ nitras fusus sul phatis paucillo mixtus.

PRUNELLE, Prunella, Pupil.

PRUNELLIER, Prunus spinosa.

PRUNELLOE, Prunum Brignolense.

PRUNEOLA SYLVESTRIS, Prunus spinosa.

PRUNES, see Prunum — p. Pulp of, Pruni Pulpa.

PRUNI PULPA, *Pulp of prunes.* Take of *prunes* a sufficient quantity, soften them in the vapour of boiling water, and having separated the stones, beat the remainder in a marble mortar and press through a hair-sieve. — Ph. U. S.

PRUNIER, Prunus domestica — *p. Sauvage,* Prunus spinosa.

PRUNUM. A *Plum,* a *Prune.* Three sorts

of plums have been usually ranked amongst the articles of the materia medica. 1. The *Prunum Brignolen'sĕ*; the *Brignole plum* or *Prunel'loe*; from Brignole in Provence. It is of a reddish-yellow colour; and has a very grateful, sweet, subacid taste. 2. The *Prunum Gal'licum*, *Prunum* (Ph. U. S.), the *French Prune*; and 3. The *Prunum Damasce'num* or *Damson*, *Brab'ylon*. All these possess the same general qualities as the other summer fruits. They are emollient and laxative.

PRUNUM STELLATUM, Averrhoa carambola.
PRUNUS ACACIA, Prunus padus.
PRUNUS ARMENIACA, *Armeni'aca vulga'ris* seu *epiroti'ca*. The *A'pricot*, *Apricock*, *Bericoc'cĕ*, βερικοκκη, *Præcoc'ia*, (F.) *Abricot*. Family, Rosaceæ. *Sex. Syst.* Icosandria Monogynia. The apricot, *Melum Armeniacum*, when ripe, is easily digested, and considered as a great delicacy.

PRUNUS A'VIUM, *P. cer'asus* seu *sylvest'ris* seu *macrophyl'la*, *Black Cherry Tree*, *Cer'asus A'vium* seu *nigra* seu *dulcis*, (F.) *Mérisier*. The fruit is eaten; and a gum exudes from the tree, the properties of which are similar to those of gum Arabic.

PRUNUS CAPULIN, (S.) *Capulies*, grows in the open fields of Peru; and is cultivated in gardens in the towns. The fruit is acid, and not often eaten; but on account of its agreeable odour it is used in making *Pucheros de flores*; or with odoriferous flowers to perfume linen. — Tschudi.

PRUNUS CER'ASUS, *Cer'asus ac"ida* seu *horten'sis* seu *vulga'ris* seu *rubra*. The *Red Cherry Tree*; (F.) *Cérisier*. The fruit *Cer'asum*, *Cera'sion*, has a pleasant, acidulous sweet flavour. It is wholesome. See Prunus avium.

PRUNUS DOMES'TICA. The *Plum* or *Damson tree*, *Coccyme'lea*, *Proune*, (F.) *Prunier ordinaire*. The damson, when perfectly ripe, affords a wholesome fruit for pies, tarts, &c. It is gently laxative. See Prunum.

PRUNUS HORTENSIS, P. cerasus.
PRUNUS INSI'TIA. The *Bullace Plum Tree*. The fruit of this tree is used like the damson.

PRUNUS LAURO-CER'ASUS, *Cer'asus lauro-cerasus*, *Padus lauro-cerasus*, *Poison Laurel*, *Cherry Laurel*, *Common Laurel*, *Lauro-cer'asus*, (F.) *Laurier-cérise*, *L. amandier*. The leaves have a bitter, styptic taste, with the flavour of bitter almonds. The flowers have a similar flavour. The powdered leaves, applied to the nostrils, excite sneezing. The flavour of the leaves has given occasion to their being employed in tarts, custards, &c.; but in large quantities they are poisonous. The poisonous principle is the prussic acid. The distilled water, called *Laurel-water*, is poisonous. (See Poisons, Table of.)

PRUNUS MACROPHYLLA, P. avium.
PRUNUS PADUS, *Padus*, *P. a'vium*, *Cer'asus Padus*, *Cer'asus racemo'sus sylves'tris*, *Wild cluster* or *Bird Cherry Tree*, (F.) *Cérisier à grappes*, *Bois puant*. The bark of the tree has a fragrant smell, and a bitter sub-astringent taste, somewhat similar to that of bitter almonds. It has been recommended in intermittents, &c. in the form of decoction. The berries have been used in dysentery.

PRUNUS SEBASTINA, Sebastina.
PRUNUS SPINO'SA. The *Sloe Tree*, *P. sylves'tris* seu *Aca'cia*, *Agriococcime'lea*, *Agru'na*, *Agrune'la*, (F.) *Prunellier*, *Prunier sauvage*. The fruit—the *sloe*—is sometimes employed in gargles, and was formerly much used in hemorrhage, owing to its astringent properties. The *Aca'cia nostras* seu *German'ica* seu *vulga'ris*, *Prune'ola sylves'tris*, *Succus acaciæ nostra'tis*, *S. Acaciæ Germanicæ inspissa'tus* is obtained from this.

PRUNUS SYLVESTRIS, P. Avium, P. Spinosa.
PRUNUS VIRGINIA'NA, *Cer'asus sero'tina*, *C. Virginia'na*, *Wild Cherry Tree*, (F.) *Cérisier de Virginie*. The bark of this tree has been found useful in intermittents. The leaves are poisonous to certain animals, and the berries intoxicate different kinds of birds. The Indians use the bark in the cure of syphilis. It is bitter and astringent, and possesses some aromatic warmth, and, likewise, a narcotic quality. It is stimulant and tonic. The leaves contain prussic acid. The distilled oil of the bark is very nearly identical with that of the bitter almond. A strong decoction of the bark is anthelmintic.

PRUNUS VULGARIS, P. Padus.
PRURIG"INOUS, *Prurigino'sus*; same etymon as the next. Relating, or belonging to, or resembling prurigo.

PRURI'GO, *Pruri'tus*, *Chris'ma*; from *pruria*, 'I itch.' The word is often used synonymously with *itching*. Willan and Bateman use the term for a genus of cutaneous diseases, the characteristic symptoms of which are a severe itching, accompanied by an eruption of papulæ of nearly the same colour as the adjoining cuticle; *Cnesmos*, *Scabies papuliform'is*, *Exor'mia pruri'go*. It affects the whole surface of the skin, under three varieties of form; — the *P. mitis*, *P. formi'cans*, *P. seni'lis*, &c. as well as some parts of the body, as the *P. pod'icis*, and *P. puden'di mulie'bris* seu *Puden'dagra pru'riens*.

PRURIGO, Heat—p. Pedicularis, Phtheiriasis.
PRURIT, Itching.
PRURITUS, Gargle, Itching, Prurigo.
PRUSSIAN BLUE, *Ferrum Zoöt'icum*, *F. Borus'sicum*, *F. Cyanogena'tum*, *F. oxydula'tum hydrocyan'icum*, *Ferri Ferrocy'anas*, *F. Ferrocyanure'tum*, *Borus'sias Ferri*, *Cæru'leum Borus'sicum*, *C. Berolinen'sĕ*, *Prussias Ferri*, *Hydrocy'anas Ferri*, *Ferri Cyanure'tum*, *Ferri percyan'idum*, *Trito-hydro-ferrocy'anate of iron*, *Ferrocyanuret of iron*, *Ferro-prus'siate of iron*, (F.) *Bleu de Prusse*. In the Pharmacopœia of the United States, the pure salt—*Ferri ferrocyanuretum*—is directed to be made as follows: *Ferri Sulph.* ℥ir. *acid sulph.* f℥iiiss, *acid nitric.* f℥vj or q. s. potassii ferrocyanuret.* ℥ivss, *aquæ*, Oij. Dissolve the sulphate in a pint of water, and having added the sulphuric acid, boil the solution. Pour into it the nitric acid, in small portions, boiling the liquid for a minute or two after each addition, until it no longer produces a dark colour; then allow the liquid to cool. Dissolve the ferrocyanuret of potassium in the remainder of the water, and add this solution gradually to the first liquid, agitating the mixture after each addition; then pour it upon a filter. Wash the precipitate with boiling water until the washings pass tasteless. Lastly, dry and rub into powder. This salt is chiefly used in the preparation of the hydrocyanic acid and the cyanuret of mercury. It has been advised in the treatment of intermittents, and in epilepsy and scrophulosis. Externally, it has been applied to ill-conditioned ulcers. (℥j to ℥j, of cerate.) Dose, four to six grains.

PSALIDIUM, Fornix.
PSALIS, Fornix, Scissors.
PSALTERIUM, Lyra.
PSAMMA, see Gravel.
PSAMMIS'MUS, *Ammis'mus*, *Gammis'mus*, from ψαμμος, 'sand.' *Arena'tio*. The application of sand to any part of the body for the cure of disease. — Paulus.

PSAMMODES, Sabulous.
PSAMMUS, see Gravel.
PSELLIS'MUS, ψελλισμος, from ψελλος, 'I stutter.' Imperfect or depraved state of the articulation. A genus in the class *Pneumatica*, order *Phonica*, of Good.

PSELLISMUS NASITAS, Rhinophonia — p. Rhetacismus, Rotacism.

PSELLOTES, Balbuties.
PSEUDACACIA ODORATA, Robinia pseudacacia.
PSEUDAC'OE, *Pseudacoï'a, Pseudecoï'a*, from ψευδής, 'false,' and ακοη, 'audition.' *Pseudacu'sis.* False hearing.
PSEUDACORUS, Iris pseudacorus.
PSEUDÆSTHE'SIA, *Sensus perver'sus*, from ψευδής, 'false,' and αισθανομαι, 'I feel.' *Parapsis illuso'ria, Pseudo'phē, Pseudaph'ia.* Depraved feeling. Imaginary sense of touch or general feeling in organs that have no existence. Common to those who have suffered amputation; and in hypochondriacs and the insane.
PSEUDALEI MORBI, Feigned diseases.
PSEUDANGUSTURINUM, Brucine.
PSEUDAPHE, Pseudæsthesia.
PSEUDARTHRO'SIS, *Pseudarticula'tio, Pseudartic'ulus, Articula'tio notha seu artificia'lis*, from ψευδής, 'false,' and αρθρον, 'a joint.' A false joint or articulation.
PSEUDARTICULATIO, Pseudarthrosis.
PSEUDECOIA, Pseudacos.
PSEUDENCEPH'ALUS, *Paraceph'alus*, from ψευδής, 'false,' and εγκεφαλον, 'the encephalon.' A monster, whose cranium is open in its whole extent, from before to behind, its base supporting a vascular tumour. — G. St. Hilaire.
PSEUDO, False — p. Asthma, Dyspnœa.
PSEUDOBLEP'SIA, *Pseudoblepsis, Pseudora'sis, Suffu'sio oc'uli*, from ψευδής, 'false,' and βλεψις, 'sight.' *Pseudops'ia, Parop'sis illuso'ria, Suffu'sio, Phantas'ma, False sight.* A generic name, used by Cullen for perversion of vision. See Metamorphopsia.
PSEUDOBLEPSIS, Paropsis.
PSEUDOCARCINOMA LABII, Cancer aquaticus.
PSEUDOCROUP, Asthma thymicum.
PSEUDOCYESIS, Pregnancy, false — p. Cyesis molaris, Mole.
PSEUDOENCEPHALITIS, Hydrencephaloid disease.
PSEUDO-FEVER, Irritation, morbid.
PSEUDOGEU'SIA, *Pseudogeu'sis, Pseudogeus'tia*, from ψευδής, 'false,' and γευσις, 'taste.' *Hallucina'tio gustûs.* False taste.
PSEUDOGEUSTIA, Pseudogeusia.
PSEUDOHELMINTHES, Ectozoa.
PSEUDOLI'EN, *Pseudosplen.* Glands situate in the neighbourhood of the spleen; probably, lymphatic glands.
PSEUDOMECHOACANA. Convolvulus panduratus.
PSEUDOMEDICUS, Charlatan.
PSEUDOMELANOTIC FORMATIONS, see Anthracosis — p. *Membrane*, Membrane, false.
PSEUDOMELANOTIC MENINX, Membrane, false — p. Metamorphosis polyposa, Polypus.
PSEUDOMEMBRANA, Membrane, false.
PSEUDONARCISSUS, Narcissus pseudonarcissus.
PSEUDOPERIPNEUMONIA, Peripneumonia notha.
PSEUDOPHLOGOSIS VENTRICULI RESOLUTIVA ET COLLIQUATIVA, Gastromalacia.
PSEUDOPHTHI'SIS. False phthisis. Emaciation occasioned by other cause than organic lesion of the lungs.
PSEUDOPLAS'MATA, from ψευδής, 'false,' and πλασσω, 'I form.' A term applied to malignant heterologous tumours. — Vogel.
PSEUDOPLEURITIS, Pleurodynia — p. Po-

lypi, see Polypi — p. Pyrethrum, Achillea ptarmica — p. Spleen, Pseudolien.
PSEUDOPNEUMONIA, Peripneumonia notha.
PSEUDOPNEUMONITIS, Peripneumonia notha.
PSEUDOPSIA, Pseudoblepsia.
PSEUDORASIS, Pseudoblepsia.
PSEUDOREX'IA, *Pseudorex'is*, from ψευδής, 'false,' and ορεξις, 'appetite.' False appetite.
PSEUDO-RHONCHUS, from ψευδής, 'false,' and ρογχος, 'rattle.' A sound heard during respiration, which appears to be produced, like the ordinary rhonchi, in the air-tubes, but is exterior to them — as in the case of *pleural pseudorhonchi.* See Rattle, and *Râle.*
PSEUDOS'MIA, *Pseudosphre'sia, Pseudosphre'sis*, from ψευδής, 'false,' and οσμη, 'smell.' False sense of smell.
PSEUDOPHRESIA, Pseudosmia.
PSEUDOSYPHILIS, Syphilis pseudosyphilis.
PSEUDOTHANATOS, Asphyxia.
PSEUDOVARIOLÆ, Varicella.
PSEUDYMEN, Membrane, false.
PSID'IUM POMIF'ERUM. The *Apple Guava, Guava, Guayava.* This plant and *P. Pyrif'erum* bear fruits; those of the former like apples, — of the latter like pears. The apple kind has an acid flavour, the other is sweet. Of the inner pulp of either, the natives of the Indies make jellies; and, of the outer rind, tarts, marmalades, &c. They are somewhat astringent; this quality, indeed, exists in every part of the tree, and abundantly in the leaf-buds, which are occasionally boiled with barley and liquorice as an excellent drink in diarrhœa. A simple decoction of the leaves is said to be useful in the itch, and most cutaneous eruptions.
PSILOSIS, Depilation.
PSILOTHRUM, Bryonia alba, Depilatory.
PSIMMYTHON, Plumbi suboarbonas.
PSOA, Dysodia.
PSOÆ, *Psoiæ, Psya, Lumbi,* 'the loins,' *Alop'eces, Nephrome'træ, Neurome'træ.* The psoas muscles.
PSOAS MAGNUS, *Psoas seu lumba'ris inter'nus, Pré-lombo-trochantin, Pré-lombo-trochantinien* (Ch.), *Femur moven'tium sextus.* A muscle, seated on the lateral parts of the lumbar portion of the vertebral column; and passing down to the superior and anterior part of the thigh. It is long, fusiform, and attached, above, to the body and transverse processes of the first four lumbar vertebræ, and last dorsal. Below, it terminates, by a very thick tendon, common to it and the iliacus muscle, — which is inserted into the top of the lesser trochanter. This muscle bends the thigh upon the pelvis, and carries it in rotation outwards. It may, also, bend the pelvis on the thigh, and the loins on the pelvis. It acts considerably in station and progression.
PSOAS PARVUS, *Pré-lombo-pubien*, (Ch.) A muscle situate anteriorly to the last. It is long, thin, flat, and narrow; and is attached, above, to the body of the last dorsal vertebra, and below, to the linea ileo-pectinea, by means of a slender tendon, which furnishes two expansions — one to the *Iliac aponeurosis*, and the other to the *pelvis.* This muscle bends the vertebral column on the pelvis; and, reciprocally, the pelvis on the vertebral column.
PSODYMUS, Gastrodidymus.
PSOLÆ, Psoæ.
PSOITE, Psoitis.
PSOI'TIS, *Inflamma'tio mus'culi Psoas, Lumba'go inflammato'ria spasmod'ica,* (F.) *Psoïte, In-*

flammation du muscle Psoas. From ψοαι, 'the loins,' and itis, denoting inflammation. Inflammation of the psoas muscles and of the parts situate before the lumbar vertebræ: accompanied, from its commencement, by considerable fever, violent pains in the part affected and in the thigh of the same side, which remains commonly half bent. Psoitis may terminate by suppuration, and form lumbar abscess.

PSOLE, ψωλη, 'the male organ.' Also, the glans when uncovered.

PSOLON, Membrosus.

PSOLON'CUS, from ψωλη, and ογκος, 'a tumour.' Swelling of the glans, or of the penis generally.

PSOLUS, from ψωλη. One who has the glans uncovered. One who has been circumcised.

PSOPHOMETER, Stethoscope.

PSOPHOS, ψοφος, 'a noise.' A loud noise; a hollow sound.

PSORA, from ψωω, 'I touch, I feel.' Sca'bies, Phlysis Scabies, Ecpye'sis Scabies, Scabiola, Itch, Scratch, Scotch fiddle, (F.) Gale, Mal Saint-Main, Rogne. A contagious eruption of very minute pimples—pustular, vesicular, papular, intermixed, and alternating, itching intolerably and terminating in scabs. It seems to be connected with an insect of the genus Acarus;—the Ac'arus seu Sarcop'tes seu Sarcop'tus seu Phthi'rium seu Cheyle'tus Scabiei, Ac'arus Ciro, Itch-insect, (F.) Ciron. The itch occupies, particularly, the spaces between the fingers, the back of the hands, wrists, elbows, axillæ, groins, hams, &c., and rarely affects the face. The best applications, for its cure, are,— the Unguentum Sulphuris or Ung. Sulph. comp. night and morning; but the unpleasant smell of the sulphur has given occasion to the use of other means;—as the White Hellebore, Potass in deliquescence, Muriate of Ammonia, Sulphuric Acid, &c. The repugnance to the smell of sulphur ought not, however, to be regarded; especially as, in the course of four or five days, it will, in almost all cases, produce a perfect cure.

PSORA AGRIA, Psoriasis inveterata—p. Leprosa, Psoriasis—p. Squamosa, Psoriasis.

PSORA'LEA GLANDULO'SA, Alvaquil'la. Family, Leguminosæ. Sex. Syst. Diadelphia Decandria. A shrub, used in Chili as a vulnerary.

PSORA'LEA PENTAPHYL'LA, Psora'lia, Contrayer'va nova, Mex'ican Contrayer'va. The root is little, if at all, inferior to the contrayerva in its medical properties; which, by the by, are unimportant.

PSORALIA, Psoralea pentaphylla.

PSORENTERIA, Cholera.

PSORI'ASIS, formerly, the state of being affected with ψωρα. Lepido'sis psori'asis, Serpe'do, Serpi'go, Impeti'go (of some), Sca'bies sic'ca, S. feri'na, Psora lepro'sa, P. squamo'sa, Scaly Tetter, Dry Scale, Dry Scall, (F.) Dartre squameuse lichenoïde, D. écailleuse, Gratelle, Gale miliare, G. canine ou sèche. A cutaneous affection, consisting of patches of rough, armorphous scales; continuous, or of indeterminate outline; skin often chappy. Psoriasis occurs under a considerable variety of forms. The surface, under the scales, is more tender and irritable than in lepra, which psoriasis, in some respects, resembles. Dr. Willan has given names to eleven varieties of psoriasis: the chief of which are the Psoriasis gutta'ta, P. diffu'sa (one form of which is the Baker's Itch and Grocer's Itch, and another, the Washerwoman's Scall), the P. gyra'ta, and P. snvetera'ta seu Psora a'gria. The treatment of psoriasis must be antiphlogistic, with the internal use of the fixed alkalies, sulphur, &c. The irritable kinds do better without any local application. The more local and less inflammatory are ameliorated by emollient and soothing applications; or by slightly stimulating means, seabathing, the Ung. hydrarg. nitrico-oxyd., Ung. oxidi zinci, &c.

PSO'RICUS. That which has the nature of itch. A medicine for curing the itch.

PSOROPHTHALMIA, Ophthalmia tarsi—p. Neonatorum, see Ophthalmia (purulenta infantum).

PSYÆ, Psoæ.

PSYCHAGOGA, Psychagogica.

PSYCHAGO'GICA, Psychago'ga, from ψυχη, 'life,' 'soul,' and αγω, 'I lead.' Medicines which resuscitate, when life seems extinct; as in syncope and apoplexy.

PSYCHE, Anima.

PSYCHIATRI'A, from ψυχη, 'mind,' and ιατρεια, 'healing.' Treatment of diseases of the mind.

PSY'CHICAL, Psy'chicus, from ψυχη, 'mind.' That which relates to the mind or mental endowments. Psychological is not unfrequently used with the like signification.

PSYCHOLOGICAL, see Psychical.

PSYCHOL'OGY, Psycholog"ia, from ψυχη 'mind,' and λογος, 'discourse.' A treatise on the intellectual and moral faculties. Also, the intellectual and moral faculties or sphere.

PSYCHONOSOL'OGY, Psychonosolog"ia, from ψυχη, 'mind,' νοσος, 'disease,' and λογος, 'a description.' The doctrine of, or a treatise on, diseases of the mind.

PSYCHOPATHIES, Psychoses.

PSYCHOR'AGES, Agoni'zans, Moribun'das, Mor'ibund, from ψυχη, 'mind,' and ραγη, 'rupture.' Dying. In Articulo Mortis. Moribund means, also, one who is dying.

PSYCHORAGIA, Agony, Death.

PSYCHORRHAGIA, Agony, Death.

PSYCHOS, Cold.

PSYCHO'SES, from ψυχη, 'mind.' Neuroses of the intellect. Diseases of the mind. Psychop'athies.

PSYCHOTICA, Analeptica.

PSYCHOTRIA, Analeptica—p. Emetica, Ipecacuanha.

PSYCHOTROPHUM, Betonica officinalis.

PSYCHROLU'SIA, Psychrolu'tron, from ψυχρος, 'cold,' and λουω, 'I wash.' A cold bath.

PSYCHROPHOB'IA, from ψυχρος, 'cold,' and φοβος, 'fear.' Dread of cold, especially of cold water. Impressibility to cold.

PSYCHTICA, Refrigerants.

PSYDRA'CIA, quasi, ψυκρα 'ιδρακια, 'cool drops.' The ancients sometimes used this term for pimples; at others, for vesicles. Willan and Bateman define Psydracium to be, a small pustule, often irregularly circumscribed, producing but a slight elevation of the cuticle, and terminating in a laminated scab. Many of the psydracia usually appear together, and become confluent; and, after the discharge of pus, they pour out a thin, watery humour; which frequently forms an irregular incrustation. Frank limits the term to a psoriform eruption, which differs from itch in not originating from an insect, and is not contagious;—perhaps the lichen. Authors have differed regarding its acceptation.

PSYDRACIA ACNE, Acne.

PSYLLIUM, Plantago psyllium—p. Erectum, Plantago psyllium.

PTARMICA, Achillea ptarmica—p. Montana, Arnica montana.

PTARMICUM, Errhine, Sternutatory.

PTARMOS, Sneezing.

PTELEA, Ulmus.

PTERIS, Polypodium filix mas.

PTERIS AQUILI'NA, *'Eagles' Wings,'* so called from its leaves. *Pter'ia, Thelyp'teris, Filix Nymphæ'a* seu *fe'mina, Asple'nium aquili'num, Common Brake* or *Female Fern; Eagle Fern, Bracken,* (F.) *Fougère femelle, La grande Fougère. Nat. Ord.* Filices. The root is considered to be anthelmintic; and as efficacious as that of the male fern in cases of tapeworm.

PTERIS PALUSTRIS, Asplenium filix fœmina.

PTERNA, Calcaneum.

PTERNIUM, Calcaneum.

PTERNOBATES, Calcigradus.

PTEROCARPUS ERINACEA, see Kino—p. Marsupium, see Kino—p. Sandalinus, P. Santalinus.

PTEROCAR'PUS SANTALI'NUS, *P. Sandali'nus, San'talum* seu *San'dalum Rubrum, Red Sanders* or *Saunders Tree,* (F.) *Santal rouge. Family,* Leguminosæ. *Sex. Syst.* Diadelphia Decandria. Red Saunders wood, *San'talum* (Ph. U. S.,) *Lignum sandali'num* is used only as a colouring matter: it gives to rectified spirit a fine deep red. The juice of this tree, like that of *P. Draco,* affords a species of *Dragon's Blood.*

PTEROS'PORA ANDROMEDEA, *Scaly Dragon claw, Dragon root, Fever root, Albany beechdrop.* An indigenous plant, *Nat. Ord.* Monotropeæ, *Sex. Syst.* Decandria Monogynia:—found in the state of New York, which blossoms in July. The root has been regarded as an anthelmintic, diuretic, emmenagogue, &c.: but it is not used.

PTERYG'ION, *Pteryg'ium, Ala,* from πτερυξ, 'a wing.' A small wing. *Onyx, Pyo'sis, Unguis,* (F.) *Drapeau, Onglet.* A varicose excrescence of the conjunctiva, of a triangular shape, and commonly occurring at the inner angle of the eye; whence it extends over the cornea. Sometimes two or three pterygia occur on the same eye, and cover the whole cornea with a thick veil, which totally prevents vision. According to Scarpa, the ancients gave the name *Pannic'ulus* to this last complication. If the pterygion cannot be dispelled by means of discutient collyria, it must be removed by the scissors.

PTERYGIUM, Pterygion, Scapula—p. Digiti, Paronychia—p. Lardaceum, Pinguecula—p. Pingue, Pinguecula.

PTERYGO-ANGULI-MAXILLAIRE, Pterygoideus internus—*p. Colli-maxillaire,* Pterygoideus externus—*p. Maxillaire, grand,* Pterygoideus internus—*p. Maxillaire, petit,* Pterygoideus externus—p. Palatine canal, Pterygoid canal—p. Pharyngeus, Constrictor pharyngis—p. Staphylinus, Circumflexus.

PTER'YGO-PAL'ATINE, *Pterygo-Palati'nus.* That which belongs to the pterygoid process and palate.

PTERYGO-PALATINE ARTERY or *Superior pharyngeal* is a very small artery, and is given off by the internal maxillary at the bottom of the zygomatic fossa: after having passed through the pterygo-palatine canal, it is distributed to the superior part of the pharynx, the sphenoid bone, and the Eustachian tube.

PTERYGO-PALATINE CANAL. A small canal, formed by the internal ala of the pterygoid process, and the palate bone. It gives passage to the vessels of the same name.

PTERYGO-STAPHYLINUS INTERNUS, Levator palati—*p. Syndesmo-staphyli-pharyngien,* Constrictor pharyngis.

PTERYGODES, Alatus.

PTER'YGOID, *Pterygoī'des, Pterygoīdeus, Alifor'mis;* from πτερυξ, 'a wing,' and ειδος, 'form.' A name given to two *processes* at the inferior surface of the sphenoid bone; the two laminæ which form them having been compared to wings. These *alæ* or *wings* or *processes,*—*Proces'sus aliform'es,*—have been distinguished, according to their position, into *internal* and *external.*

PTERYGOID ARTERY, *Vid'ian Artery, Ram'ulus Ductûs Pterygoīdei, Arte'ria pharynge'a supre'ma,* arises from the internal maxillary artery, at the bottom of the zygomatic fossa, and enters the pterygoid canal with the nerve of the same name, to proceed to be distributed on the Eustachian tube and velum palati. The name, *pterygoid arteries,* is likewise given to the branches, which the internal maxillary and some of its divisions, as the meningea media, and posterior temporalis profunda, furnish to the pterygoid muscles, behind the neck of the lower jaw.

PTERYGOID BONE, Sphenoid.

PTERYGOID CANAL, *Vid'ian canal, Ductus pterygoīdeus, Cana'lis Vidia'nus,* (F.) *Conduit ptérygoīdien* ou *Vidien, Pterygo-palatine canal,* is a narrow channel, which traverses, in a direction from before to behind, the base of the pterygoid process, and gives passage to the pterygoid nerve. The *foramina* of the sphenoid, which terminate the canals, have the same epithets applied to them.

PTERYGOID FOSSA, *Fossa Pterygoīdea,* (F.) *Fosse ptérygoīdienne* ou *ptérygoīde,* is the depression which separates the two laminæ or alæ of the pterygoid process.

PTERYGOID MUS'CLES, *Ala'res mus'culi, Aliform'es mus'culi,* are two in number. 1. The *Pterygoīdeus externus, P. minor,* (F.) *Ptérygocolli-maxillaire, Petit Ptérygo-maxillaire* (Ch.) *Petit ptérygoīdien, Ptérygoīdien externe,* is a thick, short muscle, which arises, by short aponeuroses, from the outer surface of the external ala of the pterygoid process, and from the outer surface of the great ala of the sphenoid bone; and is inserted at the anterior part of the neck of the lower jaw-bone, and the corresponding part of the inter-articular fibro-cartilage. This muscle draws the condyle of the lower jaw and the interarticular ligament forwards. It carries the chin forwards, and to the opposite side. If the two external pterygoids act together, the jaw is carried directly forwards. 2. The *Pterygoīdeus internus, P. major, Masse'ter intern'us, Latens in Ore,* (F.) *Grand Ptérygo-maxillaire, Ptérygoanguli-maxillaire, Grand Ptérygoīdien* ou *Ptérygoīdien interne.* A thick, quadrilateral muscle, which is attached by short and very strong aponeuroses; above, to the pterygoid fossa, whence it proceeds downwards, backwards, and outwards, to be inserted into the inner surface of the ramus of the lower jaw, near its angle. This muscle raises the lower jaw, and carries it a little forwards. It also performs the grinding motion.

PTERYGOID NERVES. These are two in number. I. The *Pterygoid* or *Vid'ian Nerve.* It arises from the posterior part of the sphenopalatine ganglion; traverses the Vidian canal of the sphenoid; and, beyond, divides into two filaments. 1. A *superior* or *cranial, Nervus superficia'lis* sive *petro'sus,* which ascends into the cranium, and enters the hiatus of Fallopius to unite with the facial nerve. 2. An *inferior* or *carotid, Nervus profundus* sive *major,* which traverses the carotid canal, and unites with the ascending branches of the superior cervical ganglion of the trisplanchnic. II. The *Pterygoid Nerve,* properly so called, *Nervus musculi pterygoīdei,* is given off by the inferior maxillary branch of the 5th pair.

PTERYGOÏDIEN GRAND ou *INTERNE*, Pterygoideus internus—p. *Externe*, Pterygoideus externus—p. *Petit*, Pterygoideus externus.

PTERYGO'MA. Same etymon. A wing; a projecting or pendulous body. A swelling of the vulva, which prevents coition.—M. A. Severinus.

PTERYX, Ala.

PTILOSIS, Deplumatio, Madarosis.

PTISANA, Tisane — p. Communis, Decoctum hordei compositum — p. Hippocratica, Decoctum hordei.

PTISSANA, Tisane.

PTOCHIA'TER, *Ptochia'trus*, same etymon as the next. A physician to the poor, or to an establishment for the poor.

PTOCHIATRI'A, from πτωχος, 'poor,' and ιατρεια, 'healing.' Practice amongst the poor. Also, an institution for the treatment of the diseases of the poor.

PTOCHOCOMI'UM, from πτωχος, 'a poor person,' and κομεω, 'I take care of;' *Ptochodochi'um*, *Ptochotrophe'um*. An almshouse.

PTOCHODOCHIUM, Ptochocomium.

PTOCHOTROPHEUM, Ptochocominm.

PTOMA, Cadaver.

PTOSIS, Prolapsus — p. Bulbi oculi, Exophthalmia.

Ptosis Ir'idis, *Iridoce'lè*, *Her'nia Ir'idis*, Iridopto'sis, Prolap'sus Iridis, from πτωσις, 'a falling.' A prolapsus of the iris through a wound of the cornea. It is known by a blackish tubercle, which projects a little from the cornea in various forms.

Ptosis Palpebræ, Blepharoptosis.

PTYALAGOGUE, Sialogogue.

PTYALIN, see Saliva.

PTYALISM, Salivation.

PTYALISME MERCURIEL, Salivation, mercurial.

PTYALISMUS, Salivation — p. Acutus mellitus, see Salivation — p. Acutus sympatheticus, see Salivation — p. Hydrargyratus, Salivation, mercurial — p. Iners, Slavering — p. Mercurialis, Salivation, mercurial — p. Pyrosicus, Pyrosis.

PTYALOGOGUE, Sialogogue.

PTYALON, Saliva.

PTYASMAGOGUE, Expectorant, Sialogogue.

PTYELON, Saliva, Sputum.

PTYSIS, Exspuition.

PTYSMA, Saliva.

PTYSMAGOGUE, Sialogogue.

PTYSMATIS'CHESIS, *Ptysmatos'chesis*, from πτυσμα, 'sputum,' and ισχω, 'to retain.' Suppression of pulmonary expectoration.

PTYSMATOSCHESIS, Ptysmatischesis.

PUANTEUR, Dysodia.

PUBENS, Ephebus.

PUBER, Ephebus.

PU'BERAL; same etymon as Puberty. Relating or appertaining to the age of puberty — as 'a puberal disease.'

PUBÈRE, Ephebus.

PUBERTAS, Ephebia.

PU'BERTY, *Pubertas*, *Hebè*, *Pubes*, *Aphrodis'ia*, *Ephebi'a*, *Ephe'bia*, *Ephe'botes*, *Ephebo'syne*, *Pubes'cence*, from *pubescere*, 'to begin to have hair on the chin and sexual organs.' The period of life at which young people of both sexes are *pubes'cent* or nubile. According to the civil law, puberty occurs at 12 years in females, and 14 in males. The period varies somewhat in different climates, and in different individuals of the same climate.

PUBES, *Epis'chion*, *Epicten'ion*, *Cteis*, *Pecten*; the *Pubic region*. Same etymon. The middle part of the hypogastric region; so called, because it is covered with hair, in both sexes, at the period of puberty. The hair is also called *Pubes*, *Lanu'go* seu *Pili*, *Pudendo'rum Planta'rum*; and, of old, *pubertas* signified the same.

PUBES, Puberty.

PUBESCENCE, Puberty.

PUBESCENT, see Puberty.

PUBIÆUS, Pubic.

PUBIC, *Pu'bian*, *Pu'bicus*, *Pubis'us*, (F.) *Pubien*. That which belongs to or concerns the pubis.

Pubic Arch or *Arch of the Pubis*, (F.) *Arcade pubienne*. The arch at the anterior part of the inferior circumference of the pelvis. It is more expanded in the female than in the male; to correspond with the additional functions which she has to execute.

Pubic Articula'tion, or *Sym'physis Pubis*, results from the junction of the ossa pubis. The medium of union is cartilage.

Pubic Lig'aments are two very solid, fibrous fasciæ, situate before and beneath the symphysis pubis, which they strengthen. The one is called the *anterior pubic ligament*; the other the *inferior* or *subpubic*.

Pubic Region, *Re'gio Pubis*. The region of the pubes.

PUBIEN, Pubic.

PUBIO-COCCYGIEN-ANNULAIRE, *Pubio-coccyge'us annula'ris*. Dumas gave this name to the levator ani and ischio-coccygeus, which he considers a single muscle.

PUBIO-COCCYGIEN-ANNULAIRE, Levator Ani — p. *Fémoral*, Pectinalis — p. *Femoralis*, Adductor longus femoris — p. *Ombilical*, Pyramidalis abdominis — p. Prostaticus, Compressor prostatæ — p. *Sous-ombilical*, Pyramidalis abdominis — p. *Sternal*, Rectus abdominis — p. *Urethral*, see Compressor Urethræ.

PUBIS, OS, *Episei'on*, *Epis'ion*, *Epis'chion*, *Share Bone*, *Bar-bone*, *Os Pec'tinis*. The anterior part of the os innominatum; so called because it corresponds to the genital organs and pubic region. The *angle of the pubis* is formed by the union of the body and rami of each side.

PUB'LICÆ PARTES. Those organs are so called, the object of whose functions is the nutrition of all the others. Such are the digestive and respiratory organs.

PUCCOON, Sanguinaria Canadensis — p. Red Sanguinaria Canadensis — p. Yellow, Hydrastis Canadensis.

PUCE, Pulex irritans — p. *Maligne*, see Anthrax — p. *Pénétrante*, *Chique*.

PUCÉLAGE, Virginity.

PUCELLE, Virgin.

PUDDING-GRASS, Mentha pulegium.

PUDENDA, Genital organs.

Pudenda Virorum, Pudibilia.

PUDEND'AGRA. A hybrid word; from *pudenda*, (*pudere*, 'to be ashamed,') 'the genital organs,' and the Greek αγρα, 'a seizure.' According to some, this term means pain in the genital parts: *Dolor pudendo'rum*, *Men'talagra*, *Eledyn'ia*; according to others, it is synonymous with syphilis.

Pudendagra Pruriens, Prurigo pudendi muliebris.

PUDEN'DAL HER'NIA. Hernia, which descends between the vagina and ramus ischii, and forms an oblong tumour in the labium; traceable in the pelvis, as far as the os uteri.

PUDENDALIS LONGUS INFERIOR, see Sciatic nerve, lesser.

PUDENDUM, FEMALE, Vulva — p. Muliebre, Vulva.

PUDENDUS, Pudic.

PUDIBIL'IA; from *pudere*, 'to be ashamed,'

The male genital organs; *Genita'lia Viri*, *Viri'lia*, *Pensil'ia*, *Instrumen'ta*, *Puden'da viro'rum*, *Pondus*.

PUDIC, *Pudi'cus*, *Puden'dus*, (F.) *Honteux*. Same etymon. That which causes shame. A name given to the genital organs as well as to different other parts.

PUDIC ARTERIES are distributed to the organs of generation. They are,—1. The *internal Pudic*, *Arteria Pudi'ca*, *A. puden'da commu'nis*, (F.) *Artère honteuse interne*, *A. Sous-pubienne* (Ch.), *Gen'ital Ar'tery*. It is furnished by the hypogastric, and divides into two branches; the one —the *inferior* or *perineal*—which gives off the inferior hemorrhoidal and the artery of the septum; and the other—the *superior*, (F.) *Ischiopénienne*—which furnishes the transverse perineal artery, and divides into two branches; the *artery of the corpus cavernosum*, and the *dorsalis penis*. This latter, in the female, has the name *Dorsa'lis Clitor'idis*. 2. The *external Pudic Arteries*, (F.) *Artères scrotales* ou *vulvaires* (Ch.), *A. honteuses externes*, which are two in number. The one is *superficial* or *subcutaneous*, and the other *deep-seated* or *subaponeurotic*. They are given off from the femoral artery, or some one of its branches; and are distributed to the external parts of generation.

PUDIC NERVE, (F.) *Nerf honteux*, *Nerf ischio-pénien* ou *Ischio-clitorien* (Ch.), is a branch furnished by the sacral plexus, which is distributed to the genital organs; and especially, to the penis in man, and the clitoris in the female.

PU'ERILE, *Pueri'lis*, from *puer*, 'a child,' (F.) *Respiration puérile*, *R. exagérée*, *R. supplémentaire*, *R. hypervésiculaire*. A term applied to the respiration when it is heard loud through the stethoscope, as in healthy children.

PUERILITAS, Dementia of the aged.

PUERITIA, see Age.

PUER'PERA, from *puer*, 'a child,' and *parere*, 'to bring forth.' *Tokas*, *Lochos*, *Enix'a*, *Lecho*, a *lying-in woman*, (F.) *Femme en Couche*, *Accouchée*. A female in child-bed. One recently delivered.

PUER'PERAL, *Puerpera'lis*; from *puerpera*. Relating to parturition and its consequences.

PUERPERAL CONVULSIONS, Eclampsia gravidarum et parturientium.

PUER'PERAL FEVER. Any fever occurring during the puerperal state—*Febris puerpera'rum*, *Lechop'yra*, *Lochiocœlii'tis*, *Lochiop'yra*, *Child-bed fever*. Most commonly restricted to a malignant variety of peritonitis.

PUERPERIUM, Child-bed state.

PUERPEROUS, Parturient.

PUFF, VEILED, see Cavernous respiration.

PUFF-BALL, Lycoperdon, Leontodon taraxacum.

PUF'FINESS, from (D.) poffen, 'to blow:' *Infla'tio*, *Suffla'tio*; *Tumefac'tio mollis*, (F.) *Bouffissure*, *Boursouflure*. A soft intumescence, without redness, which may be partial or general, and be produced by accumulation of serous fluid, extravasation of blood, effusion of air into the subcutaneous areolar tissue, &c. Puffiness is most frequently seen in the face and legs; and sometimes appears around a wound.

PUGIL'LUS, *Drax*, *Dra'chion*, from *pugnus*, 'the fist.' *Dragma*, *Dragmis*, (F.) *Pincée*. The quantity of any substance, which may be taken with the end of two or three fingers. The eighth part of a handful.

PUISSANCE DU MOULE INTÉRIEUR, Plastic force.

PUKE, Emetic.

PUKEWEED, Lobelia inflata.

PUKING, Vomiting, Regurgitation.

PULEGIUM, Mentha pulegium—p. Cervinum, Mentha cervina.

PULEX IRRI'TANS. The *common flea*, (F.) *Puce*. A parasitic insect found on the bodies of man and animals.

PULEX PENETRANS, *Chique*.

PULICARIA DYSENTERICA, Inula dysenterica.

PULICA'RIS, *Puricula'ris*, from *pulex*, 'a gnat.' An epithet given to cutaneous eruptions resembling gnat-bites;—and, also, to diseases in which such eruptions occur.

PULICARIS HERBA, Plantago psyllium.

PÜLLNA, MINERAL WATERS OF. These Bohemian springs contain sulphates of soda and magnesia, and chloride of magnesium.

PULMO, *Pulmo'nes*, by transposition of the letter *l* from *pleumon*, πλευμων; *Pneumon*, *Pleumon*, *Spiramen'tum an'imœ*, *Ergaste'rion spir'itûs*, *Flabell'um et ventila'brum cordis*, the Lung. The essential organ of respiration, which is double, and occupies the two sides of the chest. The lungs, which are of a spongy, soft, flexible, compressible, and dilatable structure, fill exactly the two cavities of the thorax, and are separated from each other by the mediastinum and the heart. The right lung, which is shorter and broader than the left, is divided, by two oblique fissures, into three unequal lobes, *Lobi seu Alæ pulmo'num*. The left has only two lobes, and consequently only one fissure. At the internal surface of those organs, which is slightly concave, there is, about the middle, a pedicle, formed by the bronchia and pulmonary vessels, and called, by anatomists, the *root of the lungs*, (F.) *Racine des Poumons*. Essentially, the lungs are composed of prolongations and ramifications of the bronchia, and of the pulmonary arteries and veins,—the divisions of which are supported by a fine, areolar tissue.

When the surface of the lungs is examined in a clear light, we may see, even through the pleura, that their parenchyma is formed by the aggregation of a multitude of small vesicles, of an irregularly spheroid or ovoid shape, full of air, and separated by white and opake septa. These vesicles are called *Air-cells*, *Spiramen'ta* seu *Spiram'ina* seu *Cell'ulæ Pulmo'num*. Along the partitions or septa is deposited, in greater or less quantity, *black pulmonary matter*, (F.) *Matière pulmonaire noire*, as it has been called, which seems to be natural. Sometimes it is seen in points; at others, in spots. The colour of the lungs varies according to age and other circumstances. In youth, it is more red; and afterwards, grayish or bluish; often, as if marbled. The pleura pulmonalis is their investing membrane. The air is carried to the lungs by means of the trachea and bronchia. The black venous blood, which requires oxygenation, is conveyed to them from the heart, by the pulmonary artery; and when it has undergone this change, it is returned to the heart by the pulmonary veins. The blood-vessels inservient to the nutrition of the lungs are the *bronchial* arteries and veins. The pulmonary lymphatics are very numerous. Some are superficial; others, deep-seated. They pass, for the most part, into the *bronchial ganglions* or *glands*. The nerves are furnished by the pulmonary plexus.

PULMONAIRE DES FRANÇAIS, Hieracium murorum.

PULMONA'RIA, *P. officina'lis*, *P. Macu'lata*, *P. Maculo'sa*, *Lungwort*, *Spotted Lungwort*, *Jerusalem Cowslip*, *Jerusalem Sage*, *Spotted Comfrey*, (F.) *Sauge de Jerusalem*. Family, Boragineæ. Sex. Syst. Pentandria Monogynia. The leaves of this plant have been used as demulcents and pectorals; partly from their resemblance to lungs, and, partly, because they have a slightly mucilaginous taste. The plant is not worthy of notice.

PULMONARIA, Pneumonia—p. Arborea, Lichen pulmonarius—p. Gallica, Hieracium murorum—p. Officinalis, Pulmonaria.

PUL'MONARY, *Pulmona'ris, Pulmona'lis.* That which relates or belongs to the lungs. A name given to various parts.

PULMONARY ARTERY, *Arte'ria pulmona'ris, Vena arterio'sa,* arises from the upper and left part of the right ventricle of the heart; whence it passes obliquely upwards and to the left side; dividing into two trunks, opposite the second dorsal vertebra—one passing to each lung. At its origin, it is furnished with three sigmoid or semilunar valves. It carries the blood to the lungs for aeration.

PULMONARY MATTER, BLACK, see Pulmo.

PULMONARY PLEXUS, *Plexus pulmona'ris.* A considerable nervous network, situate behind the bronchia, which is formed by the filaments of the pneumogastric nerve or par vagum, and by other filaments from the inferior cervical ganglion and the first thoracic ganglia. This plexus forms a kind of areolar web, with numerous meshes of different sizes, in which vessels are lodged, surrounded by much areolar tissue. This plexus sends filaments to the bronchia, which they accompany to their extremities.

PULMONARY VEINS, *Venæ pulmona'res, Arte'riæ veno'sæ.* These arise in the lungs from the final terminations of the arteries of the same name; collect in ramusculi and rami of greater and greater size, and ultimately unite in four trunks; two of which issue from each lung to open into the left auricle of the heart. The pulmonary veins have the same structure as the other veins of the body; from which they differ, in containing arterial blood, as the pulmonary artery differs from the others in conveying venous blood. They carry the blood back to the heart after aeration.

PULMONES TARTARIZATI, Lithiasis pulmonum.

PULMONIA, Phthisis pulmonalis, Pneumonia.

PULMON'IC, *Pulmon'icus, Pneumon'icus, Pulmona'rius, Pneumon'ic.* One affected with phthisis —one labouring under diseases of the lungs. Any thing relating or belonging to the lungs. A medicine for the lungs.

PULP, *Pulpa, Pulpa'men, Sarx.* The soft and parenchymatous parts of vegetables reduced to a paste by the operation of pulping.

PULP OF THE TOOTH, Dental pulp.

PULPA CASSIÆ, see Cassia fistula—p. Dentis, Dental pulp—p. Pruni, see Pruni pulpa—p. Prunorum sylvestrium condita, Conserva pruni sylvestris—p. Tamarindi, see Tamarindi pulpa.

PULPA TESTIS, *Paren'chyma testis.* The parenchyma of the testis.

PULPAMEN, Pulp.

PULPE DENTAIRE, Dental pulp.

PULPEZIA, Apoplexy.

PULPING, *Pulpa'tion, Pulpa'tio.* An operation — the object of which is to reduce certain vegetable substances to a pulp. For this purpose, they are bruised in a mortar, and then passed through a hair sieve, by the aid of a wooden spatula, called a *Pulper,* (F.) *Pulpoir.*

PULPOIRE, see Pulping.

PULQUE, see Agave Americana.

PULS EX OVIS et LACTE, Oogala.

PULSATILLA NIGRICANS, Anemone pratensis—p. Pratensis, Anemone pratensis—p. Vulgaris, Anemone pulsatilla.

PULSATILLE NOIRE, Anemone pratensis —p. *des Prés,* Anemone pratensis.

PULSATIO, Pulsation—p. Cordis, Palpitation.

PULSA'TION, *Pulsa'tio, Sphygmos, Sphyxis, Pede'sis, Pedeth'mos,* (F.) *Battement.* The beating of the heart and arteries. Also, the beating felt in an inflamed part.

PULSATIVUS, Throbbing.

PULSATORY, Throbbing.

PULSE, from *pulso,* 'I beat;' *Pulsus, Pulsa'tio, Pulsus cordis et arteria'rum, Ictus cordis et arteria'rum, Incur'sus arteria'rum, Sphygmos, Sphygma, Diasphyx'is,* (F.) *Pouls.* Beating of the arteries, produced by the afflux of the blood propelled by the heart in its contractions. For the sake of convenience, we choose the radial artery at the wrist to detect the precise character of the pulse. These characters relate to the number of pulsations in a given time; to their degrees of quickness; hardness and strength; to the equality or inequality either of the pulsations themselves or of their intervals; to the development or fulness of the artery, and to the different impressions it may produce on the finger.

The following estimates have been made of the pulse at various ages:

Ages.	Number of Beats per minute, according to		
	HEBERDEN.	SÖMMERING.	MÜLLER.
In the embryo			150
At birth	130 to 140		Do.
One month	120		
One year	120 to 108	120	115 to 130
Two years	108 to 90	110	100 to 115
Three years	90 to 80	90	90 to 100
Seven years	72		85 to 90
Twelve years	70		
Puberty		80	60 to 65
Adult age		70	70 to 75
Old age		60	50 to 65

It does not appear that the pulse of the aged is less frequent, but the contrary. In general it is more frequent in females and in irritable persons, than in males and those of an opposite temperament. In the healthy state, the pulse, besides having the proper number of pulsations, is neither hard nor unusually soft; it is moderately developed; of a medium strength; and perfectly equal, both as regards the pulsations and their intervals. In diseases it wanders, more or less, from these physiological conditions. The different characters of the pulse that have been recorded, are remarkably numerous. In a dictionary, it is necessary to detail them, although many of them are not now regarded, and some are ridiculous.

PULSE, ARDENT, *Pulsus ardens,* (F.) *Pouls ardent, Pouls élevé.* One which seems to raise itself to a point in order to strike the finger.

PULSE, CAP'RIZANT, *Pulsus Capri'zans, P. dor-*

cadis'eans, P. gazell'ane, P. fusa'lis, Goatleap *pulse,* (F.) *Pouls caprisant.* One which seems to leap, as it were; an imperfect dilatation of the artery being succeeded by a fuller and a stronger one.

PULSE, COMPLEX, (F.) *Pouls combiné* ou *composé, P. compliqué.* A pulse which has the character of several critical pulses united.

PULSE, CONTRACT'ED, (F.) *Pouls serré, P. concentré.* One whose pulsations are narrow, deep, and slightly hard.

PULSE, CONVUL'SIVE, *Pulsus convulsi'vus,* (F.) *Pouls convulsif.* That which is unequally frequent or unequally hard; in short, which resembles the irregular pulsations of a muscular fibre in a state of convulsion.

PULSE, CRIT'ICAL, *Pulsus crit'icus.* A pulse which, after having possessed the characters of irritation, becomes free, open, soft, &c.

PULSE, DECURTATE, Pulsus myurus: see, also, Myurus.

PULSE, DEEP, *Pulsus profun'dus,* (F.) *Pouls profond.* One which cannot be felt without difficulty, and without strong pressure by the finger.

PULSE, DEFIC"IENT, *Pulsus defic"iens, P. Flickering, Pulsus an'nuens et circum'nuens,* (F.) *Pouls défaillant, P. insensible.* One which seems, every instant, about to cease.

PULSE, DEPRESSED, *Pulsus depressus,* (F.) *Pouls déprimé.* That which is deep and weak.

PULSE, DEVEL'OPED, (F.) *Pouls développé.* That which is broad, full, strong, and frequent.

PULSE, DICROT'IC, *Pulsus Di'crotus, P. bi'crotus, P. intestina'lis, P. bife'riens, P. mallea'ris, P. interci'sus,* (F.) *P. dicrote, P. rebondissant, P. redoublé.* That in which the finger is struck twice at each pulsation; once lightly, the other time more strongly.

PULSE, EQUAL, *Pulsus æqua'lis.* That in which the pulsations resemble each other, and return at equal intervals.

PULSE, FEBRILE, *Pulsus febri'lis.* One very frequent.

PULSE, FEEBLE, WEAK, *Pulsus deb'ilis,* (F.) *Pouls faible.* One which strikes the finger feebly.

PULSE, FIL'IFORM, *P. thready.* One which resembles a thread slightly vibrating.

PULSE, FLICKERING, Pulse, deficient.

PULSE, FORM'ICANT, *Pulsus formi'cans,* (F.) *Pouls formicant.* One which resembles, by being small and scarcely perceptible, the motion of an ant.

PULSE, FREQUENT, (F.) *P. agité, P. précipité.* One which strikes more frequently than usual in a given time.

PULSE, FULL, *Pulsus plenus,* (F.) *Pouls plein.* One which gives the notion of great repletion in the vessel.

PULSE, GOAT-LEAP, P. Caprisant.

PULSE, GUT'TURAL, *Pulsus guttura'lis,* (F.) *Pouls guttural.* A pulse which has been supposed to indicate the termination of affections of the throat.

PULSE, HARD, *Pulsus durus,* (F.) *Pouls dur.* That in which the pulp of the finger seems to yield to the pulsation.

PULSE, HECTIC, *Pulsus hec'ticus.* The weak, frequent pulse observed in hectic fever.

PULSE, HEMORRHOID'AL, (F.) *Pouls des Hémorrhoïdes.* A critical pulse, announcing the appearance of the hemorrhoidal flux. It is described as unequal; — the pulsations not being alike in force, and still less the intervals.

PULSE, HEPAT'IC, (F.) *Pouls du Foie.* A pulse imagined to indicate affections of the liver. It is not worthy of description.

PULSE, INFERIOR, (F.) *Pouls inférieur, P. abdominal, P. ventral.* One supposed to announce evacuations below the diaphragm.

PULSE, INTERCUR'RENT, *Pulsus intercur'rens seu inter'cidens.* One in which a superfluous pulsation seems to occur from time to time.

PULSE, INTERMITTENT, (F.) *Pouls intercadent.* One in which the pulsations fail from time to time.

PULSE, INTES'TINAL, (F.) *Pouls des intestins, P. de la diarrhée.* A critical pulse, presumed to announce an evacuation by the intestines.

PULSE, IN'TRICATE, *Pulsus intrica'tus,* (F.) *Pouls embarrassée.* That which is but little developed and unequally slow.

PULSE, IRREG'ULAR, *Pulsus anorma'lis.* One whose pulsations are unequal, and return at unequal intervals.

PULSE OF IRRITA'TION, *Pulsus ab irritatio'ne seu nervi'nus seu acrit'icus.* One which is frequent, hard, and contracted.

PULSE, JARRING, P. vibrating — p. Jerking, Pulse, sharp.

PULSE, LANGUID, (F.) *Pouls languissant.* A slow and feeble pulse.

PULSE, LARGE, *Pulsus crassus, P. magnus,* (F.) *Pouls grand, P. large.* That which is large and full.

PULSE, LONG. One which strikes the finger to a great extent in length.

PULSE, LOW, *Pulsus hu'milis,* (F.) *Pouls bas.* One in which the pulsations are scarcely perceptible.

PULSE, NASAL, (F.) *Pouls nasal, P. capital, P. du Nez.* One supposed to announce the end of an irritation in the nasal fossæ.

PULSE, NAT'URAL, (F.) *Pouls naturel des adultes, P. parfait, P. des adultes, P. modéré.* One that is equal and regular in strength and frequency; compressible, and devoid of hardness.

PULSE, ORGANIC, (F.) *Pouls organique.* One which indicates the affected organ, or the organ by which an evacuation will take place.

PULSE, PEC'TORAL, (F.) *Pouls de l'expectoration.* A critical pulse, announcing the termination of some pulmonary irritation.

PULSE, QUICK. One which strikes sharply, but not forcibly, against the finger.

PULSE, REG'ULAR, *Pulsus norma'lis* aut *regula'ris.* One whose pulsations are equal, and succeed each other at equal intervals.

PULSE, RESIST'ING, (F.) *Pouls résistant.* One a little tense, a little hard.

PULSE, SHARP, (F.) *Pouls prompt, P. vite, P. vif.* One which strikes the finger sharply, rapidly. When to a greater extent, it is called a *jerking pulse.*

PULSE, SHARP-TAILED, Pulsus myurus: see Myurus.

PULSE, SIMPLE, *Pulsus simplex.* A critical pulse, indicating an evacuation by one organ only.

PULSE, SLOW, *Pulsus tardus, P. rarus,* (F.) *Pouls lent, P. tardif, P. rare.* One which strikes the finger slowly.

PULSE, SMALL, *Pulsus parvus,* (F.) *Pouls petit.* One whose pulsations are slender and weak.

PULSE, SOFT, *Pulsus mollis,* (F.) *Pouls mou.* One which yields under the finger.

PULSE, STOM'ACHAL, (F.) *Pouls stomacal, P. de l'estomac.* One supposed to announce an evacuation by the stomach.

PULSE, STRONG, *Pulsus fortis,* (F.) *Pouls fort, P. véhément.* One which strikes the finger strongly.

PULSE, SUPE'RIOR, *Pulsus Superior,* (F.) *Pouls supérieur.* A critical pulse, supervening on irritation of organs situate above the diaphragm.

PULSE, SUPPLE, *Pulsus elas'ticus,* (F.) *Pouls souple.* One in which the pulsations have strength without hardness.

PULSE OF SWEAT, *Pulsus Sudora'lis,* (F.) *Pouls*

Sudoral, P. de la sueur. A critical pulse, indicating an approaching perspiration.

PULSE, TENSE, *P. Cordy, Pulsus tensus,* (F.) *Pouls tendu, P. roide.* One in which the artery resembles a cord fixed at its two extremities. When resembling a wire, it is called *wiry*.

PULSE, THREADY, P. filiform.

PULSE, TREM'ULOUS, *Pulsus trem'ulus,* (F.) *Pouls tremblant, P. palpitant.* One in which each pulsation oscillates.

PULSE, UN'DULATING, *Pulsus fluctuo'sus, P. fluens, P. in'cidens Sola'ni,* (F.) *Pouls ondulant, P. ondoyant.* One which resembles, in its movements, those of the waves.

PULSE, UNE'QUAL, *Pulsus inæqua'lis,* (F.) *Pouls inégal.* One whose pulsations are not alike, or return at unequal intervals.

PULSE, U'RINAL, *Pulsus urina'lis,* (F.) *Pouls de l'Urine.* A critical pulse, fancied to denote an approaching evacuation of urine.

PULSE, U'TERINE, *Pulsus uteri'nus,* (F.) *Pouls Utérine, P. de la Matrice, P. des Règles.* One which indicates the flow of the menses, or the occurrence of metrorrhagia.

PULSE, VENOUS, Pulsus venarum.

PULSE, VERMIC'ULAR. That which imitates the movement of a worm.

PULSE, VI'BRATING, *Jarring Pulse.* One in which the artery seems to vibrate like a musical string.

PULSE, WIRY, see Pulse, tense.

PULSELESS, *Asphyc'tos,* Devoid of pulsation.

PULSELESSNESS, Asphyxia.

PULSIF'IC, *Pulsif'icus;* from *pulsus,* 'pulse.' That which causes or excites pulsation.

PULSILE'GIUM, *Pulsilo'gium, Pulsim'eter,* from *pulsus,* 'the pulse,' and *lego,* 'I tell.' *Sphygmom'eter, Sphygmoscop'ium.* Any instrument for measuring the quickness or force of the pulse.

PULSIMANTI'A; from *pulsus* and μαντεια, 'divination.' The art of predicting or prognosticating by the pulse.

PULSIMETER, Pulsilegium.

PULSUS, Pulse—p. Acriticus, Pulse of irritation—p. Æqualis, Pulse, equal—p. Annuens et circumnuens, Pulse, deficient—p. Anormalis, Pulse, irregular—p. Bicrotus, Pulse, dicrotic—p. Biferiens, P. dicrotus—p. Caprizans, Pulse, caprizant—p. Crassus, Pulse, large—p. Debilis, Pulse, feeble—p. Deficiens, Pulse, deficient—p. Dicrotus, Pulse, dicrotic—p. Dorcadissans, Pulse, caprizant—p. Durus, Pulse, hard—p. Elasticus, Pulse, supple—p. Fluctuosus, Pulse, undulating—p. Fluens, Pulse, undulating—p. Formicans, Formicant, and Pulse, formicant—p. Fortis, Pulse, strong—p. Fusalis, Pulse, caprizant—p. Gazellans, Pulse, caprizant—p. Heterochronicus, see Heterochronicus—p. Humilis, Pulse, Low—p. Incidens Solani, Pulse, undulating—p. Intercidens, Pulse, intercurrent—p. Mallearis, Pulse, dicrotic—p. Intercisus, Pulse, dicrotic—p. Intercurrens, Pulse, intercurrent—p. Intestinalis, Pulse, dicrotic—p. Intricatus, Pulse, intricate—p. Magnus, Pulse, large—p. Mollis, Pulse, soft.

PULSUS MYU'RUS, *Pulse, decurtate; P. sharp-tailed,* (F.) *Pouls myure.* One which goes on diminishing. See Myurus.

PULSUS NERVINUS, Pulse of irritation—p. Normalis, Pulse, regular—p. Parvus, Pulse, small—p. Plenus, Pulse, full—p. Rarus, Pulse, slow.

PUL'SUS SERRI'NUS, (F.) *Pouls serrin,* P. serratile. One which strikes, sometimes strongly, at others feebly, and recalls the idea of a saw.

PULSUS STRIATUS, (F.) *Pouls étroit.* One that strikes the finger to a small extent in breadth.

PULSUS SUDORALIS, Pulse of sweat—p. Tardus, Pulse, slow—p. Urinalis, Pulse, urinal—p. Uterinus, Pulse, uterine.

PULSUS VAC'UUS, (F.) *Pouls vide.* One which gives the idea of emptiness of the artery.

PULSUS VENA'RUM, *Venous Pulse, Phlebopa'lia.* A pulsation occasionally noticed in the jugular veins. It is owing to some of the blood of the right ventricle reflowing into the right auricle, and communicating an impulse to the venous blood arriving in the auricle through the descending cava. It is often a sign of impediment to the flow of blood along the pulmonary artery.

PULTATIO, Atheroma.

PULTICE, Cataplasm.

PULTICULA, *Bouillie.*

PULVERES EFFERVESCENTES, Powders, soda.

PULVERI'ZABLE, *Pul'verable.* Capable of being reduced to powder.

PULVERIZA'TION, *Pulverisa'tio, Pulveri'tio,* (F.) *Pulvérisation,* from *pulvis,* 'dust;' *Coniosto'sis.* The operation of dividing substances, so as to reduce them to powder.

Most drugs are reduced to powder by persons who make it a special business, and who are called *drug-grinders*. This is done on a large scale in *drug mills;* and the implements used are the *grinding mill* and the *stamping mill*. In the shop of the apothecary, pulverization is effected by the pestle and mortar, and the sieve. Where substances require the addition of other bodies to facilitate their reduction to powder,—as where camphor needs a few drops of alcohol—the process is called *pulverization by mediation.*

PULVILLUS, Pad, *Bourdonnet*—p. e Linamentis confectus, *Bourdonnet*—p. Rotundus, *Bourdonnet.*

PULVI'NAR, *Pulvina'rium.* A pillow.

PULVINAR HUMULI, see Humulus lupulus.

PULVINAR MEDICA'TUM seu MEDICINA'LE, *Seculus medicina'lis.* A medicated pillow; as of hops.

PULVINAR PARVUM, Pad—p. Ventriculi, Pancreas.

PULVINULUS, Pad.

PULVIS, *Conis,* (F.) *Poudre.* A substance, reduced into small particles by pulverization. *Simple powders* are those of a single substance; *compound,* those which result from a mixture of several different powders. An *impalpable powder* is one which is so fine that it can scarcely be felt under the finger. A compound powder was, formerly, called *Spe'cies,* (F.) *Espèce.*

PULVIS ABSORBENS, P. de magnesiâ compos—p. Adspersorius, Catapasma—p. Alexiterius, P. contrayervæ comp.—p. Alexiterius, P. ipecacuanhæ compositus—p. Algarothi, Algaroth.

PULVIS ALOES COMPOS'ITUS, *Compound powder of Aloes, Pulvis Aloës cum Guai'aco, P. aloet'icus cum Guaiaco.* (*Aloës epicat. ext.* ʒiss, *guaiac. gum. ros.* ʒj, *pulv. cinnam. comp.* ʒss. Rub the aloes and guaiacum separately, then mix the whole. *Ph. L.*) Cathartic, stomachic, and sudorific. Dose, gr. x to ʒj.

PULVIS ALOES CUM CANEL'LA, *Pulvis aloës et canellæ,* (Ph. U. S.,) *Powder of Aloes with Canella. Species Hi'eræ picræ, Hiera picra, Pulvis Aloëticus.* (*Aloës* ℔j. *canell.* ʒiij. Rub separately into a powder, and mix. Ph. U. S.) A warm cathartic. Dose, gr. x. to ʒj.

PULVIS ALOES CUM GUAIACO, P. A. compositus—p. Aloeticus, P. aloes cum canellâ—p. Aloeticus, Hiera picra—p. Aluminosus, P. sulphatis aluminæ compositus—p. Aluminis compositus, P. sulphatis aluminæ compositus—p. Aluminis kinosatus, see P. sulphatis aluminæ compositus.

PULVIS DE AMA'RIS COMPOS'ITUS, *Pulvis antiarthrit'icus ama'rus,* (F.) *Poudre antiarthritique* ambre. (*Rad. gentian., aristoloch. rotund.*, ǎǎ p. 3, *flor. centaur. min.* p. 4, *fol. chamædr., chamapith.* manipul.—f. pulvis, *Ph. P.*) In gouty affections, dyspepsia, &c. Dose, gr. xx.

PULVIS ANGELICUS, Algaroth—p. Anodynus, P. ipecacuanhæ comp.—p. Antiacidus, P. cretæ sompositus—p. Antiacidus, P. de magnesiâ sompos.—p. Antiarthriticus amarus, P. de amaris compositus—p. Antiarthriticus purgans, P. de sennâ, scammoneâ et lignis—p. Antiasthmaticus, P. de sulphure et scillâ.

PULVIS ANTILYS'SUS, *Mead's Powder against the bite of a mad dog.* It consisted of *ash-coloured l'verwort* in powder, with an equal quantity of *black pepper*; a drachm and a half of the two forming a dose for an adult.

PULVIS ANTIMONIALIS, Antimonial powder.

PULVIS DE ARO COMPOS'ITUS, *Compound Powder of Arum*, (F.) *Poudre de Birckmann*, (*Rad. ari, acori veri, pimpinell. saxifrag.* ǎǎ 40 p. *ocul. cancror. ppt.* 12 p., *cinnam.* 7 p., *potassæ sulph.* 6 p., *ammoniæ muriat.* 2 p.—f. pulv. *Ph. P.*) Sternutatory.

PULVIS AROMATICUS, P. cinnamomi compositus.

PULVIS AS'ARI COMPOS'ITUS, *P. sternutato'rius, P. errhi'nus, P. capita'lis Sancti An'geli, Cephal'icus, Cephalic snuff; Compound powder of Asarabac'ca*, (F.) *Poudre d'asarum composée dite sternutatoire, P. de Saint-Ange.* (*Folior. asar. Europ.* p. tres., *fol. origan. majoranæ, flor. lavand. spic.*, sing. p. 1. Rub into powder. *Ph. L.*) Sternutatory.

PULVIS AURI, see Gold—p. e. Bolo compositus cum opio, P. cretæ compositus cum opio—p. e. Bolo compositus sine opio, see P. cretæ compositus—p. Cambogiæ compositus, P. e. gummi guttâ—p. Capitalis Sancti Angeli, Pulvis asari compositus—p. Carbonatis calcis compositus, P. cretæ compositus—p. Cardiacus, P. contrayervæ comp.—p. Carthusianorum, Antimonii sulphuretum rubrum—p. Catharticus, P. scammoneæ comp.—p. Cephalicus, P. asari compositus.

PULVIS CINNAMO'MI COMPOS'ITUS, *Compound Powder of Cin'namon, Pulvis seu Spe'cies Imperato'ris, P. vitæ Imperato'ris, P. Diaro'maton, Species diacinnamo'mi, S. lætifican'tes Rhasis, Tra'gea aromat'ica, Species Diam'bræ sine odora'tis, Species aromat'ica, Pulvis aromaticus* (Ph. U. S.), *Aromatic powder*, (F.) *Poudre de canelle composée ou aromatique.* (*Cinnam., singib.* ǎǎ ℥ij, *cardam., myrist.* ǎǎ ℥j. Rub to a fine powder. Ph. U. S.) Stimulant and carminative. Dose, gr. x to ∋j.

PULVIS COBBII seu TUNQUINEN'SIS. The famous Tonquin powder, introduced into England by a Mr. Cobb. It was composed of 16 grains of *musk*, and 48 grains of *cinnabar*; and was mixed in a gill of *arrack*. It was formerly regarded as a specific in hydrophobia.

PULVIS COMITIS WARWICENSIS, P. Cornachini—p. Comitissæ, Cinchona.

PULVIS CONTRAYER'VÆ COMPOS'ITUS, *Lapis contrayervæ, Contrayerva balls, Compound Powder of Contrayer'va, Pulvis cardi'acus, P. alexite'rius, P. Mantua'nus.* (*Contrayerv. rad. contrit.* ℥v, *test. præp.* ℔ss. Mix. *Ph. L.*) Stimulant and sudorific. Dose, gr. xv to ℨss.

PULVIS CORNACHI'NI, *Diaceltates'son Paracelsi, Earl of Warwick's powder, Pulvis Ox'ydi Stib'ii compos'itus, Pulvis Com'itis Warwicen'sis, Pulvis de Tribus, Cer'berus Triceps, Pulvis Scammo'nii antimonia'lis*,(F.) *Poudre Cornachine.* (*Scammon. Alep., potass. supertart., antim. diaph.* ǎǎ p. æ. f. pulv. *Ph. P.*) Cathartic. Used chiefly in cutaneous diseases. Dose, ℨss to ℨj.

PULVIS CORNU USTI CUM O'PIO, *Pulvis opia'tus, Powder of Burnt Hartshorn with opium*, (F.) *Poudre de corne brulée avec l'opium.* (*Opii duri* cont. ℨj, *corn. ust. præp.* ℨj, *coccor.* cont. ℨj. Mix. *Ph. L.*) Ten grains contain one of opium. Anodyne.

PULVIS CRETACEUS, P. cretæ compositus.

PULVIS CRETÆ COMPOS'ITUS, *P. Carbona'tis Calcis compositus, Compound Powder of chalk, P. creta'ceus, Spe'cies e Scordio sine opio, Diasordium, Pulvis antac"idus, P. terres'tris, Species Diacre'tæ*, (with Bole Armeniac in place of chalk—the *Pulvis e Bolo compositus sine opio*), (F.) *Poudre de craie composée.* (*Cretæ ppt.* ℔ss, *cinnam. cort.* ℥iv, *tormentill. rad., acaciæ gum.*, sing ℥iij, *pip. long. fruct.* ℨiv. Reduce separately to a fine powder, and mix. *Ph. L.*) Antacid, stomachic, absorbent. Dose, gr. xx to ∋ij.

PULVIS CRETÆ COMPOS'ITUS CUM O'PIO, *Compound Powder of Chalk with opium, Pulvis e Oretâ compositus cum opio* (with Bole Armeniac instead of chalk—*Pulvis e Bolo compositus cum opio*,) *Species e Scordio cum opio*, (F.) *Poudre de craie composée avec l'opium.* (*Pulv. cret. c.* ℥vjss, *opii duri* cont. ∋iv. Mix. *Ph. L.*) Contains one grain of opium in 40. Anodyne and absorbent. Dose, ∋j to ∋ij.

PULVIS DIAPHORETICUS, P. ipecacuanhæ comp.—p. Diapnoicus, P. ipecacuanhæ comp.—p. Diaromaton, P. cinnamomi compositus—p. Diasensæ P. sennæ compos.—p. Diaturpethi compositus, P. jalapæ compositus.

PULVIS DUCIS PORTLAN'DIÆ, *Duke of Portland's Gout Powder.* (*Rad. aristoloch., gentianæ, summit. chamædr., centaur. min.* ǎǎ p. æ.) Dose, ℨss to ℨj.

PULVIS EMMENAGOGUS, P. myrrhæ compositus—p. Epilepticus Marchionum, P. de magnesiâ compositus—p. Errhinus, P. asari compositus—p. Galactopœus, P. de magnesiâ compos.

PULVIS E GUMMI GUTTÂ, *P. Cambo'giæ compositus, P. hydrago'gus, Camboge Powder*, (F.) *Poudre hydragogue ou de gomme gutte, P. de Querceta'nus.* (*Rad. jalap.* 24 p., *rad. mechoacan.* 12 p., *cinnam., rhei.* ǎǎ 8 p., *gum. cambog.* 3. p., *fol. soldanellæ* sicc. 6 p., *semin. anisi* 12 p., fiat pulvis. *Ph. P.*) A drastic cathartic. In anasarca and in worms. Dose, gr. xv to xxx.

PULVIS GUMMO'SUS ALKALI'NUS, *Sapo vegeta'bilis*, (F.) *Poudre de savon végétal.* (*Guaiac. pulv.* 32. p., *potass. carb.* 4 p. Make into a powder. *Ph. P.*) Antacid.

PULVIS EX HELMINTHOCORT'O COMPOS'ITUS, *P. vermif'ugus absque mercu'rio*, (F.) *Poudre vermifuge sans mercure.* (*Fuc. helminthocort., sem. contra., summitat. absinth., tanaceti, fol. scordii, sennæ, rhei.* ǎǎ p. æ, fiat pulvis. *Ph. P.*) Dose, ∋j to ℨj.

PULVIS HYDRAGOGUS, P. e gummi guttâ—p. Hydrargyri cinereus, see Hydrargyri oxydum cinereum—p. Hypnoticus, Hydrargyri sulphuretum nigrum—p. Imperatoris, P. cinnamomi compositus—p. Incisivus, P. de sulphure et scillâ—p. Pro infantibus, P. de magnesiâ compos.—p. Infantum, P. de magnesiâ compos.—p. Infantum antacidus, P. de magnesiâ compositus.

PULVIS IPECACUAN'HÆ COMPOS'ITUS, *P. alexite'rius, P. anod'ynus, P. diaphoret'icus, P. diapno'icus, P. sudorif'icus Dove'ri, Compound powder of Ipecacuanha, P. Ipecacuanhæ et Opii* (Ph. U. S.), *Dover's Powder*, (F.) *Poudre de Dover ou d'ipecacuanha et d'opium, P. de Dover.* (*Ipecacuanh. pulv., opii pulv.*, sing ℨj, *potassæ sulphat.* ℨj. Mix.) Diaphoretic. Dose, gr. v to gr. xij.

PULVIS IPECACUANHÆ ET OPII, P. ipecacuanhæ compos.

PULVIS JALAP'Æ COMPOS'ITUS, *P. Diaturpe'thi compositus, Compound powder of Jalap, Pulvis laxans, P. Purgans, P. laxati'vus vegetab'ilis, P. laxans cum salâ, P. Jalap'æ sali'nus, P. j. tartar'icus, Spe'cies Diajalapæ*, (F.) *Poudre de jalap composée. (Pulv. jalap.* ℨj, *potass. bitart.* ℨij. Mix.) Cathartic. Dose, ϶j to ʒij.

PULVIS JALAPÆ SALINUS, P. jalapæ compositus—p. Jalapæ tartaricus, P. jalapæ compositus—p. de Jalapâ et scammonio compositus, P. scammoneæ comp.—p. Jamesii, Antimonial powder—p. Jesuiticus, Cinchona—p. Joannis de Vigo, Hydrargyri nitrico-oxydum.

PULVIS KINO COMPOS'ITUS, *Compound Powder of kino,* (F.) *Poudre de kino composée.* (*Kino* ʒxv, *cort. cinnam.* ʒiv, *opii duri* ʒj. Rub each to powder, and mix. *Ph. L.*) Astringent. Dose, gr. v to xx.

PULVIS LAXANS, P. jalapæ compositus—p. Laxans cum sale, P. jalapæ compositus—p. Laxativus vegetabilis, P. jalapæ compositus.

PULVIS DE MAGNE'SIÂ COMPOS'ITUS, *P. Galactopœ'us, P. Nutri'cum, P. Infan'tum, P. Infantum antac'idus, P. pro Infan'tibus, P. antiac'idus, P. absor'bens, P. epilep'ticus Marchio'num, Compound powder of Magne'sia,* (F.) *Poudre absorbante et anti-acide.* (*Magnesiæ, sacchar.* ăă p. æ. Mix. *Ph. P.*)

PULVIS MANTUANUS, P. contrayervæ comp.— p. Marchionis, Marchionis Pulvis—p. Mercurialis cinereus, Hydrargyri oxidum cinereum—p. ad Mucum pulmonalem liberius ciendum, P. de sulphure et scillâ.

PULVIS MYRRHÆ COMPOS'ITUS, *P. e Myrrhâ composita, Compound Myrrh Powder, Pulvis ad ul'cera tend'inum, P. Emmenago'gus,* (F.) *Poudre Balsamique.* (*Myrrhæ, sabinæ, rutæ, castor. Russ.* ăă ʒj.) A stimulant, antispasmodic, and emmenagogue. Dose, gr. xv to xl.

PULVIS NUTRICUM, P. de magnesiâ compositus—p. Opiatus, P. cornu usti cum opio—p. Oxydi stibii compositus, P. cornachini—p. Parturiens, Ergot—p. de Phosphate calcis et stibii compositus, Antimonial powder—p. Principis, Hydrargyri nitrico-oxydum—p. Purgans, P. jalapæ compositus—p. Quercetanus, Hydrargyri submurias.

PULVIS QUERCÛS MARI'NÆ, *Powder of Yellow Bladder-Wrack.* (The wrack in fruit, dried, cleaned, exposed to a red heat in a crucible, with a perforated lid, and then reduced to powder. *Ph. D.*) Virtues dependent on iodine: used, consequently, in bronchocele, &c. Dose, gr. x to xl. See Fucus vesiculosus.

PULVIS SCAMMO'NEÆ COMPOS'ITUS, *Compound Powder of Scammony, Pulvis e Scammonio compositus, Pulvis Scammonii, Pulvis de Jalapâ et Scammo'nio compositus dictus Cathar'ticus,* (F.) *Poudre cathartique* ou *Poudre de Scammonée composée.* (*Scammon., ext. jalap. dur.,* sing., ʒij, *singib. rad.* ʒss. Rub separately to powder and mix. *Ph. L.*) Cathartic. Dose, gr. viij to gr. xv.

PULVIS SCAMMO'NII CUM ALOË, *P. e Scammonio cum Aloë, Scammony and Aloes Powder.* (*Scammon.* ʒvj, *ext. jalap. dur., aloës Socotr.* ăă ʒiss, *sing.* ʒss.) Cathartic. Dose, gr. x to xv.

PULVIS SCAMMONII ANTIMONIALIS, P. cornachini.

PULVIS SENNÆ COMPOS'ITUS, *Compound powder of Senna, Pulvis e Sennâ compositus, P. e Sennâ compositus, Pulvis Diasse'næ,* (F.) *Poudre de séné composée.* (*Sennæ folior., potass. supertart.* sing. ʒij, *scammon.* ʒss, *rad. singib.* ʒij. *Ph. L.*) Cathartic, hydragogue. Dose, ϶j to ʒj.

PULVIS DE SENNÂ, SCAMMO'NIO ET LIGNIS COMPOS'ITUS *dictus* ANTIARTHRIT'ICUS PURGANS, (F.) *Poudre de Pérard.* (*Gum Arab., potass. supertart., fol. sennæ, chinæ,* ăă 4 p., *scammon., rad. sarsapar., chinæ, guaiac. lign.* ăă 2 p., fiat pulvis. *Ph. P.*) Purgative. Used to obviate gout. Dose, ʒj.

PULVIS STANNI, see Tin—p. Sternutatorius, P. asari compositus—p. Stibiatus, Antimonial powder—p. Stypticus, P. Sulphatis aluminæ compositus—p. Sudorificus, P. ipecacuanhæ comp.—p. Sudorificus Doveri, P. Ipecacuanhæ compositus.

PULVIS SULPHA'TIS ALU'MINÆ COMPOS'ITI, *P. alumino'sus, P. alu'minis kinosa'tus, Pulvis styp'ticus, Pulvis aluminis compositus, Alu'men kinosa'tum, Compound Alum Powder,* (F.) *Poudre styptique* ou *d'alun composée.* (*Sulphatis aluminæ,* p. iv, *kino,* p. 1. *Ph. E.*) Astringent. In intestinal hemorrhage and diarrhœa. Dose, gr. x to xv.

PULVIS DE SUL'PHURE ET SCILLÂ, *P. Antiasthmat'icus, P. Incisi'vus, P. ad mucum pulmona'lem libe'rius cien'dum,* (F.) *Poudre incisive ou anti-asthmatique.* (*Sacchar. alb.* p. 3, *sulphur. lot.* p. 2, *scillæ.* siccat. p. j. *Ph. P.*) Dose, gr. v to ʒss.

PULVIS DE SULPHA'TE POTAS'SÆ COMPOS'ITUS, *P. tem'perans Stah'lii,* (F.) *Poudre tempérante de Stahl.* (*Potass. sulph., P. nitrat.* ăă 9 p., *hydrarg. sulph. rubr.* 2 p. Mix. *Ph. P.*) As an antiphlogistic, and in acidity of the first passages. Dose, ϶j to ʒij.

PULVIS E SULPHURE'TO HYDRAR'GYRI NIGRO ET SCAMMO'NIO, *dictus* VERMIF'UGUS MERCURIALIS, (F.) *Poudre vermifuge mercurielle.* (*Pulv. cornachin., hydrarg. sulphuret. nigr.* recent. præp. ăă p. æ. Mix. *Ph. P.*) Dose, ϶j to ʒj.

PULVIS SYMPATHETICUS, Sympathetic powder—p. Temperans Stahlii, P. de sulphate potassæ compositus—p. Terrestris, P. cretæ compositus.

PULVIS TRAGACAN'THÆ COMPOS'ITUS, *Species Diatragacan'thæ frig"idæ, Pulvis e Tragacan'thâ compositus, Compound Powder of Tragacanth,* (F.) *Poudre de gomme adragant composée.* (*Tragacanth. contus., acaciæ gummi cont., amyli,* sing. ʒiss, *sacch. purif.* ʒiij. *Ph. L.*) Demulcent. In coughs, &c. Dose, ʒss to ʒij.

PULVIS DE TRIBUS, P. cornachini—p. Tuquinensis, P. Cobbii—p. ad Ulcera tendinum. P. myrrhæ compositus—p. Vermifugus abeque mercurio, Pulvis ex helminthocorto comp.—p. Vermifugus mercurialis, P. e sulphureto hydrargyri nigro et scammonio—p. Vitæ Imperatoris, P. cinnamomi compositus.

PUMEX, *Lapis pu'micis, Pumice,* (F.) *Pierre Ponce.* This was formerly employed as a desiccative and dentifrice.

PUMICE, Pumex.

PUMILIO, Nanus.

PUMILUS, see Nanus.

PUMP, BREAST, Antlia lactea—p. Stomach Antlia gastrica.

PUNA, Veta, Sorocco, Soroche, Mareo. A sickness common in the elevated districts of South America and elsewhere, which attacks those unaccustomed to breathe the rarefied atmosphere. It strongly resembles sea-sickness, with a most acute and depressing throbbing in the head. It does not often affect the respiration considerably.

PUNAISE, Cimex.

PUNAISIE, Ozæna.

PUNCH, *Rhi'sagra,* from *pungere,* 'to pinch,' *Repulso'rium,* (F.) *Repoussoir.* A surgical instrument used for extracting the stumps of teeth. See Lever.

Also, an agreeable alcoholic drink, made of spirit, wine, sugar, lemon-juice, and water. Ice is sometimes substituted in part for the water: it then forms *Milk Punch.*

PUNCTA OSSIFICATIONIS, Ossification, points of.

PUNCTÆ MUCOSÆ, see Acne.

PUNCTICULA, Petechiæ.

PUNCTIO, Paracentesis, Puncture—p. Nervi Neuronygme.

PUNCTUM, Stitch.

PUNCTUM AU'REUM, *Punc'tura aurea.* Formerly, when an intestinal hernia was reduced by an incision made through the integuments down to the upper part of the spermatic vessels, a golden wire was fixed and twisted, so as to prevent the descent of any thing down the tunica vaginalis. Hence the term.

PUNCTUM SA'LIENS, *P. sanguin'eum sa'liens, Glob'ulus sanguin'eus, Punctus ruber sa'liens.* The first moving *point* which makes its appearance after the fecundation of the germ. It has been generally, but erroneously, applied to the heart of the embryo.

PUNCTURA, Paracentesis — p. Aurea, Punctum aureum.

PUNCTURE, *Punctu'ra, Punc'tio, Cente'sis, Paracente'sis, Nyxis,* from *pungere,* 'to prick;' *Tresis Punctura,* (F.) *Piqure.* A wound made by a pointed instrument, as a sword, bayonet, needle, thorn, &c. A puncture is, generally, of trifling consequence; but, sometimes, it becomes important from the parts implicated, and the after consequences.

PUNCT'URING. Same etymon. *Compunc'tio, Paracente'sis,* (F.) *Ponction.* The operation of opening, by means of a trocar, lancet, &c., any natural or accidental cavity, with the view of evacuating any fluid, effused or accumulated therein. *Paracentesis* is a sort of puncturing.

PUNCTUS RUBER SALIENS, Punctum saliens.

PUNGENT, (F.) *Pongitif.* Pain is said to be pungent, when it seems as if a pointed instrument were forced into the suffering part.

PU'NICA GRANA'TUM. The *Pomegranate, Rhoa, Rhœa, Grana'tum, Malograna'tum,* (F.) *Grenadier: Family,* Myrtoideæ. *Sex. Syst.* Icosandria Monogynia. The rind of the fruit, called *Malicho'rium, Malacorium,* or *Malicorium;* and the flowers—called *Balaustine flowers*—are used in medicine. They have been employed both internally and externally as astringents. The seeds are called *Cocco'nes,* κοκκωνες. The portion, however, of the plant, that has attained most celebrity, is the bark of the root, *Grana'ti Radi'cis Cortex,* which appears to be very efficacious in tænia. It is given in decoction, (*Granat. rad. cort.* ℨij; *Aquæ* Oij, boiled to Oiss.) Dose, fℨij, every half hour. Three or four doses are usually sufficient to expel the worm.

The bark contains a peculiar matter called *Grenadin.*

PUNK, Boletus igniarius.

PUOGENIA, Pyogenia.

PUPIL, *Pupil'la, Pu'pula, Pupil'io, Vis'io, Opsis, Corē, Cora, Rhox, Fenes'tra* seu *Nigrum* seu *Fora'men Oc'uli, Prunel'la, Lumen; Glenē, Sight of the eye,* (F.) *Pupille, Prunelle.* The aperture of the iris, through which the rays of light pass that have to impress the image of an object on the retina. This aperture can be dilated or contracted so as to allow a greater or smaller quantity of luminous rays to penetrate. The pupil, in man, is round, and by it the anterior and posterior chambers of the eye communicate with each other. In the fœtus, during the first six months of gestation, it is closed by the pupillary membrane.

PUPIL, CLOSURE OF THE, Synezizis.

PUPIL, PINHOLE. A condition of the pupil in typhus, in which it is so contracted as to resemble a pinhole. It indicates a dangerous form of brain affection.

PUPILLÆ VELUM, Pupillary membrane.

PUPILLARIS HERBA, Lapsana.

PU'PILLARY, *Pupilla'ris.* That which belongs to the pupil.

PUPILLARY MEMBRANE, *Membrana Pupilla'ris, Pupil'læ velum, Membra'na Wachendorfia'na.* The central aperture of the iris is closed, in the fœtus, during a certain period of gestation, by a very thin membrane. It disappears in the seventh month.

PUPPET ROOT, Veratrum viride.

PUPPIS OS, Frontal bone.

PUPULA, Pupil.

PU'PULÆ, *A'pices digito'rum.* The pulps or extremities of the fingers.

PURBLIND, Myopic.

PURBLINDNESS, Myopia.

PURGAMENT, Purgative.

PURGAMENTA, Excrement — p. Alba, Leucorrhœa—p. Infantis, Meconium — p. Puerperii, Lochia—p. Uteri, Lochia.

PURGANS MEDICAMENTUM, Cathartic.

PURGATIO, Catharsis — p. Alvi, Catharsis— p. Muliebris alba, Leucorrhœa — p. Puerperii, Lochia.

PURGATION, Catharsis.

PURGATIONES, Menses — p. Menstruæ, Menses.

PURGATIONS, Menses.

PUR'GATIVE, *Purgati'vus, Purgans, Moch'licus, Catoret'icus, Cutoter'icus, Cathar'tic, Pur'gament, Purge,* (F.) *Purgatif,* from *purgare,* 'to cleanse. A medicine which operates more powerfully on the bowels than a laxative, stimulating the muscular coat, and exciting increased secretion from the mucous coat.

PURGE, Purgative—p. Root, Euphorbia corollata.

PURGING, Diarrhœa.

PURIF'ICANS, *Purif'icus,* from *purificare,* 'to make pure or clean.' Purifying: hence:—

PURIFICANTIA; Medicines that cleanse or purify the blood.

PURIFICUS, Purificans.

PU'RIFORM, *Puriform'is;* from *pus,* and *forma.* Having the appearance of pus.

PURL. A medicated malt liquor, in which wormwood and aromatics are infused.

PURO-HEPATITIS, see Hepatitis.

PURO-MUCOUS, *Puro-muco'sus,* from *pus, puris,* and *mucus.* Having the character or appearance of pus and mucus.

PURPLES, Purpura hæmorrhagica.

PUR'PURA, *Por'phyra,* 'a purple colour.' This word has been employed in many senses. It generally means, livid spots on the skin from extravasated blood, with languor and loss of muscular strength, pains in the limbs. — (F.) *Pourpre.*

In PURPURA SIMPLEX, *Porphyra simplex, Petechiæ sinè febrè, Pelio'sis, Phœnig'mus Petechia'lis, Profu'sio subcuta'nea, Pete'chial Scurvy,* the spots are numerous, but small and flea-bite-shaped; chiefly on the breast, arms, and legs; with paleness of countenance. At times, the affection is accompanied by severe pains in the extremities, constituting *Pelio'sis rheumat'ica.*

In PURPURA HÆMORRHAG''ICA, *Porphyra hæmorrhagica, Stomac'ace universalis, Hæmorrhagia universa'lis, Petechiano'sis, Morbus maculo'sus hæmorrhag''icus Werlhof''ii, Pelio'sis hæmorrhag''ica, Scorbu'tus, Schorbu'tus, Hæmorrhœ'a petechia'lis, Hæmatospil'ia, Land Scurvy, Purples,* (F.) *Scorbut, S. de Terre, Maladie de Werlhof, Hémacelinose, Peliose hémorrhagique*—the spots are circular, and of different sizes; often in stripes or patches, irregularly scattered over the thighs, arms, and trunk; with occasional hæmorrhage from the mouth, nostrils, or viscera, and great debility and depression of spirits.

In PURPURA NAU'TICA, *Porphyra nautica, Scorbu'tus, Pechytyrbē, Gingibra'chium, Gingipe'-*

dium, Scelotyr'bē, Stomac'acē, Scorbu'tus nau'ticus or *Sea scurvy*, (F.) *Scorbut*, there are spots of different hues, intermixed with the livid, principally at the roots of the hair; the teeth are loose; the gums are spongy and bleeding; the breath is fetid, and the debility universal and extreme. This occurs chiefly at sea, after exposure to a moist, cold, foul atmosphere; with long use of one kind of food and of stagnant water.

All these varieties of purpura resemble each other considerably. In the first two, however, there seems, at times, to be some excitement, which has led to the employment of purgatives, and even of bleeding, with advantage. They are dependent upon a peculiar diathesis, which has been termed *Scorbu'tic Cachex'ia, Lues Scorbu'tica*, and *Cacochym'ia Scorbu'tica*. Generally speaking, the use of the mineral acids will be indicated; and, in sea scurvy, vegetable acids must be regarded as the best antiscorbutics. Nitre is, also, a good antiscorbutic, and in cases of great prostration it may be united with Peruvian bark or turpentine. Tamarinds and cream of tartar, made into drink, are also serviceable. But the great remedy is change from low to cheerful spirits; from filth to cleanliness; and from a cold and damp, to a temperate and dry climate, with change of food, and especially the use of green vegetables.

The general principles of management are the same in sea, as in land scurvy.

PURPURA, Scarlatina—p. Alba benigna et maligna, Miliary fever—p. Maligna, Petechiæ—p. Miliaris, Miliary fever—p. Puerperarum, Miliary fever—p. Urticata, Urticaria.

PURPURIC URINE, see Porphyruria.

PURPURINE, see Porphyruria.

PURPURISSUM, Hydrargyri sulphuretum rubrum.

PURRING TREMOR, *Frémissement cataire.*

PURSE, Scrotum — p. Shepherd's, Thlaspi bursa.

PUR'SINESS, *Dyspnœ'a pinguedino'sa*, (F.) *Pousse*. Dyspnœa accompanied with oppressive fatness. The word is, also, applied to dyspnœa of every kind. One so affected is said to be *pursy* or *short-winded*.

PURSLAIN, Portulaca — p. Milk, Euphorbia corollata — p. Speedwell, Veronica peregrina—p. Water, Veronica beccabunga.

PURSY, see Pursiness.

PURULENCE, Pus, Suppuration.

PURULENCY, Pus, Suppuration.

PU'RULENT, *Purulen'tus, Em'pyos, Pyo'des, Py'icus.* That which has the character of pus or consists of pus; as *purulent matter, a purulent collection*, &c.

PURULENT DEPOSIT, Pus.

PURULENTIA, Suppuration.

PURVAIN, Verbena officinalis.

PUS, *Humor purulen'tus, Pyon, Pyono'ma, Matter, Pu'rulent depos'it, Pu'rulence, Pu'rulency.* A secretion from inflamed textures, and especially from the areolar membrane. It is, almost always, of the same nature, whatever may be the part it proceeds from. Pus of a good quality,—*laudable pus, Pus bonum seu laudab'ilē seu nutriti'vum seu verum*, (F.) *Pus louable*,—is of a yellowish-white colour, opake, inodorous, and of a creamy appearance. Heat, acids, and alcohol coagulate it. When analyzed by Schwilgué, it afforded albumen and water, a particular extractive substance, and a small quantity of soda, phosphate of lime, and other salts. Normal pus consists essentially of two distinct parts, *pus corpuscles* or *pus globules*, and a colourless, aqueous fluid, *liquor puris*, in which the corpuscles are suspended. A variety of the pus corpuscles is described by M. Lebert under the name *pyoid*.

PUS BONUM, see Pus—p. Corpuscles, see Pus—p. Corrosivum, Sanies—p. Globules, see Pus—p. Laudabile, see Pus—p. Louable, see Pus—p. Malignum, Ichor—p. Malignum, Sanies—p. Nutritivum, see Pus—p. Verum, see Pus.

PUSILLA'TUM, *Pusula'tum*, from *pusilla*, 'small.' A coarse powder.

PUSILLUS, Nanus.

PUSTULA, Pustule—p. Ardens, Ecsema—p. Oris, Aphthæ—p. Gangrænosa, see Anthrax—p. Livida Esthoniæ, see Anthrax.

PUSTULÆ SICCÆ, Lichen.

PUSTULAR, *Pustulous, Pustula'ris, Pustulo'sus.* Of or belonging to pustules. Affected with pustules.

PUSTULA'TION, *Pustula'tio*, from *pustule*, 'a pustule.' The formation of pustules.

PUSTULE, *Pus'tula*, from *pus. Ecpye'sis, Ecthy'ma, Benath, Bubē, Epanas'tasis.* An elevation of the cuticle, with an inflamed base, containing pus. Willan and Bateman reckon four varieties of pustules: *Phlyza'cium, Psydra'cium, Achor*, and *Favus*. The variolous pustule is often called, by the French, *Grain;* by us, *Pock*.

PUSTULE MALIGNE, see Anthrax.

PUSTULOUS, Pustular.

PUSULATUM, Pusillatum.

PUTIUM, Prepuce.

PUTREDO, Hospital Gangrene, Putrefaction.

PUTREFAC'TION, *Putrefac'tio, Putrescen'tia, Sepsis, Sap'rotes, Putrid fermenta'tion, Putrefact'ive fermentation*, from *putris, putre*, 'rotten,' and *facere*, 'to make.' A decomposition, experienced by animal substances, when deprived of life, and placed under particular circumstances. The presence of water is indispensable. The temperature most favourable to it, is from 60° to 90° of Fahrenheit. The most common products of putrefaction are, water, carbonic acid, acetic acid, ammonia, carburetted hydrogen, and a semi-putrid substance, which is volatilized, and has an infected odour. It has been supposed that something like putrefaction may occur in the living body, as in case of putrid fever. To this condition, Piorry has given the name *Typhohe'mie*, conceiving it to be owing to alteration of the blood by putrid animal matters. *Putrefaction* signifies the state of becoming putrid: whilst *Putridity, Putre'do, Putrid'itas, Pu'tridness*, (F.) *Pourriture*, is the state of rottenness.

PUTRESCENT, Hyposapros — p. Poison, see Poison.

PUTRESCENTIA, Putrefaction — p. Uteri gravidi, Hystero-malacia.

PUTRID, *Pu'tridus, Sapros*, (F.) *Putride*, from *putrere*, 'to rot.' An epithet for some affections, in which the matters excreted and the transpiration itself exhale a smell of putridity. It is particularly applied to typhus.

PUTRIDITAS, see Putrefaction.

PUTRIDITY, see Putrefaction.

PUTRILA'GO, *Putror*, (F.) *Putrilage.* Same etymon. The pultaceous matter or *slough*, which forms in certain gangrenous and other ulcers, and is thrown off.

PUTROR, Putrilage.

PUTZOCHILL, see Myroxylon Peruiferum.

PYÆ'MIA, Pyohæmia.

PYARTH'RUM, from πυον, 'pus,' and αρθρον, 'joint.' A suppurated joint.

PYCNAN'THEMUM INCA'NUM, *Common Mountain Mint, Wild Basil.* An indigenous plant of the mint *family* — Labiatæ — which flowers in August. It has the aromatic properties of the mints.

PYCNANTHEMUM LINIFOLIUM, *Virginia Thyme*, has like virtues.
PYCNICMASTICA, Incrassantia.
PYCNOSIS, Inspissatio.
PYCNOTICA, Incrassantia.
PYEC'CHYSIS, from πυον, 'pus,' and εκχυσις, 'effusion.' An effusion of pus.
PYELI'TIS, from πυελος, 'pelvis,' and *itis*, denoting inflammation. Inflammation of the pelvis and calices of the kidney.
PYELOMETER, Pelvimeter.
PYELONEPHRI'TIS, from πυελος, 'pelvis,' νεφρος, 'kidney,' and *itis*, denoting inflammation. Inflammation of the kidney, and of the pelvis and calices.
PYELOS, Pelvis.
PYEMESIS, Pyoemesis.
PYESIS, Suppuration.
PYETIA, Colostrum.
PYGE, Nates.
PYGMÆUS, Pygmy.
PYGME, Fist, Forearm.
PYGMÉE, Pygmy.
PYGMY, *Pigmy*, *Pygmæ'us*, (F.) *Pygmée*, from πυγμη, 'the fist; as big as the fist.' A dwarf. The Pygmæi were a fabulous nation of dwarfs in the extreme parts of India; or, according to others, in Ethiopia.
PYGODIDY'MUS, *Did'ymus symphyoperina'us*, *Pygop'ages*, from πυγη, 'the nates,' and διδυμος, 'a twin.' A monstrosity, in which twins are united by the sacrum and coccyx.
PYGOPAGES, Pygodidymus.
PYICUS, Purulent.
PYLE, Porta.
PYLEMPHRAX'IS, from πυλη, 'porta,' 'a gate,' and εμφραξις, 'obstruction.' Obstruction of the vena portæ.
PYLOR'IC, *Pylor'icus*. Same etymon as pylorus. That which relates to the pylorus. An epithet given to different parts.
PYLORIC ARTERY, *Arte'ria Corona'ria dextra*, (F.) *Petite artère gastrique droite*, arises from the hepatic, and is distributed to the pylorus and to the lesser curvature of the stomach, anastomosing, particularly, with the A. coronaria ventriculi and A. gastro-epiploïca dextra.
PYLORIC VEIN follows the same distribution as the artery.
PYLO'RUS, *Jan'itor*, *Portona'rium*, from πυλη, 'a gate,' and ουρος, 'a guardian.' *Os'tium ventric'uli duodena'lā seu pylor'icum seu dextrum seu infe'rius, Orific'ium dextrum seu inferius seu Egres'sus seu Os infe'rius seu An'nulus seu Sphincter ventri'culi, Ostia'rius, Hostia'rius*, (F.) *Pylore*. The lower or right orifice of the stomach—*Orifice intestinal* (Ch.)—is called *Pylorus*, because it closes the entrance into the intestinal canal, and is furnished with a circular, flattened, fibro-mucous ring, which occasions the total closure of the stomach during digestion in that organ. This ring has been called the *Valve of the Pylorus*, *Sphincter Pylo'ri*, *Pylo'rus proprie sic dictus*, (F.) *Valvule du pylore*. It is a fold of the mucous and muscular membranes of the stomach; and is the *Pyloric muscle* of some authors.
PYOBLENNICUS, Mucopurulent.
PYOBLENNORRHŒ'A, from πυον, 'pus,' βλεννα, 'mucus,' and ρεω, 'I flow.' A discharge of puriform mucus.
PYOCENO'SIS, from πυον, 'pus,' and κενωσις, 'evacuation.' Evacuation of pus.
PYOCHEZ'IA, *Diarrhœ'a purulen'ta*, from πυον, 'pus,' and χιζω, 'I go to stool.' Discharge of pus by stool. Purulent diarrhœa.
PYOCŒ'LIA, *Asci'tes purulen'tus*, from πυον,
'pus,' and κοιλια, 'the belly.' Pus in the abdominal cavity.
PYOCYSTIS, Vomica.
PYODES, Purulent.
PYŒDE'MA, from πυον, 'pus,' and οιδημα, 'swelling.' Tumefaction of the surface owing to effusion of pus.
PYOÉM'ESIS, *Pyem'esis*, *Vom'itus purulentus*, from πυον, 'pus,' and εμεσις, 'the act of vomiting.' Vomiting of pus.
PYOGENESIS, Pyogenia.
PYOGEN'IA, *Puogen'ia*, *Pyogen'esis*, *Pyopoë'sis*, from πυον, 'pus,' and γενεσις, 'generation.' Generation of pus. The theory or mechanism of the formation of pus. Some have believed that pus is formed by the arterial system, and is deposited, by way of excretion, in the inflamed parts; others, that it is formed by the destruction of solid parts. These opinions are, however, inadmissible; and pus is now regarded as mainly the product of a particular secretion in the diseased part.
PYOGENIA CORROSIVA, Ulceration—p. Simplex, Suppuration.
PYOGEN'IC, *Pyogen'icus*. Same etymon. Having relation to the formation of pus.
PYOHÆ'MIA, *Pyæ'mia*, from πυον, 'pus,' and 'αιμα, 'blood.' Alteration of the blood by pus.
PYOID CORPUSCLES or GLOBULES, see Pus.
PYOME'TRA, *P. purulen'ta*, from πυον, 'pus,' and μητρα, 'womb.' A collection of pus in the uterus.
PYOMETRA PURULENTA, Pyometra.
PYON, Pus.
PYONÉPHRITE, see Nephritis.
PYONOMA, Pus.
PYOÖTORRHŒA, Otirrhœa.
PYOPERICAR'DIA, *Pyopericar'dium*, from πυον, 'pus,' περι, 'about,' and καρδια, 'the heart.' A collection of pus in the pericardium.
PYOPHTHALMIA, Hypopyon—p. Neonatorum, see Ophthalmia (puralenta infantum).
PYOPLEURITE, Empyema.
PYOPOËSIS, Pyogenia.
PYOP'TYSIS, from πυον, 'pus,' and πτυω, 'I spit.' Spitting of pus.
PYORRHAG"IA, from πυον, 'pus,' and ραγη, 'violent rupture.' A sudden discharge of a large collection of matter.
PYORRHŒ'A, from πυον, 'pus,' and ρεω, 'I flow.' A discharge of pus.
PYORRHŒA ALVINA, Pyochezia—p. Aurium, Otirrhœa—p. Nasalis, Ozœna—p. Palpebræ, Blepharopyorrhœa—p. Urinalis, Pyuria—p. Viarum lacrymalium, Dacryopyorrhœa.
PYOSIS, Hypopyon, Pterygion, Suppuration—p. Pectoris, Empyema.
PYOTHORAX VERUS, Empyema.
PYOTORRHÉE, Otorrhœa.
PYOTURIA, Pyuria.
PYR, Fever.
PYRA, Anthrax—p. Crustumina, Crustumintum—p. Crustumerina, Crustuminatum.
PYR'AMID, *Pyr'amis*, *Eminen'tia pyramida'lis tym'pani*, from πυρ, 'flame,' which has a conical appearance. (?) A small bony projection in the cavity of the tympanum, which is excavated, to lodge the muscle of the stapes. Also, the *Centre-pin* of the trephine. Also, a small, obtusely pointed eminence of the inferior vermiform process of the cerebellum.
PYRAMID, see Calumba—p. of Malacarne, Vermiform process, inferior.

PYRAMIDAL DE L'ABDOMEN, Pyramidalis abdominis—*p. de la Cuisse,* Pyramidalis—*p. du Nez,* Pyramidalis nasi—*p. Stapédien,* Stapedius.

PYRAMIDALE, (OS,) Cuneiform, (bone.)

PYRAMIDA'LIS ABDOM'INIS, *Mus'culus Fallo'pii* vel *succenturia'tus* vel *auxilia'rius,* (F.) *Pubio-ombilical, Pubio-sous-umbilical,* (Ch.,) *Pyramidal de l'abdomen.* A small, fleshy, pyramidal fasciculus, whose existence is not constant; and which is inserted, by its base, into the upper part of the pubis, and terminates, by its summit, at the inferior part of the linea alba. When it contracts, it stretches the linea alba.

PYRAMIDA'LIS, *P. Fem'oris, Ili'acus exter'nus, Pyriform'is, Piriformis, Primus et superior quadrigem'inus,* (F.) *Sacro-trochantérien* (Ch.), *Pyramidal de la cuisse.* A flat, triangular muscle, situate at the posterior part of the pelvis. By its base, it is attached to the anterior surface of the sacrum; to the corresponding surface of the great sacro-sciatic ligament and to the posterior part of the ilium. It terminates by a tendon, which is attached to the inner surface of the great trochanter. This muscle is a rotator of the thigh outwards, or of the pelvis in an opposite direction.

PYRAMIDALIS FEMORIS, Pyramidalis.

PYRAMIDA'LIS NASI, *Proc''erus nasi, Nasum dila'tans,* (F.) Fronto nasal (Ch.), *Pyramidal du nez.* A thin, triangular muscle, which has its summit upwards. Above, it is continuous with the occipito-frontalis. It descends vertically before the root of the nose, on which it terminates; becoming confounded with the transversalis. This muscle wrinkles the skin of the root of the nose transversely, and stretches that which covers the tip.

PYRAMIDES, Corpora pyramidalia.

PYRAMIDES ANTÉRIEURES, Corpora pyramidalia—*p.* Ferreini, Ferrein, pyramids of —*p.* Malpighianæ, Papillæ of the kidney—*p. Postérieures du cervelet,* Corpora restiformia.

PYRAMIDS OF MALPIGHI, Papillæ of the kidney—*p.* Posterior, Corpora restiformia—*p.* of Wistar, Sphenoidal cornua.

PYRAMIS, Penis, Pyramid—*p.* Cochleæ, Modiolus—*p.* Trigona, see Temporal bone.

PYRŒBA, Incendium.

PYREC'TICA, 'febrile;' from πυρετος, 'fever.' Fevers: the first order in the class *Hæmatica* of Good.

PYRENOIDES, Odontoid.

PYRÈTHRE, Anthemis pyrethrum.

PYRETHRUM, Anthemis pyrethrum, Urtica —*p.* Parthenium, Matricaria parthenium—*p.* Sylvestre, Achillea ptarmica.

PYRETICO'SIS, from πυρ, 'fire,' πυρετος, 'fever;' *Morbus febri'lis.* A febrile affection.

PYRETICUS, Febrifuge.

PYRETOGRAPH'IA, from πυρετος, 'fever,' and γραφη, 'a description.' A description of fever.

PYRETOL'OGY, *Pyretolog''ia,* from πυρετος, 'fever,' and λογος, 'a discourse.' *Pyrol'ogy.* A treatise on fevers. A title sometimes given to a monograph on fever.

PYRETOS, Fever.

PYRETOTYPOSIS, Intermittent.

PYREX'IA, *Pyrex'is.* Same etymon as the next. Fever. The febrile condition. Also, a paroxysm of fever—*Paroxysmus febri'lis.*

PYREX'IÆ, from πυρ, 'fire.' *Febrile diseases.* The first class of Cullen's Nosology.

PYRI MARTIALES, Ferrum tartarizatum.

PYRIA, Fomentation, Vaporarium.

PYRIATERIUM, Vaporarium.

PYRICAUSTUM, Burn.

PYRIFORMIS, Pyramidalis.

PYRIPH'LEGES, πυριφλεγης, from πυρ, 'fire,' and φλεγω, 'I burn.' One who has a burning fever.

PYRITES, IRON, Ferri sulphuretum.

PYRMONT, MINERAL WATERS OF. A celebrated mineral spring, on the Weser, in Westphalia, four leagues from Hamelet. The waters are tonic, and contain chlorides of sodium and magnesium, sulphates of soda and magnesia, and carbonates of iron, lime, and magnesia dissolved in carbonic acid, with some resinous principles. It is a highly carbonated chalybeate.

ARTIFIC''IAL PYRMONT WATER may be formed of *Epsom salt,* gr. xv; *common salt,* gr. v; *magnesia,* gr. x; *iron-filings,* gr. v; *water,* Oiij. Impregnated with the gas from *marble-powder* and *sulphuric acid,* āā Ʒvij.

PYRŒNUS, Spiritus rectificatus.

PYR'OLA, *P. rotundifo'lia, Round-leaved Wintergreen.* Order, Pyrolaceæ. This plant was once used as a gentle astringent and tonic.

PYR'OLA MACULA'TA, *Spotted Pipsis'ewa, Spotted Wintergreen, Whiteleaf, White Pipsissewa, King cure, Ground holly, Rheumatism weed,* &c., has similar properties.

PYROLA UMBELLA'TA, *Chimaph'ila* vel *Chimoph'ila umbella'ta, C. Corymbo'sa, Ground-holly, Pipsissewa, Wintergreen, Rheumatism weed, Herb a pisser* (Canada). This common American plant is allied to the uva ursi, in botanical as well as medical qualities. It is tonic and diuretic. The bruised leaves irritate the skin. From the decoction or infusion an agreeable beverage may be formed by adding sugar, ginger to flavour it, and yeast to produce fermentation. Under the name *Pipsis'sewa Beer* it has been used in scrofulous affections.

PYROLEUM OSSIUM RECTIFICATUM, Oleum animale Dippelii.

PYROLIG'NEOUS ACID, *Ac''idum pyroace'ticum, A. pyroligno'sum* seu *pyroxyl'icum, A. ligni pyro-oleo'sum, A. ace'ticum empyreumat'icum, A. lig'neum, Pyrolig'nic acid,* (F.) *Acide pyroligneux, Vinaigre de bois.* An acid, obtained by distillation, from wood, coal, &c., which was once believed to be of a peculiar character. It is now known to be formed of acetic acid and an empyreumatic oil, from which it may be freed; and, in this state, is sold in commerce for *Acetum distillatum.* It is used for similar purposes as distilled vinegar, and for preserving animal substances. It has also been used as an antiseptic in gangrene and sphacelus, and to foul ulcers; wherever indeed creasote is indicated.— The dose of the impure pyroligneous acid internally is from five to thirty drops, three or four times a day.

PYROMA'NIA, *Incen'diary monoma'nia,* from πυρ, 'fire,' and *mania.* Insanity, with an irresistible desire to destroy by fire.

PYROPH'AGUS, *Ignis'orus,* from πυρ, 'fire,' and φαγω, 'I eat.' One who eats fire. A juggler, who eats bodies in a state of ignition.

PYROS, Triticum.

PYRO'SIS, from πυρ, 'fire,' 'the act of burning.' *Ptyalis'mus pyros'icus, Limo'sis cardia'gia sputato'ria, Ardor stom'achi, A. ventric'uli,* (Ch.) *dial'gia sputatoria, Pyrosis Suec''ica, Apocen'osis vom'itus pyrosis, Dyspepsia pyrosis, Cuimorsymia, Ebullit''io stom'achi, Orex'is* (of some), *Waterbrash, Waterqualm, Black-water,* (F.) *Ardeur de l'estomac, Fer chaud, Cremason, Soda, Gossement.* This affection consists of a hot sensation in the stomach, with eructations of an acrid, burning liquid, that causes a distressing sensation in the parts over which it passes. Attention to diet, and the use of bitter absorbents, will usually relieve, when the disease is functional. Occasionally, it is symptomatic of organic disease of the stomach.

Pyrosis also signified, of old, inflammation, gangrene, and a burn.

PYROSIS SUECICA, Pyrosis.

PYROSOPHIA, Chymistry.

PYROTECHNIA, Chymistry.

PYROTECHNY, *Pyrotech'nè*, from πυρ, 'fire,' and τεχνη, 'art.' Art of making fire-works, &c. Also, chymistry. M. Percy has used the term *Pyrotechnie Chirurgicale* for the art of applying fire or the actual cautery in surgery.

PYROTHONIDE, from πυρ, 'fire,' and οθονη, 'linen.' *Liquor pyro-oleo'sus e lin'teo para'tus.* A kind of pyrogenous or empyreumatic oil, produced by the combustion of textures of hemp, linen, or cotton in a copper vessel. The brown product is acid. Its medical properties probably resemble those of creasote. Diluted with three or four times its weight of water, it has been used as a gargle in cynanche tonsillaris, but is not now employed.

It is said, also, to be a popular remedy for toothach and skin diseases. When prepared from rags, it is called *Rag oil;* when from paper, *Paper oil.*

PYROTICUS, Caustic.

PYRUS CYDONIA, *Cydo'nia malifor'mis* seu *vulga'ris, Sorbus Cydo'nia, Cydo'nia, Coto'nia, Quince Tree,* (F.) *Coignassier. Family,* Rosaceæ. *Sex. Syst.* Icosandria Pentagynia. The fruit is termed *Cydo'nium malum, Malum canum, Malum coto'neum, Melum cydo'nium, Quince,* (F.) *Coign.*

Quince-seeds—*Cydo'nium* (Ph. U. S. 1851)—are sometimes used in decoction as a demulcent. The fruit makes a pleasant preserve.

PYRUS DOMESTICA, Sorbus domestica.

PYRUS MALUS, *Malus, M. dasyphyl'la* seu *commu'nis* seu *sylves'tris, Sorbus malus, Melea,* the *Apple Tree,* (F.) *Pommier.* The apple—(F.) *Pomme*—is an agreeable fruit when ripe. When unripe, it disagrees, especially with those of weak digestive powers. The same may be said of the pear, (F.) *Poire;* the fruit of the *Pyrus commu'nis, Apios, P. Sorbus, P. Sati'va,* (F.) *Poirier.*

Apple Brandy is a spirituous liquor obtained from the juice of the apple, and much used in the United States.

PYTIA, Colostrum.

PYTISMA, Sputum, Sperm.

PYUL'CON, from πυον, 'pus,' and ἑλκω, 'I extract.' (F.) *Tire-pus.* A surgical instrument for extracting pus from any cavity. Many pyulca have been employed, all of which act as exhausting syringes.

PYU'RIA, *Pyotu'ria, Pyorrhœ'a urina'lis,* from πυον, 'pus,' and ουρον, 'urine.' Discharge of purulent urine: a symptom which occurs in many diseases; particularly in cases of renal calculi, and in organic affections of the bladder. It receives various epithets, according to the part whence the pus proceeds:—as *Pyuria urethra'lis, P. rena'lis,* and *P. vesica'lis.*

PYURIA CHYLOSA, Chyluria—p. Lactea, Chyluria—p. Mucosa, Cystirrhœa—p. Serosa, Cystirrhœa—p. Viscida, Cystirrhœa.

PYXIS, πυξις. A box; a pill-box. Also, an emollient ointment.—Aëtius, and Paulus.

PYXIS, *Boite,* see Cotyloid.

Q.

Q., see Abbreviation.

QUABEBE, Piper cubeba.

QUACK, Charlatan.

QUACK-MEDICINE, Arcanum.

QUACKSALVER, Charlatan.

QUADRANS, *Quarta pars libræ.* A quarter of a pound. Three ounces (Troy).

QUADRANTAL, Amphora.

QUADRATUS, Depressor labii inferioris—q. Dorsi, Q. lumborum.

QUADRA'TUS FEM'ORIS, *Quadratus,* from *quadra,* 'a square.' *Quartus quadrigem'inus quadratus,* (F.) *Tuber-ischio-trochantérien* (Ch.), *Ischio-sous-trochantérien, Carré de la Cuisse.* A muscle situate at the posterior and upper part of the thigh. It is thin, flat, and quadrilateral, and is attached to the outer part of the tuberosity of the ischium; whence it proceeds transversely to the inferior part of the posterior margin of the great trochanter. It rotates the limb, turning the toe outwards.

QUADRATUS GENÆ, Platysma myoides—q. Radii, Pronator radii quadratus.

QUADRATUS LUMBO'RUM, *Quadratus* seu *Lumba'ris externus, Flectens par lumbo'rum, Quadra'tus dorsi,* (F.) *Ilio-costal,* (Ch.) *Ilio-lombi-costal, Carré des lombes.* A flat, somewhat thick, irregularly quadrilateral muscle, situate in the loins, at the sides of the vertebral column. It is attached, below, to the crista ilii and ilio-lumbar ligament; and above, to the inferior margin of the last rib; and besides, to the base of the transverse processes of the last four lumbar vertebræ. This muscle inclines the loins to its side; depresses the last rib, and is thus a muscle of respiration. It can also raise the hip.

QUADRIGEM'INA TUBER'CULA, *Eminen'tiæ Quadrigem'inæ* seu *Bigem'inæ, Optic Lobes, Optic Ganglia, Pons Syl'vii, Cor'pora quadrigem'ina, Nates et Testes, Cor'pora bigem'ina,* (F.) *Tubercles quadrijumeaux, Éminences bigéminées.* Four medullary tubercles, situate at the posterior surface of the tuber annulare. They are white, externally; gray, internally; oblong; rounded; connected by pairs, and separated by two grooves, which divide them crucially. Of these tubercles—the superior, called *nates, Tuber'cula anterio'ra, Glu'tia,* are larger and more prominent than the lower, called *testes, Tuber'cula posterio'ra.* The pineal gland corresponds exactly to the point of intersection of the two furrows that separate them.

QUADRIGEMINUS PRIMUS ET SUPERIOR, Pyramidalis—q. Quadratus quartus, Quadratus femoris—q. Secundus et tertius, Ischiotrochanterianus.

QUADROON, see Mulatto—q. Black, see Mulatto.

QUAFADIL, Melanthium Virginicum.

QUAHOIL, Cacao.

QUAIL, Tetrao coturnix.

QUAMASH, EASTERN, Scilla esculenta.

QUANDROS. Ancient name for a precious stone, believed to exist in the brain of the val ture; and to which was attributed the property of augmenting the secretion of milk, and preserving from deadly accidents. No such stone exists.

QUAR'ANTINE, *Quar'entine, Quarentaine*, from (I.) *Quaranti'na*, itself from *quaranta*, 'forty.' (F.) *Quarantaine*. The time during which travellers, returning from a country where the plague or any other pestilential disease exists, are compelled to remain on board ship or in a lazaretto. They, as well as the ship, are said '*to perform quarantine.*' Quarantine is sometimes extended beyond forty days, whilst its duration is frequently much less. It is sometimes enforced by land; for example, when contagious diseases require the establishment of *cordons sanitaires*, and when persons are desirous of leaving infected districts. During quarantine, no communication is allowed between the travellers and the inhabitants of the country. Quarantine is a great impediment to commerce; and is, doubtless, very frequently enforced when there is but little danger of contagion. The evils, however, that might arise from the introduction of a widely-spreading contagious disease, are so disastrous, as to induce legislators to maintain these laws in perhaps an unnecessary degree of rigour.

QUARTAN, 'of or belonging to the fourth.' *Quarta'na Febris, An'etus Quarta'nus, Tetarta'us, Quartan Ague*, (F.) *Quarte*. An intermittent, the paroxysms of which recur every fourth day, leaving between them two days' interval. We speak also of the *Quartan Type*. A *Double Quartan* is one in which one paroxysm occurs on the third and another on the second day, so that there is only one day of apyrexia and two of paroxysms in succession; — the paroxysms of every fourth day resembling each other. A *Triple Quartan* is one in which there is a paroxysm every day; and on every three days the paroxysms correspond. A *redoub'ling* or *repeating quartan*, (F.) *Fièvre quarte doublée*, is one in which there are two paroxysms every fourth day. See Intermittent.

QUARTANUS REMITTENS, Tetartophia.
QUARTA'RIUS. An ancient measure, equal to one-fourth of the sextarius. See Weights and Measures.
QUARTE, Quartan.
QUARTERON, see Mulatto — q. Black, see Mulatto.
QUARTIO, Astragalus.
QUARTI-STERNAL, *Quadristerna'lis*. The fourth osseous portion of the sternum, corresponding to the fourth intercostal space. — Béclard.
QUASSATIO, Conquassation.
QUASSATURA, Conquassation.
QUAS'SIA, *Quassia ama'ra, Quassy, Quassia excel'sa, Picræ'na excel'sa, Febrif'ugum lignum, Lofty Bitterwood Tree, Bitter-ash*, (F.) *Quassie*. A West India tree, from which is obtained the *Lignum Quassia, Quassia*, (Ph. U. S.) It is an intensely durable bitter, without astringency; and has been employed as a tonic and stomachic. It is generally given in the form of infusion. The bitter principle is called *Quassin*.

QUASSIA SIMAROU'BA, *Simarouba, Simaruba, S. officina'lis, Euon'ymus, Bitter Simaruba, Mountain Damson*. The bark of the Simarouba is bitter, and not unpleasant. Both water and alcohol extract its virtues. It is not astringent. It is exhibited wherever a simple tonic is required.

QUASSIN, see Quassia.
QUATERNIO, Astragalus.
QUATRE ÉPICES, see Myrtus pimenta.
QUATRIO, Astragalus.
QUEASINESS, Nausea.

QUEEN'S DELIGHT, Stillingia — q. of the Meadows, Spiræa ulmaria — q. Root, Stillingia.
QUERCINI HERBA, Lichen plicatus.
QUERCULA MINOR, Teucrium chamædrys.
QUERCUS ALBA, the *White Oak*; QUERCUS ROBUR, the *Common Oak*; Q. TINCTO'RIA, the *Black Oak*; Q. RUBRA MONTA'NA, the *Red Oak* or *Spanish Oak*; *Family*, Amentaceæ; *Sex. Syst.* Monœcia Polyandria; (F.) *Chêne*. The bark of all these varieties is, probably, alike in medicinal properties. It is powerfully astringent and tonic, and has been used internally in intermittents, and externally in decoction, as an astringent wash, where such is indicated.

Acorns, Oeces, Nuces Quercûs, (F.) *Glands*, were at one time much used as food; and a decoction of them was once recommended in dysentery and diarrhœa, in glandular obstructions, &c. A pessary made of them has been advised in immoderate flow of the menses. They are not now used.

QUERCUS INFECTO'RIA. A tree of Asia Minor, which affords *Turkey Galls, Nut Galls, Galla Tur'cica, G. Querci'na, G. Tincto'ria, Nux Galla, Galla max'ima orbicula'ta, Cicis, Cassenoles, Gallæ, Galls, Gall-nut*, (F.) *Noix de Galle*. The *nut-gall — Galla* (Ph. U. S.) — is a morbid protuberance or tubercle, produced by the puncture of the *Diplo'lepis Gallæ Tincto'ria* or *Cynips Quercûs folii*. It is powerfully astringent and tonic, and has been employed in diarrhœa, intestinal hemorrhage, and intermittents: but is chiefly used, externally, in gargles and injections. The powder, made into an ointment with lard, is used in piles.

QUERCUS COCCIFERA, see Kermes — q. Marina, Fucus vesiculosus — q. Suber, see Suber.

QUEUE DE CHEVAL, Cauda equina, see Medulla spinalis — *q. de la Moëlle épinière*, Cauda equina — *q. de Pourceau*, Peucedanum.
QUICK-IN-THE-HAND, Impatiens.
QUICKEN TREE, Sorbus acuparia.
QUICK'ENING, from Sax. cpicean, 'to make alive.' The period of gestation when th[...] of the fœtus first becomes perceptible. This usually occurs about the eighteenth week, and was at one time erroneously believed to mark the time at which the fœtus becomes alive — *Anima'tio fœtûs*. It need scarcely be said, that it possesses the principle of life from the moment of the union of the materials furnished by the sexes at a fecundating copulation. When the motion is felt, the female is said to be 'quick with child.'
QUICKENS, Triticum repens.
QUICKLIME, Calx viva.
QUICKSILVER, Hydrargyrum.
QUIES, Acinesia.
QUINA, Quinine — q. Quina, Cinchona.
QUINÆ ACETAS, SULPHAS, &c., see Quiniæ Acetas, &c.
QUINCE, see Pyrus cydonia — q. Tree, Pyrus cydonia.
QUINIA, Quinine — q. Acetate of, Quiniæ acetas — q. Amorphous, see Quinia, extract of — q. Arseniate of, Quiniæ arsenias — q. and Cinchonia, tannate of, Quiniæ et Cinchoniæ tannas — q. Arsenite of, Quiniæ arsenis — q. Citrate of, Quiniæ citras.

QUINIA, EXTRACT OF, *Qui'niæ sulphas impu'rus*. A preparation which consists in evaporating the liquor poured off the crystals of sulphate of quinia to the consistence of a pilular mass.

It has the properties of sulphate of quinia, and its active principle appears to be *amorphous quinia*. Twenty-four grains will generally arrest ague.

QUINIA, FERROCYANATE OF, Quiniæ ferrocyanas — q. Hydriodate of, Quiniæ hydriodas — q. Impure sulphate of, Quinia, extract of — q. Iodhydrate of, Quiniæ hydriodas—q. Iodide of, Quiniæ hydriodas—q. Iodide of, Iodhydrate of, see Quiniæ hydriodas—q. Ioduret of, Quiniæ hydriodas—q. and Iron, Hydriodate of, see Quinia, Iodide of Iodhydrate of—q. Lactate of, Quiniæ lactas—q. and Mercury, protochloride of, Hydrargyri et Quiniæ Protochloridum—q. Muriate of, Quiniæ murias—q. Nitrate of, Quiniæ nitras—q. Phosphate of, Quiniæ phosphas—q. Sulphate of, Quinine, sulphate of.

QUI'NIÆ ACE'TAS, *Chi'nium ace'ticum, Ace'tas Chi'nii* seu *Chini'ni* seu *chi'nicus* seu *Qui'niæ* seu *Quinæ* seu *Quini'ni* seu *Kini'ni, Quina ace'tica, Acetate of Qui'nia* or of *Quinine.* Prepared by saturating *Quinia* with diluted *acetic acid.* Has the properties of the other salts of Quinia.

QUINIÆ ARSEN'IAS, *Quini'næ* seu *Qui'niæ Arsen'ias, Chini'num Arsenico'sum* seu *Arsenic''icum, Arseniate of Quinia* or of *Quina* or of *Quinine.* Formed by the union of *arsenic acid* and *quinia.* Employed as an antiperiodic in the dose of from three quarters of a grain to a grain and a half in the twenty-four hours.

QUINIÆ AR'SENIS, *Q. Diar'senis, Ar'senite of Qui'nia.* A salt resulting from the double decomposition of *arsenite of potassa* and *sulphate of quinia.* It has been used in chronic cutaneous diseases; and as an antiperiodic in ague, neuralgia, &c. Dose, one-third of a grain, three times a day.

QUINIÆ CITRAS, *Quiniæ* seu *Chini'ni citras, Citras chi'nicus* seu *qui'nicus, Chi'nium* seu *Chi'ni'num Ci'tricum, Citrate of Quinia,* of *Quina,* or of *Quinine.* Formed from the union of *citric acid* and *quinia.* It has the same properties as the sulphate.

QUINIÆ ET CINCHONIÆ TANNAS, *Chini'num* seu *Chi'nium tan'nicum, Tannate of Quinia* and *Cincho'nia.* This salt has the same properties as the salts of quinia in general.

QUINIÆ DIARSENIS, Quiniæ Arsenis.

QUINIÆ FERROCY'ANAS, *Chi'nium ferrocyanogena'tum* seu *ferrohydrocyan'icum, Ferrocy'anate* or *hydrocyanoferrate of Quinia* or of *Quinine.* This salt is obtained by the decomposition of *sulphate of quinia* by means of a solution of *ferrocyanuret of potassium.* It has all the properties of sulphate of quinia, and, according to some, in a superior degree.

QUINIÆ HYDRI'ODAS, *Chini'num hydriod'icum, Hydriodate* or *Iodhydrate of Quinia;* called, also, *Iodure'tum* seu *Iod'idum Qui'niæ, Iod'uret* or *l'odide of Qui'nia,* (F.) *Hydriodate* ou *Iodhydrate de Quiuine, Iodure de Quinine.* This is formed by precipitating *sulphate of quinia* by means of *iodide of potassium.* Given in scrofulous affections; half a grain to a grain, three times a day, to a child.

An *iodide* and a *biniodide* have been formed; the latter made by mixing double the quantity of the iodide of potassium with the sulphate of quinia.

An IODIDE OF IODHY'DRATE OF QUI'NIA, (F.) *Iodure d'Iodhydrate de Quinine,* is prepared by pouring into an acid solution of *quinia* a solution of *iodide of iron,* containing a slight excess of iodine. The precipitate is treated with boiling alcohol: the liquor filtered, and crystals suffered to form. The salt possesses all the properties of the other salts of quinia. Under the name, *Hydriodate of Iron and Quinia,* a preparation has been introduced by Mr. Battley. It is possessed of tonic and antiperiodic virtues.

QUINIÆ IODIDUM, Quiniæ hydriodas—q. Ioduretum, Quiniæ hydriodas.

QUINIÆ LACTAS, *Quinæ lactas, Chini'num lac'ticum, Lactate of Qui'nia* or of *Quinine.* Made by the action of *lactic acid* on *quinia.* Used in the same cases as the other salts of quinia.

47

QUI'NIÆ MU'RIAS, *Chi'nium muriat'icum* seu *sali'tum* seu *hydrochlo'ricum, Mu'rias chi'nicus, Muriate of Quinia* or of *Quinine.* May be prepared by dissolving *quinia* in dilute *muriatic acid.* Given as an antiperiodic. Dose, half a grain to a grain.

QUINIÆ NITRAS, *Chi'nium* seu *Chini'num ni'tricum, Nitrate of Quinia* or of *Quinine.* May be formed by the addition of *nitric acid* to *quinia.* Its properties are those of the sulphate of quinia.

QUINIÆ PHOSPHAS, *Chi'nium* seu *Chini'num phosphor'icum, Phosphate of Quinia* or of *Quinine;* may be prepared by the addition of dilute *phosphoric acid* to *quinia.* It is thought by many to be next to the sulphate of quinia in its remedial powers.

QUINIÆ SULPHAS, Quinine, sulphate of.

QUINIÆ VALERIA'NAS, *Chini'num* seu *Chi'nium Valerian'icum, Valerianate of Quinia,* of *Quina,* or of *Quinine;* may be formed by the union of *valerianic acid* with *quinia.* It has the properties of the salts of quinia.

QUININE, *Qui'nia, Quina, Kini'num, Chini'num, Quinina.* An alkaline, uncrystallizable substance; under the form of a porous, whitish mass; almost insoluble in water, soluble in alcohol and ether. It forms, with acids, salts that are in general soluble. It is obtained from different cinchonas, but chiefly from the yellow, and is the active principle of those valuable drugs.

QUININE, ACETATE OF, Quiniæ acetas — q. Arseniate of, Quiniæ arsenias—q. Arsenite of, Quiniæ arsenis — q. Citrate of, Quiniæ citras — q. Ferrocyanate of, Quiniæ ferrocyanas—q. Hydriodate de, Quiniæ hydriodas—q. Iodhydrate de, Quiniæ hydriodas—q. Iodide of, Quiniæ hydriodas—q. Iodure de, Quiniæ hydriodas—q. Iodure d'iodhydrate de, Quinia, iodide of iodhydrate of—q. Lactate of, Quiniæ lactas—q. Muriate of, Quiniæ murias—q. Nitrate of, Quiniæ nitras—q. Phosphate of, Quiniæ phosphas.

QUININE, QUINA or QUINIA, SULPHATE OF, QUINIÆ seu *Qui'næ* seu *Quini'næ Sulphas, Quinæ Disul'phas, Chi'nium* seu *Chini'num Sulphu'ricum,* (F.) *Sulfate de Quinine* — the salt usually employed in medicine—occurs in needles of a pearly and satiny appearance. It is employed with great success in the treatment of intermittents; and is available in many cases, where the bark in substance could not be retained, or would be injurious. Dose, as a tonic from 3 to 10 grains in the 24 hours. As an antiperiodic it may be carried much farther. Its action, in a large dose, is decidedly sedative. It is obtained, by treating the yellow bark with sulphuric acid. The following form is adopted in the Pharmacopœia of the United States,—*Cinchon. flar.* in pulv. crass. ℔iv; *Acid. muriat.* f℥iij; *Calcis,* in pulv. ℥v; *Aquæ,* cong. v; *Acid. Sulphur., Alcohol; Carbon. animal,* āā q. s. Boil the bark in one-third of the water mixed with the one-third of the muriatic acid, and strain through linen. Boil the residue twice successively with the same quantity of acid and water as before, and strain. Mix the decoctions, and, while the liquor is hot, gradually add the lime, previously mixed with two pints of water, stirring constantly, until the quinia is completely precipitated. Wash the precipitate with distilled water, and having pressed and dried it, digest it in boiling alcohol. Pour off the liquor and repeat the digestion several times, until the alcohol is no longer rendered bitter. Mix the liquors, and distil off the alcohol, until a brown viscid mass remains. Upon this substance, removed from the vessel, pour about half a gallon of distilled water, and having heated the mixture to the boiling point, add as much sulphuric acid as may be necessary to dissolve the impure alkali.

Then add an ounce and a half of animal charcoal; boil for two minutes; filter the liquor while hot, and set it aside to crystallize. Should the liquor, before filtration, be entirely neutral, acidulate it very slightly with sulphuric acid. Should it, on the contrary, change the colour of litmus paper to a bright red, add more animal charcoal. Separate the crystals from the liquor, dissolve them in boiling water slightly acidulated with sulphuric acid, add a little animal charcoal, filter and set aside to crystallize. Wrap the crystals in bibulous paper, and dry with a gentle heat. The mother-waters may be made to yield an additional quantity of sulphate of quinia by precipitating the quinia with solution of ammonia, and treating the precipitated alkali with water, sulphuric acid, and animal charcoal, as before.

QUININE, TANNATE OF, Quiniæ et cinchoniæ tannas—q. Valerianate of, Quiniæ valerianas.

QUINI'NISM, *Quininis'mus, Quinism, Cin'choniem.* The aggregate of encephalic or neuropathic phenomena induced by over-doses of quinia.

QUINOIDINE, Chinioidine.

QUINQUEFOLIUM, Potentilla reptans—Quinquefolium majus, Potentilla reptans.

QUINQUINA, Cinchona—q. Aromatique, Croton cascarilla—q. Bicolor, Cinchonæ Caribææ cortex—q. Faux de Virginie, Cusparia febrifuga—q. Gris de Loxa, Cinchonæ lancifoliæ cortex—q. Jaune, Cinchonæ cordifoliæ cortex—q. Orange, Cinchonæ lancifoliæ cortex—q. Piton, Cinchonæ Caribææ cortex—q. Rouge, Cinchonæ oblongifoliæ cortex.

QUINSEY, Cynanche tonsillaris—q. Nervous, Angone—q. Wolf, Lycanche.

QUINTAN, *Febris quinta'na, F. pemptæ'a, F. quinta;* from *quintus,* 'a fifth.' A fever whose paroxysms return only every five days inclusively; and between which there are, consequently, three days of apyrexia.

QUINTE, (F.) This word is used synonymously with *paroxysm* or *fit,* when speaking of cough,—as *une Quinte de Toux*—'a fit of coughing.' Also, the influenza.

QUINTEFEUILLE, Potentilla reptans.

QUINTERON, see Mulatto—q. black, see Mulatto.

QUINTES, see Pertussis.

QUINTES'SENCE, *Quinta Essen'tia.* A name formerly given to alcohol, impregnated with the principles of some drug. It was, consequently, often synonymous with *Alcohol'ic tincture.* The most volatile principles of bodies were, also, called *Quintes'sences.*

QUINTI'STERNAL. The fifth osseous portion of the sternum. It corresponds to the 5th and 6th intercostal spaces.

QUINUA, Chenopodium quinoa.

QUOTID'IAN, *Quotidia'nus, Ephe'merus,*—itself from *quotidiè,* 'daily.' That which takes place every day.

QUOTID'IAN FEVER, *Febris quotidia'na seu hemere'sia seu hemer'ina, Q. ague, An'etus quotidia'nus, Cathe'merus, Cathemer'inus, Methcmer'inus, Amphemer'inos, Amphimer'inus, Amphe'merus, Febris amphe'mera* seu *methemer'ina* seu *methemic'ria, Quotidia'nus,* (F.) *Fièvre quotidienne,* is an intermittent, the paroxysms of which recur every day.

A *simple, double,* or *triple quotidian,* is a quotidian, which has one, two, or three paroxysms in the 24 hours.

R.

R is placed at the commencement of a prescription, as a contraction of *Rec"ipè.* (See Abbreviation.) Originally, it was the sign ♃ of Jupiter, and was placed at the top of a formula, to propitiate the king of the gods, that the compound might act favourably.

RABDOIDES, (SUTURA,) Sagittal suture.

RABID, *Rab'idus,* (F.) *Rabique, Rabiéique,* from *rabies,* 'canine madness.' That which belongs to hydrophobia; as *rabid virus,* &c.

RABIÉIQUE, Rabid.

RABIES CANINA, Hydrophobia.

RABIQUE, Rabid.

RACAHOUT, Amylum querneum. A name given by the Arabs to the starch prepared from an edible acorn obtained from *Quercus Ilex,* but, according to Plagge, the so called *Racahout* of the Arabs, sold in Paris, is a compound of potatoe starch, chocolate, and aromatics,—as vanilla.

RACCOON BERRY, Podophyllum montanum.

RACE, from *radice,* abl. of *radix,* 'root,' breed. The union or aggregate of individuals whose conformation or particular condition differs perceptibly from those of neighbouring varieties. In the human species, several races are designated. See Homo.

RACEMEUX, Racemosus.

RACEMO'SUS, *Rac"emous, Rac"emose,* (F.) *Racemeux.* In clusters, like grapes.

RACE'MUS. A cluster—as of grapes.

RACHAMEL'CA, from Hebr. רחם (*rechem*) 'the womb,' and מלך (*molech,*) 'a king:' Recha- *mal'ca.* A peculiar formative principle, supposed, by Dolæus, to exist in the uterus.

RACHE, Porrigo.

RACHIÆI, Rachiæi.

RACHIALGIA, Colic, metallic, Rhachiodynia, Vertebral disease—r. Mesenterica, Tabes mesenterica—r. Pictoniensium, Colic, metallic—r. Pictonum, Colic, metallic.

RACHIALGIE MÉSENTÉRIQUE, Tabes mesenterica.

RACHIALGITIS, Rhachialgitis.

RACHIDIAN ARTERIES, Spinal arteries—r. Bulb, see Medulla oblongata—r. Canal, Vertebral canal.

RACHIOPHYMA, Rachiphyma.

RACHIPHY'MA, *Rhachiphy'ma, Rachiophyma, Tumor Dorsi,* from 'ραχις, 'the spine,' and φυμα, 'a tumour.' A tumour on the spine or on the back.

RACHIS, Vertebral column.

RACHIS'AGRA, *Rhachis'agra, Rhach'iagra, Rhach'eagra, Rhachid'agra, Rhachi'tis spina'li,* from 'ραχις, 'the spine,' and αγρα, 'a seizure.' A gouty or rheumatic affection of the spine.

RACHITÆ, Rhachitæ.

RACHIT'IC, *Rachit'icus, Rhachit'icus,* (F.) *Rachitique.* Same etymon as the next. Relating or appertaining to, or affected with rickets Weak, feeble in the joints; defective in development.

RACHI'TIS, *Rhachi'tis,* from 'ραχις, 'the spine,' and *itis,* a suffix denoting inflammation. Inflammation of the spine. Also, *Cyrto'sis Ra'-*

ekia, Cyrton'osus, Morbus Ang'licus, Osteomala'cia Infan'tum, Tabes pectorea; Innutritio ossium, Spina nodo'sa, Rachitis'mus, English disease, Rickets; from '*ραχις,*' 'the spine.' (F.) *Rachitisme, Nouure.* A disease characterized by crookedness of the long bones; swelling of their extremities; crooked spine; prominent abdomen; large head; and often precocity of intellect. It is accompanied by leanness, general debility, indigestion; and frequently induces atrophy and hectic. Rickets occurs, particularly, during the first years of existence, in weakly children, born of rickety or scrofulous parents; brought up in damp or confined situations; who are badly nourished, and do not take sufficient exercise. The progress and termination of the disease are very variable. Some children gradually recover their health: others become more and more deformed, and ultimately die of consumption, dropsy, or other organic disease. The treatment is almost wholly *hygienic.* Pure air; a healthy situation; nourishing diet; exercise; sea or common cold bathing, and tonics, afford the best prospect of success.

RACHITIS ADULTORUM, Mollities ossium.

RACHITISME, Rachitis.

RACHO'SIS, *Rhacho'sis, Rako'sis,* from '*ραχοω,*' or '*ρακοω,*' 'I wrinkle.' A relaxation of the scrotum. *Propto'ma* sou *lax'itas Scroti, Scrotum pen'dulum.* An excoriation of the relaxed scrotum. — Dictionaries.

RACINE À BECQUET, Geranium moschatum — *r. de Bengal,* Cassumuniar — *r. de Charcis,* Dorstenia contrayerva — *r. de Dracke,* Dorstenia ontrayerva — *r. des Philippines,* Dorstenia contrayerva — *r. de Safran,* Curcuma longa — *r. de Saint Esprit,* Angelica — *r. Salivaire,* Anthemis pyrethrum — *r. de Turbeth,* Convolvulus turpethum.

RACINES DU CERVELET, Corpora restiformia.

RACLURES DES BOYAUX, Ramenta intestinorum.

RACORNISSEMENT, (F.) from *se racornir,* 'to shrivel in the fire as leather does.' *Cor'nification.* A physical property, possessed by animal substances, which consists in a kind of contractility, accompanied with sudden corrugation and curling. It is produced by heat, and by chemical agents, especially by the strong mineral acids.

RADCLIFFE'S ELIXIR, see Tinctura aloes composita.

RADESYGE, Radzyge.

RADEZYGE, Radzyge.

RADIAD, see Radial aspect.

RA'DIAL, *Radia'lis,* from *radius,* a bone of the forearm. That which relates to the radius.

RADIAL ANTÉRIEUR, Palmaris magnus.

RADIAL ARTERY, *A. extern'a Cu'biti.* It arises from the brachial, at the upper and anterior part of the forearm; descends on the outer side as far as the lower part of the radius, and proceeds downwards and backwards towards the superior extremity of the space which separates the first two metacarpal bones. It then buries itself in the palm of the hand, where it forms the *profound* or *radial* palmar arch. The radial artery gives off the *recurrent radial,* several *radio-muscular* branches, the *transverse palmar radio-carpal artery,* the *external superficial artery of the palm of the hand,* the *external dorsal of the thumb,* the *dorsalis carpi, dorsal interosseous artery of the index,* &c.

RADIAL ASPECT. An aspect towards the side on which the radius is situated. — Barclay. *Radiad* is used by the same writer, adverbially, to signify 'towards the radial aspect.'

RADIAL EXTERNE PREMIER, see Radialis — *r. Externe second,* see Radialis — *r. Grand,* see Radialis.

RADIAL NERVE, *Radio-digital* (Ch.), *Spiral Nerve, Spiral muscular N., Musculo-spiral nerve,* arises from the four inferior branches of the brachial plexus. It is, at first, situate behind the other nerves of the plexus. It then becomes engaged between the three portions of the triceps brachialis, passes behind the humerus, and descends between the supinator longus and brachialus internus, as far as opposite the upper extremity of the radius. In its course it gives numerous filaments to the triceps, supinator longus, extensor carpi radialis longior, and to the integuments. Opposite the upper extremity of the radius it divides into two branches; — the one *posterior,* which turns backwards into the substance of the supinator brevis, and when it has reached the space between the two layers of muscles on the posterior surface of the forearm, divides into a great number of filaments, which are distributed to those muscles, and to the integuments of the hand. The other branch is *anterior:* it descends before the supinator brevis and the radius; until, near the inferior third of that bone, it engages itself between the tendons of the supinator longus and extensor carpi radialis longior; and, becoming afterwards subcutaneous, divides into two branches, whose filaments are distributed to the integuments of the thumb, index, middle finger, to the outside of the ring finger, and to the first interosseous muscle of the back of the hand.

RADIAL PETIT, see Radialis.

RADIAL VEINS, DEEP-SEATED, follow the same course as the radial artery.

RADIA'LIS EXTER'NUS BRE'VIOR, *Exten'sor Carpi Radialis Bre'vior, Radialis secundus,* (F.) *Second radial externe, Petit radial, Épicondylo-sus-métacarpien,* (Ch.) An extensor muscle of the wrist, situate beneath the extensor carpi radialis longior. It is attached, above, to the external tuberosity of the humerus, and terminates below, by a long tendon, inserted into the posterior part of the upper extremity of the third bone of the metacarpus. It has the same uses as the next muscle.

RADIA'LIS EXTER'NUS LON'GIOR, *Extensor Carpi Radia'lis Lon'gior, Radialis externus primus,* (F.) *Premier radial externe, Grand radial, Huméro sus-métacarpien,* (Ch.) It is seated at the outer part of the forearm; is thin, but thicker on the outside than on the inside. It is attached, above, to the inferior part of the outer edge, and to the corresponding tuberosity, of the humerus; and terminates, below, by a long tendon, which is attached to the superior extremity of the second bone of the metacarpus. It extends the hand on the forearm.

RADIALIS EXTERNUS BREVIOR, see Radialis — *r.* Externus primus, see Radialis — *r.* Extensor longior, see Radialis — *r.* Internus, Palmaris magnus — *r.* Secundus, see Radialis.

RAD'IATED, *Radia'tus,* from *radius,* 'a ray;' (F.) *Rayonné.* That which is arranged in rays; in lines, diverging from a common centre. An epithet given to several ligaments, &c., as to those which unite the ribs to the sternum; those which unite the tibia and fibula at their inferior extremity, &c.

RADIATED SUBSTANCE OF THE KIDNEY, see Kidney.

RAD'ICAL, *Radica'lis,* from *radix,* 'a root.' A radical cure, *cura radica'lis,* is one in which the disease is destroyed, as it were, from the root. It is used in opposition to *palliative cure.*

RADICAL MOISTURE, Humidum radicale

RADICAL VESSELS, *Vas'cular Rad'icles*, (F.) *Radicules vasculaires*, are the small vessels that take their origin in the tissues, and by their union form larger vessels.

RADICES OSSIS HYOIDEI, Cornua ossis hyoidei.

RADICIS'ECA, from *radix*, *radicis*, 'a root,' and *secare*, 'to cut.' One employed in collecting and preparing plants was formerly so called.

RADICULA, Raphanus hortensis.

RADICULES VASCULAIRES, Radical vessels.

RADII CILIARES, Ciliary processes.

RADII FRONTIS. The folds or wrinkles of the forehead.

RADIO-CARPAL, *Radio-carpia'nus*. That which relates to the radius and carpus.

RADIO-CARPAL ARTICULATION is the *wrist joint*, or articulation of the os scaphoides, os semilunare, and os cuneiforme of the carpus with the inferior surface of the radius, and the fibro-cartilage, situate below the ulna. It is strengthened by lateral, anterior, and posterior ligaments.

RADIO-CARPAL TRANSVERSE PALMAR ARTERY, (F.) *Artère Radio-carpienne-transversale-palmaire*. A transverse branch, given off by the radial artery, opposite the lower edge of the pronator quadratus, which sends several branches to the anterior or palmar surface of the carpus.

RADIO-CUTANÉ (NERF,) see Cutaneous—r. *Phalangettien du pouce*, Flexor longus pollicis manus.

RADIOLUS, Sound.

RADIO-MUS'CULAR, *Radio-muscula'ris*. A name given to the branches sent off from the radial artery to the muscles of the forearm in the first part of its course; as well as to the nervous filaments which the radial nerve sends to the same muscles.

RADIS, Raphanus hortensis.

RADISH, Raphanus hortensis—r. Water, Nasturtium amphibium.

RADIUS, 'a spoke:'—so called from its shape. *Cercis, Foc"ilè minus* seu *superius*, *Canna minor, Os adcubita'lè, Additamen'tum ulnæ, Manu'brium manûs, Parape'chyon, Arun'do bra'chii minor,* (F.) *Os du Rayon.* A long, prismatic bone, the upper and lesser extremity of which is called the *head*. This is supported by a *cervix* or neck. At the part where the neck is confounded with the *body* of the bone is the *tubercle* or *bicipital tuberosity* or eminence for the insertion of the biceps. The radius is articulated, above, with the os humeri and with the lesser sigmoid cavity of the ulna: below, with the scaphoides, semilunare, and the head of the ulna. Its inferior extremity, which is larger than the superior, is flattened before and behind: is irregularly quadrilateral; and has, below, a double facette to be articulated with the first two bones of the carpus. On the outer side is the styloid process; and, on the inner, a concave facette, which joins the ulna. Behind, are grooves for the passage of the extensor tendons. The radius is developed from three points of ossification; one for the body, and one for each extremity.

RADIUS, COL DU, Collum radii.

RA'DIX, *Rhiza*. A root: also, the male organ.

Radix, Root or *fang* of a tooth, is the part contained in the alveolus. The *radix* or *root* of the nail is the portion hidden under the skin, &c. Surgeons give the name to the prolongations, sent by scirrhous, cancerous, or other tumours into the neighbouring parts.

Five Aperient Roots, Quinque radi'ces aperien'tes, were, of old, asparagus, butchers' broom, fennel, parsley, and smallage.

Five Lesser Aperient Roots, Quinque radi'ces aperien'tes mino'res,—were caper, dandelion, eryngo, madder, and rest-harrow.

RADIX ASCLEPIADIS CRISPA, see Gomphocarpus crispus—r. Braziliensis, Ipecacuanha.

RADIX CORDIS, *Basis Cordis*. The base of the heart.

RADIX INDICA LOPEZIANA, Lopez radix—*B* Linguæ, see Tongue—r. Lopeziana, Lopez radix —r. Ninsi, Sium ninsi—r. Rubra, Rubia—r. Serpentum, see Ophiorrhiza mungos—r. Unguis, Nail, root of—r. Ventris, Umbilicus.

RADULA, Raspatorium.

RADZYGE, *Radzygin, Radesyge, Radesyge, Thæ'ria*, properly *Theria*, from θηριον, ('ελκος,) 'a malignant ulcer.' *Lepra borea'lis* seu *Norregica*, *Norwe'gian Lep'rosy*. A name given, in Norway, to a disease, bearing considerable analogy to the yaws. Some have esteemed it a species of lepra or elephantiasis.

Another form — the *Spedalske*, or *Spedalskhed* —of Norway, appears to be a variety of elephantiasis Græcorum.

RAGE, *Ira, Furor brevis, Orgè, Thymos*, (F.) *Colère.* Violent passion, characterized by contraction of the muscles of the face, violence in every movement, extreme irritation of the nervous system, acceleration of the blood's motion, and redness and swelling of the face.

RAGE, Rhage.

RAGE, Hydrophobia.

RAGWEED, Ambrosia elatior—r. Great, Ambrosia trifida.

RAGWORT, Senecio Jacobæa.

RAIDEUR CADAVÉRIQUE, Rigor mortis.

RAIFORT, Raphanus hortensis—r. *Sauvage*, Cochlearia armoracia.

RAINBOW-WORM, Herpes iris.

RAINURE, Groove—r. *Digastrique*, Mastoid groove.

RAISIN, see Vitis vinifera—r. *d'Amérique*, Phytolacca decandra—r. *de Bois*, Vaccinium myrtillus—r. *d'Ours*, Arbutus uva ursi—r. *de Renard*, Paris.

RAISINIÈRE (F.) A name given to a small granular, brownish or blackish tumour, which forms occasionally at the surface of the cornea, in consequence of ulcers or accidental wounds of that membrane.—Nysten.

RAISINS, Uvæ passæ, see Vitus vinifera—a. *de Corinthe*, see Vitus Corinthiaca.

RAISON, Reason.

RAKASIRA. An American balsam; of a brownish or brownish-red colour; semi-transparent; brittle; softening and becoming tenacious by heat; inodorous when cold, but exhaling a very agreeable smell when heated; and possessing a balsamic and slightly bitter taste. The precise vegetable that furnishes it is not known. It has been used chiefly as a balsam in gonorrhœa and urinary affections.

RAKIA, see Spirit.

RAKOSIS, Rachosis.

RÂLE, Rattle, *Rhonchus, Rhenchus, Rhenzis*, from (D.) R a t e l; *Rhoncus, Cerchnus, Rhogmos*, (F.) *Râle.* Noise produced by the air in passing through mucus, of which the lungs are unable to free themselves. This condition is chiefly observed at the approach of death, and is commonly called, "*the rattles.*"

The term *Râle* has been given to different sounds during respiration, caused by the air passing through fluid contained in the bronchi, or areolæ of the pulmonary tissue; which are perceived by the stethoscope.

RÂLE BRONCHIQUE SEC, Râle sonore—r. *Bronchique humide*, *R. muqueux*—r. *Caverneux*, *Gurgling*—r. *Cavernuleux*, see *Gurgling*—r. *Cré-*

pitant, Rhonchus crep'itans, see Crepitant—*r. c. Redux*, see Crepitant.

RÂLE MUQUEUX, *Rhon'chus muco'sus, Mucous Rattle, R. bronchique humide.* The sound produced by the passage of air through mucus accumulated in the larger bronchi or trachea, or through softened tubercular matter. This *râle* occurs in catarrh, and in softened tubercle. When carried to a very high degree, it constitutes *gurgling,* (F.) *Gargouillement.* The *sub-crep'itant rhonchus,* (F.) *Râle sous-crépitant*, is produced by the bubbling of air through liquid of variable consistence in the minute bronchial tubes. When heard at the base of both lungs, it is a sign of capillary bronchitis. When heard at one base only, it is generally connected with tuberculosis higher up.

RÂLE SIBILANT, *Rhon'chus sib'ilus seu sib'-ilans, Sib'ilant Rattle.* A slight, though prolonged, whistling sound, occurring either at the commencement of inspiration, or of expiration, owing to the presence of mucus, thin and viscid, but not abundant, which obstructs, more or less completely, the smaller bronchial ramifications. It is seated in the small tubes, and occurs in the first stage of bronchitis. The *clicking* and *whistling* varieties differ, in the former being short, the latter prolonged. The former is a quick sharp sibilus or whistle, which ceases almost instantaneously; the latter a prolonged sibulus, of less sharpness, lasting almost the whole time of the movement which it accompanies. To these may be added the *hissing* variety, the name sufficiently indicating its character.

RÂLE SONORE, *Râle bronchique sec, R. ronflant, Rhonchus sono'rus, Sonorous Rattle.* A sound resembling at times the snoring—(F.) *Ronflement*—of a person asleep; at others the sound of the bass string of an instrument when rubbed with the finger, and not unfrequently the cooing —(F.) *Roucoulement*—of a dove. It seems to be caused by a contraction of the bronchial tubes, and is characteristic of chronic catarrh.

RÂLE SOUS-CRÉPITANT, see *Râle muqueux.*

RÂLE VÉSICULAIRE, see Crepitation.

RAMEAU, Ramus.

RAMEN'TA INTESTINO'RUM, (F.) *Raclures des Boyaux.* The shreds or scrapings, as it were, of the mucous membrane of the bowels, often discharged in malignant dysentery. The evacuation in which these are contained has been termed *Diachore'ma xysmato'des.*

RAMENTUM, Fragment, Scobs.

RAMEX, Hernia—r. Varicosus, Varicocele.

RAMIFICA'TION, *Ramifica'tio,* from *ramus,* 'a branch,' and *fio,* 'to become.' A division of arteries, veins, or nerves into branches. Also, a branch itself.

RAMILLE, Ramusculus.

RAMOLLISSEMENT, Mollities—*r. du Cerveau*, Mollities cerebri—*r. du Cœur*, Cardiomalacia—*r. de l'Estomac*, Gastromalacia—*r. du Foie*, Hepatomalacia—*r. Gris*, see Hepatization—*r. de la Moelle épinière*, Mollities medullæ spinalis—*r. Rouge*, see Hepatization—*r. de l'Intestin*, Entero-malacia—*r. des Os*, Mollities ossium.

RAMPANT, (F.) *ramper,* 'to climb.' *Repens. Reptans.* That which creeps or drags on the earth. The French *Bandage rampant* has the folds arranged spirally around the part, leaving intervals between them. It is a retentive bandage, but is easily displaced, and, therefore, not employed.

RAMPES DU LIMAÇON, Scalæ of the cochlea.

RAMPHOS, Rostrum.
RAMULUS, Ramusculus.
RAMUNCULUS, Ramusculus.
RAMUS, *Clados*, a branch, (F.) *Rameau*. A division of an artery, vein, or nerve. Also, the male organ.

RAMUS DURIOR SEPTIMÆ CONJUGATIONIS, Facial nerve.

RAMUS'CULUS, *Ram'ulus, Ramun'culus, Sur'culus, Cladis'cos,* diminutive of *ramus*. A division of a ramus. (F.) *Ramuscule, Ramille.*

RANA ESCULEN'TA, (F.) *Grenouille*. This frog and the bull-frog, *Rana Tauri'na*—are eaten as a delicacy. They are nutritious, and easily digested.

RANA, Ranula.
RANCE, Rancid.

RANCID, *Ran'cidus, Sapros,* (F.) *Rance*, from *rancere,* 'to be stale.' An epithet given to fatty bodies, which have become acrid from age or the contact of air. Mild ointments may thus become very irritating, and unfit for the purposes for which they were originally intended.

RANINE, *Rani'na;* from *Rana*, 'a frog.' The termination of the lingual artery is so called; that is, the portion of the artery which advances horisontally between the genio-glossus and lingualis muscles as far as the point of the tongue. The ranine vein follows the same course as the artery, and opens into the internal jugular or into the superior thyroid.

RAN'ULA, from *Rana*, 'a frog,' so called from its resemblance; *Dyspha'gia Ranula, Emphrag'ma saliva'rë, Frog Tongue, Ba'trachos, Batra'-chium, Hydroglos'sa, Hypoglossis, Hypoglossum, Hypoglot'tis, Hypoglos'sium, Rana,* (F.) *Grenouillette.* A small, soft, fluctuating, and semi-transparent tumour, which forms under the tongue, owing to the accumulation of saliva in Wharton's duct. In order to give exit to the accumulated fluid, and to establish a permanent opening for the discharge of the saliva, the cyst may be punctued, and the opening maintained by a minute cylinder, with a button at each extremity, as has been recommended by Dupuytren; or a portion of the cyst may be removed by the scissors, and the mouth be frequently washed by any astringent lotion. Sometimes, the salivary duct is found plugged by a small calculus.

RANULA LAPIDEA, see Calculi, salivary.

RANUN'CULUS, (F.) *Renoncule. Family* Ranunculaceæ. *Sex. Syst.* Polyandria Polygynia. A genus of plants, most of the species of which, when taken internally, act as acrid poisons. See Poison. They are, also, acrid and vesicant, when applied to the skin, and have accordingly been often used as counter-irritants. The following species answer to this description.

RANUNCULUS ABORTIVUS, *Small flowered Crowfoot*, Chicken-pepper.

RANUNCULUS ACRIS, *R. praten'sis seu Stevenii seu ru'fulus seu sylvat'icus seu Sic'ulus, Upright Meadow Crowfoot, Butter Cups, Yellow-weed, Blister-weed, Pilewort, Burwort, Meadow-bloom, Yellows,* (F.) *Bouton d'or.*

RANUNCULUS ALBUS, Anemone nemorosa.

RANUNCULUS AQUATICUS, R. sceleratus.

RANUNCULUS BULBO'SUS, *R. lætus, Ranunculus* (Ph. U. S.), *Bulbous-rooted Crowfoot,* (F.) *Renoncule bulbeuse, Bassinet.*

RANUNCULUS DIGITATUS, R. sceleratus.

RANUNCULUS DECLINATUS, R. flammula.

RANUNCULUS FICA'RIA, *Chelido'nium minus, Scrophula'ria minor, Fica'ria ranunculoï'des, seu verna seu commu'nis, Chelido'nia rotundifo'lia minor, Cur'cuma hæmorrhoida'lis herba, Ranun-*

RADICAL VESSELS, *Vas'cular Rad'icles*, (F.) *Radicules vasculaires*, are the small vessels that take their origin in the tissues, and by their union form larger vessels.

RADICES OSSIS HYOIDEI, Cornua ossis hyoidei.

RADICIS'ECA, from *radix*, *radicis*, 'a root,' and *secare*, 'to cut.' One employed in collecting and preparing plants was formerly so called.

RADICULA, Raphanus hortensis.

RADICULES VASCULAIRES, Radical vessels.

RADII CILIARES, Ciliary processes.

RADII FRONTIS. The folds or wrinkles of the forehead.

RADIO-CARPAL, *Radio-carpia'nus*. That which relates to the radius and carpus.

RADIO-CARPAL ARTICULATION is the *wrist joint*, or articulation of the os scaphoides, os semilunare, and os cuneiforme of the carpus with the inferior surface of the radius, and the fibro-cartilage, situate below the ulna. It is strengthened by lateral, anterior, and posterior ligaments.

RADIO-CARPAL TRANSVERSE PALMAR ARTERY, (F.) *Artère Radio-carpienne-transversale-palmaire*. A transverse branch, given off by the radial artery, opposite the lower edge of the pronator quadratus, which sends several branches to the anterior or palmar surface of the carpus.

RADIO-CUTANÉ (NERF,) see Cutaneous—r. *Phalangettien du pouce*, Flexor longus pollicis manus.

RADIOLUS, Sound.

RADIO-MUS'CULAR, *Radio-muscula'ris*. A name given to the branches sent off from the radial artery to the muscles of the forearm in the first part of its course; as well as to the nervous filaments which the radial nerve sends to the same muscles.

RADIS, Raphanus hortensis.

RADISH, Raphanus hortensis—r. Water, Nasturtium amphibium.

RADIUS, 'a spoke:'—so called from its shape. *Cercis, Foc"ilĕ minus seu superius, Canna minor, Os adcubita'lĕ, Additamen'tum ulnœ, Manu'brium manûs, Parape'chyon, Arun'do bra'chii minor*, (F.) *Os du Rayon*. A long, prismatic bone, the upper and lesser extremity of which is called the *head*. This is supported by a *cervix* or *neck*. At the part where the neck is confounded with the *body* of the bone is the *tubercle* or *bicipital tuberosity* or eminence for the insertion of the biceps. The radius is articulated, above, with the os humeri and with the lesser sigmoid cavity of the ulna: below, with the scaphoides, semilunare, and the head of the ulna. Its inferior extremity, which is larger than the superior, is flattened before and behind: is irregularly quadrilateral; and has, below, a double facette to be articulated with the first two bones of the carpus. On the outer side is the styloid process; and, on the inner, a concave facette, which joins the ulna. Behind, are grooves for the passage of the extensor tendons. The radius is developed from three points of ossification; one for the body, and one for each extremity.

RADIUS, COL DU, Collum radii.

RA'DIX, *Rhiza*. A root: also, the male organ. *Radix, Root* or *fang* of a tooth, is the part contained in the alveolus. The *radix* or *root* of the nail is the portion hidden under the skin, &c. Surgeons give the name to the prolongations, sent by scirrhous, cancerous, or other tumours into the neighbouring parts.

Five Aperient Roots, Quinque radi'ces aperien'tes, were, of old, asparagus, butchers' broom, fennel, parsley, and smallage.

Five Lesser Aperient Roots, Quinque radi'ces aperien'tes mino'res,—were caper, dandelion, eryngo, madder, and rest-harrow.

RADIX ASCLEPIADIS CRISPA, see Gomphocarpus crispus — r. Braziliensis, Ipecacuanha.

RADIX CORDIS, *Basis Cordis*. The base of the heart.

RADIX INDICA LOPEZIANA, Lopez radix—r. Linguæ, see Tongue—r. Lopeziana, Lopez radix —r. Ninsi, Sium ninsi—r. Rubra, Rubia—r. Serpentum, see Ophiorrhiza mungos—r. Unguis, Nail, root of—r. Ventris, Umbilicus.

RADULA, Raspatorium.

RADZYGE, *Radzygia, Radesyge, Radesyge, Thæ'ria*, properly *Theria*, from θηριον, ('ελκος,) 'a malignant ulcer.' *Lepra borea'lis seu Norvegica, Norwe'gian Lep'rosy*. A name given, in Norway, to a disease, bearing considerable analogy to the yaws. Some have esteemed it a species of lepra or elephantiasis.

Another form—the *Spedalske*, or *Spedalskhed* —of Norway, appears to be a variety of elephantiasis Græcorum.

RAGE, *Ira, Furor brevis, Orgē, Thymos*, (F.) *Colère*. Violent passion, characterized by contraction of the muscles of the face, violence in every movement, extreme irritation of the nervous system, acceleration of the blood's motion, and redness and swelling of the face.

RAGE, Rhage.

RAGE, Hydrophobia.

RAGWEED, Ambrosia elatior—r. Great, Ambrosia trifida.

RAGWORT, Senecio Jacobæa.

RAIDEUR CADAVÉRIQUE, Rigor mortis.

RAIFORT, Raphanus hortensis—r. *Sauvage*, Cochlearia armoracia.

RAINBOW-WORM, Herpes iris.

RAINURE, Groove—r. *Digastrique*, Mastoid groove.

RAISIN, see Vitis vinifera—r. *d'Amérique*, Phytolacca decandra—r. *de Bois*, Vaccinium myrtillus—r. *d'Ours*, Arbutus uva ursi—r. *de Renard*, Paris.

RAISINIÈRE (F.) A name given to a small granular, brownish or blackish tumour, which forms occasionally at the surface of the cornea in consequence of ulcers or accidental wounds of that membrane.—Nysten.

RAISINS, Uvæ passæ, see Vitus vinifera—a. *de Corinthe*, see Vitus Corinthiaca.

RAISON, Reason.

RAKASIRA. An American balsam; of a brownish or brownish-red colour; semi-transparent; brittle; softening and becoming tenacious by heat; inodorous when cold, but exhaling a very agreeable smell when heated; and possessing a balsamic and slightly bitter taste. The precise vegetable that furnishes it is not known. It has been used chiefly as a balsam in gonorrhœa and urinary affections.

RAKIA, see Spirit.

RAKOSIS, Rachosis.

RÂLE, Rattle, *Rhonchus, Rhenchus, Rhexeris*. from (D.) Ratel; *Rhoncus, Cerchnus, Rhogmos*. (F.) *Râle*. Noise produced by the air in passing through mucus, of which the lungs are unable to free themselves. This condition is chiefly observed at the approach of death, and is commonly called, "*the rattles*."

The term *Râle* has been given to different sounds during respiration, caused by the air passing through fluid contained in the bronchi, or areolæ of the pulmonary tissue; which are perceived by the stethoscope.

RÂLE BRONCHIQUE SEC, Râle sonore—r. Bronchique humide, R. muqueux—r. Caverneux, Gurgling—r. *Cavernuleux*, see Gurgling—r. *Cré-*

RASU'RA, *Xysma, Xysmos*, (F.) *Râpure*, from *radere, rasum*, 'to scrape.' A rasure, or scratch, or erosion. Also, the rasping or shaving of any substance; as *Rasu'ræ Cornu Cervi, Hartshorn shavings*.
RASURA, Scobs.
RATAFI'A. A liquor prepared by imparting to ardent spirits the flavour of various kinds of fruits, adding sugar.
RATANHY, Krameria ratanhia—r. of the Antilles, Krameria ixina.
RATE, Spleen.
RATÉLEUX, Spleneticus.
RATÉLIER, see *Dentier*.
RATIO, *Rationa'litas*, from *reor, ratus*, 'to think.' A reason, a cause, an explanation, a mode or manner; as *Ratio symptom'atum*, an explanation of the symptoms,—*Ratio meden'di, Genus curatio'nis, Via curandi*; the mode or manner of cure.
RATIO, Reason—r. Medendi, see Ratio—r. Symptomatum, see Ratio.
RAT"IONAL, *Rationa'lis*. That which is conformable to reason. This epithet is often opposed to *empirical; as rational treatment*. The French, also, say *Signes rationales*, in opposition to *Signes sensibles*. See Organic.
RATIONALITAS, Ratio.
RATSBANE, Arsenious acid.
RATTLE, *Râle*.
RATTLES, THE, see *Râle*.
RATTLEBUSH, Sophora tinctoria.
RATTLESNAKE, Crotalus horridus—r. Leaf, Goodyera pubescens—r. Plantain, Goodyera pubescens—r. Root, Nabalus albus, Polygala senega, Trillium latifolium—r. Weed, Hieracium venosum.
RATTLESNAKE'S MASTER, Agave Virginica, Liatris scariosa, Nabalus albus.
RATTLEWEED, Actæa racemosa.
RATULA, Raspatorium.
RAUCE'DO, *Rau'citas, Parapho'nia rauca, Asper'itas Arte'riæ as'peræ, Vox rauca, Branchus, Hoarseness*, (F.) *Enrouement, Raucité*. A change in the voice, which loses its smoothness and becomes low and obscure. It is a common symptom in diseases of the larynx and trachea.
RAUCEDO CATARRHA'LIS. Hoarseness from cold.
RAUCITAS, Raucedo.
RAUCITÉ, Raucedo.
RAUCOUS, *Raucus*. Hoarse; as a raucous voice—*Vox rauca seu raucis'ona*.
RAVE, Brassica rapa.
RAYONNÉ, Radiated.
RAYONS SOUS-IRIENS, Ciliary processes.
RAZOR, *Culter Tonsor'ius, Machæ'ris, Norac'ula, Xyrum, Xyrus*, (F.) *Rasoir*, from *radere, rasum*, 'to shave.' An instrument for shaving. Used in surgery to remove hairs, where they would interfere with any operation.
REACHING, Vomiturition.
REAC'TION, *Reac'tio*, from *re*, 'again,' and *agere, actum*, 'to act.' An action of resistance to a power applied. A species of vital movement or excitement, tending to prevent or destroy the effects of any noxious power applied to the animal economy, and which, by some, has been attributed to the *vis medicatrix naturæ*. It is certainly dependent on the organic instinctive actions of the frame. It is the state of activity which succeeds the action on the nervous system of certain morbific influences.
REAL'GAR, *Realgal, Arlada, Arladar, Auripigmen'tum rubrum, Arsen'icum rubrum facti"'ium, Abessi, Sandara'cha Græco'rum, Red Sulphuret of Mercury*. A violent poison. See Poison.
REASON, *Ra'tio, Logos*, (F.) *Raison*. Same etymon as Ratio. The faculty or property of the mind by means of which man perceives the distinction between right and wrong, in physics as well as in morals. *Reason* is a just conclusion resulting from the comparison of two ideas, by virtue of which we form a judgment.
REBOLEA, Mummy.
REBONA, Mummy.
REBOUTEUR, Renoueur.
RECEIV'ER, *Ampulla*, (F.) *Ballon, Récipient*. In pharmacy, a wide-necked globular vessel, the neck of which widens gradually outwards, to receive the tapering beak of the retort in distillation. Like the retort, the receiver may be *plain* or *tubulated*.
A *quilled receiver* is one that has a tapering tube from its lower surface, which is inserted into a graduated bottle through a cork joint, when it is desirable to know accurately the amount of fluid that has passed over.
RECEPTACULA DURÆ MATRIS, Sinuses of the dura mater.
RECEPTAC'ULUM CHYLI, 'receptacle of the chyle;' *R. Pecquet'i seu Pecquetia'num, Diverso'rium Chyli, Stagnum chyli, Sac'culus chy'lifer seu ro'rifer, Saccus lac'teus, Al'veus ampullo'sus seu ampulles'cens, Utric'ulus lacteus, Vesic'ula chyli, Ampul'la chylif'era seu chyli, Cister'na lumba'ris, C. Chyli, Chylocys'tis, Chylodochi'um, Lat'ices lactei, Lumbar cistern, Reservoir of Pecquet*, (F.) *Réservoir du chyle, R. de Pecquet, Citerne lombaire*. A considerable dilatation of the thoracic duct, in front of the lumbar region of the vertebral column. It is the commencement of the duct.
RECEPTAC'ULUM COTUN'NII. A triangular space, formed by a separation of the two laminæ of the dura mater of the internal ear, near the middle of the posterior surface of the pars petrosa of the temporal bone, where the aquæductus vestibuli terminates. It is always filled with the *Fluid of Cotugno*.
RECEPTACULUM PECQUETI, R. Chyli—r. Sellæ equinæ lateribus appositum, Cavernous sinus.
RECEPTIV'ITY, *Receptiv'itas*, (F.) *Réceptivité*, from *recipere, receptum*, 'to receive.' A word used by Tissot to express the susceptibility of certain organs to receive morbific impressions.
RECEPTUM, Prescription.
RECESSIO, Paroxysm.
RECESSUS, Abscess, Sinus—r. Sulciformis, see Fovea vestibuli.
RECHAMALCA, Rachamelca.
RECHUTE, see Relapse.
RECIDIVA MORBI, Relapse.
RÉCIDIVE, see Relapse.
REC"IPÈ, (L.) (*re*, and *capere*, 'to take.') A Latin word which signifies 'take,' (F.) *Prenez*, and with which prescriptions are commenced. It is, often, represented by R, ℞, and was formerly by ♃, the symbol of Jove. See Abbreviation.
RÉCIPIENT, Receiver.
RECIPROCATION, VIBRATIONS OF, see Sound.
RECLINATIO, Reclination—r. Palpebrarum, Ectropion.
RECLINA'TION, *Reclina'tio*, from *reclinare*, (*re*, and *clinare*, 'to bend,') 'to bend back.' A mode of operating for the cataract, which consists in applying the needle in a certain manner to the anterior surface of the cataract and depressing it into the vitreous humour, in such a way, that the front surface of the cataract is the upper one and its back surface the lower one.

RECLUSOR PALPEBRARUM, Levator palpebræ superioris.
RECOMPOSITION, Metasynchrisis.
RECONVALESCENTIA, Convalescence.
RECORDATIO, Memory.
RECORDATUS, Memory.
RECORPORATIVUS, Metasyncritic.
RECOVERY, Restauratio.
RECREATIO, Restauratio.
REC'REMENT, *Recremen'tum,* from *re,* and *cernere, cretum,* 'to sift.' A humour, which, after having been separated from the blood, is again returned to it; such as the saliva, the secretion of serous membranes, &c. Such fluid is said to be *recrementitial,* (F.) *Récrémenteux, Récrémentitiel.*

RECREMENTA VESICÆ, Urine.
RECREMEN'TO-EXCREMENTIT"IAL. Applied to secreted fluids, as the saliva, bile, &c., which are in part reabsorbed and in part excreted.
RECREMENTUM, Recrement.
RECRUDESCEN'TIA, *Palincote'sis, Recrudes'cence,* from *re,* 'again,' and *crudus,* 'raw.' An increase of a disease after a temporary remission.
RECTAL, *Recta'lis.* Appertaining, or relating to, the rectum, — as 'rectal tube.' See Tube, rectal.
RECTIFICA'TION, *Rectifica'tio,* from *rectum facere,* 'to make right.' An operation by which certain liquids are purified by distilling them either singly or after admixture with other substances.

RECTI'TIS. A hybrid word, from *rectum,* and *itis,* denoting inflammation; properly *architis,* or *proctitis.* Inflammation of the rectum. *Proctitis, Proctal'gia inflammato'ria.*
RECTOSTENOSIS, Stricture of the rectum.
RECTO-VAG"INAL, *Recto-vagina'lis.* That which relates or belongs to the rectum or vagina.
RECTO-VAGINAL FISTULA is owing to a preternatural communication between the rectum and vagina, through the above septum.
RECTO-VAGINAL SEPTUM, (F.) *Cloison rectovaginale,* is formed by the junction — back to back — (or by what the French term *adossement*) of the rectum and vagina. It separates these two canals from each other.
RECTO-VES'ICAL, *Recto-vesica'lis.* Having relation to the rectum and bladder; as the "*rectovesical fold* or *pouch*" of the peritoneum, between the rectum and bladder.
RECTUM; so called from a notion that it is straight. It is not so. *Intesti'num Rectum, Apeuthys'menos, Euthyen'teron, Longaon, Longas, Longanon, Archos, Cys'saros, Princeps, Monoco'lon* (?). The third and last portion of the great intestine. It forms the continuation of the sigmoid flexure of the colon, occupies the posterior part of the pelvis, and extends from the left side of the sacro-vertebral articulation to the coccyx, before which it opens outwards by the orifice called the *anus.* It is cylindrical, but *saccated,* as it were, at its inferior portion, where it is consequently larger, and is attached to the sacrum by the mesorectum. Like the other portions of the canal it is formed of three membranes. Towards the lower extremity, some parallel and longitudinal wrinkles are observable on its inner surface: these are the *Columns, Colum'næ car'neæ of the Rectum* or *of Morgagni,* (F.) *Colonnes du rectum* ou *de Morgagni.* They are merely folds of the mucous membrane, between which is a number of *Lacunæ.* The arteries of the rectum are numerous. They proceed from the inferior mesenteric, hypogastric, and internal pudic, and are called *hemorrhoidal.* The veins open, partly into the hypogastric vein, partly into the inferior mesenteric. The nerves proceed from the sciatic and hypogastric plexuses. The rectum receives the fæcal matters, as they pass from the colon, which serves as a reservoir.

RECTUS ABDOM'INIS, (F.) *Pubio-sternal, Sterno-pubien* (Ch.), *Droit de l'abdomen.* A long flat muscle, situate at the anterior part of the abdomen, and separated from that of the opposite side by the linea alba. It is attached, above, to the cartilages of the last three true ribs; and, below, to the pubis by a very strong tendon, the outer edge of which is continuous with the fascia transversalis. This muscle is enclosed in an aponeurotic sheath; and, in its course, has three or four transverse aponeurotic intersections. It bends the chest on the pelvis, and conversely.

RECTUS ANTERIOR BREVIS, Rectus capitis internus minor — r. Anterior longus, R. capitis internus major — r. Capitis anticus longus, R. c. internus major.

RECTUS CAPITIS INTERNUS MAJOR, *R. internus major, R. anterior longus, Rectus capitis anti'cus longus,* (F.) *Trachélo-basilaire, Grand droit antérieur de la tête.* This muscle is long in proportion to its breadth, flat, and broader above than below. It is situate at the anterior and lateral part of the neck, and arises from the transverse processes of the third, fourth, fifth, and sixth cervical vertebræ. It is inserted into the basilary process of the occipital bone.

RECTUS CAPITIS INTERNUS MINOR, *R. internus minor, Ren'uens, An'nuens, R. anterior brevis,* (F.) *Petit trachélo-basilaire, Petit droit antérieur de la tête.* This is situate deeper than the last. It is thin, flattened, irregularly quadrilateral, and passes from the anterior surface of the body of the first vertebra, near the origin of the transverse process, to be inserted into the basilary process.

RECTUS CAPITIS LATERA'LIS, *R. lateralis Fallo'pii, Transversa'lis anti'cus primus, Rectus lateralis,* (F.) *Trachélo-atloïdo-basilaire, Atloïdo-sous-occipital* (Ch.), *Droit latéral de la tête.* There is a muscle of this name on each side of the head. It is flat, quadrilateral, and passes from the transverse process of the atlas to the occiput, behind the jugular fossa. It inclines the head to one side.

RECTUS CAPITIS POSTI'CUS MAJOR, *R. Major. R. Capitis posti'cus minor* (Albinus), *Spini-axoïdo-occipita'lis,* (F.) *Axoïdo-occipitale* (Ch.), *Grand droit postérieur de la tête.* A flat, triangular muscle, situate at the posterior and superior part of the neck. It extends from the spinous process of the second cervical vertebra to the external surface of the lower semicircular ridge of the occipital bone. This muscle extends the head, inclines it to one side, and causes it to experience a rotary motion, which directs the face to its side.

RECTUS CAPITIS POSTI'CUS MINOR, *R. minor,* (F.) *Tuber-atloïdo-occipital, Atloïdo-occipital* (Ch.), *Petit droit postérieur de la tête.* A flat triangular muscle, situate beneath the last, which passes from the posterior arch of the atlas to the occipital bone. It extends the head.

RECTUS CAPITIS POSTICUS MINOR, R. e. p. major — r. Cruris, R. femoris.

RECTUS EXTERNUS OCULI, *Abductor oculi, Indignabun'dus, Indignato'rius, Iracun'dus, Oc'ulum movens secun'dus, Orbito-extus-sclérotícien.* All the recti muscles of the eye, four in number, arise from the bottom of the orbit, and are inserted into the sclerotic coat of the eye. The *Rectus externus,* (F.) *Droit externe, Irascible* ou *Abducteur,* is divided, at its posterior extremity, into two portions, one of which is attached to the outer part of the foramen opticum, and the other to the sphenoid bone.

RECTUS FEM'ORIS, *Rectus* sive *Grac"ilis anterior*, *Rectus cruris*, (F.) *Ilio-rotulien, Droit antérieur de la cuisse*. A straight muscle, seated at the anterior part of the thigh. It extends from the anterior and inferior spine of the ilium and the cotyloid cavity of the patella. This muscle extends the leg upon the thigh, and conversely. It can, also, bend the thigh upon the pelvis or carry the pelvis forward.

RECTUS INFERIOR OCULI, *Depres'sor oculi, Tim'idus, Dep'rimens, Hu'milis, Oc'ulum movens quartus*, (F.) *Sous-optico-sphéno-scléroticien, Droit inférieur* ou *abaisseur de l'œil, Muscle humble,* arises below the optic foramen, from the sphenoid bone. It depresses the eye.

RECTUS INTERNUS OC'ULI, *Addu'cens oculi, Bibito'rius, Oculi adductor, Oculum movens primus,* (F.) *Orbito-intus-scléroticien, Droit interne de l'œil* ou *adducteur* ou *buveur.* It arises from the sphenoid at the inferior part of the foramen opticum. It turns the eye towards the nose.

RECTUS SUPERIOR OCULI, *Attol'lens oculi, Attol'lens oc'ulum, Leva'tor oculi, Superbus, Eleva'tor oculi, Oculum movens tertius,* (F.) *Sus-opticosphéno-scléroticien, Droit supérieur* ou *élévateur de l'œil, Dédaigneur,* is attached to the circumference of the foramen opticum.

All the recti muscles are concerned in the voluntary motions of the eye. The oblique muscles have been supposed by Sir C. Bell to execute the involuntary.[?]

RECTUS INFERIOR FEMORIS, Gracilis — r. Internus major, R. capitis internus major — r. Internus minor, R. capitis internus minor — r. Lateralis, R. capitis lateralis — r. Lateralis Fallopii, R. capitis lateralis — r. Major, R. capitis posticus major — r. Minor, R. capitis posticus minor.

RECUBITORIUM, Anaclinterium.
RECUPERATION, Restauratio.
RECU'PERATIVE, *Recu'peratory,* from *recuperatio,* 'recovery.' Restorative. Recovering. Belonging to recovery.

RECUR'RENT, *Recur'rens,* from *recurrere,* (*re*, and *currere*), 'to run back.' A name given to several arterial and nervous branches, which seem to re-ascend towards the origin of the trunk whence they emanate.

RECURRENT ARTERIES. This name has been given to several arteries of the forearm, and to one of the leg. In the *forearm,* there are, 1. The *Radial recurrent, Artère récurrente de l'épicondyle* (Ch.), which arises from the superior part of the radial, and ascends between the supinator longus, s. brevis, and the brachialis internus. 2. The *anterior cubital recurrent, A. récurrente de l'épitrochlée* (Ch.), which arises from the upper and inner part of the cubital, and ascends between the pronator teres and brachialis internus. 3. The *posterior cubital recurrent,* which arises from the preceding artery, or from the cubital itself, and ascends between the olecranon and internal tuberosity of the humerus. 4. The *posterior radial recurrent, A. récurrente olécranienne* (Ch.). It arises from the posterior interosseous, and ascends between the posterior cubital and anconeus muscles. In *the leg,* — the *Arteria recurrens tibia'lis, A. récurrente du genou* (Ch.), is furnished by the anterior tibial, and ascends to the tibialis anticus muscle.

RECURRENT BANDAGES are formed by convolutions of the bandages, which make a kind of cap for the part — as the head — to which they are applied.

RECURVATIO, see Hump.
RECUTITUS, Apella.
REDBEAN, Abrus precatorius.

REDBERRY, Arbutus uva ursi, Gaultheria, Panax quinquefolium — r. Bitter, Cornus Florida
RED HEAD, Asclepias Carassavica — r. Root, Celastrus, Sanguinaria Canadensis — r. Swamp, Vaccinum oxycoccos.
REDIMICULUM, Diadema.
REDINGOTES ANGLAISES, see Condom.
REDINTEGRATIO, Regeneration, Restauratio.
REDIVIA, Paronychia.
RÉDONDANCE, Plethora.
REDOUBLEMENT, Exacerbation, Paroxysm.
REDS, Menses.
REDUCTIO, Taxis — r. Præputii Impedita, Phimosis.
REDUC'TION, *Reduc'tio, Reposit"io, Restitu"tio, Diap'lasis, Diaplas'mus, Syntax'is,* from *re,* and *ducere, ductum,* 'to lead.' A surgical operation, the object of which is to restore displaced parts to their original situation. Thus, we say the reduction of a luxation, when the displaced parts are again brought to their proper relative situation. The reduction of a hernia is the restoration of the protruded parts to the cavity of the abdomen. This is, also, called *Taxis.* In pharmacy, the process of restoring oxides, chlorides, sulphurets, &c., to the metallic state.
REDUNDANTIA, Plethora.
REDUVIA, Paronychia.
REED MACE, Typha latifolia.
REFECTIO, Restauratio.
REFECTIVA, Analeptica.
REFECTUS, Restauratio.
REFICIENTIA, Analeptica.
REFLECTION, Duplicature.
REFLEC'TOR EPIGLOT'TIDIS. A muscle, which arises from the arytenoid cartilage and inner part of the thyroid, and is inserted into the lateral edges of the epiglottis.
REFLEX SYSTEM OF NERVES, see Nerves.
REFLEXIO PALPEBRARUM, Ectropion.
REFRAC'TION, *Refrac'tio, Photocamp'sis, Dia'clasis,* from *re,* and *frango,* 'I break.' The change of direction which rays of light experience when they pass obliquely from one medium into another of different density. If the light passes from a rarer to a denser medium, it approaches the perpendicular raised at the point of immersion. The contrary occurs, when it goes from a denser to a rarer medium. The theory of lenses, telescopes, and of the eye, rests entirely on this property of light.
RÉFRAICHISSANTS, Refrigerants.
RÉFRIGÉRANT, see Alembic.
REFRIG"ERANTS, *Refrigeran'tia, Psych'tica, Antither'ma, Frigefacien'tia,* (F.) *Réfraichissans, Réfrigératifs,* from *re,* and *frigere,* 'to cool.' Medicines which depress the morbid temperature of the body. The chief reputed refrigerants are the Potassæ Nitras(?), the Sodæ Boras(?), but chiefly the abstraction of caloric by ice and ice-drinks, cold water, cold lemonades, soda-water, and effervescing draughts internally; and externally, cool air, cold water, evaporating lotions, and frigorific mixtures.
RÉFRIGERATIFS, Refrigerants.
REFRIGERATOR, see Alembic.
REGENERATIO, Reproduction.
REGENERA'TION, *Regenera'tio, Palingene'sia, Redintegra'tio,* from *re,* and *generare,* 'to beget.' Reproduction of a part of the body, which has been destroyed.
REG"IMEN, from *regere,* 'to govern.' The rational and methodical use of food, and of every thing essential to life; both in a state of health and disease. It is often restricted, in its mean-

ing, to *Diet*. It is sometimes used synonymously with hygiene.

REGINA PRATI, Spiræa ulmaria.

REGIO, Region.

REGIO AURICULARIS. The region of the ear.
REGIO BUCCA'LIS. The region of the cheeks.
REGIO CARDIACA, Epigastric region.
REGIO CERVICA'LIS. The region of the neck. The cervical region.
REGIO EPIGASTRICA, Epigastrium.
REGIO FACIA'LIS. The facial region.
REGIO FRONTALIS. The frontal region.
REGIO GASTRICA, Umbilical region — r. Hypogastrica, see Hypogastrium—r. Hypochondriaca, Hypochondre—r. Iliaca, Iliac region—r. Inguinalis, Inguinal region — r. Ischiadica, Ischiadic region — r. Jugalis, Jugal region — r. Lumbalis, Lumbi—r. Mentalis, Mental region—r. Mesogastrica, Umbilical region—r. Nasalis, Nasal region —r. Nuchæ, Nuchal region—r. Nuchalis, Nuchal region—r. Occipitalis, Occiput—r. Occipitalis inferior, Nuchal region — r. Perinæi, Perinæum — r. Præcordiaca, Præcordial region — r. Pubis, Pubic region — r. Stomachalis, Epigastric region —r. Stomachica, Epigastric region—r. Temporalis, Temple — r. Umbilicalis, Umbilical region.

RE'GION, *Re'gio*. Same etymon. Anatomists have called *regions*, determinate spaces on the surface of the body or of different organs. Thus, the abdomen has been divided into several; to which different names have been given. See Abdomen, Epigastrium, Hypochondrium, Hypogastrium.

RÉGION OMBILICALE, Umbilical region.

REGIONAL ANATOMY, see Anatomy.

RÈGLES, Menses — *r. Déviés*, Menstruation, vicarious—*r. Difficiles*, Dysmenorrhœa.

RÉGLISSE, Glycyrrhiza.

REGLUTINATIO, *Décollement*.

RÈGNE ANIMAL, see Animal.

REG'ULAR, *Regula'ris*, from *regula*, 'a rule.' According to rule. Applied to the types of a disease, and to the pulse, when according to rule.

REGULAR PRACTIT"IONER. One who practises his profession according to the rules established by law or custom.

REGULUS ANTIMONII, Antimonium.

REGURGITA'TION, *Regurgita'tio*. The act by which a canal or reservoir frees itself, without effort, from substances accumulated in it. Usually, it is applied to the *puking* or *possetting* of infants; and to the *rising* of solids or fluids into the mouth in the adult,—from *re*, and *gorge*, 'the throat.' What is called "vomiting at pleasure" is regurgitation.

The substances brought into the mouth by regurgitation, the French call *Renvois*.

REIN, Kidney.

REINE DES PRÈS, Spiræa ulmaria.

REINERZ, MINERAL WATERS OF. Reinerz is a small town in Silesia, three German miles from Glatz. The waters are acidulous chalybeates. The principal springs are the tepid drinking spring, the cold spring, and three bathing springs.

REÏNFORCE'MENT, FASCIC'ULUS OF, *F. Cuneʾtus*. A band of fibres from the *corpus innominatum*, or lateral part of the antero-lateral column of the medulla, which is continued up behind and around the corpus olivare, is lined on its inner or central surface with cineritious substance, enlarges as it ascends, passes over the upper surface of the pons Varolii, and is expanded into the optic thalamus. It thus forms, in its course, the anterior paries of the fourth ventricle, and is brought into view by brushing away the *tuberculum cinereum* or gray matter of the ventricle. The band has received these names owing to its constantly increasing as it ascends, and being mixed up with gray matter on its inner face, from which it seems to derive new fibres.

REINS, Kidneys, Lumbi.

REJEC'TIO, *Anago'gē*, from *re*, and *jacere*, 'to cast.' Every excretion by the mouth; spitting, expectoration, regurgitation, or vomiting.

REJECTIO SANGUINIS E PULMONIBUS, Hæmoptysis.

REJUVENES'CENCE, *Rejuvenescen'tia*, from *re*, 'again, and *juvenescens*, 'growing young;' (*juvenis*, 'a youth'). A renewal of youth. The state of being young again. The assumption of the characteristics of youth by the aged.

RELACHEMENT, Relaxation.

RELAPSE, *Hypot'ropē, Epis'trophē, Hypodtrophē, Morbi recidi'va, Hypotropius'nous*, from *re*, 'again,' and *labor*, 'I fall down.' The return of a disease, during, or shortly after, convalescence. The French use *Rechute* in this sense: and *Récidive* (*Morbus recidi'vus*) for the return of a complaint, at a greater or less period after the complete restoration of health.

The terms *Relapsing fever, Short fever, Fiveday fever, Seven-day fever, Bil'ious Remitt'ent fever, Remitting Icteric fever*, and *Mild Yellow fever*, have been given to a form of continued fever, which has occasionally appeared epidemically, as in Edinburgh, in 1843 and 1847, and was generally attended with icteric symptoms. The main phenomena disappeared at about the end of a week; but in many cases a relapse occurred about the end of a fortnight. Few died of the affection.

RELAPSING FEVER, see Relapse.

RELATIO, *Rapport*.

RELATION, FUNCTIONS OF, see Function.

RELAX'ANT, *Laxans, Malactʾicum, Chalasʾticum, Paretʾicum*, (F.) *Relachant*, from *re*, and *laxare*, 'to loose.' A medicine which diminishes the tension of organs. Mucilaginous and fatty substances are relaxants.

RELAXANTIA, Emollients.

RELAXATIO CORDIS ET ARTERIARUM, Diastole.

RELAXA'TION, *Relaxa'tio*. Same etymon. *Chala'sis, Chalas'mos*, (F.) *Relachement*. In *Physiology*, relaxation is opposed to contraction. In *Pathology*, it means great looseness of a part.

RELEVEUR DE L'ANUS, Levator ani— *r. de la Lèvre inférieure*, Levator labii inferioris — *r. du Menton*, Levator labii inferioris — *r. de l'Omoplate*, Levator scapulæ — *r. de la Prostate*, Levator prostatæ — *r. de l'Urèthre*, Levator urethræ.

RELIQUAT, (F.) The remnant or remains of a disease.

REMAK FIBRES, see Fibres, Remak.

REMANSIO MENSIUM, Amenorrhœa.

REMÈDE, Clyster, Medicament — *r. du Capuchin*, Liquor hydrargyri nitrici—*r. de Duvand*, Liquor anodynus terebinthinatus — *r. du Duc d'Antin*, Liquor hydrargyri nitrici.

REMEDIAL, Medicinal.

REMEDIATE, Medicinal.

REMEDILESS, Incurable.

REMEDIUM, Juvans, Medicament — r. Dentifricium, Dentifrice.

REMEDY, Medicament—r. English, Cinchona.

REMISSIO, Decline, Remission — r. Cordis et Arteriarum, Diastole — r. Morbi, Remission — r. Virium, Atony.

REMIS'SION, *Remisʾsio, Epanʾesis, Anʾesis, Submisʾsio, Aphʾesis, Enʾdosis, Remisʾsio, Meiosis*, from *remittere*, (*re*, and *mittere*, 'to send'), 'to relax. In a more extensive signification, a temporary diminution of the symptoms of a disease, either acute or chronic, *Remis'sio morbi.* Diminution in the febrile symptoms, such as occurs in a remittent fever, between the exacerbations.

REMITTENS ICTERODES, Fever, yellow.
REMIT'TENT, *Remit'tens.* Same etymon. Any disease which presents *remissions.*
REMITTENT OF CHILDREN, Fever, infantile remittent.
REMITTENT FEVER, *Febris remit'tens, Epan'etus, Exac"erbating, paroxysmal, sub-continual, endem'ic, endem'ial* or *endem'ical fever,* (F.) *Fièvre rémittente,* is one which strikingly exacerbates and remits, but without intermission. The ordinary bilious fever of the United States is a simple remittent—*Epanetus mitis,* (F.) *Fièvre rémittente simple.*
REMITTENT FEVER, BILIOUS, Remittent fever, see Relapse.
REMITTING ICTERIC FEVER, see Relapse.
REM'ORA, from *remorari,* (*re,* and *mora,* 'delay,') 'to arrest.'. The name of two surgical instruments, intended to retain parts *in situ.* The one was used, formerly, in castration, to prevent the intestines from protruding at the inguinal ring; the other, called *Remora Hilda'ni,* (F.) *Arrêt d'Hildan, Echene'is,* was employed to maintain fractures and luxations reduced. It is not now used.
REMORA ARATRI, Ononis spinosa.
REN, Kidney.
RENAL, *Rena'lis,* from *Ren,* 'the kidney.' That which relates to the kidney.
RENAL ARTERIES, *Emulg"ent Arteries,* are very large and short, and commonly two in number— one to each kidney. They arise from the sides of the abdominal aorta, forming with it a right angle. The left is commonly a little more anterior and elevated than the right. After a short course, they arrive at the fissure of the kidney, where they divide, before entering it, into three or four very considerable branches.
RENAL CAPSULE, Capsule, renal—r. Nerve, see Splanchnic Nerves.
RENAL PLEX'USES, *Emulgent Plexuses.* These are two:—one on each side. They proceed from fasciculi of the solar and cœliac plexuses; from the outer side of the semilunar ganglion and the final expansion of the small splanchnic nerves. These plexuses begin by three or four ganglions, situate at the commencement of the renal artery; and they give off from their circumference many fine, straight filaments, which do not anastomose, and which enter the kidney with the divisions of the renal artery. These divisions they accompany.
RENAL VEINS, *Emulgent Veins.* These are very large. Their roots follow the same course as the arteries in the substance of the kidney. In the fissure or pelvic portion of the kidney, they unite into a single trunk, which passes transversely inwards, and opens at the side of the vena cava descendens.
RENCHUS, Snoring, Stertor.
REN'CULUS, *Renic'ulus, Ren'ulus,* diminutive of *Ren,* 'a kidney.' A small kidney. A lobe of the kidney.
RENES SUCCENTURIATI, Capsules, renal.
RENICULUS, Renculus.
RENIFORM, Nephroid.
RENNES, MINERAL WATERS OF. Thermal salines in the department of Aube, France, containing carbonic acid and chloride of magnesium. Temperature 103 to 121°, of Fahr.

RENNET, *Runnet,* from (G.) g e r i n n e n, 'to coagulate.' (?) When the fourth stomach or *Abomasus* of the calf is salted and dried, it possesses the property of coagulating milk, when a portion of it is soaked in water, and the infusion—*Rennet*—is added to milk.
RENNET WHEY, see Serum lactis.
RENNSELÆRIA, Leptandra Virginica.
RENONCULE, Ranunculus—*r. Bulbeuse,* Ranunculus bulbosus.
RENOUÉE, Polygonum aviculare.
RENOUEUR, (F.) *Rebouteur, Rhabilleur.* A *bone-doctor:*—a *bone-setter.* One who makes a trade of reducing fractures and dislocations.
RENOVATIO, Ananeosis.
RENUENS, Rectus capitis internus minor.
RENULUS, Renculus.
RENUM ATONIA, Nephratonia—r. Paralysis, Nephratonia.
RENUNCIATIO, *Rapport.*
RENVERSEMENT DE LA LANGUE, Paraglossa—*r. de la Matrice,* Uterus, inversion of the—*r. des Paupières,* Ectropion—*r. du Rectum,* Proctocele—*r. de la Vessie,* Exocyste, Exstrophia of the bladder.
RENVOIS, see Regurgitation.
REPANDATIO, Lordosis.
REPARATION, Restauratio.
REPAR'ATIVE, *Repar'atory.* Having the power of restoring or repairing.
REPELLENTIA, Repellents.
REPEL'LENTS, *Repellen'tia, Repercutien'tia, Apocrus'tica, Repercus'sives,* (F.) *Répercussifs,* from *re,* and *pellere,* 'to drive.' Medicines which, when applied to a tumefied part, cause the fluids, that render it tumid, to recede, as it were, from it. Astringents, cold water, ice, &c., are repellents.
RÉPERCUSSIFS, Repellents.
REPERCUSSIO, Contra-fissura, Repercussion.
REPERCUS'SION, *Repercus'sio, Anac'lasis,* from *re, per,* and *quatere,* 'to shake or batter.' Disappearance of a tumour or cutaneous eruption, in consequence of the application of a repellent. The action of a repellent remedy. The French writers use the term *Délitescence, Delitescen'tia,* for the sudden disappearance of a tumour, inflammation, eruptive disease, or purulent collection, without the disease occurring in any other part of the body: in this respect delitescence differs from metastasis: *Délitescence* of an inflammation or 'sudden disappearnce' is distinguished by certain French pathologists from *Resolution.* Repercussion also means *Ballottement.*
REPERCUSSIVES, Repellents.
REPERCUTIENTIA, Repellents.
REPLETION, Fulness, Plethora.
REPLI LONGITUDINAL DE LA MENINGE, Falx cerebri.
REPOSITIO, Anaplasis, Reduction, Taxis.
REPOUSSOIR, Punch—*r. d'Arêtes,* Probang.
REPRIMENS, Epischeticus.
REPRODUC'TION, *Reproduc'tio, Regenera'tio,* from *re,* and *producere,* (*pro,* and *ducere.*) The function by which living bodies produce bodies similar to themselves. See Generation. As a general remark, it will be found true, that the larger animals are uniparous; and the smaller, which are more exposed to destruction, multiparous. The mammalia being of the same natural class as man, it may be useful to compare them in this respect.

COMPARATIVE TABLE OF REPRODUCTION IN THE CLASS MAMMALIA.

Species.	Age capable of engendering.	Duration of gestation.	Number of young at each birth.	Period of cessation of the function.
Primates.				
Man	14 years	9 months	1 to 3	At a somewhat advanced age.
Monkeys (large)	3 years	7 months	Do.	
Do. (long tailed)	2 years	6 months	Do.	
Carnivora.				
Bear	2 years	112 days	1 to 4	25 to 30 years.
Badger	....	....	3 to 4	20 to 25 years.
Hedgehog	1 year	1 mo. and 10 days	3 to 5	
Ferret...............	11 months	Do.	5 to 9 twice a year	Produces during life.
Otter................	....	3 months	3 to 4	
Pole-cat, Marten, Weasel, and Ermine,	before 1 year	56 days	3 to 6	8 to 10 years.
Didelphus, Opossum, and Philander,	....	....	4 to 6	10 years. (?)
Lion	2 years	3 to 4 months	3 to 4	20 to 25 years.
Tiger, Leopard	Do.	3 months	4 to 5	Do.
Lynx	....	9 weeks	3 to 4	
Wild Cat............	before 1 year	56 days	4 to 6	9 years.
Wolf	2 years	73 days	5 to 9	15 to 20 years.
Dog, in the most natural state,	10 months	63 days	3 to 6	15 years.
Fox	1 year	2 months	Do.	10 or 12 years.
Jackall	....	Do.	5 to 8	
Isatis	....	63 days	6 to 7	
Phoca	....	3 months (?)	2 to 3	
Rodentia.				
Squirrel.............	1 year	45 days	3 to 4 twice a year	Produces during life.
Flying Squirrel......	....	....	3 to 4	Do.
Ondatra	....	....	3 to 5	Lives 6 years.
Beaver...............	....	4 months	2 to 3	
Hare	1 year	30 days	2 to 4 several times a year	Lives 8 years.
Rabbit	6 months	Do.	4 to 8 do.	Lives 8 or 9 years.
Rat	Do.	5 or 6 weeks	5 to 6 do.	Produces during life.
Mouse	Do.	1 month	Do.	Do.
Marmot	....	6 weeks	2 to 4	Do.
Guinea Pig...........	5 to 6 weeks	3 weeks	5 to 8 times a year	Do.
Dormouse	1 year	....	3 to 5	
Edentata.				
Armadilla	....	....	4 times a year	7 to 8 years. (?)
Ruminantia.				
Camel................	4 years	11 months or 1 y'r	1	40 to 50 years.
Dromedary	Do.	Do.	1	Do.
Buffalo	3 years	9 months	1	15 to 18 years.
Beef.................	2 years	Do.	1 to 2	9 years.
Lama	3 years	....	Do.	12 years.
Reindeer	2 years	8 months	1	Lives 16 years.
Buck and Doe	1½ year	Do.	1 to 2	Lives 25 or 30 years.
Roebuck	Do.	5 months	Do.	Lives 12 or 15 years.
Saiga (Antelope).....	1 year	Do.	Do.	Lives 15 or 20 years.
Chamois and Wild Goat	Do.	Do.	1, 2, and 3	Lives 18 or 20 years.
Goat	Do.	Do.	Do.	7 years.
Musimon	1½ year	Do.	1 to 2	8 or 10 years.
Sheep	1 year	Do.	Do.	8 years.
Solipedes.				
Horse	2½ years	290 days	1 to 2	25 or 30 years.
Ass	Do.	Do.	Do.	Do.
Zebra	Do.	Do.	Do.	Do.
Pachydermata.				
Hog	9 months or 1 year	4 months	10 to 20	15 years.
Elephant.............	16 years (?)	9 to 11 months	1 or 2	Lives 70 years. (?)
Rhinoceros	5 years (?)	....	1 or 2 (?)	Lives 60 years. (?)
Hippopotamus	....	....	1	
Morse	....	9 months	1	

REPULSORIUM, Punch.

REPURGA'TIO, *Anacathar'sis*, from *re*, and *purgare*, 'to cleanse.' According to Castelli — purgation by transpiration or by expectoration. Medicines producing this effect are called *Repurgan'tia*.

REQUIES, Acinesia.

REQUIETIO, Acinesia.

RES CONTRA-NATU'RAM. 'Things against nature,' (F.) *Choses contre-nature*, are those things which tend to destroy man; — as disease, and every thing connected with it.

RES CULINARIA, Culinary art — r. Medica, Medicina.

RES NATURA'LES, (F.) *Choses naturelles*. Those things, which, by their union, were conceived to constitute the nature of man; such as the elements, temperaments, humours, spirits, &c.

RES NON NATURA'LES, (F.) *Choses non-naturelles.* Those things which, anciently, formed the matter of hygiene. See Non-naturals.

RES VENEREA, Coition — r. Vestiaria, Vestitus.

RÉSEAU, Rete — r. *Admirable*, Rete mirabile — *r. Merveilleux*, Rete mirabile.

RESECTIO, Resection — r. Articulorum, see Resection.

RESECTION, *Resec'tio*, from *resecare*, (*re*, and *secare*,) 'to cut off.' A name, given, especially by the French surgeons, to operations in which the carious extremities of long bones, or the unconsolidated extremities of fractured bones forming irregular joints, are removed with the saw — *Resectio articulo'rum, Decapita'tio articulo'rum.*

RESECTION, see Amputation.

RESEDA CRISPATA — r. luteola — r. Lanceolata — r. luteola.

RESE'DA LUTE'OLA, *R. lanceola'ta seu crispa'ta, Lute'ola, Weld, Dyer's Weed.* A European plant naturalized in the United States, which was at one time used as a diaphoretic and diuretic.

RESERANS, Aperient.

RESERVE AIR, see Respiration.

RESERVOIR DE LA BILE, Gall-bladder — r. *du Chyle,* Receptaculum chyli — r. *des Larmes,* Lachrymal sac — r. of Pecquet, Receptaculum chyli — r. *de Pecquet,* Receptaculum chyli — r. of the Thymus, see Thymus.

RESIDENTIA, Sediment.

RESIDUAL AIR, see Respiration.

RESIMUS, Camus.

RESIN, *Resi'na, Rheti'nē.* A vegetable product, commonly dry and concrete, more or less brittle, inodorous or slightly odorous, insipid, or of an acrid warm taste; of a smooth, glassy fracture, heavier than water, inflammable, insoluble in water, soluble in alcohol, ether, and yolk of an egg, and negatively electrifiable by friction. Many resins are used in medicine; the greater part are purgative and irritating. Some act like acrid poisons.

RESIN, CAYENNE, Caoutchouc — r. of the Spruce fir, see Pinus abies.

RESINA, Resin — r. Abietis, Pinus Abies, Pinus picea — r. Abietis humida, Pinus abies — r. Abietis sicca, see Pinus abies — r. Alba, see Pinus sylvestris — r. Alba humida, see Pinus Abies — r. Cayennensis, Caoutchouc — r. Copal, Copal — r. Elastica, Caoutchouc — r. Flava, see Pinus sylvestris — r. Fluida Canadensis, see Pinus balsamea — r. Juniperi, Sandarac — r. Laricis, see Pinus larix — r. Lentiscina, see Pistachia lentiscus — r. Liquida pini balsameæ, see Pinus balsamea — r. Liquidi pini laricis, see Pinus larix — r. Nigra, Colophonia — r. Pini, see Pinus sylvestris — r. Pini empyreumatica liquida, see Pinus sylvestris — r. Pini abietis sponte concreta, see Pinus abies — r. Strobilina, see Pinus balsamea, and Pinus mughos — r. Terebinthi, see Pistachia terebinthus.

RESINA'TUM, *Rhetino'ton.* An epithet for wine impregnated with resin, and used by the ancients as a stomachic.

RESINE DE GAÏAC, see Guaiacum — r. *Gomart,* see Bursera gummifera — r. *de Lierre,* see Hedera helix.

RESINOCE'RUM, *Rhetinoce'ron*, from ῥητίνη, 'resin,' and κηρός, 'wax.' A mixture of resin and wax. — Galen.

RESOLUTIO, Resolution — r. Membrorum, Paralysis.

RESOLUTIO MORBI. The resolution or disappearance of a disease; especially when without any critical evacuation.

RESOLUTIO ET DIABROSIS VENTRICULI, Gastromalacia — r. Nervorum, Paralysis — r. Ventriculi autopeptica, Gastromalacia — r. Virium, Dialysis.

- RESOLU'TION, *Resolu'tio, Discus'sio,* from *resolvere,* (*re* and *solvere,* 'to loosen.') Removal or disappearance, as of a disease. Resolution is one of the terminations of inflammation, in which the inflamed part returns gradually, and without suppuration, to the healthy condition.

RÉSOLUTION DES MEMBRES, Paralysis.

RESOLVENTIA, Discutients.

RES'ONANCE, (F.) *Retentissement, Résonnance, Résonnement,* from *re,* 'again,' and *sono,* 'I sound.' 'A return of sound.' A resounding; a reverberation of sounds. A thrilling of the voice more loud than natural; or its existence in a part where it is not heard in health, — as detected by auscultation. A thickened and hardened state of the lungs, caused either by a mass of crude tubercles, or by inflammation, is generally considered to produce this phenomenon, by rendering the lung a better conductor of the murmur of the voice in the bronchi. Hence the origin of the term *Bronchoph'ony,* from βρόνχος, 'bronchus,' and φωνή, 'the voice;' (F.) *Voix bronchique, Voix tubaire, V. bourdonnante.*

RESONANCE, VIBRATIONS OF, see Sound.

RESONITUS, Contra-fissura.

RES'ONANT, *Res'onans, Res'onus,* (F.) *Retentissant, Resonnant,* Resounding, see Resonance.

RÉSONNANCE, Resonance.

RÉSONNEMENT, Resonance.

RESORBENS, Absorbent.

RESORPTIO, Absorption, Resorption — r. Cutanea, see Absorption — r. Cutis, see Absorption.

RESORP'TION, *Resorp'tio,* from *resorbere,* (*re,* 'again,' and *sorbere,*) 'to absorb again.' Absorption of a fluid which has been previously deposited in a part by the exhalants, — as of pus, blood, serum, &c.

RES'PIRABLE, *Respirab'ilis.* Same etymon as Respiration. Capable of being breathed. Adapted for respiration.

RESPIRAMEN, Respiration.

RESPIRAMENTUM, Respiration.

RESPIRATIO, Respiration — r. Abolita, Apnœa — r. Brevis, Dyspnœa — r. Difficilis, Dyspnœa — r. Stertens, Stertor — r. Stertuosa, Stertor.

RESPIRA'TION, *Respira'tio, Anap'noē,* from *respiro,* (*re,* and *spiro,*) 'I take breath.' *Anapneu'sis, Pneu'sis spira'tio, Respira'men, Respiramentum, Respira'tus, Respir'itus, Spir'itus.* A function proper to animals, the object of which is, to place the materials of the blood — the mixture of the venous blood with lymph and chyle — in contact with atmospheric air, in order that it may acquire the vivifying qualities that belong to arterial blood. The organs for executing this function are, in the mammalia, birds, and reptiles, the *lungs.* In man, the respiration consists of mechanical and chymical phenomena. The mechanical are *Inspiration* and *Expiration.* The evident chymical phenomena consist in the formation of a certain quantity of carbonic acid, the absorption of a part of the oxygen of the air, and the disengagement of a quantity of water in the state of vapour. In the healthy condition the respiration is easy, gentle, regular, and without noise. In man, the respirations are generally about 35 per minute in the first year of life; 25 during the second; 20 at puberty; and 18 in the adult age.

The air of respiration has been divided into, *first,* the *residual air* or that which cannot be expelled from the lungs but remains after a full and forcible expiration, estimated at 120 cubic inches: *secondly,* the *supplementary* or *reserve* air or that which can be expelled by a forcible expiration, after an ordinary outbreathing, valued at 130 cubic inches: *thirdly,* the *breath, tidal* or *breathing* air, valued at 26 cubic inches: and *fourthly,* the *complementary* or *complemental* air, or that which can be inhaled after an ordinary inspiration, which amounts to 100 cubic inches. This estimate gives 250 cubic inches as the average volume of air which the chest contains after an ordinary expiration.

RESPIRATION BRONCHIQUE, see Murmur, respiratory — r. *Exagérée*, see Puerile — r. *Hypervésiculaire*, see Puerile.

RESPIRATION, JERKING, (F.) *R. saccadée*. When the murmur of inspiration, in place of being continuous, is interrupted as by starts, it is called 'jerking.' It is a concomitant of incipient pleurisy, pleurodynia, spasmodic asthma, and tuberculosis of the lung with corresponding pleuritic adhesion.—Walshe.

RESPIRATION OF THE CELLS, Murmur, respiratory—r. Metallic, *Tintement métallique*—r. *Nulle*, see Murmur, respiratory — r. Proof, Docimasia pulmonum—r. *Puérile*, see Puerile—r. *Râpeuse*, see Murmur, respiratory — r. *Rude*, see Murmur, respiratory—r. *Silencieuse*, see Murmur, respiratory—r. *Saccadée*, R. jerking—r. *Soufflante*, Murmur, respiratory—r. *Supplémentaire*, see Puerile —r. Tubal, see Murmur, respiratory.

RESPIRA'TOR, same etymon. Various instruments, under this name, have been devised for the purpose of tempering the air before it reaches the lungs in winter. One of the best is that of Jeffrey, which is made of several layers of fine wire tissue.

RESPIRATORIUM VENTRIS, Diaphragm.
RESPIRATORIUS, Respiratory.
RES'PIRATORY, *Respirato'rius*, same etymon. Appertaining to respiration. An epithet applied to the *murmur* heard by auscultation in a healthy adult, during inspiration and expiration. It marks the entrance of the air into the cells, and its passage out of them. See Murmur.

RESPIRATORY, EXTERNAL, NERVE, see Thoracic nerves — r. Internal, nerves, Diaphragmatic Nerves — r. Nerve of the face, Facial Nerve — r. Superior, nerve, Spinal Nerve.

RESPIRATORY TRACT, *Tractus respirato'rius*. The middle column of the spinal marrow, described by Sir Charles Bell as that whence the respiratory nerves originate. See Nerves.

RESPIRATUS, Respiration.
RESPIRITUS, Respiration.
RESSERRÉ, (VENTRE,) Constipation.
RESTA BOVIS, Ononis spinosa.
RESTAGNATIO, Eructation.
RESTAURANS, Corroborant.
RESTAURA'TIO, *Refec'tio, Refec'tus, Analep'sis, Anatrep'sis, Anacom'idè, Analte'sis, Anacte'sis, Apocatas'tasis*. Restoration of strength, after disease or great fatigue; *Epanortho'sis, Recrea'tio, Redintegra'tio, Restaura'tio virium*. Return of the organs to their normal condition. *Recov'ery, Recupera'tion, Repara'tion*.

RESTAURATIO VIRIUM, see Restauratio.
REST HARROW, Ononis spinosa.
RESTIFORM'IS, from *restis*, 'a rope,' and *forma*, 'shape.' Shaped like a rope, as the 'Corpora restiformia.'

RESTIFORMIS PROCESSUS, Coracoid.
RESTITUTIO, Reduction—r. Organica, Morioplastice—r. Partium deperditarum, Morioplastice.
RESTLESSNESS, Agitation.
RESTORATION, Restauratio.
RESTORATIVE, Corroborative.
RESTRICTIO INTESTINI RECTI vel ANI, Stricture of the rectum.

RESUMPTI'VUS, *Resumpto'rius;* from *re*, 'again,' and *sumere*, 'to take.' Causing to resume. *Resumpti'vum*. Any agent calculated to restore flesh and strength to one who has been reduced.

RESUMPTORIUS, Resumptivus.
RESURRECTION-MAN, Resurrectionist.
RESURREC'TIONIST, *Resurrection-man, Body snatcher:* from *re*, and *surgere*, 'to arise.' An individual who violates the sanctuary of the grave to obtain subjects for dissection.

RESUSCITA'TION, *Resuscita'tio*, from *resuscita're*, (re, and *suscitare, sursum citare* seu ri---, 'to move up,' 'to stir up anew.' *Reviri*---. The restoration of persons, apparently dead, to life. See Asphyxia and Suffocation.

RETCHING, Vomiturition.
RETE, Plexus — r. Malpighii, Corpus mucosum.

RETE, *Retic'ulum ;* 'a net;' *Dict'yon.* (F.) *Réseau*. A name given to the interlacing and decussation of blood-vessels, lymphatics, fibres, and nerves when they form a kind of network.

RETE has also been applied to the *epiploon*—Castelli.

RETE MAJUS, Epiploon, gastro-colic.
RETE MIRAB'ILE, (F.) *Réseau admirable, P. merveilleux*. A name given to the ramification and anastomoses of the internal carotid and vertebral arteries at the base of the brain.

RETE MIRABILE vel RETE VASCULO'SUM MALPIG'HII is the plexus formed on the cells of the lungs by the minute ramifications of the pulmonary artery.

RETE MUCOSUM, Corpus mucosum.
RETE seu RETE VASCULO'SUM TESTIS. An irregular plexus or network, formed by the communication of the *Vasa recta* at the upper and back part of the testicle. These Vasa recta are sent out at the back part of the testicle, from the convoluted seminal tubes. The Rete Vasculosum testis sends out from twelve to eighteen straight tubes, called *Vasa efferentia*, which convey the semen from the testes to the epididymis.

RETENTIO, Retention—r. Aerea, Dyspnœa —r. Alvina, Constipation—r. Bilis, Ischuch--
RETENTIO FLUXUS HÆMORRHOIDALIS. Suppression of the hæmorrhoidal flux.
RETENTIO FŒTUS, Dystocia—r. Lactis, Ischolactia—r. Lochiorum, Ischiolochia—r. Mensium see Amenorrhœa—r. Spermatis, Ischosperm----
r. Sudoris, Hydroschesis.

RETEN'TION, *Reten'tio, Apolep'sia, Ap----sis*, from *retinere*, (re, and *tenere*,) 'to hold back.' Accumulation of a solid or liquid substance, in canals intended for its excretion, or in a reservoir, intended to contain it for a short period.

RETENTION OF URINE; *Paru'ria Reten---- vesica'lis, Ischu'ria vesica'lis, Retentio* ----, (F.) *Rétention d'urine*. A disease in which the urine accumulated in the bladder cannot be evacuated; or, at least, cannot be passed without extreme difficulty. In the former case, the retention is said to be *complete ;* in the latter, incomplete. Many writers have distinguished the degrees of this affection, to which they have given the names *Dysury, Strangury*, and *Ischury*. Retention of urine may depend upon loss of contractility, paralysis of the bladder, &c., or cases of pressure of the womb on the bladder, tumours in its vicinity, foreign bodies in it, ---- inflammation of the urethra, swelling of the prostate, stricture, &c. The pain is extremely ---- and the bladder may be found distended above the pubis. The treatment consists in introducing the catheter, or puncturing the bladder, and in combating the cause, which has produced the retention, by particular means adapted to each case.

RETENTISSANT, Resonant.
RETENTISSEMENT, Resonance—r. *Autophonique*, see Autophonia.
RETIA UTERI, see Uterus.

RETIC'ULAR, *Re'tiform, Reticula'ris, Ret'- inus, Amphiblestroi'des, Dyctoï'des, Retifor'mis,* from *rete,* 'a net.' That which resembles a net. An epithet applied to many structures in the body.

RETICULAR BODY, Corpus mucosum — r. Substance, Cellular tissue.

RETICULARIA OFFICINALIS, Lichen pulmonarius.

RETIC'ULUM: diminutive of *rete,* 'a net.' The *Bonnet* or *Honeycomb bag*— the second stomach of the ruminant animal. See also, Epiploon, and Rete.

RETICULUM CUTANEUM, Rete mucosum — r. Mucosum, Rete mucosum.

RETIFORM, Reticular.

RET'INA, from *rete,* 'a net:' *Tu'nica ret'ina seu reticula'ris seu retifor'mis seu in'tima oc'uli, Involu'crum reti compara'tum, Verricula'ris membra'na, Amphiblestroi'des membrana.* A soft, pulpy, grayish, semi-transparent, very thin membrane; extending from the optic nerve to the crystalline, embracing the vitreous humour, and lining the choroid; without, however, adhering to either of those parts. It terminates by a defined edge — *margo denta'tus* — at the posterior extremities of the ciliary processes. It is constituted, according to most anatomists, by the expansion of the optic nerve. The retina appears to be formed of two laminæ; so joined together, that it is almost impossible to separate them. The one — the innermost — is medullary, and pulpy; the other — the outer — is stronger, and fibro-vascular. The retina is the essential organ of vision; on it the images of objects are impressed. Both it and the optic nerve are devoid of general sensibility. They may be punctured or lacerated without pain being experienced. The nerve of general sensibility distributed to the eye is the fifth pair.

RETINACULA, see Retinaculum — r. Morgagnii, see Fræna of the valve of Bauhin.

RETINAC'ULUM, from *retinere,* (re, and *tenere,*) 'to hold back.' A surgical instrument, formerly used in the operation of castration; and in that of hernia, to prevent the intestines from falling into the scrotum. — Scultet. *Retinacula* are also band-like extensions of a cellulo-membranous structure, which seem to suspend the ovum in the Follicle of De Graaf. They appear to correspond to the chalazæ of the egg of the bird.

RETINACULUM, *Bride.*

RETINAC'ULUM TEN'DINUM PERONEO'RUM, *Vagi'na malleola'ris extern'a.* The ligamentous sheaths that retain in situ at the outer ankle the tendons of the peroneal muscles.

RETINI'TIS, *Inflamma'tio Ret'inæ, Amphi- blestroidi'tis, Dictyi'tis,* from *retina* and *itis,* a suffix denoting inflammation, — a term of hybrid formation. Inflammation of the retina; an uncommon affection, except as an accompaniment of other forms of ophthalmia.

RETINOS'COPY, *Retinoscop'ia,* from *retina,* and σκοπεω, 'I view.' Examination of the retina.

RETINUS, Reticular.

RETORT', *Retor'ta, Batia, Cornu, Cornu'ta, Cornes'ta, Cornumusa,* (F.) *Cornue,* from *retorqueo,* (re, and *torqueo, tortum,*) 'I bend back.' A vessel, commonly of glass or earthenware, employed in distillation. It may be *plain,* or have a *tubulure* for admitting substances whilst the distillation is going on. In the latter case, it is said to be *tu'bulated,* (F.) *Cornue tubulée.*

RETRAC'TION, *Retrac'tio,* from *retrahere,* (re and *trahere,*) 'to draw back.' State of a part, when drawn towards the centre of the body or backwards; — as retraction of the testicles. Sometimes it is used synonymously with *shortening* or *drawing up;* as in *retraction* of the thigh.

RÉTRACTION DE LA MATRICE, Retroversio uteri.

RETRACTOR ANGULI ORIS, Buccinator.

RET'RAHENS AURIS, *Poste'rior Auris, Tri- cauda'lis, Triceps Auris, Retrahens Auric'ulæ, R. Auriculam, Secun'dus proprio'rum Auric'ulæ, Bi- cauda'lis, Dep'rimens Auric'ulæ, Proprius Auris externæ,* (F.) *Mastoïdo-conchinien, Mastoïdo-ori- culaire* (Ch.), *Auriculaire postérieur.* It consists of one or more small fasciculi or fleshy, thin, somewhat irregular fibres, situated behind the ear. These are attached to the mastoid process, and pass horizontally forwards, to terminate at the convexity formed by the concha of the ear. If this muscle had any use, it would carry the ear backwards.

RÉTRÉCISSEMENT, Arctatio, Stricture.

RETRIMENTA VESICÆ, Urine.

RETRIMENTUM, Excrement.

RETROCES'SION, *Retroces'sio, Retroces'sus, Retrogres'sus,* from *retrocedere,* (retro, 'backwards,' and *cedere,* 'to give place.') The act of going back. A disappearance or metastasis of a tumour, eruption, &c., from the outer part of the body to the inner.

RETROCESSUS, Retrocession.

RETROFLEXIO UTERI, Retroversio uteri.

RETROGRESSUS, Retrocession.

RETROPHARYNGE'AL, *Retropharynge'us,* from *retro,* 'backwards,' and *pharynx,* 'the pharynx. Relating to parts behind the pharynx, — as '*retropharyngeal* abscess,' — an abscess behind the pharynx.

RÉTROPULSION DE LA MATRICE, Retroversio uteri.

RETROVACCINA'TION; from *retro,* 'backwards,' and *vaccination.* Vaccination with matter obtained from the cow, after inoculating the animal with vaccine matter from the human subject.

RETROVER'SIO U'TERI, *Retroversion of the Uterus, Ædopto'sis Uteri retrover'sa, Retroflex'io Uteri, Anapod'isis seu Anapodis'mus Uteri,* (F.) *Rétroversion, Rétraction, Obliquité* ou *Rétropulsion de la Matrice.* A change in the position of the uterus, so that the fundus of the organ is turned towards the concavity of the sacrum, whilst the neck is directed towards the symphysis pubis. This displacement is commonly attended with constipation, tenesmus, and retention of urine. Its usual period of occurrence is between the third and fourth months of pregnancy; before the uterus has escaped above the superior aperture of the pelvis. In the treatment, the catheter must be regularly used twice a day, until the uterus, by its growth, rises above the pelvis. The catheter should be small, flat, and curved considerably more than common, in consequence of the distorted course of the urethra. The bowels must be kept open; and absolute rest, in a recumbent posture, be enjoined. Should it be impracticable to draw off the urine, attempts must be made to replace the uterus. The woman being on her hands and knees, the fore and middle fingers of the accoucheur's left hand are to be passed up the rectum to the fundus uteri; which they must elevate, whilst the cervix uteri is carefully depressed by two fingers of the right hand in the vagina. Should the fingers employed to elevate the fundus not be long enough to effect this object, a piece of whalebone may be substituted, having a small piece of sponge attached to one extremity as a pad.

RÉTROVERSION DE LA MATRICE, Retroversio uteri.

REUNIO, Synthesis—r. Partium separatarum, see Synthesis —r. per Primam intentionem, see Intention—r. per Secundam intentionem, see Intention—r. Vasorum, Anastomosis.

RÉUNION PRIMITIVE, see Intention — r. *Secondaire*, see Intention.

RÉVASSERIE, Incoherence; see Somnium.
RÊVE, Somnium.
REVEIL, see Sleep—r. *en Sursaut*, see Sleep.
REVELLENT, Derivative.
REVERY, Aphelxia.
REVIVIFICATION, Resuscitation.
RÉVULSIF, Derivative.

REVUL'SION, *Revul'sio*, from *re*, and *vellere*, 'to pluck;' *Antis'pasis*. The act of turning the principle of a disease from the organ in which it seems to have taken its seat. Rubefacients, vesicatories, bleeding in the foot, &c., are often used for this purpose. See Derivation.

REVULSIVE, Derivative—r. Bleeding, see Bloodletting.
REVULSORIUS, Derivative.
REX METALLORUM, Aurum.
REYNOLDS'S SPECIFIC, see Vinum colchici.
RHA, Rheum.
RHABARBARUM, Rheum—r. Album, Convolvulus mechoachan — r. Antiquorum, Rheum Rhaponticum—r. Dioscoridis, Rheum Rhaponticum—r. Monachorum, Rumex patientia—r. Nigrum, Convolvulus jalapa—r. Pauperum, Thalictron—r. Sibericum, Rheum—r. Tartaricum Rheum—r. Turcicum, Rheum.

RHABARBE, Rheum — *r. Blanche*, Convolvulus mechoacan— *r. des Moines*, Rumex Alpinus.

RHABDOIDES (SUTURA), Sagittal suture.
RHABILLEUR, Renoueur.
RHACHETÆ, Rhachitæ.
RHACHETRUM, Medulla spinalis.
RHACHIÆI, Rhachitæ.
RHACHIAGRA, Rachisagra.
RHACHIALGIA, Rachialgia, Rhachiodynia, Spinal irritation.
RHACHIALGITIS, Spinal irritation, Myelitis.
RHACHIDAGRA, Rachisagra, Rachialgia, Rhachiodynia.
RHACHIOCYPHOSIS, Gibbositas.
RHACHIODYN'IA; from ραχις, 'the vertebral column,' and οδυνη, 'pain;' *Rhachial'gia*. Pain in the vertebral column.
RHACHIOMYELITIS, Myelitis.
RHACHIOPLEGIA, Paraplegia.
RHACHIOSCOLIOMA, Scoliosis.
RHACHIOSCOLIOSIS, Scoliosis.
RHACHIOSTROPHO'SIS; from ραχις, 'the vertebral column,' and στρεφω, 'I turn;' *Contor'tio colum'næ vertebra'lis*. Deviation of the vertebral column.
RHACHIOT'OMUS, *Rhachiot'omum*; from ραχις, 'the vertebral column,' and τομη, 'incision.' An instrument for opening the vertebral column.
RHACHIPARALYSIS, Paraplegia.
RHACHIPHYMA, Rachiphyma.
RHACHIRRHEUMA, Lumbago.
RHACHIS, Vertebral column—r. Nasi, see Nasus.
RHACHISAGRA, Rachisagra.
RHACHI'TÆ, from ραχις, 'the vertebral column;' *Rhachia'i, Rachi'tæ, Rhache'tæ*, or *Rachia'i*. The muscles of the spine.
RHACHITES, Medulla spinalis.
RHACHITICUS, Rachiticus.
RHACHITIS, Rachitis—r. Adultorum, Mollities ossium—r. Spinalis, Rachisagra.
RHACHITISMUS, Rachitis.

RHACHOSIS, Rachosis.
RHACHUS, *Rhacus, Rhagus;* from ρασσω, 'to tear.' A wrinkle. A laceration of the skin. A lacerated ulcer—*ulcus lac"erum*.
RHACUS, Rhachus, Wrinkle.
RHÆBOCRANIA, Torticollis.
RHAG'ADES, ραγαδες, *Rhaga'dia;* from ρηγνυμι, 'to break or rend;' *Scissu'ra, Fissu'æ, Fimæ*. Ruptures, chaps, or narrow and long ulcers, which form near the origin of mucous membranes, especially around the anus, and which are generally owing to the syphilitic virus.
RHAGADES, see Fissure.
RHAGÈ, *Ragè;* ραγη. Same etymon. A suffix denoting violent rupture or discharge, as in Hemorrhage, Menorrhagia, &c.
RHAGE, Fissure.
RHAGES, Uvæ passæ.
RHAGODEITIS, Uveitis.
RHAGOÏ'DES, *Rhago'des, Rhagoïdeus, Rhagicus*, from ραξ, 'a grape.' Grape-like; as Tunica *Rhagoides*: the uvea. Also, the choroid coat of the eye.
RHAGUS, Rhachus, Wrinkle.
RHAMNUS, *Rhamnus cathar'ticus, Spina cervi'na* seu *domes'tica, Rhamnus soluti'vus, Spina infecto'ria, Cervispi'na, Buckthorn, Purging thorn*, (F.) *Nerprun purgatif*. Family, Rhamnoideæ. *Sex. Syst.* Pentandria Monogynia. The berries — *Rhamni Baccæ* — have a faint and disagreeable odour; and bitterish, nauseous taste. They are cathartic, and are apt to excite griping, which must be obviated by the use of diluents.
RHAMNUS ALATER'NUS, *R. Hispan'icus, Alaternus latifo'lius, Common alaternus*, (F.) *Alaterne*. The leaves have been used as detergents and astringents, in the form of gargle especially.
RHAMNUS FRAN'GULA. The *Black Alder, Frangula Alnus, Alnus Nigra,* (F.) *Aune noir, Bourdane, Bourgène*. All the parts of this tree, as well as of the common alder, are astringent and bitter. The bark is most so. The inner yellow bark of the trunk or root acts as a cathartic. It has also been employed as an anthelmintic.
RHAMNUS HISPANICUS, R. alaternus—r. Jujuba, see Jujube—r. Lotus, see Jujube—r. Ziziphus, see Jujube.
RHANTER, Canthus, (greater.)
RHAPHANEDON, Raphanedon.
RHAPHANIA, Raphania.
RHAPHANIS, Raphanus hortensis.
RHAPHANUS, Raphanus hortensis.
RHAPHE, Raphe, Suture.
RHAPHOSYMPH'YSIS; from ραφη, 'suture' and συμφυσις, 'union.' Union by suture,—as of the bones of the cranium.
RHAPHYS, Raphanus hortensis.
RHAPONTICUM, Rheum Rhaponticum—r. Vulgare, Centaurea centaurium.
RHAPONTIQUE, Rheum rhaponticum.
RHAPS, Raphanus hortensis.
RHAPYS, Raphanus hortensis.
RHATANIA, Krameria ratanhia.
RHAX, see Vitis vinifera.
RHEGE, Cramp, Contusion, Laceration.
RHEGMA, Cramp, Contusion, Laceration. Rhexis — r. Ligamentare, Apospasma.
RHEGMUS, Cramp, Contusion, Laceration.
RHEMBASMUS, Somnambulism.
RHEMBÈ, *Rhembus;* from ρεμβω, 'to wander about.' Irregularity in the return of febrile paroxysms.
RHEMBUS, Rhembe.
RHENCHUS, Rattle, Snoring.
RHEXXIS, Rattle, Snoring.

RHEON, Rheum.
RHETINE, Resin.
RHETINOCERON, Resinatum.
RHETINOTON, Resinatum.
RHEUM, (pronounced *room*,) *Rheu'ma*, (F.) *Rhume;* from ρεω, 'to flow.' Any thin watery discharge from the mucous membranes or skin; as the thin discharge from the air passages arising from cold.

RHEUM, SALT. A popular name in the United States, like 'tetter,' for various cutaneous affections of the eczematous and herpetic forms more especially. It is at times applied to a kind of chronic psoriasis; and likewise to cutaneous affections in those who immerse the hands in metallic or acid solutions. Webster defines it "a vague and indefinite popular name, applied to almost all the non-febrile cutaneous eruptions which are common among adults, except ringworm and itch."

RHE'UM, *Rhabor'barum, Rheon, Rha, Rhœum, Lap'athum orienta'lē, L. Chinen'sē, Rhabar'barum ve'rum, R. Tartar'icum, R. Siber'icum, R. Tur'-cicum, Rhubarb*, (F.) *Rhabarbe*. Family, Polygoneæ. *Sex. Syst.* Enneandria Trigynia. The root—*Rheüm*—is the part used in medicine. Its odour is aromatic, peculiar, and rather nauseous; taste, somewhat aromatic, subacrid, bittorish, and astringent. It colours the saliva and the urine yellow. It is easily pulverized, and forms a powder of a bright buff-yellow colour. Both water and spirit extract its virtues. Rhubarb root is purgative, stomachic and astringent. (?) It is chiefly used for the properties first mentioned. Externally, the powder is sometimes sprinkled over ulcers, to assist their granulation. Dose, ℈j to ʒss of the powder. In a smaller dose, it is stomachic.

Numerous species of Rheum, *Rh. palmatum, Rh. undulatum,* and *Rh. compactum,* have purgative roots.

The rhubarbs most used in the United States are the *Chinese* or *India Rhubarb — Rheum Sinen'sē* vel *In'dicum;* the *Russian, Turkey,* or *Bucharian Rhubarb—Rheum Rus'sicum* vel *Tur'cicum;* and *European Rhubarb*.

RHEUM COMPACTUM, Rheum — r. Indicum, see Rheum—r. Palmatum, Rheum.

RHEUM RHAPON'TICUM, *Rhapon'tic Rhubarb; Rhapon'ticum, Rhabar'barum Dioscor'idis, R. Antiquo'rum*, (F.) *Rhapontique, Rhapontic.* The root of this seems to have been the rhubarb of the ancients. It is more astringent than that of the rheum palmatum, and less purgative; for the latter purpose, two or three drachms being required for a dose. *French, Rhapontic,* or *Krimea Rhubarb,* is obtained from this species, as well as from *Rh. undulatum,* and *Rh. compactum.*

RHEUM RUSSICUM, see Rheum—r. Sinense, see Rheum—r. Turcicum, see Rheum—r. Undulatum, see Rheum.

RHEUMA, Catarrh, Diarrhœa, Rheum, Rheumatism. Also, inflammation of a fibrous tissue, as in rheumatism and gout.—Fuchs.

RHEUMA CATARRHALE, Bronchitis, (chronic) — r. Epidemicum, Bronchitis, chronic, Catarrh, epidemic — r. Pectoris, Catarrh — r. Uteri, Leucorrhœa.

RHEUMAPYRA, Rheumatism, acute.
RHEUMARTHRITIS, see Rheumatism, acute.
RHEUMARTHROSIS, see Rheumatism, acute.
RHEUMATALGIA, Rheumatism, chronic—r. Arthritica, see Rheumatism, acute.

RHEUMAT'IC, *Rheumat'icus, Rheumatis'mal,* (F.) *Rhumatismale, Rhumatique.* Belonging to rheumatism; as rheumatic fever. Also, applied to one affected with rheumatism; (F.) *Rhumatisant.*

RHEUMAT'IC DIATH'ESIS, *Diath'esis rheumat'ica.* The special condition of the body that gives occasion to rheumatism. It may exist without presenting the usual phenomena in the joints; whilst the heart may be seriously affected.

RHEU'MATISM, *Catarrhœ'a;* from ρευμα, 'a defluxion, catarrh.' *Dolor Rheumat'icus et arthrit'icus,* (Hoffman,) *Rheumato'sis, Myoso'tis, Rheuma, Myodyn'ia,* (F.) *Rhumatisme.* A kind of shifting phlegmasia, sometimes seated in the muscles, sometimes in the parts surrounding the joints; and at others, within them. Hence the names *Muscular, Articular,* and *Synovial,* which have been applied to it. The disease may be *acute,* or *chronic.*

RHEUMATISM OF THE ABDOMEN, Cœliorrheuma.
RHEUMATISM, ACUTE, *Rheumatis'mus acu'tus, Rh. articulo'rum acu'tus, Rh. universa'lis febri'lis, Arthro'sia acuta, Rheumatismus, Rh. inflammato'rius* seu *hyperethen'icus, Rheumat'ic Fever, Rheumatop'yra, Rheumap'yra, Febris rheumat'ica inflammato'ria, Syn'ocha rheumat'ica, Myoso'tis, Myi'tis, Cauma rheumatis'mus, Arthri'tis rheumatismus, Arthro-rheumatis'mus, Synovi'tis rheumatisma'lis, Hæmo-arthri'tis,* (F.) *Rhumatisme aigu*, *Fièvre rhumatismale,* usually comes on with the ordinary symptoms of fever; soon after which, or simultaneously, or even before the appearance of febrile signs, excruciating pains are felt in different parts of the body, particularly in the larger joints, which are more or less red and swollen; the pain shifting from one to the other, at times with great rapidity. The disease rarely terminates in less than six weeks, during the greater part of which period the febrile symptoms remain severe; and what is peculiar to the disease, the skin may be covered daily with a profuse perspiration, although it feels extremely hot, and the pulse appears in no way modified by it. It is one of the essential symptoms of the affection, and consequently affords no relief. The only danger to be apprehended from acute rheumatism, notwithstanding the apparent severity of the symptoms, is the translation or extension of the disease (*metastat'ic rheu'matism*) to some internal part, especially to the heart. This tendency must always be borne in mind. *Acute rheumatism* seldom terminates in *chronic;* they who are liable to the former are rarely so to the latter, and conversely. The disease will generally run its course in spite of treatment. The usual antiphlogistic plan had better be pursued during the first days of the disease. Blood-letting may be employed, if the vigour of the patient and of the disease seem to require it; but, although the blood is generally buffy, bleeding does not usually seem to afford much relief. The bowels must be kept open; effervescent draughts be administered, and opium be given in full doses to allay pain. This is, generally, all that is necessary during the first week; after which, advantage will usually be obtained from the exhibition of the sulphate of quinia with sulphuric acid. It does not augment the excitement, and will be found proper in almost all cases. Rheumatic inflammation is very different from other varieties, and this may account for the anomaly. After a few weeks, the disease usually goes off, but leaves the patient very liable to a recurrence on slight exposures or errors of diet: at times, acute rheumatism of the joints puts on the appearance of gout, and seems to be a complication of the two affections. It is then called *Gouty or Arthrit'ic rheumatism* or *Rheumatic gout, Rheumatal'gia arthrit'ica, Rheumarthro'sis, Rheum ar.thri'tis, Arthri'tis rheumat'ica* seu *juveni'lis.*

RHEUMATISM OF THE ARM, Brachiorrheuma—r. Arthritic, see Rheumatism, acute — r. of the

Bladder, Cystorrheuma—r. of the Bowels, Enterorrheuma.

RHEUMATISM, CAP'SULAR, *Rheumatis'mus capsula'ris.* Rheumatism seated in the lining membrane of the joints and bursæ of the tendons. The parts most liable to its attacks are the feet and hands, where it is generally easily recognised by the enlargement of the joints; but the peculiar characters of the disease are, perhaps, most strikingly seen when it attacks the knee.

RHEUMATISM OF THE CHEST, Pleurodynia.

RHEUMATISM, CHRONIC, *Arthro'sia chron'ica, Rheumatismus chronicus seu nonfebri'lis, R. vulga'ris seu invetera'tus seu habitua'lis seu frig''idus, Rheumatal'gia, Rheumatodyn'ia, Arthrodyn'ia, Arthritis arthrodynia,* (F.) *Rhumatisme chronique, Rhumatalgie,* is attended with pains in the hips, shoulders, knees, and other large joints. These are, sometimes, confined to one joint; at others, shift from one to another, without occasioning inflammation, or fever. In this manner, the complaint often continues for a great length of time, and then goes off. There is no danger attendant upon it; but the patient may become lame, and is always liable to painful recurrences. Neither variety generally terminates in suppuration; but effusion of coagulable lymph is apt to occur, so as to occasion permanent thickening of the parts. The great preventive of chronic rheumatism, and one of the most valuable curative agents, is flannel, worn next the skin. The whole class of rubefacients may, also, be used with advantage. The warm bath, especially the natural warm bath, the temperature of which does not vary, is perhaps the most successful remedy of all.

RHEUMATISM OF THE EXTREMITIES, Acrorrheuma—r. of the Face, Prosoporrheuma—r. Gouty, see Rheumatism, acute—r. of the Heart, Cardiorrheuma—r. Lead, see Lead rheumatism—r. of the Leg, Scelorrheuma—r. of a Limb, Merorrheuma—r. Local, Merorrheuma—r. of the Loins, Lumbago—r. Metastatic, see Rh. acute—r. of the Neck, Torticollis—r. Partial, Merorrheuma.

RHEUMATISM, PREÆBDOM'INAL, (F.) *Rhumatisme pré-abdominal.* Rheumatism of the muscles of the anterior and lateral portions of the abdomen; supposed by MM. Génest and Requin to be the same as the *nervous affection of the peritoneum* of Gooch.

RHEUMATISM OF THE SKIN, see Dermalgia—r. Topical, Merorrheuma—r. of the Uterus, Metrorrheuma.

RHEUMATISM, VISCERAL. Rheumatism affecting the muscular or fibrous tissues of the viscera.

RHEUMATISM WEED, Pyrola maculata, P. umbellata.

RHEUMATISMAL, Rheumatic.

RHEUMATISMUS, Abdominis, Cœliorrheuma—r. Acutus, Rheumatism, acute—r. Articulorum acutus, Rheumatism, acute—r. Brachii, Brachiorrheuma—r. Cancrosus, Neuralgia faciei—r. Cervicis, Torticollis—r. Colli, Torticollis—r. Cordis, Cardiorrheuma—r. Cruris, Scelorrheuma—r. Dorsalis, Lumbago—r. Extremitatum, Acrorrheuma—r. Faciei, Prosoporrheuma—r. Febrilis, Dengue—r. Inflammatorius seu hypersthenicus, Rheumatismus acutus—r. Intestinorum, Enterorrheuma—r. Intestinorum cum ulcere, Dysentery—r. Larvatus, Neuralgia faciei—r. Localis, Merorrheuma—r. Membrorum singulorum, Merorrheuma—r. Non febrilis, Rheumatism, acute--r. Partialis, Merorrheuma—r. Pectoris, Pleurodynia—r. Phlegmonodes, Myositis—r. Spurius nervosus, Neuralgia—r. Universalis febrilis. Rheumatism, acute—r. Uteri, Metrorrheuma—r. Vesicæ urinariæ, Cystorrheuma

r. Vulgaris seu inveteratus seu habitualis seu frigidus, Rheumatism, chronic.

RHEUMATODYNIA, Rheumatism, chronic.

RHEUMATOPHTHAL'MIA, *Rheumophthalmia;* from ρευμα, 'rheumatism,' and οφθαλμια, 'inflammation of the eyes.' Rheumatic ophthalmia.

RHEUMATOPYRA, Rheumatism, acute.

RHEUMATOSIS, Rheumatism.

RHEUMOPHTHALMIA, Rheumatophthalmia, Sclerotitis.

RHEXIS, *Rhegma, Dirup'tio, Rup'tio, Ruptu'ra, Rupture.* Rupture of a vessel or organ. Spontaneous opening of an abscess.

RHEXIS OC'ULI. Bursting of the eye from any cause; spontaneous or excited.

RHICNO'SIS, from ρικνοομαι, 'to become wrinkled;' *Cutis corruga'tio.* Wrinkling of the skin from extenuation of the body; opposed to *rarum,* or distension from repletion.

RHIGOS, Rigor.

RHIN, Nasus.

RHINAL'GIA, *Rhinodyn'ia,* from ριν, 'the nose,' and αγλος, 'pain.' Pain in the nose.

RHINAL'GIA AB INTRU'SIS. Pain in the nose from foreign bodies.

RHINAL'GIA VERMINO'SA. Pain in the nose from worms.

RHINAN'CHONE, *Rhinan'gia, Rhinostegnosis;* from ςιν, 'the nose,' and αγχειν, 'narrowness.' Contraction of the nose. Snuffles.

RHINANGIA, Rhinanchone, Snuffles.

RHINCHOS, Rostrum.

RHINENCEPHALIA, Cyclopia.

RHINEN'CHYSIS, *Rhinenchys'ia,* from ριν, 'the nose,' εν, 'in,' and χυω, 'I pour.' An infusion or injection, made into the nostrils, with a syringe called *Rhinen'chites.*

RHINES, Nares.

RHINI'TIS, *Nasi'tis,* from ριν, ρινος, 'the nose,' and *itis,* denoting inflammation. Inflammation of the nose. Coryza.

RHINITIS ULCEROSA, Ozæna.

RHINOBLENNORRHŒA, Rhinorrhœa.

RHINOC'ACÈ, *Cory'za scarlatino'sa;* from ριν, 'the nose,' and κακος, 'evil.' The offensive discharge from the nose, and other symptoms indicating a morbid condition of the Schneiderian membrane that accompany the worst forms of scarlatina.

RHINOCATARRHUS, Coryza.

RHINOCNES'MUS, from ριν, 'the nose,' and κνησμος, 'itching.' Itching of the nose.

RHINODYNIA, Rhinalgia.

RHINOPHO'NIA, from ριν, 'the nose,' and φωνη, 'the voice.' A nasal voice, called, also, *Dyspho'nia immodula'ta nasa'lis, Parapho'nia nasalis, Paraphonia res'onans, Psellis'mus na'tas, Mycteropho'nia, Na'sitas, Vox nasa'lis. Parala'lia nasa'lis.* Speaking through the nose.

RHINOPLAS'TIC, *Rhinoplas'tica* (arts). from ριν, 'the nose,' and πλασσω, 'I form.' An epithet applied to the operation for forming a new nose. The *Taliacotian operation,* so called because described by Tagliacozzi. It consists in bringing down a portion of flesh from the forehead, and causing it to adhere to the anterior part of the remains of the nose.

RHINOP'TIA, from ριν, 'the nose,' and οροµαι, 'I see.' The act of seeing over the nose. Squinting over the nose.

RHINORRHAGIA, Epistaxis.

RHINOR'RHAPHY, *Rhinorrhaph'ia,* from ριν, 'nose,' and ραφη, 'a suture.' An operation for the removal of epicanthis, which consists in pinching up a longitudinal fold of the skin, including this fold in two elliptical incisions, removving it, and bringing together the edges of the wound by harelip suture.

RHINORRHŒ'A, *Rhinoblennorrhœ'a*, from ριν, ρινος, 'the nose,' and ρεω, 'I flow.' A discharge of limpid mucus from the nose without any inflammatory symptom. A gleet from the nose.

RHINO'SIS, from ρινος, 'a skin, leather,' or from ρικνος, 'rugous.' The state of looseness and excess of skin observed in phthisis. — Vogel.

RHINOSTEGNOSIS, Rhinanchone.
RHIPTASMOS, Jactation.
RHIPTOLUSIA, Affusion.
RHIS, Nasus.
RHIZA, Radix.
RHIZAGRA, Punch.

RHIZO'MA, *Rhizome*, from ριζα, 'a root.' The part of the root of a plant, which consists of wood or flesh, as in the carrot.

RHIZOPH'AGUS, from ριζα, 'a root,' and φαγω, 'I eat.' One who lives on roots.

RHIZOTOMIST, see Simples.
RHIZOTOMUS, Apothecary.
RHOA, Punica granatum.
RHODELÆ'ON, *Oleum rosa'rum*. Oil of roses, or oil impregnated with roses.

RHO'DIA, *Rhodi'ola ro'sea, Rosea, Rosewort*, (F.) *Rhodiole*. *Sex. Syst.* Diœcia Octandria. The root, *Roseroot*, when dry, has a very pleasant smell, and is slightly astringent. It is not used.

RHO'DINUS, *Rho'dius, Rosa'ceus, Ro'seus, Rosa'tus*. Rosy. Formed of, or containing, roses.
RHODIOLA ROSEA, Rhodia.
RHODIOLE, Rhodia.
RHODITES VINUM. Wine in which roses have been macerated.

RHO'DIUM LIGNUM, *Rhodium* or *Rosewood*. The wood or root of a tree supposed to be *Genis'ta Canarien'sis* of Linnæus. (F.) *Bois de rose, Bois de Chypre*. *Family*, Leguminosæ. *Sex. Syst.* Diadelphia Decandria. The essential oil is a perfume, and possesses cordial and tonic virtues. Its smell is attractive to fish, rats, &c.

RHODIUS, Rhodinus.
RHODODAPHNIS, Nerium oleander.

RHODODEN'DRON CHRYSAN'THEMUM, *R. chrysan'thum seu au'reum seu officina'lē*, the *Olean'der, Rose-bay, Yellow rhododendrum, Mountain Laurel*, (F.) *Rosage, R. chrysanthe*. *Nat. Ord.* Ericaceæ. *Sex. Syst.* Decandria Monogynia. This plant has been recommended in rheumatism, gout, and syphilis. In an overdose, it produces acro-narcotic symptoms.

RHODODEN'DRON MAX'IMUM, *Great Laurel, American Rose-bay*. An indigenous shrub, *Order*, Ericaceæ, which flowers in July. It is stimulant and astringent, and has been used by the Indians in gout and rheumatism.

RHODOME'LA PALMA'TA, *Dulse, Sac'charine Fucus*. One of the Algæ, eaten in large quantities throughout the maritime countries of the north of Europe, and in the Grecian Archipelago.

RHODOMELI, Mel rosæ.
RHODON, Rosa centifolia.
RHODOSACCHARUM, Confectio rosæ gallicæ.
RHODOSTACTON, Mel rosæ.
RHODOSTAGMA, Aqua rosæ.
RHŒA, Punica granatum.
RHŒAS, Papaver rhœas.
RHOEBDESIS, Absorption.
RHŒUM, Rheum.
RHOGMOS, Rattle.

RHOI'TES, ροιτης, a wine impregnated with the pomegranate; from ροις, *Pomegranates*,— Dioscorides. A confection, made by boiling the juice of the pomegranate in honey. — Paulus of Ægina.

RHOMBOÏDEUS, from ρομβος, 'a rhombus,' whose sides are equal, with two obtuse and two acute angles. *Rhomboïdeus major* and *minor, Rhomboi'des, Cervici-dorso-scapulaire*. A muscle situate at the posterior inferior part of the neck, and at the posterior part of the back. It has a rhomboidal shape, and is attached, by its inner edge, to the posterior cervical ligament, and to the spinous processes of the last cervical vertebra, and of the first four or five dorsal. By its outer edge, it is attached to the spinal or posterior edge of the scapula. It is divided into two fasciculi, constituting the *Rhomboideus major* and *minor*, the latter being situate higher than the other. This muscle draws the scapula backwards and upwards, and impresses upon it a rotatory motion, which brings its inferior angle nearer to the spine; and, consequently, depresses the anterior angle and the shoulder.

RHOMBOS, ρομβος. A bandage mentioned by Galen, so called on account of its rhomboidal shape.

RHONCHAL, *Roncha'lis*, from *ronchus*, 'rattle.' Relating or appertaining to rhonchus;—as '*rhonchal* fluctuation,' the fremitus that occurs through the influence of respiration as an attendant on cavernous rhonchi. — Walshe.

RHONCHUS, Rattle, Snoring, Stertor—r. Cavernous, see Gurgling —r. Cavernulous, see Gurgling—r. Crepitans, *Râle crépitant*—r. Crepitans Redux, see Crepitant — r. Mucous, see *Râle muqueux*—r. Sibilans, see *Râle crépitant*—r. Sibilus, *Râle sibilant*— r. Sonorus, *Râle sonore*—r. Subcrepitant, see *Râle muqueux*.

RHOPALISMUS, Priapismus.
RHOPALOSIS, Plica, Pupil, Uvea.
RHOPE, Congestion.
RHOTACISMUS, Rotacism.

RHUBARB, Rheum—r. Chinese, see Rheum — r. French, Rheum Rhaponticum — r. India, see Rheum — r. Krimea, Rheum Rhaponticum —r. Monk's, Rumex Alpinus, Rumex patientia—r. Poor man's, Thalictron—r. Rhapontic, Rheum Rhaponticum—r. Russia, see Rheum—r. Turkey, see Rheum—r. Wild, Convolvulus panduratus.

RHUBARBE FAUSSE, Thalictron — r. *des Pauvres*, Thalictron.
RHUE, Ruta.
RHUMATALGIE, Rheumatism, chronic.
RHUMATIQUE, Rheumatic.
RHUMATISANT, Rheumatic.
RHUMATISMALE, Rheumatic.
RHUMATISME, Rheumatism — r. *Aigu*, Rheumatism, acute—r. *Chronique*, Rheumatism, chronic — r. *Préabdominale*, Rheumatism, præabdominal — r. *de l' Utérus*, Metrorrheuma.
RHUME, Rheum — r. *de Cerveau*, Coryza —r. *de Poitrine*, Catarrh.

RHUS CORIA'RIA, *Sumach, Shumach, Rhus Glabrum, Adu'rion, Elm-leaved Sumach*, (F.) *Sumac des Corroyeurs*. *Family*, Terebinthaceæ. *Sex. Syst.* Pentandria Monogynia. This is the only species of the genus rhus that is innocent. Both the leaves and berries have been used as astringents and tonics.

RHUS GLABRUM, Rh. coriaria.

RHUS RADI'CANS, *Rhus vernix, Poison vine (America)*. This plant is poisonous (see Poisons, Table of), and is extremely acrid, when applied to the skin, producing erysipelas and vesications, and has been used, like the next variety, in paralysis and other nervous affections.

RHUS SYLVESTRIS, Myrica gale.

RHUS TOXICODEN'DRON, *Toxicoden'dron, Poison Oak (America)*, (F.) *Sumac vénéneux*. This plant has been used in paralytic affections and cutaneeous eruptions. It is poisonous, like the last. Dose, gr. ss to gr. iv.

RHUS VERNIX, Rh. radicans.
RHYPARIA, Rupia, Sordes primarum viarum.
RHYPOS, Sordes.
RHYPTICA, Detergents.
RHYPTICUS, Abstergent.
RHYSIS, Flux.
RHYSMUS, Rhythm.
RHYSSEMA, Wrinkle.
RHYTHM, *Rhythmus, Rhysmus*, 'measured movement.' The order or proportion, as regards time, which reigns between the different movements of an organ — as of the heart; — or of the organism in health and disease. Thus, rhythm is applied to the diurnal variations of the pulse; and to the paroxysmal movements of an intermittent.

RHYTHMICAL, Periodical.
RHYTHMICAL CONTRACTIONS OF MUSCLES, are those that succeed one another after regular intervals.
RHYTHMUS, Rhythm.
RHYTIDOSIS, Rutidosis.
RIB, Costa—r. False, see Costa—r. Floating, see Costa — r. Sternal, see Costa — r. True, see Costa.
RIBES NIGRUM, *R. ol'idum, Grossula'ria nigra, Cassis*. The *Black currant*, (F.) *Groseillier noir. Sex. Syst.* Pentandria Monogynia. The berries have been recommended in sore-throat, as diuretics. The leaves have been advised for the same purpose. They are chiefly used as preserves.
RIBES OLIDUM, R. nigrum — r. Officinale, R. rubrum.
RIBES RUBRUM, *R. officina'lē* seu *vulga'rē, Grossula'ria non spino'sa* seu *rubra*, the *Red currant*, (F.) *Groseillier rouge;* of which the *White* is only a variety. It is cultivated, and affords an agreeable fruit. It possesses the qualities of the subacid fruits in general, and makes an excellent preserve.
RIBES VULGARE, R. rubrum.
RIBS, NECK OF THE, Collum costarum — r. Short, see Costa.
RICE, Oryza—r. Disease, Cholera—r. Ground, see Oryza—r. Jelly, see Oryza.
RICE WATER, see Oryza. The evacuations of cholera have been termed — from their resemblance to rice-water — '*rice-water* discharges;' and in India, '*congee* discharges;' — *congee* in Hindoostanee meaning 'rice-water.'
RICE, WILD, Zizania aquatica.
RICHARDSONIA, see Ipecacuanha.
RICHLEAF, Collinsonia Canadensis.
RICHWEED, Actæa racemosa, Ambrosia trifida, Collinsonia Canadensis, Pilea pumila.
RICIN, Ricinus communis.
RICINOIDES, Jatropha curcas.
RIC"INUS COMMU'NIS. The *Castor oil plant, Catapu'tia major, Ricinus vulga'ris* seu *vir'idis, Palma Christi, Faba purga'trix, Cerua, Kerua, Cici*, (F.) *Ricin, Fève purgatif. Family*, Euphorbiaceæ. *Sex. Syst.* Monœcia Monadelphia. Castor-oil seeds, whence the oil is obtained, are inodorous; taste acrid and slightly sweetish. One or two seeds—*Sem'ina Catapu'tiæ majoris* seu *Ric"ini vulga'ris* — will act as a cathartic; but the oil is alone used. It is obtained by bruising the castor-seeds, previously decorticated, and then expressing the oil without the application of heat. Recently-drawn castor oil, *Oleum de kerva, O. kervi'num, Alker'va, Oleum Ric"ini, O. Cic"inum, O. Palmæ liq'uidum, O. de Palmâ Christi,* (F.) *Huile de Ricin,* is inodorous and nearly insipid. It is cathartic, operating speedily, and may be used in all cases where powerfully stimulating purgatives would be injurious. Dose, f℥j to f℥iss. Hufeland recommends that a drop of croton oil shall be added to an ounce of the oil of poppy, and that the mixture shall be called *O'leum Ric"ini Officina'lē*.

At the Cape of Good Hope the oil is obtained from *Ricinus liv'idus*.

A variety of Ricinus at Cape Verd is employed by the inhabitants to increase the secretion of milk. It is applied in the form of poultice, made with the green leaves, to the mammæ, or of a strong decoction, with which the mammæ and the external parts of generation are washed.

RICINUS LIVIDUS, see Ricinus communis—r. Major, Jatropha curcas—r. Minor, Jatropha manihot—r. Viride, R. communis—r. Vulgaris, R. communis.
RICKETS, Rachitis.
RICKETY, Rachiticus.
RICTUS LUPINUS, see Harelip.
RIDE, Wrinkle.
RIDÉ, Wrinkled.
RIDING (of Bones). *Ossĕum superposit"io,* (F.) *Chevauchement.* Displacement of the fragments of a bone, chiefly produced by the contraction of muscles, which occasions shortening of the limb; the fractured extremities *riding over* each other, instead of being end to end.
RIGIDITAS, Rigidity.
RIGIDITAS ARTICULO'RUM, *Ancylo'sis spu'ria.* Stiffness of the joints. False ancylosis.
RIGIDITY, *Rigid'itas*, from *rigere*, 'to stiffen.' Great stiffness of fibre, or want of suppleness. The stiffness of the dead body, (F.) *Roideur cadavérique*, is one of the most certain signs of the cessation of life.
RI'GOR, *Rhigos, Algor, Coldness, Chris"is,* (F.) *Frisson.* Same etymon. Sensation of cold, with involuntary shivering of the whole body:—a symptom of fever. A slighter degree, and at times full rigor, is occasionally termed a *chill, frigus ten'uē, perfrigera'tio*.
RIGOR ARTUUM, Contractura—r. Cadaverosus, Rigor mortis — r. Corporis mortui, Rigor mortis —r. Emortualis, Rigor mortis — r. Maxillæ inferioris, Trismus.
RIGOR MORTIS, *R. cor'poris mor'tui, R. cadavero'sus, R. emortua'lis, Necromarcis'ma*, (F.) *Roideur ou Raideur cadavérique.* 'Stiffness of death.' Death stiffening. The rigidity of limbs that occurs on dissolution.
RIGOR NERVORUM, Tetanus — r. Nervosus, Tetanus.
RIMA, *Schisma, Schiza*. A fissure, a cleft; as *Rima*, or *Ri'mula Glot'tidis* seu *Laryn'gis*, 'the opening of the glottis.' *Rima vulvæ, R. moyen, Intro'itus, Sinus vulvæ, Scapha, Scaphus* seu *Fossu'ra magna* seu *Scissu'ra vulvæ, Schiza*, 'the opening of the vulva.' See Vulva.
RIMA CANALIS ORBITARII, Suborbitar fissure—r. ad Infundibulum, Vulva cerebri—r. Laryngis, Rima glottidis—r. Magna, Vulva, see Rima—r. Transversa Magna Cerebri, Fissure, transversa of the brain.
RIMÆ, Rhagades.
RIMULA GLOTTIDIS, Rima glottidis—r. Laryngis, Rima glottidis.
RINÆUS, Compressor naris.
RINCHOS, Rostrum.
RING, Sax. hping, ping, Germ. Ring, Crisis, (F.) *Anneau*. A name given to natural, circular, or roundish apertures, with muscular or aponeurotic parietes, which serve for the passage of some vessel or canal: — as the *umbilical ring, inguinal ring,* &c.
RINGWORM, Herpes circinatus—r. of the

Scalp, Porrigo scutulata.—r. Ulcerative, Herpes exedens—r. Vesicular, Herpes præputii.

RIRE ou *RIS*, Risus—*r. Canin*, Canine laugh—*r. Moqueur*, Canine laugh—*r. Sardonien*, Canine laugh, Risus sardonicus—*r. Sardonique*, Canine laugh.

RISAGON, Cassumuniar.

RISIGALLUM, Orpiment.

RISING, see Regurgitation—r. of the Lights, Cynanche trachealis.

RISING or ELEVA'TION OF THE PULSE, *Pulsûs eleva'tio*. The pulse is said to rise, when it becomes more full and frequent, as occurs in the exacerbation of acute diseases.

RISO'RIUS NOVUS. Santorini gives this name to a portion of the platysma myoides, which passes from the cheek towards the commissure of the lips.

RISSIGALLUM, Orpiment.

RISUS, from *ridere*, *risum*, 'to laugh.' *Gelus*, *Laughing*, *Laughter*, *Laugh*, (F.) *Rire* ou *Ris*. An involuntary movement of the muscles of the face, and of the lips in particular, accompanied with a sonorous and interrupted respiration, commonly indicating mirth and satisfaction.

RISUS APIUM, Ranunculus sceleratus—r. Caninus, Canine laugh—r. Involuntarius, Canine laugh—r. Sardonicus, Canine laugh—r. Spasticus, Canine laugh.

RITA-CRISTINA. A celebrated double monster, born in Sardinia, in 1829. It lived to be nearly nine months old. Two distinct bodies were united at the pelvis. Below, the monster was single.

RIVER WEED, Conferva rivalis.

RIZ, Oryza.

ROAN TREE, Sorbus acuparia.

ROB, *Roob, Robub, Rohob, Rohab*, (F.) *Extrait des fruits*. This word, of Arabic extraction, means the juice of any fruit thickened to the consistence of honey by evaporation, before it has fermented. The juice of the grape, boiled to this consistence, was called *Sapa*, and, when not quite so thick, *Defru'tum*.

ROB CYNOSBATOS, Confectio rosæ caninæ—r. ex Moris, Diamorion—r. Nucum, Diacaryon.

ROBIN RUN-AWAY, Glechoma hederacea.

ROBIN'IA AMA'RA, *Family*, Leguminosæ. *Sex. Syst*. Diadelphia Decandria. The roots of the *Robinia amara* of Cochin China are bitter, and have been recommended, especially in that country, in diarrhœa and dyspepsia.

ROBINIA PSEUDO-ACA'CIA, *Pseudaca'cia odora'ta, False Aca'cia, Black Locust, Locust-tree*; native of America. The flowers are said to possess antispasmodic properties.

ROBORANS, Corroborant.

ROBORANTIA, Tonics.

ROBUB, Rob.

ROCCELLA, Lichen roccella—r. Tinctoria, Lichen roccella.

ROCHE'S EMBROCATION FOR HOOPING-COUGH. An empirical preparation, composed of *ol. oliv.* ℥xvj, *ol. succin.* ℥viij, *ol. caryoph.*, q. s. to scent it strongly.

ROCHER, see Temporal bone.

ROCHETTA ALEXANDRINA, Soda.

ROCKET, GARDEN, Brassica eruca—r. Roman, Brassica eruca.

ROCK ROSE, Helianthemum Canadense, H. Corymbosum.

ROCOU, Terra Orleana.

RODSCHIEDIA BURSA PASTORIS, Thlaspi bursa.

ROGNE, Psora.

ROHAB, Rob.

ROHENA BARK, Swietenia.

ROHOB, Rob.

ROHUN, see Strychnos nux vomica.

ROIDEUR CADAVÉRIQUE, Rigor mortis.

ROISDORFF, MINERAL WATERS OF. Alkaline waters in Germany, which contain carbonic acid and carbonate of soda.

ROLLER, Bandage, Fascia.

ROMARIN, Rosmarinus—*r. Sauvage*, Ledum sylvestre.

ROME, (CLIMATE OF.) The climate of Rome, as regards its physical qualities, is considered to be one of the best in Italy. It is peculiarly still; and, hence, has been esteemed favorable as a winter climate in pulmonary diseases, and for invalids generally, as it admits of their taking exercise in the open air at a lower temperature than they otherwise could do. In the early stages of consumption, Sir James Clark generally found the climate favourable.

ROMPEURE, Hernia.

RONCE, Rubus idæus—*r. Bleue*, Rubus cæsius—*r. de Montagne*, Rubus chamæmorus—*r. Noire*, Rubus fruticosus.

RONCHUS, Snoring, Stertor.

ROND, Round—*r. Grand*, Teres major—*r. Petit*, Teres minor.

RONFLEMENT, Snoring, Stertor, see Rattle —*r. de Diable, Bruit de Diable*.

ROOB, Rob.

ROOF OF THE MOUTH, Palate.

ROOT, Radix—r. Ague, Aletris farinosa—r. Bitter, Apocynum androsæmifolium—r. Canada, Asclepias tuberosa—r. Red, Celastrus—r. Rough, Liatris—r. of Scarcity, Beta hybrida—r. Squaw, Actæa racemosa—r. Sweet, Acorus calamus—r. Unicorn, Aletris farinosa—r. Yellow, Xanthoriza apiifolia—r. Yellow, Jeffersonia Bartoni.

ROPE BARK, Dirca palustris.

ROQUETTE, Brassica eruca, Soda.

RORELLA, Drosera rotundifolia.

RORIF'EROUS, *Ror'ifer*, (F.) *Rorifère*, from *ros*, 'dew,' and *ferro*, 'to carry.' An epithet given to vessels which pour exhaled fluids on the surface of organs.

RORIFEROUS DUCT, Thoracic duct.

ROS, Sperm—r. Calabrinus, Fraxinus ornus—r. Solis, Drosera rotundifolia.

ROSA, R. centifolia—r. Afzeliana, R. canina.

ROSA ALBA, *R. usitatis'sima, R. leucan'tha. The White Rose*, (F.) *Rosier blanc. Family*, Rosaceæ. *Sex. Syst*. Icosandria Polygynia. The flowers of this species possess similar but inferior qualities to the damask.

ROSA ARMATA, R. canina—r. Austriaca, R. Gallica—r. Calycina, R. canina.

ROSA CANI'NA, *R. sylves'tris seu sentico'sa seu Swartzia'na seu Afzelia'na seu arma'ta seu calyci'na seu rubra vulga'ris, Cynor'rhodon, Caniru'bus, Cani'nus Sentis, Cynocyt'isus, Cynospas'tum, Cynos'batos, Dog Rose, Wild Briar, Hip Tree*, (F.) *Rose du chien, Eglantier de chien, E. sauvage*. The fruit of this variety, called *Heps* or *Hips*, has a sourish taste, and is formed into a conserve. See Confectio cynosbati. It is seldom employed, except to give form to more active remedies; as to pills, boluses, linctuses, &c.

ROSA CENTIFO'LIA; *Hecatomphyl'la, Damask Rose, Rosa Damasce'na, R. Pal'lida*, (F.) *Rosier à cent feuilles, Rhodon, Rosa*. The petals of this rose have an extremely fragrant odour, and subacidulous taste. They are laxative; but are scarcely used for any purposes except for the distillation of rose water, *Oil of Roses, Oleum Rosæ*, and the formation of a syrup.

ROSA DAMASCENA, R. centifolia.

ROSA GAL'LICA, *R. Austriaca, Rosa rubra, Red Rose*, (F.) *Rosier de Provins*. The petals of this variety are astringent; and are used in infusion, conserve, &c.

ROSA LEUCANTHA, R. alba—r. Pallida, R. centifolia—r. Rubra, R. Gallica—r. Rubra vulgaris, R. canina—r. Saltans, Essera—r. Senticosa, R. canina—r. Swartziana, R. canina—r. Sylvestris, R. canina—r. Usatitissima, R. alba.
ROSACE, Roseola.
ROSACEUS, Rhodinus.
ROSAGE, Rhododendron chrysanthemum.
ROSAGO, Nerium oleander.
ROSALIA, Scarlatina.
ROSALIÆ, Scarlatina.
ROSATUS, Rhodinus.
ROSE, Erysipelas—r. Christmas, Helleborus niger—r. Corn, Papaver rhœas—r. Damask, Rosa centifolia—r. Dog, Rosa canina—r. Dog, conserve or confection of, Confectio rosæ caninæ—r. du chien, Rosa canina—r. Rash, Roseola—r. Red, Rosa Gallica—r. Rock, Helianthemum Corymbosum—r. Spots, Spots, red—r. White, Rosa alba.
ROSEA, Rhodia.
ROSEBALM, SCARLET, Monarda coccinea.
ROSEBAY, AMERICAN, Rhododendron maximum.
ROSE DROP, Gutta rosea.
ROSELLINA, Roseolæ.
ROSEMARY, Rosmarinus—r. Marsh, Statice limonium, and S. Caroliniana—r. Wild, Eriocephalus umbellulatus.
ROSENHEIM, MINERAL WATERS OF. Rosenheim is 34 miles S. E. from München, in Bavaria. The waters contain sulphuretted hydrogen, carbonic acid, carbonate of lime, chlorides of calcium and magnesium, carbonate of soda, and oxide of iron. They are used as tonics.
ROSE'OLA, *Exanthe'sis Roseola, Rose Rash,* (F.) *Roséole, Éruption anomale, Roeace, Fièvre rouge, Efflorescence érysipélateuse*. An efflorescence in blushing patches, gradually deepening to a rose-colour, mostly circular or oval; often alternately fading and reviving; sometimes, with a colourless nucleus; and chiefly on the cheeks, neck, or arms. It is frequently found, as a symptom, in dentition, dyspepsia, rheumatism, &c., and is of no consequence. See Roseola, Rubeola, and Scarlatina.
ROSEOLA ACNOSA, Gutta rosea.
ROSEOLA ÆSTI'VA. The affection which prevails in summer. The eruption is of a darker colour, and is attended with more itching.
ROSEOLA ANNULA'TA. Characterized by patches in the form of rose-coloured rays, with central areas of the colour of the skin.
ROSEOLA FICOSA, Sycosis—r. Variolosa, Roseolæ.
ROSE'OLÆ, *Roseola, Roselli'na, False measles, French measles,* (F.) *Roséole, Fausse rougéole*. This name is also given by some to an acute exanthem, midway between measles and scarlatina, and which belongs to neither one nor the other, as it affords no protection against either. It is, also, termed *Rubeolæ* by some. An eruption which often precedes that of small-pox is termed *Roseola Varioło'sa*.
ROSÉOLE, Roseola, Roseolæ.
ROSE PINK, Chironia angularis.
ROSES, MILK OF. A cosmetic wash, formed, according to one method, of *subcarbonate of potass*, gr. vj; *oil of almonds*, ℥j; *essence of bergamot*, ℨij; *aquæ rosæ*, ℨiij; *orange flower water*, ℨij. Mix.
ROSEUS, Rhodinus.
ROSEWOOD, Rhodium lignum.
ROSEWORT, Rhodia.
ROSIER BLANC, Rosa alba—r. *à Cent feuilles*, R. centifolia—r. *de Provins*, Rosa Gallica.
ROSIN, BLACK, Colophonia—r. Brown, Colophonia—r. Weed, Silphium terebinthaceum—r. White, see Pinus sylvestris—r. Yellow, see Pinus sylvestris.
ROSIO STOMACHI, Cardialgia—r. Ventriculi, Cardialgia.
ROSMARINUM, Rosmarinus.
ROSMARI'NUS, *R. officina'lis seu latifo'lius seu horten'sis, Alchachil, Libano'tis corona'ria, Dendrolib'anus, Rosemary,* (F.) *Romarin*. *Fam.* Labiatæ. *Sex. Syst.* Diandria Monogynia. The tops of this plant, *Rosmarinus*, (Ph. U. S.) *Herba Anthos*, have a fragrant, grateful smell; and an aromatic, warm, bitterish taste, which is dependent upon an essential oil, combined with camphor. Rosemary has been recommended in nervous headachs, in the form of infusion. It is now rarely used, except for its odour. The flower is called *Anthos, ανθος*. Its oil—*Oleum Rosmarini*—is officinal. From two to six or ten drops are given in nervous complaints, rubbed up with sugar.
ROSMARINUS HORTENSIS, Rosmarinus—r. Latifolius, Rosmarinus—r. Officinalis, Rosmarinus—r. Stæchadis facie, Teucrium creticum—r. Sylvestris, Ledum sylvestre.
ROSSALIA, Scarlatina—r. Squamosa, Scarlatina.
ROSSIG'NOL. A name given, in France, to an affection to which pressmen are subject. It is a sprain, followed by tumefaction of the radiocarpal joint.
ROSSOLIO, see Spirit.
ROSTRUM, *Rhinchos, Rinchos, Romphos,* 'a beak.' (F.) *Bec*. A name given to several old forceps, on account of their resemblance to the beaks of different birds. The principal were the *Rostrum corvi'num, anati'num, psittaci'num, vulturi'num, cyg'neum* vel *olori'num, gruʼinum, lacerti'num,* &c.
ROSTRUM EXTERNUM, Olecranon—r. Porcinum, Acromion—r. Posterius, Olecranon—r. Sphenoidale, Azyges processus.
ROSY BUSH, Spiræa tomentosa—r. Drop, Gutta rosea—r. Whelk, Gutta rosea.
ROT, Eructation.
ROT, Grinders', Asthma, grinders'.
ROT'ACISM, *Rotacism'us, Rhotacis'mus, Psellis'mus rhotacis'mus,* (F.) *Grasseyement*. A vicious pronunciation of the Greek, P, Rho, common in the northern parts of England; especially near Newcastle.
ROTACISMUS, *Grasseyement*.
ROTA'TOR, from *rota*, 'a wheel.' A name given to several muscles that turn the parts to which they are attached upon their axes;—such as, the oblique muscles of the eye, the pronators, supinators, &c.
ROTATOR, Trochanter.
ROTATO'RES DORSI. Eleven small muscles on each side of the dorsal vertebræ, which arise from the point or upper edge of each transverse process, and pass to the lower edge of the arch of the vertebra above, as far as the base of the transverse process. Their action is to rotate the individual vertebræ on each other.
ROTATORES FEMORIS, Obturatores—r. Oculi Oblique muscles of the eye.
ROTULA, Patella, Trochiscos—r. Genu, Patella.
ROTULAD, see Rotular aspect.
ROT'ULAR; from *rotula,* 'the patella.' Relating or appertaining to the patella.
ROT'ULAR ASPECT. An aspect towards the side on which the rotula is situated.—*Barclay*. *Rot'ulad* is used by the same writer, adverbially, to signify 'towards the rotular aspect.'
ROTULE, Patella.
ROTUNDUS, Round.
ROUCOU, Terra Orleana.

ROUEN, MINERAL WATERS OF. This water, known under the name, *Eau des fontaines de la Maréguerie*, is cold, and contains carbonate of iron, carbonic acid, carbonate of lime, chloride of calcium, &c. It is tonic.

ROUGE, Colcothar — *r. d'Angleterre*, Colcothar.

ROUGÉOLE, Rubeola — *r. Fausse*, Roseolæ.

ROUGEURS, Flush.

ROUGH ROOT, Liatris.

ROUILLÉ, Rubiginous.

ROUND, *Teres, Rotun'dus*, (F.) *Rond.* Anatomists have given this name to many organs whose fibres are collected in round fasciculi. See Teres.

ROUND FORAMEN, *Fora'men rotund'um.* A foramen of the sphenoid bone, a little behind the *foramen lacerum superius*, which gives passage to the second branch of the fifth pair of nerves, called *superior maxillary*.

ROUND HEART, Thaspium atropurpureum.

ROUND LIGAMENTS OF THE UTERUS, *Ligamen'ta rotund'a U'teri*, (F.) *Cordons sus-pubiens* (Ch.), *Cordons vasculaires, Ligaments ronds de l'utérus.* Two cords, which arise from the lateral and superior parts of the uterus, whence they proceed towards the abdominal rings, which they pass through, and terminate by vanishing in the areolar tissue of the groins, mons veneris, and labia majora. These cords are whitish, flattened, and narrower in the middle than at the extremities. According to Mr. Rainey, they are composed chiefly of the striped muscular fibre.

ROUTINE PRACTITIONER, Routinist.

ROUTINIST, pronounced *routeen'ist;* (F.) *Routinier;* from (F.) *routine;* 'a regular habit or practice, unvaried by circumstances.' One who practises in such an unvaried manner: — a *routine practitioner*.

RUBBER, INDIAN, Caoutchouc.

RUBBING SOUNDS, *Bruit de Frottement.*

RUBE'DO, *Rubor*, Redness; from *rubere*, 'to be red.' A diffused, but not spotted, redness on any part of the skin; like that which arises from blushing. Blushing.

RUBEFA'CIENT, *Erethis'ma, Erethis'ticum, Rubefa'ciens*, from *ruber*, 'red,' and *fa'cio*, 'I make.' (F.) *Rubéfiant.* That which produces redness. A medicine which causes redness of the skin. The action is called *Rubefaction*.

RUBÉFIANT, Rubefacient.

RUBE'OLA, *Rubeola vulga'ris*, from *rubere*, 'to be red.' *Ross'olæ, Exanthe'sis Rubeola, Vetera'na, Blac'ciæ, Bovil'læ, Morbil'li, Scarlati'na pustulo'sa, S. Milia'ris, Febris morbillo'sa, Typhus morbillosus, Phœnicis'mus, Ecphy'mata, Measles;* (F.) *Rougéole, Fièvre morbilleuse.* One of the major exanthemata; generally affecting individuals but once, and produced by specific contagion. The rash usually appears on the fourth, but sometimes on the third, fifth, or sixth day of a febrile disorder; and, after a continuance of four days, gradually declines with the fever. The disease commonly commences from ten to fourteen days after the contagion has been received. The eruption first shows itself in distinct, red, and nearly circular spots, somewhat less than the ordinary areolæ of flea-bites. As these increase in number, they coalesce; forming small patches of an irregular figure, but approaching nearest to that of semicircles or crescents. These patches are intermixed with single, circular dots and with interstices of the natural colour of the skin. On the face they are slightly raised, so as to give the sensation of inequality of surface to the finger passed over the cuticle. The disappearance of the eruption is followed by desquamation of the cuticle. Measles is not dangerous of itself; but it is liable to induce pneumonia in winter, and dysentery in summer, which are, at times, very fatal. These are apt to come on at the time of, or soon after, the disappearance of the eruption. When they supervene, they must be treated as idiopathic affections. It demands a general antiphlogistic treatment. Willan has pointed out a kind of RUBEOLA SPU'RIA, which he calls RUBEOLA *sine* CATAR'RHO. In this the rash runs its regular course, with little fever or catarrhal affection; affording no certain security against the common or regular disease. He also gives the name, RUBEOLA NIGRA or BLACK MEASLES, to an unusual appearance of the measles about the seventh or eighth day, when the rash becomes suddenly livid, with a mixture of yellow. It is devoid of inconvenience or danger; and is removed in a week or ten days by the mineral acids and tonics.

RUBEOLÆ, Roseolæ.

RU'BIA, *R. Tincto'rum seu peregri'na seu sylves'tris, Erythrod'anum, Rubia major, Radix rubra, Dyer's Madder, Madder*, (F.) *Garance.* Family, Rubiaceæ. *Sex. Syst.* Tetrandria Monogynia. The roots of this plant have a bitterish, somewhat austere, taste, and a slight, not agreeable, smell. They were formerly considered deobstruent, detergent, and diuretic.

RUBIG"INOUS, *Rubigino'sus*, from *rubigo*, 'rust.' (F.) *Rouillé.* Rusty. Having the colour of rust. An epithet given to the sputa in certain cases of pneumonia.

RUBINUS VERUS, Anthrax.

RUBOR, Rubedo.

RUBRI'CA FABRI'LIS. A red, heavy, earthy matter, formerly employed for making drying plasters; *Hard Ruddle, Red Chalk.*

RUBRICA SINOP'ICA. A heavy, compact, reddish earth: formerly used in diarrhœa.

RUBRIN, Hæmatin.

RUBUS AFFINIS, R. fruticosus.

RUBUS ARC'TICUS. The *Shrubby Strawberry, Baccæ Norland'icæ.* Family, Rosaceæ. *Sex. Syst.* Icosandria Polygynia. The fruit is recommended by Linnæus as possessing antiseptic, refrigerant, and antiscorbutic qualities.

RUBUS BATUS, R. Cæsius.

RUBUS CÆ'SIUS, *R. batus;* the *Dewberry plant*, (F.) *Ronce bleue.* The fruit resembles the blackberry in appearance and properties. The bark of the root of *R. Trivia'lis, American Dewberry*, is astringent.

RUBUS CHAMÆMO'RUS; the *Cloudberry Tree, Chamæmo'rus, C. Norwegica, Chamædrys, Cloudberries, Knot-berries*, (F.) *Ronce de Montagne.* The ripe fruit is sometimes prepared like a jam, and used in fevers, &c., to allay thirst. It has been much extolled as an antiscorbutic.

RUBUS FRAMBŒSIANUS, R. Idæus.

RUBUS FRUTICO'SUS, *R. affi'nis seu panicula'tus seu niger seu vulga'ris;* the *Common Bramble*, which affords *Blackberries*, (F.) *Ronce noire.* The berries are eaten as a summer fruit, of which they form a poor variety. The bark of the root of the *Rubus villo'sus, American Blackberry, High or standing blackberry, Hairy American Bramble*, is astringent, and has been used in the last stages of dysentery, and in cholera infantum.

RUBUS IDÆ'US, *R. framboesia'nus, Batos;* the *Raspberry*, (F.) *Framboise, Ronce.* The fruit of the best varieties is extremely agreeable; and is much used. It was, formerly, called *Batinos moron.*

RUBUS NIGER, R. fruticosus — *r.* Paniculatus, R. fruticosus.

RUBUS STRIGO'SUS, *Wild red raspberry*, of the United States. The leaves are often used as a mild astringent.

RUBUS TRIVIALIS, see Rubus cæsius — r. Villosus, see Rubus fruticosus — r. Vulgaris, R. fruticosus.

RUCTAMEN, Eructation.
RUCTATIO, Eructation.
'RUCTUATIO, Eructation.
RUCTUOSITAS, see Eructation.
RUCTUS, Eructation — r. Acidus, Oxyregmia — r. Nidorosus, Cnissoregmia.
RUDDLE, HARD, Rubrica fabrilis.
RUDOLPHIA FRONDOSA, Butea frondosa.
RUE, Ruta — r. Common, Ruta — r. *de Chèvre*, Galega officinalis — r. Goat's, Galega officinalis — r. Goat's, Virginia, Galega Virginiana — r. Meadow, Thalictron — r. *des Murailles*, Asplenium ruta muraria — r. *des Prés*, Thalictron — r. *Sauvage*, Ruta.

RUFT, Eructation.
RUGA, Wrinkle.
RUGINE, Raspatorium.
RUGISSEMENT, Rugitus.
RUGI'TUS, *Brycheth'mos*, from *rugire, rugitum*, 'to roar.' (F.) *Rugissement*. A Latin word, which ordinarily expresses the roaring of the lion: and which is used, by some medical writers, to designate a particular species of borborygmus compared to it.

RUGOSE, Wrinkled.
RUGOUS, Wrinkled.
RUM, *Tafia, Molas'ses Spirit.* A spirit distilled from sugar, or molasses. See Spirit.
RUMA, Mamma.
RUMEN, Hypogastrium.
RUMEX ACETO'SA, *R. tubero'sus* seu *interme'dius, Lap'athum pratense*, Common Sorrel, *Ox'alis Aceto'sa, Acetosa vulga'ris* seu *praten'sis, Anax'yris, A. arven'sis,* Sorrel, Sour dock, *Acetosa nostras,* (F.) *Oseille.* Family, Polygoneæ. *Sex. Syst.* Hexandria Trigynia. The leaves are sour, and are used in cookery, and also as a refrigerant.

RUMEX ACU'TUS; *Sharp-pointed Wild dock, Oxylap'athum, Lap'athum, L. sylves'trē* seu *acu'tum, Rumex, R. paludo'sus* seu *pusil'lus, Lap'athos,* (F.) *Patience sauvage*. The decoction of the root has long been used in cutaneous affections. It is, sometimes, employed for the cure of the itch.

RUMEX ÆTNENSIS, R. scutatus.
RUMEX ALPI'NUS, *Aceto'sa Alpi'na*. The systematic name of the plant that affords the *Monk's Rhubarb,* (F.) *Rhabarbe des Moines.* See Rumex patientia.

RUMEX AQUATICUS, Rumex hydrolapathum — r. Britannica, Rumex hydrolapathum — r. Confertus, R. patientia — r. Digynus, Oxyria reniformis — r. Glaucus, R. scutatus — r. Hastatus, R. scutatus — r. Hastifolius, R. scutatus.

RUMEX HYDROLAP'ATHUM, *Water-Dock, Hydrolapathum, Rumex aquat'icus, Herba Britan'nica, Rumex Britan'nica, Lap'athum aquat'icum,* (F.) *Parelle, Patience d'eau.* The leaves of this plant are subacid, and said to be laxative. The root has been used as a tonic, astringent, and antiscorbutic. It has also been employed externally in some cutaneous affections.

RUMEX INTERMEDIUS, R. acetosa.
RUMEX OBTUSIFO'LIUS, *Lap'athum sylvestrē, Blunt-leaved Dock.* The root of this, as well as of *R. crispus,* has similar virtues to that of the other species.

RUMEX OXYOTUS, R. scutatus — r. Paludosus, R. acutus.
RUMEX PATIEN'TIA, *R. confer'tus, Lap'athum horten'sē, Rhabar'barum monacho'rum, Hippolap'athum, Patien'tia, Garden Patience, Monk's Rhubarb,* (F.) *Patience.* This root, which is supposed to possess the virtues of rhubarb, but in an inferior degree, is, according to Linnæus, obtained from the *Rumex patientia;* according to Murpy, from the *Rumex alpi'nus.*

RUMEX PUSILLUS, R. acutus.
RUMEX SANGUIN'EUS. The root of the *bloody dock* has an austere and astringent taste; and has been employed in dysentery. It is called, also, *Lap'athum sanguin'eum,* (F.) *Oseille ou Patience Rouge, Sangdragon.*

RUMEX SCUTA'TUS, *R. glaucus* seu *hastifo'lius* seu *Ætnen'sis* seu *oxyotus* seu *hasta'tus,* French Sorrel, *Aceto'sa rotundifo'lia* seu *Roma'na* seu *Rotundifolia horten'sis* seu *scuta'ta, Lap'athum scuta'tum* seu *rotundifo'lia, Roman* or *Garden Sorrel, Green Sauce,* (F.) *Oseille boucher, Oseille ronde, Petite O.* Virtues the same as those of the common sorrel.

RUMEX TUBEROSUS, R. acetosa.
RUMINA'TION, *Rumina'tio,* from *rumen* or *rumeu,* 'the gullet.' *Merycis'mus*. A function peculiar to ruminating animals, by which they chew a second time the food they have swallowed. An analogous phenomenon is sometimes seen in man.

RUMP, *Croupion* — r. Bone, Coccyx.
RUNCINA, Raspatorium.
RUNCINULA, Raspatorium.
RUNNET, Rennet.
RUNNING, *Cursus,* (F.) *Course.* A succession of leaps, executed with rapidity, to transport the body quickly from one place to another.
RUNUNCULA, Raspatorium.
RUPES, Lips of the Vulva.
RU'PIA, *Ulcus aton'icum, Ecphly'sis Rhy'pia, Rhypa'ria,* from *ῥύπος,* 'filth.' An eruption of large flattish blebs, which contain a fluid — at first serous, afterwards puriform, and often bloody, which rapidly concretes into crusts, at the base of which are ulcers of variable depths.

It requires the use of tonics internally, and of stimulating ointments externally.

RUPTIBILITAS, Fragilitas.
RUPTIO, Rhexis.
RUPTORIUM, Cauterium — r. Commune, Potassa fusa.
RUPTURA, Ecrexis, Hernia, Laceration, Rhexis — r. Corneæ, Ceratorrhexis — r. Herniosa, Hernia — r. Ovarii, Oariorrhexis — r. Uteri, Uteri, rupture of the — r. Vaginæ, Colporrhexis.
RUPTURE, Hernia, Rhexis — r. *du Cœur,* Cardiorrhexis — r. of the Groin, Bubonocele — r. *de la Matrice,* Uterus, rupture of the — r. *War,* Herniaria glabra.

RUPTURED, see Hernia.
RUSCUS, *R. aculea'tus, Bruscus, Oxymyr'rhinē, Oxymyr'sinē, Myrtacan'tha, Catas'pois, Myacan'tha, Sco'pia re'gia, Wild Myrtle, Centromyrinē, Butcher's Broom,* (F.) *Petit houx, Fragon.* Family, Smilaceæ. *Sex. Syst.* Diœcia Monadelphia. The root has been recommended as an aperient and diuretic.

RUSCUS ACULEATUS, Ruscus.
RUSCUS HYPOGLOS'SUM; *Uvula'ria, Hypoglossum, Bislin'gua, Bonifa'cia, Laurus Alexandri'na angustifo'lia,* (F.) *Laurier Alexandrin.* Formerly used against relaxed uvula.
RUSH, SWEET, Acorus calamus, Juncus odoratus.
RUSMA, see Orpiment.
RUSPINI'S STYPTIC, see Styptic, Ruspini's.
RUSPI'NI'S TINCTURE FOR THE TEETH. An empirical preparation, composed of *Florentine orris* ℥viij, *cloves* ʒj, *rectified spirit* Oij, *ambergris* ℈j.

RUT, Heat.
RUTA, *Ruta graveolens* seu *horten'sis* seu *el'tera,* Common Rue, *Peg'anum, Besa'sa,* (F.) *Rue, Rhue, Rue sauvage.* Family, Rutaceæ. *Sex. Syst.* Decandria Monogynia. The plant has a

strong, ungrateful odour, and bitter pungent taste. It is acrid, so as to blister the skin. Its properties are reputed to be tonic, stimulant, antispasmodic, and emmenagogue. Dose, gr. xv to ℈ij.

Oleum Rutæ, distilled Oil of Rue, is antispasmodic; and, externally, rubefacient. Dose, gtt. ij to vj.

RUTA ALTERA, Ruta—r. Capraria, Galega officinalis—r. Graveolens, Ruta—r. Hortensis, Ruta—r. Muraria, Asplenium ruta muraria.

RUTABULUM, Penis.

RUTA'CEUM, from *Ruta*, 'rue.' Vinegar of rue.

RUTIDOMA, see Rutidosis.

RUTIDO'SIS, *Rytido'sis, Rhytido'sis*, from ρυτιδοω, 'I wrinkle.' The act of wrinkling; as *Rutido'ma* means a shrivelled or wrinkled body. A destruction or atrophy of the eye. Corrugation and subsidence of the cornea.

RUYSCHIA'NA TU'NICA, (F.) *Lame* ou *Membrane Ruyschienne*. According to Ruysch, and the greater part of his disciples, the choroid coat of the eye is formed of two laminæ. His son gave to the inner the name *Tunica Ruyschia'na* or *Membrana Ruyschia'na* seu *Ruysch'ii*.

Tu'nica Cellulo'sa Ruyschia'na is the areolar substance under the peritoneal covering of the stomach. It is not numbered among the coats of that organ.

RYE, Secale — r. Horned, Ergot — r. Spurred, Ergot.

RYTIDOSIS, Rutidosis.

RYTIS, Wrinkle.

S.

S. A. &c., see Abbreviation.

SABADILLA, Veratrum sabadilla, see Veratrina.

SABADILLIN, see Veratrina.

SABATILLA, Veratrum sabadilla.

SABBATIA, Chironia angularis—s. Angularis, Chironia angularis.

SABINA, Juniperus sabina.

SABINE, Juniperus sabina.

SABLÉ, Maculo'sus, 'sanded.' Having the appearance as if strewed with sand. The terms *sablé* and *piqueté* are sometimes applied to the brain, when a slice of it exhibits red points as if it had been strewed with red sand. Such is the case in cerebral hyperæmia.

SABOT DE VÉNUS JAUNE, Cypripedium luteum.

SABUCUS, Sambucus.

SAB'ULOUS, *Sabulo'sus, Areno'sus, Psammo'des*. The sandy deposit often seen in the urine.

SABULUM CONARII, see Pineal gland.

SABURA, Saburra.

SABUR'RA, *Sabu'ra, Sordes*. This word signifies, by derivation, coarse sand, or ballast. In its common acceptation, it means *foulness of the stomach*, as it is sometimes called;—vitiated matters supposed to be retained and accumulated in the stomach—the result of imperfect digestion—and which have been sometimes considered as a morbid product of the mucous secretion of that organ, or of the biliary secretion; at others, as a residuum from alimentary substances badly digested. The *Saburral state, Collu'vies gas'trica, Crudita'tes ventric'uli, Gastris'mus*, (F.) *Embarras gastrique, État saburral*, is an accumulation of saburræ, (F.) *Saburres gastriques*, in the stomach, which the Humourists considered to be the cause of a number of diseases.

SABURRA VERMINOSA, Helminthiasis.

SABURRATIO, Arenatio.

SABURRES GASTRIQUES, see Saburra.

SAC HERNIAIRE, Hernial sac.

SACCATUS, Encysted.

SACCHAR, Saccharum.

SACCHARINA, *Saccharolés*.

SACCHAROLÉS (F.), *Sacchari'na*, from *saccharum*, 'sugar.' A name given by MM. Henry and Guibourt to medicines which have sugar or honey for excipient, or for predominant principle. M. Béral so calls an exact mixture of pulverized sugar with other substances also in powder, but in less quantity.

SACCHAROM'ETER, (F.) *Saccharomètre, Pèsesirop*, from *saccharum*, 'sugar,' and μετρον, 'measure.' A hydrometer adapted for determining the density of syrups.

SACCHAROMYCES, Torula cerevisiæ.

SACCHARORRHŒA, Glycyrrhœa — s. Cutanea, Sudor dulcis.

SACCHARORRHŒ'A LAC'TEA, *Galactorrhœ'a sacchara'ta*. A secretion of unusually sweet milk.

SACCHARORRHŒA PULMONA'LIS, *Sputum dulcè* seu *sacchara'tum*. The copious expectoration of unusually sweet matter from the lungs.

SACCHARORRHŒA URINOSA, Diabetes mellitus.

SAC'CHARUM, Sacchar. From Arabic, or rather Sanscrit, *Sa-kar*, 'white earth;' *Suchar, Succhar, Sutter, Zuchar, Zu'caro, As'sakur, Tigala, Zac'charum, Zozar, Zu'charum, Zuc'carum, Zuchra, Mel arundina'ceum*, Sugar, (F.) *Sucre*. The produce of the juice of the *Sac'charum officina'rum* vel *officinalè* of Linnæus, *Cal'amus In'dicus, Cal'amus Sacchari'nus*, Sugar Cane, (F.) *Canne à Sucre, Cannamelle; Arun'do saccharif'era* of Sloane. *Family*, Gramineæ. *Sex. Syst.* Triandria Digynia) and also of the beet, maple, &c.

True Sugars are those with which alcoholic fermentation *may be* effected, by the addition of yeast and water. They are:—

Species.	Varieties.
1............	Hard sugar of the cane, maple, beet, chestnut, &c.
2............	Liquid sugar, sugar of malt, of the sweet potato, molasses, honey, &c.
3............	Hard sugar of the grape, ripe fruits, starch, diabetes, &c.
4............	Hard sugar of the mushroom.

Imperfect sugars are those in which alcoholic fermentation *cannot be* effected by means of yeast and water.

Species.	Varieties.
1............	Manna.
2............	Sugar of Milk.
3............	Sugar of jelly or glue.
4............	Liquorice.
5............	Picromel.

Sugar is prepared from the expressed juice of the sugar-cane, boiled with the addition of quicklime or common vegetable alkali. It is used, in pharmacy, for the preparation of syrups, conserves, lozenges, &c. It is very nutritious, and is employed as an aliment, and as a demulcent and antiseptic. Dissolved in small quantities in water, as in tea, it is apt to disagree with dyspeptics; an evil which does not always occur when the same substance is taken more largely.

SACCHARUM ACER'NUM, S. Canaden'sĕ, Maple Sugar, is often used as a demulcent.

SAC'CHARUM ALBUM, S. purifica'tum, Saccharum (Ph. U. S.), White Sugar, Refi'ned Sugar, Sal Indus, is the Loaf Sugar. Double-refined Sugar has been called Tabarset.

SACCHARUM CAN'DIDUM, S. candum seu cantum seu canthum, Al'phenic, Nabot, Sugar candy, (F.) Sucre Candi, is the crystallized juice of the cane.

SACCHARUM CANDUM, S. Candidum—s. Cantum, S. Candidum—s. Canthum, S. Candidum—s. Commune, Saccharum non-purificatum.

SACCHARUM HORDEA'TUM, Barley Sugar, Penides, Penid'ium, Sac'charum penid'ium, is a variety of sugar candy.

SACCHARUM LACTIS, Sugar of milk.

SACCHARUM NON-PURIFICA'TUM, Muscova'do, raw or brown or moist sugar, is the S. commu'nĕ, S. rubrum, Mel cannæ, or coarse sugar.

SACCHARUM OFFICINARUM, see Saccharum—s. Penidium, Hordeatum—s. Rosaceum, Confectio rosæ gallicæ—s. Saturni, Plumbi superacetas.

SACCHARURE, from saccharum, 'sugar.' A medicine resulting from the intimate union of sugar with the medicinal principles of alcohol or ethereal tinctures.—Béral.

SACCULATED, Encysted.

SACCULATUS, Encysted.

SACCULI ADIPOSI, Fatty vesicles—s. Chalicophori, see Lacunæ of Bone—s. Laryngei, Ventricles of the larynx.

SAC'CULI MEDICINA'LES. Bags containing medicinal substances.

SACCULI MEDULLARES, see Medullary membrane.

SAC'CULUS, diminutive of saccus, 'a little sac.' This name has been given to two sacs formed by the membranous vestibule, which open into each other, and contain the otolithes and otoconies: one of these is termed the sacculus vestib'uli, the other sacoulus. See Semicircular canals.

SACCULUS, Marsupion—s. Cephalicus, Cucupha—s. Chylifer seu rorifer, Receptaculum chyli —s. Cordis, Pericardium—s. Ellipticus, see Semicircular canals.

SAC'CULUS LARYN'GIS. A cæcal pouch, of variable size, formed by the mucous membrane in the ventricles of the larynx.—Hilton.

SACCULUS MEDICINALIS, Pulvinar medicatum — s. Sphericus, see Semicircular canals—s. Vestibuli, Semicircular canals.

SACCUS, Sac—s. Coli, Cæcum—s. Cordis, Pericardium—s. Herniosus, Hernial sac—s. Epiploicus, Epiploon—s. Intestini crassi, Cæcum— s. Lacrymalis, Lachrymal sac—s. Lacrumalis, Lachrymal sac—s. Lacteus, Receptaculum chyli —s. Mucosus, see Bursæ mucosæ—s. Pleuræ, Pleura—s. Venarum cavarum, Sinus dexter cordis —s. Venarum pulmonalium, Sinus pulmonalis.

SACER, Sacral—s. Ignis, Herpes zoster—s. Morbus, Epilepsy—s. Musculus, Transversalis dorsi.

SACERDOTIS PENIS, Arum maculatum.

SACHET (F.), Sac'culus, 'a bag.' A small bag containing perfumes to be placed among clothes to communicate to them an agreeable odour. The following is a formula for the powder they contain. Powdered cloves and powdered cassia, each one ounce, powdered orris root, an ounce and a half; powdered yellow sandal wood, one drachm; otto of roses, twenty-four drops; oil of lavender, oil of bergamot, each one drachm; musk, six grains. A scent-bag.

SACK. A wine used by our ancestors; Vinum. Probably Sherry.

SACK, Saccus, Secluso'rium; Sax. ɼæc. A bag or pouch.

SACK, HER'NIAL, Saccus hernio'sus, (F.) Sac herniaire. An envelope or pouch, formed by the serous membrane of the cavity, whence a viscus has escaped. We distinguish, in a hernial sac, its orifice or the opening by which it communicates with the great cavity lined by the serous membrane: its cervix or neck, (F.) Col'et, the narrow portion on the outside of the orifice, where strangulation sometimes occurs: the isthmus, (F.) Corps, which is the round prominent part; and the fundus or bottom,—the part opposite to the orifice.

SACK POSSET; from sack, 'the wing,' and posset. A posset made of sack, milk and other ingredients.

SACK, SEROUS. The shut cavity formed by any serous membrane, as by the pleura or peritoneum.

SACRAD, see Sacral.

SACRA FISTULA, Vertebral column.

SACRAL, Sacer, (F.) Sacré. That which belongs or relates to the sacrum. A name given to several parts.

SACRAL ARTERIES are distinguished into 1. The anterior or middle sacral. Median Artery of the Sacrum of Chaussier, which arises from the posterior part of the abdominal aorta, in front of the 4th lumbar vertebra. It descends, in a serpentine manner, upon the sacro-vertebral articulation, and on the anterior surface of the sacrum. It furnishes many lateral branches, which anastomose with the lateral sacral arteries, and enter the anterior sacral foramina, to be distributed to the membranes of the marrow, &c. 2. The lateral sacral arteries, which are two in number: one on each side. They arise from the hypogastric, from the ilio-lumbar, or from the gluteal; and descend before the anterior sacral foramina, anastomosing in an arched manner, towards the coccyx, with the middle sacral. They give off external and posterior branches, which enter the sacral foramina; and internal branches, which are distributed to the pyramidalis, sacrum, &c.

SACRAL ASPECT. An aspect towards the region where the sacrum is situated.—Barclay. Sacrad is used by the same writer adverbially to signify 'towards the sacral aspect.'

SACRAL EXTREMITIES. The lower limbs.

SACRAL GROOVES, (F.) Gouttières sacrées. Two longitudinal excavations, slightly marked, at the posterior surface of the sacrum; which appear to terminate the vertebral grooves or gutters.

SACRAL NERVES, (F.) Nerfs sacrés, are generally six in number. They arise from the termination of the spinal marrow. The first, united with the great cord which descends from the lumbar plexus, concurs with the three others in the formation of the sacral or sciatic plexus. The third and fourth, with branches of the great sympathetic, form the hypogastric plexus. The fifth and sixth (coccyge'al nerve) are distributed to the ischio-coccygeous muscle, and to the sphincter and levator ani.

SACRAL PLEXUS, Sciat'ic plexus,—the sacral portion of the crural plexus of Chaussier, constituted as just mentioned, is situate in front of the pyramidalis. It gives off, backwards, two branches, called the pudic, (F.) honteux, and the lesser sciatic. It terminates in the great sciatic nerve.

SACRÉ, Sacral.

SACROCOCCYGE'AL, Sacro-coccygeus. Relating to the sacrum and coccyx.

SACROCOCCYGE'AL ARTICULA'TION is that of

the lower extremity of the sacrum with the superior *facette* of the coccyx. It is closed by two ligaments;—an *anterior* and a *posterior sacro-coccygeal*.

SACROCOSTALIS, Sacro-lumbalis—*s. Fémoral*, Glutæus major.

SACROCOXAL'GIA, from *sacrum*, 'the os sacrum,' *coxa*, 'the hip,' and αλγος, 'pain;' a hybrid term. Some authors have called thus a rheumatic affection of the sacro-iliac symphysis.

SACROIL'IAC, *Sacro-ili'acus.* That which relates to the sacrum and ilium.

SACROÏLIAC ARTICULA'TION, SYM'PHYSIS, or SYNCHONDRO'SIS, *Ilio-sacral articula'tion, symphysis* or *synchondrosis*, is the union of two surfaces;—two inclined planes, broader above than below; one formed by the sacrum, the other by the ilium. Both surfaces are incrusted by an articular cartilage. The bands which strengthen them are the two *sacro-sciatic ligaments*, the *sacro-spinal*, a *sacro-iliac* ligament, and some irregular fibres. The *sacro-iliac* ligament is a very thick assemblage of short, dense, irregular fibres, occupying the space which the sacrum and ilium leave between them, behind their articular surface. Some authors have termed some irregular fibres, situate in front of the sacro-iliac articulation, *anterior sacro-iliac ligaments*, in opposition to the preceding fasciæ, which they call *posterior sacro-iliac*.

SACROISCHIATICUS, Sacro-sciatic.

SACROLOMBAIRE, Sacro-lumbalis.

SACROLUMBAR, *Sacro-lumba'lis, Sacro-lombaire.* That which belongs to the sacrum and loins.

SACROLUMBAR, *Sacro-lumba'lis, Sacro-lumba'ris Muscle, Sacro-costa'lis, Dorso-trache'lian portion of the Sacro-spinal* of Chaussier, (F.) *Lombo-costo-trachélien, Sacro-lombaire*, is seated at the posterior part of the trunk; is thick and triangular below; flat and thin in the remainder, and terminates in a point at its upper extremity. It is attached to the posterior surface of the sacrum; to the corresponding portion of the crista ilii; to the extremities of the transverse processes of the lumbar vertebræ; to the angles of the eleven inferior ribs; to the tuberosity of the first, and the posterior tubercle of the transverse processes of the last five cervical vertebræ. The sacro-lumbalis straightens the vertebral column when bent forwards, and maintains it straight. By means of its insertion into the ribs, it can elevate or depress these bones, according as it contracts from above to below, or from below to above. It acts, consequently, sometimes as an inspiratory, at others as an expiratory muscle.

From six or eight of the lower ribs arises an equal number of fleshy portions, which terminate at the inner side of this muscle, and are called *Mus'culi Accessor'ii* vel *Additamen'tum ad Sacrolumba'lem*, (F.) *Accessoires du Sacro-lombaire*.

From the upper part of the sacro-lumbalis, a fleshy slip, called *Cervica'lis descen'dens, Cervicalis descendens Diemerbroeck'ii, Transversa'lis collatera'lis colli, Accesso'rius ad Sacro-lumbalem*, (F.) *Transversaire grêle*, runs up, to be fixed to the transverse processes of the fourth, fifth, and sixth cervical vertebræ, by three distinct tendons. These last parts, though separated by some anatomists, belong to the sacro-lumbalis.

SACROSCIAT'IC, *Sacro-ischiat'icus.* That which belongs to the sacrum and ischium.

SACROSCIATIC LIGAMENTS are two ligaments, which assist in securing the sacro-iliac articulation. The *great* or *posterior sacro-sciatic ligament* extends from the crista ilii and the sides of the sacrum and coccyx to the tuberosity of the ischium. The *less* or *anterior sacro-sciatic ligament* arises from the same point, and terminates in the spine of the ischium.

SACROSPINAL, Dorso-trachelian portion of the sacro-lumbalis.

SACROSPINA'LIS. That which relates to the sacrum and spine. Under this name, Chaussier describes the sacro-lumbalis, longissimus dorsi, transversalis, transverso-spinalis, and intertransversalis. He divides it into three portions.

SACROTROCHANTÉRIEN, Pyramidalis.

SACROVERT'EBRAL, *Sacro-vertebra'lis.* That which relates to the sacrum and the vertebræ.

SACROVERTEBRAL ARTICULATION is the junction of the last vertebræ of the loins with the sacrum. The angle which these two bones form at the anterior part has been called the *Prom'ontory of the Sacrum*, or the *Sacro-vertebral Angle*.

SACROVERTEBRAL LIGAMENT is a strong ligament, which passes from the anterior part of each of the transverse processes of the last lumbar vertebra to be attached to the base of the sacrum. Its *use* is to maintain the articulation of those two bones *in situ*.

SACRUM, *Os sacrum, Os basila'rē, Os Alagas, Os latum, Os clun'ium, Ver'tebra magna, Albagiasi, Hi'eron ost'eon, Clunis, Subver'tebra, Subver'tebrum, Vet'ula;* from *sacer*, 'sacred;' because it contributes to protect the genital organs, which were considered sacred, or because it was offered in sacrifice. The bone, which forms the posterior part of the pelvis, and is a continuation of the vertebral column. The sacrum is symmetrical and triangular, situate at the posterior part of the pelvis, and concave anteriorly. It has, —
1. A *pelvic* or *anterior surface*, which corresponds to the pelvic cavity, and has four transverse furrows, that point out the parts where the primitive portions of the bone were separated from each other. On each side there are four foramina, called *anterior sacral;* these are oblique, and decrease in size, from above downwards. Through these pass the anterior branches of the sacral nerves. 2. A *spinal* or *posterior surface*, which is convex, rough, and covered by muscles. Upon the median line are four horizontal, tubercular eminences, forming a continuation of the spinous processes of the vertebræ; and below, a triangular notch, where the *sacral canal* terminates. On each side of the surface are four foramina, called *posterior sacral*, which are smaller than the anterior, and give passage to the posterior branches of the sacral nerves. 3. The *vertebral surface* or *base*. Its greatest extent is transversely. It is articulated with the last lumbar vertebra. On it is seen the orifice of the *sacral canal*, of a triangular shape, which decreases in width from above downward; terminates the vertebral canal; is lined by a prolongation of the cerebral membranes; contains the fasciculi of the sacral nerves; communicates, externally, by the sacral foramina; and terminates at the triangular notch on the posterior surface of the bone. At the sides of the upper orifice of the sacral canal are two articular processes, which receive the articular processes of the last lumbar vertebra. The projection formed by the union of the base of the sacrum with the last lumbar vertebra, is called the *Prom'ontory, Promonto'rium Ossis Sacri, Great Angle of the Sacrum* or *Sacro-vertebral Angle*. 4. A *coccygeal face* or *apex*, (F.) *Face coccygienne* ou *Sommet*, which is very narrow, and is articulated with the coccyx. 5. *Two lateral margins*, which have, above, a broad, oblique surface, articulated with the ilium.

The sacrum is developed by 30 to 35 points of ossification.

SADDLE, TURKISH, Sella Turcica.
SÆPES, Sepes.
SAFFLOW, Carthamus tinctorius.
SAFFLOWER, Carthamus tinctorius.
SAFFRON, Crocus — s. Bastard, Carthamus tinctorius — s. Dyers', Carthamus tinctorius — s. Flower, Carthamus tinctorius — s. Meadow, Colchicum autumnale.
SAFRAN BÂTARD, Carthamus tinctorius, Colchicum autumnale — *s. des Indes,* Curcuma longa — *s. de Mars apéritif,* Ferri subcarbonas — *s. de Mars astringent,* Colcothar — *s. des Prés,* Colchicum autumnale — *s. Racine de,* Curcuma longa.
SAFRANUM, Carthamus tinctorius.
SAFRE, Smalt.
SAGA, Sago.
SAGAPE'NUM, *Sag'apin, Serapi'non,* (F.) *Gomme séraphique.* A gum-resin, supposed to be obtained from the *Fer'ula Per'sica.* Family, Umbelliferæ. *Sex. Syst.* Pentandria Digynia. Its odour is fetid and alliaceous; taste pungent, bitterish, nauseous. It is in small, agglutinated masses of a yellow colour; tenacious; breaking with a horny fracture. It is a reputed antispasmodic and emmenagogue. Dose, gr. x to ʒss.
SAGAPIN, Sagapenum.
SAGE, Salvia — s. Indian, Eupatorium perfoliatum — s. Jerusalem, Pulmonaria — s. Tree, Lantana — s. Wild, Salvia Africana.
SAGE-FEMME, Midwife.
SAGENA, Epiploon.
SAGESSE DES CHIRURGIENS, Sisymbrium Sophia.
SAGIMEN VITRI, Soda, subcarbonate of.
SAGIT'TAL, *Sagitta'lis, Sagitta'tus,* from *sagitta,* 'an arrow.'
SAGITTAL FURROW, *Sagittal Groove,* (F.) *Gouttière sagittale,* is a channel on the median line of the inner surface of the skull-cap. It is excavated in the os frontis, in the two parietal and occipital bones, and extends from the crista galli to the internal occipital protuberance. It lodges the longitudinal sinus, which has been called the *sagittal sinus.*
SAGITTAL SUTURE, *Obelæ'a sutu'ra, O. Raphē, Sutura Virga'ta, S. juga'lis, S. Rabdoï'des, Rhabdoï'des, Rhabdo'des, Rhabdoïdeus* seu *Biparieta'lis.* The suture which unites the two parietal bones, and which extends, from before to behind, on the median line, from the coronal suture to the lambdoidal. It is so called, from *sagitta,* 'an arrow,' because it seems to meet the coronal suture as an arrow meets the string of a bow.
SAGITTA'RIA VARIAB'ILIS, *Arrowhead, Arrowleaf, Wapata* of Oregon; *Nat. Ord.* Alismaceæ; esculent, yielding fecula like arrow-root. The roots are cooling and sub-astringent, and are at times applied to the feet in cases of yaws and dropsical swellings of the legs. The leaves are applied to the breasts to dispel milk.
SAGITTA'RIUM ALEXIPHAR'MACUM, *Malac'ces radix, Canna In'dica, Arun'do Indica.* A root cultivated in the West Indies, and supposed to be a remedy for wounds by poisoned arrows.
SAGITTATUS, Sagittal.
SAGO, *Sagus, Saga, Sagu, Segu, Am'ylum palma'ceum,* (F.) *Sagou, Sague.* A fecula, obtained from the pith of the *Sagus rumph'ii, Cycas circina'lis, C. revolu'ta,* &c., growing in the Moluccas, Philippine Isles, &c., and which is brought to us in small grains. The same substance is, also, obtained from the West Indies, but it is inferior to that from the East. By boiling in water or milk, sago becomes soft and transparent, and forms an agreeable and nutritious food in febrile, calculous, and other disorders. It is made palatable by sugar, lemon-juice, or wine, where the last is not contra-indicated.

To make sago into a proper mucilage for the sick, a tablespoonful of it should be macerated in a pint of water for two hours, and then boiled for fifteen minutes, stirring assiduously. Care must be taken, that the grains are perfectly dissolved by long boiling and constant stirring.

Sago posset is made by putting *sago,* ʒij.; *water,* Oij; boiling until the mucilage is formed, then rubbing *sugar,* ʒss, on the rind of a lemon, and putting it with *tincture of ginger,* fʒj.; *sherry,* Oss; adding this mixture to the mucilage and boiling for five minutes. — It is a good restorative.

SAGO, FRENCH, see Solanum tuberosum, and Arrow-root, common — s. Portland Island, see Arum maculatum.
SAGOU, Sago.
SAGU, Sago.
SAGUE, Sago — *s. Petit,* see Solanum tuberosum.
SAGUS, Sago — s. Rumphii, see Sago.
SAHARA, Insomnia.
SAIGNÉE, Blood-letting — *s. Spoliative, Spoliativa phlebotomia.*
SAIGNEMENT DU NEZ, Epistaxis.
SAILORS, DISEASES, &c., OF. Sailors, by nature of their occupation, are liable to many diseases. Several of these may, however, be warded off by proper attention to cleanliness and ventilation.
SAIN BOIS, Daphne gnidium — s. *Doux,* Adeps præparatus.
SAINT AMAND, MINERAL WATERS OF. Sulphuretted waters, in the department of Nord, France. They contain carbonic and sulphohydric acids. The *Boue* or deposit contains sulphohydric acid, and salts of iron and magnesia. Temperature, 64° to 82° Fahr.
SAINT AUGUSTINE, CLIMATE OF. This sea-port of Florida is a frequent retreat during the winter season for the valetudinarian from the more northern parts of the United States. The climate is certainly comparatively mild and equable; but it is liable to frequent north-east storms. There are only a few days, however, in winter, in which the invalid cannot take exercise in the open air. Tampa Bay, and Pensacola, in Florida, and Mobile, in Alabama, which are somewhat visited by the consumptive, are less liable to the storms in question.
SAINT CHARLES'S ROOT, Carlo Santo (Radix).
SAINT CROIX, Santa Cruz.
SAINT JAMES'S WORT, Senecio Jacobæa.
SAINT JOHN'S DANCE, see Mania, dancing — St. John's Wort, Hypericum perforatum.
SAINT KITTS, see West Indies.
SAINT LEONARD'S, CLIMATE OF. The place, which is situate about a mile to the westward of Hastings, in Sussex, England, is less sheltered than it, and is therefore a less favourable retreat, during the winter months, for the phthisical valetudinarian.
SAINT MYON, MINERAL WATERS OF. Some cold, acidulous waters at Saint Myon, near Riom, in the department of Puy-de-Dôme. They contain free carbonic acid, subcarbonate of soda, chloride of sodium, and carbonate and sulphate of lime.
SAINT NECTAIRE, MINERAL WATERS OF. Springs in the department of Puy-de-Dôme, France. They contain carbonic acid, bicarbonate of soda, and chloride of sodium. Temperature, 75° to 103° Fahr.
SAINT PARDAUX, MINERAL WATERS

OF. Chalybeate springs in the department of Allier, France. They contain carbonic acid and iron.

SAINT SAUVEUR, MINERAL WATERS OF. Sulphurous waters in the department of Hautes-Pyrénées, France. Temperature, 76° to 93° Fahr.

SAINT VINCENT'S, see West Indies.

SAINT VITUS'S DANCE, Chorea, see Mania, dancing — s. Vitus's Dance of the Voice, Balbuties.

SAIRE, Essera.

SAL, Salt—s. Absinthii, Potassæ subcarbonas, see Potash — s. Acetosellæ, Potass, oxalate of — s. Acetosus ammoniacalis, Liquor ammoniæ acetatis — s. Acidum benzoes, Benjamin — s. Albus, Soda, muriate of — s. Alembroth, Alembroth salt — s. Alkali, Soda, subcarbonate of — s. Alkalinus fixus fossilis, Soda — s. Amarum, Magnesiæ sulphas — s. Ammoniac, volatile, Ammoniæ carbonas — s. Ammoniacum, Ammoniæ murias — s. Ammoniacum martiale, Ferrum ammoniatum — s. Ammoniacum secretum Glauberi, Ammoniæ sulphas — s. Ammoniacum tartareum, Ammoniæ tartras — s. Ammoniacum vegetabile, Liquor ammoniæ acetatis — s. Ammoniacus nitrosus, Ammoniæ nitras — s. Ammoniæ, Ammoniæ murias — s. Anglicanum, Magnesiæ sulphas — s. Antiepilepticus of Weissman, Cuprum ammoniatum — s. Antimonii, Antimonium tartarizatum — s. Ammoniacum, Ammoniæ murias—s. Artis, Alembroth salt—s. Asphaltitis, Bit noben—s. Catharticus amarus, Magnesiæ sulphas—s. Catharticus Glauberi, Soda, sulphate of—s. Communis, Soda, muriate of — s. Cornu cervi, volatile, Ammoniæ carbonas — s. Culinaris, Soda, muriate of—s. Digestivus Sylvii, Potossæ murias — s. Diureticus, Potassæ acetas — s. de Duobus, Potassæ sulphas — s. Ebsdamense, Magnesiæ sulphas — s. Enixum, Potassæ supersulphas—s. Epsomensis, Magnesiæ sulphas — s. Essentiale Benzoes, Benjamin — s. Febrifugus of Lemery, Potassæ supersulphas — s. Febrifugus Sylvii, Potassæ murias—s. Fontium, Soda, muriate of—s. Fossilis, Soda, muriate of—s. Fuliginis, Ammoniæ carbonas—s. Gemmæ, Soda, muriate of—s. Herbarum, Potassæ subcarbonas — s. Indus, Saccharum album — s. Lixiviosum, see Lixivium—s. Lucidum, Soda, muriate of — s. Marinus, Soda, muriate of — s. Martis, Ferri sulphas — s. Martis muriaticum sublimatum, Ferrum ammoniatum—s. Mirabile perlatum, Soda, phosphate of—s. Mirabilis Glauberi, Soda, sulphate of — s. Muriaticum baroticum, Baryta, muriate of — s. Nitrum, Potassæ nitras — s. Osium, Ammoniæ carbonas—s. Panchrestum, Potassæ tartras—s. Petræ, Potassæ nitras—s. Tartarum, Potassæ subcarbonas—s. Plumbi, Plumbi superacetas—s. Polychrestus, Potassæ sulphas— s. Polychrestus Glaseri, Potassæ sulphas cum sulphure — s. Polychrestum Seignetti, Soda, tartrate of — s. Prunellæ, Potassæ nitras fusus sulphatis paucillo mixtus—s. Rupellensis, Soda, tartrate of — s. Sapientiæ, Alembroth salt, Potassæ sulphas — s. Saturni, Plumbi superacetas — s. Scientiæ, Alembroth salt — s. Secretus Glauberi, Ammoniæ sulphas — s. Sedativus Hombergi, Boracic acid — s. Sedlicensis, Magnesiæ sulphas — s. Seignetti, Soda, tartrate of — s. Sennerti, Potassæ acetas — s. Seydschutzense, Magnesiæ sulphas — s. Sodæ, Soda, subcarbonate of — s. Sodomenus, Bit noben — s. Succini, Succinic acid — s. Tartari, Potassæ subcarbonas, see Potash— s. Tartari essentiale, Tartaric acid — s. Tartari sulphuratum, Potassæ sulphas — s. Urinæ, Microcosmicum Sal — s. Urinosum, Urea — s. Vegetabilis, Potassæ tartras—s. Vitæ, Alembroth salt — s. Vitrioli, Zinci sulphas — s. Vitrioli narcoticum, Boracic acid — s. Volatile, Ammoniæ car-

bonas, Spiritus ammoniæ aromaticus — s. Volatile Benzoes, Benjamin — s. Volatile boracis, Boracic acid — s. Volatile oleosum Sylvii, Spiritus ammoniæ aromaticus — s. Volatile succini, Succinic acid — s. Volatilis salis ammoniaci, Ammoniac carbonas — s. Vomitorium vitrioli, Zinci sulphas.

SALAAM CONVULSION, see Convulsion, Salaam.

SALAB, Salep.

SALACITAS, Satyriasis — s. Vulvæ, Nymphomania.

SALAD, CORN, Valeriana dentata.

SALAP, Salep.

SALCOMBE, (CLIMATE OF.) A small place — the Montpelier of Huxham — which is one of the warmest spots on the S. W. coast of England, and, therefore, in this respect adapted for the phthisical invalid as a winter retreat.

SALEP, *Saloop'* (so pronounced.) *Salab, Salap.* The prepared bulb of the *Orchis mas'cula* and other species of Orchis. The salep of Cachmere is from a species of *Euloph'ia.* Salep is in small, irregular, hard masses. In its composition in relation to water, it is closely analogous to tragacanth. It is possessed of similar virtues with sago, tapioca, &c. The mucilage is prepared by dissolving the powdered salep in hot water, with assiduous stirring, and adding to the solution sugar and milk.

SALER'NUM, (SCHOOL OF.) An ancient school of medicine at Salerno in Italy. It was established by Charlemagne, in 802; and was the first Christian university at which medicine was taught. It was much celebrated, especially in the 12th century. The work on hygiene, "*De Conservandâ Valetudine,*" which bears its name, has passed through several editions in various languages. It is supposed to have been written by John of Milan, in 1100, and is in Leonine verses.

SALICARIA, Lythrum salicaria.

SALICINE, see Salix.

SALICORNIA ARABICA, &c., see Soda.

SALINE', *Sali'nus, Salina'cius, Sulinac''idus, Sali'tus, Salsus, Hali'nus, Halmy'rus, Halico'des, Sali'nous,* from *sal.* That which contains a salt, or has the properties of a salt.

SALINE DRAUGHT OR MIXTURE. This may be made as follows:—*Potass. carbon.* ℨj, *acid. citric. vel tartar. gr.* xv, *vel succ. limon. recent.* ℨss, *aquæ* f ℨ viij, *syrup. cujusvis* ℨj. M. Given in divided doses as a febrifuge.

SALINE EFFERVESCING DRAUGHT OR MIXTURE is made by adding a due proportion of either of the acids above mentioned, or of lemon-juice, to the proper proportion of the carbonate of soda or potassa. About 25 grains of the acid saturate 30 grains of the carbonate. See Powders, soda.

SALINOUS, Saline.

SALIS AMMONIACI FLORES, Ammoniæ carbonas.

SALITIO, Leap.

SALITUS, Saline.

SALIUM, Saliva.

SALIUNCA, Valeriana Celtica.

SALI'VA, *Si'alon, Si'elon, Sialo'ma, Ptysma, Pty'alon, Pty'elon, Sa'lium, Sputa'men, Sputamen'tum, Sputum, Spittle.* An inodorous, insipid, transparent, slightly viscid fluid; secreted by the parotid, submaxillary and sublingual glands, and poured into the mouth by the ducts of Steno, Wharton and Rivinus; the use of which is to mix with the alimentary bolus, and to serve in the process of digestion. It is composed, according to Berzelius, of 992.2 parts of water, 2.9 of a particular animal matter, soluble in water, and insoluble in alcohol, *pty'alin, princip'ium saliva'l'*, *mate'ria siali'na*, of 1.4 of mucus, 1.7 of chlorides of potassium and sodium, 0.9 of lactate of soda and animal matter, and 0.2 of soda.

SALIVÆ FLUXUS CIBO VISO, see Salivation.

SALIVAIRE, Salivary.

SALIVAL, Salivary.

SALIVANS, Sialagogue.

SALIVANT, Sialagogue.

SALIVARIS, Salivary — s. Herba, Anthemis pyrethrum.

SAL'IVARY, *Saliva'rius, Saliva'ris, Salivo'sus, Sali'val, Sali'vous*, from *saliva*, (F.) *Salivaire*. That which belongs to the saliva.

SALIVARY CALCULI, see Calculi, salivary.

SALIVARY FIS'TULÆ, *Sialosyrin'ges*, are such as depend upon an accidental opening into the excretory ducts of the salivary glands. Fistulæ are most commonly met with in the duct of Steno.

SALIVARY GLANDS, *Secreting organs of the saliva, Salival glands*, are situate symmetrically, to the number of four, on each side of the face. Their form is very irregular, and their extent varies according to individuals. Their excretory ducts — *Ductus Saliva'rii*, (F.) *Canaux ou Conduits salivaires*, carry the saliva directly into the mouth, without pouring it into any intermediate reservoir, as happens in the case of some of the other glands. The salivary glands have been distinguished into,—1. The *parotid* ; 2. The *submaxillary* ; 3. The *sublingual* ; and 4. The *intralingual* or *lingual*, seated at the inferior surface of the tongue, where the mucous membrane forms a fringed fold.

SALIVATIO, Salivation—s. Mercurialis, Salivation, mercurial.

SALIVA'TION, *Saliva'tio, Saliva'tio cal'ida, Epiph'ora ptyalis'mus, Sialis'mus, Sputum Oris, Sial'achus, Sieliamos, Sialorrhœ'a, Sialose'mia, Ptyalis'mus, Pty'alism, Fluxus sali'væ*, (F.) *Flux de Bouche, Flux salivaire*. A superabundant secretion of saliva; occasioned either locally, by the mode of irritating masticatories, or under the influence of some cause which acts on the whole economy, and especially of mercurial preparations. In this last case it is accompanied by a coppery taste in the mouth, by swelling of the gums, and sometimes by looseness of the teeth. Salivation may usually be diminished by the use of astringents, laxatives, &c.

Ptyalismus acu'tus sympathet'icus, Salivæ fluxus cibo viso, Mouth watering, the increased flow of saliva produced by the sight, smell, or thought of agreeable food, is a species of ptyalism, as well as the *Ptyalismus acutus melli'tus, Apoceno'sis ptyalis'mus mellitus*, or *Sweet spittle*. In this the saliva has a sweet or mucilaginous taste.

SALIVATION, MERCU'RIAL, *Saliva'tio mercuria'lis, Sialoze'mia mercurialis, Ptyalis'mus mercuria'lis, P. hydrargyra'tus*, (F.) *Ptyalisme mercuriel, Salivation mercurielle*. Salivation produced by mercury. The stomatitis that accompanies it is termed *mercurial, Hydrar'gyro-stomati'tis*, (F.) *Stomatite mercurielle*.

SALIVATION MERCURIELLE, Salivation, mercurial.

SALIVATUM, Sialagogue.

SALIVOSUS, Salivary.

SALIVOUS, Salivary.

SALIX. The *Willow, l'tea*, (F.) *Saule*. A genus of plants in the Linnæan system.

SALIX FRAG''ILIS, *S. pen'dula* seu *decip'iens* seu *amygdali'na* seu *persicifo'lia* seu *Russelia'na* seu *pippoph'æfolia* seu *Trevira'nii*, or Crack willow (Ph. D.) SALIX ALBA, *S. cœru'lea* seu *virtelli'na*, or White willow (Ph. D. and Ph. U. S.) SALIX LATIFO'LIA, or broad-leaved willow. SALIX CA'PREA, *S. sphacela'ta* seu *tomento'sa*, or Great round-leaved willow (Ph. L.) SALIX PENTAN'DRIA seu HERMAPHRODITI'CA. SALIX HUMI'LIS, SALIX ERIOCEPH'ALA. The bark of these has a slightly aromatic odour, and a bitter astringent taste, which is nearly the same in all the species. It is tonic and astringent. It has been used in intermittents, and in dyspepsia, worms, &c. The active principle has been separated, and called *Sal'icine*. It is said the quinia in medicinal efficacy. Dose, of the powder. Dose of *Salicine* from 4 grains.

SALIX ÆGYPTIACA, Calaf.

SALLOW, Lurid.

SALMIAC, Ammoniæ murias.

SALOOP, Salep.

SALPETRA, Soda, nitrate of.

SALPINGEMPHRAX'IS, from *salpinx*, Eustachian tube,' and *εμφραξις*, 'obstruction of the Eustachian tube;—a deafness.

SALPINGI'TIS, from *σαλπιγξ*, 'a tube,' *itis*, 'denoting inflammation.' Inflammation of the Eustachian tube.

SALPINGOCYE'SIS, *Paracye'sis Gravid'itas tuba'ria*, from *σαλπιγξ*, 'a trumpet,' and *κυησις*, 'pregnancy.' Tubal pregnancy.— See Pregnancy.

SALPINGOMALLEEN, Tensor tympani— s. Staphylinus internus, Levator palati.

SALPINGOPHARYNGÆ'US, from *salpinx* 'a trumpet,' and *φαρυγξ*, 'the pharynx.' Valsalva and Douglas have given this name to a bundle of fibres, which passes from the Eustachian tube to the pharynx.

SALPINGOSTAPHYLINUS, Circumflexus muscle.

SALPINGOSTENOCHO'RIA, from *salpinx* 'a tube,' *στενος*, 'narrow,' and *χωρα*. Narrowness or stricture of the Eustachian tube.

SALPINX, Tuba.

SALSAFI, Tragopogon.

SALSAMENTUM CRUDUM, Omotarichos.

SALSAPARILLA GERMANICA, Sarsaparilla Germanica.

SALSEDO MUCRUM, Potassæ nitras.

SALSEPAREILLE, Smilax sarsaparilla—*d'Allemagne*, Sarsaparilla Germanica.

SALSILAGO, Muria.

SALSOLA DECUMBENS, S. Kali.

SALSO'LA KALI, *S. Decum'bens, Kali spino'sum, Prickly Saltwort, Kali spino'sum* com'., *Tragus* sive *Tragum Matthi'oli*. This plant, as well as the *Salsola sati'va* and the *Salsola* seu *longifo'lia, Kali iner'mis* seu *soda, Herba* produces the alkaline salt, commonly called *rilla, Soda*, or *Kelp*.

SALSOLA LONGIFOLIA, S. Kali — s. Sativa, see S. Kali, and Soda — s. Soda, see S. Kali.

SALSUGINOSUS, Halmyrodes.

SALSUS, Saline.

SALT, *Sal, Hal, Hals, 'αλς*, (F.) *Sel*. A name formerly given to a considerable number of substances of very different nature. At present chemists apply the term *Salts* exclusively to the combination of an acid with one or more bases. *Neutral salts* are those in which the acid and base reciprocally saturate each other. *Acid salts* or *supersalts*, (F.) *Sur-sels*, are those in which the acid predominates over the base. *Alkaline salts* or *subsalts*, (F.) *Sous-sels*, those in which the base is, on the contrary, predominant. The different denominations of the salts are compounded of the name of the acid; the termination of which is changed into *ite*, when the name of the acid in *ous;—ate,* when it is in *ic.* Thus the salts formed by the *sulphurous* acid are *sulphites;* those by the *sulphuric, sulphates.* 2. This name is followed up by that of the oxyd, that enters into the composition of the salt. Thus, the *sulphate of protoxyd of iron* is a combination of sulphuric acid with the protoxyd of that metal. Frequently, to shorten the name, the word *oxyd* is suppressed; and *proto, deuto, trito,* &c., put before the acid:—as *protosulphate of iron. Simple salts* are those resulting from the combination of an acid with a single base: *double salts* with two different bases: *triple* with three, &c. A *haloid salt* is one constituted after the type of common salt, or which contains a metal and a *salt-radical,* as chlorine, iodine, &c. An *oxysalt* is formed from the combination of an acid with an oxide.

When *salt* is used in an abstract sense, it means the chloride of sodium.

SALT APERIENT, OF FREDERICK, Soda, sulphate of—s. Baker's, Ammoniæ carbonas—s. of Barilla, Soda, subcarbonate of—s. Bay, Soda, muriate of—s. Bitter purging, Magnesiæ sulphas—s. Common, Soda, muriate of—s. Epsom, Magnesiæ sulphas—s. Glauber's, Soda, sulphate of—s. Glauber's, Lymington, see Soda, sulphate of—s. Rochelle, Soda, tartrate of—s. Rock, Soda, muriate of—s. Sea, Soda, muriate of—s. Secondary, Neutral salt—s. Seignette's, Soda, tartrate of—s. Smelling, Ammoniæ carbonas—s. of Soda, Soda, subcarbonate of—s. Sore-throat, Potassæ nitras fusus sulphatis paucillo mixtus—s. of Tartar, see Potassæ subcarbonas, and Potash—s. Tasteless purging, Soda, phosphate of—s. of Urine, Ammoniæ carbonas—s. White, Soda, muriate of—s. of Woodsoot, Ammoniæ carbonas—s. of Wormwood, see Potash.

SALTANS ROSA, Urticaria.
SALTATIO, Dancing—s. Sancti Viti, Chorea.
SALTERTON. A village about four miles to the eastward of Exmouth, England, frequented as a winter abode by invalids. It is in a small, open valley on the seashore, and is well protected from winds, particularly the northerly.
SALTISH, Halmyrodes.
SALTPETRE, Potassæ nitras.
SALTUS, Leap, Vulva—s. Tendinum, Subsultus tendinum.
SALTWORT, PRICKLY, Salsola kali.
SALUBRIOUS, Salutary.
SALUBRIOUSNESS, Salubrity.
SALUBRIS, Salutary.
SALU'BRITY, *Salu'britas, Salu'briousness,* (F.) *Salubrité,* from *salus,* 'health.' Any thing which contributes to the health of individuals or of communities. Situations differ materially from each other in this respect; and the cause of the difference is often an interesting topic of inquiry.
SALUS, Sanitas.
SALUTAIRE, Salutary.
SAL'UTARY, *Peries'ticos, Saluta'ris, Salu'ber, Salu'bris, Hygiei'nus, Hygiasticus, Hygie'rus, Salu'brins,* (F.) *Salutaire.* Same etymon. Healthy. That which is favourable to health. Some diseases have been considered salutary; but this is doubtful.
SALUTIF'EROUS, *Salu'tifer;* from *salus,* 'health,' and *fero,* 'I bear.' Bringing health; health-bearing.
SALVATEL'LA; same etymon, (?) *Vena salvatel'la,* is situate on the back of the hand, near its inner margin. It begins on the posterior surface of the fingers and dorsal surface of the hand, by a plexus, formed of a number of radicles, frequently anastomosing with each other; it then ascends to the inner part of the forearm, where it takes the name—*posterior cubital.* The ancients recommended this vein to be opened in certain diseases, as in melancholic and hypochondriacal affections; and they attributed to such abstraction of blood considerable efficacy in the cure of disease: hence its name.

SALVE, BLISTERING, Unguentum lyttæ—s. Eye, Unguentum oxidi zinci impuri—s. Eye, Singleton's, Unguentum hydrargyri nitrico-oxydi —s. Healing, Cerate of calamine.

SAL'VIA, *S. officina'lis* seu *horten'sis* seu *vulga'ris* seu *minor, Elelis'phacos,* (F.) *Sauge, Petite Sauge, Thé d'Europe, Thé de France.* Family, Labiatæ. *Sex. Syst.* Diandria Monogynia. Sage has a peculiar, aromatic odour, and a warm, aromatic, bitterish taste. Its virtues depend upon an essential oil. It is tonic, stimulant, and carminative. In the form of a weak infusion, it is occasionally used as a diluent, and as a wash for sore mouth. Dose, gr. xv to xxx or more.

SALVIA AFRICA'NA, *Wild Sage,* a South African species, has the same medical properties as Salvia.

SALVIA COLORATA, Salvia.
SALVIA HORMI'NUM, *Hormi'num, S. colora'ta, Hormi'num colora'tum* seu *sativum,* (F.) *Saugehormin,* of the Pharmacopœias, is used in similar cases.

SALVIA HORTENSIS, Salvia—s. Minor, Salvia—s. Officinalis, Salvia.
SALVIA SCLA'REA, *Sclarea, Gallit'richum, Æthio'pis, Biser'mas, Colus Jovis, Common Clary,* (F.) *Sauge sclarée, Grande sauge, Orvale ou Toutebonne.* The leaves have been recommended as corroborants and anti-spasmodics.

SALVIA VITÆ, Asplenium ruta muraria—s. Vulgaris, Salvia.
SAMBU'CUS, *Sabu'cus, Sambucus nigra, S. vulga'ris, S. Arbo'rea, Actē, Infe'lix lignum; the Elder,* (F.) *Sureau commun.* Family, Caparifoliaceæ. *Sex. Syst.* Pentandria Digynia—(The flower and bark were formerly called *Cuno'pum.*) The flowers, berries, and bark of the elder have been used in medicine. The *flowers* have been reputed diaphoretic and discutient: the *berries,* aperient and sudorific: the *bark,* purgative, and, in small doses, deobstruent. The flowers are sometimes used in fomentations, and to form a cooling ointment.

SAMBUCUS ARBOREA, Sambucus—s. Chamæacte, S. ebulus.
SAMBUCUS EB'ULUS, *Ebulus, Chamæac'tē, Od'ocos, Sambucus Chamæac'tē* seu *He'lion, Sambucus hu'milis* seu *Herba'cea, Dwarf-elder, Danewort,* (F.) *Hièble.* The root, interior bark, leaves, flowers, berries, (*Baccæ* seu *Grana Actes,*) and seeds have all been given in moderate doses as resolvents and deobstruents; and in large doses as hydragogues. The berries of *Sambucus Canaden'sis,* the *Common Elder* of America, are made officinal in the American Pharmacopœia.

SAMBUCUS HELION, Sambucus ebulus—s. Herbacea, S. ebulus—s. Humilis, S. ebulus—s. Nigra, Sambucus—s. Vulgaris, Sambucus.
SAMI TERRA, *Sa'mian Earth.* An argillaceous earth, found in the island of Samos, to which were ascribed virtues similar to those of the Terra Lemnii.—Galen, Dioscorides.
SAMIUS LAPIS. A stone found in the Isle of Samos, which the ancients believed to be astringent and refrigerant.
SAMPHIRE, Crithmum maritimum.
SAMPSON, BLACK, Echinacea purpurea.
SAMPSUCHUS, Thymus mastichina.
SAMPSUCUS, Origanum majorana.
SAMPSYCH'INON, *Sampsu'chinum.* An ointment composed of σαμψυχον; which was perhaps marjoram.—Dioscorides.
SANABILIS, Curable.

SANABLE, Curable.
SANAMUNDA, Geum urbanum.
SANATIO, Curation, Cure.
SANATIVE, Curative.
SAN GIULIANO, MINERAL WATERS OF. At the foot of the mountain San Giuliano, a league and a half from Pisa, are several mineral springs; temperature from 84° to 107° Fahr.
The spring, *Pozzetto*, contains carbonic acid, sulphates of soda, lime, and magnesia; chlorides of sodium and magnesium; carbonates of lime and magnesia; argil and silica.—Santi.
SAND, see Gravel.
SANDALUM CÆRULEUM, Guilandina moringa—s. Rubrum, Pterocarpus santalinus.
SAN'DARAC, *Sandara'cha, Gum Ju'niper, Gum Sandarach, Pounce, Gummi Junip'eri, Sandara'ca, Vernix sicca, Resina Junip'eri*. A name given, by the Arabs, to an odorous resin, that flows from the *Thuya aphyl'la*. Family, Coniferæ. Sex. Syst. Monœcia Monadelphia. It is stimulant, like all the resins; but is very little used.
SANDARACHA GRÆCORUM, Realgar.
SAND-BLIND. A defect of vision, in which small particles seem to fly before the eyes. See Metamorphopsia.
SANDERS, see Saunders.
SANDIVER, see Vitrum.
SANDIX, Plumbi oxydum rubrum.
SANDYX, Plumbi oxydum rubrum.
SANG, Blood—*s. Artériel*, Arterial blood—*s. Dragon*, Rumex sanguineus—*s. Dragon*, see Calamus rotang—*s. Globules du*, Globules of the blood—*s. Perte de*, Hæmorrhagia.
SANGAREE'. Wine and water, sweetened and spiced.
SANGLOT, Sob.
SANGSUE, Hirudo.
SANGUIDUCTUS DURÆ MATRIS, Sinuses of the dura mater.
SANGUIFICATIO, Hæmatosis — s. Debilior, Hyphæmatosis.
SANGUIFLUXUS, Hæmorrhagia — s. Uterinus, Metrorrhagia.
SANGUIMOTION, Circulation.
SANGUIMOTORY, Circulatory.
SANGUIN, (Vaisseau,) Blood-vessel.
SANGUINALIS CORRIGIOLA, Polygonum aviculare.
SANGUINA'RIA, *S. Canaden'sis seu acau'lis, Bloodroot, Bloodwort, Puccoon, Red Puccoon, Red Root, Indian Paint, Tur'meric*. Nat. Ord. Papaveraceæ. Sex. Syst. Polyandria Monogynia. A North American plant, the rhizoma and seeds of which are used in medicine. They are emetic. Dose of the powder, 8 to 20 grains. They are said to reduce the velocity of the pulse, like digitalis.
SANGUINARIA, Polygonum aviculare.
SANGUINE, *Sanguin'eus, Sanguino'sus, Hæmat'icus, Hæmato'des, Hæmate'rus, Hæmati'nus, Hæmo'des, Hæmoï'des, Sanguineous;* (F.) *Sanguin*. Bloody, blood-like; having the colour of blood, as 'a sanguine countenance.' Relating to, or containing blood—as 'sanguine temperament.' Plethoric.
SANGUINEA, Potassæ nitras.
SANGUINENESS, Plethora.
SANGUINEOUS, Plethoric, Sanguine.
SANGUINEUS, Sanguine.
SANGUINIS ABSORPTIO, Hæmorrhophesis—s. Congestio, Congestion—s. Dissolutio, Hæmatoclysis—s. Fluor, Hæmoptysis—s. Fluor Vesicæ, Cystorrhagia — s. Ictus, Apoplexy — s. Missio, Blood-letting—s. Profluvium copiosum, Hæmorrhagia—s. Profluvium ex Ore, Stomatorrhagia—s. Stagnatio, Hæmostasis.

SANGUIN'OLENT, *Sanguinolen'tus*, from *sanguis*, 'blood.' Tinged with blood. An epithet applied, particularly, to the sputa when so tinged. Bloody.
SANGUINOSUS, Sanguine.
SANGUIPUR'GIUM, from *sanguis*, 'blood,' and *purgare*, 'to cleanse.' Purgation of the blood. A name given by some authors to mild fevers, from an idea that they purged the blood of noxious matters.
SANGUIS, Blood, Sperm—s. Concretus, Coagulum—s. Draconis, see Calamus rotang—s. Horridus siccatus, see Blood—s. Menstruus, see Menses—s. in Urinâ, Hæmaturia.
SANGUISOR'BA CANADEN'SIS, *Canada Burnett*. A tall indigenous plant—family, Rosaceæ—with white, sometimes purple, flowers, which appear from August to October. It has the same virtues as
SANGUISOR'BA OFFICINA'LIS, *S. car'nea seu rubra, Ital'ian Pim'pinel, Pimpinel'la Ital'ica seu officina'lis,* (F.) *Pimprenelle noire*. It was formerly used as an astringent and tonic, in hemorrhages, dysentery, &c.
SANGUISUGA, Hirudo.
SANGUISU'GUM. A barbarous term, to denote too great an accumulation of blood in the heart.—Bonetus.
SANICLE, Sanicula, S. Marilandica—s. American, Heuchera cortusa—*e. de Mariland, Sanicula Marilandica*—s. Yorkshire, Pinguicola vulgaris.
SANIC'ULA, *S. Europæ'a seu officina'ra, Astran'tia diapensia, Cauca'lis Sanic'ula, Cordala'ta, Dodeca'theon, Sym'phytum petræ'um, Sanic'ula mas, Diapen'sia, D. cortu'sa, Sanicle,* (F.) *Toute-saine.* Family, Umbelliferæ. Sex Syst. Pentandria Digynia. This herb was formerly used as a mild astringent. It is bitterish and somewhat austere.
SANICULA, Saxifraga granula—s. Eboracensis, Pinguicola vulgaris—s. Europæa, Sanicula.
SANIC'ULA MARILAN'DICA, *San'icle, Ma'ryland Sanicle, Black Snakeroot,* (F.) *Sanicle de Mariland*. This indigenous plant grows in marshes, or low and shaded ground. It is possessed of tonic virtues; and the powdered root is employed in popular practice as a favourite remedy in intermittent fever. It has been recommended also, in chorea.
SANICULA MONTANA, Pinguicola vulgaris—s. Officinarum, Sanicula.
SANIDO'DES, *Sanio'des*, 'resembling a board;' from *σανις*, gen. *σανιδος*, 'a board,' and *ωδος*, 'resemblance.' One whose thorax is narrow, and, as it were, contracted.
SANIE, Sanies.
SA'NIES, *Ichor, Tabum, Virus, Pus ma'nium, P. corrosi'vum,* (F.) *Sanie*. A thin, serous fluid, presenting some of the qualities of pus and blood, and commonly exhaled at the surface of ulcers.
SANIODES, Sanidodes.
SANIOSUS, Ichorous.
SANIOUS, Ichorous.
SAN'ITORY, *San'atory*, Healing. (F.) *Sanitaire*. That which relates to health, and especially to public health; as *établissement sanitaire, police sanitaire*.
SANITA'RIUM, *Sanato'rium;* from *sanitas*, 'health.' A retreat selected for valetudinarians in consequence of its salubrity. Also, an establishment for the treatment of the sick.
SAN'ITAS, *Hygiē'a, Hygē'a, Hygian'sis, Eugi'asis, Integ'ritas, Prosper'itas Valetu'dinis, Salus, Hygiei'a, Valetu'do, Valen'do, bona seu secun'da seu com'moda, Hygē'ia, Euōdyna'mia, Health,* (F.) *Santé*, from

'sound.' Health has been defined,—a state, in which all the functions are exerted with regularity and harmony. A person may, however, be in health, although certain functions are not performed. A blind man, for example, has health when all his functions, except sight, proceed with regularity. *Sanity* is often used for soundness of mind.

SANITAS, Cure.
SANITY, Sanitas.
SANKIRA, Smilax China.
SANS PAIRE, (*Veine*,) Azygos vein.
SANTA CRUZ, (CLIMATE OF.) This West India island is frequently selected as a winter retreat for the phthisical valetudinarian from the United States; but it does not seem entitled to any preference, in such cases, over the other islands of the West Indies, whilst its general salubrity is said to be less than that of many.

SANTAL BLANC, Santalum album — *s.* Rouge, Pterocarpus santalinus.
SANTALUM, see Pterocarpus santalinus.
SAN'TALUM ALBUM, *S. cit'rinum* seu *pal'lidum* seu *myrtifo'lium*, *Sir'ium myrtifo'lium*, *Yellow Saunders*, (F.) *Santal blanc*. *Sex. Syst.* Tetrandria Monogynia. The virtues of the wood of the white saunders reside in a volatile oil and resinous principle. The odour is fragrant, and resembles a mixture of ambergris and roses. It has been used as a stimulant and sudorific, but it is not now employed. The saunders woods are called, collectively, in French, *Santaux*.

SANTALUM MYRTIFOLIUM, S. album — s. Rubrum, Pterocarpus santalinus.
SANTÉ, Sanitas.
SANTONICUM, Artemisia santonicum.
SAN'TONINE, *San'tonin*, *Cinin*. A peculiar crystalline substance obtained from Artemisia Santonica. It possesses the anthelmintic properties of the plant. Dose, five or six grains.
SANTORI'NI, FISSURES OF, (F.) *Incisures ou Scissures de Santorini*. Clefts at the upper and back part of the fibro-cartilaginous portion of the external ear.
SANTORINI, TU'BERCLES OF. Small cartilaginous projections at the top of the arytenoid cartilages, which support the ligaments of the glottis. See Corniculum Laryngis.
SANVE, Sinapis.
SAP, Sax. ɼæpe, (G.) S a f t, *Arborum Succus* seu *Lympha*, (F.) *Sève*. The circulating fluid of the vegetable, which corresponds to the blood of the animal.
SAPA, see Rob.
SAPHA'DA. Paracelsus has given this name to reddish scales adherent to the hair in some eruptions of the hairy scalp.
SAPHÆNA, Saphena.
SAPHE'NA, *Saphæ'na*, from σαφης, 'manifest,' 'evident.' (F.) *Saphène*. A name given to two subcutaneous veins of the lower limb. These are: 1. The GREAT SAPHENA VEIN, *Saphena interna*, *Tibio-malleolar*, (Ch.,) (F.) *Grande Veine Saphène ou Saphène interne*. Its radicles occupy the inner part of the great toe, and form a transverse arch on the back of the foot, which unites with the saphena externa, and receives at its convex part, which is turned forwards, a number of branches coming from the toes. These radicles, when united, ascend before the inner ankle, and form a trunk, the size of which is farther increased by several branches that proceed from the region of the tarsus, and that of the metatarsus. This trunk ascends vertically at the inner part of the leg; passes behind the inner condyle of the femur; proceeds along the inner part of the thigh; receives other subcutaneous veins, such as the abdominal subcutaneous, the external pudic, &c., and passes through the inferior opening of the crural canal to empty itself into the femoral vein. 2. The LESSER VENA SAPHENA or *Saphena externa; the Peroneomalleolar Vein* of Chaussier, (F.) *Petite Veine Saphène ou Saphène externe*, commences by several roots, which are spread over the dorsum and outer side of the foot, and embrace the outer ankle. Behind this, they unite into a single trunk, which ascends obliquely, approaching the tendo Achillis, and proceeds vertically towards the ham to open into the popliteal vein.

SAPHÈNE, Saphena.
SAPHE'NOUS, *Sapheno'sus*; from *Saphène*. Of or belonging to the saphena.
SAPHENOUS NERVES are two in number, and are branches of the crural or femoral nerve. They are the *short saphenous — nervus cutaneous internus;* and the *long saphenous, — nervus cutaneous internus longus.*

The *external saphenous*, formed by the union of the communicans popliteal and communicans peronei, passes down the leg by the side of the external saphenous vein of the foot.
SAPID, *Sa'porous*, *Sap'idus*, (F.) *Savoureux.* Possessed of sapidity. Having the power of affecting the organs of taste.
SAPID'ITY, *Sap'idness*, *Saporos'ity*, *Sapor*, (F.) *Sapidité*, from *sapere*, 'to taste.' The quality of bodies that gives them taste.
SAPIN COMMUN, Pinus picea.
SAPIN'DUS, *S. Sapona'ria*, *Sapona'ria*, *Soap Tree*, (F.) *Savonnier commun*. The name of the plant that affords the *Soap Nuts*, *Sapona'riæ Nu'culæ*, *Bac'cæ Bermuden'ses*, *Soap-berries*. A spherical fruit about the size of a cherry, the cortical part of which is yellow, glossy, and so transparent as to show the spherical black nut that rattles within, and includes a white kernel. The cortical part of this fruit, which has similar effects with soap in washing, has been recommended in chlorosis, and as a stomachic and deobstruent.

SAPO, *Soap*, Sax. ɼape, *Smegma*, (F.) *Savon*. A product obtained by treating fatty bodies with caustic alkalies dissolved in water. In the Pharmacopœia of the United States, it means Soap made with soda and olive oil.

YELLOW SOAP is formed of turpentine, oil, and alkali.

Castile Soap, being made of fine olive oil, is generally used internally. The yellow and soft soaps are the most stimulating; and are, consequently, best adapted for particular cutaneous eruptions.

Internally, soap is purgative and diuretic; externally, it is detergent and stimulant. Soapy water is used with the greatest success, in cases of poisoning by acids. It is mostly applied externally to bruises and sprains. In *Pharmacy*, it is used to favour the solution of resins.

SAPO AC''IDUS, *Acid Soap*, is a combination of a fixed oil with an acid.
SAPO AMMONIACALIS, Linimentum ammoniæ fortius—s. Ammoniæ oleaceus, Linimentum ammoniæ fortius — s. Amygdalinus, Sapo medicinalis — s. Cacaotinus, Sapo cocaneus — s. Calcarius, Linimentum aquæ calcis — s. Castiliensis, see Sap Medicinalis.
SAPO COCO'NEUS, *Soap of Cocoa-Nut Oil, S. cacaoti'nus*, (F.) *Savon de cacoa*, has been much used in Germany in herpetic affections.
SAPO DURUS, S. Hispanicus — s. Hispanicus, see S. medicinalis.
SAPO KALICUS, S. Mollis.
SAPO LIQ'UIDUS, *Liquid Soap*, *Lotio sapona'cea*, is a cosmetic which is composed of olive oil

℥iv, ol. tartari per deliquium ℥ss. Rub together, and add aquæ rosarum ℥xij.

SAPO MEDICINA'LIS, *Medic"inal Soap, Sapo amygdali'nus*, (F.) *Savon médicinal*, is made with oil of sweet almonds and half its weight of caustic alkali, or, like the *Sapo Hispani'cus* seu *Castilien'sis*, Spanish or *Castile soap, Sapo durus*, (F.) *Savon dur*, of olive oil and soda.

SAPO MOLLIS, *Common* or *Soft Soap, S. vir'idis, S. ni'ger, S. ka'licus*, (F.) *Savon mou, Savon noir*, is made of potass and oil or tallow. The *Sapo vulgaris*, or 'common soap' of the Pharm. U. S. is made with soda and animal oil.

SAPO NIGER, *Black Soap, Melanosmeg'ma*, is a composition of train oil and an alkali: and GREEN SOAP, *Sapo vir'idis*, of hempseed, linseed, or rape oil, with an alkali. See Sapo mollis.

SAPO VEGETABILIS, *Pulvis gummosus alkalinus* — s. Viridis, Sapo mollis — s. Vulgaris, see Sapo mollis.

SAPONA'CEOUS; *Sapona'ceus;* from *Sapo*, 'soap.' Soapy. Containing soap, as *Linimentum saponaceum*, Soap liniment.

SAPONAIRE, Saponaria.

SAPONA'RIA, from *Sapo*, 'soap.' *Soap-wort, Bruise-wort, Stru'thium, Luna'ria, Lychnis sylves'tris, Ibix'uma, Bootia vulga'ris Lychnis officina'lis*, (F.) *Saponaire. Family*, Caryophylleæ. *Sex. Syst.* Decandria Digynia. A decoction of the leaves of this plant has been recommended in scrofula, cancer, old syphilis, cutaneous eruptions, jaundice, visceral obstructions, &c. It is hardly ever used.

SAPONARIA, Sapindus saponaria.

SAPONARIÆ NUCULÆ, see Sapindus saponaria.

SAPO'NEA, from *Sapo*, 'soap.' A pectoral medicine, prepared with sweetened syrup of violets, and oil of sweet almonds.

SAPON'ULES, *Sapon'uli*, (F.) *Savonules*. Same etymon. Combinations of volatile or essential oils with different bases.

ACID SAPONULES are combinations of such oils with different acids.

SAPOR, Sapidity, Savour.
SAPOROSITY, Sapidity.
SAPOROUS, Sapid.

SAPO'TA, *Achras Sapota* seu *austra'lie* seu *Zapota, Sapota alchras, El nispero, Oval-fruited Sapota*, (F.) *Sapotier, Sapotillier, Sapotilla. Fam.* Sapoteæ. *Sex. Syst.* Hexandria Digynia. A tree which grows in the Antilles, and particularly at St. Domingo. Its fruit is much esteemed. It resembles the marmalade of quinces; and hence has been called *natural marmalade*. The seeds make an emulsion, which has been given in nephritic affections. The bark has been recommended as a febrifuge.

SAPOTA ALCHRAS, Sapota.
SAPOTIER, Sapota.
SAPOTILLA, Sapota.
SAPOTILLIER, Sapota.
SAPROPYRA, Typhus gravior.
SAPROS, Putrid, Rancid.

SAPROS'TOMUS, from σαπρος, 'foul, of a bad odour,' and στομα, 'mouth.' One who has an offensive breath.

SAPROTES, Putrefaction.

SAR'APUS, *Sarapous*. One who has a large foot; whose toes are largely separated, or whose feet are much asunder in walking; from σαιρω, 'I grin,' and πους, 'the foot.' See Kyllosis.

SARATO'GA, MINERAL WATERS OF. The Saratoga springs in New York are ten miles north-east from Ballston. They contain the same ingredients as those of the latter place; and are much frequented by visitors from every part of the United States. The following analysis has been given of the *Congress spring*. In a wine gallon — *gaseous contents*: carbonic acid, 311 cubic inches; atmospheric air, 7. *Solid contents*. Chloride of sodium, gr. 385; iodide of sodium, gr. 3.5; bicarbonate of soda, gr. 8.952; bicarbonate of magnesia, 95.788; carbonate of lime, 98.098; carbonate of iron, 5.075; silica, 1.5; bromide of potassium, a trace. Total gr. 597.943. — Steel.

The *Walton* or *Iodine spring* contains chloride of sodium, carbonate of magnesia, and iodide of sodium.

SARCEPIPLOCELE, Sarcoëpiplocele.
SARCEPIPLOMPHALOCELE, Sarcoëpiplomphacele.
SARCEPIPLOMPHALUS, Sarcoëpiplomphalus.
SARCIDIUM, Caruncle.
SARCINA, Fœtus.

SAR'CINA VENTRIC'ULI, *Sarcina*, 'a pack, a woolpack.' A microscopic cryptogamous plant found in the fluid of waterbrash.

SARCION, Caruncle.
SARCITES, Anasarca — s. Flatuosus, Emphysema.
SARCITIS, Myositis.

SARCOCE'LE, *Hernia carno'sa, Scirrhus Testic'uli*, from σαρξ, 'flesh,' and κηλη, 'a tumour,' *Sarco'ma scroti*, (F.) *Hernie charnue*. Scirrhus or cancer of the testicle. This disease affects adults particularly; and appears most commonly after an inflammatory swelling of the testicle. Sometimes it is dependent upon a blow; at others, it makes its appearance without any appreciable cause. It is well known by a hard, heavy, ovoid or spherical swelling of the testicle, which is, at first, slightly, or not at all painful, and merely causes an unpleasant traction on the spermatic cord. There is no heat or change of colour of the skin; the spermatic cord is swollen, and participates in the affection; very painful shootings occur; the lymphatic glands of the abdomen become swollen, and form a tumour, which may, at times, be felt through the abdomen; and the patient, at length, dies with every sign of the cancerous diathesis. The prognosis is very unfavourable. The only means, indeed, that can save life is the extirpation of the testicle.

SARCOCOL'LA, (F.) *Colle-chair*, from σαρξ, 'flesh,' and κολλα, 'glue.' A resinous matter, obtained from *Pena'a Sarcocol'la, P. mucronata* and other species of Penæa. An African shrub which has been so called from a belief that it facilitates the consolidation of flesh. It is in the form of small, oblong, semitransparent globules of a yellowish or reddish blue, and smells like aniseed. It was once employed as an astringent and detergent.

SARCODES, Carneous.

SARCOËPIPLOCE'LE, *Sarcepiploce'le*, from σαρξ, 'flesh,' επιπλοον, 'the epiploon,' and κηλη, 'a tumour.' Epiplocele, complicated with sarcoma or sarcocele.

SARCOËPIPLOM'PHALUS, *Sarcepiplomphalus, Sarcepiplomphaloce'le*, from σαρξ, 'flesh,' επιπλοον, 'the epiploon,' and ομφαλος, 'the navel.' Umbilical hernia, formed by scirrhous epiploon or complicated with sarcoma.

SARCOHYDROCELE, Hydro-sarcocele.

SARCOLEM'MA, *Sarcole'ma*, from σαρξ, 'flesh,' and λεμμα, 'a coat.' The sheath which surrounds the fibrils of muscle that form a fibre. It is quite distinct from the areolar membrane that binds the fibres into fasciculi. — BOWMAN. See Perymisium.

SARCOLOGIA, Myology.

SARCOL'OGY, *Sarcolog"ia*, from σαρξ, 'flesh,' and λογος, 'a discourse.' The part of anatomy which treats of the soft parts. It comprises myology, angiology, neurology, and splanchnology.

SARCO'MA, *Emphy'ma Sarcoma, Sarcom'atous tumour, Sarco'sis, Porrus, Sarcophy'ia, Ecsarco'ma, Exsarco'ma, Tumor car'neus, Excrescen'tia carno'sa, Pol'ypus carno'sus*, from σαρξ, 'flesh.' Any species of excrescence having a fleshy consistence.

SARCOMA, CARCINOMATOUS, Scirrhus — s. Cercosis, see Cercosis — s. Epulis, Epulis — s. Mastoid, Mammary sarcoma — s. Medullare, see Encephaloid — s. Medullary Encephaloid, Hæmatodes fungus — s. Pulpy, Hæmatodes fungus — s. Scroti, Sarcocele.

SARCOMA, COMMON VASCULAR or ORGANIZED of Abernethy, *Emphy'ma Sarcoma Vasculo'sum*, is vascular throughout: texture simple: when bulky, napped on the surface with arborescent veins. Found over the body and limbs generally.

SARCOMATEUX, Sarcomatous.
SARCOMATODES, Sarcomatous.
SARCOMATOSUS, Sarcomatous.
SARCOM'ATOUS, *Sarcomato'sus, Sarcomato'des*, (F.) *Sarcomateux*. Belonging to, or having the characters of sarcoma.

SARCOMPHALUM, Sarcomphalus.
SARCOM'PHALUS, *Sarcom'phalum*, from σαρξ, 'flesh,' and ομφαλος, 'the navel.' A scirrhous or *fleshy* tumour, developed at the navel.

SARCOMYCES, Sarcospongus.
SARCOPHAGUS, Carnivorous, Catheretic.
SARCOPHYIA, Excrescence, Sarcoma.
SARCOPTE, Acarus.
SARCOPTES SCABIEI, see Psora.
SARCOPYO'DES, from σαρξ, 'flesh,' πυον, 'pus,' and ειδος, 'resemblance.' Having the appearance of pus mixed with flesh. An epithet given to certain excreted matters, and particularly to the sputa of those labouring under consumption.

SARCO'SIS, from σαρξ, 'flesh.' The formation of flesh. Also, sarcoma.
SARCO'SIS BULBI, *Exophthal'mia fungo'sa seu sarcomat'ica*. A fleshy growth from the lobe of the eye.

SARCOSIS UTERI, Metrauxe.
SARCOSPONG'US, *Sarcomy'ces*, from σαρξ, 'flesh,' and σπογγος, 'fungus.' A fleshy fungus.
SARCOSTOSIS, Osteo-sarcoma.
SARCOTIC, Incarnans.
SARCOUS, from σαρξ, 'flesh.' Of, or belonging to, flesh or muscle — as '*sarcous tissue*.'
SARCOUS ELEMENTS, *Prim'itive par'ticles*. The elementary particles, which, by their union, form the mass of muscular fibre. — Bowman.
SARDIASIS, Canine laugh, Risus sardonicus.
SARDONIASIS, Canine laugh, Risus sardonicus.
SARE, Essera.
SARRASIN, Polygonum fagopyrum.
SARRÊTE, Trismus infantum.
SARRIETTE, Satureia hortensis — *s. de Crête*, Satureia capitata.
SARSA, Smilax sarsaparilla.
SARSAPARILLA, Smilax S. — s. False, Aralia nudicaulis.
SARSAPARIL'LA GERMAN'ICA, *Gramen major, G. rubrum, Salsaparil'la Germanica, Carex Arena'ria*, (F.) *Laiche, L. des Sables, Salsepareille d'Allemagne*. Family, Cyperoideæ. *Sex. Syst*. Monœcia Triandria. A plant, which grows plentifully on the sea-coasts of Europe. It has been recommended in some mucous affections of the trachea, in rheumatism, gout, &c.

SARSAPARILLA, INDIAN, Hemidesmus Indicus.
SARTAPARILLA, Smilax sarsaparilla.
SARTO'RIUS, from *sartor*, 'a tailor,' because used in crossing the legs. *Suto'rius, Longis'simus Fem'oris, Fascia'lis, F. Longus* seu *suto'rius*, (F.) *Il'io-cresti-tibial, Ilio-prétibial* (Ch.), *Couturier*. A muscle, situate at the anterior part of the thigh. It is long, small, and flattened, and extends, obliquely, from the anterior and superior spine of the ilium to the superior and inner part of the tibia. This muscle can, also, bend the pelvis on the thigh, and conversely.

SARX, Flesh, Pulp.
SARZA, Smilax sarsaparilla.
SASSAFRAS, Laurus sassafras — s. Medulla, see Laurus sassafras — s. Radicis cortex, see Laurus sassafras — s. Swamp, Magnolia glauca.
SAT'ELLITE, *Satelles*. That which guards. That which is placed near.
SATELLITE VEINS are those that accompany arteries.
SATHE, Penis.
SATIES, Satiety.
SATIETAS, Plesmone.
SATI'ETY, *Sati'etas, Satu'ritas, Sa'ties, Satura'tio, Plethos, Plesmonē*, from *satiare* (itself from *satis*, 'enough'), 'to give enough.' Disgust for food; commonly produced by repletion.
SATIN, Lunaria rediviva.
SATURANS, Absorbent (medicine).
SATURATIO, Satiety, Saturation.
SATURA'TION, *Satura'tio*, from *satis*, 'enough.' The state of a compound in which its elements are combined in such proportions that a fresh quantity of either cannot be added without producing excess.
SATUREI'A CAPITA'TA, *Cil'iated Sa'vory, Thymus, .Thymus sylves'tris* seu *capita'tus, Thymus Cret'icus, Cuni'la*, (F.) *Sarriette de Crète*. Possesses similar properties to thyme.
SATUREI'A HORTEN'SIS, *Satureia, S. sati'va, Cuni'la sativa Plin'ii, Thymbra, Summer Sa'vory*, (F.) *Sarriette. Family*, Labiatæ. *Sex. Syst*. Didynamia Gymnospermia. An aromatic plant, cultivated for culinary purposes. It has been used, as an excitant, in anorexia, anaphrodisia, &c.
SATUREIA ORIGANOIDES, Cunila mariana — s. Sativa, S. hortensis.
SATURITAS, Satiety.
SATURNI DULCEDO, Plumbi superacetas.
SAT'URNINE, *Saturni'nus*, from *saturnus*, 'lead.' Containing or caused by lead.
SATURNINE BREATH. The peculiar odour of the breath in one labouring under Saturnismus.
SATURNISM'US, *Intoxica'tio* seu *Cachex'ia saturni'na*, from *saturnus*, 'lead.' Poisoning by lead; lead-poisoning; saturnine cachexy.
SATURNUS, Plumbum.
SATYRI'ASIS, from Σατυρος, 'a Satyr;' because the Satyrs are said to have been greatly addicted to venery. *Satyrias'mus, Satyri'mus, Priapis'mus, Salac"itas, Brachu'na, Aras'con, Satyri'asis furens, Lagne'sis Salac"itas, Lagnesis furor masculi'nus, Lagne'a, Lagni'a, Lagno'sis, Lasciv'ia, Lasciv'itas, Tenti'go vere'tri*. An irresistible desire, in man, to have frequent connexion with females, accompanied by the power of doing so without exhaustion. The causes are commonly obscure. Sometimes, the abuse of aphrodisiacs has occasioned it. The principal symptoms are: — almost constant erection; irresistible and almost insatiable desire for venery; frequent nocturnal pollutions. Cold lotions; the cold bath; a mild diet; active exercise, &c., are the only means that can be adopted for its removal.

SATYRIASIS FURENS, Satyriasis.

SATYRIASMUS, Satyriasis.
SATYRION, Orchis mascula.
SATYRISMUS, Satyriasis.
SATYRIUM, Goodyera pubescens.
SAUCE-ALONE, Alliaria.
SAUCE, GREEN, Rumex scutatus.
SAUER KRAUT (G.), 'sour cabbage,' (F.) *Chou-croûte*. A culinary preparation, made with chopped cabbage, left to attain an incipient state of acetous fermentation. It is reputed by the Germans to be salubrious, easy of digestion, and eminently antiscorbutic.

SAUGE, Salvia — *s. des Bois*, Teucrium scordium — *s. Grande*, Salvia sclarea — *s. Hormin*, Salvia horminum — *s. de Jérusalem*, Pulmonaria — *s. Petite*, Salvia — *s. Sclarée*, Salvia sclarea.

SAULE, Salix.
SAUMURE, Muria.
SAUNDERS, RED, Pterocarpus santalinus — *s.* Tree, Pterocarpus santalinus — *s.* Yellow, Santalum album.

SAURA, Lizard.
SAURU'RUS CER'NUUS, *Lizard's Tail*. Indigenous; Order, Saururaceæ; flowering in June. It has been used in lumbago.

SAUSAGE POISON, Allantotoxicum.
SAUT, Leap.
SAUVE-VIE, Asplenium ruta muraria.
SAVEUR, Savour.
SAVINE, Juniperus sabina.
SAVINIER, Juniperus sabina.
SAVON, Sapo — *s. Ammoniacal*, Linimentum ammoniæ fortius — *s. Cacao*, Sapo cocoeneus — *s. Oulcaire*, Linimentum aquæ calcis — *s. Dur*, Sapo durus — *s. Médicinal*, Sapo medicinalis — *s. Mou*, Sapo mollis — *s. Noir*, Sapo mollis.

SAVONNIER COMMUN, Sapindus saponaria.
SAVONULE, Saponulus.
SAVONULUS, Saponulus.
SAVORY, CILIATED, Satureia capitata — *s.* Summer, Satureia hortensis.

SA'VOUR, *Sapor*, *Taste*, (F.) *Saveur*. Quality of bodies, by which they act upon the sense of taste. Chymists, at times, avail themselves of this quality to analyze an unknown substance.

SAVOUREUX, Savoury.
SA'VOURY, *Sap'idus*, (F.) *Savoureux*. An epithet given to bodies that have taste; and particularly to those that excite a very agreeable impression on the organ of taste.

SAVOYAN, Galium verum.
SAW, *Prion*, *Serra*, (Da.) *Sawe*, (Sax.) ɼaga, (F.) *Scie*. A surgical instrument, made like a common saw; and used for sawing the bones in amputations, or for removing exostoses, &c. Saws of different sizes and shapes are used in surgery. The crown of the trepan is nothing more than a species of circular saw.

SAW, AMPUTA'TION, *Serra amputato'ria*. The saw used in amputation.

SAW, HEY'S. An instrument used by Mr. Hey, of Leeds, in fractures of the cranium. It consists of a long handle, to which a small saw with a convex or straight edge is attached, and by which a piece of bone of any shape may be removed. With the trephine, the saw must always be circular.

SAW PALMETTO, Chamærops serratula — *s.* Wort, Liatris.

SAXIFRAGA, Pimpinella saxifraga — *s.* Anglica, Peucedanum silaus.

SAXIF'RAGA CRASSIFO'LIA. *Family*, Saxifrageæ. *Sex. Syst.* Decandria Digynia. The root of this species of saxifrage has been extolled by Pallas, as pre-eminently antiseptic.

SAXIFRAGA GRANULA'TA, *S. alba*, *Sanic'ula*, *Sedum*, *White sax'ifrage*, (F.) *Saxifrage granulée*. Recommended as diuretic and lithontriptic; but not used.

SAXIFRAGA RUBRA, Spiræa filipendula — *s.* Vulgaris, Peucedanum silaus.

SAXIFRAGE, BURNET, Pimpinella saxifraga — *s. Granulée*, Saxifraga granulata — *s.* Meadow, Peucedanum silaus — *s.* White, Saxifraga granulata.

SAXIFRAGUS, Lithontriptic.
SAXON'ICUS PULVIS. A powder, prepared with the roots of the wild and cultivated angelica; the asclepias vincetoxicum, &c. It was considered formerly as an antidote.

SCAB, from *Sca'bies*, and *scabere*, 'to dig.' An incrustation, which forms upon a sore, owing to the concretion of the fluid discharged from it. An eschar.

SCABBY or SCABBED. Covered or diseased with scabs.

SCABIES, Psora — *s.* Agria, Lichen — *s.* Capitis, Porrigo lupinosa, Porrigo scutulata — *s.* Capitis favosa, Porrigo favosa — *s.* Fera, Ecthyma.

SCA'BIES FERI'NA, *Itch of animals*, *Mange*. A cutaneous disease, which affects almost all domestic animals, but especially the horse, sheep, dog, and cow. It is said to have been transmitted to man; but this is questionable.

SCABIES FERINA, Psoriasis — *s.* Papuliformis, Prurigo — *s.* Sicca, Lichen, Psoriasis — *s.* Venerea contagiosa, Scherlievo.

SCABIEUSE ORDINAIRE, Scabiosa.
SCABIOLA, Scabies.
SCABIO'SA, *S. arven'sis*, *Tri'chera arven'sis*, *Field Sca'bious*, (F.) *Scabieuse ordinaire*. *Family*, Dipsaceæ. *Sex. Syst.* Tetrandria Monogynia. The plant is bitter and sub-astringent, and was formerly used in the cure of leprous affections and diseased lungs.

SCABIOSA ARVENSIS, Scabiosa — *s.* Cardifolia, Echinops.

SCABIOSA SUCCI'SA, *Succisa*, *S. praten'sis*, *Asteroceph'alus succisa*, *Morsus Diab'oli*, *Devil's bit*, (F.) *Mors du Diable*, has similar properties.

SCABIOUS, Erigeron Philadelphicum — *s.* Field, Scabiosa — *s.* Sweet, Erigeron heterophyllum.

SCABISH, Œnothera biennis.
SCABRITIES, Lichen.
SCALA, 'a ladder.' A machine formerly used for reducing dislocations of the humerus.

SCALÆ OF THE COCH'LEA, *Gyri* seu *Ductus spira'les* seu *Cana'les cochleæ*, (F.) *Rampes* or *Échelles du Limaçon* — are the cavities in the cochlea, separated from each other by the spiral septum. The one — *Scala inter'na* seu *poste'rior* seu *inferior coch'leæ*, *S. tym'pani* — would communicate with the cavitas tympani by the fenestra rotunda, were it not for the membrane that closes it. The other — *Scala exter'na* seu *anterior* seu *superior coch'leæ*, *S. vestib'uli* — opens into the cavity of the vestibule. The scalæ communicate with each other by an opening at the top of the partition.

SCALA ANTERIOR COCHLEÆ, see Scala — *s.* Clausa, see Scala — *s.* Externa cochleæ, see Scala — *s.* Inferior cochleæ, see Scala — *s.* Interior cochleæ, see Scala — *s.* Posterior cochleæ, see Scala — *s.* Superior cochleæ, see Scala — *s.* Tympani, see Cochlea, and Scala — *s.* Vestibuli, see Cochlea, and Scala.

SCALE, Sax. ꞅcale, from ꞅcylan, 'to divide, separate;' (G.) Schale, 'shell, peel;' schälen, 'to shell, to peel.' *Squama*, *Lepis*, (F.) *Écaille*, *Écaille*. An opake and thickened lamina of cuticle; commonly produced by some degree of

Inflammation of the true skin, over which it is formed.

SCALE, DRY, Psoriasis.

SCALÈNE ANTÉRIEUR, Scalenus anticus —s. Postérieur, Scalenus posticus.

SCALE'NUS, 'irregular or unequal.' Geometers employ this word to designate a triangle whose three sides are unequal. Anatomists have given the name to two muscles. 1. SCALENUS ANTI'CUS, *Portion of the Costo-trachelian* (Ch.), (F.) *Scalène antérieur*, is situate at the internal and inferior parts of the neck. It is long and triangular; and is inserted, below, at the upper surface of the first rib; and, above, at the anterior tubercle of the transverse processes of the 3d, 4th, 5th, and 6th cervical vertebræ. This muscle bends the neck, and draws it to its side. It can also raise the first rib. 2. SCALENUS POSTI'CUS, (F.) *Scalène postérieur, Portion of the Costo-trachelian* (Ch.), is situate behind the last. It is, also, long and triangular; but more bulky than the *S. anticus*. It is attached, below, to the outer surface of the first two ribs; and terminates, above, at the summit of the transverse processes of the last six vertebræ of the neck. This muscle bends the neck laterally, and can elevate the first two ribs. Some anatomists, as Albinus and Sömmering, have described five scaleni muscles on each side, and have called them *Scalenus prior, S. min'imus, S. latera'lis, S. me'dius, S. posti'cus*. Riolan and Chaussier only describe one scalenus muscle on each side. Cowper and Douglas, and the generality of the English anatomists, admit three, *S. anti'cus, me'dius*, and *posti'cus;* or, *primus, secuu'dus*, and *ter'tius;* Winslow, Boyer, and many of the French anatomists, — two, as above described.

SCALING—same etymon as Scale—in dentistry, is an operation, which consists in removing the tartar from the teeth.

SCALL, Impetigo—s. Asbestos, see Eczema of the hairy scalp—s. Dry, Psoriasis—s. Honeycomb, Porrigo favosa—s. Milky, Porrigo larvalis —s. Running, Impetigo—s. Running, Eczema—s. Washerwoman's, Psoriasis diffusa.

SCALLED HEAD, Porrigo scutulata.

SCALP, Teut. Schelpe, 'a shell.' The integuments covering the head. The *hairy scalp* is called, also, *Capillit''ium, Tricho'ton*, (F.) *Chevelure.*

SCALPEL, *Scalpel'lum, Scalpel'lus, Culter, Inciso'rium, Smi'leon;* from *scalpo*, 'I rasp, I cut.' A cutting instrument, formed of a blade of well-tempered steel, very sharp, of variable shape and size, and fixed solidly in a handle. Its use is to divide the soft parts in operations, dissection, &c.

SCALPELLUM, Scalpel—s. Lenticulare, Phacopis.

SCALPELLUS, *Bistouri*, Scalpel.

SCALPEUM, *Bistouri.*

SCALPRUM, Raspatorium — s. Chirurgicum, Lancet.

SCALPRUM DENTA'RIUM, *Lima denta'ria.* A tooth-file. A file used by the dentist.

SCALPRUM RASORIUM, Raspatorium.

SCALY, Squamous.

SCALY DISEASES or SQUAMÆ, *Lepido'ses*, form the second order in Willan and Bateman's system of cutaneous diseases.

SCAMMA, Fossa.

SCAMMONÉE D'ALEP, Convolvulus scammonia.

SCAMMONIUM, see Convolvulus scammonia —s. Syriacum, Convolvulus scammonia.

SCAMMONY, Convolvulus scammonia—s. of Montpellier, Cynanchum Monspeliacum.

SCAMNON HIPPOC'RATIS, *Bathron Hippocrati'on* of Galen, (F.) *Banc d'Hippocrate.* A machine invented by Hippocrates for reducing fractures. It was a sort of bed, six feet long, on which the patient was fixed. Straps were attached above and below the fracture or luxation, and extension and counter-extension were effected by a winch. It is described in Galen, Oribasius, Scultetus, &c. See Bathron.

SCANDIX, S. cerefolium.

SCANDIX BULBOCASTANUM, Bunium bulbocastanum.

SCANDIX CEREFO'LIUM, *Scandix, Scandyx, Pecten Ven'eris, Cerefolium, Daucus Seprin'ius, Chærophyl'lum*, Ch. *Sati'vum* seu *Cerefo'lium, Anthris'cus cerefolium, Chærefo'lium, Chervil*, (F.) *Cerfeuil. Family*, Umbelliferæ. *Sex. Syst.* Pentandria Digynia. A culinary herb, which is slightly aromatic and grateful. It is said to be gently aperient and diuretic.

SCANDIX ODORA'TA, *Sweet Cic''ely.* Properties the same as the other. Also, Chærophyllum odoratum.

SCANDULARIUS MUSCULUS, Parathenar, Transversus pedis.

SCANDYX, Scandix cerefolium.

SCAPHA, *Scaphus,* 'a skiff or cock-boat,' from σκαπτω, 'I make hollow.' The excavation or cavity of the external ear, between the helix and anthelix. The meatus auditorius externus. The rima vulvæ. Also the name of a bandage for the head, mentioned by Galen, and called, likewise, *Tholus Diocle'us.*

SCAPHIA, Nates.

SCAPHION, Cranium, Papaver (Capsule).

SCA'PHIUM OCULA'RE, *Pelvis Ocula'ris, Eye-glass*, (F.) *Bassin oculaire, Gondole oculaire, Œillière.* A small porcelain, glass or metallic vessel, used for applying lotions to the eye.

SCAPHO - CARPO - SUPER-PHALANGEUS POLLICIS, Abductor pollicis brevis.

SCAPHOID, *Scaphoï'des*, from σκαφη, 'a skiff,' and ειδος, 'form.' A name given to several parts.

SCAPHOID FOSSA, *Fossa Scaphoï'des*, (F.) *Enfoncement Scaphoïde.* A small cavity at the upper part of the internal ala of the pterygoid process, in which the peristaphylinus internus is attached.

SCAPHOID BONE OF THE HAND, *Os Scaphoïdes Manûs, Os navicula'rē, Os cymbifor'mē, Boat-like bone,* (F.) *Scaphoïde de la main.* The first bone of the first row of the carpus. The upper surface is convex, and articulated with the radius. The under and outer surfaces are also convex,—to be articulated with the trapezium and trapesoides. Between the upper and under cartilaginous surfaces there is a *rough fossa* for the insertion of the capsular ligament. The anterior and inner surface has an *oval cavity*, where it is articulated with the os magnum, which gives name to the bone. There is a *process* on the outer end of the bone, for the attachment of part of the anterior transverse ligament of the wrist.

SCAPHOID BONE OF THE FOOT, *Os Scaphoïdes Pedis, Os navicula'rē, Os cymbifor'mē, Boat-like bone*, (F.) *Scaphoïde du Pied.* This bone is situate at the forepart of the astragalus and inner part of the foot. The *posterior surface* forms a cavity, somewhat like that of a boat, for receiving the head of the astragalus. There is a prominence at the inner side of the bone, for the insertion of tendons, muscles, and strong ligaments. The forepart of the bone is convex, and divided into three articular surfaces for articulation with the ossa cuneiformia. Between the os naviculare and astragalus, the foot has its principal lateral and rotary motions; although each of the other joints of the tarsus contributes a little. Part of the tibialis posticus is inserted into it.

SCAPHOÏDE DE LA MAIN, Os scaphoides manûs—s. du Pied. Os scaphoides pedis.

SCAPHOÏDO-ASTRAG'ALAN, *Scaphoïdo-astragala'nus.* That which relates to the scaphoid bone and astragalus. The articulation of these bones is so called; and the ligament which strengthens it is termed the *Scaphoïdo-astragalan ligament.*

SCAPHOÏDO-CUBOID, *Scaphoïdo-cuboïdæ'us.* That which relates to the scaphoid and cuboid bones. The articulation of those bones is so called.

SCAPHULA, Navicularis fossa.

SCAPHUS, Auditory canal, external, Rima vulvæ, Scapha.

SCAP'ULA, *Scap'ulum, Plata, Omopla'ta, Homoplata, Scop'tula, Epino'tion, Latitu'do hu'meri, Omop'latē, Os latum hu'meri, Scutum thora'cis seu cordis, Spath'ula, Pteryg'ium, Chelo'nium, Spat'ula;* the Blade-bone, the Shoulder-blade, (F.) *Omoplate.* An irregular, broad, flat bone, of a triangular shape, situate at the posterior part of the shoulder. It has, 1. A *posterior* or *dorsal surface* or *Dorsum, Testu'do scap'ulæ,* divided transversely into two parts, by a triangular process, called *Spine of the Scapula;* which terminates by a considerable eminence, called *Acromion.* Above the spine, is the *Fossa supra-spinata;* below it, the *F. infra-spinata.* 2. An *anterior* or *costal surface,* or *venter,* forming the *Fossa subscapularis.* 3. A *superior* or *cervical edge,* which is thin, and terminates, anteriorly, by a strong, curved apophysis, called the *coracoid process.* 4. A *posterior* or *vertebral edge,* called, also, the *base.* 5. An *outer* or *axillary* or *inferior edge,* having a thick, truncated angle, in which is the *glenoid cavity.* With this is articulated the head of the humerus. The glenoid cavity is separated from the body of the bone by a narrower part, called the *cervix* or *neck.* The edges or margins are, also, called *costæ.* The scapula has three angles — an *inferior, superior,* and *anterior.*

SCAPULA, Humerus.

SCAPULÆ NASI, *Partes latera'les nasi.* The lateral parts of the nose.

SCAPULAL'GIA; from *scapula,* 'the shoulder-blade,' and αλγος, 'pain.' Arthralgia of the shoulder-joint.

SCAP'ULAR, *Scap'ulary, Scapula'ris,* from *scapula,* 'the shoulder-blade.' That which relates or belongs to the scapula.

SCAPULAR APONEURO'SIS. A broad, thin aponeurosis, with decussating fibres; which is attached, *above,* to the spine of the scapula; *below,* to a crest between the teres major and infra-spinatus; *within,* to the spinal edge of the scapula; and which, at its middle, unites with the thin aponeurosis that covers a part of the external surface of the deltoid.

SCAPULAR ARTERIES. These are several. a. The *Superior scapular, Superficial scapular* of Sömmering, *Dorsa'lis scapulæ superior, Transversa'lis scapulæ, T. Hu'meri.* This arises from the subclavian; and often from the inferior thyroid, or from a trunk common to it and the *posterior scapular* or *transverse scapular* or *cervical.* It passes behind the clavicle, above the superior edge of the scapula, and buries itself between the dorsal surface of that bone and the muscles inserted into it. b. The *inferior scapular* or *common scapular* or *internal scapular* or *subscapular artery, A. Thorac''ica axilla'ris* vel *ala'ris,* is of considerable size. It arises from the inferior part of the axillary artery, behind the brachial plexus gives off severa' branches to the armpit, and divides into two branches:—the one, *Scapula'ris interna,* and the smaller of the two, is distributed, almost entirely, to the serratus major anticus, and latissimus dorsi; the other, the larger of the two, the *Dorsa'lis Scap'ulæ inferior* vel *Circumflex'a Scapula'ris,* which distributes its branches to the subscapular and supra-spinal, and infra-spinal regions.

SCAPULAR NOTCH, see Notch, scapular.

SCAPULAR VEINS follow the same course as the arteries, which they accompany.

SCAPULARE, Scapulary.

SCAP'ULARY, *Scapula'rē, Fascia Scopula'ris,* from *scapula.* A broad, linen bandage, divided into two tails for three quarters of its length, the undivided extremity of which is attached to the posterior and middle part of a bandage carried round the body; the tails passing over the shoulders; and being attached to the anterior part of the body bandage, to prevent it from slipping down.

SCAP'ULO-HU'MERAL. An epithet given to the *shoulder-joint.* It is an orbicular articulation, resulting from the reception of the head of the humerus into the glenoid cavity of the scapula. To keep the bones in connexion, there are: 1. A very strong, conoidal capsular ligament; passing from the circumference of the glenoid cavity around the neck of the humerus. 2. A *fibro-cartilaginous ring,* called the glenoid ligament, and a synovial capsule.

SCAPULO-HUMÉRAL, Teres major—s. Huméro-olécranien, Triceps extensor cubiti—s. Hyoïdien, Omohyoideus — s. *Radial,* Biceps flexor cubiti—s. *Trochitérien, grand,* Infra-spinatus.

SCAPUS, Penis, see Hair.

SCAR, Cicatrix.

SCAR, Seam. To mark with a cicatrix or seam.

SCARABÆO'LUS HEMISPHÆRICUS, Cœcus cacti.

SCAR'BOROUGH, MINERAL WATERS OF. *Scarborough Spa.* A celebrated English chalybeate, at Scarborough, in Yorkshire. One of the springs is a simple, carbonated chalybeate, like that of Tunbridge: the other has an admixture of purging salt. Scarborough, having the additional advantage of sea-bathing, is much frequented by invalids.

SCARDAMYG'MUS, *Scardamyx'is,* (F.) *Clignement,* from σκαρδαμυσσειν, 'to wink.' Winking, nictation.

SCARIFICA'TION, *Scarifica'tio* (Galen.) *Amyx'is, Schasis, Catacas'mus, Catachas'rus, Amyg'mus, Schasmus, Encharax'is,* from σκαριφεομαι, 'to make a slight scratch.' The act of scarifying. Also, a small incision, *Am'ychē,* made into the skin with a lancet, bistoury, or scarificator, for different therapeutical purposes,—as to draw blood, or to discharge some effused fluid. When the scarifications are very superficial, and do not go farther than the skin, they are termed by the French, *Mouchetures.*

SCARIFICA'TOR, *Scarificato'rium, Schasterium.* An instrument for making scarifications. It consists of a small brass box, of a cubical shape, in which 10 or 12 lancet points turn upon a common pivot. By means of a spring, all these blades can be made to issue at once, and make as many scarifications.

SCARIFICATORIUM, Scarificator.

SCARIOLA, Cichorium endivia, Lactuca scariola.

SCARIOLE, Cichorium endivia.

SCARLATA, Scarlatina.

SCARLATI'NA, from *scarlatto* (I.) 'a deep red.' *Scarlata, Enanthe'sis Rosa'lia, Rosa'lia, Rossa'lia, R. squamo'sa, Rosa'lia, Rube'ola,* d some, *Morbil'li ig'nei*, *M. confluen'tes*, *Morbus scarlatino'sus*, *Febris scarlatino'sa*, *Gut'turis morbus epidem'icus Forest'i*, *Pur'pura*, *Typhus scarlati"nus*, *Febris rubra*, *Scarlet Fever*, *Rash-fever*, *Porphyris'mus*, *Porphyris'ma*, (F.) *Fièvre rouge*, *F. pourprée*. The characteristic symptoms of scarlatina are:—a scarlet flush, appearing about the second day of fever on the face, neck, and fauces; and progressively spreading over the body; terminating about the 7th day. Two great varieties may be reckoned;—the *S. simplex*, *S. febris*, *S. benig'na*, *S. sine angi'nâ*, in which the fever is moderate and terminates with the efflorescence; prostration of strength being trifling, and the contagious property slight;—and the *S. Angino'sa*, *S. Paristhmit'ica*, *S. Cynanch'ica*, *S. mit"ior*, in which the fever is severe; the throat ulcerated; the eruption later in its appearance, and less extensive; often changing to a livid hue; the fever being highly contagious. *Scarlati'na malig'na*, *S. gra'vior*, has been reckoned a variety of this, in its worst degree. It agrees with the Cynanche maligna of Cullen.

Scarlatina belongs to the *Major exanthemata*, and is a disease, chiefly, of children. The eruption differs from that of measles, in being an efflorescence not raised above the cuticle. Measles, too, is attended with catarrhal symptoms, whilst the complication, in scarlatina, is cynanche. The treatment of simple scarlatina need not be much. It must be antiphlogistic. If the throat be very much ulcerated, acid gargles and counter-irritants must be employed; and if the affection become manifestly typhoid, and the sore throat of a malignant character, the case must be treated like typhus gravior; with antiseptic gargles of bark, acid, &c. Anasarca sometimes supervenes on scarlatina, and requires attention Purgatives are here demanded as well as the use of sorbefacients, such as mercury and squill, &c.

SCARLATINA ANGINOSA, see Scarlatina—s. Benigna, see Scarlatina—s. Cynanchica, see Scarlatina—s. Febris, see Scarlatina—s. Gravior, see Scarlatina—s. Miliaris, Rubeola—s. Mitior, see Scarlatina—s. Paristhmitica, see Scarlatina—s. Pustulosa, Rubeola—s. Rheumatica, Dengue—s. sine Anginâ, see Scarlatina—s. Urticata, Urticaria.

SCARLATI'NOUS, *Scarlati'nal*, *Scarlatino'sus*. Relating or appertaining to scarlatina.

SCARLET BERRY, Solanum dulcamara.

SCARLET FEVER, Scarlatina.

SCATACRASIA, Scoracrasia.

SCATACRATIA, Scoracrasia.

SCELAL'GIA, from σκελος, 'the leg,' and αλγος, 'pain.' Pain of the leg.

SCELALGIA ANTICA, Neuralgia femoro-pretibialis—s. Postica, Neuralgia femoro-poplitea—s. Puerperarum, Phlegmatia dolens.

SCELETEU'SIS. Mummification. Also, the mode of making a skeleton, *Skeletopœ'a, Syntax'is*.

SCELETOLOGIA, Skeletology.

SCELETON, Skeleton.

SCELETOPŒA, Sceletensis.

SCELETUM, Skeleton—s. Artificiale, see Skeleton—s. Naturale, see Skeleton.

SCELONCUS, Phlegmatia dolens.

SCELORRHEUMA, *Rheumatis'mus cruris*, from σκελος, 'the leg,' and ρευμα, 'defluxion, rheumatism.' Rheumatism of the leg.

SCELOS, Leg.

SCELOTYRBE, Chorea, Porphyra nautica—s. Febrilis, see Subsultus tendinum—s. Festinans, Paralysis agitans—s. Tarantismus, Chorea.

SCEPARNON, Amnios, Ascia.

SCEPASTERIUM, *Couvrechef*.

SCEPASTRUM, *Couvrechef*.

SCEPTRUM, Penis.

SCHASIS, Scarification.

SCHASMUS, Scarification.

SCHASTERION, Fleam, Lancet, Scarificator.

SCHEBA ARABUM, Artemisia santonica.

SCHERBET', *Sherbet'*, *Scrbet'*, *Tscherbet'*, *Sorbe'thum*, *Sorbet'tum*, *Sorbe'tum*. A drink prepared by the Turks, Persians, &c., with sugar and the juice of acid fruits.

SCHERLIEVO, *Mal di Scherliero*, *Mal di Breno*, *Mal di Fiume*, *Margaretizza*, *Morbus Croatus*, *Frambœ'sia Illyr'ica*, *M. fluminien'sis*, *Falcadina*, *Malo di Scarliero*, *Scabies venerea contagio'sa*. A name given to a particular form of syphilis, observed in Illyria. It is said to be capable of being communicated without immediate contact; and, that its principal symptoms are:—pains in the bones, ulceration of the fauces, pustules, and fungous growths in different parts of the body.

SCHERO'MA. A dryness of the eye from the want of lachrymal secretion.—Dictionaries.

SCHIAS, Neuralgia femoro-poplitæa.

SCHIDAKE'DON, *Schidace'dum*, *Schindace'dum*, *Schindal'amus*, *Schindal'mus*, from σκιζω, 'I cleave.' A longitudinal fracture of a bone.—Galen.

SCHINDACEDUM, Schidakedon.

SCHINDALAMUS, Schidakedon,Schindylesis.

SCHINDALESIS, Schindylesis.

SCHINDALMUS, Schidakedon, Schindylesis.

SCHINDYLE'SIS, *Schindale'sis*, *Schindal'amus*, *Schindal'mus*. An articulation of bones—by furrowing, as it were; as in that of the vomer, which constitutes, in part, the septum narium. Also, the act of splitting into small pieces; from σχινδυλεω, 'I split into small pieces.—Hippocrates.

SCHINELÆ'ON, from σχινος, 'the mastic tree,' and ελαιον, 'oil;' *Oleum lentis'cinum*. Oil of mastic.—Dioscorides.

SCHINOCEPHALUS, Scillocephalus.

SCHINOS, Scilla.

SCHINZNACH or HAPSBURG, MINERAL WATERS OF. These springs are situate three leagues from Baden, and are amongst the most celebrated bathing-places in Switzerland. The waters are of the saline sulphurous kind; and have a high reputation in cutaneous and rheumatic affections, visceral obstructions, and glandular enlargements. They contain sulphate of lime, sulphate of soda, chloride of sodium, chloride of magnesium, sulphate of magnesia, sulphate of lime, carbonate of magnesia, and oxide of iron; sulphohydric acid, and carbonic acid gases.

SCHISMA, Fissure, Rima.

SCHISTOCEPH'ALUS, from σχιστος, 'cleft, separated,' and κεφαλη, 'head.' A monster having some part of the head cleft or fissured.—Gurlt.

SCHISTOCOR'MUS, from σχιστος, 'cleft, separated,' and κορμος, 'trunk.' A monster having some part of the trunk cleft or fissured.—Gurlt.

SCHISTOM'ELUS, from σχιστος, 'cleft, separated, and μελος, 'a limb.' A monster whose limbs are fissured.

SCHISTORRHACHIS, Hydrorachis.

SCHISTOSO'MUS, from σχιστος, 'cleft,' and σωμα, 'body.' A malformation of the abdomen, in which the fissure and eventration extend over the entire length of the abdomen; the lower extremities being absent, or very little developed, so that the body appears as if truncated inferiorly.—Vogel.

SCHIZA, Rima, Rima vulvæ.

SCHIZATRICH'IA, *Trichos'chisis*, *Schiso-*

trich'ia, from σχιζα, 'a cleft,' 'a split,' and θριξ, 'a hair.' The splitting of the hairs at their extremities. — J. P. Frank.

SCHLANGENBAD, MINERAL WATERS OF. Schlangenbad is a much-frequented watering-place in Germany. The waters contain a little carbonic acid, and carbonate of soda. Temperature 86° Fahrenheit.

SCHNEIDERIAN MEMBRANE, Pituitary membrane.

SCHŒNANTHUS, Juncus odoratus.

SCHOLA, School.

SCHOLLERA OXYCOCCOS, Vaccinium oxycoccos.

SCHOOL, *Schola*. A place of education. (F.) *École*. In Europe the large Medical Schools are usually attached to the universities. In England, however, there has been no medical school of celebrity at either of the universities of Oxford or Cambridge; owing greatly to their provincial situation. Of late, two schools have existed in London, attached to the London University — University College and King's College. Excellent private schools have, however, long existed in that metropolis. The medical schools of Europe which have been most celebrated, are those of Edinburgh, Leyden, Berlin, Halle, Tubingen, Paris, Montpellier, Bologna, Padua, Pavia, and Pisa. In the United States, the medical schools are numerous; at this time not fewer than 30 or 40. Those most numerously attended, are the medical department of the University of Pennsylvania, Jefferson Medical College of Philadelphia, the University of the City of New York, and the Louisville Medical Institute.

SCHOOLEY'S MOUNTAIN, MINERAL WATERS OF. The waters of this New Jersey Spring are chalybeate. According to Dr. McNevin, they contain extractive, chloride of sodium, chloride of calcium, chloride of magnesium, carbonate of lime, sulphate of lime, carbonate of magnesia, silex, and carbonate, and oxide of iron.

SCHORBUTUS, Purpura.

SCHOUSBÆA COCCINEA, Cacoucia coccinea.

SCHWALBACH, MINERAL WATERS OF. Schwalbach is a town of Germany, seated on the Aa, 32 miles west of Frankfort. The waters contain chloride of sodium, carbonates of lime and magnesia, iron, sulphate of lime, carbonic acid, oxygen, &c. Employed as a tonic.

SCHWANN, WHITE SUBSTANCE OF, see Substance, white, of Schwann.

SCHWENDECK, MINERAL WATERS OF. These waters are about 5 leagues from Münich, in Bavaria. They contain carbonic acid; carbonate and sulphate of lime, chloride of calcium; chloride of magnesium; carbonate of soda, and oxide of iron, and are much used for cutaneous affections.

SCIAT'IC, *Ischiat'ic*, *Ischiat'icus*, *Sciat'icus*, from ισχιον, 'the haunch.' A word formed by contraction from *ischiatic*, which latter is still used. See Ischiatic.

SCIATIC NERVE, GREAT, *Nervus ischiad'icus, Great fem'oro-poplite'al*, (Ch.) (F.) *Grand nerf sciatique*, ought to be esteemed a continuation of the sacral plexus. It issues from the pelvis between the pyramidalis and superior gemellus; descends along the posterior part of the thigh; and after having given branches to the gemini, quadratus, obturator externus, glutæus maximus, semi-membranosus, semi-tendinosus, biceps and third abductor muscles, it divides, about the inferior third of the thigh, into two branches; the one, named the *external popliteal;* the other, the *internal*.

SCIATIC NERVE, LESSER, *Inferior gla'teal branch of the sacral plexus*, *Lesser fem'oro-poplite'al nerve*, (Ch.) (F.) *Nerf petit sciatique*, which seems especially formed by the 2d and 3d sacral, is given off from the lower part of the plexus, and escapes from the pelvis beneath the pyramidalis muscle. It gives branches — *nervi cuta'nei cis'nium inferio'res* — to the glutæus maximus; a *sciatic branch* or *infra-pelvic cutaneous* or *perineal cutaneous*, *Pudenda'lis longus infe'rior*, which passes under the tuberosity of the ischium, and furnishes filaments to the glutæus maximus, and to the muscles of the perinæum, urethra, penis, scrotum, &c.; and *a posterior femoral cutaneous branch* — *middle posterior cutaneous nerve* — the filaments of which traverse the femoral aponeurosis, to be distributed on the skin of the posterior part of the thigh. The principal branch of the lesser sciatic nerve divides, near the ham, into two or three filaments, which descend under the integuments almost as far as the inferior part of the leg.

SCIATIC NOTCH, GREAT, *Sciatic Fora'men, Ischiu'ra ischiad'ica major*, (F.) *Grande échancrure sciatique ou grand trou sciatique*, is a large notch at the posterior edge of each os innominatum, below the posterior and inferior iliac spine, which is converted into a foramen by the sacrum and sacro-sciatic ligaments. The *lesser sciatic notch, Incisu'ra ischiad'ica minor, Luna Albi'ni,* (F. *Petite échancrure ischiatique*, is much smaller than the last, from which it is separated by the sciatic spine. It gives passage to the tendon of the obturator internus, and to the internal pudic vessels and nerves.

SCIATIC REGION, Ischiadic region.

SCIATIC SPINE, *Spine of the Ischium, Spinous Proc''ess of the Ischium*, is a short, flat, pyramidal eminence on the os innominatum, above the preceding foramen; which gives insertion to the lesser sacro-sciatic ligament.

SCIATICA, Neuralgia femoro-poplitæa.

SCIATIQUE, Neuralgia femoro-poplitæa.

SCIE, Saw.

SCIENTIA HERMETICA, Alchymy—s. Medendi, Medicina — s. Medica, Medicina.

SCIERO'PIA, from σκιερος, 'shady,' and ωψ 'the eye.' A defect of vision, in which all objects have a darker hue than natural.

SCILLA, *Scilla marit'ima, Scylla, Aschil' Schinos, Oc'ulus Typho'nis, Ornithog'alum marit'imum* seu *squil'la, Stella'ris scilla. Squill, Squill* or *sea onion, Eye of Typhon,* (F.) *Ognon marin*. Family, Liliaceæ. *Sex. Syst*. Hexandria Monogynia. Native of Spain, Austria, &c. The bulb or root of the squill has a bitter, nauseous taste, and is extremely acrid; inflaming the skin when rubbed on it. Its acrimony, on which its virtues depend, is destroyed by heat, drying, and keeping. It is extracted by vinegar, spirit, and water. In large doses, squill is emetic and purgative; in small doses, diuretic and expectorant. Its active principle has been called *scillitin*. Dose, gr. j to v of the dried root, united or not with mercury.

SCILLA ESCULEN'TA, *Phalan'gium esculentum, Eastern Quamash, Wild Hy'acinth*; indigenous; flowering in May. An article of diet amongst the Western Indians. It is made into bread and poultices for inflamed breasts.

SCILLOCEPH'ALUS, *Schinoceph'alus*, from σκιλλα, 'a bulbous-rooted plant, the squill,' and κεφαλη, 'head.' One who has a large bulbous head.

SCINCUS, σκιγκος or σκιγγος. A species of *Saurus* or *Lacer'ta*, common in Egypt, and much extolled by the ancients, as alexipharmic and aphrodisiac.

SCINTIL'LA VEN'ERIS, 'a relic of Venus.' A name given, by Paracelsus, to the impotence and loss of power in the limbs, produced by syphilis.

SCIOM'ACHY, *Skioma'chia, Skiamachia;* from σκια, 'a shade,' and μαχη, 'a fight.' An exercise with the ancients, which consisted in a mock encounter at boxing and jumping with one's own shadow.

SCIRRHE, Scirrhus.

SCIRRHOBLEPHARONCUS, see Scleriasis.

SCIRRHOCELE, Orcheocele scirrhosa.

SCIRRHOGAS'TRIA, (F.) *Squirrogastrie; Scirrhus ventric'uli;* from σκιρρος, 'hard,' and γαστηρ, 'stomach.' Scirrhus of the stomach.

SCIR'RHOID, *Scirrhoi'des, Scirrho'des,* from σκιρρος, 'scirrhus,' and ειδος, 'resemblance.' Resembling scirrhus.

SCIRRHOMA, Scirrhus.

SCIRRHOPHTHAL'MIA, *Scirrhophthal'mus,* from σκιρρος, 'scirrhus,' and οφθαλμος, 'the eye,' *Cancer oc'uli.* Cancer of the eye.

SCIRRHOPHTHALMIA PALPEBRARUM, see Scleriasis.

SCIRRHOSARCA NEONATORUM, Induration of the cellular tissue.

SCIRRHOSIS, Scirrhus.

SCIRRHOUS, *Scirrho'sus;* same etymon as scirrhus. Of or belonging to scirrhus.

SCIRRHOUS SARCO'MA OF AB'ERNETHY, *Em'phy'ma sarco'ma scirrho'sum.* Hard, rigid, vascular infarction of glandular follicles; indolent, insentient, glabrous; sometimes shrinking and becoming more indurated. Found in glandulous structures.

SCIRRHUS, *Squirrhus, Scirrho'ma, Scirrho'sis, Cancer scirrho'sus, Carcino'ma simplex, C. fibro'sum, Indura'tio malig'na, Schirrus, Sclerus, Carcinom'atous sarco'ma, Hard cancer, Fibrous cancer;* from σκιρρος, 'hard,' 'indurated;' (F.) *Squirre, Schirre, Skirre.* A disease, so called from the hardness that characterizes it. It is a state of induration, of a peculiar kind, affecting glandular structures generally, but capable of occurring in other textures. It usually precedes carcinoma, of which it may, indeed, be considered as the first stage. Scirrhus must not be confounded with the induration which succeeds inflammation, although the two states are often complicated, and may stand, occasionally, in the relation of cause and effect to each other. Scirrhus is ordinarily accompanied by violent shooting pains. It is also irregular on its surface; and when cut into has a bluish or grayish white colour. When the surgeon is satisfied of the existence of scirrhus, he had better remove it at once. No other treatment seems to possess much advantage.

Galen uses the term *Scirrho'sis* for a livid excrescence caused by inflammation.

SCIRRHUS ET CARCINOMA VENTRICULI, see Gastrostenosis cardiaca et pylorica—s. Hepatis, Hepatoscirrhus—s. Intestinorum, Enteropathia cancerosa—s. Palpebrarum, see Scleriasis—s. Testiculi, Sarcocele—s. Uteri, Metroscirrhus—s. Ventriculi, Gastroscirrhus.

SCISSIPARITÉ, see Generation.

SCISSORS, *Forfex, Forpex, Psalis, Tomis,* (F.) *Ciseaux.* A well-known instrument in common use, and often employed in surgery. Scissors are composed of two cutting blades, crossing each other and moving upon an axis. They are *straight* or *curved.* Sometimes the curve is on the flat side, when they are called, in France, *Ciseaux à cuiller;* at others, on their edges. The scissors, bent so that the blades make an obtuse angle with the handles, are also much used. They are called in France *Ciseaux coudés.* Scissors are used for dividing soft, loose, isolated parts, which it would be difficult to reach and to cut with the bistoury. They are employed, likewise, in the operation for harelip, and for removing warts, fungous excrescences, &c.

SCISSURA, Fissure—s. Vulvæ, see Rima.

SCISSURÆ, Rhagades.

SCISSURE DE GLASER, Fissure, glenoid—s. *Grand médiane du Cervelet,* Valley—*s. de Santorini,* Santorini, fissure of.

SCLAREA, Salvia sclarea.

SCLEREMA, Induration of the cellular tissue.

SCLÉRÈME, Induration of the cellular tissue.

SCLEREMIA, Induration of the cellular tissue.

SCLEREMUS, Induration of the cellular tissue.

SCLERENCEPHA'LIA, *Indura'tio cer'ebri,* from σκληρος, 'hard,' and εγκεφαλον, 'the brain.' (F.) *Endurcissement du cerveau.* Induration of the brain.

SCLERIA, Scleriasis.

SCLERI'ASIS, *Sclero'ma, Sclero'sis, Scle'ria, Sclerys'mus, Scph'irus,* from σκληρος, 'hard.' Any kind of hardness or induration. Sometimes hardness of the eyelids, *Callo'sitas palpebra'rum, Scirrhoblepharon'cus, Scirrhophthal'mia palpebra'rum, Scirrhus palpebra'rum;* at others, hardness of the genital organs of the female; probably synonymous with scirrhus.— Galen. Paulus. Hardness of bones, *Fragil'itas Os'sium.*

SCLERITIS, Sclerotitis.

SCLERODERMA, Induration of the cellular tissue.

SCLERODES, Sclerotic.

SCLEROMA, Induration of the cellular tissue, Scleriasis.

SCLEROMENINX, Dura mater.

SCLERONYXIS, Scleroticonyxis.

SCLEROPHTHALMIA, Hordeolum.

SCLEROS, Hard.

SCLEROSARCO'MA, from σκληρος, 'hard,' and σαρκωμα, 'a fleshy tumour.' A hard, fleshy tumour, seated on the gums, and resembling a cock's comb.

SCLEROSIS, Induration of the cellular tissue, Scleriasis.

SCLEROSTENOSIS CUTANEA, Induration of the cellular tissue.

SCLEROT'IC, *Sclerot'ica,* from σκληροω, 'I harden.' *Cornea opa'ca, Sclero'des, Tunica dura seu albugin'ea* seu *du'rior et crass'ior* seu *ex'tima* seu *alba* seu *can'dida* seu *innomina'ta oc'uli, Sclero'tis,* (F.) *Sclérotique.* A hard, resisting, opake membrane, of a pearly white colour and fibrous nature, which covers nearly the posterior four-fifths of the globe of the eye, and has the form of a sphere truncated before. It is strengthened by the expansion of the muscles of the eye, to which expansion many anatomists have given the name *Tu'nica albugin'ea.* It forms the *white of the eye, Albu'men, Album oc'uli, Lon'chades, Log'ades, Loch'ades, Leu'cades.* The sclerotic is penetrated posteriorly by a round opening, for the passage of the optic nerve; and, anteriorly, it has a much larger opening, into which the transparent cornea is received. There are, besides, many small oblong apertures in it for the passage of nerves and vessels, proceeding to the interior of the eye. In the fœtus, the sclerotic may be separated into two very distinct laminæ.

SCLEROTICA CERATOIDES, Cornea.

SCLEROTICITIS, Sclerotitis.

SCLEROTICONYX'IS, *Scleronyx'is, Scleroton'yx'is,* from σκληρος, 'hard,' and νυξις, 'punctur

ing.' Perforation of the sclerotica in the operation for cataract by depression.
SCLEROTICUS, Indurans.
SCLÉROTIQUE, Sclerotic.
SCLEROTIS, Sclerotic.
SCLEROTI'TIS, *Inflamma'tio Sclerot'icæ, Leuci'tis, Lonchadi'tis, Logadi'tis, Scleri'tis, Sclerociti'tis, Rheumat'ic ophthal'mia, Ophthal'mia arthrit'ica,* from sclerotica, and *itis,* denoting inflammation. Inflammation of the sclerotic coat of the eye.
SCLEROTIUM CLAVUS, see Ergot.
SCLERUNTICUS, Indurans.
SCLERUS, Induration, Scirrhus.
SCLERYNTICUS, Indurans.
SCLERYS'MA, from σκληρος, 'hard.' Induration; also, induration of the liver.
SCLERYSMUS, Scleriasis.
SCLIRUS, Scirrhus.
SCLOPETA'RIUS, from *sclopetum,* 'a gun.' Relating to a gun. Hence, *Aqua sclopeta'ria,* a water for gunshot wounds. *Vul'nera sclopeta'ria,* gunshot wounds, &c.
SCLOPETOPLAGÆ, Wounds, gunshot.
SCOBS, *Prisma, Xysma, Ramen'tum, Rasu'ra.* A shaving, also, an alkali; and the scoria of any metal.
SCŒNANTHUM, Juncus odoratus.
SCOLECESIS, Helminthiasis.
SCOLECIASIS, Helminthiasis.
SCOLEX, Ascaris lumbricoides.
SCOLIOMA, Scoliosis.
SCOLIO'SIS, *Scolio'ma, Rhachio-scolio'ma,* from σκολιος, 'crooked.' A distortion of the spine to one side. See Hump.
SCOLOPENDRA, Asplenium scolopendrium.
SCOLOPENDRIA, Asplenium ceterach, and A. scolopendrium.
SCOLOPENDRIUM LINGUA, Asplenium scolopendrium — s. Officinarum, Asplenium scolopendrium — s. Phyllitis, Asplenium scolopendrium—s. Ruta muraria, Asplenium ruta muraria —s. Vulgare, Asplenium scolopendrium.
SCOLOPOMACHÆ'RION, from σκολοπαξ, 'the woodcock,' and μαχαιρα, 'a knife;' so called because it is bent a little at the extremity like a woodcock's bill. A sort of blunt-pointed bistoury. — Scultetus.
SCOLYMUS SATIVUS, Cynara scolymus.
SCOOP, Teut. Schoepe, *Cochlea'rē,* (F.) *Curette.* A surgical instrument of the shape of a spoon, which is used for the extraction of certain foreign bodies. The scoop is often employed to extract balls impacted in the soft parts; to remove calculi from the urinary bladder in lithotomy, &c. A small scoop is sometimes used to extract foreign bodies from the meatus auditorius externus, nasal fossæ, &c.
SCOPA REGIA, Ruscus.
SCOPARIUS, see Spartium scoparium.
SCOPE, σκοπη, *Scop'ia, Scopos,* from σκοπεω, 'I look around.' A common suffix to words meaning 'view, inspection,' as oranioscopy, stethoscopy, &c.
SCOPOLINA ATROPOIDES, Hyoscyamus scopolia.
SCOPTULA, Scopula.
SCOPULA, Brush.
SCOR, Excrement.
SCORACRATI'A, *Scoracra'sia, Scatacra'sia, Scatacrati'a, Copracrati'a, Copracra'sia, Incontinen'tia Alvi,* from σκωρ, 'excrement,' and ακρασια, 'want of control.' Want of power to retain the fæces. Involuntary evacuation of the fæces.
SCORBUT, Porphyra nautica, Purpura hæmorrhagica—s. des Alpes, Pellagra—s. de Terre, Purpura hæmorrhagica.

SCORBU'TIC, *Scorbu'ticus.* That which belongs to scurvy. One affected with scurvy.
SCORBUTUS, Purpura—s. Alpinus, Pellagra —s. Nauticus, Porphyra nautica—s. Oris, Cancer aquaticus.
SCORDINEMA, Carebaria, Pandiculation.
SCORDINISMUS, Carebaria, Pandiculation.
SCORDIUM, Teucrium scordium.
SCORDON, Allium.
SCORITH, Sulphur.
SCORODON, Allium.
SCORPIODEX'IS, from σκορπιος, 'the scorpion,' and δηξις, 'bite:'—more properly, Scorpiostig'ma; from σκορπιων, and στιγμα, 'puncture.' The sting of the scorpion.
SCOR'PION, *Scor'pio, Scorpius,* from σκορπιω, 'I puncture.' A genus of insects having a sting at the extremity of their tail, with which they make dangerous wounds. An *Oil of Scor* was once made from them, which is not now used.
SCORPIOSTIGMA, Scorpiodexis.
SCORPIUS, Scorpion.
SCORTUM, Scrotum.
SCORZONE'RA, *S. hu'milis* seu *lana'ta* seu *nervo'sa, Escorzone'ra, Vipera'ria, Serpenta'ria Hispan'ica, Offic'inal viper's grass, Viper's grass, Goat's grass.* Family, Cichoraceæ. *Sex. Syst.* Syngenesia Polygamia. The roots have been used as alexipharmics, and in hypochondriacal disorders and obstructions of the viscera. The root of the *Scorzonera Hispan'ica* is esculent, but inefficacious as a drug.
SCOTAS'MA, *Scoto'ma, Scoto'dia, Scota'sis, Scotos;* from σκοτος, 'darkness.' Obscurity of vision, darkness, *Suffu'sio ra'dians.* Also Scotodinia.
SCOTCH FIDDLE, Psora.
SCOTODIA, Scotasma, Scotodinia.
SCOTODIN'IA, *Scoto'ma, Dinus Scoto'ms, Scotodi'nē, Tenebrico'sa verti'go, Scotos, Scotasma, Scoto'sis, Scot'omy,* from σκοτος, 'darkness,' and δινεω, 'I turn round.' Giddiness, with impaired sight, often succeeded by headach. See Vertigo.
SCOTOMA, Scotasma, Scotodinia.
SCOTOMY, Scotodinia.
SCOTOS, Scotasma, Scotodinia.
SCOTOSIS, Scotodinia.
SCOTT'S ACID BATH, *Nitro-muriatic acid bath.* A bath of dilute aqua regia, employed by Dr. Scott, of India, as a remedy in hepatic diseases. Three pints by measure of muriatic acid and two of nitric acid, are mixed to form the aqua regia. In preparing this for use, a pint of it is mixed with an equal quantity of water. The acid bath consists of three ounces of this dilute acid to every gallon of water.
SCRATCH, Psora.
SCREATUS, Excreation.
SCRIPTULUM, Scruple.
SCRIPULUM, Scruple.
SCRIPULUS, Scruple.
SCRIVENER'S CRAMP, Cramp, writers'.
SCROBIC'ULUS, *Scrobic'ulum,* (F.) *Fossette.* A little ditch or furrow; diminutive of *scrobs,* 'a ditch.'
Scrobic'ulus Cordis, *Anticar'dium, Præcor'dium,* (F.) *Fossette du cœur, Avant-cœur, Ante-cœur.* The pit of the stomach. The depression at the anterior part of the abdomen, below the xiphoid cartilage.
Scrobiculus Variolæ, Pockmark.
SCROFFÆ, Scrofula.
SCROF'ULA, *Scroph'ula, Scroph'ula:* from *scrofa,* 'a sow;' because swine were presumed to be subject to a similar complaint. *Scroph'ulosis, Morbus scrophulo'sus, Vit"ium scrophuloʻsum, Cacochym'ia* seu *Cachex'ia* seu *Dyscra'sia scrophulo'sa, Pædatroph'ia glandulo'sa, Struma*

Chœrus, Coiras, Tabes Glandula'ris, Adeno'sis scrofulo'sa, Scroffæ, Chrœas, King's evil, The Evil, Cruels (Scottice), (F.) Scrophules, Scrofules, Strumes, Écrouelles, Humeurs froides, Tubercules des glandes lymphatiques, Mal du Roi. A state of the system characterized by indolent, glandular tumours, chiefly in the neck; suppurating slowly and imperfectly, and healing with difficulty; the disease ordinarily occurring in those of a sanguine temperament, with thick upper lip, &c. The tumours, after suppuration, degenerate into ulcers; which, in process of time, cicatrize, leaving scars. The internal organs are apt to be attacked in those disposed to scrofula; hence they are often the subjects of phthisis and mesenteric affections. Scrofula is hereditary; and is frequently excited by insufficient or improper regimen, and by a close, confined air during the first years of existence. The best treatment is:—to strengthen the system by animal diet; pure air, and exercise, cold bathing, or sea-water bathing, &c.

SCROFULA ABDOMINALIS INTERNA, Physconia strumosa.

SCROFULAIRE, Scrophularia nodosa—*s. Aquatique*, Scrophularia aquatica.

SCROFULARIA, Scrophularia.

SCROFULEUX, Scrofulous.

SCROF'ULOUS, *Serophulo'sus, Scrophula'rius, Strumous, Strumo'sus,* (F.) *Scrofuleux, Strumeux*. Suffering from, or relating to, scrofula.

SCROPHULA, Scrofula—s. Mesenterica, Tabes mesenterica—s. Moluccana, Frambœsia.

SCROPHULÆ, Scrofula—s. Gonorrhoicæ, Gonorrhœa impura.

SCROPHULARIA, S. Nodosa.

SCROPHULA'RIA AQUAT'ICA, *Beton'ica aquat'-ica, Fica'ria, Ferra'ria, Castran'gula,* Greater Water Figwort, Water Bet'ony, (F.) *Scrofulaire aquatique*. The leaves are celebrated as correctors of the bad flavour of senna. They were at one time regarded as eminently antiscrofulous, stomachic, and carminative.

SCROPHULARIA FŒTIDA, Scrophularia nodosa—s. Lanceolata, S. Nodosa—s. Marilandica, S. Nodosa—s. Minor, Ranunculus ficaria.

SCROPHULA'RIA NODOSA, Figwort, *Kennelwort, Holmesweed,* Heal-all, *Scrophula'ria fœ'tida seu vulga'ris seu lanceola'ta, seu Marilan'dica, Millemor'bia, Scrophula'ria,* (F.) *Scrofulaire, Herbe aux écrouelles*. The root and leaves of this plant have been celebrated, both as an internal and external remedy, against inflammations, piles, scrofulous tumours, ulcers, &c.

SCROPHULARIA VULGARIS, Scrophularia nodosa.

SCROPHULARIUS, Scrofulous.

SCROPHULES, Scrofula—*s. Mésentériques,* Tabes mesenterica.

SCROPHULOSIS, Scrofula.

SCROPHULOSUS, Scrofulous.

SCROTAL, *Scrota'lis;* from *scrotum*. Relating to the scrotum,—as *Hernia scrota'lis,* scrotal hernia.

SCROTAL NERVE, see Genito-crural Nerve.

SCROTOCE'LE. A hybrid term; from (L.) *scrotum,* and κηλη, 'a tumour.' *Hernia Scrota'lis,* Scrotal *her'nia*. Inguinal hernia, descending into the scrotum; Oscheocele.

SCROTUM, from *scorteus, scorteum,* 'made of leather.' (?) *Oschē, Os'cheus, Os'chus, Os'cheon, Och'eus, Perin, Scortum, Marsu'pium, Bur'sula, Bursa tes'tium seu viri'lis, Cap'ulus,* (?) *Orchas, Os'eus, Follic'ulus genita'lis, Her'nia, the Purse, the Cod,* (F.) *Les bourses*. The integuments which cover the testes. These are nothing more than a prolongation of the skin of the inner part of the thighs, perinæum, and penis. The skin is remarkable for its brown colour, for the numerous rugæ, especially when the scrotum is contracted; for the great number of sebaceous follicles it contains; and for the long and few hairs which issue from it in the adult. The scrotum is divided into two equal parts by a raphe, which extends from the anus to the root of the penis. Its organization is similar to that of the skin of other parts of the body, except that the chorion is thinner.

SCROTUM CORDIS, Pericardium—s. Pendulum, Rhachosis.

SCRUPLE, *Diob'olon, Gramma'rium, Scru'pulus, Scru'pulum, Scrip'tulus, Scrip'ulum, Scrip'-ulus*. A weight of twenty grains, Troy; twenty-four grains, Poids de marc.

SCUDAMORE'S MIXTURE, see Mixture, Scudamore's.

SCULL, Cranium—s. Cap, Calvaria.

SCURF, Sax. ῥcurf, Teut. Schorft; *Fur'-fura*. Small exfoliations of the cuticle are so called.

SCURFY, Furfuraceous.

SCURVY OF THE ALPS, Pellagra—s. Grass, Sisyrinchium Bermudianum—s. Land, Purpura hæmorrhagica—s. Petechial, Purpura simplex—s. Sea, Porphyra nautica—s. Grass, common, Cochlearia officinalis—s. Grass, lemon, Cochlearia officinalis—s. Grass, wild, Cochlearia coronopus.

SCUTELLA, Cup.

SCUTELLA'RIA GALERICULA'TA, *Cassida galaricula'ta, Tertiana'ria, Skull-cap,* (F.) *Caside bleue*. Family, Personeæ. *Sex. Syst*. Didynamia Angiospermia. This plant has a bitter taste and a garlic smell. It has been esteemed especially serviceable in tertian ague.

SCUTELLA'RIA LATERIFLO'RA, Skull-cap, *Madweed, Hoodwort, Blue Pimp'ernel*. An indigenous plant, which grows in all parts of the United States in moist places. It was at one time esteemed a preventive of hydrophobia, but is probably possessed of little virtue of any kind.

SCUTELLARIA INTEGRIFO'LIA,—another indigenous variety,—is an intense bitter.

SCUTICULA DIGITORUM MANÛS, Phalanges of the fingers.

SCUTULÆ DIGITORUM MANÛS, Phalanges of the fingers.

SCUTUM, Thyroid cartilage—s. Cordis, Scapula, Sternum—s. Genu, Patella—s. Pectoris, Thorax.

SCUTUM STOMACH'ICUM. A large plaster, applied to the breast or stomach.

SCUTUM THORACIS, Scapula.

SCYB'ALA, plural of σκυβαλον, 'dung.' *Enterol'ithus Scyb'alum, Excrementa Alvi siccio'ra, Fæces indura'tæ*. Hard fecal matters discharged in round lumps.

SCYLLA, Scilla.

SCYPHOPHORUS PYXIDATUS, Lichen pyxidatus.

SCYPHUS AUDITORIUS, Infundibulum of the cochlea—s. Cerebri, Infundibulum of the brain—s. Vieussenii, Infundibulum of the cochlea.

SCYROS, Callosity.

SCYTALIDES DIGITORUM MANÛS, Phalanges of the fingers.

SCYTHICA, (RADIX,) Glycyrrhiza.

SCYTHROPASMUS, from σκυθρος, 'gloomy;' σκυθρωπαζειν, 'to look gloomy;' *Vultus tet'ricus et mœstus*. A gloomy, depressed countenance, of bad augury in serious diseases.

SCYTITIS, Cytitis.

SCYTODEPSIUM, Tannin.

SEA AIR. The air in the neighbourhood of the sea contains saline particles commingled with it, which render it a valuable change for scrofulous and debilitated individuals. The sea and sea-coast are usually, also, more equable in their temperature than places inland.

SEA SICKNESS, Nausea marina — s. Water, see Water, Sea.

SEAL, GOLDEN, Hydrastis Canadensis — s. Solomon's, Convallaria polygonatum.

SEAM, Cicatrix.

SEARCHING, *Sounding;* from (F.) *chercher*, 'to seek.' The operation of ascertaining, by the introduction of a metallic instrument, whether a patient has a stone in the bladder.

SEASONING, Acclimation — s. Fever, Fever, stranger's.

SEAT, Anus — s. Bone, Ischion.

SÉBACÉ, Sebaceous.

SEBA'CEOUS, *Seba'ceus*, (F.) *Sébacé;* from *sebum*, 'suet.' That which has the nature of suet.

SEBACEOUS FLUX, Stearrhœa.

SEBACEOUS or SEBIP'AROUS GLANDS, *Sebaceous Fol'licles, Sebaceous Crypts, Follic'uli seba'cei, Cryptæ seba'ceæ, Oil Glands, Mil'iary glands,* are small hollow organs, of a rounded or pyriform shape, seated in the substance of the skin, and opening on its surface by a small, excretory duct; furnishing a yellow, unctuous humour, *Smegma cuta'neum, Sebum cuta'neum,* having some analogy with suet, which is destined to lubricate the surface of the body. Follicles of a similar nature exist around the corona glandis of the male, and under the skin of the labia majora and nymphæ of females. They secrete a sebaceous matter, which emits a peculiar odour; and hence, after the name of one who described them, have been called *Gland'ulæ odorif'eræ Tyso'ni, G. Tyso'ni, Tyson's glands.*

SEBESTE'NA, *Cordia myxa* seu *sebeste'na* seu *Africa'na* seu *domes'tica* seu *obli'qua, Sebeste'na officina'lis, Sebes'ten, Sebsten, Myxa, Cornus sanguin'ea, Prunus sebesti'na, Smooth-leaved Cor'dia, Assyr'ian plum*, (F.) *Sebestier myxa.* The dark, black fruit of the *Sebestina* possesses glutinous and aperient qualities, and is exhibited, in decoction, in various diseases of the chest.

SEBESTIER MYXA, Sebestena.

SEBIPAROUS, see Sebaceous.

SEBORRHAGIA, Stearrhœa.

SEBORRHŒA, Stearrhœa.

SEBSTEN, Sebestina.

SEBUM, Pinguedo, Sevum — s. Cutaneum, see Sebaceous glands.

SECA'LE, *S. cerea'le* seu *barba'tum*. The Rye plant. (F.) *Seigle*. Rye is chiefly used as an article of diet, particularly in the northern parts of Europe, where a spirit is also extracted from it. The grain is disposed to acescency: and hence its internal use at first generally produces a laxative effect.

SECALE BARBATUM, Secale — s. Cornutum, Ergot — s. Luxurians, Ergot.

SECALIS MATER, Ergot.

SECERNENT, Secreting.

SECERNING, Secreting — s. Substance, of the kidney, see Kidney.

SECESSIO FÆCUM, Defecation.

SECESSUS NIGER, Melæna.

SÈCHE, Sepia.

SECLUSORIUM, Sac.

SEC'ONDARY, from *secundus*, 'the second.' Something that acts subordinately to another; as the *secondary symptoms* of a disease; that is, those which supervene on the *primary.*

SECONDINES, Secundines.

SECRETA. Same etymon as Secretion. Things or matters secreted or separated from the blood.

SECRE'TING, *Secreto'rius, Secer'ning, Se'cern'ent, Excer'nent.* Same etymon as Secretion. That which secretes, — as a secreting organ.

SECRETIO, Secretion — s. Lactis, Galactosis — s. Lotii, Uropoesis — s. Urinæ, Uropoesis — s. Urinaria, see Vicarious.

SECRE'TION, *Secre'tio, Apoc'risis;* from *secernere,* 'to separate.' An organic function. It is chiefly executed in the glands, and consists in an elaboration or separation of the materia of the blood, at the very extremities of the arterial system, or rather of the vascular secretory system; and which differs in each organ according to its particular structure; hence the formation of different fluids; — bile, saliva, urine, milk &c. The secretions are of three kinds: — *exhalans, licular,* and *glandular.*

SECRETORIUS, Secreting.

SECT, METHODICAL, Methodists.

SEC'TIO, *Section.* The act of cutting. Division.

SECTIO ALTA, see Lithotomy — s. Anatomica, Dissection — s. Cadaveris, Autopsia cadaverica — s. Cadaveris legalis, Autopsia cadaverica — s. Cæsarea, Cæsarean section — s. Franconiana, Lithotomy — s. Hypogastrica, see Lithotomy — s. Lateralis, see Lithotomy — s. Legalis. Obstetri — s. Mariana, see Lithotomy — s. Nymphæ, Nymphotomy — s. Rectovesicalis, see Lithotomy — s. Renalis, Nephrotomy — s. Tendinum. Tenotomy — s. Vagino-vesicalis, Colpocystotomy, Vesicalis, Lithotomy.

SECTION, Sectio — s. Sigaultian, Symphysiotomy.

SECUNDÆ, Secundines.

SECUNDINÆ, Secundines.

SEC'UNDINES, *Hys'tera, Deuter'ion, birth, Secun'dæ, Secundi'næ,* (F.) *Arrière-Secondines, Délivre.* All that remains in the uterus after the birth of the child, — viz. the placenta, a portion of the umbilical cord, and membranes of the ovum. These are occasionally not expelled till some time after the birth of the fœtus; hence their name. See *Délivrance.*

SECUNDUS PROPRIORUM AURICULÆ Retrahens auris.

SEDANTIA. Sodatives.

SED'ATIVES, *Sedati'va, Pauon'ta. Sedadec'ta, Catastal'tica, Deprimen'tia,* (F.) *Calmants, Tempérants,* from *sedo,* 'I settle or suage.' Medicines which directly depress the vital forces, and which are consequently employed whenever it is necessary to diminish preternaturally increased action. The chief reputed sedatives are: Acidum Hydrocyanicum, Acidum Hydro-sulphuricum, Tabacum, Missio Sanguinis, certain gases by inhalation, as azote, carbonic acid, (?) carburetted and sulphuretted hydrogen.

SEDEM ATTOLLENS, Levator ani.

SEDES, Anus, Excrement — s. Cruenta, Dysentery, Hæmatochezia — s. Lactescentes, Lienteria — s. Procidua, Proctocele.

SEDHEE, Bangue.

SED'IMENT, *Sédimen'tum, Lemma, Resisentia.* Same etymon. (F.) *Dépôt.* A deposit formed by the precipitation of some one or more substances, held in solution or suspension in a liquid. That which is formed in urine, at the time of cooling, has been called *Hypos'tema, poste'ma, Residen'tia, Subsiden'tia.* (F.) *De l'urine.* This sediment or deposit varies in different states of the system. In calculous affections, it is one of the most important objects of attention.

SEDIMENTUM, Sediment — s. Urinæ lateritium, see Lateritious — s. Urinæ pityroides, Furfuraceous.

SEDITIA, Nates.

SEDLITZ, MINERAL WATERS OF. Sedlitz, *Seidschütz* or *Seydschütz water.* Springs in Bohemia, near Prague, which are simple saline

They contain a large quantity of sulphate of magnesia, a little sulphate of soda and sulphate of lime, carbonic acid, carbonates of lime and magnesia, and a resinous matter.(?) They are employed as purgatives in a multitude of diseases.

SEDLITZ POWDERS may be formed of *Soda tartarizata* ℨij, *Sodæ carbon.* ℈ij, in one paper; *Acid tartaric.* gr. xxxv, in another. For half a pint of water.

SEDON BRÛLANT, Sedum — *s. Reprise*, Sedum telephium.

SEDUM, *Sedum acrĕ* seu *glacia'lĕ* seu *minus* seu *vermicula'rĕ*, *Illec''ebra*, *Hellec''ebra*, *Illec'ebrum Vermicula'rĕ*, *Vermicula'ris*, *Piper mura'lĕ*, *Sempervi'vum acrĕ*, Wall pepper, Stone crop, Biting Stone crop, Small Houseleek, *Aei'chryson*, *Æo'nion*, (F.) *Joubarbe âcre*, *Orpin brûlant*, *Vermiculaire brûlante*, *Sédon brûlant*. Family, Crassulaceæ. *Sex. Syst.* Decandria Pentagynia. In its recent state it is very acrid, and proves both emetic and cathartic. Externally, in the form of cataplasm, it produces vesications and erosions. It has been recommended in cancerous and malignant ulcers.

SEDUM, Saxifraga granulata — s. Glaciale, Sedum—s. Minus, Sedum—s. Majus, Sempervivum tectorum—s. Minus, Sedum.

SEDUM TELE'PHIUM, *S. telephoīdes*, *Faba crassa*, *Cras'sula*, *O. Major*, *Illec''ebra major*, *Tele'phium*, *Faba'ria cras'sula*, *Faba crassa*, *Anacamp'seros*, *A. al'bicans* seu *triphyll'a* seu *vulga'ris*, Orpine, (F.) *Sédon reprise*, *Grand orpin*, *Fève épaisse*, *Joubarbe des vignes*, &c. Formerly used as a cataplasm in cuts, hemorrhoids, corns, whitlows, &c.

SEDUM TELEPHOIDES, S. Telephium—s. Vermiculare, Sedum.

SEED, Sperm.

SEGMENTA CARTILAGINEA, see Trachea.

SEGNIT''IA, *Segnit''ies*, from *segnis*, 'sluggish.' Sluggishness or torpor in the exercise of a function: — as SEGNITIES ALVI, Torpor of the bowels: SEGNITIES VIRIUM, Languor.

SEGNITIES, Segnitia.

SEGRAY, MINERAL WATERS OF. Near Pithiviers, in Gâtinais, in the French department of Loiret, there is a chalybeate spring, which has some reputation.

SEGU, Sago.

SEIDLITZ, Sedlitz.

SEIDSCHUTZ, Sedlitz.

SEIGLE, Secale—*s. Ergotté*, Ergot.

SEIN, Uterus, see Mamma.

SEIRIASIS, *Coup de Soleil*.

SEIZURES, HIDDEN, see Seizures.

SEKISKAYAVODKA, see Spirit.

SEL, Salt—*s. Admirable de Lémery*, Magnesiæ sulphas—*s. Admirable perlé*, Soda, phosphate of —*s. de Cuisine*, Soda, muriate of—*s. de Déroene*, Narcotine—*s. d'Égra*, Magnesiæ sulphas—*s. Marin*, Soda, muriate of—*s. d'Opium*, Narcotine—*s. de Saturne*, Plumbi superacetas—*s. de Verre*, see Vitrum—*s. Volatil d'Angleterre*, Ammoniæ carbonas.

SELAGO, Camphorosma Monspeliaca, Lycopodium selago.

SELENE, Moon, see Nail.

SELENIASIS, Somnambulism.

SELENIASMUS, Somnambulism.

SELENOBLETUS, Lunatic.

SELENOGAMIA, Somnambulism.

SELERY, Apium graveolens.

SELFABUSE, Masturbation.

SELF-HEAL, Prunella.

SELF-LIM'ITED. An epithet applied to diseases which appear to run a definite course, but little modified by treatment, — small-pox, for example-

SELF-POLLUTION, Masturbation.

SELI'BRA, *Semili'bra*, *Sembella*, half a pound. Six ounces, Troy; eight, Avoirdupois.

SELINI'TES, σελινιτης. Wine impregnated with the seeds of the σελινον or *smallage*. — Dioscorides.

SELINUM ANGELICA, Angelica Sylvestris — s. Galbanum, Bubon galbanum — s. Imperatoria, Imperatoria—s. Opoponax, Pastinaca opoponax— s. Oreoselinum, Athamanta aureoselinum — s. Ostruthium, Imperatoria—s. Pastinaca, Pastinaca sativa — s. Peucedanum, Peucedanum — s. Pubescens, Angelica sylvestris — s. Sylvestre, Angelica sylvestris.

SELLA, S, Turcica — s. Equina, S. Turcica — s. Familiarica, Lasanum—s. Obstetricia, Diphrus —s. Sphenoidalis, S. Turcica.

SELLA TUR'CICA, *Ephip'pium*, *Fossa Pituita'ria*, *Sella*, *S. equi'na* seu *sphenoida'lis*, Turkish Saddle, (F.) *Selle Turcique* ou *du Turc*. A depression at the upper surface of the sphenoid bone, which is bounded, anteriorly and posteriorly, by the clinoid processes; and lodges the pituitary gland. It is so called from its resemblance to a *Turkish saddle*.

SELLA TURCICA, Pituitaria fossa.

SELLE TURCIQUE, Sella Turcica — *s. du Turc*, Sella Turcica.

SELS NEUTRES, Neutral salts.

SELTZ or SELTZER, MINERAL WATERS OF. Cold, acidulous springs, the source of which is at Seltz, nine leagues from Strasburg, and in the Department of the Bas-Rhin. They contain carbonates of lime, magnesia, and soda, chloride of sodium, and much carbonic acid. They are refrigerant, tonic, diuretic, and aperient.

ARTIFICIAL SELTZER WATER may be made from *muriat. acid.* gr. xxxv, *water* Oj, *white marble* gr. iij. Stop up till dissolved. Add *carbonate of Magnesia*, gr. v, and, after some time, *subcarbonate of soda*, gr. xxxij. Close it till used.

SEMBELLA, Selibra.

SEMECARPUS ANACARDIUM, Avicennia tomentosa.

SEMEIOG'RAPHY, *Semeiograph'ia*, *Semiography*, *Semiogra'phia*, from σημειον, 'a symptom,' and γραφη, 'a description.' A description of symptoms or signs of disease.

SEMEIOL'OGY, *Semeiot'icĕ*, *Semiology*, *Semiotica*, *Phænomenolog''ia*, from σημειον, 'a symptom,' and λογος, 'a discourse.' (F.) *Séméiotique*. The branch of pathology whose object is the doctrine of the symptoms or signs of disease.

SEMEION BOETHEMATICUM, Indication.

SEMEIOSIS, Semeiology.

SÉMÉIOTIQUE, Semeiology.

SEMEN, Sperm — s. Badian, Illicium anisatum — s. Cinæ, Artemisia santonica — s. Contra, Artemisia santonica — s. Contra vermes, Artemisia santonica—s. Masculinum seu virile seu genitale, Sperm — s. Muliebre, Sperm (of the female) —s. Sanctum, Artemisia santonica—s. Zedoariæ, Artemisia santonica.

SEMENCE, Sperm.

SEMENTINA, Artemisia santonica.

SEMI, from 'ημισυ, 'half.' *Semi* or *demi*, in composition, universally signifies 'half;' both in French and English.

SEMIAN'IMIS, *Semimor'tuus*, *Sem'inex*, *Semivi'vus*; from *semi*, 'half,' and *animus*, 'soul.' Half-living. Half-dead.

SEMI-BULB OF THE FEMALE, Bulbus vestibuli.

SEMICANALICULUS, Sulcus.

SEMICANALIS, Sulcus.

SEMICEPHALUS, Hemicephalus.

SEMICIRCULI OSSEI, Semicircular canals.

SEMICIR'CULAR, *Semicircula'ris*. That which represents the half of a circle.

SEMICIRCULAR CANALS, *Cana'les* seu *Ductus semicircula'res* seu *tubæform'es* seu *circula'res, Semicir'culi os'sei, Funes* seu *Canalic'uli semiannula'res labyrin'thi*, (F.) *Canaux demicirculaires*, are seated in the pars petrosa of the temporal bone, and open into the vestibule, behind which they are situate. They are three in number, of which one is *superior* or *vertical, cana'lis semicircula'ris vertica'lis supe'rior*; another *posterior* or *oblique, cana'lis semicircula'ris vertica'lis poste'rior*, and the third *exterior* or *horizontal, canalis semicircula'ris horizonta'lis*. Their parietes are formed of a bony, compact, hard plate. Their uses in audition are not known: at their termination they have the elliptical arrangements called *ampul'læ;* and by both extremities they open into the vestibule, in the sac at its superior part—the *Sac'culus Ellip'ticus, Al'veus* seu *Utric'ulus commu'nis, Utricle, Sinus* or *Alveus utriculo'sus, Sacculus vestibuli* or *Median sinus*. In front of the S. ellipticus, nearer the cochlea, and opposite the foramen ovale, is the *Sac'culus spher'icus* or *sacculus*.

SEMICIRCULUS EXSCULPTUS, Hiatus diaphragmatis aorticus.

SEMICON'GIUS. Half a gallon, or four pints.

SEMICU'BIUM, *Semicupium, Insee'sio, Incee'sio, Encathis'ma, Excathis'ma*, (F.) *Demibain*, from *semi*, 'half,' and *cubare*, 'to lie down.' A half-bath, or such as receives only the hips or extremities.

SEMICUPIUM, Bath, half, Semi-cubium—Semi-fibulæus, Peronæus brevis—Semi-interosseus indicis, Abductor indicis—Semi-interosseus pollicis, Opponens pollicis.

SEMILIBRA, Selibra.

SEMILLA DEL GUACHARO. Various kinds of hard and dry fruits, found in the stomachs of the young Guacharoes, a sort of nocturnal bird. The fruits are a celebrated South American remedy in ague.

SEMILU'NAR, *Semiluna'ris*, (F.) *Demi-lunaire* ou *Semi-lunaire*, from *semi*, 'half,' and *luna*, 'the moon.' Having the shape of a half-moon.

SEMILUNAR CART'ILAGES, *Semilunar fibro-cartilages, Sigmoid car'tilages, Cartilag''ines sigmoïdeæ* seu *semiluna'res*, are two fibro-cartilages, which exist between the condyles of the os femoris and the articular surfaces of the tibia. The innermost, which is longer from before to behind than transversely, is nearly semicircular. The outermost forms almost an entire circle; an arrangement, in both cases, corresponding to the different surfaces of the tibia. They are thicker at their outer circumference, which is convex, than at the inner, which is concave and very thin. Both are inserted, before and behind, into the spine of the tibia, by means of fibrous fasciæ.

SEMILUNAR GANGLION,—*Ganglion abdomina'lē* seu *splanch'nicum* seu *transver'sum* seu *sola'rē, G. surrénal*, (Ch.), belongs to the great sympathetic. These ganglia present considerable variety, and are deeply situate in the abdomen, above and behind the supra-renal capsules. They correspond, posteriorly, to the pillars of the diaphragm and the aorta. They have the shape of a crescent reversed, often surrounded by other ganglia of a smaller size. From their periphery the numerous filaments proceed, which go to the formation of the solar plexus.

SEMILUNAR NOTCH OF THE STERNUM, Fourchette —s. Valves, Sigmoid valves—s. Masculatus, Eunuch.

SEMILUNULA UNGUIUM, see Nail.

SEMI-MAS, Eunuch.

SEMIMASCULUS, Eunuch.

SEMIMEMBRANEUS, Semimembranosus.

SEMIMEMBRANO'SUS, *Semimembra'neus*, (F.) *Ischio-popliti-fémoral, Ischio-popliti-tibial*, (Ch.) *Demimembraneux*. A muscle situate at the posterior part of the thigh. It is flat, thin, narrow, and aponeurotic in its upper third; broader and fleshy in the middle, and tendinous below. It is attached above to the tuberosity of the ischium; and below—by a tendon, which has three divisions—to the outer condyle of the femur, and to the posterior and inner part of the internal tuberosity of the tibia. This muscle is a rotator inwards, and a flexor of the leg. It can also bend the thigh upon the leg. In standing it maintains the pelvis in position, and can even draw it downwards.

SEMIMORTUUS, Semianimis.

SEMINA CATAPUTIÆ MAJORIS, see Ricinus communis.

SE'MINA FRIG'IDA MAJO'RA. The *greater cold seeds*. The ancients gave this name to the emulsive seeds of the cucumber, melon, gourd, and water-melon.

SEMINA FRIGIDA MINORA. The *lesser cold seeds*. The ancients gave this name to the seeds of the lettuce, purslane, endive, and cichory.

SEMINA RICINI VULGARIS, see Ricinus communis.

SEMINAL, Spermatic—s. Filaments, Spermatozoa—s. Fluid, Sperm—s. Granules, see Granule.

SEMINALE MEMBRUM, Penis.

SEMINALIS, Spermatic.

SEMINERVOSUS, Semi-tendinosus.

SEMIORBICULARIS, Orbicularis oris.

SEMIPESTIS, Typhus.

SEMINEX, Semianimis.

SEMINIA MORBORUM, Predisposition.

SEMINIF'EROUS, from *semen*, 'sperm,' and *fero*, 'I carry.' *Spermatoph'orous*. An epithet given to the vessels which secrete and convey the seminal fluid.

SEMINIUM, Sperm.

SEMIOGRAPHY, Semeiography.

SEMIOLOGY, Semeiology.

SEMIOTICE, Semeiotice—s. Faciei, Physiognomy.

SEMIPLEGIA, Hemiplegia.

SEMISEXTUM, Hemiecton.

SEMISICIL'ICUS. A weight of one drachm or three scruples.—Rhodius.

SEMISIDERATIO, Hemiplegia.

SEMISIDERATUS, see Hemiplegia.

SEMISOMNIS, Coma.

SEMISOPITUS, Coma.

SEMISOPORUS, Coma.

SEMISPEC'ULUM. An instrument used for dilating the incision made into the neck of the bladder in the operation of lithotomy.—Fabricius Hildanus.

SEMISPINA'LIS COLLI, *Semispina'tus colli, Artic'ulo-spina'lis, Transver'so-spinalis Colli, Spinalis cervi'cis, Spinalis Colli, Transversa'lis Colli, Transverso-spinal*, (F.) *Demi-épineux* ou *transversaire-épineux du cou*. This muscle arises from the transverse processes of the six uppermost dorsal vertebræ, by an equal number of distinct tendons, which run obliquely under the complexus, and is inserted in the spinous processes of all the cervical vertebræ, except the first and last. Its *action* is, to extend the neck obliquely backwards and to one side.

SEMISPINALIS DORSI, *Semi-spinalis externus, Transver'so-spinalis dorsi, Semi-spina'tus*, (Riolan), *Transverso-spinal*, (F.) *Demi-épineux du dos, Transversaire-épineux du dos*. This muscle arises from the transverse processes of the seventh, eighth, ninth, and tenth dorsal vertebræ, by as many distinct tendons, which soon grow fleshy; and then again become tendinous, and are inserted into the spinous processes of the sixth or seventh uppermost dorsal, and two lowest cervical vertebræ, by as many tendons. Its action is, to extend the spine obliquely backwards.

SEMISPINALIS EXTERNUS, Semi-spinalis dorsi— s. Internus, Transversalis dorsi — s. Spinatus, Longissimus dorsi, Semi-spinalis dorsi.

SEMISPINATUS COLLI, Semispinalis colli.

SEMIS'SIS, *Semis.* The half of a pound, ounce, drachm, &c.

SEMITENDINO'SUS, *Semi-nervo'sus*, (F.) *Ischio-créti-tibial, Ischio-prétibial,* (Ch.) *Demitendineux.* This muscle is situate at the posterior part of the thigh. It extends obliquely, downwards and inwards, from the tuberosity of the ischium—to which it is attached by a flat tendon, common to it and the biceps—as far as the posterior and inner part of the tibia, to which it is attached by means of another round tendon. Its fibres are commonly interrupted by an aponeurosis. Its *uses* are the same as those of the semimembranosus.

SEMITERTIANA, Hemitritæa — *s. Tierce*, Hemitritæa.

SEMIUNCIA, Hemiuncion.

SEMIVIR, Eunuch.

SEMIVIVUS, Semianimis.

SEM'OLA, BULLOCK'S, a farinaceous article of diet, which is recommended as highly nutritious and easily digestible, consequently well adapted for infants and invalids, is said to consist of the gluten of wheat, with a small proportion of starch. Semola and Semolina resemble each other greatly. They appear, indeed, to be identical.

SEMOLI'NA, *Manna croup.* This may be made by grinding wheat in an apparatus, separating the flour from the middlings, dressing the latter four different times in a bolting mill, and sifting through parchment sieves, until the product is perfectly freed from bran. In Poland it is called *Cracow groats.*

Semolina is generally imported into England from the Baltic, and in Russia is said to be manufactured from buckwheat. It has a granular form like some kinds of oatmeal, a dingy white colour, a farinaceous, somewhat insipid, taste, and is well adapted for the diet of children affected with derangement of the bowels. A recent analysis makes it consist of the gluten of wheat with a certain proportion of the starch, part of the latter having been removed.

SEMPERVIVUM ACRE, Sedum.

SEMPERVIVUM TECTO'RUM, *S. majus, House-Leek, Sedum Majus* seu *Tecto'rum, Aizoön, Beiahalalen, Buphthalmus, Barba Jovis, Sengreen, Agriosin'ara, Andrachahara, Chrysosper'mum,* (F.) *Joubarbe des toits.* The leaves have a mild, subacid austerity, and are often applied to bruises and old ulcers.

SEMUNCIA, Hemiuncion.

SENA, Cassia senna.

SÉNÉ, Cassia senna— *s. d'Amérique,* Cassia Marilandica—*s. Faux,* Colutea arborescens.

SENEBIERA CORONOPUS, Cochlearia coronopus.

SENE'CIO, *S. vulga'ris, Erig''erum, Cortalon, Erigeron, Groundsel, Fireweed,* (F.) *Seneçon commun. Family,* Corymbiferæ. *Sex. Syst.* Syngenesia Polygamia Superflua. A common plant in Europe; frequently applied, bruised, to inflammations and ulcers, as refrigerant and anti-scorbutic.

SENECIO HIERACIFOLIUS, Erechthites hieracifolius.

SENECIO JACOBÆ'A, *Jacobæ'a, St. James' Wort, Ragwort,* (F.) *Jacobée.* The leaves have a roughish, bitter, subacid, and extremely nauseous taste. A decoction has been used in dysentery. A poultice of the leaves has been recommended in rheumatic affections; und a decoction of the root has often been employed in cases of wounds and bruises.

SENEÇON COMMUN, Senecio.

SENECTA, Senectus.

SENEC'TA AN'GUIUM. The cast skin of a serpent. A decoction of it is said to cure deafness!

SENECTA DECREPITA, Decrepitude — s. Extrema, Decrepitude — s. Summa, Decrepitude —*s.* Ultima, Decrepitude.

SENEC'TUS, *Senec'ta,* from *senere,* 'to be old.' *Geras, Se'nium, Ætas seni'lis* seu *provec'ta* seu *mala, Old age, Senil'ity,* (F.) *Viellesse.* The last period of life, commencing, according to some, at 60 years of age, but varying according to numerous circumstances. It is characterized by progressive diminution of the physical and moral faculties.

SENECTUS ULTIMA, Decrepitude.

SENEGA, Polygala senega.

SEN'EGAL, GUM, *Gummi Senegalen'sè* seu *Sen'eca* seu *Sen'ega* seu *Sen'ica.* The exudation from the *Aca'cia* seu *Mimo'sa Senegal—Family,* Leguminosæ, *Sex. Syst.* Polygamia Monœcia— which grows in the country of Africa through which the river Senegal runs. It is in loose or single drops, much larger than gum Arabic, or the gum which exudes from the cherry tree; and is much more difficult of solution than the former.

SENEGINE, see Polygala senega.

SENEKA, Polygala senega.

SÉNEVÉ, Sinapis.

SENGREEN, Sempervivum tectorum.

SENILE, *Seni'lis,* from *senere,* 'to be old.' Relating or belonging to old age:—as *'senile* delirium;' dotage.

SENILITY, Senectus.

SENNA, Cassia senna—s. Alexandrina, Cassia senna—s. American, Cassia Marilandica—s. Bladder, Colutea arborescens—s. Essence of, prepared, Selway's, see Infusum sennæ compositum — s. Germanica, Colutea—s. Italica, Cassia senna—s. Prairie, Cassia chamæcrista—s. Wild, Cassia chamæcrista, Cassia Marilandica.

SENS, Sense.

SENSA'TION, *Sensa'tio,* from *sentire, sensum,* 'to feel;' *Æsthe'ma.* The consciousness or cognizance by the brain of an impression caused by an external body on the organs of the senses. (F.) *Sentiment.* It is not necessarily, however, confined to bodies external to us; for we can receive an impression by touching any part of our own body. The body which communicates the impressions needs but to be external to the part impressed. Sensations are divided into *external, internal* and *morbid.* The *external* are communicated by the five organs of the senses. The *internal* are such as occur within the body, and arise from some alteration in the function of the part, for the time being. Hunger and thirst are internal sensations, as well as all the natural wants. *Morbid* sensations may be either internal or external. *Objec'tive sensations* are produced by impressions on the peripheral nerves; as in vision, audition, &c. *Subjective sensations,* such as originate centrically, or in the encephalon, — as tinnitus aurium.

SENSATIONAL, Sentient.

SENSE, *Sensus, Sen'sio, Æsthe'sis,* (F.) *Sens.* Same etymon as Sensation. A faculty, possessed by animals, of appreciating impressions from external objects. The senses are five in number: sight, hearing, smell, taste, and touch. Of these, the first two and the last administer more to the intellect; and, hence, have been called by some, the *intellectual senses:* the other two seem more destined for the nutrition of the body: and, hence, have been termed *corporeal* or *nutritive senses.* Other senses have been suggested — as the intense sensation experienced during the venereal act; a sense of heat and cold; a muscular sense, a common sense or cœnæsthesis, &c.

SENSES, NERVOUS SYSTEM OF THE, Medulla oblongata.

SENSIBILITAS, Sensibility—s. Anomala, see Irritable — s. Aucta, see Irritable — s. Morbosa, see Irritable.

SENSIBIL'ITY, *Sensibil'itas.* Same etymon as Sensation; *Æsthe'ma.* The faculty of receiving impressions, and having the consciousness of them. Bichat defines it as the property possessed by living bodies, of receiving impressions, whether the individual be conscious of them or not. In the former case, where conscious, he calls the sensibility *animal:* in the latter, where not, he terms it *organic.* This last is common to vegetables and animals, and presides over nutrition, absorption, exhalation, secretion, &c. The other does not exist in vegetables: it is the origin of the sensations—olfaction, vision, gustation, audition, thirst, hunger, pain, &c. There are few parts of the animal body, but what are sensible — if not in health — in disease. The free extremities of the hair and nails, and the epidermis, are not so. See Insensibility.

SENSIFEROUS, Sentient.

SENSIO, Sense.

SENSITORIUM, Sensorium.

SENSORI-VOLIT"IONAL. A term applied to nervous fibres which pass to and from the cerebro-spinal axis, and are respectively concerned in sensation and volition.

SENSO'RIAL, Sentient.

SENSORIAL POWER, according to Dr. Wilson Philip, is composed of the two functions of sensation and volition. Dr. Darwin included in it the power of muscular contraction; but it ought not to be extended to acts in which there is not consciousness.

SENSO'RIUM, *Senso'rium commu'nè, Or'ganon senso'rium internum, Sensito'rium, Empo'rium spiritunm, Æsthete'rion, Sen'sory.* The common centre of sensations.

SENSORY, Sensorium, Sentient.

SENSORY GANG'LIA. A name given by Dr. Carpenter to a series of ganglionic masses at the base of the brain, which are in direct communication with the nerves of sensation—as the *olfactory, optic, auditory* and *gustatory.*

SENSORY NERVES, *Nerves of sensation,* are so called in contradistinction to *Motor* nerves. There are *general sensory nerves* — as those connected with the posterior part of the spinal marrow, and the fifth pair; and *special sensory,* as those of the senses.

SENSUS ÆGRITUDINIS, Indisposition—s. Osmometricus, Olfaction—s. Perversus, Pseudæsthesia.

SEN'TIENT, *Sen'tiens, Sen'sory, Ideülq"enous, Senso'rial, Sensa'tional, Sensif'erous.* Feeling, causing feeling.

SENTIENT EXTREMITIES OF NERVES are their minute terminations in the organs.

SENTIMENT, see Sensation.

SEPARATO'RIUM, from *separo,* 'I separate.' A surgical instrument, for separating the pericranium from the skull.

A *Sep'aratory, Vitrum Hypoclep'ticum,* is a pharmaceutical vessel for separating fluids of different densities from each other.

SEPEDOGENESIS, Sepedonogenesis.

SEPEDONOGEN'ESIS, *Sepedogen'esis,* from σηπεδων, 'putrescency,' and γενεσις, 'generation.' A septic disposition or tendency; such as is met with in typhus gravior.

SEPES, *Sæ'pes,* 'A hedge,' 'a row:' as *Sæpes* seu *Se'ries* seu *Pecten den'tium :* —a row of teeth.

SEPES DENTIUM, See Sepes.

SEPHIRUS, Scleriasis.

SE'PIA, *S. officina'lis, Se'pium, Cuttle-Fish,* (F.) *Sèche.* The osseous part of the cuttle-fish—*Præcip'itans mag'num*—has been used as an absorbent, and is often added to tooth-powders.

SEPLASIA'RIUS. A name formerly given to one who sold perfumes, ointments, &c. It is derived from *Seplasia,* the name of a public place at Capua, where such preparations were frequently sold. A druggist.

SEPSICHYMIA, Septochymia.

SEPSIS, Putrefaction.

SEPTÆ'MIA; from σηπτος, 'rotten,' and 'αἱμα, 'blood.' A morbid condition of the blood produced by septic or putrid matters.

SEPTANA FEBRIS, Fever septan.

SEP'TENARY, *Septena'rius,* (F.) *Septénaire,* from *septem,* 'seven.' 'Consisting of seven.' The sept*e*nary years of the old believers in mystical periods were times at which, it was supposed, important changes might be expected to take place. The grand climacteric was fixed at 63, and it was considered that if a person passed that age, he had well-founded expectations that his life might be protracted to 90.

SEPTENNIAD, Climacteric, (years.)

SEPTFOIL, UPRIGHT, Tormentilla.

SEPTIC, *Sep'ticus, Septus,* from σηπω, 'a rot,' σηπτος, 'rotten.' That which produces putrefaction. A substance which corrodes and disorganizes the soft parts without causing much pain.

SEPTIC POISON, see Poison.

SEPTICÆMIA, Septæmia.

SEPTIMESTRIS FŒTUS, see Fœtus septimestris.

SEPTINERVIA, Plantago.

SEPTOCHYM'IA, *Sepsichym'ia;* from σηψις, 'putrefaction,' and Χυμος, 'juice.' Putrescence or putrescency of the humours.

SEPTOPYRA, Typhus gravior.

SEPT'ULUM; diminutive of *septum,* 'a partition.' A division between small spaces or cavities — as the *septula* or fibrous cords given off by the mediastinum testis to be inserted into the inner surface of the tunica albuginea.

SEPTUM, (F.) *Cloison.* A part intended to separate two cavities from each other, or to divide a principal cavity into several secondary cavities.

These septa are numerous in the human body. The chief are the following : —

SEPTUM CEREBELLI, Falx cerebelli—s. Cerebri, Falx cerebri—s. Cochleæ auditoriæ, Lamina spiralis.

SEPTUM CORDIS, *Septum me'dium cordis.* The partition which separates the two ventricles of the heart.

SEPTUM ENCEPHALI, Tentorium.

SEPTUM LU'CIDUM seu *pelluci'dum* seu *tra'ia d pellucidum* seu *medium* seu *Spec'ulum lucens* seu *Lapis specula'ris* seu *Mediasti'num* seu *Diaphragma ventriculo'rum latera'lium cer'ebri, Speculum,* (F.) *Septum médian,* (Ch.) *Cloison transparente.* The soft portion or medullary substance, which separates the two lateral ventricles of the brain from each other. This septum is composed of two laminæ; between which a small cavity exists, filled by a serous fluid, and called the *Fossa of Syl'vius, 5th ventricle of Cuvier. Sinus of the median septum,* (Ch.) The brothers Wen-sel are of opinion that this cavity is lined by a peculiar membrane.

SEPTUM MÉDIAN, S. lucidum—*s. Médian du cervelet*, Falx cerebelli—*s. Medium cerebri*, S. lucidum.

SEPTUM NA'RIUM, *Interseptum seu Dissepimen'tum seu Interst'nium seu Discri'men seu Imbrex seu Diaphrag'ma na'rium*, (F.) *Cloison des Fosses nasales*. The partition between the nares. It is formed by the vomer, the perpendicular plate of the ethmoid bone, and a cartilage of a triangular shape. These parts are lined by the pituitary membrane, which receives a considerable number of nerves and vessels.

SEPTUM NASI, see Nares.

SEPTUM PARVUM OCCIPITALE, Falx cerebelli—s. Pectiniforme, see Cavernous bodies—s. Pellucidum, S. Lucidum—s. Scalæ, Lamina spiralis—s. Staphylin, Velum pendulum palati—s. Tenue et pellucidum, S. lucidum—s. Thoracis, Mediastinum—*s. Transverse*, Tentorium—s. Transversum, Diaphragm—s. Vestibuli nervoso-membranaceum, see Labyrinth.

SEPTUS, Septious.

SEPUM, Sevum.

SEQUES'TRUM, from *sequestro*, 'I separate.' The portion of bone, in necrosis, which is dead, and separated from the living bone; acting, whilst retained, as an extraneous body. When the sequestrum is superficial and small, it is called *Exfolia'tion*.

SERAPEUM, Syrup.

SERAPINON, Sagapenum.

SERAPIUM, Syrup.

SERBET, Scherbet.

SER'ICUM, *Silk;* from *Seres*—the Thibetans probably—from whom it was first obtained. (F.) *Soie*. The thread spun by the *Bombyx Mori* or *Silkworm*. Silk is used by surgeons for ligatures, &c.

SERICUM ANGLICUM, see Sparadrapum adhæsivum.

SERIES DENTIUM, see Sepes.

SÉRIEUX, Serious.

SERINGUE, Syringe.

SERIOLA, Cichorium intybus.

SE'RIOUS, (F.) *Sérieux, Grave*. A term applied to a disease, *Dyspathi'a, Morbus gravis*, and to a symptom that is attended with danger.

SERIS, Cichorium intybus.

SERMOUNTAIN, Laserpitium album.

SERO-COLITIS, see Colitis.

SERO-CYSTIC, *Sero-cyst'icus*. An epithet to tumours of the female breast, which consist, in the first stage, of one or more membranous cysts, produced perhaps by dilatation of portions of the lactiferous tubes.

SERO-HEPATITIS, see Hepatitis.

SER'OLIN, from *serum*, 'whey.' A fatty matter detected in the blood by Boudet, Lecanu, Sanson, and others.

SÉROSITÉ, Serum.

SEROSITY, Serum.

SEROUS, *Sero'sus*, (F.) *Séreux*. Thin; watery. Relating to the most watery portion of animal fluids, or to membranes that secrete them. See Serum.

SEROUS LAYER, see *Tache embryonnaire*.

SEROUS MEMBRANES, Membranes, serous.

SERPEDO, Psoriasis.

SERPENT, *Serpens, Anguis, Ophis;* from *serpo*, 'I creep.' A snake.

SNAKE BROTH was, at one time, recommended as a restorative.

Many serpents are venomous: and the bites of some fatal. See Poisons, Table of.

SERPENTAIRE NOIRE, Actæa racemosa.

SERPENTARIA, Aristolochia serpentaria—s. Gallorum, Arum dracunculus—s. Hispanica, Scorzonera—s. Minor, Arum maculatum—s. Nigra, Actæa racemosa.

SERPENTARIÆ BRAZILIENSIS RADIX, Caincæ radix.

SERPENTIN, see Alembic.

SERPENTINE, Ophites.

SERPENTINUS, Ophites.

SERPES, Herpes.

SERPIG"INOUS, from *serpere*, 'to creep.' An epithet given to certain affections, which creep, as it were, from one part to another,—'*Serpiginous* erysipelas,' (F.) *Érysipèle serpigineux*.

SERPIGO, Herpes circinatus, Lichen psoriasis.

SERPILLUM, Thymus serpyllum.

SERPOLET, Thymus serpyllum.

SERPULLUM, Thymus serpyllum.

SERPYLLUM, Thymus serpyllum—s. Citratum, see Thymus serpyllum.

SERRA, Saw—s. Amputatoria, Saw, amputation—s. Versatilis, Trepan.

SERRAT'ULA AMA'RA, *Family*, Cynarocephaleæ. *Sex. Syst.* Syngenesia Polygamia æqualis. A species of *Sawwort*, recommended in ague.

SERRATULA BEHEN, Centaurea behen.

SERRATUS ANTICUS MINOR, Pectoralis minor—s. Major, Serratus magnus.

SERRA'TUS MAGNUS. So called from its serrated appearance; from *serra*, 'a saw.' *Serratus major anti'cus, Serratus major*, (F.) *Costobasi-scapulaire, Costo-scapulaire*, (Ch.,) *Grand dentelé*. A very broad (especially anteriorly,) thin, flat, irregularly quadrilateral muscle, situate at the sides of the thorax. It is attached, before, to the external surface of the first 8 or 9 ribs, by as many distinct digitations; and, behind, to the spinal edge of the scapula. The superior fibres are almost horizontal; the lower become gradually more and more oblique upwards and backwards. This muscle carries the scapula forwards, and causes it to execute a movement of rotation, which directs its inferior angle forwards, and the anterior upwards. When the shoulder is fixed, it raises the ribs.

SERRATUS POSTI'CUS INFERIOR, (F.) *Dorso-lombo-costal, Lombo-costal*, (Ch.,) *Petit dentelé postérieur et inférieur*. A broader and thinner muscle than the following, but nearly of the same shape. It is situate obliquely at the lower part of the back; and extends from the spinous processes of the last two or three dorsal vertebræ, and the first two or three lumbar, to the inferior margin of the last four false ribs. This muscle depresses the ribs, and thus concurs in expiration. It is an antagonist to the next.

SERRATUS POSTI'CUS SUPE'RIOR, (F.) *Cervici-dorso-costal, Dorso-costal*, (Ch.) *Petit dentelé supérieur*. A flat, thin, quadrilateral muscle; situate obliquely at the posterior inferior part of the neck, and the superior part of the back. It passes from the posterior cervical ligament, the spinous process of the last cervical vertebra; from the spinous processes of the first two or three dorsal, to the second, third, fourth, and fifth ribs; into which it is inserted by as many digitations. It raises the ribs, and is, consequently, an inspiratory muscle.

SERTULA CAMPANA, Trifolium melilotus.

SERUM, Sperm.

SERUM, 'whey.' *Orrhos, Oros, Seros'ity,* (F.) *Sérosité*. The most watery portion of animal fluids, exhaled by serous membranes. It is a constituent part of blood, milk, &c.

SERUM OF THE BLOOD, *Hæ'mydor, Orr'hos, Ichor san'guinis,* (F.) *Sérum du Sang*, is the liquid which separates from the blood, when coagulated at rest. It is of a greenish-yellow colour; viscid, slightly coagulable by heat, acids, and alcohol. It is composed of water; chloride of sodium; certain phosphates; and albumen, constantly united to soda, almost in a saponaceous combination.

The fluid which exudes from the albumen of the serum of the blood, when coagulated by heat, is by some called *serosity*.

SÉRUM DU SANG, S. of the blood.

SERUM LACTIS, *Aqua lactis; Serum of Milk, Whey*, (F.) *Sérum du lait, Petit lait.* That part of milk, from which the butter and caseous matter have been separated. It is a transparent, citrine-coloured liquid, containing sugar of milk, mucilage, acetic acid, phosphate of lime, and some other saline substances. It is used as a slightly nutritious diluent and refrigerant.

SERUM LACTIS HOFFMAN'NI, (F.) *Petit-lait d'Hoffmann*, is a name given to the liquid resulting from treating with boiling water milk which has been evaporated to an almost solid consistence. It is not much used.

RENNET WHEY is made thus: milk 2 pints; rennet ℨss, infused in a little hot water; mix and keep in a gentle heat for some hours, then strain.—Gray.

SERUM OF SEROUS MEMBRANES, *Serum membranarum serosa'rum, Water of Dropsy*, (F.) *Sérum des membranes séreuses, Eau des hydropiques.* It resembles the serum of the blood,—especially in cases of hydrocele. The water of hydrothorax and ascites contains much less albumen:—sometimes enough to coagulate on the application of heat: at others, not.

SERVICE, MOUNTAIN, Sorbus acuparia—s. Tree, Sorbus domestica.

SERVIETTE EN CARRÉ, Couvrechef.

SES'AMOID, *Sesamoï'des, Sesamo'des, Sesamoïdeus*, from σησαμη, 'a grain of sesamum,' and ειδος, 'resemblance.'

SESAMOID BONES, *Ossa seu Ossic'ula sesamoï'dea*, are small bones, situate in the substance of tendons, near certain joints. Their number is various. They are commonly more in the male than female. Two are constantly met with beneath the metatarso-phalangal articulations of the great toe. Sometimes, the articulations of other bones of the metatarsus with the phalanges of the toes have them likewise. In the hand, there are two before the metacarpo-phalangal joint of the thumb. At times, they are met with in the other metacarpo-phalangal articulations. Occasionally, two exist behind the condyles of the femur, in the tendons of the gastrocnemii muscles. A considerable os sesamoideum is also met with in the tendon of the peronæus longus. These bones are commonly round, and flattened only on one surface, which is incrusted with cartilage. Their size is very variable, according to the joints in which they exist. Traces of sesamoid bones are not observed in infants: in them, they are replaced by small, cartilaginous concretions. They are developed by a single point of ossification: and are, like the patella (which is a true sesamoid bone,) composed of much cellular substance, covered by a thin layer of compact tissue. The use of these bones is,—to allow the tendon to be inserted into the lever at a greater angle; and thus enable the power to act more advantageously.

Riolan has given the name *Ossa sesamoïdea* to two bony points sometimes met with;—the one at the outer side of the carotid canal of the temporal bone; and the other at the edge of the cavernous sinus, at the side of the internal carotid artery.

SESAMUM, see Sesamum orientale.

SES'AMUM ORIENTA'LE, *S. edu'lè seu oleif'erum, Bennè, Oily Grain*. The seeds of this African plant are cultivated in Georgia and South Carolina, where the negroes use them with Indian corn as an article of food. They yield a larger proportion of oil than any other vegetable; one hundred weight producing ninety pounds of oil, which is, at least, equal to Florence oil.

Benne oil, Oleum Ses'ami, is used in the Southern States as a laxative. The leaves—*Sesamum* (Ph. U. S.)—afford, by infusion, an excellent mucilage.

SESCUN'CIA, *Sesquiun'cia, Hemiol'ion.* An ounce and a half. See Sesqui.

SESELI, Laserpitium siler—s. Ægopodium, Ligusticum podagraria—s. Annuum, S. tortuosum—s. Carum, Carum—s. Carvi, Carum—s. Creticum, Tordylum officinale—s. Fœniculilium, Sison ammi—s. Graveolens, Apium graveolens—s. Meum, Æthusa meum—s. Patens, S. tortuosum—s. Pratense, Peucedanum silaus—*des Prés*, Peucedanum silaus.

SES'ELI TORTUO'SUM, *Seseli Massilien'sè seu an'nuum seu patens, Œnan'thè stria'ta rigida, Hartwort of Marseilles*. The seeds have a warm taste; and a greater degree of pungency than those of Laserpitium siler, which is the *Seseli* of the Pharmacopœias.

SESQUI. This word, joined with any number, weight, measure, &c., signifies one and a half; as *sesquigranum*, 'a grain and half.'

SESQUIUNCIA, Sescuncia.

SETA EQUI'NA, 'a horse's hair.' *Hairworm, Helmin'thus Gor'dii*. A kind of worm, found in stagnant water, from 4 to 6 inches long, and twisted into various knots and contortions; colour pale-brown, with dark extremities. It is common in the intestines of the Laplanders, causing the *Col'ica Lappon'ica*, in which the gripings are, at times, exceedingly severe.

SETA'CEUM, *Seto, Seton*, from *seta*, 'a bristle.' A long strip of fine linen or cotton twist, passed through the skin and areolar membrane, to keep up an issue; or through suppurating canals between the fragments of fractured bones, &c. to fulfil certain indications. The term is also applied to the issue so established. The operation is simple. It consists in laying hold of a fold of skin, and passing a seton-needle through it, with the thread attached. Every day a fresh portion of the thread is drawn through the skin. Setons are established in many diseases,— in obstinate ophthalmiæ, cephalalgiæ; epidemic, thoracic and abdominal affections, &c.; but they are not as much used as formerly.

SETARIA ROCCELLA, Lichen roccella.
SETFAST, see Furunculus.
SETO, Setaceum.
SETON, Setaceum.
SETTERWORT, Helleborus fœtidus.
SEVADILLA, Veratrum sabadilla.
SEVATIO, Steatoma.
SÈVE, Sap.
SÉVRAGE, Weaning.
SEVUM, Pinguedo.

SEVUM, *Sebum, Sepum, Stear, Adeps* or *Sevum verveci'num*. Suet, mutton suet, Pinguedo.

SEVUM PRÆPARA'TUM, *Serum* (Ph. U. S.) *Ovil'li Sevum Præpara'tum, Prepared suet,* (F.) *Graisse de Mouton, Suif*, is formed by cutting suet in pieces; melting over a slow fire and straining through linen. It is excellent.

and is sometimes boiled in milk (ℨij to Oj), and is used in diarrhœa and dysentery. Its principal employment is in the formation of plasters.

SEVUM VERVECINUM, Sevum.

SEX, *Sexus, Genos, Physis.* The physical difference between male and female in animals and vegetables;—as the *Male sex, Sexus po'tior* seu *for'tior* seu *viri'lis;* and the *Female sex, Sexus seq'uior, S. mulie'bris, Alter Sexus, 'The Sex.'*

SEXTANS, *Sexta pars libræ.* The sixth part of a pound.—Galen.

SEXTA'RIUS. An ancient measure for liquid and solid substances. See Weights and Measures.

SEX'TULA, *Hexagium, 'εξαγιον.* The sixth part of an ounce.

SEX'UAL, *Sexua'lis,* from *sexus,* 'sex.' That which relates to the sex; which characterizes the sex.

SEXUAL DISEASES, *Morbi sexua'les,* are the diseases of the genital organs; as SEXUAL FUNCTIONS are the genital functions.

SEXUAL INTERCOURSE, Coition—s. Organs, Genital organs.

SEXUS, Sex—s. Alter, see Sex—s. Fortior, see Sex—s. Muliebris, see Sex—s. Potior, see Sex—s. Sequior, see Sex—s. Virilis, see Sex.

SEYDSCHÜTZ WATER, Sedlitz water.

SHALLOT, Echalotte.

SHAMPOO'ING, *Massing,* (F.) *Massage, Massement.* A Hindoo process, which consists in pressing the body of the bather in a peculiar manner; cracking the various joints, and employing blows and friction.

'Kneading' consists in pressing alternately upon a part of the body to arouse the muscles to more energetic action. It is employed at times in dyspepsia.

SHAMROCK, INDIAN, Trillium latifolium—s. Water, Menyanthes verna.

SHANKER, *Chancre.*

SHARON SPRINGS, NEW YORK. These springs, which are situate about 10 or 12 miles south of Canajoharie, N. Y., and 45 miles west of Albany, are much frequented. They contain, according to the analysis of Dr. Chilton, sulphate of magnesia, sulphate of lime, chloride of sodium, chloride of magnesium, sulphohydrate of sodium, sulphohydrate of calcium, vegetable extractive matter, and free sulphohydric acid gas. Their temperature is 48° Fahr.

SHEATH, Vagina.

SHEEP POISON, Kalmia latifolia.

SHELLBARK, see Hickory.

SHELL FLOWER, Trillium latifolium—s. Liquid, see Calcis murias—s. Membrane, Membrana testæ.

SHEPHERD'S PURSE, Thlaspi bursa.

SHERBET, Scherbet—s. Orange, see Syrupus aurantii.

SHERMAN'S WORM LOZENGES, see Worm lozenges, Sherman's.

SHERRY, Sack, see Wine.

SHIELD, WATER, Nelumbium luteum.

SHIN, *O'crea, Crista tib'iæ.* The *spine* or anterior part of the tibia or leg. It is, also, called *Anticne'mion,* and *Crea.*

SHINGLES, Herpes zoster.

SHIP FEVER, see Typhus.

SHOCK, see Concussion.

SHORT, Sax. ꞅceoꞃꞇ, from ꞃcinan, 'to cut, to *shear,' shored, shor'd, short,* (F.) *Court.* A word used, by anatomists, in opposition to *long;* and to distinguish parts from each other that have otherwise the same name.

SHORT BONES, for example, are those in which the three dimensions—length, breadth, and thickness—are nearly alike; such are the vertebræ, bones of the carpus, tarsus, &c.

SHORT RIBS, see Costa.

SHORTSIGHTED, Myopic.

SHORTSIGHTEDNESS, Myopia.

SHORTWINDED, Pursy.

SHOTBUSH, Aralia spinosa.

SHOULDER-BLADE, Scapula.

SHOVEL PICKEREL WEED, Unisema deltifolia—s. Pond, Unisema deltifolia.

SHOW, see Parturition.

SHOW-CHOO, see Spirit.

SHOWER-BATH, see Bath.

SHRUB, perhaps, from Arabic, *sharab,* 'syrup.' A compound of spirits, lemon-juice, and sugar.

SHRUB, SWEET, Calycanthus—s. Sweet-scented, Calycanthus.

SHUD'DERING, *Frem'itus, Phryag'ma,* from (G.) Schauder, Schauer, (F.) *Frémissement, Tressaillement.* A peculiar sensation, felt either externally or internally; and which seems to be the result of a spasmodic movement of the parts in which it occurs. A slight feeling of cold sometimes accompanies it. It is, at times, the result of a moral cause, and is often the precursor of shivering.

SHUMAC, Rhus coriaria.

SIAGANTRI'TIS, from σιαγων, 'the jaw,' αντρον, 'a cavity,' and *itis,* denoting inflammation. Inflammation of the lining membrane of the antrum of Highmore.

SIAGON, Maxillary bone.

SIAGO'NAGRA, from σιαγων, 'the jaw,' and αγρα, 'a seizure.' *Arthri'tis maxilla'ris.* A gouty or rheumatic affection of the joint of the lower jaw.

SIALACHUS, Salivation.

SIAL'AGOGUE, *Sialago'gus, Sial'ogogue, Ptyal'agogue, Ptyas'magogue, Sali'vans, Saliva'tum, Sialocinet'icus, Apophlegmat'isans per os,* (F.) *Salivant;* from σιαλον, 'saliva,' and αγω, 'I expel.' That which provokes the secretion of saliva. Pyrethrum and mercury are sialogogues. Sialagogues may be of two kinds,—those which act through the circulation, and those which act immediately on the salivary organs. Mercury belongs to the former,—pyrethrum to the latter class. The chief sialagogues are armoraci, calamus, mezereum, pyrethrum, tabacum, and zingiber.

SIAL'ICA, from σιαλον, 'saliva.' Medicines, which affect the salivary glands.—Pereira.

SIALISMUS, Salivation.

SIALOCINETICUS, Sialagogue.

SIALOLITHI, Calculi, salivary.

SIALOLOG"IA, from σιαλον, 'saliva,' and λογος, 'a discourse.' A treatise on saliva.

SIALOMA, Saliva.

SIALON, Saliva.

SIALORRHŒA, Salivation.

SIALOS'CHESIS, from σιαλον, 'saliva,' and σχεσις, 'retention.' Retention or suppression of the saliva.

SIALOSYRINGES, Salivary fistulæ.

SIALOZEMIA, Salivation—s. Mercurialis, Salivation, mercurial.

SIAMESE TWINS, see Twins, Siamese.

SIBARE, Phrenitis.

SIBBENS, *Sivvens, Frambœ'sia Sco'tica.* An infectious disease in the mountainous parts of Scotland, viewed to be of the venereal kind. *Sivin,* in the Keltic, means raspberry; and it is said that, in this affection, fungi appear like raspberries. From *sivin,* the inhabitants have made *sievin, sibben, sibbens,* and *sivvens.* By some, this affection is regarded as a complication of the venereal and itch. In the Orkneys, *sibbens* means itch.—Jamieson.

SIBILANT, *Sib'ilus, Sib'ilans*, from *sibilo*, 'I hiss or whistle.' Making a hissing or whistling sound. See *Râle sibilant*.

SIBILISMUS AURIUM, Tinnitus aurium.

SIBILUS AURIUM, Tinnitus aurium.

SICCAN'TIA, from *siccare*, 'to dry.' *Xeran'tica*, (F.) *Siccatifs*. Drying medicines.—Galen.

SICCANTIA, Desiccativa.

SICCATIFS, Siccantia.

SICCATIO, Drying.

SICCHA'SIA, σιχχασια, 'disgust.' A distressing disgust for food; such as is experienced by women with child.

SICIL'ICUM. A Roman weight of about two drachms.

SICK, Sax. ɼeoc, *Æger, Ægro'tus, Nos'eros, Noso'des, Jacens, Laborio'sus, Laborans*, (F.) *Malade*. Labouring under disease. Such is its acceptation in old English, and generally in the United States. In England, it most commonly means,—affected with disorder of the stomach or nausea.

A sick person, *Æger, Ægro'tus*, (F.) *Malade*, who is under the charge of a physician is said to be a *patient*, or the patient of the physician. At times, but rarely, patient is used for a sick person in the abstract.

SICK STOMACH, Milk sickness.

SICKLY, *Morbo'sus, Valetudina'rius, Adyn'atos, Nosac'eros, Noso'des, Morbose*, (F.) *Maladif*. One who is subject to be sick, or is in feeble health.

SICKNESS, Disease—s. Falling, Epilepsy—s. River, Milk sickness—s. of the Stomach, Vomiting—s. Swamp, Milk sickness.

SICLIUM, Sicilicum.

SICUA, Cupping-glass.

SICULA, Beta, Penis.

SICYEDON, Cauledon.

SIDA ABUTILON, Abutilon cordatum.

SIDE, PAIN IN THE, Pleurodynia.

SIDERA'TIO, *Sydera'tio, Sidera'tion*, from *sidus*, 'a star;' because the condition was thought to be produced by the influence of the stars. The state of one struck suddenly, without apparent cause, and as if by the influence of the stars or planets—*Planet-struck*. The ancients comprised, under this name, different morbid conditions, such as paralysis, apoplexy, and gangrene.

SIDERATIO, Apoplexy, Asphyxia, Phrenitis—s. Ossis, Spina ventosa.

SIDERATION, Astrobolismos, Sideratio.

SIDERION, Ferramentum.

SIDERITES, Magnet.

SIDERITIS, Magnet, Teucrium chamæpitys.

SIDEROS, Ferrum.

SIDEROXYLON, Chrysophyllum cainito.

SIDHEE, see Gunjah.

SIDMOUTH (CLIMATE OF). Sidmouth is in Devonshire, England, on the sea-beach, at the mouth of the Sid. It is much frequented by invalids, both during the summer and winter. The climate is, however, damp, and subject to sea-fogs.

SIÉGE, Anus.

SIELISMOS, Salivation.

SIELON, Saliva.

SIEVE, see Cribration—s. Drum, see Cribration.

SIFFLEMENT (F.), from *siffler*, 'to whistle.' Whistling.

SIFFLEMENT MODULÉ, Chant des artères, Bruit musical, 'modulated whistling, or music of the arteries.' A kind of sound heard on auscultation, resembling, at times, the humming of certain insects.

The sound is chiefly met with in those labouring under chlorosis.

SIGAULTIAN SECTION, Symphyseotomy.

SIGE, Taciturnity.

SIGH, Suspirium.

SIGHT, Vision—s. Askew, Dysopia lateralis —s. False, Metamorphopsia, Pseudoblepsis—s. Feebleness of, Amblyopia.

SIGILLUM SALAMONIS, Convallaria polygonatum—s. Virginitatis, Hymen.

SIGMATOID, Sigmoid.

SIGMOID, *Sigmoid'al, Sig'matoid, Sigmoï'des, Sigmoï'deus*. That which has the form of the Greek S or C; from *sigma*, and *eid*, 'resemblance.'

SIGMOID CARTILAGES, Semilunar cartilages.

SIGMOID CAVITIES OR FOSSÆ OF THE ULNA. *Cavités ou Fosses sigmoïdes*, are two notches at the upper part of that bone,—one for the reception of the humerus; the other for that of the radius.

SIGMOID FLEXURE OF THE COLON, *Flexion sigmoï'dea*, is a turn the colon takes immediately before its termination in the rectum.

SIGMOID or SEMILUNAR VALVES, *Valvulæ Sigmoï'deæ, Proces'sus Sigmoï'des*, (F.) *Valvules sigmoïdes ou semilunaires*, are three valvulæ found at the commencement of the pulmonary artery and aorta. These valves have the form of a crescent, when applied against the parietes of the vessel. When the blood is sent from the ventricles by their contraction, the valves are applied against the sides of the vessel; but, during the diastole of the ventricle, they are depressed, and prevent the blood from returning to the heart. At the middle of the convexity of each valve is a small, hard, triangular granulum, called *Corpus'culum seu Glob'ulus Arant'ii*, which completely closes up the passage. It is, also, called *Corpusculum Morgagn'ii*, and *C. Sesamodeum*, (F.) *Globule d'Arantius*.

SIGN, *Signum, Semi'on*, (F.) *Signe*. Any present or past circumstance, afforded by the examination of a patient, or of matters concerning him, whence a conclusion may be drawn regarding the nature and seat of his disease. The phenomena which precede the disease are called *amnes'tic* or *commem'orative signs*;—those which accompany it are termed *diagnos'tic*, if they reveal the nature or seat of the disease.—*prognos'tic*, when they indicate its probable duration and termination.

SIGNA ASSIDENTIA, see Assidens.

SIG'NATURE, *Signatu'ra, Signa'tio, hoc signum*, 'a sign;' *Episphagism'os*. This term was applied in the Eastern countries, in the middle ages, to mystic characters of good or ill augury, with which it was pretended that every one was marked by the star under which he was born.

SIGNATURES OF PLANTS meant certain peculiarities in their external formation or colour, which indicated that they were adapted for particular diseases:—as in the case of the *Lungwort, Liverwort*, &c.

SIGNES AVANT-COUREURS, Precursory signs—*s. Précurseurs*, Precursory signs.

SIGNUM, see Parturition—s. Characteristicum, see Pathognomonic—s. Conjunctum— Pathognomonic—s. Diacriticum, see Diacritic—sigma—s. Morbi essentiale, see Pathognomonic.

SILACH, *Silac*. An Arabic word, used to designate thickening of the eyelids, *Crassitudo Palpebra'rum;* and, also, *Alopecia*.—Forestus Stephanus.

SILENCE, see Murmur, respiratory.

SILENE CRASSIFOLIA, Cucubalus behen—

s. Inflata, Cucubalus behen — s. Thorei, Cucubalus behen.

SILE'NE VIRGIN'ICA, *Ground Pink, Wild Pink, Catch Fly.* The root has been employed, in decoction, as an efficacious anthelmintic.

SILER LANCIFOLIUM, Laserpitium siler — s. Montanum, Laserpitium siler.

SIL'IQUA, *Cera'tion;* the carat. A weight of about four grains. A pod.

SILIQUA ARABICA, Tamarindus—s. Araci aromatici, see Vanilla—s. Banillæ, see Vanilla—s. Dulcis, Ceratonium siliqua—s. Vaniglise, see Vanilla—s. Vanilliæ, see Vanilla.

SILIQUASTRUM PLINII, Capsicum annuum.

SILK, Sericum—s. Weed, Asclepias Sullivantii, Asclepias tuberosa—s. Weed, common, Asclepias Syriaca — s. Worm, see Sericum.

SILLON, Sulcus — *s. Horizontal de la veine ombilicale,* see Liver — *s. Transversale,* see Liver — *s. de la Veine cave inférieur,* see Liver — *s. de la Veine porte,* see Liver.

SILO, Camus.

SILPHIUM, Laserpitium.

SIL'PHIUM PERFOLIA'TUM, *Cup Plant, Turpentine Sun Flower,* and

SILPH'IUM TEREBINTHINA'CEUM, *Pra'irie Burdock, Rosin Weed; Nat. Order,* Compositæ; indigenous in Ohio and Michigan, and flowering from July to September; yield a fragrant gum, which is esteemed stimulant and antispasmodic.

SILUS, Camus.

SILVER, Argentum—s. Ammonio-chloride of, see Argentum — s. Chloride of, see Argentum — s. Chloruret of, see Argentum—s. Cyanide of, see Argentum — s. Cyanuret of, see Argentum — s. Iodide of, see Argentum — s. Ioduret of, see Argentum—s. Leaf, Magnolia macrophylla—s. Muriate of, see Argentum — s. Nitrate of, Argenti nitras—s. Oxide of, see Argentum — s. and Ammonia, Chloride of, see Argentum — s. and Ammonia, Chloruret of, see Argentum.

SILYBUM, Carduus marianus—s. Maculatum, Carduus marianus — s. Marianum, Carduus marianus.

SIMAROUBA, Quassia simarouba — s. Bitter, Quassia simarouba—*s. Faux,* Malpighia mourella.

SIMARUBA, Quassia simarouba.

SIMARUBA CEDRON. A South American tree, the seeds of which — *cedron seeds* — have been used as an antidote for snake-bites. They have, also, been proposed in mental diseases and in epilepsy. The scrapings of the wood have been used as a substitute for sulphate of quinia.

SIMARUBA OFFICINALIS, Quassia simarouba.

SIMILATIO, Assimilation.

SIMITIUM, Plumbi subcarbonas.

SIMO, Camus.

SIMONEA FOLLICULORUM, Acarus folliculorum.

SIMOTRACHELUS, Bysauchen.

SIMPLES. Medicinal herbs. One skilled in simples is called a *Simplist,* a *Rhizot'omist.*

SIMPLIST, see Simples.

SIMULATED DISEASES, Feigned diseases.

SIMULATI MORBI, Feigned diseases.

SIMUS, Camus.

SINA LEVANTICA, Artemisia santonica.

SINAPELÆ'ON, from σιναπι, 'mustard,' and ελαιον, 'oil.' Oil impregnated with mustard.

SINAPI, Sinapis.

SINA'PIS, *Sinapis nigra seu cer'nua seu Olivera'na, Bras'ica nigra, Napus, Eru'ca, Sina'pâ, Sina'pi, Na'pium, Napy, Common Black Mustard,* (F.) *Moûtarde noire, Sénevé, Sanve. Family,* Cruciferæ. *Sex. Syst.* Tetradynamia Siliquosa. The seeds are inodorous, when entire; but, when bruised, the odour is very pungent; taste bitterish and acrid. They yield their virtues to water, and afford a bland oil by expression. The seeds are stimulant, diuretic, emetic, and rubefacient. They are sometimes recommended to be swallowed whole, in dyspepsia, torpor of the bowels, &c. Externally, they are applied in the form of cataplasm. See Sinapism.

SINAPIS ALBA, *S. folio'sa, Bonannia officina'lis, White Mustard, Napus Leucosina'pis,* is also used medicinally. It is somewhat less pungent than the black. The distilled oil—*Oleum Sinapis*—is a powerful stimulant and rubefacient.

Whitehead's Essence of Mustard consists of *oil of turpentine, camphor,* and a portion of *spirit of Rosemary:* to which is added a small quantity of *flour of mustard.* It is a celebrated embrocation for rheumatism, &c.

Whitehead's Essence of Mustard Pills consist of *yellow resin* and *balsam of tolu* enough to make into pills.

Mustard Whey is made by taking bruised *mustard seeds* ℥ss, and *milk* Oj. Boil together until the milk is curdled, and strain.

This whey is used in dropsy.

SINAPIS ARVEN'SIS, *S. Timoria'na, Charlock, Wild Mustard,* has the seeds sometimes substituted for black mustard.

SINAPIS CER'NUA, Sinapis — s. Eruca, Brassica eruca—s. Foliosa, S. alba—s. Oliveriana, Sinapis—s. Tamoriana, S. arvensis—s. Tuberosa, Brassica rapa.

SINAPISIS, Bole Armenian.

SIN'APISM, *Sinapis'mus,* from σιναπι, 'mustard.' A cataplasm, of which mustard forms the basis, which is used for exciting redness, and acting as a counter-irritant. It is prepared by mixing flour of mustard and vinegar together to the due consistence. See Cataplasma sinapis.

SIN'CIPUT, *Sincip'ital Region, Bregma, Syn'ciput, Mesocra'nium, Mesoc'ranum, Hemicephalæ'um, Hemicephal'ium, Hemiceph'alum;* the top of the head. The French use it synonymously with *vertex.* By some it is applied to the frontal region or fore-part of the cranium. The parietal bones have been called *sincipital bones, Ossa sincip'itis,* (F.) *Os du sinciput.*

SINDON, σινδων, very fine linen. A small piece of rag, or a round pledget, supported by a thread at its middle, and introduced into the opening in the cranium made by the trephine.

SINEW, Tendon.

SINGLETON'S GOLDEN OINTMENT is formed of *sulphuret of arsenic* (realgar,) and *lard* or *spermaceti ointment.*

SINGULT'OUS, *Lygmo'des, Lygo'des, Lyngo'des, Lynggo'des;* from *Singultus,* 'hiccough.' Relating to or affected with hiccough.

SINGULT'US, *Lynx, Lygmus, Spasmolyg'mus, Clonus singul'tus, Pneusis singul'tus, Hiccough, Hiccup,* (F.) *Hoquet.* A noise made by the sudden and involuntary contraction of the diaphragm, and the simultaneous contraction of the glottis, which arrests the air in the trachea. It is a symptom of many morbid conditions, and especially of gangrene, but occurs, frequently, in persons otherwise in good health.

SIN'ISTRAD, from *sinister,* 'to the left hand.' A term used by Dr. Barclay, adverbially, to signify 'towards the sinistral aspect.' See Mesial.

SINISTRAL ASPECT, see Mesial.

SINUEUX, Sinuous.

SINUOSITAS, Sinus.

SIN'UOUS, *Sinuo'sus,* (F.) *Sinueux,* from *sinus,* 'a bay or curve.' An epithet given to certain ulcers, and especially to certain fistulæ, which are tortuous.

SINUS, *Sinuo'sitas, Colpos, Abscon'sio, Eurycho'ria, Reces'sus,* (F.) *Golfe.* Any cavity, the interior of which is more expanded than the entrance. In this sense, anatomists have applied the term to cavities in certain bones of the head and face. It has been, also, applied to certain venous canals, into which a number of vessels empty themselves; such as the sinuses of the dura mater and of the spine; the sinus of the vena porta; uterine sinuses, &c.;—and to the bosom.

In *surgery*, it means a long, narrow, hollow track, leading from some abscess, diseased bone, &c., (F.) *Clapier.*

Sinuses of bones form part of the nasal cavities. They are the frontal, sphenoidal, maxillary, &c. The name has also been given, occasionally, to the ethmoid and mastoid cells.

SINUS ACUSTICUS, Auditory canal, internal — s. Ampullaceus, Cavitas elliptica — s. Aortici, Sinuses of Valsalva — s. Arteriosus, S. pulmonalis — s. Basilar, Sinus transversus — *s. Caverneux,* Cavernous sinus — s. Cavernosi uteri, Sinus uterini — s. Cavernosus, Cavernous sinus — s. Cerebri, Ventricles of the brain — *s. Choroïdien,* S. quartus — s. Circular, of Ridley, Sinus coronarius — s. Circularis, S. coronarius — *s. Coronaire du cœur,* see Cardiac veins.

SINUS CORONA'RIUS, *Sinus circula'ris, S. circula'ris Ridleyi, Circular sinus of Ridley, Cor'onary sinus.* A venous canal, which surrounds, in a more or less regular manner, the pituitary fossa and gland, emptying itself into the corresponding cavernous sinus by each of its extremities.

SINUS, CORONARY, Sinus coronarius — s. Coronary of the heart, Sinus coronary, venous.

SINUS CORONARY, VENOUS, *Coronary sinus of the heart.* A name given, on account of its great size, to that portion of the great coronary vein which embraces the left auriculo-ventricular furrow.

SINUS COXÆ, see Cotyloid — *s. Droit,* S. quartus.

SINUS DEXTER CORDIS, *Sinus vena'rum cava'rum, S. veno'sus, Saccus vena'rum cava'rum.* The right auricle of the heart : — *A'trium cordis dextrum.* See Auricula.

SINUSES OF THE DURA MATER, *Sinus seu Fis'tulæ seu Cavita'tes seu Ventric'uli seu Tu'buli seu Sanguiduc'tus seu Receptac'ula Duræ matris,* are formed by a separation of the layers of the dura mater, which acts as a substitute for the outer membrane of veins. Bichat admits only four great sinuses, of which all the others seem to be dependencies ; — the *two lateral sinuses,* the *straight sinus,* and the *longitudinal sinus.* To the lateral sinuses belong, — the *petrous sinuses,* superior and inferior; the *transverse sinus ;* the *cavernous sinuses ;* the *coronary sinus,* and the *occipital sinuses.* To the straight sinus belongs the *inferior longitudinal.* The longitudinal sinus, properly so called, has no sinus under its dependence.

SINUS FALCIFORMIS INFERIOR, S. longitudinal, inferior — s. Falciformis superior, S. longitudinal, superior — s. Fourth, Torcular Herophili — s. Genæ pituitarius, Antrum of Highmore — s. of the Jugular vein, see Jugular veins — s. Lacrymalis, Lachrymal sac.

SINUSES OF THE LARYNX, Ventricles of the larynx.

SINUSES, LAT'ERAL, *Sinus transver'si, S. magni, S. latera'les,* (F.) *Sinus latéraux.* Each of these sinuses, distinguished into right and left, begins at the torcular Herophili, or confluence of the sinuses, and terminates at the sinus of the jugular vein.

SINUS LATÉRAUX, Sinuses, lateral.

SINUSES, LONGITU'DINAL, *S. Longitudina'les.* These are two in number. 1. SUPERIOR LONGITUDINAL SINUS, *S. falcifor'mis superior, S. triangula'ris, Sinus médian,* (Ch.) A long, triangular canal; convex above, concave below; which occupies the whole of the upper edge of the falx cerebri. It is broad behind, and much narrower before, where it commences by a *cul-de-sac,* at the cristi galli of the ethmoid bone. It passes along the frontal or coronal crest, sagittal suture and the vertical groove of the occipital bone. It receives several veins from the dura mater; and all those that are spread over the convex and plain surfaces of the two hemispheres of the brain. It discharges itself into the upper part of the torcular Herophili. 2. INFERIOR LONGITUDINAL SINUS, *Sinus falcifor'mis inferior, Falcis cer'ebri.* This is much narrower than the last, and occupies the inferior edge of the falx cerebri, from its anterior third to the tentorium cerebelli, where it terminates, commonly by its branches, in the straight sinus.

SINUS MAGNI, Sinuses, lateral — s. Maxillaris, Antrum of Highmore — *s. Médian,* Sinus longitudinal superior — s. Median, see Semicircular canals — s. Muliebris, Vagina.

SINUS, OCCIP'ITAL, *Sinus occipita'lis.* These sinuses commence at the sides of the foramen magnum ossis occipitis, and ascend — becoming broader and nearer each other — into the substance of the falx cerebelli, where they frequently unite. Each opens into the inferior part of the torcular Herophili. They receive the veins of the falx cerebelli, of the dura mater which line the fossæ cerebelli, and of the posterior part of the cerebellum. Haller and Sömmering have given them the name of *posterior occipital sinus,* to distinguish them from the transverse sinus which they have called *anterior occipital sinus.*

SINUS OCCIPITALIS ANTERIOR, Sinus transversus — s. Ophthalmic, see Cavernous sinus — s. pendicularis, S. quartus — s. Pituitarii fossa, Frontal sinuses — s. Pocularis, see Ejaculatory ducts — s. Polymorphus, Cavernous sinus — s. Portarum, see Liver.

SINUS, PROSTAT'IC, *Sinus prostat'icus.* A fossa on each side of the verumontanum, in which are seen the numerous openings of the ducts of the prostate.

SINUS PUDENDI, Vagina — s. Pudoris, Vagina, Vulva.

SINUS PULMONALES, Sinuses of Valsalva.

SINUS PULMONA'LIS, *S. sinis'ter cordis, Atrium cordis sinis'trum, S. vena'rum pulmona'lis, arterio'sus, Saccus vena'rum pulmona'lium.* The left auricle of the heart. See Auricula.

SINUS OF THE PULMONARY VEINS, Auricle, left.

SINUS QUARTUS, *S. perpendicula'ris,* (F.) *Sinus choroïdien* (Ch.), *Sinus droit, Straight sinus.* A sinus — triangular throughout; wide posteriorly, narrower anteriorly; slightly oblique downwards and backwards — passes along the base of the falx cerebri, from the termination of the inferior longitudinal sinus to the torcular Herophili. It receives the inferior longitudinal sinus, the veins of the lateral ventricles or *venæ Galeni,* the superior cerebellous veins, &c.

SINUS RENUM, Pelvis of the kidney — s. Rhomboideus, see Ventricles of the brain — s. of the Septum lucidum, Ventricle, fifth — s. Sinister cordis, S. pulmonalis — s. Sphenoidalis, Cavernous sinus — s. Straight, S. quartus — s. Superciliaris, Frontal sinuses — s. Terminalis, Circulus terminalis — s. Transversi, Sinuses, lateral.

SINUS TRANSVER'SUS, *S. occipita'lis anterior, Bas'ilar sinus.* This sinus lies transverse to the anterior part of the basilary process of the occipital bone. It forms a communication between the two petrous sinuses, and the cavernous sinus of one side, and those of the other. Its breadth is commonly very great. It is situate between two layers of the dura mater, and presents, internally, a kind of cavernous tissue.

SINUS TRIANGULARIS, S. longitudinal, superior—s. Urogenitalis, Urogenital sinus.

SINUS UTERI'NI, *Sinus caverno'si U'teri, U'terine sinuses*. A name given to cavities, formed by the uterine veins in the substance of the uterine parietes. They are very large during pregnancy.

SINUS UTRICULOSUS, see Semicircular canals—s. *des Vaisseaux séminifères*, Corpus Highmori.

SINUSES OF VALSAL'VA are three depressions in the aorta—*Sinus aor'tici*—and pulmonary artery—*Sinus pulmona'les*—immediately opposite the semilunar valves. Their use is to leave the edges of the valves free, so that they can be caught by the refluent blood. Where the aorta is about to send off the first of its large branches, at the top of the thorax, it is of great size, and has been called the *Large sinus of Valsalva*.

SINUS OF THE VENA CAVA, Auricle, right—s. Venarum cavarum, S. dexter cordis—s. Venarum pulmonalium, S. pulmonalis—s. Venosus, S. dexter cordis.

SI'NUSES, VER'TEBRAL, (F.) *Sinus vertébraux*. Two great venous sinuses, different from those of the dura mater, which extend the whole length of the vertebral canal, from the occipital foramen to the end of the sacrum, behind the bodies of the vertebræ, before the dura mater, and at the sides of the posterior vertebral ligament. At their inner side they communicate with each other by means of branches, which form true *transverse sinuses*. They are situate at the middle of the body of each vertebra, passing under the posterior vertebral ligament. They receive, at their middle part, the veins that arise in the spongy tissue of the vertebræ. By their external side, the vertebral sinuses communicate with the posterior branches of the vertebral, intercostal, and lumbar veins. At their posterior side they receive the veins, which creep on the prolongation of the dura mater that envelops the marrow.

SINUS VULVÆ, Rima vulvæ.
SIPEERI, Bebeeru.
SIPEERINE, see Bebeeru.
SIPHAR, Peritoneum.
SIPHILIS, Syphilis.
SIPHITA, Somnambulism—s. Parva, Chorea.
SIPHO, Siphon—s. Urinæ, Diabetes.
SIPHON, *Sipho, σιφων*, 'a tube.' A bent tube, whose limbs are of unequal length, employed in pharmacy for transferring liquids from one vessel to another. With this view, the shorter limb is plunged into the fluid; and air is sucked from the extremity of the lower limb. The pressure of the atmosphere forces the fluid through the tube; and the flow will continue as long as the extremity of the longer limb is below the level of the fluid in which the shorter limb is immersed.

An exhausting syringe is, at times, attached to the longer extremity of the siphon by means of which the air can be drawn from it.

SIPHON, PLUNGING. An instrument, used in pharmacy for obtaining a specimen,—at times, a measured specimen,—of any liquid. With this view, the instrument is immersed into liquid, and allowed to remain there until full. The opening at the top is then closed with the thumb; and the contents, thus removed, are allowed to flow out by removing the thumb and permitting the entrance of air. It is a form of the *pipette*.

SIPHONIA CAHUCHU, see Caoutchouc—s. Elastica, see Caoutchouc.
SIPHUNCULUS, Syringe.
SIRA, Orpiment.
SIRENS, Symmeles.
SIRIASIS, *Coup de Soleil*, Insolation, Phrenitis—s. Ægyptiaca, *Coup de Soleil*.
SIRIUM MYRTIFOLIUM, Santalum album.
SIRIUS, Canicula.

SIROP DE CAPILLAIRE, see Adiantum capillus veneris—s. *de Coralline*, see Corallina Corsicana.
SIRUP, Syrup.
SISON AMMI, *Æthu'sa ammi, Cnid'ium tenuifolium, Pimpinella laterifo'lia, Ses'eli fœniculifo'lium. Family,* Umbelliferæ. *Sex. Syst.* Pentandria Digynia. The plant that affords the *Ammi verum* of the shops; (F.) *Ammi des Boutiques*. The seeds—*Semen Am'mios cretici seu veri*—were once used as a carminative.

SISON AMO'MUM, (F.) *Amome faux*, is considered to be excitant and diuretic. It is the *field honewort*.

SISON ANISUM, Pimpinella anisum—s. Podagraria, Ligusticum podagraria.
SISTENS, Epischeticus.
SISYMBRIUM ALLIARIA, Alliaria—s. Barbarea, Erysimum barbarea—s. Erucastrum, Brassica eruca—s. Menthastrum, Mentha aquatica.

SISYM'BRIUM NASTUR'TIUM, *Nasturtium aquat'icum seu officina'lē, Laver odora'tum, Cratcva'sium, Cressi, Cardami'nē fonta'na seu nastur'tium, Water Cress,* (F.) *Cresson de fontaine. Family,* Cruciferæ. *Sex. Syst.* Tetradynamia Siliquosa. Water-cresses are commonly used in salad. They have obtained a place in the materia medica for their antiscorbutic qualities.

SISYMBRIUM OFFICINALE, Erysimum—s. Parviflorum, S. sophia.
SISYMBRIUM SO'PHIA, *S. parviflo'rum, Herb Sophia, Sophia Chirurgo'rum, Flix* or *Flux-weed*, (F.) *Sagesse des Chirurgiens*. It was once reputed to be anthelmintic, and valuable in hysterical affections. It is not used.

Other species of *Nasturtium*, as N. PALUS'TRE, *Marsh water-cress;* and *N. amphib'ium, Water-radish*, possess similar virtues with Nasturtium officinale.

SISYRIN'CHIUM BERMUDIA'NUM, *Blue-eyed grass, Lily grass, Physic grass, Scurvy grass;* indigenous; *Order*, Iridaceæ; flowering from June to August. Used as a cathartic by the Thompsonians. A decoction of the root is acrid and cathartic.

SITICULOSUS, Dipsodes, see Alterative.
SITIENS, Dipsodes.
SITIS, Thirst—s. Intensa, Polydipsia—s. Morbosa, Polydipsia.
SITKA, MINERAL WATERS OF. See Archangel, New, mineral waters of.
SITOS, Aliment.
SITUS ANOMALUS seu PERVERSUS INTESTINORUM, Splanchnectopia—s. Mutatus, see Monster.
SITZBATH, see Bath, half.
SIUM, *Sium nodiflo'rum seu angustifo'lium seu Ber'ula seu erec'tum seu inci'sum, A'pium sium, Ber'ula angustifo'lia, Ber'ula, Creeping Water-parsnep,* (F.) *Berle nodiflore. Family,* Umbelliferæ. *Sex. Syst.* Pentandria Digynia. It is stimulant, and supposed to be diuretic and lithontriptic. It is, sometimes, employed in cutaneous eruptions.

SIUM ANGUSTIFOLIUM, S. nodiflorum—s. Apium, Apium graveolens—s. Berula, S. nodiflorum—s. Bulbocastanum, Bunium bulbocastanum—s. Carvi, Carum—s. Erectum, S. nodiflorum—s. Graveolens, Apium graveolens—s. Incisum, S. nodiflorum.

SIUM LATIFO'LIUM is the common *Water-parsnep* of the United States. It is said to be poisonous.

SIUM NINSI. The plant whose root is called *Radix Ninsi, Ninzin, Nindsin*. This root was long supposed to be the same as ginseng, and it possesses similar, though weaker properties.

SIUM SILAUS, Peucedanum silaus.

SIUM SIS'ARUM, *Skirret*, is used as a salad in Europe; and has been supposed a useful diet in chest affections.

SIUM VULGARE, Ligusticum podagraria.

SIVVENS, Sibbens.

SKELETIA, Emaciation.

SKELETOL'OGY, *Sceletolog"ia*, (F.) *Squelettologie*, from σκελετος, 'a skeleton,' and λογος, 'a discourse.' A treatise on the solid parts of the body. This part of anatomy comprehends *Osteology* and *Syndesmology*.

SKEL'ETON, *Scel'etum*, from σκελετος, *Cadav'er exsicca'tum;* (F.) *Squelette, Sceleton*, a dried body; from σκελλω, 'I dry.' The aggregate of the hard parts of the body, or the bones. A skeleton is found in almost all animals, although it may not always be formed in the same manner. In some, as in the crustacea and testacea, it is wholly or partly *external, Exo-skeleton, Dermo-skeleton*. In others, as in birds, the mammalia, &c., it is *internal, Endo-skeleton, Neuro-skeleton*. It serves as a support for other organs. On it the general shape of the body and of its various parts is greatly dependent. When the bones are united by their natural ligaments, the skeleton is said to be *natural, Scel'etum natura'lĕ;* when articulated by means of wires, *artificial, Scel'etum artificia'lĕ*.

SKELETOPŒIA, *Sceletopœ'a, Sceleteu'sis*, from σκελετος, 'a skeleton,' and ποιεω, 'I make.' The part of practical anatomy which treats of the preparation of bones, and the construction of skeletons. Bones are prepared to exhibit their conformation, structure, chymical composition, mode of development, and changes; the different cavities formed by the union; and to demonstrate their connexions, relations, modes of union, &c.

SKEVISCH, Erigeron Philadelphicum.

SKEVISH, FLEABANE, Erigeron Philadelphicum.

SKIN, Cutis.

SKIN-BOUND DISEASE, Induration of the cellular tissue.

SKIOMACHIA, Sciomachy.

SKIRRET, Sium sisarum.

SKIRSE, Scirrhus.

SKOKE, Phytolacca decandra.

SKOLEMORA FERNAMBUCENSIS, Geoffræa vermifuga.

SKUE-SIGHT, Dysopia lateralis.

SKULL, Cranium.

SKULL-CAP, Calvaria, Scutellaria galericulata.

SKUNK-CABBAGE, Dracontium fœtidum.

SKUNK-WEED, Dracontium fœtidum.

SLATE, IRISH, Hibernicus lapis.

SLATERS, Onisci aselli.

SLATKAIA TRAVA, see Spirit.

SLAV'ERING, from *saliva. Ptyalis'mus iners, Driv'elling*, (F.) *Bave*. Involuntary flow of saliva, from sluggishness of deglutition, without increased secretion. It is seen in the infant, the aged, and the idiot.

SLEEP, Sax. ꞃlep; *Somnus, Sompnus, Sopor, Dormit"io, Hypnos,* (F.) *Sommeil*. Temporary interruption of our relations with external objects. A repose of the organs of sense, intellectual faculties, and voluntary motion.

The act of quitting this condition is called *awaking,* (F.) *Évigilation, Reveil*. Sometimes this is progressive and natural; at others, sudden and starting; (F.) *Reveil en sursaut,*—as in nightmare, affections of the heart, hypochondriasis, &c.

SLEEP, MAGNET'IC, *Hypno'sis biomagnet'ica*, is the sleep induced by the so called animal magnetism. See Magnetism, animal.

SLEEP, NERVOUS, see Magnetism, animal.

SLEEPLESSNESS, Insomnia.

SLEEP-WALKING, Somnambulism.

SLIACS, MINERAL WATERS OF. Slias is a favourite bathing-place in Hungary, a few miles from Neusohl. Some of the waters are cold; others, thermal: the former are carbonated chalybeates; the latter are much used in the same cases as thermal springs in general.

SLING, (G.) Schlinge, *Mitel'la, Mit'rum.* A bandage employed to keep the forearm bent on the arm, in cases of injury done to those parts, in fracture of the clavicle, injury of the hand, &c. A handkerchief is often sufficient for this purpose. It must be folded diagonally, and be tied, by the extremities, round the neck. The French surgeons have used many varieties of *Écharpes* or *slinge;* as the *Grande écharpe, Écharpe moyenne, Petite écharpe, Écharpe de J. L. Petit*, &c.

SLIPPERS, Impatiens.

SLIT AND TAIL BANDAGE, Invaginated bandage.

SLOE-TREE, Prunus spinosa.

SLOUGH, Eschar.

SLOWS, Milk-sickness.

SLUG, Limax — s. Sea, *Biche de Mer*.

SLUMBER, Somnolency.

SMALLAGE, Apium graveolens.

SMALL-POX, Variola—s. Modified, Varioloid.

SMALT, *Protox'ide of Cobalt, Smaltum. S., Azur, Blue Starch*. This oxyd has been given in rheumatism, in the dose of ten to twenty grains. A larger quantity excites vomiting.

SMARAG'DUS, (F.) *Émeraude*. The emerald. It was formerly regarded as a tonic.

SMARTWEED, Polygonum punctatum.

SMECTICA, Detergents.

SMECTIS, Cimolia terra.

SMECTRIS, Cimolia terra.

SMEGMA, σμηγμα, from σμηχω, 'to wipe, rub off.' Soap, grease, a salve, a liniment. Also the secretion from the sebaceous follicles of the skin.

SMEGMA ARTICULARE, Synovia—s. Cutaneum, see Sebaceous glands.

SMEGMA PRÆPU'TII. The fatty secretion from the sebaceous follicles of the glans penis.

SMEGMATORRHŒA, Stearrhœa.

SMEGMORRHŒA, Stearrhœa.

SMELL, SENSE OF, Olfaction.

SMELLING, Olfaction.

SMELLOME'S OINTMENT FOR THE EYES, Ceratum resinæ.

SMILAX, Taxus baccata — s. Aspera Chinensis, Smilax China — s. Aspera Peruviana, Sarsaparilla—s. Canellæfolia, S. pseudo-China.

SMILAX CHINA, *Smilax as'pera Chinen'. Family,* Smilaceæ. *Sex. Syst.* Diœcia Hexandria. The root — *China, Ch. orienta'lis* seu *ponderosa* seu *vera, Sankira, Gauquara, China root, Squine, Esquine*. Formerly much used in scrofulous and venereal affections.

SMILAX GLAUCA, S. sarsaparilla—s. Hederacea, *Sarsaparilla*—s. Indica Spinosa, S. sarsaparilla pseudo-China—s. Officinalis, Smilax sarsaparilla.

SMILAX PSEUDO-CHINA, *Smilax In'dica spinosa* seu *canellæfo'lia* seu *hederæfo'lia, China denta'lis, China spu'ria nodo'sa, American West India China*. In scrofulous disorders the root has been often preferred to the oriental kind. In other cases, it possesses similar virtues.

SMILAX SARSAPARIL'LA, *S. officina'lis* seu *ca, Sarsaparil'la, Sartaparil'la, Smilax officina'lis Peruvia'na, Sarsa, Sarsa, Osirvillas'di, Juncan'ga, Macapatli, Zarza, Zarzaparil'la*. (F.) *Separeille*. The root of the Sarsaparilla is inodorous; taste bitterish, feculaceous, and fibrous; a dark colour externally; white within. It is possessed of diuretic and demulcent properties, and has been often employed in the sequelæ of syphilis; when, after a mercurial course, nocturnal pains, ulceration, &c., continue. It has, also, been advised in scrofula, chronic rheumatism, &c.; but its efficacy is, to say the least of it, a matter of doubt. Dose, ℈j to ʒj of the powder.

SMILE, σμίλη. A curved, two-edged bistoury. A knife.

SMILEON, Scalpel.

SMYRNA, Myrrha.

SMYRNISMOS, Embalming.

SMYR'NIUM OLUSA'TRUM, *Hipposeli'num, Smyr'nium, Macero'na, Macedonis'ium, Herba Alexandri'na, Gri'elum, Agrioseli'num, Alexan'ders, Alsanders*. A plant formerly cultivated for culinary purposes. The seeds are bitter and aromatic, and the roots more powerfully bitter. They have been recommended as resolvents, diuretics, emmenagogues, &c.

SNAGREL, Aristolochia serpentaria.

SNAIL, Limax — s. Shell, Cochlea.

SNAKEHEAD, Chelone glabra.

SNAKEROOT, Garuleum bipinnatum — s. Birthwort, Aristolochia serpentaria — s. Black, Actæa racemosa, Sanicula Marilandica — s. Button, Eryngium aquaticum, Liatris spicata — s. Canada, Asarum Canadense — s. Dewitt, Prenanthes — s. Evergreen, Polygala paucifolia — s. Heart, Asarum Canadense — s. Virginiana, Aristolochia serpentaria — s. White, Eupatorium ageratoides.

SNAKEWEED, Aristolochia serpentaria, Helenium autumnale, Polygonum bistorta—s. American, Cicuta masculata.

SNEEZING, from Sax. nieꞅan, (G.) Niesen, *Clonus Sternuta'tio, Sternuta'tio, Sternutamen'tum, Sternumen'tum, Ptarmos*, (F.) *Éternuement*. A convulsive motion of the expiratory muscles, by which the air is driven rapidly, and rushes sonorously, through the nasal fossæ, carrying with it the mucus and foreign bodies, which adhere to the pituitary membrane, and have occasioned the movement.

SNEEZEWORT, Achillea ptarmica, Helenium autumnale.

SNORING, *Rhenchus, Rhenxis, Ronchus, Rhonchus, Stertor, Renchus,* (F.) *Ronflement,* from (G.) Scharnen. Noise made in the posterior part of the mouth and nasal fossæ during the movements of inspiration, particularly in sleep, both when the person is in health, and in disease, as in apoplexy. In certain affections of the chest— in some cases of pulmonary catarrh — a kind of snoring may be distinctly heard by applying the ear or the stethoscope to the chest.

SNOT, Nasal mucus.

SNOUT, Nasus.

SNOW, Sax. ꞅnaꞅ, *Nix, Chion,* (F.) *Neige*. Water in a solid state, which falls from the atmosphere in white flakes. It is used externally as a tonic and discutient.

SNOWBALL, Cephalanthus occidentalis.

SNOWBERRY, Symphoricarpus racemosus.

SNUFF, CEPHALIC, Pulvis asari compositus.

SNUFFLES, Teut. Snuffeln, *Grave'do neonato'rum, Rhinan'gia, Rhinanch'oné*. Breathing hard through the nose, often owing to accumulation of the mucous secretions,—an affection to which infants are liable, and which is relieved by oiling the interior of the nostrils.

SOAP, Sapo — s. Acid, see Sapo — s. Berries, Sapindus saponaria—s. Black, see Sapo—s. Castile, Sapo durus — s. of the Cocoa-nut oil, see Sapo — s. Common or soft, see Sapo — s. Liquid, see Sapo — s. Medicinal, see Sapo — s. Spanish, Sapo durus — s. Yellow, see Sapo.

SOAPWORT, Saponaria.

SOB, from Sax. reoꞅiaꞃ, 'to grieve;' (F.) *Sanglot*. A spasmodic, sudden, and momentary contraction of the diaphragm, immediately followed by relaxation, by which the little air, that the contraction has caused to enter the chest, is driven out with noise. It is an evidence of corporeal or mental suffering.

SOBOLES, Epigone.

SOBRIETAS, Temperance.

SOCIA PAROTIDIS, see Parotid.

SOCI'ETY, *Soci'etas,* (F.) *Société*, from *sociare*, 'to associate.' An association for the promotion of some common object.

SOCIETIES, MEDICAL. Associations of medical gentlemen for the promotion of science have been numerous, and productive of valuable results. In the United States, societies exist in many of the states, possessing the power of examining into the qualifications of every one who may be desirous of practising within their particular jurisdiction. In some of the states, however, the qualified and unqualified are permitted to exercise their profession with equal privileges and immunities.

Amongst the medical associations that have issued from time to time useful transactions or publications, are the following: IN AMERICA, — The *Massachusetts Medical Society;* the *Physico-medical,* and *Medical Societies of the State of New York;* the *College of Physicians of Philadelphia,* and the *American Medical Association.* IN EUROPE, — The *Association of Fellows and Licentiates of the King's and Queen's College of Physicians of Ireland;* 'the *Medico-Chirurgical* and *Phrenological Societies of Edinburgh;* the *College of Physicians,* the *Medico-Chirurgical,* the *Medical* and the *Sydenham Societies of London;* the *Associated Apothecaries and Surgeon Apothecaries of England and Wales,* and the *Provincial Medical and Surgical Association;* the *Royal Academy of Surgery,* the *Royal Society of Medicine,* the *Société Médicale d'Émulation,* the *Société de Médecine,* the *Royal Academy of Medicine,* and the *Société Médicale d'Observation,* of *Paris;* the *Médico-Chirurgical Academy of Vienna;* the *Medical Societies of Berlin and Copenhagen,* &c., &c. IN ASIA.— The *Medical and Physical Society of Calcutta*.

Valuable medical essays are likewise contained in the published *Transactions of the American Philosophical Society;* of the *Royal Societies of London, Edinburgh, Göttingen,* &c.; of the *Royal Academy of Sciences of Paris;* the *Imperial Society of Sciences of St. Petersburg;* the *Royal Academy of Sciences of Turin;* the *Academia Imperialis Leopoldina Naturæ Curiosorum,* &c.

SOCORDIA, Hallucination.

SODA. An Arabic word. *Protox'ide of sodium,* (F.) *Soude,* is obtained by adding *caustic lime* to a solution of *carbonate of soda*. The soda in solution may be obtained by evaporation as hydrate of soda. Its action is like that of potassa; but it is not officinal.

Soda impu'ra, Baril'la, Barig'lia, Baril'lor, Soda Hispan'ica, Ana'tron, Natron, Ana'ton, Nitrum Antiquo'rum, Kelp, Aphroni'trum, Sal alkali'nus fixus fos'silis, Car'bonas Sodæ im'purus, Subcar'bonas Sodæ impūra, Anachron. The *mineral alkali* is obtained from several sources; —naturally, in Egypt: artificially, from the incineration of marine plants; and from the decomposition of sulphate of soda, &c. It is principally, however, derived from plants growing on the sea-coast; — as the *Salso'la sati'va, S. soda, S. tragus, Salicor'nia herba'cea, Salicornia Arab'ica,* &c. The *Barilla ashes* are from the ashes of the *Salicor'nia Europæ'a*: the *Kelp*, *Soude de Varecq*, from the *Fucus vesiculo'sus* and other varieties;—the *Turkey Barilla*, *Roquette*, *Cendre du Levant*, *Rochet'ta Alexandri'na*, from the *Mesembryan'themum Cop'ticum*;—the *Al'icant Barilla*, *Soda Alicanti'na*, *S. Alonen'sis*, from the *Mesembryan'themum nodiflo'rum*;—and the *Carthage'na Barilla*, from the *Salicor'nia* and *Salso'la*.

Impure subcarbonate of soda, (F.) *Soude du commerce*, consists of subcarbonate of soda, potash, chloride of sodium, clay and other earthy substances. It is chiefly used for preparing the pure subcarbonate.

SODA, Cardialgia, Cephalalgia, Pyrosis.

SODA ACETA'TA, *Sodæ Acetas*, *Ac"etate of Soda*, *Terra folia'ta minera'lis*, (F.) *Acétate de soude*. This salt is used in similar cases with the acetate of potass.

SODA AËRATA, Sodæ carbonas — s. Alonensis, Soda — s. Biborate of, Borax — s. Bicarbonate of, Sodæ carbonas — s. Borate of, Borax — s. Boraxata, Borax.

SODA, CAR'BONATE OF, *Sodæ Car'bonas*, *Carbonas Na'tricum*, *Soda Aëra'ta*, *Sodæ Bicar'bonas*, *Bicar'bonate of Soda*, *Carbonate of protox'ide of So'dium*, (F.) *Carbonate de Soude*, *S. effervescente*, *S. aërée*, *S. Crayeuse*. (*Sodæ subcarb*, ℔j, *aquæ destill.* Oiij. Dissolve the subcarbonate of soda, and pass carbonic acid through the solution; set it aside to crystallize.) Its use is the same as the subcarbonate, than which it is less caustic, and better adapted for effervescing draughts.

SODA CAU'STICA, *Protox'ide of So'dium*, *Caustic Soda*, (F.) *Soude caustique*, *S. à la Chaux*, *Soude pure*. The impure subcarbonate, treated by quicklime, and consequently deprived of its carbonic acid. It may be used as a caustic, like the *Potassa fusa*, and is even preferable to it, as it does not deliquesce and run.

SODA, CHLORIDE OF, *S. Chlorina'ta*, *Sodæ Chlo'ridum*, *Chlo'rinated Soda*, *Natrum Oxymuriat'icum*, *Sodæ Chlorure'tum*, *Oxymu'riate of Soda*, (F.) *Chlorure de Soude*, *Chlorure d'oxide de Sodium*. This salt is used as a disinfecting agent; both to remove offensive smells in chambers, and to alter the condition of fetid ulcers. See Liquor Sodæ Chlorinatæ.

SODA, CHLORINATED, Soda, chloride of — s. Hispanica, Soda — s. Hydrochlorate of, Soda, muriate of.

SODA, HYPOSULPH'ITE OF, *Sodæ hyposulph'is*, (F.) *Hyposulfite de Soude*. This salt has been lately extolled in chronic cutaneous, and scrofulous affections. It is given in syrup.

SODA, LITHATE OF, Urate of soda — s. Mephite of, Soda, subcarbonate of.

SODA, MU'RIATE OF, *Sodæ murias*, *Soda muria'ta*, *S. muriat'ica*, *Al'kali minera'lē sali'num*, *Sal commu'nis*, *Sal culina'ris*, *Sal fon'tium*, *Sal gemmæ*, *Sal mari'nus*, *Natron muria'tum*, *Sal albus*, *Natrum muriat'icum*, *Common salt*, *Sea salt*, *Hydrochlo'rinas Na'tricus*, *Sal fos'silis*, *Sal lu'cidum*, *Muria*, *Rock salt*, *Bay salt*, *White salt*, *Quadrichlo'ruret of Sodium*, *Hydrochlo'rate of protox'ide of Sodium*, *Hydrochlo'rate of Soda*, *Chlorure'tum So'dii*, *So'dii Chlo'ridum*, *Chloride of Sodium*, (F.) *Chlorure de Sodium*, *Sel marin*, *Sel de Cuisine*. In an impure state, this salt is one of the most abundant of natural productions. It is soluble in 3 parts of water, and is tonic, purgative, and anthelmintic. Externally, stimulant. It is a well-known and useful culinary substance.

SODA, NITRATE OF, *Sodæ Nitras*, *Natron ni'tricum*, *Al'kali minera'lē nitra'tum*, *Nitrum Cu'bicum*, *Nitrate of protox'ide of Sodium*, *Protoni'trate of Sodium*, *Nitrum Rhomboida'lē*, *Nitrum Natricum*, *Salpe'tra*, *Cubic Nitre*. Its virtues are similar to those of the nitrate of potass, for which it has been substituted.

SODA, OXYMURIATE OF, Soda, chloride of.

SODA, PHOSPHATE OF, *S. Phosphora'ta*, *Sodæ phos'phas*, *Subphosphate of protox'ide of Sodius*, *Phosphas Na'tricum*, *Natrum Oxyphosphoro'des*, *Subprotophosphate of Sodium*, *Subphos'phate of Soda*, *Sal mirab'ilē perla'tum*, *Triba'sic phosphate of Soda*, *Alkali minera'lē phosphora'tus*. *Tasteless purging salt*, (F.) *Phosphate de Soude*, *Sel admirable perlé*. (*Bone* burnt to whiteness and powdered, ℔x; *Sulphuric acid*, ℔vj; *Carbonate of soda*, q. s. Mix the bone with the acid in a covered vessel, add a gallon of water, and stir. Digest for three days, occasionally adding a little water to that lost by evaporation, and frequently stirring the mixture. Pour it now a gallon of boiling water, and strain through linen, gradually adding more boiling water, until the liquor passes nearly tasteless. Set the strained liquor by, that the dregs may subside; from which pour off the clear solution, and boil down to a gallon. To this solution, poured off from the dregs and heated in an iron vessel, add by degrees the carbonate of soda previously dissolved in hot water, until effervescence ceases, and the phosphoric acid is completely neutralized; then filter the liquor, and set it aside to crystallize. Having removed the crystals, add, if necessary, a small quantity of carbonate of soda to the liquor, so as to render it slightly alkaline; then alternately evaporate and crystallize so long as crystals are produced. Lastly, preserve the crystals in a well stopped bottle.—Ph. U. S.) Cathartic, in the dose of from ʒss to ʒj.

SODA, PHOSPHATE OF, TRIBASIC, S. Phosphate of.

SODA, SUBCARB'ONATE OF, *Sodæ Subcarbonas*, *Sodæ Carbonas* (Ph. U. S.), *Subcarbonate of protox'ide of Sodium*, *Memphite of Soda*, *Natron præpara'tum*, *Sal Soda*, *Salt of Soda*, *Flos Salis*, *Sagi'men Vitri*, *Salt of Baril'la*, *Sal al'kali*, *Carbonas Sodæ* of some, (F.) *Sous-carbonate de Soude*. The impure subcarbonate, dissolved in water; the solution filtered and crystallized. Soluble in two parts of water at 60°. It is much used as an antacid; and also as a deobstruent in scrofulous and other affections. Dose, gr. x to ʒss.

The dried Subcar'bonate of Soda, *Soda Subcar'bonas exsiccata*, *Sodæ carbonas exsicca'ta*, (Ph. U. S.) *Carbonas Sodæ sicca'tum*, (F.) *Souscarbonate de Soude desséché*, is employed as an antacid and lithontriptic. Dose, gr. x to xv.

SODA, SUBPHOSPHATE OF, S. phosphate of.

SODA, SULPHATE OF, *Sodæ Sulphas*, *Natron vitriola'tum*, *Sal cathar'ticus Glaube'ri*, *Alcali minera'lē sulphu'ricum*, *Natrum sulpha'ricum*, *Soda vitriola'ta*, *Sulphas na'tricus*, *Sal mirab'ilis Glaube'ri*, *Ape'rient Salt of Frederick*, *Glauber's Salts*, (F.) *Sulfate de Soude*. Obtained from the salt that remains after the distillation of muriatic acid; the superabundant acid being saturated with subcarbonate of soda. It is soluble in three parts of water at 60°; is purgative, and in small doses, diuretic. Dose, ʒvj to ʒx.

The *Lymington Glauber's Salts* is a *Sulphate of Magnesia and Soda*, and is obtained from the mother liquor of sea-water, or by dissolving Epsom salt in a solution of Glauber's salt.

SODA, TARTRATE OF, *Tartrate of potass and Soda*, *Soda Tartariza'ta*, *Tar'tarized Soda*, *S. Rupellen'sis*, *Rochelle Salt*, *Sal Polychres'tus Seignet'ti*, *S. Seignetti*, *Seignette's Salt*, *Natron tartariza'tum*, *Tartris potas'sæ et Sodæ*, *Soda et Potas'sæ Tartras* (Ph. U. S.), *Sodæ potassio-tartras*, *Tartras Potas'sæ et Sodæ*, *Tartrate de potasse*

tasse et de Soude. (*Sodæ carb.* ℔i; *potass. bitart.* in pulv. ℥xvj, *Aq. bullient.* Ov. Dissolve the carbonate in water; and add, gradually, the bitartrate. Filter the solution and crystallize, Ph. U. S.) It is a gentle cathartic. Dose, ℨss to ℨj.

SODA, URATE OF, Urate of Soda — s. Vitriolata, S. sulphate of — s. Water, Acidulous water, simple.

SODÆ ACETAS, Soda, acetate of — s. Biboras, Borax — s. Bicarbonas, Soda, carbonate of — s. Boras, Borax — s. Boras alcalescens, Borax — s. Boras supersaturus, Borax — s. Carbonas, Soda — s. Carbonas, Soda, subcarbonate of — s. Carbonas exsiccatus, see Soda, subcarbonate of — s. Carbonas impurus, Soda—s. Chloras, Soda, chlorate of — s. Hyposulphis, Hyposulphite of soda — s. Murias, Soda, muriate of — s. Nitras, Soda, nitrate of — s. Phosphas, Soda, phosphate of — s. et Potassæ tartras, Soda, tartrate of—s. Potassiotartras Soda, tartrate of— s. Subboras, Borax — s. Subcarbonas impura, Soda.

SODII AURO-TERCHLORIDUM, see Gold — s. Chloridum, Soda, muriate of — s. Chloruretum, Soda, muriate of.

SO'DIUM, *Na'trium, Natro'nium.* The metallic basis of soda.

SODIUM, CARBONATE OF PROTOXIDE OF, Sodæ carbonas — s. Chloride of, Soda, muriate of — *s. Chlorure de,* Soda, muriate of—s. *Chlorure d'Oxide de,* Soda. chloride of — s. Protonitrate of, Soda, nitrate of— s. Protoxide of, Soda — s. Protoxide of, hydrochlorate of, Soda, muriate of — s. Protoxide of, nitrate of, Soda, nitrate of—s. Protoxide of, phosphate of, Soda, phosphate of — s. Protoxide of, subcarbonate of, Soda, subcarbonate of — s. Quadri-chloruret of, Soda, muriate of — s. Subborate of protoxide of, Borax—s. Subprotoborate of, Borax—s. Subprotophosphate of, Soda, phosphate of.

SODOMA GALLORUM, Syphilis.
SODOMIA, Buggery.
SODOMY, Buggery.
SOFTENING, Mollities.
SOI-POUR-SOI, Homœozygy.
SOIE, Sericum.
SOIF, Thirst—*s. Excessive,* Polydipsia.
SOL, Gold.
SOL-LUNAR, *Sol-luna'ris;* from *sol,* 'the sun,' and *luna,* 'the moon.' An epithet applied to a fancied influence exerted by the sun and moon on man in a state of health and disease.

SOLAMEN INTESTINORUM, Pimpinella anisum—s. Scabiosorum, Fumaria.

SOL'ANOID, *Solanoï'des;* from *solanum,* 'the potato,' and ειδος, 'resemblance.' Resembling a potato; potato-like. An epithet applied to a form of cancer, which appears to be intermediate between scirrhus and encephaloid, increasing more rapidly than the former, yet approaching it in firmness.

SOLA'NUM, *S. nigrum seu vulga'rē seu vulga'tum, Common Nightshade, Garden Nightshade,* (F.) *Morelle à fruit noir. Family,* Solaneæ. *Sex. Syst.* Pentandria Monogynia. A narcotic poison. The *Huile de Morelle* is made, by macerating in oil, for several days, the leaves and fruit of this plant. The oil is anodyne and discutient.

SOLANUM DULCAMA'RA, *Dulcamara, D. flexuo'sa, Solanum Scandens, Glycipi'cros, Ama'ra dulcis, Solanum ligno'sum,* Στρυχνος of Theophrastus, *Bittersweet, Woody Nightshade, Bittersweet Nightshade, Bittersweet Vine, Nightshade Vine, Violet bloom,* (F.) *Douce-amère, Morelle grimpante.* The taste of the stalks is bitter, followed by sweetness; hence its name. It has been used in many diseases, as a diuretic and sudorific, especially in chronic rheumatism, humoral asthma, dropsy, various skin diseases, scrofula, and jaundice. Dose, in powder, ℈j to ℨj.

SOLANUM ESCULENTUM, S. tuberosum — s. Fœtidum, Datura stramonium—s. Furiosum, Atropa belladonna—s. Humboldtii, S. Lycopersicum — s. Lethale, Atropa belladonna — s. Lignosum, S. dulcamara.

SOLANUM LYCOPER'SICUM; *Lycoper'sicon esculent'um, Lycoper'sicum pomum amo'ris, S. Humbold'tii seu pseudolycoper'sicum, Malum lycoper'sicum, Love-apple plant.* The fruit of this, called *Toma'ta* or *Love-apple,* (F.) *Pomme d'Amour,* is much eaten in the United States; and, with the French, Spaniards, Portuguese, &c., forms an esteemed sauce.

SOLANUM MAGNUM VIRGINIANUM RUBRUM, Phytolacca decandra — s. Maniacum, Atropa belladonna, Datura stramonium — s. Melanocerasus, Atropa belladonna.

SOLANUM MELON'GENA, *Melongena, Egg-plant, Mud Apple plant;* (F.) *Aubergine.* A native of Asia, Africa, and America. Its oblong, eggshaped fruit, *Ponum Melon'genæ, Malum insa'num,* is prepared in soups and sauces in those countries, like the tomata.

SOLANUM NIGRUM, Solanum.
SOLANUM NIV'EUM. A South African plant, the leaves of which, applied to foul ulcers, cleanse them. The fresh juice of the berries and leaves, made into an ointment with lard or fat, is used by the farmers for the same purpose.

SOLANUM PARMENTERII, S. tuberosum — s. Pseudolycopersicum, S. Lycopersicum — s. Quadrifolium, Paris — s. Racemosum Americanum, Phytolacca decandra.

SOLANUM SANCTUM; *Palestine Nightshade.* The fruit of this is globular, and is much eaten in the countries where it is a native.

SOLANUM SCANDENS, S. Dulcamara.
SOLANUM TUBEROS'UM, *Bata'bas, Solanum esculen'tum seu Parmente'rii, Lycoper'sicum tubero'sum, Papas America'nus, Pappus America'nus, America'num Tubero'sum, Batta'ta Virginia'na;* the *Pota'to,* (F.) *Pomme de Terre.* A native of Peru. A nutritious and wholesome vegetable; one of the most useful, indeed, that exists. One hundred pounds of potatoes afford ten pounds of starch, which is equal to arrow-root, as a nutrient and demulcent. It is called *Potato Flour, P. Starch, French Sago, Petit Sague, Common Arrowroot,* &c.

SOLANUM URENS, Capsicum annuum — s. Vesicarium, Physalis—s. Vulgare, Solanum.

SOLAR, *Sola'ris,* from *sol,* 'the sun.' Relating to the sun; having rays like the sun.

SOLAR PLEXUS, *Plexus sola'ris, Centrum commu'nē, Cer'ebrum abdomina'lē.* A collection of ganglions and filaments, interweaving and anastomosing with each other repeatedly, and belonging to the system of the great sympathetic. This vast plexus, lying on the vertebral column, the aorta, and the pillars of the diaphragm, has a very irregular shape. The ganglions and filaments composing it are soft, reddish, and almost all issue from the semilunar ganglions. It receives, also, branches from the pneumogastric. It seems to be chiefly intended for the aorta, and accompanies all its branches; furnishing many secondary plexuses, which are called the *infradiaphragmatic, cœliac, superior mesenteric, inferior mesenteric, renal* or *emulgent, spermatic,* &c.

SOLDANELLA, Convolvulus soldanella.
SOLDIER'S WEED, Matico.

SOLE, *Solum, Solea, Basis cor'poris, Ichnus, Superfic''ies planta'ris pedis, Peti'na, Vestig''ium, Pe'dion, Peza, Pelma, Planta'ris superficies pedis, Fa'cies conca'va* seu *infe'rior* seu *Planum* seu *Concavum* seu *Pars inferior* seu *Planit''ies* seu *Planta* seu *Vola pedis*, (F.) *Plante du Pied*. The sole of the foot; the under surface of the foot.

SOLEA, Sole — s. Ipecacuanha, see Ipecacuanha.

SOLÉAIRE, Soleus.

SOLEN, Cradle, see Vertebral column.

SOLENA'RIUM, from σωλην, 'a canal.' An instrument of surgery, representing a kind of gutter, in the cavity of which the penis was placed, like a limb in a *cradle*. — Galen. The word *Solen* itself—σωλην, *Cana'lis*—was used, in antiquity, for a grooved channel, in which a fractured limb was placed.

SOLENOSTEMMA ARGEL, Cynanchum oleæfolium.

SOLE'US, *Gastrocne'mius inter'nus, Tibiocalcanien*, (Ch.;) (F.) *Soléaire*, from *solea*, 'a sole of a shoe.' A muscle situate at the posterior part of the leg. It is broad, flat, and almost oval; and is attached, above, to the posterior edge of the fibula, to the oblique line on the posterior surface, and to the inner edge of the tibia. It terminates, below, by a large tendon, which unites to that of the gastrocnemius externus, to form the tendo Achillis. This muscle extends the foot on the leg, and conversely.

SOLID, *Sol'idus, Ste'reos*. A body whose integrant molecules are so united by the force of cohesion, that they will not separate by their own weight. The solids, in the human body, are the bones, cartilages, tendons, muscles, ligaments, arteries, veins, nerves, membranes, skin, &c. The anatomy, or rather study of the solids, is called *Stereol'ogy*, from στερεος, 'solid,' and λογος, 'a discourse.'

SOLIDAGO, see Solidago virgaurea — s. Saracenica, S. virgaurea.

SOLIDA'GO RIG''IDA, *Rigid Goldenrod, Bones' styptic*; indigenous; of the Composite *family*, flowering in August and September; is astringent and tonic.

SOLIDA'GO VIRGAU'REA, *S. vulga'ris* seu *Saracen'ica, Virga aurea, Herba do'rea, Cony'sa coma aurea, Sym'phytum Petræ'um, Elichry'sum, Consol'ida* seu *Saracen'ica, Golden rod. Nat. Ord.* Compositæ Corymbiferæ. *Sex. Syst.* Syngenesia superflua. (F.) *Verge d'or*. The leaves of *Solida'go odo'ra — Solida'go* (Ph. U. S.) — and the flowers have been recommended as aperients and tonics, in urinary diseases, and in internal hemorrhage.

SOLIDAGO VULGARIS, S. virgaurea.

SOL'IDISM, *Patholog''ia solida'ris*. The doctrine of those physicians who refer all diseases to alterations of the solid parts of the body. To the believers in this doctrine, the appellation *Sol'idists* has been given. The solidists think that the solids alone are endowed with vital properties; that they alone can receive the impression of morbific agents, and be the seat of pathological phenomena. Solidism has been the prevalent doctrine. It is scarcely necessary to say, that in all our investigations, the condition of both solids and fluids must be regarded.

SOLIUM, *Baignoire*, Tænia solium — s. Pedis, Metatarsus.

SOLUBIL'ITY, *Solubil'itas*, from *solvere, solutum*, 'to dissolve.' That property of a body by virtue of which it can be dissolved in a menstruum.

TABLE OF THE SOLUBILITY OF SOME SUBSTANCES IN WATER.

NAMES OF SALTS.	Solubility in 100 parts water.	
	at 60°	at 212°
Acids.		
Benzoic	0.208	4.17
Citric	133	200
Oxalic	50	100
Tartaric	very soluble	
Salts.		
Acetate of Potassa	100	
——— Soda	35	
Bitartrate of Potassa	1.5	33
Borate of Soda	8.4	16.3
Carbonate of Ammonia	50	
——— Magnesia	2	
——— Potassa	25	
——— Soda	50	
Chlorate of Potassa	6	40
——— Soda	35	35
Chloride of Lime	200	
——— Magnesium	100	
——— Potassium	33	
——— Sodium	35.42	36.16
Muriate of Ammonia	33	100
Nitrate of Potassa	14.25	100
——— Soda	23	100
Phosphate of Soda	25	50
Sulphate of Ammonia	50	100
——— Copper	25	50
——— Iron	50	100
——— Magnesia	100	132
——— Potassa	6.25	20
——— Soda	37	125
Supersulphate of Potassa	5.0	100
Tartrate of Potassa	25	
——— Potassa and Soda	20	
——— Antimony & Potassa	6.6	23

SOLUM, Sole.

SOLUTÉ, Solution.

SOLUTIO, Solution — s. Alexiteria Gaubiana, see Disinfection — s. Ammoniæ subcarbonatis, Liquor ammoniæ subcarbonatis — s. Arsenicalis, Liquor arsenicalis — s. Arsenicata, Liquor arsenicalis — s. Arsenitis kalicæ, Liquor arsenicalis — s. Calcis, Liquor calcis — s. Camphoræ æthera, Tinctura ætherea camphorata — s. Camphoræ oleosa, Linimentum camphoræ — s. Continui, Solution of continuity — s. Ferri nitratis, Liquor Ferri nitratis — s. Guaiaci gummosa, Mistura guaiaci — s. Muriatis barytæ, Baryta, muriate of — s. Muriatis calcis, see Calcis murias — s. Muriatis ferrici ætherea, Tinctura seu alcohol sulphurico-æthereus ferri — s. Muriatis hydrargyri oxygenati, Liquor hydrargyri oxymuriatis — s. Potassii iodidi iodureta, Liquor iodini compositus — s. Resinæ guaiaci aquosa, Mistura guaiaci — s. Subcarbonatis ammoniaci spirituosa, Spiritus ammoniæ.

SOLUTIO SULPHA'TIS CUPRI COMPOS'ITA, *Aqua vitriol'ica cœru'lea, Sydenham's Styptic Water*. (*Sulph. cupri*, ʒiij; *alum., acid. sulph.,* ää ʒij; *aquæ*, ʒviij : dissolve, and filter.) A styptic, and largely diluted, an astringent collyrium.

SOLU'TION, *Solu'tio, Lysis*, (F.) *Dissolution*. An operation which consists in dissolving a solid body in a menstruum. Likewise, the product of such operation—*Solu'tum*, (F.) *Soluté*. It means, also, with many, the termination of a disease:— with others, a termination accompanied by critical signs;—and, with others, again, it is synonymous with crisis.

SOLUTION OF ACETATE OF AMMONIA, Liquor ammoniæ acetatis — s. of Acetate of morphia, Liquor morphiæ acetatis — s. Alkaline, see *Pelligokali* — s. of Alkaline iron, Liquor ferri alkalini — s. of Alum, compound, Liquor aluminis compositus — s. of Ammoniated copper, Liquor cupri ammoniati — s. Arsenical, Liquor arsenicalis — s. of Charcoal, concentrated, see Tinctura catechu

—s. of Chlorinated soda, Liquor sodæ chlorinatæ —s. of Citrate of magnesia, see Magnesiæ citras —s. of Citrate of potassa, Liquor potassæ citratis —s. of Continuity, see Continuity—s. of Corrosive sublimate, Liquor hydrargyri oxymuriatis — s. Donovan's, see Arsenic and Mercury, Iodide of — s. Fowler's, Liquor arsenicalis — s. of Hydriodate of potass, Liquor potassæ hydriodatis — s. of Iodide of iron, Liquor ferri iodidi—s. of Iodine, compound, Liquor iodini compositus—s. of Iron, nitrated, see Tinctura ferri muriatis — s. Labarraque's *Eau de Javelle*—s. of Lime, Liquor calcis — s. Lugol's, Liquor iodini compositus — s. of Magnesia, condensed, Magnesia, fluid — s. of Monro, Liquor of Monro — s. of Nitrate of iron, Liquor ferri nitratis — s. of Oxymuriate of mercury, Liquor hydrargyri oxymuriatis—s. Plenck's, see Hydrargyri oxydum cinereum—*s. de Potasse*, Liquor potassæ—s. of Potassa, Liquor potassæ— s. of Sesquinitrate of iron, Liquor ferri nitratis—s. of Subacetate of Lead, Liquor plumbi subacetatis —s. of Subacetate of lead, diluted, Liquor plumbi subacetatis dilutus—s. of Subcarbonate of potass, Liquor potassæ subcarbonatis—s. of Sulphate of morphia, Liquor morphiæ sulphatis—s. of Tartarized antimony, Vinum antimonii tartarisati—s. of Ternitrate of sesquioxide of iron, Liquor ferri nitis — s. of Van Swieten, Liquor hydrargyri oxymuriatis.

SOLUTIVUS, Laxative.
SOLUTUM, Solution.
SOLVENS, Solvent — s. Minerale, Liquor arsenicalis.
SOLVENT, *Solvens*, (F.) *Fondant*, from *solvere*, 'to dissolve.' A medicine supposed to possess the property of dissolving or removing obstructions and extraneous substances. Thus we have *solvents* of the stone in the bladder, &c. See Dissolventia.
SOLVENT, MINERAL, Liquor arsenicalis.
SOMA, Body, Corpus.
SOMACETICS, Gymnastics.
SOMAT'IC, *Somat'icus;* from σωμα, 'the body.' That which concerns the body;—as *somatic* death, or death of the body, in contradistinction to *molecular* death or the death of a part.
SOMATODYM'IA, from σωμα, σωματος, 'the body,' and δυω, 'I enter into.' A double monstrosity in which the trunks are united. Of this, there are several varieties; — *Vertebrodym'ia*, where the union is by the vertebræ; *Ischiodym'ia*, by the ossa ischii; *Sternodym'ia*, by the sternum; *Supraomphalodym'ia*, (F.) *Sus-omphalodymie*, by the super-umbilical regions; *Supra et infra-omphalodymia*, by the superior and inferior umbilical regions; and *Sterno-omphalodym'ia*, where the union is by both the sternal and the umbilical regions. — Cruveilhier.
SOMATOL'OGY, *Somatolog"ia*, from σωμα, 'the body,' and λογος, 'a discourse.' A treatise on the human body. Anatomy.
SOMATOTOMY, Anatomy.
SOMMEIL, Sleep.
SOMNAMBULATION, Somnambulism.
SOMNAM'BULISM, *Somnambula'tio*, *Hypnobate'sis*, *Hypnobata'sis*, *Hypnobati'a*, *Rhembas'mus*, *Lunatis'mus*, *Hypnoner'gia*, *Selenoga'mia*, *Nyctobate'sis*, *Autonyctobati'a*, *Seleni'asis*, *Seleniae'mus*, *Somnambulis'mus*, *Nyctob'asis*, *Noctambula'tio*, *Noctambulis'mus*, *Nyctoba'dia*, *Nyctoba'tia*, *Siph'ita*, *Syph'ita*, *Paroni'ria am'bulans*, *Noctisur'gium*, *Oneirodym'ia acti'va*, *Somno-vigil*, *Somnambula'tion*, *Sleep-walking*, from *somnus*, 'sleep,' and *ambulare*, 'to walk.' A condition of the brain which occasions the individual to execute, during sleep, some of those actions that commonly take place when awake. It has been imagined that the somnambulist is guided solely by his internal senses; but there are many facts which induce the belief that the external senses are not always entirely suspended. The causes of somnambulism are very obscure; and the principal indication of treatment is, — so to arrange the bed-chamber of the somnambulist, that he cannot get out of it during sleep; and to avoid suppers, as well as all bodily and mental excitement.

SOMNAMBULISM, MAGNET'IC MESMERIC, or ARTIFIC"IAL, *Somnambulis'mus artificia'lis*, *Cataph'ora magnet'ica*, *Hyp'notism*, *Somnip'athy*, is that peculiar condition, into which individuals have been thrown by the *Animal Magnetizer*. It has occurred only in those of weak nervous temperament; in hysterical females, &c.
SOMNAMBULISMUS, Somnambulism—s. Artificialis, Somnambulism, magnetic.
SOMNAM'BULIST, *Somnam'bulus*, *Hypnob'ates*, *Noctam'bulus*, *Lunat'icus*, *Noctam'bulo*, *Somnam'bulo*. A sleep-walker.
SOMNAMBULIS'TIC. Relating or appertaining to somnambulism, — as the '*somnambulis'tic state.*'
SOMNAMBULO, Somnambulist.
SOMNIA'TIO, from *somnium*, 'a dream.' The act of dreaming.
SOMNIATIO MORBOSA, Oneironosus—s. in Statu Vigili, Hallucination.
SOMNIF'EROUS, *Som'nifer*, *Sopor'ifer*, *Hypnot'icus*, *Hypnopæ'us*, *Soporati'vus*, *Soporif'ic*, *Soporif'erous*. A medicine which causes sleep.
SOMNIL'OQUIST; same etymon as the next. One who talks in his sleep.
SOMNILO'QUIUM, *Somniloquis'mus*, *Somnil'oquism*, from *somnus*, 'sleep,' and *loquor*, 'I speak.' Talking in the sleep.
SOMNOPATHY, Somnambulism, magnetic.
SOM'NIUM, *Enyp'nion*, *Insom'nium*, *a Dream*, (F.) *Rêve*, *Songe*. A confused assemblage, or accidental and involuntary combination of ideas and images, which present themselves to the mind during sleep. Dr. S. Mitchell, of New York, used the word *Somnium* to signify the state between sleeping and waking, in which persons perform acts of which they are unconscious.
For 'waking dreams,' see Hallucination.
Those distressing dreams which occur during a state of half sleep, are called, by the French, *Rêvasseries*.
SOMNO-VIGIL, Somnambulism.
SOM'NOLENCY, *Somnolen'tia*, *Hypnæsthe'sis*, *Hypno'dia*, *Dormita'tio*, *Heav'iness*, *Carus Lethar'gus Cataph'ora*, *Cataphora*, *Coma Somnolen'tum*, *Caro'sis*, *Slumber*, (F.) *Assoupissement*. Sleepiness. Also a state intermediate between sleeping and waking. It is often a symptom of disease.
SOMNUS, Sleep.
SOMPNUS, Sleep.
SON, Furfur, Sound.
SONCHUS, *S. Olera'ceus*, *Hiera'cium olera'ceum*, *Cicer'bita*, *Sow Thistle*, (F.) *Laiteron doux*. *Family*, Cichoraceæ. Most of the species of Sonchus abound with a milky juice, which is very bitter, and said to possess diuretic virtues.
SONCHUS FLORIDANUS, Mulgedium Floridanum.
SONDE, Sound, Specillum — *s. Cannlée*, Director.
SONDE D'ANEL. A very fine stylet of silver, awl-shaped at one end. It is used for probing the lachrymal passages through the punctum lacrymale.
SONDE DE BELLOC. An instrument invented by Belloc for plugging the nasal fossæ, in cases of hemorrhage. It consists of a curved silver canula, open at both ends, and furnished with a button. The instrument is passed through the nares to the throat; and a plug is attached

to the button, so that, when the instrument is drawn forwards through the nose, the posterior nostril is stopped.

SONDE BRISÉE, (F.), *Eyed probe.* A long, straight stylet, composed of two parts, which may be screwed to each other; blunt at one end, and furnished at the other with an eye, so that it may be used either as a probe for punctured wounds, or for a seton needle.

SONDE À CONDUCTEUR, (F.) A modification of the ordinary catheter;—to facilitate the changing of catheters, without the fear of making false passages. It is a common catheter, open at its beak. The *Stylet* or *Mandrin* is one half longer than that of the ordinary catheter. To use the instrument, the stylet is pushed into the cavity of the bladder through the catheter. The latter is then withdrawn by slipping it over the stylet, which is kept in its place, and serves as a guide to a fresh catheter.

SONDE À DARD, see Lithotomy (high operation.)

SONDE DE LAFOREST. A small, crooked canula, used for probing the nasal duct from below upwards, and for throwing injections into it.

SONDE ou *PINCE DE HUNTER.* A cylindrical silver canula; of the size of a common catheter; open at both extremities, and containing a wire of iron, one of the ends of which is split into two parts; each being terminated by a small silver scoop, and separating from each other by virtue of their elasticity, when pushed out of the canula, and again approximating when drawn in. It has been used for laying hold of small calculi in the urethra.

SONDE DE VARECQ, Soda.

SONGE, Somnium.

SONITUS AURIUM, Tinnitus aurium — s. Fluidi, Hygrechema — s. Hepaticus, Hepatechema — s. Intestinalis, Enterechema — s. Stomachicus, Gasterechema.

SONOROUS RHONCHUS, *Râle sonore.*

SONUS, Sound—s. Vocis, Accent.

SOOJA, see Dolichos.

SOOJIE, BASTER'S, a farinaceous article of diet, is said to consist of wheat flour sweetened with sugar.

SOOL, Gastroperiodynia.

SOOT, Fuligo — s. Tea, see Fuligokali — s. Wart, Cancer, chimney-sweeper's.

SOPHIA, Sisymbrium sophia — s. Chirurgorum, Sisymbrium sophia.

SOPHISTICATION, Falsification.

SOPHO'RA HEPTAPHYL'LA, *Anticholer'ica.* Family, Leguminosæ. *Sex. Syst.* Decandria Monogynia. The root and seeds of this shrub are intensely bitter, and are said to have been found useful in cholera, colic, dysentery, &c.

SOPHORA TINCTO'RIA, *Baptis'ia tincto'ria, Podalyr'ia Tincto'ria, Indigof'era, Wild Indigo, Indigo Weed, Broom, Indigo Broom, Horsefly Weed, Yellow Broom, Clover Broom, Rattle Bush, Yellow Indigo.* An American plant, the taste of whose root is unpleasant, sub-acrid, and nauseous — very similar to ipecacuanha. In a large dose, the bark of the root acts both as an emetic and cathartic. It has been considered antiseptic and febrifuge, and has been used, in the form of fomentation or cataplasm, in phagedenic and gangrenous ulcers. A liniment, prepared by simmering the *cortical part* of the root in cream, has been found an efficacious application to sore nipples and to ulcerated breasts.

Baptis'ia Leucan'tha, Tall white false Indigo, an indigenous plant, has the same properties.

SOPHRONISTÆ DENTES, see Dentition.

SOPHRONISTERES DENTES, see Dentition.

SOPHROSYNE, Temperance.

SOPIENS, Paregoric.

SOPIO, Opium.

SOPOR. A profound sleep, from which the person can be roused with difficulty. It is a symptom in many of the neuroses.

SOPOR CAROTICUS, Carus.

SOPORARIÆ ARTERIÆ, Carotids.

SOPORATIVUS, Somniferous.

SOPORIFEROUS, Somniferous.

SOPORIFIC, Somniferous.

SO'POROUS, *So'porus*, from *sopor*, 'sleep.' Sleepy: causing sleep.

SORA, Essera.

SORB TREE, Sorbus domestica.

SORBASTRELLA, Pimpinella saxifraga.

SORBEFA'CIENT, *Sorbefa'ciens*, from *sorbere*, 'to suck in,' and *facere*, 'to make.' A remedy that promotes absorption.

The following are the chief sorbefacients:—Acida Vegetabilia; Alkalia; Ammoniacum: Bromium; Galbanum; Hydrargyri Præparata; Iodinum; Liquor Calcii chloridi; Spongia usta; Compression, (methodical;) Friction; Mesa Sorbefacients, (Imagination, Emotions.)

SORBETHUM, Sherbet.

SORBETTUM, Sherbet.

SORBETUM, Sherbet.

SORBIER DES OISELEURS, Sorbus acuparia.

SORBITIO, Jus.

SORBITIO CARNIS seu EX CARNE. Broth or soup made of meat.

SORBITUM, Jus.

SORBUM, see Sorbus domestica.

SORBUS, Cratægus aria, S. domestica.

SORBUS ACUPA'RIA, seu *Aucupa'ria, Mes'pilus M. acupa'ria, Mountain Service, Mountain Ash, Quicken tree, Roan tree*, (F.) *Sorbier des oiseleurs.* The berries of this tree are employed for similar purposes as the last.

SORBUS ALPINA, Cratægus aria—s. Aria, Cratægus aria—s. Aucuparia, S. acuparia—s. Cydonia, Pyrus cydonia.

SORBUS DOMEST'ICA, *Sorbus, Pyrus domest'ica, Mes'pilus domes'tica, Oie, Service* or *Sorb Tree*, (F.) *Cormier. Family*, Rosaceæ. *Sex. Syst.* Icosandria Trigynia. The fruit of this tree, *sorbum*, is astringent, and has been recommended in diarrhœa and dysentery. It is given in the form of rob. A kind of cider is made from it, and is brandy.

SORBUS MALUS, Pyrus malus.

SORDES, *Rhypos.* A dirty-looking matter discharged from ulcers. Also, accumulations of the secretions of the mouth, on the teeth in asthenic fevers more especially, and of foul matters in the stomach—*Sordes prim'arum via'rum. Epipa'ria.* The French call an ulcer, exhibiting such an appearance, *sordid.* Also dirt of any kind.

SORDES, Ichor, Saburra — s. Acidæ, Acid first — s. Aurium, Cerumen — s. Primarum viarum, Embarras gastrique, see Sordes — s. Ventris, Excrement.

SORDICULÆ AURIUM, Cerumen.

SORE, Ulcer.

SORE, BAY. A disease which Mosely considers to be a true cancer. It is endemic in the Bay of Honduras.

SORE MOUTH, Stomatitis — s. Clergyman's, Pharyngitis, follicular — s. Gangrenous, Cancer aquaticus — s. Inflammatory, Cynanche vesicularis — s. Putrid, Cynanche maligna — s. Threatened, Cynanche — s. Throat, tubercular, Pharyngitis follicular — s. Throat, ulcerous, Cynanche maligna.

SORENESS, from Teut. *seer*, (G.) **Sehr**, 'very.' Sax. ꞅáp, *Parap'sis acris teneritu'do*. Painful uneasiness or tenderness, local or general, on being touched with a pressure that does not usually excite distressing feeling. Often, a febrile symptom. Also, the tenderness of a wound, ulcer, &c.

SORGHUM, Panicum Italicum.

SOROCCO, Puna.

SOROCHE, Puna.

SORORIA'TIO. The period at which the breasts of the female become developed. The act of becoming thus developed. A young maiden, whose mammæ begin to show, was formerly called *sororians virgo*.—Plautus.

SORREL, COMMON, Rumex acetosa — s. French, Rumex scutatus — s. Garden, Rumex scutatus — s. Mountain, Oxalis acetosella, Oxyria reniformis — s. Salt of, Potass, oxalate of — s. Roman, Rumex scutatus — s. Tree, Andromeda arborea — s. White, Oxalis acetosella — s. Welsh, Oxyria reniformis.

SOSTRUM, improperly *Sotrum*; from σωζειν, 'to save.' A reward given to one who saves the life of another. A physician's fee or *honorarium*.

SOTERIA DOCTRINA, Medicina.

SOTERIÆ AQUÆ, Waters, mineral.

SOTIREL'LA. Ancient name of a medicine composed of *opium*, several *narcotics*, *nutmeg*, *saffron*, *camphor* and *soot*. It was used in certain diseases of the teeth.

SOTRUM, Sostrum.

SOUBRESAUT, Subsultus tendinum.

SOUCHERLOON, Bit noben.

SOUCHET DES INDES, Curcuma longa — s. *Odorant*, Cyperus longus — s. *Rond*, Cyperus rotundus.

SOUCI, Calendula officinalis, Panophobia — s. *des Champs*, Calendula arvensis — s. *Ordinaire*, Calendula officinalis.

SOUDE, Soda — s. *Acétate de*, Soda, acetate of — s. *Aéré*, Sodæ carbonas — s. *Borate de*, Borax — s. *Borate sursaturé de*, Borax — s. *Carbonate de*, Sodæ carbonas — s. *Caustique*, Soda caustica — s. *à la Chaux*, Soda Caustica — s. *Chlorure de*, Soda, chloride of — s. *du Commerce*, Soda — s. *Crayeuse*, Sodæ carbonas — s. *Effervescente*, Sodæ carbonas — s. *Hyposulfite de*, Soda, hyposulphite of — s. *Phosphate de*, Soda, phosphate of — s. *et de Potasse, Tartrate de*, Soda, tartrate of — s. *Pure*, Soda caustica — s. *Sousborate de*. Borax — s. *Souscarbonate de*, Soda, subcarbonate of — s. *Sulfate de*, Soda, sulphate of.

SOUFFLE, see Murmur, respiratory — s. *Amphorique*, see Cavernous respiration — s. *Métallique*, see Cavernous respiration — s. *Placentaire*, *Bruit placentaire* — s. *Tubaire*, see Murmur, respiratory — s. *Utérin*, *Bruit placentaire* — s. *Voilé*, see Cavernous respiration.

SOUFRE, Sulphur — s. *Iodure de*, Sulphuris iodidum — s. *Sublimé*, Sulphur sublimatum.

SOUND, *Specill'um*, *Stylus*, *Explorato'rium*, *Radi'olus*, (F.) *Sonde*. An instrument used by surgeons to discover whether there be a stone in the bladder. It is usually made of highly polished steel, and is shaped like the catheter. The operation is termed sounding.

The French *Sonde* has, however, a more extensive signification. It means different instruments introduced into cavities of certain organs, or into wounds, fistulas, &c., to investigate their condition, or to fulfil some therapeutical indication. See *Sonde*.

SOUND, *Sonus*, *Echos*, *Noise*, (F.) *Son*, *Bruit*. The sensation produced on the auditory nerve by the vibrations of a sonorous body. Sounds may be propagated in three modes. 1. By *reciproca'tion* or *con'sonance*, as when a sounding body, of a definite pitch, produces a musical tone when another body of the same pitch is sounded near it. 2. By *res'onance*, as when a sounding body is placed in connection with another, one or more of whose parts may be thrown into reciprocal vibration; and 3. By *conduc'tion*, as where the vibrations are transmitted through fluid, liquid, or solid media.

SOUND, Catheterize, S. Auricular, Apyromele — s. Bellows, friction, rasp, saw, lancet, &c., see *Bruit* — s. Crumpling, pulmonary, *Froissement pulmonaire* — s. Laryngeal, Laryngecho.

SOUNDING, Searching, see Sound.

SOUNDNESS OF MIND, Sanity.

SOUPIR, Sigh.

SOUR BERRY, see Oxycantha Galeni, Vaccinium oxycoccos — s. Dock, boreal, Oxyria reniformis — s. Leaf, Andromeda arborea — s. Tree Andromeda arborea — s. Wood, Andromeda arborea.

SOURCIL, Supercilium.

SOURCILIER, Corrugator supercilii, 'Superciliary.

SOURDS MUETS, see Mutitas surdorum.

SOURIS, Nictation.

SOUS-ACROMIO-CLAVI-HUMÉRAL, Deltoid — s. *Atloïdien*, Subatloidæus — s. *Axoïdien*, Subaxoidæus — s. *Clavier*, Subclavius — s. *Costaux*, Intercostal — s. *Cutané*, Subcutaneous — s. *Épineux*, Infra-spinatus — s. *Lingual*, Sub-lingual — s. *Maxillaire*, Submaxillary — s. *Maxillo-Labial*, Depressor anguli oris — s. *Mental*, Submental — s. *Métacarpo-latéri-phalangien*, Prior annularis — s. *Optico-sphéno-sclérotieien*, Rectus inferior oculi — s. *Orbitaire*, Suborbitar — s. *Pubio-coccygien*, Levator ani — s. *Pubio-créti-tibial*, Gracilis — s. *Pubio-prétibial*, Gracilis — s. *Pubio-trochantérien-externe*, Obturator externus — s. *Pubio-trochantérien-interne*, Obturator internus — s. *Scapulaire*, Subscapularis — s. *Scapulo-trochinien*, Subscapularis — s. *Sels*, see Salt.

SOUTHERNWOOD, Artemisia abrotanum — s. Field, Artemisia campestris — s. Maritime, Artemisia maritima — s. Tartarian, Artemisia santonica.

SOWBREAD, Arthanita, Cyclamen.

SOWENS, Flummery.

SOY, see Dolichos soja.

SOYMIDA, Swietenia febrifuga.

SPA, MINERAL WATERS OF. A town seven leagues southeast of Liège, where there are several springs, possessing a sharp acidulous taste; containing much carbonic acid, carbonates of iron, lime, and magnesia; carbonate of soda, and chloride of sodium. The water is much used as a tonic.

SPA WATER, ARTIFICIAL. *Sodæ subcarb.*, gr. vij; *magnesiæ carbon.*, ℨj; *limat. ferri.*, gr. iij; *sodii chlorid.*, gr. j; *aquæ*, Oiij. Impregnate with gas from *marble powder* and *sulph. acid.*, āā ℨx.

SPACE, INTERPEDUNCULAR, Tarini pons — s. Perforated, anterior, Locus perforatus anticus — s. Perforated, posterior, Tarini pons.

SPADO, Castratus, Eunuch, Spasm.

SPAGYRIA, Chymistry.

SPAG"YRISTS, from σπαω, 'I separate,' and αγιιρω, 'I assemble;' because they reduced compounds into elements, and formed the latter into compounds (?). A sect of physicians, who pretended to account for the changes that occur in the human body in health and disease, in the same manner as the chymists of their day explained those of the inorganic kingdom. — *Medici'na Paracelsis'tica seu Spagyr'ica*, was likewise called *Hermet'ica*, because it was believed that the

SPANÆMIA 800 SPASME

means of cure adopted in it had been found in the books of Hermes.

SPANÆ'MIA, from σπανος, 'poor,' and 'αιμα, 'blood.' Poverty of the blood. Diminution in the quantity of fibrin and red corpuscles of the blood, — as where bleeding has been carried beyond certain limits.—Simon.

SPANÆ'MIC, Spanæ'micum (remedium), Dysplas'ticum, Plastilyt'icum et erethilyt'icum, Hæmatolyt'icum, Dyscrasiacum. Same etymon as the last. Relating to spanæmia.

A medicine whose protracted use is said to impoverish the blood, — as iodine, bromine, &c.

SPANDARAPUM, Sparadrapum.

SPANISH FLY, Cantharis.

SPANOPO'GON, from σπανος, 'rare,' and πωγων, 'beard.' One who has lost his beard, or has a thin beard.

The Greeks called those who had little beard, or who had lost it, Spanopogo'nes.

SPARADRAPA, Sparadrapum.

SPARADRAPIER. The name of a machine for spreading sparadraps. A Plaster machine. It consists of a table, with two raised pieces, movable, and furnished with points, by which the cloth can be stretched, and of a lamina or blade of metal to extend the plaster over it.

SPARADRA'PUM, Sparadra'pa, Sparadrapus, Tela emplas'tica, Spandara'pum, (F.) Sparadrap. Any adhesive plaster spread upon linen or paper. The chief sparadraps are the following:—

SPARADRAPUM ADHÆSI'VUM, Adhe'sive Plaster. A spread plaster of the Emplastrum adhæsivum. It is also called Strapping.

English Court Plaster is a Sparadrap, (F.) Taffetas agglutinatif, T. gommé, Tuffetas d'Angleterre; Ser'icum An'glicum, Emplas'trum Anglicum, E. Anglica'num, E. Adhæsi'vum Woodstock'ii, E. Ichthyocol'læ telæ indue'tum, E. Glutino'sum, Tela Ichthyocol'læ glu'tinans, Isinglass Plaster. It is made by stretching black silk, and brushing it over with a solution of isinglass ℥j, in proof spirit ℥xij, to which tinct. benzoin ℥ij, are added. When dry, this is repeated five times; after this, two coats are given it of a solution of tereb. Chiæ ℥iv, in tinct. bens. ℥vj, which render it less liable to crack.

Liston's Isinglass Plaster is made by spreading several coats of strong solution of isinglass in weak spirit over oiled silk, or, still better, over animal membrane previously prepared for the purpose from the peritoneal coat of the cæcum of the ox.

SPARADRAPUM PRO FONTIC'ULIS, Issue Plaster, is sometimes made of simple diachylon, ℔ij; Burgundy pitch and sarcocolla, each ℥iv; common turpentine, ℥j. Spread upon linen and polished with a moistened calendering glass rubber.

SPARADRAPUM seu TELA GALTERI, Defensive Plaster, (F.) Toile de Gautier. This is made of olive oil, ℔ss; suet, ℥iv; wax, ℥x; litharge, common turpentine, thus, and mastich, āā ℥ij; bole armeniac, flour, āā ℥j. Pour it, while liquid, upon cloth, and spread. Used for issues and to keep on dressings.

SPARADRA'PUM VESICATO'RIUM. Several substances have been introduced as substitutes for blistering plaster, (see Emplastrum Lyttæ,) under the names, Tela vesicato'ria, Blistering Tissue, &c., and other forms of which are the Taffetas vésicant, Papier épispastique, Charta vesicato'ria, Taffetas épispastique. They are made of an ethereal or alcoholic extract of cantharides, or of cantharidin, mixed with wax and spread, in a very fine layer, on silk or paper previously oiled or waxed. They are efficient agents.

SPARADRAPUM VIR'IDE, Corn Plaster. This may be made of yellow wax, ℔ij; Burgundy pitch, ℥xij; common turpentine, ℥vj; verdigris, ℥iij; spread on cloth and polished.

Kennedy's Corn Plaster is made of yellow wax, ℔j; Venice turpentine, ℥ij; verdigris, ℥j.

SPARADRAPUS, Sparadrapum.

SPARAGMA, Laceration.

SPARAGMOS, Spasm.

SPARAGUS, Asparagus.

SPARAL'LIUM, Clyster uteri'nus. An injection into the vagina.—Ruland and Johnson.

SPAREDIA. A ligature covered with the white of egg.—Paracelsus.

SPARGA'NIUM RAMO'SUM, Great Burreed. Indigenous; Order, Typhaceæ; flowering in July and August. The roots are subastringent, but esculent; yielding a fine fecula, similar to salep. They are sometimes made into a poultice for inflamed mammæ.

SPAR'GANON, Spar'ganum, from σπαργω, 'I swathe,' 'I wrap.' 'Swathing clothes;' a kind of bandage, with which children were formerly surrounded.—Foësius. Also, a fascia.

SPARGANO'SIS, Sparga'sis, Intumescen'tia lac'tea mamma'rum, Mastodyn'ia polyg'ala, from σπαργαω, 'I am ready to burst.' Extreme distention of the breasts by milk. Sparganosis also means the wrapping of a child in swathing clothes.

SPARGANOSIS PUERPERARUM, Phlegmatia dolens.

SPARGANUM, Sparganon.

SPARROWGRASS, Asparagus.

SPARSUS, Sporadic.

SPAR'TIUM JUN'CEUM, Spanish broom. A small European shrub, cultivated in the gardens of the United States, on account of its yellow flowers. The seeds are diuretic and emetic in small doses; emetic and cathartic in large. They have been used in dropsy—10 or 15 grains three times a day.

SPARTIUM SCOPA'RIUM, Cyt'isus scopa'rius, Genis'ta, G. scopa'ria, Genis'ta hirsu'ta, Broom, Cytiso-genista, (F.) Génêt à balai. Family, Leguminosæ. Sex. Syst. Diadelphia Decandria. Broom Tops, Spartii Cacumina, Scopa'rius, Ph. U. S. have a bitter taste, and are possessed of diuretic properties. They have been used in dropsies. Dose, of the powder, ℈j to ℥j. All the genista have similar virtues. A decoction of genista, along with the cauterization of the pustules under the tongue, has been recommended in hydrophobia.

SPARTIUM TINCTORIUM, Genista tinctoria.

SPASM, Spasmus, Sparag'mos, Synol'ci, Spasis, from σπαω, 'I draw.' The Greeks gave this name to all kinds of convulsions. It is now usually applied to involuntary muscular contractions; and these, again, have been divided into tonic spasm, Paraton'ia, which consists in permanent rigidity and immobility of the muscles that are the seat of it (see Tetanus); and clonic spasm, which consists in alternate contractions and relaxations (see Convulsion).

Cullen has a class, Spasmi — the neuroposes of Fuchs.

SPASM, CLONIC, Convulsion — s. Cynic, see Canine laugh — s. of the Glottis, Asthma thymicum — s. of the Larynx, Asthma thymicum — s. with Rigidity, Tetanus.

SPASM, WRITERS'. Involuntary spasms of the muscles of the thumb and index finger, observed at times, in those who are much accustomed to writing. See Cramp, writers'.

SPASMATICUS, Spasmoticus.

SPASMATODES, Spasmoticus.

SPASME, DE LA GLOTTE ET DU THO-

RAX, Asthma thymicum — *s. de la Vessie,* Cystospasmus.

SPASMI, see Spasm.

SPASMODES, Convulsive.

SPASMODIC, Spasmoticus.

SPASMOL'OGY, *Spasmolog"ia,* from σπασμος, 'spasm, and λογος, 'a treatise.' A treatise on spasms.

SPASMOLYGMUS, Singultus.

SPASMOT'ICUS, *Spasmat'icus, Spasmato'des, Spas'ticus, Spastic, Spasmod'ic.* Any thing relating to spasm. Also, an antispasmodic.

Morbi constricto'rii, M. spasmot'ici, &c., are diseases accompanied with spasm.

SPASMUS, Convulsion, Spasm — s. Aurium, Otalgia — s. Caninus, see Canine laugh — s. Clonicus, Convulsion — s. Cynicus, see Canine laugh — s. Facialis, Tic — s. Glottidis, Asthma thymicum — s. Linguæ, Glossospasmus — s. Maxillæ inferioris, Trismus — s. Muscularis, Cramp — s. Musculorum Faciei, Canine laugh — s. Universalis, Synclonus — s. Ventriculi, see Cardialgia — s. Vesicæ, Cystospasmus.

SPAS'NIA, same etymon as Spasm. A term, used by Mercurialis, to designate the lancinating pain produced, at times, in the chest by violent fits of coughing.

SPASTIC, Spasmoticus, Tonic spasm.

SPASTICUM, Tetanic.

SPATHA, Hypaleiptron.

SPATHES'TER, from σπαω, 'I draw.' (?) A surgical instrument, used for drawing the prepuce over the glans, when too short.—P. Amman.

SPATHOMELE, Spatula.

SPATHULA, Scapula, Spatula — s. Fœtida, Iris fœtidissima.

SPATHYEMA FŒTIDA, Dracontium fœtidum.

SPAT'ILĒ, σπατιλη, 'human excrement.' A liquid fecal evacuation. Excrement. — Hippocrates.

SPATIUM ORIS, Mouth — s. Trigonum, Lyra.

SPAT'ULA, *Spath'ula,* diminutive of *Spatha,* σπαθη, 'a broad-sword.' *Spathome'lē, Specill'um latum.* An instrument used for spreading plasters, stirring ointments, holding down the tongue, &c. Also, the scapula.

SPATULA PRO ORE, Glossospatha.

SPEARWORT. Ranunculus flammula.

SPEAUTER, Zinc.

SPECIES, Powders, compound — s. Aromaticæ, Pulvis cinnamomi compositus — s. Diacinnamomi, Pulvis cinnamomi compositus — s. Diacretæ, Pulvis cretæ compos. — s. Diajalapæ, Pulvis jalapæ compositus — s. Diambræ sine odoratis, Pulvis cinnamomi compositus — s. Diatragacanthæ frigidæ, Pulvis tragacanthæ compositus — s. Hieræ picræ, Pulvis aloes cum canellā — s. Lætificantes Rhazis, Pulvis cinnamomi compositus — s. e Scordio cum opio, Pulvis cretæ compositus cum opio — s. e Scordio sine opio, Pulvis cretæ compositus.

SPECIF'IC, *Specif'icus,* from *species,* 'a form or fashion,' and *facere,* 'to make.' A substance to which is attributed the property of removing, directly, one disease rather than any other. Probably no such remedy exists. *Mercury* in syphilis, and *sulphur* in the itch, have been regarded as the strongest examples.

SPECIFIC OF HERRENSCHWAND. A once celebrated German vermifuge. It is said to have consisted of 10 grains of *Gamboge,* with 20 of *Carbonate of Potassa.* It is affirmed, that mercury and arsenic have also been found in it. — Paris.

SPECIFICUM PARACELSI, Potassæ sulphas.

SPECIL'LUM, *Melē, Stylus, Explorato'rium,* from *specio,* 'I examine,' *Specla'rion,* a probe, (F.) *Stylet, Sonde.* A surgical instrument, employed for examining wounds, fistulas, and for passing setons, &c. It is usually formed of silver; and is terminated, at one end, by an olive-shaped button. The *eyed probe* has an aperture at the other extremity.

SPECILLUM, Everriculum, Hypaleiptron, Sound — s. Auricularium, Apyromele — s. Cereum, *Bougie* — s. Excavatum, Stylus excavatus — s. Latum, Spatula — s. Minus, Melotis.

SPECLARION, Specillum.

SPEC'TACLES, from *spectare,* 'to behold;' *Conspicil'la,* (F.) *Besicles, Lunettes ordinaires, Conserves.* Glasses to assist the sight; arranged so as to be adapted to both eyes. These glasses are more or less *concave* or *convex,* according as the sight is more or less short, (*myopic,*) or long, (*presbyopic.*) When the glass is adapted to one eye, it is called an *Eyeglass, Conspicil'lum, Perspicil'lum, Vitrum ocula'rē.*

SPECULA'RIS LAPIS. A transparent mineral, but of what nature is not clear, which was formerly employed in epilepsy. In old times it was used for glass. — Pliny.

SPEC'ULUM, *Catop'ter, Catop'tron, Diop'tron.* In Latin, 'a mirror;' from *specio,* 'I see.' In surgery, it means different instruments for dilating cavities, and facilitating their examination. See Dilator. There are various instruments of this kind, — the *S. Ani, S. Auris, S. Vaginæ, (Colpeuryn'ter, Elytreurynter,) S. Matri'cis, S. Oculi, S. Oris* ((F.) *Baillon,) S. Gutturis, S. Vesicæ.*

SPECULUM CITRINUM, Orpiment — s. Indicum, Ferri limatura — s. Lucidum, Septum lucidum — s. Oris, Glossocatochus — s. Veneris, Achillea millefolium.

SPECUS, Vulva — s. Cordis, Ventricle of the Heart — s. Pro medullā spinali, see Vertebral column — s. Vertebralis, see Vertebral column.

SPEDALSKE, see Radzyge.

SPEDALSKHED, see Radzyge.

SPEECH, Voice, articulated.

SPEECHLESSNESS, Mutitas.

SPEEDIMAN'S PILLS, see Pilulæ aloes et myrrhæ.

SPEEDWELL, BROOKLIME, Veronica beccabunga — s. Female, Antirhinum elatine — s. Officinal, Veronica — s. Purslain, Veronica peregrina — s. Water, Veronica beccabunga.

SPELTRUM, Zincum.

SPERAGUS, Asparagus.

SPERM, from σπειρω, 'I sow.' *Spermat'ic fluid* or *liquor, Sem'inal fluid,* Seed, *Semen, S. viri'lē* seu *masculi'num* seu *genita'lē, Semin'ium, Genita'lē, Medul'læ, Rytis'ma, Ros, Sanguis, Serum, Humor genita'lis* seu *semina'lis* seu *vene'reus, Uri'na genita'lis, Genitu'ra, Sperma, S. viri'lē, Spermi'um, Tho'rē, Tho'rus, Lac marīs, Lagne'a, Lagni'a, Lagneu'ma, Germen, Male's milk, Prop'agatory* or *genital liquor, Vita'lē virus, Vital* or *quickening venom,* (F.) *Semence, Fluide seminal.* A whitish, viscid fluid, of a peculiar smell, secreted by the testicles, whence it is carried by the vasa deferentia to the vesiculæ seminales, to be thrown into the vagina, during coition, through the ejaculatory ducts and the urethra. It is the fecundating fluid, and must come into actual contact with the germ of the female. The *Aura sem'inis, Gonau'ra,* is incapable of effecting fecundation. The semen, at the time of emission, is composed of two different fluids; the one liquid and transparent, which is considered to be the secretion of the prostate, — the other, white, and as thick as mucilage; the product of the testicular secretion. The sperm contains, according to Vauquelin, 900 parts of water, 50 of animal mucilage, 10 of soda, and 30 of calcareous phosphate. The animal matter is peculiar, and by some termed *spermatin*.

Microscopic observations show that it contains *spermatozo'a*, or more properly *spermatozo'ids;* for their animalcular nature is not demonstrated. They are produced in cells — *sperm-cells* — and have probably no more title to be considered animalcular, than the cilia of the ciliated epithelium. By careful examination, other minute, round, granulated bodies may almost always be detected, which are in all cases much less numerous than the spermatozoa. These bodies are the *seminal granules, gran'ula sem'inis.* Pure sperm, in its most perfect state, consists principally of spermatozoids and seminal granules; both of which are enveloped in a small quantity of fluid, *liquor sem'inis.*

It has been imagined, but erroneously, that during coition there is a secretion of female sperm — *Semen mulie'brē, Thelyg'onum.* The increased secretion that takes place is chiefly from the glands of Duverney.

Sperm also means spermaceti.

SPERM CELL, see Sperm.

SPERMA, Sperm — s. Mercurii, Hydrargyrus acetatus.

SPERMA RANA'RUM, *Sperni'ola seu Sperni'olum seu Spermi'ola seu Spermi'olum rana'rum.* Frog's spawn. Once used in medicine.

SPERMACETI, Cetaceum — s. Whale, see Cetaceum.

SPERMACRASIA, Spermatorrhœa.

SPERMATACRASIA, Spermatorrhœa.

SPERMATACRATIA, Spermatorrhœa.

SPERMAT'IC, *Spermat'icus, Semina'lis, Sem'inal.* That which relates to the sperm. A name given to different parts connected with the organs of generation.

SPERMATIC ARTERIES, *A. Spermat'icæ, A. præparan'tes,* (F.) *Artères testiculaires, A. de l'ovaire* (Ch.), are two in number—one on each side—and arise from the sides of the aorta, sometimes from the renal arteries. They descend, almost vertically, at the sides of the vertebral column, and are distributed differently in the two sexes. In man, the spermatic artery, situate at the side of the vas deferens, issues by the abdominal ring; gives numerous ramifications to the spermatic chord, and divides into two fasciculi of branches, one of which goes to the testicle,—the other to the epididymis. In the female, the spermatic artery, *ova'rian artery,* dips into the pelvis, and passes to the ovarium, Fallopian tube, and round ligament.

SPERMATIC CHORD, *Testic'ular Chord, Funic'ulus Spermaticus, Corpus varico'sum,* (F.) *Cordon spermatique ou testiculaire.* The vascular and nervous chord, by which the testicle is suspended. It is composed of the spermatic artery and veins; of other small vessels; of lymphatics; of nervous filaments from the spermatic plexus, and from the genito-crural branch of the lumbo-abdominal plexus; of the vas deferens, and, very often, of a fibro-cellular chord, which unites the peritoneum to the upper part of the tunica vaginalis, and in which encysted hydrocele of the spermatic chord occurs. All these parts are united together by a very lax, areolar tissue, and surrounded by coats, which, reckoning from without, are:—1. The skin and areolar membrane. 2. A fibro-cellular membrane, formed by the fascia superficialis. 3. A very thin layer, formed by fibres of the cremaster muscle, united archwise before, and often also behind, the chord. 4. The proper sheath of the spermatic vessels, or the tubular prolongation furnished by the fascia transversalis to the chord, on a level with the superior orifice of the inguinal canal. The spermatic chord is commonly shorter on the right side than on the left; and of a different size in different individuals. It ascends, almost vertically, from the superior margin of the testicle as far as the lower orifice of the inguinal canal; passes through this canal and enters the abdomen, crossing the epigastric artery. Here it forms an evident elbow, directing its course backward. At this part, also, the organs composing it separate from each other :— the vas deferens descending into the pelvis to pass behind the bladder ;—the blood-vessels and lymphatics ascending towards the lumbar region, &c.

SPERMATIC FLUID, Sperm.

SPERMATIC GANGLION. A large ganglion, formed by branches from the hypogastric ganglion, and from the spermatic plexus. It supplies the fundus uteri. Besides these ganglia, D. Robt. Lee describes *ves'ical* and *vag''inal gan;* and anterior and posterior *subperitone'al gan;* and *plexuses*, which communicate with the preceding, and constitute an extensive nervous net over the entire uterus.

SPERMATIC LIQUOR, Liquor, Sperm.

SPERMATIC PASSAGES OR WAYS, *Viæ Spermaticæ*, are the canals concerned in the excretion of semen.

SPERMATIC PLEXUSES of nerves, *Plexus testiculares*, are two in number, and are furnished by the renal plexuses. Their filaments, called *spermatic nerves*, follow the arteries of the same name to the testicle in man; and to the ovary and Fallopian tube in the female,—*ova'rian nerves*. They cannot be traced into the substance of these organs.

SPERMATIC VEINS are two or three in number on each side. They accompany the spermatic artery, and open — those of the right, into the vena cava inferior; those of the left, into the corresponding renal vein. These veins form above the testicle, a kind of venous network, called, by some, the *Spermatic Plexus*; and another plexus before the psoas muscle, called the *Corpus pampiniforme*.

SPERMATIN, see Sperm.

SPERMATIS'MUS, *Emis'sio sem'inis*, from σπερμα, 'sperm.' The emission of sperm.

SPERMATOCE'LĒ, *Hernia semina'lis seu Oscheoce'lē semina'lis, Gonoce'lē*, from σπερμα, 'sperm,' and κηλη, 'a tumour.' The ancients gave this name to certain swellings of the testicle which were regarded as produced by an accumulation of sperm in the organ. Also, varicocele.

SPERMATOCLEMMA, see Pollution.

SPERMATOCLEPSIS, see Pollution.

SPERMATOCYSTIDORRHAG''IA, *Cystirhag''ia ejaculato'ria, Hæmatu'ria ejaculato''ria, H. semina'lis*, from σπερμα, σπερματος, 'sperm,' κυστις, 'bladder,' and ρηγ, 'a breaking forth.' A discharge of blood from the urethra, or that of ejaculation of sperm.

SPERMATODES, Gonoides.

SPERMATOGON'IA, *Spermogon'ia, Spermatopæ'ia, Spermatopoē'sis, Spermi'um*, from σπερμα, 'sperm,' and γενναω, 'to beget.' The preparation or secretion of sperm.

SPERMATOID, Gonoides.

SPERMATOLEPSIS, see Pollution.

SPERMATOLIPSIS, see Pollution.

SPERMATOL'OGY, *Spermatolog''ia*, from σπερμα, 'sperm,' and λογος, 'a discourse.' A treatise on sperm.

SPERMATOPH'OROUS, *Seminif'erous*, from σπερμα, 'sperm,' and φερω, 'I carry.' Sperm-bearing. The cells or granules in the sperm have been so called.

SPERMATOPŒIA, Spermatogonia.

SPERMATOPOESIS, Spermatogonia.
SPERMATOPOETIC, Spermatopœus.
SPERMATOPŒ'US, *Spermatopoët'icus, Spermatopoiet'icus, Spermatopoët'ic, Gonepœ'us, Gonepoiet'icus, Gonopoiet'icus*, from σπερμα, 'sperm,' and ποιειν, 'to make.' Food, to which has been attributed the property of augmenting the secretion of semen; and, consequently, of exciting the venereal act. Very succulent and very nutritious substances have been so considered.

SPERMATORRHŒ'A, *Spermorrhœ'a, Spermacra'sia, Spermatoze'mia, Spermatacra'sia, Gonacra'sia, Gonacrati'a, Spermatacrati'a, Gonorrhœ'a vera*, (F.) *Flux de Sperme, Pollutions, Pertes séminales;* from σπερμα, 'sperm,' and ρεω, 'I flow.' An emission of sperm, without copulation. See Gonorrhœa, and Pollution.
SPERMATORRHŒA ATONICA, Gonorrhœa laxorum.

SPERMATOS'CHESIS, from σπερμα, 'sperm,' and σχισις, 'retention.' Retention or suppression of the spermatic secretion.

SPERMATOZEMIA, Spermatorrhœa.

SPERMATOZO'A, *Zooëper'mata*, from σπερμα, 'sperm,' and ζωον, 'animal.' *Zoöspermes, Spermatozoüires, Spermatozo'ïds, Animal'cula semina'lia* seu *spermat'ica, Vermic'uli spermat'ici, Seminal filaments, Spermatic* or *seminal animalcules* (?). Reputed animalcules seen in the sperm; by most physiologists supposed to be the formative agents in generation. See Sperm.
SPERMATOZOAIRES, Spermatozoa.
SPERMATOZOIDS, Spermatozoa.
SPERMIOLUM RANARUM, Sperma ranarum.
SPERMIUM, Sperm, Spermatogonia.
SPERMOBOLE, see Ejaculation, Spermatismus.
SPERMOEDIA CLAVUS, Ergot.
SPERMOGONIA, Spermatogonia.
SPERMORRHŒA, Spermatorrhœa.
SPERNIOLUM RANARUM, Sperma ranarum.
SPEWING, Vomiting.
SPHACELATION, Mortification.
SPHACÈLE, Sphacelus — *s. de la Bouche,* Cancer aquaticus.
SPHACELIA SEGETUM, see Ergot.
SPHACELISMUS, Sphacelus — s. Cerebri, Phrenitis.
SPHAC"ELUS, *Gangræ'na Sphacelus, Sphacelis'mus, Cold mortification,* (F.) *Sphacèle, Gangrène froide,* from σφαζω, 'I slay.' This word is used, by some, synonymously with gangrene; by others, with gangrene when it occupies the whole substance of a limb. Commonly, it means the disorganized portion, in cases of mortification, *anthraconecro'sis*, which must be thrown off—or is, in other words, totally dead. The foul disorganized portion of an ulcer—called the *slough*—must be considered a kind of sphacelus.
Sphacelus was formerly used to denote excessive pain; and for agitation from excessive pain, or violent emotion.
SPHACELUS CEREALIS, Ergotism — s. Nosocomialis, Hospital gangrene.
SPHÆRA, Pila — s. Marina, Pila marina — s. Thalassia, Pila marina.
SPHÆRANTHUS INDICUS, Adaca.
SPHÆRIDION, Pilula.
SPHÆRION, Globule, Pilula.
SPHÆROCEPHALA ELATIOR, Echinops.
SPHÆROCOCCUS CRISPUS, Fucus crispus — s. Helminthochortus, Corallina Corsicana — s. Lichenoides, Fucus amylaceus.
SPHÆRULÆ SANGUINIS, Globules of the blood.

SPHAGE, Throat.
SPHENDONE, Funda.
SPHENOID, *Sphenoï'des, Spheno'des, Sphenoïdeus, Sphenoïda'lis,* from σφην, 'a wedge,' and ειδος, 'resemblance.' Wedge-shaped. Hence,
SPHENOID BONE, *Sphenoïdes os, Os basila'rē* seu *cuneifor'mē* seu *cu'neo compara'tum* seu *sphenoïda'lē* seu *multifor'mē* seu *as'ygos* seu *papilla'rē* seu *polymor'phon* seu *paxilla'rē* seu *baxilla'rē* seu *alæfor'mē* seu *sphecoï'des* seu *vespifor'mē* seu *inconjuga'tum, Pter'ygoid bone*. An azygous bone, situate on the median line, and at the base of the cranium. It articulates with all the other bones of that cavity; supports them, and strengthens their union. Its form is singular, and resembles a bat with its wings extended. It has, 1. An *inferior* or *guttural surface*, on which is situate the crista, that joins the vomer; a channel, which concurs in forming the pterygo-palatine foramen; the pterygoid process; the pterygoid fossa; the scaphoid depression; the Vidian or pterygoid canal; the foramina — ovale, spinale, &c. 2. A *superior* or *cerebral surface*, on which are: — the clinoid processes; the pituitary fossa; the foramina (ovale, rotundum, and spinale); the *Apophysis of Ingrassias* or lesser wing; the foramen opticum, &c. 3. An *occipital* or *posterior surface*, which is articulated with the basilary process of the occipital bone. 4. An *anterior* or *orbitarnasal surface*; having, anteriorly, a crista to unite with the ethmoid bone; and, on each side, a round aperture, which leads into two cavities in the substance of the bone, separated by a middle septum, and called the *sphenoïdal sinuses*. 5. Two *zygomato-temporal* or *external surfaces*, which correspond to the temporal and zygomatic fossæ.
Some divide the sphenoid into *body* or *middle portion;* and *alæ*, which are four in number, and are subdivided into *great (Temporal Plates* or *Wings)* and *little (Apophyses of Ingrassias)*. The *Sphenoid suture* surrounds the bone.
SPHENOID, SPINOUS PROCESS OF THE, Sphenoid spine.

SPHENOÏD'AL, *Sphenoïda'lis*. That which belongs or relates to the sphenoid bone.
SPHENOIDA'LIA COR'NUA, (F.) *Cornets sphénoïdaux, Cornets de Bertin; Ossic'ula Berti'ni, Ossa triangula'ria, Pyr'amids of Wistar*. Two small, thin, and curved bones, situate between the sphenoid and ethmoid, with which they are confounded in the adult. They have the shape of a hollow pyramid, with the base turned backwards; and are developed by a single point of ossification. They are articulated with the sphenoid, ethmoid, palate bone, and vomer.
SPHENOIDAL or SUPE'RIOR OR'BITARY FISSURE, *Fora'men lac"erum supe'rius*, (F.) *Fente sphénoïdale*, is a large fissure, situate between the great and little ala of the sphenoid. It is seen at the upper and back part of the orbit between which and the cranium it is a means of communication.
SPHENOIDAL SPINE, (F.) *Épine sphénoïdale, Spinous Process of the Sphenoid;* — 1. A projecting crista at the inferior surface of the sphenoid bone, for articulation with the vomer. 2. A triangular process, *Apophyse sous-temporale* (Ch.), met with near the posterior margin of the same bone, behind the foramen spinale. At the point of the spinous process, a *styloid process* is frequently met with.
SPHENOIDES, Cuneiform, Sphenoid — s. Os, Sphenoid bone.
SPHENOMAX'ILLARY, *Spheno-maxilla'ris*. That which relates to the sphenoid and maxillary bones.
SPHENOMAXILLARY FISSURE, *Inferior or'bitar*

Fissure, (F.) *Fente sphéno-maxillaire* ou *orbitaire inférieure;* called, also, *Fora'men lac"erum inferius, F. spheno-maxilla're,* is situate at the posterior part of the angle formed by the union of the internal and inferior parietes of the orbit. It is constituted, above, by the sphenoid bone; below, by the superior maxillary and palate bones; and, before, by the malar bone. It is narrower at the middle than at the extremities, and forms a communication between the orbital cavity and the zygomatic fossa.

SPHENOMAXILLARY FOSSA is a name given by some anatomists, to a depression at the union of the sphenomaxillary and pterygomaxillary fissures.

SPHENO-OR'BITAR. A name given, by Béclard to the anterior part of the body of the sphenoid bone, which is developed by a variable number of points of ossification.

SPHENOPAL'ATINE, *Sphenopalati'nus.* That which relates to the sphenoid and palate bones.

SPHENOPALATINE ARTERY, *Large lateral nasal A.,* is the termination of the internal maxillary. It enters at the posterior part of the superior meatus of the nose, through the spheno-palatine foramen, and spreads its numerous branches on the pituitary membrane covering the septum, the cornua, and the meatus.

SPHENOPALATINE FORA'MEN is a round aperture, formed by the vertical portion of the os palati and the sphenoid. It establishes a communication between the nasal fossae and the zygomatic fossa.

SPHENOPALATINE GANGLION, *Ganglion of Meckel, Spheno'id'al G.* (Ch.) A small, nervous, cordiform, or triangular ganglion, of variable size, situate without the foramen sphæno-palatinum, in the pterygomaxillary fissure. It seems suspended by several nervous filaments to the trunk of the superior maxillary nerve, and gives off *internal* or *sphenopalatine filaments, inferior* or *palatine filaments,* and a *posterior filament,* which is the *Vidian* or *pterygoid nerve.*

SPHENOPALATINE NERVES,*Lat'eral nasal nerves,* arise from the ganglion — just described — at its inner part, and enter the nasal fossae by the sphenopalatine foramen. They are five or six in number, and distribute their filaments to the outer and inner parietes of the nasal fossae. One of the most remarkable branches is the *Naso-palatine.*

SPHENOPALATINUS, Levator palati.

SPHENOPARI'ETAL, *Spheno-parieta'lis.* That which belongs or relates to the sphenoid and parietal bones.

SPHENOPARIETAL SUTURE is formed by the articulation of the extremity of the greater ala of the sphenoid with the anterior and inferior angle of the parietal bone.

SPHENO-PTERYGO-PALATINUS, Circumflexus — s. Salpingostaphylinus, Circumflex — s. Salpingo-mallien, Laxator tympani.

SPHENOSIS, see Wedged.

SPHENOSTAPHYLINUS, Levator palati.

SPHENOTEMP'ORAL, *Spheno-tempora'lis.* That which belongs to the sphenoid and temporal bones.

SPHENOTEMPORAL SUTURE is the suture at the articulation of the great alae of the sphenoid bone with the squamous portion of the temporal. Béclard gives the name *sphenotemporal* to the posterior part of the body of the sphenoid, which is developed by distinct points of ossification.

SPHEX, Wasp.

SPHINCTER, *Constric'tor, Musc'ulus constricto'rius,* from σφιγγω, 'I constrict.' A name given to several annular muscles, which constrict or close certain natural openings.

SPHINCTER ANI, *Annula'ris Ani.* Many anatomists have described two sphincter muscles of the anus: — 1. The *S. exter'nus, Aspidis*[?], *S. cuta'neus, Coccygio-cutané-sphincter, Orbicularis Recti, Constric'tor Ani, Coccygio-anal,* (Ch.) is situate around the anus; is elliptical from before to behind; flattened, and pierced at its middle. Its fibres describe concentric arcs, which are attached, behind, to the extremity of the coccyx, by a dense, areolar substance; and are confounded, anteriorly, with the bulbo-cavernosi and transversi perinaei muscles. This muscle contracts and closes the anus. 2. The *inner* or *internal Sphincter Ani, Sphincter intestina'lis* of Winslow, is by many anatomists considered as the termination of the circular fibres of the rectum. It is annular, and situate around the inferior extremity of the rectum, to the extent of about a finger's breadth. It has the same use as the other.

SPHINCTER GULÆ, Constrictores pharyngis — s. Ilei, Bauhin, valve of — s. Intestinalis, Sphincter ani internus — s. Labiorum, Orbicularis oris — s. Oculi, Orbicularis palpebrarum — s. Palpebrarum, Orbicularis palpebrarum — s. Pylori, see Pylorus — s. Vaginae, Constrictores cunni — s. Ventriculi, Pylorus.

SPHINCTER VESI'CÆ, *Sphincter of the bladder.* Some anatomists have given this name to white, elastic, and circular fibres, which surround the neck of the bladder, but do not constitute a particular muscle. Morgagni has given the name PSEUDO-SPHINCTER to the anterior fibres of the levator ani, which pass beneath the neck of the bladder, and, by their contraction, close that opening. See Compressor urethrae.

SPHONDYLIUM, Heracleum spondylium.

SPHONGUS, Spongia.

SPHRAGIDONYCHARGOCOME'TA, from σφραγις, 'a seal,' ονυξ, 'the nail,' αργυρος, 'silver,' or perhaps αργυρος, 'silver,' and κομη, 'I adorn.' A charlatan who adorned his fingers to the very nails with rings. — Aristophanes, Hippocrates.

SPHYGMA, Pulse.

SPHYG'MICA ARS, *Sphygmic art,* from σφυγμος, 'the pulse.' The art of judging by the pulse in health or disease.

SPHYGMICA DOCTRINA, Sphygmologia.

SPHYGMICUS, Throbbing.

SPHYGMOCEPHALUS, Crotaphe.

SPHYGMODES, Throbbing.

SPHYGMOLOG"IA, *Sphyg'mica Doctri'na,* from σφυγμος, 'the pulse,' and λογος, 'a description.' The doctrine of the pulse.

SPHYGMOMETER, Pulsilegium.

SPHYGMOS, Pulsation, Pulse.

SPHYGMOSCOPIUM, Pulsilegium.

SPHYRA, Malleolus.

SPHYXIS, Pulsation.

SPIC, Lavendula.

SPICA, *Fas'cia repens,* the *Spica bandage.* *Epi.* A bandage so called in consequence of its somewhat resembling a *spike* of barley. The turns of the bandage cross like the letter V: each leaving a third of the roller uncovered. It is distinguished into *ascending* and *descending*. It may be applied over various parts of the body, and in a different manner in each case; thus, there is the *Spica* seu *Fascia inguina'lis, Spica inguina'lis duplex,* the spica for the shoulder, and another for the thumb.

SPICA, Lavendula.

SPICA ALPINA, Valeriana Celtica — s. Celtica, Valeriana Celtica — s. Indica, Nardus Indica — s. Nardi, Nardus Indica.

SPICEBERRY, Gaultheria, Laurus Benzoin.

SPICEBUSH, Laurus Benzoin.

SPICES, FOUR, see Myrtus pimenta.
SPICEWOOD, Laurus Benzoin.
SPICILLUM, Specillum.
SPIDER, see Araneæ tela.
SPIDERWORT, Liliago, Tradescantia Virginica.
SPIGELIA, S. Marilandica.
SPIGE'LIA MARILAN'DICA, *Anthel'mia, Spige'lia Lonic''era, Lonic''era Marilan'dica, Peren'nial Wormgrass* or *Indian Pink, Caroli'na Pink, Starbloom, Wormroot. Nat. Ord.* Gentianeæ. *Class,* Pentandria. *Order,* Monogynia. Indigenous. The root — *Spigelia* (Ph. U. S.) — is celebrated as an anthelmintic, particularly in cases of lumbrici. It is, also, asserted to have been found serviceable in remittent fever. It is a narcotico-acrid. Dose, gr. x to ʒss.
SPIGNEL, Æthusa meum.
SPIKENARD, Conyza squarrosa, Nardus Indica — s. American, Aralia racemosa — s. Small, Aralia nudicaulis — s. Tree, Aralia spinosa.
SPILANTHES ACMELLA, Spilanthus acmella.
SPILAN'THUS ACMEL'LA, *S, cilia'ta* seu *fimbria'ta, Spilan'thes acmel'la, Bidens acmella, Achmella, Acmella, A. Mauritiana, Verbesi'na acmella, Balm-leaved Spilanthus. Family,* Corymbiferæ. *Sex. Syst.* Syngenesia Polygamia æqualis. This plant possesses a glutinous, bitter taste, and fragrant smell. The herb and seed are said to be diuretic and emmenagogue. They have been used in dropsies, jaundice, fluor albus, and calculous complaints; given in infusion.
SPILANTHUS, BALM-LEAVED, Spilanthus acmella — s. Ciliata, S. acmella — s. Fimbriata, S. acmella.
SPILANTH'US OLERA'CEUS, *Spear-leaved Spilanthus,* (F.) *Cresson de Para.* A tincture of the plant has been recommended in toothach.
SPILI, see Nævus.
SPILOMA, see Nævus.
SPILOSIS, Epichrosis — s. Ephelis, Ephelides s. Poliosis, Poliosis.
SPILSBURY'S ANTISCORBUTIC DROPS. An empirical preparation, formed of *hydrarg. oxymur., rad. gentian., cort. aurant. sicc.* āā ʒij; *antimon. crud., santal. rubr.* āā ʒj; *spiritus vini rectif., aquæ,* āā ʒviij.
SPINA, 'a thorn;' *Spine,* (F.) *Épine.* A process on the surface of a bone, which has been compared to the spines or thorns on certain vegetables. The chief processes of this name are: — the *nasal spine,* the *spine of the scapula,* the *spine of the ischium,* the *four iliac spines,* the *palatine spine,* the *maxillary,* the *sphenoid,* &c. The *spine of the back* is the collection of vertebræ constituting the *vertebral column.*
SPINA, Penis — s. Acida, Oxycantha Galeni — s. Ægyptiaca, see Acaciæ gummi — s. Alba, Carduus marianus, Mespilus oxycantha. Onopordum acanthium — s. Bifida, Hydrorachis — s. Cervina, Rhamnus — s. Domestica, Rhamnus — s. Dorsi, Vertebral column, see Nasus — s. Dorsi introrsum Flexa, Lordosis — s. Ferrea, Pin — s. Helmontii, *Aiguillon* — s. Hirci, Astragalus verus — s. Infectoria, Rhamnus — s. Nodosa, Rachitis.
SPINA VENTO'SA, *Spinæ ventos'itas, Tere'do, Fungus Artic'uli, Ostarthroc'acē, Tumor fungo'sus artic'uli, Lu'pia junctu'ræ, Hyperepon'gia, Flatus spinæ, Arthroc'acē, Pædarthroc'acē, White Swelling* (of some,) *Sidera'tio Ossis, Cancer Ossis, Gangræ'na Ossis, Exosto'sis.* A term of no definite meaning, as is obvious from these various words having been considered its synonymes. By some, it is defined to be — a disease of the osseous system, in which the texture of the bone dilates, seeming to be distended with air, and constituting a variety of osteo-sarcoma. By others, it is considered to be a tumour arising from an internal caries of a bone; occurring most frequently in the carpus or tarsus. The term itself is a translation from the Arabic of Rhazes. See, also, Hydrarthrus, and Mollities Ossium.
SPINA VERTEBRALIS, Vertebral column.
SPINACH, Spinacia.
SPINACHIA, Spinacia.
SPINA'CIA, *Spina'chia, Spina'cia olera'cea, Spin'age,* Spinach, (F.) *Épinard. Family,* Atriplicæ. *Sex. Syst.* Diœcia Pentandria. A plant which resembles the cabbage in its dietetic powers. The leaves boiled, with the addition of oil, form a good emollient cataplasm. It has been used in phthisical complaints; but its medicinal properties, if it have any, are not now regarded.
SPINACIA OLERACEA, Spinacia.
SPINÆ, Spinous processes — s. Ventositas, Spina ventosa.
SPINAGE, Spinacia.
SPINAL, *Spina'lis, Spino'sus, Spina'tus,* (F.) *Épinière,* from *spina,* 'the spine.' That which relates to the vertebral column.
SPINAL ARTERIES are two in number, viz: 1. The *posterior spinal, Artère médiane postérieure du Rachis,* (Ch.) It arises from the vertebral, near the corpora pyramidalia, and descends on the posterior surface of the spinal marrow, distributing its ramifications to it. 2. The *anterior spinal artery, A. médiane antérieure,* (Ch.,) is larger than the last, and arises, also, from the vertebral. It descends, in a serpentine manner, upon the anterior surface of the marrow; furnishes ramusculi to it, and unites with that of the opposite side, opposite the foramen magnum occipitis. A very tortuous branch arises from this union, which descends as far as the inferior extremity of the marrow, to which it sends numerous divisions.
The term *Spinal Arteries* or *Rachinian Arteries* is also given, in the abstract, to all the arteries of the spinal marrow and vertebral canal. The same may be said of the veins and nerves.
SPINAL CORD, Medulla spinalis.
SPINAL FORAM'INA, (F.) *Trous rachidiens,* in the abstract, are the foramina formed by every two contiguous vertebræ, through which the spinal nerves issue. See Vertebral. The term *Foramen Spina'lē* is especially applied, however, to a small foramen, in front of the spinous process of the sphenoid bone, through which the middle artery of the dura mater enters the cranium. It is, likewise, called *Foramen spheno-spino'sum,* (F.) *Trou Sphéno-épineux* ou *petit rond, Trou épineux.*
SPINAL IRRITA'TION, *Rhachialgi'tis, Rhachial'gia, Neural'gia spina'lis, Notal'gia.* A modern pathological view, which refers most nervous diseases to irritation of the spinal cord. This irritation is presumed to be indicated by tenderness on pressure over the spinous process of one or more vertebræ, or over the nerves proceeding from the cord and distributed to the parts at the sides of the spine. Such tenderness, however, by no means indicates the pathological condition in question, as it is often met with in those enjoying perfect health. The treatment advised is cupping and counter-irritation on each side of the spine, which may be beneficial in such diseases, no matter what part of the frame may be in a morbid state, by exciting a new and revellent impression on a very sensible portion of the cutaneous surface.
SPINAL NERVE, *Ac'cessory of the Par vagum* or *8th pair, Accessory nerve of Willis, Spinal Accessory, Spino-cranio-trapézien, Superior res'pira-tory N., Eleventh pair of encephalic nerves, Trachélo-dorsal* (Ch.), arises from the medulla spi-

nalis, within the vertebral canal, between the anterior and posterior roots of the cervical nerves at a greater or less distance from the cranium. The roots unite to form the nerve, which ascends into the cranium through the foramen magnum of the occipital bone, and issues by the foramen lacerum posterius, crossing the sterno-cleido-mastoideus, to which it gives filaments, and losing itself entirely on the trapezius muscle. The pneumogastric and spinal accessory nerves together—*nercus vagus cum accesso'rio*—resemble the spinal nerves; the former, with its ganglion, being the posterior root; the latter, the anterior.

SPINAL NERVES, Vertebral nerves—s. Prolongation, Medulla spinalis.

SPINAL SYSTEM OF NERVES, see Nerves.

SPINALES COLLI MINORES, Interspinales colli — s. et Transversales lumborum, Transversalis dorsi.

SPINALIS CERVICIS, Semi-spinalis colli — s. Colli, Semi-spinalis colli.

SPINALIS DORSI, *Grand épineux du dos, Spinalis Dorsi major.* Winslow calls thus some fleshy fasciculi, which are situate on the lateral surfaces of the spinous processes; from the third dorsal vertebra to the first or second lumbar; and which form part of the transverso-spinalis of most authors. The same anatomist calls—*Spina'lis Dorsi minor, Petit épineux du dos*—some small, fleshy fibres, situate on each side of the interspinal ligament. They are short, flat, and pass from one spinous process to the other. Like the preceding, they form part of the transverso-spinalis. All these fleshy fasciculi strengthen the vertebral column.

SPINATI, Interspinales colli.

SPINATUS, Spinal.

SPINDLE TREE, Euonymus Americanus.

SPINE, Vertebral column — s. Curvature of the, Gibbositas—s. Hæmal, Sternum—s. Neural, Spinous process.

SPINI-AXOIDO-OCCIPITALIS, Rectus capitis posticus major—*s. Axoido-trachéli-atloïdien*, Obliquus inferior capitis.

SPINITIS. Myelitis.

SPINO-DORSITIS, Myelitis.

SPINOLA, see Hydrorachis.

SPINOSUS, Spinal.

SPINOUS, *Spino'sus,* (F.) *Épineux.* Having the shape of a spine or thorn.

SPINOUS PROC"ESSES or APOPH'YSES *of the Ver'tebræ, Acan'thæ, Spinæ, Cynol'ophoi, Neural Spines* of Mr. Owen, (F.) *Apophyses épineuses,* are situate at the posterior part of each vertebra, and afford attachment to the muscles, whose office it is to extend the spine. See Vertebra.

SPIRAC'ULA, (F.) *Spiracules,* from *spiro,* 'I breathe.' Respiratory pores of the skin.

SPIRÆ CEREBRI, Convolutions, cerebral.

SPIRÆA DENUDATA, S. ulmaria.

SPIRÆA FILIPEN'DULA, *Filipendula, Sarif'raga rubra, Dropwort,* (F.) *Filipendule. Family,* Rosaceæ. *Sex. Syst.* Icosandria Pentagynia. The root of this plant is said to possess astringent and lithontriptic virtues.

SPIRÆA TOMENTOSA, *Hardhack, Red meadowsweet, Steeple bush, Rosy bush, White leaf.* This indigenous species, which is abundant in the northern States of the Union, is tonic and astringent; and is usually administered either in the form of extract or decoction, (Spiræa ʒss; aquæ Oj.)

SPIRÆA TRIFOLIATA, Gillenia trifoliata.

SPIRÆA ULMA'RIA, *S. denuda'ta, Ulmaria, U. palus'tris, Regi'na Prati, Barba capræ, Meadow Sweet, Queen of the Meadows, Bar'bula capri'na,* (F.) *Ulmaire, Reine des Prés.* The leaves have been recommended as mild astringents:—the flowers as antispasmodics and diaphoretics.

SPIRAMENTA PULMONUM, see Pulmo.

SPIRAMENTUM ANIMÆ, Pulmo.

SPIRAMINA PALPEBRARUM, Lachryma puncta — s. Pulmonum, see Pulmo.

SPIRATIO, Respiration.

SPIRIT, *Spir'itus;* from *spirare,* 'to exhale,' (F.) *Esprit.* A name given to every liquid product of distillation. Spirits were formerly distinguished into — *inflammable, acid,* and *oleose* and consequently a number of substances were crowded together, which often resembled each other in no other property than in being volatile. The term is now confined to alcoholic liquors, of which the following are the chief:

Arrack. Distilled from coarse palm sugar named jaggery, fermented with the bark of the Mimosa *leucophlea*; also from rice and the fermented juice of the Palm; made in India. Its varieties are :—

1. *Mahwah Arrack.* Made in India from the flowers of the Madhuca tree, Bassia *butyracea.*

2. *Tuba.* Made from palm wine, in the Philippine Islands.

Araka. Distilled, by the Tartars, from koumis, fermented mares' milk.

Araki. Distilled from dates, by the Egyptians

Arika. A variety of koumis, distilled from fermented mares' milk, in Tartary and Iceland.

Brandy. Distilled from wine, figs, peaches, persimmon, apple, mulberries, and sometimes other fruits, in Europe, Asia, North and South America, wherever wine is made. The best brandy is that of Cognac; the next, that of Bordeaux and Rochelle. The varieties are—

1. *Aguardiente,* (S.) In Peru, the coarse brandy obtained from grapes is the *Aguardiente de Pisco,* so called, because shipped at the port of Pisco. Another kind, much dearer, and of excellent flavour, is made from Muscatel grapes and is called *Aguardiente de Italia.* It is sometimes seen in the United States.

2. *Lau.* Made from rice, in Siam.

3. *Rakia.* Made in Dalmatia from the husks of grapes mixed with aromatics.

4. *Rossolio.* Made at Dantzic, from a compound of brandy, rossolis, and other plants.

5. *Troster.* Made on the Rhine, from the husks of grapes, fermented with barley and rye.

6. *Sekis-kayarodka.* Made from the lees of wine and fruit at Scio.

Geneva Hollands, (genièvre, French for juniper.) Distilled from malted barley and rye, rectified on juniper berries, in Holland. Its varieties—

Gin. Made in England, from malted barley, rye, potatoes; rectified with turpentine.

Goldwasser. Distilled at Dantzic, from wheat barley, and rye, rectified with aniseed, cinnamon and other spices.

Kirschwasser. Distilled from the Mahaleb cherry, in Switzerland.

Maraschino. Distilled from the Marasca cherry, at Zara, the capital of Dalmatia.

Rum, (supposed to be derived from the terminal syllable of the word *saccharum*: but the original Americans call this liquor Rum.) Distilled, in the West Indies and South America from cane-sugar and molasses, and in North America from maple-sugar. Its variety is—

Slatkaia trava. Made in Kamtschatka, from a sweet grass.

Show-choo. Distilled, in China, from the lees of mandarin, a wine made from boiled rice.

Whisky, (supposed to be derived from *usque,* the first two syllables of *usquebagh,* the original name in Ireland.) Distilled, in Scotland and Ireland

land, from malted and raw barley, rye, oats, and potatoes; and in the south of France, from aloes. In Ireland it was called *buil-ceaun*, or madness of the head. The best Scotch whisky is *Glenlivet*, the best Irish, *Ennishowen.*
Y-wer-a. Distilled, in the Sandwich Islands, from the root of the Tee-root, baked, pounded, and fermented.

To these may be added an intoxicating liquor made by the Affghanistans, from ewes' milk; and that made in Kamtschatka, from a species of mushroom, named muchumer.

SPIRIT OF ANISEED, Spiritus anisi—s. Bathing, Freeman's, see Linimentum saponis compos.—s. Bathing, Jackson's, see Linimentum saponis compos.—s. Bezoardic of Bussius, see Bussii spiritus Bezoarticus—s. Bone, Liquor volatilis cornu cervi—s. of Burrhus, Burrhi spiritus matricalis—s. of Carraway, Spiritus carui—s. of Ether, aromatic, Spiritus ætheris aromaticus — s. Fuming, of Beguin, Ammoniæ sulphuretum — s. Fuming, of Boyle, Ammoniæ sulphuretum — s. of Hartshorn, Liquor cornu cervi — s. of Horseradish, compound, Spiritus armoraciæ compositus—s. of Lavender, Spiritus lavandulæ — s. of Lavender, compound, Spiritus lavandulæ compositus—s. of Mindererus, Liquor ammoniæ acetatis—s. of Nitre, sweet, Spiritus ætheris nitrici—s. of Nitric ether, Spiritus ætheris nitrici—s. of Pennyroyal, Spiritus pulegii—s. of Peppermint, Spiritus menthæ piperitæ — s. Proof, Spiritus tenuior — s. of Salt, Muriaticum acidum — s. of Scurvygrass, golden, see Spiritus armoraciæ compositus—s. of Spearmint, Spiritus menthæ viridis — s. of Sulphuric ether, Spiritus ætheris sulphurici — s. of Sulphuric ether, compound, Spiritus ætheris sulphurici compositus—s. of Turpentine, Oleum terebinthinæ rectificatum — s. Verdigris, Aceticum acidum—s. of Vitriol, Sulphuric acid—s. of Wine and camphor, Spiritus camphoræ.

SPIRITS, ANIMAL, Nervous fluid.
SPIRITUOUS, Alcoholic.
SPIRITUS, Breath, Life, Respiration, Spirit — s. Æthereus nitrosus, Spiritus ætheris nitrici — s. Æthereus vitriolicus, Spiritus ætheris sulphurici.

SPIR'ITUS ÆTHERIS AROMAT'ICUS, *Æther Sulphu'ricus cum alcoho'lē aromat'icus, Elix'ir vitrio'll dulcē, Sweet Elix'ir of Vit'riol, Viga'ni's Elixir of Vitriol, Aromat'ic Spirit of Ether.* (*Cinnam. cort.* contus. ʒiij. *cardam. sem.* contus. ʒiss. *piperis longi fruct.* cont., *zingib. rad.* concis., sing. ʒj. *spiritûs ætheris sulphuric.* Oj. Macerate, for 14 days, in a stopped glass vessel and strain. Ph. L.) It is used as a stimulant in nervous affections. Dose, f ʒss to f ʒj.

SPIRITUS ÆTHERIS NIT'RICI, *Sp. Ætheris nitro'si, Sp. nitri dulcis, Sp. Æthe'reus nitro'sus, Sweet Spirit of Nitre, Nitre drops, Spiritus nitricus alcoolisa'tus, Spirit of Nitric Ether.* (*Nitrate of Potassa*, in coarse powder, ℔ij, *Sulphuric acid*, ℔iss; *Alcohol*, Oixss; *Diluted Alcohol*, Oj; *Carbonate of Potassa*, ʒj. Mix the nitrate of potassa and the alcohol in a large glass retort, and having gradually poured in the acid, digest with a gentle heat for two hours; then raise the heat, and distil a gallon. To the distilled liquor add the diluted alcohol and carbonate of potassa, and again distil a gallon. — Ph. U. S.) It is refrigerant, diuretic, antispasmodic, and diaphoretic. Dose, gtt. xxv to f ʒj. Specific gravity, 0.834.

SPIRITUS ÆTHERIS SULPHU'RICI, *Æther Sulphuricus cum Alcoho'lē, Liquor Æthe'reus Sulphuricus, Spiritus Vitrioli dulcis, Spiritus Ætheris vitriol'ici, Liquor Sulphuricus alcoolisa'tus, Spirit of Sulphuric Ether.* (*Æther. sulphuric.* Oss; *sp. rec.* Oj. Mix. *Ph. L.*) Stimulant,

diaphoretic, diuretic, and antispasmodic. Dose, f ʒss to f ʒiij.

SPIRITUS ÆTHERIS SULPHURICI COMPOS'ITUS, (Ph. U. S. 1842), *Sp. ætheris vitriol'ici compositus, Spiritus Æ'theris compositus* (Ph. U. S. 1851), *Liquor anod'ynus Hoffmanni, Compound Spirit of Sulphuric Ether, Hoffmann's Anodyne Liquor.* (*Æther Sulphuric.* Oss; *Alcohol*, Oj; *Ol. Æther.* f ʒiij. Ph. U. S. Ph. L.) Mix. A stimulant and antispasmodic. Specific gravity, 0.816.

SPIRITUS ÆTHERIS VITRIOLICI COMPOSITUS, Spiritus ætheris sulphuric. comp.

SPIRITUS AMMO'NIÆ, *Al'kali ammoni'acum spirituo'sum, Al'cohol ammonia'tum, Sp. salis ammoni'aci, Ammoni'aca alcoholisa'ta, Liquor ammo'nii vino'sus, L. ammoniæ spirituo'sus, Lixiv'ium ammoniaca'lē vino'sum, Spiritus salis ammoni'aci vino'sus seu dulcis seu dulcifica'tus, Solu'tio subcarbona'tis ammoni'aci spirituo'sa,* (F.) *Esprit d'ammoniaque.* (*Ammon. muriat.* in *pulv. subtilissim., calcis,* āā ℔j; *alcohol.* f ʒxx; *aquæ*, f ʒix. The water is employed to slake the lime; the muriate of ammonia is then well mixed with it, and by means of heat, the ammonia is made to pass into the distilled water contained in a quart bottle. Ph. U. S.) Stimulant and antispasmodic. Dose, f ʒss to f ʒj.

SPIRITUS AMMONIÆ AROMAT'ICUS, *Alcohol ammonia'tum aromaticum, Aromatic ammonia'ted Alcohol, Sal volat'ilē Drops, Spiritus salis volat'ilis oleo'sus, Sp. volatilis aromaticus, Sal volatile oleosum Sylvii, Sp. ammoniæ compos'itus, Tinctu'ra aromatica ammoniata, Liquor oleo'sus Sylvii, Lixiv'ium ammoniaca'lē aromaticum.* (*Ammon. muriat.* ʒv; *Potass. carb.* ʒviij, *cinnam.* cont., *caryophyll.* cont. āā ʒij; *Limon. cort.* ʒiv; *alcohol., aquæ* āā, Ov. M. Distil Ovijss. Stimulant. Dose, f ʒss to f ʒj.

SPIRITUS AMMONIÆ COMPOSITUS, Spiritus aromaticus.

SPIRITUS AMMONIÆ FŒ'TIDUS, *Sp. volat'ilis fœtidus, Fit Drops, Al'cohol ammonia'tum fœtidum, Tinctu'ra asafœtidæ ammoniata, Fetid Spirit of Ammonia.* (*Sp. ammoniæ* Oij, *asafœtidæ* ʒij. Macerate for 12 hours, and distil Oiss. *Ph. L.*) Stimulant and antispasmodic. Dose, f ʒss to f ʒj.

SPIRITUS AMMONIÆ SUCCINA'TUS, *Succinated Spirit of Ammonia, Common Eau de Luce, Ammoni'acum succina'tum, Aqua Lu'ciæ, Liquor ex Ammoniâ et Oleo Suc'cini, Liquor ex'citans, Spiritus Ammoniæ cum Suc'cino, Sp. Salis Ammoni'aci lactes'cens seu lacteus.* (*Mastich.* ʒiij, *sp. rect.* f ʒix, *ol. lavand,* gtt. xlv, *ol. succin.* gtt. iv *liq. ammon.* f ʒx. Macerate the mastich in the alcohol, and pour off the clear tincture: add the rest and shake. *Ph. L.*) Stimulant and antispasmodic. Dose, gtt. x to f ʒss, or f ʒj.

SPIRITUS ANIMALES, see Nervous fluid.
SPIRITUS ANI'SI, *Spiritus Anisi compos'itus, Aqua anisi for'tis, Aqua Sem'inum Anisi composita, Spirit of An'iseed,* (F.) *Esprit d'anis.* (*Anisi sem.* cont. ℔ss, *spirit tenuior.* cong., *aquæ* quod satis sit ad prohibendum empyreuma. *Ph. L.*) Carminative. Dose, f ʒss to f ʒss. In the compound spirit, angelica is usually an ingredient.

SPIRITUS ANTHOS, Spiritus rosmarini.

SPIRITUS ARMORA'CIÆ COMPOS'ITUS, *Sp. Raph'ani compositus, Aqua Raphani composita, Compound Spirit of Horseradish,* (F.) *Esprit de raifort composé.* (*Armorac. rad.* recent. concis., *aurant. cort. exsicc.,* sing. ℔j, *myrist. nuc.* contus. ʒss, *spirit. ten.* cong. *aquæ* q. s. ad prohibendum empyreuma. *Ph. L.*) Stimulant and antiscorbutic. (?) Dose, f ʒj, to f ʒiv.

The *Golden Spirit of Scurvy grass* — an empirical preparation — is formed by adding *gamboge* ʒviij, to one gallon of the *sp. armoraciæ compositus.*

Greenough's Tincture for the teeth, is formed of amygd. amar. ℨij, lig. Bresil., cassiæ bacc., āā ℨiv, irid. Florent. ℨij, coccinell., sal. acetosellæ, alum. āā ℨj, sp. vin. rect. Oij, sp. armoraciæ comp. f℥ss.

SPIRITUS BEGUINIS, Ammoniæ sulphuretum—s. Bellidis, see Osmitopsis asterisooides.

SPIRITUS CAMPH'ORÆ, *Sp. camphora'tus, Sp. vino'sus camphoratus, Tinctu'ra Camphoræ*, (Ph. U. S.) *Spirit of Wine and Camphor, Spirit of Camphor*, (F.) *Esprit de Camphre, Alcool camphré, Eau de Vie camphrée.* (*Camphor.* ℨiv, alcohol. Oij. Dissolve.) Stimulant, anodyne and discutient. Used only externally.

SPIRITUS CAR'UI, *Sp. Cari Carui, Spirit of Car'raway, Aqua Sem'inum Carui fortis, A. Sem'inum Carui, Strong Carui Waters*, (F.) *Esprit de Carvi.* (*Carui sem.* cont. ℔iss, *sp. tenuior.* cong., aquæ q. s. Distil a gallon. *Ph. L.*) Carminative. Dose, f℥j to f℥ss.

SPIRITUS CINNAMO'MI, *Sp. Lauri Cinnamomi, Spirit of Cin'namon, Aqua Cinnamomi fortis, Aqua Cinnam. spirituo'sa, Strong Cinnamon Water*, (F.) *Esprit de Cannelle.* (*Cort. cinnam.* ℈v, *sp. rect.* Oivss.) Stimulant and carminative. Dose, f℥j to f℥ss.

SPIRITUS COL'CHICI AMMONIA'TUS, *Ammoniated Spirit of Colchicum.* (*Sem. colchic.* cont. ℨij, *sp. ammon. aromat.* Oj. *Ph. L.*) Narcotic, cathartic, and diuretic. Used in gout, rheumatism, and dropsy. Dose, from gtt. xxx to f℥j.

SPIRITUS CORNU CERVI, Liquor C. C. — s. Fumans Beguini, Ammoniæ sulphuretum—s. Genitalis, Aura seminis.

SPIRITUS JUNIP'ERI COMPOS'ITUS, *Compound Spirit of Juniper, Aqua Junip'eri composita*, (F.) *Esprit de genièvre composé.* (*Ol. junip.* ℨiss, *Ol. carui, Ol. fœnicul.*, āā ℨx; *Alcohol dilut.* cong. Solve. Ph. U. S.) Stimulant and diuretic. Dose, f℥j to f℥ss.

SPIRITUS LAURI CINNAMOMI, Spiritus cinnamomi.

SPIRITUS LAVAN'DULÆ, *Sp. Lavandulæ spicæ, Spirit of Lav'ender, Sp. Lavand. simpl., Lavender Water*, (F.) *Esprit de Lavande.* (*Lavand.* recent. ℔ij, *Alcohol.* cong., aquæ Oij. Distil a gallon.) Usually made by adding the oil to rectified spirit. Used as a perfume chiefly.

SPIRITUS LAVANDULÆ COMPOS'ITUS, *Tinctu'ra Lavandulæ composita, Red Hartshorn, Lavender drops, Compound Spirit of Lavender*, (F.) *Esprit de Lavande composé.* (*Sp. Lavand.* Oiij, *sp. rosmarin.* Oj, *cinnam.* contus. ℨj, *myristic.* cont. ℨss. *caryophyll.* cont. ℨij, *santali* conc. ℨiij. Macerate for 14 days, and filter through paper. Stimulant. Dose, gtt. xl to f℥j.

SPIRITUS LETHALIS, Carbonic acid — s. Lumbricorum, Liquor volatilis cornu cervi.

SPIRITUS MENTHÆ PIPERI'TÆ, *Spirit of Peppermint, Aqua Menthæ piperit'idis spirituo'sa, Sp. Menthæ piperit'idis* (F.) *Esprit de Menthe poivrée.* (*Olei menth. pip.* ℈vjss, *sp. rectif.* Oivss, aquæ, q. s. distil a gallon. *Ph. L.*) Carminative and stimulant. Dose, f℥ss to f℥iij.

SPIRITUS MENTHÆ SATIVÆ, Spiritus menthæ viridis.

SPIRITUS MENTHÆ VIR'IDIS, *Spearmint, Spiritus menthæ sati'væ, Aqua Menthæ vulga'ris spirituo'sa*, (F.) *Esprit de Menthe verte.* (*Olei Menth. virid.* ℈vjss, *sp. rectif.* Oivss, aq. q. s. Distil a gallon. *Ph. L.*) Like the last in properties and dose.

SPIRITUS MILLEPEDARUM, Liquor cornu cervi.

SPIRITUS MYRIS'TICÆ, *Spiritus Myristicæ Moscha'tæ, Sp. Nucis Moschatæ, Aqua Nucis Moschatæ, Nutmeg Water, Aqua Nephrit'ica*, (F.)

Esprit de Muscade. (*Myrist.* cont. ℨij, *Alcohol dil.* cong., aquæ Oj. Distil a gallon.) Cordial and carminative. Dose, f℥j to f℥iv.

SPIRITUS MYRTI PIMENTÆ, Spiritus pimentæ — s. Nitri acidus, Nitric acid — s. Nitri dulcis, Spiritus ætheris nitrici — s. Nitri duplex, Nitri acid — s. Nitri fumans, Nitric acid — s. Nitri Glauberi, Nitric acid — s. Nitri simplex, see Nitric acid — s. Nitri vulgaris, see Nitric acid — s. Nucis moschatæ, Spiritus myristicæ — s. Ophthalmicus Mindereri, Liquor ammoniæ acetatis.

SPIRITUS PIMEN'TÆ, *Sp. Myrti Pimentæ, Spiritus Pimento, Spirit of Pimento, Aqua Mirabilis.* (*Ol. Piment.* f. ℨij, *Alcohol. dilut.* q st. Solve. Ph. U. S.) Cordial and carminative. Dose, f℥j to f℥iv.

SPIRITUS PULE'GII, *Spirit of Pennyroyal, Aqua Pulegii spirituo'sa, Spirituous Pennyroyal Water*, (F.) *Esprit de Pouliot.* (*Olei pulegii* ℈vij, *sp. rect.* Oivss, aquæ, q. s. Distil a gallon. *Ph. L.*) Same as spirit of spearmint in properties and dose.

SPIRITUS PYRO-ACETICUS, Acetone.

SPIRITUS RECTIFICA'TUS, *Sp. Vini rectifica'tum Œnostag'ma, Œnelæ'um, Pyræ'nus, Sp. Vinosus rectificatus, Al'cohol, A. Vini, Spirit of Wine*, (F.) *Esprit de Vin rectifié.* Rectified spirit is much used in Pharmacy to dissolve resins and other substances. It is seldom exhibited internally; although it exists in the diluted state in all vinous and spirituous liquors. Externally, it is employed as a discutient. — S. g., according to the London Pharmacopœia, 0.838; according to that of Dublin, 0.840; of Edinburgh and United States, 0.835, (see Alcohol,) and of Paris, 0.818 to 0.827.

SPIRITUS RECTOR, Aroma — s. Raphani compositus, Spiritus armoraciæ compositus.

SPIRITUS ROSMARI'NI, *Sp. Rosmarini officinalis, Spirit of Rosemary, Spiritus Anthos, Hungary Water*, (F.) *Esprit de Romarin.* (*Ol. rosmarini* ℨiv, *Alcohol.* cong. Solve. Ph. U. S. Stimulant. Dose, f℥j to f℥iv.

SPIRITUS SALIS ACIDUS seu FUMANS, Muriaticum acidum — s. Salis ammoniaci, Spiritus ammoniæ — s. Salis ammoniaci aquosus, Liquor ammoniæ — s. Salis ammoniaci lactescens — s. Salis lacteus, Spiritus ammoniæ succinatus — s. Salis ammoniaci sulphuratus, Ammoniæ sulphuretum — s. Salis Glauberi, Muriaticum acidum — s. Salis marini, Muriaticum acidum — s. Salis marini coagulatus, Potassæ murias — s. Salis marini oleosus, Spiritus ammoniæ aromaticus — s. Sulphurico-æthereus camphoratus, Tinctura ætherea composita — s. Sulphurico-æthereus martis, Tinctura seu Alcohol sulphurico-æthereus ferri — s. Sulphuris, Sulphurous acid — s. Sulphuris per campanam, Sulphurous acid — s. Sulphuris volatilis, Ammoniæ sulphuretum — s. Sulphurosus volatilis, Sulphurous acid.

SPIRITUS TENU'IOR, *Alcohol dilu'tum, Spiritus vino'sus tenu'ior, Proof Spirit* (F.) *Esprit de réi délayé.* Generally made for pharmaceutical purposes, by mixing equal parts of rectified spirit and water. S. g. Lond. 0.920; Edinb. and United States, 0.935. It is employed in the same cases as those in which the alcohol is used — chiefly, as a solvent of vegetable matter in the form of tinctures.

SPIRITUS VENERIS, Aceticum acidum — s. Tartari rectificatus, Spiritus rectificatus — s. Vinosus camphoratus, Spiritus camphoræ — s. Vinosus tenuior, Spiritus tenuior — s. Vitalis, Nervous fluid — s. Vitrioli, Sulphuric acid — s. Vitrioli acidus leri, Sulphuricum acidum dilutum — s. Vitrioli coagulatus Mynsichti, Potassæ sulphas — s. Vitrioli dulcis, Spiritus ætheris sulphurici — s. Vitrioli phlogisticatus, Sulphurous acid — s. Volatilis aromatious, Spiritus ammoniæ aromaticus — s. Volatilis fœtidus, Spiritus ammoniæ fœtidus.

SPIROID CANAL, Aquæductus Fallopii.

SPIROM'ETER; badly compounded from *spiro*, 'I breathe,' and μετρον, 'a measure:'—properly *Anapnom'eter, Pneusom'eter, Pneumom'eter, Pneumatom'eter*. Any instrument for measuring the quantity of air concerned in respiration, and, consequently, the capacity of the lungs.

SPIROPTERA HOMINIS, see Worms.

SPISSANTIA, Incrassantia.

SPIT, Sputum.

SPIT'AL, MINERAL WATERS OF. The village of Spital is situate on the south side of the Tweed, near Tweedmouth. The springs there contain chloride of calcium, sulphate of soda, sulphate and carbonate of lime. They act as saline cathartics.

SPITH'AMA, *Dorans*. A measure of twelve fingers' breadth.

SPITTING, Exspuition.

SPITTLE, Saliva—s. Sweet, see Salivation.

SPLANCHNA, Entrails.

SPLANCHNECTOP'IA, *Splanchnodias'tasis, Situs perver'sus* seu *anom'alus intestino'rum;* from σπλαγχνον, 'an intestine,' εκ, 'out of,' and τοπος, 'place.' Misplacement or ectopia of the intestines.

SPLANCHNELMINTHA, Worms.

SPLANCHNEURYS'MA, from σπλαγχνον, 'an intestine,' and ευρυνω, 'I dilate.' Morbid dilatation of the intestines.

SPLANCHNIC, *Splanch'nicus, Vis'ceral*, from σπλαγχνον, 'viscus.' Relating or belonging to the viscera.

SPLANCHNIC CAV'ITIES are the three great cavities of the body;—those of the cranium, chest, and abdomen.

SPLANCHNIC NERVES belong to the great sympathetic, and are two in number on each side. They are distinguished into:—1. The *great splanchnic nerve*, (F.) *Grand surrénal* (Ch.), Its roots—four or five in number, come from the 6th, 7th, 8th, 9th, and sometimes the 10th, thoracic ganglia. They descend inwards, on the sides of the vertebral column, beneath the pleura, and unite into a single trunk, which enters the abdomen through a separation of the fleshy fibres of the pillars of the diaphragm; passes behind the stomach, and divides into several branches, which pass into the semilunar ganglion. 2. The *lesser splanchnic nerve*, *Renal nerve*, (F.) *Splanchnique accessoire* of Walther, *Petit surrénal*, (Ch.), is composed of two distinct branches, proceeding from the 10th and 11th thoracic ganglion, which unite on the 12th dorsal vertebra into a cord, that pierces the diaphragm singly; enters the abdomen, and divides into two branches, one of which anastomoses with the greater splanchnic nerve, whilst the other sends its filaments to the renal and solar plexuses.

SPLANCH'NICA. Medicines adapted to diseases of the bowels. Also, the 2d order of the class *Caliaca* of Good; defined,—diseases affecting the collatitious viscera, and characterized by disquiet or diseased action in the organs auxiliary to the digestive process, without primary inflammation.

SPLANCHNODIASTASIS, Splanchnectopia.

SPLANCHNOD'YNÊ, from σπλαγχνον, 'a viscus,' and οδυνη, 'pain.' Pain in the bowels.

SPLANCHNOGRAPHIA, Splanchnography.

SPLANCHNOG'RAPHY, *Splanchnogra'phia*, from σπλαγχνον, 'a viscus,' and λογος, 'a description.' The part of anatomy which treats of the viscera.

SPLANCHNOLITHI'ASIS; from σπλαγχνον, 'a viscus,' and λιθος, 'a stone.' The formation of a calculous concretion in any viscus.

SPLANCHNOL'OGY, *Splanchnolog''ia*, from σπλαγχνον, 'a viscus,' and λογος, 'a discourse.' A treatise on the viscera:—also, Splanchnography.

SPLANCHNOPATHI'A, from σπλαγχνον, 'a viscus,' and παθος, 'suffering.' A disease of the intestines.

SPLANCHNOSCLERO'SIS, from σπλαγχνον, 'a viscus,' and σκληρος, 'hard.' Induration of a viscus.

SPLANCHNOT'OMY, *Splanchnotom'ia, Splanchnot'omê*, from σπλαγχνον, 'a viscus,' and τεμνω, 'I cut.' Dissection or anatomy of the viscera.

SPLAYFOOT, see Kyllosis.

SPLEEN, *Lien, Hepar sinis'trum* seu *adulteri'num*, (F.) *Rate*. A soft, spongy, parenchymatous organ; of a more or less deep violet red, situate deeply in the left hypochondrium, below the diaphragm, above the colon, between the great tuberosity of the stomach and the cartilages of the false ribs, and above and anterior to the kidney. Its ordinary length is $4\frac{1}{2}$ inches; its thickness $2\frac{1}{4}$; and its weight 8 ounces. Its parenchyma, which is bathed in blood, contains a multitude of grayish, soft, and semi-transparent granulations — *splenic corpuscles* or *Malpighian bodies of the spleen*. It is covered by a serous membrane, furnished by the peritoneum; and by a proper coat, of a fibrous nature, which is intimately united with it, and transmits into its interior delicate, solid, and very elastic prolongations — *trabeculæ*. At its inner edge is a fissure, by which the vessels and nerves enter the organ. The functions of the spleen are unknown. One of the latest opinions is, that it belongs to the lymphatic system; and acts as a diverticulum to the vascular system.

SPLEEN, Hypochondriasis — s. Malpighian bodies of the, see Spleen—s. Supernumerary, Lienculus.

SPLEENWORT, Asplenium, A. filix fœmina, Asplenium scolopendrium — s. Bush, Comptonia asplenifolia.

SPLENAL'GIA, *Neural'gia lie'nis, Sple'nica, Splenodyn'ia*, from σπλην, 'the spleen,' and αλγος, 'pain.' Pain in the spleen.

SPLENALGIA BENGALENSIS, see Cachexia, splenic — s. Phlegmonodea, Splenitis — s. Subinflammatoria chronica, Splenoncus.

SPLENATROPH'IA, *Atroph'ia Lie'nis*, from σπλην, 'spleen,' and *atrophia*, 'atrophy.' Wasting or atrophy of the spleen.

SPLENAUXE, Splenoncus.

SPLENECTAMA, Splenoparectama.

SPLENECTASIS, Splenoparectama.

SPLENECTOM'IA, *Splenec'tomê*, from σπλην, 'the spleen,' εκ, 'out of,' and τεμνω, 'I cut.' Extirpation of the spleen.

SPLENECTOP'IA, *Disloca'tio lie'nis* seu *splenis;* from σπλην, 'the spleen,' and εκτοπος, 'out of place.' Dislocation of the spleen. Not a common occurrence.

SPLENEMPHRAX'IS, *Splenophrax'ia*, from σπλην, 'the spleen,' and εμφρασσω, 'I obstruct.' Obstruction of the spleen.—Vogel. See Splenoncus.

SPLENES, Hypochondriasis.

SPLENET'ICUS, *Sple'nicus, Splenit'icus, Lieno'sus*, (F.) *Ratéleux*. That which relates to the spleen: one labouring under diseased spleen. A medicine adapted for diseases of the spleen.

SPLENIC, *Sple'nicus, Sple'nius*, from σπλην, 'the spleen.' That which relates to the spleen.

SPLENIC ARTERY. It arises from the cœliac; and passes from right to left, forming many windings along the upper edge of the pancreas, which lodges it in a special groove. It reaches the fissure of the spleen, and divides into several branches that enter the organ. In its course it furnishes the pancreatic, left gastro-epiploic, and the vasa brevia.

SPLENIC CACHEXIA, see Cachexia splenica—s. Corpuscles, see Spleen.

SPLENIC PLEXUS is a nervous network, which proceeds from the cœliac plexus, and accompanies the splenic artery, sending secondary plexuses to each division.

SPLENIC VEIN arises from the spleen, and accompanies the splenic artery; proceeding from left to right, to unite with the superior mesenteric vein, and to form, with it, the abdominal vena porta. In its course, it receives veins corresponding to the vasa brevia, the right and left gastro-epiploic, the duodenal, pancreatic, coronaria ventriculi, and inferior mesenteric veins.

SPLENICA, Splenalgia. Also, medicines which affect the spleen.— Pereira.

SPLENICUS, Spleneticus, Splenic.
SPLENIOLA, Compress.
SPLENIS TUMOR, Ague cake.
SPLÉNISATION, Splenization.
SPLENISCUS, Compress.
SPLENITICUS, Splenic.
SPLENI'TIS, from σπλην, 'the spleen,' and *itis*, denoting inflammation. Inflammation of the spleen. *Empres'ma splenitis, Inflamma'tio lie'nis, I. splenis, Splenal'gia phlegmono'dea*, (F.) *Inflammation de la Rate*. A rare disease, characterised by local pain, swelling, and heat, which sometimes terminates by suppuration. It must be treated like other inflammations.

SPLENIUM, Compress — s. Corporis Callosi, see Corpus callosum — s. Cruciatum, *Croix de Malte.*

SPLE'NIUS, *S. Cap'itis, S. Colli,* (F.) *Cervicodorso-mastoïdien et dorso-trachélien, Cervico-mastoïdien* (Ch.), *Posterior mastoid muscle.* So called from its resemblance to the *spleen* of certain animals. A muscle situate at the posterior part of the neck, and upper part of the back. It is much broader above than below, where it terminates in a point. It is attached, by its inner edge, to the spinous processes of the first five dorsal vertebræ; to that of the 7th cervical, and to the inferior part of the posterior cervical ligament. By its upper extremity, it is attached to the transverse processes of the first two cervical vertebræ, to the mastoid process, and to the posterior surface of the occipital bone. Some have considered this muscle to be formed of two portions, which they have called *Splenius colli,* and *Splenius cap'itis.* The splenius extends the head, inclines it, and rotates it. If the splenii of each side act together, they extend the head.

SPLENIZA'TION, *Splenizatio,* (F.) *Splénisation,* from σπλην, 'the spleen.' A term applied to the state of the lung in the first or second stage of pneumonia in which its tissue resembles that of the spleen.

SPLENOCE'LE, *Her'nia liena'lis,* from σπλην, 'the spleen,' and κηλη, 'a tumour.' Hernia formed by the spleen.

SPLENODYNIA, Splenalgia.
SPLENOG'RAPHY, *Splenograph'ia,* from σπλην, 'the spleen,' and γραφη, 'a description.' A description of the spleen.

SPLENOHÆ'MIA, (F.) *Splénohémie,* from σπλην, 'the spleen,' and 'αιμα, 'blood.' Congestion or hyperæmia of the spleen, a common phenomenon in many diseases, especially in typhoid and intermittent fevers.

SPLENOID, *Splenoï'des, Spleno'des,* from σπλην, 'spleen,' and ειδος, 'resemblance.' Spleenlike. Having the appearance of the spleen.

SPLENOL'OGY, *Splenolog''ia,* from σπλην, 'the spleen,' and λογος, 'a discourse.' A treatise on the spleen.

SPLÉNONCIE, Splenoncus.

SPLENON'CUS, *Megalosple'nia, Hypertroph'ia seu Supernutrit''io splenis seu lie'nis, Intumescen''tia seu Infarc'tus seu Physco'nia lienis, Splenaf'gia subinflammato'ria chron'ica, Splenemphrax'is, Splenaux'e, Hypersplenotroph'ia, Lien ingens,* (F.) *Splénoncie, Hypertrophie de la Rate;* from σπλην, 'the spleen,' and ογκος, 'a tumour.' Tumefaction of the spleen. See Ague cake.

SPLENOPAREC'TAMA, *Splenec'tama, Splenoparec'tasis, Splenec'tasis,* from σπλην, 'the spleen,' and παρεκταμα, 'excessive volume.' Excessive enlargement of the spleen.—Ploucquet.

SPLENOPARECTASIS, Splenoparectama.
SPLENOPHRAXIA, Splenemphraxis.
SPLENORRHAG''IA, from σπλην, 'the spleen,' and ῥαγη, 'rupture.' Hemorrhage from the spleen.

SPLENOSCIR'RHUS, from σπλην, 'the spleen,' and σκιρρος, 'hardness.' Scirrhus or cancer of the spleen.

SPLENOT'OMY, *Splenotom'ia, Splenot'ome,* from σπλην, 'the spleen,' and τεμνω, 'I cut.' Dissection of the spleen.

SPLINT, Teut. S p l i n t e r, from s p l i j t e n, 'to split;' *Hastel'la, Ass'ula, Asser'culum, Plag'ula, Narthex, Fer'ula,* (F.) *Attelle, Éclisse.* A flexible and resisting lamina of wood, used in the treatment of fractures, to keep the fragments in apposition, and prevent their displacement. Splints are made of iron, wood, bark of trees, leather, gutta percha, pasteboard, &c. They are generally padded, and are fixed by a roller or by tapes, according to circumstances.

SPLINTER, (F.) *Esquille.* Same etymon. This term is sometimes applied to a small portion of wood, which occasionally enters the skin, and gives occasion to much irritation until it is removed,—*Acu'leus lig'neus,* (F.) *Écharde.*
It is also applied to fragments that separate from a fractured or diseased bone.

SPLITROCK, Heuchera cortusa.
SPODIUM GRÆCORUM, Album græcum.
SPOLIARIUM, Apodyterium.
SPO'LIATIVE, *Spoliati'va,* from *spolio,* 'I take away.' *Phlebotom'ia spoliati'va,* (F.) *Saignée spoliative.* Blood-letting, used for the purpose of diminishing the mass of blood.

SPOLIATORIUM, Apodyterium.
SPONDYLAL'GIA, *Spondylodyn'ia,* from σπονδυλος, 'a vertebra,' and αλγος, 'pain.' Pain in the vertebræ. Cacorrhachitis. See Vertebral Disease.

SPONDYLARTHRI'TIS, from σπονδυλος, 'a vertebra,' αρθρον, 'a joint,' and *itis,* denoting inflammation. Gouty or rheumatic inflammation of the spinal column.

SPONDYLARTHROCACE, Vertebral disease.
SPONDYLI, Vertebræ.
SPONDYLIS, Coccyx.
SPONDYLI'TIS, *Inflamma'tio ver'tebræ,* from σπονδυλος, and *itis,* denoting inflammation. Inflammation of the vertebræ.

SPONDYLIUM, Coccyx, Heracleum spondylium.

SPONDYLOCACE, Vertebral disease.
SPONDYLODYNIA, Spondylalgia.
SPONDYLOPATHI'A, from σπονδυλος, 'a vertebra,' and παθος, 'a disease.' A disease of the vertebral column.

SPONDYLOPYOSIS, Vertebral disease.

SPOND'YLUS, σπονδυλος. A *vertebra;* and, especially, the two large cervical vertebræ. Also, the vertex.

SPONGE, BASTARD, Alcyonium.

SPONGI. The tumefied glands of the neck.

SPON'GIA, *Spongos, Sphongus, Spongia officina'lis, Spon'gia Mari'na, Sponge,* (F.) *Éponge.* An organized marine substance, of the great class of Zoophytes, met with in many seas, but especially in the Mediterranean and Arabian. It is supple, elastic, porous, and capable of absorbing fluids in which it may be placed, and of thus increasing in size. It is employed in *surgery,* for cleansing or washing; for absorbing acrid discharges from ulcers; suppressing hemorrhage when the mouth of the vessel can be compressed by it, and for forming tents for dilating wounds; in which case, the sponge is immersed in melting wax, and cooled before being used. It is then called *Prepared Sponge* or *Sponge Tent.*

SPONGIA ASSA, S. Usta—s. Cynosbati, Bedegar.

SPONGIA USTA, *S. Assa, Carbo spon'giæ, Burnt Sponge,* contains carbonate and phosphate of lime, carbonate of soda, charcoal, and iodine. It is used in bronchocele, scrofulous affections, and herpetic eruptions; and its good effects seem to be dependent upon iodine. It is made by cutting sponge into pieces, and heating it, that any extraneous matter may be separated; burning it in a close iron vessel until it becomes black and friable, and, lastly, rubbing it into very fine powder. — Ph. U. S.

SPON'GIÆ LAPIS. A name given to small friable stones found in sponge. They were formerly esteemed lithontriptic.

SPONGIODES, Spongoid.

SPONGIOLE, Spongiolum: from σπογγιον, 'a small sponge.' The soft succulent extremity of the fibrils or true roots of a plant, by which it absorbs or sucks up fluid. Similar spongioles have been supposed to exist at the terminations of the absorbents in animals.

SPON'GION. Ancient name of an epithem made of goats' dung: and also of a malagma, which was considered capable of absorbing the serum in dropsies, like a sponge. — Paulus, Gorræus.

SPONGIOSUM (OS), Ethmoid bone.

SPONGIOSUS, Spongoid.

SPONGOID, *Spongoides, Spongio'des, Spongio'sus,* from σπογγια, 'sponge,' and ειδος, 'resemblance.' Resembling sponge. Of the nature of sponge.

SPONGOID INFLAMMATION, Hæmatodes fungus.

SPONGOID TISSUE, (F.) *Tissu spongoïde.* An adventitious spongy tissue, found in cases of rickets. — Guérin.

SPONGOS, Tonsil.

SPONSA SOLIS, Calendula officinalis.

SPONTA'NEOUS, *Sponta'neus,* from *sponte,* 'voluntarily.' That which occurs of itself, or without any manifest external cause. Evacuations are termed *spontaneous,* which are not produced by medicine. *Sponta'neous las'situde* is that which is not the result of fatigue. Diseases are also *spontaneous* which supervene without apparent cause. *Sponta'neous Amputa'tion* is the separation of a limb from the fœtus in utero.

SPONTANEOUS EVOLUTION, see Evolution — s. Version, Evolution, spontaneous.

SPONTÉPARITÉ, Generation, spontaneous.

SPOONWOOD, Kalmia latifolia, Tilia.

SPORAD'IC, *Spor'ades, Sporad'ici, Morbi disper'si, Morbi sparsi,* from σπειρειν, 'to spread.' Diseases are so called which supervene indifferently in every season and situation, from accidental causes, and independently of any epidemic or contagious influence.

SPORE, *Spor'ule, Sporum, Spor'ulum,* from σπειρω, 'I sow.' The reproductive body in cryptogamous plants, which is analogous to the seed of phanerogamous plants.

SPORID'IUM; same etymon. The reproductive body in algaceous plants, which resembles the spore of other plants.

SPORULE, Spore.

SPORUM, Spore.

SPOTS, GERMINAL, see Molecule.

SPOTS, RED, (F.) *Taches rouges, Rose spots.* Small red spots which appear in typhoid fever, from the 8th to the 15th day of the disease. They are most frequently seen on the lower and middle portions of the chest, and upper part of the abdomen.

SPOTS, ROSE, Spots, red.

SPRAIN, corrupted from *strain:* — *Subluxa'tio, Distor'tio, Dias'trophē, Diastrem'ma, Luxa'tio imperfec'ta, Exarthre'ma, Exarthro'sis, Stremma, Thlasma Stremma;* a *wrench,* (F.) *Détorse, Entorse, Foulure.* A violent straining or twisting of the soft parts surrounding the joints. According to the degree of the sprain, the fibrous parts of the joint may be simply stretched, or they may be ruptured. This affection, which has been regarded as incomplete luxation, occurs, particularly, in the ginglymoid joints; — as in the foot, wrist, knee, &c. The violence causes an afflux of blood; the serum of the blood is poured out, and often the blood itself, owing to the rupture of vessels; and inflammation arises, which ends in resolution or induration. Local, antiphlogistic applications are required, with perfect rest; and, when the inflammatory action has subsided, cold pumping and friction, with the application of a plaster and bandage, will afford support till the parts affected recover their due tone.

SPRAT, YELLOW-BILLED, Clupea thryssa.

SPRUCE BEER, *White Spruce Beer.* A beer made as follows: To 10 gallons of *water,* add 6 pounds of *sugar,* and 4 oz. of *essence of spruce.* Add yeast, and bottle, when ready. It is grateful and antiscorbutic.

SPRUCE BEER POWDERS may be formed of *white sugar,* ℨj, and ℈ij; *sodæ subcarb.,* gr. xxvj; *essence of spruce,* gr. x, in each blue paper; and *acid of tartar,* ℨss in each white paper. For half a pint of water.

SPUITIO, Exspuition.

SPUMA ARGENTI, Plumbi oxydum semi-vitreum—s. Cerevisiæ, Yest—s. Trium draconum, Antimonium muriatum.

SPUMEUX, Frothy.

SPUMOSUS, Frothy.

SPUNK, Boletus igniarius.

SPUR, Sax. rpur, (F.) *Éperon des Artères.* The angle at which the arteries leave a cavity or trunk.

SPUR, Ergot.

SPURGE, CAPER, Euphorbia lathyris — s. Cypress, Euphorbia Cyparissias—s. Flax, Daphne gnidium — s. Flowering, large, Euphorbia corollata—s. Garden, Euphorbia lathyris—s. Greater, Euphorbia palustris — s. Ipecacuanha, Euphorbia ipecacuanha — s. Laurel, Daphne laureola — s. Marsh, Euphorbia palustris — s. Olive, Cneorum tricoccum — s. Olive, Daphne mezereum — s. Sea, Euphorbia paralias.

SPUTA, PRUNE JUICE, see Prune Juice.

SPUTAMEN, Saliva, Sputum.

SPUTAMENTUM, Saliva, Sputum.

SPUTATIO, Exspuition.

SPUTATION, Exspuition.

SPUTUM, Plural, *Sputa, Apochrem'ma, Chremma, Emptys'ma, Sputa'men, Pty'elon, Pytis'ma,*

Spit, from *spuere*, *sputum*, 'to spit.' (F.) *Crachat*. The secretions ejected from the mouth in the act of spitting. It is composed of saliva, and of the mucus secreted by the mucous membrane of the nasal fossæ and fauces, and often by the membrane of the larynx and bronchia. The sputa are, sometimes, called *eruginous*, when of a greenish-yellow colour; *gummy*, when they resemble a thick solution of gum; *frothy*, (F.) *mousseux*, when covered with froth; *rubiginous*, (F.) *rubigineux* ou *rouillés*, when of a reddish-yellow; and *streaked*, (F.) *striés*, when mixed with lines of blood. Also, saliva.

SPUTUM CRUENTUM, Hæmoptysis — s. Dulce, Saccharorrhœa pulmonalis — s. Oris, Salivation — s. Saccharatum, Saccharorrhœa pulmonalis — s. Sanguinis, Hæmoptysis.

SQUALLING, Vagitus.
SQUAMA, Scale, Table.
SQUAMÆ, Scaly diseases.
SQUAMARIA, Plumbago Europæa.
SQUAMEUX, Squamous.
SQUAMIFORMIS, Squamous.
SQUAMOUS, *Squamo'sus*, *Lepidoï'des*, *Lepido'des*, *Squamifor'mis*, *Scaly*; from *squama*, 'a scale.' That which relates to or resembles a scale.

SQUAMOUS PORTION of the temporal bone, (F.) *Portion squameuse* ou *écailleuse du Temporal*, is the upper part of the temporal, so called from a fancied resemblance to a scale.

SQUAMOUS SUTURE, *Sutu'ra squamo'sa*, *S. mendo'sa* seu *lepidoeï'des* seu *lepido'des*, *Sutu'ra cra'nii squamo'sa*, (F.) *Suture squameuse* ou *écailleuse*. The suture which unites the squamous portion of the temporal bone to the parietal.

Certain *scaly* cutaneous affections are also called *squamous*, (F.) *squameux*. See Scale.
SQUARE STALK, Monarda coccinea.
SQUAW-MINT, Hedeoma.
SQUAW-ROOT, Actæa racemosa, Caulophyllum thalictroïdes.
SQUAW-WEED, Erigeron Philadelphicum.
SQUEAMISHNESS, Fastidium cibi.
SQUEAZINESS, Nausea.
SQUELETTE, Skeleton.
SQUELETTOLOGIE, Skeletology.
SQUILL, Scilla — s. Vinegar of, Acetum scillæ.
SQUILLA, Scilla.
SQUINANCIE, Cynanche, Cynanche tonsillaris.
SQUINANCY, COMMON, Cynanche tonsillaris.
SQUINANTHIA, Cynanche.
SQUINANTHUS, Juncus odoratus.
SQUINE, Smilax China.
SQUINSY, Cynanche tonsillaris.
SQUINT-EYED, see Strabismus.
SQUINTER, see Strabismus.
SQUINTING, Strabismus.
SQUIRRE, Scirrhus.
SQUIRREL CORN, Dicentra Canadensis.
SQUIRROGASTRIE, Scirrhogastria.
SQUIRRUS, Scirrhus.
SQUIRT, Syringe.
STACHELBERG, MINERAL WATERS OF. Stachelberg Springs are far down in the valley of the Linth, in Switzerland. The waters are sulphureous, and are much visited by gouty and rheumatic invalids.

STACHYS FŒTIDA, Galeopsis.
STACTE, Myrrha.
STADE, Stage.
STADIUM, Period, Stage.
STA'DIUM ACMES seu STA'SEOS. The period of the height of a disease.
STA'DIUM ANNIHILATIO'NIS seu CONVALESCEN'TIÆ seu RECONVALESCENTIÆ. The period of recovery from disease.
STADIUM AUGMEN'TI seu INCREMEN'TI MORBI. The period or stage of increase of a disease.

STADIUM CALORIS, Stage, (hot) — s. Convalescentiæ, S. annihilationis.
STADIUM DECREMEN'TI. The period or stage of decrease of a disease.
STADIUM FRIGORIS, Stage, (cold) — s. Incrementi Morbi, S. Augmenti morbi — s. Latentis Catagii, Prodromus — s. Opportunitatis, Prodromus — s. Prodromorum, Prodromus — s. Reconvalescentiæ, S. Annihilationis.

STAFF, (D.) S t a f. An instrument of great importance in lithotomy, — being the director for the gorget or knife. It is made of steel; and its handle is flat and rough, in order that it may be more securely held. The groove is on its convex surface.

STAFF TREE, CLIMBING, Celastrus scandens.
STAFFA, Stapes.
STAG'S PIZZLE, see Cervus.
STAGE, *Sta'dium*, (F.) *Estage*, *Étage*, *Stade*. The period or degree of a disease; especially the period of an intermittent: — as the *cold stage*, — *sta'dium fri'goris* — *hot stage*, &c.
STAGGERWEED, Delphinium.
STA'GIUM. The sixth part of an ounce.
STAGMA, from σταζω, 'I distil;' *Staley'ma*. Any distilled liquid or liquor.
STAGMA, Gutta.
STAGNA'TION, *Stagna'tio*, from *stagnare*, 'to form a pond.' Accumulation and retardation of fluids in any part of the body.
STAGNUM CHYLI, Receptaculum chyli.
STAHLIAN. One who follows the doctrine of Stahl.
STAHL'IANISM. The doctrine of Stahl, which considered every vital action under the direction and presidency of the soul. See Animist.
STALAGMA, Stagma.
STALAGMI'TIS CAMBOGIOÏ'DES, *S. Cambo'gia*. Gamboge was long ascribed to this fancied Ceylonese plant. It is now known, that the name was given by Murray to specimens of two distinct trees of different genera. See Cambogia.
STALAGMOS, Distillation.
STALTICUS, Incarnans.
STAMMERING, Balbuties — s. of the Fingers, Cramp, writers'.
STAMPING MILL, see Pulverization.
STANGOS, Tin.
STANNI MURIAS, Tin, muriate of — s. Oxyduli murias, Tin, muriate of — s. Pulvis, see In
STANNIOLUM, Tinfoil.
STANNUM, Tin — s. Cinereum, Bismuth — s. Foliatum, Tinfoil — s. Glaciale, Bismuth — s. Granulatum, see Tin — s. Indicum, Zincum.
STAPÉDIEN, Stapedius.
STAPE'DIUS, Stapes, (F.) *Stapédien*, *Pyramidal-stapédien*. A muscle of the middle ear which draws the stapes obliquely upwards.
STAPES, *Stapha*, *Staffa*, 'a stirrup.' (F.) *Étrier*. The innermost of the small bones of the ear, so called because it resembles a *stirrup*. It is situate horizontally in the cavity of the tympanum. Its head, which is directed outwards, is articulated with the os orbiculare. Its base fits inwards, and is applied to the fenestra ovalis, which it closes imperfectly, and to the membrane of which it is united. Its *branches* are one *anterior*, and the other *posterior*. They are curved; and the space between them is parabolic. Surgeons have given the name *Stapes* to a bandage used in bleeding from the foot; which forms a figure of 8 around the ankles.

STAPHA, Stapes.
STAPHIS, Delphinium staphisagria.
STAPHISAGRIA, Delphinium staphisagria.
STAPHISAIGRE, Delphinium staphisagria.

STAPHYLÆMATO'MA, from σταφυλη, 'the uvula,' and hæmatoma. A tumour formed by effusion of blood beneath the mucous membrane of the uvula.

STAPHYLAGRA, Staphylepartes.

STAPHYLE, Uvula, see Vitis vinifera.

STAPHYLEPAR'TES, from σταφυλη, 'the uvula,' and εταιρω, 'I lift up.' Staph'ylagra. An instrument for laying hold of, and removing the uvula.— Paulus.

STAPHYLINI, see Azygos muscle — s. Medii, see Azygos muscle.

STAPHYLINO-PHARYNGEUS, Palato-pharyngeus.

STAPHYLINUS EXTERNUS, Circumflexus.

STAPHYLIS, Nipple.

STAPHYLITIS, Uvulitis.

STAPHYLIUM, Nipple.

STAPHYLODIALYSIS, Cionis, Staphyloedema.

STAPHYLŒDE'MA, Angi'na uvula'ris, Dyspha'gia uvulo'sa, Hypostaph'ylē, Hypostaphyli'tis, Staphylodial'ysis, Prolapsus seu Propto'sis u'vulæ, Casus u'vulæ, Himas, Himanto'ma, Himanto'sis, Staphylon'cus, Staphylon'cia, Œde'ma u'vulæ, Produc'tio uvulæ à pitui'tā, U'vula decid'ua seu relaxa'ta, Oras'pedon. Relaxation and tumefaction of the uvula, which, either from inflammation or infiltration, hangs down so as to occasion difficult deglutition, cough, &c. Scarification, astringent gargles, and, if necessary, excision, constitute the treatment.

STAPHYLO'MA, from σταφυλη, 'a grape.' Uva'tio, Myoceph'alon, Myĭoceph'alum, Parop'sis Staphylo'ma, Staphylo'sis, Polygro'ma. A name given to different tumours of the anterior surface of the globe of the eye.

STAPHYLOMA CONICUM, Staphyloma of the cornea—s. Pellucidum conicum, Staphyloma of the cornea.

STAPHYLOMA OF THE CORNEA, Sugar-loaf Cornea, Con'ical Cornea, Con'ical hydrophthal'mia, Staphylo'ma con'icum, S. pellu'cidum con'icum, Conophthal'mia, Prolap'sus cor'neæ, Ceraton'cus, Hypercerato'sis, Hypercer'asis, is an unequal, embossed, bluish or whitish, round or conical tumour; of variable size; formed by the projection of the transparent cornea, which is sometimes extenuated and distended, at others thickened.

STAPHYLOMA OF THE IRIS is the disease described by Scarpa under the name Procidentia Iridis. It is hernia of the iris, through an accidental opening of the cornea. Also, iridauxesis.

STAPHYLOMA OF THE SCLEROT'IC differs from the last, in the prominence existing on a part of the eye covered by the sclerotic, which is much thinner.

STAPHYLOMA UVEÆ, Iridauxesis.

STAPHYLONCIA, Staphyloedema.

STAPHYLONCUS, Staphyloedema.

STAPHYLOPLAS'TIC, Staphyloplas'ticus, from σταφυλη, 'the uvula,' and πλασσω, 'I form.' An epithet applied to the operation for replacing the soft palate, when it has been lost.

STAPHYLOR'RAPHY, Velosynth'esis, Staphylorrha'phia, Kionorrha'phia, Cionorrhaph'ia, Uranor'rhaphē, Uranorrha'phia, Uraniscorrha'phia, Uraniscor'rhaphē, from σταφυλη, 'the uvula,' and ραφη, 'a suture.' The operation for uniting a cleft palate. It consists in paring the edges of the cleft; passing ligatures through them, and bringing them together.

STAPHYLOSIS, Staphyloma.

STAPHYLOT'OMY, Staphylotom'ia, from σταφυλη, 'the uvula,' and τομη, 'incision.' Amputation of the uvula.

STAR-APPLE, BROAD-LEAVED, Chrysophyllum cainito—s. Blazing, Aletris farinosa—s. Bloom, Spigelia Marilandica — s. Grass, Aletris farinosa, Hypoxys erecta — s. Knap-weed, Centaurea calcitrappa—s. Stroke, Coup-de-soleil — s. Wort, Aletris farinosa — s. Wort, golden, Bubonium.

STARBECK SPA. A chalybeate spring at Harrogate.

STARCH, Amylum — s. Blue, Smalt.

STARCH, IODIDE OF, Iod'idum seu Iodure'tum Am'yli, Am'ylum ioda'tum, (F.) Iodure d'Amidon; prepared by triturating iodine and starch, is said to have the eutrophic effects of iodine; but, by some, is esteemed inert. Dose, four to six grains.

STARCH, POTATO, see Solanum tuberosum — s. Sugar, Glucose.

STARKEY'S PILLS, see Pilulæ ex helleboro et myrrhâ.

STASE, Stasis.

STASIS, στασις, from στaω, 'I stop,' (F.) Stase. This word has nearly the same signification as stagnation. Stagnation, however, sometimes includes a morbid condition of the fluids, — Stasis never.

STASIS, Station.

STATIC. An epithet applied to the physical phenomena presented by organized bodies in contradistinction to the organic or vital.

STAT'ICA SEPTI NA'RIUM, Appen'dix cuta'nea septi na'rium. The cutaneous appendage to the septum narium.

STAT'ICE CAROLINIA'NA of the United States, Amer'ican Thrift, Marsh Rose'mary, Marsh Root, Seaside Thrift, Inkroot, Sea Lavender, is considered to be a mere variety of the statice limonium.

STAT'ICE LIMO'NIUM, S. Marit'imum, Behen rubrum, Limo'nium, L. majus seu vulga'rē, Behen, Sea Lav'ender, Red Behen, Behmen Ackmar, Marsh Rosemary, Lavender Thrift, (F.) Behen rouge. Family, Plumbagineæ. Sex. Syst. Pentandria Pentagynia. The roots have been esteemed astringent, tonic, and eminently antiseptic.

STATICE MARITIMUM, S. limonium—s. Vulgare, S. limonium.

STA'TION, Sta'tio, Stasis, Status, from stare, 'to stand.' The act of standing.

STA'TIONARY, Stationa'rius, from stare, 'to stand.' A name given by Sydenham and Stoll to certain diseases, which depend upon a particular state of the atmosphere; and which prevail in a district for a certain number of years, and then give way to others.

STATIS'TICS, MEDICAL, Vital Statistics, Biostat'ics, (F.) Statistique médicale. That part of medicine which relates to details — medico-statistical — connected with the mortality, salubrity, &c., of different countries and situations.

It has, also, been used in a wider sense to signify the same as Numerical method, (F.) Méthode numérique; which is applied to the systemization of medical facts, or to the use of numbers in the investigation of disease.

STATISTICS, VITAL, Statistics, medical.

STATURE, Statu'ra, Meg'ethos, Magnitu'do cor'poris, from sto, statum, 'I stand.' The height of the human figure. The following table exhibits the results of several admeasurements, with the heights of some of the monkey species, on the authority of Mr. Lawrence.

STATURE.

	Feet.	In.
An Englishman,	{ 6 to 5	4½ 00
An Englishwoman,	{ 5 to 5	4 00
European male skeleton,	5	8
Do.	5	5
A Negro at the Lunatic Hospital, Liverpool,	5	10½
Another from Virginia,	5	5½
Another from the Gold Coast,	5	8
Another,	5	00
Negro skeleton,	4	11
Another,	5	7½
A Lascar,	5	4
Venus de Medici,	5	00
Tyson's Chimpansé (*Simia Troglodytes*)	2	2
Mr. Abel's Orang Otang,	2	7
Camper's Do.	less than	30
Mr. White's Monkey,	2	2

STATUS, Acme — s. Cruditatis, Crudity — s. Erethiticus, Nervous diathesis—s. Gastricus, Embarras gastrique—s. Nervosus, Nervous diathesis — s. Sthenicus, Sthenia — s. Verminosus, Helminthiasis.

STAVESACRE, Delphinium staphisagria.

STAXIS, *Apostax'is*. A slight epistaxis or nasal hemorrhage. — Hippocrates.

STEAM-DOCTOR. A term applied to one who treats all or most diseases by steam.

STEAR, Pinguedo, Sevum.

STEARIN, see Pinguedo.

STEARINUM CETACEUM, Cetaceum.

STEARRHŒ'A, *Steatorrhœ'a*, *Seborrhœ'a*, *Seborrhag''ia*, *Smegmatorrhœ'a*, *Smegmorrhœ'a*, *Seba'ceous Flux*, from στεαρ, 'suet,' and ρεω, 'I flow.' Augmentation of secretion from the sebaceous follicles of the skin.

STEATITES, Polysarcia.

STEATOCE'LE, from στεαρ, 'suet,' and κηλη, 'a tumour.' A tumour formed by a collection of steatomatous matter in the scrotum.

STEATO'MA, *Tumor lar'deus*, from στεαρ, 'suet.' *Secu'tio*, *Steato'sis*, *Emphy'ma encys'tis steatoma*. An encysted tumour, whose contents are similar to fat.

STEATOP'YGA, from στεαρ, 'fat,' and πυγη, 'buttocks.' *Buttock-hump*. Fat buttocks; such as exist in the Hottentot females.

STEATORRHŒA, Stearrhœa.

STEATO'SIS, Steatoma.

STEATO'SIS CORDIS, *Degenera'tio adipo'sa cordis*, *Cardiethmolipo'sis* and *Cardiomyolipo'sis* (Piorry), *Fatty heart*. Unusual deposition of fat on the heart:—by some presumed to be occasionally a true adipous degeneration of the substance of the heart, which is probably incorrect.

STEATOZOON FOLLICULORUM, Acarus Folliculorum.

STEEL, Chalybs.

STEEPLE-BUSH, Spiræa tomentosa.

STEER'S OPODELDOCH, see Opodeldoch, Steer's.

STEGANOP'ODES, στεγανοποδες, *Planip'edes*. They who have flat feet, or are web-footed, from στεγανος, 'covered,' and πους, 'foot.'

STEGNO'SIS, *Steno'sis*, *Constipa'tio*, *Stipa'tio*, *Condensa'tio*, *Obstruc'tio*, from στεγνοω, 'I constrict.' Constriction or narrowness of the pores and vessels. Stricture. Constipation. Suppression of the evacuations. See Arctatio.

STEGNOTICA, Astringents.

STEIROSIS, Sterilitas.

STELENGIS, Stridor dentium.

STELLA, *Fas'cia stella'ta*, (F.) *Étoile*. A bandage, improperly compared to a star, because it is crossed like the letter X. This bandage is applied upon one or both shoulders. In the first case, it is called *simple*; in the second, *d..* It was employed in cases of fractures of the sternum, clavicle, and scapula; in luxations of the humerus, &c.

STELLA TERRÆ, Plantago coronopus.

STELLARIA MEDIA, Alsine media—s. Scilla, Scilla.

STELLATA RUPINA, Centaurea calcitrapa.

STELOCHITIS, Osteocolla.

STENAGMUS, Suspirium.

STENAXIS, Suspirium.

STENIA, Sthenia.

STENICUS, Active.

STENOBREGMATE. see Cranium.

STENOCARDIA, Angina pectoris, Cardiostenosis.

STENOCHO'RIA, *Stenochori'asis*. Ang..a Employed by some for contraction of the va..

STENOCHORIA INTESTINI RECTI, Stricture of the rectum — s. Œsophagi, Dysphagia constricta.

STENOMYCTE'RIA, from στενος, 'narrow' and μυκτηρ, 'nose.' Contraction of the nasal passages.

STENOSIS, Stegnosis.

STENOSTEGNOSIS, Stenostenosis.

STENOSTENO'SIS, *Stenostegno'sis*, from στενος, and στενωσις, 'contraction.' Obstruction of the *Stenonia'na*. Narrowness or contraction of the duct of Steno.

STENOSTOM'IA, from στενος, 'narrow,' and στομα, 'mouth.' Contraction of the mouth.

STENOTHORA'CES, from στενος, 'narrow,' and θωραξ, 'the chest.' They who have narrow chests.

STENTOROPHO'NUS, from Στεντωρ, Stentor, a Greek in the army before Troy; and φωνη 'voice.' One who has a strong voice.

STEPHANE, Crown.

STEPHENS, MRS., REMEDY FOR THE STONE. This consisted of lime, prepared by calcining the shells of eggs and snails, made into pills with soap. A decoction was. also administered, consisting of chamomile, fennel, parsley and burdock, with a portion of Alicant soap. Its virtues were dependent upon the lime and the tonic properties of the decoction. Hales, Hartley, Kirkpatrick, Lobb, and others, wrote in favour of this nostrum; and it was ultimately bought by the British parliament for £5000.

STERA, Uterus.

STERCORA'CEOUS, *Stercora'rius*, *Dejectitius*, *Ster'coral*, from *stercus*, 'dung.' *Fæces*, *Fæcal*, (F.) *Stercoraire*, *Stercoral*.

The French use the term. *Fistules stercoraires* for those which are kept up by the constant passage of fecal or *stercora'ceous matter*. The name *Stercoraires* is sometimes given, in derision, to those physicians who are fond of purging their patients: *à posteriori* has been similarly used.

STERCORAIRE, Stercoraceous.

STERCUS, Excrement, Fimus—s. America Fimus anserie—s. Caninum album, Album Græcum—s. Diaboli, Asafœtida—s. Equi non caccum Fimus.

STERCUS HUMA'NUM, Homerda. Human excrement.

STERCUS LACERTÆ, Crocodilia.

STEREOCYST'IS, from στερεος, 'hard,' and κυστις, 'cyst.' A hard steatoma.

STEREOS, Solid.

STEREOT'ICA, from στερεος, 'hard.' Fortifying

tous lesions or deformities affecting the hard parts. The 2d order, class *Tychica* of Good.

STER'ILE, *Ster'ilis, A'gonos, Aph'orus, Aph-o'ricus, Ablast'es, Infecun'dus*, (F.) *Stérile*. Same etymon as Sterilitas. Not producing fruit: infecund.

STERILIS, Sterile.

STERIL'ITAS, *Agon'ia, Steiro'sis, Stiro'sis, Agenne'sia, Agenne'sis, Infecun'ditas, Steril'ity, Acye'sis, Bar'renness, Infecun'dity, Apho'ria, Atec'nia, Atoc'ia*, from στερρος, or στερος, 'hard, barren.' Quality of that which is barren. Sterility may be *absolute* or *relative*. The former depends upon some vicious conformation of the genital organs, apparent or concealed, and occasionally admits of cure. Sterility is *relative* when a female does not conceive with one individual, but does with another. Sterility in females is often dependent upon a condition of the uterus characterized by membranous menstruation.

STERNAD, see Sternal.

STERNAL, *Sterna'lis*, from *sternum*, 'the breast bone.' Relating or appertaining to the sternum or breast bone.

STERNAL ASPECT. The aspect of the body where the sternum is situate.—Barclay. *Sternad* is used by the same writer adverbially to signify towards the sternal aspect.

STERNALGIA, Angina pectoris.

STERNO-CLAVIC'ULAR, *Sterno-clavicula'ris*. That which relates to the sternum and clavicle.

STERNO-CLAVIC'ULAR ARTICULA'TION is the union of the inner extremity of the clavicle with a round facette at each side of the superior extremity of the sternum. In this articulation there are, besides the incrusting cartilages, two *radiated sterno-clavicular*, (F.) *Sterno-claviculaires rayonnées; one* anterior, and *one* posterior —an *inter-clavicular ligament*, extending between the two clavicles, and two synovial capsules, separated by an *inter-articular fibro-cartilage*. The costo-clavicular ligament may also be considered to belong to this articulation.

STERNO-CLAVIO-MASTOÏDIEN, Sterno-cleido-mastoideus — s. Cleido-hyoideus, Sterno-hyoideus.

STERNO-CLEIDO BRACHIALIS, Pectoralis major.

STERNO-CLEIDO-MASTOIDEUS, *Sterno-mastoïdeus, Cleido-mastoïdeus, Mastoïdeus, Mastoïdeus anterior, Nuta'tor cap'itis;* (F.) *Sterno-clavio-mastoïdien, Sterno-mastoïdien;* from στερνον, 'the sternum,' κλεις, 'the clavicle,' and μαστος, 'the mastoid process.' A muscle situate at the anterior and lateral part of the neck. It is long and flattened: simple, above: and divided into two portions below; where it is inserted into the anterior and superior part of the sternum, and the inner quarter of the clavicle. Above, it terminates at the mastoid process, which it embraces, at the neighbouring part of the temporal bone, and at the outer third of the upper curved line of the occipital bone. It carries the head forward; inclines, and rotates it to one side. When both contract, they bend the head directly forwards.

STERNO-COSTAL, Triangularis sterni—*s. Costo-clavio-huméral*, Pectoralis major—*s. Dynia*, see Somatodynia—*s. Huméral*, Pectoralis major.

STERNO-HYOÏDEUS, *Sterno-cleido-hyoideus, Sterno-hyoïdes, Hyoïdes primus;* from στερνον, 'the sternum,' and 'νοειδης, 'the os hyoides.' A muscle situate at the anterior part of the neck; inserted, above, at the inferior edge of the body of the hyoid bone; below, into the upper part of the posterior surface of the sternum;—at the posterior part of the sterno-clavicular articulation, and sometimes into the cartilage of the first rib. It depresses the os hyoides.

STERNO-MASTOÏDIEN, Storno-cleido-mastoideus—*s. Pubien*, Rectus abdominis.

STERNO-THYROÏDEUS, *Sterno-thyroïdes, Bron'chius*. A muscle, situate at the anterior part of the neck. It is attached, above, to the oblique line seen on the outer surface of the thyroid cartilage; and terminates, below, at the upper part of the posterior surface of the sternum, and the cartilage of the second rib. When it contracts, it depresses the thyroid cartilage and os hyoides, by the medium of the thyro-hyoid membrane.

STERNODYNIA SYNCOPALIS, Angina pectoris—*s*. Syncoptica et Palpitans, Angina pectoris.

STERNO-OMPHALODYMIA, see Somatodymia.

STERNUM, *Sternon*, from στερρος, 'solid;' *Pectus, Os asser* seu *pec'torie* seu *xiphoïdes* seu *gladi'oli* seu *ensifor'mē, Scutum cordis, Breast Bone, Hæmal Spine* of Owen. An azygous symmetrical bone, situate at the fore-part of the chest. It is flat; broad above; narrower in the middle; and terminates, below, by a pointed cartilage— the xiphoid. It has an *anterior* or *cutaneous surface,* a *posterior* or *mediastinal* — a *superior* or *clavicular extremity*, and an *inferior* or *abdominal*. It is articulated with the clavicles and the seven upper ribs on each side, by means of their cartilages. According to Béclard, it is formed of six principal bones, which he names, from their position, 1. *Primi-sternal* or *clavi-sternal:* 2. *Duo-sternal:* 3. *Tri-sternal:* 4. *Quarti-sternal:* 5. *Quinti-sternal:* 6. *Ultimi-sternal* or *ensisternal*.

STERNUMENTUM, Sneezing.

STERNUTAMENTORIA, Achillea ptarmica.

STERNUTAMENTUM, Sneezing.

STERNUTATIO, Sneezing.

STERNUTATOIRE, Sternutatory.

STER'NUTATORY, *Sternutato'rius*, from *sternutare*, 'to sneeze.' *Sternutamen'tum, Errhi'num, Ptar'micum, Anarrhi'num*, (F.) *Sternutatoire*. A substance which provokes sneezing; as tobacco, &c.— See Errhine.

STERTEUR, Stertor.

STERTOROUS, see Stertor.

STERTOR, *Ronchus* or *Rhonchus, Renchus, Rhencus*, (F.) *Sterteur, Ronflement*, from *stertere*, 'to snore.' The deep snoring which accompanies inspiration in some diseases, particularly in apoplexy. Such respiration is said to be *ster'torous; Respira'tio stertuo'sa* seu *stertens* seu *stertoro'sa*.

STETHÆ'MIA, *Hyperæ'mia Pulmo'num* seu *Pec'toris, Conges'tio Pulmonum* seu *Pectoris,* (F.) *Hyperémie des Poumons, Congestion des Poumons.* Hyperæmia of the lungs. Congestion or accumulation of blood in the pulmonary vessels.

STETHOCATHARSIS, Expectoration.

STETHOCHYSIS, Hydrothorax.

STETHODESMIS, Corset.

STETHODESMIUM, Corset.

STETHODESMUS, Corset.

STETHOM'ETER, from στηθος, 'the chest,' and μετρον, 'measure.' An instrument, proposed by Mr. Richard Quain, for measuring the extent of movement of the walls of the chest, as a means of diagnosis in thoracic diseases. It consists of a flat case, not unlike a watch-case, having on its upper surface a graduated dial and index, which is acted on by a simple mechanism. A silk cord, long enough to surround one-half the chest, passes through an aperture in the case. The dial is graduated into fifty equal parts, each of which represents the 1-200th of an inch. In using the instrument, the dial is placed firmly against the spine, and the point of the tape over the sternum, or at any other spot according to the part to be examined. The extension of the string, as indicated by the dial, shows the amount of elasticity of the parietes of the thorax.

STETHOPARAL'YSIS, *Paral'ysis nervo'rum thora'cis, phrenicorum*, &c.; from στηθος, 'the chest,' and παραλυσις, 'paralysis.' Palsy of the muscles of the chest.

STETHORRHEUMA, Pleurodynia.

STETH'OSCOPE, *Stethoscop'ium, Stethos'copum, Echoscop'ium, Psophom'eter, Thoracoscop'ium*, from στηθος, 'the chest,' and σκοπεω, 'I examine.' An instrument invented by Laënnec, of Paris, for exploring the chest. The stethoscope, sometimes called *Pectoriloque*, is a cylinder of wood, from four inches to a foot long; pierced through and through by a longitudinal canal about a quarter of an inch in diameter. The longer are generally composed of two portions, that fit together by means of a screw, one of which is hollowed at the extremity, in the shape of a funnel. These two portions being screwed to each other, the physician lays hold of the instrument, as he would of a pen, puts the funnel-shaped extremity on the chest of the patient, and applies his ear to the other. To explore the pulsations of the heart, the funnel is plugged up by a piece of the same kind of wood accurately adapted to it, and pierced by a canal of the same width as that in the body of the instrument. Stethoscopes are sometimes flexible, like the flexible ear-trumpet.

This mode of examining affections of the chest, *Steth'oscopy, Stethoscop'ia*, &c., is what Laënnec terms *Auscultation médiate, Mediate Auscultation*.

STETHOSCOPIA, see Auscultation, and Stethoscope.

STETHUS, Thorax.

STEW, Stove.

STHENI'A, *Steni'a, Diath'esis sthen'ica, Status sthen'icus, Vis aucta*, from σθενος, 'strength,' 'power.' Excess of strength; excitement of the organic actions. A word used, especially by the Brunonians, as well as *Asthenia*,— its antitheton. *Sthenic* or *dynamic diseases* are such as depend upon excessive excitement.

STHENICUS, Active.

STHENOPYRA, Synocha.

STIBI, Antimonium.

STIBIALIS, Antimonial.

STIBIATUS TARTRIS LIXIVIÆ, Antimonium tartarizatum.

STIBII BUTYRUM, Antimonium muriatum — s. Deuto-murias sublimatus, Antimonium muriatum—s. et Potassæ deuto-tartras, Antimonium tartarizatum—s. Hydrosulphuretum rubrum, Antimonii sulphuretum rubrum — s. Oxidum acido muriatico oxygenato paratum, Algaroth—s. Oxidum album mediante nitro confectum, Antimonium diaphoreticum — s. Oxidum præcipitando paratum, Algaroth — s. Oxodes album, Antimonium diaphoreticum — s. Oxodes sulphuretum, Antimonii sulphuretum præcipitatum — s. Oxydi sulphurati hydro-sulphuretum luteum, Antimonii sulphuretum præcipitatum—s. Oxydulati sulphuretum, Antimonii sulphuretum præcipitatum — s. Oxydulum vitreatum, Antimonii vitrum—s. Oxydum semivitreum, Antimonii vitrum—s. Oxydum sulphuratum, Oxydum stibii sulphuratum — s. Subhydrosulphas, Antimonii sulphuretum rubrum — s. Submurias præcipitando paratum, Algaroth — s. Sulphurati hydrosulphuretum rubrum, Antimonii sulphuretum rubrum — s. Sulphuretum nigrum, Antimonium — s. Vitrum, Antimonii vitrum.

STIBIOSUM HYDROSULPHURETUM CUM SULPHURE, Antimonii sulphuretum præcipitatum — s. Oxidum, Antimonium diaphoreticum.

STIBIUM, Antimonium.
STICHAS ARABICA, Lavendula stœchas.
STICKWORT, Agrimony.
STICTA PULMONACEA, Lichen pulmonarius.
STIFF JOINT, MUSCULAR, Contractura.
STIFF JOINTS, Milk sickness.
STIFFNECK, Torticollis.
STIGMA, Cicatricula.
STIGMATA, see Nævus. The breathing pores of insects are so called.
STIG'MATA OVARIO'RUM, *Cicatri'ces Ovario'rum*. The cicatrices left in the ovary after the escape of ova.
STILBOMA, Cosmetic.
STILL, Alembic.
STILLA, Gutta.
STILLATIO SANGUINIS E NARIBUS, Epistaxis.

STILLICID'IUM, *Substil'lum*, from *stillare*, 'to drop.' This term is often used synonymously with *Strangury*. It means the flow of any fluid. — particularly the urine — drop by drop. Also, a kind of embrocation, *Stillicid'ium supra partem*, effected by dropping a liquid upon a part.
STILLICIDIUM LACRYMARUM, Epiphora—s. Narium, Coryza — s. Sanguinis e naribus, Epistaxis — s. Supra partem, see Stillicidium.

STILLIN'GIA, *S. sylvat'ica, Queen's Root, Queen's delight, Yaw root, Mar'cory, Cork*: An indigenous plant, which grows in pine barrens, from Virginia to Florida. *Sex. Syst.* Monœcia Monadelphia. *Nat. Ord.* Euphorbiaceæ. The root is said to be used in syphilis, obstinate cutaneous affections, &c., like sarsaparilla.

STIMATO'SIS, *Stymatosis, Hemorrhagia Penis, Stymatorrhag'ia, Phallorrhag'ia*, from ερυμα, 'priapism,' itself from ερυω, 'to erect.' Hemorrhage from the male organ, accompanied or not with priapism.

STIMMI, Antimonium.
STIM'ULANT, *Stim'ulans, Ex'citans, Excitant, In'citans, Incenti'vum, Irri'tans, Incitans, Hypersthen'ic*, from *stimulare*, 'to goad.' A medicine which has the power of exciting the organic action of the different systems of the economy. Some stimulants are *diffusible*,— that is, have a prompt but temporary action; others are *permanent* or *persistent*. The action of stimulants is called *Stimula'tion, Stimula'tio, Incita'tio*.

The chief stimulants are the following: Æther Sulphuricus, Ammonia, Asafœtida, Brucia, Camphora, Capsicum, Castoreum, Cinnamomum, Copaiba, Cubeba, Guaiacum, Hydrargyri Præparata, Iodinum, Nux Vomica, Olea Essentialia, Opium (in small dose), Piper, Sinapis, Serpentaria, Zingiber,— Alcohol, Caloric, Electricity, Mental Emotions, (the Impetuous.)

STIM'ULUS, 'a goad.' *Incitamen'tum, Irrita'men, Irritamen'tum, Poten'tia Irri'tans.* Anything which excites the animal economy.

STINK POKE, Dracontium fœtidum—s. Weed, Chenopodium anthelminticum, Datura stramonium, Polanisia graveolens.

STIPATIO, Stegnosis.
STIPATIO TELÆ CELLULO'SÆ INFANTIUM, Induration of the cellular tissue of children.

STIROSIS, Sterilitas.
STITCH, same root as *stick, Sax. ρτεκαν, (G.) steeken*, (F.) *Point,* (L.) *Punctum;* (from *pungere, punctum*, 'to prick or sting.') A lancinating pain, like that produced by the puncture of a sharp needle.

STITCH, COMMON, Suture, common — s. Royal, Suture, common — s. in the Side, Pleurodynia.
STIZOLOBIUM, Dolichos pruriens.

STLENGIS, Stridor dentium.

STOBÆ'A RUBRICAU'LIS. A South African plant, *Nat. Ord.* compositæ. A tincture of the bruised roots is diuretic, and of great service in gravel.

STOCHEION, Element.

STOCKING, LACED, (F.) *Bas lacé.* A bandage used by surgeons, which consists of a stocking made of firm cloth or dog-skin, admitting of being tightly laced anteriorly. It is employed in varices and ulcers of the legs.

STŒCHAS ARABICA, Lavendula stœchas.

STOMA, Mouth.

STOMAC'ACE, *Stomatoc'acē, Stomal'gia, Labrisul'cium, Cheiloc'acē, Uloc'acē, Cheilomala'cia, Stomatono'ma, Stomatonecro'sis,* from στομα, 'the mouth,' and κακος, 'evil:' *Cancer Oris, Canker.* Fœtor of the mouth with a bloody discharge from the gums. (F.) *Cancer aquatique;* see *Cancer Aquaticus.* Also, Scurvy.

STOMACACE, Porphyra nautica—s. Gangrænosum, Cancer aquaticus—s. Universale, Purpura hæmorrhagica.

STOMACAL, Stomachal.

STOMACALGIA, Cardialgia.

STOMACH, *Stom'achus, Ventric'ulus, Nedys, Anocœ'lia, Gaster,* (F.) *Estomac,* from στομα, 'a mouth.' One of the principal organs of digestion. It is a musculo-membranous reservoir; continuous, on the one side, with the œsophagus; on the other, with the duodenum. It is situate beneath the diaphragm, between the liver and the spleen; and occupies the epigastrium and a part of the left hypochondrium. In it the food is converted into chyme. When viewed externally, the stomach has, 1. An *anterior face,* which looks a little upwards. 2. An *inferior face,* directed downwards. 3. An *inferior* or *colic margin,* which is convex and extensive, and is called the *greater curvature,* (F.) *Grand courbure.* It gives origin to the omentum majus. 4. A *superior* or *diaphragmatic margin,* which is shorter, concave, and is called the *lesser curvature,* (F.) *Petit courbure.* The lesser omentum is attached to this. 5. A *left* or *œsophageal orifice,* called, also, the *cardia, Os ventric'uli* or *upper orifice.* 6. A *right* or *intestinal,* or *inferior orifice,* called the *pylorus.* 7. A considerable dilatation, situate to the left of the cardia and greater curvature—the *great tuberosity of the stomach;* and, 8. A less extensive dilatation, situate to the right of the greater curvature,— *the lesser tuberosity* or *lesser cul-de-sac, Antrum Pylo'ri.* The inner surface of the stomach is of a reddish-white colour, and has a marbled appearance. It is constantly covered by thick mucus, and is lined by a mucous membrane, which presents numerous wrinkles. The parietes of the stomach consist of three membranes in superposition. The outermost is serous, and is an extension of the peritoneum; the middle coat is *muscular,* — some of its fibres running longitudinally; others, transversely, and others obliquely; the innermost membrane is of a mucous nature, *Crusta villo'sa ventric'uli, Gastro-mycod'eris,* but not exactly a continuation of the membrane that lines the œsophagus. The mucous and muscular membranes form, at the pylorus, a valve, called the *Pyloric valve.* These three coats are united by a dense, close, areolar membrane; and, between the mucous and muscular coats, along the two curvatures especially, is a quantity of muciparous glands, called *Glands of Brunner.* The arteries of the stomach are very numerous, and proceed from the coronaria ventriculi, the pyloric, splenic, and right and left gastro-epiploic. The veins have the same name, and pursue the same course as the arteries. They pour their blood into the trunk

of the vena porta. Its lymphatic vessels are very numerous, and pass into ganglia, situate along the two curvatures. The nerves of the stomach proceed from the pneumogastric, and three divisions of the cœliac plexus.

STOMACH CELL, see Favulus—s. Disease, Limosis—s. First, Ingluvies.

STOMACH PUMP, *Gastren'chyta, Antli'a gas'trica.* A useful instrument for conveying fluids to the stomach, when deglutition is impracticable, and for pumping out the contents of that organ. It consists of a forcing syringe, to the bottom and nozzle of which flexible tubes can be attached. When the object is to force fluids into the stomach, the stomach-tube must be attached to the nozzle, and passed down the throat,—the tube connected with the bottom of the syringe being placed in the fluid to be injected. To empty the stomach, the stomach-tube must be attached to the bottom of the instrument. This instrument has been of great service where poisons have been taken. The antidote, when any exists, and is at hand, should be administered immediately prior to its use.

The stomach pump was first employed in America by Dr. Physick, in the year 1812.

STOMACH, SECOND, Proventriculus—s. Sick, Milk sickness—s. Third, Ventriculus callosus—s. Tube, see Tube, œsophageal.

STOM'ACHAL, *Stomach'ic, Stomach'ical, Cardi'acus, Stomach'icus, Stomacha'lis, Viscera'lis,* (F.) *Stomacal, Stomachique.* That which belongs to the stomach; that which is good for the stomach; which strengthens the stomach. A medicine that gives tone to the stomach.

STOMACHALGIA, Cardialgia.

STOMACHI RESOLUTIO, Dyspepsia.

STOMACHIC, Stomachal.

STOMACHICAL, Stomachal.

STOMACHIQUE Stomachal.

STOM'ACHUS, from στομα, 'mouth.' This word has been used in several different acceptations; for example, for the œsophagus, for the cardiac orifice of the stomach, (see Cardia,) and for the stomach itself. Hippocrates calls the neck of the bladder στομαχος κυστεως; and the neck of the uterus της μητρας στομαχος.

STOMAL'GIA, *Stomatal'gia, Stomatodyn'ia,* from στομα, 'mouth,' and αλγος, 'pain.' Pain in the mouth; *Stomac'acē.*

STOMAPYRA, Aphthæ—s. Aphtha, Aphthæ.

STOMATALGIA, Stomalgia.

STOMAT'IC, *Stomat'icus,* from στομα, 'mouth.' A medicine used in diseases, &c., of the mouth. Dentifrices, masticatories, &c., are stomatics.

STOMATITE APHTHEUSE, Stomatitis, aphthous — *s. Charbonneuse,* Cancer aquaticus — *s. Couenneuse,* Stomatitis, pseudo-membranous— *s. Crêmeuse pultacée,* Aphthæ — *s. Folliculeuse,* Stomatitis, aphthous — *s. Gangréneuse,* Cancer aquaticus— *s. Mercurielle,* see Salivation, mercurial — s. *Ulcéreuse,* Stomatitis, aphthous.

STOMATI'TIS, from στομα, 'the mouth,' and *itis,* denoting inflammation. (F.) *Inflammation de la Bouche;* Inflammation of the mouth.

STOMATITIS, APHTHOUS, *S. follic'ular, S. ul'cerous, Emphly'sis Aphthæ, A. Adulto'rum,* (F.) *Stomatite, S. aphtheuse, S. folliculeuse, S. ulcéreuse.* An inflammation of the follicles of the mouth, constituting the aphthæ of the adult, which is generally accompanied by cephalic, gastric, and general disturbance. It may be either descrete or confluent, and requires general and local treatment, adapted to the case.

STOMATITIS, ERYTHEM'ATOUS. Simple inflammation of the mouth.

STOMATITIS, EXSUDATIVA, Aphthæ—s. Follicular, S. aphthous — s. Gangrenous, Cancer aquaticus.

STOMATITIS, MERCU'RIAL, *Hydrargyrostom'atis, Hydrargyrostomati'tis, Stomati'tis mercuria'lis.* Inflammation of the mouth induced by mercury.

STOMATITIS OF NURSING-WOMEN appears to be a variety of S. aphthous.

STOMATITIS, PSEUDOMEM'BRANOUS, (F.) *Stomatite couenneuse, Diphthérite buccale, Pseudomembranous inflammation of the mouth;* — in its worst form, *Stomatyphus,* (F.) *Fégarite.* Inflammation of the mouth accompanied by the exudation of a false membrane, — a disease which is rarely seen except in large foundling establishments.

STOMATITIS, ULCEROUS, S. aphthous — s. Vesiculosa infantum, Aphthæ.

STOMATOCACE, Stomacace.

STOMATODYNIA, Stomalgia.

STOMATO-GAS'TRIC, *Sto'mato-gas'tricus,* from στομα, 'the mouth,' and γαστηρ, the stomach.' Appertaining to the mouth and stomach,—as the *stomato-gastric* ganglia of the lower animals.

STOMATOMALACIA PUTRIDA, Cancer aquaticus.

STOMATONECROSIS, Cancer aquaticus, Stomacace.

STOMATONOMA, Stomacace.

STOMATOPA'NUS, from στομα, 'the mouth,' and πανος, 'a glandular tumour.' *Stomatophy'ma glandulosum, Panus Fau'cium.* Tumefaction of the glands of the mouth.

STOMATOPHY'MA, from στομα, 'the mouth,' and φυμα, 'a swelling.' A swelling in the mouth.

STOMATOPHYMA GLANDULOSUM, Stomatopanus.

STOMATOPLAS'TIC, *Stomatoplas'ticus;* from στομα, 'the mouth,' and πλασσω, 'I form.' The operation of forming a mouth, where the aperture has been contracted from any cause.

STOMATORRHAG''IA, *Stomatorrhœ'a, Hæmorrhag''ia oris, H. fau'cium, San'guinis proflu'vium ex Orē, Hæmorrhoi'des Oris, Stomato'sis, Stomorrhag''ia,* (F.) *Hémorrhagie buccale,* from στομα, 'the mouth,' and ρηγνυμι, 'I break out.' Hemorrhage from the mouth.

STOMATORRHAGIA ALVEOLORUM, Phatnorrhagia — s. Gingivarum, Ulorrhagia.

STOMATORRHŒA, Stomatorrhagia.

STOMATOSCOPE, from στομα, 'mouth,' and σκοπεω, 'I view.' Any instrument for keeping the mouth open, so as to permit the parts within to be inspected; *Speculum oris.*

STOMATOSEPSIS, Cancer aquaticus.

STOMATOSIS, Stomatorrhagia.

STOMATOSPASMUS, Trismus.

STOMATYPHUS, Stomatitis, pseudomembranous.

STOMOMANICON, Platysma myoides.

STOMORRHAGIA, Stomatorrhagia.

STONE IN THE BLADDER, Calculi, vesical — s. Binder, Osteocolla — s. Crop, Sedum — s. Crop, biting, Sedum — s. Mint, Cunila mariana — s. Pock, Acne — s. Root, Collinsonia Canadensis.

STONES, THE, Testes.

STOOL, Dejectio.

STOOL, CALOMEL, see Calomel.

STORAX, Styrax — s. Liquida, Liquidambar styraciflua.

STOREY'S WORM CAKES. An empirical preparation, formed of *calomel* ℈j, *jalap.* ℈j, *zinyib.* ℈ij, *sacch.* ℥j, *cinnab. antim.* q. s. to colour them; *syrup. simpl.* q. s. to make into cakes.

STORKBILL, Geranium maculatum.

STOVE. Old French *Estuve, Stupha;* a Stew, *Æstua'rium,* (F.) *Étuve.* A limited space, warmed artificially, and in which the air is slowly renewed. It is used for drying various substances, as plants, extracts, conserves, &c., or for taking vapour baths. In this case, the stew or stove is said to be *wet* or *humid;* in the opposite case, it is said to be *dry,* (F.) *sèche.* The latter, which is used by the Turks, is the *Lacon'icum* or *Calida'rium* of the Romans. The former is their *Tepida'rium* or *Vapora'rium.* These kinds of [...] greatly excite the cutaneous transpiration; and are valuable agents in rheumatic and other affections.

STRABI, see Strabismus.

STRABILISMOS, Strabismus.

STRABIS'MUS, *Strabilis'mos, Parop'sis Strabismus,* from στραβος, 'twisted,' 'one who squints,' *Strabos'itas, Loxophthal'mus, Distor'sio,* [...] *Illo'sis, Ilo'sis, Helo'sis,* Squinting, *Goggle E[.]* (F.) *Strabisme, Vue louche, Louchement.* Want of concordance of the optic axes. It may be dependent upon natural or acquired inequality in the action of the motor muscles of the eye; or a convulsive state of one of those muscles; a difference in the sensibility of the two eyes; or a cerebral affection. In the treatment, if the disease seem to depend upon an excess of strength in one of the motor muscles, we must endeavour to give tone to that which is too weak, by placing before the eye a mask having a small aperture on the side to which it is necessary to direct the pupil; or by wearing glasses, provided with a piece of looking-glass, on the side to which the eye is vitiously turned; so that the reflection may be inconvenient, and occasion the organ to be turned in an opposite direction; or by putting a black patch on the angle opposite to that to which the eye is turned. If owing to weakness the organ must be strengthened by being exerted alone, and by leaving the other at rest. If the disease be symptomatic of cerebral affection, attention must, of course, be directed to the latter.

Strabismus may be *single* or affect one eye only, or *double,* and it may be *convergent* or *divergent.*

Those affected with Strabismus are called *Strabi, Strabo'nes, Strabo'ni, Strobli, Illi,* Squinters, *Squint-eyed;* in French, *Louches, Bigles.*

STRABISMUS, CONVERGENT, see Strabismus — s. Divergent, see Strabismus — s. Double, see Strabismus — s. Single, see Strabismus.

STRABONES, see Strabismus.

STRABONI, see Strabismus.

STRABOSITAS, Strabismus.

STRABOT'OMY, *Strabotom'ia,* from στραβος, 'one who squints,' and τομη, 'incision.' The operation for the removal of squinting by the division of the muscle or muscles that distort the eye-ball.

STRAIN, Sprain.

STRAIN, *colare,* (F.) *couler,* from *stringere,* (F.) *estreindre,* 'to constrict or squeeze.' To pass decoctions, infusions, &c., forcibly through linen; also, to exert an effort. This is accomplished by fixing firmly the parts where the muscles to be exerted originate, in order that their full power may be developed.

STRAINING, Nisus.

STRAITS OF THE PELVIS, see Pelvis.

STRAMOINE, Datura stramonium.

STRAMONIA, Datura stramonium.

STRAMONIUM, Datura stramonium — s. Fœtidum, Datura stramonium — s. Majus album, Datura stramonium — s. Spinosum, Datura stramonium — s. Vulgatum, Datura stramonium.

STRANGAL'IDES, from στραγγω, 'I bind.' Small, hard tumours, which form in the breast, when the milk does not find issue.

STRANGALION, Tubercle.
STRANGALIS, Tubercle.
STRANGALISMUS, Strangulation.
STRANGERS' FEVER, see Fever, strangers'.
STRANGULATIO, Orthopnœa, Strangulation — s. Uterina, Angone.
STRANGULA'TION, *Strangula'tio, Pnix, Pnig'mos, Strangalis'mus,* (F.) *Étranglement, Strangulation.* State of a part too closely constricted. Thus we say that there is *strangulation* of an intestinal hernia, when the opening that gives passage to the portion of protruded intestine contracts, so as to intercept the continuity of the digestive canal. In *Legal Medicine*, it means the forcible obstruction of the air passages, by a ligature or by the hand, for criminal purposes. See Suffocation.
STRANGULATOR, see Lycoides.
STRANGURIA, Enuresis—s. Cruenta, Cystorrhagia.
STRANGURIE, Strangury — *s. Menstruelle,* Dysmenorrhœa.
STRANGU'RIOUS; same etymon as the next. Affected with, or of the nature of, strangury.
STRAN'GURY, *Strangu'ria, Paru'ria stillati'tia,* from στραγγειν, 'to squeeze,' and ουρον, 'urine:' *Dysu'ria, Uri'næ Stillicid'ium* vel *Substil'lum,* (F.) *Strangurie.* Extreme difficulty in evacuating the urine, which issues only drop by drop, and is accompanied with heat, pain, tenesmus at the neck of the bladder, &c. See Ischuria, and Retention.
STRATHPEFFER, MINERAL WATERS OF. A sulphuretted water, at Strathpeffer, a few miles west from Dingwall, in Ross-shire, Scotland. It contains sulphate of soda, sulphate of lime, chloride of sodium, sulphate of magnesia, and sulpho-hydric acid.
STRATIOTES, Achillea millefolium.
STRATUM BACILLATUM, see Tunica Jacobi—s. Malpighii, Corpus mucosum—s. Pigmenti, see Choroid—s. Proligerum, Proligerous disc.
STRAWBERRY, Fragaria—s. Bush, Euonymus Americanus—s. Shrubby, Rubus arcticus—s. Tree, Euonymus Americanus—s. Wild, Fragaria Virginiana.
STREAK, PRIMITIVE, Groove, primitive.
STREATHAM, MINERAL WATERS OF. Streatham is a village near London. The waters are saline and cathartic.
STREBLI, see Strabismus.
STREBLOSIS, Luxation.
STREMMA, Luxation, Sprain.
STREPITO'SUS MORBUS. 'Noisy disease.' A kind of flatulent disease, said by Sorbait to be not uncommon in the Austrian Alps, in which emphysematous tumours form on different parts of the body, — accompanied by sonorous excretion of gas by the mouth and anus.
STREPITUS AURIUM, Tinnitus aurium.
STRETCHING, Pandiculation.
STRIÆ, Vibices—s. Ciliares, Ciliary processes —s. Corneæ, Tenia semicircularis—s. Longitudinales Lancisii, see Corpus callosum — s. Medullares, see Processus teretes — s. Retinæ subjectæ ligamento ciliari, Halo signatus—s. Semilunares, Tænia semicircularis—s. Terminales, Tænia semicircularis—s. Transversæ Willisii, see Corpus callosum.
STRIATED MUSCULAR FIBRE, see Muscular fibre.
STRIATUS, *Cannelé,* Grooved, see Corpora striata.
STRIBILIGO, Efflorescence.
STRICTURA, Stricture—s. Ani, Stricture of the rectum—s. Intestini recti, Stricture of the rectum—s. Intestini recti spasmodica, Stricture of the rectum, spasmodic—s. Œsophagi callosa,

Dysphagia constricta—s. Œsophagi spasmodica, Œsophagismus—s. Pharyngis seu œsophagi vera, Dysphagia constricta—s. Præputii, Phimosis—s. Urethræ, Urethrostenosis—s. Ventriculi, Stricture of the stomach.
STRICTURE, *Strictu'ra,* from *stringere, strictum,* 'to tie hard.' *Çoarcta'tio, Stegno'sis,* (F.) *Rétrécissement.* A diminution or contracted condition of some tube or duct, as the œsophagus, rectum, urethra, &c. This must be dilated by appropriate bougies. Strictures may, also, occur in the intestines: they are unmanageable, with the exception of those of the rectum, which admit of topical applications.
STRICTURE OF THE ŒSOPHAGUS, Dysphagia constricta — s. of the Pharynx, Dysphagia constricta.
STRICTURE OF THE RECTUM, SPASMOD'IC, *Strictu'ra Intesti'ni Recti spasmod'ica, Obstruc'tio Recti spas'tica.* An affection occurring in the nervous especially, which subsides spontaneously, after a longer or shorter continuance.
Stricture of the rectum, *Strictu'ra Ani seu Intesti'ni Recti, Archostegno'ma, Rectosteno'sis, Euthyenterosteno'ma, Archostegno'sis, Archosteno'sis, Proctoëneli'sis, Angusta'tio et Restric'tio intestini recti vel ani, Stenocho'ria intesti'ni recti, Proctosteno'sis organ'ica,* occurs also organically, and is a very serious affection; being generally dependent upon scirrhus.
STRICTURE OF THE STOMACH, *Gastrosteno'sis, Coarcta'tio* seu *Strictu'ra ventric'uli.* See Gastrostenosis cardiaca, &c.
STRICTURE OF THE URETHRA, Urethrostenosis — s. of the Urinary bladder, Cystostenochoria — s. Vesicæ urinariæ, Cystostenochoria.
STRIDOR DENTIUM, Brygmus.
STRIGA CARTILAGINOSA CORDIS, Isthmus of the fossa ovalis.
STRIGIL, *Strig'ilis, Stlen'gis, Stelen'gis.* A flesh-brush. Also, an instrument, anciently used in the baths, for scraping off the sweat.
STRIPED MUSCULAR FIBRE, see Muscular fibre.
STROBILITI'TES, from στροβιλος, *stro'bilus,* 'a cone of the pine.' Wine impregnated with the cones of the pine.
STROEMIA, Cadaba.
STROKE, APOPLEC'TIC. An apoplectic seizure.
STROKE, BACK, OF THE HEART, Impulse, diastolic.
STROKE, PARALYT'IC. A sudden attack of encephalo-spinal paralysis.
STROMA, *Strag'ulum, Stramen'tum;* from στρωννυω, στρωννυμι, 'to spread out; to cover.' The bed or foundation-texture of an organ,— as the stroma of the ovary. Applied, also, to the bed or base of any deposit— as the 'amorphous stroma' of scrofulous deposits.
STROMBULOUS, Forceps (bullet.)
STRONGLE, Strongylus—s. *Géant,* Strongylus gigas.
STRON'GYLUS, from στρογγυλος, 'round.' Hippocrates, Chabert, and others, mean the *Ascaris lumbricoi'des* by this term. The *Strongylus Gigas,* (F.) *Strongle, S. géant,* is, however, distinct. It has an obtuse, flat head; mouth surrounded with six flattish papillæ: the whole burns of the male truncated: the tail of the female rounded. It is sometimes met with,—five inches, a foot, a foot and a half, and even three feet long, —and from two lines to half an inch in diameter. It is occasionally found in the human kidney; rarely in other viscera, and still more rarely in the intestinal tube.
STRONGYLUS, Teres.
STROPHOS, Tormina.
STROPHULE, Strophulous.

STROPH'ULUS, *Licheni"asis stroph'ulus, Ebullit"io, Exanthe'ma strophulus, Exor'mia strophulus,* Red Gum, Red Gown, Tooth Rash, White Gum, Milk-spots, (F.) *Strophule, Feux de dents.* It consists of an eruption of red, or sometimes whitish pimples; occurring in early infancy, chiefly about the face, neck, and arms, surrounded by a reddish halo; or interrupted by irregular patches of cutaneous blush. All the varieties under this genus arise in consequence of the extreme vascularity and irritability of the skin at this period of life, when the constitution is liable to be disturbed by irritation, either in the alimentary canal, gums or other parts. None of these eruptions are of any importance, and no medical treatment is usually necessary. If the stomach seem at all disordered, a little rhubarb and magnesia may be administered occasionally. Willan and Bateman reckon five species,— *Strophulus intertinc'tus,* Red gum or gown; *S. al'bidus* or white gum; *S. confer'tus* or rank red gum, Tooth rash; *S. volat'icus* or *Erythe'ma volat'icum,* and *S. can'didus.*

STROPHULUS SYLVESTRIS, Ignis sylvaticus—s. Volaticus, Ignis sylvaticus.

STROPHUS, Tormina.

STRUCTIO, Structura.

STRUC'TURAL; same etymon as the next. Of, or belonging to, structure.

STRUCTURE, *Structu'ra, Struc'tio, Conforma'tio, Catasceu'ē,* from *struere, structum,* 'to build.' The arrangement of the different tissues or organic elements of which animals and vegetables are composed.

STRUMA, Bronchocele, Scrofula.

STRUMA ADIPO'SA, *Obes'itas colli.* Fatty neck. Prominence of the neck from obesity.

STRUMES, Scrofula.

STRUMEUX, Scrofulous.

STRUMOSIS CEREBRI, Encephalophymata —s. Pulmonum, Tubercles of the lungs.

STRUMOSUS, Scrofulous.

STRUMOUS, Scrofulous.

STRUTHIOPH'AGUS, from στρουθιον, 'a young ostrich,' and φαγω, 'I eat.' Struthiophagous tribes still exist in some parts of Africa.

STRUTHIUM, Saponaria.

STRUVE'S LOTION FOR HOOPING-COUGH, see Lotion, Struve's, for hooping-cough.

STRYCHNIA, *Strychni'na, Strych'nine, Strych'nium, Strych'nium, Vauqueline.* An alkaline principle; solid, crystalline, inodorous, bitter, and excessively poisonous, which has been discovered in the *Strychnos nux vomica.* (*Nucis vomicæ.* rasur. ℔iv; *calcis* pulv. ℨvj; *acid. muriat.* f ℨiij; *alcohol., acid. sulphuric. dil., liquor. ammoniæ, carbon. animal. purif., aquæ,* āā q. s. Digest the nux vomica in two gallons of water, acidulated with a fluidounce of muriatic acid, for 24 hours: then boil for two hours, and strain with expression through a strong linen bag. Boil the residuum twice successively in the same quantity of acidulated water, each time straining as before. Mix the decoctions, and evaporate to the consistency of thin syrup; then add the lime previously mixed with a pint of water, and boil for ten minutes, frequently stirring. Pour the mixture into a double linen bag, and having washed the precipitate well with water, press, dry, and powder it. Treat the powder repeatedly with boiling alcohol, until deprived of its bitterness; mix the liquors, and distil off the alcohol by means of a water-bath. Mix the residue with water, and having applied heat, drop in sufficient diluted sulphuric acid to neutralize and dissolve the strychnia; then add purified animal charcoal; boil for a few minutes, filter, evaporate, and crystallize. Dissolve the crystals in water, and add sufficient solution of ammonia to precipitate the strychnia. Lastly, dry the precipitate on bibulous paper. Ph. U. S.) The medical action of strychnia on man and animals is exactly like that of the alcoholic extract of nux vomica. It is, however, more active. An eighth of a grain is sufficient to kill a large dog; and a quarter of a grain produces marked effects on the human body, when in health. It has been given in paralysis and other cases like the nux vomica. Dose, one twelfth to one eighth of a grain.

STRYCHNIA, ACETATE OF, Strychniæ acetas—s. Hydriodate of, Strychniæ hydriodas—s. Iodate of, Strychniæ iodas — s. Iodide of, Strychniæ hydriodas.

STRYCH'NIA, I'ODIDE OF IODHYDRATE OF, *Iodure d'Iodhydrate de Strychnine,* is made by a solution of *iodouretted iodide of potassium* into a solution of *a salt of strychnia;* treating the precipitate with *boiling alcohol,* and crystallizing. Used in the same cases as strychnia. Dose, a sixth of a grain.

STRYCHNIA, NITRATE OF, Strychniæ nitras—s. Sulphate of, Strychniæ sulphas.

STRYCHNIA and ZINC, DOUBLE IODIDE OF, double Iodide of Zinc and Strychnia.

STRYCH'NIÆ ACE'TAS, *Strych'nium strychni'num ace'ticum, Ace'tas strych'nii, strych'nicus, Ac"etate of Strychnia* or *Strychn.* This salt is formed by the direct combination of strychnia with *acetic acid.* It is given in the same cases as pure strychnia.

STRYCH'NIÆ HYDRI'ODAS, *S. iodhy'dras, Strych'nium hydroiod'icum, Hydri'odas seu hy'dras strych'nicus, Hydri'odate* or *Iodhydrate Strychnia,* is prepared by mixing a solution of *iodide of potassium* with a concentrated solution of *acetate of strychnia.*

STRYCH'NIÆ I'ODAS, *Strychni'næ Iodas, Strychni'na Ioda'ta, Strych'nium seu Strychni'nium icum, I'odas Strych'nii seu Strych'nicus, Iodide of Strych'nia* or *Strychnine.* This salt may formed by adding a concentrated solution of *iodic acid* to *strychnia;* treating with boiling *alcohol;* filtering, and leaving it to spontaneous evaporation.

STRYCHNIÆ NITRAS, *Strych'nium ni'tricum. Nitrate of Strychnia* or *Strychnine.* Used in the same cases as strychnia.

STRYCH'NIÆ SULPHAS, *Strych'nium sulphuricum,* Sulphate of Strychnia or Strychnine. Has the same properties.

STRYCHNINA, Strychnia.

STRYCHNINE, Strychnia.

STRYCHNINUM, Strychnia.

STRYCHNIUM, Strychnia—s. Aceticum Strychniæ acetas—s. Nitricum, Strychniæ nitras —s. Sulphuricum, Strychniæ sulphas.

STRYCHNOS, Solanum dulcamara—s. Guianensis, see Curare — s. Ignatii, Ignatia amara.

STRYCHNOS NUX VOM'ICA, *Nux Vomica, Metel'la, Caniram, Koochla tree. Family. Strychnoideæ. Sex. Syst.* Pentandria Monogynia. *Vomiquier.* A tree of the family *Strychnoideæ* which grows in India, and the seeds of which have been long sold in the shops, under the names, *Nux Vomica, Vomic nut, Poison Bachelors' buttons,* &c., (F.) *Noix vomique.* For a long time, these seeds were used only for poisoning rats; but of late years, an alcoholic extract has been prepared from them, which has been administered in paralytic affections, in small doses. Dose of the *Alcoholic Extract, Extractum nucis vom'icæ spirituo'sum, E. nucis vomicæ no'sum, E. n. v. alcohol'icum,* (F.) *Extrait alcoholique de noix vomique,* one or two grains. It produces a kind of tetanic convulsion in the paralyzed parts, when given to the requisite extent. It has, also, been administered in chronic diarrhoea rhœa and dysentery. The following is the formula for the preparation of the EXTRAC'TUM NUCIS VOM'ICÆ of the Pharm. U. S. Take of *Nux vomica*, ℔j; *Alcohol*, a sufficient quantity. Expose the Nux Vomica to steam till it is softened; then, having sliced and dried it, grind it into powder. Introduce it into an apparatus for displacement, and pour alcohol upon it gradually, until the liquid passes without bitterness. Distil off the greater part of the alcohol from the filtered liquor, and evaporate the residue to the proper consistence.

The bark is the *false angustura* or false *cusparia bark; Rohun*.

The wood of *Strychnos colubri'na*, an Indian tree, contains strychnia. It was formerly considered a specific against the bites of venomous animals; and was recommended by Boerhaave in intermittents. It is the *Lignum Colubri'num*, (F.) *Bois de Couleuvre*.

STRYCHNOS TOXICARIA, see Curare.
STRYPHNA, Astringents.
STRYPHNOS, Acerb.
STUDIOSUS MEDICINÆ, Philiatros.
STUDIUM INANE, Aphelxia otiosa.
STUDY, BROWN, Aphelxia otiosa.
STUFFING, Cynanche trachealis.
STULTITIA, Fatuitas.
STUMP, (G.) **Stumpf**, (D.) *Stomp*, 'a stump;' also, 'blunt.' (F.) *Moignon*. The part remaining from which a limb or other part has been amputated or removed in any manner.

STUNNED. Old French, *Estonné*, (L.) *attonitus*, 'astonished.' (F.) *Étonné*. An epithet, applied to one who, in consequence of a fall or other accident, has received such a concussion of the brain as to deprive him, for a time, of his mental manifestations.

STUPA, *Stupha, Stuppa, Stupei'on*. Tow, used in certain surgical apparatuses and dressings. Also, a *Stupe*, that is, cloth or tow used in fomentations. A flannel or other article wrung out of hot water, plain or medicated, applied to a part, is a *stupe*. The act of applying such stupe is called *stuping*.

STUPE, Stupa.
STUPEFACIENTIA, Narcotics.
STUPÉFACTIFS, Narcotics.
STUPEFACTIO, Narcosis.
STUPÉFIANTS, Narcotics.
STUPEION, Stupa.
STUPEUR, Stupor.
STUPHA, Stove, Stupa.
STUPIA, Tin.
STUPIDITAS, Idiotism, Imbecility.
STUPING, see Stupe.
STUPOR, *Ecplex'is, Ecplex'ia, Consterna'tio*, (F.) *Stupeur*, from *stupere*, 'to be stupified.' Diminished activity of the intellectual faculties; often amounting to lethargy. It occurs in many affections, especially in the neuroses.

STUPOR, Narcosis—s. Artuum, Obdormitio—s. Dentium, Hæmodia—s. Formicans, Formication—s. Mentis, Fatuitas—s. Vigilans, Catalepsy.

STUPPA, Stupa.
STUPRATION, Stuprum.
STUPRUM, *Rape, Stupra'tion*, (F.) *Défloration, Viol*. Forcible and illicit enjoyment of a married or unmarried female. When committed upon the latter, which is most commonly the case, it is also called, *Deflora'tion, Deflora'tio, Devirgina'tio, Vitia'tio, Apanthis'mus*, &c. In judging whether rape has been committed under such circumstances, the state of the genital organs; the age of the individual; and the possibility of accidents and diseases of the parts, will have to be considered. It will be necessary, also, to be acquainted with the evidences of virginity; and to determine,—if signs of virginity no longer exist, — whether its loss be attributable to copulation, or to the introduction into the vagina of any other body than the male organ, &c. *Recent deflowering* can, of course, be much more readily distinguished than that which has taken place some time.

STUTTERING, Balbuties.
STYAN, Hordeolum.
STYE, Hordeolum.
STYMATES. M. J. Cloquet has proposed this word, or *Stigmates*, from στιγμα, 'a mark,' to designate the marks, in form of cicatrices, which remain on the peritoneum after the obliteration of the neck of the hernial sac. They are, commonly, radiated folds, of a whitish appearance, more or less thick, and of a fibrous or fibrocartilaginous nature.

STYLET, Specillum.
STYLI, Styloid processes.
STYLIFORM, Styloid.
STYLO-CERATOIDES, Stylo-hyoideus — s. Cerato-hyoideus, Stylo-hyoideus.
STYLO-CHONDRO-HYOÏDEUS. A name given, by Douglas and Albinus, to a fleshy fasciculus which the stylo-hyoid muscle sometimes presents, and which is attached to the lesser cornu of the os hyoides. It is the same fasciculus which Santorini calls *Stylo-hyoï'des novus, Stylo-hyoïdeus alter*.

STYLO-GLOSSUS. A muscle situate at the anterior and superior part of the neck. It is narrow behind, much broader before; is attached to the styloid process of the temporal bone, and to the stylo-maxillary ligament; and is inserted into the side of the tongue. It raises the base of the tongue and carries it backwards.

STYLO-HYOÏDEUS, *Stylo-hyoïdien, Stylocer'ato-hyoïdeus, Stylo-ceratoï'des, Stylo-hyoïdes major*. A muscle, situate at the superior, anterior, and lateral part of the neck. It is thin and narrow, — especially posteriorly: anteriorly, it opens to give passage to the tendon of the digastricus. It is attached to the styloid process of the temporal bone, and to the body of the os hyoides. It raises the os hyoides, and carries it backwards.

STYLO-HYOID LIGAMENT is a fibrous, flattened cord, which passes from the styloid process to the lesser cornu of the os hyoides.

STYLO-HYOID NERVE is the second branch given off by the facial nerve.

STYLOID, *Sty'liform, Styloï'des, Graphioï'des, Graphoï'des, Graphio'des, Graphidoï'des, Belonoï'des*, from στυλος, 'a style,' 'a peg,' 'a pin,' and ειδος, 'shape.' Shaped like a peg or pin.

STYLOID CORNUA, see Hyoides os.
STYLOID PROC"ESSES, *Pencil-like Processes, Proces'sus Beloïdes* seu *Belemnoïdes* seu *Belonoï'des* seu *Graphioïdes* seu *Graphoï'des, Styli*, are, 1. A long and slender process of the temporal bone, to which are attached the stylo-glossus, stylo-pharyngeus, and stylo-hyoideus muscles, and the stylo-hyoid and stylo-maxillary ligaments. 2. Two slender and pyramidal processes at the inferior extremities of the radius and ulna.

STYLO-MASTOID, *Stylo-mastoïdeus*. That which relates to the styloid and mastoid processes.

STYLO-MASTOID ARTERY arises from the posterior auricular, and, in some subjects, from the occipital. It enters the stylo-mastoid foramen; passes along the aqueduct of Fallopius, and spreads its ramifications on the mucous membrane of the tympanum, and in the mastoid cells, and semi-circular canals; and terminates by anastomosing with a branch of the *Arteria meningæa media*, which enters by the *Hiatus Fallopii*. Murray has given the name — *Stylo-mastoid* — to the posterior auricular artery itself.

STYLO-MASTOID FORA'MEN, *Foramen Stylo-mastoideum* or *F. Aquæduc'tus Fallo'pii*, (F.) *Trou anonyme*, is situate at the inferior surface of the petrous portion of the temporal bone, between the styloid and mastoid processes. It terminates the aqueduct of Fallopius, and gives passage to the facial nerve.

STYLO-MAX'ILLARY, *Stylo-maxilla'ris.* That which relates to the styloid processes and jaw.

The STYLO-MAXILLARY LIGAMENT is a ligamentous, flat cord, extending between the styloid process and the angle of the jaw.

STYLO-PHARYNGEUS, (F.) *Stylo-thyropharyngien.* A muscle, situate at the anterior and lateral part of the neck. It is slender; thin above; attached to the styloid process of the temporal bone, and terminates in the parietes of the pharynx, as well as at the posterior margin of the thyroid cartilage. It raises the pharynx and carries it backwards. Professor Chaussier has united, under the name *Stylo-pharyngien*, the three constrictor muscles of the pharynx, the stylo-pharyngeus, and palato-pharyngeus.

STYLOPH'ORUM DIPHYL'LUM, *Meconop'sis diphyl'la, Cel'andine Poppy, Horn Poppy, Bruise root.* An indigenous plant, of the *family* Papaveraceæ, growing from western Pennsylvania to Wisconsin, which flowers from May to August. The juice is fetid and narcotic. Infused in wine, it has been given internally in gravel; and has been applied externally to contusions, &c.

STYLO-THYRO-PHARYNGIEN, Stylopharyngeus.

STYLUS, Sound.

STYLUS EXCAVA'TUS, *Specil'lum excava'tum.* A hollow sound.

STYMA, Erection, Priapismus.

STYMATOSIS, Stimatosis.

STYM'MATA, from στυμμα, 'that which constricts or thickens.' The most solid ointments. Also, the ingredients proper for increasing their consistence.

STYPSIS, Astriction, Constipation.

STYPTERIA, Alumen, Styptics.

STYPTIC, EATON'S. A name first given to *Helvetius's Styptic*, when introduced into Great Britain. It is now usually made of *calcined green vitriol*, ʒj; *proof spirit*, tinged with a little oak bark, Oij.

STYPTIC, HELVETIUS'S, see Ferrum tartarisatum.

STYPTIC, RUSPINI'S, *Liquor Stypt'icus Ruspini.* A nostrum, said to consist of *gallic acid*, a small quantity of *sulphate of zinc* and *opium*, dissolved in a mixture of *alcohol* and *rose-water*, which has had much reputation as an internal and external astringent.

STYPTICS, *Contrahen'tia, Constricti'va Medicamen'ta, Constringen'tia, Anastal'tica, Stypte'ria*, from στυπω, 'I constringe.' Sometimes used synonymously with astringent, but generally applied to a substance employed to arrest hemorrhage, — *Enæ'mon.* A *mechanical styptic* is one that arrests the flow of blood, by being applied immediately to the mouth of the bleeding vessel, or by inducing a coagulum, *mechanically*, in it. A *chymical styptic* is one which coagulates, *chymically*, the blood around a bleeding orifice.

STYRAC"INUM O'LEUM. Oil obtained by boiling storax in good olive oil.

STYRAX, from στυραξ, 'a reed,' in which it was preserved. A resin obtained from the *Styrax officina'lis* and *S. calami'ta.* It is the *s..i storax*; — *officinal storax.* There are two kinds of storax met with: 1. The *Red Storax*, *Storax, Thus Judæo'rum, Styrax rubra, S., bal'samum, Balsamum styracis officinalis*, is obtained by incision from the *Styrax officinalis* and, perhaps, from the *Liquidam'bar orientalis* The purest is in tears; but it has lost some of its smell in drying. 2. *Common Storax, Syrax calami'ta.* That which has been received in casks or vessels, and has had saw-dust added immediately to thicken it. The odour of storax is fragrant; the taste aromatic. It is considered like the other balsams, to be stimulant and expectorant, but is rarely used long.

PU'RIFIED STORAX, *S. cola'ta, S. purificata* prepared by dissolving storax in alcohol; straining the solution; then distilling off the alcohol with a gentle heat, until the storax acquires a proper consistence. — Ph. U. S. Dose, gr. to xxx.

STYRAX ALBA, see Myroxylon Peruiferum — s Benzoin, see Benjamin — s. Calamita, see Styrax — s. Liquida, Liquidambar styraciflua — s. Officinalis, see Styrax.

STYSIS, Erection, Priapismus.

SUAVEOLENS, Beneolens.

SUB. A common Latin prefix, signifying 'beneath.'

SUBAC'TIO, *Chiro'sis, Cheirosis.* The operation of making plasters, extracts, &c., with the hand, or with the pestle and mortar.

SUBAFFECTIO, Hydropathia.

SUBAGITATRIX, *Tribade.*

SUB-ATLOÏDEUS, *Infra-atloïdeus*, (F.) *Sous-atloïdien.* That which is situate beneath the atlas or first cervical vertebra. Chaussier has given this name to the second pair of cervical nerves.

SUB-AXOÏDEUS, *Infra-axoïdeus*, (F.) *Sous-axoïdien.* That which is below the *axis* or vertebra dentata. Chaussier has given this name to the third pair of cervical nerves.

SUBBORAS NATRICUM, Borax.

SUBCARTILAGINEUM, Hypochondre.

SUBCLA'VIAN, *Subcla'vius, Subclavien*, from *sub*, 'under,' and *clavis*, 'the clavicle.' That which is under the clavicle.

SUBCLAVIAN ARTERIES, (F.) *Artères souclavières*, are situate at the upper part of the chest and the lateral and lower parts of the neck. The right arises at the corresponding side of the trachea, and comes off from the arteria innominata or brachio-cephalic trunk. The left leaves the aorta at the end of the arch. Both extend as far as the superior surface of the first rib. In the space between the scaleni muscles, beyond which they take the name *axillary arteries.* The subclavian arteries run, for some distance without sending off any branch. In the neighbourhood of the first rib, however, they give off 1. *Upwards*, the *vertebral* and *inferior thyroid*. 2. *Downwards*, the *internal mammary* and superior intercostal. 3. *Outwards*, the *transverse cervical* or *posterior scapular*, the *superior scapular* and the *posterior cervical* or *profunda*.

SUBCLAVIAN or SUBCLAVIUS MUSCLE, *Subclavia'nus*, (F.) *Costo-claviculaire* (Ch.), *Sous-clavier*, is situate at the superior and anterior part of the chest. It is attached, by its inner extremity, to the superior surface of the cartilage of the first rib; and by its superior margin and outer extremity to the inferior surface of the clavicle. This muscle depresses the clavicle, and carries it forward. When the shoulder is fixed it can raise the first rib.

SUBCLAVIAN VEINS, (F.) *Veines sous-clavières*

are continuations of the axillary, and extend from the inferior extremity of the scalenus anticus, in front of which they pass, to the vena cava superior, which they form by their union. The right subclavian vein is very short; the left, longer and broader. These veins receive the mouths of the internal and external jugulars, vertebral and superior intercostal. The left subclavian receives two veins more than the right,—the left internal mammary and left inferior thyroid. The thoracic duct opens into the left subclavian:—the corresponding great lymphatic vessel into the right.

SUBCLAVIC'ULA, from *sub*, 'under,' and *clavicula*, 'the clavicle.' The first rib.

SUBCLAVICULARIS, Subclavian.

SUBCLAVIUS, Subclavian muscle.

SUBCRUEN'TUS, 'somewhat bloody;' from *sub*, and *cruentus*, 'bloody;' *Hyphœ'mos*. That which has the colour and nature of blood. An epithet given to certain excreted substances, which are mixed with blood, or have the appearance of blood.

SUBCRURÆI, see Crurœus.

SUBCUTA'NEOUS, *Subcuta'neus*, from *sub*, 'under,' and *cutis*, 'the skin;' *Intercuta'neus*, (F.) *Sous-cutané*. That which is placed immediately under the skin.

SUBCUTANEUS COLLI, Superficialis colli — s. Malæ (Nervus), Orbitar nerve.

SUBDELIRIUM, Typhomania.

SUB'DITA, *Subditit"ia*, from *subdere*, 'to put under;' *Pros'theta*. Medicines introduced into some one of the natural apertures;—as suppositories, pessaries, &c.

SUBDITITIA, Subdita.

SUBDUCTIO, Dejection.

SUBER, *Cork:*—the bark of the *Quercus Suber* or *Cork Tree*. (F.) *Liége*. Family, Amentaceæ. *Sex. Syst.* Monœcia Polyandria. Cork, when burnt, is applied as a mechanical styptic to bleeding piles, &c. Surgeons use it for making tents; and it has been recommended to be worn as an amulet to suppress the secretion of milk!

SUBETH, Coma.

SUBFRONTA'LIS SUTU'RA. A suture resulting from the articulation of the os frontis with the nasal process of the superior maxillary bone, and the proper bones of the nose.

SUBGRONDATION, Depression.

SUBHUMERATIO, Catomismos.

SUBIGATOR, *Tribade*.

SUBINFLAMMATIO, Subinflammation — s. Hepatis, Hepatitis, chronic.

SUBINFLAMMA'TION, *Subinflamma'tio*, from *sub*, 'under,' and *inflammatio*. *Inflammatiun'cula*, *Hypophlegma'sia*. A mild degree of inflammation, so slight as hardly to deserve the name *inflammation*. Broussais understood by the term, an augmentation in the vital phenomena of the vessels that convey white blood. Lymphatic engorgements, scrofula, herpes, and cancer he considered subinflammations.

SUBINTRAN'TES FEBRES, from *sub*, 'under,' and *intrare*, 'to enter.' *Communican'tes febres*. Fevers primarily intermittent, whose paroxysms approximate, so that one paroxysm begins before that which preceded it has gone through its stages.— L. Bellini.

SUBJECTIVE SENSATIONS, see Sensation.

SUBJEE, Bangue.

SUBLIGACULUM, Truss.

SUBLIGATURA, Truss.

SUBLIMAMENTUM, Enæorema.

SUBLIMATE, CORROSIVE, Hydrargyri oxymurias.

SUBLIMA'TION, *Sublima'tio*, *Meteoris'mus*, *Hypeo'sis*, from *sublimo*, 'I raise up.' An operation by which dry and solid matters are volatilized and condensed at the upper part of a subliming apparatus. Calomel, sal ammoniac, &c., are commonly obtained by sublimation. The product of sublimation is a *Sub'limate Sublima'tum*, (F.) *Sublimé*.

SUBLIMATUS CORROSIVUS, Hydrargyri oxymurias.

SUBLIME, Sublimis.

SUBLIMÉ, Enæorema, Sublimate — s. *Corrosif*, Hydrargyri oxymurias.

SUBLI'MIS, (F.) *Sublime*, 'high, elevated, superficial.' Anatomists have given the name *sublimis* to certain muscles, which are situate more superficially than their kindred muscles. These last they have called *profundi*. Of the former, the *flexor sublimis digitorum* is an example.

The French use the term '*respiration sublime*' for the respiration which is accompanied by considerable elevation of the ribs, and with separation of the alæ nasi at the time of inspiration.

SUBLINGUA, Uvula.

SUBLIN'GUAL, *Sublingua'lis*, (F.) *Souslingual*, from *sub*, 'under,' and *lingua*, 'the tongue.' That which is seated under the tongue.

SUBLINGUAL ARTERY, with some, is the *Lingual*. With others, it is a branch given off by the lingual opposite the genio-glossus muscle, which is distributed particularly to the sublingual gland, to the mylo-hyoid, and genio-glossus muscles, &c.

SUBLINGUAL GLAND, *Glan'dula sublingua'lis*, *G. Bartholinia'na*, *G. Rivinia'na*, is seated in the substance of the inferior paries of the mouth, beneath the anterior part of the tongue. It is smaller than the submaxillary, of which it frequently seems to be only a prolongation. It is oblong, flattened, amygdaloid, and is covered by the mucous membrane of the mouth, beneath which it projects. This gland has 10 or 12 excretory ducts — *Ductus Rivinia'ni* seu *Waltheria'ni*—some of which open beneath the frænum linguæ, joining Wharton's duct, whilst others pierce the mucous membrane of the mouth separately. It has the same structure as the parotid.

SUBLINGUIUM, Uvula.

SUBLINGUUM, Epiglottis.

SUBLOB'ULAR, *Sublobula'ris*; from *sub*, 'under,' and *lobus*, 'a lobe.' That which is placed under a lobe.

SUBLOBULAR VEINS OF THE LIVER. The veins in which the intra-lobular veins terminate. By their union, the sublobular veins form the hepatic veins.

SUBLUXATIO, Sprain.

SUBMAX'ILLARY, *Submaxilla'ris*, *Inframaxilla'ris*, (F.) *Sous-maxillaire*, from *sub*, 'under,' and *maxilla*, 'the jaw.' That which is seated beneath the jaw.

SUBMAXILLARY GANGLION is a small nervous ganglion, situate opposite the gland. It seems to be formed by the superior branch of the Vidian nerve, and communicates with the lingual nerve of the inferior maxillary. Its filaments form a plexus which penetrates the submaxillary gland.

SUBMAXILLARY GLAND, *Max'illary Gland*, *Hypognath'aden*, is a salivary gland, less than the parotid, seated at the inner side of the ramus and body of the inferior maxillary bone, in the triangular space between the two bellies of the digastricus. Irregularly ovoid, and flattened on three surfaces, it has the same aspect and organization as the other salivary glands. Its excretory duct is called *Wharton's Duct*, and terminates at the side of the frænum linguæ, by a very small orifice. It is also called *Ductus inferior*.

SUBMEN'TAL, *Submenta'lis*, (F.) *Sousmental*,

from *sub*, 'under,' and *mentum*, 'the chin.' Situate under the chin.

SUBMENTAL ARTERY is furnished by the facial, near the base of the jaw. It passes forwards along the attachment of the mylo-hyoideus, to which it furnishes branches that cross it to anastomose with those of the sublingual. Near the median line it bifurcates, to be distributed to the chin and muscles of the infra-hyoid region.

SUBMENTAL VEIN, which accompanies the artery, opens into the labial.

SUBMER'SION, *Submer'sio*, from *sub*, 'under,' and *mergere, mersum*, 'to plunge.' The act of plunging, or being entirely plunged, in a liquid.

Asphyx'ia by submersion, Drowning, Asphyxia Immerso'rum, is not owing to a certain quantity of liquid being introduced into the alimentary or air-passages; but simply to the interception of air, and of the respiratory phenomena. It is a case of suffocation, the signs of which, on dissection, are equivocal, without circumstantial evidence.

SUBMISSIO, Remission—s. Cordis, Systole.

SUBMU'COUS, *Submuco'sus;* from *sub*, 'under,' and *mucus*. Under a mucous membrane, — as the '*submucous* areolar tissue.'

SUBMURIAS AMMONIACO-HYDRARGYRICUS, Hydrargyrum præcipitatum.

SUBMUS'CULAR, *Submuscula'ris;* from *sub*, 'under,' and *musculus*, 'a muscle.' Seated beneath muscles or a muscular layer.

SUBOCCIP'ITAL, *Suboccipita'lis;* from *sub*, 'under,' and *occiput*. That which is situated under the occiput.

SUBOCCIP'ITAL NERVE, Occipital nerve.

SUBOR'BITAR, *Suborbita'rius, Infra-or'bitar, Infra-orbita'lis*, (F.) *Sous-orbitaire*, from *sub*, 'under,' and *orbita*, 'the orbit.' That which is seated beneath the orbitar cavity.

SUBORBITAR ARTERY, *Infra-orbitar, A.*, proceeds from the internal maxillary, from which it separates near the anterior and superior part of the zygomatic fossa. It enters the infra-orbitar canal, and passes through it, giving branches to the anterior and superior dental canal; issues by the foramen infra-orbitarium; and divides, in the fossa canina, into a number of branches, which lose themselves in the neighbouring parts. The infra-orbitar vein follows the same course.

SUBORBITAR CANAL, *Infra-orbitar Canal*, (F.) *Canal ou Conduit sous-orbitaire*, is a small canal, which runs obliquely through the substance of the inferior paries of the orbit. It begins, behind, by a simple gutter, and divides, anteriorly, into two branches, one of which descends into the anterior paries of the maxillary sinus, whilst the other passes out, in the canine fossa, by an orifice, called *Foramen-infra-orbitarium*, (F.) *Trou sous-orbitaire*. The infra-orbitar artery and nerve pass along it.

SUBORBITAR FISSURE, *Infra-orbitar Fissure, Rima cana'lis orbita'rii, Fissu'ra infra-orbita'lis*. A fissure in the superior maxillary bone; the superior commencement of the suborbitar canal.

SUBORBITAR FOSSA, Canine fossa.

SUBORBITAR NERVES, *Infra-orbitar Nerves*, seem to terminate the superior maxillary. They issue from the infra-orbitar canal by the foramen of the same name, and spread out in a radiated manner in the fossa canina, to divide into *superior* or *palpebral filaments, inferior* or *labial, internal* or *nasal*, and *external* or *buccal*.

SUBPERITONE'AL, *Subperitonea'lis;* from *sub*, 'under,' and *peritoneum*. That which lies under the peritoneum.

SUBPERITONEAL APONEUROSIS, Fascia, subperitoneal — s. Ganglia, see Spermatic ganglion.

SUBPLACENTA, Decidua membrana.

SUBPOPLITÆUS, Popliteus muscle.

SUBPUBIC ARCH, *Arcus subpu'bicus*. A strong arch of the superior pelvic aponeurosis, which completes the posterior orifice of the obturator or subpubic canal.

SUBPUBIC MEMBRANE, Obturator membrane.

SUBPUBIO-FEMORALIS, Abductor brevis —s. Prostaticus, Compressor prostatæ.

SUBPUTRIS, Hyposapros.

SUBSCAP'ULAR, *Subscapula'ris*, (F.) *Sous-capulaire, Sous-scapulo-trochinien*, from *sub*, 'under,' and *scapula*, 'the shoulder-blade.' That which is beneath the scapula.

SUBSCAPULAR FOSSA, *Fossa Subscapula'ris*. A considerable excavation at the anterior surface or venter of the scapula, in which the subscapularis is seated.

SUBSCAPULAR MUSCLE, *Subscapula'ris Musc. Immer'sus, Infra-scapula'ris*, (F.) *Sous-scapulotrochinien* (Ch.), *Porte-feuille, Muscle sous-scapulaire*. A muscle situate in the above-mentioned fossa. It is flat, broad, and triangular; is attached, by its base, to the subscapulary fossa and to the anterior lip of the edge of the spine of the scapula, and is inserted into the lesser tuberosity of the humerus. It carries the arm in rotation inwards. It can also depress it, and bring it towards the body.

SUBSCAP'ULAR NERVES are two in number. One arises from the brachial plexus above the clavicle; the other from the posterior aspect of the plexus within the axilla. They are distributed to the subscapularis muscle.

SUBSE'ROUS, *Subsero'sus;* from *sub*, 'under,' and *serous*. Under a serous membrane, — as the '*subserous* areolar tissue.'

SUBSIDENTIA, Sediment.

SUBSTANCE ÉMAILLÉE DES DENTS, Enamel of the teeth — s. Horny, see Tooth.

SUBSTANCE, HYALINE, Cytoblastema—s. Intercellular, Cytoblastema—s. *Vitrée des Dents*, Enamel of the teeth.

SUBSTANCE, WHITE, OF SCHWANN. A hollow cylinder within the tubular nervous fibre, which differs in composition and refracting power from the matter that occupies the centre of the tube.

SUBSTANTIA ADAMANTINA DENTIUM, Enamel — s. Filamentosa dentium, Enamel — Hyalina, Cytoblastema — s. Ossea dentium, Tooth—s. Ostoidea, see Tooth.

SUBSTANT'IA PERFORA'TA ME'DIA. When the pia mater has been removed from the space between the crura cerebri termed the *interval*, or *interpedunc'ular*, the surface appears criblé from the perforations of the numerous minute vessels which penetrate it. This is the *substantia perfora'ta me'dia* of Vicq d'Azyr.

SUBSTANTIA PULPOSA DENTIS, Dental pulp — Rhomboidea, Corpus dentatum — s. Spongio Urethræ, Corpus spongiosum urethræ—s. Vitrea dentium, Enamel of the teeth — s. Vitrea, Cytoblastema.

SUB'STANTIVE, *Substanti'vus;* from *subero* (*sub* and *stare*,) 'to stand under or subsist.' An epithet applied by Dr. Paris to aliments which are nutritious, in contradistinction to adjunctive aliments, which are themselves not possessed of nutritive virtues, but impart to the digestive organs greater energy, so as to enable them to extract more nutriment from the substantive aliments. Meat, for example, is a substantive aliment: the condiment, as mustard, eaten with it, an *adjective* aliment.

SUBSTILLUM, Stillicidium.

SUBSULTIO, Palpitation.

SUBSUL'TUS TEN'DINUM. *Saltus tendinum, Clonus subsultus, Subsultus, Corphology spasmod'ica, Myopal'mus, Twitching of the Tendons*

dons, (F.) *Soubressaut*, from *subsilire, subsultum,* (*sub* and *salire,*) 'to make short leaps.' Twitching, communicated to the tendons by the involuntary and instantaneous contraction of the muscular fibres. It is more observable at the wrist than elsewhere; and is an evidence of great cerebral irritability, and debility, when it occurs at an advanced period of fever.

The muscular agitations or twitchings observed in febrile diseases, especially of children, have been termed *Convulsibil'itas, Sclerotyr'bē febri'lis,* and *Irritabil'itas morbo'sa.*

SUBSURDITAS, Deafness.

SUB'UBERES, from *sub,* 'under,' and *ubera,* 'the breasts.' *Infan'tes sugen'tes, Sucking children.* Infants at the breast, in contradistinction to the *Exu'beres, αποψαλακτοι,* or those which have been weaned.

SUBUN'GUIAL, *Subun'guical,* (F.) *Sous-ungéale,* from *sub,* 'under,' and *unguis,* 'a nail.' Belonging to parts under the nail; — as *subungnial exostosis,* (F.) *Exostose sous-ungéale,* an exostosis under the nail of the great toe especially.

SUBVERSIO STOMACHI, Vomiturition.

SUBVERTEBRA, Sacrum.

SUBVERTEBRUM, Sacrum.

SUBVOLA, Hypothenar.

SUC, Succus — s. de Citron, see Citrus medica — *s. Gastrique,* Gastric juice — *s. Médullaire,* Marrow — *s. du Limon,* see Citrus medica.

SUCCA'GO, from *succus,* 'juice.' The inspissated juice of plants; robs, jellies, &c.

SUCCEDA'NEUM, *Succida'neum, Substitu'tum, Antiballom'enum, Surroga'tum, Antemballom'enum, Quid pro quo,* from *succedere,* (*sub,* and *cedere*), 'to go under, to come in place of another.' An epithet for medicines that may be substituted for others possessing similar properties.

SUCCENTURIA'TUS, from *succenturiare* (*snb,* and *centuria*), 'to supply a soldier to fill a vacancy;' and hence, 'to substitute or put in the room of.' That which is a substitute for another; as Renes *succenturiati,* Ventriculus *succenturiatus,* &c.

SUCCHAR, Saccharum.

SUCCIDANEUM, Succedaneum.

SUCCIN, Succinum.

SUCCINCTURA, Diaphragm.

SUCCINCTUS, Diaphragm.

SUCCINI RESINA, Musk, artificial.

SUCCIN'IC ACID, *Ac''idum Suc'cini, A. Succin'icum, Acor Succin'eus, Sal Succini, Sal volat'ilē Succini,* has been considered antispasmodic and diaphoretic, in the dose of from five to twenty grains.

SUC'CINUM, *Elec'trnm, Ambra, Ambram, Ampar, Bereni'cē, Amber, Yellow Amber,* (F.) *Succin, Ambre jaune.* This substance, which is found on the shores of the Baltic, is composed of a resinous matter, of essential oil, and an acid *sui generis.* It is inodorous, except when heated or rubbed; insipid; in fragments of a pale golden-yellow colour; transparent, and has a shining lustre. S. g. 1.08; insoluble in water, and slightly acted on by alcohol. It is used for affording its essential oil—the *O'leum* or *Bal'samum Suc'cini,* (F.) *Huile de Succin.* This oil possesses stimulant, antispasmodic, diuretic, and rubefacient properties.

The *O'leum Suc'cini rectifica'tum, Rectified Oil of Amber,* is made as follows:—*Oil of Amber,* Oj; *water,* Ovj. Mix in a glass retort, and distil until Oiv of the water have passed with the oil into the receiver; separate the oil from the water, and keep it in well-stopped bottles.—(Ph. U. S.)

The *White amber, Leuceleo'trum,* (F.) *Ambre blanc,* is a variety.

SUCCINUM CINEREUM, Ambergris — *s. Griseum,* Ambergris.

SUCCION, Sucking.

SUCCISA, *Scabiosa succisa* — *s. Pratensis, S.* succisa.

SUCCOLATA, Chocolate.

SUCCORY, WILD, Cichorium intybus, Chironia angularis.

SUC'CUBUS, from *sub,* and *cubare,* 'to lie.' Some authors have used this word synonymously with nightmare. Others mean by it a female phantom, with which a man in his sleep may believe he has intercourse; — as *Incubus* has been applied to the male phantom, with which a female may dream she is similarly situate.

SUCCUS, *Chylus, Opos, Opis'ma, Chylis'ma, Ecchylo'ma, Apothlim'ma, Juice,* (F.) *Suc.* The fluid obtained by pressing plants, flesh, &c.; *succus expres'sus.* It is, also, applied to certain animal fluids, as *S. Gastricus,* &c.

SUCCUS ACACIÆ GERMANICÆ INSPISSATUS, see Prunus spinosa—*s.* Acaciæ nostratis, see Prunus spinosa — *s.* Arborum, Sap — *s.* Cicutæ spissatus, Extractum conii — *s.* Cyrenaicus, Laserpitium.

SUCCUS ENTER'ICUS, *S. Intestina'lis, Intes'tinal Juice.* The fluid secreted from the lining membrane of the small intestines.

SUCCUS EXPRESSUS, Apothlimma — *s.* Gastricus, Gastric juice — *s.* Glycyrrhizæ, Extractum glycyrrhizæ — *s.* Hypocistidis, see Cytinus — *s.* Intestinalis, Succus entericus — *s.* Japonicus, Catechu — *s.* Limonis, see Citrus medica — *s.* Liquiritiæ, Extractum glycyrrhizæ — *s.* Nerveus, Nervous fluid — *s.* Nutritius, Chyle — *s.* Orni concretus, see Fraxinus ornus — *s.* Pancreaticus, see Pancreas — *s.* Spissatus Aconiti Napelli, Extractum aconiti — *s.* Spissatus atropæ belladonnæ, Extractum belladonnæ — *s.* Spissatus conii maculati, Extractum cicutæ — *s.* Spissatus hyoscyami nigri, Extractum hyoscyami — *s.* Spissatus lactucæ sativæ, Extractum lactucæ.

SUCCUS'SION, *Hippocrat'ic Succus'sion, Succus'sio,* from *succutio* (*sub,* and *quatio*), 'I shake from beneath.' A mode of ascertaining the existence of a fluid in the thorax, (*fluctuation by succussion,*) by giving the body one or more slight shakes.

SUCCUSSION, *Ballottement.*

SUCHOR, Saccharum.

SUCKING, *Suc'tio, Suctus, Athelx'is, Bdalsis, Myze'sis,* (F.) *Succion,* from *sugere, suctum,* 'to suck.' The act of drawing liquid into the mouth, by forming a vacuum with the tongue acting as a piston, during inspiration.

SUCKING BOTTLE. A bottle so formed, that, when filled with milk, it can be sucked from instead of the breast.

SUCKING CHILD, *Lactens.* A suckling.

SUCKLE, *Lactare, γαλακτοτροφειν, τιθηνυειν,* (F.) *Allaiter* ou *Alaiter.* To give suck. To nurse.

SUCKLING, Lactation, Sucking child.

SUCRE, Saccharum — *s. Candi,* Saccharum candidum — *s. de Lait,* Sugar of milk — *s. de Saturne,* Plumbi superacetas.

SUCTIO, Exsuctio, Sucking,

SUCTION POWER. The force exerted on the blood in the veins, by the active dilatation of the heart. See Derivation.

SUCTO'RIA, from *sugo,* 'I suck.' Animals provided with mouths for sucking. Also, organs for sucking or adhesion,—hence termed *suctorial* — as '*suctorial oscula.*'

SUCTORIAL, see Suctoria.

SUCTUS, Sucking.

SUDAM'INA, *Hydro'ata, Hidro'ta, Pap'ulæ sudora'les, Suffersu'ræ, Alha'sef, Planta noctis, Boa,* from *sudor,* 'sweat.' Small vesicles, which appear upon the skin, especially in the summer time, in hot countries, and in diseases attended with much sweating. It is a miliary eruption. See Miliary fever.

SUDAMINA, Desudatio, *Échauboulures*, Lichen tropicus.

SUDARIUM, Achicolum.
SUDATION, Hidrosis.
SUDATORIA, Hidrosis — s. Maligna, see Sudor Anglicus.
SUDATORIUM, Achicolum.
SUDOR, *Hidros*, (F.) *Sueur*, 'sweat.' The product of cutaneous transpiration, when visible on the surface of the body. It is colourless; of an odour more or less strong and variable; and of a saline taste. It is composed, according to Berselius, of water, lactic acid, lactate of soda united with a little animal matter, chloride of sodium, and a little chloride of potassium, an atom of earthy phosphate, and some oxyd of iron.

SUDOR, Miliary fever.
SUDOR AN'GLICUS, *Hidron'osos, Hidrop'yra, Hidropyr'etos, Febris sudato'ria, Milia'ris sudato'ria, Sudor milia'ris, Morbus sudatorius, Ephem'era malig'na, E. sudatoria, E. Britan'nica, Pestis Britannica, Sudato'ria malig'na, E. An'glica pestilens, Sweating Sickness, Sweating Fever*, (F.) *Suette, S. Miliare, S. épidémique, Sueur Anglaise*. A very severe epidemic disease, characterized by profuse sweating, which appeared in England in 1486; and recurred, at different times, until about the middle of the 16th century. It was accompanied with coldness, excessive prostration of strength, palpitation, frequency and inequality of the pulse, &c., and terminated favourably or unfavourably in the course of 24 hours. The French have given the name SUETTE DE PICARDIE, *Suette des Picards, Fièvre suante; Miliaris sudatoria, Sudor Picard'icus*, to an epidemic disease, which has appeared several times in that province; the principal symptoms of which were profuse sweats and a miliary eruption. The disease recurred in 1821, and has been described, at length, by M. Rayer, who considers it to consist of a simultaneous state of inflammation of various tissues; and proposes to class it with variola, scarlatina, and measles.

SUDOR COLLIQUATIVUS, S. Profusus.
SUDOR CRUEN'TUS, *S. sanguin'eus, Hæmatidro'sis, Hæmathidro'sis, Epidro'sis cruen'ta, Hæmorrhag''ia per Cutem*, (F.) *Hématidrose, Sueur de Sang; Sweating of blood, Bloody sweat, Hem'orrhage from the skin*. Cutaneous perspiration intermixed with blood: — a very uncommon affection.

SUDOR DULCIS, *Saccharorrhœ'a cuta'nea, Ephidro'sis sacchara'ta*. A discharge of saccharine matter by perspiration.

SUDOR LOCALIS, Meridrosis—s. Miliaris, Miliary fever, Sudor Anglicus—s. Partialis, Meridrosis.
SUDOR PERFU'SUS, *S. Colliquati'vus*. A profuse or immoderate sweat.
SUDOR SANGUINEUS, Sudor cruentus — s. Universalis, Panhidrosis.
SUDORIFER, Sudoriferous, Sudorific.
SUDORIF'EROUS, *Sudor'ifer, Hydroph'orus*, from *sudor*, 'sweat,' and *fero*, 'I carry.' That which carries sweat, as the *sudoriferous* ducts or glands.
SUDORIF'IC, *Sudorif'icum, Sudor'ifer, Hidrot'icum, Hydrote'rium, Hydrotopœ'um, Hidropoët'icum*, from *sudor*, 'sweat,' and *facio*, 'I make.' A medicine which provokes sweating. See Diaphoretic.
FOUR SUDORIFIC WOODS, *Quat'uor ligna sudorifica*, were, formerly, *guaiacum, perfumed cherry, sarsaparilla*, and *sassafras*.
SUDORIPAROUS, see Perspiration.

SUDORIS NULLITAS, Anidrosis — s. Privatio, Anidrosis — s. Suppressio, Ischidrosis.
SUET, Sevum.
SUETTE, Sudor Anglicus — s. Ép[...], Sudor Anglicus — s. *Miliaire*, Sudor Ang. — s. *de Picardie*, Sudor picardicus—s. [...], Sudor picardicus.
SUEUR, Sudor— s. *Anglaise*, Sudor A[...] — s. *d'Expression*, Expression, sweat of — s. *Sang*, Diapedesis, Sudor cruentus.
SUFFERSURÆ, Sudamina.
SUFFIMEN, Suffimentum.
SUFFIMENT'UM, *Hypocapnis'ma, S[...] Thymi'ama, Suffi'tus, Suffumiga'tio, S[...] tion*, (F.) *Parfum*. A perfume; suffum[...] gation.
SUFFITIO, Fumigation.
SUFFITUS, Fumigation, Suffimentum.
SUFFLATIO, Puffiness.
SUFFOCATIO, Suffocation, Orthop[...] Hypochondriaca, Hypochondriasis—s. H[...] Angone — s. Stridula, Cynanche trache[...] Uterina, Angone.
SUFFOCA'TION, *Suffoca'tio, Pre[...] Apopnix'is, Asphyx'ia, Melanæ'ma*, from 'under,' and *fucus*, 'a fire-place.' Death suspended animation from impeded resp[...] whether caused by the *inhalation of noxi[...] drowning, hanging, strangling*, or *smothe[...] principal morbid appearances in such ca[...]—the lungs of a deep-blue colour, with the extravasated in the air-cells; right aur[...] ventricle filled with dark blood, as well [...] neighbouring veins; lividity of the count[...] turgescence, and, perhaps, rupture of the [...] of the brain.

Treatment of suspended animation by m[...] in general. The patient must be conve[...] a room not too warm. Blood-letting m[...] used, if at all, with caution; — friction m[...] employed with salt, or warm flannels; stim[...] fluids, in a dilute state, be poured into th[...] mach by means of a tube, and attempts be m[...] to inflate the lungs. Laryngotomy, if nece[...]
SUFFOCATION, *Pnigopho'bia*, (F.) Étou[...] is used for threatened suffocation, as one [...] is. It means the state of dyspnœa and [...] sion experienced when a sufficient quantity[...] does not enter the lungs, or when the chem[...] phenomena of respiration are imperfectly [...] cuted; as in cases of asthma.

SUFFOCATION UTÉRINE, Hysteria.
SUFFRAGO, Poples.
SUFFUMIGATION, Suffimentum.
SUFFUMIGE, Suffimentum.
SUFFUMIGIUM, Fumigation.
SUFFUMINATIO, Fumigation.
SUFFUSIO, Pseudoblepsia — s. Aurigi[...] Icterus—s. Bilis, Icterus—s. Colorans, Chrom[...] sia—s. Dimidians, Hemiopia—s. Exclaran[...] opia — s. Fellis, Icterus — s. Lentis crys[...] Cataract — s. Metamorphosis, Metamorph[...] s. Multiplicans, see Diplopia — s. Myodes [...] morphopsia—s. Nigra, Amaurosis—s. Ocu[...] taract, Pseudoblepsia — s. Oculorum, Me[...] phopsia — s. Radians, Scotasma — s. Sang[...] Ecchymoma.

SUGAR, Saccharum — s. Barley, Pen[...] s. Candy, Saccharum candidum — s. C[...] Saccharum—s. Diabetic, Glucose—s. Fru[...] cose — s. Grape, Glucose — s. Honey, Gluc[...] s. of Lead, Plumbi superacetas.
SUGAR OF MILK, *Sac'charum lactis, G[...] sac'charum, Lactine*, (F.) *Sucre de Lait*, [...] tained from whey by evaporation and cry[...] zation. It possesses the demulcent properti[...] the sugars.

SUGAR, PINE, see Arrowroot — s. Starch, Glucose.

SUGARS, VARIOUS, see Saccharum.

SUGARBERRY, Celtis occidentalis.

SUGGILLA'TION, *Sugilla'tio, Livor, Sugillation, Œde'ma cruentum;* a *bruise;* from *sugillare,* 'to give a black eye.' By most authors used synonymously with ecchymosis and ecchymoma. It is, also, applied to the spots, or ecchymoses which occur in consequence of intrinsic causes,— in disease and in incipient putrefaction. It is common in dead bodies. To this last case it is, indeed, restricted by some medico-legal writers; and an interesting question sometimes arises :— Whether the appearance have been induced before death or afterwards? Whether it be a case of *ecchymosis* or of *suggillation*? In the former, the extravasated blood will usually be coagulated; not so in the latter. It is often, however, difficult to form a correct judgment without reference to the history of the case.

SUGGRUN'DIUM, perhaps from *suggredi,* 'to go under.' The cave of a house.

SUGGRUNDIUM OCULI, Superciliary arch — s. Superciliorum, Frontal protuberance.

SUICIDA, Autochir.

SUICIDAL INSANITY, Suicide.

SU'ICIDE, *Suici'dium:* from *sui cædes,* 'murder of one's self.' The act of killing one's self. *Autochi'ria, Autocton'ia, Idiocton'ia, Autophon'ia.* Suicide is very frequently the result of disease of the mind; the individual seeming, at times, to be irresistibly impelled to self-destruction. — *Melancho'lia Suicid'ium, M. autochi'ria, Suici'dal Insanity.* Also, one who commits self-murder.

SUIE, Fuligo.

SUIF, Sevum.

SUITES DE COUCHES, Lochia.

SULCATUS, Cannelé, Grooved.

SULCULUS LABII SUPERIORIS, Lacuna Labii superioris.

SULCUS, *Semicana'lis, Semicanalic'ulus.* A furrow. A groove. (F.) *Sillon.* Anatomists have given this name to grooves on the surface of bones and other organs.

French writers on anatomy often use the term *Sillons* for the grooves which lodge the arteries and creep on the surface of bones; whilst those that receive veins are called *gouttières*, 'gutters.' Also, the vulva.

SULCUS ANTERO-POSTERIOR JECORIS, see Liver — s. Labii superioris, Lacuna Labii superioris.

SULCUS, LAT'ERAL, ANTE'RIOR, OF THE SPINAL MARROW. A mere trace on the marrow, marked only by the attachment of the filaments of the anterior roots of the spinal nerves.

SULCUS, LATERAL, POSTERIOR, OF THE SPINAL MARROW, corresponds with the attachment of the posterior roots of the spinal nerves.

SULCUS TRANSVERSALIS, see Liver— s. Umbilicalis, see Liver.

SULFATE D'AMMONIAQUE, Ammoniæ sulphas.

SULFIDUM CARBONII, Carbonis sulphuretum.

SULFUR, Sulphur.

SULFURE DE CARBON, Carbonis sulphuretum.

SULPHAS ALUMINARIS, Alumen—s. Ammoniacus Cupratus, Cuprum ammoniatum—s. Cadmicus, Cadmii Sulphas — s. Kalico-aluminicum, Alumen—s. Natricus, Soda, sulphate of—s. Zincicum, Zinci sulphas.

SULPHUR, *Sulfur, Scorith, Thei'on, Thion, Averich, Terra folia'ta, Fumus cit'rinus, Aq'uila, Brimstone,* (F.) *Soufre.* The *Native Sulphur* is called *Rock Sulphur, Sulphur vivum,* &c. Sulphur, as we meet with it, is in *rolls, Sulphur in rot'ulis, S. rotun'dum, Roll Brimstone.* It is a volcanic production, and is obtained, in large quantities, from Solfatara, in Italy. *Roll Sulphur* is impure sulphur, melted, and run into moulds. It is unpleasantly odorous, when heated or rubbed; insipid; solid, and brittle. S. g. 1.99. Fusible at 226°; volatilizable by heat, and condensing unchanged.

SULPHUR ANTIMONIATUM, Antimonii sulphuretum præcipitatum—s. Carburet of, Carbonis sulphuretum—s. Chloratum, Sulphur, Chloride of.

SULPHUR, CHLORIDE OF, *Sul'phuris Chlo'ridum, Sul'phuris Dichlo'ridum, Dichlo'ride of Sulphur, Protochlo'ride of Sulphur, Hypochlo'ride of Sulphur, Subchlo'ride of Sulphur, Sulphur chlora'tum, Hypochlore'tum sulphuro'sum, Bisulph'uret of Chlorine, Chlorum hypersulphura'tum,* is obtained by passing *dry chlorine gas* over washed and dried *flowers of sulphur,* until they are for the most part dissolved, and distilling the decanted fluid from the excess of dissolved sulphur. One drachm of the liquid to an ounce of lard has been used in lepra, psoriasis, and other chronic cutaneous diseases. Ten drops, dissolved in ether, have been given in adynamic fever.

SULPHUR, DICHLORIDE OF, Sulphur, chloride of—s. Hypochloride of, Sulphur, chloride of — s. Iodatum, Sulphuris iodidum — s. Iodide of, Sulphuris iodidum—s. Ioduret of, Sulphuris iodidum — s. Liver of, Potassæ sulphuretum.

SULPHUR LOTUM, *Sulphur sublima'tum lotum, Washed Sulphur, Magiste'rium Sulph'uris, Sulphuris Flores loti,* is prepared by pouring boiling water on sublimed sulphur, so as to wash away any acid it may contain, and then drying it.

SULPHUR PRÆCIPITA'TUM, *Lac Sulph'uris, Milk of Sulphur, Precip'itated Sulphur,* (F.) *Crème de Soufre,* is prepared by boiling sublimed sulphur and lime together, and adding muriatic acid to precipitate the sulphur.

SULPHUR, PROTOCHLORIDE OF, Sulphur, chloride of—s. Subchloride of, Sulphur, chloride of.

SULPHUR SUBLIMA'TUM, *Sulphur,* (Ph. U. S.) *Sublimed Sulphur, Flowers of Sulphur,* (F.) *Soufre sublimé, Fleurs de Soufre,* is the sulphur of commerce, sublimed in close vessels.

Sulphur is possessed of stimulant, laxative, and diaphoretic properties. As a laxative, it is used in hæmorrhoidal and other affections. In the itch, applied externally and taken internally, it has been considered as a specific (?), and it is a valuable remedy in most cutaneous affections that are local. Dose, ʒss to ʒij.

The fæces or dregs, left in the purification or sublimation of sulphur, are called *Horse Brimstone, Dregs of Sulphur vivum, Sulphur caballi'num, S. vivum, Sulphuris vivi recremen'ta.* They are very impure, and are only used externally.

SULPHUR, VEGETABLE, Lycopodium—s. Wort, Peucedanum.

SULPHURATUS, Sulphureous, Sulphurated.

SULPHU'REOUS, *Sulphuro'sus, Sulphu'rius, Sulphura'tus, Sulph'uretted.* Possessing the properties of, or relating to, or containing sulphur.

SULPHURETTED, Sulphureous — s. Hydrogen, see Hydrogen, sulphuretted.

SULPHURETUM AMMONIACÆ, Ammoniæ sulphuretum—s. Ammoniæ hydrogenatum, Liquor fumans Boylii—s. Kalicum, Potassæ sulphuretum —s. Lixiviæ, Potassæ sulphuretum.

SULPH'URIC ACID, *Ac''idum Sulphu'ricum* vel *Sulfuricum, Oleum Vitrio'li, Spir'itus Vitrioli, S. v. fortis, Acidum vitriol'icum, Oil of Vitriol, Spirit of Vitriol, Vitriol'ic Acid, Acidum Vitrioli dephlogistica'tum, Acor Sulphuris,* (F.) *Acide Sulphurique* ou *Sulfurique.* Sulphuric acid is inodorous; has a strong acid taste, and is corrosive. S. g. 1.845 (Ph. U. S.) It is escharotic, stimulant, and rubefacient. Mixed with lard, it is sometimes used in local pains, and certain cutaneous affections.

SULPHURIC ACID, AROMAT'IC, *Ac''idum Sulphu'ricum Aromat'icum, A. vitriol'icum aromat'icum, A. vitriolicum alcoho'lĭ aromaticum, Elixir vitri-o'li, E. v. aromaticum, E. vitrioli Mynsich'ti, E. vitrioli Edinburgen'sium, E. vitrioli cum tinctu'râ aromaticâ, E. vitrioli dulcĕ seu acido-aromat'icum, Alcohol cum aromat'ibus sulphurica'tus, Tinctu'ra acidi sulphurici*, is formed of *sulphuric acid*, f℥iijss; *ginger*, bruised, ℨj; *cinnamon*, bruised, ℨiss; *Alcohol*, Oij.—Ph. U. S. Dose, gtt. x to xxx.

SULPHURIC ACID, DILU'TED, *Ac''idum Sulphu'ricum Dilu'tum, Acidum vitriol'icum dilutum, Elixir of Vitriol, Elixir vitrio'li, Spir'itus vitrio'li ac''idus Vogle'ri*, (F.) *Acide sulfurique délayé*, is formed, according to the Pharmacopœia of the United States, by adding *aq. destillat.* f℥xij, to *acid. sulph.* f℥j. It is tonic, astringent, and refrigerant. Dose, gtt. x to xx, largely diluted. When used as a gargle, half a drachm may be added to ℨvj of water.

Very dilute sulphuric acid was formerly termed *Phlegma vitrioli*.

SULPHURIS CHLORIDUM, Sulphur, chloride of—s. Dichloridum, Sulphur, chloride of.

SULPH'URIS IO'DIDUM, *S. Iodure'tum, Sulphur Ioda'tum, Ioduret* or *l'odide of Sulphur*, (F.) *Soufre Ioduré, Ioduré de Soufre*. It is thus directed to be prepared in the Pharmacopœia of the U. S. (*Iodin.* ℨiv; *sulphur.* ℨj.) Rub the iodine and sulphur together in a glass, porcelain, or marble mortar, until they are thoroughly mixed. Put the mixture into a matrass, close the orifice loosely, and apply a gentle heat, so as to darken the mass without melting it. When the colour has become uniformly dark throughout, increase the heat so as to melt the iodide; then incline the matrass in different directions, in order to return into the mass any portions of iodine which may have condensed on the inner surface of the vessel: lastly, allow the matrass to cool, break it, and put the iodide into bottles, which are to be well stopped.

SULPHURIUS, Sulphureous.
SULPHUROSUS, Sulphureous.
SULPHUROUS, Sulphureous.

SUL'PHUROUS ACID, *Ac''idum sulphuros'icum, A. sulph'uris volat'ilĕ, A. Sulphuro'sum* vel *Sulfurosum, Spir'itus sulphuris, Spiritus sulphuro'sus volat'ilis, Sp. sulphuris per campa'nam, Sp. vitrio'li phlogistica'tus, Gas sulphuris*, (F.) *Acide Sulfureux, Air Acide Vitriolique*. Obtained by treating mercury with concentrated sulphuric acid, or by burning sulphur. It is sometimes used in the gaseous,—at others, in the liquid state. Sulphurous acid gas is used to disinfect cloths, confined air, letters coming from infected places, &c. It is also exhibited, with great success, in the form of fumigation, in the treatment of certain chronic cutaneous affections, and of sciatic and rheumatic pains in general. If respired pure, it acts in the manner of violent irritants; and is not long in producing death.

SULTZMALT, MINERAL WATERS OF. Sultzmalt is a village in the department of the Upper Rhine; where are several sources of cold, acidulous waters, which seem to contain carbonic acid, subcarbonate of soda, subcarbonate of lime, sulphate of lime, and a little bitumen. They are refrigerant, aperient, and alterative.

SUMAC DES CORROYEURS, Rhus coriaria—*s. Vénéneux*, Rhus toxicodendron.

SUMACH, Rhus coriaria.

SUMBUL. The name of a root, *Sum'buli radix, Jatamansi, Musk-root*, presumed to belong to the Umbelliferæ family, much employed in Russia and Germany against cholera. Its exact botanical history is not determined. It contains a strongly odorous principle like that of musk; and is regarded as an antispasmodic.

SUMBULI RADIX, Sumbul root.
SUMEN, Hypogastrium.

SUMMER COMPLAINT. A popular term in the United States, for diarrhœa occurring in summer. It is often, also, made to include dysentery and cholera infantum. With some it means cholera infantum only.

SUMMER DISEASES, see Estival—s. Rash, Lichen tropicus.

SUMMITAS CUTIS, Epidermis.
SUMMUS HUMERUS, Acromion.

SUNBURN, Ephelides—s. Dew, Drosera rotundifolia—s. Flower, false, Helenium autumnale—s. Flower, swamp, Helenium autumnale—s. Flower, tickweed, Coreopsis trichosperma—s. Flower, turpentine, Silphium perfoliatum—s. Pain, see Hemicrania—s. Rash, Lichen—s. Stroke, *Coup de Soleil*—s. Egyptian, *Coup de Soleil*.

SUPELLECTILE DIOGENIS, Palm.
SUPELLEX ANATOMICA, Museum anatomicum—s. Diogenis, Palm.

SUPER. A common Latin prefix; in composition, signifying 'above.'

SUPERBUS, Rectus superior oculi.
SUPERCHLORIDUM FORMYLICI Chloroform.

SUPERCILIARIS, Corrugator supercilii.

SUPERCIL'IARY, *Supercilia'ris*, from 'above,' and *cilium*, 'the edge of the eyelid.' That which relates to the supercilia or eyebrows. (F.) *Sourcilier* ou *Surcilier*.

SUPERCIL'IARY ARCHES, *Superciliary Arcus supercilia'res, Suggrun'dia oculi—*Arcades sourcilières*, are two slightly raised apophyses, situate at the anterior surface of os frontis, above the superior margin of the orbits. They are separated by the nasal bone; covered by the superciliaris muscle, to which they give attachment.

SUPERCILIARY RIDGES, Superciliary arches.

SUPERCIL'IUM, *Ophrys, Oph'rys*, (F.) *Sourcil*. Same etymon. The eyebrow is two arched eminences,—convex above, and more or less prominent, according to the individual, which lie on the superciliary arch of the frontis, above the eyelids, and extend from the root of the nose to the temple. The inner extremity or *head* is more prominent than the outer or *tail*. The eyebrows are covered with short and stiff hairs, which are directed obliquely, from within outwards, and are, commonly, of the colour of the hair. The skin in which these hairs are implanted, rests on the *bicularis palpebrarum, frontalis*, and *superciliary* muscles, which move the eyebrows in different directions. The eyebrows serve as an ornament to the countenance; and by covering the eye defend it from the impression of too strong a light. They direct the perspiration away from the eye.

SUPERCILIUM ACETAB'ULI. The edge of the cotyloid cavity of the os innominatum.

SUPERCONCEPTION, see Superfœtation.
SUPEREVACUATIO, Hypercrisis.
SUPERFECUNDATION, see Superfœtation.

SUPERFICIA'LIS COLLI, *Nervus Colli*. A nerve formed by communicating branches from the second and third cervical nerves. It is distributed to the superficial parts of the neck.

SUPERFICIES PLANTARIS PEDIS, Sole.
SUPERFŒCUNDATIO, Superfœtation.

SUPERFŒTATIO, Superfœtation.
SUPERFŒTA'TION, *Superfœta'tio, Epicye'sis, Hypercye'sis, Superimprægna'tio, Epig'onè, Superfecunda'tio, Superfecunda'tion, Superimpregna'tion,* from *super,* 'upon,' and *fœtare,* 'to bring forth young.' Conception of a fœtus—*epicye'ma*—in a uterus which already contains one. The impregnation of a female already pregnant. The possibility of this has been denied; but there is abundant evidence to show, that it is possible at a very early period of pregnancy. Twin cases may be of this kind of *superconception.*
SUPERGEMINALIS, Epididymis.
SUPERGENUALIS, Patella.
SUPERHUMERALE, Epomis.
SUPERIMPRÆGNATIO, Superfœtation.
SUPERIOR AURIS, Attollens aurem—s. Rotundus clitoridis, Ischio-cavernous.
SUPERLABIA, Clitoris.
SUPERLIGAMEN, Epidesmus.
SUPERLIGULA, Epiglottis.
SUPERNUTRITIO LIENIS, Splenoncus—s. Splenis, Splenoncus.
SUPEROXALAS KALICUM, Potass, oxalate of.
SUPERPURGATIO, Hypercatharsis.
SUPERSCAPULARIS, Supraspinatus—s. Inferior, Infra-spinatus.
SUPINATEUR COURT ou *PETIT,* Supinator radii brevis — *s. Grand* ou *long,* Supinator radii longus.
SUPINA'TION, *Supina'tio,* from *supinus,* 'lying on the back.' The movement in which the forearm and hand are carried outwards, so that the *anterior* surface of the latter becomes *superior.*
In Pathology, *Supination, Supinatio, Hyptias'ma, Hyptias'mus,* means the horizontal position on the back, with the head thrown back, and the legs and arms extended. It is often a sign of great weakness in disease.
SUPINA'TOR. Same etymon. That which produces supination. A name given to two muscles of the forearm.
SUPINATOR BREVIS seu MINOR, Supinator radii brevis — s. Longus seu major, Supinator radii longus.
SUPINATOR RADII BREVIS, *S. brevis* seu *minor,* (F.) *Épicondylo-radial* (Ch.), *Supinateur court* ou *petit supinateur.* A muscle, seated at the outer and back part of the forearm. It is flattened, triangular, and curved upon itself, in such a manner that it embraces the superior extremity of the radius. It is attached, on the one hand, to the external tuberosity of the humerus, and to a small portion of the posterior surface of the ulna, and is inserted into the upper third of the outer and upper surfaces of the radius. It produces, by contracting, the motion of supination.
SUPINATOR RADII LONGUS, *S. longus* sive *major, Bra'chio-radia'lis,* (F.) *Huméro-sus-radial* (Ch.), *Long* ou *grand supinateur,* is seated at the anterior and outer part of the forearm. It arises from the inferior part of the outer edge of the os humeri, and from the external intermuscular aponeurosis; and is inserted, by a long tendon, into the outer edge of the radius, near the base of the styloid process. It causes the supination of the forearm, which it can likewise bend on the arm.
SUPPEDANEA, Hypopodia.
SUPPLANTALIA, Hypopodia.
SUPPLEMENTA EPIPLOICA, Epiploic appendages.
SUPPLEMENTARY AIR, see Respiration.
SUPPORTER, ABDOMINAL, Belt, Russian —s. Utero-Abdominal, see Belt, Russian.

SUPPOSITION DE PART, Pregnancy, pretended.
SUPPOSITORIUM, Suppository — s. Uterinum, Pessary.
SUPPOS'ITORY, *Supposito'rium, Hypoth'eton, Bacil'lus, Balanis'mus, Bal'anus, Glans,* from *supponere,* (*sub,* and *ponere,* 'to put,') 'to put under.' Any solid medicine, in the form of a cone or cylinder, intended to be introduced into the rectum;—either for the purpose of favouring intestinal evacuations, or to act as an anodyne. Purgative suppositories are made of soap, aloes, or any other irritating substance.
SUPPRESSIO ALVI, Constipation — s. Lochiorum, Ischolochia—s. Lotii, Ischuria—s. Mensium, Amenorrhœa — s. Menstruationis, Amenorrhœa—s. Sudoris, Ischidrosis.
SUPPRESSION DU FLUX MENSTRUEL, Amenorrhœa—*s. de Part,* see Parturition— *s. d' Urine,* Ischuria.
SUPPURANS, Suppurative.
SUPPURA'TION, *Suppura'tio, Ecpye'ma, Purulen'tia, Pyo'sis, Pye'sis, Diapye'ma, Diapye'sis, Pyogen'ia simplex, Pu'rulence, Pu'rulency,* (F.) *Aboutissement.* Formation or secretion of pus, (see, also *Pyogenia,*) from *sub,* 'under,' and *pus.* It is a frequent termination of inflammation, and may occur in almost any of the tissues. This termination is announced by slight chills, by remission of the pain, which, from being lancinating, becomes heavy; by a sense of weight in the part, and, when the collection of pus can be easily felt, by fluctuation. When pus is thus formed in the areolar membrane, and is collected in one or more cavities, it constitutes an *abscess.* If it be formed from a surface exposed to the air, it is an *ulcer:* and such ulcers we are in the habit of establishing artificially in certain cases of disease.
SUP'PURATIVE, *Suppu'rans, Suppurati'vus, Diapye'ticus, Ecpyo'ticus, Ecpyiscon'tus.* That which facilitates suppuration. Suppuratives are, generally, vesicants mixed with lard.
SUPRA. A common Latin prefix: in composition, signifying 'above.'
SUPRA-COSTA'LES, *Levato'res Costa'rum,* (F.) *Sur-costaux,* from *supra,* 'above,' and *costa,* 'a rib.' A name given to twelve small, fleshy fasciculi, which are flattened, triangular, and with radiating fibres. They pass from the transverse processes of the dorsal vertebræ to the superior margin of the rib beneath. Spigelius, Cowper, Boyer, Chaussier, and others consider them to form part of the intercostales externi.
SUPRA-OMPHALODYMIA, see Somatodymia — s. et Infra-omphalodymia, see Somatodymia.
SUPRA-OR'BITAR, *Supra-orbita'lis, Supraorbita'rius,* (F.) *Sus-orbitaire,* from *supra,* 'above,' and *orbita,* 'the orbit.' That which is situate above the orbit.
SUPRA-OR'BITAR FORA'MEN, *Fora'men Supraorbita'rium, F. orbitarium supe'rius,* (F.) *Trou sus-orbitaire* ou *orbitaire supérieur,* is a foramen or notch completed by a ligament at the inner third of the orbitar arch. It gives passage to the *supra-orbitar* or *superciliary artery,* a branch of the ophthalmic, which ascends the forehead, and is distributed thereto.
SUPRA-PU'BIAN, *Supra-pubic, Supra-pubia'nus,* from *supra,* and *pubes.* That which is seated above the pubis.
SUPRA-PUBIAN NERVE, (F.) *Nerf sus-pubien,* is the internal ramus of the inguino-cutaneous branch of the first lumbar nerve. It is the *genitocrural* branch of Bichat. It descends almost vertically before the psoas muscle; and, near the crural arch, divides into two branches. One of

these accompanies the spermatic cord, and is distributed to the cremaster, scrotum, and integuments on the inner part of the thigh. The other issues from the pelvis with the femoral filaments; traverses the aponeurosis of the thigh, and is distributed to the integuments of the upper and anterior part of the limb.

SUPRA-RE'NAL, *Supra-rena'lis*, (F.) *Surrénal*, from *supra*, 'above,' and *ren*, 'the kidney.' Seated above the kidney—as the *supra-renal* capsule.

SUPRA-SCAPULAR; *Supra-scapula'ris*; from *supra*, 'above,' and *scapula*. Seated above the scapula;—as

SUPRA-SCAPULAR NERVE. This arises from the fifth cervical; passes through the supra-scapular notch, and is distributed to the supra-spinatus and infra-spinatus muscles.

SUPRA-SCAPULARIS, Supra-scapular, and Supraspinatus muscle.

SUPRA-SEMIORBICULARIS, Orbicularis oris.

SUPRA-SPINA'TUS, *Supra-spino'sus*, (F.) *Sur-épineux, Sus-épineux*, from *supra*, and *spina*. That which is seated above the spine.

SUPRA-SPINATA FOSSA, (F.) *Fosse sus-épineuse*, is a triangular depression above the spine of the scapula.

SUPRA-SPINATUS MUSCLE, *Super-scapula'ris, Supra-scapularis*, (F.) *Sus-spino-scapulo-trochitérien, Petit sus-scapulo-trochitérien* (Ch.), is situate in the fossa supra-spinata. It is elongated, thick, and triangular, and is attached, on the one hand, to the two inner thirds of the fossa supra-spinata; and terminates, on the other, at the anterior part of the great tuberosity of the humerus. This muscle raises the arm.

SUPRA-SPINO'SA LIGAMEN'TA, *Supra-spinal lig'amenta*, are two in number. 1. The *Dorso-lumbo-supra-spinal ligament*, (F.) *Ligament sur-épineux dorso-lombaire*, extending above the spinous processes of the dorsal and lumbar vertebræ from the 7th cervical as far as the median crista of the sacrum. 2. *Cervical-supra-spinal ligament*, (F.) *Ligament-sur-épineux cervical*, which extends above all the cervical spinous processes, and is attached, above, to the outer occipital protuberance.

SUR, *Supra*. A French prefix, signifying 'above.'

SURA, *Gastrocne'mē, Gastrocne'mia, Gastrocne'mium*; calf of the leg, (F.) *Mollet, Gras de Jambe*. The projection, formed at the posterior part of the leg by the gastrocnemii muscles. Also, the fibula.

SURCILIER, Corrugator supercilii, Superciliary.

SURCOSTAUX, Supracostales.
SURCULI FELLEI, Pori biliarii.
SURCULUS, Ramusculus.

SURDENT (F.), *supra*, 'above,' and *dens*, 'a tooth.' When a milk-tooth does not fall out at the period of the second dentition, but is merely forced to one side by the new tooth, it is called a *surdent*.

SURDITAS, Cophosis, Deafness.
SURDITÉ, Cophosis, Deafness.
SURDOMUTITAS, Deaf-dumbness.
SUREAU COMMUN, Sambucus.
SURELLE, Oxalis acetosella.
SURÉPINEUX, Supra-spinatus.
SUR-EXCITATION, see Excitement, and Super-excitation.
SURFEIT, Colica crapulosa.

SURGEON, *Chirur'geon*; old French, *Surgien, Chiro'nax, Chirur'gus, Vul'nerum med'icus, Oheiria'ter, Ohiria'ter, Iätrus*, (F.) *Chirurgien*, from χείρ, 'the hand,' and εργον, 'work.' One who practises surgery. The surgeon, says Celsus, ought to be young, or, at all events, not advanced in life. His hand must be steady, expert, and never tremulous: he must use the right or left with equal facility: his sight must be clear and penetrating: his mind intrepid; and although not moved when he proceeds to operate, he must not be in haste, nor cut less than is necessary, to finish his operation, as if the cries of the patient made no impression upon him.

In the middle ages, the Universities of Italy and Spain sent out educated surgeons, as well as physicians, under the name *chirurgi-physici*.

SURGEON-APOTH'ECARY. One who unites the practice of surgery with that of the apothecary. A *general practitioner*.

SURGEON-DENTIST, Dentist.
SUR'GEONCY. The office of a surgeon.

SUR'GERY, *Chirur'gia, Chiriatri'a, Cheirisis, Chi'risis, Chirix'is, Chirie'mus, Metachirisis, Metachi'risis, Metachiris'mus, Tracta'tio manuaria, Medici'na operati'va, Medici'na ef'ficax. Chirurgie*. The part of the healing art which relates to external diseases; their treatment, and, especially, to the manual operations adapted for their cure. Also, the office of a surgeon.

SURGERY, ANAPLASTIC, Morioplastice — Autoplastic, Morioplastice — s. Dental, Dentistry.

SURGERY, MIL'ITARY, (F.) *Chirurgie militaire*, is that which relates to the operations to be performed on the field of battle, or subsequently:— with the attention to be paid to the wounded, &c.

SURGERY, OP'ERATIVE, is termed *Acivrgia, Acur'gia*, and *Acidur'gia*, (F.) *Médecine opératoire*.

SURGERY, PLASTIC, Morioplastica.

SUR'GICAL, *Chirur'gicus*, (F.) *Chirurgical, Chirurgique*. That which relates to surgery, as surgical anatomy, surgical operations, surgical instruments, &c.

SURGIEN, Surgeon.
SURINAMINE, see Geoffræa Surinamensis.
SUR-IRRITATION, see Irritation.

SUROXYGÉNÈSES. A name given by Baumes to diseases attributed by him to superabundance of oxygen.

SURPEAU, Epidermis.
SURRECTA ALBA, Ranunculus flammula.
SUR-RENAL, Supra-renal.
SURROGATUM, Succedaneum.
SURSELS, see Salt.

SURTOUTS LIGAMENTEUX DE LA COLONNE VERTÉBRALE, Vertebral ligaments.

SURUMPE (S.) A disease to which the traveller in the Cordilleras is liable. It consists in a violent inflammation of the eyes, caused by the reflection of the bright rays of the sun. The eyes become highly inflamed, and the lids swell and bleed. The pain is intense, and frequently produces delirium. — Tschudi.

SURVIE, Survivorship.

SURVI'VORSHIP, (F.) *Survie*, from super-vivere, (*super*, and *vivere*,) *survivere*, 'to live longer.' In *legal medicine*, this word means probably that any individual has survived others in an accident, which has been fatal. This is often an important question, connected with the inheritance of property, and on which physiology can rarely afford more than presumptive grounds for conclusion.

SUS, *Supra*. A French prefix, signifying 'above.'

SUS-ACROMIO-HUMÉRAL, Deltoid.

SUS-CARPIEN; from *sus*, (F.) 'above,' and *carpe*, 'the wrist.' Above the wrist. An epithet given by Chaussier to the dorsal artery of the wrist — *Artère sus-carpienne* — a branch of the radial.

SUS-ÉPINEUX, Supra-spinatus—s. *Maxillo-labial*, Levator anguli oris—s. *Maxillo-labial, grand*, Levator labii superioris alæque nasi—s. *Maxillo-labial moyen*, Levator labii superioris proprius—s. *Maxillo-nasal*, Compressor naris—s. *Omphalodymie*, see Somatodymia—s. *Optico-sphéno-scléroticien*, Rectus superior oculi—s. *Orbitaire*, Supra-orbitar—s. *Phalangien du pouce*, Abductor pollicis brevis—s. *Pubio-fémoral*, Pectinalis—s. *Scapulo-trochitérien, le plus petit*, Teres minor—s. *Scapulo-trochitérien, petit*, Supra-spinatus—s. *Spino-scapulo-trochitérien*, Supra-spinatus.

SUSCEPTIBIL'ITY, *Facilè suscipiens*, (sub or *sus*, and *capio*, 'I take,') 'easily taking, or undertaking.' Sensibility, in its most enlarged acceptation. Impressibility. This term, with the epithet *nervous*, is sometimes used for that increase in the moral sensibility which is particularly observed in nervous affections.

SUSCEPTIO INTESTINORUM, Intussusception.

SUSPENDICULUM, Cremaster.

SUSPENSA, Enæorema.

SUSPENSOIRE, Suspensory.

SUSPENSORIUM, Suspensory—s. Testis, Cremaster.

SUSPEN'SORY, *Suspenso'rius*, from *suspendere*, (sub or *sus*, 'under,' and *pendere*, 'to hang,') 'to hang under.' (F.) *Suspensoire*. That which sustains or suspends.

SUSPENSORY BANDAGE, *Suspenso'rium*, is a bandage intended to support the scrotum, in cases of disease of the testicle or of scrotal hernia. It consists of a kind of bag, fixed above to a cincture, and retained below by strings passing between the thighs, and fixed to the cincture behind.

SUSPENSORY LIGAMENT OF THE LIVER, *Ligamen'tum suspenso'rium he'patis, Perpendic'ulum he'patis*, is a triangular duplicature of the peritoneum, between the inferior surface of the diaphragm and the upper surface of the liver, which is continuous with the great falx of the umbilical vein.

SUSPENSORY LIGAMENT OF THE PENIS is a fibro-cellular fascia, of a triangular shape, which extends from the anterior part of the symphysis pubis to the corpus cavernosum, which it sustains. A similar ligament belongs to the clitoris.

SUSPENSUM, Enæorema—s. Urinæ, Enæorema.

SUSPIRATION, Suspirium.

SUSPIRATUS, Suspirium.

SUSPIRITUS, Suspirium.

SUSPIR'IUM, *Suspira'tio, Suspira'tus, Suspir'itus*, from *sub* or *sus*, 'under,' and *spiro*, 'I breathe ;' *Mygmus, Mych'mus, Mychthis'mus, Stenag'mus, Stenax'is, Sigh, Suspira'tion*, (F.) *Soupir*. A short breathing. A slow, voluntary contraction of the diaphragm and intercostal muscles, the effect of which is to restore the due relation between the circulation and respiration, or to free ourselves from an inconvenient sense of weight felt in the chest, when we are much depressed,—a weight, which appears to be chiefly dependent on the functions of the heart being disturbed through the moral influence. The sigh differs from the *sob:*—the latter being involuntary and spasmodic. Sighing, occurring in fevers to a great extent, indicates considerable depression. When accompanied with a vocal sound, it constitutes a *groan*.

SUSPIRIUM CARDIACUM, Angina pectoris.

SUSTENTACULUM, Aliment.

SUSTENTATOR CLITORIDIS, Erector-clitoridis—s. Penis, Erector penis.

SUSURRATION, Whispering.

SUSURRUS, *Bourdonnement:*—s. Aurium, Tinnitus aurium.

SUTELA, Suture.

SUTERBERRY, Xanthoxylum fraxineum.

SUTORIUS, Sartorius.

SUTTER, Saccharum.

SUTURA ABDOMINALIS, Gastroraphy—s. Arcualis, Coronal suture—s. Biparietalis, Sagittal suture—s. Clavata, Suture, quilled—s. Corporis callosi externa, see Raphe—s. Cranii squamosa, Squamous suture—s. Dentata, see Suture—s. Frontoparietalis, Coronal suture—s. Jugalis, Sagittal suture—s. Lambdoidalis, Lambdoid suture—s. Limbosa, see Suture—s. Lepidoides, Squamous suture—s. Mendosa, Squamous suture—s. Notha, see Suture—s. Obelæa, Sagittal suture—s. Ossium Spuria, Harmony—s. Proræ, Lambdoid suture—s. Punctata, Suture, common—s. Puppis, Coronal suture—s. Rhabdoides, Sagittal suture—s. Serrata, see Suture, Sagittal suture—s. Vera, see Suture.

SUTURAL, *Sutura'lis;* same etymon as the next. Relating to a suture.

SUTURE, *Sutu'ra, Sute'la, Armê, Rhaphê,* from *suere, sutum*, 'to stitch ;' *Dove-tail joint*, (F.) *Engrenure*. A kind of immovable articulation, in which the bones unite by means of serrated edges, which are, as it were, *dove-tailed* into each other. The articulations of the greater part of the bones of the skull are of this kind. The coronal, lambdoidal, and sagittal sutures are called *true sutures*, the two temporal are called *false sutures, suturæ nothæ*.

A *dentated suture — Sutu'ra denta'ta —* is one in which the processes are long and dentiform, as in the interparietal suture. In a *serrated suture — sutu'ra seu syntax'is serra'ta —* the indentations and processes are small and fine, like the teeth of a saw, as in the suture between the two portions of the frontal bone. In the *sutu'ra limbo'sa* there is along with the dentated margins a degree of bevelling of one, so that one bone rests on the other, as in the occipito-parietal suture.

SUTURE, in *Surgery, Rha'phê*, means an operation which consists in stitching the lips of a wound to procure their union. The suture was, at one time, largely employed; but, in modern times, its use has been wisely restricted. There are few wounds in which the edges may not be brought together by adhesive plaster appropriately applied. This kind of union, by adhesive plaster simply, has been absurdly termed *Sutura sicca* or *dry suture*, in opposition to the *Sutura cruenta* or suture properly so called. The suture is generally performed with waxed thread and straight or curved needles, according to the arrangement of parts.

The chief sutures are the *interrupted suture*, the *quilled suture*, the *glover's suture*, and the *twisted suture*. 1. The INTERRUP'TED SUTURE, (F.) *Suture à points séparés, Suture entrecoupée*, is performed by passing a needle, armed with a ligature, through the lips of the wound previously brought into contact; and then tying the extremities of the thread. The other stitches are made in the same manner. They are separate or interrupted. It is the suture most commonly used. 2. The QUILLED SUTURE, *Sutura clava'ta*, (F.) *Suture enchevillée* ou *emplumée* ou *empennée, Compound Suture*, is merely the interrupted suture, with this difference, that the ligatures are not tied over the face of the wound, but over two quills or rolls of plaster, or bougies, which are laid along the sides of the wound. It is used by some surgeons, on account of there being less danger of the stitches tearing out. It is not much employed. 3. The GLOVER'S SU-

TURE, *Contin'ued Suture, Uninterrup'ted Suture,* (F.) *Suture de Pelletier, Suture en surget,* is executed by introducing the needle first into one lip of the wound from within outwards, then into the other in the same way; and, in this manner, sewing up the whole extent of the wound. It has been chiefly used in wounds of the intestinal canal. It is now rarely employed except for stitching up dead bodies. The common stitch or suture, *Sutura puncta'ta,* (F.) *Suture à points passés,* has been used in similar cases. 4. The ROYAL STITCH or SUTURE is the name of an old operation for the cure of bubonocele. It consisted in putting a ligature under the hernial sac, close to the abdominal ring, and then tying that part of the sac, so as to render it impervious by the adhesive inflammation thus excited. 5. The TWISTED SUTURE, (F.) *Suture entortillée,* is employed, chiefly, to unite wounds of the cheeks and of the free edges of the lips. To perform it, a pin or needle is passed through the edges of the wound, so as to keep them accurately in contact. A piece of thread is then wound accurately around the pin, from one side of the division to the other, in the form of the figure ∞. The number of pins and sutures must, of course, correspond with the extent of the wound. This is the suture used in cases of harelip. 6. The *SUTURE À ANSE,* of Le Dran, has only been employed in cases of wounds of the intestines. For this purpose, the edges of the wound are brought together, and as many needles, with unwaxed threads, used as there are to be stitches. Each stitch is then made by passing a needle through the edges; and all the ligatures which belong to one side of the wound are tied together, and twisted so as to form a thread, which is fixed externally.

SUTURE, COMPOUND, Suture, quilled — s. Continued, Suture, glover's — s. *Écailleuse,* Squamous suture — s. *Empennée,* Suture, quilled — s. *Emplumée,* Suture, quilled — s. *Enchevillée,* Suture, quilled — s. *Entortillée,* Suture, twisted — s. *Entrecoupée,* Suture, interrupted — s. False, Harmony — s. *Occipitale,* Lambdoid suture — s. Occipito-parietal, Lambdoid suture — s. *de Pelletier,* Suture, glover's — s. *à Points passés,* Suture, common — s. *à Points séparés,* Suture, interrupted — s. Sagittal, see Sagittal suture — s. *Squameuse,* Squamous suture — s. *en Surget,* Suture, glover's — s. Superficial, Harmony — s. Uninterrupted, see Suture, glover's.

SWAB, from Sax. ꞃpebban, 'to clean with a mop.' A piece of sponge or rag tied to a rod of whalebone or wood, for cleansing the mouth of the sick, or applying remedial agents to deep-seated parts.

SWADDLING CLOTHES, Swathing clothes.

SWAGBELLY, Physconia.

SWALLOW, Hirundo — s. Wort, Asclepias vincetoxicum — s. Wort, orange, Asclepias tuberosa — Wort, tuberous-rooted, Asclepias tuberosa — s. Wort, white, Asclepias vincetoxicum.

SWALLOW'S NEST, Nidus hirundinis.

SWAMP CABBAGE, Dracontium foetidum — s. Dogwood, Petela trifoliata — s. Sickness, Milk sickness — s. Wood, Cephalanthus occidentalis, Dirca palustris.

SWATHING CLOTHES, *Swaddling Clothes, Incunab'ula, Fasciæ, Panni,* from Sax. ꞃbeban, 'to bind.' (F.) *Maillot.* The kind of clothing or bandaging formerly applied to children during the first year of life. It is now, properly, laid aside, and every freedom allowed to muscular exertion.

SWEAT, Sudor — s. Bloody, Sudor cruentus — s. Glands, see Perspiration — s. Root, Polemonium reptans — s. Scab, Crusta genu equinæ.

SWEATING, Hidrosis — s. Bath, Achicolum — s. of Blood, see Diapedesis, and Sudor cruentus — s. House, Achicolum — s. Plant, Eupatorium perfoliatum — s. Room, Achicolum — s. Sickness, Sudor Anglicus.

SWEATING SICKNESS, MALWAH. A disease which appears to be allied to the worst form of cholera, and to bear a close relation to malignant congestive fever. As its name imports, it occurs in Malwah in India.

SWEET BITTER, Triosteum — s. Bush, Cyptonia asplenifolia — s. Fern, Comptonia asplenifolia — s. Flag, Acorus calamus — s. Pod, Cassia nium siliqua — s. Root, Aralia nudicaulis.

SWELLING, *Epanaste'ma, Exar'ma, Exuvisis, Presis, Preuma, Oncus, Extumefac'tio, Tumefac'tio,* (F.) *Enflure, Gonflement,* from the rpellan, (D.) s w e l l e n (G.) s c h w e l l e n, 'to swell.' Morbid increase of bulk in the whole, a part, of the body. See Tumour.

SWELLING, WHITE, Hydrarthrus.

SWERTIA CHIRAYITA, Gentiana chirayita — s. Difformis, see Calumba — s. Frasera, see Calumba — s. Lutea, Gentiana lutea.

SWIETE'NIA FEBRIF'UGA, *S. S. ... Soym'ida, S. Febrif'uga, Feb'rifuge Swietenia,* (F.) *Mahogan fébrifuge. Family,* Meliaceæ. *Syst.* Decandria Monogynia. The bark of this tree, which is a native of the East Indies, and called there *Rohena Bark,* has an aromatic and bitter taste. It is tonic and stomachic, and has been used in intermittents, and in diseases where bitter tonics are indicated. Dose, ℈ij of the powder.

SWIETE'NIA MAHOG'ANI, *Cedrus Mahogany, Mahogany Tree,* grows in the West Indies and tropical America, and is possessed of similar properties.

SWIETENIA SOMIDA, S. Febrifuga.

SWIMBLADDER, Airbladder.

SWIMMING, Natation — s. Bladder, Airbladder — s. of the Head, Vertigo.

SWOON, Syncope.

SWOONING, Syncope.

SYALADENI'TIS, *Inflamma'tio glandularum saliva'lium,* from σιαλον, 'saliva, also, 'a gland,' and *itis,* denoting inflammation. Inflammation of the salivary glands.

SYCAMINOS, Morus nigra.

SYCAMINUM, see Morus nigra.

SYCE, Ficus, Ficus carica.

SYCEA, Ficus.

SYCEPH'ALUS, from συν, 'with,' and κεφαλη, 'head.' A monster having two heads united together.

SY'CION, συκιον, from συκον, 'a fig.' A decoction of dried figs.

SY'CIOS ANGULA'TUS. *One-seeded cucumber, Wild Bry'ony.* The roots and seeds of this indigenous plant, *Order* Cucurbitaceæ, are bitter, purgative and diuretic. It is used in dropsy in the same cases as bryony.

SYCI'TES, from συκον, 'a fig.' Wine, in which figs have been infused.

SYCITES, Catorchites.

SYCOMA, Ficus.

SYCO'SIS. Same etymon. A tumour of the shape of a fig. Also, a fungous ulcer. A large excrescence about the eyelids. Dr. Bateman defines it: — an eruption of inflamed but not very hard tubercles occurring on the bearded parts of the face and on the scalp, in adults; and usually clustering together in irregular patches. — *Phyma Sycosis, Rose'ola fico'sa.* Of this he has given two species: 1. *Sycosis Menti, S. hirsuta Men'tagra, Menti'go, Varus Men'tagra, (Chinese) Barber's Itch,* (F.) *Dartre pustuleuse mentagre;*

and, 2. *Sycosis Capil'li, S. Capillit'ii.* The treatment, in both cases, resembles that for porrigo favosa.

SYCOSIS, Ficus.
SYCUM, Ficus.
SYDERATIO, Sideratio.
SYLLEPSIS, Conception.
SYLLEPSIOLOG'IA, from συλληψις, 'conception,' and λογος, 'a description.' The doctrine of conception.

SYM, SYN, συν, 'with, together,' like the *cum, con, col, cor,* &c., of the Latins. A common prefix. Before *b, p, ph, ps,* and *m,—sym,* or *xyn,* is changed into *sym* or *xym,* (com;) before *c, ch, g, k,* and *x,* into *syn* or *xyn, συy, ξυy,* (con;) before *l* into *syl* or *xyl,* (col;) before *r* into *syr* or *xyr* (cor;) and before *s* into *sy* or *xy,* and *sys,* (co and cos.

SYMBLEPHARON, Ankyloblepharon.
SYMBLEPHARO'SIS, *Concre'tio palpebra'rum cum bulbo oc'uli,* from συν, 'with,' and βλεφαρον, 'an eyelid.' A preternatural adhesion between the eyelids; and especially between the upper eyelid and globe of the eye.

SYMBLEPHAROSIS, Ankyloblepharon.
SYMBOL, *Sym'bolum, Charac'ter,* (F.) *Caractère,* from συμβαλλω (συν, 'with,' and βαλλω, 'I throw'), 'I compare.' A sign or representation of something else.

The following are the symbols used in prescriptions:

℞, Recipe. See R.
gr., *Granum,* a grain.
Ɗ, *Scrupulus* seu *scrupulum,* a scruple.
℥, *Drachma,* a drachm.
℥, *Uncia,* an ounce.
℔, *Libra,* a pound.
♏, *Minimum,* a minim.
f℥, *Fluidrachma,* a fluidrachm.
f℥, *Fluiduncia,* a fluidounce.
O, *Octarius,* a pint.
C, *Congius,* a gallon.

SYMBOLE, Commissure.
SYMBOLEUSIS, Consultation.
SYMBOLISMUS, Sympathy.
SYMBOLIZATIO, Sympathy.
SYMBOLOGICA, Symptomatology.
SYMBOLUM, Sympathy.
SYM'MELES, from συν, 'with, and μελος, 'an extremity.' *Mon'opus.* A genus of monsters whose extremities are joined together: *Sirens.*— I. G. St. Hilaire.

SYMMETRIA, Symmetry.
SYMMET'RICAL, *Symmet'ricus, συμμετρος,* from συν, 'with,' and μετρειν, 'to measure.' An epithet given to those parts of the body, which, if seated on the median line, may be divided into two equal, and perfectly like halves; or which— if situate, the one to the right, the other to the left of this line — have a similar conformation, and a perfectly analogous arrangement.

SYMMETRICAL DISEASES, see Symmetry.
SYM'METRY, *Symmet'ria, Commen'sum, Membro'rum Om'nium Competen'tia, Propor'tio.* The regularity in form, observed in many parts, situate on the median line; and, also, the resemblance which exists between many organs that are situate on each side of the median line. Bichat first noticed that this symmetry was confined to the organs of animal life; as the head, brain, spine, organs of sense, locomotion, &c.

It has been affirmed — and there is evidence in favour of the assertion — to be a law of the animal economy, that, when uninfluenced by disturbing agents, all general or constitutional diseases affect equally and similarly the corresponding parts of the two sides of the body. This has been called the *Symmetry of Diseases;* and the resulting diseases are said to be *symmetrical.*

SYMMETRY OF DISEASES, see Symmetry.
SYMPARATERESIS, Observation.
SYMPASMA, Catapasma.
SYMPATHESIS, Sympathy.
SYMPATHET'IC, *Sympath'icus, Sympa:'leticus,* (F.) *Sympathique,* from συν, 'with,' and παθος, 'suffering.' That which depends on sympathy. Sympathetic affections of an organ are those morbid phenomena that supervene without any morbific cause acting directly on it, and by the reaction of another organ primarily affected. Thus, itching of the nose is a *sympathetic affection,* produced by irritation in the intestinal canal.

The epithet *sympathetic* is, also, given to different nerves. See Trisplanchnic, Pneumogastric, and Facial.

SYMPATHETIC, GREAT, Trisplanchnic nerve—s. Middle, Pneumogastric.

SYMPATHETIC POWDER, *Pulvis sympathet'icus* of Sir Kenelm Digby, was composed of *calcined sulphate of iron,* prepared in a particular manner. It was long supposed to be able to cure a wound, if applied to the weapon that inflicted it; or even to a portion of the bloody clothes. It is proper to remark, however, that the wound itself was carefully excluded from the air, and from all irritation.

SYMPATHETICUS MINOR, Facial nerve.
SYMPATHETISMUS, Sympathy.
SYMPATHIA, Consent of parts.
SYMPATHICUS, Sympathetic.
SYMPATHIQUE, Sympathetic.
SYM'PATHY, *Sympathi'a, Sympathe'sis, Compas'sio, Consensus, Sympathetis'mus, Xympathi'a, Conflux'io, Conspira'tio, Commer'cium, Consor'tium, Homoiopathi'a, Homoëth'nia, Adelphix'is, Symbolis'mus, Symboliza'tio, Sym'bolum.* The connexion that exists between the action of two or more organs, more or less distant from each other; so that the affection of the first is transmitted, secondarily, to the others, or to one of the others, by means unknown. A knowledge of the particular sympathies between different organs throws light on the etiology of diseases, their seat, and the particular organ towards which our therapeutical means should be directed. See Irritation.

SYMPEPSIS, Coction.
SYMPEXIS, Concretion.
SYMPHORA, Congestion.
SYMPHOREMA, Congestion.
SYMPHORESIS, Congestion.
SYMPHORICAR'PUS RACEMO'SUS, *Snowberry.* An indigenous plant, *Order* Caprifoliaceæ, *Tribe* Loniceræ, whose berries are large, bright white, and remain till winter; flowering from June to September. The root is tonic and astringent, and has been used in ague; and by the Indians in syphilis.

SYMPHYIA, Symphysis.
SYMPHYOCEPH'ALUS, *Metop'ages, Cephalop'ages,* from συμφυης, 'united together,' and κεφαλη, 'head.' A monstrosity in which twins are united by the head.

SYMPHYSEOT'OMY, *Symphyseot'omy, Synchondrot'omy, Symphyseotom'ia, Symphysiotom'ia,* from συμφυσις, and τεμνω, 'I cut.' The *operation* or *section of the Symphysis, Sigaultian operation, Sigaultian section.* This operation is performed with the view of augmenting the diameter of the pelvis, in order to facilitate delivery in certain cases of faulty conformation of that cavity, with wedging of the head of the child therein. To perform the operation, (F.) *Désymphyser,* the female is placed on her back; the pubes is shaved; and, with a strong scalpel, the soft parts are divided on the median line. The articulation is then cut. As soon as the fibrous parts, which hold the bones together, are divided, they separate to a certain distance from each other; and the delivery may be accomplished. The knife, with which the operation is performed, is called, by the French, *Couteau symphysien*.

SYMPHYS'IA, from συμφυσις, 'a growing together.' A malformation consisting in the union of parts that are usually divided. — Breschet.

SYMPHYSIOTOMIA, Symphyseotomy.

SYM'PHYSIS, *Symphy'ia, Coalescen'tia, Coal'itus*, from συμφυω (συν, 'with,' and φυω, 'I grow'), 'I unite together.' A union of bones. The bond of such union. The aggregate of means used for retaining bones *in situ* in the articulations. The name symphysis has, however, been more particularly appropriated to certain articulations; as to the *symphysis pubis, sacro-iliac symphysis*, &c. See Monster.

SYMPHYSIS, Coalescence, Commissure, Insertion — s. Cartilaginea, Synchondrosis — s. Ligamentosa, Syndesmosis — s. Ossium muscularis, Syssarcosis — s. Pubis, Pubic articulation.

SYMPHYSOTOMY, Symphyseotomy.

SYMPHYTOS, Hereditary.

SYM'PHYTUM. Same etymon. *Symphytum officina'lis seu album seu Bohe'micum, Consol'ida major, Comfrey, Alum, Alus*, (F.) *Grande Consoude*. Family, Boragineæ. Sex. Syst. Pentandria Monogynia. The roots of this European plant are very mucilaginous, and are employed as emollients. They are used in decoction in hæmoptysis, dysentery, chronic diarrhœa, &c.

SYMPHYTUM, Solidago virgaurea — s. Album, Symphytum — s. Bohemicum, Symphytum — s. Minimum, Bellis — s. Minus, Prunella — s. Officinale, Symphytum.

SYMPHYTUM PETRÆ'UM, *Coris Monspelien'sis, Montpel'lier Coris*. An intensely bitter and nauseous plant, which is said to have been useful in syphilis. See, also, Sanicula.

SYMPLOCARP'US ANGUSTISPATHA, Dracontium angustispatha — s. Fœtida, Dracontium fœtidum.

SYMPOD'IA, *Monopod'ia*, from συν, 'together,' and πους, ποδος, 'a foot.' A monstrosity in which there is coalescence of the lower extremities.

SYMPTOM, *Sympto'ma, Ac'cidens, Casus*, from συν, 'with,' and πτωμα, 'a fall,' from πιπτω, 'I fall.' Any change, perceptible to the senses, in any organ or function, which is connected with morbific influence. It is by the aggregate and succession of symptoms that a disease is detected. The term *symptoms of symptoms* has been used for the effects which result from the symptoms of a disease; but which effects are not essentially connected with the disease itself. Thus, the debility arising from the frequency of evacuations in dysentery is a symptom of symptoms. See Sign.

SYMPTOMA TURPITUDINIS, Nymphomania.

SYMPTOMAT'IC, *Symptomat'icus*. That which is a symptom of some other affection. Thus we speak of a symptomatic disease, in opposition to one that is idiopathic.

SYMPTOMATOL'OGY, *Symptomatolog''ia, Symbolog''ica*, from συμπτωμα, 'a symptom,' and λογος, 'a treatise.' The branch of pathology, the object of which is the knowledge of symptoms.

SYMPTO'SIS, from συν, 'with,' and πιπτω, 'I fall.' Depression or collapse, emaciation or atrophy, either of the whole body or of a part.

SYNÆREMA, Corrugation.
SYNÆTION, Concausa.
SYNANCHE, Cynanche, Cynanche tonsillaris.
SYNANCIE, Cynanche.
SYNAPHYMENITIS, see Ophthalmia.
SYNAPTASE, see Amygdalin.
SYNARTHRODIA, Synarthrosis.

SYNARTHRO'DIAL, *Synarthrodia'lis*, from συν, 'with,' and αρθρωσις, 'articulation.' That which belongs to synarthrosis; as *Synarthrodial articulation*.

SYNARTHRO'SIS, *Synarthro'dia, Akentia'tio, Coarticula'tio*. An immovable articulation. Synarthrosis includes three species: *Sutura, Harmony*, and *Gomphosis*.

SYNATHROESIS, Congestion.
SYNATHROISMUS, Congestion.

SYNCAN'THUS, from συν, 'with,' and κανθος, 'the corner of the eye.' A morbid adhesion between the globe of the eye and the orbit.

SYNCHONDRO'SIS, *Sym'physis seu Coitus seu Connex'io cartilagin'ea, Chondrosyndes'mus*, from συν, 'with,' and χονδρος, 'a cartilage.' Union or articulation of bones by means of cartilage: — as the articulations of the ribs with the sternum, by means of their cartilages of prolongation.

SYNCHONDROTOMY, Symphyseotomy.
SYNCHRONIUS, Synchronous.

SYN'CHRONOUS, *Syn'chronus, Synchro'nus, Isoch'ronous*, from συν, 'with,' and χρονος, 'time.' That which occurs at the same time. Thus the pulsations of an artery may be synchronous with those of the heart.

SYNCHRONUS, Synchronous.
SYNCHYSIS, Confusion.
SYNCIPUT, Sinciput.
SYNCLONESIS, Synclonus.

SYN'CLONUS, *Synclone'sis*, from συγκλονεω (συν, 'with,' and κλονεω, 'I shake,') 'I shake together.' *Clon'ici universa'les, Clonus*, (Ploucquet.) Tremulous, simultaneous, and chronic action of various muscles, especially when excited by the will. Also, general spasm, σπασμος universa'lis. See Tremor, Chorea, &c.

SYNCLONUS BALLISMUS, Paralysis agitans — s. Beriberia, Beriberi — s. Chorea, Chorea — s. Epiphania, Raphania — s. Saltans, Chorea — s. Tremor, Tremor.

SYNCOMIS'TUS, from συγκομιζω, (συν, κομιζω,) 'I bring together.' *Autop'yros, Panis domes'ticus, secundarius, ciba'rius, confusa'neus*. Bread of the whole wheat or of the unsifted. *Household bread*. Also, a cataplasm made of the same.

SYN'COPAL, *Syncopa'lis, Syncop'ticus, Syncop'tus*. Same etymon as Syncope; as *Syncopal Fever, Febris Syncopa'lis*. A pernicious remittent, characterised by repeated attacks of syncope.

SYN'COPE, from συγκοπτω, 'I fall down,' *An'imi defec'tio, Animi deli'quium, Leipopsych'ia, Lipopsych'ia, Apsych'ia, Apsyx'ia, Lipopsyx'ia, Asphyx'ia, Apopsych'ia, Lipothym'ia, Leipothym'ia, Eclipsis, Su'bitus animi casus, Swooning, Fainting, Fainting fit, Faintness, Ermäktung*, (F.) *Evanouissement, Défaillance, Pamoison*. Complete and, commonly, sudden loss of sensation and motion, with considerable diminution or entire suspension of the pulsations of the heart and the respiratory movements. Syncope is, commonly, an affection of no consequence: but, sometimes, it is an index of diseased heart. Placing the patient in the horizontal posture, sprinkling cold water over the face, and the application of volatile substances to the nose, are all that will be required during the fit. See Asphyxia, and Suffocation.

An approach to this condition is termed *faintishness*.

SYNCOPE ANGINA, Angina pectoris — s. Anginosa, Angina pectoris.
SYNCOPTICUS, Syncopal.
SYNCOPTUS, Syncopal.
SYNCRITICA, Astringents.
SYNDACTYLUS, Aschistodactylus.
SYNDESMI'TIS, see Ophthalmia. Also, inflammation of articular ligaments; *Inflamma'tio ligamento'rum*.
SYNDESMOG'RAPHY, *Syndesmograph'ia*, from συνδεσμος, 'a ligament,' and γραφη, 'a description.' A description of the ligaments. The part of anatomy which describes the ligaments.
SYNDESMOL'OGY, *Syndesmolog"ia*, from συνδεσμος, 'a ligament,' and λογος, 'a treatise, discourse.' A treatise on the ligaments.
SYNDES'MO-PHARYNGEUS. A fasciculus of the constrictor pharyngis superior.
SYNDESMOS, Ligament.
SYNDESMO'SIS, *Synneuro'sis, Synymen'esis, Connex'io* seu *Sym'physis ligamento'sa, Commis'su'ra ner'vea, Connerva'tio, Colliga'tio*, from συνδεσμος, 'ligament.' The articulation of two or more bones by means of ligament; — as of the radius with the ulna.
SYNDESMOT'OMY, *Syndesmatom'ia*, from συνδεσμος, 'ligament,' and τεμνω, 'I cut or dissect.' Dissection of the ligaments.
SYNDESMUS, Bandage, Ligament.
SYN'DROME, from συν, 'with,' and δρομος, 'a course.' *Concur'sus, Concourse.* A name given by the Empirical Sect to the union of symptoms which takes place in diseases. *Syndromē pletho'rica*, for example, meant the union of symptoms produced by plethora.
SYNDYASMUS, Coition.
SYNECHES, see Continued fever.
SYNECHI'A, from συν, 'with,' and εχειν, 'to have,' or 'to hold.' Adhesion between the iris and transparent cornea, or between the iris and crystalline lens. The former case is called *Synechia ante'rior*: the latter, *S. poste'rior.*
SYNENERGIA, Synergy.
SYNERGIA, Synergy.
SYNERGIE, Synergy.
SYN'ERGY, *Synergi'a, Synenergi'a,* (F.) *Synergie*; from συν, 'with,' and εργον, 'work.' A correlation or concourse of action between different organs in health; and, according to some, in disease.
SYNESIS, Intellect.
SYNEUROSIS, Syndesmosis.
SYNEZI'ZIS, *Synize'sis, Considen'tia*, from συν, 'with,' and ζυγνυειν, 'to join.' *Parop'sis Synizesis, Cali'go a Synizesi, Caligo Pupil'læ, Imperfora'tio pupillæ, Closure* or *occlu'sion* or *oblitera'tion of the Pupil, Phthisis Pupil'læ, Amyo'sis.* This disease is sometimes faulty conformation, depending upon the continued existence of the membrana pupillaris, or the absence of the pupil. It is, in other words, *congenital.* At other times, it is owing to accident, and supervenes on violent ophthalmia, or on the operation for cataract. They who are affected with synezixis are completely blind; — the iris having no central aperture. In certain cases, a remedy may be obtained by making an opening in the iris, which may supply the place of the pupil, and through which the rays of light may reach the retina. This operation is called the *operation for artificial pupil.*
SYNGENES, Hereditary.

SYNGENICUS, Congenital.
SYNHYMENESIS, Synymenesis.
SYNIMENESIS, Synymenesis.
SYNIZESIS, Considentia, Synezisis.
SYNNEUROSIS, Syndesmosis.
SYN'OCHA, from συνεχω, (συν, and εχω, 'I have or hold,') 'I continue.' *Inflam'matory Fever, Dynam'ic Fever, Angiop'yra, Sthenŏp'yra, Febris causo'des, F. caumato'des, Febris deu'rens, F. ardens, Febris contin'ua sanguin'ea, Febris contin'ua non putris, Syn'ochus* (Vogel), *Febris acmas'tica, Synochus impu'tris* (Galen,) *Febris acu'ta, F. acu'ta sanguin'ea, F. con'tinens, F. continens non pu'trida, F. angioten'ica, F. sthenica, F. sanguin'ea, Homot'onos, F. inflammato'ria, Ene'cia cauma, Enecia, F. ton'ica, Phlogop'yrus, Cauma, Calentura continua,* (F.) *Fièvre ardente, F. continente inflammatoire, F. sanguine, F. irritative, F. angeioténique, F. inflammatoire, Gastro-entérite intense, General inflammation.* A species of continued fever, characterized by increased heat; and by quick, strong, and hard pulse; urine high-coloured; disturbance of mind slight. It requires, of course, the most active treatment.
SYNOCHA RHEUMATICA, Rheumatism, acute—s. Vaccina, Vaccina.
SYN'OCHAL, *Synocha'lis;* same etymon. Relating to, or having the characters of, synocha.
SYN'OCHUS, *Ene'cia syn'ochus, Febris lenta,* (Linnæus,) same etymon. Continued fever, compounded of synocha and typhus: — in its commencement often resembling the former; in its progress, the latter: *Mixed fever, Common continued fever, Syn'ochoid fever.* See Continued fever, Fever, and Typhus.
SYNOCHUS, Synocha—s. Biliosa, Fever, gastric, Fever, bilious—s. Catarrhalis, Influenza—s. Icterodes, Fever, yellow—s. Imputris, Synocha—s. Miliaria, Miliary fever—s. Varicella, Varicella.
SYNOLCE, Spasm.
SYNONIA, Synovia.
SYNOSTEOG'RAPHY, *Synosteogra'phia*, from συν, 'with,' οστεον, a 'bone,' and γραφω, 'I describe.' The part of anatomy which describes the joints.
SYNOSTEOL'OGY, *Synosteolog"ia*, from συν, 'with,' οστεον, 'a bone,' and λογος, 'a treatise.' A treatise on the joints.
SYNOSTEO'SIS, *Synosto'sis*, from συν, 'with,' and οστεον, 'a bone. Union by means of bone.
SYNOSTEOT'OMY, *Synosteotom'ia*, from συν, 'with,' οστεον, 'a bone,' and τεμνειν, 'to cut.' Dissection of the joints.
SYNOSTOSIS, Synosteosis.
SYNO'VIA, from συν, 'with,' and ωον, 'an egg.' *Mucila'go, Un'guen articula'rē, Syno'nia, Axun'gia articula'ris, Unguen'tum* seu *Smegma articula'rē, Mucila'go articulo'rum* seu *functura'rum, Humor articula'ris, Hydrarthrus, Humor* seu *Hu'midum nati'vum* seu *Gluten articulo'rum* (F.) *Synovie.* A fluid resembling the white of egg, which is exhaled by the synovial membranes surrounding the moveable articulations. The synovia has been found, on analysis, to consist of water, a little albumen, soda, chloride of sodium, phosphate of lime, and—Fourcroy fancied —uric acid. Its use is to lubricate the joints, and the sheaths in which tendons play.
SYNO'VIAL, *Synovia'lis.* That which relates to the synovia.
SYNOVIAL GLANDS, *Havers's Glands, Gland'ulæ articula'res, G. Synovia'les, G. Haversia'næ*, are the secretory fringes, which float in the interior of the synovial capsules (see Capsules.) They do not seem to be glandular. They have been

called *Syno'vial fim'briæ*, (F.) *Franges synoviales.*

SYNOVI'TIS; from *Synovia*, and *itis*, a termination denoting inflammation. A term, badly compounded, applied at times to inflammation of the synovial membrane.

SYNOVITIS RHEUMATISMALIS, Rheumatism, (acute.)

SYN'TASIS, *συντασις*, from *συντεινω*, (*συν*, and *τεινω*, 'I stretch,') 'I strain.' Tension of parts: hence *συντατικα*, are medicines which render parts tense. *Syntex'is*, on the other hand, means *Colliqua'tio*, or wasting of the body; from *συντηκω*, 'I melt together.'

SYNTAXIS, Articulation, Reduction, Taxis—s. Serrata, see Suture.

SYNTECOPYRA, Hectic fever.

SYNTECTYCOPYRA, Hectic fever.

SYNTENO'SIS, from *συν*, 'with,' and *τενων*, 'a tendon.' A species of articulation in which two bones are joined by means of tendon; as the sesamoid bones with the toes, the rotula with the tibia, &c.

SYNTERESIS, Prophylaxis.

SYNTERETICUS, Prophylactic.

SYNTEXIS, Colliquation, Consumption.

SYNTHENA. A term employed by Paracelsus to designate a species of epilepsy, accompanied by cardialgia and tormina.

SYN'THESIS, *Reu'nio*, 'composition or putting together,' from *συν*, and *τιδημι*, 'I place.' A surgical operation, which consists in uniting parts that are divided; and approximating such as are separated or distant from each other, *Reu'nio par'tium separata'rum*, *Syn'thesis of continu'ity*, means the union of the edges of a wound, or the approximation of the extremities of a fractured bone. *Synthesis of contigu'ity* is the reduction of displaced organs; as in cases of hernia and luxations.

SYNTHESIS, Composition.

SYNTHETIS'MUS, same etymon. The aggregate of operations and means for reducing a fracture, and maintaining it reduced:—comprising extension, counter-extension, coaptation, and bandaging.

SYNTRIMMA, Contritio.

SYNTRIPSIS, Contritio.

SYNTROPHOS, Connutritus.

SYNULOSIS, Cicatrization.

SYNULOTICA, Cicatrisantia.

SYNUSIA, Coition.

SYNYME'NESIS, *Synhyme'nesis, Synime'nesis*, from *συν*, 'with,' and '*υμην*, 'a membrane.' Union of bones by membrane, as in the case of the bones of the head in the fœtus.

SYNYMENESIS, Syndesmosis.

SYPHAR, Peritoneum.

SYPHILIDES, *Syphili'da*, (F.) *Dermo-syphilides, Dermatosies véroleuses*. Same etymon as Syphilis. The cutaneous eruptions that accompany constitutional syphilis are so denominated by the French writers.

SYPHILIDIA'TER, *Syphilidia'trus*, from *Syphilis*, and *ιατρος*, 'a physician.' A pox doctor. One who occupies himself in treating syphilis.

SYPHILIDOMANIA, Syphilomania.

SYPHYLIPHO'BIA; from *Syphilis* and *φοβος*, 'dread,' A morbid dread of syphilis, giving rise to fancied symptoms of the disease: a form of hypochondriasis.

SYPH'ILIS, *Morbus Gal'licus, Siphilis, Syphili'mus, Cachex'ia venerea, Cachochym'ia Vene'rea, Malum vene'reum, Mor'bus Ital'icus, M. Hispan'icus, Puden'dagra, Lues, Me'vium, Lues vene'rea, Lues syphilis, Morbus aphrodis'ius, Sy- philis venerea, S. maligna, Morbus Neapolitanus, Morbus In'dicus, Patursa, Basilid'um, Bea. Sod'oma Gallo'rum; Venereal, Venereal Disease. Fr. French Pox;* (F.) *Vérole, Maladie vénérienne, Mal de Naples, Mal Françoria, Maladie de Vénus.* The etymology of syphilis is unknown. Some consider it to proceed from *συς*, 'a hog,' and others, from *σιφος*,—formed, by contraction, from *σιχαλος*, 'shameful,' 'dirty,' &c. It is an infectious disease, communicable by coition, or by the contact of parts that are only lined with a thin epidermis; as the lips, nipple, &c. It generally makes its first appearance by a chancre, followed sooner or later by a bubo. The chancre is a primary symptom or sore; but there are others which are *secondary* or *constitutional*. These are:—ulcers in the throat; copper-colored blotches on the skin; pains in the bones, nodes, &c.: the last are sometimes termed *tertiary* phenomena. The origin of syphilis is not known. It is believed to have been introduced into Europe from America, at the end of the 15th century [?]. Its progress is extremely various, as well as its duration, which is often unlimited, if left to itself. Mercury may be esteemed the best remedy, but the disease admits of cure without it. Almost every antisyphilitic composition, whose use is attended with success, probably retains mercury united with diaphoretics or other medicines. It is generally sufficient to keep the mouth sore for a fortnight for the cure of chancre. for venereal sore throat, and other recent constitutional symptoms, eight or ten weeks will be required; and, of course, a longer time, if these symptoms have persisted longer. Sometimes after mercury has been given for a time, the symptoms continue stationary; and do not yield until the mercury has been discontinued, and tonics and eutrophics have been administered. The preparations of iodine have been much used of late, in the revellent treatment of this disease.

SYPHILIS INDICA, Framboesia.

SYPHILIS PSEUDO-SYPHILIS, *Lues Syphili'des, Pseudo-syphilis*. A term given to ulcers or other affections that resemble syphilis, but are indeterminate in their character,—the symptoms being irregular in their appearance, and usually yielding spontaneously, or under the use of tonics, change of air, &c. The condition has not been at all well defined. The *Sievens, Radesyge*, &c., have been referred to this head.

SYPHILISMUS, Syphilis.

SYPHILOG'RAPHER, from *syphilis*, and *γραφω*, 'I describe.' A writer on syphilis.

SYPH'ILOID, *Syphiloi'des*; from *syphilis*, and *ειδος*, 'resemblance.' Resembling syphilis: as 'a *syphiloid* affection.'

SYPHILOMA'NIA, *Syphilidoma'nia*,—vulgarly, *Noddle Pox*. A mania, with which some persons are affected, so that they subject themselves to antivenereal treatment, under the notion that they are affected with syphilis.

SYPHITA, Somnambulism.

SYPHOAURICULARIS, Otenchytes.

SYPHON, see Siphon.

SYRIGMOPHO'NIA, from *συριγμος*, 'whistling,' and *φωνη*, 'voice.' A piping state of the voice.

SYRIGMUS, Tinnitus aurium.

SYRINGA, Eustachian Tube, Fistula, Syringe, Trachea.

SYRINGA CLYSMATICA, Syringe, (Clyster.)

SYRIN'GA VULGA'RIS, *Lilac vulga'ris*, Common Lilac. The leaves and fruit are bitter and somewhat acrid, and have been used as a tonic and antiperiodic.

SYRINGE, *Syr'inx, Syrin'ga, Sipho Siphun'culus, Squirt*, (F.) *Seringue*, from *συριγξ*, 'a pipe

A familiar apparatus through which any liquid is squirted.
Various forms of syringe are used in medicine and surgery.
SYRINGE, CLYSTER, *Syrin'ga clysmat'ica, Clysantli'um*, (F.) *Clysopompe.* A syringe for administering clysters.
SYRINGE, CUPPING, Antlia sanguisuga.
SYRINGICUS, Fistulous.
SYRINGI'TIS EUSTA'CHII, Inflammation of the Eustachian tube.
SYRINGMOS, Tinnitus aurium.
SYRINGODES, Fistulous.
SYRINGOTOME, Syringot'omus, Syringot'-omum, from συριγξ, 'a pipe,' 'a fistula,' and τεμνειν, 'to cut.' A surgical instrument, formerly used in the operation for *fistula in ano.* It is a bistouri, concave at its edge, and terminated by a long, flexible, probe-pointed stylet. This stylet or probe was first introduced by the external opening of the fistula into the rectum, whence it was drawn externally through the anus, carrying with it the cutting edge of the instrument, which divided the intermediate parts. The operation for fistula in ano has been called *Syringotomy.*
SYRINGOT'OMY, *Syringotom'ia.* Same etymon as the last. The operation for fistula in ano by incision.
SYRINX, Eustachian tube, Fistula, Syringe, Trachea—s. Hiera, Vertebral column.
SYRMAIS'MOS, from συρμαιζω, 'I evacuate.' A gentle evacuation by vomiting or stool.
SYROP, Syrup — *s. d'Ail*, Syrupus allii — *s. d'Armoise composé*, Syrupus aromaticus — *s. de Chicorée composé,* Syrupus de cichorio compositus — *s. des Cinq racines,* Syrupus e quinque radicibus — *s. de Cuisinier,* Syrupus de sarsaparillâ et senna compositus — *s. d'Éther,* Syrupus cum æthere sulphurico paratus — *s. de Gingembre,* Syrupus zingiberis—*s. de Guimauve,* Syrupus althæeæ — *s. de Longue vie,* Mellitum de mercuriali compositum — *s. de Mercure,* Syrupus de mercurio mediante gummi—*s. de Mûres,* Syrupus mori—*s. de Nerprun,* Syrupus rhamni — *s. de Pavots blancs,* Syrupus papaveris — *s. de Pommes composé,* see Syrupus sennæ — *s. de Quinquina avec le Vin,* Syrupus de kinâ kinâ cum vino — *s. de Roses pâles,* Syrupus rosæ — *s. de Roses rouges,* Syrupus rosæ—*s. de Vinaigre,* S. aceti.
SYRUP, *Sirup, Syr'upus, Serapi'um, Serape'-um,* (F.) *Syrop ;* derived, according to some, from συρω, 'I draw,' and οπος, 'juice ;' but more probably, from the Arabic *Siruph, Sirab,* or *Scharab,* which signifies 'a potion.' A saturated solution of sugar in water, either simply, or united with some vegetable or other principle. Syrups, in general, require two pounds of sugar to the pint, and they are judged to be sufficiently boiled when a portion, taken up in a spoon, flows like oil. In the Pharmacopœia of the United States, it is directed, that syrups, whose density is not precisely determined by the process, should have the s. g. 1.261, when boiling, and of about 1.319 at ordinary temperatures. Syrups should be kept in small bottles in a cool place. They are chiefly used to render medicines palatable. See Syrupus simplex.
SYRUP, see Syrupus — s. of Almonds, Syrupus amygdalæ—s. Antiscorbutic, Syrupus antiscorbuticus — s. of Buckthorn, Syrupus rhamni — s. of Capillaire, common, Syrupus simplex—s. of Cinchona with wine, Syrupus de kinâ kinâ cum vino — s. of Citric acid, Syrupus acidi citrici — s. of Clove July flower, Syrupus caryophylli rubri — s. of Clove pinks, Syrupus Caryophylli rubri — s. of Ether, Syrupus cum æthere sulphurico paratus—s. of Five roots, Syrupus e quinque radicibus—s. of Garlic, Syrupus allii — s. of Ginger,

Syrupus zingiberis — s. of Gum Arabic, Syrupus acaciæ — s. Hive, Syrupus scillæ compositus — s. of Honey, Mellitum simplex—s. of Iodide of iron, Liquor Ferri iodidi—s. of Ipecacuanha, Syrupus ipecacuanhæ — s. of Lemon, Syrupus limonis — s. of Marshmallows, Syrupus althææ—s. of Meadow saffron, Syrupus colchici autumnalis — s. of Mugwort, compound, Syrupus aromaticus—s. of Mulberries, Syrupus mori—s. of Orange juice, see Syrupus aurantii — s. of Orange peel, Syrupus aromaticus — s. of Orgeat, Syrupus amygdalæ — s. of Poppies, Syrupus papaveris — s. of Poppy, red, Syrupus rhœados — s. of Rhatany, Syrupus krameriæ — s. of Rhubarb, Syrupus rhej — s. of Rhubarb, aromatic, Syrupus rhei aromaticus — s. of Rhubarb, spiced, Syrupus rhej aromaticus — s. of Saffron, Syrupus croci — s. of Squills, Syrupus scillæ—s. of Squill, compound, Syrupus scillæ compositus — s. of Succory, compound, Syrupus de cichorio compositus—s. of Tolu, Syrupus tolutanus — s. of Vinegar, Syrupus aceti — s. of Violets, Syrupus violæ—s. of Wild cherry bark, Syrupus Pruni Virginianæ.

SYRUPUS, S. simplex.
SYRUPUS ACA'CIÆ, *Syrup of Gum Arabic,* (*Acaciæ* ℥ij, *Sacchar.* ℥xv, *Aq.* f℥viij. Dissolve the gum in the water; add the sugar, and strain. Ph. U. S.) A good pectoral syrup. Dose, f℥j to ℥iij.

SYRUPUS ACE'TI, *S. Ac"idi Aceto'si, Syrup of Vinegar,* (F.) *Syrop de Vinaigre.* (*Aceti* Oiiss, *sacch. purif.* ℔iiiss. Boil to form a syrup. Ph. E.) It is refrigerant and antiseptic. Dose, f℥j to f℥ij.

SYRUPUS ACIDI ACETOSI, S. aceti.
SYRUPUS AC"IDI CIT'RICI, *Syrup of Citric Acid.* (*Acid. citric.* pulv. ℨij; *Ol. Limon.* ♏iv; *Syrup.* Oij. Rub the acid and oil with an ounce of the syrup; add the rest of the syrup, and dissolve with a gentle heat. Ph. U. S.) Virtues the same as those of the Syrupus Limonis.

SYRUPUS CUM Æ'THERE SULPHU'RICO PARATUS, *Syrup of Ether,* (F.) *Sirop d'éther.* (Very pure sugar, 1000 p.; *distilled water,* 500 p.; dissolve in the cold, and strain; add *sulphuric ether,* 48 p. Shake for five or six days, and draw off the limpid syrup. Ph. L.) Properties like those of ether.

SYRUPUS AL'LII, *Syrup of Garlic,* (F.) *Syrop d'ail.* (*Allii recent.* concis. ℥vj, *acet. destillat.* Oj, *sacchar.* ℔ij. Macerate the garlic in the vinegar, in a glass vessel, for four days; then express the liquor and set it by, that the dregs may subside; lastly, add the sugar to the clear liquor, and proceed in the manner directed for syrup. Ph. U. S.) Use, same as that of garlic. Dose, f℥j to f℥iv.

SYRUPUS ALTHÆ'Æ, *Syrup of Marshmallow, Syrupus ex Althæ'â, S. de Althæâ, S. Althææ officina'lis,* (F.) *Syrop de Guimauve.* (*Althææ rad. recent.* cont. ℔ss, *sacch. pur.* ℔ij, *aquæ* Oiv. Boil the root in the water to one-half, and press out the liquor; when cold, defecate; add the sugar, and boil. Ph. L.) Emollient and demulcent. Dose, f℥j to f℥iij.

SYRUPUS AMOMI ZINGIBERIS, S. zingiberis.
SYRUPUS AMYG'DALÆ, *Syrup of Almonds, Syrup of Orgeat, Orgeat.* (*Amygdal. dulc.* ℔j, *amygdal. amar.* ℥iv, *aquæ,* Oiij, *sacchar.* ℔vj. Blanch the almonds, and rub them in a mortar to a very fine paste, adding, during the trituration, three fluidounces of the water, and a pound of the sugar. Mix the paste thoroughly with the remainder of the water; strain with strong expression; add the remainder of the sugar to the strained liquor, and dissolve it with the aid of a gentle heat. Strain the syrup through fine linen, and having allowed it to cool, put it into bottles

which must be well stopped, and kept in a cool place. *Ph. U. S.*)

SYRUPUS ANTICAUSOTICUS, see Anticausodic.

SYRUPUS ANTISCORBU'TICUS, *S. de Armora'ciâ compositus, Antiscorbu'tic Syrup.* (*Leaves of cochlearia, buckbean, water-cresses, horse-radish root* and *bitter oranges*, each ℔j, *cinnamon*, ℥iss. Cut, and pour on *white wine* ℔iv. Macerate for two days; distil over Oj in a sand-bath; add to this of *sugar*, ℔ij, and form a syrup. Again, take what remains in the cucurbit: pass it through cloth; let it rest; decant, and add *sugar* ℔ij; make into a syrup, and clarify with white of egg. Mix it with the first while yet warm. *Ph. P.*) Antiscorbutic, alterative, tonic, stomachic, &c. Dose, f℥ij to f℥ij.

SYRUPUS AROMAT'ICUS, *S. de Artemis'iâ compositus, Compound Syrup of Mugwort,* (F.) *Syrop d'armoise composé.* (*Tops of artemisia vulgaris*, in flower, ℥vj, *inula root, ligusticum levisticum*, and *fennel*, each ℥ss, *pennyroyal, catmint, savine leaves*, each ℥vj, *marjoram, hyssop, pyrethrum, rue, basil*, each ℥iij, *aniseed* and *cinnamon*, each ℥ix; bruise and macerate in *hydromel* ℔xviij; distil over Oss; add to this a pound of sugar. Again, take the liquid that remains in the cucurbit, strain it gently; and add *sugar* ℔iv. Then mix the two. *Ph. P.*) Tonic, emmenagogue, &c.

SYRUPUS DE ARMORACIÂ COMPOSITUS, S. antiscorbuticus—s. de Artemisiâ compositus, S. antiscorbuticus—s. Asparagi, see Asparagus.

SYRUPUS AURAN'TII, *S. Aurantio'rum, S. Citri Aurantii, S. Cor'ticis Aurantii, S. Aurantii Corticis* (Ph. U. S.), *S. e Cortic"ibus Aurantio'rum, S. de Corticâ Aurantio'rum, Syrup of Orange peel.* (*Aurant. cort. cont.* ℥ij, *aq. ferv.* Oj, *sacch.* ℔ijss. Macerate the peel in the water for twelve hours. Add the sugar. *Ph. U. S.*) Stomachic. Dose, f℥j to f℥ij.

A *Syrup of Orange Juice, Orange Sherbet, Syrupus e succo Aurantiorum*, may be made by adding *white sugar* ℔ij to ℔j of the juice of oranges, strained and clarified.

SYRUPUS BALSAMICUS, S. tolutanus.

SYRUPUS CARYOPHYL'LI RUBRI, *S. Dianthi Caryophylli, Syrup of Clove July flower, Syrup of Clove Pinks, Syrupus infusio'nis florum caryophyllo'rum.* (*Petalorum dianth., caryoph. recent.* unguibus resectis ℔j, *aquæ bull.* Oiv, *sacch. purif.* ℔vij. *Ph. E.*) Aromatic.

SYRUPUS CASSIÆ SENNÆ, S. sennæ.

SYRUPUS DE CICHO'RIO COMPOS'ITUS, *S. de Rheo, Compound Syrup of Succory,* (F.) *Syrop de chicorée composé.* (*Root of succory* ℥vj, *leaves of succory* ℥ix, *leaves of fumitory* and *scolopendrium*, each ℥iij, *Alkekengi berries* ℥ij. Boil in *water* Oxiv to Oxij: pass through cloth, and dissolve in *white sugar* ℔v. Boil till it has the consistence of syrup. Again, take *water* Oviij, *rhubarb* ℥vj, *yellow sanders* and *cinnamon*, each ℥ss. Infuse for twenty-four hours; pass through linen, and add the preceding syrup. *Ph. P.*) It is laxative and stomachic. Dose, f℥j to f℥ss.

SYRUPUS CINCHONÆ CUM VINO, S. de kinâ kinâ cum vino.

SYRUPUS CINCHO'NIÆ, *Syrup of Cincho'nia.* (*Simple syrup* one pound; *sulphate of cinchonia* nine grains. Mix.) Six spoonfuls are commonly sufficient to arrest an intermittent.

SYRUPUS CITRI AURANTII, S. aromaticus.

SYRUPUS COL'CHICI AUTUMNA'LIS, *S. Colchici, Syrup of Meadow Saffron.* (*Rad. colch. autumn. recent.* ℥j, *acidi acetosi* f℥xvi, *sacch. pur.* ℥xxvj. Macerate the root in the vinegar for two days, occasionally shaking the vessel; then strain, with gentle expression. T ·me strained fluid add the sugar, and boil to a syrup. *Ph. E.*) Diuretic, antiarthritic. Dose, f℥j to f℥ss, or more.

SYRUPUS CORTICIS AURANTII, S. aromaticus—s. Citri medicæ, S. limonum—s. e Succo citronum, S. limonum.

SYRUPUS CROCI, *Syrup of Saffron.* (*Croci stigmat.* ℥j, *aquæ fervent.* Oj, *sacch. purif.* ℔iiss. *Ph. L.*) Cardiac. Chiefly used for colouring.

SYRUPUS DIACODION, Diacodion—s. Dianthi Caryophylli, S. caryophylli rubri.

SYRUPUS EMETI'NÆ, *Syrup of Em'etine.* (*Simple syrup* ℔j, *emetine* 16 gr.) In small doses, expectorant; and in large, emetic.

SYRUPUS EMPYREUMATICUS, Melasses—s. Ferri iodidi, Liquor Ferri iodidi—s. Hydrargyri, Syrupus de mercurio mediante gummi—s. Infusi ex florum caryophyllorum, Syrupus caryophyllirubri.

SYRUPUS IPECACUAN'HÆ, *Syrup of Ipecacuanha.* (*Ipecac.* in pulv. crass. ℥j, *alcohol. dilut.* Oj, *sacchar.* ℔iiss, *aquæ* q. s. Macerate the ipecacuanha in the alcohol for 14 days, and filter. Evaporate the filtered liquor to 6 fluidounces, again filter, and add sufficient water to make the [b...] measure a pint; add the sugar, and evaporate by a water-bath to a proper consistence. *Ph. U. S.*) It may also be prepared by displacement.

SYRUPUS DE JALAP'Â, *Syrup of Jalap.* (*Pulv. Jalapæ* ℥x, *sem. coriandr., fœnicul. dulc.* āā ℥s: *aquæ* f℥xijss, *sacch.* ℥xxv. *Ph. P.*) Cathartic. Dose, f℥ij to f℥ss for children.

SYRUPUS DE KINÂ KINÂ CUM VINO, *S. Cincho'na cum vino, Syrup of Cinchona with wine,* (F.) *Syrop de quinquina avec le vin.* (*Cort. cinchonæ officinalis* ℥ij, *ext. cinchonæ* ℥vj, *vini albi* (Fin. Lunel. vel cujusvis ei similis,) Oj, *alcohol* s [.] .985, to .915.) f℥j, *sacchar. alb.* ℔iss. Bruise the cinchona; gradually add the alcohol, so as to form a soft mass; pour on the wine; macerate for two days, and strain. Dissolve the extract, add the sugar, and make a syrup. *Ph. P.*) Dose, f℥ss to f℥j.

SYRUPUS KRAME'RIÆ, *Syrup of Rhatany.* (*Ext. Kramer.* ℥ij, *aquæ* Oj, *sacchar.* ℔ijss. Dissolve the extract in the water, and filter; then add the sugar, and form into syrup. *Ph. U. S.* It may also be made by displacement from *Kramer.* in pulv. crass. ℔j, *sacchar.* ℔iiss; *aq.* q. s.) An adjunct to astringent mixtures; or given in diarrhœa, a tea-spoonful to a child.

SYRUPUS LIMONIS, S. Limonum—s. Succi limonis, S. limonum.

SYRUPUS LIMO'NUM, *S. limonis,* (Ph. U. S.) *S. citri med'icæ, S. e succo citro'num, S. e succo limo'num, S. succi limo'nis, Syrup of Lemon, Lemon Syrup.* (*Limon. succ. colat.* Oj, *sacchar.* ℔j. Cooling, antiseptic.

SYRUPUS E MECONIO, S. papaveris—s. de Melle, Mellitum simplex.

SYRUPUS DE MERCU'RIO MEDIAN'TE GUMMI, *Mercu'rius gummo'sus Plenck'ii, Syrupus Hydrargyri,* (F.) *Syrop de mercure ou Mercure gommeux de Plenck.* (*Hydrargyri pur.* ℥j, *p. gum. acaciæ,* ℥ij, *syrup diacod.* ℥ss. Rub together till the mercury is extinguished. *Ph. P.*) Possesses the properties of the blue pill. Dose, gr. ij to viij, or more.

SYRUPUS MORI, *S. e succo moro'rum, S. mori, Syrup of Mul'berries,* (F.) *Syrop de mûres.* (*Mori succ. colat.* Oj, *sacchar. purif.* ℔ij. *Ph. L.*) Gratefully refrigerant.

SYRUPUS E SUCCO MORORUM, S. mori.

SYRUPUS MORPH'IÆ ACETA'TIS, *Syrup of acetate of morphia.* (*Syrup*, one pint, *acetate of morphia*, gr. iv.) Dose, two tea-spoonfuls, as an opiate. It is about the strength of the same quantity of syrup of poppies.

SYRUPUS MORPHIÆ SULPHA'TIS is made in the same way.

SYRUPUS NIGER, Melasses.

SYRUPUS PAPAV'ERIS, *S. papaveris somnif'eri,*

S. papaveris albi, S. e meco'nio, S. de meconio, Diaco'dion, Syrup of poppies, (F.) Syrop de pavots blancs ou diacode. (Papav. capsul. exsiccat. et contus. exemptis seminibus, ℥xiv, sacch. pur. ℔ij, aq. fervent. cong. ijss. Macerate the capsules in water for 12 hours; boil to a gallon, and express strongly. Boil the liquor to Oij; and strain while hot. Defecate by rest, and boil to Oj, adding the sugar so as form a syrup. Ph. L.) One ounce contains about one grain of opium. Anodyne and demulcent.

The Dublin college has a SYRUPUS OPII, called Common Syrup of Poppies, which is made by dissolving 18 grains of the Watery Extract of Opium in 18 ounces of boiling water. Properties, those of opium and syrup.

SYRUPUS DE PAPAVERE ERRATICO, S. rhœados —s. de Pomis compositus, see S. sennæ.

SYRUPUS PROTEÆ, see Protea mellifera. Syrupus Pruni Virginia'næ, Syrup of Wild cherry bark. (Pruni Virginia. in pulv. crass. ℥v, sacchar. ℔ij, Aquæ q. s. Moisten the bark with water; let it stand for 24 hours; transfer it to a percolator; pour water gradually upon it, until a pint of filtered liquor has passed. Add the sugar in a bottle, and dissolve by agitation. Ph. U. S., 1851.) Dose, as a demulcent expectorant, f℥j to f℥ij.

SYRUPUS QUI'NIÆ, Syrup of Quinia. (Simple syrup, 2 pints, sulphate of quinia, 64 grains.) Six spoonfuls are commonly sufficient to arrest an intermittent.

SYRUPUS E QUINQUE RADI'CIBUS, Syrup of five roots, (F.) Syrop des cinq racines. (Rad. apii, fœniculi, apii petroselini, āā ℥v. Infuse for 24 hours in boiling water Oiiss, and strain. Rad. asparag., rusci aculeati, āā ℥v, aquæ, Ovij. Boil and reduce to half; adding, towards the end, the residue of the preceding infusion. Boil again for some minutes; strain, and add white sugar, ℔vj. Ph. P.) Aperient and diuretic. Used in obstructions of the liver, spleen, and mesentery; and in dropsy, &c. Dose, f℥ss to f℥j, or more.

SYRUPUS RHAMNI, S. Rhamni cathar'tici, S. de Spinâ cervi'næ, S. spinæ cervi'næ, Syrup of Buckthorn, (F.) Syrop de nerprun. (Rhamn. baccar. succ. recent. Oiv, singib. rad. concis., pimentæ bacc. contrit. āā ℥ss, sacch. purif. ℔iiiss. Defecate the juice for 3 days, and strain. To a pint of this, add the ginger and pimento; macerate for 4 hours, and strain; boil what remains to Oiss. Mix the liquors and add sugar, so as to form a syrup. Ph. L.) Cathartic, but apt to gripe. Dose, f℥iv to f℥ij.

SYRUPUS RHEI, Syrup of Rhubarb. (Rhei, in pulv. crass. ℥ij; Alcohol, Oss; Aquæ Oiss; sacchar. ℔ij. Mix the alcohol and water; pour f℥iv on the rhubarb, mixed with an equal bulk of sand, and allow the whole to stand four hours; put the mass into a percolator, and gradually pour on the remainder of the alcohol and water. By means of a water-bath, evaporate to f℥xiij; add the sugar, and make a syrup. Ph. U. S.) Dose to a child, as a laxative, one or two teaspoonfuls.

SYRUPUS RHEI AROMAT'ICUS, Aromatic Syrup of Rhubarb, Spiced Syrup of Rhubarb. (Rhej, cont. ℥iiss; Caryophyl. cont., Cinnam. cont. āā ℥ss; Myrist. cont. ℥ij; Alcohol. dilut. Oij; Syrup Ovj. Macerate the rhubarb and aromatics in the diluted alcohol for 14 days, and strain; then, by means of a water-bath, evaporate the liquor to a pint, and while still hot, mix with the syrup previously heated. Ph. U. S.) It may also be made by the process of displacement.

The aromatic syrup of rhubarb is a gentle carminative cathartic. Dose to a child, f℥j; to an adult, f℥j.

SYRUPUS DE RHEO, Syrupus de Cichorio compositus.

SYRUPUS RHŒ'ADOS, S. de papav'eri errat'ico, S. papaveris erratici, Syrup of Red Poppy, (F.) Syrop de coquelicot. (Rhœad. petal. recent. ℔j, aq. fervent. f℥xviij, sacch. purif. ℔iiss. To the water, heated in a water-bath, add the petals. Remove the vessel; macerate for 12 hours; express; defecate, and add sugar to form a syrup. Ph. L.) Chiefly used to give colour.

A factitious syrup is often made of aloes, dissolved in simple syrup.

SYRUPUS ROSÆ, Syrupus rosa'rum soluti'vus, S. e rosis siccis, S. rosæ centifo'liæ, S. rosa'ceus soluti'vus, Syrup of Roses, (F.) Syrop de roses pâles. (Rosæ centif. petal. exsicc. ℥vij, sacch. purif. ℔vj, aq. fervent. Oiv. Macerate the petals for 12 hours. Evaporate the strained liquor to ℔iiiss. Add the sugar. Ph. L.) Gently laxative. Dose, f℥ij to f℥iss, or more.

SYRUPUS ROSÆ GAL'LICÆ, Syrup of Red Roses, (F.) Syrop de roses rouges. (Rosæ Gallic. petal. exsicc. ℥vij, aquæ bull. Ov, sacch. purif. ℔vj; prepared like the last. Ph. E.) Mildly astringent. Added to stomachic infusions.

SYRUPUS SACCHARI, S. Simplex.

SYRUPUS SARSAPARIL'LÆ, Syrup of Sarsaparilla. (Rad. Sarsap. cont. ℔j, aquæ bullient. cong., sacch. purif. ℔j. Macerate the root for 24 hours; boil to Oiv. Strain while hot; add the sugar, and boil. Ph. L.) Used in the same cases as the root. Dose, f℥j to f℥iv, and more.

SYRUPUS DE SARSAPARIL'LÂ ET SENNÂ COMPOS'ITUS, Compound Syrup of Sarsaparilla and Senna, (F.) Syrop de Cuisinier. (Rad. Sarsap. concis. ℔ij. Infuse for 24 hours in warm water Oxij; boil for a quarter of an hour; pass with expression, and boil again the residuum in Ox of water. Reduce this to Ovj, and repeat the operation 2 or 3 times. Mix all the liquors and boil them together with flowers of borage, white roses, senna leaves and aniseed, each ℥ij; reduce to half, pass, and add honey ℔ij. Boil to a syrup. Ph. P.) It is considered to be alterant, depurative, and sudorific. Dose, f℥ss to f℥ij.

A similar syrup, under the name SYRUPUS SARSAPARIL'LÆ COMPOS'ITUS, Compound Syrup of Sarsaparilla, is directed in the Pharmacopœia of the United States. (Sarsaparill. cont. ℔ij; Lign. guaiac. rasur. ℥iij; Rosæ centifol., Sennæ, Glycyrrhiz. cont. āā ℥ij; Ol. Sassafras, Ol. Anisi. āā m. v.; Ol. Gaultheriæ m. iij; Alcohol. dilut. Ox.; Sacchar. ℔viij. Macerate the sarsaparilla, guaiacum wood, roses, senna, and liquorice root in the diluted alcohol for 14 days; express and filter. Evaporate the tincture in a warm bath to four pints; filter, add the sugar, and form into syrup. Lastly, having rubbed the oils with a small quantity of the syrup, mix them thoroughly with the remainder. Ph. U. S.)

It may also be made by the process of displacement.

SYRUPUS DE SCAMMO'NIO, Syrup of Scam'mony. (Pulv. Scammon. ℥ss, sacch. alb. ℥iv, alcohol. (s. g. .985 to .915) f℥viij. Heat the mixture moderately: then set fire to the alcohol with a lighted taper; agitate constantly, until the flame is extinguished. Suffer it to cool; pass through cloth, and add Syrup of Violets, f℥iv. Ph. P.) ℥j contains 18 grains of scammony. Dose, f℥j to f℥ss.

SYRUPUS SCILLÆ, S. scillit'icus, S. scillæ marit'imæ, Syrup of Squills. (Acet. scillæ. Oj, sacch. ℔ij.) Diuretic, expectorant, and emetic. Used in the same cases as the oxymel.

SYRUPUS SCILLÆ COMPOS'ITUS, Mel Scillæ Compositum, Compound Honey of Squill, Compound Syrup of Squill, Hive Syrup. (Scillæ cont.; *Senegæ* cont. ̅ss ʒiv; *Antim. et Potassæ Tart.* gr. xlviij; *Aquæ* Oiv; *Sacchar.* ℔iiss. Pour the water upon the squills and seneka, and, having boiled to one-half, strain and add the sugar. Then evaporate to three pints, and while the syrup is still hot, dissolve in it the tartrate of antimony and potassa.)

It may also be made by the process of displacement. *Ph. U. S.*

It is often given as an emetic in cases of croup, and in catarrh, especially in children. Dose, to infants, 10 drops to a drachm, repeated every 15 minutes, if vomiting be desirable.

SYRUPUS SEN'EGÆ, *Syrup of Seneka.* (*Senegæ* cont. ʒiv; *Aquæ* Oj; *Sacchar.* ℔j. Boil the water with the seneka to one-half, and strain; then add the sugar, and form into syrup. *Ph. U. S.*)

It may also be formed by the process of displacement. *Ph. U. S.*

This is a favourite stimulant expectorant (?) with many practitioners. Dose, f ʒj or f ʒij.

SYRUPUS SENNÆ, *S. cassiæ sennæ, Syrup of Senna,* (*Sennæ* ʒij, *sem. fœnicul.* cont. ʒj, *sacch. pur.* ʒxv, *aquæ bullient.* Oj. Macerate the senna leaves and fennel-seeds with a gentle heat for an hour. Strain; add the sugar, and make into a syrup. *Ph. U. S.*) Cathartic. Dose, f ʒij to f ʒiss, or more.

The Parisian Codex has a *Syrupus de Senná* of a compound character, called *Syrupus de pomis compos'itus,* (F.) *Syrop de pommes composé.* It contains, also, borage, bugloss, &c. Dose, f ʒss to f ʒij.

SYRUPUS SIMPLEX, *Syrupus* (Ph. U. S.), *S. Sac'chari, Sac'charum clarifica'tum, Liqua'rium, Simple Syrup, Syrup, Common syrup of capillaire.* (*Sacch. purif.* ℔iiss, *aquæ* Oj. Dissolve the sugar; set aside for 24 hours; remove the scum, and pour off the clear liquid.) Used to cover nauseous tastes, &c.

SYRUPUS DE SPINÁ CERVINÁ, *Syrupus rhamni* —s. de Stœchade communis, see Lavendula.

SYRUPUS TOLUTA'NUS, *S. Toluta'ni, S. toluif'eræ bal'sami, S. balsam'icus, Balsam'ic syrup, Syrup of tolu.* (*Tinct. Tolut.* f ʒiss; *Aquæ* Oj; *Sacchar.* ℔iiss. Mix the tincture with the sugar in coarse powder; expose it on a shallow dish to a gentle heat, until the alcohol has evaporated; pour the water upon it; heat gradually until the sugar is dissolved, and strain. *Ph. U. S.*) Used to give flavour.

SYRUPUS VI'OLÆ, *S. violæ odora'tæ, S. viola'rum, S. e succo viola'rum, Syrup of Violets.* (*Flor. recent. viol. odorat.* ℔ij, *aq. bull.* Oviij, *sacch. pur.* ℔xv. Macerate in a covered vessel, for 24 hours; pass, without expression, through linen; add the sugar so as to form a syrup. *Ph. E.*) Very gently laxative. Dose, f ʒj to f ʒij.

SYRUPUS E SUCCO VIOLARUM, S. violæ.

SYRUPUS ZINGIB'ERIS, *S. amo'mi singiberis, Syrup of Ginger,* (F.) *Syrop de gingembre.* (*Tinct. Zingib.* f ʒiv; *Aquæ* Oiv; *Sacchar.* ℔x. Mix the tincture with four pounds of the sugar in coarse powder; and expose it in a shallow dish to a gentle heat until the alcohol has evaporated. Add the rest of the sugar, and then the water in a covered vessel; heat gradually until the sugar is dissolved, and strain. *Ph. U. S.*) To the strained liquor add the sugar, and form a syrup.

N. B. The Parisian Codex contained a few other compound syrups besides those enumerated; amongst these is a *Syrup of calf's lungs, Syrupus e pulmon'ibus vituli'nis,* (F.) *Syrop de mou de veau,* as an expectorant.

These syrups are made according to the usual rule, and possess the virtues of the substances after which they are named.

SYSPA'SIA, from σνσπαω, (συν, and σπαω, 'draw,') 'I contract.' Clonic spasm, with diminished sensibility and inability of utterance. A genus in Good's Nosology, which includes convulsion, epilepsy, and hysteria.

SYSPASIA CONVULSIO, Convulsion — s. Epilepsia, Epilepsy — s. Hysteria, Hysteria.

SYSSARCO'SIS, from συν, 'with,' and σαρξ, 'flesh.' *Commissu'ra ossium car'nea, Symphysis ossium muscula'ris, Connex'io ossium carnos ̄̄na'tio, Concarna'tio.* Union of bones by means of muscles; such as the union of the os hyoides with the lower jaw, of the scapula with the ribs, &c.

SYSTALCIS, Systole.

SYSTAL'TIC, *Systal'ticus, Peristal'tic:* from συστελλω, (συν, and στελλω,) 'I contract.' A taltic motion in a part is one in which there is alternate contraction and dilatation. See Systole.

SYSTAT'ICA, from συνιστημι, (συν, and ιστημι, 'I place,') 'I associate.' Diseases affecting several or all of the sensorial powers simultaneously; irritation or inertness of mind, extending to the muscles, or external senses; or of the muscles or external senses, extending to the mind:— the 4th order, class *Neurotica,* of Good.

SYSTEM, *Syste'ma,* from συν, 'together,' and ιστημι, 'I place.' This word, taken in a general sense, means the collection and arrangement of different matters having an analogy to each other or working towards the same end. In natural history, it means a methodical arrangement of beings for the purpose of facilitating their study. System is, however, sometimes used in an unfavourable sense in physical science, and then means, — a purely gratuitous supposition, by which the march of nature is attempted to be universally explained, and to which every thing is made to bend. In anatomy, system is an assemblage of organs, composed of the same tissues, and intended for similar functions; for instance the *nervous system, muscular system,* &c.

SYS'TEMATISM. A method, according to which every fact of a science is collected around an opinion, true or false. One who reduces things to such a method is called a *Sys'tematist.*

SYS'TEMATIST, see Systematism.

SYSTEMATOL'OGY, *Systematolog"ia,* from συστημα, 'system,' and λογος, 'a discourse.' The doctrine or a treatise of systems.

SYSTÈME VASCULAIRE À SANG NOIR, see Vascular — s. *Vasculaire à sang rouge,* see Vascular.

SYSTEMIC. Belonging to the general system — as '*systemic circulation*' in contradistinction to the '*pulmonic.*'

SYS'TOLE. Same etymon as SYSTALTIC. *Systal'sis, Constric'tio, Contrac'tio* seu *Anguste'tio, Submissio* seu *Mica'tio cordis.* The movement of constriction or contraction of the heart, to give impulse to the blood, or to cause its progress. It is opposed to the *Diastole* of the organ.

SYS'TOLIC, *Systol'icus;* same etymon. Relating to the systole of the heart, — as '*systolic murmur.*'

SYZYGIUM NERVORUM, Par nervorum

T.

T BANDAGE, *T. fas'cia, Fas'cia T. formis* seu *Heliodo'ri, Cru'cial Bandage*. A bandage shaped like the letter T. It consists of a strip of linen, of variable length and breadth, the middle of which is attached, at right angles, to the extremity of another strip, also of variable length and breadth. When two such strips are attached, at a distance from each other, the bandage is called a *double T*. This bandage is used, principally, for supporting the dressings after the operation for fistula in ano, in diseases of the perinæum, groin, anus, &c.

T FASCIA, T Bandage.

TABAC, Nicotiana tabacum—*t. des Savoyards*, Arnica montana—*t. des Vosges*, Arnica montana.

TABACUM, Nicotiana tabacum.

TABARZET, Saccharum album.

TAB'ASHEER, *Tabaschir, Tabaxir*. A substance found in the knots of the bamboo, in the East Indies, as a consequence of a morbid condition of the part. It is distinguished for its great proportion of silicic acid, in combination with a small quantity of mineral and vegetable matters; as well as for its slight refractive property. It has been used in obstruction of the bowels. The sweet juice of the bamboo stalks has also been called *Tabasheer*.

TABEFACTION, Emaciation.

TABEFY, Emaciate.

TABEL'LA, *Tab'ula, Tabula'tum, Lozan'ga, Lozan'gia, Mor'sulus, Morsel'lus*, a lozenge; *Tes*sel'la, (F.) *Tablette*, 'a small table.' A solid medicine, composed of a powder, sugar, and mucilage; and generally shaped like a disk. See Pastil, and Troch.

TABELLA, Table.

TABELLÆ ABSORBENTES, T. de Magnesiâ.

TABELLÆ AC''IDI OXAL'ICI, *T. ad sitem, Lozenges of Oxalic Acid*. (*Acid. oxalic*. ℨj, *sacch. alb.* ℨss, *ol. limonis*, gtt. xviij vel gtt. xij. Make into lozenges with *mucilage of gum tragacanth*. *Ph. P.*) Lozenges are made in the same way with the citric and tartaric acids. They are refrigerant.

TABELLÆ DE ALTHÆ'Â, *Lozenges of Marsh*mallows. (*Rad. althææ*, pulv., ℨiss, *sacchar. alb.* pulv. ℨivss; f. massa. *Ph. P.*) Demulcent; expectorant.

TABELLÆ ANTIMONIA'LES KUNCKE'LII, *Tabellæ de stib'ii sulphure'to, Lozenges of Sulph'uret of Ant'imony, Mor'suli antimonia'les, M. stibii, M. stibia'ti, Trochis'ci stibiati.* (*Amygdal. dulc.* ℨj, *sacch.* ℔ss, *sem. cardam., cinnam. pulv., sulph. antim. præpar.*, āā ℨj; fiant tabellæ. *Ph. P.* Each to weigh 10 grains.) Recommended in cutaneous diseases, blennorrhagia, arthritic pains, &c. Dose, 4 or more.

TABELLÆ AD ARDOREM VENTRICULI, Trochisci carbonatis calcis—t. Cardialgicæ, Trochisci carbonatis calcis.

TABELLÆ DE CAT'ECHU ET MAGNE'SIÂ, *Lozenges of Catechu and Magnesia*, (F.) *Tablettes de cachou et de magnésie*. (*P. catech.* ℨvj, *p. magnes.* ℨiv, *p. cinnam.* ℨiij, *sacch. alb.* ℔ss, *g. tragac.* gr. xij, *aq. cinnam.* q. s. ut f. massa. *Ph. P.* Each to weigh 12 gr.) Antacid, absorbent, and stomachic. Dose, 5 to 10 lozenges.

TABELLÆ CINCHO'NÆ, *T. de kinâ kinâ*, Bark Lozenges. (*Ext. cinchon.* slcc. ℨss, *sacch.* ℨiv, *cinnam.* ℨss, *mucilag. g. trag.* q. s. ut f. massa. *Ph. P.*) Tonic.

TABELLÆ DE CITRO ET DIACARTHAMO, T. de Scammonio et Sennâ.

TABELLÆ DE FERRO, *Steel lozenges, Tabulæ martia'les, T. instauran'tes, T. antichlorot'icæ*. (*Ferri limat. porphyris.* ℨss, *p. cinnam.* ℨj, *p. sacch.* ℨv, *g. trag. et aq. cinnam.* q. s., ut fiat massa. Each lozenge to weigh 12 gr. *Ph. P.*) Tonic, stomachic. Dose, v to x.

Aromatic lozenges of steel. These consist of sulphate of iron, with a small proportion of the *Tincture of Cantharides*.

TABELLÆ DE KINÂ KINÂ, T. cinchonæ.

TABELLÆ DE MAGNESIÂ, *P. absorben'tes, Magnesia lozenges*. (*Magnes.* ℨj, *sacchar. alb.* ℨiv, *mucil. g. tragac.* q. s. *Ph. P.*) Absorbent and antacid.

TABELLÆ DE RHEO, *Rhubarb lozenges*. (*P. rhej* ℨss, *sacch.* ℨv, *mucilag. gum. tragac.* q. s.; f. massa. Each to contain 12 grains. *Ph. P.*) Stomachic and laxative.

TABELLÆ DE SCAMMO'NIO ET SENNÂ COMPOS'ITÆ, *Compound lozenges of scammony and senna, T. de citro et diacar'thamo*. (*Scammon.* ℨiij, *Sennæ* ℨivss, *rhej.* ℨiss, *caryoph.* ℨj, *corticis limon. confect.* ℨj, *sacch.* ℨvj; f. massa. *Ph. P.*) Purgative. Dose, ℨij to ℨvj, or more.

TABELLÆ AD SITEM, T. acidi oxalici — t. ad Sodam, Trochisci carbonatis calcis — t. de Stibii sulphureto, T. antimoniales Kunckelii.

TABELLÆ DE SUL'PHURE SIM'PLICES, *Simple sulphur lozenges*. (*Sulphur lot.* ℨss, *sacch.* ℨiv, *muc. g. tragac.* cum aquâ rosâ præpar. q. s. *Ph. P.*) Expectorant, demulcent, &c. Used in diseases of the chest, and in cutaneous affections. Dose, a lozenge.

TABELLÆ DE SULPH'URE COMPOS'ITÆ, *Compound sulphur lozenges*. (*Sulph. lot.* ℨij, *acid. benzoic.* gr. xij, *rad. irid. p.* ℨss, *ol. anisi*, gtt. viij, *sacch.:* ℨvss, *g. trag.* q. s. *Ph. P.*) Aperient, expectorant, and stimulant. (?) Dose, 4 a day.

TABERNA MEDICA, Pharma copolium.

TABES, *Maras'mus Tabes, Tabum, Tab'idness*, from *tabere*, 'to consume;' *Te'kedon, Atroph'ia, Decline*. Emaciation of the whole body, with general languor, hectic fever, and, for the most part, depressed spirits.

TABES, Atrophy, Phthisis — t. Coxaria, Ischiophthisis — t. Diabetica, Diabetes mellitus — t. Diuretica, Diabetes mellitus.

TABES DORSA'LIS, *T. Dorsua'lis, Maras'mus tabes dorsa'lis, Phthisis no'tias* seu *dorsa'lis* seu *sicca, Myelophthi'sis, Myelatroph'ia, Tabes ossis sacri*. By this term is meant a wasting of the body, attended at first with a pain in the back or loins, and afterwards in the neck or head, — caused, it has been conceived, by too early or too frequent addiction to venery.

TABES GLANDULARIS, T. mesenterica, Scrofula — t. Ischiadica, Ischiophthisis — t. Lactea, Atrophia lactantium, see Galactia.

TABES MESENTER'ICA, *Atroph'ia mesenter'ica, Atroph'ia Infant'um, A. glandula'ris, A. infanti'lis, A. dorsi, Parabys'ma mesenter'icum, Ma'cies Infan'tum, Pædatroph'ia, Tabes glandula'ris, T. Scrofulo'sa, Scrof'ula mesenterica, Rachial'gia mesenterica, Myelophthi'sis sicca, Febris hec'tica infan'tum, Phthisis mesara'ica, Physco'nia mesenterica, Mesenteri'tis, Mesenter'ic Disease*, (F.) Carreau, Chartre, Scrofules ou Écrouelles mésentériques, Étisie mésentérique, Rachialgie mésentérique, Atrophie mésentérique, Physconie mésentérique, Entéro-mésentérite, Tubercles des ganglions mésentériques, Phthisie mésentérique. An engorgement and tubercular degeneration of the mesenteric glands, followed by emaciation and general disorder of the nutritive functions. The disease is often owing to inflammation or irritation of the lining membrane of the intestines, giving occasion to enlargement of the glands of the mesentery,—as injury to the upper or lower extremities causes inflammation, and enlargement of the lymphatic glands of the axilla and groin. It occurs, particularly, in children of a scrofulous diathesis; and in those who are weaned too early, or fed on indigestible substances. Diarrhœa, emaciation, anorexia, or immoderate appetite; hardness and swelling of the abdomen; and, towards the end, hectic fever, are the chief symptoms of this affection; the prognosis of which is usually unfavourable. On opening the bodies of those who die of the disease, the mesenteric glands are found disorganized, tubercular, or in a more or less advanced state of suppuration. The treatment is the same as in scrophulosis. Frictions may be added over the abdomen and spine; and mercury, in small doses, so as to excite a new action in the system. The food must be easy of digestion, and the bowels be kept soluble.

TABES NUTRICUM, Atrophia lactantium, see Galactia—t. Ossis sacri, Tabes dorsalis—t. Pectorea, Rachitis—t. Pulmonalis, Phthisis pulmonalis—t. Scrofulosa, T. mesenterica—t. Senum, Marasmus senilis.

TABESCERE, Emaciate.

TABID, *Tab'idus*, (F.) *Tabide*. Same etymon as Tabes. Relating or appertaining to tabes. Wasted by disease.

TABIDNESS, Tabes.

TABLE, *Tab'ula, Tabell'a, Tabula'tum, Lam'ina, Paries, Squama*. A name given to the plates of compact tissue, which form the bones of the cranium. Of these, one is external; the other *internal*, and called *Tab'ula vi'trea*, on account of its brittleness.

TABLES DE MORTALITÉ, Mortality, bills of.

TABLET, Trochiscus.

TABLETTE, Tabella.

TABLETTES DE CACHOU ET DE MAGNÉSIE, Tabellæ de catechu et magnesiâ.

TABLIER, Ventrale cutaneum.

TABOURET, Thlaspi bursa.

TABULA, Tabella, Table.

TABULÆ ANTICHLOROTICÆ, Tabellæ de ferro—t. Instaurantes, Tabellæ de ferro—t. Martiales, Tabellæ de ferro.

TABULATUM, Tabella, Table.

TABUM, Ichor, Sanies, Tabes.

TAC, Influenza.

TACAMAHACA, Fagara octandra—t. Caragna, Carànna.

TACHE, Macula.

TACHE EMBRYONNAIRE, 'Embryonic spot;' *Cu'mulus, Ger'minal cu'mulus, Cu'mulus germinati'vus seu prolig''erus, A'rea germinati'va, Nu'cleus cicatric'ulæ seu blastoderm'atis*. A name given by M. Coste to a spot seen on the blastoderma about the end of the first week, from which the development of the embryo proceeds.

According to Bischoff, the blastodermic vesicle consists here of a double layer—the upper one the *serous or animal*; the lower, the *mucous or vegetative*; and between these is afterwards formed the *vascular layer*.

TACHE GERMINATIVE, see Molecule—t. *de Naissance*, Nævus.

TACHENCAUSIS, Combustion, human.

TACHES HÉPATIQUES, Chloasma.

TACHES LAITEUSES, Plaques laiteuses,

'milky spots or patches.' White spots occasionally seen on the heart, and regarded by many pathologists as the results of previous pericarditis.

TACHES DE ROUSSURE, Ephelides—t. *Rouges*, Spots, Red.

TACHYIA'TER, *Tachyiatrus*. Same etymon as the next. One who cures speedily.

TACHYIATRI'A, from *ταχυς*, 'quick,' and *ιατρεια*, 'healing.' The art of curing quickly.

TACH'YTOMY, *Tachytom'ia*, from *ταχυς*, 'quick,' and *τομη*, 'incision.' The art of cutting or operating rapidly.

TACITUR'NITY, *Tacitur'nitas, Sigê*, 'silence,' from *tacere*, 'to be silent.' 'State of a person who does not speak.' Morbid taciturnity sometimes exists as a symptom of the neuroses, especially of melancholy.

TACT, *Tactus*, from *tangere, tactum*, 'to touch.' A modification of the sense of touch. Passive judgment by the cutaneous nerves regarding bodies exterior to the skin. Tact is passive: Touch, active.

TACTILE, *Tac'tilis*; same etymon. Relating or appertaining to touch.

TACTION, Touch.

TACTUS, Tact, Touch—t. Dolorificus, Hypodysphoria.

TÆDA, *Das, δαις*. A term used for a medicine employed under the form of fumigation, pessary, or troch.

TÆ'NIA, *Te'nia, Fas'cia*, from *ταινια*, 'a fillet, a riband.' See Bandage. Also a genus of intestinal worms, characterized by an elongated, flattened, and articulated body, with four such lateral oscula on the head. Of this genus, two only inhabit the human body—the *Tænia lata*, (see Bothriocephalus latus,) and *Tænia solium*.

TÆNIA ACEPHALA, Bothriocephalus latus—t. *Anneaux courts*, Bothriocephalus latus—t. *Anneaux longs*, Tænia solium—t. Articulis dentens, Tænia solium—t. Cucurbitina, Tænia solium—t. Dentata, Bothriocephalus latus—t. Grisea, Bothriocephalus latus—t. Hippocampi, Corpus fimbriata—t. Humana armata, Tænia solium—t. Humana inermis, Bothriocephalus latus—t. Bidatigena, Hydatid—t. Lata, Bothriocephalus latus—t. *à Longues articulations*, Tænia solium—t. Membranacea, Bothriocephalus latus—t. Nervosa Halleri, Ganglion of Gasser—t. *Nes corporis*, Bothriocephalus latus—t. Osculi lateralibus geminis, Bothriocephalus latus—t. Osculis lateralibus solitariis, Bothriocephalus latus—t. Osculis marginalibus solitariis, Tænia solium—t. Osculis superficialibus, Bothriocephalus latus—t. Prima, Bothriocephalus latus—t. *Sans épine*, Tænia solium—t. Secunda, Tænia solium.

TÆNIA SEMICIRCULA'RIS, *T. striata, Geminum centrum semicircula'rê, Limbus poste'rior corporis stria'ti, Stria cor'nea seu semiluna'ris seu termina'les, Frænulum novum, Fascia semicircularis*, (F.) *Bandelette des éminences pyramidales* (Ch.), *Bandelette, B. demicirculaire, Lame cornée*. A medullary, grayish, semitransparent layer, situate in the groove that separates the thalamus opticus from the corpus striatum in the lateral ventricle.

TÆNIA SO'LIUM, *T. os'culis marginal'ibus cœta'riis, Tænia cucurbiti'na, Tænia humana ar*ma'ta, *Hal'ysis solium, Vermis cucurbitinus, Lumbri'cus latus, Ténia sans épine, Tænia osculos demit'tens, So'lium, T. secunda, Tænia à longues articulations, Ténia à anneaux longs, Ténia solitaire, V. cucurbitain, Long Tape Worm*. Has an almost hemispherical, discrete head: about the neck full anteriorly; all the joints slightly obtuse, the anterior very short; the next almost square, and the rest oblong; the maxpos-

foramina vaguely alternated. The tænia solium is commonly a few feet long: sometimes its length is enormous. It is said to have been met with 600 feet long. It principally inhabits the small intestines, and is not common. The oil of turpentine, in some form, largely exhibited, is perhaps the best remedy.

TÆNIA STRIATA, T. semicircularis — t. Tarini, Lamina cornea—t. Tenella, Bothriocephalus latus —t. Vulgaris, Bothriocephalus latus.

TÆNIÆ COLI, see Colon.

TÆ'NIAFUGE, *Tæniaf'ugum*, from *tænia*, and *fugo*, 'I drive off.' A remedy calculated to expel tænia.

TÆNIOLA, *Bandelette.* Used by Gerber for a simple, band-like, or flat fibre, *Filum tæniaforme*, seen under the microscope.

TAFFETAS AGGLUTINATIF, Sparadrapum adhæsivum — t. *d'Angleterre*, see Sparadrapum adhæsivum — t. *Épispastique*, Sparadrapum vesicatorium — t. *Gommé*, see Sparadrapum adhæsivum — t. *Vésicant*, Sparadrapum vesicatorium.

TAFIA, Rum.

TAILLADE, Incision, see *Entaille.*

TAILLE, Lithotomy — t. *Hypogastrique*, Hypogastric operation of lithotomy, see Lithotomy —t. *Par le rectum*, see Lithotomy—t. *Postérieure*, see Lithotomy — t. *Recto-vésicale*, see Lithotomy — t. *Sus-pubiénne*, see Lithotomy.

TAKAMAHAKA, Fagara octandra.

TAL. A word formerly employed for alkali. It also meant the dung of the peacock.

TALC EARTH, Magnesia.

TALCUM NEPHRITICUM, Nephreticus lapis.

TALEN'TUM, ταλαντον. An ancient weight equal to 54 pounds, 2 oz., 5 dr., and 24 grains *Poids de Marc*. See Weights and Measures.

TALEOLUS, Malleolus.

TALIACOTIAN OPERATION, Rhinoplastic.

TALINUM UMBELLATUM, see *Mistura.*

TALIPES, Kyllosis (Clubfoot) — t. Equinus, see Kyllosis — t. Valgus, see Kyllosis — t. Varus, see Kyllosis.

TALON, see Calcaneum.

TALPA, 'a mole.' *Topina'ria, Tupina'ria, Talpa'ria, Testu'do*, (F.) *Taupe*. A tumour situate on the head, which has been supposed to burrow like a mole.

TALPARIA, Talpa.

TALUS, Astragalus, Malleolus, see Calcaneum.

TAMARA CONGA, Averrhoa carambola.

TAMARÆA ZECLA, Tamarindus.

TAMARIN, Tamarindus.

TAMARIN'DI PULPA, *Pulp of tamarinds*, (*Tamarinds*, q. s. Digest them with a small quantity of water, until they become of a uniform consistence; then separate the seeds and filaments, by pressing through a hair-sieve. Ph. U. S.)

TAMARINDS, PULP OF, Tamarindi pulpa.

TAMARIN'DUS, *T. In'dica, Thamarindus, Oxiphœnicon, Sil'iqua Arab'ica, Balampul'li, Tamarœ'a zecla, Oxyphœni'cia, Aca'cia Indica, Tamarind tree*, (F.) *Tamarin*. Family, Leguminosæ. *Sex. Syst*. Triandria Digynia. The pulp of the tamarind with the seeds connected by numerous tough strings, is exported from the West Indies, preserved in syrup, — *Tamarindus*, (Ph. U. S.) It is refrigerant and laxative. *Tamarind whey* is made by boiling ℥ij of the pulp with ℔iss of milk. When strained, it is used as a diluent in fever.

TAMARISCUS, Tamarix Gallica.

TAM'ARIX, *T. Gal'lica, T. Pentan'dra, Tamaris'cus. The Tamarisk tree. Family*, Portulaceæ. *Sex. Syst*. Pentandria Pentagynia. The bark, wood, and leaves were formerly employed medicinally;—the former for its aperient and corroborant virtues, in obstructions of the liver; the latter in icterus, hæmoptysis, and some cutaneous affections.

TAMBOUR, CAVITÉ DU, Tympanum.

TAMPA BAY, see Saint Augustine.

TAMPON, see Plugging.

TAMPONNEMENT, Plugging.

TANACE'TUM, *T. vulga'rē, Tana'sia, Athana'sia, Parthe'nium mas, Tansy*, (F.) *Tanaisie vulgaire. Family*, Corymbiferæ. *Sex. Syst*. Syngenesia Polygamia. The leaves and flowers of tansy have a peculiar, strong odour, and warm, bitter taste. They are tonic, deobstruent(?), and anthelmintic. Dose, ʒss to ʒj. The infusion is usually drunk as tea.

TANACE'TUM BALSAMI'TA, *Balsami'ta mas* seu *vulga'ris, B. suaveolens, B. major, Tanacetum horten'sē, Costus horto'rum, Mentha Roma'na* seu *Saracen'ica, Costmary, Alecost, Cock-mint*, (F.) *Menthe coq, Herbe au coq, Grand Baume*. A fragrant-smelling herb, somewhat resembling mint, and formerly much esteemed as a corroborant, carminative, and emmenagogue.

TANACETUM HORTENSE, T. balsamita.

TANACE'TUM MULTIFLO'RUM. A South African plant, which is used as a tonic, antispasmodic and anthelmintic. It is given in flatulency, gout, amenorrhœa and dropsy: but is especially prescribed in cases of ascarides lumbricoïdes and other entozoa. It is administered in the form of powder or infusion; the latter acting also, as a diaphoretic and diuretic. It is used likewise as a resolvent and anodyne fomentation.

TANAISIE VULGAIRE, Tanacetum.

TANASIA, Tanacetum.

TANGE, ταγγη, 'rancidity.' A putrescent tumour.

TANINUM, Tanninum.

TANNIC ACID, Tannin.

TANNICUM PURUM, Tannin.

TANNIN, from (F.) *tanner*, 'to tan.' *Tan'nicum purum, Tanni'num, Tani'num, Princip'ium adstringens* seu *Scytodep'sicum* seu *Byrsodep'sicum* seu *Coria'ceum, Scytodep'sium, Acidum Tan'nicum, A. Quercitan'nicum, Tannic acid*, (F.) *Acide tannique*. A principle obtained from oak bark and other astringent vegetables, so called from its forming the principal agent in the process of *tanning*. Pure tannin, obtained from galls, by the action of ether, (see Ph. U. S.) has been employed as an excellent and powerful astringent. Dose, two grains repeated several times a day.

TANSY, Tanacetum — t. Wild, Potentilla anserina.

TAPER, HIGH, Verbascum nigrum.

TAPE'TUM, *Ta'pestry, Tape'tum choroideæ*. A shining spot, on the outside of the optic nerve, in the eyes of certain animals, which is owing to the absence of the pigmentum nigrum, occasioning the reflection of a portion of the rays from the membrana Ruyschiana. Its use appears to be, by reflecting the rays, to cause a double impression on the retina, and thus add to the intensity of vision.

TAPETUM, see Corpus Callosum.

TAPETUM ALVE'OLI, *Membra'na exter'na den'tium*. The outer membrane of thé teeth. The lining membrane or periosteum of the alveoli.

TAPEWORM, BROAD, Bothriocephalus latus — t. Long, Tænia solium.

TAPIOCA, see Jatropha manihot — t. Pearl, see Jatropha manihot.

TAPSUS BARBATUS, Verbascum nigrum.

TAPSARIA, Decoctum hordei.

TAR, see Pinus sylvestris — t. Barbadoes, Petroleum — t. Mineral, Pissasphaltum.

TAR'ACHĒ, *Tarax'is, Tarag'ma, Tarag'mus,* 'disorder.' A disorder of sight, which arises from a blow, compression of the eye, or the action of dust, smoke or other external cause. By some, it is understood to signify mild or incipient ophthalmia.

Ταραχη της κοιλιας, 'disturbance of the belly.' Diarrhœa.

TARAGMA, Tarache.
TARAGMUS, Tarache.
TARAGON, Artemisia dracunculus.
TARANTALISMUS, Tarantismus.
TARANTISM'US, *Tarentis'mus, Tarantalis'mus, Dinoma'nia, Chore'a Sancti Valenti'ni, Taren'tulism, Tar'antism.* A feigned or imaginary disease in Apulia, characterized by excessive avidity for dancing at the sound of instruments, and which was ascribed, by the vulgar, to the bite of the tarantula. A sort of tarantismus, considered peculiar to Africa, and believed to be spontaneous, has been called *Tarentismus Tangita'nus, Janon-tarentisme.*

TARAN'TULA, from Tarentum or Tarento, a town of Italy where it abounds; *Taren'tula,* (F.) *Tarentule.* A species of spider—the *Ara'nea Tarentula* of Linnæus, *Lyco'sa Tarentula* of Latreille, whose bite has been looked upon as dangerous. Music has been thought to cure it.

TARASCON, MINERAL WATERS OF. Chalybeate springs in the department of Arriège, France. They contain iron and carbonic acid.

TARAXACUM, Leontodon taraxacum — t. Dens leonis, Leontodon taraxacum.

TARAXIS, Tarache, see Ophthalmia.
TARCHON SYLVESTRIS, Achillea ptarmica.
TARENTISMUS, Tarantismus — t. Tangitanus, Tarantismus.
TARENTULA, Tarantula.
TARENTULISM, Tarantismus.
TARGAR, Juniperus communis.

TARI. Palm or cocoa wine, from which sugar was obtained, called *Jagre.* It was once used as a tonic.

TARI'NI PONS, *Interpedun'cular space, Posterior perforated space, Locus perfora'tus posti'cus.* A cineritious substance, between the corpora albicantia, which assists in forming the bottom of the third ventricle.

TARO, Arum esculentum.
TARQUETTE, Horniaria glabra.
TARSAL, *Tar'seus.* That which relates to the tarsus.

TARSAL ARTICULATIONS result from the union of the bones of the tarsus with each other.

TAR'SEA LATA (LIGAMENTA). Three ligaments, described by Winslow as stretching from the edge of the orbit to that of the tarsi, with which, he thought, they formed a complete layer of the eyelids. Zinn could not trace the ligaments all the way to the tarsi; whilst Haller doubted altogether their ligamentous texture, and Zeis regards them as merely areolar substance.

TARSEUS, Tarsal.

TARSO-METATARSAL, *Tarso-metatar'seus.* That which relates to tarsus and metatarsus.

TARSO-METATARSAL ARTICULATIONS are those between the bones of the second row of the tarsus and the metatarsal bones. The term *Tarso-metatarsal* is likewise applied to ligaments connected with these joints, some of which are *dorsal,* and others *plantar.*

TARSO-MÉTATARSI-PHALANGIEN DU I OUCE, Adductor pollicis pedis—*t. Phalangien du pouce,* Flexor brevis pollicis pedis — *t. Sous-phalangien du petit orteil,* Flexor brevis minimi digiti pedis—*t. Sous-phalangettien du premier orteil,* Flexor brevis pollicis pedis.

TARSOPHY'MA, from *Tarsus,* and φυμα, 'a tumour.' A swelling of the tarsus.

TARSOR'RHAPHY, *Tarsorraph'ia,* from *tarsus,* 'the tarsal cartilage,' and ραφη, 'suture.' An operation for diminishing the size of the opening between the eyelids, when it is enlarged by surrounding cicatrices.

TARSOT'OMY, *Tarsotom'ia,* from *tarsus,* and τομη, 'incision.' The section or removal of the tarsal cartilages.

TARSUS, *Planta prima pedis, Rasce'ta Rasce'ta pedis, Pe'dium, Cavic'ulæ pedis.* 1. The posterior part of the foot. The tarsus consists of 7 bones, arranged transversely in two rows, between which amputation is sometimes performed. The *first* or *Tibial row,* (F. *première rangée, R. jambière,* consists of the astragalus and os calcis; the *second* or *metatarsal, seconde rangée, R. métatarsienne,* of the scaphoides, cuboides, and three ossa cuneiformia. 2. The *Tarsi,* Tarsal cartilages, *Tarsal fibrocartilages, Orchoi, Crepid'ines* seu *Coro'næ tabulæ* seu *Un'gulæ Palpebra'rum, Tharsi,* are small cartilaginous layers, seated in the substance of the free edge of each eyelid. The upper is larger and broader than the lower. Both commence at the bifurcated extremity of the tarsi of the orbicularis palpebrarum, and pass to the opposite commissure of the eyelids. They are broader in the middle than at their extremities.

TARTAR, Antimonium tartarizatum (improperly), Potassæ supertartras impurus—t. Calcareous, Potassæ subcarbonas — t. Crystals, Potassæ supertartras — t. Emetic, Antimonii tartarizatum — t. Soluble, Potassæ tartras et Potash.

TARTA'REI MORBI. A term employed by Paracelsus to designate certain diseases which he attributed to tartar.

TARTARI CRYSTALLI, Potassæ supertartras.

TARTAR'IC ACID, *Ac"idum tartari'cum, tartaro'sum, Acor tartar'icus, Acidum tartari essentia'lē, Tarta'reous acid, Sal tartari essentialē.* (Potassæ bitart. ℔iiss, aq. destillat. cong. iij, cretæ ppt. ℔j, acidi sulph. ℔j. Bitartrate with two gallons of the water, and gradually add the prepared chalk, until no more bubbles appear; let the tartrate of lime subside then pour off the fluid and wash the tartrate of lime with distilled water, until it is tasteless. Pour upon it the sulphuric acid, diluted with a gallon of boiling distilled water; and set the mixture aside for 24 hours, occasionally stirring it. Filter and evaporate to crystallize. Ph. E.) It is refrigerant and antiseptic, but it is chiefly used for making effervescent draughts with soda.

TARTARUM, Potassæ supertartras impurus— t. Vitriolatum, Potassæ sulphas.

TARTARUS AMMONIÆ, Ammoniæ tartras — t. Chalybeatus, Ferrum tartarizatum — t. Crudus, Potassæ supertartras impurus — t. Dentis, Odontolithos — t. Emeticus, Antimonium tartarizatum—t. Kalicoferricus, Ferrum tartarizatum, t. Kalinus, Potassæ tartras—t. Lixivius, Potassæ tartras — t. Martialis, Ferrum tartarizatum — Potassæ ferruginosus, Ferrum tartarizatum — t. Subpotassicus, Potassæ supertartras—t. Supertassicus, Potassæ supertartras — t. Tartarisatus, Potassæ tartras.

TARTRATE D'AMMONIAQUE, Ammoniæ tartras.

TARTRE BRUT, Potassæ supertartras impurus—*t. Cru,* Potassæ supertartras impurus—*t. Dents,* Odontolithos— *t. Emétique,* Antimonium

tartarisatum — t. *Stibié*, Antimonium tartarizatum.
TARTRUM SOLUBILE, Potassæ tartras.
TASIS, Extension, Tension.
TASTE, *Gustus, Geusis, Geuma, Geuthmos*, (F.) *Goût*. One of the five external senses, which instructs us of the savours of bodies, and of which the tongue is the principal organ.
Gustation, Gustatio, is the exercise of this faculty. In disease, the taste frequently becomes variously vitiated. The nerves of taste are probably the lingual branch of the fifth pair and the glosso-pharyngeal.
TASTE, Savour.
TAUPE, Talpa.
TAUROCOL'LA, from ταυρος, 'a bull,' and κολλα, 'glue.' Glue made of the ears and genitals of the bull. It was formerly much esteemed.
TAURUS, Penis, Perineum.
TAXIS, 'arrangement;' from τασσω, 'I order,' 'I arrange;' *Reposit''io, Reduc'tio, Syntax'is*. A methodical pressure exerted by the hand on a hernial tumour, for the purpose of reducing it. This operation is generally easy in herniæ that are free from adhesions, of small size, and with a large opening into the sac; but it is very difficult and frequently impracticable in those that are adherent or strangulated. To perform the taxis, the patient should be put in the horizontal posture, and in one in which the parietes of the abdomen are relaxed. The manual procedure varies in each species of hernia. In all cases, too strong pressure of the parts must be avoided; as inflammation and gangrene might be induced. The displaced organs must be pushed into the abdomen, according to the direction of the axis of the hernial sac. The reduction is sometimes favoured by blood-letting *ad deliquium;* the warm bath; warm fomentations; tobacco; emollient glysters; and, at times, by cold applications, as ice, &c. In a case of strangulated hernia, should the taxis fail, an operation becomes necessary.
TAXUS BACCA'TA. The Yew tree, *Smilax, Smilax, Thym'alos*, (F.) *If. Family*, Coniferæ. *Sex. Syst.* Diœcia Monadelphia. The ancients believed the yew to be poisonous; but the fruit may be eaten without inconvenience. The leaves have been often recommended in epilepsy. The resin, obtained from the bark, has been called *albir*.
TAYE, Caligo.
TAYLOR'S REMEDY FOR DEAFNESS, see Allium.
TEA, Thea — t. Apple, see Apple tea — t. Bahama, Lantana camara — t. Beef, see Beef tea — t. Berried, Gaultheria — t. Berry, Gaultheria — t. Blankenheim, see Galeopsis grandiflora — t. Brazil, Lantana pseudothea — t. Bushman's, Methyscophyllum glaucum — t. Caffre, Helichrysum nudifolium — t. Chicken, see Chicken tea — t. Flaxseed, Infusum Lini compositum — t. Ginger, Infusum Zingiberis — t. Hottentots', Helichrysum serpyllifolium — t. Labrador, Ledum latifolium — t. Lemon-peel, see Citrus medica — t. Marsh, Ledum palustre — t. Mexico, Chenopodium ambrosioides — t. Mountain, Gaultheria — t. Mutton, see Mutton tea — t. New Jersey, Celastrus — t. Oswego, Monarda coccinea — t. Redberry, Gaultheria — t. Slippery elm, Infusum Lini compositum — t. Soot, see Fuligokali — t. South sea, Ilex vomitoria — t. Spanish, Chenopodium ambrosioides — t. Veal, see Veal tea.
TEAR, Sax. teap, *Lac'ryma, Lach'ryma, Lac'rima, Lac'ruma, Dacry, Dae'ryma, Dac'ryon, Humor lacryma'lis, Eyedrop*, (F.) *Larme*. An excrementitious humour, secreted by the lachrymal gland, and poured between the globe of the eye, and the eyelids, to facilitate the motions of those parts. The tears are saline, inodorous, and colourless. They turn the syrup of violets green; and contain chloride of sodium, with excess of base, phosphates of lime and soda, and albumen.
TEARS, DEERS', Bezoar of the deer.
TEASEL, CULTIVATED, Dipsacus sylvestris.
TEAT, Nipple.
TEAZEL, Eupatorium perfoliatum.
TECEDON, Phthisis.
TECNOCTONIA, Infanticide.
TECOLITHOS, Judæus (lapis.)
TECO'MA RADI'CANS, *Bigno'nia radi'cans, Trumpet flower, Trumpet creeper, Virgin'ia creeper*. Indigenous; the orange and scarlet flowers appearing in July. *Order*, Bignoniaceæ. The leaves are acrid.
TECTARIA CALAHUALA, see Calagualæ radix — t. Ferruginea, see Calagualæ radix.
TEETH, see Tooth — t. Eye, Canine teeth — t. Jaw, Molar teeth — t. Milk, see Dentition — t. Neck of the, Collum dentium — t. Vitreous substance of the, Enamel of the teeth.
TEETHING, Dentition.
TEGIMEN, Integument.
TEGMEN, Integument.
TEGULA HIBERNICA, Hibernicus lapis.
TEGUMEN, Integument.
TÉGUMENT, Integument.
TEGUMEN'TARY. Relating or appertaining to the integument.
TEGUMEN'TUM, Integument — t. Auris, see Tympanum — t. Ventriculorum cerebri, Centre, oval, of the brain.
TEIGNE, Pityriasis, Porrigo, Porrigo lupinosa — t. *Annulaire*, Porrigo scutulata — t. *en Anneau*, Porrigo scutulata — t. *Faveuse*, Porrigo favosa — t. *Furfuracée*, Porrigo furfurans — t. *Nummulaire*, Porrigo scutulata.
TEINESMOS, Tenesmus.
TEINODYN'IA; from τεινειν, 'to extend,' and οδυνη, 'pain.' Pain of the sinews or tendons.
TEINOPHLOGO'SIS; from τεινειν, 'to extend,' and φλογωσις, 'inflammation.' Inflammation of the sinews or tendons.
TEINTURE, Tincture — t. *Éthérée*, Æthereal — t. *Rubéfiante*, Tinctura cantharidis.
TEKEDON, Tabes.
TELA, Texture, Tissue — t. Accidentalis Medullaris, Encephaloid — t. Cellulosa, Cellular tissue — t. Emplastica, Sparadrapum — t. Erectilis, Erectile tissue — t. Galteri, Sparadrapum Galteri — t. Hippocratis cribrosa, Cellular tissue — t. Hymenochondroides, Tissue, cartilaginous — t. Hymenochondrodes, Tissue, cartilaginous — t. Ichthyocollæ glutinans, see Sparadrapum adhæsivum — t. Inodularis, Tissue, inodular — t. Organica, Histos — t. Vesicatoria, Sparadrapum vesicatorium.
TELAMON, Habena.
TELAMO'NES, τελαμωνες, 'bandages.' Charpie, used for wounds; or linen, employed for bandages.
TELANGECTASIS, Telangiectasia.
TELANGIECTA'SIA, *Telangiec'tasis, Telangec'tasis, Angeotelecta'sia, Hæmatotelangio'sis, Hæmotelangio'sis, Angiecta'sia, Anastomu'sis aneurysmat'ica;* from τελος, 'far,' αγγειον, 'vessel,' and εκτασις, 'dilatation.' Dilatation of vessels. Nævus maternus. Aneurism by anastomosis. According to some, fungus hæmatodes. See Hæmatodes fungus.
TELANGIECTASIA OCULI, Cirsophthalmus.
TELEPH'IUM, *Ulcus telephium*. The ancients gave this name to any ulcer of a very bad kind, and difficult to cure, because the wound, which

Achilles inflicted on Telephus, degenerated into a similar ulcer.

TELEPHIUM, Sedum telephium.
TELLURISMUS, Magnetism, animal.
TELUM, Penis.
TEMPE, Temple.
TEM'PERAMENT, *Temperamen'tum, Temperatu'ra, Tempera'tio, Tempe'ries;* originally from *tempus,* 'time;' the great *temperer; Complex'io, Crasis, Euora'sia.* A name given to the remarkable differences that exist between individuals, in consequence of the variety of relations and proportions between the constituent parts of the body. Thus, of old, it was supposed that, according to the predominance of any one of the four humours then generally admitted,—blood, lymph, bile, and atrabilis or black bile,—the manifestations of the functions were tempered or modified so as to give rise to a *sanguine, lymphatic, choleric,* or *atrabilious* or *melancholic* predominance or temperament. The idea of the existence of certain of these humours has been banished; yet the influence of some, as of the blood, lymph, and bile, is still admitted by many. Too much influence has, doubtless, been assigned to temperament in the sense in which it was formerly and still is generally understood, although there can be no question that difference of organization occasions a difference in the activity of organs.

TEMPERAMENT, BILIOUS, Choleric temperament.
TEM'PERANCE, *Sophros'ynē, Nephal'iotes, Sobrietas, Sobri'ety.* Moderation, opposed to gluttony and drunkenness. The advantage of temperance, in a hygienic point of view, requires no comment.

TEMPÉRANTS, Sedatives.
TEMPERATIO, Temperament.
TEMPERATURA, Temperament.
TEMPERIES, Temperament.
TEMPLE, *Tempus, Re'gio Tempora'lis, Crot'aphus,* (F.) *Tempe.* A depression, on each side of the head, between the forehead and eye anteriorly, and the ear posteriorly. The *temples,* distinguished into *right* and *left,* correspond to the temporal fossa on each side. The word is said to be from the Latin *tempus,* 'time,' because in this part the hair first begins to turn white, and to indicate age.

TEMPORAL, *Tempora'lis.* That which relates to the temples.

TEMPORAL APONEURO'SIS is a very strong aponeurosis, of a bluish, shining colour, which is attached to the whole of the curved line of the temporal bone; to the posterior edge of the malar bone; to the superior margin of the zygomatic arch; and forms an envelope for the temporal muscle.

TEMPORAL ARTERIES, *Crot'aphite Arteries,* are several:—1. The *Temporal Artery,* properly so called, arises from the outer side of the superior part of the external carotid. It ascends between the ramus of the jaw, the meatus auditorius externus, and the parotid gland, which covers it as far as the zygomatic arch. Above this it becomes subcutaneous; and, when it has attained the middle of the temporal region, it divides into two branches; the one anterior—*A. tempora'lis fronta'lis* seu *inter'na* seu *ante'rior;* the other posterior—the *A. temporalis occipita'lis* seu *exter'na* seu *supe'rior.* The temporal artery, before its division, gives off, 1. Branches to the parotid; to the joint of the lower jaw; to the meatus auditorius, and to the masseter. 2. The *transverse artery of the face.* 3. The *middle temporal,* which arises beneath the cheek-bone, and traverses the temporal aponeurosis, immediately beneath that bone. II. The *Deep-seated Tem'porales. A. tempora'les profun'dæ.* These are two in number. They arise from the internal maxillary, and have been distinguished, from their position, into anterior and posterior. They send their principal divisions to the temporal muscle.

TEMPORAL BONE, *Os tem'poris* seu *temporis* seu *arcua'lē* seu *arma'lē* seu *parieta'lē* seu *crotaphit'icum* seu *memen'to mori* seu *squamosum* seu *crot'aphus,* is seated at the lateral and inferior part of the cranium, of which it forms part; and contains, within it, the special organ of audition. It is usually divided into three portions:—1. The *squamous, Pars squamosa* seu *lepidoï'des* seu *squamo'sum* seu *squamiformis,* Portion *écailleuse* ou *squameuse.* 2. The *mastoid portion,* and, 3. The *Petrous portion, Pars Proc''ess, Pars petro'sa, Pyr'amis trique'tra lapideum* seu *lapido'sum* seu *saxeum* seu *petrosum* seu *lithoïdes* seu *durum* seu *prærupta rupis mila'tum* seu *nervalē, Pars pyramidalis ossis pori,* (F.) *Portion pierreuse, Rocher, Os petreux, Apophyse pyramidale, A. pétrée.*

It has, *first,* an auricular or external face, which is a surface that makes part of the temporal fossa; the zygomatic process; the glenoid cavity; the fissure of Glaser; the meatus auditorius externus; the mastoid process; the tric groove; the canalis caroticus; the jugular fossa; the styloid process; the stylo-mastoid ramen, &c. 2. A cerebral or internal face, which corresponds to the cavity of the cranium, and on which is the *Pars petrosa,* the hiatus Fallopii, the meatus auditorius internus, the orifice of the aquæductus vestibuli, a portion of the gutter for the lateral sinus, &c. 3. A circumference, on which is observed the orifice of the bony portion of the Eustachian tube and the aqueduct of the cochleæ, &c. The temporal bone is articulated with the sphenoid, occipital, parietal, malar, and inferior maxillary bones. It is developed by five points of ossification.

TEMPORAL FOSSA is an excavation, observed at each side of the head. It is filled by the muscle whose name it bears, and is formed by the temporal and sphenoid, below; by the parietal and frontal bones, above; is separated by a transverse crista, from the zygomatic fossa, and completed, before, by the cheek-bone.

TEMPORAL MUSCLE, *Tempora'lis, Crotaphites,* (F.) *Arcadi-temporo maxillaire, Temporo maxillaire* (Ch.), is a broad, flattened, triangular muscle, which fills the temporal fossa. Its fibres attached to the temporal aponeurosis and the bone; and all converge into a strong tendon, which passes under the zygomatic arch, and is inserted into the coronoid process of the lower jaw. This muscle raises the lower jaw, and applies the teeth against each other.

TEMPORAL NERVES. These are distinguished into the *superficial temporal,* furnished by the inferior maxillary branch of the fifth pair, near the condyle of the jaw; and the *temporales profundi,—anterior* and *posterior,—furnished by the same nerve, at its exit from the cranium. Sömmering has given the name *temporales* to divisions sent by the facial nerve to the temporal regions.

TEMPORAL VEINS were formerly called Jugulares or *Aëtoï Phlebes, Aq'uilæ Venæ.*

TEMPORO-AURICULAIRE, Attollens aurem.

TEM'PORO-FA'CIAL, *Tem'poro-facia'lis,* belonging to the temple and face.

TEMPORO-FACIAL NERVE, *Nervus temporofacia'lis.* A branch of the facial nerve distributed to the face and temple.

TEMPORO-MAXILLAIRE, Temporal muscle.

TEMPORO-MAX'ILLARY, *Tem'poro-maxilla'ris*. That which belongs to the temporal bone and lower jaw.

TEMPORO-MAXILLARY ARTICULATION or joint of the lower jaw, is seated between the glenoid cavity and transverse process of the temporal bone on the one hand, and the condyle of the lower jaw on the other. Two thin cartilages cover the surfaces of these bones. The one is common to the transverse process and the portion of the glenoid cavity, anterior to the fissure of Glaser; the other belongs to the condyle. This articulation is furnished with an inter-articular fibro-cartilage, two synovial capsules, and two lateral ligaments:— the one internal, and the other external.

TEMPORO-MAXILLARY NERVES of Bichat are the divisions of the facial nerve, distributed to the temporal and maxillary regions.

TEMPUS, Temple — t. Intercalare, Apyrexia, Intermission.

TEMULENCE, Temulentia.

TEMULEN'TIA, *Ebri'etas, Ebrios'itas, Methys'mus, Tem'ulence, Tem'ulency, Inebria'tion, Intoxica'tion, Drunk'enness*: — from wine, *Œnophlyg''ia, Œnophlyx'is, Vinolen'tia, Vi'nolence*, (F.) *Ivresse*. Plater gave this name to delirium; Ettmuller, to an apoplectic condition, depending upon drunkenness; the *Apoplex'ia Temulen'ta* or dead drunkenness. Commonly, *Temulentia* is used synonymously with drunkenness, *Methê*; and is often employed in the description of diseases to indicate a state resembling drunkenness. *Mania e Timulentiâ* is the same as *Delirium Tremens*.

TENACULA, Bone-nippers— t. Volsella, Forceps (lithotomy).

TENAC'ULUM, from *teneo*, 'I hold.' A kind of fine hook attached to a handle which is thrust through the parietes of a blood vessel to draw it out and enable it to be tied.

TENACULUM, ASSALINI'S. An ingenious instrument, invented by Assalini. It consists of a forceps, or double tenaculum, the points of which are fine, sharp, and bifurcated, so as to be readily received into each other when the instrument is closed on the artery, which it is by a spring. It is of great use when the surgeon has no assistant at hand. The instrument is figured in S. Cooper's "First Lines."

TENAILLE INCISIVE, Bone-nippers.

TENASMUS, Tenesmus.

TENDON, *Tendo, Pronerva'tio*, from *τεινω*, 'I stretch.' *Tenon*, a *Sinew*. A fibrous cord, more or less round, long, or flattened; of a white, pearl colour, and composed of very close parallel fibres. The tendons are attached to the bones, by one extremity; by the other, they receive the insertions of the fleshy fibres: sometimes they afford attachment to fleshy fibres at both ends;— as in the digastric muscle. The tendons must be considered as so many cords, for transmitting the motion of muscles to the bones or levers.

TENDON D'ACHILLE, Achillis tendo.

TENDON, CORDIFORM, OF THE DIAPHRAGM, Centre, phrenic.

TENDONS, TWITCHING OF THE, Subsultus tendinum.

TENEOTOMIA, Tenotomy.

TÉNESME, Tenesmus — t. *de l'Œsophage*, Œsophagismus — t. *Vésical*, Bradysuria.

TENES'MUS, *Teines'mos, Tenas'mus*, from *τεινω*, 'I stretch.' *Proc'tica Tenesmus, Proctospas'mus, Obstipa'tio Tenesmus, Tinag'mus*, (F.) *Ténesme, Épreintes*. Frequent, vain, and painful desires to go to stool;— one of the chief symptoms of inflammation of the lining membrane of the digestive tube, as of dysentery.

TENESMUS VESICÆ, Bradysuria — t. Vesicæ mucosus, Cystirrhœa.

TENETTES, Forceps (craniotomy).

TÉNIA, Tænia.

TENNESSEE', MINERAL WATERS OF. On the waters of the French Bread River, in this state, is a large, clear, thermal spring. The heat is so great that, on first going into the water, it is almost insupportable.

TENON, Tendon.

TENONT'AGRA, from *τενων*, 'tendon,' and *αγρα*, 'seizure.' A variety of gout, which affects the tendinous parts of muscles, or the tendinous ligaments which strengthen certain articulations.

TENONTOTOMIA, Tenotomy.

TENONTOTRO'TI, from *τενων*, 'tendon,' and *τιτρωσκω*, 'I wound.' They who are wounded in the tendons. — Galen.

TENOT'OMY, *Tenotom'ia, Teneotom'ia, Tenontom'ia, Sec'tio seu Dissec'tio ten'dinum*, from *τενων*, 'a tendon,' and *τομη*, incision.' The operation of dividing a tendon, often practised for the removal of loxarthrus, or deviation of the joints — as in club-foot.

TENSEUR DE L'APONÉVROSE FÉMORALE, Fascia lata muscle.

TEN'SION, *Ten'sio, Tensu'ra, Tasis, Diat'asis, Entonia*, (*Enton'ia* is, also, used for overtension,) *Conten'sio, Disten'sio*, from *tendere*, 'to stretch.' State of a part, which is stretched, when its textures are distended by the afflux of fluids, or the accumulation of gas; or when its fibres are drawn, as it were, in an opposite direction, and are, consequently, more resisting than usual.

TENSOR CHOROIDEÆ, Ciliary muscle — t. Palati, Circumflexus musculus.

TENSOR TARSI. A small muscle, belonging to the inner commissure of the eyelids, well described by Professor Horner, of Philadelphia, and hence termed *Muscle of Horner*. It is about three lines broad and six long; arises from the posterior flat surface of the os unguis, near its junction with the ethmoid bone, and passes forwards and outwards, lying on the posterior face of the lachrymal ducts. As it approaches the commissure of the lids, it splits into two nearly equal parts, each of which is appropriated to a duct, and inserted along its course, almost to the punctum lacrymale. Its chief office seems to be, to influence the position of the puncta lacrymale, and to regulate the course of the tears through the lachrymal ducts.

TENSOR TYM'PANI, *Inter'nus Auris, Internus Mal'lei*, (F.) *Salpingo-malléen*. A small muscle, which arises from the petrous portion of the temporal bone, and the cartilage of the Eustachian tube, and terminates by a tendon, which is reflected over the processus cochleaformis, and is inserted into the apophysis of the handle of the malleus.

TENSOR VAGINÆ FEMORIS, Fascia lata muscle.

TENSURA, Tension.

TENSUS, Penis.

TENT, *Tenta, Turun'da*, and its diminutive, *Turun'dula, Penic'ulus, Penicil'lus, Penicil'lum, Motos, Lemnis'cus*, (F.) *Tente, Mèche*, from *tentare*, 'to try or explore.' In surgery, tents are small rolls of lint, of a cylindrical or pyramidal shape, which are introduced into wounds and deep ulcers, to prevent them from closing before they are filled up from the bottom. Tents are sometimes, also, made of prepared sponge, gentian root, &c. They are not so much used as they formerly were.

TENTACULARIA, Filaria hominis bronchialis.
TENTACULUM CEREBELLI, Tentorium.
TENTA'MEN MED'ICUM. 'A medical trial.' An examination in medicine, in the Prussian universities, which is conducted both in writing and vivâ voce before the Dean of the Medical Faculty.

TENTE, Tent — t. du Cervelet, Tentorium.
TENTIGO VENEREA, Nymphomania — t. Veretri, Satyriasis.
TENTIPEL'LUM, from tendo, 'I stretch,' and pellis, 'the skin.' Ancient name of a cosmetic, with which, it was pretended, wrinkles could be effaced.

TENTO'RIUM, T. cerebel'lo super-exten'sum, T. cerebelli, Tentac'ulum cerebelli, Septum transverse (Ch.), Transversæ septum, Septum enceph'ali, Intersep'ta horizonta'lia Pacchio'ni, Proces'sus transver'sus duræ matris, Lateral Processes of the Dura Mater, Diaphrag'ma cer'ebri, (F.) Tente du cervelet, Plancher du Cerveau, from tendere, tentum, 'to stretch.' A process of the dura mater, which separates the cerebrum from the cerebellum. It extends from the internal horizontal spine of the occipital bone, directly forwards to the sella Turcica of the sphenoid.

TENTORIUM CEREBELLI, Tentorium.
TENTUM, Penis.
TENTWORT, Asplenium ruta muraria.
TENUIS MATER, Pia mater.
TENUITAS AQUOSA, Predominium aquæ.
TEPHROSIA VIRGINIANA, Galega Virginiana.
TEPIDARIUM, see Stove.
TEPLITZ, Töplitz.
TERAS, Monster.
TERATOG"ENY, Teratogen'ia, from τερας, τεραος, 'a monster,' and γινεσις, 'generation.' The formation of monsters.
TERATOL'OGY, Teratolog"ia, from τερας, τεραος, 'a monster,' and λογος, 'a discourse.' A description, or the doctrine of monsters.
TERATOSIS, see Monster.
TERCERON, see Mulatto — t. Black, see Mulatto.
TEREBELLA, Trepan.
TÉRÉBENTHINE, Terebinthina—t. de Bordeaux, see Pinus sylvestris — t. de Chio, see Pistacia terebinthus—t. de Copahu, Copaiba—t. Commune, see Pinus sylvestris—t. d'Égypte, see Amyris opobalsamum—t. de Giléad, see Amyris opobalsamum — t. du Grand Caire, see Amyris opobalsamum—t. de Judée, see Amyris opobalsamum —t. de Melèze, see Pinus larix.
TEREBIN'THINA, from τερμινθος, or τερεβινθος, 'the turpentine tree.' Tur'pentine, Botin, Albotim, Altilibat, Brutino, (F.) Térébenthine. A substance, of the consistence of honey, which flows from many trees of the terebinthaceæ and coniferæ families. It is viscid; shining; more or less transparent; inflammable; of a warm, pungent taste; strong smell; and is entirely composed of resin and essential oil, without benzoic acid. It is soluble in alcohol. See Turpentine, Pinus palustris and Pinus sylvestris. All the turpentines are stimulant, diuretic, and cathartic.

TEREBINTHINA ARGENTORATENSIS, see Pinus picea — t. Balsamea, see Pinus balsamea — t. Canadensis, see Pinus balsamea — t. Chia, see Pistacia terebinthus — t. Communis, see Pinus sylvestris — t. Cypria, see Pistacia terebinthus — t. Empyreumatica, see Pinus sylvestris — t. Laricina, see Pinus larix—t. Veneta, see Pinus larix— t. Vera, see Pistacia terebinthus—t. Vulgaris, see Pinus sylvestris — t. de Vénise, see Pinus larix.

TEREBINTHUS, Terminthus—t. Gummifera, Bursera gummifera — t. Lentiscus, Pistacia lentiscus — t. Vulgaris, Pistacia terebinthus.
TEREBRA, Trepan.
TEREBRATIO, Trepanning.
TEREDO OSSIUM, Caries, Spina ventosa.
TERES, Stron'gylus, Cylindroi'des, 'long and round.' An epithet given to many organs, the fibres of which are collected into round fasci

TERES LIGAMEN'TUM, (F.) Ligament rond. This name is given to the round ligament in the cotyloid cavity of the os innominatum, which is attached to the head of the bone, and to the bottom of the cavity. It is, also, given to a small fibrous fascia, which extends from the coronoid process of the ulna to below the bicipital tubercle of the radius.

TERES MAJOR, (F.) Anguli - scapulo - huméral, Scapulo-huméral (Ch.), Grand rond, is situate at the inferior and posterior part of the shoulder. It is attached, on the one hand, to the outer surface of the scapula; to the corresponding part of its axillary margin; and, on the other, to the posterior margin of the bicipital groove of the humerus. It carries the arm backwards and inwards, and carries it, also, inwards in rotating. When it acts with the longissimus dorsi and pectoralis major, it applies the arm against the lateral part of the chest, and keeps it forcibly there.

TERES MINOR, (F.) Le plus petit sus-scapulo-trochitérien, (Ch.) Petit rond, Margini-sus-scapulo-trochitérien, Nonus hu'meri Placenti'ni, is situate at the posterior and inferior part of the shoulder; it is narrow and flattened, from above to below, in its inner half; and, from before to behind, in the outer. It is attached, on the one part, to the outer surface of the scapula, near its inferior angle; and, on the other, to the inferior part of the great tuberosity of the humerus. It depresses the arm, and causes it to turn on its axis from within outwards. It also carries it backwards.

TERESIS, Observation.
TERETRIUM, Trepan.
TERETRON, Trepan.
TERGAL, Dorsal.
TERGEMINI, Trigemini.
TERGUM, Dorsum, Vertebral column.
TERMINALIA, see Myrobalanus.
TERMINOLOGY, Nomenclature.
TERMIN'THUS, Terebin'thus, from τερμινθος, 'the turpentine tree.' Phyma Anthrax, Terminthus, Berry or Fungous carbuncle. The ancients gave this name to a tumour, surmounted by a black pustule, and resembling the fruit of the turpentine tree.

TERMINTHUS, Pistacia terebinthus.
TERMINUS SUPERIOR ASPERÆ ARTERIÆ, Larynx.
TERMONOLOGY, Nomenclature.
TERMS, Menses.
TERRA ABSORBENS MINERALIS, Magnesiæ carbonas—t. Aluminis, Argilla pura—t. Amara aërata, Magnesiæ carbonas—t. Amara salsibrica, Magnesiæ sulphas—t. Bolaris, Argilla —t. Foliata, Sulphur—t. Foliata mineralis, Soda acetata — t. Foliata tartari, Potassæ acetas — t. Fornacum, see Bricks — t. Fullonica, Cimolia purpurescens — t. Japonica, Catechu, Nux gambir.

TERRA LEM'NIA, Argilla bolus flava, Lem'n-a Earth, Lemp'nias. A name given by the ancients to a solid, reddish, astringent, substance, compared with the pulp of the fruit of the Ba—, an African tree, according to Prosper Alpinus. It seems, however, to be an argillaceous earth. It has been employed as an astringent.

TERRA LIVON'ICA. A *terra sigilla'ta* or *sealed earth* from Livonia, redder than that from Silesia, and very astringent.

TERRA MERITA, Curcuma longa.

TERRA NOCERIA'NA. A whitish, soft, and astringent earth, found in the environs of Nocera, in Italy.

TERRA ORLEA'NA, *Pigmen'tum urucu, Urucu,* (F.) *Rocou, Roucou, Bichet.* A pigmental matter obtained from the seeds of *Bixa Orleana* seu *Orella'na* seu *America'na, Orella'na, Orlea'na.* In Jamaica, it is recommended in dysentery, and is considered to possess astringent and stomachic qualities. It is called, according to its shape, *Flag, Roll,* or *Egg Annotto.*

Spanish Annotto, Bixa, is in small, oblong cakes. It is chiefly employed as a colouring matter.

TERRA OS'SEA, *Mate'ria ossea.* Bony matter. The earthy portion of bones.

TERRA PONDEROSA, Baryta—t. Ponderosa muriata, Baryta, muriate of— t. Ponderosa salita, Baryta, muriate of — t. Saponaria, Cimolia purpurescens.

TERRA PORTUGAL'LICA, *Barros, Bucaros.* A reddish, astringent, styptic earth, obtained from Portugal.

TERRA SIGILLA'TA, *Sealed Earth.* A bole or earthy matter, made into little cakes or flat masses, and stamped with certain impressions, as with the head of the Grand Seignior. To these belong the *Terra Silesiaca, Terra Lemnia, T. Turcica.* See Bolus alba.

TERRA SILESIACA, see Terra sigillata— t. Talcosa oxyanthracodes, Magnesiæ carbonas — t. Turcica, see Terra sigillata.

TERRA URI'NÆ. The earthy deposit in the urine.

TERRA VITRIOLI DULCIS, Colcothar.

TERRAPIN, Emys palustris.

TERRE BOLAIRE, Bolus—*t. Noix,* Bunium bulbocastanum — *t. Pesante,* Baryta — *t. Sigillée,* Bolus alba.

TERRETTE, Glechoma hederacea.

TERTIAN FEVER, *Febris tertia'na, An'etus tertianus, Trita'us, Tertian Ague,* (F.) *Fièvre tierce.* An intermittent, whose paroxyms recur every *third* day, or every 48 hours. The *mildest,* and the most *pernicious,* intermittents belong to this head. As a general rule, it is the most manageable form of ague.

TERTIANARIA, Scutellaria galericulata.

TESSARA, Cuboid.

TESSELLA, Tabella.

TEST, DANIEL'S, see Docimasia pulmonum — t. Hydrostatic, see Docimasia pulmonum — t. Ploucquet's, see Docimasia pulmonum—t. Static, see Docimasia pulmonum.

TESTA, see Ostrea.

TESTA PRÆPARA'TA, *Prepared Oyster-shell.* Oyster-shell, freed from extraneous matter, washed with boiling water, reduced to powder, and prepared in the same manner as Creta præparata.

TESTA'CEOUS, from *testa,* 'a shell.' A powder, consisting of burnt shells. These contain carbonate of lime chiefly, and hence the term has been applied to cretaceous substances. See Creta.

TESTÆ FORNACEÆ, Bricks—t. Ostreæ, see Ostrea.

TESTES. The *Testicles.* Vulgarly, the *Stones.* A name, also, given to the inferior tubercles of the corpora quadrigemina, to distinguish them from the superior, called *Nates.*

TESTES CEREBRI, see Quadrigemina corpora.

TES'TICLE, *Testis, T. viri'lis, Testic'ulus, Orchis, Pomum amo'ris, Did'ymus, Her'nia, Gem'ini* (pl.), *Gemelli* (pl.), *Ovum,* (F.) *Testicule,* from *testis,* 'a witness;' because the testicles are evidences of virility. The name of two glandular organs, contained in the scrotum, whose office is to secrete sperm. The substance of the testicle consists of numerous conical, flattened lobules — *lob'uli testis —* whose bases are directed towards the surface of the organ, and the apices towards the corpus Highmorianum. They are formed of a gray and softish substance, composed of tortuous canals, called *Tu'buli seminif'eri* vel *Vasa semina'lia,* folded on each other, and of extreme fineness; the number of which, according to the estimate of Monro, is 62,500, and the total length 5,208 feet. All these canals, uniting in their course, pass through the corpus Highmorianum, concur in forming the epididymis, and give origin to the vas deferens. The testicles are covered, immediately, by a fibrous membrane, of an opake white colour, and very tough, called *Tu'nica Albugin'ea,* or, simply, *Albugin'ea, Perites'tis,* of which the corpus Highmorianum is only an enlargement. Over this, again, is the tunica vaginalis, the second envelope of the testis.

TESTICLE, SWELLED, Hernia humoralis.

TESTICONDUS, Crypsorchis.

TESTICULE, Testicle.

TESTICULUS, Testicle—t. Accessorius, Epididymis — t. Caninus, Orchis mascula.

TESTIMO'NIUM MATURITA'TIS. 'Evidence of fitness.' A certificate of complete education, required, in the Prussian universities, of a candidate, before he can be admitted to examination for the degree of Doctor of Medicine.

TESTIS FEMINEUS, Ovary — t. Irritable, Orchidalgia — t. Minor, Prostate — t. Muliebris, Ovary — t. Virilis, Testiclo.

TESTUDINATIO CRANII, Camarosis.

TESTU'DO, *Chelo'nē,* (F.) *Tortue.* A genus of reptiles, including the turtle, the flesh of which is much esteemed as an article of diet.

Also, an encysted tumour, which has been supposed to resemble the shell of a turtle; *Emphy'ma encys'tis gang'lion.* See Talpa.

TESTUDO CEREBRI, Fornix — t. Scapulæ, see Scapula.

TETAN'IC, *Tetan'icum, Spas'ticum, Convulsi'vum, Convul'sive,* from τεινω, 'I stretch.' A remedy, which acts on the nerves, and, through them, on the muscles, occasioning, in large doses, convulsions. The chief agents of this class are *Nux Vomica, Strychnia, Brucia, Arnica,* and *Toxicodendron.*

Also, an epithet for a tonic convulsion.

TETANOMAṬA, Tetanothra.

TETANO'THRA, *Tetanom'ata, Erugato'ria,* from τεταυος, 'free from wrinkles.' Medicines which remove wrinkles. — Gorræus.

TÉTANOS, Tetanus.

TET'ANUS, from τεινω, 'I stretch.' *Spasm with rigidity, Convul'sio In'dica, Holoton'ia, Holoton'icus, Holotet'anus, Tet'anus universa'lis, Rigor nervo'sus* seu *nervo'rum, Exten'sio* seu *Dieten'sio, Enta'ria tetanus, Cat'ochus cervi'nus, Catochus holoton'icus,* (F.) *Tétanos.* A disease which consists in a permanent contraction of all the muscles or merely of some, without alternations of relaxation. It is characterized by closure of the jaws; difficulty or impracticability of deglutition; rigidity and immobility of the limbs and trunk, which is sometimes curved forwards (*Emprosthot'onos*), sometimes backwards (*Opisthot'onos*), and sometimes to one side (*Pleurothot'onos*). When tetanus is confined to the muscles of the jaws, it is called *Trismus.* It is a most formidable affection. The means of treatment are: — copious and repeated blood-let'ing; bathing, cold and warm; powerful doses of opium, and other narcotics. In *Traumat'ic Tetanus*, or that which supervenes on a wound, every extraneous matter must, of course, be removed from the wound, and soothing applications be made to it.

TETANUS ANTICUS, Emprosthotonos — t. Dolorificus, Cramp — t. Dorsalis, Opisthotonos — t. Lateralis, Pleurothotonos — t. Maxillæ inferioris, Trismus — t. Posterganeous, Opisthotonos — t. Posticus, Opisthotonos — t. Universalis, see Tetanus.

TETARTÆUS, Quartan.

TETARTOPHI'A, from τέταρτος, 'the fourth,' and φυω, 'I arise.' *Quarta'nus remit'tens*. A quartan, in which the intermission is inordinately short or imperfect.

TÊTE, Caput, Head — t. *de Veau*, Elephantiasis of the Greeks.

TETRADRACH'MON, from τέτρας, 'four,' and δραχμη, 'a drachm.' A weight of four drachms or half an ounce.

TETRAGONUS, Platysma myoides.

TETRAHIT LONGIFLORUM, Galeopsis grandiflora.

TETRAMY'RON, from τέτρας, 'four,' and μυρον, 'an ointment.' An ointment of four ingredients. — Galen.

TETRANGURIA, Cucurbita citrullus.

TETRANTHE'RA PICHU'RIM, *Faba Pichurim, F. Pechu'rei*. The seeds of this Brazilian plant have been used in diarrhœa, dysentery, flatulent colic, &c. Dose, ℨij.

TETRA'O COTUR'NIX, *Coturnix*, the Quail, (F.) *Caille*. The quail is an esteemed article of diet. The Greek name is ορτυξ; and the places, called *Ortygia*, are named after it. The excrements of the quail were formerly extolled in epilepsy, and the fat in specks of the eye.

TETRAPHAR'MACUM, from τέτρας, 'four,' and φαρμακον, 'a medicine.' A medicine consisting of four ingredients.

TETRAS'CELUS, from τέτρα, 'four,' and σκελος, 'leg.' A monster having four legs. — Gurlt.

TETROB'OLON. The weight of four oboli, or two scruples. — Gorræus.

TETROROS, Astragalus.

TETTER, Herpes — t. Crusted, Impetigo — t. Honeycomb, Porrigo favosa — t. Humid, Eczema impetigo — t. Milky, Porrigo larvalis — t. Pustular, Impetigo — t. Running, Impetigo — t. Scaly, Psoriasis.

TETTERWORT, Chelidonium majus.

TEUCRIUM ÆGYPTIACUM, T. capitatum — t. Belium, T. capitatum.

TEUCRIUM CAPITA'TUM, *Poley Mountain of Montpel'lier, T. Bel'ium seu Ægypti'acum, Po'lium Capita'tum*, is, generally, substituted for the last. The common *Poley Mountain* is the *Teucrium monta'num*; and the *Golden Poley Mountain*, the *Teucrium Po'lium, Po'lion*.

TEU'CRIUM CHAMÆ'DRYS, *T. officina'lis, Chamædrys, C. minor repens, C. vulga'ris, Quer'cula minor seu Calamandri'na, Trissa'go, Chamæ'drops, Trixa'go, Common German'der, Creeping Germander, Small Germander, English Treacle*, (F.) *Petit chêne, Germandrée officinale*. Family, Labiatæ. *Sex. Syst*. Didynamia Gymnospermia. This is possessed of aromatic and bitter properties. The dose of the dried powder is from ʒss to ʒj.

TEUCRIUM CHAMÆP'ITYS, *Chamæpitys, Arthet'ica. Arthretica, Aju'ga, A. Chamæp'itys, Bu'gula Chamæ'pitys, Abiga, Chamæmo'rus, Iva arthrit'ica, Holoc'yron, Io'nia, Sideri'tis, Common Groundpine*, (F.) *Petite Ivette*. Properties like the last. The tops or leaves have been recommended as aperients and tonics; especially in female obstructions, and in paralytic disorders.

TEUCRIUM CRET'ICUM, *T. hyssopifo'lium seu Rosmarinifo'lium, Rosmari'nus cta'chadis [?], Poley-mountain of Candy, Po'lium Cret[?]*. The tops and whole herb enter into the old compounds, *Mithridate* and *Theriaca*. It has a moderately aromatic smell; and a nauseous, [?] taste, and is placed among the aperients and coroborants.

TEUCRIUM FLAVUM has similar properties to T. chamædrys.

TEUCRIUM HYSSOPIFOLIUM, T. Creticum.

TEUCRIUM IVA, *Chamæ'pitys moscha'ta, [?] moscha'ta Monspelien'sium, Iva, Chamæpitys [?] thyl'lus, French Groundpine*, (F.) *Ivette [?]*. It has similar virtues to T. Chamæpitys, but is weaker.

TEUCRIUM MARITIMUM, T. Marum.

TEUCRIUM MARUM, *T. marit'imum, Marum syriacum, Marum Cret'icum, Majora'na Syron, Marum verum, M. Cortu'si, Chamæ'drys [?] marit'ima seu marum, Marum germander, Syron herb mastich, Cat thyme, Orig'anum Syriacum*, (F.) *Marum ou Germandrée maritime, Herbe [?] chats*. A very aromatic plant, of a camphor[?] smell; formerly much used in medicine as a tonic, antispasmodic, emmenagogue, &c.

TEUCRIUM OFFICINALE, T. chamædrys — t. Palustre, T. scordium — t. Pyramidale, Ajuga — t. Rosmarinifolium, T. Creticum.

TEUCRIUM SCOR'DIUM, *T. palus'tre, Water Germander, Scordium, Trissa'go palus'tris, [?] drys palustris seu scor'dium, Al'lium red* — (F.) *Germandrée Scorodone, Sauge des bois, [?] mandrée aquatique*. The leaves have a garlic smell, and bitterish, slightly pungent taste. It has the tonic properties of the other Teucria.

TEXTUM INTERLOBULARE, Interlobular tissue.

TEXTURA, Texture — t. Organica, Histus.

TEX'TURAL. Same etymon as Texture. Relating or appertaining to a texture.

TEXTURE, *Textu'ra, Textus*, from *texere, textum*, 'to weave.' *Tela, Hypha, Hyphé*. The particular arrangement of the tissues that constitute an organ.

TEXTUS, Texture, Tissue — t. Cellulosus, Cellular tissue — t. Desmosus, Desmoid tissue — t. Nervorum, Plexus nervorum — t. Organicus, Cellular tissue — t. Papillaris, Corpus papillare — t. Parenchymalis, Cellular tissue.

THÆRIA, Radzyge.

THAL'AMUS, Θαλαμος, (F.) *Couche*. 'A [?] or chamber; a bed.' The place at which a nerve originates, or has been considered to originate.

THAL'AMI NERVO'RUM OPTICO'RUM see [?] *Eminen'tiæ magnæ cer'ebri, Ganglia cerebri posti'ca, Crura medul'læ oblonga'tæ* (of some), *a'ta cor'pora super'na posterio'ra, Colli[?] vo'rum optico'rum, Optic thal'ami, Poster[?] ebral gan'glion*, (F.) *Couches des nerfs optiques, Couches optiques* (Ch.) *Couches des nerfs optiques, Couches optiques*. Two rounded and irregular surfaces, which are seen exposed in the lateral ventricles of the brain, and in the third ventricle, the inferior surface of which presents two projections, called (F.) *genicula'ta*, that furnish several filaments to the optic nerves. The name was given from a belief that the optic nerves originate from them. They, however, arise more posteriorly, and adhere more to the inner margin of those bodies. Gall considers, that the thalami act as ganglions of the nerves; and, hence, he calls them *Grand ganglion cérébral inférieur*. They are, also, called *posterior ganglion of the cerebrum*. From the thalami and corpora striata fibres proceed upwards to constitute the convolutions of the brain, and the various bands that connect the different parts of the brain together. The upper and inner parts of the thalami are so closely connected as to form one continued surface, called *Commissu'ra mollis.* The posterior parts turn downwards and outwards; after which they are elongated to form the two white cords, termed *Tractus op'tici.*

THALAMUS REGALIS, Pericardium.

THALIC'TRON, *Thalictrum, T. magnum,* seu *flavum* seu *flaves'cens* seu *praten'sě* seu *ni'gricans* seu *rugo'sum* seu *vagina'tum, Meadow-rue, Poor Man's Rhubarb, Rhabar'barum pau'perum,* (F.) *Pigamon jaunâtre, Rue des prés, Fausse-Rhubarbe, Rhabarbe des pauvres.* Family, Ranunculaceæ. *Sex. Syst.* Polyandria Polygynia. The root resembles rhubarb in its properties.

THALIC'TRUM ANEMONOI'DES, *Meadow Rue, Rue-leaved Anem'ony;* an indigenous plant, flowering in April and May.

THAMARINDUS, Tamarindus.

THANASIMUS, Mortal.

THANATODES, Mortal.

THAN'ATOID, *Thanatoï'des;* from θανατος, 'death,' and ειδος, 'resemblance.' Resembling death. Apparently dead.

THANATOL'OGY, *Thanatolog"ia, Thnescolog"ia,* from θανατος, 'death,' and λογος, 'a discourse.' A description, or the doctrine, of death.

THANATOS, Death.

THAP'SIA, from the island Thapsus. The *deadly carrot, Thapsia ascle'pias.* Family, Umbelliferæ. *Sex. Syst.* Pentandria Digynia. The root operates violently, both upwards and downwards. It is not used.

THAPSUS BARBATUS, Verbascum nigrum.

THARSI, see Tarsus.

THASPIUM ATROPURPU'REUM, *Th. corda'tum, Round heart.* The flowers, which appear in June, are of a dark purple.

THAS'PIUM BARBINO'DE, *Meadow Parsnep.* An indigenous plant, of the Northern and Western States, — *Order,* Umbelliferæ,—which flowers in June. Flowers, yellow.

Both plants have been esteemed vulnerary, antisyphilitic, and diaphoretic; and as antidotes to the bite of a rattlesnake.

THASPIUM CORDATUM, Th. atropurpureum.

THÉ, Thea — *t. des Apalaches,* Ilex vomitoria — *t. de France,* Salvia—*t. d'Europe,* Salvia veronica—*t. de la Mer du sud,* Ilex vomitoria—*t. du Mexique,* Chenopodium ambrosioides — *t. de Simon Pauli,* Myrica gale — *t. Suisse,* Falltranck.

THEA, *Chaa, Tea,* (F.) *Thé.* There are two principal species of tea-plant; the *Thea Bohe'a,* and *Thea vir'idis;* the *black tea,* and the *green.* Family, Hesperideæ. *Sex. Syst.* Polyandria Monogynia. In commerce, many kinds of tea are met with. Several of the differences between these appear to result from the age at which the leaves have been collected, and the mode of their desiccation.

Tea-drinking was introduced into Europe about the year 1666; since which time its use has become almost universal; and, in spite of the assertions of medical terrorists, it is, except in particular idiosyncracies, entirely harmless.

By an analogical transference, very common in language, the word *Tea* has been used almost synonymously with infusion, as *Beef tea, Mint tea,* &c.

THEA GERMANICA, Veronica.

THEBE'SIUS, VEINS OF. A name given to supposititious branches of the coronary veins, which Christopher Adam Thebesius, a German anatomist, described as opening into the heart by small depressions observable in the right auricle; and which have been called *Foram'ina Thebe'sii.* No such veins can be demonstrated. The valve, at the orifice of the coronary vein, in the right ventricle, is called *Valvula Thebe'sii, V. Guiffartia'na, V. venæ magnæ.*

THECA, Case, Vagina, Sheath — t. Cerebri, Cranium—t. Cordis, Pericardium—t. Vertebralis, see Vertebral canal.

THEION, Sulphur.

THEIOPEGÆ, Water, mineral (sulphureous.)

THEIOTHERMÆ, Waters, mineral, sulphureous.

THELASIS, Lactation.

THELASMUS, Lactation.

THELASTRIA, Nurse.

THELE, Nipple, Papilla.

THELI'TIS, from θηλη, 'the female nipple,' 'the female breast,' and *itis,* denoting inflammation. Inflammation of the nipple.

THELON'CUS, Mastoncus.

THELOS, Mamma.

THELYGON'IA, from θηλος, 'pertaining to the female sex,' and γενη, 'generation.' The part taken by the female in the act of generation. Also, nymphomania.

THELYGONUM, Sperm (of the female.)

THELYPTERIS, Pteris aquilina.

THENAD, Thenal.

THENAL, *Thenar;* same etymon as *thenar.* Relating or appertaining to the thenar.

THENAL ASPECT. An aspect towards the side on which the thenar is situated.—Barclay. *Thenad* is used, adverbially, by the same writer, to signify 'towards the thenal aspect.'

THENAR, θεναρ, from θεινω, 'I strike.' The palm of the hand, or sole of the foot.

THENAR, Flexor brevis pollicis manus, Palm.

THENAR or THENAL EM'INENCE is the projection at the anterior and outer part of the hand, formed by the abductor brevis, opponens, and flexor brevis pollicis.

THENAR or THENAL MUSCLE. Riolan and Winslow give this name to the fleshy mass, formed of the abductor brevis, opponens pollicis and the anterior part of the flexor brevis pollicis In the foot, Winslow gives the name *Thenal muscle* to the abductor and flexor brevis pollicis pedis.

THEOBROMA CACAO, Cacao.

THEOMANIA, Demonomania.

THEOPLEGIA, Apoplexy.

THEOPLEXIA, Apoplexy.

THEORET'ICAL, *Theoret'icus, Theo'ricus.* from θεωρεω, 'I contemplate.' (F.) *Théorétique, Théorique.* That which is confined to theory, or is connected with it. An epithet also applied to a sect of physicians, who founded their doctrine chiefly on reasoning.

THEORIA, Theory.

THÉORIQUE, Theoretical.

THE'ORY, *Theo'ria,* from θεωρεω, 'I contemplate.' The speculative part of a science. The connexion established in the mind between a general fact, or the least possible number of general facts, and all the particular facts dependent thereon: for example, the motions of the heavenly bodies, and the most important natural phenomena are connected with a single fact, previously known by observation; viz. that the force of gravity acts inversely according to the square of the distance. This constitutes the theory of universal gravitation. *Theory* must not be confounded with *system.* Theory regards nature as it is, and is a rigid deduction from facts. *System* is too often the creature of the imagination, to which nature is made to bend.

THEORY OF MEDICINE, *Institutes of Medicine, Theoretical Medicine,* is that part of the science

THEIOTHERMÆ 852 THIRST

which attempts philosophically to account for the various phenomena that present themselves during health as well as in disease. It is the philosophy of Medicine. The *Institutes of Medicine* are generally considered to comprise Physiology and its applications to Pathology, Hygiene, and Therapeutics. By some, it is considered to include General Pathology and General Therapeutics.

THEIOTHERMÆ, Waters, mineral, sulphureous.

THERAPEIA, Curation, Therapeutics.
THERAPEUSIS, Therapeutics.
THERAPEUTA, Therapeutist.
THERAPEUTICE, Therapeutics.
THERAPEU'TICS, *Therapeu'ticè, Therapeun'sia, Therapeu'sia, Iatrotech'nicè, Practice of Physic, Therapei'a, Therapi'a, Curato'ria Meth'odus, Methodus Meden'di*, from θεραπεύω, 'I wait upon, I alleviate, I attend upon the sick.' (F.) *Thérapeutique.* That part of medicine, the object of which is the treatment of disease. With others, the department which comprises an explanation of the *modus operandi* of medicines.

THÉRAPEUTIQUE, Therapeutics.
THERAPEU'TIST, *Therapeu'ta.* Same etymon. One who practises therapeutics. A practitioner of medicine. To be a good therapeutist, a man must be well versed in every department of medicine, and be capable of observing and reasoning well. He may be a good *observer*, and yet a bad *reasoner.* He cannot practise well unless he is both. Hence, the comparatively small number of good therapeutists.

THERAPIA, Therapeutics.
THERIA, Radzyge.
THERIAC, Theriaca — t. of Antipater, Antipatri theriaca.

THERIACA, Θηριακα, *The'riac*, from θηρ, 'a ferocious or venomous animal,' and ακεομαι, 'I cure.' Treacle. (F.) *Thériaque.* A medicine, believed to be capable of curing or preventing the effects of the bite of a venomous animal. In this sense it is chiefly used by writers. *Theriac* and *Theriacal* have been used adjectively for medicinal.

THERIACA ANDROM'ACHI, Venice Treacle, is an ancient *alexipharmic electuary;* consisting of a farrago of 61 different ingredients, which possessed the most opposite properties. It was invented by Andromachus of Crete, and prepared by order of Nero. It has received various modifications; and, to the discredit of the *Faculté de Médecine* of Paris, has held its place in their Codex, with even an additional number of ingredients. The *Electua'rium Opia'tum polyphar'macum* of the Codex has contained *acid ingredients*, 5; *astringent*, 5; *bitter*, 22; *indigenous aromatics*, 10; *umbelliferous aromatics*, 7; *balsams and resinous substances*, 8; *fetid ingredients*, 6; *narcotics*, 1; *earthy substances*, 1; *gummy or amylaceous*, 4; *saccharine*, 3; total 72! and one of these the *flesh of the viper!* A little more than a grain of opium is contained in each drachm of the compound.

THERIACA CELESTIS, Tinctura opii — t. Communis, Melasses — t. Edinensis, Confectio opii.
THERIACA GERMANO'RUM. An extract or rob, prepared from juniper berries. Used as a stomachic.
THERIACA LONDINEN'SIS, *Cataplasma Cymi'ni.* A cataplasm of *cumin seed, bay berries, germander snakeroot, cloves, honey*, and sometimes *opium*, or *syrup of poppies.*
THERIACA RUSTICORUM, Allium.
THÉRIAQUE, Theriaca.
THERIAKI. In Turkey, *opium-eaters*, or they who indulge largely in the use of opium, are so called.

THERIATRICA, Veterinary art.
THERIODES, Ferine.
THERIO'MA, *Therion*, from θηρ, 'a venomous animal.' Any extremely malignant ulcer. Sometimes confined to ulcers of the lungs.
THERION, Therioma.
THERIOTOMY, Zootomy.
THERMA, Heat — t. Emphytum, Animal heat.
THERMÆ, θερμαι, *Ther'mata.* Warm baths or springs. See WATERS (mineral.)
THERMÆ FABARIÆ, Pfeffers Mineral Waters of — t. Piperinæ, Pfeffers, Mineral Waters of — t. Plumbariæ, Plombières, Mineral Waters of.
THERMAL, *Therma'lis;* from θερμη, 'heat,' θερμος, 'hot.' Relating or appertaining to heat. Hot, warm. As 'a *thermal* mineral water.'
THERMANTICA, Calefacientia.
THERMASMA, Fomentation.
THERMATA, Thermæ.
THERMUM EMPHYTUM, Animal heat, Ellychnium.

THESIS, θεσις, from τιθημι, 'to place.' 'A position or proposition.' *Disputa'tio, Inaugural Disserta'tion.* The name usually given to an essay composed by a candidate for graduation in medicine, which he is at times required to defend publicly. Often, however, it is a mere form, giving useless labour and trouble to the student, inasmuch as it is executed as a task, and never afterwards regarded by the preceptor or by others. Sandifort, Haller, Smellie, and Stoll, have published collections of these.

Also, a suffix denoting 'arrangement;' hence *Diathesis.*

THEVE'TIA A'HOUAI, *Ahouai.* The kernel of the nut of this Brazilian tree are said to be a violent poison. At the Antilles, its nuts are called *Noix de Serpent;* and they are used against the bites of serpents.

THIGH, Sax. ðeoh, *Femur, Femen*, Crus, *Merus, Me'rium*, (F.) *Cuisse.* The part of the lower limb which extends from the pelvis to the knee. The thigh is larger at its superior than inferior part, and has the form of an inverted and truncated cone, slightly depressed from within outwards. Above, it is bounded, *anteriorly,* by the groin; *externally*, by the hip; *behind*, by the fold of the nates; and *within*, by the perineal region. Below, it is bounded, *anteriorly*, by the prominence of the knee; *posteriorly*, by the ham. It is formed of a considerable number of muscles, blood-vessels, lymphatics, nerves, &c.; and covered by a strong aponeurosis.

THIGHBONE, Femur — t. Neck of the, Collum femoris.
THION, Sulphur.
THIRST, Sax. ðyrst, (D.) *Dorst, Dipsa, Potio'nis deside'rium*, (F.) *Soif.* A desire or an absolute want for liquids. Physiologists are not entirely agreed regarding the seat of thirst; some place it in the fauces; others the stomach. Its immediate cause is not known. It has been attributed to a dry condition of the nervous papillæ of the pharynx, produced by suppression of the salivary and mucous secretions. This is probably true; but, again, it is owing to the wants of the system, — a supply of fluid being required to compensate the numerous losses that are constantly taking place. Thirst is an *internal sensation*, — an *instinctive want*, arising from organization, and inexplicable. It is an urgent symptom in many diseases, particularly in those of vascular excitement.

THIRST, EXCESSIVE, Polydipsia — t. Morbid, Dipsosis.

THIRSTY, Dipsodes.

THISTLE, BLESSED, Centaurea benedicta — t. Cotton, Onopordium acanthium — t. Globe, Echinops — t. Holy, Centaurea benedicta—t. Ladies', Carduus Marianus—t. Milk, common, Carduus Marianus — t. Pine, Atractylus gummifera — t. Sow, Sonchus oleraceus — t. Star, Centaurea calcitrapa — t. Yellow, Argemone Mexicana.

THLADIAS, Eunuch

THLASIAS, Eunuch.

THLASIS, Contusion — t. Depressio, Depression.

THLASMA, Contusion—t. Concussio, Concussion — t. Stremma, Sprain.

THLASPI, *Pennycress*. *Family*, Cruciferæ. *Sex. Syst.* Tetradynamia Siliculosa. Two species of thlaspi are directed, in some pharmacopœias, for medical use:—the *Thlaspi arven'sĕ* or *Treacle mustard*, and the *Thlaspi campes'trĕ* seu *hirsu'tum* seu *vulga'tius, Lepid'ium campes'trĕ, Lep'ia campes'tris, Ibe'ris campes'tris, Mith'ridate mustard*. The pharmaceutical properties of both kinds resemble those of common mustard.

THLASPI BURSA, *Th. bursa'tum, Capsell'a bursa pasto'ris, Ibe'ris bursa pastoris, Nastur'tium bursa pastoris, Rodschie'dia bursa pasto'ris, Bursa pasto'ris*, (F.) *Bourse à berger, Bourse à pasteur, Tabouret, Shepherd's purse*. A common European plant, introduced into this country. It is slightly astringent, but is little used.

THLASPI BURSATUM, Thlaspi bursa — th. Nasturtium, Lepidium sativum—th. Sativum, Lepidium sativum.

THLIBIAS, Eunuch.

THLIPSENCEPH'ALUS, from θλιψις, 'compression,' and εγκεφαλος, 'the encephalon.' A monster in whom the skull is open, not merely in the frontal and parietal, but also in the occipital regions — a distinct fontanelle not existing.

THLIP'SIS, θλιψις, *Compres'sio*. Compression, and especially constriction of vessels by an xternal cause. Oppression.

THNESCOLOGIA, Thanatology.

THOLUS, Achicolum—t. Diocleus, Scapha.

THOMPSO'NIAN. One who practises or believes in Thompsonianism.

THOMPSO'NIANISM, *Thomp'sonism*. A fanciful doctrine, of which a person of the name of Thompson, of New York, is the founder. One of its leading principles is, that the human body is composed of four *elements* (?), earth, air, fire and water; and one of its apothegms, — that metals and minerals are in the earth, and, being extracted from the depths of the earth, have a tendency to carry all down into the earth who use them; that the tendency of all vegetables is to spring up from the earth, and therefore to uphold mankind from the grave.

The Thompsonians are Botanic Physicians.

THORACENTE'SIS, *Paracente'sis Thora'cis*, from θωραξ, 'the thorax,' and κεντησις, 'perforation.' Tapping the thorax. Perforation of the thorax.

THORACHIQUE, Thoracic.

THORAC''IC, *Thorac''icus*, from *thorax*, 'the chest;' (F.) *Thoracique* ou *Thorachique*. That what relates or belongs to the chest; as *Thoracic vis'cera*, &c.

THORACIC INFERIOR ARTERY, *Arte'ria Thorac''ica Exter'na Infe'rior* vel *Longa, A. mamma'ria externa, A. Thoracica inferior*, (F.) *Deuxième des Thoraciques* (Ch.), arises from the axillary, a little below the preceding, and descends vertically over the lateral part of the thorax, and the serratus major anticus. It afterwards bends inwards; becomes subcutaneous, and divides into several branches, which embrace the breast. It gives numerous ramifications to the pectoralis major, serratus anticus, intercostals, ganglions of the axilla, mamma, &c.

THORACIC SUPERIOR ARTERY, *Arte'ria Thoracica Exter'na Superior*, (F.) *Artère thoracique supérieure, Première des Thoraciques* (Ch.), arises from the axillary artery or from the acromial; and descends forwards between the pectoralis major and P. minor, to which it distributes itself by a great number of branches. In some subjects, there are two or three *Arteriæ thoracicæ externæ superiores*.

THORACIC DUCT, *Ductus thorac''icus* seu *chy'lifer* seu *chyli* seu *lac'teus* seu *ro'rifer* seu *Pecqueti* seu *Pecquetia'nus, Vena alba thora'cis, Alveus ampullæ'cens, Distributo'ria lactea thoracica, Ductus thoracicus poste'rior* seu *vertebra'lis, Galax'ia, Duct of Pecquet, Alimen'tary Duct*, (F.) *Canal* ou *Conduit Thoracique*, is the duct in which the lymphatics of the lower limbs, abdomen, left superior extremity, left side of the head, neck, and thorax terminate. It begins at the *receptaculum chyli*, which is formed by the union of five or six large lymphatic trunks,—themselves formed from the union of all the absorbent plexuses of the abdomen. The duct ascends into the chest through the pillars of the diaphragm, and by the side of the aorta and vena azygos. It contracts in dimension, as far as the 6th dorsal vertebra, when it inclines towards the left hand; ascends behind the arch of the aorta; passes behind the left internal jugular vein, and opens at the posterior part of the subclavian vein of the same side. Its embouchure is furnished with two valves, which prevent the blood from passing from the vein into the duct.

THORACIC LIMBS are the upper limbs; so called because they are articulated with the lateral and upper parts of the chest.

THORACIC, LONG or INFERIOR, Mammary inferior external artery.

THORACIC NERVES. The *short* or *anterior thoracic nerves* are two in number. They arise from the brachial plexus, and divide into an anterior and a posterior branch :— the former distributed to the pectoralis major muscle; the latter uniting with a branch of the other to form a loop, from which numerous branches are given off to the pectoralis major and p. minor.

The *long thorac''ic nerve, Poste'rior thorac''ic, External respiratory* of Sir Charles Bell, is a long branch, which arises from the fourth and fifth cervical nerves, immediately after their escape from the intervertebral foramina, and passes downwards to be distributed upon the serratus magnus muscle.

THORACIC REGIONS are the different regions of the chest. Thus we say, *anterior, lateral*, and *superior thoracic*, &c.

THORACICA, Pectorals.

THORACICS, FIRST OF THE, Mammary superior external artery.

THORACIQUE, Thoracic.

THORACOCENTE'SIS, from θωραξ, 'the chest,' and κεντησις, 'puncture.' *Paracente'sis thora'cis*. Puncture of the chest to evacuate contained fluid — as in empyema.

THORACOCYSTIS, Thoracystis.

THOR'ACO-GASTRODID'YMUS, *Did'ymus sym'phyo-thoracogas'trius, Xyphŏdid'ymus*: from θωραξ, 'the chest,' γαστηρ, 'the belly,' and διδυμος, 'a twin.' A monstrosity in which twins are united by the chest and abdomen.— Gurlt.

THORACO-FACIAL, Platysma myoides — t. Maxillo-facial, Platysma myoides.

THORACODID'YMUS, from θωραξ, 'the chest,' and διδυμος, 'a twin.' A monstrosity in which twins are united by the thorax.— Gurlt.

THORACODYNE, Pleurodynia.

THORACOPATHI'A, from θωραξ, 'the chest,' and παθος, 'disease.' Disease or suffering in the chest.

THORACOSCOPIA, see Auscultation.

THORACOSCOPIUM, Stethoscope.

THORACYST'IS, *Thoracocystis*, from θωραξ, 'the chest,' and κυστις, 'a bladder.' Encysted dropsy of the chest. Hydatids in the chest.

THORAX, θωραξ, 'a cuirass, a coat of mail.' *Cith'arus, Venter me'dius, Pectus, Stethus, Scutum pec'toris*, the Breast, the Chest, Bir, *Chelys, Cassa*, (F.) *Poitrine*. One of the splanchnic cavities; bounded, posteriorly, by the vertebræ; laterally, by the ribs and scapula; anteriorly, by the sternum; above, by the clavicle; and below, by the diaphragm. It is destined to lodge and protect the chief organs of respiration and circulation — the lungs and the heart.

THORAX, Corset.

THORE, Sperm.

THORN APPLE, Datura stramonium — t. Red, Datura Sanguinea.

THOROUGHSTEM, Eupatorium perfoliatum.

THOROUGHWAX, Eupatorium perfoliatum.

THOROUGHWORT, Eupatorium perfoliatum.

THOROW-WAX, Bupleurum rotundifolium.

THORULUS STRAMINEUS, *Fanon*.

THREADWORM, Dracunculus — t. Long, Trichocephalus.

THREPSIS, Assimilation, Nutrition.

THREPSOL'OGY, *Threpsolog"ia*, from θρεψις, 'nutrition,' and λογος, 'a description.' The doctrine of, or a treatise on, the nutrition of organized bodies.

THREPTICE, Assimilation.

THRIDACE, Lactucarium.

THRIDAX, Lettuce.

THRIFT, LAVENDER, Statice limonium — t. American, Statice Caroliniana — t. Sea-side, Statice Caroliniana.

THRIX, Capillus, Hair.

THROAT, βροτε, δηοτα, *Jugulum, Interstit"ium Jugula'rē, Guttur, Sphagē*. The anterior part of the neck. (F.) *Gorge*. Also, the *Fauces*, (F.) *Gosier*.

THROATROOT, Geum Virginianum, Liatris.

THROATWORT, Campanula trachelium.

THROBBING, *Pulsati'vus, Sphyg'micus, Sphygmo'des, Pul'satory*. A *throbbing pain*, (F.) *Douleur pulsative*, is a kind of pain which is, or seems to be, augmented by the pulsation of arteries.

THROE, Agony, Pains, labour.

THROMBI LACTEI, Infarctus mammæ lacteus.

THROMBOCYS'TIS, from θρομβος, 'a clot,' and κυστις, 'a cyst.' The cyst occasionally surrounding a clot of blood — as in encephalic hemorrhage.

THROMBOSIS, Coagulation, Thrombus.

THROMBUS, θρομβος, 'a clot,' from τρεφειν, 'to coagulate;' *Thrombo'sis, Trumbus, Hæmato'ma*. A small, hard, round, bluish tumour; formed by an effusion of blood in the vicinity of a vein which has been opened in the operation of bloodletting. The thrombus is most commonly owing to the opening in the vein and that of the skin not corresponding; to excessive smallness of the cutaneous orifice; or to small, fatty granules, which prevent the discharge of the blood. Compresses, dipped in salt water; camphorated spirit, and slight compression, usually disperse it. See Blood.

THROMBUS NEONATORUM, Cephalæmatoma.

THROTTLE, Trachea.

THROW, Agony, Pains, labour.

THROWORT, Leonurus cardiaca.

THRUSH, Aphthæ — t. Milk, Aphthæ — t. White, Aphthæ.

THRYPSIS, Comminution.

THUJA OCCIDENTALIS, Thuya occidentalis.

THUREA, Juniperus lycia — t. Virga, Juniperus lycia.

THUS, see Pinus abies — t. Fœmininum. see Pinus abies — t. Judæorum, Croton cascarilla. Syrax, Thymiama — t. Libanotos, Juniperus lycia. t. Masculum, Juniperus lycia — t. Verum, Juniperus lycia — t. Vulgare, see Pinus abies.

THUYA APHYLLA, see Sandarac.

THU'YA seu THUJA OCCIDENTA'LIS, *T. obtu. Cupres'sus Arbor Vitæ, Arbor Vitæ, Tree of Life*. Nat. Family, Coniferæ. The leaves and wood were formerly in high repute as resolvents, sudorifics, and expectorants, and were given in phthisical affections, intermittent fevers, and dropsies. The expressed juice has been applied to condylomata. The arrangement of the medullary matter of the cerebellum, termed *Arbor Vitæ*, is also called *Thuya*.

THYLACIITIS, Gutta rosea.

THYM, Thymus.

THYMA, Thymion.

THYMALOS, Taxus baccata.

THYMASTHMA, Asthma thymicum.

THYMBRA, Satureia hortensis — t. Hispanica, Thymus mastichina.

THYME, CAT, Teucrium Marum — t. Common. Thymus — t. Lemon, see Thymus serpyllum — t. Mother of, Thymus serpyllum — t. Virginia Pycnanthemum linifolium — t. Wild, Thymus serpyllum.

THYMELÆA, Daphne gnidium — t. Laureola, Daphne laureola — t. Mezereum, Daphne mezereum — t. Monspeliaca, Daphne gnidium.

THYMELCO'SIS, from θυμος, 'thymus,' and 'ελκος, 'an ulcer.' Ulceration of the thymus gland.

THYMI'AMA, θυμιαμα, 'a perfume;' *Maiwood, Thus Jadæo'rum*, (F.) *Narcaphte*. A bark from Syria, Cilicia, &c., supposed to be the product of the liquid storax tree. It has an agreeable, balsamic smell; approaching that of liquid storax.

THYMIAMA, Fumigation, Suffimentum.

THYMIASIOTECHNIA, Thymiatechny.

THYMIASIS, Fumigation.

THYMIATECH'NY, *Thymiatech'nia, Thymasiotech'nia, Cura fumigato'ria*, from θυμιαμα, 'odour,' and τιχνη, 'art.' The art of employing perfumes in medicine.

THYM'ION, *Thyma, Thymus, Porrum. Parra. Verru'ca rhagoi'dea, Verru'ca minor*, from θυμος, 'thyme.' A small wart on the skin, resembling a bud of thyme.

THYMIOSIS, Frambœsia — t. Indica, Frambœsia.

THYMI'TES. Wine impregnated with thyme.

THYMI'TIS, from θυμος, 'thymus,' and *itis* denoting inflammation. Inflammation of the thymus gland.

THYMOPATHI'A, *Psychopathi'a*, from θυμος, 'the mind,' and παθος, 'affection.' A disease of the mind.

THYMOS, Rage.

THYMOXAL'ME, from θυμος, 'thyme,' δξυς, 'acid,' and 'αλς, 'salt.' A compound of thyme, vinegar, and salt.

THYMUS, θυμος, *Gland'ula Thymus. (F.) Thymiamum seu Thy'micum, Glan'dium. Figue gland, Corpus incomprehensib'ile* of Jos. Frank. An organ, the uses of which are totally unknown, and which is seated in the upper separation of the anterior mediastinum. The thymus has the appearance of a glandular body. It is oblong; bilobate; soft, and very variable in size and colour. In the fœtus, it is very large, and contains in a central cavity — *reservoir of the thymus* — a milky fluid; but it gradually disappears, and in old age is scarcely discernible. The arteries, called *thymic*, are from the inferior thyroid, internal mammary, bronchial, and mediastinal. The veins have the same arrangement. It receives some nervous filaments from the pneumogastric nerves, the phrenic, and the inferior cervical ganglia.

THYMUS, *T. vulga'ris* seu *tenuifo'lius* seu *horten'sis*, Common Thyme, (F.) *Thym, T. ordinaire.* Family, Labiatæ. *Sex. Syst.* Didynamia Gymnospermia. This herb has an agreeable, aromatic smell; and a warm, pungent taste. It is reputed to be resolvent, emmenagogue, tonic, and stomachic. It is not much used.

THYMUS, Satureia capitata, Thymion—t. Calaminthus, Melissa calamintha—t. Capitatus, Satureia capitata—t. Ciliatus, T. mastichina—t. Creticus, Satureia capitata—t. Hortensis, Thymus—t. Includens, T. serpyllum.

THYMUS MASTICH'INA, *T. cilia'tus*, Common herb *Mastich, Marum vulga're, Samp'suchus, Clinopo'dia, Mastich'ina Gallo'rum, Thymbra Hispan'ica, Jaca In'dica.* A low, shrubby, Spanish plant, used as an errhine. It has a smell like mastich. Its virtues resemble those of the *Marum Syriacum;* but it is said to be less powerful.

THYMUS MULTIFLORUS, Melissa nepeta—t. Nepeta, Melissa nepeta.

THYMUS SERPYL'LUM, *T. inolu'dens, Mother of Thyme, Wild Thyme, Her'pylos, Herpyl'los, Serpyl'lum, Serpul'lum, Serpil'lum, Gila'rum, Serpyl'lum vulga'rē minus*, (F.) *Serpolet.* This plant has the same sensible properties as the garden thyme; but has a milder, and rather more grateful flavour. *Lemon Thyme*, the *Serpyllum citra'tum*, is merely a variety of the *Thymus Serpyllum*. It is very pungent; and has a particularly grateful odour, approaching that of lemons.

THYMUS SYLVATICUS, Clinopodium vulgare — th. Sylvestris, Satureia capitata — th. Tenuifolius, Thymus.

THYRA, θυρα, 'a gate, folding-door.' In composition, *Thyreo* and *Thyro*, θυρεος, 'a shield resembling a folding-door,' mean the thyroid cartilage.

THYREMPHRAXIS, Bronchocele.

THYREO, *Thyro*, in composition, relate to the thyroid cartilage or gland.

THYREOADENITIS, Thyreoitis.

THYREO-ARYT'ENOID, *Thyro-arytenoideus*, or *Thyro-arytenoïdes*. That which relates to the thyroid and arytenoid cartilages.

THYREO-ARYTENOID LIGAMENTS, *Inferior Ligaments of the Larynx, Lips of the Glottis, Vocal Cords*, are two ligaments about two lines broad, formed of elastic and parallel fibres, which are contained in a duplicature of the mucous membrane of the larynx. They extend horizontally from the anterior projection at the base of each arytenoid cartilage to the middle of the angle of union of the thyroid cartilage. They are the essential organs of voice. See Glottis.

THYREO-ARYTENOID MUSCLES, THYREO-ARYTENOIDEI, are thin muscles, which arise from the middle and inferior part of the posterior surface of the thyroid cartilage; whence they proceed backwards and outwards, to be inserted into the outer part of the base of the arytenoid cartilage. They give the necessary tension to the ligaments of the glottis, in the production of the voice.

Santorini has given the name *Thyreo-arytenoideus obliquus* to a portion of the *arytenoïdeus* muscle.

THYREO-EPIGLOT'TIC, *Thyreo-epiglottideus, Thyrepiglott'icus.* Sabatier and Santorini have given this name to the outer portion of the thyro-arytenoid muscle; because it passes from the thyroid cartilage to the anterior part of the epiglottis.

THYREO-HYOID, *Thyro-hyoïdeus, Thyrohyoïdes, Hyodeothyreo'des.* That which belongs or relates to the thyroid cartilage and os hyoides.

THYREO-HYOID or HYO-THYROID MEMBRANE is a very broad, yellowish, fibrous membrane, thicker at the middle than at the extremities, which is attached above to the posterior surface of the body and great cornu of the os hyoides; and, below, to the whole superior edge of the thyroid cartilage.

THYREO-HYOÏDEUS or *Hyo-thyreoïdeus Muscle* is situate at the anterior and superior part of the neck. It is attached to the oblique line on the anterior surface of the thyroid cartilage; to the inferior edge of the body of the os hyoides, and to the anterior portion of its great cornu. It approximates the thyroid cartilage and os hyoides to each other, by raising the cartilage, and with it the whole larynx: or, it can depress the os hyoides.

THYREO-PHARYNGEUS, Thyro-Pharyngeus.

THYREOID, Thyroid.

THYREOIDEUS, Thyroideal.

THYREOI'TIS, *Thyreoädeni'tis, Angi'na thyreoïdea*, from θυρεος, 'a shield,' and *itis*, denoting inflammation. Inflammation of the thyroid gland.

THYREONCUS, Bronchocele.

THYREOPHRAXIA, Bronchocele.

THYREPIGLOTTICUS, Thyreoëpiglottic.

THYRO, see Thyreo.

THYRO-ARYTENOID, Thyreo-arytenoid.

THYRO-CRICO-PHARYNGEUS, see Crico-pharyngeal.

THYRO-HYOIDEUS, Thyreo-hyoid.

THYRO-PHARYNGEUS, *Thyreo-pharyngeus.* Valsalva, Morgagni, Santorini, and Winslow have given this name to the portion of the constrictor pharyngis inferior, which is attached to the thyroid cartilage.

THYRO-PHARYNGEUS, Constrictor pharyngis, see Crico-pharyngeal.

THYRO-PHARYNGO-STAPHYLINUS, Palato-pharyngeus.

THYROCELE, Bronchocele.

THYROID, *Thy'reoid, Thyroï'des*, from θυρα, 'a gate or folding-door,' or from θυρεος, 'a shield,' and ειδος, 'form.' That which has the shape of a folding-door.

THYROID CAR'TILAGE, *Cartila'go Scutifor'mis, C. Scuta'lis, C. Clypea'lis, Coöpertorium, C. Pelta'lis* seu *pelta'tus, Scutum, Ada'mi Morsūs Os*, is the largest of the cartilages of the larynx, at the anterior part of which it is situate. It is larger transversely than vertically; broader above than below; and seems formed by the junction of the two quadrilateral plates, which produce, by their union, an angle that projects forwards. Its two posterior margins terminate above, and on each side, by an ensiform prolongation, called the *greater cornu of the thyroid cartilage;* and, below, by a less prominent eminence, the *lesser cornu*, which is articulated with the cricoid.

THYROID GLAND, *Corpus Thyreoïdeum, Glan'dula Thyreoïdea*, (F.) *Gland ou Corps Thyroïde*, is an organ, the uses of which are not known. It covers the anterior and inferior part of the larynx, as well as the first rings of the trachea, and seems to be composed of two lobes, flattened from before to behind, which are united by a transverse prolongation of the same nature as themselves, called the *Isthmus of the Thyroid Gland.* The tissue of the thyroid is soft, spongy, and of a brownish colour; but its intimate structure is unknown. It is formed of several distinct lobules; collected in lobes of greater or less size. These are composed of granulations, some of which contain a yellowish or milky fluid. The thyroid gland receives four large arteries, called *Thyroideal,* as well as corresponding veins. Its nerves proceed from the pneumogastric, and from the cervical ganglia. No excretory duct has ever been found in it. Its uses are not known.

THYROIDEAL, *Thyroideus, Thyreoideus,* (F,) *Thyroïdien.* That which concerns the thyroid gland or cartilage.

THYROIDEAL ARTERIES are two on each side. 1. The *superior Thyroideal, superior laryngeal, superior guttural,* arises from the anterior part of the external carotid, and proceeds to the upper part of the thyroid gland, after having given off a *laryngeal branch* and a *crico-thyroid*. 2. The *inferior Thyroideal, infe'rior gut'tural,* much larger than the last, arises from the upper part of the subclavian. It passes, in a serpentine manner, to the inferior part of the thyroid gland, to which it is distributed, after having given a number of branches to the neighbouring parts, among which is the *cervicalis ascendens.*

THYROIDEAL VEINS are, 1. A *superior thyroideal,* and several *middle thyroideal,* which open into the internal jugular vein. 2. An *inferior thyroideal,* much larger than the preceding, whose branches form — by anastomosing with those of the opposite side, in front of the trachea — a very remarkable venous plexus, which J. Cloquet calls the *infra-thyroideal plexus.* The inferior thyroideal veins open,—the left into the corresponding subclavian;—the right, into the vena cava superior.

THYROÏDIEN, Thyroideal.

THYROPHRAXIA, Bronchocele.

THYRSUS, Penis.

TIBI-PÉRONÉO-TARSIEN, Peronæus longus.

TIB'IA. A Latin word, which signifies a *flute* or *pipe. Cnemē, Procne'mē, Procne'mium, Fo'cilē majus, Arun'do major, Canna major, Canna major seu domes'tica cruris.* The largest bone of the leg. A long, irregular, and triangular bone, situate on the inner side of the fibula. It has, 1. A *Superior* or *femoral extremity,* which is very large, rounded, and has two eminences at the sides, called *Tuberos'ities of the Tibia,* or *Tibial tuberosities.* The outermost is articulated with the fibula. On its head are two articular, oval, concave surfaces, separated by a process, called *Spine of the tibia,* which are articulated with the condyles of the *Os femoris.* 2. An *inferior* or *tarsal extremity,* having an articular surface beneath, which joins the astragalus; within, a triangular eminence, which forms the malleolus internus; and, on the outside, a triangular surface, which articulates with the fibula. 3. The body or shaft of the tibia has three faces, separated by three angles, the anterior of which is the most prominent, and is called the *spine* or *crista of the tibia* or *tibial spine.* It is the *shin.* The tibia is articulated with the femur, fibula, and astragalus. It is developed by three points of ossification, one for the body, and one for each extremity.

TIBIA MINIMA, Fibula.

TIBIÆUS, Tibial.

TIB'IAL, *Tibia'lis, Tibiæ'us,* (F.) *Tibial, Jambier.* That which relates to the tibia or to the leg.

TIBIAL APONEURO'SIS, (F.) *Aponévrose Jambière,* surrounds the muscles of the leg. It is continuous, above, with the femoral aponeurosis, and arises, also, from the head of the fibula, and from several fibrous expansions which detach themselves from the tendons of the triceps, sartorius, gracilis, and semitendinosus. Thence it descends around the leg, attaching itself to the whole extent of the anterior and inner edges of the tibia. It sends, below, an expansion, which passes before the tendo Achillis, and is continuous with the anterior annular ligament of the tarsus. It is attached, also, to the sheath of the peronei muscles.

TIBIAL ARTERIES are two in number. 1. The *Tibia'lis Anti'ca,* which arises from the popliteal artery, before its bifurcation; passes immediately through the opening in the upper part of the interosseous ligament, and reaches the anterior part of the leg; when it turns downwards, and descends obliquely, between the extensor communis digitorum pedis and the tibialis anticus, anterior to the interosseous ligament; glides under the anterior annular ligament of the tarsus, and takes the name *Dorsalis tarsi.* Amongst the numerous branches, given off by the tibialis antica, may be distinguished — the *Tibialis recur'rens, A. malleola'ris interna,* and *A. malleolaris externa.* 2. The *Tibialis posti'ca,* arises from the bifurcation of the popliteal artery; and, slightly torn ?? descends between the two planes of the posterior muscles of the leg; until it arrives under the arch of the calcaneum, where it divides into two branches — the *Plantar arteries.*

TIBIAD, see Tibial aspect.

TIB'IAL ASPECT. An aspect towards the side on which the tibia is situated.—Barclay. *Tibiad* is used adverbially by the same writer, to signify, 'towards the tibial aspect.'

TIBIAL NERVES are two in number. 1. The *anterior tibial nerve, Prétibio-susplantaire,* (Ch.) One of the two branches in which the external popliteal terminates. It accompanies the artery tibialis antica. 2. The *posterior tibial nerve, Branche tibiale du nerf fémoro-poplité,* (Ch.) is the internal popliteal.

TIBIAL VEINS, ANTERIOR AND POSTERIOR, have the same arrangement as the arteries which they accompany.

TIBIA'LIS ANTI'CUS, *Cate'na muscul??,* (F.) *Tibio-sus-métatarsien, Tibio-sustarsi??,* (Ch.) *Jambier antérieur.* A muscle situate at the anterior part of the leg. Above, it has the shape of a triangular prism; below, it is slender and tendinous. It is attached, above, to the anterior part of the external tuberosity of the tibia, to the superior half of the outer surface of this bone; and to the anterior surface of the interosseous ligament. Below, its tendon terminates at the base of the first cuneiform bone, and at the posterior extremity of the first metatarsal bone. This muscle bends the foot on the leg, and directs its point inwards, at the same time that it raises its inner edge. It can, also, bend the leg on the foot, and prevent it from falling backwards in standing.

TIBIALIS GRACILIS, Plantar muscle.

TIBIALIS POSTI'CUS, (F.) *Tibio-tarsien, Tibio-sous-tarsien,* (Ch.) *Jambier postérieur.* This muscle is situate at the posterior and deep part of the leg. It is thicker above than below; and is attached, above, to the posterior surface of the fibula; to the posterior surface of the tibia, and to the interosseous ligament. Its tendon terminates, below, at the tuberosity on the inferior extremity of the os scaphoides. This muscle extends the foot on the leg; at the same time rai??

ing its inner edge. It, likewise, extends the leg on the foot.

TIBIO-CALCANIEN, Soleus—t. Phalangettien, Flexor longus digitorum pedis profundus perforans — t. Sous-tarsien, Tibialis posticus — t. Sus-métatarsien, Tibialis anticus — t. Sus-tarsien, Tibialis anticus.

TIB'IO-TARSAL, Tibio-tar'seus, (F.) Tibiotarsienne. What relates to the tibia and tarsus.

TIBIO-TARSAL ARTICULA'TION is the articulation of the foot with the leg. It is formed by the tibia and the astragalus; and is strengthened by lateral, and by anterior and posterior ligaments.

TIBIO-TARSIEN, Tibialis posticus.

TIC, Twitching, Vellication. A local and habitual convulsive motion of certain muscles; and, especially, of some of those of the face. It is, sometimes, called in France Tic convulsif ou Tic non douloureux, to distinguish it from Tic douloureux or neuralgia faciei, and has been termed a partial chorea or form of chronic chorea, Spasmus facia'lis, Chore'a fa'ciei.

TIC DOULEUREUX, Neuralgia, facial — t. non douloureux, see Tic.

TICKLE WEED, Veratrum viride.

TICKLING, (F.) Chatouillement. This word, sometimes, means the action of tickling (titilla'tio, titillation;) at others, the sensation produced by this action (pruri'tus). A vivid sensation, which commonly causes laughter, and a state of general spasm that may be dangerous if too long protracted. There are some parts of the body, where we are easier tickled than others; for example, the sole of the feet, and the hypochondriac regions.

TICKSEED SUNFLOWER, Coreopsis trichosperma.

TICKWEED, Hedeoma — t. Sunflower, Coreopsis trichosperma.

TIDAL AIR, see Respiration.

TIERCE, see Tertian.

TIGE PITUITAIRE, Infundibulum of the brain — t. Sus-sphénoïdale, Infundibulum of the brain.

TIGILLUM, Crucible.

TIGLIA SEU TIGLII GRANA, see Croton Tiglium.

TIGRETIER, see Mania, dancing.

TIGULA, Saccharum.

TIKIMMA, Cacoucia coccinea.

TILBURY, MINERAL WATERS OF. A saline chalybeate at West Tilbury, in Essex, England. It is not much frequented.

TILIA, T. Europæ'a seu grandiflo'ra seu cordifo'lia seu paucifo'ra seu platyphyll'a, Phil'yra. The Lime tree or Linden tree, Basswood, Whitewood, Spoonwood, (F.) Tilleul. Family, Tiliaceæ. The flowers have been supposed to possess anodyne and antispasmodic virtues.

TILLEUL, Tilia.

TILLICHERRY CORTEX, Nerium antidysentericum.

TILMA, Linteum.

TILMOS, Evulsion.

TILMUS, Carphologia.

TILY, OF THE INDIANS, Viburnum dentatum.

TIMAC. The name of an East India root, but of what vegetable is not clear. It is said to possess diuretic properties; and hence has been given in dropsies.

TIMIDUS, Rectus inferior oculi.

TIN, (D.) T e n. Stannum, Cassit'eros, Cattit'eros, Stangos, Ju'piter, Stu'pia, Laos, Plumbum album seu can'didum, Plumbum candidum, (F.) Étain. A solid metal; of a peculiar odour when rubbed; insipid; colour whitish; s. g. 7.291; giving a peculiar tinkling sound when struck. It is used, in medicine, only as a mechanical anthelmintic. Dose, ʒj of the Pulvis Stanni, Stannum granula'tum or Granular tin, in molasses. This is made by melting tin in an iron vessel over the fire, and, while it is cooling, stirring until it is reduced to a powder, which is passed through a sieve.—Ph. U. S.

TIN, BUTTER OF, Tin, muriate of—t. Chloruret of, Tin, muriate of—t. Deutohydrochlorate of, T. muriate of.

TIN-FOIL, Stannum folia'tum, Stanni'olum, is used for plugging carious teeth, &c.

TIN-GLASS, Bismuth — t. Granular, see Tin — t. Muriate of, superoxygenated, T. muriate of.

TIN, MURIATE OF, Butter of Tin, Fuming liquor of Liba'vius, Mu'rias Stanni, Murias Oxyd'uli Stanni, Chlor'uret of Tin, Deu'to-hydro-chlorate of Tin, Superoxygena'ted Muriate of Tin. This is formed of Tin, one part; concentrated muriatic acid, three parts. To be crystallized by the aid of heat. A violent cathartic. Dose, gr. ij or iij.

TIN, SULPHURET OF, Aurum musivum.

TINAGMUS, Concussion.

TINASMUS, Tenesmus.

TINCTU'RA, from tingere, tinctum, 'to dye.' Tincture, Essen'tia, (F.) Teinture, Alcoolat, Alcohol. The term tincture is generally restricted to spirituous solutions of vegetable, animal, and some saline substances. It corresponds, therefore, with the word Quintes'sence, in one of its old significations; and with the Alcoola'tum of the Codex of Paris. It is not unusual, however, to speak of aqueous tincture, ethereal tincture, &c. Tinctures are made either with pure alcohol or proof spirit. The former are precipitated by water: and, therefore, are seldom used internally; the latter are common additions to infusions, decoctions, &c. They ought not, of course, to be united with any vehicle which can decompose them, or separate any thing from them in a palpable form; unless such decomposition is desired by the prescriber. In making tinctures, the ingredients should be reduced to a coarse powder; and the maceration be made in close vessels, exposed to a heat of about 80°, and frequently shaken. When completed, they must be filtered, and put away for use in close bottles. When the process of displacement is employed, great care must be taken, so that the substances treated may be, as far as possible, exhausted of their soluble principles, and a perfectly clear tincture be obtained. To those who are not familiar with the process, the plan of maceration is preferable. —Ph. U. S.

TINCTURA ABSIN'THII COMPOS'ITA, Compound Tincture of wormwood, Essen'tia absin'thii composita seu amara. (Absinth., artem. pontic., caryoph. āā ℥ss, sacch. ʒij. alcohol. Oss. Macerate for fifteen days. Ph. P.) Tonic, stomachic, vermifuge, and carminative. Dose, f ʒij to f ℥ss.

TINCTURA ACACIÆ CATECHU, T. catechu — t. Acetatis ferri cum alcohole, see T. ferri acetatis — t. Acidi sulphurici, Sulphuricum acidum aromaticum.

TINCTURA ACONI'TI, (Ph. U. S. 1842.) Tinctu'ra Aconi'ti folio'rum, (Ph. U. S. 1851.) Tincture of Aconite, (Aconit. folior. ℥iv, alcohol. dilut. Oij. Macerate for 14 days, express, and filter through paper. It may also be made by displacement. Ph. U. S.) Dose, gtt. v. It is rubbed on the seat of neuralgia.

TINCTURA ACONI'TI RADI'CIS, Tincture of Aconite root, (Aconit. radicis, contus. ℔j, Alco'ol. Oij. Macerate for 14 days; express and filter. It may also be prepared by displacement. Ph. U. S.) Uses same as the last.

TINCTURA ÆTHE'REA CAMPHORA'TA, *Solu'tio eam'phoræ æthe'rea, Liquor nervinus Bangii, Spiritus sulphu'rico-æthereus camphora'tus, Naphtha vitrioli camphora'ta.* (Camphor. p. i. Æther sulphuric. p. ii.) Stimulant in atonic diseases, arthritic cardialgia and spasm. Dose, 20 to 30 drops in white wine.

TINCTURA ÆTHEREA FERRI, Alcohol (seu Tinctura) sulphurico - æthereus ferri — t. Alcoholica Chinæ composita, T. cinchonæ composita—t. Alcoholica corticum aurantiorum Whyttii, Tinctura cinchonæ amara — t. Alexipharmaca Huxhami, Tinctura cinchonæ composita.

TINCTURA AL'OES, *T. Al'oes Socotori'næ, Essen'tia Aloes, Al'cohol cum Aloë perfolia'tâ, Tincture of Aloes.* (Aloes, pulv. ʒj, ext. glycyrrh. ʒiij, aquæ Oiss, alcohol. Oss. Macerate for 14 days, and filter. Ph. U. S.) Properties, those of aloes. Dose, fʒss to fʒiss.

TINCTURA ALOES ÆTHE'REA, *Æthe'real Tincture of Aloes, Tinctura aloes vitriola'ta.* (Aloes Socot., Myrrh, āā ʒiss, croci ʒj, sp. ætheris sulph. Oj. Digest the myrrh in the ether for 4 days; then add the aloes and saffron. Ph. E.) Stimulant and cathartic. Dose, fʒj to fʒij.

TINCTURA ALOES COMPOS'ITA, *Elix'ir Proprieta'tis, E. aperiti'vum, E. Aloes, Tinctura Aloes cum Myrrhâ, T. Aloës et Myrrhæ,* (Ph. U. S.,) *T. Aloes et Myrrhæ croca'ta, Elixir of long life, Compound Tincture of Aloes,* (F.) *Elixir de longue vie, Baume de vie de Lelièvre,* (Aloes, in pulv. ʒiij, croci, ʒj, Tinct. Myrrhæ, Oij.) Macerate for 14 days, and filter. Purgative and stomachic. Dose, fʒj to fʒij.

Boerhaave's Elixir consisted of *aloes, myrrh, saffron,* and *tartrate of potassa,* digested in *alcohol* and *water.*

Rudcliffe's Elixir is formed of *Aloes Socotr.* ʒvj, *cort. cinnam., rad. zedoar,* āā ʒss, *rad. rhei* ʒj, *coccinell.* ʒss, *syrup. rhamni* ʒij, *sp. tenuior.* Oj. *aquæ puræ* fʒv.

TINCTURA ALOES ET MYRRHÆ, T. aloës composita — t. Aloes et myrrhæ crocata, T. A. composita — t. Aloes vitriolata, T. A. ætherea — t. Amara, T. gentianæ composita — t. Amomi repentis, T. cardamomi — t. Amomi zingiberis, T. zingiberis.

TINCTURA ANGUSTU'RÆ, *Tincture of Angustura.* (Cort. cuspar. in pulv. crass. redact. ʒij, sp. vin. ten. Oij. Digest. Ph. D.) Dose, fʒj to fʒij.

TINCTURA ANTIFEBRILIS WARBURGI, see Bebeeru.

TINCTURA ANTIODONTAL'GICA, *Toothache Tincture.* (Tannin. ℈j, Mastich, gr. v, æther. ʒij. M.) To be applied on cotton wool, to the tooth previously dried.

TINCTURA ARISTOLOCHIÆ SERPENTARIÆ, T. serpentariæ — t. Aromatica, T. cinnamomi composita — t. Aromatica ammoniata, Spiritus ammoniæ aromaticus.

TINCTURA ASSAFŒ'TIDÆ, *T. Fer'ulæ Assafœtidæ, Tincture of Assafœtida, T. fœtida, T. assafœtidæ,* (Assafœtid. ʒiv, alcohol. Oij. Macerate for 14 days and filter.) Dose, gtt. xv to fʒj.

TINCTURA ASSAFŒTIDÆ AMMONIATA, Spiritus Ammoniæ fœtidus.

TINCTURA AURAN'TII, *T. Cor'ticis Aurantii, Tincture of Orange Peel.* (Aurant. cort. recent. ʒiij, sp. rect. Oij. Digest for 14 days.) Stomachic. Used as an adjunct to stomachic draughts. Dose, fʒss to ʒij.

TINCTURA AUREA, Alcohol seu tinctura sulphurico-æthereus ferri.

TINCTURA BELLADON'NÆ, *Tincture of Belladonna.* (Belladonnæ, ʒiv, alcohol. dilut. Oij. Macerate for 14 days; express, and filter through paper. It may, also, be prepared by displacement. Ph. U. S.)

TINCTURA BENZO'INI COMPOS'ITA, *Compound Tincture of Benzoin, T. Benzoes composita, Balsamum Cathol'icum, B. Per'sicum, Balsamum traumat'icum, Elixir traumaticus, Friar's Balsam, Vervain's Balsam, Wade's Drops,* [...] *drops, Commander's Balsam, Wound Balsam, Balsam for cuts.* (Benzoin. ʒiij, styrac. [...] ʒij, Balsam. tolut. ʒj, aloes, in pulv. ʒss. [...] Oij. Macerate for 14 days and filter. Stimul[...] Used chiefly to wounds and ulcers.

The basis of *Turlington's Balsam of Life* is [...] Compound Tincture of Benzoin. The follow[...] form is recommended by a committee of the P[...]ladelphia College of Pharmacy: — Alcoh[...] Benzoin. ʒxij, Styrac. liquid, ʒiv, Aloes S[...] ʒj, Balsam Peruvian. ʒij, Myrrhæ, ʒj, R[...] gelic. ʒss, Balsam Tolut., Ext. Glycyrrh. [...] Digest for 10 days, and strain.

The *Essence of Coltsfoot* consists of equal part of the *Compound Tincture of Benzoin* and *Balsam of Tolu,* to which is added double the [...]tity of *Rectified Spirit of Wine.* It is sold as pectoral.

TINCTU'RA CALUM'BÆ, *T. Columbæ, T. C[...] Tincture of Columbo, Columbo Bitters,* ([...] rad. cont. ʒiv, alcohol. dilut. Oij. Macerate 14 days; express, and filter. Ph. U. S.) D[...] fʒss to ʒiv. It may, also, be made by displ[...]ment.

TINCTURA CAMPHORÆ, Spiritus camphoræ.

TINCTURA CAM'PHORÆ COMPOS'ITA. *T. [...] Camphora'ta,* (Ph. U. S.,) *Compound Ti[...] Camphor, Camphorated Tincture of Opium, [...] Paregor'icum, Paregor'ic Elixir.* (Opii. in p[...] Acid Benzoic. āā ʒj, ol. anisi, fʒj, mellis op[...]mat. ʒij, Camphor. ʒj, alcohol. dilut. Oij. M[...]cerate for 14 days, and filter through paper. [...] U. S.) One fluidounce contains nearly gr. [...] opium. Anodyne. Dose, fʒj to fʒiij.

Squire's Elixir, an empirical carminative [...]paration, is thus made, according to one form[...] (Opii ʒiv, camphor. ʒj, coccinell. ʒj, [...] dulc. ʒij, tinct. serpent. Oj, sp. anisi. [...] aquæ Oij, auri musivi, ʒvj.)

TINCTURA CANTHAR'IDIS, *T. C. Vesicato[...] Lyttæ, T. Meloës vesicato'rii, Tincture of [...]ing Flies, T. of Spanish Flies,* (F.) *Teinture [...] fiante.* (Cantharid. cont. ʒij, alcohol. di[...] Macerate for 14 days; express, and filter. [...] may, also, be prepared by displacement. [...] U. S.) Stimulant and diuretic, but not [...] used internally. Externally, stimulant. D[...] gtt. x.

Matthew's Injection, a once celebrated n[...] for fistula in ano, consisted wholly of a [...] *Tincture of Cantharides.*

TINCTURA CAP'SICI, *Tincture of Caps[...]* (Capsic. ʒj. alcohol. dil. Oij. Macerate [...] days, and filter. It may, also, be prepared [...] displacement.) Stimulant. Dose, fʒss to ʒ[...]

TINCTURA CARDAMO'MI, *T. amo'mi [...] Tincture of Car'damoms.* (Cardam. cont. [...] alcohol. dilut. Oij. Macerate for 14 days, [...] and filter. It may, also, be made by disp[...]ment.) Use, the same as the seeds. Dose [...] to fʒiv.

Solomon's Balm of Gil'ead, an empirical p[...]ration, seems to be an aromatic tinctur[...] which *Cardamoms* form a leading ingred[...] made with brandy. Some affirm that it co[...] *cantharides.*

TINCTURA CARDAMOMI COMPOS'ITA, *Co[...] Tincture of Card'amoms, Stomach Tinctu[...] tura Stomach'ica.* (Cardamom. cont. ʒij [...] cont. ʒij. cinnam. cont. ʒv, Uvæ passæ [...] acinis, ʒv, cocci. cont. ʒj, alcohol. dilut. [...]

Macerate for 14 days; express and filter. *Ph. U. S.*) Stomachic and carminative. Dose, f₃ij to f₃v.

TINCTURA CARMINATI'VA SYL'VII, *Alcoola'tum Carminati'vum Sylvii, Carminative Elixir of Sylvius.* (*Rad. angelic.* 4 p., *rad. imperator., galang.* āā 6 p., *fol. rosmarin., majoran., rutæ, basilic.* āā 48 p., *baccar. laur. nobil.* 12 p. *sem. angelic., ligust. levist., anis.* āā 16 p., *zingib., nuc. moschat.* āā 6 p., *cinnam.* 12 p., *caryoph., cort. limon.* āā 4 p. Add *alcohol* 1500 p. Macerate and distil, 1000 p. *Ph. P.*) A warm stomachic, carminative, &c. Dose, ₃ss to f₃ss.

TINCTURA CASCARIL'LÆ, *T. Croto'nis Eleuthe'riæ, Al'cohol cum Croto'nē Cascarillā, Tincture of Cascarilla.* (*Cascarill. cort.* cont. ₃iv, *sp. ten.* Oij. *Ph. L.*) Dose, f₃j to f₃iv.

TINCTURA CASTO'REI, *T. Castorei Ros'sici, Essen'tia Castorei, Al'cohol castoria'tum, T. Castorei Canaden'sis, Tincture of Castor.* (*Castor* cont. ₃ij, *alcohol.* Oij. Macerate for 7 days, express, and filter.) Tonic and antispasmodic. Dose, gtt. xx to f₃ij, or more.

TINCTURA CASTOREI COMPOS'ITA, *Compound Tincture of Castor.* (*Cast.* ₃j, *g. asafœtid.* ₃ss, *alcohol. ammoniat.* Oj. *Ph. E.*) Antispasmodic. Dose, f₃j to f₃iv. Called, also, *Elixir fœ'tidum, Tinctura castorei fœtida seu fœtida ammonia'ta.*

TINCTURA CAT'ECHU, *Tinctura Japon'ica, T. Mimo'sæ Catechu, T. Aca'ciæ Catechu, Tincture of Catechu.* (*Catech.* ₃iij, *cinnam. contus.* ₃ij, *alcohol. dilut.* Oij. Macerate for 14 days, express and filter. *Ph. U. S.*) Astringent. Dose, f₃j to f₃ij.

The *Concentrated Solution of Charcoal*, sold for cleaning the teeth, seems to be little more than the tincture of catechu.

TINCTURA CICUTÆ, T. conii maculati.

TINCTURA CINCHO'NÆ, *T. Cor'ticis Peruvia'ni Simplex, T. Cort. Peruvia'ni, Tincture of Cinchona, Tincture of Bark.* (*Cinchon. flav.* in pulv. ₃vi, *alcohol. dilut.* Oij. Macerate for 14 days, express, and filter through paper. It may, also, be made by displacement. *Ph. U. S.*) Dose, f₃j to ₃iv or more.

TINCTURA CINCHO'NÆ AMA'RA, *Elixir antihypochondri'acum, E. rob'orans Whyt'tii, E. Whyttii, Essen'tia Cor'ticis Peruvia'ni Composita, Tinctu'ra alcohol'ica corticum aurantio'rum Whyttii, T. Kinki'næ ama'ra, Elixir stomach'icus spirituo'sus.* (*Cinch.* p. viij, *Gentian. Rad., Cort. Aurant.* p. iij. *Alcohol* (.900) 96 p. Digest. Dose, one or two teaspoonfuls.

TINCTURA CINCHONÆ AMMONIA'TA, *T. Cor'ticis Peruvia'ni volat'ilis, Ammoniated Tincture of Bark, Volatile Tincture of Bark.* (*Cinchon. lancifol. cort.* cont. ₃iv, *sp. ammon. aromat.* Oij. *Ph. L.*) In dyspepsia, combined with acidity and languor.

TINCTURA CINCHONÆ ÆTHE'REA COMPOS'ITA, *T. Kinæ Kinæ æthe'rea compos'ita, Elixir'ium Antisep'ticum Docto'ris Chaussier, Chaussier's Antisep'tic Elixir.* (*Cinchon. officin.* ₃ij, *cascarill.* ₃ss, *cinnam.* ₃iij, *croci* ₃ss, *sacch. alb.* ₃xxxviij. Put these bruised into a matrass, and add *vin. alb. Hispanic. vel vin. muscat., alcohol.* āā Oj. Macerate for two days, and add *sulphuric ether* f₃iss. *Ph. P.*) Topic, stimulant, and antiseptic. Dose, f₃ss to f₃j.

TINCTURA CINCHONÆ COMPOS'ITA, *Compound Tincture of Cinchona or Bark, Huxham's Tincture of Bark, T. Cor'ticis Peruvia'ni Composita, T. febrif'uga Docto'ris Huxha'mi, Essen'tia Chinæ, E. Cor'ticis Peruvia'ni Alexiphar'maca Huxhami, Essen'tia antisep'tica Huxhami, Tinctu'ra Alexiphar'maca Huxhami, Tinctu'ra Alcohol'ica Chinæ Compos'ita.* (*Cinchon. rubr. pulv.* ₃ij, *aurant. cort.* cont. ₃iss, *serpent.* cont. ₃iij, *croci, santal.* āā ₃j, *alcohol. dilut.* Oij. f₃xx. Macerate for 14 days, express, and filter. *Ph. U. S.*) It may, also, be made by displacement. More grateful than the simple tincture. Dose, f₃j to f₃iij.

TINCTURA CINNAMO'MI, *Tincture of Cinnamon, Essen'tia Cinnamomi, T. Lauri Cinnamomi,* (*Cinnam.* cont. ₃iij, *alcohol. dilut.* Oij. Macerate for 14 days, express, and filter. *Ph. U. S.*) It may, also, be prepared by displacement. Stomachic. Dose, f₃j to f₃ij.

TINCTURA CINNAMO'MI COMPOS'ITA, *Compound Tincture of Cinnamon, Tinctu'ra Aromat'ica, Essen'tia Aromatica, Alcoöl cum Aromat'ibus Compos'itus, Eau de Bonferme ou d'Armagnac.* (*Cinnam.* cont. ₃j, *cardam.* cont. ₃ss, *zingib.* cont. ₃iij, *alcohol. dilut.* Oij. Macerate for 14 days, express, and filter. *Ph. U. S.*) It may, also, be prepared by displacement. Use, same as the last. Dose, f₃j to f₃ij.

TINCTURA DE COCHLEA'RIIS, *Alcoola'tum de Cochlea'riis, A. antiscorbu'ticum.* (*Fol. cochlear. recent.* 2500 p., *rad. armoraciæ,* 230 p., *alcohol.* (22° to 32° Beaumé) 3000 p., distil off 2000 p. *Ph. P.*) Antiscorbutic. Dose, f₃ij to ₃j.

TINCTURA COL'CHICI, *T. C. Sem'inis,* (*Ph. U. S.*), *Tincture of Colchicum Seed.* (*Colchic. sem.* cont. ₃iv, *alcohol. dilut.* Oij. Macerate for 14 days, express, and filter. *Ph. U. S.*) It may, also, be prepared by displacement. Dose, ten to sixty drops.

TINCTURA COLCHICI SEMINIS, T. colchici—t. Colombæ, T. Calumbæ.

TINCTURA CONI'I, *T. C. Macula'ti, T. Cicu'tæ, Tincture of Hemlock.* (*Conii fol.* ₃iv, *alcohol. dil.* Oij. Macerate for 14 days, express, and filter. *Ph. U. S.*) It may also be made by displacement. Use;—the same as that of the leaves.

TINCTURA CONII MACULATI, T. conii — t. Convolvuli Jalapæ, T. jalapii — t. Corticis aurantii, T. aurantii — t. Corticis Peruviani composita, T. cinchonæ comp.— t. Corticis Peruvianni simplex, T. cinchonæ — t. Corticis Peruvianni volatilis, T. cinchonæ ammoniata.

TINCTURA CROCI SATI'VI, *T. Croci, Tincture of Saffron.* (*Croci Angl.* cont. ₃j, *alcohol. dilut.* ₃xv. *Ph. E.*) Slightly stomachic (?). Dose, f₃j to f₃iij.

TINCTURA DE CROCO COMPOS'ITA, *Elixir'ium de Garus, Alcoola'tum de Croco Compos'itum, Compound Tincture of Saffron, Elixir of Garus.* (*Aloes Socotr.* 320 p., *myrrh.* 64 p., *croci.* 32 p., *cinnam., nuc. moschat., caryoph.* āā 16 p. *alcohol.* 1000 p. *aq. flor. aurant.* 5000 p. Digest for two days, distil 4000 p. and add *syrup of capillaire*, 5000 p. *Ph. P.*) Aromatic, cordial, stomachic. It is also called *Elixir cordia'lē et stomach'icum*, and *E. anticol'icum croça'tum.*

TINCTURA CROTONIS ELEUTHERIÆ, T. cascarillæ.

TINCTURA CUBEB'Æ, *Tincture of Cubebs.* (*Cubeb.* cont. ₃iv, *alcohol. dilut.* Oij. Macerate for 14 days, express, and filter. *Ph. U. S.*) It may, also, be prepared by displacement. Dose, one or two fluidrachms.

TINCTURA DIGITA'LIS, *Tincture of Digitalis, T. Digitalis purpu'reæ.* (*Digital.* ₃iv, *alcohol. dilut.* Oij. Macerate for 14 days, express, and filter.) It may, also, be prepared by displacement. Use, same as that of the leaves. Dose, gtt. x.

TINCTURA FEBRIFUGA DOCTORIS HUXHAMI, T. cinchonæ composita.

TINCTURA FERRI ACETA'TIS, *Tincture of Acetate of Iron.* (*Potass. acetat.* ₃ij, *sulph. ferri* ₃j, *sp. rectif.* Oij. Rub the acetate and sulphate into a soft mass. Dry and rub with the spirit. Digest for 7 days, and pour off. *Ph. D.*) Tonic and astringent. Dose, gtt. xx to f₃j. The Dublin college directs a *Tinctura Acutatis Ferri cum Alcoho'lē*, which differs from the other, in having half the quantity, only, of the *Acetate of Potass.*

TINCTURA FERRI AMMONIA'TA, *Tincture of Ammoniated Iron,* T. *Ferri Ammoniaca'lis,* T. *Florum martia'lium,* T. *Martis Mynsich'ti.* (*Ferri ammon.* ℥iv, *sp. ten.* Oj. *Ph. L.*) *Use* — same as that of the ammoniated iron. Dose, f℥ss to f℥ij.

TINCTURA FERRI CHLORIDI, T. ferri muriatis.

TINCTURA FERRI MURIA'TIS, T. *Ferri chlo'ridi,* (Ph. U. S.), T. *Ferri sesqui-chlo'ridi, Liquor Ferri muria'tis, Tincture of Muriate of Iron,* T. *Martis in Spiritû Salis,* T. *M. cum Spiritû Salis,* T. *Ferri Muria'ti, Tincture of Steel, Alcohol ferra'tus.* (*Ferri subcarb.* ℔ss, *acid. muriat.* Oj, *alcohol.* Oiij. Add the acid to the subcarbonate in a glass vessel, and shake during three days. Pour off and add the spirit. *Ph. U. S.*) Tonic and styptic. Dose, gtt. x to xx.

Bestucheff's Tincture or *Klaproth's Tincture* is an ethereal tincture of chloride of iron. It is composed of dry *perchloride* of iron, one part; *Hoffmann's anodyne liquor,* seven parts.

The *Antivenereal Drops,* at one time so celebrated at Amsterdam, were examined by Scheele, and found to be a tincture of chloride of iron and corrosive sublimate.

TINCTURA FERRI SESQUICHLORIDI, T. Ferri muriatis — t. Ferulæ Asafœtidæ, T. Asafœtidæ — t. Florum martialium, T. ferri ammoniata — t. Fœtida, T. asafœtidæ — t. Fœtida ammoniata, T. castorei composita — t. Fuliginis, see Fuligo.

TINCTURA GAL'BANI, *Tincture of Galbanum.* (*Galb.* ℥ij, *sp. tenuior.* Oij. *Ph. D.*) Stimulant and antispasmodic. Dose, f℥j to f℥ij.

TINCTURA GALLA'RUM, T. *Gallæ,* (Ph. U. S.) *Tincture of Galls.* (*Gall. contus.* ℥iv, *alcohol. dilut.* Oij. Macerate for 14 days, express and filter. *Ph. U. S.*) It may, also, be prepared by displacement. Astringent. Dose, f℥j to ℥iij.

TINCTURA GENTIA'NÆ COMPOS'ITA, *Compound Tincture of Gentian,* Tinct. *Ama'ra, Spirit Bitters, Elix'ir Stomach'icum.* (*Gent. concis.* ℥ij, *aurant. cort.* ℥j, *cardam. cont.* ℥ss, *alcohol. dilut.* Oij. Macerate for 14 days, express, and filter. It may, likewise, be prepared by displacement. *Ph. U. S.*) Tonic and stomachic. Dose, f℥j to f℥iij.

Brodum's Nervous Cordial consists of the *Tinctures of Gentian, Columba, Cardamom,* and *Bark,* with the *Compound Spirit of Lavender,* and *Wine of Iron.*

Stoughton's Elixir is a compound tincture of gentian. The *Elixir'ium Docto'ris Stoughton* seu *Tinctu'ra Ama'ra* of the Parisian Codex is prepared as follows: — *Absinth. summit. exsiccat., Teucri chamædrys., Rad. gentian., cort. aurant.* ā ā ℥vj, *cascarillæ* ℥j, *rhei* ℥ss, *aloes socotr.* ℥j, *alcohol.* Oij.) Digest.

TINCTURA GUAI'ACI, T. *G. Officina'lis, Tincture of Guai'acum.* (*Guaiac.* ℔ss, *alcohol.* Oij. Macerate for 14 days, and filter.) Stimulant and sudorific. Used especially in rheumatic and arthritic cases. Nearly the same as *Hill's Essence of Bardana* or *Burdock.*

TINCTURA GUAI'ACI AMMONIA'TA, *Ammoniated Tincture of Guai'acum,* T. *Guaiaci'na Volat'ilis, Elixir Guai'aci Volatilis, Al'cohol cum Guai'aco officina'le ammonia'tus, Al'cohol ammoniæ et Guai'aci,* T. *Guai'aci,* (*P. L.* 1788,) *Vol'atile Tincture of Guai'acum.* (*Guaic.* pulv. ℥iv, *sp. ammon. arom.* Oiss. Macerate for 14 days, and filter.) Properties same as the last. Dose, f℥j to f℥ij.

Hatfield's Tincture — a nostrum — consists of Guaiacum and Soap, ā ā ℥ij, rectified spirit, Oiss.

TINCTURA HELLEB'ORI, T. H. *Nigri, Tincture of Black Hellebore,* T. *Melampo'dii.* (*Helleb. nigr. cont.* ℥iv, *alcohol. dilut.* Oij. Macerate for 14 days, express and filter. It may also be prepared by displacement. *Ph. U. S.*) Dose, f℥ss to f℥j.

TINCTURA HIERA, Vinum aloes.

TINCTURA HU'MULI, *Tincture of Hops.* (*Humuli,* ℥v, *alcohol. dilut.* Oij.) Tonic and sedative. Dose, f℥ss to f℥iij.

TINCTURA HYOSCY'AMI, T. *Hyoscyami sicci, Tincture of Henbane.* (*Hyoscyam. fol.* ℥iv, *alcohol. dilut.* Oij. Macerate for 14 days, express and filter. It may also be prepared by displacement. *Ph. U. S.*) Narcotic, anodyne. Dose, gtt. x to f℥j.

TINCTURA IO'DINI, (Ph. U. S., 1842,) *Tinctura Iodin'ii,* (Ph. U. S., 1851,) *Alcohol Io'dii, Tincture of Iodine.* (*Iodin.* ℥j, *alcohol.* Oj. Dissolve. *Ph. U. S.*) The tincture spoils by keeping. With least, deposits the iodine. It has been much used in goître, &c. Dose, ten drops three times a day.

TINCTURA IODINI COMPOS'ITA, (Ph. U. S., 1842) *Tinctura Iodin'ii Composita,* (Ph. U. S., 1851,) *Compound Tincture of Iodine.* (*Iodin.* ℥ss, *potassii iodid.* ℥j, *Alcohol.* Oj. Dissolve. *Ph. U. S.*) Dose, 10 to 30 drops.

TINCTURA JALA'PII, T. *Jala'pæ,* (Ph. U. S.) *Convol'vuli Jalapæ, Tincture of Jalap.* (*Jalap.* pulv. ℥vi, *Alcohol. dilut.* Oij. Macerate for 14 days, express, and filter. *Ph. U. S.* It may also be made by displacement. Cathartic. Dose, f℥j to f℥iv.

TINCTURA JALA'PII COMPOS'ITA, *Elixir Jalap'æ Compos'itum, Elixir purgans, Emetocathol'ica purgans Roth'ii, Elixir antheleminticum Sueco'rum, Eau de vie Allemande.* (*Jalap.* ℔ss, *Scammon.* ℥j, *Alcohol.* (22°) Oij. Macerate for eight days. *Ph. P.*) Dose, 60 to 100 drops.

TINCTURA JAPONICA, Tinctura catechu — t. Kinæ kinæ ætherea composita — t. Cinchonæ ætherea composita — t. Kinkinæ amara, Tinctura cinchonæ amara.

TINCTURA KINO, *Tincture of Kino.* (*Kino in* pulv., ℥vj; *Alcohol. dilut.* q. s. Put the kino mixed with an equal bulk of sand, into a percolator, and gradually pour on diluted alcohol until f℥viij of filtered liquor pass. The tincture should be renewed frequently, and kept in closely stopped bottles. *Ph. U. S.*) Astringent. Dose f℥j to f℥ij.

TINCTU'RA KRAME'RIÆ, *Tincture of Rhatany.* (*Kramer.* in pulv. ℥vj, *alcohol. dilut.* Oij. Macerate for 14 days, express, and filter. *Ph. U. S.* It may also be prepared by displacement. Dose, f℥j to f℥ij.

TINCTURA LAURI CINNAMOMI, Tinctura cinnamomi — t. Lavandulæ composita, Spiritus lavand. comp. — t. Lyttæ, Tinctura cantharidis — t. Martis Glauberi, see Ferrum tartarizatum — t. Martis in spiritû salis, Tinctura ferri muriatis — t. Martis Mynsichti, Tinctura ferri ammoniata — t. Martis vinosa, Vinum ferri — t. Melampodii, Tinctura hellebori nigri — t. Meloes vesicatorii, Tinctura cantharidis — t. Metallorum, Lilium Paracelsi — Mimosæ catechu, Tinctura catechu.

TINCTU'RA LOBE'LIÆ, *Tincture of Lobelia.* (*Lobel.* ℥iv, *alcohol. dilut.* Oij. Macerate for 14 days, express, and filter. *Ph. U. S.*) It may also be prepared by displacement. Dose, f℥ss to f℥ij.

TINCTU'RA LUPULI'NÆ, *Tincture of Lupuline.* (*Lupulin.* ℥iv, *alcohol.* Oij. Macerate for 14 days and filter. *Ph. U. S.*) Dose, f℥j to f℥ij.

TINCTURA MELOES VESICATORII, Tinctura cantharidis.

TINCTURA MOSCHI, *Tincture of Musk.* *Essentia of Musk.* (*Mosch.* in pulv. redact. ℈j, *sp. rect.* Oj.) Dose, f℥j to f℥iv.

TINCTURA MYRRHÆ, *Tincture of Myrrh,* *Spiritus Tincture of Myrrh.* (*Myrrhæ contusæ* ℥ij, *alcohol.* Oiij. Macerate for 14 days, and filter. *Ph.*

U. S.) Tonic, deobstruent, antiseptic, and detergent. It is chiefly used in gargles, and applied to foul ulcers, spongy gums, &c.

Hudson's Preservative for the Teeth and Gums consists of Tinct. myrrh., tinct. cinch., aq. cinnam. āā ℥iij, eau d'arquebusade, ℥j, pulv. gum. Arab. ℥ss. M.

TINCTURA NERVINA BESTUCHEFFII, Tinctura seu alcohol sulphurico-æthereus ferri—t. Nervina Halensis, Tinctura seu alcohol sulphurico-æthereus ferri—t. Nervino-tonica, Lamotte's, Alcohol seu tinctura sulphurico-æthereus ferri.

TINCTURA NUCIS VOM'ICÆ, *Tincture of Nux Vomica.* (Alcohol. s. g. .837, f℥j; *Dry Extract of Nux Vomica*, 3 gr.) Dose, gtt. v to xxx, in cases where the nux vomica is indicated.

It is directed, in the last edition of the Ph. U. S. (1851), to be prepared as follows:— *Nucis vomicæ* rasur., ℥viij; *alcohol*, Oij. Macerate for 14 days, express, and filter. It may also be prepared by the process of displacement. Dose, gtt. v to xx.

TINCTURA OLEI MENTHÆ PIPERI'TÆ, *Tincture of Oil of Peppermint, Essence of Peppermint.* (Ol. menthæ piperitæ, f℥ij, alcohol. Oj. Dissolve. Ph. U. S.) Dose, 5 drops, as a carminative.

TINCTURA OLEI MENTHÆ VIR'IDIS, *Tincture of Spearmint, Essence of Spearmint*, is made in the same manner. Ph. U. S.

TINCTURA OPII, *Tincture of Opium, Liquid Laudanum, Theriaca cœles'tis, Al'cohol cum Opio, Tinctura Theba'ica, Tinctura Sedati'va.* (Opii pulv. ℥ijss, alcohol. dilut. Oij. Macerate for 14 days, express, and filter. Ph. U. S.) Nineteen minims contain about one grain of opium. Properties, those of opium. Dose, gtt. xx to lx and more. By macerating the dregs remaining after making the *Tinctura Opii* in a solution of *Tartaric Acid*, a solution is obtained, which is said to be devoid of the exciting and constipating properties of the tincture of opium. Gray calls it *Haden's Liquor Opii Sedati'vus.*

TINCTU'RA OPII ACETA'TA, *Ac"etated Tincture of Opium.* (Opii ℥ij; aceti, f℥xij; alcohol. Oss. Rub the opium with the vinegar; add the alcohol, and having macerated for 14 days, express and filter. Ph. U. S.) Twenty drops are equivalent to a grain of opium.

TINCTURA OPII AMMONIA'TA, *Ammo'niated Tincture of Opium, Edinburgh Paregor'ic Elix'ir.* (Flor. benz., croci, āā ℥iij, opii ℥j, ol anisi ℥ss, alcohol. ammoniat. f℥xvj. Digest. Ph. E.) f℥j contains one grain of opium. Used like the *Tinctura Camphoræ Composita.*

TINCTURA OPII CAMPHORATA, Tinctura camphoræ composita—t. Plumbosa, Liquor plumbi subacetatis dilutus.

TINCTURA QUAS'SIÆ, *T. Quassiæ excel'sæ, Tincture of Quassia.* (Quassiæ rasur. ℥ij, alcohol. dilut. Oij. Macerate for 14 days, express, and filter. Ph. U. S.) It may also be prepared by displacement. Tonic. Dose, f℥j to ℥j.

TINCTURA QUI'NIÆ SULPHA'TIS, *Tincture of Sulphate of Qui'nia.* (Sulphate of Quinia, gr. vj; alcohol, (.847) f℥j. M.) Dose, f℥j to ℥iv, in the day.

A *Tinctura Cincho'niæ Sulpha'tis* may be made in a similar manner.

TINCTURA RHABARBARI, Tinctura rhei—t. Rhabarbari composita, Tinctura rhei—t. Rhabarbari vinosa, Vinum rhei palmati.

TINCTURA RHEI, *T. Rhabarb'ari, T. Rhabarbari spirituo'sa, T. Rhæi, T. Rhei palma'ti, Tincture of Rhubarb.* (Rhei, contus. ℥iij, cardam. cont. ℨss, alcohol. dilut. Oij. Macerate for 14 days, express, and filter. It may also be prepared by displacement. Ph. U. S.) Stomachic or purgative, according to the dose employed:

f℥j to ℥ij, as a stomachic; f℥iv to ℥j, as a purgative.

TINCTURA RHEI COMPOS'ITA, *T. Rhabarbari composita, Compound Tincture of Rhubarb.* (Rhei rad. concis. ℥ij, glycyrrhiz. rad. cont. ℨss, zingib. rad. concis., croci stigmat. āā ℨj, aquæ f℥xlj, sp. ten. Oj. Ph. L.) Properties same as the last.

TINCTURA RHEI ET AL'OES, *Tincture of Rhubarb and Aloes, Elixir sacrum.* (Rhei concis ℨx, aloes, pulv. ℨvj, cardam. cont. ℨss, alcohol dilut. Oij. Macerate for 14 days, express, and filter. Ph. U. S.) Properties like the last.

Rymer's Car'diac Tincture consists of an infusion of *Capsicum, Camphor, Cardamom seeds, Rhubarb, Aloes* and *Castor* in *Proof Spirit*, with a very small quantity of *Sulphuric Acid*.

TINCTURA RHEI ET GENTIA'NÆ, *Tincture of Rhubarb with Gen'tian, Tinctura Rhei Ama'ra.* (Rhei cont. ℥ij, gentian. cont. ℨss, alcohol. dilut. Oij. Macerate for 14 days, express and filter. Ph. U. S.) It may also be prepared by displacement. Properties same as the last.

TINCTURA RHEI ET SENNÆ, *Tincture of Rhubarb and Senna, Warner's Gout Cordial.* (Rhei cont. ℨj, sennæ, ℨij, coriandr. cont., fœnicul. cont. āā ℨj, santal. rasur. ℨij, croci ext. glycyrrhiz. rad. āā ℨss, uvar. passar. acinis exemptis, ℔ss, alcohol. dilut. Oiij. Macerate for 14 days; express and filter. Ph. U. S.) Dose, f℥ss to f℥ij.

TINCTURA RHŒI, Tinctura rhei — t. Rhœi amara, Tinctura rhei et gentianæ—t. Sacra, Vinum aloes.

TINCTURA SANGUINA'RIÆ, *Tincture of Bloodroot.* (Sanguinar. cont. ℥iv, alcohol. dilut. Oij. Macerate for 14 days, express, and filter. Ph. U. S.) It may also be prepared by displacement. Dose, 30 to 60 drops.

TINCTURA SAPONIS CAMPHORATA, Linimentum saponis — t. Saponis et opii, Linimentum saponis et opii.

TINCTURA SCILLÆ, *Tincture of Squill.* (Scillæ ℥iv, alcohol. dilut. Oij. Macerate for 14 days, express, and filter. It may also be made by displacement. Ph. U. S.) Dose, gtt. xv to lx.

TINCTURA SEDATIVA, Tinctura opii.

TINCTURA SENNÆ, *T. Sennæ Compos'ita, Elixir Salu'tis, Daffy's Elixir, Tincture of Senna.* (Sennæ fol. ℥iij, carui sem. cont. ℨiij, cardam. sem. cont. ℨj, uvarum passarum demptis acinis, ℥iv, sp. ten. Oij. Ph. L. & D.) Stomachic, carminative and cathartic. Dose, f℥ij to f℥j.

TINCTURÆ SENNÆ ET JALA'PÆ, *Tincture of Senna and Jalap.* (Sennæ ℥iij, jalap. pulv. ℥j, coriandr. cont., carui cont., āā ℨss, cardam. cont ℨij, sacch. ℥iv, alcohol. dilut. Oiij. Macerate for 14 days, express, and filter. Ph. U. S.) It may also be prepared by displacement. Dose, f℥ij to f℥j.

TINCTURA SERPENTA'RIÆ, *T. S. Virginia'næ, T. Aristolochi'æ Serpentariæ, Tincture of Snakeroot.* (Rad. serpent. ℥iij, alcohol. dilut. Oij. Macerate for 14 days, express, and filter. Ph. U. S.) It may also be prepared by displacement. Tonic. Dose, f℥ss to f℥ij.

TINCTURA STOMACHICA, Tinctura cardamomi composita.

TINCTURA STRAMO'NII, *Tincture of Stramo'nium.* (Stramon. sem. cont. ℥iv, alcohol. dilut. Oij. Macerate for 14 days, express, and filter. Ph. U. S.) It may also be prepared by displacement. Dose, ten to twenty minims.

TINCTURA STRYCH'NIÆ. *Tincture of Strych'nia.* (Alcohol. s. g. .837, Oj, strychniæ gr. iij.) Dose, 6 drops to 24. Properties, those of strychnia.

TINCTURA seu AL'COHOL SULPHU'RICO-ÆTHEREUS FERRI, *Guttæ nervi'næ, Liquor Anod'ynus Martia'lis, Al'cohol æthe'reus ferra'tus, Naph'tha*

Vitrioli Martia'lis, Solutio Muriatis ferrici æthe'rea, Spir'itus sulphurico-æthe'reus martialis, Tinctu'ra nervi'na Halen'sis, T. Ton'ico-nervi'na Halen'sis, Tinctura au'rea, T. nervina Bestucheffii, T. nervino-ton'ica (Lamotte's), T. æthe'rea ferri, Æther Martia'lis, De La Motte's Golden Drops, Bestucheff's Nervous Tincture, Elixir d'Or de M. le Général De La Motte. An ethereal solution of muriate of iron. It is much used in gout, hypochondriasis, &c.

TINCTURA SULPHURIS VOLATILIS, Liquor fumans Boylii — t. Thebaica, Tinctura opii, Vinum opii.

TINCTURA TOLUIF'ERÆ BAL'SAMI, *Tincture of Balsam of Tolu, T. Bal'sami Toluta'ni, T. Toluta'ni*, (Ph. U. S., 1842.) *T. Toluta'na*, Ph. U. S., 1851), (*Bals. Tolutan.* ℥iij, alcohol Oij.) Reputed to be expectorant and corroborant. Dose, f℥ss to f℥j, or more.

TINCTURA TONICA NERVINA HALENSIS, Alcohol (seu Tinctura) sulphurico-æthereus ferri.

TINCTURA VALERIA'NÆ, *Tincture of Valerian.* (*Valerian.* cont. ℥iv, *alcohol. dilut.* Oij. Macerate for 14 days, express, and strain. It may also be prepared by displacement. *Ph. U. S.*) Stimulant and antispasmodic. Dose, f℥ss to ℥ij.

TINCTURA VALERIANÆ AMMONIA'TA, *Ammo'niated or Volatile Tincture of Valerian, T. Valerianæ Volat'ilis.* (*Valerianæ* cont. ℥iv, *sp. ammon. arom.* Oij. Macerate for 14 days, express, and filter. It may also be made by displacement. *Ph. U. S.*) Like the former. Dose, f℥ss to f℥ij.

TINCTURA VERA'TRI, *T. Veratri albi, Tincture of White Hellebore.* (*Rad. veratri alb.* cont. ℥viij, *alcohol. dilut.* Oijss. *Ph. E.*) Emetic and cathartic; but not very manageable. Dose, gtt. v to x.

TINCTURA ZINGIB'ERIS, *T. Amo'mi Zingiberis, Tincture of Ginger.* (*Zingib.* cont. ℥viij, *alcohol.* Oij. Macerate for 14 days, express, and filter. It may also be made by displacement. *Ph. U. S.*) Stimulant and carminative. Dose, f℥ss to f℥j.

TINCTURE OF ACETATE OF IRON, Tinctura ferri acetatis—t. of Aconite, Tinctura aconiti —t. of Aconite root, Tinctura aconiti radicis — t. of Balsam of Tolu, Tinctura toluiferæ balsami — t. of Bark, Tinctura cinchonæ — t. of Bark, ammoniated, Tinctura cinchonæ ammoniata — t. of Bark, compound, Tinctura cinchonæ composita —t. of Bark, Huxham's, Tinctura cinchonæ composita — t. of Bark, volatile, Tinctura cinchonæ ammoniata—t. of Belladonna, Tinctura belladonnæ—t. Bestucheff's, see Tinctura ferri muriatis— t. of Blistering Fly, Tinctura cantharidis — t. Cardiac, Rymer's, Tinctura rhei et aloes — t. of Colchicum seeds, Tinctura colchici — t. of Colombo, Tinctura Calumbæ — t. of Cubebs, Tinctura cubebæ — t. of Galls, Tinctura gallarum — t. of Ginger, Tinctura zingiberis — t. for the Gout, Dr. Wilson's, see Colchicum autumnale—t. Hatfield's, see Tinctura guaiaci ammoniata — t. of Hellebore, white, Tinctura veratri — t. of Hemlock, Tinctura conii maculati — t. of Henbane, Tinctura hyoscyami — t. of Hops, Tinctura humuli — t. of Iodine, compound, Tinctura iodini composita—t. of Iron, ammoniated, Tinctura ferri ammoniata — t. of Iron, muriated, Tinctura ferri muriatis—t. Klaproth's, see Tinctura ferri muriatis — t. of Lobelia, Tinctura lobeliæ — t. of Ludwig, see Ferrum tartarizatum — t. of Lupuline, Tinctura lupulinæ — t. of Musk, Tinctura moschi — t. Nervous, Bestucheff's, Tinctura seu alcohol sulphurico-æthereus ferri — t. of Oil of Peppermint, Tinctura Olei menthæ piperitæ — t. of Oil of Spearmint, Tinctura olei menthæ viridis — t. of Opium, acetated, Tinctura opii acetata — t. of Orange-peel, Tinctura aurantii — t. of Rhatany, Tinctura krameriæ — t. of Rhubarb, Tinctura rhei — t. of Rhubarb and aloes, Tinctura rhei et aloes — t. of Rhubarb and gentian, Tinctura rhei et gentianæ—t. of Rhubarb and senna, Tinctura rhei et sennæ — t. of Saffron, Tinctura croci—t. of Saffron, compound, Tinctura de croco composita — t. of Senna and jalap, Tinctura sennæ et jalapæ—t. of Snakeroot, Tinctura serpentariæ— t. of Soap, camphorated, Linimentum saponis—t. of Spanish Fly, Tinctura cantharidis—t. of S...— Tinctura scillæ — t. of Steel, Tinctura ferri ...— ridi—t. Stomach, Tinctura cardamomi composita — t. of Stramonium, Tinctura stramonii — t. for the Teeth, Greenough's, see Spiritus armoraciæ compositus — t. Toothach, Tinctura antiodontalgica — t. of Wormwood, compound, Tinctura absinthii composita.

TINDER, Boletus igniarius.

TINEA, Porrigo—t. Faciei, Porrigo larvalis — t. Favosa, Porrigo favosa — t. Ficosa, Porrigo scutulata — t. Furfuracea, Porrigo furfurans — t. Granulata, Porrigo scutulata, Porrigo lupinosa — t. Lactea, Porrigo larvalis — t. Lupina, Porrigo lupinosa—t. Mucosa, Porrigo lupinosa—t. Pruriginosa, Porrigo furfurans — t. Tondens, Porrigo decalvans.

TINKER'S WEED, Triosteum.

TINKLING, METALLIC, *Tintement métallique.*

TINNIMENTUM METALLICUM, *Tintement métallique.*

TINNI'TUS AU'RIUM, *Fluctua'tio seu Sonitus au'rium, Paracu'sis imagina'ria, Susurrus au'rium, Ote'chus, Syrig'mus, Syring'mus, Syrilus aurium, S. clango'sus, Strep'itus seu Sonimus aurium, Echos, Eneche'ma, Bombus.* Noise, 'ringing of the ears,' from *tinnire*, 'to ring.' (F.) *Tintement, Tintouin, Bourdonnement, Bruissement.* An imaginary sound, like the ringing of a bell, the noise of wind, the murmur of water, &c., heard in health and in sickness. It is, often, an accompaniment of cerebral disorder.

TINTEMENT, Tinnitus aurium—t. B... T. *métallique.*

TINTEMENT MÉTALLIQUE (F.), *Tintement bullaire, Tinnimen'tum metal'licum, (F.) stethoscop'icus, Metallic Respiration, Metallic Voice, Metallic Tinkling.* A particular sound heard by the stethoscope when applied to the chest, and which, according to Laënnec, resembles that caused by striking glass, metal, porcelain, with a pin; but is, perhaps, more akin to the sound of the keys of a musical snuff-box. The *tintement métallique* or *metallic tinkling* is heard on causing the patient to speak or breathe; but is more distinct when he coughs. When the phenomenon is not so strongly marked, it produces only the *metallic resonance.* The 'metallic tinkling,' is a pathognomonic symptom of a communication between the bronchia and cavity of the chest; in other words, of *Pneumothorax.*

TINTINNABULUM, Uvula.

TINTOUIN, Tinnitus aurium.

TIPSARIA, Decoctum hordei.

TIRE-BALLE, Forceps (bullet.)

TIRE-FOND, (F.) A surgical instrument formerly used to elevate the piece of bone sawed off by the trephine.

TIRE-PUS, Pyulcon.

TIRE-TÊTE, (F.) A name given to different instruments used for extracting the head of the child when left in the uterus, and in certain cases of difficult labour. The crotchet is one of these, as well as the *Tire-tête à bascule* of Levret, &c.

TIRES, Milk sickness.

TISANE, *Pti'sana* or *Ptis'ana, Ptisane,* from πτισανη, 'pearl barley,' itself from πτισσω, 'I corticate.' A name given to aqueous or vinous, containing but little, if any, medicinal agent.

The ancients gave the name particularly to the decoction of barley.
TISANE COMMUNE, Decoctum hordei.
TISIC, Phthisis.
TISICAL, Phthisicus.
TISSU, Tissue — *t. Accidental*, see Accidental, and Tissue, accidental — *t. Caverneux*, Cavernous texture — *t. Celluleux des os*, Cancelli — *t. Indulaire*, Tissue, inodular — *t. Lardacé*, Lardaceous — *t. Spongoïde*, Spongoid tissue.

TISSUE, *Textus, Tela*, (F.) *Tissu*. By this term, in anatomy, is meant the various parts, which, by their union, form the organs; and are, as it were, their anatomical elements. Histological anatomy is the anatomy of the tissues, which are the seat of the investigations of the pathological anatomist. The best division, indeed, of diseases would be according to the tissues mainly implicated. For the elementary tissues, see Fibre. The compound tissues, which, by associating or combining variously, form every organ of the body, have been variously classed: but every division is imperfect and liable to objection. The following, by Messrs. Todd and Bowman, is one of the most recent.

TABULAR VIEW OF THE TISSUES OF THE HUMAN BODY.

	Examples.
1. Simple membrane, homogeneous, or nearly so, employed alone, or in the formation of compound membranes.	Posterior layer of the cornea. — Capsule of the lens. — Sarcolemma of muscle, &c.
2. Filamentous Tissues, the elements of which are real or apparent filaments.	White and yellow fibrous tissues. — Areolar tissue.
3. Compound membranes, composed of simple membrane and a layer of cells of various forms, (epithelium or epidermis,) or of areolar tissue and epithelium.	Mucous membrane — Skin. — True or secreting glands — Serous and synovial membranes.
4. Tissues which retain the primitive areolar structure as their permanent character.	Adipose tissue. — Cartilage. — Gray nervous matter.
5. Sclerous or hard tissue.	Bone. — Teeth.
6. Compound tissues.	
a. Composed of tubes of homogeneous membrane, containing a peculiar substance.	Muscle. — Nerve.
b. Composed of white fibrous tissues and cartilage.	Fibro-cartilage.

TISSUE, ACCIDENTAL or ADVENTITIOUS, consists of every substance — foreign to the primitive organization of the economy, but yet organized and living — which may be developed in the anterior or at the surface of organs. Laënnec divides the accidental issues into two sections: 1. Those that resemble others in the animal economy, or *analogous accidental tissues;* and, 2. Those that have nothing analogous in the body, and which are always the result of a morbid process — the *heterologous* or *heteroclite accidental tissues*. To the first class belong, ossifications; accidental fibrous, fibro-cartilaginous, cartilaginous, areolar, and corneous tissues; hairs; the serous membranes of certain encysted tumours; the mucous membranes of fistulous canals, and accidental synovial membranes. To the second belong tubercles, scirrhi, melanosis, &c.

TISSUE, AREOLAR, Cellular tissue.
TISSUE, CARTILAG"INOUS, *Hymenochondro'des seu Hymenochondroï'des (Textura seu Tela.)*
TISSUE, CRIBRIFORM, Cellular tissue — t. Fibrous, see Fibrous — t. Filamentous, Cellular tissue.
TISSUE, INOD'ULAR, *Tela inodula'ris*, (F.) *Inodule, Tissu inodulaire*. A name given by Delpech to an accidental fibrous tissue developed in suppurating wounds, which is the principal agent in cicatrization. It has, at first, the appearance of a reddish cellulo-fibrous layer; but soon loses its vascularity; and its fibres, which pass in all directions, become of a dull white colour, and of a consistence and hardness, that may be compared to those of the strongest articular ligaments. It is well seen in the cicatrix left after burns.

TISSUE, LAMINATED, Cellular tissue — t. Ligamentous, Desmoid tissue — t. Mucous, Cellular tissue — t. Porous, Cellular tissue — t. Reticulated, Cellular tissue.
TIT, Nipple.
TITHENE, Nurse.
TITHYMALUS CYPARISSA, Euphorbia cyparissias — t. Lathyris, Euphorbia lathyris — t. Latifolius, Euphorbia latifolius — t. Palustris, Euphorbia palustris — t. Paralias, Euphorbia paralias.
TITILLAMENTUM, Gargarism.
TITILLATION, Tickling.
TITTHE, Nipple.
TITTHION, Nipple.
TITTHIS, Nipple.
TITTHOS, Mamma, Nipple.
TITUBANTIA, *Bredouillement*.
TITUBATIO, Fidgets, Vacillatio.
TO-AND-FRO-SOUND, *Bruit de frottement*.
TOAD-FLAX, Antirrhinum linaria — t. f. Bastard, Comandra umbellata.
TOAST-WATER, *Aqua tostæ panis*. Toast well half a slice of a stale quartern loaf; put it into a pitcher, and pour over it a quart of water. After two hours, decant the water from the bread. It is a common drink in febrile affections.
TOBACCO, Nicotiana tabacum — t. English, Nicotiana rustica — t. Indian, Lobelia inflata — t. Poison, Hyoscyamus niger — t. Wild, Lobelia inflata.
TOCETOS, Parturition.
TOCODOMYCODORITIS MALIGNA VAGINALIS, Colpocace puerperarum.
TOCOLOGY, Obstetrics.
TOCOS, Parturition.
TODDY TREE, Mamei.
TOE, Digitus pedis.
TOEPLITZ, see Toplitz.
TOFUS, Tophus.
TOILE D'ARAIGNEE, Araneæ tela — *t. Choroïdienne*, see Choroid — *t. de Gaultier*, Sparadrapum Galteri.
TOKAS, Puerpera.
TOKOLOGY, Obstetrics.
TOLA, Tonsil.
TOL'ERANCE, *Toleran'tia ;* from *tolerare*, 'to bear.' The power of bearing. A word used by the Italian school of Rasori, to signify the power of bearing large doses of certain potent remedies, as tartrate of antimony and potassa. See Contro-stimulus.
TOLES, Tonsil.
TOLIUM, Tonsil.
TOLLES, Tonsil.
TOLLUM, Tonsil.
TOLUIF'ERA BAL'SAMUM, *Myrox'ylon To-luif"erum*. Family, Terebinthaceæ. *Sex. Syst.* Decandria Monogynia. The name of the tree which affords the *Balsam of Tolu, Balsamum Toluta'num, Toluta'num, Toluif'eræ Balsami Balsamum, Goac'onax, Red Balsam of Peru,* (F.) *Baume de Tolu, B. de Carthagène*. It has a very fragrant odour, and warm, sweetish taste; is thick, and of a reddish-yellow colour. It is stimulant and expectorant, (?) and is used in coughs. It is chiefly, however, employed on account of its flavour.
TOLUTANUM, see Toluifera balsamum.
TOMATA, Solanum lycopersicum.
TOMĔ, *Tom'us*, τομη, τομος, 'incision.' A common suffix, as in Litho*tomy*, Broncho*tomy*, &c.

TOME, Cut, Incision.
TOMEION, Knife.
TOMEN'TUM CER'EBRI, from *tomentum*, 'a flock of wool.' The infinite number of small vessels which pass between the pia mater and convolutions of the brain. They enter the substance of the brain at right angles.
TOMEUS, Knife.
TOMIS, Scissors.
TOMOTOCIA, Cæsarean section.
TONE, *Tonus*, from τεινω, 'I stretch.' The state of tension or firmness proper to each organic tissue. It is the effect of tonicity.
TONE, Elasticity.
TONGA, see Datura sanguinea.
TONGRES, MINERAL WATERS OF. The town of Tongres is about a league from Maestricht in the Low Countries. The springs, of which there are several, are chalybeate, containing carbonates of iron and magnesia.
TONGUE, Sax. τung, (D.) T o n g, *Lingua, Glossa, Glotta,* (F.) *Langue*. The tongue is a muscular, symmetrical, and very mobile organ; situate in the mouth, from the os hyoides and epiglottis to the incisor teeth. Its particular use is, to procure the sensation of savours; and it aids in the acts of sucking, mastication, deglutition, pronunciation, and expuition. It has the shape of a pyramid, flattened above and below; rounded at its angles, and terminated, anteriorly, by a blunt point. Its *upper surface*, called the *dorsum*, is free, flat, and divided into two portions by a median furrow, *lin'ea media'na;* at the posterior extremity of which is the *foramen cæcum* or *Fora'men of Morgagni*. The *inferior surface* is free, and covered by the mucous membrane on its anterior third and sides: but behind and in the middle it is attached to the lower jaw by means of the genio-glossus; and to the hyoides by the hyoglossus. Its *margins* are rounded; thick behind, thinner anteriorly. Its *tip, or point, or dental extremity* is rounded and free: — the *root, base,* or *hyoid extremity, Radix linguæ,* is continuous with the epiglottis and velum palati. It is very thick at the foramen cæcum; but thinner as it approaches the hyoid bone. The tongue is composed of muscles, and covered by a mucous membrane— *Periglot'tis, Involu'crum linguæ, Membra'na seu Tu'nica cagina'lis seu Cutis seu Epider'mis seu Tunica seu Involu'crum muco'sum seu Crusta villo'sa linguæ* —which forms also the frænum beneath the tongue. On this membrane are seen the different *papillæ*. The nerves of the organ proceed from the *inferior maxillary, glosso-pharyngeal* and *hypoglossal*. The first and second are connected with taste; the last with the motions of the organ. Some recent observers, however, consider the glosso-pharyngeal to be the special nerve of gustation. The arteries are the *lingual*, from the external carotid; and the *palatine* and *tonsillar*, from the labial. The veins are the *superficialis linguæ, ranina, lingualis,* and *submentalis.* They open into those of the pharynx and larynx. Its lymphatic vessels pass into ganglia, situate at the edge of the hyoglossi muscles.
TONGUE, BLACK. A fever which prevailed in the western States in the winter of 1842–3; probably typhoid fever. According to some, an epidemic erysipelas.
TONGUE, HERNIA OF THE, Glossocele — t. Inflammation of the, Glossitis — t. Red, fever, see Typhus — t. Scraper, *Cure-langue* — t. Tie, see Ankyloglossum.
TON'IC, *Ton'icus*. Same etymon as *Tone*. Relating to tone.
Tonic, Ton'icus, Tono'ticus, Antasthen'icus, (F.) *Tonique, Fortifiant,* in Therapeutics, means a medicine, which has the power of exciting slowly, and by insensible degrees, the organic actions of the different systems of the animal economy, and of augmenting their strength in a durable manner. Bitter, vegetable substances which are not associated with an acrid or narcotic principle; preparations of iron; cold water, &c., act as tonics. They are also called *Comfortan'tia, Confortati'va, Corroboran'tia, Confirman'tia, Euboran'tia,* &c.
The following are the chief Tonics: — Acidum Arseniosum, Acidum Nitricum, Acidum Sulphuricum, Argenti Nitras, Bismuthi Subnitras, Cort. Ligni, Cascarilla, Cinchona, Cinchonia, Colomba, Cornus Florida, Cupri Acetas, Cupri Sulphas, Cuprum ammoniatum, Cusparia, Eupatorium perfoliatum, Ferri Præparata, Gentiana, Lignum dron, Lupulina, Piperina, Prunus Virginia, Quassia, Quinia, Salix, Salicina, Serpentaria. Liquor præparata; Aquæ minerales acidulæ et ferrugineæ, Mental Tonics, (Confidence, Hope, Amusement.)
TONIC POWER, Irritability.
TONIC SPASM, *Spasmus ton'icus, Convul'sio tonica, Conductio, Spas'ticus, Tonos, Ento'nia, Estasis, Enta'sia.* A rigid contraction of muscle without relaxation, as in trismus, tetanus, &c. See Tetanus and Spasm.
TONIC"ITY, *Tonic''itas*. The faculty that determines the general tone of the solids. Excessive tonicity causes *er'ethism* or *crispness*; deficient tonicity, *atony* or *weakness. Tonicity has* been used in the same sense as irritability.
TONIQUE, Tonic.
TONOS, Tonic spasm — t. Trismus, Trismus.
TONOTICUS, Tonic.
TONSIL, *Tonsil'la, Amyg'dala, Parisi* e *Paristh'mium, Amphibran'chium, Glan'du* a *Tola, Tolles, Toles, To'lium, Tollum, Spongra, tias,* Pl. *Anti'ades, Almond of the ear, Almond of the throat,* (F.) *Amygdale, Tonsille*. An ovoid collection of follicles, about half an inch in length, similar in shape to an almond, and situate, on each side, between the pillars of the velum palati. The inner surface, projecting into the isthmus of the throat, is covered by the mucous membrane, in which are the orifices of a dozen cells, whence a transparent, viscid mucus oozes on pressure. This mucus is destined to facilitate deglutition by lubricating the isthmus faucium; and is forced out during the passage of the alimentary bolus.
TONSILLÆ PESTILENTES, Cynanche maligna.
TONSILLARUM GANGRÆNA, Cynanche maligna.
TONSILLE, Tonsil.
TONSILLIT'IC, *Tonsillit'icus*. Belonging or relating to the tonsils; as the '*tonsillitic branches* of the glosso-pharyngeal nerve.'
TONSILLITIS, Cynanche tonsillaris.
TONSORIUS CULTER, Razor.
TOOTH, Sax. τοδ, *Dens, Odous,* (F.) *Dent*. The teeth, *Dentes, Mord'ices,* are small, hard bones, fixed in the alveoli of each jaw, and serving to lay hold of, and to cut, tear, and triturate alimentary substances. True teeth are found only in man, the mammalia, reptiles, and fish. The teeth have, in general, the shape of an irregular cone, the base of which is towards the interior of the mouth; and the apex, single or divided, towards the bottom of the alveoli. Each tooth has a part situate out of the alveolus and covered by a vitriform substance. This part is called the *crown* or *coro'na*. It is bounded by a narrower portion, called the *cervix,* (F.) *collet*, which separates it from the portion in the alveolus—the *fang* or *root,* (F.) *racine*. In the adult the teeth are 32 in number; 16 to each jaw:

these consist of 4 *incisors*, 2 *canine*, 4 *bicuspidati*, and 6 *molares*. (See these various terms.) The teeth enclose a vascular and nervous pulp, in a central cavity, *Cav'itas Pulpæ*, *Cavum Dentis*, *Antrum denta'lě*. They are formed of a very hard, compact tissue; and the corona is covered by a vitreous substance called *Enam'el*. The incisor and canine teeth are developed by a single point of ossification; the lesser molares, by two; and the larger, by four or five. See Dentition. Researches by Retzius, Müller and others, have led them to believe that the *ivory* of the tooth or *Dentine*, *Substan'tia os'sea* of Malpighi, *proper tooth substance*, *bone of the tooth*, *osseous substance of tooth*, *tooth bone*, consists of tubular fibres, which contain organic deposits of calcareous salts; and of intertubular substance, in which are observed corpuscles or osseous cells of the tooth, called by Professor Owen *calcig"erous cells*, which also contain earthy salts. At the part where the enamel terminates at the cervix of the tooth, the *crusta petro'sa*, *cemen'tum* or *cortical substance*, commences in an extremely thin stratum, passes down and gradually increases in thickness towards the extremity of the root, where it is generally the thickest. It is said by Nasmyth to have been traced on the enamel, and Purkinje and Fränkel thought that it lined the cavitas pulpæ. They gave it the name *Substantia ostoidea*. It is the *mate'ria tarta'rea* of Malpighi. It has been found, however, that the hard substance deposited on the inner surface of the dentine, at the age of twenty years or later, and which encroaches on the cavity, has a distinct structure from the cement, and resembles in part dentine, and in part bone. It is the *horny substance* of Blumenbach, the *osteodentine* of Owen, and the *secondary dentine* of Tomes. In the compound teeth of the herbivorous animal, a deposition is found on the surface of the enamel, which has been called *cementum*. Müller, however, regards it to be a deposit from the salts and the saliva, and to be essentially the same as what is called tartar in the human subject.

TOOTH-ACH, Odontalgia—t. Bone, see Tooth — t. Bush, Xanthoxylum fraxineum — t. Tree, Aralia spinosa, Xanthoxylum clava Herculis.

TOOTH EDGE, *Agacement des dents*, Hæmodia—t. Paste, Dentifricium—t. Rash, Strophulus —t. Shell, dog-like, Dentalium.

TOPHACEOUS CONCRETION, Tophus.

TOPHUS, *Tofus*, *Osteot'ophus*, *Topha'ceous Concretion*. A collection of hard, calcareous matter, which forms, particularly, at the surface of joints affected with gout; (see Calculi, arthritic,) and occasionally, in the interior of organs, around the teeth, &c. It likewise meant gravel and chalaza.

TOP'IC, *Top'ical*, *Top'icus*. A local application; (F.) *Topique*. See Local.

TOPICUS, Local.

TOPINARIA, Talpa.

TOPIQUE, Topic.

TÖPLITZ or TEPLITZ, MINERAL WATERS OF. Töplitz is a town of Bohemia, celebrated for its numerous thermal springs. The water contains chloride of sodium, carbonate, and sulphate of soda; and carbonates of lime and iron, &c. Temp. 114° to 122° Fahr.

TOPLITZ. Töplitz.

TOPOGRAPHICAL ANATOMY, see Anatomy.

TORCULAR, Tourniquet.

TOR'CULAR HEROPH'ILI, The *Press of Heroph'ilus*, *Lechenei'on*, *Lenos*, *Lenum*, *Fourth Sinus*, (F.) *Confluent des Sinus*, *Pressoir d'Hérophile*. A smooth and polished cavity, of irregular shape, in which several sinuses of the dura mater meet.

It is situate before the internal occipital protuberance, at the union of the three great duplicatures of the dura mater. It has six openings into it: —one above, that of the superior longitudinal sinus; two below, answering to the occipital sinuses; one anterior, belonging to the straight sinus; and two lateral, and very broad, which lead into the lateral sinuses; and convey from the cavity the blood that has been poured into it by the others.

TORCULUM, Tourniquet.

TORDY'LIUM, *T. Officina'lě*, *Ses'eli Cret'icum* seu *Monta'num*, (F.) *Séseli de Crète*. Family, Umbelliferæ. Sex. Syst. Pentandria Digynia. The seeds and roots of this Southern European plant are considered carminative and diuretic. They enter into the theriaca.

TORE'NIA ASIAT'ICA, *Cœla-dolo*. A small Malabar plant, the juice of whose leaves, sweetened with sugar, is said to cure gonorrhœa.

TORMENTIL, Geranium maculatum, Tormentilla.

TORMENTIL'LA, *T. erec'ta* seu *sylves'tris* seu *officina'lis* seu *tubero'sa*, *Fraga'ria tormentil'la officina'lis*, *Potentill'a tormentill'a*, *Common Tormen'til*, *Upright Septfoil*, *Heptaphyl'lum*, *Consol'ida rubra*, (F.) *Tormentille*. Family, Rosaceæ. Sex. Syst. Icosandria Polygynia. The root has a slightly aromatic odour; and austere, styptic taste. It is astringent. Dose, of the powder, gr. x to ʒj.

TORMENTUM, Ileus, Intussusceptio.

TOR'MINA, *Strophos*, *Cœlial'gia*, *Encœlial'gia*, *Anile'ma*, *Anile'sis*, *Gripes*, *Mulligrubs*, (F.) *Tranchées*. Acute colicky pains. Dysentery.

TORMINA CELSI, Dysentery—t. Parturientium, Pains, labour—t. Post partum, see Pains, labour.

TORNACULUM, Tourniquet.

TOROS'ITAS, *Corpulen'tia carno'sa*, *Hab'itus athlet'icus*. Muscular strength; from *torosus*, 'brawny,'—*tori*, 'brawn.'

TOROSUS, Muscular.

TORPEDO, Narcosis.

TORPEFACTIO UNIVERSALIS, Holonarcosis.

TORPID, *Tor'pidus*, (F.) *Engourdi*; from *torpeo*, 'I am benumbed.' Numb. Incapable of exertion and of feeling. Dull, stupid, inactive.

TORPIDITAS, Torpor.

TORPIDUS, Narcotized, Torpid.

TORPOR, *Torpid'itas*, *Noth'rotes*, *Parap'sis expers*, (F.) *Engourdissement*, from *torpere*, 'to be numbed.' State of a part which becomes numb, and almost incapable of motion. *Torpor*, *Torpid'ity*, *Torpid'ness*, *Tor'pitude* are also applied to a debilitated, sluggish condition of a part or of the whole of the body; *Aër'gia*, (F.) *Accablement*.

TORPOR, Narcosis—t. of the Colon, see Colon, torpor of the—t. Intestinorum, Constipation—t. Soporificus, Nocar.

TORQUAY. A town in Devonshire, England, which, on account of the mildness of its climate, and its sheltered situation from the bleaker winds, is a frequent retreat for the phthisical invalid.

TOR'SION, *Tor'sio*. The act of twisting. Torsion of the extremities of bleeding vessels, *Angios'trophě*, until the blood ceases to flow, is sometimes used to arrest hemorrhage from divided vessels.

TORTELLE, Erysimum.

TORTICOL'LIS, *Obstip'itas*, *Caput obsti'pum*, *Obsti'pa cervix*, *Obstip'itas cap'itis* seu *Colli*, *Collum obsti'pum*, *Trachel'agra*, *Enta'sia Loxia*, *Lox'ias*, *Cephalox'ia*, *Ancylode'rē*, *Ancylode'ris*, *Rhæbocra'nia*, *Auchenorrheu'ma*, *Rheumatis'mus colli*, *Rh. Cervi'cis*, *Stiffneck*, *Wryneck*; from *torquere*, *tortum*, 'to twist,' and *collum*, 'the neck.'

A variety of rheumatism, seated in the muscles of the neck, which prevents the motion of the head, and causes the patient to hold it inclined to the side affected. It is, commonly, of short duration; usually disappearing in a few days. Rubefacients are the best topical applications. The term is also applied to permanent contraction of the muscles of the neck, which causes the head to be held to one side. The remedy is the division of the contracted muscles.

TORTOISE, FRESHWATER, GREAT, Hydraspis expansa.

TORTUE, Testudo.

TORTURA ORIS, Canine laugh, Neuralgia faciei—t. Oris paralytica Linnæi, Paralysis, Bell's.

TOR'ULA CEREVIS'IÆ, *Saccharom'yces* seu *Mycoder'ma cerevisiæ, Cryptococ'cus ferment'um, Yeast plant*. One of the simplest forms of vegetation, capable, under favourable circumstances, of vegetating rapidly, and assisting in producing the fermentation of saccharine substances. The plant has been found in vomited fluids, and in fæces.

TORULUS GLANDIS, Crown of the glans.

TORUS, Muscle — t. Manûs, Metacarpus.

TOTA BONA, Chenopodium bonus Henricus.

TOTUM CARNOSUM, Pancreas.

TOUCH, *Tactus, Tac'tio, Haphē, Hapsis, Tac'tion, Palpa'tion*, (F.) *Toucher*. One of the five senses, and that which makes known to us the palpable qualities of bodies, such as their consistence, quality, &c. It is seated, particularly, in the hands; and differs from tact in being active.

TOUCH-ME-NOT, Impatiens fulva.

TOUCH, ROYAL. It was at one time almost universally believed, in England, that the royal touch would remove *Scrofula* or *King's Evil*, (as it was thence called.) This superstition is now entirely exploded. Edward, the Confessor, was the first English king who *touched* for the Evil.

TOUCHER, Esaphe, Touch.

TOUCHWOOD, Boletus igniarius.

TOUR DE MAÎTRE, Coup de maître.

TOURBILLON VASCULAIRE, Vasa vasorum.

TOURNESOL, Heliotropium Europæum.

TOURNIOLE, Paronychia.

TOUR'NIQUET, *Tor'cular, Tor'culum, Tornac'ulum, Præ'linm, Præ'lium, Præ'linm* seu *Prælum arteria'lē, Verticil'lum, Fae'cia tor'tilis*, from (F.) *tourner*, 'to turn.' A surgical instrument for stopping the course of blood in the limbs, by exerting a strong compression upon the principal artery. It was invented by a French surgeon, Morel, in the middle of the 17th century; and was modified subsequently, by Nuck, Verduc, Monro, Petit, and Louis. It is used to suspend, for a time, the circulation in a limb, during great operations; to arrest arterial hemorrhage in cases of wounds; to compress certain aneurismal and other tumours, &c.

TOUS-LES-MOIS, *Am'ylum canna'ceum*. A fecula obtained from the root of *Canna coccin'ea*. It resembles potato starch, and may be substituted for arrow-root. It is obtained from St. Kitts.

TOUTE BONNE, Salvia sclarea.

TOUTE ÉPICE, see Myrtus pimenta — t. *Saine*, Sanicula.

TOUX, Tussis—t. Bleue, Pertussis — t. *Bronchique*, Bronchial cough, Cough, tubal—t. *Caverneuse*, see Cavernous respiration — t. *Convulsive*, Pertussis — t. *Quinteuse*, Pertussis — t. *Tubaire*, Bronchial cough, Cough, tubal.

TOXICÆMIA, Toxicohæmia.

TOXICAL, Poisonous.

TOXICATIO, Poisoning.

TOXICODENDRON, Rhus toxicodendron.

TOXICOHÆ'MIA, *Toxica'mia*, from *τοξικον*, 'a poison,' and '*αιμα*, 'blood.' Poisoning of the blood.—Piorry.

TOXICOL'OGY, *Toxicolog"ia*, from *τοξικον* (itself from *τοξον*, 'a bow,') 'a poison,' and *λογος*, 'a description.' A treatise on poisons.

TOXICO'SES, (G.) Toxikosen, from *τοξικον*, 'a poison.' A family of diseases, according to the classification of Fuchs, caused by the reception of poisons into the system.

TOXICUM, Poison, Venom.

TRABECULA CEREBRI, Corpus callosum—t. Cordis, Columnæ carneæ.

TRABECULÆ SPLENIS, see Spleen—t. Willisii, Chordæ Willisii.

TRABES CORDIS, Columnæ carneæ.

TRABS, Penis—t. Cerebri, Corpus callosum—t. Medullaris, Corpus callosum.

TRACE, PRIMITIVE, Groove, primitive.

TRACHE'A, (generally, however, accented *Tra'chea*,) *Trache'a arte'ria, Bronchus*, *Aspera arteria, Fis'tula spiritua'lis, F. pulmona'lis*, (F.) *Trachée artère*, from *τραχυς*, 'rough,' *αρτηρια*, 'artery,' composed of *αηρ*, 'air,' and *τηρειν*, 'to keep.' The trachea is a cylindrical fibro-cartilaginous and membranous tube, flattened behind, and situate on the median line, before the vertebral column, from the inferior part of the larynx, as far as the third dorsal vertebra. There it divides into two branches, the bronchi, which separate to go to each lung. The trachea, the function of which is to convey air to the lungs during respiration, is composed, 1. Of cartilaginous rings, *An'nuli cartilagin'ei, Sygma cartilagin'ea, Orbes cartilagino'si*, incomplete behind; situate one above the other, and kept in situ by a fibrous membrane. 2. Of a mucous membrane, which lines it internally, and contains numerous mucous follicles. 3. Of transverse muscular fibres, not well-marked, which occupy its posterior surface. 4. Of vessels, which proceed from the superior and inferior thyroideals; and, 5. Of nerves, that are given off by the pneumogastric and the cervical ganglia. The breathing tubes of insects are termed *Trachea*.

TRACHEA ARTERIA, Trachea.

TRACHEÆ, see Trachea.

TRA'CHEAL, *Trachea'lis*. Appertaining to the trachea. An epithet applied to respiration as heard through the stethoscope opposite the trachea, larynx, and root of the bronchi; the air appearing as if sucked in from the cyrist during inspiration, and expelled during expiration.

TRACHEAL GLANDS. Mucous follicles on the posterior surface of the trachea. They are small, flattened ovoid bodies.

TRACHÉE ARTÈRE, Trachea.

TRACHEITIS, Cynanche trachealis.

TRACHELAGRA, Torticollis.

TRACHELIAN, Cervical.

TRACHELISM'US, from *τραχηλος*, 'the neck.' A term proposed by Dr. Marshall Hall, for a fancied spasmodic action of the muscles of the neck which he esteems to be the cause of many nervous phenomena, by inducing compression of the veins of the neck and an impeded return of blood from the head.

TRACHELITIS, Cynanche trachealis.

TRACHELIUM AMERICANUM, Lobelia cardinalis.

TRACHÉLO-ATLOIDO-OCCIPITAL, Obliquus superior capitis—t. *Atloïdo-basilaire*, Rectus capitis lateralis — t. *Basilaire*, Rectus capitis anticus.

ternus major — t. *Basilaire, petit*, Rectus capitis internus minor.

TRACHE'LO-DIAPHRAGMAT'IC, *Trachelo-diaphragmat'icus*. The fourth pair of cervical nerves, whence the phrenic nerve chiefly arises. — Chaussier.

TRACHÉLO-MASTOÏDIEN, Complexus minor — t. *Occipital*, Complexus — t. *Phyma*, Bronchocele — t. *Scapulaire*, Levator scapulæ.

TRACHELOS, Collum.

TRACHEOCELE, Bronchocele.

TRACHEOPHONY, Laryngophony.

TRACHEOPHTHISIS, see Phthisis laryngea.

TRACHEORRHAG''IA, *Hæmop'toë seu Hæmop'tysis larynge'a et trachea'lis*, from τραχεια, 'the trachea,' and ρηγνυμι, 'to break forth.' Hæmorrhage from the trachea.

TRACHEOSTENO'SIS, from τραχεια, 'the trachea,' and στενωσις, 'contraction.' Contraction or narrowness of the trachea.

TRACHEOTOMY, see Bronchotomy.

TRACHITIS, Cynanche trachealis.

TRACHO'MA, *Aspre'do*, from τραχυς, 'rough.' *Gran'ular conjuncti'va, Gran'ular eyelid*, (F.) *Asperité des Paupières*. A roughness of the inner surface of the eyelids; granular eyelids. A variety of ophthalmia, of which three kinds have been designated : — *T. sabulo'sum*, from sand, &c., getting between the eyelids; *T. carunculo'sum, Phadaro'des, Phadaro'sis, Morum pal'pebræ inter'næ*, from fleshy excrescences; and *T. herpet'-icum*, from hard pustules on the inner surface of the eyelids. This last is, also, called *Fico'sis*, and *Pal'pebra fico'sa*.

TRACT, OPTIC, see Optic nerves — t. Respiratory, see Respiratory tract.

TRACTATIO MANUARIA, Surgery.

TRACTORATION, Perkinism, see Tractors, metallic.

TRACTORS, METAL'LIC. Metallic agents, introduced by Dr. Elisha Perkins, of Connecticut, about the end of the last century, to cure diseases. The parts were rubbed with these tractors, and hundreds of thousands of cases were reported to have been cured by the *Tractora'tion*. The affections, in which they were chiefly used, were local inflammations, and pains in different parts. The good effects were, doubtless, owing to the influence exerted by the mind over the body. The bubble did not exist long. See Perkinism.

TRACTUS INTESTINORUM, Intestinal Tube — t. Opticus, see Optic nerves — t. Respiratorius, Respiratory tract.

TRACTUS SPIRA'LIS FORAMINULEN'TUS. Minute openings at the base of the modiolus, arranged in a spiral manner, which transmit the filaments of the cochlear nerve. The central canal of the Tractus is longer than the rest, and is called *Tu'-bulus centra'lis modi'oli*.

TRADESCAN'TIA VIRGIN'ICA, *Spiderwort;* indigenous; *Order*, Commelynaceæ; flowering from May to August. The roots are demulcent.

TRAGACAN'THA, *Gummi Tragacan'tha, G. Astrag'ali Tragacanthæ, Gum Tragacanth, Gum Dragon*. The concrete juice of the *Astragalus Tragacantha* or *Astragalus Verus*, a native of Persia. *Family*, Leguminosæ. *Sex. Syst.* Diadelphia Decandria. (F.) *Gomme Adragant, Adragant.* This gum is inodorous; nearly insipid; of a whitish colour; semi-transparent, and striated. It is in thin, vermiform pieces; and does not form a smooth, uniform mucilage with water. It is demulcent, but is rarely used alone.

TRAGEA AROMATICA, Pulvis cinnamomi compositus.

TRAG''ICUS, *Tragien* (Ch.), from Tragus. A small, flat, triangular muscle which almost wholly covers the outer surface of the tragus, arising from its base, and terminating at the top of the eminence.

TRAGIEN, Tragicus.

TRAGOMASCHA'LIA, *Tragomas'chalē*, from τραγος, 'a goat,' and μασχαλη, 'axilla.' The strong, unpleasant odour of the armpits.

TRAGOPHONIA, Egophony.

TRAGOPO'GON, *Barba hirci*, from τραγος, 'a goat,' and πωγων, 'beard.' A genus of plants; *Family*, Cichoraceæ. *Sex. Syst.* Syngenesia Polygamia Æqualis. (F.) *Barbe de Bouc;* of which the roots of the *Tragopogon porrifo'lium, Salsifi, Oyster-root*, and the young shoots of the *T. praten'se, Meadow Salsifi, Common Goat's Beard*, (F.) *Salsifis des prés*, are eaten as food. The root of the latter has been used as a diuretic.

TRAGOSELINUM, Pimpinella saxifraga — t. Angelica, Ligusticum podograria — t. Magnum, Pimpinella magna — t. Majus, Pimpinella magna — t. Saxifraga, Pimpinella magna.

TRAGUS, τραγος, 'a goat;' from its being furnished, in some persons, with hair, like the beard of a goat. *Hircus, Hirquus*. A small, flattened, triangular nipple, situate before the meatus auditorius externus, which it appears to conceal. It is covered with hair in old people, whence its name. Also, the peculiar goat-like smell of the axillæ.

TRAGUS MATTHIOLI, Salsola kali.

TRAINASSE, Polygonum aviculare.

TRAMIS, Perinæum.

TRANCE, Catalepsy, Ecstasis.

TRANCHÉES, Tormina — t. *Utérines*, Pains, after.

TRANSFIGURATIO, Transformation.

TRANSFORMA'TION, *Transforma'tio, Transfigura'tio, Transmuta'tio, Metab'olē*, from *trans*, 'beyond,' and *forma*, 'form.' Change of form.

TRANSFORMATIONS DE TISSU, (F.) The French pathologists designate thus the change that occurs in an organ, the tissue of which becomes similar to that of another organ. The chief transformations are cartilaginous, osseous, and adipous. See Tissue.

TRANSFU'SION, *Transfusio*, from *transfundere (trans*, and *fundere*, 'to pour'), 'to pour from one vessel into another.' *Transfusio San'guinis, Cura Medea'na, Methæmachym'ia, Hæmatometach'ysis, Hæmometach'ysis, Diach'ysis, Transplanta'tio med'ica nova, Chirur'gia transfuso'ria, Exotichæmato'sis*. The act of passing the blood of one animal into the veins of another; an operation which was formerly used to fulfil various therapeutical intentions. It has been revived in cases of uterine hemorrhage; and, apparently, with some success.

The operation can only be performed safely on animals having like kinds of blood. See Globule.

TRANSLATION, Metastasis.

TRANSMUTATIO, Transformation.

TRANSPIRATIO, Perspiration — t. Unilatera, Hemidiaphoresis.

TRANSPLANTA'TIO, *Metaphytei'a*. A pretended method of curing diseases, devised by Paracelsus — by making them pass from one individual to another, either animal or vegetable.

TRANSPLANTATIO, Morioplastice — t. Medica nova, Transfusion.

TRANSPLANTA'TIO DENTIS, *Insit''io dentis*. The act of transplanting a tooth from one person to another.

TRANSPORT, Delirium.

TRANSPOSITIO, Metathesis.

TRANSPOSIT"ION, *Transpositio,* from *trans,* 'over,' and *ponere,* 'to put.' *Metath'esis.* Change of situation.

TRANSPOSITION OF THE VIS'CERA, *Polype'ria promis'cua translati'va, Intus inver'sus,* is a congenital vice of conformation, which consists in the viscera being found out of the situations they ordinarily occupy: the heart, for example, being on the right side; the liver on the left, &c.

TRANSUDATIO, Diapedesis.

TRANSUDA'TION, *Transuda'tio,* from *trans,* 'through,' and *sudare, sudatum,* 'to sweat.' The passage of a fluid through the tissue of any organ, which may collect in small drops on the opposite surface, or evaporate from it.

TRANSUDATION, Exosmose.

TRANSVERSAIRE ÉPINEUX, Transversalis dorsi — *t. Épineux du cou,* Semispinalis colli — *t. Grêle,* see Sacro-lumbalis — *t. Épineux du dos,* Semi-spinatus dorsi.

TRANSVERSAL DE LA CONQUE, Transversalis auris — *t. du Nez,* Compressor nasi — *t. des Orteils,* Transversus pedis.

TRANSVERSALIS, Transverse.

TRANSVERSA'LIS ABDOM'INIS, (F.) *Lombo-abdominal,* (Ch.) *Transverse de l'Abdomen.* This muscle is seated, deeply, on the lateral parts of the abdomen. It is flat, thin, and broader before than behind. It is attached, above, to the cartilage of the last true rib, and to those of every false rib; and, below, to the inner lip of the crista of the ilium; to the two outer thirds of the crural arch, and to the upper part of the pubis. Its fibres, moreover, are inserted, behind, by means of broad aponeuroses, into the top of the transverse and spinous processes of the first four lumbar vertebræ; and, before, into the linea alba, and the ensiform cartilage. This muscle, all of whose fibres have a transverse direction, constricts the belly, and diminishes the base of the chest, by drawing inwards the ribs to which it is attached.

TRANSVERSALIS ANTICUS PRIMUS, Rectus capitis lateralis — t. Collateralis colli, see Sacro-lumbalis.

TRANSVERSA'LIS COLLI, *Transversalis Major colli,* Portion of the Sacro-spinal (Ch.), (F.) *Transversaire.* A muscle, seated at the posterior and lateral part of the neck and upper part of the back. It is attached to the transverse processes of the five or six lowest vertebræ of the neck; and to those of the four or five first dorsal. It extends the vertebræ of the neck, and inclines them to its side.

TRANSVERSALIS COLLI, Semi-spinalis colli.

TRANSVERSALIS DORSI, *Transverso-spinalis, Multif'idus Spinæ, Lumbo-cervical portion of the Spinal* (Ch.), (*Transverso-spinalis Lumbo'rum, Transverso-spinalis Dorsi, Transverso-spinalis Colli,*) *Mus'culus sacer, Spinales et transversales lumborum, Semi-spinalis internus* sive *Transverso-spinalis colli pars interna* (Winslow), *Lombo-dorsi-spinal,* &c., (F.) *Transversaires épineux.* This muscle, usually called, by English anatomists, *Multifidus spinæ,* and including all the *transverso-spinales,* is situate in the vertebral gutters, extending from the posterior part of the sacrum to the second cervical vertebræ. It is thicker in the neck and loins than in the back and behind the sacrum. Its use is—to straighten the vertebral column, and to impress upon it a slight rotary motion.

TRANSVERSALIS NASI, Compressor naris.

TRANSVERSARIUS, Transverse.

TRANSVERSE, *Transver'sus, Transversa'lis, Transversa'rius,* from *trans,* 'over,' and *vertere,* 'to turn.' That which runs across: also, that which relates to the transverse processes of the vertebræ.

TRANSVERSE ARTERY OF THE FACE, arises from the temporal; passes transversely across the face, in front of the condyle of the lower jaw, and gives its branches to the different muscles of the cheek.

TRANSVERSE FISSURE, see Liver—t. Ligament of the Atlas, Annular ligament.

TRANSVERSE PERINEAL ARTERY, *Urethro-bulbar* (Ch.), is given off from the upper branch of the internal pudic; and passes inwards and forwards above the transversus perinæi muscle, as far as the bulb of the urethra, into which it dips, subdividing into numerous branches.

TRANSVERSE PROC"ESSES OF THE VERTEBRÆ, *Diapophyses,* of Owen, (F.) *Apophyses transverses des vertèbres,* are the bony eminences that jut out transversely and posteriorly from the sides of the vertebræ.

TRANSVERSE SUTURE, *Sutu'ra transversa'lis,* runs across the face, and sinks into the orbit: joining the bones of the skull to those of the face, but with so many irregularities and interruptions, that it can scarcely be recognised as a suture.

TRANSVERSE DE L'ABDOMEN, Transversalis abdominis — *t. de l'Oricule,* Transversus auris — *t. du Périnée,* Transversus perinæi.

TRANSVERSO-SPINAL, Semi-spinalis colli, Semi-spinalis dorsi — t. Spinalis, Transversus dorsi — t. Spinalis colli. Semi-spinalis colli — t. Spinalis dorsi, Semi-spinalis dorsi.

TRANSVER'SUS AURIS, *Transver'sus Auric'ulæ,* (F.) *Transverse de l'Oricule* (Ch.), *Transversal de la Conque,* is often wanting. It is formed of some transverse fibres, situate transversely, behind the projection of the helix which divides the concha into two portions.

TRANSVERSUS PEDIS, *Scandula'rius,* (F.) *Transversal des Orteils, Métatarso-sous-phalangien transversal du premier orteil* (Chaussier). A muscle, which arises by fleshy slips from the heads of the metatarsal bones of the three outer toes. Its tendon is inserted into the base of the first phalanx of the great toe, being blended with that of the adductor pollicis.

TRANSVERSUS PERINÆI, *Leva'tor Ani parvus, Ischio-périneal* (Ch.,) (F.) *Transverse du Périnée,* is placed at the posterior part of the perinæum. It is thin, triangular, and situate transverse. Its external extremity is attached to the ramus and tuberosity of the ischium: its inner extremity is confounded with its fellow of the opposite side, and with the anterior part of the sphincter ani and posterior part of the bulbo-cavernosus. The use of this muscle is, — to compress the urethra and to support the rectum and bladder. To a fasciculus of this muscle, Santorini has given the name *Ure'thræ Eleva'tor* seu *Ejacula'tor.*

TRANSVERSUS PERINÆ'I ALTER, *Prostaticus inferior.* A small muscle which occasionally accompanies the last.

TRAPA NATANS, (F.) *Macre flottant, Noix d'Eau, Chataigne d'Eau. Sex. Syst.* Tetrandria Monogynia. The plant which affords the *Nux Aquat'icæ, Trib'uli aquatici, Caltrops.* The nut is considered nutrient and demulcent, and is said to be useful in diarrhœa from abrasion of the bowels, and in calculus. A poultice is sometimes made of it to discuss hard and indolent tumors.

TRAPÈZE, Trapezium, Trapezius.

TRAPE'ZIUM OS, τραπεζιον. So called from its shape. *Os multan'gulum majus,* (F.) *Os trapèze.* The first bone of the second row of the carpus. It is articulated, above, with the scaphoides; below, with the first bone of the metacarpus; within, with the trapezoides, and second metacarpal bone. Anteriorly, posteriorly, and externally, it gives attachment to ligaments.

TRAPE'ZIUS, *Cuculla'ris*, (F.) *Dorso-susacromien* (Ch.), *Trapèse, Capuchon*. A muscle, seated at the posterior part of the neck and shoulder, and at the upper part of the back. It has the shape of a trapezium; is attached, on the one hand, to the inner third of the upper curved line of the occipital bone; to the posterior cervical ligament; to the spinous process of the 7th cervical vertebra; and to those of all the dorsal vertebræ; and, on the other hand, to the spine of the scapula; the acromion and the outer third of the posterior margin of the clavicle. Its upper fibres are situate obliquely downwards and outwards; the transverse and inferior, obliquely outwards and inwards. This muscle elevates the shoulder; carries it backwards, or depresses it, according as its upper, middle, or lower fibres contract separately. It straightens the head, also, and inclines it to one side.

TRAP'EZOID LIGAMENT. The anterior part of the coraco-clavicular ligament. It is a very strong, fibrous fasciculus, which has the shape of a trapezium, and is situate obliquely, between the acromion process and clavicle.

TRAPEZOI'DES, OS, *Os multan'gulum minus, Os pyramida'lē carpi*, from τραπεζιον, 'a trapezium,' and ειδος, 'shape or resemblance.' The second bone of the second row of the carpus,—so called from its shape. It is smaller than the trapezium, on the inside of which it is situate. It is articulated, above, with the os naviculare; below, with the second metacarpal bone; on the outside, with the trapezium; and internally, with the magnum. Anteriorly and posteriorly, it affords attachment to ligaments.

TRAUBENOUR, Grape cure.
TRAULISMUS, see Balbuties and Blæsitas.
TRAULOTES, see Blæsitas.
TRAUMA, Wound.
TRAUMAT'IC, *Traumat'icus, Vulnera'rius, Vul'nerary*; from τραυμα, 'a wound.' Any thing relating to a wound.
TRAUMATICA, Detergents, Vulneraries.
TRAUMATICUS, Traumatic, Vulnerary.
TRAUMATOP'YRA, *Febris traumat'ica*; from τραυμα, 'a wound,' and πυρ, 'fire.' A wound fever, or fever consecutive to a wound.
TRAVAIL, Parturition.
TRAVAIL D'ENFANT, Parturition.
TRAVELLER'S JOY, Clematis vitalba.
TREACLE, Melasses, Theriaca—t. English, Teucrium chamædrys—t. Venice, Theriaca.
TREAD, Cicatricula—t. of the Cock, Molecule.
TREE, ELK, Andromeda arborea—t. of Life, Thuya occidentalis—t. Sour, Andromeda arborea.
TRÈFLE D'EAU, Menyanthes trifoliata.
TREFOIL, Hepatica triloba—t. Bean, stinking, Anagyris—t. Marsh, Menyanthes verna—t. Sour, Oxalis acetosella—t. Shrubby, Ptelea trifoliata—t. Water, Menyanthes trifoliata.
TREMA, Foramen.
TREMBLEMENT, Tremor—t. *Métallique*, see Tremor.
TREMBLES, Milk-sickness.
TREMBLING, Tremor.
TREMELLA AURICULA, Peziza auricula.
TREMOR, *Trepida'tio, Syn'clonus Tremor, Tromo-spasmus, Tromus, Trembling*, (F.) *Tremblement*, from *tremere*, 'to tremble.' Involuntary agitation of the body, or of some part of it, without any obstacle to voluntary motion. It depends, generally, upon debility of the muscular, or of the nervous system; and, hence, is observed in convalescence, and in typhoid affec-

tions. It occurs, also, in old people; in hard drinkers; workers in mercury, lead, &c.: in the last case, it is called by the French, *Tremblement métallique, Tremor metal'licus*. Tremor seems to resemble paralysis more than convulsion. See Paralysis agitans and Pavitatio.

TREMOR CORDIS, Hippus, Palpitation—t. Metallicus, see Tremor—t. Purring, *Frémissement cataire*.

TREPAN, *Trep'anum, Terebel'la, Trip'anon, Pereter'ium, Peretor'ium, Serra versat'ilis, Chœn'icis, Chœnic'ion, Ter'ebra, Ter'etron, Tere'trium, Vertib'ulum, Try'panon*, (F.) *Trépan*, from τρυπαω, 'I perforate.' A surgical instrument resembling a wimble, and worked in the same manner. It is used for removing portions of bone, and particularly of the bones of the skull. The term *trepan* is given more particularly to the part of the instrument that makes the perforation. The handle is so constructed as to receive different bits, as the Crown, the *Trépan perforatif* or *Perite'rion*, the *T. exfoliatif* or *Desquamato'rium trep'anum*, and the *T. abaptis'ta*.

In Great Britain and the United States, this instrument has been superseded by the trephine, which is more manageable.

TREPANATIO, Trepanning.
TRÉPANATION, Trepanning.
TREPAN'NING, *Terebra'tio, Anatre'sis, Cephalotripe'sis, Trepana'tio, Trype'sis, Tresis, Prisis, Prismus, Fora'tio*, (F.) *Trépanation*. Same etymon as Trepan. The methodical application of the trepan.
TREPANON, Trepan.
TREPANUM, Trepan.
TREPHINE. The instrument which has replaced the trepan in some countries. It consists of a simple, cylindrical saw; with a handle placed transversely like that of a gimlet, and from the centre of the circle, described by the teeth of the saw, a sharp little perforator projects, called the *Centre-pin*. The centre-pin is capable of being removed, at the surgeon's option, by means of a key for the purpose. It is used to fix the instrument until the teeth of the saw have made a circular groove, sufficiently deep for it to work steadily. The pin must then be removed. Sometimes the pin is made to slide up and down, and to be fixed in any position, by means of a screw.
TREPHOUSA, Nurse.
TREPIDATIO, Tremor—t. Cordis, Cardiotromus.
TREPON'DO. A weight of three pounds.—Scribonius.
TRE'SIS, τρησις, from τρεω, 'I bore.' Properly, a perforation. A wound. A forcible solution of continuity in a soft part, commencing externally. A genus in the nosology of Good.
TRESIS, Trepanning, Wound—t. Causis, Burn—t. Punctura, Puncture—t. Vulnus, Wound—t. Vulnus laceratum, see Laceration—t. Vulnus simplex, Cut.
TRESSAILLEMENT, Shuddering.
TRESSO'RIA, *Επισι'ον, εποιον*. A term formerly applied to the hair covering the mons veneris, the absence of which has, by the vulgar, been esteemed a matter of reproach.
TRI, τρι, in composition, 'three.' Hence:
TRIANGLE MÉDULLAIRE, Fornix.
TRIANGLE, VESICAL, see Urinary Bladder.
TRIAN'GULAR, *Trigo'nos, Triangula'ris*, from *tris*, for *tres*, 'three,' and *angulus*, 'an angle.' That which has three angles.
TRIANGULAR LIGAMENT or INFRA-PUBIAN IS a ligamentous fascia with short fibres, situate transversely beneath the symphysis pubis, which it strengthens.

TRIANGULARIS, Depressor anguli oris — t. Coccygis, Coccygeus — t. Nasi, Compressor naris.

TRIANGULA'RIS STERNI, *Sterno-costal* (Ch.,) *Pectora'lis inter'nus*. A muscle situate at the anterior and inner part of the chest, behind the cartilages of the ribs. It has the shape of a lengthened triangle, the base of which is directed downwards. It is attached to the posterior, lateral, and inferior part of the sternum, whence its fibres pass upwards and outwards, and terminate by as many distinct digitations at the cartilages of the 3d, 4th, 5th, and 6th true ribs. This muscle depresses the ribs and contributes to expiration.

TRIBAS, (F.) *Tribade*, from τριβω, 'I rub.' *Frictrix, Frica'trix, Futu'tor, Mas'cula, Subagita'trix, Subiga'tor*. A female whose clitoris is so large as to cause her to be regarded as an hermaphrodite. One who acts as a male with another female.

TRIBULI AQUATICI, see Trapa natans.

TRIBUTUM LUNARE, Menses — t. Menstruum, Menses.

TRICÆ, Plica — t. Incuborum, Plica — t. Scroforum, Plica.

TRICAGO, Teucrium chamædrys.

TRICAUDALIS, Retrahens auris.

TRICEPS, from *tris* for *tres*, 'three,' and *caput*, 'head.' A name given to muscles that have three fleshy bundles at one of their extremities.

TRICEPS ADDUC'TOR FEM'ORIS. Under this appellation are comprehended three distinct muscles; *Adductor brevis, A. longus*, and *A. magnus*.

TRICEPS AURIS, Retrahens auris — t. Brachialis, Triceps extensor cubiti.

TRICEPS CRURIS, *Femora'lis*, (F.) *Trifémororatulien* (Ch.,) *Orural, Trifémoro-tibi-rotulien, Triceps crural, T. de la cuisse*, is situate at the anterior, inner, and outer part of the thigh. It is formed of three bundles at its superior extremity, viz. 1. A middle fasciculus (the *crura'lis* of most anatomists.) 2. An external fasciculus (the *vastus externus*) and 3. An inner fasciculus (the *vastus internus*.) It is attached, above, to the anterior, inner, and outer surfaces of the femur, and to the two edges of the linea aspera, from the base of the trochanter to within four fingers' breadth of the knee. Below, it terminates by a large tendon, which is attached to the base and edges of the patella, as well as to the inner and outer tuberosities of the tibia. The triceps extends the leg on the thigh, and conversely.

TRICEPS DE LA CUISSE, Triceps cruris — t. *Crural*, Triceps cruris.

TRICEPS EXTEN'SOR CU'BITI, *Triceps brachia'lis*, (F.) *Scapulo-huméro-olécranien* (Ch.), *Triceps brachial*. This muscle, which occupies all the posterior part of the os humeri, is described as two muscles by Douglas, and as three by Winslow. It arises by three heads. The first or long head, — *long head of the biceps externus* of Douglas, *Anconeus major* of Winslow, — arises from the anterior extremity of the inferior costa of the scapula, near its neck, and below the origin of the teres minor The second head, or *short head of the biceps externus* of Douglas, *Anconeus externus* of Winslow, arises from the upper and outer part of the os humeri, at the base of the great tuberosity; and the third head, — *Brachialis externus* of Douglas, *Anconeus internus* of Winslow, — the shortest of the three, arises from the back part of the os humeri, behind the flat tendon of the latissimus dorsi. These three portions unite about the middle of the arm, so as to form one thick and powerful muscle, which is inserted at the upper part of the olecranon. It extends the forearm on the arm, and conversely.

TRICEPS MAGNUS, Adductor magnus — t. Minor, Adductor longus femoris — t. Secundus, Adductor brevis.

TRICHÆ INCUBORUM, Plica.

TRICHANGIECTA'SIA, *Angidiecta'sia, Trichocireus*, from θριξ, τριχος, 'a hair,' αγγειον, 'a vessel,' and εκτασις, 'dilatation.' Morbid dilatation of the capillary vessels.

TRICHAUX'E; from θριξ, τριχος, 'hair,' and αυξη, 'increase.' Increase in the quantity and size of the hair, without change of texture.

TRICHERA ARVENSIS, Scabiosa.

TRICHIA, Entropion.

TRICHI'ASIS, *Trichio'sis, Tricho'sis*, from θριξ, τριχος, 'hair.' *Morbus pila'ris*. This name has been given to several affections. 1. To a disease of the kidneys or bladder, in which filamentous substances, resembling hairs, are passed in the urine. This is also called *Pilimic'sis*. It must be regarded as a variety of *Cater'rus vesi'cæ*. 2. To a painful swelling of the breast in child-bed women, when the milk is excreted with difficulty: — a disease attributed, by Aristotle, to a hair swallowed by accident and carried to the breasts through the circulation; and 3dy. To inversion of the eye-lashes. See Entropion.

TRICHIASIS LACTEA, Infarctus mammae lacteus.

TRICHILIA, Cathartica.

TRICHI'NA SPIRA'LIS. Same etymon. A small species of entozoa discovered in the muscle of voluntary motion. Trichinæ consist of very minute cysts, of an oblong figure, having considerable resemblance, in size and colour, to young pediculi, and are somewhat allied to the rich found in paste and vinegar. No symptoms have as yet been observed to be pathognomonic of their presence.

TRICHIOSIS, Trichiasis — t. Districh, Pitii.

TRICHIS'MUS. Same etymon. *Capillis—Fissu'ra pila'ris*. A capillary fracture, issue, or crack.

TRICHIURIA, Trichocephalus.

TRICHOCEPH'ALUS, *Tricheceph'alus impar*: from θριξ, τριχος, 'a hair,' and κεφαλη, 'head.' *Trichu'ris, Trichuris vulgaris, Trichuris intestina'lis, As'curis trichu'ria, Trichio'ris. Trichocephalus hom'inis, Mastigo'des hominis*, Long *thread-worm*. A worm, from an inch and a half to two inches long; the head acute; the body spirally involuted in the male, almost straight in the female. The *trichocephalus dispar* generally inhabits the cæcum and colon, and is rarely met with in the small intestines. It gives rise to no peculiar symptoms, and requires the usual anthelmintic treatment.

TRICHOCIRSUS, Trichangiectasia.

TRICHOLABIS, Madisterium.

TRICHOLABIUM, Madisterium.

TRICHOLOGIA, Carphologia.

TRICHOMA, Capillamentum, Plica.

TRICHOMANES, Asplenium trichomanoides — t. Crenata, Asplenium trichomanoides.

TRICHOMATION, Capillamentum.

TRICHOMATOSE HAIR, Plica.

TRICHOM'ONAS, *Trichom'onas*; from θριξ, τριχος, 'a hair,' and μονας, μοναδος, 'unity.' It animalcule found by by M. Donné in the mucus of the vagina, where cleanliness has not been attended to, and to which he has given the name *Trichom'onas vagina'lis*. By some it is considered to be nothing more than separated ciliated epithelium from the uterus.

TRICHON'OSUS, from θριξ, τριχος, 'hair,' and νοσος, 'disease.' A disease of the hair.

TRICHOPHY'IA, *Trichophyt'ica*, from θριξ

τριχος, 'hair,' and φυειν, 'to grow. Remedies that promote the growth of the hair.

TRICHOPHYTON TONSURANS, see Porrigo decalvans.

TRICHOSCHISIS, Schizatrichia.

TRICHO'SIS, *Pila'ri malum;* from θριξ, τριχος, 'hair.' Morbid organization or deficiency of hair. A genus in the system of Good.

TRICHOSIS, Entropion, Trichiasis—t. Area, Porrigo decalvans—t. Athrix, Alopecia—t. Distrix, Distrix—t. Furfuracea, Porrigo furfurans—t. Hirsuties, Hirsuties—t. Plica, Plica—t. Poliosis, Poliosis—t. Setosa, Hystriciasis.

TRICHOTON, Scalp.

TRICHURIS, Trichocephalus.

TRICLISPERMA GRANDIFLORA, Polygala paucifolia.

TRICUS'PID, *Tricus'pis, Tricuspida'lis, Tricuspida'tus,* from *tris* for *tres,* 'three,' and *cuspis,* 'a point.' That which has three points.

TRICUSPID VALVES, *Val'vulæ Tricus'pides* seu *triglo'chines* seu *trisul'cæ,* are three triangular, valvular duplicatures, formed by the inner membrane of the right cavities of the heart, around the orifice by which the auricle communicates with the ventricle. The elongated and pointed top of each of these valves is continuous with the chordæ tendineæ, which set out from the columnæ carneæ of the heart. These valves are depressed to allow the blood to flow from the auricle into the ventricle; and are raised to prevent its reflux into the auricle.

TRIENS, *Un'ciæ qua'tuor.* The third part of a pound. Four ounces, Troy.— Galen.

TRIFACIAL, Trigemini.

TRIFÉMORO-ROTULIEN, Triceps cruris—t. *Tibi-rotulien,* Triceps cruris.

TRIFOLIUM ACETOSUM, Oxalis acetosella—t. Aquaticum, Menyanthes trifoliata—t. Aureum, Hepatica triloba—t. Cervinum, Eupatorium cannabinum—t. Fibrinum, Menyanthes trifoliata—t. Hepaticum, Hepatica triloba.

TRIFO'LIUM MELILO'TUS OFFICINA'LIS, *T. offic''- ina'lē, Melilo'tus cit'rina, Melilotus, Lotus sylves'- tris, Ser'tula Compa'na, Trifo'lium caballi'num, Coro'na regia, Trifolium odora'tum,* Common *mel'ilot,* (F.) *Mélilot.* Family, Leguminosæ. Sex. Syst. Diadelphia Decandria. The infusion or distilled water of this plant has been employed in cases of ophthalmia. It has also been used in fomentations, glysters, &c.

TRIFOLIUM OFFICINALE, T. melilotus officinalis—t. Paludosum, Menyanthes trifoliata—t. Palustre, Menyanthes trifoliata.

TRIGAS'TRIC, *Trigas'tricus, Triven'ter;* from τρεις, 'three,' and γαστηρ, 'belly.' That which has three bellies. An epithet for muscles so circumstanced.

TRIGEM'INI, *Tergem'ini,* from *tris,* 'three,' and *gem'inus,* 'double;' 'threefold,' 'triplets.' *The fifth pair of nerves, Par trigem'inum, Nervi divi'si, N. gustato'rii, Nervus quintus, Par quintum nervorum cerebra'lium, N. tremellus, N. mixtus, N. sympathet'icus me'dius, N. sympath'icus mediua, N. anon'ymus, N. innomina'tus, Par trium funiculo'rum, Trifa'cial,* (F.) *Nerf gustatif innominé, Nerf à trois cordes, Nerf trijumeau.* This nerve arises below the tuber annulare by one large posterior root from the corpora restiformia, and by two small anterior roots from the corpora olivaria, whence, proceeding forwards to the side of the sella Turcica, the filaments composing the large root form a ganglion — the Gasserian. Emerging from this ganglion, the filaments, of which the large root consists, form, with those constituting the small roots, form, and which had not passed through the ganglion, two flattened trunks, each of which is soon divided into three branches, in such a manner, however, that the *first,* or *ophthalmic branch,* and the *second* or *upper maxillary,* are composed exclusively of the filaments that arose from the corpora restiformia and passed through the Gasserian ganglion; whilst the *third* or *lower maxillary branch* is composed in part of those filaments, and in part of those that arose from the corpora olivaria, and passed on one side of the ganglion without going through it. The whole, therefore, of the first and second branches, and a part of the third are sensiferous nerves, whilst the remaining part of the third—the *man'ducatory* or *mas'ticatory* — is wholly motiferous, and passes to the pterygoid and other muscles concerned in mastication.

TRIGONE CÉRÉBRAL, Fornix—*t. Vésical,* see Urinary Bladder.

TRIGONEL'LA FŒNUM, *T. Fœ'num Græ'cum, Fen'ugreek, Fœ'nugreek, Fœnum Græ'cum, Bu'ceras, B. Fœnum Græ'cum, Carphos, Ægoc''- eras,* (F.) *Fénugrec.* Family, Leguminosæ. Sex. Syst. Diadelphia Decandria. A native of the south of France. The seeds have a strong, disagreeable smell, and an unctuous, farinaceous taste; accompanied by a slight bitterness. They are chiefly used in poultices.

TRIGONOS, Triangular.

TRIGONUS VESICÆ, see Urinary bladder—t. Lieutaudi, see Urinary bladder.

TRIJUMEAUX, Trigemini.

TRIL'LIUM LATIFO'LIUM, *Broadleaf Bethroot, Bethroot, Rattlesnake root, Wakerobin, Coughroot, Indian Balm, Ground Lily, Jews' Harp, Indian Shamrock, Pariswort, Truelove.* Sex. Syst. Hexandria Trigynia. A plant peculiar to North America, which blossoms in the spring. The root is astringent.

There are many species of Trillium, all of which possess the same properties.

TRIOCEPHALIA, Aprosopia.

TRIOR'CHIS, from τρεις, 'three,' and ορχις, 'a testicle.' One who has three testicles.

TRIOSTEOSPERMUM, Triosteum.

TRIOS'TEUM, *T. Perfolia'tum* seu *majus, Triosteosper'mum, Bastard Ipecacuan'ha, Fever Root, Feverwort, Tinker's weed, Horse ginseng, Ipecac., Wild Coffee, White ginseng, Gen'tian, White Gentian, Sweet Bitter.* In very large doses, the bark of the root proves emetic. It is a good cathartic, in doses of twenty or thirty grains. It sometimes operates as a diuretic.

TRIPE DE ROCHE. Different lichens of the species Gyrophora, inhabiting the arctic regions of America, bear this name. They are eaten as food by the hunters.

TRIPHAR'MACUM. τριφαρμακον. A medicine composed of three ingredients.

TRIPLET, from *triplex,* 'triple.' One of three children born at the same accouchement or gestation. Also, relating to triplets — as a '*triplet* conception.'

TRIPLET MONSTERS, *Monstra trip'lica* seu *trigem'ina,* are such as have parts of the body tripled. They are rare.

TRIPSIS, Contusio, Trituration.

TRIPUDIATIO SPASTICA, Chorea.

TRIQUETRUM, (OS,) Cuneiform (bone.)

TRISIS, Brygmus.

TRISMUS, from τριζω, 'I gnash.' *Enta'sia Trismus, Capis'trum, Tonos Trismus, Locked Jaw, Spasmus* seu *Rigor* seu *Tet'anus maxill'æ inferio'ris, Gnathospas'mus, Stomatospas'mus,* (F.) *Mal de Machoire.* Spastic closure of the under jaw; a partial tetanus. Cullen makes two varieties—*T. nascen'tium, T. neonato'rum, Nineday fits,* (F.) *Sarrête,* attacking infants during two weeks from birth; and *T. traumaticus,* originating from a wound.

TRISMUS CAPISTRATUS, *Brédissure*—t. Catarrhalis maxillaris, Neuralgia maxillaris—t. Clonicus, Neuralgia faciei—t. Cynicus, see Canine laugh—t. Diastrophe Sauvagesii, Paralysis, Bell's—t. Dolorificus, Neuralgia faciei—t. Maxillaris, Neuralgia faciei—t. Nascentium, see Trismus—t. Neonatorum, see Trismus—t. Sardonicus, Risus sardonicus.

TRISPER'MUM, from τρεις, 'three,' and σπερμα, 'a grain or seed.' A cataplasm, consisting of three seeds,—*cumin, bay,* and *smallage.* Gorræus.

TRISPLANCHIA, Cholera.

TRISPLANCH'NIC, *Trisplanch'nicus;* from τρεις, 'three,' and σπλαγχνον, 'viscus.' That which relates to three orders of viscera.

TRISPLANCHNIC NERVE, *Great sympathet'ic, Intercos'tal, Ganglion'ic nerve, Nerve of organ'ic life, Ver'tebral nerve;*—named by Bichat the *organic nervous system,* in opposition to the other nervous parts, called the *animal nervous system.* Gall terms it, the *nervous system of the automat'ic functions.* It has also been called the *organic nervous system,* and *ganglionic nervous system.* It is called *Trisplanchnic,* because it distributes its branches to the organs in the three great splanchnic cavities — the head, chest and abdomen. It is composed of a series of ganglia, united by intermediate branches, and passing along the side of the spine to the lowest part of the trunk; communicating, by a branch, with each of the thirty pairs of spinal nerves and several of the cerebral nerves; and detaching nerves from its several ganglia, which accompany the arteries, and are distributed, particularly, to the organs of involuntary functions. At its upper part, it is concealed in the canalis caroticus and cavernous sinus, and is joined there by a branch of the 6th pair of nerves, and by a twig from the Vidian nerve of the 5th pair. In passing down by the side of the spine, it forms three ganglia in the neck:—the *superior, middle,* (*thyroid ganglion,*) and *inferior,* (*ver'tebral ganglion*); 12 in the back — the *thoracic;* 5 in the loins—the *lumbar;* and three or four *sacral.* When it reaches the coccyx it unites with its fellow from the opposite side, forming a small ganglion — the *coccygeal, Gan'glion impar, az'ygous gan'glion.* Meckel divides it into two portions — 1. The *central ganglions* or *central part,* composed of the numerous ganglionic plexuses in the abdomen; the centre of which is the *semilunar* and *solar plexuses.* 2. The *external ganglions, Limitrophes* or *external part,* which comprise the series of ganglions situate at the sides of the spine, from the base of the cranium to the sacrum. The great sympathetic seems to form a distinct nervous system, destined for the organs of involuntary motion; for although communicating with both brain and spinal marrow, it does not seem to be immediately under the influence of either.

TRISPLANCHNITIS, Cholera, (spasmodic.)

TRISSAGO, Teucrium chamædrys—t. Palustris, Teucrium scordium.

TRISTEMANIA, Melancholy.

TRISTERN'AL. Béclard has given this name to the third bony portion of the sternum;—that which corresponds to the third intercostal space.

TRISTITIA, Athymia, Mœror.

TRITÆOPHYA AMERICANA, Fever, yellow.

TRITÆOPH'YES, *Tritæoph'ya,* from τριταιος, 'tertian,' and φυω, 'I originate.' A fever, whose type approaches the tertian. Sauvages gave the name *Tritæophya Vratislavien'sis,* to an epidemic, which broke out in the Prussian army at Breslav, in the middle of the last century.

TRITÆUS, Tertian fever.

TRIT'ICUM ÆSTI'VUM, *T. cerea'li* seu *Cavallos* seu *compac'tum* seu *erina'ceum* seu [?] *neria'num* seu *Linnæa'num* seu *pruino'um,* 'Summer wheat;' and TRIT'ICUM HYBERN'UM seu *[?]cum* seu *Mu'ticum* seu *Sic'ulum, Winter wheat,* F. Froment. Family, Gramineæ. *Sex. Syst.* Triandria Digynia. From these plants our wheaten flour is obtained, by grinding the seeds—*Wheat, Pyrus, Frumen'tum*—and to them we are indebted for our bread and pastry. The nutritive properties of wheaten flour are so well known as not to need comment.

Bread, (F.) *Pain,* mixed with milk, constitutes the ordinary emollient poultice;—and the *crumb of bread, Micæ panis,* are a common excipient for pills and boluses.

TRITICUM ARVENSE, T. repens — t. Cereale, t. æstivum — t. Cevallos, T. æstivum—t. Compactum, T. æstivum — t. Faginum, Polygonum fagopyrum — t. Gaertnerianum, T. æstivum—t. Glaucum, T. hybernum, and T. repens—t. Hybernum, see T. æstivum—t. Muticum, T. hybernum—t. Linnæanum, T. æstivum — t. Pruinosum, T. æstivum.

TRIT'ICUM REPENS, *T. arven'sè* seu *glauca, Agrop'yrum lævis'simum, Bromus glaber,* Grown *cani'num, Gramen dioscor'idis, G. repens,* La-*iceum radi'cè repen'tè, Dog-grass, Couch-grass, Quickens,* (F.) *Chiendent.* The roots are sweet, and possess aperient properties. They are said, also, to be diuretic.

TRITICUM SICULUM, T. hybernum.

TRITIO, Contritio, Trituration.

TRITON PALUSTRIS, see Ectosos.

TRITURA, Contritio.

TRITURA'TION, *Tritura'tio, Trits'ra, Trina, Tri'tio, Tripsis,* from *terere, tritum,* 'to bruise.' The act of reducing a substance to powder.

TRITURATION, Contritio.

TRITUS, Contritio, Trituration.

TRIVELIN, see Liver.

TRIVENTER, Trigastric.

TROCAR, *Trochar, Acus paracent'ica* seu *paracentet'ica, A. triq'uetra vulga'ris, Paraventcion, Paracentete'rion.* Corrupted from the F. *Troisquarts* or *Trocart,* 'three quarters;' so called from the triangular shape of the point—*Injectrum.* An instrument used for evacuating fluids from cavities, particularly in ascites, hydrocele, &c. A trocar consists of a perforator or stylet and a cannula, which is so adapted to the perforator, that, when the puncture is made, both enter the wound with facility; after which the stylet being withdrawn, the cannula remains in the wound and affords the fluid a ready passage outwards.

TROCART, Trocar.

TROCH, Trochiscos.

TROCHAN'TER, *Trokanter, Rota'tor,* from τροχαω, 'I turn.' Anatomists have given the names *great* and *little trochanter* to two processes at the upper extremity of the femur. The *great trochan'ter, glutus,* is the one on the outside; the *less* is lower down and more internally. Both afford attachment to rotator muscles of the thigh, and hence their name. Chaussier, by the name *trochanter,* means the larger process, the smaller he calls *trochantin.*

TROCHANTER'IAN, *Trochanteria'nus, Trokanter'ian.* That which belongs or relates to the great trochanter. — Chaussier.

TROCHANTIN'IAN, *Trokantin'ion, Trochantinia'nus.* That which belongs or relates to the trochantin or lesser trochanter.

TROCHAR, Trocar.

TROCHES OF CARBONATE OF LIME, Trochisci carbonatis calcis — t. of Chalk, Trochisci carbonatis calcis — t. Escharotic, Trochisci escharotici — t. Gum, Trochisci gummosi — t. of Ipecacuanha, Trochisci ipecacuanhæ — t. Liquorice, Trochisci glycyrrhizæ — t. Liquorice, with opium, Trochisci glycyrrhizæ cum opio — t. of Magnesia, Trochisci magnesiæ — t. Nitre, Trochisci nitratis potassæ — t. of Peppermint, Trochisci menthæ piperitæ.

TROCHIA, Orbit.

TROCHILIA, Trochlea.

TROCHIN, from τροχυν, 'to turn.' Chaussier has given this name to the smaller of the tuberosities at the upper extremity of the os humeri; because it gives attachment to one of the rotator muscles of the arm,— the subscapularis.

TROCHIN'IAN, *Trochinia'nus.* That which belongs or relates to the trochin.

TROCHIS'CUS, *Phthois, Artis'cus, Collix, Colix, Phthois'cos, Rot'ula, Cyclis'mos,* diminutive of τροχος, 'a wheel.' A *troch* or *round* table, (F.) *Trochisque.* See Pastil, and Tabella. A solid medicine, prepared of powders, incorporated by means of mucilage, crumb of bread, juices of plants, &c. In French nomenclature, the *trochisque* differs from the *tablette,*—the former containing no sugar. This form of preparation is adapted for the purpose of allowing the medicines of which the troch is composed to dissolve slowly in the mouth, and to pass gradually into the stomach.

The Parisian Codex has two formulæ for troches for external use.

TROCHISCI BECHICI NIGRI, T. glycyrrhizæ glabræ.

TROCHISCI CARBONA'TIS CALCIS, *Troches of Oar'bonate of lime, T. of chalk, Tabellæ ad ardo'rem ventric'uli, Lozenges for the heartburn, Tabel'læ cardial'gicæ, T. ad sodam, Trochis'ci e cretâ, T. cretæ* (Ph. U. S.) (*Cret.* ppt. ℨiv; *acaciæ,* in pulv. ℨj; *myrist.* in pulv. ℨj; *sacch.* in pulv. ℨvj. M. Form into troches with *water.*) Antacid and absorbent.

TROCHISCI E CRETÂ, Tr. carbonatis calcis — t. Cretæ, T. carbonatis calcis.

TROCHISCI vel PASTIL'LI EMETI'NÆ PECTORA'LES, *Pectoral Lozenges of Em'etine.* (*Sugar,* ℨiv; *emetine,* 32 grains. Form into lozenges of nine grains each.) One is a dose.

TROCHISCI ESCHAROT'ICI, *Escharot'ic Troches.* (*Hydrarg. oxymur.* p. 8; *amyli,* p. 16; *mucilag. g. tragac.* q. s. Make into troches, to which a few drops of laudanum may be added.— Ph. P.) Used in foul ulcers, to remove excrescences, &c.

TROCHISCI ESCHARQT'ICI DE MIN'IO. (*Oxyd. plumbi. rubr.* p. 16; *hydrarg. oxymur.* p. 32; *mic. panis,* p. 128; *aq. rosæ,* q. s.— Ph. P.) Used like the last.

TROCHISCI GLYCYRRI'ZÆ GLABRÆ, *Liq'uorice troches, Black pectoral lozenges, Trochis'ci bech'ici nigri.* (*Ext. glyc. glabr., gum. acac.* ää p. j; *sacch. purif.* p. ij. Dissolve in warm water; strain; evaporate, and form into troches.— Ph. E.) Demulcent. To allay cough.

TROCHISCI GLYCYRRHI'ZÆ CUM O'PIO, *T. G. et opii* (Ph. U. S.), *Trochisci Theba'ici, T. sedati'vo-balsam'ici, T. pectora'les regis Dano'rum, Liquorice Troches with Opium, Wistar's Lozenges.* (*Opii,* in pulv. ℨss; *ext. glycyrrh.* in pulv., *sacchar.* in pulv., *acaciæ,* in pulv., ää ℨx; *ol. anisi,* fℨj. Make into troches.— Ph. U. S.) Demulcent and anodyne.

Spitta's Lozenges for coryza, hoarseness, and sore-throat, are composed as follows: — (*Cubeb. recent.* in pulv. ℨij; *extract. glycyrrhis.* ℨj; *myr-*

oxyl. ℨj; *acaciæ,* ℨiv; *syrup,* q. s. ut fiant trochisci gr. x singulis.

TROCHISCI GUMMO'SI, *Gum Troches.* (*G. acac.* p. v; *amyli,* p. i; *sacch. pur.* p. xij. Make up the troches with rose-water.— Ph. E.) Demulcent.

TROCHIS'CI IPECACUAN'HÆ, *Troches of Ipecacuanha.* (*Ipecacuanh.* in pulv. ℨss; *sacchar.* in pulv. ℨxiv; *marantæ,* in pulv. ℨiv; *mucilag. tragacanth.* q. s. Make into troches.— Ph. U. S.)

TROCHISCI MAGNE'SIÆ, *Troches of Magne'sia.* (*Magnes.* ℨiv; *sacchar.* ℔j; *myrist.* pulv. ℨj; *mucilag. tragacanth.* q. s. Make into troches.— Ph. U. S.) Useful in acidity of the stomach, with constipation.

TROCHISCI MENTHÆ PIPERI'TÆ, *Troches of Peppermint.* (*Ol. menth. piperit.* fℨj; *sacchar.* in pulv. ℔j; *mucilag. tragacanthæ,* q. s. Make into troches.— Ph. U. S.) Used as a carminative.

TROCHISCI NITRA'TIS POTAS'SÆ, *Nitre Troches.* (*Nitrat. potassæ,* p. j; *sacch. pur.* p. iij. Make into troches with mucilage of tragacanth. — Ph. E.) In slight inflammatory sore-throat and fever.

TROCHISCI PECTORALES REGIS DANORUM, Tr. glycyrrhizæ cum opio — t. Sedativo-balsamics, Tr. glycyrrhizæ cum opio.

TROCHIS'CI SODÆ BICARBONA'TIS, *Troches of Bicar'bonate of Soda.* (*Sodæ bicarb.* ℨiv; *sacchar.* in pulv. ℔j; *mucilag. tragacanth.* q. s. To be made into a mass, and divided into troches, each weighing ten grains.— Ph. U. S.)

The *Pastilles de Vichy, Pastilles digestives d'Hauterive-Vichy, Pastil'li digesti'vi Darcet'ii,* composed of *bicarbonate of soda, oil of peppermint,* and *sugar,* are much used in France, like the Vichy waters, in cardalgia, gout, and lithiasis.

TROCHISCI STIBIATI, Tabellæ antimoniales Kunckelii — t. Thebaici, T. glycyrrhizæ cum opio.

TROCHISQUE, Trochiscos.

TROCH'ITER, from τροχιν, 'to turn.' The larger of the two tuberosities at the upper extremity of the os humeri; so called because it affords insertion to rotator muscles. — Chaussier.

TROCHITER'IAN, in the language of Chaussier, means any thing belonging or relating to the trochiter.

TROCH'LEA, *Trochil'ia,* (F.) *Trochlée* ou *Troklée.* A pulley; from τροχαω, 'I turn,'— for example, the articular surface at the lower extremity of the os humeri; so called from its forming a kind of pulley on which the ulna moves, in flexion and extension of the forearm. Also, the cartilaginous pulley over which the tendon of the trochlearis muscle passes, at the upper and inner part of the orbit.

TROCHLEA LABYRINTHI, Cochlea.

TROCHLEARIS, Obliquus superior oculi.

TROCHLÉATEUR, GRAND, Obliquus superior oculi— t. *Petit,* Obliquus superior oculi.

TROCHLÉE, Trochlea.

TRO'CHOID, from τροχος, 'a wheel,' and ειδος, 'resemblance.' *Trochoï'des, Ax'ea commissu'ra.* An articulation, in which one bone turns upon another, like a wheel upon its axle; as the *Atlo-ïdo-axoïd articulation.*

TROCHOIDES, Axea commissura.

TROËNE, Ligustrum vulgare.

TROISQUARTS, Trocar.

TROKANTER, Trochanter.

TROKANTERIAN, Trochanterian.

TROKANTINIAN, Trochantinian.

TROKLÉE, Trochlea.

TROMOMANIA, Delirium tremens.

TROMOPARANŒA, Delirium tremens.

TROMOS, see Paralysis agitans.
TROMOSPASMUS, Tremor.
TROMPE, Tuba.— *t. d'Eustache*, Eustachian tube—*t. de Fallope*, Tuba Fallopiana—*t. Utérine*, Tuba Fallopiana.
TROMUS, Tremor.
TRONC, Trunk — *t. Brachial*, Brachial artery —*t. Basilaire*, Basilary artery.
TROPÆ'OLUM MAJUS, *Indian Cress, Nastur'tium Indicum, Acrivi'ola, Flos sanguin'eus monar'di, Nastur'tium Peruvia'num, Cardamin'dum majus, Car'damum majus.* Family, Geraniaceæ. *Sex. Syst.* Octandria Monogynia. (F.) *Cresson des Indes, Cresson du Mexique, Capucine.* An antiscorbutic.
TROPÆ'OLUM TUBERO'SUM, *Ulluco.* A tuberous plant, cultivated in the Sierra, Peru. It is smaller than the potato.
TROPHALIS, Colostrum.
TROPHE, Aliment, Cibatio, Pabulum.
TROPHI. Same etymon as Trophy. In insects, the parts of the mouth that are employed in receiving and preparing the food.
TROPH'ICAL, *Troph'icus.* Same etymon as Trophy. Relating to nourishment or nutrition.
TROPH'ICAL NERVES. The organic nerves, or nerves of the sympathetic system, have been so termed, from a belief that they were concerned in nutrition.
TROPHIMOS, Nutrition.
TROPHONEURO'SIS, from τροφη, 'nourishment,' and *neurosis.* A morbid condition of the process of nutrition owing to diminished nervous influence.
TROPHON'OSI, *Trophonu'si*, from τροφη, 'nourishment,' and νοσος, 'a disease.' Diseases of nutrition.
TROPH'Y, *Troph'ia*, τροφη, a suffix denoting 'nourishment or nutrition;' as hypertrophy, 'excess of nourishment or nutrition.'
TROPONU'SI, *Morbi trop'ici*, from τροπη, the solstitial or tropical point where the sun turns or alters its course, and νουσος, 'a disease.' Diseases that prevail in the tropics.
TROSTER, see Spirit.
TROU, Foramen—*t. Anonyme*, Foramen stylomastoideum—*t. Aveugle ou Borgne*, Cæcum foramen — *t. Borgne* of the Medulla oblongata, Foramen cæcum of the medulla oblongata—*t. de Botal*, Botal foramen, Ovale foramen—*t. Déchiré antérieur*, Lacerum anterius foramen—*t. Déchiré postérieur*, Lacerum posterius foramen — *t. Épineux*, Spinale foramen — *t. Mentonnier*, Mental foramen — *t. Optique*, Foramen opticum — *t. Orbitaire supérieur*, Foramen supra-orbitarium — *t. Orbitaire supérieur*, Orbitar foramen superior — *t. Ovale*, Ovale foramen — *t. Rond, petit*, Spinale foramen — *t. Sous-orbitaire*, see Suborbitar canal — *t. Sous pubien*, Obturatorium foramen—*t. Sphéno-épineux*, Spinale foramen — *t. Sus-orbitaire*, Foramen supra-orbitarium.
TROUS CAROTIDIENS, Carotica foramina —*t. Condyloïdiens*, Condyloidea foramina—*t. de Conjugaison*, Conjugationis foramina—*t. de Conjugaison*, see Vertebræ — *t. Olfactifs*, Olfactory foramina—*t. Rachidiens*, Spinal foramina.
TROUSSE-GALANT, Cholera morbus.
TROUSSEAU, Fasciculus.
TROUSSEAUX ARRIÈRE-MÉSENTÉRIQUES, (F.) A name given by Winslow to the nervous plexus situate between the two mesenteric plexuses, of which it is a dependence, and which descends into the pelvis to concur in the formation of the hypogastric plexus.
TRUBS, Lycoperdon tuber.
TRUCULENTUS, Homicidal.
TRUELOVE, Paris, Trillium latifolium.

TRUFFE, Lycoperdon tuber.
TRUFFLE, Lycoperdon tuber.
TRUMBUS, Thrombus.
TRUMPET CREEPER, Tecoma radicans—t. Flower, Tecoma radicans—t. Weed, Eupatorium purpureum.
TRUNCUS, Trunk.
TRUNK, *Truncus*, (F.) *Tronc.* The principal part of the body, to which the limbs are articulated. The trunk has been divided into three parts : — a *superior*, the *head;* a *middle*, the *thorax*, and an *inferior*, the *pelvis*. These three regions contain the great splanchnic cavities. They are united by a common *stalk* — the vertebral column. To the *middle* are articulated the superior extremities; and, to the *inferior*, the lower extremities.
The *trunk* of an artery, vein, nerve, or lymphatic, is its largest part, which has not yet given off branches. It is, also, applied to the parent vessel, after branches have been sent off.
TRUSS, from (F.) *trousser*, 'to tie up.' *Brachirium, Brachie'rium, Brachi'lè, Brachi'rium Brackeri'olum, Amma, Hamma, Subligatorium, Subligatu'ra*, (F.) *Brayer.* A hernial bandage for keeping hernia reduced. The ancient trusses were inelastic. They consisted simply of a pad and strap. At the present day, elastic bandages are alone employed. They possess the advantage of making an equable and continuous pressure at the aperture of the sac; and of yielding to the changes of form in the abdominal parietes. In most important part of these bandages is a piece of narrow steel, flat, and adapted to the shape of the body. This is the *spring*, (F.) *Ressort*. It embraces the body on the side affected: extends from beyond the spine, and terminates opposite the ruptured part, by an iron plate to which is riveted. The posterior surface of this plate is furnished with a convex *pad*, (F.) *Pelote*, adapted in shape and size to the aperture which it has to close. The spring is covered with leather, and the inner surface is padded; a strap extends from the posterior extremity; passes round the sound side and is attached to the plate of the pad. The strap is pierced with numerous holes, which allow the patient to tighten or slacken it at pleasure. Trusses have been variously constructed; and different patents obtained for the modification. They all act upon the above principle. Sometimes they have a double pad.
TRYGODES, Feculent.
TRYPANON, Trepan.
TRYPESIS, Trepanning.
TRYPSIS, Friction.
TSCHERBET, Sherbet.
TSIANA, Costus.
TSJAMPACA, Michelia champaca.
TUBA, Tube—t. Aristotelica, Eustachian tube — t. Cæca, Tuba, Fallopiana — t. Uterina, Itu Fallopiana — t. Vocalis, Tube, vocal.
TUBAL RESPIRATION, see Murmur, respiratory.
TUBE, *Tuba, Trumpet, Salpinx*, (F.) *Trompe.* A name given to some parts which are hollow and have the shape of a trumpet.
TUBE, ALIMENTARY, Canal, alimentary — Eustachian, Eustachian tube.
TUBE, FALLO'PIAN, *Tuba Fallopia'na* see *Fallopii, Hys'terosalpinx, Oviduc'tus mulie'bris, Def'erens mulie'ris, Tuba uteri'na, T. cæca, Iter vario'sum* seu *Proces'sus latera'lis* seu *Meatus semina'lis* seu *Mea'tus semina'rius utei* —t. *Trompe de Fallope, T. utérine*, is a canal, found in the abdomen, and extending on each side to the superior angles of the uterus as far as the sides of the brim of the pelvis. They are four inches long. Near the uterus, they are straight

and very narrow; but, in their course, they widen, become tortuous, and terminate by a free, expanded, and *fim'briated extremity;* called, also, *Folia'ceum ornamen'tum, Morsus diab'oli, Infundib'ulum* seu *Digitatio'nes* seu *Fim'briæ* seu *Vexillæ tuba'rum Fallo'pii, Lacin'iæ tuba'rum Fallopii*, (F) *Morceau frangé, Pavillon de la trompe, Morceau du diable.* Within, the tubes are hollow and lined by a mucous membrane: the tissue exterior to which is spongy and erectile. The use of the Fallopian tubes is to conduct the sperm to the ovarium, and the fecundated ovum back to the uterus. They establish a communication between the cavity of the peritoneum and that of the uterus, the abdominal termination being termed *Os'tium abdomina'lē;* the uterine, *Os'tium uteri'num.*

TUBE, INTESTINAL, Canal, alimentary.
TUBE, ŒSOPHAGE'AL, *Stomach Tube.* A long elastic gum tube, capable of being passed into the œsophagus or stomach.
TUBE, RECTAL, *Defeca'tion tube.* An elastic gum tube, similar to the last, which is sometimes passed into the colon, to remove air from that intestine, or to enable enemata to be thrown up into it.
TUBE, STOMACH, see Tube, œsophageal.
TUBE, VOCAL; *Tuba voca'lis.* The part of the air-passages above the inferior ligaments of the larynx, including the passages through the nose and mouth.
TUBER, Hump, Lycoperdon tuber, Tubercle — t. *Atloïdo-occipital,* Rectus capitis posticus minor — t. Cibarium, Lycoperdon tuber.
TUBER CINE'REUM. A grayish tubercle, seen at the base of the brain behind the commissure of the optic nerves, which is continuous with the infundibulum.
TUBER FRONTALE, Frontal protuberance — t. Gulosorum, Lycoperdon tuber — t. Gutturosum, Bronchocele — t. *Ischio-trochantérien,* Quadratus femoris — t. Ischii, see Ischiatic — t. Nigrum, Lycoperdon tuber — t. Pellagra, Pellagra — t. Tympani, Promontory of the tympanum.
TUBERA TERRÆ, Lycoperdon tuber.
TU'BERCLE, *Tuber'culum, Tuber, Strangal'ion, Stran'galis, Tuber'culous depos'it,* a *Kernel,* (vulg.), a *Knot* (vulg.), (F.) *Tubercule.* A tumour in the substance of organs, from the production of new matter: — sensation null; growth sluggish. In *Pathological Anatomy,* the term is generally given to a species of degeneration which consists of an opake matter, of a pale yellow colour: this, in its crude condition, has a consistence analogous to that of concrete albumen: it subsequently becomes soft and friable, and gradually acquires a consistence and appears analogous to those of pus. Tubercles may be developed in different parts of the body; but they are most frequently observed in the lungs and mesentery. Pulmonary tubercles, *Pneumophy'mata, Tuber'cula Pulmo'num,* (F.) *Tubercules pulmonaires,* are the cause of *Tuber'cular Phthisis. Mesenteric tubercles* are often met with in the same affection, but particularly in *Tabes Mesenterica.* Laënnec classes tubercles among the accidental tissues which have no resemblance to the natural tissues, and which never exist except in consequence of morbid action. Others consider them as a scrofulous degeneration. Broussais conceives that they are produced exclusively by inflammation of the white vessels, whose existence, however, is more than questionable. When tubercles in any organ are few in number, they may pass to the state of permanent induration without danger to the patient; but when they are very numerous, they usually cause serious mischief. Dr. Baron considers that they are produced by hydatids. The morbid condition which gives rise to the development of tubercles, *Tuberculisa'tion,* is termed *Tuberculo'sis, Morbus tuberculo'sus, Strumosis* seu *Phymato'sis pulmonum,* and *Dyscra'sia Tuberculo'sa.* Tubercles are seen of various forms, — to wit, in fine points, ((F.) *Poussière tuberculeuse,*) gray and yellow granulations, miliary tubercles; and gray or yellow tubercular masses, softened, and cretaceous.

TUBERCLE, BLACK, Melanosis.
TUBERCLES OF THE AREOLA, see Mamma.
TUBER'CULA ARAN'TII, *Cor'pora Arantii, Corpus'cula Aran'tii, Tubercles of Arantius* or *Aransi.* Small eminences at the middle part of the convex edge of the semilunar valves of the pulmonary artery and aorta.
TUBERCULA ARTHRITICA, Calculi, arthritic — t. Cerebri, Encephalophymata — t. Gonorrhoica, Gonorrhœa impura — t. Hepatis, *Hépato-strumosie* — t. Intestinorum, Enterophymata — t. Nervorum nodosa, Ganglions, nervous — t. Parva duræ matris, Glandulæ Pacchioni — t. Peritonæi, Cœliophymata — t. Pulmonum, see Tubercles, (of the lungs) — t. Quadrigemina, Quadrigemina Tubercula.
TUBER'CULAR, *Tuber'culous, Tuberculo'sus, Tuber'culate,* (F.) *Tuberculeux.* That which relates to tubercles, or which is formed by tubercles.
TUBERCULAR or TUBERCULOUS CONSTITUTION or DIATHESIS, *Phthisio'sis,* is the habit of body which predisposes to tubercular phthisis; as *Tuberculous Cachex'ia, Tuberculo'sis, Morbus tuberculo'sus, Dyscra'sia tuberculo'sa,* is the condition of one labouring under tuberculosis.
TUBERCULAR MATTER. A morbid production, contained in cysts, or loose in the tissue of organs. It varies, in its consistence, at the different periods of the tubercular affection: being, at first, compact, and yellowish; at times, calcareous; afterwards pultaceous, semi-fluid, and curdy. See Tubercle.
TUBERCULAR PHTHISIS, is that produced by the development of tubercles in the lungs.
TUBERCULAR SORE THROAT, Pharyngitis, follicular.
TUBERCULATE, Tubercular.
TUBERCULATE SARCO'MA OF AB'ERNETHY, *Emphy'ma Sarcoma tuberculo'sum, Tumor tuberculosus.* Tubercles, firm, round, and clustering; pea-sized or bean-sized; yellowish or brownish-red; when large, disposed to ulcerate, and produce a painful, malignant, and often fatal sore. Found chiefly in the lymphatic glands of the neck; often, simultaneously, in other glands and organs.
TUBERCULATED LIVER, Cirrhosis.
TUBERCULE, Tubercle.
TUBERCULES DES GLANDES LYMPHATIQUES, Scrofula — t. *du Foie, Hépatostrumosie* — t. *des Ganglions mésentériques,* Tabes mesenterica — t. of the Larynx and Fauces, Pharyngitis, follicular — t. Miliary, see Granulation — t. *Pisiformes,* Mamillary tubercles — t. *Pulmonaires,* see Tubercle — t. *Quadrijumeaux,* Quadrigemina corpora.
TUBERCULEUX, Tubercular.
TUBERCULIZATION, see Tubercle.
TUBERCULOSIS, see Tubercle, and Tubercular Cachexia — t. Laryngis et Tracheæ, Phthisis laryngea — t. Pulmonum, Phthisis pulmonalis — t. Vertebrarum, Vertebral disease.
TUBERCULOSUS, Tubercular.
TUBERCULOUS, Tubercular — t. Deposit, Tubercle — t. Disease of the Lungs, Phthisis pulmonalis — t. Dust, *Poussière tuberculeuse.*
TUBER'CULUM CINE'REUM, 'Ash-coloured tubercle,' diminutive of *tuber; Fasci'cu-*

cine'rea. A mass of cineritious substance at the top of the calamus scriptorius, which is continuous below with the posterior horn of cineritious substance in the cord, and upon the sides with the corpus restiforme.

TUBERCULUM LACRYMALE, see Lachrymal puncta — t. Loweri, Lower, tubercle of.

TUBEROSITAS, Tuberosity — t. Tympani, Promontory of the tympanum.

TUBÉROSITÉ BICIPITALE, Bicipital tubercle—*t. Sciatique*, see Ischiatic.

TUBEROS'ITY, *Tuberos'itas*, from *tuber*, 'a bump.' Anatomists have given this name to an eminence or process, the surface of which is unequal and rough; and which gives attachment to muscles or ligaments.

TUBI MEMBRANACEI, see Villous membranes.

TU'BULAR, *Tubula'ris*, (F.) *Tubulaire*. Same etymon as the next. Relating to or having the form of a small tube.

TUBULAR BLOWING SOUND, see Murmur, respiratory—t. Neurine, see Neurine—t. Substance of the Kidney, see Kidney.

TUBULE, *Tu'bulus*; diminutive of *Tuba*. A small tube.

TUBULI BELLINI, Uriniferous tubes — t. Duræ matris, Sinuses of the dura mater—t. Nervei, Nerve fibres — t. Pelvis renum, see Calix — t. Uriniferi Bellini, Uriniferous tubes.

TUBULUS, Cannula — t. Centralis Modioli, see Tractus spiralis foraminulentus.

TUBUS ACUSTICUS, Ear-trumpet — t. Alimentaris, Canal, alimentary — t. Intestinorum, Canal, alimentary—t. Nervorum, Neurilemma—t. Vermicularis cæci, Appendix vermiformis cæci.

TUCKAHO, Lycoperdon tuber.

TUE-CHIEN, Colchicum autumnale.

TULBAG'HIA ALLIA'CEA. A South African plant, *Nat. Ord.* Asphodeleæ, the bulbs of which, boiled in milk, are recommended in phthisis and as an anthelmintic.

Tulbaghia cepa'cea and *T. viola'cea* serve the same purpose.

TULIP TREE, Liriodendron.

TULIPIER, Liriodendron.

TULIPIFERA LIRIODENDRON, Liriodendron tulipifera.

TUMEFACTIO, Swelling—t. Mollis, Puffiness.

TUMESCENTIA PITUITOSA, Leucophlegmatia.

TUMEUR, Tumour — *t. Anomale*, see Hæmatodes fungus — *t. Blanche*, Hydrarthrus — *t. Caverneuse*, see Hæmatodes fungus — *t. Encéphaloïde*, Encephaloid — *t. Erectile*, see Hæmatodes fungus—*t. Hémorrhagiale circonscrite*, see Aneurism — *t. Lymphatique des articulations*, Hydrarthrus—*t. Variqueuse*, see Hæmatodes fungus.

TUMOR, Swelling, Tumour—t. Albus, Hydrarthrus—t. Anomalus, Hæmatodes fungus—t. Artuum, Obdormitio—t. Capitis Sanguineus, Cephalæmatoma — t. Carneus, Sarcoma—t. Cysticus, Encystis—t. Cysticus serosus, Hygroma—t. Fibrosus, Tumour, fibrous—t. Ficoosus, Ficus—t. Flatulentus, Emphysema — t. Fugax, see Fugacious — t. Fungosus articuli, Spina ventosa — t. Fungosus sanguineus, Hæmatodes fungus — t. Gangliformis, Ganglion, nervous — t. Genarum, Meloncus — t. Genu albus, Genocace — t. Glandulæ parotideæ, Parotidoncus—t. Lacteus, Galactocele — t. Lardeus, Steatoma—t. Malarum, Meloncus—t. Ovarii, Oarioncus — t. Parotidis, Parotidoncus — t. Prostatæ, Prostatoncus—t. Renalis, Nephroncus — t. Sanguineus, Hæmatoma — t. Squamiformis carnosus, Lepidosarcoma — t. Tuberculosus, Tuberculate sarcoma — t. Tunicatus, Encystis — t. Uteri, Hysteroncus.

TUMOUR, from *tumeo*, 'I swell,' *Tumor, Oncos, Oncus, Epar'ma, Eparsis, Em'plys, Excescen'tia* (Sauvages,) *Ecphy'ma*. F. *Tumeur.* A rising or prominence, of greater or less size... ed by a morbific cause in some part of the... Cullen defines a tumour to be "a partial swelling without inflammation." Sauvages restricts the term to a rising formed by the congestion of a fluid; and he calls *excrescences* those which have a fleshy or osseous consistence. Boyer admits: "any preternatural eminence developed in any part of the body." Good uses it synonymously with tubercle. Boyer's is the best general definition. Tumours differ greatly from each other according to their seat, the organs interested, their nature, &c.

The French use the term *Tumeur blanche* nonymously with *White Swelling*;—see Hydrarthrus. The term is, however, applied by the generality of surgeons to swellings of the extremity joints, without change of colour of the skin, of a more or less firm consistence, which are dependent upon disease of the osseous or of the soft parts about the joint.

Scrofula is the most common cause of these affections.

TUMOUR, EREC'TILE. A tumour produced by the development of a soft, vascular tissue, which is susceptible of elevation and depression. See Erectile.

TUMOUR, FIBROUS, *Fibrous growth*, F... *Tumour fibro'sus, Inchylo'ma*. A tumour or growth formed of fibrous tissue.

TUMOUR, LAMINATED, NACREOUS FATTY, Cholesteatoma — t. Milk-like, Encephaloid.

TUMOUR, VAR'ICOSE, *Tumor varico'sus*. A circumscribed, bluish tumour, formed by the dilatation and turgescence of the capillary vessels of a part.

TUMOUR, VASCULAR, see Hæmorrhois.

TUNAS, see Cactus opuntia.

TUNBRIDGE, MINERAL WATERS OF. A celebrated acidulous chalybeate in Kent, England, a few miles distant from the village of Tunbridge, and thirty-six miles south of London, which is much frequented. It contains carbonic acid, bicarbonate of iron, and sulphate of magnesia.

TUNDA OCULI, Conjunctiva membrana.

TUNDUS CORDIS, Mucro cordis.

TUNIC, *Tu'nica, Chi'ton*, a coat. An envelope. A name given to different membranes which envelop organs; as the tunics or coats of the eye, stomach, bladder, &c.

TUNICA ACINALIS, Uvea — t. Aciniformis Uvea — t. Acinosa, Uvea — t. Adnata, Conjunctiva — t. Agnata, Conjunctiva — t. Alba... Sclerotic — t. Albuginea, Albuginea — t. Albuginea oculi, Sclerotic — t. Allantoides, Allantois—t. Arachnodes, Arachnoid membrane—t. Aranea Arachnoid membrane — t. Caduca, Decidua—t. Candida oculi, Sclerotic — t. Carnosa, Panniculus carnosus — t. Conjunctiva, Conjunctiva—t. Cristalis, Pleura—t. Crassa, Decidua—t. Crystallina Arachnoid membrane — t. Dura oculi, Sclerotic — t. Durior et crassa, Sclerotic — t. Elytroides Vaginalis tunica — t. Erythroides, Cremaster—t. Exterior ovi, Decidua — t. Extima oculi, Sclerotic — t. Farciminalis, Allantois — t. Filamentosa Decidua

TUNICA GRANULO'SA. An investment of the ovum exterior to the zona pellucida, described by Dr. Barry, but the existence of which, as a structure, distinct and independent from the membrana granulosa, is denied.

TUNICA HORTENSIS, Dianthus caryophyllus — t. Innominata oculi, Sclerotic — t. Interna oculi, Retina.

TUNICA JACO'BI. A highly delicate serous

membrane, interposed between the retina and the choroid coat, discovered by Dr. Jacob, of Dublin. Its structure is curious, being composed of cylindrical, transparent, highly refractive staff-shaped bodies, and hence called *Stratum bacilla'tum*, which are arranged perpendicularly to the surface of the retina, their outer extremities being imbedded, to a greater or less depth, in a layer of the pigmentum nigrum.

TUNICA MUSCULARIS, Dartos — t. Nervorum, Neurilemma — t. Perforata, Uvea — t. Prætensa abdominis, Peritonæum — t. Reticularis, Retina — t. Retiformis, Retina — t. Rhagoides, Choroidea tunica, Uvea — t. Rubicunda scroti, Dartos — t. Rubra, Dianthus caryophyllus — t. Ruyschiana, see Choroid — t. Subcostalis, Pleura — t. Thoracis, Corset — t. Uvalis, Uvea — t. Uvea, Uvea — t. Uviformis, Uvea — t. Vaginalis, see Vaginal — t. Vaginalis Linguæ, see Tongue — t. Vaginalis Propria, Vaginal coat of the Testicle — t. Vaginalis reflexa, Vaginal coat of the Testicle — t. Vasculosa oculi, Choroid, see Eye.

TUNICA VASCULO'SA TESTIS, *Pia mater testis*. An extremely delicate membrane, consisting of minute ramifications of the spermatic vessels united by areolar tissue, which separates the lobules of the testis from each other. It is situate immediately within the tunica albuginea, and encloses the substance of the gland. It sends processes inward that separate the lobules, in the same manner as the pia mater is reflected between the convolutions of the brain.

TUNICA VITREA, Hyaloid membrane.
TUNICULA, Clitoris.
TUNIQUE ALBUGINÉE, Albuginea.
TUNNYFISH, SALTED, Omotarichos.
TUPHLO-ENTERITIS, Typhlo-enteritis.
TUPHUS, Typhus.
TUPINARIA, Talpa.
TURBA HÆMORRHOIDALIS, see Hæmorrhois

TURBATIONES ANIMI, Affections of the mind.

TUR'BINATED BONES, *Ossa turbina'ta*. Bones shaped like a top; from *turbo* or *turben*, 'a top.' *Ossa spongio'sa*, *Cornua*, *Concha na'rium*, *Tur'bines nasi seu na'rium*, *Conchyl'ia*, *Bucci'na*, *Lam'inæ spongio'sæ nasi*, *Ossa tertia maxilla superio'ris*. Very thin, bony plates, rolled up in the form of horns, and situate in the nasal fossa. 1. *Os spongio'sum supe'rius* or *Cornet de Morgagni*;—the highest. 2. *Os spongiosum me'dium*, the *middle cornu* of French anatomists, — the *ethmoid'al cornu* or *Os spongiosum superius*, *Os turbinatum*, of English anatomists, *Os convolu'tum superius*, *Concha*, *C. na'rium superius*, *C. Morgagnia'na*, (F.) *Cornet Moyen*. This bone projects inwards and downwards into the cavity of the nose, from the ethmoid cells at the side of the nasal lamella, and serves to enlarge the organ of smell. It is convex towards the septum, and concave outwards. 3. *Os spongiosum vel turbinatum inferius*, *Concha inferior*, *Convolu'tum inferius os*, *Os sous-ethmoïdal*, (Ch.), projects at the under part of the side of the nose, is convex towards the septum, and concave outwards. It is connected to the os maxillare, os palati, and os unguis. 4. *Sphenoid'al cornu*.

All the turbinated bones extend the olfactory surface.

TURBINES NASI SEU NARIUM, Turbinated bones.

TURBITH BLANC, Globularia alypum — t. Mineral, Hydrargyrus vitriolatus — t. Montpellier, Globularia alypum — t. Plant, Convolvulus turpethum.

TURBO CEREBRI, Pineal gland.

TURGENTIA, Turgescence.
TURGES'CENCE, *Turges'cency*, *Turgid'ity*, *Tur'gidness*, *Turgescen'tia*, *Turgen'tia*, *Orgas'mus*, from *turgescere*, 'to swell.' Superabundance of humours in a part. The term *Turgescence of Bile* was formerly used to denote the passage of that fluid into the stomach, and its discharge by vomiting. A vital action of turgescence or expansibility — *Turgor vita'lis* — has been presumed to exist in certain organs, as in the capillaries; but the generality of physiologists do not admit it.

TURGESCENTIA, Turgescence.
TURGESCEN'TIA VESIC'ULÆ FELL'EÆ, *Asci'tes Hep'ato-cys'ticus*, *Physco'nia bilio'sa*, *Hepatal'gia Petitia'na*, *Cystocè'lè bilio'sa*, *Hydrocholecys'tis*, *Hydrops vesi'cæ fell'eæ*, (F.) *Hydropisie de la Vésicule du Fiel*, *Distension de la Vésicule du Fiel*, *Cholicystiectasie*. Distension of the gall-bladder by bile.

TURGIDITY, Turgescence.
TURGIDNESS, Turgescence.
TURGOR VITALIS, see Turgescence.
TURMERIC, Curcuma longa, Sanguinaria Canadensis.
TURN OF LIFE, see Menses.
TURNING, *Versio*, *V. fœtûs*, from (F.) *tourner*, 'to turn.' (F.) *Version*. The operation of bringing down the feet, or some part of the lower extremity, when the presentation of the child is such that it cannot be delivered by the natural efforts.

TURNIP, Brassica rapa — t. Dragon, Arum triphyllum — t. Indian, Arum triphyllum — t. Pepper, Arum triphyllum.

TURNS, Menses.
TURPENTINE, Terebinthina — t. Bordeaux, see Pinus sylvestris — t. Briançon, see Pinus cembra — t. Chio, see Pistacia terebinthus — t. Common, see Pinus sylvestris — t. Common, American, see Pinus sylvestris — t. Cyprus, see Pistacia terebinthus — t. Damarra, see Pinus damarra — t. Dombeya, see Dombeya excelsa — t. Horse, see Pinus sylvestris — t. Strasburg, see Pinus picea — t. Tree, Pistacia terebinthus — t. Venice, see Pinus larix — t. Venice, true, see Pistacia terebinthus — t. White, see Pinus sylvestris.

TURPETHUM, Convolvulus turpethum — t. Minerale, Hydrargyrus vitriolatus — t. Nigrum, Hydrargyri oxydum cinereum.

TURQUOISE. This stone has been long imagined to change its colour, according as the wearer is at the time in good or bad health: — a superstitious notion.

TURTLE BLOOM, Chelone glabra — t. Green, Chelonia mydas — t. Head, Chelone glabra.
TURUNDA, Tent.
TURUNDULA, Tent.
TUSSACA RETICULATA, Goodvera pubescens.
TUSSEDO, Tussis.
TUSSICULA, Tussis.
TUSSIC'ULAR, *Tussicula'ris*, *Tussiculo'sus*, from *tussis*, 'a cough.' Relating to a cough, or to a slight cough.

TUSSICULOSUS, Tussicular.
TUSSILA'GO, *T. Far'fara seu vulga'ris*, *Be'chium*, *Be'chion*, *Cal'ceum equi'num*, *Chamæleu'cè*, *Chamægei'ron*, *Fi'lius ante patrem*, *Farfarel'la*, *Galliomarchus*, *Farfara*, *Farfara Be'chium*, *Un'gula caballi'na*, *Coltsfoot*, (F.) *Pas d'âne*. *Family*, Corymbiferæ. *Sex. Syst.* Syngenesia Polygamia Superflua. It is demulcent and expectorant, and has been used in coughs, and pulmonary affections in general, and in some cutaneous diseases.

TUSSILAGO FARFARA, Tussilago — t. Hybrida, T. pelasites.

TUSSILAGO PETASI'TES, T. hy'brida seu Petasites hermaphrodita, Butterbur, Pestilent-wort, Petasites, Petasites major seu rubens seu officina'lis seu hy'bridus seu vulga'ris. The roots of this plant have been recommended as aperient and alexipharmic. — They have a strong smell; and a bitterish, acrid taste, of the aromatic kind, but not agreeable.

TUSSILAGO PETASITES HERMAPHRODITA, T. petasites — t. Vulgaris, Tussilago.

TUSSIS — diminutive, Tussic'ula; Cough, Coughing, Begma, Bex, Tusse'do, Bexis, Tussis nervo'sa, Catar'rhus, Pneusis Tussis, (F.) Toux. Violent, sonorous, frequent, and short expirations, by means of which the air, in passing rapidly through the bronchia and trachea, carries along with it the mucus of the parts, which forms the sputa. The cough is said to be dry, when unaccompanied by expectoration. It is symptomatic of many diseases. See Bronchitis.

TUSSIS AMPHEMERINA, Pertussis — t. Asinina, Pertussis — t. Bronchica, Cough, tubal, see Bronchitis — t. Canina, Pertussis — t. Catarrhalis Simplex, Catarrh — t. Clamosa, Pertussis — t. Clangosa, Pertussis — t. Convulsiva, Pertussis — t. Delassans, Pertussis — t. Ferina, Pertussis — t. Pueros strangulans, Pertussis — t. Quinta, Pertussis — t. Senilis, Bronchitis (chronic) — t. Spasmodica, Pertussis — t. Stomachalis, Pertussis — t. Suffocans, Pertussis — t. Suffocativa, Pertussis — t. Tussiculosa, Pertussis.

TUSSIVE; Tussi'vus; from tussis, 'cough.' Belonging or relating to cough: — as tussive vibration; the vibration of the parietes of the chest, caused by coughing.

TUTAM'INA, pl. of Tuta'men, 'a defence,' 'a protection,' from tutare, 'to defend.' Parts are so called which defend or protect each other.

TUTAMINA CER'EBRI are the scalp, pericranium, bones of the skull, and the meninges.

TUTAMINA OC'ULI are the eyebrows, eyelids, and lachrymal apparatus.

TUTENAG, Zincum.

TUTHIA, Tutia.

TU'TIA, Pom'pholyx, Cadmi'a, Alfasa, Meseru, Capni'tis, Tuthia, Ox'ydum zinci impu'rum. The oxyd of zinc that attaches itself to the chimneys of furnaces in which ores of zinc are smelted. It is in the form of gray incrustations; and is sometimes used for making an eye-salve. It is prepared, for this purpose, by levigation.

TWIN, Gemellus.

TWINKLING OF THE EYE, Nictation.

TWINLEAF, COMMON, Jeffersonia Bartoni.

TWINROOT, Orchis.

TWINS, SIAMESE. Two brothers, Chang and Eng, connected by means of a ligamentous band passing from the epigastrium of one to that of the other, who were exhibited in various parts of Europe and America, about the year 1830. They are now [1851] living in North Carolina: both are married, and have children. See Xiphopages.

TWITCHING, Tic.

TYCH'ICA, from τυχη, 'accident.' Fortuitous lesions or deformities. The 7th class of Good's Nosology.

TYLE, Callosity.

TYLOMA, Callosity.

TYLOSIS, Callosity.

TYLUS, Callosity.

TYMMA, Wound.

TYMPAN, Tympanum.

TYMPANAL, Tympanic.

TYMPANIA, Tympanites.

TYMPANIAS, Tympanites.

TYM'PANIC, Tympan'icus, Tym'panal; same etymon as tympanum. Relating to the tympanum, as 'tympanic canal.'

TYMPANIC NERVE, see Petrous ganglion.

TYMPANITA, Tympanites.

TYMPANITE, Tympanites.

TYMPANI'TES, Emphyse'ma Abdom'inis, Hydrops Tympanites, Affec'tio tympaniti'ca, Ectympano'sis, Pneumato'sis Abdom'inis, Hydrops abdominis aëreus, Aëro'sis, Aero-enterecta'sis, Physocæ'lia, Tympano'sis, Physe'ma, Physe'sis, Hydrops siccus et flatulentus, Tympa'nia, Tympa'nia, Tympani'ta, Tympani'tis, Emphyse'ma Tympanites, E. Tympanit'icum, Meteorismus, Tympany, Me'teorism, Wind dropsy, (F.) Tympanite, Pneumatose péritonéale, Ballonnement, from τύμπανον, 'a drum;' so called because the abdomen is distended with wind, and sounds like a drum when struck. A swelling of the abdomen, caused by accumulation of air in the intestinal tube or in the peritoneum. Tympanites may be idiopathic or symptomatic. The former depends upon exhalation of air from the inner surface of the intestine, or from the decomposition of substances contained in it; the latter is the result of some organic affection, and often depends upon obliteration of the digestive tube, which prevents the gas from escaping. Idiopathic tympanites may be more readily cured. The symptomatic is usually fatal. On dissection in such cases, the stomach and intestines are found enormously distended; with strangulation or disorganization of some part of the mucous membrane of the intestine. Carminatives may be proper when tympanites depends upon atony of the digestive organs: but, in cases of the symptomatic kind, they cannot be productive of advantage, and may do harm.

Sometimes the air is contained in the cavity of the peritoneum — constituting Tympani'tes abdomina'lis, Aëropéritonie, of some: — the accumulation in the intestines being called Tympani'tes intestina'lis.

TYMPANITES, UTERINE, Physometra.

TYMPANI'TIS, Inflamma'tio tym'pani: from τύμπανον, 'a drum,' and itis, denoting inflammation. Inflammation of the lining membrane of the middle ear, Also, tympanites.

TYMPANOSIS, Tympanites.

TYM'PANUM, τύμπανον, 'a drum.' The Drum or barrel of the ear. The names Cavity of the Tympanum or Cavity of the Drum, Cav'itas Tympani, Antrum seu cavitas antro'sa Auris, Cavum Tym'pani, (F.) Tympan, Cavité du tympan, Caisse du tambour — have been given to a cavity of an irregular shape, which constitutes the middle ear, and has been compared to a drum. It is situate in the pars petrosa of the temporal bone, between the meatus auditorius externus and the labyrinth. This cavity is lined by a mucous membrane: and communicates, externally, by means of the Eustachian tube, which is situate between it and the pharynx. The tympanum has six parietes. 1. An external, which is almost entirely formed of the Membrane of the Drum, Membrana tympani, Diaphrag'ma auris, Mediasti'num seu Tegumentum auris, Myrin'ga, Myrinx, (F.) Membrane de tympan — a species of thin, transparent, circular septum; convex within, and concave without, which closes the inner extremity of the meatus auditorius. 2. An internal, on which are the fenes'tra ova'lis, Prom'ontory, and Fora'men rotundum. 3. A superior. 4. An inferior, on which is the glenoid fissure. 5. A posterior, on which is the opening of the mastoid cells, and the pyramid. 6. An anterior, on which are the Proces'sus cochleaform'is and the inner orifice of the Eustachian tube. The cavity of the tympanum is crossed by a series of four small bones, articulated with each other by diarthrosis, moved by certain muscles, and representing a kind of bent lever extending from the membrana tympani to the fenestra ovalis. They are called the *Bones* or *Ossicles of the Ear*, and are the malleus, incus, os orbiculare, and stapes.

For the nervous plexus of the tympanum, see Petrosal Ganglion, and Otic Ganglion.

TYMPANUM MINUS, see Fenestra — t. Secundarium, see Fenestra.

TYMPANY, Tympanites — t. of the Womb, Physometra.

TYPE, *Typus, Periodus morbi,* from τυπος, 'a stamp,' itself from τυπτω, 'I strike.' The *type* is the order in which the symptoms of a disease exhibit themselves, and succeed each other. It may be continued, intermittent, or remittent.

TYPHA ANGUSTIFOLIA has the same proties as

TYPHA AROMATICA, Acorus calamus.

TYPHA LATIFOLIA, *Cattail, Reed mace,* (F.) *Massette, Masse d' Eau,* (τιφος, 'a marsh,' [?]). A plant common in marshes and ponds, in this country and in Europe. *Family,* Typhaceæ. *Sex. Syst.* Monœcia triandria. Its roots have been used in dysentery and blennorrhagia. The young shoots, before they reach the surface of the water, taste like asparagus, when boiled.

The down, (F.) *Aigrette, Poils,* which accompanies the flowers, has been applied to burns like cotton.

TYPHICUS, Typhoid.

TYPHIQUE, Typhoid.

TYPHLITIS, Typhlo-enteritis.

TYPHLO-ENTERI'TIS, *Typhlo-enteritis, Typhli'tis, Typhloteri'tis, Inflamma'tio Cæci, Phleg'monous Tumour of the Cæcum,* (F.) *Inflammation du Cæcum,* from τυφλος, *cæcus,* and *enteritis,* 'inflammation of the intestines.' Inflammation of the cæcum, occasionally leading to perforative ulceration.

TYPHLOENTERUM, Cæcum.

TYPHLOPS, Cæcus.

TYPHLOSIS, Cæcitas.

TYPHLOTERITIS, Typhlo-enteritis.

TYPHLOTERON MONOCOLON, Cæcum.

TYPHLOTERUM, Cæcum.

TYPHLOTES, Cæcitas.

TYPHODES, Typhoid.

TYPHOÉMIE ENTÉRIQUE, see Typhus.

TYPHOHÆMIA, see Putrefaction.

TYPHOID, *Typhoïdes, Typho'des, Ty'phicus, Typho'sus, Lac'tica,* (F.) *Typhique, Typhoïde, Typhode.* Appertaining to or resembling typhus; as *Typhoid Fever.* Also, according to some, *Typhous Fever,* typhus. Fuchs has employed the word *Typhoïde* for a family of diseases, to distinguish them from *phlogoses;* of this family, *Stomacace, Pharyngocace,* and *Pneumocace* are examples.

TYPHOID AFFECTION, see Typhus—t. Fever of India, Cholera.

TYPHOMA'NIA, from τυφος, 'stupor,' and μανια, 'delirium.' *Delirium with stupor, Subdelir'ium.* The kind of delirium common in typhus.

TYPHOMANIA, Coma vigil, Insomnia.

TYPHONIA, Coma vigil.

TYPHOSEPSES, Typhoseptoses.

TYPHOSEPTO'SES, *Typhosep'ses,* from τυφος, 'stupor,' and σηψις, 'putrefaction.' Typhous affections.

TYPHOSUS, Typhoid.

TYPHOUS, *Typho'sus;* same etymon as Typhus. Belonging or relating to typhus.

TYPHOUS DEPOS'IT. A peculiar substance of new formation found in the areolar membrane between the mucous and muscular coats of the patches of Peyer in typhoid fever.

TYPHOUS FEVER, see Typhoid.

TYPHUS, *Semipes'tis, Typhus, Febris Typho'des, Febris asthen'ica seu adynam'ica, Asthenop'yra,* (F.) *Fièvre adynamique, F. ataxique, F. adynamique ataxique, Typhus d'Europe,* from τυφος, 'stupor.' A fever characterised by small, weak, and unequal, but usually frequent pulse, with great prostration of strength, and much cerebral disturbance; its duration being usually from a fortnight to three weeks or longer. It is continued fever, accompanied with great cerebral irritation and prostration. (See Fever.) By most writers, this disease has been divided into two varieties—the *Typhus mitior* and *Typhus gravior.*

TYPHUS MIT'IOR, *T. simplex, T. nervo'sus, T. comato'sus, Fe'bris lenta nervosa, Blechrop'yrus, F. pu'trida nervosa, F. hec'tica malig'na nervosa, Nervous Fever, Neurop'yra, Neuropyr'etus,* (F.) *Fièvre nerveuse,* is characterised by slight shiverings, heavy, vertiginous headach; great oppression, peculiar expression of anxiety, nausea, sighing, despondency, and coma or quiet delirium. TYPHUS GRA'VIOR, *Typhus car'cerum, T. castren'sis, T. anthropophthor'aous, True Typhus, Exanthemat'ic typhus, Nervous fever with exanthem'atous erup'tion, Conta'gious typhus, Febris nervo'sa epidem'ica, F. nervo'sa exanthemat'ica, F. malig'na cum sopo're, F. nervo'sa petechia'lis, F. pestilentia'lis Euro'pæ, Typhus contagio'sus exanthemat'icus, T. nostras, T. Europæ'us, T. commu'nis, T. bel'licus, T. exanthemat'icus, T. Hiber'nicus, Pestis bel'lica, Febris pes'tilens malig'na, Febris nau'tica pestilentia'lis, Febris petechia'lis, Typhus petechia'lis, Porphyro-typhus, Pulicula'ris morbus, Febris puncticula'ris, F. Saprop'yra, F. oss'cerum et nosocomio'rum, F. Putrida, F. con'tinens pu'trida, F. contin'ua pu'trida, Septop'yra, Putrid Fever, Jail Fever, Hospital Fever, Ship Fever,* (F.) *Fièvre des Camps, F. nautique, F. d'Hôpital, F. nosocomiale, F. des Prisons, F. lenticulaire, Typhus contagieux,* is attended with rigors and heat, alternating; little or no perspiration; pulse, tense and hard, usually quick, but fluttering; pain over the forehead and vertex; a '*mulberry rash,*' appearing on the fifth to the seventh day of the disease, and lasting till the end; delirium, succeeded by stupor, signs of incipient putrescency,—as true petechiæ, vibices, hemorrhages, &c. Typhus, under particular circumstances, seems to be communicable by contagion; but if proper attention be paid to cleanliness and ventilation, there is not much danger of communication. The general principles of treatment, laid down under the head of Fever, are applicable here. All the varieties of continued fever resemble each other in the cardinal points, although they may differ in many of their characters. Ventilation and cleanliness; warm or cold ablation or sponging; keeping the bowels free; and attending to symptoms as they may rise, with the avoiding of all irritation of every kind, are the main indications. When symptoms of great prostration occur, the strength must be supported by wine; and tonics be exhibited, with the mineral acids. Of the tonics, the sulphate of quinia is perhaps as good as any, whilst it is free from the objection which applies to most others,—of being too bulky. In the whole management of this affection, however, the physician has to discriminate carefully between oppression and prostration. The former may require evacuants; the latter cannot.

Of late, certain observers have endeavoured to show, that there is an essential difference between typhoid fever and typhus; that the former is an abdominal affection, and dependent upon, or con-nested with, an inflamed or ulcerated condition of the mucous follicles of the intestines; hence it has received the names *Fièvre mésentérique, F. typhoïde, Maladie* ou *Affection typhoïde, F. entéro-mésentérique, Entérite typho-hémique, Typhoémie entérique, Entéro-mésentérite typhoïde, Exanthème intestinale, Dothinentérie, Dothinentérite*, &c., *Ileodiclidite, Entérite folliculeuse, Gastro-entérite* with nervous affection of the brain, *Follicular gastroenteritis, F. enteritis, Enteri'tis folliculo'sa, Typhus abdomina'lis, T. intestina'lis, T. Sporad'icus, Enterotyphus, T. gangliona'ris abdomina'lis, Febris intestina'lis ulcero'sa, F. nervo'sa gas'trica, F. nervo'sa enter'ica, F. enter'ica, F. nervo'sa mesenter'ica, Enterhelio'sis nervo'sa, Typhus enter'ious, Ileop'yra, Ileotyphus, Typhoid affection, Enteric fever.* Accompanying this form of fever there is generally a typhoid eruption, consisting of rose-red papulæ, (see Spots, red,) which appear mostly on the abdomen. They are distinct from true petechiæ, as they can be removed by pressure; and distinct also from sudamina, which are perhaps the universal accompaniments of sweating, and are consequently a variety of miliaria. The common continued fever or synochus of Great Britain, and of this country, has been presumed by some to be this variety: but farther observations are needed to establish the distinctions which have been attempted; and there is reason to believe, that the abdominal affection is a complication, existing in certain cases and epidemics of adynamic fever, and not in others. The *Red Tongue Fever* of Kentucky is considered by Professor Bartlett to be typhoid fever.

Certain modern French writers have considered the Typhus of the European continent, *Typhus of Europe, Peste d'Europe, pestilential fever, contagious typhus, Hungary fever, Hospital fever, camp fever, jail fever, lenticular petechial fever,* &c., to be identical with the typhoid affection. They admit but one fever on the European continent — the typhoid. Typhus, they maintain — but by no means establish the position — to be peculiar to England.

TYPHUS ABDOMINALIS, see Typhus — *t. d'Amé-rique*, Fever, yellow — *t.* Anthracicus, Plague — *t.* Anthropophthoracus, Typhus — *t.* Aphthides, Aphthæ — *t.* Bellicus, Typhus — *t.* Bengalens, Cholera — *t.* Bubonicus, Plague — *t.* Camerin, Typhus gravior — *t.* Castrensis, Typhus gra— *t.* Comatosus, Typhus mitior — *t.* Communis, Typhus — *t.* Contagieux, Typhus — *t.* Contagns, Typhus — *t.* Contagiosus exanthematicus, Typhus — *t. d'Europe*, Typhus — *t.* of Europe, see Typhus — *t.* Exanthematicus, Typhus — *t.* Gangl—*t.* abdominalis, see Typhus — *t.* Gravissimus, P— *t.* Hibernicus, T. gravior — *t.* Icterodes, F— yellow — *t. Jaune*, Fever, yellow — *t.* Intermit see Typhus — *t. Miasmatique ataxique p— jaune*, Fever, yellow — *t.* Morbillosus, Rubeola— *t.* Nervosus, Typhus mitior — *t.* Nostras, Typhus — *t. d'Orient*, Plague — *t.* Pestilentialis, Plague — *t.* Pestis, Plague — *t.* Petechialis, Typhus grav— *t. Puerpéral*, see Peritonitis — *t.* Scarlatinosus — Scarlatina — *t.* Simplex, Typhus mitior — *t.* Sporadicus, see Typhus — *t.* Tropicus, Fever, yellow — *t.* True, Typhus — *t.* Vesicularis, Pemphigus.

TYP'IC, *Typ'ical, Typ'icum*, (F.) *Typ— .* Same etymon as *Type*. Characterized by periodicity, — as a '*typical fever*;' or one which observes a particular type.

TYPOSES, see Periodicity.

TYPUS, Type.

TYRANNUS, see Critical days.

TYRBASIA, Agitation.

TYRBE, Agitation.

TYREM'ESIS, *Tyrotem'esis*, from τυ '*cheese*,' and εμεσις, '*vomiting*;' *Tyre'si. reu'sis*. Vomiting of curdy matter, in infa— especially.

TYREUSIS, Tyremesis, Tyrosis.

TYRIA, Porrigo decalvans.

TYRIASIS, Elephantiasis Arabica.

TYRODES, Cheesy.

TYROMA, Porrigo decalvans.

TYROS, Cheese.

TYROSIS, Tyremesis. Also, the curding of milk in the stomach; *Tyreu'sis*.

TYROTEMESIS, Tyremesis.

U.

UBERIS APEX, Papilla.

ULA, Gingivæ.

ULATROPH'IA, from ουλον, '*the gum*,' and *atrophia*, atrophy. Shrinking of the gums; falling away of the gums.

ULCER, *Ulcus*, (diminutive *Ulcus'culum*,) *Helcos, Elco'sis, Elco'ma, Helcus, Helco'ma*, a *Sore*, (F.) *Ulcère.* A solution of continuity in the soft parts, of longer or shorter standing, and kept up by some local disease or constitutional cause. Richerand makes four great distinctions between a wound and an ulcer. 1. A wound arises from the action of an extraneous body : — the cause of an ulcer is inherent in the economy. 2. A wound is always idiopathic : — an ulcer is always symptomatic. 3. A wound has essentially a tendency to heal, because the action of its cause has been momentary : — an ulcer, on the contrary, has a tendency to enlarge, because its cause persists. 4. The treatment of a wound is purely surgical; that of an ulcer is medical as well. The immediate cause of an ulcer is an augmented action of the absorbents; and a specific action of the small vessels, which secrete pus from the blood. Ulcers have been variously divided, according to their nature; — into *simple, sinuous, fistulous, fungous, gangrenous, scorbutic, syphilitic, cancerous, inveterate, scrofulous, phagedenic, virulent, corro— sordid, carious, varicose,* &c. The treatment consists in removing, by appropriate means, the internal and the local causes which keep up the ulceration, and in exciting the vessels of the part where necessary, by appropriate bandaging, &c.

ULCER, MALIGNANT, Hospital gangrene — *t.* Putrid, Hospital gangrene.

ULCERA INTESTINALIA, Gastrelcosis — *t.* Laryngis, Phthisis laryngea — *u.* Serpentia seu 'Aphthæ — *u.* Uteri, see Metrophthisis — *u.* Vesiculi, Gastrelcosis — *u.* Vesicæ, Cystophthisis.

UL'CERATED, *Ulcera'tus, Exulcera'tus, co'des*, (F.) *Ulcéré.* In the state of an ulcer. Affected with ulcers.

ULCERATIO INTESTINALIS, Enteroleosi — *u.* Ventriculi, Gastrelcosis.

ULCERA'TION, *Ulcera'tio, Exulcerati., gen'ia corrosi'va.* A superficial ulcer. The formation of an ulcer — *Exelco'sis, Elco'sis, co'sis.*

ULCÈRE, Ulcer — *u. du Larynx*, Phthisis laryngea.

UL'CEROUS, *Ulcero'sus, Helco'des, Helco—*

Having the character of an ulcer. Affected with ulcers.

ULCERS, EGYPTIAN, Ægyptia ulcera.

ULCUS, Ulcer — u. Atonicum, Rupia — u. Cacoethes, see Cacoethes — u. Cancrosum, Cancer, Chancre — u. Dacryodes, see Dacryodes — u. Depascens, Phagedenic ulcer — u. Ferinum, Phagedenic ulcer — u. Fistulosum, Hypophora — u. Hypulum, see Hypulus — u. Narium fœtens, Ozæna — u. Obambulans, Phagedenic ulcer — u. Pulmonum, Phthisis pulmonalis — u. Sinuosum, Hypophora — u. Syriacum, Cynanche maligna — u. Telephium, Telephium — u. Tuberculosum, Lupus — u. Uteri, Hysterelcosis, Leucorrhœa.

ULCUSCULA PRÆPUTII, Herpes præputii.

ULCUSCULUM, Ulcer — u. Cancrosum, Chancre.

ULE, Cicatrix.

ULETICUS, Gingivalis.

ULICUS, Gingivalis.

ULI'TIS, from ουλος, 'solid,' (σαρξ ουλη, 'solid flesh:') hence, ουλον, 'the gum.' *Inflamma'tio gingi'væ, Periodonti'tis gingiva'rum*, (F.) *Gengivite, Inflammation des gencives*, from ουλον, 'the gum,' and *itis*, denoting inflammation. Inflammation of the gums.

ULITIS SEPTICA, Cancer aquaticus.

ULLUCO, Tropæolum tuberosum.

ULMAIRE, Spiræa ulmaria.

ULMARIA, Spiræa ulmaria — u. Palustris, Spiræa ulmaria.

ULMUS, *U. campes'tris* seu *glabra* seu *monta'na* seu *nuda* seu *sati'va* seu *scabra*, Ptelea, Common Elm, (F.) *Orme. Family*, Amentaceæ. *Sex. Syst.* Pentandria Digynia. The inner, rough bark of this tree is inodorous; and has a bitter, austere, and mucilaginous taste. It is considered tonic, alterative, and diuretic; and has been used, chiefly, in lepra and other cutaneous affections.

ULMUS ALA'TA, *Lynn Wahoo*. The bark of the root has been used successfully as a cataplasm in phlegmonous inflammation.

ULMUS AMERICA'NA, *U. fulva, Rough-leaved Elm, Red Elm, Slippery Elm*. The inner bark is highly mucilaginous, and is used in coughs, diarrhœas, and dysenteries; also, as a poultice for tumours; lacerated and contused wounds, &c.

ULMUS CAMPESTRIS, Ulmus — u. Fulva, U. Americana — u. Glabra, Ulmus — u. Montana, Ulmus — u. Nuda, Ulmus — u. Sativa, Ulmus — u. Scabra, Ulmus.

ULNA, *O'lenē, Foc''ilē infe'rius* seu *majus*, *Canna Bra'chii, Os cu'biti infe'rius, Os procubita'lē, Cu'bitus, Cubit, Arun'do bra'chii major.* Anatomists have given this name to the bone of the forearm which forms the prominence of the elbow, during the flexion of that joint. It is the longer and larger of the two bones, and is inserted at the inner side. Its upper and larger extremity has, behind, a considerable process, called *olecranon*; and, before, a smaller one, called *coronoid*. These two eminences are separated from each other by the greater *sigmoid* or *semilunar fossa* or *olec'ranoid cavity*, which receives the articular trochlea of the humerus. The tubercle of the ulna is a small, rough spot, under the root of the coronoid process, for the insertion of the *Brachialis internus*. On the outside of this extremity of the bone is the *lesser sigmoid cavity*. It is articulated with the head of the radius. The inferior extremity of the cubitus, which is much smaller than the superior, and articulated with the radius, has a surface that corresponds to the fibro-cartilage which separates it from the os cuneiforme; and a pointed process, called *styloid*. The body of the ulna is manifestly triangular. It is articulated with the os humeri and radius, and, mediately, with the os cuneiforme. It is developed by three points of ossification.

Also, the elbow.

ULNAD, see Ulnar aspect.

ULNAR, Cubital.

ULNAR ASPECT. An aspect towards the side on which the ulna is situated. — Barclay. Ulnad is used adverbially by the same writer, to signify 'towards the ulnar aspect.'

ULNARIS, Cubital — u. Externus, see Cubital muscles — u. Gracilis, Palmaris longus — u. Internus, see Cubital muscles.

ULOCACE, Cancer aquaticus, Stomacace.

ULON'CUS, from ουλον, 'the gum,' and ογκος, 'tumour.' Swelling of the gums; epulis.

ULORRHAG''IA, *Stomatorrhag''ia, Hæmorrhag''ia gingivarum, Ulorrhœ'a*, from ουλον, 'the gum,' and ρηγνυμι, 'I break forth.' Bleeding from the gums.

ULORRHŒA, Ulorrhagia.

ULOTICA, Cicatrisantia.

UL'TIMI-STERNAL. Professor Béclard has given this appellation to the sixth or last bony portion of the sternum. He calls it also *Ensisternal*.

UL'TIMUM MO'RIENS, 'last dying.' A term given to the part of the economy which dies last.

ULVA CRISPA, Fucus crispus.

UMBIL, YELLOW, Cypripedium luteum.

UMBILIC, Umbilical, Umbilicus.

UMBIL'ICAL, *Um'bilic, Umbilica'lis, Umbilica'tus*, from *umbilicus*, 'the navel.' That which belongs or relates to the navel.

UMBILICAL ARTERIES, which exist only in the fœtus, seem, as it were, continuations of the primitive iliacs. They clear the umbilical ring, and proceed to the placenta, to which they carry the residuum of the blood sent to the fœtus by the umbilical vein. As soon as respiration is established, the blood ceases to pass by the umbilical arteries, which become obliterated, as well as the vein, and are transformed into two very strong ligamentous cords, — the vein forming the *Ligamen'tum rotun'dum* of the liver.

UMBILICAL CORD, Funiculus umbilicalis.

UMBILICAL REGION, *Re'gio umbilica'lis, Mesogas'trium Re'gio gas'trica* seu *Mesogastrica*, (F.) *Région ombilicale*, is the middle region of the abdomen, in which the umbilicus is placed. The sides of this are called the *flanks* or *lumbar regions*. In the umbilical region are the omentum majus; the inferior extremity of the duodenum; the jejunum; and the greater part of the mesentery; the aorta; vena cava; the trunks of the renal arteries and veins; the origin of the spermatic arteries, &c.

UMBILICAL RING, *An'nulus umbilica'lis*, (F.) *Anneau ombilical*, is a fibrous ring which surrounds the aperture of the umbilicus, and through which umbilical hernia occurs in children.

UMBILICAL VESICLE, Vesicula umbilicalis.

UMBILICAL VESSELS, (F.) *Vaisseaux ombilicaux*, include the two arteries, and umbilical vein. The umbilical vein arises from the placenta, and terminates at the fissure on the inferior surface of the liver of the fœtus, to which it conveys the blood necessary for its nutrition.

UMBILICALIS, Umbilical.

UMBILICATUS, Umbilical.

UMBILI'CUS, *Umbo, Om'phalos, Umbili'cum, Radix ventris, Mesompha'lium, Mesom'phalum, Protme'sis, (navel of a new-born child;)* the *umbilic*, the *navel;* from *umbo*, 'the button or prominence in the midst of a buckler,' or from υμφαλος, or rather ομφαλος, which signifies the same, as well as the navel; (F.) *Ombilic, Nombril* round cicatrix, about the median line of the abdomen. It is in the situation of an aperture, which, in the fœtus, affords passage to the vessels of the umbilical cord.

UMBILICUS MARI'NUS, *Cotyle'don marina, Andro'sacē, Acetab'ulum marinum, Andro'sacē Matthi'oli, Fungus petræ'us marinus.* A submarine production, found on the rocks and the shells of fishes, in the south of France. It is reputed to be anthelmintic and diuretic.

UMBO, Elbow, Umbilicus.

UMBRELLA TREE, Magnolia tripetala.

UMSCHLAG, see Compress.

UNBOWELING, Exenterismus.

UNCARIA GAMBIR, Nauclea Gambir.

UNCAS, INDIAN, Veratrum viride.

UNCIA, Ounce.

UN'CIFORM, *Unciform'is, Uncina'tus*, from *uncus*, 'a hook,' and *forma*, 'shape.' That which has the shape of a hook.

UNCIFORM BONE, *Os unciform'ĕ, Os hama'tum, Os uncina'tum*, (F.) *Os crochu.* The fourth bone of the second row of the carpus. Its shape is very irregular. Inwards and forwards, it has a considerable eminence, which is curved upon itself, and gives attachment to the annular ligament of the carpus. It is articulated with the os semilunare, os magnum, os cuneiforme, and the fourth and fifth metacarpal bones. It is developed from a single point of ossification.

UNCIFORM EMINENCE, Hippocampus minor.

UNCINATUS, Unciform.

UNCINUS, Hook.

UNCTION, Inunction, Unguentum, Unguentum hydrargyri.

UNCUS, Hook.

UNDERCLIFF, ISLE OF WIGHT, ENGLAND, (CLIMATE OF.) The Undercliff comprehends a tract of country from Dunnose to St. Catherine's Hill, on the southeast coast, about six miles in length, and from a quarter to half a mile in breadth. It is well protected from the colder winds; and the climate is remarkably equable, as well as mild and dry, so that there are not many days during the winter in which the invalid cannot take some exercise in the open air. It is an excellent climate for the pulmonary valetudinarian.

UNDIM'IA. A name given, by Paracelsus, to a tumour, filled with a gelatinous matter, like the white of an egg.

UNDOSUS, Cymatodes.

UNDULATIO, Fluctuation.

UNEDO, Arbutus unedo — u. Papyracea, Arbutus unedo.

UNGUEAL MATRIX, see Nail.

UNGUEN, Unguentum — u. Articulare, Synovia.

UNGUÉNT, ARMATORY, Hoplochrysma.

UNGUENTARIA, see Myristica moschata.

UNGUENTA'RIUS, *Myropœ'us, Myrep'sus, Myropo'les, Myropo'lus, Pigmenta'rius;* from *unguen'tum*, 'an ointment.' One who makes and sells ointments. A perfumer.

UNGUEN'TUM, *Unguen, Myron, Unction*, (F.) *Onguent*, from *ungere*, 'to anoint.' Ointment. Ointments are topical applications, of a consistence more or less analogous to that of lard. They are used, chiefly, as local applications to ulcers and wounds; but are sometimes rubbed upon a part in cutaneous affections; and, especially, where it is desired that the constituents of the ointment should be absorbed. Ointments are of less consistence than cerates, although the terms are often used indiscriminately.

UNGUEN'TUM AC"IDI NITRO'SI, *Ointment of Nitrous Acid, Poma'tum vel Unguen'tum Ni'tricum vel Oxygena'tum*, (F.) *Pommade oxygénée, Graisse oxygénée, Pommade d'Alyon.* (Adip. *suillæ*, ℔j; *acid. nitros.* ℨvj. Melt the fat, and rub in the acid gradually, till cold. *Ph. E.*) Stimulant. Used in itch and other cutaneous eruptions, and in foul ulcers.

UNGUENTUM ADIPOCERÆ CETORUM, Ceratum cetacei — u. Ægyptiacum, Linimentum æruginis — u. Ægyptium album, Crinomyron — u. Albæ, Unguentum cetacei — u. Album Resolvens, Linimentum ammoniæ fortius.

UNGUENTUM DE ALTHÆA, *Marsh mallow Ointment, U. de Terebin'thinâ et cerâ, Cera'tum u Althæâ, Emplas'trum mucilagino'sum, E. *nalieus, E. cit'rinum, E. flavum, E. de Althæa.* (*Unguentum flavum, U. Cit'rinum, U. resi'næ pinnves'tris compos'itum seu resumptivum seu lentivum,* (F.) *Onguent de guimauve, O. d'althéa.* (Uno *de mucilaginibus*, 1000 p., *ceræ flavæ*, 250 p. re*sinæ terebinthin.*, āā 125 p. Liquefy: strain and stir till cold. *Ph. P.*) *Common Olive Oil* may be substituted for the *Oil of Mucilage.*

UNGUENTUM AMYGDALINUM, Ceratum Galeni.

UNGUENTUM ANTIMO'NII, *U. A. Tartarisa'i, U. A. Potassio-tar'tratis, U. tar'tari emet'ici, (ointment of tar'tarised an'timony.* (*Antimon. et potass. tartrat.* in pulv. subtiliss. ℨij, *adipis* ℨ. If a drachm of this ointment be rubbed upon any part, night and morning, it will excite, in a few days, a painful pustular eruption. Hence, it is employed as a counter-irritant. This preparation is also called *Ung. Tar'tari stibia'ti* see *eme* — *Ung. e Tar'taro stibia'to. Adeps Tartari stibiti medica'tus, Ung. Tar'tratis Potass'æ stibia'ti, Pommade d'Autenrieth, Pommade stibiée.*

UNGUENTUM ANTIMONII POTASSIO-TARTRATIS, Unguentum antimonii — u. Antimonii tartarisati, U. antimonii — u. Antipernium, see Antipernium.

UNGUENTUM AQUÆ ROSÆ, *Ointment of Rose water, Cold Cream.* (Aq. Rosæ, f℥j; *ol. amygd.* f℥ij; *cetacei*, ℨss; *ceræ albæ*, ℨj. Melt together in a water-bath, the oil, spermaceti. and will then add the rose-water, and stir until it is cold. *Ph. U. S.*) Cooling to irritated surfaces.

UNGUENTUM ARMARIUM, Hoplochrysma — u. Arthanitæ, see Arthanita — u. Articulare, Synovia — u. Basilicon flavum, Ceratum resinæ — u. Basilicon nigrum, Unguentum resinæ nigræ — u. Basilicum viride, Unguentum subacetatis cupri.

UNGUENTUM BELLADON'NÆ, *Ointment of belladonna.* (Ext. belladonnæ ℨj; *adipis* ℨj. *Ph. U. S.*) An anodyne application to irritable ulcers, &c.

UNGUENTUM CANTHARIDIS, Unguentum lyttæ.

UNGUEN'TUM CERÆ (*albæ* vel *flavæ*), *Wax ointment, Unguentum simplex*, (Ph. U. S.) *Linimentum simplex, Oil and Bees' Wax*, (F.) *Onguent cire.* (Ceræ ℔j, adipis ℔iv, Ph. U. S. or — aā ℨij, *ol. oliv.* ℥v.) Emollient. A mild dressing. Also, the basis of most of the compound ointments.

UNGUENTUM CERATUM, Ceratum Galeni — u. Cerussæ, Unguentum oxidi plumbi albi. Unguentum plumbi subcarbonatis — u. Cerussæ acetatæ, Ceratum plumbi superacetatis, U. plumbi superacetatis — u. Citrinum, U. de althæa, U. hydrargyri nitratis.

UNGUENTUM CETA'CEI, *Unguentum Spermatis Ceti, U. album, Linimen'tum album, Sperma'ceti ointment*, (F.) *Onguent de blanc de baleine.* (*Cetacei* ℨvj, *ceræ albæ* ℨiv, *ol. oliv.* f℥iij. *Ph. U. S.*) The ordinary dressing for blisters and excoriations.

UNGUEN'TUM CREASO'TI, *Ointment of Creasote.* (*Creasot.* fℨss; *adipis*, ℨj. Add the creasote to the lard previously melted with a moderate heat, and stir constantly till cold. *Ph. U. S.*) Used in chronic cutaneous affections.

UNGUENTUM Cupri Subacetatis, Unguentum subacetatis cupri.
UNGUENTUM Digesti'vum Simplex, U. Terebin'thinæ et ovo'rum vitel'li, Simple digestive ointment, (F.) Onguent digestif simple. (Terebinthin. pur. 64 p. Vitell. ovor. No. 2, vel 32 p. Mix, for a long time, in a glass mortar, and add, gradually, enough of the Oil of Hypericum (Millepertuis) to make a soft ointment. Ph. P.) Detergent. It may be rendered more so by adding a little of the Acetate of copper.
UNGUENTUM Elemi, Balsam of Arcæus, Unguentum elemi compositum.
UNGUENTUM El'emi Compos'itum, Linimen'tum Arcæ'i, Unguentum e gummi elemi, Ung. de Terebin'thinâ et adip'ibus, U. elemi, Ointment of Elemi, (F.) Baume d'Arcéus. (Elemi ℔ij, terebinthinæ vulgaris ʒx, sevi præparati ℔ij, olivæ olei f ℥ij. Melt the elemi with the suet; remove it from the fire; and mix in the turpentine and oil. Strain the mixture through a linen cloth. Ph. L.) Stimulant and digestive. To keep open issues, &c.
UNGUENTUM Epispas'ticum de Daphne Gnidio, Adeps Cor'ticâ daphnes gnidii medica'tus, (F.) Pommade de Garou. (Adip. præpar, 320 p., ceræ, 32 p., cort. daphn. gnid. 128 p. Melt the fat and wax; and add the bark softened in water. Boil until the water is evaporated; then pass through cloth. Ph. P.) To keep open blisters, issues, &c. See Unguentum Mezerei.
UNGUENTUM Epispasticum Fortius, Cerate of cantharides—u. Epispasticum mitius, Unguentum lyttæ—u. Epispasticum viride, Unguentum lyttæ medicatum—u. Flavum, Unguentum de althææ—u. e Gummi elemi, Unguentum compositum — u. Hellebori albi, Unguentum veratri.
UNGUENTUM Gallæ, Ointment of Galls, (Gallæ in pulv. ℥j; adipis. ℥vij. M. Ph. U. S.) As an astringent in piles, indolent ulcers, &c.
UNGUEN'TUM Hydrar'gyri, U. cæru'leum, U. Neapolita'num, Blue ointment, Cera'tum mercuria'lê, Adeps Hydrar'gyro medica'tus, Mercurial Ointment, Unction, (F.) Onguent mercuriel ou Napolitain.
The Strong Mercurial Ointment, Unguentum Hydrargyri fortius of the London Pharmacopœia, Unguen'tum Hydrar'gyri (Ph. U. S.), is thus made —Hydrarg. ℔ij, adipis ℥xxiij, sevi ℥j. Rub till the globules entirely disappear.
The Milder Mercurial Ointment, — Unguentum Hydrargyri Mitius, —is made by adding, to one pound of the strong, two pounds of lard.
Mercurial ointment is antisyphilitic and discutient. It is rubbed on the inside of the thigh, in venereal affections; especially in those cases where mercury, given internally, runs off by the bowels. The stronger ointment is used for this purpose. The weaker is employed as a dressing, or as an application to cutaneous eruptions.
UNGUENTUM Hydrargyri Ammoniati, Unguentum hydrargyri præcipitati albi — u. Hydrargyri calcis albæ, Unguentum hydrargyri præcipitati albi—u. Hydrargyri compositum, Unguentum hydrargyri nitratis—u. Hydrargyri deutoxydi nitrati, Unguentum hydrargyri nitrico-oxydi—u. ex Hydrargyro mitius diuton cinereum, Unguentum oxydi hydrargyri cinereum.
UNGUENTUM Hydrargyri Nitra'tis, U. H. nitrati, U. supernitra'tis hydrargyri, Ointment of Nitrate of Mer'cury, Citrine Ointment, Bal'samum mercuria'lê, Ung. hydrar'gyri compos'itum, U. mercurialê cit'rinum, Adeps nitra'tê hydrargyri medica'tus, Unguentum citrinum ad scabiem, (F.) Onguent de nitrate de mercure, O. citrin contre la gale. (Hydrarg. ℥j, acid. nitric. f ʒxiv, olei bubuli f ℥ix, adipis ℥iij. Dissolve the mercury in the acid; and, while hot, add the oil and melted lard. Ph. U. S.

A milder ointment,—Ung. Nitratis Hydrargyri mitius, — is made with triple the quantity of oil and lard. It is stimulant and detergent, and is much used as an application to herpes, porrigo, and cutaneous eruptions. The weaker ointment is sometimes used in ophthalmia tarsi, &c.
UNGUENTUM Hydrargyri Ni'trico - ox'ydi, Ung. subnitra'tis hydrargyri, Ung. Oxydi Hydrargyri rubri, U. H. oxidi rubri (Ph. U. S.), Ointment of Nitric Oxyd of Mercury, Bal'samum ophthal'micum rubrum, Unguentum deutox'ydi hydrarg. nitrati, Red Precip'itate Ointment, Golden Ointment, Singleton's Eye Salve, U. Hydrargyri rubri, U. ex Hydrargyro oxyda'to rubro, U. mercurii rubrum, U. ophthal'micum rubrum, U. subnitra'tis hydrargyr'ici. (Hydrarg. oxid. rubr. in pulv. subtiliss. ʒj; Ung. simpl. ℥j. Add the oxyd, reduced to a fine power, to the melted ointment. Ph. U. S.) Stimulant and escharotic. Applied to foul ulcers, to inflammation of the tarsi, &c. &c.
Belleville's Cerate, which has been long used in cases of scalled head, and of chronic cutaneous diseases in general, is made as follows : —Plumbi acet. ʒj; hydrarg. oxid. rubr. ʒss; hyd. chlorid. mit. ʒij; ceræ albæ ℥iv; ol. oliv. ʒvj. Melt the last two, and add the others in fine powder.
UNGUENTUM Hydrargyri Oxidi Rubri, Unguentum hydrargyri nitrico-oxydi — u. ex Hydrargyro oxydato rubro, Unguentum hydrargyri nitrico-oxydi—u. Hydrargyri oxydi rubri, Unguentum hydrargyri nitrico-oxydi.
UNGUENTUM Hydrargyri Præcipita'ti Albi, U. Hydrar'gyri ammonia'ti, (Ph. U. S.), U. submuria'tis hydrargyri ammonia'ti, Unguentum ad scabiem Zelleri, U. mercuria'lê album, U. mundif'icans Zelleri, Ointment of white precipitate, Ung. e mercu'rio præcipita'to, Ung. calcis hydrargyri albæ. (Hyd. ammon. ʒj, ung. simpl. ℥iss. Melt the fat, and add the precipitate.) Detergent. Used in cutaneous eruptions, to destroy vermin, &c.
UNGUENTUM Hydrargyri Rubri, U. Hydrargyri nitrico-oxydi — u. Hydrargyri submuriatis ammoniati, U. Hydrargyri præcipitati albi — u. Hydrargyri subnitratis, U. hydrargyri nitrico-oxydi—u. Hydrargyri subnitratis, U. hydrargyri nitrico-oxydi—u. Hydrargyri supernitratis, U. hydrargyri nitratis—u. Infusi meloes vesicatorii, U. lyttæ—u. Irritans, U. lyttæ.
UNGUEN'TUM Io'DINI, U. Iodin'ii, Ointment of Iodine. (Iodin. ℈j; Potass. iodid. gr. iv; Aquæ ♏vj; Adipis. ℥j. Rub the iodine and iodide first with the water until liquified, and then with the lard until mixed. Ph. U. S.) Used as a local application to goîtrous and other swellings.
UNGUENTUM Io'DINI Compos'itum, U. Iodin'ii compositum, Compound Ointment of Iodine. (Iodin. ʒss; Potassii iodid. ʒj; Alcohol, f ʒj; adipis ℥ij. Rub the iodine and iodide first with the alcohol and then with the lard until they are well mixed. Ph. U. S.)
UNGUENTUM Lau'rinum, O'leum lau'rinum, Adeps lauro-medica'tus, Bay Ointment, (F.) Onguent ou Huile de laurier. (Fol. lauri, 500 p., adip. suillæ, 1000 p. Bruise in a marble mortar; evaporate all humidity by boiling; and add Bay berries, in powder, 500 p. Digest and pass through linen. Ph. P.) Reputed to be corroborant and nervine. It is simply emollient.
UNGUENTUM Lenitivum, U. de althææ—u. Liliaceum, Crinomyron.
UNGUENTUM Lyttæ, Ung. canthar'idis, U. vesicato'rium, U. irri'tans, U. ad vesica'ta, Blistering Salve, Ung. infu'si mel'oes vesicato'rii, Ointment of Spanish Flies, Ointment of Infusion of Spanish Flies, Unguentum epispas'ticum mit''ius, Milder blis'tering Ointment. (Canthar'id. in pulv.

℥ij; *aquæ destillat.* Oss; *cerat. resin.* ℥viij. Boil down the water with the Spanish flies to one-half, and strain; then mix the cerate with the strained liquor, and evaporate to the proper consistence. *Ph. U. S.*) It is stimulant and epispastic; and is chiefly used for keeping up the discharge from a blistered surface.

UNGUENTUM LYTTÆ MEDICA'TUM, *Adeps cantharid'ibus medica'tus, Poma'tum* seu *Unguentum epispas'ticum vir'idē stim'ulans ac'ribus,* Green blis'tering Ointment, (F.) *Pommade épispastique verte.* (*Pomati unguenti cantharid.* 64 p., *unguent. populei* 168 p., *ceræ albæ* 256 p., *cupri acetat., ext. opii,* āā 24 p. Melt the unguentum populeum, and wax, and add, as they cool, the oxyd of copper, cantharides, and opium. *Ph. P.*) Use, same as the last.

UNGUENTUM LYTTÆ MEDICA'TUM A'LIUD, *Adeps cantharid'ibus medica'tus alius, Poma'tum epispas'ticum flavum et mit''ius,* Yellow Blistering Ointment, (F.) *Pommade épispastique jaune.* (*Pulv. cantharid.* 120 p., *adip. præp.* 1680 p., *aquæ* 250 p. Melt the lard; mix the cantharides, and add the water at the same time; place the whole on a gentle fire; stir continually for two hours, and add a little water to replace that which has been evaporated. Pass through linen and strain. Keep it in a water-bath, and add powdered *turmeric,* 8 p. Let it cool till the superfluous liquid separates; pour off and add *yellow wax,* 250 p., *Oil of Lemon,* 8 p. *Ph. P.*) A complex preparation. Use, same as the last.

An ointment, not very philosophically combined, was used by Dr. Physick, which is known by the name of "*Dr. Physick's Issue Ointment.*" It is made by boiling half an ounce of powdered *cantharides* in two ounces of *rose-water,* and evaporating until one-half of the fluid is driven off, having previously added 15 grains of *tartar emetic.* The decoction is to be strained, and three ounces of *olive oil,* an ounce and a half of *white wax,* and one ounce of *spermaceti* added to it, and the mixture then boiled till all the water is evaporated.

UNGUENTUM MELANICUM CAUSTICUM, Causticum Æthiopicum.

UNGUENTUM MERCURIALE ALBUM, Unguentum hydrargyri præcipitati albi — u. Mercuriale citrinum, Unguentum hydrargyri nitratis—u. e Mercurio præcipitato, Unguentum hydrargyri præcipitati albi — u. Mercurii rubrum, Unguentum hydrargyri nitrico-oxydi—u. Mundificans Zelleri, Unguentum hydrargyri præcipitati albi.

UNGUENTUM MEZ'EREI, Ointment *of Mezereon.* (*Mezer.* incis. transversim, ℥iv; *adipis,* ℥xiv; *ceræ albæ,* ℥ij; moisten the mezereon with a little alcohol, and beat in an iron mortar, until reduced to a fibrous mass; then digest it with the lard, in a salt-water bath, for 12 hours; strain forcibly, and allow the strained liquor to cool slowly, so that any undissolved matters may subside; from these separate the medicated lard; melt it with the wax at a moderate heat, and stir constantly till they are cold. Ph. U. S.) To keep open blisters, issues, &c.

UNGUENTUM MURIA'TIS HYDRARGYRI OXYGENA'TO MEDICA'TUM, *Adeps muria'tē hydrargyri oxygena'to medica'tus, Cyrillo's* Ointment, (F.) *Pommade de Cyrillo.* (*Hydrar. oxymur.* 4 p.; *adipis suillæ præp.* 32 p.— Ph. P.) Antivenereal and alterative. Used in friction, ʒss at a time.

UNGUENTUM NARDINUM, see Nardus Indica— u. Neapolitanum, Unguentum hydrargyri — u. Nervinum, Unguentum Sambuci — u. Nitricum vel oxygenatum, Unguentum acidi nitrosi.

UNGUENTUM OPHTHAL'MICUM, *Adeps ox'ido hydrargyri rubro et plumbi aceta'tē medica'tus, Regent's Pommade ophthalmique,* (F.) *Pommade ophthalmique.* (*Butyr. recent., aq. rosar. lavat.* 4½ p.; *camphor., oxyd. hydrarg. rubr., acetatis plumbi,* āā 0.25 p. Mix intimately.—Ph. P.) In chronic inflammation of the conjunctiva or tarsi.

UNGUENTUM OPHTHALMICUM, Unguentum oxidi zinci impuri—u. Ophthalmicum rubrum, Unguentum hydrargyri nitrico-oxydi.

UNGUENTUM OX'IDI HYDRARGYRI CINE'REI, *Adeps* seu *Unguentum ex hydrargyro mit'iss dotum cinereum,* Ointment *of gray oxide of mercury,* (F.) *Onguent gris.* (*Oxyd. hydrarg. ciner.* p.j; *adipis suilli,* p. iij. — Ph. E.) Properties like the mercurial ointment. It is not much used.

UNGUENTUM OX'IDI PLUMBI ALBI, *Ung. ceruleæ, Ung. album, Ung. subaceta'tis plumbi,* Ointment *of white oxide of lead,* White ointment. (*simplicis,* p. v; *oxyd. plumb. alb.* p. j.—Ph. L. and P.) Cooling and desiccative. Applied to excoriated and burnt surfaces.

UNGUENTUM OXIDI PLUMBI CARBONATI, Plumbi subcarbonatis — u. Oxidi zinci, Unguentum zinci.

UNGUENTUM OX'IDI ZINCI IMPU'RI, *Unguentum tu'tiæ, Ung. ophthal'micum, Eye-salve, Adeps ex'idi zinci medica'tus, Tutty ointment, Ointment of impure oxide of zinc.* (*Linim. simpl.* p. v; *oxid. zinc. imp. præp.* p. j.— Ph. E.) Generally used in ophthalmia tarsi and atonic ophthalmia.

UNGUENTUM PICIS LIQ'UIDÆ, *Ung. Picis, e Picē, Tar* Ointment. (*Picis liquid., acri,* ℔j. Melt, and stir till cold.) Stimulant and detergent. Used in tinea capitis, and other cutaneous eruptions.

UNGUENTUM PICIS NIGRÆ, Unguentum resinæ nigræ — u. Plumbi acetatis, Ceratum plumbi superacetatis — u. Plumbi carbonatis, Unguentum plumbi subcarbonatis — u. Plumbi oxydi carbonati, Unguentum plumbi subcarbonatis—u. Plumbi subacetatis, Unguentum oxidi plumbi albi—u. Plumbici carbonatis, Unguentum plumbi subcarbonatis.

UNGUENTUM PLUMBI SUBCARBONA'TIS, *Unguenti carbona'tis, Cera'tum de cerus'ā, Ung. a'cetis U. album simplex, U. carbona'tis plumbici, Unguent. ceruseæ, U. oxidi plumbi carbona'ti,* (F.) *Ongue*nt *blanc de Rhases, O. de ceruse, O. de Rhases.* (*Plumbi carbonat.* in pulv. subtiliss. ʒj; *Unguent. simpl.* ℔j. Add the carbonate of lead to the ointment previously softened over a gentle fire, and mix.— Ph. U. S.) Chiefly used as a dressing for burns.

UNGUENTUM PLUMBI SUPERACETA'TIS, *Unguenta'tis plumbi,* Ointment *of sugar of lead, Unguentum saturni'num, U. ceruseæ aceta'tæ, Balsamum universa'lē.* (*Olive oil,* ℔ss; *white wax,* ℥ss; *superacetate of lead,* ℥ij.) Cooling, desiccative. Called, also, *Balsamum saturni'num, Butyrum satur'ni, Linimen'tum plumba'tum, Poma'tum satur'ni, Ung. triphar'macum.*

UNGUENTUM POPULE'UM, *Adeps papav'erē hyoscy'amo, et belladon'nā medica'tus.* (Fresh *buds* of the *populus nigra,* 500 p., macerated in *olive suillus præp.* melted, 1500 p., for 24 hours. Preserve this. Take *black poppy leaves, belladonna hyoscyamus, black nightshade,* āā 128 p.; bruise in a mortar with the former preparation until all the humidity is evaporated, and strain.— Ph. P.) Anodyne. Applied to local inflammations, hemorrhoids, sore nipples, cancer, &c. Green elder ointment is often sold for this.

UNGUENTUM POPULEUM, see Populus.

UNGUENTUM POTAS'SÆ HYDRIODA'TIS, *Unguenta'sii io'didi,* Ointment *of hydri'odate of potass. (Potass. iodid.* in pulv. subtil. ʒj; *ag. ferv.* fʒj; *adipis,* ℥j. Dissolve the iodide in the water and mix the solution with the lard.— Ph. L.) Half a drachm of this ointment is rubbed on scrofulous glands, goitre, &c.

UNGUENTUM POTASSII IODIDI, Unguentum Potassæ

tassæ Hydriodatis — u. Pulvis meloes vesicatorii, Cerate of cantharides—u. Resinæ flavæ, Ceratum resinæ flavæ.

UNGUENTUM RESI'NÆ NIGRÆ, *Ung. resinæ nigrum, Ung. basil'icon nigrum, Ung. tetrapharm'acum, Black basilicon, Black resin ointment, Unguentum picis nigræ.* (*Resin. nigr., ceræ flavæ, resinæ flav.* āā ʒix; *olei olivæ,* Oj.—Ph. L. *Uses,* the same as the *Ceratum resinæ* or *Yellow basilicon.*

UNGUENTUM RESINÆ PINI SYLVESTRIS COMPOSITUM, Unguentum de Althææ—u. Resinosum, Ceratum resinæ flavæ — u. Resumptivum, Unguentum de althææ.

UNGUENTUM SABINÆ, Ceratum Sabinæ.

UNGUENTUM SAMBU'CI, *Ung. sambu'cinum, Green ointment, Unguentum nervi'num, Elder ointment,* (F.) *Onguent de sureau.* (*Sambuci flor.* ℔ij; *adipis præp.* ℔ij. Boil.— Ph. L. and D.) Emollient.

UNGUENTUM SATURNINUM, Unguentum plumbi superacetatis—u. ad Scabiem Zelleri, Unguentum hydrargyri præcipitati albi—u. Simplex, Ceratum Galeni, Unguentum ceræ — u. Solidum de cicutâ, Emplastrum cicutæ — u. Spermatis ceti, Unguentum cetacei.

UNGUENTUM STRAMO'NII, *Ointment of Stramo'nium.* (*Ext. stramon. fol.* ʒj; *adipis,* ʒj. Rub the extract with a little water until uniformly soft, and then with the lard.— Ph. U. S.) An anodyne ointment to irritable ulcers, hemorrhoids, &c.

UNGUENTUM SUBACETA'TIS CUPRI, *U. cupri subaceta'tis* (Ph. U. S.), *Ung. deter'gens, Ung. basil'icum vir'idè, Ung. æru'ginis, Bal'samum viridè, Ointment of subacetate of copper, Ver'digris ointment.* (*Cupri subacet.* in pulv. subtiliss. ʒj; *ung. simpl.* ʒxv. Add the subacetate to the ointment previously melted with a moderate heat, and stir till cold.— Ph. U. S.) Detergent and escharotic.

UNGUENTUM SULPHURA'TUM AD SCA'BIEM, *Adeps sul'phurē et ammo'niæ muria'tē medica'tus.* (*Adipis,* 120 p.; *sulph. lot.* 60 p.; *ammoniæ muriat., aluminæ sulphat.* āā 4 p.; fiat unguentum.— Ph. P.) Antipsoric.

Bailey's Itch Ointment is composed of *olive oil, lard, nitre, alum, sulphate of zinc,* and *cinnabar;* scented with *oil of aniseed, oil of origanum,* and *oil of spike,* and coloured with *alkanet-root.*

UNGUENTUM SULPHURA'TUM ALCALI'NUM AD SCA'BIEM, *Adeps sul'phurē et carbona'tē potassæ medica'tus, Hel'merick's Alcaline Sulphura'ted Itch Ointment.* (*Adip. præp.* 800 p.; *sulphur. lot.* 200 p.; *carbonat. potass. pur.* 100 p.; fiat ung.— Ph. P.) Use, same as the last.

Bateman's Itch Ointment resembles this. It is coloured with *cinnabar,* and scented with *essence of bergamot.*

UNGUENTUM SUL'PHURIS, *Ung. e sulph'urē, Sulphur ointment.* (*Sulph.* ℔j; *adip.* ℔ij. — Ph. U. S.) Used chiefly in itch, and some herpetic affections.

UNGUENTUM SULPHURIS COMPOS'ITUM, *Compound Sulphur Ointment, Itch Ointment, Unguentum Antipsor'icum, Jackson's Itch Ointment, Pommade Antipsorique de Jasser.* (*Sulph. sublim.* ℔ss; *veratri rad.* contus. ʒij; *potassæ nitrat.* ʒj; *saponis mollis,* ℔ss; *adipis,* ℔ss; *ol. bergamot.* ℟xxx. — Ph. L.) The UNGUENTUM SULPHURIS COMPOSITUM of the Pharm. U. S., is made as follows:—*Sulphur.* ʒj; *hydrargyri ammoniat., acid. benzoic.* āā ʒj; *ol. bergamot., acid. sulphuric.* āā fʒj; *potassæ nitrat.* ʒij; *adipis,* ℔ss. To the melted lard add the other ingredients, and stir till cold. Use, the same as the last; but it is more stimulating.

UNGUENTUM SULPHE'URIS IOD'IDI, *Ointment of Iodide of Sulphur.* (*Sulphur. iodid.* ʒss; *adipis,* ʒj. Rub the iodide with a little of the lard; add the remainder, and mix.—Ph. U. S.) An excellent application in chronic cutaneous affections.

UNGUENTUM SUBINUM, Crinomyron.

UNGUENTUM TAB'ACI, *Tobacco Ointment.* (*Tabac. recent.* concis. ʒj; *adipis,* ℔j. Boil the tobacco in the lard, over a gentle fire, till it becomes friable; then strain through linen. — Ph. U. S.) Applied to irritable ulcers, tinea capitis, &c.

UNGUENTUM TARTARI EMETICI, U. antimonii tartarizati — u. Tartari stibiati, U. antimonii tartarizati — u. e Tartaro potassæ stibiati, U. antimonii tartarizati — u. Tartratis potassæ stibiati, U. antimonii tartarizati — u. de Terebinthinâ et adipibus, U. elemi compositum — u. de Terebinthinâ et cerâ, U. de althææ — u. Terebinthinæ et ovorum vitelli, U. digestivum simplex—u. Tetrapharmacum, Basilicon, U. resinæ nigræ — u. Tripharmacum, U. plumbi superacetatis — u. Tutiæ, U. oxidi sinci impuri.

UNGUENTUM VERA'TRI, *U. V. albi, Unguentum helleb'ori albi, White hellebore ointment.* (*Veratr.* pulv. ʒij; *adipis,* ʒviij; *olei limon.* ℟xx.) Used in cases of itch, where sulphur is objected to. It is not equally efficacious.

The principal ingredients in the EDINBURGH OINTMENT are *white hellebore* and *muriate of ammonia.*

UNGUENTUM AD VESICATA, U. lyttæ—u. ad Vesicatoria, Cerate of cantharides — u. Vesicatorium.

UNGUENTUM ZINCI, *Ung. ox'idi sinci, U. sinci oxidi* (Ph. U. S.), *Zinc ointment.* (*Zinci oxid.* ʒj; *adipis,* ʒvj. Use, the same as that of the *Unguentum tutiæ.*

UNGUENTUM ZINCI OXIDI, U. zinci.

UNGUIS, Hippocampus minor, Nail, Pterygion—u. Avis, Hippocampus minor—u. Halleri, Hippocampus minor — u. Odoratus, Blatta Byzantia.

UNGUIS OS, *Os lachryma'lē.* A small, quadrilateral, very thin, and semi-transparent bone, which has been compared to a human *nail,* and is situate at the anterior and inner part of the orbit. It aids in the formation of the lachrymal gutter and the nasal duct. It is articulated with the frontal, superior maxillary, ethmoid, and inferior spongy bones, and is developed by a single *punctum ossificationis.*

UNGULA CABALLINA, Tussilago.

UNGULÆ PALPEBRARUM, see Tarsus.

UNILOC'ULAR, *Unilocula'ris,* from *unus,* 'one,' and *loculus,* 'a cell.' Having one cell or cavity, as *Biloc'ular* means having two cells or cavities; *multiloc'ular,* having many.

UNIO, Pearl.

UNIOCULUS, Cyclops, Monoculus.

UNIPARIENS, Uniparous.

UNIPARIENT, Uniparous.

UNIP'AROUS, *Unipa'rient, Unipariens,* from *unus,* 'one,' and *pario,* 'I bring forth.' Producing one at a birth.

UNISE'MA DELTIFO'LIA, *Pontede'ria corda'ta, Shovel Pickereelweed, Pond Shovel, Shovelleaf, Water Plantain.* An indigenous plant, Ord. Pontederiaceæ, *Sex. Syst.* Hexandria Monogynia, which grows in water, and flowers from June to August. The root is emollient and astringent.

UNI'TING BANDAGE, (F.) *Bandage unissant.* A bandage for bringing the edges of a wound into approximation. The arrangement of such a bandage differs according as the wound is transverse or longitudinal.

UNIVOCAL GENERATION, see Generation.

UNOCULUS, *Borgne,* Cyclops, Monoculus.

UNORGANIZED, Inorganic.

UNSTRIPED MUSCULAR FIBRE, see Muscular fibre.

UNWELL, see Menstruation.

UPAS. A word used in the Archipelagos of Molucca and Sunda, and signifying *Vegetable Poison, Ipo, Bohon Upas, Boa Upas, Pohon Antiar, Boon Upas*. A substance used by the natives of those places for poisoning their arrows. The smallest quantity is capable of destroying the largest animal. The tree which produces it is said to be the *Antia'ris Toxica'ria*. Another species of upas, the *U. Tieuté*, is the produce of a *Strychnos*. Many idle stories are told regarding the upas, most of which are fabulous.

U'RACHUS, *U'racus, Urinac'ulum*, from ουρον, 'urine,' and εχω, 'I contain.' (F.) *Ouraque*. The urachus, in certain animals, is a long membranous canal, which arises from the bladder, makes its exit from the abdomen by the umbilicus, and terminates in the pouch called *allantois*. According to Sabatier, this is the arrangement of the urachus in the human fœtus; but Bichat and other anatomists consider, that when the canal exists in it, it is a malformation. They regard it as a kind of suspensory ligament of the bladder, extending from the top of that organ to the umbilicus; and, at the umbilicus, confounded with the abdominal aponeurosis.

URACRATIA, Enuresis.

URACUS, Urachus.

URÆ'MIA, from ουρον, 'urine,' and 'αιμα, 'blood.' A condition of the blood in which it contains urine or urea.

URALI, Curare.

URANA, Ureter.

URANE, Urinal.

URANISCONI'TIS, from ουρανισκος, 'the palate,' and *itis*, denoting inflammation. *Palati'tis*. Inflammation of the palate.

URANISCOPLAS'TICÉ, from ουρανισκος, 'the roof of the mouth,' and πλαστικος, 'forming.' The operation of engrafting in case of deficiency of the soft palate.

URANISCORRHAPHIA, Staphylorraphy.

URANISCOS, Palate.

URANORRHAPHIA, Staphylorraphy.

URAPOSTE'MA, *Absces'sus urino'sus, Urasde'ma*. A tumefaction produced by the escape of urine. An abscess containing urine.

URARI, Curare.

URAS, Urate.

URATE, *Uras, Lithate, Lithas*; from ουρον, 'urine.' A generic name for salts, formed by the combination of uric or lithic acid with different bases. *Urate* or *Lithate of Soda* is found in arthritic calculi :— *Urate* or *Lithate of Ammo'nia* in some urinary calculi.

URE'A, *Uron, Uren'ium, U'ricum, Mate'ria urino'sa,. Princip'ium seu Sal urino'sum*, (F.) *Urée*. Same etymon. A white, pearly, brilliant substance, in transparent plates, inodorous, and of a cool taste; very soluble in water; deliquescent, and soluble in alcohol. It exists, in great quantity, in the urine; and is an essential part of it. It has been used as a diuretic. Dose, gr. xv to ʒj.

UREC'CHYSIS, *Urech'ysis*, from ουρον, 'urine,' and εκχυσις, 'effusion.' Effusion of urine into the cellular membrane.

UREDO, Urticaria.

URÉE, Urea.

UREMA, Urine.

UREN, Urea.

URENIUM, Urea.

URENS, Caustic.

UREORRHŒA, Diabetes.

URESIÆSTHESIS, Diuresiæsthesis.

URESIS, Micturition.

URE'TER. Same etymon as Urate. *Urus, Vena alba renum, Cana'lis ner'veus fistulo[sus?] num, Ductus seu Ductor Uri'næ, Vas urinarium*, (F.) *Uretère*. A long, excretory canal—membranous and cylindrical—which conveys the urine from the kidney to the bladder. It enters obliquely, between the pelvis of the kidney, viz. which it is continuous, and the base fond of the bladder, into which it opens. It enters at the posterior and inferior part, for some distance between the coats, and opens into the cavity of the bladder, at the posterior angle of the *[tri-?]vesical*. The ureter is formed of an external, white, opake, and fibrous membrane; and of a inner, which is mucous.

URETERAL'GIA, from ουρητηρ, 'the ureter,' and αλγος, 'pain.' Pain in the course of the ureter,—as from calculus, *Ureteral'gia calc[ulosa?]*

URETERALGIA CALCULOSA, see *Ureteralgia*. u. Inflammatoria, Ureteritis.

URETÈRE, Ureter.

URETER'ICUS. An epithet for ischury, &c. arising from an affection of the ureter.

URETERI'TIS, *Ureteral'gia infl[am]matoria, Ureterophlegma'sia*. Inflammation of the ureter generally caused by calculus.

URETERO-LITH'ICUS, from ουρητηρ, 'the ureter,' and λιθος, 'a stone.' An epithet applied to ischury or other affection caused by a stone in the ureter.

URETEROL'ITHUS. Same etymon. Calculus in the ureter.

URETEROPHLEGMASIA, Ureteritis.

URETERO-PHLEGMAT'ICUS, from ουρητηρ, 'the ureter,' and φλεγμα, 'phlegm or mucus.' Any affection caused by mucus accumulated in the ureter.

URETERO-PY'ICUS, from ουρητηρ, 'the ureter,' and πυον, 'pus.' An epithet applied to affections caused by the presence of pus in the ureter.

URETERORRHAG"IA, from ουρητηρ, 'the ureter,' and ρηγη, 'rupture.' Hemorrhage from the ureter.

URETERO-STOMAT'ICUS, from ουρητηρ, 'the ureter,' and στομα, 'orifice.' That which is dependent upon obstruction of the orifice of the ureter.

URETERO-THROMBOI'DES, from ουρητηρ, 'the ureter,' θρομβος, 'grumous blood,' and ειδος, 'resemblance.' Ischury from grumous blood in the ureter.

URE'THRA, ουρηθρα, *Cana'lis seu Mea'tus Ductus urina'rius, Urias, Ure'tra, Fis'tula urinaria, Iter urina'rium seu Uri'næ*; (F.) *Urètre*, from ουρον, 'urine.' The excretory canal for the urine in both sexes; and for the sperm in man. In the latter, it is 8 or 10 inches long. It extends from the neck of the bladder to the extremity of the penis, in which its external aperture is situate. In the male urethra, three portions are distinguished :—1. *A Prostatic portion*, near the bladder, about an inch and a quarter in length, which traverses the prostate gland:— 2. *A membranous portion, Isthmus ure'thræ Pars ure'thra membrana'cea*, from 8 to 10 lines long, which is separated from the rectum by the cellular tissue only :—3. *A spongy portion*, which expands, anteriorly, to form the glans, and commences at the *bulb of the urethra*. Before opening externally, the canal has a dilatation called the *Fossa* or *Fossic'ula navicula'ris*. In the interior of the urethra two white lines are perceptible—the one above, the other below. The latter commences at the *verumontanum*, and at the surface of this, the *ejaculatory* and *prostatic ducts* open. The urethra is lined, in its whole extent, by a mucous membrane; on which are seen, particularly at the bulb, the orifices of a number of follicular ducts, *Lacunæ* or *Sinuses of Morgagni*. At about an inch and a half from the opening of the meatus, one of these lacunæ is generally found, much larger than the rest, and is named *Lacuna Magna*. The arteries of the urethra are numerous, and proceed from the internal pudic, — the largest branches entering the bulb. The veins follow the course of the arteries. The lymphatics pass into the inguinal and hypôgastric plexuses. The nerves come from the pudic and gluteal. In the *female*, the urethra is only about an inch long. It is wider than in man, and susceptible of great dilatation. It is very wide at its commencement; and descends obliquely forwards, to terminate at the top of the external aperture of the vagina by the *mea'tus urina'rius*. In its course, it is slightly curved, the concavity being forwards.

URETHRA, BLIND DUCTS OF THE, see Cæcus — u. Mucous lacunæ of the, see Cæcus.

URE'THRAL, *Urethra'lis. Ure'thricus*, from ουρηθρα, 'the urethra.' Relating to the urethra.

URETHRAL'GIA, from ουρηθρα, 'the urethra,' and αλγος, 'pain.' Pain in the urethra. Gonorrhœa.

URÈTHRE, Urethra.

URETHREMPHRAXIS, Urethrophraxis.

URETHRITIS, Gonorrhœa.

URETHROBLENNORRHŒ'A, from ουρηθρα, 'the urethra,' βλεννα, 'mucus,' and ρεω, 'I flow.' Gonorrhœa; gleet.

URETHROCYSTAUCHENOTOMIA, see Lithotomy.

URETHROCYSTEOANEURYSMATOTOMIA, see Lithotomy.

URETHROCYSTEOTRACHELOTOMIA, see Lithotomy.

URETHROHÆMORRHAGIA, Urethrorrhagia.

URETHROPHRAX'IS, *Urethremphrax'is*, from ουρηθρα, 'the urethra,' and φρασσω, 'I obstruct.' Obstruction of the urethra.

URETHROPLAS'TIC, *Urethroplas'ticus*; from ουρηθρα, 'the urethra,' and πλασσω, 'I form.' An epithet given to the operation *urethroplasty* which supplies defects in the canal of the urethra through which the urine escapes.

URETHRORRHA'GIA, *Urethrohæmorrha'gia, Caulorrha'gia stillatit"ia, Hæmatu'ria stillatit"ia*, from ουρηθρα, 'the urethra,' and ρηγνυμι, 'I break out.' Hemorrhage from the urethra. Frank.

URETHRORRHŒ'A, from ουρηθρα, 'the urethra,' and ρεω, 'I flow.' A discharge of any kind from the urethra.

URETHROSTENO'SIS, *Strictu'ra ure'thræ, Urosteno'sis*, from ουρηθρα, 'the urethra,' and στενωσις, 'narrowness.' Stricture of the urethra.

URETHROT'OMUS, (F.) *Uréthrotome*, from ουρηθρα, 'the urethra,' and τεμνω, 'I cut.' An instrument so called by Le Cat, with which he divided the skin, and laid open the urethra, in the operation for lithotomy. Also, an instrument for dividing strictures of the urethra.

URETHROT'OMY, *Urethrotom'ia*; same etymon. An operation, which consists in opening the urethra for the removal of stricture. See *Boutonnière*.

URETHRYMENO'DES, from ουρηθρα, 'the urethra,' and 'υμην, 'a membrane.' That which is caused by a membrane formed in the urethra.

URETICUS, Diuretic, Urinary.

URETRA, Urethra.

URÈTRE, Urethra.

URETRIS, Urinal.

URIAS, Fistula, (urinary,) Urethra.

URIASIS, Lithia, Uresis.

URIC ACID, *Ac"idum u'ricum, Ac"idum urolith'icum, Acidum lith'icum, Lithic Acid, Urylic Acid*. An acid which exists in human urine, chiefly, if not wholly, in the form of urate of soda or urate of ammonia, and which in combination constitutes the greater part of urinary calculi. It is often deposited from the urine in health. See Calculi, urinary.

URIC OXIDE, *Ox'idum u'ricum, Xanthic oxide, Xanthine, Urous acid*. A substance not discovered in healthy urine, although probably bearing some relation to the yellow colouring matter. It is a very rare ingredient of calculous concretions, and little is known either of its chemical or pathological history.

URICUM, Urea.

URICUS, Urinary.

URINA CEREBELLA, see Cerebella—u. Chyli, see Urine — u. Cibi, see Urine — u. Diabetica, Urine, diabetic — u. Febrilis, Urine, febrile — u. Furfuracea, see Furfuraceous—u. Galactodes, see Galactodes—u. Genitalis, Sperm—u. Jumentosa seu Jumentaria, Urine, jumentous — u. Mucosa, Cystirrhœa — u. Nephelodes, see Nepheloid — u. Oroboides seu Orobodes, see Oroboides — u. Pericardii, see Pericardium — u. Potûs, see Urine — u. Sanguinis, see Urine—u. Vaccæ, Urine, cows'.

URINACULUM, Urachus, Urinal.

URINÆ PROFLUVIUM, Diabetes — u. Suppressio, Ischuria—u. Stillicidium, Strangury—u. Substillum, Strangury.

U'RINAL, *Urinato'rium, Chernib'ium, U'rané, Ure'tris, Urinac'ulum, Urodochi'um, Urod'oché, Urodoche'um, Uratra'cium, Matra'cium, Mat'ula, Matel'la*; from *urina*, 'urine.' A name given, 1. To certain vessels, used to pass the urine into. 2. To reservoirs, of different shapes and character, which are adapted to the penis, in cases of incontinence of urine, and which are intended to receive the urine as it flows off.

URINALIS, Diuretic, Urinary.

URINARIA, Antirhinum linaria, Leontodon taraxacum.

U'RINARY, *Urina'rius, Urina'lis, Urino'sus, U'ricus, Uret'icus*. Same etymon. That which relates to the urine.

URINARY BLADDER, *Vesi'ca Urina'ria, Cystis, Urocys'tis*, (F.) *Vessie*. A musculo-membranous reservoir, intended for the reception of the urine, until the accumulation of a certain quantity solicits its excretion. The bladder is situate in the hypogastric region, between the rectum and pubis in man; and between the pubis and vagina in the female. Its upper region is not covered, except by the peritoneum, posteriorly. From its centre arises the *urachus*. Its lower region is bounded, anteriorly, by the prostate, in man; and rests on the vesiculæ seminales and rectum. In the female, it corresponds to the vagina. The lowest portion of this region bears the name *Bas-fond*. The anterior surface of the organ is not covered by peritoneum. It is attached to the symphysis pubis by a fibro-cellular expansion called the *anterior ligament*. The posterior ligaments are duplicatures of the peritoneum on its posterior surface, which extend from this surface to the rectum in the male, and to the uterus in the female. The bladder is composed of a serous membrane, formed by the peritoneum;—of a muscular membrane; of a somewhat thick layer of areolar tissue; and is lined on its inner surface, by a mucous membrane, which is, sometimes, raised up, here and there, in long prominences or *columnæ* by the muscular fibres beneath. To this condition, the French anatomists give the term—*vessie à colonnes*. In the *bas-fond* the two ureters open, and the urethra commences; and the triangular space, which the apertures of these three canals leave between them, is called, by the French, the *Trigône vésical* or *Vesical Triangle, Trigo'nus seu Trigo'num vesi'cæ seu Lieutau'di*. In the orifice of the urethra, which is also called the neck of the bladder, there is, at its lower part, a more or less prominent tubercle, which is formed by the anterior angle of the *Trigone vésical*, and is called the *Vesical uvula, U'vula vesi'cæ*, (F.) *Luette vésicale*.

The arteries of the bladder proceed from the hypogastric, umbilical, sciatic, middle hemorrhoidal, and internal pudic. Its veins, which are more numerous than the arteries, open into the hypogastric venous plexus. Its nerves emanate from the sciatic and hypogastric plexuses; and its lymphatic vessels pass into the hypogastric ganglia.

URINARY CALCULI. The calculi which form in the urinary passages. See Calculi, urinary.

URINARY PASSAGES, (F.) *Voies urinaires*. The aggregate of canals and cavities intended to contain the urine and convey it externally. These *ways* are composed of excretory ducts, which form the tubular portion of the kidney; of calices; pelvis; ureters; bladder; and urethra.

URINATORIUM, Urinal.

URINE, *Uri'na, U'ron, Ure'ma, Lot'ium, Lot, Lapis au'reus, Omich'ma, Recremen'ta seu Retrimen'ta vesi'cæ, Aqua pedum, Aqua*. An excrementitial fluid; secreted by the cortical part of the kidney; filtered through the tubular portion; poured *guttatim* from the apices of the tubular papillæ into the pelvis of the kidney; and transmitted by it to the ureters; which convey it slowly, but in a continuous manner, into the bladder, where it remains deposited, until its accumulation excites a desire to void it. The excretion of the fluid takes place through the urethra; and is caused by the action of the abdominal muscles and diaphragm and the contraction of the fibrous coat of the bladder. Urine is transparent; of a citron-yellow colour; of a peculiar odour, and of an acid, saline, and slightly bitter taste. That which is passed some time after taking fluid, is less coloured, and less odorous and dense than that which is voided 7 or 8 hours after eating. The first is the *Uri'na potûs*, (F.) *Urine de la Boisson, Urine from drink*:— the latter *Uri'na san'guinis*, (F.) *Urine de la digestion, Urine de la coction, Urine cuite, Oocted urine, Urine of digestion*. Three distinct varieties of urine may, according to Dr. Golding Bird, be recognised: *First*. That passed some little time after drinking freely of fluids, which is generally pale, and of low specific gravity—1.003 to 1.009—*Urina potûs*. *Secondly*, That secreted after the digestion of a full meal; s. g. 1.020 to 1.028, or even 1.030 —*Urina chyli* vel *cibi*. *Thirdly*, That secreted independently of the immediate stimulus of food and drink, as after a night's rest, which is usually of average density—1.015 to 1.025, and presents the essential characters of urine—*Urina sanguinis*.

The following are the ordinary constituents of healthy human urine:—urea, uric acid, [hippuric acid;] extractive matters, embracing alcohol extract, spirit extract, and water extract, with their respective constituents; mucus; brown colouring matter of the urine, (hæmaphæin;) red colouring matter of the urine, (uroërythrin;) carbonic, lactic, hydrochloric, sulphuric, phosphoric, silicic, and hydrofluoric acids; soda; potassa; ammonia: lime; magnesia; and peroxide of iron. The proportion of solid matters in 1000 parts of urine may vary from 20 to 70. The following table expresses the relative amounts of the different components in every 100 parts of the solid matter, according to the analysis of different observers:

	Berzelius	Lehmann	Simon	Marchand
Urea,	45.10	49.68	32.50	4.91
Uric Acid,	1.50	1.61	1.40	1.2
Extractive matter, Ammonia, Salts, and Chloride of Sodium,	36.30	28.25	42.99	2.6
Alkaline Sulphates,	10.30	11.58	8.14	10.19
Alkaline Phosphates,	6.88	5.96	6.58	4.7
Phosphates of lime and magnesia,	1.50	1.97	1.50	1.21

Its average specific gravity is about 1.015. Its quantity passed by the adult in the 24 hours varies. On the average it may amount to two pounds and a half. Sometimes, the urine, in health and disease, exhibits appearances that have received special names. Thus, that which is characterized by a deficiency of solid matter generally, has been called *Hydru'ria*, ('water;') by a deficiency of urea, *Anazotu'ria*, (a privative, and *azote*;) by a superabundance of urea, *Azotu'ria*. Urine in which the deposit consists of lithic acid, and the lithates, has been termed *Lithu'ria*; and that in which the deposit consists of the earthy and earthy-alkaline phosphates, *Phosphu'ria Ceramu'ria*, (κεραμος, 'potter's earth,') &c. &c. At times, a *pellicle* forms on the surface (*Cremor urinæ*) which consists of mucus and some salts: at others, there is a cloud, (*nubec'ula, nubes*,) towards its upper part, which is called *Eneore'ma* when it is suspended, as it were, about the middle of the liquid. Occasionally, there is a sediment, to which the names *Hypos'tasie, Sedimen'tum*, &c., have been given. (see these various words.) The urine is often deserving of attention in disease; but it has been considered a matter of more importance than it merits. Some empirics have presumed to pronounce on the nature of disease by simply inspecting it. See Uroscopy.

Human urine was, at one time, considered aperient; and was given in jaundice, in the dose of one or two ounces. Cow's urine, *Urina Vacca, Allflower water*, was once used, warm from the cow, as a purge, in the dose of Oss.

Urine has been variously designated by pathologists, according to its appearance, &c.; for example:—

URINE, ANÆ'MIC, *Uri'na anæ'mica*. [Æd. ls not felicitously, for the form of urine that occurs in anæmia, chlorosis, &c.— Becquerel.

URINE ARDENTE, Ardent urine—u. Bloody, Hæmaturia—u. *de la Boisson*, Urine, hysterical see Urine—u. *de la Coction*, see Urine.

URINE, CRUDE, (F.) *Urine crue*. Urine that is thin, transparent, and but little coloured, affording neither cloud nor deposite.

URINE CRUE, Urine, crude— u. Cuite, see Urine.

URINE, CYSTINIC, *Cystinu'ria*. Urine containing cystine or cystic oxide in solution, or as a deposite.

URINE, DIABETIC, *Uri'na diabe'tica*. Urine passed in *Diabetes mellitus, Melitu'ria*. It contains a large quantity of sugar analogous to that of the grape, which may be separated in the form of crystals. In other respects, the urine is very abundant and very limpid in that affection.

URINE DE LA DIGESTION, see Urine.

URINE, DROP'SICAL, is an ammoniacal urine often containing much albumen and scarcely any urea.

URINE, DYSPEP'TIC, has been found to precipitate tannin abundantly, and to soon putrefy.

URINE ÉPAISSE, Urine, mucilaginous.

URINE, FEBRILE, *Uri'na febri'lis*. Urine discharged in inflammation and inflammatory fever.

URINE, FILAMENTOUS, see Filamentous.

URINE, FLOC'CULENT, (F.) *Urine floconneuse*, is when the fluid is troubled by flocculi, suspended in it.

URINE, FURFURA'CEOUS, see Furfuraceous—u. Floconneuse, Urine, flocculent—u. des Goutteux, Urine, gouty.

URINE, GOUTY, (F.) *Urine des goutteux*, contains much phosphate of lime, and, after severe attacks of gout, precipitates a mixture of the uric and rosacic acids.

URINE HUILEUSE, Urine, oily.

URINE, HYSTER'ICAL, is clear, colourless, and similar to the *Urine de la Boisson*.

URINE, ICTER'ICAL, contains bile.

URINE, INCONTINENCE OF, Enuresis.

URINE OF INFLAM'MATORY DISEASES. This is, generally, small in quantity, and very high-coloured.

URINE, INVOLUNTARY DISCHARGE OF, Enuresis.

URINE, JUMEN'TOUS, *Uri'na jumento'sa* seu *jumenta'ria*, (F.) *Urine Jumenteuse*. A term used, by the French, for ammoniacal urine, rendered turbid by a substance similar to small grains of dust, which causes it to resemble the urine of herbivorous animals.

URINE LACTESCENTE, U. milky—u. Laiteuse, Urine, milky.

URINE, MILKY, (F.) *Urine lactescente* ou *laiteuse*. White and troubled urine.

URINE, MUCILAG"INOUS, (F.) *Urine épaisse*. Urine containing much mucus.

URINE, NERVOUS. Thin and very liquid urine; such as is passed shortly after the attack of nervous diseases.

URINE OF NERVOUS FEVERS is generally very thin; and often deposits a mixture of uric and rosacic acids.

URINE, OILY, (F.) *Urine huileuse*, is that which pours like oil, or which has an oily pellicle at its surface.

URINE, OXAL'IC, *Oxalu'ria*. Urine containing a salt of the oxalic acid.

URINE, PHOSPHORES'CENT, *Phosphoru'ria, Phosphu'ria*. Urine which is luminous or phosphorescent.

URINE, PUR'PURIC, see Porphyruria.

URINE, RICK'ETY, contains much phosphate of lime.

URINE, SANDY, Arenosa urina—u. Stoppage of, Ischuria—u. Ténue, Urine, thin.

URINE, THIN, (F.) *Urine ténue*. Urine that is transparent, slightly coloured, and but little dense.

URINIF'EROUS, *Urinifer*, from ουρον, 'urine,' and *fero*, 'I carry.' That which carries urine.

URINIFEROUS SUBSTANCE OF THE KIDNEY, see Kidney.

URINIF'EROUS TUBES or DUCTS OF BELLI'NI, *Tu'buli vel duc'tus urinif'eri Belli'ni, Tu'buli Belli'ni, Bellinia'ni Ductus, Bellinia'næ Fis'tulæ*. The collection of small tubes, converging from the cortical part of the kidney to the apices of the papillæ.

URINODES, Urinous.

URINOM'ETER, from ουρον, 'urine,' and μετρον, 'measure.' A small hydrometer for taking the specific gravity of urine. The urinometer suggested by Dr. Prout is divided into 60 degrees, the zero being the point at which it floats in distilled water. The numbers on the scale added to 1000, the specific gravity of water, give the particular specific gravity: thus, supposing the number cut by the surface of the liquid to be 30, it would indicate a s. g. of 1.030. The letters H. S. on the back of the scale mean "healthy standard," which ranges from 10° to 20°.

U'RINOUS, *Urino'sus, Urino'des*. Having the character of urine. Similar to urine.

UROCE'LE, *Œde'ma scroti urino'sum, Uroscheoce'lè, Oscheoce'lè urina'lis*, from ουρον, 'urine,' and κηλη, 'a rupture.' A tumour of the scrotum, owing to the effusion of urine into the same, and into the areolar tissue.

UROCHES'IA, *Uroches'ia*, from ουρον, 'urine,' and χεζειν, 'to go to stool.' A discharge of urine by the bowels.

UROCRASIA, Enurosis.

UROCRIS'IA, from ουρον, 'urine,' and κρινω, 'I judge.' *Urocrite'rion*. A judgment formed either of the urine, or of disease after inspecting the urine.

UROCRITERION, Urocrisia.

UROCYSTIS, Urinary bladder.

UROCYSTITIS, Cystitis.

UROCYSTOCATARRHUS, Cystirrhœa.

URODIAL'YSIS, from ουρον, 'urine,' and διαλυσις, 'dissolution, loss of strength.' A partial and temporary suspension of the function of the kidney, such as occurs in the course of most acute diseases. A condition of the function of the kidney and of the urine, similar to that observed in acute diseases, but without local mischief or preceding inflammatory fever, has been termed, when occurring in children, *Urodial'ysis Neonato'rum*; in the aged, *Urodialysis Senum*.—Schönlein.

URODOCHIUM, Urinal.

URODYN'IA, from ουρον, 'urine,' and οδυνη, 'pain.' Pain during the excretion of the urine.

URŒDEMA, Urapostema.

UROGEN'ITAL, *Urogenita'lis, Gen'ito-u'rinary, Gen'ito-urina'rius*. Relating or appertaining to the urinary and genital apparatuses.

UROGENITAL SINUS, *Sinus uro-genita'lis*. A cavity or canal in the embryo of the mammalia opening externally, in which the excretory ducts of the Wolffian bodies, the ureters and the efferent parts of the generative apparatus, terminate internally. It is prolonged into the urachus. Subsequently it becomes separated by a process of division into a *pars urina'ria* and a *pars genita'lis*. The former, extending towards the urachus, is converted into the urinary bladder; whilst from the latter are formed the *vesiculæ seminales* in the male, and the middle portion of the uterus in the female.—J. Müller.

UROLITHI, Calculi, urinary.

UROLITHIASIS, Lithia.

UROLITHOLOG"IA; from ουρον, 'urine,' λιθος, 'a stone,' and λογος, 'a description.' A description of urinary calculi.

UROLITHOTOMIA, Lithotomy.

UROMANTI'A, from ουρον, 'urine,' and μαντεια, 'divination.' The art of divining diseases by simple inspection of the urine; *Urosco'pia*. One professing to be able to do this is called *Uroman'tes*. Vulgarly, a water-doctor.

UROMPH'ALUS, *Her'nia U'rachi*. A monstrosity, which consists in the protrusion of the urachus at the umbilicus.

URON, Urine.

URON'CUS, from ουρον, 'urine,' and ογκος, 'a swelling.' A urinary swelling.

URONOL'OGY, *Uronolog"ia*, from ουρον, 'urine,' and λογος, 'a description.' The part of medicine which treats of the urine.

UROPHTHISIS, Diabetes mellitus.

UROPLA'NIA, from ουρον, 'urine,' and πλανη, 'wandering.' The presence of urine in other parts than the urinary organs.

UROPOE'SIS, *Uropoïe'sis*, from ουρον, 'urine,' and ποιεω, 'I make.' *Secre'tio uri'næ* seu *lo'tii*. The secretion of urine by the kidney.

UROPOIESIS, Uropoesis.

UROPYGION, Coccyx.

UROPYGIUM, *Croupion.*
URORRHAGIA, Diabetes.
URORRHŒA, Enuresis, Diabetes.
UROSCHEOCELE, Urocele.
UROSCOPIA, see Uromantia.
URO'SES, from *ουρον*, 'urine.' Diseases of the urinary organs.—Alibert.
UROS'TEALITH, *Urosteal'ithos*, from *ουρον*, 'urine,' *στεαρ*, 'suet,' and *λιθος*, 'stone.' A peculiar fatty ingredient of urinary calculi, discovered by Heller.
UROSTENOSIS, Urethrostenosis.
UROUS ACID, Uric oxide.
UROZEMIA, Diabetes — u. Albuminosa, Kidney, Bright's disease of the—u. Mellita, Diabetes mellitus.
URTI'CA, *U. Dioi'ca* seu *major* seu *his'pida*, *Pyr'ethrum*, the *Common stinging nettle*, *Ad'icè*, (F.) *Ortie*. *Family*, Urticeæ. *Sex. Syst.* Monœcia Tetrandria. This plant has been long used for medical and culinary purposes. The young shoots, in the spring, are considered to possess diuretic and antiscorbutic properties.
URTICA BALEARICA, U. pilulifera — u. Dioica, Urtica — u. Hispida, Urtica — u. Iners magna fœtidissima, Galeopsis — u. Major, U. dioica — u. Minor, U. uréns — u. Mortua, Lamium album.
URTICA PILULIF'ERA, *Pill-bearing Nettle*, *U. Pilulo'sa* seu *Roma'na* seu *Balea'rica*, (F.) *Ortie Romaine*. The seed was formerly given in diseases of the chest.
URTICA PILULOSA, U. pilulifera—u. Roman, U. pilulifera.
URTICA URENS, *U. minor*, *Dwarf nettle*, (F.) *Ortie brulante*. A lesser variety of the nettle, possessing similar virtues.
Nettles have been used as stimulants to paralytic limbs.
URTICAIRE, Urticaria.
URTICA'RIA, from *urtica*, 'a nettle;' *Enanthe'sis urtica'ria*, *Ure'do*, *Scarlati'na urtica'ta*, *Cnido'sis*, *Urtica'ria porcell'ana*, *Exanthe'ma urtica'tum*, *Epinyc'tis prurigino'sa*, *Febris urtica'ta*, *Pur'pura urticata*, *Febris rubra prurigino'sa*, *Saltans rosa*, (F.) *Urticaire*, *Fièvre Ortie*, *Porcelaine*, *Nettle-rash;* vulgarly *Hives*, *Bold Hives;* from *urtica*, 'a nettle,' because the eruption resembles that produced by the stings of a nettle. A disease distinguished by those elevations of the cuticle called *wheals*. They have a white top, and are often surrounded by a diffuse redness. They excite intolerable itching, especially when the person is warm in bed. The eruption frequently goes and comes once or more in the 24 hours, and is generally dependent upon gastric derangement. In some people, nettle-rash is induced by shell-fish, eggs, nuts, &c. It is not usually a disease of any consequence, and its treatment is limited to the use of absorbent laxatives, and simple general means. Willan has described six varieties of the complaint;—*Urtica'ria febri'lis*, *U. evan'ida*, *U. perstans*, *U. confer'ta*, *U. subcuta'nea*, and *U. tubero'sa*.
URTICARIA PORCELLANA, Essera, Urticaria.
URTICA'TIO, *Cnido'sis*, *Urtica'tion*, from *urtica*, 'a nettle.' A sort of flagellation, with nettles;—used with the intention of exciting the skin.
URUCU, Terra Orleana.
URYLIC ACID, Uric acid.
USNEA, Lichen saxatilis — u. Florida hirta, Lichen plicatus — u. Hirta, Lichen plicatus — u. Plicata, Lichen plicatus
USSACU, Hura Braziliensis.
USTILAGO, Ergot.
USTIO, Burn, Ustion.
USTION, *Us'tio*, *Causis*, from *urere*, *ustum*, 'to burn.' The act of burning or of applying the actual cautery. Also the effect of cauterisation; a burn.

USTULA'TIO, *Ustula'tion*. A pharmaceutical operation by which a substance is dried by heat.
USUALIA, Officinals.
USUS, Habit.
UTER, Uterus.
UTERI ADSCENSUS, Hysteria—u. Antiversio, Hysteroloxia anterior—u. Carcinoma, Metrocarcinoma—u. Convulsivus morbus, Lorind mercis—u. Coryza, Leucorrhœa—u. Exulceratio, Hysterelcosis—u. Flexio, Hysteroloxia — u. Inclinatio, Hysteroloxia—u. Obliquitas, Hysteroloxia—u. Pronatio, Hysteroloxia anterior — u. Prurus Nymphomania — u. Reflexio completa, Hysteroloxia posterior — u. Retroversio, Hysteroloxia posterior — u. Rheuma, Leucorrhœa — u. Ulcus Hysterelcosis — u. Versio incompleta, Hysteroloxia.
U'TERINE, *Uteri'nus*, from *uterus*, 'the womb.' That which belongs or relates to the womb.
UTERINE ARTERY, *Arte'ria uteri'na hypogastrica*. Its size is always in a ratio with the greater or less state of development of the uterus. It arises from the hypogastric, either separately or with the umbilical, or from the interna, passes upon the lateral parts of the vagina, which it gives branches; and afterwards on the sides of the uterus, and divides into a considerable number of very tortuous branches which enter the tissue of the organ.
UTERINE MUSCLE OF RUYSCH consists of the fleshy fibres at the fundus of the uterus which he regarded as forming a particular muscle.
UTERI'NUS FRATER. In law, a brother by the mother's side.
UTERO-ABDOMINAL SUPPORTER, a Belt, Russian.
UTERO-GESTATION, Pregnancy.
UTEROMANIA, Nymphomania.
U'TERUS, *Uter*, *Utric'ulus*, *Loci*, *Luci*, *Umbres*, *Vulva*, *Venter*, *Arvum natu'ra*, *Cœnum*, *ulum*, *Matrix*, *Ager natu'ræ*, *Hys'tera*, *Stera*, *An'gus*, *Delphys*, *Alvus*, *Eporo*, *Gaster*, *Mater*, *Nedys*, *Postrema*, the *Womb*, *Matrice*, *Sein*. The uterus, destined to lodge the fœtus from the commencement of conception to birth, is a hollow symmetrical organ, having the shape of a truncated conoid: it is situate in the pelvis, between the bladder and the rectum, above the vagina, and below the convolutions of the small intestine. The uterus is flattened from fore to behind, and is nearly an inch in thickness. It is two inches broad at its highest part. It becomes narrower towards the vagina; terminating in a contracted portion, called the *cervix* or *neck*, to distinguish it from the rest of the organ called the *body*. From its *fundus* or upper portion, the Fallopian tubes pass off. The small cavity called *Os U'teri* or *Os Tincæ*. The cavity is very small, and its parietes are thick. The portion of the cavity corresponding with the body is triangular and flattened. Its superior angles present the extremely fine orifices of the Fallopian tubes. The cavity of the neck is slightly dilated towards opening into the vagina. The uterus is composed—
1. *Of a serous membrane*. This is external, furnished by the peritoneum; which is reflected upon the uterus from the posterior surface of the bladder and the anterior surface of the rectum. It forms, also, the *broad ligaments of the uterus*, *Ligamen'ta lata*, *Alæ vespertilio'nis*, *Retinæ uteri*. These contain, above, the Fallopian tubes; beneath and anteriorly, the round ligaments; and behind, the ovary. They are two membranous productions or duplicatures of the peritoneum sent from the edges of the uterus and passing to the extremity of the vagina, in a transverse direction to be fixed to, and line, the side of the pelvis.
2. *Of a mucous membrane*, which is a prolongation—

tion of that of the vagina, and extends into the tubes. 3. Of a *proper tissue*, whose thickness is considerable. It is of a close texture; is grayish and elastic; and resists the instrument that divides it. Its intimate nature is but little known. During gestation it is truly muscular. The arteries of the uterus proceed from the spermatic and hypogastric. Its veins follow the same course, and bear the same name as the arteries. They are very tortuous, and form large sinuses in the parietes of the organ, called *U'terine Si'nuses.* Its nerves proceed from the sciatic and hypogastric plexuses. Its lymphatic vessels are very multiplied; and during pregnancy acquire enormous dimensions. The changes experienced by the uterus during gestation, and after delivery, are very numerous and important to be known. They regard its situation, direction, size, shape, texture, connexions, vital properties, &c.

UTERUS, Abdomen — u. Anteversion of the, Hysteroloxia anterior.

UTERUS BIF'IDUS. A double uterus. One separated into two cavities.

UTERUS DUPLEX, Dihysteria — u. Hour-glass contraction of the, *Chaton* — u. Inclinatus, Hysteroloxia.

UTERUS, IR'RITABLE, *Neural'gia of the Uterus.* A disease characterized by deep-seated pain in the lower part of the abdomen, and in the back and loins; generally diminished by lying down, and increased by exercise, and more severe for a few days preceding and during menstruation. On examination *per vaginam,* the uterus is found to be tender on pressure; and the cervix and body slightly swollen, but not usually indurated. It is an obstinate affection, but frequently ends of itself after years of suffering. The treatment must be, — the horizontal posture; local bloodletting to the uterus; emollients; soothing injections; narcotics, warm bath, &c. See Hysteralgia.

UTERUS, INVERSION OF THE, *Inver'sio U'teri, Metranas'trophé, Ædopto'sis Uteri inver'sa,* (F.) *Inversion de la Matrice, Renversement de la Matrice.* The uterus, displaced and turned inside out. This can only happen through want of caution on the part of the medical practitioner. It is a fatal accident, unless speedily reduced. This must be done by gradually returning the superior part, by grasping it with the hand, and making the rest follow.

UTERUS MASCULINUS, see Ejaculatory ducts — u. Obliquus, Hysteroloxia — u. Retroversion of the, Hysteroloxia posterior.

UTERUS, RUPTURE OF THE, *Metrorrhex'is, Hysterorrhex'is, Ruptu'ra Uteri, Perfora'tio Uteri, Laceration of the Womb,* (F.) *Rupture de la Matrice.* This dreadful accident occurs during labour, and is known to have taken place, when the child's head suddenly recedes during a pain, with vomiting, sinking of the pulse, cold sweats, &c. When it is evident that this has occurred, the hand must be passed into the uterus, and the feet of the child be brought down.

Cases are on record, in which partial lacerations of the uterus have healed, and the patient has done well. This is a rare event, and not to be anticipated.

UTRICLE, see Semicircular canals.

UTRIC'ULAR, *Utricula'ris;* from *utriculus,* 'a small bag or bottle.' Relating to or resembling a small bag or bottle.

UTRICULAR GLANDS, *Glan'dulæ utricula'res.* The glands or follicles in the interior of the uterus, which are concerned in the formation of the decidua.

UTRICULUS, see Ejaculatory ducts, Uterus — u. Communis, see Semicircular canals — u. Lacteus, Receptaculum chyli.

UVA, Uvula, see Vitis vinifera — u. Inversa, Paris — u. Lupina, Paris — u. Ursi, see Arbutus uva ursi — u. Vulpina, Paris.

UVÆ CORINTHIACÆ, see Vitis Corinthiaca.

UVÆ PASSÆ, *Rhages, Dried Grapes, Raisins,* see Vitis vinifera.

UVÆ PASSÆ MAJORES, see Vitis vinifera — u. Passæ minores, see Vitis Corinthiaca — u. Passæ sole siccatæ, see Vitis vinifera.

UVATIO, Ceratocele, Staphyloma.

U'VEA, from *uva,* 'an unripe grape.' *Tu'nica acino'sa* seu *aciniformis* seu *uva'lis* seu *acina'lis* seu *uviformis, Rhagoï'des, Tu'nica rhagoïdes* seu *uvea* seu *perfora'ta, Membrana uvea, Rhox,* (F.) *Uvée.* Some anatomists have given this name to the choroid coat of the eye; others, to the posterior layer of the iris, on account of the black and very thick varnish that covers it.

UVEA, COMMISSURE OF THE, Ciliary ligament.

UVÉE, Uvea.

UVEI'TIS; a word of hybrid formation; from *uvea,* 'the uvea,' and *itis,* denoting inflammation; properly, *Rhagoeï'tis.* Inflammation of the uvea.

UVIGENA, Uvula.

UVIGERA, Uvula.

UVULA, diminutive of *uva,* 'a grape.' *Pinnac'ulum for'nicis guttura'lis, Uva, Staph'yle, Tintinnab'ulum, Columel'la, Cion, Ci'onis, Garga'reon, Colum'na oris, Gurgu'lio, Intersep'tum, Processus* seu *Cartila'go U'vifer, Uvig''ena, Uvig''era, Pap of the Throat, Himas, Plectrum, Sublin'gua, Sublin'guium,* (F.) *Luette.* A fleshy appendix or prolongation, which hangs from the middle or free edge of the velum palati. The uvula has a conical shape, and is of a greater or less size in individuals. It is formed, especially, by the mucous membrane of the velum palati; and contains, within it, the azygos uvulæ muscle. Its use is not clear.

Also, a small prominence or lobule in the portion of the cerebellum that forms the posterior boundary of the fourth ventricle. It is on the median line, and behind the nodulus.

UVULA, see Vermiform process inferior — u. Decidua, Staphylœdema — u. Relaxata, Staphylœdema — u. Vesicæ, see Urinary bladder — u. Vesical, see Urinary bladder.

U'VULAR, *Uvula'ris,* from *uvula.* That which belongs to the uvula.

UVULAR GLANDS are small follicles, belonging to the mucous membrane covering the uvula.

UVULARIA, Ruscus hypoglossum.

UVULA'RIA PERFOLIA'TA, *Smaller Bellwort;* indigenous: *Order,* Melanthaceæ; flowering in May and June. The root, when fresh, is subacrid and mucilaginous. A decoction of the plant is used in sore mouth. It is said to cure the bites of rattlesnakes.

UVULI'TIS, a word of hybrid formation, from *uvula,* and *itis,* denoting inflammation. *Angi'na uvula'ris, Staphyli'tis, Cioni'tis, Inflamma'tio u'vulæ,* (F.) *Inflammation de la Luette, Falling down of the Palate.* Inflammation of the uvula.

V.

VACCIN, see Vaccina.

VACCI'NA, *Vaccin'ia, Vari"ola vaccina, V. vaccin'ica, V. tuto'ria, V. tutrix, Exanthe'ma vaccina, E. antivariolo'sum, Syn'ocha vaccina, Vacci'ola, Vacci'ola vera, Vacci'na primig"ena seu vaccinato'ria seu antivariolo'sa, Vacciola scutella'ta, Vari'olæ tuto'riæ, Cow-pox, Kine Pock, Inoc'ulated Cow-pox, Emphly'sis vaccina inser'ta,* from *vacca,* 'a cow;' (F.) *Vaccine.* The cow-pox is a disease of the cow, arising spontaneously, which, if transmitted to man by means of inoculation, may preserve him from small-pox contagion. The promulgation of this valuable property of the vaccine virus is due to Dr. Jenner. When inoculating for small-pox in Gloucestershire, in 1775, he was surprised to meet with a number of persons in the same district, on whom the insertion of the virus produced no effect, although they had never passed through the small-pox. On investigation, he found that all these persons had previously been affected by a pustular eruption of the cow, which they had taken by milking the animal; and which eruption they called *Cow-pox.* This discovery induced him to institute experiments, and he found that such preservative effect actually existed. The *Vaccine Virus, Virus Vacci'num,* (F.) *Vaccin,* or the fluid of the eruption, is not now usually taken immediately from the cow; experience having demonstrated, that it is nearly as efficacious when obtained from the human vesicle. The characteristic of cow-pox eruption is:— a semi-transparent, pearl-coloured vesicle, with a circular or somewhat oval base; its upper surface, until the end of the 8th day, being more elevated at the margin than in the centre; and the margin itself being turgid, shining, and rounded, so as often to extend a little over the line of the base. This vesicle is filled with clear lymph; contained in numerous little cells, that communicate with each other. After the 8th or 9th day from the insertion of the virus, it is surrounded by a bright red, circumscribed areola, which varies in its diameter, in different cases, from a quarter of an inch to two inches; and is usually attended with a considerable tumour, and hardness of the adjoining areolar membrane. This areola declines on the 11th or 12th day; the surface of the vesicle then becomes brown in the centre; and the fluid in the cells gradually concretes into a hard, rounded scab or crust, of a reddish-brown colour, which at length becomes darker, contracted, and dry, but is not detached till three weeks after vaccination. It leaves a permanent, circular cicatrix, about five lines in diameter, and a little depressed; the surface being marked with very minute pits or indentations, denoting the number of cells of which the vesicle had been composed. This is the progress of the *genuine cow-pox.* At times, fever occurs about the 9th or 11th day; but, at others, not the slightest indisposition is felt. Aberrations from this progress occur, which must be attended to; as the same preservative influence is not exerted by *irregular* or *spurious cow-pox.* If the eruption runs speedily to a height, has an aureola too early, is irregular at its edges, and contains pus instead of a limpid fluid,— it cannot at all be depended upon.

Small-pox occurs, at times, as an epidemic after vaccination. For a while, the enthusiastic advocates of vaccination would not admit the affection to be small-pox; and, accordingly, they gave it the name Varioloid. It is unquestionably small-pox, but modified, and greatly divested of its terrors by previous vaccination; and it is said to happen less frequently after vaccination than after *small-pox inoculation.* Vaccination is now practised every where, except among those in whom ignorance and prejudice exclude the lights of reason and philanthropy. There is ground, however, for the belief, that for full protection revaccination may be occasionally necessary.

VACCINA ANTIVARIOLOSA, Vaccina— v. Primigena, Vaccina— v. Tutoria, Vaccina— v. Tutrix, Vaccina— v. Vaccinatoria, Vaccina.

VACCINAL, Vaccine.

VACCINA'TION, *Vaccina'tio,* from *vacca,* 'a cow;' *Cow-pox inoculation, Jenne'rian inoculation.* An operation which consists in inserting the vaccine virus under the cuticle, so that it may come in contact with the absorbents. It is extremely simple, and requires merely that the point of the lancet should be held under the cuticle for a short time. The best time for taking the matter from the *Cow-pox vesicle,* for vaccination, is about the 7th or 8th day, before the appearance of the aureola, when it ought to be limpid and transparent. The most certain method is, to pass it from arm to arm; but this is not always convenient; and, hence it is used upon *points* or pieces of quill, or between glasses. It must, of course, be softened for use. This is done by means of a little water, which does not destroy its efficiency. The scab, too, which is off about the end of three weeks—sooner or later —is capable of communicating the affection, if dissolved in water; and this is the most common method of transmitting the vaccine virus in some countries.

VAC'CINATOR, *Vac'cinist,* one who inoculates for the cow-pox.

VACCINE, Vaccina.

VACCINE, *Vacci'nus, Vaccina'lis,* (F.) *Vaccinal:* same etymon. Relating or appertaining to vaccination, as the '*vaccine vesicle,*' 'a *vaccine* physician.'

VACCINEL'LA. A term employed by some to designate spurious cow-pox.— *Vaccis"ois, Vacci'ola spu'ria seu lepro'sa.*

VACCINIA, Vaccina—v. Palustris, Vaccinium oxycoccos.

VACCINIST, Vaccinator.

VACCINIUM MACROCARPON, see V. oxycoccos.

VACCIN'IUM MYRTIL'LUS, *Vitis idæ'a myrtil'lus.* The *Myrtle Berry, Vaccin'ia myrtil'lus, Bilberry, Blea-berry, Whortle-berry, Black Whorts, Vaccin'ium nigrum,* (F.) *Airelle Anguleuse, Raisin de Bois.* Family, Vaccineæ. Sex. Syst. (Octandria Monogynia. The berries— *Baccæ Myrtillo'rum*— are esteemed to be antiscorbutic, when prepared with vinegar. They are also said to possess antiseptic and sub-astringent properties when dried. They are not used in medicine; but are frequently eaten with milk and sugar.

VACCINIUM NIGRUM, V. myrtillus.

VACCINIUM OXYCOC'COS, *Oxycoc'cos, O. palustris, Schollera oxycoccos, Vaccinia palus'tris, Vitis Idæ'a palus'tris, Moorberry, Cranberry, Marberry, Swamp Redberry, Sourberry,* (F.) *Canneberge.* The berries are pleasantly acid and cooling. They make an agreeable preserve. The common American Cranberry is from *Vaccinium macrocarpon.*

VACCIN'IUM PUNCTATUM, V. vitis idæa — v. Resinosum, Gaylussacia resinosa.

VACCINIUM STAMIN'EUM, *Buckberry, Squaw Huckleberry, Deerberry.* The leaves of these plants are astringent.

VACCINIUM VITIS IDÆ'A, *V. puncta'tum, Vitis Idæ'a puncta'ta, Red Bilberry, Am'pelos Idæ'a, Whortleberry, Cowberry,* (F.) *Airelle* ou *Canneberge ponctuée.* A decoction of the leaves has been used in calculous affections. They are astringent. The ripe berries are pleasantly acid, and refrigerant. *Whortleberries* are furnished by different species of Vaccinium.

VACCINOIS, Vaccinella.

VACCINUS, Vaccine.

VACCIOLA, Vaccina — v. Leprosa, Vaccinella — v. Scutellata, Vaccina — v. Spuria, Vaccinella — v. Vera, Vaccina.

VACILLA'TIO, *Tituba'tio,* from *vacillare,* 'to waver.' Staggering; waddling — *claudica'tio anat'ica.*

VACILLATIO DENTIUM, Odontoseisis.

VAGIN, Vagina.

VAGI'NA, 'a sheath,' *Vagi'na mulie'bris* seu *uteri'na* seu *U'teri* seu *Penis, Sinus mulie'bris* seu *Pudo'ris* seu *Puden'di, Col'eus, Peris, Perin, Colpos, Vulvo-uterine canal,* (F.) *Vagin.* A cylindrical canal, five or six inches long; situate within the pelvis, between the bladder and rectum. It communicates by one extremity, *Aulos,* with the vulva; by the other, with the womb, the neck of which it embraces. The vagina is lined, internally, by a mucous membrane; and is partly closed, in young females, by the hymen, and carunculæ myrtiformes. — Around the mucous membrane is a layer of spongy, erectile tissue; and a cellulo-vascular membrane. A constrictor muscle; numerous vessels furnished by the vaginal artery, particularly; veins and nerves, proceeding from the sciatic plexus, also, enter into the composition of the organ.

The term Vagina or sheath, *Theca,* is extended to many parts, which serve as envelopes to others.

Sheath, (F.) *Gaine,* is sometimes applied to the fascia enveloping the limbs; to areolar membrane, enveloping the muscles, and entering between their fibres; to that which surrounds the blood-vessels; to the synovial membranes surrounding tendons, and lining the gutters of bones, &c.

VAGINA CORDIS, Pericardium — v. Femoris, Fascia lata aponeurosis — v. Funiculi Umbilicalis, see Funiculus umbilicalis — v. Glissonii, Capsule of Glisson — v. Malleolaris externa, Retinaculum tendinum perinæorum — v. Muliebris, Vagina — v. Muscularis, Perimysium — v. Nervorum, Neurilemma — v. Penis, Vagina — v. Portæ, Capsule of Glisson — v. Uterina, Vagina.

VAGINA OF THE VENA PORTA, *Sheath of the Vena Porta,* (F.) *Gaine de la Veine-porte,* is the areolar membrane that accompanies the divisions of the vena porta into the substance of the liver.

VAGINÆ SYNOVIALES, Bursæ mucosæ.

VAG"INAL, *Vagina'lis,* from *vagina,* 'a sheath.' — Relating or pertaining to a sheath.

VAGINAL ARTERY. This exists, as a matter of course, only in the female. It arises from the hypogastric or from the uterine, vesical, internal pudic, umbilical, &c., and sends its branches, first to the lateral parts of the vagina, and afterwards to the anterior and posterior surfaces.

VAGINAL BIL'IARY PLEXUS. A plexus of ramifications of the hepatic duct through the capsule of Glisson.

VAGINAL BRANCHES OF THE VENA PORTA are those which have to pass through the sheath of the capsule of Glisson, previous to entering the interlobular spaces. In this course, they form the *vaginal plexus.* There are, also, *vaginal branches,* and a *vaginal plexus* formed by the hepatic artery.

VAGINAL COAT OF THE EYE, see Eye.

VAGINAL COAT OF THE TESTICLE, *Tu'nica Vagina'lis, T. Elytroï'des* vel *Elytro'des,* is the serous membrane which envelops the testicle. Before the descent of the testicle, the tunica vaginalis does not exist. It is formed by a prolongation, furnished by the peritoneum to the testicle when it issues from the abdomen. The tunica vaginalis forms a close sac, investing the testicle and epididymis, without containing them in its cavity, and reflected so as to form a bag around the circumference of the testis; hence it is divided into *Tu'nica vagina'lis pro'pria* and *Tu'nica vagina'lis reflex'a.* Between the two layers, the inner surface is smooth, and lubricated by a serous fluid.

VAGINAL GANGLIA, see Spermatic ganglion.

VAGINAL PLEXUS, see Vaginal branches of the vena porta.

VAGINAL PROCESS OF THE TEMPORAL BONE, (F.) *Apophyse vaginale* ou *engaînante, Gaine de l'apophyse styloïde, Chaton,* is a bony crista, which embraces the base of the styloid process.

VAGINITIS, Leucorrhœa (vaginal.)

VAGISSEMENT, Cry, Vagitus.

VAGI'TUS, (F.) *Vagissement.* The cry of the new-born child. *Squalling.*

VAGI'TUS UTERI'NUS. The cry of the child in utero.

VAGUS NERVUS, Pneumogastric.

VAIRON (F.), *Dispar oc'ulus.* One who has eyes of different colours. It also means a *wall-eyed* animal, or one whose iris is surrounded by a whitish circle.

VAISSEAU, Vessel — *v. Sanguin,* Blood-vessel.

VAISSEAUX CAPILLAIRES, Capillary vessels — *v. Chylifères.* Chyliferous vessels — *v. Lactés,* Chyliferous vessels — *v. Lactifères,* Lactiferous vessels — *v. Ombilicaux,* Umbilical vessels.

VALANIDA, Fagus sylvatica.

VALANTIA APARINE, Galium aparine.

VALERIAN, AMERICAN, Cypripedium luteum, Valeriana pauciflora — v. Garden, Valeriana phu — v. Greek, Polemonium reptans — v. Officinal, Valeriana — v. Wild, Valeriana.

VALERIA'NA, *V. officina'lis, Wild Vale'rian, Valeriana minor, Offic"inal Valerian. Family,* Dipsaceæ. *Sex. Syst.* Triandria Monogynia. The root, *Valeria'na,* (Ph. U. S.) has been long extolled as an efficacious remedy in epilepsy, and in a variety of nervous complaints. It has been also advised as a tonic, antispasmodic, and emmenagogue. It has a strong, fetid odour; bitterish, subacrid, and warm taste; and its virtues are extracted by water and alcohol.

VALERIANA CAPEN'SIS, a South African species, has similar virtues.

VALERIANA CELT'ICA, *V. Saxat'ilis, Celtic Nard, Spica Cel'tica, S. Alpi'na, Nardus Cel'tica, Saliun'ca, Nardum Gall'icum, Spica Cel'tica Dioscor'idis,* (F.) *Nard Celtique.* The roots of this Alpine plant have been recommended as a stomachic, carminative and diuretic. It has a moderately strong smell, and a warm, bitterish, subacrid taste.

VALERIANA DENTA'TA, *V. locus'ta, Corn Salad.* A wholesome, succulent plant, cultivated in Europe as a salad. It is antiscorbutic and gently aperient.

VALERIANA MAJOR, V. phu — v. Locusta, V. dentata — v. Minor, Valeriana — v. Officinalis, Valeriana.

VALERIANA PAUCIFLO'RA, *American Vale'rian,* has the properties of the other Valerians.

VALERIANA PHU, V. major, Garden Valerian, (F.) Grand Valériane. The root has been recommended in rheumatism; especially in sciatica, and in epilepsy.

VALERIANA SAXATILIS, V. celtica.

VALÉRIANE GRAND, Valeriana phu.

VALET À PATIN (F.), Volsel'la Pati'ni. The common ligature forceps is a modification of this instrument invented by one Patin. It consists of two branches, united at the middle by a hinge, which may be separated or approximated by means of a screw or running ring. It is used for seizing hold of vessels that are to be tied.

VALETUDINARIUM, Hospital.

VALETUDINARIUS, Sickly, Valetudinary.

VALETU'DINARY, Valetudina'rian, Valetudina'rius, Inval'idus, from valetudo, 'health.' — One of delicate health. One subject to frequent diseases. An Invalid.

VALETUDO, Sanitas—v. Adversa, Disease—v. Bona, Sanitas — v. Commoda, Sanitas — v. Secunda, Sanitas.

VALGUS, see Kyllosis

VALIGA, Tinctura jalapii.

VALITUDO, Sanitas.

VALLECULA, Valley.

VALLEY, Vallec'ula, (F.) Grand Scissure Médiane du Cervelet. The deep fissure on the inferior part of the cerebellum, which divides it into two symmetrical portions.

VALLUM. The eyebrow or supercilium. Also, a species of bandage.—Galen.

VALS, MINERAL WATERS OF. A French acidulous chalybeate at Vals, six leagues from Viviers, in the department of Ardèche. There are five springs, containing carbonic acid, sulphate of iron, and alum. They are employed in passive hemorrhages, leucorrhœa, &c.

VALVE, Val'vula, Dictis, (F.) Valvule, from valvæ, 'folding-doors,' itself from volvo, 'I fold up.' A small door. Any membrane or duplicature of a membrane, which prevents a reflux of humours or other matters in the vessels and canals of the animal body. There are some valves, whose functions appear to be, — to retard or to modify the course of substances along canals, &c. See mitral, sigmoid, tricuspid, ileo-cœcal valve, &c.

VALVE OF FALLOPIUS, Bauhin, valve of — v. Ileo-cœcal, Bauhin, valve of — v. Ileo-colic, Bauhin, valve of—v. of Tulpius, Bauhin, valve of—v. of Varolius, Bauhin, valve of

VALVES, SEMILUNAR, Sigmoid valves.

VALVULA, Valve—v. Cæci, Bauhin, valve of —v. Cerebelli, Valvula Vieussenii—v. Coli, Bauhin, valve of—v. Foraminis ovalis, Ovalis fossa —v. Guiffartiana, see Thebesius, veins of — v. Ilei, Bauhin, valve of — v. Magna Cerebri, V. Vieussenii.

VALVULA SEMILUNA'RIS, Plica Semiluna'ris, Membran'ula semiluna'ris conjuncti'va, Plica luna'ta. A small doubling of the tunica conjunctiva, which lies between the caruncula lacrymalis and the ball of the eye. In birds, this is large, and called Membra'na nic'titans vel Pal'pebra ter'tia.

VALVULA TARINI, Velum medullare posterius — v. Thebesii, see Thebesius, veins of — v. Vaginæ, Hymen — v. Venæ magnæ, see Thebesius, valve of.

VALVULA VIUESSE'NII, Velum Vieussenii, Val'vula cerebel'li seu Willisia'na seu magna cer'ebri, Velum interjec'tum cerebelli, V. apoph'ysi vermiformi obtentum, Lacu'nar ventric'uli quarti superior, Velum medulla'rē seu medulla'rē anti'orum seu ante'rius, (F.) Valvule de Vieussens, Voile médullaire supérieure. A thin, medullary lamina, over the under end of the Aquæductus Sylvii and upper part of the fourth ventricle. At the side of the valves are two medullary tracts, called Process'us ad Testes, Colum'næ Val'vulæ Viessenii, or Oblique intercer'ebral Com'missure.

VALVULA WILLISIANA, Valvula Vieussenii.

VALVULÆ BICUSPIDALES, Mitral valves.

VALVULÆ CONNIVEN'TES. Numerous circular folds in the intestinal canal from the pyloric orifice through the greater part of the small intestine. They are folds of the mucous membrane and their chief use appears to be, to retard the course of the alimentary mass, and to afford a larger surface for the origin of chyliferous vessels.

VALVULÆ CORDIS, Ostiola cordis — v. Cordis mitrales, Mitral valves — v. Triglochines, Tricuspid valves — v. Trisulcæ, Tricuspid valves.

VALVULE, Valve—v. d' Eustache. Eustachian valve—v. de Pylore, see Pylorus—v. de Vieussens, Valvula Vieussenii.

VALVULES, V. Épiscopales, Mitral valves—v. Sigmoïdes ou Semilunaires, Sigmoid valves.

VANELLOE, Vanilla.

VANIL'LA, Banil'ia, Banilas, Banillœa, banilla, Benzo'ënil, Ar'acus aromat'icus, (F.) Vanille, Baume de Vanille. The Vanelloe—Siliqua vanill'æ seu Banill'æ seu Vaniglia seu racemus seu Ar'aci aromat'ici — is a long, flattish pod containing, under a wrinkled, brittle shell, a reddish-brown pulp, with small, shining, black seeds. The parasitic plant which affords this pod is the Epiden'drum Vanilla, Vanill'a aromat'ica seu Mexica'na. Family, Orchideæ. Sex. Syst. Gynandria Monandria. Vanelloes have an unctuous aromatic taste, and a fragrant smell, like that of some of the finer balsams, heightened with musk. Although chiefly used as perfumes, they are reputed to possess aphrodisiac virtues.

VANILLA AROMATICA, see Vanilla.

VAPEURS, Hypochondriasis, Hysteria.

VAPORA'RIUM, Atmiste'rion, Laconicum, Py'ria, Pyriate'rium, Vapour bath. A useful remedy in rheumatic and cutaneous affections and wherever it is important to relax the cutaneous capillaries. In the Russian Vapour Bath the vapour is produced by throwing water over hot stones. Its temperature is from 122° to 140°.

VAPORARIUM, Hypocaustum, see Stove.

VAPORATIO, Evaporation.

VAPORES UTERINI, Hysteria.

VAPOUR, Flatulence—v. Bath, Vaporarium.

VAPOURISH, Hypochondriac, Hysterical.

VAPOUROUS, Windy.

VAPOURS, Hypochondriasis, Hysteria.

VAPOURY, Hypochondriacal, Hysterical.

VARA, Barre.

VAREC, Kelp — v. Vésiculeux, Fucus vesiculosus.

VARENI, Ambulo-flatulentus, Gout (wandering.)

VARICE, Varix.

VARICELL'A, (diminutive of Variola, Smallpox,) Em'phlysis varicella, Exanthe'ma varicella, Syn'ochus varicella, Chicken pox, Variole volante, V. spu'ria, V. sylves'tris, Variole notha, V. illegit'ima, Pseudo-variole. V. volatica, V. pusilla, Æoli'ion, Æoli'ium, (F.) Variole, Petite vérole volante, Vérolette. A disease characterized by vesicles scattered over the body, which are glabrous, transparent, and about the size of peas. They appear in successive crops are covered by a thin pellicle, and, about the third, fourth, or fifth day from their appearance, burst at the top, and concrete into small puckered scabs, which rarely leave a pit in the skin. Three varieties have, sometimes, been designated. 1. The V. lentiformes, or lenticular chicken pox which are irregularly circular, and flattened on the top; the fluid being at first whitish, and afterwards straw-coloured. This is the *common chicken pox*. 2. The *Varicella conifor'mis, Conoi'dal Chicken Pox, Pem'phigus variolo'des, Variola lymphat'ica, Hydrach'nis, Swine Pox, Water Pox, Water Jags,* in which the vesicles are generally acuminated, and the fluid pellucid throughout; and, 3dly, the *Varicel'la globula'ris* or *Hives*, in which the vesicles are globular and larger; the fluid being, at first, whey-coloured, and afterwards yellowish. These divisions are, however, very arbitrary, for they are generally confounded.

Variola has been, sometimes, mistaken for this disease, and conversely. A little attention to the history of the eruption in the two affections will prevent error. Varicella is not contagious. At times, it prevails epidemically. It cannot be propagated by inoculation. The treatment is extremely simple; rest, abstinence, and the antiphlogistic regimen, being all that is generally required.

VARICELLA VARIOLOIDEA, Varioloid.

VARICIFOR'MES PARAS'TATÆ. A name given, by some authors, to the ducts of the epididymis, because they seem knotty and varicose.

VARICOBLEPH'ARON, from *varix*, and βλέφαρον, 'eyelid.' A varicose tumour of the eyelid.

VARICOCE'LE, from *varix*, and κηλη, 'a tumour;' *Oscheoce'lē varico'sa, Her'nia varico'sa, Ramex varico'sus, Spermatoce'lē, Cirsocele.* A varicose dilatation of the veins of the scrotum and spermatic cord. This latter variety of the disease is more common on the left side than the right. It appears under the form of a soft, doughy, unequal, knotty, compressible, and indolent tumour, situate in the course of the cord, and increasing from below upwards. It is less when the individual is in the recumbent posture, and increases when he is erect. It is, ordinarily, an affection of no moment, and is very common, requiring merely the use of a proper suspensory bandage. It has been advised, in bad cases, to tie the enlarged vein, but the operation is not free from danger induced by phlebitis. Sir A. Cooper has proposed the removal of a portion of the scrotum, so as to render the remainder of the scrotum a natural bandage. This plan has been found effectual.

VARICOM'PHALUS, from *varix*, and ομφαλος, 'the umbilicus.' Varicose tumour of the umbilicus; cirsomphalus.

VAR'ICOSE, *Varico'sus*, (F.) *Variqueux.* Affected with varix; or belonging to, or connected with, varix;—as a *varicose vein*, a *varicose ulcer*, that is, one kept up by *varices.*

VARICOSITAS CONJUNCTIVÆ, Cirsophthalmia.

VARIC'ULA, *Varix parva.* A diminutive of *varix.* Also, a varicose swelling of the veins of the tunica conjunctiva.—M. A. Severinus.

VARI'OLA, *Variolæ, V. vera, Varioli, Small-Pox, Empye'sis Variola, Euphlog''ia, Charpā, Evlec'thyma, Pox* (N. of England), *Pestis variolo'sa, Febris variolo'sa;* from *varius*, 'spotted,' or from *vari*, 'pimples;' (F.) *Variole, Petit Vérole, Picote.* A disease, now of somewhat less interest than before the discovery of vaccination. It is of a very contagious nature, and is supposed to have been introduced into Europe from Asia, at an early period of the middle ages. It is characterised by fever, with pustules, appearing from the third to the fifth day, and suppurating from the eighth to the tenth, and it possesses all the distinctive properties of the major exanthemata. It is capable of being produced by inoculation, but this *inoculated small-pox—Vari'ola inser'ta*—communicates the disease as readily through the air as the *natural small-pox*, or that received without inoculation.

Small-pox is distinguished into two classes, according to the character of the eruption, the *discrete* or *distinct*, and the *confluent*. 1. In VARIOLA DISCRE'TA, *Empyesis variola discreta, Variola discreta benig'na, Variolæ regulares seu discretæ, Distinct Small-pox,* the pustules are usually of the size of peas; distinct, distended, and circular; the intervening spaces being red; the fever inflammatory throughout, and ceasing when the eruption is complete. 2. In VARIOLA CON'FLUENS, *Empyesis variola confluens, Variolæ regula'res confluen'tes, Vesic'ulæ Divæ Bar'baræ, Vésicules de Sainte-Barbe* or *Confluent Small-pox,* the pustules are confluent, or run together; flaccid and irregularly circumscribed; the intervening spaces being pale, and the accompanying fever typhoid. In children, diarrhœa, and, in adults, ptyalism, with swelling of the hands and feet, generally appear, towards the period of the *sec'ondary fever,* which occurs from the tenth to the thirteenth day. The fever that precedes and accompanies the eruption is called the *Eruptive fever.* The prognosis is favourable in the distinct kind, if properly managed. The confluent is always dangerous,—the unfavourable symptoms being—flattening of the pustules, or subsidence of the eruption; the breathing becoming much obstructed or oppressed; or marks of inflammatory and congestive affections occurring in the different viscera. The treatment of the distinct kind is very simple: the antiphlogistic regimen, with cathartics, being all that is necessary. The confluent kind requires the same management as typhus fever.

When the pimples are confluent in patches, the patches, being, however, separated by intervals of unaffected skin; it constitutes the clustered, coherent, or corymbose variety—*Vari'ola corymbo'sa.*

VARIOLA AMBOINENSIS, Frambœsia—v. Corymbosa, see Variola—v. Inserta, Variola (by inoculation)—v. Lymphatica, Varicella—v. Mitigata, Varioloid.

VARI'OLA sine VARI'OLIS, *Vari'olous Fever.* These terms are applied to cases occasionally observed during the prevalence of variola, in which the constitutional phenomena are present without the cutaneous eruption.

VARIOLA SPURIA, Varicella—v. Vaccina, Vaccina—v. Vaccinatorum, Varioloid.

VARIOLÆ, Variola—v. Equinæ, see Grease—v. Illegitimæ, Varicella—v. Modificatæ, Varioloid—v. Nothæ, Varicella—v. Pucellæ, Varicella—v. Sylvestris, Varicella—v. Tutoriæ, Vaccina—v. Veræ, Variola—v. Volaticæ, Varicella.

VARIOLATION, Inoculation (Small-pox.)

VARIOLE, Variola.

VARIOLI, Variola.

VAR'IOLOID, *Variolois, Varioloi'des, Vari'ola modifica'ta, V. mitiga'ta, V. vaccinato'rum, Varicel'la, Varioloïdea,* from *variola*, small-pox, and ειδος, 'form,'—resembling small-pox. This is, really, small-pox, modified by previous inoculation or vaccination; and hence it has been properly called *modified small-pox.* That it is small-pox is proved by the fact, that matter, taken from a varioloid pustule, will communicate small-pox to one who has never had it naturally or by inoculation, or who has never been vaccinated. It is, almost always, a milder disease than small-pox; and this circumstance, with its shorter duration, exhibits the salutary effects of previous vaccination or inoculation. It has appeared epidemically.

VARIOLOIS, Varioloid.
VARIQUEUX, Varicose.
VARIX, *Phlebeurys'ma, Phlebec'tasis, Her'nia seu Ecta'sia vena'rum, Angiecta'sia veno'sa, Ix'ia, Cirsus, Cedma, Var'icose Vein*, (F.) *Varice*, is considered, by some, to come from the verb *variare*, 'to turn,' to twist,'—on account of the sinuosities of varicose veins. Dilatation of a vein. Varices are owing to local retardation of the venous circulation; and, in some cases, to relaxation of the parietes of the veins. They are very common in the superficial veins of the lower limbs, especially of pregnant females. The tumour or tumours, formed by varices, are soft, knotty, unequal, indolent, and livid; without pulsation, and yielding readily to the impression of the finger; but returning as soon as the compression is discontinued. Sometimes, the vein bursts and gives rise to hemorrhage. The treatment is usually palliative, and consists in exerting a uniform and constant pressure upon the part, by means of an appropriate bandage. The radical cure has, also, been obtained by extirpation, division of the vein, or ligature. The second course is apt to be followed by phlebitis.

VAROLI, BRIDGE OF, Pons Varolii.
VARUS, Acne, Ionthus, see Kyllosis—v. Mentagra, Sycosis.
VAS, Vessel, Penis—v. Deferens mulieris, Tuba Fallopiana—v. Urinarium, Ureter.
VASA ABSORBENTIA, Absorbent vessels—v. Capillaria, Capillary vessels.
VASA CHYLOPOIËT'ICA URINIF'ERA. Bloodvessels, which, according to Lippi, convey drinks from the chyliferous vessels to the renal veins.
VASA EFFERENTIA, see Efferent — v. Exhalantia, Exhalant vessels—v. Hydragoga, Lymphatic vessels—v. Lactea, Chyliferous vessels, Lactifereus vessels—v. Meningea, Meningeal vessels—v. Sedalia, Hæmorrhoidal vessels — v. Lymphatica, Lymphatic vessels—v. Nutritia, Vasa vasorum—v. Recta, see Rete testis—v. Resorbentia, Absorbent vessels, Lymphatic vessels.
VASA VASO'RUM, *V. nutrit"ia*. Small vessels that supply larger. However minutely a vessel is traced, its parietes will be found supplied with blood for its nutrition by a smaller vessel.
VASA VORTICO'SA, (F.) *Tourbillon vasculaires*. The contorted vessels which creep on the choroid coat of the eye; ciliary veins.
VASCOA AMPLEXICAU'LIS. A South African shrub, *Nat. Ord.* Leguminosæ, the roots of which taste like liquorice. They are used, in decoction, in catarrh and phthisis, and are a good substitute for liquorice.
VAS'CULAR, *Vascula'ris, Vasculo'sus, Angei'al*, from *vas*, 'a vessel.' That which belongs or relates to vessels; — arterial, venous, or lymphatic; but generally restricted to blood-vessels only. Full of vessels. Bichat gave the name *Vascular system* to the blood-vessels, and of this he made two divisions. 1. The *Arterial system*, or *System of red blood*, (F.) *Système vasculaire à sang rouge*, which commences with the radicles of the pulmonary veins; and includes the pulmonary veins, the left cavities of the heart and the aorta with all its ramifications. The blood, in this system, is distributed to the general capillary system, where it loses its arterial quality and becomes venous. 2. The *Venous system* or *Vascular system of black blood*, (F.) *Système vasculaire à sang noir*, carries the blood from every part of the system to the lungs. It takes its origin in the general capillary system; continues in the veins, right auricle, and ventricle of the heart and the pulmonary artery and its branches, and is finally lost in the capillary system of the lungs. See Circulation.

VASCULAR LAYER, see Tache embryonnaire—v. Radicals, Radical vessels—v. Substance of the Kidney, see Kidney — v. System, intermediate, Capillary system — v. System, peripheral, Capillary system—v. Tumour, see Hæmorrhois.
VASCULAR'ITY. The state of being vascular, or largely supplied with vessels.
VASCULUM, Penis, Vessel.
VAS'CULUM ABER'RANS, *Appendix to the Epididymis*. A small convoluted duct, of varied length, generally connected with the duct of the epididymis, immediately before the commencement of the vas deferens.
VASE À SAIGNER, Cup.
VASTUS. That which is *vast* or has a great extent.
VASTUS EXTERNUS and VASTUS INTERNUS are two considerable, fleshy masses, which form part of the Triceps cruris.
VASUM, Vessel.
VATERIA INDICA, see Copal.
VATICINIUM CHIROMANTICUM, Chiromancy.
VAULT, (old F. *Voulte*,) 'a round or turn, from *volvere, volutum*, 'to turn;' *Fornix, Camera* (F.) *Voûte*. A name given by anatomists several parts which are rounded superiorly; concave and arched inferiorly,—as the *Vault of the cranium* or the upper part of the skull,—the *palatine vault* or *roof of the mouth*, &c., &c.
VAUQUELINE, Strychnina.
VEAL TEA. This may be made in the same manner as beef tea, by using a pound of silk *veal*, free from fat and sliced, and a pint and a half of *boiling water*; and boiling for half an hour. It may also be made with the same quantity of the fleshy part of a knuckle of veal.
VECORDIA, Idiotism.
VECTIS, Lever—v. Elevatorius, Elevator—t. Triploides, Elevator, triploid.
VEGETARIAN, see Vegetarianism.
VEGETA'RIANISM. Same etymon as Vegetation. A modern term, employed to designate the view, that man, for his full mental and corporeal developement, ought to subsist on the direct productions of the vegetable kingdom, and totally abstain from flesh and blood. An embracer and practiser of this doctrine is called a vegetarian.
VÉGÉTATIF, Vegetative.
VEGETA'TION, *Vegeta'tio*, 'growing like a plant,' from *vigeo*, 'I flourish.' A morbid process which rises as an excrescence in syphilis, &c. as the *Cauliflower excrescence*, &c. The term is also applied to the fleshy granulations or *fungous sarcoses*, which sometimes arise at the surface of wounds or ulcers.
VEG"ETATIVE, *Vegetati'vus*, (F.) *Végétatif*; same etymon as the last. Having relation to growth or nutrition; hence, the *vegetative or nutritive functions*.
VEGETATIVE LAYER, see Tache embryonnaire.
VEGETATIVUS, Vegetative.
VE'HICLE, *Vehic'ulum, Oche'ma, Commitiva* (F.) *Véhicule*, from *vehere*, 'to carry.' Anything which serves to carry; thus air is the vehicle of sound; the arteries are the *vehicles of the blood*, &c. In *Pharmacy*, the name *vehicle* is given to any excipient; or to substances which serve as the media of administration for any medicine.
VÉHICULE, Vehicle.
VEILED PUFF, see Cavernous respiration.
VEIN, *Vena*, diminutive *ven'ula, Phleps, Phleb* (F.) *Veine*. The veins are vessels for the conveyance of black blood from every part of the body to the heart. They are found wherever there are arteries, and, altogether, form the *venous system*.

which may be subdivided into two distinct secondary systems. 1. The *General venous system*, which commences in all the organs, by very minute radicles; and terminates in the heart by the vena cava and the coronary vein. 2. The *Abdominal venous system*, which is limited to the abdominal cavity; commences, also, by a great number of branches, and terminates in the liver by a single trunk, which subdivides in that organ. It is called, also, the *System of the Vena Porta*, or the *Portal System*. See Porta. The veins form two sets, one *deep-seated, Venæ satel'lites, V. concom'ites*, which accompany the arteries; the other *superficial* or *subcutaneous*. Their parietes, which are thinner than those of the arteries, are composed of two coats; the one, external, loose, extensible, and with parallel, longitudinal fibres — the *proper membrane*; the other, the *common* or *inner membrane*, which is thin, polished, and has numerous duplicatures or folds forming parabolic valves. These valves are most numerous in the veins of the lower extremities. The coats of the veins are supplied with small arteries or *vasa vasorum*, veins, and lymphatics. They have not as many nervous filaments as the arteries. These filaments are from the great sympathetic.

TABLE OF THE VEINS.

1. VEINS WHICH FORM THE SUPERIOR VENA CAVA.

1. Subclavian {
  - Receive the Axillary which
    1. Basilic, formed of the — { 1. Posterior ulnar. 2. Anterior ulnar. 3. Median basilic. }
    2. Cephalic, forming the { 1. Superficial radial. 2. Median cephalic. }
    3. Circumflex veins.
    4. Inferior scapular.
    5. Long thoracic.
    6. Superior thoracic.
    7. Acromial veins.
  - External Jugular
    1. Internal maxillary, composed of the { 1. Pterygoid. 2. Spheno-palatine. 3. Alveolar. 4. Infra-orbitar. 5. Mental. 6. Inferior dental. 7. Deep temporal. }
    2. Superficial Temporal, composed of the { 1. Middle temporal. 2. Anterior auriculars. 3. Transverse of the face. }
    3. Posterior Auricular. The trunk then takes the name of *External Jugular*, and in its course along the neck, receives —
    4. Cervical cutaneous.
    5. Trachelo-scapular, &c.
  - Internal Jugular — Receives
    1. Superior Cerebral Veins.
    2. Veins of the Corpus Striatum.
    3. Veins of the Choroid plexus.
    4. Superior Cerebellar Veins.
    5. Inferior Cerebellar Veins.
    6. Lateral and inferior Cerebral Veins.
    7. Ophthalmic Vein, composed of the { 1. Lachrymal. 2. Central of the retina. 3. Infra-orbitar. 4. Ciliary. 5. Ethmoidal. 6. Palpebral, and 7. Nasal Veins. }
    8. Facial Vein, called *angular*, near the eye, receiving the { 1. Palpebral and 2. Superciliary Veins. 3. Dorsals of the nose. 4. Superior & 5. Inferior Coronaries of the lip. 6. Several Buccal and 7. Masseteric Veins. 8. Ranine. 9. Submental, and 10. Inferior Palatine. }
    9. Lingual and Pharyngeal Veins.
    10. Superior thyroid.
    11. Occipital, and
    12. Veins of the Diploë.

2. Right Internal Mammary Vein.
3. Inferior Thyroid Vein, opening into the Vena Cava, between the two Subclavians.

4. Vena Azygos, which receives the { 1. Right Bronchial. 2. Intercostal Veins. 3. Semi-azygos. }

2. VEINS WHICH FORM THE INFERIOR VENA CAVA.

1. Common Iliacs —
  - Receive the
    1. External Iliacs, formed by the — { 1. Femoral or Crural, which is a continuation of the 2. Popliteal, commencing by 3. veins which accompany the fibular arteries, and receiving the — { 1. External Saphena and 2. Internal Saphena, which receive — { 1. Several abdominal veins. 2. Circumflex Iliac, and 3. External pudic veins. } } }
    2. Internal Iliacs which receive the — { 1. Vesical Veins, commencing with the 2. Sacro-lateral Veins. { 1. Dorsal veins of the penis of the male. 2. Veins of the clitoris, in the female. } }
  3. Middle Sacral Vein.
  4. Lumbar Veins — four in number on each side, commencing by an — { 1. Abdominal branch. 2. Dorsal branch. }
  5. Spermatic Veins, commencing with the { 1. Spermatic plexus in the male. 2. Ovarium, Fallopian tube, &c. in the female. }
  6. Renal Veins.
  7. Capsular and Adipose Veins.
  8. Hepatic Veins.
  9. Middle,
  10. Left, and } Hepatic Veins.
  11. Right
  12. Inferior Diaphragmatic Veins, two in number

3. VEINS OF THE HEART.

1. Great right Coronary.
2. Small right Coronary.
3. Left Coronary Veins.

4. VEINS WHICH FORM THE VENA PORTÆ.

1. Splenic Vein. { Receives the 1. Veins which correspond to the vasa brevia. 2. Right and left gastro epiploic. 3. Duodenal, and 4. Pancreatic veins. 5. Coronary Vein of the Stomach, and 6. Small mesenteric vein. }
2. Superior Mesenteric Vein.

VEIN, BRONCHIAL, LEFT, see Azygos — v. Demi-azygous, see Azygos — v. Frontal, see Facial vein — v. Semi-azygous, see Azygos, (vena) — v. Superior intercostal, left, see Azygos — v. Tibio-malleolar, Saphena, great — v. Palato-labial, Facial vein — v. Peroneo-malleolar, Saphena minor — v. Varicose, Varix.

VEINE, Vein — *v. Cave*, Cava vena — *v. Céphalique*, Jugular vein, internal — *v. Céphalique du pouce*, Cephalic vein of the thumb — *v. Cubitale cutanée*, Basilic vein — *v. Fessière*, Gluteal vein — *v. de Médine*, Dracunculus — *v. Porte*, Porta vena — *v. Prélombo-thoracique*, Azygos, (vena) — *v. Préparate*, Cephalic vein — *v. Radiale cutanée*, Cephalic vein — *v. Sans paire*, Azygos, vein — *v. Trachélo-sous-cutanée*, Jugular vein, external.

VEINES ARTÉRIELLES, Arterial veins — *v. Ciliaires*, Ciliary veins — *v. Sous-clavières*, Subclavian veins — *v. Sus-hépatiques*, Hepatic veins.

VEINS, CORONARY, Cardiac veins — v. Intralobular, Hepatic veins — v. Supra-hepatic, Hepatic veins.

VEINSTONE, Phlebolite.
VELAMEN NATIVUM, Integument.
VELAMENTA BOMBYCINA, Villous membranes — v. Cerebralia, Meninges — v. Infantis, Membranes of the fœtus.
VELAMENTUM ABDOMINALE, Peritoneum — v. Corporis commune, Integument — v. Nativum, Integument.

VELAR, Erysimum.

VELLICATION, Tic.

VELOSYNTHESIS, Staphylorraphy.

VELUM, Velum pendulum palati—v. Apophysi vermiformi obtentum, Valvula Vieussenii—v. Interjectum cerebelli, Valvula Vieussenii—v. Medullare anticum, Valvula Vieussenii.

VELUM MEDULLA'RE INFERIUS, (F.) *Voile médullaire inférieur*. A name given, by Reil, to the medullary band or strip, by which the cerebellum communicates with the medulla.

VELUM MEDULLA'RE POSTE'RIUS seu POSTI'CUS seu SEMILUNA'RE, *Val'vula Tari'ni*. The small posterior valve of the cerebellum; a thin medullary plate, situate between the medulla oblongata and vermis inferior, in front of the nodulus.

VELUM PALATI, Velum pendulum palati—v. Palatinum, Velum pendulum palati.

VELUM PEN'DULUM PALA'TI, 'Pendulous veil of the palate.' *Velum, Velum Palati'num, Velum Palati, Velum Pen'dulum, Velum Staphyli'num, Pala'tum pen'dulum, Pen'dulum pala'ti, Claustrum Palati, Soft Palate, Palatum Mollé*, (F.) *Septum Staphylin* (Ch.), *Voile du Palais*. A moveable, soft, and broad septum, attached to the posterior extremity of the palatine arch, and separating the mouth from the pharynx. Its form is nearly quadrilateral. Its *anterior surface* corresponds to the mouth; the *posterior* to the pharynx. Its *superior edge* is fixed to the palatine arch; the inferior is free, floating, and has an appendix at its middle — the *uvula*. The lateral margins of the velum are held down by two folds, separated from each other by a triangular space; these are called the *pillars;* the anterior passes to the base of the tongue, the posterior to the sides of the pharynx. The velum palati is formed of a mucous coat, which contains numerous follicles, and of a muscular stratum, in which are the peristaphylini interni and p. externi muscles, the glosso-staphylini, the pharyngo-staphylini and the palato-staphylinus. The arteries of the velum palati are furnished by the internal maxillary, the labial and the superior pharyngeal. Its veins open into the internal jugular. Its nerves are sent off from the ganglion of Meckel, and come from the palatine branches. The glosso-pharyngeal nerve, likewise, sends it some filaments.

VELUM STAPHYLINUM, Velum pendulum palati —v. Vieussenii, Valvula Vieussenii.

VELVET LEAF, Pareira.

VENA, Vein, Penis—v. Alba renum, Ureter—v. Alba thoracis, Thoracic duct — v. Apoplectica, Jugular vein, internal—v. Arteriosa, Porta vena, Pulmonary artery—v. Capitis, Cephalic vein—v. Cava, Cava vena—v. Cubiti interior, Basilic vein —v. Demiazygos, see Azygos—v. Falcis cerebri, Sinus longitudinal inferior—v. Hemiazygus, see Azygos—v. Lactea, Porta vena—v. Magna, Porta vena—v. Medina Arabum, Dracunculus—v. Medinensis, Dracunculus—v. Ostiaria, Porta vena—v. Pari carens, Azygos, (vena)—v. Portalis, Porta vena— v. portarum, Porta vena — v. ad Portas, Porta vena—v. quæ ad Portas est, Porta vena—v. Ramalis, Porta vena — v. sine Pari, Azygos, (vena)—v. Stelechiæa, Porta vena—v. Subalaris, Vena axillaris—v. Terminalis, Circulus venosus.

VENÆ APOPLECTICÆ, Jugular veins — v. Cavæ hepatis, Hepatic veins—v. Centrales, Intralobular veins—v. Concomites, see Vein—v. Galeni, Choroid, (veins)—v. Innominatæ, see Innominatum — v. Intralobulares, Intralobular veins—v. Lacteæ, Chyliferous vessels — v. Lymphaticæ, Lymphatic vessels — v. Micantes, (arteries,) see Artery — v. Pulsatiles, (arteries,) see Artery—v. Satellites, see Vein—v. Soporales, Jugular veins —v. Sphagitidæs, Jugular veins.

VENÆSECTIO, see Blood-letting—v. Revulsoria, see Blood-letting.

VENÆ VORTICO'SÆ. The veins which principally form the external or venous layer of the choroid coat of the eye; so called from their peculiar arrangement; from *vertex* seu *vortex*, 'a whirlpool.'

VENAL, Venous.

VENEFICIUM, Poisoning.

VENENATION, Poison, Poisoning, Venom.

VENENATUS, Venomous.

VENENOSE, Venomous.

VENENUM, Poison, Venom.

VENE'REAL, *Vene'reus, Aphrodisiacus, ne'rean*, (F.) *Vénérien*, from *Venus*, 'the goddess of pleasure.' That which relates to the pleasure of love. In a more restricted sense, the word *venereal* is synonymous with *syphilitic*, as it is with *syphilis*. Some authors have proposed that those diseases should be called *venereal* which are produced by excess in venery; and the *syphilitic* should be limited to those which are the result of impure connexion. It is, also, used in the same sense as aphrodisiac, — adapted to excite venereal desire.

VENEREAL DESIRE, Libido — v. Disease, Syphilis.

VÉNÉRIEN, Venereal. This term also means one labouring under syphilis; as *Hôpital des vénériens*.

VENERIVAGUS, Libidinous.

VEN'ERY. Same etymon. The pleasures of love. Sexual communication. Coition.

VENESECTION, see Blood-letting.

VENIMEUX, Venomous.

VENIN, Venom.

VENOM, *Vene'num, Tox'icum, Venena'tio*, *Venin*. A poisonous fluid secreted by certain animals, as the viper, in a state of health, and which they preserve in a particular reservoir for use as a means of attack or defence. It is not, according to some, from *virus*, as the latter is always the result of a morbid process, which must be produced by the individuals who receive it, in their turn, and be transmitted to others.

VENOM, QUICKENING, Sperm—v. Vital, Sperm.

VEN'OMOUS, *Venena'tus, Ven'enose*, *Venimeux*. An epithet applied to animals which have a secretion of venom, as the viper, the snake, &c.; and, by some, to liquids in the animal body, which have been so perverted by previous disease, that their contact occasions serious mischief in sound individuals; as happens in hydrophobia. Virus is more commonly used in this case.

VENOSITAS, Venosity — v. Sanguinis, Prædominium sanguinis venosi.

VENOS'ITY, *Venos'itas, Ve'nousness, Venous state, Venous cachex'ia, Melanæ'mia, Melanosis universa'lis*, from *vena*, 'a vein.' A condition which, it has been supposed, the blood is at times slowly; is more venous; and the venous blood itself in greater quantity. This state is said to be chiefly observed in hemorrhoids, gout, hypochondriasis, melancholia, &c. — Puchelt.

VENOUS, *Venal, Veno'sus*. Same etymon. Appertaining to a vein, or to the blood in the veins; as *venous* cachexia, *venous* pulse.

VENOUS CACHEXIA, Venosity—v. Hue Pale de Diable — v. State, Venosity—v. System, Abdominal, Porta vena— v. System, see Vascular.

VENOUSNESS, Venosity.

VENT, Wind.

VENTER, Abdomen, Belly, Uterus. In law, venter designates the maternal parentage of children. Thus, if A were B's child by his first wife, he would be described in law as "by the first *venter.*" "A died seised, leaving two infant daughters by different *venters.*"

VENTER IMUS, Abdomen, Hypogastrium, Neisera — v. Inferius, Abdomen — v. Infimus, Abdomen — v. Magnus, Ingluvies — v. Medius, Thorax — v. Parvus, Hypogastrium — v. Propendens, Hysteroloxia anterior — v. Renum, Pelvis of the kidney — v. Supremus, Cavum cranii.

VENTEUX, Windy.

VENTILA'TION, *Ventila'tio*, from *ventus*, 'wind.' The act of renewing the air of vessels, hospitals, and apartments, or of situations where many people are collected together. The utility of such renewal must be evident, when it is considered that atmospheric air loses its oxygen during respiration, and that carbonic acid supplies its place. Stagnant air, also, becomes loaded with numerous impurities; and hence one of the greatest hygienic improvements, of modern times, has been a proper attention to circulation of air. It is, moreover, one of the most valuable additions to our stock of therapeutical agencies in many diseases.

Instruments used for the purpose of renewing the air, in ships, apartments, &c., have been called *ventilators*.

VENTOSITÉ, Flatulence.

VENTOSITY, Flatulence.

VENTOUSES SCARIFIÉES, Cupping with the scarificator.

VENTOUSES SÈCHES, Cupping, dry.

VENTRAL, Abdominal.

VENTRAL HER'NIA, *Her'nia ventra'lis*. Direct hernia accurring in any part of the abdomen. It is most frequently found between the recti muscles.

VENTRALE, Belt (Russian).

VENTRALE CUTA'NEUM, 'Cutaneous apron.' (F.) *Tablier*. An elongation of the nymphæ in the Bosjesman female, which hangs down before the vulva like an apron.

VENTRE, Abdomen — *v. Inférieur*, Abdomen — *v. Resserré*, Constipation.

VENTRE INSPICIENDO DE, see De ventre inspiciendo.

VEN'TRICLE, *Ventric'ulus*, diminutive of *venter*, 'belly.' Literally, a *little belly*. A name given, in anatomy, to various parts.

VENTRICLE OF ARAN'TIUS. A small cavity, lined with gray substance, at the point of the calamus scriptorius.

VENTRICLES OF THE BRAIN, *Ventric'uli* seu *Cavita'tes* seu *Sinus Cer'ebri*, (F.) *Ventricules du cerveau*, are five cavities in the interior of that organ, which are distinguished into the *lateral ventricles*, *middle ventricle*, *fourth ventricle* or *ventricle of the cerebellum*, and *fifth ventricle*. The *middle ventricle* or *third ventricle*, (F.) *Ventricule moyen du cerveau*, is situate in front of the pineal gland. It is bounded, *above*, by the tela choroidea and the fornix; *below*, by a portion of cerebral substance, which separates it from the base of the cranium; *laterally*, by the thalami nervorum opticorum; *anteriorly*, by a medullary cord, called the *anterior commissure;* and, *posteriorly*, by another medullary cord, called the *posterior commissure*. It communicates with the lateral ventricles by two openings, situate behind the anterior pillar or crus of the fornix. The *Lateral ventricles*, *Ventric'uli latera'les*, *V. magni*, *V. majo'res*, *V. prio'res*, *V. superio'res*, *V. tricor'nes*, (F.) *Ventricules latéraux*, are two in number. They are large, and, owing to their considerable curvature, occupy a great part of the cerebral centre. They are bounded, *above*, by the inferior surface of the corpus callosum; *anteriorly*, by the curved portion of the same body; *posteriorly*, by a considerable mass of cerebral substance; and, *internally*, they are separated from each other by the septum of the ventricles, — a medullary plate, which is given off from the lower part of the corpus callosum. The lateral ventricles have, in their upper and anterior portion, the *Corpora striata*, *Thalami optici*, and *Tænia semicircularis:* — their inferior portion contains the *corpus fimbriatum*, cornu Ammonis, &c. The *Fourth ventricle*, *Ventriculus cerebelli* seu *quartus*, *V. Aran'tii*, *Sinus rhomboï'deus*, (F.) *Quatrième ventricule*, is situate beneath the *aqueduct of Sylvius*, by which it communicates with the third ventricle. It extends from this aqueduct to the upper part of the medulla; and is seated in the substance of the tuber annulare. The *Fifth ventricle*, *Ventric'ulus septi pellu'cidi*, *Incisu'ra septi*, (F.) *Cinquième ventricule*, is the small serous cavity between the laminæ of the septum lucidum; called, also, *Fissure* or *Fossa of Sylvius* or *Sinus of the septum lu'cidum*.

VENTRICLES OF THE HEART, *Ventric'uli cordis*, *Specus cordis*, (F.) *Ventricules du cœur*, are two in number. The *Right ventricle*, *Pulmonary ventricle*, *Ventric'ulus anterior*, *V. primus*, *V. pulmona'lis*, (F.) *Ventricule droit* ou *pulmonaire*, is situate at the fore-part of the heart, the base and apex corresponding to those of the heart. In it are seen the *Columnæ carneæ* and *Cordæ tendineæ*. The right ventricle communicates with the right auricle by the *Ostium venosum*, and from it the *Pulmonary artery* arises. Around the auricular orifice is a tendinous margin or ring, from which the tricuspid valve is given off. The use of the ventricle is to send the blood, by its contraction, along the pulmonary artery to the lungs. The *Left ventricle*, *Ventric'ulus aor'ticus*, *V. posterior*, *V. secundus*, (F.) *Ventricule gauche* ou *aortique*, is situate at the posterior and left part of the heart. Its parietes are much thicker and stronger than those of the right, owing to its having to send the blood over the whole system. The inner surface has the same general appearance as that of the right. The *Columnæ carneæ* and *Cordæ tendineæ* are, however, much stronger. It communicates with the left auricle by means of the *Mitral valve;* and from it proceeds the largest blood-vessel of the body — the aorta.

VENTRICLES OF THE LARYNX, *Sac'culi laryngei*, *Sinuses of the larynx*, (F.) *Ventricules* ou *Sinus du larynx*, are two depressions in the larynx, comprised between the superior and inferior ligaments.

VENTRICLE, PULMONARY, V. right.

VENTRIC'ULAR, *Ventricula'ris*. Same etymon as Ventricle. Relating to a ventricle.

VENTRICULE AORTIQUE, Ventricle, left — *v. Cinquième*, Ventricle, fifth — *v. Droit*, Ventricle, right — *v. Gauche*, Ventricle, left — *v. Moyen du Cerveau*, Ventricle, middle, of the brain — *v. Pulmonaire*, Ventricle, right — *v. Quatrième*, Ventricle, fourth.

VENTRICULES DU CERVEAU, Ventricles of the brain — *v. du Cœur*, Ventricles of the heart — *v. Latéraux*, Ventricles, lateral.

VENTRICULI CORDIS, Ventricles of the heart — v. Dilatatio, Gastrectasis — v. Dissolutio, Gastro-malacia — v. Duræ matris, Sinuses of the dura mater — v. Emollitio, Gastro-malacia — v. Exulceratio, Gastrelcosis — v. Fluxus, Gastrorrhœa — v. Inflammatio, Gastritis — v. Laterales, see Ventricles, lateral of the brain — v. Magni, Ventricles, lateral, of the brain — v. Majores, Ventricles, lateral — v. Metamorphosis gelatiniformis, Gastro-malacia — v. Perforatio, Gastro-brosis — v. Priores, Ventricles, lateral — v. Pseudophlogosis resolutiva et colliquativa, Gastro-malacia — v. Superiores, Ventricles, lateral — v. Tricornes, Ventricles, lateral — v. Ulceratio, Gastrelcusia.

VENTRICULUS, Stomach, Ventricle—v. Anterior, Ventricle, right—v. Aorticus, Ventricle, left—v. Arantii, see Ventricles of the brain.

VENTRICULUS CALLOSUS, 'Callous stomach.' The *gizzard* or *third stomach* of the gallinaceous bird. It consists of a double-bellied or *digastric* muscle; is lined by a firm cuticle, and forms a kind of pouch, depending from the alimentary tube, in which the second stomach terminates, and from which the duodenum or *Ventriculus succenturia'tus* issues. In the interior of the gizzard there are numerous pebbles, which seem to be destined to aid in the trituration of the food. The gizzard is an organ of mastication, and is possessed of great muscular power.

VENTRICULUS CEREBELLI, see Ventricles of the brain—v. Posterior, Ventricle, left—v. Primus, Ventricle, right—v. Pulmonalis, Ventricle, right—v. Quartus, see Ventricles of the brain—v. Secundus, Ventricle, left—v. Septi Pellucidi, see Ventricles of the brain—v. Succenturiatus, Duodenum.

VENTRILOQUE, Engastrimythos.
VENTRILOQUISM, see Engastrimyth.
VENTRILOQUIST, Engastrimythos.
VENTRILOQUY, see Engastrimyth.
VENTROSITAS, Physconia.
VENTUS, Wind.
VEN'ULA, *Phlebion*, diminutive of *Vena*. See Vein. A small vein. Hippocrates seems to use it in the same sense as *Arteria*.

VENULÆ CENTRALES, Intralobular veins—v. Intralobulares, Intralobular veins.

VENUS, Clitoris, Coition, Cuprum—v. Crystals of, Cupri subacetas—v. *Oryateux de*, Cupri subacetas.

VER CUCURBITAIN, Tænia solium—v. *Cutané*, Dracunculus—v. *Filaire*, Dracunculus—v. *de Guinée*, Dracunculus—v. *Luisant*, Cicindela—v. *de Médine*, Dracunculus—v. *Solitaire*, Bothriocephalus latus, Tænia solium.

VERATRIA, Veratrina.
VERATRI'NA, *Vera'tria, Ver'atrine*. A vegetable alkali, found in the seeds of *Vera'trum sabadil'la, V. officina'lĕ, Helo'nias officina'lis*, and *Asagræ'a officina'lis*, which are known in commerce under the names *Cebadill'a, Cevadill'a*, and *Sabadill'a*, and are imported from Mexico. They usually occur, in commerce, mixed with the fruit of the plant, are two or three lines long, of a black colour, and are shining, flat, shriveled, winged, and elastic seeds. *Veratrine* is solid, white, pulverulent, and inodorous; of a very acrid taste; decomposable by heat; very soluble in water, and soluble in alcohol. When prepared in the usual manner, it still contains other substances,—*Sabadil'lin, Ver'atrin*, gum resin of the sabadilla, and black greasy matter. It is extremely poisonous, and but little used internally in medicine. Magendie has given it as an emetic and drastic in very small doses. It has been recommended to be applied in the way of friction, or endemically, (from gr. v to xx to ʒj of lard or cerate,) in various neuralgic affections. The following is the formula for its preparation in the Pharmacopœia of the United States:—Take of *cevadilla*, ℔ij; *alcohol*, 2 gallons; *sulphuric acid, solution of ammonia, purified animal charcoal*, and *magnesia*, each a sufficient quantity. Boil the cevadilla in a gallon of the alcohol, in a retort with a receiver attached, for an hour, and pour off the liquor. To the residue add another gallon of the alcohol, together with the portion recently distilled; again boil for an hour, and pour off the liquor. Repeat the boiling a third time with the remaining alcohol, and with that distilled in the previous operation. Press the cevadilla, mix and strain the liquors, and, by means of a water-bath, distil off the alcohol. Boil the residue three or four times in water acidulated with sulphuric acid, and strain the liquors, and evaporate to the consistence of syrup. Add magnesia in slight excess, shake the mixture frequently, then express and wash what remains. Repeat the express and washing two or three times, and having dried the residue, digest it with a gentle heat several times in alcohol, and strain after each digestion. Distil off the alcohol from the liquor, boil the residue for fifteen minutes in water with a little sulphuric acid and purified animal charcoal, and strain. Having thoroughly washed what remains, mix the washings with strained liquor, evaporate with a moderate heat to the consistence of syrup, and then drop in much solution of ammonia as may be necessary to precipitate the veratria. Lastly, separate and dry the precipitate. See Colchicum autumnale.

VERA'TRUM ALBUM, *Helleb'orus*, *Elleb'orum album, Elleborus albus, Chert..., White hellebore*, (F.) *Hellébore blanc.* &c. Polygamia Monœcia. *Nat. Ord.* Melanthaceæ (Lindley.) The root or rhizoma of this common European plant is indebted to the veratrine for its properties. It is inodorous; has a bitter, acrid, nauseous taste, and is violently emetic, purgative, even when applied to an ulcerated surface. It is, also, possessed of errhine properties and acts, externally, as a stimulant. It is now exhibited internally. Sometimes it is given as a sneezing powder; but it operates with great violence. It forms, also, an itch ointment. See Ung. Veratri.

VERATRUM LUTEUM, Chamælirium luteum.
VERATRUM SABADIL'LA, *Sabadilla, Schœnocanlon Interfec'tor, Caus'ticum America'nus, Cevadil'la Hispano'rum, Sevadilla, Hor'deum cau'cum*, (F.) *Cévadille*. The seeds of this plant have been used, mostly as anthelmintics. Dose to a child, four years old. It possesses the general properties as the veratrum album.

VERATRUM VIR'IDE, *American Hellebore, Swamp hellebore, Indian poke, Indian Poke weed, Bear weed, Itch weed, Tickleweed, Earth gall, Devilbit, Wolfsbane, Puppet root*, indigenous in the swampy districts of almost every part of the United States. Its properties are like those of the genus.

VERBASCULUM, Primula veris.
VERBASCUM ALBUM, V. thapsus—v. Latum, V. thapsus—v. Collinum, V. thapsus—Crassifolium, V. thapsus—v. Elongatum, V. thapsus—v. Lychnitis, V. thapsus—v. Montanum, thapsus.

VERBAS'CUM NIGRUM, *Black Mullein, Cave re'gia, Thapsus barba'tus, Tapsus barbe'tus, dela'ria, Lana'ria;* and VERBAS'CUM TE...
V. thapsoi'des seu *ala'tum* seu *colli'num* ...
seu *crassifo'lium* seu *elonga'tum* seu *Lychnitis*, seu *monta'num* seu *simplex, Phlogmos. Phlox, great broad-leaved Mullein, High Taper, Cow's Lungwort*, or *Yellow Mullein*, (F.) *Bouillon blanc; Family*, Solaneæ; &c. Pentandria Monogynia,—especially the leaves, have been used as emollient, applied externally in the form of fomentation. The large leaves have been chosen for this purpose. Occasionally, the mucilage which they contain has been extracted by decoction or infusion, and administered in pectoral affections.

VERBASCUM SIMPLEX, V. thapsus—v. Thapsoides, V. thapsus—v. Thapsus, see V. nigrum.
VERBE'NA HASTA'TA, an American species, is more bitter than the European, and said to be emetic.

VERBE'NA OFFICINA'LIS, *Verbena, Dichrum*

Verbena'ca, Periste'rium, Hierobot'ani, Herba sacra, Vervain, Purvain, (F.) *Verveine.* Family, Pyrenaceæ. *Sext. Syst.* Diandria Monogynia. A plant formerly held sacred; used in sacrifices, and suspended round the neck as an amulet. In the form of cataplasm, it is said to have relieved obstinate headachs, and to have been of service in scrofula. It is not used.

VERBE'NA URTICIFO'LIA, an indigenous species, has been used in poisoning from Rhus Toxicodendron.

VERBENACA, Verbena officinalis.

VERBESINA ACMELLA, Spilanthus Acmella.

VERBUS, Penis.

VERCOQUIN, Phreni'tis vermino'sa. A form of phrenitis, attributed to the presence of a worm in the brain!

VERDET, Cupri subacetas.

VERDIGRIS, Cupri subacetas.

VERENDA, Genital organs.

VERETRUM, Penis.

VERGE, Penis — *v. d'Or,* Solidago virgaurea.

VERGERETTE DE PHILADELPHIE, Erigeron Philadelphicum.

VERGETURES, Vibices.

VERJUICE, *Ompha'cium,* (F.) *Verjus, Verdjus.* A sour kind of grape. Also, an acid liquor, prepared from very sour grapes or crab-apples. It is principally used in culinary preparations; although, occasionally, an ingredient in medicinal compounds. See Vitis vinifera.

VERJUS, Verjuice.

VERMES, Worms—v. Cerebri, Choroid plexus.

VERMICULAIRE BRULANTE, Sedum.

VERMICULAR, Vermiform.

VERMICULARIS, Lumbricalis, Sedum.

VERMICULI SPERMATICI, Spermatozoa.

VERMIC'ULUM, *Vermyc'ilum.* An elixir; a tincture. — Ruland and Johnson.

VERMICULUS CAPILLARIS, Dracunculus.

VER'MIFORM, *Vermic'ular, Vermicula'ris, Vermifor'mis,* from *vermis,* 'a worm,' and *forma,* 'form.' That which resembles a worm.

VERM'IFORM PROC"ESSES, *Proces'sus Vermiform'es, Protuberan'tiæ vermiformes, Montic'uli cerebel'li, Appen'dices vermiformes, Vermis, Worm,* (F.) *Éminences vermiformes du cervelet,* are two medullary projections, at the surface of the cerebellum. The *superior vermiform process, Vermis superior cerebelli,* is an elongated projection, at the anterior and middle part of the superior surface of the cerebellum;—and the *inferior vermiform process, Vermis inferior cerebelli, Pyr'amid of Malacarne,* is a somewhat large projection, situate in the depression at the inferior surface of the same organ. The inferior vermiform process is usually described as consisting of three portions—the *pyramid,* the *uvula,* and the *nodulus.* The anterior portion of the superior vermiform process is elevated, and termed *Montic'ulus.*

VERMIFUGE, Anthelmintic.

VERMIFUGE, MATHIEU'S. This consisted of two distinct electuaries; the one for killing, the other for expelling tape-worm. The former is made of an ounce of *tin filings,* and six drachms of *fern* root.

VERMIFUGUS, Anthelmintic.

VERMILION, Hydrargyri sulphuretum rubrum.

VERMILLON DE PROVENCE, Antimonii sulphuretum rubrum.

VERMINATIO, Helminthiasis.

VERMINATION, CUTANEOUS, Malis.

VERMINEUX, Verminous.

VERM'INOUS, *Vermino'sus,* (F.) *Vermineux.* That which is caused by worms; as a *verminous affection.*

VERMIS, Vermiform processes—v. Bombycinus, Cornu ammonis — v. Cerebelli, Vermiform process—v. Cerebri, Fever, Hungary—v. Cucurbitinus, Tænia solium — v. Digiti, Paronychia.

VERMITIO, Helminthiasis.

VERNIX CASEO'SA, 'cheesy varnish.' The fatty varnish, or deposit, often found on the fœtus, which is secreted by the sebaceous follicles of the skin.

VERNIX SICCA, Sandarac.

VERNO'NIA ANTHELMIN'TICA, *Ascari'cida anthelmin'tica, Calagirah, Calageri.* A plant which is indigenous in India. Family, Compositæ. *Sex. Syst.* Syngenesia Polygamia superflua. It has great celebrity in the East Indies, and is a bitter tonic; but the seeds are chiefly used as an anthelmintic, in cases of ascarides and lumbrici in children.

VERNO'NIA NOVEBORACEN'SIS, *Iron weed, Flat top;* an indigenous plant; whose purple flowers appear in August and September, is reported to possess cathartic properties.

VÉROLE, Syphilis — *v. Petite,* Variola — *v. Petite volante,* Varicella.

VÉROLETTE, Varicella.

VERONI'CA, *Veronica officina'lis* seu *Tournefor'tii, Veronica mas, Thea German'ica, Beton'ica Pauli, Chamæ'drys, Male Veronica, Fluellin, Offioinal Speedwell,* (F.) *Véronique, Thé d'Europe.* Family, Rhinanthodeæ. *Sex. Syst.* Diandria Monogynia. This plant was once used as a pectoral.

VERONICA AQUATICA, V. beccabunga.

VERONICA BECCABUN'GA, *Beccabunga, Anagal'lis aquat'ica, Laver German'icum, Veronica aquat'ica, Cepæ'a, Water Pim'pernel, Brooklime, Brooklime Speedwell, Water Speedwell, Neckweed, Water Purslain,* (F.) *Véronique cressonée.* This plant was formerly used in a variety of diseases. It is, however, almost insipid and inodorous; and has been long banished from practice.

VERONICA MAS, Veronica — v. Officinalis, Veronica.

VERONICA PEREGRI'NA, *Neckweed, Purslain, Speedwell;* indigenous; flowering from April to June, is given internally in scrofulosis, and is applied as a wash to scrofulous tumours.

VERONICA PURPUREA, Betonica officinalis—v. Tournefortii, Veronica—v. Virginica, Leptandra Virginica.

VÉRONIQUE, Veronica—v. *Cressonée,* Veronica beccabunga.

VERPA, Penis.

VERRE, Vitrum — *v. d'Antimoine,* Antimonii vitrum.

VERRU'CA, diminutive *Verru'cula, Ecphy'ma verruca, Phymato'sis verruco'sa,* a *Wart,* (F.) *Verrue.* A small, hard, mamillary tumour, which forms at the surface of the skin, and particularly on that of the hands and face. Warts are generally rugous at the surface, and broad at the base; their roots being implanted in the derma by whitish filaments, which are dense, semifibrous, and very numerous.

Warts may be destroyed by caustic, or removed by excision. Their vitality is, generally, not great.

VERRUCA CARNOSA, Condyloma — v. Formicaria, Formica — v. Minor, Thymion—v. Palpebrarum, see Hydatid—v. Pensilis, Acrochordon—v. Rhagoidea, Thymion.

VERRUCARIA, Calendula officinalis, Heliotropium Europæum.

VERRUCOSE, Warty.

VERRUCOUS, Warty.

VERRUCULA, Verruca.

VERRUE, Verruca.

VERS, Worms.

VERSE-CHARMS, see Charm.
VERSIO, Turning — v. Fœtûs, Turning — v. Spontanea, Evolution spontaneous — v. Uteri, Hysteroloxia.
VERSION, Turning.
VERT-DE-GRIS, Cupri subacetas.
VERTEBRA DENTATA, Axis — v. Dorsi Prima, Lophia — v. Lumborum Prima, Asphaltites — v. Magna, Sacrum.
VER'TEBRÆ, Spon'dyli, (F.) *Vertèbres;* from *vertere,* 'to turn.' This name has been given to the bones, which by their union form the vertebral or spinal column. The vertebræ are short, thick, very angular bones; twenty-four in number, and situate one above another. The *body—centrum,* of Owen — of the vertebra is the middle and anterior portion. Above and below it is articulated, by means of a fibro-cartilage, with the contiguous vertebræ. The *Processes,* (F.) *Masses apophysaires,* of each vertebra are: — 1. The *spinous process,* situate behind, and in the median line. 2. The two *transverse processes,* standing off from each side. 3. The *four articular* or *oblique processes* — *zygapophyses,* of Owen — two *superior,* and two *inferior* — which serve to unite the vertebræ with each other. These transverse and articulating processes are made continuous with the lateral and posterior parts of the body of the vertebra by narrow bony portions or pedicles, on each of which are notches. These, by their union with similar notches in the contiguous vertebra, form the lateral foramina, (F.) *Trous de conjugaison,* through which the spinal nerves leave the vertebral canal. The different processes are united with each other, so as to form a kind of ring of the lateral and posterior parts of the vertebra; and the foramen, within this,—that is, between the body and processes,—concurs in forming the vertebral canal. The vertebræ have particular characters, according to the regions they occupy. They are divided into seven *cervical,* twelve *dorsal,* and five *lumbar.* The first cervical is called *atlas;* the second, *axis* or *vertebra dentata;* and the seventh, *vertebra proëminens.* The vertebræ are articulated with each other. Those of the back are joined, moreover, to the ribs. The first or atlas is articulated with the occipital bone; and the last lumbar vertebra with the sacrum. The cervical vertebræ are developed by nine points of ossification; the dorsal and lumbar by eight.

VER'TEBRAL, *Vertebra'lis.* That which relates or belongs to the vertebræ.

VERTEBRAL ARTERY, *Posterior cerebral artery,* (Ch.,) is the largest of the branches of the subclavian. It arises from the posterior part of that vessel; is lodged in a canal, (F.) *Petit canal vertébral,* formed by the foramina in the transverse processes; enters the cranium, and proceeds to anastomose with its fellow of the opposite side, and to form the *Basilary artery.* Besides the branches sent to the neck, the vertebral artery gives off the *anterior* and *posterior spinal arteries,* and the *inferior cerebellous,* in the cavity of the cranium.

VERTEBRAL COLUMN, *Rachis, Rhachis, Notos, Acnes'tis;* the *Spine;* the back bone, *Cari'na, C. hom'inis, Spina dorsi* seu *vertebra'lis, Colum'na spina'lis, C. vertebra'lis, C. dorsi, Spina Dorsum, Tergum, Compa'ges Vertebra'rum, Acan'tha, Sacra fis'tula, Hi'era Syrinx,* (F.) *Colonne vertébrale, Épine du dos, Échine.* A kind of bony column, situate at the posterior and central part of the trunk; extending from the head to the sacrum; flexible in every direction, yet very solid and hollowed by a *canal* called *vertebral,* which gives it lightness without diminishing its strength, and runs through its whole length. The vertebral column is formed by the superposition of the vertebræ. It represents a pyramid, whose base is below. Anteriorly, it is convex in the neck, concave in the back, and convex, again, in the loins. Behind, the curvatures are of course the reverse of these. There is also, in the dorsal region, a lateral curvature, the concavity of which is towards the left side. Considered as a whole, the vertebral column has an *anterior* or *prosurface;* a *posterior* or *spinal;* two *laterals base;* and an *apex* or top. In the nomenclature of Chaussier, the anterior surface, in the neck, is called *trachelian;* in the back, *predorsal;* in the loins, *prelumbar.* The dorsal surface at its middle, the spinous processes; and at sides, the *vertebral gutters,* (F.) *Gouttières vertébrales,* formed by the succession of the vertebral *plates,* (F.) *Lames vertébrales,* which, by their junction, constitute the spinous processes. These are filled by the sacro-spinalis muscle. The inner or lateral surfaces present the foramina resulting from the union of the *vertebral notches,* (F.) *Échancrures vertébrales.* These are called *vertebral foramina,* (F.) *Trous de conjugaison* and give passage to the *vertebral nerves.* The base of the vertebral column is oblique, to unite with the sacrum; and forms with it an angle, called *sacro-vertebral angle* or *promontory.* The apex or top of the vertebral column is articulated with the occipital bone. Sometimes, the term *vertebral column* includes the whole of the column from the occipital bone to the extremity of the coccyx. The *Vertebral* or *Spinal Canal, Rachid'ian Canal, Solen, Cana'lis medulla spinalis, Specus pro medull'a Spina'li* seu *vertebrali,* exists through the whole of the vertebral column, whose curvatures it follows. It is continuous, above, with the cranium; below, with the sacral canal, if we consider the vertebræ to terminate at the sacrum. It is lined by a prolongation of the meninges, forming the *Theca vertebralis* and lodges the spinal marrow.

The vertebral column, which unites lightness with solidity, serves to support the head and chest. It is the seat of all the movements of the trunk, the weight of which it transmits to the pelvis. It lodges and protects the spinal marrow, and gives passage to the vertebral nerves, and to numerous vessels.

VERTEBRAL DISEASE, *Rachial'gia* (of some), *Caries of the Ver'tebræ, Spondylartroc'acè, Spondyloc'acè, Kypho'sis inflammato'ria, L. polyt'ica, Gibbos'itas cario'sa, Ca'ries vertebrarum, Spondylal'gia, Spondylopyo'sis, Tubercula Vertebra'rum.* The spinal column is liable to distortion, (see Hump,) at times, without the vertebræ being much, if at all, diseased. At other times, a more formidable affection is induced, the vertebræ becoming carious, and the intervertebral cartilages ulcerated; followed by a more or less complete loss of power over the lower extremities. In such case, on examining the spine, one or more of the spinous processes is found to project beyond the rest. The disease was first well described by Mr. Percival Pott; and hence it has been called, by the French, *Maladie Pott, (Malum Pot'tii, Gibbus Pot'tii,* or *Pott's disease.*) It usually occurs in scrofulous subjects, and the treatment consists in establishing a counter-irritation by blisters, issues, or the moxa, opposite the transverse processes of the diseased vertebræ. The sore must be suffered remain open and the patient kept in the horizontal posture until the use of the limbs is recovered; employing tonics, the free admission of fresh air, &c., at the same time.

VERTEBRAL LIG'AMENTS, (F.) *Ligaments vertébraux, Surtouts ligamenteux de la colonne vertébrale tèbrale*, are distinguished into *anterior* and *posterior*. They consist of long, ligamentous coverings; the *anterior* occupying the anterior part of the vertebral column; and the *posterior* seeming to arise from the occipito-axoid ligament, and seated behind the bodies of the vertebræ, from the axis to the sacrum.

VERTEBRAL NERVE, Trisplanchnic.

VERTEBRAL NERVES, *Spinal Nerves*, spring successively from the spinal marrow; from its origin to its termination. These nerves—30 pairs in all—arise by two roots; one *anterior*, from the *anterior* or *an'tero-lat'eral column* of the spinal marrow, and the other *posterior*, from the *posterior column*, and afterwards issue by the vertebral and sacral foramina. Each of these roots seems to have a distinct function; the *posterior* being destined to convey sensation to parts; the *anterior*, motion. On the posterior root, before its junction with the anterior, there is a ganglion. Of the 30 pairs, 7 are *cervical nerves*, 12 *dorsal*, 5 *lumbar*, and 6 *sacral*. See Nerves.

VERTÈBRES, Vertebræ.

VERTEBRODYMIA, see Somatodymia.

VERTEBRO-ILIAC LIGAMENT, Ileo-lumbar ligament.

VERTEX, *Cor'yphĕ*, *Acrori'a*, *Spon'dylus*. The top or highest part of the head. See Sinciput.

VERTEX CORDIS, Mucro Cordis — v. Cubiti, Olecranon —v. Palpitans, Fontanella.

VERTIBULUM, Trepan.

VERTICULA, Articulation.

VERTICULUM, Articulation.

VERTICULUS, Articulation.

VERTIGE, Vertigo.

VERTIG"INOUS, *Vertigino'sus*, (F.) *Vertigineux*. Relating or pertaining to vertigo. Giddy.

VERTI'GO, from *vertere*, 'to turn;' *Dinos*, *Ilin'gos*, *Gid'diness*, *Diz'ziness*, *Dinus verti'go*, *Hallucina'tio vertigo*, *Autal'gia vertigo*, *Circumgyra'tio*, *Swimming of the head*, (F.) *Vertige*, *Étourdissement*. A state in which it seems that all objects are turning round; or that the individual himself is performing a movement of gyration. Two varieties have been designated;— *simple vertigo*, where the objects are seen; and *scotodynia*, in which the sight is obscured, and the individual often falls. Vertigo is dependent upon the condition of the brain; and often announces an attack of apoplexy or epilepsy.

VERTIGO TENEBRICOSA, Scotodynia.

VERUGAS (S.), from *verruca*. A peculiar disease affecting certain localities of Peru, which manifests itself by sore-throat, pains in the bones, and other febrile symptoms. In the course of a few days, an eruption of red pimples or boils appears. These sometimes increase in magnitude till they become nearly as large as an egg, and discharge blood copiously. It is ascribed to the water of certain springs in the valleys, and especially in that of Surea: called *Agua de Veruga*. — Tschudi.

VERUMONTANUM, Gallinaginis caput.

VERVAIN, Verbena officinalis.

VERVEINE, Verbena officinalis.

VESA'NIA, *Vesa'niæ*, 'madness.' Derangement of the intellectual and moral faculties, without coma or fever. Many nosologists have used this as a generic term; under which they have included the different species of mental alienation, hypochondriasis, somnambulism, and even hydrophobia. See Nosology.

VESANIA MANIA, Mania.

VESANIÆ, Insanity.

VESICA BILIARIA, Gall-bladder—v. Cordis, see Pericardium—v. Fellea, Gall-bladder—v. Intestinales, Vesicula umbilicalis—v. Prostatica, see Ejaculatory Ducts—v. Saccata, Stricture of the urinary bladder — v. Urinaria, Urinary bladder.

VESICÆ IRRITABILITAS, Cysterethismus — v. Unguinosæ tendinum, Bursæ mucosæ.

VES'ICAL, *Vesica'lis*, from *vesica*, 'the bladder.' That which belongs or relates to the bladder.

VESICAL ARTERIES vary in number and origin. The umbilical artery always sends off two or three: the middle hemorrhoidal, internal pudic, and obturator furnish others, which ramify and anastomose in the parietes of the bladder; the hypogastric furnishes one which is somewhat larger, the *Vesico-prostatic* (Ch.), and proceeds to the *bas-fond* of the bladder, sending numerous ramifications to it as well as to the surrounding parts.

VESICAL GANGLIA, see Spermatic Ganglion — v. Triangle, see Urinary Bladder.

VESICAL VEINS, much more numerous than the arteries, open into the hypogastric plexus.

VESICANT, Blister, Epispastic.

VESICARIUM, Ovarium.

VESICA'TION, *Vesica'tio*; same etymon, (F.) *Ve'sication*. The action of a vesicant. The formation of blisters.

VÉSICATOIRE, Blister — v. *Magistral*, Magistral.

VESICATORIUM, Blister.

VESICLE, Vesicula—v. Allantoid, Allantois—v. Blastodermie, see Molecule — v. Cowpox, see Vaccination.

VESICLE OF DEVELOPMENT, V. *of Evolution*. A vesicle or cyst concerned in histogeny.

VESICLE OF EVOLUTION, V. of Development — v. Germinal, see Molecule — v. Purkinjean, see Molecule — v. Umbilical, Vesicula umbilicalis.

VESICLES OF DE GRAAF, Folliculi Graafiani.

VES'ICO-VAG"INAL, *Vesi'co-vagina'lis*. Relating to the bladder and the vagina; as *vesico-vaginal fistula*.

VESIC'ULA, *Cystinx*, *Ves'icle*; diminutive of *vesica*, 'a bladder.' A small bladder or cyst.

VESICULA, *Ves'icle*, *Ecphly'sis*, *Cystinx*, in pathology, means a small orbicular elevation of the cuticle containing lymph, which is sometimes clear and colourless, but often opake and whitish or pearl-coloured. It is succeeded, either by a scurf, or by a laminated scab.

VESICULA ÆNIGMATOSA, Vesicula umbilicalis — v. Alba, Vesicula umbilicalis — v. Bilis, Gallbladder — v. Blastodermatica, see Molecule — v. Chyli, Receptaculum chyli—v. Erythroidea, Erythroid vesicle—v. Fellis, Gall-bladder— v. Gangrænescens, see Anthrax — v. Germinativa, see Molecule—v. Omphalo-mesenterica, Vesicula umbilicalis—v. Ovalis, Vesicula umbilicalis— v. Prolifera, see Molecule — v. Prostatica, see Ejaculatory Ducts.

VESIC'ULA UMBILICA'LIS, *Umbil'ical Ves'icle*, *Vesicula alba* seu *om'phalo-mesenter'ica* seu *ænigmato'sa* seu *ova'lis*, *Vesi'ca intestinalis*, *Intestinal Vesicle*, *Vit'elline Pouch*. A small, pyriform, round, or spheroidal sac, which, about the fifteenth or twentieth day after fecundation, is of the size of a common pea, and probably acquires its greatest dimensions in the course of the third or fourth week. After the seventh week, it becomes shrivelled and disappears insensibly. It seems to be situate between the chorion and amnion, and is commonly adherent either to the outer surface of the amnion, or to the inner surface of the chorion, but at times is loose between them. The *vitelline ped'icle*, which attaches the vesicle to the embryo, is continuous with the intestinal canal; and, up to twenty or thirty days of embryonic life, is hollow;—*Ductus om'phalo-mesenter'icus* seu *vitello-intestina'lis* seu *vitella'rius*, *vitelline Duct.* Its arteries are the omphalo-mesenteric. The *vitelline fluid*, contained in the vesicle, has been compared, from analogy, to the *vitellus* or yolk of birds; and, like it, is an oleaginous substance, and presumed to be inservient to the nutrition of the embryo.

VESICULÆ constitute the 6th order of Bateman's classification of *Cutaneous Diseases*.

VESICULÆ, see Villous membranes — v. Divæ Barbaræ, Variola confluens — v. Gingivarum, Aphthæ—v. Pulmonales, see Cellule—v. Rotundæ cervicis uteri, Nabothi glandulæ — v. Sanguinis, Globules of the blood — v. Seminales mulierum, Nabothi glandulæ—v. Spermaticæ, Vesiculæ seminales.

VESICULÆ SEMINA'LES, *V. Semina'ria seu spermat'icæ, Cap'sulæ semina'les, Conceptac'ula seminaria, Gonecys'tides,* (F.) *Vésicules séminales, Gardouches, Greniers,* are two small membranous sacs, which serve as reservoirs for the sperm, and probably secrete a fluid to be mixed with the sperm. They are situate beneath the bladder, and above the rectum, behind the prostate and to the outer side of the vasa deferentia. They are of an irregular conoidal shape; flattened from above to below; embossed on their surface, and of a grayish tint. Their *posterior extremity* or *fundus* terminates by a round cul-de-sac. Their *anterior extremity* or *neck* is narrow and elongated, and is continuous with the excretory duct of the vesicula. This duct joins the vas deferens, and forms with it the ejaculatory duct. The interior of the vesiculæ exhibits several cells, which communicate with each other, and are lined by a very thin, mucous membrane.

VESIC'ULAR, *Vesicula'ris.* Of or belonging to a vesicle:—full of or containing small vesicles or cells. The cortical or gray matter of the brain is sometimes termed *vesicular*. See Cortex cerebri and Neurine.

VÉSICULE BILIAIRE, Gall-bladder—*v. du Fiel,* Gall-Bladder—*v. Germinative,* see Molecule —*v. Ovulifère,* see Folliculi Graafiani.

VÉSICULES DE GRAEF, Folliculi Graafiani —*v. de Sainte Barbe,* Variola confluens—*v. Séminales,* Vesiculæ seminales.

VESPA, Wasp.

VESSEL, *Vas, Vasum,* diminutive *Vasculum, Angei'on, Angos, Conceptac'ulum,* from (L.) *vas, vasculum,* (F.) *Vaisseau.* A canal, more or less elastic, formed by the superposition of membranes, and distinguished, according to its uses and general arrangement, into *Artery, Vein,* and *Lymphatic.* See, also, Vascular.

VESSELOUP, Lycoperdon.

VESSIE, Urinary bladder—*v. à Colonnes,* see Urinary bladder — *v. Col de la,* Collum vesicæ.

VESSIE NATATOIRE, Air-bladder.

VESTIBULAR NERVE, see Auditory Nerve.

VES'TIBULE, *Vestib'ulum,* from *vestio,* 'to cover.' The porch or entrance to a house.

VESTIBULE, *Vestib'ulum, V. Vagi'næ, Prona'us, Atrium Vagi'næ, Amb'itus genita'lis mulie'bris,* is a smooth cavity between the perinæum and nymphæ in the female, which leads to two passages — to the urethra above, and to the vagina below.

VES'TIBULE OF THE EAR, *Vestib'ulum, V. labyrin'thi,* (F.) *Vestibule.* A cavity of an irregular shape, which forms part of the labyrinth or internal ear. The vestibule is situate on the inner side of the tympanum; on the outer side of the meatus auditorius internus; before the semicircular canals, and behind the cochlea. It is lined by a particular membrane, and contains the liquor of Cotunnius and branches of the auditory nerve. There is also another membrane, constituting the *mem'branous vestibule,* but it is not an exact imitation of the osseous cavity. It is composed of two distinct sacs, which open into each other—the *sac'culus vestib'uli,* and the *sacculus.* There are three contiguous *cavities* in the vestibule; one of which, the *semi-oval,* is situate above; another, the *hemispherical,* below; and the third, of oval form, which is the orifice of the aquæductus vestibuli, behind.

VESTIBULUM LABYRINTHI, Vestibule of the ear—v. Vaginæ, Vestibulæ.

VESTIGE (F.), *Vestig"ium,* 'a vestige, a trace.' A kind of fracture of flat bones, consisting of a simple incision having the mark of the instrument that caused it. The term is also applied to a part of the body, which may have evident use in man, and yet may be greatly employed in animals. For example, the muscles of the external ear in man are almost devoid of use, or are *vestiges* of what they are in certain animals.

VESTIGIUM, Sole, *Vestige* — v. Fossa ovalis, Ovalis fossa—v. Pedis, Metatarsus.

VESTI'TUS, *Esthe'ma, Esthe'sis, Chlaina, Investia'ria, Dress, Vestura,* (F.) *Vêtement, vestire, vestitum,* 'to clothe.' Any substance used for the purpose of covering nakedness, or preserving from atmospheric temperature by being worn on the body. The best clothing in winter is composed of articles that are bad conductors of caloric, and do not admit of ready evaporation of the matter of perspiration. In this respect woollen vestments deserve the first place, cotton the second. Colour has likewise to be regarded — the darkest hues transmitting the heat most readily through them. It has been found that the same rule applies to odours—the darker colours retaining a greater amount of odoriferous particles than the lighter. Hence the necessity of white walls, white bed-clothes, &c., in the ward of hospitals; for it is probable that the like law applies to contagious miasms.

VESTURE, Vestitus.

VETA, Puna.

VÊTEMENT, Vestitus.

VETERANA, Rubeola.

VETERINARIUS, see Hippiater and Veterinary.

VET'ERINARY, *Veterina'rius,* (F.) *Vétérinaire,* from *veterinus,* 'that which bears burdens; itself from *vetere,* 'to carry.' That which appertains to beasts of burden: hence, *veterinary surgeon,* (see Farrier,) *veterinary college,* and *veterinary medicine.*

VETERINARY ANATOMY, see Anatomy.

VETERINARY ART, *Ars seu Medici'na veterina'ria, Zoöi'asis, Zoiatri'a, Theriat'rica, Medici'na, Zoötherapi'a, Zoötherapeu'tice, Ars veterina'rica, Far'riery.* The art of treating the diseases &c., of cattle.

VETERNOSITAS, Coma vigil.

VETERNUS, Coma vigil.

VETONICA CORDI, Betonica officinalis.

VETULA, Sacrum.

VEXILLA TUBARUM FALLOPII, see Tuba Fallopian.

VEXILLUM, *Drapeau.*

VIA, Way — v. Curandi, Ratio medendi—v. Stomachi et ventris, Œsophagus.

VIABILITY, see Viable.

VI'ABLE, *Viab'ilis,* from *vie,* 'way.' (F.) *vie,* 'life,' (Orfila.) A word, which has been introduced with great advantage from the French into our language. It is an epithet applied to a fœtus whose organs are properly formed, and developed as to permit its continued existence. Every fœtus is not *viable.* Anencephali have lived ten or twelve days, yet they are not viable, a part or the whole of the brain being wanting.

The older the fœtus, the more viable is it. It is an idle prejudice that a child, born at the end of eight months, is less likely to live than one born at the end of seven. The signs of *viability* are drawn from the weight, length, external conformation, &c., of the fœtus. It may be laid down as a general rule, that no fœtus born before the end of the seventh month is viable.

VIÆ CHYLIFERÆ, Chyliferous vessels.

VIÆ CLANDES'TINÆ, *Clandestine Passages.* Supposititious secret ways or passages or 'royal roads,' to account for the rapid transmission of substances taken into the stomach to the kidneys or bladder.

VIÆ EXTRAORDINARIÆ LACTIS, Galactoplania —v. Lacrymales, Lachrymal passages — v. Primæ, Ways, digestive—v. Secundæ, Ways, second.

VIAL, Phiala.

VIBI'CES, *Mol'opes, Striæ,* (F.) *Vergetures.* Large purple spots, like the marks produced by the strokes of a whip, which appear under the skin in certain malignant fevers. They are unfavourable indications, as they denote great prostration.

VIBRAMEN, Oscillation.

VIBRANS, Vibratory.

VIBRATILE, Vibratory.

VIBRATIL'ITY, *Vibratil'itas,* from *vibrare,* 'to oscillate.' Capability of being thrown into vibration.

VIBRATIO, Oscillation—v. Cardiaca, Palpitation—v. Cordis, Palpitation.

VIBRATION, PECTORAL, see Fremitus—v. Tactile, see Fremitus—v. Tussive, see Tussive.

VIBRATIONS OF SOUND, see Sound.

VIBRATOR, Deferens vas.

VI'BRATORY, *Vi'brative, Vibrans,* (F.) *Vibratile,* from *vibrare,* 'to quiver.' An epithet applied to the pain that accompanies some neuralgiæ, which seems to the patient to vibrate among the nerves.

VIBRATORY MOTION, see Cilia.

VIBRATUS, Oscillation.

VIB'RIO; from *vibrare,* 'to quiver.' A genus of infusory animalcules, of which different species are met with,—for example, *Vib'rio pro'lifer* in almost all putrescent fluids containing protein, and in the pus of chancres; in which last the *V. lineola* has likewise been found.

VIBRIS'SÆ, from *vibrare,* 'to quiver.' The hairs which grow at the entrance of the nostrils and of other outlets. In the feline tribe, the whiskers.

VIBURNUM CASSINOIDES, Ilex Paraguensis.

VIBUR'NUM DENTA'TUM, *Arrow Wood, Mealy Tree, Tily* of the Indians. A high indigenous shrub, of the same family as V. lentago; the bark of which has been used by the Indians as a diuretic.

VIBURNUM LÆVIGATUM, Ilex Paraguensis.

VIBURNUM LENTA'GO, *Sweet Viburnum, Nannyberry.* A handsome indigenous tree, of the honeysuckle *family*—Caprifoliaceæ—which flowers in May and June. It has been used as an antiperiodic.

VIBUR'NUM PRUNIFO'LIUM, *Black Haw, Sloe-leaved Viburnum.* Indigenous: flowering in May. The leaves have been used as tea.

VIBURNUM, SLOW-LEAVED, V. prunifolium—v. Sweet, V. lentago.

'VIC-LE-COMPTE, MINERAL WATERS OF. Vic-le-Compte is a small village in the department of Puy de Dôme, three leagues from Issoire; where there is an acidulous chalybeate, which is aperient.

VICA'RIOUS, *Vica'rius,* from *vicis,* 'change, place.' Taking the place of another:—as 'vicarious secretion,' *Secre'tio vica'ria;* a secretion which takes place in one part instead of another.

VICAR'S BRAY, MINERAL WATERS OF. This spring is situate in Perthshire, Scotland, about two miles from Dollor, and near to Blarngone. The water is one of the strongest chalybeates known.

VICE, Cachosis.

VICHY, MINERAL WATERS OF. Carbonated alkaline chalybeates, the sources of which are at Vichy, six leagues from Moulins, in the department of Allier. The springs are seven in number. Almost all are thermal; give off bubbles of carbonic acid gas, and have a slightly sulphureous odour. They deposite carbonates of lime and magnesia, and a little oxide of iron; and afford, on analysis, carbonates of lime, soda, iron, and magnesia, carbonic acid, sulphate of soda, and chloride of sodium. They are employed as tonics, particularly in chronic affections of the abdominal viscera, in old catarrhs, diseases of the joints, &c.

VICHY WATER, FACTIT"IOUS, *Aqua Vicien'sis,* (F.) *Eau de Vichy,* is made of simple *acidulous water,* impregnated with twice its bulk of *carbonic acid,* ℥xxss; *subcarbonate of soda,* gr. xxij; *sulphate of soda,* gr. xvj; *chloride of sodium,* gr. iv; *subcarbonate of magnesia,* gr. ss; *chloride of iron,* gr. ¼. Mix. *Ph. P.*)

VICIA ERVILIA, Ervum.

VIC"IA FABA, *Faba, F. major seu vulgaris, Or'obus faba.* The *Common Garden Bean,* (F.) *Fève* ou *fève des marais. Family,* Leguminosæ. *Sex. Syst.* Diadelphia Decandria. A native of Egypt, of which there are many varieties. Beans are not easy of digestion. They are proverbially flatulent, especially when old. When young, they are more digestible and wholesome. Bean meal was one of the four resolvent meals of the ancients.

VICINITRACTUS, Erysipelas.

VICINITRAHA, Erysipelas.

VICTORIALIS FEMINEA, Gladiolus vulgaris — v. Longa, Allium victoriale — v. Rotunda, Gladiolus vulgaris.

VICTÛS RATIO, Diet.

VIDANGES, Lochia.

VIDIAN CANAL, Pterygoid canal.

VIE, Life—v. *Durée de la,* see Longevity—*v. Moyenne,* see Longevity.

VIEILLESSE, Senectus.

VIERGE, Virgin.

VIF ARGENT, Hydrargyrum.

VIGILANCE, Insomnia.

VIGILANTIA, Egregorsis.

VIGILATIO, Egregorsis.

VIGILIA, Egregorsis.

VIGILIÆ, Egregorsis—v. Nimiæ, Coma vigil.

VIGILIUM, Egregorsis.

VIGNE, Vitis vinifera — v. *Blanche,* Bryonia alba—v. *du Nord,* Humulus lupulus — v. *Vierge,* Bryonia alba.

VIGOR, Acme.

VILLA FRANCA, (CLIMATE OF.) This little town is situate immediately to the eastward of Montalbano, which separates the bay of Villa Franca from that of Nice. It is on the southern declivity of a steep and lofty range of mountains; and is more effectually sheltered from the north and north-west winds than Nice, with the climate of which that of Villa Franca closely corresponds.

VILLI, see Villous membranes.

VILLOUS, *Villo'sus,* from *villus,* a hair.'

VILLOUS MEMBRANES or COATS, *Velamen'ta Bombyc"ina,* (F.) *Membranes villeuses, Membranes veloutés,* are such as are covered with soft papillæ or *Villi, Flocci, Floc'culi, Vesic'ulæ, Cylin'dri, Tubi Membrana'cei,* constituted of blood-vessels, nerves, and absorbents; or such as are covered with fine down, so as to cause them to feel soft and velvety. The term is, however, chiefly restricted to the former. Chaussier gives the name *simple villous membranes* to the serous membranes; and that of *complicated* or *follicular villous membranes* to the mucous membranes. On these membranes there are bodies endowed with *ciliary motion.*

VIN, Wine — *v. de Bordeaux,* Claret — *v. de Poulet,* see *Poulet*—*v. de Quinquina composé,* Vinum de kinâ kinâ compositum—*v. Sec,* Sack.

VINAIGRE, Acetum, see Aceticum acidum—*v. Scillitique,* Acetum scillæ — *v. de Bois,* Pyroligneous acid.

VINAIGRES MÉDICINAUX, Acetica.

VINCA MINOR, *Vinca pervin'ca, Clem'atis daphnoi'des major, Lesser periwinkle,* (F.) *Pervenche, Violette des Sorciers.* It has bitter and astringent properties, and has been used in gargles and diseases of the chest.

VINCETOXICUM, Asclepias vincetoxicum.

VINCTURA, Fascia.

VINCULA, Fascia.

VINCULUM, Bandage, Lien — v. Caninum, Frænum penis—v. Linguæ, Frænum linguæ—v. Præputii, Frænum penis—v. Umbilicale, Funiculus umbilicalis.

VINE, Vitis vinifera—v. Grape, Vitis vinifera —v. Poison, Rhus radicans—v. Wild, Pareira.

VINEGAR, AROMATIC SPIRIT OF, see Aceticum acidum — v. of Cantharides, Acetum cantharidis—v. Common, Acetum — v. Distilled, see Aceticum acidum—v. Marseilles, Acetum aromaticum—v. of Meadow saffron, Acetum colchici —v. of Opium, Guttæ nigræ—v. Radical, Aceticum acidum — v. of Squills, Acetum scillæ — v. :f the Four Thieves, Acetum aromaticum — v. Thieves', Acetum aromaticum — v. Whey, see Acetum—v. of Wood, see Aceticum acidum.

VINETTIER, Oxycantha Galéni.

VINEUX, Vinous.

VINOLENTA, see Temulentia.

VINOLENTIA, Temulentia.

VINOSUS, Vinous.

VINOUS, *Vino'sus, Œno'des, Œnol'des.* Relating to wine. Having the character of, or resembling, wine. Made of wine.

VINUM, Wine, Sherry wine, (Ph. U. S. 1842,) see Wine.

VINUM ABSINTHI'TES, *Wine of Wormwood.* (*Fol. absinth. exsic., absinth. Pontic.,* āā ℥vj, *vini albi* Oiv. Macerate for 24 hours, and strain. *Ph. P.*) Stimulant, tonic, febrifuge, vermifuge.

VINUM ADUSTUM, Brandy—v. Album, Sherry wine, (Ph. U. S. 1851,) see Wine—v. Album Hispanicum, see Wine—v. Album Montanum, see Wine.

VINUM AL'OES, *V. aloës Socutori'næ, Vinum aloët'icum, V. aro'mo-aloët'icum, Wine of Aloes, Tinctu'ra hi'era, Tinctura sacra.* (*Aloës* in pulv. ℥j, *cardam.* cont., *Zingib.* cont., āā ʒj; *vini alb.* Oj. Macerate for 14 days, and filter. *Ph. L.*) Purgative and stomachic, according to the dose. Dose, f℥j to f℥ij.

VINUM AMARUM, V. Gentianæ comp.—v. Amarum scilliticum, &c., V. diureticum amarum—v. Amarum cum spiritû vini, V. gentianæ compositum — v. Antimoniale, V. antimonii tartarizati—v. Antimoniatum Huxhami, V. antimonii tartarizati—v. Antimonii potassio-tartratis, V. antimonii tartarizati.

VINUM ANTIMONII, *V. antimo'nii tartariza'ti, V. tart'ratis antimonii, V. antimo'nii potas'sio-tartratis, Liquor tar'tari emet'ici, Solution of tar'tarized antimony, Essen'tia antimonii* seu *stib'ii, Antimonial wine, Vinum benedic'tum, Vinum antimonia'tum Huxha'mi, V. antimonialé, Aqua benedic'ta Rulan'di, Vinum emet'icum.* (*Ant. et*

Potass. tart. ʒj, *vini albi* f℥j. Dissolve the tartarized antimony in the wine. Ph. U. S.) Each fluidounce contains two grains of the tartrate.

The ordinary *Antimonial wine* is made with a *glass of antimony* ℥j, *sherry* Oiss.

Ward's Red Drop consists of a strong wine solution of tartarized antimony.

VINUM ANTISCORBU'TICUM, *Antiscorbu'tic wine.* (*Rad. armoracia recent.* ℥j, *fol. cochlear. recent., nasturtii aquat., trifol. aquatic.,* semin. sem. āā ℥ss, *ammoniæ muriat.* ʒij, *vin. albi* Oj. Macerate for 36 hours; filter, and add *tincturæ cochlear.* ℥ss. *Ph. P.*) Stimulant and tonic. Dose f℥ss to f℥ij.

VINUM AROMAT'ICUM, *Aromatic wine.* (*Spec. aromatic.* ℥iv, *vin. rubr.* Oij. Macerate for 6 days and filter. *Ph. P.*) Stimulant and tonic. Used externally, in fomentations, embrocations, &c.

VINUM AROMO-ALOETICUM, V. aloes—v. Benedictum, V. antimonii tartarizati.

VINUM CAMPA'NUM, *V. Campana'cum. Champagne wine.* A well-known sparkling wine of France.

VINUM CANARINUM, see Wine—v. Chalybeatum V. ferri — v. Cinchonæ compositum, V. de kinâ kinâ comp.

VINUM COL'CHICI, *Wine of Colchicum, V. Colchici Radi'cis, Want's Eau d'Husson.* (*Colchici rad.* bene contus. ℔j, *vini alb.* Oij. Macerate for 14 days, with occasional agitation, and then express strongly, and filter. Ph. U. S.) It may also be prepared by displacement. Diuretic, sedative, and purgative. Chiefly used in gout. Dose, gtt. 40 to f℥j.

Reynold's Specific for gout and rheumatism consisted of the fresh bulb of *Colchicum* ʒj, *Sherry wine,* f℥xvj. The colchicum was macerated for eight or ten days in the wine, at a gentle heat; coloured with *syrup of poppies* and flavoured with *rum.* Reynolds is said to have killed himself by taking an over-dose of it.

VINUM COLCHICI RADICIS, V. colchici.

VINUM COLCHICI SEM'INIS, *Wine of Colchicum seed.* (*Colchic. sem.* cont. ℥iv; *vini alb.* 1) Macerate for 14 days, with occasional agitation then express and filter. *Ph. U. S.*) Dose, f℥j.

VINUM CREMATUM, Brandy.

VINUM DIURET'ICUM AMA'RUM, *Vinum amarum scillit'icum compos'itum in Charita'te Numerii usurpa'tum, Bitter diuret'ic wine.* (*Cort. cinch.,* Winteran., limon., āā ℥ij, *rhus toxicodendr.* cacumin. angelicæ, āā ℥ss, *fol. absinth., rutæ,* āā ℥j, *baccar. junip., macis,* āā ℥ss, *rad. iridis,* Oviij. Macerate and filter. *Ph. P.*) Stimulant, tonic, and diuretic. Dose, f℥ss to f℥iss.

VINUM EMETICUM, V. antimonii tartarizati.

VINUM ER'GOTÆ, *Wine of Ergot.* (*Ergotæ* cont., ℥ij; *vini alb.* Oj. Macerate for 14 days with occasional agitation; then express, and filter. Ph. U. S.) Dose, ♏︎xx to f℥j to produce the peculiar effects of ergot.

VINUM FERRATUM, V. Ferri.

VINUM FERRI, *V. chalybea'tum, Steel wine Wine of Iron, Vinum ferra'tum, V. Martis, V. Martis, Tinctura Martis vino'sa, Tinctura Martis cum vino.* (*Iron,* ℥j, *super-tartrate of Potass,* in powder, ℥vj, *distilled water,* Oij × 1 *proof spirit,* f℥xx. Rub the iron and super-tartrate of potass together, and expose them to the air in a flat vessel, moistened with a sufficient of water, for a fortnight; agitating every morning with a spatula, and sprinkling them with water to keep them moist. Then dry with a gentle heat, and mix with ℥xxx of *distilled water.* Filter the fluid and add the spirit. *Ph. L.*) Iron. Dose, f℥j to f℥iv.

It is sometimes made by adding two parts of

wine to two ounces of iron filings; macerating and filtering.

VINUM GENTIA'NÆ COMPOS'ITUM, *V. Ama'rum, Compound wine of gentian, Infu'sum ama'rum vino'sum, Vinum amarum cum spiritû vini, Wine bitters.* (*Rad. gentian. luteæ* ℥ss, *cort. cinchon. offic.* ʒj, *cort. aurant.* ʒij, *canellæ alb.* ʒj, *alcohol. dilut.* f℥iv, *vini alb. Hispanic.* Oijss. *Ph. E,*) Dose, f ʒj to f ʒvj.

VINUM HIPPOCRATICUM, Claret—v. Hispanicum, Vinum, see Wine—v. Hordeaceum, Cerevisia—v. Hydatodes, see Hydatoid.

VINUM IPECACUAN'HÆ, *Ipecacuan'ha wine.* (*Ipecacuan.* cont. ʒij, *vini alb.* Oij.) Macerate for 14 days, express, and filter. Emetic and diaphoretic. Dose, as an emetic, f ʒiv to f ʒx.

VINUM DE KINÂ KINÂ COMPOS'ITUM, *V. cincho'næ compositum, Compound bark wine,* (F.) *Vin de quinquina composé.* (*Cort. cinchon.* pulv. ℔ss, *quassiæ, cort. Winteran., cort. aurant.* sicc., āā ʒss, *alcohol.* (12° to 22° Beaumé) Oj. Macerate for 24 hours; and add *vini albi* Ovj. Macerate for four days, and filter. *Ph. P.*) Tonic, febrifuge, and stomachic. Dose, f ʒss to f ʒij.

VINUM MARTIATUM, V. ferri—v. Martis, V. ferri — v. Medicatum, see Claret.

VINUM MEDICINA'LE, *Medicated Wine.* Wine, holding in solution one or more medicines. Medicinal wines are obtained by macerating or digesting medicinal substances in wine. They differ, of course, according to the nature of the medicine employed, the strength of the wine, &c. In a late Pharmacopœia of the London College, all the wines were changed into weak tinctures; but the old names were left unaltered. Sherry is the wine usually employed. The following are medicated wines.

VINUM MERUM, Acratum—v. Nicotianæ tabaci, V. tabaci — v. Opiatum fermentatione paratum, Laudanum abbatis Rousseau.

VINUM O'PII, *Wine of Opium, Vinum de opio compos'itum, Laud'anum liq'uidum Sydenha'mi, Laudanum liquidum Hoffman'ni, Tinctu'ra Theba'ica, Ford's laudanum.* (*Opii* in pulv. ʒij; *cinnam.* cont. *caryophyll.* cont. āā ʒj; *vini albi* Oj. Macerate for 14 days; express and filter.— Ph. U. S.) Narcotic. Dose, gtt. xv to f ʒj.

VINUM DE OPIO COMPOSITUM, V. opii—v. Picatum, Pissites.

VINUM PORTUGAL'LICUM, *V. rubrum,* (Ph. U. S. 1851.) Wine of Portugal or of Oporto. Port wine. A strong astringent wine, not much drunk in the United States; but greatly used in England.

VINUM QUI'NIÆ, *Wine of Quinia.* (*Wine* ℔ij, *sulphate of quinia* gr. x. Mix.) Dose, f ʒiss or more; according as it is used as a stomachic, or to arrest ague. A *Vinum Cincho'niæ* may be made in the same way.

VINUM RHEI, *V. R. palma'ti, Rhubarb Wine, Tinctura Rhabar'bari Vino'sa, Vinum Rhabarbari, Elixir Rhei dulcé, E. R. Compos'itum.* (*Rhei* cont. ʒij, *canellæ* cont. ʒj, *alcohol. dilut.* f ʒij, *vini albi,* Oj. Macerate for 14 days; express and filter. — *Ph. U. S.*) Laxative and stimulant. Dose, f ʒiv to f ʒiss.

VINUM RHEI PALMATI, V. Rhei—v. Rhenanum, see Wine — v. Rhabarbari, V. rhei palmati — v. Rubrum, V. Portugallicum — v. Rubrum Portugallicum, see Wine.

VINUM TAB'ACI, *Vinum Nicotia'næ Tabaci, Tobac'co Wine.* (*Tabac.* incis. ʒj, *vini albi,* Oj. Macerate for 14 days; express and strain. Ph. U. S.) Narcotic, diuretic, and antispasmodic. In dropsical cases, colica pictonum, and ileus. Not used. Dose, gtt. xx to xxxvj.

VINUM VERA'TRI, *V. V. albi, Wine of White Hel'lebore.* (*Veratri* cont. ʒiv; *Vini albi,* Oj. Macerate for 14 days, express and filter.—*Ph. U. S.*) In cutaneous affections, and in gout. Dose, ten minims.

VINUM VERATRI ALBI, V. Veratri.

VIOL, Stuprum.

VI'OLA, *Viola odora'ta* seu *mar'tia, Ion, Matrona'lis, Viola'ria, the Sweet Violet,* (F.) *Violette à bouquets, V. odorante.* The flowers of the sweet violet have a pleasant, peculiar odour, and scarcely any taste. They are slightly laxative.

VIOLA CANI'NA, *V. sylves'tris.* The *Dog Violet.* The root of this plant is emetic and cathartic. Dose, ℈j.

VIOLA IPECACUANHA, see Ipecacuanha—v. Lutea, Cheiranthus cheiri—v. Martia, Viola—v. Odorata, Viola—v. Palustris, Pinguicola vulgaris.

VIOLA PEDA'TA, *Viola,* (Ph. U. S.) This indigenous violet, which grows from New England to Carolina, is regarded by some as a useful demulcent in pectoral affections.

VIOLA SYLVESTRIS, V. Canina.

VIOLA TRI'COLOR, *Heart's ease, Pansies, Jace'a tricolor, Herba* seu *Flos Trinita'tis,* (F.) *Pensée, P. sauvage.* The decoction of this beautiful little plant has been recommended in diseases of the skin, &c. Its roots are, also, emetic and cathartic.

VIOLARIA, Viola.

VIOLET, DOG, Viola canina — v. Bloom, Solanum dulcamara—v. Sweet, Viola.

VIOLETTE À BOUQUETS, Viola—*v. Odorante,* Viola—*v. des Sorciers,* Vinca minor.

VIOLIER JAUNE, Cheiranthus cheiri.

VIORNA, Clematis vitalba.

VIPER, EGYPTIAN, Aspis — v. Grass, Scorsonera—v. Ten inch long, Echidna ocellata.

VIPERA, Coluber berus.

VIPERARIA, Aristolochia serpentaria, Scorsonera.

VIPERINA VIRGINIANA, Aristolochia serpentaria.

VIR, Penis—v. Effœminatus, Gynæcaner.

VIRAGO, see Pogoniasis.

VIRGA, Penis—v. Cerea, Bougie—v. Cerebri, Pineal gland.

VIRGILIA, Cladrastis tinctoria.

VIRGIN, *Virgo, Par'thenus, Expers nuptia'rum,* (F.) *Vierge, Pucelle.* A female who has never had sexual intercourse. Applied, also, occasionally to the male so circumstanced.

VIR'GINAL, *Virgina'lē,* from *virgo,* 'a virgin.' The external genital organs of the virgin.

VIRGINAL MEMBRANE, Hymen.

VIRGIN'IA, MINERAL WATERS OF. There are several celebrated mineral springs in Virginia, on the western side of the Blue Ridge. Two *Thermal* springs exist in Bath county. The *Warm Spring,* as it is called, issues with a bold stream, sufficient to turn a mill, and to keep the water of its basin at the temperature of 97°. The *Hot Spring* is a few miles from the Warm. Its temperature is 107°. They are both slightly sulphureous. The *Sweet Springs* are at the eastern foot of the Allegheny, in Botetourt county; 42 miles from the Warm Springs. The water has a temperature of 70°, and is highly impregnated with carbonic acid. The *White Sulphur,* as well as the *Red Sulphur,* and *Salt Sulphur Springs,* are also much celebrated. The Red Spring is affirmed to exert a sedative influence on the pulse, diminishing the number of its beats. About 15 miles from Staunton are *Stribling's Springs* — a sulphuretted water; and near Warrenton, in Fauquier county, there is a sulphureous water, called *Lee's Springs,* which is much frequented. *Berkley* and *Capon Springs* are likewise celebrated.

VIRGINIA, Hymen.

VIRGIN'ITY, *Virgin'itas, Parthenei'a, Integ'-*

vitæ, Maid'enhood, Maid'enhead, (F.) *Virginité, Pucélage.* The state of one who has never had carnal commerce.

VIRGIN'S BOWER, COMMON, Clematis vitalba, Clematis Virginica—v. Bower, upright, Clematis recta—v. Sweet-scented, Clematis flammula.

VIRGIN'S MILK, *Lac Vir'ginis, Lac Virgina'lis,* (F.) *Lait virginal.* A tincture of benjamin or of any other balsam, precipitated by the addition of water, which gives it a milky appearance. Also, sub-acetate of lead precipitated by water. It has been used as a cosmetic to remove freckles, &c.

VIRGINITAS DEFLORATA, Defloration.
VIRGO, Virgin—v. Aurea, Solidago virgaurea.
VIRGULA, Penis.
VIRIDE ÆRIS, Cupri subacetas — v. Montanum, Cuprum.
VIRILE, Penis.
VIRILES'CENCE; from *vir,* 'a man.' The state of the aged female in which she assumes certain of the characteristics of the male.—Mehliss.
VIRILIA, Pudibilia.
VIRILITY, Adult age.
VIROSUS, Virulent.
VIRTUE, Faculty.
VIRTUS FORMATRIX, Plastic force — v. .lastica, Plastic force.

VIR'ULENT, *Virulen'tus, Viro'sus,* from *virus.* That which is of the nature of a virus or which is caused by a virus. Highly noxious.

VIRUS, from *vis,* 'force.' A Latin word, which signifies poison; but which, in medicine, has a somewhat different acceptation. By it is understood a principle, unknown in its nature and inappreciable by the senses, which is the agent for the transmission of infectious diseases. Thus we speak of the *variolic, vaccine,* and *syphilitic viruses.* Virus differs from *venom* in the latter being a secretion natural to certain animals, whilst the former is always the result of a morbid process; —a morbid poison.

VIRUS, Ichor, Poison, Sanies — v. Vaccine, see Vaccina — v. Vitale, Sperm.

VIS, Force — v. Adhæsionis, Cohesion (force of) — v. Attractionis, Cohesion (force of) — v. Aucta, Sthenia — v. Cohæsionis, Cohesion (force of) — v. Conservatrix, V. medicatrix naturæ — v. Elastica, Elasticity — v. Essentialis, Plastic force.

VIS EXPUL'TRIX. The organic force by which, it was supposed, the useless was removed from the body.

VIS FORMATIVA, Plastic force — v. Generatrix, Potentia generandi — v. Imminuta, Asthenia — v. Insita, Irritability — v. Irritabilitatis, Irritability.

VIS MEDICA'TRIX NATU'RÆ, *Vis conserva'trix, Autocrati'a, Autonom'ia, Autocrato'ria, Authygian'sis, Autotherapei'a, Physiat'rice, Physioautocrati'a, Physiautocrati'a.* A term, employed by some, to express that instinctive healing power, in an animal or vegetable, by virtue of which it can repair injuries inflicted upon it, or remove disease.

VIS MOR'TUA. Under this name Haller included the mechanical properties of membrane, —flexibility, extensibility, elasticity, &c.—which are totally independent of the vital properties. They remain some time after the complete extinction of life in all its functions; seem to be connected with the mechanical arrangement of particles and the chymical composition of the substance in which they reside, and not to be affected until the progress of decomposition has become sensible.

VIS MUSCULARIS, Myodynamia — v. Nervorum, Nervous power — v. Nervosa, Nervous power — Plastica, Plastic force — v. Reproductiva, ... force — v. Vitæ, Irritability.

VIS VITA'LIS, *Vis seu Fac'ultas Zo'tic...*, *Force vitale.* The vital force—*Biod* ... Von Reichenbach — which distinguishes ... matter from the dead. Also, Irritability.

VIS ZOTICA, Vis vitalis.
VISAGE, Countenance.
VISCAGO BEHEN, Cucubalus behen.
VISCERA, Entrails.
VISCERAL, Splanchnic.
VISCERALIS, Stomachal.
VISCERATION, Exenterismus.
VISCÈRES, Entrails.
VISCONIA, Physconia.

VISCUM ALBUM, *Mis'tletoe, Ixos,* Ir... bach, (F;) *Gui.* A parasitic plant, which ... on a number of trees. *Family,* Capri... *Sex. Syst.* Diœcia Tetrandria. That of the ... *Viscum querci'num* — has been most cele... but it does not differ from the others. It ... at one time, much used in epilepsy and ... neuroses; the wood or leaves being g... powder, in the dose of ʒss or ʒj. The ... also called *Pommes hæmorrhoidales,* from ... supposed virtues, are drastic; and, when ... externally, are maturative.

VISCUM CAPEN'SE. A South African pa... shrub, which grows on the stems of sever... cies of Rhus and Euclea.

VISCUM FLAVES'CENS, *Yel'lowish* M... indigenous, has been given in similar c... the *Viscum album.*

VISIO, Pupil, Vision.
VIS'ION, *Vis'io, Visus,* from *videre,* ... 'to see;' *Opsis, Omma,* (F.) *Vue.* The ... of seeing. The *sight.* The sight is c... five senses, and the eye is its organ. By ... distinguish colours, and appreciate most ... physical qualities of external objects. The ... composed of different transparent med... curvatures and refractive powers are so ... as to render insensible the aberrations of ... city and refrangibility, and to concentr... numerous rays proceeding from more ... distant objects. These rays travers... ively, the transparent cornea, the aque... mour, the crystalline, the vitreous humo... strike upon the retina, on which they ... the figure of the object whence they h... ceeded; and, in order that no obscurity ... from the reflections that might otherwi... the anterior of the eye is lined by a m... the choroid—which is itself covered inter... a dark pigment. This absorbs the light ... dark pigment in the interior of telescop... thus obviates confusion. As the rays p... from an object must cross each other ... course to the retina, it follows that th... ceeding from the upper part of an ob... fall upon the lower part of the retina, ... versely; so that the object must be imp... upon the retina in an inverted position: ... perience teaches us to appreciate the pos... curately.

VISION, BINOCULAR, see Binocular — v. ... loured, Chromopsia — v. Double, Dipl... Single, see Binocular.

VISORIUM ORGANUM, Eye.
VISORIUS, Visual.
VIS'UAL, *Visua'lis, Viso'rius.* Same ... That which concerns the sight or belongs ...

VISUAL ANGLE is the angle formed ... crossing of two rays, proceeding from ... points of any body, in their passage thro... pupil. It is by the size of this angle that ... to a certain extent, of the dimensions of ...

VISUS, Vision—v. Acris, Oxydercia—v. Acrior, Nyctalopia—v. Coloratus, Chromopsia—v. Debilitas, Asthenopia—v. Decolor, Achromatopsia—v. Dimidiatus, Hemiopia—v. Diurnus, Hemeralopia—v. Duplicatus, Diplopia—v. Hebetado, Amblyopia—v. Juvenum, Myopia—v. Lucidus, Photopsia—v. Muscarum, see Metamorphopsia—v. Nocturnus, Nyctalopia—v. Senilis, Presbytia.

VITA, Life—v. Propria, Irritability.

VITAL, *Vita'lis, Biot'ic, Biot'icus*, (F.) *Vital,* from *vita,* 'life.' Relating or appertaining to life;—as

VITAL DYNAMICS, see Dynamic—v. Force, Vis vitalis.

VITAL PRIN'CIPLE, *Flam'mula seu Aura vita'lis, Microcosme'tor*, (F.) *Flamme vitale, Vital Flame*. The principle which, in association with matter, as in organized bodies, controls its manifestations and properties, and distinguishes organized matter from the inorganic. We know nothing of this principle, except in its connexion with organization.

VITAL PROPERTIES, see Properties, vital — v. Statistics, Statistics, medical.

VITALBA, Clematis vitalba.

VITAL'ITY, *Vital'itas,* from *vita,* 'life.' The vital principle: also used in the sense of vital action or movement.

VITALIZE, To endow with life.

VITALS, *Vita'lia*. Parts that are necessary for life—the heart, lungs, and nervous centres more especially.

VITARO'BORANT, PALMER'S. A farinaceous preparation, which appears to consist of a mixture of the red or Arabian lentil and wheat flour, the latter in considerable amount, sweetened with sugar. It bears considerable resemblance to Revalenta.

VITELLARY, Vitelline—v. Membrane, Zona pellucida.

VITELLINE, Zona pellucida.

VIT'ELLINE, *Vitel'linus, Vit'ellary,* from *vitellus,* 'the yolk of an egg.' Appertaining to or resembling the vitellus or yolk.

VITELLINE DISC, Proligerous Disc — v. Fluid, see Vesicula umbilicalis.

VITELLINE PED'ICLE or APOPH'YSIS, is the pedicle which attaches the umbilical vesicle to the embryo. See Vesicula umbilicalis.

VITELLINE POUCH, Vesicula umbilicalis — v. Vessels, Omphalo-mesenteric.

VITELLO-MESENTERIC, Omphalo-mesenteric.

VITELLUM OVI, see Ovum.

VITELLUS OVI, see Ovum.

VITEX, *V. Agnus Castus seu verticilla'ta, Agnus Castus,* (F.) *Gattilier, Petit Poivre, Poivre sauvage.* Family, Pyrenaceæ. *Sex. Syst.* Didynamia Angiospermia. The *Chaste Tree*. The seeds, when fresh, have a fragrant smell, and an acrid, aromatic taste. Formerly, they were celebrated as antaphrodisiacs.

VITI SALTUS, Chorea.

VITIA PRIMÆ CONFORMATIONIS, see Monster.

VITIATIO, Stuprum.

VITILIGINES, Ephelides.

VITILIGO, Lepra—v. Alphus, Lepra alphoides—v. Melas, Lepra nigricans—v. Nigra, Lepra nigricans.

VITIS ALBA SYLVESTRIS, Bryonia alba—v. Apyrena, see V. Corinthiaca.

VITIS CORINTHIACA. *Family* of the Vines. *Sex. Syst.* Pentandria Monogynia. This plant affords the *Uvæ passæ mino'res, Passæ Corinthiacæ, Pas'sulæ mino'res, Uvæ Corinthiacæ, Corinthiacæ, Currants,* (F.) *Raisins de Corinthe;* which are the dried fruit of the *Vitis Corinthiaca* or *Vitis apyre'na;* and are similar, in their properties, to the raisin.

VITIS IDÆA MYRTILLUS, Vaccinium myrtillus—v. Idæa Palustris, Vaccinium oxycoccos—v. Idæa punctata, Vaccinium vitis idæa—v. Sativa, V. vinifera.

VITIS VINIF'ERA, *V. sati'va, Am'pelos, A. Œnoph'oros*. The *Grape vine, the Vine,* (F.) *Vigne*. Vine leaves and the tendrils have an astringent taste, and were formerly used in diarrhœa, hemorrhage, &c. The juice or sap, called *Lac'ryma,* has been recommended in calculous disorders and in cases of chronic ophthalmia. The juice of the unripe fruit is called *Verjuice*. The *Grape, Uva, Botrys, Staph'ylé, Rhax,* (F.) *Raisin,* when ripe, is a wholesome delicious fruit; and, when dried, forms the *Uvæ passæ majo'res, Pass'ulæ majo'res, Uvæ passæ solè sicca'ta, Zibebæ, Raisins*. These are inodorous; and to the taste, sub-acidulous, sweet, and mucilaginous. They are demulcent and nutritive.

VITIUM, Disease—v. Caducum, Epilepsy.

VITIUM CONFORMA'TIONIS. A disease or fault of conformation.

VITIUM DIVINUM, Epilepsy — v. Herculeum, Epilepsy—v. Scrophulosum, Scrofula.

VITRARIA, Parietaria.

VITREOUS, Hyaline—v. Humour, Corpus vitreum—v. Humour of the ear, *Vitrine auditive*.

VITREUS, Hyaline.

VITRINE AUDITIVE (F.), from *vitrum,* 'glass;' *End'olymph, Liquor of Scarpa, Fluid of Scarpa, Vitreous Humour of the Ear*. The fluid contained in the *membranous labyrinth* of the ear, so called from its resemblance to the *vitreous* humour of the eye.

VITRIOL, Ferri sulphas—v. Blue, Cupri sulphas—v. Cæruleum, Cupri sulphas—v. Green, Ferri sulphas—v. Roman, Cupri sulphas—v. White, Zinci sulphas.

VITRIOLUM ALBUM, Zinci sulphas—v. Ammoniacale, Ammoniæ sulphas—v. Cupri, Cupri sulphas—v. Cyprium, Cupri sulphas—v. Ferri, Ferri sulphas—v. Goslariense, Zinci sulphas—v. Martis, Ferri sulphas — v. Romanum, Cupri sulphas—v. Veneris, Cupri sulphas—v. Viride, Ferri sulphas—v. Zinci, Zinci sulphas.

VITRUM, *Hy'alos, Glass, Brancia,* (F.) *Verre,* from *videre,* 'to see.' Glass, coarsely powdered, has been sometimes used to remove specks of the cornea.

Powdered glass has been regarded, but erroneously, as a poison. It acts only mechanically.

The saline scum, which swims on glass when first made, has been used in tooth-powders. It is called *Sandiver, Sel de verre, Glass Gall, Fel vitri,* &c.

VITRUM ANTIMONII, see Antimonii vitrum—v. Hypoclepticum, Separatorium — v. Oculare, see Spectacles—v. Sublimatorium, Aludel.

VITTA, *Bandelette,* Caul.

VIVÆSECTIO, Vivisection.

VIVERRA CIVETTA, see Civetta.

VIVIPARITÉ, see Viviparous.

VIVIP'AROUS, from *vivus,* 'alive,' and *pario,* 'I bring forth.' An epithet applied to animals whose young are brought forth detached, without requiring to be hatched, as in the *Oviparous*. The condition may be termed *Vivip'arousness,* (F.) *Viviparité*. See Generation.

VIVIPAROUSNESS, see Viviparous.

VIVISECTION, *Vivisec'tio, Vivæsec'tio, Biotom'ia,* from *vivus,* 'alive,' and *secare, sectum,* 'to cut.' The act of opening or dissecting living animals. One who performs vivisections is a vivisector.

VOCAL, Oral—v. Tube, see Tube, vocal.

VOCALIS, Vowel.

VOCE DI PETTO, see Voice—v. di Testa, see Voice.

VOICE, *Vox, Audā, Phonē,* (F.) *Voix,* from *vocare,* 'to name, to call.' An appreciable sound produced by the air, when driven from the lungs, throwing the inferior ligaments of the glottis into vibration. The function by which this is effected has been called *Phona'tion*. It is a function of *animal* life; and, in animals, is limited to the production of the *simple* or *instinct'ive voice,* as well as in the idiot; but, in intellectual man, becomes much more complicated and articulated,—an evidence of his intellectual superiority.

VOICE, ARTIC'ULATED, Speech, *Loque'la, Glossa, Glotta, La'lia, Phrasis,* (F.) *Parole, Voix articulée,* is the voice as produced by the glottis, modified by the motions of the tongue, lip, and other parts of the vocal tube. Most physiologists agree in regarding the glottis, or the space between the thyro-arytenoid ligaments plus the ligaments themselves, as the part where vocal sounds are formed; but the mechanism of this formation is a matter of dispute. The greater part of individuals regard the glottis and its ligaments, with the *vocal tube,* or the space which the sound has to traverse after it is produced in the glottis, as a reed instrument, like the clarionet, the inferior ligaments of the glottis constituting the reed. In speech, as ordinarily effected, the tongue, lips, teeth, &c., are concerned, but there are some authentic cases on record, where it has been accomplished after the tongue has been removed. In such cases, the articulated voice must have been produced in the glottis alone, or in it aided by an obscure action of the parts above it.

The singing voice is not limited to the larynx; the pharynx would seem to be concerned also. The notes that are produced in the latter have been termed *supra-laryngeal,* or *notes of the second register.* They constitute the *pharyngeal voice, falsetto* or *faucette voice* or *voce di testa,* (I.) The *laryngeal voice* or *voice of the first register,* is the *Voce di Petto,* (I.)

VOICE, BLEATING, Egophony—v. Cavernous, Pectoriloquy.

VOICE, CHOL'ERIC, *Vox Choler'ica*. The peculiar husky voice of those affected with cholera.

VOICE, CONVUL'SIVE, *Vox convulsi'va,* (F.) *Voix convulsive*. A neurosis of the voice, consisting in the production of discordant sounds—acute and grave—which cannot be brought to the natural tones by any effort of volition. It seems to be caused by disordered contraction of the muscles of the larynx.

VOICE, FALSETTO, see Voice—v. Goat's, Egophony—v. Laryngeal, Laryngophony, see Voice—v. Pharyngeal, see Voice—v. Tracheal, Laryngophony.

VOIE, Way.

VOIES DIGESTIVES, Ways, digestive—v. *Lachrymales,* Lachrymal passages—v. *Premières,* Ways, digestive—v. *Secondes,* Ways, second—v. *Urinaires,* Urinary passages.

VOILE DU PALAIS, Velum pendulum palati—v. *Médullaire inférieure,* Velum medullare inferius—v. *Médullaire supérieure,* Valvula Vieussenii.

VOIX, Voice—v. *Aigre,* see Acid—v. *Articulée,* Voice, articulated, Pectoriloquy—v. *Bourdonnante,* see Resonance—v. *Bronchique,* Resonance—v. *Caverneuse,* Pectoriloquy—v. *Chévrotante,* Egophony—v. *Égophonique,* Egophony—v. *de Polichinelle,* Egophony—v. *Sénile,* Egophony—v. *Tubaire,* see Resonance.

VOLA, Palm—v. Manûs, Palm—v. Pedis, Sole.

VOLATICA, Lichen.

VOLATILIZA'TION, *Volatilisa'tio, Volatica'-tio,* from *volare,* 'to fly.' The operation of reducing volatilizable substances into gas or vapor.

VOLATISATIO, Volatilization.

VOLIT"ION, *Volit"io,* from *volo,* 'to will.' The act of willing. Hence:

VOLIT"IONAL, relating to volition. Its the muscles may be moved by a *volition*; it is an *emotional* impulse.

VOLNUS, Wound.

VOLSELLA, Acanthobolos, Forceps, Muserium—v. Patini, *Valet à Patin*.

VOLTAISM, Galvanism.

VOLTUS, Countenance, Face.

VOL'UNTARY, *Hecu'sius, Voluntā'rius, voluntas,* 'will.' Relating to the will; as *tary* muscles;' muscles which act in obedience the will.

VOLUNTAS, *Volen'tia, Arbit'rium, itas, Boule'sis, Bule'sis, Thele'ma,* (F.) Will or desire.

VOLUN'TAS SEU CUPID'ITAS DESIDENT'I *do intesti'ni.* The desire to go to stool.

VOLVULUS, Ileus—v. Intestinorum. Intussusceptio.

VOMENDI CONAMEN INANE, Vexation.

VOMER, 'a ploughshare;' *Os vomeris, trum, Os maxill'æ superio'ris undec"imus,* of the bones of the face, so called from its resemblance. It is an azygous bone, forming the terior part of the septum narium. It is thin and quadrilateral; and is articulated below the superior maxillary and palatine bones; above, to the sphenoid, ethmoid, and cornu of Bertin. It is developed by a single point of ossification. Also, the penis.

VOM'ICA, *Pyocys'tis,* from *vomere,* 'to cast up.' (F.) *Vomique, Crachemet.* A term used by some authors for any collection of purulent matter in the interior of a viscus. The acceptation is commonly restricted to purulent collections in the encysted or not, which may be discharged by the mouth, by breaking into the bronchia. Two kinds of vomicæ are distinguished: one caused by the softening or breaking of pulmonary tubercles; the other, of more rare occurrence, formed by a circumscribed of the lungs. Instead of opening into the chia, the abscess is sometimes discharged into the cavity of the pleura, causing empyema.

VOMICINE, Brucia.

VOMIQUE, Vomica.

VOMIQUIER, Strychnos nux vomica.

VOMISSEMENT, Vomiting—v. *de Sang,* Hæmatemesis.

VOMIT, Emetic—v. Black, Fever, Yellow; Melæna.

VOMIT, DRY, OF MARRIOTT. A once celebrated emetic, called 'dry,' from its having been given without solution. It consisted of equal parts of tartrate of antimony and potassa, and sulphate of copper.

VOMITIF, Emetic.

VOMITINE, Emetine.

VOM'ITING, *Vom'itus, Vomit"io, Vomit"itum, Evomit"io, Ana'trope, Em'esis, Palmus vom'itus, Ægritu'do ventric'uli,* Spewing, Puking, Sickness of *the Stomach,* (F.) *Vomissement,* from *vomere,* 'to cast up.' The act by which solids and liquids, contained in the stomach, are ejected by the mouth. Vomiting is the effect of some special irritation of the coats of the stomach, calling, by reflex action, on the appropriate muscles to expel the contents of the viscus. It is not accomplished solely by the contraction of the stomach, as was for a long time believed. That organ, indeed, assists the process; but the main cause is the compression exerted upon the parietes of the viscus by the diaphragm and abdominal muscles. Vomiting is a symptom common to numerous diseases. At times, it is sympathetic, as in affections of the kidney, uterus, brain, &c. At others, it is symptomatic, as in gastritis, peritonitis, &c. When very troublesome, it may often be palliated by effervescent draughts, aromatics, sinapisms, or blisters to the epigastric region, &c.

VOMITING AT PLEASURE, Regurgitation — v. of Blood, Hæmatemesis — v. Stercoraceous, Copremesis.

VOMITIO, Vomiting—v. Sanguinis, Hæmatemesis.

VOMITIUM, Vomiting.

VOMITO NEGRO, Fever, yellow — v. Prieto, Fever, yellow.

VOMITORIUM, Emetic.
VOMITORY, Emetic.
VOMITUM, Vomiting.

VOMITURIT''ION, *Vomituri'tio, Emes'ia, Dysemes'ia, Subver'sio stom'achi*. Same etymon as Vomiting. Ineffectual efforts to vomit; *Vomen'di cona'men ina'nē, Retching, Reaching, Heav'ing*. Some authors mean, by this term, a vomiting of but little matter, or that which is effected almost without effort. The first acceptation is the most general.

VOMITUS, Vomiting — v. Cruentus, Hæmatemesis—v. Fæculentus, Copremesis—v. Marinus, Nausea marina—v. Navigantium, Nausea marina —v. Niger, Fever, yellow—v. Pituitosus, Blennemesis—v. Profusus, Hyperemesis—v. Purulentus, Pyemesis—v. Sanguinis, Hæmatemesis—v. Stercoris, Copremesis.

VOORARA, Curare.

VOUACAPUA AMERICANA, Geoffræa inermis.

VOÛTE, Vault—*v. Médullaire*, Corpus callosum — *v. à Trois Piliers*, Fornix.

VOWEL, *Voca'lis*, from Latin *vox*, 'the voice,' and *voco*, 'to call.' (F.) *Voyelle*. Physiologically, a continuous breath or sound, produced in the glottis; but more or less modified by the form of the vocal tube, through which it has to pass. In the English language, a, e, i, o, u, w, and y are vowels.

VOX, Voice — v. Cholerica, Voice, choleric — v. Clangosa, Oxyphonia — v. Convulsiva, *Voix Convulsive*—v. Nasalis, Rhinophonia—v. Rauca, Raucedo, Raucous voice—v. Raucisona, Raucous voice.

VOYELLE, Vowel.

VUE, Vision — *v. Courte*, Myopia—*v. Diurne*, Hemeralopia—*v. Faible*, Amblyopia—*v. Longue*, Presbytia—*v. Louche*, Strabismus—*v. Nocturne*, Nyctalopia.

VULGA, Vulva.

VULNÉRAIRE, Vulnerary—*v. Suisse*, see Falltranck.

VULNERARIUS, Traumatic.

VUL'NERARY, *Vulnera'rius, Traumat'icus, Traumatic*, from *vulnus, vulneris*, 'a wound.' (F.) *Vulnéraire*. A name applied by the ancients to medicines, which they considered capable of favouring the consolidation of wounds. The property has been ascribed to various plants.

VULNERATIO NERVI, Neurotrosis.

VULNUS, Wound — v. Laceratum, see Laceration — v. Sclopetarium, Wound, gun-shot — v. Simplex, Cut.

VULNUSCULUM, Wound.

VULPIS MORBUS, Alopecia.

VULTUEUX (F.), *Vultuo'sus*. Corvisart has used the expression, *Face vultueuse, Fa'cies vultuo'sa*, for the face, when it is more florid and swollen than in the natural state. This appearance, which is observed in active aneurism of the heart, according to Corvisart, is owing to the afflux of blood into the arterial capillaries, and hence differs from the livid and swollen appearance caused by the accumulation of blood in the venous capillaries, constituting the *Face injectée*.

VULTUS, Countenance, Face — v. Tetricus et Mœstus, Scythropasmus.

VULVA, Uterus, see Vulva.

VULVA, from *valva*, 'a door.' *Hortus, Cunnus, Puden'dum mulie'brē, Sinus pudo'ris, Choiros, Arvum, Bucca, Bulga, Cadur'cus, Custos, Femen, An'nulus, Femur summum, Follic'ulus, Fundus, Gre'mium, Hia'tus, Lanu'vium, Navis, Oppid'ulum, Specus, Vulga, Cymba, Saltus, Clitor'ium, Os'tium, Sulcus, Amphicaus'tis, Concha, Porcus, Porta, Interfemineum, Mulie'bria, Fossa magna mulie'bris, Episei'on, Es'chara, Hor'tulus cupid'inis, Bouba'lios, Byssos, Cava, Caver'na, Delphys, Delta, Fovea, Gynœce'um*, the *Female puden'dum*, the *Female organs of generation*, the *Female parts, Loci mulie'bres*, (F.) *Vulve*. A longitudinal opening between the projecting parts of the external organs of generation in the female, extending from the mons veneris to the perineum, and which is called, also, *Fossa magna*. Some anatomists mean, by this term, the whole of the external genital organs of the female:—mons veneris; labia majora, and the cleft or vestibule separating them; the clitoris; nymphæ; meatus urinarius; entrance of the vagina; with the hymen or the carunculæ myrtiformes, fossa navicularis and fourchette.

VULVA, *Fora'men commu'nē ante'rius, Iter ad infundib'ulum, Iter seu Ad'itus ad ter'tium ventric'ulum, Rima ad infundib'ulum, Apertu'ra ante'rior ventric'uli ter'tii cerebri*. An opening situate at the junction of the optic thalami, in the third ventricle of the brain, and immediately beneath the anterior crus of the fornix.

VULVAIRE, Chenopodium vulvaria.

VULVAR, *Vulva'ris*, from *vulva*. That which relates to the vulva. Chaussier gives this name to the external pudic arteries, because they are distributed to the vulva.

VULVARIA, Chenopodium vulvaria.

VULVE, Vulva.

VULVI'TIS, a hybrid word, from *vulva*, and *itis*, denoting inflammation. Inflammation of the vulva.

VULVO-UTERINE CANAL, Vagina.

W.

WAD, Graphites.
WAHOO, see Euonymus.
WAISTCOAT, STRAIT, *Indu'cula*, (F.) *Camisole, Gilet de force*. A dress, used for restraining maniacs, or those labouring under violent delirium. It has long sleeves, which are tied behind the body, so that the arms cannot be extricated from them. It ought, of course, to be made of very resisting materials.
WAKE-ROBIN, Arum maculatum, Trillium latifolium.
WALE, Wheal.
WALKING, *Gressus, Inces'sus, Deambula'tio, Ambula'tio, Bad'isis,* (F.) *La marche*. The action by which we change place, by means of a succession of steps in the same direction. In walking forwards, the centre of gravity is constantly altered; and a series of small, parabolic curves is described on the heads of the thigh-bones, the extent of which is regulated by volition, under the guidance of vision.
WALLA'CHIA, MINERAL WATERS OF. There are many excellent sulphureous springs in this country, especially those at Bobotsch, Fincesohti, Sibitchiudi Sus, Bräsa, Otschin, Serboneschte, Kimpalungi, Kosia, and Oloneschti. Chalybeate and saline springs have, also, been found at Sibitschiudi Sus. — Siller.
WALLFLOWER, Cheiranthus cheiri.
WALLRUE, Asplenium ruta muraria.
WALNUT, Juglans regia — w. White, Juglans cinerea.
WALTON, MINERAL WATERS OF. A mineral spring near Tewkesbury, in Gloucestershire, England. It is an acidulous chalybeate.
WANT, from past participle of Sax. panian, 'to wane,' 'to fall away.' 'Need of that which is necessary.' (F.) *Besoin*. This word is sometimes used to express the imperious necessity which compels us to take food, drink, &c. (See Hunger and Thirst.) In a more general sense, it means the impressions transmitted by the organs to the brain, when it is necessary that they should act: these wants are called *instinctive desires* and *internal sensations* or *stimuli*. Such are the desires or wants to eat, drink, void the urine, breathe (*besoin de respirer*), &c.
WANT, in the sense of indigence, (L.) *Egestas, Indigen'tia*, is the cause of a number of diseases.
WARBURG'S FEVER-DROPS, see Bebeeru.
WARD'S ESSENCE FOR THE HEADACH, Linimentum camphoræ compositum — w. White Drops, see Hydrargyri nitras.
WARMBRUNN, MINERAL WATERS OF. Much frequented springs in Silesia, about a league from Hirschberg. They are thermal, 95° to 100° Fah., and are chiefly used as baths. The impregnating materials are carbonate of soda, sulphate of soda, sulphate of lime, chloride of sodium, carbonate of magnesia, and sulphohydric acid gas.
WARM SPRINGS, see Virginia, mineral waters of.
WARNERA CANADENSIS, Hydrastis Canadensis.
WART, Verruca — w. Corneous, Cornu.
WARTY, *Ver'rucose, Ver'rucous, Verruco'sus*, from Sax. peapt. Full of warts. Resembling, relating, or belonging to warts.
WARTY TUMOUR OF CICATRICES. A name given by Mr. Howship to the tumour, which sometimes appears on an old scar, many years, perhaps, after the injury that caused it.
WASH, BLACK, see Hydrargyri submuria— w. Preventive, Lotion, Hannay's — w. White, Liquor plumbi subacetatis dilutus.
WASHERWOMAN'S SCALL, Psora diffusa.
WASP, *Vespa, Sphex*, (F.) *Guêpe*. A genus of gregarious insects, like the bee and the ant. They are armed with a sting, which pours a poisonous fluid into the puncture made by it. (See Poisons, Table of.) The best application is a sp. ammoniæ aromaticus, or some preparation of ammonia.
WASSERBURG, MINERAL WATERS OF. Wasserburg is a town of Bavaria, seated on the Inn, 28 miles east of Münich. The water, called also, *Aqua Aga'tii*, contains carbonic acid; carbonates of lime and magnesia; sulphates of lime and magnesia; chloride of sodium, carbonate of soda and oxide of iron.
WASSERCUR, Hydrosudotherapeia.
WATER, Sax. pæten, (G.) *Wasser, Aqua, ύδωρ, Alma*, (F.) *Eau, Protox'ide of hydrogen*. Water was at one time regarded as a simple element. It is now known to consist of eight parts by weight of oxygen, and one of hydrogen. It freezes at 32°, and boils at 212° of Fahrenheit; and is taken as the unit in all tables of specific gravity of solid and liquid substances. Water, as we meet with it, is very different in its state of purity; generally, it contains small quantities of saline matter; at other times, as in sea-water and mineral waters, it is largely impregnated. The characters of water, as met with under ordinary circumstances, are well compared by the words "*Aqua levissima pluvialis est; deinde fontium ex flumine; tum ex puteo; post hæc ex aut glacie; gravior his ex lacu; graviorissima e palude.*" Pure water is one of the best diluents that can be used. When cold, and especially when iced, it is one of the most useful refrigerants; and, in the form of the cold, tepid, or warm bath, it is serviceable in numerous diseases.
WATER OF AIX-LA-CHAPELLE, see Aix-la-Chapelle — w. Allflower, Urine, cow's — w. Apple-tea — w. Barley, Decoctum hordei.
WATER BED. A bed, contrived by Dr. Arnott, which, in consequence of its being placed in water, is well adapted for the bedridden.
WATER, BINELLI, Aqua Binellii — w. of Bitter Almonds, Aqua Amygdalarum concentrata — w. Brash, Pyrosis — w. Brocchieri, Aqua Brocchierii — w. Camphor, Mistura Camphoræ.
WATER CANKER, Cancer aquaticus.
WATER, CARUI, STRONG, Spiritus carui — w. Chicken, Chicken-tea — w. Cinnamon, Aqua Cinnamomi — w. Cinnamon, strong, Spiritus cinnamomi — w. Cologne, *Eau de Cologne*.
WATER CURE, Hydrosudotherapeia.
WATER, DISTIL'LED, *Aqua destilla'ta*, (F.) *Eau distillée, Holy water*, is generally ordered in extemporaneous prescriptions, but is rarely used. In some cases, however, it is absolutely necessary; as water, containing any saline impregnation — hard water, for example — decomposes certain substances. Distilled water has been recommended as a diet-drink in cancerous affections; and it is used in the religious ceremonies of the Catholic church. In the Pharmacopœia of the United States, it is directed to be made as follows: — Take of *water*, ten gallons. First distil

two pints, and throw them away; then distil eight gallons. Keep the distilled water in glass bottles.

WATER-DOCTOR, see Uromantia.

WATER-DRESSING. The treatment of wounds and ulcers by the application of water. It generally consists in dipping folds of lint in water, and placing them on the part:—the whole being covered with oiled silk or elastic gum.

WATER, EPILEPTIC, of Langius, Langii aqua epileptica.— w. Fennel, Aqua fœniculi.

WATER FLAG, YELLOW, Iris pseudacorus.

WATER, FLORIDA,—a celebrated perfume,—may be made of *Ol. Bergami* f$\mathbb{Z}$iv; *Tinct. bensoin. c.* f$\mathbb{Z}$ij; *Alcohol.* cong.

WATER, GOULARD, Liquor plumbi sub-acetatis dilutus.

WATER, HARD. Common water, which decomposes and curdles soap; in contradistinction to *soft water*, which is readily miscible with soap. The hardness of water depends upon the presence in it of earthy salts, the most common of which is sulphate of lime.

WATER, HOLY, Water, distilled — w. Honey, see Mel — w. in the Head, Hydrocephalus — w. Hungary, Spiritus rosmarini.

WATER JAGS, see Varicella.

WATER, LAKE, *Aqua ex lacu*, (F.) *Eau de lac*, is apt to be impure, from decayed animal and vegetable matters. A great deal will, however, depend upon the magnitude of the collection, and the degree of stagnation.

WATER, LAUREL, see Prunus lauro-cerasus — w. Lavender, Spiritus lavandulæ — w. Lemonpeel, see Lemonpeel Tea — w. Lime, Liquor calcis — w. Lime, compound, Liquor calcis compositus — w. Magnesia, aerated, Magnesia, fluid — w. Magnesia, carbonated, Magnesia, fluid.

WATER, MARSH, *Aqua paludo'sa*, (F.) *Eau de Marais*, is the most impure of all. It is generally more stagnant, and of course more loaded with decomposing animal and vegetable matters.

WATER, MINERAL, *Aqua minera'lis, A. salu'bris, A. medica'ta, Fons saluta'rius, F. medica'tus, F. sote'rius, Aqua sote'ria*, (F.) *Eau minérale*. Water, holding in solution different saline and gazeous substances in sufficient quantity to be possessed of medicinal properties, or of a temperature different from that of the ordinary springs of the country.

Mineral waters may be divided into four classes: — 1. *Gazeous* or *Acidulous*. 2. *Chalybeate*. 3. *Saline*. 4. *Sulphureous*. These may be *thermal*, or *cold*,—*natural*, or *artificial*. Many of these divisions, however, run into each other; some of the substances, which they hold dissolved, belonging to one class as well as to another.

1. *Ga'zeous, Acid'ulous* or *Car'bonated Min'eral Waters, Aquæ minera'les acid'ulæ*, (F.) *Eaux minérales gazeuses* ou *acidules*. The waters referred to this class are those that contain carbonic acid gas in such quantity as to communicate to it certain sensible qualities. Waters impregnated with free carbonic acid, sparkle when drawn from the spring, or when poured into a glass. They have a sharp, acidulous taste; but become vapid from exposure to the air. Along with the carbonic acid, there are generally present portions of saline, earthy or metallic matter, chiefly carbonates of lime, magnesia, and iron. Waters, highly impregnated with carbonic acid gas, are grateful to the stomach; increase the appetite, and are diuretic; hence, their utility in dyspepsia, hypochondriasis, and gout. Their properties are, of course, modified by the saline matter that may be also contained in them. The most celebrated amongst the acidulous waters are those of Bar, Chateldon, St. Myon, Mont d'Or, Langeac, Seltzer, Schlangenbad, Sultzmatt, Pyrmont, Spa, Carlsbad, Cheltenham, Scarborough, Saratoga, Ballston, and the Sweet Springs of Virginia.

2. *Chalyb'eate* or *Ferru'ginous Mineral Waters, Aquæ minera'les ferrugino'sæ, A. Chalybea'tæ, A. Martia'les*, (F.) *Eaux minérales ferrugineuses*, contain iron — sulphate, chloride or carbonate, generally the latter — held in solution by an excess of acid. Chalybeate waters have a peculiar styptic taste. They are transparent when taken from the spring; but, when exposed for some time to the air, a pellicle forms on the surface, and a deposite of the iron takes place. Chalybeate waters are used as tonics in debility of all kinds; in all cases, in fact, where iron is considered to be indicated. They are the most numerous of all the classes of mineral waters. In this dictionary, those only are specified which have some celebrity; yet there are upwards of ninety; whilst there are more than sixty of the saline, and upwards of thirty-five of the sulphureous. The most celebrated chalybeates are those of Tunbridge, Scarborough, Spa, Bussang, Forges, Vichy, Pyrmont, Passy, Provins, and Vals.

3. *Saline Mineral Waters, Aquæ minerales sali'næ, Amna alcaliza'ta* (Paracelsus,) *Hydralmæ*, (F.) *Eaux minérales salines*. Waters, holding in solution different saline substances in greater quantity than the acidulous waters. They differ in properties, according to the salts contained in them. The salts usually present are sulphates, chlorides, and carbonates; and the bases, with which the acids forming these are combined, are soda, magnesia, and lime. Saline mineral waters are usually aperient; and the most noted are those of Seltzer, Sedlitz, Balaruc, Bourbonne-les-Bains, Baden, Epsom, Cheltenham, &c.

To this class may also be added *Sea water*.

4. *Sulphu'reous Mineral Waters, Aquæ minerales sulphu'reæ*; when warm, termed *Theiothermæ, Theiopegæ, Theother'mæ, Fontes sulphu'rei cal'idi*, (F.) *Eaux minérales sulfureuses, Eaux sulfurées, E. sulfureuses, E. hépatiques*, &c. These waters owe their distinguishing character to an impregnation of sulphuretted hydrogen, and are at once recognized by their peculiar fetid smell, resembling that of rotten eggs. They usually contain saline substances, which modify their powers. From the action of the sulphuretted hydrogen, they are useful in cutaneous affections; and, from the combined action of this and the saline matter, they are valuable agents in diseases of the digestive organs. They are also employed in cutaneous eruptions; and the warm sulphur baths have been especially celebrated in such cases, as well as in rheumatic affections. The most renowned sulphureous waters are those of Baréges, Bagnères-de-Luchon, Cauterets, Bonnes, Aix in Savoy, Aix-la-Chapelle, Enghien, Harrogate, Moffat, Virginia Springs, &c.

Some springs, as those of Bath, Buxton, Dax, Matlock, Warm and Hot Springs of Virginia, &c., are almost pure *Thermal Mineral Waters*. They are valuable agents in rheumatic affections; the warmth being equable during the whole period the individual is immersed in them; which cannot be the case in the artificial thermal bath.

The following Table by Dr. Pereira exhibits the composition of some of the principal mineral waters.

FIXED CONSTITUENTS

ENTERING INTO THE COMPOSITION OF SOME OF THE MORE CELEBRATED MINERAL SPRINGS.

PROPORTIONS IN 10,000 PARTS OF WATER.

NOTE.— In reducing the analyses contained in this Table to a uniform measure, in order to render them susceptible of direct comparison with each other, the old English gallon is assumed to be as = 58,338 grains; the wine pint = 7305 grains; the imperial gallon = 70,000 grains; and the German 16-ounce measure = 7368 grains.

The different salts have been reduced to their elementary constituents by Wollaston's scale of chemical equivalents.

Name.	Country.	Acids.			Bases.			Oxide of Iron.	Silica.	Sum.	Authority and Date.	Remarks.
		Carbonic.	Sulphuric.	Muriatic.	Soda.	Lime.	Magnesia.					
San Restituta	Ischia	0	19.30	29.05	34.50	2.08	2.35	3.19	0.40	94.44	Giudice	Iron in the state of ferruginous alumina; sub-borate of soda 2.79.
Gurgitello	Ditto	14.55	9.05	11.18	31.45	2.95	2.38	1.39	0.56	74.03	Ditto	Iron as in San Restituta.
Wiesbaden	Nassau	1.38	0.87	33.09	31.99	5.29	0.92	0.05	0.26	57.63	Kastner, 1823	Free carbonic acid 18.9; azote; pot-ash 0.83; alumina 0.56; organic extract 2.37.
Carlsbad Sprudel	Bohemia	7.45	14.50	6.40	24.55	1.75	0.85	0.02	0.75	54.59	Berzelius, 1822	Minute traces of phosphoric and fluoric acids, strontian, alumina, and manganese.

THERMAL.

St. Nectaire	France	15.13	0.87	13.00	23.90	2.45	1.14	0.14	1.00	53.94	Berthier	
Vichy	Ditto	15.81	1.55	0.72	24.47	0.27	0	0.01	0	42.75	Ditto	[nese 2.42.
Ems (Krünchenquelle)	Nassau	20.32	0.76	2.43	14.87	2.65	1.45	0.65	trace	42.74	Kastner, 1830	Alumina, a trace; oxide of manga-
Olmitello	Ischia	0	6.91	5.95	5.98	0	1.80	0	0.42	24.43	Giudice	Potash 2.73.
Bath (King's Bath)	England	2.38	8.71	2.05	2.79	5.29	0.77	0.03	0.37	20.53	Phillips	Magnesia, by Scudamore.
Mont d'Or	France	2.86	0.36	1.32	4.74	0.90	0.28	0.01	2.10	13.39	Berthie	
Geyser	Iceland	0	0.81	0.86	2.74	0	0	0	5.40	10.75	Black, 1791	Alumina 0.48.
Chaudes Aigues	France	3.07	0	0	3.12	1.01	0.59	0.15	1.16	9.96	Berthier	
Rycum [Reikum]	Iceland	0	0.71	1.55	2.43	0	0	0	3.73	8.47	Black, 1791	Alumina .005.
Bristol Hot well	England	1.02	2.25	1.17	1.17	0.82	0.43	0	0	8.19	Carrick, 1797	Free carbonic acid 12.99.
Schlangenbad	Nassau	3.50	0.40	0.80	2.42	0.90	0.53	0	0	6.96	Kastner, 1823	Free carbonic acid 6.0.
Teplitz	Bohemia	1.89	0.29	0.29	2.62	0.36	0.18	0.03	0.42	6.24	Berzelius, 1822	Phosphoric acid; potash; alumina.
Buxton	England	0.78	0.06	0.28	0.19	1.04	0.04	0	0	2.70	Scudamore, 1830	Azote 2.01, by Pearson.

WATER, MINERAL

COLD.

Spring	Country									Total	Analyst, Date	Remarks
Vicar's Bridge	Scotland	0	203.00	0.18	0.16	2.56	13.20	103.00	0	563.10	Connell, 1831	Potash, a trace.
Pullna	Bohemia	4.63	182.83	17.20	75.00	20.38	45.45	0	0.24	341.1	Struve	Potash 3.55.
Seidschutz	Ditto	4.81	97.43	1.43	14.20	6.02	41.92	trace	0.16	177.4	Ditto	Nitric acid 7.75; phosphoric acid; potash 3.61; strontian 0.03; alumina; oxide of manganese.
Leamington (Royal Pump)	England	0	20.80	71.90	57.90	12.00	4.95	1.09	0	153.9	Thomson, 1830	Traces of iodine and bromine by Daubeny.
Harrowgate (old sulphur well)	Ditto	1.20	0.80	76.83	60.50	4.47	1.94	0	0	145.4	Scudamore, 1819	
Airthrey (first spring)	Scotland	0	4.25	76.46	32.10	32.50	0.31	0	0	127.4	Thomson, 1825	
Cheltenham (old well)	England	0	11.05	50.65	45.80	4.26	1.22	0	0	111.6	Scudamore, 1819	Trace of iodine by Daubeny. Alumina 5.10.
Hartfell aluminous chalybeate	Scotland	0	63.23	2.95	0	5.68	0	trace	0	101.3	Thomson, 1828	
Isle of Wight	England	0	48.58	9.50	6.85	2.87	0.82	14.60	0.96	88.21	Marcet	Alumina 7.77.
Marienbad (Ferdinandsquelle)	Bohemia	9.52	27.60	9.50	38.05	2.87	1.67	0.12	0.50	86.18	Steinmann, 1820	Phosphoric acid, lithion, strontian, alumina, manganese, by Berzelius.
Dunblane (north spring)	Scotland	0.30	2.23	33.55	15.30	14.04	0	0.23	0	63.21	Murray, 1814	
Vals	France	22.48	0.29	3.00	33.34	1.60	0.22	0.06	0.45	61.17	Berthier	
Bilin	Bohemia	20.51	3.40	1.44	28.47	2.47	1.60	0.10	0	57.46	Reuss, 1788	
Franzenbad (Franzensbrunn)	Ditto	5.44	18.50	6.21	26.70	1.26	0	0.37	0.48	55.80	Tromsdorff, 1820	Phosphoric acid, lithian, strontian, alumina, manganese, by Berzelius.
Pitcaithly	Ditto	0.30	0.73	27.20	8.50	13.99	0	trace	trace	46.95	Murray, 1814	
Roisdorf	Rhenish Prussia	6.76	2.50	9.70	16.00	1.78	1.33	0.07	0.21	38.11	Bischoff, 1826	Potash.
Epsom	England	2.50	14.80	4.21	5.64	11.80	0	0	0	37.94	Daubeny, 1830	Trace of bromine.
Selters (Nieder)	Nassau	5.37	0.18	9.92	16.06	1.37	1.00	0.12	0.38	34.00	Bischoff, 1826	Phosphoric acid 0.19.
Fachingen	Ditto	11.49	0.12	2.63	15.63	1.83	1.09	0.07	0.11	32.98		Phosphoric acid 000.5.
Soden	Ditto	3.35	0.07	12.30	10.72	4.08	0.06	0.08	0.06	30.89	Meyer, 1820	
Moffat	Scotland	0	2.80	13.60	12.75	0.68	0.26	0	0	30.03	Thomson, 1828	
Pyrmont	Germany	4.03	9.83	0.99	1.29	85.6	1.98	0.36	0.68	27.89	Struve	Phosphoric acid, potash, strontian, manganese.
Marienfels	Nassau	4.83	0.18	1.88	3.42	2.20	1.27	0.10	trace	15.99	Kastner	Potash 1.19; strontian, manganese, phosphoric acid.
Strathpeffer (pump-room)	Scotland	0	9.32	2.17	6.18	2.33	0.30	0	0	15.36	Thomson, 1828	Potash.
Geilnau	Nassau	6.00	0.07	0.18	5.08	1.46	1.40	0.13	0.14	14.66	Bischoff, 1826	Phosphoric acid .012.
Weilbach	Ditto	3.61	0.81	1.31	4.60	1.55	2.05	0	0	14.40	Creve, 1810	Sulphur-resin 0.18.
Hartfell Spa	Scotland	0	2.76	3.05	0	2.30	0	2.49	0	9.95	Thomson, 1828	Alumina a trace.
Langenschwalbach (Weinbrunn)	Nassau	3.84	0.12	0.12	0.34	1.55	1.95	0.67	trace	8.58	Kastner, 1829	Potash, lithion, iodine, strontian, alumina, manganese, phosphoric acid.
Spa	Belgium	6.63	0.51	0.33	0.92	0.74	0.72	7.90	0.68	5.92	Struve	Phos. acid; potash 0.58; manganese.
Carlsbad (Sauerling)	Bohemia	0.28	0.13	0.07	0.28	0.16	0.06	0.06	0.61	1.42	Berzelius, 1822	Phosphoric acid, fluate of lime, alumina, oxide or manganese.
Tunbridge	England	0.20	0.14	0.29	0.19	0.39	0.02	0.38	0.07	1.32	Scudamore, 1816	Oxide of manganese.
Malvern	Ditto	0.32	0.14	0.08	0.55	0.03	0.02	0.04	0	1.01	Phillip, 1805	

WATER, MINERAL, Acidulous water, simple.
WATERS, MINERAL, ARTIFICIAL, (F.) *Eaux minérales artificielles* ou *factices*. These are imitations of the natural; and some of them — as the factitious Cheltenham water, and Sedlits water — answer the purpose of the natural water tolerably well. The acidulous and chalybeate waters are, however, most easily imitated.

WATER, NUTMEG, Spiritus myristicæ — w. Parsnep, creeping, Sium — w. Pennyroyal, spirituous, Spiritus pulegii — w. Peppermint, Aqua menthæ piperitæ.

WATER POX, see Varicella.

WATER, PROTOXIDE OF NITROGEN, Aqua nitrogenii protoxydi.

WATER QUALM, Pyrosis.

WATER, RAIN, *Aqua pluvia'lis*, *A. plu'via*, *A. Im'brium*, (F.) *Eau de pluie*, when collected at a distance from houses or other elevated objects, is the purest natural water, and has the least specific gravity. The only bodies which it usually holds in solution, are carbonic acid, and minute traces of carbonate of lime and chloride of calcium.

WATER, RICE, see Oryza.

WATER, RIVER, *Aqua fluviat'ilis*, is derived from the conflux of numerous springs and rain water. It is, generally, pretty pure.

WATER, ROSE, Aqua rosæ.

WATER, SEA, *Aqua Mari'na*, *Humor Dor'idis*, (F.) *Eau de Mer*. This contains chlorides of sodium, magnesium and calcium, and sulphate of magnesia. It is cathartic, and forms the usual glyster at sea. It makes an excellent tonic bath; superior in most cases — especially in scrofula — to the fresh water-bath.

WATER, SEARLE'S PATENT OXYGENOUS AERATED, Aqua Nitrogenii protoxydi — w. Seydschutz, Sedlits water.

WATER SHIELD, Brasenia hydropeltis.

WATER, SNOW, *Aqua niva'ta*, (F.) *Eau de neige*, has usually been deemed unwholesome. It exactly resembles rain water in composition, and is equally salubrious.

WATER, SODA, Acidulous water, simple — w. Soft, see Water, hard — w. Spearmint, Aqua menthæ viridis.

WATER, SPRING, *Aqua fonta'na*, *Hydrope'gē*, (F.) *Eau de fontaine*, contains, in addition to the substances detected in rain water, more or less sulphate of lime. When this is to such an extent as to curdle soap, the water is said to be *hard*; if not, *soft*. Hard water is, of course, inferior to soft, for domestic and medicinal purposes.

WATER, STYPTIC, Sydenham's solutio sulphatis cupri composita — w. Tar, see Pinus sylvestris — w. Toast, see Toast-water.

WATER, WELL, *Aqua putea'lis* seu *Putea'na*, *A. ex pu'teo*, (F.) *Eau de puit*, *Eau de source*, is the same as spring water, but liable to impregnation, owing to the land springs filtering into the wells, and conveying impurities into them.

WATERS, DISCHARGED OR BROKEN, Profusio aquæ — w. Distilled, Aquæ destillatæ — w. First, Primitiæ.

WATTWEILER, MINERAL WATERS OF. Wattweiler is a small town in the department of Haut-Rhin, at the foot of the Vosges. The waters are acidulous chalybeates, and contain carbonates of iron, lime, and soda; chloride of sodium, and free carbonic acid.

WAX, Cera — w. Ear, Cerumen.

WAX, MYRTLE. A wax obtained from the fruit of *Myri'ca cerif'era*. It has been prescribed in dysentery.

WAX, YELLOW AND WHITE, Cera flava et alba.

WAXING KERNELS, *Crescen'tiæ*, (F.) *Croissances*, *Croissants*, *Glandes de croissance*. A popular term for small tumours, formed by an enlargement of the lymphatic glands — in the groin of children particularly. They have been looked upon as connected with the growth of the body. — hence their name.

WAY, Saxon wæg, Via, *Passage*, *Odos*, *Voie*. A name given to different canals.

WAYS, DIGESTIVE, *Digestive Pa'nym Prima Via*, (F.) *Voies digestives*, *Premières* are the series of hollow organs of digestion, composed of mouth, œsophagus, stomach, and small and large intestines. The term is often restricted to the first three of these.

WAYS, SECOND, *Second Passages*, *Secundæ via*, (F.) *Secondes voies*, comprise the chyliferous lymphatic and blood vessels.

WEAKSIGHTEDNESS, Asthenopia.

WEAL, Wheal.

WEANING, from Saxon ᵹeneᵹan, 'to wean' *Ablacta'tio*, *Apogalactis'mus*, (F.) *Sevrage*. The act of depriving the infant, permanently, of the breast, in order to feed it on other and more solid nourishment.

WEANING BRASH, see Brash, weaning.

WEATHERCOCKS, Impatiens.

WEB, MUSCULAR, Panniculus carnosus.

WEB-EYE, Caligo.

WEDGED, (D.) w e g g h e, *Inclu'sa*, *hierens*, (F.) *Enclavée*. The head of the fœtus is said to be wedged in the pelvis, when it remains fixed, notwithstanding the uterine efforts.

The condition is called *Incuneа'tio seu hæsitа'tio fœtūs*, *Spheno'sis*, *Inhærens*, (F.) *Enravement*. See Paragomphosis.

WEED, see Mastitis — w. in the Breast, Mastitis — w. Dyer's, Reseda luteola — w. Fly, Anthemis cotula — w. Horsefly, Sophora tinctoria — w. Milk, Apocynum androsæmifolium — w. Soldiers', Matico — w. Silver, Potentilla anserina.

WEEPING, Fletus.

WEIGHT, from Saxon pæᵹan, 'to weigh' (F.) *Pésanteur*. A sensation of heaviness or pressure over the whole body, or over a part — the stomach or head, for example.

WEIGHTS AND MEASURES, *Pondera et Mensu'ra*, (F.) *Poids et Mésures*. The importance of possessing a uniform system of weights and measures has impressed the scientific of all countries, and numerous endeavours have been made to accomplish the object. It is, however, a matter of considerable difficulty, and one not likely to be attained. The new French measures are upon decidedly the best footing, but they are not adopted out of France. The greatest diversity prevails over Europe in the measures of weight and capacity. Some of the following tables will show, that every subdivision of the pound, as well as the pound itself, differs in England and in France.

WEIGHTS.

Troy Weight, as used by the British Apothecary. — Pondus pharmaceu'ticum seu medicina.

The pound ℔	contains	12 ounces.
The ounce ℥		8 drachms.
The drachm ʒ		3 scruples.
The scruple ℈		20 grains.
The grain gr.		

These, and the signs by which they are denoted, are the same in all the British Pharmacopœias as well as in the American.

℔	Oz.	Drm's.	Scrup.	Grs.
1	— 12	— 96	— 288	— 5760
	1	— 8	— 24	— 480
		1	— 3	— 60
			1	— 20

WEIGHTS

Poids de Marc.

The *pound* ⎫   ⎧ 16 ounces.
The *ounce* ⎪   ⎪ 8 drachms.
The *drachm* ⎬ contains   ⎨ 3 scruples.
The *scruple*⎪   ⎪ 24 grains.
The *grain* ⎭   ⎩

Avoirdupois.

Pound.	Ounces.	Drachms.	Troy grains.
lb. 1.	16	256	7000
	1	16	437.5
		1	27.34375

The avoirdupois drachm is sometimes divided into three scruples, and the scruple into ten grains. The pound of 7680 grains avoirdupois = 7000 grains troy, and hence 1 grain troy = .97 grain avoirdupois.

The *Poids de Marc* is that employed by the French Pharmaciens, when the new weights are not. The Avoirdupois is now used by the Dublin College.

The following tables exhibit the relative value of the old French and English weights:

Poids de Marc.	Troy Wt.	Avoird.	Troy grs.
1 pd. (livre) =	1.31268 lb	1.080143 lb =	7561
1 oz. (once) =	.984504 oz	1.080143 oz =	472.5625
1 dr. (gros.) =	.954504 dr	=	59.0703125
1 gr. =			.820421

Troy.		Poids de Marc.	French grains.
1 pound	=	0.76180 lb.	7561
1 ounce	=	1.01574 onces	585.083
1 drachm	=	1.01574 gros	73.135
1 grain	=		1.219

Avoirdupois.		Poids de Marc.	French grains.
1 pound	=	0.925803 lb.	8532.3
1 ounce	=	0.925803 once	533.27

To convert		
" French grains into Troy grains, divide by		
" Troy grains into French grains, multiply by		1.2189
" French ounces into Troy ounces, divide by		
" Troy ounces into French ounces, multiply by		1.015734
" French pounds (*poids de marc*) into Troy pounds, multiply by		
" Troy pounds into French pounds, divide by		1.31268

Troy grains.		Poids de Marc or French grain.
1	=	1.219
2	=	2.438
3	=	3.657
4	=	4.876
5	=	6.095
6	=	7.314
7	=	8.533
8	=	9.752
9	=	10.971

French grain.		Troy grain.
1	=	0.8203
2	=	1.6406
3	=	2.4609
4	=	3.2812
5	=	4.1015
6	=	4.9218
7	=	5.7421
8	=	6.5624
9	=	7.3827

New French Decimal or Metrical Weights.

		Troy grains.		lb.	oz.	dr.	gr.
Milligramme	=	.0154					
Centigramme	=	.1543					
Decigramme	=	1.5434					
Gramme	=	15.4340					
Decagramme	=	154.3402	=	0	0	2	34.4
Hectogramme	=	1543.4023	=	0	3	1	44.4
Kilogramme	=	15434.0234	=	2	8	1	24
Myriagramme	=	154340.2344	=	26	9	6	0

Comparative Value of the French Medicinal Pound and that of other Places.

	lbs.	oz.	dr.	gr.	
Germany	0	15	4	48	
Amsterdam	1	00	0	42	
Belgium	1	00	0	42	
Berne	1	00	0	00	
Copenhagen	0	15	3	20¼	
Florence	0	11	0	50	divided into 12 oz.
Genoa	0	10	5	60	do. into 12 oz.
Geneva	1	00	0	18	
Hamburg	0	15	2	15	
Lisbon	0	16	7	68	
London	0	12	3	12	divided into 12 oz.
Madrid	0	15	0	16	
Milan	0	9	3	00	
Monaco	0	15	2	23	
Naples	0	10	7	54	divided into 12 oz.
Paris	1	00	0	00	divided into 16 oz.
Rome	0	11	0	50	do. into 12 oz.
Stockholm	0	13	7	8	
United States	0	12	3	12	divided into 12 oz.
Warsaw	1	10	4	24	
Venice	0	8	6	00	
Vienna	1	2	2	32	

MEASURES OF CAPACITY.

English Measure of Fluids.

The *gallon* (congius) . . . . . O ⎫   ⎧ 8 pints.
The *pint* (octarius) . . . . . . O ⎪   ⎪ 16 fluidounces.
The *fluidounce* . . . . f℥   ⎬ contains   ⎨ 8 fluidrachms.
The *fluidrachm* . . . . fℨ   ⎪   ⎪ 60 minims.
The *minim* . . . . ♏   ⎭   ⎩

Proportions of the Apothecaries' and Wine Gallon.

Gal.	Pints.	Fluidoz.	Fluidr.	Minims.	Cub. inches.
1 =	8 =	128 =	1024 =	61440 =	231
	1 =	16 =	128 =	7680 =	28.875
		1 =	8 =	480 =	1.8047
			1 =	60 =	.2256

Imperial Measure, adopted by the London College in their Pharmacopœia of 1836.

Gallon.	Pints.	Fluidounces.	Fluidr.	Minims.
1 =	8 =	160 =	1280 =	76800
	1 =	20 =	160 =	9600
		1 =	8 =	480
			1 =	60

Comparative Value of the Proportions of the Wine and Imperial Gallons.

Wine.			Imperial.		
		Pints.	Fluidoz.	Fluidr.	Minims.
1 gallon	=	6	13	2	23
1 pint			16	5	18
1 fluidounce	=		1	0	20
1 fluidrachm	=			1	2¼

Imperial.			Wine.		
		Gallon.	Pint.	Fluidoz. Fluidr.	Minims.
1 gallon	=	1	1	9 5	8
1 pint	=		1	3 1	38
1 fluidounce	=			7	41
1 fluidrachm	=				58

French Measures of Capacity.

		English cubic inches.		Wine Measure.
Millilitre	=	.061028	=	16.2318 minims.
Centilitre	=	.610280	=	2.7053 fluidrachms.
Decilitre	=	6.102800	=	3.3816 fluidounces.
Litre	=	61.028000	=	2.1135 pints.
Decalitre	=	610.280000	=	2.6419 gallons.
Hectolitre	=	6102.800000		
Kilolitre	=	61028.000000		
Myrialitre	=	610280.000000		

Approximate comparison between the ancient French Measures of Capacity, and the new, and conversely.

		Grammes.		Litres.	Decilitres.	Centilitres.
1 *poisson*	=	125	or	0	1	2
1 *demi-setier*	=	250	or	0	2	5
1 *chopine*	=	500	or	0	5	0
1 *pinte*	=	1000	or	1	0	0

WEIGHTS 918 WEIGHTS

Grammes.	lbs. oz. dr. gr.
1 centilitre =	10 or 0 0 2½ 00
1 decilitre =	100 or 0 3 2 00 [pints.
1 litre =	1000 or 2 0 3 36 = 2.113 Eng. wine

Measures of Length.

	Inches.
1 line, the 12th part of an inch.	
3 barleycorns	1.000
A palm or hand's breadth (Scripture measure)	3.648
A hand (horse measure)	4.000
A span (Scripture measure)	10.944
A foot	12.000
A cubit (Scripture measure for common purposes)	18.000
A cubit (Scripture measure for sacred purposes)	21.888
A Flemish ell	27.000
A yard	3 ft. 00
An English ell	3 " 09
A fathom or toise	6 " 00

New French Measures of Length.

	English Inches.
Millimètre	0.039
Centimètre	0.393
Decimètre	3.937
Mètre	39.371 — 1 yd. 0 ft. 3.37 inch.

VALUES OF THE GRECIAN, ROMAN, AND ARABIAN WEIGHTS AND MEASURES IN POIDS DE MARC.

1. Weights of the Ancient Greeks.

	lbs. oz. dr. gr.
The talent (τάλαντον)	54 2 5 2
The mina (μνα)	14 3 2
The drachm (δραχμη)	1 11
The obolus (ὀβολος)	
The ceration (κερατιον)	4
The chalcus (χαλκους)	2
The septon (σεπτον)	

2. Weights of the Ancient Romans.

	oz. dr. gr.
The pound (libra)	10 6
The ounce (uncia)	7
The duella	5
The sicilicus	2
The sextula	1
The consular denier, denarius	1
The imperial denier or drachm, drachma	
The victoriatus	
The scriptulum or scruple	
The obolus	
The siliqua	4

The Greeks divided their obolus into chalci and lepta: some divided it into 6 chalci, each chalcus into 7 lepta; others into 8 chalci, and every chalcus into 8 lepta or minuta.

Dr. Milligan, in his edition of Celsus, gives the following table, exhibiting the Troy weight measures of capacity and of weight in use amongst the Romans.

	Urna.	Libra.	Uncia.	Denarius.	Scrupulus.	Sextans.	Chalcus.	Grm.
Amphora	2	80	960	6720	20160	40320	403200	
Urna	1	40	480	3360	10080	20160	210600	
Congius	¼	10	120	840	2540	5040	50400	
Sextarius	12-3	20	140	420	840	8400		
Libra	1	12	84	252	504	5040		
Hemina	8 4-7	60	180	360	3600			
Acetabulum	2 1-7	15	45	90	900			
Sesqui-cyathus	2 1-7	15	45	90	900			
Cyathus	1 3-7	10	30	60	600			
Sescuncia	1½	10½	31¼	63	630			
Uncia	1	7	21	42	420			
Cochleare		2¼	7½	15	150			
Drachma		1	3	6	60			
Denarius		1	3	6	60			
Scrupulus			1	2	20			
Scrupulus dimidiatus			½	1	10			
Obolus				1	10			
Sextans				1	10			
Chalcus					1			

He gives also the following 'Carmen Mnemonicum,' which exhibits the analogies of the Roman and British imperial weights.

To the congius and gallon, each, ten pounds allow,
On the bushel and amphora eighty bestow;
Rome's pound, as in Troy weight, twelve ounces obtains,
But her ounce is Avoirdupois, strictly, in grains:
Denarii drams, scruples scrupli define,
Septarius answers to our bottle of wine,
And the mna's a short pint — fourteen ounces in fine.

3. Weights said to be of the Arabians, Modern Greeks, and Latins of the barbarous periods of the Middle Ages.

	oz. dr. gr.
The alchemion	14 3 40
The manes or omines	10 6 28
sacros, augbhen, adar, assatil	7 16
The great or royal nut	3 44
The sextarius, stater	3 44
The lesser nut	2 50
Aliovanus	2 29
Aureus, Alcobolus	2 14
The hazel nut, bendacats, holca, alchi, darchimi, atogochiloe, eloginat, nabach	1 11
The acorn, lupine, Egyptian or Syrian bean, the bachil	42

	oz. dr. gr.
The Alexandrian bean or tremessis	3
The Greek bean or gramme, the karmet, genam, harmi, gracchus	2
The ring, cumulus, sominat, omolocich, omolocoat	
The denich	
The kirat, alkilat, kararit	4

1. Greek Measures.

	lbs. oz. dr. gr.
The metretes (μετρητης)	84 4 3 0
The chus, choa, congius (χους)	7 0 2 0
The xestes (ξεστης)	1 1 7 8
The cotyla (κοτυλη)	8 7 3
The tetarton (τεταρτον)	4 3 0
The oxybaphon (οξυβαφον)	2 1 4
The cyathus (κυαθος)	1 4 0
The concha (κογχη)	6 0
The mystron (μυστρον)	3 0
The chama minor (χαμη)	2 4
The cochliarion (κοχλιαριον)	1 2

2. Roman Measures of Capacity.

	lbs. oz. dr. gr.
The amphora or cadus	56 2 2 0
The urna	28 1 3 0
The congius	7 0 2 0
The sextarius	1 4 0 0
The hemina	10 1 2
The quartarius	5 0 6
The acetabulum	2 4 2
The cyathus or small glass	1 5 2
The ligula or spoonful	3 2

3. *Measures said to be of the Arabian, Arabist, and Latin Physicians of the Middle Ages.*

	lbs.	oz.	dr.	gr.
The *missokaos* weighed	3	8	1	33
Aben. kirt, ejub, sberia, or *Roman mina*	1	6	0	00
The *phial, hasflius,* or *hassitinus*	10	1	18	
The *calix* or *rejelati*		5	0	44
The *handful, pugillum, cornusum*		3	2	68
The *hassuf, assasse,* or *anesims*		2	4	20
The *conos* or *coatus, alcantus* or *almunessi, briale cuabus*		1	5	34
The *lesser bachates*			5	56
The *largest spoonful*			4	44
A *spoonful*			1	52
The *colanos* or *reclanarium*			1	28
A *small spoonful* or *flagerina,* or *cyanes*			1	11
The *smallest spoonful* or *fahaliel*				42

A good section on weights and measures is contained in the edition of "The Seven Books of Paulus Ægineta," by Mr. Francis Adams, published by the Sydenham Society of London, vol. iii, p. 609, London, 1847.

Besides the weights and measures above mentioned, employed by the moderns, there are modes of estimating the quantities of substances by approximation. For example:—

A *glassful* or *cupful,* ((F.) *Verre,*) is reckoned to contain 4 or 5 fluidounces.

A *wine-glassful*, 1½ ounce or two ounces.

A *table-spoonful,* ((F.) *Cuiller à bouche,*) about half an ounce.

A *coffee* or *dessert-spoonful,* about 3 drachms.

A *tea-spoonful,* a fluidrachm.

A *handful, manipulus,* ((F.) *Poignée,*) as much as can be held in the hand.

The *Pugillus* ((F.) *Pincée*) is as much as can be held by the three fingers.

These last quantities are occasionally prescribed by the French practitioners. Their weights must, of course, vary, according to the article. The authors of the Parisian codex have valued them, as regards certain substances.

		French.	
		oz.	dr.
A *Manipulus* of barley weighs		3	2¼
"	linseed	1	4
"	linseed meal	3	3
"	dried mallow leaves	1	3
"	dried cichory leaves	1	0
"	flowers of the tilia	1	2¼

		dr.	scr.	gr.
A *Pugillus* of chamomile flowers weighs	2			
"	arnica	1	2	
"	marsh-mallow	1	1	
"	mallow			60
"	fennel seeds		1	60
"	aniseed	1	½	60

A *hen's egg,* newly laid, weighs about 2 ounces and 2 drachms: when deprived of its shell, 2 ounces. The *white* weighs 1 ounce, 2 drachms, and 57 grains: the *yolk,* 5 drachms and 15 grains.

WEILBACH, MINERAL WATERS OF. The village of Weilbach is in the plain between the Maine and the southern extremity of the Taunus hills. It has in its neighbourhood a cold sulphureous alkaline spring, the water of which is bottled and exported, although not of great efficacy. Its use is at times combined with that of the saline springs in Nassau, and of Baden-Baden, in various chronic abdominal and thoracic affections.

WELD, Reseda luteola.

WELK, *Whelk.* An inequality; a protuberance; a cutaneous eruption of this character. Acne.

WEMDING, MINERAL WATERS OF. These waters are situate about four leagues from Donawert in Bavaria. They contain sulphuretted hydrogen; carbonates of lime, magnesia, and soda; sulphates of lime and magnesia; a little chloride of calcium, and oxide of iron; and are much used in asthenic diseases.

WEN, Sax. ꝥen, *Lu'pia, Tumour,* (F.) *Loupe.* A name given to circumscribed, indolent tumours, without inflammation or change of colour of the skin. They may be met with in almost every part of the body. Their magnitude, as well as nature, is very variable. The term is sometimes given to an encysted tumour, and to bronchocele.

WESTERN ISLANDS, Azores.

WEST INDIES, (CLIMATE OF.) The climate of the West Indies has long been regarded as favourable to the consumptive. In confirmed consumption, it appears, however, to be positively injurious. As a prophylactic for those predisposed to consumption, it is generally favourable. The nature of the patient's constitution, in regard to the effects of elevated temperature, has always to be taken into account. In diseases that are benefited by warm climates, the West Indies afford an appropriate residence. The islands in which the invalid can best obtain all the advantages of the climate, are Jamaica, Barbadoes, St. Vincents, Antigua, St. Kitts, and Santa Cruz.

WHAHOO, see Euonymus.

WHEAL, *Weal, Wale.* A ridge, or elevation of the skin, produced by a rod or whip; or as if produced in that manner. Such elevations are seen in urticaria.

WHEAT, Triticum—w. Indian, Zea mays—w. Turkey, Zea mays.

WHELK, Acne, Welk — w. Chin, Sycosis—w. Rosy, Gutta rosea.

WHEY, Serum lactis—w. Mustard, see Sinapis —w. Rennet, see Serum lactis—w. Tamarind, see Tamarindus—w. Vinegar, see Acetum—w. Wine, Wine whey.

WHIFFING MURMUR, see Murmur, respiratory.

WHISKY, see Spirit. A spirituous liquor obtained from oats, potatoes, &c., by distillation.

WHISKY LIVER, Liver, nutmeg.

WHIS'PERING; evidently an onomatopœia (*hooisp'ering*), *Susurra'tio, Susurra'tion.* Articulation of the air sent through the vocal tube without any action of the glottis.

WHISTLING, *Sifflement,* see *Râle sibilant.*

WHITE, Flake, Plumbi subcarbonas.

WHITE BALL, Cephalanthus occidentalis — w. Leaf, Pyrola maculata, Spiræa tomentosa — w. Leg, Phlegmatia dolens—w. Matter of the brain, see Cerebrum — w. Root, Angelica lucida, Asclepias tuberosa.

WHITE, SPANISH, Bismuth, subnitrate of.

WHITE SWELLING, Hydrarthrus — w. Swelling of lying-in women, Phlegmatia dolens —w. Substance of Schwann, see Nerve fibre—w. Sulphur, see Virginia, mineral waters of—w. Weed, Chrysanthemum leucanthemum — w. Wood, Liriodendron, Tilia.

WHITENESS OF COMPLEXION, Paleness.

WHITES, THE, Leucorrhœa.

WHITLEYA STRAMONIFOLIA, Anisodus luridus.

WHITLOW, Paronychia.

WHOOPING-COUGH, Pertussis.

WHORLYWORT, Leptandria purpurea.

WHORTLEBERRY, Vaccinium myrtillus, Vaccinium vitis idæa — w. Bears', Arbutus uva ursi.

WHORTS, BLACK, Vaccinium myrtillus.

WIDOW-WAIL, Cneorum tricoccum, Daphne Alpina.

WIESBADEN, MINERAL WATERS OF, see Wisbaden.

WIESSAU, MINERAL WATERS OF. These waters are situate about four leagues from the convent of Waldsassen in Bavaria. They contain carbonic acid; carbonates of lime and magnesia; chlorides of calcium, magnesium, and aluminum; carbonate of soda, and much oxide of iron. The Bavarians consider them to resemble the waters of Pyrmont.

WILD, Sax. pild, (D.) Wild. An epithet given to the countenance, when not in harmony with the condition of the individual, and indicating strong mental emotion;—a *wild look*, (F.) *Physiognomie égarée*.

WILDBAD, MINERAL WATERS OF. Wildbad is a small town of Wurtemberg, three German miles from Baden-Baden. It is much frequented as a watering-place. The water is thermal, from 95° to 100° of Fahr., and is much employed in cases in which thermal waters are indicated. It is used internally, a pint not containing more than a grain of solid ingredients, which consist of salts of soda and lime. The proportion of carbonic acid gas is very small.

WILDUNGEN, MINERAL WATERS OF. Wildungen is situate a few miles from Cassel in Germany. In its neighbourhood are several mineral springs; the chief of which, according to Stucke, contain a bituminous matter; chloride of sodium and sulphate of soda; carbonate and sulphate of lime, &c. They are used, chiefly, as refrigerants.

WILL, Voluntas.

WILLOW, Salix.

WILLOW HERB, common, Lythrum salicaria — w. Herb, great, Epilobium augustifolium — w. Herb, purple, Lythrum salicaria — w. Herb, purple veined, Epilobium coloratum.

WILLOW, LOW-BUSH, Salix humilis — w. Speckled, Salix humilis — w. Red, Cornus sericea — w. Rose, Cornus sericea — w. Sweet, Myrica gale.

WIND, Sax. pind, *Ventus*, *An'emos*, (F.) *Vent*. Winds exert considerable influence on the animal economy; acting by their temperature, which necessarily modifies that of the circumambient air, as well as by their moisture or dryness, and by the emanations of different kinds, which they transport to greater or less distances. The winds which blow over a considerable extent of country, are dry and serene: those which come from the ocean are moist and chilly.

WIND DROPSY, Emphysema, Tympanites — w. Flower, Anemone — w. Pipe, Trachea — w. Root, Asclepias tuberosa.

WINDINESS, Flatulence.

WINDY, *Flatulen'tus*, *Flat'ulent*, *Va'pourous*, (F.) *Venteux*. That which causes wind or flatulence; also, that which is caused by wind or flatulence; as *windy food*, *windy colic*, &c. Also, one affected with flatulence, or who is 'troubled with the wind.'

WINE, Sax. pin, (G.) Wein, originally, perhaps, from *œvos*, *Œnos*, *Vinum*, (F.) *Vin*. A name given by chymists to all liquors that have become spirituous by fermentation. The term is generally, however, restricted to the fermented juice of the grape, or of fruits, the product of whose fermentation resembles, in almost all respects, that of the juice of the grape. Wine is composed of alcohol; saccharine matter; malic acid; tartaric acid; bitartrate of potass; acetic acid; an extractive colouring matter, more or less bitter, and partly resinous; and sometimes of an aromatic substance. The extractive colouring matter is chiefly met with in red wines. All these constituents, except the alcohol, are found ready formed in the grape. The alcohol proceeds from the decomposition of the saccharine matter. A part of the acetic acid is also formed during fermentation.

The following table, drawn up by Mr. Brande, exhibits the quantity of spirit in different kinds of wine and liquors. It is proper, however, to remark, that many of these wines are prepared for the London market, and are more brandied or "reinforced," than the same varieties sold in the United States. This is strikingly the case with port. Dr. Henderson, too, has remarked, that some of the wines analyzed by Mr. Brande were mixed with a considerable quantity of adventitious alcohol. Dr. Henderson's additions and corrections have the letter H. affixed.

PROPORTION OF ALCOHOL, S. G. 0.825, IN ONE HUNDRED PARTS BY MEASURE OF THE FOLLOWING WINES, AND MALT AND SPIRITUOUS LIQUORS.

1. Lissa
   Do.
   Average.
2. Raisin Wine
   Do.
   Do.
   Average.
3. Marsala
   Do.
   Average.
4. Port — average of six kinds
   Do. — highest
   Do. — lowest
5. Madeira
   Do.
   Do. (Sercial)
   Do.
   Average.
6. Currant Wine
7. Sherry
   Do.
   Do.
   Do.
   Average.
8. Teneriffe
9. Colares
10. Lacryma Cristi
11. Constantia — white
    " — red
12. Lisbon
13. Malaga
14. Bucellas
15. Red Madeira
    Do.
    Average.
16. Cape Muscat
17. Cape Madeira
    Do.
    Do.
    Average.
18. Grape Wine
19. Calcavella
    Do.
    Average.
20. Vidonia
21. Alba Flora
22. Malaga
23. White Hermitage
24. Roussillon
    Do.
    Average.
25. Claret
    Do.
    Do.
    Do.
    Average.
26. Malmsey Madeira
27. Lunel
28. Scheraaz
29. Syracuse
30. Sauterne
31. Burgundy
    Do.
    Do.
    Do.
    Average.
32. Hock
    Do.
    Do. (old in cask)
    Average.
    Rudesheimer (1811) .... H
    Do.   (1800) .... H
    Average. H
    Johannisberger .... H
33. Nice
34. Barsac

(a) 15.90 H. (b) 18.40 H. (c) 14.50 H. (d) 12.91 H

35. Tent	13.30
36. Champagne (still)	13.80
Do. (sparkling)	12.80
Do. (red)	12.56
Do.	11.30
Average,	12.61
37. Red Hermitage	12.32
38. Vin de Grave	13.94
Do.	12.80
Average,	13.37
39. Frontignac	12.79
40. Côte Rotie	12.32
41. Gooseberry Wine	11.84
42. Orange Wine—average of six samples made by a London manufacturer	11.26
43. Tokay	9.88
44. Elder Wine	9.87
45. Rhenish Wine...........H.	8.71
46. Cider — highest average	9.87
Do. lowest	5.21
47. Perry — average of four samples	7.26
48. Mead	7.32
49. Ale (Burton)	8 88
Do. (Edinburgh)	6.90
Do. (Dorchester)	5.56
Average,	6.87
50. Brown Stout	6.80
51. London Porter — average	4.20
Do. Small Beer — average	1.26
52. Brandy	53.39
53. Rum	53.68
54. Gin	51.60
55. Scotch Whisky	54.32
56. Irish do.	53.90

The only wine recommended in some pharmacopœias is *Sherry, Vinum, Vinum album Hispan'icum, Leucus'nus*. It is a *dry wine*; the least variable in its properties, and agrees best with the dyspeptic. Other wines used officinally are—*Canary* or *Sack wine, Vinum Canari'num; Mountain wine, Vinum album monta'num; Tent wine; Rhenish wine, Vinum Rhena'num;* and *Port wine, Vinum rubrum Portugal'licum*.

The wines habitually drunk are almost innumerable. Those that are sweet, or contain a large portion of free, saccharine matter, are decidedly the least wholesome to the dyspeptic.

When wine is good, and of a proper age, it is tonic and nutritive; when new, flatulent and cathartic, disagreeing with the stomach and bowels. In medicine, it is a valuable tonic in the last stage of typhus, when the skin is not too hot and dry. Its use, however, requires great caution; and when once commenced under proper circumstances, it cannot be suddenly dropped without mischief. It is, perhaps, the best permanent stimulus in the catalogue of the materia medica.

Mulled Wine is made as follows: — Take of bruised *cinnamon* ʒiß; half a *nutmeg* grated; and ten bruised *cloves*. Infuse in boiling *water* Oss for an hour; strain and add *sugar* ʒj. Pour the whole into a pint of hot *Port* or *Sherry*. Useful in adynamic conditions.

WINE, AMINÆAN, Aminæum vinum — w. of Aloes, Vinum aloes—w. Antimonial, Vinum antimonii tartarizati—w. Antiscorbutic, Vinum antiscorbuticum — w. Aromatic, Vinum aromaticum —w. Bark, compound, Vinum de kinâ kinâ compositum—w. Barley, Cerevisia—w. Bitter, diuretic, Vinum diureticum amarum.

WINE BITTERS, *Vinum gentia'næ compositum.* The formulæ for these may be various. The following is as good and as agreeable as any. (*Rad. gentian.* ℔j, *cort. aurant.* ʒx, *sem. cardam.* cont. ʒiv, *cinnam. cort.* ʒiv, *wine*, foreign or domestic, three gallons and a half.) Tonic and stomachic.

WINE, CEDAR, Cedrinum vinum — w. Champagne, Vinum campanum—w. Chian, Chium vinum — w. of Colchicum, Vinum colchici — w. of Colchicum seed, Vinum colchici seminis—w. of Ergot, Vinum ergotæ—w. of Gentian, compound,

Vinum gentianæ compositum — w. of Hellebore, white, Vinum veratri — w. Ipecacuanha, Vinum ipecacuanhæ—w. of Iron, Vinum ferri—w. Medicated, Vinum medicinale — w. Mulled, see Wine — w. of Opium, Vinum opii — w. Port, Vinum Portugallicum — w. Pullet, *Poulet, vin de*—w. of Quinia, Vinum quiniæ—w. Rhubarb, Vinum rhei palmati — w. Sherry, Vinum — w. Steel, Vinum ferri — w. Tobacco, Vinum tabaci.

WINE WHEY, *White Wine Whey*. Take of good *milk* two-thirds of a pint, and add *water* to make a pint. Take of *sherry*, or any other good white *wine*, two glasses, and of *sugar* a dessert-spoonful. Place the milk and water in a deep pan on the fire; and the moment it boils, pour into it the wine and sugar. Stir assiduously for 12 or 15 minutes, whilst it boils. Lastly, strain through a sieve.

It is a good mode of giving wine in adynamic states.

WINE, WHITE, see Wine — w. of Wormwood, Vinum absinthites.

WING-SEED, Ptelea trifoliata.

WINKING, Scardamygmus.

WINTER-BARK TREE, Wintera aromatica —w. Berry, Virginia, Prinos—w. Berry, smooth, Prinos lævigatus — w. Berry, whorled, Prinos.

WINTER BLOOM, Hamamelis Virginiana — w. Cough, Bronchitis, chronic — w. Green, Gaultheria — w. Green, round-leaved, Pyrola—w. Green, spotted, Pyrola maculata.

WINTERA, see Wintera aromatica.

WIN'TERA AROMAT'ICA, *Drimys Winteri, Wintera'na aromat'ica, Winter-bark Tree*. The bark, Wintera (Ph. U. S.), *Cortex Wintera'nus, Cortex Winteranus Magellan'icus, Cortex Magellan'icus, Cinnamo'mum Magellan'icum,* (F.) *Écorce de Winter, Cannelle poivrée,* is very much allied in its properties to Canella alba.

WINTERANA AROMATICA, Wintera aromatica.

WISBADEN, MINERAL WATERS OF. Wisbaden is a town of Germany, about 6 miles north of Mains, and 22 west of Frankfort. It has been long celebrated for its hot springs; and is much frequented. There are numerous cold and thermal springs, — the former containing sulphohydric acid; the latter being saline and acidulous. The temperature of the hot springs varies from 117° to 160° Fahr.

WISMUTHUM, Bismuth.

WOAD, Isatis tinctoria.

WOLFBANE, Veratrum viride.

WOLFSBANE, Aconitum — w. Wholesome, Aconitum anthora.

WOLFSCLAW, Lycopodium.

WOLFSJAW, see Harelip.

WOMANHOOD, Mulieritas.

WOMB, Uterus—w. Falling down of the, Prolapsus uteri.

WOMB GRAIN, Ergot.

WOMB, LACERATION OF THE, Uterus, rupture of the—w. Tympany of the, Physometra.

WOOD, BRAZIL, Cæsalpinia echinata — w. Elk, Andromeda arborea — w. Fernambuco, Cæsalpinia echinata.

WOOD-LICE, Onisci aselli—w. Nicaragua, see Cæsalpinia — w. Peach, see Cæsalpinia—w. Pernambuco, Cæsalpinia echinata—w. Sampfen, Cæsalpinia sappan—w. Sappaa, Cæsalpinia sappan — w. Sorrel, Oxalis acetosella — w. Sour, Andromeda arborea — w. Waxen, Genista tinctoria.

WOODBINE, COMMON, Lonicera periclymenum.

WOODROOF, SWEET-SCENTED, Asperula odorata.

WOODS, SUDORIF'IC, (F.) *Bois sudorifiques.* This term is applied, collectively, to the grain-eum, sassafras, china, and sarsaparilla; which are often used together to form the sudorific decoction.

WOORARA, Curare.

WORM, see Alembic, Vermiform process — w. Bark tree, Geoffrœa inermis — w. Cakes, Story's, see Cakes, worm, Story's — w. Disease, Helminthiasis — w. Goosefoot, Chenopodium anthelminticum — w. Grass, perennial, Spigelia Marilandica.

WORM, GUINEA, Dracunculus.

WORM LOZ'ENGES, CHING'S. Empirical preparations, which consist of yellow and brown lozenges. The former are directed to be taken in the evening; the latter on the following morning. The *Yellow Lozenges*. (*Saffron*, ℥ss, *water*, Oj; boil, and strain; and add of *white panacea of mercury*, (calomel washed in spirit of wine,) ℔j, *white sugar*, 28 ℔s, *mucilage of gum tragacanth* q. s., to make a mass. Divide, so that each lozenge may contain a grain of the panacea.) The *Brown Lozenges*. (*Panacea* ℥vij, *resin of jalap* ℔iijss, *white sugar* ℔ix, *mucilage of gum tragac.* q. s. Each lozenge to contain gr. ss of the panacea.)

WORM LOZENGES, SHERMAN'S, are said to be composed of *calomel, gamboge*, and *sugar*.

Peters's Worm Lozenges are said to be composed in a similar manner.

WORM ROOT, Spigelia Marilandica — w. Seed, Artemisia santonica, Chenopodium anthelminticum — w. Seed, goosefoot, Chenopodium anthelminticum — w. Weed, Corsican, Corallina Corsicana, Polanisia graveolens — w. Weed, white, Corallina — w. Wood, biennial, Artemisia biennis — w. Wood, common, Artemisia absinthium — w. Wood, creeping, Artemisia rupestris — w. Wood, lesser, Artemisia Pontica — w. Wood, Roman, Artemisia Pontica — w. Wood, Sea, Artemisia maritima — w. Wood, silky, Artemisia glacialis.

WORMIA'NA OSSA seu OSSIC'ULA, *O. epacta'lia, O. raphogeminan'tia, O. triq'uetra, O. triungula'ria Bla'sii, Claves calva'riæ, O. sutura'rum*, (F.) *Os Wormiens, Clefs du crâne, Os épactaux, Os surnuméraires*, (Ch.), *Os intercalés, Os triangulaires*. Small bones, which are sometimes observable in the sutures of the bones of the cranium, of which they form a part. They were called *Wormiana*, from Olaus Wormius, who is said to have first described them. They had been previously, however, mentioned by G. Andernach, a physician at Strasburg. The Ossa Wormiana exist more commonly in the sutures of the vault of the skull; especially in the lambdoidal, sagittal, and squamous. They are uncommon at the base of the skull. Their size is very variable, and shape irregular. Their structure and development are similar to those of the other bones of the cranium; and, like them, they are bounded by sutures.

WORMS, originally from (L.) *Vermes; Intestinal Worms, Entozo'a, Entozoa'ria, Enterozo'a, Endozo'a, Vermes intesti'ni, Entelminth'a, Enthelmin'thes, Helmin'thi, Helminth'ia Alvi, H. pod'icis, Splanchnelmin'tha, Entoparasites*, (F.) *Vers, Vers intestinaux, Entozoaires.* Animals whose common character is that of existing only in other animals; hence their name *entozoa*, from ἐντός, 'within,' and ζῶον, 'animal.' They are met with, not only in the natural cavities, but even in the tissue of the organs. Cuvier, Rudolphi, Brera, Bremser, Laënnec, and others, have endeavoured to classify them, — some according to their shape; others, according to their anatomical characters.

The following table exhibits the entozoa, which have been met with in the human body, and their usual habitat: —

Entozoa.	*Where found.*
Trichoceph'alus dispar,	
Oxyu'ris vermicula'ris,	
As'caris lumbricoi'des,	
Bothrioceph'alus latus,	Intestines.
Tæ'nia so'lium,	
Ditrachyo'eras rudis,	
Diploso'ma crena'ta,	
Spirop'tera hom'inis,	Urinary bladder.
Dactyl'ius aculea'tus,	
Dis'toma hepat'icum,	Gall bladder.
Stron'gylus gigas,	Kidney.
Fila'ria oc'uli,	Eye.
Acephalocyst'is endog"ena,	Liver.
Echinococ'cus hom'inis,	Liver, Spleen, and Omentum.
Polys'toma pinguic'ola,	Ovary.
Polys'toma vena'rum seu sanguic'ola, Hexathyrid'ium vena'rum,	Veins.
Fila'ria bronchia'lis,	Bronchial glands.
Trichi'na spira'lis,	Muscles.
Cysticer'cus cellulo'sæ,	
Acephalocyst'is multif'ida,	Brain.
Fila'ria medinen'sis,	Cellular texture.

The most common of these are: — the Oxyuris vermiculares, Ascarides lumbricoides, and Tænia, which are found in the intestines. The origin of these worms is extremely singular, and is favourable than any other fact to the hypothesis of spontaneous generation in the lowest tribes of animated nature. They are certainly not identical with any worms out of the body. They are most commonly met with in children improperly fed; but their presence cannot be positively detected by any symptom, except that of the discharge of the worms themselves in the evacuations. They may, of course, give rise to every kind of irritation in the intestinal tube, and to sympathetic disturbance in most of the functions; but all these signs may be produced by internal irritation resulting from other causes.

Anthelmintics or *vermifuges*, employed, as the name imports, for their removal, may be of two kinds — *mechanical* and *true*. To the first class the *mechanical* — belong *Emetics, Purgatives, Picuna, powdered Tin*, &c. To the latter — the *anthelmintics*, — *Turpentine, Chenopodium anthelminticum, Pink-root, Semina Santonici*, &c. Of these, the best is turpentine. See Oleum terebinthinæ. The great object, however, is to prevent their generation. This must be done by generous diet, fresh air, and tonics, where necessary.

WORT, Sax. ꝥꝩꞃꞇ, *Mustum, Infu'sum Byne seu Bra'sii seu Malti*, (F.) *Moût de la Bière*. An infusion of malt. This has been recommended in scurvy. One measure of ground malt is added to three equal measures of boiling water. The mixture must be well stirred, and left to stand covered three or four hours. Dose, one to four pints, daily. It has, also, been recommended in other cases, where a strong putrescent disposition appeared to prevail in the fluids, as in cancer and phagedenic ulcers. It is not now employed.

WOUND, Sax. ꝩund, *Vulnus, Velnus*, (diminutive *Vulnus'culum,*) *Plaga, Trauma, Troma, Tresis Vulnus, Blabá, Tymma*, (F.) *Plaie*. A *sure*. A solution of continuity in the soft parts produced by some mechanical agent. Wounds present innumerable differences, as regards the situation; the parts interested; their direction; size; shape; the nature of the instrument or agent by which they are produced; their more or less simple or complex character, duration, &c. A wound is called *incised*, (F.) *Coupure, incisure*, when made by a cutting instrument; — *punctured*,

Nygma, (F.) *Piqure*, when made by a pointed instrument; — *lacerated*, (F.) *Déchirure, Plaie par arrachement*, when the parts are lacerated or torn by the wounded body; *poisoned, Celluli'tis venena'ta, Necu'sia*, (F.) *Plaie envenimée*, when some virulent or venomous substance has been introduced;—and *contused*, (F.) *Plaie contuse*, when produced by a blunt body. *Gunshot wounds, Sclopetopla'gæ, Vul'nera sclopeta'ria*, (F.) *Plaies d'armes à feu ou d'arquebusade, Coup de feu*, belong to the last division.

WOURALI, Curare.
WOURARI, Curare.
WOURARU, Curare.
WRACK, SEA, Fucus vesiculosus.
WRACK, BLADDER, YELLOW, Fucus vesiculosus.
WRAPPING UP, (OF THE HYDROPATHISTS,) *Emaillottage*.

WRENCH, Sprain.
WRIGHTIA ANTIDYSENTERICA, Nerium antidysentericum.
WRINKLE, Sax. ppincle, *Ruga, Rytis, Rhacus, Rhachus, Rhagus, Rhysse'ma, Corruga'tio cutis*, (F.) *Ride*. A furrow or fold in the skin of the face, forehead, vagina, &c. See Corrugation.
WRINKLED, *Rugo'sus, Rugous, Rugose*, (F.) *Ridé*. Full of wrinkles.
WRIST, Carpus.
WRIST-DROP. Paralysis of the muscles of the forearm, induced by the poison of lead.
WRITERS' SPASM, see Spasm, writers'.
WURALI, Curare.
WURSTGIFT, Allantotoxicum.
WRONG HEIR, Cancellus.

X.

XALAPPA, Convolvulus jalapa.
XANTHIC OXIDE, Uric oxide.
XANTHINE, Uric oxide.
XAN'THIUM, *X. struma'rium* seu *Orienta'lē* seu *Vulga'rē, Barda'na minor, Lappa minor, Lesser Burdock, Burweed, Burthistle, Clotbur*, (F.) *Lampourde, Petit Glouteron, Petite Bardane*. This herb, as one of its names imports, was once esteemed for the cure of scrofula. The seeds have been administered in cutaneous affections.
XANTHIURIA, Xanthuria.
XANTHOP'SIA, from ξανθος, 'yellow,' and οψις, 'vision.' Yellow vision, — as sometimes occurs in jaundice.
XANTHORRHIZA, Xanthorrhiza apiifolia.
XANTHORRHI'ZA APIIFO'LIA, *Xanthorrhiza, X. simplicis'sima, X. Marboī'ca, Zanthorrhiza tincto'ria, Yellow Root, Parsley-leaved Yellow Root or Yellow wort, Shrub yellow root*. The root of this American plant — *Xanthorrhiza*, (Ph. U. S.) — is a strong and pleasant bitter; and, in the dose of two scruples, sits easy upon the stomach.
XANTHOS, Yellow.
XANTHO'SIS. A term applied to the yellow discoloration often observed in cancerous tumours — especially in encephaloid of the testicle. — Lebert.
XANTHOXYLUM CLAVA HER'CULIS, *Prickly Ash, Toothach Tree*, (F.) *Clavalier à feuilles de frêne, Frêne épineux*. The bark — *Xanthoxylum*, (Ph. U. S.) — is a very strong stimulant and powerful sialagogue. It has been given, internally, in rheumatism. Another species — *Xanthoxylum fraxinifo'lium, Xanthoxylum fraxin'eum, Shrubby prickly ash, Toothach bush, Pell'itory, Yellow wood, Suterberry*, — possesses active powers. A spirituous infusion of the bark has been highly recommended in cases of violent colic. The fresh juice, expressed from the roots of the xanthoxylum, is said to afford relief in the dry bellyache of the West Indies. A decoction of the bark is sometimes used as a wash to foul ulcers.
XANTHU'RIA, *Xanthiu'ria*, from ξανθος, 'yellow,' and ουρον, 'urine.' A condition of the system and of the urine, in which xanthic oxide is deposited from the urine.
XANTICA, Carminatives.
XANTOLINA, Artemisia santonica.
XENODOCEUM, Hospital.

XENODOCHEUM, Hospital.
XERANSIS, Arefaction, Drying.
XERANTIA, Siccantia.
XERA'SIA. Same etymon; from ξηρος, 'dry.' A disease of the hairs, which become dry, cease to grow, and resemble down covered with dust. — Galen.
XERION, Catapasma.
XEROCOLLYR'IUM, from ξηρος, 'dry,' and κολλυριον, 'a collyrium;' *Collyr'ium siccum*. A dry collyrium.
XERODER'MA, from ξηρος, 'dry,' and δερμα 'skin.' Diminution of secretion of the sebaceous glands.
XEROMA, Xerophthalmia—x. Conjunctival, Xerophthalmia.
XEROMA, LACHRYMAL. Suppression of the lachrymal secretion.
XEROMYCTER, Xeromycteris.
XEROMYCTE'RIA, *Xeromycter*, from ξηρος, 'dry,' and μυκτηρ, 'the nose.' Dryness of the nose.
XEROMYRON, *Unguen'tum siccum;* from ξηρος, 'dry,' and μυρον, 'an ointment.' A dry ointment. — Gorræus.
XEROPHA'GIA, from ξηρος, 'dry,' and φαγω, 'I eat.' Excessive use of dry aliment. A kind of regimen to which the ancient athletæ subjected themselves, with the view of increasing their strength.
XEROPHTHAL'MIA, *Ophthal'mia sicca, Ophthalmoxero'sis, Xero'ma*, from ξηρος, 'dry,' and οφθαλμια, 'inflammation of the eye.' An inflammation of the eye, without discharge. The term — as well as *Conjuncti'val Xero'ma*, and *Cutic'ular Conjuncti'va* — has been given to cases in which the conjunctiva is so changed, that it presents more of the characters of skin than of mucous membrane. It is incapable of radical cure. Also, lippitudo.
XEROTRIBIA, see Friction.
XEROTRIPSIS, Friction, dry.
XIPHISTERNUM, Xiphoid.
XIPHODES, Xiphoid.
XIPHODYMUS, Thoraco-gastrodidymus.
XIPHOID, *Xiphoī'des, Xipho'des, Ensifor'mis*, from ξιφος, 'a sword,' and ειδος, 'shape;' *Cartila'go Xiphoīdes, C. Xiphoīdea, C. Scuta'lis, C. Ensiformis, C. Pelta'lis* seu *pelta'tus, En'siform cartilage, Furcel'la infe'rior, Mucrona'tum os*,

Mucrona'ta Cartila'go, Chondros, Processus xiphosterna'lis seu xiphoïdes seu sterni xiphoïdeus, Xiphisternum, (F.) Appendice ou cartilage xiphoïdes, C. Mucroné, Appendice sous-sternale, Palette. The name of the appendix which terminates the sternum beneath; and which is so called from some resemblance to a sword.

XIPHOID LIG'AMENT, Costo-xyphoid L. (F.) Ligament xiphoïdien ou costo-xiphoïdien, is a small, very thin, ligamentous fasciculus, which passes from the cartilage of prolongation of the 7th rib to the anterior surface of the xiphoid cartilage, into which it is inserted by its fibres decussating with those of the opposite ligament.

XIPHOP'AGES, Did'ymus, Symphyo-epigas'trius; from ξιφος, 'a sword,' and πηγνυμι, 'I fix.' A monstrosity, in which twins are united by the epigastrium, as in the case of the Siamese twins.

XYLO-ALOES, Agallochum — x. Balsamum, see Amyris opobalsamum — x. Cassia, Laurus cassia — x. Cinnamomum, Laurus cinnamomum.
XYLUM, Gossipium.
XYMPATHIA, Sympathy.
XYRIS, Iris foetidissima.
XYRIS BULBO'SA, X. In'dica, X. Carolinia'na, Yellow-eyed Grass; indigenous; Order, Xyridaceæ; flowering from July to September. The roots and leaves are said to be used by the Hindoos in lepra, and chronic cutaneous diseases in general.
XYRUM, Novacula.
XYRUS, Novacula.
XYSMA, Linteum, Rasura, Scobs.
XYSMOS, Rasura.
XYSTER, Raspatorium.
XYSTOS, Linteum.
XYSTRUM, Raspatorium—x. Ophthalmicum, Ophthalmoxyster.

Y.

YAM. This esculent root is principally obtained from three species of Diosco'rea, — ala'ta bulbif'era, and sati'va. They grow spontaneously in both the Indies, and their roots are eaten promiscuously, as the potato is with us. Their taste is somewhat like the potato.

YAM ROOT, WILD, Dioscorea villosa.
YARD, Penis.
YARROW, COMMON, Achillea millefolium.
YAUPON, Ilex vomitoria.
YAWNING, from Sax. geonan, Chasmã, Chasmus, Hia'tus, Osce'do, Oscita'tio, Clonus pandicula'tio maxilla'rum, Gaping, (F.) Baillement. Yawning consists of a deep inspiration, with considerable separation of the jaws, executed slowly and in an involuntary manner, and followed by a prolonged and more or less sonorous expiration. This respiratory movement is preceded by a feeling of oppression in the epigastric region, and in the muscles of respiration and mastication. Yawning has been conceived to be owing to torpor in the pulmonary circulation; the causes producing it being commonly ennui, fatigue, sleepiness, monotonous sounds, hunger, sympathy, &c. Yawning often precedes the invasion of certain intermittents, attacks of hysteria, &c., and it may, by its frequency, and obstinacy, become a true disease.

YAWROOT, Stillingia.
YAWS, Frambœsia.
YEAST, Yest—y. Plant, Torula cerevisiæ.
YELK, see Ovum.
YELLOW, Flavus, Lu'teus, Xanthus, from past participle of Sax. ʒemlan, 'to burn.' One of the seven primitive colours.

YELLOW ASH, Cladrastis tinctoria — y. Berry, Podophyllum montanum — y. Fever, see Fever, Yellow—y. Fever, mild, see Relapse.
YELLOW LIGAMENTS, (F.) Ligaments jaunes, occupy the spaces between the vertebral plates, from the interval, which separates the second vertebra from the third, to that which separates the last vertebra from the sacrum. They are so called in consequence of their colour.

YELLOW PAINT, Hydrastis Canadensis — y. Root, Jeffersonia Bartoni — y. Root, Parsley-leaved, Xanthorrhiza apiifolia — y. Root, Shrub, Xanthorrhiza apiifolia — y. Star, Helenium autumnale—y. Weed, Ranunculus acris—y. Wood, Xanthoxylum fraxineum — y. Wort, Parsley-leaved, Xanthorrhiza apiifolia.

YELLOWS, Cypripedium luteum, Icterus, Ranunculus acris.
YERBA DEL SOLDADA, Matico — y. de Huaca, Datura sanguinea.
YEST, Yeast, Sax. ʒeɼt, from ýɼt, 'a storm,' ýɼtiȝ, 'stormy;' Cerevis'iæ Fermen'tum, Spuma Cerevis'iæ, Barm, (F.) Levure, Levure de la Bière. The scum, which collects on the surface of beer whilst fermenting. Yest is antiseptic and tonic. It has been much extolled in putrid fevers, — a table-spoonful being given as a dose, in porter, wine, &c. It is, also, applied, in the form of cataplasm, to foul ulcers. In all these cases, it acts by virtue of the generation of carbonic acid gas.

YEUX ARDENS, Ardent eyes — y. d'Ecrevisse, Cancrorum chelæ.
YEW TREE, Taxus baccata.
YLECH, Ilech.
YLIATHR, Ilech.
YOLK, see Ovum.
YOUTH, Adolescence.
YOPON, Ilex vomitoria.
YPSELOGLOSSUS, Basioglossus.
YRIDES, Orpiment.
YSAM'BRA, Pedigam'bra. An ancient Spanish poison, of which hellebore formed the greatest part.
YUCCA, Jatropha manihot.
Y-WER-A, see Spirit.

Z.

ZACCHARUM, Saccharum.
ZAEL, Borosail.
ZAFFRAN, Crocus.
ZAMBO, see Mulatto.
ZAMIA INTEGRIFOLIA, see Arrowroot—z. Pumila, see Arrowroot.
ZANNA. A kind of Armenian bole, used by the ancients as a desiccative. It was also called Zarnacha.
ZANTHORRHIZA APIIFOLIA, Xanthorrhiza apiifolia.
ZANTHOXYLUM CLAVA HERCULIS, Xanthoxylum clava Herculis.
ZAPANIA NODIFLORA, Anacoluppa.

ZARNACHA, Zanna.
ZARSA, Smilax sarsaparilla.
ZARZAPARILLA, Smilax sarsaparilla.
ZEA MAYS, *Z. vulga'rē, Mays zea seu America'na, Mays, Indian Corn, Corn, Turkey Wheat, Maize, Ador, Indian Wheat,* (F.) *Mais, Graine de Turquie, Blé d'Inde, Blé d'Espagne, Blé d'Italie, Blé de Turquie.* A native of America, and much used over the whole of the continent as an article of diet. It is ground for the same purposes as wheat, and forms an excellent bread.
ZÉDOAIRE ROND, Kæmpferia rotunda.
ZEDOARIA, Kæmpferia rotunda — z. Longa, see Kæmpferia — z. Rotunda, see Kæmpferia.
ZEDOARY, Kæmpferia rotunda.
ZELOSIS, Zelotypia.
ZELOTYP'IA, from ζηλος, 'love,' and τυπος, 'form,' 'model;' *Zelo'sis.* It has been proposed to apply this name to the violent mental affection produced by the acknowledged or presumed infidelity of a beloved object; and to the consequences of such affection; — melancholy, mania, &c.
ZEMA, Decoction.
ZEN'ICON, ζενικον. Ancient name of a Keltic poison, used for poisoning arrows.
ZEPHACH, Peritonæum.
ZERMA, Zerna.
ZERNA, *Zerna.* Amongst the barbarous Latin writers it signified ulcerated impetigo, *Impeti'go ulcera'ta.*
ZERUMBET, Cassumuniar.
ZESIS, Effervescence, Decoction.
ZEST, see Citrus medica.
ZESTOLUSIA, Bath, hot.
ZIBEBÆ, see Vitis vinifera.
ZIBETHUM, Civetta.
ZIGNITES, Zingrites.
ZINC, *Zincum, Zinkum, Speltrum, Speauter, Tutenag, Zinchum, Zint, Stannum In'dicum.* Perhaps formed etymologically from (G.) Zin, 'Tin.' A metal obtained from calamine and blende. Its colour is bluish-white; lustre of the fresh surface considerable, but soon dulled, from the facility with which it oxidates; hard; texture striated. S. g. 7.190. Melts at 700° Fah., burns with a bright flame in a higher temperature, and is volatilized in the form of a white, flocculent oxyd. Its use, in medicine, is in the formation of the following preparations.
ZINC, ACÉTATE DE, Zinci acetas—z. Butter of, Zinci chloridum — z. Chloride of, Zinci chloridum — z. *Chlorure de,* Zinci chloridum — z. Ferrohydrocyanate of, Zinci cyanuretum — z. Flowers of, Zinci oxydum — z. Hydrocyanate of, Zinci cyanuretum — z. Iodide of, Zinci Iodidum —z. Ioduret of, Zinci Iodidum.
ZINC AND MORPH'IA, DOUBLE I'ODIDE OF. (F.) *Iodure double de Zinc et de Morphine.* This salt is prepared by boiling *iodide of iodhydrate of morphia with water and zinc,* after they have acted on each other for some days; filtering and crystallizing. It is considered to combine the properties of morphia and the salts of zinc, and has been prescribed as an anodyne and antispasmodic. Dose, a quarter of a grain.
ZINC, OXIDE DE, Zinci oxydum—z. Oxyd of, Zinci oxydum.
ZINC AND STRYDI'NIA, DOUBLE I'ODIDE OF. This salt is prepared by digesting for several days in hot water, *iodide of iodhydrate of strychnia and zinc;* filtering and crystallizing. It has been proposed in the same cases as strychnia.
ZINC, SULFATE DE, Zinci sulphas—z. Sulphate of, Zinci Sulphas—z. Valerianate of, Zinci Valerianas.
ZINCHUM, Zincum.

ZINCI ACE'TAS, *Ac"ètate of Zinc,* (F.) *Acétate de Zinc.* (*Plumbi acet.* ℔j, *zinc. granul.* ℥ix, *aquæ destillat.* Oiij. Dissolve the acetate of lead in the water, and filter. Add the zinc to the solution, and agitate them occasionally together, in a stopped bottle, for five or six hours, or until the liquid yields no precipitate, with a solution of iodide of potassium. Filter the liquor, evaporate it with a moderate heat to one-fifth, and set it aside to crystallise. Pour off the liquid, and dry the crystals on bibulous paper.
Should the crystals be coloured, dissolve them in distilled water, and having heated the solution, drop into it, while hot, a filtered solution of chlorinated lime, until it ceases to let fall sesquioxide of iron; filter the liquor, acidulate it with a few drops of acetic acid, evaporate, and crystallise.—*Ph. U. S.*)
Frequently used to form a gently astringent wash in ophthalmia and other local inflammations; and as an injection in gonorrhœa.
ZINCI CARBONAS IMPURUS, Calamina.
ZINCI CAR'BONAS PRÆCIPITA'TUS, *Precip'itated carbonate of Zinc.* (*Zinci sulphat., sodæ carbonat.* ᴀᴀ ℔j; *aq. bullient.* cong. Dissolve the sulphate of zinc and carbonate of soda respectively in Oiv of water. Mix the solutions; stir, and set the mixture by, that the powder may subside. Having poured off the liquid, wash the precipitated carbonate of zinc with hot water, until the fluid of the washings is nearly tasteless, and dry with a gentle heat.— Ph. U. S.) Used to prepare the Zinci oxidum.
ZINCI CARBONAS PRÆPARATUS, Calamina præparata.
ZINCI CHLO'RIDUM, *Z. chlorure'tum, Zincum chlora'tum, Z. muriat'icum* (*oxydatum*), *Chloride* or *Chloruret of Zinc, Butter of Zinc,* (F.) *Chlorure de Zinc.* (*Zinc.* in frustulis, ℥ijss; *acid. nitric., cretæ præparat.* ᴀᴀ ℨj; *acid. muriat.* q. s. To the zinc, in the porcelain vessel, add gradually sufficient muriatic acid to dissolve it; strain, add the nitric acid, and evaporate to dryness. Dissolve the dry mass in water, add the chalk, allow the mixture to stand for 24 hours, filter, and again evaporate to dryness.— Ph. U. S.) It is very deliquescent in the air, forming the *Butter of Zinc, Buty'rum Zinci.*
Chloride of Zinc is a powerful escharotic, and has been lately employed as an effective antiseptic.
ZINCI CHLORURETUM, Z. chloridum.
ZINCI CYANURE'TUM, *Hydrocy'anas Zinci, Zincum Cyanogena'tum, Z. Borus'sicum, Z. Zoöticum, Hydrocy'anate of Zinc.* This salt is formed by adding sulphate of zinc to hydrocyanate of potassa so long as any precipitate is thrown down. When dried and calcined at a low heat, the product is a mixture of cyanuret of zinc and of potassium. It has been recommended in nervous cardialgia. Dose, from one-sixteenth to one-twelfth of a grain.
It is chiefly used as a caustic; one part of the chloride being mixed with four, three, or two parts of flour, according to the desired strength, and a few drops of water being added to form a paste.
ZINCI FERROHYDROCY'ANAS, *Cyanure'tum Ferrosin'cicum, Zincum Ferrohydrocyan'icum, Ferrohydrocyanate of Zinc.* Made by the mutual decomposition of boiling-hot solutions of sulphate of zinc and ferrocyanate of potassa. It has been recommended in the same cases as the last preparation.
ZINCI HYDROCYANAS, Zinci cyanuretum.
ZINCI IOD'IDUM, *Z. Iodure'tum, Zincum Ioda'tum, Iode'tum Zinci seu Zin'cicum, Protoiodure'tum Zinci, I'odide* or *Iod'uret of Zinc.* This salt

is made by boiling together *iodine* and *zinc* to dryness, and subliming. An ointment, composed of a drachm to an ounce of lard, has been used in cases where the external use of iodide of potassium is indicated.

ZINCI IODURETUM, Z. iodidum — z. Nix, Zinci oxydum.

ZINCI OX'YDUM, *Zincum calcina'tum, Oxyd of Zinc, Flowers of Zinc, Nihil Album, Lana Philosopho'rum,* L. *Philosoph'ica, Nix Zinci, Nihil Gris'eum, Pom'pholyx,* (F.) *Oxide de Zinc.* (Procured by burning zinc in a long, deep, crucible, placed so as to collect the sublimate. Also, by exposing the precipitate thrown down from a solution of *sulphate of zinc* by *carbonate of ammonia* to a strong heat, so as to drive off the carbonic acid.—Ph. U. S.) It is tonic and antispasmodic; externally, detergent and desiccative. Employed in epilepsy, chorea, &c. For its external use, see Ung. Zinci.

ZINCI OXYDUM IMPURUM, Tutia.

ZINCI SULPHAS, *Sulphate of Zinc, Zincum Vitriola'tum, Vitrio'lum Album, White Vitriol,* V. *Goslarien'sè,* V. *Zinci, Sulphas Zin'cicum, Gilla Vitrioli, Gilla Theophras'ti, Sal Vomito'rium Vitrioli, Chalcan'thum Album, White Copperas, Sal Vitrioli,* (F.) *Sulfate de Zinc.* (Zinc. in frustul. ℥iv; acid. sulphuric. ℥vj; aquæ destillat. Oiv. To the zinc and water, previously introduced into a glass vessel, add by degrees the sulphuric acid, and, when the effervescence shall have ceased, filter the solution through paper; then boil it down till a pellicle begins to form, and set aside to crystallize.—Ph. U. S.) The sulphate of zinc is inodorous; taste, styptic. It is in white, semi-transparent, efflorescent crystals; soluble in three parts of water at 60°. It is emetic, tonic, antispasmodic, and, externally, astringent. A nostrum, sold under the name *Antipertus'sis,* and, as its title imports, given in hooping-cough, contains this salt as its chief ingredient. It is emetic. Dose, as an emetic, gr. x to ℨss; as a tonic, gr. j to ij. Used externally as a collyrium, gr. j to water f℥j.

ZINCI VALERIA'NAS, *Valerianate of Zinc.* A salt formed by saturating valerianic acid with freshly prepared carbonate of zinc. It is in pure white, pearly scales, and has been recommended as a tonic in neuralgic diseases, epilepsy, &c. The dose is one or two grains several times a day.

ZINCUM, Zinc — z. Borussicum, Zinci cyanuretum — z. Calcinatum, Zinci oxydum — z. Chloratam, Zinci chloridum — z. Cyanogenatam, Zinci cyanuretum — z. Ferrohydrocyanicum, Zinci ferrohydrocyanas — z. Iodatum, Zinci iodidum — z. Muriaticum, Zinci chloridum — z. Vitriolatum, Zinci sulphas — z. Zooticum, Zinci cyanuretum.

ZINGIBER, Amomum zingiber — z. Cassumuniar, see Cassumuniar — z. Cliffordia, see Cassumuniar — z. Germanicum, Arum maculatum — z. Officinale, Amomum zingiber — z. Purpureum, see Cassumuniar — z. Spurium, see Cassumuniar — z. Zerumbet, see Cassumuniar.

ZINGIBERIN, Piperoid.

ZINGRI'TES, *Zigni'tes.* A stone, resembling glass; to which the ancients attributed marvellous properties.

ZINKUM, Zincum.

ZINT, Zincum.

ZINZIBER, Amomum zingiber.

ZIPHAC, Peritonæum.

ZIRBUS, Epiploon — z. Adipinus, Epiploon, gastro-colic.

ZIZA'NIA AQUAT'ICA, *Wild Rice;* called by the Indians, *Menomene,* grows abundantly on the marshy margins of the northern lakes and waters of the upper branches of the Mississippi. The grain resembles oats. It furnishes the northern savages and the Canadian traders and hunters with their annual supplies of grain.

ZIZYPHUM, Jujube.

ZIZYPHUS JUJUBA, see Jujube — z. Nidi, see Jujube — z. Sativa, see Jujube — z. Sylvestris, see Jujube.

ZOA'GRIA, from ζωη, 'life,' and αγρεω, 'I catch up.' The saving and preservation of life. *Zoöris.* A reward for preserving life; *Sacra.* A votive offering hung up in the temples for b saved.

ZOANTHRO'PIA, *Melancho'ia zoäethro'pia,* from ζωον, 'an animal,' and ανθρωπος, 'a man.' A species of monomania, in which the patient believes himself transformed into an animal. Lycanthropia and cynanthropia belong to this species of monomania.

ZOARA, Insomnia.

ZOE, Life.

ZOGRAPHIA, Zoographia.

ZOIATRIA, Veterinary art.

ZOIATRUS, Hippiater.

ZOMIDIUM, Jus.

ZOMOS, *Consommé,* Jus.

ZONA, Herpes zoster — z. Castitatis, Hymen — z. Ciliaris, Ciliary zone — z. Ignea, Herpes zoster.

ZONA PELLU'CIDA, *Oolem'ma pellu'cides,* V. *tellary membrane,* (F.) *Vitelline, Membrane vitelline.* The membrane that surrounds the yolk in the mammalia is so called on account of its thinness and peculiar transparency.

ZONA SERPIGINOSA, Herpes zoster — z. Virginitatis, Hymen.

ZONA TENDINO'SA. The whitish circle around the auriculo-ventricular orifice of the right side of the heart.

ZONE, Cingulum.

ZONULA CILIARIS, see Ciliary, and Ciliary zone — z. Cochleæ, see Lamina spiralis — z. Hildani, Cingulum Hildani — z. Zinnii, see Ciliary.

ZOÖCHEMIA, Chymistry, animal.

ZOÖCHEM'ICAL, *Zoöchym'ical, Zoöchem'us* seu *Zoöchym'icus.* Appertaining or having relation to animal chymistry.

ZOÖCHEMY, Chymistry, animal.

ZOÖCHYMY, Chymistry, animal.

ZOÖGENIUM, Azote.

ZOÖG"ENY, *Zoögen'ia, Zoögen'esis,* from ζωον 'animal,' and γενεσις, 'generation.' The doctrine of animal formation.

ZOÖG'RAPHY, *Zoögra'phia, Zogra'phia,* from ζωον, 'an animal,' and γραφη, 'a description.' A description of animals. The natural history of animals.

ZOÖHEMATINE, Hæmatine.

ZOÖHY'LAS, from ζωον, 'an animal,' and υλη, 'matter.' Animal matter.

ZOÖHY'LICA CONCREMEN'TA. Concretions formed of animal matter.

ZOÖIASIS, Veterinary art.

ZOÖL'OGIST, *Zoölogis'ta, Zoölogus,* from ζωον, 'an animal,' and λογος, 'description.' One skilled in the natural history of animals.

ZOÖL'OGY, *Zoölog''ia.* Same etymon. The natural history of animals.

ZOÖMAGNETISMUS, Magnetism, animal.

ZOÖMYCUS, Mucus.

ZOÖMYXA, Mucus.

ZOÖN, Animal.

ZOÖNOM'IA, *Organozoönom'ia, Zoön'omy,* from ζωον, 'an animal,' and νομος, 'law.' The laws which govern the organic actions of animals in general: — *Animal Physiology, Zoöphysiology.*

ZOONOSOLOG"IA, from ζωον, 'an animal,' νοσος, 'a disease,' and λογος, 'description.' The nosology of animals.

ZOOPATHOLOG"IA, from ζωον, 'an animal,' παθος, 'a disease,' and λογος, 'a description.' The pathology of animals.

ZOÖPH'AGOUS, *Zoöph'agus*, (F.) *Zoöphage.* from ζωον, 'an animal,' and φαγω, 'I eat.' Feeding on animals. Carnivorous.

ZOÖPHTHALMUS, Hydrophthalmia.

ZOÖPHYSIOLOGIA, Physiology, animal, Zoonomia.

ZO'ÖPHYTE, *Zoöph'ytum, Phytozo'ön, Animal plant*, from ζωον, 'an animal,' and φυτον, 'a plant.' A name given to the lowest class of animals, which seem to form the transition between the animal and the vegetable kingdoms.

ZOÖSIS, Animation, Zoagria.

ZOÖSPERMATA, Spermatozoa.

ZOÖSPERMES, Spermatozoa.

ZOOTHAP'SIS, from ζωη, 'life,' and θαπτω, 'I inter.' Burial alive. Premature interment.

ZOOT'OMIST, *Zootom'icus.* Same etymon as the next. One who dissects animals.

ZOÖT'OMY, *Zoötom'ia*, from ζωον, 'an animal,' and τεμνω, 'I cut.' *Theriot'omy, Anatom'ia anima'lis seu comparati'va seu compara'ta, Compar'ative Anatomy.* The anatomy of animals. Animal anatomy.

ZOPISSA, see Pinus sylvestris.

ZOPYRON, Fomites.

ZOSTER, Herpes zoster.

ZOSTERA MARINA, Pila marina — s. Maritima, Pila marina.

ZOZAR, Saccharum.

ZUCARO, Saccharum.

ZUCCARUM, Saccharum.

ZUCHAR, Saccharum.

ZUCHARUM, Saccharum.

ZUCHRA, Saccharum.

ZULAPIUM, Julep.

ZYGAPOPHYSES, see Vertebræ.

ZYGOMA, Malæ os.

ZYGOMAT'IC, *Zygomat'icus, Juga'lis, Jugal.* That which relates to the *zygoma* or cheek-bone.

ZYGOMATIC ARCH, see Zygomatic process — s. Bone, Malæ os.

ZYGOMATIC FOSSA is the space included between the posterior margin of the outer ala of the pterygoid process, and the crista which descends from the malar tuberosity to the superior alveolar margin.

ZYGOMATIC MUSCLES are two in number. 1. *Zygomat'icus major, Distort'or Oris,* (F.) *Zygomato-labial* (Ch.), *Muscle grand zygomatique*, which is situate obliquely at the fore-part and sides of the face. It is a small, rounded muscle; arises from the outer surface of the os malæ, and is inserted at the commissure of the lips, which it raises and draws outwards. It acts principally in laughing. 2. *Zygomat'icus minor,* (F.) *Petit Zygomato-labial* (Ch.), *Petit Zygomatique*, does not always exist. It is situate on the inner side of the last; arises from the outer surface of the os malæ, and is inserted at the corner of the mouth, or rather into the upper lip, which it raises and draws outwards.

ZYGOMATIC PROCESS, *Proces'sus zygomat'icus, Apoph'ysis Zygomat'ica, Malar process, Jugal process*, arises from the outer surface of the temporal bone by two roots, one of which is transverse, (*Condyle du temporal*, Ch.,) and the other longitudinal: between them is the glenoid cavity. The process passes forwards, and is articulated with the posterior angle of the os malæ, with which it forms a bony bridge, called the *Zygomat'ic arch, Pars zygomat'icus, Arcus zygomat'icus*, (F.) *Arcade Zygomatique.* The cavity, beneath this bridge, is sometimes called *Zygo'ma.*

ZYGOMATIC SUTURE is placed between the zygomatic parts of the temporal and cheek bones; and slants obliquely downwards and backwards.

ZYGOMATIQUE GRAND, Zygomaticus major—s. Petit, Zygomaticus minor.

ZYGOMATO-LABIAL, Zygomaticus major —s. *Labial, petit*, Zygomaticus major—s. *Maxillaire*, Masseter—s. *Oriculaire*, Anterior auris.

ZYGOPHYL'LUM FABA'GO, (F.) *Fabagelle.* A Syrian and Mauritanic plant, possessed of an acrid and bitter taste. It has vermifuge properties. The Arabs believe that the recently expressed juice of *Zygophyllum simplex*, is capable of removing specks from the cornea.

ZYMA, Ferment.

ZYMOMA, Ferment.

ZYMOSIS, Fermentation, see Zymotic.

ZYMOT'IC, *Zymot'icus*, from ζυμοω, 'to ferment.' An epithet proposed for any epidemic, endemic, or contagious affection. *Zymosis* is used to signify such an affection.

ZYTHOGALA, Posset.

ZYTHUM, Cerevisia.

ZYTHUS, Cerevisia.

THE END.

CATALOGUE
OF
BLANCHARD & LEA'S
MEDICAL AND SURGICAL PUBLICATIONS.

TO THE MEDICAL PROFESSION.

In submitting the following catalogue of our publications in medicine and the collateral sciences, we beg to remark that no exertions are spared to render the issues of our press worthy a continuance of the confidence which they have thus far enjoyed, both as regards the high character of the works themselves, and in respect to every point of typographical accuracy, and mechanical and artistical execution. Gentlemen desirous of adding to their libraries from our list, can in almost all cases procure the works they wish from the nearest bookseller, who can readily order any which may not be on hand; and who, as well as ourselves, will be happy to answer any inquiries as to price, &c.

BLANCHARD & LEA.

PHILADELPHIA, February, 1855.

TWO MEDICAL PERIODICALS, FREE OF POSTAGE,
FOR FIVE DOLLARS PER ANNUM.

THE AMERICAN JOURNAL OF THE MEDICAL SCIENCES, subject to postage, when not paid for in advance, - - - - - - - $5 00

THE MEDICAL NEWS AND LIBRARY, invariably in advance, - - 1 00

or, BOTH PERIODICALS furnished, FREE OF POSTAGE, for Five Dollars remitted in advance.

THE AMERICAN JOURNAL OF THE MEDICAL SCIENCES,
EDITED BY ISAAC HAYS, M. D.,

is published Quarterly, on the first of January, April, July, and October. Each number contains at least two hundred and eighty large octavo pages, appropriately illustrated, wherever necessary, by engravings. It has now been issued regularly for a period of THIRTY-FIVE years, during a quarter of a century of which it has been under the control of the present editor. Throughout this long space of time, it has maintained its position in the highest rank of medical periodicals both at home and abroad, and has received the cordial support of the entire profession in this country. Its list of Collaborators will be found to contain a large number of the most distinguished names of the profession in every section of the United States, rendering the department devoted to

ORIGINAL COMMUNICATIONS

full of varied and important matter, of great interest to all practitioners.

As the aim of the Journal, however, is to combine the advantages presented by all the different varieties of periodicals, in its

REVIEW DEPARTMENT

will be found extended and impartial reviews of all important new works, presenting subjects of novelty and interest, together with very numerous

BIBLIOGRAPHICAL NOTICES,

including nearly all the medical publications of the day, both in this country and Great Britain, with a choice selection of the more important continental works. This is followed by the

QUARTERLY SUMMARY,

being a very full and complete abstract, methodically arranged, of the

IMPROVEMENTS AND DISCOVERIES IN THE MEDICAL SCIENCES.

This department of the Journal, so important to the practising physician, is the object of especial care on the part of the editor. It is classified and arranged under different heads, thus facilitating the researches of the reader in pursuit of particular subjects, and will be found to present a very full and accurate digest of all observations, discoveries, and inventions recorded in every branch of medical science. The very extensive arrangements of the publishers are such as to afford to the editor complete materials for this purpose, as he not only regularly receives

ALL THE AMERICAN MEDICAL AND SCIENTIFIC PERIODICALS,

but also twenty or thirty of the more important Journals issued in Great Britain and on the Continent, thus enabling him to present in a convenient compass a thorough and complete abstract of everything interesting or important to the physician occurring in any part of the civilized world.

An evidence of the success which has attended these efforts may be found in the constant steady increase in the subscription list, which renders it advisable for gentlemen desiring the Journal, to make known their wishes at an early day, in order to secure a year's set with certainty, the publishers having frequently been unable to supply copies when ordered late in the year. To their old subscribers, many of whom have been on their list for twenty or thirty years, the publishers feel that no promises are necessary; but those who may desire for the first time to subscribe can rest assured that no exertion will be spared to maintain the Journal in the high position which it has occupied for so long a period.

By reference to the terms it will be seen that, in addition to this large amount of valuable and practical information on every branch of medical science, the subscriber, by paying in advance, becomes entitled, without further charge, to

THE MEDICAL NEWS AND LIBRARY,

a monthly periodical of thirty-two large octavo pages. Its "NEWS DEPARTMENT" presents current information of the day, while the "LIBRARY DEPARTMENT" is devoted to presenting standard works on various branches of medicine. Within a few years, subscribers have thus received without expense, the following works which have passed through its columns:—

WATSON'S LECTURES ON THE PRACTICE OF PHYSIC.
BRODIE'S CLINICAL LECTURES ON SURGERY.
TODD AND BOWMAN'S PHYSIOLOGICAL ANATOMY AND PHYSIOLOGY OF MAN
724 pages, with numerous wood-cuts, being all that has yet appeared in England.
WEST'S LECTURES ON THE DISEASES OF INFANCY AND CHILDHOOD.
MALGAIGNE'S OPERATIVE SURGERY, with wood-cuts.
SIMON'S LECTURES ON GENERAL PATHOLOGY.
BENNETT ON PULMONARY TUBERCULOSIS, with wood-cuts, and
WEST ON ULCERATION OF THE OS UTERI.

While the year 1855, presents

BROWN ON THE SURGICAL DISEASES OF FEMALES.
HANDSOMELY ILLUSTRATED ON WOOD.

The diseases treated in this volume have hitherto not received from writers of system works the attention to which their importance entitles them. In treatises on female diseases have been but little noticed, as belonging more properly to the surgeon, while our surgical texts have in like manner referred them to the writer on midwifery and female affections. In supplying this palpable vacancy in medical literature, Mr. Brown has brought to his subject the result of many years of observation and experience, and his labors will prove of much value to all practitioners. The publishers therefore flatter themselves that in securing this volume for the "LIBRARY DEPARTMENT" of the "MEDICAL NEWS" they will meet the wishes of their numerous subscribers, who will thus receive this highly important work free of all expense.

It will thus be seen that for the small sum of FIVE DOLLARS, paid in advance, the subscriber will obtain a Quarterly and a Monthly periodical,

EMBRACING ABOUT FIFTEEN HUNDRED LARGE OCTAVO PAGES,

mailed to any part of the United States, free of postage.

These very favorable terms are now presented by the publishers with the view of removing difficulties and objections to a full and extended circulation of the Medical Journal to the office of every member of the profession throughout the United States. The rapid extension of mail facilities, will now place the numbers before subscribers with a certainty and dispatch not heretofore attainable; while by the system now proposed, every subscriber throughout the Union is placed upon an equal footing, at the very reasonable price of Five Dollars for two periodicals, without further expense.

Those subscribers who do not pay in advance will bear in mind that their subscription of Five Dollars will entitle them to the Journal only, without the News, and that they will be at the expense of their own postage on the receipt of each number. The advantage of a remittance when ordering the Journal will thus be apparent.

As the Medical News and Library is in no case sent without advance payment, its subscribers will always receive it free of postage.

It should also be borne in mind that the publishers will now take the risk of remittances by mail, only requiring, in cases of loss, a certificate from the subscriber's Postmaster, that the money was duly mailed and forwarded.

Address, BLANCHARD & LEA, PHILADELPHIA.

ANALYTICAL COMPENDIUM

OF MEDICAL SCIENCE, containing Anatomy, Physiology, Surgery, Midwifery, Chemistry, Materia Medica, Therapeutics, and Practice of Medicine. By JOHN NEILL, M. D., and F. G. SMITH, M. D. Second and enlarged edition, one thick volume royal 12mo. of over 1000 pages, with 350 illustrations. ☞ See NEILL.

ABEL (F. A.), F. C. S.
Professor of Chemistry in the Royal Military Academy, Woolwich.
AND
C. L. BLOXAM,
Formerly First Assistant at the Royal College of Chemistry.

HANDBOOK OF CHEMISTRY, Theoretical, Practical, and Technical, with a Recommendatory Preface by Dr. HOFMANN. In one large octavo volume of 662 pages, with illustrations. (*Now Ready.*)

"The present volume is a synopsis of their (the authors') experience in laboratory teaching; it gives the necessary instruction in chemical manipulation, a concise account of general chemistry as far as it is involved in the operations of the laboratory, and lastly, qualitative and quantitative analysis. It must be understood that this is a work fitted for the earnest student, who resolves to pursue for himself a steady search into the chemical mysteries of creation. For such a student the 'Handbook' will prove an excellent guide, since he will find in it, not merely the approved modes of analytical investigation, but most descriptions of the apparatus necessary, with such manipulatory details as rendered Faraday's 'Chemical Manipulations' so valuable at the time of its publication. Beyond this, the importance of the work is increased by the introduction of much of the technical chemistry of the manufactory."—*Dr Hofmann's Preface.*

ASHWELL (SAMUEL), M. D.,
Obstetric Physician and Lecturer to Guy's Hospital, London.

A PRACTICAL TREATISE ON THE DISEASES PECULIAR TO WOMEN. Illustrated by Cases derived from Hospital and Private Practice. Third American, from the Third and revised London edition. In one octavo volume, of over 500 pages. (*Now Ready.*)

The most able, and certainly the most standard and practical, work on female diseases that we have yet seen.—*Medico-Chirurgical Review.*

We commend it to our readers as the best practical treatise on the subject which has yet appeared.—*London Lancet.*

The young practitioner will find it invaluable, while those who have had most experience will yet find something to learn, and much to commend, in a book which shows so much patient observation, practical skill, and sound sense.—*British and Foreign Med. Review.*

With no work are we acquainted, in which the pleasant and the useful are more happily blended. It combines the greatest elegance of style with the most sound and valuable practical information. We feel justified in recommending it, in unqualified terms, to our readers, as a book from which they can scarcely fail to derive both pleasure and improvement. It is truly a model for medical compositions.—*Southern Med. and Surg. Journal.*

ARNOTT (NEILL), M. D.

ELEMENTS OF PHYSICS; or Natural Philosophy, General and Medical. Written for universal use, in plain or non-technical language. A new edition, by ISAAC HAYS, M. D. Complete in one octavo volume, of 484 pages, with about two hundred illustrations.

BENNETT (HENRY), M. D.

A PRACTICAL TREATISE ON INFLAMMATION OF THE UTERUS, ITS CERVIX AND APPENDAGES, and on its connection with Uterine Disease. Fourth American, from the third and revised London edition. In one neat octavo volume, of 430 pages, with wood-cuts. *Just Issued.*)

This edition will be found materially improved over its predecessors, the author having carefully revised it, and made considerable additions, amounting to about seventy-five pages.

This edition has been carefully revised and altered, and various additions have been made, which render it more complete, and, if possible, more worthy of the high appreciation in which it is held by the medical profession throughout the world. A copy should be in the possession of every physician.—*Charleston Med. Journal and Review.*

We are firmly of opinion that in proportion as a knowledge of uterine diseases becomes more appreciated, this work will be proportionably established as a text-book in the profession.—*The Lancet.*

When, a few years back, the first edition of the present work was published, the subject was one almost entirely unknown to the obstetrical celebrities of the day; and even now we have reason to know that the bulk of the profession are not fully alive to the importance and frequency of the diseases of which it takes cognizance. The present edition is so much enlarged, altered, and improved, that it can scarcely be considered the same work.—*Dr. Ranking's Abstract.*

BROWN (ISAAC BAKER).,
Surgeon-Accoucheur to St. Mary's Hospital, &c.

ON SOME DISEASES OF WOMEN ADMITTING OF SURGICAL TREATMENT. With handsome illustrations. One vol. 8vo. (*At Press.*)

Publishing in the "Medical News and Library" for 1855. See preceding page.

Mr. Brown has earned for himself a high reputation in the operative treatment of sundry diseases and injuries to which females are peculiarly subject. We can truly say of his work that it is an important addition to obstetrical literature. The operative suggestions and contrivances which Mr. Brown describes, exhibit much practical sagacity and skill, and merit the careful attention of every surgeon-accoucheur.—*Association Journal.*

We have no hesitation in recommending this book to the careful attention of all surgeons who make female complaints a part of their study and practice.—*Dublin Quarterly Journal.*

BENNETT (J. HUGHES), M. D., F. R. S. E.,
Professor of Clinical Medicine in the University of Edinburgh, &c.

THE PATHOLOGY AND TREATMENT OF PULMONARY TUBERCU-
LOSIS, and on the Local Medication of Pharyngeal and Laryngeal Diseases frequently mistaken for or associated with, Phthisis. In one handsome octavo volume, with beautiful wood-cuts. (*Now Ready*.)

BILLING (ARCHIBALD), M. D.

THE PRINCIPLES OF MEDICINE. Second American, from the Fifth and Improved London edition. In one handsome octavo volume, extra cloth, 250 pages.

BLAKISTON (PEYTON), M. D., F. R. S., &c.

PRACTICAL OBSERVATIONS ON CERTAIN DISEASES OF THE CHEST, and on the Principles of Auscultation. In one volume, 8vo., pp. 384.

BURROWS (GEORGE), M. D.

ON DISORDERS OF THE CEREBRAL CIRCULATION, and on the Connection between the Affections of the Brain and Diseases of the Heart. In one 8vo. vol., with colored plates, pp. 216.

BUDD (GEORGE), M. D., F. R. S.,
Professor of Medicine in King's College, London.

ON DISEASES OF THE LIVER. Second American, from the second and enlarged London edition. In one very handsome octavo volume, with four beautifully colored plates, and numerous wood-cuts. pp. 468. New edition. (*Just Issued*.)

The reputation which this work has obtained as a full and practical treatise on an important class of diseases will not be diminished by this improved and enlarged edition. It has been carefully and thoroughly revised by the author; the number of plates has been increased, and the style of its mechanical execution will be found materially improved.

The full digest we have given of the new matter introduced into the present volume, is evidence of the value we place on it. The fact that the profession has required a second edition of a monograph such as that before us, bears honorable testimony to its usefulness. For many years, Dr. Budd's work must be the authority of the great mass of British practitioners on the hepatic diseases. It is satisfactory that the subject has been taken up by so able and experienced a physician.—*British and Foreign Medico-Chirurgical Review.*

BUSHNAN (J. S.), M. D.

THE PHYSIOLOGY OF ANIMAL AND VEGETABLE LIFE; a Popular Treatise on the Functions and Phenomena of Organic Life. To which is prefixed a Brief Exposition of the great departments of Human Knowledge. In one handsome royal 12mo. vol., with over one hundred illustrations.

Though cast in a popular form and manner, this work is the production of a man of science. It presents its subject in its latest development, based on truly scientific and accurate principles. It may therefore be consulted with interest by those who wish to obtain in a concise form, and at a very low price, a résumé of the present state of animal and vegetable physiology.

BLOOD AND URINE (MANUALS ON).

BY JOHN WILLIAM GRIFFITH, G. OWEN REESE, AND ALFRED MARKWICK. One thick volume, royal 12mo., extra cloth, with plates. pp. 460.

BRODIE (SIR BENJAMIN C.), M. D., &c.

CLINICAL LECTURES ON SURGERY. 1 vol. 8vo., cloth. 350 pp.

BIRD (GOLDING), A. M., M. D., &c.

URINARY DEPOSITS: THEIR DIAGNOSIS, PATHOLOGY, AND THERAPEUTICAL INDICATIONS. A new and enlarged American, from the last improved London edition. With over sixty illustrations. In one royal 12mo. volume, extra cloth.

The new edition of Dr. Bird's work, though not increased in size, has been greatly modified, and much of it rewritten. It now presents, in a compendious form, the gist of all that is known and reliable in this department. From its terse style and convenient size, it is particularly applicable to the student, to whom we cordially commend it.—*The Medical Examiner.*

It can scarcely be necessary for us to say anything of the merits of this well-known Treatise, which so admirably brings into practical application the results of those microscopical and chemical researches regarding the physiology and pathology of the urinary secretion, which have contributed so much to the increase of our diagnostic powers, and to the extension and satisfactory employment of our therapeutic resources. In the preparation of this new edition of his work, it is obvious that Dr. Golding Bird has spared no pains to render it a faithful representation of the present state of scientific knowledge on the subject it embraces.—*The British and Foreign Medico-Chirurgical Review.*

BY THE SAME AUTHOR.

ELEMENTS OF NATURAL PHILOSOPHY; being an Experimental Introduction to the Physical Sciences. Illustrated with nearly four hundred wood-cuts. From the third London edition. In one neat volume, royal 12mo. pp. 402.

BARTLETT (ELISHA), M. D.,
Professor of Materia Medica and Medical Jurisprudence in the College of Physicians and Surgeons, New York.

THE HISTORY, DIAGNOSIS, AND TREATMENT OF THE FEVERS OF THE UNITED STATES. Third edition, revised and improved. In one octavo volume, of six hundred pages, beautifully printed, and strongly bound.

In preparing a new edition of this standard work, the author has availed himself of such observations and investigations as have appeared since the publication of his last revision, and he has endeavored in every way to render it worthy of a continuance of the very marked favor with which it has been hitherto received.

The masterly and elegant treatise, by Dr. Bartlett is invaluable to the American student and practitioner.—*Dr. Holmes's Report to the Nat. Med. Association.*

We regard it, from the examination we have made of it, the best work on fevers extant in our language, and as such cordially recommend it to the medical public.—*St. Louis Medical and Surgical Journal.*

Take it altogether, it is the most complete history of our fevers which has yet been published, and every practitioner should avail himself of its contents.—*The Western Lancet.*

Of the value and importance of such a work, it is needless here to speak; the profession of the United States owe much to the author for the very able volume which he has presented to them, and for the careful and judicious manner in which he has executed his task. No one volume with which we are acquainted contains so complete a history of our fevers as this. To Dr. Bartlett we owe our best thanks for the very able volume he has given us, as embodying certainly the most complete, methodical, and satisfactory account of our fevers anywhere to be met with.—*The Charleston Med. Journal and Review.*

BUCKLER (T. H.), M. D.,
Formerly Physician to the Baltimore Almshouse Infirmary, &c.

ON THE ETIOLOGY, PATHOLOGY, AND TREATMENT OF FIBRO-BRONCHITIS AND RHEUMATIC PNEUMONIA. In one handsome octavo volume, extra cloth. (*Just Issued.*)

BOWMAN (JOHN E.), M. D.
PRACTICAL HANDBOOK OF MEDICAL CHEMISTRY. In one neat volume, royal 12mo., with numerous illustrations. pp. 288.

BY THE SAME AUTHOR.

INTRODUCTION TO PRACTICAL CHEMISTRY, INCLUDING ANALYSIS. With numerous illustrations. In one neat volume, royal 12mo. pp. 350.

BARLOW (GEORGE H.), M. D.
A MANUAL OF THE PRINCIPLES AND PRACTICE OF MEDICINE. In one octavo volume. (*Preparing.*)

BEALE (LIONEL JOHN), M. R. C. S., &c.
THE LAWS OF HEALTH IN RELATION TO MIND AND BODY. A Series of Letters from an old Practitioner to a Patient. In one handsome volume, royal 12mo., extra cloth.

COLOMBAT DE L'ISERE.
A TREATISE ON THE DISEASES OF FEMALES, and on the Special Hygiene of their Sex. Translated, with many Notes and Additions, by C. D. MEIGS, M. D. Second edition, revised and improved. In one large volume, octavo, with numerous wood-cuts. pp. 720.

The treatise of M. Colombat is a learned and laborious commentary on these diseases, indicating very considerable research, great accuracy of judgment, and no inconsiderable personal experience. With the copious notes and additions of its experienced and very erudite translator and editor, Dr. Meigs, it presents, probably, one of the most complete and comprehensive works on the subject we possess.—*American Med. Journal.*

M. Colombat De L'Isere has not consecrated ten years of studious toil and research to the frailer sex in vain; and although we regret to hear it is at the expense of health, he has imposed a debt of gratitude as well upon the profession, as upon the mothers and daughters of beautiful France, which that gallant nation knows best how to acknowledge.—*New Orleans Medical Journal.*

COPLAND (JAMES), M. D., F. R. S., &c.
OF THE CAUSES, NATURE, AND TREATMENT OF PALSY AND APOPLEXY, and of the Forms, Seats, Complications, and Morbid Relations of Paralytic and Apoplectic Diseases. In one volume, royal 12mo., extra cloth. pp. 326.

CLYMER (MEREDITH), M. D., &c.
FEVERS; THEIR DIAGNOSIS, PATHOLOGY, AND TREATMENT. Prepared and Edited, with large Additions, from the Essays on Fever in Tweedie's Library of Practical Medicine. In one octavo volume, of 600 pages.

CARSON (JOSEPH), M. D.,
Professor of Materia Medica and Pharmacy in the University of Pennsylvania.

SYNOPSIS OF THE COURSE OF LECTURES ON MATERIA MEDICA AND PHARMACY, delivered in the University of Pennsylvania. In one very neat octavo volume, of 208 pages.

CARPENTER (WILLIAM B.), M.D., F.R.S., &c.,
Examiner in Physiology and Comparative Anatomy in the University of London.

PRINCIPLES OF HUMAN PHYSIOLOGY; with their chief applications to
Psychology, Pathology, Therapeutics, Hygiene, and Forensic Medicine. Fifth American, from the fourth and enlarged London edition. With three hundred and fourteen illustrations. Edited with additions, by FRANCIS GURNEY SMITH, M. D., Professor of the Institutes of Medicine in the Pennsylvania Medical College, &c. In one very large and beautiful octavo volume, of about 1100 large pages, handsomely printed and strongly bound in leather, with raised bands. New edition. (*Lately Issued.*)

The most complete work on the science in our language.—*Am. Med. Journal.*

The most complete exposition of physiology which any language can at present give.—*Brit. and For. Med.-Chirurg. Review.*

We have thus adverted to some of the leading "additions and alterations," which have been introduced by the author into this edition of his physiology. These will be found, however, very far to exceed the ordinary limits of a new edition, "the old materials having been incorporated with the new, rather than the new with the old." It now certainly presents the most complete treatise on the subject within the reach of the American reader; and while, for availability as a text-book, we may perhaps regret its growth in bulk, we are sure that the student of physiology will feel the impossibility of presenting a thorough digest of the facts of the science within a more limited compass.—*Medical Examiner.*

The greatest, the most reliable, and the best book on the subject which we know of in the English language.—*Stethoscope.*

The most complete work now extant in our language.—*N. O. Med. Register.*

The changes are too numerous to admit of an extended notice in this place. At every point where the recent diligent labors of organic chemists and micrographers have furnished interesting and valuable facts, they have been appropriated, and no pains have been spared, in so incorporating and arranging them that the work may constitute one harmonious system.—*Southern Med. and Surg. Journal.*

The best text-book in the language on this extensive subject.—*London Med. Times.*

A complete cyclopædia of this branch of science.—*N. Y. Med. Times.*

The standard of authority on physiological subjects. * * * In the present edition, to particularize the alterations and additions which have been made, would require a review of the whole work. scarcely a subject has not been revised and altered, added to, or entirely remodelled to adapt it to the present state of the science.—*Charleston Med. Journ.*

Any reader who desires a treatise on physiology may feel himself entirely safe in ordering this.—*Western Med. and Surg. Journal.*

From this hasty and imperfect allusion it will be seen by our readers that the alterations and additions to this edition render it almost a new work, and we can assure our readers that it is one of the best summaries of the existing facts of physiological science within the reach of the English student and physician.—*N. Y. Journal of Medicine.*

The profession of this country, and perhaps also of Europe, have anxiously and for some time awaited the announcement of this new edition of Carpenter's Human Physiology. His former editions have for many years been almost the only text-book on Physiology in all our medical schools, and its circulation among the profession has been unsurpassed by any work in any department of medical science. It is quite unnecessary for us to speak of this work as its merits would justify. The mere announcement of its appearance will afford the highest pleasure to every student of Physiology, while its perusal will be of infinite service in advancing physiological science.—*Ohio Med. and Surg. Journ.*

BY THE SAME AUTHOR. (*Now Ready.*)

PRINCIPLES OF COMPARATIVE PHYSIOLOGY. New American, from
the Fourth and Revised London edition. In one large and handsome octavo volume, with over three hundred beautiful illustrations.

The delay which has existed in the appearance of this work has been caused by the very thorough revision and remodelling which it has undergone at the hands of the author, and the large number of new illustrations which have been prepared for it. It will, therefore, be found almost a new work, and fully up to the day in every department of the subject, rendering it a reliable text-book for all students engaged in this branch of science. Every effort has been made to render its typographical finish and mechanical execution worthy of its exalted reputation, and creditable to the mechanical arts of this country. A few notices of the last edition are appended.

Without pretending to it, it is an Encyclopedia of the subject, accurate and complete in all respects—a truthful reflection of the advanced state at which the science has now arrived.—*Dublin Quarterly Journal of Medical Science.*

A truly magnificent work—in itself a perfect physiological study.—*Ranking's Abstract.*

This work stands without its fellow. It is one few men in Europe could have undertaken; it is one no man, we believe, could have brought to so successful an issue as Dr. Carpenter. It required for its production a physiologist at once deeply read in the labors of others, capable of taking a general,

critical, and unprejudiced view of those labors and of combining the varied, heterogeneous materials at his disposal, so as to form an harmonious whole. We feel that this abstract can give the reader a very imperfect idea of the fulness of this work, and no idea of its unity, of the admirable manner in which material has been brought, from the most various sources, to conduce to its completeness, of the lucidity of the reasoning it contains, or of the clearness of language in which the whole is clothed. Not the profession only, but the scientific world at large, must feel deeply indebted to Dr. Carpenter for this great work. It must, indeed, add largely even to his high reputation.—*Medical Times.*

BY THE SAME AUTHOR. (*Preparing.*)

THE MICROSCOPE AND ITS REVELATIONS. In one handsome volume,
beautifully illustrated with plates and wood-cuts.

BY THE SAME AUTHOR. (*Preparing.*)

GENERAL PHYSIOLOGY. In one large and very handsome octavo volume.
with several hundred illustrations.

The subject of general physiology having been omitted in the last edition of the author's "Comparative Physiology," he has undertaken to prepare a volume which shall present it more thoroughly and fully than has yet been attempted, and which may be regarded as an introduction to his other works.

CARPENTER (WILLIAM B.), M. D., F. R. S.,
Examiner in Physiology and Comparative Anatomy in the University of London.

ELEMENTS (OR MANUAL) OF PHYSIOLOGY, INCLUDING PHYSIO-
LOGICAL ANATOMY. Second American, from a new and revised London edition. With one hundred and ninety illustrations. In one very handsome octavo volume.

In publishing the first edition of this work, its title was altered from that of the London volume, by the substitution of the word "Elements" for that of "Manual," and with the author's sanction the title of "Elements" is still retained as being more expressive of the scope of the treatise. A comparison of the present edition with the former one will show a material improvement, the author having revised it thoroughly, with a view of rendering it completely on a level with the most advanced state of the science. By condensing the less important portions, these numerous additions have been introduced without materially increasing the bulk of the volume, and while numerous illustrations have been added, and the general execution of the work improved, it has been kept at its former very moderate price.

To say that it is the best manual of Physiology now before the public, would not do sufficient justice to the author.—*Buffalo Medical Journal.*

In his former works it would seem that he had exhausted the subject of Physiology. In the present, he gives the essence, as it were, of the whole.—*N. Y. Journal of Medicine.*

Those who have occasion for an elementary treatise on Physiology, cannot do better than to possess themselves of the manual of Dr. Carpenter.—*Medical Examiner.*

The best and most complete exposé of modern Physiology, in one volume, extant in the English language.—*St. Louis Medical Journal.*

With such an aid in his hand, there is no excuse for the ignorance often displayed respecting the subjects of which it treats. From its unpretending dimensions, it may not be so esteemed by those anxious to make a parade of their erudition; but whoever masters its contents will have reason to be proud of his physiological acquirements. The illustrations are well selected and finely executed.—*Dublin Med. Press.*

BY THE SAME AUTHOR.

A PRIZE ESSAY ON THE USE OF ALCOHOLIC LIQUORS IN HEALTH
AND DISEASE. New edition, with a Preface by D. F. CONDIE, M. D., and explanations of scientific words. In one neat 12mo. volume. (*Now Ready.*)

This new edition has been prepared with a view to an extended circulation of this important little work, which is universally recognized as the best exponent of the laws of physiology and pathology applied to the subject of intoxicating liquors, in a form suited both for the profession and the public. To secure a wider dissemination of its doctrines the publishers have done up copies in flexible cloth, suitable for mailing, which will be forwarded through the post-office, free, on receipt of fifty cents. Societies and others supplied in quantities for distribution at a liberal deduction.

CHELIUS (J. M.), M. D.,
Professor of Surgery in the University of Heidelberg, &c.

A SYSTEM OF SURGERY. Translated from the German, and accompanied
with additional Notes and References, by JOHN F. SOUTH. Complete in three very large octavo volumes, of nearly 2200 pages, strongly bound, with raised bands and double titles.

We do not hesitate to pronounce it the best and most comprehensive system of modern surgery with which we are acquainted.—*Medico-Chirurgical Review.*

The fullest and ablest digest extant of all that relates to the present advanced state of surgical pathology.—*American Medical Journal.*

As complete as any system of Surgery can well be.—*Southern Medical and Surgical Journal.*

The most learned and complete systematic treatise now extant.—*Edinburgh Medical Journal.*

A complete encyclopædia of surgical science—a very complete surgical library—by far the most complete and scientific system of surgery in the English language.—*N. Y. Journal of Medicine.*

The most extensive and comprehensive account of the art and science of Surgery in our language.—*Lancet.*

CHRISTISON (ROBERT), M. D., V. P. R. S. E., &c.

A DISPENSATORY; or, Commentary on the Pharmacopœias of Great Britain
and the United States; comprising the Natural History, Description, Chemistry, Pharmacy, Actions, Uses, and Doses of the Articles of the Materia Medica. Second edition, revised and improved, with a Supplement containing the most important New Remedies. With copious Additions, and two hundred and thirteen large wood-engravings. By R. EGLESFELD GRIFFITH, M. D. In one very large and handsome octavo volume, of over 1000 pages.

It is not needful that we should compare it with the other pharmacopœias extant, which enjoy and merit the confidence of the profession : it is enough to say that it appears to us as perfect as a Dispensatory, in the present state of pharmaceutical science, could be made. If it omits any details pertaining to this branch of knowledge which the student has a right to expect in such a work, we confess the omission has escaped our scrutiny. We cordially recommend this work to such of our readers as are in need of a Dispensatory. They cannot make choice of a better.—*Western Journ. of Medicine and Surgery.*

There is not in any language a more complete and perfect Treatise.—*N. Y. Annalist.*

In conclusion, we need scarcely say that we strongly recommend this work to all classes of our readers. As a Dispensatory and commentary on the Pharmacopœias, it is unrivalled in the English or any other language.—*The Dublin Quarterly Journal.*

We earnestly recommend Dr. Christison's Dispensatory to all our readers, as an indispensable companion, not in the Study only, but in the Surgery also.—*British and Foreign Medical Review.*

CONDIE (D. F.), M. D., &c.

A PRACTICAL TREATISE ON THE DISEASES OF CHILDREN. Fourth edition, revised and augmented. In one large volume, 8vo., of nearly 750 pages. (Just Issued.)

FROM THE AUTHOR'S PREFACE.

The demand for another edition has afforded the author an opportunity of again subjecting the entire treatise to a careful revision, and of incorporating in it every important observation made since the appearance of the last edition, in reference to the pathology and therapeutics of the several diseases of which it treats.

In the preparation of the present edition, as in those which have preceded, while the author has appropriated to his use every important fact that he has found recorded in the works of writers having a direct bearing upon either of the subjects of which he treats, and the numerous valuable observations—pathological as well as practical—dispersed throughout the pages of the medical journals of Europe and America, he has, nevertheless, relied chiefly upon his own observations, experience, acquired during a long and somewhat extensive practice, and under circumstances peculiarly well adapted for the clinical study of the diseases of early life.

Every species of hypothetical reasoning has, as much as possible, been avoided. The author has endeavored throughout the work to confine himself to a simple statement of well-ascertained pathological facts, and plain therapeutical directions—his chief desire being to render it what its title imports it to be, A PRACTICAL TREATISE ON THE DISEASES OF CHILDREN.

Dr. Condie's scholarship, acumen, industry, and practical sense are manifested in this, as in all his numerous contributions to science.—*Dr. Holmes's Report to the American Medical Association.*

Taken as a whole, in our judgment, Dr. Condie's Treatise is the one from the perusal of which the practitioner in this country will rise with the greatest satisfaction.—*Western Journal of Medicine and Surgery.*

One of the best works upon the Diseases of Children in the English language.—*Western Lancet.*

Perhaps the most full and complete work now before the profession of the United States; indeed, we may say in the English language. It is vastly superior to most of its predecessors.—*Transylvania Med. Journal.*

We feel assured from actual experience that no physician's library can be complete without a copy of this work.—*N. Y. Journal of Medicine.*

A veritable pædiatric encyclopædia, and must to American medical literature.—*Ohio Medical & Surgical Journal.*

We feel persuaded that the American medical profession will soon regard it not only as a good but as the VERY BEST "Practical Treatise on Diseases of Children."—*American Medical Journal.*

We pronounced the first edition to be the best work on the diseases of children in the English language, and, notwithstanding all that has been published, we still regard it in that light.—*Medical Examiner.*

COOPER (BRANSBY B.), F. R. S.,
Senior Surgeon to Guy's Hospital, &c.

LECTURES ON THE PRINCIPLES AND PRACTICE OF SURGERY. In one very large octavo volume, of 750 pages. (*Lately Issued.*)

For twenty-five years Mr. Bransby Cooper has been surgeon to Guy's Hospital; and the volume before us may be said to consist of an account of the results of his surgical experience during that long period. We cordially recommend Mr. Bransby Cooper's Lectures as a most valuable addition to our surgical literature, and one which cannot fail to be of service both to students and to those who are actively engaged in the practice of their profession.—*The Lancet.*

COOPER (SIR ASTLEY P.), F. R. S., &c.

A TREATISE ON DISLOCATIONS AND FRACTURES OF THE JOINTS. Edited by BRANSBY B. COOPER, F. R. S., &c. With additional Observations by Prof. J. WARREN. A new American edition. In one handsome octavo volume, with numerous illustrations on wood.

BY THE SAME AUTHOR.

ON THE ANATOMY AND TREATMENT OF ABDOMINAL HERNIA. One large volume, imperial 8vo., with over 130 lithographic figures.

BY THE SAME AUTHOR.

ON THE STRUCTURE AND DISEASES OF THE TESTIS, AND ON THE THYMUS GLAND. One vol. imperial 8vo., with 177 figures, on 29 plates.

BY THE SAME AUTHOR.

ON THE ANATOMY AND DISEASES OF THE BREAST, with twenty-five Miscellaneous and Surgical Papers. One large volume, imperial 8vo., with 252 figures, 36 plates.

These last three volumes complete the surgical writings of Sir Astley Cooper. They are all handsomely printed, with a large number of lithographic plates, executed in the best style, and are presented at exceedingly low prices.

CHURCHILL (FLEETWOOD), M. D., M. R. I. A.

ON THE THEORY AND PRACTICE OF MIDWIFERY. A new American, from the last and improved English edition. Edited, with Notes and Additions, by D. FRANCIS CONDIE, M. D., author of a "Practical Treatise on the Diseases of Children," &c. With 139 illustrations. In one very handsome octavo volume, pp. 510. (*Lately Issued.*)

To bestow praise on a book that has received such marked approbation would be superfluous. We need only say, therefore, that if the first edition was thought worthy of a favorable reception by the medical public, we can confidently affirm that this will be found much more so. The lecturer, the practitioner, and the student, may all have recourse to its pages, and derive from their perusal much interest and instruction in everything relating to theoretical and practical midwifery.—*Dublin Quarterly Journal of Medical Science.*

A work of very great merit, and such as we can confidently recommend to the study of every obstetric practitioner.—*London Medical Gazette.*

This is certainly the most perfect system extant. It is the best adapted for the purposes of a text-book, and that which he whose necessities confine him to one book, should select in preference to all others.—*Southern Medical and Surgical Journal.*

The most popular work on midwifery ever issued from the American press.—*Charleston Med. Journal.*

Were we reduced to the necessity of having but *one* work on midwifery, and *permitted to choose*, we would unhesitatingly take Churchill.—*Western Med. and Surg. Journal.*

It is impossible to conceive a more useful and elegant manual than Dr. Churchill's Practice of Midwifery.—*Provincial Medical Journal.*

Certainly, in our opinion, the very best work on the subject which exists.—*N. Y. Annalist.*

No work holds a higher position, or is more deserving of being placed in the hands of the tyro, the advanced student, or the practitioner.—*Medical Examiner.*

Previous editions, under the editorial supervision of Prof R. M. Huston, have been received with marked favor, and they deserved it; but this, reprinted from a very late Dublin edition, carefully revised and brought up by the author to the present time, does present an unusually accurate and able exposition of every important particular embraced in the department of midwifery. * * The clearness, directness, and precision of its teachings, together with the great amount of statistical research which its text exhibits, have served to place it already in the foremost rank of works in this department of remedial science.—*N. O. Med. and Surg. Journal.*

In our opinion, it forms one of the best if not the very best text-book and epitome of obstetric science which we at present possess in the English language.—*Monthly Journal of Medical Science.*

The clearness and precision of style in which it is written, and the great amount of statistical research which it contains, have served to place it in the first rank of works in this department of medical science. —*N. Y. Journal of Medicine.*

Few treatises will be found better adapted as a text-book for the student, or as a manual for the frequent consultation of the young practitioner.—*American Medical Journal.*

BY THE SAME AUTHOR.

ON THE DISEASES OF INFANTS AND CHILDREN. In one large and handsome volume of over 600 pages.

We regard this volume as possessing more claims to completeness than any other of the kind with which we are acquainted. Most cordially and earnestly, therefore, do we commend it to our professional brethren, and we feel assured that the stamp of their approbation will in due time be impressed upon it. After an attentive perusal of its contents, we hesitate not to say, that it is one of the most comprehensive ever written upon the diseases of children, and that, for copiousness of reference, extent of research, and perspicuity of detail, it is scarcely to be equalled, and not to be excelled, in any language.—*Dublin Quarterly Journal.*

After this meagre, and we know, very imperfect notice of Dr. Churchill's work, we shall conclude by saying, that it is one that cannot fail from its copiousness, extensive research, and general accuracy, to exalt still higher the reputation of the author in this country. The American reader will be particularly pleased to find that Dr. Churchill has done full justice throughout his work to the various American authors on this subject. The names of Dewees, Eberle, Condie, and Stewart, occur on nearly every page, and these authors are constantly referred to by the author in terms of the highest praise, and with the most liberal courtesy.—*The Medical Examiner.*

The present volume will sustain the reputation acquired by the author from his previous works. The reader will find in it full and judicious directions for the management of infants at birth, and a compendious, but clear account of the diseases to which children are liable, and the most successful mode of treating them. We must not close this notice without calling attention to the author's style, which is perspicuous and polished to a degree, we regret to say, not generally characteristic of medical works. We recommend the work of Dr. Churchill most cordially, both to students and practitioners, as a valuable and reliable guide in the treatment of the diseases of children.—*Am. Journ. of the Med. Sciences.*

We know of no work on this department of Practical Medicine which presents so candid and unprejudiced a statement or posting up of our actual knowledge as this.—*N. Y. Journal of Medicine.*

Its claims to merit both as a scientific and practical work, are of the highest order. Whilst we would not elevate it above every other treatise on the same subject, we certainly believe that very few are equal to it, and none superior.—*Southern Med. and Surgical Journal.*

BY THE SAME AUTHOR.

ESSAYS ON THE PUERPERAL FEVER, AND OTHER DISEASES PECULIAR TO WOMEN. Selected from the writings of British Authors previous to the close of the Eighteenth Century. In one neat octavo volume, of about four hundred and fifty pages.

To these papers Dr. Churchill has appended notes, embodying whatever information has been laid before the profession since their authors' time. He has also prefixed to the Essays on Puerperal Fever, which occupy the larger portion of the volume, an interesting historical sketch of the principal epidemics of that disease. The whole forms a very valuable collection of papers, by professional writers of eminence, on some of the most important accidents to which the puerperal female is liable.—*American Journal of Medical Sciences.*

CHURCHILL (FLEETWOOD), M. D., M. R. I. A., &c.

ON THE DISEASES OF WOMEN; including those of Pregnancy and Childbed. A new American edition, revised by the Author. With Notes and Additions, by Francis Condie, M. D., author of "A Practical Treatise on the Diseases of Children." In one and handsome octavo volume, with wood-cuts, pp. 684. (*Just Issued.*)

From the Author's Preface.

In reviewing this edition, at the request of my American publishers, I have inserted several new sections and chapters, and I have added, I believe, all the information we have derived from recent researches; in addition to which the publishers have been fortunate enough to secure the services of an able and highly esteemed editor in Dr. Condie.

We now regretfully take leave of Dr. Churchill's book. Had our typographical limits permitted, we should gladly have borrowed more from its richly stored pages. In conclusion, we heartily recommend it to the profession, and would at the same time express our firm conviction that it will not only add to the reputation of its author, but will prove a work of great and extensive utility to obstetric practitioners.—*Dublin Medical Press.*

Former editions of this work have been noticed in previous numbers of the Journal. The sentiments of high commendation expressed in those notices, have only to be repeated in this; not from the fact that the profession at large are not aware of the high merits which this work really possesses, but from a desire to see the principles and doctrines therein contained more generally recognized, and more universally carried out in practice.—*N. Y. Journal of Medicine.*

We know of no author who deserves that approbation, on "the diseases of females," to the same extent that Dr. Churchill does. His, indeed, is the only thorough treatise we know of on the subject; and it may be commended to practitioners and students as a masterpiece in its particular department. The former editions of this work have been commended strongly in this journal, and they have won their way to an extended, and a well-deserved popularity. This fifth edition, before us, is well calculated to maintain Dr. Churchill's high reputation. It was revised and enlarged by the author. American publishers, and it seems to us that scarcely any species of desirable information subjects that may not be found in this work.—*Western Journal of Medicine and Surgery.*

We are gratified to announce a new and improved edition of Dr. Churchill's valuable work on the diseases of females. We have ever regarded it as one of the very best works on the subjects embraced within its scope, in the English language. The present edition, enlarged and revised by the author, renders it still more entitled to the confidence of the profession. The valuable notes of Prof. Huston have been retained, and contribute, in no small degree, to enhance the value of the work. It is a source of congratulation that the publishers have permitted the author to be, in this instance, his own editor, thus securing all the revision that an author alone is capable of making.—*The N. O. Med. Lancet.*

As a comprehensive manual for students, and work of reference for practitioners, we can, with common justice when we say that it stands before any other that has ever issued on the subject from the British press.—*The Dublin Quarterly Journal.*

DEWEES (W. P.), M. D., &c.

A COMPREHENSIVE SYSTEM OF MIDWIFERY. Illustrated by occasional Cases and many Engravings. Twelfth edition, with the Author's last Improvements and Corrections. In one octavo volume, of 600 pages. (*Just Issued.*)

BY THE SAME AUTHOR.

A TREATISE ON THE PHYSICAL AND MEDICAL TREATMENT OF CHILDREN. Tenth edition. In one volume, octavo, 548 pages. (*Just Issued.*)

BY THE SAME AUTHOR.

A TREATISE ON THE DISEASES OF FEMALES. Tenth edition. In one volume, octavo, 532 pages, with plates. (*Just Issued.*)

DICKSON (S. H.), M. D.,
Professor of Institutes and Practice of Medicine in the Medical College of South Carolina; late Professor of the Institutes and Practice of Medicine in the Medical Department of the University of New York, &c. &c.

ELEMENTS OF MEDICINE; A Treatise on Pathology and Therapeutics. In one large and handsome octavo volume. (*Preparing.*)

DANA (JAMES D).

ZOOPHYTES AND CORALS. In one volume, imperial quarto, extra cloth with wood-cuts.

ALSO,

AN ATLAS TO THE ABOVE, one volume, imperial folio, with sixty-one magnificent plates, colored after nature. Bound in half morocco.

ALSO,

ON THE STRUCTURE AND CLASSIFICATION OF ZOOPHYTES. Sold separate, one vol., cloth.

DE LA BECHE (SIR HENRY T.), F. R. S., &c.

THE GEOLOGICAL OBSERVER. In one very large and handsome octavo volume, of 700 pages. With over three hundred wood-cuts. (*Lately Issued.*)

DRUITT (ROBERT), M. R. C. S., &c.

THE PRINCIPLES AND PRACTICE OF MODERN SURGERY. A new American, from the improved London edition. Edited by F. W. SARGENT, M. D., author of "Minor Surgery," &c. Illustrated with one hundred and ninety-three wood-engravings. In one very handsomely printed octavo volume, of 576 large pages.

Dr. Druitt's researches into the literature of his subject have been not only extensive, but well directed; the most discordant authors are fairly and impartially quoted, and, while due credit is given to each, their respective merits are weighed with an unprejudiced hand. The grain of wheat is preserved, and the chaff is unmercifully stripped off. The arrangement is simple and philosophical, and the style, though clear and interesting, is so precise, that the book contains more information condensed into a few words than any other surgical work with which we are acquainted.—*London Medical Times and Gazette*, February 18, 1854.

No work, in our opinion, equals it in presenting so much valuable surgical matter in so small a compass.—*St. Louis Med. and Surgical Journal.*

Druitt's Surgery is too well known to the American medical profession to require its announcement anywhere. Probably no work of the kind has ever been more cordially received and extensively circulated than this. The fact that it comprehends in a comparatively small compass, all the essential elements of theoretical and practical Surgery—that it is found to contain reliable and authentic information on the nature and treatment of nearly all surgical affections—is a sufficient reason for the liberal patronage it has obtained. The editor, Dr. F. W. Sargent, has contributed much to enhance the value of the work, by such American improvements as are calculated more perfectly to adapt it to our own views and practice in this country. It abounds everywhere with spirited and life-like illustrations, which to the young surgeon, especially, are of no minor consideration. Every medical man frequently needs just such a work as this, for immediate reference in moments of sudden emergency, when he has not time to consult more elaborate treatises.—*The Ohio Medical and Surgical Journal.*

The author has evidently ransacked every standard treatise of ancient and modern times, and all that is really practically useful at the bedside will be found in a form at once clear, distinct, and interesting.—*Edinburgh Monthly Medical Journal.*

Druitt's work, condensed, systematic, lucid, and practical as it is, beyond most works on Surgery accessible to the American student, has had much currency in this country, and under its present auspices promises to rise to yet higher favor.—*The Western Journal of Medicine and Surgery.*

The most accurate and ample resumé of the present state of Surgery that we are acquainted with.—*Dublin Medical Journal.*

A better book on the principles and practice of Surgery as now understood in England and America, has not been given to the profession.—*Boston Medical and Surgical Journal.*

An unsurpassable compendium, not only of Surgical, but of Medical Practice.—*London Medical Gazette.*

This work merits our warmest commendations, and we strongly recommend it to young surgeons as an admirable digest of the principles and practice of modern Surgery.—*Medical Gazette.*

It may be said with truth that the work of Mr. Druitt affords a complete, though brief and condensed view, of the entire field of modern surgery. We know of no work on the same subject having the appearance of a manual, which includes so many topics of interest to the surgeon; and the terse manner in which each has been treated evinces a most enviable quality of mind on the part of the author, who seems to have an innate power of searching out and grasping the leading facts and features of the most elaborate productions of the pen. It is a useful handbook for the practitioner, and we should deem a teacher of surgery unpardonable who did not recommend it to his pupils. In our own opinion, it is admirably adapted to the wants of the student.—*Provincial Medical and Surgical Journal.*

DUNGLISON, FORBES, TWEEDIE, AND CONOLLY.

THE CYCLOPÆDIA OF PRACTICAL MEDICINE: comprising Treatises on the Nature and Treatment of Diseases, Materia Medica, and Therapeutics, Diseases of Women and Children, Medical Jurisprudence, &c. &c. In four large super royal octavo volumes, of 3254 double-columned pages, strongly and handsomely bound.

⁂ This work contains no less than four hundred and eighteen distinct treatises, contributed by sixty-eight distinguished physicians.

The most complete work on Practical Medicine extant; or, at least, in our language.—*Buffalo Medical and Surgical Journal.*

For reference, it is above all price to every practitioner.—*Western Lancet.*

One of the most valuable medical publications of the day—as a work of reference it is invaluable.—*Western Journal of Medicine and Surgery.*

It has been to us, both as learner and teacher, a work for ready and frequent reference, one in which modern English medicine is exhibited in the most advantageous light.—*Medical Examiner.*

We rejoice that this work is to be placed within the reach of the profession in this country, it being unquestionably one of very great value to the practitioner. This estimate of it has not been formed from a hasty examination, but after an intimate acquaintance derived from frequent consultation of it during the past nine or ten years. The editors are practitioners of established reputation, and the list of contributors embraces many of the most eminent professors and teachers of London, Edinburgh, Dublin, and Glasgow. It is, indeed, the great merit of this work that the principal articles have been furnished by practitioners who have not only devoted especial attention to the diseases about which they have written, but have also enjoyed opportunities for an extensive practical acquaintance with them, and whose reputation carries the assurance of their competency justly to appreciate the opinions of others, while it stamps their own doctrines with high and just authority.—*American Medical Journ.*

DUNGLISON (ROBLEY), M. D.,
Professor of the Institutes of Medicine in the Jefferson Medical College, Philadelphia.

HUMAN HEALTH; or, the Influence of Atmosphere and Locality, Change of Air and Climate, Seasons, Food, Clothing, Bathing, Exercise, Sleep, &c. &c., on Healthy Man; constituting Elements of Hygiene. Second edition, with many modifications and additions. In one octavo volume, of 464 pages.

DUNGLISON (ROBLEY), M. D.,
Professor of Institutes of Medicine in the Jefferson Medical College, Philadelphia.

MEDICAL LEXICON; a Dictionary of Medical Science, containing a concise Explanation of the various Subjects and Terms of Physiology, Pathology, Hygiene, Therapeutics, Pharmacology, Obstetrics, Medical Jurisprudence, &c. With the French and other Synonymes; Notices of Climate and of celebrated Mineral Waters; Formulæ for various Officinal, Empirical and Dietetic Preparations, etc. Eleventh edition, revised. In one very thick octavo volume, of over nine hundred large double-columned pages, strongly bound in leather, with raised bands. (*Just Issued.*)

Every successive edition of this work bears the marks of the industry of the author, and of his determination to keep it fully on a level with the most advanced state of medical science. Thus nearly FIFTEEN THOUSAND WORDS have been added to it within the last few years. As a complete Medical Dictionary, therefore, embracing over FIFTY THOUSAND DEFINITIONS, in all the branches of the science, it is presented as meriting a continuance of the great favor and popularity which have carried it, within no very long space of time, to an eleventh edition.

Every precaution has been taken in the preparation of the present volume, to render its mechanical execution and typographical accuracy worthy of its extended reputation and universal use. The very extensive additions have been accommodated, without materially increasing the bulk of the volume by the employment of a small but exceedingly clear type, cast for this purpose. The press has been watched with great care, and every effort used to insure the verbal accuracy so necessary to a work of this nature. The whole is printed on fine white paper; and, while thus exhibiting in every respect so great an improvement over former issues, it is presented at the original exceedingly low price.

We welcome it cordially; it is an admirable work, and indispensable to all literary medical men. The labor which has been bestowed upon it is something prodigious. The work, however, has now been done, and we are happy in the thought that no human being will have again to undertake the same gigantic task. Revised and corrected from time to time, Dr. Dunglison's "Medical Lexicon" will last for centuries.—*British and Foreign Med. Chirurg. Review*, July, 1853.

The fact that this excellent and learned work has passed through eight editions, and that a ninth is rendered necessary by the demands of the public, affords a sufficient evidence of the general appreciation of Dr. Dunglison's labors by the medical profession in England and America. It is a book which will be of great service to the student, in teaching him the meaning of all the technical terms used in medicine, and will be of no less use to the practitioner who desires to keep himself on a level with the advance of medical science.—*London Medical Times and Gazette.*

In taking leave of our author, we feel compelled to confess that his work bears evidence of almost incredible labor having been bestowed upon its composition.—*Edinburgh Journal of Med. Sciences*, Sept. 1853.

A miracle of labor and industry in one who has written able and voluminous works on nearly every branch of medical science. There could be no more useful book to the student or practitioner, in the present advancing age, than one in which would be found, in addition to the ordinary meaning and derivation of medical terms—so many of which are of modern introduction—concise descriptions of their explanation and employment; and all this and much more is contained in the volume before us. It is therefore almost as indispensable to the other learned professions as to our own. In fact, to all who may have occasion to ascertain the meaning of any word belonging to the many branches of medicine. From a careful examination of the present edition, we can vouch for its accuracy, and for its being brought quite up to the date of publication; the author states in his preface that he has added to it about four thousand terms, which are not to be found in the preceding one.—*Dublin Quarterly Journal of Medical Sciences.*

On the appearance of the last edition of this valuable work, we directed the attention of our readers to its peculiar merits; and we need do little more than state, in reference to the present reissue, that, notwithstanding the large addition previously made to it, no fewer than four thousand terms, not to be found in the preceding edition, are contained in the volume before us. Whilst it is a wonderful monument of its author's erudition and industry, it is also a work of great practical utility, as we can testify from our own experience; for we keep it constantly within our reach, and make very frequent reference to it, nearly always finding in it the information we seek.—*British and Foreign Med.-Chirurg. Review.*

It has the rare merit that it certainly has no rival in the English language for accuracy and extent of references. The terms generally include also physiological and pathological descriptions, so that, as the author justly observes, the reader does not possess in this work a mere dictionary, but a book which, while it instructs him in medical etymology, furnishes him with a large amount of useful information. The author's labors have been properly appreciated by his own countrymen; and we can only confirm their judgment, by recommending this most useful volume to the notice of our transatlantic readers. No medical library will be complete without it.—*London Med. Gazette.*

It is certainly more complete and comprehensive than any with which we are acquainted in the English language. Few, in fact, could be found better qualified than Dr. Dunglison for the production of such a work. Learned, industrious, persevering, and accurate, he brings to the task the peculiar talents necessary for its successful performance; while, at the same time, his familiarity with the writings of the ancient and modern "masters of our art," renders him skilful to note the exact usage of the several terms of science and the various modifications which medical terminology has undergone with the change of theories or the progress of improvement.—*American Journal of the Medical Sciences.*

One of the most complete and copious known to the cultivators of medical science.—*Boston Med. Journal.*

The most comprehensive and best English Dictionary of medical terms extant.—*Buffalo Med. Journal.*

BY THE SAME AUTHOR.

THE PRACTICE OF MEDICINE. A Treatise on Special Pathology and Therapeutics. Third Edition. In two large octavo volumes, of fifteen hundred pages.

Upon every topic embraced in the work the latest information will be found carefully posted up.—*Medical Examiner.*

The student of medicine will find, in these two elegant volumes, a mine of facts, a gathering of precepts and advice from the world of experience, that will nerve him with courage, and faithfully direct him in his efforts to relieve the physical sufferings of the race.—*Boston Medical and Surg. Journal.*

It is certainly the most complete treatise of which we have any knowledge.—*Western Journal of Medicine and Surgery.*

One of the most elaborate treatises of the kind we have.—*Southern Med. and Surg. Journal.*

DUNGLISON (ROBLEY), M. D.,
Professor of Institutes of Medicine in the Jefferson Medical College, Philadelphia.

HUMAN PHYSIOLOGY. Seventh edition. Thoroughly revised and extensively modified and enlarged, with nearly five hundred illustrations. In two large and handsomely printed octavo volumes, containing nearly 1450 pages.

It has long since taken rank as one of the medical classics of our language. To say that it is by far the best text-book of physiology ever published in this country, is but echoing the general testimony of the profession.—*N. Y. Journal of Medicine.*

There is no single book we would recommend to the student or physician, with greater confidence than the present, because in it will be found a mirror of almost every standard physiological work of the day. We most cordially recommend the work to every member of the profession, and no student should be without it. It is the completest work on Physiology in the English language, and is highly creditable to the author and publishers.—*Canadian Medical Journal.*

The most complete and satisfactory system of Physiology in the English language.—*Amer. Med. Journal.*

The best work of the kind in the English language.—*Silliman's Journal.*

The most full and complete system of Physiology in our language.—*Western Lancet.*

BY THE SAME AUTHOR. (*Just Issued.*)

GENERAL THERAPEUTICS AND MATERIA MEDICA; adapted for a Medical Text-book. Fifth edition, much improved. With one hundred and eighty-seven illustrations. In two large and handsomely printed octavo vols., of about 1100 pages.

The new editions of the United States Pharmacopœia and those of London and Dublin, have rendered necessary a thorough revision of this work. In accomplishing this the author has spared no pains in rendering it a complete exponent of all that is new and reliable, both in the departments of Therapeutics and Materia Medica. The book has thus been somewhat enlarged, and a like improvement will be found in every department of its mechanical execution. As a convenient text-book for the student, therefore, containing within a moderate compass a satisfactory resumé of its important subject, it is again presented as even more worthy than heretofore of the very great favor which it has received.

In this work of Dr. Dunglison, we recognize the same untiring industry in the collection and embodying of facts on the several subjects of which he treats, that has heretofore distinguished him, and we cheerfully point to these volumes, as two of the most interesting that we know of. In noticing the additions to this, the fourth edition, there is very little in the periodical or annual literature of the profession, published in the interval which has elapsed since the issue of the first, that has escaped the careful search of the author. As a book for reference, it is invaluable.—*Charleston Med. Journal and Review.*

It may be said to be *the* work now upon the subjects upon which it treats.—*Western Lancet.*

As a text-book for students, for whom it is particularly designed, we know of none superior to it.—*St. Louis Medical and Surgical Journal.*

It purports to be a new edition, but it is rather a new book, so greatly has it been improved, both in the amount and quality of the matter which it contains.—*N. O. Medical and Surgical Journal.*

We bespeak for this edition, from the profession, an increase of patronage over any of its former ones, on account of its increased merit.—*N. Y. Journal of Medicine.*

We consider this work unequalled.—*Boston Med. and Surg. Journal.*

BY THE SAME AUTHOR.

NEW REMEDIES, WITH FORMULÆ FOR THEIR ADMINISTRATION. Sixth edition, with extensive Additions. In one very large octavo volume, of over 750 pages.

One of the most useful of the author's works.—*Southern Medical and Surgical Journal.*

This well-known and standard book has now reached its sixth edition, and has been enlarged and improved by the introduction of all the recent gifts to therapeutics which the last few years have so richly produced, including the anæsthetic agents, &c. This elaborate and useful volume should be found in every medical library, for as a book of reference, for physicians, it is unsurpassed by any other work in existence, and the double index for diseases and for remedies, will be found greatly to enhance its value.—*New York Med. Gazette.*

The great learning of the author, and his remarkable industry in pushing his researches into every source whence information is derivable, has enabled him to throw together an extensive mass of facts and statements, accompanied by full reference to authorities; which last feature renders the work practically valuable to investigators who desire to examine the original papers.—*The American Journal of Pharmacy.*

DURLACHER (LEWIS).

A TREATISE ON CORNS, BUNIONS, THE DISEASES OF NAILS, AND THE GENERAL MANAGEMENT OF THE FEET. In one 12mo. volume, cloth. pp. 134.

DE JONGH (L. J.), M. D., &c.

THE THREE KINDS OF COD-LIVER OIL, comparatively considered, with their Chemical and Therapeutic Properties. Translated, with an Appendix and Cases, by EDWARD CAREY, M. D. To which is added an article on the subject from "Dunglison on New Remedies." In one small 12mo. volume, extra cloth.

DAY (GEORGE E.), M. D.

A PRACTICAL TREATISE ON THE DOMESTIC MANAGEMENT AND MORE IMPORTANT DISEASES OF ADVANCED LIFE. With an Appendix on a new and successful mode of treating Lumbago and other forms of Chronic Rheumatism. One volume, octavo, 226 pages.

ELLIS (BENJAMIN), M. D.

THE MEDICAL FORMULARY: being a Collection of Prescriptions, derived from the writings and practice of many of the most eminent physicians of America and Europe. Together with the usual Dietetic Preparations and Antidotes for Poisons. To which is added an Appendix, on the Endermic use of Medicines, and on the use of Ether and Chloroform. The whole accompanied with a few brief Pharmaceutic and Medical Observations. Tenth edition, revised and much extended by ROBERT P. THOMAS, M. D., Professor of Materia Medica in the Philadelphia College of Pharmacy. In one neat octavo volume, of two hundred and ninety-six pages. (*Now Ready. Revised and enlarged to 1854.*)

After an examination of the new matter and the alterations, we believe the reputation of the work built up by the author, and the late distinguished editor, will continue to flourish under the auspices of the present editor, who has the industry and accuracy, and, we would say, conscientiousness requisite for the responsible task.—*American Journal of Pharmacy*, March, 1854.

It will prove particularly useful to students as young practitioners, as the most important prescriptions employed in modern practice, which are scattered through our medical literature, are here collected and conveniently arranged for reference—*Charleston Med. Journal and Review.*

ERICHSEN (JOHN),
Professor of Surgery in University College, London, &c.

THE SCIENCE AND ART OF SURGERY; BEING A TREATISE ON SURGICAL INJURIES, DISEASES, AND OPERATIONS. Edited by JOHN H. BRINTON, M. D. Illustrated with three hundred and eleven engravings on wood. In one large and handsome octavo volume of over nine hundred closely printed pages. (*Now Ready.*)

This is a new work, brought up to May, 1854.

It is, in our humble judgment, decidedly the best book of the kind in the English language. Strange that just such books are not oftener produced by public teachers of surgery in this country and Great Britain. Indeed, it is a matter of great astonishment, but no less true than astonishing, that of the many works on surgery republished in this country within the last fifteen or twenty years as text-books for medical students, this is the only one, that even approximates to the fulfilment of the peculiar wants of young men just entering upon the study of this branch of the profession.—*Western Jour. of Med. and Surgery.*

Embracing, as will be perceived, the whole surgical domain, and each division of itself almost complete and perfect, each chapter full and explicit, each subject faithfully exhibited, we can only express our estimate of it in the aggregate. We consider it an excellent contribution to surgery, as probably the best single volume now extant on the subject, and with great pleasure we add it to our text-books—*Nashville Journal of Medicine and Surgery.*

Its value is greatly enhanced by a very complete, well-arranged index. We regard this as one of the most valuable contributions to modern surgery. To one entering his novitiate of practice, we recommend the most serviceable guide which he can consult. He will find a fulness of detail leading him through every step of the operation, and not deserting him till the final issue of the case is decided. For the same reason we recommend it to those whose routine of practice lies in such parts of the country that they rarely encounter cases requiring surgical management.—*Stethoscope.*

Prof. Erichsen's work, for its size, has never been surpassed; his nine hundred and eight pages, profusely illustrated, are rich in physiological, pathological, and operative suggestions, doctrines, and processes; and will prove a reliable resource for information, both to physician and surgeon in the hour of peril.—*N. O. Med. and Surg. Journal.*

FOWNES (GEORGE), PH. D., &c.

ELEMENTARY CHEMISTRY; Theoretical and Practical. With numerous illustrations. A new American, from the last and revised London edition. Edited, with additions, by ROBERT BRIDGES, M. D. In one large royal 12mo. volume, of over 550 pages, with wood-cuts, sheep, or extra cloth. (*Now Ready.*)

The lamented death of the author has caused the revision of this edition to pass into the hands of those distinguished chemists, H. Bence Jones and A. W. Hofmann, who have fully sustained the reputation by the additions which they have made, more especially in the portion devoted to Organic Chemistry, considerably increasing the size of the volume. This labor has been so thoroughly performed, that the American Editor has found but little to add, his notes consisting chiefly of such matters as the rapid advance of the science has rendered necessary, or of investigations which have apparently been overlooked by the author's friends.

The volume is therefore again presented as an exponent of the most advanced state of chemical science, and as not unworthy a continuation of the marked favor which it has received as an elementary text-book.

We know of no better text-book, especially in the difficult department of organic chemistry, upon which it is particularly full and satisfactory. We would recommend it to preceptors as a capital "office book" for their students who are beginners in Chemistry. It is copiously illustrated with excellent wood-cuts, and altogether admirably "got up."—*N. J. Medical Reporter*, March, 1854.

A standard manual, which has long enjoyed the reputation of embodying much knowledge in a small space. The author has achieved the difficult task of condensation with masterly tact. His book is concise without being dry, and brief without being too dogmatical or general.—*Virginia Med. and Surgical Journal.*

The work of Dr. Fownes has long been before the public, and its merits have been fully appreciated as the best text-book on chemistry now in existence. We do not, of course, place it in any way superior to the works of Brande, Graham, Turner, Gregory, or Gmelin, but we say that, as a text-book for students, it is preferable to any of them.—*London Journal of Medicine.*

A work well adapted to the wants of the student. It is an excellent exposition of the chief doctrines and facts of modern chemistry. The size of the work and still more the condensed yet perspicuous style in which it is written, absolve it from the censure very properly urged against most manuals of popular.—*Edinburgh Monthly Journal of Medical Science.*

FRICK (CHARLES), M. D.

RENAL AFFECTIONS; their Diagnosis and Pathology. With illustrations. One volume, royal 12mo., extra cloth.

FERGUSSON (WILLIAM), F. R. S.,
Professor of Surgery in King's College, London, &c.

A SYSTEM OF PRACTICAL SURGERY. Fourth American, from the third and enlarged London edition. In one large and beautifully printed octavo volume, of about seven hundred pages, with three hundred and ninety-three handsome illustrations. (*Just Issued.*)

The most important subjects in connection with practical surgery which have been more recently brought under the notice of, and discussed by, the surgeons of Great Britain, are fully and dispassionately considered by Mr. Fergusson, and that which was before wanting has now been supplied, so that we can now look upon it as a work on practical surgery instead of one on operative surgery alone. There was some ground formerly for the complaint before alluded to, that it dwelt too exclusively on operative surgery; but this defect is now removed, and the book is more than ever adapted for the purposes of the practitioner, whether he confines himself more strictly to the operative department, or follows surgery on a more comprehensive scale.—*Medical Times and Gazette.*

No work was ever written which more nearly comprehended the necessities of the student and practitioner, and was more carefully arranged to that single purpose than this.—*N. Y. Med. and Surg. Journal.*

The addition of many new pages makes this work more than ever indispensable to the student and practitioner.—*Ranking's Abstract.*

Among the numerous works upon surgery published of late years, we know of none we value more highly than the one before us. It is perhaps the very best we have for a text-book and for ordinary reference, being concise and eminently practical.—*Southern Med. and Surg. Journal.*

GRAHAM (THOMAS), F. R. S.,
Professor of Chemistry in University College, London, &c.

THE ELEMENTS OF CHEMISTRY. Including the application of the Science to the Arts. With numerous illustrations. With Notes and Additions, by ROBERT BRIDGES, M. D., &c. &c. Second American, from the second and enlarged London edition

PART I. (*Lately Issued*) large 8vo., 430 pages, 185 illustrations.
PART II. (*Preparing*) to match.

The great changes which the science of chemistry has undergone within the last few years, render a new edition of a treatise like the present, almost a new work. The author has devoted several years to the revision of his treatise, and has endeavored to embody in it every fact and inference of importance which has been observed and recorded by the great body of chemical investigators who are so rapidly changing the face of the science. In this manner the work has been greatly increased in size, and the number of illustrations doubled; while the labors of the editor have been directed towards the introduction of such matters as have escaped the attention of the author, or as have arisen since the publication of the first portion of this edition in London, in 1850. Printed in handsome style, and at a very low price, it is therefore confidently presented to the profession and the student as a very complete and thorough text-book of this important subject.

GROSS (SAMUEL D.), M. D.,
Professor of Surgery in the Louisville Medical Institute, &c.

A PRACTICAL TREATISE ON THE DISEASES AND INJURIES OF THE URINARY ORGANS. In one large and beautifully printed octavo volume, of over seven hundred pages. With numerous illustrations.

A volume replete with truths and principles of the utmost value in the investigation of these diseases.—*American Medical Journal.*

Dr. Gross has brought all his learning, experience, tact, and judgment to the task, and has produced a work worthy of his high reputation. We feel perfectly safe in recommending it to our readers as a monograph unequalled in interest and practical value by any other on the subject in our language.—*Western Journal of Med. and Surg.*

It has remained for an American writer to wipe away this reproach; and so completely has the task been fulfilled, that we venture to predict for Dr. Gross's treatise a permanent place in the literature of surgery, worthy to rank with the best works of the present age. Not merely is the matter good, but the getting up of the volume is most creditable to transatlantic enterprise; the paper and print would do credit to a first-rate London establishment; and the numerous wood-cuts which illustrate it, demonstrate that America is making rapid advances in this department of art. We have, indeed, unfeigned pleasure in congratulating all concerned in this publication, on the result of their labours; and experience a feeling something like what animates a long-expectant husbandman, who, oftentimes disappointed by the produce of a favorite field, is at last agreeably surprised by a stately crop which may bear comparison with any of its former rivals. The grounds of our high appreciation of the work will be obvious as we proceed; and we doubt not that the present facilities for obtaining American books will induce many of our readers to verify our recommendation by their own perusal of it.—*British and Foreign Medico-Chirurgical Review.*

Whoever will peruse the vast amount of valuable practical information it contains, and which we have been unable even to notice, will, we think, agree with us, that there is no work in the English language which can make any just pretensions to be its equal.—*N. Y. Journal of Medicine.*

BY THE SAME AUTHOR. (*Now Ready.*)

A PRACTICAL TREATISE ON FOREIGN BODIES IN THE AIR-PASSAGES. In one handsome octavo volume, with illustrations.

No complete monograph on this interesting and difficult subject has hitherto appeared in any language. The profession will therefore find a want supplied by the present volume, containing an elaborate investigation of the nature, symptoms, and treatment of this class of accidents, founded on the details of more than two hundred cases, carefully analyzed and compared. Besides the experience gathered from the author's practice, and that of numerous friends and correspondents, he has laboriously collected all the scattered information embodied in medical periodicals, reports of learned societies, and other sources; and, examining the whole by the aid of the most recent pathological and anatomical investigations, he has presented a complete and systematic view of the subject in all its bearings.

BY THE SAME AUTHOR. (*Preparing.*)

A SYSTEM OF SURGERY; Diagnostic, Pathological, Therapeutic, and Operative. With very numerous engravings on wood.

GRIFFITH (ROBERT E.), M. D., &c.

A UNIVERSAL FORMULARY, containing the methods of Preparing and Administering Officinal and other Medicines. The whole adapted to Physicians and Pharmaceutists. SECOND EDITION, thoroughly revised, with numerous additions, by ROBERT P. THOMAS, M. D., Professor of Materia Medica in the Philadelphia College of Pharmacy. In one large and handsome octavo volume, of over six hundred pages, double columns. (*Just Issued*.)

It was a work requiring much perseverance, and when published was looked upon as by far the best work of its kind that had issued from the American press, being free of much of the trashy, and embracing most of the non-officinal formulæ used or known in American, English, or French practice, arranged under the heads of the several constituent drugs, placing the receipt under its more important constituent. Prof. Thomas has certainly "improved," as well as added to this Formulary, and has rendered it additionally deserving of the confidence of pharmaceutists and physicians.—*American Journal of Pharmacy*.

We are happy to announce a new and improved edition of this, one of the most valuable and useful works that have emanated from an American pen. It would do credit to any country, and will be found of daily usefulness to practitioners of medicine; it is better adapted to their purposes than the dispensatories.—*Southern Med. and Surg. Journal*.

A new edition of this well-known work, edited by R. P. Thomas, M. D., affords occasion for renewing our commendation of so useful a handbook, which ought to be universally studied by medical men of every class, and made use of by way of reference by office pupils, as a standard authority. It has been much enlarged, and now condenses a vast amount of needful and necessary knowledge in small compass. The more of such books the better for the profession and the public.—*N. Y. Med. Gazette*.

It is one of the most useful books a country practitioner can possibly have in his possession.—*Medical Chronicle*.

The amount of useful, every-day matter, for a practicing physician, is really immense.—*Boston Med. and Surg. Journal*.

This is a work of six hundred and fifty one pages, embracing all on the subject of preparing and administering medicines that can be desired by the physician and pharmaceutist.—*Western Lancet*.

In short, it is a full and complete work of the kind, and should be in the hands of every physician and apothecary.—*O. Med. and Surg. Journal*.

We predict a great sale for this work, and we especially recommend it to all *medical* teachers.—*Richmond Stethoscope*.

This edition of Dr. Griffith's work has been greatly improved by the revision and ample additions of Dr. Thomas, and is now, we believe, one of the most complete works of its kind in any language. The additions amount to about seventy pages, and no effort has been spared to include in them all the recent improvements which have been published in medical journals, and systematic treatises. A work of this kind appears to us indispensable to the physician, and there is none we can more cordially recommend.—*N. Y. Journal of Medicine*.

BY THE SAME AUTHOR.

MEDICAL BOTANY; or, a Description of all the more important Plants used in Medicine, and of their Properties, Uses, and Modes of Administration. In one large octavo volume, of 704 pages, handsomely printed, with nearly 350 illustrations on wood.

GLUGE (GOTTLIEB), M. D.,
Professor of Physiology and Pathological Anatomy in the University of Brussels, &c.

AN ATLAS OF PATHOLOGICAL HISTOLOGY. Translated, with Notes and Additions, by JOSEPH LEIDY, M. D., Professor of Anatomy in the University of Pennsylvania. In one volume, very large imperial quarto, with three hundred and twenty figures, plain and colored, on twelve copperplates.

This being, as far as we know, the only work in which pathological histology is separately treated of in a comprehensive manner, it will, we think, for this reason, be of infinite service to those who desire to investigate the subject systematically, and who have felt the difficulty of arranging in their mind the unconnected observations of a great number of authors. The development of the morbid tissues, and the formation of abnormal products, may now be followed and studied with the same ease and satisfaction as the best arranged system of physiology.—*American Med. Journal*.

GREGORY (WILLIAM), F. R. S. E.,
Professor of Chemistry in the University of Edinburgh, &c.

LETTERS TO A CANDID INQUIRER ON ANIMAL MAGNETISM. In one neat volume, royal 12mo., extra cloth.

GARDNER (D. PEREIRA), M. D.

MEDICAL CHEMISTRY, for the use of Students and the Profession: being a Manual of the Science, with its Applications to Toxicology, Physiology, Therapeutics, Hygiene, &c. In one handsome royal 12mo. volume, with illustrations.

HASSE (C. E.), M. D.

AN ANATOMICAL DESCRIPTION OF THE DISEASES OF RESPIRATION AND CIRCULATION. Translated and Edited by SWAINE. In one volume, octavo.

HARRISON (JOHN), M. D.

AN ESSAY TOWARDS A CORRECT THEORY OF THE NERVOUS SYSTEM. In one octavo volume, 292 pages.

HUNTER (JOHN).

TREATISE ON THE VENEREAL DISEASE. With copious Additions, by DR. PH. RICORD, Surgeon to the Venereal Hospital of Paris. Edited, with additional Notes, by F. J. BUMSTEAD, M. D. In one octavo volume, with plates. (*Now Ready*.) ☞ See RICORD.

ALSO, HUNTER'S COMPLETE WORKS, with Memoir, Notes, &c. &c. In four neat octavo volumes, with plates.

HUGHES (H. M.), M. D.,
Assistant Physician to Guy's Hospital, &c.

A CLINICAL INTRODUCTION TO THE PRACTICE OF AUSCULTATION, and other Modes of Physical Diagnosis, in Diseases of the Lungs and Heart. Second American from the Second and Improved London Edition. In one royal 12mo. vol. (*Now Ready*.)

It has been carefully revised throughout. Some small portions have been erased; much has been, I trust, amended; and a great deal of new matter has been added; so that, though fundamentally it is the same book, it is in many respects a new work.—*Preface*.

HORNER (WILLIAM E.), M. D.,
Professor of Anatomy in the University of Pennsylvania.

SPECIAL ANATOMY AND HISTOLOGY. Eighth edition. Extensively revised and modified. In two large octavo volumes, of more than one thousand pages, handsomely printed, with over three hundred illustrations.

This work has enjoyed a thorough and laborious revision on the part of the author, with the view of bringing it fully up to the existing state of knowledge on the subject of general and special anatomy. To adapt it more perfectly to the wants of the student, he has introduced a large number of additional wood-engravings, illustrative of the objects described, while the publishers have endeavored to render the mechanical execution of the work worthy of the extended reputation which it has acquired. The demand which has carried it to an EIGHTH EDITION is a sufficient evidence of the value of the work, and of its adaptation to the wants of the student and professional reader.

HOBLYN (RICHARD D.), A. M.

A DICTIONARY OF THE TERMS USED IN MEDICINE AND THE COLLATERAL SCIENCES. Second and Improved American Edition. Revised, with numerous Additions, from the second London edition, by ISAAC HAYS, M. D., &c. In one large royal 12mo. volume, of over four hundred pages, double columns. (*Nearly Ready*.)

In passing this work a second time through the press, the editor has subjected it to a very thorough revision, making such additions as the progress of science has rendered desirable, and supplying any omissions that may have previously existed. As a concise and convenient Dictionary of Medical Terms, at an exceedingly low price, it will therefore be found of great value to the student and practitioner.

HOPE (J.), M. D., F. R. S., &c.

A TREATISE ON THE DISEASES OF THE HEART AND GREAT VESSELS. Edited by PENNOCK. In one volume, octavo, with plates, 572 pages.

JONES (C. HANDFIELD), F. R. S., & EDWARD H. SIEVEKING, M.D.,
Assistant Physicians and Lecturers in St. Mary's Hospital, London.

A MANUAL OF PATHOLOGICAL ANATOMY. First American Edition, Revised. With three hundred and ninety-seven handsome wood engravings. In one large and beautiful octavo volume of nearly seven hundred and fifty pages.

In a work like the present, intended as a text-book for the student of pathology, accurate engravings of the various results of morbid action are of the greatest assistance. The American publishers have, therefore, considered that the value of the work might be enhanced by increasing the number of illustrations, and, with this object, many wood-cuts, from the best authorities, have been introduced, increasing the number from one hundred and sixty-seven, in the London Edition, to three hundred and ninety-seven in this. The selection of these wood-cuts has been made by a competent member of the profession, who has supervised the progress of the work through the press, with the view of securing an accurate reprint, and of correcting such errors as had escaped the attention of the authors.

With these improvements, the volume is therefore presented in the hope of supplying the acknowledged want of a work which, within a moderate compass, should embody a condensed and accurate digest of the present state of pathological science, as extended by recent microscopical, chemical, and physiological researches.

A comprehensive English work on pathological anatomy has long been a desideratum in medical literature. The progress of pathological science has been so rapid, and the contributions of pathologists have been so numerous, that the learner has been compelled to resort to various books in different languages, and to monographs on special subjects, in order to become acquainted with the morbid affections of the human body. The present work fills up in a great measure the deficiency which has hitherto existed, and Drs. Jones and Sieveking deserve great credit for the manner in which they have performed their task. They have availed themselves of the best existing sources of information, and they have confirmed or contested the conclusions of preceding authors by observations made by themselves. The book is also abundantly illustrated by well-executed wood-engravings, many of which are drawn from specimens examined by the authors.—*Med. Times and Gazette*.

JONES (T. WHARTON), F. R. S., &c.

THE PRINCIPLES AND PRACTICE OF OPHTHALMIC MEDICINE AND SURGERY. Edited by ISAAC HAYS, M. D., &c. In one very neat volume, large royal 12mo., of 529 pages, with four plates, plain or colored, and ninety-eight wood-cuts.

The work amply sustains, in every point the already high reputation of the author as an ophthalmic surgeon as well as a physiologist and pathologist. The book is evidently the result of much labor and research, and has been written with the greatest care and attention. We entertain little doubt that this book will become what its author hoped it might become, a manual for daily reference and consultation by the student and the general practitioner. The work is marked by that correctness, clearness, and precision of style which distinguish all the productions of the learned author.—*British and Foreign Medical Review*.

KIRKES (WILLIAM SENHOUSE), M. D.,
Demonstrator of Morbid Anatomy at St. Bartholomew's Hospital, &c.; and

JAMES PAGET, F. R. S.,
Lecturer on General Anatomy and Physiology in St. Bartholomew's Hospital.

A MANUAL OF PHYSIOLOGY. Second American, from the second and improved London edition. With one hundred and sixty-five illustrations. In one large and handsome royal 12mo. volume. pp. 550. (*Just Issued.*)

In the present edition, the Manual of Physiology has been brought up to the actual condition of the science, and fully sustains the reputation which it has already so deservedly attained. We consider the work of MM. Kirkes and Paget to constitute one of the very best handbooks of Physiology we possess—presenting just such an outline of the science, comprising an account of its leading facts and generally admitted principles, as the student requires during his attendance upon a course of lectures, or for reference whilst preparing for examination. The text is fully and ably illustrated by a series of very superior wood-engravings, by which a comprehension of some of the more intricate of the subjects treated of is greatly facilitated.—*Am. Medical Journal.*

We need only say, that, without entering into discussions of unsettled questions, it contains all the recent improvements in this department of medical science. For the student beginning this study, and the practitioner who has but leisure to refresh his memory, this book is invaluable, as it contains all that it is important to know, without special detail, which are read with interest only by those who would make a specialty, or desire to possess a critical knowledge of the subject.—*Charleston Medical Journal.*

One of the best treatises that can be put into the hands of the student.—*London Medical Gazette.*

The general favor with which the first edition of this work was received, and its adoption as a favorite text-book by many of our colleges, will insure a large circulation to this improved edition. It will fully meet the wants of the student.—*Southern Med. and Surg. Journal.*

Particularly adapted to those who desire to possess a concise digest of the facts of Human Physiology.—*British and Foreign Med.-Chirurg. Review.*

We conscientiously recommend it as an admirable "Handbook of Physiology."—*London Journal of Medicine.*

KNAPP (F.), PH. D., &c.

TECHNOLOGY; or, Chemistry applied to the Arts and to Manufactures. Edited with numerous Notes and Additions, by Dr. EDMUND RONALDS and Dr. THOMAS RICHARDSON. First American edition, with Notes and Additions, by Prof. WALTER R. JOHNSON. In two handsome octavo volumes, printed and illustrated in the highest style of art, with about five hundred wood-engravings.

LEHMANN.

PHYSIOLOGICAL CHEMISTRY. Translated by GEORGE E. DAY, M. D. (*Preparing.*)

LEE (ROBERT), M. D., F. R. S., &c.

CLINICAL MIDWIFERY; comprising the Histories of Five Hundred and Forty-five Cases of Difficult, Preternatural, and Complicated Labor, with Commentaries. From the second London edition. In one royal 12mo. volume, extra cloth, of 238 pages.

LA ROCHE (R.), M. D., &c.

PNEUMONIA; its Supposed Connection, Pathological and Etiological, with Autumnal Fevers, including an Inquiry into the Existence and Morbid Agency of Malaria. In one handsome octavo volume, extra cloth, of 500 pages.

A more simple, clear, and forcible exposition of the groundless nature and dangerous tendency of certain pathological and etiological heresies, has seldom been presented to our notice.—*N. Y. Journal of Medicine and Collateral Science*, March, 1854.

This work should be carefully studied by Southern physicians, embodying as it does the reflections of an original thinker and close observer on a subject peculiarly their own.—*Virginia Med. and Surgical Journal.*

The author had prepared us to expect a treatise from him, by his brief papers on kindred topics in the periodical press, and yet in the work before us he has exhibited an amount of industry and learning, research and ability, beyond what we are accustomed to discover in modern medical writers; while his own extensive opportunities for observation and experience have been improved by the most laudable diligence, and display a familiarity with the whole subject in every aspect, which commends both respect and confidence. As a corrective of prevalent and mischievous error, sought to be propagated, novices and innovators, we could wish that Dr. La Roche's book could be widely read.—*N. Y. Medical Gazette.*

BY THE SAME AUTHOR. (*In Press.*)

YELLOW FEVER, considered in its Historical, Pathological, and Etiological Relations. In one very large and handsome octavo volume.

LONGET (F. A.)

TREATISE ON PHYSIOLOGY. With numerous Illustrations. Translated from the French by F. G. SMITH, M. D., Professor of Institutes of Medicine in the Pennsylvania Medical College. (*Preparing.*)

LAWRENCE (W.), F. R. S., &c.

A TREATISE ON DISEASES OF THE EYE. A new edition, edited, with numerous additions, and 243 illustrations, by ISAAC HAYS, M. D., Surgeon to Wills Hospital, &c. In one very large and handsome octavo volume, of 950 pages, strongly bound in leather with raised bands. (*Now Ready*.)

This work is thoroughly revised and brought up to 1854.

This work is so universally recognized as the standard authority on the subject, that the publishers in presenting this new edition have only to remark that in its preparation the editor has carefully revised every portion, introducing additions and illustrations wherever the advance of science has rendered them necessary or desirable. In this manner it will be found to contain over one hundred pages more than the last edition, while the list of wood-engravings has been increased by sixty-seven figures, besides numerous improved illustrations substituted for such as were deemed imperfect or unsatisfactory. The various important contributions to ophthalmological science, recently made by Dalrymple, Jacob, Walton, Wilde, Cooper, &c., both in the form of separate treatises and contributions to periodicals, have been carefully examined by the editor, and, combined with the results of his own experience, have been freely introduced throughout the volume, rendering it a complete and thorough exponent of the most advanced state of the subject.

In a future number we shall notice more at length this admirable treatise—the safest guide and most comprehensive work of reference, which is within the reach of all classes of the profession.—*Stethoscope*, March, 1854.

This standard text-book on the department of which it treats, has not been superseded, by any or all of the numerous publications on the subject heretofore issued. Nor with the multiplied improvements of Dr. Hays, the American editor, is it at all likely that this great work will cease to merit the confidence and preference of students or practitioners. Its ample extent—nearly one thousand large octavo pages—has enabled both author and editor to do justice to all the details of this subject, and condense in this single volume the present state of our knowledge of the whole science in this department, whereby its practical value cannot be excelled. We heartily commend it, especially as a book of reference, indispensable in every medical library. The additions of the American editor very greatly enhance the value of the work, exhibiting the learning and experience of Dr. Hays, in the light in which he ought to be held, as a standard authority on all subjects appertaining to this specialty, to which he has rendered so many valuable contributions.—*N. Y. Medical Gazette*.

BY THE SAME AUTHOR.

A TREATISE ON RUPTURES; from the fifth London edition. In one octavo volume, sheep, 480 pages.

LUDLOW (J. L.), M. D.,
Lecturer on Clinical Medicine at the Philadelphia Almshouse, &c.

A MANUAL OF EXAMINATIONS upon Anatomy and Physiology, Surgery, Practice of Medicine, Chemistry, Obstetrics, Materia Medica, Pharmacy, and Therapeutics. Designed for Students of Medicine throughout the United States. A new edition, revised and extensively improved. In one large royal 12mo. volume, with several hundred illustrations. (*Preparing*.)

LISTON (ROBERT), F. R. S., &c.

LECTURES ON THE OPERATIONS OF SURGERY, and on Diseases and Accidents requiring Operations. Edited, with numerous Additions and Alterations, by T. D. MÜTTER, M. D. In one large and handsome octavo volume, of 566 pages, with 216 wood-cuts.

LALLEMAND (M.).

THE CAUSES, SYMPTOMS, AND TREATMENT OF SPERMATORRHŒA. Translated and edited by HENRY J. McDOUGAL. In one volume, octavo, 320 pages. Second American edition. (*Just Issued*.)

LARDNER (DIONYSIUS), D. C. L., &c.

HANDBOOKS OF NATURAL PHILOSOPHY AND ASTRONOMY. Revised, with numerous Additions, by the American editor. FIRST COURSE, containing Mechanics, Hydrostatics, Hydraulics, Pneumatics, Sound. and Optics. In one large royal 12mo. volume, of 750 pages, with 424 wood-cuts. SECOND COURSE, containing Heat, Electricity, Magnetism, and Galvanism, one volume, large royal 12mo. of 450 pages, with 250 illustrations. THIRD COURSE (*now ready*), containing Meteorology and Astronomy, in one large volume, royal 12mo. of nearly eight hundred pages, with thirty-seven plates and two hundred wood-cuts. The whole complete in three volumes, of about two thousand large pages, with over one thousand figures on steel and wood.

The various sciences treated in this work will be found brought thoroughly up to the latest period.

The work furnishes a very clear and satisfactory account of our knowledge in the important department of science of which it treats. Although the medical schools of this country do not include the study of physics in their course of instruction, yet no student or practitioner should be ignorant of its laws. Besides being of constant application in practice, such knowledge is of inestimable utility in facilitating the study of other branches of science. To students, then, and to those who, having already entered upon the active pursuits of business, are desirous to sustain and improve their knowledge of the general truths of natural philosophy, we can recommend this work as supplying in a clear and satisfactory manner the information they desire.—*The Virginia Med. and Surg. Journal*.

The present treatise is a most complete digest of all that has been developed in relation to the great forces of nature, Heat, Magnetism, and Electricity. Their laws are elucidated in a manner both pleasing and familiar, and at the same time perfectly intelligible to the student. The illustrations are sufficiently numerous and appropriate, and altogether we can cordially recommend the work as well-deserving the notice both of the practising physician and the student of medicine.—*The Med. Examiner*.

MEIGS (CHARLES D.), M. D.,
Professor of Obstetrics, &c. in the Jefferson Medical College, Philadelphia.

ON THE NATURE, SIGNS, AND TREATMENT OF CHILDBED
FEVER. In a Series of Letters addressed to the Students of his Class. In one handsome octavo volume, of three hundred and sixty-five pages. (*Now Ready.*)

The instructive and interesting author of this work, whose previous labors in the department of medicine which he so sedulously cultivates, have placed his countrymen under deep and abiding obligations, again challenges their admiration in the fresh and vigorous, attractive and racy pages before us. It is a delectable book. * * * This treatise upon child-bed fevers will have an extensive sale, being destined, as it deserves, to find a place in the library of every practitioner who scorns to lag in the rear of his brethren.—*Nashville Journal of Medicine and Surgery.*

This book will add more to his fame than either of those which bear his name. Indeed we doubt whether any material improvement will be made in the teachings of this volume for a century to come, since it is so eminently practical, and based on a profound knowledge of the *science* and consummate skill in the *art* of healing, and ratified by an intense and extensive experience, such as few men have the industry or good fortune to acquire.—*N. Y. Med. Gazette.*

BY THE SAME AUTHOR.

WOMAN: HER DISEASES AND THEIR REMEDIES. A Series of Lectures to his Class. Third and Improved edition. In one large and beautifully printed octavo volume. (*Just Issued. Revised and enlarged to 1854.*)

The gratifying appreciation of his labors, as evinced by the exhaustion of two large impressions of this work within a few years, has not been lost upon the author, who has endeavored in every way to render it worthy of the favor with which it has been received. The opportunity thus afforded for a second revision has been improved, and the work is now presented as in every way superior to its predecessors, additions and alterations having been made whenever the advance of science has rendered them desirable. The typographical execution of the work will also be found to have undergone a similar improvement and the work is now confidently presented as in every way worthy the position it has acquired as the standard American text-book on the Diseases of Females.

It contains a vast amount of practical knowledge, by one who has accurately observed and retained the experience of many years, and who tells the result in a free, familiar, and pleasant manner.—*Dublin Quarterly Journal.*

There is an off-hand fervor, a glow, and a warm-heartedness infecting the effort of Dr. Meigs, which is entirely captivating, and which absolutely hurries the reader through from beginning to end. Besides, the book teems with solid instruction, and it shows the very highest evidence of ability, viz., the clearness with which the information is presented. We know of no better test of one's understanding a subject than the evidence of the power of lucidly explaining it. The most elementary, as well as the obscurest subjects, under the pencil of Prof. Meigs, are isolated and made to stand out in such bold relief, as to produce distinct impressions upon the mind and memory of the reader.—*Charleston Med. Journal.*

Professor Meigs has enlarged and amended his great work, for such it unquestionably is, has it passed the ordeal of criticism at home and abroad, but been improved thereby; for in this new edition the author has introduced real improvements, and increased the value and utility of the book very measurably. It presents so many novel, bold, and sparkling thoughts; such an exuberance of new ideas on almost every page, that we confess ourselves to have become enamored with the book and its author; and cannot withhold our congratulations from our Philadelphia confreres, that so able a teacher is in their service.—*N. Y. Med. Gazette.*

BY THE SAME AUTHOR.

OBSTETRICS: THE SCIENCE AND THE ART. Second edition, revised and improved. With one hundred and thirty-one illustrations. In one beautifully printed octavo volume, of seven hundred and fifty-two large pages. (*Lately Published.*)

The rapid demand for a second edition of this work is a sufficient evidence that it has supplied a desideratum of the profession, notwithstanding the numerous treatises on the same subject which have appeared within the last few years. Adopting a system of his own, the author has combined the leading principles of his interesting and difficult subject, with a thorough exposition of its rules of practice, presenting the results of long and extensive experience and of familiar acquaintance with all the modern writers on this department of medicine. As an American Treatise on Midwifery, which has at once assumed the position of a classic, it possesses peculiar claims to the attention and study of the practitioner and student, while the numerous alterations and revisions which it has undergone in the present edition are shown by the great enlargement of the work, which is not only increased as to the size of the page, but also in the number.

BY THE SAME AUTHOR. (*Now Ready.*)

A TREATISE ON ACUTE AND CHRONIC DISEASES OF THE NECK OF THE UTERUS. With numerous plates, drawn and colored from nature in the highest style of art. In one handsome octavo volume, extra cloth.

The object of the author in this work has been to present in a small compass the practical results of his long experience in this important and distressing class of diseases. The great changes introduced into practice, and the accessions to our knowledge on the subject, within the last few years resulting from the use of the metroscope, brings within the ordinary practice of every physician numerous cases which were formerly regarded as incurable, and renders of great value a work like the present combining practical directions for diagnosis and treatment with an ample series of illustrations, copied accurately from colored drawings made by the author, after nature.

BY THE SAME AUTHOR.

OBSERVATIONS ON CERTAIN OF THE DISEASES OF YOUNG CHILDREN. In one handsome octavo volume, of 214 pages.

MILLER (JAMES), F. R. S. E.,
Professor of Surgery in the University of Edinburgh, &c.

PRINCIPLES OF SURGERY. Third American, from the second and revised Edinburgh edition. Revised, with Additions, by F. W. SARGENT, M. D., author of "Minor Surgery," &c. In one large and very beautiful volume, of seven hundred and fifty-two pages, with two hundred and forty exquisite illustrations on wood.

This edition is far superior, both in the abundance and quality of its material, to any of the preceding. We hope it will be extensively read, and the sound principles which are herein taught treasured up for future application. The work takes rank with Watson's Practice of Physic; it certainly does not fall behind that great work in soundness of principle or depth of reasoning and research. No physician who values his reputation, or seeks the interests of his clients, can acquit himself before his God and the world without making himself familiar with the sound and philosophical views developed in the foregoing book.—*New Orleans Med. and Surg. Journal.*

Without doubt the ablest exposition of the principles of that branch of the healing art in any language. This opinion, deliberately formed after a careful study of the first edition, we have had no cause to change on examining the second. This edition has undergone thorough revision by the author; many expressions have been modified, and a mass of new matter introduced. The book is got up in the finest style, and is an evidence of the progress of typography in our country.—*Charleston Medical Journal and Review.*

We recommend it to both student and practitioner, feeling assured that as it now comes to us, it presents the most satisfactory exposition of the modern doctrines of the principles of surgery to be found in any volume in any language.—*N. Y. Journal of Medicine.*

BY THE SAME AUTHOR. (*Now Ready.*)

THE PRACTICE OF SURGERY. Third American from the second Edinburgh edition. Edited, with Additions, by F. W. SARGENT, M. D., one of the Surgeons to Will's Hospital, &c. Illustrated by three hundred and nineteen engravings on wood. In one large octavo volume, of over seven hundred pages.

No encomium of ours could add to the popularity of Miller's Surgery. Its reputation in this country is unsurpassed by that of any other work, and, when taken in connection with the author's *Principles of Surgery*, constitutes a whole, without reference to which no conscientious surgeon would be willing to practice his art. The additions, by Dr. Sargent, have materially enhanced the value of the work.—*Southern Medical and Surgical Journal.*

It is seldom that two volumes have ever made so profound an impression in so short a time as the "Principles" and the "Practice" of Surgery by Mr. Miller—or so richly merited the reputation they have acquired. The author is an eminently sensible, practical, and well-informed man, who knows exactly what he is talking about and exactly how to talk it.—*Kentucky Medical Recorder.*

The two volumes together form a complete exposé of the present state of Surgery, and they ought to be on the shelves of every surgeon.—*N. J. Med. Reporter.*

By the almost unanimous voice of the profession, his works, both on the principles and practice of surgery have been assigned the highest rank. If we were limited to but one work on surgery, that one should be Miller's, as we regard it superior to all others.—*St. Louis Med. and Surg. Journal.*

The author, distinguished alike as a practitioner and writer, has in this and his "Principles," presented to the profession one of the most complete and reliable systems of Surgery extant. His style of writing is original, impressive, and engaging, energetic, concise, and lucid. Few have the faculty of condensing so much in small space, and at the same time so persistently holding the attention; indeed, he appears to make the very process of condensation a means of eliminating attractions. Whether as a text-book for students or a book of reference for practitioners, it cannot be too strongly recommended.—*Southern Journal of the Medical and Physical Sciences.*

MALGAIGNE (J. F.).

OPERATIVE SURGERY, based on Normal and Pathological Anatomy. Translated from the French, by FREDERICK BRITTAN, A. B., M. D. With numerous illustrations on wood. In one handsome octavo volume, of nearly six hundred pages.

We unhesitatingly pronounce it the very best guide in surgical operations that has come before the profession in any language.—*Charleston Med. and Surg. Journal.*

MOHR (FRANCIS), PH. D., AND REDWOOD (THEOPHILUS).

PRACTICAL PHARMACY. Comprising the Arrangements, Apparatus, and Manipulations of the Pharmaceutical Shop and Laboratory. Edited, with extensive Additions, by Prof. WILLIAM PROCTER, of the Philadelphia College of Pharmacy. In one handsomely printed octavo volume, of 570 pages, with over 500 engravings on wood.

It is a book, however, which will be in the hands of almost every one who is much interested in pharmaceutical operations, as we know of no other publication so well calculated to fill a void long felt.—*Medical Examiner.*

The book is strictly practical, and describes only manipulations or methods of performing the numerous processes the pharmaceutist has to go through, in the preparation and manufacture of medicines, together with all the apparatus and fixtures necessary thereto. On these matters, this work is very full and complete, and details, in a style uncommonly clear and lucid, not only the more complicated and difficult processes, but those not less important ones, the most simple and common.—*Buffalo Medical Journal.*

The country practitioner who is obliged to dispense his own medicines, will find it a most valuable assistant.—*Monthly Journal and Retrospect.*

MACKENSIE (W.), M. D.,
Surgeon Oculist in Scotland in ordinary to Her Majesty, &c. &c.

A PRACTICAL TREATISE ON DISEASES OF THE EYE. To which is prefixed an Anatomical Introduction explanatory of a Horizontal Section of the Human Eyeball. By THOMAS WHARTON JONES, F. R. S. From the Fourth Revised and Enlarged London Edition. With Notes and Additions by ADDINELL HEWSON, M. D., Physician to Wills Hospital, &c. &c. In one very large and handsome octavo volume, with plates and numerous wood-cuts. (*Preparing.*)

The reputation which this work has universally attained will be enhanced by the present edition. Besides the thorough revision by the author which it has enjoyed in recently passing through the press in London, the additions by the editor will embrace whatever is necessary to adapt it completely to the wants of the American practitioner, constituting it a library of Ophthalmic Medicine and Surgery.

MACLISE (JOSEPH), SURGEON.

SURGICAL ANATOMY. Forming one volume, very large imperial quarto. With sixty-eight large and splendid Plates, drawn in the best style and beautifully colored, containing one hundred and ninety Figures, many of them the size of life. Together with ample and explanatory letter-press. Strongly and handsomely bound in extra cloth, being one of the cheapest and best executed Surgical works as yet issued in this country.

Copies can be sent by mail, in five parts, done up in stout covers.

This great work being now concluded, the publishers confidently present it to the attention of the profession as worthy in every respect of their approbation and patronage. No complete work of the kind has yet been published in the English language, and it therefore will supply a want long felt in this country of an accurate and comprehensive Atlas of Surgical Anatomy to which the student and practitioner can at all times refer, to ascertain the exact relative position of the various portions of the human frame towards each other and to the surface, as well as their abnormal deviations. The importance of such a work to the student in the absence of anatomical material, and to the practitioner when about attempting an operation, is evident, while the price of the book, notwithstanding the large size, beauty, and finish of the very numerous illustrations, is so low as to place it within the reach of every member of the profession. The publishers therefore confidently anticipate a very extended circulation for this magnificent work.

One of the greatest artistic triumphs of the age in Surgical Anatomy.—*British American Medical Journal.*

Too much cannot be said in its praise; indeed, we have not language to do it justice.—*Ohio Medical and Surgical Journal.*

The most admirable surgical atlas we have seen. To the practitioner deprived of demonstrative dissections upon the human subject, it is an invaluable companion.—*N. J. Medical Reporter.*

The most accurately engraved and beautifully colored plates we have ever seen in an American book—one of the best and cheapest surgical works ever published.—*Buffalo Medical Journal.*

It is very rare that so elegantly printed, so well illustrated, and so useful a work, is offered at so moderate a price.—*Charleston Medical Journal.*

Its plates can boast a superiority which places them almost beyond the reach of competition.—*Medical Examiner.*

Every practitioner, we think, should have a work of this kind within reach.—*Southern Medical and Surgical Journal.*

No such lithographic illustrations of surgical regions have hitherto, we think, been given.—*Boston Medical and Surgical Journal.*

As a surgical anatomist, Mr. Maclise has probably no superior.—*British and Foreign Medico-Chirurgical Review.*

Of great value to the student engaged in dissecting, and to the surgeon at a distance from the means of keeping up his anatomical knowledge.—*N. Y. Times.*

The mechanical execution cannot be excelled.—*Transylvania Medical Journal.*

A work which has no parallel in point of accuracy and cheapness in the English language.—*N. Y. Journal of Medicine.*

To all engaged in the study or practice of the profession, such a work is almost indispensable.—*Dublin Quarterly Medical Journal.*

No practitioner whose means will admit it, fail to possess it.—*Ranking's Abstract.*

Country practitioners will find these plates of immense value.—*N. Y. Medical Gazette.*

We are extremely gratified to announce to the profession the completion of this truly magnificent work, which, as a whole, certainly stands unrivalled, both for accuracy of drawing, beauty of coloring, and all the requisite explanations on the subject in hand.—*The New Orleans Medical and Surgical Journal.*

This is by far the ablest work on Surgical Anatomy that has come under our observation. We know of no other work that would justify a student, in any degree, for neglect of actual dissection. In those sudden emergencies that may arise, and which require the instantaneous recall of minute anatomical knowledge, a work of this kind keeps the details of the dissecting-room perfectly fresh in the memory.—*The Western Journal of Medicine and Surgery.*

☞ The very low price at which this work is furnished, and the beauty of its execution require an extended sale to compensate the publishers for the heavy expenses incurred.

MULLER (PROFESSOR J.), M. D.

PRINCIPLES OF PHYSICS AND METEOROLOGY. Edited, with additions, by R. EGLESFELD GRIFFITH, M. D. In one large and handsome octavo volume, extra cloth, with 550 wood-cuts, and two colored plates.

The Physics of Müller is a work superb, complete, unique: the greatest want known to English Science could not have been better supplied. The work is of surpassing interest. The value of this contribution to the scientific records of this country may be duly estimated by the fact that the cost of the original drawings and engravings alone has exceeded the sum of £2,000.—*Lancet.*

MAYNE (JOHN), M. D., M. R. C. S.

A DISPENSATORY AND THERAPEUTICAL REMEMBRANCER. Comprising the entire lists of Materia Medica, with every Practical Formula contained in the British Pharmacopœias. With relative Tables subjoined, illustrating, by upwards of six hundred and sixty examples, the Extemporaneous Forms and Combinations suitable for the different Medicines. Edited, with the addition of the Formulæ of the United States Pharmacopœia, by R. EGLESFELD GRIFFITH, M. D. In one 12mo. volume, extra cloth, of over 300 large pages.

MATTEUCCI (CARLO).

LECTURES ON THE PHYSICAL PHENOMENA OF LIVING BEINGS. Edited by J. PEREIRA, M. D. In one neat royal 12mo. volume, extra cloth, with cuts, 388 pages.

NEILL (JOHN), M. D.,
Surgeon to the Pennsylvania Hospital, &c.; and
FRANCIS GURNEY SMITH, M. D.,
Professor of Institutes of Medicine in the Pennsylvania Medical College.

AN ANALYTICAL COMPENDIUM OF THE VARIOUS BRANCHES OF MEDICAL SCIENCE; for the Use and Examination of Students. Second edition, revised and improved. In one very large and handsomely printed royal 12mo. volume, of over one thousand pages, with three hundred and fifty illustrations on wood. Strongly bound in leather, with raised bands.

The speedy sale of a large impression of this work has afforded to the authors gratifying evidence of the correctness of the views which actuated them in its preparation. In meeting the demand for a second edition, they have therefore been desirous to render it more worthy of the favor with which it has been received. To accomplish this, they have spared neither time nor labor in embodying in it such discoveries and improvements as have been made since its first appearance, and such alterations as have been suggested by its practical use in the class and examination-room. Considerable modifications have thus been introduced throughout all the departments treated of in the volume, but more especially in the portion devoted to the "Practice of Medicine," which has been entirely rearranged and rewritten. The authors therefore again submit their work to the profession, with the hope that their efforts may tend, however humbly, to advance the great cause of medical education.

Notwithstanding the enlarged size and improved execution of this work, the price has not been increased, and it is confidently presented as one of the cheapest volumes now before the profession.

In the rapid course of lectures, where work for the students is heavy, and review necessary for an examination, a compend is not only valuable, but it is almost a sine qua non. The one before us is, in most of the divisions, the most unexceptionable of all books of the kind that we know of. The newest and soundest doctrines and the latest improvements and discoveries are explicitly, though concisely, laid before the student. Of course it is useless for us to recommend it to all last course students, but there is a class to whom we very sincerely commend this cheap book as worth its weight in silver—that class is the graduates in medicine of more than ten years' standing, who have not studied medicine since. They will perhaps find out from it that the science is not exactly now what it was when they left it off.—*The Stethoscope*

Having made free use of this volume in our examinations of pupils, we can speak from experience in recommending it as an admirable compend for students, and as especially useful to preceptors who examine their pupils. It will save the teacher much labor by enabling him readily to recall all of the points upon which his pupils should be examined. A work of this sort should be in the hands of every one who takes pupils into his office with a view of examining them; and this is unquestionably the best of its class. Let every practitioner who has pupils provide himself with it, and he will find the labor of refreshing his knowledge so much facilitated that he will be able to do justice to his pupils at very little cost of time or trouble to himself.—*Transylvania Med. Journal.*

NELIGAN (J. MOORE), M. D., M. R. I. A., &c.

A PRACTICAL TREATISE ON DISEASES OF THE SKIN. In one neat royal 12mo. volume, of 334 pages.

OWEN (PROF. R.),
Author of "Lectures on Comparative Anatomy," "Archetype of the Skeleton," &c.

ON THE DIFFERENT FORMS OF THE SKELETON, AND OF THE TEETH. One vol. royal 12mo., with numerous illustrations. (*Now Ready.*)

The name of the distinguished author is a sufficient guarantee that this little volume will prove a satisfactory manual and guide to all students of Comparative Anatomy and Osteology. The importance of this subject in geological investigations will also render this work a most valuable assistant to those interested in that science.

PHILLIPS (BENJAMIN), F. R. S., &c.

SCROFULA; its Nature, its Prevalence, its Causes, and the Principles of its Treatment. In one volume, octavo, with a plate.

PANCOAST (J.), M. D.,
Professor of Anatomy in the Jefferson Medical College, Philadelphia, &c.

OPERATIVE SURGERY; or, A Description and Demonstration of the various Processes of the Art; including all the New Operations, and exhibiting the State of Surgical Science in its present advanced condition. Complete in one royal 4to. volume, of 380 pages of letter-press description and eighty large 4to. plates, comprising 486 illustrations. Second edition, improved.

Blanchard & Lea having become the publishers of this important book, have much pleasure in offering it to the profession.

This excellent work is constructed on the model of the French Surgical Works by Velpeau and Malgaigne; and, so far as the English language is concerned, we are proud as an American to say that, OF ITS KIND IT HAS NO SUPERIOR.—*N. Y. Journal of Medicine.*

PARKER (LANGSTON),
Surgeon to the Queen's Hospital, Birmingham.

THE MODERN TREATMENT OF SYPHILITIC DISEASES, BOTH PRIMARY AND SECONDARY; comprising the Treatment of Constitutional and Confirmed Syphilis, by a safe and successful method. With numerous Cases, Formulæ, and Clinical Observations. From the Third and entirely rewritten London edition. In one neat octavo volume. (*Now Ready.*)

(*Now Complete.*)
PEREIRA (JONATHAN), M. D., F. R. S., AND L. S.

THE ELEMENTS OF MATERIA MEDICA AND THERAPEUTICS.

Third American edition, enlarged and improved by the author; including Notices of most of the Medicinal Substances in use in the civilized world, and forming an Encyclopædia of Materia Medica. Edited, with Additions, by JOSEPH CARSON, M. D., Professor of Materia Medica and Pharmacy in the University of Pennsylvania. In two very large octavo volumes of 2100 pages, on small type, with over four hundred and fifty illustrations.

VOLUME I.—Lately issued, containing the Inorganic Materia Medica, over 800 pages, with 15 illustrations.

VOLUME II.—Now ready, embraces the Organic Materia Medica, and forms a very large octavo volume of 1250 pages, with two plates and three hundred handsome wood-cuts.

The present edition of this valuable and standard work will enhance in every respect its well-deserved reputation. The care bestowed upon its revision by the author may be estimated by the fact that its size has been increased by about five hundred pages. These additions have extended to every portion of the work, and embrace not only the materials afforded by the recent editions of the pharmacopœias, but also all the important information accessible to the care and industry of the author in treatises, essays, memoirs, monographs, and from correspondents in various parts of the globe. In this manner the work comprises the most recent and reliable information respecting all the articles of the Materia Medica, their natural and commercial history, chemical and therapeutical properties, preparation, uses, doses, and modes of administration, brought up to the present time, with a completeness not to be met with elsewhere. A considerable portion of the work which preceded the remainder in London, has also enjoyed the advantage of a further revision by the author expressly for this country, and in addition to this the editor, Professor Carson, has made whatever additions appeared desirable to adapt it thoroughly to the U. S. Pharmacopœia, and to the wants of the American profession. An equal improvement will likewise be observable in every department of its mechanical execution. It is printed from new type, on good white paper, with a greatly extended and improved series of illustrations.

Gentlemen who have the first volume are recommended to complete their copies without delay. The first volume will no longer be sold separate.

When we remember that Philology, Natural History, Botany, Chemistry, Physics, and the Microscope, are all brought forward to elucidate the subject, one cannot fail to see that the reader has here a work worthy of the name of an encyclopedia of Materia Medica. Our own opinion of its merits is that of its editors, and also that of the whole profession, both of this and foreign countries—namely, " that in copiousness of details, in extent, variety, and accuracy of information, and in lucid explanation of difficult and recondite subjects, it surpasses all other works on Materia Medica hitherto published." We cannot close this notice without alluding to the special additions of the American editor, which pertain to the prominent vegetable productions of this country, and to the directions of the United States Pharmacopœia, in connection with all the articles contained in the volume which are referred to by it. The illustrations have been increased, and this edition by Dr. Carson cannot well be regarded in any other light than that of a treasure which should be found in the library of every physician.—*New York Journal of Medical and Collateral Science*, March, 1854.

The third edition of his "Elements of Materia Medica, although completed under the supervision of others, is by far the most elaborate treatise in the English language, and will, while medical literature is cherished, continue a monument alike honorable to his genius, as to his learning and industry.—*American Journal of Pharmacy*, March, 1854.

The work, in its present shape, and so far as we be judged from the portion before the public, forms the most comprehensive and complete treatise on materia medica extant in the English language. Dr. Pereira has been at great pains to instruct into his work, not only all the information on the natural, chemical, and commercial history of medicines, which might be serviceable to the physician and surgeon, but whatever might enable his readers to understand thoroughly the mode of preparing and manufacturing various articles employed either for preparing medicines, or for certain purposes in the arts connected with materia medica and the practice of medicine. The accounts of the physiological and therapeutic effects of remedies are given with great clearness and accuracy, and in a manner calculated to interest as well as instruct the reader.—*The Edinburgh Medical and Surgical Journal*.

PEASLEE (E. R.), M. D.,
Professor of Anatomy and Physiology in Dartmouth College, &c.

HUMAN HISTOLOGY, in its applications to Physiology and General Pathology;
designed as a Text-Book for Medical Students. With numerous illustrations. In one handsome royal 12mo. volume. (*Preparing.*)

The subject of this work is one, the growing importance of which, as the basis of Anatomy and Physiology, demands for it a separate volume. The book will therefore supply an acknowledged deficiency in medical text-books, while the name of the author, and his experience as a teacher for the last thirteen years, is a guarantee that it will be thoroughly adapted to the use of the student.

PIRRIE (WILLIAM), F. R. S. E.,
Professor of Surgery in the University of Aberdeen.

THE PRINCIPLES AND PRACTICE OF SURGERY. Edited by JOHN
NEILL, M. D., Demonstrator of Anatomy in the University of Pennsylvania, Surgeon to the Pennsylvania Hospital, &c. In one very handsome octavo volume, of 780 pages, with 316 illustrations. (*Just Issued.*)

We know of no other surgical work of a reasonable size, wherein there is so much theory and practice, or where subjects are more soundly or clearly taught.—*The Stethoscope*.

There is scarcely a disease of the bone or soft parts, fracture, or dislocation, that is not illustrated by accurate wood-engravings. Then, again, every instrument employed by the surgeon is thus represented. These engravings are not only correct, but really beautiful, showing the astonishing degree of perfection to which the art of wood-engraving has arrived. Prof. Pirrie, in the work before us, has elaborately discussed the principles of surgery, in a safe and effectual practice predicated upon them. Perhaps no work upon this subject heretofore issued is so full upon the science of the art of surgery.—*Nashville Journal of Medicine and Surgery*.

One of the best treatises on surgery in the English language.—*Canada Med. Journal*.

Our impression is, that, as a manual for students, Pirrie's is the best work extant.—*Western Med. and Surg. Journal*.

RAMSBOTHAM (FRANCIS H.), M.D.

THE PRINCIPLES AND PRACTICE OF OBSTETRIC MEDICINE AND SURGERY, in reference to the Process of Parturition. A new and enlarged edition, thoroughly revised by the Author. With Additions by W. V. KEATING, M. D. In one large and handsome imperial octavo volume, with sixty-four beautiful Plates, and numerous Wood-cuts in the text, containing in all nearly two hundred large and beautiful figures. (*Now Ready.*)

In calling the attention of the profession to the new edition of this standard work, the publishers would remark that no efforts have been spared to secure for it a continuance and extension of the remarkable favor with which it has been received. The last London issue, which was considerably enlarged, has received a further revision from the author, especially for this country. Its passage through the press here has been supervised by Dr. Keating, who has made numerous additions with a view of presenting more fully whatever was necessary to adapt it thoroughly to American modes of practice. In its mechanical execution, a like superiority over former editions will be found. The plates have all been re-engraved in a new and beautiful style; many additional illustrations have been introduced, and in every point of typographical finish it will be found one of the handsomest issues of the American press. In its present improved and enlarged form the publishers therefore confidently ask for it a place in every medical library, as a text-book for the student, or a manual for daily reference by the practitioner.

From Prof. Hodge, of the University of Pa.
To the American public, it is most valuable, from its intrinsic undoubted excellence, and as being the best authorized exponent of British Midwifery. Its circulation will, I trust, be extensive throughout our country.

We recommend the student who desires to master this difficult subject with the least possible trouble, to possess himself at once of a copy of this work.—*American Journal of the Med. Sciences.*

It stands at the head of the long list of excellent obstetric works published in the last few years in Great Britain, Ireland, and the Continent of Europe. We consider this book indispensable to the library of every physician engaged in the practice of midwifery.—*Southern Med. and Surg. Journal.*

When the whole profession is thus unanimous in placing such a work in the very first rank as regards the extent and correctness of all the details of the theory and practice of so important a branch of learning, our commendation or condemnation would be of little consequence; but regarding it as the most useful of all works of the kind, we think it but an act of justice to urge its claims upon the profession.—*N. O. Med. Journal.*

RICORD (P.), M. D.,
Surgeon to the Hôpital du Midi, Paris, &c.

ILLUSTRATIONS OF SYPHILITIC DISEASE. Translated from the French, by THOMAS F. BETTON, M. D. With the addition of a History of Syphilis, and a complete Bibliography and Formulary of Remedies, collated and arranged, by PAUL B. GODDARD, M. D. With fifty large quarto plates, comprising one hundred and seventeen beautifully colored illustrations. In one large and handsome quarto volume.

BY THE SAME AUTHOR. (*Now Ready.*)

A TREATISE ON THE VENEREAL DISEASE. By JOHN HUNTER, F. R. S. With copious Additions, by PH. RICORD, M. D. Edited, with Notes, by FREEMAN J. BUMSTEAD, M. D. In one handsome octavo volume, with plates.

Every one will recognize the attractiveness and value which this work derives from thus presenting the opinions of these two masters side by side. But, it must be admitted, what has made the fortune of the book, is the fact that it contains the "most complete embodiment of the veritable doctrines of the Hôpital du Midi," which has ever been made public. The doctrinal ideas of M. Ricord, ideas which, if not universally adopted, are incontestably dominant, have heretofore only been interpreted by more or less skilful secretaries, sometimes accredited and sometimes not.

In the notes to Hunter, the master substitutes himself for his interpreters, and gives his original thoughts to the world, in a summary form it is true, but in a lucid and perfectly intelligible manner. In conclusion we can say that this is incontestably the best treatise on syphilis with which we are acquainted, and, as we do not often employ the phrase, we may be excused for expressing the hope that it may find a place in the library of every physician —*Virginia Med. and Surg Journal.*

BY THE SAME AUTHOR.

LETTERS ON SYPHILIS, addressed to the Chief Editor of the Union Médicale. With an Introduction, by Amédée Latour. Translated by W. P. Lattimore, M. D. In one neat octavo volume.

Blanchard & Lea are now the publishers of this valuable work.

From the Translator's Preface.
To those who have listened to the able and interesting lectures of our author at the Hôpital du Midi, this volume will need no commendation; while to those who have not had the pleasure to which we allude, the book will commend itself by the truths it contains, told as they are in the same inimitable style in which M. Ricord delivers his clinical lectures.

BY THE SAME AUTHOR.

A PRACTICAL TREATISE ON VENEREAL DISEASES. With a Therapeutical Summary and Special Formulary. Translated by SIDNEY DOANE, M. D. Fourth edition. One volume, octavo, 340 pages.

RIGBY (EDWARD), M. D.,
Physician to the General Lying-in Hospital, &c.

A SYSTEM OF MIDWIFERY. With Notes and Additional Illustrations. Second American Edition. One volume octavo, 422 pages.

ROYLE (J. FORBES), M. D.

MATERIA MEDICA AND THERAPEUTICS; including the Preparations of the Pharmacopœias of London, Edinburgh, Dublin, and of the United States. With many new medicines. Edited by JOSEPH CARSON, M. D., Professor of Materia Medica and Pharmacy in the University of Pennsylvania. With ninety-eight illustrations. In one large octavo volume of about seven hundred pages.

This work is, indeed, a most valuable one, and will fill up an important vacancy that existed between Dr. Pereira's most learned and complete system of Materia Medica, and the class of productions on the other extreme, which are necessarily imperfect from their small extent.—*Brit. and Foreign Medical Review.*

SKEY (FREDERICK C.), F. R. S., &c.

OPERATIVE SURGERY. In one very handsome octavo volume of over 650 pages, with about one hundred wood-cuts.

Its literary execution is superior to most surgical treatises. It abounds in excellent moral hints, and is replete with original surgical expedients and suggestions.—*Buffalo Med. and Surg. Journal.*

With high talents, extensive practice, and a long experience, Mr. Skey is perhaps competent to the task of writing a complete work on operative surgery.—*Charleston Med. Journal.*

We cannot withhold from this work our highest recommendation. Students and practitioners will find it an invaluable teacher and guide upon every topic connected with this department.—*N. Y. Medical Gazette.*

A work of the very highest importance—a work by itself.—*London Med. Gazette.*

SHARPEY (WILLIAM), M. D., JONES QUAIN, M. D., AND RICHARD QUAIN, F. R. S., &c.

HUMAN ANATOMY. Revised, with Notes and Additions, by JOSEPH LEIDY, M. D. Complete in two large octavo volumes, of about thirteen hundred pages. Beautifully illustrated with over five hundred engravings on wood.

It is indeed a work calculated to make an era in anatomical study, by placing before the student every department of his science, with a view to the relative importance of each; and so skilfully have the different parts been interwoven, that no one who makes this work the basis of his studies, will hereafter have any excuse for neglecting or undervaluing any important particulars connected with the structure of the human frame; and whether the bias of his mind lead him in a more especial manner to surgery, physic, or physiology, he will find here a work at once so comprehensive and practical as to defend him from exclusiveness on the one hand, and pedantry on the other.—*Monthly Journal and Retrospect of the Medical Sciences.*

We have no hesitation in recommending this treatise on anatomy as the most complete on that subject in the English language; and the only one, perhaps, in any language, which brings the sum of knowledge forward to the most recent discoveries.—*The Edinburgh Med. and Surg. Journal.*

Admirably calculated to fulfil the object for which it is intended.—*Provincial Medical Journal.*

The most complete Treatise on Anatomy in the English language.—*Edinburgh Medical Journal.*

There is no work in the English language to be preferred to Dr. Quain's Elements of Anatomy.—*London Journal of Medicine.*

SMITH (HENRY H.), M. D., AND HORNER (WILLIAM E.), M. D.

AN ANATOMICAL ATLAS, illustrative of the Structure of the Human Body. In one volume, large imperial octavo, with about six hundred and fifty beautiful figures.

These figures are well selected, and present a complete and accurate representation of that wonderful fabric, the human body. The plan of this Atlas, which renders it so peculiarly convenient for the student, and its superb artistical execution, have been already pointed out. We must congratulate the student upon the completion of this Atlas, as it is the most convenient work of the kind that has yet appeared; and we must add, the very beautiful manner in which it is "got up" is so creditable to the country as to be flattering to our national pride.—*American Medical Journal.*

SARGENT (F. W.), M. D.

ON BANDAGING AND OTHER POINTS OF MINOR SURGERY. In one handsome royal 12mo. volume of nearly 400 pages, with 128 wood-cuts.

The very best manual of Minor Surgery we have seen; an American volume, with nearly four hundred pages of good practical lessons, illustrated by about one hundred and thirty wood-cuts. In these days of "trial," when a doctor's reputation hangs upon a clove hitch, or the roll of a bandage, it would be well, perhaps, to carry such a volume as Mr. Sargent's always in our coat-pocket, or, at all events, to listen attentively to his instructions at home.—*Buffalo Med. Journal.*

We have carefully examined this work, and it is well executed and admirably adapted to the use of the student. Besides the subjects usually embraced in works on Minor Surgery, there is a short chapter on bathing, another on anæsthetic agents, and an appendix of formulæ. The author has given us an excellent work on this subject, and his publishers have illustrated and printed it in most beautiful style.—*The Charleston Medical Journal.*

STANLEY (EDWARD).

A TREATISE ON DISEASES OF THE BONES. In one volume, octavo, extra cloth, 286 pages.

STILLÉ (ALFRED), M. D.
PRINCIPLES OF THERAPEUTICS. In one handsome volume. (*Preparing*.)

SIMON (JOHN), F. R. S.
GENERAL PATHOLOGY, as conducive to the Establishment of Rational Principles for the Prevention and Cure of Disease. A Course of Lectures delivered at St. Thomas's Hospital during the summer Session of 1850. In one neat octavo volume.

SMITH (TYLER W.), M. D.,
Lecturer on Obstetrics in the Hunterian School of Medicine.
ON PARTURITION, AND THE PRINCIPLES AND PRACTICE OF OBSTETRICS. In one large duodecimo volume, of 400 pages.

SIBSON (FRANCIS), M. D.,
Physician to St. Mary's Hospital.
MEDICAL ANATOMY. Illustrating the Form, Structure, and Position of the Internal Organs in Health and Disease. In large imperial quarto, with splendid colored plates. To match "Maclise's Surgical Anatomy." (*In Press*.)

SOLLY (SAMUEL), F. R. S.
THE HUMAN BRAIN; its Structure, Physiology, and Diseases. With a Description of the Typical Forms of the Brain in the Animal Kingdom. From the Second and much enlarged London edition. In one octavo volume, with 120 wood-cuts.

SCHOEDLER (FRIEDRICH), PH. D.,
Professor of the Natural Sciences at Worms, &c.
THE BOOK OF NATURE; an Elementary Introduction to the Sciences of Physics, Astronomy, Chemistry, Mineralogy, Geology, Botany, Zoology, and Physiology. First American edition, with a Glossary and other Additions and Improvements; from the second English edition. Translated from the sixth German edition, by HENRY MEDLOCK, F. C. S., &c. In one thick volume, small octavo, of about seven hundred pages, with 679 illustrations on wood. Suitable for the higher Schools and private students. (*Now Ready*.)

This volume, as its title shows, covers nearly all the sciences, and embodies a vast amount of information for instruction. No other work that we have seen presents the reader with so wide a range of elementary knowledge, with so full illustrations, at so cheap a rate.—*Silliman's Journal*, Nov. 1853.

TAYLOR (ALFRED S.), M. D., F. R. S.,
Lecturer on Medical Jurisprudence and Chemistry in Guy's Hospital.
MEDICAL JURISPRUDENCE. Third American, from the fourth and improved English Edition. With Notes and References to American Decisions, by EDWARD HARTSHORNE, M. D. In one large octavo volume, of about seven hundred pages. (*Just Issued*.)

We know of no work on Medical Jurisprudence which contains in the same space anything like the same amount of valuable matter.—*N. Y. Journal of Medicine*.

The American editor has appended several important facts, the whole constituting by far the best, most reliable, and interesting treatise on Medical Jurisprudence, and one that we cannot too strongly recommend to all who desire to become acquainted with the true and correct exposition of this department of medical literature.—*Northern Lancet*.

No work upon the subject can be put into the hands of students either of law or medicine which will engage them more closely or profitably; and none could be offered to the busy practitioner of either calling, for the purpose of casual or hasty reference, that would be more likely to afford the aid desired. We therefore recommend it as the best and safest manual for daily use.—*American Journal of Medical Sciences*.

We have heretofore had reason to refer to it in terms of commendation, and need now only state that, in the edition before us, the author has completely revised the whole work, making many additions and alterations, and brought it fully up to the present state of knowledge. The task of the American editor has been to present all the important facts and cases that have recently occurred in our own country, bearing on the subjects treated of. No better work can be placed in the hands of the physician or jurist.—*St. Louis Medical and Surgical Journal*.

BY THE SAME AUTHOR.
ON POISONS, IN RELATION TO MEDICAL JURISPRUDENCE AND MEDICINE. Edited, with Notes and Additions, by R. E. GRIFFITH, M. D. In one large octavo volume, of 688 pages.

The most elaborate work on the subject that our literature possesses.—*British and Foreign Medico-Chirurgical Review*.

It contains a vast body of facts, which embrace all that is important in toxicology, all that is necessary to the guidance of the medical jurist, and all that can be desired by the lawyer.—*Medico-Chirurgical Review*.

One of the most practical and trustworthy works on Poisons in our language.—*Western Journal of Medicine*.

It is, so far as our knowledge extends, incomparably the best upon the subject; in the highest degree creditable to the author, entirely trustworthy, and indispensable to the student and practitioner.—*N. Y. Annalist*.

THOMSON (A. T.), M. D., F. R. S., &c.
DOMESTIC MANAGEMENT OF THE SICK ROOM, necessary in aid of Medical Treatment for the Cure of Diseases. Edited by R. E. GRIFFITH, M. D. In one large royal 12mo. volume, with wood-cuts, 360 pages.

TOMES (JOHN), F. R. S.
A MANUAL OF DENTAL PRACTICE. Illustrated by numerous engravings on wood. In one handsome volume. (*Preparing.*)

TODD (R. B.), M. D., AND BOWMAN (WILLIAM), F. R. S.
PHYSIOLOGICAL ANATOMY AND PHYSIOLOGY OF MAN. With numerous handsome wood-cuts. Parts I, II, and III, in one octavo volume, 552 pages. Part IV will complete the work.

The distinguishing peculiarity of this work is, that the authors investigate for themselves every fact asserted; and it is the immense labor consequent upon the vast number of observations requisite to carry out this plan, which has so long delayed the appearance of its completion. The first portion of Part IV, with numerous original illustrations, was published in the Medical News and Library for 1853, and the completion will be issued immediately on its appearance to those. Those who have subscribed since the appearance of the preceding portion of the work can have the three parts by mail, on remittance of $2 50 to the publishers.

WATSON (THOMAS), M. D., &c.
LECTURES ON THE PRINCIPLES AND PRACTICE OF PHYSIC. Third American, from the last London edition. Revised, with Additions, by D. Francis Condie, M. D., author of a "Treatise on the Diseases of Children," &c. In one octavo volume, of eleven hundred large pages, strongly bound with raised bands.

To say that it is the very best work on the subject now extant, is but to echo the sentiment of the medical press throughout the country.—*N. O. Medical Journal.*

Of the text-books recently republished Watson is very justly the principal favorite.—*Holmes's Rep. to Nat. Med. Assoc.*

By universal consent the work ranks among the very best text-books in our language.—*Illinois and Indiana Med. Journal.*

Regarded on all hands as one of the very best, if not the very best, systematic treatise on practical medicine extant.—*St. Louis Med. Journal.*

Confessedly one of the very best works in any other language.—*Med. Examiner.*

As a text-book it has no equal; as a compend of pathology and practice no superior.—*N. Y. Annalist.*

We know of no work better calculated to be placed in the hands of the student, and the book; on every important point the author is to have posted up his knowledge to the present.—*Amer. Med. Journal.*

One of the most practically useful books that ever was presented to the student.—*N. J. Med. Journal.*

WALSHE (W. H.), M.D.,
Professor of the Principles and Practice of Medicine in University College, London.
DISEASES OF THE HEART, LUNGS, AND APPENDAGES; their Symptoms and Treatment. In one handsome volume, large royal 12mo., 512 pages.

We consider this as the ablest work in the English language, on the subject of which it treats; the author being the first stethoscopist of the age.—*Charleston Medical Journal.*

WHAT TO OBSERVE
AT THE BEDSIDE AND AFTER DEATH, IN MEDICAL CASES. Published under the authority of the London Society for Medical Observation. A new American from the second and revised London edition. In one very handsome volume, royal 12mo., extra cloth. (*Now Ready.*)

The demand which has so rapidly exhausted the first edition of this little work, shows the advantages it offers to the profession have been duly appreciated, and has stimulated the author to render it more worthy of its reputation. It has therefore been thoroughly revised, and improvements (among which is a section on TREATMENT) have been made as further experience its use has shown to be desirable.

We hail the appearance of this book as the grand desideratum.—*Charleston Medical Journal.*

This is truly a very capital book. The whole medical world will reap advantages from its publication. The medical journals will soon show its influence on the character of the "Reports of Cases" which they publish. Drs. Ballard and Walshe have given to the world, through a small but well medical organization, a cheap but invaluable work. We do advise every reader of this notice to buy and use it. Unless he is so vain as to imagine himself superior to the ordinary human capacity, he will in six months see its inestimable advantages.—*Stethoscope.*

WILDE (W. R.),
Surgeon to St. Mark's Ophthalmic and Aural Hospital, Dublin.
AURAL SURGERY, AND THE NATURE AND TREATMENT OF DISEASES OF THE EAR. In one handsome octavo volume, with illustrations. (*Now Ready.*)

So little is generally known in this country concerning the causes, symptoms, and treatment of aural affections, that a practical and scientific work on that subject, from a practitioner of Mr. Wilde's great experience, cannot fail to be productive of much benefit, by attracting attention to this obscure class of diseases, which too frequently escape attention until past relief. The immense number of cases which have come under Mr. Wilde's observation for many years, afforded him opportunities rarely enjoyed for investigating this branch of medical science. His work may therefore be regarded as of the highest authority.

This work certainly contains more information on the subject to which it is devoted than any other with which we are acquainted. We feel grateful to the author for his manful effort to rescue this department of surgery from the hands of the empirics who nearly monopolize it. We think he has successfully shown that aural diseases are not beyond the resources of art; that they are governed by the same laws, and amenable to the same general mode of treatment as other morbid processes. The work is not written to supply the cravings of popular magazines, but it is wholly addressed to the profession and bears on every page the impress of the labors of a sagacious and practical surgeon.—*Va. Surg. and Med. Journal.*

WILSON (ERASMUS), M.D., F.R.S.,
Lecturer on Anatomy, London.

A SYSTEM OF HUMAN ANATOMY, General and Special. Fourth American, from the last English edition. Edited by PAUL B. GODDARD, A.M., M.D. With two hundred and fifty illustrations. Beautifully printed, in one large octavo volume, of nearly six hundred pages.

In many, if not all the Colleges of the Union, it has become a standard text-book. This, of itself, is sufficiently expressive of its value. A work very desirable to the student; one, the possession of which will greatly facilitate his progress in the study of Practical Anatomy.—*New York Journal of Medicine.*

Its author ranks with the highest on Anatomy.—*Southern Medical and Surgical Journal.*

It offers to the student all the assistance that can be expected from such a work.—*Medical Examiner.*

The most complete and convenient manual for the student we possess.—*American Journal of Medical Science.*

In every respect, this work as an anatomical guide for the student and practitioner, merits our warmest and most decided praise.—*London Medical Gazette.*

BY THE SAME AUTHOR.

THE DISSECTOR; or, Practical and Surgical Anatomy. Modified and Rearranged, by PAUL BECK GODDARD, M. D. A new edition, with Revisions and Additions. In one large and handsome volume, royal 12mo., with one hundred and fifteen illustrations.

In passing this work again through the press, the editor has made such additions and improvements as the advance of anatomical knowledge has rendered necessary to maintain the work in the high reputation which it has acquired in the schools of the United States, as a complete and faithful guide to the student of practical anatomy. A number of new illustrations have been added, especially in the portion relating to the complicated anatomy of Hernia. In mechanical execution the work will be found superior to former editions.

BY THE SAME AUTHOR.

ON DISEASES OF THE SKIN. Third American, from the third London edition. In one neat octavo volume, of about five hundred pages, extra cloth. (*Just Issued.*)

Also, to be had done up with fifteen beautiful steel plates, of which eight are exquisitely colored; representing the Normal and Pathological Anatomy of the Skin, together with accurately colored delineations of more than sixty varieties of disease, most of them the size of nature. The Plates are also for sale separate, done up in boards.

The increased size of this edition is sufficient evidence that the author has not been content with a mere republication, but has endeavored to maintain the high character of his work as the standard text-book on this interesting and difficult class of diseases. He has thus introduced such new matter as the experience of the last three or four years has suggested, and has made such alterations as the progress of scientific investigation has rendered expedient. The illustrations have also been materially augmented, the number of plates being increased from eight to sixteen.

The "Diseases of the Skin," by Mr. Erasmus Wilson, may now be regarded as the standard work in that department of medical literature. The plates by which this edition is accompanied leave nothing to be desired, so far as excellence of delineation and perfect accuracy of illustration are concerned.—*Medico-Chirurgical Review.*

Of these plates it is impossible to speak too highly. The representations of the various forms of cutaneous disease are singularly accurate, and the coloring exceeds almost anything we have met with in point of delicacy and finish.—*British and Foreign Medical Review.*

BY THE SAME AUTHOR.

ON CONSTITUTIONAL AND HEREDITARY SYPHILIS, AND ON SYPHILITIC ERUPTIONS. In one small octavo volume, beautifully printed, with four exquisite colored plates, presenting more than thirty varieties of syphilitic eruptions.

Dr. Wilson's views on the general subject of Syphilis appear to us in the main sound and judicious, and we commend the book as an excellent monograph on the subject. Dr. Wilson has presented us a very faithful and lucid description of Syphilis and has cleared up many obscure points in connection with its transmissibility, pathology and sequelæ. His facts and references will, we are satisfied, be received as decisive, in regard to many questions vexatæ. They appear to us entitled to notice at some length.—*Medical Examiner.*

BY THE SAME AUTHOR. (*Now Ready.*)

HEALTHY SKIN; A Popular Treatise on the Skin and Hair, their Preservation and Management. Second American, from the fourth London edition. One neat volume, royal 12mo., with numerous illustrations.

Copies can be had done up in paper covers for mailing, price 75 cents.

WHITEHEAD (JAMES), F.R.C.S., &c.

THE CAUSES AND TREATMENT OF ABORTION AND STERILITY; being the Result of an Extended Practical Inquiry into the Physiological and Morbid Conditions of the Uterus. Second American Edition. In one volume, octavo, 368 pages. (*Now Ready.*)

The simple title of this work gives a very imperfect idea of its contents. The subject of sterility occupies a mere fraction of space, and upwards of one-half of the whole volume is taken up with an elaborate account of menstruation as a physiological process, and of the disorders which its deviations from health are apt to produce.—*Medical Chirurg. Review.*

Such are the advances made from year to year in this department of our profession, that the practitioner who does not consult the recent works on the complaints of females, will soon find himself in the rear of his more studious brethren. This is one of the works which must be studied by those who would know what the present state of our knowledge is respecting the causes and treatment of abortion and sterility.—*The Western Journal of Medicine and Surgery.*

WEST (CHARLES), M. D.,
Physician to the Hospital for Sick Children, &c.

LECTURES ON THE DISEASES OF INFANCY AND CHILDHOOD
Second American, from the Second and Enlarged London edition. In one volume, octavo, of nearly five hundred pages. (*Now Ready*.)

From the Preface to the Second Edition.

In the preparation of the second edition of these Lectures, the whole work has been carefully revised. A few formulæ have been introduced and a minute alphabetical index has been appended, while additions amounting altogether to fifty pages, have been made, wherever I felt that my extended observation, or more careful reflection had enabled me to supply some of those deficiencies which I am well aware, are still far too numerous. The work now contains the result of all observations, and 199 post-mortem examinations, chiefly made among 16,276 children who came under my notice during the ten years of my connection with the Children's Infirmary in Lambeth.

We take leave of Dr. West with great respect for his attainments, a due appreciation of his acute powers of observation, and a deep sense of obligation for this valuable contribution to our professional literature. His book is undoubtedly in many respects the best we possess on diseases of children. The extracts we have given will, we hope, satisfy our readers of its value; and yet in all candor we must say that they are even inferior to some other parts, the length of which prohibited our entering upon them. That the book will shortly be in the hands of most of our readers we do not doubt, and it will give us much pleasure if our strong recommendation of it may contribute towards the result.—*The Dublin Quarterly Journal of Medical Science.*

Dr. West has placed the profession under deep obligation by this able, thorough, and finished work upon a subject which almost daily taxes to the utmost the skill of the general practitioner. He has with singular felicity threaded his way through all the tortuous labyrinths of the difficult subject he has undertaken to elucidate, and has in many of the darkest corners left a light, for the benefit of succeeding travellers, which will never be extinguished. Not the least captivating feature in this admirable performance is its easy, conversational style, which acquires force from its very simplicity, and leaves an impression upon the memory, of the truths it conveys, as clear and refreshing as its own pages. The author's position secured him extraordinary facilities for the investigation of children's diseases, and his powers of observation and discrimination have enabled him to make the most of these great advantages.—*Nashville Medical Journal.*

BY THE SAME AUTHOR. (*Now Ready.*)

AN ENQUIRY INTO THE PATHOLOGICAL IMPORTANCE OF ULCERATION OF THE OS UTERI. Being the Croonian Lectures for the year 1854. In one neat octavo volume, extra cloth.

WILLIAMS (C. J. B.), M. D., F. R. S.,
Professor of Clinical Medicine in University College, London, &c.

PRINCIPLES OF MEDICINE; comprising General Pathology and Therapeutics, and a brief general view of Etiology, Nosology, Semeiology, Diagnosis, Prognosis, and Hygienics. Edited, with Additions, by MEREDITH CLYMER, M. D. Fourth American, from the last and enlarged London edition. In one octavo volume, of 476 pages. (*Now Ready.*)

This new edition has been materially enlarged and brought up by the editor.

It possesses the strongest claims to the attention of the medical student and practitioner, from the admirable manner in which the various inquiries in the different branches of pathology are investigated, combined, and generalized by an experienced practical physician, and directly applied to the investigation and treatment of disease.—EDITOR'S PREFACE.

The best exposition in our language, or, we believe, in any language, of rational medicine, in its present improved and rapidly improving state.—*British and Foreign Medico-Chirurg. Review.*

Few books have proved more useful, or met with a more ready sale than this, and no practitioner should regard his library as complete without it. —*Ohio Med. and Surg. Journal.*

BY THE SAME AUTHOR.

A PRACTICAL TREATISE ON DISEASES OF THE RESPIRATORY ORGANS; including Diseases of the Larynx, Trachea, Lungs, and Pleuræ. With numerous Additions and Notes, by M. CLYMER, M. D. With wood-cuts. In one octavo volume, pp. 500.

YOUATT (WILLIAM), V. S.

THE HORSE. A new edition, with numerous illustrations; together with a general history of the Horse; a Dissertation on the American Trotting Horse; how Trained and Jockeyed; an Account of his Remarkable Performances; and an Essay on the Ass and the Mule. By J. S. SKINNER, formerly Assistant Postmaster-General, and Editor of the Turf Register. One large octavo volume.

BY THE SAME AUTHOR.

THE DOG. Edited by E. J. LEWIS, M. D. With numerous and beautiful Illustrations. In one very handsome volume, crown 8vo., crimson cloth, gilt.

B. & L. subjoin a condensed list of their publications in general and educational literature, of which more detailed catalogues will be furnished on application.

HISTORY AND BIOGRAPHY.

BROWNING'S HISTORY OF THE HUGUENOTS. 1 vol. 8vo.
CAMPBELL'S (LORD) LIVES OF THE LORD CHANCELLORS OF ENGLAND, from the earliest Times to the Reign of George IV. In seven handsome crown octavo volumes, extra cloth or half morocco.
CAMPBELL'S (LORD) LIVES OF THE CHIEF JUSTICES OF ENGLAND, from the Norman Conquest. In two handsome crown octavo vols., to match the "Chancellors."
DIXON'S LIFE OF WILLIAM PENN. A new work. 1 vol. royal 12mo., extra cloth.
GRAHAME'S COLONIAL HISTORY OF THE UNITED STATES. 2 vols. 8vo. A new edition.
GUIZOT'S LIFE OF CROMWELL. Two large vols., royal 12mo. (Now ready.)
HERVEY'S MEMOIRS OF GEORGE II. 2 vols. royal 12mo., extra cloth.
HUGHES'S OUTLINES OF SCRIPTURE GEOGRAPHY AND HISTORY, 1 vol., royal 12mo., with colored maps. (Just issued.)
INGERSOLL'S HISTORY OF THE LATE WAR. 2 vols 8vo.
KENNEDY'S LIFE OF WILLIAM WIRT. 2d edition, 2 vols. royal 12mo., extra cloth, with Portrait.
Same work. library edition, 2 vols. 8vo.
KAVANAGH'S WOMAN IN FRANCE IN THE EIGHTEENTH CENTURY. 1 vol. royal 12mo., extra cloth.
LOUIS BLANC'S FRANCE UNDER LOUIS PHILIPPE, 1830–1840. 2 vols. crown 8vo., extra cloth.

LOUIS BLANC'S FRENCH REVOLUTION. 1 vol. crown 8vo , extra cloth.
MARSH (MRS.) ROMANTIC HISTORY OF THE HUGUENOTS. 2 vols. royal 12mo., extra cloth.
NIEBUHR'S ANCIENT HISTORY. By LEONHARD SCHMITZ. In three handsome crown octavo vols., (Lately Issued.)
PARDOE'S FRANCIS THE FIRST. 2 vols. royal 12mo., extra cloth.
PALGRAVE'S NORMANDY AND ENGLAND. In three vols. crown 8vo., (Preparing.)
RUSH'S COURT OF LONDON. 1 vol. 8vo.
RANKE'S HISTORY OF THE REFORMATION IN GERMANY. To be complete in 1 vol. 8vo.
RANKE'S HISTORY OF THE OTTOMAN AND SPANISH EMPIRES. 8vo. Price 50 cents.
RUSSEL'S LIFE OF CHARLES JAMES FOX. 2 vols., handsome royal 12mo. (Now ready.)
Same Work, Second Series. (Preparing)
STRICKLAND'S LIVES OF THE QUEENS OF ENGLAND, from the Norman Conquest. Complete in 6 handsome crown 8vo. volumes, various styles of binding.
STRICKLAND'S LIVES OF THE QUEENS OF HENRY VIII. In one handsome crown 8vo. vol., extra cloth, various styles.
STRICKLAND'S LIFE OF QUEEN ELIZABETH. In one handsome crown 8vo. volume, extra cloth, various styles.
STEINMETZ'S HISTORY OF THE JESUITS. 2 vols. crown 8vo., extra cloth.

MISCELLANEOUS.

ACTON (MRS.) MODERN COOKERY. Edited by Mrs. S J. HALE. 1 handsome volume, royal 12mo., extra cloth, with illustrations.
ADDISON ON CONTRACTS, and on Parties to Actions, ex contractu. 1 large octavo volume, law sheep.
BUFFUM'S SIX MONTHS IN THE GOLD MINES. 1 vol. royal 12mo., extra cloth or paper, 50 cents.
BAIRD'S WEST INDIES AND NORTH AMERICA. 1 vol. royal 12mo., extra cloth.
CLATER ON THE DISEASES OF HORSES. By SKINNER. 1 vol 12mo.
CLATER'S CATTLE AND SHEEP DOCTOR. 1 vol. 12mo., cuts.
DON QUIXOTE. With numerous illustrations by Johannot. 2 vols. 8vo. cloth, or half morocco.
ENCYCLOPÆDIA OF GEOGRAPHY. In three octavo vols., many cuts and maps, various bindings.
ENCYCLOPÆDIA AMERICANA. 14 vols. 8vo., various bindings.
Vol. 14. bringing the work up to 1846, sold separate.
EXPLORING EXPEDITION, NARRATIVE OF. In six vols., imperial quarto, with several hundred plates, maps, and wood-cuts.
EVANS'S SUGAR-PLANTER'S MANUAL. 1 vol. 8vo , extra cloth. plates.
ERMAN'S TRAVELS IN SIBERIA. 2 vols. royal 12mo., extra cloth.
FIELDING'S SELECT WORKS. In one vol. 8vo. cloth. or 4 parts. paper.
FLETCHER'S NOTES FROM NINEVEH. 1 vol. royal 12mo., extra cloth.
HAWKER ON SHOOTING. Edited by PORTER. With plates and cuts. 1 vol. 8vo., beautiful extra cloth, new edition, (Just Issued.)
HOLTHOUSE'S LAW DICTIONARY. By PENINGTON. 1 vol. large 12mo., law sheep.
JOHNSON'S DICTIONARY OF GARDENING. By LANDRETH. 1 vol. large royal 12mo., 650 pages, many cuts.
LANGUAGE OF FLOWERS. 8th edition. 1 vol. 18mo., colored plates, crimson cloth. gilt.
LEWIS'S HINTS TO SPORTSMEN. 1 vol. royal 12mo., extra cloth, illustrated.

LYNCH'S NARRATIVE OF THE U. S. EXPEDITION TO THE DEAD SEA AND RIVER JORDAN. 1 large octavo volume, with numerous plates and maps.
Same work, condensed edition, in neat royal 12mo.
MACFARLANE'S TURKEY AND ITS DESTINY. 2 vols. royal 12mo., extra cloth.
MACKAY'S TRAVELS IN THE UNITED STATES. 2 vols. royal 12mo., extra cloth.
MARTINEAU'S EASTERN LIFE. 1 vol. crown 8vo., extra cloth.
MARTINEAU'S HOUSEHOLD EDUCATION. 1 vol. royal 12mo., extra cloth.
PAGET'S HUNGARY AND TRANSYLVANIA. 2 vols. royal 12mo., extra cloth.
PULSZKY'S HUNGARIAN LADY. 1 vol. royal 12mo., extra cloth.
PICCIOLA—The Prisoner of Fenestrella. Illustrated edition, with cuts, royal 12mo., beautiful crimson cloth.
Same work. fancy paper. price 50 cents.
READINGS FOR THE YOUNG FROM SIR WALTER SCOTT, 2 vols. royal 18mo., extra crimson cloth. plates.
SELECT WORKS OF TOBIAS SMOLLETT Cloth or paper.
SHAW'S OUTLINES OF ENGLISH LITERATURE. 1 large vol. royal 12mo., extra cloth.
SMALL BOOKS ON GREAT SUBJECTS. In three neat volumes, royal 18mo., extra cloth.
SAM SLICK'S NEW WORK—WISE SAWS AND MODERN INSTANCES. 1 vol. 12mo., (Now Ready.)
THOMSON'S DOMESTIC MANAGEMENT OF THE SICK ROOM. 1 vol. 12mo.
WHEATON'S INTERNATIONAL LAW. 1 vol. large 8vo., law sheep, or extra cloth. 3d edition, much improved.
YOUATT ON THE HORSE, &c. By SKINNER. 1 vol. 8vo., many cuts.
YOUATT ON THE DOG. With plates. 1 vol. crown 8vo., beautiful crimson cloth.
YOUATT ON THE PIG. 1 vol. 12mo., extra cloth, with cuts.
Same work in paper, price 50 cents.

NATURAL SCIENCE.

AMERICAN ORNITHOLOGY. By PRINCE CHARLES BONAPARTE. In four handsome folio volumes, with beautiful colored plates.
ARNOTT'S ELEMENTS OF PHYSICS. New Edition. By ISAAC HAYS, M. D. In one octavo volume, with 200 illustrations.

BRODERIP'S ZOOLOGICAL RECREATIONS. 1 vol. royal 12mo., extra cloth.
BOWMAN'S PRACTICAL CHEMISTRY. 1 vol. royal 12mo., extra cloth ; cuts.
BIRD'S NATURAL PHILOSOPHY. 1 vol. royal 12mo., with many cuts.

NATURAL SCIENCE.—Continued.

BEALE ON THE LAWS OF HEALTH IN RELATION TO MIND AND BODY. 1 vol. royal 12mo., extra cloth.
BREWSTER'S TREATISE ON OPTICS. 1 vol. 12mo., cuts.
CARPENTER'S GENERAL AND COMPARATIVE PHYSIOLOGY. With numerous woodcuts. 1 vol. large 8vo, new edition. (Preparing.)
CARPENTER ON THE MICROSCOPE. Handsomely illustrated. (Preparing.)
DANA ON CORALS. 1 vol. royal 4to., extra cloth, with wood-cuts.
Atlas to do., large imperial folio, half morocco, with over 60 magnificent colored plates.
DE LA BECHE'S GEOLOGICAL OBSERVER. 1 large vol. 8vo. over 300 cuts. (Now Ready.)
FOWNES'S RECENT WORK ON CHEMISTRY. New edition. By Bridges. 1 vol. 12mo., many cuts, sheep or extra cloth.
GRAHAM'S ELEMENTS OF CHEMISTRY. Large 8vo., many cuts. (Part I, lately issued, Part II, preparing.)
GREGORY ON ANIMAL MAGNETISM. 1 vol. royal 12mo.
GRIFFITH'S CHEMISTRY OF THE FOUR SEASONS. 1 vol. 12mo., many cuts.
GRIFFITH'S MEDICAL BOTANY. 1 vol. large 8vo., extra cloth, nearly 400 cuts.
HERSCHEL'S OUTLINES OF ASTRONOMY. 1 vol. crown 8vo., ex. cl., with plates and wood-cuts.
HUMBOLDT'S ASPECTS OF NATURE. 2d edition. 1 large vol. royal 12mo., extra cloth.
HANDBOOKS OF NATURAL PHILOSOPHY AND ASTRONOMY. By Dionysius Lardner. 3 thick vols. royal 12mo., with 1000 wood-cuts.

HALE'S ETHNOLOGY AND PHILOLOGY OF THE U. S. EXPLORING EXPEDITION. 1 vol. royal 4to., extra cloth.
JOHNSTON'S PHYSICAL ATLAS OF NATURAL PHENOMENA. In one large and handsome imperial 4to. vol., half bound in morocco, with 26 maps, beautifully colored.
KNAPP'S TECHNOLOGY, OR CHEMISTRY APPLIED TO THE ARTS AND TO MANUFACTURES. Translated by Ronalds. Edited by Johnson. Vol. I., with 244 large wood engravings. Vol. II., large 8vo., with 250 wood engravings.
MULLER'S PHYSICS AND METEOROLOGY. 1 vol. large 8vo., 2 colored plates, and 550 wood-cuts.
MILLWRIGHT'S AND MILLER'S GUIDE. By Oliver Evans. In one vol. 8vo., sheep, many plates.
MATTEUCCI ON PHYSICAL PHENOMENA OF LIVING BEINGS. 1 vol. royal 12mo., ex. cl., cuts.
ORR'S CIRCLE OF THE SCIENCES, royal 12mo. with numerous illustrations, containing Animal and Vegetable Physiology, by Dr. Bushnan. The Different Forms of the Skeleton, by Prof. Owen. Physical Geography and Geology, by Prof. Ansted. Natural Philosophy, by Rev. W. Mitchell, &c. &c.
SOMERVILLE'S PHYSICAL GEOGRAPHY. New edition. 1 large vol. royal 12mo., extra cloth.
SCHOEDLER AND MEDLOCK'S BOOK OF NATURE. With Additions and Improvements. 1 one thick volume, crown 8vo., with over 679 illustrations.
WEISBACH'S PRINCIPLES OF THE MECHANICS OF MACHINERY AND ENGINEERING. 2 large octavo volumes, extra cloth, 900 beautiful wood engravings.

EDUCATIONAL WORKS.

ARNOTT'S ELEMENTS OF PHYSICS. New edition. Complete in 1 vol. 8vo., many illustrations.
BOLMAR'S FRENCH SERIES, consisting of:—
LEVIZAC'S FRENCH GRAMMAR, 1 volume, 12mo., sheep.
PERRIN'S FABLES, with Key. 1 vol. 12mo., half bound.
COLLOQUIAL PHRASES, 1 vol. 18mo., hf. bound.
AVENTURES DE TELEMAQUE, 1 vol. 12mo., half bound.
KEY to do. do. do.
FRENCH VERBS, 1 vol. 12mo., half bound.
BAIRD'S CLASSICAL MANUAL. An Epitome of Ancient Geography, Mythology, Antiquities, and Chronology. 1 vol. royal 18mo., extra cloth.
Same work, half bound, embossed leather backs.
BUSHNAN'S PHYSIOLOGY OF ANIMAL AND VEGETABLE LIFE. A new and popular work. 1 vol. royal 12mo. with illustrations. (Just Ready.)
BIRD'S ELEMENTS OF NATURAL PHILOSOPHY. 1 vol. royal 12mo., sheep, or ext. cl. 372 cuts.
BUTLER'S ATLAS OF ANCIENT GEOGRAPHY. Revised edition. 1 vol. 8vo. half bound, 21 colored maps.
BUTLER'S GEOGRAPHIA CLASSICA. Revised edition; 1 vol. 12mo., half bound.
BREWSTER'S TREATISE ON OPTICS. With additions. By Bache. 1 vol. 12mo., half bound, cuts.
BROWNE'S GREEK CLASSICAL LITERATURE. 1 vol. crown 8vo., extra cloth.
BROWNE'S ROMAN CLASSICAL LITERATURE. 1 vol. crown 8vo., ex. cloth. (Now Ready.)
FOSTER'S HANDBOOK OF MODERN EUROPEAN LITERATURE. 1 vol. royal 12mo., ex. cl.
FOWNE'S CHEMISTRY FOR STUDENTS. New edition. By Bridges. 1 vol. royal 12mo., many cuts, extra cloth, or sheep.
GRAHAM'S ELEMENTS OF CHEMISTRY. 2d edition, enlarged. Edited by Bridges. 8vo. many cuts. Part I., lately issued. Part II., preparing.
HERSCHEL'S OUTLINES OF ASTRONOMY. A new edition. With numerous plates and woodcuts. 1 vol. crown 8vo., extra cloth.
HUGHES'S OUTLINES OF SCRIPTURE GEOGRAPHY AND HISTORY, 1 vol., royal 12mo., with colored maps. (Just issued.)

JOHNSTON'S ATLAS OF PHYSICAL GEOGRAPHY. 1 vol., with 26 colored plates. hf. bound.
LARDNER'S HANDBOOKS OF NATURAL PHILOSOPHY AND ASTRONOMY.
First Course, containing Mechanics, Hydrostatics, Hydraulics, Pneumatics, Sound, and Optics. 1 very large vol., royal 12mo., sheep, 424 cuts.
Second Course, containing Heat, Electricity, Magnetism, and Galvanism. 1 vol. royal 12mo., sheep, 250 cuts.
Third Course, containing Astronomy and Meteorology. 1 very large vol., royal 12mo., 37 plates and 216 wood-cuts. (Now ready.)
MULLER'S PHYSICS AND METEOROLOGY. 1 vol. 8vo., over 500 beautiful cuts and two colored plates, extra cloth.
NATIONAL SCHOOL MANUAL. 4 parts. 12mo.
SOMERVILLE'S PHYSICAL GEOGRAPHY. 3d and enlarged edition, with American notes. 1 large vol. royal 12mo., extra cloth.
SHAW'S OUTLINES OF ENGLISH LITERATURE. 2d ed. With Sketch of American Literature. By Tuckerman. 1 vol. royal 12mo., ext c.
SCHOEDLER AND MEDLOCK'S BOOK OF NATURE. Edited and revised. 1 large vol., crown 8vo., with 679 wood cuts. (Now ready.)
SCHMITZ AND ZUMPT'S CLASSICAL SERIES FOR SCHOOLS. In neat royal 18mo. volumes as follows:—
KALTSCHMIDT'S LATIN DICTIONARY Complete, handsome embossed leather.
SCHMITZ'S ELEMENTARY LATIN GRAMMAR AND EXERCISES.
SCHMITZ'S ADVANCED LATIN GRAMMAR.
ADVANCED LATIN EXERCISE BOOK, with Selections for Reading. (Now Ready.)
CÆSAR, extra cloth, with a Map.
SALLUST, extra cloth, with a Map.
VIRGIL, extra cloth.
OVID, extra cloth.
HORACE, extra cloth.
LIVY, extra cloth, two colored Maps.
CICERO, extra cloth.
QUINTUS CURTIUS, extra cloth, with a Map.
CORNELIUS NEPOS, now ready, extra cloth.
OTHER WORKS OF THE SERIES PREPARING.

ILLUSTRATED MEDICAL CATALOGUE.

BLANCHARD & LEA have now ready a Catalogue of their Medical, Surgical, and Scientific Publications, containing descriptions of the works, with Notices of the Press, and specimens of the Illustrations, making a pamphlet of sixty-four large octavo pages. It has been prepared with great care, and without regard to expense, forming one of the most beautiful specimens of typographical execution as yet issued in this country. Copies will be sent by mail, and the postage paid, on application to the Publishers, by inclosing two three cent postage stamps.

Ingram Content Group UK Ltd.
Milton Keynes UK
UKHW010023040723
424490UK00008B/582